PRINCIPLES OF NEURAL SCIENCE

THIRD EDITION

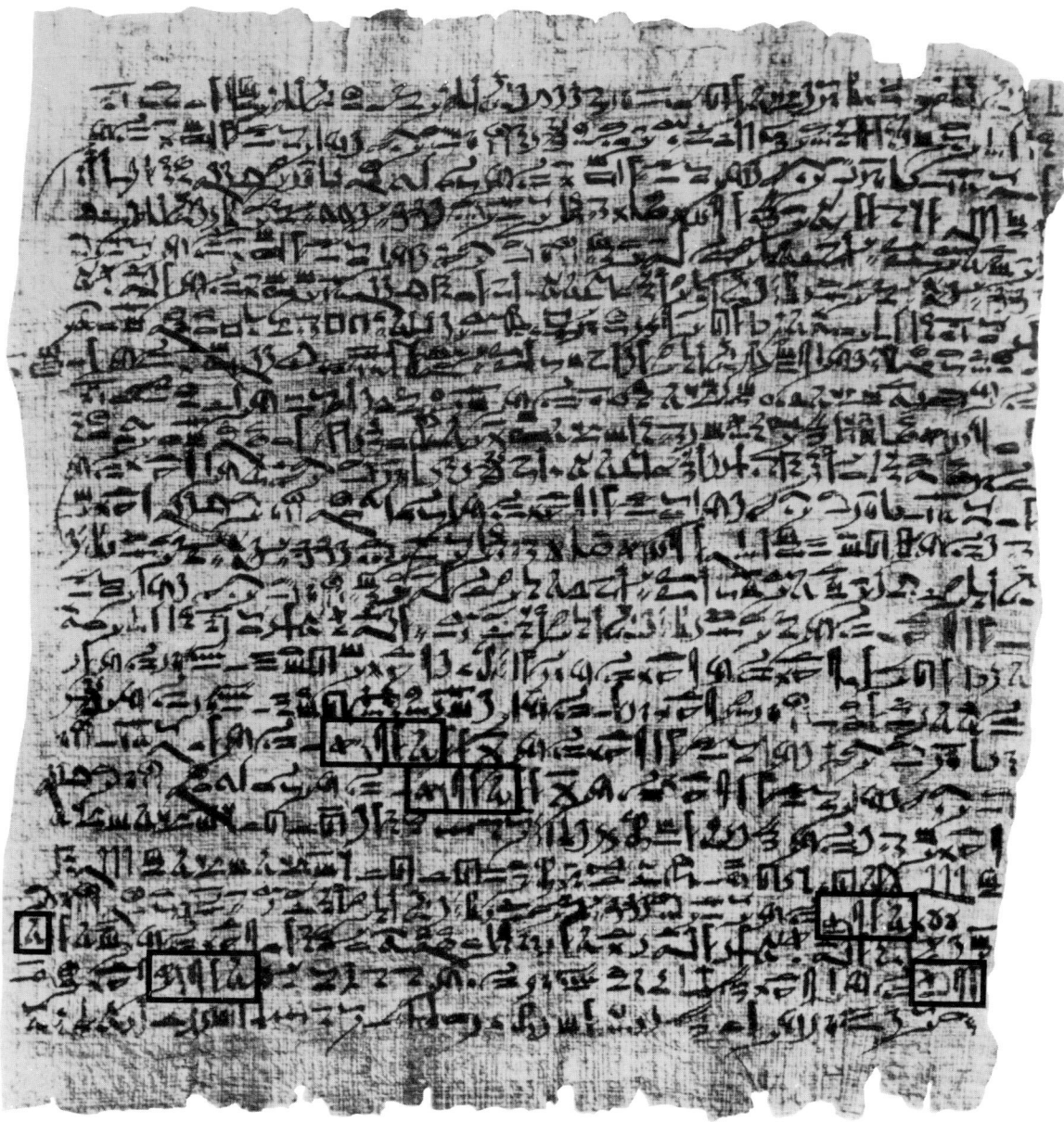

Columns II (left) and IV (right) of the Edwin Smith Surgical Papyrus

This papryus, written in the Seventeenth Century B.C., contains the earliest reference to the brain anywhere in human records. According to James Breasted, who translated and published the document in 1930, the word brain ('ys) occurs only 8 times in ancient Egyptian, 6 of them on these pages of the Smith Papyrus describing the symptoms, diagnosis and prognosis of two patients, wounded in the head, who had compound fractures of the skull. The entire treatise is now in the Rare Book Room of the New York Academy of Medicine.

Reference: Breasted, James Henry. The Edwin Smith Surgical Papyrus, 2 volumes. The University of Chicago Press, Chicago. 1930.

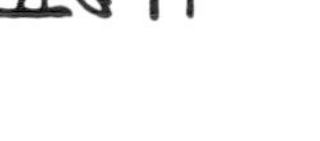

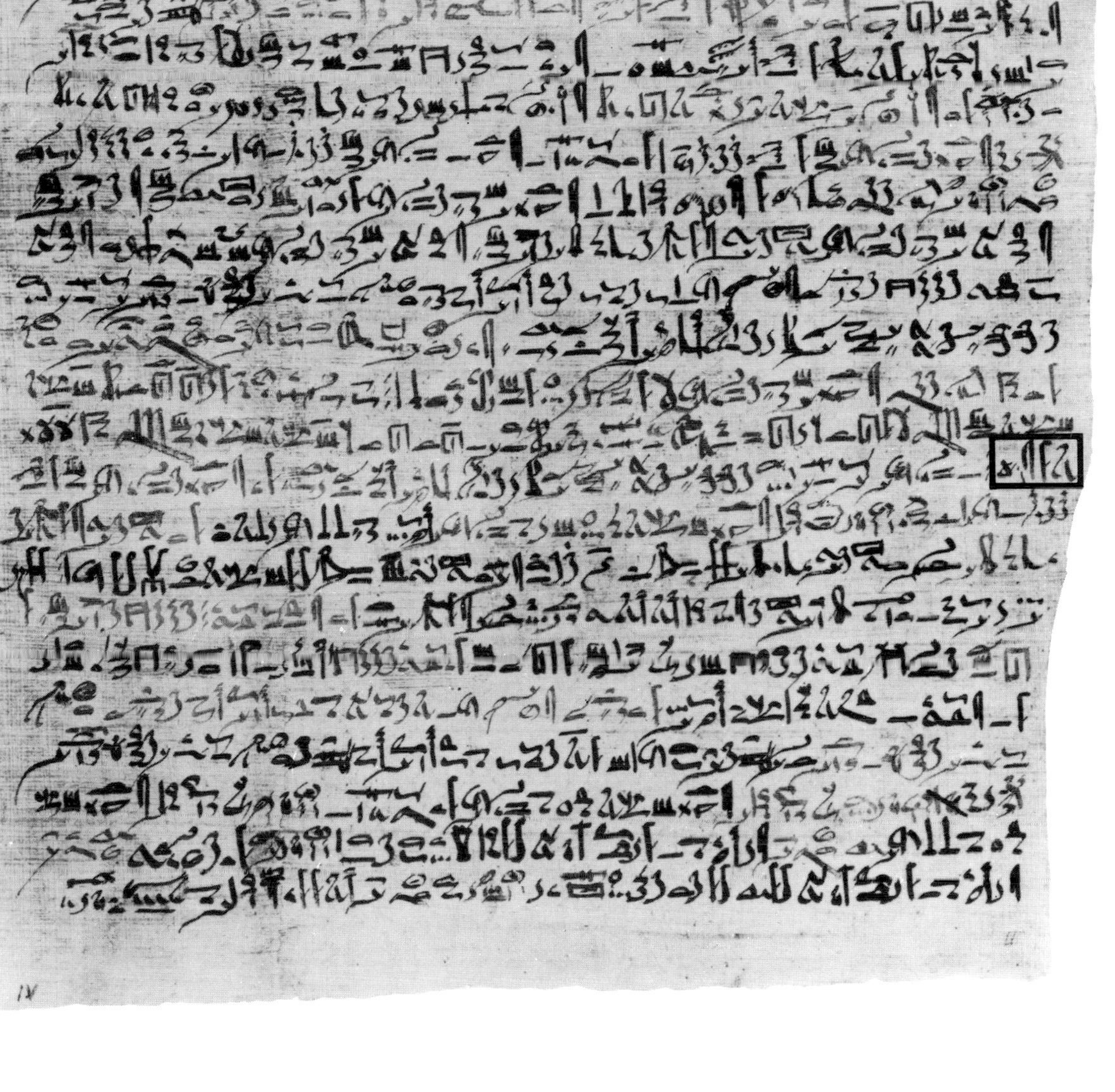

Men ought to know that from the brain, and from the brain only, arise our pleasures, joys, laughter and jests, as well as our sorrows, pains, griefs and tears. Through it, in particular, we think, see, hear, and distinguish the ugly from the beautiful, the bad from the good, the pleasant from the unpleasant . . . . It is the same thing which makes us mad or delirious, inspires us with dread and fear, whether by night or by day, brings sleeplessness, inopportune mistakes, aimless anxieties, absent-mindedness, and acts that are contrary to habit. These things that we suffer all come from the brain, when it is not healthy, but becomes abnormally hot, cold, moist, or dry, or suffers any other unnatural affection to which it was not accustomed. Madness comes from its moistness. When the brain is abnormally moist, of necessity it moves, and when it moves neither sight nor hearing are still, but we see or hear now one thing and now another, and the tongue speaks in accordance with the things seen and heard on any occasion.
But all the time the brain is still, a man can think properly.

attributed to Hippocrates,
Fifth Century, B.C.

PRINCIPLES OF NEURAL SCIENCE

THIRD EDITION

Edited by

ERIC R. KANDEL
JAMES H. SCHWARTZ
THOMAS M. JESSELL

Center for Neurobiology and Behavior
College of Physicians & Surgeons of Columbia University
and
The Howard Hughes Medical Institute

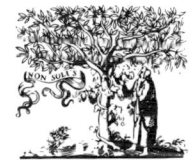

ELSEVIER

New York · Amsterdam · London · Tokyo

Elsevier Science Publishing Co., Inc.
655 Avenue of the Americas, New York, New York 10010

Sole distributors outside the United States and Canada:
Elsevier Science Publishers B.V.
P.O. Box 211, 1000 AE Amsterdam, The Netherlands

This book is printed on acid-free paper.

Library of Congress Cataloging-in-Publication Data

Principles of neural science / edited by Eric R. Kandel, James H.
Schwartz, Thomas M. Jessell.—3rd ed.
p. cm.
Includes bibliographical references and index.
ISBN 0-444-01562-0 (hardcover: alk. paper)
1. Neurology. 2. Neurons. I. Kandel, Eric R. II. Schwartz,
James H. III. Jessell, Thomas M.
[DNLM: 1. Behavior. 2. Nervous System Diseases.
3. Neurochemistry. 4. Neurons. 5. Neurophysiology. WL 102 P9547]
QP355.2.P76 1991
612.8—dc20
DNLM/DLC
for Library of Congress
91-24678   CIP

Illustration by Jonathan Dimes and Terese Winslow, AMI

Frontispiece quotation from *Hippocrates*, Vol. 2, translated by W.H.S. Jones,
London and New York: William Heinemann and Harvard University Press, 1923,
Chapter XVII: "The Sacred Disease," p. 175.

Current printing (last digit)
10 9 8 7 6 5 4 3 2 1

Manufactured in the United States of America

We dedicate the third edition of this book to our many colleagues
in the neurobiology community throughout the world who have read earlier
versions of these chapters critically and who have offered
many useful and important suggestions for their improvement.

Contents in Brief

Contents xiii
Preface xxxix
Acknowledgments xli
Contributors xliii
How to Use This Book xlv

Part I
An Overall View 2

1 Brain and Behavior 5
2 Nerve Cells and Behavior 18

Part II
Cell and Molecular Biology of the Neuron 34

3 The Cytology of Neurons 37
4 Synthesis and Trafficking of Neuronal Proteins 49
5 Ion Channels 66
6 Membrane Potential 81
7 Passive Membrane Properties of the Neuron 95
8 Voltage-Gated Ion Channels and the Generation of the Action Potential 104

Part III
Elementary Interactions Between Neurons: Synaptic Transmission 120

9 Synaptic Transmission 123

10 Directly Gated Transmission at the Nerve–Muscle Synapse 135
11 Directly Gated Transmission at Central Synapses 153
12 Synaptic Transmission Mediated By Second Messengers 173
13 Transmitter Release 194
14 Chemical Messengers: Small Molecules and Peptides 213
15 Synaptic Vesicles 225
16 Diseases of Chemical Transmission at the Nerve–Muscle Synapse: Myasthenia Gravis 235
17 Diseases of the Motor Unit 244
18 Reactions of Neurons to Injury 258

Part IV
Functional Anatomy of the Central Nervous System 270

19 Anatomical Organization of the Nervous System 273
20 The Neural Basis of Perception and Movement 283
21 Development as a Guide to the Regional Anatomy of the Brain 296
22 Imaging the Living Brain 309

Part V
Sensory Systems of the Brain: Sensation and Perception 326

23 Coding and Processing of Sensory Information 329
24 Modality Coding in the Somatic Sensory System 341
25 Anatomy of the Somatic Sensory System 353
26 Touch 367
27 Pain and Analgesia 385
28 Phototransduction and Information Processing in the Retina 400
29 Central Visual Pathways 420
30 Perception of Motion, Depth, and Form 440
31 Color Vision 467
32 Hearing 481
33 The Sense of Balance 500
34 Smell and Taste: The Chemical Senses 512

Part VI
Motor Systems of the Brain: Reflex and Voluntary Control of Movement 530

35 The Control of Movement 533
36 Muscles: Effectors of the Motor Systems 548
37 Muscle Receptors and Spinal Reflexes: The Stretch Reflex 564
38 Spinal Mechanisms of Motor Coordination 581
39 Posture 596
40 Voluntary Movement 609
41 The Cerebellum 626
42 The Basal Ganglia 647
43 The Ocular Motor System 660

Part VII
The Brain Stem and Reticular Core: Integration of Sensory and Motor Systems 680

44 The Brain Stem: Cranial Nerve Nuclei and the Monoaminergic Systems 683

45 Trigeminal System 701
46 Clinical Syndromes of the Spinal Cord and Brain Stem 711

Part VIII
Hypothalamus, Limbic System, and Cerebral Cortex: Homeostasis and Arousal 732

47 Hypothalamus and Limbic System: Peptidergic Neurons, Homeostasis, and Emotional Behavior 735
48 Hypothalamus and Limbic System: Motivation 750
49 The Autonomic Nervous System 761
50 The Collective Electrical Behavior of Cortical Neurons: The Electroencephalogram and the Mechanisms of Epilepsy 777
51 Sleep and Dreaming 792
52 Disorders of Sleep and Consciousness 805

Part IX
Localization of Higher Functions and the Disorders of Language, Thought, and Affect 820

53 Localization of Higher Cognitive and Affective Functions: The Association Cortices 823
54 Disorders of Language: The Aphasias 839
55 Disorders of Thought: Schizophrenia 853
56 Disorders of Mood: Depression, Mania, and Anxiety Disorders 869

Part X
Development, Critical Periods, and the Emergence of Behavior 884

57 Control of Cell Identity 887
58 Cell Migration and Axon Guidance 908
59 Neuronal Survival and Synapse Formation 929

60 Early Experience and the Fine Tuning of Synaptic Connections 945

61 Sexual Differentiation of the Nervous System 959

62 Aging of the Brain: Dementia of the Alzheimer's Type 974

Part XI
Genes, Environmental Experience, and the Mechanisms of Behavior 984

63 Genetic Determinants of Behavior 987

64 Learning and Memory 997

65 Cellular Mechanisms of Learning and the Biological Basis of Individuality 1009

Appendices

A Current Flow in Neurons 1033

B Cerebral Circulation: Stroke 1041

C Cerebrospinal Fluid: Blood–Brain Barrier, Brain Edema, and Hydrocephalus 1050

Index 1061

Contents

Preface   xxxix
Acknowledgments   xli
Contributors   xliii
How to Use This Book   xlv

Part I
An Overall View   2

1 **Brain and Behavior**   5
Eric R. Kandel

Two Alternative Views Have Been Advanced on
the Relationship Between Brain and Behavior   6

Regions of the Brain Are Specialized for
Different Functions   7

Language and Other Cognitive Functions Are
Localized Within the Cerebral Cortex   7

Affective and Character Traits Are Also
Anatomically Localized   12

Mental Processes Are Represented in the Brain by
Their Elementary Operations   15

Selected Readings   16

References   16

2 **Nerve Cells and Behavior**   18
Eric R. Kandel

The Nervous System Has Two Classes
of Cells   19
Nerve Cells   19
Glial Cells   22

Nerve Cells Are the Signaling Units of
Behavioral Responses   24

Signaling Is Organized in the Same Way in All
Nerve Cells   26

Signals Represent Changes in the Electrical
Properties of Neurons   26
*The Input Component Produces Graded Local
Signals*   27
*The Integrative Component Makes the Decision
to Generate an Action Potential*   28
*The Conductile Component Propagates an All-or-
None Action Potential*   29
The Output Component Releases Transmitter   29

The Information Carried by a Signal Is
Transformed As It Passes from One Component to
the Next   30

Nerve Cells Differ Most at the
Molecular Level   31

Patterns of Interconnection Allow Relatively
Stereotyped Nerve Cells to Convey
Unique Information   31

Selected Readings   32

References   32

Part II
Cell and Molecular Biology of the Neuron   34

3 **The Cytology of Neurons**   37
James H. Schwartz

The Neurons That Mediate the Stretch Reflex
Differ in Their Morphology and Transmitter
Substance   38

The Sensory Neuron   38
The Motor Neuron   38

The Axons of Both Sensory and Motor Neurons Are Ensheathed in Myelin   43

A Major Function of the Neuron's Cell Body Is the Synthesis of Macromolecules   45

An Overall View   47

Selected Readings   47

References   47

4 **Synthesis and Trafficking of Neuronal Proteins**   49
James H. Schwartz

Messenger RNA Gives Rise to Three Classes of Proteins   49
Cytosolic Proteins   51
Nuclear, Mitochondrial, and Peroxisomal Proteins   52
Cell Membrane Proteins and Secretory Proteins   52
Fate of Major Membrane Proteins   55

Axonal Transport Controls the Distribution of Membranes and Secretory Proteins in the Neuron   57
Fast Anterograde Transport   57
Slow Axonal Transport   58
Fast Retrograde Transport   59

Fibrillar Proteins of the Cytoskeleton Are Responsible for the Shape of Neurons   60

The Dynamics of Polymerization   62

An Overall View   64

Selected Readings   65

References   65

5 **Ion Channels**   66
Steven A. Siegelbaum and John Koester

Ions Cross the Cell Membrane Through Channels   67

Ion Channels Can Now Be Investigated by Functional and Structural Methods   68
Single-Channel Recording Can Measure the Activity of a Single Protein Molecule   68
Ion Channels Can Now Be Studied Through Molecular Biological Approaches   69

Ion Channels Share Several Characteristics   73

Ion Channels Facilitate the Passive Flux of Ions Across the Cell Membrane   73
The Opening and Closing of a Channel Involves Conformational Changes   75
Variants of Each Type of Ion Channel Are Found in Different Tissues   78
Genes That Encode Ion Channels Can Be Grouped into Families   78

An Overall View   78

Selected Readings   79

References   79

6 **Membrane Potential**   81
John Koester

Membrane Potential Results from the Separation of Charge Across the Cell Membrane   82

The Resting Membrane Potential Is Determined by the Relative Abundance of Different Types of Nongated Ion Channels   82
Nongated Channels in Glial Cells Are Selective Only for Potassium   84
Nongated Channels in Nerve Cells Are Selective for Several Ion Species   84
The Passive Fluxes of Sodium and Potassium Through Nongated Channels Are Balanced by Active Pumping of Sodium and Potassium Ions   86
Chloride Ions Are Often Passively Distributed   88

The Action Potential Is Generated by the Sequential Opening of Voltage-Gated Channels Selective for Sodium and Potassium   88

The Resting and Action Potentials Can Be Quantified by the Goldman Equation   88

The Neuron Can Be Represented by an Electrical Equivalent Circuit   89
Each Ion Channel Acts as a Conductor and Battery   89
An Equivalent Circuit Model of the Membrane Includes Batteries, Conductors, a Capacitor, and a Current Generator   90

An Overall View   92

Postscript   92
Calculation of Membrane Potential from the Equivalent Circuit Model of the Neuron   92
The Equation for Membrane Potential Can Be Written in a More General Form   93
The Sodium–Potassium Pump Counteracts the Passive Fluxes of Sodium and Potassium   94

Selected Readings   94

References   94

7 **Passive Membrane Properties of the Neuron** 95

John Koester

Membrane Capacitance Prolongs the Time Course of Electrical Signals 95

Membrane and Axoplasmic Resistance Affect the Efficiency of Signal Conduction 97

Axon Diameter Affects the Current Threshold 100

Passive Membrane Properties and Axon Diameter Affect the Velocity of Action Potential Propagation 100

An Overall View 102

Selected Readings 103

8 **Voltage-Gated Ion Channels and the Generation of the Action Potential** 104

John Koester

The Action Potential Is Generated by the Flow of Ions Through Voltage-Gated Sodium and Potassium Channels 105

Voltage-Gated Channels Can Be Studied by Use of the Voltage Clamp 105

The Voltage-Gated Sodium and Potassium Channels Have Different Kinetics 105
Sodium and Potassium Membrane Conductances Are Calculated from Their Currents 108

The Action Potential Can Be Reconstructed from the Known Electrical Properties of the Neuron 109

The Hodgkin–Huxley Model of Excitability Is Universally Applicable: Modifications Reflect the Diversity and Distribution of Voltage-Gated Channels 110

The Basic Mechanism of Action Potential Generation Is the Same in All Neurons 110
The Nervous System Expresses a Rich Variety of Voltage-Gated Ion Channels 111
Gating of Voltage-Sensitive Ion Channels Can Be Influenced by Changes in Intracellular Ion Concentrations 111
Excitability Properties Vary Among Neurons 111
Excitability Properties Vary Within Regions of the Neuron 112

Voltage-Gated Channels Have Characteristic Molecular Properties 112

Voltage-Gated Sodium Channels Are Sparsely Distributed 112

Voltage-Gated Channels Open in an All-or-None Fashion 113
Charges Are Redistributed Within the Membrane When Voltage-Gated Sodium Channels Open 113
The Voltage-Gated Sodium Channel Selects for Sodium on the Basis of Size, Charge, and Energy of Hydration of the Ion 115
The Voltage-Gated Potassium, Sodium, and Calcium Channels Belong to One Gene Family 115

An Overall View 118

Selected Readings 118

References 118

Part III
Elementary Interactions Between Neurons: Synaptic Transmission 120

9 **Synaptic Transmission** 123

Eric R. Kandel, Steven A. Siegelbaum, and James H. Schwartz

Synaptic Transmission Can Be Electrical or Chemical 124

Electrical Synapses Can Be Either Unidirectional or Bidirectional 124

Electrical Transmission Allows for Rapid and Synchronous Firing of Interconnected Cells 125
In Electrical Synapses the Pre- and Postsynaptic Elements Are Bridged by Gap Junctions 129

At Chemical Synapses the Pre- and Postsynaptic Elements Are Separated by a Synaptic Cleft 131

Chemical Transmission Involves Transmitter Release and Receptor Activation 131
Chemical Receptors Use Two Major Molecular Mechanisms to Gate Ion Channels 132

An Overall View 133

Selected Readings 134

References 134

10 **Directly Gated Transmission at the Nerve–Muscle Synapse** 135

Eric R. Kandel and Steven A. Siegelbaum

The Neuromuscular Junction Is a Simple Synapse for Studying Directly Gated Transmission 135

Synaptic Excitation of Skeletal Muscle by
Motor Neurons Involves Directly Gated
Ion Channels   138

The Ion Channel at the End-Plate Is Permeable to
Both Sodium and Potassium   139

Transmitter-Gated Channels Are Fundamentally
Different from Voltage-Gated Channels   140

The Action of a Single Transmitter-Gated Channel
Can Be Studied Experimentally   142
*Individual Transmitter-Gated Channels Conduct
a Unitary Current   144*
*Current Flow Depends on the Number of Open
Channels, Concentration of the Transmitter,
Channel Conductance, and Membrane
Potential   144*

The Nicotinic Acetylcholine Receptor Is
an Intrinsic Membrane Protein with
Five Subunits   146

An Overall View   148

Postscript: The End-Plate Current Can Be
Calculated from an Equivalent Circuit   149

Selected Readings   152

References   152

11   Directly Gated Transmission at
Central Synapses   153
Eric R. Kandel and James H. Schwartz

The Spinal Stretch Reflex Illustrates the Major
Features of Synaptic Transmission Between
Central Neurons   154

Excitatory Synaptic Action Is Mediated by
Receptor-Channels Selective for Sodium
and Potassium   155
*The Current Flow During the EPSP Can Be
Measured Experimentally   155*
*Glutamate Is a Major Excitatory Transmitter in
the Brain   158*

Inhibitory Synaptic Action Is Mediated by
Receptor-Channels Selective for Chloride   160
*The Current Flow During the IPSP Can Also Be
Readily Analyzed   160*
*GABA and Glycine Are Inhibitory
Transmitters   162*

Receptors for GABA, Glycine, and Glutamate Are
Multisubunit Transmembrane Proteins   162

Transmitter-Gated Ion Channels Are Structurally
Similar to Voltage-Gated Channels   164

Common Ionic Mechanisms Are Used in All
Neuronal Signaling   164

Excitatory and Inhibitory Synaptic Actions Are
Integrated at a Common Trigger Zone   166

Synapses onto a Single Central Neuron Are
Grouped According to Function   168
*Synapses on Cell Bodies Are Often
Inhibitory   168*
*Synapses on Dendritic Spines Are Often
Excitatory   170*
*Synapses on Axon Terminals Are Often
Modulatory   170*
*Excitatory and Inhibitory Synapses Have
Distinct Ultrastructures   170*

An Overall View   171

Selected Readings   172

References   172

12   Synaptic Transmission Mediated By
Second Messengers   173
James H. Schwartz and Eric R. Kandel

Different Second-Messenger Pathways Share a
Common Molecular Logic   175
*The Cyclic AMP Pathway Involves a Polar and
Diffusible Cytoplasmic Messenger   177*
*Some Second Messengers Are Generated Through
Hydrolysis of Phospholipids   179*

Second-Messenger Pathways Can Interact with
One Another   182

Second Messengers Often Act Through Protein
Phosphorylation to Open or Close
Ion Channels   182

Second Messengers and G-Proteins Can
Sometimes Act Directly on Ion Channels   185

Second Messengers Can Alter the Properties of
Transmitter Receptors: Desensitization   186

Second Messengers Can Regulate Gene Expression
and Thereby Endow Synaptic Transmission with
Long-Lasting Consequences   187

Other Second-Messenger Pathways: Tyrosine
Kinases and Cyclic GMP   191

An Overall View   191

Selected Readings   192

References   192

13   Transmitter Release   194
Eric R. Kandel

Transmitter Release Is Controlled by
Calcium Influx   194
Sodium Influx Is Not Necessary   195

Potassium Efflux Is Not Necessary   196
Calcium Influx Is Essential   197

Transmitter Is Released in Quantal Units   198
Calcium Influx Affects the Probability That a Quantum of Transmitter Will Be Released   199
Each Quantum of Transmitter Is Stored in a Specialized Organelle Called a Synaptic Vesicle   201

Transmitter Is Discharged from Synaptic Vesicles by Exocytosis at the Active Zone   203

The Docking of Synaptic Vesicles, Fusion, and Exocytosis Are Controlled by Calcium Influx   203
Calcium Influx Is Greatest in the Region of the Active Zone   206
Calcium Mobilizes Vesicles from the Cytoskeleton   206

The Number of Transmitter Vesicles Released Can Be Modulated by Altering Calcium Influx   206
Intrinsic Cellular Mechanisms Regulate the Concentration of Free Calcium   206
Synaptic Connections on Presynaptic Terminals Also Regulate Intracellular Free Calcium   207

An Overall View   209

Postscript: Calculating the Probability of Transmitter Release   210

Selected Readings   211

References   212

14 **Chemical Messengers: Small Molecules and Peptides**   213
James H. Schwartz

Chemical Messengers Should Fulfill Four Criteria to Be Considered Transmitters   214

There Are a Limited Number of Small-Molecule Transmitter Substances   215
Acetylcholine   215
Biogenic Amine Transmitters   215
Amino Acid Transmitters   217

There Are Many Neuroactive Peptides   217

Peptides and Small-Molecule Transmitters Differ in Several Presynaptic Aspects   221

Peptides and Small-Molecule Transmitters Can Coexist and Be Coreleased   221

An Overall View   224

Selected Readings   224

References   224

15 **Synaptic Vesicles**   225
James H. Schwartz

Transmitters Are Stored in Vesicles   225
Subcellular Fractionation Allows Biochemical Study of Vesicles   226
Transmitter Is Actively Taken up into Vesicles   226

Vesicles Are Involved in Transmitter Release   227

Synaptic Vesicle Membranes Contain Specific Proteins   227

Synaptic Vesicles Are Recycled   228

Vesicle Membranes Differ with the Type of Neuron   231

Transmitter Can Be Released by Carrier Mechanisms   232

Removal of Transmitter from the Synaptic Cleft Terminates Synaptic Transmission   232

An Overall View   233

Selected Readings   233

References   233

16 **Diseases of Chemical Transmission at the Nerve–Muscle Synapse: Myasthenia Gravis**   235
Lewis P. Rowland

Myasthenia Gravis Affects Transmission at the Nerve–Muscle Synapse   236
Physiological Studies Showed a Disorder of Neuromuscular Transmission   236
Immunological Studies Indicated That Myasthenia Is an Autoimmune Disease   236

Identification of Antibodies to the Acetylcholine Receptor Initiated the Modern Period of Research   237

Immunological Changes Cause the Physiological Abnormality   238

The Basis of Antibody Binding in Myasthenia Gravis Has Been Defined   239

The Molecular Basis of the Autoimmune Reaction Has Been Defined   241

Myasthenia Gravis May Be More than One Disease   241

Current Therapy for Myasthenia Gravis Is
Effective But Not Ideal 242

Other Disorders of Neuromuscular
Transmission: Presynaptic (Facilitating)
Neuromuscular Block 242

An Overall View 242

Selected Readings 243

References 243

17 Diseases of the Motor Unit 244
Lewis P. Rowland

The Motor Unit Includes the Neuron, Peripheral
Nerve, and Muscle Cell 244

Neurogenic and Myopathic Diseases Are
Distinguished by Clinical and
Laboratory Criteria 245
Clinical Criteria Help to Identify Neurogenic and
Myopathic Conditions 245
Laboratory Criteria 246

Diseases of Motor Neurons Are Acute
or Chronic 248
Motor Neuron Diseases Do Not Affect Sensory
Neurons 248
Motor Neuron Disease Is Characterized by
Fasciculation and Fibrillation 250

Diseases of Peripheral Nerves Are Also Acute
or Chronic 250
Neuropathies Can Have Positive or Negative
Symptoms 251
Demyelination Leads to a Slowing of Conduction
Velocity 251

Diseases of Skeletal Muscle Can Be Inherited
or Acquired 252
Muscular Dystrophies Are the Most Common
Inherited Myopathies 252
Dermatomyositis Is an Acquired Myopathy 253
Weakness in Myopathies Need Not Be Due to
Loss of Muscle Fibers 253

Molecular Genetics Illuminates the
Physiology and Pathology of Duchenne
Muscular Dystrophy 253

An Overall View 257

Selected Readings 257

References 257

18 Reactions of Neurons to Injury 258
Thomas M. Jessell

Severing the Axon Causes Degenerative Changes
in the Neuron 259
Synaptic Transmission Is Lost Rapidly 259
The Distal Axon Segment Degenerates
Slowly 260
The Membrane Compartments of the Cell Body
Are Disrupted 260
Glial Cells and Macrophages Scavenge the Debris
Caused by Injury 260

Cells That Have Synaptic Connections with
Injured Neurons Also Degenerate 261

Neurons in the Peripheral Nervous System Can
Regenerate Their Axons 262
Trophic Factors Prevent the Degeneration of
Peripheral Neurons after Axotomy 262
Schwann Cells Contribute to the Regeneration of
Peripheral Axons 264

Neurons in the Adult Central Nervous System
Have Only Limited Capacity to Regenerate
Their Axons 264

Several Potential Manipulations Can Promote the
Recovery of Function after Damage to the Central
Nervous System 265
Peripheral Nerve Grafts Promote the Growth of
Central Axons 265
Transplantation of Embryonic Neurons into Adult
Brain Promotes Recovery of Function after
Damage 266
In Some Animals New Neurons Can Be
Generated in the Adult Brain 268

An Overall View 268

Selected Readings 268

References 268

Part IV
Functional Anatomy of the
Central Nervous System 270

19 Anatomical Organization of the
Nervous System 273
James P. Kelly and Jane Dodd

The Nervous System Has Peripheral and
Central Components 273
The Peripheral Nervous System 273
The Central Nervous System 274

The Central Nervous System Consists of Six
Main Regions 275

The Cerebral Cortex Is Divided into Four Lobes
Concerned with Different Functions 276

The Motivational System Influences Behavior by Acting on the Somatic and Autonomic Motor Systems 279

Even Simple Behavior Involves the Activity of the Sensory, Motor, and Motivational Systems 279

Four Principles Govern the Organization of the Major Functional Systems 279
Each System Contains Synaptic Relays 279
Each System Is Composed of Several Distinct Pathways 280
Each Pathway Is Topographically Organized 280
Most Pathways Cross the Midline 281

An Overall View 282

Selected Readings 282

References 282

20 The Neural Basis of Perception and Movement 283
James P. Kelly
The Spinal Cord Provides Sensory and Motor Innervation to the Trunk and Limbs 283
The Internal Structure of the Spinal Cord Varies at Different Levels 284
Sensory Axons Innervating the Trunk and Limbs Originate in the Dorsal Root Ganglia 286
Central Axons of Dorsal Root Ganglion Neurons Are Arranged Somatotopically in the Dorsal Column 287
The Dorsal Column–Medial Lemniscal System Is the Principal Pathway for Somatosensory Perception 287

The Thalamus Is the Principal Synaptic Relay for Information Reaching the Cerebral Cortex 287

The Highest Level of Information Processing Occurs in the Cerebral Cortex 292

The Corticospinal Tract Is a Direct Pathway for Voluntary Movement 293

Voluntary Movements Recruit the Actions of the Entire Motor System 294

Selected Readings 295

References 295

21 Development as a Guide to the Regional Anatomy of the Brain 296
John H. Martin and Thomas M. Jessell

The Neural Tube Is the Embryonic Precursor of the Six Brain Regions 296
The Neural Tube Develops from the Neural Plate 297
The Neural Epithelium Gives Rise to the Entire Nervous System 297

The Spinal Cord and Brain Stem Follow Similar Developmental Plans 300

The Brain and Spinal Cord Become Segmented by Different Mechanisms 302

The Cavities of the Brain Vesicles Become the Ventricular System of the Brain 303

The Ventricular System Provides a Guide to Understanding the Regional Anatomy of the Diencephalon and Cerebral Hemispheres 304
The Caudate Nucleus Becomes C-Shaped Like the Lateral Ventricles 306
The Major Components of the Limbic System Also Develop into a C Shape 307

An Overall View 308

Selected Readings 308

References 308

22 Imaging the Living Brain 309
John H. Martin, John C. M. Brust, and Sadek Hilal
Imaging the Brain with X-Rays Depicts Structures with Large Differences in Absorbency of Radiation 309
Brain Asymmetry Is Revealed on Conventional Radiographs 310
Computerized Tomography Has Improved the Depiction of Brain Structures within the Skull 311

Positron Emission Tomography Localizes Biochemical Processes in the Three-Dimensional Living Brain 312

Magnetic Resonance Imaging Reveals the Structure and the Functional State of the Central Nervous System 314
Proton Images Show Structural Lesions in the Brain 321
The Paramagnetic Effects of Iron Allow Imaging of Specific Neural Systems 321
Sodium and Phosphorus Scans Reveal Cerebral Infarcts, Neoplastic Changes, and Metabolism 323

An Overall View 323

Selected Readings 324

References 324

Part V
Sensory Systems of the Brain: Sensation and Perception 326

23 Coding and Processing of Sensory Information 329
John H. Martin

Sensory Information Underlies Motor Control and Arousal As Well As Sensation 330

Sensory Systems Mediate Four Attributes of a Stimulus That Can Be Quantitatively Correlated with a Sensation 331
Modality 331
Intensity 331
Duration 333
Location 333

Sensory Systems Have a Common Plan 333
Sensory Receptors and Sensory Neurons in the Central Nervous System Have a Receptive Field 334
Sensory Information Is Processed by the Thalamus and Transmitted to the Cerebral Cortex 335
Sensory Systems Are Organized in Both a Hierarchical and Parallel Fashion 335
Sensory Systems Are Topographically Organized 335

Sensory Receptors Translate Stimulus Features into Neural Codes 336
Stimulus Intensity Is Encoded by Frequency and Population Codes 336
Stimulus Duration Is Encoded in the Discharge Patterns of Rapidly and Slowly Adapting Receptors 337
Modality Is Encoded by a Labeled Line Code 338

Stimulus Information Is Transmitted to the Central Nervous System by Conducted Action Potentials 338

An Overall View 339

Selected Readings 339

References 339

24 Modality Coding in the Somatic Sensory System 341
John H. Martin and Thomas M. Jessell

The Dorsal Root Ganglion Neuron Is the Sensory Receptor in the Somatic Sensory System 342

Different Sensory Receptors Have Distinguishing Anatomical Features 342

Pain Is Mediated by Nociceptors 343

Warmth and Cold Are Mediated by Thermal Receptors 343

Touch Is Mediated by Mechanoreceptors in the Skin 344
Glabrous and Hairy Skin Have Different Types of Mechanoreceptors 345
Mechanoreceptors Differ in Their Ability to Resolve Spatial and Temporal Features of Stimuli 346

Limb Proprioception Is Mediated by Muscle Afferent Fibers 347

Afferent Fibers of Different Diameters Conduct Action Potentials at Different Rates 349

An Overall View 352

Selected Readings 352

References 352

25 Anatomy of the Somatic Sensory System 353
John H. Martin and Thomas M. Jessell

Afferent Fibers Enter the Spinal Cord Through the Dorsal Roots 353

The Spinal Cord Is the First Relay Point for Somatic Sensory Information 354
Spinal Gray Matter Contains Nerve Cell Bodies 354
Spinal White Matter Contains Myelinated Axons 356
Dorsal Root Fibers Branch in the White Matter and Terminate in the Gray Matter 356
Afferents Conveying Different Somatic Sensory Modalities Have Distinct Terminal Projections 357

Two Major Ascending Systems Convey Somatic Sensory Information to the Cerebral Cortex 359
The Dorsal Column–Medial Lemniscal System Mediates Tactile Sense and Arm Proprioception 360
The Anterolateral System Mediates Pain and Temperature Sense 362

The Primary Somatic Sensory Cortex Is Divided into Four Functional Areas 364

Pyramidal Cells in Layers 2, 3, 5, and 6 Are the Output Cells of the Primary Somatic Sensory Cortex 364

An Overall View 365

Selected Readings   365

References   366

26 Touch   367
Eric R. Kandel and Thomas M. Jessell

Sensory Information About Touch Is Processed by a Series of Relay Nuclei   367

The Body Surface Is Represented in the Brain in an Orderly Fashion   370
Somatic Sensations Are Localized to Specific Regions of Cortex   370
Electrophysiological Studies Have Correlated Body Areas and Cortical Areas   370

Each Central Neuron Has a Specific Receptive Field   374
Sizes of Receptive Fields Vary in Different Areas of the Skin   374
Receptive Fields of Central Neurons Have Inhibitory and Excitatory Components   374
Lateral Inhibition Can Aid in Two-Point Discrimination   374

Inputs to the Somatic Sensory Cortex Are Organized into Columns by Submodality   377

Detailed Features of a Stimulus Are Communicated to the Brain   378
In the Early Stages of Cortical Processing the Dynamic Properties of Central Neurons and Receptors Are Similar   378
In the Later Stages of Cortical Processing the Central Nerve Cells Have Complex Feature-Detecting Properties and Integrate Various Sensory Inputs   380

An Overall View   381

Selected Readings   383

References   383

27 Pain and Analgesia   385
Thomas M. Jessell and Dennis D. Kelly

Noxious Insults to the Body Activate Nociceptors   386
Nociceptors Are Activated by Mechanical, Thermal, or Chemical Stimuli   386
Tissue Damage Can Sensitize Nociceptors   386
Local Pain Can Be Sensed Even When Nociceptive Pathways Are Damaged   387
Pain Syndromes Can Result From Surgery Intended to Alleviate Pain   388

Primary Afferent Fibers Synapse with Dorsal Horn Neurons   389

Primary Afferent Fibers Use Amino Acids and Peptides As Transmitters   389

Nociceptive Information Is Conveyed to the Brain Along Several Ascending Pathways   390

Pain Can Be Modulated by the Balance of Activity Between Nociceptive and Other Afferent Inputs   392

Pain Can Be Controlled by Central Mechanisms   393
Direct Electrical Stimulation of the Brain Produces Analgesia   393
Nociceptive Control Pathways Descend to the Spinal Cord   393
Opiate Analgesia Involves the Same Pathways As Stimulation-Produced Analgesia   394
Endogenous Opioid Peptides and Their Receptors Are Located at Key Points in the Pain Modulatory System   394
Supraspinal and Spinal Networks Coordinately Modulate Nociceptive Transmission   396
Local Dorsal Horn Circuits Modulate Afferent Nociceptive Input   396

Behavioral Stress Can Induce Analgesia Through Both Opioid and Nonopioid Mechanisms   397

An Overall View   398

Selected Readings   398

References   398

28 Phototransduction and Information Processing in the Retina   400
Marc Tessier-Lavigne

The Retina Contains the Eye's Receptor Sheet   401
There Are Two Types of Photoreceptors: Rods and Cones   402
Light Is Absorbed by Visual Pigments in the Outer Segments of Rods and Cones   403

Phototransduction Results from a Cascade of Biochemical Events in the Outer Segment of Photoreceptors   403
Light Activates Pigment Molecules in Photoreceptors   404
Activated Pigment Molecules Affect the Cytoplasmic Concentration of Cyclic GMP   406
Cyclic GMP Gates Specialized Ion Channels in the Plasma Membrane of the Photoreceptor   406
Closing of Cyclic GMP-Gated Ion Channels in the Outer Segment Hyperpolarizes the Photoreceptor   406
Changes in Intracellular Calcium Underlie Light Adaptation in Photoreceptors   408

Ganglion Cells Are the Output Neurons of the Retina 408

Ganglion Cell Receptive Fields Have a Center and Antagonistic Surround 409

The Properties of Ganglion Cells Enhance the Ability to Detect Weak Contrasts and Rapid Changes in the Visual Image 411

Ganglion Cells Are Also Specialized for Processing Specific Aspects of the Visual Image 412

Bipolar Cells and Other Interneurons Relay Signals from Photoreceptors to Ganglion Cells 412

Cone Signals Are Conveyed to Ganglion Cells Through Direct or Lateral Pathways 412

Bipolar Cells Also Have Center-Surround Receptive Fields 412

Each Class of Bipolar Cells Has Excitatory Connections with Ganglion Cells of the Same Class 414

Different Pathways Convey Rod Signals to Ganglion Cells in the Moderately and Extremely Dark-Adapted Eye 414

Some Chemical Synapses in the Retina Have Distinctive Morphologies 415

An Overall View 416

Selected Readings 416

References 416

29 Central Visual Pathways 420
Carol Mason and Eric R. Kandel

The Retinal Image Is an Inversion of the Visual Field 420

The Retina Projects to Three Subcortical Regions in the Brain 423

The Pretectal Area of the Midbrain Controls Pupillary Reflexes 424

The Superior Colliculus Controls Saccadic Eye Movements 424

The Lateral Geniculate Nucleus Processes Visual Information 425

Neurons in the Lateral Geniculate Nucleus Have Concentric Receptive Fields 426

The Primary Visual Cortex Transforms Concentric Receptive Fields into Linear Segments and Boundaries 427

Simple and Complex Cells Decompose the Outlines of a Visual Image into Short Line Segments of Various Orientation 430

Some Feature Abstraction Can Be Accomplished by Progressive Convergence Within the Primary Visual Cortex 431

The Primary Visual Cortex Is Organized into Vertical Columns 431

Columnar Units Are Linked by Horizontal Connections 434

The Visual and Somatic Sensory Cortices Are Functionally Similar 436

Lesions in the Retino-Geniculate-Cortical Pathway Cause Predictable Changes in Vision 436

An Overall View 438

Selected Readings 438

References 438

30 Perception of Motion, Depth, and Form 440
Eric R. Kandel

Visual Perception Is a Creative Process 441

Vision Is Thought to Be Mediated by Three Parallel Pathways That Process Information for Motion, Depth and Form, and Color 445

Psychological Evidence Supports the Idea That Separate Pathways Carry Different Visual Information 448

Clinical Evidence Is Also Consistent with Parallel Processing of Visual Information 448

Motion in the Visual Field Is Analyzed by a Special Neural System 449

Motion Is Represented in the Middle Temporal Area (V5) and Medial Superior Temporal Area (V5a) 450

Lesions of the Middle Temporal Area Selectively Impair the Ability to Analyze Motion 452

The Perceptual Judgment of Motion Direction Can Be Influenced by Microstimulation of Cells Within the Middle Temporal Area 452

Three-Dimensional Vision Depends on Monocular Depth Cues and Binocular Disparity 454

Monocular Cues Create Far-Field Depth Perception 454

Stereoscopic Cues Create Near-Field Depth Perception 455

Information from the Two Eyes Is First Combined in the Primary Visual Cortex 457

Recognition of Faces and Other Complex Forms Occurs in the Inferior Temporal Cortex 458

Visual Attention Focuses Perception by Facilitating Coordination Between Separate Visual Pathways 459

The Analysis of Visual Attention May Provide Important Clues Toward Understanding Conscious Awareness 462

An Overall View   464

Selected Readings   464

References   465

31   Color Vision   467
Peter Gouras

Three Separate Cone Systems Respond Best to
Different Parts of the Visible Spectrum   468

Color Discrimination Requires at Least Two
Types of Photoreceptors with Different
Spectral Sensitivities   468

Color Opponency, Simultaneous Color Contrast,
and Color Constancy Are Key Features of
Color Vision   470
In the Retina and Lateral Geniculate Nucleus
Color Is Coded by Color Opponent Cells   471
In the Cortex Color Information Is Processed by
Double-Opponent Cells in the Blob Zones   473
Double-Opponent Cells Help Explain Color
Opponency, Color Contrast, and Color
Constancy   476

Color Experience Is Based on Impressions of Hue,
Saturation, and Brightness   476

Color Blindness Can Be Caused by Genetic
Defects in Photoreceptors or by
Retinal Disease   477

An Overall View   479

Selected Readings   479

References   479

32   Hearing   481
James P. Kelly

Sound Is Produced by Vibrations and
Is Transmitted Through Air by
Pressure Waves   481

Vibrations of the Conductive Apparatus Generate
Fluid Waves in the Cochlea   482

Fluid Waves in the Cochlea Vibrate
Hair Cells   483
Different Regions of the Cochlea Respond
Selectively to Different Frequencies of
Sound   486
Individual Hair Cells at Different Points Along
the Cochlea Are Tuned to Different Frequencies
of Vibration   487

Vibrations of Hair Cells Are Transformed into
Electrical Signals in the Auditory Nerve   489

Central Auditory Neurons Are Specialized
Physiologically to Preserve Time and
Frequency Information   491

Bilateral Auditory Pathways Provide Cues to
Localize Sound   493

The Auditory Cortex Is Composed of Separate
Functional Areas   494

An Overall View   498

Selected Readings   498

References   498

33   The Sense of Balance   500
James P. Kelly

The Organs of Balance Are Located in the
Inner Ear   501
The Vestibular Labyrinth Is Filled with
Endolymph   501
Specialized Regions of the Vestibular Labyrinth
Contain Hair Cells   501

Vestibular Hair Cells Respond to Changes in
Movement or Position of the Head   503
The Hair Cells Are Polarized Structurally and
Functionally   503
The Semicircular Ducts Respond to Angular
Acceleration in Specific Directions   506
The Utricle Responds to Linear Acceleration in
All Directions   506

The Central Connections of the Vestibular
Labyrinth Reflect Its Dynamic and
Static Functions   508
The Lateral Vestibular Nucleus Participates in the
Control of Posture   508
The Medial and Superior Vestibular Nuclei
Mediate Vestibulo-Ocular Reflexes   509
The Inferior Vestibular Nucleus Integrates Inputs
from the Vestibular Labyrinth and the
Cerebellum   510

An Overall View   510

Selected Readings   510

References   511

34   Smell and Taste: The Chemical
Senses   512
Jane Dodd and Vincent F. Castellucci

Smell and Taste Result from the Activation of
Specific Receptors   513

The Sensation of Smell Is Transduced by Neurons
Within the Olfactory Epithelium   513

*Presentation of Odorants to the Receptor Cell
May Involve an Olfactory Binding Protein*   514

*Olfactory Transduction Involves Second
Messenger-Regulated Ion Channels*   515

*Individual Olfactory Neurons Respond to a
Variety of Odorants*   515

**Olfactory Information Is First Encoded in the
Paleocortex and Then Projects to the Neocortex
via the Thalamus**   516

**Abnormalities of Olfaction Can Give Rise to Both
Sensory Loss and Hallucination**   518

**The Sensation of Taste Is Transduced by
Gustatory Receptor Cells**   518

*Taste Receptor Cells Are Innervated by Primary
Afferent Neurons*   519

*Four or Five Basic Stimulus Qualities Can Be
Distinguished*   521

**There Are Distinct Representations of Taste in the
Thalamus and Cortex**   524

*Afferents from Taste Buds Project to the
Gustatory Nucleus*   524

*Taste Sensations Are Encoded by Specific
Pathways and by Patterns of Activity Across
These Pathways*   525

**Both Inborn and Learned Taste Preferences Are
Important for Behavior**   527

An Overall View   527

Selected Readings   528

References   528

Part VI
Motor Systems of the Brain:
Reflex and Voluntary Control
of Movement   530

35 **The Control of Movement**   533
Claude Ghez

**Sensory Information Is Necessary for the Control
of Movement**   534

*Sensory Information Is Used to Correct Errors
Through Feedback and Feed-forward
Mechanisms*   535

*Patients with Impaired Sensation in the Limbs
Show Deficits in Both Feedback and Feed-forward
Control of Movement*   535

**There Are Three Levels in the Hierarchy of
Motor Control**   537

*The Spinal Cord, the Brain Stem, and Cortical
Motor Areas Are Organized Hierarchically and in
Parallel*   537

*The Cerebellum and Basal Ganglia Control the
Cortical and Brain Stem Motor Systems*   539

**Motor Neurons in the Spinal Cord Are Subject to
Afferent Input and Descending Control**   539

*Spinal Motor Neurons Are Topographically
Organized into Medial and Lateral Groups That
Innervate Proximal and Distal Muscles*   539

*The Terminations of Medial and Lateral
Interneurons and Propriospinal Neurons Have
Different Distributions*   540

**The Brain Stem Modulates Motor Neurons and
Interneurons in the Spinal Cord Through
Four Systems**   540

*Medial Pathways Control Axial and Proximal
Muscles*   541

Lateral Pathways Control Distal Muscles   541

*Aminergic Pathways Modulate the Excitability of
Spinal Neurons*   541

**The Motor Cortex Acts on Motor Neurons
Directly Via the Corticospinal Tract and Indirectly
Through Brain Stem Pathways**   542

*The Corticospinal Tract Is the Largest Descending
Fiber Tract from the Brain*   543

*Cortical Control of Movement Is Achieved Only
Late in Phylogeny*   543

**Lesions of the Cortical Motor Areas and Their
Projections Cause Characteristic Symptoms**   543

*Muscle Weakness May Result from Disturbances
in Descending Motor Pathways or in the Spinal
Motor Neurons Themselves*   545

*Parallel Control of Motor Neurons Allows
Recovery of Function Following Lesions*   546

An Overall View   546

Selected Readings   547

References   547

36 **Muscles: Effectors of the Motor
Systems**   548
Claude Ghez

**Movement and Force Are Produced by the
Contraction of Sarcomeres**   548

*Contraction Results from the Sliding of
Filamentous Proteins within the Muscle
Fiber*   548

*The Force of Contraction Depends on the Length
of the Muscle*   551

*The Force of Contraction Also Depends on the
Relative Rates of Movement of the Thick and
Thin Filaments*   552

*Muscles Contract Slowly and the Force Generated
by a Train of Impulses Summates*   553

*Repeated Activation of Muscles Causes
Fatigue*   555

**A Single Motor Neuron and the Muscle Fibers It
Innervates Constitute a Motor Unit**   555

*Three Types of Motor Units Are Distinguished by
the Properties of Their Muscle Fibers*   555

*The Properties of Motor Neurons Are Closely
Matched to Muscle Fibers*   556

**The Nervous System Grades the Force of Muscle
Contraction in Two Ways**   556

*Motor Units Are Recruited in a Fixed Order from
Weakest to Strongest*   556

*Increases in Firing Rate of Motor Units Produce
Increasing Force Output*   559

**Muscle Properties Limit the Strategies Available
to Control Movement**   560

*Several Strategies Can Produce a Given Joint
Angle*   560

*Skeletal Muscles Are Low-Pass Filters of Neural
Input*   561

An Overall View   562

Selected Readings   563

References   563

37   Muscle Receptors and Spinal Reflexes: The Stretch Reflex   564

James Gordon and Claude Ghez

**Muscles Contain Specialized Receptors That
Sense Different Features of the State of
the Muscle**   565

*Muscle Spindles Respond to Stretch of Specialized
Muscle Fibers*   566

*Golgi Tendon Organs Are Sensitive to Changes in
Tension*   567

*Functional Differences Between Spindles and
Tendon Organs Derive from Their Different
Anatomical Arrangements within Muscle*   568

**Muscle Spindles Are Sensitive to
Muscle Stretch**   569

*The Primary and Secondary Endings of Spindle
Afferents Respond Differently to Phasic Changes
in Length*   569

*Two Types of Gamma Motor Neurons Alter the
Responsiveness of Spindles*   570

*Spindle Afferents and Efferents Innervate Different
Types of Intrafusal Fibers*   570

**The Central Nervous System Can Control
Sensitivity of the Muscle Spindles Through the
Gamma Motor Neurons**   571

*The Fusimotor System Maintains Spindle
Sensitivity During Muscle Contraction*   571

*Fusimotor Output Can Be Adjusted
Independently of Motor Output*   573

**Discharge of Muscle Spindle Afferents Produces
Stretch Reflexes**   574

*The Stretch Reflex Has Phasic and Tonic
Components*   574

*Group Ia Afferents Make Monosynaptic
Connections to Motor Neurons*   575

*The Main Connections of Group II and
Group Ib Afferents to Motor Neurons Are
Polysynaptic*   576

Stretch Reflexes Contribute to Muscle Tone   577

*Stretch Reflexes Regulate Muscle Tone Through
Negative Feedback*   577

*Stretch Reflexes Allow Muscles to Respond
Smoothly to Stretch and Release*   578

An Overall View   578

Selected Readings   579

References   580

38   Spinal Mechanisms of Motor Coordination   581

James Gordon

**Interneurons Are the Building Blocks of
Spinal Reflexes**   582

*Convergent and Divergent Connections Are the
Basis of Reflex Pathways*   582

*Networks of Interneurons Coordinate the Timing
of Reflex Components*   582

**Inhibitory Interneurons Coordinate Muscle Action
Around a Joint**   584

*Group Ia Inhibitory Interneurons Coordinate
Opposing Muscles*   585

*Renshaw Cells Are Part of a Negative Feedback
Loop to Motor Neurons*   585

*Group Ib Inhibitory Interneurons Receive
Convergent Input from Several Types of
Receptors*   586

**Cutaneous Stimuli Elicit Complex Reflexes That
Serve Protective and Postural Functions**   586

*Cutaneous Stimuli Modulate the Excitability of
Specific Motor Neuron Pools*   586

*Flexion Reflex Pathways Coordinate Whole Limb
Movements*   587

*Certain Reflexes Consist of Rhythmic
Movements*   589

*Certain Reflexes Adapt to Different Body
Postures*   590

**Spinal Circuits Generate Rhythmic
Locomotor Patterns**   591

Tonic Descending Signals from the Brain Stem Activate the Spinal Circuits Responsible for Locomotion 591

NMDA Receptors Are Involved in Generating the Locomotor Pattern 593

Goal-Directed Locomotion Requires Intact Supraspinal Systems 593

Afferent Information Modifies the Rhythmic Locomotor Pattern 593

An Overall View 594

Selected Readings 594

References 594

39   Posture   596
Claude Ghez

Postural Stability During Standing and Walking Is Maintained by Both Feedforward Control and Rapid Feedback Compensatory Corrections 597

Three Classes of Sensory Input Are Important for Triggering Postural Responses but Are Normally Used in Different Ways 597

The Topography of Rapid Postural Responses Is Dependent on Context 598

Postural Responses Are Triggered Centrally Before Voluntary Movements 599

Vestibular and Neck Reflexes Stabilize the Head and Eyes 600

Vestibulocollic and Vestibulospinal Reflexes Maintain the Head Vertical with Respect to Gravity 600

Neck and Vestibular Reflexes Are Synergistic in the Neck but Antagonistic in the Limbs: Cervicocollic and Cervicospinal Reflexes 601

Vestibular and Neck Afferents Converge on the Vestibular Nuclei and Propriospinal Neurons 602

Brain Stem and Spinal Mechanisms Play a Major Role in the Control of Posture 602

The Pontine Reticular Nuclei Facilitate Motor Neurons Whereas Medullary Reticular Nuclei Produce Both Facilitation and Inhibition 602

Section of the Brain Stem above the Vestibular Nuclei Produces Decerebrate Rigidity 604

Lesions of the Cerebellum Modify Vestibular and Reticular Influences on Posture 604

Spasticity Is a Common Manifestation of Supraspinal Lesions in Humans 606

An Overall View 606

Selected Readings 606

References 607

40   Voluntary Movement   609
Claude Ghez

The Motor Areas of the Cerebral Cortex Are Organized Somatotopically 610

The Primary Motor, Supplementary Motor, and Premotor Areas Contribute the Majority of Axons in the Corticospinal Tract 611

Inputs to Motor Areas from the Periphery, Cerebellum, and Basal Ganglia Are Mediated by Other Areas of Cortex and the Thalamus 611

Corticospinal Axons Influence Segmental Motor Neurons Through Direct and Indirect Connections 612

Neurons of the Primary Motor Cortex Encode the Direction of the Force Exerted 613

Individual Corticospinal Neurons Control Small Groups of Muscles 613

Neurons in the Primary Motor Cortex Encode the Amount of Force to Be Exerted 613

Movement Direction Is Encoded by Populations of Neurons, Not By Single Cells 614

Neurons in the Motor Cortex Are Informed of the Consequences of Movements 616

Premotor Cortical Areas Prepare the Motor Systems for Movement 619

Motor Preparation Time Is Longer Than the Response Time to Stimuli 619

Lesions of the Premotor Cortex, Supplementary Motor, and Posterior Parietal Areas Impair the Ability to Execute Purposeful Movements 619

The Supplementary Motor Area Is Important in Programming Motor Sequences and in the Coordination of Bilateral Movements 619

The Premotor Cortex Controls the Proximal Movements that Project the Arm to Targets 620

The Posterior Parietal Lobe Plays a Critical Role in Providing the Visual Information for Targeted Movements 622

An Overall View 624

Selected Readings 624

References 624

41   The Cerebellum   626
Claude Ghez

The Regional Organization of the Cerebellum Reflects Its Different Functions 627

The Cerebellum Is Divided into Three Lobes 627

Two Longitudinal Furrows Divide the Cerebellum into Medial and Lateral Regions 628

The Cellular Organization of the Cerebellum Is Highly Regular 630

The Cerebellar Cortex Is Divided into Three Distinct Layers 630

The Purkinje Cells Provide the Output of the Cerebral Cortex and Receive Excitatory Input from Three Fiber Systems 631

Purkinje Cells Are Inhibited by Local Interneurons 632

The Cerebellum Has Three Functional Divisions 632

The Vestibulocerebellum Controls Balance and Eye Movements 634

The Vestibulocerebellum Receives Input Directly from the Vestibular Nuclei 634

Diseases of the Vestibulocerebellum Cause Disorders in the Control of Eye Movements and Disturbances of Equilibrium 634

The Spinocerebellum Adjusts Ongoing Movements 634

The Spinocerebellum Contains Complete Somatosensory Maps of the Body 634

Somatic Sensory Information Reaches the Spinocerebellum Mainly Through Direct and Indirect Mossy Fiber Pathways 635

Efferent Spinocerebellar Projections Control the Medial and Lateral Descending Systems in the Brain Stem and Cerebral Cortex 635

The Spinocerebellum Uses Sensory Feedback to Control Muscle Tone and the Execution of Movement 637

The Cerebrocerebellum Coordinates the Planning of Limb Movements 637

The Cerebrocerebellum Is the Center of a Complex Feedback Circuit That Modulates Cortical Motor Commands 637

Lesions of the Cerebrocerebellum Produce Delays in Movement Initiation and in Coordination of Limb Movement 637

The Cerebellum Participates in Motor Learning 642

Cerebellar Diseases Have Distinctive Symptoms and Signs 644

An Overall View 645

Selected Readings 645

References 645

42 The Basal Ganglia 647

Lucien Côté and Michael D. Crutcher

The Basal Ganglia Consist of Five Nuclei 648

The Basal Ganglia Receive Input from and Project to the Cortex By Way of the Thalamus 648

Internuclear Connections in the Basal Ganglia Are Topographically Organized 650

The Basal Ganglia Project to Nuclei in the Thalamus 650

The Neostriatum Is Organized into Modules Called Striosomes and Matrix 651

The Motor Portion of the Basal Ganglia Is Somatotopically Organized and Involved in Higher-Order Aspects of Movement 651

The Basal Ganglia Are Linked to Cortex for Behavioral Functions Unrelated to Voluntary Movements 652

The Circuits within the Basal Ganglia Use Different Neurotransmitters 652

Diseases of the Basal Ganglia Have Characteristic Disorders in Transmitter Metabolism 653

Loss of Dopaminergic Cells Leads to Parkinson's Disease 654

The Neurotoxin MPTP Produces a Parkinsonian Syndrome 655

Huntington's Disease Results from the Loss of Striatal Neurons 656

There Are Now Genetic Markers for Huntington's Disease 656

Tardive Dyskinesia Is a Response to Long-Term Treatment with Antipsychotic Drugs 657

Glutamate-Induced Neuronal Cell Death Contributes to Huntington's Disease 657

An Overall View 658

Selected Readings 658

References 659

43 The Ocular Motor System 660

Michael E. Goldberg, Howard M. Eggers, and Peter Gouras

Five Neuronal Control Systems Keep the Fovea on Target 661

The Vestibulo-ocular and Optokinetic Reflexes Compensate for Head Movement 661

The Smooth Pursuit System Keeps Moving Targets in the Fovea 663

The Saccadic System Points the Fovea Toward Objects of Interest 664

The Vergence Movement System Aligns the Eyes to Look at Targets with Different Depths 664

The Eye Is Moved by Three Complementary Pairs of Muscles 664

Eye Position and Velocity Are Signaled by Extraocular Motor Neurons 665

The Vestibulo-ocular Reflex Is Coordinated in the Brain Stem   667

The Semicircular Canals Send an Eye Velocity Signal to Brain Stem Oculomotor Centers   667

Disease of the Vestibular System Causes Nystagmus   668

A Brain Stem Network Coordinates the Horizontal Vestibulo-ocular Reflex   668

A Neural Integrator Maintains Eye Position After the Head Has Stopped Moving   669

Modulation of the Vestibulo-ocular Reflex Requires the Cerebellum   670

Subcortical and Cortical Structures Contribute to the Optokinetic Reflex   671

Saccades and Smooth Pursuit Are Organized in Pontine and Mesencephalic Reticular Centers   671

Horizontal Saccades Are Generated in the Pontine Reticular Formation   671

Vertical Saccades Are Generated in the Mesencephalic Reticular Formation   672

Modulation of the Saccadic System by Experience Requires the Cerebellum   672

Smooth Pursuit Requires the Cerebral Cortex, Cerebellum, and Pons   672

Vergence Is Organized in the Midbrain   673

Patients with Brain Stem Lesions Have Characteristic Deficits in Eye Movements   673

The Saccade Generator in the Brain Stem Is Controlled in the Cerebral Cortex   674

The Superior Colliculus Transmits Cortical Oculomotor Signals to the Brain Stem   674

The Frontal Eye Field Sends a Specific Movement Signal to the Superior Colliculus   675

An Overall View   675

Selected Readings   676

References   676

**Part VII
The Brain Stem and Reticular Core:
Integration of Sensory
and Motor Systems**   680

44   **The Brain Stem: Cranial Nerve Nuclei and the Monoaminergic Systems**   683
Lorna W. Role and James P. Kelly

Most Cranial Nerves Are Located in the Brain Stem   683

Cranial Nerves Contain Motor, Visceral, and Somatic Afferent Fibers   684

There Are Three Classes of Motor Neurons in the Brain Stem   686

There Are Four Classes of Sensory Neurons   687

The Cranial Nerve Nuclei Are Organized into Columns   687

The Motor Nuclei   687

The Sensory Nuclei   690

Several Principles Govern the Organization of the Brain Stem   691

Most Motor Nuclei in the Brain Stem Project to Their Targets Through a Single Cranial Nerve   691

The Sensory Nuclei in the Brain Stem Receive Input from Several Cranial Nerves   691

Somatic Sensory and Motor Tracts Traverse the Brain Stem   691

Cranial Nerve Fiber Types May Intermingle in the Periphery   691

Nuclei in the Reticular Formation Form Widespread Networks   692

There Are Three Major Monoaminergic Systems in the Brain Stem   693

The Noradrenergic System Originates in Two Nuclear Groups: The Locus Ceruleus and the Lateral Tegmental Nucleus   696

The Dopaminergic System Originates in the Midbrain and Projects to the Striatum, Limbic System, and Neocortex   697

The Serotonergic System Originates in the Raphe Nuclei   698

An Overall View   698

Selected Readings   699

References   699

45   **Trigeminal System**   701
Jane Dodd and James P. Kelly

The Trigeminal Nerve Has Three Major Branches That Innervate the Face, Oral Cavity, and Dura Mater   701

Trigeminal Nerve Fibers Ascend to the Principal Sensory Nucleus and Descend to the Spinal Nucleus   702

Tactile Sensation from the Face Is Mediated by the Principal Sensory Nucleus   702

Pain and Temperature Sensation Are Mediated by the Spinal Nucleus   702

Lesions of the Trigeminal Sensory System Have Elucidated the Functional Organization of the Spinal Nucleus   705

Proprioceptive Responses from the Jaw Muscles Are Mediated by the Mesencephalic Nucleus   705

The Trigeminal Motor Nucleus Controls the Activity of the Jaw Muscles   706

Trigeminal Sensory Information Is Mapped Somatotopically in the Cortex   707

Whiskers Are Represented in the Unique Modular Organization in the Cortex   707

An Overall View   708

Selected Readings   710

References   710

46 Clinical Syndromes of the Spinal Cord and Brain Stem   711
Lewis P. Rowland

The Clinically Important Anatomy of the Spinal Cord Involves Four Descending or Ascending Tracts   712

Somatotopic Organization of the Spinothalamic Tract Is an Aid to Diagnosis and Treatment of Chronic Pain   713

Function Is Lost Below a Transverse Spinal Lesion   714
The Site of a Spinal Cord Lesion May be Indicated by Focal Weakness (the Motor Level)   715
The Site of a Spinal Cord Lesion Is More Often Indicated by the Pattern of Sensory Loss (the Sensory Level)   715

It Is Important to Distinguish Intra-Axial from Extra-Axial Spinal Lesions   715

Lesions of the Spinal Cord Often Give Rise to Characteristic Syndromes   716
Complete Transection   717
Partial Transection   717
Hemisection (Brown-Séquard Syndrome)   718
Multiple Sclerosis   718
Syringomyelia   718
Subacute Combined Degeneration   719
Friedreich's Ataxia   719

The Brain Stem Is the Site of a Number of Essential Functions   719

Extra-Axial Lesions of the Brain Stem Are Illustrated by the Acoustic Neuroma and Other Tumors of the Cerebellopontine Angle   719

Intra-Axial Lesions of the Brain Stem Often Cause Gaze Palsies and Internuclear Ophthalmoplegia   720
Gaze Palsies   720

Syndrome of the Median Longitudinal Fasciculus: Internuclear Ophthalmoplegia   721

Vascular Lesions of the Brain Stem and Midbrain May Cause Characteristic Syndromes   722
Medial Syndromes of the Medulla and Pons   724
Lateral Syndromes of the Medulla and Pons   726
Midbrain Syndromes   728
Coma and the Locked-In Syndrome   728

An Overall View   729

Selected Readings   729

References   730

**Part VIII
Hypothalamus, Limbic System, and Cerebral Cortex: Homeostasis and Arousal**   732

47 Hypothalamus and Limbic System: Peptidergic Neurons, Homeostasis, and Emotional Behavior   735
Irving Kupfermann

The Anatomy of the Hypothalamus and Limbic System Reflects Their Interrelated Functions   736
Higher Cortical Centers Communicate with the Hypothalamus via the Limbic System   737
The Structure of the Hypothalamus Reflects Its Diverse Functions   739

The Hypothalamus Contains Various Classes of Peptidergic Neuroendocrine Cells   740
Peptidergic Neurons Control Endocrine Function   740
Magnocellular Neurons Secrete Oxytocin and Vasopressin   741
Parvocellular Neurons Secrete Inhibiting and Releasing Hormones   742
Both Magnocellular and Parvocellular Neurons Contain Multiple Peptides that Are Found Throughout the Nervous System   743

Hypothalamic Neurons Participate in Four Classes of Reflexes   744
Milk Ejection and Uterine Contraction Are Regulated by Neural Input and Humoral Output   744
Urine Flow Is Regulated by Humoral Input and Output   744
Feedback Loops Involve Humoral Input and Output   744
Central Effects of Hormones on Behavior Involve Humoral Input and Neural Output   745

Neurons in the Hypothalamus Undergo Structural and Biochemical Changes in Response to Behavioral Demands   746

The Hypothalamus Helps Regulate the Autonomic Nervous System and Is Involved in Emotional Behavior   746

An Overall View   747

Selected Readings   748

References   748

48   Hypothalamus and Limbic System: Motivation   750
Irving Kupfermann

Motivation Is an Inferred Internal State Postulated to Explain Variability of Behavioral Responses   750

Homeostatic Processes Such as Temperature Regulation, Feeding, and Thirst Correspond to Motivational States   751

Temperature Regulation Involves Integration of Autonomic, Endocrine, and Skeletomotor Responses   752

Feeding Behavior Is Regulated by a Great Variety of Mechanisms   753
Body Weight Is Regulated Around a Set Point   753
Dual Controlling Elements Are Involved in the Control of Food Intake   754
Chemical Stimulation of the Hypothalamus Alters Feeding Behavior   756

Thirst Is Regulated by Tissue Osmolality and Vascular Volume   757

Motivational States Can Be Regulated by Factors Other Than Tissue Needs   758
Ecological Constraints   758
Anticipatory Mechanisms   758
Hedonic Factors   759

Intracranial Stimulation Can Simulate Motivational States and Reinforce Behavior   759

An Overall View   759

Selected Readings   759

References   760

49   The Autonomic Nervous System   761
Jane Dodd and Lorna W. Role

The Autonomic Nervous System Is a Visceral and Largely Involuntary Motor System   762

The Autonomic Nervous System Is Organized into Three Divisions   763
The Sympathetic (Thoracolumbar) Division   764
The Parasympathetic (Craniosacral) Division   766
The Enteric Division   766

The Hypothalamus and the Nucleus of the Solitary Tract Play a Major Role in Controlling the Output of the Autonomic Nervous System   766

The Autonomic Nervous System Has Been Studied at the Cellular Level   768
Synaptic Transmission in Autonomic Ganglia Is Predominantly Cholinergic   768
Autonomic Targets Are Regulated by Both Cholinergic and Noradrenergic Input   769
Autonomic Control of Target Function Is Coordinately Regulated   770

An Overall View   774

Selected Readings   774

References   775

50   The Collective Electrical Behavior of Cortical Neurons: The Electroencephalogram and the Mechanisms of Epilepsy   777
John H. Martin

The Collective Behavior of Neurons Can Be Studied Noninvasively in Humans with Macroelectrodes   778

The Cellular Mechanisms Underlying Electroencephalography   779
The EEG Is Generated in the Cortex by the Flow of Synaptic Currents Through the Extracellular Space   781
The EEG Reflects Primarily Synaptic Potentials in Pyramidal Cells   784

Epilepsy Interrupts Normal Brain Function   785
Partial and Generalized Seizures Have Different Clinical and EEG Features   785
Large Populations of Neurons Are Activated Synchronously During an Epileptic Seizure   786
A Depolarization Shift Underlies Focal Seizures   787

Excitatory Connections Between Cortical Neurons Synchronize Discharges in an Epileptic Focus 789

Synaptic Inhibition May Limit Seizure Spread 789

Generalized Epilepsy Can Be Produced Experimentally 789

An Overall View 790

Selected Readings 790

References 791

51 **Sleep and Dreaming** 792
Dennis D. Kelly

Sleep Is an Active and Rhythmic Neural Process 793

Normal Sleep Is Composed of a Recurring Succession of Identifiable Stages 793

Slow-Wave Sleep Stages Are Distinguished Principally by Electroencephalographic Criteria 793

An Active Sleep Stage Can Be Distinguished by Rapid Eye Movements (REM Sleep) 794

Sleep Architecture Refers to the Pattern of Sleep Stages Throughout the Night 795

There Are Several Clues to the Biological Importance of REM Sleep 795

Selective Deprivation of REM Sleep Results in a REM Rebound 795

The Need for REM Sleep Steadily Declines During Early Development 795

The Need for REM Sleep Differs Markedly Across Species 796

REM Sleep Can Occur Without Atonia Following Damage to the Pons 797

The Mental Content of Dreams Is Linked to the Physiology of Sleep 797

Several Neural Mechanisms May Be Responsible for the Sleep–Wake Cycle 798

Sleep Factors Interact with the Immune System 798

Early Concepts of the Reticular Activating System Cast Sleep as a Passive Process 799

Active Sleep-Inducing Neurons Reside in the Brain Stem 799

The Suprachiasmatic Nucleus Serves as the Biological Clock for the Sleep–Wake Cycle 800

Distinct Regions of the Brain Stem May Trigger REM Sleep 801

An Overall View 802

Selected Readings 803

References 803

52 **Disorders of Sleep and Consciousness** 805
Dennis D. Kelly

Insomnia Is a Symptom with Many Causes, Not a Unitary Disease 806

The Sleep of Insomniacs Differs Physiologically from That of Normal Sleepers 806

Anticipation of Insomnia May Cause Insomnia 807

Psychopathology Is Often Mirrored in Disturbed Sleep 807

Temporary Insomnia Is a Natural Consequence of Altered Circadian Rhythms 807

Sleep Problems Are Magnified in the Elderly 808

The Barbiturates: Earlier Sleep Medications Initially Helped, Then Harmed Sleep 808

The Benzodiazepines: Subjective Benefits to Insomniacs May Exceed Objective Improvements in Sleep Measures 809

Parasomnias Are Behavioral Dysfunctions Associated with Sleep, Sleep Stages, or Partial Arousals 810

Nocturnal Enuresis Is Not Caused by Dreaming 810

Sleepwalking Is Triggered by Arousal from Slow-Wave Sleep 810

REM Behavior Disorder: REM Sleep Without Atonia Causes Violent Episodes in Human Sleepers 811

Night Terrors, Nightmares, and Terrifying Dreams Occur in Different Stages of Sleep 811

Sleep Apnea: Persistent Nocturnal Arousals Can Result from Lapses in Breathing 812

Narcolepsy: Irresistible Sleep Attacks Are Accompanied by Several REM-Related Symptoms 813

Loss of Consciousness: Coma Is Not Deep Sleep 815

Transient Losses of Consciousness Can Result from Decreased Cerebral Blood Flow 815

Coma Has Many Causes 815

The Determination of Cerebral Death Constitutes a Medical, Legal, and Social Decision 817

Selected Readings 818

References 818

Part IX
Localization of Higher Functions and
the Disorders of Language, Thought, and
Affect   820

53 Localization of Higher Cognitive and Affective Functions: The Association Cortices   823
Irving Kupfermann

The Three Association Areas Are Involved in Different Higher Functions   825

The Association Areas of the Frontal Region Are Thought to Be Involved in Cognitive Behavior and Motor Planning   826

Lesions of the Principal Sulcus in Monkeys Interfere with Specific Motor Tasks   827

Lesions of the Inferior Prefrontal Convexity Interfere with Appropriate Motor Responses   829

The Association Areas of the Limbic Cortex Are Involved in Memory and in Aspects of Emotional Behavior   829

The Orbitofrontal Cortex and Cingulate Gyrus Are Concerned with Emotional Behavior   829

The Temporal Lobe Portion of the Limbic Association Cortex Is Thought to Be Concerned with Memory Functions   830

The Association Areas of the Parietal Lobes Are Involved in Higher Sensory Functions and Language   831

The Two Hemispheres Are Not Fully Symmetrical and Differ in Their Capabilities   832

Split-Brain Experiments Reveal Important Asymmetries and Show That Consciousness and Self-Awareness Are Not Unitary   833

Why Is Function Lateralized to One Hemisphere?   835

Cognitive Functions Can Be Simulated by Connectionist Networks Capable of Parallel Distributed Processing   836

An Overall View   837

Selected Readings   838

References   838

54 Disorders of Language: The Aphasias   839
Richard Mayeux and Eric R. Kandel

Language Is Distinctive from Other Forms of Communication   840

Animal Models of Human Language Have Been Largely Unsatisfactory   840

What Is the Origin of Human Language?   841

Is the Capability for Language an Innate Skill or Learned?   842

Aphasias Are Disorders of Language that Also Interfere with Other Cognitive Functions   843

The Wernicke–Geschwind Model for Language Is a Useful Clinical Model for Distinguishing Damage to the Two Major Language Regions of the Brain   843

Recent Cognitive and Imaging Studies of Normal Subjects and Aphasic Patients Have Clarified the Interconnections of the Two Language Regions   845

Seven Types of Aphasia Can Be Distinguished and Related to Different Anatomical Systems   846

Wernicke's Aphasia   846

Broca's Aphasia   847

Conduction Aphasia   847

Anomic Aphasia   848

Global Aphasia   848

Transcortical Aphasias   848

Subcortical Aphasia   848

Certain Affective Components of Language Are Affected by Damage to the Right Hemisphere   848

Some Disorders of Reading and Writing Can Be Localized   849

Alexias and Agraphias Are Acquired Disorders of Reading and Writing   849

Dyslexia and Hyperlexia Are Developmental Disorders of Reading   850

An Overall View   850

Selected Readings   850

References   851

55 Disorders of Thought: Schizophrenia   853
Eric R. Kandel

Defining a Psychiatric Syndrome Poses Unusual Difficulties   853

There Are Now Reliable Clinical Criteria for Classifying Mental Illnesses   854

Schizophrenia Has Been Studied Extensively to Improve Classification and Diagnosis of the Illness   854

Schizophrenia Is Characterized by Psychotic Episodes Preceded by Prodromal Signs and Followed by Residual Symptoms   855

Schizophrenia Has an Important Genetic Predisposition   856

Some People with Schizophrenia Have Prominent Anatomical Changes in the Brain   857

Antipsychotic Drugs Are Effective in the Treatment of Schizophrenia   858

Antipsychotic Drugs Block Dopamine Receptors   860

Excess Dopaminergic Transmission May Contribute to the Development of Schizophrenia   861

Schizophrenic Symptoms Have Been Associated with Distinct Anatomical Components Within the Dopaminergic System   863

Abnormalities in Dopaminergic Transmission Do Not Account for All Aspects of Schizophrenia   865

An Overall View   866

Selected Readings   867

References   867

56 **Disorders of Mood: Depression, Mania, and Anxiety Disorders**   869
Eric R. Kandel

The Major Affective Disorders Can Be Either Unipolar or Bipolar   870

Unipolar Depression Is Most Likely Several Disorders   870

Bipolar Depressive (Manic-Depressive) Disorders Give Rise to Euphoria and Depression   871

There Is a Strong Genetic Predisposition for Affective Disorders   871

Depressive and Manic-Depressive Disorders Can Now Be Treated Effectively   872

Drugs Effective in Depression Act on Serotonergic and Noradrenergic Pathways   875

An Abnormality in Biogenic Amine Transmission May Contribute to the Affective Disorders   875

Depression May Involve Disturbances of Neuroendocrine Function   879

There Are Two Major Types of Anxiety Disorders   880

Panic Attacks Are Brief Episodes of Terror   881

Generalized Anxiety Disorder Is Long-Lasting   881

An Overall View   882

Selected Readings   882

References   882

Part X
Development, Critical Periods, and the Emergence of Behavior   884

57 **Control of Cell Identity**   887
Thomas M. Jessell and Samuel Schacher

Cell Lineage Can Control the Fate of Neural Cells   888

In Most Species the Fate of Neural Cells Is Not Determined by Cell Lineage   891

Neural and Epidermal Cell Fate Is Regulated by Local Cell Interactions   891

Induction of the Neural Plate from the Ectoderm Is Dependent on Interactions with the Adjacent Mesoderm   891

Regional Differentiation Within the Neural Plate Is Also Controlled by the Mesoderm   896

Studies of Invertebrate Embryos Have Identified Genes that Control the Fate of Ectodermal Cells   896

Diffusible Factors Control Glial Cell Differentiation in the Central Nervous System   898

Cell Position Controls the Identity of Photoreceptors in the *Drosophila* Eye   899

The Fate of Neural Crest Cells Is Controlled by the Local Environment   902

The Transmitter Choice of Peripheral Neurons Is Controlled by Signals from Neighboring Cells   904

An Overall View   905

Selected Readings   906

References   906

58 **Cell Migration and Axon Guidance**   908
Thomas M. Jessell

The Migration Pattern of Neurons Establishes the Basic Plan of the Central Nervous System   908

The Birthday of a Neuron Defines Its Eventual Position and Properties   909

Immature Neurons in the Brain Migrate on a Scaffold of Radial Glial Cells   909

The Growth Cone Guides the Axon to Its Target   911

The Pathways of Developing Axons Are Accurate   914

Studies in Invertebrates Reveal the Precision of Axon Pathfinding and the Existence of Specific Cellular Cues   915

Guidance Cues Can Be Inhibitory   916

Some Growth Cones Are Guided by Chemotropic Molecules   916

Adhesion Molecules Are Involved in Axon Extension   917

Several Major Classes of Glycoproteins Are Involved in Neural Cell Adhesion   918

Many Glycoproteins Involved in Axon Fasciculation Are Members of the Immunoglobulin Superfamily   921

Axons Often Pause As They Project to Their Targets   921

Molecular Gradients May Help Axons Find Their Correct Location Within a Target Field   921

Pruning of Axons Focuses Their Projection to Targets   922

The Initial Formation of Synaptic Connections Is Often Accurate   923

An Overall View   926

Selected Readings   926

References   926

59   **Neuronal Survival and Synapse Formation**   929
Thomas M. Jessell

The Survival of Neurons Is Regulated by Interactions with Their Targets   929

The Survival of Many Classes of Neurons Depends on Nerve Growth Factor   930

The Activity of Target Muscle Regulates the Survival of Motor Neurons   933

Synapse Formation Is a Gradual Process   935

The Presynaptic Nerve Terminal Triggers Biochemical and Morphological Changes in the Postsynaptic Membrane   936

The Distribution and Stability of Nicotinic Acetylcholine Receptors Change After Innervation of Skeletal Muscle   937

The Functional Properties of Nicotinic Acetylcholine Receptors in Muscle Change After Innervation   939

Other Components of the Nerve–Muscle Synapse Are Also Regulated by Innervation of Muscle   940

Innervation Changes the Contractile Properties of Muscle   941

Presynaptic Neurons Also Regulate the Development of Nicotinic Receptors in Neurons   941

The Postsynaptic Muscle Cell Regulates the Differentiation of the Motor Nerve Terminal   941

Some Synapses Are Eliminated During Development   942

An Overall View   943

Selected Readings   943

References   943

60   **Early Experience and the Fine Tuning of Synaptic Connections**   945
Eric R. Kandel and Thomas Jessell

Normal Development Depends on Sensory Experience and Social Interaction   946

There Is an Early Critical Period in the Development of Social and Perceptual Competence   946

Isolated Young Monkeys Do Not Develop Normal Social Behavior   946

Early Sensory Deprivation Alters Perceptual Development   947

Early Sensory Deprivation Alters the Development of Neural Circuits   947

The Development of Ocular Dominance Columns Is an Important Example for Understanding the Development of Behavior   949

Cooperation and Competition Are Important for Segregating Afferent Inputs into the Ocular Dominance Columns   950

Cooperation Requires Synchronous Activity   953

Different Regions of the Brain Have Different Critical Periods of Development   956

Studies of Development Are Important Clinically   957

An Overall View   957

Selected Readings   957

References   958

61   **Sexual Differentiation of the Nervous System**   959
Dennis D. Kelly

The Gene for the Testes Determining Factor Is Located on the Y Chromosome   960

The Developing Gonads Are Embryologically Bipotential, Becoming Testes If the TDF Gene Is Present and Ovaries If It Is Not   961

Sexual Differentiation Is Regulated by
Gonadal Hormones from Both Mother and
Male Fetus   962

Gonadal Hormones Exert Both Organizational and
Regulatory Effects upon Nervous Tissue
Depending upon the Stage of the Life Cycle   962

Perinatal Hormones Impose a Permanent Sex-
Specific Blueprint upon the Developing
Nervous System   963
*Fetal Exposure to Male Hormones Causes
Pseudohermaphroditism in Genetic Females*   963
*Steroid Hormones Influence Perinatal
Development Only During Critical Periods*   964
*The Brain Can Be Masculinized Not Only by
Male Hormones But Also by Many Other
Compounds*   964

Alpha-Fetoprotein Binds Estrogen in the
Rat and Thus Protects Female Fetuses
from Masculinization   965

Receptors in the Cell Nucleus Mediate the Effects
of Gonadal Steroid Hormones   965

Sexually Differentiated Brains Have
Different Physiological Properties and
Behavioral Tendencies   967
*Perinatal Hormones Also Determine the Degree to
Which Sex-Linked Behaviors Are Expressed by
Normal Males and Females*   968
*Sexual Differentiation Is Reflected in the
Structure of Certain Neurons*   968
*The Cellular Mechanisms Involved in the
Development of Sex Differences in the Brain Can
Be Studied in Vitro*   969

A Wide Range of Behaviors Is Influenced by Sex
Differences in the Organization of the Brain   970
*Sexual Dimorphism Is Evident in Cognitive
Development in Monkeys*   970
*Human Cerebral Asymmetry Is Sexually
Dimorphic*   971

An Overall View   971

Selected Readings   972

References   972

62   Aging of the Brain: Dementia of the
Alzheimer's Type   974
James Goldman and Lucien Côté
Several Hypotheses Have Been Proposed for the
Molecular Mechanisms of Aging   974

Normal Aging Produces Characteristic Changes in
the Brain and Behavior   976

Progressive Decline in Mental Function Is Not An
Inevitable Consequence of Aging   976

Alzheimer's Disease Is the Most Common Form
of Dementia   976
*There Is a Genetic Component to Certain Forms
of Alzheimer's Disease*   977
*Extracellular Plaques Containing Amyloid
Deposition Are a Prominent Feature of
Alzheimer's Disease*   977
*Neurofibrillary Tangles Are an Intracellular
Characteristic of Alzheimer's Disease*   979
*There Are Neurotransmitter Deficits in
Alzheimer's Disease*   981

Other Degenerative Diseases Also
Produce Dementia   981

An Overall View   982

Selected Readings   982

References   982

Part XI
Genes, Environmental Experience,
and the Mechanisms of Behavior   984

63   Genetic Determinants of
Behavior   987
Irving Kupfermann
Are Aspects of Behavior
Genetically Determined?   987
*Ethologists Define Instincts as Inborn Motor
Patterns*   988
Can a Behavior Be Inherited?   988

Some Species-Specific Behaviors Are Elicited by
Sign Stimuli   989

Each Species Has a Repertory of Fixed-Action
Patterns Generated by Central Programs   989

The Role of Genes in the Expression of Behavior
Can Be Studied Directly   991

Higher Mammals and Humans Seem to Have
Certain Innate Behavioral Patterns   993
*Certain Human Behavioral Traits Have a
Hereditary Component*   993
Many Human Behaviors Are Universal   993
*Stereotyped Sequences of Movements Resemble
Fixed-Action Patterns*   993
*Certain Complex Patterns Require Little or No
Learning*   994

The Brain Sets Limits on the Structure
of Language   994

An Overall View   995

Selected Readings   996

References   996

64 **Learning and Memory**   997
Irving Kupfermann

Certain Elementary Forms of Learning Are Nonassociative   998

Classical Conditioning Involves Associating a Conditioned and an Unconditioned Stimulus   998

Conditioning Involves the Learning of Predictive Relationships   999

Operant Conditioning Involves Associating an Animal's Own Behavior with a Subsequent Reinforcing Environmental Event   1000

Food-Aversion Conditioning Illustrates How Biological Constraints Influence the Efficacy of Reinforcers   1001

Conditioning Is Used as a Therapeutic Technique   1001

Learning and Memory Can Be Classified as Reflexive or Declarative on the Basis of How Information Is Stored and Recalled   1002

The Neural Basis of Memory Can Be Summarized in Four Generalizations   1003

Memory Has Stages   1003

Long-Term Memory May Be Represented by Plastic Changes in the Brain   1004

The Plastic Changes Encoding Memory Are Often Localized in Different Places Throughout the Nervous System   1005

Reflexive and Declarative Memories May Involve Different Neuronal Circuits   1005

An Overall View   1007

Selected Readings   1007

References   1007

65 **Cellular Mechanisms of Learning and the Biological Basis of Individuality**   1009
Eric R. Kandel

Simple Forms of Reflexive Learning Lead to Changes in the Effectiveness of Synaptic Transmission   1010

Habituation Involves Depression of Synaptic Transmission   1010

Sensitization Involves Enhancement of Synaptic Transmission   1012

Long-Term Memory Requires Synthesis of New Proteins and the Growth of New Synaptic Connections   1014

Classical Conditioning Involves an Associative Enhancement of Presynaptic Facilitation That Is Dependent on Activity   1016

Long-Term Potentiation in the Hippocampus Is an Example for Both Associative and Nonassociative Learning in the Mammalian Brain   1019

Long-Term Potentiation in the CA1 Region Is Associative   1019

Associative Long-Term Potentiation Is Thought to Be Important for Spatial Memory   1022

Long-Term Potentiation in the CA3 Region Is Nonassociative   1023

Is There a Molecular Grammar for Learning?   1023

The Somatotopic Map in the Brain Is Modifiable by Experience   1024

Changes in the Somatotopic Map Produced by Learning May Contribute to the Biological Expression of Individuality   1025

Changes in the Somatotopic Map May Reflect Common Cellular Mechanisms for Associative Plasticity   1026

Studies of Neuronal Changes with Learning Provide Insights into Psychiatric Disorders   1027

An Overall View   1028

Selected Readings   1030

References   1030

Appendices

A **Current Flow in Neurons**   1033
John Koester

Definition of Electrical Parameters   1033

Potential Difference (V or E)   1033

Current (I)   1034

Conductance (g)   1034

Capacitance (C)   1034

Rules for Circuit Analysis   1036

Conductance   1036

Current   1036

Capacitance   1037

Potential Difference   1037

Current Flow in Circuits with Capacitance   1038

Circuit with Capacitor   1038

Circuit with Resistor and Capacitor in Series   1038

Circuit with Resistor and Capacitor in Parallel   1039

B   Cerebral Circulation: Stroke   1041
John C. M. Brust

The Blood Supply of the Brain Can Be Divided into Arterial Territories   1041

The Cerebral Vessels Have Unique Physiological Responses   1043

A Stroke Is the Result of Disease Involving Blood Vessels   1045

Clinical Vascular Syndromes May Follow Vessel Occlusion, Hypoperfusion, or Hemorrhage   1045

Infarction Can Occur in the Middle Cerebral Artery Territory   1045

Infarction Can Occur in the Anterior Cerebral Artery Territory   1046

Infarction Can Occur in the Posterior Cerebral Artery Territory   1046

The Anterior Choroidal and Penetrating Arteries Can Become Occluded   1046

The Carotid and Basilar Arteries Can Become Occluded   1047

Diffuse Hypoperfusion Can Cause Ischemia or Infarction   1047

The Rupture of Microaneurysms Causes Intraparenchymal Stroke   1047

The Rupture of Saccular Aneurysms Causes Subarachnoid Hemorrhage   1048

Stroke Alters the Vascular Physiology of the Brain   1048

Selected Readings   1049

C   Cerebrospinal Fluid: Blood–Brain Barrier, Brain Edema, and Hydrocephalus   1050
Lewis P. Rowland, Matthew E. Fink, and Lee Rubin

Cerebrospinal Fluid Is Secreted by the Choroid Plexus   1050

Cerebrospinal Fluid Has Several Functions   1053

Specific Permeability Barriers Exist Between Blood and Cerebrospinal Fluid and Between Blood and Brain   1053

The Properties of the Brain Capillary Endothelial Cells Account for the Blood–Brain Barrier   1054

The Blood–Brain Barrier Develops Early   1055

Some Areas of the Brain Do Not Have a Blood–Brain Barrier   1055

Why Is a Blood–Brain Barrier Necessary?   1056

Disorders of the Blood–Brain Barrier   1056

Drug Delivery to the Brain   1057

The Composition of Cerebrospinal Fluid May Be Altered in Disease   1057

Increased Intracranial Pressure May Harm the Brain   1057

Brain Edema Is a State of Increased Brain Volume Due to Increased Water Content   1058

Vasogenic Edema Is a State of Increased Extracellular Fluid Volume   1058

Cytotoxic Edema Is the Swelling of Cellular Elements   1058

Interstitial Edema Is Attributed to Increased Sodium in Periventricular White Matter   1058

Hydrocephalus Is an Increase in the Volume of the Cerebral Ventricles   1059

Selected Readings   1060

References   1060

Index   1061

Preface

The goal of neural science is to understand the mind, how we perceive, move, think, and remember. In the two previous editions of this book we stressed that important aspects of behavior could be examined at the level of individual nerve cells by seeking answers to four questions: How does the brain develop? How do nerve cells in the brain communicate with one another? How do different patterns of interconnections give rise to different perceptual and motor acts? How is neural communication modified by experience? In the first two editions the approach to these problems was for the most part framed in cell biological terms. Now it is also possible to address these questions directly on the molecular level.

It was already clear a decade ago that molecular studies would make interesting contributions to the understanding of how ion channels in the membrane of nerve cells produce the resting potential, the action potential, and the various synaptic potentials. But it was not certain how rapidly these contributions would come and how important they would be. In fact, for many years the molecular study of nerve cell signaling progressed slowly, until suddenly neurobiologists realized that a great deal of information about the structure of membrane proteins could be inferred from simply inspecting the protein's amino acid sequence. Specifically, the sequences contain important clues as to how proteins are arranged in the membrane. In addition, the sequences often reveal unexpected similarities to other proteins, which provide novel insights into function. Moreover, the methods of *reverse genetics* made it possible for neurobiologists to test ideas about molecular structure and function. The resulting analysis, on the molecular level, has provided a completely new view of both voltage-gated and transmitter-gated channels involved in neuronal signaling.

Similar molecular approaches have also deepened our understanding of the nature of the membrane receptors that are coupled to intracellular second-messenger systems and how these receptors modulate physiological responses of nerve cells. In addition, there has been dramatic progress in understanding the molecular basis of neural development. Characterization of the genes encoding transcriptional regulatory factors, diffusible signals, and cell and substrate adhesion molecules has changed a cellular field into a molecular one. We now can identify mechanisms important in the development of the nervous system, including the generation of cell lineages, cell–cell adhesion, axon outgrowth, target recognition, and synapse formation.

Finally, molecular biology has made it possible to probe the pathogenesis of a variety of disorders that effect neural function, including several devastating genetic disorders: muscular dystrophy, retinoblastoma, and neurofibromatosis. For these diseases the mutant gene has now been identified, sequenced, and characterized. The genetic analysis of Huntington's disease, Alzheimer's disease, and even depression and schizophrenia soon may reach a similar level of understanding. These remarkable new insights into the genetic basis of these diseases are useful for genetic counseling, developing new drugs, and perhaps even gene therapy. As a result, we think it is time to stress even more vigorously a belief advocated in previous editions: that the future of clinical neurology and psychiatry is intimately tied to that of molecular neural science.

What has made the past six years particularly remarkable is that the progress in molecular neural science has been matched by advances in the biology of higher brain functions. These advances are particularly evident in the mapping of mental functions ranging from perception to selective attention to specific regions of the brain. This progress owes much to the collaboration of cognitive psychology with neural science, a collaboration we encouraged in the previous editions of this text. Until recently, ascribing a particular aspect of behavior to an unobservable mental process—such as selective attention—removed the problem from direct experimental analysis. The ability to locate mental functions to particular regions of the brain whose activities can be monitored allows even complex cognitive processes to be studied directly. As a result, higher mental functions no longer need be completely inferred.

Despite the complexity of recent advances in neural science, our aim remains to write a coherent introduction to the nervous system for a broad range of students of behavior, biology, and medicine. Because this is a textbook for students with different backgrounds and different academic goals, we try to make clear the major principles that have emerged from studying the nervous system without becoming lost in detail. As neurobiology takes a central position within the biological sciences, students interested in biology increasingly want to become familiar with neural science in their undergraduate years. Likewise, more students in psychology are interested in the biological basis of behavior. Thus, we have made a special effort in this new edition to write a text useful to undergraduate students of biology and psychology, as well as to graduate and medical students. We do this by providing comprehensive introductions to each of the major topics in neural science: ion channels, synaptic transmission, perception, motor control, development, motivation, and learning. We also have added didactic boxes to explain clearly the importance of certain key methodological and conceptual issues.

We hope, through this third edition, to encourage the next generation of undergraduate, graduate, and medical students to see the study of behavior in a new way, a way that unites both its social and biological dimensions. Engraved at the entrance to the Temple of Apollo at Delphi was the famous maxim "Know thyself." From ancient times understanding human behavior has been central to Western culture. Thus, the study of the mind and consciousness defines the frontier of biology. Throughout this book we both document the central principle that all behavior is an expression of neural activity and illustrate the insights into behavior that neural science provides.

Eric R. Kandel
James H. Schwartz
Thomas M. Jessell

Acknowledgments

A book by a single faculty reflects its university. Columbia has provided a stimulating intellectual environment that encourages interaction between basic science and clinical departments, an essential condition for writing an interdisciplinary book. It is therefore a pleasure again to express our indebtedness to our colleagues at the College of Physicians & Surgeons of Columbia University, to Donald Tapley who, as Dean of the College, founded the Center of Neurobiology and Behavior, and to Herbert Pardes, our current Dean, whose efforts continue to strengthen it.

We were fortunate in this edition to have recruited Howard Beckman who edited the several versions of this text with his characteristic demand for clarity and logic of argument. We are again indebted to Kathrin Hilten, who has been with the Center for Neurobiology and Behavior since its inception, for the initial preparation and final editing of the artwork. As always she took on this difficult and time consuming task by combining expertise with judgment, taste, and good humor. We also benefitted greatly from the help of Sarah Mack. For the final version of the figures, we are grateful to Terese Winslow and Jonathan Dimes.

Many colleagues read portions of the manuscript critically. We are particularly indebted to Ronald Calabrese for his careful reading of the first third of the book and to John H. Martin for helping us again with the anatomical drawings. In addition, the following friends and colleagues have made constructive comments on various chapters: Tom Abrams, George Aghajanian, Albert Aguayo, Richard Aldrich, David Anderson, Nancy Andreasen, Samuel Barondes, Barbara Barres, Allan Basbaum, Denis Baylor, Floyd Bloom, Dianne Broussard Belknap, James Bloedel, Robert Burke, John Byrne, Tom Carew, Greg Clark, Martha Constantine-Paton, David Corey, Maxwell Cowan, Lee Crews, Antonio Damasio, Mahlon Delong, Marc Dichter, John Dowling, Anke Ehrhardt, Howard Fields, Marion Frank, Esther Gardner, Michael Gazzaniga, M. Felice Ghilard, Charles Gilbert, Alexander Glassman, Mitchell Glickstein, André Golard, Jay Goldberg, Jack Gorman, Roger Gorski, Ann Graybiel, Amiran Grinvald, Charles Gross, Murray Grossman, Jeffrey Hall, Ziaul Hasan, Robert Hawkins, Fritz Henn, Bertil Hille, Stephen Ho, J. Allan Hobson, John Horn, Robert Horvitz, James Houk, Ronald Hoy, David Hubel, Albert Hudspeth, Richard Huganir, Bruce Johnson, Kenneth Johnson, Edward Jones, Bela Julesz, John Kauer, Charles Kaufmann, Darcy Kelley, Gerald Klerman, Mark Konishi, Edward Kravitz, Arnold Kriegstein, Yves Lamarre, Donald Lawrence, M. Charles Lieberman, Jeff Lichtman, Steven Lisberger, Margaret Livingstone, Arthur Loewy, Jennifer Lund, Robert McBurney, Susan McConnell, Bruce McEwan, Jack McMahan, Richard Masland, Gary Mawe, John Maunsell, Lorne Mendell, Frederick Miles, Christopher Miller, Robert Moore, Kent Morest, Richard Morimoto, Adrian Morrison, Anthony Movshon, William Newsome, Roger Nicoll, Keir Pearson, Edward Perl, Gian Poggio, Michael Posner, Tom Powell, Donald Price, David Prince, Arthur Prochazka, Ed Pugh, Efraim Racker, Martin Raff, Marcus Raichle, Stanley Rapaport, Elio Raviola, Steven Rayport, Robert Rescorla, Frances Richmond, Howard Roffwarg, John Rush, David Sabatini, Joshua Sanes, Peter Sargent, Peter Schiller, Howard Schulman, Dennis Selkoe, Michael Selzer, Carla Shatz, Ann-Judith Silverman, Jerome Siegel, Solomon Snyder, David Sparks, Larry Squire, Peter Sterling, Charles Stevens, Peter Strick, Thomas Sudhof, Nobuo Suga, Larry Swanson, Terry Takahashi, John Tallman, C. Dominique Toran-Allerand, Allan Wagner, B. Timothy Walsh, Elizabeth Warrington, Stanley Watson, Daniel Weinberger, Myrna Weissman, William Willis, Jeffery Winer, Steven Wise, Robert Wong, Robert Wurtz, and Semir Zeki.

We also are greatly indebted to Seta Izmirly, who patiently and with great effectiveness coordinated the production of all aspects of the book at Columbia, and to Erilyn Riley, who read both the galleys and the page proofs. We thank Harriet Ayers and Andrew Krawetz for typing the many versions of the manuscript, Mildred Bobrovich for checking the bibliography and Judy Cuddihy for preparing the index. Finally, we are indebted to Susan Schmidler of Elsevier for her imaginative participation in producing this edition, to her artist assistant Gregg Eisenberg, and to Kimberly Quinlan, our desk editor.

Contributors

College of Physicians and Surgeons of Columbia University

John C. M. Brust, M.D.
Professor, Department of Neurology; Director of Neurology Service, Harlem Hospital

Vincent F. Castellucci, Ph.D.
Director, Department of Neurobiology, Institut de Recherches de Montreal, Montreal, Quebec, Canada

Lucien Côté, M.D.
Professor, Departments of Neurology and Rehabilitation Medicine

Michael Crutcher, Ph.D.
Assistant Professor, Department of Neurology, Emory University, Atlanta, Georgia

Jane Dodd, Ph.D.
Assistant Professor, Department of Physiology and Cellular Biophysics; Center for Neurobiology and Behavior

Howard Eggers, M.D.
Assistant Professor, Department of Ophthalmology

Matthew E. Fink, M.D.
Assistant Professor of Clinical Neurology, Department of Neurology; Director, Neurological Intensive Care Unit, Columbia Presbyterian Medical Center

Claude Ghez, M.D., Ph.D.
Professor, Department of Neurology and Department of Physiology and Cellular Biophysics; Center for Neurobiology and Behavior; New York State Psychiatric Institute

Michael E. Goldberg, M.D.
Laboratory of Sensorimotor Research; National Eye Institute, National Institutes of Health, Bethesda, Maryland

James E. Goldman, M.D., Ph.D.
Associate Professor, Department of Pathology; Center for Neurobiology and Behavior

James Gordon, Ed.D.
Assistant Professor, Program in Physical Therapy; Center for Neurobiology and Behavior

Peter Gouras, M.D.
Professor, Department of Ophthalmology

Sadek Hilal, M.D.
Professor, Department of Radiology

Thomas M. Jessell, Ph.D.
Professor, Department of Biochemistry and Molecular Biophysics; Center for Neurobiology and Behavior; Investigator, The Howard Hughes Medical Institute

Eric R. Kandel, M.D.
University Professor, Department of Physiology and Cellular Biophysics and Department of Psychiatry; Center for Neurobiology and Behavior; Senior Investigator, The Howard Hughes Medical Institute

Dennis D. Kelly, Ph.D.
Associate Professor, Department of Psychiatry; New York State Psychiatric Institute

James P. Kelly, Ph.D.
Associate Research Scientist, Departments of Anatomy and Cell Biology and Otolaryngology

John Koester, Ph.D.
Associate Professor of Clinical Neurobiology and Behavior in Psychiatry; Acting Director, Center for Neurobiology and Behavior; New York State Psychiatric Institute

Irving Kupfermann, Ph.D.
Professor, Department of Psychiatry and Department of Physiology and Cellular Biophysics; Center for Neurobiology and Behavior

John H. Martin, Ph.D.
Assistant Professor, Department of Psychiatry; Center for
Neurobiology and Behavior

Carol Ann Mason, Ph.D.
Associate Professor, Departments of Pathology and Anatomy
and Cell Biology; Center for Neurobiology and Behavior

Richard Mayeux, M.D.
Professor, Departments of Neurology and Psychiatry

Lorna W. Role, Ph.D.
Assistant Professor, Department of Anatomy and Cell Biology;
Center for Neurobiology and Behavior

Lee L. Rubin, Ph.D.
Adjunct Associate Professor, Department of Pathology; Athena
Neurosciences, San Francisco, California

Lewis P. Rowland, M.D.
Professor and Chairman, Department of Neurology; Director of
Neurological Service, Neurological Institute, Columbia
Presbyterian Medical Center

Samuel Schacher, Ph.D.
Associate Professor, Department of Anatomy and Cell Biology
and Department of Psychiatry; Center for Neurobiology and
Behavior; New York State Psychiatric Institute

James H. Schwartz, M.D., Ph.D.
Professor, Departments of Physiology and Neurology; Center
for Neurobiology and Behavior; Investigator, The Howard
Hughes Medical Institute

Steven Siegelbaum, Ph.D.
Associate Professor, Department of Pharmacology; Center for
Neurobiology and Behavior; Associate Investigator, The
Howard Hughes Medical Institute

Marc Tessier-Lavigne, Ph.D.
Assistant Professor, Department of Anatomy, University of
California, San Francisco, California

How to Use This Book

The book originated as a textbook for the 65 lectures in neurobiology and behavior for medical students, graduate students, and house officers in neurology and psychiatry at the College of Physicians & Surgeons of Columbia University. Here at Columbia the book was read in sequence in its entirety, with one lecture devoted to each chapter.

With this edition we have expanded the original contents of the book so that it can also be used as a primary textbook in undergraduate and graduate courses. First, this new edition can be used by undergraduates in a single semester neurobiology course in which the focus is on five topics: the cell biology of signaling, motor perception, organization, development, and higher mental functions. For this undergraduate course we recommend using appropriate parts of the following 25 chapters: Chapters 1 and 2 to provide an overall view; Chapters 6, 9, 10, 11, 12, 13, 14, 15, and 16 to cover the cell biology of signaling; Chapters 20, 22, 23, 24, 25, 26, 27, and Chapters 35 and 40 for a coverage of perception and motor coordination; Chapters 53, 60, 61, 64, and 65 to serve as an introduction to higher mental functions.

Second, this book can be used by undergraduates in an introduction to neuropsychology: the neurobiology of behavior. Here we would suggest using Chapters 1 and 2 as an introduction, Chapters 5, 9, 10, 11, 12, 13, and 14 for coverage of neuronal signaling, Chapters 19 to 35 for perception and movement, and Chapters 47 to 56 and 60, 61, 63, 64 and 65 for motivation, learning, and other higher mental functions.

Finally, the book can serve as text in an advanced graduate course in neurobiology. Here, Chapter 1 can be used as a general introduction to contemporary ideas in neural science and Chapters 2 through 4 as a brief refresher on the cell biology of nerve cells. Chapters 5 through 15 describe neuronal signaling: the excitable properties of nerve cells, impulse initiation, and synaptic transmission. Chapters 23 through 31 illustrate the neural basis of sensation, focusing on the somatosensory and visual systems. Chapters 35 and 40 describe the principles of motor organization. An overview of the development of the nervous system is given in Chapters 57 through 60, and cellular approaches to learning and memory are described in Chapter 65.

We invite comments on how the text might be changed to make it better suited for nonmedical undergraduate courses and for medical students.

PRINCIPLES
OF NEURAL
SCIENCE

THIRD EDITION

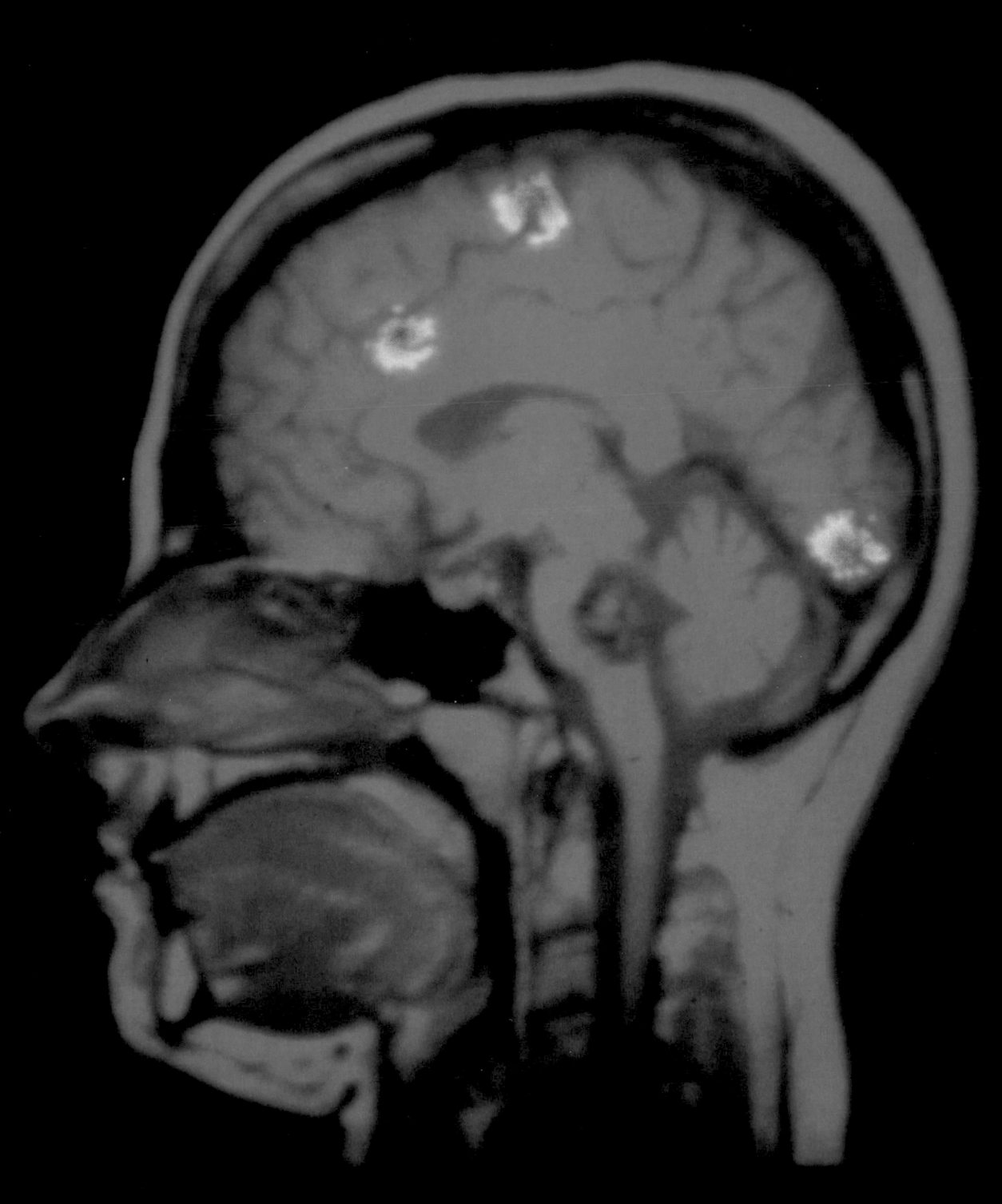

An Overall View

Perhaps the last frontier of science—its ultimate challenge—is to understand the biological basis of consciousness and the mental processes by which we perceive, act, learn, and remember. Are these processes localized to specific regions of the brain, or do they represent a collective and emergent property of the whole brain? If various mental processes can be localized to different brain regions, what rules relate the anatomy and physiology of a region to its specific function in perception, thought, or movement? Can these rules be understood better by examining the region as a whole or by studying its individual nerve cells? How do genes contribute to behavior, and how is gene expression in nerve cells regulated by developmental and learning processes? Can experience alter the way the brain processes and perceive subsequent events? In Part I of this book we introduce the study of the nervous system by considering to what degree mental functions can be located to specific regions of the brain. Within those regions we shall want to know to what degree behavior can be understood in terms of the properties of specific nerve cells and their interconnections.

Behaviorism dominated experimental psychology for a good part of the 20th Century. Behaviorists thought that the only way to study behavior was by examining a subject's observable actions. They regarded the brain as an unapproachable black box and denied the usefulness of studying mental processes because they were basically unobservable. The current view of psychology is very different. Most psychologists now want to look into the black box and understand how mental processes function. Toward that end, Michael Posner, a psychologist at the University of Oregon, and Marcus Raichle, a neurologist at Washington University in St. Louis, have combined the techniques of cognitive psychology and positron emission tomography (PET) to study mental processes such as cognition and affect by making them observable in the living brain. In this illustration PET scanning was used to visualize thought and language in action. These PET scans of brain function have been laid over a magnetic resonance image of the brain's anatomy. Bright spots generated by the PET scans show three areas in the left brain that are metabolically active during a language task. The back of the head lights up when the subject reads. The area in the middle is active during speech. And the area at the front brightens when the subject thinks about the meaning of a word. (From *DISCOVER*, March 1989.)

PART I

Chapter 1:   Brain and Behavior
Chapter 2:   Nerve Cells and Behavior

Eric R. Kandel

1

Brain and Behavior

Two Alternative Views Have Been Advanced on the Relationship Between Brain and Behavior

Regions of the Brain Are Specialized for Different Functions

Language and Other Cognitive Functions Are Localized Within the Cerebral Cortex

Affective and Character Traits Are Also Anatomically Localized

Mental Processes Are Represented in the Brain by Their Elementary Operations

The central tenet of modern neural science is that all behavior is a reflection of brain function. According to this view, a view that we shall try to document in this text, what we commonly call mind is a range of functions carried out by the brain. The action of the brain underlies not only relatively simple motor behaviors such as walking, breathing, and smiling, but also elaborate affective and cognitive behaviors such as feeling, learning, thinking, and composing a symphony. As a corollary, the disorders of affect (feelings) and cognition (thought) that characterize neurotic and psychotic illness can be seen as disturbances of brain function.

The brain is made up of individual units—nerve cells (or neurons) and glial cells. The task of neural science is to explain how the brain marshalls these units to control behavior and how, in turn, the functioning of the constituent cells in an individual's brain is influenced by that person's environment, including the behavior of other people. In this chapter and the next we provide an overall view of this task. In this chapter we examine the strategies used by the human brain to represent language, the most elaborate cognitive behavior. We shall focus on the cerebral cortex, the part of the brain that has expanded most in recent primate evolution and that is concerned with higher aspects of human behaviors. We illustrate how large groups of neurons are organized within the nervous system and how even highly complex behaviors can be localized to specific regions of the brain. In the next chapter we shall consider nervous system function at the cellular level, using a simple reflex behavior to examine how sensory signals are transformed into motor acts.

Two Alternative Views Have Been Advanced on the Relationship Between Brain and Behavior

Current views of nerve cells, the brain, and behavior have emerged over the last century from the coalescence of five experimental traditions: anatomy, embryology, physiology, pharmacology, and psychology.

The anatomical complexity of nervous tissue was not appreciated before the invention of the compound microscope. Until the eighteenth century nervous tissue was thought to be glandular in function, an idea that was based on Galen's proposal that nerves are ducts conveying fluid secreted by the brain and spinal cord to the periphery of the body. Toward the end of the nineteenth century, the histology of the nervous system became a more precise science, culminating in the investigations of Camillo Golgi and Santiago Ramón y Cajal. Golgi developed a silver impregnation method that allowed microscopic visualization of the anatomy of the whole neuron, including the cell body and its two major processes, the dendrites and the axon. Ramón y Cajal used this staining technique to label individual cells, thus showing that the nervous system is not a syncytium (a continuous mass of fused cells sharing a common cytoplasm) but an intricate network of discrete cells. In the course of this work Ramón y Cajal developed some of the key conceptual insights and much of the early empirical support for the *neuron doctrine*—the principle that the nervous system is made up of individual signaling elements, the neurons, which contact one another only at specialized points of interaction, called *synapses*.

Final experimental support for the neuron doctrine was provided by embryology, the second discipline. The embryologist Ross Harrison devised tissue culture methods that showed directly that the major processes of the nerve cell, the dendrites and the axon, are continuous with the cell body and extend from it. Harrison found further, as Ramón y Cajal had suggested, that the tip of the axon gives rise to the *growth cone*, which leads the advancing axon to its targets.

Neurophysiology, the third scientific discipline fundamental to the modern analysis of neural function, began in the late eighteenth century when Luigi Galvani discovered that muscle cells produce electricity. During the nineteenth century the foundations of electrophysiology were laid by Emil DuBois-Reymond, Johannes Müller, and Hermann von Helmholtz, who discovered that the electrical activity of nerve cells provides a means of carrying the signal that conveys information from one end of a cell to the other and from one nerve cell to the next.

The impact of the fourth discipline, pharmacology, started at the end of the nineteenth century when Claude Bernard, Paul Ehrlich, and John Langley demonstrated that drugs interact with specific receptors on cells. This discovery later became the basis of the modern study of chemical synaptic transmission.

Psychology, the fifth discipline important for understanding the brain, has the longest history. Western ideas about mind were first formulated by the classical Greek philosophers and received further definition in the writings of René Descartes, David Hume, and John Locke. The scientific study of behavior as the observable actions of an individual did not begin, however, until Charles Darwin's investigations on evolution in the second half of the nineteenth century had paved the way for behavior to be studied scientifically, giving rise to experimental psychology, the study of behavior in the laboratory, and to ethology, the study of behavior in nature.

The merging of anatomy, developmental biology, physiology, and the study of behavior began in a preliminary way in the nineteenth century with the phrenologists, led by the Austrian physician and neuroanatomist Franz Joseph Gall. Gall appreciated that the functions of the mind have a biological basis and, specifically, that they are carried out by the brain. He postulated that the brain is not a unitary organ but a collection of at least 35 domains or centers (others were added later), each corresponding to a specific mental function. Gall thought that even the most elaborate and abstract mental functions—generosity, mother love, and secretiveness—occur in discrete areas of the cerebral cortex. He further believed that the center for each mental function could develop and increase in size as a result of use, much as the size of a muscle is increased by exercise. As each center grew, it was thought to cause the overlying surface to protrude. Therefore the location of cranial bumps would indicate which regions of the brain are most developed (Figure 1–1). By correlating the personality of individuals with the bumps on their skulls, Gall sought to develop a new objective science for describing character based on the anatomy of the brain: *anatomical personology*.

This extreme and fanciful view was subjected to experimental analysis by Pierre Flourens at the beginning of the nineteenth century. Flourens attempted to determine the specific contribution to behavior of different parts of the nervous system by removing various portions of the brains of experimental animals. From these experiments Flourens concluded that mental functions are not localized, but that all regions of the brain, especially the cerebral hemispheres of the forebrain, participate in all mental function. He proposed that any part of the cerebral hemisphere is able to perform all of the functions of the hemisphere. Injury to one area of the cerebral hemisphere would therefore affect all higher functions equally. Thus, in 1823 Flourens wrote, "All perceptions, all volitions occupy the same seat in these (cerebral) organs; the faculty of perceiving, of conceiving, of willing merely constitutes therefore a faculty which is essentially one." The rapid and fairly general acceptance of this belief (later called the *aggregate field* view of the brain) was based only partly on Flourens's experimental work. It also represented a philosophical reaction against the materialistic basis of mind—the idea that mind is completely biological—implied by the view that specific parts of the brain are dedicated to such human emotions as benevolence, hope, and self-esteem.

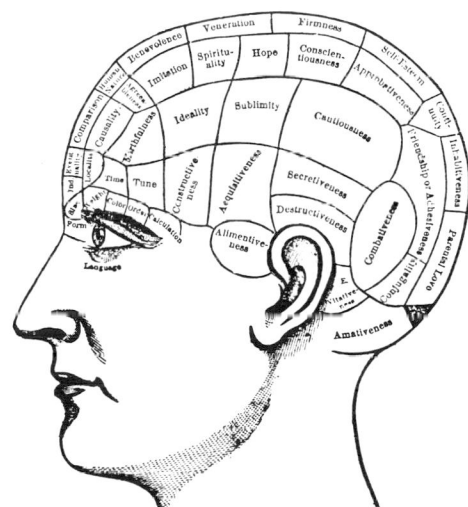

FIGURE 1–1
Phrenologists attempted to associate higher brain functions with bumps and ridges on the human skull. This map, taken from an early nineteenth-century drawing, distinguishes 35 intellectual and emotional faculties in distinct areas of the skull and the underlying cortex. (Adapted from Spurzheim, 1825.)

The aggregate field view prevailed until the middle of the nineteenth century, when it was first seriously challenged by the British neurologist J. Hughlings Jackson. Jackson's clinical studies of focal epilepsy, a disease characterized by convulsions that begin in one part of the body, showed that different motor and sensory activities are localized in different parts of the cerebral cortex. These studies were later elaborated systematically by the German neurologist Karl Wernicke and by Ramón y Cajal into an alternative view of brain function called *cellular connectionism*. According to this view, individual neurons are the signaling units of the brain; they are generally situated together in functional groups and connect to one another in a precise fashion. Wernicke's work in particular showed that different behaviors are mediated by different brain regions that are interconnected by discrete neural pathways.

The history of the dispute between the proponents of the aggregate field and cellular connection views of cortical function can best be illustrated by the analysis of language, the highest and certainly the most characteristic human mental function. Before we consider the relevant clinical and anatomical studies concerned with the localization of language, let us briefly survey the structure of the brain.

Regions of the Brain Are Specialized for Different Functions

The central nervous system, which is bilateral and essentially symmetrical, consists of six main parts: the spinal cord, the medulla oblongata, the pons (and cerebellum), the midbrain, the diencephalon, and the cerebral hemispheres (Figures 1–2 and 1–3). The modern revolution in imaging techniques has made it possible to visualize these structures in the living human brain (Figure 1–3). Through a variety of experimental methods, specific functions have been assigned to these brain regions (Table 1–1). As a result, the idea that different regions are specialized for different functions is now accepted as one of the cornerstones of modern brain science. One of the reasons that this conclusion eluded Flourens and other investigators for so many years lies in another organizational principle of the nervous system known as *parallel processing*. As we shall see below, many sensory, motor, and other mental functions are subserved by more than one neural pathway. When one region or pathway is damaged, others often are able to compensate partially for the loss, thereby obscuring the behavioral evidence for localization. However, the precision with which certain higher functions are actually localized emerges clearly from a consideration of language, to which we now turn.

Language and Other Cognitive Functions Are Localized Within the Cerebral Cortex

Brain functions relating to language are located primarily in the cerebral cortex, which overlies the cerebral hemispheres. In each of the brain's two hemispheres the overlying cortex is divided into four anatomically distinct lobes: *frontal*, *parietal*, *occipital*, and *temporal* (Figure 1–2). Originally named for overlying bones of the skull, the lobes have specialized functions. The frontal lobe is largely concerned with the planning for future action and with control of movement; the parietal lobe with somatic sensation and body image, the occipital lobe with vision, and the temporal lobe with hearing as well as aspects of learning, memory, and emotion. Each lobe has several

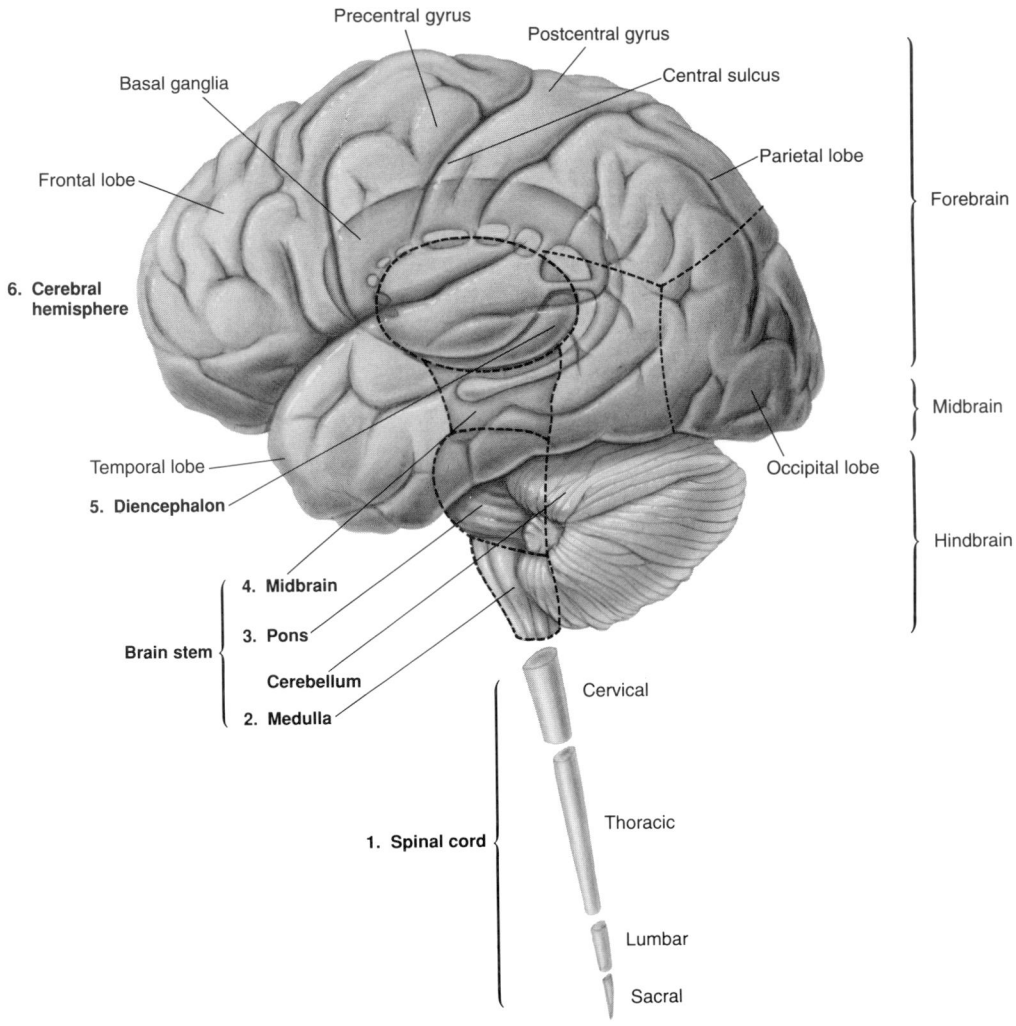

FIGURE 1–2

The central nervous system is divided into six main parts, indicated on the left: **(1)** the spinal cord, subdivided into cervical, thoracic, lumbar, and sacral regions; **(2)** the medulla; **(3)** the pons with the overlying cerebellum; **(4)** the midbrain; **(5)** the diencephalon (the hypothalamus and thalamus); and **(6)** the cerebral hemispheres. The cerebral hemisphere has three deeply-lying structures; only one, the basal ganglia, is illustrated here.

Overlying the cerebral hemispheres is the cerebral cortex, which is divided into four lobes: frontal, parietal, temporal, and occipital. The brain is also commonly subdivided into three broader regions, indicated on the right: the hindbrain (medulla, pons, and the cerebellum), the midbrain, and the forebrain (diencephalon and cerebral hemispheres). The brainstem includes the structures of the hindbrain and midbrain, except the cerebellum.

characteristic convolutions or infoldings (an evolutionary strategy to increase surface area). The crests of the convolutions are called *gyri*. The intervening grooves are called *sulci* or *fissures*. The more prominent gyri and sulci are quite similar in all individuals and therefore have specific names. For example, the *precentral gyrus*, concerned with motor function, is separated from the *postcentral gyrus*, concerned with sensory function, by the *central sulcus* (Figure 1–4).

The organization of the cerebral cortex is characterized by two important features, both of which we shall con-

sider in this chapter. First, each hemisphere is concerned primarily with sensory and motor processes on the *contralateral* side of the body. Sensory information that enters the spinal cord from the left side of the body crosses over to the right side of the nervous system (either within the spinal cord or in the brainstem) before being conveyed to the cerebral cortex. Similarly, the motor areas in one hemisphere exert control over the movements of the opposite half of the body. Second, the hemispheres, although they appear to be similar, are not completely symmetrical in structure, nor are they equivalent in function.

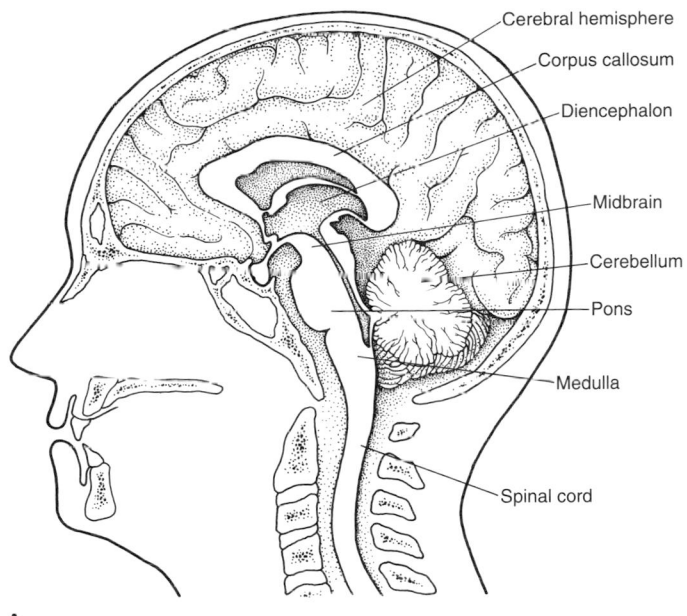

Cerebral hemisphere
Corpus callosum
Diencephalon
Midbrain
Cerebellum
Pons
Medulla
Spinal cord

A

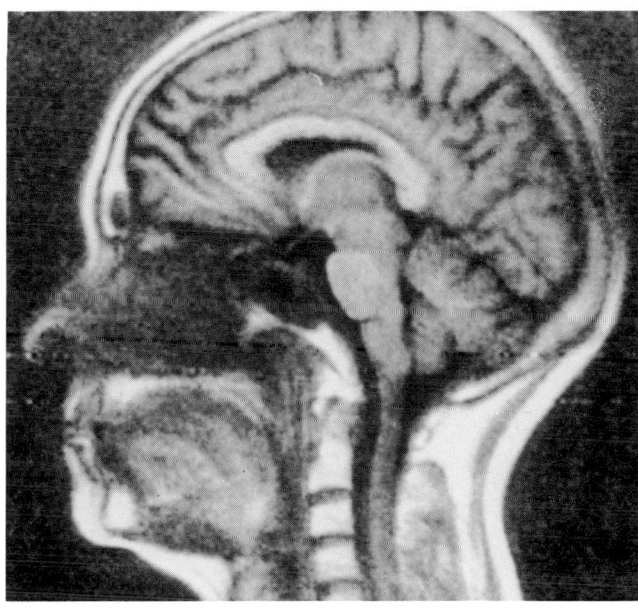

B

FIGURE 1–3

When the brain is cut between the two hemispheres down the midline (a midsagittal section) the six main divisions illustrated in Figure 1–2 can be seen clearly.

A. This schematic midsagittal section shows the position of the six major brain structures in relation to external landmarks.

The corpus callosum is a large fiber bundle that interconnects the left and right hemispheres.

B. The same section in **A** is illustrated in this magnetic resonance image of the living brain.

TABLE 1–1. Functions of the Six Main Parts of the Central Nervous System (See Figures 1–2 and 1–3)

1. The *spinal cord*, the most caudal part of the central nervous system, controls movement of the limbs and the trunk. It receives and processes sensory information from the skin, joints, and muscles of the limbs and trunk.

   The spinal cord continues rostrally as the *brain stem*. The brain stem receives sensory information from the skin and muscles of the head and provides the motor control for the muscles of the head; it also contains several collections of cell bodies, called *cranial nerve nuclei*. Some of these nuclei receive information from the skin and muscles of the head; others control motor output to muscles of the face, neck, and eyes. Still others are specialized for information from the special senses: for hearing, balance, and taste. In addition, the brain stem conveys information from the spinal cord to the brain and from the brain to the spinal cord; and it regulates levels of arousal and awareness. This is accomplished by the diffusely organized reticular formation. The brain stem consists of three parts, the *medulla, pons,* and *midbrain.*

2. The *medulla oblongata,* which lies directly above the spinal cord, includes several centers responsible for such vital autonomic functions as digestion, breathing, and the control of heart rate.

3. The *pons,* which lies above the medulla, conveys information about movement from the cerebral hemisphere to the cerebellum.

   The *cerebellum* lies behind the pons and is connected to the brain stem by several major fiber tracts called *peduncles.* The cerebellum modulates the force and range of movement and is involved in the learning of motor skills.

4. The *midbrain,* which lies rostral to the pons, controls many sensory and motor functions, including eye movement and the coordination of visual and auditory reflexes.

5. The *diencephalon* lies rostral to the midbrain and contains two structures. One, the *thalamus,* processes most of the information reaching the cerebral cortex from the rest of the central nervous system. The other, the *hypothalamus,* regulates autonomic, endocrine, and visceral function.

6. The *cerebral hemispheres* consist of the *cerebral cortex* and three deep-lying structures: the *basal ganglia,* the *hippocampus,* and the *amygdaloid nucleus.* The basal ganglia participate in regulating motor performance; the hippocampus is involved with aspects of memory storage, and the amygdaloid nucleus coordinates autonomic and endocrine responses in conjunction with emotional states.

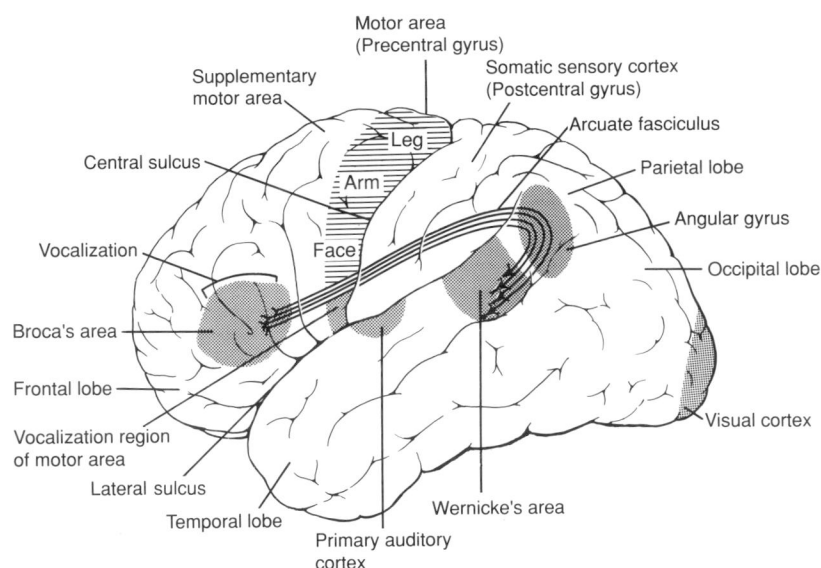

FIGURE 1–4

This lateral view of the cerebral cortex of the left hemisphere shows some of the areas involved in language. Wernicke's area, near the primary auditory cortex, is important to the understanding of spoken language. Wernicke's area lies near the angular gyrus, which combines auditory input with information from other senses. The arcuate fasciculus is a fiber tract that connects Wernicke's area to Broca's area. Broca's area initiates grammatical speech. It, in turn, lies near the vocalization region of the motor area, which issues the specific commands that cause the mouth and tongue to form words. (Adapted from Geschwind, 1979.)

Much of what we know about the localization of normal language comes from the study of *aphasia*, a disorder of language that is found most often in patients who have suffered a stroke (an occlusion of a blood vessel supplying a portion of the cerebral hemisphere). Many of the important discoveries in the study of aphasia occurred in rapid succession during the last half of the nineteenth century and form one of the most exciting chapters in the study of human behavior.

The first advance occurred in 1861 when the French neurologist Pierre Paul Broca described the case of a patient who could understand language but could not speak. The patient did not have conventional motor deficits of his tongue, mouth, or vocal cords that would affect speech. In fact, he could utter isolated words and sing a melody without difficulty; but he could not speak grammatically or in full sentences, nor could he express his ideas in writing. Postmortem examination of his brain showed a lesion in the posterior region of the frontal lobe (an area now called *Broca's area*; Figure 1–4). Broca studied eight similar patients, all of whom showed lesions in this region. In each of these patients the lesion was located in the left cerebral hemisphere. This discovery led Broca to announce, in 1864, one of the most famous principles of brain function: *"Nous parlons avec l'hémisphère gauche!"* ("We speak with the left hemisphere!")

Broca's work stimulated a search for the cortical sites of other specific behavioral functions—a search that was soon rewarded. In 1870, nine years after Broca's initial discovery, Gustav Fritsch and Eduard Hitzig galvanized the scientific community with their discovery that characteristic movements of the limbs can be produced in dogs by electrically stimulating a certain region of the brain. They also found that individual movements are represented in small, quite discrete regions of the cortex and that movements of a limb are produced by stimulating the precentral gyrus in the *contralateral* motor cortex (Figure 1–4). Thus, the right hand, commonly used for writing and skilled movements, is controlled by the *same* hemisphere that controls speech. In most people, therefore, the left hemisphere is regarded as being *dominant*.

The next step was taken in 1876 by Carl Wernicke. At the age of 26 Wernicke published a now classic paper entitled "The Symptom Complex of Aphasia: A Psychological Study on an Anatomical Basis." In this paper he described a new type of aphasia, involving an impairment of comprehension rather than execution (a *receptive* as opposed to an *expressive* malfunction). Whereas Broca's patients could understand but not speak, Wernicke's patient could speak but not understand. Wernicke found that this new type of aphasia had a different locus from that described by Broca: The cortical lesion is located in the posterior part of the temporal lobe where it joins the parietal and occipital lobes (Figure 1–4).

In addition to making this discovery, Wernicke formulated a theory of language that attempted to reconcile and extend the two existing theories of brain function. Phrenologists had argued that the cortex is a mosaic of specific functions and that even abstract mental attributes are localized to single, functionally specific cortical areas. The opposing aggregate field school argued that mental functions are distributed homogeneously throughout the cerebral cortex. Based on his discoveries and those of Broca, Fritsch, and Hitzig, Wernicke proposed that only the most basic mental functions, those concerned with simple perceptual and motor activities, are localized to single cortical areas. According to Wernicke, interconnections between these functional sites make more complex intellectual functions possible. By placing the principle of localized function within a connectionist framework, Wernicke appreciated that different components of a single behavior are processed in different regions of the brain.

He thus advanced the first evidence for the idea of *distributed processing*, which is now central to current thinking on brain function.

Wernicke postulated that language involves separate motor and sensory regions. He proposed that Broca's area controls the *motor* program for coordinating mouth movements for speech—a task for which Broca's area is suitably located, immediately in front of the motor area that controls the mouth, tongue, palate, and vocal cords (Figure 1-4). He attributed word perception, the *sensory* component of language, to the temporal lobe area that he had discovered. This area is also suitably located, being surrounded by the auditory cortex as well as by areas of cortex called *association cortex* that integrate auditory, visual, and somatic sensation into complex perception.

Thus, Wernicke formulated a coherent model of language perception that, with certain modifications we shall learn about later, is still useful today. According to this model, the initial auditory and visual perceptions of language are formed in their respective primary and secondary cortical sensory areas. The neural representations of these perceptions are then conveyed to the angular gyrus, an area of association cortex specialized for both visual and auditory information, where spoken or written words are transformed into a common neural representation in the form of an auditory code important for both speech and writing. From the angular gyrus this neural representation is conveyed to Wernicke's area, where it is registered as language and associated with meaning. Without that associative recognition, the ability to comprehend language is lost. Once registered, the neural representation is relayed from Wernicke's to Broca's area by the arcuate fasciculus, where it is transformed from a sensory (auditory) representation into a motor representation that can be used as spoken or written language. When this transformation cannot take place, the ability to express language (either as spoken words or in writing) is lost.

Using this model, Wernicke predicted a new type of aphasia, later to be demonstrated clinically. This form of aphasia is produced by a type of lesion different from those in Broca's and Wernicke's aphasias: The receptive and motor speech zones are spared, but the fiber pathways that connect them (the arcuate fasciculus in the lower parietal region) are destroyed (Figure 1-4). The resulting disconnection syndrome, now called *conduction aphasia*, is characterized by an incorrect use of words (*paraphasia*). Patients with conduction aphasia can understand words that are heard and seen but cannot repeat simple phrases. Although they speak fluently, they cannot speak correctly; they omit parts of words and substitute incorrect sounds in the words. Painfully aware of their own errors, they are unable to correct them.

Inspired in part by Wernicke, a new school of cortical localization arose in Germany at the beginning of the twentieth century, led by the anatomists Vladimir Betz, Theodore Meynert, Oskar Vogt, and Korbinian Brodmann. This school attempted to distinguish different functional areas of the cerebral cortex based on *cytoarchitectonics*, the occurrence in each region of nerve cells with dis-

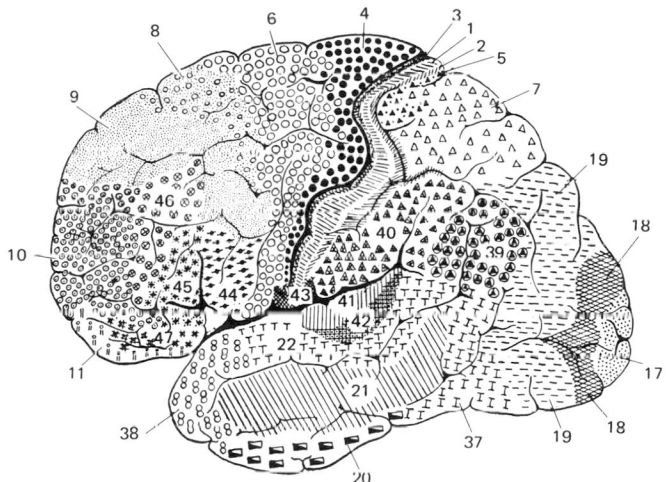

FIGURE 1-5

Based on cell structure and arrangement, Brodmann divided the human cerebral cortex into 52 discrete areas, a number of which are illustrated in this lateral view. Each symbol represents a distinct area, numbered as shown. Area 4, the motor cortex, occupies most of the precentral gyrus. The postcentral gyrus, where the primary somatic sensory cortex is found, is divided into three distinct areas (3, 1, 2). Area 17 is the primary visual cortex. The primary auditory cortex is composed of areas 41 and 42. The prefrontal association cortex (8, 9, 10, and 11) and the parietal–temporal–occipital association cortex (19, 21, 22, 37, 39, and 40) are also composed of distinct cytoarchitectonic areas.

tinctive structure and the characteristic arrangement of these cells into layers. Using this method, Brodmann distinguished 52 areas in the human cerebral cortex and suggested that each area is functionally distinct (Figure 1-5).

By the beginning of the twentieth century there was compelling functional and anatomical evidence for many discrete areas in the cortex, and some could be specifically assigned a role in certain behaviors. Surprisingly, however, the view that dominated experimental thinking and clinical practice during the first half of this century was not cellular connectionism but the aggregate field view. Most neural scientists, including such major figures as the British neurologist Henry Head, the German neuropsychologist Kurt Goldstein, the Russian behavioral physiologist Ivan Pavlov, and the Americans Jacques Loeb and Karl Lashley, continued to advocate the aggregate field view.

Most influential of this group was Lashley, Professor of Psychology at Harvard. Lashley was deeply skeptical of the cortical subdivisions determined by the cytoarchitectonic approach. "The 'ideal' architectonic map is nearly worthless," Lashley wrote. "The areal subdivisions are in large part anatomically meaningless, and . . . misleading as to the presumptive functional divisions of the cortex."[1]

---

[1] Lashley and Clark, 1946, p. 298

Lashley's skepticism was reinforced by his attempts, in the tradition of Flourens's work, to find a specific locus of learning by studying the effects of various brain lesions on the ability of rats to master a maze. Rather than finding a specific learning center, Lashley found that the severity of the learning defect produced by brain lesions seemed to depend on the extent of the damage, not on its precise location. This observation and his later disappointment with cortical cytoarchitectonics led Lashley—and, after him, many other psychologists—to conclude that learning and other mental functions have no special locus in the brain and consequently cannot be related to specific collections of neurons. Lashley therefore reformulated the aggregate field view in a theory of brain function called *mass action*, which further belittled the importance of individual neurons, of specific neuronal connections, and of discrete, functionally specific regions of the brain. According to this view, brain mass, not neuronal architecture, is important to brain function.

Applying this logic to aphasia, Head and Goldstein argued that disorders of language cannot be attributed to lesions at specific sites, but could result from injury to almost any cortical area. They asserted that cortical damage, regardless of site, caused the patient to regress from abstract symbolic language to the concrete language characteristic of aphasia.

The work of Lashley and of Head has gradually been reinterpreted. A variety of studies have demonstrated that maze learning, the task used by Lashley, is unsuitable for studying localization of function because it involves so many complex motor and sensory capabilities. Deprived of one sensory capability (such as vision), an animal can still learn with another (by following tactile or olfactory cues). In addition, the evidence for localization of function has been greatly strengthened. Beginning in the late 1930s, Edgar Adrian in England and Wade Marshall, Clinton Woolsey, and Philip Bard in the United States discovered that tactile stimuli elicit responses that can be recorded from discrete regions of the cerebral cortex. Shortly thereafter, Jerzy Rose and Clinton Woolsey, and others after them, reexamined the concept of the architectonic field rigorously. Together, these studies established that cortical fields could be defined unambiguously according to several independent criteria, including cell type and cell layering, input and output connections, and, most important, physiological function. Indeed, as we shall see in later chapters, recent studies lead us to believe that regional specialization is a key principle of cortical organization and that the brain is divided into even more functional regions than Brodmann had identified.

By combining studies of brain localization with progressively more sophisticated observations of behavior, it has been possible to learn a great deal about the localization of mental functions in the brain. For example, in the 1950s Wilder Penfield used small electrodes to stimulate the cortex of awake patients during brain surgery for epilepsy (carried out under local anesthesia). Penfield tested the cortex specifically for areas that produce disorders of language to ensure that the surgery would not damage the patient's communication skills. Based on the verbal reports of his conscious patients, he confirmed directly the localization assigned by Broca's and Wernicke's studies.

Until recently almost everything we knew about the anatomical organization of language came from clinical studies of patients with lesions of the brain. These studies have now been extended to normal individuals by Michael Posner, Steven Peterson, and Marcus Raichle and their colleagues using positron emission tomography (PET scanning). PET is a noninvasive imaging procedure that visualizes local changes in the cerebral blood flow and metabolism that accompany mental activity, including reading, speaking, and even thinking. Posner and his colleagues discovered that language is processed by parallel components in addition to Wernicke's serial processing. Recall that according to Wernicke's model, both visual and auditory information are transformed into a common neural code, as an auditory representation of language. This information is then conveyed to Wernicke's area, where it becomes associated with meaning before being coded for output as written or spoken language.

Posner and his colleagues asked: Does a word that is read also have an auditory representation before it can be associated with a meaning? Or can visual information be transferred directly to Broca's area? Using PET imaging, they determined how individual words are coded in the brain when the words are read or heard. They found that when words are heard, Wernicke's area becomes active, but when words are seen but not heard or spoken, there is no activation of Wernicke's area. The visual information from the occipital cortex is conveyed directly to Broca's area without first being transformed into an auditory representation in the posterior temporal cortex. From this Posner and his colleagues concluded that perceptions of words presented visually or orally use different brain pathways with separate sensory modality-specific codes, and that these pathways have independent access to higher-order regions concerned with the assignment of meaning and the expression of language (Figure 1–6). When subjects think about the meaning of a word, a still different area in the left frontal cortex becomes active.

Thus, the processing of language is both *serial* and *parallel*. As we shall see later, a similar conclusion has also been reached from studies of sensory perception and the control of movement. These studies demonstrate that information processing requires a specific pattern of interconnection, and that individual cells respond to, and therefore code for, only certain aspects of specific sensory stimuli or motor movement and not for others.

Affective and Character Traits Are Also Anatomically Localized

Even with the evidence for localization of cognitive functions related to language, the idea persisted that affective or emotional functions are not localized. Emotion, it was believed, must be an expression of the activity of the whole brain. Only recently has this view been modified. Although the emotional aspects of behavior have not been

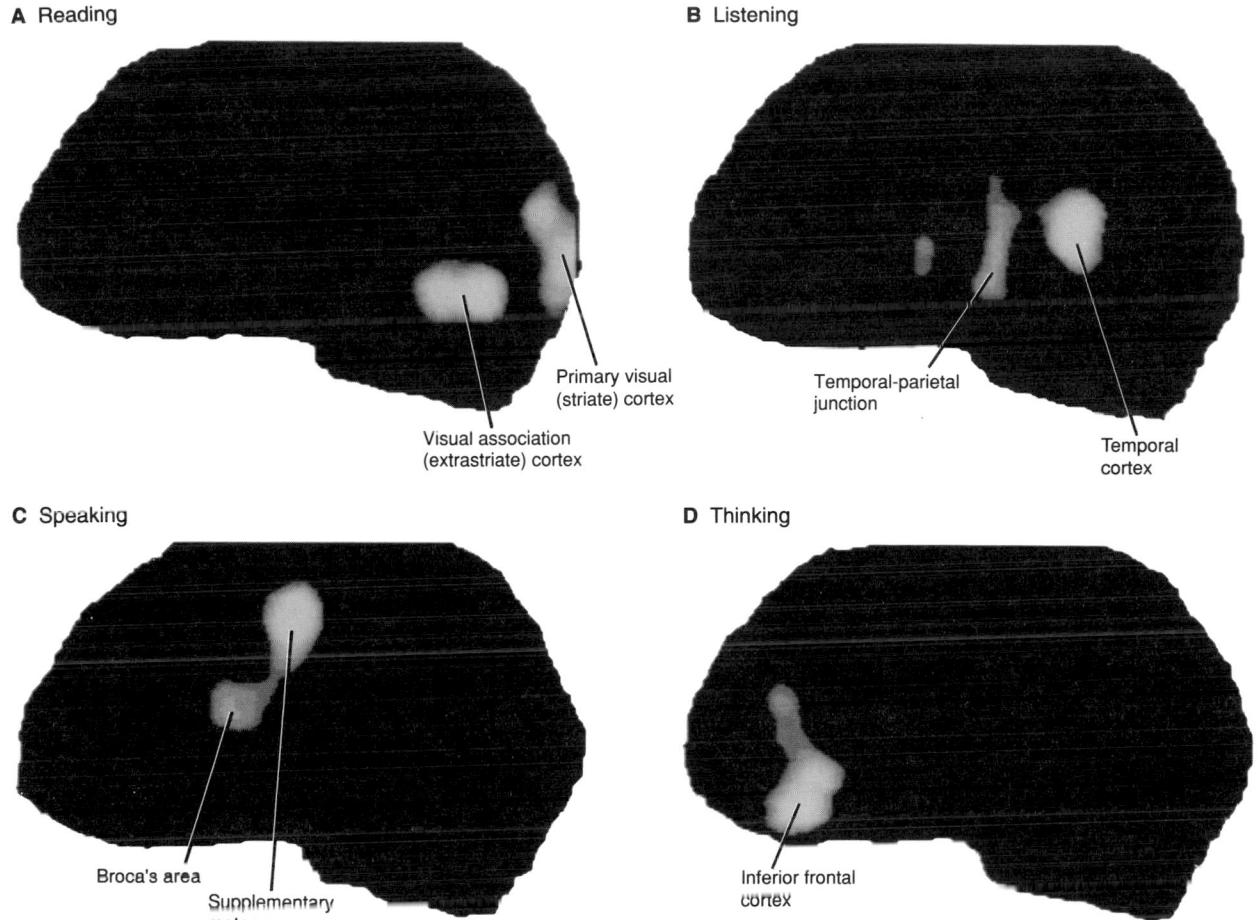

A Reading

Primary visual
(striate) cortex

Visual association
(extrastriate) cortex

B Listening

Temporal-parietal
junction

Temporal
cortex

C Speaking

Broca's area

Supplementary
motor area

D Thinking

Inferior frontal
cortex

FIGURE 1–6

The brain uses different pathways to process recognition of a word, depending on whether the word is read or heard. By averaging PET images it is possible to isolate cortical regions concerned with the processing of words. The four lateral views of the human brain shown here are averages of the brain activities of nine normal subjects. The input component of language—visually scanning a word or hearing it—activates the regions of the brain shown in **A** and **B**. The motor output component activates the regions shown in **C** and **D**. (Courtesy of Marcus Raichle.)

A. The regions active while reading. Only one word was read and it produced a response both in the primary visual cortex and in the visual association cortex.

B. The regions active while hearing words. The same words used in the reading task were used for this listening test. The spoken word activates an entirely different set of areas in the temporal cortex and at the junction of the temporal–parietal

cortex. Thus, the visual responses are not transformed into an auditory code but have their own areas for processing language.

C. The regions active while speaking. Subjects were presented with repeated words, either spoken through earphones or displayed on a screen. (The visual and auditory activity that occurred when there was no word on the screen has been subtracted from the active responses in this image.) Speaking a word activates the supplementary motor area of the medial frontal cortex. In addition, Broca's area is activated whether the words are seen or heard. Thus, both visual and auditory pathways converge on Broca's area, the common site for motor programming and output.

D. The anterior inferior frontal cortex becomes active during mental operations such as analyzing the meaning of a word. The subjects were asked to respond to the word brain with an appropriate verb (e.g., think).

as precisely localized as have cognitive functions, distinctive emotions have been elicited by stimulating specific parts of the brain in humans or experimental animals. Localization of affect has been demonstrated dramatically in the temporal lobe in studies of three types of patients: those with certain types of language disorders, those who have a particular form of epilepsy, and those with acute anxiety disorders (panic attacks).

Patients with aphasia manifest not only cognitive defects in language, but also defects in the affective components of language, consisting of the intonation of speech (called *prosody*) and emotional gesturing. Elliott Ross and Kenneth Heilman have found that these affective aspects of language are represented in the *right* hemisphere and that their anatomical organization mirrors the organization of the cognitive content of language in the left hemisphere. Damage to the right temporal area homologous to Wernicke's in the left hemisphere leads to disturbances in *comprehending* the emotional content of language, in appreciating from the intonation whether a person speaking is telling about a sad or happy event. In contrast, damage to the right frontal area homologous to Broca's area leads to difficulty in *expressing* emotional aspects of language. These studies also show that some linguistic functions exist in the right hemisphere. Moreover, some disorders of affective language can be localized to the right hemisphere, and these disorders, called *aprosodias*, can be classified as sensory, motor, and conduction aprosodias, in the same way as the aphasias are classified. Furthermore, although this pattern of localization appears to be inborn, it is by no means completely determined. Young children in whom the left cerebral hemisphere is severely damaged early in life can develop an essentially normal range of language functions.

Patients with chronic temporal lobe epilepsy manifest characteristic emotional changes that also provide clues to the localization of affect. Some of these changes are present during the seizure itself and are called *ictal phenomena* (Latin *ictus*, a blow or a strike). Among the frequent ictal phenomena experienced by patients during temporal lobe seizures are feelings of unreality and déjà vu (the sensation of having been in a place before, or having had a particular experience before); transient visual or auditory hallucinations; feelings of depersonalization, fear, or anger; delusions; sexual feelings; and paranoia.

The more enduring changes, however, are those that occur when the patient is not having seizures. These *interictal phenomena* are interesting because they represent a chronic change in personality, a true psychiatric syndrome. A detailed description of the personality of patients with temporal lobe epilepsy has been compiled by David Bear. He found that many patients with temporal lobe epilepsy lose all interest in sex. This decrease in sexual interest often is paralleled by an increase in social aggressiveness. Most patients also have one or more characteristic personality traits: They can be intensely emotional, ardently religious, extremely moralistic, or lacking in humor. In contrast, patients with epileptic foci outside the temporal lobe do not generally show abnormalities in emotion and behavior. Bear has argued that the consequences of the irritative lesions of epilepsy are exactly the opposite of those of destructive lesions. Whereas destructive lesions bring about loss of function, often through the disconnection of specialized areas, epileptic processes may entail excessive activity in the affected regions, leading to excessive expression of emotion or an overelaboration of ideas.

Panic attack is a third clearly defined affective disorder that has been localized to the temporal lobe. Panic attacks are brief, spontaneously recurrent episodes of terror that generate a sense of impending disaster without a clearly identifiable cause. A form of acute anxiety disorder, they are characterized by a racing heart and shortness of breath. Using PET scanning, Eric Reiman, Eli Robins, and their colleagues have found that patients with panic attacks have a circumscribed abnormality in the right parahippo-

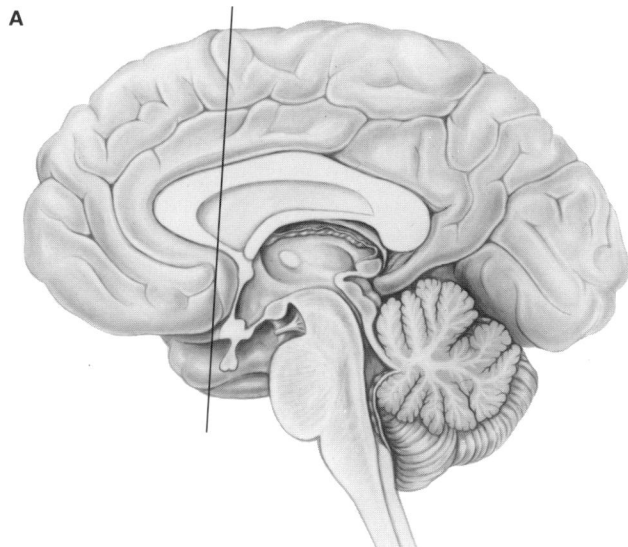

A

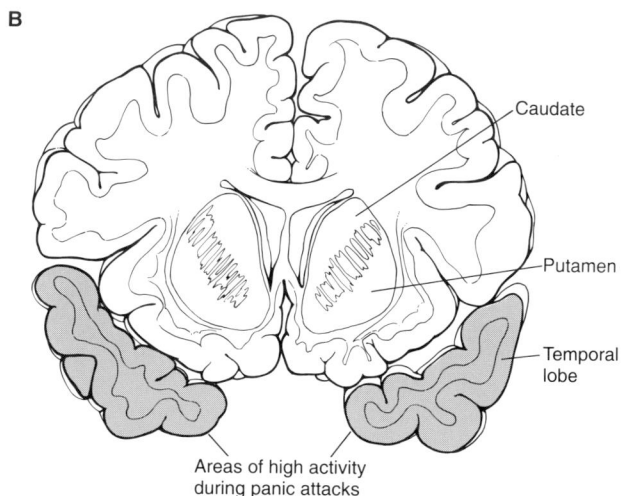

B

Caudate

Putamen

Temporal lobe

Areas of high activity during panic attacks

FIGURE 1–7

Neuroanatomical correlates of normal anticipatory anxiety. During anxiety blood flow increases significantly in the poles of both temporal lobes, indicating increased neural activity. The activity in this region is also disturbed in patients with panic attacks and thus seems to be involved in both normal and pathological anxiety. (Adapted from Reiman et al., 1989.)

A. Midsagittal section of a human brain. The vertical line indicates the plane of the figure in part **B.**

B. A frontal (coronal) section through the temporal poles. The right hemisphere is on the reader's left. The shaded areas are the sites of maximal increase in blood flow.

campal gyrus. Blood flow to this area is abnormally high and appreciably higher than that in the corresponding area in the left hemisphere. The increased flow indicates a high level of cellular activity in this region. This abnormality is present in susceptible subjects, even when panic attacks are not actually occurring. Thus, a predisposition to this particular emotional disorder can be traced to a permanent abnormality in a local anatomical region of the brain. During the panic attack itself blood flow to *both* temporal poles increases significantly. This may occur because the increased activity spreads electrically from the chronic focus in the right parahippocampal gyrus to the homologous region on the left. When normal subjects experience anxiety, they show a transient increase in blood flow in these areas (Figure 1–7). Thus, both normal anxiety and panic attacks stem from the same bilateral site.

Such clinical studies and their counterparts in experimental animal studies suggest that all behavior, including higher mental functioning (affective as well as cognitive), can be localized to specific regions or constellations of regions within the brain. Descriptive neuroanatomy provides us with a functional guide to local sites within the brain that correspond to specific behaviors. With such a map we can infer from a clinical examination of a patient's behavior where the dysfunctional regions in the patient's brain are located.

Mental Processes Are Represented in the Brain by Their Elementary Operations

This discussion brings up one final point. Why has the evidence for localization, which seems so obvious and compelling in retrospect, been rejected so often in the past? The reasons are several.

First, the phrenologists introduced the idea of localization in an extreme form and without adequate evidence. They thought of each region of the cerebral cortex as an independent mental organ used for a *distinct, complex mental function* (much as the pancreas and the liver are independent digestive organs). The subsequent rebuttal by Flourens and the ensuing dialectic between proponents of the aggregate field view (against localization) and the cellular connectionists (for localization) were responses to a theory of localization that, although correct in a general sense, was extreme in principle and wrong in detail. The concept of localization that ultimately emerged, and that has prevailed, is much more complex than Gall (or even Wernicke) had envisioned.

The functions localized to discrete regions in the brain are not complex faculties of mind, but *elementary operations*. More elaborate faculties are constructed from the serial and parallel (distributed) interconnections of several brain regions. As a result, damage to a single area need not lead to the disappearance of a specific mental function as Flourens, Lashley, and many later neurologists had predicted. Even if the function does disappear, it may partially return because the undamaged parts of the brain can reorganize to some extent to perform the lost function. Thus, interrelated local brain functions do not represent a series of links in a single chain, for in such an arrangement all related functions stop when one link is disrupted. Rather, interrelated functions are processed by many neural pathways distributed in parallel. The interruption of a single link within a pathway disrupts only the one pathway, but this need not interfere permanently with the performance of the system as a whole. The remaining parts of the system can modify their performance following the breakage of a link.

Models of localized function were slow to be accepted because there was, and to some extent still is, great diffi-

culty in demonstrating what aspects of a given mental operation are actually localized to a particular region or pathway. Only during the last decade, with the convergence of modern cognitive psychology and the brain sciences, have we begun to appreciate that *all* mental functions are divisible into subfunctions. Each mental process—perceiving, thinking, learning, remembering—seems continuous and indivisible. We experience mental processes as essentially instantaneous, smooth operations. Actually these processes are composed of several independent information-processing components, and even the simplest cognitive task requires the coordination of several distinct brain areas.

To illustrate this point, consider how we store and recall the representation of objects and of people, or of even the simplest event in our environment. We sense intuitively that we store each piece of knowledge—each object or fact about the world—as one unified representation that can be recalled by sensory stimuli or even by the imagination alone. For example, we feel that our knowledge about our grandmother is stored in one unified representation as grandmother, a representation that is equally accessible to us whether we see grandmother, hear her voice, or simply think about her. Elizabeth Warrington and her colleagues have found that this intuitive belief is incorrect. Knowledge is not stored as general representations, but is subdivided into distinct categories. Accordingly, selected lesions in the association areas of the left temporal lobe can lead to the loss of one specific knowledge category— to a loss of knowledge of living things, especially people, without loss of knowledge of inanimate objects. Moreover, this kind of loss is specific for each sensory modality. Thus a left temporal lobe lesion can destroy verbal knowledge of living things without affecting visual knowledge (Table 1–2).

The most astonishing example of the divisible nature of mental processes is the finding that our very sense of ourselves as a *self*—a coherent being—is achieved by connecting, neurally, a family of distinct operations carried out independently in the two cerebral hemispheres. Roger Sperry and Michael Gazzaniga studied epileptic patients in whom the two cerebral hemispheres had been surgically separated by cutting the corpus callosum, a fiber tract that interconnects the two hemispheres. They found that each hemisphere carries an independent awareness of the self. For example, each hemisphere is aware of tactile stimuli applied to the contralateral hand, but is unaware of those given to the ipsilateral hand. Thus, when identical objects are placed in both hands, the object in the left

TABLE 1–2. Deficits in a Patient with a Limited Left Temporal Lobe Lesion

	Pictures	Words
Inanimate objects	98%	89%
Living things	94%	33%

The values indicate the percent of normal function in each category. The patient had selective impairment in processing information about animate objects and use and understanding of spoken language but not in perceiving images. Otherwise he had no neurological abnormality.

hand can be identified by the right hemisphere. But, because the corpus callosum is cut, this object cannot be compared with the same object placed in the right hand because that object can be identified only by the left hemisphere, which is no longer in communication with the right hemisphere. Even more dramatic is the demonstration that in most cases the right hemisphere cannot understand language that is well understood by the isolated left hemisphere. As a result, contravening and opposing commands can be given selectively to each hemisphere!

As these several examples illustrate, perhaps the primary reason it has taken so long to appreciate that mental activities are localized within the brain is that we are dealing here with some of the deepest questions in biology: the neural representation of consciousness and self-awareness. Given the dimensions of the problem, it is important to appreciate that we have only begun to understand how complex behavior is represented in the brain. To study the relationship between a mental process and specific regions of the brain, we must be able to identify the components and properties of the behavior that we are attempting to explain. Yet, of all behaviors, higher mental processes are the most difficult to describe and measure objectively. Similarly, the brain is immensely complex anatomically, and the structure and interconnections of many of its parts are still not fully understood. To analyze how a specific mental activity is represented we need to discern *which* aspects of a mental activity are represented in *which* regions of the brain.

Only recently have we been able to combine cognitive psychology with brain imaging to visualize the regional substrates of complex behaviors, and to see how these behaviors can be fractionated into simpler mental operations and localized to specific interconnected brain regions. As a result of this convergence, there is a new excitement in neural science today, an excitement that is based on the conviction that the proper conceptual and methodological tools—cognitive psychology, brain imaging techniques, and new anatomical methods—are at last in hand to explore the organ of the mind. With these tools and this conviction comes the optimism that the principles underlying the biology of mental function will now be understood.

Selected Readings

Bear, D. M. 1979. The temporal lobes: An approach to the study of organic behavioral changes. In M. S. Gazzaniga (ed.), Handbook of Behavioral Neurobiology, Vol. 2. Neuropsychology. New York: Plenum Press, pp. 75–95.

Churchland, P. S. 1986. Neurophilosophy, Toward a Unified Science of the Mind-Brain. Cambridge, Mass.: MIT Press.

Cooter, R. 1984. The Cultural Meaning of Popular Science: Phrenology and the Organization of Consent in Nineteenth-Century Britain. Cambridge, England: Cambridge University Press.

Cowan, W. M. 1981. Keynote. In F. O. Schmitt, F. G. Worden, G. Adelman, S. G. Dennis (eds.), The Organization of the Cerebral Cortex: Proceedings of a Neurosciences Research Program Colloquium. Cambridge, Mass.: MIT Press, pp. xi–xxi.

Ferrier, D. 1890. The Croonian Lectures on Cerebral Localisation. London: Smith, Elder.

Geschwind, N. 1974. Selected Papers on Language and the Brain. Dordrecht, Holland: Reidel.

Harrington, A. 1987. Medicine, Mind, and the Double Brain: A Study in Nineteenth-Century Thought. Princeton, N.J.: Princeton University Press.

Harrison, R. G. 1935. On the origin and development of the nervous system studied by the methods of experimental embryology. Proc. R. Soc. Lond. [Biol.] 118:155–196.

Jackson, J. H. 1884. The Croonian Lectures on Evolution and Dissolution of the Nervous System. Br. Med. J. 1:591–593; 660–663; 703–707.

Kandel, E. R. 1976. Cellular Basis of Behavior: An Introduction to Behavioral Neurobiology. San Francisco: Freeman, chap. 1, "The Study of Behavior: The Interface Between Psychology and Biology."

Kosslyn, S. M. 1988. Aspects of a cognitive neuroscience of mental imagery. Science 240:1621–1626.

Marshall, J. C. 1988. Cognitive neurophysiology: The lifeblood of language. Nature 331:560–561.

Marshall, J. C. 1988. Cognitive neuropsychology: Sensation and semantics. Nature 334:378.

Posner, M. I., Petersen, S. E., Fox, P. T., and Raichle, M. E. 1988. Localization of cognitive operations in the human brain. Science 240:1627–1631.

Ross, E. D. 1984. Right hemisphere's role in language, affective behavior and emotion. Trends Neurosci. 7:342–346.

Shepherd, G. M. 1991. Foundations of the Neuron Doctrine. New York: Oxford University Press.

Sperry, R. W. 1968. Mental unity following surgical disconnection of the cerebral hemispheres. Harvey Lect. 62:293–323.

Young, R. M. 1970. Mind, Brain and Adaptation in the Nineteenth Century. Oxford: Clarendon Press.

References

Adrian, E. D. 1941. Afferent discharges to the cerebral cortex from peripheral sense organs. J. Physiol. (Lond.) 100:159–191.

Bernard, C. 1878–1879. Leçons sur les phénomènes de la vie communs aux animaux et aux végétaux, 2 vols. Paris: Baillière.

Boakes, R. 1984. From Darwin to Behaviourism: Psychology and the Minds of Animals. Cambridge, England: Cambridge University Press.

Broca, P. 1865. Sur le siége de la faculté du langage articulé. Bull. Soc. Anthropol. 6:377–393.

Brodmann, K. 1909. Vergleichende Lokalisationslehre der Grosshirnrinde in ihren Prinzipien dargestellt auf Grund des Zeelenbaues. Leipzig: Barth.

Darwin, C. 1872. The Expression of the Emotions in Man and Animals. London: Murray.

DuBois-Reymond, E. 1848–1849. Untersuchungen über thierische Elektricität, Vols. 1, 2. Berlin: Reimer.

Ehrlich, P. 1913. Chemotherapeutics: Scientific principles, methods, and results. Lancet 2:445–451.

Flourens, P. 1823. Recherches expérimentales. Archiv. gén. de Méd. Vol II, 321–370. Cited and translated in Pierre Flourens, J. M. D. Olmsted. In E. A. Underwood (ed.), Science, Medicine and History. London: Oxford University Press, 1953, Vol. 2, pp. 290–302.

Flourens, P. 1824. Recherches expérimentales sur les propriétés et les fonctions du système nerveux, dans les animaux vertébrés. Paris: Chez Crevot.

Fritsch, G., and Hitzig, E. 1870. Ueber die elektrische Erregbarkeit des Grosshirns. Arch. Anat. Physiol. Wiss. Med., pp. 300–332. G. von Bonin (trans.) In: Some Papers on the Cerebral Cortex. Springfield, Ill.: Thomas, 1960, pp. 73–96.

Gall, F. J., and Spurzheim, G. 1810. Anatomie et physiologie du système nerveux en général, et du cerveau en particulier, avec des observations sur la possibilité de reconnoître plusieurs dispositions intellectuelles et morales de l'homme et des animaux, par la configuration de leurs têtes. Paris: Schoell.

Galvani, L. 1791. Commentary on the Effect of Electricity on Muscular Motion. R. M. Green (trans.) Cambridge, Mass.: Licht, 1953.

Gazzaniga, M. S., and LeDoux, J. E. 1978. The Integrated Mind. New York: Plenum Press.

Geschwind, N. 1979. Specializations of the human brain. Sci. Am 241(3):180–199.

Goldstein, K. 1948. Language and Language Disturbances: Aphasic Symptom Complexes and Their Significance for Medicine and Theory of Language. New York: Grune & Stratton.

Golgi, C. 1906. The neuron doctrine—Theory and facts. In: Nobel Lectures: Physiology or Medicine, 1901–1921. Amsterdam: Elsevier, 1967, pp. 189–217.

Head, H. 1921. Release of function in the nervous system. Proc. R. Soc. Lond. [Biol.] 92:184–209.

Head, H. 1926. Aphasia and Kindred Disorders of Speech, 2 vols. Cambridge, England: Cambridge University Press. Reprint, New York: Hafner, 1963.

Heilman, K. M., Scholes, R., and Watson, R. T. 1975. Auditory affective agnosia. Disturbed comprehension of affective speech. J. Neurol. Neurosurg. Psychiatry 38:69–72.

Helmholtz, H. von. 1850. On the rate of transmission of the nerve impulse. Monatsber. Preuss. Akad. Wiss. Berl., pp. 14–15. Translated in W. Dennis (ed.), Readings in the History of Psychology. New York: Appleton-Century-Crofts, 1948, pp. 197–198.

Langley, J. N. 1906. On nerve endings and on special excitable substances in cells. Proc. R. Soc. Lond. [Biol.] 78:170–194.

Lashley, K. S. 1929. Brain Mechanisms and Intelligence: A Quantitative Study of Injuries to the Brain. Chicago: University of Chicago Press.

Lashley, K. S., and Clark, G. 1946. The cytoarchitecture of the cerebral cortex of Ateles: A critical examination of architectonic studies. J. Comp. Neurol. 85:223–305.

Loeb, J. 1918. Forced Movements, Tropisms, and Animal Conduct. Philadelphia: Lippincott.

Marshall, W. H, Woolsey, C. N., and Bard, P. 1941. Observations on cortical somatic sensory mechanisms of cat and monkey. J. Neurophysiol. 4:1–24.

McCarthy, R. A., and Warrington, E. K. 1988. Evidence for modality-specific meaning systems in the brain. Nature 334:428–430.

Nieuwenhuys, R., Voogd, J., and van Huijzen, Chr. 1988. The Human Central Nervous System: A Synopsis and Atlas, 3rd rev. ed. Berlin: Springer.

Pavlov, I. P. 1927. Conditioned Reflexes: An Investigation of the Physiological Activity of the Cerebral Cortex. G. V. Anrep (trans.). London: Oxford University Press.

Penfield, W. 1954. Mechanisms of voluntary movement. Brain 77:1–17.

Penfield, W., and Rasmussen, T. 1950. The Cerebral Cortex of Man: A Clinical Study of Localization of Function. New York: Macmillan.

Penfield, W., and Roberts, L. 1959. Speech and Brain Mechanisms. Princeton, N. J.: Princeton University Press.

Ramón y Cajal, S. 1892. A new concept of the histology of the central nervous system. D. A. Rottenberg (trans.). (See also historical essay by S. L. Palay, preceding Ramón y Cajal's paper.) In D. A. Rottenberg and F. H. Hochberg (eds.), Neurological Classics in Modern Translation. New York: Hafner, 1977, pp. 7–29.

Ramón y Cajal, S. 1906. The structure and connexions of neurons. In: Nobel Lectures: Physiology or Medicine, 1901–1921. Amsterdam: Elsevier, 1967, pp. 220–253.

Ramón y Cajal, S. 1908. Neuron Theory or Reticular Theory? Objective Evidence of the Anatomical Unity of Nerve Cells. M. U. Purkiss and C. A. Fox (trans.) Madrid: Consejo Superior de Investigaciones Científicas Instituto Ramón y Cajal, 1954.

Ramón y Cajal, S. 1852–1937. Recollections of My Life. E. H. Craigie (trans.) Philadelphia: American Philosophical Society. Republished in 1989. Cambridge, Mass.: MIT Press. Cambridge, Mass.: MIT Press.

Reiman, E. M., Fusselman, M. J., Fox, P. T., and Raichle, M. E. 1989. Neuroanatomical correlates of anticipatory anxiety. Science 243:1071–1074.

Reiman, E. M., Raichle, M. E., Butler, F. K., Herscovitch, P., and Robins, E. 1984. A focal brain abnormality in panic disorder, a severe form of anxiety. Nature 310:683–685.

Reiman, E. M., Raichle, M. E., Robins, E., Mintun, M. A., Fusselman, M. J., Fox, P. T., Price, J. L., and Hackman, K. A. 1989. Neuroanatomical correlates of a lactate-induced anxiety attack. Arch. Gen. Psychiatry 46:493–500.

Rose, J. E., and Woolsey, C. N. 1948. Structure and relations of limbic cortex and anterior thalamic nuclei in rabbit and cat. J. Comp. Neurol. 89:279–347.

Ross, E. D. 1981. The aprosodias: Functional-anatomic organization of the affective components of language in the right hemisphere. Arch. Neurol. 38:561–569.

Spurzheim, J. G. 1825. Phrenology, or the Doctrine of the Mind, 3rd ed. London: Knight.

Swazey, J. P. 1970. Action proper and action commune: The localization of cerebral function. J. Hist. Biol. 3:213–234.

Wernicke, C. 1908. The symptom-complex of aphasia. In A. Church (ed.), Diseases of the Nervous System. New York: Appleton, pp. 265–324.

Eric R. Kandel

Nerve Cells and Behavior

The Nervous System Has Two Classes of Cells
  Nerve Cells
  Glial Cells

Nerve Cells Are the Signaling Units of Behavioral Responses

Signaling Is Organized in the Same Way in All Nerve Cells

Signals Represent Changes in the Electrical Properties of Neurons
  The Input Component Produces Graded Local Signals
  The Integrative Component Makes the Decision to Generate an Action Potential
  The Conductile Component Propagates an All-or-None Action Potential
  The Output Component Releases Transmitter

The Information Carried by a Signal Is Transformed As It Passes from One Component to the Next

Nerve Cells Differ Most at the Molecular Level

Patterns of Interconnection Allow Relatively Stereotyped Nerve Cells to Convey Unique Information

I nformation coming from peripheral receptors that sense the environment is analyzed by the brain into components that give rise to perceptions, some of which are stored in memory. On the basis of this information, the brain gives commands for the coordinated movements of muscles. The brain does all this with nerve cells and the connections between them. Despite the simplicity of the basic units, the complexity of behavior—evident in our capability for perception, information storage, and action—is achieved by the concerted signaling of an enormous number of neurons. The best estimate is that the human brain contains about 10^{11} neurons. Although nerve cells can be classified into perhaps as many as 10,000 different types, they share many common features. A key discovery in the organization of the brain is that nerve cells with basically similar properties are able to produce very different actions because of precise connections with each other and with sensory receptors and muscle.

Since only a few principles of organization give rise to considerable complexity, it is possible to learn a great deal about how the nervous system works by paying attention to four general features:

1. The mechanisms by which neurons produce their relatively stereotyped signals.
2. The ways in which neurons are connected.
3. The relationship of different patterns of interconnections to different types of behavior.
4. The means by which neurons and their connections are modified by experience.

In this chapter we shall introduce the basic features of neuronal signaling by considering some structural and functional properties of neurons and their surrounding glial support cells. We shall examine how the interconnections between nerve cells produce a simple behavior, the knee jerk, and then briefly describe the location and function of the various signaling mechanisms, and how signaling is transformed within the neural circuit to mediate the behavior.

The Nervous System Has Two Classes of Cells

There are two distinct classes of cells in the nervous system: nerve cells (or neurons) and glial cells (or glia). We shall first consider nerve cells.

Nerve Cells

A typical neuron has four morphologically defined regions (Figure 2–1): the cell body (also called the soma, consisting of the nucleus and perikaryon), dendrites, axon, and presynaptic terminals. As we shall see later, each of these regions has a distinct function in the generation of signals.

The *cell body* is the metabolic center of the neuron. The cell body usually gives rise to two types of processes called the *dendrites* and the *axon*. A neuron usually has several dendrites; these branch out in tree-like fashion and serve as the main apparatus for receiving the input to the neuron from other nerve cells. Often the cell body is triangular or pyramidal in shape. Pyramidal-shaped cells typically have two sets of dendrites—a long slender set of *apical* dendrites emerging from the apex of the cell body and two or more sets of stubbier *basal* dendrites emerging from the base.

The cell body also gives rise to one axon, a tubular process with a diameter ranging from 0.2 to 20 μm that can ramify and extend for up to 1 meter. The axon is the main conducting unit of the neuron; it is capable of conveying information great distances by propagating in an all-or-none way a transient electrical signal called the *action potential*. The axon arises from a specialized region of the cell body called the *axon hillock*, where the action potential is initiated once a critical threshold is reached.

FIGURE 2–1

The main features of a typical vertebrate neuron. This neuron is drawn to illustrate its various regions and its points of contact with other nerve cells. The cell body contains the nucleus and perikaryon. The cell body gives rise to two types of processes—dendrites (both apical and basal) and axons. The axon is the transmitting element of the neuron. Axons vary greatly in length, with some extending more than 1 meter. Most axons in the central nervous system are very thin (between 0.2 and 20 μm) compared with the diameter of the cell body (up to 50 μm or more in diameter). The axon hillock, the region of the cell body where the axon emerges, is where the action potential is initiated. Many axons are insulated by a fatty myelin sheath, which is interrupted at regular intervals by regions known as the nodes of Ranvier. Branches of the axon of one neuron (the presynaptic neuron) form synaptic connections with the dendrites or cell body of another neuron (the postsynaptic cell). The branches of the axon may form synapses with as many as 1000 other neurons.

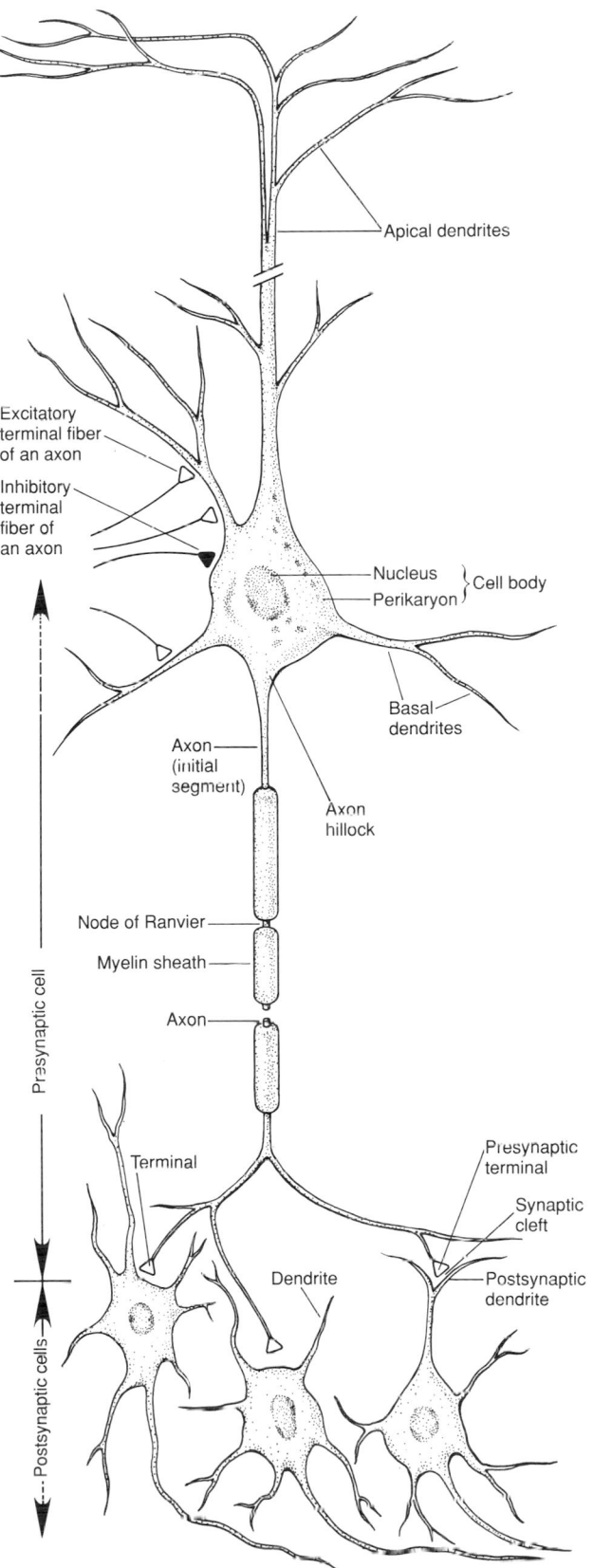

The axon hillock and the axon lack ribosomes and cannot synthesize proteins. Newly synthesized macromolecules are assembled into organelles within the cell body and moved along the axon to presynaptic terminals by a process called axoplasmic transport, which we shall consider in Chapter 4. When severed from the cell body, the axon degenerates and dies (a topic we shall consider in Chapter 18). Large axons are surrounded by a fatty insulating sheath called *myelin*, which is essential for high-speed conduction of action potentials. The myelin sheath is formed not by the axon but by neighboring glial cells. The sheath is interrupted at regular intervals by *nodes of Ranvier*, named after the neuroanatomist Louis Antoine Ranvier, who first described them toward the end of the nineteenth century. We shall learn more about myelination in Chapter 3.

Near its end the axon divides into fine branches that have specialized swellings called *presynaptic terminals*; these are the transmitting elements of the neuron. By means of its terminals, one neuron transmits information about its own activity to the receptive surfaces (the dendrites and cell bodies) of other neurons. The point of contact is known as a *synapse*. The cell sending out the information, therefore, is called the *presynaptic cell*; the cell receiving the information is called the *postsynaptic cell*. The space separating the presynaptic from the postsynaptic cell at the synapse is called the *synaptic cleft*; it communicates freely with the extracellular space. Most presynaptic neurons terminate near the postsynaptic neuron's dendrites, but communication may occur with the cell body or, less often, with the initial segment or terminal portions of axons.

As we saw in Chapter 1, Ramón y Cajal provided much of the evidence for the *neuron doctrine*, which holds that neurons are the basic signaling units of the nervous system and that each neuron is a discretely bounded cell whose several processes arise from its cell body. In retrospect, it is hard to appreciate how difficult it was for Ramón y Cajal and others to obtain the evidence for this elementary idea. After Jacob Schleiden and Theodor Schwann put forward the cell theory in the early 1830s, the idea that cells are the structural units of all living matter became the central dogma for studying tissues and organs. For years, however, most anatomists believed that the cell theory did not apply to the brain. Unlike other tissues, whose cells are simple in shape and fit into a single field of the compound microscope, the cells of the nervous system are large and have complex shapes with processes that appear to extend endlessly and were therefore thought to be unrelated to the cell body.

The coherent structure of the neuron did not become clear until late in the nineteenth century, following the introduction of a special histological technique in 1873 by Camillo Golgi. Golgi's silver impregnation method, which is still used today, has two advantages: (1) for unknown reasons the silver solution stains, in a random manner, only about 1% of the cells in any particular region of the brain, making it possible to study a single nerve cell in relative anatomical isolation from its neigh-

bors, and (2) the neurons that do take up the stain are delineated in their entire extent, including cell body, axon, and full dendritic tree.

Ramón y Cajal applied Golgi's method to the embryonic nervous systems of many organisms, including the human brain. By carefully examining the structure of nerve cells and their contacts with other cells in histological sections of almost every region of the nervous system, Ramón y Cajal described the differences between classes of nerve cells and delineated the precise connections between many of them. He thereby gained important insights not only into neuronal structure but also into neuronal function. In addition to the fundamental principles of the neuron doctrine, Ramón y Cajal grasped two other principles that proved particularly important and form the cellular basis of the modern connectionist approach to the brain that we discussed in Chapter 1.

First, the *principle of dynamic polarization* states that information flows in a predictable and consistent direction within each nerve cell. The flow is from the receiving sites of the neuron (usually the dendrites and cell body) to the trigger zone at the axon hillock. There the action potential is initiated and propagated unidirectionally along the axon to the presynaptic release sites in the axon terminal. Although neurons vary greatly in shape and function, most adhere to this pattern of information flow.

Second, the *principle of connectional specificity* entails three important considerations: (1) there is no cytoplasmic continuity between nerve cells (even at the synapse, a synaptic cleft separates the presynaptic terminal from the postsynaptic cell); (2) nerve cells do not connect indiscriminately to one another to form random networks; rather (3) each cell makes specific connections at precise and specialized points of synaptic contacts—with *some* postsynaptic target cells but not with others.

Ramón y Cajal and the neuroanatomists who followed him also found that the feature that most dramatically distinguishes one neuron from another is shape, specifically the number and form of a neuron's processes. On the basis of the number of processes that arise from the cell body, neurons are classified into three large groups: unipolar, bipolar, and multipolar (Figure 2–2).

Unipolar cells have one primary process that may give rise to many branches. One branch is the axon and other branches serve as dendritic receiving structures. Unipolar cells have no dendrites emerging from the soma. These cells predominate in the nervous systems of invertebrates (Figure 2–2A), but they also occur in certain ganglia of the vertebrate autonomic nervous system.

Bipolar neurons have an ovoid soma that gives rise to two processes: a peripheral process or dendrite, which conveys information from the periphery, and a central process or axon, which carries information toward the central nervous system. Many bipolar neurons are sensory, such as the bipolar cells of the retina and of the olfactory epithelium (Figure 2–2C). The sensory cells of spinal ganglia—that carry information about touch, pressure, and pain—are special examples of bipolar cells. They initially develop as bipolar cells, but the two processes fuse to form

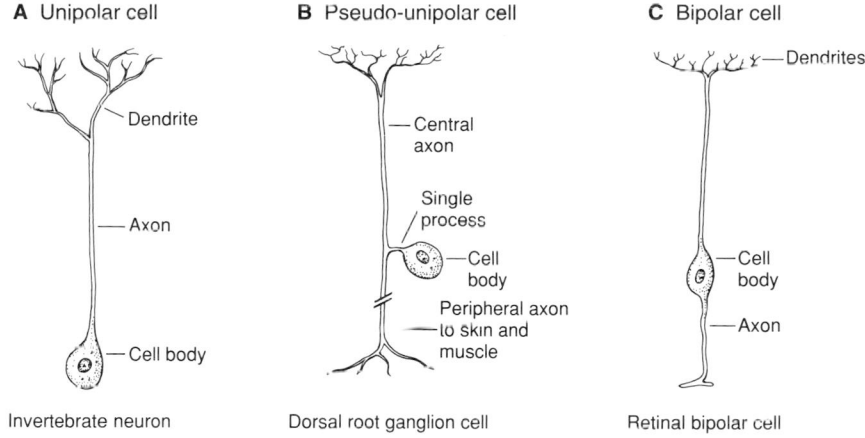

A Unipolar cell

Dendrite

Axon

Cell body

Invertebrate neuron

B Pseudo-unipolar cell

Central axon

Single process

Cell body

Peripheral axon to skin and muscle

Dorsal root ganglion cell

C Bipolar cell

Dendrites

Cell body

Axon

Retinal bipolar cell

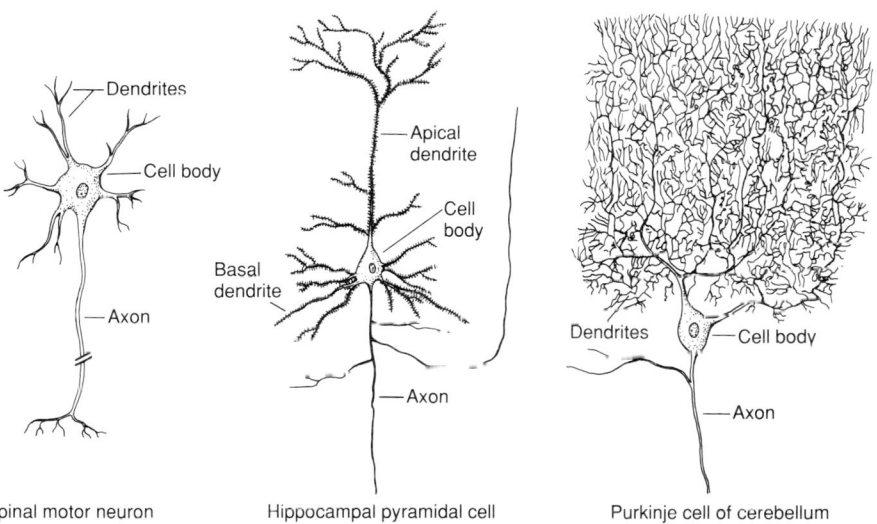

D Three types of multipolar cells

Dendrites

Cell body

Axon

Spinal motor neuron

Apical dendrite

Cell body

Basal dendrite

Axon

Hippocampal pyramidal cell

Dendrites

Cell body

Axon

Purkinje cell of cerebellum

FIGURE 2–2

Neurons can be classified as unipolar, bipolar, or multipolar according to the number of processes that originate from the cell body. (Adapted from Ramón y Cajal, 1933.)

A. Unipolar cells, which have a single process, are characteristic of the invertebrate nervous system. In invertebrates different segments of a single axon serve as receptive surfaces or releasing terminals.

B, C. Bipolar cells have two processes: the dendrite, which carries information toward the cell, and the axon, which transmits information away from the cell. Neurons in the dorsal root ganglia of the spinal cord (**B**), which carry sensory information to the central nervous system, belong to a subclass of bipolar cells called pseudo-unipolar. As such cells develop, the two processes of the embryonic bipolar cell become fused and emerge from the cell body as a single process. This process then splits into

two processes, both of which function as axons, one going peripherally to skin or muscle, the other going centrally to the spinal cord. Bipolar cells of the retina (**C**) or of the olfactory epithelium represent typical bipolar cells.

D. Multipolar cells, which have an axon and many dendritic processes, are the most common type of neuron in the mammalian nervous system. Three examples show the large diversity of shape and organization. The spinal motor neuron innervates skeletal muscle fibers. The pyramidal cell has a pyramid shaped cell body. Dendrites emerge from both the apex (the apical dendrite) and base (the basal dendrites). Pyramidal cells are found in the hippocampus and throughout the cerebral cortex. The Purkinje cell of the cerebellum is characterized by its rich and extensive dendritic tree in one plane. This structure is designed to accommodate an enormous synaptic input.

a single process that emerges from the cell body and splits into two processes; one runs to the periphery (to skin and muscle), the other to the spinal cord. As a result, sensory cells are called *pseudo-unipolar* (Figure 2–2B).

Multipolar neurons predominate in the vertebrate nervous system. These cells have a single axon and one or more dendritic branches that typically emerge from all parts of the cell body (Figure 2–2D). Even within the category of multipolar neurons, the size and shape of cells vary greatly. Multipolar cells vary in the number and length of their dendrites and the length of their axons. The number and extent of dendritic processes in a given cell correlate with the number of synaptic contacts that other neurons make onto it. A spinal motor cell, whose dendrites are moderate in both number and extent, receives about 10,000 contacts—2000 on the cell body and 8000 on the dendrites. The larger dendritic tree of the Purkinje cell of the cerebellum receives approximately 150,000 contacts!

The neurons of the brain can be classified functionally into three major groups: afferent, motor, and interneuronal. Afferent or sensory neurons carry information into the nervous system both for conscious perception and for motor coordination.[1] Motor neurons carry commands to muscles and glands. Interneurons constitute by far the largest class and consist of all the remaining cells in the nervous system that are not specifically sensory or motor. Interneurons process information locally or convey information from one site within the nervous system to another. The distinction between these two signaling functions of interneurons is in part determined by the length of their axon. Interneurons with long axons (sometimes called *Golgi type I cells*) relay information over great distances, from one brain region to another; they are therefore called *relay* or *projection interneurons*. Interneurons with short axons (*Golgi type II cells*) process information within specific regions of the brain; they are therefore called *local interneurons*.

Glial Cells

Nerve cell bodies and axons are surrounded by glial cells (Greek *glia*, "glue"). There are between 10 and 50 times more glial cells than neurons in the central nervous system of vertebrates. Glial cells are probably not essential for processing information, but they are thought to have several other roles:

1. They serve as supporting elements, providing firmness and structure to the brain. They also separate and occasionally insulate groups of neurons from each other.
2. Two types of glial cells, the oligodendrocyte in the central nervous system and the related Schwann cell in the peripheral nervous system, form myelin, the insulating sheath that covers most large axons.
3. Some glial cells are scavengers, removing debris after injury or neuronal death.
4. Glial cells buffer the K^+ ion concentration in the extracellular space and some take up and remove chemical transmitters released by neurons during synaptic transmission.

5. During development certain classes of glial cells guide the migration of neurons and direct the outgrowth of axons.
6. Certain glial cells induce formation of the impermeable tight junctions in endothelial cells that line the capillaries and venules of the brain, causing the lining of these vessels to create the *blood–brain barrier*.
7. There is suggestive evidence that some glial cells have nutritive functions for nerve cells, although this has been difficult to demonstrate conclusively.

Glial cells in the vertebrate nervous system are divided into two major classes: *microglia* and *macroglia*. Microglia are phagocytes that are mobilized after injury, infection, or disease. They arise from macrophages and are physiologically and embryologically unrelated to the other cell types of the nervous system. We shall therefore not consider the microglia further. The macroglia consist of three predominant types: oligodendrocytes, Schwann cells, and astrocytes (Figure 2–3).

Oligodendrocytes and *Schwann cells* are small cells with relatively few processes (Figure 2–3A, B). These cells insulate axons by forming a myelin sheath, which greatly enhances the conduction of electrical signals. They form this sheath by wrapping their membranous processes concentrically around the axon in a tight spiral. Oligodendrocytes, which occur in the central nervous system, may envelop several axons (on average 15). Schwann cells, which occur in the peripheral nervous system, envelop only one axon (Figure 2–3B). Oligodendrocytes and Schwann cells also differ to some degree in their chemical makeup. Myelination is considered in greater detail in Chapter 3.

Astrocytes, the third major class of glial cell, are the most numerous and, at the same time, the most enigmatic. They have irregularly shaped cell bodies and often relatively long processes (Figure 2–3C). In the optic nerve, astrocytes extend two sets of processes. Some of them form *end-feet* on the surface of the nerve, brain, and spinal cord, giving rise to the *glial membrane* (or *limiting sheath*) that surrounds the central nervous system as a protective covering. Others contact blood vessels and cause the endothelial cells to form tight junctions. This impenetrable seal between cells lining the capillaries forms the blood–brain barrier that protects the brain by preventing toxic substances in the blood from entering the brain (Figure 2–4).

Oligodendrocytes produce the myelinated segments (internodes) and maintain the integrity of the myelinated axon.

Astrocytes also serve additional functions. First, astrocytes that surround synaptic regions take up certain neurotransmitters with high affinity, thus removing them from the synaptic cleft. Second, the fact that astrocytes have end-feet that contact both blood capillaries and neurons has led to the suggestion that astrocytes have a nutritive function. Third, astrocytes may, along with microglia, remove neuronal debris and help seal off damaged brain tissue after injury. Finally, as first shown by Stephen Kuffler, John Nicholls, and their colleagues, the resting potential of astrocytes is exclusively determined by their high permeability to K^+. As a result, astrocytes take up and buffer the excess K^+ released by neurons when their activity is high.

---

[1]Afferent neurons are also commonly called primary sensory neurons, and we use these two terms interchangeably in this chapter. The term afferent (carried *toward* the nervous system) applies to all information reaching the central nervous system from the periphery, whether or not this information leads to conscious sensation. The term sensory should, strictly speaking, be applied only to that component of afferent input that enters the brain to generate a conscious perception.

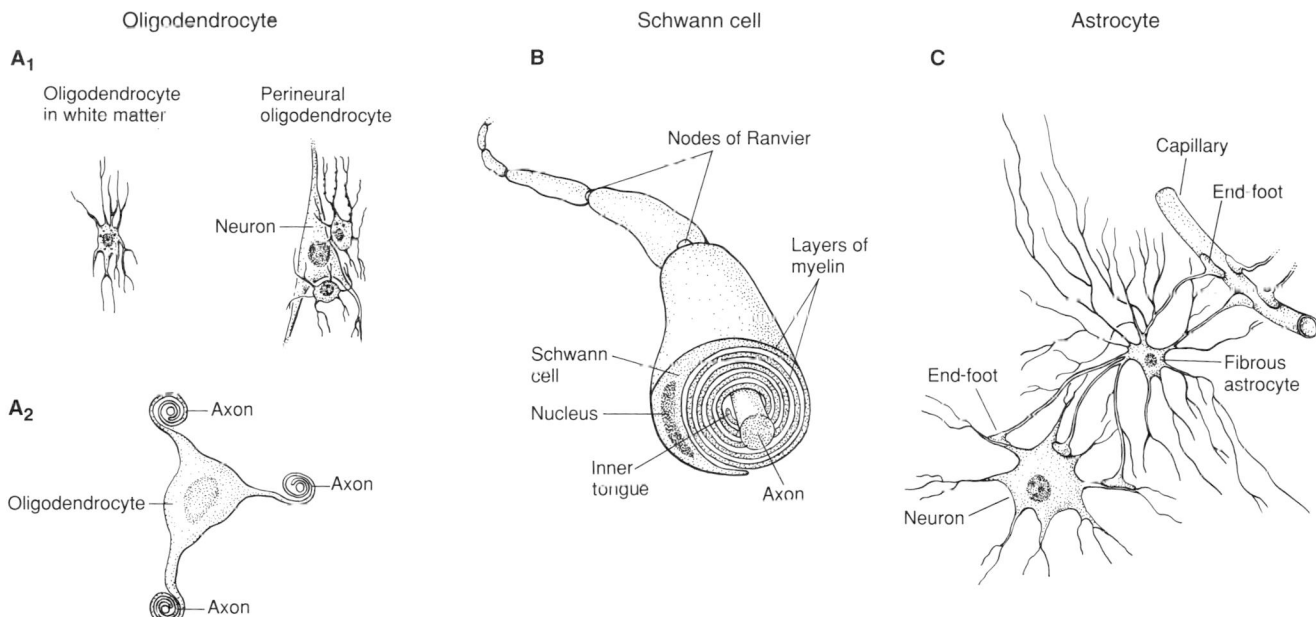

| Oligodendrocyte | Schwann cell | Astrocyte |

A₁

Oligodendrocyte in white matter

Perineural oligodendrocyte

Neuron

A₂

Axon

Oligodendrocyte

Axon

Axon

B

Nodes of Ranvier

Layers of myelin

Schwann cell

Nucleus

Inner tongue

Axon

C

Capillary

End-foot

Fibrous astrocyte

End-foot

Neuron

FIGURE 2–3

The principal types of macroglia in the nervous system are the astrocytes and oligodendrocytes in the central nervous system and the Schwann cells in the peripheral nervous system.

A. Oligodendrocytes are small cells with many processes and are found in the central nervous system. **1.** In white matter (**left**) they participate in myelination; in gray matter (**right**) they surround the cell bodies of neurons. **2.** A single oligodendrocyte forms myelin sheaths around many axons by wrapping its plasma membrane around the axons. (Adapted from Penfield, 1932.)

B. Schwann cells are found in the peripheral nervous system. Each of several Schwann cells lined up along the length of a single axon at regular intervals forms a segment of myelin sheath about 1 mm long. The intervals between the segments of myelin become the nodes of Ranvier. The myelin sheath is formed when the inner tongue of the Schwann cell turns around the axon several times, thereby adding concentric layers of membrane to the axon. In reality, the layers of myelin are more compact than shown here. (Adapted from Alberts et al., 1989.)

C. Astrocytes are star shaped. They have end-feet that contact both capillaries and neurons and are therefore thought to have a nutritive role as well as a role in inducing endothelial cells to form the blood–brain barrier.

FIGURE 2–4

The optic nerve of the adult rat contains two types of glial cells: oligodendrocytes and astrocytes. The nerve is composed of the axons of many ganglion cells (the optic nerve fibers). Oligodendrocytes form the myelin sheath for the axons of ganglion cells. Astrocytes form the glial membrane at the surface of the nerve and have processes that terminate on blood vessels. The astrocytes also serve to buffer high extracellular K⁺ (which results from the extrusion of K⁺ with high rates of neuronal activity) by taking it up and extruding it in regions of low K⁺ concentration. In cultures of optic nerve, two types of astrocytes are apparent. Only type 1 astrocytes are illustrated in the figure; type 2 are discussed in Chapter 57. In culture, type 2 astrocytes contact the axon at the initial segment and the nodes of Ranvier, but their existence *in vivo* remains to be established. (Adapted from Raff, 1989.)

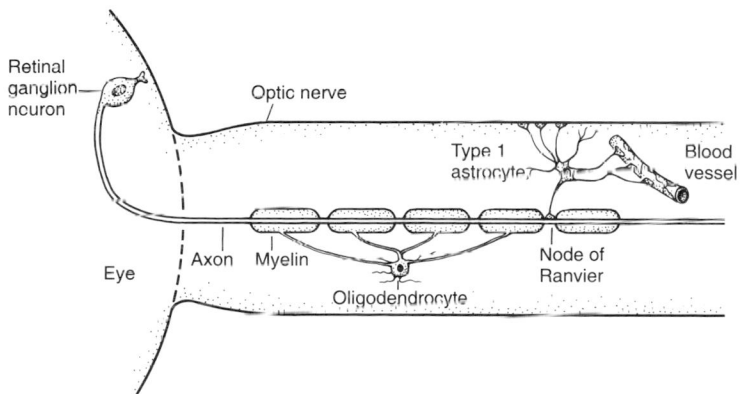

Retinal ganglion neuron

Optic nerve

Type 1 astrocyte

Blood vessel

Eye

Axon Myelin

Oligodendrocyte

Node of Ranvier

When neurons fire repeatedly, K$^+$ accumulates in the extracellular space. Because of their high permeability, astrocytes can take up the excess K$^+$ and store it so as to protect the neighboring neurons from the depolarization that might result if the K$^+$ accumulated. To maintain electrical neutrality, astrocytes can gain an amount of Cl$^-$ equal to that of K$^+$. The movement of Cl$^-$ will therefore neutralize the charge.

In addition, since astrocytes are connected to each other through cytoplasmic bridges (electrical synapses we shall learn more about later), they form large syncytia—sheets of interconnected cells—and therefore can also lose the K$^+$ they gain at one site to a distal site. Eric Newman has found that the K$^+$ conductance is not uniformly distributed along the surface of astrocytes. The end-feet of astrocytes that contact blood vessels and the pial membrane, the surface covering that surrounds and protects the brain, have a much higher K$^+$ conductance than the remainder of the astrocyte cell surface. The astrocytes therefore extrude from their end-feet the excess K$^+$ they have taken up anywhere along their surface. Depending upon neuronal activity, the K$^+$ concentration in the extracellular space can vary from 3 to 10 mM. This is the range of K$^+$ concentration that is critical for controlling the diameter of the arteries and arterioles of the cerebral vasculature, on which the astrocytes end. When neuronal activity drives the K$^+$ concentration to 10 mM, the diameter of the vessels increase by 50%! The siphoning capabilities of astrocyte end-feet and the sensitivity of the cerebral vessels to K$^+$ therefore provide a mechanism for autoregulation of the vasculature, so that blood flow and oxygen consumption can keep pace with neuronal activity. When neural activity increases, K$^+$ accumulates, the vessels dilate, and blood flow increases.

Although the electrical properties of some glial cells can be altered by changes in external K$^+$ concentration, and even though many glia have a variety of ion channels in their plasma membranes that can be affected by voltage and even by chemical transmitters, there is no evidence that glia are directly involved in electrical signaling. Signaling is the function of nerve cells.

Nerve Cells Are the Signaling Units of Behavioral Responses

The critical signaling functions of the brain—the processing of sensory information, the programming of motor and emotional responses, learning and memory—are carried out by interconnected sets of neurons. We shall examine in general terms how these interconnections produce a behavior by considering a simple involuntary stretch reflex, the knee jerk. We shall use this behavior to illustrate the two basic principles of neuronal functioning delin-

FIGURE 2–5

The knee jerk reflex is an example of a monosynaptic reflex system. Each extensor and flexor motor neuron in the drawing represents a population of many cells. Tapping the knee pulls on the tendon of the quadriceps femoris muscle, an extensor muscle that extends the lower leg. When the muscle stretches in response to the pull of the tendon, information regarding this change in the muscle is conveyed by afferent (sensory) neurons to the central nervous system. In the spinal cord the sensory neurons act directly on motor neurons that contract the quadriceps. In addition, they act indirectly, through interneurons, to inhibit motor neurons that contract the antagonist muscle, the hamstring. These actions combine to produce the reflex behavior. Other signals convey information about the reflex to higher regions of the brain.

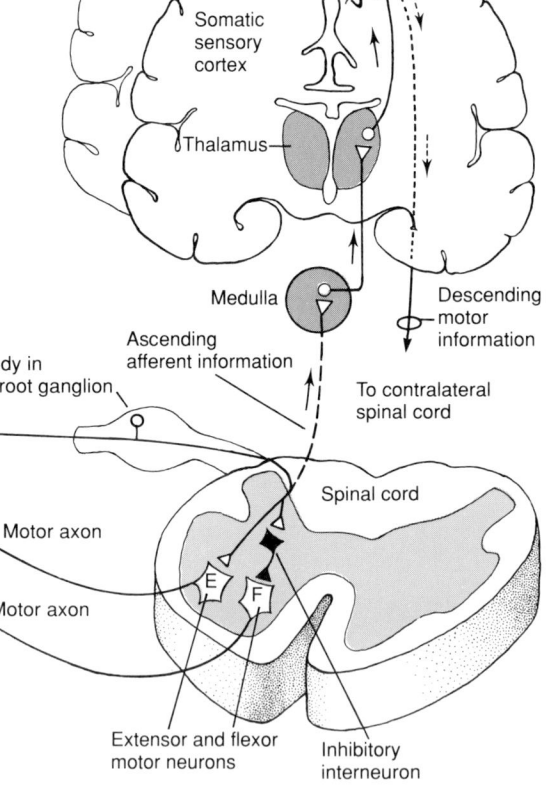

eated by Ramón y Cajal: dynamic polarization and connectional specificity.

The patella (kneecap) is the site of attachment for the tendon of the quadriceps femoris, an extensor muscle that moves the lower leg. By tapping the patellar tendon, the quadriceps femoris is pulled by the tendon and briefly stretched. This initiates a kick, a reflex contraction of the quadriceps femoris and the concomitant relaxation of the antagonist flexor muscles, the hamstrings (Figure 2–5). The stretch reflex changes the position of the body and limb by increasing the tension of selected groups of muscles. It also maintains muscle tone, a background level of tension.

The stretch reflex is called a *monosynaptic reflex* because it is mediated in large part by a single set of synaptic connections between two types of neurons in the spinal cord—sensory (afferent) neurons, which send information to the central nervous system, and motor neurons, which send information from the central nervous system to muscles. The cell bodies of the sensory neurons of this reflex are clustered near the spinal cord in the *dorsal root ganglia* (Figure 2–5). They are an example of a bipolar cell: one branch of the cell's axon goes out to the muscle and the other runs into the spinal cord (see Figure 2–2). The branch that innervates the muscle makes contact with receptors in the muscle, called *muscle spindles*, which are sensitive to stretch. The branch in the spinal cord forms excitatory connections both with the motor neurons that innervate the extensor muscles and control their contrac-

tion, and with local interneurons that inhibit the motor neurons that innervate the antagonist flexor muscles.

Although only two types of nerve cells are involved, the stretching of a single muscle activates several hundred sensory neurons, each of which innervates between 100 and 150 motor neurons. This type of connection, where a single neuron branches many times and terminates on many target cells, is common especially in the input stages of the nervous system and allows for *divergence* of information flow (Figure 2–6A). As a result of *neuronal divergence*, a single neuron can exert a widespread influence by distributing its signals to many target cells. Because there are usually five to ten times more sensory neurons than motor neurons, many sensory cells terminate on a single motor cell. This type of connection allows for *convergence* of information flow, common at the output of the nervous system (Figure 2–6B). *Neuronal convergence* allows a target cell to integrate diverse information from many sources.

In summary, the stretch reflex is mediated by a simple, direct connection between sensory and motor neurons. Sensory neurons are excited when an extensor muscle is stretched. In turn, the sensory neurons excite motor neurons, which cause the extensor muscle to contract. Concurrently, the sensory neurons end on projection interneurons that transmit information about the local neural activity to higher regions of the brain concerned with movement. Thus, the electrical signals that produce the stretch reflex convey four kinds of information: (1) sen-

FIGURE 2–6

Divergence and convergence of neuronal connections illustrate a key principle in the organization of the brain. In the sensory systems, the neurons at the input stages usually branch and make divergent connections with the second stage of processing, and this divergence is carried forward to the third and subsequent stages. In turn, the motor neurons at the output of the nervous system receive a progressive convergence of connections.

This convergence induces not only excitatory influences as illustrated here, but inhibitory influences as illustrated in Figure 2–10.

A. Two consecutive stages of divergence illustrate how the divergence of a single cell can exert influence on many target cells.

B. Two stages of convergence illustrate the focusing on one target cell of the influence of many presynaptic neurons.

A Divergence

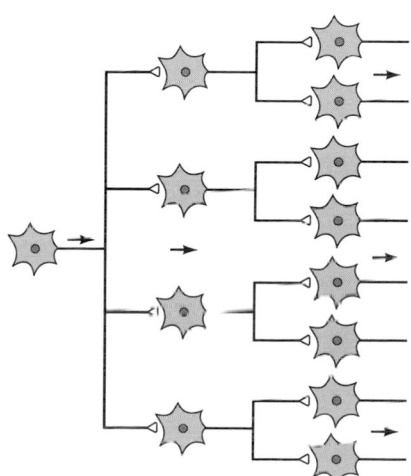

B Convergence

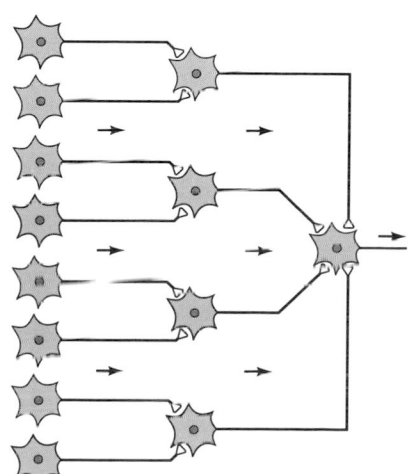

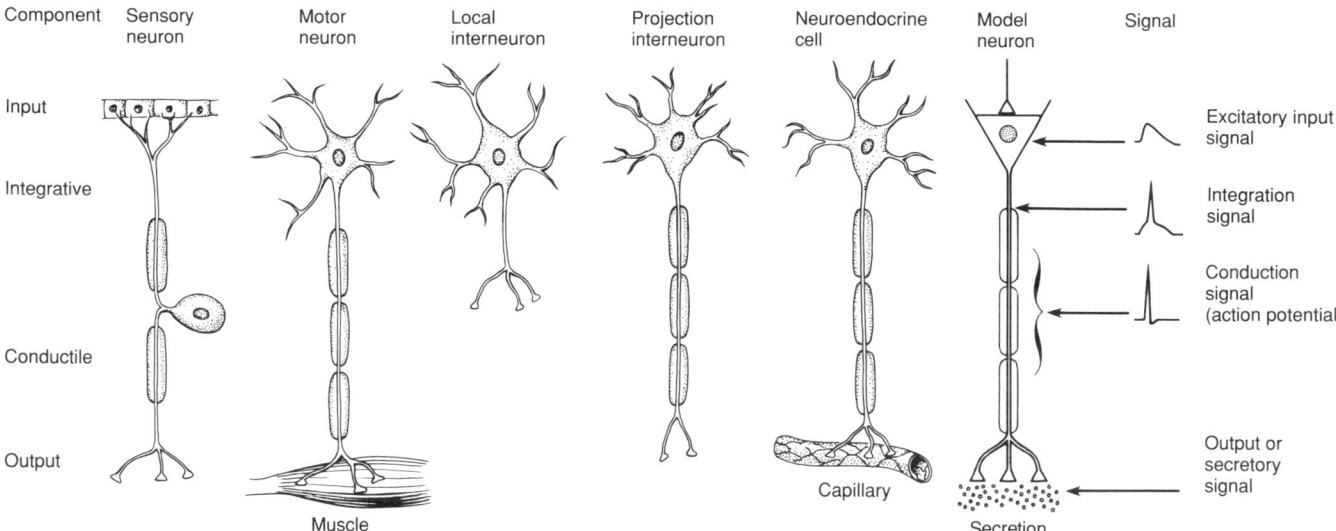

FIGURE 2–7
Most neurons, whether they are sensory, motor, interneuronal, or neuroendocrine, have four functional components in common: an input component, an integrative component, a conductile component, and an output component. On the basis of these common features, the functional organization of neurons in general can be represented by a model neuron. The functional components of the neuron are represented in distinct regions, with unique shapes and properties, and each produces a characteristic signal. Not all neurons share all of these features; for example, local interneurons often lack conductile components.

sory information from the body surface to the central nervous system (the spinal cord), (2) motor commands from the central nervous system to muscles, the end organs of effector behavior, (3) complementary motor commands (excitation and inhibition of different motor neurons) leading to coordinated muscle action, and (4) sensory information about local neuronal activity related to behavior to other parts of the central nervous system. In our example a transient imbalance of the body produces sensory information that is conveyed to motor cells, which convey commands to the muscles to contract so that balance will be restored.

Signaling Is Organized in the Same Way in All Nerve Cells

To produce a behavior, each participating sensory and motor nerve cell generates, in sequence, four types of signals at four different sites within the neuron: an *input signal* (called a *receptor potential* in the sensory neuron, and a *synaptic potential* in the interneuron or motor neuron), an *integration signal*, a *conducting signal*, and an *output signal*. Indeed, regardless of size, shape, transmitter biochemistry, or behavioral function, almost all neurons can be described by a generalized model neuron that has four components: an input or receptive component, an integrative or summing component, a long-range signaling or conductile component, and an output or secretory component (Figure 2–7). Each component is located at a particular region in the neuron and carries out a special function in signaling. All of these signals depend on the electrical properties of the cell membrane.

This model neuron is a modern restatement of Ramón

y Cajal's principle of dynamic polarization. The type of message conveyed by a neuron is determined not so much by the properties of the signal but by the neuron's specific connections. To understand the mechanism by which neurons produce signals and how these signals are transformed by one component after another, it is first necessary to understand the electrical properties of the cell membrane.

Signals Represent Changes in the Electrical Properties of Neurons

Neurons, like other cells of the body, maintain a potential difference of about 65 mV across their external membrane. This potential is called the *resting membrane potential*. It results from an unequal distribution of Na^+, K^+, Cl^-, and organic anions across the membrane of cells, which leaves the inside of the nerve cell membrane negative in relation to the outside. Because the outside of the membrane is arbitrarily defined as zero, we say the resting membrane potential is −65 mV. In different nerve cells the resting membrane potential may range from −40 to −80 mV. In muscle cells the resting potential is higher still, about −90 mV.

The unequal distribution of ions is maintained by a metabolically driven pump, the Na^+–K^+ pump, which we shall learn more about in Chapter 6. The pump establishes the ionic gradients for Na^+ and K^+ that characterize the nerve cell. By transporting Na^+ out of the cell and K^+ into it, this pump keeps the Na^+ concentration low within the cell (about 10 times lower than outside) and the K^+ concentration within the cell high (about 50 times higher than outside). The resting membrane potential results from two properties of the cell: (1) the concentration gradients established by the Na^+–K^+ pump, and (2) the membrane's high leakiness (permeability) to K^+ and relatively low permeability to Na^+ in its resting state. Because of its high concentration inside the cell, K^+ tends to be driven out of the cell under the influence of the concentration gradient. As K^+ moves out of the cell, it leaves behind a cloud of unneutralized negative charge on the inside surface of the membrane, which makes the membrane more negative on the inside (by about 65 mV) than on the outside (see Figure 6–1).

Excitable cells, such as nerve and muscle cells, are different from most other cells in the body in that their resting membrane potential can be significantly altered and therefore can serve as a signaling mechanism. When the membrane potential of a nerve cell is reduced by 10 mV (from about −65 to −55 mV), an all-or-none action potential is initiated. During the action potential the permeability characteristics of the resting nerve cell membrane suddenly reverse—the membrane becomes highly permeable to Na^+ and, after a delay, returns to its resting state permeability to K^+. We shall learn more about the mechanisms underlying the resting and action potential in Chapters 6 and 8.

Other types of neuronal signaling, such as receptor potentials and synaptic potentials, also involve changes in potential across the membrane. The resting membrane potential therefore provides the baseline against which *all* other signals are expressed. These signals result from perturbations of the membrane, which cause the membrane potential either to increase or decrease with respect to the resting potential. An increase in membrane potential (e.g., from −65 to −75 mV) is called *hyperpolarization*. A reduction in membrane potential (e.g., from −65 to −55 mV) is called *depolarization*. As we shall see later, hyperpolarization decreases a cell's ability to generate an action potential (the conducting signal transmitted along the axon) and is therefore *inhibitory*. Depolarization increases a cell's ability to generate a transmittable signal and is therefore *excitatory*.

Using the sensory and motor neurons involved in the simple knee jerk as an example, we shall now examine how neural information is generated and transformed both within and between neurons by the four components essential for signaling.

The Input Component Produces Graded Local Signals

In most neurons the resting potential is the same throughout the cell, so that no current flows from one part of the neuron to another in the resting state. Typically, current flow is initiated at the input component of the neuron, where appropriate sensory or chemical stimuli activate special protein molecules, thereby giving rise to an input signal—a change in membrane potential. In sensory neurons the protein molecules are called *transducing receptor proteins*; in motor or interneurons they are called *synaptic receptor proteins*.

The input signal of sensory neurons, the receptor potential, is generated at a specialized region of the sensory cell called the receptive surface. In the example of the stretch reflex the transducing proteins are stretch-sensitive ion channels we shall learn more about in Chapter 23. These transducing proteins transform the sensory stimulus into a flow of ionic current that produces a change in the resting potential of the cell membrane: the receptor potential. The magnitude of the receptor potential is graded in both amplitude and duration. The larger or longer-lasting the stretch of the muscle, the larger and longer-lasting are the resulting receptor potentials (Figure 2–8A). Most receptor potentials are depolarizing. As we shall learn later in considering vision, however, some receptor potentials are hyperpolarizing.

The receptor potential is the first representation of stretch to be coded in the nervous system, but it alone would not cause any signals to appear in the rest of the nervous system. This is because the transducing proteins are restricted to the receptive surface of the sensory neurons and the receptor potential is a purely local signal that spreads only passively along the axon. It decreases in amplitude with distance and cannot be conveyed much farther than 1 or 2 mm. At about 1 mm down the axon the amplitude of the signal is only about one-third what it was at the site of generation. For the signal to be conveyed to the rest of the nervous system, it must be further amplified.

The input signal of motor neurons (or interneurons), the synaptic potential, has properties that are similar to those of the receptor potential. Synaptic potentials are the perturbations of membrane potential in one neuron (the postsynaptic neuron) caused by the output of another cell (the presynaptic neuron). They are the means by which one cell influences the activity of another. The presynaptic sensory neuron releases a chemical transmitter that interacts with synaptic receptor molecules at the surface of the postsynaptic motor cell. In the postsynaptic cell the synaptic receptor molecule transforms chemical potential energy into an electrical signal: the synaptic potential. Like the receptor potential, the synaptic potential is graded; its amplitude and duration are functions of the amount of transmitter and the time period over which it is released. The synaptic potential can be either depolarizing (excitatory) or hyperpolarizing (inhibitory), depending on the receptor molecule.

Receptor molecules for transmitters also are typically highly localized. For example, the receptors for inhibitory synapses are often segregated from those for excitatory synapses. Inhibitory synapses are often located on the cell body of the neuron, whereas excitatory synapses are often located on the dendrites or on dendritic specializations called *spines* (see below). Synapses are not usually found along the main portion of the axon, but some neurons have synaptic receptors on their presynaptic terminals and occasionally at nodes of Ranvier. Synaptic potentials, like receptor potentials, spread passively from one region of the neuron to another. The features of receptor and synaptic potentials are summarized in Table 2–1.

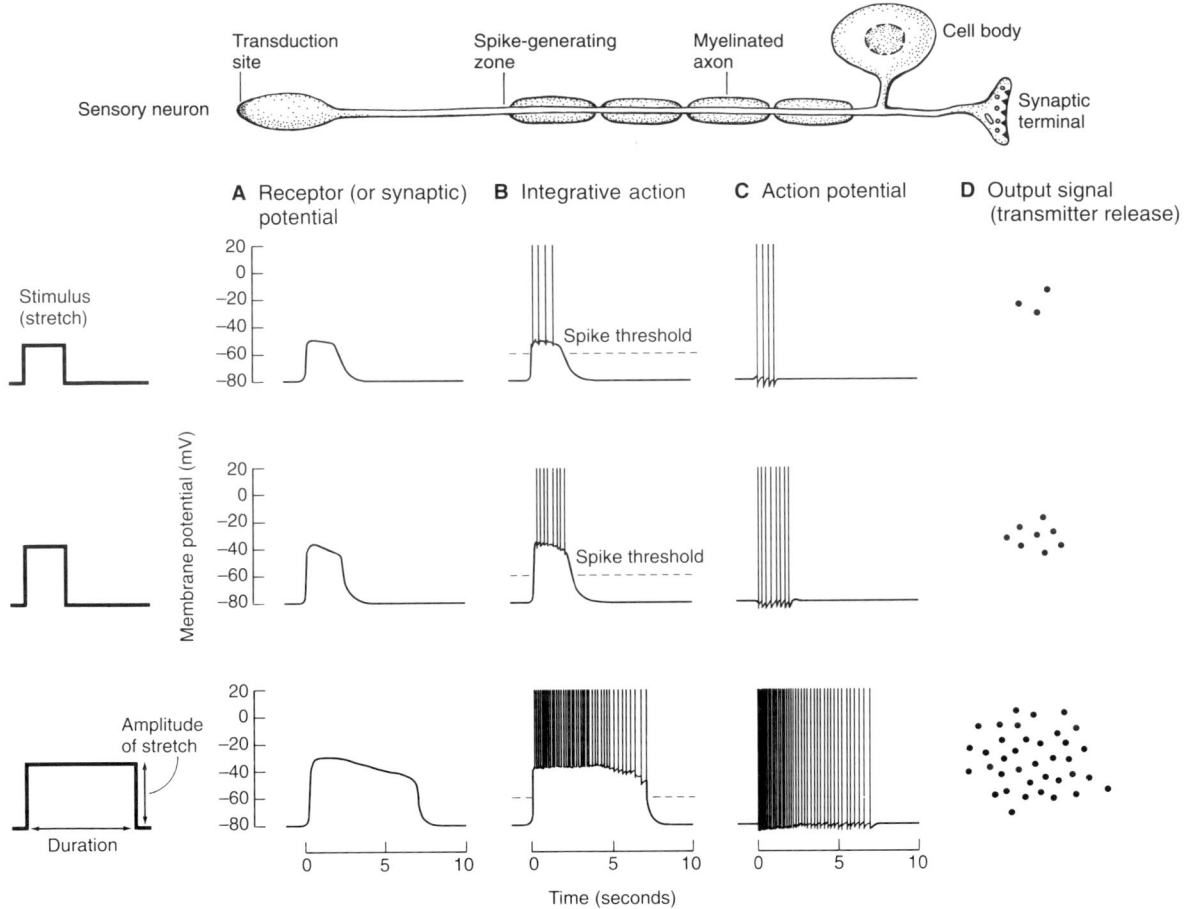

FIGURE 2–8

Transformation of information within a neuron. Each of the four components of an afferent neuron produces a characteristic signal.

A. The input signal, the receptor potential, is graded in amplitude and duration, proportional to the amplitude and duration of the stimulus.

B. The integrative action transforms the information in the input signal into action potentials that are actively propagated down the axon. An action potential is generated only if the receptor (or synaptic) potential is greater than a certain threshold. Once the receptor potential surpasses this threshold, any further increase in amplitude increases the frequency with which the action potentials are generated. The graded nature of input signals is translated into a frequency code of action potential at the trigger zone. The *duration* of the input signal determines the duration of the train of action potentials.

C. Action potentials are all-or-none: Every potential has the same shape, amplitude, and duration. These action potentials are conducted without fail along the full length of the axon, which can be 1-2 meters. The information in the signal therefore continues to be coded in the frequency and number of spikes. The greater the amplitude of the stimulus, the greater the frequency of spikes. The greater the duration of the stimulus, the longer the burst of potentials and therefore the greater the number of spikes.

D. The output signal, the release of transmitter substance onto the postsynaptic cell, results when the action potential reaches the synaptic terminal. The total number of action potentials per unit time determines exactly how much transmitter (**black dots**) will be released.

The Integrative Component Makes the Decision to Generate an Action Potential

Action potentials, the conducting signals of neurons, are generated by a sudden inrush of Na^+ through voltage-sensitive Na^+ channels. These channels are absent in the input region of the neuron (the membrane of the receptor terminal of sensory neurons or the synaptic membrane of interneurons and motor neurons). In most neurons the functional properties of the membrane change and the density of Na^+ channels increases dramatically within 1 mm of the input component. In sensory neurons these changes occur at the first node of Ranvier in the myelinated axon; in motor neurons or interneurons they occur at the axon hillock, the initial segment of the axon as it emerges from the cell body. These axon regions have the *highest density* of voltage-gated Na^+ channels in the neuron and therefore the *lowest threshold* for generating an

TABLE 2–1. Features of Receptor, Synaptic, and Action Potentials

Feature	Receptor potential	Synaptic potential	Action potential
Amplitude	Small (0.1–10 mV)	Small (0.1–10 mV)	Large (70–110 mV)
Duration	Brief (5–100 ms)	Brief to long (5 ms–20 min)	Brief (1–10 ms)
Summation	Graded	Graded	All-or-none
Signal	Hyperpolarizing or depolarizing	Hyperpolarizing or depolarizing	Depolarizing
Propagation	Passive	Passive	Active

action potential. When the input signal spreads passively to this region it will, if it is larger than the threshold, give rise to one or more action potentials. At the integrative component the activity of all receptor (or synaptic) potentials is summed and the decision is reached as to whether or not to generate an all-or-none signal (Figures 2–7 and 2–8). Consequently, this region in the axon is called the *trigger zone* or *integrative component*.

Many cell bodies also have the capability of generating action potentials, but the threshold of the cell body is usually higher than that of the initial segment of the axon. Some neurons also have a trigger zone in the dendrites, where the threshold for an action potential also is relatively low. Dendritic trigger zones serve to amplify the effectiveness of synapses distant from the cell body. The action potentials produced at these dendritic trigger zones then discharge the final common trigger zone in the initial segment of the axon.

The Conductile Component Propagates an All-or-None Action Potential

Once the threshold of the integrative component has been exceeded, an action potential is initiated. Unlike input potentials, which are graded, the conducting signal is *all-or-none*. This means that stimuli below the threshold will not produce a signal, whereas all stimuli above the threshold produce the same signal —the amplitude and duration of the signal are always the same regardless of variations in the stimuli. Moreover, unlike input potentials, which spread passively and thus decrease in amplitude with distance, the action potential does not decay as it travels the length of the axon from the initial segment to the terminal of the neuron, a distance that can be 1 meter or more in length (Table 2–1). The action potential is a large depolarizing signal up to 110 mV in amplitude (Figure 2–8C). It often lasts only 1 ms and can be conducted at rates that vary between about 1 and 100 meters per second.

The remarkable feature of action potential signaling is that it is so stereotyped that it varies only subtly (although in some cases importantly) from nerve cell to nerve cell. This feature was demonstrated by Edgar Adrian, who was the first to study the nervous system on the cellular level in the 1920s. Adrian, and subsequently Joseph Erlanger and Herbert Gasser, found that the shape of all action potentials is similar whatever their function and wherever they occur in the nervous system. Indeed, action potentials carried into the nervous system by a sensory axon often are indistinguishable from those carried out of the nervous system by a motor axon. What determines the intensity of sensation or the speed of movement is not the magnitude or duration of individual action potentials, but their *frequency*. In turn, the duration of a sensation or movement is determined by the period during which action potentials are generated (Figure 2–8C).

Only two features of neuronal firing are critical for signaling in the axon: the number of action potentials and the time intervals between them. As Adrian put it in 1928, summarizing his work on sensory fibers: ". . . all impulses are very much alike, whether the message is destined to arouse the sensation of light, of touch, or of pain; if they are crowded together the sensation is intense, if they are separated by long intervals the sensation is correspondingly feeble."

Adrian's comments point to one of the deep questions on the organization of the brain. If the signaling mechanisms are stereotyped and do not reflect properties of the stimulus, how do neural messages carry specific meaning? How is a message that carries visual information distinguished from one that carries information about a bee sting, or both of these from message commands for voluntary movement? As we shall learn in later chapters, the *meaning* of a signal is determined entirely by the neural *pathway* activated by the stimulus. The pathways activated by photoreceptor cells responding to light are completely different from those activated by sensory cells that respond to touch. The meaning of the signal—be it visual or tactile, sensory or motor—is determined not by the signal itself, but by the specific pathway along which it travels.

The Output Component Releases Transmitter

When the action potential reaches the terminal region of the neuron, it stimulates the release of packets of chemical transmitter. Transmitters can be small molecules related to amino acids, such as L-glutamate or acetylcholine, or they can be peptides like enkephalin. These transmitter molecules are packaged in subcellular organelles called *vesicles*, and are loaded into specialized release sites in the presynaptic terminals called *active zones*. The transmitter is released at these sites from its vesicles by fusion of the vesicle with the surface membrane, a process known as *exocytosis*. The release of chemical transmitter serves as the *output signal*. The amount of transmitter release is a graded function of the number and the frequency of the action potentials (Figure 2–8D). The transmitter released by the presynaptic neuron diffuses across the synaptic cleft to the postsynaptic cell, where it causes the postsynaptic cell to generate either an excitatory or an inhibitory synaptic potential, depending on the postsynaptic receptor and the current flow initiated by this protein.

The Information Carried by a Signal Is Transformed As It Passes from One Component to the Next

A critical feature of neuronal signaling is that the neural information is *transformed* as it passes from one component of the neuron to the next. The information is even more elaborately transformed as it passes from one neuron to the next. In the stretch reflex we can see aspects of these transformations in their most elementary form.

The particular features of the stimulus of a stretch of muscle—its amplitude and duration—are reflected in the graded amplitude and duration of the receptor potential in the afferent neuron. If the receptor potential exceeds the threshold for initiating an action potential, the graded signal is transformed at the initial segment of the afferent neuron into an all-or-none signal, a pattern of action potentials, or frequency code. The action potential guarantees that the signal will be propagated faithfully and without fail to the terminals of the neuron. Moreover, any increase in the amplitude of the receptor potential beyond threshold increases the frequency of the action potentials, and any increase in the duration of the input signal increases the duration of the train of action potentials. The digitally coded information—the frequency and number of action potentials—is conveyed along the entire extent of the axon. At the presynaptic terminals of the sensory neurons the frequency of action potentials determines the amount of transmitter released. In this way the digital signal (frequency of action potentials) is retransformed into an analog signal (a graded amount of transmitter).

These sets of transformation are recapitulated in the motor neuron. The transmitter released by the sensory neurons interacts with receptor molecules on the motor neurons to initiate a graded synaptic potential, which spreads to the initial segment of the axon. There it can initiate an action potential, which propagates without fail to the motor cell's terminals, where it causes transmitter release. This then triggers a synaptic potential in the muscle. This synaptic potential in the muscle fiber produces an action potential that leads to the final transformation of this reflex—muscle contraction and the generation of a behavioral act. The sequence of signal transformations from sensory to motor neuron to muscle is illustrated in Figure 2–9.

The stretch reflex is a very simple behavior, produced by two classes of neurons connected to each other through excitatory connections. Half the neurons of the brain are inhibitory, however. They release transmitter that hyperpolarizes the membrane potential of the postsynaptic cell and thus reduces the likelihood of firing. For example, in

FIGURE 2–9

This diagram summarizes the sequence of signals that produces a reflex action. Graded stretching of a muscle produces a graded (proportional) *receptor potential* in the terminal fibers of the sensory neuron (the dorsal root ganglion cell). This potential then spreads passively to the integrative segment, or trigger zone, at the first node of Ranvier. If the receptor potential is sufficiently large, it will trigger an *action potential* at the integrative segment, and the action potential will propagate actively and without change along the axon to the terminal region. At the terminal of the afferent neuron the action potential leads to an output signal: the release of a transmitter substance. The trans-mitter diffuses across the synaptic cleft and interacts with receptor molecules on the external membranes of the motor neurons that innervate the stretched muscle. This interaction initiates a synaptic potential in the motor cell. The synaptic potential then spreads passively to the axon hillock or initial segment of the motor neuron axon, where it may initiate an action potential that propagates actively to the terminal of the motor neuron. At the terminal the action potential causes transmitter release, which triggers a synaptic potential in the muscle. This signal produces an action potential in the muscle, causing contraction of the muscle fiber.

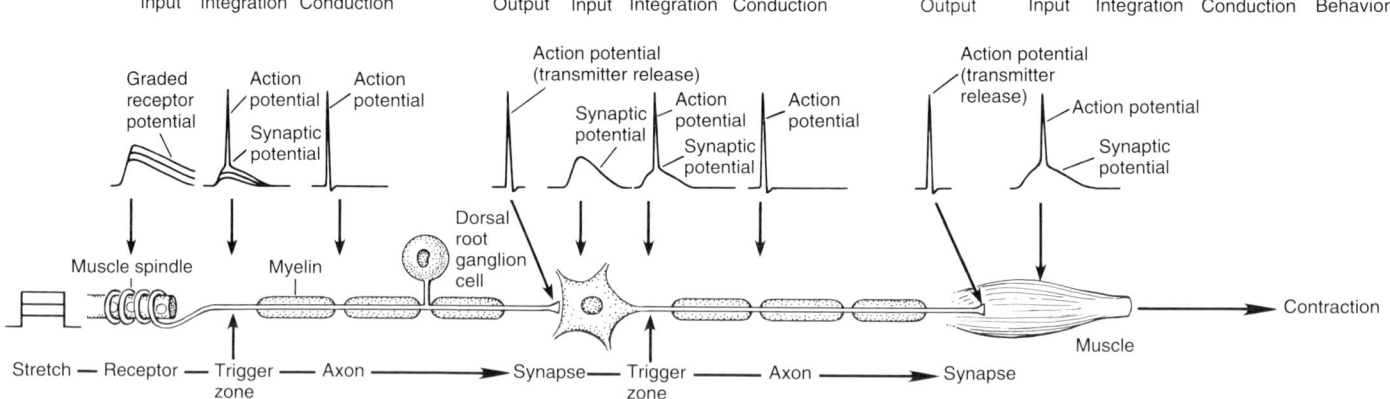

A   Feed-forward inhibition

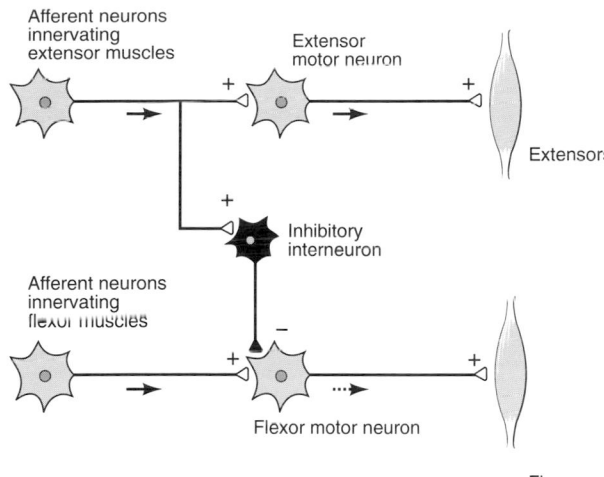

B   Feedback inhibition

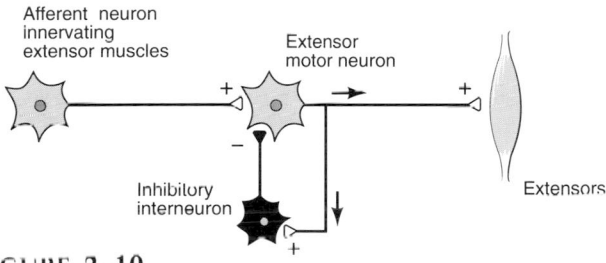

FIGURE 2–10

Inhibitory interneurons can make either feed-forward or feed-back connections.

A. Feed-forward inhibition is common in monosynaptic reflex systems, such as the knee jerk reflex system (see Figure 2–5). Afferent neurons from extensor muscles excite not only the extensor motor neurons but also inhibitory neurons that inhibit the firing of the motor cells that innervate the antagonistic flexor muscles. Feed-forward inhibition enhances the activity of the active synergistic pathway by suppressing the activity of other antagonistic pathways.

B. In negative feedback (recurrent) inhibition the extensor motor neurons activate inhibitory interneurons that reduce the probability of firing in the extensor motor neurons themselves. Negative feedback is self-regulating and prevents activity within the active pathway from exceeding a certain critical maximum.

the knee jerk reflex the afferent neurons that contract the extensor muscles of the leg also activate inhibitory interneurons that prevent the antagonist flexor muscles from being brought into action. This type of inhibition is a form of *feed-forward* inhibition designed to suppress other competitive actions (Figure 2–10A). Inhibition can also be self regulating and of the *feedback* variety. In this type a neuron that excites a target cell also acts on an inhibitory interneuron that feeds back and inhibits the active neu-

ron, thereby limiting its ability to excite the target (Figure 2–10). We will repeatedly encounter both types of inhibitory arrangements when we examine more complex behaviors in later chapters.

Nerve Cells Differ Most at the Molecular Level

The four-component model we have outlined here, although applicable to the vast majority of neurons, is a simplification and is not accurate in detail for all neurons. For example, some neurons do not generate action potentials; typically, these are local interneurons that lack a conductile component— they have no axon or only a very short one. In these neurons the input signals are summed and spread passively to the terminal region, where they directly affect secretion. Other cells do not have a steady resting potential and consequently are spontaneously active. Even cells that appear similar can differ in important details at the molecular level. For example, different neurons use different combinations of ion channels in their membranes. As we shall learn in Chapter 8, the diversity of ion channels results in neurons having different thresholds, excitability properties, and firing patterns. For example, neurons with different ion channels can encode the same synaptic potential into different patterns of firing.

Neurons also differ in their chemical transmitters and receptors. These differences have physiological importance, but they also account for the fact that a disease may strike one class of neurons but not others. Certain diseases strike motor neurons only (for example, amyotrophic lateral sclerosis or poliomyelitis), whereas others, such as tabes dorsalis, affect primarily sensory neurons. A motor disorder called Parkinson's disease affects a particular population of interneurons, which are located in the substantia nigra of the basal ganglia and use dopamine as a chemical transmitter. Some diseases are selective even within the neuron: Some only affect the receptive elements, others the cell body, and still others the axon. Indeed, because there are so many cell types and each type has molecularly distinct molecular components, the nervous system is attacked by a greater number and variety of diseases, both neurological and psychiatric, than any other organ in the body.

Despite these differences, the basic electrical signaling properties of nerve cells are surprisingly similar. Given the large number of different nerve cells in the brain, this simplicity is fortunate. If we understand in detail the molecular mechanisms that produce signaling in any one kind of cell, we shall be well along the way to understanding these mechanisms in many other kinds of nerve cells.

Patterns of Interconnection Allow Relatively Stereotyped Nerve Cells to Convey Unique Information

We have seen how a limited number of nerve cells can interact to produce simple behaviors by activating certain movements and inhibiting others. But can more complex behaviors be related so specifically to individual neurons?

In invertebrate animals a single (command) cell can initiate a complex behavioral sequence. However, as far as we know, in the human brain no such complex functions are initiated by a single neuron. Rather, every behavior is generated by many cells. The neural mediation of behavior is subdivided into discrete aspects of sensory input, motor output, and intermediate processing. Each of these aspects is conveyed by a group of neurons, and even a single aspect can involve several groups of neurons. The deployment of several groups of neurons or several pathways to convey the same information is called *parallel processing*. This probably increases both the richness and the reliability of function within the central nervous system.

Subdivision and localization of function are key strategies in the nervous system. Specific aspects of information processing are restricted to particular regions within the brain. For example, each sensory modality is processed to a distinct region where the sensory connections represent precisely a map of the appropriate surface of the body—the skin, tendons and joints, retina, basilar membrane of the cochlea, or olfactory epithelium. Muscles and movements are also represented in an orderly arrangement of connections. Thus, the brain contains at least two classes of maps: one class for sensory perceptions and the other for motor commands. The two types of maps are interconnected in ways that we do not as yet fully understand.

Most neurons, whether motor, sensory, or interneuronal, do not differ greatly in their electrical properties. Neurons with similar properties carry out different functions because of the connections they make in the nervous system. These connections are established during development and determine the cell's role in behavior. In those regions of the brain in which we understand how the components of a mental process are represented, the logical operations performed by a group of neurons only becomes comprehensible when the flow of information through the interconnections of the network is specified.

A similar conclusion about the importance of connections has now been recognized by scientists attempting to construct computational models of brain function. Scientists working in this field, a branch of computer science called *artificial intelligence*, initially used serial processing models to simulate the higher-level cognitive processes of the brain—processes such as pattern recognition, the acquisition of new information, memory, and motor performance. They soon realized that although these serial models solved many problems rather well, including such difficult tasks as playing chess, they performed poorly and slowly on other computations that the brain does rapidly and well, such as the almost immediate recognition of faces or the comprehension of speech.

As a result, most modelers of neural function have turned from serial systems to parallel distributed systems, which they call *connectionistic models*. Connectionistic models use interconnected computational elements that, like neural circuits, process information simultaneously and in parallel. The preliminary insights that have emerged from such models are consistent with physiological studies, and illustrate that individual elements in the model do not transmit large amounts of information. It is the connections between the many elements, not the contribution of individual components, which make complex information processing possible. Individual neurons can carry out important computations because they are wired together in organized and different ways. It is the distinctiveness of the wiring and the ability to modify this wiring through learning that create a brain in which relatively stereotyped units can endow us with individuality.

Selected Readings

Adrian, E. D. 1928. The Basis of Sensation: The Action of the Sense Organs. London: Christophers.

Jones, E. G. 1988. The nervous tissue. In L. Weiss (ed.), Cell and Tissue Biology: A Textbook of Histology, 6th ed. Baltimore: Urban and Schwarzenberg, pp. 277–351.

Katz, B. 1966. Nerve, Muscle, and Synapse. New York: McGraw-Hill.

Paulson, O. B., and Newman, E. A. 1987. Does the release of potassium from astrocyte endfeet regulate cerebral blood flow? Science 237:896–898.

Posner, M. I. (ed.) 1989. Foundations of Cognitive Science. Cambridge, Mass.: MIT Press.

Ramón y Cajal, S. 1852–1937. Recollections of My Life. E. H. Craigie (trans.) Philadelphia: American Philosophical Society. Republished 1989. Cambridge, Mass.: MIT Press.

Rumelhart, D. E., McClelland, J. L., Asanuma, C., Crick, F. H. C., Elman, J. L., Hinton, G. E., Jordan, M. I., Kawamoto, A. H., Munro, P. W., Norman, D. A., Rabin, D. E., Sejnowski, T. J., Smolensky, P., Stone, G. O., Williams, R. J., and Zipser, D. 1986. Parallel Distributed Processing: Explorations in the Microstructure of Cognition, Vol. 1: Foundations. Cambridge, Mass.: MIT Press.

References

Adrian, E. D. 1932. The Mechanism of Nervous Action: Electrical Studies of the Neurone. Philadelphia: University of Pennsylvania Press.

Alberts, B., Bray, D., Lewis, J., Raff, M., Roberts, K., and Watson, J. D. 1989. Molecular Biology of the Cell, 2nd ed. New York: Garland.

Erlanger, J., and Gasser, H. S. 1937. Electrical Signs of Nervous Activity. Philadelphia: University of Pennsylvania Press.

Kuffler, S. W., Nicholls, J. G., and Martin, A. R. 1984. From Neuron to Brain: A Cellular Approach to the Function of the Nervous System, 2nd ed. Sunderland, Mass.: Sinauer.

Martinez Martinez, P. F. A. 1982. Neuroanatomy: Development and Structure of the Central Nervous System. Philadelphia: Saunders.

Newman, E. A. 1986. High potassium conductance in astrocyte endfeet. Science 233:453–454.

Penfield, W. (ed.) 1932. Cytology & Cellular Pathology of the Nervous System, Vol. 2. New York: Hoeber.

Raff, M. C. 1989. Glial cell diversification in the rat optic nerve. Science 243:1450–1455.

Ramón y Cajal, S. 1933. Histology, 10th ed. Baltimore: Wood.

Sears, E. S., and Franklin, G. M. 1980. Diseases of the cranial nerves. In R. N. Rosenberg (ed.), The Science and Practice of Clinical Medicine, Vol. 5: Neurology. New York: Grune & Stratton, pp. 471–494.

5'---CAGCUAUCAGCUGUCGCUGAGACAGGUGGCAUAAGAGUGGAACAGAGAGUUGAAAAGGCAGGAAACUGGCUUAUCUCUUCACUAGAAAAGAGCUGAACACAGAAGUCCAGAAGAU
     -240   -220   -200   -180   -160

                                                    -20
                                               Met Ile Leu Cys Ser Tyr Trp His Val Gly Leu Val
CUAACAAGUUCAUCGUUUAGUUAUUAGAAGUGGCAGAUUUGCUUGAAAAGCCAAUUAUUGAAAGCUGAAGA AUG AUU CUG UGC AGU UAU UGG CAU GUA GGG UUG GUG
     -140   -120   -100   -80   -60   -40

    -10   -1 1   10   10
Leu Leu Leu Phe Ser Cys Cys Gly Leu Val Leu Gly Ser Glu His Glu Thr Arg Leu Val Ala Asn Leu Leu Glu Asn Tyr Asn Lys Val
CUA CUG UUA UUU UCG UGU UGU GGU CUG GUA CUA GGU UCU GAA CAU GAA ACA CGU UUG GUU GCU AAU UUA UUA GAA AAU UAU AAC AAG GUG
              -20   -1 1   20   40

   20   30   40
Ile Arg Pro Val Glu His His Thr His Phe Val Asp Ile Thr Val Gly Leu Gln Leu Ile Gln Leu Ile Ser Val Asp Glu Val Asn Gln
AUU CGU CCA GUG GAG CAU CAC ACC CAC UUU GUA GAU AUU ACA GUG GGG CUA CAG CUG AUA CAA CUC AUC AGU GUG GAU GAA GUA AAU CAA
    60   80   100   120   140

   50   60   70
Ile Val Glu Thr Asn Val Arg Leu Arg Gln Gln Trp Ile Asp Val Arg Leu Arg Trp Asn Pro Ala Asp Tyr Gly Gly Ile Lys Lys Ile
AUU GUG GAA ACA AAU GUG CGC CUA AGG CAG CAA UGG AUU GAU GUG AGG CUU CGC UGG AAU CCA GCC GAU UAU GGU GGA AUU AAA AAG AUC
               160   180   200   220

   80   90   100
Arg Leu Pro Ser Asp Asp Val Trp Leu Pro Asp Leu Val Leu Tyr Asn Asn Ala Asp Gly Asp Phe Ala Ile Val His Met Thr Lys Leu
AGA CUG CCU UCU GAU GAU GUU UGG CUG CCA GAU UUA GUU CUG UAC AAC AAU GCU GAU GGU GAU UUU GCC AUU GUU CAC AUG ACC AAA CUG
     240   260   280   300   320

  110   120   130
Leu Leu Asp Tyr Thr Gly Lys Ile Met Trp Thr Pro Pro Ala Ile Phe Lys Ser Tyr Cys Glu Ile Ile Val Thr His Phe Pro Phe Asp
CUU UUG GAU UAU ACG GGA AAA AUA AUG UGG ACA CCU CCA GCA AUC UUC AAA AGC UAU UGU GAA AUU AUU GUA ACA CAU UUC CCA UUU GAU
             340   360   380   400

  140   150   160
Gln Gln Asn Cys Thr Met Lys Leu Gly Ile Trp Thr Tyr Asp Gly Thr Lys Val Ser Ile Ser Pro Glu Ser Asp Arg Pro Asp Leu Ser
CAA CAA AAU UGC ACU AUG AAG UUG GGA AUC UGG ACG UAC GAU GGG ACA AAA GUU UCC AUA UCC CCG GAA AGU GAC CGU CCG GAU CUG AGU
     420   440   460   480   500

  170   180   190
Thr Phe Met Glu Ser Gly Glu Trp Val Met Lys Asp Tyr Arg Gly Trp Lys His Trp Val Tyr Tyr Thr Cys Cys Pro Asp Thr Pro Tyr
ACA UUU AUG GAA AGU GGA GAG UGG GUA AUG AAA GAU UAU CGU GGA UGG AAG CAC UGG GUG UAU UAU ACC UGC UGU CCU GAC ACU CCU UAC
             520   540   560   580

  200   210   220
Leu Asp Ile Thr Tyr His Phe Ile Met Gln Arg Ile Pro Leu Tyr Phe Val Val Asn Val Ile Ile Pro Cys Leu Leu Phe Ser Phe Leu
CUG GAU AUC ACC UAC CAU UUU AUC AUG CAG CGU AUU CCU CUU UAU UUU GUU GUG AAU GUC AUC AUU CCU UGU CUG CUU UUU UCA UUU UUA
     600   620   640   660   680

  230   240   250
Thr Gly Leu Val Phe Tyr Leu Pro Thr Asp Ser Gly Glu Lys Met Thr Leu Ser Ile Ser Val Leu Leu Ser Leu Thr Val Phe Leu Leu
ACU GGA UUA GUA UUU UAC UUA CCA ACU GAU UCA GGU GAG AAG AUG ACU UUG AGU AUU UCC GUU UUG CUG UCU CUG ACU GUG UUC CUU CUG
             700   720   740   760

  260   270   280
Val Ile Val Glu Leu Ile Pro Ser Thr Ser Ser Ala Val Pro Leu Ile Gly Lys Tyr Met Leu Phe Thr Met Ile Phe Val Ile Ser Ser
GUU AUU GUU GAG CUG AUC CCC UCA ACU UCC AGC GCU GUG CCU UUG AUU GGC AAA UAC AUG CUU UUU ACA AUG AUU UUU GUC AUC AGU UCA
     780   800   820   840   860

  290   300   310
Ile Ile Ile Thr Val Val Val Ile Asn Thr His His Arg Ser Pro Ser Thr His Thr Met Pro Gln Trp Val Arg Lys Ile Phe Ile Asp
AUC AUC AUU ACU GUU GUU GUA AUU AAU ACU CAC CAU CGC UCU CCA AGU ACA CAU ACA AUG CCA CAA UGG GUA CGA AAG AUC UUU AUU GAU
             880   900   920   940

  320   330   340
Thr Ile Pro Asn Val Met Phe Phe Ser Thr Met Lys Arg Ala Ser Lys Glu Lys Gln Glu Asn Lys Ile Phe Ala Asp Asp Ile Asp Ile
ACU AUA CCC AAU GUU AUG UUU UUC UCA ACA AUG AAA CGA GCU UCU AAG GAA AAG CAA GAA AAU AAG AUA UUU GCU GAU GAC AUU GAU AUC
     960   980   1,000   1,020   1,040

  350   360   370
Ser Asp Ile Ser Gly Lys Gln Val Thr Gly Glu Val Ile Phe Gln Thr Pro Leu Ile Lys Asn Pro Asp Val Lys Ser Ala Ile Glu Gly
UCU GAC AUU UCU GGA AAG CAA GUG ACA GGA GAA GUA AUU UUU CAA ACA CCU CUC AUU AAA AAU CCA GAU GUC AAA AGU GCU AUU GAG GGA
             1,060   1,080   1,100   1,120

  380   390   400
Val Lys Tyr Ile Ala Glu His Met Lys Ser Asp Glu Glu Ser Ser Asn Ala Ala Glu Glu Trp Lys Tyr Val Ala Met Val Ile Asp His
GUC AAA UAU AUU GCA GAG CAC AUG AAG UCU GAU GAG GAA UCA AGC AAU GCU GCA GAG GAA UGG AAG UAU GUU GCA AUG GUG AUU GAU CAC
             1,140   1,160   1,180   1,200   1,220

  410   420   430
Ile Leu Leu Cys Val Phe Met Leu Ile Cys Ile Ile Gly Thr Val Ser Val Phe Ala Gly Arg Leu Ile Glu Leu Ser Gln Glu Gly
AUU CUG CUG UGU GUC UUC AUG CUG AUU UGU AUA AUU GGU ACA GUU AGC GUG UUU GCU GGC CGU CUC AUU GAA CUC AGU CAA GAG GGC UAA
             1,240   1,260   1,280   1,300

AUCUUCAUUGUGAGCAAAAAAGGCAAUACUGGAAUAAGGGAUGGAUAUCACUCCACAGAAAAGAUGUGUGGGUUUAGUGUUGCAAUUGUAGUCUGUUUUAUGAGAUAUAUAGUUUGCUUU
   1,320   1,340   1,360   1,380   1,400   1,420

GUUUUACAAUGAAAGUGACUUAAGGUAUUUGAAUAUGUAAAAAAAAGUAAUGAAAUAACAGUAAGUGAAAAAUGUUAUUAUGCAAGUACCUGAAACGUGUAAUAAGUGGAACAACUUUUU
   1,440   1,460   1,480   1,500   1,520   1,540

AAUACAUUACUAUAAAAGUAAGCAAAAAAAUAAGUUUAACAAAUAUGAGGGUAGUCAUUUGAAAUGUAACAGAGAAAUGAAAAUUAUUAAAUAUAAACAGUAUAUUAUUAAGUUAAACAA
   1,560   1,580   1,600   1,620   1,640   1,660

AGUUAAUCCAUUCUUUUAUAUCCAAAGUUUGUAUUAUACAUUUAGAAGUGUAGUUCUAUUGUAUAAUUUAAAGUAUGUUUUACAGAUCAUUAAUAAAAUAUUCAAUGCAUUACU---3'
   1,680   1,700   1,720   1,740   1,760   1,780

II

Cell and Molecular Biology of the Neuron

From modern cell biology we learn that complex biological systems are built from similar, repeating units. These units, or modules, may be relatively undifferentiated, as in primitive organisms like sponges or in simple organs of the body like liver and spleen, or they may be extraordinarily specialized, as in higher metazoan animals. Perhaps the most complex biological system is the vertebrate brain, which, as we shall see in the following chapters, is also constructed of repeating modules. In all biological systems, from the most simple to the most complex, these modules are composed of cells.

Biological systems also show another morphological feature: The construction of its modules is architectonic. The anatomy and fine structure of the body repetitively mirror its function. Thus, behavior is reflected in the construction of the brain, and is mirrored in the cytology, biophysics, and biochemistry of the neurons of which it is composed.

Despite their diversity, all nerve cells are built on a single basic plan. Indeed, nerve cells share many features with other cells of the body. At the same time, nerve cells have the unique ability to communicate precisely, rapidly, and over long distances with one another and with target cells, such as muscles and gland cells. This ability derives from membrane proteins, such as ion channels and receptors, that allow specific inorganic ions—Na^+, K^+, Ca^{2+}, or Cl^-—to pass rapidly through the membrane. In this part of the book we shall be especially concerned with ion channels that open in response to changes in potential across the cell membrane. Other kinds of ion channels are opened by the neurotransmitters released by other nerve cells. We shall examine in particular the responses to external stimuli, the integrative actions of the various subcellular components of nerve cells, and the variety and distribution of ion channels.

The complete nucleotide base sequence of the messenger RNA that encodes the α subunit of the nicotinic acetylcholine receptor. Shosaku Numa and his colleagues also cloned and sequenced the β, γ, and δ subunits. This information has permitted specific and detailed models for the conformation and function of the receptor. (From Numa, S., Noda, M., Takahashi, T., Tanabe, M., Toyosato, Y., Furutani, Y., and Kikyotani, S. 1983. Molecular structure of the nicotinic acetylcholine receptor. Cold Spring Harbor Symp. Quant. Biol. 48:57–69.)

PART II

Chapter 3: **The Cytology of Neurons**
Chapter 4: **Synthesis and Trafficking of Neuronal Proteins**
Chapter 5: **Ion Channels**
Chapter 6: **Membrane Potential**
Chapter 7: **Passive Membrane Properties of the Neuron**
Chapter 8: **Voltage-Gated Ion Channels and the Generation of the Action Potential**

James H. Schwartz

3

The Cytology of Neurons

**The Neurons That Mediate the
Stretch Reflex Differ in Their Morphology
and Transmitter Substance**

   The Sensory Neuron

   The Motor Neuron

**The Axons of Both Sensory and Motor Neurons
Are Ensheathed in Myelin**

**A Major Function of the Neuron's Cell Body
Is the Synthesis of Macromolecules**

An Overall View

The cells of the nervous system are more varied than cells in any other part of the body. Although neurons differ from one another, they all share features that distinguish them from liver cells, fibroblasts, and cells in other tissues. For example, they typically are highly polarized. The cell body, which contains the nucleus and the organelles for making RNA and protein, is only one of the four important regions of the neuron, and in most neurons the cell body contains less than a tenth of the cell's total volume. The remaining cell volume is contained in the dendrites and axon that originate from the cell body. As shown in Chapter 2 (Figure 2–1), dendrites are thin processes that branch several times and are specially shaped to receive synaptic input from other nerve cells. The cell body usually gives off a single axon, another thin process that carries electrical impulses often considerable distances to the neuron's terminals or synaptic endings on other nerve cells or on target organs. Neurons differ from most other cells in being excitable. Excitability results from specific and characteristic proteins in neuronal membranes (ion channels and pumps) that will be described in later chapters.

Neuronal diversity is well illustrated in the cerebellum, a part of the brain described in Chapter 41 that is important in controlling motor behavior and whose five types of nerve cells have been completely cataloged. At one extreme are the Purkinje cells, among the largest neurons in the vertebrate nervous system. Their cell bodies are 80 μm in diameter and their dendrites arborize extensively over relatively long distances to receive diverse inputs. At the other extreme are the small granule neurons, whose cell bodies are only 6–8 μm in diameter and consist of a nucleus surrounded by the thinnest shell of cytoplasm; the dendritic processes of these cells remain much closer to the cell body.

Cytological diversity is the result of the process developmental biologists call differentiation. By the genes it expresses, each type of cell synthesizes only certain macromolecules—enzymes, structural proteins, membrane constituents, and secretory products—and avoids making others. In essence, each cell is the macromolecules that it makes. Nevertheless, not all constituents of a neuron are specialized. Many molecules are common to all cells in the body; some are characteristic of all neurons, others of large classes of neurons, and still others are restricted to only a few nerve cells. Thus, each neuron consists of a combination of specific as well as general molecules.

In this chapter and the next we shall consider the cytology of the nerve cell, describing both distinctive and general constituents. Although the details of neuronal cytology might be illustrated by different nerve cells that exhibit particular features in a striking manner, we have chosen to illustrate these features with the two types of neurons that mediate the simple behavior discussed in Chapter 2, the stretch reflex operating in the knee jerk. In this way the relationship between structure and function should be more easily appreciated. The monosynaptic component of the reflex consists only of the large sensory neurons of the dorsal root ganglion that are connected to muscle spindles and the motor neurons in the spinal cord that cause the thigh muscle to contract (the role of this reflex in motor control is discussed in Chapters 36 and 37). These two types of nerve cells differ in function and structure as well as in certain macromolecular components. They also display some cytological and biochemical features that are typical of other neurons. In addition, they have many parts that are common to all cells of the body.

Organelles and macromolecular components are not randomly distributed throughout the neuron but are situated in specific regions of the cell. Indeed, this regional specialization of subcellular parts often determines the functions of regions within the cell. Because of the great polarity of nerve cells, the location of the various regions of a neuron within the nervous system is of obvious functional importance. In this chapter we shall describe how these sensory and motor neurons are situated in the nervous system as well as discuss differences in the location of their subcellular parts, paying special attention to the regional distribution of receptors, ion channels, pumps, and insulating myelin. In the next chapter we shall consider some of the mechanisms by which these macromolecules are distributed within the cell.

The Neurons That Mediate the Stretch Reflex Differ in Their Morphology and Transmitter Substance

The knee jerk reflex is produced by two types of cells: an afferent (or sensory) neuron and a motor neuron upon which it synapses. The anatomical arrangement of these neurons and their connections is shown in Figure 2–5.

The Sensory Neuron

The sensory neuron's receptor is formed from a coil around a fine, specialized muscle fiber (*intrafusal fiber*) that lies within the larger stretch receptor called the *muscle spindle* (Figure 3–1, and see Figures in Chapter 37). From the muscle, the sensory axon travels within the femoral nerve to the cell body in the dorsal root ganglion in the lumbosacral region of the spinal cord (see Figure 20–2). In the nerve the sensory process is 14–18 μm in diameter and is coated with a white, insulating sheath of myelin. This sheath, which is 8–10 μm thick, is regularly interrupted along the length of the axon by gaps that are less than 0.5 μm and are called nodes of Ranvier (Figure 3–2). At these gaps the plasma membrane of the axon, called the *axolemma*, is exposed to the extracellular space. This nodal arrangement of myelin is important for the speed at which the nerve impulse is conducted along the axon, as explained in Chapter 8.

The cell bodies of the primary afferent (sensory) fibers are round and large in diameter (60–120 μm) (Figure 3–3). As we saw in Chapter 2, these dorsal root ganglion cells are classified as pseudo-unipolar neurons because they give rise to only one process that bifurcates into two branches a short distance from the cell body. One, the peripheral branch of the Ia afferent, is the sensory process that leads from the muscle spindle; the other, the central branch of the Ia afferent, extends through the dorsal root to the spinal cord, where it synapses on the motor neurons that control the reflex (Figure 3–4).

The Motor Neuron

The sensory axon projects directly to two kinds of motor neurons: those that innervate the same muscle from which the sensory fiber emerges, and those that innervate synergistic muscles (muscles that work together to stretch

FIGURE 3–1
Primary sensory nerve endings in the cat soleus muscle. The naked endings of the Ia (primary) afferent axon coil around specialized muscle fibers within the muscle spindle. **B** designates bag fibers, and **Ch**, chain fibers. This structure, which is the sensory organ for stretch, is described in detail in Chapters 36 and 37. (From Boyd and Smith, 1984.)

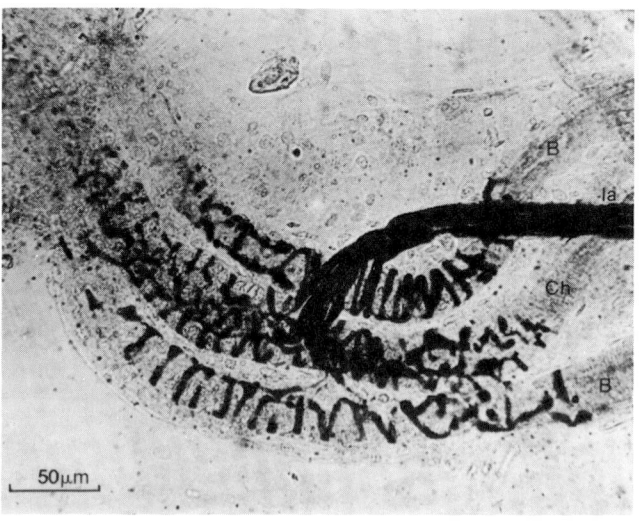

50μm

A Peripheral   **B** Central

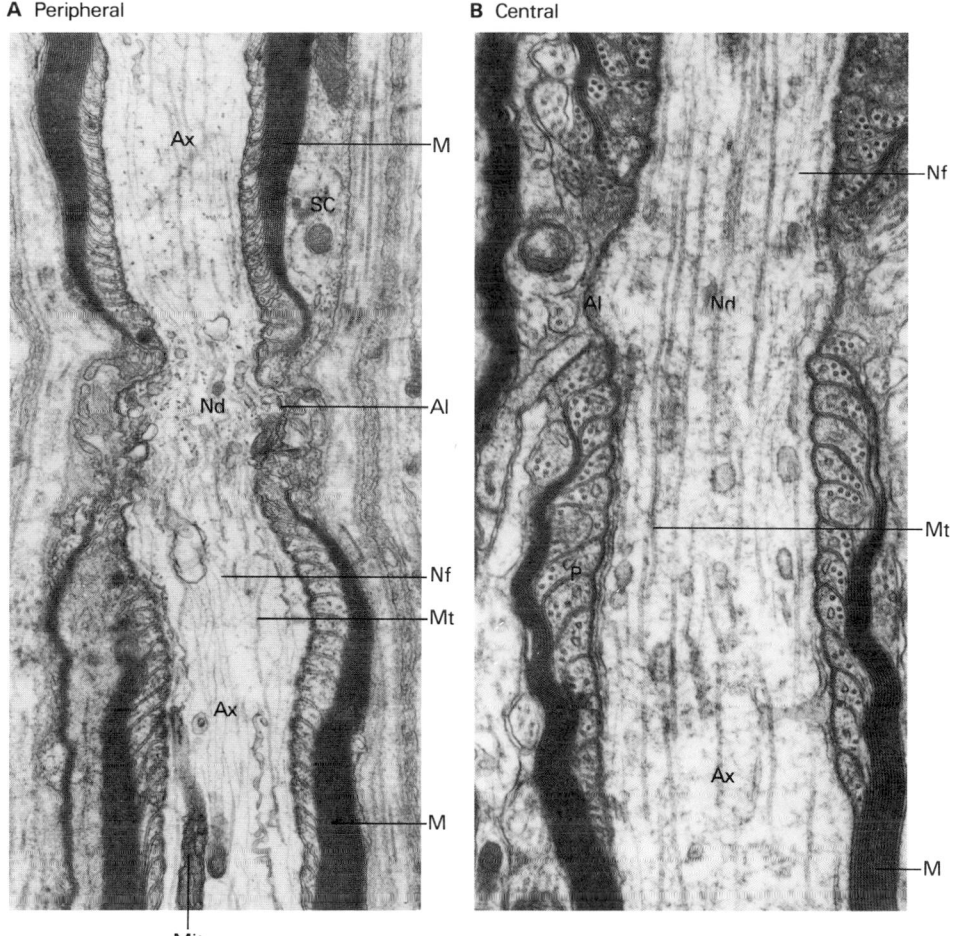

FIGURE 3–2

The insulating myelin sheath of the axon has regularly spaced gaps called the nodes of Ranvier. Axon segments from the peripheral nervous system (**A**) and the central nervous system (**B**) are shown in the region of a node. The axon (**Ax**) runs from the top to the bottom in both pictures. The axon is coated with many layers of myelin (**M**), which is periodically terminated at the nodes (**Nd**) in pockets of paranodal cytoplasm (**P**) of the supporting glial cell. In the peripheral nervous system the support cell is called a Schwann cell (**SC**), and in the central nervous system it is an oligodendrocyte. At the node the axolemma (**Al**) is exposed. The elements of the cytoskeleton that can be seen within the axon are microtubules (**Mt**) and neurofilaments (**Nf**). Mitochondria (**Mit**) are also seen. (From Peters, Palay, and Webster, 1991.)

the knee joint). These motor neurons are located in the anterior horn of the spinal cord (see Figures 2–5, 3–3C, 3–4). They have large cell bodies, up to 80 μm in diameter, whose nucleus is distinctive because of its large size and prominent nucleolus (Figure 3–3D). Unlike dorsal root ganglion cells, which have no dendrites, motor neurons have extensive dendritic trees (Figure 3–5). Dendrites differ from axons in several ways. They are typically smaller in diameter and shorter in length. Whereas the axon conducts the output signal of a cell, dendrites receive synaptic input from other neurons, often at specialized regions called *spines*.

Most of the protein made in neurons is synthesized in the cell body. But some synthesis occurs in dendrites also. Unlike axons, especially the parts close to the cell body, dendrites contain the subcellular organelles needed for protein synthesis (ribosomes, endoplasmic reticulum, and Golgi apparatus, which are discussed in the next chapter).

These organelles frequently are situated just beneath a spine. The cytoskeleton of the dendrite (composed predominantly of the fibrous polymeric proteins, neurofilaments, microtubules, and microfilaments, also discussed in Chapter 4) differs to some degree from that in the axon. Its molecular composition is similar to the cytoskeleton of the cell body. In particular, the kinds of tubulin monomers from which microtubule polymers are formed, and the specific proteins associated with the microtubules (also to be described in the next chapter), differ from those of the axon.

The number of primary or first-order dendrites of a motor neuron ranges from 7 to 18, and each ramifies four to six times, usually by bifurcating but sometimes by even more extensive branching. Because each primary dendrite gives rise to about 10 or more terminal branches, the total number of terminal dendritic branches per cell is commonly over 100. The average length of a dendrite from the

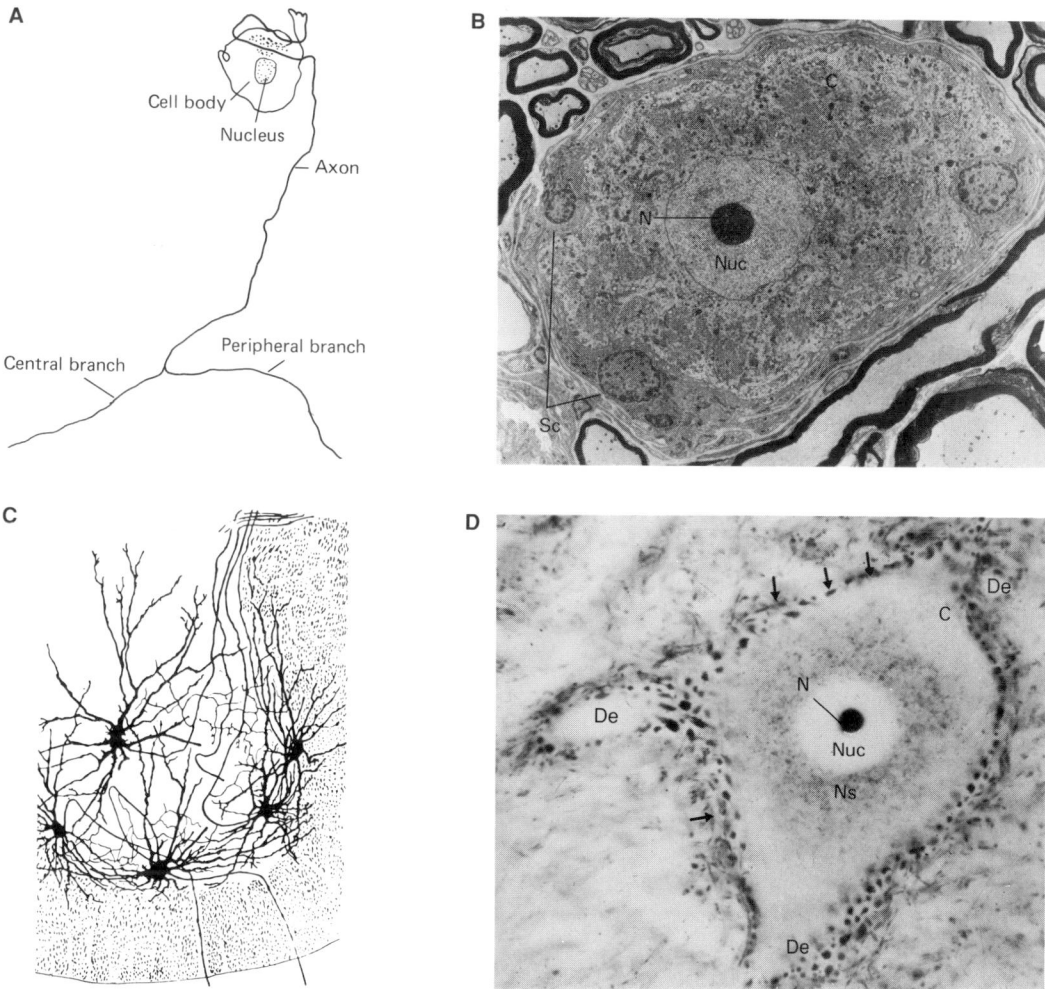

FIGURE 3–3

The appearance of the two types of cells that participate in the knee jerk stretch reflex: the afferent (sensory) dorsal root ganglion cell and the spinal motor neuron.

A. The dorsal root ganglion cell. The cell body contains a prominent nucleus. The axon typically is quite convoluted before it bifurcates into a central and a peripheral branch. (From Dogiel, 1908.)

B. This low-power electron micrograph shows the cell body (**C**) of a large dorsal root ganglion cell. Within the nucleus (**Nuc**) a prominent nucleolus (**N**) can be seen. The cell body of the neuron is surrounded by glial support cells (**Sc**). (Courtesy of R. E. Coggeshall and F. Mandriota.)

C. A drawing of five spinal motor neurons in the ventral horn of a kitten. These neurons were stained with Golgi's silver method (see Chapter 4), which reveals the many dendritic processes arborizing from the cell bodies. (From Ramón y Cajal, 1909.)

D. This photomicrograph of the cell body (**C**) of a motor neuron shows an enormous number of nerve endings from presynaptic neurons (**arrows**). These terminals, called synaptic boutons, appear as knob-like enlargements on the cell membrane. Three dendrites (**De**) are also shown. The nucleus and its nucleolus are surrounded by Nissl substance (**Ns**), clumps of ribosomes associated with the membrane of the endoplasmic reticulum. The synaptic boutons are prominent in this micrograph because the tissue is specially impregnated with silver. (Courtesy of G. L. Rasmussen.)

cell body to its termination is about 20 cell-body diameters, but some branches are twice as long (mean path length about 1.5 mm). Because the branches project radially, the dendritic tree of a single motor neuron can extend over an area within the spinal cord about 2–3 mm in diameter. Amazingly, the total surface area of the membrane of the dendrites and cell body can reach 1 mm²! Such extensive dendritic branching permits cells to receive many inputs over a large area.

Although each motor neuron has many dendrites, it gives rise to only one axon, which originates from a specialized region of the cell body called the *axon hillock* (Figure 3–6). The first portion of the axon is called the *initial segment*. Together, the axon hillock and initial segment extend the length of about one cell-body diameter, at which point the axon becomes ensheathed in myelin. The axon hillock and initial segment of the axon function as a *trigger zone* that integrates the many incoming signals from other cells and initiates the signal that the neuron sends to the muscle.

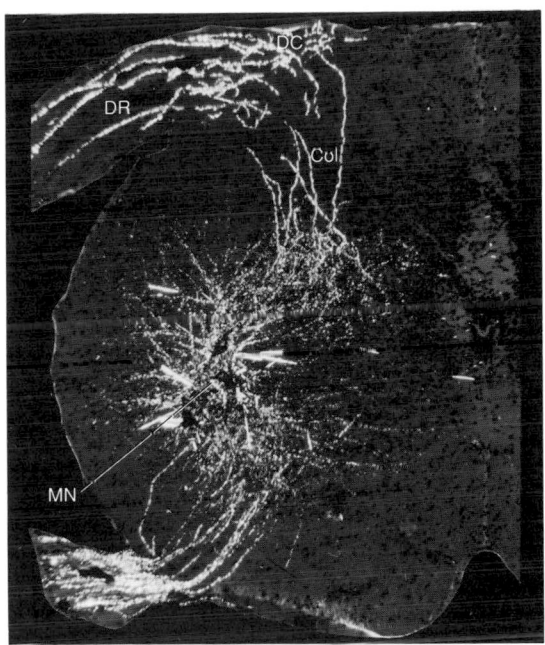

FIGURE 3–4

This micrograph shows the connections between sensory neurons of the triceps muscle and motor neurons in the brachial spinal cord of a bullfrog. The triceps nerve was labeled with horseradish peroxidase. The sensory axons enter the spinal cord through the dorsal root (**DR**) and then run longitudinally in the dorsal columns (**DC**). Collaterals (**Col**) descend from the dorsal columns to the spinal gray matter, where they arborize and make synaptic contact with the dendrites of brachial motor neurons (**MN**). Dorsal is up, lateral is to the left. × 50. (Courtesy of E. Frank.)

FIGURE 3–5

The dendritic structure of a spinal motor neuron.

A. Light micrograph of a motor neuron in the lumbosacral region of a cat's spinal cord. The cell body is shown in the lower left of the picture. The boxed area shows distal dendritic branches receiving contacts (**arrows**) from sensory (Ia afferent) neurons. Both sensory and motor neurons were identified by injection of the enzyme horseradish peroxidase, which serves as an intracellular marker (see Chapter 4). Since this is one of a set of serial sections, the complete dendritic branching pattern of this motor neuron can be reconstructed. The **upper arrow** identifies a presynaptic contact on a fifth-order dendritic branch, and the **lower arrow** points to a contact on a third-order branch. (From Brown and Fyffe, 1981.)

B. Presynaptic contacts (**arrows**) on primary dendrites within 45 μm of the cell body of the motor neuron shown in **A**. (From Brown and Fyffe, 1984.)

A

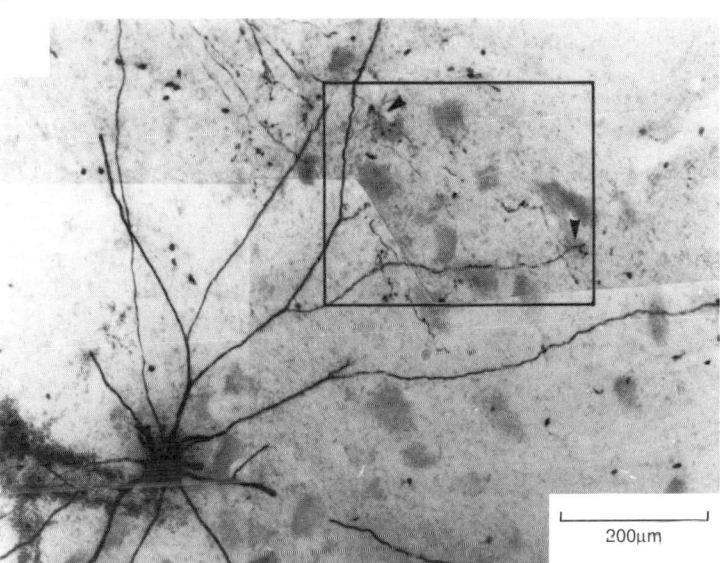

200μm

B

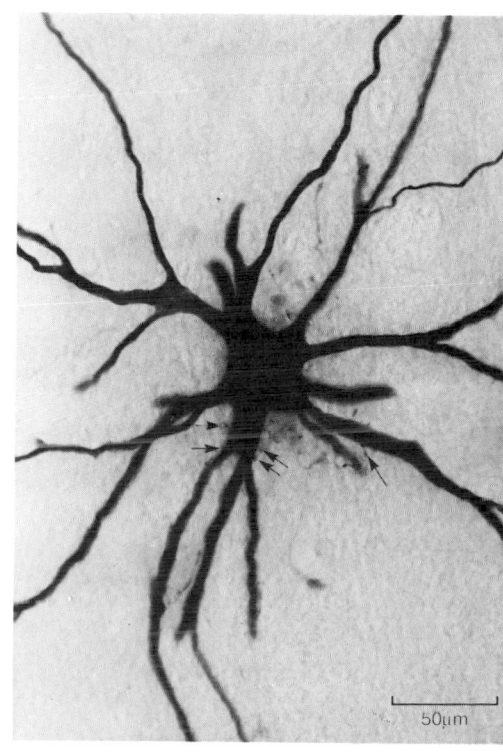

50μm

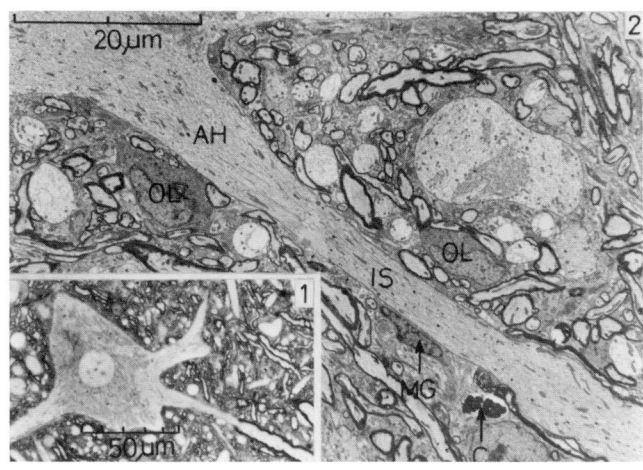

A

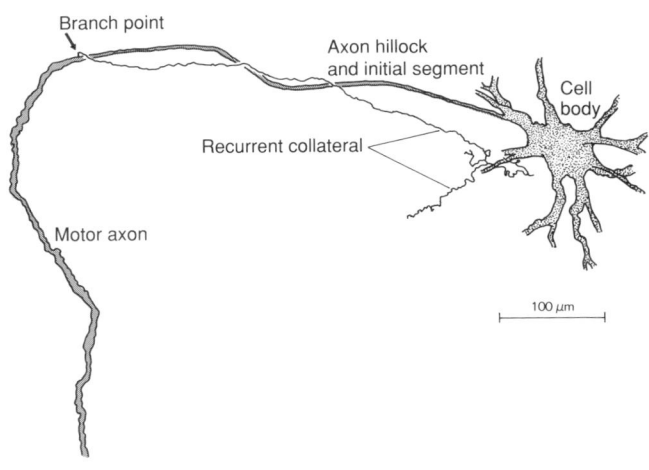

B

FIGURE 3–6

The axon of a spinal motor neuron branches to make synaptic contact with several interneurons, and, rarely, a recurrent (feedback) connection on the motor neuron.

A. Two electron micrographs, **(1)** and **(2)**, show the cell body, axon hillock **(AH)**, initial segment **(IS)**, and the first part of the myelinated portion of a cat's spinal motor neuron. Glial cells (**OL**, oligodendrocytes; **MG**, microglial cell) surround the initial part of the axon. **C** is a cross section of a capillary. The inset **(1)** shows two dendrites emerging from opposite sides of the cell body. (From Conradi, 1969.)

B. This camera lucida diagram of the cell body and initial part of the axon of a motor neuron shows recurrent axonal branching. The axons of motor neurons typically give off from one to five recurrent branches that usually make synaptic contact with inhibitory interneurons. In this rare example the recurrent axonal branch makes direct contact with its own cell body. This neuron was identified by injection with horseradish peroxidase. (Courtesy of R. E. Burke.)

Close to the cell body, the motor axon itself gives off one to five collateral branches (Figure 3–6). These branches are called *recurrent* because, as a rule, they synapse on inhibitory interneurons called *Renshaw* cells, which in turn project axons back to the motor neurons. (A rare recurrent branch from the motor neuron can end directly on neighboring motor neurons without synapsing on interneurons; sometimes it even ends directly on its own cell body.) There also are several other kinds of inhibitory interneurons. Inhibitory interneurons are thought to use glycine or γ-aminobutyric acid (GABA) as transmitter substances. The biosynthesis of these neurotransmitters is discussed in Chapter 14.

About half the surface area of the axon hillock and cell body and three-quarters of the dendritic membrane are covered by knob-like enlargements, called *synaptic boutons*, that are the nerve endings of other neurons (Figure 3–3B). The motor neuron receives excitatory input from the primary sensory neurons, excitatory and inhibitory inputs from interneurons that control motor behavior, and feedback inhibition from Renshaw and other inhibitory interneurons. All of these synaptic inputs are tallied by mechanisms described in Chapter 11. The resultant change in membrane potential is sensed at the trigger zone, whose membrane is rich in voltage-gated Na⁺ channels. When these channels are sufficiently activated, a propagated action potential is initiated (as described in Chapter 8).

One striking difference between the motor neuron and the sensory cell is the location of synaptic inputs. While the sensory neuron has few if any synaptic boutons on its cell body or axons within the dorsal root ganglion, the primary and modifying inputs to the motor neuron occur on the cell body and dendrites. In addition to the primary input from muscle spindles, the sensory neuron receives modifying inputs near its terminals onto motor neurons within the spinal cord. (In Chapter 12 we consider these axoaxonic, modulatory connections from higher levels of the central nervous system, many of which cause presynaptic inhibition.) Sebastian Conradi, Alan Brown, and Robert Burke and their colleagues examined many individual cat motor neurons and found that only 5% of the synaptic boutons from all sources are located on the cell body itself and the rest on dendritic branches (Figure 3–5). The synaptic input to the motor cell is arranged in an orderly fashion: Most inhibitory synapses are close to the cell body, while excitatory ones are further out on dendrites. Each motor neuron receives two to six contacts from a single sensory neuron, and each sensory neuron contacts 500 to 1000 motor neurons. The neurotransmitter used by the primary sensory cell has not been identified with certainty, but much evidence indicates that it is the amino acid L-glutamate.

The axon of the motor neuron, about 20 μm in diameter, leaves the spinal cord in the ventral root. In our example the axon leaves the lumbosacral region of the spinal cord to enter the femoral nerve. Thus, the motor axon travels along the same peripheral path as the sensory fiber from the muscle. When it enters the muscle, the motor axon ramifies into many branches that become increasingly thinner, reaching a diameter of only a few micrometers. Eventually, each branch loses its myelin sheath and runs along the surface of a muscle fiber to make synaptic contacts called *neuromuscular junctions*, at which the neurotransmitter acetylcholine is released by the motor neuron. The neuromuscular junction is the most completely characterized and best understood of all synapses and is discussed in detail in Chapter 10.

In summary, the sensory and motor neurons that mediate the knee jerk use similar signaling mechanisms but differ in many ways—in their appearance, in their location in the nervous system, and in the distribution of their processes. All of these cytological features have important behavioral consequences, which are discussed in Part VI in the context of the control of movement. In addition, the two types of cells use different neurotransmitters (although both transmitters are excitatory in function) and receive markedly different kinds of input. Synaptic transmission by the motor neuron, which occurs through the release of acetylcholine, requires not only the biosynthetic enzyme choline acetyltransferase, but also at least one special membrane protein that is not made in the sensory cell or in other noncholinergic neurons: a specific transporter or pump protein for choline, which is an essential precursor of the transmitter.

The Axons of Both Sensory and Motor Neurons Are Ensheathed in Myelin

The signal-conducting processes of both sensory and motor neurons are ensheathed in myelin along much of their length. Electron microscopy has revealed that this myelin sheath is arranged in concentric layers (Figures 3–2, 3–3B, and 3–7). Early microscopists were impressed with the high degree of regularity of myelin, and used X-ray diffraction and polarized light (techniques appropriate for analyzing crystal structure) to investigate its structure. In 1939 Francis Schmitt concluded that the sheath consists of repeating bimolecular layers of lipids interspersed between adjacent protein layers. Biochemical analysis shows that myelin has a composition similar to that of plasma membranes, consisting of 70% lipid and 30% protein, with a high concentration of cholesterol and phospholipid.

Both the regularity and the biochemical composition of myelin can now be explained because we understand how the sheath is formed (Figure 3–7). During development, before myelination takes place, the sensory cell axon lies along a peripheral nerve in a trough formed by a series of glia called *Schwann cells*. Schwann cells line up along the axon with intervals between them that will eventually become the nodes of Ranvier. The plasmalemma (external cell membrane) of each Schwann cell then surrounds a single axon, and forms a double-membrane structure called the *mesaxon*, which then elongates and spirals around the axon in concentric layers. The cytoplasm of the Schwann cell appears to be squeezed out during this ensheathing process. The Schwann cell's processes then condense into the compact lamellae of the mature myelin sheath. Because the primary sensory axon in the femoral nerve is about 0.5 m long and the internodal distance is 1–1.5 mm, it can be estimated that approximately 300–500 nodes of Ranvier occur along a primary afferent fiber between the thigh muscle and the dorsal root ganglion, where the cell body lies. And since each internodal segment is formed by a single Schwann cell, as many as 500 Schwann cells participate in the myelination of a single peripheral sensory axon.

The central axonal branch of the dorsal root ganglion cell in the spinal cord and the axon of motor neurons are also myelinated. The myelin in the central nervous system differs from its peripheral counterpart to some degree, however, because the glial cell responsible for elaborating central myelin is the *oligodendrocyte*, which typically ensheaths several axon processes. Schwann cells and oligodendrocytes differ developmentally and biochemically. The genes in Schwann cells that encode myelin are turned on by the presence of axons. In contrast, expression of the genes in oligodendrocytes that encode myelin appears to depend on the presence of astrocytes, the other major glial cell type in the central nervous system.

Early during myelination in the periphery, the Schwann cell expresses myelin-associated glycoprotein (MAG), a protein that is destined to become only a minor component of mature (compact) myelin. This protein is situated primarily at the margin of the mature myelin sheath just adjacent to the axon. Its early expression, subcellular location, and structural similarity to other surface recognition proteins have led to the idea that it is an adhesion molecule important for the initiation of the myelination process. Two isoforms of MAG with molecular weights of 68,900 and 64,000 can be produced from a single gene through alternative RNA splicing. MAG belongs to a superfamily that is related to the immunoglobulins and includes several important cell-surface proteins thought to be involved in cell-to-cell recognition (for example, the major histocompatability complex of antigens, T-cell surface antigens, and the neural cell adhesion molecule, NCAM).

The major protein in mature peripheral myelin, P_o, has a molecular weight of 28,000 and spans the plasmalemma of the Schwann cell once. It has a basic intracellular domain; like myelin-associated glycoprotein, P_o is also a member of the immunoglobulin superfamily. The glycosylated extracellular part of the protein, which contains the immunoglobulin domains, is thought to play a role in the compaction of myelin by interacting with identical domains on the surface of the apposed membrane. Central myelin (which lacks P_o) contains a characteristic *proteolipid*. The proteolipid has a molecular weight of 30,000 and constitutes more than half of the total protein in central myelin. Like many biochemical terms, the name proteolipid was originally introduced by Jordi Folch-Pi on the basis of a property of the molecule that is easy to demonstrate experimentally and which distinguishes it from

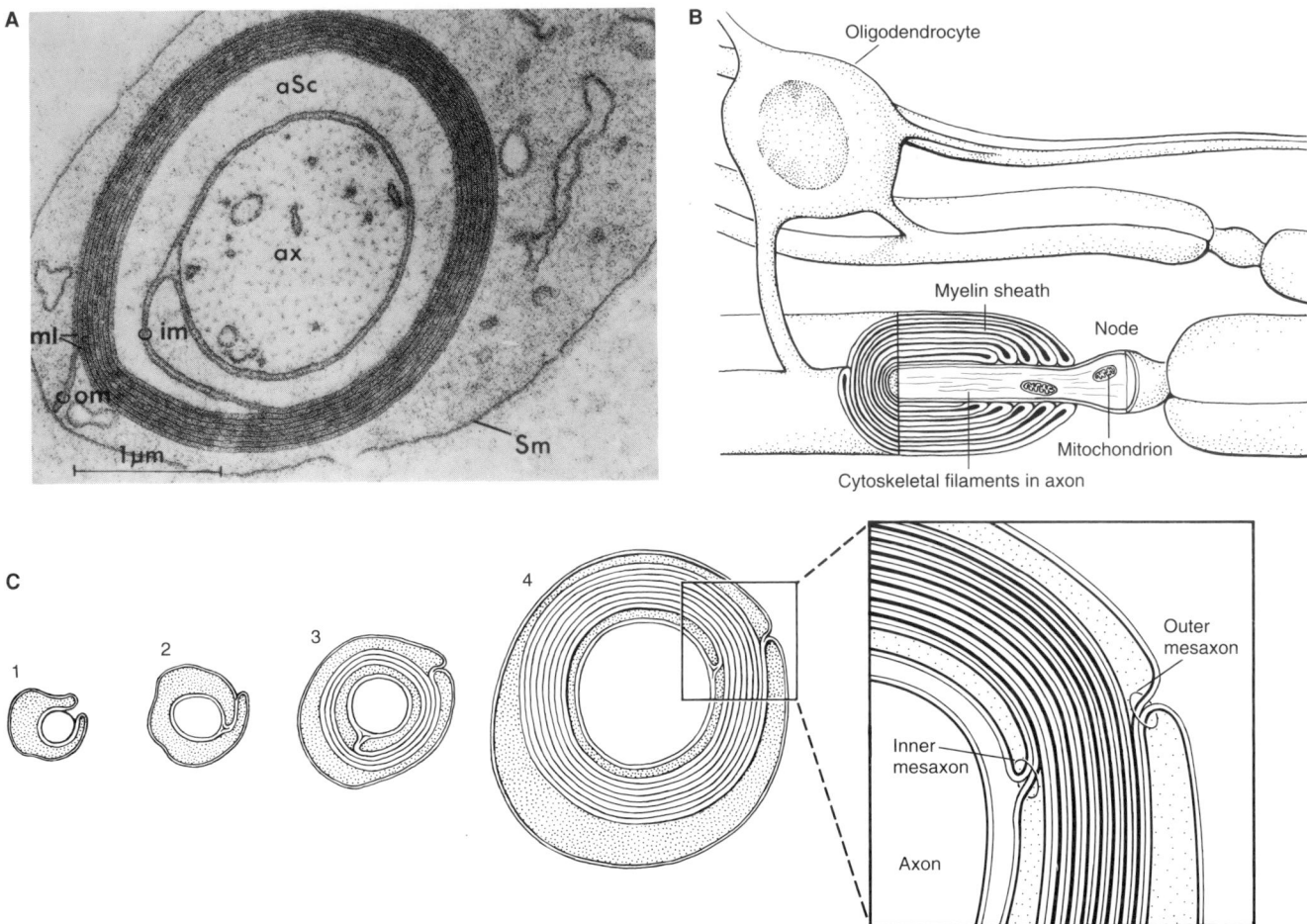

FIGURE 3–7
The axons of both motor and sensory neurons are insulated by a myelin sheath.

A. An electron micrograph of a transverse section through an axon (**ax**) in the sciatic nerve of a mouse. The spiraling lamellae of the myelin sheath (**ml**) start at the internal mesaxon (**im**). The spiraling sheath is still developing and is seen arising from the surface membrane (**Sm**) of the Schwann cell, which is continuous with the outer mesaxon (**om**). In this micrograph the Schwann cell cytoplasm is still present close to the axon (**aSc**).

Eventually the Schwann cell cytoplasm is withdrawn and the sheath becomes compact. (From Dyck et al., 1984.)

B. The processes of an oligodendrocyte are shown forming a myelin sheath around an axon in the central nervous system. (Adapted from Bunge, 1968.)

C. The development and organization of the myelin sheath of a peripheral nerve fiber are shown in this diagram. During formation of the sheath myelin formed by the Schwann cell progressively surrounds the axon. (From Williams et al., 1989.)

molecules that appear to be somewhat similar. Operationally, proteolipids differ from lipoproteins because they are insoluble in water. Through modern structural studies, it is now clear that proteolipids are soluble only in organic solvents because they contain long chains of fatty acids that are covalently bound to amino acid residues throughout the proteolipid molecule. Covalent addition of the lipid chains is a post-translational modification that occurs during processing of certain membrane proteins in the endoplasmic reticulum and Golgi apparatus (described in the next chapter). In contrast, lipoproteins are noncovalent complexes of proteins with lipids so structured that many serve as soluble carriers of the lipid moiety in the blood.

Both central and peripheral myelin contain the same group of proteins, originally called *myelin basic protein*. Although once thought to be a single molecule, this group has been shown by gene cloning to consist of at least seven related proteins with molecular weights from 14,100 to 21,400 that are produced from a single gene by alternative splicing. These proteins are highly antigenic. When injected into animals, myelin basic proteins produce a cellular autoimmune response called *experimental allergic encephalomyelitis*, characterized by focal inflammation and demyelination in the central nervous system. This experimental disease has been used by some investigators as a model for *multiple sclerosis*, a relatively common human disease. Multiple sclerosis manifests itself primarily as impaired sensory or motor performance because the demyelination of axons interferes with impulse conduction and therefore with sensory perception and proper motor coordination (see Chapter 35).

Another disease affecting myelination is found in mice with the shiverer (or shi) mutation, which experience coarse tremors and frequent convulsions and die young. This recessive mutation results from deletion of five of the six exons of the gene for myelin basic proteins on chromosome 18. In mice that are homozygous for the shiverer mutation (shi/shi), myelination is greatly deficient and abnormal in the central nervous system (less than 10% of the myelin basic proteins found in normal mice is present in shiverer mice). Carol Readhead and her collaborators have shown definitively that expression of the myelin basic protein gene in shiverer mice is impaired. When the wild-type gene is injected into fertilized eggs of the shiverer mutant, the resulting transgenic mice express the wild-type gene at the right time during development (during the first month after birth) and produce about 20% of the normal amounts of myelin basic proteins and their alternatively spliced messenger RNAs. Examination by electron microscopy reveals much improvement in the myelination of central neurons in the transgenic mice. Thus, these experiments are early examples of successful gene therapy. As shown in Figure 3–8, the introduction of the wild-type gene partially restores these animals to health: Although they still have occasional tremors, they do not convulse and have a normal life span.

A Major Function of the Neuron's Cell Body Is the Synthesis of Macromolecules

One of the important differences between sensory and motor neurons is the role played by the motor neuron's cell body in the transmission of synaptic signals. Under normal circumstances, an action potential in the peripheral branch of the sensory neuron axon is transmitted directly to the central branch, although it can be detected in the cell body by a recording microelectrode. The invasion of the action potential into the cell body can be slowed or completely blocked if the cell body is hyperpolarized, but this blockade in no way affects the passage of the signal along the axons. What, then, is the function of the sensory neuron's cell body? The answer to this question was suggested by a critical series of experiments dating from the mid-nineteenth century in which the English physiologist Augustus Waller cut the various roots and nerves of the spinal cord and studied the distribution of fibers that degenerated as a result. From the patterns of degeneration, Waller concluded that the dorsal root ganglion cell body maintains the vitality of the axon and dendrites attached to it. In a lecture delivered to the Royal Institution of Great Britain in 1861, he said, "A nerve-cell would be to its effluent nerve fibers what a fountain is to the rivulet which trickles from it—*a centre of nutritive energy*." For the most part this nourishment is provided in the form of proteins.

A Shiverer

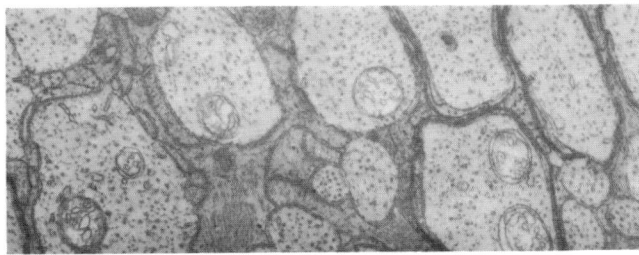

B Normal

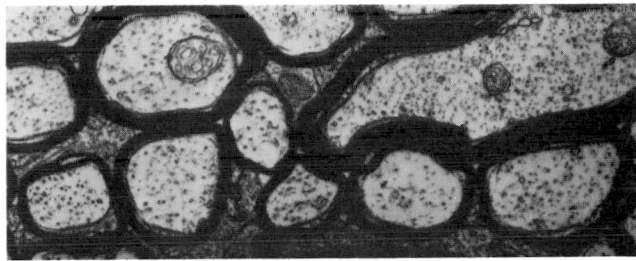

C Transfected

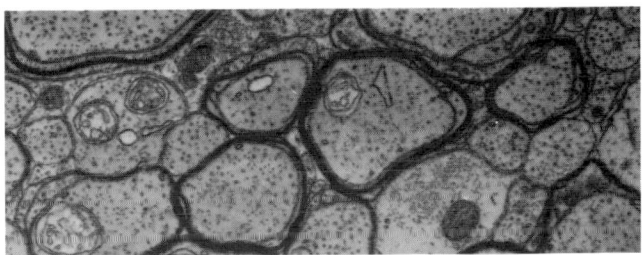

D

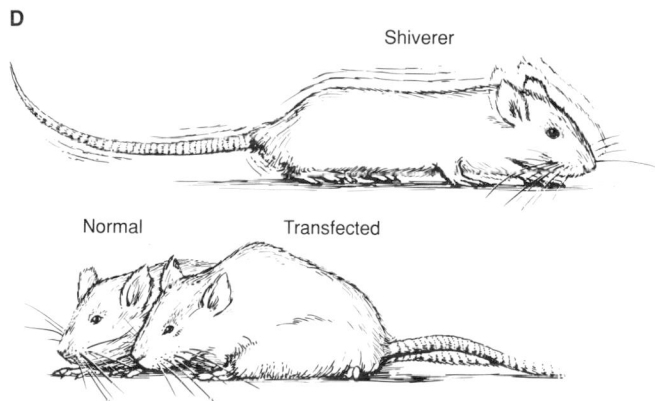

FIGURE 3–8

A genetic disorder of myelination in mice (*shiverer* mutant) can be partially cured by transfection of the normal gene encoding myelin basic protein. (From Readhead et al., 1987.)

Electron micrographs show the state of myelination in the optic nerve of the shiverer mutant (**A**), a normal mouse (**B**), and a shiverer mutant transfected with the gene for myelin basic protein (**C**). Myelination is incomplete in the shiverer mutant and greatly improved in the transfected animal.

D. The shiverer mutant exhibits poor posture and evident weakness. A normal mouse and a transfected shiverer mutant look perky.

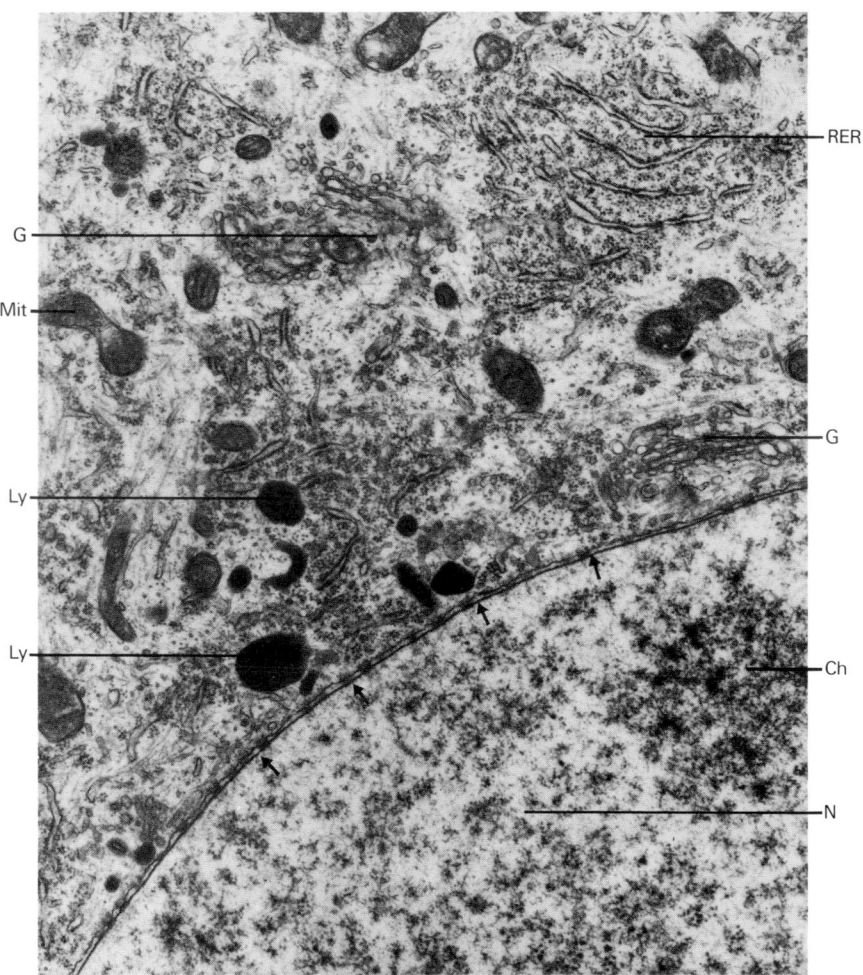

FIGURE 3–9

Some of the components of a spinal motor neuron that participate in the synthesis of macromolecules. The nucleus **(N)**, containing masses of chromatin **(Ch)**, is bounded by a double-layered membrane, the nuclear envelope, which contains many nuclear pores **(arrows)**. The mRNA leaves the nucleus through these pores and attaches to polyribosomes that either remain free in the cytoplasm or attach to the membranes of the endoplasmic reticulum to form the granular or rough endoplasmic reticulum **(RER)**. Several parts of the Golgi apparatus **(G)** are seen. Also present in the cytoplasm are lysosomes **(Ly)** and mitochondria **(Mit)**. (From Peters, Palay, and Webster, 1991.)

From modern cell biology we now know that information for the synthesis of proteins is encoded in the DNA of the chromosomes within the cell's nucleus (Figure 3–9). In all cell types there are two important ways in which this information can be processed: (1) the genetic information is passed from parent to daughter cell during cell division (heredity), and (2) a selected portion of the genetic information is *transcribed* into RNA and *translated* into proteins (gene expression). In most mature nerve cells, and in the two cells that we have been discussing in this chapter, cell division is no longer possible. A cell in this state is said to be terminally differentiated—the chromosomes function only in gene expression.

Because mature neurons cannot divide, the chromosomes are not arranged in compact structures, but exist in a relatively uncoiled state. Thus, the neuronal nucleus, even when viewed in the electron microscope, has a rather amorphous appearance, except for a prominent spherical body called the *nucleolus* (Figure 3–3B and D). The nucleolus contains the specific portion of DNA encoding the RNA (rRNA) of future *ribosomes*. During development, this part of the genetic material is reduplicated many times and is especially prominent in secretory cells, like neurons, that make large quantities of proteins. The nucleolus appears as a distinct structure because it contains many repetitive sequences of DNA and RNA that cohere in a more compact organization than do the components of the rest of the chromosomes.

In addition to the ribosomal genes of the nucleus, many other genes are also actively transcribed into the nuclear precursors of mRNA. These are then selectively processed or spliced to form mature mRNA. The mRNA is transported across the double-layered nuclear envelope through pores 65 nm in width arranged in rows with a center-to-center spacing of about 150 nm (Figure 3–9). Because the pores in adjacent rows are staggered, the pattern of pores appears as a roughly hexagonal array in tangential views of the nuclear membrane. The two leaflets of the nuclear envelope are continuous only at the margin of the pores. The outer leaflet of the nuclear envelope is continuous with the highly folded membrane of the endoplasmic reticulum, an extensive system of sheets, sacs, and tubules that extends throughout the cytoplasm around the nucleus.

Although most of the genetic information for the synthesis of proteins is encoded in the cell's nucleus, a small amount is contained in circular DNA molecules within mitochondria (Figure 3–9). It is in these organelles, each of which is about the size of a bacterial cell, that the energy generated by the metabolism of sugars and fats is transformed into ATP by oxidative phosphorylation. The sequence of the 16,569 nucleotides in the human mitochondrial genome has been determined; it encodes information for mitochondrial transfer RNAs (tRNAs) and rRNAs (which differ from those in the rest of the cell), and for a small number of the mitochondrion's proteins (cytochrome oxidase, cytochrome b, a subunit of ATP synthetase, subunits of NADH-coenzyme Q reductase, and an ATPase). The rest of the mitochondrion's proteins are encoded by genes in nuclear chromosomes, synthesized on cytoplasmic ribosomes, and then taken up into the mitochondrion, as discussed in the next chapter.

An Overall View

As in all other cells, in neurons the genetic information for encoding proteins and the complex apparatus for synthesizing them are contained in the cell's DNA. In common with other cells, neurons have mitochondria and enzymes both for biosynthesis of small molecules and for intermediary metabolism—the major pathways that convert carbohydrates and other substances into usable energy. Since nerve cells are excitable, they share some membrane constituents with cells in other excitable tissues, but many components are highly specialized and are restricted to specific classes of nerve cells. Thus, only certain neurons contain one or another transmitter substance, special ion channels, membrane transport mechanisms, or receptors for neurotransmitters. Our understanding of neural function ultimately depends on identifying and characterizing these molecules, both general and neuron specific. In the next chapter we shall examine how proteins are synthesized and processed in nerve cells.

Selected Readings

Baldissera, F., Hultborn, H., and Illert, M. 1981. Integration in spinal neuronal systems. In V. B. Brooks (ed.), Handbook of Physiology, Section 1: The Nervous System, Vol. II. Motor Control, Part 1. Bethesda, Md.: American Physiological Society, pp. 509–595.

Burke, R. E. 1990. Spinal cord: Ventral horn. In G. M. Shepherd (ed.), The Synaptic Organization of the Brain, 3rd ed. New York: Oxford University Press, pp. 88–132.

Jones, E. G. 1988. The nervous tissue. In L. Weiss (ed.), Cell and Tissue Biology: A Textbook of Histology, 6th ed. Baltimore: Urban & Schwarzenberg, pp. 277–351.

Peters, A., Palay, S. L., and Webster, H. deF. 1991. The Fine Structure of the Nervous System: Neurons and Their Supporting Cells, 3rd ed. New York: Oxford University Press.

Siegel, G. J., Agranoff, B. W., Albers, R. W., and Molinoff, P. B. (eds.) 1989. Basic Neurochemistry: Molecular, Cellular, and Medical Aspects, 4th ed. New York: Raven Press.

Williams, P. L., Warwick, R., Dyson, M., and Bannister, L. H. (eds.) 1989. Gray's Anatomy, 37th ed. Edinburgh: Churchill Livingstone, pp. 859–919.

References

Albers, R. W., Siegel, G. J., and Stahl, W. L. 1989. Membrane transport. In G. J. Siegel, B. W. Agranoff, R. W. Albers, and P. B. Molinoff (eds.), Basic Neurochemistry: Molecular, Cellular, and Medical Aspects, 4th ed. New York: Raven Press, pp. 49–70.

Attardi, G., and Schatz, G. 1988. Biogenesis of mitochondria. Annu. Rev. Cell Biol. 4:289–333.

Boyd, I. A., and Smith, R. S. 1984. The muscle spindle. In P. J. Dyck, P. K. Thomas, E. H. Lambert, and R. Bunge (eds.), Peripheral Neuropathy, 2nd ed., Vol. I. Philadelphia: Saunders, pp. 171–202.

Brown, A. G., and Fyffe, R. E. W. 1981. Direct observations on the contacts made between Ia afferent fibres and α-motoneurones in the cat's lumbosacral spinal cord. J. Physiol. (Lond.) 313: 121–140.

Brown, A. G., and Fyffe, R. E. W. 1984. Intracellular Staining of Mammalian Neurones. London: Academic Press.

Bunge, R. P. 1968. Glial cells and the central myelin sheath. Physiol. Rev. 48:197–251.

Burke, R. E. 1981. Motor units: Anatomy, physiology, and functional organization. In V. B. Brooks (ed.), Handbook of Physiology, Section 1: The Nervous System, Vol. II. Motor Control, Part 1. Bethesda, Md.: American Physiological Society, pp. 345–422.

Burke, R. E., Dum, R. P., Fleshman, J. W., Glenn, L. L., Lev-Tov, A., O'Donovan, M. J., and Pinter, M. J. 1982. An HRP study of the relation between cell size and motor unit type in cat ankle extensor motoneurons. J. Comp. Neurol. 209:17–28.

Conradi, S. 1969. Ultrastructure and distribution of neuronal and glial elements on the motoneuron surface in the lumbosacral spinal cord of the adult cat. Acta Physiol. Scand. [Suppl.] 332: 5–48.

Davidoff, R. A. (ed.) 1983. Handbook of the Spinal Cord (ed.), Vol. 1: Pharmacology. New York: Marcel Dekker.

Dogiel, A. S. 1908. Der Bau der Spinalganglien des Menschen und der Säugetiere. Jena: Fischer.

Dyck, P. J., Thomas, P. K., Lambert, E. H., and Bunge, R. (eds.) 1984. Peripheral Neuropathy, 2nd ed., 2 vols. Philadelphia: Saunders.

Folch, J., Ascoli, I., Lees, M., Meath, J. A., and Le Baron, F. N. 1951. Preparation of lipide extracts from brain tissue. J. Biol. Chem. 191:833–841.

Lemke, G. 1988. Unwrapping the genes of myelin. Neuron 1:535–543.

Mikoshiba, K., Okano, H., Tamura, T., and Ikenaka, K. 1991. Structure and function of myelin protein genes. Annu. Rev. Neurosci. 14:201–217.

Ochs, S. 1975. Waller's concept of the trophic dependence of the nerve fiber on the cell body in the light of early neuron theory. Clio Med. 10:253–265.

Ramón y Cajal, S. 1909. Histologie du Système Nerveux de l'Homme & des Vertébrés, Vol. 1. L. Azoulay (trans.). Paris: Maloine. Republished in 1952. Madrid: Instituto Ramón y Cajal.

Readhead, C., Popko, B,. Takahashi, N., Shine, H. D., Saavedra, R. A., Sidman, R. L., and Hood, L. 1987. Expression of a myelin basic protein gene in transgenic Shiverer mice: Correction of the dysmyelinating phenotype. Cell 48:703–712.

Schmitt, F. O., Worden, F. G., Adelman, G., and Dennis, S. G. (eds.) 1981. The Organization of the Cerebral Cortex: Proceedings of a Neurosciences Research Program Colloquium. Cambridge, Mass.: MIT Press.

Thomas, P. K., and Ochoa, J. 1984. Microscopic anatomy of peripheral nerve fibers. In P. J. Dyck, P. K. Thomas, E. H. Lambert, and R. Bunge (eds.), Peripheral Neuropathy, 2nd ed., Vol. I. Philadelphia: Saunders, pp. 39–96.

Ulfhake, B., and Kellerth, J.-O. 1981. A quantitative light microscopic study of the dendrites of cat spinal α-motoneurons after intracellular staining with horseradish peroxidase. J. Comp. Neurol. 202:571–583.

4

James H. Schwartz

Synthesis and Trafficking of Neuronal Proteins

Messenger RNA Gives Rise to Three Classes of Proteins

Cytosolic Proteins

Nuclear, Mitochondrial, and Peroxisomal Proteins

Cell Membrane Proteins and Secretory Proteins

Fate of Major Membrane Proteins

Axonal Transport Controls the Distribution of Membranes and Secretory Proteins in the Neuron

Fast Anterograde Transport

Slow Axonal Transport

Fast Retrograde Transport

Fibrillar Proteins of the Cytoskeleton Are Responsible for the Shape of Neurons

The Dynamics of Polymerization

An Overall View

T he brain expresses more of the total genetic information encoded in DNA than does any other organ in the body. About 200,000 distinct mRNA sequences are thought to be expressed, 10–20 times more than in the kidney or liver. In part, this diversity results from the greater number and variety of cell types in the brain as compared to cells in the more homogeneous body tissues. But many neurobiologists also believe that each of the brain's 10^{11} nerve cells actually expresses a greater amount of its genetic information than does a liver or kidney cell. What sort of proteins are encoded by these mRNAs, and where are they synthesized?

Messenger RNA Gives Rise to Three Classes of Proteins

Before describing the types of proteins made in neurons, it is first necessary to discuss briefly the three distinct membrane systems within a cell. The most extensive is the *major membrane system of the cell*. This system extends from the nucleus to the plasma (external) membrane. It consists of the nuclear membrane, which is continuous with the endoplasmic reticulum, the membranes of the Golgi apparatus, the secretory granules, the lysosomes, the endosomes, and the plasma membrane surrounding the neuron (Figures 4–1 and 4–2). The inside (luminal) surfaces of all the membrane-bound organelles of the cell can be considered topologically to be continuous with the extracellular space (as explained in Figure 4–1). The two other distinct and independent membrane systems are the *mitochondria* and *peroxisomes*, organelles chiefly dedicated to the use of molecular oxygen. These two organelles differ from the subcellular components that make up the major membrane system. They are thought to have developed from symbiotic organisms that invaded the eukaryotic cell very early in evolution.

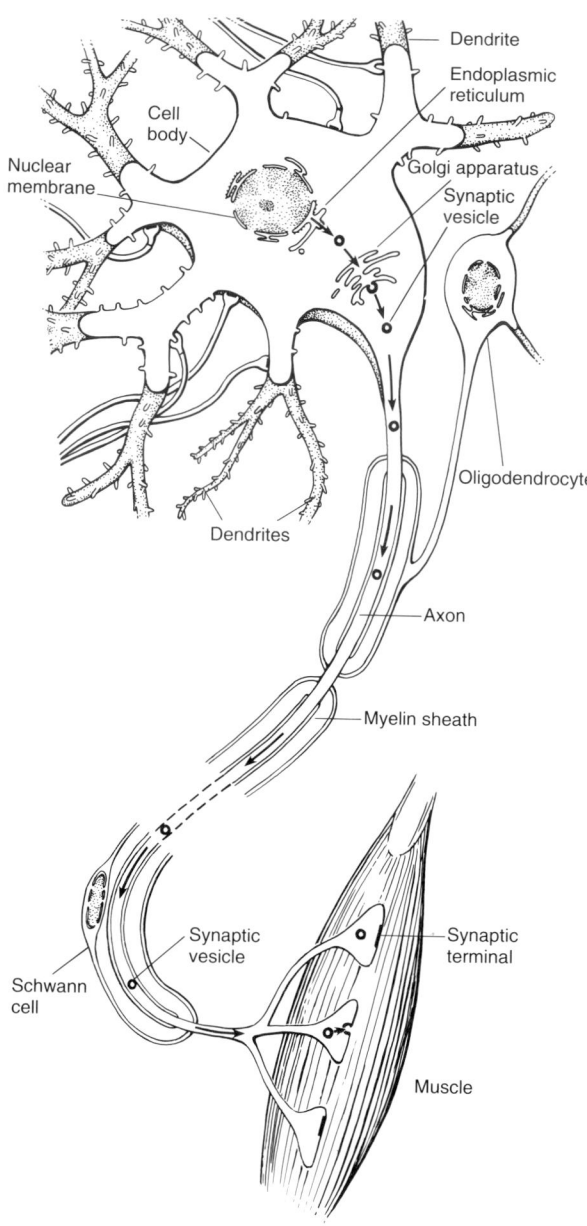

All three membrane systems constitute separate compartments within the neuron, are made up of different proteins, and serve separate functions within the cell. They are all embedded in the cytosol, which, far from being a homogeneous solution, actually is a gel within a matrix formed from a variety of filaments and associated proteins that make up the *cytoskeleton*.

With the exception of the few proteins encoded by the mitochondrial genome enumerated in Chapter 3, essentially all of the macromolecules of a neuron are made in the cell body from mRNAs that are transcribed and spliced in the nucleus. Like other cells, each nerve cell makes only three classes of proteins:

1. Proteins that are synthesized in the cytosol and remain there.
2. Proteins that are synthesized in the cytosol but are later incorporated into the nucleus, mitochondria, or peroxisomes.
3. Proteins that are synthesized in association with the cell membrane system. These include at least three categories of protein molecules.
   a. Proteins that remain attached to the membranes of the endoplasmic reticulum, Golgi apparatus, and the vesicles that later bud off from the Golgi apparatus. These are of three types: *membrane-spanning, anchored,* and *associated.*[1] Some proteins are loosely associated with the membrane through weak protein–protein or protein–lipid interactions. Others are anchored by covalent bonds to membrane constituents. Both anchored and associated proteins typically are easier to extract than membrane-spanning proteins, because they do not traverse the lipid bilayer.
   b. The second category includes proteins that remain within the lumen of the endoplasmic reticulum or Golgi sacs but are not attached to the membrane.
   c. The third category includes proteins that are synthesized in association with the cell's membrane system and are later distributed by means of a variety of vesicles that bud off from the *trans* face of the Golgi apparatus (to be described later in this chapter) for distribution to other organelles, for example, lysosomes and secretory vesicles. We shall be interested especially in the proteins of this category that are destined to become secretory products.

The mRNAs that encode the proteins of the first two classes (cytosolic proteins and the proteins destined to be imported into the nucleus, mitochondria, or peroxisomes)

FIGURE 4–1

The topological continuity of the cell's major membrane system. The space between the two membranes that constitute the nuclear envelope is continuous with the extracellular space. The figure shows the cell body of a spinal neuron containing the nucleus surrounded by the nuclear envelope, which is continuous with the rough and smooth endoplasmic reticulum. Vesicles, which bud off the endoplasmic reticulum, shuttle to the *cis* face of the Golgi apparatus. These vesicles maintain the topological relationship between the inside of the cell (the cytosol) and the space within the membrane system. Various kinds of vesicles bud off the *trans* face of the Golgi apparatus. In this diagram a precursor of a synaptic vesicle is shown making its way down the axon by fast axonal transport. At the nerve ending the synaptic vesicle fuses with the external (synaptic) membrane to release acetylcholine. During this exocytotic process the inside of the vesicle's membrane faces the extracellular space. (From Williams et al., 1989.)

---

[1]Membrane-spanning proteins are also called *integral,* a term that was first introduced as an experimental definition for molecules that cannot be extracted from membranes by dilute aqueous salt solutions buffered at a mildly alkaline pH (7–8), but rather require strong *chaotropic* conditions that disrupt the lipid bilayer (for example, detergents, extremely alkaline pH, or high concentrations of certain salts). More recent usage reserves the term for a protein molecule whose polypeptide chain traverses the lipid bilayer at least once. All other proteins associated with membrane were called *peripheral.* Many proteins are now known to be linked covalently (anchored) to membrane constituents (as is discussed later in this chapter) and are frequently also called integral proteins.

are translated on free polyribosomes (polysomes). The mRNAs that encode the third class (proteins incorporated into the major membrane system of the cell) form polysomes that become attached to the flattened sheets of the endoplasmic reticulum (Figure 4–2). What determines the class to which a particular protein will belong? In addition to encoding the primary sequence of the finished protein, the mRNAs contain information that, when translated into polypeptide sequences, targets the new protein to its final destination.

As in other cells, most of the protein formed in neurons is cytosolic. Nevertheless, secretory products constitute a substantial proportion of the macromolecules synthesized. Moreover, although most of the macromolecules made by nerve cells do not appear to differ from those made by other cells, some cytosolic, cell membrane, and secretory proteins are specific to groups of neurons and even to single cells. We shall consider each of the three classes of proteins in turn.

Cytosolic Proteins

Cytosolic proteins comprise the two most abundant groups of proteins in the cell: (1) the *fibrillar elements* that make up the cytoskeleton (neurofilaments, tubulins, and actins and their associated proteins, which together account for at least 25% of the total protein in the neuron), and (2) the numerous *enzymes* that catalyze the various metabolic reactions of the cell. Some of these enzymes are characteristic of specific types of neurons. For example, in the spinal motor neurons that we considered in Chapters 2 and 3, choline acetyltransferase catalyzes the synthesis of acetylcholine. After they are synthesized in the cell body, both the soluble components of the cytoplasm and fibrillar elements of the cytoskeleton move into the dendrites and axons of the neuron by slow transport, which will be discussed later in this chapter.

Messenger RNA molecules for cytosolic proteins emerge through the nuclear pores and become associated with ribosomes to form free polysomes in the neuron's cytoplasm (Figure 4–2). Proteins are polypeptides or polymers of amino acids. One end has a free amino (N-terminal) group and the other a carboxyl (C-terminal). Translation of the peptide chain begins at the N-terminal end.

Cytosolic polypeptides are little modified or processed, in contrast to the proteins made in association with the endoplasmic reticulum and Golgi apparatus. Modifications that are important can be classified as *cotranslational*, occurring while the polypeptide chain is being synthesized, or *posttranslational*, occurring after the chain is completed. The most important cotranslational modification is *N*-acetylation, the transfer of an acyl group to the N-terminus of the growing polypeptide chain.

$$\overset{O}{\underset{}{R-\overset{\|}{C}-CoA}} + H_2N\sim \rightarrow R-\overset{\overset{O}{\|}}{C}-\overset{H}{N}\sim + CoA$$

The acyl group is activated by being coupled to CoA, the universal metabolic intermediate for transferring acyl

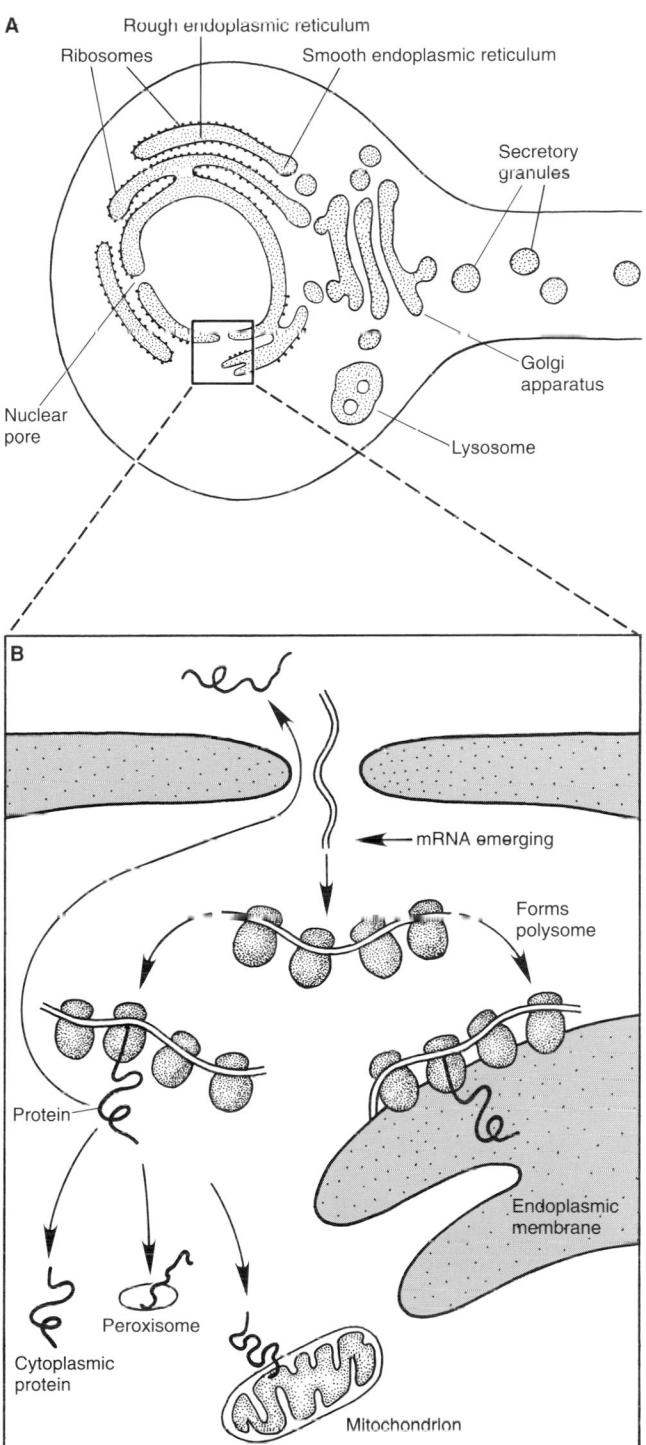

FIGURE 4–2

A. The organelles responsible for the synthesis and processing of proteins.

B. Enlargement of **A** in the region of a nuclear pore. Messenger RNAs, transcribed from genomic DNA in the neuron's nucleus, emerge through nuclear pores to form polysomes by attaching to ribosomes. Three classes of proteins are formed. The class of protein formed depends on the fate of the particular polysome and this, in turn, is determined by information encoded in the particular mRNA.

groups. One of the most common acyl groups is the acetyl group.

$$CH_3-\overset{\overset{\displaystyle O}{\|}}{C}-$$

Another is a myristoyl group, a 14-carbon saturated fatty acid (designated 14:0, i.e., 14 carbons, no double bonds). In proteins that are *N*-acetylated the initiator methionine is removed and the next residue becomes the new N-terminus of the growing chain. While the chain elongates, an acyl group is enzymatically transferred to the new N-terminus of the protein. *N*-myristoylated proteins include the α subunit of the GTP-binding protein (G_s) that stimulates adenylyl cyclase, the catalytic subunit of the cAMP-dependent protein kinase, and calcineurin, a major Ca^{2+}-dependent protein phosphatase. The fatty acid moiety may help to locate the protein within the cell; in some instances these modified proteins become loosely associated with the inner leaflet of the plasma membrane or with the cytoplasmic surface of organelles. The presence of an N-terminal acyl group is not sufficient for this type of association, however.

Addition of other functional groups to specific amino acid residues occurs posttranslationally. Probably the most important example of this kind of modification is the phosphorylation of serine, threonine, or tyrosine residues by special protein kinases that are discussed in Chapter 12. Phosphorylation, which is reversible, can change the activity of a protein and is probably the most common mechanism for altering the biochemical function of proteins in all cells. Another important posttranslational modification is the addition of *ubiquitin*, a highly conserved protein with 76 amino acid residues, to the ε amino group of lysine residues throughout the protein molecule. This isopeptide linkage of ubiquitin occurs in three enzymatic steps, and each ubiquitin molecule linked consumes the energy of ATP. Addition of ubiquitin is a mechanism for tagging proteins for degradation by special proteases, one of the most important ways cells turn over their proteins.

Nuclear, Mitochondrial, and Peroxisomal Proteins

Nuclear and peroxisomal proteins, as well as the mitochondrial proteins that are encoded by the cell's nucleus, are also formed on free polysomes. Soon after synthesis they are targeted to their proper organelle by a mechanism called *posttranslational importation*. Specific receptors around nuclear pores bind and translocate these recently synthesized polypeptide chains. The nuclear receptors recognize structural features of the polypeptides that permit transport from the cytoplasm into the nucleus through nuclear pores. Similar membrane receptors insert or translocate the proteins into mitochondria, and probably into peroxisomes.

The distribution of these and other proteins to the various membrane compartments of the cell depends on the presence of certain sequences of amino acids, often situated at the N-terminal end of the protein (*presequences*),

but also located within the polypeptide chain. Regardless of the location of the amino acid sequence, the information that specifies the protein's final destination is not contained in consensus sequences of specific amino acid residues; rather, these sequences endow the polypeptide with a common secondary (conformational) structure that targets the protein. Thus, the presequences marking a protein for mitochondria differ in conformation from target sequences directing a protein to the endoplasmic reticulum and hence to the cell's major membrane system.

Nuclear uptake of proteins depends on sequences rich in basic amino acid residues. These sequences are not removed from the mature protein. In addition to basic amino acid residues, mitochondrial presequences contain hydroxylated amino acids as well as long stretches of hydrophobic residues. In contrast to the targeting sequences of nuclear proteins, the presequences of most of the proteins destined for mitochondria are cleaved off after importation. Experiments with genetically engineered chimeric polypeptides containing mitochondrial presequences joined to proteins not normally found in mitochondria have shown that the presequence is both necessary and sufficient for targeting proteins to mitochondria. The specific type of presequence also determines whether a portion of the protein remains within the inner mitochondrial membrane (as a membrane-spanning protein) or is completely translocated through the membrane into the *matrix* (interior) of the mitochondrion.

Although nuclear, mitochondrial, and peroxisomal proteins represent only a small fraction of the total protein produced by the neuron, they illustrate an important feature of cell biology. This group of proteins reaches its destination in the cell *after* synthesis has been completed on free ribosomes. In contrast, most membrane and secretory proteins reach their destination by cotranslational transfer, which is discussed next.

Cell Membrane Proteins and Secretory Proteins

Messenger RNAs encoding proteins destined to become secretory products or constituents of the organelles of the cell's major membrane systems are formed on polysomes that attach to the endoplasmic reticulum (Figure 4–2). These sheets of membrane, when studded with ribosomes, have a granular appearance in the electron microscope and are therefore called *rough endoplasmic reticulum*. Rough endoplasmic reticulum is usually most dense in the region nearest the nucleus but is differently distributed in different neurons (Figure 4–3). For example, in motor neurons it is densely distributed around the nucleus in highly ordered parallel arrays (Figure 4–3A), but is also found in primary dendrites, especially where the dendrites emerge from the cell body. In contrast, in sensory cells of the dorsal root ganglion the rough endoplasmic reticulum has a more disorderly appearance (Figure 4–3B).

Ribosomal RNA in the rough endoplasmic reticulum stains intensely with basic histological dyes (toluidine blue, cresyl violet, and methylene blue). Under the light microscope this basophilic material is called *Nissl sub-*

A Motor neuron

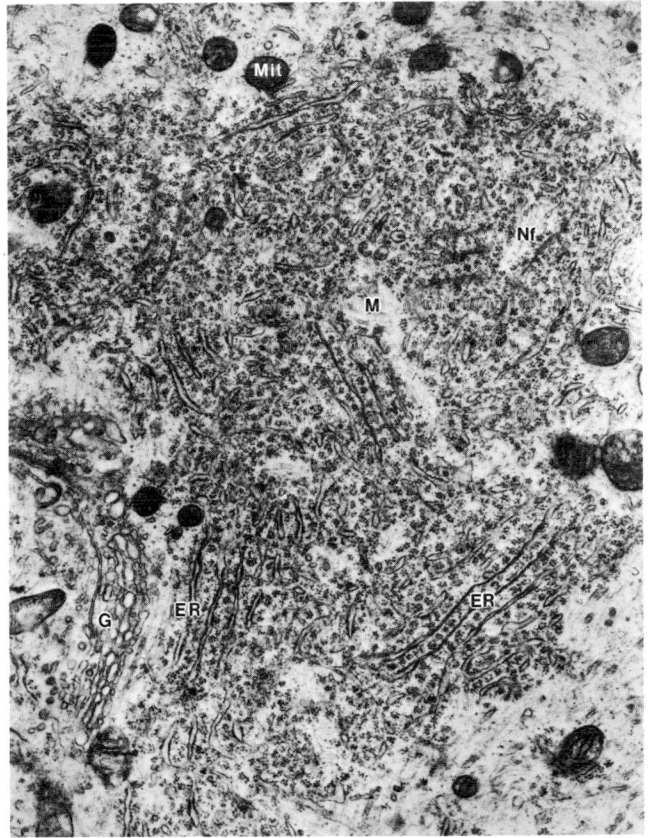

B Dorsal root ganglion cell

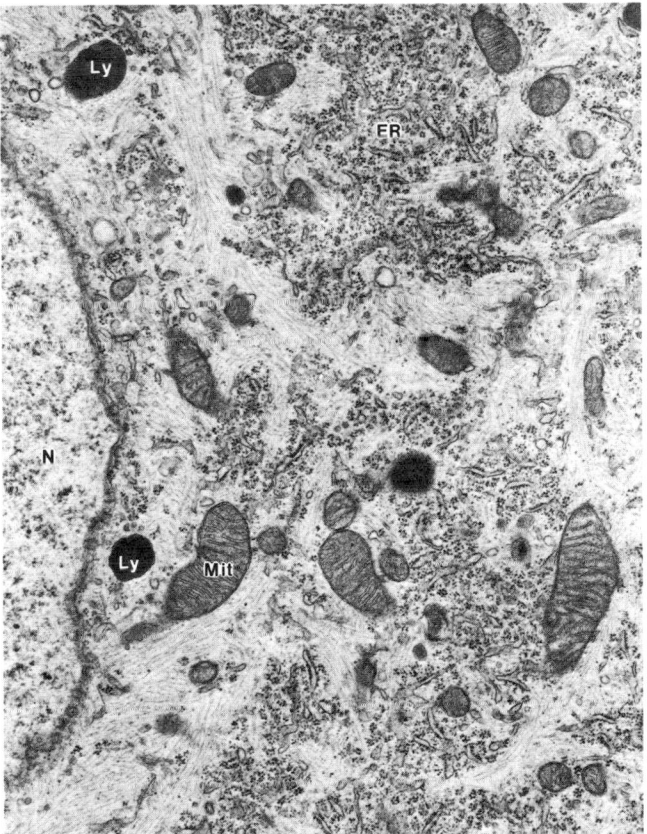

FIGURE 4–3

These electron micrographs show the organelles in the cell body that are chiefly responsible for synthesis and processing of proteins. Through the double-layered nuclear envelope that surrounds the nucleus (**N**), mRNA enters the cytoplasm to form polyribosomes. Some of these polyribosomes elaborate proteins in the cytoplasm, some of which remain soluble and some of which are transported after they are synthesized into mitochondria (**Mit**). One major class of proteins is formed after the polysomes attach to the membrane of the endoplasmic reticulum

(**ER**). In the light microscope this is called Nissl substance. Both cells have similar kinds of organelles, but the particular region of the motor neuron shown in **A** also contains membranes of the Golgi apparatus (**G**), in which membrane and secretory proteins are further processed. Some of the newly synthesized proteins leave the Golgi in vesicles that move by rapid axonal transport down the axon to the synapses; other membrane proteins are incorporated into lysosomes (**Ly**). (From Peters, Palay, and Webster, 1991.)

stance after the Bavarian histologist who, in 1892, first described changes in the intensity and distribution of staining in neurons after their axons are cut. (These changes, which reflect alterations in the patterns of protein synthesis in injured and regenerating neurons, are discussed in Chapter 18.) A large portion of the endoplasmic reticulum lacks attached ribosomes and is therefore called *smooth endoplasmic reticulum*.

The polysomes that produce membrane and secretory proteins are formed from the same population of ribosomes as those that produce the other proteins in the cell. Polysomes for membrane and secretory proteins, however, attach themselves to the cytoplasmic face of the endoplasmic reticulum. An N-terminal portion of the nascent polypeptide typically acts as a *signal sequence*; as a rule, this sequence is cleaved off and does not remain in the mature protein. Signal sequences of proteins destined for

the cell's major membrane system differ in secondary structure from the presequences of proteins targeted to the nucleus, mitochondria, or peroxisomes. Signal sequences have several specific functions. One is to cause the polysome to bind to a small ribonucleoprotein body called the *signal receptor particle*, which arrests translation of the mRNA at the end of the signal peptide sequence. The complex then binds to a receptor, called the *docking protein*, on the cytoplasmic surface of the endoplasmic reticulum. Binding to this protein displaces the signal receptor particle from the polysome bearing the nascent polypeptide chain and translation begins again.

In an energy-dependent process, the growing peptide is transported through the lipid bilayer into the lumen of the endoplasmic reticulum, where the signal peptide usually is removed by proteolytic cleavage catalyzed by an enzyme, the *signal peptidase*. The polypeptide continues to

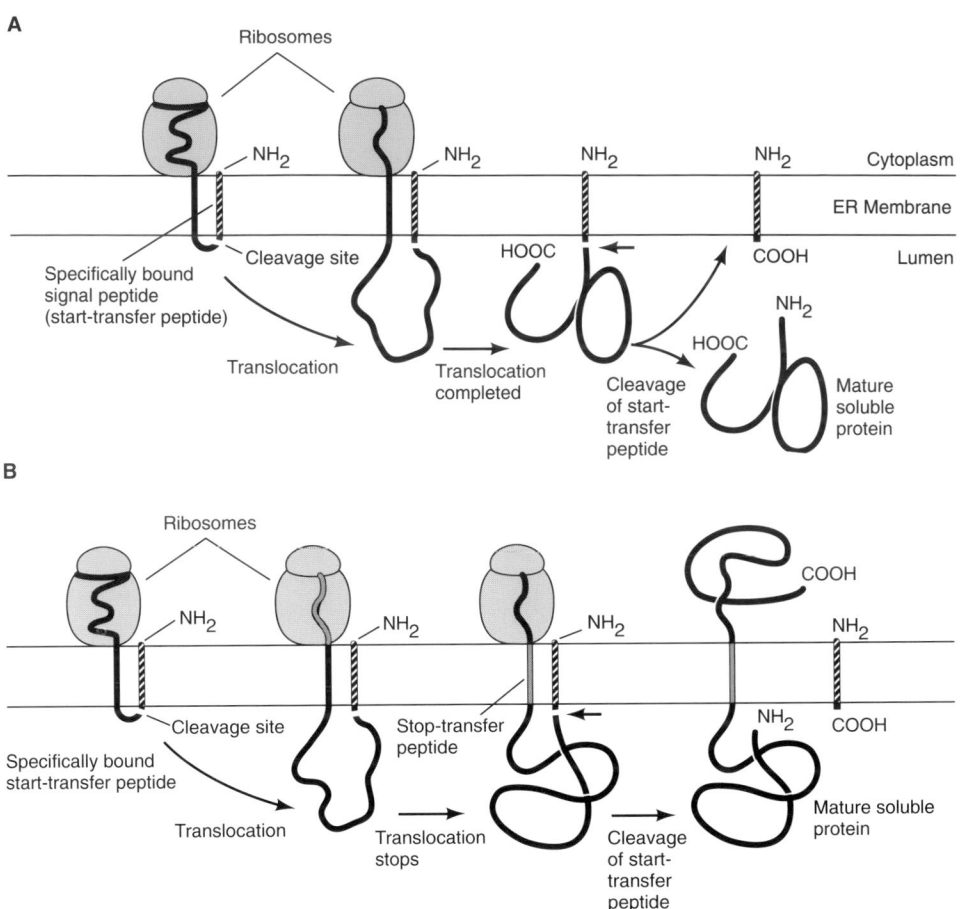

FIGURE 4-4

Examples of how proteins are formed in association with the endoplasmic reticulum. Several configurations of cell membrane proteins can be produced by variations of the cotranslational transfer process. All of these proteins start with an N-terminal signal sequence with three functionally distinct portions. The first is a short, hydrophilic segment that is important for the initiation of insertion, but which plays little or no part in the association of the polysome to the signal receptor particle or its release from the docking protein. This segment is not itself translocated through the membrane. The second segment is a stretch of 8–16 hydrophobic residues that is essential for translocation of the protein through the membrane. The mechanism of translocation is not yet well understood, but probably requires that some of this hydrophobic segment assume an α-helical structure and that part be extended, since a stretch of 8 hydrophobic residues, if fully extended, is sufficient to span the 3-nm width of the membrane, but would be too short in the helical configuration. The third segment, consisting of a few C-terminal amino acids of the signal sequence, usually begins with a glycine or proline (residues that interrupt α-helices), and is known to be important for removing the signal sequence by the *signal peptidase* located on the luminal side of the endoplasmic reticulum. (Adapted from Alberts, 1989.)

A. A secretory protein with both ends of the molecule free within the endoplasmic reticulum results if the entire polypeptide chain is translocated through the membrane of the endoplasmic reticulum. Note that the N-terminus is free because of the cleavage of the signal sequence, and the C-terminus, because the translocation of the rest of the polypeptide chain is complete.

B. A membrane-spanning protein results if the translocation of the polypeptide chain through the membrane is incomplete. Incomplete translocation occurs because of the presence of a stop-transfer sequence (shown in gray). As in the example shown in **A**, the N-terminal signal sequence is cleaved while the polypeptide chain is being synthesized. The C-terminal end of the completed protein remains on the cytoplasmic side of the endoplasmic reticulum.

grow in length at its C-terminal end. *Cotranslational transfer* through the membrane continues until a *halt* or *stop transfer* segment is reached within the nascent polypeptide chain. Stop transfer sequences are about 20 residues in length, contain hydrophobic or uncharged amino acids followed by several basic residues, and may occur anywhere along the polypeptide.

Transport of the nascent polypeptide through the membrane can result in four configurations of proteins: three integral membrane proteins and one secretory (Figure

4–4). The most common configuration occurs if transfer through the membrane stops before the message is fully translated; the result is an integral membrane protein with its C-terminus on the cytoplasmic side and its N-terminus on the luminal side of the endoplasmic reticulum. If the signal sequence is not cleaved and translocation continues, the result is an integral membrane protein with its N-terminus on the cytoplasmic side and its C-terminus within the lumen.

If there are alternating series of insertion and stop transfer sequences within a single chain, the result is an integral membrane protein with multiple membrane-spanning regions because the nascent polypeptide can then transverse the membrane several times. In these proteins, the original N-terminal signal sequence also serves to fix the protein in the membrane. Although the presence of multiple membrane-spanning domains governed by repeating insertion and stop transfer signals may seem complex, in many instances it is merely repetitive, since each segment with its pair of start and stop signals is similar in sequence. These repeating segments are thought to arise during evolution by reduplication of the same base sequences within an ancestral gene with subsequent divergence. Important examples of this type of intrinsic membrane protein are receptors for neurotransmitters that form ion channels through the plasma membrane, which are discussed in Chapters 5 and 10. Finally, if the C-terminus is completely transferred into the lumen of the endoplasmic reticulum after cleavage of the signal sequence, a secretory or lysosomal protein will result.

Transfer into the endoplasmic reticulum requires the energy of ATP and occurs at different rates for different constituents. To be transferred, proteins must have a suitable conformation, one that is different from their final secondary structure. Attainment of proper secondary structure in the endoplasmic reticulum is fostered by special protein factors now called *foldases* or *chaperonins*.

Fate of Major Membrane Proteins

Although the organelles that contribute to the major membrane system of the cell (nuclear membrane, endoplasmic reticulum, Golgi apparatus, plasma membrane, secretory granules, and endosomes) can be considered topologically a connected membrane system, they each have biochemically distinct membranes. These differences result from the fates of the proteins that we have been describing. Thus, some of the proteins remain in the endoplasmic reticulum, both as membrane-spanning proteins and as soluble luminal constituents, some are distributed to the other organelles of the system, and others are destined to be secreted. The mechanisms of sorting, modification, and distribution of these proteins are diverse and are just beginning to be understood. We shall describe only some of these mechanisms that are now known to be important to neuronal function. Our primary concern in this chapter will be mechanisms that operate in secretion.

Cell membrane and secretory proteins, unlike those made in the cytosol, are extensively modified after trans-lation. For example, secretory products typically are synthesized as part of larger precursor polypeptide chains, which undergo sequential and specific tailoring by the process of proteolytic cleavage. This process begins in the lumen of the endoplasmic reticulum, both rough and smooth, and continues in the Golgi apparatus. Indeed, modification can continue within finished organelles—secretory granules, endosomes, lysosomes, and the plasma membrane. Processing of neuropeptide transmitters is discussed in Chapter 14 in greater detail.

Production of smaller proteins from a larger polypeptide can have several physiological consequences. One consequence is its configuration. For example, as we have just discussed, the final orientation of the protein in the membrane depends on how the N-terminal signal sequence is removed. Another consequence is the masking of a potential activity that would be undesirable within the cell. Production of large proteins also permits amplification or diversification of secreted peptide products, a feature important for hormones and neuroactive peptides (see Chapter 14). For example, in the processing of opioid peptides more than one copy of the same peptide and several different peptides are cut from the same large precursor molecule. When this occurs, the polypeptide precursor is called a *polyprotein* because it contains more than one active peptide.

In addition to being processed by proteolytic cleavage, membrane proteins and secretory products are also glycosylated by the addition of oligosaccharide chains, or conjugated to *complex* (amino sugar-containing) *lipids*. Sugars are continuously being added through glycosidic linkage both with the ε amino group of asparagine residues (N-linked) and, less commonly, through hydroxyl groups of serine and threonine (O-linked). These polymers are trimmed enzymatically in a specific manner both in the endoplasmic reticulum and in the Golgi apparatus. Within the endoplasmic reticulum, just after the polypeptide has been synthesized, the C-terminal end of certain proteins is anchored to the membrane by the addition of a complex sugar. Several proteins known to be important to neuronal function—a form of acetylcholinesterase and the neuronal cell adhesion molecule, NCAM—are anchored in this manner, and it is certain that more will be discovered.

Anchoring through a complex sugar linkage occurs with a certain type of polypeptide just after it has been synthesized and transported through the membrane of the endoplasmic reticulum (in the way described above for secretory proteins). These proteins bear a *C-terminal recognition sequence* some 20–40 residues long. These signals, like the N-terminal signals already discussed, do not have a unique primary sequence of amino acids but rather share common conformational features. In the lumen of the endoplasmic reticulum, this sequence is cleaved off, exposing a new C-terminus (Figure 4–5). This free carboxyl group forms a peptide bond with phosphorylethanolamine, which in turn is anchored to the inner leaflet of the membrane through the diacylglycerol moiety of a complex inositol phospholipid. Conjugation occurs rapidly, presumably in one or two enzymatic steps.

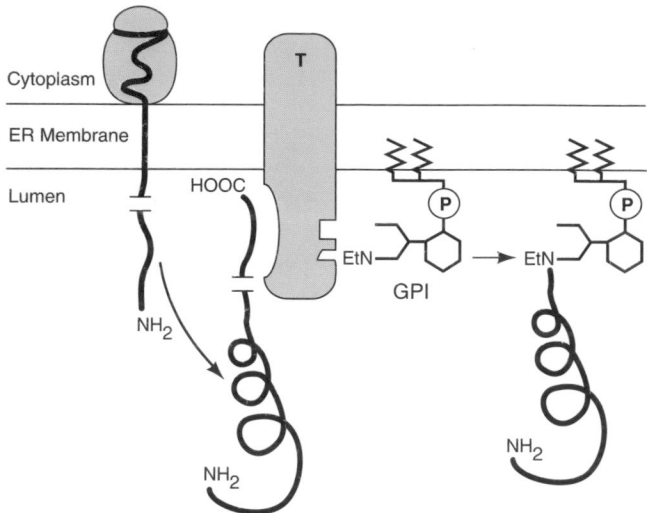

FIGURE 4–5

Hypothetical model for the anchoring of protein to membrane by a complex sugar linkage. The nascent polypeptide is translocated through the membrane of the rough endoplasmic reticulum (**ER**) as diagramed in Figure 4–4A. Soon after completion the polypeptide binds to an enzyme or complex of enzymes (**T**), which removes a short segment from the C-terminal end of the polypeptide and attaches the new C-terminus (**COOH**) to a phosphatidyl inositol glycan (**GPI**) anchor through a peptide linkage with the amine group of ethanolamine (**EtN**) in the glycan moiety. (From Ferguson and Williams, 1988.)

Conjugation through a phosphoinositol linkage is undoubtedly of functional importance, not only because it is still another way of attaching proteins to the membrane, but also because proteins so anchored to the *inner* leaflet of the cell's membrane system ultimately will become linked to the *outer* leaflet of the plasma membrane. Thus, this type of linkage is particularly well suited for proteins that will function in adhesion. Furthermore, this linkage to the cell's membrane might be broken at specific times during development by environmental signals. Since these peripheral proteins are linked at the third position of a phosphatidyl inositol moiety (see Chapter 12), activation of a specific phospholipase could release them into the extracellular space.

Because of the great chemical specificities of the oligosaccharide and complex sugar moieties, these modifications can have other physiological consequences. Mechanisms that require intermolecular recognition—for example, cell-to-cell adhesion that occurs during development and in the formation of synapses—could be mediated by binding of proteins at these moieties. Moreover, since the same protein can have somewhat different oligosaccharide chains (a phenomenon called *microheterogeneity*), glycosylation can diversify the function of a given protein. For example, the same polyprotein with sugar residues at different sites along the molecule may be cut into different products by the same processing protease because the sugars can protect sites of cleavage.

From the smooth endoplasmic reticulum, new membrane and secretory proteins pinch off in transport vesicles that shuttle to the Golgi apparatus. The Golgi apparatus, which is found in the cell bodies of all neurons, consists of several interconnected membranous cisternae arranged in flattened stacks (Figure 4–2A). In some cells these cisternae are quite long, extending almost concentrically around the nucleus. In other cells the Golgi apparatus is arranged so that one of its broad aspects (the *cis* or *forming* face) faces the nucleus and the other (the *trans* face) faces the plasma membrane, axons, and dendrites. The mechanisms by which new and specific membrane is produced in the Golgi apparatus are quite complex. Proteins destined for incorporation into the organelles of the cell's major membrane system all pass through the endoplasmic reticulum and the Golgi stacks where they are biochemically tailored by processes involving specific glycosylation, proteolytic cleavage, and the addition of other functional groups, such as the saturated fatty acid (16:0) palmitate.

How these biochemical steps finally result in the precise and orderly segregation of membrane constituents within the neuron is still being elucidated. These membrane components leave the Golgi apparatus in a variety of vesicles. Especially important to the neuron are secretory granules or synaptic vesicles and their precursors. In all cells the membranous and secretory material is conveyed to the plasma membrane and extracellular space by one of two pathways. As discussed further in Chapter 15, these pathways are called *constitutive* and *regulated*.

Vesicles moving in the constitutive pathway continuously renovate the plasmalemma by bringing newly formed membranous constituents to it, and by cycling existing constituents back into the cell, primarily through endosomes. After they are retrieved from the plasmalemma, these constituents enter lysosomes to be degraded or to be recycled and reappear in the external membrane. Secretory and synaptic vesicles follow the regulated pathway, so called because they fuse with the plasma membrane and release their contents not continuously, but only in response to external stimuli, for example, the influx of Ca^{2+} induced by depolarization, hormones, or neurotransmitters. In both pathways the vesicles fuse with the plasma membrane and their contents are secreted into the extracellular space by the process of exocytosis. (How vesicles in these two pathways participate in the release of neurotransmitter and the recycling of synaptic membrane are discussed in Chapter 15.)

Other vesicles, particularly those associated with the *trans*-most cisternae and that are not secretory, can be identified as precursors of lysosomes because cytochemical stains reveal that they contain acid hydrolase activity. Lysosomal hydrolases are glycoproteins. Proteins destined for lysosomes bind to membrane receptors that, at a neutral pH, recognize mannose 6-phosphate residues. Because the pH in lysosomes is low, these glycoproteins dissociate from the receptors and are incorporated into lysosomes.

Axonal Transport Controls the Distribution of Membranes and Secretory Proteins in the Neuron

Although the secretory process in neurons is formally similar to that in other cells, it is actually quite different because of the extreme polarity of the nerve cell. Typically, cell bodies and nerve terminals are at considerable distances from each other. Consider, for example, a spinal motor neuron that innervates muscles around the knee joint. The separation between cell body and nerve terminals calls for the existence of a special transport system to bring newly formed membrane and secretory products from the Golgi apparatus to the end of the axon.

There are three ways by which constituents move within the axon: by fast anterograde (forward moving) axonal transport, by slow axoplasmic flow, and by fast retrograde axonal transport. Essentially all newly synthesized membranous organelles within axons and dendrites (except in the regions of primary dendrites nearest the cell body) are exported to the axon from the cell body by fast anterograde axonal transport. In adult warm-blooded animals, the organelles transported move at a rate in excess of 400 mm/day. A large proportion of this material consists of synaptic vesicles or their precursors for delivery to the terminals (Figure 4–6).

At the nerve terminals the vesicle membranes are recycled many times, through exocytosis, for reuse in synaptic transmission (see Chapter 15). Membrane is constantly being replaced by new components arriving from the cell body. At a compensating rate, existing membrane components are returned from nerve terminals to the cell body, where they are either degraded or reused (Figure 4–6).

Ever since the cell theory was accepted, there has been considerable speculation about the factors that maintain the far-reaching structure of the neuron. One curious but incorrect theory is that the three-dimensional structure of the neuron is maintained by a hydrodynamic mechanism in which the perikaryon acts as a pressure head that keeps the cell's processes extended. This notion prompted the first experiment in axoplasmic transport. In 1948 Paul Weiss tied off a sciatic nerve and observed that axoplasm in the nerve fiber accumulated with time on the proximal side of the ligature. He concluded that axoplasm moves distally at a slow, constant rate from the cell body toward the terminals in a process called axoplasmic flow. Today we know that the flow Weiss observed consists of several kinetic components, both fast and slow.

Fast Anterograde Transport

Direct microscopic analysis of the movement of large particles (probably mitochondria) in living axons in culture started as early as 1920, but more recently it has been used to examine the movement of particles in a variety of nerve fibers. Continuous direct observation using video-enhanced light microscopy, developed independently by Robert D. Allen and Shinya Inoue, has revealed that large

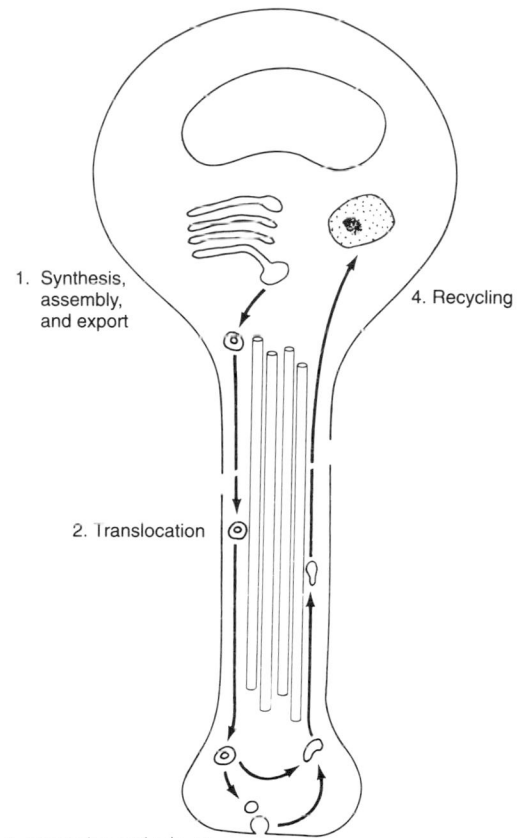

1. Synthesis, assembly, and export

2. Translocation

3. Maturation and release

4. Recycling

FIGURE 4–6

Synaptic vesicles and other membranous organelles involved in synaptic transmission at the nerve terminal are returned to the cell body for recycling after they are used at the synapse. **1.** Proteins and lipids are synthesized and incorporated into membranes within the endoplasmic reticulum and Golgi apparatus in the neuron's cell body. **2.** Organelles are then assembled from these components and exported from the cell body into the axon, where they are rapidly moved toward terminals by fast axonal transport. **3.** Synaptic vesicles and their precursors reach the neuron's terminals, where they participate in the release of transmitter substances by exocytosis. At random, a small proportion of the membrane becomes degraded, and this material is returned to the cell body by fast retrograde axonal transport. **4.** The degraded membrane is partly recycled; its residue is progressively accumulated in large, end-stage lysosomes that are characteristic of neuronal cell bodies.

particles move in a stop-and-go (saltatory) fashion in both the anterograde and retrograde directions (from and to the cell body).

To trace transport, proteins synthesized in dorsal root ganglion cell bodies can be labeled by radioactive amino acids (as constituents of proteins) injected into the ganglion. Transport is then measured by counting the amount of radioactivity in uniform sequential segments along a nerve. Transport profiles showing the distribution of la-

FIGURE 4–7

The distribution of radioactive proteins along the sciatic nerve of the cat at various times after injection of [³H]leucine into dorsal root ganglia in the lumbar region of the spinal cord. In order to display transport curves from various times (2, 4, 6, 8, and 10 hours after the injection) in one figure, several ordinate scales (in logarithmic units) had to be used. Large amounts of labeled protein stay in the ganglion cell bodies. With time, protein moves out along axons in the sciatic nerve. Since the advancing front of the labeled protein (**arrows**) is displaced progressively farther from the cell body with time, the velocity of transport can be calculated from the distances displaced at the various times. From experiments of this kind, Sidney Ochs found that the rate of fast transport is constant at 410 mm per day at body temperature. (Adapted from Ochs, 1972.)

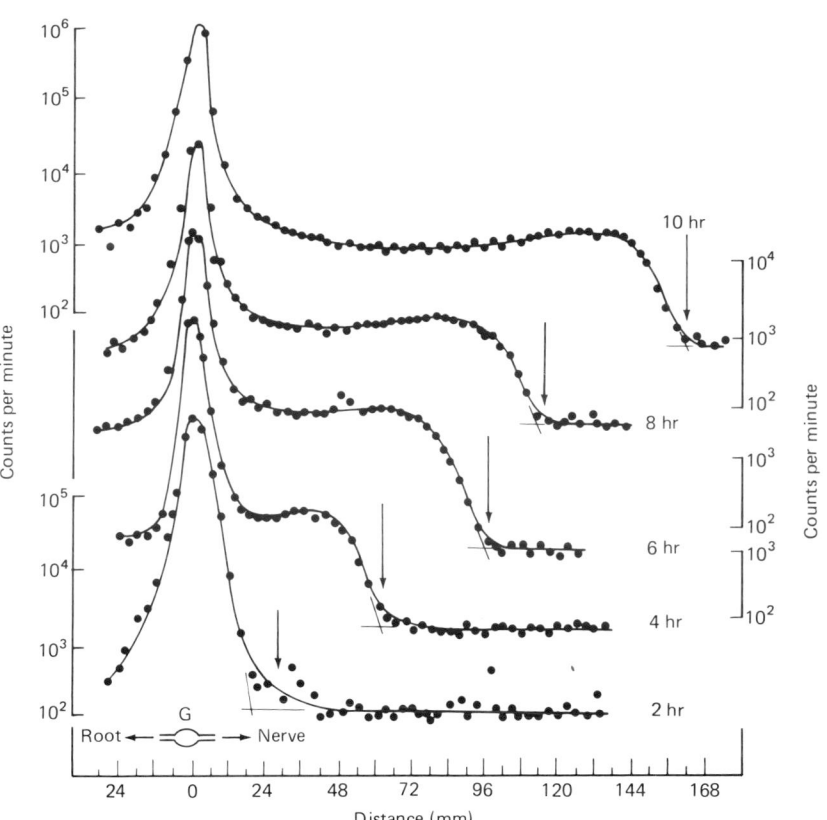

beled protein along the nerve are obtained from different specimens at various times after the injection (Figure 4–7). Studies using this system have shown that fast antero-grade transport depends critically on oxidative metabolism, is not affected by inhibitors of protein synthesis (once the label is incorporated), and in fact is independent of the cell body, because it occurs in nerves actually severed from their cell bodies in the ganglion.

Fast anterograde transport depends on one or more of the filaments that make up the neuron's cytoskeleton (which is discussed later in this chapter). Fast anterograde transport in the axon is based on microtubules that provide an essentially stationary track on which specific organelles move in a saltatory fashion. Evidence for this idea is that colchicine and vinblastin, alkaloids that cause the disruption of microtubules and block mitosis (which is known to depend on microtubules) also interfere with fast transport. Current work has implicated one or more microtubule-associated ATPases: the motor molecule for anterograde movement is thought to be *kinesin*, an ATPase that consists of two large subunits (α), each with a molecular weight of about 125,000, and two small subunits (β). The holoenzyme (α₂β₂) has a molecular weight of about 270,000. About 20 years ago, electron microscopists observed cross-bridges between microtubules and vesicular particles that were thought to play a role in moving the particles. Kinesins, which differ somewhat among species, form the cross-bridges between the moving membranous

organelles, which have the appearance of little feet walking along the microtubules (Figure 4–8). In nonneuronal cells cellular and intracellular motility is based either on the protein *actin* (for example, in contraction of muscle, cell division, and amoeboid motion) or on *dynein*, a microtubule-associated ATPase (used in the beating of cilia and the movement of chromosomes during cell division). An attractive idea is that the kinesin molecule is analogous to myosin in structure, with light and heavy chains. This idea implies that kinesin would operate in association with other proteins, perhaps like actin.

Slow Axonal Transport

Whereas subcellular organelles are moved down the axon by fast transport, the cytosol (cytoskeletal elements and soluble proteins) is transported down the axon by *slow axoplasmic flow*. Slow transport is somewhat more complex than fast anterograde transport. It consists of at least two kinetic components that can be distinguished both by their relative rates of movement along the axon and by the proteins that each transports. The slower component travels at a rate of 0.2–2.5 mm/day and carries the proteins used to make up the fibrillar elements of the cytoskeleton: the subunits that make up neurofilaments and the α and β tubulin subunits that make up the microtubule. These fibrous proteins constitute about 75% of the total protein

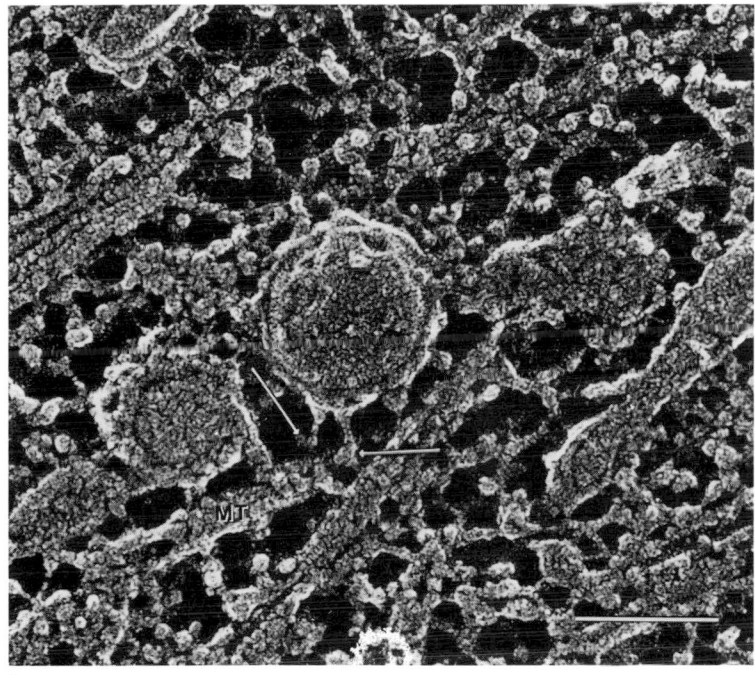

A

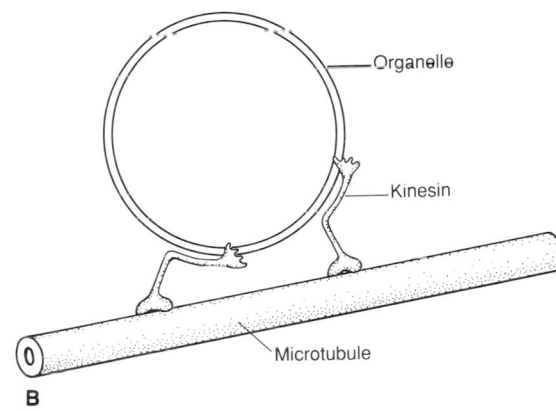

B

FIGURE 4–8
Structures with the morphology of kinesin appear to cross-link membrane-bound organelles to microtubules.

A. Many rod-shaped structures bridge between organelles (large round structures) and microtubules (**MT**) in this quick-freeze, deep-etched electron micrograph from rat spinal cord. Several of these rod-shaped cross-bridges have globular ends that appear to contact the microtubules (**arrows**) Bar, 100 nm.

B. Model for how kinesin moves organelles along microtubules. Kinesin appears to contain a pair of globular heads that bind to microtubules and a fan-shaped tail that binds the organelle to be moved. A hinge region is present near the center of the kinesin molecule. The similarities between kinesin and muscle myosin suggest that movement is produced by the sliding of the kinesin molecules along microtubular tracks. (From Hirokawa et al., 1989.)

moved by the slower component. The neurofilaments and microtubules are thought to move in polymerized form as a network along with the regulatory and cross-linking proteins that are tightly associated with them (Figure 4–9).

The faster component of slow axoplasmic flow is about twice as fast as the slower component. Its protein composition is more complex. Except for actin (the 43,000-molecular-weight protein that polymerizes to form microfilaments and constitutes 2%–4% of the protein carried by this component), all of the other proteins are present in much smaller amounts. These include neural myosin or a myosin-like protein and clathrin. Clathrin is a 180,000-molecular-weight protein that forms a highly ordered polyhedral coat around coated vesicles; it plays a critical role in the recycling of synaptic vesicle membrane (see Chapter 15).

In addition to these cytoarchitectural and cytoskeletal proteins, the enzymes of intermediary metabolism that are formed on free ribosomes also move by the faster component. Calmodulin, the 17,000-molecular-weight Ca^{2+}-binding protein, has also been identified in this component. In the presence of Ca^{2+} this highly conserved protein binds reversibly to many enzymes and other proteins, thereby regulating their function.

Fast Retrograde Transport

Rapid transport also occurs in the retrograde direction from nerve endings toward the cell body, returning materials from terminals to the cell body either for degradation or for restoration and reuse. These materials are packaged in large membrane-bound organelles that are part of the lysosomal system. The rate of fast retrograde transport is about one-half to two-thirds that of fast anterograde transport. As in fast anterograde transport, particles move along microtubules. The motor molecule for fast retrograde transport is a form of *dynein*, which also is a microtubule-associated ATPase (MAP-1C).

Although transport in the retrograde direction serves a scavenger function, the movement of materials from nerve endings back to the cell body also has clinically important functions. An interesting example is the transport of nerve growth factor, a peptide synthesized by the target cell that stimulates the growth of certain neurons. There is strong evidence from developmental neurobiology that retrograde transport has a role in informing the cell body (the site of macromolecular synthesis) about events that occur at the distant ends of axonal processes (Chapter 18).

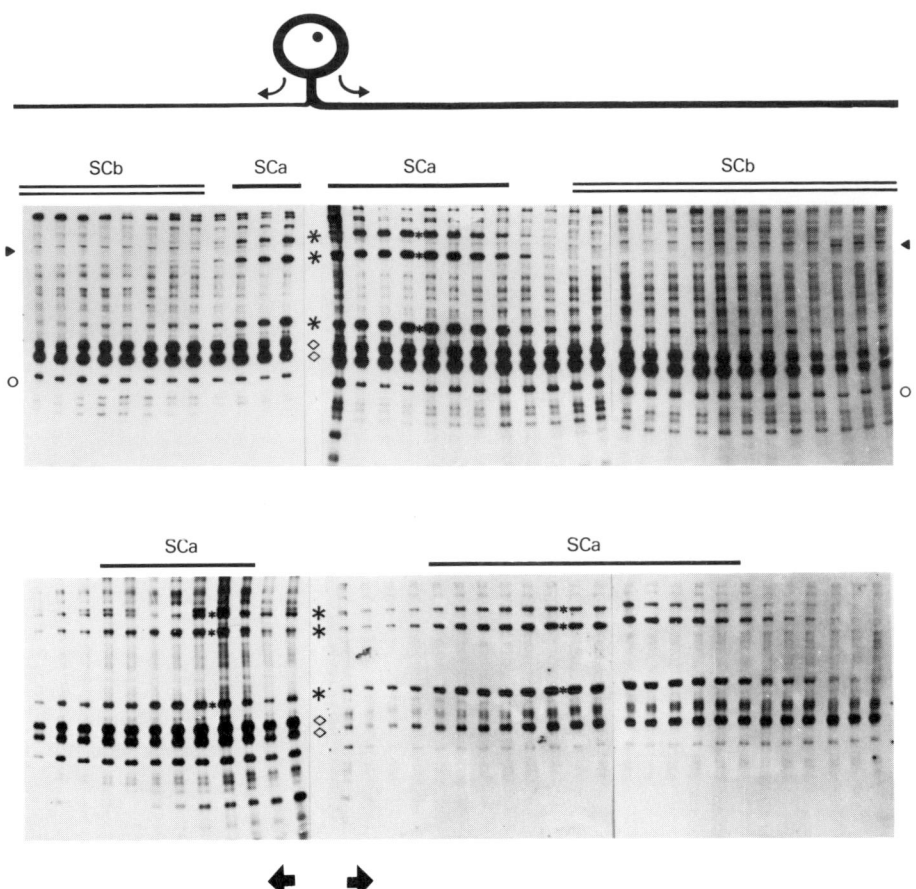

FIGURE 4–9

Slow axoplasmic transport of proteins in the neuron. The auto-radiographs illustrate the differences in the rate and amount of the two components of slow transport in the axon of dorsal root ganglion (DRG) cells. Each lane represents the electrophoretic separation on a polyacrylamide gel of proteins in consecutive 2-mm segments of the central branch (**left**) or peripheral branch (**right**) of the axon of DRG cells in adult rats. In the top panel the axon was retrieved 7 days after injecting [^{35}S]methionine into the L5 DRG; in the bottom panel a 14-day interval had elapsed. The major proteins that constitute the SCa wave of slow transport are the neurofilament proteins (**stars**) with molecular weights of 200,000, 145,000, and 68,000, and the tubulin subunits of the microtubule (**diamonds**), α-tubulin (mol wt 53,000), and β-tubulin (mol wt 57,000). The advance of the SCa wave over one week can be seen by the location of the peak of the neurofilament radioactivity (indicated by **small stars**) at the two time intervals. The composition of the fast-moving SCb wave is more complex but three identified proteins are indicated. These include clathrin (**arrowhead**), actin (**open circle**), and tubulin (**diamonds**). (Courtesy of M. Oblinger.)

Not everything transported in the axon benefits the cell: Some neurotropic viruses and toxins reach the central nervous system by ascending from peripheral nerve terminals to cell bodies by fast retrograde transport. This has been demonstrated for several viruses, including herpes simplex, rabies, polio viruses, and for tetanus toxin.

Extracellular components transported in the retrograde direction are taken up at the terminals by *endocytosis*, a process that can be considered the reverse of exocytosis. Adsorbed material is readily engulfed and packaged into large vesicular organelles, which presumably are the means by which membrane components are returned to the cell body. Unadsorbed particles (fluid-phase particles) and substances not bound are also transported back to the cell body within vesicles but are not taken up as rapidly by endocytosis. The most familiar experimental example of an unadsorbed particle is the enzyme horseradish peroxidase, useful in histochemical tracing (Box 4–1).

Fibrillar Proteins of the Cytoskeleton Are Responsible for the Shape of Neurons

The bulk of axoplasm moves by slow transport. The fibrillar elements of the cytoskeleton all move by slow transport. As we have seen, the proteins that constitute the cytoskeleton mediate the movement of organelles from one region of the cell to another and serve to anchor membrane constituents, for example receptors, at appropriate locations on the cell's surface. They also determine the shape of the neuron. Still another important feature of these fibrillar proteins is that they undergo profound

Neuroanatomical Tracing Based on Fast Axonal Transport   BOX 4–1

In the past 20 years the experimental use of fast axonal transport to trace neural projections has revolutionized neuroanatomy. Previously, the projections of neurons were mapped by cutting axons, allowing them to degenerate, and then locating the affected cell bodies or axons. These studies relied on difficult and sometimes unreliable histochemical staining procedures.

Making use of anterograde transport, neuroanatomists can now locate axons and terminals of specific nerve cell bodies by autoradiographically tracing labeled protein soon after administering radioactively labeled amino acids, certain labeled sugars (fucose or amino sugars, precursors of glycoprotein), or by tracing specific transmitter substances. Similarly, the location of the cell bodies belonging to specific terminals can be identified by making use of particles, proteins, or dyes that are taken up at nerve terminals and transported back to cell bodies. Horseradish peroxidase has been most widely used for this type of study because it is transported in the retrograde direction and its reaction product is conveniently visualized histochemically. In the experiment illustrated in Figure 4–10, the marker enzyme, horseradish peroxidase, is used to study fast axonal transport.

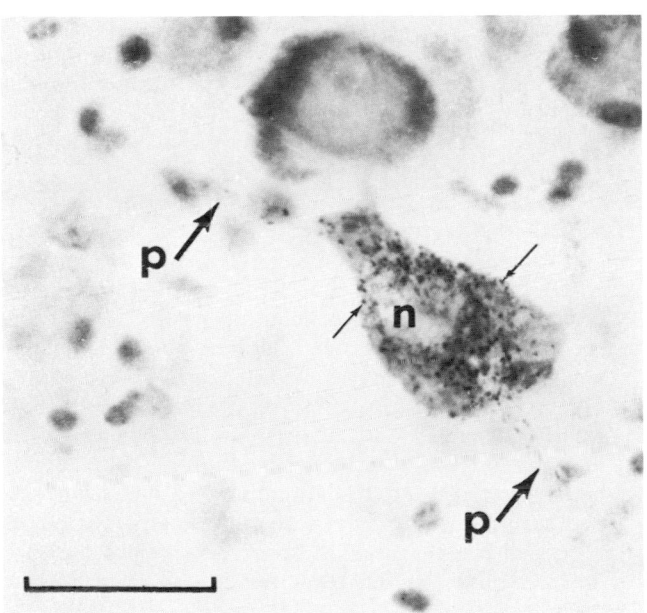

FIGURE 4–10

Fast retrograde transport can be used to study the axon distribution of a neuron in the central nervous system. This photomicrograph is taken from an experiment investigating the sources of afferents to the inferior parietal lobule of the cerebral cortex (association cortex, Brodmann's area 7) in the rhesus monkey. A cell body in the magnocellular nucleus of the basal forebrain was found to be labeled 2 days after injection of horseradish peroxidase (HRP) into the cortex. The HRP, taken up by the cell's terminals in the cortex, was transported in the retrograde direction, to mark the cell body. **Thin arrows** indicate HRP reaction product in the cell body; **thick arrows** indicate processes (**p**) in which some reaction product can be seen. The neuron's nucleus (**n**) does not contain any label. Bar, about 25 μm. This neuron in the limbic forebrain is part of a pathway through which the forebrain is thought to influence directly the cortex in accordance with motivational and emotional states. (From Divac et al., 1977.)

changes in diseased or aging nerve cells (described in Chapter 62). The organization of the cytoskeleton in an axon is revealed in the photomicrograph of a freeze-etched preparation shown in Figure 4–11. Three types of fibrillar elements of varying thickness are the chief constituents of the cytoskeleton of neurons: microtubules, neurofilaments, and microfilaments together with their associated proteins (Figure 4–12).

Microtubules, the thickest of the neuron's cytoskeletal fibers, are long polar polymers usually constructed of 13 protofilaments (linearly arranged α- and β-tubulin dimers) packed in a tubular array with an outside diameter of 25–28 nm (Figure 4–12A). Each monomer binds two guanosine triphosphate (GTP) molecules, or one GTP and one GDP molecule. In the axon they are oriented longitudinally with polarity always in the same direction. This arrangement is presumably important for the directional specificities of the two forms of fast axonal transport. Although axonal or dendritic microtubules can be as long as 0.1 mm, they usually do not extend the full length of the axon or dendrite, and are not continuous with microtubules in the cell body. The tubulins are encoded by a multigene family (there are six or more genes for both the α and β subunits). More than 20 isoforms in the brain result from expression of the different genes and from posttranslational modifications.

Microtubule-associated proteins (MAPs) regulate the stability of microtubules and promote their oriented polymerization or assembly. MAP-1, MAP-2, and *tau* promote assembly. MAP-2 and *tau* are substrates for both the cAMP-dependent and the Ca^{2+}/calmodulin-dependent protein kinases. Protein phosphorylation of these MAPs

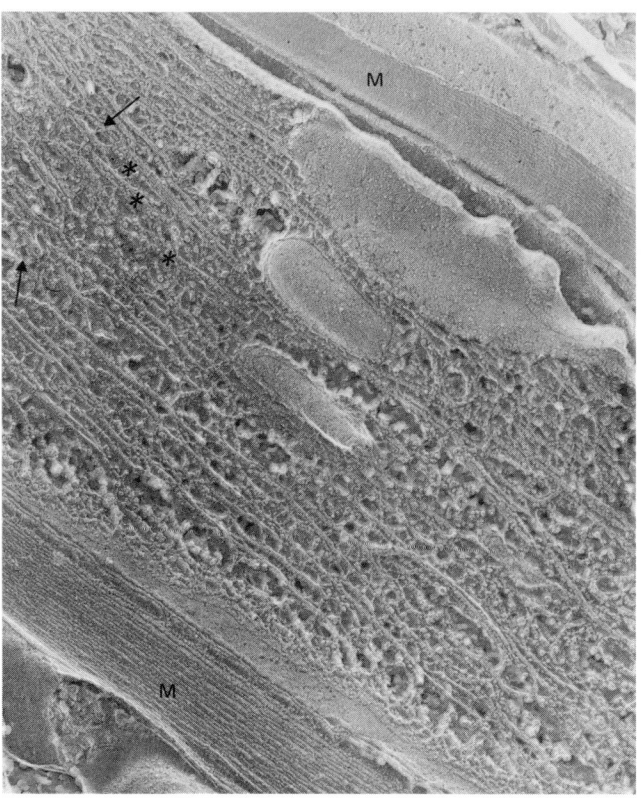

FIGURE 4–11
The zone near the axolemma where filamentous material contacts particles on the inner axolemma surface. At the top of the figure are two sausage-shaped organelles that probably correspond to components moving by retrograde transport. The left end of the large one is associated with a gap in the axoplasm. These organelles are in a microtubule domain of the axoplasm (bracketed by **arrows at left**) that passes obliquely through the plane of fracture and consequently has a very irregular outline. Pieces of at least five microtubules (**stars**) are evident in the vicinity of the organelles. **M,** myelin sheath. × 105,000. (Courtesy of B. Schnapp and T. Reese.)

diminishes their ability to promote assembly, thereby producing depolymerization. MAP-2 is abundant in the cell body and dendrites of neurons, but is absent in axonal processes. In contrast, MAP-3 is present only in axons and glial cells.

Neurofilaments, 10 nm in diameter, typically are the most abundant fibrillar components in axons and are the bones of the cytoskeleton (Figure 4–12B). Bundles of these filaments, which are often referred to as neurofibrils, were first observed by Robert Remak in 1843. These fibrils were important in verifying the neuron theory because they are the elements that retain silver nitrate, the stain first applied by Golgi in 1873 and later used extensively by Ramón y Cajal. Neurofilaments are related to the *intermediate filaments* of other cell types, all of which belong to a family of proteins called *cytokeratins,* which includes vimentin, glial fibrillary acidic protein, desmin, and keratin. Neurofilaments are essentially totally polymerized in the cell: like hair, to which they are related, there is hardly any physiological condition under which these pro-

teins can exist in solution. They also are oriented along the length of the axon. On average, there are three to ten times more neurofilaments than microtubules in an axon; indeed, some small axons have few, if any, microtubules. In Alzheimer's disease and some other degenerative disorders these proteins appear to be modified, forming a characteristic lesion called the neurofibrillary tangle (discussed in Chapter 62).

Microfilaments, 3–5 nm in diameter, are the thinnest of the three types of fibers that make up the cytoskeleton (Figure 4–12C). Like the thin filaments of muscle, microfilaments are polar polymers of globular actin monomers (each bearing an ATP or ADP) wound into a two-stranded helix. Actins are a major constituent of all cells (perhaps the most abundant animal protein in nature). They are encoded by a gene family that includes, in addition to the α-actin of skeletal muscle, at least two other molecular forms (β and γ). Neural actin, first described by Sol Berl, is a mixture of the β and γ species, which differ from α-actin at a few amino acid residues. Despite these differences, most of the actin molecule is highly conserved, not only in different cells of an animal but also in organisms as distant as humans and protozoa.

Much of the actin in neurons is associated with the plasma membrane; in cortical dendrites it is concentrated at the dendritic spines, specialized outpocketings upon which most synapses occur. Some axonal microfilaments are oriented longitudinally. As in other cells, these filaments are attached to the plasma membrane through several associated proteins linked to actin (spectrin, ankyrin, vinculin, and talin). These structural proteins are all tightly associated with membrane, but they are not integral membrane proteins because their polypeptide chains do not extend through the lipid bilayer. The principal anchoring protein in neurons and other cells of the body is *fodrin* (or *neural spectrin*), some of which is transported down the axon at the same velocity as actin. Microfilaments are also able to interact with proteins in the extracellular matrix (for example, *laminin* and *fibronectin*) through their association with a family of membrane-spanning proteins called *integrins.*

The Dynamics of Polymerization

Unlike the bones that make up the skeleton of the body, the fibers of the neuronal cytoskeleton are in a dynamic state, growing longer or shorter. Microfilaments and microtubules are in a state of continuous flux in the neuron. At any one time, about half of the total actin in neurons may exist as unpolymerized monomers. The state of actin within the cell is controlled by several different binding proteins that block polymerization by capping the end at which the filament grows or severing the filament, or both. Other binding proteins cross-link or bundle microfilaments. The dynamics of polymerization varies with each type of fiber (Figure 4–13).

The simplest way all filamentous proteins polymerize is *self-assembly.* Self-assembly requires no input of energy but instead depends on an equilibrium between the concentration of monomers and the polymer, which is more

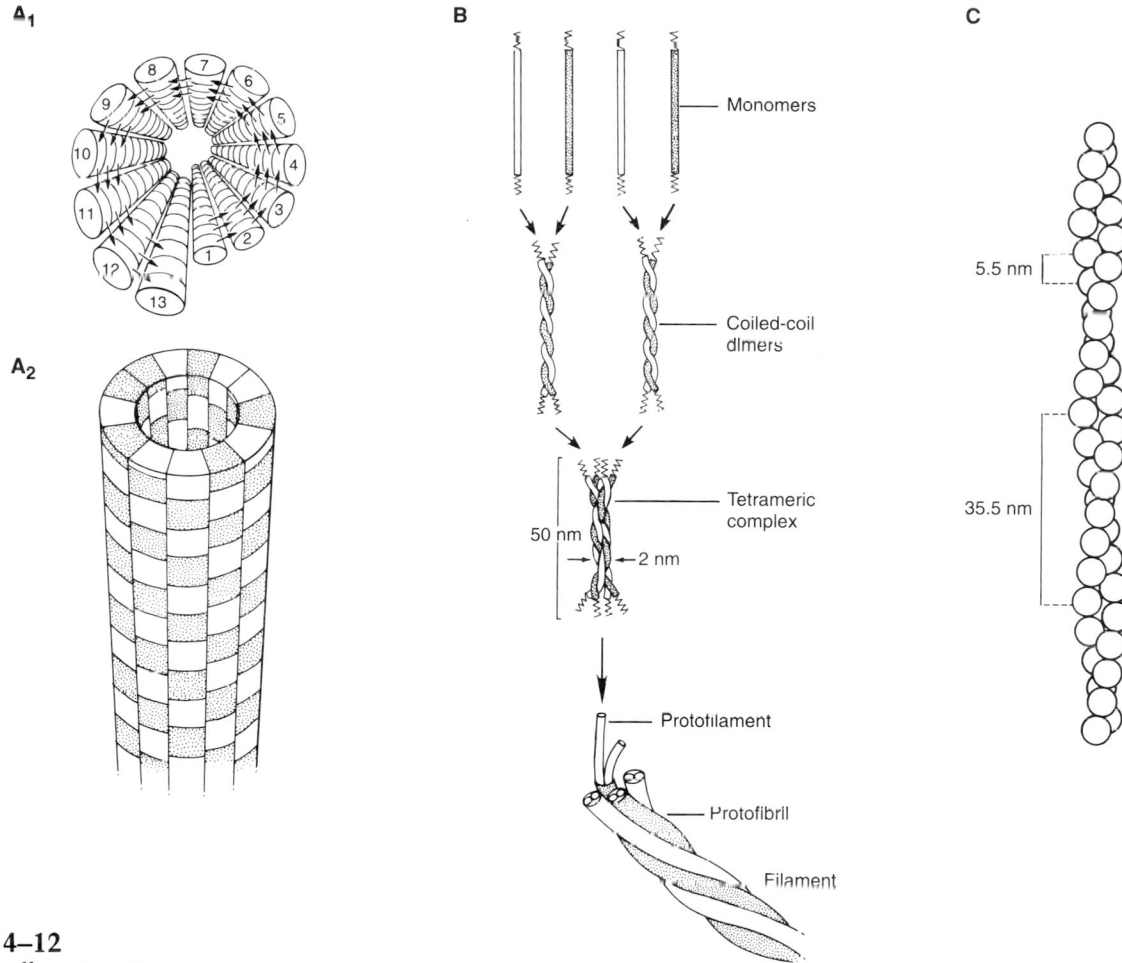

FIGURE 4–12

Atlas of fibrillary structures.

A. Microtubules, the largest-diameter fibers (25 nm), are helical cylinders composed of 13 protofilaments each 5 nm in width. Protofilaments are linearly arranged pairs of alternating α- and β-tubulin subunits (each subunit with a molecular weight of about 50,000). A tubulin molecule is a heterodimer consisting of one α- and one β-tubulin subunit. **1.** An exploded view up a microtubule with arrows indicating the direction of the right-handed helix. **2.** Diagram of a side-view of a microtubule showing alternate α- and β-subunits (different shading).

B. Neurofilaments are built with fibers that twist around each other to produce coils of increasing thickness. The thinnest units are monomers that form coiled-coil heterodimers. These dimers form a tetrameric complex that becomes the protofilament. Two protofilaments become a protofibril, and four proto-

fibrils are helically twisted to form the 10-nm neurofilament. (From Bershadsky and Vasiliev, 1988.)

C. Microfilaments, the smallest diameter fibers (about 7 nm), are composed of two strands of polymerized globular (G) actin monomers arranged in a helix. There are several isoforms of G-actin encoded by families of actin genes. In mammals there are at least six different (but closely related) actins, two of which are classified as nonmuscle, cellular or β and γ. Each variant is encoded by a separate gene. Microfilaments are polar structures, since the globular monomers actually are asymmetric. Each monomer can be thought of as an arrowhead with a pointed tip and a chevron-shaped (barbed) end. These monomers polymerize tip to tail.

stable than are the free monomers. For example, the neurofilament polymer is essentially stable in the cell and is at a lower energy level than the free monomers and protofilaments (Figure 4–13A). Polymerization of microfilaments and microtubules is both more complex and more dynamic.

In addition to the equilibrium conditions imposed by self-assembly, microfilaments and microtubules can also consume the energy of a nucleotide triphosphate during polymerization. In microfilaments, the hydrolysis of ATP to ADP permits the molecule to polymerize at one end

and depolymerize at the other. This process of directional polymerization is called *treadmilling* (Figure 4–13B). Rapid growth or disappearance of microtubules plays a crucial role in many cellular processes, for example in the movement of chromosomes during cell division and in the nervous system during the growth and extension of axons and dendrites.

In microtubules, each monomer of tubulin can act as a GTPase that hydrolyzes only one of the two nucleotide triphosphates bound. This process is called *dynamic instability* (Figure 4–13C). In addition to self-assembly and

FIGURE 4–13

Three states of polymerization. All three fibers (microtubules, neurofilaments, and microfilaments) are more stable than the free monomers from which they are formed at the concentrations present within the neuron.

A. A true equilibrium between the polymer and monomers. Above a critical concentration, more monomers will exist in polymers than as free molecules. Nevertheless, as with all other chemical equilibria, the components will be in a dynamic state, monomers adding and dissociating from both ends of the polymer.

B. Treadmilling. Addition of monomers to one end of the polymer with dissociation at the other (treadmilling or directional polymerization) can be imposed on the true equilibrium described in A if some source of energy is available. With microtubules (GTP) and microfilaments (ATP), the energy is available in the form of nucleotide triphosphates that are bound to the monomers. Energy is put into the system when a nucleotide triphosphate is hydrolyzed to a nucleotide diphosphate. The **shaded** monomers in the diagram signify molecules with bound nucleotide triphosphates.

C. In addition to true equilibrium and treadmilling, microtubules and microfilaments can also change in length abruptly. Again, the energy needed for these changes, which are called dynamic instability, is provided in the form of the nucleotide triphosphates. Dynamic instability is a transient (nonequilibrium) process that depends on the amounts of monomers with nucleotide triphosphates at the ends of the polymer. Any condition that increases the number of monomers with unhydrolyzed nucleotide triphosphates at the ends of the polymer (called caps) will increase the rate of polymerization by stabilizing its growth. Any condition that decreases the number of monomers with nucleotide triphosphates in the caps leads to rapid shortening of the polymer.

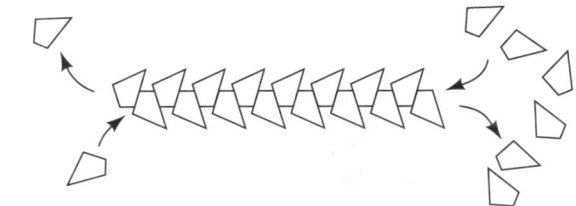

A True equilibrium

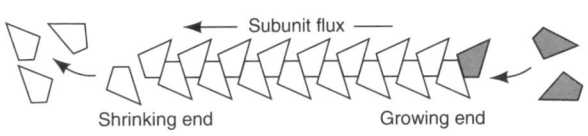

B Treadmilling

Subunit flux

Shrinking end   Growing end

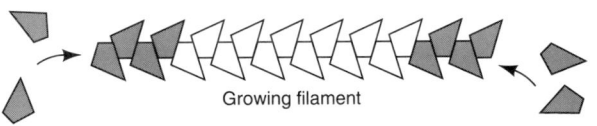

C Dynamic instability

Growing filament

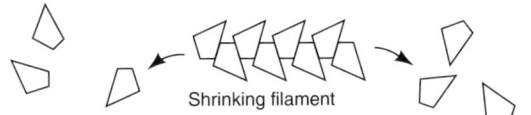

Shrinking filament

treadmilling, microtubules can also undergo rapid alterations in length. At the growing ends of microtubules, the GTP bound to the recently added monomers is not yet hydrolyzed, and these monomers do not readily depolymerize, a situation that favors continued elongation. In the mid-region of the polymer, each monomer binds one GTP and one GDP (only one of the two bound GTPs can be hydrolyzed). Depolymerization is dependent on the nature of the nucleotides at the ends of the polymer; the rate of polymerization is related to the length of the caps bearing monomers that bind unhydrolyzed GTP. If for any reason polymerization is physically blocked or delayed, more of the GTP at the capped ends is hydrolyzed, and the polymer shortens rapidly. Alternatively, microtubules can be stabilized by capping the ends of the polymer.

An Overall View

Genetic information from the nucleus is transcribed into mRNA and carried through nuclear pores into the cytoplasm, where it is translated into one of the three major classes of proteins: 1) cytosolic, 2) nuclear, mitochondrial, and peroxisomal, and 3) proteins for the major membrane system of the neuron. Each of these classes of macromolecules has distinctive physiological roles in the biology of the neuron.

Cytosolic proteins, which are distributed throughout the neuron primarily by slow axoplasmic transport, include the fibrillar elements of the cytoskeleton that determine the shape of the cell and cytosolic enzymes. These enzymes, which are used both for intermediary metabolism and for special biosynthetic pathways, consume or transform the many low-molecular-weight substances in the cell.

Proteins destined for the nucleus include the important enzymes that synthesize DNA and RNA and various transcription factors that regulate gene expression. The two organelles that are independent of the major membrane system of the neuron—mitochondria and peroxisomes—serve similar functions in all cells of the body. The primary function of mitochondria, which are also distributed throughout the neuron in one phase of slow transport, is to generate ATP, the major molecule by which cellular energy is transferred or spent. Peroxisomes, whose function is detoxification through peroxidation reactions, also prevent the accumulation of the strong oxidizing agent hydrogen peroxide, because almost half of its protein content is the enzyme *catalase*.

Finally, membrane and secretory proteins, which are moved along axons and dendrites by fast axonal transport, act in the signaling function of the neuron and in its interaction with the environment, through secretion by exocytosis and maintenance of the plasma membrane by recycling of membrane and endocytosis.

Which proteins are crucial to the signaling properties of nerve cells? Proteins in each of the three classes have properties that, while not *directly* relevant to axonal conduction and synaptic transmission, contribute indirectly. Thus, cytosolic enzymes catalyze the synthesis of the small molecule transmitter substances; the energy of the ATP formed in mitochondria is needed in synaptic transmission. Still further, one of the chief products of the class of cell membrane and secretory proteins in neurons is the synaptic vesicle and, in peptidergic neurons, its neurosecretory contents. Finally, this class includes most of the membrane-spanning proteins that are destined to become ion channels and receptors.

Selected Readings

Alberts, B., Bray, D., Lewis, J., Raff, M., Roberts, K., and Watson, J. D. 1989. Molecular Biology of the Cell, 2nd ed. New York: Garland.

Bershadsky, A. D., and Vasiliev, J. M. 1988. Cytoskeleton. New York: Plenum.

Burgess, T. L., and Kelly, R. B. 1987. Constitutive and regulated secretion of proteins. Annu. Rev. Cell Biol. 3:243–293.

Darnell, J., Lodish, H., and Baltimore, D. 1990. Molecular Cell Biology, 2nd ed. New York: Scientific American Books.

Evans, W. H., and Graham, J. M. 1989. Membrane Structure and Function. Oxford: IRL Press.

Fawcett, D. W. 1981. The Cell, 2nd ed. Philadelphia: Saunders.

Grafstein, B., and Forman, D. S. 1980. Intracellular transport in neurons. Physiol. Rev. 60:1167–1283.

Holtzman, E. 1989. Lysosomes. New York: Plenum.

Spudich, J. A. (ed.) 1989. Molecular Genetic Approaches to Protein Structure and Function: Applications to Cell and Developmental Biology. New York: Liss.

Warner, F. D., and McIntosh, J. R. 1989. (eds.) Cell Movement, Vol. 2. Kinesin, Dynein, and Microtubule Dynamics. New York: Liss.

Warner, F. D., Satir, P., and Gibbons, I. R. (eds.) 1989. Cell Movement, Vol. 1. The Dynein ATPases. New York: Liss.

References

Berl, S., Puszkin, S., and Nicklas, W. J. 1973. Actomyosin-like protein in brain. Science 179:441–446.

Cross, G. A. M. 1990. Glycolipid anchoring of plasma membrane proteins. Annu. Rev. Cell Biol. 6:1–39.

Divac, I., LaVail, J. H., Rakic, P., and Winston, K. R. 1977. Heterogeneous afferents to the inferior parietal lobule of the rhesus monkey revealed by the retrograde transport method. Brain Res. 123:197–207.

Dokas, L. A. 1983. Analysis of brain and pituitary RNA metabolism: A review of recent methodologies. Brain Res. Rev. 5:177–218.

Ferguson, M. A. J., and Williams, A. F. 1988. Cell-surface anchoring of proteins via glycosyl-phosphatidylinositol structures. Annu. Rev. Biochem. 57:285–320.

Finley, D., and Chau, V. 1991. Ubiquitination. Annu. Rev. Cell Biol. 7. In press.

Hirokawa, N., Pfister, K. K., Yorifuji, H., Wagner, M. C., Brady, S. T., and Bloom, G. S. 1989. Submolecular domains of bovine brain kinesin identified by electron microscopy and monoclonal antibody decoration. Cell 56:867–878.

Hoffman, P. N., and Lasek, R. J. 1975. The slow component of axonal transport: Identification of major structural polypeptides of the axon and their generality among mammalian neurons. J. Cell Biol. 66:351–366.

McIlhinney, R. A. J. 1990. The fats of life: The importance and function of protein acylation. Trends Biochem. 15:387–391.

McIntosh, J. R., and Porter, M. E. 1989. Enzymes for microtubule-dependent motility. J. Biol. Chem. Sci. 264:6001–6004.

Mitchison, T., and Kirschner, M. 1988. Cytoskeletal dynamics and nerve growth. Neuron 1:761–772.

Mori, H., Komiya, Y., and Kurokawa, M. 1979. Slowly migrating axonal polypeptides: Inequalities in their rate and amount of transport between two branches of bifurcating axons. J. Cell Biol. 82:174–184.

Oblinger, M. M., and Lasek, R. J. 1985. Selective regulation of two axonal cytoskeletal networks in dorsal root ganglion cells. In P. O'Lague (ed.), Neurobiology: Molecular Biological Approaches to Understanding Neuronal Function and Development. UCLA Symposium on Molecular and Cellular Biology, new series, Vol. 24. New York: Liss, pp. 135–143.

Ochs, S. 1972. Fast transport of materials in mammalian nerve fibers. Science 176:252–260.

Peters, A., Palay, S. L., and Webster, H. deF. 1991. The Fine Structure of the Nervous System: Neurons and Their Supporting Cells, 3rd ed. New York: Oxford University Press.

Puszkin, S., Berl, S., Puszkin, E., and Clarke, D. D. 1968. Actomyosin-like protein isolated from mammalian brain. Science 161:170–171.

Rothman, J. E. 1989. Polypeptide chain binding proteins: Catalysts of protein folding and related processes in cells. Cell 59:591–601.

Sabatini, D. B., and Adesnik, M. B. 1989. The biogenesis of membranes and organelles. In C. R. Scriver, A. L. Beaudet, W. S. Sly, and D. Valle (eds.), The Metabolic Basis of Inherited Disease, 6th ed. New York: McGraw-Hill, Vol. 1, pp. 177–223.

Schnapp, B. J., and Reese, T. S. 1982. Cytoplasmic structure in rapid-frozen axons. J. Cell Biol. 94:667–679.

Towler, D. A., Gordon, J. I., Adams, S. P., and Glaser, L. 1988. The biology and enzymology of eukaryotic protein acylation. Annu. Rev. Biochem. 57:69–99.

Vallee, R. B., and Bloom, G. S. 1991. Mechanisms of fast and slow axonal transport. Annu. Rev. Neurosci. 14:59–92.

Weiss, P., and Hiscoe, H. B. 1948. Experiments on the mechanism of nerve growth. J. Exp. Zool. 107:315–395.

Steven A. Siegelbaum
John Koester

Ion Channels

Ions Cross the Cell Membrane Through Channels

Ion Channels Can Now Be Investigated by Functional and Structural Methods

  Single-Channel Recording Can Measure the Activity of a Single Protein Molecule

  Ion Channels Can Now Be Studied Through Molecular Biological Approaches

Ion Channels Share Several Characteristics

  Ion Channels Facilitate the Passive Flux of Ions Across the Cell Membrane

  The Opening and Closing of a Channel Involves Conformational Changes

  Variants of Each Type of Ion Channel Are Found in Different Tissues

  Genes That Encode Ion Channels Can Be Grouped into Families

An Overall View

Neuronal signaling depends on rapid changes in the electrical potential difference across nerve cell membranes. During an action potential the membrane potential changes quickly, up to 500 volts per second. These rapid changes in potential are made possible by *ion channels*, a class of integral proteins that traverse the cell membrane. These channels have three important properties: (1) they conduct ions, (2) they recognize and select among specific ions, and (3) they open and close in response to specific electrical, mechanical, or chemical signals.

Ion channels in nerve and muscle conduct ions across the cell membrane at extremely rapid rates of up to 100,000,000 ions per second, thereby providing a large flow of ionic current. This current flow causes the rapid changes in membrane potential required for signaling, as will be discussed in Chapters 8 and 10. The high rate of ionic flow in channels is extraordinary—the turnover rates of even the most active enzymes are slower by several orders of magnitude.

In addition to having a high permeation rate, ion channels are highly selective for one or more types of ions. For example, the membrane potential of nerve cells at rest is largely determined by ion channels that are selectively permeable to K^+. Typically, these channels are a hundred-fold more permeable to K^+ than to other cations, such as Na^+. During the action potential, however, ion channels selective for Na^+ are activated; these channels are 10- to 20-fold more permeable to Na^+ than to K^+. Thus, a key feature of neuronal signaling is the activation of different classes of ion channels, each of which is selective for specific ions.

Finally, channels involved in neuronal signaling are also *gated*: They open and close in response to various stimuli. Nongated channels that are always open contribute significantly to the resting potential (see Chapter 6). In contrast, gated channels that can open or close rapidly in response to different signals are very useful for rapid neuronal signaling. Three major signals can gate ion channels: voltage (voltage-gated channels), chemical transmitters (transmitter-gated channels), and pressure or stretch (mechanically gated channels). Individual channels are usually most sensitive to only one type of signal.

In this chapter we consider four questions: Why do cells have channels? How do channels conduct ions at such high rates and yet remain selective? How are channels gated? How are the properties of these channels modified by various intrinsic and extrinsic signals? Later, in Chapters 6 and 8, we shall consider how nongated channels generate the resting potential and how voltage-gated channels generate the action potential. In Chapters 9 to 11 we shall examine how transmitter-gated channels produce synaptic potentials.

Ions Cross the Cell Membrane Through Channels

To appreciate why cells need channels, we need to understand the nature of the plasma membrane and the physical chemistry of ions in solution. The plasma membrane of all cells, including nerve cells, is about 6–8 nm thick and consists of a mosaic of lipids and proteins. The surface of the membrane is formed by a double layer of lipids. Embedded within this continuous lipid sheet are proteins, including ion channels. The lipids within the membrane are hydrophobic—they are immiscible with water. In contrast, the ions of the extracellular and intracellular space are hydrophilic—they attract water molecules strongly.

Although the net charge on a water molecule is zero, charge is separated within the molecule: Water molecules are *dipolar*. The oxygen atom in a water molecule tends to attract electrons and so bears a small net negative charge, whereas the hydrogen atoms tend to lose electrons and have a small net positive charge. As a result of this distribution of charge, water creates a polar environment. Cations are strongly attracted electrostatically to the oxygen atom of water, and anions to the hydrogen atoms. Because they attract water, ions become surrounded by electrostatically bound water, called the *waters of hydration* (Figure 5–1). For an ion to move from water into the nonpolar hydrocarbon tails of the lipid bilayer in the membrane, a large amount of energy has to be supplied to overcome the attractive forces between the ions and the surrounding water molecules. For this reason, it is extremely unlikely for an ion to move from solution into the lipid bilayer, and therefore the bilayer itself is almost completely impermeable to ions. Ions cross the membrane only through specialized proteins such as ion channels, where, as we shall see, the energetics favor ion movement.

The fact that ion channels are made up of protein and are not simply holes in the lipid membrane has been known with certainty for only about 15 years. The idea of ion channels, however, dates to the end of the nineteenth century. At that time, physiologists knew that cells are

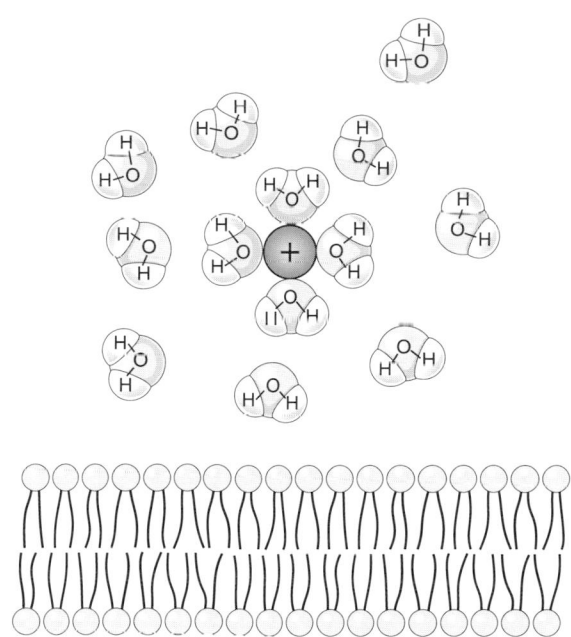

FIGURE 5–1
Ions in solution are surrounded by a cloud of water molecules (waters of hydration) that are attracted by the net charge of the ion. This cloud is carried along by the ion as it diffuses through the solution, adding to its effective size. It is extremely energetically unfavorable, and therefore improbable, for the ion to leave this polar environment to enter the nonpolar environment of the lipid bilayer.

permeable to many small solutes, including some ions, despite the barrier that the cell membrane presents. To explain osmosis (water flow) across biological membranes, the Viennese physiologist Ernst Brucke proposed that membranes contain channels that allow water to flow across membranes but exclude larger solutes. Later, William Bayliss, a British physiologist, suggested that a water-filled channel would also permit ions to cross membranes since the ions would not need to be stripped of their waters of hydration.

The idea that ions move through channels leads to a question: How can a water-filled channel conduct at high rates and yet be selective? How does a channel allow K^+ to pass while excluding Na^+ ions? The explanation cannot be based solely on ionic diameter, because K^+ has a crystal radius of around 0.133 nm, which is larger than the Na^+ crystal radius of 0.095 nm. As we have seen, however, an ion in solution is surrounded by the waters of hydration. Thus, the ease with which an ion moves in solution (its mobility or diffusion constant) is not related simply to the size of an isolated ion; rather it is determined by the size of the shell of water surrounding the ion. The smaller an ion, the more highly localized its charge and the stronger its electric field. As a result, a smaller ion such as Na^+ has a stronger effective electric field surrounding it than a larger ion like K^+, and thus exerts a stronger attraction on its waters of hydration. As Na^+ moves through solution,

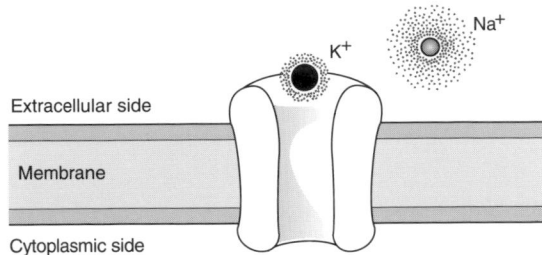

Extracellular side

Membrane

Cytoplasmic side

FIGURE 5–2

A model for K^+ selectivity based on ion diffusion in a water-filled pore. Although a Na^+ ion is smaller than a K^+ ion, its effective diameter in solution is larger because its local field strength is more intense, causing it to attract a larger cloud of water molecules. Thus, a K^+-selective channel can, in principle, select for K^+ over Na^+ by excluding hydrated ions larger than a given diameter (determined by the pore diameter).

its extra electrostatic attraction for water tends to slow it down relative to K^+; thus, Na^+ behaves as if it has a larger water shell. In fact, there is an inverse relation between the size of an ion and its mobility in solution. We therefore can model a channel selective for K^+ simply on the basis of interactions of the ion with water in a water-filled channel (Figure 5–2).

Whereas this idea provides a possible explanation for how a channel can select K^+ and exclude Na^+, it cannot explain how a channel could select Na^+ and exclude K^+. The difficulty in explaining a Na^+-selective channel led many physiologists in the 1930s and 1940s to abandon the channel theory in favor of the idea that ions cross cell membranes by first binding to a specific carrier protein that then transports the ion through the membrane. In this carrier model, selectivity is achieved through a specific chemical binding between the ion and the polar or charged amino acid residues of the carrier protein, not on the basis of mobility in solution. In fact, we now know that ions can cross membranes by means of carriers, or transport proteins, the Na^+–K^+ pump being a well-characterized example (see Chapter 3).

However, many observations on ion conductance across the cell membrane do not fit the carrier model. One of the most telling pieces of evidence is the rate of ion transfer across membranes. This was first examined in the early 1970s in acetylcholine-activated ion channels located in the membrane of skeletal muscle at the synapse between nerve and muscle (see Chapter 10). Using measurements of membrane current noise (small statistical fluctuations in the mean ionic current induced by acetylcholine), Bernard Katz and Ricardo Miledi, and later Charles Anderson and Charles Stevens, inferred that a single acetylcholine-activated channel can transport 10^7 ions per second. In contrast, the Na^+–K^+ pump can transport at most 10^3 ions per second. If the acetylcholine receptor acted as a carrier, it would have to shuttle an ion across the membrane in 0.1 μs, a physically implausible rate. Therefore, the acetylcholine receptor (and similar li-

gand-gated receptors) must conduct ions through a protein channel. Later measurements on many voltage-gated channels selective for K^+, Na^+, and Ca^{2+} demonstrated similar large single-channel conductances, indicating that they too are channels.

But we are still left with the crucial problem: How does a channel achieve ion selectivity? To explain selectivity, the original pore theory was extended first by Loren Mullins, and later by George Eisenman and Bertil Hille, who proposed that channels have a narrow region that acts as a molecular sieve (Figure 5–3). At this *selectivity filter*, an ion sheds most of its waters of hydration and forms a weak chemical bond (electrostatic interaction) with charged or polar amino acid residues that line the walls of the channel. Since the shedding of waters of hydration is energetically unfavorable, an ion will permeate a channel only if the energy of interaction with the selectivity filter compensates for the loss of waters of hydration. Permeant ions remain bound to the selectivity filter for a short time (less than 1 μs), after which the electrochemical gradient propels the ion through the channel. In some channels the pore diameter is large enough to accommodate several water molecules. An ion traversing such a channel need not be stripped *completely* of all of its water shell. Thus, a variety of physical interactions between the ion and the channel molecule produces a wide range of ion selectivities (Figure 5–3).

These interactions in voltage-gated and transmitter-gated ion channels are described in detail in Chapters 8 and 10.

Ion Channels Can Now Be Investigated by Functional and Structural Methods

To understand fully how channels work, we ultimately will need three-dimensional structural information that has proven so informative in the study of enzymes and other cytoplasmic proteins. So far X-ray crystallographic and other structural analyses have not been generally applied to integral membrane proteins, such as ion channels, because their hydrophobic regions make them difficult to crystallize. However, two other powerful methods, single-channel recording and gene cloning, have taught us a good deal about ion channels.

Single-Channel Recording Can Measure the Activity of a Single Protein Molecule

Before it became possible to resolve the small unitary currents through single ion channels in biological membranes, it was already possible to study channel function in artificial planar lipid bilayers. In the early 1960s, Paul Mueller and Donald Rudin developed a technique for making functional lipid bilayers by painting a thin drop of lipid over a small hole in a nonconducting chamber that separates two salt solutions. Because lipids are impermeable to ions, these lipid membranes have a very low con-

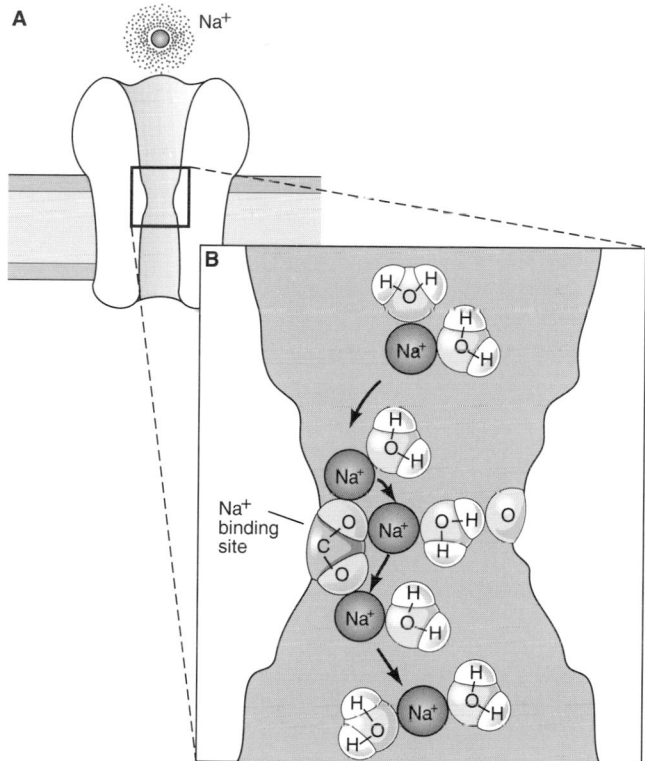

FIGURE 5–3

Sodium channels have a selectivity filter somewhere along the length of the channel, with a site that weakly binds Na$^+$ ions. (From Hille, 1984.)

A. Schematic diagram of the Na$^+$ channel.

B. Schematic diagram of the site within the channel that selects which ions will permeate. According to the hypothesis developed by Bertil Hille and colleagues, as a Na$^+$ ion moves through the filter it binds transiently at the active site. Here, the positive charge of the ion is stabilized by a hydrophilic (polar) amino acid residue lining the channel and also by a water molecule that is attracted to a second polar amino acid residue lining the other side of the channel wall. It is thought that, for steric reasons, a K$^+$ ion with its associated water molecules cannot be stabilized as effectively and therefore will be excluded from the filter. (From Hille, 1984.)

ductance to ions (high resistance). When Mueller and Rudin added certain bacterial proteins to the salt solution in the bath, the membrane underwent a dramatic increase in ion conductance.

Based on this remarkable finding, Stephen Hladky and Dennis Haydon, in 1970, studied in detail the conductance changes produced by the antibiotic gramicidin A, a peptide only 15 amino acids long that consists of alternating hydrophobic d and l amino acids. Surprisingly, Hladky and Haydon, followed by Olaf Anderson and his colleagues, found that when they applied a low concentration of gramicidin A to the planar bilayer, the antibiotic induced small unitary, step-like changes in current flow across the membrane (Figure 5–4A). These reflected the

all-or-none opening and closing of an ion channel formed by the peptide.

The unitary current depends on membrane potential in a linear manner (Figure 5–4A, B). Thus, the channel behaved as a simple resistor; the amplitude of the single channel current could be obtained from Ohm's law, $I = V/R$. The slope of the relation between current (I) and voltage (V) yielded a value for the resistance of a single open channel of around 8×10^{10} ohms (Figure 5–4B). However, in dealing with channels, we generally speak of its *conductance*, the reciprocal of *resistance*, which provides an electrical measure of ion permeability. The unitary conductance of the gramicidin A channel is around 12×10^{-12} siemens or 12 picosiemens (pS), where 1 siemen = 1/ohm.

Biochemical and X-ray crystallographic analyses have shown that the unusual alternating d and l amino acid composition of gramicidin allows the peptide to form a β-helical structure (Figure 5–4C2). The polar carbonyl oxygen atoms of the peptide bonds (with a slight negative charge) all tilt inward toward the center of the helix, where they form the walls of the channel and interact with the permeant cations. The hydrophobic amino acid side chains all point outward from the center of the helix and interact with the lipid membrane. Two gramicidin peptides are thought to form a channel by dimerizing end-to-end (Figure 5–4C1). The opening and closing of the gramicidin channel corresponds to the dimerization and dissociation of the gramicidin monomers, respectively.

Although such artificial systems provided the first insights into the basic principles of channel properties, these principles had yet to be demonstrated in biological membranes. In 1976 Erwin Neher and Bert Sakmann developed the patch-clamp technique for recording current flow from single channels in biological membranes (Box 5–1). Neher and Sakmann used the same frog skeletal muscle preparation that Katz and Miledi examined using noise analysis. A glass micropipette containing acetylcholine, the neurotransmitter that activates channels in the membrane of skeletal muscle, was pressed tightly against the muscle membrane. Small unitary current events, representing the opening and closing of single acetylcholine-activated ion channels, were observed in the area of the membrane under the pipette tip. As with the gramicidin A channels, these acetylcholine receptor-channels also displayed a linear relation between current and voltage and had a single-channel conductance of around 25 pS.

Ion Channels Can Now Be Studied Through Molecular Biological Approaches

What do biological channels look like? How does the channel protein span the membrane? What happens to the structure of the channel when it changes conformation from its closed to its open state? Where along the length of the channel do drugs and transmitters bind? Definitive answers to these questions will require X-ray crystallographic analysis of purified ion channel proteins. How-

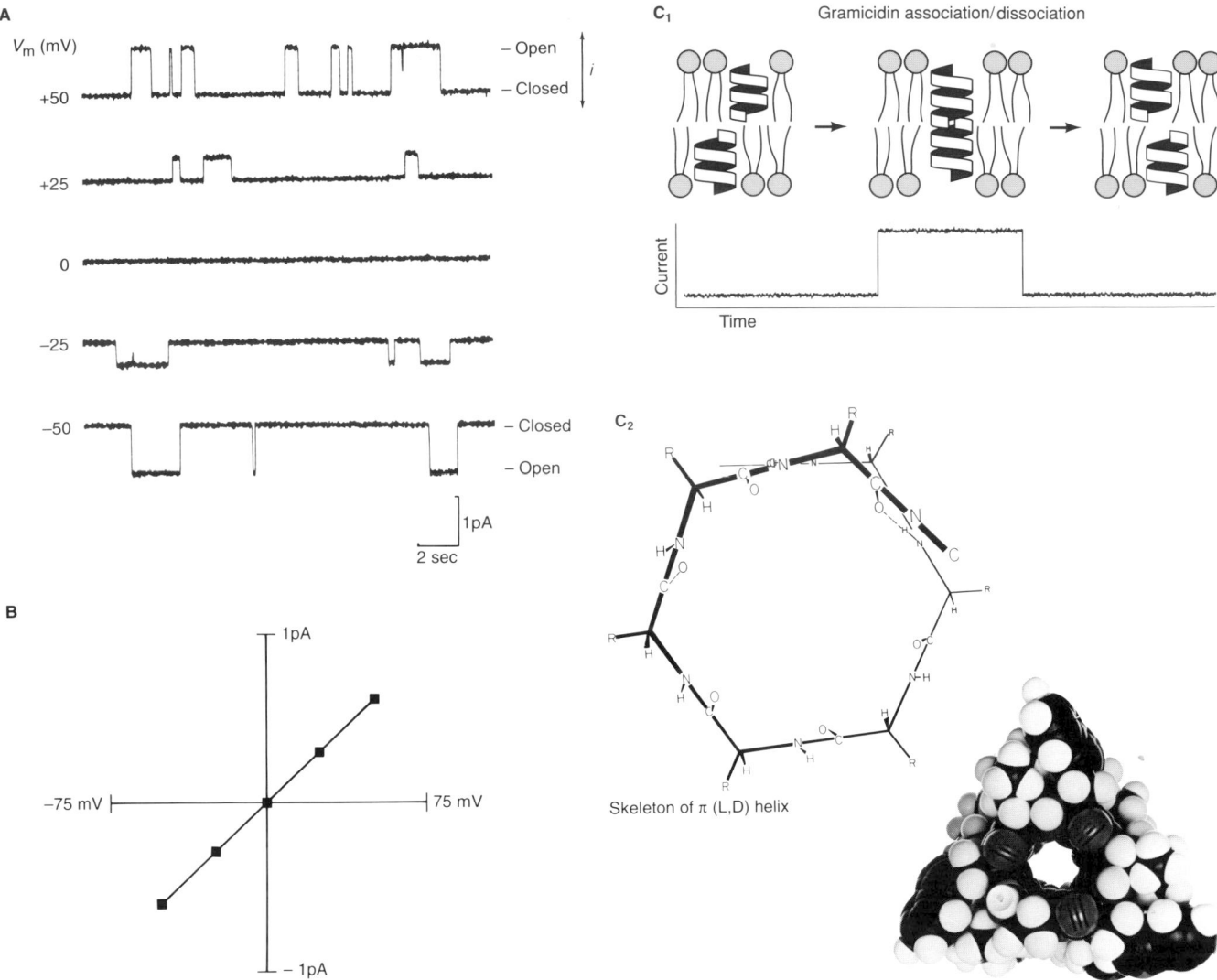

FIGURE 5–4

Characteristics of the current that flows through gramicidin channels.

A. Channels formed by a few gramicidin molecules in a lipid bilayer open and close in an all-or-none fashion, resulting in brief current pulses of quantal size through the membrane. If the electrical potential (Vm) across the membrane is varied, the current through the channels changes proportionally due to the altered electrical driving force.

B. A plot of the current through the channel versus the potential difference across the membrane reveals that the current is

linearly related to the driving force, i.e., the channel behaves as an electrical resistor that follows Ohm's law $(I = V/R)$. (Data in **A** and **B** courtesy of Olaf Anderson and Lyndon Providence.)

C. Proposed structure of the gramicidin A channel. **1.** A functional channel is formed by end-to-end dimerization of two gramicidin peptides. (From Sawyer et al., 1989.) **2.** The helical structure of gramicidin A peptide. The carbonyl and amide groups of the peptide backbone form the hydrophobic channel lining. The hydrophobic side chains **(R)** point outward into lipid. The space-filling model shows how the pore is formed in the center of the helix. (From Urry, 1971.)

ever, over the past several years biochemical and molecular biological approaches have resulted in considerable progress in understanding channel structure and function.

Ion channels are large integral membrane glycoproteins, ranging in molecular weight from 25,000 D to 250,000 D. All channels have a central aqueous pore that spans the entire width of the membrane. Many ion channels are made up of two or more subunits, which may be identical or distinct (Figure 5–6).

The genes for six or seven major classes of ion channels have now been cloned and sequenced. The primary amino acid sequence of the channel inferred from the nucleotide sequence has been used to suggest the structure of different channel proteins. These models rely on computer programs that predict regions of secondary structure (α-helices or β-sheets) that are likely to correspond to transmembrane domains of the channel, based on existing information on proteins whose actual three-dimensional structure is known from electron and X-ray diffraction

Recording Current Flow from Single Ion Channels

BOX 5–1

The patch-clamp technique was developed in 1976 by Erwin Neher and Bert Sakmann to record current flow from single ion channels. This technique is a refinement of voltage clamping (see Box 8–1). A small fire-polished glass micropipette with a tip diameter of around 1 μm is pressed against the membrane of a frog skeletal muscle fiber that has been treated with proteolytic enzymes to remove connective tissue from the muscle surface. The pipette is filled with a physiological salt solution. A metal electrode in contact with the electrolyte in the micropipette connects it to a special electrical circuit that measures the current that flows through channels in the membrane under the pipette tip.

A

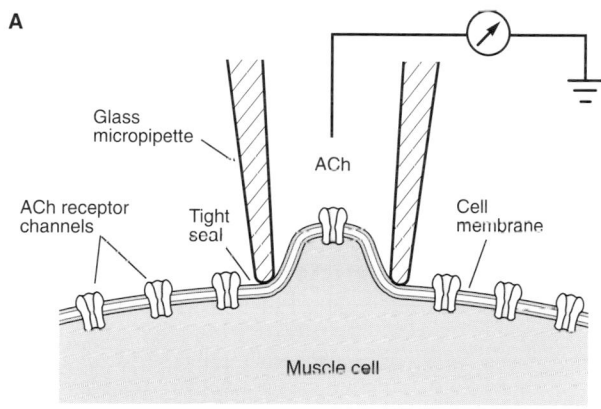

FIGURE 5–5A
Patch-clamp setup. (Adapted from Alberts et al., 1989.)

In 1980 Neher discovered that applying a small amount of suction to the patch pipette greatly tightens the seal between the pipette and the membrane. The result is a seal with extremely high resistance between the inside and outside of the pipette. This dramatically lowers electronic noise and extends the utility of the technique to the whole range of channels involved in electrical excitability, including those with small conductance. Since this discovery, Neher and Sakmann, and many others, have used the patch-clamp technique to study all three major classes of ion channels—voltage-gated, transmitter-gated, and mechanically gated channels—in a variety of neurons and other cells.

B

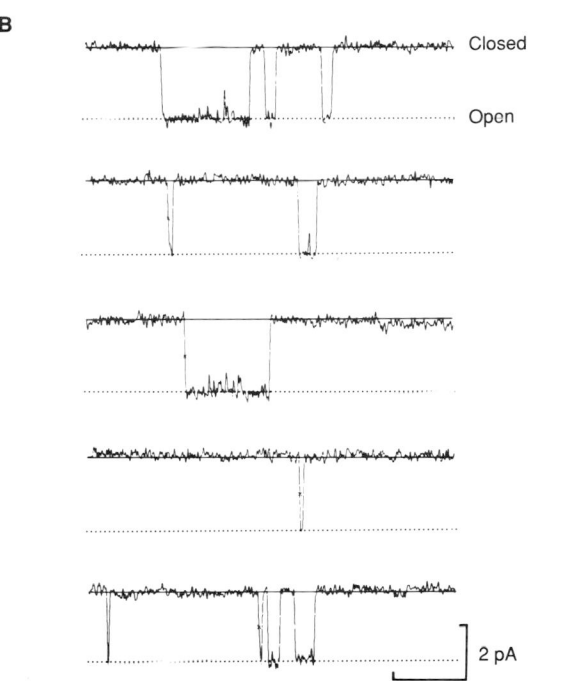

Closed

Open

2 pA

20 msec

FIGURE 5–5B
Record of the current flowing through a single ion channel as the channel switches between closed and open states. (Courtesy of B. Sakmann.)

Independently Christopher Miller developed a method for incorporating channels from biological membranes into planar lipid bilayers. With this technique, biological membranes are first homogenized and a membrane vesicle fraction is isolated by differential centrifugation. Under appropriate ionic conditions these vesicles fuse with a planar lipid membrane. Any ion channel in the vesicle will thus be incorporated into the planar membrane. This technique has two experimental advantages. First, it allows ion channels to be studied from regions of cells that are inaccessible to patch clamp. For example, Miller has successfully studied a K^+ channel isolated from the internal membrane of skeletal muscle sarcoplasmic reticulum. Second, it allows the study of how the composition of the membrane lipids influences channel function.

---

analysis. The first membrane protein whose structure was well understood is the bacterial photo-pigment bacteriorhodopsin (Figure 5–7A). This protein has a molecular weight of 25,000. It contains regions with polar (hydrophilic) amino acids, such as the acidic amino acids glutamate and aspartate, and basic amino acids, such as lysine, and regions with nonpolar or uncharged (hydrophobic) amino acids, such as glycine, alanine, and phenylalanine.

There are, in all, seven hydrophobic regions. Each hydrophobic region is about 15–20 amino acids long, has an α-helical secondary structure, and spans the membrane. These membrane-spanning regions are in turn linked by three cytoplasmic and three extracellular hydrophilic loops.

Efforts to understand the secondary structure of channels are based largely on information from bacteri-

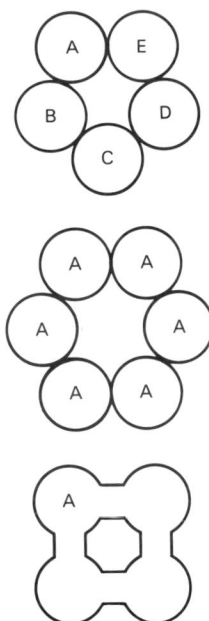

FIGURE 5–6
Subunit basis of channel structure. Channels can be constructed as hetero-multimers from distinct subunits (**top**), homo-oligomers from a single type of subunit (**middle**), or from a single polypeptide chain organized into repeating motifs that act as pseudo-subunits (**bottom**).

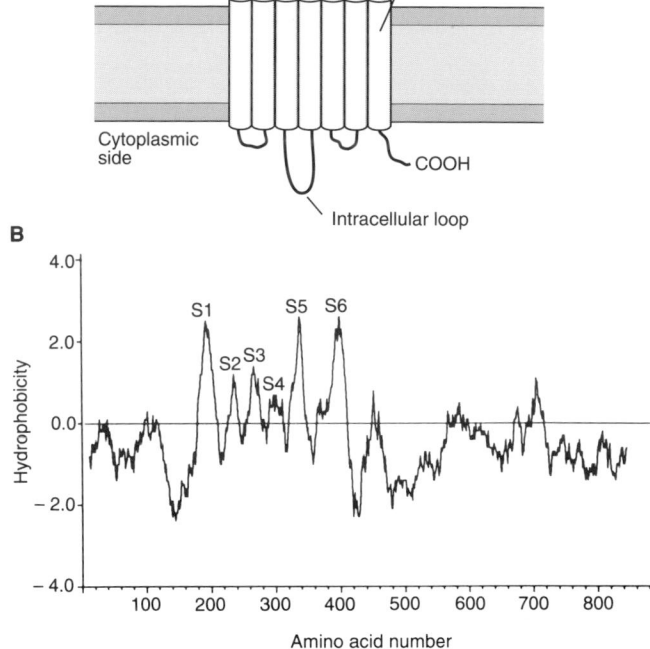

FIGURE 5–7
Secondary structure of membrane-spanning proteins.

A. A proposed secondary structure for bacteriorhodopsin. Each cylinder represents a membrane-spanning α-helix containing around 20 hydrophobic amino acids residues. The membranes are connected by segments (loops) of hydrophilic residues. (From Huang et al., 1982.)

B. The membrane-spanning regions of an ion channel can be identified using a hydrophobicity plot. A running average of the hydrophobicity is plotted for the entire amino acid sequence for a K^+ channel from rat brain. Each point in the plot represents the average hydrophobic index of a 19-amino-acid-long window plotted at the amino acid residue position corresponding to the midpoint of this window. This plot is based on the inferred amino acid sequence obtained from the nucleotide sequence of the cloned K^+ channel gene. (From Frech et al., 1989.)

orhodopsin and more recent information from the X-ray diffraction studies of the photosynthetic reaction center (an important plant membrane protein). Regions of a protein that are nonpolar can be identified using a *hydrophobicity plot*, in which each amino acid residue is assigned a hydrophobicity index based on the nature of its side chain. Amino acids with hydrophobic side chains are given large positive numbers; amino acids with hydrophilic side chains are given large negative numbers. The hydrophobic index for several amino acids around a given residue is then averaged and this number is plotted as a function of position in the primary sequence (Figure 5–7B). Since an α-helix made of 15–20 amino acids can span the lipid bilayer of a biological membrane (with a thickness of 4 nm), a stretch of 15–20 or more amino acids with a large hydrophobic index is a candidate for a membrane-spanning region. To form a complete channel whose walls completely surround an aqueous pore, four to six transmembrane α-helices are required.

In principle, a membrane-spanning α-helix could also be constructed from an amphipathic peptide consisting of alternating polar and nonpolar amino acids. If the polar amino acids are placed at every third or fourth position, all the polar side chains will line up on one side of that helix (which makes a complete turn every 3.5 amino acid residues). This is an attractive model for an ion channel, since the polar side chains could form the walls of the water-filled pore while the nonpolar side chains would face the lipid bilayer or hydrophobic interior of the protein.

Additional insight into channel structure and function can be obtained by comparing the primary amino acid sequence of related channels from different species and identifying regions with high degrees of sequence homology. The fact that such regions have been highly conserved through evolution points to the importance of that region in channel structure and function. Further insight into structure-function relationships can be obtained from sequence homologies among different, but related, channels. Such homologous regions are likely to underlie a common biophysical function shared by the different channels. For example, all voltage-gated channels contain a putative α-helix membrane-spanning domain that contains positively charged amino acids (lysine or arginine) spaced at every third position along the α-helix. The fact that this motif is observed in all voltage-gated Na^+, K^+, and Ca^{2+}

channels, but not in ligand-gated channels, lends support to the view that this charged region may play an important role in voltage-dependent gating (see Chapter 8).

Once a structure for a channel has been proposed, it can be tested in several ways. First, antibodies can be raised against synthetic peptides corresponding to different hydrophilic regions in the protein sequence. Using immunocytochemistry, one can then determine whether the antibody binds to the extracellular or cytoplasmic surface of the membrane, thus defining whether a particular region of the channel is extracellular or intracellular.

Second, genetic engineering can be used to produce chimeric channels, channels with selected parts derived from the genes of different species. This technique takes advantage of the fact that channels in different species have somewhat different properties. For example, the bovine acetylcholine-gated receptor channel has a slightly higher single-channel conductance than the same channel in electric fish. By comparing the properties of a chimeric channel to those of the original channels, it is possible to assess which regions of the channel are involved in different functions. For example, Sakmann and Shosaku Numa and their colleagues have been able to identify a specific membrane-spanning segment of the acetylcholine-gated channel as the region that forms the lining of the pore (see Chapter 10). Finally, the roles of different amino acid residues or stretches of residues can also be tested using *site-directed mutagenesis*, a type of genetic engineering in which specific amino acid residues are substituted or deleted.

Ion Channels Share Several Characteristics

All cells make use of local intercellular signaling processes, but only nerve and muscle cells are specialized for rapid signaling over long distances. Although nerve and muscle cells have a particularly rich variety and high density of membrane ion channels, their channels do not appear to differ fundamentally from those in other cells in the body. In this section we describe the general properties of ion channels found in a wide variety of cell types.

Ion Channels Facilitate the Passive Flux of Ions Across the Cell Membrane

The flux of ions through ion channels is passive, requiring no expenditure of metabolic energy. The direction and eventual equilibrium for this flux is determined not by the channel itself, but rather by the electrochemical driving force across the membrane.

Ion channels select the types of ions that they allow to cross the membrane. Each channel type discriminates between possible permeant ions on the basis of ionic charge, allowing either cations or anions to permeate. Some cation-permeable channel types are relatively nonselective for the cations present in extracellular fluid—they will pass Na^+, K^+, Ca^{2+}, and Mg^{2+}. However, most cation-selective channels are more selective; each one is permeable primarily to a single type of ion, either Na^+, K^+, or Ca^{2+}. All known types of anion-selective channels are permeable to only one physiological ion, Cl^-.

The kinetics of ion flow through a channel are characterized by the size and voltage-dependence of the channel's conductance. The kinetic properties of ion permeation are best described by the channel's conductance, which is determined by measuring the current (ion flux) that flows through the open channel in response to a given electrochemical driving force. The net electrochemical driving force is determined by two factors—the electrical potential difference and the concentration gradient of the permeant ions across the membrane. Changing either one can change the net driving force (see Chapter 6). In some channels, the current through the open channel varies linearly with driving force, i.e., the channels behave as simple resistors. In others the current flow through the open channel is a nonlinear function of driving force. This type of channel behaves like a rectifier—it conducts ions more readily in one direction than in the other when the direction of the driving force is reversed. It is customary to characterize the conductance of a rectifying channel not by a single value but rather by plotting current versus voltage for the channel over the physiological voltage range (Figure 5–8).

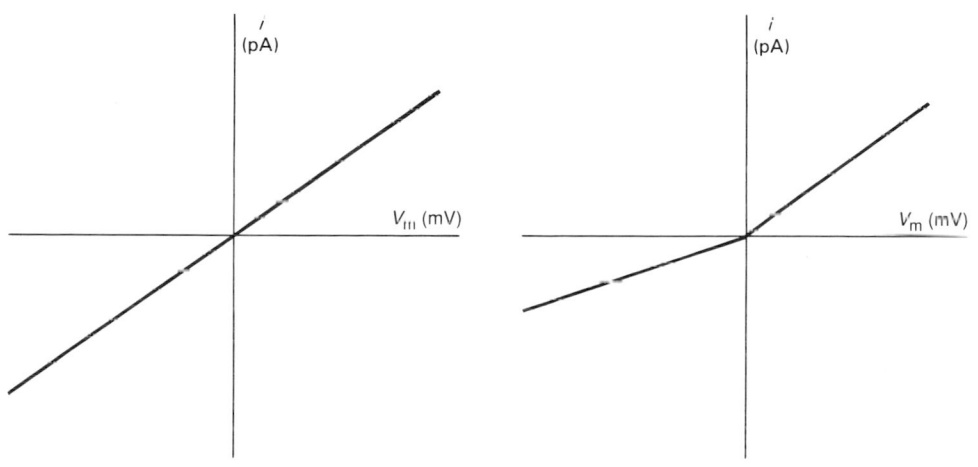

FIGURE 5–8
Single-channel current–voltage relationships. In many channels the relation between current flow through an open channel (*I*) and the applied membrane voltage (V_m) is linear, as illustrated in the plot at **left**. Such channels are said to be ohmic, as they follow Ohm's law, $I = V_m/R$. In other channels the relation between current and membrane potential is nonlinear, as shown on the **right**. This kind of channel is said to rectify.

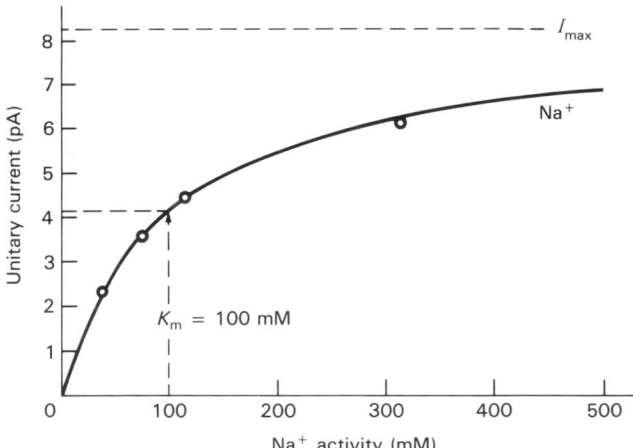

FIGURE 5–9
The relation between single channel current and ionic concentration saturates. Here the size of the outward ionic current through an ACh-activated channel is plotted as a function of internal Na⁺ concentration (actually Na⁺ activity is plotted). The data (**open points**) are fitted by the equation for a simple one-to-one binding relation, for which a dissociation constant (K_m) of 100 mM defines the affinity of the channel for Na⁺, at which concentration the binding sites are half-occupied. (Adapted from Horn and Patlak, 1980.)

Ionic flow through an ion channel may saturate. The rate at which ions flow through a channel (i.e., current) varies with the concentration of the ions in the surrounding solution. At low concentrations the current increases almost linearly with concentration. At higher ion concentrations the current tends to saturate, even though the electrochemical driving force is greater (Figure 5–9).

This saturation effect is consistent with the idea that ion permeation involves binding of ions to specific polar sites within the pore of the channel, rather than obeying

FIGURE 5–10
Ion channels can be blocked.

A. Permeating ions readily pass through the selectivity filter.

B. Blocking particles (**larger circles**) enter the mouth of the channel but become stuck, as they are too wide to pass through the selectivity filter. If the blocking particle entering the membrane is electrically charged, its binding kinetics will be influenced by the membrane potential. For example, a positively charged blocker is forced toward the binding site when the inside of the cell is made more negative.

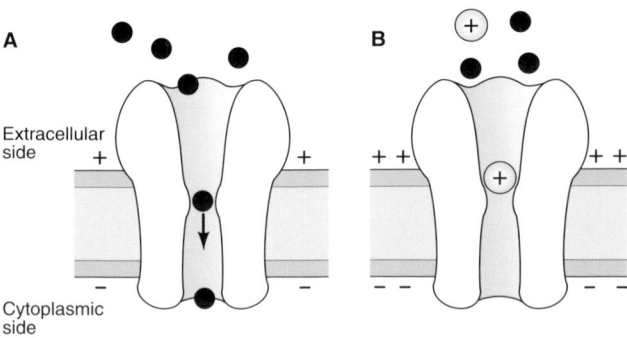

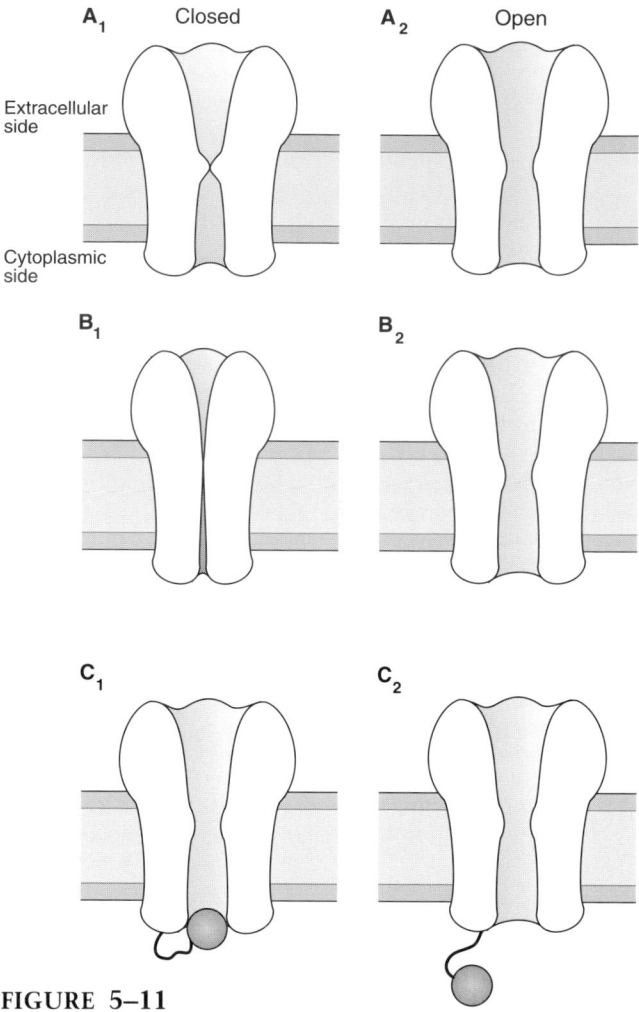

FIGURE 5–11
Three different physical models for channel gating.

A. A discrete conformational change occurs in one region of the channel.

B. A generalized conformational change results in changes in structure along the length of the channel.

C. A blocking particle swings into and out of the channel mouth.

the laws of electrochemical diffusion in free solution. A simple electrodiffusion model would predict that the ionic current should continue to increase as the ionic concentration is increased—the more charge carriers in solution, the greater the current flow. But with nearly all channels, current flow begins to saturate at high ionic concentrations. The relation between current and ionic concentration for a wide range of ion channels is often well fitted by a simple one-to-one binding equation (rectangular hyperbola), suggesting that a single ion binds to a channel during permeation. The ionic concentration at which current flow is half-maximal defines the dissociation constant for ion binding in the channel. One striking feature of these plots is that the dissociation constant is typically quite high—around 100 mM—indicating a weak binding compared with the dissociation constants for typical enzyme-substrate interactions. This weak interaction indicates that the bonds between the ion and the channel are rapidly formed and broken. In fact, an ion typically stays bound in the channel for less than 1 μs. This rapid off-rate for ion binding ensures that channels achieve a very high conduction rate (on the order of 10^7 ions per second).

Permeation through the ion channel can be inhibited by blocking access to or plugging the pore. Permeation through an ion channel can be inhibited by a blocking molecule that binds either to a site at the mouth of the pore or somewhere within the pore (Figure 5–10). If the inhibitor is an ionized molecule that binds to a site within the pore, binding will be influenced by membrane potential, because the charged inhibitor molecule will sense the membrane electric field as it enters the channel. For example, if a positively charged channel blocker enters the channel from outside the membrane, making the membrane potential more negative will drive the blocker into the channel, increasing the degree of the block. Although most blocking molecules are typically exogenous drugs or toxins, some are present under physiological conditions. For example, common ions such as Mg^{2+}, Ca^{2+}, and Na^+ can act as channel blockers in certain types of channels.

The Opening and Closing of a Channel Involves Conformational Changes

All ion channels so far studied that open and close are *allosteric proteins*. Each channel protein has two or more conformational states that are relatively stable. Each of these stable conformations represents a different functional state. For example, each allosteric channel has at least one open state and one closed state, and may have more than one of each. The transition of a channel between closed and open states is called gating.

Relatively little is known about gating mechanisms, other than that they involve a conformational change in channel structure. Although the picture of a gate swinging open and shut is a convenient image, it probably is accurate only for certain channels (for example, the inactivation of Na^+ and K^+ channels, which we shall consider in Chapter 8). More commonly, channel gating involves widespread changes in channel conformation. For example, evidence from high-resolution electron microscopy and image analysis of the gap junction type of ion channel (that we shall consider in Chapter 9) suggests that the opening and closing of this channel involves a concerted twisting and tilting of the six subunits that make up the channel. Three general physical models of channel gating are illustrated in Figure 5–11.

Because the primary function of ion channels in neurons is to mediate rapid signaling, several specialized allosteric control mechanisms have evolved that influence the amount of time a channel spends in each of its different conformations. Some ion channels are regulated by the noncovalent binding of chemical ligands. These ligands may be neurotransmitters or hormones in the extracellular environment that bind to the extracellular side of the channel (Figure 5–12A), or they may be intracellular second messengers that are activated by transmitters. As

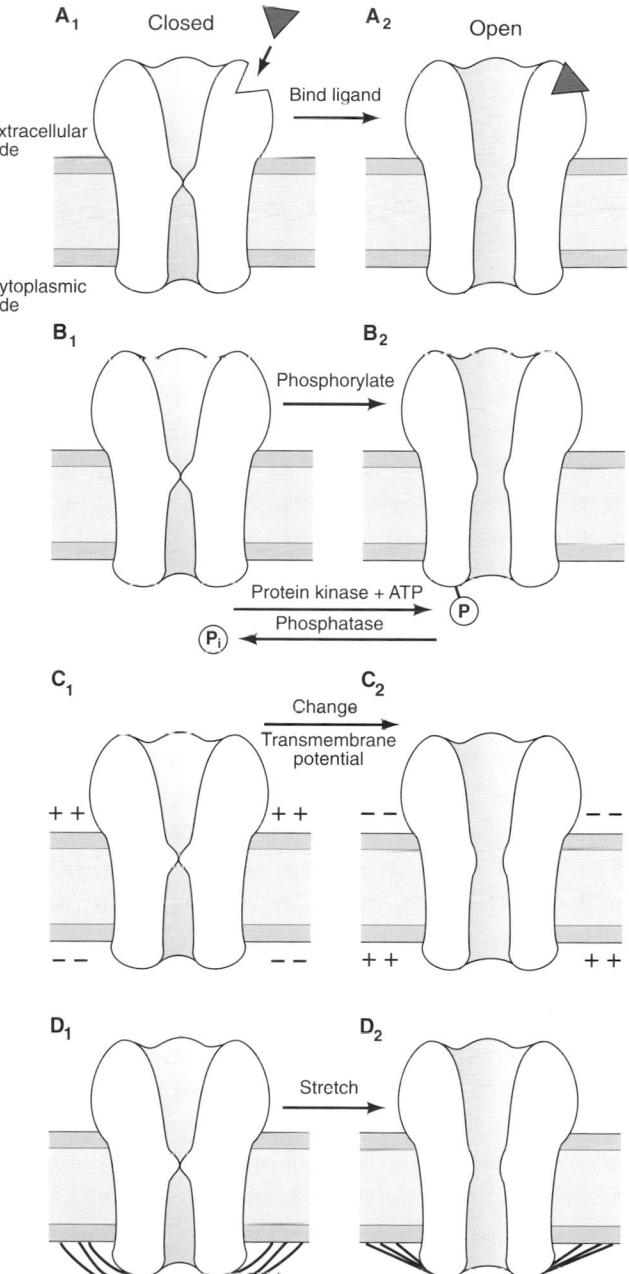

FIGURE 5–12

Channel gating is controlled by several types of stimuli.

A. Ligand-gated channels open in response to binding of the ligand to its receptor. The energy from ligand binding drives channel gating toward an open state.

B. Protein phosphorylation and dephosphorylation regulate the opening and closing of some channels. The energy for channel opening comes from the transfer of the high-energy phosphate, P.

C. Changes in membrane voltage can open and close some channels. The energy for channel gating comes from changes in the electrical potential difference across the membrane.

D. Other channels are activated by stretch or pressure. The energy for gating may come from mechanical forces due to channel–cytoskeleton interactions.

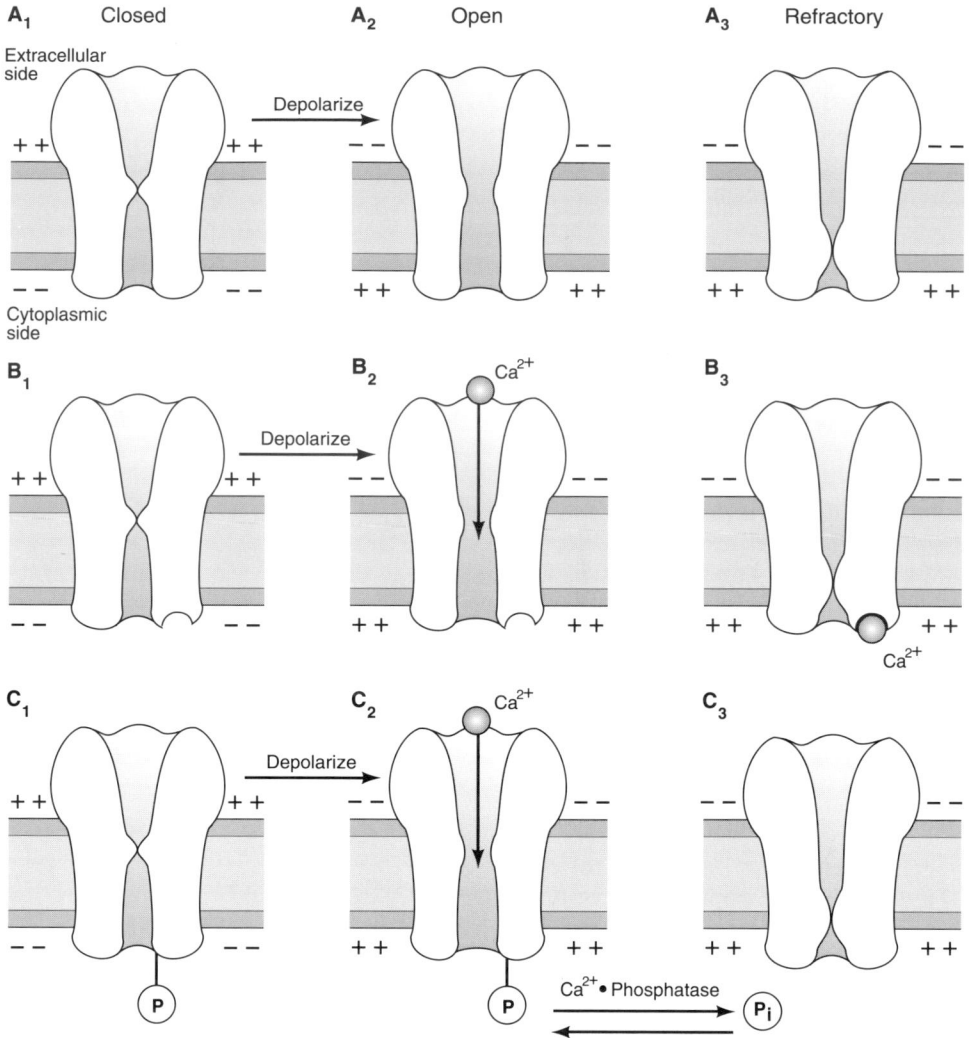

FIGURE 5–13

Three mechanisms by which channels can enter refractory states in which they are closed and incapable of being activated.

A. Voltage-gated channels often respond to a change in membrane potential by first going from a closed resting state (**1**) to a transient open state (**2**). The channel then enters a prolonged refractory or inactivated state (**3**). Only after the potential difference across the membrane is restored to its original value can the channel recover from inactivation, returning to the resting state (**1**).

B. Intracellular Ca^{2+} causes inactivation in some channels by directly binding to the channel. The internal Ca^{2+} level rises as

a result of the opening of voltage-dependent Ca^{2+} channels in response to depolarization. The internal Ca^{2+} then can act in a *cis* manner, inactivating the channel that permitted its entry. Alternatively, internal Ca^{2+} can act in a *trans* fashion, causing inactivation of other types of ion channels.

C. An increase in internal Ca^{2+} concentration may also activate phosphatases (calcineurin) and produce inactivation through dephosphorylation of Ca^{2+} channels. At high concentrations, Ca^{2+} may even produce an irreversible, nonspecific inactivation of channels due to recruitment of Ca^{2+}-activated proteases.

we shall consider in more detail in Chapter 12, the second messenger may act on the inside of the channel either directly, by binding to the channel, or indirectly, by initiating protein phosphorylation that is mediated by enzymes called *protein kinases* (Figure 5–12B). This covalent modification of the channel is reversed by dephosphorylation, a reaction catalyzed by protein phosphatases. Covalent modification results in relatively long-lasting changes in the functional states of ion channels called *modulatory changes*. Because ion channels are integral membrane proteins, some are subject to the influence of two other classes of allosteric regulators: the electric field

across the membrane and the mechanical stretch of the membrane (Figure 5–12C, D). Under the influence of allosteric regulators, ion channels can enter one of three functional states: closed and activatable (resting); open (active); closed and nonactivatable (refractory).

How does a given stimulus, such as a voltage change or ligand binding, produce a change in conformation of a channel? For voltage-gated channels, such as the Na^+ channel, the opening and closing is associated with a movement of a charged region of the channel through the electric field of the membrane. Changes in the membrane voltage tend to move this charged region back and forth

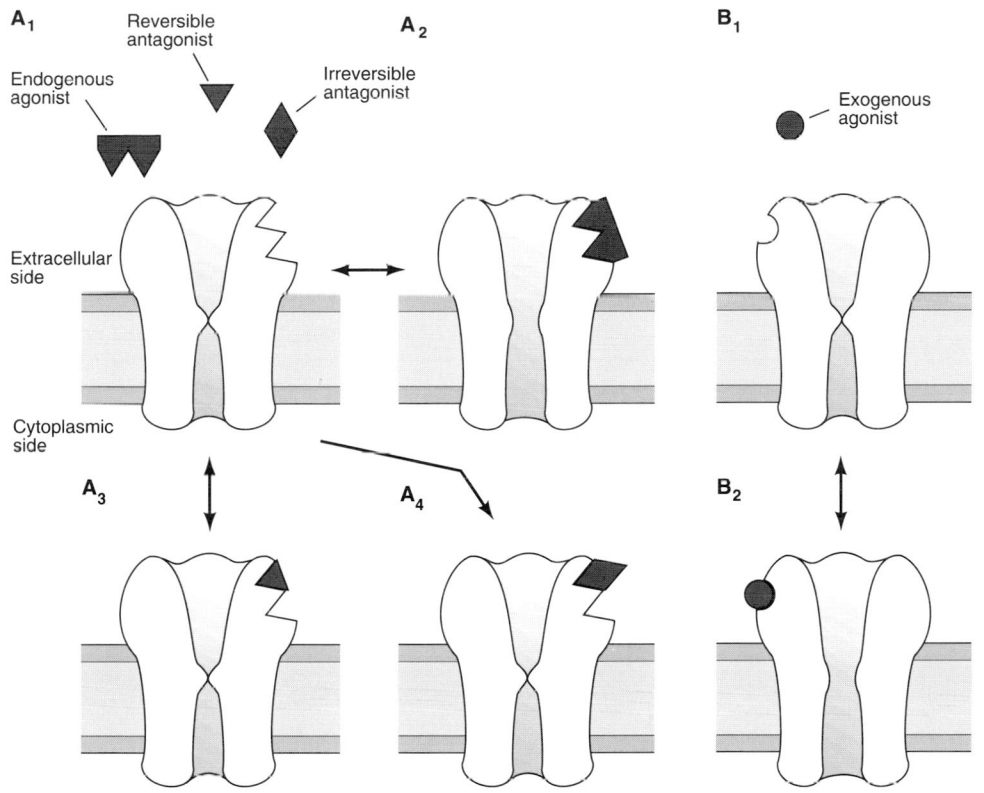

FIGURE 5–14
The binding of exogenous ligands to a channel can bias the channel to either an open or a closed state by a variety of mechanisms.

A. For a channel that normally is opened by the binding of an endogenous ligand (**1, 2**), a drug or toxin may block the binding of the activator by either a reversible (**3**) or irreversible (**4**) reaction.

B. Some exogenous regulators can bias a channel to the open state by binding to a regulatory site.

through the electric field, and thus drive the channel between closed and open states. For transmitter-gated channels, the change in free energy of the ligand bound to its site on the channel as compared to the ligand in solution leads to channel opening. For mechanically activated channels the energy associated with membrane stretch is thought to be transferred to the channel through the cytoskeleton (Figure 5–12).

The rates at which transitions occur between open and closed states of a channel depend on the signals that gate the channel. For a voltage-gated channel, the rates are steeply dependent on membrane potential. Although these rates can vary from the microsecond to minute time scale, on average they tend to require a few milliseconds. Thus, once a channel opens, it stays open for a few milliseconds before closing, and after it closes it stays closed for a few milliseconds before opening again. This time scale of gating is much slower than the rate of ion permeation through an open channel, which occurs in less than a microsecond. Once a transition between an open and closed state begins, it proceeds virtually instantaneously (in less than 10 μsec, the present limits of experimental measurements), giving rise to abrupt, all-or-none step-like changes in single channel current as the channel goes from a fully closed to a fully open state.

Ligand-gated and voltage-gated channels enter refractory states through different processes. Ligand-gated channels can enter the refractory state when they are exposed to a high concentration of the ligand. This process is called *desensitization*. At present, desensitization is not com-

pletely understood. In some channels it appears to be an intrinsic property of the channel, whereas in others it is due to phosphorylation of the channel molecule by a protein kinase. Many, but not all, voltage-gated channels can enter a refractory state following activation. This process is termed *inactivation*. Inactivation of voltage-gated Na^+ and K^+ channels is thought to be due to a conformational change in the channels, controlled by a subunit or region of the channel separate from that which controls activation. For example, intracellular application of certain proteolytic enzymes can eliminate the ability of voltage-gated Na^+ channels to inactivate without affecting the ability of the channel to be activated. In contrast, inactivation of certain voltage-gated Ca^{2+} channels is thought to be a consequence of Ca^{2+} influx. In this case, an increase in internal Ca^{2+} concentration inactivates the Ca^{2+} channel either directly, by binding to an allosteric control site on the inside of the channel, or indirectly, by activating an intracellular enzyme that inactivates the channel by protein dephosphorylation (Figure 5–13).

Exogenous factors, such as drugs and toxins, can modulate the allosteric control sites of an ion channel. Most of these agents bias the channel toward the closed state (Figure 5–14). Some compounds act as competitive inhibitors, binding to the same site at which the normal gating ligand binds. This binding may be either of low energy and reversible—as in the blockade of the nicotinic acetylcholine (ACh) receptor-channel by the poison curare—or of high energy and not reversible—as in the blockade of the ACh receptor-channel by the snake venom poison α-bunga-

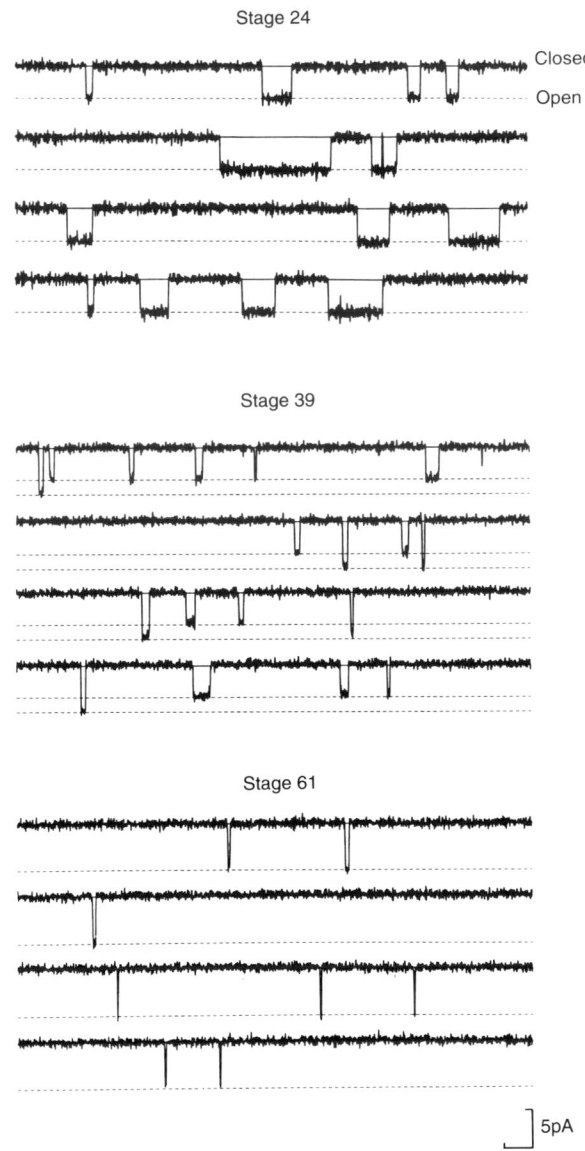

Stage 24

Closed

Open

Stage 39

Stage 61

5pA

10 msec

FIGURE 5–15
The functional properties of ion channels can change over the course of development. These examples of conductance in individual ACh-activated channels were recorded from *Xenopus* myotomal muscle at early, intermediate, and late stages of development. In immature muscle the single channels have a small conductance and a relatively long open time. In mature muscle the channel conductance is larger and the average open time is smaller. At intermediate stages of development the population of channels is mixed, exhibiting both types of gating behavior and both classes of conductance. (From Owens and Kullberg, 1989.)

rotoxin. Other exogenous substances act in a noncompetitive or allosteric manner and affect the normal gating mechanism only indirectly. This type of inhibition can work not only on gating transitions normally controlled by ligand binding, but also on those controlled by voltage and by stretch. A few exogenous allosteric modulators bias the channel to the open state.

Variants of Each Type of Ion Channel Are Found in Different Tissues

More than a dozen basic channel types are known to exist in neurons, and each type includes several closely related isoforms that differ in their rate of opening or closing and sensitivity to different regulators of gating. This variability is generated either by differential expression of two or more homologous genes, or by alternative splicing of the mRNA from the same gene. As with isozymes of a particular enzyme, variants of a channel type are expressed at different developmental stages, in different cell types and even in different regions within a cell (Figure 5–15). These subtle variations in structure and function of an ion channel type are presumed to adapt the channel to its specific function. The rich variety of cell-specific subtypes of ion channels may make it possible to develop drugs that can activate or block channels in selected regions of the nervous system. Such drugs can, in principle, be selected to have maximum therapeutic effectiveness with a minimum of side effects.

Genes That Encode Ion Channels Can Be Grouped into Families

Three gene families encode most of the ion channels that have been described to date. The members of a given gene family show substantial amino acid sequence homology with one another. Each family is thought to have evolved from a common ancestral gene by gene duplication and divergence. The genes that encode voltage-gated ion channels, selective for either Ca^{2+}, Na^+, or K^+, belong to one of these families. Similarly, transmitter-gated ion channels that are sensitive to either ACh, γ-aminobutyric acid (GABA), or glycine belong to another. Like the family of voltage-gated ion channels, the members of the transmitter-gated ion channel family can differ from each other in ion selectivity. The genes coding for the different gap junction channels, specialized channels that bridge the cytoplasm of two cells, form the third class of channel gene families (see Chapter 9). Because the genes for only a few ion channels have been sequenced, it remains to be seen how many additional channel families exist.

An Overall View

Ion channels are an important class of membrane-spanning glycoproteins that exist in all cells and govern the flow of ions across the membrane. In nerve and muscle cells they are important for controlling the rapid changes in membrane potential associated with the action potential and postsynaptic potentials. The Ca^{2+} influx controlled by these channels can alter many metabolic processes within cells, leading to activation of various enzymes and proteins. As described in Chapter 13, Ca^{2+} influx also acts as a trigger for the release of neurotransmitter.

Channels can be distinguished from each other on the basis of their ion selectivity and the factors that control their opening and closing, or gating. Ion selectivity is achieved through physical-chemical interaction between the ion and various amino acid residues that line the walls of the channel pore. Gating involves a conformational change of the channel in response to various external stimuli, including voltage, ligands, and stretch or pressure.

Two methodological advances in the past several years have greatly increased our understanding of channel function. First, the patch-clamp technique has made it possible to measure directly the activity of single ion channel molecules by recording the unit current flow through single open channels. Second, gene cloning and sequencing have determined the primary amino acid sequences of many ion channels. From these results, many of the channels described so far can be grouped into two gene families: the voltage-gated channels (including channels selective for Na^+, K^+, and Ca^{2+}) and the transmitter-gated channels.

The activity of channels can be modified by cellular metabolic reactions, including protein phosphorylation, by various ions that act as blockers, and by toxins, poisons, and drugs. Channels are also important targets in various diseases. Certain autoimmune neurological disorders, such as myasthenia gravis and the Lambert–Eaton syndrome (which we will discuss in Chapter 16), are thought to result from the actions of specific antibodies interfering with channel function. Cystic fibrosis is thought to involve a genetic defect in the control of a certain type of chloride channel. With our increasing understanding of channel structure and function it seems likely that other diseases of channel function will soon be identified. Through a detailed knowledge of the genetic basis of channel structure and function, it may one day be possible to devise new pharmacological therapies for certain neurologic and psychiatric disorders.

Selected Readings

Catterall, W. A. 1988. Structure and function of voltage-sensitive ion channels. Science 242:50–61.

Hille, B. 1984. Ionic Channels of Excitable Membranes. Sunderland, Mass.: Sinauer

Miller, C. 1987. How ion channel proteins work. In L. K. Kaczmarek and I. B. Levitan (eds.), Neuromodulation: The Biological Control of Neuronal Excitability. New York: Oxford University Press, pp. 39–63.

Miller, C. 1989. Genetic manipulation of ion channels: A new approach to structure and mechanism. Neuron 2:1195–1205.

References

Alberts, B., Bray, D., Lewis, J., Raff, M., Roberts, K., and Watson, J. D. 1989. Molecular Biology of the Cell, 2nd ed. New York: Garland.

Anderson, C. R., and Stevens, C. F. 1973. Voltage clamp analysis of acetylcholine produced end-plate current fluctuations at frog neuromuscular junction. J. Physiol. (Lond.) 235:655–691.

Armstrong, C. M. 1981. Sodium channels and gating currents. Physiol. Rev. 61:644–683.

Armstrong, D. L. 1989. Calcium channel regulation by calcineurin, a Ca^{2+}-activated phosphatase in mammalian brain. Trends Neurosci. 12:117–122.

Bayliss, W. M. 1918. Principles of General Physiology, 2nd ed., rev. New York: Longmans, Green.

Eisenman, G. 1962. Cation selective glass electrodes and their mode of operation. Biophys. J. 2 (Suppl. 2):259–323.

Frech, G. C., Van Dongen, A. M. J., Schuster, G., Brown, A. M., and Joho, R. H. 1989. A novel potassium channel with delayed rectifier properties isolated from rat brain by expression cloning. Nature 340:642–645.

Guharay, F., and Sachs, F. 1984. Stretch-activated single ion channel currents in tissue-cultured embryonic chick skeletal muscle. J. Physiol. (Lond.) 352:685–701.

Hamill, O. P., Marty, A., Neher, E., Sakmann, B., and Sigworth, F. J. 1981. Improved patch-clamp techniques for high-resolution current recording from cells and cell-free membrane patches. Pflügers Arch. 391:85–100.

Henderson, R., and Unwin, P. N. T. 1975. Three-dimensional model of purple membrane obtained by electron microscopy. Nature 257:28–32.

Hladky, S. B., and Haydon, D. A. 1970. Discreteness of conductance change in bimolecular lipid membranes in the presence of certain antibiotics. Nature 225:451–453.

Horn, R., and Patlak, J. 1980. Single channel currents from excised patches of muscle membrane. Proc. Natl. Acad. Sci. U.S.A. 77:6930–6934.

Huang, K. -S., Radhakrishnan, R., Bayley, H., and Khorana, H. G. 1982. Orientation of retinal in bacteriorhodopsin as studied by cross-linking using a photosensitive analog of retinal. J. Biol. Chem. 257:13616–13623.

Imoto, K., Methfessel, C., Sakmann, B., Mishina, M., Mori, Y., Konno, T., Fukuda, K., Kurasaki, M., Bujo, H., Fujita, Y., and Numa, S. 1986. Location of a δ-subunit region determining ion transport through the acetylcholine receptor channel. Nature 324:670–674.

Katz, B., and Miledi, R. 1970. Membrane noise produced by acetylcholine. Nature 226:962–963.

Katz, B., and Thesleff, S. 1957. A study of the 'desensitization' produced by acetylcholine at the motor end-plate. J. Physiol. (Lond.) 138:63–80.

Kyte, J., and Doolittle, R. F. 1982. A simple method for displaying the hydropathic character of a protein. J. Mol. Biol. 157:105–132.

Miller, C. (ed.) 1986. Ion Channel Reconstitution. New York: Plenum Press.

Mueller, P., Rudin, D. O., Tien, H. T., and Wescott, W. C. 1962. Reconstitution of cell membrane structure in vitro and its transformation into an excitable system. Nature 194:979–980.

Mullins, L. J. 1961. The macromolecular properties of excitable membranes. Ann. N.Y. Acad. Sci. 94:390–404.

Neher, E., and Sakmann, B. 1976. Single-channel currents recorded from membrane of denervated frog muscle fibres. Nature 260:799–802.

Noda, M., Takahashi, H., Tanabe, T., Toyosato, M., Kikyotani, S., Furutani, Y., Hirose, T., Takashima, H., Inayama, S., Miyata, T., and Numa, S. 1983. Structural homology of Torpedo californica acetylcholine receptor subunits. Nature 302:528–532.

Owens, J. L., and Kullberg, R. 1989. In vivo development of nicotinic acetylcholine receptor channels in Xenopus myotomal muscle. J. Neurosci. 9:1018–1028.

Sawyer, D. B., Koeppe, R. E. II, and Andersen, O. S. 1989. Induction of conductance heterogeneity in gramicidin channels. Biochemistry 28:6571–6583.

Tempel, B. L., Papazian, D. M., Schwarz, T. L., Jan, Y. N., and Jan, L. Y. 1987. Sequence of a probable potassium channel component encoded at Shaker locus of Drosophila. Science 237:770–775.

Urry, D. W. 1971. The gramicidin A transmembrane channel: A proposed $\pi_{(L,D)}$ helix. Proc. Natl. Acad. Sci. U.S.A. 68:672–676.

John Koester

Membrane Potential

Membrane Potential Results from the Separation of Charge Across the Cell Membrane

The Resting Membrane Potential Is Determined by the Relative Abundance of Different Types of Nongated Ion Channels

Nongated Channels in Glial Cells Are Selective Only for Potassium

Nongated Channels in Nerve Cells Are Selective for Several Ion Species

The Passive Fluxes of Sodium and Potassium Through Nongated Channels Are Balanced by Active Pumping of Sodium and Potassium Ions

Chloride Ions Are Often Passively Distributed

The Action Potential Is Generated by the Sequential Opening of Voltage-Gated Channels Selective for Sodium and Potassium

The Resting and Action Potentials Can Be Quantified by the Goldman Equation

The Neuron Can Be Represented by an Electrical Equivalent Circuit

Each Ion Channel Acts as a Conductor and Battery

An Equivalent Circuit Model of the Membrane Includes Batteries, Conductors, a Capacitor, and a Current Generator

An Overall View

Postscript

Calculation of Membrane Potential from the Equivalent Circuit Model of the Neuron

The Equation for Membrane Potential Can Be Written in a More General Form

The Sodium–Potassium Pump Counteracts the Passive Fluxes of Sodium and Potassium

The flow of information within and between neurons is conveyed by electrical and chemical signals. Transient electrical signals are particularly important for transferring information rapidly and over long distances. These electrical signals—receptor potentials, synaptic potentials, and action potentials—are all produced by temporary changes in the current flow into and out of the cell that drives the electrical potential across the cell membrane away from its resting value.

Current flow into and out of the cell is controlled by ion channels embedded in the cell membrane. There are two types of ion channels in membrane—gated and nongated. Nongated channels are always open and are not influenced significantly by extrinsic factors. They are primarily important in maintaining the resting membrane potential—the electrical potential across the membrane in the absence of signaling activity. Gated channels, in contrast, can open and close. Most gated channels are closed when the membrane is at rest, and their probability of opening is greatly enhanced by the three influences that we considered in the last chapter—change in membrane potential, ligand binding, or stretch of the membrane.

An analysis of the mechanisms underlying the resting membrane potential is a first step toward understanding how transient electrical signals are generated. Therefore, in this chapter we shall first discuss how the nongated ion channels establish the resting potential and how the flux of ions through gated channels generates the action potential. We shall then illustrate how the channels, along with other components important for nerve cell signaling, can be represented by an electrical equivalent circuit. The circuit approach is commonly used in neurobiology because it provides a complete quantitative description of the electrical signaling properties of the neuron. An understanding of this equivalent circuit model provides basic insights into the principles of signaling in excitable cells and serves as an essential foundation for interpreting all clinical tests of the electrical function of nerve and muscle. The equivalent circuit approach is extended in Chapter 7 to describe how the passive, nonchanging electrical properties of the neuron influence the active signals—action potentials, synaptic potentials, and receptor potentials. The gating mechanisms of ion channels that mediate these three types of signals are then described in Chapters 8–11 and 23, respectively.

Membrane Potential Results from the Separation of Charge Across the Cell Membrane

Every neuron has a separation of electrical charge across its cell membrane consisting of a thin cloud of positive and negative ions spread over the inner and outer surfaces of the membrane (Figure 6–1). A nerve cell at rest has an excess of positive charges on the outside of the membrane and an excess of negative charges on the inside. This separation of charge is maintained because the lipid bilayer acts as a barrier to the diffusion of ions, as explained in Chapter 5. The charge separation gives rise to an electrical potential difference across the membrane. The potential difference, or voltage, is called the *resting membrane potential*. It is directly proportional to the charge separation across the membrane. In most neurons the resting membrane potential ranges from about 60 mV to 70 mV. All electrical signaling results from brief changes away from the resting membrane potential (Box 6–1).

The term resting membrane potential applies only to the potential across the membrane when the cell is at rest. The more general term *membrane potential* refers to the electrical potential difference across the membrane at any moment in time—at rest or during signaling. By convention, the potential outside the cell is arbitrarily defined as zero, so membrane potential (V_m) is defined as

$$V_m = V_{in} - V_{out}$$

where V_{in} is the potential on the inside of the cell and V_{out} the potential on the outside. According to this convention the resting potential (V_R) is negative

$$V_R = -60 \text{ to } -70 \text{ mV}.$$

In an ionic solution electrical current is carried by ions—both anions and cations. By convention, the direction of current flow is defined as the direction of *net* movement of *positive* charge. Thus, in an ionic solution cations move in the same direction as the current, and anions move in the opposite direction. The charge separation across the membrane is disturbed whenever there is a net flux of ions into or out of the cell, thus altering the polarization of the membrane. A reduction of the charge separation is called *depolarization*; an increase in charge separation is called *hyperpolarization* (see Box 6–1). Passive depolarizing or hyperpolarizing responses of the membrane potential to current flow are called *electrotonic potentials*. Hyperpolarizing responses are purely passive. Small depolarizations are also passive. However, at a critical level of depolarization, called the *threshold*,

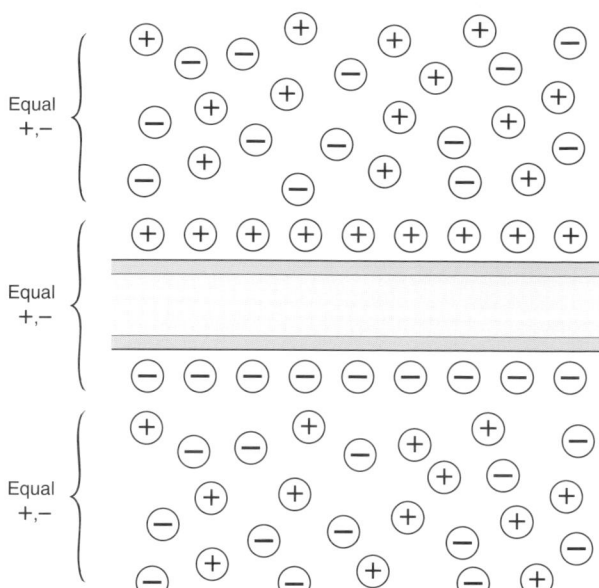

FIGURE 6–1
The membrane potential results from a separation of positive and negative charges across the cell membrane. The excess of positive charges outside and negative charges inside the membrane of a nerve cell at rest represents a small fraction of the total number of ions inside and outside the cell.

the cell responds actively with an all-or-none *action potential* (Box 6–1).

We shall begin our examination of the membrane potential by analyzing how the passive flux of individual ion species through nongated membrane channels generates the resting potential. We shall then be able to understand how the selective gating of different types of ion channels generates the action potential, as well as the receptor and synaptic potentials.

The Resting Membrane Potential Is Determined by the Relative Abundance of Different Types of Nongated Ion Channels

No single ion species is distributed equally on the two sides of a nerve cell membrane. Of the four most abundant types of ions found on either side of the cell membrane, Na^+ and Cl^- are more concentrated outside the cell, and K^+ and organic anions (A^-) are more concentrated inside. The organic anions are primarily organic acids and proteins. The distribution of these ions inside and outside the membrane of the giant axon of the squid, which is a popular experimental preparation for neurophysiology, is shown in Table 6–1. In vertebrate nerve cells the absolute values of the concentration of various ions in nerve cells are two- to threefold lower, but the concentration gradients are about the same.

The unequal distribution of ions raises two important questions. First, how do these ionic gradients contribute

Recording the Membrane Potential

BOX 6–1

Reliable techniques for intracellular recordings were developed in the late 1940s. These allowed measurement across the membrane of both the resting and the action potentials. To measure the resting potential, an intracellular electrode is inserted into the nerve cell. The electrode is a glass pipette drawn out to a tip about 0.5 μm in diameter and filled with a concentrated salt solution (usually 3 M KCl). The pipette acts as a salt bridge, providing an electrical connection between the cytoplasm and a metal electrode that is connected to the electronic apparatus. A second salt bridge of the same ionic composition, connected to a metal electrode, is used as the extracellular electrode. The two metal electrodes inserted into the back ends of the two salt bridges are connected to a voltage amplifier, which in turn is connected to an oscilloscope that displays the amplitude of the membrane potential as the vertical deflection of a spot of light on the screen.

FIGURE 6–2A

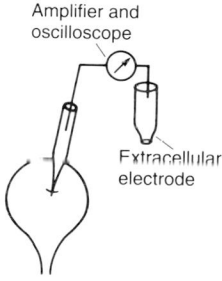

Amplifier and oscilloscope

Extracellular electrode

When both electrodes are outside the cell, no electrical potential difference is recorded; but as soon as one electrode is inserted into the cell, the oscilloscope displays a steady deflection of about −65 mV, the resting membrane potential.

FIGURE 6–2B

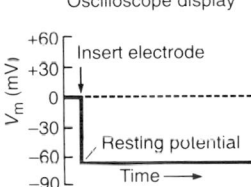

Oscilloscope display

Insert electrode

Resting potential

The membrane potential can be changed using a current generator connected to a second pair of electrodes—one intracellular and one extracellular. By making the intracellular current electrode positive with respect to the external electrode, the current generator delivers a pulse of current that depolarizes the cell. Current flows into the neuron from the intracellular electrode causing a net accumulation of

positive charge on the inside of the membrane; at the same time, net positive charge is withdrawn from the outside of the membrane by the extracellular electrode. The result is a progressive decrease in the normal separation of charge or *depolarization*.

FIGURE 6–2C

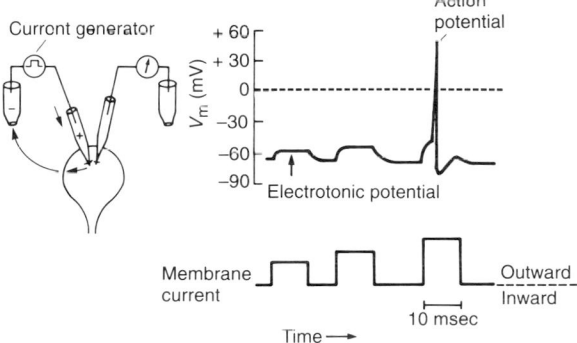

Current generator

Action potential

Electrotonic potential

Membrane current

Outward

Inward

Time →   10 msec

Reversing the direction of current flow—by making the intracellular electrode negative with respect to the extracellular electrode—makes the membrane potential more negative. This results in an increase in charge separation or *hyperpolarization.*

FIGURE 6–2D

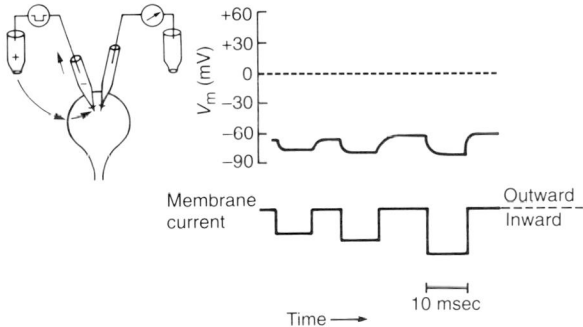

Membrane current

Outward

Inward

Time →   10 msec

The membrane can respond to current injections either passively or actively. The responses to hyperpolarization are purely passive (electrotonic). As the size of the current pulse increases, the hyperpolarization increases proportionately. Likewise, small depolarizing current pulses evoke purely electrotonic potentials, and the size of the potential change is proportional to the size of the current pulses. However, depolarizing current eventually drives the membrane potential to a critical level called the *threshold*, where an active response, the all-or-none *action potential*, is triggered (Figure 6–2C). The action potential differs from the electrotonic potential in magnitude, duration, and the way in which it is generated.

TABLE 6–1. Distribution of the Major Ions Across the Membrane of the Squid Giant Axon

Ion	Cytoplasm (mM)	Extracellular fluid (mM)	Nernst potential* (mV)
K^+	400	20	-75
Na^+	50	440	$+55$
Cl^-	52	560	-60
A^-	385	—	—

*The membrane potential at which there is no net flux of an ion across the cell membrane.

to the resting membrane potential? Second, how are they maintained? What prevents the ionic gradients from being dissipated by passive diffusion of ions across the membrane through the passive (nongated) channels? These two questions are interrelated, and we shall answer them by considering two examples of membrane permeability: the resting membrane of glial cells, which is selectively permeable to only one species of ions, and the resting membrane of nerve cells, which is permeable to three species of ions. In this discussion we shall consider only the nongated ion channels, which are always open.

Nongated Channels in Glial Cells Are Selective Only for Potassium

A membrane's selectivity for permeant ions is determined by the relative proportions of various types of ion channels. The membranes of glial cells have nongated channels that for the most part are selectively permeable to K^+, and thus are almost exclusively permeable to K^+ ions when the cell is at rest. A glial cell has a high concentration of K^+ and organic anions on the inside and a high concentration of Na^+ and Cl^- on the outside. Assume that initially there is no potential difference across the membrane. Since the glial cell membrane is selectively permeable to K^+, the K^+ diffuses down its *concentration gradient* out of the cell, leaving nonpermeant anions behind (Figure 6–3).[1] The result is a surplus of cations outside the cell and a surplus of anions inside the cell. The electrostatic attraction between the excess cations on the outside of the membrane and the excess anions on the inner surface generates a thin cloud of positive charges on the exterior surface of the membrane and an equal density of negative charge on the interior surface (Figure 6–1).

The diffusion of K^+ out of the cell is self-limiting. The buildup of positive charge outside the cell and negative charge inside impedes the efflux of K^+ by electrostatic repulsion and attraction. Thus, two opposing forces act on each K^+ ion, one chemical and the other electrical. The

---

[1]If there is no electrical potential difference across the membrane, the permeability of the membrane to an ion (P_i) is defined as the net flux (J_i) of that ion divided by the product of the concentration difference of that ion across the membrane (ΔC_i) times the membrane area (A):

$$P_i = J_i / (\Delta C_i A).$$

driving force of the chemical concentration gradient tends to drive K^+ out of the cell through the K^+ channels. As the outside of the cell membrane becomes positive relative to the inside, the electrostatic force due to the charge separation results in an *electrical potential difference* that tends to push K^+ back into the cell. The difference in electrical potential across the membrane increases as the diffusion of K^+ continues to increase the separation of charge. It continues to increase until it reaches a value that has an effect on K^+ equal and opposite to the effect of the concentration gradient. At this value of membrane potential, which in most glial cells is about -75 mV, the K^+ concentrations inside and outside the cell are in equilibrium. In a cell permeable only to K^+ ions the resting membrane potential is therefore the K^+ *equilibrium potential*.

In a cell that has only K^+ channels in its membrane, no metabolic energy is required to maintain the ionic concentration gradients shown in Table 6–1. The membrane potential automatically settles at the K^+ equilibrium potential. The gradients for other ions are not important, because these ions cannot pass through the membrane. Thus, once the ionic gradients are established, they will persist indefinitely with no expenditure of metabolic energy.

The membrane potential at which K^+ ions are in equilibrium across the membrane can be calculated from an equation derived in 1888 from basic thermodynamic principles by the German physical chemist Walter Nernst:

$$E_K = \frac{RT}{ZF} \ln \frac{[K^+]_o}{[K^+]_i} \qquad \textbf{Nernst Equation}$$

where E_K is the value of membrane potential at which K^+ is in equilibrium (the K^+ *Nernst potential*), R is the gas constant, T the temperature in degrees Kelvin, Z the valence of K^+, F the Faraday constant, and $[K^+]_o$ and $[K^+]_i$ the concentrations of K^+ on the outside and inside of the cell. To be precise, chemical activities should be used rather than concentrations. For K^+, $Z = +1$, and at 25°C RT/ZF is 26 mV. The constant for converting from natural logarithms to base 10 logarithms is 2.3. Substituting the values of K^+ concentration given in Table 6–1, we have

$$E_K = 26 \text{ mV} \times 2.3 \log_{10} \frac{20}{400} = -75 \text{ mV}.$$

The Nernst equation can be used to find the equilibrium potential of any ion that is present on both sides of a membrane permeable to that ion. The Na^+, K^+, and Cl^- Nernst potentials for the distributions of ions across the squid axon are given in Table 6–1.

Nongated Channels in Nerve Cells Are Selective for Several Ion Species

In 1902 Julius Bernstein used the Nernst equation as the theoretical framework on which to develop the hypothesis that the resting potential of neurons is based on the selective permeability of the membrane to K^+. Bernstein's idea

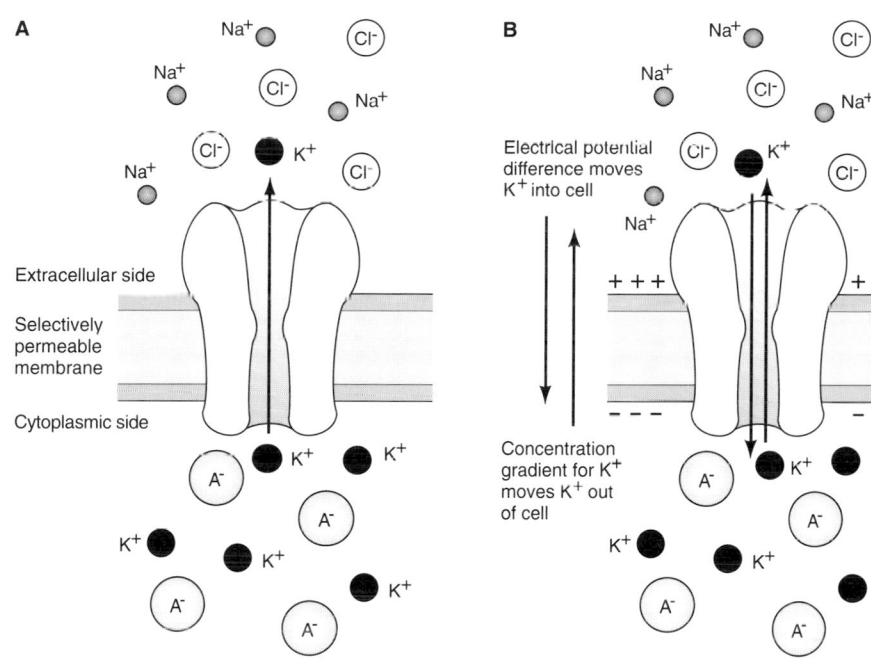

FIGURE 6–3
The flux of K$^+$ across the membrane is determined by both the K$^+$ concentration gradient and the electrical potential across the membrane.

A. In a cell permeable only to K$^+$ the resting potential is generated by the efflux of K$^+$ down its concentration gradient.

B. The continued efflux of K$^+$ builds up an excess of positive charge on the outside of the cell and leaves behind on the inside an excess of negative charge. This buildup of charge acts to impede the further efflux of K$^+$, so that eventually an equilibrium is reached, at which the electrical and chemical driving forces are equal and opposite.

could not be tested quantitatively until the 1940s, when techniques for intracellular recording were developed. It then became possible to compare the measured resting membrane potential to the value of E_K predicted from the Nernst equation. The observed values of membrane potentials in neurons deviate from the theoretical curve for a Nernst potential for K$^+$, particularly at relatively low values of [K$^+$]$_o$ (Figure 6–4). This suggests that neurons at rest have significant numbers of open channels that are selective to ions other than K$^+$. In contrast, the fit between theoretical and observed curves is much better for glial cells, with good agreement down to quite low values of [K$^+$]$_o$. Thus, glial cell membranes can be described to a first approximation as having only open K$^+$ channels when the membrane potential is at its resting value.

Measurements of the resting membrane potential with intracellular electrodes and flux studies using radioactive tracers have verified that, unlike glial cells, nerve cells at rest are permeable to Na$^+$ and Cl$^-$ in addition to K$^+$. Of the most abundant ion species in nerve cells, only the large organic anions, such as amino acids and proteins, are nonpermeant. How can three concentration gradients (for Na$^+$, K$^+$, and Cl$^-$) be maintained across the cell membrane, and how do these three concentration gradients interact to determine the resting membrane potential?

To answer these questions, it will be easiest to examine first only the diffusion of K$^+$ and Na$^+$. Let us return to the simple example of a cell having only K$^+$ channels, with unequal concentration gradients of K$^+$, Na$^+$, Cl$^-$, and A$^-$ as shown in Table 6–1. Under these conditions the resting membrane potential, V_R, is determined solely by the K$^+$ concentration gradient, so that $V_R = E_K$. Now consider what happens if a few Na$^+$ channels are added to the membrane, making it slightly permeable to Na$^+$. Two forces act

on Na$^+$ to drive it into the cell. First, Na$^+$ is more concentrated outside than inside and therefore tends to flow into the cell down its concentration gradient. Second, Na$^+$ is driven into the cell by the electrical potential difference across the membrane. The equilibrium potential for Na$^+$, calculated from the Nernst equation, is

$$E_{Na} = \frac{RT}{ZF} \ln \frac{[Na^+]_o}{[Na^+]_i}.$$

FIGURE 6–4
The relationship between membrane potential and external K$^+$ concentration (log scale) in nerve cells and glia. The calculated Nernst potential for K$^+$ (**solid line**) matches the observed membrane potential in glia (**open circles**) over a wide range of extracellular K$^+$ concentration. In nerve cell membranes, however, the observed potential deviates from the theoretical curve at relatively low values of extracellular K$^+$ (**dashed line**). (Adapted from Orkand, 1977.)

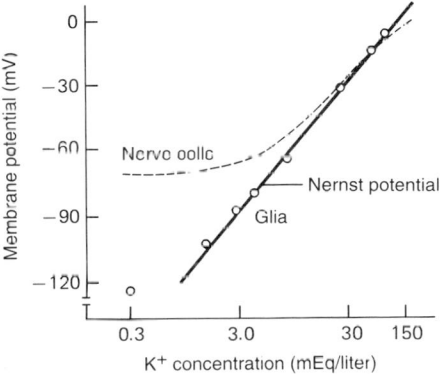

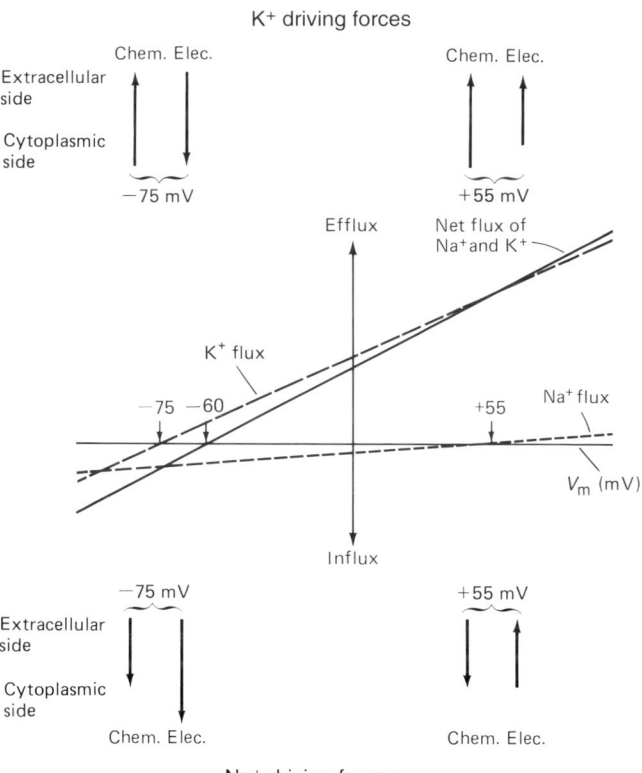

FIGURE 6–5

The resting potential of a cell with nongated Na⁻ and K⁻ channels is defined as the potential at which K⁻ efflux is balanced by Na⁺ influx. The direction and amplitude of the chemical and electrical driving forces acting on Na⁻ and K⁻ are shown for two different values of V_m. They result in the flux curves shown for each ion (**broken lines**) and the net flux curve for Na⁻ and K⁻ combined (**solid line**). The changes in driving force are the same for Na⁺ and K⁻ for a given change in V_m. The difference in the slopes of the Na⁻ and K⁺ flux curves reflects the fact that the resting membrane is more permeable to K⁻ than to Na⁻. The shapes of the Na⁻ and K⁻ flux curves in the plot are simplified considerably. These curves become quite nonlinear as voltage-gated channels begin to open at values of V_m more positive than about −50 mV, as described in Chapter 8.

For the value given in Table 6–1,

$$E_{Na} = 26 \text{ mV} \times 2.3 \log_{10} \frac{440}{50} = +55 \text{ mV}.$$

At a resting membrane potential of −75 mV, Na⁺ will be 130 mV away from equilibrium, and a strong electrochemical force will drive Na⁺ through the open Na⁺ channels.

The influx of Na⁺ (driven by both the concentration and electrical gradients) depolarizes the cell, moving V_m toward E_{Na}. However, since many more K⁺ channels than Na⁺ channels are open in the resting membrane, V_m actually moves only slightly away from E_K and does not come close to approaching E_{Na}. For once V_m begins to diverge from E_K, K⁺ flows out of the cell, tending to counteract the Na⁺ influx. The more V_m differs from E_K, the greater is the electrochemical force driving K⁺ out of the cell, and consequently the greater the K⁺ efflux. Eventually, V_m reaches a resting potential at which the outward movement of K⁺ just balances the inward movement of Na⁺. This balance point (−60 mV) is more positive than E_K (−75 mV), but still far from E_{Na} (+55 mV). Thus, if the resting membrane is only slightly permeable to Na⁺, V_R shifts slightly away from E_K toward E_{Na} (Figure 6–5).

To understand how this balance point is determined, bear in mind that the flux of an ion across a cell membrane is the product of its electrochemical force times the permeability of the membrane to the ion. In a cell at rest ($V_m = V_R$), relatively few Na⁺ channels are open, so the permeability to Na⁺ is quite low. As a result, the influx of

Na⁺ is small, despite the large chemical and electrical forces driving Na⁺ into the cell. The K⁺ concentration gradient driving K⁺ out is only slightly greater than the electrical force acting to hold it in. Nevertheless, because the membrane permeability to K⁺ is relatively large, the small net outward force acting on K⁺ is enough to produce a K⁺ efflux that balances the Na⁺ influx (Figure 6–6).

The Passive Fluxes of Sodium and Potassium Through Nongated Channels Are Balanced by Active Pumping of Sodium and Potassium Ions

For the cell to have a steady resting membrane potential, the charge separation across the membrane must be constant: The influx of positive charge must be balanced by the efflux of positive charge. If these fluxes were not equal, the charge separation across the membrane, and thus the membrane potential, would vary continually. Therefore, for the cell to achieve a resting state, the movement of K⁺ out of the cell must balance the movement of Na⁺ into the cell (Figure 6–5). Although these steady ion leaks cancel each other, they cannot be allowed to continue unopposed for any appreciable length of time. Otherwise, [K⁺]ᵢ would be depleted, [Na⁺]ᵢ would increase, and the ionic gradients would gradually run down, reducing the resting membrane potential.

Dissipation of ionic gradients is prevented by the Na⁺–K⁺ pump, which extrudes Na⁺ from the cell while

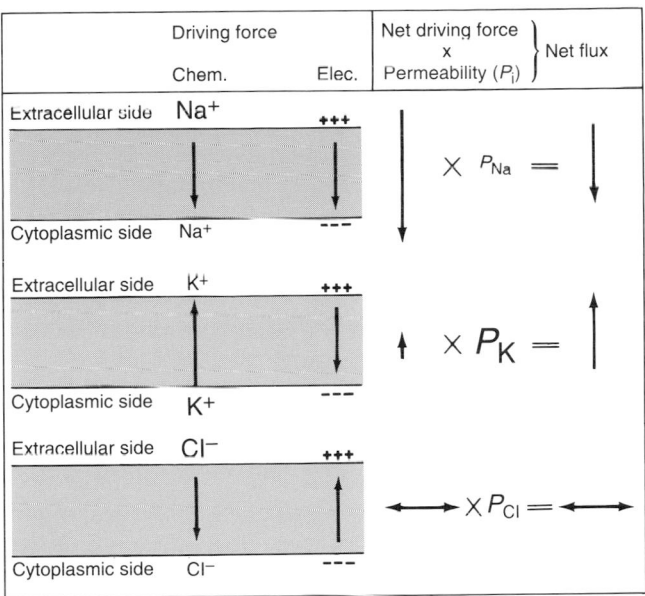

| | Driving force | | Net driving force | |
| | Chem. | Elec. | × Permeability (P_i) | Net flux |

FIGURE 6–6
The fluxes for Na^+, K^+, and Cl^- across the cell membrane are a result of their chemical and electrical driving forces and the permeability of the membrane. The fluxes shown here are for a cell with a membrane potential of -60 mV and the ionic gradients shown in Table 6–1. (**Horizontal arrows** signify no net driving force or no net flux.)

taking in K^+ (Figure 6–7). Because the pump moves Na^+ and K^+ against their net electrochemical gradients, energy must be provided to drive these actively transported fluxes. The energy comes from the hydrolysis of ATP.

The Na^+–K^+ pump is an integral membrane protein. It is a multimeric complex consisting of two different polypeptides: a transmembrane catalytic subunit (α) and a glycoprotein regulatory subunit (β). The probable structure of the holoenzyme is $\alpha_2\beta_2$ with a molecular weight of 270,000. The catalytic subunit has binding sites for Na^+ and ATP on its intracellular surface and sites for K^+ and ouabain, a poison that specifically and irreversibly inhibits the pump, on its extracellular surface. ATP transfers its terminal phosphate group to the catalytic subunit (E)

forming a covalent intermediate (E-P) at a specific β-aspartic acid residue. This reaction depends on the presence of Na^+ ions:

$$E + ATP \xrightleftharpoons{Na^+} E\text{-}P + ADP.$$

Protein phosphorylation changes the conformation of the complex, which leads to the removal of three Na^+ ions from the inside of the cell to the outside in exchange for two extracellular K^+ ions. The phosphorylated catalytic subunit is hydrolyzed in the presence of K^+ ions:

$$E\text{-}P + H_2O \xrightarrow{K^+} + P_i.$$

Thus, the overall reaction results in the hydrolysis of ATP.

When the cell is at rest, the active fluxes (driven by the pump) and the passive fluxes (due to diffusion) are balanced for Na^+ and K^+, so that the net flux of each of these two ions is zero. Thus, at the resting membrane potential the cell is not in equilibrium, but rather in a *steady state*: Metabolic energy must be used to maintain the ionic gradients across the membrane.

Because the pump extrudes three Na^+ ions for every two K^+ ions it brings in, it is said to be electrogenic. This outward flux of positive charge tends to hyperpolarize the membrane. The greater the hyperpolarization, the greater the inward electrochemical force driving Na^+ into the cell, and the smaller the force driving K^+ out. Thus, Na^+ current (I_{Na}) and K^+ current (I_K) that result from passive diffusion are no longer in balance, and there is a net inward current through the nongated channels. The steady state for such a cell is achieved when a membrane potential is reached at which there is a net passive inward current through the ion channels that exactly counterbalances the active outward current driven by the pump. This balance occurs when three Na^+ ions diffuse in for every two K^+ ions that diffuse out. When this condition is met, the active and passive fluxes of Na^+ are equal and opposite, as are the corresponding K^+ fluxes, so the concentration gradients for Na^+ and K^+ remain constant. The resting potential for a cell with an electrogenic pump is typically a few millivolts more negative than would be expected from the purely passive diffusion of ions.

FIGURE 6–7
When the cell is at rest the passive fluxes of Na^+ and K^+ into and out of the cell are balanced by active transport driven in the opposite direction by the ATP-dependent Na^+–K^+ pump.

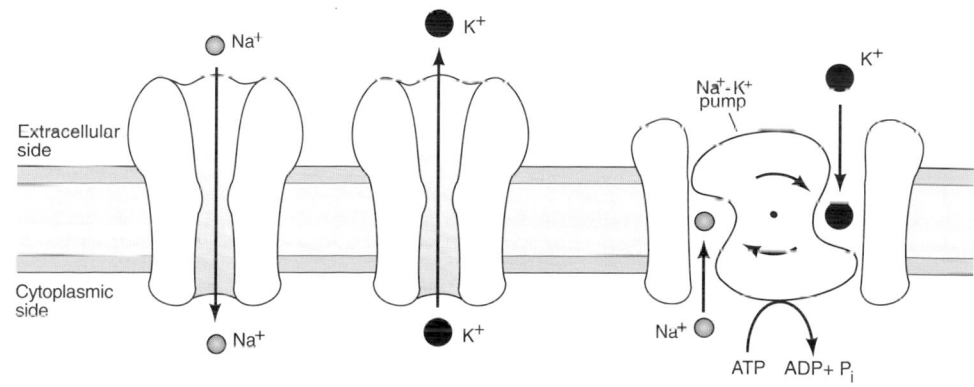

Chloride Ions Are Often Passively Distributed

In the discussion above we have ignored the contribution of Cl^- to the generation of the resting potential, even though all nerve cells have nongated Cl^- channels. Whether this simplification is valid for a particular type of cell depends on whether the cell membrane has a Cl^- pump. In cells without a Cl^- pump V_R is ultimately determined by K^+ and Na^+ fluxes, because their intracellular concentrations are fixed by the Na^+–K^+ pump. The Cl^- concentration inside the cell is free to change, because it is acted on only by passive forces (electrical potential and concentration gradient). In a cell with no Cl^- pump, therefore, Cl^- ions must be in equilibrium across the membrane and the concentration ratio of intracellular and extracellular Cl^- settles at a value such that $E_{Cl} = V_R$.

In nerve cells that do have a Cl^- pump the active transport is directed outward, so that $[Cl^-]_o/[Cl^-]_i$ is greater than the ratio that would result from passive diffusion alone. The effect of increasing the Cl^- gradient is to make E_{Cl} more negative than V_m. This difference between E_{Cl} and V_R results in a steady inward leak of Cl^- that is balanced by active extrusion of Cl^- by the Cl^- pump.

The Action Potential Is Generated by the Sequential Opening of Voltage-Gated Channels Selective for Sodium and Potassium

In the nerve cell at rest, the steady Na^+ influx through nongated channels is balanced by a steady K^+ efflux, so that the membrane potential is constant. This steady-state balance changes, however, when the cell is depolarized sufficiently to trigger an action potential. A transient depolarizing potential, such as an excitatory synaptic potential, causes some voltage-gated Na^+ channels to open, and the resultant increase in membrane Na^+ permeability allows Na^+ influx to outstrip the K^+ efflux. Thus, a net influx of positive charge flows through the membrane, and positive charges accumulate inside the cell, causing further depolarization. The increase in depolarization causes more voltage-gated Na^+ channels to open, resulting in a greater influx of positive charge, which accelerates the depolarization still further.

This regenerative, positive feedback cycle develops explosively, driving the membrane potential toward the Na^+ equilibrium potential of +55 mV. Because K^+ efflux continues through the K^+ channels, the membrane potential at the peak of the action potential never actually reaches E_{Na}. A slight diffusion of Cl^- into the cell also counteracts the depolarizing tendency of the Na^+ influx. Nevertheless, so many voltage-gated Na^+ channels open during the rising phase of the action potential that the permeability to Na^+ is much greater than that to Cl^- or K^+. To a first approximation, the membrane potential approaches E_{Na} at the peak of the action potential, just as it approaches E_K at rest, when the K^+ permeability is predominant.

The membrane potential would remain at this large positive value indefinitely but for two processes that re-

polarize the membrane, terminating the action potential. First, as the depolarization continues, it slowly turns off, or *inactivates*, the voltage-gated Na^+ channels. That is, the Na^+ channels have two types of gating mechanisms: activation, which rapidly opens the channel in response to depolarization, and inactivation, which slowly closes the channel if the depolarization is maintained. The second repolarizing process results from the delayed opening of voltage-gated K^+ channels. As K^+ channels begin to open, K^+ efflux increases. The delayed increase in K^+ efflux combines with a decrease in Na^+ influx to produce a net efflux of positive charge from the cell, which continues until the cell has repolarized to its resting value of V_R.

The Resting and Action Potentials Can Be Quantified by the Goldman Equation

Although Na^+ and K^+ fluxes set the value of the resting potential, V_R is not equal to either E_K or E_{Na}, but lies between them. As a general rule, when V_m is determined by two or more species of ions, the influence of each species is determined both by its concentrations inside and outside the cell and by the permeability of the membrane to that ion. This relationship is given quantitatively by the *Goldman equation*[2]:

$$V_m = \frac{RT}{F} \ln \frac{P_K[K^+]_o + P_{Na}[Na^+]_o + P_{Cl}[Cl^-]_i}{P_K[K^+]_i + P_{Na}[Na^+]_i + P_{Cl}[Cl^-]_o} \quad \textbf{Goldman Equation}$$

This equation applies only when V_m is not changing. It states that the greater the concentration of a particular ion species and the greater its membrane permeability, the greater its role in determining the membrane potential. In the limiting case, when permeability to one ion is exceptionally high, the Goldman equation reduces to the Nernst equation for that ion. For example, if $P_K \gg P_{Cl}, P_{Na}$, as in glial cells, the equation becomes

$$V_m \approx \frac{RT}{F} \ln \frac{[K^+]_o}{[K^+]_i}.$$

In 1949 Alan Hodgkin and Bernard Katz first applied the Goldman equation systematically to changes in membrane potential evoked by altering external ion concentrations in the squid giant axon. They measured the variation of V_R while changing extracellular concentrations of Na^+, Cl^-, and K^+. Their results showed that if V_R is measured shortly after the concentration change, before the internal ionic concentrations are altered, $[K^+]_o$ has a strong effect

---

[2]There are three basic steps in the derivation of this equation:
1. Express the flux (J) of each species of ion (Na^+, K^+, Cl^-) across the membrane as a function of V_m, concentration, and membrane permeability: $J_i = f(V_m, conc_i, P_i)$.
2. Convert these fluxes to membrane currents, I (e.g., an influx of Na^+ or an efflux of Cl^- is an *inward* membrane current). Since V_m is constant, the charge separation across the membrane is not changing, so that $I_{Cl} + I_{Na} + I_K = 0$.
3. Substitute the equations from step 1 into the equation in step 2; rearrange terms and solve for V_m.

on the resting potential, $[Cl^-]_o$ has a moderate effect, and $[Na^+]_o$ has little effect. Their data could be fit accurately to the Goldman equation by assuming the following permeability ratios for the membrane at rest:

$$P_K : P_{Na} : P_{Cl} = 1/0.04/0.45.$$

For the membrane at the peak of the action potential, however, the variation of V_m with external ionic concentrations could be fit best by assuming a quite different set of permeability ratios:

$$P_K : P_{Na} : P_{Cl} = 1/20/0.45.$$

For this set of permeabilities $(P_{Na} \gg P_K, P_{Cl})$, the Goldman equation reduces to

$$V_m \approx \frac{RT}{F} \ln \frac{[Na^+]_o}{[Na^+]_i} = +55 \text{ mV}.$$

Thus, at the peak of the action potential, when the membrane is much more permeable to Na^+ than to any other ion, V_m approaches E_{Na}, the Nernst potential for Na^+.

The Neuron Can Be Represented by an Electrical Equivalent Circuit

A simple mathematical model derived from electrical circuits is helpful for describing the three critical features used by the nerve cell for electrical signaling the ion channels, the concentration gradients of relevant ions, and the ability of the membrane to store charge. In this model, called an *equivalent circuit*, all of the important functional properties of the neuron are represented by an electrical circuit consisting only of conductors (resistors), batteries, and capacitors. This model provides an intuitive understanding as well as a quantitative description of how current flow due to the movement of ions generates signals in nerve cells. The first step in developing the model is to relate the discrete physical properties of the membrane to its electrical properties. A review of elementary circuit theory in Appendix A may be helpful before proceeding.

Each Ion Channel Acts as a Conductor and Battery

As described in Chapter 5, ions do not enter the lipid bilayer of the membrane; the bilayer is therefore a poor conductor of ionic current. Even a large potential difference will produce practically no current flow across a pure lipid bilayer. Consider the cell body of a typical spinal motor neuron, which has a membrane area of about 10^{-4} cm². If that membrane were composed solely of lipid bilayer, its electrical conductance would be only about 1 pS. But because thousands of nongated ion channels are embedded in the membrane, ions constantly diffuse across it, so that its actual resting conductance is about 40,000 times greater, or about 40 nS.

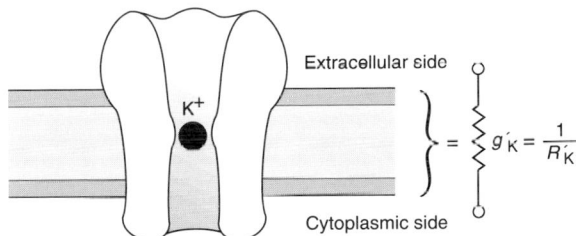

FIGURE 6–8

A single K^+ channel can be represented by the electrical symbol for a conductor, g'_K.

In the equivalent circuit model each K^+ channel can be represented by the symbol for a conductor (Figure 6–8). An ion going through an ion channel is likely to interact with the walls of the channel, as explained in Chapter 5. For this reason the conductance of the lumen of the channel is less than that of an equivalent volume of extracellular fluid. The conductance of a single channel (e.g., g'_K) is typically used in describing channel properties because it provides a direct measure of how efficiently the channel can conduct ions. But since conductance is inversely proportional to resistance, the resistance of the channel to current flow provides an equally valid description of this property:

$$g'_K = 1/R'_K.$$

Each open ion channel also contributes to the generation of an electrical potential difference across the membrane. For example, K^+, which is present at a higher concentration inside the cell, tends to diffuse out of the resting cell through nongated channels selective for K^+. This diffusion leads to a net separation of charge across the

FIGURE 6–9

A channel selectively permeable to K^+ ions gives rise to an electromotive force with a value equal to the K^+ Nernst potential. This can be represented by a battery, E_K, in series with a conductor, g'_K.

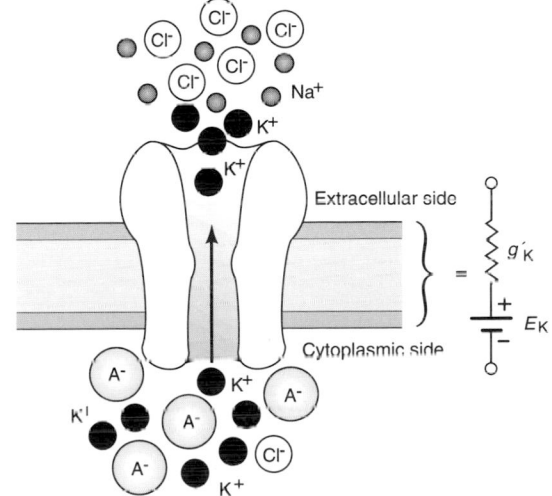

FIGURE 6–10
All of the passive K⁺ channels in a nerve membrane can be lumped into a single equivalent electrical structure: a battery (E_K) in series with a conductor, g_K; $g_K = N_K \times g'_K$, where N is the number of passive K⁺ channels and g'_K is the conductance of a single K⁺ channel.

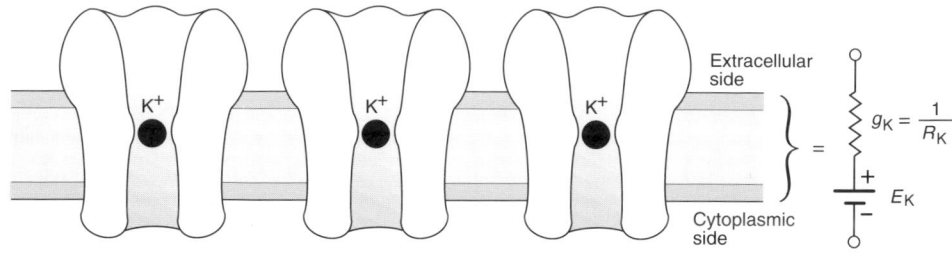

membrane—positive charges accumulate on the outside, leaving an excess of negative charges on the inside—resulting in an electrical potential difference. A source of electrical potential is called an electromotive force. An electromotive force generated by a difference in chemical potentials is called a battery. We may therefore represent the electrical potential generated across each K⁺ channel as a battery in series with the conductance of the channel (Figure 6–9). The potential generated by this battery is equal to E_K, which is typically about −75 mV.

All of the passive K⁺ channels in the membrane can be combined into a single equivalent structure, consisting of a conductor in series with a battery (Figure 6–10).[3] The value of the K⁺ conductance in this equivalent structure is determined by the fact that the total K⁺ conductance (g_K) of the cell membrane in its resting state is equal to the number of passive K⁺ channels (N_K) multiplied by the conductance of an individual K⁺ channel (g'_K):

$$g_K = N_K \times g'_K.$$

The value of the battery for this circuit equivalent of all the passive K⁺ channels is determined by the concentration gradient for K⁺ and is independent of the number of K⁺ channels. Therefore its value is simply E_K.

An Equivalent Circuit Model of the Membrane Includes Batteries, Conductors, a Capacitor, and a Current Generator

As we have seen, the entire population of passive K⁺ channels can be represented by a single conductor in series with a single battery. By analogy, all the passive Cl⁻ channels can be represented by a similar combination, as can the passive Na⁺ channels (Figure 6–11). These three types

of channels account for the bulk of the passive ionic pathways through the membrane in the cell at rest.[4]

We can incorporate these electrical representations of the total population of passive Na⁺, K⁺, and Cl⁻ channels into a simple equivalent circuit of a neuron to calculate the membrane potential. To construct this circuit we need only connect the elements representing each type of channel at their two ends by elements representing the extracellular fluid and cytoplasm. (These channels are, of course, in parallel with the conductance of the lipid bilayer. But, because the conductance of the bilayer is so much lower than that of the ion channel pathways, virtually all transmembrane current flows through the channels, and the negligible conductance of the bilayer can be ignored.) The extracellular fluid and cytoplasm are both excellent conductors because they have relatively large cross-sectional areas and many ions available to carry charge. The extracellular fluid and the cytoplasm can each be approximated by a short circuit—a conductor with zero resistance (Figure 6–12). The relationship between the electrical properties of the circuit in Figure 6–12 and membrane potential can be described by the following general equation (see the appendix at the end of this chapter for the derivation of this equation):

$$V_m = \frac{g_K \times E_K + g_{Cl} \times E_{Cl} + g_{Na} \times E_{Na}}{g_K + g_{Cl} + g_{Na}}.$$

In this equation the membrane potential is a weighted sum of the different ionic batteries, with each battery weighted according to the value of its membrane conductance. Note the similarity between this equation and the Goldman equation: Both equations state that V_m is determined by the ions with the greatest conductance or permeability.

The circuit model can be made more complete by adding a current generator. As described above, steady fluxes of Na⁺ and K⁺ ions through the passive membrane channel are exactly counterbalanced by active ion fluxes driven by the Na⁺–K⁺ pump, which extrudes Na⁺ ions and pumps in K⁺ ions. This ATP-dependent Na⁺–K⁺ pump, which keeps the ionic batteries charged, can be added to the

---

[3]Although the membrane conductance to K⁺ is related to the permeability of the membrane to K⁺, the two terms are not interchangeable. Permeability is determined by the state of the membrane, but conductance depends on both the state of the membrane and the concentration of surrounding ions. Consider a limiting case in which K⁺ concentration is very low on both sides of the membrane. Even if a large number of open K⁺ channels were present, g_K would be low because relatively few K⁺ ions would be available to carry current across the membrane in response to a potential difference. At the same time, K⁺ permeability would be quite high, since it depends only on how many K⁺ channels are open. Under most physiological conditions, however, a membrane with high K⁺ permeability also has a high K⁺ conductance.

---

[4]Although there is good evidence that the membrane has separate *gated* channels for Na⁺, K⁺, Cl⁻, and Ca²⁺, it is not clear whether the different ion species have separate nongated channels or whether they all share a common (leakage) pathway. For convenience, we shall assume separate nongated channels.

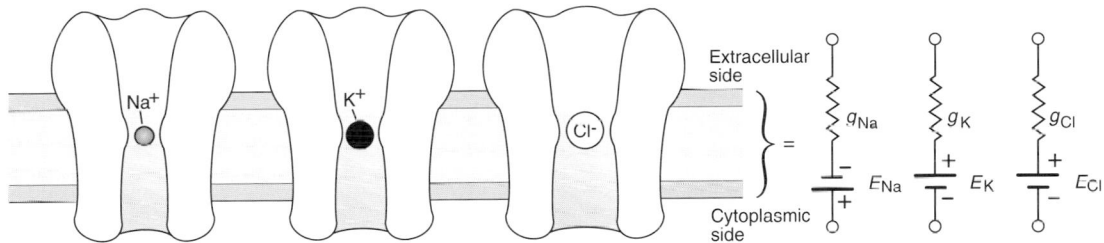

FIGURE 6–11
Each population of ion channels selective for Na$^+$, K$^+$, or Cl$^-$ can be represented by a battery in series with a conductor.

equivalent circuit in the form of a current generator (Figure 6–13).

In addition to electromotive force and conductance, the third important passive electrical property of the neuron is capacitance. In general, an electrical capacitor is defined as two conducting materials separated by an insulating material. For the neuron the conducting materials are the cytoplasm and the extracellular fluid; the insulating material is the cell membrane, specifically the lipid bilayer. Because the bilayer is penetrated by ion channels, the membrane acts as a leaky capacitor. Nevertheless, since the density of ion channels is low, the capacitor portion of the membrane occupies at least 100 times the area of all the ion channels combined. Membrane capacitance is included in the equivalent circuit in Figure 6–13.

The fundamental property of a capacitor is the ability to store charges of opposite sign on its two surfaces. The excess of positive and negative charge stored on either side of a capacitor gives rise to an electrical potential difference, as expressed in the following equation:

$$V = \frac{Q}{C}$$

where V is the potential difference between the two sides, Q is the excess of positive or negative charges on either side of the capacitor, and C is the capacitance.

A typical value of membrane capacitance for a nerve cell is about 1 μF/cm^2 of membrane area. The excess of positive and negative charges separated by the membrane of a spherical cell body with a resting potential of -60 mV and a diameter of 50 μm is 29×10^6 ions. Although this number may seem large, it represents only a tiny fraction (1/200,000) of the total number of positive or negative charges within the cytoplasm. The bulk of the cytoplasm and the bulk of the extracellular fluid are electroneutral (see Figure 6–1).

Changes in local charge separation, not in bulk concentration, are required to change membrane potential. During the action potential, the membrane potential changes from -60 to $+50$ mV, a total excursion of 110 mV. The total number of Na$^+$ ions that must flow into the cell to change the charge on the membrane can be determined by calculating the amount of charge required to produce this change in V_m. Given that 29×10^6 charges must be separated across the membrane to produce a 60 mV potential difference, the change in charge separation required to change the potential by 110 mV is

$$29 \times 10^6 \text{ ions} \times \frac{110 \text{ mV}}{60 \text{ mV}} = 53 \times 10^6 \text{ ions.}$$

In other words, for a cell body 50 μm in diameter, 53 million Na$^+$ ions must diffuse across the membrane to

FIGURE 6–12
The current flow in a neuron can be modeled by an electrical equivalent circuit that includes elements representing the ion-selective membrane channels and the short-circuit pathways provided by the cytoplasm and extracellular fluid.

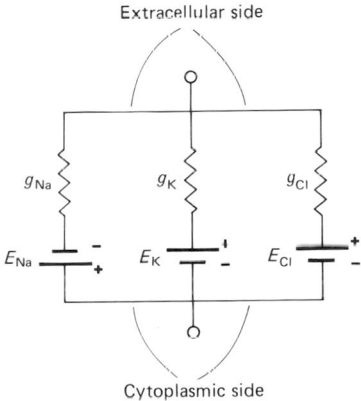

FIGURE 6–13
This electrical equivalent circuit of a neuron at rest includes the most abundant types of ion channels in parallel. Under steady-state conditions, Na$^+$ and K$^+$ currents resulting from passive diffusion through membrane channels are balanced by active Na$^+$ and K$^+$ fluxes (I'_{Na} and I'_K) driven by the Na$^+$–K$^+$ pump. The lipid bilayer endows the membrane with electrical capacitance (C_m).

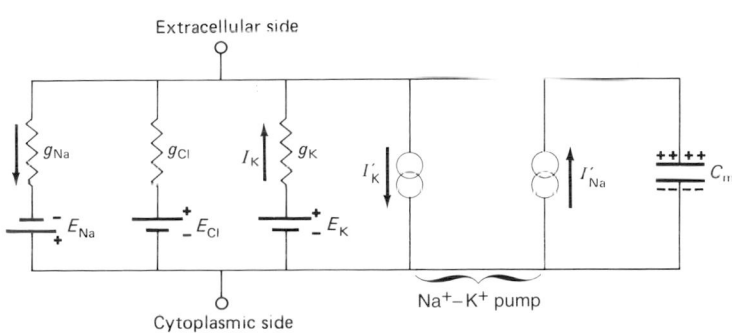

depolarize it from −60 to +50 mV. The influx of this number of Na⁺ ions produces only a 0.012% change in internal Na⁺ concentration from its typical value of 12 mM.

An Overall View

The membrane at rest is a leaky capacitor. The lipid bilayer, which is virtually impermeant to ions, is an insulator separating two conductors, the cytoplasm and the extracellular fluid. Nevertheless, ions leak across the lipid bilayer through the ion channels. When the cell is at rest, these passive ionic fluxes into and out of the cell are balanced, so that the charge separation across the membrane remains constant and the membrane potential remains at its resting value.

The value of the resting membrane potential is determined primarily by nongated channels selective for K⁺, Cl⁻, and Na⁺. In general, the membrane potential will be closest to the Nernst potential of the ion or ions with the greatest membrane conductance. The conductance for an ion species is proportional to the number of open channels permeable to that ion.

At rest, the membrane potential is close to the Nernst potential for K⁺, the ion to which the membrane is most permeable. However, the membrane is also somewhat permeable to Na⁺, and an influx of Na⁺ drives the membrane potential slightly positive to the K⁺ Nernst potential. At this potential the electrical and chemical driving forces acting on K⁺ are no longer in balance, so K⁺ diffuses out of the cell. These two passive fluxes are each balanced by active fluxes driven by the Na⁺–K⁺ pump.

Chloride is actively pumped out of some, but not all, cells. When it is not, it is passively distributed so as to be at equilibrium. Under most physiological conditions the bulk concentrations of Na⁺, K⁺, and Cl⁻ inside and outside the cell are constant. The changes in membrane potential that occur during signaling (action potentials, synaptic potentials, and receptor potentials) are caused by the substantial changes in the relative membrane permeabilities to these three ions, not by changes in the bulk concentrations of ions, which are negligible. These changes in permeability, caused by the opening of gated ion channels, in turn cause changes in the net charge separation across the membrane.

Postscript

Calculation of Membrane Potential from the Equivalent Circuit Model of the Neuron

We shall illustrate with a simple example how the equivalent circuit of the neuron may be used to analyze neuronal properties quantitatively. The equivalent circuit model of the resting membrane will be used to calculate the resting potential. To simplify calculation of the membrane potential, we shall initially ignore Cl⁻ channels and begin with just two types of passive channels, K⁺ and Na⁺, as illustrated in Figure 6–14. Because there are more passive channels for K⁺ than for Na⁺, the membrane conduc-

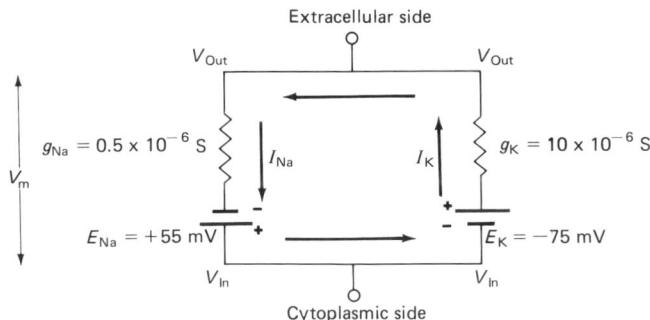

FIGURE 6–14
This electrical equivalent circuit for calculating resting membrane potential omits the Cl⁻ pathway for simplicity.

tance for current flow carried by K⁺ is much greater than that for Na⁺. In Figure 6–14, g_K is 20 times higher than g_{Na} (10×10^{-6} S compared to 0.5×10^{-6} S). Given these values and the values of E_K and E_{Na}, we can calculate the membrane potential V_m as follows.

Since V_m is constant in the resting state, the net current must be zero, otherwise the separation of positive and negative charges across the membrane would change, causing V_m to change. Therefore, I_{Na} is equal and opposite to I_K[5]:

$$I_{Na} = -I_K \tag{6–1}$$

or

$$I_{Na} + I_K = 0.$$

We can easily calculate I_{Na} and I_K in two steps. First, we add up the separate potential differences across the Na⁺ and K⁺ branches of the circuit. As one goes from inside to outside across the Na⁺ branch, the total potential difference is the sum of the potential differences across E_{Na} and across g_{Na}[6]:

$$V_m = E_{Na} + I_{Na}/g_{Na}.$$

Similarly, for the K⁺ conductance branch

$$V_m = E_K + I_K/g_K.$$

Next, we rearrange and solve for I:

$$I_{Na} = g_{Na} \times (V_m - E_{Na}). \tag{6–2a}$$

$$I_K = g_K \times (V_m - E_K). \tag{6–2b}$$

As these equations illustrate, the ionic current through each conductance branch is equal to the conductance of that branch multiplied by the net electrical driving force.

---

[5]This equality is true only if one makes the simplifying assumption that the Na⁺–K⁺ pump is electroneutral.

[6]Because we have defined V_m as $V_{in} - V_{out}$, the following convention must be used for these equations. Outward current (in this case I_K) is positive and inward current (I_{Na}) is negative. Batteries with their positive poles toward the inside of the membrane (e.g., E_{Na}) are given positive values in the equations. The reverse is true for batteries that have their negative poles toward the inside, such as the K⁺ battery.

For example, the conductance for the K$^+$ branch is proportional to the number of open K$^+$ channels, and the driving force is equal to the difference between V_m and E_K. If V_m is more positive than E_K (-75 mV), the driving force is positive (outward); if V_m is more negative than E_K, the driving force is negative (inward).

In Equation 6–1 we saw that $I_{Na} + I_K = 0$. If we now substitute Equations 6–2a and 6–2b for I_{Na} and I_K in Equation 6–1, we obtain the following expression:

$$g_{Na} \times (V_m - E_{Na}) + g_K \times (V_m - E_K) = 0.$$

Multiplying through we see that

$$(V_m \times g_{Na} - E_{Na} \times g_{Na}) + (V_m \times g_K - E_K \times g_K) = 0.$$

This can now be rearranged to yield

$$V_m \times (g_{Na} + g_K) = (E_{Na} \times g_{Na}) + (E_K \times g_K).$$

Solving for V_m, we obtain an intuitively useful expression for the resting membrane potential:

$$V_m = \frac{(E_{Na} \times g_{Na}) + (E_K \times g_K)}{g_{Na} + g_K}. \qquad (6-3)$$

This equation allows us to calculate V_m for the equivalent circuit. Using the circuit values of Figure 6–14, we can calculate V_m to be

$$V_m = \frac{(+55 \times 10^{-3}\ \text{V})(0.5 \times 10^{-6}\ \text{S})}{0.5 \times 10^{-6}\ \text{S} + 10 \times 10^{-6}\ \text{S}}$$

$$+ \frac{(-75 \times 10^{-3}\ \text{V})(10 \times 10^{-6}\ \text{S})}{0.5 \times 10^{-6}\ \text{S} + 10 \times 10^{-6}\ \text{S}}$$

$$= \frac{-722.5 \times 10^{-9}\ \text{V} \times \text{S}}{10.5 \times 10^{-6}\ \text{S}}$$

$$= -69\ \text{mV}.$$

Equation 6–3 states that V_m will approach the value of the ionic battery that is associated with the greater conductance. This principle can be illustrated with another example as we consider what happens during the action potential. At the peak of the action potential, total membrane g_K is essentially unchanged from its resting value, but g_{Na} increases by as much as 500-fold. This increase in g_{Na} is caused by the opening of voltage-gated Na$^+$ chan-

nels. In the example shown in Figure 6–14 a 500-fold increase would change g_{Na} from 0.5×10^{-6} S to 250×10^{-6} S. If we substitute this new value of g_{Na} into Equation 6–3 and solve for V_m, we obtain $+50$ mV, a value much closer to E_{Na} than to E_K. V_m is closer to E_{Na} than to E_K at the peak of the action potential because g_{Na} is now 25-fold greater than g_K, so the Na$^+$ battery becomes much more important than the K$^+$ battery in determining V_m.

The Equation for Membrane Potential Can Be Written in a More General Form

The resting membrane has open conductance channels not only for Na$^+$ and K$^+$, but also for Cl$^-$. It is useful therefore to have a general equation to describe the resting potential as a function of all three permeant ions. If one constructs an equivalent circuit that includes a conductance pathway for Cl$^-$ with its associated Nernst battery (Figure 6–8), one can derive a more general equation for V_m by following the same sequence of steps outlined above:

$$V_m = \frac{(E_K \times g_K) + (E_{Na} \times g_{Na}) + (E_{Cl} \times g_{Cl})}{g_K + g_{Na} + g_{Cl}}. \qquad (6-4)$$

This equation is similar to the Goldman equation presented earlier in this chapter. As in the Goldman equation, the contribution to V_m of each ionic battery is weighted in proportion to the conductance (or permeability) of the membrane for that particular ion. In the limit, if the conductance for one ion is much greater than that for the other ions, V_m will approach the value of that ion's Nernst potential.

The contribution of Cl$^-$ ions to the resting potential can now be determined by comparing V_m calculated for the circuits in Figures 6–14 and 6–15. For most nerve cells, the value of g_{Cl} ranges from one-fourth to one-half of g_K. In addition, E_{Cl} is typically quite close to E_K, but slightly less negative. For the example shown in Figure 6–15, Cl$^-$ ions are passively distributed across the membrane, so that E_{Cl} is equal to the value of V_m, which is determined by Na$^+$ and K$^+$. Note that if $E_{Cl} = V_m$ (-69 mV in this case), no net current flows through the Cl$^-$ channels. If one includes g_{Cl} and E_{Cl} from Figure 6–15 in the calculation of V_m (i.e., Equation 6–4), the calculated value of V_m does not differ from that for Figure 6–14. On the other hand, if Cl$^-$ were

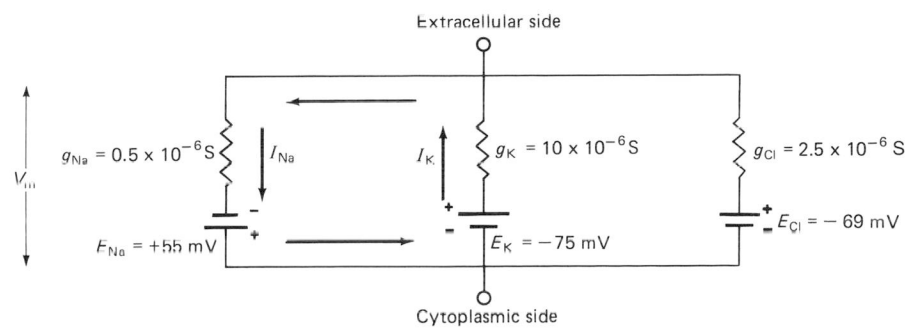

FIGURE 6–15

The electrical equivalent circuit of a neuron in which Cl$^-$ is passively distributed across the membrane. No current flows through the Cl$^-$ channels in this example because V_m is at the Cl$^-$ equilibrium (Nernst) potential.

not passively distributed but actively pumped out of the cell, then E_{Cl} would be more negative than -69 mV. Adding the Cl^- pathway to the calculation would then shift V_m to a slightly more negative value.

The Sodium–Potassium Pump Counteracts the Passive Fluxes of Sodium and Potassium

An important feature of the resting membrane is the steady leakage of Na^+ into the cell and of K^+ out of the cell, even when the cell is in its resting state. Referring back to the circuit in Figure 6–14, we can calculate these currents from Equations 6–2a and 6–2b:

$$I_{Na} = g_{Na} \times (V_m - E_{Na})$$
$$I_K = g_K \times (V_m - E_K).$$

Substituting the values from Figure 6–14 and the value of V_m calculated above yields

$$I_{Na} = (0.5 \times 10^{-6}\ S) \times [(-68.8 \times 10^{-3}\ V) - (+55 \times 10^{-3}\ V)]$$
$$= -62 \times 10^{-9}\ A$$
$$I_K = (10 \times 10^{-6}\ S) \times [(-68.8 \times 10^{-3}\ V) - (-75 \times 10^{-3}\ V)]$$
$$= +62 \times 10^{-9}\ A.$$

These steady fluxes of Na^+ and K^+ ions through the passive membrane channels are exactly counterbalanced by active ion fluxes driven by the Na^+–K^+ pump, as illustrated in Figure 6–13. To prevent the ionic batteries from running down, the Na^+–K^+ pump continually extrudes Na^+ ions and pumps in K^+, even when the cell is at rest. The actively driven Na^+ current (I'_{Na}) is equal and opposite to the passive Na^+ current (I_{Na}), and the actively driven K^+ current (I'_K) is equal and opposite to the passive K^+ current (I_K).

The equality between I_{Na} and I_K holds only for the simplified case in which the Na^+–K^+ pump is electroneutral. If the pump is electrogenic—pumping three Na^+ ions out for every two K^+ ions that it pumps in—the membrane will be in a steady state when $V_m = -70.8$ mV (for the example shown in Figure 6–13). Thus, the effect of the electrogenic pump is to generate a resting membrane po-

tential slightly more negative than the value that would result for passive diffusion alone. At this more negative potential

$$I_{Na}/I_K = I'_{Na}/I'_K = 3/2,\quad I_{Na} = I'_{Na},\ \text{and}\ I_K = I'_K\ .$$

Selected Readings

Finkelstein, A., and Mauro, A. 1977. Physical principles and formalisms of electrical excitability. In E. R. Kandel (ed.), Handbook of Physiology, Section 1: The Nervous System, Vol. I. Cellular Biology of Neurons, Part 1. Bethesda, Md.: American Physiological Society, pp. 161–213.

Hille, B. 1984. Ionic Channels of Excitable Membranes. Sunderland, Mass.: Sinauer.

Hodgkin, A. L. 1976. Chance and design in electrophysiology: An informal account of certain experiments on nerve carried out between 1934 and 1952. J. Physiol. (Lond.) 263:1–21.

References

Albers, R. W., Siegel, G. J., and Stahl, W. L. 1989. Membrane transport. In G. J. Siegel, B. W. Agranoff, R. W. Albers, and P. B. Molinoff (eds.), Basic Neurochemistry: Molecular, Cellular, and Medical Aspects, 4th ed. New York: Raven Press, pp. 49–70.

Bernstein, J. 1902. Investigations on the thermodynamics of bioelectric currents. Translated from Pflügers Arch. 92:521–562. In G. R. Kepner (ed.), Cell Membrane Permeability and Transport. Stroudsburg, Pa.: Dowden, Hutchinson & Ross, 1979, pp. 184–210.

Fambrough, D. M., and Bayne, E. K. 1983. Multiple forms of (Na$^+$ + K$^+$)-ATPase in the chicken: Selective detection of the major nerve, skeletal muscle, and kidney form by a monoclonal antibody. J. Biol. Chem. 258:3926–3935.

Goldman, D. E. 1943. Potential, impedance, and rectification in membranes. J. Gen. Physiol. 27:37–60.

Hodgkin, A. L., and Katz, B. 1949. The effect of sodium ions on the electrical activity of the giant axon of the squid. J. Physiol. (Lond.) 108:37–77.

Nernst, W. 1888. On the kinetics of substances in solution. Translated from Z. physik. Chemie 2:613–622, 634–637. In G. R. Kepner (ed.), Cell Membrane Permeability and Transport. Stroudsburg, Pa.: Dowden, Hutchinson & Ross, 1979, pp. 174–183.

Orkand, R. K. 1977. Glial cells. In E. R. Kandel (ed.), Handbook of Physiology, Section 1: The Nervous System, Vol. I. Cellular Biology of Neurons, Part 2. Bethesda, Md.: American Physiological Society, pp. 855–875.

John Koester

Passive Membrane Properties of the Neuron

Membrane Capacitance Prolongs the Time Course of Electrical Signals

Membrane and Axoplasmic Resistance Affect the Efficiency of Signal Conduction

Axon Diameter Affects the Current Threshold

Passive Membrane Properties and Axon Diameter Affect the Velocity of Action Potential Propagation

An Overall View

Neurons have passive electrical properties that do not change during signaling. These *constant* properties are determined by three features of the cell that were described in Chapter 6—the conductance of nongated ion channels, the membrane capacitance, and the conductance of the cytoplasm. Although these properties are constant, they influence the effectiveness of active signaling processes within the neuron. For example, they affect the time course of synaptic potentials as well as how efficiently the synaptic potentials are conducted from their site of origin to the trigger zone. In turn, these properties of synaptic potentials contribute to *synaptic integration*, the process by which a nerve cell adds up all incoming signals and determines whether or not it will generate an action potential. Once an action potential is generated, the speed with which it is conducted from the trigger zone to the axon terminals also depends on the passive electrical properties of the axon.

Membrane Capacitance Prolongs the Time Course of Electrical Signals

During signaling the rate of change in the membrane potential, which is important in determining the rate of information transfer within a neuron, is critically dependent on membrane capacitance. We shall illustrate how membrane capacitance exerts this effect by referring to the equivalent circuit model of the membrane developed in Chapter 6, with one important difference. In Chapter 6 we described the conducting pathways of the equivalent circuit (the ion channels) in terms of conductance, because we were interested in which ion species flow most readily across the nerve cell membrane and because conductance across the membrane is directly proportional to the number of open channels. Since conductance and resistance are reciprocally related ($g = 1/R$), either term can be used

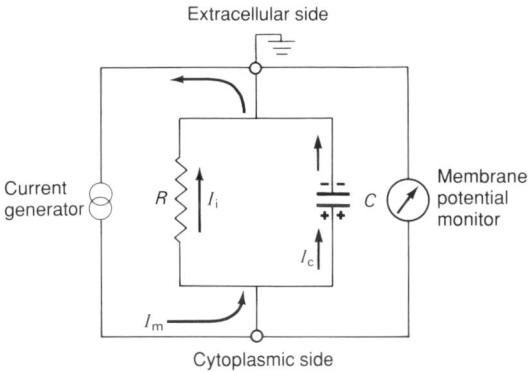

FIGURE 7–1

A simplified electrical equivalent circuit is used to examine the effects of membrane capacitance (C) on the rate of change of membrane potential in response to current flow. All conductance channels are lumped into a single resistance element (R). Batteries representing the electromotive forces generated by ion diffusion are not included because they affect only the absolute value of membrane potential, not the rate of change. This equivalent circuit represents the experimental setup shown in Figure 6–2, in which pairs of electrodes are connected to the current generator and the membrane potential monitor.

to describe a conducting pathway in an equivalent circuit. In this chapter we shall describe the conducting pathways of the equivalent circuit in terms of *resistance* because we wish to introduce a few simple concepts dealing with current flow in neurons that include resistive elements. These concepts were first developed in physics and engineering, and, by tradition, their mathematical expression uses resistance rather than conductance.

When current flows into or out of a cell through ion channels in the membrane, the membrane voltage always changes more slowly than the current. To understand why this is so, let us refer to the equivalent circuit in Figure 7–1, a simplified equivalent circuit of the experimental preparation described in Chapter 6 (Figure 6–2A). In Figure 7–1 the cell membrane is represented by a capacitor (C) in parallel with a resistor (R). The resistance element represents the parallel combination of the nongated K^+, Na^+, and Cl^- conductance (or resistive) elements described in Chapter 6 (Figure 6–12). We can ignore the ionic batteries included in the circuits in Chapter 6 because they affect only the absolute value of V_m, not its rate of change. As a further simplification, we shall focus on the passive membrane properties by considering only the effects of depolarizing current pulses that are too small to open a significant number of voltage-gated Na^+ and K^+ channels.

When a rectangular step of current is injected into the cell, the change in voltage lags behind the change in current (Figure 7–2A). To account for this lag, we must first understand the two types of current that flow across the nerve cell membrane: ionic current (I_i) and capacitive current (I_c). The sum of these two components is the total membrane current (I_m):

$$I_m = I_i + I_c .$$

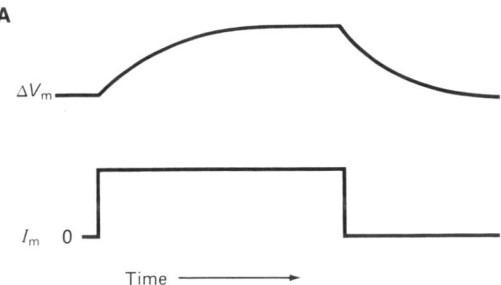

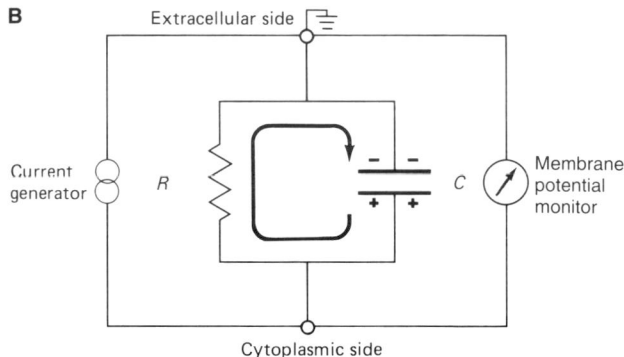

FIGURE 7–2

The rate of change in the membrane potential is slowed by the membrane capacitance.

A. When V_m is changed by current injected into the cell, ΔV_m lags behind the current pulse (I_m). Outward membrane current is represented by an upward deflection of the current trace; inward current is represented by a downward deflection.

B. At the end of the pulse the capacitance is discharged by an inward capacitive current that drives an outward current through the membrane resistance, R.

Ionic (or resistive) *membrane current* is carried by ions flowing across the membrane through ion channels—for example, Na^+ ions moving through Na^+ channels from outside to inside the cell. *Capacitive membrane current* is carried by ions that change the net charge stored on the membrane. For example, an outward capacitive current adds positive charges to the inside of the membrane and removes an equal number of positive charges from the outside of the membrane (Figure 7–1).

The cause of the delay between I_m and ΔV_m is revealed by examining the time courses of I_c and I_i. Recall that the potential (V) across a capacitor is proportional to the charge (Q) stored on the capacitor:

$$V = \frac{Q}{C} .$$

For a change in potential (ΔV_m) to occur across the membrane, there must be a change in the amount of charge (ΔQ) stored on the membrane:

$$\Delta V_m = \frac{\Delta Q}{C} . \tag{7–1}$$

This ΔQ is brought about by the flow of capacitive current (I_c). Current is defined as the net movement of positive charge per unit time. The larger the current and the longer it flows, the greater the value of ΔQ and thus of ΔV_m. Conversely, the larger the value of membrane capacitance (C), the smaller the change in the membrane potential (ΔV_m) for a given amplitude and duration of capacitive current (I_c).

The shape of the change in potential in Figure 7–2A is determined by the fact that the membrane capacitance and resistance are in parallel (see Figures 6–13 and 7–1); therefore, the potential across these two elements must be equal at all times. Initially, most of the membrane current flows into the capacitor to change the charge on its plates. As the pulse continues and ΔQ increases, however, more and more current must flow through the resistor, because at any instant the voltage drop across the membrane resistance ($\Delta V_m = I_rR$) must be equal to the voltage across the membrane capacitance ($\Delta V_m = \Delta Q/C$). As a larger fraction of the total membrane current flows through the resistor, less is available for charging the capacitor; thus the *rate of change* of V_m decreases with time. When ΔV_m reaches its plateau value, all of the membrane current is flowing through the resistor and $\Delta V_m = I_mR$. After the current turns off, current flows around the RC loop as the capacitor discharges and drives current through the resistor (Figure 7–2B).

The capacitance of the membrane has the effect of reducing the rate at which the membrane potential changes in response to a current pulse (Figure 7–2A). If the membrane had only resistive properties, a step pulse of outward current passed across it would change the membrane potential instantaneously (Figure 7–3, line a). On the other hand, if the membrane had only capacitive properties, the membrane potential would change slowly, in a ramp-like manner, in response to the same step pulse of current (Figure 7–3, line b). Because the membrane has *both* capacitive and resistive properties in parallel, the actual change in membrane potential resulting from a rectangular current pulse combines features of the two pure responses. Thus, the initial slope of V_m as a function of time is the same as that for a purely capacitive element, whereas the final slope and amplitude are the same as those for a purely resistive element (Figure 7–3, line c).

The rising phase of the potential change shown in Figure 7–2A can be described by the following equation:

$$\Delta V_m(t) = I_mR(1 - e^{-t/\tau})$$

where e, which has the value of 2.72, is the base of the system of natural logarithms, and τ equals RC, the product of the resistance and capacitance of the membrane. The parameter τ, called the *membrane time constant*, can be measured experimentally. For the response of the membrane to a rectangular step of current (Figure 7–3), τ is the time that it takes V_m to move 63% of the way toward its final value $(1 - 1/e \times 100)$. The time constants of different neurons typically range from 1 to 20 ms.

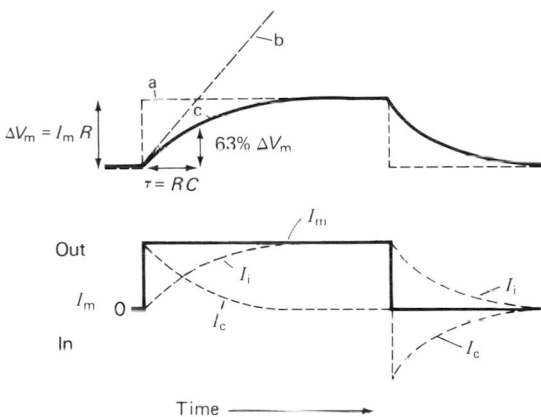

FIGURE 7–3

The time course of the change of membrane potential in response to a step of current combines features of a purely capacitive and a purely resistive element. The response of the membrane potential (ΔV_m) to a rectangular current pulse is shown in the **upper plot**. The actual shape of the response (**line c**) combines the properties of a purely resistive element (**line a**) and a purely capacitive element (**line b**). In the lower plot the total membrane current (I_m) is shown by the **solid line**; the **broken lines** show the time course of the ionic (I_i) and capacitive (I_c) currents.

The effect of the time constant on integration of synaptic input is especially important. Most synaptic potentials are caused by brief synaptic currents triggered by the opening of ligand-gated channels. The time course of the rising phase of a synaptic potential is determined by both active and passive properties of the membrane, but the falling phase is purely a passive process. Its time course is a function of the membrane time constant. The longer the time constant, the longer the duration of the synaptic potential. When synaptic potentials overlap in time, they add together in a process known as *temporal summation*. In this way individual excitatory postsynaptic potentials that alone might be too small to trigger an action potential can sum to reach threshold. If a postsynaptic cell has a long membrane time constant, the synaptic potential lasts longer and there is more chance for temporal summation (Figure 7–4). Temporal summation of receptor potentials in receptor cells takes place in a similar fashion.

Membrane and Axoplasmic Resistance Affect the Efficiency of Signal Conduction

A voltage signal decreases in amplitude with distance from its site of initiation within a neuron. To understand why this decrement occurs, we must first consider an equivalent circuit that shows how the three-dimensional geometry of a neuron determines the distribution of current flow. Consider a dendrite. The cytoplasmic core of a dendrite offers significant resistance to the longitudinal flow of current because it has a relatively small cross-sectional area. The greater the length of the cytoplasmic

A

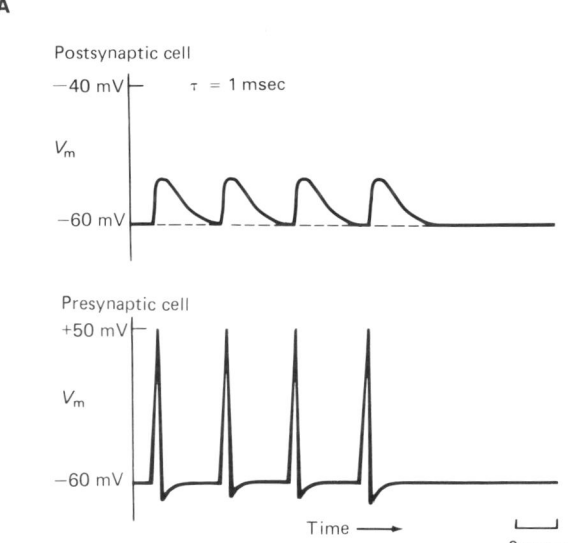

B

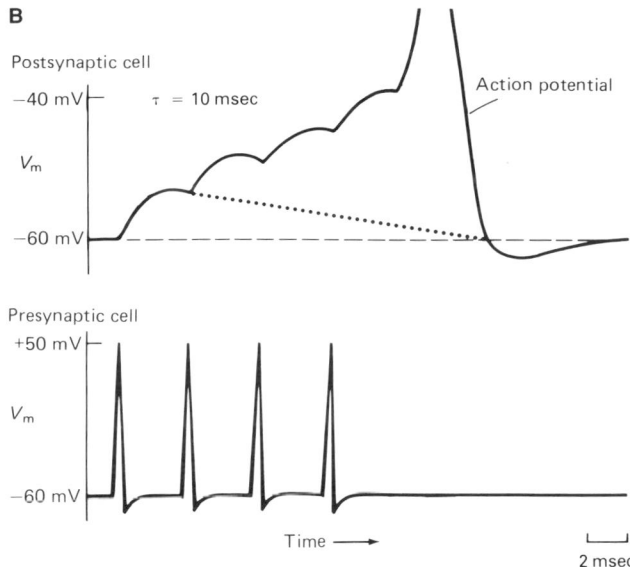

FIGURE 7–4

When the time course of individual postsynaptic potentials is longer than the interval between spikes in the presynaptic cell, the postsynaptic potentials overlap and their temporal summation can drive the membrane potential to the threshold for an action potential. The larger the membrane time constant (τ) of the postsynaptic cell, the longer the postsynaptic potential lasts

and the greater the extent of temporal summation. Here the consequences of different time constants in two postsynaptic cells are compared. In **A** the time constant is 1 ms; in **B** it is 10 ms. The **dotted line** shows the extrapolated falling phase of an individual excitatory postsynaptic potential.

core, the greater the resistance, because ions experience more collisions as they flow down the length of the dendrite. To represent the incremental increase in resistance along the length of the dendritic core, the dendrite can be thought of as a series of identical cytoplasm-containing membrane cylinders. Each unit cylinder can then be represented separately in the equivalent circuit (Figure 7–5).

The *axial resistance* (r_a) of the cytoplasmic core is expressed in units of Ω/cm. The *membrane resistance* per unit length of cylinder, which is defined as r_m, is expressed in units of $\Omega \cdot cm$. For a dendrite of a uniform diameter, r_m is the same for equal lengths of membrane cylinder. Because the extracellular fluid has such a large volume, it has a negligible resistance that can be ignored for this discussion.

If current is injected into the dendrite at one point, how will the membrane potential change with distance along the dendrite? For simplicity, let us consider the variation of membrane potential with distance after a constant-amplitude current pulse has been on for some time ($t \gg \tau$). Under these conditions the membrane potential will have reached a steady value, so capacitive current will be zero. When $I_c = 0$, all of the membrane current is ionic, $I_m = I_i$. The variation of the potential thus depends solely on the relative values of r_m and r_a.

The current that is injected flows out across the membrane by several pathways along the length of the process (Figure 7–6A). Each of these pathways is made up of two resistive components in series: a total axial resistance, R_a, and a membrane component, r_m. The total axial resistance

FIGURE 7–5

A neuronal process, either an axon or dendrite, can be divided into unit lengths, which can be represented in an electrical equivalent circuit. Each unit length of the process is a circuit with its own membrane resistance (r_m) and capacitance (c_m). All the circuits are connected by resistors (r_a), which represent the axial resistance of segments of cytoplasm.

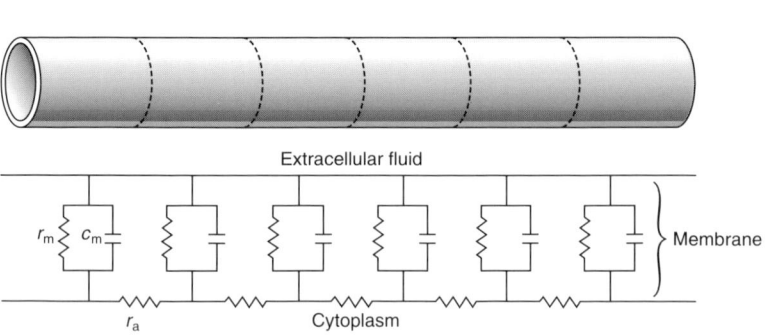

A

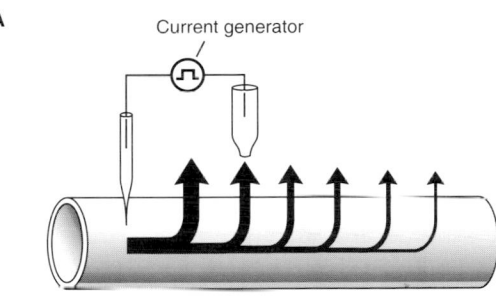

Current generator

B

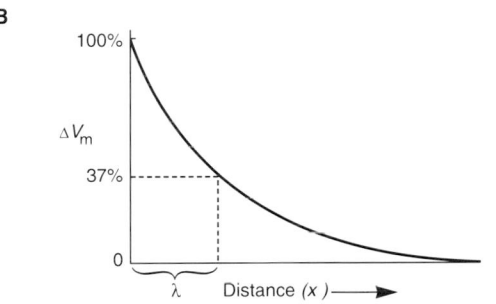

100%

ΔV_m

37%

0

λ Distance (x) ——→

FIGURE 7–6
Current injected into a neuronal process by a microelectrode follows the path of least resistance to the return electrode in the extracellular fluid (**A**). Under these conditions the change in V_m decays exponentially with distance along the length of the process (**B**).

for each current pathway is the cytoplasmic resistance between the site of current injection and any point along the dendrite. Since resistors in series add, $R_a = r_a x$, where x is the distance along the dendrite from the site of current injection. The membrane component, r_m, has the same value for each of these current pathways.

More current flows across the membrane near the site of injection than at more distant regions because current always tends to follow the path of least resistance, and the total axial resistance, R_a, increases with distance from the

site of injection (Figure 7–6A). Because $V_m = I_m r_m$, the change in membrane potential, $\Delta V_m(x)$, produced by the current becomes smaller as one moves down the dendrite away from the current electrode. This decay with distance has an exponential shape (Figure 7–6B), expressed by the following equation:

$$\Delta V_m(x) = \Delta V_0 e^{-x/\lambda},$$

where λ is the membrane *length constant*, x is the distance from the site of current injection, and V_0 is the change in membrane potential produced by the current flow at the site of the current electrode ($x = 0$).

The length constant, λ, which is the distance along the dendrite to the site where ΔV_m has decayed to $1/e$, or 37% of its value at $x = 0$, is determined by the ratio of r_m to r_a, where

$$\lambda = \sqrt{\frac{r_m}{r_a}}.$$

The better the insulation of the membrane (the higher r_m is) and the better the conducting properties of the inner core (the lower r_a is), the greater the length constant of the dendrite. That is, current is able to spread further along the inner conductive core of the dendrite before leaking across the membrane. Typical length constant values fall in the range of 0.1–1.0 mm.

Such passive spread of voltage changes along the neuron is called *electrotonic conduction*. The efficiency of this process, which is measured by the length constant, has two important effects on neuronal function. First, it influences *spatial summation*. This is the process by which synaptic potentials generated in different regions of the neuron are added together at the trigger zone, the decision-making component of the neuron. For a cell with a short length constant, synaptic potentials that are initiated at the distal ends of dendrites will diminish considerably as they are passively conducted to the trigger zone, so they contribute relatively little to spatial summation (Figure 7–7).

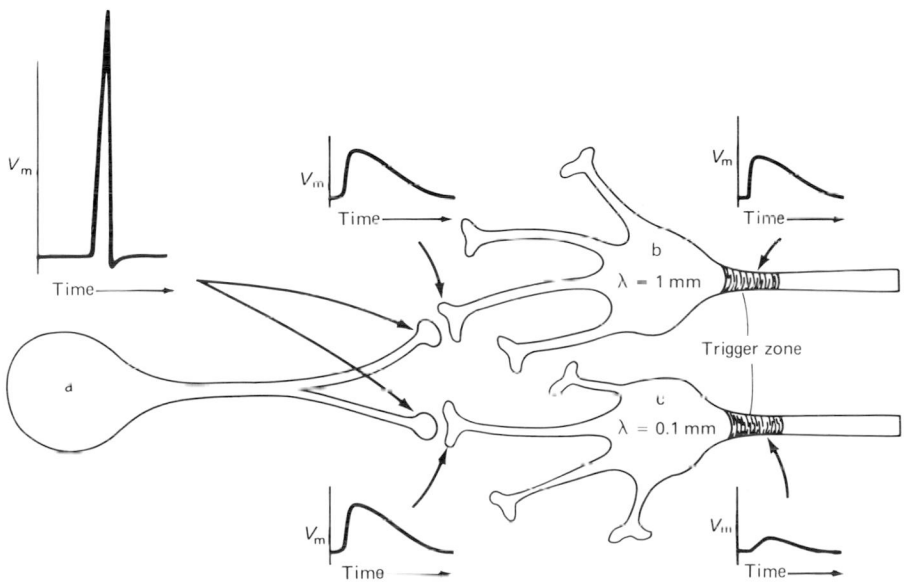

FIGURE 7–7
The length constant (λ) affects the efficiency of electrotonic conduction of synaptic potentials. An action potential in cell a elicits synaptic potentials in cells b and c. The two synaptic potentials are equal in amplitude at their sites of initiation and travel the same distance in both cells b and c. However, the amplitude of the synaptic potential that arrives at the trigger zone in cell b is much larger than in c because the length constant of the dendrites of b is much greater (1 mm) than that of cell c (0.1 mm).

A

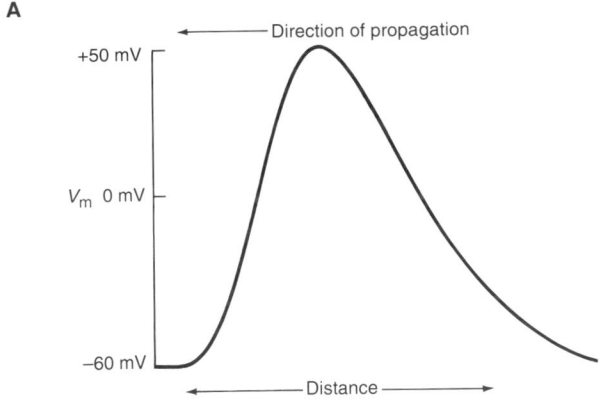

B

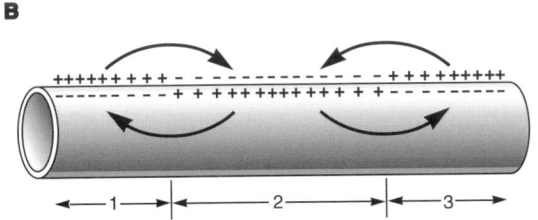

FIGURE 7–8

Passive conduction of depolarization along the axon contributes to action potential propagation.

A. The waveform of an action potential propagating from right to left.

B. The difference in potential along the length of the axon creates a local-circuit current flow that causes the depolarization to spread passively from the active region (**2**) to the inactive region (**1**) ahead of the action potential, as well as to area **3** behind the action potential. However, because there is also an increase in g_K in the wake of the action potential (see Chapter 8), the buildup of positive charge along the inside of membrane in area **3** is more than balanced by the local efflux of K^+, allowing this region of membrane to repolarize.

A second important feature of electrotonic conduction is its role in the propagation of the action potential. Once the membrane at any point along an axon has been depolarized beyond threshold, an action potential is generated in that region in response to the opening of voltage-gated Na^+ channels (see Chapter 8). This local depolarization then spreads electrotonically along the axon, causing the adjacent region of the membrane to reach the threshold for generating an action potential (Figure 7–8). The depolarization is spread by "local-circuit" current flow resulting from the potential difference between the active and the inactive regions of the axon membrane. Once the depolarization of the inactive region of the membrane approaches threshold, the voltage-gated Na^+ channels in this region of membrane open up, Na^+ rushes down its electrochemical gradient into the cytoplasm, and the depolarization becomes greater. This increase in depolarization causes more Na^+ channels to open, so that more Na^+ comes in, and so forth. Thus, as the local membrane potential approaches threshold, the depolarization changes from a pas-

sive to an active regenerative process. This actively generated depolarization then spreads by passive, local-circuit flow of current to the next region of membrane, and the cycle is repeated.

Axon Diameter Affects the Current Threshold

When a peripheral nerve is stimulated by passing current through a pair of extracellular electrodes, the total number of axons that generate action potentials varies with the amplitude of the current pulse. To drive a cell to threshold, the current must pass through the cell membrane. But for any given axon, most of the stimulating current bypasses the fiber, moving instead through other axons or through the low-resistance pathway provided by the extracellular fluid. In the vicinity of the positive electrode only a small fraction of the total stimulating current flows across the membrane of any one axon. Once current passes into an axon, it flows along the axoplasmic core, and then out again through more distant regions of axonal membrane, to the second (negative) electrode in the extracellular fluid. In general, the *largest diameter axons have the lowest current threshold.* The larger the diameter of the axon, the lower the resistance of its axoplasm to the flow of longitudinal current because of the greater number of intracellular charge carriers (ions) per unit length of the axon. As a result, a greater fraction of total current enters the larger axon, so it is depolarized more effectively than a smaller axon.[1] Thus, a gradual increase in current strength will recruit (excite) the larger axons first (at low values of current); smaller diameter axons will be recruited only at relatively larger current strengths.

Passive Membrane Properties and Axon Diameter Affect the Velocity of Action Potential Propagation

The passive spread of depolarization during conduction of the action potential is not instantaneous. In fact, it is a rate-limiting factor in the propagation of the action potential. We can understand this limitation by considering a simplified equivalent circuit of two adjacent membrane segments connected by a segment of axoplasm, r_a (Figure 7–9). As described above, an action potential generated in one segment of membrane supplies depolarizing current to the adjacent membrane, causing it to depolarize gradually toward threshold. According to Ohm's law, the larger the axoplasmic resistance, the smaller the current flow around the loop ($I = V/R$), and thus the longer it takes to change the charge on the membrane of the adjacent segment.

---

[1] A greater fraction of total current enters and leaves the larger axon because of its lower r_a. On the other hand, the greater membrane area per unit length in the larger diameter axon means that these larger axons have a lower r_m and a larger c_m across which the current must flow to produce a depolarization. Therefore, the larger the axon diameter, the more current is required to produce a given depolarization. However, r_m decreases and c_m increases linearly with axon diameter, whereas r_a decreases with the square of the diameter, so r_a is dominant. The net effect is that larger axons have lower current thresholds.

A

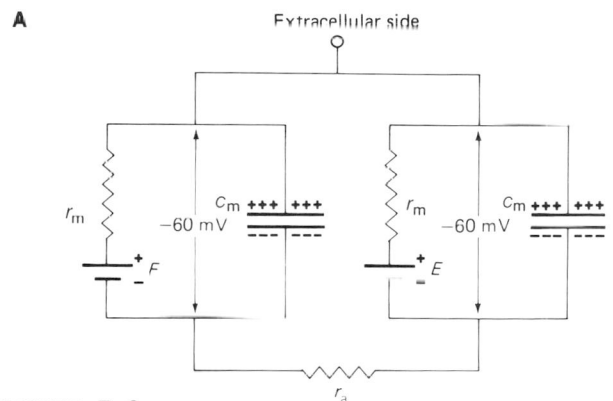

B

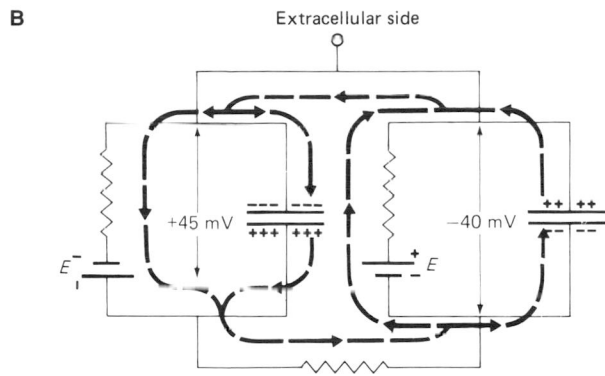

FIGURE 7–9

An electrical equivalent circuit representing two adjacent membrane segments of an axon connected by a segment of axoplasm. In **A** both membrane segments are at rest. In **B** an action potential is spreading from the membrane segment on the left to the segment on the right. **Broken lines** indicate pathways of current flow.

Recall that since $\Delta V = \Delta Q/C$, membrane potential will change slowly if the current is small because ΔQ will change slowly. Similarly, the larger the membrane capacitance, the more charge must be deposited on the membrane to change the potential across the membrane, so the current must flow for a longer time to produce a given depolarization. Therefore, the time it takes for depolarization to spread along the axon is determined by both the axial resistance and the capacitance per unit length of the axon (r_a and c_m). The rate of passive spread varies inversely with the product $r_a c_m$. If this product is reduced, the rate of passive spread of a given depolarization will increase and the action potential will propagate faster.

Rapid propagation of the action potential is functionally important, and two distinct mechanisms have evolved to increase it. One adaptive strategy is to increase conduction velocity by *increasing the diameter of the axon core*. Because the axial resistance (r_a) decreases in proportion to the square of axon diameter, while the capacitance per unit length of the axon (c_m) increases in direct proportion to diameter, the net effect of an increase in diameter is a decrease in $r_a c_m$. This adaptation has been carried to its extreme in the giant axon of the squid, which can be as large as 1 mm in diameter. No larger axons have evolved, presumably because of the opposing need to keep neuronal size small (so that many cells can be packed into a restricted space).

A second mechanism for increasing conduction velocity by reducing $r_a c_m$ is *myelination*, the wrapping of glial cell membranes around an axon as described in Chapter 3. This process is functionally equivalent to increasing the thickness of the axonal membrane by as much as 100 times. Because the capacitance of a parallel-plate capacitor such as the membrane is inversely proportional to the thickness of the insulating material, myelination decreases c_m and thus $r_a c_m$. The increase in total fiber diameter achieved by myelination causes a much larger percentage decrease in $r_a c_m$ than if the same increase in fiber diameter were achieved by increasing the diameter of the axon core. For this reason, conduction in myelinated axons is typically faster than in nonmyelinated axons of the same diameter.

Although myelin is quite effective in increasing conduction velocity, it interferes with the normal regenerative mechanism for actively propagating the action potential. In a neuron with a myelinated axon the action potential is triggered at the bare membrane of the axon hillock. The inward current that flows through this region of membrane is then available to discharge the capacitance of the myelinated axon ahead of it. Even though the thickness of myelin makes the capacitance of the axon quite small, the amount of current flowing down the core of the axon from the trigger zone is not enough to discharge the capacitance along the entire length of the myelinated axon. Therefore, the action potential gradually diminishes as it spreads passively down the axon.

To counteract this decrement and prevent the action potential from dying out completely, the myelin sheath is interrupted every 1–2 mm by the nodes of Ranvier. The bare patches of axon membrane at the nodes are only about 2 μm in length. Although the area of each nodal membrane is quite small, it contains a relatively high density of voltage-gated Na^+ channels and thus can generate an intense depolarizing inward Na^+ current in response to the passive spread of depolarization from the axon upstream. These regularly distributed nodes thus boost the amplitude of the action potential periodically, preventing it from dying out.

The action potential, which spreads quite rapidly along the internode because of the low capacitance of the myelin sheath, slows down as it crosses the high capacitance region of each bare node. Consequently, as the action potential moves down the axon, it seems to jump quickly from node to node (Figure 7–10). For this reason, the action potential in a myelinated axon is said to move by *saltatory conduction* (from the Latin *saltare*, to leap). Because ionic membrane current flows only at the nodes in myelinated fibers, saltatory conduction is also favorable from a metabolic standpoint. Less energy must be expended by the Na^+–K^+ pump in restoring the Na^+ and K^+

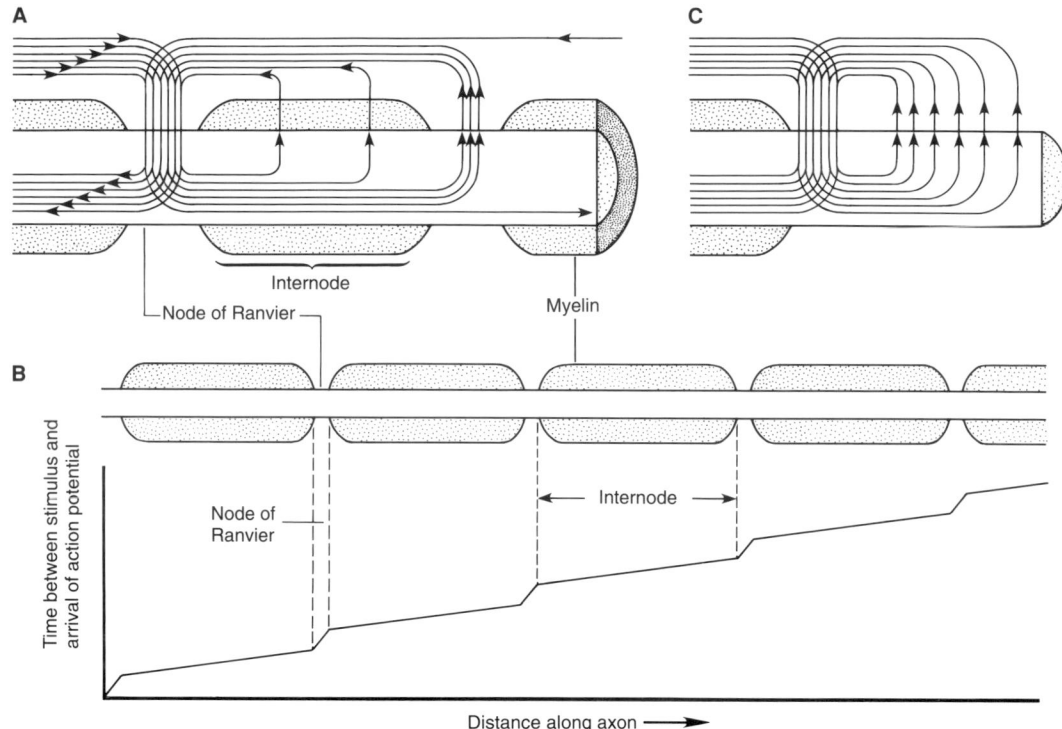

FIGURE 7–10

Saltatory conduction in myelinated nerves.

A. Capacitive and ionic membrane current densities (membrane current per unit area of membrane) are much higher at the nodes of Ranvier than in the internodal regions of the axon. Membrane current density is represented by the distribution of the lines depicting current flow (**arrows**).

B. Because of the low capacitance of the myelin sheath, the action

potential skips rapidly from node to node. It slows down at the nodes because of their high capacitance.

C. Action potential conduction is slowed down or blocked at axon regions that have lost their myelin. The local-circuit currents must charge a larger area of membrane capacitance, and, because of the low r_m, they do not spread effectively along the length of the axon.

concentration gradients, which tend to run down as a result of action potential activity.

Several diseases of the nervous system, such as multiple sclerosis and Guillain–Barre syndrome, cause demyelination (see Chapter 18). Because the lack of myelin slows down the conduction of the action potential, these diseases can have devastating effects on behavior. As an action potential goes from a myelinated region to a bare stretch of axon, it encounters a region of relatively high c_m and low r_m. For this unmyelinated segment of membrane to reach the threshold for an action potential, the inward current generated at the node just before this area has to flow for a longer time. In addition, this local-circuit current does not spread as far as normal because it is flowing into a segment of axon that, because of its low r_m, has a short length constant (Figure 7–10C). These two factors can combine to slow, and in some cases actually block, the conduction of action potentials.

An Overall View

Two competing pressures determine the functional design of neurons. First, to maximize the computing power of the

nervous system, neurons must be small, so that large numbers of them can fit into the available space. Second, to maximize the ability of the organism to respond to changes in its environment, neurons must conduct signals rapidly. In meeting these two design objectives, evolution has been constrained by the materials from which neurons are made. Because the nerve cell membrane is very thin and is surrounded by a conducting medium, it has a very high capacitance and thus slows down the conduction of voltage signals. In addition, the currents that change the charge on the membrane capacitance must flow through a relatively poor conductor—a thin column of cytoplasm. The nongated ion channels that give rise to the resting potential also degrade the signaling function of the neuron. They make the cell leaky and, together with the high membrane capacitance, they limit the distance that a signal can travel without being actively amplified.

A number of features in the nervous system have evolved to compensate for these constraints. (1) The long time constant of a neuron is exploited at the integrative zone, where inputs to the cell are time-averaged over a period of several milliseconds (temporal integration). (2) The integrative zone of a neuron is compact, so that receptor or synaptic potentials are generated fairly close to the trigger zone, thus optimizing spatial integration. (3) The spatially decrementing inputs to the neuron (synaptic potentials or receptor potentials) are converted into a pulse code for long distance signaling. The voltage-gated channels generate the all-or-none action potential, which is conducted without decrement. (4) For pathways in which rapid signaling is particularly important, the conduction velocity of the action potential is enhanced by either myelination or an increase in axon diameter, or both.

Selected Readings

Barrett, J. N. 1975. Motoneuron dendrites: Role in synaptic integration. Fed. Proc. 34:1398–1407.

Graubard, K., and Calvin, W. H. 1979. Presynaptic dendrites: Implications of spikeless synaptic transmission and dendritic geometry. In F. O. Schmitt and F. G. Worden (eds.), The Neurosciences: Fourth Study Program. Cambridge, Mass.: MIT Press, pp. 317–331.

Hodgkin, A. L. 1964. The Conduction of the Nervous Impulse. Springfield, Ill.: Thomas, chap. 4.

Hubbard, J. I., Llinás, R., and Quastel, D. M. J. 1969. Electrophysiological Analysis of Synaptic Transmission. Baltimore: Williams & Wilkins, chap. 2, pp. 91–109, 257–264.

Jack, J. 1979. An introduction to linear cable theory. In F. O. Schmitt and F. G. Worden (eds.), The Neurosciences: Fourth Study Program. Cambridge, Mass.: MIT Press, pp. 423–437.

Jack, J. J. B., Noble, D., and Tsien, R. W. 1975. Electric Current Flow in Excitable Cells. Oxford: Clarendon Press, chaps. 1–5, 7; pp. 276–277.

Khodorov, B. I. 1974. The Problem of Excitability. New York: Plenum Press, chap. 3.

Moore, J. W., Joyner, R. W., Brill, M. H., Waxman, S. D., and Najar-Joa, M. 1978. Simulations of conduction in uniform myelinated fibers: Relative sensitivity to changes in nodal and internodal parameters. Biophys. J. 21:147–160.

Rall, W. 1977. Core conductor theory and cable properties of neurons. In E. R. Kandel (ed.), Handbook of Physiology, Section 1: The Nervous System, Vol I. Cellular Biology of Neurons, Part 1. Bethesda, Md.: American Physiological Society, pp. 39–97.

John Koester

Voltage-Gated Ion Channels and the Generation of the Action Potential

The Action Potential Is Generated by the Flow of Ions Through Voltage-Gated Sodium and Potassium Channels

Voltage-Gated Channels Can Be Studied by Use of the Voltage Clamp

The Voltage-Gated Sodium and Potassium Channels Have Different Kinetics

Sodium and Potassium Membrane Conductances Are Calculated from Their Currents

The Action Potential Can Be Reconstructed from the Known Electrical Properties of the Neuron

The Hodgkin–Huxley Model of Excitability Is Universally Applicable: Modifications Reflect the Diversity and Distribution of Voltage-Gated Channels

The Basic Mechanism of Action Potential Generation Is the Same in All Neurons

The Nervous System Expresses a Rich Variety of Voltage-Gated Ion Channels

Gating of Voltage-Sensitive Ion Channels Can Be Influenced by Changes in Intracellular Ion Concentrations

Excitability Properties Vary Among Neurons

Excitability Properties Vary Within Regions of the Neuron

Voltage-Gated Channels Have Characteristic Molecular Properties

Voltage-Gated Sodium Channels Are Sparsely Distributed

Voltage-Gated Channels Open in an All-or-None Fashion

Charges Are Redistributed Within the Membrane When Voltage-Gated Sodium Channels Open

The Voltage-Gated Sodium Channel Selects for Sodium on the Basis of Size, Charge, and Energy of Hydration of the Ion

The Voltage-Gated Potassium, Sodium, and Calcium Channels Belong to One Gene Family

An Overall View

Signals can be conveyed over long distances within the nervous system because, as we saw in Chapter 7, nerve cells generate and conduct action potentials that do not decrease in amplitude as they travel away from the site of initiation.

The generation of action potentials by nerve axons and muscle fibers was first described in 1849 by the German physiologist Emil DuBois-Reymond. It was not until more than a 100 years later, however, that the underlying mechanism could be explained in terms of the properties of specific membrane proteins—the voltage-gated ion channels for Na$^+$ and K$^+$.

The Action Potential Is Generated by the Flow of Ions Through Voltage-Gated Sodium and Potassium Channels

An important early clue about how action potentials are generated came from an experiment done in 1938 by Kenneth Cole and Howard Curtis. Recording from the squid giant axon, they found that conductance of the membrane to ions increases during the action potential. This demonstration provided an early indication that the action potential results from the movement of ions through channels in the membrane. It also raised a question: Which ions are responsible for the action potential? A decade later, Alan Hodgkin and Bernard Katz found that the amplitude of the action potential is reduced when the external Na$^+$ concentration is lowered.

On the basis of their own observations and those of Cole and Curtis, Hodgkin and Katz proposed that the depolarization that initiates an action potential causes a transient change in the membrane that briefly switches its predominant permeability from K$^+$ to Na$^+$. We now know that these permeability changes occur because of the opening of voltage-sensitive channels in the membrane that allow Na$^+$ to move down its concentration gradient into the cell. These Na$^+$ channels are normally kept closed by a voltage-sensitive gating mechanism. Depolarization opens these Na$^+$ channels, allowing increased Na$^+$ influx into the cell, thereby producing the rising phase of the action potential. The falling phase of the action potential is caused by the subsequent closing of the Na$^+$ channels, which reduces Na$^+$ influx, and by the opening of voltage-gated K$^+$ channels, which allows increased K$^+$ efflux from the cell.

To test this hypothesis, it is necessary to vary membrane potential systematically and measure the resulting changes in the conductance through the Na$^+$ and the K$^+$ channels. This is difficult to do experimentally because there is mutual coupling between membrane potential and the Na$^+$ and K$^+$ channels. For example, if the membrane is depolarized sufficiently to open some of the voltage-gated Na$^+$ channels, inward Na$^+$ current flows through these channels and causes additional depolarization. The added depolarization causes still more Na$^+$ channels to open and consequently induces more inward

Na$^+$ current. A regenerative cycle is thereby initiated that makes it impossible to achieve a stable membrane potential. This positive feedback cycle, which eventually drives V_m to the peak of the action potential, can be depicted as follows:

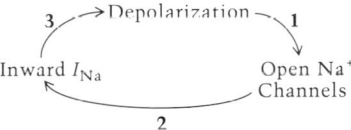

A similar technical difficulty hinders the study of the active K$^+$ conductance channels that are responsible for the falling phase of the action potential. In 1949 Cole designed an apparatus known as the voltage clamp to overcome these problems. By using the voltage-clamp technique on the squid giant axon in the early 1950s, Hodgkin and Andrew Huxley provided the first complete description of the ionic mechanisms underlying the action potential.

Voltage-Gated Channels Can Be Studied by Use of the Voltage Clamp

The basic function of the voltage clamp is to interrupt the interaction between the opening and closing of voltage-gated channels and membrane potential. By recording the current that must be generated by the voltage clamp to keep the membrane potential from changing, one obtains a direct measure of the membrane current (Box 8–1). The membrane current that is recorded can then be separated into ionic and capacitive components. Recall that V_m at any time is proportional to membrane capacitance (C_m). When V_m is not changing, C_m is constant and no capacitive current flows. Capacitive current flows *only* when V_m is changing (Chapter 7). Therefore, if the membrane potential changes in response to a very rapid step of command potential, capacitive current flows only at the beginning and the end of the step. This capacitive current is essentially instantaneous, and it can be separated easily from the later ionic currents by inspection of the oscilloscope record. Having eliminated the capacitive current, one is in the position to analyze the ionic currents that flow through the membrane channels.

From the ionic membrane current and the membrane potential one can calculate the voltage- and time-dependence of the changes in membrane conductances caused by the opening and closing of Na$^+$ and K$^+$ channels. This information provides insights into the properties of the channels for these two ions.

The Voltage-Gated Sodium and Potassium Channels Have Different Kinetics

Let us consider the results of a typical voltage-clamp experiment (Figure 8–2). We start with the membrane po-

The voltage-clamp technique, first developed by Kenneth Cole in 1949, was used by Alan Hodgkin and Andrew Huxley in 1952 to study the squid giant axon. When an axon is voltage-clamped, voltage-gated ion channels are able to open or close in response to imposed changes in membrane potential, but the voltage clamp prevents the resultant changes in membrane current from influencing the membrane potential. The conductance of the membrane to different ions can then be measured as a function of membrane potential.

The voltage clamp is a current source connected to two electrodes, one inside and the other outside the cell. By passing current across the cell membrane, the membrane potential can be stepped rapidly to various predetermined levels of depolarization.

FIGURE 8–1A

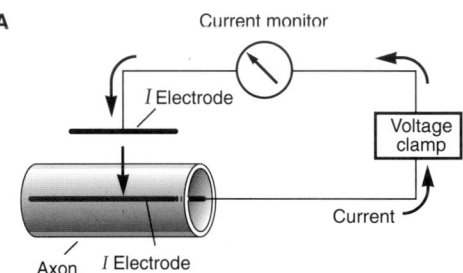

These depolarizations open voltage-gated Na^+ and K^+ channels. The resulting movement of Na^+ and K^+ across the membrane would ordinarily change the membrane potential, but the voltage clamp holds or "clamps" the membrane potential at a commanded level. For example, when Na^+ channels open in response to a depolarizing voltage step, an inward membrane current develops because Na^+ ions flow through these channels. This Na^+ influx tends to depolarize the membrane by increasing the positive charge on the inside of the membrane and reducing the positive charge on the outside. The voltage clamp prevents the membrane potential from depolarizing further by simultaneously withdrawing positive charges out of the cell into the external solution. The voltage-clamp circuit automatically counteracts the flow of any membrane current that would tend to change the membrane potential from its commanded value by generating an equal and opposite current (Figure 8–1A). As a result there is no change in the *net* amount of charge separated by the membrane and therefore no significant change in V_m.

Under voltage-clamp conditions the first two steps in the regenerative cycle described above are not affected directly: An imposed depolarization still causes Na^+ channels to open, which still results in an increased inward Na^+ current. The third step, however, the further depolarization caused by this extra Na^+ influx, is prevented by the clamp.

The voltage clamp is a negative feedback system. A negative feedback system is one in which the value of the output of the system (V_m in this case) is "fed back" to the input of the system, where it is compared to a command signal for the desired output. Any difference between the command potential and the output signal activates a "controller" device that automatically reduces the difference. Thus, the membrane potential *automatically* follows the command potential exactly (Figure 8–1B).

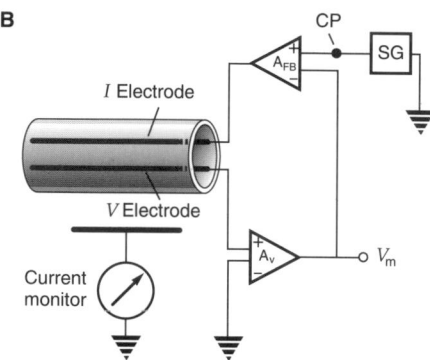

FIGURE 8–1B

Membrane potential is measured by the voltage amplifier (A_v), which is connected to an intracellular (V) electrode and to the system ground, which is connected to the bath. The membrane potential signal (V_m) is displayed on an oscilloscope and is also fed into one terminal of the "feedback" amplifier (A_{FB}). This amplifier has two inputs—one for membrane potential and the other for the command potential (CP). The command potential, which comes from a signal generator (SG), is selected by the experimenter and can be of any desired amplitude and waveform. The feedback amplifier subtracts the membrane potential from the command potential. Any difference between these two signals is amplified several thousand times at the output of the feedback amplifier. The output of this amplifier is connected to a thin wire, the current-passing electrode (I), which runs the length of the axon. For the measured membrane current-voltage relationship to be meaningful, it is important that the membrane potential be uniform along the entire surface of the membrane. This condition can be maintained because the highly conductive current-passing wire short circuits the axoplasmic resistance, reducing the axial resistance to zero. The presence of this low-resistance pathway within the axon makes it impossible for a potential difference to exist between different points along the axon core.

For example, assume that an inward Na^+ current through the voltage-gated Na^+ channels causes the membrane potential to become more positive than the command potential. The resulting voltage at the output of the feedback amplifier will be negative. This output voltage will make the internal current electrode negative, withdrawing net positive charge from the cell through the voltage clamp circuit. As current flows around the circuit, an equal amount of net positive charge will be deposited into the external solution through the other current electrode.

A refinement of the voltage clamp, the patch-clamp technique described in Chapter 5, allows the functional properties of individual ion channels to be determined.

tential clamped at its resting value. If a 10 mV, depolarizing potential step is commanded, we observe that an initial, very brief outward capacitive current (I_c) instantaneously discharges the membrane capacitance by the amount required for a 10 mV depolarization. This capacitive current is followed by a smaller, steady outward ionic current that persists for the duration of this pulse. At the end of the pulse there is a brief inward capacitive current, and the ionic current returns to zero (Figure 8–2A). The steady ionic current, the current that flows through the nongated ion channels of the membrane (Chapter 7), is called the *leakage current*, I_l. The total conductance of this population of channels is called the *leakage conductance* (g_l). These nongated leakage channels, which are always open, are responsible for generating the resting potential (Chapter 6). In a typical neuron, most of the nongated leakage channels are permeable to K^+ ions; the remaining leakage channels are permeable to Cl^- or Na^+ ions.

If a larger depolarizing step is commanded, the current records become more complicated (Figure 8–2B). The capacitive and leakage currents are both increased in amplitude. In addition, shortly after the end of the capacitive current and the start of the leakage current, an inward current develops; it reaches a peak within a few milliseconds, declines, and gives way to an outward current. This outward current reaches a plateau that is maintained for the duration of the pulse.

A simple interpretation of these findings is that the depolarizing voltage step sequentially turns on active conductance channels for two separate ions: one type of channel for inward current and another for outward current. Because these two oppositely directed currents partially overlap in time, the most difficult part of the analysis of voltage-clamp experiments is to determine their separate time courses.

Hodgkin and Huxley achieved this separation by changing ions. By substituting a larger, impermeant cation (choline) for Na^+ in the external bathing solution, they eliminated the inward Na^+ current. Since then a simpler technique has been developed for separating inward and outward currents: selective pharmacological blockade of the separate voltage-sensitive conductance channels. Tetrodotoxin blocks the voltage-gated Na^+ channel and tetraethylammonium blocks the voltage-gated K^+ channel.

To measure I_{Na}, the current flowing through the voltage-gated Na^+ channels, as a function of V_m, various command pulses are given to change V_m to different levels. When tetraethylammonium is applied to the axon to block the K^+ channels, the total membrane current consists of I_c, I_l, and I_{Na}. The leakage conductance, g_l, is constant; it does not vary with V_m or with time. Therefore, I_l may be readily calculated and subtracted from I_m, leaving I_{Na} and I_c. Because I_c occurs only briefly at the beginning and end of the pulse, it can be eliminated easily by inspection, leaving a pure I_{Na}. By a similar process, I_K may be measured when the Na^+ channels are blocked by tetrodotoxin (Figure 8–2C).

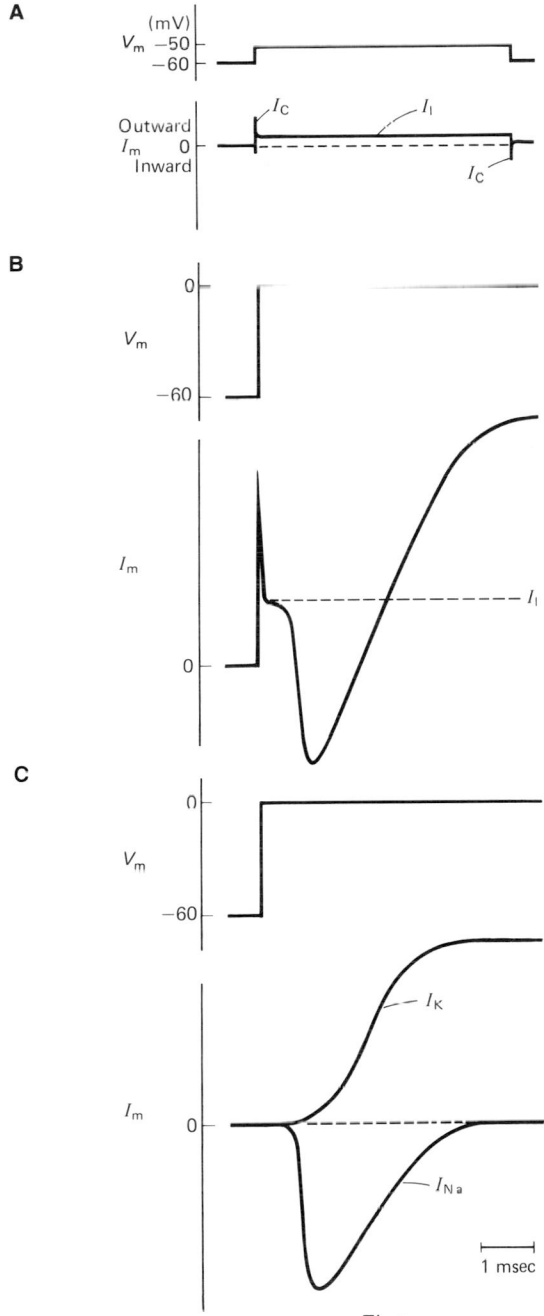

FIGURE 8–2
This record from a squid axon voltage-clamp experiment demonstrates the existence of two types of voltage-gated channels.

A. A small depolarization is accompanied by capacitive and leakage currents (I_c and I_l, respectively).

B. A larger depolarizing step results in larger capacitive and leakage currents plus additional currents caused by the opening of voltage-gated Na^+ and K^+ channels.

C. When the voltage step shown in **B** is repeated in the presence of tetrodotoxin (which blocks the Na^+ current) and again in the presence of tetraethylammonium (which blocks the K^+ current), records of the pure K^+ and Na^+ currents (I_K and I_{Na}, respectively) are obtained by subtraction of I_c and I_l.

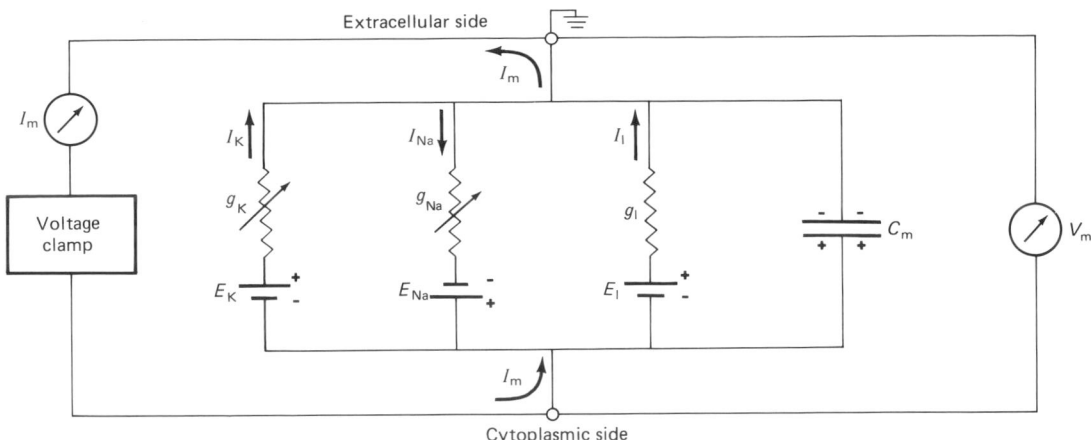

FIGURE 8–3

Electrical equivalent circuit of a nerve cell under voltage-clamp conditions. The voltage-gated conductance pathways are repre-   sented by the symbol for a variable conductance—a conductor (resistor) with an arrow through it.

Sodium and Potassium Membrane Conductances Are Calculated from Their Currents

Once the Na^+ and the K^+ currents have been separated (Figure 8–2C), the kinetics of opening and closing of the entire population of voltage-gated Na^+ and K^+ channels can be calculated. This analysis is illustrated with an equivalent circuit of the membrane that includes the membrane capacitance (C_m) and leakage conductance (g_l), as well as g_{Na} and g_K (Figure 8–3). In this context g_l represents the conductance of all of the nongated K^+, Na^+, and Cl^- channels (see Chapter 6); g_{Na} and g_K represent the conductances of the voltage-gated Na^+ and K^+ channels. The ionic battery of the passive (leakage) channels, E_l, is equal to the resting potential (see Equation 6–4). The voltage-sensitive Na^+ and K^+ conductances are in series with their appropriate ionic batteries.

The current through each class of active conductance channel may be calculated from Ohm's law, written in the same form used to calculate the currents through the passive channels (see Equations 6–2a and 6–2b):

$$I_K = g_K \times (V_m - E_K) \qquad (8\text{–}1a)$$

$$I_{Na} = g_{Na} \times (V_m - E_{Na}) \qquad (8\text{–}1b)$$

Rearranging and solving for g gives two equations that can be used to compute the conductances for the active Na^+ and K^+ channel populations[1]:

$$g_K = \frac{I_K}{(V_m - E_m)}$$

$$g_{Na} = \frac{I_{Na}}{(V_m - E_{Na})}$$

Measurements of Na^+ and K^+ conductances at various levels of membrane potential reveal two basic similarities and two differences between them. They are alike in that both populations of channels open in response to depolarizing steps of membrane potential, and they both do so more rapidly and to a greater extent for larger depolarizations (Figure 8–4). They differ, however, in their rates of onset and offset and their responses to prolonged depolarization. At all levels of depolarization, Na^+ channels open more rapidly than do K^+ channels (Figure 8–4). They also close more rapidly when the depolarizing pulse is very brief (Figure 8–5, line a). In addition, when depolarization is maintained, the Na^+ channels begin to close, or inactivate (Figures 8–4 and 8–5), leading to a decay of inward current. In contrast, the K^+ channels remain open as long as the membrane is depolarized (Figure 8–5).

Each Na^+ channel can exist in three different states thought to represent three different conformations of the Na^+ channel protein—resting, activated, or inactivated (see chapter 5). Upon depolarization the channel goes from the resting (closed) to the activated (open) state. If the depolarization is brief, the channels go directly back to the resting state. If the depolarization is maintained, the channel switches to the inactivated (closed) state. Once the channel is inactivated it cannot be activated (opened) by depolarization. The inactivation can be removed only by repolarizing the membrane, which allows the channel to switch from the inactivated to the resting state. This switch takes time because channels leave the inactivated state relatively slowly (Figure 8–6). In other words, each Na^+ channel acts as if it has two kinds of gates, both of which have to be open for this channel to conduct Na^+ ions. There is an *activation gate*, which is closed when the membrane is at its resting potential and is rapidly activated by depolarization, and an *inactivation gate*, which is open at the resting potential and closes slowly in response to depolarization. The channel conducts only for the brief

---

[1]To solve these equations for g_K and g_{Na}, one must know V_m, E_K, E_{Na}, I_K, and I_{Na}. The independent variable V_m is set by the experimenter. The dependent variables I_K and I_{Na} can be obtained from the current records of voltage-clamp experiments by the ionic separation techniques described above (Figure 8–2C). E_K and E_{Na} are constants; they can be calculated from the Nernst equation or determined empirically by finding the values of V_m at which I_K and I_{Na} reverse their polarities. For example, if V_m is stepped to very positive values, I_{Na} becomes less inward. At E_{Na} it goes to zero, and for values of V_m more positive than E_{Na}, I_{Na} is outward (Equation 8–1b).

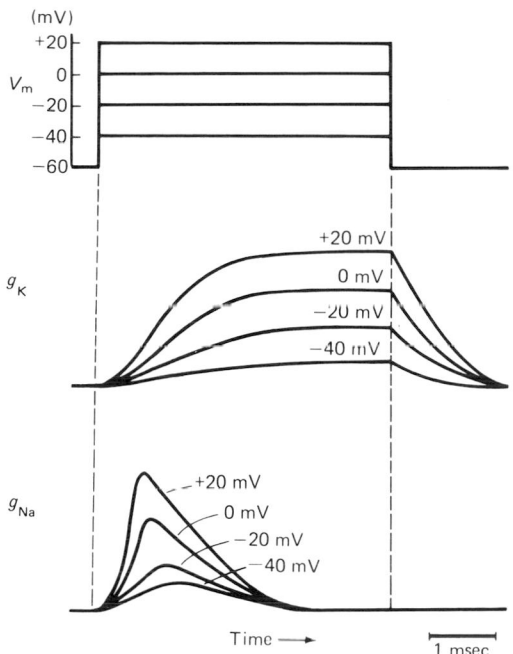

FIGURE 8–4

Voltage-clamp experiments show that g_{Na} turns on and off more rapidly than g_K over a wide range of membrane potentials. The gradual increases and decreases in total Na⁺ and K⁺ conductances shown here reflect the shifting of thousands of voltage-gated channels between the open and closed states.

period during depolarization when both gates are open. Repolarization reverses the two processes (see Figure 8–10). After the channel has returned to the resting state, it is again available for activation by depolarization.

The Action Potential Can Be Reconstructed from the Known Electrical Properties of the Neuron

After measuring the conductance changes for depolarizing pulses of various amplitudes and durations, Hodgkin and Huxley fit their data to a set of empirical equations that describe completely the variations of membrane Na⁺ and K⁺ conductances as functions of membrane potential and time. Using these equations and measured values for the passive properties of the axon, they computed the shape and the conduction velocity of the propagated action potential. The calculated waveform of the action potential matched almost perfectly the waveform recorded in the unclamped axon. This close agreement indicates that the voltage- and time-dependence of the active Na⁺ and K⁺ channels, calculated from the voltage-clamp data, accurately describe the properties of these channels that are essential for the generation and propagation of the action potential.

According to the Hodgkin–Huxley model, an action potential involves the following sequence of events. A depolarization of the membrane causes a rapid opening of Na⁺ channels (an increase in g_{Na}), resulting in an inward Na⁺ current. This current, by discharging the membrane capacitance, causes further depolarization, causing more

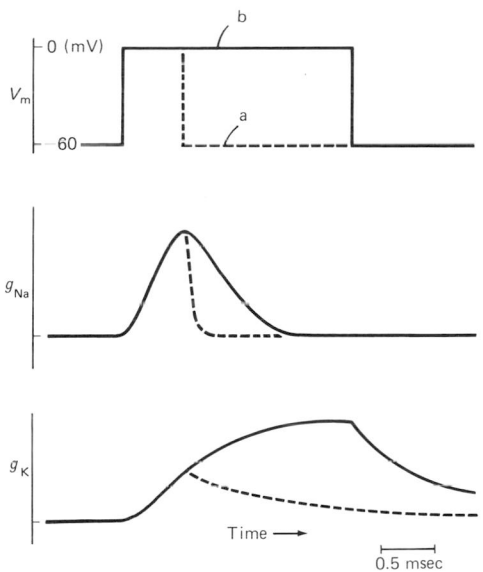

FIGURE 8–5

For a brief depolarizing step (**a**) both g_{Na} and g_K return to their initial values when the cell repolarizes. For a longer step (**b**), g_{Na} inactivates even though the depolarization is maintained, while g_K reaches a plateau level that is constant for the duration of the depolarization.

FIGURE 8–6

Time course of recovery of Na⁺ channels from inactivation and return to the resting state. If the interval between two depolarizing pulses is brief, the second pulse (P₂) produces a smaller increase in g_{Na} because inactivation of Na⁺ channels persists for a few milliseconds after the end of the first activating pulse. The longer the interval between pulses, the greater the fraction of channels that will have switched from the inactivated to the resting state when P₂ begins.

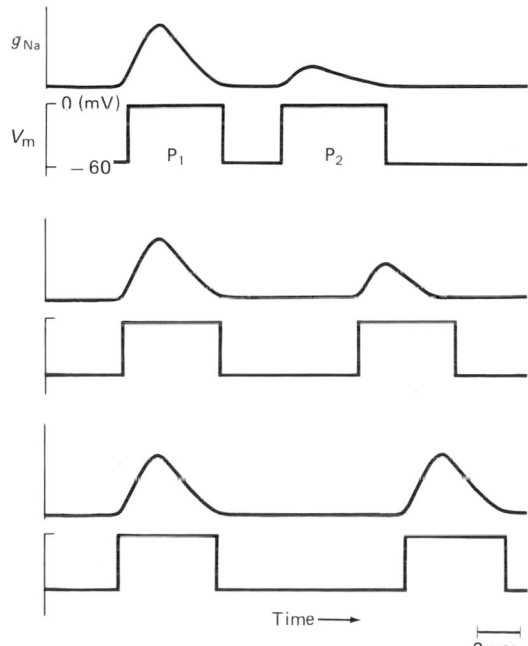

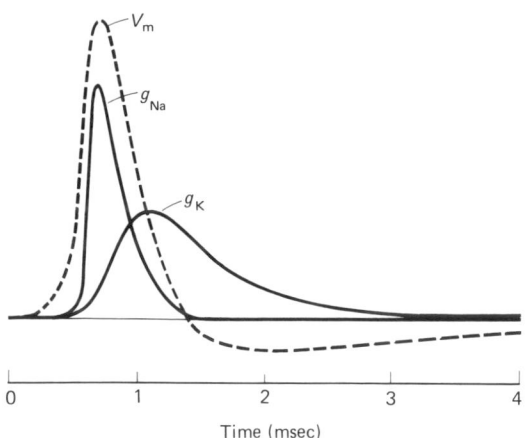

FIGURE 8–7
The shape of the action potential can be calculated from the changes in g_{Na} and g_K that result from the opening and closing of voltage-gated Na$^+$ and K$^+$ channels. The calculated shape shown here (**dashed line**) matches quite closely the shape recorded empirically. (Adapted from Hodgkin, 1964.)

Na$^+$ channels to open, resulting in more inward current. This regenerative process generates the action potential. Two factors limit the duration of the action potential. (1) The depolarization of the action potential gradually inactivates the Na$^+$ channels (g_{Na}). (2) The depolarization also opens, with some delay, the voltage-gated K$^+$ channels, thereby increasing g_K (Figure 8–7). Consequently, the Na$^+$ current is followed by an outward K$^+$ current that tends to repolarize the membrane.

In most nerve cells, action potentials are followed by a transient hyperpolarization, the hyperpolarizing *afterpotential*. This brief increase in membrane potential occurs because the K$^+$ channels that open during the later phase of the action potential close some time after V_m has returned to its resting value. It takes a few milliseconds for all of the voltage-gated K$^+$ channels to return to the closed state. During this time the efflux of K$^+$ from the cell is greater than during the resting state. As a result, V_m is hyperpolarized slightly with respect to its normal resting value (Figure 8–7).

The action potential is also followed by a brief period of refractoriness, which can be divided into two phases. The *absolute refractory period* comes immediately after the action potential; during this period it is impossible to excite the cell no matter how large a stimulating current is applied. This phase is followed directly by the *relative refractory period*, during which it is possible to trigger an action potential, but only by applying stimuli that are stronger than normal. These periods of refractoriness, which together last just a few milliseconds, are caused by the residual inactivation of Na$^+$ channels and opening of K$^+$ channels.

Another feature of the action potential predicted by the Hodgkin–Huxley model is its all-or-none behavior. A fraction of a millivolt may be the difference between a subthreshold depolarizing stimulus and a stimulus that generates a full-blown action potential. This all-or-none phenomenon may seem surprising when one considers that Na$^+$ conductance (proportional to the number of Na$^+$ channels that are open) increases in a strictly graded manner as depolarization is increased (Figure 8–4). With each increment of depolarization, the number of voltage-gated Na$^+$ channels that switch from the closed to the open state increases in a gradual fashion, thereby causing a gradual increase in Na$^+$ influx. Why then is there a threshold for action potential generation?

Although a small subthreshold depolarization increases the inward I_{Na}, it also increases two *outward* currents, I_K and I_l, by changing the electrochemical driving forces that determine their values (see e.g., Equation 8–1a). At the same time, the depolarization also causes a slow increase in g_K by gradually increasing the number of open K$^+$ channels (Figure 8–4). As I_K and I_l increase with depolarization, they tend to resist the depolarizing action of the Na$^+$ influx. However, the great voltage sensitivity and rapid kinetics of the Na$^+$ channel activation process ensure that the depolarization will eventually reach a point—the threshold—where the increase in inward I_{Na} exceeds the increase in outward I_K and I_l, and becomes regenerative. The threshold, V_T, is therefore the specific value of V_m at which the *net* ionic current ($I_{Na} + I_K + I_l$) just changes from outward to inward, depositing positive charge on the inside of the membrane.

The Hodgkin–Huxley Model of Excitability Is Universally Applicable: Modifications Reflect the Diversity and Distribution of Voltage-Gated Channels

The original analysis of the action potential by Hodgkin and Huxley was performed on an invertebrate preparation—the giant axon of the squid. To what degree does their model for action potential generation apply to the other components of the neuron—the cell body, dendrites, and presynaptic terminals—and to the neurons of vertebrates? Five fundamental conclusions have emerged from studies designed to test the general applicability of the Hodgkin–Huxley model of voltage-gated channels and their role in generating the action potential.

The Basic Mechanism of Action Potential Generation Is the Same in All Neurons

Hodgkin and Huxley proposed that the action potential in the squid axon is caused by an inward membrane current followed by an outward current, and that the currents flow through voltage-gated membrane conductance channels. This mechanism of excitability has been found to be universally applicable in all excitable cells despite the fact that dozens of different types of voltage-gated ion channels have been described. Although different types of ion channels have important consequences for membrane excitability, the basic mechanism by which the all-or-none action potential is generated is the same in virtually all nerve and muscle cells.

The Nervous System Expresses a Rich Variety of Voltage-Gated Ion Channels

The Na^+ and K^+ channels described by Hodgkin and Huxley in the squid axon have been found in almost every type of neuron examined. Nevertheless, many other kinds of channels have been identified as well. Most neurons have voltage-gated Ca^{2+} channels that open in response to membrane depolarization. Because Ca^{2+} has a strong electrochemical gradient driving it into the cell, Ca^{2+} influx contributes to the upstroke of the action potential. Some neurons also have voltage-gated Cl^- channels.

Each type of ion-selective channel has many variants. For example, several types of voltage-gated K^+ channels are found in neurons. They differ from each other in their kinetics of activation, voltage activation range, and sensitivity to various ligands. Four types of K^+ channel variants are particularly common in the nervous system. (1) The slowly activating channel described by Hodgkin and Huxley is called the *delayed rectifier*. (2) The Ca^{2+}-activated K^+ channel is activated by depolarization but its voltage sensitivity is a function of the intracellular Ca^{2+} concentration. (3) The fast, transient (A-type) K^+ channel is activated rapidly by depolarization, as rapidly as the Na^+ channel; it also inactivates rapidly, but only if the depolarization is maintained. (4) The M-type K^+ channel is activated by depolarization but inactivated by acetylcholine. There are at least three types of voltage gated Ca^{2+} channels and two types of voltage gated Na^+ channels. Thus, a single ion species can cross the membrane through several distinct types of ion channels, each with its own characteristic kinetics and voltage sensitivity. Moreover, many types of voltage-gated channels can be classified into subtypes. For example, there are several types of fast, transient K^+ channels.

Gating of Voltage-Sensitive Ion Channels Can Be Influenced by Changes in Intracellular Ion Concentrations

In its most basic form a change in membrane potential involves the flow of ionic current through membrane channels, which leads to a change in the net charge stored on the membrane. This process does not require a change in intracellular ionic concentrations, and in general any such changes are negligible. However, in some neurons current flow through ion channels does lead to changes in the intracellular concentration of ions, and such changes have important modulatory influences on voltage-gated channels. The ion that most commonly has such a modulatory effect is Ca^{2+}. The concentration of free Ca^{2+} in the cytoplasm of a resting cell is extremely low, about 10^{-7} M, which is several orders of magnitude below that for Na^+, Cl^-, or K^+. For this reason the intracellular Ca^{2+} concentration is particularly likely to increase as the result of current flow through Ca^{2+} channels in the membrane. In fact, a number of cellular mechanisms exploit the increase in Ca^{2+} concentration that results when voltage-gated Ca^{2+} channels open and Ca^{2+} rushes into the cell.

For example, even the amount of Ca^{2+} that comes into the cell through voltage-gated Ca^{2+} channels during a single action potential may briefly saturate the Ca^{2+} buffering systems of the cell. When this occurs, the transient increase in Ca^{2+} concentration near the inside of the membrane increases the probability of opening of a Ca^{2+}-sensitive K^+ channel, so more of these channels enter the open state. A train of action potentials will have an even more significant effect on these Ca^{2+}-sensitive K^+ channels. Some Ca^{2+} channels are themselves sensitive to levels of intracellular Ca^{2+} and are inactivated when incoming Ca^{2+} binds to their internal surfaces. In other Ca^{2+} channels Ca^{2+} influx activates a Ca^{2+}-sensitive protein phosphatase, calcineurin, which dephosphorylates the channel, thereby inactivating it.

Thus, in some cells the Ca^{2+} influx during an action potential can have opposing effects—the positive charge that it carries into the cell contributes to the regenerative depolarization, while the increase in Ca^{2+} concentration results in the opening of more K^+ channels and the turning off of Ca^{2+} channels. As a result of the latter two effects, outward ionic current increases, inward ionic current decreases, and the cell tends to repolarize as the net efflux of positive charge increases. Thus, the influx of Ca^{2+} through voltage-gated Ca^{2+} channels is self-limited by two processes that aid repolarization—an increase in K^+ efflux and a decrease in Ca^{2+} influx.

Excitability Properties Vary Among Neurons

Although the function of each neuron is determined to a great extent by its position in a specific circuit, its function is also determined by its biophysical properties; these determine the relation between the synaptic input to the cell and the action potential train that it generates. How a neuron responds to synaptic input is determined by the proportions of different types of voltage-gated channels in the cell's integrative and trigger zones. Some cells respond to a constant excitatory input with a decelerating train of action potentials, others respond with an accelerating train, and others maintain a constant firing frequency. In certain neurons small changes in the strength of synaptic inputs produce a large increase in firing rate, whereas in others the firing rate responds only to large changes in synaptic input. In some neurons a steady hyperpolarizing input reduces the responsiveness of the cell to excitatory input by removing the inactivation of the fast, transient voltage-gated K^+ channels; in other neurons such a steady hyperpolarization makes the cell more excitable because it removes the inactivation of a particular class of voltage-gated Ca^{2+} channels (Figure 8–8).

As Hodgkin and Huxley clearly showed, only two types of ion channels are required to generate an action potential. The great diversity of voltage-gated ion channel types that have evolved and their expression in various combinations in different cells results in a vastly enriched range of excitability properties. As a result, different types of neurons encode the same synaptic input into different temporally patterned spike trains, which in turn are encoded into unique patterns of synaptic output.

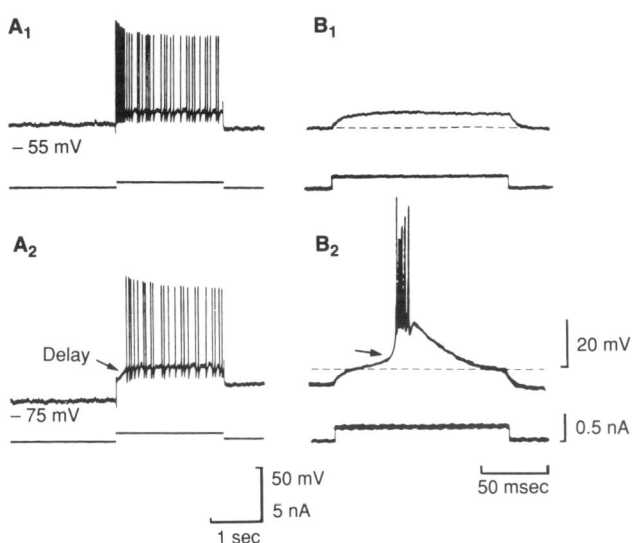

FIGURE 8–8

Repetitive firing properties vary widely among different types of neurons.

A. Injection of a depolarizing current pulse into a neuron from the nucleus tractus solitarius normally triggers an immediate train of action potentials (**1**). If the cell is first held at a hyperpolarized membrane potential, the same depolarizing pulse triggers a spike train after a delay (**2**). The delay is caused by the fast, transient K$^+$ channels that are activated in response to depolarizing synaptic input. The opening of these channels generates a transient, outward K$^+$ current that briefly drives V_m away from threshold. The fast, transient (type A) K$^+$ channels typically are inactivated at the resting potential (V_R), but steady hyperpolarization removes the inactivation, allowing the channels to become available for activation by depolarization. (From Dekin and Getting, 1987.)

B. When a small depolarizing pulse is injected into a thalamic neuron that is at rest, only an electrotonic, subthreshold depolarization is generated (**1**). If the cell is held at a hyperpolarized level, the same depolarizing pulse triggers a burst of action potentials (**2**). The effectiveness of depolarization is enhanced because the hyperpolarization removes the inactivation of a type of voltage-gated Ca^{2+} channel that is normally inactivated at V_R. The dotted line indicates the level of the resting potential. (From Jahnsen and Llinás, 1982.)

These data demonstrate that steady hyperpolarization, such as might be produced by inhibitory synaptic input to a neuron, can profoundly affect the spike train pattern that a neuron generates. This type of effect varies greatly among cell types.

Excitability Properties Vary Within Regions of the Neuron

In addition to variations in the type and density of ion channels in cells throughout the nervous system, important differences also exist in the distribution of channel types within individual cells. These topographic variations have important functional consequences. For example, the membranes of the dendrites, cell body, axon hillock, and nerve terminals have a greater variety of channels than does the axon membrane. The simple array

of channel types in the axon may be a function of the role of the axon as a simple relay line between the input and output zones of a cell, whereas the input and output zones must transform the signals they receive. The input zone converts synaptic or sensory input into a temporally patterned train of action potentials. The output zone converts this train of potentials into a series of synaptic potentials, the amplitudes of which depend critically on the ion fluxes across the presynaptic membrane (Chapter 13).

Voltage-Gated Channels Have Characteristic Molecular Properties

The empirical equations derived by Hodgkin and Huxley were remarkably successful in describing how the flow of ions through the Na$^+$ and K$^+$ channels generates the action potential. However, these equations describe the process of excitation primarily in terms of changes in membrane conductance and current flow. The data of Hodgkin and Huxley tell us little about the molecular nature of the voltage-gated conductance channels and the mechanisms by which they are activated. Technical advances, such as those described in Chapter 5, have made it possible to examine in detail the molecular structure and function of the voltage-gated Na$^+$, K$^+$, and Ca^{2+} channels.

Voltage-Gated Sodium Channels Are Sparsely Distributed

Characterization of the distribution of the voltage-gated Na$^+$ channel has been aided greatly by the availability of several naturally occurring neurotoxins that bind tightly to the channel and therefore can be used as specific probes for labeling the channel molecules. These include tetrodotoxin from the puffer fish, saxitoxin from a dinoflagellate that infects shellfish, batrachotoxin from South American poisonous frogs, and the venom from the North African scorpion. For example, the density of voltage-gated Na$^+$ channels per unit area of axon membrane has been estimated from the binding of radiolabeled tetrodotoxin molecules to the axon membrane. These studies indicate that tetrodotoxin binds to a small number of specific sites on the membrane. These specific sites are thought to represent the Na$^+$ channels, because the binding constant and the kinetics of tetrodotoxin binding to these sites correspond to the values determined by electrophysiological measurement of the tetrodotoxin blockade of Na$^+$ conductance.

Murdoch Ritchie and his colleagues estimated the number of voltage-gated Na$^+$ channels by measuring the total amount of tetrodotoxin that was bound when these specific binding sites were saturated. They found that the greater the density of Na$^+$ channels in the membrane of an axon, the greater the velocity at which the axon conducts action potentials. This result is to be expected. During an action potential, a greater density of voltage-gated Na$^+$ channels allows more current to flow through the excited membrane and along the axon core, thus discharging the capacitance of the unexcited membrane downstream (see

Figure 7–9). The density is quite low in nonmyelinated axons, ranging in different cell types from 35 to 500 Na$^+$ channels per μm^2 of axon membrane. Even if one includes the thick channel wall surrounding the pore, the channel area taken up by 500 Na$^+$ channels per μm^2 is only 1/100 of the total membrane area. Despite this small number, quite large Na$^+$ currents can flow during the action potential because the ion flux through each channel is quite high. Patch-clamp recordings demonstrate that a single Na$^+$ channel can pass up to 10^7 Na$^+$ ions per second.

Voltage-Gated Channels Open in an All-or-None Fashion

The current flow through a single channel cannot be measured in ordinary voltage-clamp experiments for two reasons. First, the voltage clamp surveys a large area of membrane in which thousands of channels are opening and closing randomly. Second, the background noise caused by current flow through passive membrane channels is much larger than the current flow through any one channel. This problem is circumvented by electrically isolating a tiny piece of membrane with the patch-clamp technique (see Figure 5–5). Patch-clamp experiments have demonstrated that voltage-gated channels generally have two conductance states, open and closed. Each channel opens in an all-or-none fashion and, when open, permits a pulse of current to flow with a variable duration but constant amplitude (Figure 8–9). In the open state the conductances of single Na$^+$ channels vary between about 8 and 18 pS, depending on the type of channel. The conductances of individual voltage-gated K$^+$ channels range from about 4 to 20 pS; in single Ca^{2+} channels, they range from about 1 to 3 pS.

Charges Are Redistributed Within the Membrane When Voltage-Gated Sodium Channels Open

In their classic study of the squid axon Hodgkin and Huxley suggested that a change in membrane potential might regulate g_{Na} and g_K by causing a conformational change in an intramembranous gating molecule. They postulated that the gating molecule would have a net charge, the *gating charge*, somewhere within its structure. A change in membrane potential, by causing the gating charge to move, could cause such a molecule to undergo a conformational change, which in turn could open the activation gate.

Hodgkin and Huxley predicted that when the membrane is depolarized a positive gating charge would move from near the inner surface to near the outer surface. Since such a displacement of positive charge is equivalent to a reduction in the net separation of charge across the membrane, they postulated that, to keep the membrane potential constant in a voltage-clamp experiment, a small extra component of outward capacitive current, called *gating current*, would have to be generated by the voltage clamp. For technical reasons, the gating current (I_g) predicted by Hodgkin and Huxley could not be detected until the early

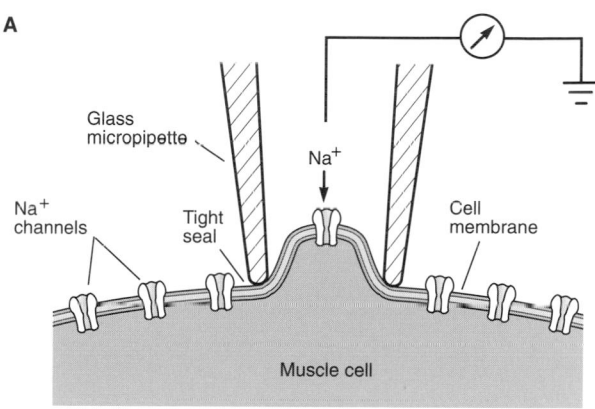

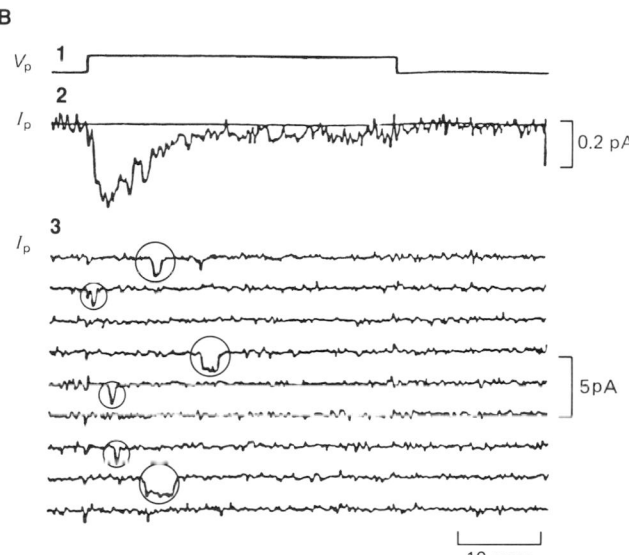

FIGURE 8–9

Individual voltage-gated channels open in an all-or-none fashion.

A. A small patch of membrane containing only a single voltage-gated Na$^+$ channel is electrically isolated from the rest of the cell by the patch electrode. The Na$^+$ current that enters the cell through these channels is recorded by a current monitor connected to the patch electrode.

B. Recordings of single Na$^+$ channels in cultured muscle cells of rats. **1.** The time course of a 10 mV depolarizing voltage step applied across the patch of membrane. V_p = potential difference across the patch. **2.** The sum of 300 trials of the inward current through the Na$^+$ channels in the patch (K$^+$ channels were blocked with tetraethylammonium and capacitive current was subtracted electronically). I_p = current through the patch of membrane. **3.** Nine individual trials from the set of 300, showing six individual Na$^+$ channel openings (**circles**). These data demonstrate that the total Na$^+$ current recorded in a conventional voltage-clamp record (Figure 8–2C) can be accounted for by the all-or-none opening and closing of individual Na$^+$ channels. (From Sigworth and Neher, 1980.)

1970s. When the membrane current was finally examined by means of very sensitive techniques, the predicted gating current was found to flow at the beginning and end of a depolarizing voltage-clamp step that opens Na$^+$ channels (Figure 8–10).

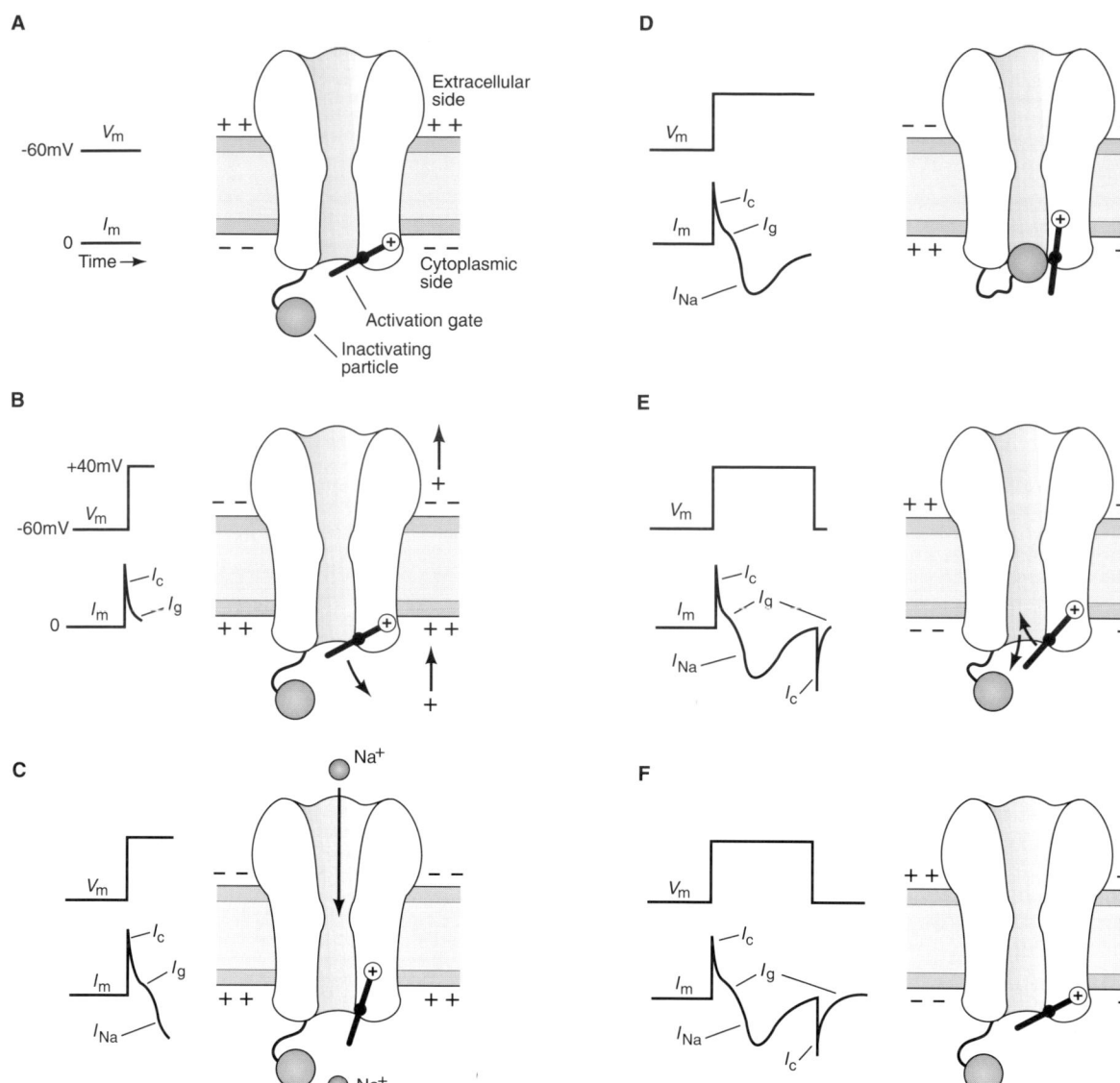

FIGURE 8–10

Changes in charge distribution within the Na$^+$ channel give rise to the gating current.

A. When the cell is in its resting state, the Na$^+$ activation gate is closed and the inactivation gate is open.

B. When the cell is stepped to a depolarized membrane potential by the voltage clamp, the standard passive capacitive current, I_c, flows only during the instant when V_m is changing. Once V_m has changed, the activation gates of the various channels begin to open, as the gating charge reorients itself with respect to the new electric field across the membrane. As the activation gate for each channel moves into the open configuration, a small outward capacitive current, the gating current (I_g), is generated by the clamp to keep the net charge separation across the membrane constant. The gates for different channels respond in a stochastic fashion—most open right away, but some take a longer time. As a result, the capacitive gating current is spread out in time, and does not occur instantaneously.

C. By the time most of the Na$^+$ channels have opened, the inward Na$^+$ current is maximal.

D. As the depolarization is maintained, channels that have opened begin to close because the inactivation gates shut. Because

no gating current is associated with the inactivation process, it is assumed that the voltage dependence of inactivation derives indirectly from some sort of coupling between the activation and inactivation processes. For example, the inactivation gate may have a tendency to close spontaneously, independent of voltage, but this tendency may be prevented when the activation gate is closed.

E. After the membrane is repolarized, the gating charges of the Na$^+$ channels again reorient, giving rise to an *inward* capacitive gating current. This off gating current is spread out over a longer time than the on gating current, perhaps because the activation gates cannot close until the inactivation gates have opened—a relatively slow process. This interpretation again is consistent with the hypothesis that there is coupling between the activation and inactivation processes.

F. The channel has returned to its resting state. The voltage sensitivity of the activation gate is postulated to arise from a rearrangement of a segment of the channel molecule that possesses a net charge. The actual sign of the gating charge is not known, but preliminary evidence (see Figure 8–13) suggests that it is positive.

Analysis of the gating current by Clay Armstrong and Francesco Bezanilla has provided two critical insights into the properties of the Na^+ channel. (1) *Gating is a multistep process.* Several steps of charge movement with different kinetics occur before the channel opens in response to depolarization. (2) *Activation and inactivation are coupled processes.* During short depolarizing pulses net movement of gating charge within the membrane at the beginning of the pulse is balanced by an opposite movement of gating charge at the end of the pulse. If the pulse lasts long enough for significant Na^+ inactivation to occur, however, the movement of gating charge back across the membrane at the end of the pulse is delayed. The gating charge is temporarily immobilized, and becomes free to move back across the membrane only as the Na^+ channels recover from inactivation. Armstrong and Bezanilla interpreted this charge immobilization to mean that the activation gate cannot close while the channel is in the inactivated state, i.e., while the inactivation gate is closed (Figure 8–10).

The Voltage-Gated Sodium Channel Selects for Sodium on the Basis of Size, Charge, and Energy of Hydration of the Ion

After the gates of the Na^+ channel have opened, how does this protein channel discriminate between Na^+ and other ions? Bertil Hille has examined the selectivity of the Na^+ channel by measuring its relative permeability to several types of organic and inorganic cations that differ in size and hydrogen-bonding characteristics. He found that the channel acts as if it contains a filter or recognition site that selects partly on the basis of size, by acting as a molecular sieve, with a pore size of 0.3×0.5 nm (see Figure 5–3). The ease with which ions with good hydrogen-bonding characteristics pass through the channel led Hille to suggest that part of the inner wall of the protein channel is made up of amino acids that are rich in oxygen atoms. Hille and Ann Woodhull also found that when the pH of the fluid surrounding the cell is lowered, the conductance of the open channel is gradually reduced, and this reduction parallels the titration curve for the carboxyl groups of amino acid residues in protein. On the basis of these results, Hille proposed the following mechanism by which the channel selects for Na^+ ions.

Negatively charged carboxylic acid groups located at the outer mouth of the pore perform the first step in the selection process by attracting cations and repelling anions. Cations that are larger than 0.3×0.5 nm in diameter are too large to pass through the pore. Cations smaller than this critical size pass through the pore, but only after losing most of the waters of hydration they normally carry in free solution. The negative carboxylic acid group, as well as the oxygen atoms that line the pore, can substitute for these waters of hydration, but the degree of effectiveness of this substitution varies for different types of ions. The more effective this substitution is for a given ion species, the more readily that ion permeates the Na^+ channel.

The Voltage-Gated Potassium, Sodium, and Calcium Channels Belong to One Gene Family

To understand fully the selection and gating functions of the Na^+ channel, it is necessary to determine its structure. The first step in this direction, biochemical identification and purification of Na^+ channel molecules, was accomplished using the naturally occurring neurotoxins that bind specifically to the channel. William Catterall labeled the Na^+ channel by treating rat brain membranes with a radioactively labeled azido nitrobenzoyl derivative of scorpion toxin. In the dark this derivative binds reversibly to the same sites in the protein as does the native toxin, but when exposed to ultraviolet light it can form a covalent bond with amino acid residues at the binding site.

With this and related approaches, Catterall isolated three subunits that are thought to be present in equal proportions in the functional channel: one large glycoprotein with a molecular weight of 270,000 (α) and two smaller polypeptides with molecular weights of 39,000 (β1) and 37,000 (β2). Although the α-subunit appears to be ubiquitous, the smaller subunits are variable in their appearance in different tissue types and in different species. For example, the electric organ of the electric eel has a Na^+ channel composed solely of the large α-subunit. By inserting only the α-subunit into an artificial lipid bilayer, William Agnew and his associates reconstituted the function of the purified Na^+ channel and showed by patch-clamp recordings that the biophysical properties of the purified channel match those of the normal channel in the membrane. These results have led to the conclusion that the α subunit forms the aqueous pore of the channel, whereas the smaller, variable subunits play a structural, stabilizing, or regulatory role.

Next, Shosaku Numa and his colleagues cloned the gene that encodes the α subunit of the Na^+ channel. Examination of the nucleotide sequence for the gene, as well as the amino acid sequence that it encodes, has revealed two fundamental structural features of the Na^+ channel. First, the ion-conducting portion of the Na^+ channel is comprised of four internal repetitions (sequences I–IV), with only slight variations, of a basic amino acid sequence that is approximately 150 amino acids in length. Each repetition of this basic motif, when analyzed by a hydrophobicity plot (see Figure 5–6), has been interpreted as having six membrane-spanning hydrophobic domains, each of which is likely to exist in the form of an α helix (Figure 8–11). The four repeated versions of the basic sequence are thought to be roughly symmetrically arranged, with the walls of the water-filled pore being formed by either one or two of the membrane-spanning helices, repeated four times around the circumference of the pore (Figure 8–12).

The second fundamental insight into the structural organization of the Na^+ channel stems from the observation that one of its putative membrane-spanning regions, called the S4 region, is highly conserved between Na^+ channels from different species. This high degree of conservation suggests that the S4 region may have a critical role in Na^+ channel function. Moreover, the S4 region is

Na⁺ channel

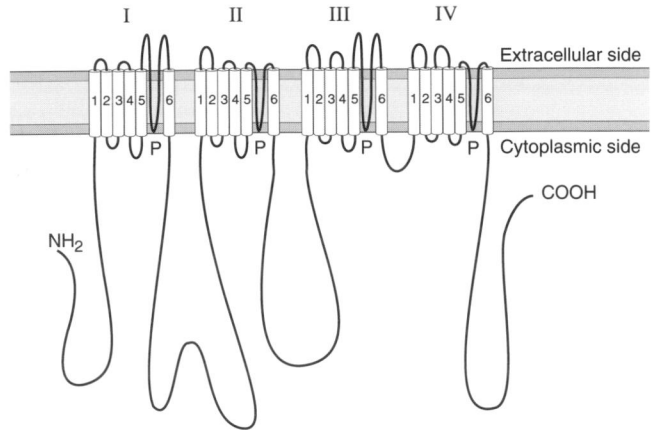

Ca²⁺ channel

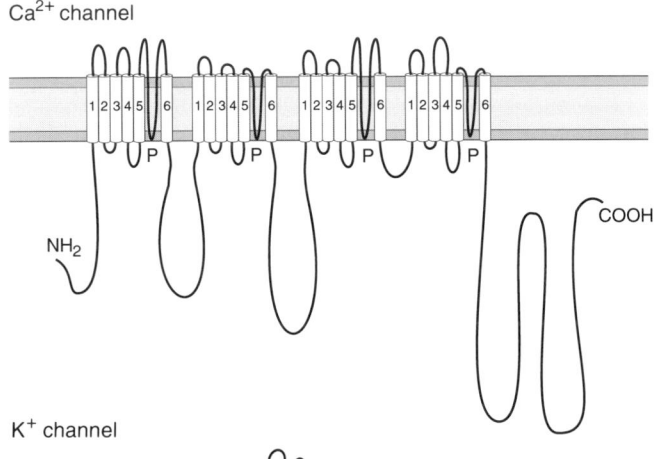

K⁺ channel

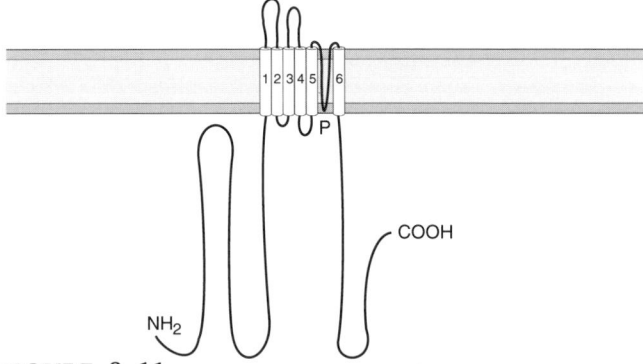

FIGURE 8–11

Hydrophobicity analysis of the primary sequence of the subunit of the voltage-gated Na⁺ channel and the corresponding segments of the voltage-gated Ca²⁺ and K⁺ channels suggests that they have the following secondary structures in the membrane. The α-subunit of the Na⁺ and Ca²⁺ channels consists of a single polypeptide chain with four repetitions of six membrane-spanning α-helical regions. Experiments correlating functional properties of the channel with specific parts of protein structure suggest that a stretch of amino acids, the *P region*, between α-helices 5 and 6, dips into the membrane in the form of two antiparallel β strands. A four-fold repetition of the P region is believed to line the pore. The gene for the K⁺ channel encodes only a single copy of the six α-helices, and the P region. It is assumed that four such subunits are assembled to form a complete channel. (Modified from Catterall, 1988 and Stevens, 1991.)

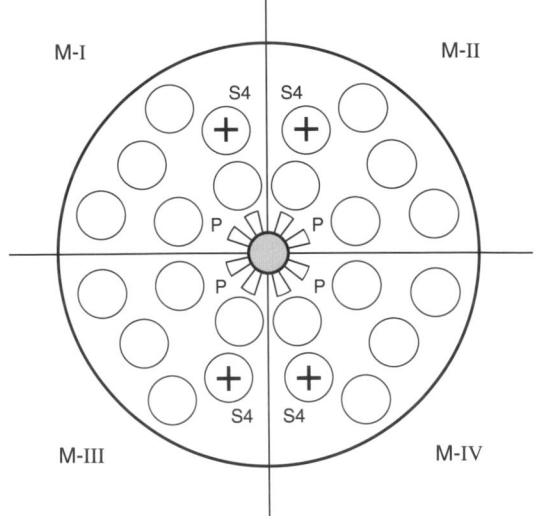

FIGURE 8–12

The postulated tertiary structure of the voltage-gated Na⁺ and Ca²⁺ channels, based on the secondary structures shown in Figure 8–11. The pore (gray circle) is surrounded by the four internally repeated domains (M-I to M-IV). Each quadrant of the channel includes six cylinders representing the six putative membrane-spanning α-helices. The S4 segment, because of its net charge, is thought to be involved in gating. The two central figures in each quadrant represents the pair of β strands (the P region) that dip into the membrane to form the wall of the pore. Voltage-gated K⁺ channels are thought to have a similar structure, with four separate subunits making up the four repeating domains. (Modified from Alsobrook and Stevens, 1988 and Stevens, 1991.)

also homologous to specific regions of the voltage-gated Ca²⁺ and K⁺ channels (Figure 8–11). Because all three channels are voltage gated, it has been suggested that this region may transduce a change in membrane potential into a gating transition within the channel that opens the activation gate. This hypothesis gains support from the fact that the S4 region, although it is hydrophobic, has a relatively high density of charged amino acid residues along the length of the postulated helical region; every third amino acid along the helix has a net positive charge. The conformation of such a highly charged structure is likely to be quite sensitive to changes in the electric field across the membrane.

One hypothesis for how the S4 region might control the activation gate of the Na⁺ channel is derived from an idea initially advanced several years ago by Armstrong. According to the current version of this scheme, the S4 region forms an α-helix. The regularly spaced, mobile positive charges on the S4 helix align with immobile negatively charged residues on adjacent regions of the membrane-spanning portions of the channel protein. When the cell is depolarized, the increase in positivity within the cell causes the positive charges on the S4 region to move outward. This movement results in a screw-like rotation as each positive charge on the S4 region moves about 60° of a turn closer to the outside of the membrane, to a position where it is stabilized by its electrostatic attraction to the neighboring negative charge that is next in line

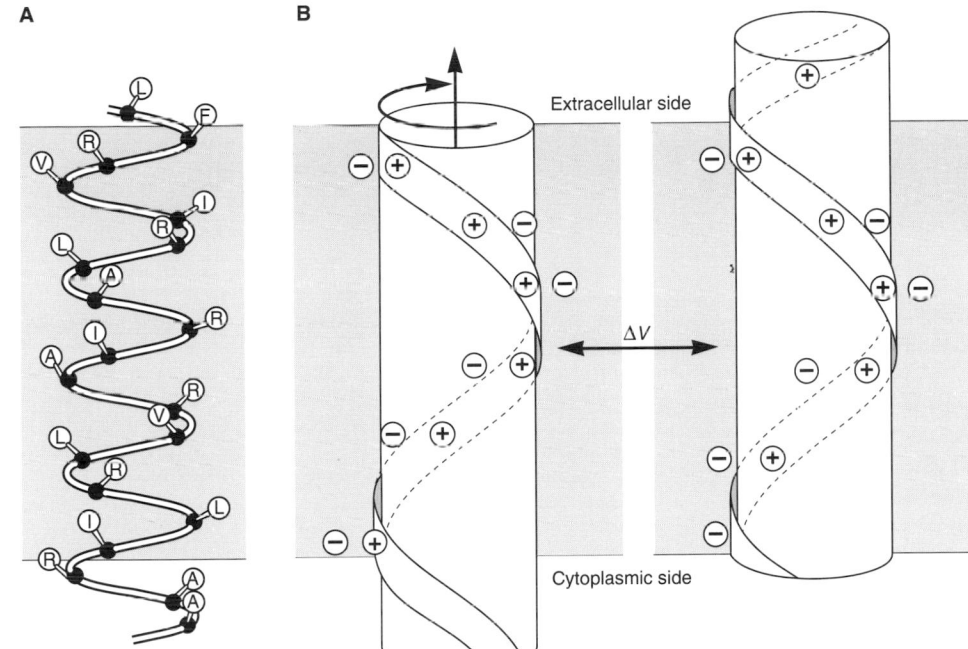

FIGURE 8–13

Postulated movement of the S4 region during gating.

A. Ball-and-chain model of the S4 region. The Rs stand for positively charged arginine residues.

B. In the resting state each net positive charge on the region (α-helix) is stabilized by a negative charge on a neighboring portion of the molecule. When the cell is depolarized, the change in electrical field across the membrane allows the positive charges on the S4 region to move toward the outer edge of the membrane. It is postulated that this movement is translated into a screw-type movement, which stops when each positive charge on S4 is again in register with a stationary negative charge on an adjacent helix, thus stabilizing the channel in a new conformation. (Catterall, 1988.)

(Figure 8–13). This type of internal redistribution of charge could also account for the gating currents recorded in voltage-clamp experiments when the activation gates open or close (Figure 8–10B,C). It is thought that before the activation gate can open, all four S4 regions in the channel must undergo the type of conformational change illustrated in Figure 8–13.

To test the hypothesis that charge movement within the S4 region is involved in gating, Numa and Walter Stühmer and their colleagues used site-directed mutagenesis to modify the gene encoding the voltage-gated Na$^+$ channel so as to reduce the positivity of the S4 region. They found that reducing the net positive charge in one of the S4 regions of the channel reduced the voltage sensitivity of the activation gate. They also showed that cleaving the region of the molecule that connects the repeating sequences III and IV on the cytoplasmic face of the membrane (see Figure 8–11) slows the rate of inactivation of the Na$^+$ channel. This result is corroborated by the finding by Vassilev and his colleagues that an antibody directed against the same region of the channel also slows inactivation. Thus, this cytoplasmic segment of the molecule may move into position to block the inner mouth of the pore after the activation gate has opened, thereby causing inactivation (Figure 8–10C,D).

The genes encoding two types of Ca^{2+} channels have also been cloned and sequenced by Numa and his colleagues. One type of Ca^{2+} channel, the dihydropyridine-binding channel, is voltage gated. Large regions of this channel are structurally homologous with both the voltage-gated Na$^+$ and fast, transient K$^+$ channels, suggesting that all three channels belong to the same gene family and have evolved from a common ancestral structure (see Figure 8–11). The second type of Ca^{2+} channel analyzed by Numa is not voltage gated. This channel, which is found in the membrane of the sarcoplasmic reticulum in muscle, is characterized by its ability to bind ryanodine, a plant alkyloid. It is not homologous to the voltage-gated Na$^+$, K$^+$, or Ca^{2+} channels that have been sequenced. The details of the mechanism that controls the gating of the ryanodine-sensitive Ca^{2+} channel are not known, except that the first step is depolarization of the t-tubules, immediately adjacent to the sarcoplasmic reticulum.

The gene for the fast, transient K$^+$ channel in Drosophila has been cloned by Lily Jan, Yuh Nung Jan, Olaf Pongs, Alberto Ferrus, Mark Tanouye, and their colleagues using a combined genetic and molecular biological approach. As mentioned above, the nucleotide sequence of the gene has significant homology with the gene for the voltage-gated Na$^+$ and Ca^{2+} channels. However, because the protein encoded by the K$^+$ channel gene has only one of the four internally repeated motifs found in the Na$^+$ and Ca^{2+} channels (see Figure 8–11), the functioning K$^+$ channel is thought to be formed by four similar, perhaps identical, subunits that aggregate around a central pore. Subsequently, a family of four genes that are homologous to the Drosophila K$^+$ channel gene have been cloned in mammals. Some of the members of this gene family also exist as subfamilies, with as many as five variants. It appears that some of the members of this gene family encode the A-type K$^+$ channel, whereas others encode the delayed rectifier K$^+$ channel described by Hodgkin and Huxley. Thus, the diversity of K$^+$ channel types in mammals is thought to have been generated primarily by gene duplication and mutation.

The stretch of amino acids that makes up the wall of the K$^+$ channel pore has been determined by Roderick MacKinnon, Gary Yellen, and others. Using genetic engineering, they were able to show that this portion of protein, which forms the conducting region of the open channel, is restricted to a stretch of amino acids, the *P region*, that connects the putative S5 and S6 α-helices. The loop of amino acids that forms the P region is thought to dip into the membrane, forming an antiparallel pair of β strands; this pair is repeated four-fold to form the lining of the channel lumen. By analogy, it is assumed that the homologous regions of primary sequence of the Na^+ and Ca^{2+} channels also form the pores of these two related channels (Figures 8–11 and 8–12).

An Overall View

According to the ionic hypothesis developed by Hodgkin and Huxley, the action potential is produced by the movement of ions across the membrane through voltage-gated channels. This movement, which occurs only after the channels are opened, changes the distribution of charges on either side of the membrane. An influx of Na^+, and in some cases Ca^{2+}, reverses the resting charge distribution, after which K^+ efflux repolarizes the membrane by restoring the initial charge distribution. Most of the more recently described ion channels are opened primarily when the membrane potential is near the action potential threshold, and thus have profound effects on the firing patterns generated by the neuron.

Three major technical advances have led to detailed explanations of the mechanisms of action of voltage-gated channels. First, the voltage-clamp technique has been extended to patch-clamp recording and gating-current analysis. Second, isolation of neurotoxins that bind selectively to different membrane channels has made it possible to estimate the density of the Na^+ channels, to purify Na^+ and Ca^{2+} channels, and to determine their primary sequences by sequencing cDNA clones of the genes that encode them. Third, a combined genetic and molecular biological approach has led to the sequence for the K^+ channel. A concerted effort involving biophysical, structural, biochemical, and molecular biological approaches is leading to a comprehensive understanding of how these channels function.

Selected Readings

Armstrong, C. M. 1981. Sodium channels and gating currents. Physiol. Rev. 61:644–683.

Catterall, W. A. 1988. Structure and function of voltage-sensitive ion channels. Science 242:50–61.

Hille, B. 1984. Ionic Channels of Excitable Membranes. Sunderland, Mass.: Sinauer.

Hodgkin, A. L. 1976. Chance and design in electrophysiology: An informal account of certain experiments on nerve carried out between 1934 and 1952. J. Physiol. (Lond.) 263:1–21.

Llinás, R. R. 1988. The intrinsic electrophysiological properties of mammalian neurons: Insights into central nervous system function. Science 242:1654–1664.

Ritchie, J. M., and Rogart, R. B. 1977. The binding of saxitoxin and tetrodotoxin to excitable tissue. Rev. Physiol. Biochem. Pharmacol. 79:1–50.

References

Alsobrook, J. P., II, and Stevens, C. F. 1988. Cloning the calcium channel. Trends Neurosci. 11:1–2.

Cole, K. S., and Curtis, H. J. 1939. Electric impedance of the squid giant axon during activity. J. Gen. Physiol. 22:649–670.

Dekin, M. S., and Getting, P. A. 1987. In vitro characterization of neurons in the vertical part of the nucleus tractus solitarius. II. Ionic basis for repetitive firing patterns. J. Neurophysiol. 58:215–229.

Hartmann, H. A., Kirsch, G. E., Drewe, J. A., Taglialatela, M., Joho, R. H., and Brown, A. M. 1991. Exchange of conduction pathways between two related K^+ channels. Science 251:942–944.

Hodgkin, A. L., and Huxley, A. F. 1952. A quantitative description of membrane current and its application to conduction and excitation in nerve. J. Physiol. (Lond.) 117:500–544.

Hodgkin, A. L., and Katz, B. 1949. The effect of sodium ions on the electrical activity of the giant axon of the squid. J. Physiol. (Lond.) 108:37–77.

Kamb, A., Tseng-Crank, J., and Tanouye, M. A. 1988. Multiple products of the Drosophila *Shaker* gene may contribute to potassium channel diversity. Neuron 1:421–430.

Llinás, R., and Jahnsen, H. 1982. Electrophysiology of mammalian thalamic neurones *in vitro*. Nature 297:406–408.

Noda, M., Shimizu, S., Tanabe, T., Takai, T., Kayano, T., Ikeda, T., Takahashi, H., Nakayama, H., Kanaoka, Y., Minamino, N., Kangawa, K., Matsuo, H., Raferty, M. A., Hirose, T., Inayama, S., Hayashida, H., Miyata, T., and Numa, S. 1984. Primary structure of *Electrophorus electricus* sodium channel deduced from cDNA sequence. Nature 312:121–127.

Papazian, D. M., Schwarz, T. L., Tempel, B. L., Jan, Y. N., and Jan, L. Y. 1987. Cloning of genomic and complementary DNA from *Shaker*, a putative potassium channel gene from *Drosophila*. Science 237:749–753.

Pongs, O., Kecskemethy, N., Müller, R., Krah-Jentgens, I., Baumann, A., Kiltz, H. H., Canal, I., Llamazares, S., and Ferrus, A. 1988. *Shaker* encodes a family of putative potassium channel proteins in the nervous system of *Drosophila*. E.M.B.O. J. 7:1087–1096.

Rosenberg, R. L., Tomiko, S. A., and Agnew, W. S. 1984. Single-channel properties of the reconstituted voltage-regulated Na channel isolated from the electroplax of *Electrophorus electricus*. Proc. Natl. Acad. Sci. U.S.A. 81:5594–5598.

Sigworth, F. J., and Neher, E. 1980. Single Na^+ channel currents observed in cultured rat muscle cells. Nature 287:447–449.

Stevens, C. F. 1991. Making a submicroscopic hole in one. Nature 349:657–658.

Stühmer, W., Conti, F., Suzuki, H., Wang, X., Noda, M., Yahagi, N., Kubo, H., and Numa, S. 1989. Structural parts involved in activation and inactivation of the sodium channel. Nature 339:597–603.

Takeshima, H., Nishimura, S., Matsumoto, T., Ishida, H., Kangawa, K., Minamino, N., Matsuo, H., Ueda, M., Hanaoka, M., Hirose, T., and Numa, S. 1989. Primary structure and expression from complementary DNA of skeletal muscle ryanodine receptor. Nature 339:439–445.

Vassilev, P. M., Scheuer, T., and Catterall, W. A. 1988. Identification of an intracellular peptide segment involved in sodium channel inactivation. Science 241:1658–1661.

Wei, A., Covarrubias, M., Butler, A., Baker, K., Pak, M., and Salkoff, L. 1990. K^+ current diversity is produced by an extended gene family conserved in *Drosophila* and mouse. Science 248:599-603.

Woodhull, A. M. 1973. Ionic blockage of sodium channels in nerve. J. Gen. Physiol. 61:687–708.

Yellen, G., Jurman, M. E., Abramson, T., and MacKinnon, R. 1991. Mutations affecting internal TEA blockade identify the probable pore-forming region of a K^+ channel. Science 251:939–942.

Yool, A. J., and Schwarz, T. L. 1991. Alteration of ionic selectivity of a K^+ channel by mutation of the H5 region. Nature 349:700–704.

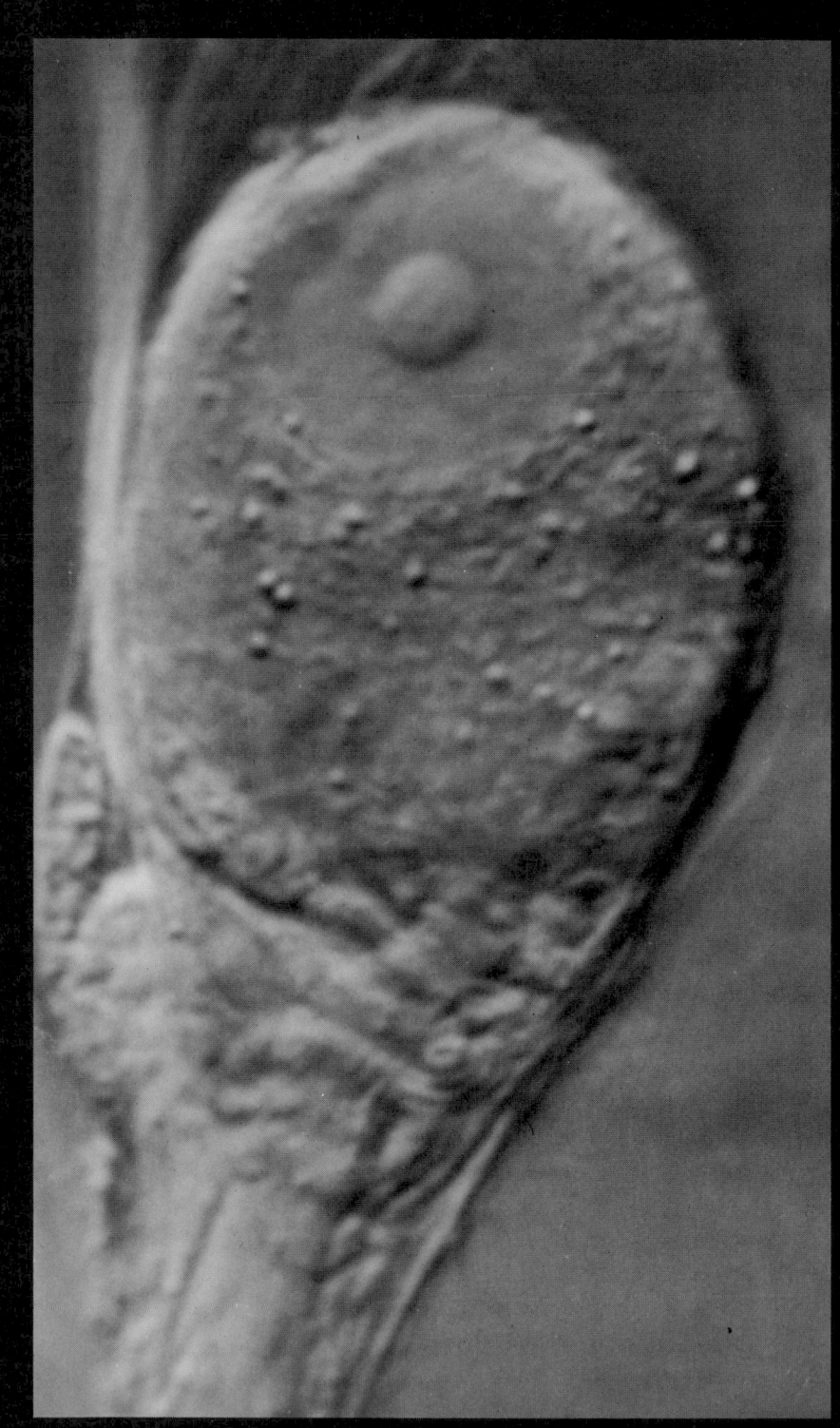

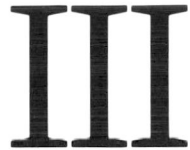

Elementary Interactions Between Neurons: Synaptic Transmission

In the first two parts of the book we considered the individual nerve cell—the elementary signaling unit of the nervous system. In this part we shall consider how one neuron communicates with another at *synapses*. The cellular mechanisms of neuronal signaling are the basis for many of the issues we shall consider throughout later sections of this text: perception, motor action, and learning.

An average neuron forms about 1000 synaptic connections and receives even more. Since the human brain contains at least 10^{11} neurons, about 10^{14} synaptic connections are formed in the brain. Thus, there are more synapses in one human brain than there are stars in our galaxy! Fortunately, only a few basic mechanisms operate to control synaptic transmission at these connections.

The common transmitters are low-molecular-weight molecules, but a wide variety of peptides also can serve as messengers at synapses. In the last several years, molecular biological techniques have helped to elucidate the structure of these peptides and to analyze how they are synthesized and processed in the presynaptic cell. The

methods of molecular biology are also being used to characterize receptor molecules in postsynaptic target cells that bind and respond to the chemical messengers, and second-messenger pathways that mediate the consequences of transducing signals within the cell.

In the first seven chapters we shall consider synaptic transmission at its most elementary level—first the communication between one presynaptic neuron and a single postsynaptic cell, then the processing by one postsynaptic cell of the signal it receives from a few presynaptic cells. We begin by analyzing the contributions of postsynaptic and presynaptic elements to synaptic transmission, and then consider the molecular machinery of synaptic actions. An understanding of the synapse is necessary for considering, in the remaining chapters, how injury and disease disrupt synaptic function by interfering with one or another component of the synapse.

How does nerve cell injury result in neurological disease? The diagnosis of a neurological disease usually involves two steps. First, the anatomical site of the lesion in

Convincing evidence for neurotransmission was obtained by Otto Loewi in 1921 when he showed acetylcholine could be released by stimulation of the vagus nerve to the frog heart. This micrograph shows cholinergic synaptic boutons ending on a parasympathetic ganglion neuron in the frog heart. The resolutions afforded in this and other simple preparations permitted Stephen Kuffler and his colleagues to study the detailed physiology and ultrastructure of vertebrate neuronal synapses. (From U. J. McMahan and S. W. Kuffler, Proc. R. Soc. Lond. [Biol.], 1971, 177:485–508.)

the nervous system is determined, and second, the cause of the lesion is inferred. Because lesions in different parts of the nervous system produce characteristic deficits, it is often possible to infer the location of the lesion within the nervous system through clinical examination. Serious in- jury to nerve cells often leads to their death, and therefore to a reduction in total numbers of nerve cells. Although most neurons do not multiply, they can regenerate parts of their axons after certain kinds of injury.

PART III

Chapter 9:	**Synaptic Transmission**
Chapter 10:	**Directly Gated Transmission at the Nerve–Muscle Synapse**
Chapter 11:	**Directly Gated Transmission at Central Synapses**
Chapter 12:	**Synaptic Transmission Mediated by Second Messengers**
Chapter 13:	**Transmitter Release**
Chapter 14:	**Chemical Messengers: Small Molecules and Peptides**
Chapter 15:	**Synaptic Vesicles**
Chapter 16:	**Diseases of Chemical Transmission at the Nerve–Muscle Synapse: Myasthenia Gravis**
Chapter 17:	**Diseases of the Motor Unit**
Chapter 18:	**Reactions of Neurons to Injury**

Eric R. Kandel
Steven A. Siegelbaum
James H. Schwartz

9

Synaptic Transmission

**Synaptic Transmission Can Be Electrical
or Chemical**

**Electrical Synapses Can Be Either Unidirectional
or Bidirectional**

Electrical Transmission Allows for Rapid and
Synchronous Firing of Interconnected Cells

In Electrical Synapses the Pre- and Postsynaptic
Elements Are Bridged by Gap Junctions

**At Chemical Synapses the Pre- and Postsynaptic
Elements Are Separated by a Synaptic Cleft**

Chemical Transmission Involves Transmitter
Release and Receptor Activation

Chemical Receptors Use Two Major Molecular
Mechanisms to Gate Ion Channels

An Overall View

Nerve cells differ from other cells in the body because of their ability to communicate rapidly with one another, sometimes over great distances and with great precision. This rapid and precise communication is made possible by two signaling mechanisms—axonal conduction and synaptic transmission. In previous chapters we examined the conduction of signals along axons. Here we shall examine in a general way the two major kinds of synaptic transmission in the nervous system—chemical and electrical. Both have been analyzed in molecular detail so that our understanding of them is now quite good.

Electrical synapses are not unique to nerve cells; they also connect other cells in the body, such as the cells of the heart and smooth muscle, and epithelial liver cells. In the brain, however, electrical synapses are less common than chemical synapses, and are characterized by rapid speed of transmission and by relatively stereotyped function. For example, electrical synapses do not readily allow inhibitory actions or long-lasting changes in effectiveness. In contrast, chemical synapses mediate either excitatory or inhibitory actions and tend to be involved in behaviors more complex than those employing electrical synapses. Chemical synapses are more flexible—they are capable of enduring changes in effectiveness, and this plasticity is important for memory and other higher functions of the brain. Most important, chemical synapses can amplify neuronal signals, allowing a small presynaptic nerve terminal to alter the potential of a large postsynaptic cell.

In this chapter we shall compare the properties of electrical and chemical synapses. Because chemical transmission is central to understanding how the nervous system works—how we perceive, move, feel, learn, and remember—we shall discuss the mechanisms of chemical transmission in detail in Chapters 10, 11, and 12.

Synaptic Transmission Can Be Electrical or Chemical

Charles Sherrington introduced the term *synapse* at the turn of the century to describe the specialized zone of contact between neurons first described histologically by Ramón y Cajal as the point at which one neuron communicates with another. Otto Loewi showed in the 1920s that a chemical, acetylcholine, mediates transmission from the vagal nerve to the heart. This provoked considerable debate in the 1930s over the mechanisms of synaptic transmission at nerve–muscle synapses and in the brain. Two schools, one physiological the other pharmacological, each took the view that only one mechanism is responsible for all synaptic transmission. The physiologists, led by John Eccles, argued that synaptic transmission is electrical, that the conduction of the action potential results from the passive flow of current from the presynaptic neuron to the postsynaptic cell. The pharmacologists, led by Henry Dale, argued that transmission is chemical and that a chemical mediator (a transmitter substance) released by the presynaptic neuron initiates current flow in the postsynaptic cell.

Later, when physiological techniques improved in the 1950s and 1960s, it became clear that not all synapses use the same mechanism. The work of Paul Fatt and Bernard Katz, Eccles and his colleagues, and Edwin Furshpan and David Potter showed that both kinds of transmission occur. Although most synapses use a chemical transmitter, some do operate by purely electrical means. Once the fine structure of synapses was made visible with the electron microscope, chemical and electrical synapses were found to have different morphologies. At electrical synapses ion channels connect the cytoplasm of the pre- and postsynaptic cells; at chemical synapses there is no cytoplasmic continuity between the cells, and the neurons are separated by a cleft.

The main functional properties of the two types of synapses are summarized in Table 9–1. Many of these differences can be illustrated by observing the consequences of injecting positive current into the presynaptic cell. In both types of synapses this current flows outward across the presynaptic cell membrane. The current deposits a positive charge on the inside of the presynaptic cell membrane, reducing its negative charge and thereby depolarizing the cell. At electrical synapses some current also flows through the low-resistance, high-conductance channels that bridge the pre- and postsynaptic cells. This current deposits a positive charge on the inside of the membrane of the postsynaptic cell, depolarizing it, and then flows out through postsynaptic nongated conductance channels (Figure 9–1A). If the depolarization is greater than threshold, an action potential is generated by voltage-gated channels in the postsynaptic cell. Because there are no channels bridging the pre- and postsynaptic cells at chemical synapses, the outward current injected into a presynaptic cell flows out of the presynaptic neuron into the extracellular fluid in the synaptic cleft, seeking the path of lowest resistance. Little or no current crosses the high resistance of the external membrane of the postsynaptic cell (Figure 9–1B). Instead, the action potential in the presynaptic neuron of a chemical synapse leads to the release of a chemical transmitter substance that diffuses across the synaptic cleft to interact with specific receptors that either depolarize or hyperpolarize the postsynaptic cell.

Electrical Synapses Can Be Either Unidirectional or Bidirectional

In a prescient review in 1954, Fatt predicted that electrical synapses most are likely to occur between a large presynaptic nerve fiber and a small postsynaptic neuron. Fatt realized that if synaptic transmission relied only on the flow of electrical current, a great deal of current would be required to depolarize the postsynaptic cell. At electrical synapses this current would have to be generated directly by the voltage-gated ion channels of the presynaptic cell. Thus, at an electrical synapse the voltage-gated channels in the presynaptic cell must fulfill two functions. First, they must depolarize the membrane of the presynaptic

TABLE **9–1.** Distinguishing Properties of Electrical and Chemical Synapses

	Property	Electrical synapses	Chemical synapses
1.	Distance between pre- and postsynaptic cell membranes	3.5 nm	30–50 nm
2.	Cytoplasmic continuity between pre- and postsynaptic cells	Yes	No
3.	Ultrastructural components	Gap junction channels	Presynaptic active zones and vesicles; postsynaptic receptors
4.	Agent of transmission	Ionic current	Chemical transmitter
5.	Synaptic delay	Virtually absent	Significant: at least 0.3 ms, usually 1–5 ms or longer
6.	Direction of transmission	Usually bidirectional	Unidirectional

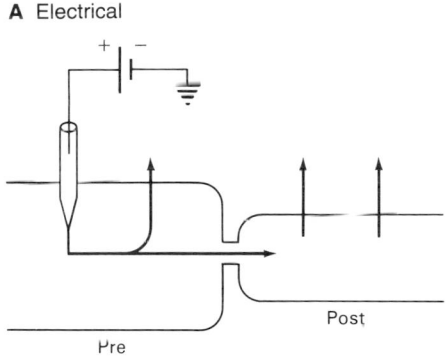

A Electrical

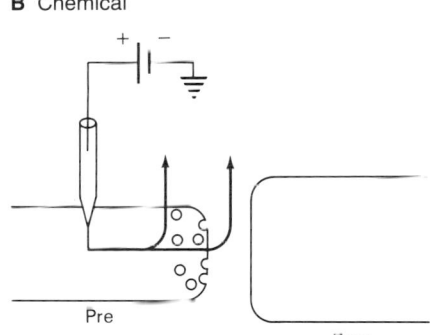

B Chemical

FIGURE 9–1

Electrical and chemical synapses differ in the path taken by current injected into the presynaptic cells.

A. In electrical synapses some of the injected current escapes through nongated channels in the presynaptic cell depolarizing it. In addition, some flows into the postsynaptic cell through channels connecting the cytoplasm of the two cells.

B. In chemical synapses none of the injected current crosses the membrane of the postsynaptic cell. Instead, the current escapes through channels in the presynaptic cell, depolarizing it, thereby activating the release of vesicles (shown as **circles**) containing chemical neurotransmitters.

cell and initiate an action potential. Second, they must generate sufficient ionic current to produce a potential change in the postsynaptic cell. To accomplish this, the presynaptic terminal would have to be large. Likewise, the postsynaptic cell would have to be small since a given change in presynaptic current (ΔI) will produce a larger voltage change across the high resistance of a small cell than across the low resistance of a large cell ($\Delta V = \Delta I \times R$).

In 1957 Furshpan and Potter provided the first evidence for electrical synaptic transmission at the giant motor synapse of the crayfish, where it is possible to place stimulating and recording electrodes in both the pre- and postsynaptic elements (Figure 9–2). At this synapse the presynaptic fiber is much larger than the postsynaptic fiber. An action potential generated in the presynaptic fiber produces a depolarizing postsynaptic potential that is often large enough to discharge an action potential. The latency between the presynaptic spike and the postsynaptic potential is remarkably short, in fact almost synchronous with the presynaptic action potential (Figure 9–2). This short latency seemed incompatible with chemical transmission, a process that requires several intervening steps (the release of a transmitter from the presynaptic neuron, diffusion of the transmitter to the postsynaptic cell, binding to a specific receptor, and subsequent gating of ion channels). It thus seemed likely that electric current flowed directly from the presynaptic to the postsynaptic cell. To test this possibility, Furshpan and Potter injected into the presynaptic neuron a depolarizing current that was less than the threshold for initiating an action potential, and found that the current does flow into the postsynaptic cell and depolarizes it (Figure 9–3A).

On the basis of the simplest model of the electrical synapse (see Figure 9–1A), one would expect electrical transmission to be bidirectional. That is, the channels bridging the presynaptic and postsynaptic neurons should

pass current equally well in both directions. However, when Furshpan and Potter depolarized the postsynaptic cell at the crayfish giant synapse, the current did not flow into the presynaptic cell. The synapse proved to be unidirectional or *rectifying* (Figure 9–3). As we shall see below, this probably results from the voltage sensitivity of the channels connecting these particular two cells. At first, this discovery placed in doubt the generality of a simple bidirectional model for electrical transmission. Since then, however, many electrical synapses have been identified in both invertebrate and vertebrate animals. The crayfish giant synapse turns out to be an unusual example of an electrical connection. Most behave as simple resistors, passing current equally well in either direction between pre- and postsynaptic cells (Figure 9–4). Thus, although some electrical synapses are rectifying, most are not.

At a nonrectifying electrical synapse the change in potential of the postsynaptic cell mimics the size and shape of the change in potential of the presynaptic cell. For example, a presynaptic action potential that has a large hyperpolarizing afterpotential will produce a biphasic (depolarizing–hyperpolarizing) change in electric potential in an electrically coupled postsynaptic cell. This is very similar to the passive propagation of subthreshold electrical signals along axons (see Chapter 7). Thus, transmission at nonrectifying electrical synapses is often referred to as *electrotonic transmission*. Electrotonic transmission now has been encountered even at junctions where the pre- and postsynaptic elements are of similar size.

Electrical Transmission Allows for Rapid and Synchronous Firing of Interconnected Cells

Why have electrical synapses? As we have seen, transmission across electrical synapses is extremely rapid because it results from the direct flow of current into the postsyn-

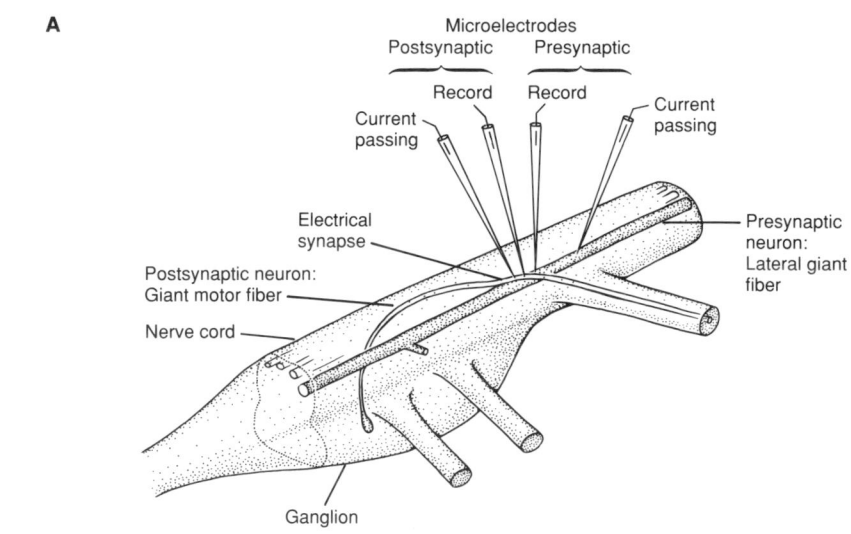

A

FIGURE 9–2

Electrical transmission was discovered at the giant synapse in the crayfish.

A. This drawing of a portion of a crayfish abdominal nerve cord and one of its ganglia shows the experimental setup for recording at an electrical synapse. The presynaptic neuron is the lateral giant fiber running down the nerve cord. The postsynaptic neuron is the motor fiber; the cell body in the ganglion projects its axon to the periphery. Current passing and recording electrodes are placed intracellularly in both the pre- and postsynaptic cells.

B. Transmission at an electrical synapse is virtually instantaneous (see Figure 9–9 for comparison to chemical synapses). **1.** An action potential in the presynaptic neuron produces a postsynaptic response that follows presynaptic stimulation in a fraction of a millisecond. **2.** Transmission is unidirectional (rectifying). When the *postsynaptic* cell is stimulated, there is only a tiny response in the presynaptic cell. (Adapted from Furshpan and Potter, 1957 and 1959.)

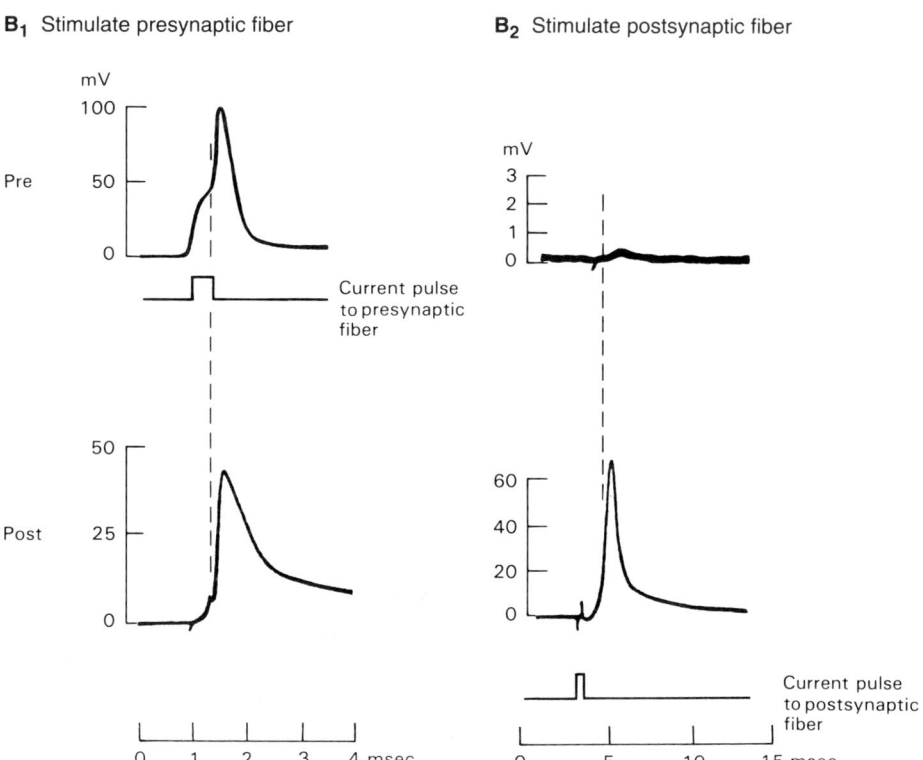

aptic cell generated by voltage-gated channels in the presynaptic neuron. Speed is important for certain escape responses. For example, the tail-flip escape response of goldfish is mediated by the giant Mauthner neuron in the brainstem, which receives input from sensory neurons through electrical synapses. These electrical synapses permit the rapid depolarization of the Mauthner cell, which in turn activates the tail motor neurons through a chemical synapse, leading to a rapid escape.

Electrical synapses are not restricted to connections between two cells; they are often found in interconnected groups of neurons, where they serve to synchronize their activity. When several neurons are electrically coupled to one another in an effective way, their threshold for generating an action potential becomes elevated. This is because the synaptic current flowing across the membrane of one cell will also flow into and out of the other electrically coupled cells. In this way several small electrically

A Current injected into the presynaptic
    axon (orthodromic)

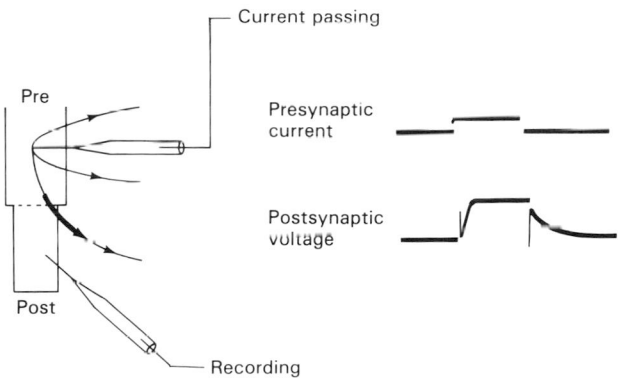

B Current injected into the postsynaptic
    axon (antidromic)

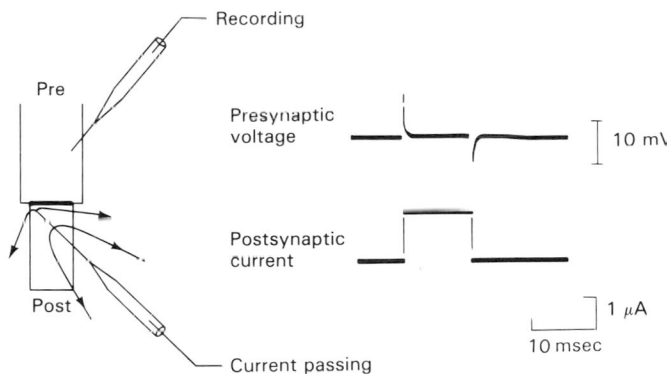

FIGURE 9–3

Current flow at the crayfish synapse is unidirectional (rectifying). This can be demonstrated by alternatively depolarizing the presynaptic or postsynaptic cell. In the two situations depicted here the positive (depolarizing) current is passed by one electrode and the membrane potential is recorded with a second electrode. Outward current and depolarization appear as upward deflections.

A. Orthodromic transmission is tested by injecting current in

the presynaptic neuron and recording the voltage response in the postsynaptic neuron. A depolarizing stimulus causes a depolarization in the postsynaptic cell.

B. Antidromic transmission is tested by injecting current in the postsynaptic neuron and recording the response in the presynaptic neuron. Here a depolarizing stimulus causes no response. This illustrates rectification at this synapse. (Adapted from Furshpan and Potter, 1957.)

FIGURE 9–4

Most electrical synapses are nonrectifying and current flow is bidirectional.

A. In nonrectifying synapses current injected into the presynaptic cell (cell A) depolarizes the cell (V_A) and also flows into the postsynaptic cell (cell B) and depolarizes it (V_B).

B. Nonrectifying coupling is typically symmetrical so that current flows equally well in the opposite direction from cell B to cell A, resulting in depolarization of cell A. (Adapted from Eckert, 1988.)

A Stimulate presynaptic cell

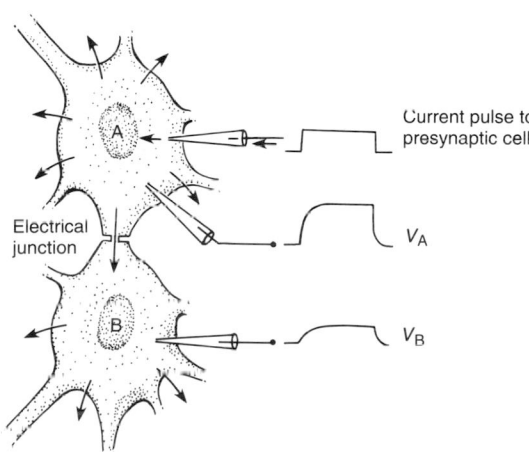

B Stimulate postsynaptic cell

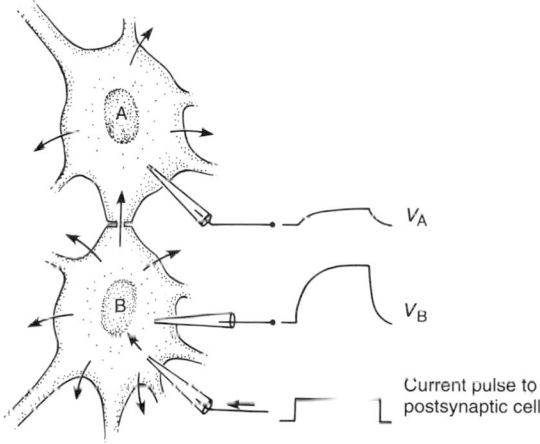

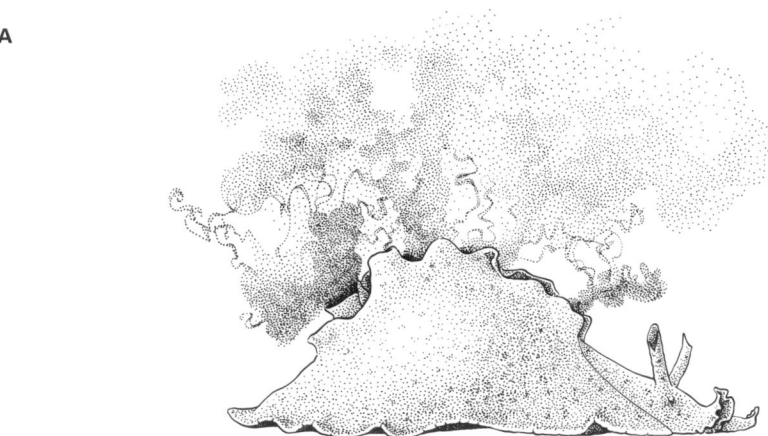

A

FIGURE 9–5

A defensive screen of ink is released from *Aplysia* when it is perturbed in a way that causes a group of motor neurons to fire together. These cells are interconnected by electrical synapses.

A. Noxious stimulation of the tail results in release of ink.

B. Neuronal circuitry underlying inking. **1.** The three motor neurons to the ink gland are interconnected by means of electrical synapses. As a result, hyperpolarization of cell A also hyperpolarizes cells B and C. **2.** Sensory neurons from the tail ganglia synapse on motor neurons that project to the ink gland.

C. A train of stimuli applied to the tail produces a synchronized discharge in all three motor neurons. **1.** The cells are at their resting potential and the stimulus triggers a train of identical action potentials in all three cells. This synchronous activity in the motor neurons results in inking. **2.** The motor neurons are hyperpolarized so that the stimulus cannot trigger action potentials because the cell is so far from threshold. When action potentials are prevented in the motor cells, the inking response is blocked. (Adapted from Carew and Kandel, 1976.)

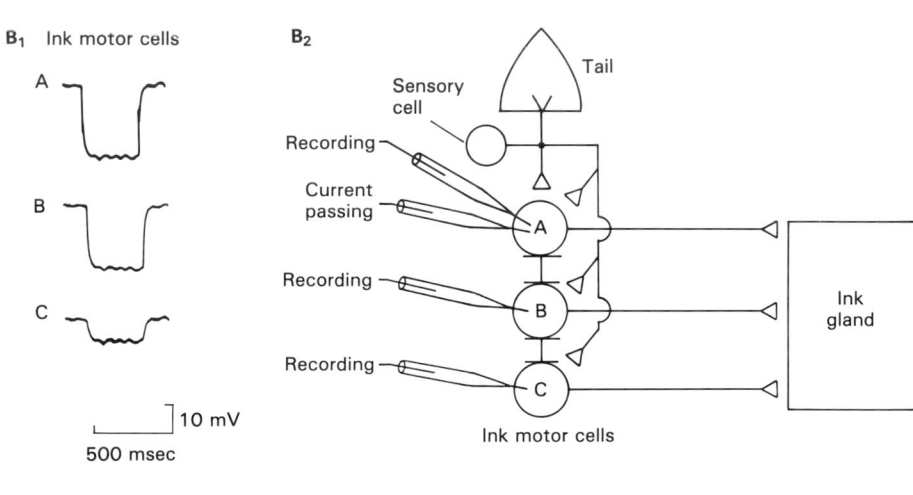

B_1 Ink motor cells

A

B

C

⌐ 10 mV

500 msec

B_2

Tail

Sensory cell

Recording

Current passing

Recording

Recording

A

B

C

Ink gland

Ink motor cells

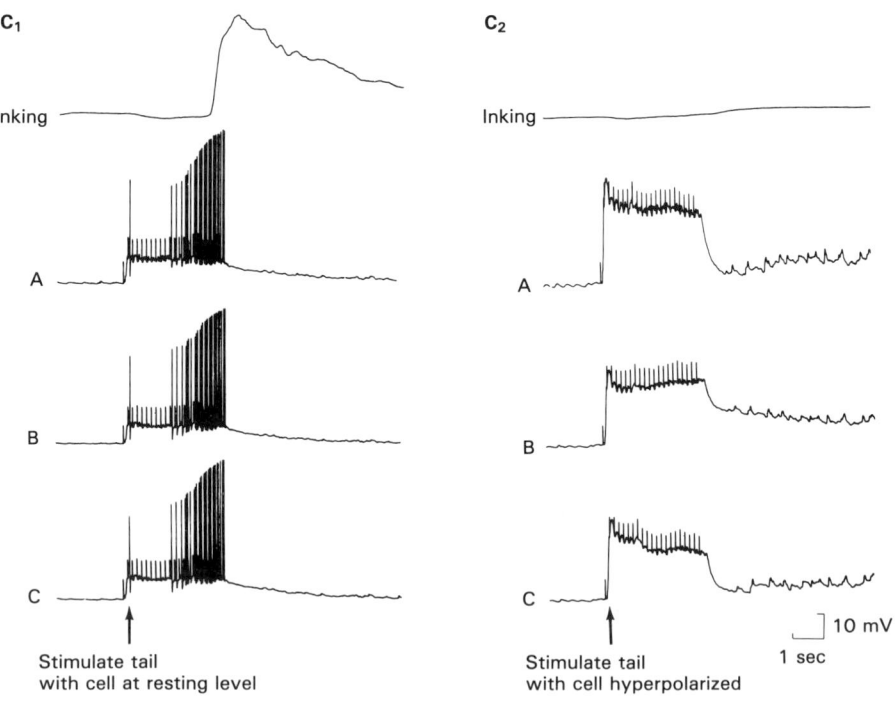

C_1

Inking

A

B

C

Stimulate tail
with cell at resting level

C_2

Inking

A

B

C

⌐ 10 mV

1 sec

Stimulate tail
with cell hyperpolarized

coupled cells act as one large cell, and thus the effective resistance of each of the coupled neurons is decreased. From Ohms law ($\Delta V = \Delta I \times R$) we can see that the lower the resistance (R) of a neuron, the smaller the depolarization (ΔV) produced by an excitatory synaptic current (ΔI). Once this high threshold is surpassed, however, groups of electrically coupled cells tend to fire synchronously.

Thus, behaviors mediated by electrical synapses often have two interesting features: they have a high threshold and they occur explosively in an all-or-none manner once the high threshold is reached. For example, the marine snail *Aplysia* exhibits a stereotypic all-or-none defensive behavior when seriously perturbed. It releases a massive amount of purple ink that screens the animal. The motor component of this behavior is mediated by three electrically coupled, high-threshold motor cells that innervate the ink gland. Once the threshold is exceeded, these motor cells fire synchronously (Figure 9–5). Similarly, in certain fish rapid saccadic eye movements produced by extraocular motor neurons are mediated by the synchronizing properties of electrical synapses.

Beyond participating in electrical communication that requires speed or synchrony, electrical synapses are thought to be important for transmitting *developmental* or *regulatory signals* between cells. This is because the diameter of the gap junction channel pore of electrical synapses is relatively large, 1.5 nm, allowing compounds with molecular weights up to 1000, such as cyclic adenosine 3′,5′-monophosphate (cAMP) and small peptides, to pass from one cell to the next. Recall that the electrical coupling between glial cells that we considered in Chapter 2 allows them to act over considerable distances to regulate K^+ buffering in the extracellular space.

In Electrical Synapses the Pre- and Postsynaptic Elements Are Bridged by Gap Junctions

What is the morphological structure of an electrical synapse? How do these structural features explain why some electrical synapses are unidirectional whereas most are bidirectional? The zone of apposition between two neurons at the site of an electrical synapse is called a *gap junction* and is bridged by channels called gap junction channels (Figure 9–6). These channels conduct the flow of ionic current and thus mediate electrical transmission. Whereas the normal extracellular space is about 20 nm, the gap separating pre- and postsynaptic cells at an electrical synapse is only 3.5 nm (35 Å). Rectifying and nonrectifying electrical synapses do not appear to differ in ultrastructure. At both types of synapses markers such as fluorescent dyes flow readily between the pre- and postsynaptic cells through the junction. The major difference between the two classes of electrical synapses may reside in the extent to which channel gating is sensitive to voltage.

Single-channel recordings by Jacques Neyton and Alain Trautmann indicate that channels at a gap junction have an elementary conductance of 100 pS. The gap junction channels are not always open, however. Michael Bennett and his colleagues found that the conductance of some gap

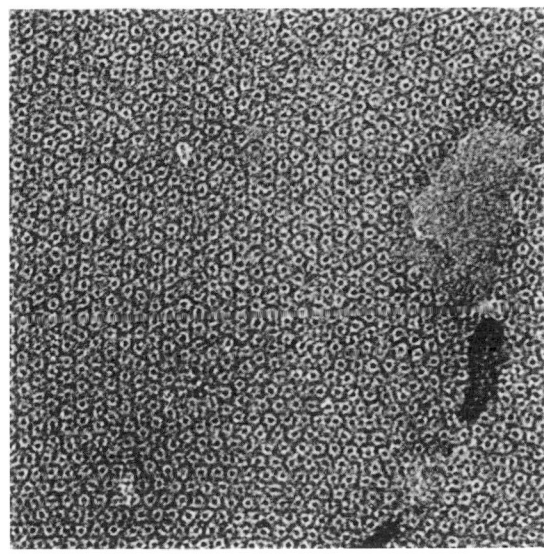

FIGURE 9–6
Electrical transmission between two cells occurs at gap junctions, shown here isolated from rat liver ($\times$ 307,800). The tissue has been negatively stained, a technique that darkens the area around the channels and in the pores. The membrane surface is shown, revealing a regular lattice of hexagonal particles. (Courtesy of N. Gilula.)

junction channels and the consequent electrical transmission can be modulated by intracellular pH, by Ca^{2+}, or even by neurotransmitters and second messengers. For example, gap junction channels at nonrectifying electrical synapses close in response to lowered pH or elevated cytoplasmic Ca^{2+}. Some nonrectifying synapses are even slightly sensitive to voltage (although not nearly as sensitive as are rectifying synapses). Finally, neurotransmitters can alter gap junctions through signal transduction pathways (see Chapter 12).

Because gap junctions can be isolated from nervous tissue (or from the liver, where they can be obtained in even greater abundance), it has been possible to characterize them in molecular and structural detail. All gap junctions consist of a pair of cylinders (hemi-channels), one in the presynaptic and the other in the postsynaptic cell. The cylinders meet in the gap between the two membranes and connect, by means of homophilic interactions, to establish a communicating channel about 1.5 nm in diameter between the cytoplasm of the two cells. Each hemichannel cylinder is called a *connexon*. Each connexon is made up of six identical protein subunits, called *connexins*, which are 7.5 nm in length and arranged hexagonally (Figure 9–7). Each connexin has two functions: It recognizes the other five subunits to assemble an effective connexon hemi-channel and it recognizes its counterpart hemi-channel in the apposed cell to form a complete conductive channel.

Nigel Unwin and his colleagues suggest that when the channel opens the six subunits of each connexon hemichannel rotate slightly with respect to each other, much like the elements of the shutter in a camera, and expose

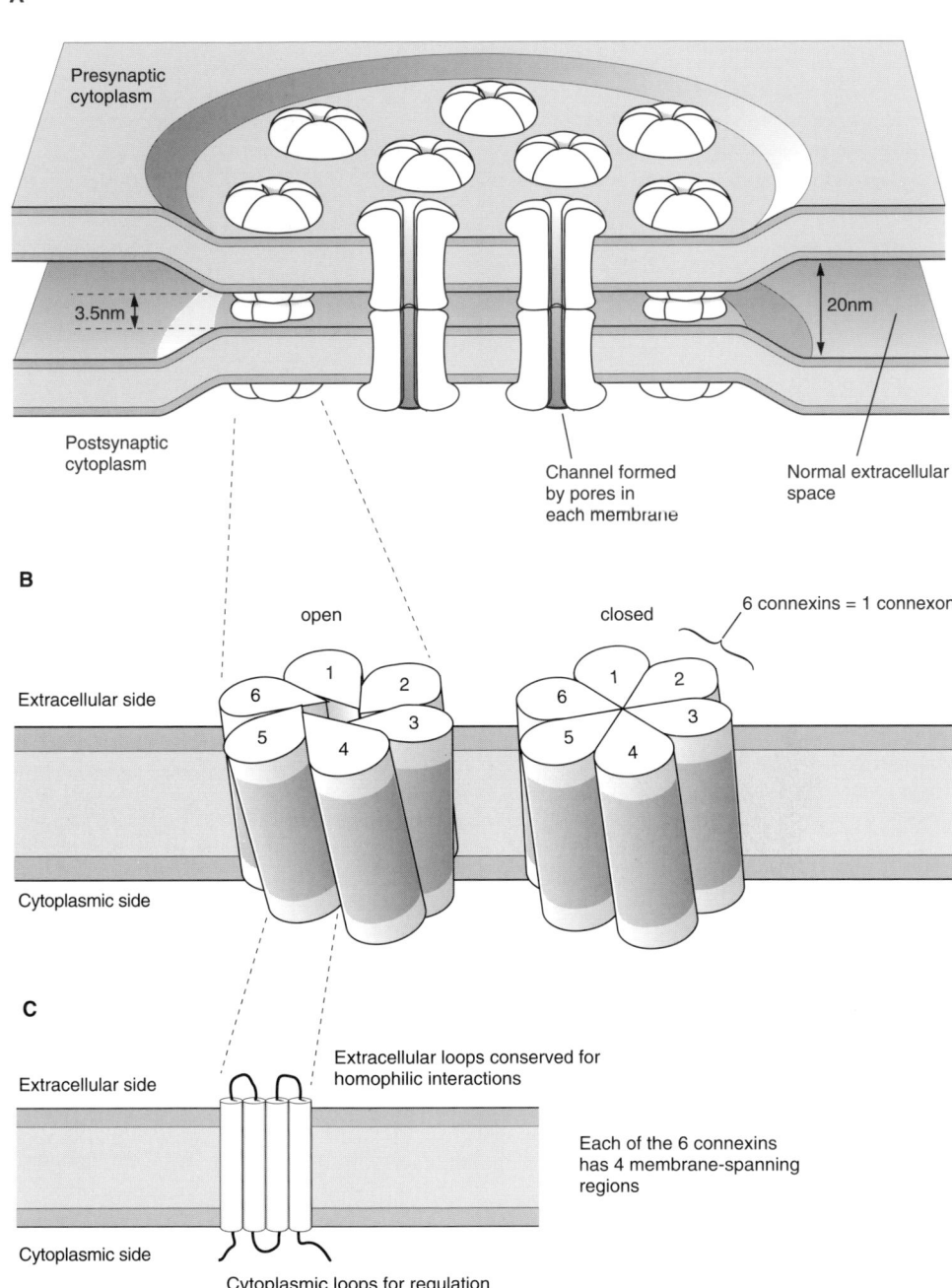

A

Presynaptic cytoplasm

3.5nm

20nm

Postsynaptic cytoplasm

Channel formed by pores in each membrane

Normal extracellular space

B

open

closed

6 connexins = 1 connexon

Extracellular side

6 1 2
5 3
4

6 1 2
5 3
4

Cytoplasmic side

C

Extracellular loops conserved for homophilic interactions

Extracellular side

Each of the 6 connexins has 4 membrane-spanning regions

Cytoplasmic side

Cytoplasmic loops for regulation

FIGURE 9–7

A three-dimensional model of the gap junction channel based on X-ray diffraction studies.

A. Each apposite cell contributes half of a channel (hemi-channel) called a connexon. Each connexon, about 1.5–2.0 nm in diameter, is formed from six protein subunits called connexins. Each connexin is about 7.5 nm long, spanning the membrane and contacting a matched connexin across the gap between the cells. At these sites the cells are only 3.5 nm apart, whereas neurons are normally separated by a 20 nm gap. (Adapted from Makowski et al., 1977.)

B. Model of a single connexon. This figure illustrates how the six connexin subunits that form the hemi-channel may change configuration to open and close the hemi-channel. Closure is achieved by the subunits sliding against each other and tilting at one end, thus rotating at the base in a clockwise direction. Each subunit is thought to move about 0.9 nm at the cytoplasmic surface. The dark shading indicates the portion of the connexon embedded in the membrane. (Adapted from Unwin and Zampighi, 1980.)

C. Model of a single membrane-spanning connexin indicating the four predicted membrane-spanning regions.

the channel's pore. The concerted tilting of each connexin by a few angstroms at one end leads to a somewhat larger tangential displacement at the other end (Figure 9–7B). Such conformational changes may be a common mechanism for opening and closing ion channels (see Chapter 5).

Connexins appear to belong to a large gene family. Several investigators have recently obtained protein or cDNA sequences of gap junctions from the lens, liver, and heart and found that, although the channels in each of these tissues are formed by distinctive protein, all have regions of similarity. In particular, four hydrophobic domains thought to span the membrane are highly conserved, as are two extracellular regions thought to be involved in the homophile matching of the two hemi-channels of adjacent cells (Figure 9–7C). The cytoplasmic regions, on the other hand, vary greatly, and this variation may be the reason why gap junctions in different tissues differ in their sensitivity to various modulatory factors.

At Chemical Synapses the Pre- and Postsynaptic Elements Are Separated by a Synaptic Cleft

Unlike electrical synapses, the pre- and postsynaptic neurons of chemical synapses are not connected structurally. In fact, the synaptic cleft in chemical synapses is slightly *wider* (20–40 nm) than the adjacent extracellular space (typically 20 nm), and in some instances substantially wider. Many pre- and postsynaptic membranes have morphologically specialized regions. The presynaptic terminals contain localized collections of vesicles, the *synaptic vesicles*, which are filled with chemical neurotransmitter (Figure 9–8). In response to the presynaptic action potential, the transmitter is released from the synaptic vesicles at the nerve terminals. After it is released, the transmitter diffuses and binds to receptor sites on the postsynaptic cell, where it causes ion channels to open (or close), thereby altering the membrane conductance and potential of the postsynaptic cell (Figure 9–9).

These several steps account for the synaptic delay at chemical synapses, a delay that is often several milliseconds or longer but can be as short as 0.3 ms. Although chemical transmission lacks the speed of electrical synapses, it has the important property of amplification. By releasing one or more synaptic vesicles, each of which contains several thousand molecules of transmitter, thousands of ion channels in the postsynaptic cell are opened. In this way a small presynaptic nerve terminal, which generates only a weak electrical current, is able to depolarize a large postsynaptic cell.

Chemical Transmission Involves Transmitter Release and Receptor Activation

Chemical synaptic transmission can be divided into two processes. The presynaptic *transmitting* process releases the chemical messenger, the postsynaptic *receptive* process determines the binding of the transmitter to the receptor molecule in the postsynaptic cell.

In some ways the presynaptic terminals of a chemical synapse resemble an endocrine gland, and chemical trans-

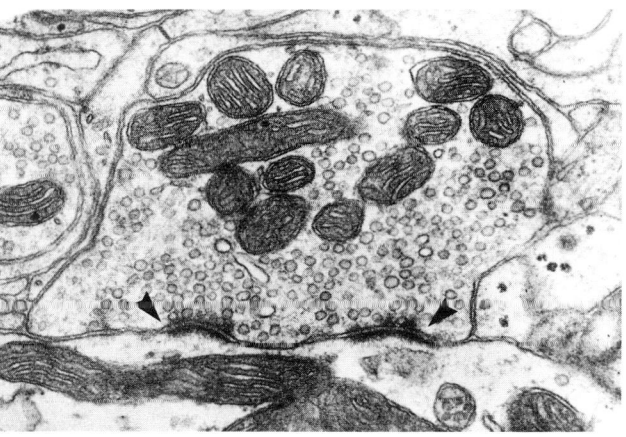

FIGURE 9–8
At the chemical synapse presynaptic and postsynaptic membranes are separated by extracellular space called the synaptic cleft. This electron micrograph of a nerve–muscle synapse shows the fine structure of a presynaptic terminal. The large dark structures are mitochondria. Together with the endoplasmic reticulum, they are thought to buffer the concentration of free Ca^{2+} in the presynaptic terminal. The many round bodies are vesicles that contain the neurotransmitter acetylcholine. The fuzzy dark thickenings (**arrows**) along the presynaptic side of the cleft are called active zones, specializations that are thought to be docking sites for vesicles. The docking sites are thought to facilitate release of vesicles by exocytosis. Active zones are discussed in Chapter 13. × 20,000. (Courtesy of J. E. Heuser and T. S. Reese.)

mission is a modified form of hormone secretion. Both endocrine glands and presynaptic terminals release a chemical agent with a signaling function. But there is one important difference between the two. Endocrine glands are usually at some distance from their target organs, and the hormone released by the gland carries the signal over this distance through the blood stream. Neurons, too, can interact over long distances, but they have axons that carry electrical signals to the point of contact with target cells. At the axon terminal the electrical signal triggers release of the chemical transmitter, which travels only a small distance to its target. Neuronal signaling, therefore, has two advantages over endocrine signaling: It is faster and more directed.

Most neurons have in their presynaptic terminals specialized secretory machinery for focused release, called *active zones*, that are absent in endocrine cells. Active zones are lacking at certain chemical synapses, and at such synapses the distinction between neuronal and hormonal transmission becomes blurred. For example, the presynaptic neurons involved in the autonomic innervation of smooth muscle are at some distance from the postsynaptic cells and do not have specialized release sites in their terminals; thus, synaptic actions between these cells are slower and more diffuse. Moreover, the same chemical messenger can serve several functions. At one locus it can be a conventional transmitter, acting directly on neighboring cells; at another locus it can be a modulator, producing a more diffuse action that fine tunes a neu-

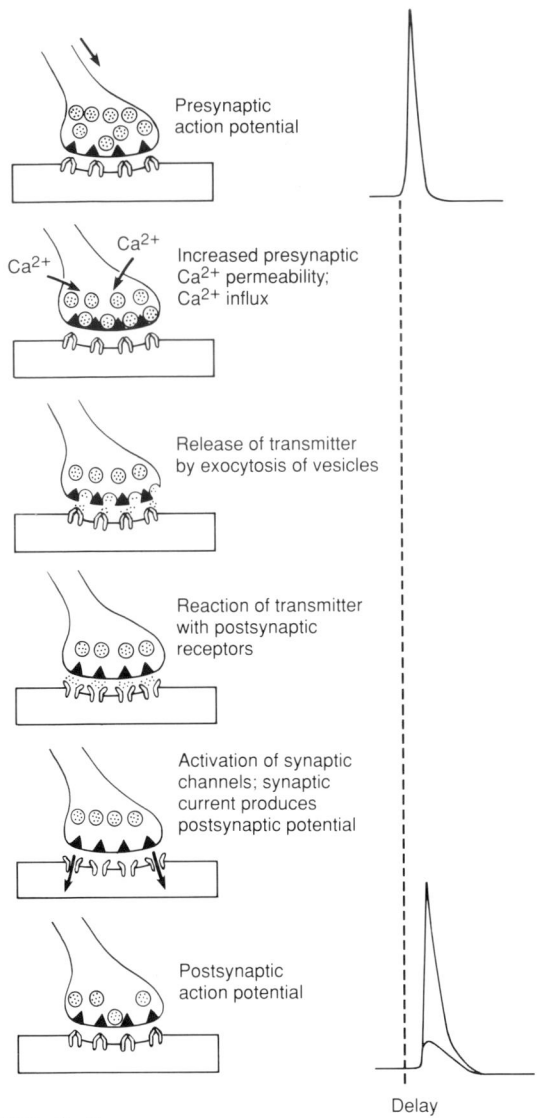

Presynaptic
action potential

Increased presynaptic
Ca^{2+} permeability;
Ca^{2+} influx

Release of transmitter
by exocytosis of vesicles

Reaction of transmitter
with postsynaptic
receptors

Activation of synaptic
channels; synaptic
current produces
postsynaptic potential

Postsynaptic
action potential

Delay

FIGURE 9–9

The general mode of transmission at chemical synapses. An
action potential arriving at the terminal of a presynaptic axon
causes vesicles containing neurotransmitter, and loaded into
active zones, to fuse with the cytoplasmic membrane. The fusion causes the vesicles to release their contents into the synapse. The released neurotransmitter substances then diffuse
across the synaptic cleft and bind to specific receptors on the
postsynaptic membrane. These receptors cause ion channels to
open (or close), thereby changing the membrane conductance
and depolarizing the cell. Whereas transmission at electrical
synapses is virtually instantaneous (see Figure 9–2B, 1), chemical synaptic transmission involves a delay between action
potentials in the pre- and postsynaptic cells.

ron's response; and at a third locus it can be released into
the bloodstream to act as a hormone.

A variety of small molecules—for example, acetylcholine (ACh), γ-aminobutyric acid (GABA), glycine, glutamate, serotonin, dopamine, and norepinephrine—can
serve as transmitters; so can various peptides. Nevertheless, the action of a specific chemical messenger in the

postsynaptic cell does not depend on the chemical nature
of the transmitter, but instead on the properties of the
receptors with which the transmitter binds. For example,
acetylcholine can excite some postsynaptic cells and inhibit others, and can do both simultaneously at still others. It is the receptor that determines whether a cholinergic synapse is excitatory or inhibitory, and whether an ion
channel will be activated directly by the transmitter or
indirectly through a second messenger. Within a group of
closely related animals a given transmitter substance
binds to conserved families of receptors and is associated
with specific physiological functions. For example, in vertebrates ACh produces synaptic excitation at the neuromuscular junction by acting on a nicotinic ACh receptor.
Similarly, ACh invariably slows the heart in vertebrates
by acting on an inhibitory muscarinic ACh receptor.

The notion of a receptor was introduced in the late
nineteenth century by the German biological chemist
Paul Ehrlich to explain the selective action of toxins and
other pharmacological agents and the specificity of immunological reactions. In his Croonian lecture of 1900 Ehrlich said that "chemical substances are only able to
exercise an action on the tissue elements with which they
are able to establish an intimate chemical relationship. . . .
[This relationship] must be specific. The [chemical] groups
must be adapted to one another . . . as lock and key." In
1906 the English pharmacologist John Langley postulated
that the sensitivity of skeletal muscle to curare and nicotine is due to a receptive molecule. Receptor theory was
subsequently developed by Langley's students—in particular, Eliot Smith and Henry Dale—and was greatly influenced by the study of both enzyme kinetics and
cooperative interactions between small molecules and
proteins. As we shall see in the next chapter, Langley's
receptive molecule has now been isolated and characterized as the ACh receptor of the neuromuscular junction.

All receptors for chemical transmitters have two common biochemical features:

1. They are membrane-spanning proteins. The region exposed to the external environment of the cell recognizes and binds the transmitter from the presynaptic
   cell.
2. They carry out an effector function within the target
   cell, either gating an ion channel directly or indirectly,
   by initiating a second-messenger cascade.

Chemical Receptors Use Two Major Molecular Mechanisms to Gate Ion Channels

The receptors for chemical neurotransmitters fall into two
classes based on whether their gating of the ion channel is
direct or indirect. The two classes of receptor proteins are
derived from two distinct gene families.

Receptors that gate ion channels *directly* such as those
mediating the action of ACh at the neuromuscular junction, consist of a single macromolecule containing several
protein subunits that form both the recognition element
and ion channel (Figure 9–10A). Such *ionophoric* receptors, when bound to a neurotransmitter, undergo a conformational change that opens the channel. A similar

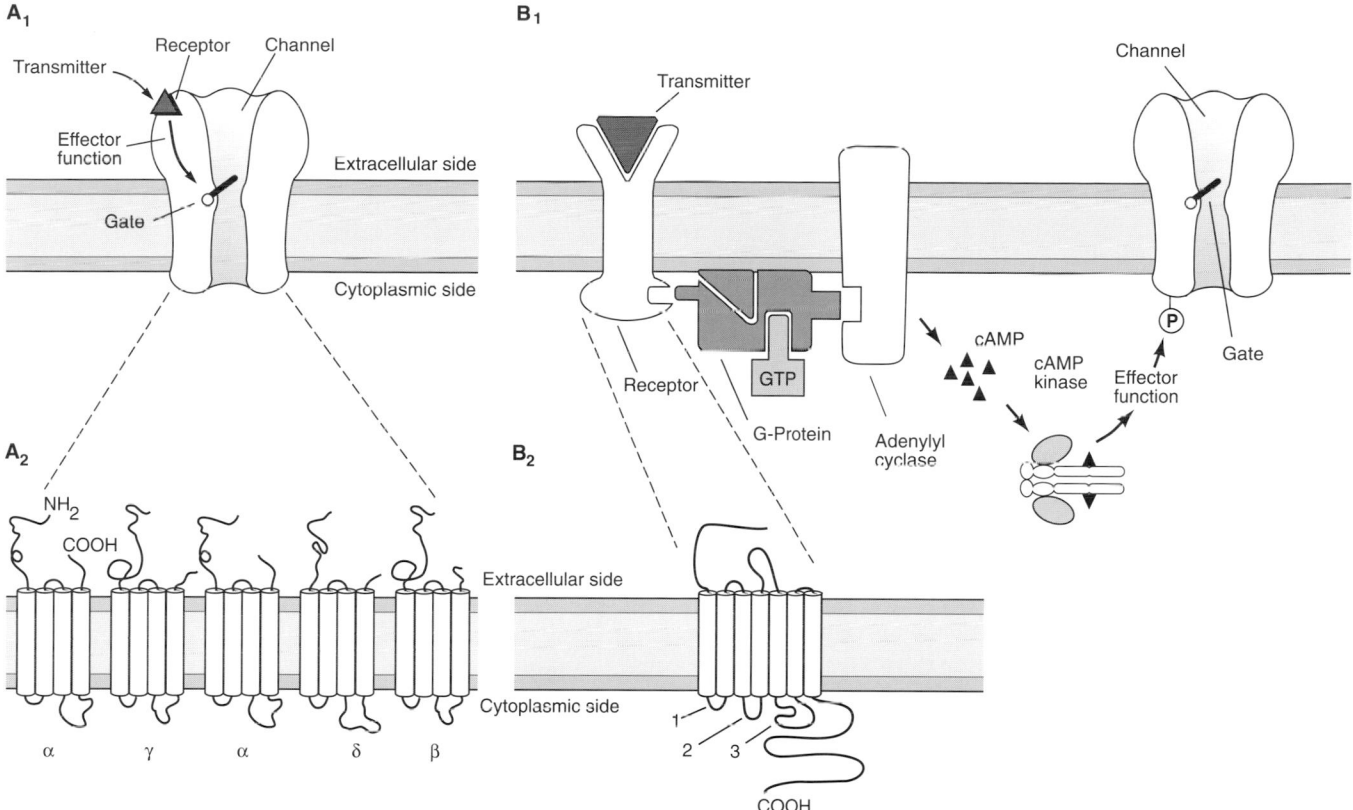

FIGURE 9–10

Two classes of neurotransmitter actions.

A. 1. Direct gating of an ion channel is mediated by a transmitter receptor that is part of the ion channel. 2. These receptors are composed of four (or five) subunits, each of which contains four or five membrane-spanning α-helical regions.

B. Indirect gating is mediated by a second messenger that couples the receptor to the ion channel. 1. The receptor activates a GTP-binding protein (G-protein), which in turn activates a sec-

ond-messenger cascade that modulates ion channel activity. The channel to be modulated and the receptor are different molecules. In this example the G-protein stimulates adenylyl cyclase, which converts ATP to cAMP. The cAMP activates the cAMP-dependent protein kinase (cAMP-kinase), which phosphorylates the channel (**P**), leading to a change in function. 2. The typical receptor of this family of proteins is composed of a single protein with seven membrane-spanning α-helical regions that bind the ligand within the plane of the membrane.

mechanism is found in certain channels in the central nervous system regulated by glutamate, glycine, and GABA (see Chapter 11).

Receptors that gate ion channels *indirectly*, like those for norepinephrine or serotonin at synapses in the cerebral cortex, involve separate receptors and ion channels that communicate through GTP-binding proteins (G-proteins). These G-proteins couple the receptors to effector enzymes that produce one or another intracellular second messenger, such as cAMP or diacylglycerol (Figure 9–10B). The second messenger then acts on a channel directly, or more commonly activates one of a family of enzymes called protein kinases, which can modulate channels by phosphorylating either the channel protein or a regulatory protein that acts on the channel. In addition, in certain cases, G proteins can also interact with ion channels directly, independent of second-messenger production. Whereas receptors that directly gate ion channels are composed of several subunits, those that activate second-messenger cascades through G-proteins consist

of a single polypeptide chain (Figure 9–10B) (see Chapter 12).

The two types of receptors have different functions. Receptors that directly gate ion channels produce relatively fast synaptic actions lasting only milliseconds. These are commonly used in the neural circuitry that produces behavior. Receptors that gate ion channels indirectly result in slow synaptic actions lasting seconds and even minutes. These slower actions often serve to modulate behavior by altering the excitability of neurons and the strength of the synaptic connections of the basic neural circuitry. For example, modulatory synaptic pathways often serve as reinforcing stimuli in learning.

An Overall View

Information is transferred between neurons by two types of synaptic transmission: electrical and chemical. Electrical transmission is mediated by the direct flow of current from the presynaptic to the postsynaptic neuron through gap junctions. Electrical synapses can be rectifying (passing current in one direction better than in the other) or nonrectifying (passing current equally well in either direction). Electrical transmission occurs by means of current flow through gap junction channels that directly connect the cytoplasm of both cells. Gap junction channels are paired hemi-cylinders in the membranes of each apposite cell and are permeable to small molecules and some second messengers. Because its mechanism is direct, electrical transmission is the most rapid form of synaptic communication between neurons. Groups of cells with electrical synapses can fire together when their collective threshold is reached. These two properties, speed and synchrony, make electrical synapses suitable for fast, stereotyped behaviors, such as escape and defensive responses.

Chemical synaptic transmission is slower than electrical transmission because the presynaptic neuron must first release a neurotransmitter, which then diffuses across the synaptic cleft and binds to receptors in the postsynaptic cell membrane. It is the receptor, not the transmitter, which determines whether the synaptic response is excitatory or inhibitory. Directly gated chemical transmission is only slightly slower than electrical transmission. This type of synaptic response is mediated by receptors that are part of the ion channel molecule. Indirectly gated chemical transmission is slower because it involves several steps; the receptors are coupled to enzymes that synthesize second messengers, which then act on the ion channels.

Although even the fastest chemical synaptic responses are slower than electrical synaptic responses, chemical synaptic transmission has the advantage that a single action potential releases thousands of neurotransmitter molecules, allowing amplification of the synaptic response. Perhaps because it is a multistep process, chemical transmission is more easily modified than electrical transmission. In the next several chapters we shall see how the nervous system makes use of diverse chemical transmission mechanisms in neuronal signaling. In addition, we shall see that many synaptic receptors are selective targets for diseases and also for drug therapy.

Selected Readings

Bennett, M. V. L., Barrio, L. C., Bargiello, T. A., Spray, D. C., Hertzberg, E., and Sáez, J. C. 1991. Gap junctions: New tools, new answers, new questions. Neuron 6:305–320.

Eccles, J. C. 1976. From electrical to chemical transmission in the central nervous system. The closing address of the Sir Henry Dale Centennial Symposium. Notes Rec. R. Soc. Lond. 30: 219–230.

Edelman, G. M., Gall, W. E., and Cowan, W. M. (eds.) 1987. Synaptic Function. New York: Wiley.

Fatt, P. 1954. Biophysics of junctional transmission. Physiol. Rev. 34:674–710.

Furshpan, E. J., and Potter, D. D. 1959. Transmission at the giant motor synapses of the crayfish. J. Physiol. (Lond.) 145:289–325.

Hertzberg, E. L., Lawrence, T. S., and Gilula, N. B. 1981. Gap junctional communication. Annu. Rev. Physiol. 43:479–491.

Ross, E. M. 1989. Signal sorting and amplification through G protein-coupled receptors. Neuron 3:141–152.

Unwin, N. 1989. The structure of ion channels in membranes of excitable cells. Neuron 3:665–676.

References

Beyer, E. C., Paul, D. L., and Goodenough, D. A. 1987. Connexin43: A protein from rat heart homologous to a gap junction protein from liver. J. Cell Biol. 105:2621–2629.

Carew, T. J., and Kandel, E. R. 1976. Two functional effects of decreased conductance EPSP's: Synaptic augmentation and increased electrotonic coupling. Science 192:150–153.

Dale, H. 1935. Pharmacology and nerve-endings. Proc. R. Soc. Med. (Lond.) 28:319–332.

Eckert, R. 1988. Animal Physiology: Mechanisms and Adaptations. 3rd ed. New York: Freeman, chap. 6, "Propagation and transmission of signals."

Ehrlich, P. 1900. On immunity with special reference to cell life. Croonian Lecture. Proc. R. Soc. Lond. 66:424–448.

Fatt, P., and Katz, B. 1951. An analysis of the end-plate potential recorded with an intra-cellular electrode. J. Physiol (Lond.) 115:320–370.

Furshpan, E. J., and Potter, D. D. 1957. Mechanism of nerve-impulse transmission at a crayfish synapse. Nature 180:342–343.

Langley, J. N. 1906. On nerve endings and on special excitable substances in cells. Proc. R. Soc. Lond. (Biol.) 78:170–194.

Lasater, E. M., and Dowling, J. E. 1985. Electrical coupling between pairs of isolated fish horizontal cells is modulated by dopamine and cAMP. In M. V. L. Bennett and D. C. Spray (eds.), Gap Junctions. Cold Spring Harbor, N.Y.: Cold Spring Harbor Laboratory, pp. 393–404.

Loewi, O., and Navratil, E. 1926. Über humorale Übertragbarkeit der Herznervenwirkung. X. Mitteilung: Über das Schicksal des Vagusstoffs. Pflügers Arch. 214:678–688. (English translation "On the humoral propagation of cardiac nerve action. Communication X. The fate of the vagus substance.") In I. Cooke and M. Lipkin, Jr. (eds.), 1972. Cellular Neurophysiology: A Source Book. New York: Holt, Rinehart and Winston, pp. 478–485.

Makowski, L., Caspar, D. L. D., Phillips, W. C., Baker, T. S., and Goodenough, D. A. 1984. Gap junction structures. VI. Variation and conservation in connexon conformation and packing. Biophys. J. 45:208–218.

Margiotta, J. F., and Walcott, B. 1983. Conductance and dye permeability of a rectifying electrical synapse. Nature 305:52–55.

Neyton, J., and Trautmann, A. 1985. Single-channel currents of an intercellular junction. Nature 317:331–335.

Neyton, J., Piccolino, M., and Gerschenfeld, H. M. 1985. Neurotransmitter-induced modulation of gap junction permeability in retinal horizontal cells. In M. V. L. Bennett and D. C. Spray (eds.), Gap Junctions. Cold Spring Harbor, N.Y.: Cold Spring Harbor Laboratory, pp. 381–391.

Pappas, G. D., and Waxman, S. G. 1972. Synaptic fine structure—morphological correlates of chemical and electrotonic transmission. In G. D. Pappas and D. P. Purpura (eds.), Structure and Function of Synapses. New York: Raven Press, pp. 1–43.

Ramón y Cajal, S. 1894. La fine structure des centres nerveux. Proc. R. Soc. Lond. 55:444–468.

Ramón y Cajal, S. 1911. Histologie du Système Nerveux de l'Homme & des Vertébrés, Vol. 2. L. Azoulay (trans.) Paris: Maloine. Republished in 1955. Madrid: Instituto Ramón y Cajal.

Sherrington, C. 1947. The Integrative Action of the Nervous System, 2nd ed. New Haven: Yale University Press.

Unwin, P. N. T., and Zampighi, G. 1980. Structure of the junction between communicating cells. Nature 283:545–549.

Eric R. Kandel
Steven A. Siegelbaum

10

Directly Gated Transmission at the Nerve–Muscle Synapse

The Neuromuscular Junction Is a Simple Synapse for Studying Directly Gated Transmission

Synaptic Excitation of Skeletal Muscle by Motor Neurons Involves Directly Gated Ion Channels

The Ion Channel at the End-Plate Is Permeable to Both Sodium and Potassium

Transmitter-Gated Channels Are Fundamentally Different from Voltage-Gated Channels

The Action of a Single Transmitter-Gated Channel Can Be Studied Experimentally

Individual Transmitter-Gated Channels Conduct a Unitary Current

Current Flow Depends on the Number of Open Channels, Concentration of the Transmitter, Channel Conductance, and Membrane Potential

The Nicotinic Acetylcholine Receptor Is an Intrinsic Membrane Protein with Five Subunits

An Overall View

Postscript: The End-Plate Current Can Be Calculated from an Equivalent Circuit

Chemical synaptic transmission is the predominant form of synaptic communication in the brain. There are two major types of chemical transmission that differ according to the postsynaptic receptor that is activated. In one type the postsynaptic receptor gates an ion channel directly; in the other it does so indirectly, by means of a second messenger. Receptors that directly gate ion channels are best understood at the synapse between the motor neuron and skeletal muscle fiber of vertebrates, where synaptic excitation is mediated by an ion channel directly gated by acetylcholine (ACh). Therefore, we begin our consideration of chemical transmission by discussing this synapse. In the next two chapters we extend this discussion, first to directly gated synaptic transmission in the central nervous system and then to synaptic actions mediated by second messengers.

The Neuromuscular Junction Is a Simple Synapse for Studying Directly Gated Transmission

The synapse between the motor neuron and skeletal muscle is convenient for examining the synaptic actions of directly gated ion channels because it is easy to study. The muscle cell is large enough to accommodate several microelectrodes for electrophysiological measurements. Unlike synapses in the central nervous system, the region of the synapse where the presynaptic terminal contacts the postsynaptic membrane can be visualized with the light microscope in a living cell. The anatomy is relatively simple: A single muscle fiber usually is innervated by only one motor axon. The transmitter released by the axon ter-

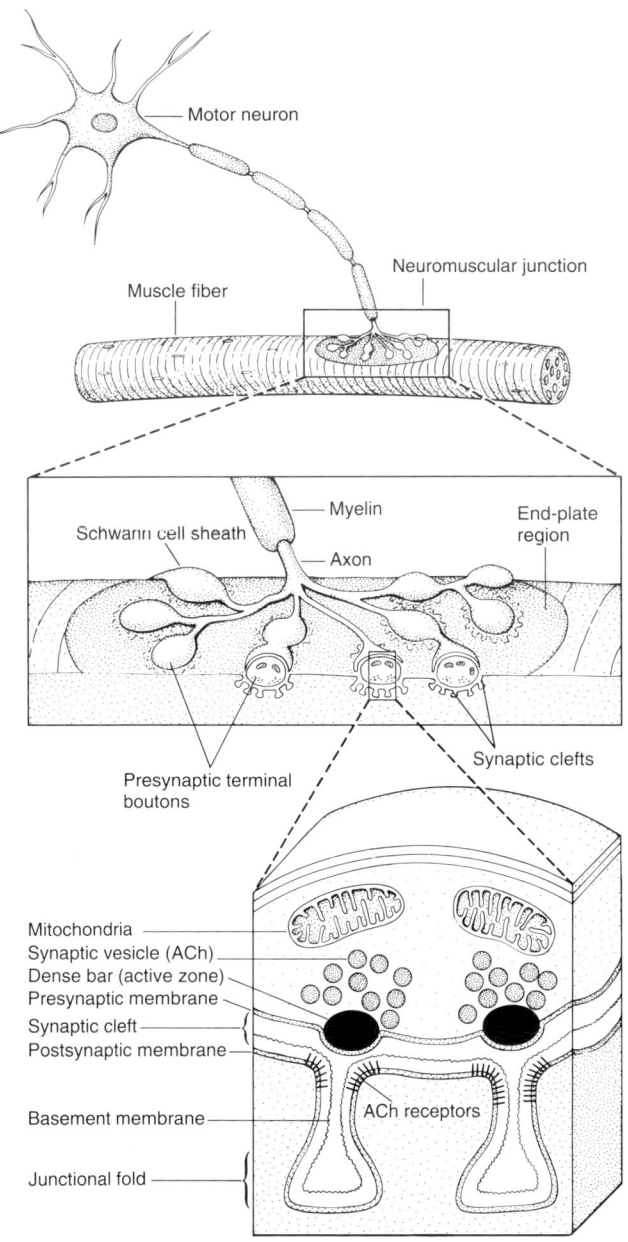

FIGURE 10–1

The neuromuscular junction. Drawings from top to bottom show progressive enlargements of segments of a neuromuscular junction. The presynaptic terminals consist of multiple swellings or varicosities called *synaptic boutons* or *terminals* covered by a thin layer of Schwann cells. The boutons are separated from the postsynaptic cell by the *synaptic cleft*, which is about 50 nm wide. Directly apposed to the motor neuron terminals is the *end-plate*, a specialized region of the muscle fiber membrane. *Junctional folds* in the end-plate contain a high density of ACh receptors. Lying over the muscle fiber is a layer of connective tissue called the *basement membrane* (basal lamina), which contains acetylcholinesterase, the enzyme that breaks down ACh. Each presynaptic bouton contains mitochondria and synaptic vesicles clustered around dense bars or *active zones* that are the site of release of the ACh transmitter. (Adapted in part from McMahan and Kuffler, 1971.)

minal is ACh, and the receptor on the muscle membrane is the nicotinic type of ACh receptor.[1]

The motor neuron's axon innervates a specialized region of the muscle membrane called the *end-plate*. As the motor axon approaches the end-plate, it loses its myelin sheath and splits into several fine branches. A fine branch is approximately 2 μm thick and forms at its end multiple grape-like varicosities, called *synaptic boutons*, where transmitter is released. Each bouton lies over a depression in the surface of the muscle fiber where the membrane of the muscle fiber forms deep *junctional folds* (Figure 10–1). These folds are lined by the *basement membrane* (or *basal lamina*), a network of connective tissue consisting of collagen and glycoproteins that covers the surface of the entire muscle fiber. Both the presynaptic terminal and the muscle fiber secrete proteins into the basement membrane at the end-plate, including the enzyme acetylcholinesterase, which inactivates the ACh released by the presynaptic terminal by hydrolyzing it to acetate and choline. The basement membrane also acts to organize the synapse by bringing appropriate pre- and postsynaptic elements into register, as discussed in Chapter 59.

Each presynaptic bouton contains all the machinery required to release transmitter. This includes (1) the *synaptic vesicles*, which contain ACh; (2) the *active zone*, a membrane specialization for transmitter release; and (3) voltage-gated Ca^{2+} channels. These channels allow Ca^{2+} to enter the terminal with each action potential; the Ca^{2+} triggers fusion of the synaptic vesicles with the terminal, and this fusion leads to the release of the vesicle's content.

Every active zone is positioned opposite a postsynaptic junctional fold. At the crest of these folds the receptors for ACh are clustered in a geometric lattice, with a density of about 10,000 receptors per $μm^2$ (Figure 10–2A, 10–3). Each receptor protein is about 8.5 nm in diameter and when appropriately stained appears as a hollow cylinder (Figure 10–2B). In the region below the crest and extending into the depths of the folds, the membrane of the muscle cell is rich in voltage-gated Na^+ channels, which convert the end-plate potential into an action potential.

When the motor axon is stimulated, ACh is released from the axon terminal and interacts with the ACh receptors in the crest of the folds of the muscle membrane to produce an excitatory postsynaptic potential called the *end-plate potential*. The amplitude of the end-plate potential is unusually large; a single motor cell produces a synaptic potential of about 70 mV. Under normal circumstances this synaptic potential is large enough to trigger an action potential in the muscle fiber. In contrast, most neurons in the central nervous system produce synaptic potentials less than 1 mV in amplitude. Because this synaptic potential is small, input from many presynaptic neu-

---

[1]There are two basic types of receptors to ACh: *nicotinic* and *muscarinic*. Both bind ACh, but the two receptors can be distinguished because there are agonists (drugs that simulate the actions of ACh, e.g., nicotine or muscarine) that bind exclusively to one type of ACh receptor or the other. We shall learn more about muscarinic ACh receptors in Chapter 12.

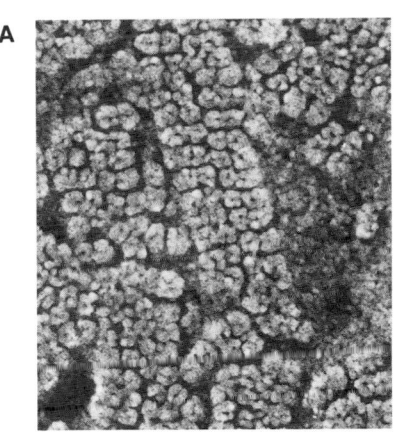

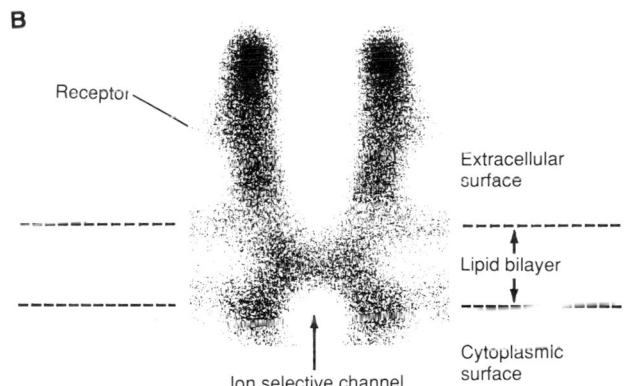

FIGURE 10–2

The clustering of ACh receptor-channels at the end-plate.

A. Acetylcholine receptors are densely packed in the postsynaptic membrane of a cell in the electric organ of *Torpedo californica*, a fish that can deliver an electric shock. This electron micrograph shows the external surface of the cell. The ACh receptors are the light areas. The pores in the receptors cannot be completely resolved. (Courtesy of J. E. Heuser and S. R. Salpeter.)

B. Reconstructed electron microscope image of the *Torpedo* ACh receptor-channel complex. The image was obtained by computer processing of negatively stained images of ACh receptors. The resolution is 1.7 nm, fine enough to see overall structures but too coarse to resolve individual atoms. The pore is wide at the external and internal surfaces of the membrane, but it narrows considerably within the lipid bilayer. The channel extends some distance into the extracellular space. (Adapted from Toyoshima and Unwin, 1988.)

FIGURE 10–3

Acetylcholine receptors in an end-plate from the sternomastoid muscle of the mouse. The receptors can be labeled with antibodies or with the snake venom neurotoxin (α-bungarotoxin), which bind to nicotinic ACh receptors. The toxin has been used extensively because it can be labeled with radioactive iodine or made fluorescent when covalently bound to rhodamine or fluorescein.

The muscle tissue was incubated with ^{125}I-labeled α-bungarotoxin until all neurally evoked muscle contractions were blocked, indicating that all ACh receptors were labeled. Labeled receptors appear black.

A. This electron microscopic autoradiograph shows that the label is not uniformly distributed throughout the postsynaptic membrane but is localized in regions of the junctional folds closest to the apposed axon. (**JF**, junctional folds; **A**, axon; **M**, muscle.) ×21,000.

B. In this autoradiograph the labeled receptors appear as dark densities along the junctional folds. The receptors are concentrated at the postjunctional membrane nearest the peaks of the fold (arrows). ×37,500. (From Fertuck and Salpeter, 1974.)

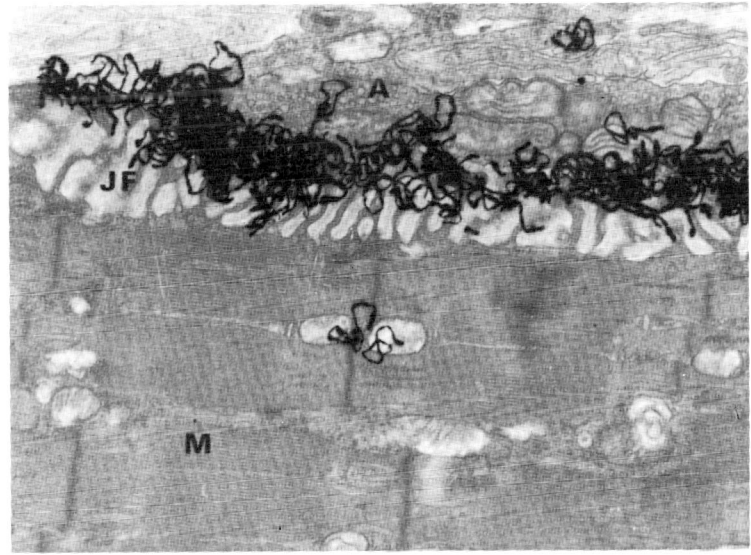

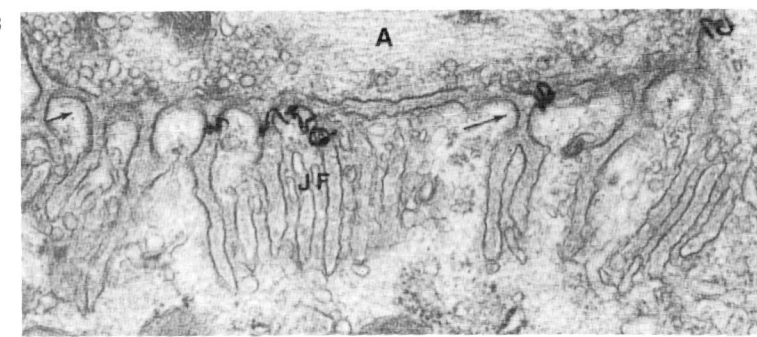

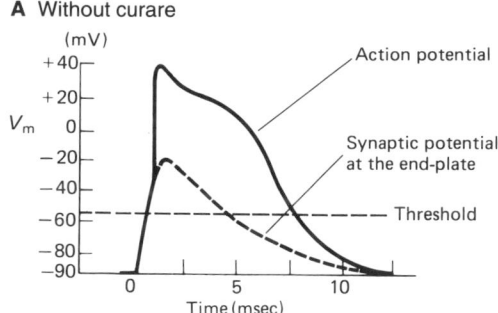

A Without curare

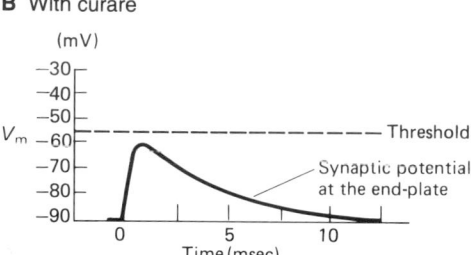

B With curare

FIGURE 10–4

The end-plate potential (EPP) can be isolated pharmacologically for study.

A. Under normal circumstances stimulation of the motor axon produces a large EPP in the muscle fiber that surpasses threshold and triggers an action potential (**solid trace**). The **dashed trace** shows the inferred time course of the underlying EPP.

B. The EPP can be isolated in the presence of curare. Curare blocks the binding of ACh to its receptor and so reduces the amplitude of the EPP below threshold. This technique is used to study the currents and channels that contribute to the EPP, which are different from those producing an action potential. The values for the resting potential, synaptic potential, and action potential shown in these intracellular recordings are typical of a vertebrate skeletal muscle.

rons is needed to generate an action potential in central neurons.

Synaptic Excitation of Skeletal Muscle by Motor Neurons Involves Directly Gated Ion Channels

The synaptic potential at the nerve–muscle synapse was first studied in detail in the 1950s by Paul Fatt and Bernard Katz. Using the drug curare, they reduced the amplitude of the synaptic potential below the threshold for the action potential and thus were able to isolate the synaptic potential in intracellular voltage recordings (Figure 10–4). Curare is a mixture of plant toxins used by South American Indians as an arrowhead poison to paralyze their quarry. Tubocurarine, the purified active agent, blocks neuromuscular transmission by binding to the receptor and preventing its activation by ACh. Fatt and Katz found that the synaptic potential produced in muscle cells by the action of the motor neuron is largest when the intracellular electrode is placed right at the end-plate. As the electrode is moved down the muscle fiber away from the end-plate region, the amplitude of the synaptic potential decreases progressively (Figure 10–5). From this analysis Fatt and Katz concluded that the synaptic potential is generated by an inward current confined to the end-plate region, which then spreads passively away from the end-plate. The current flow is confined to the end-plate region because the ACh receptor proteins are localized in that region, opposite the presynaptic terminal from which transmitter is released (Figure 10–1).

At the end-plate the synaptic potential rises rapidly but decays more slowly. The rapid rise is due to the sudden increase in concentration of ACh after its release into the synaptic cleft by the action potential in the presynaptic nerve terminal. Once released, ACh diffuses rapidly to the receptors at the end-plate. Not all the released ACh

FIGURE 10–5

The synaptic potential is largest at its site of origin at the end-plate region and propagates away from it passively.

A. Recordings from the end-plate and along the muscle fiber at various distances show that the peak amplitude of the synaptic potential decays and its time course becomes slower with increasing distance from the end-plate region.

B. The decay illustrated in **A** results from the leakiness of the muscle fiber membrane. Since current flow must complete a circuit, the inward synaptic current at the end-plate region gives rise to a return flow of outward current through nongated channels and across the capacitor of the membrane. It is this outward flow of current across the capacitor that produces the depolarization. Since current leaks out all along the membrane, the current flow decreases with distance from the end-plate. Thus, unlike the regenerative action potential, the local depolarization produced by the synaptic potential of the membrane also decreases with distance. (Adapted from Miles, 1969.)

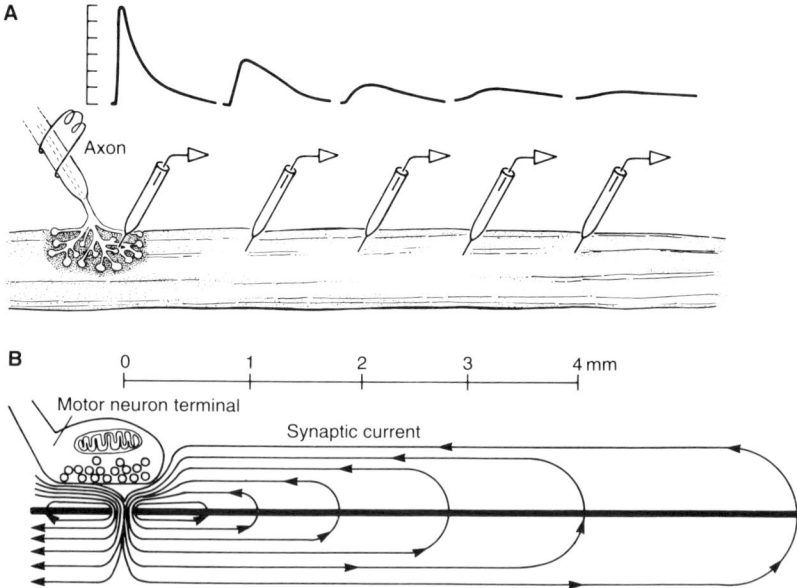

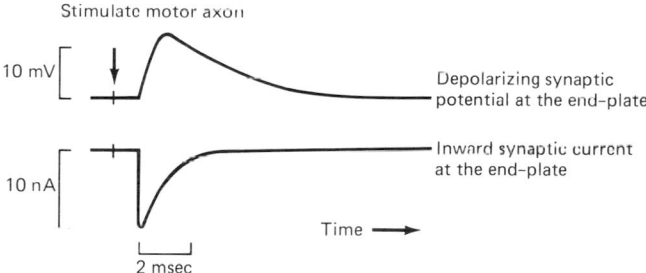

Stimulate motor axon

Depolarizing synaptic potential at the end-plate

Inward synaptic current at the end-plate

Time ⟶

2 msec

FIGURE 10–6

The time course of the end-plate potential is considerably slower than the underlying inward current. The end-plate potential changes slowly because synaptic current must first alter the charge on the membrane capacitance of the muscle. As we have seen in Chapter 7, only when capacitance is charged can the membrane potential change. The synaptic current is measured at a constant membrane potential (e.g., −90 mV) using the voltage-clamp technique.

reaches the postsynaptic receptors, however, because two processes act quickly to remove ACh from the cleft: (1) ACh is hydrolyzed by the *acetylcholinesterase* localized in the basement membrane and (2) ACh diffuses away, out of the synaptic cleft. Because the ACh concentration falls rapidly, it does not contribute to the time course of decay of the synaptic potential.

The time course and properties of the current that generates the end-plate potential were first studied in voltage-clamp experiments by Akira Takeuchi and Norika Takeuchi. The Takeuchis found that this current rises and decays more rapidly than the resultant depolarizing change in end-plate potential (Figure 10–6). The time course of the end-plate current is thought to reflect the rapid opening and closing of the ion channels activated by ACh. The slower time course of the synaptic potential is partly determined by the passive time constant of the muscle membrane. As we saw in Chapter 7 (Figure 7–3) it takes time for an ionic current to charge or discharge the muscle membrane capacitance (see the Postscript at the end of this chapter).

The Ion Channel at the End-Plate Is Permeable to Both Sodium and Potassium

Which ions move through the membrane to produce this synaptic action? An important clue can be obtained by systematically changing the membrane potential and determining the *reversal potential* for the synaptic action, much as Alan Hodgkin and Andrew Huxley determined the reversal potential for the inward and outward current responsible for the action potential (Chapter 8). The reversal potential of the end-plate potential is the membrane potential at which the synaptic potential or synaptic current has zero amplitude. At the reversal potential there is no net current because an equal amount of current flows in both directions. Does the reversal potential of the synaptic potential at the end-plate coincide with the equilibrium potential for a specific ion species in the muscle

fiber, such as −100 mV for K⁺ or +55 mV for Na⁺? If so, either of these ion species might carry the end-plate current.

At the resting potential of the muscle (−90 mV) the synaptic current is inward (Figure 10–6). To determine the reversal potential, we need to examine the synaptic current at different values of membrane potential. The change in current flowing through transmitter-gated channels at different membrane potentials can be calculated from Ohm's law, as was done in Chapter 8 for the change in ionic currents through the voltage-gated channels responsible for the action potential. According to Ohm's law, the current responsible for the excitatory postsynap-

FIGURE 10–7

The end-plate potential is produced by simultaneous Na⁺ and K⁺ flow.

A. The ionic currents responsible for the end-plate potential can be determined by examining the reversal potential of the end-plate potential. The reversal potential is the potential at which inward and outward currents are in equilibrium. To measure the postsynaptic current flow across the membrane, the membrane is voltage clamped at different potentials and the nerve is stimulated. When the membrane potential is held at the equilibrium potential for the ion involved, no current results. If only Na⁺ were responsible for the end-plate current, its reversal potential would occur at +55 mV, the equilibrium potential for Na⁺ (E_{Na}).

B. The end-plate current actually reverses at 0 mV because the ion channel is permeable to both Na⁺ and K⁺, which thus are able to move into and out of the cell simultaneously.

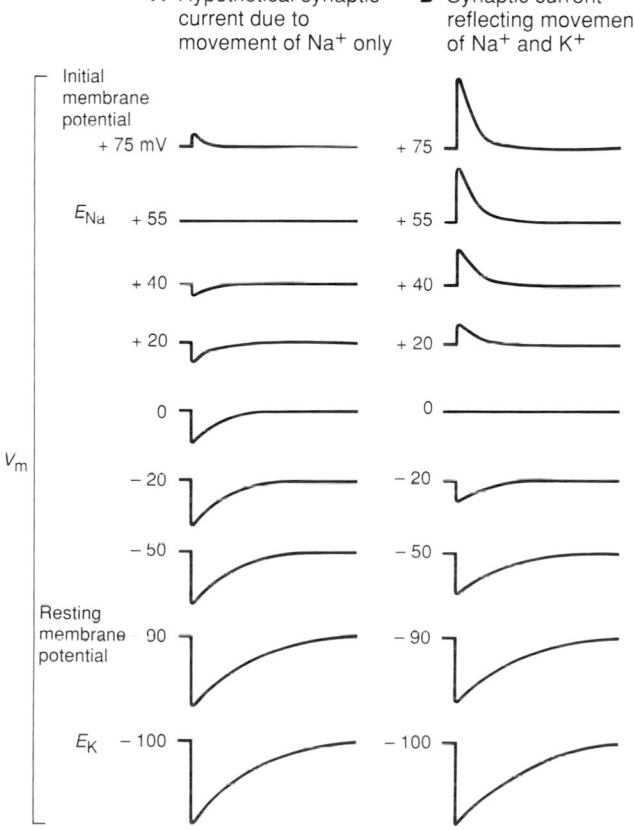

A Hypothetical synaptic current due to movement of Na⁺ only

B Synaptic current reflecting movement of Na⁺ and K⁺

Initial membrane potential

+75 mV

E_{Na} +55

+40

+20

0

V_m

−20

−50

Resting membrane potential −90

E_K −100

tic potential (I_{EPSP}) is given by

$$I_{EPSP} = g_{EPSP} \times (V_m - E_{EPSP}).$$

Here g_{EPSP} represents the conductance of the channels activated by ACh (the synaptic conductance), and the term $V_m - E_{EPSP}$ represents the electrochemical driving force for the ionic current flowing through the channel (where V_m is the membrane potential and E_{EPSP} is the reversal potential for the excitatory postsynaptic potential).

If an influx of Na$^+$ were solely responsible for the end-plate potential, E_{EPSP} would be the same as the equilibrium potential for Na$^+$, or +55 mV. Thus, by altering the membrane potential experimentally from −100 mV to +55 mV, the end-plate current should diminish progressively because the electrochemical driving force on Na$^+$ ($V_m - E_{EPSP}$) is reduced. At +55 mV the inward current flow should be abolished, and at values more positive than +55 mV the end-plate current should reverse in direction and become outward.

Instead, Fatt and Katz and the Takeuchis found something quite different and unexpected. As the membrane potential was reduced, the inward current rapidly became smaller and was abolished at 0 mV! At values more positive than 0 mV the end-plate current reversed direction

and became outward (Figure 10–7B). Since this particular value of membrane potential is not equal to the equilibrium potential for any of the major cations or anions, these experiments raised an intriguing question: Could some unidentified ion be responsible for the synaptic potential at the end-plate? Fatt and Katz, who first determined the reversal potential, soon appreciated that this potential must be produced not by a single ion species but by a combination of ions. In fact, as was found later by the Takeuchis, the synaptic channel at the end-plate is almost equally permeable to both major cations, Na$^+$ and K$^+$. Thus, during the synaptic potential Na$^+$ flows into the cell and K$^+$ flows out. The combined fluxes of these ions explains why the reversal potential is at 0 mV, which is a weighted average of E_{Na} and E_K (see Box 10–1 and Figure 10–14).

Transmitter-Gated Channels Are Fundamentally Different from Voltage-Gated Channels

The chemical mechanism that generates an excitatory synaptic potential thus appears to be similar to the voltage-gated mechanism that generates the action potential. In both mechanisms Na$^+$ and K$^+$ move down their concentration gradients through channels formed by mem-

---

Reversal Potential of the Excitatory Postsynaptic Potential　　　　　　　　　**BOX 10–1**

The reversal potential of a particular membrane current, such as the end-plate current through the ACh receptor-channel, is determined by two factors: the relative conductance for the permeant ions (g_{Na} and g_K), and the equilibrium potentials of the ions (here E_{Na} and E_K). At the reversal potential for the ACh receptor-channel, inward current carried by Na$^+$ is balanced by outward current carried by K$^+$. Thus

$$I_{Na} + I_K = 0. \tag{1}$$

The individual Na$^+$ and K$^+$ currents can be obtained from

$$I_{Na} = g_{Na} \times (V_m - E_{Na}) \tag{2a}$$

$$I_K = g_K \times (V_m - E_K). \tag{2b}$$

Remember that these currents are not due to Na$^+$ and K$^+$ flowing through separate channels (as occurs during the action potential), but represent Na$^+$ and K$^+$ movement through a single ACh receptor-channel. Since $V_m = E_{EPSP}$ at the reversal potential, substituting Equations 2a and 2b for I_{Na} and I_K in Equation 1 we can write:

$$g_{Na} \times (E_{EPSP} - E_{Na}) + g_K \times (E_{EPSP} - E_K) = 0. \tag{3}$$

Solving this equation for E_{EPSP} yields

$$E_{EPSP} = \frac{(g_{Na} \times E_{Na}) + (g_K \times E_K)}{g_{Na} + g_K}. \tag{4}$$

If we divide the top and bottom of the right side of this equation by g_K, we obtain

$$E_{EPSP} = \frac{\dfrac{g_{Na}}{g_K} \times E_{Na} + E_K}{\dfrac{g_{Na}}{g_K} + 1}. \tag{5}$$

Thus, if $g_{Na} = g_K$, then $E_{EPSP} = (E_{Na} + E_K)/2$.

These equations can also be used to obtain the ratio g_{Na}/g_K if one knows E_{EPSP}, E_K, and E_{Na}. Thus, rearranging Equation 3 yields

$$\frac{g_{Na}}{g_K} = \frac{(E_{EPSP} - E_K)}{(E_{Na} - E_{EPSP})}. \tag{6}$$

At the neuromuscular junction $E_{EPSP} = 0$ mV, $E_K = -100$ mV, and $E_{Na} = +55$ mV. Thus, from Equation 6, g_{Na}/g_K has a value around 1.8, indicating that the conductance of the ACh receptor-channel for Na$^+$ is slightly higher than for K$^+$. A similar approach can be used to analyze the reversal potential and the movement of ions during excitatory and inhibitory synaptic potentials in the central neurons (Chapter 11).

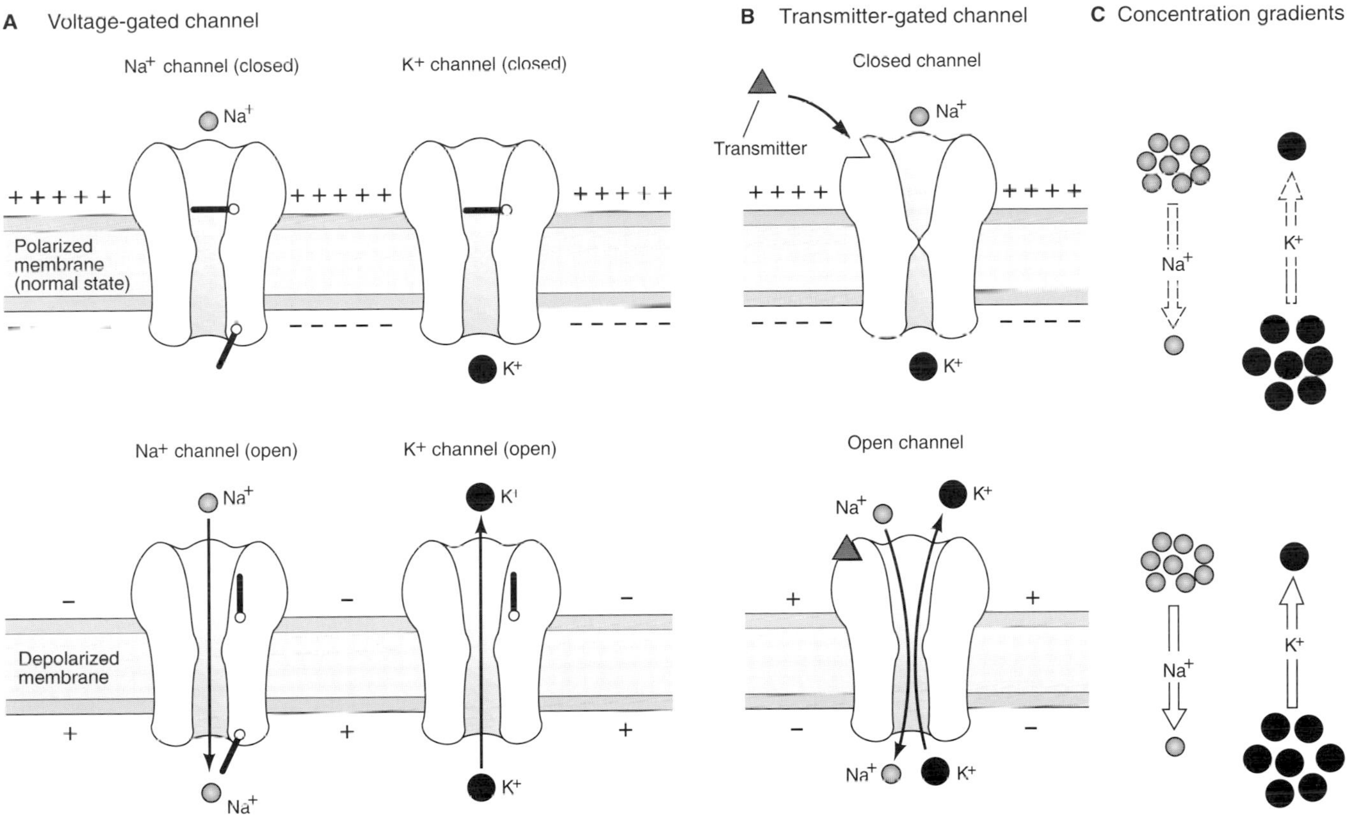

A Voltage-gated channel

Na$^+$ channel (closed)   K$^+$ channel (closed)

B Transmitter-gated channel

Closed channel

C Concentration gradients

Polarized membrane (normal state)

Na$^+$ channel (open)   K$^+$ channel (open)

Depolarized membrane

Open channel

FIGURE 10–8

Voltage-gated and transmitter-gated channels operate by different mechanisms. (Adapted from Alberts et al., 1989.)

A. Voltage-gated channels, which contribute to the action potential, are selective for different cations. There are separate channels for Na$^+$ and K$^+$.

B. Transmitter-gated channels, which contribute to the synaptic potential, are permeable to *both* Na$^+$ and K$^+$.

C. The concentration gradients for the ions are the same for both classes of channels.

brane-spanning proteins. The channels, however, differ in three important ways.

One difference is that Na$^+$ and K$^+$ move through two distinctly different classes of voltage-gated channels, one selective for Na$^+$ and another for K$^+$, which are activated sequentially. In contrast, there is only one type of transmitter-gated channel at the end-plate, the ACh-activated channel, and this channel is large enough to allow either Na$^+$ or K$^+$ to pass with nearly equal selectivity (Figure 10–8). Indeed, the channel is so large that it also allows divalent cations, such as Ca^{2+}, and even certain organic cations to pass. Anions are excluded, however, because the channels contain fixed negative charges.

Bertil Hille and his co-workers have suggested that the pore diameter of the ACh activated channel is substantially larger than that of the voltage-gated Na$^+$ or K$^+$ channels. At its narrowest point in cross section the ACh-activated channel pore is approximately 0.65 nm in diameter. This estimate was obtained from the dimensions of the largest organic cation that is able to permeate the channel. In contrast, the voltage-gated Na$^+$ channel is thought to be about 0.5 nm in its largest diameter, and the voltage-gated K$^+$ channel is only 0.3 nm in diameter (Figure 10–9).

FIGURE 10–9

A comparison of the dimensions of the narrowest points in voltage-gated K$^+$ and Na$^+$ channels, and in the ACh activated channel. The grid size is 0.1 nm (1 Å). Sizes were evaluated by testing channel permeability to several cations and measuring the dimensions of the ions from space-filling models. Note that the ACh-activated channel is quite large compared to the two voltage-gated channels. This explains why the voltage-gated channels are selective for one ion whereas the ACh-activated channel is permeable to both Na$^+$ and K$^+$. (From Hille, 1984.)

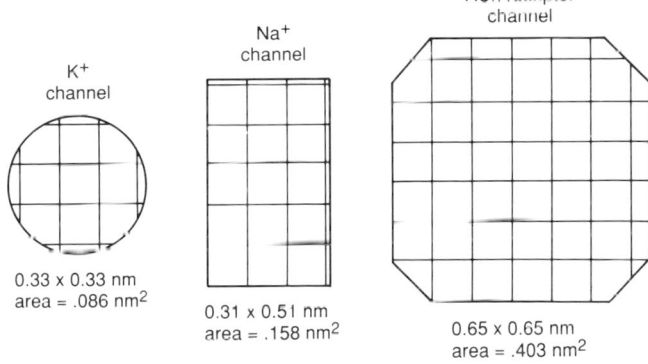

K$^+$ channel
0.33 x 0.33 nm
area = .086 nm^2

Na$^+$ channel
0.31 x 0.51 nm
area = .158 nm^2

ACh receptor channel
0.65 x 0.65 nm
area = .403 nm^2

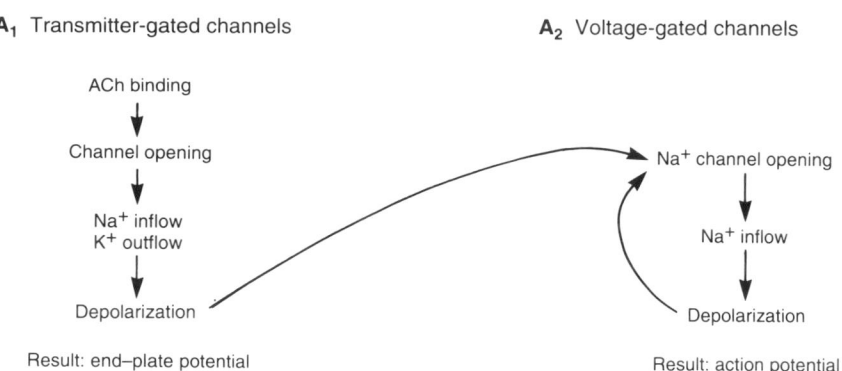

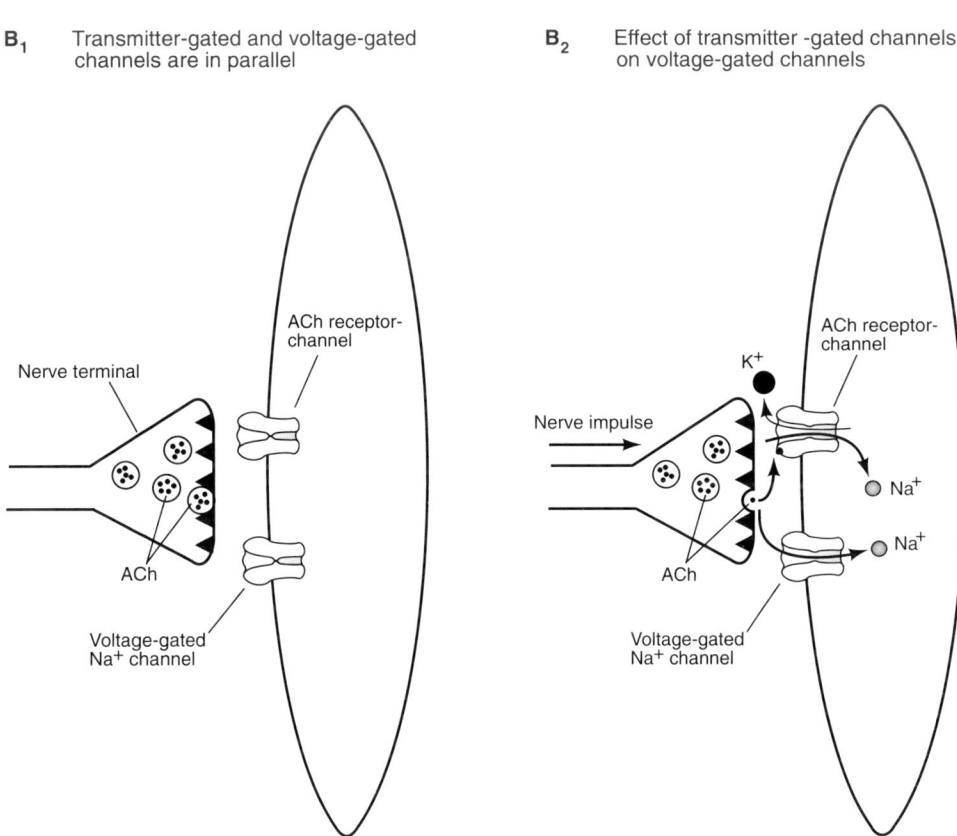

FIGURE 10–10

The binding of a chemical transmitter (ACh) at transmitter-gated channels opens channels permeable to both Na^+ and K^+. The flow of these ions into and out of the cell depolarizes the cell membrane, producing the end-plate potential. This depolarization opens neighboring voltage-gated Na^+ channels. To elicit an action potential, the depolarization produced by the end-plate potential must open sufficient Na^+ channels to reach the threshold for initiating the action potential. (Adapted from Alberts et al., 1989.)

A second difference between transmitter-gated and voltage-gated channels is that Na^+ flux through voltage-gated channels is regenerative. The increased depolarization of the cell caused by the Na^+ influx opens more voltage-gated Na^+ channels. This regenerative capacity underlies the all-or-none property of the action potential. In contrast, the number of ACh-activated channels opened during the synaptic potential is limited by the amount of ACh available. The depolarization produced by Na^+ influx through these channels does not lead to the opening of more transmitter-gated channels and, because it is limited, cannot produce an all-or-none action potential. To trigger an action potential, an end-plate potential must recruit neighboring voltage-gated channels (Figure 10–10).

Third, as might be expected from these two differences in physiological properties, there are also pharmacological differences between transmitter-gated and voltage-gated channels. Tetrodotoxin, which blocks the voltage-gated Na^+ channel, does not block the influx of Na^+ through the nicotinic ACh-activated channels. Similarly, α-bungarotoxin, a protein that binds to the nicotinic receptors and blocks the action of ACh, does not interfere with voltage-gated Na^+ or K^+ channels.

In Chapter 11 we shall learn about still another type of channel, the NMDA receptor, which is found in certain neurons of the brain. This channel is doubly gated, responding to *both* a chemical transmitter and voltage.

The Action of a Single Transmitter-Gated Channel Can Be Studied Experimentally

The current underlying an end-plate potential flows through several hundred thousand transmitter-gated

A

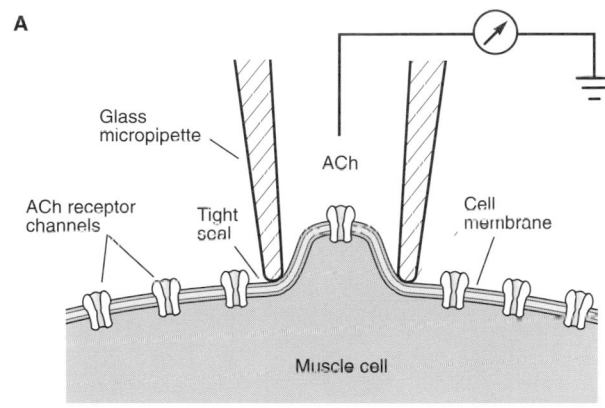

B_1

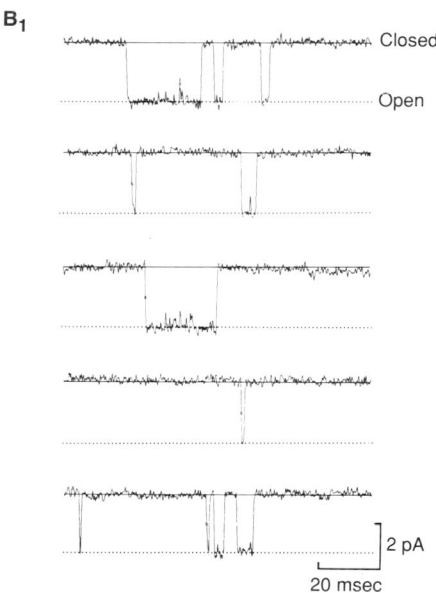

Closed

Open

2 pA

20 msec

FIGURE 10–11

Acetylcholine channels open in an all-or-none fashion and add current linearly.

A. To record single channels a small fire-polished glass microelectrode filled with salt solution and a low concentration of ACh is brought into close contact with the surface of the muscle membrane. Gentle suction is then applied to the distal end of the electrode so that the membrane forms a tight seal on the open tip of the pipette. (Adapted from Alberts et al., 1983.)

B. Single-channel currents in frog muscle fiber recorded in the presence of 100 nM ACh at a resting membrane potential of −90 mV. **1.** The opening of a channel results in a pulse of inward current, which is recorded as a downward deflection.
2. When plotted in a histogram, the distribution of the amplitudes of these rectangular pulses has a single peak. This distribution indicates that the patch of membrane contains only a single type of active channel and that the size of the elementary current through this channel varies randomly around a mean of 2.69 pA (1 pA = 10^{-12} A). This mean is called the *elementary current*. It is equivalent to an elementary conductance of about 30 pS, obtained by dividing the elementary current by the electrochemical driving force $(V_m - E_{EPSP})$ of −90 mV.

C. Single-channel currents in frog muscle fiber recorded in the presence of 100 nM ACh at a membrane potential of −130 mV. The individual channel currents give rise to all-or-none increments of −3.9 pA, equivalent to 30 pS. Simultaneous channel openings cause the individual current pulses to add linearly. In this record up to three channels are open at any instant. (Parts **B** and **C** courtesy of B. Sakmann.)

B_2

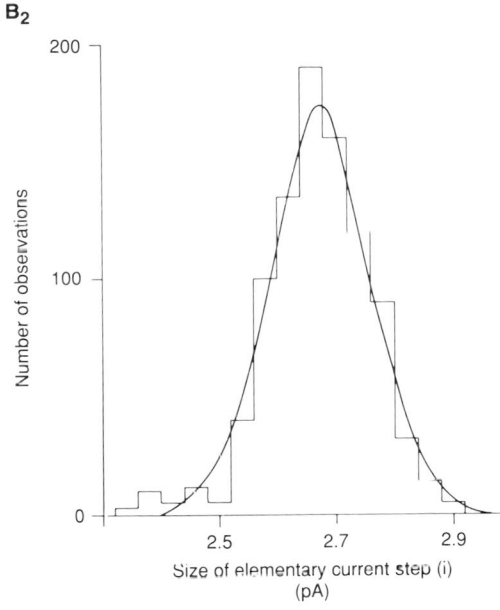

Number of observations

200

100

0

2.5   2.7   2.9

Size of elementary current step (i)
(pA)

C

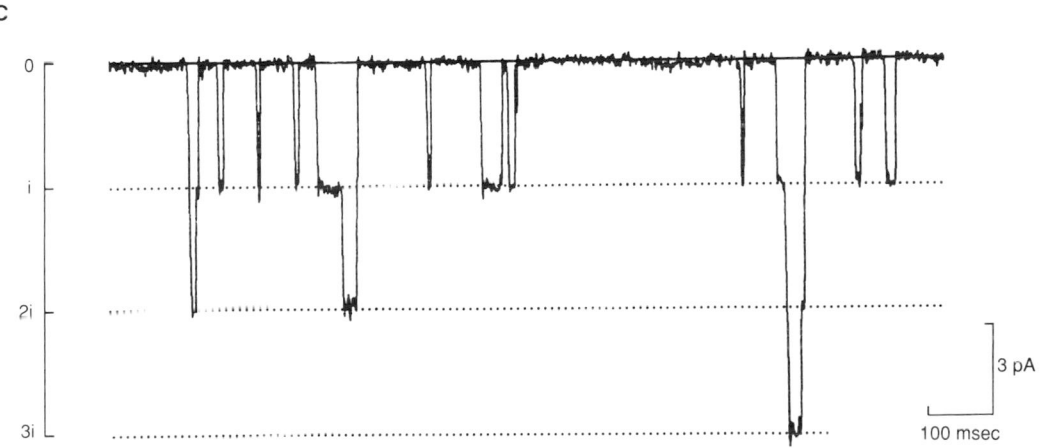

0

i

2i

3i

3 pA

100 msec

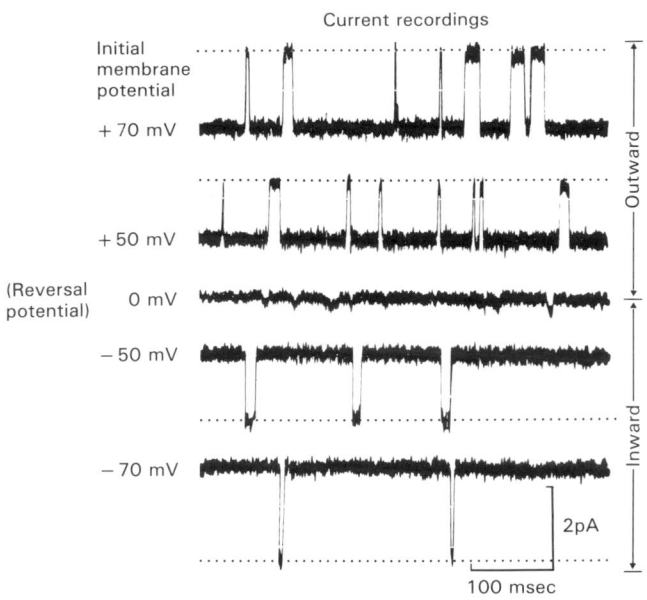

Current recordings

Initial membrane potential

+70 mV

+50 mV

(Reversal potential) 0 mV

−50 mV

−70 mV

Outward

Inward

2pA

100 msec

FIGURE 10–12

A single-channel current has the same reversal potential (0 mV) as does the total end-plate current. The voltage across the patch of membrane where this recording was made was systematically varied prior to exposure to 2 μM ACh. The current is inward below 0 mV and outward above 0 mV.

channels. This macroscopic current can be analyzed by reducing it to its fundamental unit, the elementary current through a *single* ACh-activated channel. This can be done using the patch-clamp technique developed by Erwin Neher and Bert Sakmann (Chapter 5, Box 5–1).

Individual Transmitter-Gated Channels Conduct a Unitary Current

Sakmann and Neher and their colleagues found that ACh opens individual channels in all-or-none steps. Thus, each time a channel opens it conducts a current of fixed amplitude. At a resting potential of −90 mV the single-channel current is around −2.7 pA, corresponding to a single-channel conductance of 30 pS (Figure 10–11B). Although the *amplitude* of the current for a single channel is relatively constant, the *duration* of the opening of the channel is governed by a stochastic (random) process and so varies from one opening to the next. The *mean open time* (measured from hundreds of individual openings) is a fixed property of the end-plate channels (under given experimental conditions) and is around 1 ms. During the opening of a single channel about 17,000 Na^+ ions flow into the cell and a somewhat smaller number of K^+ ions flows out.

Changing the membrane potential changes the magnitude of the current through the channels (Figure 10–12). This happens because a change in driving force ($V_m - E_{EPSP}$) has the same effect on single channels that it has on the total current at the end-plate. Recall that Ohm's law applied to synaptic current is

$$I_{EPSP} = g_{EPSP} \times (V_m - E_{EPSP}).$$

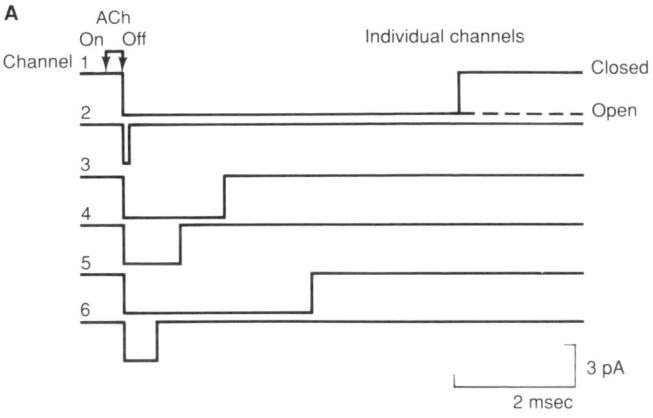

A

ACh
On Off

Channel 1

2

3

4

5

6

Individual channels

Closed

Open

3 pA

2 msec

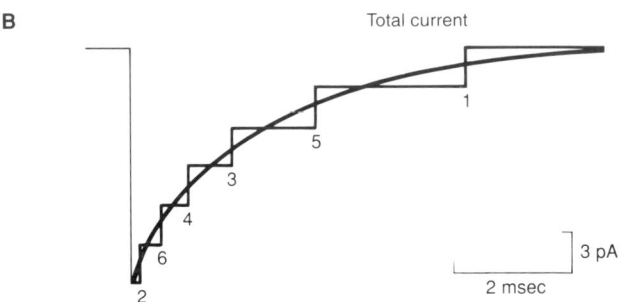

B

Total current

1

5

3

4

6

2

3 pA

2 msec

FIGURE 10–13

The total end-plate current is the summed average of the currents in thousands of individual ion channels.

A. Individual ACh-activated channels respond to a brief pulse of ACh. All channels open rapidly in response to ACh but remain open for varying times.

B. Summation of the current from the individual ion channels shown in **A** yields a net current with a smoother continuous decay. This idealized record is equivalent to the time course of the ACh-activated current in a whole muscle fiber (with thousands of channels). The stepped trace reflects the closing of each channel (the number indicates which channel has closed); in the final period of net current flow only channel **1** is open. (Adapted from D. Colquhoun, 1981.)

The equivalent expression for current flow through a single channel is

$$i_{EPSP} = \gamma \times (V_m - E_{EPSP})$$

where i_{EPSP} is the amplitude of current flow through a single open channel and γ is the conductance of the channel.

Current Flow Depends on the Number of Open Channels, Concentration of the Transmitter, Channel Conductance, and Membrane Potential

The total synaptic conductance, g_{EPSP}, of a large population of ACh channels results from the summed conductance of all open channels. It is given by $g_{EPSP} = n \times \gamma$, where n is the average number of channels opened by the ACh released from a presynaptic terminal. For an end-plate that contains a large number of ACh channels, the average number of open channels is $n = N \times p_o$, where p_o is the

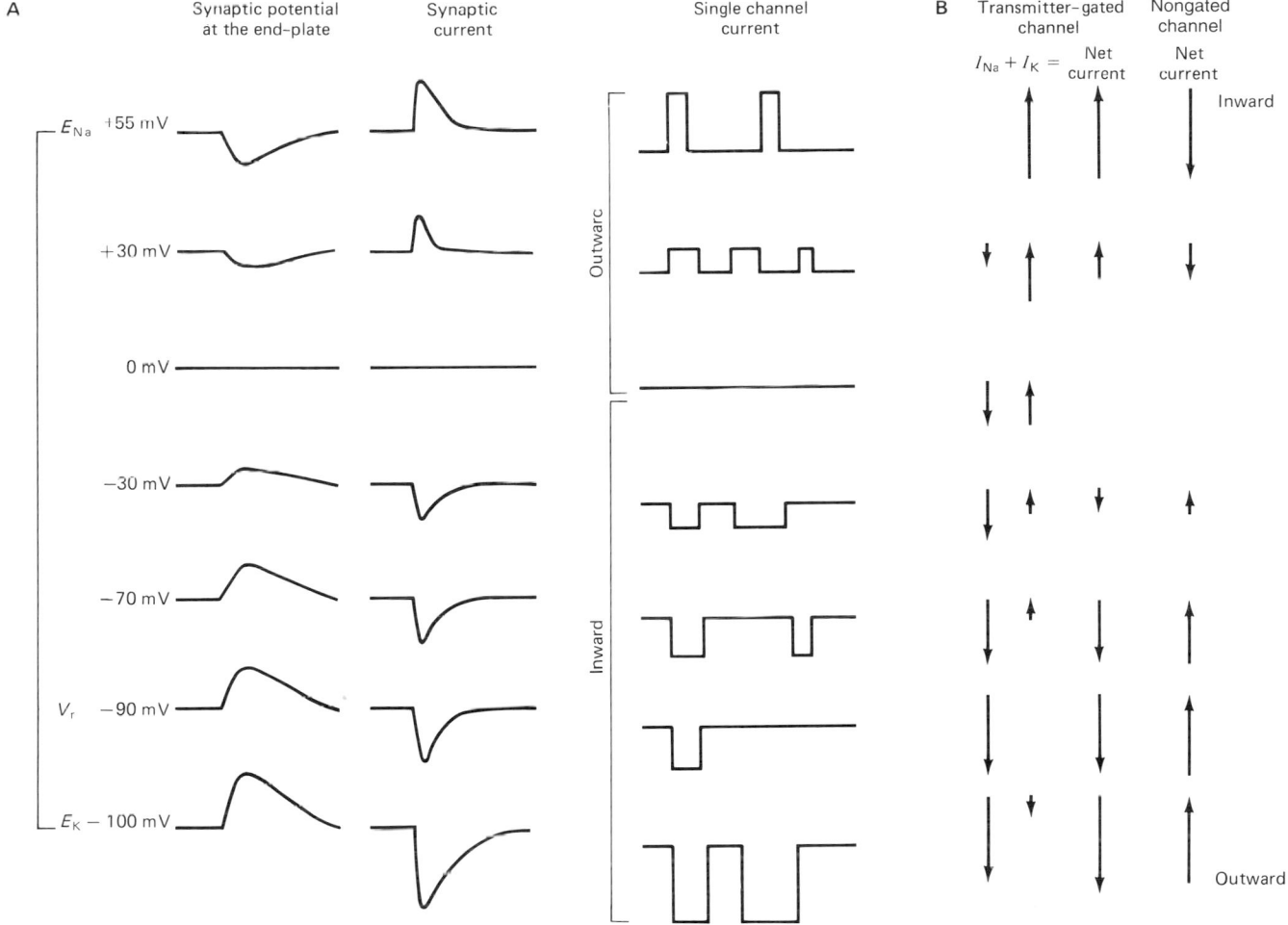

FIGURE 10–14

The ACh-activated end-plate potential, total synaptic current, and single channel current are all affected in a similar way by the membrane potential.

A. At the normal muscle resting potential of −90 mV the single-channel currents and total synaptic current (made up of currents from more than 200,000 single channels) are large and inward because of the large inward driving force on current flow through the ACh-gated channels. This large inward current produces a large depolarizing end-plate potential. At more positive levels of membrane potential (increased depolarization) the inward driving force on Na$^+$ is less and the outward driving force on K$^+$ is greater. This results in a decrease in the size of the single-channel currents and the magnitude of the synaptic currents, thus reducing the size of the end-plate potential. At the reversal potential (0 mV), the inward Na$^+$ flux is balanced by the outward K$^+$ flux, so there is no inward synaptic current flow and no change in V_m. Further depolarization to +30 mV inverts the direction of the synaptic current, as there is now a large outward driving force on K$^+$ and a small inward driving force on Na$^+$. On either side of the reversal potential the synaptic current drives the membrane potential toward the reversal potential.

B. The direction of Na$^+$ and K$^+$ fluxes in individual channels is altered by changing V_m. The algebraic sum of the Na$^+$ and K$^+$ fluxes gives the *net current* that flows through the transmitter-gated channels. This net synaptic current is equal in size and opposite in direction to that of the net extrasynaptic current flowing in the return pathway of the nongated channels and membrane capacitance (see Appendix A). (The relative magnitude of a current is represented by the length of the arrow.)

probability that any given ACh channel is open and N is the total number of ACh channels in the end-plate membrane. The total end-plate current is therefore given by:

$$I_{EPSP} = n \times \gamma \times (V_m - E_{EPSP})$$

or

$$I_{EPSP} = N \times p_o \times \gamma \times (V_m - E_{EPSP})$$

This equation shows that the current for the end-plate potential depends on four factors: (1) the total number of end-plate channels (N); (2) the probability that a channel is open (p_o); (3) the conductance (γ) of each open channel; and (4) the driving force ($V_m - E_{EPSP}$) that acts on the ions. The probability that a channel is open depends largely on the concentration of the transmitter at the receptor, not on the value of the membrane potential, because the channels are opened by the binding of ACh, not by voltage.

The normal end-plate current is the sum of the opening of more than 200,000 channels. This number is estimated by comparing the synaptic potential of 70 mV to the de-

A

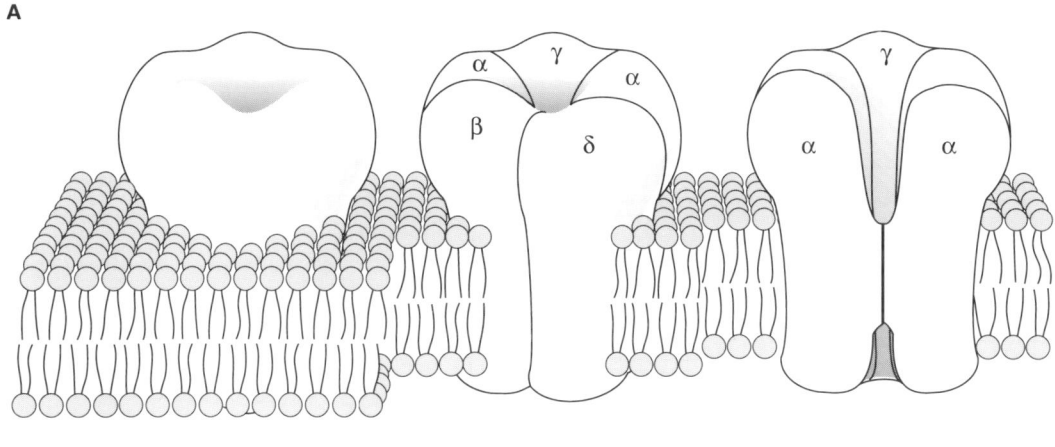

B₁ No ACh bound:
Channel closed

B₂ 2 ACh molecules bound:
Channel open

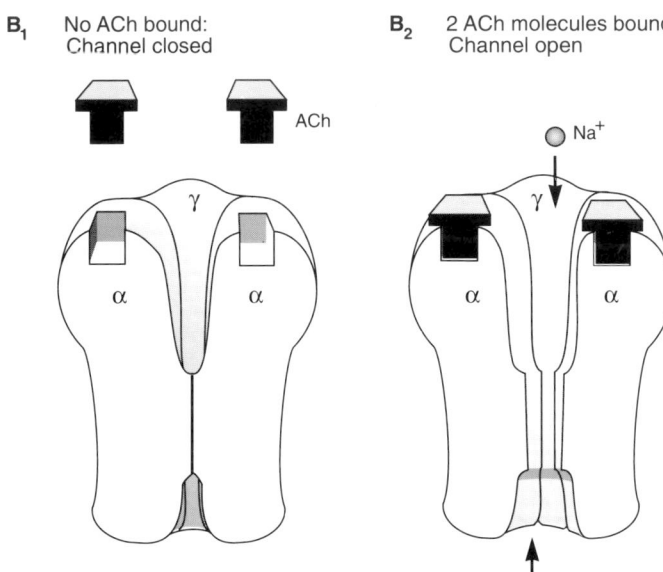

FIGURE 10–15

The molecular structure of the ACh-activated receptor-channel.

A. Three-dimensional model of the nicotinic ACh-activated ion channel based on the model of Karlin and co-workers. The receptor-channel complex consists of several subunits. One ACh molecule binds to each α-subunit prior to channel opening. All subunits contribute to the pore.

B. When two molecules of ACh bind to the portions of the α-subunits exposed to the membrane surface, the receptor-channel changes conformation, opening a pore in the portions of the receptor embedded in the lipid bilayer. Both K^+ and Na^+ flow through the open channel down their individual electrochemical gradients.

polarization of only 0.3 μV caused by the opening of a single channel. The rapid rising phase of the end-plate current is due to the nearly synchronous opening of these channels in response to the rapid rise in ACh concentration in the synaptic cleft. The ACh concentration then rapidly falls (in less than 1 ms) due to hydrolysis of ACh and diffusion. Following the fall in ACh concentration, the ACh-gated channels begin to close; each closure produces a unitary decrease in the inward synaptic current. The apparently smooth decay of the total synaptic current and the synaptic potential results from the closing of many thousands of channels at random intervals, each contributing only a small step of current (Figure 10–13).

The relationship between single-channel current, total end-plate current, and end-plate potential is shown in Figure 10–14 for a wide range of membrane potentials.

The Nicotinic Acetylcholine Receptor Is an Intrinsic Membrane Protein with Five Subunits

As we saw in Chapter 9, a directly gated receptor-channel has two functions: (1) it recognizes and binds the chemical

transmitter, and (2) it opens a channel in the membrane through which ions flow. Where in the receptor molecule is the binding site located? Where does the channel lie? What are its properties? Insights into these questions have been obtained from molecular studies of the ACh-activated receptor-channel proteins and their genes.

Biochemical studies by Arthur Karlin, Jean-Pierre Changeux, and Michael Raftery and their colleagues indicated that the nicotinic ACh receptor is a membrane glycoprotein with a molecular weight of about 275,000. The receptor is formed from five subunits, with the stoichiometry $\alpha_2\beta\gamma\delta$ (Figure 10–15). The four polypeptide chains have apparent molecular weights of 40,000 (α), 48,000 (β), 58,000 (γ), and 64,000 (δ). Only the α-subunit binds ACh with high affinity. Indeed, one molecule of ACh must bind to each of the two α-subunits for the channel to open efficiently (Figure 10–15B). The cDNAs coding for each of the subunits of the receptor have been cloned. Both site-directed mutagenesis and chemical labeling experiments have identified the binding site for ACh near two cysteine residues localized on a hydrophilic region of the α-subunit exposed to the extracellular space. The inhibitory snake

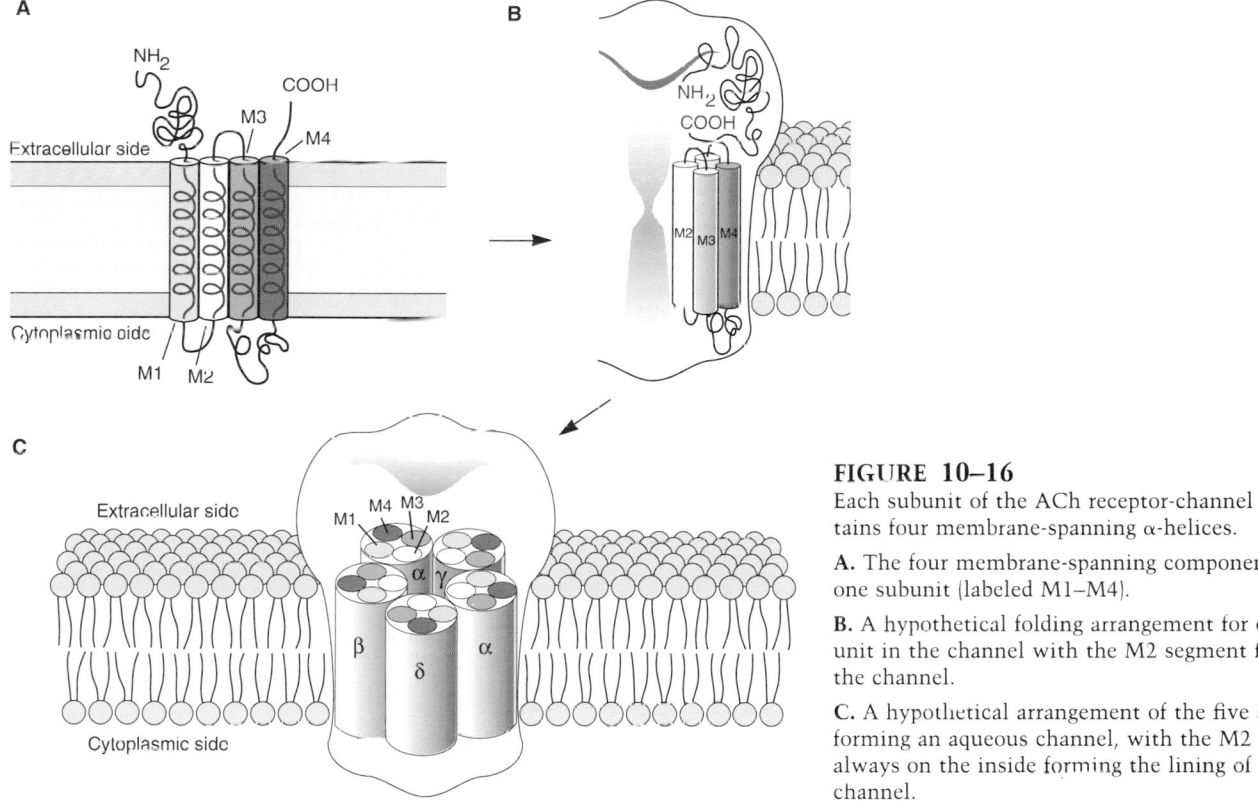

FIGURE 10-16

Each subunit of the ACh receptor-channel contains four membrane-spanning α-helices.

A. The four membrane-spanning components of one subunit (labeled M1–M4).

B. A hypothetical folding arrangement for one subunit in the channel with the M2 segment facing the channel.

C. A hypothetical arrangement of the five subunits forming an aqueous channel, with the M2 segment always on the inside forming the lining of the channel.

venom α-bungarotoxin, which is recognized by and binds specifically to the receptor, binds to the α-subunit.

Insight into the nature of the channel has come from analysis of the nucleotide sequences encoding the four types of receptor subunits as well as biophysical studies of the receptor-channel. Shosaku Numa and his colleagues found that the four subunit types are encoded by distinct but related genes. Sequence comparison of the subunits shows a high degree of similarity among them—50% of the amino acid residues are identical or conservatively substituted. This similarity suggests that the functions of all subunits are similar. Like the voltage-gated channels discussed in Chapter 8, all four of the modern genes for the subunits are thought to be derived from a single ancestral gene.

Important clues as to how the subunits are threaded through the membrane bilayer were obtained by examining the distribution of the polar and nonpolar amino acids. Each of the four subunit types contains four hydrophobic regions of about 20 amino acids. Numa and his colleagues proposed that each of the four hydrophobic regions forms an α-helix traversing the membrane. The four candidate membrane-spanning regions are called M1, M2, M3, and M4 (Figure 10–16). Their amino acid sequences suggest that the subunits are symmetrically arranged in such a way that they create a central membrane-spanning channel (Figure 10–16).

Further analyses by Numa and Sakmann and their colleagues indicate that the lining of the channel pore is formed by the M2 region and the segment connecting M2

to M3. Moreover, the channel's cation selectivity is thought to derive from three rings of negative charge that flank the M2 region (Figure 10–17). Each ring is made up of three or four negative charges contributed by negatively charged amino acids (primarily glutamate) of the different subunits. One ring, near the internal mouth, is formed by amino acids in the cytoplasmic region connecting the M1 and M2 segments; a central ring is formed by amino acids within the M2 transmembrane segment itself; a third ring, beyond the external side of the membrane, is formed by amino acids in the extracellular region connecting the M2 and M3 segments (Figure 10–17A). Evidence from site-directed mutagenesis experiments suggests that replacing the critical glutamate residues with a neutral amino acid decreases the single-channel conductance.

A similar conclusion about the role of the M2 segment in forming the lining of the pore has been reached independently by Changeux and his colleagues. They used a blocker that penetrates the open channel about two-thirds of the way and then plugs it by binding to a ring of serine resides on the M2 region within the channel pore.

A three-dimensional image of the receptor has now been obtained at a resolution of 1.7 nm by Chikashi Toyoshima and Nigel Unwin. Their reconstructed electron microscopic images confirm that the channel has a long vertical wall made up of the encircling receptor subunits (Figures 10–2B and 10–17A). A surprisingly large component of this channel, about 6.0 nm in length, extends into the extracellular space. At its external surface the channel has a wide mouth about 2.5 nm in diameter.

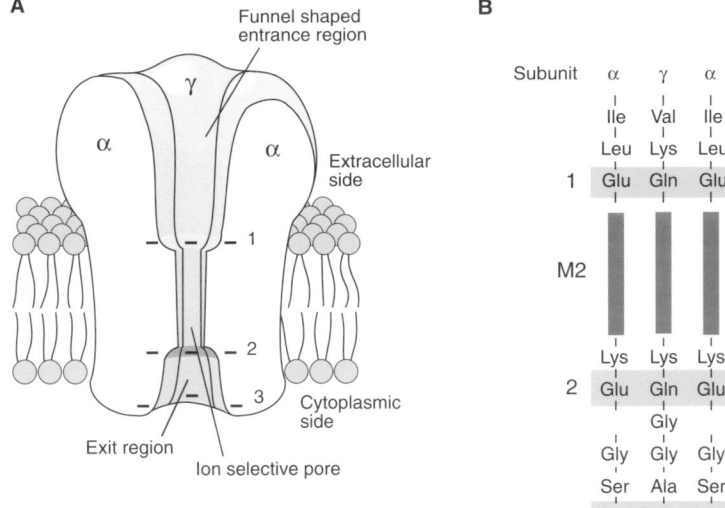

FIGURE 10–17

A model of the ACh receptor-channel.

A. Model of the ACh receptor-channel based on experiments by Numa, Unwin and their colleagues. According to this model negatively charged amino acids on each subunit form three rings of charge around the pore. As a permeant ion traverses the channel it encounters this series of three such negatively charged rings. The external (**1**) and internal (**3**) rings may serve as prefilters and divalent blocking sites; the central site (**2**) in the part of the channel embedded in the bilayer may function as a selectivity filter for cations. This model is based on the *Torpedo* ACh receptor-channel reconstructed electron microscope image we saw in Figure 10–2B (dimensions are not to scale).

B. Aligned sequences of the M2 regions and the flanking sequences of each of the five subunits. The shaded areas **1**, **2**, and **3** identify the three rings of negative charge (aspartate or glutamate residues) that flank the M2 region and may account for the selectivity of the channel for cations.

But within the bilayer of the membrane the channel abruptly narrows so markedly that it cannot be resolved. It is presumably here, where the M2 segments are thought to line the pore, that the selectivity filter lies (Figure 10–17A). This narrow region is quite short, only 2.5–3.0 nm in length, corresponding to the lengths of both the M2 segment and the hydrophobic core of the bilayer (Figure 10–17B). As the channel emerges from the inner surface of the membrane, it suddenly widens again. Thus, the receptor-channel complex is divided into three regions: a large entrance region at the external membrane surface, a narrow transmembrane pore that may determine cation selectivity, and a large exit region at the internal membrane surface.

An Overall View

In response to an action potential in the presynaptic motor neuron, ACh is released from the terminals of the motor neuron. It then diffuses across the synaptic cleft and activates nicotinic ACh receptor-channels. Binding of ACh to the receptor leads to the opening of a channel that is an integral part of the receptor protein. This channel is permeable to cations (Na^+, K^+, and Ca^{2+}) and its opening leads to a net influx of Na^+ ions, producing a depolarizing synaptic potential called the end-plate potential. Acetyl-choline-activated channels also allow the passage of much larger molecules than do the voltage-dependent Na^+ and K^+ channels.

Because the number of ACh-activated channels opened is limited by a fixed amount of ACh released onto the postsynaptic cell, these channels by themselves cannot produce a regenerative action potential. Instead, by depolarizing the postsynaptic cell they activate voltage-dependent Na^+ channels outside the end-plate. Because the Na^+ channels are voltage regulated, more of them open as depolarization of the postsynaptic cell increases, and in this way the Na^+ channels are able to generate the amount of current needed to produce an action potential.

Voltage- and transmitter-gated channels also differ in their sensitivity to various drugs and toxins. The nicotinic ACh-activated channel has been purified and its genes have been cloned and sequenced. The receptor is an integral membrane protein composed of five subunits (four homologous types). Each subunit has four hydrophobic regions that are thought to form membrane-spanning α-helices, called M1–M4. The M2 membrane-spanning segments of each of the five subunits are thought to form the walls of the channel. Negatively charged amino acids in these membrane-spanning regions, in particular the M2 region, appear to be responsible for the selectivity of the channel for cations.

Receptors have two functions: (1) the recognition and binding of neurotransmitter from the presynaptic cell, and (2) the gating of the ion channel. The two functions of the ACh-activated receptor have been localized in their molecular structure. The steps that link the binding of a transmitter (ACh) to the opening of the ion channel are under investigation. Thus, we should be able soon to answer the question: How does the detailed molecular structure of the ACh receptor account for its various physiological functions?

Acetylcholine is one of many neurotransmitters used by the nervous system, and the end-plate potential is one of many examples of postsynaptic transmitter actions. Do other neurotransmitters produce actions similar to those of ACh at the nerve-muscle synapse? Do the same principles also apply to transmitter actions in the central nervous system, or are other mechanisms involved? In the past these questions were difficult to answer because of the small size and great complexity of nerve cells in the central nervous system. Recent advances in experimental technique (patch clamping) have made a new range of neurotransmitter actions available for study. It is already clear that although many neurotransmitters operate in a way similar to that of ACh at the end-plate, other types of transmitters do not. In the next two chapters we shall explore some of this rich variety in synaptic transmission in the central and peripheral nervous systems.

Postscript: The End-Plate Current Can Be Calculated from an Equivalent Circuit

As we have seen in this chapter the flow of current through a population of end-plate channels can be described simply by Ohm's law. However, to understand fully how the flow of electrical current during the synaptic potential generates the end-plate potential, we need to consider not only the ACh-activated end-plate channels but also all the nongated channels in the surrounding membrane that can serve as the return pathway for current flow. Since channels are proteins that span the bilayer of the membrane, we must also take into consideration the capacitive properties of the membrane and the ionic batteries determined by the distribution of Na^+ and K^+ inside and outside the cell.

A circuit model will allow us to explain the flow of current at the end-plate region of the muscle fiber by using rules governing the flow of current in passive electrical devices that consist only of resistors, capacitors, and batteries (see Chapter 7). We can represent the end-plate region with an equivalent circuit that has three parallel branches: (1) a branch representing the flow of synaptic current through the transmitter-gated channels; (2) a branch representing the return current flow through nongated channels (the nonsynaptic membrane); and (3) a third branch representing current flow across the lipid bilayer, which acts as a capacitor (Figure 10–18).

Since the end-plate current is carried by both Na^+ and K^+, we could represent the synaptic branch of the equivalent circuit as two parallel branches, each representing

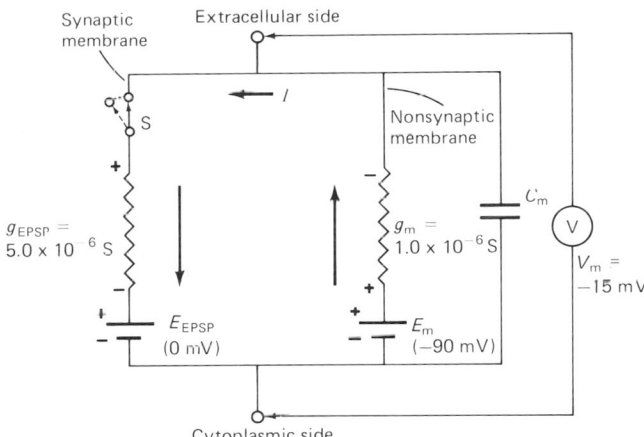

FIGURE 10–18

The equivalent circuit of the end-plate potential with two parallel current pathways. One consists of a battery representing the synapse, E_{EPSP}, in series with a conductance through ACh-gated channels, g_{EPSP}. The other pathway consists of the battery representing the resting potential (E_m) in series with the conductance of the nongated channels (g_m). In parallel with both of these conductance pathways is the membrane capacitance (C_m). When no ACh is present the gated channel is closed and no current flows through it. This is depicted as an open electrical circuit in which the synaptic conductance is not connected to the rest of the circuit. The binding of ACh opens the synaptic channel. This event is electrically equivalent to throwing the switch (S) that connects the gated conductance pathway (g_{EPSP}) with the nongated pathway (g_m). As a result, in the steady state, current flows inward through the gated channels and outward through the nongated channels. The voltmeter (V) measures the potential difference between the inside and the outside of the cell. With the indicated values of conductances and batteries, the membrane will depolarize from −90 mV (its resting potential value) to −15 mV (the peak of the synaptic potential).

the flow of a different ion species. This is the approach we used in the equivalent circuit for the axonal membrane (Chapter 7). At the end-plate, however, Na^+ and K^+ flow through the same ion channel. It is therefore more convenient (and correct) to combine the Na^+ and K^+ current pathways into a single conductance, representing the channel gated by ACh. The conductance of this pathway depends on the number of channels opened, which in turn depends on the concentration of transmitter. In the absence of transmitter, no channels are open and the conductance is zero. When a presynaptic action potential causes the release of transmitter, the conductance of this pathway rises to a value of around 5×10^{-6} S (or a resistance of $2 \times 10^5\ \Omega$). This is about five times the conductance of the parallel branch representing the nongated channels (g_m).

The end-plate conductance is in series with a battery (E_{EPSP}), whose value is given by the reversal potential for synaptic current flow (0 mV) (Figure 10–18). As discussed earlier in this chapter, this value is the weighted algebraic sum of the Na^+ and K^+ equilibrium potentials.

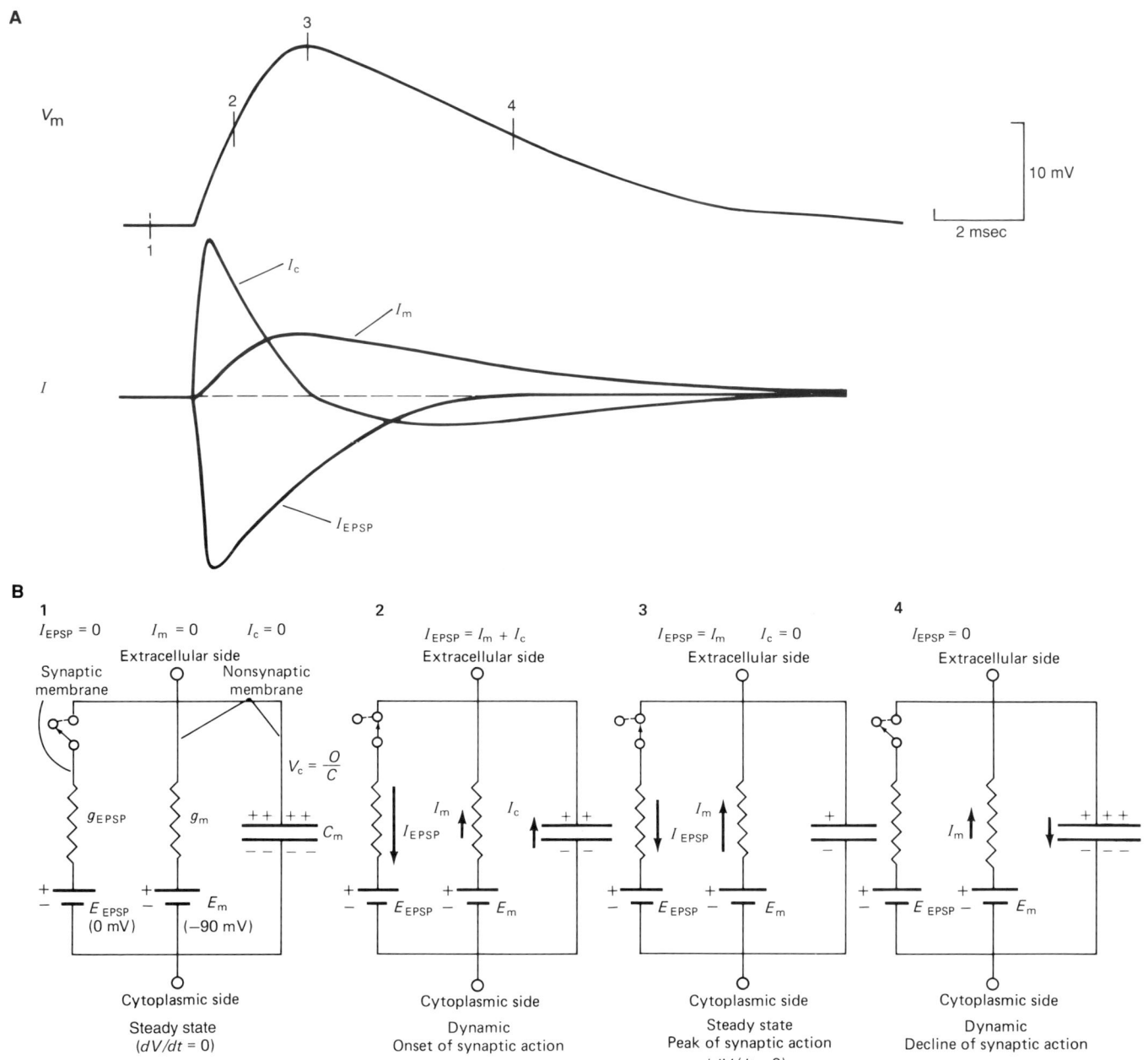

FIGURE 10–19

Both the active synaptic conductance and passive membrane properties determine the time course of the end-plate potential. Capacitive current flows only when the membrane potential is changing. In the steady state, such as at the peak of the synaptic potential, the inward flow of ionic current through the gated channels (g_{EPSP}) is exactly balanced by the outward flow of ionic current across the nongated channels (g_m) and there is no flow of capacitive current.

A. Comparison of the time course of the end-plate potential (top trace) with the time courses of the components of the current: through the ACh-gated channels (I_{EPSP}), the nongated channels (I_m), and the capacitor (I_c).

B. Equivalent circuits for the current at times **1, 2, 3,** and **4** during the synaptic potential shown in **A.** (The relative magnitude of a current is represented by the length of the arrow.)

The current flowing during the excitatory postsynaptic potential (I_{EPSP}) is given by

$$I_{EPSP} = g_{EPSP} \times (V_m - E_{EPSP}).$$

Using this equation and the equivalent circuit of Figure 10–18, we can now analyze the end-plate potential in terms of the flow of ionic current. At the onset of the excitatory synaptic action (the dynamic phase) an inward current flows through the ACh-activated channels because of the increased conductance to Na^+ and K^+ and the large inward driving force at the initial resting potential (−90 mV). Since current flows in a closed loop, the inward synaptic current (I_{EPSP}) must leave the cell as outward current. From the equivalent circuit we see that there are two parallel pathways for outward current flow: a conductance pathway (I_m) representing current flow through the nongated channels and a capacitive pathway (I_c) representing current flow across the membrane capacitance. Thus,

$$I_{EPSP} = -(I_m + I_c).$$

During the earliest phase of the end-plate potential the membrane potential, V_m, is still close to its resting value, E_m. As a result, the outward driving force on current flow through the nongated channels ($V_m - E_m$) is small. Therefore, most of the current leaves the cell as capacitative current, and the membrane depolarizes rapidly (Figure 10–19). As the cell depolarizes, the outward driving force on current flow through the nongated channels increases while the inward driving force on synaptic current flow through the ACh-activated channels decreases. Concomitantly, as the concentration of ACh in the synapse falls, the ACh-activated channels begin to close, and eventually the flow of inward current through the gated channels is exactly balanced by outward current flow through the nongated channels, $I_{EPSP} = -I_m$. At this point there is no current flow into or out of the capacitor (i.e., $I_c = 0$), and since the rate of change of membrane potential is directly proportional to I_c (i.e., $I_c = dV/dt$), the membrane potential will have reached a peak steady-state value ($dV/dt = 0$). As the gated channels close, I_{EPSP} decreases further. Now I_{EPSP} and I_m are no longer in balance and the membrane potential starts to repolarize because the outward current flow due to I_m becomes larger than the inward synaptic current (Figure 10–19). During most of the declining phase of the synaptic action, current no longer flows through the ACh-activated channels, since they are all shut, but instead flows only out through g_m and in across C_m.

A convenient feature of the synaptic potential at its peak or steady-state value is that $I_c = 0$ and therefore the value of the membrane potential (V_m) can be easily calculated. The inward current flow through the gated channels (I_{EPSP}) must be exactly balanced by outward current flow through the nongated channels (I_m):

$$I_{EPSP} + I_m = 0. \tag{10-1}$$

The current flowing through the active ACh-gated channels (I_{EPSP}) and through the nongated membrane channels (I_m) is given by Ohm's law:

$$I_{EPSP} = g_{EPSP} \times (V_m - E_{EPSP}),$$

and

$$I_m = g_m \times (V_m - E_m).$$

By substituting these two expressions into Equation 10–1 we obtain

$$g_{EPSP} \times (V_m - E_{EPSP}) + g_m \times (V_m - E_m) = 0.$$

To solve for V_m we need only expand the two products in the equation and rearrange them so that all terms in voltage (V_m) appear on the left side:

$$(g_{EPSP} \times V_m) + (g_m \times V_m) = (g_{EPSP} \times E_{EPSP}) + (g_m \times E_m).$$

By factoring out V_m on the left side, we finally obtain

$$V_m = \frac{g_{EPSP} \times E_{EPSP} + g_m \times E_m}{g_{EPSP} + g_m}. \tag{10-2}$$

This equation is similar to that used to calculate the resting and action potentials (Chapter 6). According to Equation 10–2, the peak voltage of the end-plate potential is a weighted average of the electromotive forces of the two batteries for gated and nongated currents. The weighting factors are given by the relative magnitude of the two conductances. If the gated conductance is much smaller than the resting membrane conductance ($g_{EPSP} \ll g_m$), $g_{EPSP} \times E_{EPSP}$ will be negligible compared with $g_m \times E_m$. Under these conditions V_m will remain close to E_m. This situation occurs when only a very few channels are opened by ACh (because its concentration is low). On the other hand, if g_{EPSP} is much larger than g_m, Equation 10–2 states that V_m approaches E_{EPSP}, the synaptic reversal potential. This situation occurs when the concentration of ACh is high and a large number of channels are opened. At intermediate ACh concentrations, with a moderate number of synaptic channels open, the peak synaptic potential lies somewhere between E_m and E_{EPSP}.

We can now use Equation 10–2 to calculate the peak end-plate potential for the specific case shown in Figure 10–18, where $g_{EPSP} = 5 \times 10^{-6}$ S; $g_m = 1 \times 10^{-6}$ S; $E_{EPSP} = 0$ mV; and $E_m = -90$ mV. Substituting these values into Equation 10–2 yields

$$V_m = \frac{(5 \times 10^{-6} \text{ S}) \times (0 \text{ mV}) + (1 \times 10^{-6} \text{ S}) \times (-90 \text{ mV})}{(5 \times 10^{-6} \text{ S}) + (1 \times 10^{-6} \text{ S})}$$

or

$$V_m = \frac{(1 \times 10^{-6} \text{ S}) \times (-90 \text{ mV})}{(6 \times 10^{-6} \text{ S})}$$

$$= -15 \text{ mV}.$$

The peak amplitude of the end-plate potential is then

$$\Delta V_{EPSP} = V_m - E_m$$

$$= -15 \text{ mV} - (-90 \text{ mV})$$

$$= 75 \text{ mV}.$$

As a check for consistency we can see whether, at the peak of the end-plate potential, the synaptic current is equal and opposite to the nonsynaptic current so that the net membrane current is zero. Thus

$$I_{EPSP} = (5 \times 10^{-6} \text{ S}) \times (-15 \text{ mV} - 0 \text{ mV})$$

$$= -75 \times 10^{-9} \text{ A}$$

and

$$I_m = (1 \times 10^{-6} \text{ S}) \times [-15 \text{ mV} - (-90 \text{ mV})],$$

$$= 75 \times 10^{-9} \text{ A}.$$

Here we see that solving Equation 10–2 ensures that $I_{EPSP} + I_m = 0$.

Selected Readings

Fatt, P., and Katz, B. 1951. An analysis of the end-plate potential recorded with an intra-cellular electrode. J. Physiol. (Lond.) 115:320–370.

Heuser, J. E., and Reese, T. S. 1977. Structure of the synapse. In E. R. Kandel (ed.), Handbook of Physiology, Section 1: The Nervous System, Vol. I. Cellular Biology of Neurons, Part 1. Bethesda, Md.: American Physiological Society, pp. 261–294.

Hulme, E. C. (ed.) 1990. Receptor Biochemistry: A Practical Approach. Oxford: IRL Press.

Imoto, K., Busch, C., Sakmann, B., Mishina, M., Konno, T., Nakai, J., Bujo, H., Mori, Y., Fukuda, K., and Numa, S. 1988. Rings of negatively charged amino acids determine the acetylcholine receptor channel conductance. Nature 335:645–648.

Katz, B., and Miledi, R. 1970. Membrane noise produced by acetylcholine. Nature 226:962–963.

Miller, C. 1989. Genetic manipulation of ion channels: A new approach to structure and mechanism. Neuron 2:1195–1205.

Neher, E., and Sakmann, B. 1976. Single-channel currents recorded from membrane of denervated frog muscle fibres. Nature 260:799–802.

Sakmann, B., and Neher, E. (eds.) 1983. Single-Channel Recording. New York: Plenum Press.

Unwin, N. 1989. The structure of ion channels in membranes of excitable cells. Neuron 3:665–676.

References

Alberts, B., Bray, D., Lewis, J., Raff, M., Roberts, K., and Watson, J. D. 1989. Molecular Biology of the Cell, 2nd ed. New York: Garland.

Changeux, J.-P. 1981. The acetylcholine receptor: An "allosteric" membrane protein. Harvey Lect. 75:85–254.

Claudio, T., Ballivet, M., Patrick, J., and Heinemann, S. 1983. Nucleotide and deduced amino acid sequences of Torpedo californica acetylcholine receptor γ subunit. Proc. Natl. Acad. Sci. U.S.A. 80:1111–1115.

Colquhoun, D. 1981. How fast do drugs work? Trends Pharmacol. Sci. 2:212–217.

Dwyer, T. M., Adams, D. J., and Hille, B. 1980. The permeability of the endplate channel to organic cations in frog muscle. J. Gen. Physiol. 75:469–492.

Fertuck, H. C., and Salpeter, M. M. 1974. Localization of acetylcholine receptor by ^{125}I-labeled α-bungarotoxin binding at mouse motor endplates. Proc. Natl. Acad. Sci. U.S.A. 71:1376–1378.

Heuser, J. E., and Salpeter, S. R. 1979. Organization of acetylcholine receptors in quick-frozen, deep-etched, and rotary-replicated Torpedo postsynaptic membrane. J. Cell. Biol. 82:150–173.

Hille, B. 1984. Ionic Channels of Excitable Membranes. Sunderland, Mass.: Sinauer.

Karlin, A. 1983. The anatomy of a receptor. Neurosci. Comment. 1:111–123.

Karlin, A. 1991. Exploration of the nicotinic acetylcholine receptor. Harvey Lect. 85. In press.

Kistler, J., Stroud, R. M., Klymkowsky, M. W., Lalancette, R. A., and Fairclough, R. H. 1982. Structure and function of an acetylcholine receptor. Biophys. J. 37:371–383.

Ko, C.-P. 1984. Regeneration of the active zone at the frog neuromuscular junction. J. Cell Biol. 98:1685–1695.

Kuffler, S. W., Nicholls, J. G., and Martin, A. R. 1984. From Neuron to Brain: A Cellular Approach to the Function of the Nervous System, 2nd ed. Sunderland, Mass.: Sinauer.

McMahan, U. J., and Kuffler, S. W. 1971. Visual identification of synaptic boutons on living ganglion cells and of varicosities in postganglionic axons in the heart of the frog. Proc. R. Soc. Lond. [Biol.] 177:485–508.

Miles, F. A. 1969. Excitable Cells. London: Heinemann.

Neher, E. 1982. Unit conductance studies in biological membranes. In P. F. Baker (ed.), Techniques in Cellular Physiology, Vol. P1/II (P 121). County Clare, Ireland: Elsevier/North Holland, pp. 1–16.

Noda, M., Furutani, Y., Takahashi, H., Toyosato, M., Tanabe, T., Shimizu, S., Kikyotani, S., Kayano, T., Hirose, T., Inayama, S., and Numa, S. 1983. Cloning and sequence analysis of calf cDNA and human genomic DNA encoding α-subunit precursor of muscle acetylcholine receptor. Nature 305:818–823.

Noda, M., Takahashi, H., Tanabe, T., Toyosato, M., Kikyotani, S., Furutani, Y., Hirose, T., Takashima, H., Inayama, S., Miyata, T., and Numa, S. 1983. Structural homology of Torpedo californica acetylcholine receptor subunits. Nature 302:528–532.

Palay, S. L. 1958. The morphology of synapses in the central nervous system. Exp. Cell. Res. Suppl. 5:275–293.

Raftery, M. A., Hunkapiller, M. W., Strader, C. D., and Hood, L. E. 1980. Acetylcholine receptor: Complex of homologous subunits. Science 208:1454–1457.

Ramón y Cajal, S. 1911. Histologie du Système Nerveux de l'Homme & des Vertébrés, Vol. 2. L. Azoulay (trans.) Paris: Maloine. Republished in 1955. Madrid: Instituto Ramón y Cajal.

Takeuchi, A. 1977. Junctional transmission. I. Postsynaptic mechanisms. In E. R. Kandel (ed.), Handbook of Physiology, Section 1: The Nervous System, Vol. I. Cellular Biology of Neurons, Part 1. Bethesda, Md.: American Physiological Society, pp. 295–327.

Tzartos, S. J., and Lindstrom, J. M. 1980. Monoclonal antibodies used to probe acetylcholine receptor structure: Localization of the main immunogenic region and detection of similarities between subunits. Proc. Natl. Acad. Sci. U.S.A. 77:755–759.

Toyoshima, C., and Unwin, N. 1988. Ion channel of acetylcholine receptor reconstructed from images of postsynaptic membranes. Nature 336:247–250.

Eric R. Kandel
James H. Schwartz

11

Directly Gated Transmission at Central Synapses

The Spinal Stretch Reflex Illustrates the Major Features of Synaptic Transmission Between Central Neurons

Excitatory Synaptic Action Is Mediated by Receptor-Channels Selective for Sodium and Potassium

The Current Flow During the EPSP Can Be Measured Experimentally

Glutamate Is a Major Excitatory Transmitter in the Brain

Inhibitory Synaptic Action Is Mediated by Receptor-Channels Selective for Chloride

The Current Flow During the IPSP Can Also Be Readily Analyzed

GABA and Glycine Are Inhibitory Transmitters

Receptors for GABA, Glycine, and Glutamate Are Multisubunit Transmembrane Proteins

Transmitter-Gated Ion Channels Are Structurally Similar to Voltage-Gated Channels

Common Ionic Mechanisms Are Used in All Neuronal Signaling

Excitatory and Inhibitory Synaptic Actions Are Integrated at a Common Trigger Zone

Synapses onto a Single Central Neuron Are Grouped According to Function

Synapses on Cell Bodies Are Often Inhibitory

Synapses on Dendritic Spines Are Often Excitatory

Synapses on Axon Terminals Are Often Modulatory

Excitatory and Inhibitory Synapses Have Distinct Ultrastructures

An Overall View

Our examination of directly gated synaptic transmission began in the last chapter with the peripheral synapse that connects vertebrate motor neurons to skeletal muscle. In this chapter we consider how directly gated synaptic transmission works in the central nervous system. We shall continue to focus on postsynaptic aspects of synaptic transmission because, as we have seen, the nature of the synaptic action is determined by the transmitter receptor and the channels that the receptor gates.

Many of the principles that govern the function of directly gated synaptic connections in the neuromuscular junction also operate in the central nervous system. The signaling mechanisms in skeletal muscle are simpler, however. First, most muscle fibers are innervated by only one motor neuron. Second, the muscle fiber receives only excitatory input (there are no inhibitory synapses onto vertebrate skeletal muscle). Third, all the excitatory connections on muscle fibers are regulated by the same neurotransmitter, acetylcholine (ACh), which activates the same kind of receptor-channel, the nicotinic ACh receptor-channel, at all connections. Finally, the neuromuscular connections are highly effective—each synaptic potential invariably produces an action potential.

In contrast, a central nerve cell such as the motor neuron in the spinal cord receives connections, both excitatory and inhibitory, not from one but from hundreds of neurons that use different chemical transmitters. This complex converging input to a single cell is mediated by different kinds of synaptic receptors sensitive to the different transmitters, and these receptors control distinct ion channels, some directly gated and some gated indirectly by second messengers. As a result, unlike a muscle fiber, a central neuron must integrate a diverse set of inputs into a coordinated response.

We shall, therefore, first examine how transmitter-gated inhibitory synaptic actions differ from excitatory

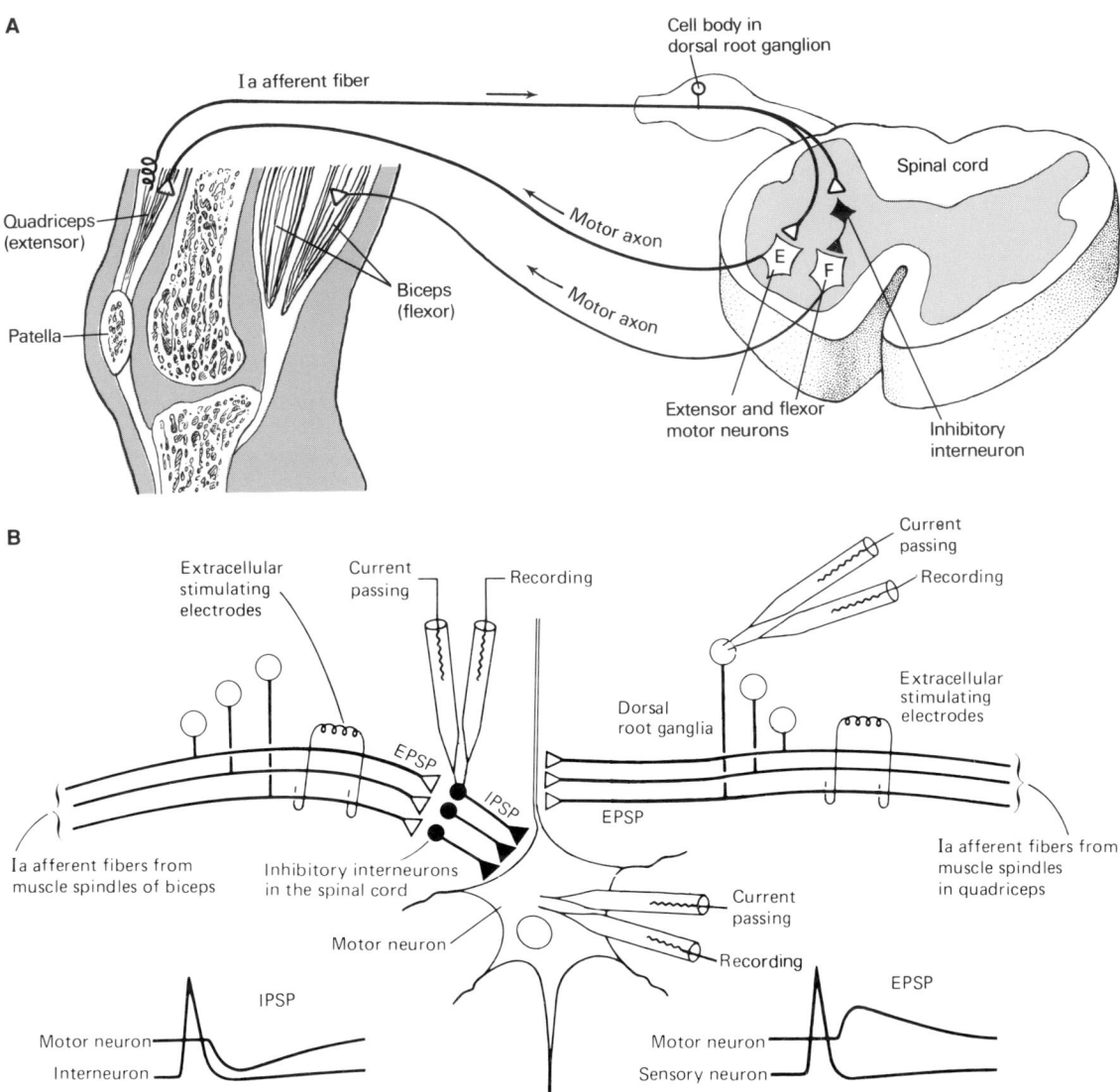

FIGURE 11–1

Synaptic connections of neurons mediating the stretch reflex of the quadriceps muscle.

A. The afferent neuron from the quadriceps muscle makes an excitatory connection with the motor neuron innervating this same muscle group. It also makes an excitatory connection with an interneuron. This interneuron makes an inhibitory connection with the motor neuron innervating the antagonist muscle group, the biceps.

B. This idealized experimental setup shows alternative approaches to studying inhibition and excitation of a motor neuron in the pathway illustrated in **A.** To study excitation, either

the whole afferent nerve from the quadriceps can be stimulated electrically with extracellular electrodes, or single axons can be stimulated with intracellular electrodes. To study inhibition, the inhibitory interneuron in the pathway from the biceps can be stimulated intracellularly. The type of signal conveyed at each synapse is shown in the idealized electrical recordings at the bottom of the figure. An action potential stimulated in the inhibitory interneuron in the *biceps* pathway causes an inhibitory (hyperpolarizing) postsynaptic potential (IPSP) in the motor neuron. In contrast, an action potential stimulated in the afferent neuron from the *quadriceps* triggers an excitatory (depolarizing) postsynaptic potential (EPSP) in the motor neuron.

ones. What distinguishes the ion channels that mediate inhibition from those that mediate excitation? We next will discuss the molecular similarities between transmitter-gated ion channels and the voltage-gated channels that we discussed in Chapter 8. Finally, we shall consider how the competing inhibitory and excitatory signals from different sources are integrated in a single cell to give a coherent response.

The Spinal Stretch Reflex Illustrates the Major Features of Synaptic Transmission Between Central Neurons

The first insight into directly gated synaptic actions in the central nervous system came from the work of John Eccles and his colleagues on spinal motor neurons, work based on the studies of the nerve–muscle synapses by Paul Fatt and Bernard Katz that we reviewed in the preceding chapter. The spinal motor neurons have large cell bodies and are useful for examining synaptic mechanisms because they receive both excitatory and inhibitory connections.

Among the first synaptic connections that Eccles and his colleagues analyzed were those that mediate the stretch reflex, the simple behavior we examined in Chapters 2 and 3 (Figure 11–1A). Using fine stimulating wires, Eccles activated the large axons of sensory cells that innervate the stretch receptor organs in the quadriceps muscle.[1] The same experiments can now be done by stimulating a *single* sensory neuron directly. Passing sufficient current through a microelectrode inserted into the cell body of one of the sensory neurons in the dorsal root ganglion produces an action potential in the cell. This in turn produces a small *excitatory* (depolarizing) *postsynaptic potential* (EPSP) in a motor neuron innervating the muscle from which the sensory neuron originates. The EPSP produced by the one sensory cell depolarizes the motor neuron by less than 1 mV (often only 0.2–0.4 mV), which is far below the threshold required for generating an action potential. A depolarization of 10 mV or more is required to reach threshold.

Stimulating a sensory neuron that innervates the hamstrings, a muscle group antagonistic to the quadriceps, produces a small *inhibitory* (hyperpolarizing) *postsynaptic potential* (IPSP) in the motor neuron of the quadriceps. The inhibition is mediated by an inhibitory interneuron, which receives input from the stretch receptor neurons and in turn connects with the motor neurons. The interneurons also can be recorded from and stimulated intracellularly (Figure 11–1B).

Although a single excitatory postsynaptic potential in the motor neuron is not nearly large enough to elicit an action potential, the convergence of many excitatory synaptic potentials from many afferent fibers can be integrated by the neuron to initiate an action potential. Inhibitory synaptic potentials, if strong enough, can counteract the sum of the excitatory actions and prevent the membrane potential from reaching threshold. Synaptic inhibition, in addition to counteracting synaptic excitation, can exert powerful control over *spontaneously active* nerve cells. Many cells in the brain are spontaneously active, like the pacemaker cells of the heart. By suppressing spontaneous generation of action potentials in these cells, synaptic inhibition can determine the pattern of firing in a cell (Figure 11–2). This function is called the *sculpturing role* of inhibition. We shall first consider the mechanisms of excitatory synaptic action.

Excitatory Synaptic Action Is Mediated by Receptor-Channels Selective for Sodium and Potassium

Eccles and his colleagues discovered that the EPSP in spinal motor cells results from the opening of transmitter-

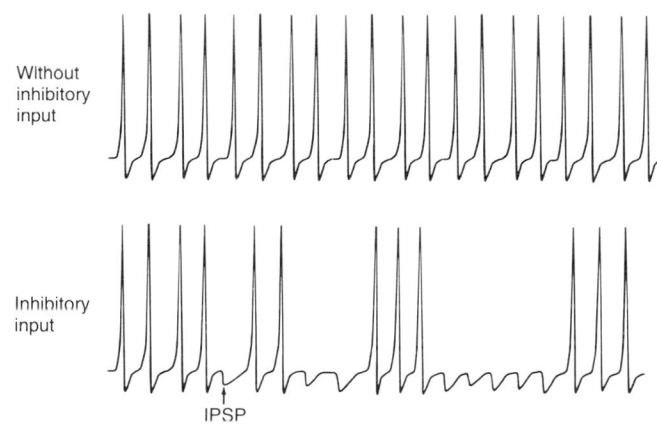

FIGURE 11–2

Inhibition can shape the firing pattern of a spontaneously active neuron. Without inhibitory input the neuron fires continuously at a fixed interval. With inhibitory input some action potentials are inhibited. This alters the pattern of impulses and is therefore called *sculpturing*.

gated ion channels permeable to both Na^+ and K^+. This mechanism is similar to the opening of the cation-selective channels in skeletal muscle by ACh. As the strength of the extracellular stimulus is increased, more afferent fibers are excited, and the depolarization produced by the excitatory synaptic potential becomes larger. The depolarization eventually becomes large enough to bring the membrane potential of the axon hillock (the integrative component) of the motor neuron to the threshold for generation of an action potential (Figure 11–3B).

The Current Flow During the EPSP Can Be Measured Experimentally

As we saw in Chapter 10, the best way to study the movement of ions responsible for the EPSP is to use the voltage clamp. This technique was applied to motor neurons by Alan Finkel and Stephen Redman. Even earlier, Eccles and his colleagues and Redman had been able to gain considerable insight into the ionic mechanism of the EPSP by measuring the size and polarity of the EPSP while varying membrane potential to obtain the reversal potential. This can be done by passing current across the membrane with an intracellular microelectrode. The size of the EPSP (V_{EPSP}) depends on the magnitude of the synaptic current (I_{EPSP}) and on the cell's nonsynaptic membrane conductance (g_m) mediated by the nongated ion channels:[2]

$$V_{EPSP} = \frac{I_{EPSP}}{g_m}.$$

Most transmitter-gated ion channels in the spinal motor neurons are not voltage dependent. As a result, the

---

[1]These axons, discussed in Chapters 2 and 3, are called primary afferent fibers; they are described more fully in Chapters 24 and 25.

[2]It also depends on the membrane capacitance (see Chapter 7), but for simplicity we omit this here.

A

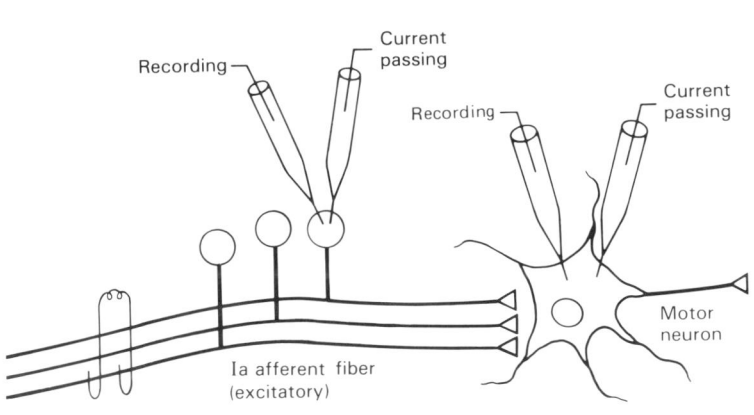

B

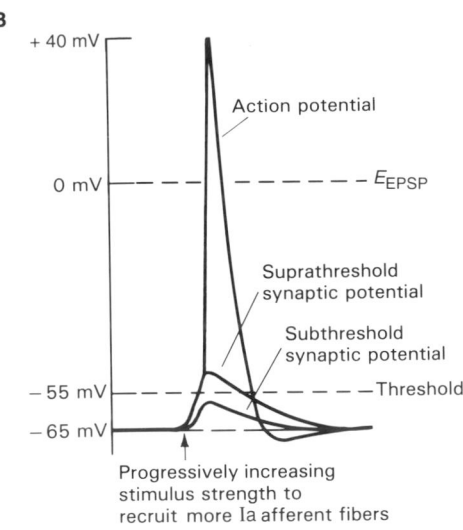

C   **D**

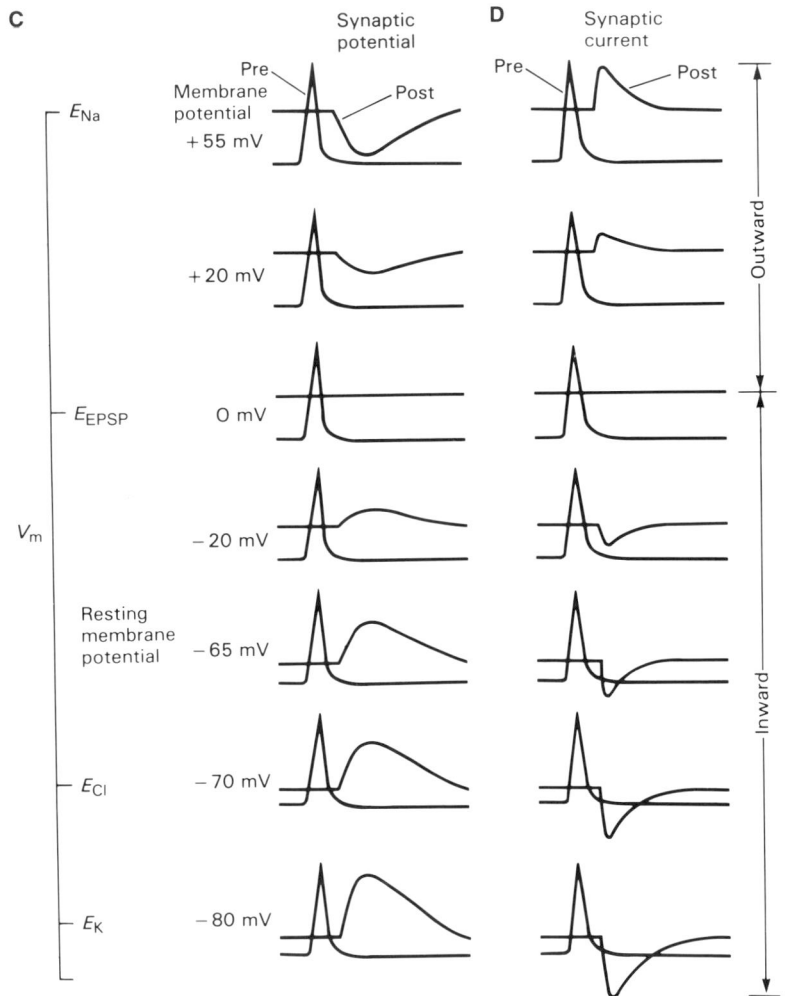

FIGURE 11–3

Chemical excitatory synaptic actions result from opening channels permeable to both Na^+ and K^+. This can be deduced by determining the reversal potential for the EPSP.

A. Intracellular electrodes are used to stimulate and record from the neurons in this experimental system. Current is passed in the motor (postsynaptic) neuron either to alter the level of the resting membrane potential prior to presynaptic stimulation (a method of membrane control called *current clamp*) or to keep the membrane potential fixed during the flow of synaptic current (*voltage clamp*).

B. A weak stimulus to the afferent nerve from the quadriceps recruits only a few afferent fibers, resulting in a subthreshold EPSP. A strong stimulus recruits more afferent fibers, driving the membrane potential toward its reversal potential, which is beyond the threshold (−55 mV) for initiating an action potential.

C. The reversal potential for the *synaptic potential* can be determined using a current clamp. When the membrane potential is at its resting value (−65 mV), a presynaptic action potential produces a depolarizing EPSP, which increases when the membrane potential is hyperpolarized to −70 and −80 mV. In contrast, when the membrane potential is depolarized to −20 mV, the EPSP becomes smaller; when the membrane potential reaches the reversal potential (0 mV), the EPSP is nullified. Further depolarization to +20 mV inverts the synaptic potential, causing hyperpolarization. Thus synaptic action, whether hyperpolarizing or depolarizing, always drives the membrane potential toward the reversal potential, E_{EPSP}.

D. The reversal potential for the *synaptic current* can be determined using a voltage clamp. At the resting membrane potential and at more negative clamped potentials (−70 and −80 mV) the synaptic current is large and inward because the electrochemical driving force ($V_m - E_{EPSP}$) is inward. This inward current generates the EPSP. When the membrane potential is made less negative (−20 mV), the magnitude of the inward synaptic current decreases; at the reversal potential (0 mV) it becomes zero. When the membrane potential is made more positive than the reversal potential (+20 or +55 mV), the synaptic current is outward. (Adapted from Finkel and Redman, 1983.)

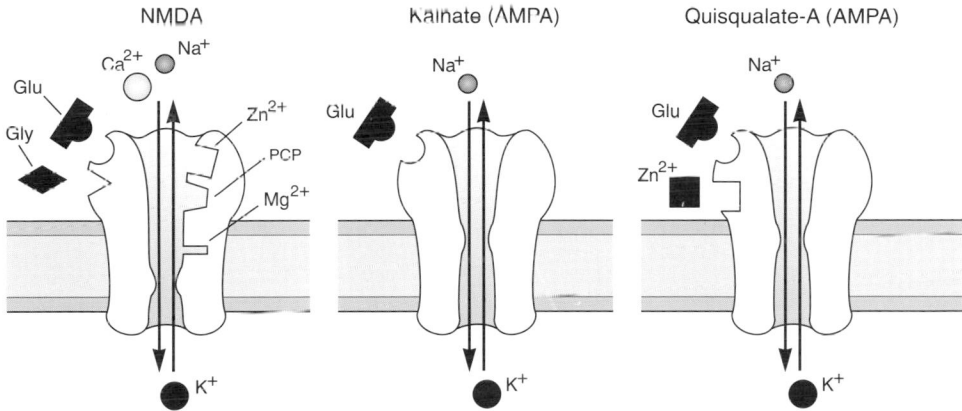

A   Directly gated receptors

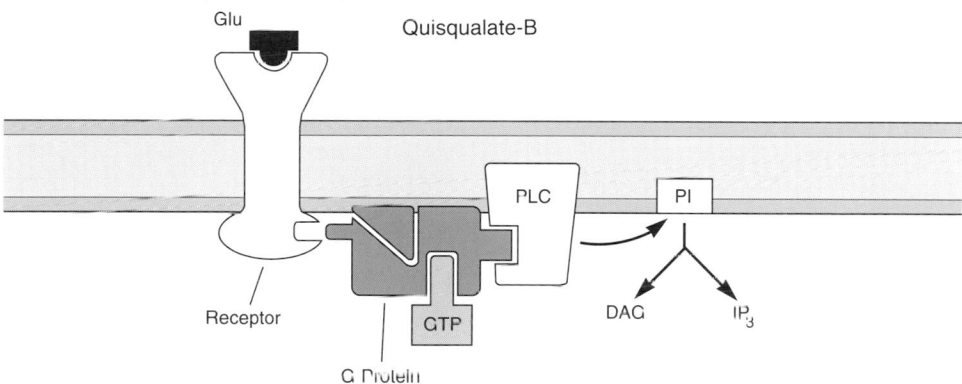

B   Second messenger linked receptor

FIGURE 11–4

Four classes of glutamate receptors regulate excitatory synaptic actions in motor and other neurons in the brain.

A. The NMDA receptor regulates a channel permeable to Ca^{2+}, K^+, and Na^+, and has several binding sites for glycine, Zn^{2+}, PCP, MK8OI (an experimental drug), and Mg^{2+}, which regulate the functioning of this channel in different ways. The kainate receptor binds the glutamate agonist AMPA and regulates a channel permeable to Na^+ and K^+. The quisqualate-A receptor

also binds AMPA and regulates a Na^+-K^+ channel very similar to the kainate-activated receptor- channel. It, too, has a binding site for Zn^{2+}.

B. The quisqualate-B receptor stimulates the activity of phospholipase C (PLC) leading to the formation of the second messengers inositol 1,4,5-triphosphate (IP_3) and diacylglycerol (DAG) from phosphatidylinositol-4,5-biphosphate (PIP_2).

number of channels opened by the transmitter depends largely on the concentration of the transmitter. Thus, changes in the amplitude of the EPSP at different membrane potentials reflect changes in the I_{EPSP} produced by changes in the driving force ($V_m - E_{EPSP}$):

$$I_{EPSP} = g_{EPSP} \times (V_m - E_{EPSP}).$$

Most nerve cells have a resting membrane potential of about −65 mV, considerably lower than that of muscle cells (−90 mV). As the membrane potential of the nerve cell is increased from −65 to −70 mV, the EPSP increases in amplitude, much like the synaptic potential in muscle (Figure 11–3C). This occurs because more inward current flows through the synaptic channels as the driving force ($V_m - E_{EPSP}$) is increased.

As the membrane is progressively depolarized, however, the EPSP diminishes, until it disappears near 0 mV,

its reversal potential. At that point the inward Na^+ current that flows through the synaptic channels is reduced because the membrane potential is now closer to E_{Na}, and the outward K^+ current is increased because it is further from E_K. The inward Na^+ current is thus balanced by the outward K^+ current, with the result that no net current flows through the synaptic channels. Additional depolarization (beyond 0 mV) produces a hyperpolarizing EPSP. The outward K^+ current now becomes greater than the inward Na^+ current, resulting in a net outward ionic current because the membrane potential is closer to E_{Na} than to E_K.

Finkel and Redman obtained similar results when they used a voltage clamp to examine synaptic current (rather than the synaptic potential) as a function of different membrane potentials. The current flow was nullified at 0 mV and reversed from inward to outward as the membrane was depolarized further (Figure 11–3D). Both the synaptic potential and the synaptic current tend to drive the membrane potential to the reversal potential from membrane voltages that are either below or above the equilibrium potential. This experiment therefore also illustrates why EPSPs actually excite the motor neuron. As the EPSP drives the membrane potential from its resting level (−65 mV) toward its reversal potential (0 mV), the membrane potential must pass through threshold (−55 mV).

Glutamate Is a Major Excitatory Transmitter in the Brain

The basic properties of the synaptic channels for excitation in motor neurons are similar to those of the channels involved in excitation of skeletal muscle. The excitatory transmitter released from the primary afferent neurons has not been definitively identified, but pharmacological evidence suggests that it is the amino acid glutamate.

There are four types of glutamate receptors, and at least some of these have subtypes. The major excitatory action of glutamate on motor neurons is produced by binding to two types of glutamate receptors, the kainate and quisqualate A receptors, so named because of the selective action on each type of receptor by the glutamate agonists

kainate and quisqualate (Figure 11–4). Although distinguished by these two ligands, the two receptor types are very similar. Both are not affected by the glutamate agonist NMDA, yet both bind the glutamate agonist AMPA (α-amino-3 hydroxy-5 methyl-4 isoxazole proprionic acid). Both directly gate a low-conductance cation channel (less than 20 pS) that is permeable to Na^+ and K^+ (but not to Ca^{2+}). Moreover, as we shall see below, the kainate receptors so far cloned all also bind quisqualate and AMPA. As a result, the two channel types are often referred to generically as the AMPA receptors.

These AMPA receptors appear to mediate the EPSP produced in motor neurons by the Ia afferent fibers. Another type of quisqualate receptor (quisqualate B) indirectly gates a channel permeable to Na^+ and K^+ by activating a phosphoinositide-linked second-messenger system (Figure 11–4B) that we shall consider further in the next chapter.

As a result of pharmacological studies by Jeffrey Watkins, we now know that glutamate also binds to still another type of receptor, the NMDA receptor, which is selectively activated by the agonist N-methyl-D-aspartate (Figure 11–4). The NMDA receptor and its channel have two exceptional properties. First, the receptor controls a cation channel of high conductance (50 pS) that is permeable to Ca^{2+} as well as to Na^+ and K^+ (Figure 11–5). Second, because the channel is plugged by extracellular Mg^{2+}

FIGURE 11–5

Magnesium blockade of the NMDA receptor-channel is dependent on voltage. These single-channel recordings were made from rat hippocampal cells in culture obtained in an outside-out configuration, where the extracellular surface of the membrane is exposed to the extracellular bathing medium. When, as on the left, the extracellular Mg^{2+} is 0 mM, the opening and closing of the channel does not depend on voltage. The channel

is open at the resting potential of −60 mV and the synaptic current reverses near 0 mV, as it does in the whole membrane current shown in Figure 11-3D. In contrast, on the right, when Mg^{2+} is present in the normal concentration (1.2 mM) the channel is largely closed (due to Mg^{2+} blockade) at the resting level of −60 mV, and needs substantial depolarization (to +30 mV) before it opens. (Courtesy of J. Jen and C. F. Stevens.)

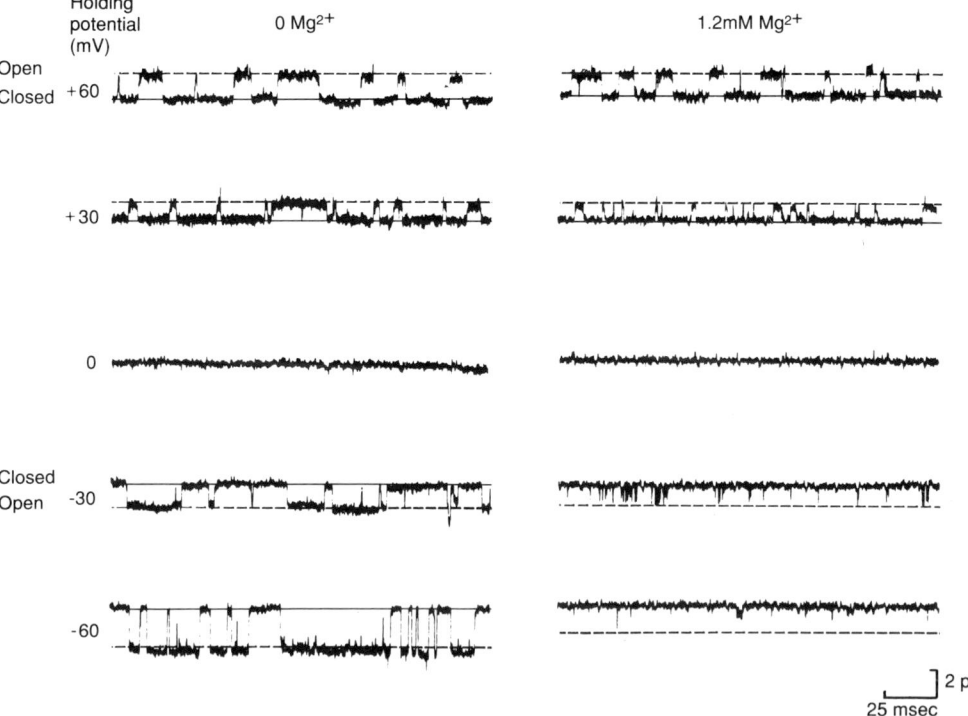

at the normal resting membrane potential (−65 mV), the channel does not conduct ions efficiently when activated by glutamate unless the membrane depolarization is large enough (Figure 11–5). Adequate depolarization of the membrane, by 20 to 30 mV, drives Mg^{2+} out of the channel, allowing Na^+ and Ca^{2+} to enter the cell if glutamate is present. In addition, for reasons that are not yet understood, the channel only functions efficiently in the presence of glycine. When the concentration of glycine is reduced, the ability of glutamate to open the channel is greatly reduced.

In most cells that have both NMDA and non-NMDA receptors, blockade of the NMDA-activated channel by Mg^{2+} prevents this channel from contributing importantly to the EPSP at the resting membrane potential. Thus, the EPSP depends largely on the activation of the non-NMDA glutamate receptors: the kainate and quisqualate receptors. Only a small late component of the EPSP is due to the NMDA receptor. However, the more the neuron is depolarized by the activation of the non-NMDA receptors, the more NMDA-activated channels are opened, and the more current flows through the NMDA-activated channels. This delayed opening of NMDA-activated channels contributes a characteristic late phase to the EPSP (Figure 11–6A).

The NMDA receptor can be distinguished pharmacologically from the kainate and quisqualate receptors. It is blocked selectively by the drug 2-amino-5-phosphonovalerate (APV) (Figure 11–6B), and is inhibited by the hallucinogenic drug phencyclidine (PCP, also known as angel dust).

The NMDA-activated receptor-channel has three other interesting features, to which we shall return in later chapters. First, because it is normally blocked by Mg^{2+} at

FIGURE 11–6

The NMDA receptor-channel contributes only a small late component to the normal excitatory synaptic current in the hippocampus. Similar receptor channels are present on motor neurons. (From Hestrin et al., 1990.)

A. The contribution of the NMDA receptor is revealed by the use of APV, a selective blocker of the NMDA receptor-channel. In this figure the synaptic current was recorded at three different membrane potentials ranging from −80 to +20 before and during the application of 50 µM of APV. At −80 mV there is no current through the NMDA receptor-channel but at −40 mV a small late current is evident. This contribution becomes larger as the membrane is depolarized to +20 mV. The shaded areas indicate the size of the NMDA (APV-sensitive) component. The vertical **dotted line** indicates 25 ms after the peak of current and is used for the calculations of the late current in part B.

B. Effect of APV on early and late components of the synaptic current. At each membrane potential the synaptic current was recorded before and during the application of 50 µM APV at membrane potentials ranging from −80 to +20 mV. To measure the early component, the peak values of current–voltage relations were obtained before (▲) and during (△) the application of APV. Both components are plotted in relation to the membrane potential. The NMDA component is small at negative potentials ranging from −15 to 50 mV because of Mg^{2+} blockade. This blockade is removed when the cell is greatly depolarized (from −20 to +20 mV). Nevertheless, the peak values are identical, because APV has no effect on the early kainate/quisqualate components of current. The NMDA-induced current is reflected in the late current measured 25 ms after the peak of the excitatory postsynaptic current before (●) and during (○) the application of APV. These curves for the late current diverge at approximately −80 mV, indicating that some of the Mg^{2+} blocking the channel is normally removed at this voltage. As the voltage decreases, more Mg^{2+} is removed.

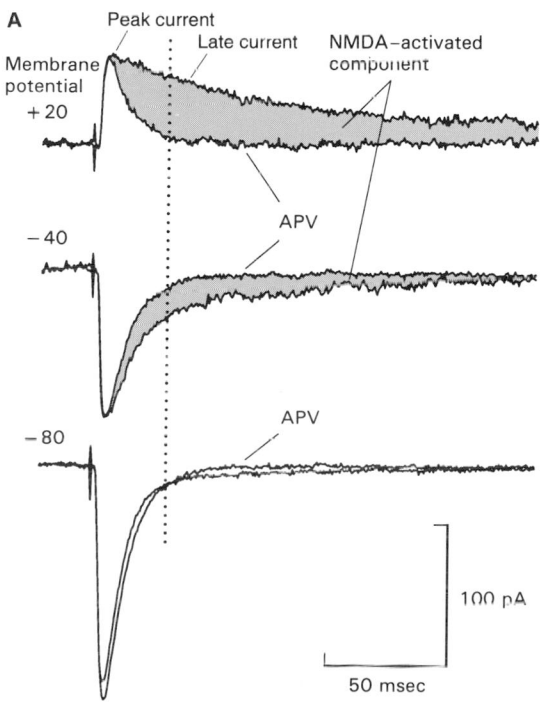

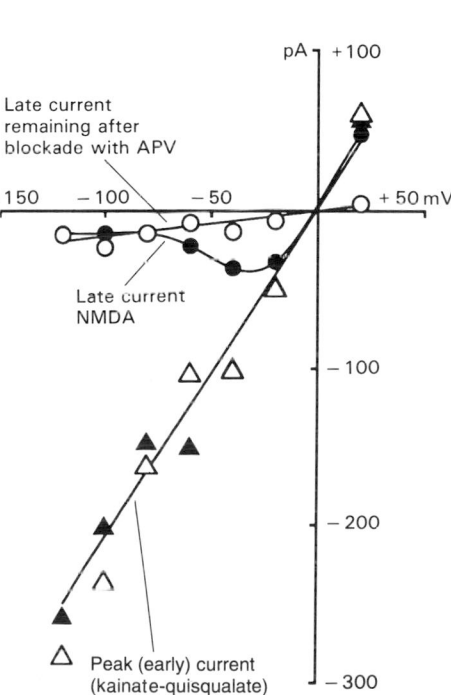

the resting level of membrane potential, the channel is unique among transmitter-gated channels thus far characterized in that it is also gated by voltage (Figure 11–6). That is, the current flow through the channel is maximal when both glutamate is present *and* the cell is depolarized. Second, Ca^{2+} entry through the NMDA-activated channel is thought to activate Ca^{2+}-dependent second-messenger cascades. These are important in triggering biochemical changes that contribute to certain forms of long-lasting synaptic modification, which are considered in Chapter 65. Finally, and most surprisingly, an imbalance in excitatory transmitters like glutamate may, under certain circumstances, contribute to disease.

Excessive amounts of glutamate are highly toxic to neurons. Since glutamate is the major excitatory transmitter in the brain, almost all cells in the brain have receptors that respond to it. In tissue culture, even a brief exposure to high concentrations of glutamate will kill many neurons, an action called *glutamate toxicity*. Although glutamate toxicity may be due in part to the other types of glutamate receptors, in many cell types it is thought to result predominantly from excessive inflow of Ca^{2+} through NMDA-activated channels. High concentrations of intracellular Ca^{2+} may activate Ca^{2+}-dependent proteases and may produce free radicals that are toxic to the cell. Glutamate toxicity may contribute to cell damage after stroke, to the cell death that occurs with persistent seizures in *status epileptics*, and to degenerative diseases, such as Huntington's chorea. Agents that selectively block the NMDA receptor may protect against the toxic effects of glutamate and are currently being tested clinically.

Inhibitory Synaptic Action Is Mediated by Receptor-Channels Selective for Chloride

Eccles and his colleagues could inhibit the firing of a motor neuron by stimulating the Ia afferent pathways from muscles that *oppose* the movements of muscle innervated by the motor neuron. The afferents from antagonist muscles produce inhibitory postsynaptic potentials that prevent the membrane potential of the initial segment of the axon from reaching the threshold for spike generation. IPSPs usually hyperpolarize the membrane; they also reduce the synaptic potentials produced by excitatory synapses.

In the spinal motor neurons studied by Eccles, and in most central neurons, the inhibitory transmitters open Cl^- channels. Inhibition mediated by second messengers can involve opening of K^+ channels as well, as we shall see in Chapter 12. Both Cl^- and K^+ ion channels are similar in that their reversal potentials (the Nernst potentials for E_K and E_{Cl}) are more negative than the resting membrane potential. In a typical nerve cell E_{Cl} is about -70 mV and E_K is -80 mV, whereas the membrane potential is -65 mV. The concentration of Cl^- is high on the outside of the cell (150 mM) and low inside (15 mM), so that opening of Cl^- channels leads to the movement of Cl^- down its concentration gradient. The influx of Cl^- adds to the

negative charge inside the cell while the efflux of K^+ removes positive charge. Thus, opening either Cl^- or K^+ channels leads to a positive or outward current and a net hyperpolarization.

The Current Flow During the IPSP Can Also Be Readily Analyzed

The flow of current due to an inhibitory synaptic potential (I_{IPSP}) can be analyzed in a way similar to that for excitatory actions—by using a current clamp to change the membrane potential (V_m) systematically and thus determine the reversal potential for the IPSP (Figure 11–7). When the membrane potential is depolarized, the IPSP becomes larger with increasing depolarization because the electrochemical force on Cl^- ($V_m - E_{Cl}$) becomes larger. The force of the Cl^- concentration gradient, which promotes the movement of Cl^- from outside to inside the cell, remains the same, but the force of the electrical gradient, which opposes the movement of Cl^-, is reduced. Therefore, more Cl^- flows in across the membrane through synaptic channels. When the membrane potential is hyperpolarized from its resting level of -65 mV to -70 mV, the IPSP decreases to zero. This null point is the reversal potential for the IPSP (E_{IPSP}). It is also the Nernst equilibrium potential for Cl^- (E_{Cl}). Thus, at -70 mV the electrical force acting on Cl^- is exactly equal and opposite to the force of the concentration gradient. Even when g_{Cl} is increased due to the opening of Cl^- channels, there is no net current through these channels. If the membrane potential is increased further to -80 mV, the electrical force exceeds the force of the concentration gradient, and Cl^- will move out of the cell. Since this is equivalent to positive current flowing into the cell, the membrane depolarizes.

The resting potential of a central neuron is usually close to E_{Cl}. Indeed, in some cells the resting potential is equal to E_{Cl}. In these cells synaptic actions that increase Cl^- conductance do not change the postsynaptic membrane potential at all—the cell does not become hyperpolarized. How then does an inhibitory transmitter that opens Cl^- channels prevent a cell from firing? When Cl^- channels are opened, the Cl^- influx drives the membrane potential toward the reversal potential for Cl^-, or holds it at E_{Cl} if it already is there. Since this reversal potential is -70 mV and therefore at some distance from the threshold (-55 mV) for generating an action potential, the opening of Cl^- channels increases the level of excitatory input needed to drive V_m toward threshold (Figure 11–7B).

In addition, the opening of Cl^- channels increases the overall conductance of the membrane of the postsynaptic cell (g_m). Since the amplitude of an excitatory synaptic potential is dependent on g_m,

$$V_{EPSP} = \frac{I_{EPSP}}{g_m},$$

the increased g_m during inhibition will reduce the amplitude of any excitatory input (V_{EPSP}) that occurs during the inhibitory action (Figure 11–7C).

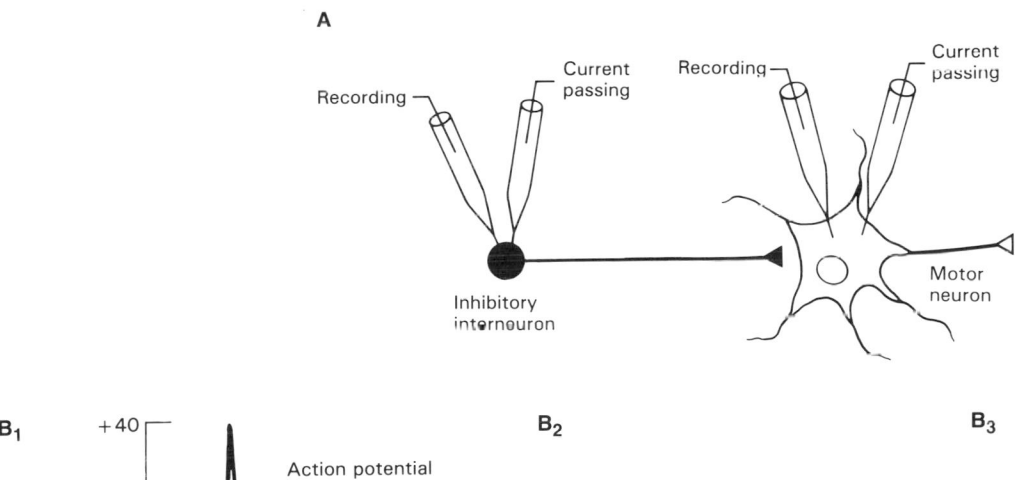

A

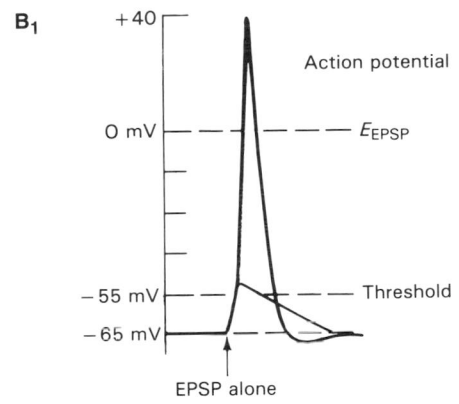

B₁

+40

0 mV ——— E_{EPSP}

Action potential

−55 mV ——— Threshold

−65 mV

EPSP alone

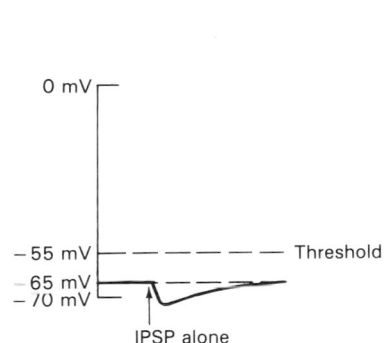

B₂

0 mV

−55 mV ——— Threshold
−65 mV
−70 mV

IPSP alone

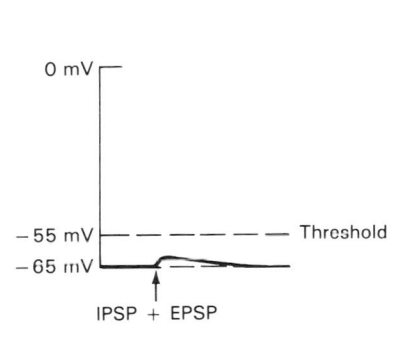

B₃

0 mV

−55 mV ——— Threshold
−65 mV

IPSP + EPSP

FIGURE 11–7

Chemical inhibitory synaptic action hyperpolarizes the postsynaptic cell by opening ion channels to Cl⁻.

A. In this hypothetical experiment two electrodes are placed in the presynaptic interneuron and two in the postsynaptic motor neuron. The current-passing electrode in the presynaptic cell is used to produce an action potential; in the postsynaptic cell it is used to alter the membrane potential systematically (current clamp).

B. Inhibitory actions counteract excitatory actions. 1. A large excitatory postsynaptic potential occurring alone moves the membrane potential toward E_{EPSP} and exceeds the threshold for generating an action potential. 2. An inhibitory potential occurring alone moves the membrane potential away from the threshold toward E_{Cl} (−70 mV). 3. When inhibitory and excitatory potentials occur together, the effectiveness of the excitatory postsynaptic potential is reduced, preventing it from reaching threshold.

C. The inhibitory synaptic potential reverses at the equilibrium potential for Cl⁻. At the resting membrane potential (−65 mV) a presynaptic spike produces a hyperpolarizing IPSP, which increases in amplitude as the membrane is artificially depolarized. However, when the membrane potential is hyperpolarized to −70 mV, the IPSP is nullified. This reversal potential for the IPSP occurs at E_{Cl}, the Nernst potential for Cl⁻. With further hyperpolarization, the IPSP is inverted to a depolarizing postsynaptic potential (−80 and −100 mV) because the membrane potential is hyperpolarized in relation to E_{Cl}. Even this depolarizing action has an inhibitory effect, however, because the inhibitory input tends to hold the membrane potential at or below −70 mV, a considerable distance from threshold (−55 mV).

C

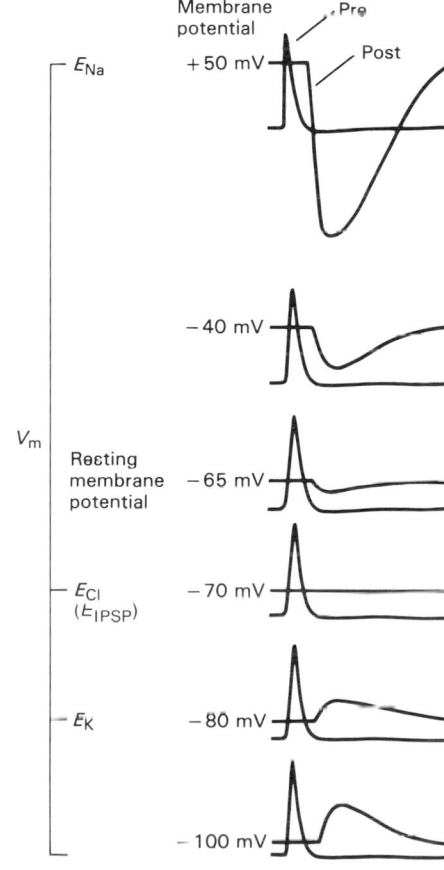

Membrane potential

E_{Na} — Pre, Post, +50 mV

−40 mV

V_m

Resting membrane potential — −65 mV

E_{Cl} (E_{IPSP}) — −70 mV

E_K — −80 mV

−100 mV

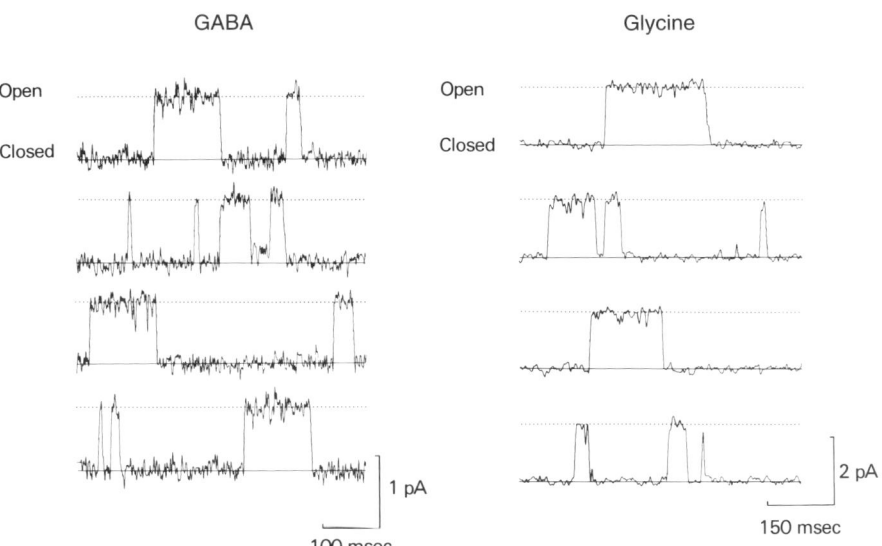

FIGURE 11–8

GABA and glycine act on different receptors that control a similar chloride channel. The recordings are of current through single transmitter-gated Cl⁻ inhibitory channels in a mouse spinal neuron at a membrane potential of 0 mV. Upward deflections indicate outward current steps. Channels opened by GABA (10 μM) and glycine (10 μM) produce similar elementary pulses of outward currents with similar size conductances, indicating that similar Cl⁻ channels are opened. (Courtesy of B. Sakmann.)

Thus the opening of Cl⁻ (or K⁺) channels inhibits the postsynaptic cell in three ways. First, an IPSP can hyperpolarize the membrane and move the membrane potential further away from threshold (Figure 11–7C). Second, by increasing the cell's permeability to Cl⁻ (or K⁺), the inhibitory transmitter acts to stabilize or clamp the membrane potential near E_{Cl} (or E_K), preventing it from reaching threshold (see Equation 6–4). Finally, an IPSP increases the membrane conductance, thereby reducing the amplitude of an EPSP. This result is called the *short-circuiting* or *shunting* action of inhibition.

The opening of Cl⁻ (or K⁺) channels has still one other important feature. As with most forms of synaptic excitation, the opening of the inhibitory channels is not influenced by membrane voltage—a change in the membrane potential does not alter the number of channels opened by the transmitter. This again demonstrates the important difference between most transmitter-gated channels (the NMDA-activated channel being an exception) and voltage-gated channels.

GABA and Glycine Are Inhibitory Transmitters

Gamma-aminobutyric acid (GABA) is a major inhibitory transmitter in the brain and spinal cord (see Chapter 3). Glycine, a less common transmitter, is used in the spinal cord by interneurons that inhibit antagonist muscles. Bert Sakmann and his colleagues have obtained single-channel recordings of elementary current steps from spinal neurons in culture and found that both GABA and glycine produce similar outward current steps, in each case because of the movement of Cl⁻ (Figure 11–8). This inhibitory action can be demonstrated on the single-channel level

by comparing the reversal potential of the elementary inhibitory currents induced by GABA to the elementary excitatory currents induced by glutamate. The glutamate current reverses at 0 mV, thereby driving the membrane past threshold. By contrast, the GABA current is nullified and begins to reverse beyond −60 mV and prevents the membrane from reaching threshold (Figure 11–9).

Receptors for GABA, Glycine, and Glutamate Are Multisubunit Transmembrane Proteins

Like the ACh-activated cation channel (Chapter 10), the GABA- and glycine-activated channels are each formed from a single transmembrane protein that consists of both a conducting pore embedded in the cell membrane and a transmitter binding site on the outer face of the membrane. The GABA-activated channel has at least two other functional regions since benzodiazepines and barbiturates act at different sites to increase the GABA-induced Cl⁻ current. The benzodiazepines are antianxiety agents and muscle relaxants that include diazepam (Valium) and chlordiazepoxide (Librium). Barbiturates are hypnotics that include phenobarbital and secobarbital.

The presence of any one of the three ligands—GABA, benzodiazepine, or barbiturate—influences the binding of the other two. For example, a benzodiazepine (or a barbiturate) will bind more tightly when GABA is bound to the receptor. Although all three sites can interact, each is distinct from the others. Indeed, analysis of the primary structure of the $GABA_A$ receptor by Eric Barnard and Peter Seeburg and their colleagues indicates that the receptor is composed of at least three subunits—α, β, and γ. All of the subunits bind GABA, although the α-subunit does so with the greatest affinity. Both the α- and the β-subunits

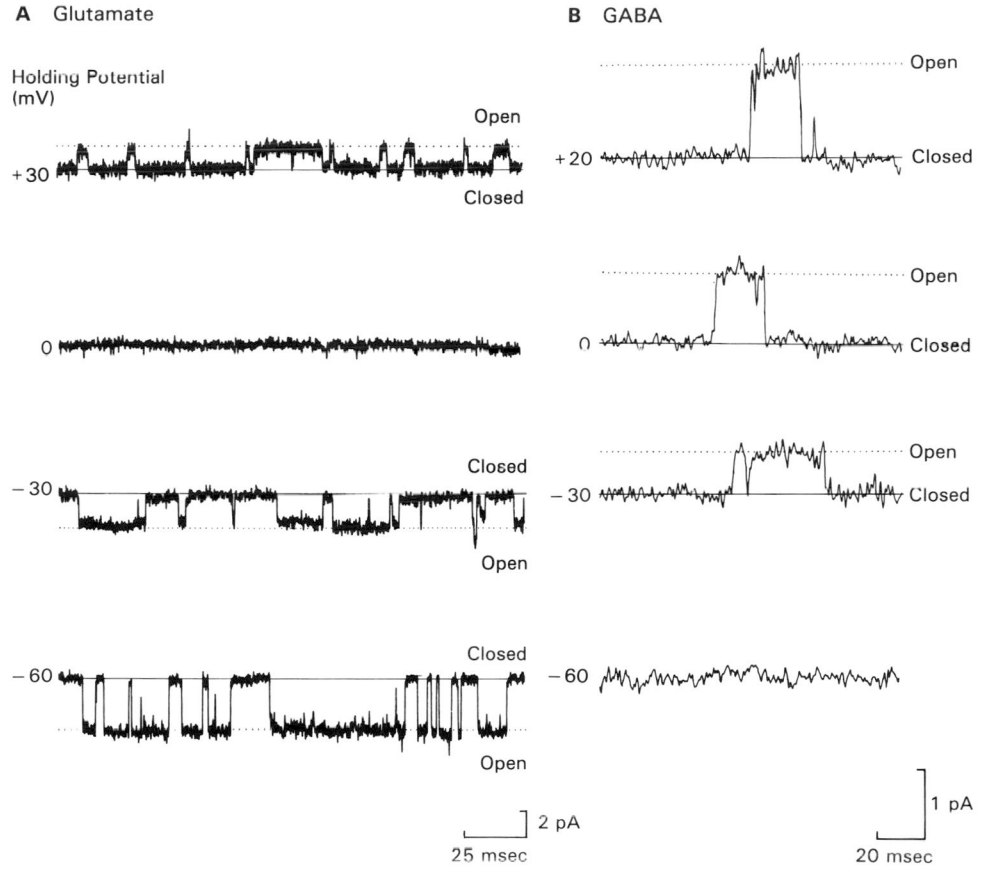

FIGURE 11-9

Single-channel currents activated by the excitatory transmitter glutamate and those activated by the inhibitory transmitter GABA have different reversal potentials. Downward deflection indicates inward current pulses; upward deflection indicates outward current pulses.

A. Elementary excitatory current activated by glutamate in a rat hippocampal neuron. As the membrane potential is moved in a depolarizing direction (from −60 to −30 mV), the current pulses become smaller. At 0 mV (the reversal potential for the EPSP) the current pulses are nullified, and at +30 mV they in-

vert and are outward. The reversal potential at 0 mV (see Figure 11–3) is the averaged equilibrium potentials for Na⁺ and K⁺, the two ions responsible for generating this current. (Courtesy of J. Jen and C. F. Stevens.)

B. Elementary inhibitory current activated by GABA (5 μM) in a rat hippocampal neuron. The current is nullified at approximately −60 mV (the reversal potential for IPSP). At more depolarized levels the current pulses are outward. This reversal potential lies near the equilibrium potential for Cl⁻, the only ion contributing to this current. (Courtesy of B. Sakmann.)

bind barbiturates, but only one, the γ-subunit, binds benzodiazepines.

This work, and similar studies by Heinrich Betz and his colleagues on a subunit of the glycine receptor, reveals that the inhibitory anion channels are similar to the ACh-activated cation channel. Together these three directly gated channels are encoded by genes that belong to a single family. All known members of this gene family have several subunits, and all the subunits are structurally similar. As with the nicotinic ACh receptor, each of the GABA and glycine subunits appears to have four membrane-spanning helixes, based on their hydrophobicity profiles (also named M1, M2, M3, and M4), and therefore may have similar transmembrane structures.

Other receptor-channels that may belong to this family are the channels gated by glutamate, the non-NMDA (AMPA) receptor-channels activated by kainate and quis-

qualate, and perhaps the NMDA receptor. For example, the four AMPA receptors that have been cloned by Steven Heineman, Seeburg, and their colleagues also have four transmembrane regions. However, these AMPA receptor-channels, even though cation selective, have only minimal sequence similarity to the nicotinic ACh receptor, even in the M2 region. Moreover, each of the four AMPA receptors has a small amino acid segment preceding the fourth membrane-spanning region, which exists in two alternatively spliced versions named *flip* and *flop*. The alternative flip and flop modules are located on adjacent exons of each receptor gene and endow the gene with the capability of transcribing two alternatively spliced mRNAs. The alternatively spliced mRNAs encode two distinct receptors with different electrophysiological and pharmacological properties and distinctive patterns of expression in the brain.

Since the subunits of the GABA and glycine receptors both form anion-selective channels, it is not surprising that they resemble each other (35–40% similarity) more than they resemble the ACh receptor (only 15–20% similarity). The M2 region, which we examined in the ACh-activated channel, is also present in the GABA- and glycine-activated channels, and is also thought to line the channel pore. The M2 region in inhibitory receptors contains clusters of basic amino acids (positively charged at neutral pH, e.g., arginine and lysine) that are thought to give these channels their anion selectivity.

Transmitter-Gated Ion Channels Are Structurally Similar to Voltage-Gated Channels

In addition to the transmitter-gated ion channels that we have considered here, there are two other major classes that we considered earlier in Chapters 8 and 9: those gated by voltage, and the gap junction channels. How are these three classes of ion channels related? To begin with, each of these three classes is encoded by a separate gene family. The transmitter-gated family of ion channels can be either cation selective (excitatory) or anion selective (inhibitory). Both types are made of several peptides. These peptides or subunits all have four membrane-spanning segments, one of which, the M2 region, is thought to line the pore. When the M2 segment is flanked by a cluster of acidic amino acids (e.g., aspartate or glutamate), as in the nicotinic ACh receptor (see Figure 10–15), the channel is selective for cations. When the M2 segment has clusters of basic residues (e.g., lysine or arginine) as in the GABA and glycine receptors, the channel is selective for anions (Figure 11–10A).

As with transmitter-gated channels, individual voltage-gated channels are also selective for ions, specifically Na^+, Ca^{2+}, or K^+. In contrast to the multiple subunits of the transmitter-gated channels, at least some of the voltage-gated channels—those for Na^+ and Ca^{2+}—form a pore by means of a single major subunit. As is evident in the Na^+ channel, this single peptide contains four internal segments with similar molecular motifs (Figure 11–10A). Each repeated segment is analogous to a single subunit of the multimeric protein that forms the transmitter-gated channel. Thus, each of the four internal motifs is thought to include six membrane-spanning α-helices (S1–S6). One of these helices, the S4 region, has a series of repeating basic amino acid residues at every third position, with hydrophobic residues in between. These charged residues may be the voltage sensor, the region of the channel that transforms changes in the membrane potential into the conformational changes in the protein that open and close the channel. Between α-helical segments 5 and 6 a stretch of amino acids called the P region dips into the membrane (as β strands) to line the pore of the voltage-gated ion channel much as the M2 region lines the pore of the ligand-gated ion channel.

The gene families for both the voltage-gated and transmitter-gated channels thus represent variations on a common structural plan, a plan shared by the third gene family, that of the gap junction channels (Figure 11–10C). All three families are membrane-spanning proteins and all have five features in common. First, they all share an architectural plan in which the segments that span the membrane are arranged around a central axis to form a gated, water-filled pathway for ions. Second, the structural units of the three types of channels are either identical protein subunits, very similar protein subunits, or several similar domains within a single polypeptide chain. Third, the ion selectivity of each type of channel appears to be roughly related to the number of subunits and the resulting diameter of the pore. Of the channels so far characterized in terms of their subunits, the most selective channels, the voltage-gated Na^+ and Ca^{2+} channels, have four structural units and the narrowest pore; the least selective channel, the gap junction channel, has six units and the widest pores. The nicotinic ACh receptor, with five units, has intermediate properties.

Fourth, even channels belonging to different gene families, and which have different numbers of subunits and different-sized central pores, seem to be similar in conformation and may therefore work by similar mechanisms. For example, in all channels the narrower portion of the pore seems to be formed by α-helices or β strands from each of the encircling subunits; the number depends mainly on the size of the pore needed to suit the task. Finally, the switch from open to closed states in all gated channels is thought to involve only a slight tilting of subunits, not a radical realignment.

Common Ionic Mechanisms Are Used in All Neuronal Signaling

Not only are the various types of membrane spanning ion channels structurally similar, but these channels also have similar actions and produce electrical signals that have features in common. All channels produce electrical signals that result from the movement of ions down their electrochemical gradients through the channels. The signals differ in the specific ions involved, in the molecular properties of the channels through which the ions move, in the state of the channels (open or closed) when the cell membrane is at rest, and in the type of stimulus that opens and closes the channel. These stimuli include voltage for the Na^+ and K^+ channels involved in generating the action potential, chemical transmitters for the channels involved in synaptic actions, mechanical pressure for the channels involved in producing the generator potentials of stretch and touch receptors, and light for the light-sensitive Ca^{2+} and Na^+ channels in the retina. Thus, by moving through different channels, the same ions can produce different actions. For example, K^+ moves through a nongated channel to generate the resting potential, through a voltage-gated channel to repolarize the membrane during the action potential, and through a second-messenger gated channel to hyperpolarize the membrane in some inhibitory synaptic actions.

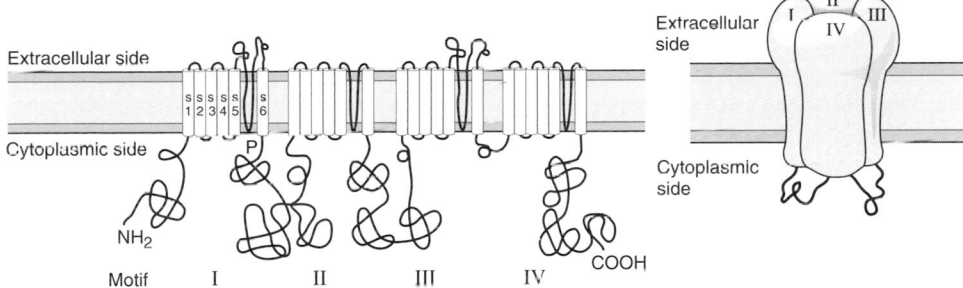

A Voltage-gated channel (Na⁺ channel)

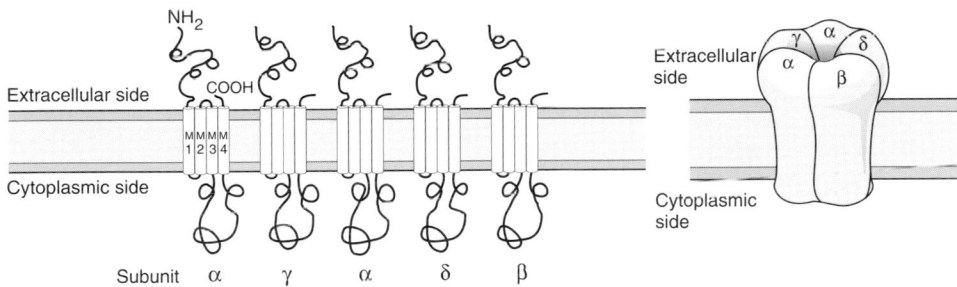

B Transmitter-gated channel (ACh receptor)

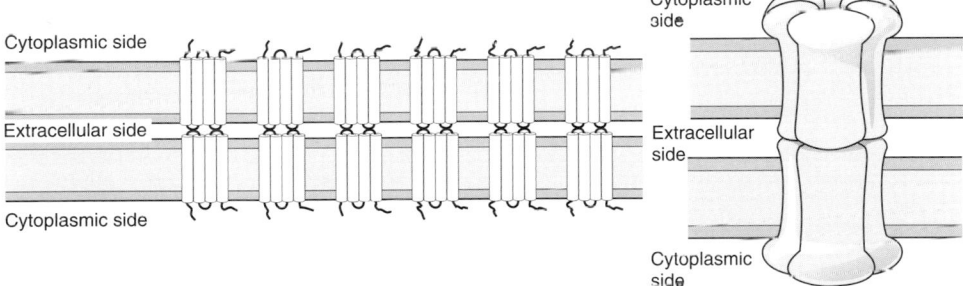

C Gap junction channel

FIGURE 11–10
All ion channels have similar molecular structures.

A. The voltage-gated Na⁺ channel is formed from a single (α) polypeptide chain thought to contain four homologous domains (I to IV), each with six α-helical membrane-spanning regions (S1–S6) and one P region thought to line the pore. Each cylinder represents a single transmembrane α-helix. The figure at the right shows a hypothetical model of the four domains.

B. Pentameric structure of the nicotinic ACh receptor-channel

shows (left) the five subunits of the receptor with each subunit consisting of four transmembrane regions. The channel is modeled on the right.

C. The gap junction channel, found at electrical synapses, is formed from a pair of channels in the pre- and postsynaptic membranes that join in the space between two cells. Each hemi-channel (left) is made of six subunits, each with four transmembrane regions. The two hemicylinders are illustrated as a continuous channel on the right.

In addition, when two ion species are involved in synaptic signaling, the type of signal depends on whether the two species move simultaneously through one channel or sequentially through two distinct channels. For example, simultaneous movement of Na⁺ and K⁺ through the same channel produces synaptic excitation; movement through independent channels in sequence produces an action po-

tential. Finally, most (but not all) of the transmitter-gated channels are not influenced by changes in membrane potential and therefore lack the regenerative link between conductance and voltage that is critical for the explosive all-or-none firing of the action potential. The features of the various signaling potentials are summarized in Table 11–1.

TABLE 11–1. Features of Different Types of Electrical Potentials in Neurons

| Potential | Ion Channels | | Signal properties |
	Type	Mechanism	
Resting potential	Mostly K$^+$ and Cl$^-$ channels; some Na$^+$ channels	Channels usually nongated (occasionally gated K$^+$ channels)	Usually steady, ranging in different cells from −35 to −90 mV
Action potential	Separate Na$^+$ and K$^+$ channels	Voltage	All or none; about 100 mV in amplitude, 1–10 ms in duration
Receptor potential	Single class of channels for both Na$^+$ and K$^+$	Sensory stimulus	Graded; fast, several milliseconds in duration; several millivolts in amplitude
Electrical PSP	Gap junctions (permeable to many ions and small organic molecules)	ΔV, ΔpH, ΔCa^{2+}	Passive spread of presynaptic potential change
Increased-conductance PSPs	EPSP depends on a single class of channels for Na$^+$ and K$^+$, IPSP depends on channels for Cl$^-$ (or K$^+$)	Chemical transmitter	Graded; fast, several milliseconds to seconds in duration; several millivolts in amplitude
Decreased-conductance PSPs (Chapter 12)	Closure of channels for K$^+$, Na$^+$, or Cl$^-$	Chemical transmitter and intracellular messenger	Graded; slow, seconds to minutes in duration; one to several millivolts in amplitude; contributes to the action potential's amplitude and duration

Excitatory and Inhibitory Synaptic Actions Are Integrated at a Common Trigger Zone

A single neuron in the central nervous system, whether in the spinal cord or in the brain, is constantly bombarded by synaptic input from other neurons. A motor neuron, for example, may have as many as 10,000 different presynaptic endings. Some are excitatory, others inhibitory; some strong, others weak. Some inputs contact the motor cell on the tips of its apical dendrites, others on proximal dendrites, some on the dendritic shaft, others on dendritic spines. The different inputs can reinforce as well as cancel one another.

No one presynaptic neuron in the central nervous system is capable of exciting a postsynaptic cell sufficiently to reach the threshold for an action potential. The synaptic potentials produced by a single presynaptic neuron typically are small. The EPSPs produced in a motor neuron by most stretch-sensitive afferent neurons are only 0.2–0.4 mV in amplitude. If the EPSPs generated in a single motor neuron were to sum linearly (which they do not), at least 75 afferent neurons would have to fire together to depolarize the trigger zone by the 10 mV required to reach threshold. However, at the same time these EPSPs are influencing the postsynaptic cell, IPSPs produced by other cells may be acting on the same cell to prevent the firing of action potentials. The relative contribution of the inputs at any individual excitatory or inhibitory synapse will therefore depend on several factors:

its location, size, and shape, and the proximity and relative strength of other synergistic or antagonistic synapses.

These competing inputs are integrated in the postsynaptic neuron by a process called *neuronal integration*. Neuronal integration, the decision to fire or not to fire an action potential, reflects at the level of the cell the task that confronts the nervous system as a whole. Charles Sherrington described the brain's ability to choose between competing alternatives—to select one and suppress the others—as the *integrative action of the nervous system*. He regarded this decision-making capability as the brain's most fundamental activity.

In motor neurons and most interneurons, the decision to initiate an action potential is made at the initial segment of the axon, the *axon hillock* (Chapter 2). This is because the membrane there has a lower threshold than does the membrane of the cell body or dendrites. The lower threshold is the result of a higher density of voltage-dependent Na$^+$ channels, so that more inward current flows for each increment of membrane depolarization (Figure 11–11). Thus, the depolarization required to reach threshold at the axon hillock is only 10 mV (from −65 mV to −55 mV). In contrast, the membrane of the cell body has to be depolarized by 30 mV (from −65 mV to −35 mV) before its threshold is reached.

Synaptic excitation will therefore first discharge the region of the membrane of the axon hillock. The action potential at the axon hillock then brings the membrane of

A

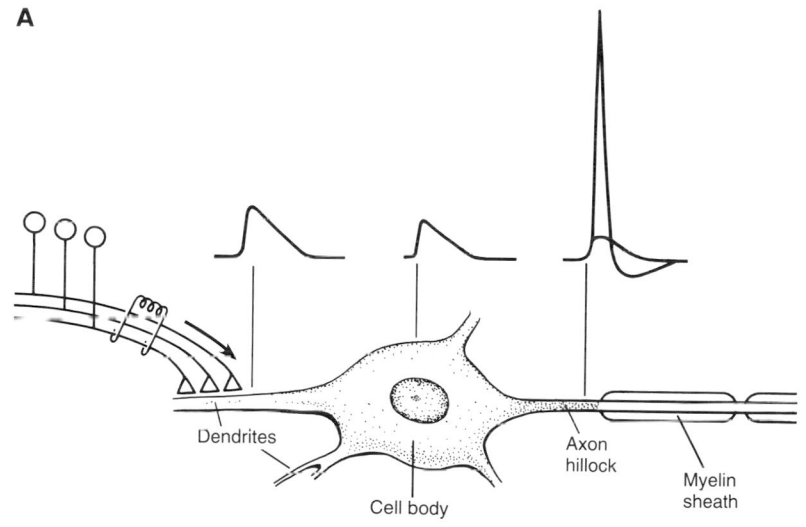

Dendrites

Cell body

Axon hillock

Myelin sheath

B

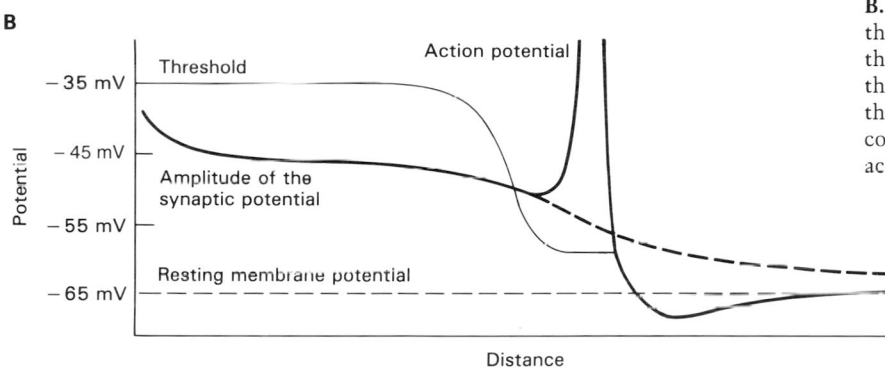

Potential

Threshold

Action potential

−35 mV

−45 mV

Amplitude of the synaptic potential

−55 mV

Resting membrane potential

−65 mV

Distance

FIGURE 11–11

Spatial decay of a synaptic potential initiated by an input onto a dendrite. (Adapted from Eckart and Randall, 1989.)

A. An excitatory synaptic potential originating in the dendrites decreases with distance as it propagates passively in the cell. Nevertheless, an action potential will be initiated at the axon hillock because the density of the Na⁺ channels in this region is high and thus the threshold is low. (The density of Na⁺ channels in the cell is indicated by the density of the stippling.)

B. Comparison of the threshold for initiation of the action potential at different points along the neuron. Action potential is generated where the amplitude of the synaptic potential crosses the threshold. The dashed line shows the course the synaptic potential would take if no action potential were generated.

the cell body to threshold and concomitantly initiates conduction along the axon. The integrative action of a neuron is thus focused on the control of the membrane potential at the trigger zone.

Some cortical neurons have one or more additional (booster) trigger zones within the dendritic tree. These dendritic trigger zones amplify weak excitatory input on remote parts of the dendrite. In neurons that have several trigger zones, each zone sums the local excitation and inhibition produced by nearby synaptic inputs and, if the net input is above threshold, a local action potential can be generated, usually by voltage-dependent Ca²⁺ channels. These local action potentials are not conducted along the dendrites in a regenerative manner. Rather, they propagate electrotonically to the cell body and axon hillock, where they are integrated with all other input signals in the cell.

Because neuronal integration depends on the summation of synaptic potentials that spread passively to the trigger zone, it is critically affected by two passive membrane properties of the neuron (see Chapter 7). First, the *time constant* helps determine the time course of the synaptic potential and thereby affects the *temporal summation*, the process by which consecutive synaptic actions produced at the same site add together in the postsynaptic cell. Neurons with a long time constant have a greater

capability for temporal summation than do neurons with a short time constant (Figure 11–12A). As a result, two consecutive inputs from an excitatory presynaptic neuron are more likely to bring a cell with a long time constant to threshold, than a cell with a short time constant (Figure 11–12A).

Second, the degree to which a depolarizing current decreases as it spreads passively is determined by the *length constant* of the cell. In cells with a long length constant the signals spread to the trigger zone with minimal decrement; in cells with a short length constant the signals decay rapidly with distance. Since the depolarization produced at one synapse is almost never sufficient to trigger an action potential at the trigger zone, the inputs from many presynaptic neurons acting at different sites on the postsynaptic neuron must be added together. This process is called *spatial summation*. Neurons with a long space constant are more likely to be brought to threshold by two different inputs that contact the neuron at different points than do neurons with a short space constant (Figure 11–12B).

Thus, to analyze neuronal integration in an individual cell, we need to know the passive properties of the postsynaptic cell, whether the synaptic inputs are excitatory or inhibitory, and where on the neuron's surface the synaptic contacts are made.

FIGURE 11-12

The effects of temporal and spatial summation on neuronal integration.

A. Temporal summation of two EPSPs produced consecutively by a single presynaptic neuron A. The synaptic current flow, I_{EPSP}, generated by the action of the presynaptic neuron is illustrated at the cell body. This same synaptic current will give rise to very different synaptic potentials depending on whether the postsynaptic cell has a long or a short time constant. In a cell with a long time constant the first EPSP will not decay totally by the time the second EPSP is triggered. Therefore the depolarizing effects of both potentials are additive, bringing the membrane potential above the threshold and triggering an action potential. In a cell with a short time constant the first EPSP decays to the resting potential before the second EPSP is triggered. The second EPSP alone does not cause enough depolarization to trigger an action potential.

B. Spatial summation of two EPSPs produced by two presynaptic neurons (A and B) assuming two different length constants for the postsynaptic cell. In this hypothetical experiment the current (I_{EPSP}) produced by each of these synaptic contacts is assumed to be the same. Both synapses are the same distance from the postsynaptic trigger zone, but in one case the postsynaptic cell has a long length constant, the other a short length constant. In the cell with a long length constant, the initial segment is only one length constant away from the site of the synaptic contacts. Therefore, the EPSPs produced by each of the two presynaptic neuron will decrease only 37% before reaching the trigger zone. This results in enough depolarization to exceed threshold, triggering an action potential. For the cell with a short length constant, the distance between the synapse and the trigger zone in the

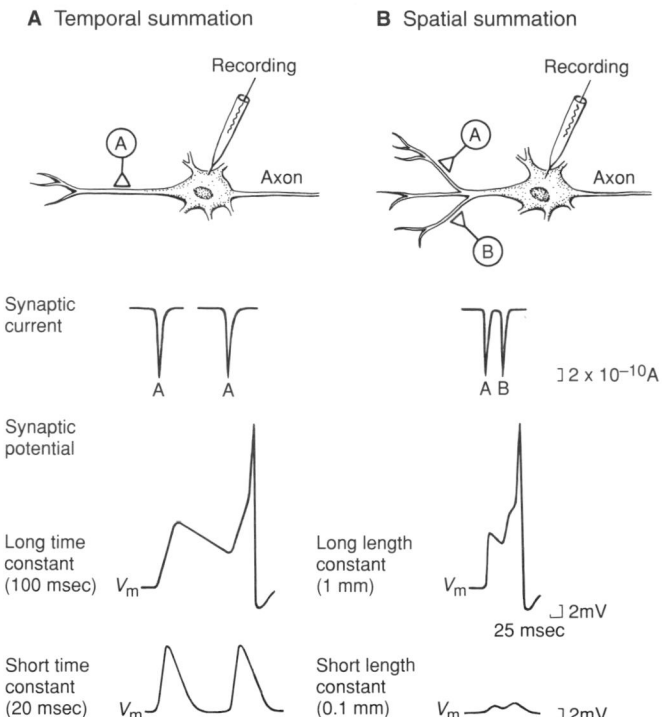

initial axon segment is equal to three length constants. Therefore, each synaptic potential is barely detectable when it arrives in the postsynaptic cell body, and even the summation of two potentials is not sufficient to trigger an action potential.

FIGURE 11-13

Synaptic contact can occur on the cell body, the dendrites, or the axon. The synapse names—axosomatic, axodendritic and axo-axonic—identify the contacting regions of both the presynaptic and postsynaptic neurons (the presynaptic element is identified first). Note that axodendritic synapses can occur on either the main *shaft* of a dendrite branch or on a specialized input zone, the *spine*.

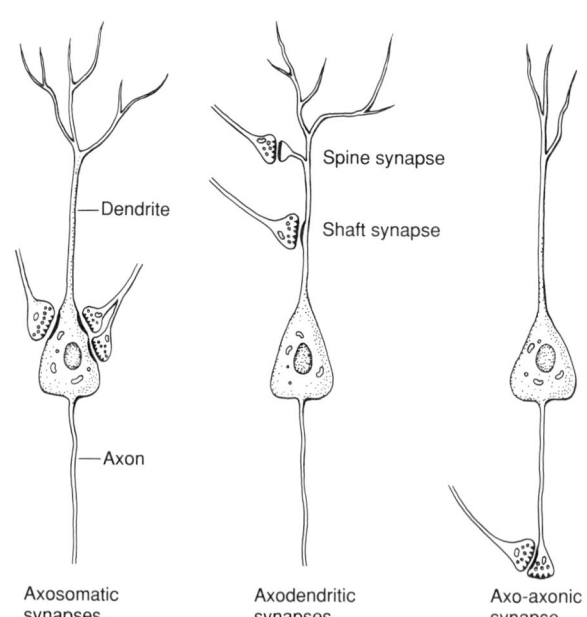

Synapses onto a Single Central Neuron Are Grouped According to Function

All three regions of the nerve cell— axon, cell body, and dendrites—can be receptive sites for synaptic contact (Figure 11-13). The most common types of contact therefore are *axo-axonic*, *axosomatic*, and *axodendritic* (by convention, the presynaptic element is identified first). Axodendritic synapses can occur at the shaft or spine of the dendrite. *Dendrodendritic* and *somasomatic* contacts are also found, but they are rare. The proximity of a synapse to the trigger zone of the postsynaptic cell is obviously important in determining its effectiveness. Synaptic current generated at an axosomatic site has a stronger signal and therefore a greater influence on the outcome at the trigger zone than current from the more remote axodendritic contacts (Figure 11-14).

Synapses on Cell Bodies Are Often Inhibitory

The location of inhibitory inputs in relation to excitatory ones is also critical for their functional effectiveness. Inhibitory short-circuiting actions of the sort that we considered earlier in this chapter are more important when they are initiated at the cell body near the initial axon segment. The depolarization produced by an excitatory current from a dendrite must pass through the cell body as it moves toward the initial axon segment. Inhibitory actions at the cell body will open Cl⁻ channels, thus increas-

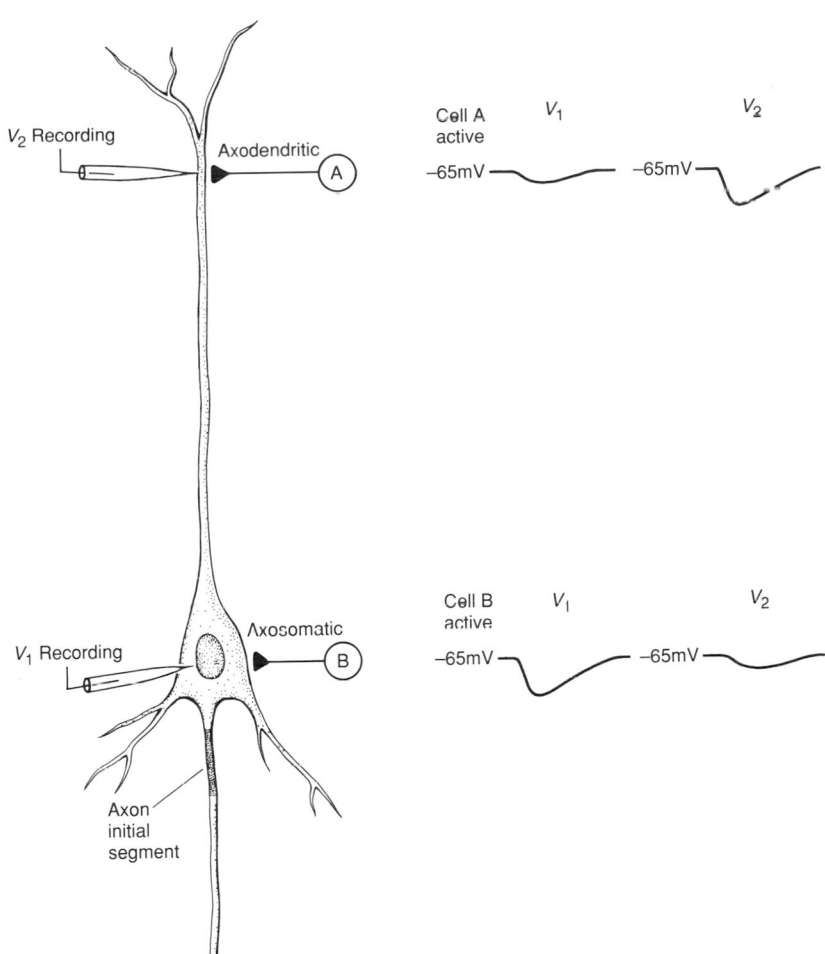

FIGURE 11-14

Comparison of electrotonic spread of inhibitory current from synapses at two different sites along the postsynaptic neuron. In this hypothetical experiment, the inputs from axosomatic and axodendritic synapses are compared by obtaining recordings from both the cell body (V_1) and the dendrite (V_2) of the postsynaptic cell. Stimulating cell **B** (axosomatic synapse) produces a large IPSP in the cell body. As a result it will have substantial influence on the trigger zone. Because the synaptic potential is initiated in the cell body it will not decay before arriving at the trigger zone in the initial segment of the axon. Stimulating cell **A** (axodendritic synapse) produces a small IPSP in the cell body because the synaptic potential is initiated in a distal dendrite. The amplitude of this IPSP decreases with distance and thus has only a minor influence on the trigger zone.

FIGURE 11-15

Interaction of excitation and inhibition on a single nerve cell. (Adapted from Eckart and Randall, 1989.)

A. An excitatory input on the base of a dendrite causes inward current to flow through cation-selective channels (Na^+ and K^+) at the dendrite that flows outward at the initial segment and produces a large depolarizing synaptic potential there.

B. An inhibitory input causes an outward (Cl^-) current at the synapse on the cell body and an inward current at other regions of the cell, producing a large hyperpolarization at the initial segment.

C. Summation of excitatory and inhibitory synaptic currents. Stimulation of separate presynaptic pathways gives rise to both excitatory and inhibitory synaptic currents. Now the channels opened by inhibitory pathway shunt the excitatory current and therefore they reduce the excitatory synaptic potential. This illustrates the shunting action of inhibition.

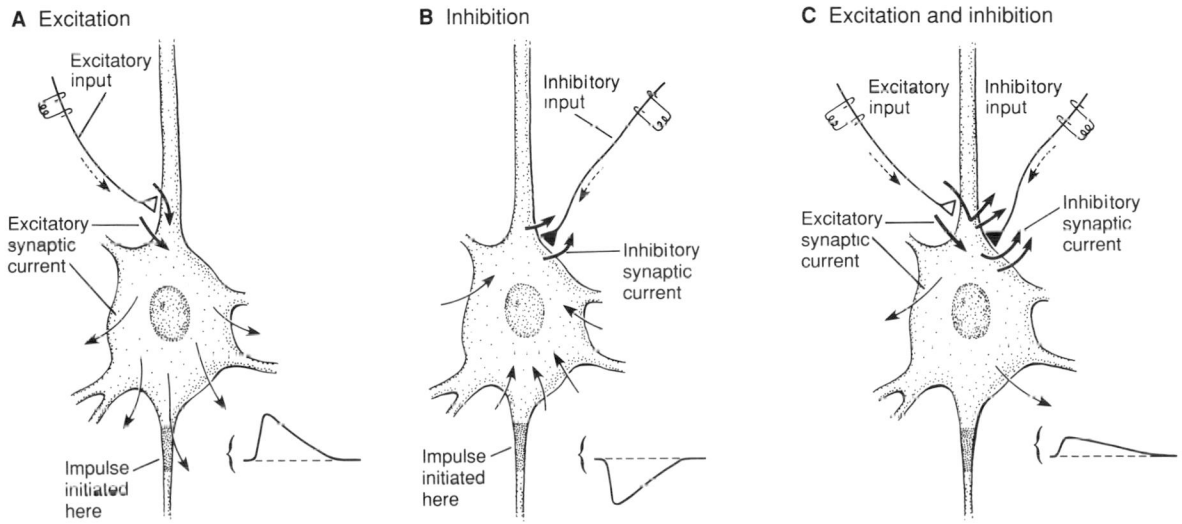

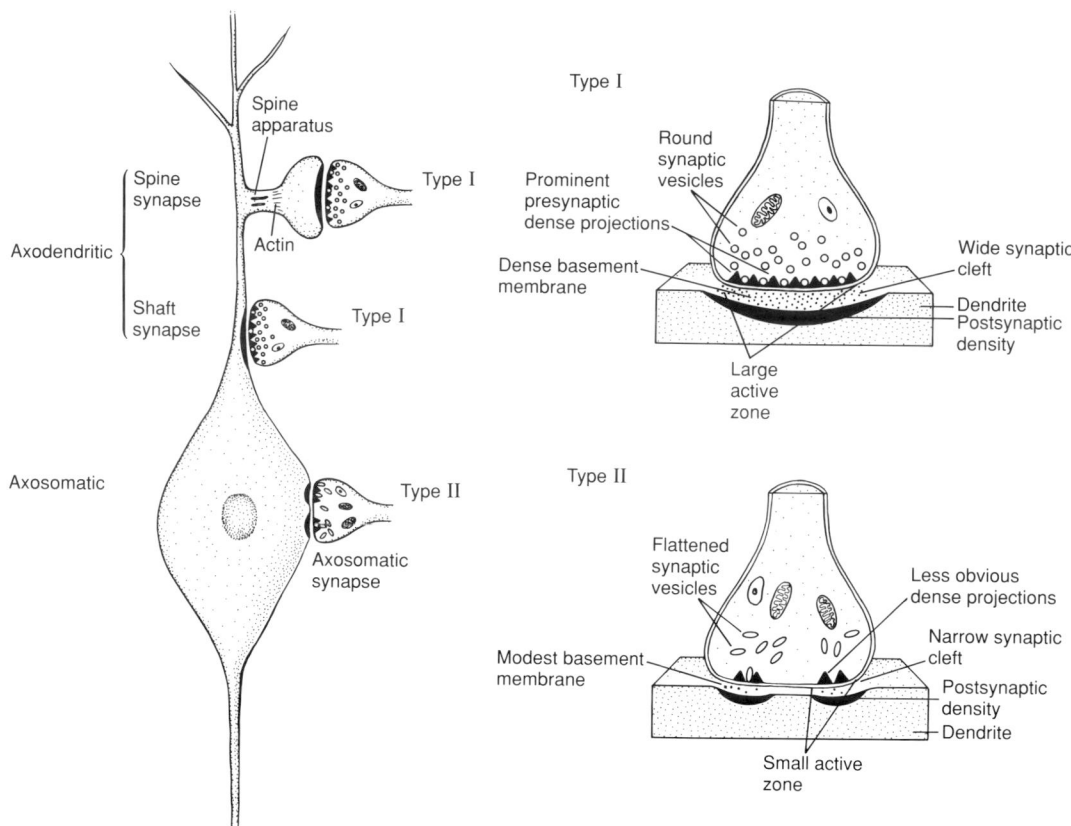

FIGURE 11–16

The two most common types of synapses in the central nervous system are Gray type I and type II synapses. Type I is usually excitatory, exemplified by glutaminergic synapses; type II is usually inhibitory, exemplified by GABAergic synapses. Differences include the shape of vesicles, prominence of presynaptic densities, total area of the active zone, width of the synaptic cleft, and presence of a dense basement membrane. Type I synapses end on dendritic shafts, but frequently contact dendritic spines. Type II synapses often end on the cell body.

ing Cl^- conductance and reducing, by shunting, much of the depolarization produced by the spreading excitatory current. As a result, the influence of the excitatory current on the potential of the membrane of the trigger zone will be strongly curtailed (Figure 11–15). In contrast, inhibitory actions at a remote part of a dendrite are much less effective in shunting excitatory actions or in affecting the more distant axonal trigger zone. Thus, in the brain important inhibitory input often occurs on the cell body of neurons.

Synapses on Dendritic Spines Are Often Excitatory

Central neurons have 20–40 main dendrites that branch into still finer dendritic processes (Chapter 3). Each branch has two major sites for synaptic inputs, the *main shaft* and the *spines* (Figure 11–13). The spine is a highly specialized input zone, typically consisting of a thin spine neck and a more bulbous spine head (Figure 11–16). Every spine has at least one synapse on its surface. In certain cortical neurons, such as the pyramidal cells of the CA1 region of the hippocampus, the spine head contains NMDA receptors.

Here the postsynaptic density is rich in Ca^{2+}/calmodulin-dependent protein kinase; this kinase can therefore be activated selectively when Ca^{2+} flows through the NMDA-activated channel. Thus, each spine represents a distinct biochemical compartment.

Synapses on Axon Terminals Are Often Modulatory

In contrast to axodendritic and axosomatic input, most axo-axonic synapses have no direct effect on the trigger zone of the postsynaptic cell. Instead, they indirectly affect the activity of the postsynaptic neuron by controlling the amount of transmitter it releases (see Chapter 13).

Excitatory and Inhibitory Synapses Have Distinctive Ultrastructures

As we learned in Chapter 9, the sign of a synaptic potential, whether it is excitatory or inhibitory, is determined not by the type of transmitter released from the presynaptic neuron, but by the type of ion channels gated by the transmitter in the postsynaptic cell. Most transmitters are recognized by several receptor-channels, and these mediate either excitatory or inhibitory potentials. Nevertheless, some transmitters act predominantly on receptors that are of one or another sign. For example, in the vertebrate brain, neurons that release glutamate typically act on receptors that produce excitation; neurons that release GABA or glycine act on inhibitory receptors. (An exception is found in the retina, which we discuss in a later chapter, and there are *many* exceptions in invertebrates.) The presynaptic terminals of excitatory and inhibitory neurons can sometimes be distinguished by their morphology.

The first studies of the ultrastructure of synaptic connections in the brain in the 1960s revealed two common morphological types. These are referred to as Gray type I and type II (after E. G. Gray, who described them). Type I synapses are often glutamatergic and therefore excitatory, whereas type II synapses are often GABAergic and therefore inhibitory. In type I synapses the cleft is slightly widened to approximately 30 nm, the presynaptic active zone is 1–2 μm^2 in area, and dense projections, the presumed release sites for the vesicles, are prominent. The synaptic vesicles tend to assume a characteristic round shape with certain electron microscopic fixatives. The dense region on the postsynaptic membrane also is extensive, and amorphous dense basement membrane material appears in the synaptic cleft. In type II synapses the cleft is 20 nm across, the active zone is smaller (less than 1 μm^2), the presynaptic membrane specializations and dense projections are less obvious, and there is little or no basement membrane within the cleft. Characteristically, the vesicles of type II synapses tend to be oval or flattened (Figure 11–16).

The morphological characteristics of type I and type II synapses proved to be only a first approximation of transmitter biochemistry. As we shall learn in Chapter 14, we have gained a much more precise and impressive morphological identification of transmitter type through the use of immunocytochemistry.

An Overall View

Chemical synaptic transmission in the central nervous system is similar in principle to that in the neuromuscular junction but differs in some essential ways. In the central nervous system, synaptic transmission can be either excitatory or inhibitory. Excitatory postsynaptic potentials in the central nervous system tend to be less than 1 mV in amplitude, compared to 70 mV in muscle. However, central neurons receive input from hundreds of presynaptic neurons, whereas only a single motor neuron innervates a single muscle fiber.

The major excitatory transmitter in the brain and spinal cord is glutamate. Four classes of postsynaptic receptors for glutamate have thus far been identified. The quisqualate and kainate receptors are very similar to each other and are thus often classified together as AMPA receptors. Like the nicotinic ACh receptor, these receptors also form channels permeable to both Na$^+$ and K$^+$, and they have reversal potentials around 0 mV. Ion flux through these channels contributes to the fast early peak of the EPSP. The third receptor, the NMDA receptor, forms a channel permeable to Ca^{2+} in addition to Na$^+$ and K$^+$. This receptor-channel is unique among transmitter-gated receptors in that it is also voltage dependent. In the resting state this channel is blocked by extracellular Mg^{2+} that is removed when the membrane is depolarized. Thus, both glutamate and depolarization are needed to open NMDA receptor-channels. Because of the delay in opening, ion flux through this channel contributes to the late component of the EPSP. Calcium influx through NMDA receptor-channels is thought to trigger cellular processes involved in certain types of memory as well as certain cell processes contributing to brain damage. The fourth class of glutamate receptor, quisqualate B, is not directly coupled to a channel but to a second-messenger pathway.

The major inhibitory transmitters in the central nervous system are GABA and glycine. The postsynaptic receptors for these transmitters form channels permeable to Cl$^-$. Gating of these channels permits Cl$^-$ influx into the cell, which hyperpolarizes the membrane. Opening these channels also increases the resting membrane conductance. Thus, opening these channels also shunts any excitatory current flowing into the cell. Two important classes of drugs, benzodiazepines and barbiturates, both bind to GABA receptors and enhance the Cl$^-$ flux through these channels in response to GABA.

All of the transmitter-gated channels thus far cloned show structural conservation. Like the ACh receptor, both the GABA and glycine receptors have multiple subunits, with each subunit containing four membrane-spanning segments. The GABA and glycine receptors are more similar to each other than to the ACh receptor, as is expected from the fact that they are anionic, not cationic, channels. Thus, where the ACh receptor has negatively charged amino acids (glutamate aspartate) in the segment lining the channel pore, the GABA and glycine receptors have positively charged residues (lysine, arginine).

Transmitter-gated and voltage-gated channels are produced by separate gene families. The voltage-dependent Na$^+$ and Ca^{2+} channels thus far cloned are all formed by a single subunit with internal repeats, whereas the transmitter-gated channel molecules have multiple subunits. Nonetheless, the overall structure of both families of molecules is similar. All classes of channels, including gap junctions, consist of several transmembrane sequences arranged symmetrically around a water-filled pore. Indeed, in the voltage-gated K$^+$ channel, where the subunit is a small protein, several subunits are thought to be required for the channel to function.

The thousands of excitatory and inhibitory inputs onto a single central neuron are not simply added together until threshold (−55 mV) is reached. The temporal and spatial summation of inputs within a single cell depends critically on the passive properties of the cell, specifically its time and length constants. The location of a particular synapse also contributes to its efficacy. Excitatory glutaminergic synapses tend to be located on the dendrites. In contrast, inhibitory synapses are found primarily on the cell body, where they can very effectively override excitatory inputs from the cell's axon and dendrites. The final integration of inputs to the cell is made at the axon hillock, the region of the cell body membrane near the initial segment of the axon. This region contains the highest density of Na^+ channels in the cell and thus has the lowest threshold for spike initiation.

Much of the discussion in this chapter has focused on the model of the neuron first outlined by Ramón y Cajal and considered in Chapters 2 and 3. According to this model, the dendritic arbor is specialized as the receptive pole of the neuron, the axon is the conducting portion, and the axon terminal is the transmitting pole. This model implies that the nervous system is composed of information receiving and transmitting units. Most brain regions are not quite this simple, however. As we shall see in considering the sensory and the motor systems, cells in many brain regions transform information in addition to transmitting it.

Selected Readings

Choi, D. W. 1988. Glutamate neurotoxicity and diseases of the nervous system. Neuron 1:623–634.

Cooper, J. R., Bloom, F. E., and Roth, R. H. 1991. The Biochemical Basis of Neuropharmacology, 6th ed. New York: Oxford University Press.

Eccles, J. C. 1964. The Physiology of Synapses. Berlin: Springer.

Heuser, J. E., and Reese, T. S. 1977. Structure of the synapse. In E. R. Kandel (ed.), Handbook of Physiology, Section 1: The Nervous System, Vol. I. Cellular Biology of Neurons, Part 1. Bethesda, Md.: American Physiological Society, pp. 261–294.

Hollmann, M., O'Shea-Greenfield, A., Rogers, S. W., and Heinemann, S. 1989. Cloning by functional expression of a member of the glutamate receptor family. Nature 342:643–648.

Masu, M., Tanabe, Y., Tsuchida, K., Shigemoto, R., and Nakanishi, S. 1991. Sequence and expression of a metabotropic glutamate receptor. Nature 349:760–765.

Nicoll, R. A., Malenka, R. C., Kauer, J. A. 1990. Functional comparison of neurotransmitter receptor subtypes in mammalian central nervous system. Physiol. Rev. 70:513–565.

Pritchett, D. B., Sontheimer, H., Shivers, B. D., Ymer, S., Kettenmann, H., Schofield, P. R., and Seeburg, P. H. 1989. Importance of a novel $GABA_A$ receptor subunit for benzodiazepine pharmacology. Nature 338:582–585.

Snyder, S. H. 1984. Drug and neurotransmitter receptors in the brain. Science 224:22–31.

Sommer, B., Keinänen, K., Verdoorn, T. A., Wisden, W., Burnashev, N., Herb, A., Köhler, M., Takagi, T., Sakmann, B., and Seeburg, P. H. 1990. Flip and flop: A cell-specific functional switch in glutamate-operated channels of the CNS. Science 249:1580–1585.

Stevens, C. F. 1987. Molecular neurobiology: Channel families in the brain. Nature 328:198–199.

References

Coombs, J. S., Eccles, J. C., and Fatt, P. 1955. The specific ionic conductances and the ionic movements across the motoneuronal membrane that produce the inhibitory post-synaptic potential. J. Physiol. (Lond.) 130:326–373.

Finkel, A. S., and Redman, S. J. 1983. The synaptic current evoked in cat spinal motoneurones by impulses in single group Ia axons. J. Physiol. (Lond.) 342:615–632.

Gray, E. G. 1963. Electron microscopy of presynaptic organelles of the spinal cord. J. Anat. 97:101–106.

Grenningloh, G., Rienitz, A., Schmitt, B., Methsfessel, C., Zensen, M., Beyreuther, K., Gundelfinger, E. D., and Betz, H. 1987. The strychnine-binding subunit of the glycine receptor shows homology with nicotinic acetylcholine receptors. Nature 328:215–220.

Hamill, O. P., Bormann, J., and Sakmann, B. 1983. Activation of multiple-conductance state chloride channels in spinal neurones by glycine and GABA. Nature 305:805–808.

Hestrin, S., Nicoll, R. A., Perkel, D. J., and Sah, P. 1990. Analysis of excitatory synaptic action in pyramidal cells using whole-cell recording from rat hippocampal slices. J. Physiol. (Lond.) 422:203–225.

Miller, C. 1989. Genetic manipulation of ion channels: A new approach to structure and mechanism. Neuron 2:1195–1205.

Olsen, R. W. 1982. Drug interactions at the GABA receptor-ionophore complex. Annu. Rev. Pharmacol. Toxicol. 22:245–277.

Palay, S. L. 1958. The morphology of synapses in the central nervous system. Exp. Cell. Res. Suppl. 5:275–293.

Peters, A., Palay, S. L., and Webster, H. deF. 1991. The Fine Structure of the Nervous System: Neurons and Their Supporting Cells, 3rd ed. New York: Oxford University Press.

Redman, S. 1979. Junctional mechanisms at group Ia synapses. Prog. Neurobiol. 12:33–83.

Sherrington, C. S. 1897. The Central Nervous System. Part III of M. Foster, A Text Book of Physiology, 7th ed. London: Macmillan.

Sigel, E., Stephenson, F. A., Mamalaki, C., and Bernard, E. A. 1983. A γ-aminobutyric acid/benzodiazepine receptor complex of bovine cerebral cortex. J. Biol. Chem. 258:6965–6971.

Stevens, C. F. 1991. Ion channels: Making a submicroscopic hole in one. Nature 349:657–658.

Unwin, N. 1989. The structure of ion channels in membranes of excitable cells. Neuron 3:665–676.

Watkins, J. C., and Evans, R. H. 1981. Excitatory amino acid transmitters. Annu. Rev. Pharmacol. Toxicol. 21:165–204.

James H. Schwartz
Eric R. Kandel

12

Synaptic Transmission Mediated By Second Messengers

Different Second-Messenger Pathways Share a Common Molecular Logic

   The Cyclic AMP Pathway Involves a Polar and Diffusible Cytoplasmic Messenger

   Some Second Messengers Are Generated Through Hydrolysis of Phospholipids

Second-Messenger Pathways Can Interact with One Another

Second Messengers Often Act Through Protein Phosphorylation to Open or Close Ion Channels

Second Messengers and G-Proteins Can Sometimes Act Directly on Ion Channels

Second Messengers Can Alter the Properties of Transmitter Receptors: Desensitization

Second Messengers Can Regulate Gene Expression and Thereby Endow Synaptic Transmission with Long-Lasting Consequences

Other Second-Messenger Pathways: Tyrosine Kinases and Cyclic GMP

An Overall View

Synaptic receptors have two major functions: recognition of specific transmitters and activation of effectors. The receptor first recognizes and binds a transmitter in the external environment of the cell; then, as a consequence of binding, the receptor alters the cell's biochemical state. Receptors for neurotransmitters so far identified can be divided into two major families according to how the receptor and effector functions are coupled (Figures 12–1 and 12–2). In one family—the receptors that gate ion channels directly—the two functions are carried out by different domains of a single macromolecule. This family contains all of the receptors that we considered in preceding chapters in which the recognition domain directly gates an ion channel. It includes the nicotinic acetylcholine (ACh), the γ-aminobutyric acid (GABA), the glycine, the AMPA (kainate-quisqualate), and the *N*-methyl-D-aspartate (NMDA) class of glutamate receptors.

In the other family—the receptors that gate channels indirectly or G-protein coupled receptors—recognition of the transmitter and activation of effectors are carried out by distinct and separate molecules. These receptors are considered in this chapter. This family includes the α- and β-adrenergic, serotonin, dopamine, and muscarinic ACh receptors, and receptors for neuropeptides as well as rhodopsin (Figure 12–2). In each member of this family, the receptor molecule is coupled to its effector molecule by a guanosine nucleotide-binding protein (G-protein). Activation of the effector component requires the participation of several distinct proteins. Typically the effector is an enzyme that produces a diffusible second messenger, for example, cyclic adenosine monophosphate (cAMP), diacylglycerol, or an inositol polyphosphate. These second messengers in turn trigger a biochemical cascade either activating specific protein kinases that phosphorylate a variety of the cell's proteins or mobilizing Ca^{2+} ions from intracellular stores, thus initiating the reactions that change the cell's biochemical state. In some instances,

174

A Directly gated ion channel receptors

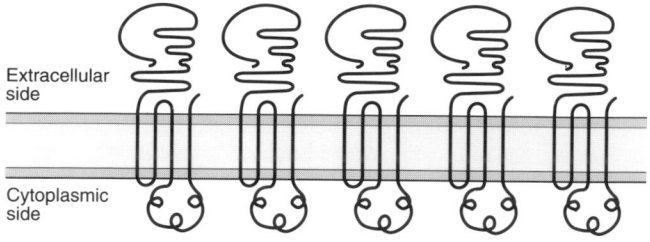

FIGURE 12–1

Structural representation of two families of neurotransmitter receptors and ion channels.

A. Directly gated ion channel receptors have several subunits. Here, the receptor and the ion channel represent different domains of the same protein.

B. G-protein coupled receptors. Here, the receptor activates ion channels and other substrates indirectly by activating a G-protein that engages an effector (second-messenger) enzyme.

B G-Protein coupled receptors

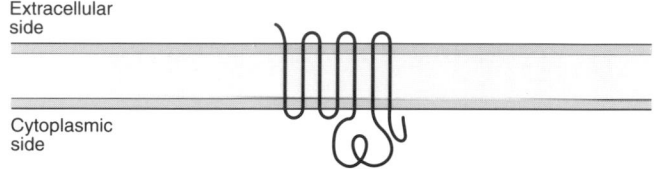

FIGURE 12–2

General scheme of synaptic second messengers. Only a few key signal transduction pathways have been identified thus far, of which three are illustrated. These all follow a common sequence of steps **(left)**. Chemical transmitters arriving at receptor molecules in the plasma membrane **(gray)** activate a closely related family of transducer proteins that activate primary effector enzymes. These enzymes produce a second messenger that activates a secondary effector or acts directly on a target (regulatory) protein. The first pathway illustrated generates the second messenger cAMP, which is produced by adenylyl cyclase when activated by a G-protein, so called because it requires GTP to function. The G-protein shown is G_s, because it stimulates the cyclase. Some receptors activate G_i, a G-protein that inhibits the cyclase. The second pathway, activated by a muscarinic ACh receptor, uses another kind of G-protein to activate phospholipase C (PLC). The enzyme hydrolyzes phosphatidyl-inositol 4,5-biphosphate (PIP_2) yielding a pair of second messengers, DAG and inositol 1,4,5-triphosphate (IP_3). IP_3 mobilizes Ca^{2+} from internal stores. This pathway is not known to recognize inhibitory external signals. DAG activates protein kinase C (PKC). The third major system activates the arachidonic acid cascade through phospholipase A_2 (PLA_2).

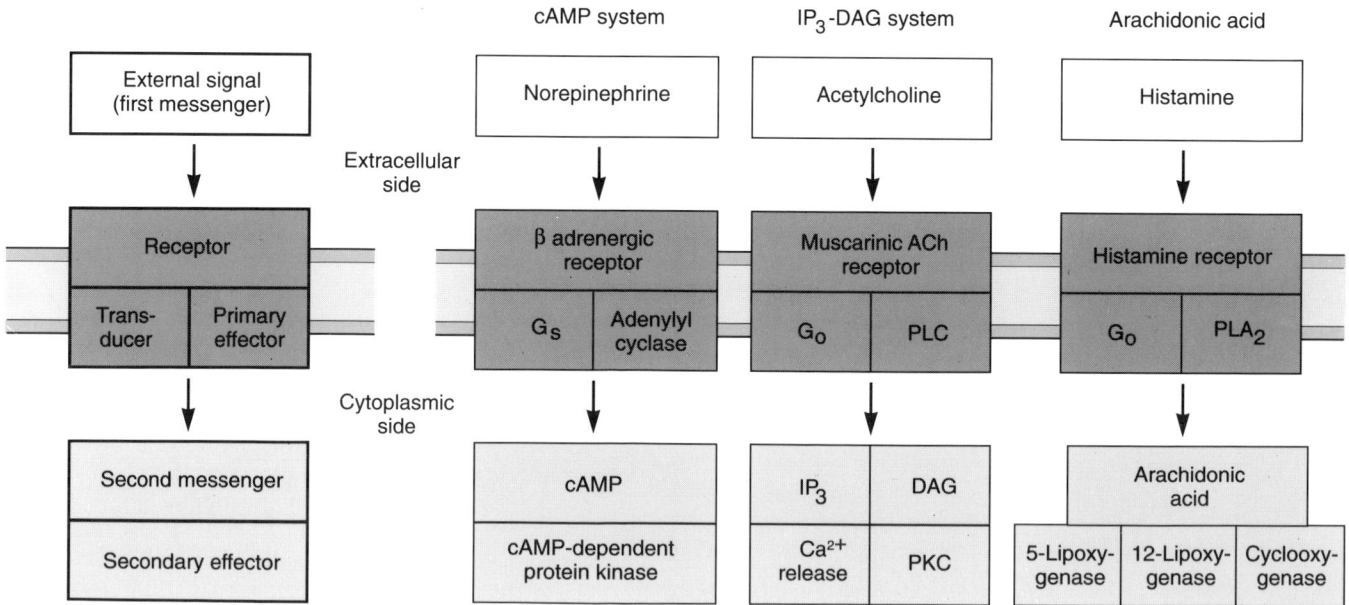

however, the G-protein or the second messenger (cAMP, cGMP, or metabolites of arachidonic acid) can act directly on an ion channel.

As might be expected, the structural differences between the two families of receptors are reflected in their functions. Thus, neurobiologists often classify the actions of transmitters on receptors as being fast or slow, a distinction that refers both to speed of onset and duration of the postsynaptic effect. Direct gating of ion channels usually is rapid—on the order of milliseconds—because it involves only a change in the conformation of a single macromolecule. In contrast, receptors linked to G-proteins are slow in onset (hundreds of milliseconds to seconds) and longer lasting (seconds to minutes) because they involve a cascade of reactions, each of which takes time.

There are perhaps 100 substances that act as transmitters, each of which activates its own specific receptors on the cell surface. But there are many fewer major second-messenger pathways. Only four of these have been well characterized. The first second messenger to be characterized was cAMP. In 1950 Earl Sutherland and his colleagues discovered that cAMP regulates carbohydrate metabolism in liver and muscle. The cAMP cascade probably is still the one best characterized, and the work on cAMP has greatly influenced our thinking about second-messenger mechanisms. Two more recently discovered cascades are initiated by the hydrolysis of phospholipids in the cell's plasma membrane. One of them produces two

messengers, *inositol polyphosphates* and *diacylglycerol;* the other starts with the release of *arachidonic acid.*

There are still other cascades. For example, there are receptors that activate guanylate cyclase and those that activate tyrosine kinases. The functions of these effectors in the nervous system are not yet as well understood. We shall briefly consider them at the end of this chapter.

Different Second-Messenger Pathways Share a Common Molecular Logic

Despite their differences, second-messenger pathways share many common features (Figure 12–2). For example, as we have seen, all receptors that initiate second-messenger actions belong to a common gene family. Unlike the receptors that directly gate channels, which consist of *several* subunits that form a channel through the membrane, receptors that are coupled to G-proteins and generate second messengers consist of a single subunit with seven characteristic membrane-spanning regions (Figure 12–3).

The binding of transmitter to a receptor with seven membrane-spanning regions activates a *transducing G-protein.* (G-proteins are discussed later in greater detail.) In the resting state a G-protein binds a molecule of GDP and is inactive. When transmitter is bound, the receptor interacts with the G-protein, producing a conformational change that causes GTP to displace GDP (Figures 12–2 and 12–4). The activated G-protein then binds

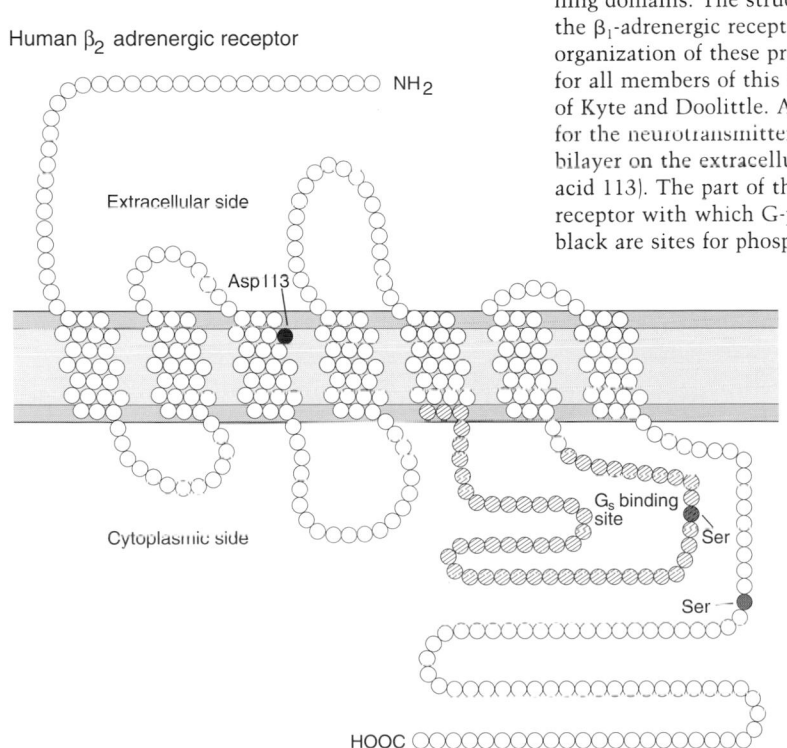

FIGURE 12 3

The structure of a G-protein coupled receptor contains seven membrane-spanning domains. The structure of the β_2-adrenergic receptor is similar to that of the β_1-adrenergic receptor, the muscarinic ACh receptor, and to rhodopsin. The organization of these protein molecules within the membrane, which is similar for all members of this family of receptors, is based on the hydrophobicity index of Kyte and Doolittle. An important functional feature is that the binding site for the neurotransmitter (in this example norepinephrine) is just within the lipid bilayer on the extracellular surface of the cell (here amino acid residue aspartic acid 113). The part of the receptor indicated by striped circles is the part of the receptor with which G-protein associates. The two serine residues indicated in black are sites for phosphorylation. (Adapted from Frielle et al., 1989.)

Human β_2 adrenergic receptor

NH$_2$

Extracellular side

Asp 113

Cytoplasmic side

G$_s$ binding site

Ser

Ser

HOOC

176

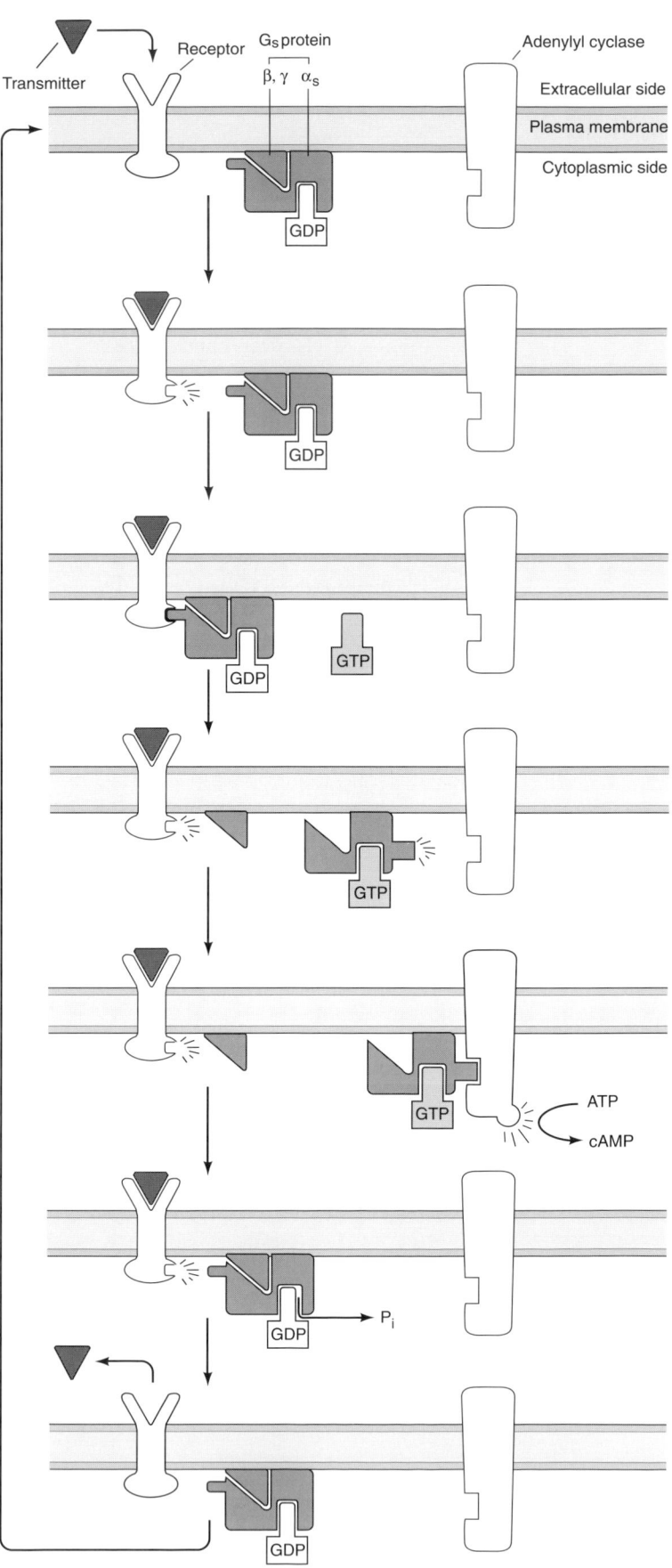

FIGURE 12–4

The cAMP cycle. Binding of a transmitter to the portion of the receptor on the external surface of the neuron allows the stimulatory G-protein (G_s) bearing GDP to bind to an intracellular domain of the receptor. This association with the transmitter–receptor complex causes GTP to replace GDP and the α_s-subunit to dissociate from the $\beta\gamma$-subunits of the G-protein. The α_s-subunit, now bearing GTP, next associates with an intracellular domain of adenylyl cyclase, thereby activating the enzyme to produce many molecules of cAMP from ATP. The α_s-subunit, when bound to the cyclase, is a GTPase. Hydrolysis of GTP to GDP and inorganic phosphate (P_i) leads to the dissociation of α_s from the cyclase and its reassociation with the $\beta\gamma$-subunits. The cyclase then stops producing the second messenger. Some time during this cycle the transmitter dissociates from the receptor. The initial inactive state of the system is restored when the ligand binding site on the receptor is empty, the three subunits of the G-protein have reassociated, and the guanine nucleotide binding site on the $\beta\gamma$-subunit is occupied by GDP. (Adapted from Alberts et al., 1989.)

to an effector enzyme with a catalytic domain on the cytoplasmic surface of the membrane: adenylyl cyclase in the cAMP system, phospholipase C in the diacylglycerol-inositol polyphosphate system, and phospholipase A_2 in the arachidonic system. In each of these systems the second messengers formed lead to changes in specific proteins within the cell. This is achieved either by binding of the second messenger to a target (or regulator) protein directly, or by activating a protein kinase that phosphorylates the target protein (a kinase is the generic term for an enzyme that uses ATP as a donor of phosphoryl groups).

What does phosphorylation of a substrate accomplish? The introduction of the negatively charged phosphoryl group can alter the conformation of a protein to modify the function of an enzyme, a cytoskeletal protein, a subunit of an ion channel, or a transcriptional activator (a DNA-binding protein that can regulate transcription). For example, by decreasing an enzyme's affinity for its substrates or by changing its location within the cell, phosphorylation can diminish the enzyme's activity. Conversely, activity can be enhanced if phosphorylation increases the affinity for its substrates, if it positions the enzyme in a more effective subcellular locale, or prevents association of the enzyme with an inhibitor. In some neurons, protein phosphorylation can lead to closure or opening of ion channels and thus modulate the signaling properties of those cells. These changes, which depend on transiently elevated concentrations of second messenger in the postsynaptic neuron, usually last from seconds to minutes, longer than the changes in membrane potential produced by receptors that directly gate ion channels. The duration of the biochemical changes is limited by intracellular enzymes that inactivate the second messengers and by protein phosphatases that hydrolyze phosphoryl groups from the protein.

The Cyclic AMP Pathway Involves a Polar and Diffusible Cytoplasmic Messenger

The cAMP pathway is the prototype of an intracellular signaling pathway that makes use of a water-soluble second messenger that diffuses within the cytoplasm. This pathway illustrates the typical steps in a neuronal second-messenger pathway (Figures 12–4 and 12–5). Binding of transmitter to receptor (for example, the β-adrenergic receptor that is discussed later in this chapter) leads to the activation of a stimulatory G-protein called G_s, which then activates the enzyme adenylyl cyclase. This enzyme has recently been cloned by Randall Reed and Alfred Gilman, and shown to be an integral membrane protein that spans the plasma membrane many times. (The inferred amino acid sequence suggests that the cyclase is distantly related to bacterial transporters). The cyclase in turn catalyzes the conversion of ATP to cAMP. The GTP–G-protein complex and the catalytic subunit of the cyclase together constitute the active form of the enzyme. When associated with the catalytic subunit, G_s also acts as a GTPase, hydrolyzing its bound GTP to GDP. As a result, the G-protein dissociates from the cyclase, stopping the synthesis of cAMP (Figure 12–4). The receptor and the

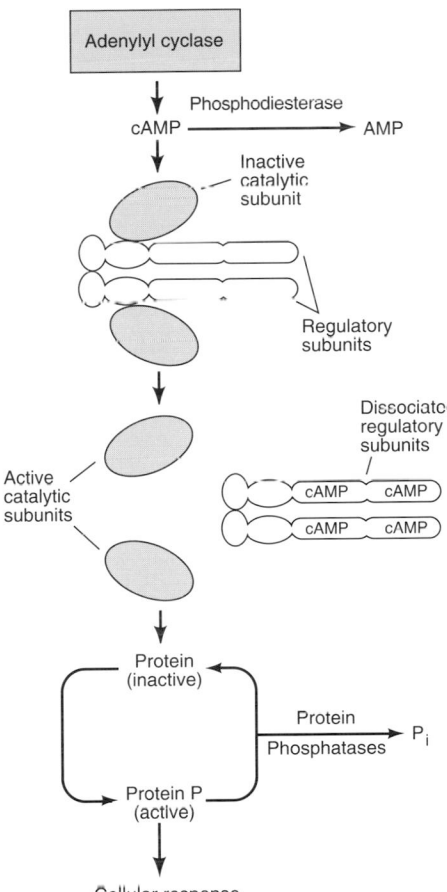

FIGURE 12–5

The cAMP pathway. Adenylyl cyclase converts ATP into cAMP. Four cAMP molecules bind to the two regulatory subunits of the cAMP-dependent protein kinase, liberating the two catalytic subunits, which are then free to phosphorylate specific substrate proteins that regulate a cellular response. Two kinds of enzymes regulate this pathway. Several phosphodiesterases convert cAMP to AMP (which is inactive), and several kinds of protein phosphatases remove phosphate groups from the regulator (substrate) proteins.

cyclase thus do not interact directly, but are coupled by a transducer protein. The duration of cAMP synthesis is regulated by the GTPase activity of the G-protein. After the GTP is hydrolyzed, the G-protein is able to bind a new transmitter–receptor complex at the surface of the cell, and thereby activate the cyclase again.

G-proteins are not integral membrane components. Rather, they are associated with the internal leaflet of the plasma membrane and consist of three subunits: α, β, and γ. The α-subunit is only loosely associated with the membrane. There are many types of α-subunits and these couple different members of the seven membrane-spanning receptor family to a variety of primary effector enzymes. In contrast to the β-adrenergic receptor, which activates the cyclase through the α-subunit of G_s, other receptors (for example, α-adrenergic receptors or certain muscarinic ACh receptors) inhibit the cyclase because they operate through G_i, another G-protein, that contains a different α-subunit. More than a dozen varieties of G-proteins that have been identified, primarily by molecular cloning studies, which differ in their α-subunit. Compared to other organs of the body, the brain contains an exceptionally high proportion of these *other* G-proteins, which now are collectively called G_o (*o* for other). These G-proteins mediate the activation of guanylate cyclase, phospholipases A_2 and C, and most probably of many other signal transduction mechanisms not yet identified (Figure 12–2).

One way the α-subunit of G_s can be distinguished from those of the other types of G-proteins (G_i and G_o) is by its response to bacterial toxins. G_s is permanently activated by an enzymatic reaction catalyzed by the toxin from the cholera vibrio. (The action of the toxin on the G_s of intestinal cells is the initial molecular step in the pathogenesis of cholera.) In contrast, G_i and G_o are inactivated by a similar reaction catalyzed by the toxin from the bacterium *Bordetella pertussis*, which causes whooping cough. Common to these reactions is the formation of a covalent ADP-ribosylated derivative of the α-subunit with NAD^+. As we have seen, all of these α-subunits bind to similar β- and γ-subunits, of which fewer isoforms exist. As a β-γ complex, these are much more tightly fixed to the membrane than the α-subunit. G-proteins outnumber the receptor molecules in a cell. In fact, the molecular stoichiometry indicates that they act to amplify the small synaptic signal (represented by the relatively few chemical transmitter and receptor molecules) into the larger number of activated cyclase complexes needed to catalyze the synthesis of an effective concentration of cAMP within the cell.

Further amplification occurs with the protein kinase reaction, the next step in the cAMP cascade (Figure 12–5). Cyclic AMP activates the cAMP-dependent protein kinase by causing its two regulatory subunits (R) to dissociate from the catalytic subunits (C) according to the reaction:

$$R_2C_2 + 4\ cAMP \rightleftharpoons 2R(2\ cAMP) + 2C.$$

When combined, the tetrameric holoenzyme, R_2C_2, is inactive. There are several isoforms of regulatory subunits. Nevertheless, all regulatory subunits contain three functional domains: (1) an N-terminal region responsible for binding to its counterpart, which is always the identical isoform; (2) an N-terminal region that is responsible for inhibiting the catalytic subunit; and (3) two similar binding sites for cAMP. When bound to these binding sites, cAMP is not chemically changed; rather, it alters the conformation of the regulatory subunits so that they dissociate from the catalytic subunits. Each catalytic subunit is then free to transfer the γ phosphoryl group of ATP to the hydroxyl groups of specific serine and threonine residues in protein:

$$\text{Protein} + \text{ATP} \xrightarrow{C} \text{Phosphoprotein} + \text{ADP}.$$

Each catalytic subunit contains a binding site for ATP that is highly conserved in other kinases, as well as a site that recognizes specific sequences of amino acids in substrate proteins. Before describing these sequences further we need to discuss the molecular mechanisms by which the catalytic subunits are regulated (Figure 12–6). An essential feature of regulation is the association with the regulatory subunits through the N-terminal domain already mentioned. Certain isoforms of the regulatory subunits can be phosphorylated in this domain by the catalytic subunits. This autophosphorylation reaction, which is intramolecular, is typical of many protein kinases. Thus the regulatory domain can serve as a substrate for an enzyme's *own* catalytic domain. When the concentration of cAMP falls within the cell, the second messenger dissociates from the free regulatory subunits, which then combine with catalytic subunits again. Ora Rosen and her colleagues found that regulatory subunits that are phosphorylated recombine with catalytic subunits at a much slower rate than do dephosphorylated regulatory subunits.

The other serine and threonine protein kinases that are discussed in this chapter—the cGMP-dependent, the Ca^{2+}/calmodulin-dependent, and protein kinase C—have regulatory and catalytic domains present within the same protein. Regulation of cAMP-dependent protein phosphorylation illustrates the molecular principle common to the regulation of almost all protein kinases, whether the regulatory domain is situated on separate subunits or is a part of the same polypeptide chain as the catalytic region. As we saw, some regulatory subunits actually are substrates for phosphorylation. To explain further how the regulatory subunits and the regulatory domains of the other protein kinases operate, it is important to know that a protein can only be a substrate for a kinase if it has a special *phosphorylation sequence*—a specific sort of amino acid sequence around the serine or threonine residues to be phosphorylated. These phosphorylation sequences are a necessary part of the binding site on the substrate protein for the catalytic subunit during the phosphorylation reaction itself. One of the suitable sequences for the cAMP-dependent protein kinase is –Arg–Arg–X–Ser–. Other residues near this sequence also contribute to the affinity of the protein substrate for the kinase.

An important feature of kinase regulatory domains is that they all contain a sequence similar to the phosphorylation sequence, except that the serine (or threonine) in the regulatory domain is replaced by an amino acid residue that does not have a hydroxyl group. Consequently, this region of the regulatory subunit serves as a *pseudosubstrate*. Even though it binds to the catalytic site with high affinity, this part of the regulatory subunit cannot be phosphorylated. Thus, the regulatory domain acts as a competitive inhibitor of the kinase reaction. Bruce Kemp and his colleagues have synthesized peptides with serine residues that act as artificial kinase substrates or with residues that cannot be phosphorylated and therefore act as pseudosubstrate inhibitors. As already mentioned, some isoforms of regulatory subunits *also* have a functioning substrate domain. In these subunits, the amino acid to be phosphorylated is masked except in the presence of cAMP.

A cAMP-dependent protein kinase

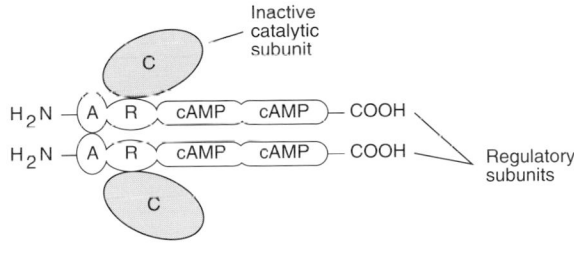

B cGMP-dependent protein kinase

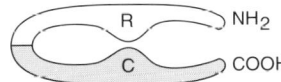

C Protein kinase C

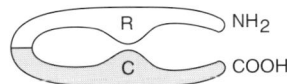

D Ca²⁺/Calmodulin-dependent protein

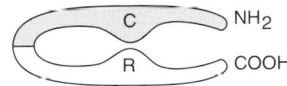

E Tyrosine protein kinase

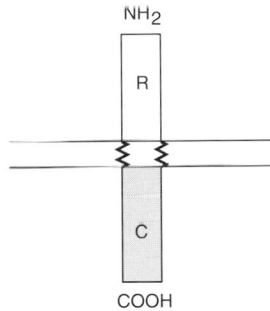

FIGURE 12–6

All protein kinases are related and are regulated in a similar way. In the absence of an activator, the kinases are enzymatically inactive because their catalytic domains are inhibited. With the serine/threonine-specific protein kinase (**A–D**), the catalytic domains are actually covered by regulatory domains that are similar in amino acid sequence to the sequences required for phosphorylation in substrate proteins, but, unlike substrate proteins, the serine or threonine residue to which a phosphoryl group would be transferred is absent. Its place is taken by an amino acid residue lacking a hydroxyl group. Thus, these regulatory domains can be regarded as *pseudosubstrate inhibitors.*

A. In the cAMP-dependent protein kinase two identical regulatory subunits associate with each other at site **A** and with the catalytic subunits at site **R**. These two sites are situated at the N-terminal of the subunit molecule. Each regulatory subunit also contains two binding sites for cAMP, which are situated toward the C-terminal of the molecule. When cAMP is bound, a conformational change in the regulatory domains (**R**) of the subunits results in their dissociation from the two catalytic subunits. Dissociated catalytic subunits then can phosphorylate substrate proteins.

B-D. In the other major protein kinases the regulatory domains (**R**) and the catalytic domains (**C**) are part of the same polypeptide chain. The cGMP-dependent protein kinase is quite similar to the cAMP-dependent protein kinase in amino acid sequence. Greatest similarity exists in their catalytic domains. The regulatory domains of both the cGMP-dependent protein kinase (**B**) and protein kinase C (**C**) are situated at the N-terminal end of the molecules. In the Ca²⁺/calmodulin-dependent protein kinase (**D**), the regulatory domain is in the C-terminal region of the molecule. Unlike the other kinases this enzyme is present in the cell as a complex of several of these kinase molecules, each with similar biochemical properties. In all of these enzymes binding of second messenger is thought to unfold the molecule, thereby exposing and activating the catalytic region.

E. Receptor-mediated regulation of tyrosine kinases is somewhat different. The regulatory domains are extracellular. Binding of a transmitter, hormone, or growth factor to the regulatory domain, as in receptors, causes a conformational change in the molecule through the plasma membrane to activate the intracellular catalytic domain.

Some Second Messengers Are Generated Through Hydrolysis of Phospholipids

A similar logic is evident in the way second messengers are generated through the hydrolysis of phospholipids in the inner leaflet of the plasma membrane. Hydrolysis is catalyzed by two specific enzymes, phospholipase C and phospholipase A₂, each of which can be activated by different G-proteins. Phospholipases are designated according to the bond that they hydrolyze in the phospholipid. Although similar in enzymatic mechanism to the soluble pancreatic lipases that digest fats in the small intestine, in neurons these specific lipases are membrane-associated proteins.

Before considering the three major second-messenger cascades that stem from these two phospholipases, it is helpful to know the structure of phosphatidyl inositol (PI)

and to understand that the fatty acid composition of this phospholipid in brain is exceptionally uniform. Almost all of the phosphoinositides of brain have the following chemical structure:

Phosphatidylinositol (PI)

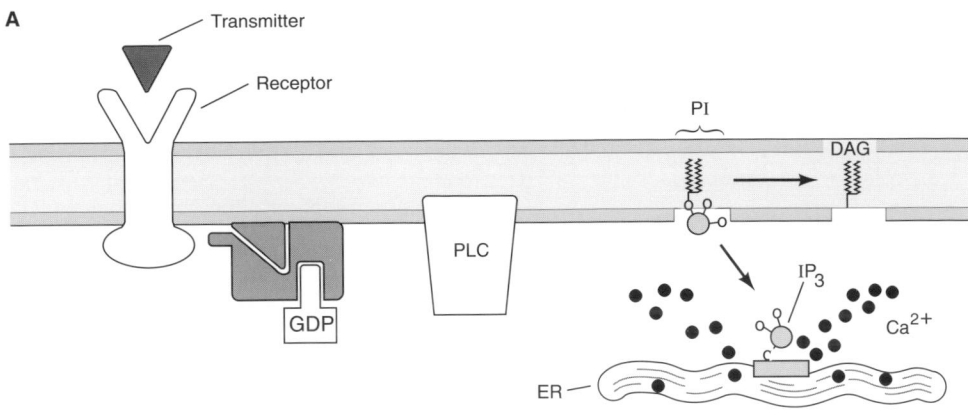

B Ca²⁺/Calmodulin-dependent protein kinase

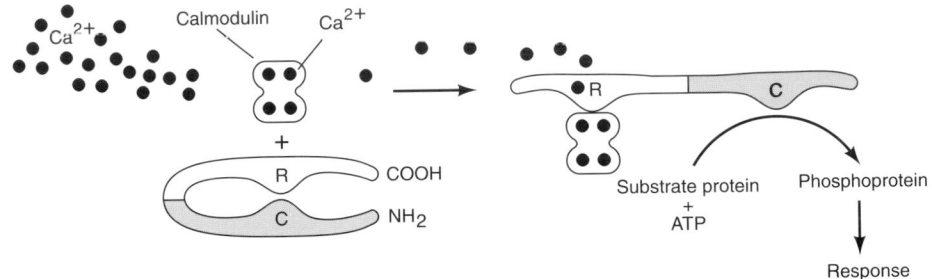

C Protein kinase C

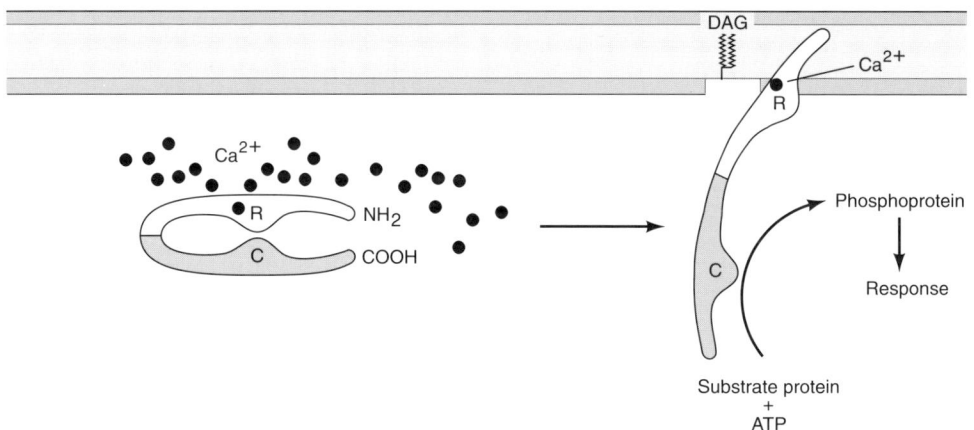

FIGURE 12–7
Activation of IP$_3$, the Ca^{2+}/calmodulin-dependent protein kinase, and PKC.

A. In the inositol-lipid pathway, binding of transmitter to a receptor, activates a G-protein, which in turn activates phospholipase C. This phospholipase cleaves the phosphatidyl inositol (PI) PIP$_2$ into two second messengers, IP$_3$ and diacylglycerol (DAG). IP$_3$ is water soluble, and can diffuse into the cytoplasm.

There it binds to a receptor on the endoplasmic reticulum to release Ca^{2+} from internal stores.

B. Ca^{2+} bound to calmodulin activates the protein kinase.

C. DAG, the other second messenger produced by the cleavage of PIP$_2$, remains in the membrane, where it activates PKC; for this activation membrane phospholipid is necessary. Thus, PKC is active only when translocated from the cytoplasm to the membrane. Some isoforms of PKC do not require Ca^{2+} for activation.

All phospholipids consist of a glycerol molecule esterified at its first and second hydroxyl group (1 and 2) to fatty acids; the third hydroxyl group (3) forms a diester of phosphoric acid and one of four special alcohols (choline, in phosphatidylcholine, PC; serine, in PS; ethanolamine, in PE; and inositol, in PI). In brain the ester bond at the first position is usually made with stearic acid (18:0; 18 carbons, no double bonds), and at the second, with arachidonic acid (20:4), an unsaturated 20-carbon fatty acid. At the third carbon of the glycerol backbone is a diester with myo-inositol, a six-carbon cyclic polyalcohol (the term *myo-* refers to one of nine possible isomers of hexahydroxycyclohexane, the only isomer present in natural membranes). The hydroxyl group designated **1** participates in the diester linking the phosphatidyl moiety; other hydroxyl groups in the inositol moiety may bear phosphoryl groups. The bonds hydrolyzed by phospholipase C and A$_2$ are also indicated in the formula.

The Diacylglycerol-IP$_3$ System Is Produced by Activating Phospholipase C. Receptor-activated phospholipase C produces diacylglycerol and inositol 1-phosphate (IP$_1$) from PI itself, inositol-1,4-*bis* phosphate (IP$_2$) from phospholipid inositol phosphate (PIP$_1$), or inositol trisphosphate (IP$_3$) from PIP$_2$. IP$_3$ can be converted to IP$_4$ and IP$_5$ by further phosphorylation with specific kinases. The 1,4,5-isomer of IP$_3$ serves as another water-soluble, diffusible second messenger. It combines with specific receptors on membranous organelles (the endoplasmic reticulum and mitochondria) to release Ca^{2+} from endogenous stores, in particular from the endoplasmic reticulum (Figure 12–7). 1,3,4,5-IP$_4$ is also suspected of being a second messenger that acts on Ca^{2+} channels in the plasma membrane. It remains to be determined whether other inositol polyphosphate intermediates also play a role in intracellular signaling.

The metabolism of the inositol phosphates is quite complex, and much still remains to be discovered. These compounds are degraded by phosphatases in several reaction sequences to the free alcohol inositol, which is reincorporated into membrane phospholipids. The final step in all of these degradative pathways is blocked by Li$^+$ ion, which inhibits the release of free inositol from the three positional isomers (1, 3, and 4) of IP$_1$. This effect may contribute to the therapeutic usefulness of Li$^+$ in the treatment of manic depressive illness (Chapter 56).

Protein Kinase C. Diacylglycerol (DAG), which is hydrophobic, remains within the membrane, where it activates protein kinase C (see Figure 12–7) In addition to DAG, activation of protein kinase C (PKC) also requires membrane phospholipids. The inactive form of this kinase is in the cytoplasm. When diacylglycerol is generated, the enzyme is translocated to the membrane to form the active complex that can phosphorylate many protein substrates in the cell, both membrane-associated and cytoplasmic.

This important kinase was discovered by Yasutomi Nishizuka. There are at least eight isoforms of protein kinase C. All forms have been found in nervous tissue. These different forms are encoded by distinct genes. One gene yields two transcripts, however, and the β$_I$ and β$_{II}$ forms are the result of alternative RNA splicing. The PKCs have molecular weights between 75,000 and 90,000. Rather than having different proteins as regulatory and catalytic elements, each holoenzyme contains regulatory and catalytic domains in a single continuous polypeptide chain (see Figure 12–6). Like the cAMP-dependent protein kinase, PKCs also can be autophosphorylated.

Two functionally interesting differences have thus far been found among these isoforms. The so-called *major* forms (α, β$_I$, β$_{II}$, and γ) all have a Ca^{2+}-binding site and are differentially dependent upon Ca^{2+} ions. The minor forms (δ, ε, ζ and η) are molecules that lack the Ca^{2+}-binding domain, and therefore their activity is independent of Ca^{2+}. The second interesting difference is that, of the major forms, only PKC γ is activated by low concentrations of arachidonic acid, while all of the isoforms respond to diacylglycerol or phorbol esters (plant toxins that bind to PKC and act as tumor promoters). The effect of arachidonic acid on the minor forms has not yet been studied.

An important aspect of the bifurcating second messenger pathway that stems from phospholipase C is that the two products of hydrolysis can act independently as well as synergistically. Some transmitter receptors cause the production of IP$_3$, and many receptors activate both. In some cases, IP$_3$ acting alone can raise the concentration of free Ca^{2+} within the cell, which can then activate a variety of cellular processes. Ca^{2+} often acts when it forms a complex with the 17,000-molecular-weight protein calmodulin. An important example is the activation of the Ca^{2+}/calmodulin-dependent protein kinase (to be discussed further in the next chapter and in Chapter 15). Although this enzyme in tissue is made up of a complex containing many similar subunits, each subunit contains regulatory and catalytic domains within the same polypeptide chain. Each subunit can be autophosphorylated by an intramolecular reaction at many sites in the enzyme molecule. The C-terminal regulatory domain behaves as a pseudosubstrate inhibitor of the catalytic portion of this kinase when Ca^{2+} and calmodulin are absent (Figure 12–6). Conformational changes of the kinase molecule caused by the binding of Ca^{2+}/calmodulin unfetter the catalytic domain for action (Figure 12–7).

The Arachidonic Acid Pathway. Because arachidonate is usually the fatty acid esterified at the second position in brain phospholipids, receptors that activate phospholipase A$_2$ cause the release of arachidonic acid from the cell membrane (Figure 12–8). The metabolism of arachidonic acid in brain tissue was first described in 1964 by Bengt Samuelsson. The arachidonic acid released is rapidly converted to a family of active *eicosanoid* metabolites. Arachidonate, which accounts for about 10% of the total fatty acids in neural phospholipids, is metabolized by three types of enzymes: cyclooxygenases (producing prostaglandins and thromboxanes), several lipoxygenases (producing a variety of metabolites to be discussed below), and the cytochrome P-450 heme-containing complex, which oxidizes both arachidonic acid itself as well as cyclooxygenase and lipoxygenase metabolites.

Most work in nervous tissue has been done with cyclooxygenase and the lipoxygenases. In other tissues, metabolites of arachidonic acid have been extensively characterized because of their potent actions in inflammation, injury, and control of smooth muscle in blood vessels

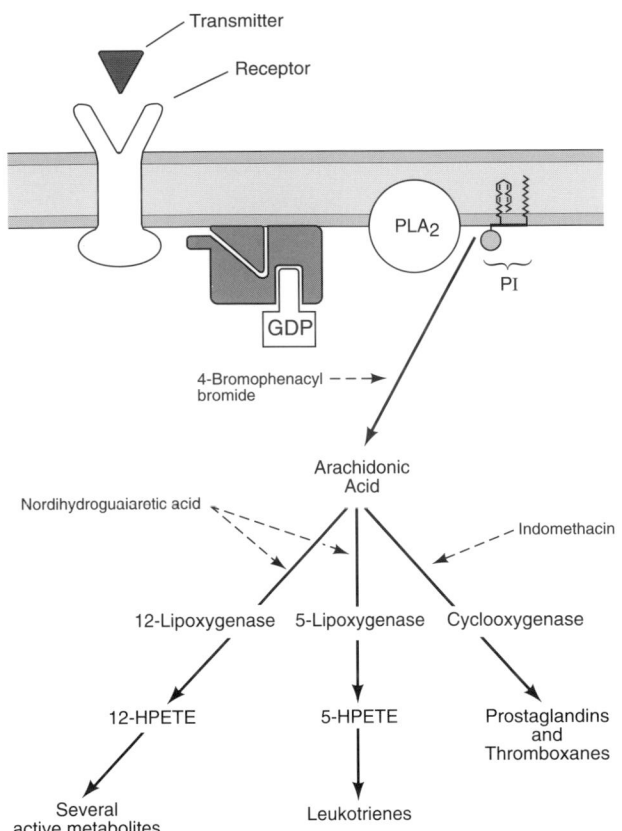

FIGURE 12–8

The arachidonic acid cascade. Arachidonic acid is released through receptor-mediated activation of a phospholipase. The phospholipase shown in the figure is phospholipase A_2, which hydrolyzes phosphoinositol (PI) in the plasma membrane. This enzyme is inhibited by alkylation with 4-bromophenacyl bromide at a histidine residue in the lipase. (Another pathway involves phospholipase C, which produces IP_3 and diacylglycerol. Arachidonic acid is then released by diacylglycerol lipase. This pathway is thought to be of minor significance.) Once released, arachidonic acid is metabolized through several pathways, three of which are shown in the figure. The two lipoxygenase pathways (12- and 5-) both produce several active metabolites. Lipoxygenases are inhibited by nordihydroguaiaretic acid (NDGA). The cyclooxygenase pathway produces prostaglandins and thromboxanes. This enzyme is inhibited by indomethacin, aspirin, and other nonsteroidal antiinflammatory drugs.

and lung. Prostaglandins and thromboxanes, the metabolites stemming from the cyclization and peroxidation catalyzed by cyclooxygenase, also are present in brain, and their synthesis is dramatically increased by relatively nonspecific stimulation, for example, electroconvulsive shock, trauma, and acute cerebral ischemia. How these eicosanoids play a specific role in modulating synaptic transmission or neuronal excitability remains to be discovered.

Lipoxygenases introduce an oxygen molecule into one of the polyunsaturated pentadiene moieties (see previous formula) of the arachidonic acid molecule resulting in a hydroperoxyeicosatrienoic acid (HPETE). The carbon

number at which the hydroxyperoxy group is introduced names the types of lipoxygenase: 5-, 12-, and 15-lipoxygenases are present in brain, but 12-lipoxygenase appears to be the most active in nervous tissue. Leonhard Wolfe and his colleagues have found that depolarization of brain slices with high concentrations of extracellular K^+ ions, glutamate or N-methyl-D-aspartate (NMDA) greatly increases 12-lipoxygenase activity. Also, 12-HPETE and some of its metabolites have been shown to modulate the actions of ion channels at specific synapses, as we describe later in this chapter.

Second-Messenger Pathways Can Interact with One Another

The three second-messenger systems—the cAMP, the diacylglycerol-IP_3, and the arachidonic acid pathways—do not always achieve their regulatory effects independently of each other. Some examples of interaction have been found, and undoubtedly many other points of intersection between these pathways remain to be discovered. Protein phosphorylation, influenced by all three second-messenger systems, has complex regulatory consequences because metabolic transformations consist of many interacting reaction sequences. These reactions are catalyzed by enzymes, many of whose activities are changed by phosphorylation.

Opportunities for interaction (also called *cross-talk*) occur because individual enzymes, channels, or cytoskeletal proteins, can be modified at more than one site in the molecule, each by a protein kinase that is dependent on a different second messenger. Specific examples are the β-adrenergic receptor, discussed later in this chapter, and synapsin I, discussed in Chapter 13.

Second Messengers Often Act Through Protein Phosphorylation to Open or Close Ion Channels

Second-messenger systems often alter the activity of ion channels by phosphorylating the channel protein (Figure 12–9). Protein phosphorylation initiated by second-messenger kinases can have two effects. First, phosphorylation can open channels that are closed at the resting membrane potential. This action appears similar to that produced by the actions of a transmitter on a directly gated ion channel. Second, kinases activated by second messengers can produce a novel synaptic action: They can close channels that are open at the resting potential. In certain cells, some leakage (nongated) K^+ channels that contribute to the resting membrane potential are also controlled by synaptically activated second-messenger actions. Transmitters that close these channels depolarize the neuron (Figure 12–9). In addition, closure of leakage K^+ channels increases the excitability of the neuron and overrides the neuron's tendency to accommodate during repetitive firing.

One well-characterized example of such a synaptic ac-

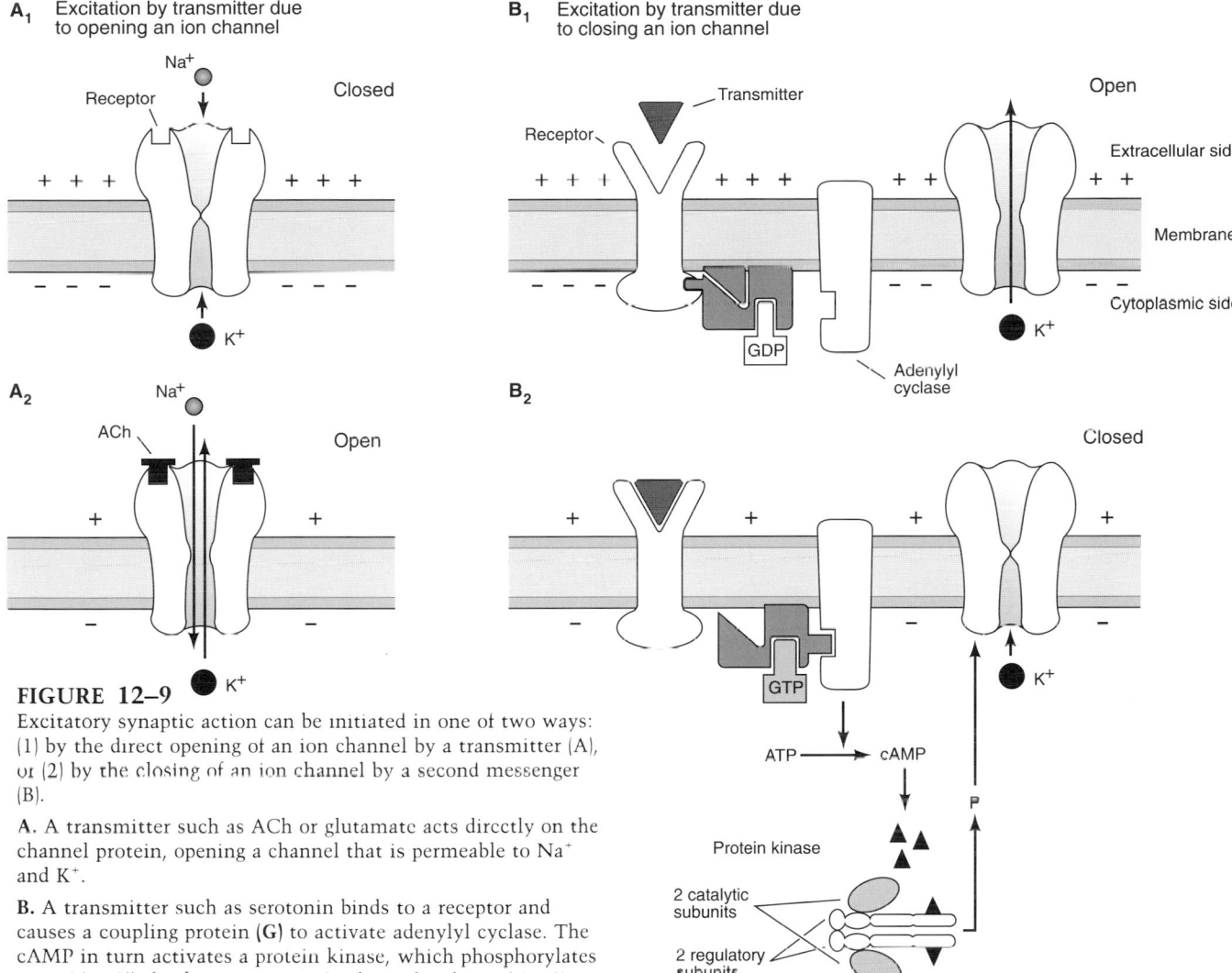

FIGURE 12–9

Excitatory synaptic action can be initiated in one of two ways: (1) by the direct opening of an ion channel by a transmitter (A), or (2) by the closing of an ion channel by a second messenger (B).

A. A transmitter such as ACh or glutamate acts directly on the channel protein, opening a channel that is permeable to Na⁺ and K⁺.

B. A transmitter such as serotonin binds to a receptor and causes a coupling protein (**G**) to activate adenylyl cyclase. The cAMP in turn activates a protein kinase, which phosphorylates an unidentified substrate protein (perhaps the channel itself or a regulatory protein that acts on the channel), causing the K⁺ channel to close.

tion is the effect of ACh on the K⁺ current in sympathetic ganglion cells. As we have seen in Chapters 10 and 11, there are two basic types of receptors for ACh: *nicotinic* and *muscarinic*. Both bind ACh, but they can be distinguished because there are agonists (nicotine or muscarine), as well as antagonists (drugs that block the receptor, e.g., curare and atropine) that bind exclusively to one type of ACh receptor or to the other. The two types of receptors differ from one another biochemically, and they serve different functions in the nervous system. The directly gated receptors in skeletal muscle, discussed in Chapter 10, are nicotinic. In sympathetic neurons and in certain neurons of the hippocampus and cerebral cortex, ACh acts on one or more muscarinic receptors. Paul Adams and David Brown found that muscarinic receptors activate an as yet unidentified second-messenger system that closes a K⁺ channel, which they call the *M (muscarinic) channel* to distinguish it from other K⁺ channels.

A slow synaptic excitation produced by serotonin in the sensory neurons of the marine snail *Aplysia* is caused by closure of a leakage K⁺ channel called the *S-type K⁺ channel*. In this synaptic action, serotonin binds to a receptor that activates the cAMP cascade. The cAMP-dependent protein kinase phosphorylates a substrate protein that is either the S-type K⁺ channel itself or a regulatory protein that acts on this K⁺ channel to close it. Norepinephrine produces a similar slow excitatory postsynaptic potential (EPSP) in certain cortical neurons. Norepinephrine-releasing terminals in the brain originate in a group of nerve cell bodies in the brain stem called the *locus ceruleus*. Neurons from this nucleus innervate the hippocampus and extend widely over the surface of the cerebral cortex (see Chapter 43). Roger Nicoll and his colleagues found that norepinephrine acts through cAMP to close a K⁺ channel that increases excitability and overrides accommodation. This channel is a Ca²⁺-activated K⁺ channel (Figure 12–10).

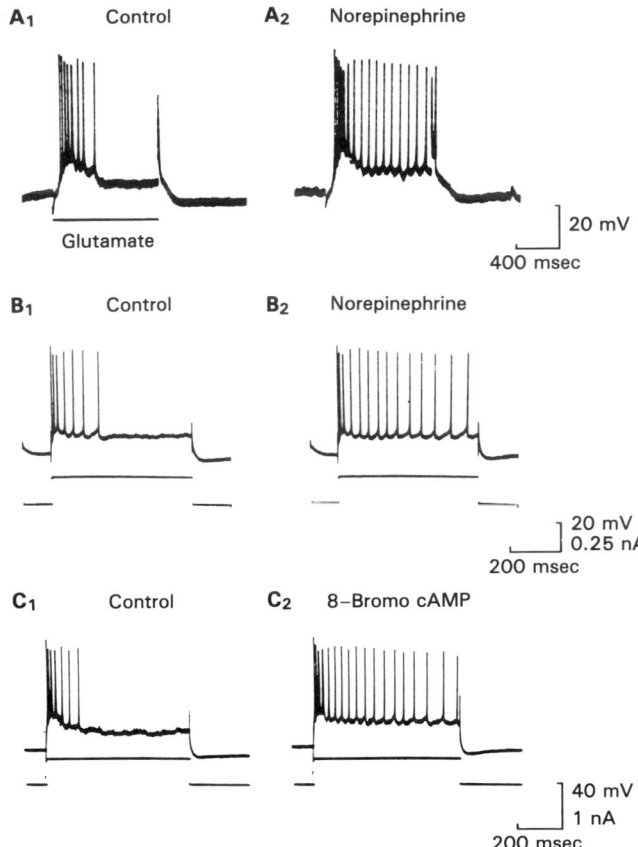

FIGURE 12–10

Norepinephrine activates cAMP and produces a modulatory excitatory action on hippocampal neurons by closing a K$^+$ channel. This action of norepinephrine increases the excitability of the neuron as evident in its overcoming the neuron's intrinsic tendency toward accommodation. In the presence of norepinephrine or an analog of cAMP the neuron fires for a longer period in response to glutamate or a constant depolarizing current pulse. (Adapted from Madison and Nicoll 1986; and Nicoll et al., 1987.)

A. Norepinephrine enhances the response of a pyramidal cell to glutamate, overcoming accommodation.

B. Norepinephrine enhances the response to intracellular depolarizing currrent pulses.

C. Cyclic AMP analog (8-bromocyclic AMP) enhances the response to depolarizing current pulses.

How does closure of K$^+$ channels that are normally open at the resting potential result in excitation? As we saw in Chapter 6, the resting membrane is permeable to K$^+$, Na$^+$, and Cl$^-$. The resting potential therefore results from a compromise among the permeabilities to the three ions. The K$^+$ channels, open at rest, hyperpolarize the membrane. Closure of some of these K$^+$ channels therefore moves V_m to a new depolarized value, somewhat closer to E_{Na}, bringing the membrane closer to the threshold for firing an action potential. In addition, decreasing the number of open K$^+$ channels reduces the effective

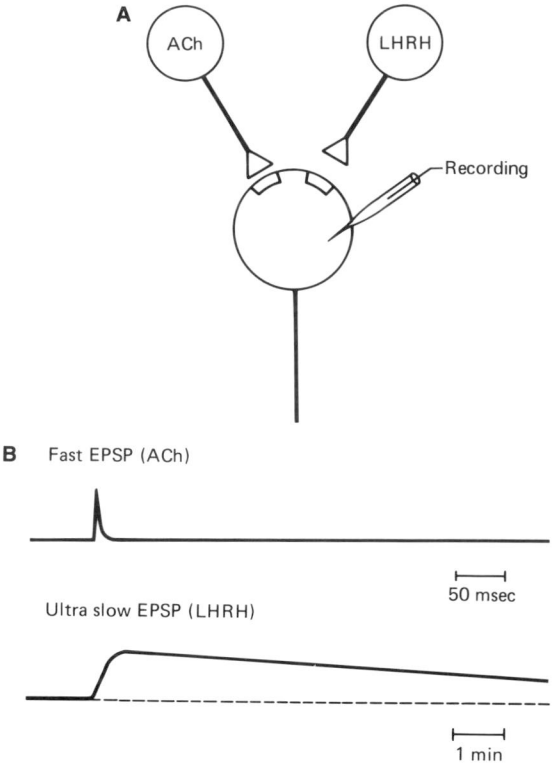

FIGURE 12–11

Certain neurons in sympathetic ganglia receive independent convergent excitatory connections from two different sets of neurons. One set of neurons uses ACh as its transmitter, the other uses a peptide, luteinizing hormone-releasing hormone (LHRH). Acetylcholine produces an EPSP through the opening of ion channels permeable to Na$^+$ and K$^+$; LHRH produces an EPSP through the closing of K$^+$ channels. (Adapted from Jan, Jan, and Kuffler, 1979.)

A. The neurons that use ACh make a conventional directed synaptic contact. The neurons that use LHRH make a nondirected contact. Their release site is some distance from the target cell.

B. In the same neuron the time course of the decreased-conductance EPSP due to the closing of a K$^+$ channel is much slower than that of an increased-conductance EPSP due to the opening of the channel. The increased-conductance EPSP induced by ACh lasts 20 ms, whereas the decreased-conductance EPSP induced by LHRH is very slow, lasting 10 min. (Note the different time scales in the two recordings.)

membrane conductance, g_m. As a result, any other excitatory input that generates a fast EPSP will produce greater depolarization ($V_{EPSP} = I_{EPSP}/g_m$). This is the reverse of the short-circuit effect of synaptic inhibition, which we considered in Chapter 11, where the opening of Cl$^-$ channels increases g_m and thus decreases the effectiveness of excitatory synaptic inputs.

The actions of second messengers are not limited to leakage channels. Some channels closed by second messengers are voltage dependent. For example, in dorsal root ganglion cells norepinephrine and enkephalin close voltage-gated Ca^{2+} channels through protein phosphorylation by PKC.

In addition to being able to close channels that are open at the resting potential, synaptic actions resulting from second-messenger-mediated protein phosphorylation differ from directly gated synaptic actions in several other ways. First, second messengers can diffuse intracellularly to affect a distant part of the cell. As a result, K^+ channels closed (or opened) by a transmitter need not be located directly beneath the receptors acted on by the transmitter, but can be at some distance.

Second, the time course of second-messenger-mediated synaptic actions is much slower—in several known instances 10,000 times slower than directly mediated actions. Stephen Kuffler and his colleagues Yuh Nung Jan and Lily Yeh Jan described an excitatory synaptic potential in sympathetic ganglion neurons that results from closure of the M species of K^+ channel and lasts about 10 minutes. A peptide similar to luteinizing hormone-releasing hormone, acting as a chemical messenger, closes the channel. In contrast, an EPSP produced in the same neurons by the nicotinic ACh receptor-channels lasts 20 ms (Figure 12–11). In *Aplysia* neurons, too, the EPSP produced when serotonin closes the K^+ channels can persist for several minutes. As we shall see in the next chapter, these slow synaptic actions modulate neuronal activity over a period of minutes (Table 12–1). Third, with the exception of the NMDA glutamate receptor-channel, directly gated channels are not activated by voltage and therefore are not affected by membrane potential. Consequently they do not contribute to the action potential. In contrast, the various K^+ channels that close in response to second messengers are voltage sensitive and do contribute to the action potential.

As these two features illustrate, the slow synaptic actions produced by second messengers typically *modulate* the excitability of neurons. Fast synaptic actions, on the other hand, are *mediating*. Mediating synaptic actions typically provide the common *detectable* synaptic actions between cells. In contrast, modulatory actions often are ineffective by themselves but act to regulate mediating synaptic actions. They do so in ways that we shall learn about in the next chapter. For example, modulatory transmitters affect not only transmitter-gated channels but also

voltage-sensitive channels that contribute to the action potential. As a result, modulatory transmitters can affect the threshold for spike generation, accommodation, as well as the amplitude and duration of the action potential. By affecting the action potential in the presynaptic terminals, modulatory transmitters can regulate Ca^{2+} influx and thereby the amount of transmitter a neuron releases.

Second Messengers and G-Proteins Can Sometimes Act Directly on Ion Channels

In several important instances modulatory actions have been discovered in which a G-protein moves within the membrane and interacts directly with an ion channel, causing it either to open or to close without the intervention of a protein kinase (Figure 12–12A). As first shown by Paul Pfaffinger, Bertil Hille, and their colleagues, and by Gerda Breitwieser and Gabor Szabo, the hyperpolarization produced by muscarinic receptors in the heart is caused by the direct action of a G-protein that opens a K^+ channel. As shown by Arthur Brown and his colleagues, it is the α-subunit of the G-protein that seems to activate the channel. Another class of G-proteins produces a depolarization by directly opening Ca^{2+} channels. In certain cells the same ion channel is modulated in two ways in response to a transmitter: directly and relatively rapidly by the binding of a G-protein and indirectly and more slowly as a result of phosphorylation by the second messenger kinase activated by the same G-protein. This illustrates that G proteins can act on different effectors, on enzymes that synthesize second messengers, as well as on ion channels.

Some channels are modulated directly by the second messengers themselves: by cGMP, cAMP, or metabolites of arachidonic acid, without requiring protein phosphorylation (Figure 12–12B). As we shall see later, the cation-selective ion channels of photoreceptors and the depolarizing bipolar cells in the retina are both opened by the direct action of cGMP on the channel. The cation-selective channel activated by the olfactory receptor is directly opened by the action of cAMP. Similarly, the transmitter Phe-Met-Arg-Phe-NH_2 (FMRFamide), a peptide found in invertebrates that is distantly related to enkephalins, produces hyperpolarization and synaptic inhibition in sensory neurons of *Aplysia* by opening the S-type K^+ channel. This action is mediated by the direct action of 12-lipoxygenase metabolites of arachidonic acid.

TABLE 12–1. Comparison of Synaptic Excitation Produced by the Opening and Closing of Ion Channels

Properties	EPSP due to opening of channels	EPSP due to closing of channels
Ion channels involved	Cation channel for Na^+ and K^+	Channel for K^+
Effect on total membrane conductance	Increase	Decrease
Contribution to action potential	None	Modulates current of action potential
Time course	Usually fast (milliseconds)	Slow (seconds or minutes)
Intracellular second messenger	None	Cyclic AMP (or other second messengers)
Nature of synaptic action	Mediating	Modulating

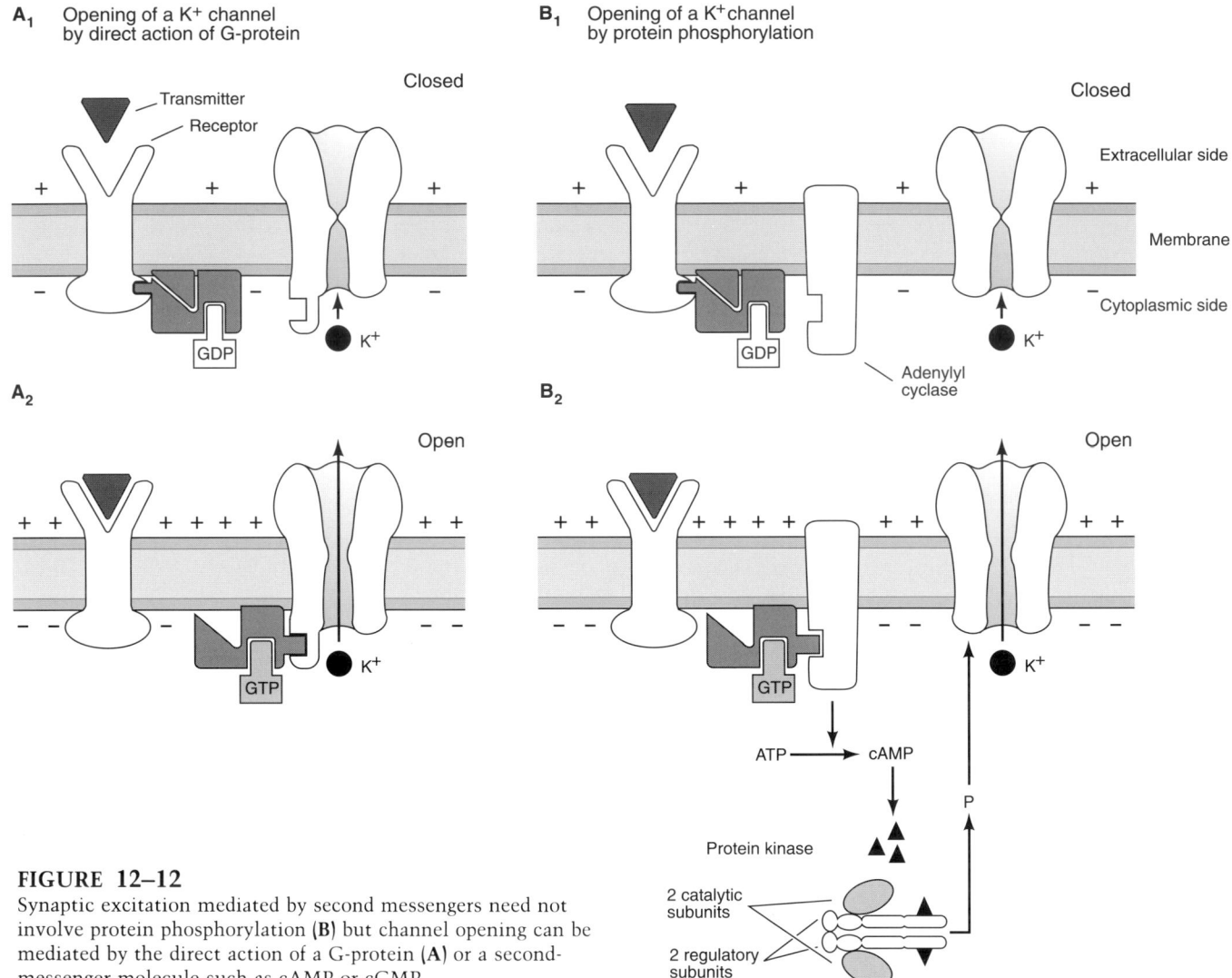

A₁ Opening of a K⁺ channel by direct action of G-protein

A₂

B₁ Opening of a K⁺channel by protein phosphorylation

B₂

FIGURE 12–12

Synaptic excitation mediated by second messengers need not involve protein phosphorylation (**B**) but channel opening can be mediated by the direct action of a G-protein (**A**) or a second-messenger molecule such as cAMP or cGMP.

Second Messengers Can Alter the Properties of Transmitter Receptors: Desensitization

Second-messenger systems also exert actions on many target proteins other than voltage-sensitive ion channels. A particularly interesting class of target proteins are the receptors for other transmitters. Second messengers can affect both types of receptors for neurotransmitters—those that gate ion channels indirectly and those that gate channels directly. In this way, the action of one receptor can regulate its own effectiveness or the effectiveness of a receptor for another transmitter. For example, after prolonged exposure to its own transmitter, a receptor can become refractory to later applications of the same transmitter, a process called *desensitization* (Figure 12–13). Although many mechanisms produce diminished responsiveness, desensitization has been shown in several instances to result from protein phosphorylation. One example, analyzed by Robert Lefkowitz, Marc Caron, and

their colleagues, is the β-adrenergic receptor, which is phosphorylated in the cytoplasmic domains of the receptor molecule that interact with G_s by a specific cAMP-dependent receptor kinase (βARK) as well as by both the cAMP-dependent protein kinase and PKC. During phosphorylation of the receptor, 2–3 mol of phosphate per mol of receptor are incorporated into the receptor protein, and the degree of desensitization correlates with the extent of phosphorylation. Phosphorylation by the cyclic AMP-dependent kinase or by βARK slows the ability of the receptor to activate G_s. But the chief inhibitory effect of βARK is to promote the binding of an inhibitory protein with a molecular weight of about 48,000 to the phosphorylated receptor. This inhibitor is similar to *arrestin*, a protein that regulates the function of rhodopsin in the retina.

Receptors that gate ion channels directly can also be modulated by phosphorylation (Figure 12–13). Richard Huganir, Paul Greengard, and Steven Scheutze found that the cAMP-dependent protein kinase phosphorylates the γ-

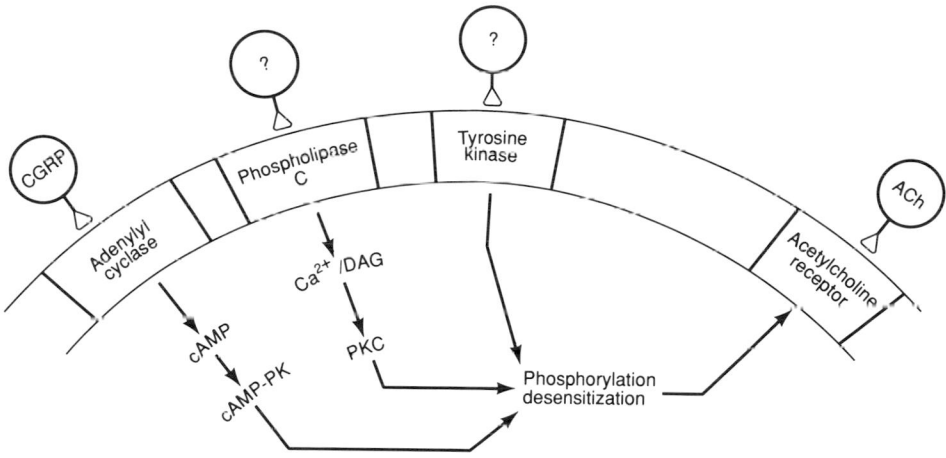

FIGURE 12–13

Second-messenger systems can affect other receptors and their directly gated ion channels. The peptide calcitonin gene-related peptide (CGRP) activates the cAMP cascade, which leads to the phosphorylation of the ACh receptor. Phosphorylation causes the receptor to respond less effectively to ACh, a process called desensitization. Phosphorylation of the ACh receptor can also be produced by PKC and by a tyrosine kinase. (Adapted from Huganir and Greengard, 1990.)

and δ-subunits of the nicotinic ACh receptor. In addition, PKC acts on the α- and δ-subunits, and tyrosine-specific protein kinases phosphorylate the β-, γ-, and δ-subunits (see below). The α-subunit of this receptor is phosphorylated by PKC, the β-subunit by tyrosine-specific kinases, the γ-subunit by the cAMP-dependent protein kinase and tyrosine-specific protein kinases, and the δ-subunit by all three kinases. Thus, three different kinases phosphorylate the ACh receptor at seven different sites, all of which are located in the major cytoplasmic domain of each subunit. Not all of these phosphorylations are known to have functional consequences, but the cAMP-dependent phosphorylation of the γ- and δ-subunits does increase the rate at which the receptor is desensitized.

Second Messengers Can Regulate Gene Expression and Thereby Endow Synaptic Transmission with Long-Lasting Consequences

So far we have considered two types of chemically mediated synaptic actions: fast, directly gated synaptic actions lasting milliseconds, and slow, second-messenger-mediated actions involving modifications of ion channels and other substrate proteins lasting seconds to minutes (Figure 12–15). Recently, a third kind of synaptic action has been discovered by which transmitters, acting through second messengers, phosphorylate transcriptional regulatory proteins and thereby alter gene expression (Figure 12–15 and Box 12–1). Thus, second-messenger kinases not only can produce covalent modification of *preexisting proteins*, but also can induce the synthesis of *new proteins* by altering gene expression. This third kind of synaptic action can lead to other changes, such as neuronal growth, that last days or even longer. These long-term changes are likely to be important for neuronal development and for long-term memory.

To illustrate the relative importance of transient modifications of proteins and the more enduring synthesis of new protein by altered gene expression, we shall consider how a cholinergic presynaptic neuron can regulate the amount of transmitter substance (norepinephrine) in a postsynaptic target cell. Norepinephrine is a common small molecule transmitter (see Chapter 14). Because synthesis of norepinephrine is highly regulated, the amount available for release can keep up with substantial variations in neuronal activity. In certain ganglia of the autonomic nervous system (a part of the central nervous system that we shall learn about later), the amount of norepinephrine synthesized is regulated transynaptically through synaptic receptors in response to activity of presynaptic neurons. If the activity in these presynaptic neurons is sufficiently prolonged, the released transmitter will induce relatively long-term changes in the postsynaptic cell. These changes will increase the supply of norepinephrine by acting on *tyrosine hydroxylase*, the first enzyme in the biochemical pathway for the synthesis of norepinephrine. These regulatory mechanisms also occur in adrenergic cells of the central nervous system.

The immediate, short-term mechanisms lead to protein phosphorylation: presynaptic activity releases ACh and a peptide transmitter that activates a receptor in the postsynaptic cell and thus the production of cAMP. Cyclic AMP activates the cAMP-dependent protein kinase, which phosphorylates tyrosine hydroxylase. Normally, tyrosine hydroxylase activity is dependent on the concentration of its substrate, tyrosine; the enzyme also requires a pteridine cofactor, tetrahydrobiopterin. Enzyme activity is reversibly inhibited by norepinephrine and dopamine, the end-products of the pathway; these feedback inhibitors compete with the binding of the oxidized form of the

Regulation of Gene Expression

With the exception of mature lymphocytes, each cell in the human body contains precisely the same complement of genes (thought to be between 100,000 and 1,000,000) that is present in every other cell. The reason cells differ from one another—why the liver cell is a liver cell and a brain cell a brain cell—is that different combinations of genes are expressed in specific cell types. This requires mechanisms both for activating and repressing the expression of specific genes. Repression and activation of genes occurs during development and often is maintained throughout the life of the differentiated cell. Moreover, in any given cell many genes are not competent for transcription and as a consequence are never transcribed.

In addition to these relatively permanent changes, the expression of many genes that are capable of being expressed within specific cell types is regulated. For example, the rate at which a gene transcribes messenger RNA can be transiently enhanced or depressed by the actions of proteins that bind to regulatory regions of the gene. The activity of these regulatory proteins is in turn controlled by receptors located within the cell or on the cell surface. These receptors recognize molecules such as steroid hormones, peptide growth factors, and neurotransmitters.

Genes can be divided into two major regions: a *coding region* and a *regulatory region*. For most genes that encode proteins, messenger RNA is transcribed from template DNA in the coding region by the actions of the enzyme RNA polymerase II. The regulatory region usually lies upstream of the coding region. Because these DNA regulatory regions are usually near the coding region they are called *cis*-regulatory elements. In contrast, the transcription regulatory proteins that bind to these regulatory regions are called *trans*-regulatory elements, because they often are encoded by genes that are not linked to the gene being regulated.

The DNA regulatory region in turn consists of two types of control elements. The first (or *proximal*) type of control element is called the *promoter region*. In many genes this element is an *eight-base pair*, AT-rich region called the *TATA box*, surrounded by a region rich in GC. The TATA box is usually located

FIGURE 12–14 Transcriptional control.
A. The typical eukaryotic gene such as the pro-opiomelanocortin gene illustrated has two regions. There is a *coding region* that is transcribed by RNA polymerase II into a messenger RNA and in turn is then translated into a specific protein, and a *regulatory region*, consisting of *enhancer elements* and a *promoter element*. The enhancers and promoter are (commonly) located upstream from the coding region and regulate the initiation of the transcription of the structural gene.

B. Transcriptional regulatory proteins bind both to the promoter and the enhancer regions. A set of proteins binds to the TATA box, to the promoter, and to the distal enhancer regions. Proteins that bind to the enhancer region cause looping of the DNA, thereby allowing the regulatory proteins that bind to distal enhancers to contact the polymerase.

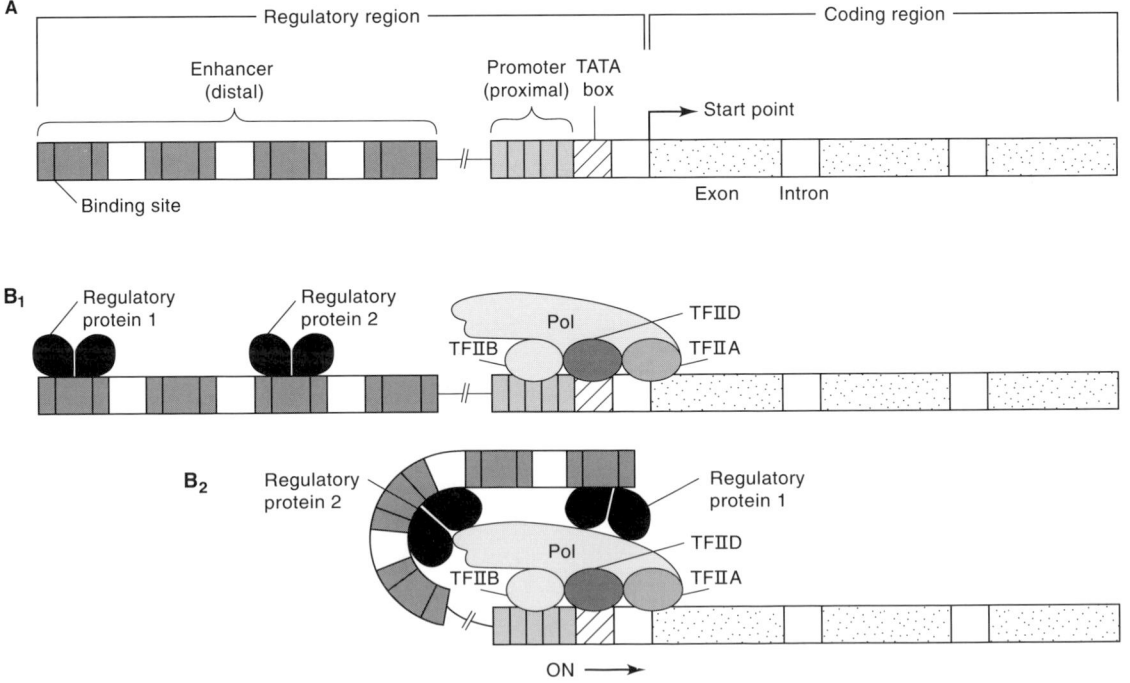

BOX 12–1

about 30-base pairs (bp) upstream from the start site for transcription (Figure 12–14).

The TATA box and adjacent DNA elements in the promoter region are involved in positioning the RNA polymerase in the region where transcription of messenger RNA begins. In eukaryotic organisms RNA polymerase II does not bind directly to the TATA box. Rather, the TATA box is occupied by a complex of other proteins called TATA box proteins. These TATA box-binding proteins are thought to interact directly with RNA polymerase II and direct its binding to a region of DNA adjacent to the site where transcription starts. In addition, there are often other DNA regulatory modules near the TATA box; these include the CAAT box and the GC-rich modules that may facilitate the initial binding of the polymerase.

The second (or *distal*) type of DNA region is called the *enhancer region*. The enhancer elements can be located within a few hundred-base pairs from the promoter, or as far as 100 kilobases away. Some enhancers are also found in introns or at sites 3' to the coding region of genes. Each of the individual control elements of the enhancer region is generally a region of DNA 7- to 20-base pairs long, and each of these modules functions as a binding site for proteins that control whether the gene will be transcribed by RNA polymerase II (Figure 12–14).

The enhancer elements that bind cell-specific regulator proteins are called *response elements*. Thus, the cyclic AMP response element (CRE) consists of the sequence ACGTCA; it recognizes CREB proteins that are activated by phosphorylation under the control of the cAMP-dependent protein kinase. The serum or phorbol ester response element (SRE or PRE) has the sequence TGACTCAG. The glucocorticoid response element (GRE) consists of the sequence TGGTA CAAATGTTCT. The GRE recognizes the protein receptor that is activated by binding of glucocorticoid hormones. Many of these DNA-binding sites have dyad (two-fold) symmetry, and the proteins bind to them as dimers.

Certain enhancer elements bind activator proteins continuously which permits basal levels of transcription. Other enhancer elements bind regulatory proteins only intermittently. This permits the gene to be regulated (induced or repressed) by appropriate protein transcriptional regulators. Thus, whether the RNA polymerase binds and transcribes a gene and how often it does so in any given period of time is determined by transcriptional regulators that bind to different control segments of the proximal region and the upstream enhancer region. In addition to the proteins (the TATA box factors) that bind to the promoter, regulatory factors need to bind to enhancer regions for the induced expression by hormones, stress, and learning. Some of these enhancers are several hundred base pairs away from the TATA box. To

explain how proteins at a distance can activate transcription by facilitating the binding of the polymerase to the TATA box, it is thought that the intervening DNA sequence loops out, thereby bringing together proteins bound to the distal enhancer and the proximal promoter (Figure 12–14).

Transcriptional factors that bind to these control regions typically have three functional domains: (1) a *DNA-binding domain*, which contains many basic residues that permit the protein to recognize and bind selectively to a specific DNA sequence; (2) an *activator domain*, which is often acidic in nature and permits the protein to contact and activate the basal transcription machinery (the TATA box-binding factors and RNA polymerase II); and (3) one or more *ligand-binding* or *phosphorylation domains*, which are required for activating the transcription factors.

Many of the DNA-binding domains of transcriptional regulators fall into one of three major families:

(1) *Helix-turn-helix proteins*, which consist of factors containing at least two alpha helices. One helix occupies the major groove of the DNA and interacts with the regulatory nucleotide backbone. A second helical region is located at an angle across the DNA and interacts less directly with DNA. The *homeobox proteins* (Chapter 58) that play important roles in developmental processes fall into this class of proteins.

(2) *Zinc finger*, so called because a stretch of about 23 amino acids containing alternating cystines and histidines forms a finger-like loop whose structure is maintained by the binding of a zinc ion. The proteins interact with DNA through the loop regions. Glucocorticoid, estrogen, vitamin A, progesterone, thyroid, and retinoic acid receptors each contain two zinc fingers.

(3) *Amphipathic helical proteins*. These include two submotifs: helix-loop-helix proteins and leucine zipper proteins. The amphipathic helical regions of these proteins serve as domains for dimer formation as well as for DNA binding.

In fact, each of these three classes of transcriptional regulatory proteins forms dimers that bind to each other through protein-protein interactions as well as binding to the DNA by means of protein DNA interactions. The transcriptional dimers can be *homodimers*, such as CREB-CREB (or *jun-jun*), or *heterodimers*, such as *fos-jun*. One important consequence of the dimerization of transcriptional regulatory proteins is that additional specificity can be achieved by forming heterodimers between related family members. Heterodimers can bind to distinct DNA sequences and can then regulate the activity of different combinations of target genes. In this way a greater diversity of regulatory interactions can be achieved by a limited number of regulatory proteins.

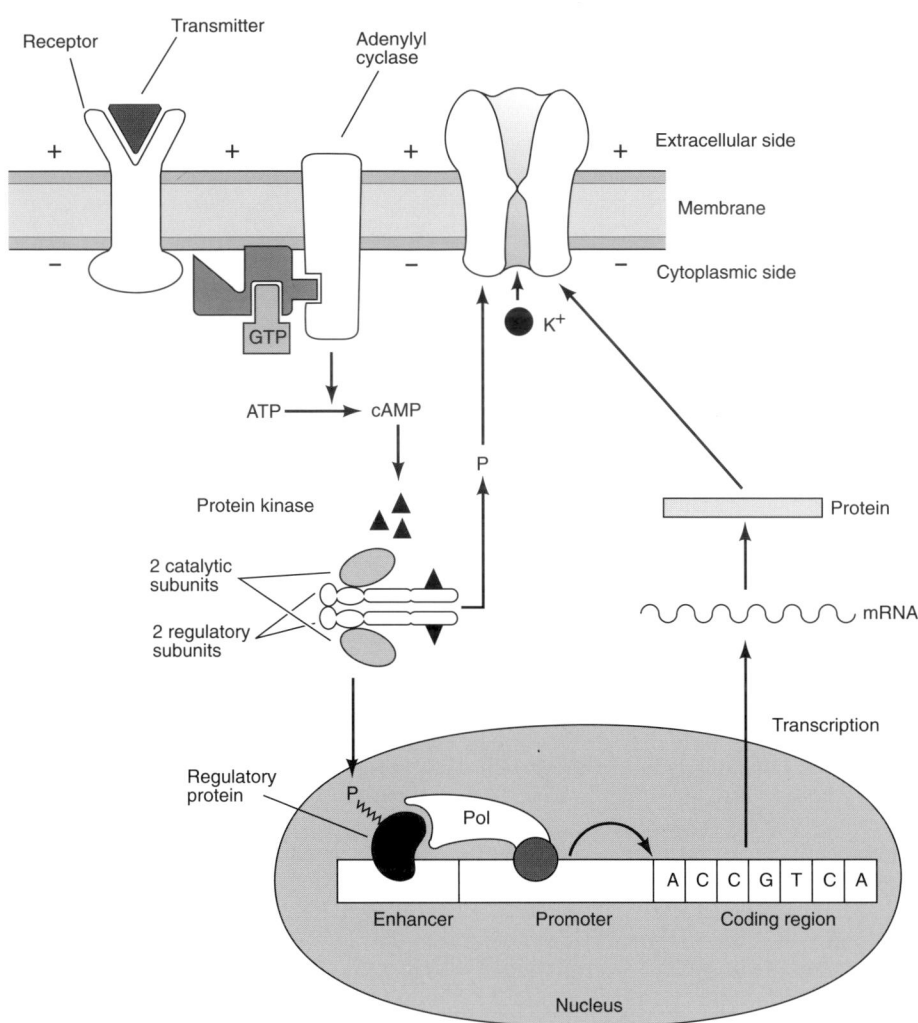

FIGURE 12–15

A single chemical transmitter can produce synaptic actions with different time courses. In this example a single exposure to the transmitter activates the cAMP second-messenger system, which in turn activates the cAMP-dependent protein kinase that phosphorylates a K+ channel to produce a synaptic potential that modifies neuronal excitability for minutes. With repeated activation, the transmitter, acting through the cAMP-dependent protein kinase, also phosphorylates one or more transcriptional activator proteins that regulate gene expression. This produces a protein that modifies the channel and results in more enduring closure of the channel and changes in neuronal excitability lasting days or weeks.

pteridine cofactor. Phosphorylation frees the hydroxylase from these inhibitory mechanisms.

The short-term increase in norepinephrine produced by covalent modification of existing enzyme molecules occurs within minutes, and is rapidly reversible. Severe or prolonged stress to the animal (cold or immobilization) results in intense presynaptic activity and consequently persistent firing of the adrenergic neuron. This puts a greater demand on transmitter synthesis and ultimately results in a long-term increase in norepinephrine. The increase is observed in the cell body within hours and later at nerve endings. The change is maintained for days after the original stress. This persistent increase in the amount of transmitter in the neuron is not the result of phosphorylation of the hydroxylase. Rather, prolonged release of peptides by the presynaptic neuron activates the cAMP pathway sufficiently, so that the kinase phosphorylates not only tyrosine hydroxylase molecules in the cytoplasm but also a transcriptional regulator, a nuclear protein that can bind to the regulatory region of a gene to alter gene expression. Once phosphorylated, this *trans*-activating protein (called the CRE-binding protein or CREB) binds to a specific DNA regulatory region (an enhancer sequence called the cAMP-response element, CRE) that is upstream

(5') of the coding region of the hydroxylase gene. Binding of the transcriptional activator to CRE facilitates the binding of RNA polymerase to the gene's promoter and increases the frequency of transcriptional initiation (Figure 12–14 and 12–15).

Other Second-Messenger Pathways: Tyrosine Kinases and Cyclic GMP

One second-messenger pathway, the tyrosine kinase pathway, often is associated with growth as well as tumor production. Certain receptors for some peptides, such as epidermal growth factor (EGF), nerve growth factor (NGF), and insulin, differ from the typical G-protein-coupled receptor because they consist of monomers or dimers that span the membrane only once and include a protein kinase that, when activated by the ligand, phosphorylates proteins on tyrosine residues within their cytoplasmic domain (Figure 12–6). Other kinases phosphorylate proteins on serine and threonine residues. Like the serine-threonine kinases that we have discussed in this chapter, tyrosine kinases also regulate the function of the neuronal proteins they phosphorylate. At present, the substrates for tyrosine kinase appear to belong to a special class dedicated to producing long-term changes in neuronal function (Figure 12–13).

Cyclic GMP also activates a specific protein kinase. Guanylate cyclase, which is presumably activated through specific receptors by neurotransmitters and hormones, converts GTP to cGMP. Cyclic GMP has been found to act directly on specific ion channels in the outer segment of retinal rod cells. This important regulatory role of cGMP is described in Chapter 27 in detail. The cGMP-dependent kinase differs from cAMP-dependent protein kinases because it is a single polypeptide that contains both *regulatory* (cGMP-binding) and *catalytic* domains. As we have seen, these domains are similar to those subunits or domains of other protein kinases with similar function, especially those that are responsible for catalysis. Because of the similarities among the cAMP-dependent, Ca^{2+}/calmodulin-dependent, and tyrosine protein kinases, all of these second-messenger enzymes are believed to be related, and to have arisen from an ancestral kinase.

The function of cGMP-dependent protein phosphorylation is not yet understood, even though it occurs throughout the brain (usually in amounts less than 10% of that of cAMP-dependent protein phosphorylation). The greatest amounts of cGMP-dependent protein phosphorylation occur in Purkinje cells of the cerebellum, and moderate amounts in the choroid plexus. Synthesis of cGMP is stimulated in neurons and glial cells of the cerebellum by nitric oxide (NO), an unstable molecule that readily diffuses through cell membranes. Nitric oxide is produced in neurons in response to glutamate, apparently acting through NMDA receptors, and requires influx of Ca^{2+} ions. Nitric oxide is formed from the amino acid L-arginine by the enzyme nitric oxide synthetase acting in con-

junction with the cofactor, reduced nicotinamide adenine dinucleotide phosphate (NADPH), and Ca^{2+} ions. In the reaction arginine

$$
\begin{array}{c}
NH \\
\parallel \\
C-NH_2 \\
\mid \\
NH \\
\mid \\
(CH_2)_3 \\
\mid \\
H_2NCHCOOH
\end{array}
$$

is converted to citrulline.

$$
\begin{array}{c}
NH_2 \\
\mid \\
C=O \\
\mid \\
NH \\
\mid \\
(CH_2)_3 \\
\mid \\
H_2NCHCOOH
\end{array}
$$

Nitric oxide was previously recognized as a local hormone released from endothelial cells of blood vessels in a variety of nonneural tissues in response to substances that cause vasodilation (histamine, for example). Release of NO by vascular endothelium causes relaxation of the smooth muscle of vessel walls also through activation of guanylate cyclase.

The action of NO illustrates a key principle of second-messenger mechanisms: The second messengers used by neurons are not specific to nerve cells, but are common to many cell types. Another important feature of this recently discovered pathway is that NO, like eicosanoid metabolites, readily passes through cell membranes. This feature permits hitherto unexpected ways of modulating neuronal signaling by transcellular (or retrograde) mechanisms in which the postsynaptic cell can influence the presynaptic neuron.

An Overall View

The molecular actions of the three receptor mechanisms that we have considered here and in the preceding chapters generally conform to the speed of the synaptic action they mediate. Thus, directly gated ion channels operate most rapidly, and are used for physiological processes that need speed. The behavior illustrating neuronal signaling in Chapters 2 and 3, the simple knee jerk reflex, is one example. Similar fast processes also include synaptic connections that produce much of the animal's perceptual and motor behavior.

In recent years it has become increasingly clear that neurons also have longer-lasting, regulatory effects in target cells. Indeed, even in muscle contraction sustained activity requires neural regulation of the muscle cell's metabolism. Regulation is achieved by receptor mechanisms that are slower in onset and that persist for longer periods of time.

In the integrating centers of the brain neurons make use of both transient and enduring forms of synaptic transmission, using receptors that gate ion channels directly or second messengers. Synaptic actions that gate ion channels directly and open channels that are closed at the resting potential invariably increase the overall conductance of the postsynaptic membrane. In contrast, synaptic actions mediated by second messengers also close ion channels that are open at the resting potential, thereby decreasing the conductance of the membrane. Finally, in addition to gating ion channels, second messengers can alter the biochemical state of a nerve cell. For example, second messengers can alter gene expression to initiate persistent changes in function.

Selected Readings

Agranoff, B. W. 1989. Phosphoinositides. In G. J. Siegel, B. W. Agranoff, R. W. Albers, and P. B. Molinoff (eds.), Basic Neurochemistry: Molecular, Cellular, and Medical Aspects, 4th ed. New York: Raven Press, pp. 333–347.

Bishop, W. R., and Bell, R. M. 1988. Assembly of phospholipids into cellular membranes: Biosynthesis, transmembrane movement and intracellular translocation. Annu. Rev. Cell Biol. 4:579–610.

Casey, P. J., and Gilman, A. G. 1988. G protein involvement in receptor-effector coupling. J. Biol. Chem. 263:2577–2580.

Comb, M., Hyman, S. E., and Goodman, H. M. 1987. Mechanisms of trans-synaptic regulation of gene expression. Trends Neurosci. 10:473–478.

Cooper, J. R., Bloom, F. E., and Roth, R. H. 1991. The Biochemical Basis of Neuropharmacology, 6th ed. New York: Oxford University Press.

Edelman, A. M., Blumenthal, D. K., and Krebs, E. G. 1987. Protein serine/threonine kinases. Annu. Rev. Biochem. 56:567–613.

Gilman, A. G. 1987. G proteins: Transducers of receptor-generated signals. Annu. Rev. Biochem. 56:615–649.

Hanks, S. K., Quinn, A. M., and Hunter, T. 1988. The protein kinase family: Conserved features and deduced phylogeny of the catalytic domains. Science 241:42–52.

Huganir, R. L., and Greengard, P. 1990. Regulation of neurotransmitter receptor desensitization by protein phosphorylation. Neuron. 5:555–567.

Kaczmarek, L. K., and Levitan, I. B. 1987. Neuromodulation: The Biochemical Control of Neuronal Excitability. New York: Oxford University Press.

Kikkawa, U., Kishimoto, A., and Nishizuka, Y. 1989. The protein kinase C family: Heterogeneity and its implications. Annu. Rev. Biochem. 58:31–44.

Lefkowitz, R. J., and Caron, M. G. 1988. Adrenergic receptors. Models for the study of receptors coupled to guanine nucleotide regulatory proteins. J. Biol. Chem. 263:4993–4996.

Nathanson, N. M., and Harden, T. K. (eds.) 1990. G Proteins and Signal Transduction. Society of General Physiologists Series, Vol. 45. New York: Rockefeller University Press.

Needleman, P., Turk, J., Jakschik, B. A., Morrison, A. R., and Lefkowith, J. B. 1986. Arachidonic acid metabolism. Annu. Rev. Biochem. 55:69–102.

Nestler, E. J., and Greengard, P. 1984. Protein Phosphorylation in the Nervous System. New York: Wiley.

Nicoll, R. A., Malenka, R. C., and Kauer, J. A. 1990. Functional comparison of neurotransmitter receptor subtypes in mammalian central nervous system. Physiol. Rev. 70:513–565.

Sternweis, P. C., and Pang, I-H. 1990. The G protein-channel connection. Trends Neurosci 13:122–126.

Taylor, S. S., Buechler, J. A., and Yonemoto, W. 1990. cAMP-dependent protein kinase: Framework for a diverse family of regulatory enzymes. Annu. Rev. Biochem. 59:971–1005.

Zigmond, R. E., Schwarzchild, M. A., and Rittenhouse, A. R. 1989. Acute regulation of tyrosine hydroxylase by nerve activity and by neurotransmitters via phosphorylation. Annu. Rev. Neurosci. 12:415–461.

References

Adams, P. 1982. Voltage-dependent conductances of vertebrate neurones. Trends Neurosci. 5:116–119.

Akita, Y., Ohno, S., Konno, Y., Yano, A., and Suzuki, K. 1990. Expression and properties of two distinct classes of the phorbol ester receptor family, four conventional protein kinase C types, and a novel protein kinase C. J. Biol. Chem. 265:354–362.

Benovic, J. L., Bouvier, M., Caron, M. G., and Lefkowitz, R. J. 1988. Regulation of adenylyl cyclase-coupled β-adrenergic receptors. Annu. Rev. Cell Biol. 4:405–428.

Benovic, J. L., Kühn, H., Weyand, I., Codina, J., Caron, M. G., and Lefkowitz, R. J. 1987. Functional desensitization of the isolated β-adrenergic receptor by the β-adrenergic receptor kinase: Potential role of an analog of the retinal protein arrestin (48-κ Da protein). Proc. Natl. Acad. Sci. U.S.A. 84:8879–8882.

Berridge, M. J. 1987. Inositol trisphosphate and diacylglycerol: Two interacting second messengers. Annu. Rev. Biochem. 56: 159–193.

Bourne, H. R., Sanders, D. A., and McCormick, F. 1990. The GTPase superfamily: A conserved switch for diverse cell functions. Nature 348:125–132.

Bredt, D. S., and Snyder, S. H. 1989. Nitric oxide mediates glutamate-linked enhancement of cGMP levels in the cerebellum. Proc. Natl. Acad. Sci. U.S.A. 86:9030–9033.

Cedar, H., and Schwartz, J. H. 1972. Cyclic adenosine monophosphate in the nervous system of Aplysia californica II. Effect of serotonin and dopamine. J. Gen. Physiol. 60:570–587.

Colbran, R. J., and Soderling, T. R. 1990. Calcium/calmodulin-dependent protein kinase. Curr. Top. Cell Regul. 31:181–221.

Dennis, E. A. (ed.) 1991. Phospholipases. Meth. in Enzymol. 197: 1–640.

Frielle, T., Kobilka, B., Dohlman, H., Caron, M. G., and Lefkowitz, R. J. 1989. The β-adrenergic receptor and other receptors coupled to guanine nucleotide regulatory proteins. In S. Chien (ed.), Molecular Biology in Physiology. New York: Raven Press, pp. 79–91.

Furch-gott, R. F., and Vanhoutte, P. M. 1989. Endothelium-derived relaxing and contracting factors. FASEB J. 3:2007–2108.

Gustafsson, B., and Wigström, H. (eds.) 1990. Associative long-lasting modifications in synaptic efficacy. Sems. Neurosci. 2:317–420.

Hockberger, P. E., and Swandulla, D. 1987. Direct ion channel gating: A new function for intracellular messengers. Cell. Mol. Neurobiol. 7:229–236.

Jan, Y. N., Jan, L. Y., and Kuffler, S. W. 1979. A peptide as a possible transmitter in sympathetic ganglia of the frog. Proc. Natl. Acad. Sci. U.S.A. 76:1501–1505.

Kemp, B. E. 1990. Peptides and Protein Phosphorylation. Boca Raton, Fla.: CRC Press.

Knowles, R. G., Palacios, M., Palmer, R. M. J., and Moncada, S. 1989. Formation of nitric oxide from L-arginine in the central nervous system: A transduction mechanism for stimulation of the soluble guanylate cyclase. Proc. Natl. Acad. Sci. U.S.A. 86:5159–5162.

Madison, D. V., and Nicoll, R. A. 1986. Cyclic adenosine 3',5' monophosphate mediates β-receptor actions of noradrenaline in rat hippocampal pyramidal cells. J. Physiol. (Lond.) 372: 245–259.

Majerus, P. W., Connolly, T. M., Bansal, V. S., Inhorn, R. C., Ross, T. S., and Lips, D. L. 1988. Inositol phosphates: Synthesis and degradation. J. Biol. Chem. 263:3051–3054.

Murphy, R. C., and Fitzpatrick, F. A. (eds.) 1990. Arachidonate related lipid mediators. Meth. Enzymol. Sci. 187:1–683.

Nestler, E. J., and Greengard, P. 1984. Protein Phosphorylation in the Nervous System. New York: Wiley.

Nicoll, R. A., Madison, D. V., and Lancaster, B. 1987. Noradrenergic modulation of neuronal excitability in mammalian hippocampus. In H. Y. Meltzer (ed.), Psychopharmacology. The Third Generation of Progress. New York: Raven Press, pp. 105–112.

Nishizuka, Y. 1988. The molecular heterogeneity of protein kinase C and its implications for cellular regulation. Nature 334:661–665.

Piomelli, D., Volterra, A., Dale, N., Siegelbaum, S. A., Kandel, E. R., Schwartz, J. H., and Belardetti, F. 1987. Lipoxygenase metabolites of arachidonic acid as second messengers for presynaptic inhibition of Aplysia sensory cells. Nature 328:38–43.

Rangel-Aldao, R., and Rosen, O. M. 1976. Dissociation and reassociation of the phosphorylated and nonphosphorylated forms of adenosine 3′:5′-monophosphate-dependent protein kinase from bovine cardiac muscle. J. Biol. Chem. 251:3375–3380.

Role, L. W., and Schwartz, J. H. 1989. Cross-talk between signal transduction pathways. Trends Neurosci. 12:centerfold.

Schaap, D., Parker, P. J., Bristol, A., Kriz, R., and Knopf, J. 1989. Unique substrate specificity and regulatory properties of PKC-ε: A rationale for diversity. FEBS Lett. 243:351–357.

Schwartz, J. H., and Greenberg, S. M. 1987. Molecular mechanisms for memory: Second messenger induced modifications of protein kinase in nerve cells. Annu. Rev. Neurosci. 7:291–301.

Schworer, C. M., and Soderling, T. R. 1983. Substrate specificity of liver calmodulin-dependent glycogen synthase kinase. Biochem. Biophys. Res. Comm. 116:412–416.

Shapiro, E., Piomelli, D., Feinmark, S., Vogel, S. S., Chin, G. J., and Schwartz, J. H. 1988. The role of arachidonic acid metabolites in signal transduction in an identified neural network mediating presynaptic inhibition in Aplysia. Cold Spring Harbor Symp. Quant. Biol. 53:425–433.

Sibley, D. R., Benovic, J. L., Caron, M. G., and Lefkowitz, R. J. 1987. Regulation of transmembrane signaling by receptor phosphorylation. Cell 48:913–922.

Siegelbaum, S. A., Camardo, J. S., and Kandel, E. R. 1982. Serotonin and cyclic AMP close single K^+ channels in Aplysia sensory neurones. Nature 299:413–417.

Eric R. Kandel

13

Transmitter Release

Transmitter Release Is Controlled by Calcium Influx

Sodium Influx Is Not Necessary

Potassium Efflux Is Not Necessary

Calcium Influx Is Essential

Transmitter Is Released in Quantal Units

Calcium Influx Affects the Probability That a Quantum of Transmitter Will Be Released

Each Quantum of Transmitter Is Stored in a Specialized Organelle Called a Synaptic Vesicle

Transmitter Is Discharged from Synaptic Vesicles by Exocytosis at the Active Zone

The Docking of Synaptic Vesicles, Fusion, and Exocytosis Are Controlled by Calcium Influx

Calcium Influx Is Greatest in the Region of the Active Zone

Calcium Mobilizes Vesicles from the Cytoskeleton

The Number of Transmitter Vesicles Released Can Be Modulated by Altering Calcium Influx

Intrinsic Cellular Mechanisms Regulate the Concentration of Free Calcium

Synaptic Connections on Presynaptic Terminals Also Regulate Intracellular Free Calcium

An Overall View

Postscript: Calculating the Probability of Transmitter Release

S ome of the most remarkable activities of the brain, such as learning and memory, are thought to emerge from elementary properties of chemical synapses. The distinctive feature of chemical synapses is that the action potentials in the presynaptic terminals lead to the secretion of chemical messengers. In the last three chapters we examined the properties of the postsynaptic receptors and the ion channels and second-messenger systems they engage. In this and the next two chapters we examine the presynaptic component of the synapse. Here we consider how the secretory process of neurotransmission is coupled to the electrical events in presynaptic terminals.

Transmitter Release Is Controlled by Calcium Influx

Several key mechanisms in the initiation of transmitter release were revealed by Bernard Katz and his collaborators, who examined the steps between the action potential in the presynaptic cell and the release of chemical transmitter. As we have seen, the action potential results from two sequential steps. First, voltage-gated Na$^+$ channels open, allowing Na$^+$ to move into the presynaptic cell. Then voltage-gated K$^+$ channels open and K$^+$ moves out of the cell. Is either of these two processes responsible for triggering the release of the transmitter substance? Katz and Ricardo Miledi answered this question by using agents that selectively block each ion channel: tetrodotoxin blocks the voltage-gated Na$^+$ channel, and tetraethylammonium blocks the voltage-gated K$^+$ channel.

As discussed in Chapter 8, these agents are amazingly selective: Tetrodotoxin does not affect K$^+$ channels, nor does it affect the slight leak of Na$^+$ that normally occurs through the nongated channels of the membrane at rest.

Tetrodotoxin also does not interfere with properties of the postsynaptic receptor or of the channel that the receptor controls. Thus, at a cholinergic synapse tetrodotoxin blocks the presynaptic Na$^+$ spike but acetylcholine (ACh) will still produce an excitatory postsynaptic potential (EPSP) when applied directly to the postsynaptic receptors. This is not surprising since, as we saw in Chapter 10, the Na$^+$ channels activated by the action potential are different from the channels permeable to both Na$^+$ and K$^+$ that generate the synaptic potential. These drugs are examples of an important principle of neuropharmacology: classes of drugs are able to act selectively at specific regions of the neuron, and in those regions they act on specific molecular components.

Sodium Influx Is Not Necessary

To explore the contribution of Na$^+$ and K$^+$ to transmitter release, Katz and Miledi used the giant synapse of the squid because it is large enough to permit insertion of two electrodes into the presynaptic terminal (one for stimulating and one for recording) and an electrode into the postsynaptic cell for recording the synaptic potential and for use as an index of transmitter release.

The presynaptic cell typically produces an action potential of 110 mV, which leads to transmitter release and the generation of a large synaptic potential in the postsynaptic cell. When tetrodotoxin is added to the extracellular solution bathing the giant synapse, the presynaptic action potential becomes progressively smaller with time, due to the progressive block of Na$^+$ channels, and the postsynaptic potential is reduced accordingly. When the amplitude of the presynaptic spike is reduced below 40 mV, the synaptic potential disappears (Figure 13–1B).

From these results it might appear that influx of Na$^+$ into the presynaptic cell is essential for transmitter release. However, while the Na$^+$ channels were still fully blocked, Katz and Miledi next artificially depolarized the

FIGURE 13–1
Blocking presynaptic voltage-gated Na$^+$ channels with TTX affects the amplitude of the presynaptic action potential and the resulting postsynaptic potential. (Adapted from Katz and Miledi, 1967a.)

A. Recording electrodes are inserted in both the pre- and postsynaptic fibers of the giant synapse in the stellate ganglion of a squid.

B. After TTX is added, the amplitudes of both the presynaptic action potential and the postsynaptic potential gradually decrease. After 7 min the presynaptic action potential can still produce a suprathreshold synaptic potential that triggers an action potential in the postsynaptic cell (1). After 14 and 15 min the presynaptic spike gradually becomes smaller and produces smaller synaptic potentials (2 and 3). When the presynaptic spike is reduced to 40 mV or less, it fails to produce a synaptic potential (4).

C. When the Na$^+$ channels for the presynaptic action potential are blocked, one can obtain an input-output curve for transmitter release. **1.** In this experiment the presynaptic spike had to be 40 mV to produce a synaptic potential. Beyond this threshold there is a steep increase in synaptic potential corresponding to small changes in the amplitude of the presynaptic potential. **2.** As illustrated on the semilogarithmic plot of these data, the relationship between the presynaptic spike and the postsynaptic potential is logarithmic; a 10 mV increase in the presynaptic spike produces a tenfold increase in the synaptic potential.

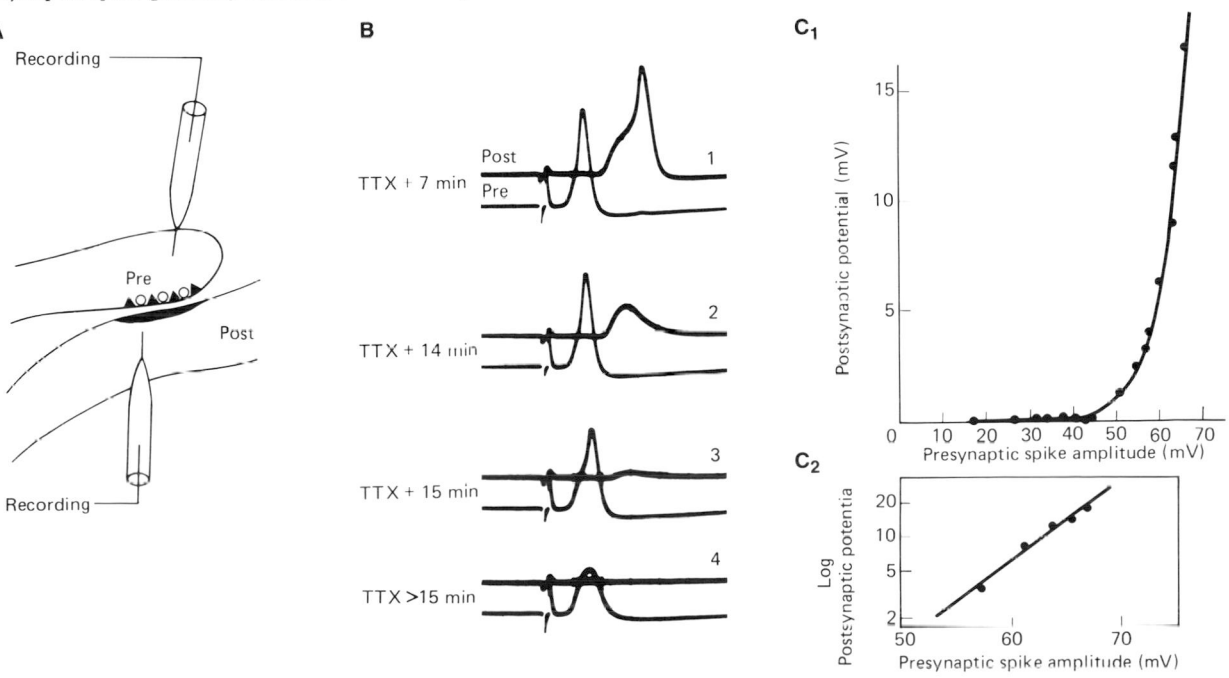

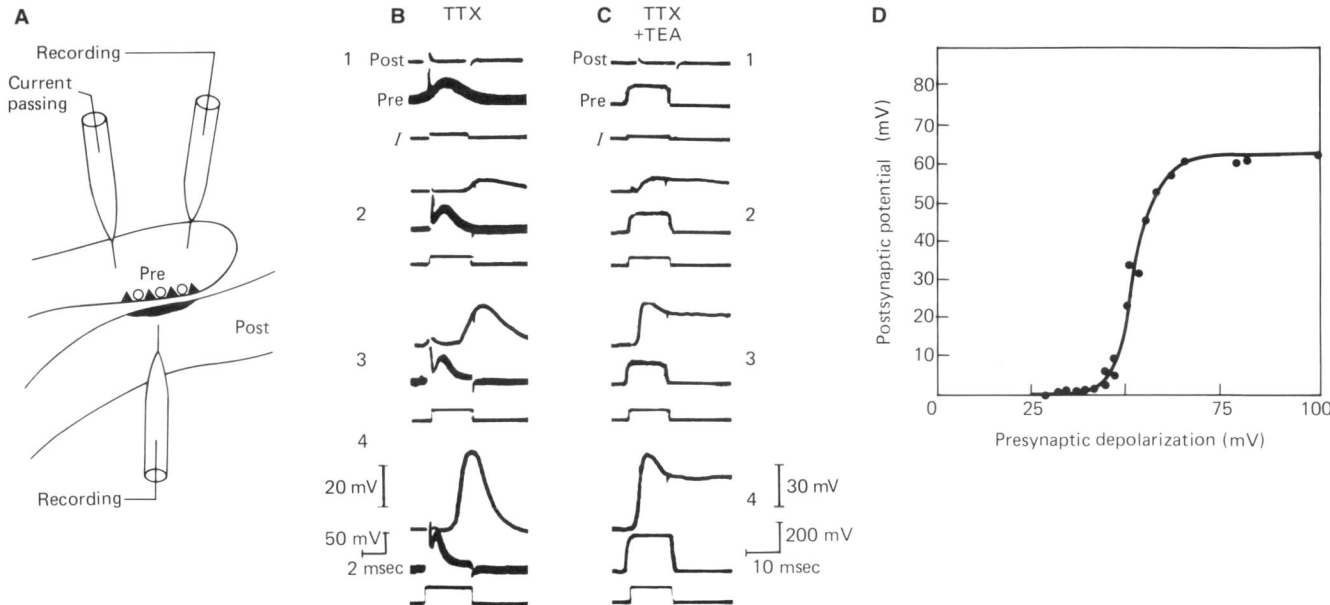

FIGURE 13–2

Transmitter release does not depend on K+ and Na+ currents. Blocking the voltage-sensitive Na+ channels and K+ channels in the presynaptic terminals with TTX and TEA affects the amplitude and duration of the presynaptic action potential and the resulting postsynaptic potential. However, as shown here, it does not block the release of transmitter, since postsynaptic potentials can still be produced by injecting depolarizing current presynaptically. (Adapted from Katz and Miledi, 1967a.)

A. The experimental arrangement is the same as in Figure 13–1, except that a current-passing electrode has been inserted into the presynaptic cell.

B. The Na+ channels of the action potentials have been blocked with TTX. **1.** The three traces represent (from bottom to top) the current pulse injected into the presynaptic terminal (*I*), the resulting potential in the presynaptic terminal (**Pre**), and the postsynaptic potential generated as a result of transmitter release in the postsynaptic cell (**Post**). **2–4.** Progressively stronger current pulses are applied to produce correspondingly greater depolarizations of the presynaptic terminal. These presynaptic depolarizations cause postsynaptic potentials even in the absence of Na+ flux. The greater the presynaptic depolarization,

the larger the postsynaptic potential. The presynaptic depolarizations are not maintained throughout the duration of the depolarizing current pulse because of the delayed activation of the voltage-gated K+ channel, which causes repolarization.

C. After the Na+ channels of the action potential have been blocked with TTX, TEA is injected into the presynaptic terminal to block the voltage-gated K+ channels. **1.** The three traces represent current pulse, presynaptic potential, and postsynaptic potential as in part B. Because K+ channels are blocked presynaptically, the electrotonic depolarization is maintained throughout the current pulse. **2–4.** Under these conditions larger presynaptic depolarizations still produce a larger postsynaptic potential. This indicates that neither Na+ nor K+ is required for effective transmitter release.

D. In the presence of TTX and TEA it is possible to generate a more complete input–output curve as a function of different depolarization steps than that shown in Figure 13–1. In addition to the steep part of the curve, there is now a plateau: a level of presynaptic depolarization above which no greater postsynaptic response is seen. (The initial level of the presynaptic membrane potential was about −70 mV.)

presynaptic membrane in steps up to 150 mV above the resting level of membrane potential by passing current out of the terminal through the second intracellular microelectrode. They found that, as the terminal was increasingly depolarized beyond a threshold of about 40 mV from the resting potential, progressively greater amounts of transmitter were released (as judged by the appearance and amplitude of the postsynaptic potential). In the range of depolarization at which chemical transmitter was released (40–70 mV above the resting level) a 10 mV increase in depolarization produced a 10-fold increase in transmitter release (Figure 13–2). Thus, they concluded that the presynaptic terminal is able to release transmitter without the influx of Na+. Some other ion flux associated with depolarization of the cell causes transmitter release.

Potassium Efflux Is Not Necessary

To examine the contribution of K+ efflux to transmitter release, Katz and Miledi blocked voltage-sensitive K+ and Na+ channels with tetraethylammonium (TEA) and tetrodotoxin (TTX) together (Figure 13–2). They then passed a depolarizing current through the presynaptic terminals and found that the postsynaptic potentials were of normal size, indicating that transmitter was released normally. Indeed, the presynaptic potential was maintained throughout the current pulse because the K+ current that normally repolarizes the presynaptic membrane was blocked. As a result, transmitter release was sustained (Figure 13–2C). By sustaining high levels of presynaptic depolarization, Katz and Miledi were also able to show that increases in the presynaptic potential above an upper limit produced no increase in postsynaptic potential (Figure 13–2D). Katz and Miledi therefore concluded that neither Na$^+$ nor K$^+$, the ions responsible for the action potential in the axon, is required for transmitter release.

Calcium Influx Is Essential

Katz and Miledi next turned their attention to Ca^{2+} ions. Earlier, José del Castillo and Katz had found that Ca^{2+} influences transmitter release. Increasing the extracellular Ca^{2+} enhances transmitter release; lowering it reduces and ultimately blocks synaptic transmission. The facilitating effect of Ca^{2+} on synaptic transmission is inhibited by Mg^{2+}, a blocker of Ca^{2+} channels.

How could external Ca^{2+} influence transmitter release, an intracellular process? An answer to this question was suggested by Alan Hodgkin and Peter Baker, who found in the squid giant axon that each action potential produces a small influx of Ca^{2+} through voltage-gated Ca^{2+} channels. Although these channels are sparsely distributed along the axon, Katz and Miledi proposed that they might be much more abundant at the axon terminal and that Ca^{2+} might serve two functions: as a carrier of charge during the action potential (like Na$^+$ and K$^+$) and as a special signal conveying information about changes in membrane potential to the intracellular machinery responsible for transmitter release.

Consistent with this prediction, Katz and Miledi found that when Na$^+$ and K$^+$ channels were blocked by TTX and TEA, any remaining current was carried by Ca^{2+} ions. Under these conditions the Ca^{2+} influx actually produces a regenerative action potential in the terminals! This was later called a *secretory potential* because it was discovered that this Ca^{2+} current is responsible for the secretion of transmitter into the synaptic cleft. The secretory potential does not occur throughout the length of the axon because of the low density of Ca^{2+} channels. Even in the axon terminal Ca^{2+} currents are small and are normally masked by Na$^+$ and K$^+$ currents, which are 10–20 times larger. However, Rodolfo Llinás and his colleagues voltage-clamped the presynaptic terminals of the squid giant synapse in the presence of TTX and TEA and showed that graded depolarizations of the terminals activate a graded inward Ca^{2+} current. The graded Ca^{2+} influx in turn results in graded release of transmitter (Figure 13–3). Unlike the voltage-gated Na$^+$ channels, the Ca^{2+} channels in the squid terminals do not inactivate quickly, but stay open as long as the presynaptic depolarization lasts.

At what stage during depolarization of the presynaptic cell does Ca^{2+} influx produce transmitter release? To answer this question, Katz and Miledi used a frog nerve-muscle preparation bathed in TTX and Ca^{2+}-free Ringer's solution. In addition to inserting a recording electrode inside the muscle fiber, they also used two external electrodes. One, filled with NaCl, was used to depolarize the terminals; the other, filled with CaCl$_2$, was used to raise the local Ca^{2+} concentration before or after the depolarizing pulse. Katz and Miledi found that Ca^{2+} must be

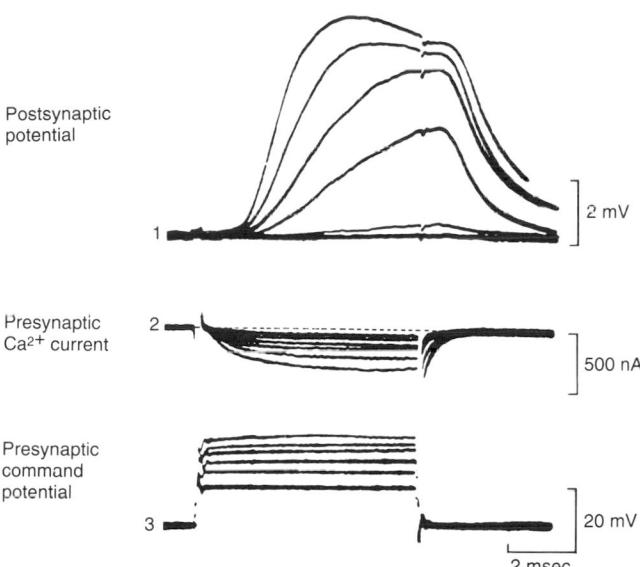

FIGURE 13–3

Transmitter release is a function of Ca^{2+} influx into the presynaptic terminal. These recordings are from a squid giant synapse in which the voltage-sensitive Na$^+$ and K$^+$ channels were blocked by TTX and TEA. The size of the postsynaptic potentials in the top traces (1), which reflects the amount of transmitter released, can be seen to correlate in a graded manner with the amount of inward Ca^{2+} current that accompanies the depolarization (2). The presynaptic terminal is voltage-clamped and the membrane potential is stepped to six different command levels of depolarization (3). Increases in depolarization produce the increases in Ca^{2+} current seen in 2. The notch in the postsynaptic potential trace is an artifact that results from turning off the presynaptic command potential. (Adapted from Llinás and Heuser, 1977.)

present *during* the depolarization to produce transmitter release (Figure 13–4B). When the Ca^{2+} pulse was delayed until the end of the depolarization, no postsynaptic potential was produced. Nor was a potential produced when Mg^{2+} was injected into the bathing solution, since Mg^{2+} blocks the Ca^{2+} channels (Figure 13–4C).

These findings suggested to Katz and Miledi that the depolarization produced by the action potential in the terminals opens voltage-dependent Ca^{2+} channels so that Ca^{2+} can then move into the cell down its steep concentration gradient and reach the sites from which transmitter is released. The normal synaptic delay characteristic of chemical synapses—the time that is required from the onset (Chapter 9) of the action potential in the presynaptic terminals to the onset of the postsynaptic potential—is due in large part to the time required for Ca^{2+} channels to open in response to depolarization. Because of this delay in channel activation, Ca^{2+} does not begin to flow until the end of the action potential in the presynaptic cell, when the membrane potential begins to return to the resting level (Figure 13–5).

We now know from the work of Llinás, that the voltage-dependent Ca^{2+} channels can act within 0.2 ms to trigger transmitter release because they are located very close to the transmitter release sites. As we shall see later

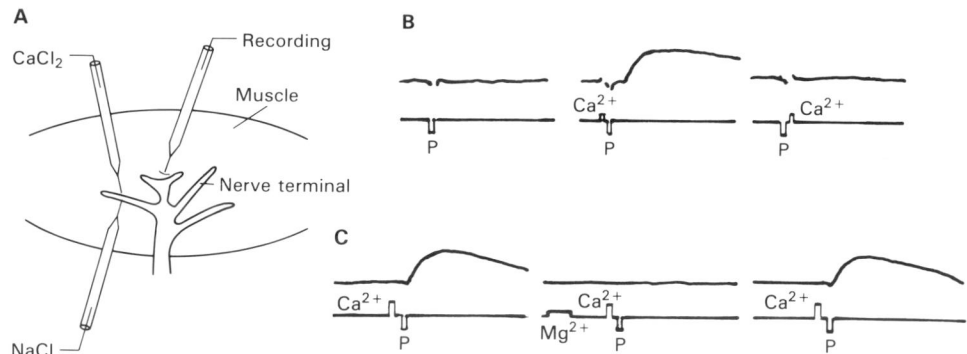

FIGURE 13–4

Calcium influx must occur during depolarization for transmitter release to occur. (Adapted from Katz and Miledi, 1967b.) (PCa²⁺)

A. In this experiment at the vertebrate neuromuscular junction, the extracellular fluid around the nerve and muscle is free of Ca^{2+} to prevent transmitter release and contains TTX to block action potentials. As a result, transmitter release is completely controlled by two external electrodes. One electrode (with NaCl) controls the membrane potential, the other electrode (with CaCl₂) determines when Ca^{2+} is available to the presynaptic neuron. The end-plate potentials resulting from transmitter release are recorded intracellularly from the muscle fiber.

B. Electrical recordings of the postsynaptic response in the muscle are shown in the top traces. A brief depolarizing pulse is applied to the presynaptic terminals through the NaCl elec-

trode in each of three conditions: depolarizing current pulse alone, (P), just after a pulse of Ca^{2+} ($Ca^{2+}P$), and just before a pulse of Ca^{2+} (PCa²⁺). The bottom traces show the depolarizing pulse (P, downward step) relative to the Ca^{2+} pulse (upward step). Transmitter is released (as indicated by the presence of a postsynaptic potential) only when the Ca^{2+} pulse precedes the depolarizing pulse. Thus, for Ca^{2+} to be an effective agent of transmitter release, it must be present during the depolarization.

C. In the first recording a postsynaptic potential is produced by depolarization preceded by a Ca^{2+} pulse. In the second recording no postsynaptic potential is produced because the influx of Ca^{2+} is blocked by a pulse of Mg^{2+} and no transmitter is released. (The Mg^{2+} is applied by a third pipette filled with MgCl₂, which is not shown in the diagram in A.). Transmitter release is again turned on by Ca^{2+} when Mg^{2+} is no longer present.

---

in this chapter, the duration of the action potential is an important determinant of the amount of Ca^{2+} that flows into the terminal. If the action potential is prolonged, more Ca^{2+} flows in and therefore more transmitter is released, causing a greater postsynaptic potential.

In most nerve cells other than the giant axon of squid, there are at least two (and probably more) classes of voltage-sensitive Ca^{2+} channels. One class (the *L type* channel) is characterized by a very slow rate of inactivation, so that it remains open during a prolonged depolarization of the membrane. This class is blocked by the dihydropyridine drugs, such as nifedipine. The second class (*N type*) inactivates more rapidly and is insensitive to dihydropyridines. In many cells other than the squid giant synapse, the influx of Ca^{2+} through this rapidly inactivating N type channel contributes most directly to transmitter release.

Transmitter Is Released in Quantal Units

How and where does Ca^{2+} produce its actions? To answer that question we must consider how transmitter substances are released. Even though the release of synaptic transmitter appears smoothly graded, it is actually quantized. Each *quantum* of transmitter produces a postsynaptic potential of fixed size, called the *unit synaptic potential*. The total synaptic potential is made up from an integral number of unit potentials. The synaptic potentials and the input–output curves in Figures 13–1 and

13–2 seem smoothly graded because each unit potential is small relative to the total postsynaptic potential. Paul Fatt and Katz discovered the quantal nature of transmission when they recorded from the nerve–muscle synapse of the frog without presynaptic stimulation and observed small spontaneous potentials of about 0.5–1.0 mV. Similar results have since been obtained in mammalian muscle and in central neurons. Because the synaptic potentials at vertebrate nerve–muscle synapses are called end-plate potentials, Fatt and Katz called these spontaneous potentials *miniature end-plate potentials*.

The time course of the miniature end-plate potentials and the effects of various drugs on them are indistinguishable from the effects on the end-plate potential evoked by nerve stimulation. Because ACh is the transmitter at the nerve–muscle synapse, the miniature end-plate potentials, like the full-sized end-plate potentials, are enhanced and prolonged by prostigmine, a drug that inhibits the hydrolysis of ACh by acetylcholinesterase. Similarly, the miniature end-plate potentials are reduced and finally abolished by agents that block the ACh receptor, such as *d*-tubocurarine. In the absence of stimulation the miniature end-plate potentials occur at random intervals; their frequency can be increased by depolarizing the presynaptic terminal. They disappear if the presynaptic nerve degenerates but reappear with reinnervation, indicating that small amounts of ACh are continuously released at the presynaptic nerve terminal.

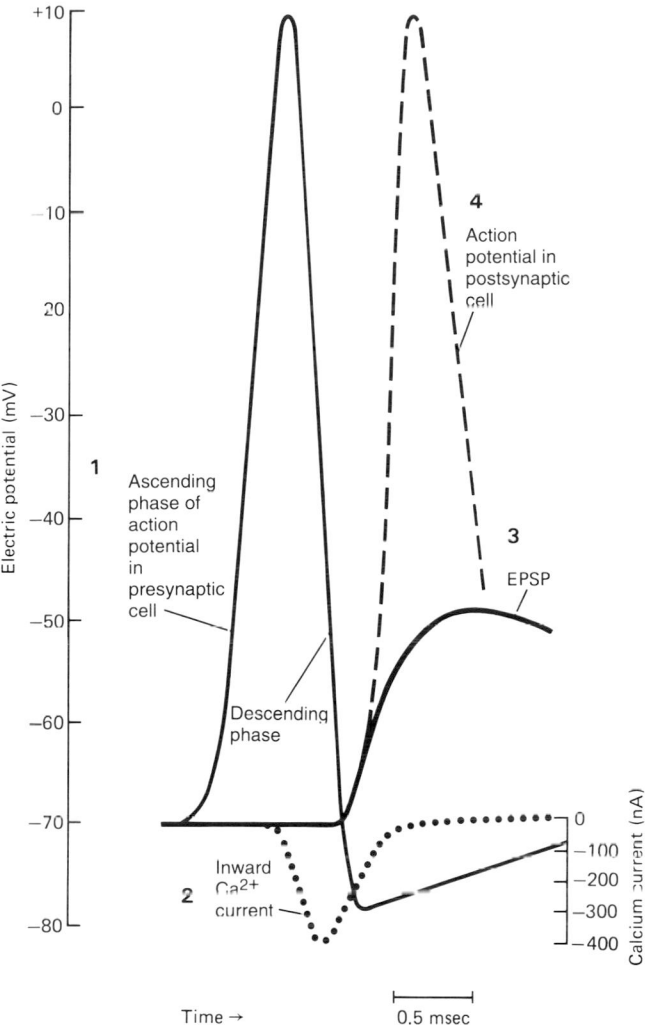

FIGURE 13–5

Time course of four events related to synaptic transmission. An action potential in the presynaptic cell (**1**) causes presynaptic Ca^{2+} channels to open and a Ca^{2+} current (**2**) to flow into the terminal leading to the release of neurotransmitter from the terminal. (Note that the Ca^{2+} current is turned on late during the falling phase of the presynaptic action potential.) The postsynaptic response to the transmitter begins soon afterward (**3**), and, if sufficiently large, will trigger an action potential in the postsynaptic cell (**4**). (Adapted from Llinás, 1982.)

What could account for the fixed size (0.5–1.0 mV) of the spontaneous miniature end-plate potential? Del Castillo and Katz first tested the possibility that the fixed size represents a fixed response of a single ACh receptor to one ACh molecule. By ejecting small amounts of ACh iontophoretically from a microelectrode applied to the frog muscle end-plate, they were able to elicit depolarizing responses smaller than 0.5 mV. From this it became clear that the miniature end-plate potential must reflect the opening of many individual ACh receptor-channels.

Later, Katz and Miledi were able to estimate the elementary ionic conductance event—the opening of a single synaptic channel caused by the interaction of ACh with a single receptor. They did this by applying small amounts of ACh to the receptor-rich membrane. The resulting fluctuations in membrane potential noise were assumed to represent the fluctuations produced by the random opening and closing of many channels. By analyzing this noise mathematically, Katz and Miledi estimated that the elementary ACh potential produced by the opening of a single ACh receptor-channel is only about 0.3 μV, or about 1/2000 of the amplitude of a spontaneous miniature potential. This was later confirmed when the currents through single channels responsive to ACh could be measured directly using patch-clamp techniques (see Chapter 10).

A miniature end-plate potential of 0.5 mV would therefore require summation of the elementary conductance of about 2000 channels. For a single channel to open, two ACh molecules must bind to the receptor. In addition, some of the ACh released is lost, either by diffusion out of the synaptic cleft or by hydrolysis by acetylcholinesterase, and never reaches the receptor molecules. Thus, about 5000 molecules are needed to produce a miniature end-plate potential. This number was confirmed by direct chemical measurement of the ACh released per unit synaptic potential. Thus, a miniature synaptic potential is produced not by a single molecule but by about 5000 transmitter molecules. As we shall see below, there is good reason to believe that ACh is stored and released from the terminal by specialized organelles called *synaptic vesicles*, which are abundant in electron micrographs of synaptic terminals.

Calcium Influx Affects the Probability That a Quantum of Transmitter Will Be Released

We can now ask some important questions: Are the spontaneously released quanta the same as the unit potentials that are released during normal synaptic transmission? If ACh is normally released in quanta, how does Ca^{2+} influence the amount of ACh released? These questions were answered by examining the results of decreasing the external concentration of Ca^{2+}. Del Castillo and Katz found that when the neuromuscular junction was bathed in a solution that was low in Ca^{2+}, the evoked end-plate potential (normally 70 mV in amplitude) was reduced markedly to about 0.5–2.5 mV. The amplitude of the evoked end-plate potential was not fixed but varied from stimulus to stimulus and often could not be detected. However, the minimum response above zero, the unit synaptic potential in response to an action potential, was identical in size and shape to the spontaneously occurring miniature end-plate potential. All end-plate potentials larger than the unit synaptic potential were integral multiples of the unit potential (Figure 13–6 and Postscript).

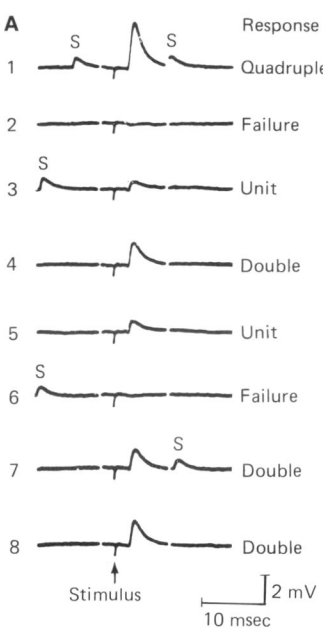

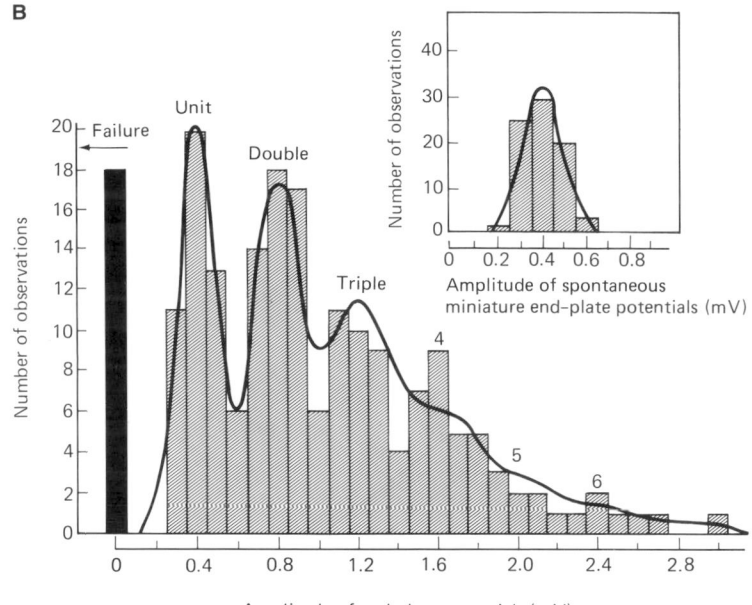

FIGURE 13–6

Transmitter is released in quanta, each of which produces a response of fixed-amplitude. Any one response is a result of the release of a certain number of quanta of transmitter and its amplitude is equal to the unit amplitude multiplied by the number of quanta of transmitter.

A. Intracellular recordings from a rat nerve–muscle synapse show the spontaneous occurrence of miniature end-plate potentials (S) as well as synaptic responses (end-plate potentials) evoked by eight consecutive stimuli to the motor nerve (1–8). To reduce transmitter output and to keep the end-plate potentials small, the tissue is bathed in a Ca^{2+}-deficient (and Mg^{2+}-rich) solution. The same size stimulus elicits some variation in response: Two impulses produce complete failures, two produce unit potentials, and still others produce responses that are approximately two to four times the amplitude of the unit potential. The spontaneous miniature end-plate potentials (S) are the same size as the unit potential. (Adapted from Liley, 1956.)

B. After many recordings similar to those shown in A, the amplitude of each potential was measured. The number of responses at each amplitude was then counted and plotted in the histogram shown here. The distribution of responses falls into a number of peaks. The first peak, at 0 mV, represents failures. The first peak of responses, at 0.4 mV, represents the unit potential, the smallest elicited response. This unit response is the same amplitude as the spontaneous miniature potentials (inset). Subsequent peaks of responses occur at amplitudes that are integral multiples of the amplitude of the unit potential. The solid line shows a theoretical distribution fitted to the data of the histogram. Each peak is slightly spread out in a Gaussian distribution, reflecting the fact that the amount of transmitter in each quantum varies slightly and in a random fashion. The distribution of amplitudes of the spontaneous miniature potentials, shown in the inset, fits the theoretical Gaussian curve (solid line) well. (Adapted from Boyd and Martin, 1956.)

When the external Ca^{2+} concentration was increased, the amplitude of the unit synaptic potential did not change. However, the number of failures decreased and the incidence of higher-amplitude responses increased. These observations illustrate that alterations in external Ca^{2+} concentration do not affect the *size* of a quantum (the number of ACh molecules) but the *probability* that it will be released. The greater the Ca^{2+} influx into the terminal, the larger the number of quanta released.

The finding that the amplitude of the end-plate potentials increases in a stepwise manner at low levels of ACh release, that the amplitude of each step increase is an integral multiple of the unit potential, and that the unit potential has the same mean amplitude as that of the spontaneous miniature end-plate potentials led del Castillo and Katz to propose that the normal end-plate potential is caused by the release of about 150 quanta,

each about 0.5 mV in amplitude. In the absence of an action potential only one quantum is released at the end-plate per second. This low probability of release is reflected in the small number of spontaneously released miniature end-plate potentials. The Ca^{2+} that enters with an action potential transiently increases the rate of quantal release 100,000-fold, resulting in the synchronous release during 1–2 ms of 150 quanta on average. The amplitude of the end-plate potential actually varies slightly in response to consecutive action potentials because the precise number of quanta released varies randomly from stimulus to stimulus.

Quantal transmission has been demonstrated at all chemical synapses so far examined, with the possible exception of the retina, which we shall consider later. However, at most synapses in the central nervous system each action potential releases between one and 10 quanta, much less than the 150 quanta at the nerve–muscle synapse. The reason for this is that a given presynaptic motor terminal ending on a muscle fiber is large (about 2000 to 6000 μm²). Distributed along this large presynaptic surface are about 300 active zones. In contrast, a typical Ia afferent excitatory fiber from a dorsal root ganglion cell has only about four endings on a motor neuron, each of which is about 2 μm² and contains only one active zone. Quantal analysis of Ia afferent neurons by Stephen Redman indicates that each terminal ending releases no more than one quantum of transmitter and alternates between 0 and 1. Similar results have been obtained for other central synapses by Henri Korn and Donald Faber. Thus, the variations in the overall response of a central neuron to a single presynaptic neuron results from the all-or-none probability of release of single quanta from a few boutons with single release sites.

Each Quantum of Transmitter Is Stored in a Specialized Organelle Called a Synaptic Vesicle

How is a quantum of transmitter released by a neuron? In 1957 the first electron micrographs of synapses revealed accumulations of small vesicles in the presynaptic terminal. This discovery coincided with the physiological observations by del Castillo and Katz that transmitter release is quantal. The electron micrographs suggested to del Castillo and Katz that the vesicles were storage organelles for the transmitter quanta. They argued that each

vesicle stored one quantum of transmitter amounting to several thousand molecules. The vesicle was thought to fuse with the inner surface of the presynaptic terminal at specific release sites, where it opened transiently and extruded its entire contents into the synaptic cleft.

Some years after del Castillo and Katz's proposal Sanford Palay obtained high-resolution electron micrographs of chemical synapses. Palay's pictures revealed that synaptic vesicles are not uniformly distributed throughout the presynaptic terminal, but rather are clustered at regions where the presynaptic membrane appears thicker and more dense than elsewhere. Using tissue treated with phosphotungstic acid, René Couteaux found that the presynaptic thickening at the nerve–muscle synapse is a membrane-associated specialization, not an actual thickening of the plasma membrane. The specialization appeared as dense bodies attached to the internal face of the presynaptic membrane directly above the junctional folds in the muscle (Figure 13–7). At the nerve–muscle synapse these dense bodies are bar-shaped; at central synapses they take the form of discrete pyramidal projections. The vesicles collect in rows along the edges of the dense bodies. Couteaux called the region the *active zone* because in occasional electron micrographs he occasionally found configurations of the presynaptic membrane, called *omega* figures within this region. These figures appeared to be vesicles undergoing exocytosis. The term active zone is now applied only to the region with dense bodies, where transmitter is actually released from small electron-lucent

FIGURE 13–7

The topography of the transmitter release site at the neuromuscular junction is shown in this thin-section micrograph (**A**) and drawing (**B**). Small synaptic vesicles (40–50 nm in diameter) containing ACh molecules are clustered around dense bars in the presynaptic neuron. The region of dense bodies is called the active zone and is located just above ACh receptors at the apexes of the junctional folds in the muscle membrane. Running through the synaptic cleft is the basement membrane, to which acetylcholinesterase attaches. (Adapted from Kuffler, Nicholls, and Martin, 1984.)

A

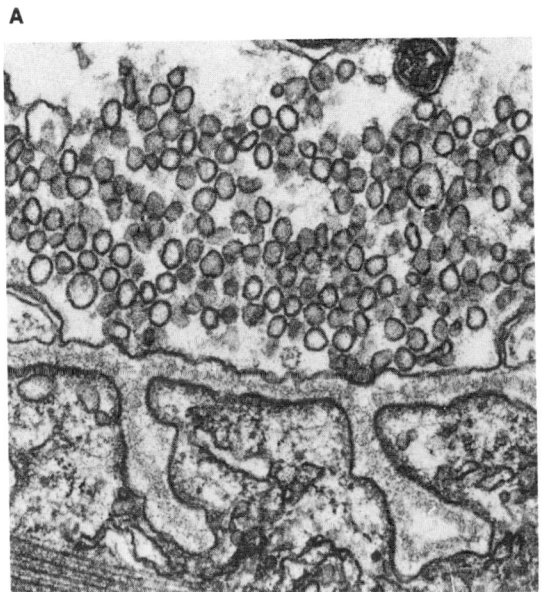

B

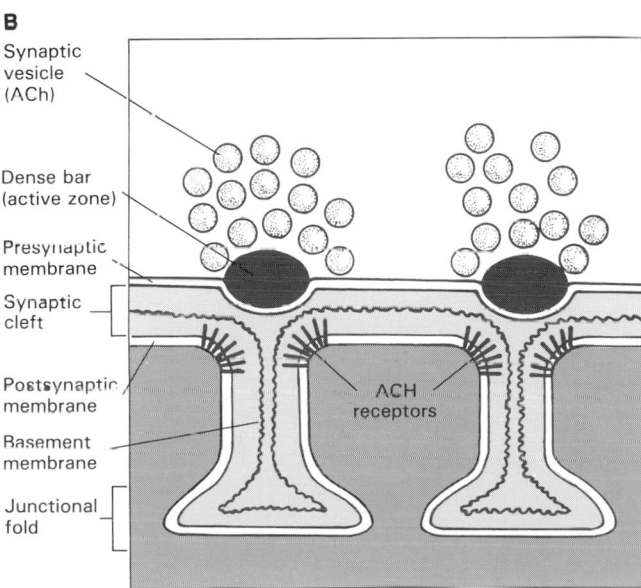

Synaptic vesicle (ACh)

Dense bar (active zone)

Presynaptic membrane

Synaptic cleft

Postsynaptic membrane

Basement membrane

Junctional fold

ACh receptors

Freeze-Fracture Technique BOX 13–1

Freeze-fracture reveals the structural details of synaptic membranes. Frozen tissue is broken open under a high vacuum and coated with platinum and carbon. The frozen membranes tend to break along the weakest plane, which is between the bimolecular layer of lipids. The membrane is weakest there because the bimolecular leaflets are held together only by noncovalent interactions between the hydrophobic heads of phospholipid molecules. Two complementary faces of the membrane are thus exposed: The leaflet nearest the cytoplasm (the interior half) is called the pro-

toplasmic (P) face, and the leaflet that borders the extracellular space is the external (E) face.

Because freeze fracture exposes a view of a large area of the presynaptic area, deformations of the membrane that occur at the active zone, where vesicles are attached, are readily apparent. The panoramic view of the region of active zones that the freeze-fracture technique affords is best appreciated by comparing this figure with the conventional transmission electron microscopic image of the active zone (see Figure 13–7).

FIGURE 13–8A

The path of membrane cleavage is along the hydrophobic interior of the lipid bilayer, resulting in two complementary fracture faces. The P face contains most of the integral membrane proteins (particles) because of their anchoring to cytoskeletal structures. The E face shows pits complementary to the integral protein particles. (Redrawn from Fawcett, 1981.)

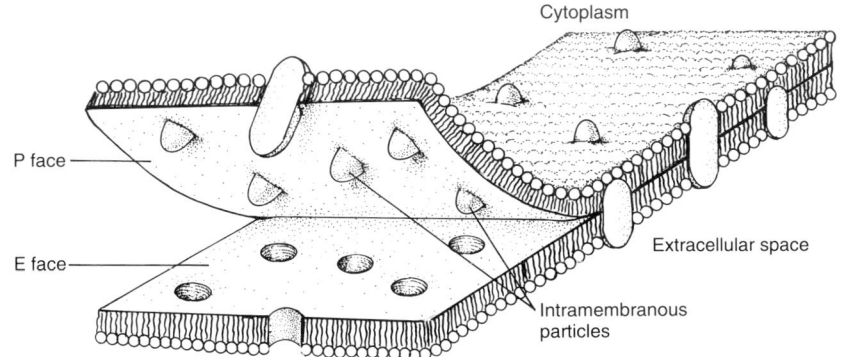

FIGURE 13–8B

This three-dimensional view of pre- and postsynaptic membranes shows active zones with adjacent rows of synaptic vesicles as well as places where the vesicles are undergoing exocytosis. The split membrane shows the predicted image of these structures in freeze-fracture. The rows of particles on either side of the active zone are intramembranous proteins thought to be Ca^{2+} channels. (Adapted from Kuffler, Nicholls, and Martin, 1984.)

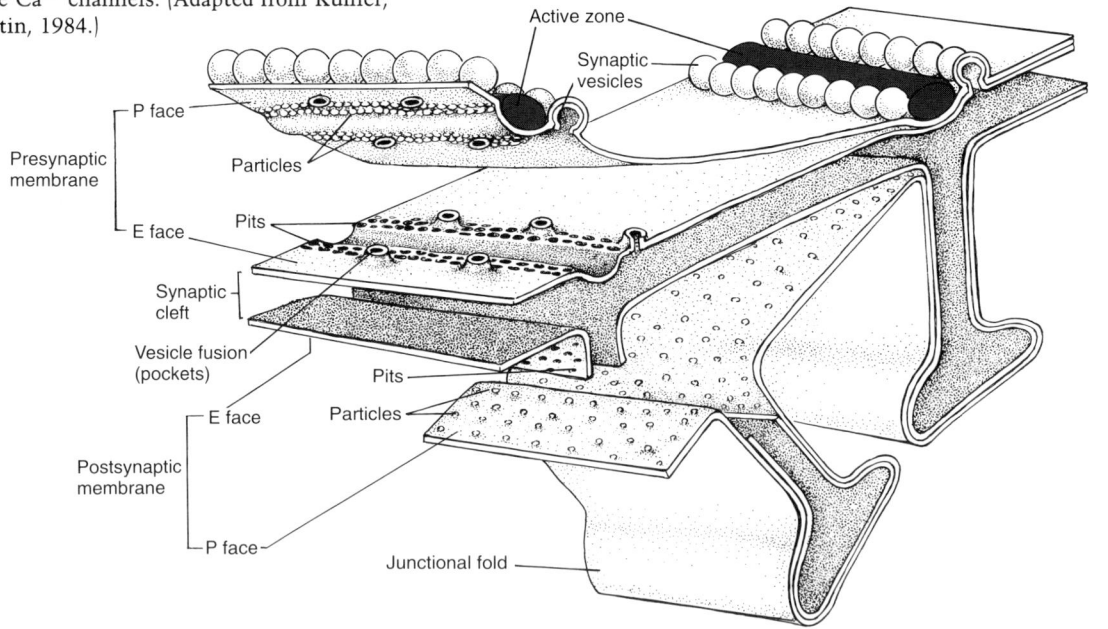

vesicles. At the frog neuromuscular junction there are about 300 active zones around which cluster about 10^6 vesicles. Here as at central synapses the vesicles are typically small and ovoid in shape with a diameter of about 50 nm. As we shall learn later and in the next chapter, biogenic amine and peptide transmitters are stored in larger vesicles that do not release their contents from active zones.

Transmitter Is Discharged from Synaptic Vesicles by Exocytosis at the Active Zone

The discovery of the dense bodies indicated that synaptic vesicles collect preferentially at specific points in the presynaptic membrane, from where they discharge their contents by *exocytosis*. But are these the only sites at which exocytosis occurs? This question is difficult to investigate in conventionally fixed tissue sections because the chance of finding a vesicle in the act of being discharged is extremely small. For example, a thin section through a terminal at the neuromuscular junction of the frog shows only 1/4000 of the total presynaptic membrane.

Because only relatively small areas of synaptic membrane can be examined in the ultrathin sections (50–100 nm) required for transmission electron microscopy, and because the exocytotic opening of each small vesicle is smaller than the thickness of the section, in the 1970s many workers began to apply freeze-fracture techniques to this problem (Box 13–1).

Using freeze fracture, Thomas Reese and John Heuser made three important observations. (1) Along both margins of each of the dense bars described by Couteaux there are one or two rows of unusually large intramembranous particles (Figures 13–8B and 13–9A). Although the function of these particles is not yet known, their density (about 1500 per μm^2) is approximately that of the voltage-gated Ca^{2+} channels essential for transmitter release. Moreover, the proximity of the particles to the release site is consistent with the short delay between the onset of the Ca^{2+} current and the release of transmitter observed by Llinás. (2) Deformations alongside the rows of intramembranous particles become apparent during synaptic activity (Figure 13–9B). These deformations coincide with the region of nerve terminal where electron microscopic thin sections show omega figures, which could represent invaginations of the cell membrane during exocytosis. (3) The deformations do not persist after the transmitter has been released; rather, they seem to be transient distortions that occur only when vesicles are discharged.

To catch vesicles in the act of exocytosis, Heuser and Reese devised a quick-freezing machine cooled by liquid helium. This device also allows stimulation of the presynaptic axon so that the tissue can be frozen at precisely defined intervals after the nerve has been stimulated. The neuromuscular junction can thus be frozen just as the action potential invades the terminal and exocytosis occurs. Using this device and the drug 4-aminopyridine (a tetraethylammonium-like substance that blocks certain voltage-gated K^+ channels, broadens the action potential, and increases the number of quanta discharged with each nerve impulse), Heuser, Reese, and their colleagues studied the morphological events accompanying exocytosis quantitatively.

Their observations of vesicles during exocytosis at the frog neuromuscular junction indicate that one vesicle undergoes exocytosis for each quantum of transmitter that is released. Statistical analyses of the spatial distribution of synaptic vesicle discharge sites along the active zones show that individual vesicles fuse with the plasma membrane independently of one another. This result is consistent with physiological studies that indicate that quanta of transmitter are released independently. These morphological studies therefore provide independent evidence that the synaptic vesicles store the transmitter and that exocytosis is the release mechanism.

Fusion of the membrane of the synaptic vesicles with the plasma membrane of the presynaptic terminal during exocytosis leads to an increase in surface area of the plasma membrane. In certain favorable circumstances this series of events can be detected in electrical measurements of membrane capacitance. As we saw in Chapter 7, the capacitance of the membrane is proportional to its surface area. In certain cell types, such as mast cells of the rat peritoneum, individual vesicles are large enough so that the increase in capacitance associated with fusion of a single vesicle can be detected (Figure 13–10). Massive release of transmitter is followed somewhat later by stepwise decreases in capacitance, which presumably reflect retrieval and recycling of the excess membrane (Figure 13–10).

The Docking of Synaptic Vesicles, Fusion, and Exocytosis Are Controlled by Calcium Influx

We saw earlier that Ca^{2+} influx affects the probability of transmitter release. Recent evidence shows that Ca^{2+} is required at two steps: (1) for fusion of the synaptic vesicle at the active zone and (2) for mobilization of vesicles into release sites at the active zone. Most vesicles in the presynaptic terminal are associated with cytoskeletal elements *near* the active zone. Only a small number of vesicles actually are positioned at the active zones (Figure 13–7). These vesicles are thought to have the highest probability of being released by exocytosis. Calcium is thought to act by allowing them to fuse with the membrane at the release site (Figure 13–11).

How does docking at the active zone and fusion of the vesicles actually occur? The mechanisms are still not known, but there is evidence from patch-clamp studies of mast cells by Lorna Breckenridge and Wolf Almers that fusion of the secretory vesicle to the plasma membrane leads to the temporary formation of an ion channel at the point of contact. These patch-clamp recordings support

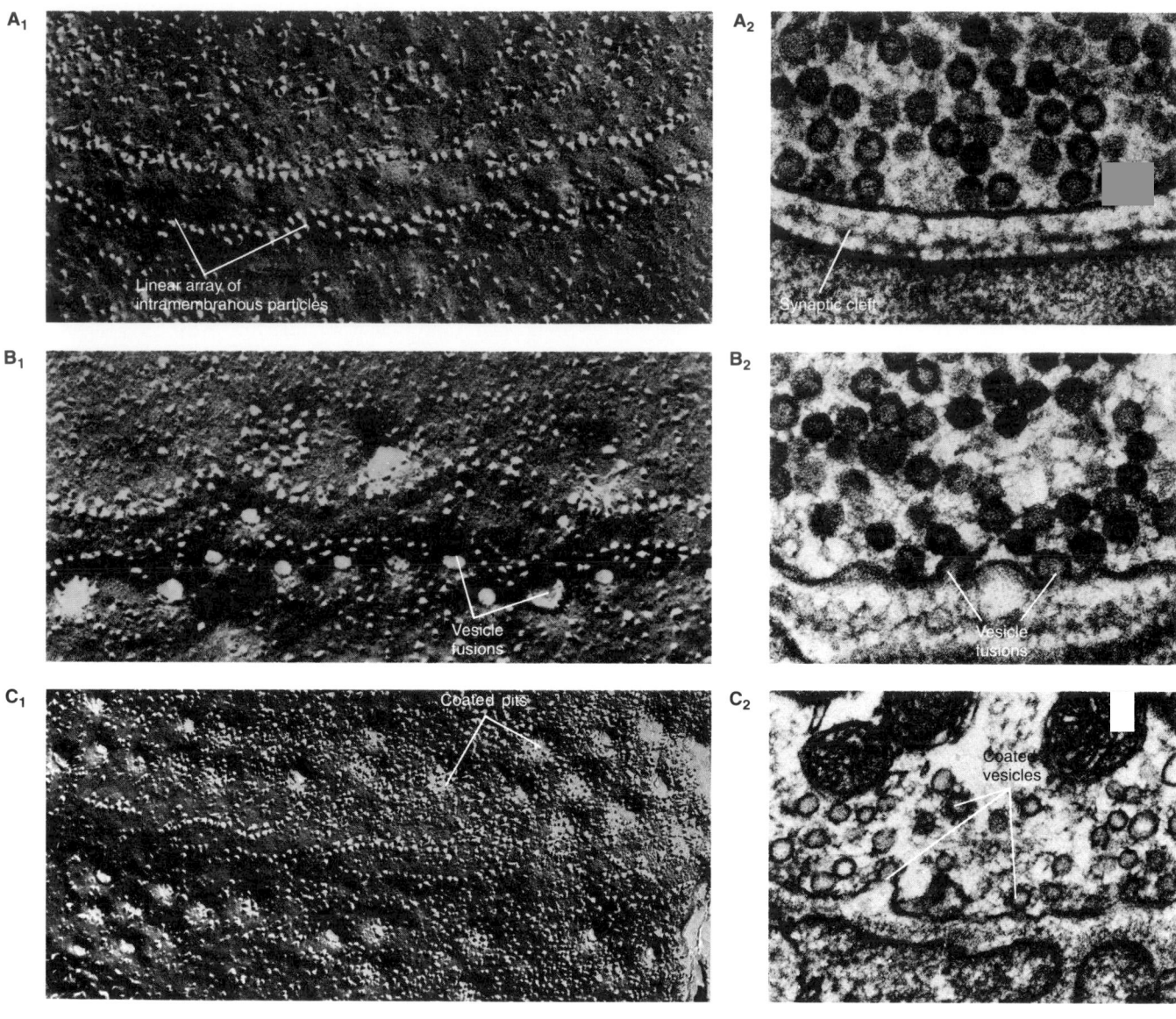

├── 100 nm ──┤

FIGURE 13–9

Exocytosis viewed with electron microscopy in the experiment of Reese and Heuser. Freeze-fracture electron micrographs of the cytoplasmic half of the presynaptic membrane are shown on the **left**; thin-section micrographs are shown on the **right**. (From Alberts et al., 1989.)

A. 1–2. The active zone in the resting state is marked by parallel arrays of intramembranous particles (See Figure 13–8).

B. 1. Synaptic vesicles begin fusing with the plasma membrane within 5 ms after the stimulus. **2.** Fusion is complete within

another 2 ms. Each opening in the plasma membrane represents the fusion of one synaptic vesicle.

C. 1. Membrane retrieval becomes apparent within about 10 s as coated pits form. After another 10 s the coated pits begin to pinch off by endocytosis to form coated vesicles. **2.** These vesicles include the original membrane proteins of the synaptic vesicle and also contain molecules captured from the external medium.

the morphological observation that early in exocytosis there is a rapid formation of a *fusion pore*, a narrow cytoplasmic bridge that unites the vesicle membrane with the plasma membrane at the active zone and connects the lumen of the vesicle with the extracellular space. This small pore initially has a mean conductance of about 230 pS, similar to that of connexons found at gap junctions,

whose typical diameter is about 1.5 nm. This pore soon dilates to reach 50 nm in size, and, in parallel, the conductance increases dramatically as exocytosis occurs.

How the fusion pore is produced is not known. Since transmitter release is so fast, Almers and Fred Tse argue that fusion must occur within a fraction of a millisecond. As a result the fusion protein that docks synaptic vesicles

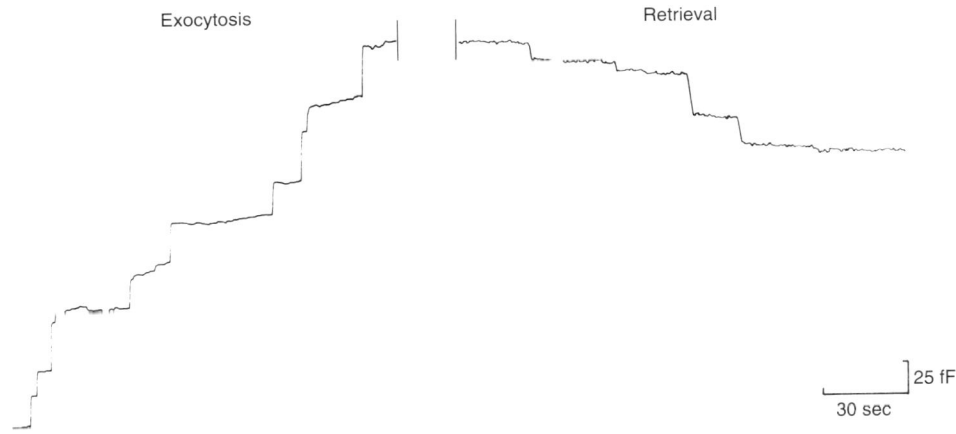

Exocytosis

Retrieval

25 fF

30 sec

FIGURE 13–10

Exocytosis of synaptic vesicles and subsequent retrieval of the excess membrane produce changes in the surface area of the membrane that can be detected by electrical measurement of membrane capacitance. The increases in capacitance occur in a stepwise fashion and reflect the fusion of individual synaptic vesicles with the cell membrane. The unequal step increases indicate a variability in the diameter of the vesicles. The increases are not associated with measurable changes in mem-

brane conductance. After transmitter is released from the vesicles, the membrane added by fusion of the synaptic vesicles is excised, retrieved, and transported to the cell body. In this way the cell maintains a constant size. The recording here is from a rat connective tissue cell, a mast cell undergoing massive exocytotic release of its large secretory granules (units are femtofarads, fF, where 1 fF ≈ 0.1 μm^2 membrane area). (From Fernandez, Neher, and Gomperts, 1984).

to the plasma membrane is most likely already present in the vesicle before fusion occurs. Much like the hemichannels of a gap junction, the fusion pore in neurons may consist of two halves, one in the vesicle membrane and the other in the plasma membrane, which join in the

course of docking the vesicles (Figure 13–11). Calcium influx would then simply cause the preexisting pore to dilate and allow release of transmitter. Indeed, there are now two candidate proteins associated with the membrane of the vesicle that might serve as fusion proteins. One of

FIGURE 13–11

Calcium influx affects both exocytosis of synaptic vesicles and mobilization of vesicles at the active zone. (From Kelly, 1988.)

A. In the resting state most vesicles are above the active zone and anchored to actin (**black bars**). A few vesicles are docked at the active zone, anchored to membrane fusion proteins. Voltage-gated Ca^{2+} channels are closed.

B. An action potential arriving at the terminals opens the Ca^{2+} channels. Calcium entering the cell affects the movement of vesicles toward the active sites by dissolving some actin filaments. It also aids the fusion of the vesicles with the plasma membrane. The transmitter is extruded through channels that appear to have properties similar to those of the gap junction channels described in Chapter 9.

A   Resting state

B   After Ca^{2+} influx

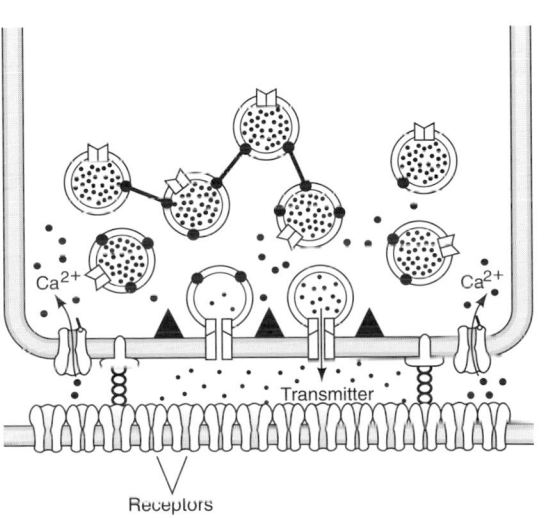

Synaptic vesicle

Vesicle fusion protein

Synaptic actin binding protein

Actin

Transmitter

Membrane fusion protein

Dense bodies

Ca^{2+} channels

Presynaptic terminal

Postsynaptic membrane

Alignment protein

Receptors

Ca^{2+}

Ca^{2+}

Transmitter

Receptors

these, synaptophysin, has been cloned by Thomas Südhof and his colleagues, and by Heinrich Betz. This protein makes up 6% of the total synaptic vesicle membrane protein and has several α-helices that are thought to span the vesicle membrane, and might function as a channel. Another vesicle protein called synaptotagmin, cloned by Südhof, also has a membrane-spanning region. The protein binds calmodulin and contains a domain homologous to the regulatory region of protein kinase C. Synaptotagmin binds phospholipids and might therefore insert into the bilayer in response to Ca^{2+} influx.

Calcium Influx Is Greatest in the Region of the Active Zone

Is the Ca^{2+} influx that initiates transmitter release localized in the neuron? Stephen Smith and his colleagues studied the distribution of voltage-sensitive Ca^{2+} channels at the squid giant synapse using the dye Fura-2, which reveals the location of intracellular Ca^{2+}. They found that Ca^{2+} influx is 10 times greater in the region of the active zone than elsewhere in the terminal. This localization is consistent with the distribution of the intramembranous particles thought to be Ca^{2+} channels (Figure 13–8). During an action potential the Ca^{2+} concentration at the active zone can rise a thousandfold within a few hundred microseconds, from a basal level of 100 nM to 100 μM. This large and rapid Ca^{2+} increase is well suited for the rapid and synchronous release of transmitter.

Calcium Mobilizes Vesicles from the Cytoskeleton

As we have seen, only a small fraction of synaptic vesicles in the synaptic terminal are positioned in active release sites. The remaining vesicles represent a reserve storage pool of transmitter. These vesicles do not move about freely in the terminal, but rather are anchored to a network of cytoskeletal filaments.

A family of proteins that may be important for anchoring vesicles to the cytoskeleton, the synapsins, were discovered by Paul Greengard and his colleagues. Four synapsins have now been characterized (synapsin Ia, Ib, IIa, and IIb). Of these, synapsin Ia and Ib are the best studied. These two proteins are substrates for both the cAMP-dependent protein kinase and the Ca^{2+}/calmodulin-dependent kinase. When synapsin I is not phosphorylated, it is thought to link the synaptic vesicles to actin filaments and other components of the cytoskeleton. When the nerve terminal is depolarized and Ca^{2+} enters, synapsin I is thought to become phosphorylated by the Ca^{2+}/calmodulin-dependent protein kinase. It is hypothesized that this frees the vesicles from the cytoskeletal constraint, making them available to move into the active zone.

What then guides or targets the vesicles to assure that they dock correctly at the active zone? There is now suggestive evidence that two low molecular weight G-proteins—rab 3A and rab 3B—of the p21^{ras} superfamily guide the vesicle to the release site and mediate recognition prior to exocytosis.

Not all transmitters are released from small (40–50 nm) vesicles, however. As we shall learn in Chapters 14 and 15, peptides and biogenic amines are packaged in large vesicles, often called dense-core vesicles because of their characteristic appearance in electron micrographs. These vesicles are 70–200 nm in diameter. Unlike small vesicles, large vesicles are not anchored to the cytoskeleton by synapsins. Some neurons that release primarily peptide or biogenic amine transmitters do not have active zones. Neurons that co-release both small-molecule transmitters, (such as ACh or glutamate) and peptides, release the peptides at unspecialized regions of the membrane, away from the active zone. In some cells the peptides or biogenic amines are released at the dendrites!

The Number of Transmitter Vesicles Released Can Be Modulated by Altering Calcium Influx

As we saw in Chapter 9, the actions of chemical synapses can be modified for both short and long periods of time, whereas the action of electrical synapses cannot. This property is called *synaptic plasticity*. Synaptic plasticity is controlled by two types of processes: (1) processes within the neuron, such as changes in the membrane potential and the firing of action potentials, and (2) extrinsic processes, such as the synaptic input from other neurons. We shall consider the long-term changes in chemical synaptic action in later chapters on development and learning (Chapters 60 and 65). Here we shall discuss the short-term changes—modifications of the influx or accumulation of Ca^{2+} within the presynaptic terminal that affect the amount of transmitter released.

Intrinsic Cellular Mechanisms Regulate the Concentration of Free Calcium

Because of the strong dependence of transmitter release on intracellular Ca^{2+} concentration, mechanisms within the presynaptic neuron that affect the concentration of free Ca^{2+} in the presynaptic terminal also affect the amount of transmitter released. In some cells there is a small steady influx of Ca^{2+} through the membrane of the presynaptic terminals, even at the resting membrane potential. This influx occurs through a class of voltage-gated Ca^{2+} channels that inactivate little, if at all. This steady-state Ca^{2+} conductance is enhanced by depolarization and decreased by hyperpolarization. A slight depolarization of the membrane can increase the steady-state influx of Ca^{2+} and enhance the amount of transmitter released by subsequent action potentials. A slight hyperpolarization has the opposite effect (Figure 13–12). By altering the amount of Ca^{2+} influx into the terminal, small changes in the resting membrane potential can make an effective synapse inoperative or a weak synapse highly effective. These changes in membrane potential can be produced experimentally by injecting current or naturally by transmitter released at axo-axonic synapses that regulate ion channels.

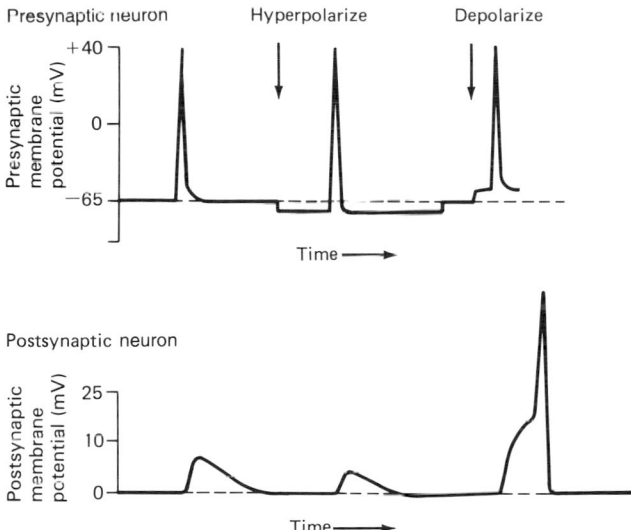

FIGURE 13-12

Changes in membrane potential of the presynaptic terminal affect the intracellular concentration of Ca^{2+} and thus the amount of transmitter released. When the presynaptic terminal is at the resting potential, an action potential (**top trace**) produces a postsynaptic potential of a given size (**lower trace**). If the presynaptic terminal is hyperpolarized by 10 mV, the steady-state Ca^{2+} influx is decreased and the same size action potential produces a smaller postsynaptic potential. In contrast, if the presynaptic neuron is depolarized by 10 mV, the steady-state Ca^{2+} influx is increased and the same size action potential produces a larger postsynaptic potential, which triggers an action potential in the postsynaptic cell.

In some nerve cells, synaptic effectiveness can be altered by intense activity. In these cells a train of high-frequency action potentials is followed by a period during which action potentials produce successively larger postsynaptic potentials. High-frequency stimulation of the presynaptic neuron (which in some cells can fire 500–1000 action potentials per second) is called *tetanic stimulation*. The increase in size of the postsynaptic potentials during tetanic stimulation is called *potentiation*; the increase that persists after tetanic stimulation is called *posttetanic potentiation*. This enhancement usually lasts several minutes, but it can persist for 1 hour or more (Figure 13–13).

Posttetanic potentiation is thought to result from a transient saturation of the various Ca^{2+} buffering systems in the terminals, primarily smooth endoplasmic reticulum and mitochondria. The excess of Ca^{2+}, called *residual Ca^{2+}*, builds up after the relatively large influx accompanying many action potentials. The resulting increase in the resting concentration of free Ca^{2+} presumably acts on Ca^{2+}-dependent mobilization steps in the terminals and enhances synaptic transmission for many minutes or longer.

The excess Ca^{2+} allows more synaptic vesicles to be freed from their cytoskeletal restraint and to be mobilized into release sites. As a result, each action potential in the

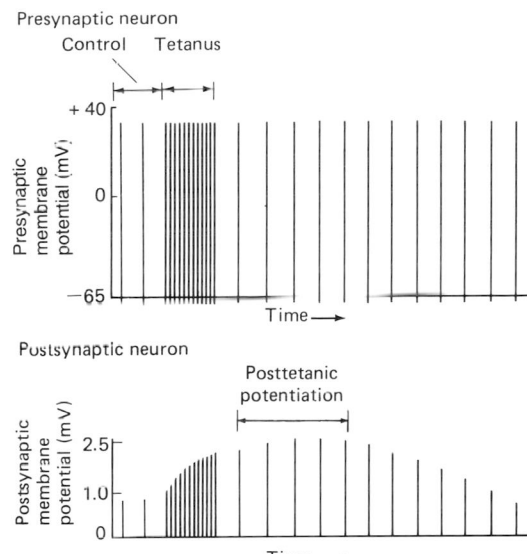

FIGURE 13-13

Following a high rate of stimulation of the presynaptic neuron, there is a successively prolonged increase in the amplitude of postsynaptic potentials. This enhancement in the strength of the synapse is a way of remembering past events in the neuron. The time scale of this experimental record has been compressed (each presynaptic and postsynaptic potential appears as a simple line indicating its amplitude). To establish a baseline (control) the presynaptic neuron is stimulated at a rate of 1 per second, producing a postsynaptic potential of about 1 mV. The presynaptic neuron is then stimulated for several seconds at a higher rate of 5 per second. During this tetanic stimulation, the postsynaptic potential increases in size, a phenomenon known as *potentiation*. After several seconds of stimulation, the presynaptic neuron is returned to the control rate of firing (1 per second). However, the postsynaptic potentials continue to increase for minutes, and in some cells for several hours. This persistent increase is called *posttetanic potentiation*.

presynaptic neuron will release more transmitter than before. Here then is a simple kind of cellular memory! The increase in free Ca^{2+} concentration produces a prolonged change in the cell's activity. In Chapter 65 we shall see how posttetanic potentiation at certain synapses is followed by an even longer-lasting process, also initiated by Ca^{2+} influx, called *long-term potentiation*, which can last for many hours and even days.

Synaptic Connections on Presynaptic Terminals Also Regulate Intracellular Free Calcium

Neurons synapse with one another not only on the cell body and dendrites where they can control impulse activity, but also at their terminals (axo-axonic synapses) where they can control transmitter release (See Figure 11–15). Axo-axonic synapses can either depress or enhance transmitter release through *presynaptic inhibition* or *presynaptic facilitation* (Figure 13–14). The presynaptic terminals of the neuron whose release is modulated con-

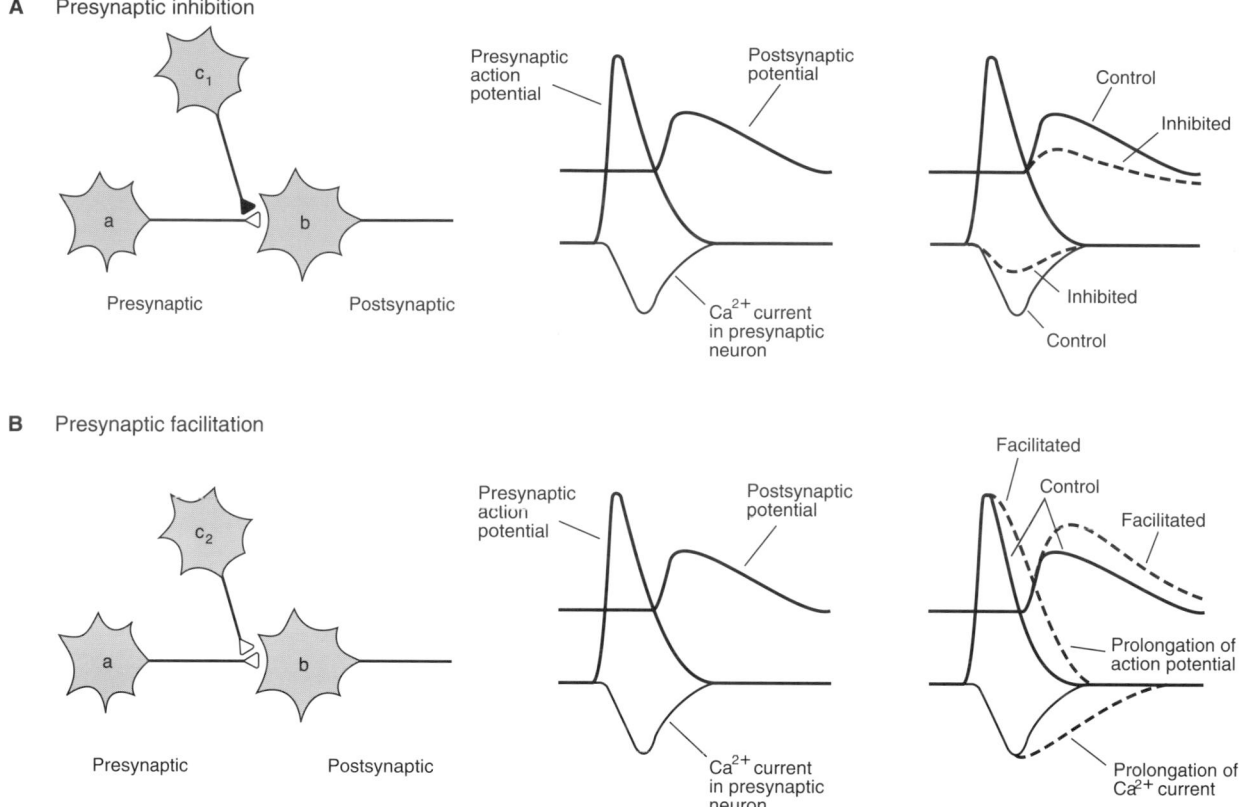

FIGURE 13–14

Axo-axonic synapses can inhibit or facilitate transmitter release by altering Ca²⁺ influx.

A. Presynaptic inhibition occurs when a presynaptic inhibitory neuron (c₁) depresses the Ca²⁺ current in the terminal of a second presynaptic neuron (a), leading to a reduction in the amount of transmitter released. As a result, the synaptic potential recorded in the postsynaptic cell (b) is depressed.

B. Presynaptic facilitation occurs when a facilitating neuron (c₂) depresses the K⁺ current in the terminal of a second presynaptic neuron (a), leading to an increase in the duration of the action potential and therefore of the Ca²⁺ current. The resulting increase in transmitter release enhances the amplitude of the synaptic potential in the postsynaptic cell (b).

tain receptors for various neurotransmitters (*presynaptic receptors*). Certain presynaptic receptors, called *autoreceptors*, are able to recognize and bind the cell's own transmitter. Axo-axonic synapses produce several actions. One important action is that they can control the Ca²⁺ influx into the terminals.

The distinction between axo-axonic and axosomatic (or axodendritic) synaptic actions is important. We shall use inhibition as an example. When one neuron hyperpolarizes the cell body (or dendrites) of another, it decreases the likelihood that the postsynaptic cell will fire. This action, which we examined earlier (Chapter 11), is called *post*synaptic inhibition. In contrast, when a neuron contacts the axon terminal of another cell, it can reduce the amount of transmitter released by the second cell onto a third cell. This action is called *pre*synaptic inhibition. Whereas axosomatic synaptic actions affect all the branches of the postsynaptic neuron (because they affect the probability that the neuron will fire an action potential), axo-axonic actions selectively control the behavior of individual branches of a neuron.

For reasons that are not well understood, presynaptic

modulation often tends to occur early in the pathway of sensory inflow. For example, presynaptic inhibition is found in relay nuclei for sensory information concerned with vision, touch, and position sense (in the retina, spinal cord, and dorsal column nuclei). The best-analyzed instances of presynaptic inhibition and facilitation are in the neurons of invertebrates and in the mechanoreceptor afferent neurons (dorsal root ganglion cells) of vertebrates. These studies have revealed three mechanisms for presynaptic inhibition. One is the simultaneous closure of Ca²⁺ channels and opening of voltage-gated K⁺ channels, which decreases the influx of Ca²⁺ and thus enhances repolarization of the cell. In certain neurons this is due to a specific type of second messenger, lipoxygenase metabolites of arachidonic acid, which we learned about in the previous chapter. The second mechanism is an increased conductance to Cl⁻, which decreases (or short-circuits) the amplitude of the action potential in the presynaptic terminal. As a result, less depolarization is produced and fewer Ca²⁺ channels are activated by the action potential. The third mechanism involves direct inhibition of the transmitter release process independent of Ca²⁺ influx.

Presynaptic facilitation, in contrast, can be caused by enhanced influx of Ca^{2+}. In molluscan neurons, the facilitatory transmitter serotonin acts through cAMP-dependent protein phosphorylation to close a class of K^+ channels, thereby broadening the action potential and allowing the Ca^{2+} influx to persist for a longer period of time (Figure 13–14).

Thus, regulation of the free Ca^{2+} concentration in the presynaptic terminal is the basis for a variety of mechanisms that give plasticity to chemical synapses. Although we know a fair amount about short-term changes in synaptic effectiveness—changes that last minutes and hours—we are only beginning to learn about long-term changes that persist days, weeks, and longer. It seems quite likely that these long-term changes, in addition to alterations in Ca^{2+} influx and enhancement of release from pre-existing synapses, require growth and an increase in the number of synapses.

An Overall View

Using the squid giant synapse, Katz and Miledi found that neither Na^+ influx nor K^+ efflux is required for synaptic transmission. Only Ca^{2+}, which enters the cell through voltage-dependent channels in the presynaptic terminal, is essential. Synaptic delay, the time between the onset of the action potential and the release of transmitter, reflects the time it takes for incoming Ca^{2+} to diffuse to its site of action and trigger the discharge of transmitter from synaptic vesicles.

The discovery of spontaneous miniature synaptic potentials in muscle greatly facilitated the analysis of synaptic transmission. Each such potential is produced by the spontaneous release of one quantum of transmitter, approximately 1000–3000 ACh molecules contained in a single synaptic vesicle. The size of these miniature synaptic potentials (0.5–1.0 mV) matches the size of a unit synaptic potential, which can be measured experimentally when extracellular Ca^{2+} is lowered. Larger synaptic potentials evoked under such conditions tend to be integral multiples of the unit potential. Increasing the extracellular Ca^{2+} does not change the size of the spontaneous miniature synaptic potentials or the unit synaptic potentials. Rather, it increases the probability that a synaptic vesicle will discharge its transmitter, so that action potentials evoke fewer failures and higher-amplitude postsynaptic potentials.

At the neuromuscular junction the normal synaptic potential (70 mV) is due to the release of about 150 quanta of transmitter. At central neuronal synapses less than 10 quanta (each producing about a 100 μV depolarization) are typically released in response to a single action potential. Analysis of central synapses indicates that a single presynaptic bouton releases a single quantum of transmitter in an all-or-none fashion.

Ultra-structural support for the quantal hypothesis of synaptic transmission comes from the finding that many small clear vesicles are clustered around dense bodies in presynaptic specializations called active zones. In contrast, as we shall learn in the next two chapters, large vesicles containing peptides are not released from active zones. Rapid freezing experiments have shown that the vesicles fuse with the presynaptic plasma membrane in the vicinity of the active zone. Freeze-fracture studies have also revealed rows of large intramembranous particles along the active zone, and these are thought to be Ca^{2+} channels. These highly localized channels may be responsible for the observed rapid increase, as much as a thousandfold, in the Ca^{2+} concentration of the axon terminal during an action potential. One hypothesis about how Ca^{2+} triggers vesicle fusion is that it gates a pore that traverses both the vesicle and plasma membrane and thus releases the contents of the vesicle into the extracellular space.

Calcium also mobilizes the small synaptic vesicles to the active zone. These vesicles appear to be bound to the cytoskeleton, and Ca^{2+} is thought to free the vesicles by triggering the Ca^{2+}/calmodulin-dependent phosphorylation of synapsin, a protein on the surface of synaptic vesicles that anchors the vesicles to the cytoskeleton. In contrast, the large dense-core vesicles that contain peptide neurotransmitters do not have synapsin on their surface and do not discharge their contents from active zones.

Finally, the amount of transmitter released from a neuron is not fixed, but can be modified by both intrinsic and extrinsic regulatory processes. High-frequency stimulation produces an increase in transmitter release called posttetanic potentiation. This potentiation, which lasts a few minutes, is caused by transient saturation of Ca^{2+} buffering in the terminal following the large Ca^{2+} influx that occurs during the action potential. Tonic depolarization or hyperpolarization of the presynaptic neuron can also modulate release by altering steady-state Ca^{2+} influx. At axo-axonic synapses, neurotransmitters acting on receptors in the axon terminal of another neuron can facilitate or inhibit transmitter release by altering the steady-state level of Ca^{2+} influx or the Ca^{2+} influx during the action potential.

In his book *Ionic Channels of Excitable Membranes*, Bertil Hille summarizes the importance of Ca^{2+} in regulating neuronal function:

Electricity is used to gate channels and channels are used to make electricity. However, the nervous system is not primarily an electrical device. Most excitable cells ultimately translate their electrical excitation into another form of activity. As a broad generalization, excitable cells translate their electricity into action by Ca^{2+} fluxes modulated by voltage-sensitive Ca^{2+} channels. Calcium ions are intracellular messengers capable of activating many cell functions . . . Ca^{2+} channels . . . serve as the only link to transduce depolarization into all the nonelectrical activities controlled by excitation. Without Ca^{2+} channels our nervous system would have no outputs.

What are the molecular mechanisms by which Ca^{2+} affects transmitter release? This is one of the pressing questions in neurobiology today. Calcium may have a direct role in the fusion of the vesicle membrane with the cell membrane, or it may act through one or more Ca^{2+}-sensitive proteins, such as calmodulin, a calmodulin-sensitive protein kinase, or a phospholipid kinase. Therefore, the next step in understanding transmitter release is clear. To follow the trail of Ca^{2+} influx, we need to move from the channel at the membrane to the regulatory machinery for release within the cell.

Postscript: Calculating the Probability of Transmitter Release

According to del Castillo and Katz, transmitter is released in quanta in a random manner. The fate of each quantum of transmitter in response to an action potential has only two possible outcomes—the transmitter is or is not released. This event resembles a binomial or Bernoulli trial (similar to tossing a coin in the air to determine whether it comes up heads or tails). The probability of a quantum being released by an action potential is independent of the probability of other quanta being released by that action potential. Therefore for a population of releasable quanta, each action potential represents a series of independent binomial trials (comparable to tossing a handful of coins to see how many coins come up heads).

In a binomial distribution p stands for the average probability of success and q (or $1 - p$) stands for the mean probability of failure. Both the average probability (p) that individual quanta are released and the store (n) from which the quanta are released are assumed to be constant. (Any reduction in the store is assumed to be quickly replenished after each stimulus.) Once n and p are known, the binomial probability law allows one to estimate the mean number of quanta (m, called the *quantal content* or *quantal output*) that are released to make up the end-plate potentials following a series of stimuli where $m = np$.

Calculation of the probability of transmitter release can be illustrated with the following example. A terminal has a releasable store of five quanta ($n = 5$). If we assume that $p = 0.1$, then q (the probability that a quantum is not released from the terminals) is $1 - p$, or 0.9. We can now determine for any given number of stimuli, say 100, the probability that a stimulus will release no quanta (failure), a single quantum, two quanta, three quanta, or any number of quanta (up to n). The probability that none of the five available quanta will be released by a given stimulus is the product of the individual probabilities that each quantum will not be released: $q^5 = (0.9)^5$, or 0.59. We would thus expect to see 59 failures in a hundred stimuli. The probabilities of observing zero, one, two, three, four, or five quanta are represented by the successive terms of the binomial expansion:

$$(q + p)^5 = q^5 \text{(failures)} + 5q^4p(1 \text{ quantum})$$
$$+ 10q^3p^2(2 \text{ quanta}) + 10q^2p^3(3 \text{ quanta})$$
$$+ 5qp^4(4 \text{ quanta}) + p^5(5 \text{ quanta}).$$

Thus, in 100 stimuli the binomial expansion would predict 33 unit responses, seven double responses, one triple response, and zero quadruple and quintuple responses.

If instead of five quanta there are n quanta, the probability of occurrence of multiunit responses is given by the expansion

$$(q + p)^n = \binom{n}{0} q^n + \binom{n}{1} pq^{n-1} + \binom{n}{2} p^2q^{n-2}$$
$$+ \binom{n}{3} p^3q^{n-3} \dots + \binom{n}{x} p^rq^{n-x} \text{ (general term)} \dots$$
$$\binom{n}{3} p^n \text{ (last term)},$$

where

$$\binom{n}{0}, \binom{n}{1}, \binom{n}{2}, \binom{n}{x}$$

denote the number of possible selections of 0, 1, 2, or x quanta from a pool of n quanta taken 0, 1, 2, or x at a time. Since

$$\binom{n}{x} = \frac{n!}{(n-x)!x!},$$

the probability that x quanta (0, 1, 2, 3, 4 ... n) will be released by a given stimulus is given by the general term of the binomial expansion, which can be expressed as

$$P_x = (q + p)^n = \binom{n}{x} p^xq^{n-x} = \frac{n!}{(n-x)!x!} p^xq^{n-x}. \quad (1)$$

With this general formulation one can also predict the probability of seeing a failure, a unit, a double, triple, quadruple, or quintuple response to a *series of stimuli*. For a series of stimuli the expected number of stimuli that release x quanta is given by $N_x = N \times P_x$, where N is the total number of stimuli.

The binomial is a *two*-parameter distribution. These predictions require that two of the three parameters n, p, or m be known. For many synapses it is difficult to determine two parameters. Although m can often be reliably estimated directly, or at least indirectly, estimates of n and p are always indirect and in some cases not highly reliable.

However, at low levels of release (in high Mg^{2+}, low Ca^{2+} solutions) p is often very low compared to n, so that p approaches zero. Further, n is often a very large number. Under these conditions the binomial distribution can be approximated by the Poisson distribution. The great advantage of the Poisson distribution is that it is a *one*-parameter distribution. Knowing the mean quantal output, m, one can describe the entire distribution. Moreover, as we will see below, the Poisson statistics provide several easy ways to estimate m.

The general expression for the probability of observing a postsynaptic potential made of x unit potentials is given by the Poisson distribution:

$$P_x = \frac{m^xe^{-m}}{x!}. \quad (2)$$

Experimentally, m can be obtained in four independent ways. A direct estimate (usually referred to as m_1) can be obtained by dividing the average amplitude of the synaptic potential in a given series (v) by the average amplitude of the spontaneously occurring miniature synaptic potential v_1 or its equivalent, the unit synaptic potential:

$$m_1 = v/v_1. \quad (3)$$

A second method of direct determination is to count

the number of quanta released by each stimulus in a series of stimuli and divide by the number of stimuli. This can be done if m is small and release occurs over time (by cooling to a low temperature), or if release consists only of unit responses and failures.

A third (less direct) method for determining m is derived from the Poisson distribution (Equation 2). Given $x = 0$, both $x!$ and m^x become 1 and the probability (P_0) of producing a failure from any single stimulus is given by

$$P_0 = e^{-m}.$$

The probability P_0 is equal to the number of failures in a series of stimuli (N_0) divided by the total number of stimuli (N) in that series:

$$\frac{N_0}{N} = e^{-m}.$$

Taking the natural log on both sides gives

$$\ln \frac{N_0}{N} = \ln e^{-m},$$

which can be rewritten as

$$\ln \frac{N_0}{N} = -m \ln e.$$

Since $\ln e = 1$, dividing by -1 and rewriting yields

$$m_0 = \ln \frac{N}{N_0}. \tag{4}$$

Thus, m_0 can be obtained from the ratio of the number of failures following presynaptic stimulation to the total number of stimuli.

A fourth estimation of m derives from the properties of the Poisson distribution that the variance is equal to the mean. Since the mean of the Poisson distribution is equal to m, the variance equals m and the standard deviation (which is the square root of the variance) is equal to $\sqrt{m}$. Thus the coefficient of variation (the ratio of standard deviation to the mean) can be expressed as

$$CV = \frac{\sqrt{m}}{m}. \tag{5}$$

By squaring both sides of the equation and solving for m we have

$$m_{CV} = \frac{1}{(CV)^2}.$$

The coefficient of variation of the quantal content can be estimated from the coefficient of variation of the synaptic potential for a series of stimuli.

These four tests for m were first carried out by Katz and his colleagues at the frog nerve–muscle synapse. Quantal analyses with essentially similar results have also been obtained at other nerve–muscle junctions in vertebrates and invertebrates, at certain peripheral synapses in sympathetic ganglia, and in the central synapses of the spinal cord of the frog and the cat.

Values for m vary, from about 100 to 300 at the vertebrate nerve–muscle synapse, the squid giant synapse, and *Aplysia* central synapses, to as few as 1 to 4 in the synapses of the sympathetic ganglion and spinal cord of vertebrates. The probability of release p is thought to be high and ranges from 0.7 at the neuromuscular junction in the frog to 0.9 in the crab. Estimates for n range from 1000 (at the vertebrate nerve–muscle synapse) to 3 (at single terminals of the crayfish).

The parameters n and p are statistical terms; the physical processes represented by them are not yet known. Although the parameter n is usually referred to as the readily releasable (or readily available) store of quanta, it may actually represent the number of release sites in the presynaptic terminals that are loaded with vesicles. The number of release sites is thought to be fixed, but the fraction loaded with vesicles is thought to be variable. The parameter p probably represents a compound probability depending on at least two functions: P_1, the probability of mobilizing a vesicle into a release site (reloading) after an impulse; and P_2, the probability that an action potential discharges a quantum from an active site.

The mean quantal content m is a measure of the amount of transmitter released and is therefore a reflection of certain properties of the presynaptic cell: (1) the size of the presynaptic terminals; (2) the number of terminal branches of a single presynaptic fiber; and (3) possible alterations of quantal release associated with changes in synaptic efficacy. On the other hand, assuming that each vesicle contains the normal number of transmitter molecules, the average quantal size (q) indicates the response of the postsynaptic membrane to a single quantum of transmitter. Quantal size therefore depends on properties of the postsynaptic cell, such as the input resistance (which can be independently estimated) and the sensitivity of the postsynaptic receptor to the transmitter substance, as measured by response to application of a constant amount of transmitter.

Selected Readings

Almers, W., and Tse, F. W. 1990. Transmitter release from synapses: Does a preassembled fusion pore initiate exocytosis? Neuron 4:813–818.

Breckenridge, L. J., and Almers, W. 1987. Currents through the fusion pore that forms during exocytosis of a secretory vesicle. Nature 328:814–817.

De Camilli, P., and Jahn, R. 1990. Pathways to regulated exocytosis in neurons. Annu. Rev. Physiol 52:624–645.

Kandel, E. R. 1981. Calcium and the control of synaptic strength by learning. Nature 293:697–700.

Katz, B. 1969. The Release of Neural Transmitter Substances. Springfield, Ill.: Thomas.

Kelly, R. B. 1988. The cell biology of the nerve terminal. Neuron 1:431–438.

Llinás, R. R. 1982. Calcium in synaptic transmission. Sci. Am. 247(4):56–65.

Reichardt, L. F., and Kelly, R. B. 1983. A molecular description of nerve terminal function. Annu. Rev. Biochem. 52:871–926.

Smith, S. J., and Augustine, G. J. 1988. Calcium ions, active zones and synaptic transmitter release. Trends Neurosci. 11:458–464.

Südhof, T. C., and Jahn, R. 1991. Proteins of synaptic vesicles involved in exocytosis and membrane recycling. Neuron. In press.

References

Bähler, M., and Greengard, P. 1987. Synapsin I bundles F-actin in a phosphorylation-dependent manner. Nature 326:704–707.

Baker, P. F., Hodgkin, A. L., and Ridgway, E. B. 1971. Depolarization and calcium entry in squid giant axons. J. Physiol. (Lond.) 218:709–755.

Boyd, I. A., and Martin, A. R. 1956. The end-plate potential in mammalian muscle. J. Physiol. (Lond.) 132:74–91.

Breckenridge, L. J., and Almers, W. 1987. Final steps in exocytosis observed in a cell with giant secretory granules. Proc. Natl. Acad. Sci. U.S.A. 84:1945–1949.

Couteaux, R., and Pécot-Dechavassine, M. 1970. Vésicules synaptiques et poches au niveau des "zones actives" de la jonction neuromusculaire. C. R. Hebd. Séances Acad. Sci. Sér. D. Sci. Nat. 271:2346–2349.

Del Castillo, J., and Katz, B. 1954. The effect of magnesium on the activity of motor nerve endings. J. Physiol. (Lond.) 124:553–559.

Erulkar, S. D., and Rahamimoff, R. 1978. The role of calcium ions in tetanic and post-tetanic increase of miniature end-plate potential frequency. J. Physiol. (Lond.) 278:501–511.

Faber, D. S., and Korn, H. 1988. Unitary conductance changes at teleost Mauthner cell glycinergic synapses: A voltage-clamp and pharmacologic analysis. J. Neurophysiol. 60:1982–1999.

Fatt, P., and Katz, B. 1952. Spontaneous subthreshold activity at motor nerve endings. J. Physiol. (Lond.) 117:109–128.

Fawcett, D. W. 1981. The Cell, 2nd ed. Philadelphia: Saunders.

Fernandez, J. M., Neher, E., and Gomperts, B. D. 1984. Capacitance measurements reveal stepwise fusion events in degranulating mast cells. Nature 312:453–455.

Heuser, J. E., and Reese, T. S. 1977. Structure of the synapse. In E. R. Kandel (ed.), Handbook of Physiology, Section 1: The Nervous System, Vol. I. Cellular Biology of Neurons, Part 1. Bethesda, Md.: American Physiological Society, pp. 261–294.

Hille, B. 1984. Ionic Channels of Excitable Membranes. Sunderland, Mass.: Sinauer.

Kandel, E. R. 1976. The Cellular Basis of Behavior: An Introduction to Behavioral Neurobiology. San Francisco: Freeman.

Katz, B., and Miledi, R. 1967a. The study of synaptic transmission in the absence of nerve impulses. J. Physiol. (Lond.) 192:407–436.

Katz, B., and Miledi, R. 1967b. The timing of calcium action during neuromuscular transmission. J. Physiol. (Lond.) 189:535–544.

Klein, M., Shapiro, E., and Kandel, E. R. 1980. Synaptic plasticity and the modulation of the Ca^{2+} current. J. Exp. Biol. 89:117–157.

Kretz, R., Shapiro, E., Connor, J., and Kandel, E. R. 1984. Post-tetanic potentiation, presynaptic inhibition, and the modulation of the free Ca^{2+} level in the presynaptic terminals. Exp. Brain Res. Suppl. 9:240–283.

Kuffler, S. W., Nicholls, J. G., and Martin, A. R. 1984. From Neuron to Brain: A Cellular Approach to the Function of the Nervous System, 2nd ed. Sunderland, Mass.: Sinauer.

Liley, A. W. 1956. The quantal components of the mammalian end-plate potential. J. Physiol. (Lond.) 133:571–587.

Llinás, R. R., and Heuser, J. E. 1977. Depolarization-release coupling systems in neurons. Neurosci. Res. Program Bull. 15:555–687.

Llinás, R., Steinberg, I. Z., and Walton, K. 1981. Relationship between presynaptic calcium current and postsynaptic potential in squid giant synapse. Biophys. J. 33:323–351.

Martin, A. R. 1977. Junctional transmission. II. Presynaptic mechanisms. In E. R. Kandel (ed.), Handbook of Physiology, Section 1: The Nervous System, Vol I. Cellular Biology of Neurons, Part 1. Bethesda, Md.: American Physiological Society, pp. 329–355.

Neher, E., and Sakmann, B. 1976. Single-channel currents recorded from membrane of denervated frog muscle fibres. Nature 260:799–802.

Nicoll, R. A. 1982. Neurotransmitters can say more than just "yes" or "no." Trends Neurosci. 5:369–374.

Peters, A., Palay, S. L., and Webster, H deF. 1991. The Fine Structure of the Nervous System: Neurons and Supporting Cells, 3rd ed. Philadelphia: Saunders.

Redman, S. 1990. Quantal analysis of synaptic potentials in neurons of the central nervous system. Physiol. Rev. 70:165–198.

Rehm, H., Wiedenmann, B., and Betz, H. 1986. Molecular characterization of synaptophysin, a major calcium-binding protein of the synaptic vesicle membrane. EMBO J. 5:535–541.

Smith, S. J., Augustine, G. J., and Charlton, M. P. 1985. Transmission at voltage-clamped giant synapse of the squid: Evidence for cooperativity of presynaptic calcium action: Proc. Natl. Acad. Sci. U.S.A. 82:622–625.

Südhof, T. C., Czernik, A. J., Kao, H.-T., Takei, K., Johnston, P. A., Horiuchi, A., Kanazir, S. D., Wagner, M. A., Perin, M. S., De Camilli, P., and Greengard, P. 1989. Synapsins: Mosaics of shared and individual domains in a family of synaptic vesicle phosphoproteins. Science 245:1474–1480.

Wernig, A. 1972. Changes in statistical parameters during facilitation at the crayfish neuromuscular junction. J. Physiol. (Lond.) 226:751–759.

Zucker, R. S. 1973. Changes in the statistics of transmitter release during facilitation. J. Physiol. (Lond.) 229:787–810.

14

James H. Schwartz

Chemical Messengers: Small Molecules and Peptides

Chemical Messengers Should Fulfill Four Criteria to Be Considered Transmitters

There Are a Limited Number of Small-Molecule Transmitter Substances

    Acetylcholine

    Biogenic Amine Transmitters

    Amino Acid Transmitters

There Are Many Neuroactive Peptides

Peptides and Small-Molecule Transmitters Differ in Several Presynaptic Aspects

Peptides and Small-Molecule Transmitters Can Coexist and Be Coreleased

An Overall View

In the last several chapters we considered a general scheme that describes chemical transmission in four steps—two presynaptic and two postsynaptic. These steps are: (1) synthesis of transmitter substance, (2) storage and release of transmitter, (3) interaction of transmitter with receptor in the postsynaptic membrane, and (4) removal of the transmitter from the synaptic cleft (Figure 14–1). In the previous chapter we considered aspects of steps 2, 3, and 4, the release of the transmitter and its interaction with the postsynaptic receptor. We now turn to the nature and synthesis of the molecules used as transmitters. In the next chapter we shall discuss how vesicle membrane systems are used by neurons to release chemical messengers.

Even though many transmitter molecules are synthesized locally at nerve endings, other parts of a neuron contribute significantly to the process. As we saw in Chapters 3 and 4, the terminal is dependent on the cell body for all of the macromolecular components needed for transmission—biosynthetic and degradative enzymes, proteins of the synaptic vesicles (both those in vesicle membranes and those that may be contained within the vesicle in soluble form), and most (but not all) of the lipid. Most of a neuron's small-molecule transmitter is synthesized locally at nerve terminals, but the cell bodies of neurons that use peptides as chemical messengers must supply the terminals with the peptide itself as well as with the vesicles in which peptides are processed and packaged (Chapter 4). After their synthesis in the cell body, these macromolecular components are rapidly moved along the axon to nerve terminals by fast axonal transport.

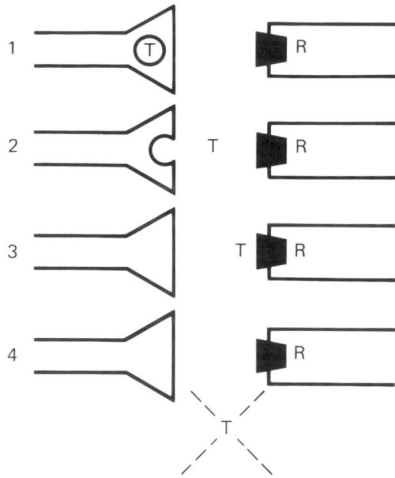

FIGURE 14–1
There are four biochemical steps in synaptic transmission.
1. Synthesis of the neurotransmitter substance (**T**). **2.** Release of transmitter into the synaptic cleft. **3.** Binding of the transmitter to the postsynaptic receptor (**R**). **4.** Removal or destruction of the transmitter substance.

Chemical Messengers Must Fulfill Four Criteria to Be Considered Transmitters

Before we consider in detail the biochemical processes involved in synaptic transmission, it is important to make clear what is meant by a *chemical transmitter*. The concept had become familiar by the early 1930s, after Otto Loewi demonstrated the release of acetylcholine (ACh) from vagus terminals in frog heart (see Box 49–1) and Henry Dale reported his work on cholinergic and adrenergic transmission. These terms are used by convention to indicate that the neuron uses ACh or norepinephrine (or epinephrine) as transmitter. Since that time, ideas about transmitters have been continually modified to accommodate new information about the cell biology of neurons and the pharmacology of receptors.

As a first approximation, we can define a transmitter as a substance that is released at a synapse by one neuron and that affects another cell (neuron or effector organ) in a specific manner. As with many other operational concepts that emerge in biology, the concept of a transmitter is quite clear at the center but can be somewhat fuzzy at the edges. Most neural scientists would agree that a small number of low-molecular-weight substances can indisputably function as transmitters, but many other transmitter candidates exist about which there are varying degrees of uncertainty. Moreover, it is often difficult to prove that one of the accepted substances actually operates as a transmitter at some synapses. Because of these difficulties, a set of experimental criteria has been developed. Strictly speaking, a substance will not be accepted as a transmitter at a particular synapse of a neuron unless the following four criteria are met:

1. It is synthesized in the neuron.
2. It is present in the presynaptic terminal and is released in amounts sufficient to exert its supposed action on the postsynaptic neuron or effector organ.
3. When applied exogenously (as a drug) in reasonable concentrations, it mimics exactly the action of the endogenously released transmitter (for example, it activates the same ion channels or second-messenger pathway in the postsynaptic cell).
4. A specific mechanism exists for removing it from its site of action (the synaptic cleft).

Needless to say, it is often difficult to demonstrate experimentally *all* of these features at a given synapse.

A great many nerve cells have been characterized with respect to their transmitter biochemistry, and an important generalization has emerged: *A mature neuron makes use of the same transmitter substance(s) at all of its synapses.* This generalization was formulated as a principle in 1957 by John Eccles based on the work and speculation of Henry Dale. Eccles had been studying the motor neuron of the spinal cord, which was then known to have a cholinergic synapse at the neuromuscular junction. He correctly predicted—on the basis of Dale's discussions of work on cholinergic and adrenergic neurons dating from the early 1930s—that the synapse from the recurrent central branch of the motor neuron onto the Renshaw cells of the cord would also be cholinergic. Since then synaptic transmission has been studied in great detail, and the number of accepted transmitter substances has increased from the two that had been recognized in the 1930s, ACh and norepinephrine. Since most of the neurons examined were found to use only one transmitter substance, Dale's principle was interpreted to mean that neurons are highly differentiated cells that use only one transmitter substance.

This strict interpretation of Dale's law is not obeyed in some developing neurons, which have been shown to synthesize and release more than one transmitter substance. Many mature neurons have also been found to contain more than one potential chemical messenger. This situation, loosely called *co-existence*, almost always involves a low-molecular-weight transmitter and a neuroactive peptide. Several different neuroactive peptides can also be released from the same cell because peptides typically are processed from larger polyprotein precursors (discussed below). As a consequence, to conserve Dale and Eccles's important cell-biological insight, this principle of neuronal specificity might be reformulated to state that *a neuron makes use of the same combination of chemical messengers at all of its synapses.* Thus, adult neurons are differentiated so that only the biochemical apparatus specific to these transmitters is present; consequently, a mature neuron contains an exclusive set of biochemical processes that endows that cell with its differentiated character. Neuronal differentiation, in this respect, is thought to resemble the specialization of cells in other body tissues (e.g., liver cells differentiate to make albu-

TABLE **14–1.** Small-Molecule Transmitter Substances and Their Key Biosynthetic Enzymes

Transmitter	Enzymes
Acetylcholine	Choline acetyltransferase (specific)
Biogenic amines	
Dopamine	Tyrosine hydroxylase (specific)
Norepinephrine	Tyrosine hydroxylase and dopamine β-hydroxylase (specific)
Epinephrine	Tyrosine hydroxylase and dopamine β-hydroxylase (specific)
Serotonin	Tryptophan hydroxylase (specific)
Histamine	Histidine decarboxylase (specificity uncertain)
Amino acids	
γ-Aminobutyric acid	Glutamic acid decarboxylase (probably specific)
Glycine	General metabolism (specific pathway undetermined)
Glutamate	General metabolism (specific pathway undetermined)

min, but not insulin; fibroblasts make collagen, but not albumin; and red blood cells make hemoglobin, but not immunoglobulin).

The nervous system makes use of two main classes of chemical substances for signaling: (1) small-molecule transmitters (Table 14–1), and (2) neuroactive peptides, which are short chains of amino acids (Table 14–2). The biochemical distinctions between these two classes are fundamental, so we shall consider each in turn.

There Are a Limited Number of Small-Molecule Transmitter Substances

There are eight classical and generally accepted low-molecular-weight transmitter substances. All are amines; seven are amino acids or their derivatives. These chemical messengers therefore share many biochemical similarities. All of them are charged small molecules that are formed in relatively short biosynthetic pathways, and all are synthesized from precursors that ultimately derive from the major carbohydrate substrates of intermediary metabolism. Like other pathways of intermediary metabolism, synthesis of these neurotransmitters is catalyzed by enzymes that, almost without exception, are cytosolic. (One exception is dopamine β-hydroxylase.)

The particular small-molecule transmitter used by a neuron is determined by a specific set of biosynthetic enzymes. A specific set of enzymes is a necessary but not a sufficient determinant of transmitter specificity, however, because other biochemical processes intervene between synthesis of the transmitter and its release at synapses, for example, packaging of the transmitter into synaptic vesicles that mediate synaptic release (described in Chapter 15). As we shall see later in this chapter, ATP, which is present in all synaptic vesicles or its metabolite, adenosine, also can serve as transmitters at some synapses.

In all transmitter pathways, as in any biosynthetic pathway, there is an enzymatic step at which the overall synthesis of the transmitter is regulated. The controlling enzyme ordinarily is characteristic of the neuron and endows the cell with the property of being cholinergic, norepinephrinergic (noradrenergic), dopaminergic, serotonergic, etc.

Acetylcholine

Acetylcholine is the only accepted low-molecular-weight transmitter substance that is not an amino acid or derived directly from one. The biosynthetic pathway for ACh has only one enzymatic reaction, that catalyzed by choline acetyltransferase (step 1 in the reaction below); this transferase is the determining and characteristic enzyme in ACh biosynthesis.

$$\text{Acetyl CoA + choline}$$

$$(1) \Big\Downarrow$$

$$CH_3-\overset{\overset{\textstyle O}{\|}}{C}-O-CH_2-CH_2-\overset{+}{N}-(CH_3)_3 + CoA$$

$$\text{Acetylcholine}$$

The biosynthesis of the cosubstrate acetyl coenzyme A (acetyl CoA) is not specific to cholinergic neurons, because this substance participates in many metabolic pathways. Nervous tissue cannot synthesize choline, which is ultimately derived from the diet and delivered to neurons through the blood stream.

Acetylcholine is the transmitter used by the motor neurons of the spinal cord, and therefore at all nerve–skeletal muscle junctions in vertebrates. In the autonomic nervous system it is the transmitter for all preganglionic neurons and for the parasympathetic postganglionic neurons as well. It is used at many synapses throughout the brain. In particular, in the nucleus basalis there are many cell bodies that synthesize ACh and these neurons have widespread projections to the cerebral cortex.

Biogenic Amine Transmitters

The term *biogenic amine*, although chemically imprecise, has been used for decades for certain neurotransmitters.

This group includes the catecholamines, derived from the amino acid tyrosine (for example dopamine, norepinephrine, and epinephrine) and the indolamine, serotonin, derived from the amino acid tryptophan. Because histamine is an imidazole, its biochemistry is remote from the catecholamines and the indolamines. Nevertheless it is often referred to as a biogenic amine.

Catecholamines are substances that have a catechol nucleus, a 3,4-dihydroxylated benzene ring. The catecholamine transmitters are dopamine, norepinephrine, and epinephrine. These three transmitters are synthesized from the amino acid tyrosine in a common biosynthetic pathway that uses five enzymes: tyrosine hydroxylase, aromatic amino acid decarboxylase, dopamine β-hydroxylase, pteridine reductase, and phenylethanolamine-N-methyl transferase.

The first enzyme, tyrosine hydroxylase (1), is an oxidase that converts tyrosine to L-dihydroxyphenylalanine (L-DOPA). This enzyme is rate limiting for the synthesis of both dopamine and norepinephrine. It is present in all cells producing catecholamines and requires a reduced pteridine (Pt-2H) cofactor, which is regenerated from pteridine (Pt) by another enzyme, pteridine reductase (4). (This reductase is not specific to neurons.)

L-DOPA is next decarboxylated by a decarboxylase (2) to give dopamine and CO_2.

The third enzyme in the sequence, dopamine β-hydroxylase (3), converts dopamine to norepinephrine.

In the central nervous system, norepinephrine is used as a transmitter by nerve cells whose cell bodies are located in the locus ceruleus, a nucleus of the brain stem (see Chapter 44). Although these neurons are relatively few in number, they project diffusely throughout the cortex, cerebellum, and spinal cord. In the peripheral nervous system norepinephrine is the transmitter in the postganglionic neurons of the sympathetic nervous system (see Chapter 49).

In the adrenal medulla, in addition to these four catecholaminergic biosynthetic enzymes, a fifth enzyme, phenylethanolamine-N-methyl transferase (5), methylates norepinephrine to form epinephrine. This reaction requires S-adenosylmethionine as methyl donor. Some neurons in the brain also are thought to use epinephrine as a transmitter.

Not all cells that release catecholamines express all five of these biosynthetic enzymes, although cells that release epinephrine do. Neurons that use norepinephrine do not express the methyltransferase, and neurons releasing dopamine do not express the transferase or dopamine β-hydroxylase. Thus, the expression of the genes encoding the enzymes that synthesize catecholamines can be independently regulated. This insight prompted Tong Joh and his colleagues and Dona Chikaraishi to examine the genetic organization of these enzymes. Using recombinant DNA technology, they found a high degree of similarity in amino acid sequence and in the nucleic acid sequences encoding three of the biosynthetic enzymes: tyrosine hydroxylase, dopamine β-hydroxylase, and phenylethanolamine-N-methyltransferase. The genes for these enzymes appear to be linked together on the same chromosome. The gene expression of these three enzymes can be regulated coordinately.

Several other naturally occurring amines derived from catecholamines are also thought to be transmitters. Tyramine and octopamine have both been found to be active in invertebrate nervous systems.

Serotonin and the amino acid tryptophan from which it is derived belong to a group of aromatic compounds called indoles with a five-membered ring containing nitrogen joined to a benzene ring. Two enzymes synthesize serotonin (5-hydroxytryptamine, 5-HT): tryptophan hydroxylase (1), an oxidase similar to tyrosine hydroxylase, puts a hydroxyl group in the 5 position on the indole ring of tryptophan to make 5-hydroxytryptophan (5-HTP); and 5-hydroxytryptophan decarboxylase (2) forms serotonin.

The controlling step is tryptophan hydroxylase, the first enzyme in the pathway. Interestingly, L-DOPA decarboxylase and 5-hydroxytryptophan decarboxylase seem to be identical. An enzyme with similar activity, L-aromatic amino acid decarboxylase, is present in many non-nervous tissues, but it is not yet certain whether these decarboxylases are identical in structure or whether different molecular forms of the enzyme (specific isozymes) exist in the different tissues.

Cell bodies of serotonergic neurons are found in and around the midline raphe nuclei of the brain stem; the projections of these cells (like those of the noradrenergic cells in the locus ceruleus) are widely distributed throughout the brain and spinal cord (see Chapter 44).

Histamine, like the amino acid histidine from which it is derived, is an imidazole containing a characteristic five-membered ring with two nitrogen atoms. It has been recognized for a long time as a local hormone or autocoid active in the inflammatory reaction, in the control of vasculature, smooth muscle, and exocrine glands (e.g., secretion of gastric juice of high acidity). (When a cell releases a substance that acts upon receptors on its own membrane, that substance is called an *autocoid*. Autocoids often act as feedback regulators of transmitter release from neurons through *autoreceptors*.) Histamine has been convincingly shown to be a transmitter in invertebrates, and binding sites for certain kinds of antihistaminic drugs have been localized to neurons in the vertebrate brain. This putative vertebrate transmitter substance is concentrated in the hypothalamus. It is synthesized from histidine by decarboxylation. Although not extensively analyzed, the decarboxylase (1) catalyzing this step appears to be characteristic of histaminergic neurons.

$$\text{Histidine} \xrightarrow{(1)} \text{[imidazole ring]} - CH_2 - CH_2 - NH_2 + CO_2$$

Histamine

Histamine also is a precursor of two dipeptides that are found in nervous tissue. A synthetase catalyzes the formation of carnosine (β-alanyl histidine) from the amino acid β-alanine and ATP. (Although β-alanine, $H_2N\text{-}CH_2\text{-}CH_2\text{-}COOH$, is normally present in tissues, only α amino acids—amino acids with both carboxyl and amino groups on the α-carbon—can be incorporated into proteins.) The same enzyme forms homocarnosine (β-aminobutyrylhistidine) from α-histidine and γ-aminobutyric acid (GABA). Although the roles of these peptides are not known, carnosine, which is highly concentrated in olfactory areas of the brain, might have a special function there.

Amino Acid Transmitters

Acetylcholine and the biogenic amines are not intermediates in general biochemical pathways, and are produced only in certain neurons. In contrast, a group of amino acids that are released as neurotransmitters also are universal cellular constituents. Glycine, glutamate, and aspartate are three of the 20 common amino acids that are incorporated into the proteins of all cells.

Glutamate and aspartate are products of the Kreb's cycle that we shall not review here. The case for glutamate as a transmitter in the brain and spinal cord is strong; aspartate's role is more tentative. Glycine, which is probably synthesized from serine, is one of the two known transmitters in spinal cord inhibitory interneurons (see

Chapter 11). Its specific biosynthesis in neurons has not been studied, but its biosynthetic pathways in other tissues are well known. GABA is synthesized from glutamate in a reaction catalyzed by glutamic acid decarboxylase (1):

$$
\begin{array}{ccc}
COOH & & COOH \\
| & & | \\
CH_2 & & CH_2 \\
| & \xrightarrow{(1)} & | \quad +CO_2 \\
CH_2 & & CH_2 \\
| & & | \\
H_2N\text{—}CH & & H_2N\text{—}CH_2 \\
| & & \\
COOH & & \\
\text{Glutamate} & & \text{GABA}
\end{array}
$$

GABA is present at high concentrations in the central nervous system, where it is widely distributed, although it is also detectable in other tissues (especially islet cells of the pancreas and the adrenal gland). In some cells GABA can serve as a substrate in intermediary metabolism in a special side pathway known as the GABA shunt. An important class of inhibitory interneurons in the spinal cord uses GABA as transmitter. In the brain GABA is thought to be the major inhibitory transmitter of various inhibitory interneurons, of the granule cells in the olfactory bulb, and to be released in amacrine cells of the retina, in Purkinje cells of the cerebellum, and in basket cells of both the cerebellum and the hippocampus.

It might at first seem puzzling that common amino acids can act as transmitters in some neurons but not in others. This phenomenon can be taken as an indication that the presence of a substance, even in substantial amounts, is insufficient evidence that the substance is used as a transmitter. To illustrate this point, consider the following example. GABA is inhibitory at the neuromuscular junction of the lobster (and of other crustacea and insects) and glutamate is excitatory. Edward Kravitz and his co-workers found that the concentration of GABA is about 20 times greater in inhibitory cells than in excitatory cells, and this supports the idea that GABA is the inhibitory transmitter. On the other hand, the concentration of glutamate (the excitatory transmitter) was found to be the same in both excitatory and inhibitory cells.

Glutamate therefore must be compartmentalized within these neurons, that is, *transmitter* glutamate must somehow be kept separate from *metabolic* glutamate. What mediates the compartmentalization of the amino acid transmitters is not yet certain. When ACh and the biogenic amines function as transmitters they are packaged in characteristic membranous vesicles. Similar vesicles are present in the terminals of neurons that use the amino acid transmitters, and, although it has not yet been proved, it is likely that these vesicles constitute the transmitter compartment (see Chapter 15).

There Are Many Neuroactive Peptides

With rare exceptions (for example, dopamine β-hydroxylase), the enzymes that catalyze the steps in the synthesis of the low-molecular-weight neurotransmitters that we considered above are cytoplasmic. These enzymes are synthesized on free polysomes in the cell body and are distributed throughout the neuron by slow axoplasmic transport (see Chapter 4). Because these biosynthetic enzymes are distributed throughout the cell, the small-molecule transmitter substances can be formed in all parts of the neuron; most important, these transmitters can be synthesized at the nerve terminals where they are released. In contrast, the neuroactive peptides are derived from the processing of secretory proteins that are formed in the cell body on polyribosomes attached to the cytoplasmic surface of the endoplasmic reticulum (discussed in Chapter 4). Like other secretory proteins, neuroactive peptides or their precursors are processed in the endoplasmic reticulum and move to the Golgi apparatus to be processed further (Chapter 4). They leave the Golgi apparatus within secretory granules and are moved to terminals by fast axonal transport.

More than 50 short peptides have been found in neurons that are pharmacologically active (Table 14–2). These peptides cause inhibition, excitation, or both when applied to appropriate target neurons. Some of these peptides had been previously identified as hormones, with known targets outside the brain (for example, angiotensin and gastrin), or as products of neuroendocrine secretion (for example, oxytocin, vasopressin, somatostatin, luteinizing hormone, and thyrotropin-releasing hormone). Neuronal localization on the one hand, and specific hormonal action on the other, spurred the idea that, in addition to being hormones in some tissues (i.e., substances released at a considerable distance from their intended sites of action), these peptides act as transmitters released close to the site of intended action. The study of neuroactive peptides is particularly important because some of them have been implicated in modulating sensibility and emotions. For example, some peptides (substance P and enkephalins) are preferentially localized in regions of the brain thought to be involved in the perception of pain; and others in regulating complex responses to stress (γ-melanocyte-stimulating hormone, adrenocorticotropin, and β-endorphin).

The diversity of neuroactive peptides is enormous. Nevertheless, with the information now at hand, we can attempt to outline the main features of the cell biology of this class of chemical messengers. A striking generality is that neuroactive peptides are grouped in families. At least 10 have already been recognized (Table 14–3). Members of each family are structurally related: They contain long stretches of similar amino acid residues. How is relatedness between peptides determined? The most direct way is to compare either the actual amino acid sequences of the peptides or the nucleotide base sequences in the genes that encode them.

Often, the *primary structure* (amino acid sequence) is determined only after the physiological activity of the

---

TABLE 14–2. Neuroactive Peptides: Mammalian Brain Peptides Categorized According to Tissue Localization

Hypothalamic-releasing hormones	Gastrointestinal peptides
Thyrotropin-releasing hormone	Vasoactive intestinal polypeptide
Gonadotropin-releasing hormone	Cholecystokinin
Somatostatin	Gastrin
Corticotropin-releasing hormone	Substance P
Growth hormone-releasing hormone	Neurotensin
	Methionine-enkephalin
Neurohypophyseal hormones	Leucine-enkephalin
Vasopressin	Insulin
Oxytocin	Glucagon
	Bombesin
Pituitary peptides	Secretin
Adrenocorticotropic hormone	Somatostatin
β-Endorphin	Thyrotropin-releasing hormone
α-Melanocyte-stimulating hormone	Motilin
Prolactin	
Luteinizing hormone	Heart — atrial naturetic peptide
Growth hormone	
Thyrotropin	Others
	Angiotensin II
Invertebrate peptides	Bradykinin
FMRFamide*	Sleep peptide(s)
Hydra head activator	Calcitonin
Proctolin	CGRP (calcitonin gene-related peptide)
Small cardiac peptides	Neuropeptide Y
Myomodulins	Neuropeptide Yy
Buccalins	Galanin
Egg-laying hormone	Substance K (neurokinin)
Bag cell peptides	

*Phe-Met-Arg-Phe-NH$_2$.
(Expanded from Krieger, 1983.)

TABLE 14–3. Some Families of Neuroactive Peptides

Opioid: opiocortins, enkephalins, dynorphin, FMRFamide

Neurohypophyseal: vasopressin, oxytocin, neurophysins

Tachykinins: substance P, physalaemin, kassinin, uperolein, eledoisin, bombesin, substance K (neurokinin A)

Secretins: secretin, glucagon, vasoactive intestinal peptide, gastric inhibitory peptide, growth hormone releasing factor, peptide histidine isoleucineamide

Insulins: insulin, insulin-like growth factors I and II

Somatostatins: somatostatins, pancreatic polypeptide

Gastrins: gastrin, cholecystokinin

peptides is discovered. Similarity in function may therefore be the first clue to structural similarity; relatedness is suspected if two peptides mediate the same or similar physiological processes. Because the types of physiological processes that we have been discussing are mediated by the interaction of a chemical messenger with specific receptors, functional similarity may indicate that the peptides are recognized by the same or similar receptors. Receptor recognition is one index of structural similarity between peptides. Family members may not have similar biological activities, however. For example, family members glucagon and secretin are functionally divergent but secretin and vasoactive intestinal peptide can recognize each other's receptor, although each binds to its own receptor with much greater affinity.

Structural analysis of neuroactive peptides, especially in studies in which recombinant DNA technology has been used, has demonstrated a third feature of this class of chemical messengers. Most eukaryotic proteins are encoded by genes in which regions that ultimately will be translated into amino acid sequences (*exons*) are interrupted by intervening, noncoding regions (*introns*). Thus, the initial RNA transcribed from the gene contains base sequences that will be read and sequences that will be excised. Transcripts are processed in the nucleus in a multistep mechanism, not yet completely understood, that results in the excision of the introns. Alternative RNA splicing occurs when specific exon sequences (in addition to the introns) are also excised. A given region of a polypeptide may be encoded by two different exons. Alternative ways of splicing the transcript can therefore result in different mature mRNAs that encode polyproteins with different amino acid sequences.

Although the mechanisms that regulate how transcripts are spliced are not yet fully understood, alternative splicing is common, and occurs with all sorts of transcripts. At present, a few examples of peptide transcripts that are alternatively spliced are those for calcitonin, FMRFamide, preprotachykin, and nerve growth factor. Splicing can occur exclusively at one or another splice junction in different cells to yield different mRNAs and, ultimately, different peptide products. Calcitonin/calcitonin gene-related protein (CGRP) and substance P/substance K are instances of this cell-specific mechanism.

Because of divergent or convergent evolution of genes, the production of the same or similar peptides from a single polyprotein can explain why some neuroactive peptides are related. In divergent evolution, the mRNA, which is the template for several copies of the same or of partly homologous peptides, is transcribed from genomic DNA that might have evolved by a series of duplications of a simpler DNA ancestor. Amplification of genes by reduplication appears to have been common. In the genes for polyproteins that contain neuroactive chemical messengers, reduplication followed by divergence could result in the production of related but diversified sets of peptides. In *convergent* evolution, independent nucleotide sequences with the potential to code for similar physiologically active peptides might originally have been located at a variety of sites in the ancestral chromosome. During evolution these sequences could have come together and been organized in a similar way in all of the genes that encode the polyproteins of a given gene family.

In most instances several different neuroactive peptides are encoded by a single continuous mRNA, which is translated into one large protein precursor (*polyprotein*) (Figure 14–2). Production from a large precursor can sometimes serve as a mechanism for amplification, since more than one copy of the *same* peptide can be produced from the one polyprotein. Examples can be found in the opioid peptide family; many distinct peptides with opioid activity all contain the sequence Tyr-Gly-Gly-Phe. Opioid peptides arise from three different polyprotein precursors, each of which is the product of a distinct gene (see Chapter 27). Another example is the precursor of glucagon, which contains two copies of the hormone. In other instances the biological purposes served are more complicated, since peptides with either *related* or *antagonistic* functional capacities can be generated from the same precursor. Processing of more than one functional peptide from a single polyprotein is a mechanism by no means unique to peptide chemical messengers, as it was first described for proteins encoded by small RNA viruses. Since several viral polypeptides are produced and all contribute to the generation of new virus particles, it seems evident that at least with the virus, the polyprotein mechanism serves a related biological purpose.

Processing of neuroactive peptide precursors takes place within vesicles, as discussed below and in Chapter 4. Several peptides are produced from a single polyprotein by limited and specific proteolytic cleavages that are catalyzed by proteases present within these internal membrane systems. Some of these enzymes are serine proteases, a class that also includes the digestive enzymes, trypsin and chymotrypsin. They are called serine proteases because they all have a serine residue at the catalytic center whose hydroxyl group participates in the cleavage reaction. As with trypsin, the peptide bond cleaved is determined by the presence of one or two dibasic amino acid residues (lysine and arginine). In neuroactive peptides this bond often is between the carboxyl of a residue N-terminal to a *pair* of dibasic residues (-*X-Lys-Lys*, -*X-Lys-Arg*, -*X-Arg-Lys*, or -*X-Arg-Arg*). Although cleavage at dibasic

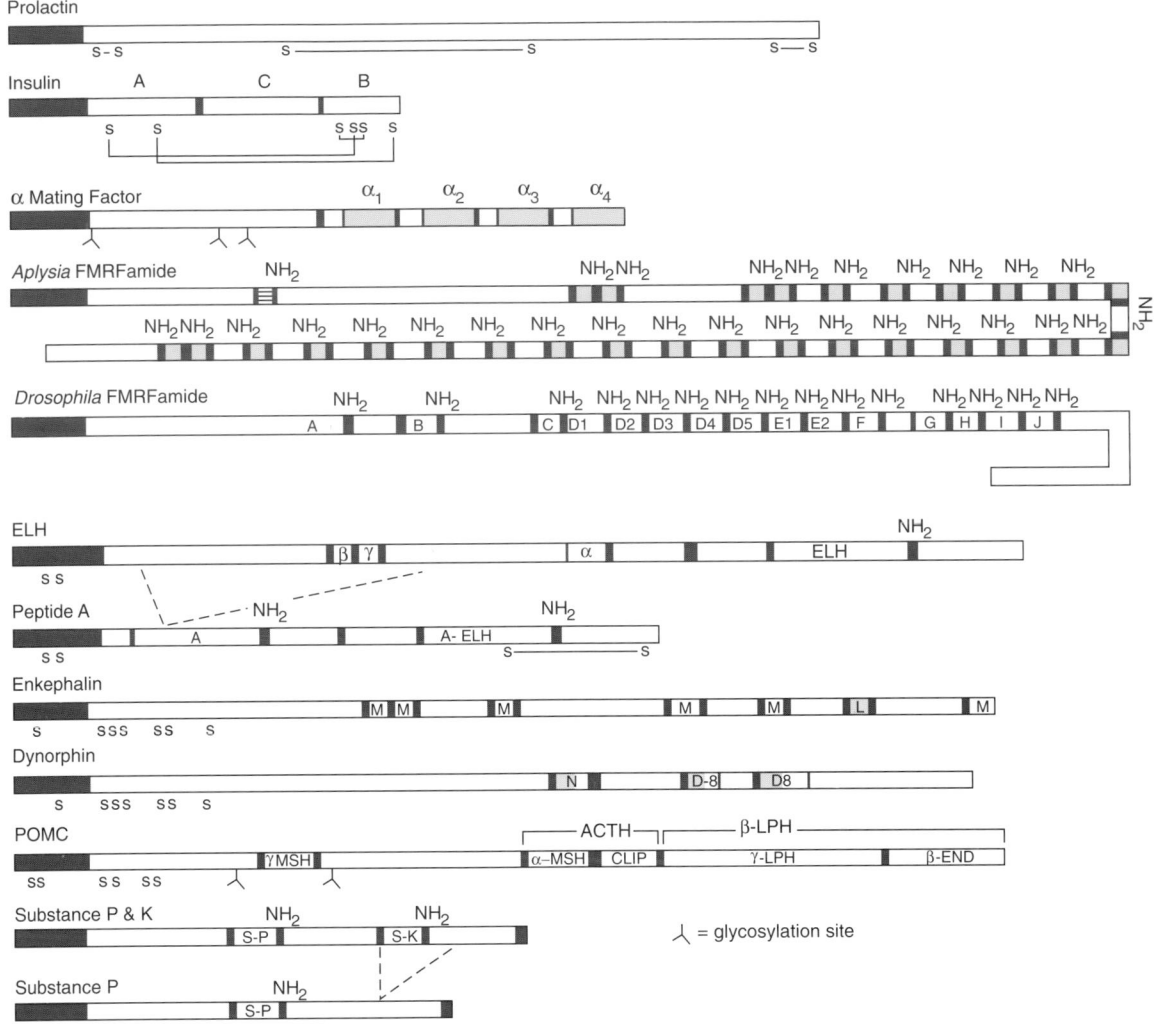

FIGURE 14–2

The structures of several hormone and neuropeptide precursors. Each of the preprohormones is initiated by a hydrophobic signal sequence (**black bars**). Internal endoproteolytic cleavages at basic residues are indicated by the **vertical lines** within the sequence and some active peptides are named. Cystine (**S**) and sugar (λ) residues are indicated below the schematic. In prolactin the mature hormone arises from the removal of the signal sequence and formation of three pairs of disulfide bonds. The **insulin** precursor is cleaved at two internal sites, resulting in the disulfide-linked A and B chains of mature insulin and the C peptide. The α mating factor from yeast is processed by endoproteolytic cleavage at dibasic residues followed by diaminopeptidyl peptidase trimming to generate four copies of the mating factor (α$_{1-4}$). The *Aplysia* FMRFamide precursor encodes 28 copies of the tetrapeptide (**light shading**) and a single copy of the related FMRFamide peptide (**dark shading**). An NH$_2$ above the cleavage site indicates a glycine signal for amidation of the C-terminus of the peptide. The *Drosophila* FMRFamide precursor encodes at least 15 predicted peptides with 10 different structures. The egg-laying hormone (ELH) precursor encodes at

least four physiologically active peptides, α, β, and γ bag cell peptides as well as ELH. The peptide A precursor is quite similar to the ELH precursor; the major differences include a 240-amino-acid deletion encompassing the β and γ bag cell peptides (indicated by **dashed lines**) as well as single base changes that affect the patterns of cleavage, amidation, and disulfide linkage. The family of peptides giving rise to the opioid peptides is illustrated. The enkephalin precursor gives rise to six Met (**M**) and one Leu (**L**) enkephalin peptides. The dynorphin precursor is cleaved to at least three peptides, which are related to Leu enkephalin. The POMC precursor is processed differently in different lobes of the pituitary gland, resulting in different peptides. The endoproteolytic cleavage within ACTH and β-lipotropin are cleaved in the intermediate lobe but not the anterior lobe. Alternative RNA splicing generates two prohormones, giving rise to the tachykinins (substance K). One prohormone includes exons encoding both substance P and substance K, while the other skips over this exon, generating a precursor that encodes only substance P. Bar represents the length of 20 amino acid residues. (Adapted from Sossin et al., 1989.)

residues is quite common, cleavage occurs at single basic residues, and polyproteins sometimes are cleaved at peptide bonds between amino acids in sequences other than -X-basic amino acid residue.

Other types of peptidases have been identified that cause the limited proteolysis required for processing polyproteins into neuroactive peptides. Among these are thiol endopeptidases (with catalytic mechanisms like that of pepsin), amino peptidases (which remove the N-terminal amino acid of the peptide), and carboxypeptidase B (an enzyme that removes an amino acid from the N-terminal end of the peptide if it is basic).

One particularly common mode of processing is through α-amidation that follows endopeptidase cleavage and removal of a basic amino acid by carboxypeptidase B.

$$\begin{array}{ccc} \text{Carboxypeptidase} & & \text{Endopeptidase} \\ (2)\downarrow & & \downarrow(1) \\ \text{N} \sim\sim\sim\sim\sim\sim \text{Gly} & \text{Lys} & \text{Arg} \sim\sim\sim\sim\sim \text{C} \\ (3)\uparrow & & \\ \alpha\text{-amidation} & & \end{array}$$

As shown in the example, the precursors of oxytocin and vasopressin contain a C-terminal glycine preceded by a pair of basic amino acids. The endopeptidase cleaves between the two basic amino acids; the terminal lysine is then removed by the carboxypeptidase, and the new C-terminal glycine is amidated by a specific Cu^{2+}-dependent enzyme that requires the C-terminal glycine as substrate.

Processing is a critical step in determining which peptides a peptidergic neuron releases. Of course, the types of peptides that can be produced depend first on the particular gene expressed by the neuron; the genetic information also specifies the positions within the polyprotein of those amino acid residues that can determine sites of possible proteolytic cleavage (two dibasic amino acids, lysine, or arginine). The polyprotein is then subject to specific processing. In addition to alternative splicing of precursor RNA (see below), a single gene can give rise to several sets of chemical messengers because the same protein precursor can be processed differently in different neurons. An example is pro-opiomelanocortin (POMC), one of the three branches of the opioid family. The same mRNA for POMC is found in the anterior and intermediate lobes of the pituitary in the hypothalamus and in several other regions of the brain, as well as in the placenta and the gut, but different peptides are produced and released in these different tissues. It is not yet known how differential processing occurs. Information about the biochemistry of membrane proteins and secretory products discussed in Chapter 4 suggests two plausible mechanisms. Two neurons might process the same polyprotein differently because each cell contains proteases with different specificities within the lumena of their internal membrane systems and vesicles. Alternatively, the two neurons might contain the same processing proteases, but each cell might glycosylate the common polyprotein at different sites, thereby protecting different regions of the polypeptide from cleavage.

Peptides and Small-Molecule Transmitters Differ in Several Presynaptic Aspects

Many of the four established criteria for identifying a substance as a neurotransmitter formulated for small-molecule neurotransmitters have been met by some neuroactive peptides, and a few have satisfied all of them. Moreover, certain features of the metabolism and action of peptides differ from those of the accepted small-molecule transmitters. Although these neuroactive peptides are present in relatively high concentrations in some neurons, they are made only in the cell body because their synthesis requires peptide bond formation on ribosomes, whereas the small-molecule transmitters can be synthesized locally at terminals. Distinguishing between the two classes of chemical messengers by mode of synthesis can present some semantic difficulty because formation of the peptide bond can also be catalyzed by cytosolic enzymes called *synthetases*. Synthesis of peptides from amino acids without the participation of mRNA, however, usually results in short polymers, many of which involve the carboxyl group in the γ position of an amino acid rather than the α position, for example, carnosine, homocarnosine, and glutathione as well as other γ-glutamyl peptides.

Furthermore, although the Ca^{2+}-dependent synaptic release of some neuroactive peptide messengers has been demonstrated, the release patterns of peptides and small-molecule substances can be expected to be quite different. Because vesicles can be refilled rapidly with the small-molecule transmitters that are resynthesized at terminals, release can be both rapid and sustained. With peptides, once release occurs, a new supply of the peptide must arrive from the cell body before release can occur again.

Peptides and Small-Molecule Transmitters Can Coexist and Be Coreleased

Peptides, small-molecule transmitters and other potentially neuroactive molecules can coexist in the same neuron, as first demonstrated by Tomas Hökfelt and Victoria Chan-Palay. In mature neurons, the combination usually consists of one of the small-molecule transmitters and a peptide or peptides derived from one kind of polyprotein. (Certain amacrine cells of the retina contain and release both ACh and GABA, but GABA may not be released by exocytosis; see Chapter 15.) As an example, Hökfelt, Jan Lundberg, and their collaborators found that ACh and vasoactive intestinal peptide (VIP) can be released together by a presynaptic neuron and work synergistically on the same target cells. Another example is CGRP, which is present in most spinal motor neurons together with ACh.

We have already considered the action of ACh on the nicotinic ACh receptor (AChR) of skeletal muscle in earlier chapters. CGRP activates adenylyl cyclase, raising cAMP to potentiate the force of contraction. Thus, at the neuromuscular junction a small-molecule transmitter (ACh) and a peptide (CGRP) are present (coexist) in the same presynaptic neuron and are both released from it.

Histochemical Detection of Chemical Messengers Within Neurons   BOX 14–1

A major task in studying the functioning of neurons is to identify the chemical messengers they might use. Powerful histochemical techniques are available for detecting both small-molecule transmitter substances and neuroactive peptides in histological sections of nervous tissue. Specific histochemical and autoradiographic methods are used to localize the biogenic amines within neurons in these tissue sections and to show that vesicles contain transmitter. Catecholamines and serotonin, when reacted with formaldehyde vapor, form fluorescent derivatives. The Swedish neuroanatomists, Bengt Falck and Nils Hillarp, found that under properly controlled conditions the reaction can be used to locate transmitters with the fluorescence (light) microscope. Because individual vesicles are too small to be resolved by the light microscope, histofluorescence can only localize transmitters to particular regions of a nerve cell. The position of the vesicles can be inferred by comparing the distribution of fluorescence under the light microscope with the position of vesicles under the electron microscope.

Histochemical analysis can be extended to the ultrastructural level under special conditions; fixation of nervous tissue intensifies the electron density of vesicles containing biogenic amines. Thus, fixation in the presence of potassium permanganate, chromate, or silver salts brings out the large number of dense-core vesicles that are characteristic of aminergic neurons.

It is also possible to identify neurons in which the gene for a particular transmitter enzyme or peptide precursor is expressed. Many methods for detecting specific mRNAs depend on the phenomenon of nucleic acid *hybridization*. One particularly elegant method is *in situ* hybridization (Figure 14–3). Two single strands of a nucleic acid polymer will pair or hybridize if their sequence of bases is complementary. In *in situ* hybridization the strand of noncoding DNA (negative or antisense strand or its corresponding RNA) is applied to tissue sections under conditions suitable for hybridizing with endogenous (sense) mRNA. If the probes are radiolabeled, autoradiography reveals the locations of neurons that contain the complex formed between the labeled complementary

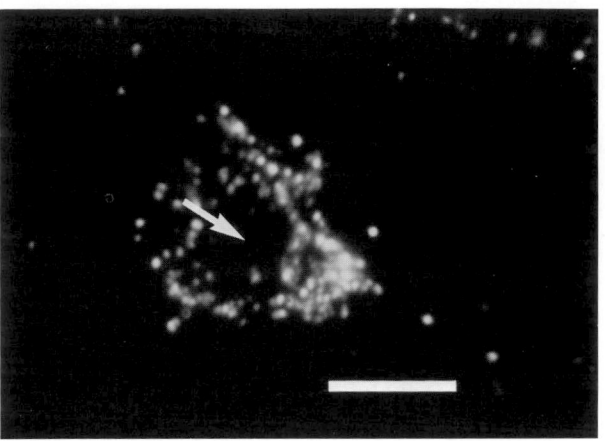

FIGURE 14–3

In situ hybridization of the periarcuate region of the rat hypothalamus with ^{35}S-labeled cRNAs encoding pro-opiomelanocortin. Because the mRNA is translated in the endoplasmic reticulum, the silver grains over neurons are predominantly localized to cytoplasm. There is a relative lack of silver grains over the nucleus (**arrow**). For visualization of the hybrids, the section was dipped in nuclear track emulsion. The section was photographed in a microscope equipped with polarized light epiluminescence. Bar = 25 μm. (From Fremeau et al., 1989.)

nucleic acid strand and the mRNA. When oligonucleotides synthesized with nucleotides containing immunoreactive base analogs are used, the hybrid can be localized immunocytochemically with even greater sensitivity and more precision than with autoradiography.

Transmitter substances can also be localized directly to vesicles by electron-microscopic autoradiography and by immunocytochemistry (Figure 14–4). Amino acid transmitters and biogenic amines can be successfully located by autoradiography because they have a primary amino group that permits their covalent fixation in place within the neuron; this group becomes cross-linked to proteins by aldehydes, the usual fixatives used in microscopy. For immunohistochemical localization, specific antibodies to the transmitter substance are necessary. Specific antibodies have been raised to serotonin, histamine, and to

Since nearby postsynaptic cells have receptors for both chemical messengers, this is also an example of *cotransmission*.

Moreover, neurons that contain peptides processed from a single polyprotein can release several neuroactive peptides with potentially different postsynaptic actions. As described in Chapter 13 and as we shall see in the next chapter, the vesicles that release peptides differ from those that mediate release of small-molecule transmitters at active zones. They are larger and do not require the presyn-

aptic membrane specialization for their exocytotic release. These peptide-containing vesicles may or may not contain small-molecule transmitter, but all vesicles do contain ATP, and ATP is coreleased with both types of chemical messengers.

At some synapses ATP and its degradation products—for example adenosine—act as chemical messengers. Adenine and guanine and their derivatives are called purines; the evidence for *purinergic* transmission is especially strong for purines released from sympathetic neurons on

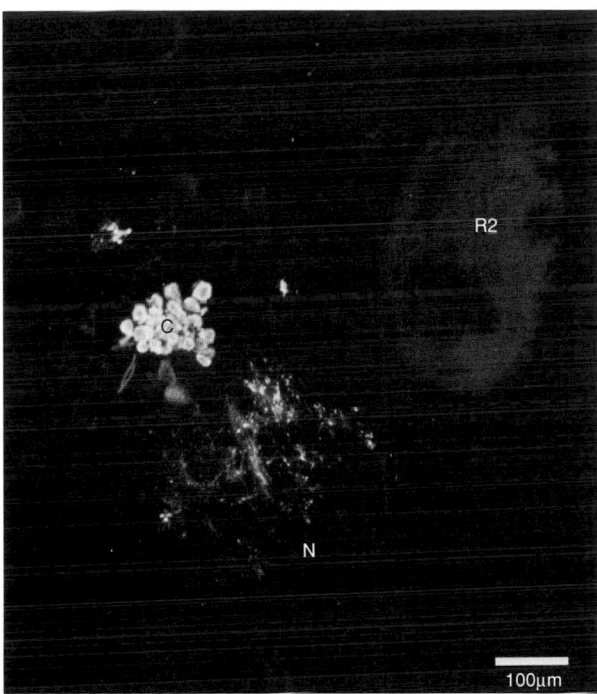

FIGURE 14–4

A cryostat section labeled with an antibody against histamine shows the distribution of histamine-containing neurons in the abdominal ganglion of *Aplysia*. A large cluster of small cells is immunostained (**C**). These cells participate in controlling respiration. The cell bodies surrounding this cluster are not immunoreactive. The cell body of **R2**, which is cholinergic, is one of the largest in the animal kingdom. The nerve (**N**) contains immunoreactive processes. Bag cells, which synthesize the prohormone for the egg-laying hormone (ELH, see Figure 14–2), lie outside the field of this micrograph, just above the right corner, and are not immunoreactive. (From Elste et al., 1990.)

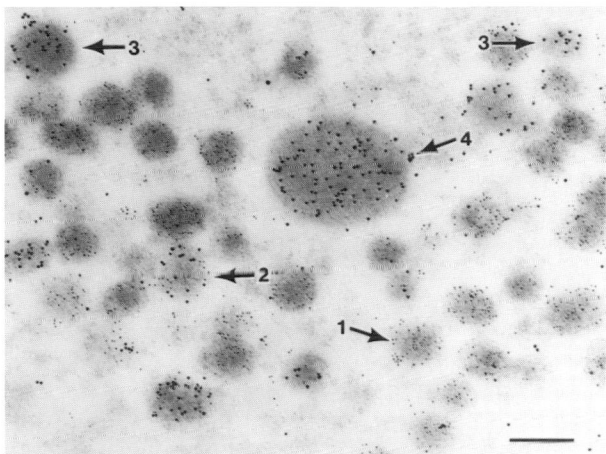

FIGURE 14–5

An electron micrograph of a section through an *Aplysia* bag cell body, treated with two antibodies against different regions of the prohormone, illustrates the use of immunogold particles of different size to locate two antigens in a single electron microscopic tissue section. The bag cells, which control reproductive behavior by releasing a group of neuropeptides cleaved from the ELH prohormone (see Figure 14–2), contain several kinds of dense-cored vesicles. One of these antibodies was raised in rabbits and the other in rats. These antibodies were detected with anti-rabbit or anti-rat immunoglobulins (secondary antibodies) raised in goats. Each secondary antibody was coupled to colloidal gold particles of a distinct size. The specific fragments cleaved from the prohormone are seen to be located in different vesicles. Bar = 240 nm. (From Fisher et al., 1988.)

many neuroactive peptides. These transmitter-specific antibodies, in turn, can be detected by a second antibody (in a technique called indirect immunofluorescence). As an example, if the first antibody is rabbit antihistamine, the second antibody can be a goat antibody raised against rabbit immunoglobulins. These antibodies are commercially available labeled with fluorescent dyes (fluorescein, rhodamine, and Texas red, for example). They can be used under the fluorescence microscope to locate antigens to regions of individual neurons—cell bodies, axons, and sometimes terminals.

Ultrastructural localization can be achieved by immunohistochemical techniques. Another method is to use antibodies linked to gold particles, which are electron-dense (Figure 14–5). Spheres of colloidal gold can be generated with precise diameters in the nanometer range and, because they are electron-dense, can be seen in the electron microscope. This technique has the additional useful feature that more than one specific antibody can be used to examine the same tissue section if each of the antibodies is linked to gold particles of a different size.

the vas deferens, on muscle fibers of the heart, from nerve plexuses on smooth muscle in the gut, and from dorsal root ganglion cells that synapse onto some neurons in the dorsal horn of the spinal cord. The amount of ATP in vesicles in some of these nerve endings appears to be considerably greater than at others. At other synapses, where ATP has been shown to be released, purines have no effect on postsynaptic targets. Presumably whether these common metabolites can act in synaptic transmission depends on the presence of receptors that are sensitive to purines.

Well-characterized *presynaptic* receptors for adenosine have also been described, where the purine may act as an autocoid.

The corelease of ATP (which after release can be degraded to adenosine) is an important instance where coexistence and corelease do not necessarily signify cotransmission. ATP, like many other substances, can be released from neurons but still not be effective when there are no receptors for them close by: They are like the unheard falling of a tree in a forest. On the other hand, receptors exist on some postsynaptic neurons for both ATP and adenosine or for one and not for the other. When the appropriate receptors are present, the crash of the tree is heard.

An Overall View

The information carried by the neuron is encoded in electrical signals that travel along the axon and into the nerve terminal. At the synapse these signals are carried by one or more chemical messengers across the synaptic cleft. None of these chemical messengers carries unique information, like RNA or DNA. Indeed, some of them have several functions within cells as metabolites in other biochemical pathways—amino acids are polymerized into proteins, glutamate and GABA act as substrates in intermediary metabolism, and ATP is the principal means of transferring metabolic energy. To fulfill a signaling function, these molecules act as allosteric ligands for membrane receptors. Once they are bound, these chemical messenger-receptor complexes transform information into new electrical or metabolic signals in the postsynaptic cell. The corelease of several neuroactive substances from a presynaptic neuron and the concomitant presence of appropriate postsynaptic receptors permit an extraordinary combinatorial diversity of information transfer.

Selected Readings

Cooper, J. R., Bloom, F. E., and Roth, R. H. 1991. The Biochemical Basis of Neuropharmacology, 6th ed. New York: Oxford University Press.

Koob, G. F., Sandman, C. A., and Strand, F. L. (eds.) 1990. A Decade of Neuropeptides: Past, present and future. Ann. N.Y. Acad. Sci. 579:1–281.

Kupfermann, I. 1991. Functional studies of cotransmission. Physiol. Rev. In press.

Martin, J. B., Brownstein, M. J., and Krieger, D. T. (eds.) 1987. Brain Peptides Update, Vol. 1. New York: Wiley.

McGeer, P. L., Eccles, J. C., and McGeer, E. G. 1987. Molecular Neurobiology of the Mammalian Brain, 2nd ed. New York: Plenum Press.

Siegel, G. J., Agranoff, B. W., Albers, R. W., and Molinoff, P. B. (eds.) 1989. Basic Neurochemistry: Molecular, Cellular, and Medical Aspects, 4th ed. New York: Raven Press.

Sossin, W. S., Fisher, J. M., and Scheller, R. H. 1989. Cellular and molecular biology of neuropeptide processing and packaging. Neuron 2:1407–1417.

References

Breitbart, R. E., Andreadis, A., and Nadal-Ginard, B. 1987. Alternative splicing: A ubiquitous mechanism for the generation of multiple protein isoforms from single genes. Annu. Rev. Biochem. 56:467–495.

Burnstock, G. 1986. Purines as cotransmitters in the adrenergic and cholinergic neurones. In T. Hökfelt, K. Fuxe, and P. Pernow (eds.), Coexistence of Neuronal Messengers: A New Principle in Chemical Transmission. Progress in Brain Research, Vol. 68. Amsterdam: Elsevier, pp. 193–203.

Cambi, F., Fung, B., and Chikaraishi, D. 1989. 5' Flanking DNA sequences direct cell-specific expression of rat tyrosine hydroxylase. J. Neurochem. 53:1656–1659.

Dale, H. 1935. Pharmacology and nerve-endings. Proc. R. Soc. Med. (Lond.) 28:319–332.

Eccles, J. C. 1957. The Physiology of Nerve Cells. Baltimore: Johns Hopkins Press.

Elste, A., Koester, J., Shapiro, E., Panula, P., and Schwartz, J. H. 1990. Identification of histaminergic neurons in Aplysia. J. Neurophysiol. 64:736–744.

Falck, B. 1962. Observations on the possibilities of the cellular localization of monoamines by a fluorescence method. Acta Physiol. Scand. 56 [Suppl. 197]:1–25.

Falck, B., Hillarp, N. Å., Thieme, G., and Torp, A. 1962. Fluorescence of catechol amines and related compounds condensed with formaldehyde. J. Histochem. Cytochem. 10:348–354.

Fisher, J. M., Sossin, W., Newcomb, R., and Scheller, R. H. 1988. Multiple neuropeptides derived from a common precursor are differentially packaged and transported. Cell 54:813–822.

Fremeau, R. T., Jr., Autelitano, D. J., Blum, M., Wilcox, J., and Roberts, J. L. 1989. Intervening sequence-specific in situ hybridization: Detection of the pro-opiomelanocortin gene primary transcript in individual neurons. Mol. Brain Res. 6:197–201.

Fuller, R. S., Brake, A. J., and Thorner, J. 1989. Intracellular targeting and structural conservation of a prohormone-processing endo-protease. Science 246:482–486.

Herbert, E., Oates, E., Martens, G., Comb, M., Rosen, H., and Uhler, M. 1983. Generation of diversity and evolution of opioid peptides. Cold Spring Harbor Symp. Quant. Biol. 48:375–384.

Hökfelt, T., and Björklund, A. 1985. Handbook of Chemical Neuroanatomy, Vol. 3: Classical Transmission and the Transmitter Receptors in the CNS, Part 2. Amsterdam: Elsevier Biomedical.

Hökfelt, T., Johansson, O., Ljungdahl, Å., Lundberg, J. M., and Schultzberg, M. 1980. Peptidergic neurones. Nature 284:515–521.

Joh, T. H., Baetge, E. E., Ross, M. E., and Reis, D. J. 1983. Evidence for the existence of homologous gene coding regions for the catecholamine biosynthetic enzymes. Cold Spring Harbor Symp. Quant. Biol. 48:327–335.

Kravitz, E. A. 1967. Acetylcholine, γ-aminobutyric acid, and glutamic acid: Physiological and chemical studies related to their roles as neurotransmitter agents. In G. C. Quarton, T. Melnechuk, and F. O. Schmitt (eds.), The Neurosciences: A Study Program. New York: Rockefeller University Press, pp. 433–444.

Loewi, O. 1960. An autobiographic sketch. Perspect. Biol. Med. 4:3–25.

Miller, R. J. 1988. Are single retinal neurons both excitatory and inhibitory? Nature 336:517–518.

Otsuka, M., Kravitz, E. A., and Potter, D. D. 1967. Physiological and chemical architecture of a lobster ganglion with particular reference to gamma-aminobutyrate and glutamate. J. Neurophysiol. 30:725–752.

Scatton, B., Javoy-Agid, F., Rouquier, L., Dubois, B., and Agid, Y. 1983. Reduction of cortical dopamine, noradrenaline, serotonin and their metabolites in Parkinson's Disease. Brain Res. 275:321–328.

Schwartz, J. H., Elste, A., Shapiro, E., and Gotoh, H. 1986. Biochemical and morphological correlates of transmitter type in C2, an identified histamineric neuron in Aplysia. J. Comp. Neurol. 245:401–421.

Tuček, S. 1988. Choline acetyltransferase and the synthesis of acetylcholine. In V. P. Whittaker (ed.), "The Cholinergic Synapse," Handbook of Experimental Pharmacology, Vol. 86. Berlin: Springer, pp. 125–165.

15

James H. Schwartz

Synaptic Vesicles

Transmitters Are Stored in Vesicles
    Subcellular Fractionation Allows
    Biochemical Study of Vesicles
    Transmitter Is Actively Taken up into Vesicles

Vesicles Are Involved in Transmitter Release

**Synaptic Vesicle Membranes
Contain Specific Proteins**

Synaptic Vesicles Are Recycled

**Vesicle Membranes Differ with
the Type of Neuron**

**Transmitter Can Be Released by
Carrier Mechanisms**

**Removal of Transmitter from the Synaptic Cleft
Terminates Synaptic Transmission**

An Overall View

In this chapter we shall consider the intracellular membrane systems that store and release chemical messengers. In almost all neurons storage and release are mediated by synaptic vesicles by the process of exocytosis. Most neurons contain at least two populations of synaptic vesicles, small (about 50 nm in diameter) and large (70–200 nm in diameter). Although the current view is that these two populations are distinct and independent of one another, the possibility that the smaller vesicles are derived from the larger ones has not been ruled out definitively. In any case, all of these vesicles originate from the cell's major membrane system that was discussed in Chapter 4.

We shall also discuss the three known mechanisms for removing chemical messengers from the synapse after they are released and how these removal mechanisms can be manipulated pharmacologically. Because the binding of transmitter to the postsynaptic receptor is a reversible process, and because removal of the transmitter from the synaptic cleft stops synaptic transmission, these removal mechanisms represent the molecular basis for punctuating the synaptic message.

Transmitters Are Stored in Vesicles

There is abundant evidence that small-molecule transmitters are located in vesicles. If free in the cytoplasm, these transmitters would be vulnerable to intracellular degradative enzymes. For example, the *monoamine oxidases*, which are situated in the outer membrane of mitochondria, degrade biogenic amines. (There are at least two types of monoamine oxidases, A and B, which can be distinguished on the basis of their substrate specificity.) Vesicular stores constitute a large reserve of transmitter that is protected from these intracellular enzymes.

Neuroactive peptides are also contained within vesicles. For example, substance P is located within vesicles in terminals of neurons from dorsal root ganglion cells in the substantia gelatinosa (see Chapter 25) of the spinal cord, and calcitonin gene-related peptide (CGRP) is known to have a similar distribution in terminals of spinal motor neurons. Because neuroactive peptides are synthesized as secretory products, it can be assumed that essentially all of the peptide within a neuron is packaged within vesicles (see Chapter 4). Unlike the small-molecule transmitters, none of these peptide transmitters are synthesized in the cytosol, and no mechanism for regulating their cytoplasmic concentration need exist. The absence of specific enzymes for controlling the intracellular store of these messengers is an important difference between small-molecule transmitters and neuroactive peptides.

Subcellular Fractionation Allows Biochemical Study of Vesicles

Transmitter vesicles have been isolated by means of *subcellular fractionation* techniques. These vesicles can be separated from other subcellular organelles because they differ in size, density, and shape. Isolation of synaptic vesicles is facilitated by an artifact produced when nervous tissue is homogenized: When neurons are ground gently in an isotonic solution, entire synaptic terminals can be pinched off. The vesicle-filled sacs were named *synaptosomes* by Victor Whittaker. Synaptosomes are fairly stable and much larger (about 1 μm in diameter) than most subcellular membrane structures. Therefore they can be isolated by *differential centrifugation* using either step or continuous density gradients created by layering or mixing viscous solutions of inert, impermeable substances such as sucrose or polysaccharide polymers.[1] Once separated from the smaller cellular components, the membrane of the isolated synaptosomes, which are large, can be broken open by osmotic shock when diluted in water. The synaptosomes first swell by the rapid influx of water, and then burst to release synaptic vesicles. Because of their small size, the free vesicles can be separated from all the other constituents of synaptosomes by another step of differential centrifugation.

After the vesicles are isolated, they can be characterized biochemically. Biochemical measurements of the amount of acetylcholine (ACh) in a single cholinergic vesicle (about 2000 molecules) are somewhat lower than those estimated from neurophysiological experiments (about 5000 molecules). This quantitative discrepancy is probably small enough to disregard. These results are consistent with the view that the vesicles are the repository of the transmitter quanta discussed in Chapter 13, where the quantal hypothesis of transmitter release is considered.

Studies of vesicles isolated from adrenergic neurons show two populations of vesicles, large and small. Less extensive work on serotonergic, dopaminergic, and histaminergic neurons suggests that these neurons, too, have more than one type of transmitter vesicle. In aminergic neurons, the large aminergic vesicle contains both a higher concentration and more transmitter than do the smaller vesicles. Nevertheless, small vesicles, which are similar in size to the cholinergic vesicles, are believed to be the ones that mediate release of biogenic amine transmitters at active zones in aminergic nerve endings. Precise electrophysiological measurements of the amount of transmitter in a single vesicle are more difficult to do in aminergic neurons than at the cholinergic neuromuscular junction because the norepinephrine released diffuses rapidly from the autonomic synapses with smooth muscle (see Chapter 49).

Isolated synaptic vesicles contain substances other than neurotransmitter. Both cholinergic and aminergic vesicles contain ATP. The large adrenergic vesicles contain at least two soluble proteins, called *chromogranins*. Large and small adrenergic vesicles also contain the enzyme dopamine β-hydroxylase, some enzyme molecules in a soluble state within the vesicle, and others bound to its membrane. Within vesicles, ATP and the chromogranins form complexes with transmitter (osmotic pressure depends on the *number* of molecules in a solution, not on their size), which could serve to decrease the osmotic activity that would otherwise result from the high intravesicular concentration of free transmitter.

Transmitter Is Actively Taken up into Vesicles

How do the vesicles concentrate small-molecule transmitters? Catecholamines have been shown to move across the membrane of aminergic vesicles because of a pH gradient. The pH within the vesicle is 5.5; that of the cytoplasm is 7. This chemiosmotic mechanism is similar to the one first proposed by Peter Mitchell in 1961 to explain oxidative phosphorylation. A transport mechanism in the vesicle membrane, powered by the hydrolysis of ATP, brings in protons. The influx of H^+ makes the inside of the vesicle more acidic than the cytoplasm—and generates an electrochemical gradient (positive inside of the vesicle).

The detailed molecular steps by which the energy stored in the proton gradient is coupled to transport of the transmitter may be explained by several plausible models. One explanation assumes that only uncharged biogenic amine molecules are transported. (Biogenic amine transmitters exist as charged and uncharged species.) The pK of the primary amine group in catecholamines is about 9; therefore, at the neutral pH of cytoplasm only about 1% of the amine exists in uncharged form. The cytoplasmic surface of the vesicle membrane contains specific receptors

---

[1]When solutions of progressively lighter density, containing lower concentrations of sucrose or polysaccharide, are layered carefully on top of one another, a step, or discontinuous, gradient results; when two solutions of different densities are mixed slowly, a continuous density gradient is formed. Naturally, the less dense regions of the gradients are situated at the top. Centrifugation is carried out at high speeds. The speed at which an organelle sediments depends upon three parameters—the centrifugal force, the size and shape of the organelle, and its density with respect to the solution in which the centrifugation is performed. If carried out long enough, the organelle will reach a position in the centrifuge tube at the point in the gradient where it is at equilibrium. This position is determined by a balance among the three parameters, centrifugal force, size, and relative density.

to which the biogenic amine binds in its protonized (cationic) form.

Once bound, the amine becomes uncharged by the dissociation of a proton. The neutral transmitter molecule is then transported by a carrier through the membrane into the vesicle. Because the pH inside the vesicle is 5.5, the proportion of uncharged (unprotonated) amine inside is about 70-fold lower than in the cytoplasm. Because of the low pH inside the vesicles, a molecule of uncharged amine coming into the vesicle is protonated and does not readily escape. According to this view, the transmitter is concentrated in the vesicle by ion trapping and by the formation of complexes with ATP and internal proteins. Uptake of ACh by small cholinergic vesicles is thought to occur by similar mechanisms. Uptake of small-molecule transmitters can be demonstrated in preparations of purified synaptic vesicles, and transporters for amine transmitters have been isolated and partially characterized.

Vesicles Are Involved in Transmitter Release

Although there is still some debate, the vesicle hypothesis has been generally accepted, and there is little doubt that synaptic vesicles are directly involved in the release of neurotransmitters (see Chapter 12). Biochemical evidence that transmitter release is an exocytotic process first came from experiments of William Douglas. Douglas stimulated cells of the adrenal medulla to release their content of biogenic amines (norepinephrine and epinephrine) into the circulation. Embryologically these cells are related to postganglionic adrenergic neurons of the sympathetic nervous system and are called chromaffin because they stain in tissue sections with salts of chromium. When Douglas assayed the materials released with the catecholamines, he found that ATP, *chromogranins* (the set of specific proteins within large adrenergic vesicles), and dopamine β-hydroxylase were also released into the blood along with the amines. Furthermore, these constituents were present in the same molar ratios in which they occurred *within* the secretory vesicles isolated from the medulla by centrifugation. Only the soluble fraction of dopamine β-hydroxylase was released: No membrane proteins were lost from the gland. Historically, these experiments were quite influential, even though these adrenal cells are not neurons.

More recent morphological and biochemical observations indicate that synaptic transmission, although an exocytotic process, differs in certain respects from glandular release. Release by the adrenal medulla involves the large dense-cored chromaffin granules that contain high concentrations of biogenic amines complexed to the chromogranins; these large vesicles interact slowly with the plasma membrane of the gland cell. Synaptic transmission, on the other hand, typically is mediated by smaller electron-lucent vesicles and is facilitated by the membrane specializations of the active zone. Transmission mediated by small vesicles at active zones in the terminals of neurons may be a highly specialized form of glandular secretion.

Large and small vesicles can be isolated by subcellular fractionation of tissue rich in true aminergic nerve endings, and this reveals that the small vesicles contain little if any core protein. In contrast, the large vesicles contain both small-molecule amine transmitters, core proteins, and peptides. Neuropeptides are not exocytosed in the small synaptic vesicles by this specialized facilitated mechanism. Since all neuropeptides are found primarily, if not exclusively, in larger vesicles of neurons, nerve terminals probably also maintain the more primitive mechanism of release used by gland cells.

Synaptic Vesicle Membranes Contain Specific Proteins

Several integral membrane proteins have been isolated from purified small synaptic vesicles (Table 15–1). Thus far we have discussed two important activities of synaptic vesicles—they move and they mediate exocytosis. We expect that some of the proteins in the membranes of synaptic vesicles might participate in these activities. Vesicles move from the Golgi apparatus to nerve terminals by fast axonal transport (described in Chapter 4). Once they arrive at terminals, they join a large pool of vesicles that are a characteristic of profiles of synapses seen in the electron microscope (see Chapter 9). In order to release transmitter by exocytosis at active zones, the vesicles must then move from this pool to the docking sites at the synaptic membrane, a process called *mobilization* (also described in Chapter 13).

Mobilization of vesicles is thought to be mediated by the elements of the cytoskeleton and by their associated proteins (see Chapter 4). One protein found in vesicle membranes, *caldesmin*, binds actin filaments and tubulin as well as Ca^{2+} ions. In addition, certain proteins are thought to inhibit mobilization. Rodolfo Llinás, Paul Greengard, and their collaborators proposed that the *synapsins* are inhibitory in the dephosphorylated form. The inhibition is reversed when the synapsins are phosphorylated. As described in Chapter 13, one of the chief multifunctional protein kinases, the Ca^{2+}/calmodulin-dependent protein kinase, phosphorylates synapsin and relieves the inhibition. It is therefore not surprising that calmodulin is associated with synaptic vesicle membranes through binding to a protein designated *p65*.

Mobilization of vesicles, their attachment to synaptic docking sites at the active zones, and their actual fusion with synaptic membrane are known to involve Ca^{2+} ions. Many of the proteins identified in the vesicle membrane bind Ca^{2+}. Calcium-binding proteins associated with membranes are called *annexins*, a group to which several of the membrane proteins in synaptic vesicles belong.

Proteins involved in membrane fusion, which have been identified and characterized by James Rothman and his collaborators from Golgi membranes, and which promote transport of membranes along constitutive pathways of secretion in a Ca^{2+}-independent manner, have not been found in nerve terminals. Since fusion with synaptic vesicles is a process that is regulated by Ca^{2+} ions, some of the Ca^{2+}-binding proteins associated with vesicle mem-

TABLE 15–1. Proteins Associated with Membranes of Synaptic Vesicles

Name	Other Names	MW_r (10^{-3})	Properties
A. *Calcium-Binding Proteins*			
Cytoskeleton-Associated Proteins			
Caldesmon	p70	70	Binds F-actin and tubulin
Annexins			
Calelectrin (mammalian)	p68, p70, protein III, synhibin, calcimedin, chromobidin	68	Evolutionary duplication of calpactin-class molecules
Calelectrin (*Torpedo*)	p34, p36	34	Promotes membrane aggregation
Calpactin I	p36, p33, protein I, lipocortin II	36	Aggregates membranes
Calpactin complex	2(p36, p10)	92	Complex aggregates membranes at lower Ca^{2+} concentrations than p36 monomer
Calpactin II	p35, lipocortin I, protein I	35	—
Endonexin I	33K calectrin	33	—
Endonexin II	p32	33	—
Protein II	—	35	—
Synexin I	—	47	Aggregrates membranes and has channel activity
Enzyme Modulators			
Calmodulin	—	17	Abundant enzyme regulator, no fusion activity
p65	synaptagmin	65	Integral membrane glycoprotein-calmodulin receptor; binds phosphatidyl serine
B. *Other Synaptic Vesicle Proteins*			
Inhibitors of Mobilization			
Synapsin Ia,b	Protein Ia,b	86,80	Phosphoproteins, binds vesicles and cytoskeleton
Synapsin IIa,b	Protein IIIa,b	74,55	Phosphoproteins
Possible Fusion Proteins			
Synaptophysin	p38	38	Membrane-spanning protein phosphorylation substrate; related to gap-junction protein
Proteins of Unknown Function			
p29	—	29	Membrane-spanning protein
VAMP-1,2	Synaptobrevin	18	Membrane-spanning protein differentially expressed in CNS
VAT-1	—	42	Membrane-spanning protein
rab 3A	—	25	GTP-binding protein
rab 3B	—	25	GTP-binding protein

branes plausibly operate in the fusion that occurs at synapses during exocytosis. *Synaptophysin* is an abundant Ca^{2+}-binding membrane protein with a molecular weight of 38,000. It is present in 10–20 copies per vesicle, and has a structure (inferred from the amino acid sequence deduced from cDNA cloning studies) that is similar to that of the gap-junction protein, connexin. These, and other proteins associated with synaptic vesicles whose functions are not yet known, are also listed in Table 15–1.

Synaptic Vesicles Are Recycled

When transmitter is released from vesicles by exocytosis, the membrane of the vesicle fuses with the membrane of the synaptic terminal in order to gain access to the extracellular space. If no process compensated for exocytosis, the membrane of a synaptic terminal would enlarge as a result of nerve activity, because vesicle membrane would be added continuously to the plasmalemma. The expected increase normally does not occur because the vesicle membrane added to the terminal membrane is retrieved rapidly and recycled.

The number of vesicles in a nerve terminal decreases but membrane is conserved. The total amount of membrane in vesicles, cisternae, and plasma membrane remains constant, indicating that membrane is retrieved from the plasmalemma into the internal organelles. Additional evidence for the recycling of terminal membranes has come from studies using the tracer enzyme horseradish peroxidase, whose reaction product can be visualized by electron microscopy. The peroxidase, which is soluble in the extracellular space, is engulfed during endocytosis. Most of the horseradish peroxidase taken up into the stimulated neurons appears first in coated vesicles. The appearance of the tracer enzyme in coated vesicles is evidence that this recycling process is part of the regulated pathway of secretion discussed in Chapter 4, in which the vesicles reentering a cell by endocytosis are coated by the protein *clathrin*. The horseradish peroxidase eventually makes its way into cisternae, and finally, after a period of rest, into the synaptic vesicles themselves. It is later released from these vesicles when the nerve is again stimulated.

The retrieval of membrane can also be shown by studies with an electron-dense iron-containing protein, cationized ferritin. Unlike the peroxidase that is in solution in the extracellular space, the ferritin marker is adsorbed to the terminal membrane. Results from these studies suggest that this recycling process is specific. The only membrane components retrieved are those of synaptic vesicles.

How recycling takes place in nerve endings has not yet been resolved. In other epithelial cells, there are three retrieval pathways through the endosomal compartment, which are discussed in Chapter 4. These pathways result in the *recycling* of receptors and other membrane constituents, the delivery of substances bound to surface receptors to specific targets within the cell, and the degradation of membrane constituents in lysosomes. Membrane constituents are removed from the plasma membrane in pits coated with clathrin that pinch off to become coated vesicles. The coated vesicles then fuse with endosomes, where the pH is low. Receptors release their ligands in the acidic environment within the endosome. The first two are called regulated pathways, because, as discussed in Chapter 4, they are under the control of external stimuli. The membrane is retrieved by the first pathway when the bit of membrane is returned to the same region of the plasma membrane from which it was originally removed. In the second pathway, *transcytosis*, endosomes return the membrane to a region of the plasma membrane some distance away from the site where it was originally lo-

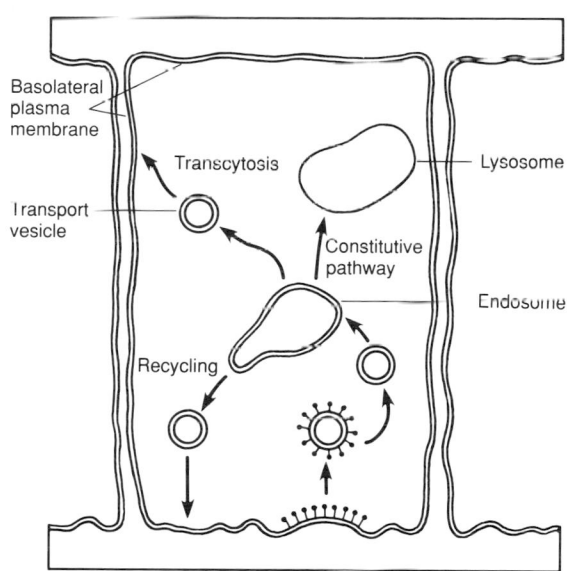

FIGURE 15–1

Three pathways for recapturing membrane in an idealized epithelial cell. Most membrane constituents that are not retrieved from endosomes follow the constitutive pathway from endosomes to lysosomes, where they are degraded. Retrieved constituents are either returned to the domain of the external membrane from which they came (*recycling*) or inserted into a different part of the plasma membrane (*transcytosis*). (Adapted from Alberts et al., 1989.)

cated. Most of the membrane proteins from coated vesicles follow the third or *constitutive pathway*, however, and are delivered to lysosomes for degradation. These three pathways are illustrated in Figure 15–1.

One mechanism suggested by Thomas Miller and John Heuser for recycling vesicle membrane proteins in neurons is shown in Figure 15–2. According to this explana-

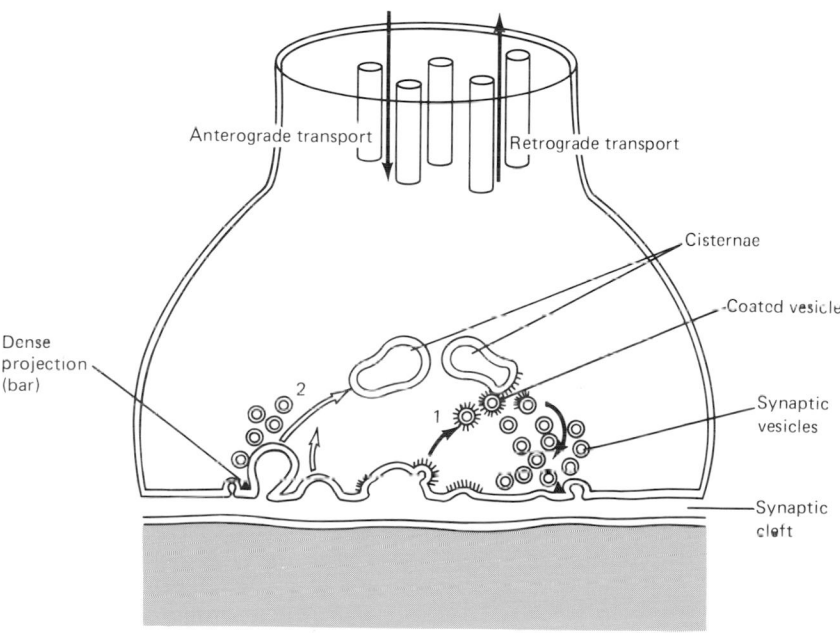

FIGURE 15–2

Vesicle membrane at the frog neuromuscular junction may be recycled by two pathways. In the first and physiologically most important pathway, excess membrane is retrieved by means of coated pits (**1**). These coated pits are selective and concentrate intramembranous particles. They are not found at the active zones but only at other areas of the terminal. As the plasma membrane enlarges with time after the beginning of the exocytotic event, more membrane invaginations have coated cytoplasmic surfaces. The path of the coated pits is shown by solid arrows. In the second pathway, excess membrane reenters the terminal by budding from uncoated pits (**2**). These uncoated cisternae are formed in highest concentration at the active zones. Nearly all of the uncoated pits form during the first few seconds after exocytosis. During the physiological functioning of the synapse, this second pathway may not be used at all. (Adapted from Miller and Heuser, 1984.)

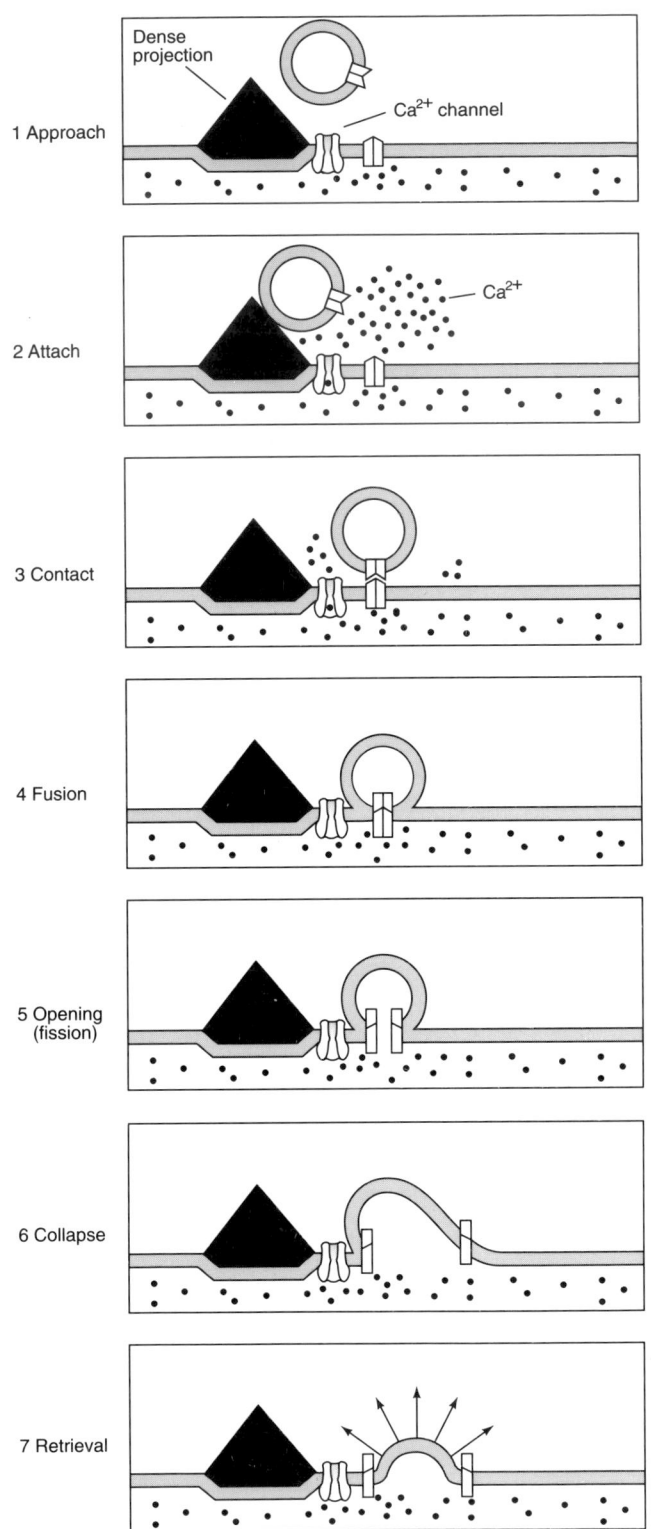

FIGURE 15–3

The exocytosis of synaptic vesicles and vesicle membrane retrieval can be divided into separate stages. The seven distinct stages have been inferred from morphological studies, which cannot resolve the molecular structure of the components here proposed to participate in the process. (Adapted from Llinás and Heuser, 1977.)

tion for the retrieval of membrane at the neuromuscular junction, excess membrane contributed to the plasmalemma of the terminal by synaptic vesicles that have undergone exocytosis is recycled by one of two routes. The first pathway, believed to be the major process for recycling membrane at normal physiological rates of stimulation, is the slower of the two, peaking at 30 seconds after exocytosis and lasting for more than 1 minute. In this pathway excess membrane anywhere in the terminal except at the active zone forms a pit coated with clathrin. The clathrin coat forms a regular lattice around the pit, which finally pinches off as a small coated vesicle. After shedding this clathrin coat, these vesicles can serve again as synaptic vesicles. This pathway would correspond to the *recycling* pathway in Figure 15–1.

Only a small portion of the membrane follows the second pathway. The amount of membrane recycled through it is thought to be significant only at unphysiologically high rates of activity. In this process membrane is taken up directly and rapidly from the plasmalemma and reenters the terminal as large, uncoated vacuoles or cisternae. Most of this uptake occurs close to the release site, but some membrane can also be retrieved away from the active zone. This pathway may correspond to *transcytosis* in Figure 15–1.

Some of the retrieved membrane is not recycled into functioning vesicles, however, and is returned to the cell body. The studies with horseradish peroxidase described above have shown that, during synaptic activity, some of the tracer ultimately winds up in lysosomes. Synaptic vesicle membrane turnover must thus involve retrograde fast axonal transport of membranes to the cell body for further processing, including lysosomal degradation. The old and used vesicles are replaced by new ones brought into the terminals by fast anterograde axonal transport (considered in Chapter 4).

According to Heuser and Thomas Reese, synaptic vesicle exocytosis and membrane retrieval can be divided into several distinct stages illustrated in Figure 15–3. The vesicles initially approach the active zone, perhaps by some energy-requiring process that may involve the dense projections that are part of the membrane specialization at active zones seen in transmission electron microscopy. These structures would consist of actin and actin-anchoring proteins, but it is thought they are artifactually condensed by almost all fixation procedures used. Vesicles closest to the dense projections appear to be attached to them and can be seen in thin-section electron micrographs to hover close to the presynaptic membrane even in the absence of a nerve impulse. The entry of Ca^{2+} with each nerve impulse (perhaps through channels represented by the intermembranous particles next to the dense projections that are mentioned in Chapter 13) leads to contact and fusion of the vesicle membrane with the synaptic membrane. Fusion is followed by fission of all the membrane components, which opens up the synaptic vesicle. The vesicle membrane then collapses and coalesces into the external membrane, presumably as a consequence of membrane fluidity. Finally, some vesicle membrane is retrieved for reuse, and some leaves the terminals within lysosomes to be degraded and returned to the cell body.

The fusion of synaptic vesicle membrane with the plasma membrane as well as the speed at which vesicle membrane is retrieved is indicated by the experiments with the frog neuromuscular junction shown in Figure 15–4. In these experiments Bruno Ceccarelli and his collaborators used an antibody to the vesicle membrane-spanning protein, synaptophysin, to trace the fate of vesicle membrane after exocytosis. They examined the distribution of synaptophysin first under conditions in which endocytosis is blocked and then after exocytosis followed by endocytosis. For these experiments, exocytosis was induced by α-latroxin, a component of black widow spider venom.

Application of this toxin produces Ca^{2+}-independent exocytosis, and, if Ca^{2+}-ion is omitted from the extracellular fluid, nerve terminals are rapidly depleted of vesicles. Depletion occurs because retrieval by endocytosis is blocked, since it too normally depends on the presence of Ca^{2+}. Analysis by immunogold electron-microscopy (see Box 14–1, Chapter 14) reveals a swollen and empty presynaptic terminal surrounded by a plasma membrane labeled by the antibody to synaptophysin. This image contrasts dramatically with the picture of the terminal at rest, which contains profiles of many synaptic vesicles, the membranes of which are the only sites labeled by immunogold particles (compare Figure 15–4A and B). Thus, when retrieval is blocked, the membranes of exocytosed synaptic vesicles add to the plasma membrane, enlarging it prodigiously.

Next, when exocytosis is induced by the toxin under conditions in which endocytosis can take place (addition of extracellular Ca^{2+}), retrieval of vesicle membrane keeps up with exocytosis, so that the profile of the terminal is essentially indistinguishable from that seen at rest: Synaptic vesicles labeled with the synaptophysin antibody cluster within undistended terminals and labeling of the plasma membrane is virtually absent (Figure 15–4C). These observations are consistent with the idea that the retrieval of vesicle membrane is efficient and rapid.

Vesicle Membranes Differ with the Type of Neuron

As we have seen, storage granules and synaptic vesicles share many biochemical characteristics, but there are differences among the vesicles in neurons of different transmitter type. In addition to the specific transmitter biosynthetic pathways discussed in Chapter 14, each type of neuron has characteristic membrane proteins for packaging and processing its particular transmitter substances. In most neurons a substance cannot be used as a transmitter unless it is packaged; thus, in addition to the specificity built into the biosynthetic enzymatic pathway, there is a specificity to the packaging apparatus in these cells. These various specificities are interesting not only theoretically, but also therapeutically because whenever a

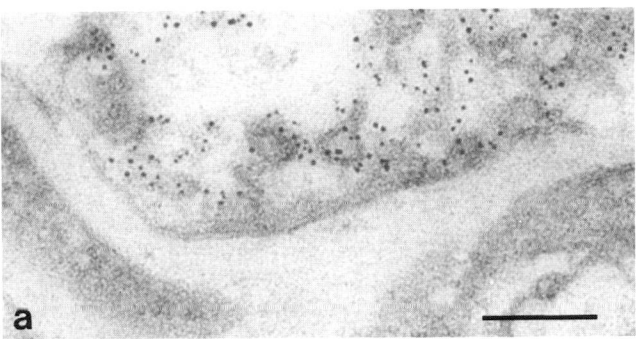
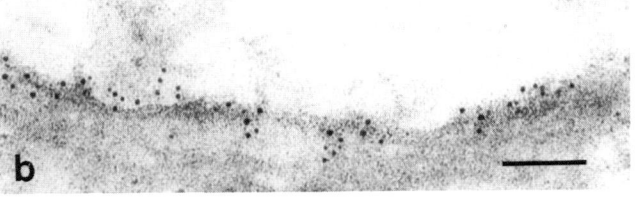
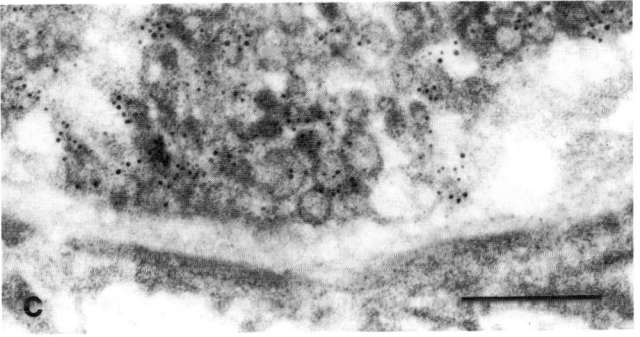

FIGURE 15–4

Membranes of synaptic vesicles are incorporated into the plasmalemma during exocytosis and then recycled. Electron micrographs of ultrathin frozen sections of frog neuromuscular junctions are stained by antibodies against synaptophysin (a protein specific to synaptic vesicle membranes) which are coupled to electron-dense gold particles. (Adapted from Torri-Tarelli et al., 1990.)

A. In the resting nerve terminal, gold particles are concentrated around synaptic vesicles, revealing the location of synaptophysin. The plasma membrane is unlabeled. Bar = 0.1 μm.

B. A nerve terminal exposed to α-latrotoxin, a spider venom toxin, for one hour in Ca^{2+}-free solution. Under these conditions exocytosis of synaptic vesicles is greatly stimulated and recycling of vesicle membrane is blocked. The terminals have been depleted of synaptic vesicles by exocytosis. Immunogold is now located on the plasmalemma, indicating the incorporation of bits of synaptophysin-containing membrane. Bar = 0.1 μm.

C. A nerve terminal exposed to α-latrotoxin for one hour in a Ca^{2+}-containing solution, a condition in which exocytosis is stimulated and recycling can take place. Synaptophysin now is restricted to synaptic vesicles. It can therefore be inferred that the synaptic vesicle membrane has been recaptured. This experiment indicates that exocytosis and endocytosis of synaptic vesicles does not result in intermixing of membrane components. Bar = 0.2 μm.

biological system has a specificity, it offers the possibility of being interfered with pharmacologically.

Presumably the specificity of packaging results from receptors or carrier molecules in vesicle membranes. Any mechanism for recognizing a specific transmitter substance within neurons can easily discriminate between naturally occurring transmitters, such as ACh and serotonin, because they are chemically quite dissimilar. Drugs that are sufficiently similar to the normal transmitter substance can act as *false transmitters*; these are packaged in the vesicles, and released as if they were true transmitters. They often bind only weakly or not at all to the postsynaptic receptor for the natural transmitter. Therefore, their release decreases the efficacy of transmission at specific synapses. Several drugs used to treat hypertension, such as phenylethylamines, are taken up into adrenergic terminals and replace norepinephrine in synaptic vesicles. When released, these drugs are not as potent as norepinephrine at postsynaptic adrenergic receptors.

Transmitter Can Be Released by Carrier Mechanisms

Not all substances that are released by neurons are released by the exocytotic mechanism. Thus, arachidonic acid and eicosanoids (prostaglandins and lipoxygenase metabolites, see Chapter 12) are membrane permeable, and can traverse the lipid bilayer by diffusion. These substances may act at synapses either as autocoids or as chemical messengers. Other substances can be moved out of nerve endings by transporter carrier proteins (pumps) if their intracellular concentration is sufficiently high. Reversal of transporters that usually function to take up transmitters from the extracellular space has been described as a mechanism for releasing glutamate and γ-aminobutyric acid (GABA). This occurs in certain retinal cells. Still other substances simply leak out of nerve terminals at a low rate. Thus, about 90% of the ACh released at the neuromuscular junction is due to continuous leakage. Because this leakage is diffuse, it is functionally ineffective.

Removal of Transmitter from the Synaptic Cleft Terminates Synaptic Transmission

Removal of transmitters after release is critical to synaptic transmission. If a released transmitter substance persisted for a long time, a new signal could not get through. The synapse would be refractory mainly because of receptor desensitization produced by the continued exposure to transmitter. There are three mechanisms by which nervous tissue disposes of soluble or unbound transmitter substances: diffusion, enzymatic degradation, and reuptake. *Diffusion* removes some fraction of *all* chemical messengers; it can be an important means by which the synaptic cleft is cleared of transmitter.

Enzymatic degradation of transmitter substance is used primarily by the cholinergic system; the extracellular enzyme involved is acetylcholinesterase. Although this enzyme is important in shortening the duration of synaptic transmission, another important role, at least at the neuromuscular junction, is to make possible the *recapture* of choline. As seen in Figure 12–1 (Chapter 12), the active zones of the presynaptic nerve terminal are located just above the tips of the muscles's junctional folds. The ACh receptors are situated only at the surface of the muscle, and do not extend deep into the folds, whereas the esterase is anchored to the basement membrane only within the folds. This anatomical arrangement of the molecules serves two functions. Since any ACh after dissociation from the receptor most likely will be diluted in the relatively large volume within the junctional folds and hydrolyzed to choline and acetate, the transmitter molecules will only be used once. Thus, one function of the esterase is to punctuate the synaptic message rapidly. The second function is to recapture the choline that otherwise might be lost by diffusion away from the synaptic cleft. Once hydrolyzed by the esterase, the choline is held at a low concentration in the reservoir provided by the junctional folds later to be taken back up into cholinergic nerve endings by a high affinity uptake mechanism (see below and Chapter 14).

There are many enzymatic pathways that degrade transmitter substances within the neuron and in nonneural tissues. These enzymes can be important for controlling the concentrations of the transmitter within the neuron or in inactivating transmitters that have diffused from the synaptic cleft, but they are not involved specifically in terminating synaptic transmission. Many of these degradative pathways are important clinically. They provide sites for drug action and opportunity for diagnosis. Monoamine oxidase inhibitors, for example, which block degradation of amine transmitters within the cell, are currently used for the control of high blood pressure and for treating depression. Another example is the intracellular enzyme catechol-O-methyltransferase, which is important for degrading biogenic amines. It is found in the cytoplasm of most cells, including neurons, but is most prominent in liver and kidney. The concentrations of this enzyme's metabolites in body fluids serve as an indirect diagnostic indication of the efficacy of drugs that affect the synthesis or degradation of the biogenic amines in nervous tissue.

A postsynaptic feature that distinguishes neuroactive peptides from small-molecule transmitters is their slow rate of removal after release. It is likely that diffusion and proteolysis by extracellular peptidases are the only mechanisms of removing peptides. The slow removal of peptides contributes to the long duration of their action and makes their metabolism seem more like that of hormones.

Reuptake of the transmitter substance from the synaptic cleft is probably the most common mechanism used for inactivation. At nerve endings there are high-affinity uptake mechanisms for the released transmitter. These mechanisms are mediated by transporter molecules in the membranes of nerve terminals or of glial cells with binding constants of 25 μM or less. High-affinity uptake mechanisms were first described for norepinephrine, dopamine, and serotonin by Julius Axelrod. Similar uptake mechanisms for amino acid transmitters, glutamate, GABA, and glycine, and for choline (but not ACh) were found later. These uptake mechanisms are characteristic of specific neurons; as an example, noncholinergic neurons do not take up choline with high affinity. Certain powerful psychotropic drugs block these uptake processes (for example, cocaine for norepinephrine and the tricyclic antidepressants like imipramine for serotonin). The application of appropriate drugs to block uptake prolongs and enhances the action of the biogenic amines and GABA.

Carrier molecules for several substances have been characterized. Among the first were the Na^+, K^+-ATPase described in Chapter 6 and several permeases of bacteria (for example, the transporter for glucose). (As mentioned in Chapter 12, adenylyl cyclase is thought to be distantly related to permeases.) These membrane-spanning proteins thread through the cell membrane many times. Like most other membrane proteins, these molecules in eukaryotes are glycosylated at several sites in the domains of the protein that are extracellular. The transporters that take up transmitters depend on exchange with ions, usually Na^+, and operate using the energy of ATP. A carrier for GABA (GABA-1) has been cloned from rat brain by Norman Davidson, Henry Lester, and their collaborators. Its molecular properties presumably are typical of this group of proteins. From its inferred amino acid sequence, the GABA-1 transporter has a molecular weight of 67,000, but is surely larger since it has four potential sites for glycosylation. Its hydrophobicity plot predicts a secondary structure with 12 membrane-spanning regions. When expressed in frog eggs, the GABA-1 transporter takes up GABA into the oocyte with a Michaelis constant between 3 and 10 μM. Because no other exogenous mRNA is needed in these experiments, it can be assumed that the protein cloned alone serves as the transporter either as a single molecule or as multiple (identical) subunits. Uptake of GABA is dependent upon both Na^+ and Cl^- ions. GABA-1 is not the only isoform, since there is evidence from other studies for several GABA transporter molecules.

An Overall View

Communication at synapses depends upon two classes of molecules: chemical messengers and chemically gated receptors. In the last two chapters, we examined a variety of small-molecule transmitters and neuroactive peptides; we also considered how the molecular properties of these messengers and their receptors might contribute to the character of the transmission that they mediate. In this chapter we have seen how these chemical messengers are packaged in vesicles within the neuron. These vesicles play different roles in the life cycle of the two major classes of chemical messengers—small-molecule transmitters and neuroactive peptides. After synthesis in the cytoplasm, small-molecule transmitters are taken up and concentrated in vesicles, where they are protected from

intracellular degradative enzymes that maintain a constant level of the transmitter substance in the cytoplasm.

Because nerve endings contain so high a concentration of synaptic vesicles into which locally synthesized transmitter is concentrated, and because the contents of the synaptic vesicles are being continuously released, from dynamic considerations it is to be expected that much of the small-molecule transmitter in the neuron must be synthesized at the terminals. In contrast, the protein precursors of neuroactive peptides are introduced only during synthesis in the cell body; they ultimately become packaged in secretory granules and synaptic vesicles that are transported from the cell body to terminals. Unlike the vesicles that contain small-molecule transmitters, these vesicles are not refilled at the terminal.

While certain aspects of vesicle function vary considerably among different types of neurons, one is shared by most neurons. With the exception of neurons that release transmitters by diffusion or by carrier mechanisms, vesicles mediate the release of the chemical messenger through exocytosis. It seems axiomatic that the understanding of the molecular strategy of chemical transmission begins with the identification of the *contents* of the synaptic vesicle: Only if a molecule can be released does it have the potential of activating a receptor. But not all of the molecules released by a neuron are chemical messengers: Only those capable of binding to appropriate receptors can serve as transmitters.

Selected Readings

Bradford, H. F. 1986. Chemical Neurobiology: An Introduction to Neurochemistry. New York: Freeman, chap. 6, "The synaptosome: An in vitro model of the synapse."

Cooper, J. R., Bloom, F. E., and Roth, R. H. 1991. The Biochemical Basis of Neuropharmacology, 6th ed. New York: Oxford University Press.

De Camilli, P., and Jahn, R. 1990. Pathways to regulated exocytosis in neurons. Annu. Rev. Physiol. 52:624–645.

Martin, J. B., Brownstein, M. J., and Krieger, D. T. (eds.) 1987. Brain Peptides Update, Vol. I. New York: Wiley.

Sossin, W. S., Fisher, J. M., and Scheller, R. H. 1989. Cellular and molecular biology of neuropeptide processing and packaging. Neuron 2:1407–1417.

Trimble, W. S., Linial, M., and Scheller, R. H. 1991. Cellular and molecular biology of the presynaptic nerve terminal. Annu. Rev. Neurosci. 14:93–122.

References

Alberts, B., Bray, D., Lewis, J., Raff, M., Roberts, K., and Watson, J. D. 1989. Molecular Biology of the Cell, 2nd Ed. New York: Garland.

Almers, W., and Tse, F. W. 1990. Transmitter release from synapses: Does a preassembled fusion pore initiate exocytosis? Neuron 4:813–818.

Block, M. R., Glick, B. S., Wilcox, C. A., Wieland, F. T., and Rothman, J. E. 1988. Purification of an N-ethylmaleimide-sensitive protein catalyzing vesicular transport. Proc. Natl. Acad. Sci. U.S.A. 85:7852–7856.

Burgess, T. L., and Kelly, R. B. 1987. Constitutive and regulated secretion of proteins. Annu. Rev. Cell Biol. 3:243–293.

Dale, H. 1935. Pharmacology and nerve-endings. Proc. R. Soc. Med. (Lond.) 28:319–332.

Douglas, W. W. 1968. Stimulus-secretion coupling: The concept and clues from chromaffin and other cells. Br. J. Pharmacol. 34:451–474.

Gilman, A. G., Goodman, L. S., Rall, T. W., and Murad, F. (eds.) 1985. Goodman and Gilman's The Pharmacological Basis of Therapeutics, 7th ed. New York: Macmillan.

Guastella, J., Nelson, N., Nelson, H., Czyzyk, L., Keynan, S., Miedel, M. C., Davidson, N., Lester, H. A., and Kanner, B. I. 1990. Cloning and expression of a rat brain GABA transporter. Science 249:1303–1306.

Heuser, J. E., and Reese, T. S. 1977. Structure of the synapse. In E. R. Kandel (ed.), Handbook of Physiology, Section 1: The Nervous System. Vol. I. Cellular Biology of Neurons, Part 1. Bethesda, Md.: American Physiological Society, pp. 261–294.

Heuser, J. E., and Reese, T. S. 1981. Structural changes after transmitter release at the frog neuromuscular junction. J. Cell Biol. 88:564–580.

Hökfelt, T., and Björklund, A. 1985. Handbook of Chemical Neuroanatomy, Vol. 3: Classical Transmission and the Transmitter Receptors in the CNS, Part 2. Amsterdam: Elsevier Biomedical.

Iversen, L. L. 1967. The Uptake and Storage of Noradrenaline in Sympathetic Nerves. Cambridge, England: Cambridge University Press.

Johnson, R. G., Carty, S., and Scarpa, A. 1982. A model of biogenic amine accumulation into chromaffin granules and ghosts based on coupling to the electrochemical proton gradient. Fed. Proc. 41:2746–2754.

Llinás, R. R., and Heuser, J. E. 1977. Depolarization-release coupling systems in neurons. Neurosci. Res. Program Bull. 15:555–687.

Marshall, I. G., and Parsons, S. M. 1987. The vesicular acetylcholine transport system. Trends Neurosci. 10:174–177.

Maycox, P. R., Declewerth, T., Hell, J. W., and Jahn, R. 1988. Glutamate uptake by brain synaptic vesicles: Energy dependence of transport and functional reconstitution in proteoliposomes. J. Biol. Chem. 263:15423–15428.

Meldolesi, J., and Ceccarelli, B. 1981. Exocytosis and membrane recycling. Phil. Trans. R. Soc. (Lond.) B. 296:55–65.

Miller, T. M., and Heuser, J. E. 1984. Endocytosis of synaptic vesicle membrane at the frog neuromuscular junction. J. Cell Biol. 98:685–698.

Mitchell, P. 1961. Coupling of phosphorylation to electron and hydrogen transfer by a chemi–osmotic type of mechanism. Nature 191:144–148.

Pearse, B. M. F., and Robinson, M. S. 1990. Clathrin, adaptors, and sorting. Annu. Rev. Cell Biol. 6:151–171.

Schwartz, E. A. 1987. Depolarization without calcium can release γ-aminobutyric acid from a retinal neuron. Science 238:350–355.

Stern-Bach, Y., Greenberg-Ofrath, N., Flechner, I., and Schuldiner, S. 1990. Identification and purification of a functional amine transporter from bovine chromaffin granules. J. Biol. Chem. 265:3961–3966.

Südhof, T. C., Czernik, A. J., Kao, H.-T., Takei, K., Johnston, P. A., Horiuchi, A., Kanazir, S. D., Wagner, M. A., Perin, M. S., De Camilli, P., and Greengard, P. 1989. Synapsins: Mosaics of shared and individual domains in a family of synaptic vesicle phosphoproteins. Science 245:1474–1480.

Südhof, T. C., and Jahn, R. 1991. Proteins of synaptic vesicles involved in exocytosis and membrane recycling. Neuron 6:665–677.

Torri-Tarelli, F., Villa, A., Valtorta, F., De Camilli, P., Greengard, P., and Ceccarelli, B. 1990. Redistribution of synaptophysin and synapsin I during α-latrotoxin-induced release of neurotransmitter at the neuromuscular junction. J. Cell Biol. 110:449–459.

Whittaker, V. P., Michaelson, I. A., and Kirkland, R. J. A. 1964. The separation of synaptic vesicles from nerve-ending particles ('synaptosomes'). Biochem. J. 90:293–303.

Winkler, H., Sietzen, M., and Schober, M. 1987. The life cycle of catecholamine-storing vesicles. Ann. N.Y. Acad. Sci. 493:3–19.

Lewis P. Rowland

16

Diseases of Chemical Transmission at the Nerve–Muscle Synapse: Myasthenia Gravis

Myasthenia Gravis Affects Transmission at the Nerve–Muscle Synapse

Physiological Studies Showed a Disorder of Neuromuscular Transmission

Immunological Studies Indicated That Myasthenia Is an Autoimmune Disease

Identification of Antibodies to the Acetylcholine Receptor Initiated the Modern Period of Research

Immunological Changes Cause the Physiological Abnormality

The Basis of Antibody Binding in Myasthenia Gravis Has Been Defined

The Molecular Basis of the Autoimmune Reaction Has Been Defined

Myasthenia Gravis May Be More than One Disease

Current Therapy for Myasthenia Gravis Is Effective But Not Ideal

Other Disorders of Neuromuscular Transmission: Presynaptic (Facilitating) Neuromuscular Block

An Overall View

I n the preceding chapters we examined the mechanisms by which chemical transmitters are synthesized and released by neurons and the functional consequences of activating neurotransmitter receptors. Many human diseases disrupt chemical transmission between neurons and their target cells. For this reason, analysis of the abnormalities in synaptic transmission that are associated with human disease has shed light on the mechanisms underlying normal synaptic function. The most prevalent and the most thoroughly studied disease that affects synaptic transmission is myasthenia gravis, a disorder of function at the synapse between cholinergic motor neurons and skeletal muscle.

Myasthenia gravis (the term means severe muscle weakness) is an autoimmune disorder in which antibodies are produced against the nicotinic acetylcholine (ACh) receptor. These antibodies interfere with synaptic transmission by reducing the number of functional receptors or by impeding the interaction of ACh with its receptors. Because ACh is the neurotransmitter at the neuromuscular junction, the skeletal muscle becomes weakened. This weakness has four special characteristics:

1. The weakness often affects cranial muscles (eyelids, eye muscles, and oropharyngeal muscles; Figure 16–1A) as well as limb muscles.
2. Unlike any other disease of muscle or nerve, the severity of the weakness varies within the course of a single day, from day to day, or over longer periods (giving rise to periods of remission or exacerbation).
3. There are no conventional clinical signs that indicate that the muscle is deprived of its innervation similar to the signs that characterize disorders of the motor unit, such as loss of tendon reflexes or atrophy of muscle, and there are no electromyographic signs of denervation.

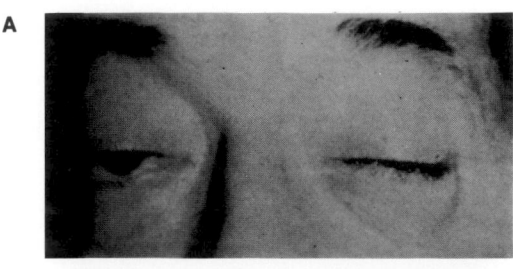

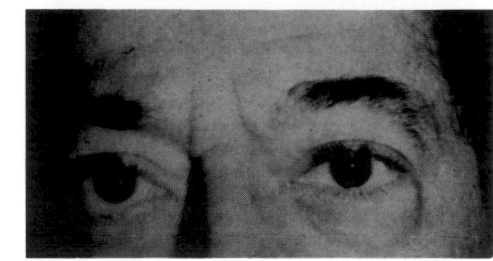

FIGURE 16–1
Myasthenia gravis typically affects the cranial muscles. (From Rowland, Hoefer, and Aranow, 1960.)

A. Severe drooping of the eyelids, or ptosis, is characteristic of myasthenia gravis. This patient also could not move his eyes to look to either side.

B. One minute after an intravenous injection of 10 mg of edrophonium, an inhibitor of cholinesterase, both eyes are open and can be moved freely.

4. The weakness is reversed by drugs that inhibit acetylcholinesterase, the enzyme that degrades ACh (Figure 16–1B).

Myasthenia Gravis Affects Transmission at the Nerve–Muscle Synapse

The first well-documented example of myasthenia gravis was reported in 1877 by Samuel Wilks. By 1900 neurologists had described the important clinical characteristics of the disease. At that time, however, diseases were still defined primarily in terms of lesions observed by microscopy at postmortem examination rather than in terms of physiological or etiological factors. In myasthenia, the brain, spinal cord, peripheral nerves, and muscles all appeared normal at autopsy, and the disease was therefore considered a disorder of function.

Physiological Studies Showed a Disorder of Neuromuscular Transmission

Two discoveries in the mid-1930s helped to identify myasthenia as a disease of neuromuscular transmission. First, Henry Dale, Wilhelm Feldberg, and Marthe Vogt demonstrated that transmission at the neuromuscular junction is mediated by a chemical transmitter that they identified as ACh. Second, Mary Walker found that inhibitors of acetylcholinesterase, such as physostigmine and neostigmine, reverse the symptoms of myasthenia gravis.

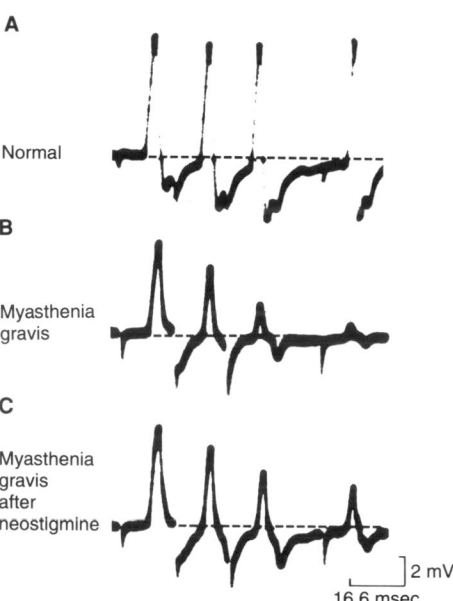

FIGURE 16–2
Neostigmine increases the duration of action of ACh and thus can compensate for the reduced ACh activity in myasthenia. (From Harvey, Lilienthal, and Talbot, 1941.)

A. In a normal person the amplitude of action potentials evoked by a train of four stimuli at 16.6 ms intervals remains constant.

B. In the myasthenic patient there is a rapid decrease in amplitude.

C. After injection of 2 mg of neostigmine into the brachial artery of the myasthenic patient, the decrease in amplitude was partially reversed. (Calibration, 2.0 mV.)

In the years between 1945 and 1960 A. McGhee Harvey and his colleagues described in detail the physiological basis of the disorder. When a motor nerve is stimulated electrically, the summed electrical activity of a population of muscle fibers (known as the compound action potential) can be measured with surface electrodes. At stimulation rates of 2–5 per sec, the amplitude of the compound action potential evoked in normal human muscle remains constant. Harvey found that in myasthenia gravis the amplitude of evoked compound action potentials decreases rapidly. This abnormality resembles the pattern induced in normal muscle by *d*-tubocurarine (curare), which blocks ACh receptors and inhibits the action of ACh at the neuromuscular junction. Neostigmine, an inhibitor of cholinesterase that increases the duration of action of ACh at the neuromuscular junction, reverses the decrease in amplitude of evoked compound action potentials in myasthenic patients (Figure 16–2).

Immunological Studies Indicated That Myasthenia Is an Autoimmune Disease

Soon after the clinical syndrome had been identified, it was recognized that about 15% of adult patients with myasthenia had a benign tumor of the thymus (thymomas). In 1939 Alfred Blalock first reported that the symptoms in myasthenic patients were improved by removal of the thymoma. Based on this finding, Blalock and Harvey in the 1950s found that removing the thymus in patients with myasthenia gravis also resulted in a reduction in symptoms, and this procedure has now become standard therapy. At that time it was not clear why these tumors were associated with myasthenia or why thymectomy was beneficial, because the immunological role of the thymus was not established until the 1960s. The neurologist John Simpson was one of the first to suggest that myasthenia was an immunological disorder, because it frequently occurs in patients with other diseases, such as rheumatoid arthritis, that are thought to have an autoimmune basis.

Identification of Antibodies to the Acetylcholine Receptor Initiated the Modern Period of Research

The modern concept of myasthenia emerged with the isolation and characterization of the nicotinic ACh receptor. The breakthrough came in 1966. Two chemists, C. C. Chang and Chen-Yuan Lee, were concerned with a local public health problem in Taiwan—poisonous snake bites. One of the toxins they isolated from snake venom, α-bungarotoxin, was found to cause paralysis by binding essentially irreversibly to ACh receptors at the motor end-plate. By 1971 Lee and Jean-Pierre Changeux, and Ricardo Miledi and Lincoln Potter had used the toxin to isolate and purify ACh receptors from the electric organ of the electric eel.

In 1973 Douglas Fambrough and Daniel Drachman used radioactive α-bungarotoxin to label the ACh receptors in human end-plates. They found fewer binding sites in myasthenic muscle than in controls (Figure 16–3). In the same year James Patrick and Jon Lindstrom injected ACh receptors purified from eel electroplax (which is related to the skeletal muscles of higher vertebrates) into

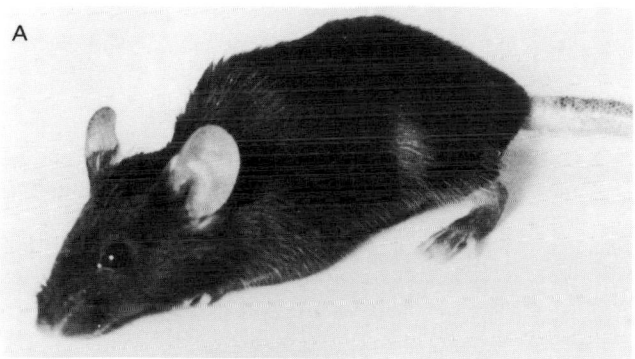

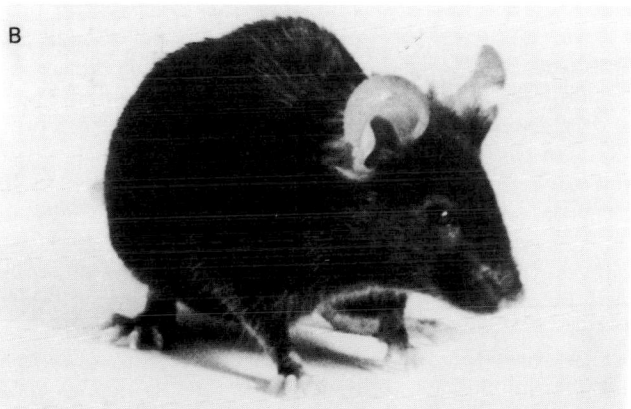

FIGURE 16–4

Posture of a myasthenic mouse before and after treatment with neostigmine. To produce the syndrome the mouse was immunized with 15 μg of ACh receptors from *Torpedo californica* and boosted 45 days later with 15 μg of the receptor. (From Berman and Patrick, 1980.)

A. Before treatment the mouse is inactive.

B. Twelve minutes after receiving an intraperitoneal injection of 37.5 μg/kg neostigmine bromide, the mouse is standing.

FIGURE 16–3

In myasthenia gravis the density of ACh receptors in human muscle fibers is reduced. ACh receptors are marked with ^{125}I-labeled α-bungarotoxin and detected in autoradiograms (drawn here). (Adapted from Fambrough, Drachman, and Satyamurti, 1973.)

A. In normal fibers there is a dense accumulation of silver grains in a limited junctional area, the end-plate, and a paucity of grains outside this region.

B. In myasthenic fiber the grains are also localized in the end-plate region, but the number per unit area is markedly reduced, indicating a reduced density of functional reactive sites.

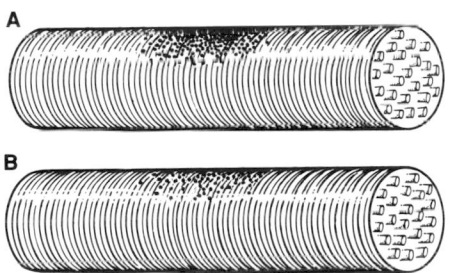

rabbits, intending to use the resulting antibodies to study the properties of eel ACh receptors. Strikingly, the generation of antibodies was accompanied by the onset of myasthenia-like symptoms in the rabbit. Moreover, the weakness was reversed by the cholinesterase inhibitors neostigmine or edrophonium. As in humans with myasthenia gravis, the animals were abnormally sensitive to neuromuscular blocking agents, such as curare, and the evoked compound action potentials in muscle decreased with repetitive stimulation. It was later shown that a similar syndrome can be induced in mice and other mammals by immunization with ACh receptor protein (Figure 16–4).

By 1975 all the essential characteristics of human disease had been reproduced in experimentally induced myasthenia gravis. These characteristics included a reduction in the amplitude of the miniature end-plate potentials, a smoothing of the normal convoluted appearance of the postjunctional folds, a loss of ACh receptors from the tips of postjunctional folds, and the deposition at postjunctional sites of antibody and complement, a serum protein that participates in antibody-mediated cell lysis. Acetylcholine receptors from electric fish induced experimental autoimmune myasthenia gravis in mice, rats, and monkeys, suggesting that the structure of ACh receptors is highly conserved across species.

After experimental myasthenia gravis was characterized, antibodies directed against ACh receptors were found in the serum of patients with myasthenia. In addition, when B lymphocytes from patients with myasthenia were cultured, the lymphocytes produced antibodies to ACh receptors. The idea that the human antibodies actually cause the symptoms of myasthenia was also supported by other observations. Repeated injection of mice with serum from patients with myasthenia reproduced the electrophysiological abnormalities in these mice by reducing the number of ACh receptors in skeletal muscle. A similar reduction in ACh receptors occurs with monoclonal antibodies to ACh receptors.

Further support for the role of antibodies against ACh receptors was provided by the detection of antibodies in infants with neonatal myasthenia. These children of myasthenic mothers have difficulty swallowing and impaired limb movements. The syndrome lasts from 7 to 10 days and, as the symptoms abate, the level of antibodies declines. Similarly, draining lymph from the thoracic lymph ducts improves myasthenia symptoms in adults. The

symptoms recur when the lymph fluid is returned to the patient, but not when lymphocytes are replaced. Furthermore, symptoms improve and antibody levels decline when patients are subjected to *plasmapheresis*, a procedure in which blood is removed from a patient, cells are separated from plasma, and the cells alone are returned to the patient (the plasma, which contains the antibodies, is discarded).

Immunological Changes Cause the Physiological Abnormality

How do the immunological observations that we have just considered account for the characteristic decrease in the response of myasthenic muscle to repetitive stimulation?

Normally, an action potential in a motor axon releases enough ACh from synaptic vesicles to induce an excitatory end-plate potential with an amplitude of about 70–80 mV (Chapter 10). Since the threshold for spike generation is about −45 mV, the normal end-plate potential is greater than the threshold needed to initiate an action potential. Thus, in normal muscle the difference between the threshold and the actual end-plate potential amplitude—the *safety factor*—is quite large (Figure 16–5A). In fact, in many muscles the amount of ACh released during synaptic transmission can be reduced to as little as 25% of normal before it fails to initiate an action potential.

FIGURE 16–5

Failure of transmission at the neuromuscular junction in myasthenia gravis. (From Lisak and Barchi, 1982.)

A. In the normal neuromuscular junction the amplitude of the end-plate potential is so large that all fluctuations in the efficiency of transmitter release occur well above the threshold for a muscle action potential (**1**). Therefore, the amplitude of a compound muscle action potential during repetitive stimulation is constant and invariant (**2**).

B. In the myasthenic neuromuscular junction postsynaptic changes reduce the amplitude of the end-plate potential in response to presynaptic release of a given amount of ACh, so that

under optimal circumstances the end-plate potential may be just sufficient to produce a muscle action potential. Fluctuations in transmitter release that normally accompany repeated stimulation now cause the end-plate potential to drop below this threshold, leading to conduction failure at that junction (**1**). When the action potential is recorded from the surface of a myasthenic muscle, the amplitude of the compound action potential—a measure of contributions from all fibers in which synaptic transmission is successful—shows a progressive decline and only a small and variable recovery (**2**), and indicates why the safety factor is reduced in myasthenia.

A Normal junction

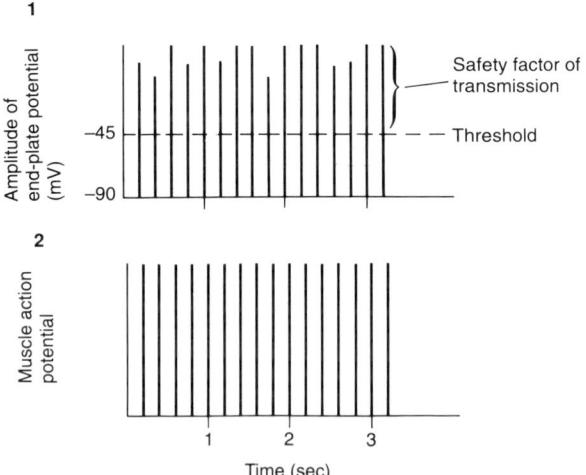

B Myasthenic junction

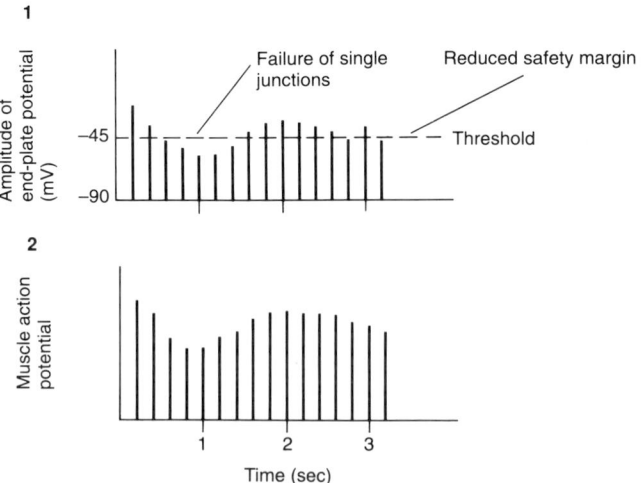

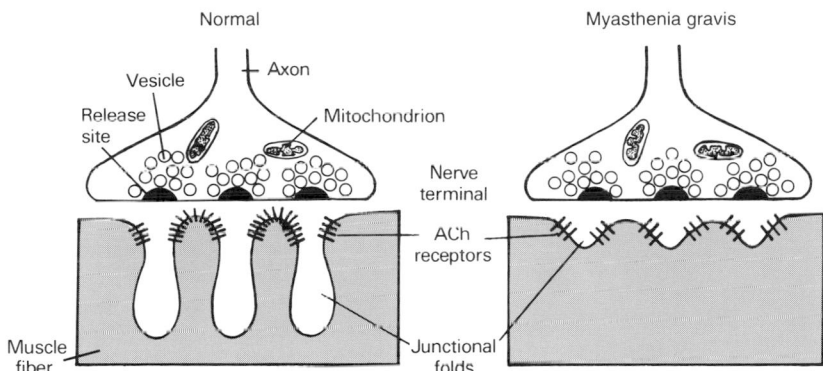

FIGURE 16–6
In myasthenia, morphological changes in the neuromuscular junction reduce the likelihood of synaptic transmission. The myasthenic junction has a normal nerve terminal but the number of ACh receptors is reduced, the junctional folds are sparse and shallow, and the synaptic space is widened. (Adapted from Drachman, 1983.)

Most of the ACh released into the synaptic cleft by an action potential is rapidly hydrolyzed by acetylcholinesterase. When the density of ACh receptors is reduced, as it is in myasthenia, it is less probable that a molecule of ACh will find a receptor before it is hydrolyzed. Moreover, the geometry of the end-plate is also disturbed in myasthenia. The normal infolding is reduced, and the synaptic cleft is enlarged (Figure 16–6). These morphological changes increase the diffusion of ACh away from the synaptic cleft and thus reduce further the probability of ACh interacting with the few remaining functional receptors. As a result, the amplitude of the end-plate potential is reduced to the point where it is barely above threshold (Figure 16–5B). Thus, transmission is readily blocked even though the vesicles in the presynaptic terminals contain normal amounts of ACh and the processes of exocytosis and release are intact. Both the physiological abnormality (the decremental response) and the clinical symptoms (muscle weakness) are partially reversed by drugs that inhibit active cholinesterase because the released ACh molecules remain unhydrolyzed for a longer time and therefore the probability that they will interact with receptors is increased.

The reduced efficacy of neuromuscular transmission in myasthenia can be assessed by the clinical technique of single-fiber electromyography, which measures the intervals between discharges of different muscle fibers innervated by the same motor neuron. The normal variation in intervals is called *jitter*. The extent of jitter depends on the velocity of conduction in nerve terminals, transmitter release, and activation of the postsynaptic membrane. Jitter may therefore increase in other neurogenic diseases, but is especially pronounced in myasthenia gravis.

The Basis of Antibody Binding in Myasthenia Gravis Has Been Defined

As discussed in Chapter 10, the genes for each of the subunits of mammalian ACh receptor have now been cloned and sequenced and peptides corresponding to specific domains of ACh receptor subunits have been synthesized. In experimental animals, antibodies that cause myasthenia are usually active against either of two peptide sequences on the native receptor—the bungarotoxin-binding site or an area on the α-subunit called the *main immunogenic region*. Circulating antibodies in humans are often directed against the main immunogenic region.

Even though it has been well established that antibodies to the α-subunit of ACh receptors have a central role in the pathogenesis of myasthenia—so much so that myasthenia is now the prototype of human autoimmune disease—several questions remain unanswered. What, for example, initiates the production of antibodies to the ACh receptor? One possibility is that persistent viral infection could alter the properties of the surface membrane, rendering it immunogenic, but this has not been shown. Another possibility is that viral or bacterial antigens may share epitopes with the ACh receptor. Thus, when a person is infected, the antibodies generated against the foreign organism may also recognize the ACh receptor.

How do antibodies cause the symptoms of myasthenia? The antibodies do not occupy the receptor site. This conclusion arises from the test used to detect anti-receptor antibodies in human serum. The circulating antibodies react with purified ACh receptors that have been labeled by radioactive α-bungarotoxin. Because the toxin itself occupies and blocks the agonist site, the antibody must react with epitopes elsewhere on the receptor molecule.

One indirect effect of the antibodies might be steric hindrance of the interaction of ACh and the receptor. The loss of receptors is, however, probably due to an increase in turnover and degradation of ACh receptors. Myasthenic antibodies are able to bind and cross-link ACh receptors, in this way triggering the internalization of the receptor (Figure 16–7). In addition, some antibodies to ACh receptors in myasthenic patients bind proteins of the complement cascade, which may result in lysis of the postsynaptic membrane.

Although the evidence implicating ACh receptor antibodies in myasthenic symptoms is compelling, the antibodies are not found in all myasthenic patients. Moreover, there is no consistent relationship between the concentration of antibodies directed against ACh receptors and the severity of symptoms. One explanation of this dissociation is that the antibodies found in the serum of myasthenic patients or in animals with experimentally induced myasthenia gravis are polyclonal; they are produced by different B cells in response to different antigenic determi-

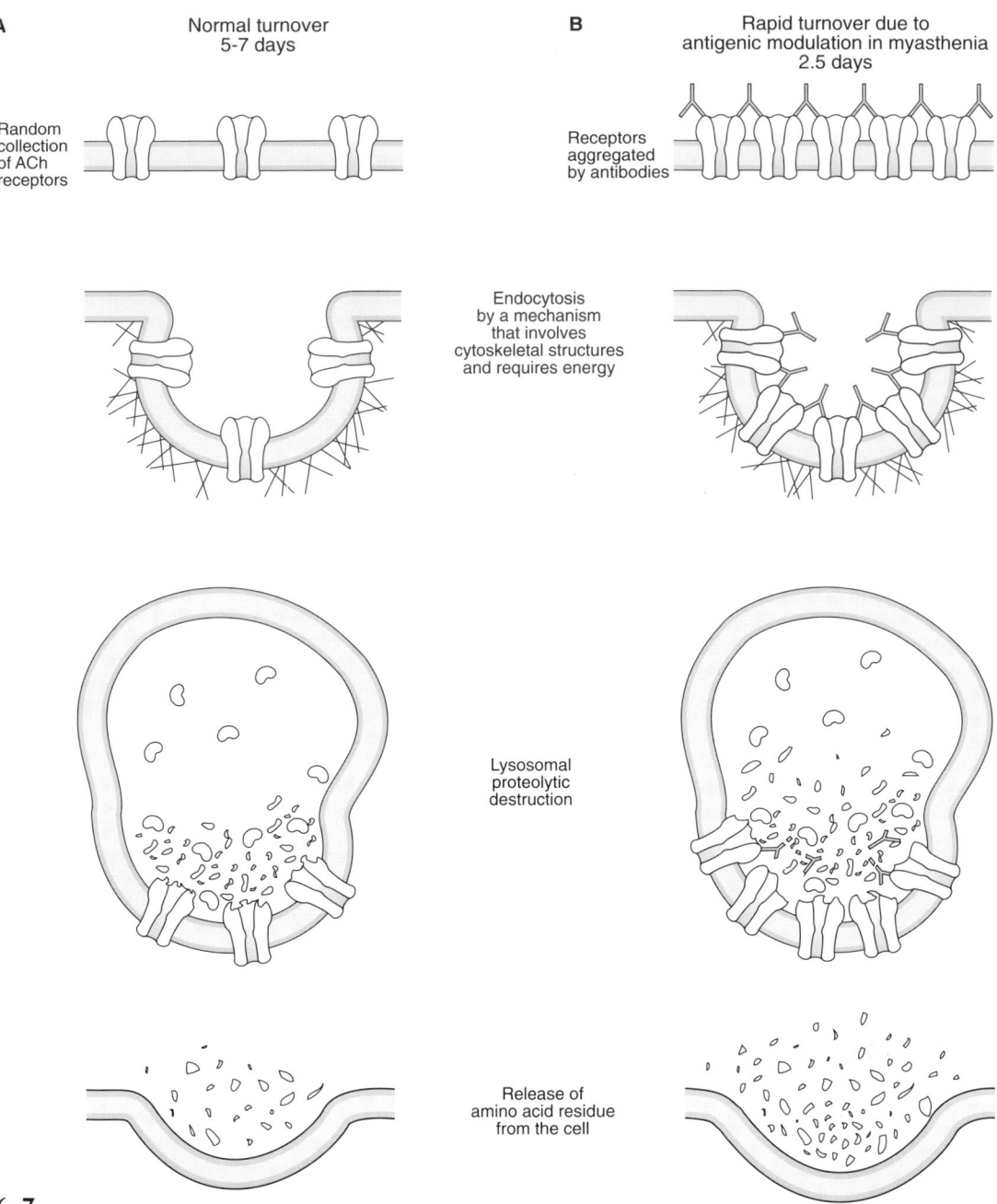

A Normal turnover 5-7 days

Random collection of ACh receptors

B Rapid turnover due to antigenic modulation in myasthenia 2.5 days

Receptors aggregated by antibodies

Endocytosis by a mechanism that involves cytoskeletal structures and requires energy

Lysosomal proteolytic destruction

Release of amino acid residue from the cell

FIGURE 16–7

The normal rate of destruction of ACh receptors is increased in myasthenia. The degradation of the receptor is schematically illustrated as occurring in consecutive steps. (Adapted from Lindstrom, 1983, and Drachman, 1983.)

A. Normal turnover of randomly spaced ACh receptors takes place every 5–7 days.

B. In myasthenia gravis and in experimental myasthenia gravis the cross-linking of ACh receptors by the antibody facilitates the

normal endocytosis and phagocytic destruction of the receptors, which leads to a two- to threefold increase in the rate of receptor turnover. Binding of anti-receptor antibody activates the complement cascade, which is involved in focal lysis of the postsynaptic membrane. This focal lysis is probably primarily responsible for the characteristic alterations of postsynaptic membrane morphology observed in myasthenia (Figure 16–6).

nants, and therefore the serum of each patient contains antibodies with distinct specificities. As a consequence, some people with high titers of antibodies to the receptor but few or no clinical symptoms might have a type of antibody that is limited in its ability to interfere with

synaptic transmission or to influence ACh receptor turnover. In contrast, other patients with severe myasthenia might have low titers of antibodies that are effective in interfering with the function of the receptor and its turnover.

The Molecular Basis of the Autoimmune Reaction Has Been Defined

The autoimmune reaction depends on the interaction of three molecules, the trimolecular complex, comprised of the following: (1) the antigen, the immunogenic peptide of the ACh receptor or a peptide that mimics the receptor; (2) an antigen-specific T cell receptor; (3) class II molecules of the major histocompatibility complex (MHC) that are expressed on the antigen-presenting cell (Figure 16–8A). The T cells become reactive against the ACh receptor. This could result from an infection in which a viral protein includes a peptide homologous to one in the ACh receptor, a form of molecular mimicry. Once activated the T cells could recognize the ACh receptors on myoid cells in the thymus. Antigen-specific T cells have actually been identified in the thymus glands of patients with myasthenia.

The class II major histocompatibility complex (MHC) genes also play a major role in determining susceptibility. Patients with myasthenia gravis show an over-representation of the histocompatibility subtypes DR3 and DQw2. The relative risk of people with HLA-DQ for myasthenia is 32 times more than that of people with other HLA haplotypes. The specific immunogenic peptides of human ACh receptor have also been identified.

These findings open new approaches to therapy for patients who do not improve sufficiently with anticholinesterase drug therapy or thymectomy. For instance, it might be possible to make antibodies against the anti-ACh receptor antibodies, or anti-idiotype antibodies. However, this has proven difficult in experimental myasthenia. Another approach is to develop peptide competitors for ACh receptors (Figure 16–8B) that might block T-cell recognition of ACh receptors or MHC binding of ACh receptor fragments. Alternatively, antibodies might be developed against either MHC class II molecules of the antigen-presenting cells or receptors on the T cells that recognize ACh receptors.

Myasthenia Gravis May Be More than One Disease

The modern analysis of myasthenia has given increased support to the idea that myasthenia gravis is more than one disease. This had been suspected earlier but is difficult to prove. For instance, it had long been recognized that congenital myasthenia (symptoms present from birth in children whose mothers do not have myasthenia) is often hereditary. Now it seems that patients with congenital myasthenia do not have antibodies to ACh receptors. Therefore, there may be two distinct categories of myasthenia: an acquired autoimmune form in older children and adults (with ACh receptor antibodies) and a nonimmune heritable congenital myasthenia (without ACh receptor antibodies). Even among adults, antibodies are much more likely to be found in patients with generalized myasthenia than among those with solely eye muscle symptoms.

Biophysical and immunocytochemical studies of con-

A   Activation of autoimmune T lymphocytes

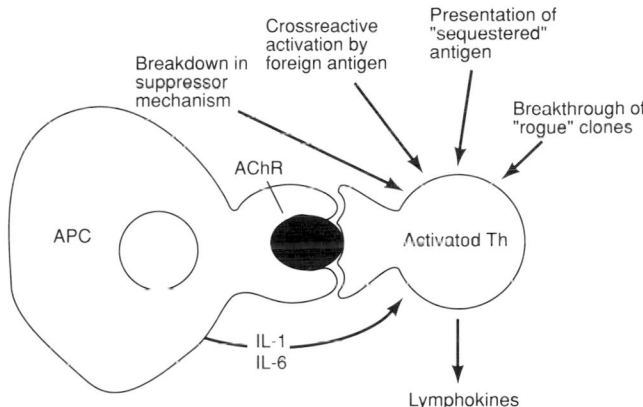

1) IFN-γ: upregulates class II MHC
2) IL-2: helps autoreactive T cells
3) IL-4,IL-5 & IL-6: help autoreactive B cells

B   Interfering with activation of autoreactive T lymphocytes

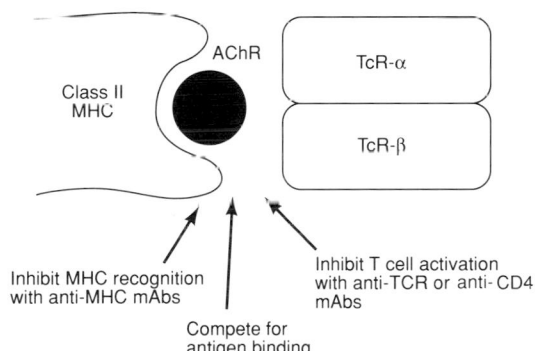

FIGURE 16–8

Mechanisms of the autoimmune reaction directed against the ACh receptor. Abbreviations: APC, antigen-presenting cell; AChR, acetylcholine receptor; Th, thymocyte; MHC, major histocompatibility complex; TcR, T-cell receptor; IFN, interferon; IL, interleukin; mAb, monoclonal antibody. (Adapted from Steinman and Mantegazza, 1990.)

A. Activation of autoimmune T lymphocytes requires three molecules: an immunogenic peptide in the ACh receptor (AChR) or one that mimics it; a specific class II molecule of the major histocompatibility complex (MHC) on the antigen-presenting cell; and an antigen-specific T-cell receptor.

B. Treatment of myasthenia gravis may be improved by molecular therapy designed to inhibit MHC recognition by use of antibodies to MHC; by administering peptides that compete with ACh receptors and so block the T cells; or by using antibodies directed against the T cells themselves.

genital myasthenia by Andrew Engel, Edward Lambert, and their colleagues, and by Angela Vincent, John Newsom-Davis, Stuart Cull-Candy, and their colleagues also indicate that myasthenia is a heterogeneous syndrome. Some cases seem to be due to abnormality in the presynaptic terminals, with impaired release of ACh from the terminals. Others are apparently due to postsynaptic disorders, including congenital lack of acetylcholinesterase, altered capacity of ACh receptors to react with ACh, or abnormally low numbers of ACh receptors. We shall here consider two illustrative examples: loss of acetylcholinesterase and the slow-channel syndrome.

Lack of acetylcholinesterase has the following characteristics. There is a decrease in response to repetitive stimulation at 2 Hz, as in myasthenia gravis, but the muscle responds repetitively to a single stimulus, a feature not seen in other conditions. End-plate potentials and miniature end-plate potentials are not small, as in myasthenia gravis, but are markedly prolonged, a feature that could explain the repetitive response. Cytochemical studies reveal that the enzyme acetylcholinesterase is absent from the postsynaptic membranes. In contrast, ACh receptors, as visualized by labeling with radioactive bungarotoxin, are preserved.

The slow-channel syndrome is characterized by prominent limb weakness with little weakness of cranial muscles (just the reverse of the pattern usually seen in myasthenia gravis, where muscles of the eyes and oropharynx are almost always affected). The end-plate potentials in the slow-channel syndrome are prolonged in a manner similar to that observed with acetylcholinesterase deficiency, and spontaneous miniature end-plate potentials are also prolonged. In contrast, acetylcholinesterase is present and shows normal enzyme kinetics. These features suggest that the opening of the ACh receptor-channel is abnormally prolonged. In addition miniature end-plate potentials are of abnormally low amplitude, which may result from the degeneration of junctional folds and a loss of ACh receptors.

It is not certain how the slow-channel syndrome arises. However, the ACh receptor-channel is slow in newly formed end-plates. Thus, it is possible that the developmental transition from slow-to-fast channels, which is accompanied by replacement of the γ-subunit of the ACh receptor by an ε-subunit, is prevented. It is also possible that a mutation has altered the ACh receptor in a way that modifies the time the channel spends in the open state. Discriminating between the several different kinds of myasthenia—congenital and adult varieties, autoimmune and those due to other mechanisms, familial and acquired—remains a major challenge.

Current Therapy for Myasthenia Gravis Is Effective But Not Ideal

Twenty-five years ago the mortality rate of myasthenia was about 33%. Now, few patients die of myasthenia and life expectancy is almost normal. This change is largely due to advances in intensive care, including mechanical ventilation and antibiotics. Years ago, respiratory-care units of hospitals were populated by many patients in myasthenic "crisis," defined by the use of a mechanical ventilator for a patient in respiratory distress. Now, the number of patients in crisis has declined drastically. Many investigators attribute this change to the practice of thymectomy. After thymectomy about half of the patients are in "remission"—they have no symptoms of myasthenia and take no drugs. Further improvement in therapy will have to be directed to patients who are not helped by thymectomy.

Other Disorders of Neuromuscular Transmission: Presynaptic (Facilitating) Neuromuscular Block

Some patients with cancer, such as small-cell cancers of the lung, show a weakness associated with a neuromuscular disorder that is the opposite of myasthenia. Instead of a decline in synaptic response to repetitive stimulation, these patients show a gradual increase in response leading to a state called *facilitating neuromuscular block*. Here, the first postsynaptic potential to stimulation is abnormally small. Subsequent responses increase in amplitude so that the final summated action potential produced by a train of five spikes per second is two to four times the amplitude of the first potential. This disorder, called the *Lambert-Eaton syndrome* after the investigators who identified it, is attributed to the presence of antibodies to voltage-gated Ca^{2+} channels in the presynaptic terminal. Because the syndrome occurs frequently in patients with lung cancer, it is relevant that cultured cells of small-cell lung cancers show functional voltage-gated Ca^{2+} channels. These channels may serve as the natural antigens for the pathogenic antibodies that distort function at the neuromuscular junction.

Mice injected with serum from Lambert-Eaton patients show electrophysiological abnormalities typical of the syndrome and morphologic evidence of loss of the presynaptic active zones and the active zone particles (see Chapter 13). Loss of voltage-gated Ca^{2+} channels might be expected to reduce the entry of Ca^{2+} when nerve terminals are depolarized and so impair release of transmitter. In addition, patients often improve after plasmapheresis or treatment with immunosuppressive drugs, consistent with the notion that circulating antibodies are the cause of the syndrome.

The Lambert-Eaton syndrome also occurs in patients who do not have cancer. In these patients the pathogenesis is still unknown. A similar presynaptic physiological abnormality is seen in human botulism, and experimental studies have indicated that blockade by botulinum toxin is associated with impaired release of ACh. Both Lambert-Eaton syndrome and botulism are treated by calcium gluconate and by guanidine, agents that promote the release of ACh.

An Overall View

Myasthenia gravis is a neuromuscular disability caused by a reduced number of ACh receptors at the nerve–muscle synapse. It is improved by drugs that inhibit cholinesterase and thereby prolong the action of the transmitter. In another neuromuscular disorder, facilitating neuromuscular block, the amount of transmitter released is reduced because of a loss of Ca^{2+} channels. In principle, these findings suggest a strategy for treatment of diseases of synaptic function. First, the origin of the disorder in either the presynaptic neuron (a disease of transmitter release) or postsynaptic neuron (a disease of the receptor) is determined. Once the cause has been identified the most effective treatment is likely to be one that corrects the affected step in transmission or eliminates the pathogenic agent. This insight emphasizes the importance of a theoretical understanding of synaptic transmission for analyzing and treating neurological diseases.

However, the history of work on myasthenia gravis also illustrates that progress in our understanding of neurological diseases often depends on the interplay of clinical and basic research. For example, it was first observed clinically that thymectomy is therapeutic; only later was the physiological evidence of the immunological role of the thymus discovered. Likewise, clinical evidence associating myasthenia with rheumatoid arthritis and other diseases of autoimmunity identified the disease as autoimmune. Similarly, the clinical observation that neostigmine is an effective treatment established myasthenia as a disease of neuromuscular transmission because the drug is an inhibitor of acetylcholinesterase.

Selected Readings

Drachman, D. B. (ed.) 1987. Myasthenia Gravis: Biology and Treatment. Ann. N.Y. Acad. Sci. 505:1–914.

Engel, A. G. 1988. Congenital myasthenic syndromes. J. Child Neurol. 3:233–246.

Lindstrom, J. 1983. Using monoclonal antibodies to study acetylcholine receptors and myasthenia gravis. Neurosci. Comment. 1:139–156.

Lisak, R. P., and Barchi, R. L. 1982. Myasthenia Gravis. Philadelphia: Saunders.

Numa, S. 1989. Molecular structure and function of acetylcholine receptors and sodium channel. In S. Chien (ed.), Molecular Biology in Physiology. New York: Raven Press, pp. 93–118.

Pachner, A. R. 1988. Myasthenia gravis. Immunol. Allerg. Clin. North Am. 8:277–293.

Rowland, L. P. 1980. Controversies about the treatment of myasthenia gravis. J. Neurol. Neurosurg. Psychiatry 43.644–659.

Swift, T. R. 1981. Disorders of neuromuscular transmission other than myasthenia gravis. Muscle Nerve 4:334–353.

Wilks, S. 1883. Lectures on Diseases of the Nervous System Delivered at Guy's Hospital, 2nd ed. Philadelphia: P. Blakiston, Son & Co.

References

Berman, P. W., and Patrick, J. 1980. Experimental myasthenia gravis: A murine system. J. Exp. Med. 151:204–223.

Berman, P. W., Patrick, J., Heinemann, S., Klier, F. G., and Steinbach, J. H. 1981. Factors affecting the susceptibility of different strains of mice to experimental myasthenia gravis. Ann. N.Y. Acad. Sci. 377:237–257.

Blalock, A., Mason, M. F., Morgan, H. J., and Riven, S. S. 1939. Myasthenia gravis and tumors of the thymic region. Report of a case in which the tumor was removed. Ann. Surg. 110:544–561.

Chang, C. C., and Lee, C.-Y. 1966. Electrophysiological study of neuromuscular blocking action of cobra neurotoxin. Br. J. Pharm. Chemother. 28:172–181.

Changeux, J.-P., Kasai, M., and Lee, C.-Y. 1970. Use of a snake venom toxin to characterize the cholinergic receptor protein. Proc. Natl. Acad. Sci. U.S.A. 67:1241–1247.

Cull-Candy, S. G., Miledi, R., and Trautman, A. 1979. End-plate currents and acetylcholine noise at normal and myasthenic human end-plates. J. Physiol. (Lond.) 287:247–265.

Dale, H. H., Feldberg, W., and Vogt, M. 1936. Release of acetylcholine at voluntary motor nerve endings. J. Physiol. (Lond.) 86:353–380.

Drachman, D. B. 1983. Myasthenia gravis: Immunobiology of a receptor disorder. Trends Neurosci. 6:446–451.

Eaton, L. M., and Lambert, E. H. 1957. Electromyography and electric stimulation of nerves in diseases of the motor unit: Observations on myasthenic syndrome associated with malignant tumors. J.A.M.A. 163:1117–1124.

Engel, A. G. 1984. Myasthenia gravis and myasthenic syndromes. Ann. Neurol. 16:519–534.

Fambrough, D. M., Drachman, D. B., and Satyamurti, S. 1973. Neuromuscular junction in myasthenia gravis: Decreased acetylcholine receptors. Science 182:293–295.

Harcourt, G. C., Sommer, N., Rothbard, J., Willcox, H. N. A., and Newsom-Davis, J. 1988. A juxta-membrane epitope on the human acetylcholine receptor recognized by T cells in myasthenia gravis. J. Clin. Invest. 82:1295–1300.

Harvey, A. M., Lilienthal, J. L., Jr., and Talbot, S. A. 1941. Observations on the nature of myasthenia gravis: The phenomena of facilitation and depression of neuromuscular transmission. Bull. Johns Hopkins Hosp. 69:547–565.

Hohlfeld, R., Toyka, K. V. Miner, L. L., Walgrave, S. L., and Conti-Tronconi, B. M. 1988. Amphipathic segment of the nicotinic receptor alpha subunit contains epitopes recognized by T lymphocytes in myasthenia gravis. J. Clin. Invest. 81:657–660.

Jaretzki, A., III, Penn, A. S., Younger, D. S., Wolff, M., Olarte, M. R., Lovelace, R. E., and Rowland, L. P. 1988. "Maximal" thymectomy for myasthenia gravis: Results. J. Thorac. Cardiovasc. Surg. 95:747–757.

Kim, Y. I., and Neher, E. 1988. IgG from patients with Lambert-Eaton syndrome blocks voltage-dependent calcium channels. Science 239:405–408.

Miledi, R., Molinoff, P., and Potter, L. T. 1971. Isolation of the cholinergic receptor protein of Torpedo electric tissue. Nature 229:554–557.

O'Neill, J. H., Murray, N. M. F., and Newsom-Davis, J. 1988. The Lambert-Eaton myasthenic syndrome. A review of 50 cases. Brain 111:577–596.

Patrick, J., and Lindstrom, J. 1973. Autoimmune response to acetylcholine receptor. Science 180:871 872.

Rowland, L. P., Hoefer, P. F. A., and Aranow, H., Jr. 1960. Myasthenic syndromes. Res. Publ. Assoc. Res. Nerv. Ment. Dis. 38:548–600.

Simpson, J. A. 1960. Myasthenia gravis: A new hypothesis. Scot. Med. J. 5:419–436.

Soliven, B. C., Lange, D. J., Penn, A. S., Younger, D., Jaretzki, A., III, Lovelace, R. E., and Rowland, L. P. 1988. Seronegative myasthenia gravis. Neurology 38:514–517.

Steinman, L., and Mantegazza R. 1990. Prospects for specific immunotherapy in myasthenia gravis. FASEB J. 4:2726–2731.

Toyka, K. V., Drachman, D. B., Pestronk, A., and Kao, I. 1975. Myasthenia gravis: Passive transfer from man to mouse. Science 190:397–399.

Vincent, A., Pinching, A. J., and Newsom-Davis, J. 1977. Circulating anti-acetylcholine receptor antibody in myasthenia gravis treated by plasma exchange. Neurology 27:364.

Walker, M. B. 1934. Treatment of myasthenia gravis with physostigmine. Lancet 1:1200–1201.

Lewis P. Rowland

Diseases of the Motor Unit

**The Motor Unit Includes the Neuron,
Peripheral Nerve, and Muscle Cell**

**Neurogenic and Myopathic Diseases Are
Distinguished by Clinical and Laboratory Criteria**
Clinical Criteria Help to Identify Neurogenic
and Myopathic Conditions
Laboratory Criteria

Diseases of Motor Neurons Are Acute or Chronic
Motor Neuron Diseases Do Not
Affect Sensory Neurons
Motor Neuron Disease Is Characterized by
Fasciculation and Fibrillation

**Diseases of Peripheral Nerves Are Also Acute
or Chronic**
Neuropathies Can Have Positive or
Negative Symptoms
Demyelination Leads to a Slowing of
Conduction Velocity

**Diseases of Skeletal Muscle Can Be Inherited
or Acquired**
Muscular Dystrophies Are the Most Common
Inherited Myopathies
Dermatomyositis Is an Acquired Myopathy
Weakness in Myopathies Need Not Be Due to
Loss of Muscle Fibers

**Molecular Genetics Illuminates the Physiology
and Pathology of Duchenne Muscular Dystrophy**

An Overall View

T he motor neuron in the ventral horn of the spinal cord plays an essential role in the mediation of voluntary motor commands and reflexes that underlie all motor behaviors. In 1925 Edward Liddell and Charles Sherrington introduced the term *motor unit* to designate the basic unit of motor function—a motor neuron and the group of muscle fibers it innervates. The experimental analysis of disorders of the motor unit advanced in 1929 when Edgar Adrian and Detlev Bronk developed a technique for recording the action potentials from single motor units in human muscles. This method established the discipline of electromyography, which now has a prominent role in the clinical diagnosis of diseases of the motor unit. These physiological approaches have been supplemented by molecular genetic analysis of disorders of the motor unit. By combining physiological and molecular methods, we now have obtained a detailed understanding of some diseases of the motor unit.

In this chapter we consider disorders that affect the cell body and axon of the motor neuron and the muscle cell. In addition we describe the impact of molecular genetics in characterizing the gene that underlies X-linked muscular dystrophies.

The Motor Unit Includes the Neuron, Peripheral Nerve, and Muscle Cell

The motor unit has four functional components: the cell body of the motor neuron, the axon of the motor neuron that runs in the peripheral nerve, the neuromuscular junction, and the muscle fibers innervated by that neuron. The number of muscle fibers innervated by a single motor neuron varies greatly depending on the function of the particular muscles. In muscles that control fine movements—for example, those of the ocular muscles or the small muscles of the hand—motor units consist of only three to six muscle fibers. In contrast, there are about 2000 muscle fibers in each motor unit of the gastrocnemius, the calf muscle that flexes the foot in the movements of walking. Motor units of other muscles, such as the trapezius, a back muscle used in postural control, also have large numbers of muscle fibers. Contraction of muscle is the final expression or output of the motor system. Variations in the range, force, or type of movement are determined by the pattern of recruitment and the frequency of firing of different motor units. The motor unit can therefore be considered the elementary unit of function in the motor system.

Most diseases of the motor unit cause weakness and wasting of skeletal muscles. The distinguishing features of these diseases depend upon which of the four components of the motor unit is primarily affected. As we saw in the last chapter, distinctions among diseases were originally established at postmortem examination. When pathologists in the nineteenth century studied patients who had died from diseases characterized by progressive weakness and wasting of limb muscles, they found different morphological changes in patients with different symptoms or signs. Some patients had pronounced changes in the nerve cell bodies or peripheral nerves but only minor changes in muscle fibers. These *neurogenic* diseases, or *neuropathies*, were subdivided into those that primarily affected the nerve cell bodies (*motor neuron diseases*) and those that primarily affected the peripheral axons (*peripheral neuropathies*). Other patients had advanced degeneration of muscles, with little change in motor neurons or their axons; these diseases were called *myopathic* diseases, or *myopathies*.

These pathological findings demonstrate two important features of neurological disease. First, disease can be functionally selective; some diseases affect only sensory systems, others only motor systems. Second, a disease may be regionally selective, affecting only one part of the neuron (for example, the axon rather than the cell body). Thus, the functional distinctions among the different components of the neuron have important clinical implications.

Neurogenic and Myopathic Diseases Are Distinguished by Clinical and Laboratory Criteria

When a peripheral nerve is cut, the muscles innervated by that nerve immediately become paralyzed and then waste progressively; tendon reflexes are lost immediately. Because the nerve carries sensory as well as motor fibers, sensation in the area innervated by the nerve is also lost. In neurogenic diseases the effects of denervation are similar but appear more slowly; that is, the muscles gradually become weak and wasted. The term *atrophy* (literally, lack of nourishment) refers to the wasting away of a once-normal muscle, and by historical accident appears in the names of several diseases that are thought to be neurogenic. Therefore, in describing the appearance of a patient's muscles, it is best to use the term wasting in general and the term atrophic only when the condition is known to be neurogenic.

Although muscle also becomes dysfunctional in myo-

pathic diseases, there is no evidence that the muscle is actually denervated. The main symptoms are due to weakness of skeletal muscle and often include difficulty in walking or lifting. Other, less common symptoms include an inability to relax (*myotonia*), cramps, pain (*myalgia*), or the appearance in the urine of the heme-containing protein that colors the muscle red (*myoglobinuria*). The *muscular dystrophies* are a group of hereditary myopathies with special characteristics: All symptoms are due to weakness, the weakness becomes progressively more severe, and degeneration and regeneration can be seen histologically.

Because both neurogenic and myopathic diseases are characterized by weakness of muscle, differential diagnosis may be difficult. Classification and diagnosis of these diseases involve both clinical and laboratory criteria.

Clinical Criteria Help to Identify Neurogenic and Myopathic Conditions

In general neurogenic and myopathic disorders tend to cause weakness in different areas of the limb: distal limb weakness indicates a neurogenic disorder, proximal limb weakness a myopathic dysfunction. But, because there are many exceptions to this generalization, location of weakness cannot be regarded as a reliable differential sign. Other signs, such as fasciculations and fibrillations, are highly reliable because they are found only in neurogenic diseases. *Fasciculations* are visible twitches of muscle that can be seen as ripples under the skin. They occur within a single motor unit and result from involuntary but synchronous contractions of the muscle fibers innervated by the same motor neuron. For reasons that are not clear, fasciculations are characteristic of slowly progressive diseases of the motor neuron itself and are rarely seen in peripheral neuropathies. *Fibrillations*, on the other hand, arise from spontaneous activity within single muscle fibers. They are not visible clinically and can be recognized only by electromyography.

Overactive tendon reflexes are evidence of disease of upper motor neurons, while weak, wasted, and twitching muscles are evidence of disease of the lower motor neuron.[1] The concurrence of these apparently incompati-

---

[1]For diagnostic purposes, clinicians have found it useful to use the terms lower and upper motor neurons. *Lower motor neurons* refer to primary motor neurons of the spinal cord and brain stem that directly innervate skeletal muscles. *Upper motor neurons* refer to neurons that originate in higher regions of the brain, such as the motor cortex, and which synapse on the lower motor neurons to convey descending commands for movement. Strictly speaking, upper motor neurons are not motor but *premotor* neurons. However, as we shall learn in Chapter 35, since they affect motor output in such a fundamental way, their functional properties are often considered together with primary motor neurons in the spinal cord. Axons of upper motor neurons make up the corticospinal (pyramidal) tract. The distinction between lower and upper motor neurons continues to be important clinically because diseases involving either class of neurons produce distinctive symptoms. Disorders of lower motor neurons result in atrophy, fasciculations and fibrillations, decreased muscle tone, and loss of tendon reflexes. Disorders of upper motor neurons and their axons result in spasticity, overactive tendon reflexes, and abnormal extensor reflexes (Babinski signs).

ble signs in the same limb is virtually diagnostic of *amyotrophic lateral sclerosis* (Lou Gehrig's disease), a condition that involves both the upper and the lower motor neurons, as we shall discuss below. When the sole manifestation of a disease is limb weakness, as often happens, clinical criteria alone rarely suffice to distinguish between neurogenic and myopathic diseases. To assist in this differentiation, clinicians rely upon several laboratory tests: measurement of serum enzyme activity, electromyography and nerve conduction studies, and muscle biopsy.

Laboratory Criteria

Measurement of serum enzyme activities is one test that helps to distinguish myopathic from neurogenic diseases. The sarcoplasm of muscle is rich in soluble enzymes that are also found in low concentrations in the serum. In many muscle diseases the concentration of these sarcoplasmic enzymes in serum is elevated, presumably because the diseases affect the integrity of surface membranes of the muscle that ordinarily retain soluble enzymes within the sarcoplasm. Slight increases in the serum levels of these enzymes are also found in some denervating diseases, but the increase is usually much less than in a myopathy. The enzyme activity most commonly measured for diagnosing myopathy is creatine kinase (CK), an enzyme that phosphorylates creatine and is important in the energy metabolism of muscle; assays for serum glutamic oxaloacetic transaminase (SGOT) and lactate dehydrogenase (LDH) are also used.

Some abnormalities can be diagnosed by *electromyography*, a routine clinical procedure in which a small needle is inserted into a muscle to record the electrical activity of several neighboring motor units. Three specific measurements are important: spontaneous activity at rest, the number of motor units under voluntary control, and the duration and amplitude of each motor unit potential (Figure 17–1). Each unit gives rise to an all-or-none potential. Normally, there is no activity in a resting muscle outside the end-plate. During a weak voluntary contraction a series of motor unit potentials is recorded as different motor units are recruited. In fully active normal muscles, these potentials overlap in an interference pattern so that it is impossible to identify single potentials. Normal values have been established for the amplitude and duration of these unit potentials. The amplitude of the unit potential is determined by the number of muscle fibers within the motor unit.

In neurogenic disease, the denervated muscle is spontaneously active even at rest. The muscle may still contract in response to voluntary motor commands but, because some motor axons have been lost, fewer motor units are under voluntary control. This loss of motor units is evident in the electromyographic records, which show a discrete pattern of motor unit potentials instead of the profuse interference pattern seen in normal muscles (Figure 17–2). The amplitude and duration of individual synaptic potentials may increase, presumably because the remaining axons give off small branches that innervate the

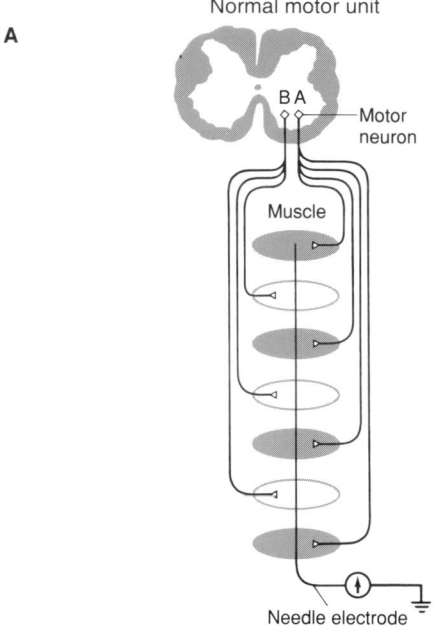

A

Normal motor unit

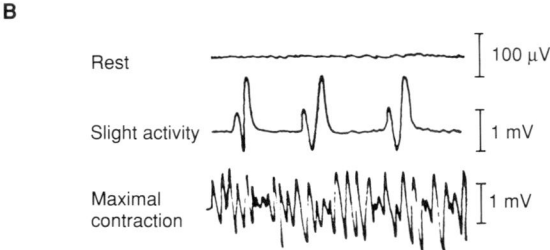

B

FIGURE 17–1

The motor unit consists of a single motor neuron and the population of muscle fibers it innervates.

A. The muscle fibers innervated by a single motor neuron are not usually adjacent to one another. When the neuron fires, a needle electrode inserted into the muscle records an all-or-none unit potential because the highly effective transmission at the neuromuscular junction ensures that each muscle fiber will contract in response to an action potential.

B. Examples of electromyogram traces of recordings from normal muscle at rest, during slight activity, and under conditions of maximal contraction.

muscle fibers denervated by the loss of other axons so that surviving units contain more than the normal number of muscle fibers.

In contrast, in myopathic diseases there is no activity in the muscle at rest and no change in the number of units firing during a contraction. But because there are fewer surviving muscle fibers in each motor unit, the motor unit potentials are smaller and of shorter duration (Figure 17–3).

Electrical stimulation and recording can also be used to measure the conduction velocities of peripheral motor axons. The conduction velocity of the motor axons is slowed in *demyelinating neuropathies*, as we shall see later, but is normal in neuropathies without demyelination (*axonal neuropathies*).

Motor neuron disease

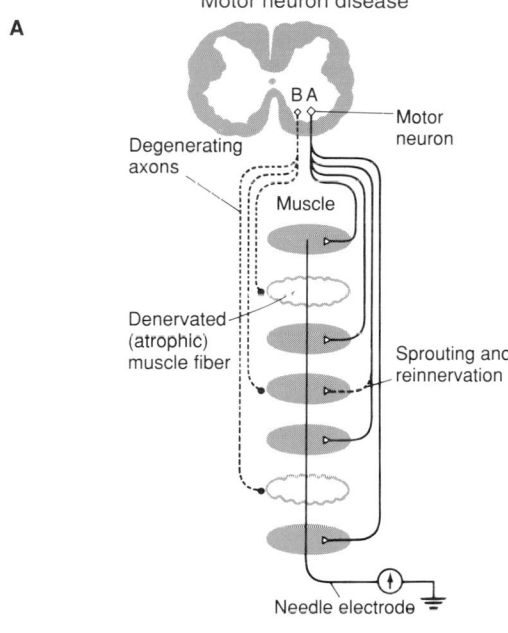

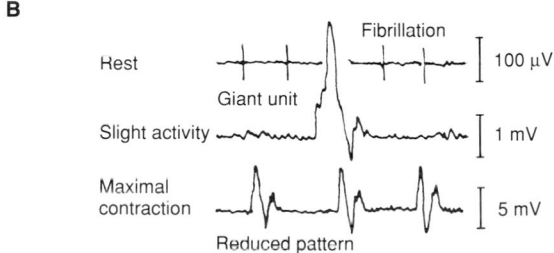

FIGURE 17–2

When motor neurons are diseased, the number of motor units under voluntary control is reduced, but individual unit synaptic potentials increase because the surviving nerve fibers sprout and reinnervate denervated muscle fibers.

A. Muscle fibers supplied by the degenerating motor neuron (**cell B**) are becoming denervated and atrophic; thus, this motor unit no longer produces unit potentials. However, the surviving neuron (**cell A**) has sprouted an axonal branch that has reinnervated one of the denervated muscle fibers.

B. Because the surviving motor neuron innervates more than the usual number of muscle fibers, it produces a unit synaptic potential that is larger than normal (**middle trace**). In addition, axons of the surviving motor unit fire spontaneously even at rest, giving rise to fasciculations (**top trace**), another characteristic of motor neuron disease. Under conditions of maximal contraction the amplitudes of the electromyogram spikes are reduced (**lower trace**).

Finally, muscle can be biopsied and the muscle fibers examined histologically. Two types of muscle fibers can be distinguished histochemically. One type corresponds to the fast-twitch (type I) fibers; the predominant metabolic enzymes present in these muscle fibers are those of anaerobic (glycolytic) metabolism. The other type corresponds to the red slow-twitch (type II) fibers, which rely primarily on oxidative metabolism. Although this distinc-

Muscle disease

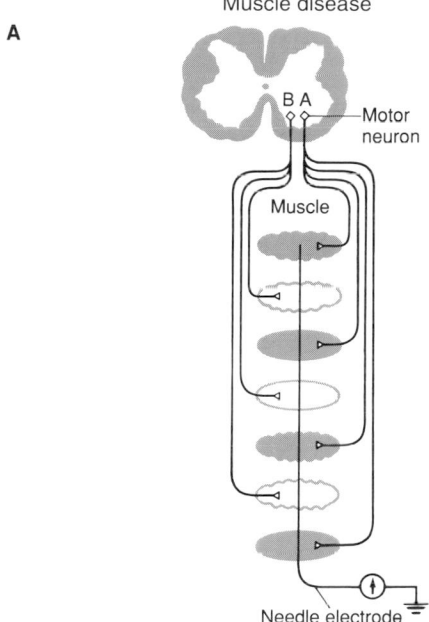

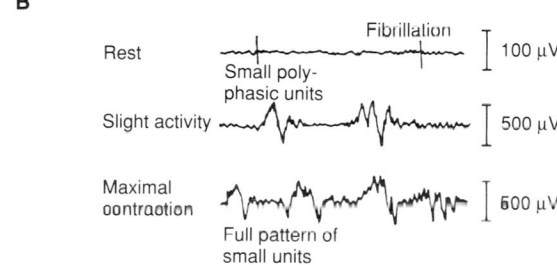

FIGURE 17–3

When muscle is diseased the number of muscle fibers in each motor unit is reduced, and thus the individual unit synaptic potentials are smaller.

A. Some muscle fibers innervated by the two motor neurons have shrunk and become nonfunctional.

B. The unit synaptic potentials have not decreased in number, but they are smaller and briefer than normal.

tion is probably an oversimplification and there may be subtypes within these major classes, the biochemical differences can be demonstrated vividly by histochemical stains for specific enzymes of either class.

Prolonged stimulation of a single motor axon in a ventral root depletes the enzyme substrate in the muscle fibers of that motor unit, as demonstrated by appropriate histochemical stains. Experiments of this kind indicate that all of the muscle fibers innervated by a single motor neuron are of the same histochemical type. However, the muscle fibers of one motor unit do not lie side by side; instead, they are interspersed among the muscle fibers of other motor units. This is easily shown in a cross section of normal muscle; when an enzyme stain selective for only one type is used, the cross section will show stained

FIGURE 17-4

Because the motor neuron determines the histochemical properties of the muscle it innervates, muscle histochemistry helps to distinguish neurogenic and myopathic diseases. (Courtesy of A. P. Hays.)

A. In this gastrocnemius muscle from a normal adult the two types of muscle fibers (types I and II) are roughly equal in number and seem to be distributed in a random fashion. (Myofibrillar [myosin] ATPase, preincubation at pH 9.4, × 100.)

B. In this gastrocnemius muscle from a patient with a chronic sensorimotor polyneuropathy the two types of muscle fibers are more distinctly separated. Neighboring muscle fibers have assumed uniform histochemical and physiological properties because axon sprouts from surviving motor units have innervated the denervated muscle fibers. (Myofibrillar ATPase, preincubation at pH 9.4, × 100.)

C. In this gastrocnemius muscle from another patient with a chronic sensorimotor polyneuropathy a large concentrated group of muscle fibers has atrophied **(center)** and is surrounded by fibers that are normal in size or hypertrophied. This so-called group atrophy of fibers is characteristic of disorders of lower motor neurons. (Modified Gomori trichrome, × 60.)

D. In this vastus lateralis muscle from a 4-year-old boy with Duchenne muscular dystrophy the focal character of the damage to muscle fibers is evident in the hypercontracted (hyaline) fibers **(large arrows)** and necrotic fibers **(small arrows)**. The **arrowheads** indicate muscle fibers with cytological signs of regeneration. (Modified Gomori trichrome, × 60.)

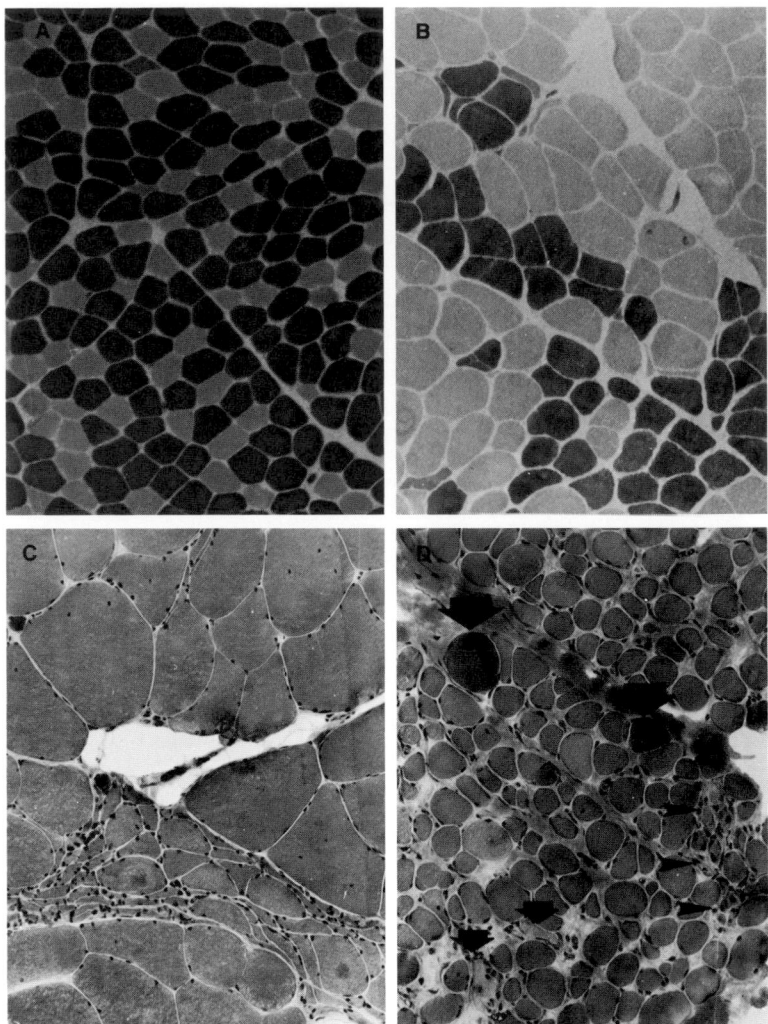

and unstained fiber types alternating in an irregular pattern (Figure 17-4A).

In chronic neurogenic diseases the muscle innervated by a dying motor neuron becomes atrophic and some muscle fibers disappear. Axons of surviving neurons tend to sprout and innervate some of the remaining muscle fibers that are denervated when neurons die. Because the motor neuron determines the histochemical type, the reinnervated fibers assume the histochemical properties of the neuron. As a result, instead of a normal checkerboard pattern, the fibers of a muscle in neurogenic disease become clustered by type (a pattern called *fiber-type grouping*) (Figure 17-4B). If the disease is progressive and the neurons in the surviving motor units also become affected, atrophy occurs in groups of adjacent muscle fibers belonging to the same histochemical type, a process called *group atrophy* (Figure 17-4C).

In myopathic diseases, the muscle fibers are affected in a more or less random fashion. Sometimes an inflammatory cellular response is evident and sometimes there is prominent infiltration of the muscle by fat and connective tissue (Figure 17-4D).

The main clinical and laboratory features that serve in the differential diagnosis of diseases of the motor unit are listed in Table 17-1. Some of the major diseases that affect the motor neuron, motor axons, or muscle are listed in Table 17-2. We shall consider each of them in turn.

Diseases of Motor Neurons Are Acute or Chronic

Motor Neuron Diseases Do Not Affect Sensory Neurons

The best-known disorder of motor neurons is amyotrophic lateral sclerosis, also called Lou Gehrig's disease. *Amyotrophy* is another word for neurogenic atrophy of muscle. *Lateral sclerosis* refers to the hardness felt when the spinal cord is examined at autopsy. This hardness is due to the proliferation of astrocytes and scarring of the lateral columns of the spinal cord. Scarring is caused by disease of the corticospinal tracts, which carry the axons of premotor cells (the upper motor neurons) from the cortex and

TABLE 17–1. Differential Diagnosis of Neurogenic and Myopathic Diseases

Finding	Neurogenic	Myopathic
Clinical finding:		
Weakness	+	+
Wasting	+	+
Loss of reflexes	+	+
Fasciculations	+ (ALS)	0
Sensory loss	+ (PN)	0
Hyperreflexia, Babinski sign	+ (ALS)	0
Laboratory finding:		
Cerebrospinal fluid protein increased	+ (PN)	0
Slow nerve conduction velocity	+ (PN)	0
Electromyography		
Duration of potentials	Increased	Decreased
Fibrillation, fasciculation	+	0
Number of potentials	Decreased	Normal
Serum enzymes increased	±	+ + + +
Muscle biopsy	Group atrophy, fiber-type grouping	Necrosis and regeneration

Abbreviations: ALS, amyotrophic lateral sclerosis; PN, peripheral neuropathy; +, present; 0, absent; + + + +, marked change; ± slight change.

brain stem to the spinal cord. Although both the upper motor neurons in the cortex and the lower motor neurons in the brain stem and spinal cord degenerate progressively, some motor neurons are spared, notably those supplying ocular muscles and those involved in voluntary control of bladder sphincters. The cause of the disease is not known and there is no effective treatment for this uniformly fatal condition.

Symptoms usually start with painless weakness of the arms or legs. Typically, the patient, often a man in his 60s, discovers that he has become awkward in executing fine movements of the hands: typing, playing the piano, playing baseball, fingering coins, or working with tools. This weakness is associated with wasting of the small muscles of the hands and feet and fasciculations of the muscles of the forearm and upper arm. These signs of lower motor neuron disease are often paradoxically associated with *hyperreflexia*, an increase in tendon reflexes that is characteristic of upper motor neuron disease. Sensation is always normal. The condition is inexorably progressive and may ultimately affect muscles of respiration. There is no effective treatment for this uniformly fatal condition.

There are other variants of motor neuron disease. Sometimes the first symptoms are restricted to muscles innervated by cranial nerves, with resulting *dysarthria* (difficulty speaking) and *dysphagia* (difficulty swallowing). When cranial symptoms occur alone, the syndrome is called *progressive bulbar palsy* (the term *bulb* is used interchangeably with *medulla*, and *palsy* means weakness). If only lower motor neurons are involved, the syndrome is called *spinal muscular atrophy*. Spinal muscular atrophy is characterized by weakness, wasting, loss of reflexes, and fasciculation. Although hyperreflexia and other signs of disease of the upper motor neuron are lacking, autopsy usually reveals some demyelination in the corticospinal tracts. Thus, spinal muscular atrophy in adults is probably the same disease as amyotrophic lateral sclerosis. Presumably, the degeneration of the lower motor neurons in spinal muscular atrophy obscures clinical expression of upper motor neuron signs. (If the extensor of the great toe is paralyzed, it is impossible to elicit the abnormal extensor reflex of Babinski. Similarly, if tendon reflexes have been lost in spinal muscular atrophy, there cannot be hyperreflexia.)

TABLE 17–2. Examples of Neurogenic and Myopathic Diseases

Neurogenic		Myopathic	
Motor neuron	Peripheral nerve	Inherited	Acquired
Amyotrophic lateral sclerosis	Guillain-Barre syndrome	Duchenne dystrophy	Dermatomyositis
		Facioscapulohumeral dystrophy	Polymyositis syndrome
	Chronic peripheral neuropathy	Limb-girdle dystrophy	Endocrine myopathies
		Myotonic dystrophy	Myoglobinurias

Amyotrophic lateral sclerosis and its variants are restricted to motor neurons; they do not affect sensory neurons or autonomic neurons. The acute viral disease poliomyelitis is also confined to motor neurons. These diseases illustrate dramatically the individuality of nerve cells and the principle of *selective vulnerability*. Although the basis of this selectivity is not understood, one possible explanation is that protein receptor molecules in the membrane of motor neurons are recognized by specific *neurotropic viruses* (viruses that attack the nervous system). For example, the receptor for poliovirus is now known to be a surface membrane protein that is a member of the immunoglobulin superfamily of adhesion and recognition molecules, which are discussed in Chapter 58.

Motor Neuron Disease Is Characterized by Fasciculation and Fibrillation

Diseases of the motor neuron lead to two types of spontaneous activity in muscle: fasciculation and fibrillation. The cause of fasciculation is not known. The electromyographic counterpart of a visible twitch is a compound motor unit potential, and these electrical changes may also be seen in disorders of nerve roots or peripheral nerves. In all of these conditions the electrical activity may persist after a nerve block produced by injection of a local anesthetic or even after cutting the nerve. Since a nerve block eliminates all activity that originates central to the site of injection (the spinal cord, dorsal and ventral roots, and proximal nerve), continued spontaneous muscle activity must arise distal to the block—in the remote axon just before it branches, in the terminals, or at the neuromuscular junction. Acetylcholine is thought to be involved in fasciculations because the activity can be abolished by *d*-tubocurarine and because neostigmine (an inhibitor of cholinesterase) can induce fasciculation in a normal mammalian nerve–muscle preparation.

Whereas fasciculations involve activation of one or more motor units and therefore produce visible twitching of the skin, fibrillations result from the discharge of a single muscle fiber, and are too small to be seen as movement through the skin; thus, fibrillations are detectable only by electromyography. In some circumstances fibrillations are thought to be due to the insertion of new voltage-dependent Na^+ and Ca^{2+} channels into the plasma membranes of denervated muscle fibers. These new channels make the fiber spontaneously active, much like the action of pacemaker cells of the heart. The appearance of new voltage-gated channels cannot be the entire explanation, however, because fibrillations are increased by intraarterial injection of ACh or epinephrine, suggesting that there may also be transmitter-gated channel systems involved.

Diseases of Peripheral Nerves Are Also Acute or Chronic

Because motor and sensory axons run in the same nerves, disorders of peripheral nerves (neuropathies) usually affect both motor and sensory functions. Some patients with peripheral neuropathy report abnormal, frequently unpleasant, sensory experiences, similar to that felt after local anesthesia for dental work; these sensations are variously called *numbness*, *pins-and-needles*, or *tingling*. When these sensations occur spontaneously without an external sensory stimulus, they are called *paresthesias*. Patients may be unable to discriminate between hot and cold. Lack of pain perception may lead to injuries. Patients with paresthesias usually have impaired perception of cutaneous sensations (pain and temperature) because the small myelinated fibers that carry these sensations are selectively affected; the sense of touch may or may not be involved. Proprioceptive sensations (position and vibration) may be lost without loss of cutaneous sensation. The sensory disorders are always more prominent distally (called a *glove-and-stocking pattern*), possibly because the distal portions of the nerves are most remote from the cell body and therefore most susceptible to disorders that interfere with axonal transport of essential metabolites and proteins.

The motor disorder of peripheral neuropathy is first manifested by weakness, which may be predominantly proximal in acute cases and is usually distal in chronic disorders. Tendon reflexes are usually depressed or lost. Fasciculation is only rarely seen, and wasting does not ensue unless the weakness has been present for many weeks. The protein content of the cerebrospinal fluid is often increased, presumably because the permeability of the nerve roots within the subarachnoid space of the spinal cord is altered.

Neuropathies may be either acute or chronic. The best-known acute neuropathy is the Guillain-Barre syndrome, which achieved notoriety in 1976 when many cases seemed to follow vaccination against the swine influenza virus. Most cases, however, follow respiratory infection or occur without preceding illness. This condition may be mild, or it may be so severe that mechanical ventilation is required. Cranial nerves may also be affected, leading to paralysis of ocular, facial, and oropharyngeal muscles. The disorder is believed to be due to an autoimmune attack on peripheral nerves by circulating antibodies. It is therefore often treated with plasmapheresis. Even when the condition is life-threatening, some improvement occurs in every survivor, and, no matter how severe the original state, return to normal function often is possible. Many patients are left with some disability, however.

The chronic neuropathies also vary from the mildest manifestations to incapacitating or even fatal conditions, and there are many varieties, including genetic diseases (acute intermittent porphyria, Charcot-Marie-Tooth disease), metabolic disorders (diabetes, B_{12} deficiency), intoxications (lead), nutritional disorders (alcoholism, thiamine deficiency), carcinomas (especially carcinoma of the lung), and immunological disorders (plasma cell diseases, amyloidosis). Some chronic disorders, such as the neuropathy of B_{12} deficiency in pernicious anemia, are amenable to therapy.

In addition to being acute or chronic, neuropathies may be categorized as *demyelinating* or *axonal*. Demyelinating neuropathies are probably more common. As might be expected from the role of the myelin sheath in saltatory conduction, the velocity of conduction is slow in axons that have lost myelin. In axonal neuropathies, the myelin sheath is not affected and conduction velocity is normal.

Neuropathies Can Have Positive or Negative Symptoms

Axonal and demyelinating neuropathies may lead to positive or negative symptoms. The positive symptoms of peripheral neuropathies consist of paresthesias that are attributed to abnormal impulse activity in sensory fibers. These paresthesias may arise from spontaneous activity of injured nerve fibers or from electrical interaction (cross-talk) between abnormal axons, a process called *ephaptic transmission* to distinguish it from normal synaptic transmission between axons. For reasons that are not known, damaged nerves also become *hyperexcitable*. This is evident in the Tinel sign, named after a French neurologist who studied nerve injuries in World War I. Tinel found that lightly tapping the site of injury evoked a burst of unpleasant sensations in the region over which the nerve is distributed. This sign is useful both for showing peripheral nerve damage and also for pinpointing the site of the lesion. The negative symptoms consist of weakness or paralysis, loss of tendon reflexes, and impaired sensation, resulting from damage to motor axons.

Demyelination Leads to a Slowing of Conduction Velocity

Negative symptoms have been studied most thoroughly in demyelinating neuropathy and can be attributed to three basic mechanisms: conduction block, slowed conduction, and impaired ability to conduct impulses at higher frequencies.

Conduction block was first recognized in 1876 by the German neurologist Wilhelm Erb, one of the first clinicians to study human nerves with electrical methods. Erb observed that stimulation of an injured peripheral nerve *below* the site of injury evoked muscular response, whereas stimulation *above* the site of injury produced no response. He concluded that the lesion blocked impulses of central origin, even when the segment of the nerve distal to the lesion was functional. Later experimental studies illustrated that diphtheria and other toxins produce conduction block by causing demyelination at the site of application.

Why does demyelination produce nerve block and how does it lead to slowing of conduction velocity? As discussed in Chapter 7, conduction velocity is much more rapid in myelinated fibers than in unmyelinated axons for two reasons. First, the axons of myelinated fibers tend to be larger in diameter, and there is a direct relationship between conduction velocity and axon diameter. Second, in myelinated axons the action potential propagates discontinuously from one node of Ranvier to the next (Figure 17–5A). The continuous propagation that occurs in unmyelinated axons is much slower than saltatory conduction.

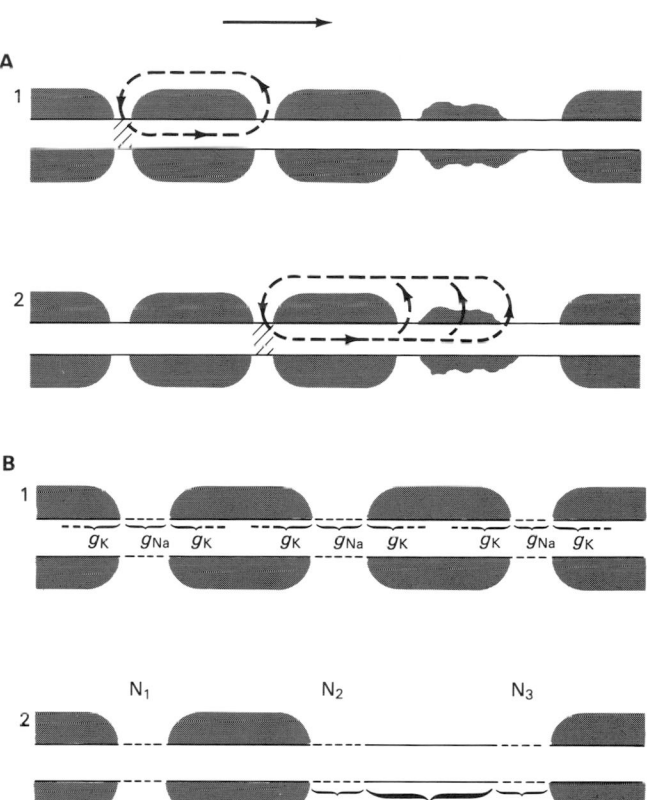

FIGURE 17–5

Conduction along demyelinated nerve fibers is impaired.

A. The demyelinated region of a nerve fiber does not conduct an impulse as well as the normal, myelinated region. The **solid arrow** indicates the direction of impulse conduction; the **hatched area** indicates the region occupied by the impulse. Current flow is indicated by the **broken line**. 1. In normal, myelinated regions the high resistance and low capacitance of the myelin shunts the majority of current to the next node of Ranvier. 2. In a demyelinated region current is lost through the damaged myelin sheath. (From Waxman, 1982.)

B. The densities of Na^+ channels and K^+ channels differ in the myelinated and demyelinated regions of the axons. 1. Sodium channels (g_{Na}) are dense at the node of Ranvier but sparse or absent in the internodal regions of the axon membrane. The K^+ channels (g_K) are located beneath the myelin sheath in internodal regions. 2. The conduction properties of the nodal regions of the axon membrane (**broken lines**) and the internodal regions (**solid lines**) are therefore different.

When demyelination along the axon is disrupted by disease, the action potentials in different axons of the nerve begin to conduct at slightly different velocities, and the nerve loses its normal synchrony of conduction. Figure 17–6 shows the arrangement for measuring conduction velocities in peripheral nerves. This slowing and the temporal dispersion are thought to account for some of the early clinical signs of neuropathy. For example, functions that normally depend upon the arrival of synchronous bursts of neural activity, such as tendon reflexes and vibratory sensation, are lost soon after the onset of a

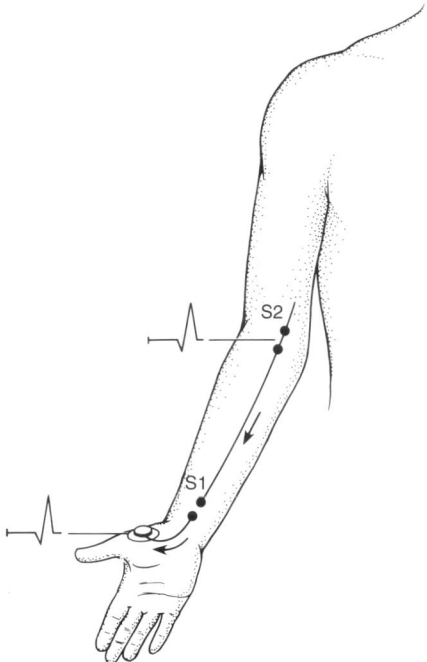

FIGURE 17–6
Motor nerve conduction velocity can be determined by recording action potentials with transcutaneous or surface electrodes along the pathway of the motor nerve. The time from S2 to the muscle is the proximal latency; the time from S1 to the muscle is the distal latency. The time S2 − S1 is divided into the distance between S1 and S2 to give the conduction velocity.

Diseases of Skeletal Muscle Can Be Inherited or Acquired

Skeletal muscle diseases are conveniently divided into those that are inherited and those that appear to be acquired.

Muscular Dystrophies Are the Most Common Inherited Myopathies

The best known inherited diseases are the *muscular dystrophies*, of which there are four major types based on clinical and genetic patterns (Table 17–3). Two types are characterized by weakness alone: the Duchenne and facioscapulohumeral dystrophies. The Duchenne type starts in the legs, affects males only (because it is transmitted as an X-linked recessive trait), and progresses relatively rapidly, so that patients are in wheelchairs by age 12 and usually die in their third decade. The facioscapulohumeral type is autosomal dominant, affects both sexes equally, starts later (usually in adolescence), affects the shoulder girdle and face early, and may be much milder, resulting in an almost normal life span. These clinical and genetic differences imply different biochemical abnormalities, which have not been identified. As discussed below, Duchenne dystrophy results from a genetic defect in a membrane-associated muscle protein.

A third type of inherited muscular dystrophy also causes weakness but has an additional and characteristic feature, *myotonia* and is therefore called myotonic muscular dystrophy. Myotonia is manifest as a delayed relaxation of muscle after vigorous voluntary contraction, percussion, or electrical stimulation. The delayed relaxation is caused by repetitive firing of muscle action potentials and is independent of nerve supply because it persists after nerve block or curarization. The mutant gene responsible has been localized to the central region of chromosome 19, but the biochemical consequence of this mutation is not known. In addition to myotonia, the dystrophy has other special characteristics: it involves cranial muscles, and the limb weakness is primarily distal rather than proximal. The symptoms are not confined to muscles; for instance, cataracts are found in almost all patients, and testicular atrophy and baldness are common in

chronic neuropathy. Although the average conduction velocity may be reduced only slightly in the early stage of neuropathy, the fact that the individual axons no longer fire synchronously leads in itself to clinical symptoms. As demyelination becomes more severe, conduction becomes blocked. This block may be either *intermittent*, occurring only at high frequencies of activity, or *complete*. Block of conduction in the largest and fastest fibers of a nerve could also contribute to *overall* slowing of the average conduction velocity in nerves that contain axons with a variety of diameters (mixed sensory and motor fibers).

TABLE 17–3. Major Forms of Muscular Dystrophy

Features	Duchenne	Facioscapulohumeral	Myotonic	Limb-girdle
Sex	Male	Both	Both	Both
Onset	Before age 5	Adolescence	Infancy or adolescence	Adolescence
Initial symptoms	Pelvic	Shoulder-girdle	Hands or feet	Either
Face involved	No	Always	Often	No
Pseudohypertrophy	80%	No	No	Rare
Progression	Rapid	Slow	Slow	Slow
Inheritance	X-linked recessive	Autosomal dominant	Autosomal dominant	Autosomal recessive
Serum enzymes	Very high	Normal	Normal	Slight increase
Myotonia	No	No	Yes	No

affected men. Like most dominant diseases, myotonic dystrophy may be so mild that the patient is literally asymptomatic, or so severe that disability occurs at an early age.

Forms of inherited muscular dystrophy that do not fit these three major types are lumped into a fourth group, *limb-girdle dystrophy*. This category certainly includes more than one type because affected families differ in the extent of limb weakness, age at onset, and patterns of inheritance.

Dermatomyositis Is an Acquired Myopathy

The prototype of an acquired myopathy is *dermatomyositis*, defined by two clinical features: rash and myopathy. The rash has a predilection for the face, chest, and extensor surfaces of joints, including the fingers. The myopathic weakness primarily affects proximal limb muscles. Both rash and weakness usually appear simultaneously and become worse in a matter of weeks. The weakness may be mild or life-threatening, and the disorder affects children or adults. The cause is not known, but about 10% of adult patients have malignant tumors. Although the pathogenesis is also not known, the fact that some lymphocytes can infiltrate muscle suggests a cell-mediated autoimmune disorder.

Weakness in Myopathies Need Not Be Due to Loss of Muscle Fibers

The weakness seen in any myopathy is attributed to degeneration of muscle fibers. At first the missing fibers are replaced by the regeneration of new fibers. Ultimately, however, renewal cannot keep pace and fibers are lost progressively. This leads to the appearance of compound motor unit potentials of brief duration and reduced amplitude. The decreased number of functioning muscle fibers would then account for the diminished strength. There may also be other contributing factors. For instance, in one form of inherited myopathy, the *glycogen storage diseases*, which are due to a lack of phosphorylase or phosphofructokinase, large amounts of glycogen accumulate within the cells because glycogen breakdown is blocked. Glycogen accumulation disrupts the normal architecture of many muscle fibers, as seen by light microscopy; at the ultrastructural level there is major distortion of the myofilaments.

Despite these severe physical changes, however, the patient may have no symptoms of weakness. Thus, physical damage to muscles does not invariably lead to weakness. Muscle weakness in some myopathies may therefore be due to a biochemical or physiological abnormality in the remaining fibers instead of, or in addition to, loss of muscle fibers.

Molecular Genetics Illuminates the Physiology and Pathology of Duchenne Muscular Dystrophy

In 1987, the techniques of recombinant DNA cloning pro-

vided the first identification of genes responsible for two human diseases, Duchenne muscular dystrophy and chronic granulomatous disease, a disease of polymorphonuclear white blood cells. Both advances came from the search for the gene involved in Duchenne muscular dystrophy. Before 1987 there were few clues to the nature of Duchenne dystrophy. For a variety of reasons it seemed that the primary problem was in the muscle cell. Even that was not certain, however, and there were alternative theories—that the muscle damage was secondary to a disorder of the nerve cell or to a metabolic problem in the liver.

The disease was recognized as being X-linked because the gene seemed to be carried by women but symptoms appeared only in boys. Moreover, the serum level of sarcoplasmic enzymes (such as creatine kinase) was very high, an observation that was the basis of the *membrane* theory of the disease. According to this theory, the normal function of the surface membranes (sarcolemma) was distorted, allowing enzyme molecules to escape into the plasma and somehow causing the weakness.

In the early 1980s a myopathy similar to Duchenne dystrophy was recognized in young girls with translocations in the second band on the short arm of the X chromosome that move the dislocated distal fragment to an autosome. In all cases, the breakpoint involved the band called Xp21. (The symbol for the short arm of a chromosome is p; the long arm, q.) That pattern implicated Xp21 as a likely site of the gene for Duchenne dystrophy.

It is possible to identify the genes responsible for human diseases using techniques for mapping DNA polymorphisms called *restriction fragment length polymorphisms* (Box 17–1). Kay Davies and her colleagues used this approach in an attempt to identify the gene for Duchenne muscular dystrophy and found restriction fragment length polymorphisms that were linked to clinical manifestations of the disease and which seemed to flank the Xp region of chromosome 21. To find probes that would be even closer to the Duchenne gene, Ronald Worton used the breakpoint for one of the translocations that involved Xp21.

A major breakthrough came when Uta Francke and her colleagues identified a large deletion of the region around Xp21 in a patient with five different X-linked conditions—Duchenne dystrophy, retinitis pigmentosa, mental retardation, an unusual abnormality of blood groups called the McLeod syndrome, and chronic granulomatous disease. Louis Kunkel, Anthony Monaco, and their associates reasoned that the missing area of the X chromosome must contain the Duchenne gene. By the end of 1987, probes had been used to identify deletions of that area in the DNA of boys with Duchenne dystrophy, reinforcing the view that this region of DNA contained the gene for the disease. At the same time, the probes were used to identify and then clone the entire gene. The results provided new information about the human genome, about human genetics, and also about Duchenne dystrophy and the other diseases carried by the young man with the deleted X chromosome.

If two genes are located near one another, they are likely to be inherited together. As a result, if abnormality of one gene produces a disease and a nearby gene encodes a phenotypic marker that is readily recognized (such as hair or eye color), or the gene encodes a readily detectable gene product (such as protein present in the blood), it should be possible to show that people who express the marker also express the disease—even though the marker may have nothing to do with the disease. These markers, called *genetic polymorphisms*, vary in the normal population. The traits encoded by these genes, such as eye color, are the expression of the particular genetic locus; both the phenotypic trait and the DNA sequence at the locus vary in the normal population.

FIGURE 17–7A

The presence of a restriction fragment polymorphism can be detected by restriction endonucleases, enzymes that cut DNA at specific nucleotide sequences (▼). In this example the b chromosome is missing a restriction site that is present on the a chromosome. Cutting with a restriction enzyme produces a larger DNA fragment with the b chromosome. A radiolabeled DNA probe against this region can be used to reveal this polymorphism after the DNA from both chromosomes have been separated by gel electrophoresis and transferred to nylon filters (a procedure called Southern blotting). Because the b fragment is larger, it runs more slowly than the a fragment.

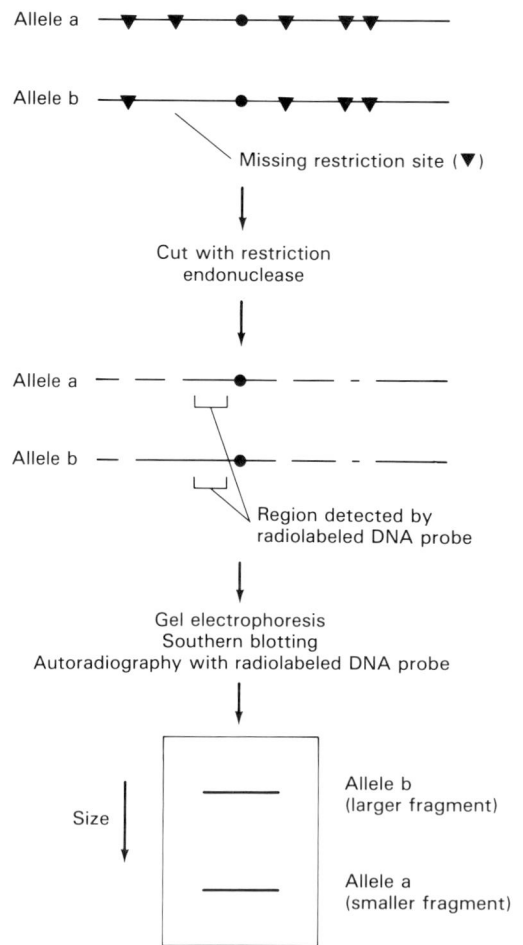

In the past, genetic markers were derived primarily from variations in the coding regions of DNA expressed as gene products, such as blood groups, enzymes, or antigens of the histocompatibility complex. However, 80% of the genome contains noncoding regions (introns); the gene products are mapped to only 20% of the total human genome. Fortunately, it is now possible to saturate the human genome with markers based on variations in DNA sequences throughout the whole genome (including noncoding as well as coding sequences). This broad coverage has made it easier to trace the inheritance of a disease to a specific region of a particular chromosome.

These new markers are based on *restriction fragment length polymorphisms* (RFLP). These polymorphisms are the result of differences in DNA sequence that are detected because they produce or eliminate a cutting site for a particular restriction enzyme—enzymes that cut DNA only at a specific nucleotide sequence. A restriction enzyme produces DNA fragments of different lengths from the two alleles on the paired chromosomes. Chromosomal DNA can be fingerprinted. The fragments that differ in length can be separated by electrophoresis in agarose gels and distinguished by specific DNA probes—a procedure called Southern blot hybridization after the originator Edward Southern (Figure 17–7A).

When a polymorphic region of the DNA is closely linked to a particular gene, inheritance of the gene can be traced by following the inheritance of a particular pattern of restriction fragments. The method can be applied to the analysis of polymorphisms in any population of subjects. Like fingerprints, which are also genetic polymorphisms, the polymorphism need not be related functionally to the genetic disease with which it happens to be linked (Figure 17–7B).

FIGURE 17–7B

Genetic linkage analysis detects the coinheritance of a mutated gene responsible for a human disease and a nearby restriction fragment length polymorphism (RFLP) marker. In this example the gene responsible for the disease is coinherited with the RFLP marker in 75% of offspring that result from the union of the mother's egg with the father's sperm. Thus, the gene responsible for the disease is located close to the RFLP marker on this chromosome. (Adapted from Alberts et al., 1989.)

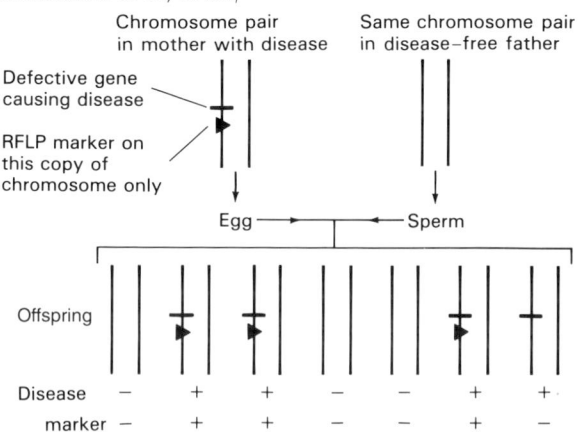

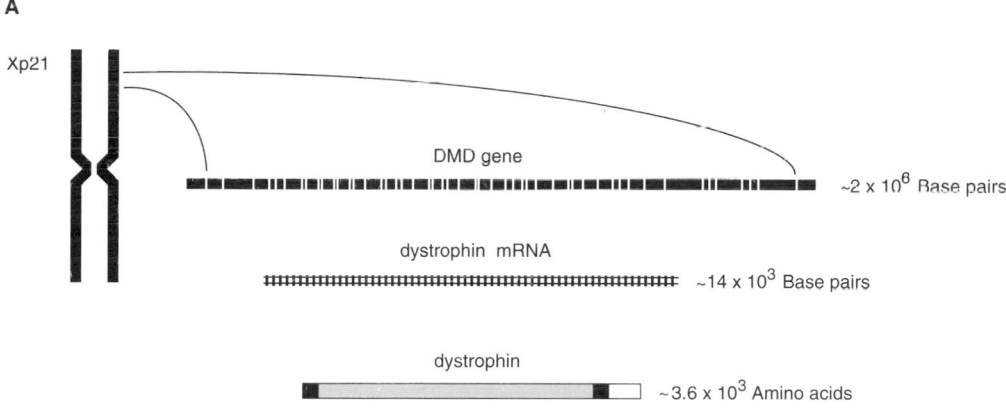

A

Xp21

DMD gene

~2 x 10⁶ Base pairs

dystrophin mRNA

~14 x 10³ Base pairs

dystrophin

~3.6 x 10³ Amino acids

B₁ Deletion resulting in severe DMD

Severely truncated dystrophin
Rapidly degraded by cell

B₂ Deletion resulting in mild BMD

Internally deleted,
semi-functional dystrophin
Allowed to persist by cell

FIGURE 17–8

The predicted effect of specific deletion mutations in the Duchenne muscular dystrophy gene on the translational reading frame and clinical phenotype. (From Hoffman and Kunkel, 1989.)

A. The top of the schematic drawing shows the relative position of the Duchenne muscular dystrophy gene within the Xp21 region of the X chromosome. An enlargement of this locus showing the 65 exons (**white lines**) defines the approximately 2.0 × 10⁶ base pairs Duchenne gene. Transcription of the Duchenne gene gives rise to a ~14 × 10³ bp Duchenne mRNA, and translation of this mRNA gives rise to the 427,000 MW protein dystrophin.

B. Examples of how two similar deletions can exhibit dramatically different clinical phenotypes. A deletion of genomic DNA encompassing only a single exon results in clinically severe Duchenne muscular dystrophy. A larger deletion encompassing four exons results in clinically milder Becker muscular dystrophy. In both cases the gene is transcribed into mRNA and the exons (**boxed areas**) flanking the deletion are brought together. In the case of the single exon deletion in the Duchenne patient (**B₁**) the exon to the right of the deletion is incorrectly translated. This causes the translational machinery to immediately encounter a nonsense (translation stop) codon, resulting in the termination of translation. This out-of-frame deletion produces a dramatically truncated dystrophin protein that is presumably nonfunctional and is quickly degraded by the cell. In the case of larger deletions (**B₂**) the exons flanking a four-exon deletion share the same phase of the reading frame. As a result, the resulting internally deleted mRNA maintains the original open reading frame over the new exon junction. Translation of the mRNA is permitted to continue, resulting in a truncated dystrophin protein. Such an altered dystrophin protein is presumably partly functional and apparently escapes degradation by cellular processes designed to eliminate abnormal proteins.

The Duchenne gene is the largest human gene so far characterized. It is about 2.5 million base pairs in length, more than 10 times larger than any other known human gene and almost as large as the entire genome of some simple bacteria. This one gene accounts for 1% of the X chromosome and about 0.1% of the total human genome. It comprises at least 65 exons that encode a 14-kilobase mRNA.

The large size of the gene explains why it is a particularly susceptible target to deletions, and why more than half of all boys with Duchenne dystrophy have deletions that can be detected with cDNA probes. The specificity of these deletions has been used to practical advantage. In more than half the cases prenatal diagnosis is relatively simple and rapid. For the other half of the cases, those with no detectable deletion, indirect diagnosis is possible using a series of probes for the Xp21 region, defining a consistent pattern called a *haplotype* that can be followed through a family. The haplotype can be used to identify carriers of the gene and to discern whether a fetus is affected. Together, detection of deletions and haplotype analysis make it possible to determine whether a boy is affected with almost 95% accuracy. That still leaves a margin of uncertainty, although this seems likely to diminish as methods improve.

The use of molecular genetics has also clarified the relationship between Duchenne and other dystrophies. For instance, it had long been known that there is another X-linked myopathy, one that resembles Duchenne dystrophy in distribution of weakness, and high serum levels of creatine kinase. It differs from Duchenne dystrophy because it starts later and the rate of progression is much slower. The gene for the myopathy, called Becker muscular dystrophy, was once thought to be located far from the Duchenne gene, implying that it was an entirely different disease. However, when DNA analysis became available, it became apparent that the two conditions were allelic, affecting the same gene.

How can the same gene account for two such different syndromes? As patients were studied the mystery seemed to deepen because no relationship between the clinical pattern and either the size of the deletion or the location within Xp21 became apparent. Identical deletions were seen in some patients with Duchenne dystrophy and others with the Becker form. Then, Monaco, working with Kunkel, suggested that there might be a difference in the

effect of the deletion on the reading frame. If the deletion shifts the translational reading frame so that a stop codon is introduced, mRNA is not synthesized and the protein is not made (Figure 17–8). If the gene product is absent, the resulting clinical syndrome is the severe early-onset Duchenne dystrophy. If, on the other hand, the reading frame is maintained (but the deleted portion includes coding region sequences), translation can proceed and a protein is made. The resulting gene product is smaller than normal and may be missing peptide segments that are essential for normal function. Under these circumstances the clinical syndrome is the milder Becker dystrophy.

Molecular genetics has made other fundamental contributions to understanding muscular dystrophies. For instance, once the nucleotide sequence was identified, it was possible to deduce the amino acid sequence of the gene product, a novel protein called dystrophin. Dystrophin has a rod-like structure and a molecular weight of 427,000. The protein shares structural features with two cytoskeletal proteins, α-actinin and spectrin (Figure 17–9). These similarities suggested that normal dystrophin is part of the cytoskeleton of muscle cells. The use of antibodies reveals that dystrophin is localized to the plasma membrane of skeletal muscle and that the protein is actually lacking in Duchenne muscle.

Working with Kunkel, Eric Hoffman used antibodies to identify the protein in extracts obtained by muscle biopsy. Dystrophin is lacking in Duchenne dystrophy patients, whereas in patients with Becker dystrophy the protein is present but is abnormal in one or both of two character-

FIGURE 17–9

A hypothetical model of the structure of dystrophin and its subcellular organization. This diagram synthesizes much of what is currently known about dystrophin's molecular organization.

A. Schematic diagram of a single dystrophin molecule. Dystrophin is thought to consist of four domains, which are schematically indicated as A, B, C, and D. Domain **A** represents the 240-amino-acid amino-terminal domain that is highly related to the analogous domains of cytoskeletal α-actinin and is thought to bind actin filaments. Domain **B** is the large (2700 amino acid), central, triple-helical domain, which is analogous to domains in both α-actinin and spectrin. Domain **C** represents a

140-amino-acid domain that is rich in cysteines and is related to the carboxy-terminus of α-actinin. Domain **D** is the carboxy-terminal domain of dystrophin (420 amino acids), which bears no apparent resemblance to any previously reported protein.

B. Membrane organization of dystrophin. One or more domains of dystrophin arranged as an antiparallel dimer are thought to be associated with the cytoplasmic domain of an (as yet unidentified) integral membrane protein (**IMP**). The peripheral association of dystrophin with the cytoplasmic face of the plasma membrane has been deduced from biochemical and immunocytochemical studies. (From Hoffman and Kunkel, 1989.)

A   Dystrophin structure

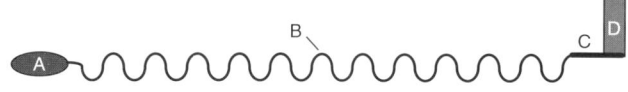

B   Dystrophin subcellular organization

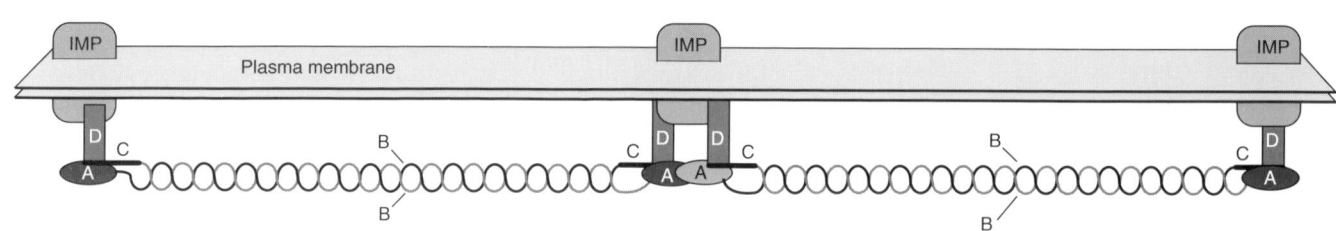

istics: It is smaller than normal or is present in low levels. The use of antibodies in biopsies has already become an essential part of the diagnosis and the definition of these diseases.

These advances have had a tremendous impact but there are still problems to be solved. We still do not know the normal function of dystrophin or understand how the lack of dystrophin leads to severe disease or how structural abnormalities in dystrophin leads to mild disease. The antibodies to dystrophin have led to the discovery of two true X-linked animal models of the disease, one in the dog (X-linked canine muscular dystrophy or CXMD) and the other in the mouse (mdx). Affected dogs are clinically weak, but mdx mice, even though lacking dystrophin in skeletal muscle, are not weak, another puzzle. The final test will be application of this new knowledge to design an effective treatment. Attempts are being made to replace the missing gene by implantation of cultured myoblasts or by injection of a plasmid that contains the gene for dystrophin.

An Overall View

The fruitful interplay of clinical observation and basic science is nowhere more evident than in the analysis of diseases of the motor unit. The application of molecular genetics to the study of Duchenne muscular dystrophy has produced information that bears upon the organization of the human genome, the nature of inherited deletions, and the physiological function of normal muscle, including the discovery of a novel muscle protein. Effective therapy may also result from these discoveries. Molecular genetic studies of Duchenne and Becker dystrophies may also point the way to effective therapy of these diseases. For instance, the injection of normal myoblasts (muscle cell precursors) into the dystrophic muscle of mdx mice is followed by the appearance of normal dystrophin in the affected animals. The notion of *muscle transplantation* for a human disease may seem far off, but plans are progressing for experimental trials of myoblast implantation under some conditions.

Selected Readings

Adrian, R. H., and Bryant, S. H. 1974. On the repetitive discharge in myotonic muscle fibres. J. Physiol. (Lond.) 240:505–515.

Barchi, R. L. 1982. A mechanistic approach to the myotonic syndromes. Muscle Nerve 5:S60–S63.

Brooke, M. H. 1977. A Clinician's View of Neuromuscular Diseases. Baltimore: Williams & Wilkins.

Culp, W. J., and Ochoa, J. (eds.) 1982. Abnormal Nerves and Muscles as Impulse Generators. New York: Oxford University Press.

Desmedt, J. E. (ed.) 1981. Motor Unit Types, Recruitment and Plasticity in Health and Disease. Basel: Karger.

Dyck, P. J., Thomas, P. K., Lambert, E. H., and Bunge, R. (eds.) 1984. Peripheral Neuropathy, 2nd ed., 2 vols. Philadelphia: Saunders.

Hoffman, E. P., and Kunkel, L. M. 1989. Dystrophin abnormalities in Duchenne/Becker muscular dystrophy. Neuron 2:1019–1029.

Rowland, L. P., and Layzer, R. B. 1977. Muscular dystrophies, atrophies, and related diseases. In A. B. Baker (ed.), Clinical Neurology, Vol. 3. New York: Harper & Row, pp. 1–109.

Rowland, L. P. (ed.) 1982. Human Motor Neuron Diseases. New York: Raven Press.

Rowland, L. P. 1988. Clinical concepts of Duchenne muscular dystrophy. The impact of molecular genetics. Brain 111:479–495.

Sumner, A. J. (ed.) 1980. The Physiology of Peripheral Nerve Disease. Philadelphia: Saunders.

Walton, J. (ed.) 1988. Disorders of Voluntary Muscle, 5th ed. Edinburgh: Churchill Livingstone.

Waxman, S. G. 1982. Membranes, myelin, and the pathophysiology of multiple sclerosis. N. Engl. J. Med. 306:1529–1533.

References

Boyd, Y., Buckle, V., Holt, S., Munro, E., Hunter, D., and Craig, I. 1986. Muscular dystrophy in girls with X; autosome translocations. J. Med. Genet. 23:484–490.

Burghes, A. H. M., Logan, C., Hu, X., Belfall, B., Worton, R. G., and Ray, P. N. 1987. A cDNA clone from the Duchenne/Becker muscular dystrophy gene. Nature 328:434–437.

Forrest, S. M., Cross, G. S., Flint, T., Speer, A., Robson K. J. H., and Davies, K. E. 1988. Further studies of gene deletions that cause Duchenne and Becker muscular dystrophies. Genomics 2:109–114.

Francke, U., Ochs, H. D., de Martinville, B., Giacalone, J., Lindgren, V., Distèche, C., Pagon, R. A., Hofker, M. H., van Ommen, G.-J. B., Pearson, P. L., and Wedgwood, R. J. 1985. Minor Xp21 chromosome deletion in a male associated with expression of Duchenne muscular dystrophy, chronic granulomatous disease, retinitis pigmentosa, and McLeod syndrome. Am. J. Hum. Genet. 37:250–267.

Hoffman, E. P., Brown, R. H., Jr., and Kunkel, L. M. 1987. Dystrophin: The protein product of the Duchenne muscular dystrophy locus. Cell 51:919–928

Hoffman, E. P., Fischbeck K. H., Brown, R. H., Johnson, M., Medori, R., Loike, J. D., Harris, J. B., Waterston, R., Brooke, M., Specht, L., Kupsky, W., Chamberlain, J., Caskey, C. T., Shapiro, F., and Kunkel, L. M. 1988. Characterization of dystrophin in muscle-biopsy specimens from patients with Duchenne's or Becker's muscular dystrophy. N. Engl. J. Med. 318:1363–1368.

Hoffman, E. P., Kunkel, L. M., Angelini, C., Clarke, A., Johnson, M., and Harris, J. B. 1989. Improved diagnosis of Becker muscular dystrophy by dystrophin testing. Neurology 39:1011–1017.

Monaco, A. P., Bertelson, C. J., Liechti-Gallati, S., Moser, H., and Kunkel, L. M. 1988. An explanation for the phenotypic differences between patients bearing partial deletions of the DMD locus. Genomics 2:90–95.

Partridge, T. A., Morgan, J. E., Coulton, G. R., Hoffman, E. P., and Kunkel, L. M. 1989. Conversion of mdx myofibres from dystrophin-negative to -positive by injection of normal myoblasts. Nature 337:176–179.

Schonk, D., Coerwinkel-Driessen, M., van Dalen, I., Oerlemans, F., Smeets, B., Schepens, J., Hulsebos, T., Cockburn, D., Boyd, Y., Davis, M., Rettig, W., Shaw, D., Roses, A., Ropers, H., and Wieringa, B. 1989. Definition of subchromosomal intervals around the myotonic dystrophy gene region at 19q. Genomics 4:384–396.

18

Thomas M. Jessell

Reactions of Neurons to Injury

Severing the Axon Causes Degenerative Changes in the Neuron

Synaptic Transmission Is Lost Rapidly

The Distal Axon Segment Degenerates Slowly

The Membrane Compartments of the Cell Body Are Disrupted

Glial Cells and Macrophages Scavenge the Debris Caused by Injury

Cells That Have Synaptic Connections with Injured Neurons Also Degenerate

Neurons in the Peripheral Nervous System Can Regenerate Their Axons

Trophic Factors Prevent the Degeneration of Peripheral Neurons after Axotomy

Schwann Cells Contribute to the Regeneration of Peripheral Axons

Neurons in the Adult Central Nervous System Have Only Limited Capacity to Regenerate Their Axons

Several Potential Manipulations Can Promote the Recovery of Function after Damage to the Central Nervous System

Peripheral Nerve Grafts Promote the Growth of Central Axons

Transplantation of Embryonic Neurons into Adult Brain Promotes Recovery of Function after Damage

In Some Animals New Neurons Can Be Generated in the Adult Brain

An Overall View

In the preceding chapters we have seen how diseases of the nervous system affect synaptic transmission between a neuron and its target cell. Diseases of the motor neuron can alter the properties of muscle, and diseases of muscle affect the motor neuron. For example, in muscular dystrophy the degeneration of the muscle fiber leads to a generalized dysfunction of the motor unit. Conversely, diseases that affect the motor neuron result in atrophy of the target muscle. Thus, the degeneration of one cell type in the nervous system can impair the function of the cells with which it forms functional contacts.

In this chapter we discuss, more generally, the serious and often irreversible functional consequences to the mammalian nervous system of damage caused by physical injuries. Injuries that destroy the cell body of a neuron invariably lead to the death of the cell. Moreover, death of neurons can also be brought about by injuries that sever the axon of a neuron. When neurons in the adult nervous system die they are not replaced, because most adult neurons have withdrawn from the cell cycle and thus are no longer capable of division. Neuronal death therefore results in long-lasting or permanent loss of function.

Injuries that sever the axon, however, do not invariably lead to the death of the neuron. Under some circumstances neurons are capable of regenerating their axonal projections and reestablishing contact with other cells. If these connections are regained, considerable function can be restored. The ability of a neuron to regenerate an axon may involve some of the same mechanisms that contribute to the initial growth of the axon during development. Thus, basic research into the mechanisms that underlie the growth and regenerative capacity of neurons is of great interest to neurology. Any insights that we gain about the molecules responsible for axonal growth and regeneration may point to ways of promoting functional recovery after damage to the central nervous system.

In this chapter we first discuss how neurons respond to injury and later consider experimental and clinical approaches to promoting axonal regeneration in the mature nervous system.

Severing the Axon Causes Degenerative Changes in the Neuron

Cutting an axon, either by sectioning a tract within the brain or by sectioning a peripheral nerve, divides it into two segments. The part of the axon that is connected to the cell body is called the *proximal segment* and the part isolated from the rest of the cell is called the *distal segment*.

Immediately after injury, axoplasm seeps out of the cut ends of both segments until the severed ends of each segment seal by fusion of the axonal membrane. The proximal and distal segments also retract from one another and begin to swell because materials that are normally carried within the axons, either by fast axonal transport or slow axoplasmic flow, now accumulate in the axonal stump (see Chapter 4). Both segments swell because axonal transport carries components both away from and toward the cell body. The swelling of the proximal end is greater, however, because the cell body continues to synthesize the components of the cytoskeleton, neurofilaments, microtubules, and microfilaments, which move down the axon by slow axoplasmic flow. Another early change that occurs after cutting axons is the entry of Ca^{2+}, which may be important in mediating the damaging effects of axonal

injury through activation of Ca^{2+}-dependent proteases or the generation of free radicals, such as superoxides that have toxic actions on neurons.

Injury to the axon triggers other alterations in the damaged neuron and eventually affects the cells that make synaptic contact with the damaged neuron. The responses of the neuron and surrounding cells to axonal injury are illustrated in Figure 18–1 and discussed in Box 18–1 and below in more detail.

Synaptic Transmission Is Lost Rapidly

As we have seen in Chapter 4, the protein synthetic capacity of a neuron is limited to its cell body and proximal dendrites. Because a nerve terminal cannot synthesize protein, its integrity depends critically on materials that are provided by transport from the cell body. Degeneration of nerve terminals has been studied in most detail in peripheral nerve rather than in the central nervous system because peripheral axons and terminals are generally more accessible. For example, severing a motor neuron axon to skeletal muscle fibers results in rapid degeneration in the nerve terminal. The effects of injury can be assessed by intracellular recording from the denervated muscle fibers. Synaptic transmission fails within hours, even before the first morphological signs of terminal degeneration become apparent. The onset of failure is variable, however, and depends on where the axon is cut. Transmission fails more rapidly if the cut is close to the synaptic terminal than if it is near the cell body. If the distal segment is long

FIGURE 18–1

When an axon is severed, degenerative changes occur in the injured neuron as well as in those neurons with which it has synaptic connections.

A. This simplified drawing illustrates the normal anatomical relationships of presynaptic and postsynaptic neurons.

B. After axotomy many reactive changes take place. In the injured neuron degeneration occurs at the nerve terminals (**1**) and

Wallerian degeneration occurs at the distal segment of the axon (**2**), myelinating cells withdraw leaving myelin debris (**3**); phagocytotic cells infiltrate the site of the lesion (**4**); and the cell body undergoes chromatolysis (**5**). In the presynaptic neuron, terminals retract from the dendrites of the injured neuron (**6**) and the cell body can undergo retrograde transneuronal degeneration (**7**). In the postsynaptic neuron anterograde transneuronal degeneration can occur (**8**).

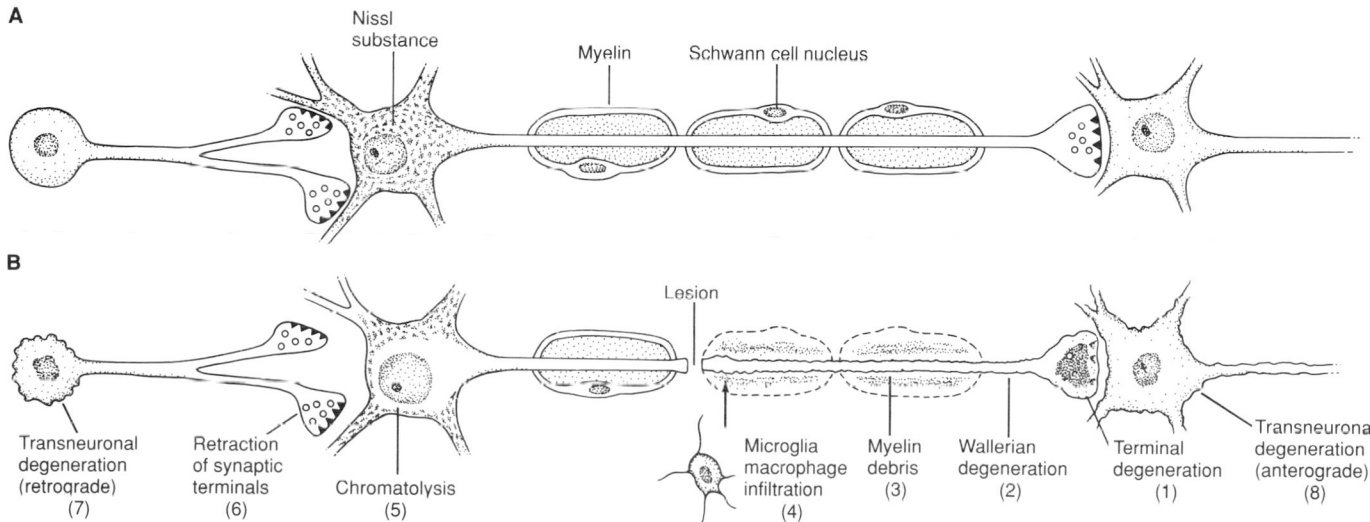

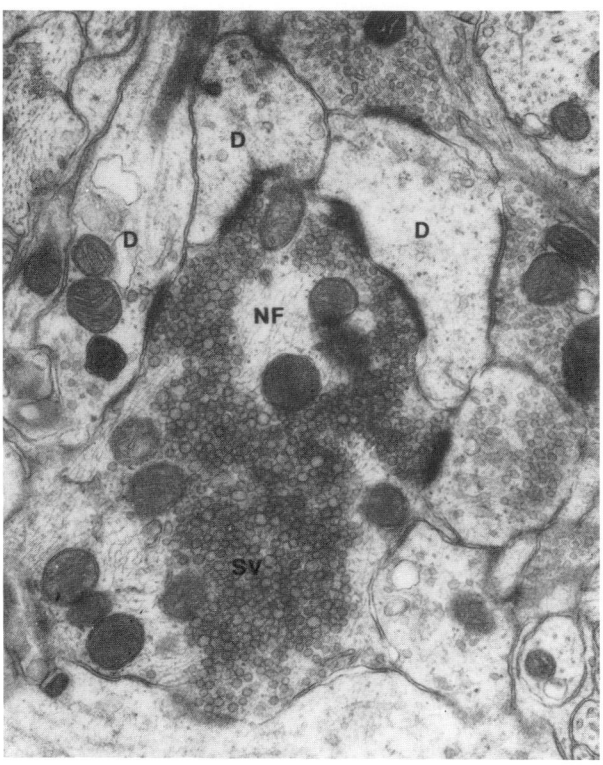

FIGURE 18–2

Early degeneration of a synaptic terminal following injury to the axon. This micrograph shows degeneration of a synaptic terminal in the dorsal horn of the spinal cord of the monkey following lesions of the axons in the dorsal roots. One early sign of degeneration is the appearance of neurofilaments (**NF**) among clumps of synaptic vesicles. The dendrites of postsynaptic neurons are also shown (**D**). (Courtesy of H. J. Ralston III.)

enough, axonal transport within the segment can continue for a short time to provide the terminal with the materials necessary to maintain synaptic transmission.

The morphological changes that occur at degenerating synapses within the central nervous system can be analyzed, although this is technically more difficult (see Box 18–1). Within a few days after cutting the axon, the terminals of some central neurons become filled with whorls of neurofilaments that surround mitochondria that have become disrupted and swollen (Figure 18–2). Others become more evenly filled with electron-dense products of degeneration. After about a week, contact between the terminal and postsynaptic neurons or peripheral target cells is disrupted by invading glial cells. During the second week the terminals formed by the distal segment withdraw completely from the postsynaptic cell.

The Distal Axon Segment Degenerates Slowly

Even if the affected neuron ultimately survives the injury, degeneration of the terminal is followed by loss of the entire distal segment (Figure 18–1). This process is termed *Wallerian degeneration* after Augustus Waller who de-

scribed it in the nineteenth century. Changes in the distal axon segment become apparent about 1 week after the terminal begins to degenerate, and continue over the next 1–2 months or until the entire distal segment is destroyed.

When the distal segment of an axon degenerates, the myelin sheath pulls away from the distal segment and breaks apart (Figure 18–1). Clumps of neurofilaments and microtubules soon fill the axon, which swells and breaks up into short beaded segments. In the peripheral nervous system the debris is degraded within a period of days to weeks, whereas in the central nervous system this process commonly lasts for several months. The reason for this difference is unclear but may be related to the classes of cells that phagocytose the debris. Demyelination is discussed in more detail later in the chapter.

The Membrane Compartments of the Cell Body Are Disrupted

Within a few days following axotomy, changes occur in the cell body of most types of neurons. For example, the cell body of a dorsal root ganglion cell or spinal motor neuron swells, and may even double in size. The nucleus swells and moves to an eccentric position, usually opposite the axon hillock. Next, the rough endoplasmic reticulum breaks apart and moves to the periphery of the swollen cell body. This phenomenon, referred to as *chromatolysis*, is a useful histological indication that the axon of a neuron has been severed. Chromatolysis can be most easily seen when the rough endoplasmic reticulum is stained with basic dyes, such as thionin, that bind to ribosomes. After injury, endoplasmic reticulum that is stained in this way (termed *Nissl substance*) can be seen around the margin of the cell, instead of around the nucleus as in uninjured cells. Chromatolysis is more pronounced in young animals, in which axotomized neurons in the peripheral nervous system usually degenerate completely after axotomy.

Chromatolysis is often accompanied by an increase in the number of free polysomes in the cell body as well as an increase in RNA and protein synthesis. These metabolic changes probably reflect the injured cell's need for proteins to rebuild the severed part of the axon. If the neuron successfully regenerates an axon and restores connections with other cells in the nervous system, the cell body usually returns to its former appearance. Failure to contact a new target cell leads to atrophy and death.

Not all neurons exhibit chromatolysis or regenerative changes after axotomy. Purkinje cells of the cerebellum, for example, do not shrink detectably after axotomy. Neurons in the thalamus shrink soon after their axons are cut but remain in this state indefinitely.

Glial Cells and Macrophages Scavenge the Debris Caused by Injury

Glial cells provide structural and functional support for the intact nervous system and also help restore damaged neurons. As we saw in Chapter 2, the central nervous system has two major categories of glial cells: the macroglia, which include oligodendrocytes and astrocytes, and the microglia, which are macrophage-like scavenger cells. Another type of glial cell, the Schwann cell, is prominent in the peripheral nervous system. In both peripheral and central tracts the glial cell processes that form the myelin sheath around the distal segment of injured axons are destroyed during Wallerian degeneration.

The role of glial cells in recovery of function after injury differs in the central and peripheral nervous systems. In the peripheral nervous system macrophages are recruited to the site of a lesion, where they help degrade the distal segment of the axon by secreting proteases and engulfing the debris. They may also promote peripheral nerve regeneration by secreting factors that are required for subsequent Schwann cell proliferation. In the central nervous system resident microglial cells and astrocytes, not macrophages, are responsible for removal of debris. Presumably, macrophages are prevented from penetrating central nervous tissue by the blood–brain barrier. The persistence of myelin and axonal debris in the central nervous system is thought to hinder the regeneration of axons.

Glial cells also change the organization of the synapses onto injured neurons. In the region near the cell body of the postsynaptic neuron the invading glial cells push apart the pre- and postsynaptic elements of the synapse (Figure 18–3). As a consequence, the number of presynaptic contacts is reduced and excitatory synaptic potentials evoked in the injured cell are smaller in amplitude. Nevertheless, the cell may still be excited at synapses on the dendrites, which in the normal cell are ineffective. One possible explanation for the enhanced efficacy of dendritic synapses is an increase in the excitability of dendrites following axotomy. If regenerated axons make connections with new target cells, the normal input to the cell body returns. If the neuron is unable to reestablish contact with its targets, the neuron dies and microglial cells in the vicinity of the disintegrating cell body scavenge the neuronal debris.

Cells That Have Synaptic Connections with Injured Neurons Also Degenerate

Degenerative changes may eventually occur in cells that had synaptic contacts with an injured neuron. These changes are called *transneuronal* or *transsynaptic*. Some transneuronal changes are mild, while others are often severe enough to cause complete degeneration of the affected cells. Transneuronal degeneration explains, at least in part, how an injury at one site in the central nervous system is able to affect sites that are some distance from the lesion. It also is an indication of the degree to which neurons are dependent on one another for survival.

Transneuronal degeneration is referred to as *anterograde* if the affected cell received synapses *from* the injured neuron, and *retrograde* if the affected cell made synapses *on* the injured neuron. As an example, both anterograde and retrograde cell loss can be illustrated in the mammalian visual system. In the intact visual system the axons of the retinal ganglion cells join to form the optic

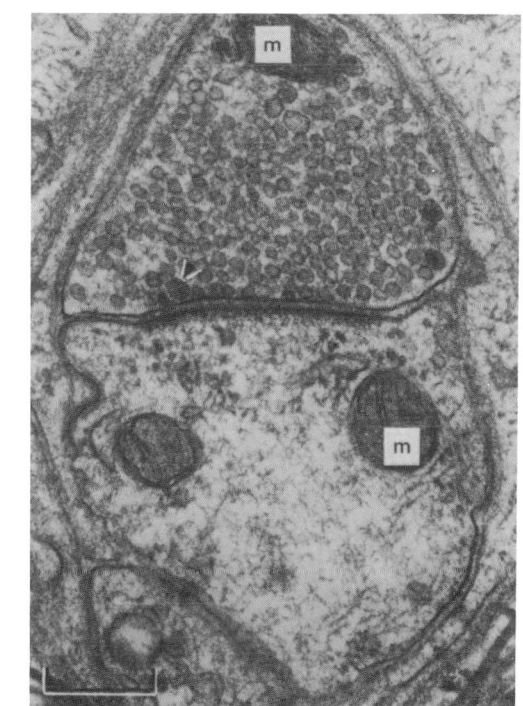

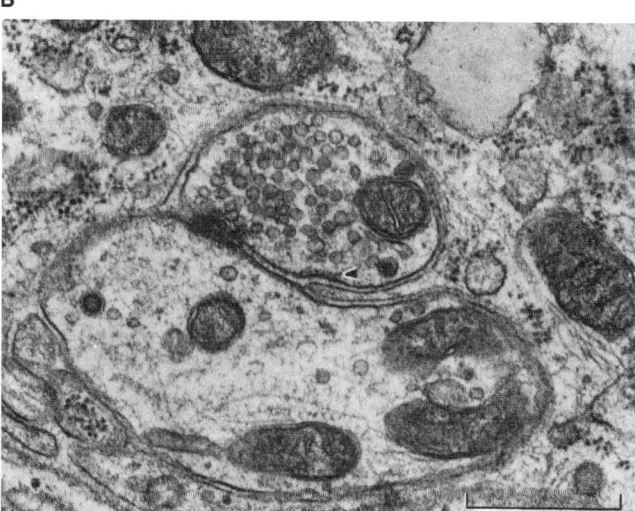

FIGURE 18–3
Glial cells interpose themselves between the synaptic terminals of an injured neuron and the postsynaptic element. (From Matthews and Nelson, 1975.)

A. Normal synaptic contact between a presynaptic nerve terminal and the dendrite of a sympathetic neuron with an intact axon. (Micrographs are of a guinea pig sympathetic ganglion neuron.) **m**, mitochondria. Scale bar = 0.3 μM.

B. Retraction of contact between a presynaptic terminal and the dendrite of an axotomized sympathetic neuron. Scale bar = 0.5 μM.

nerve, which terminates in a region of the thalamus called the *lateral geniculate nucleus*. In higher animals these postsynaptic thalamic neurons send their axons to the visual cortex in the occipital lobe. When the optic nerve is

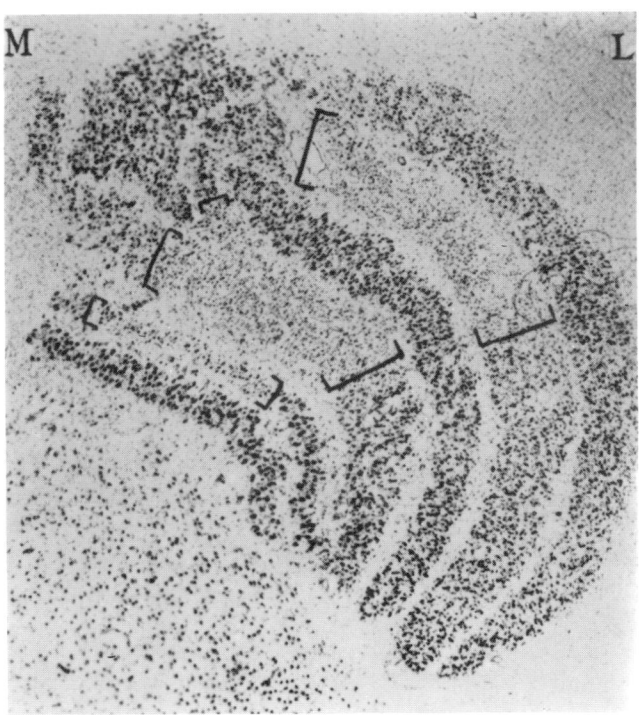

FIGURE 18–4
Following a retinal lesion, degeneration of retinal ganglion cells causes degeneration of the postsynaptic cells in the thalamus. This photomicrograph of a Nissl preparation of monkey tissue shows transneuronal degeneration of nerve cells in three laminae of the lateral geniculate nucleus after a retinal lesion. (From Le Gros Clark and Penman, 1934.)

cut, the terminals of the retinal ganglion cells undergo rapid anterograde degeneration and the postsynaptic neurons atrophy in the lateral geniculate nucleus (Figure 18–4). Retrograde degeneration also occurs in the visual system and may spread across more than one synapse. For example, lesions in the visual cortex cause neurons in the lateral geniculate nucleus to degenerate; in turn, retinal

ganglion cells that synapse on these thalamic neurons may atrophy after a few months.

Neurons in the Peripheral Nervous System Can Regenerate Their Axons

Damage to the peripheral nervous system is frequently reversible. Neurons are able to regenerate and eventually restore functional connections of their peripheral axons. This contrasts sharply with the responses of neurons to damage of the central nervous system. We next compare the factors that contribute to the differential regenerative capacities of central and peripheral neurons.

Trophic Factors Prevent the Degeneration of Peripheral Neurons after Axotomy

Some of the molecules involved in the survival of neurons after injury may be the same as those needed by immature neurons as they develop. Studies on neural development have identified several neurotrophic factors that are released by the targets of neurons and which trigger biochemical changes in the neuron that are important for its survival and growth. Nerve growth factor (NGF) is the best-characterized neurotrophic factor, and is discussed in more detail in Chapter 59. Here we focus on its role in supporting the survival of neurons after injury. Three major classes of neurons are sensitive to the trophic actions of NGF: sympathetic neurons, primary sensory neurons of the dorsal root ganglion, and cholinergic neurons of the septum and nucleus basalis of the forebrain. Many neurons that are not sensitive to NGF are dependent on other related trophic factors, such as brain-derived neurotrophic factor (BDNF) and neurotrophin-3.

The availability of trophic factors determines whether injured neurons are maintained. For example, when the axons of sympathetic neurons are cut, the presynaptic autonomic neurons withdraw their terminals (Figure 18–5B). The withdrawal of the terminals is due to the deprivation

---

Neuroanatomical Tracing Based on Degenerative Changes in Neurons   **BOX 18–1**

The classical methods for tracing neuronal pathways are histological methods that detect degenerative changes in neurons following damage. These staining methods provide a remarkably accurate picture of neuronal projections in the central nervous system. Today it is possible to trace projections among intact neurons using the label horseradish peroxidase, autoradiography, and fluorescent dye tracers (see Box 14–1).

Four major degenerative staining techniques, each named after the anatomists who first developed them, have been particularly useful in tracing connections: the Weigert, Nauta, Bodian, and Fink-Heimer methods.

The Weigert method uses chromium salts and hematoxylin to stain myelin. When a nerve tract is cut, the myelin surrounding the distal portion of the fibers disappears and the demyelinated fibers are not marked by the Weigert stain. The pale regions devoid of staining thus reveal axonal pathways disrupted by the lesion.

The Nauta, Bodian, and Fink-Heimer methods all use the degenerative neurofilaments to bind silver selectively (the argyrophilic reaction), because neurofilaments in degenerating fibers are intensely labeled after silver staining.

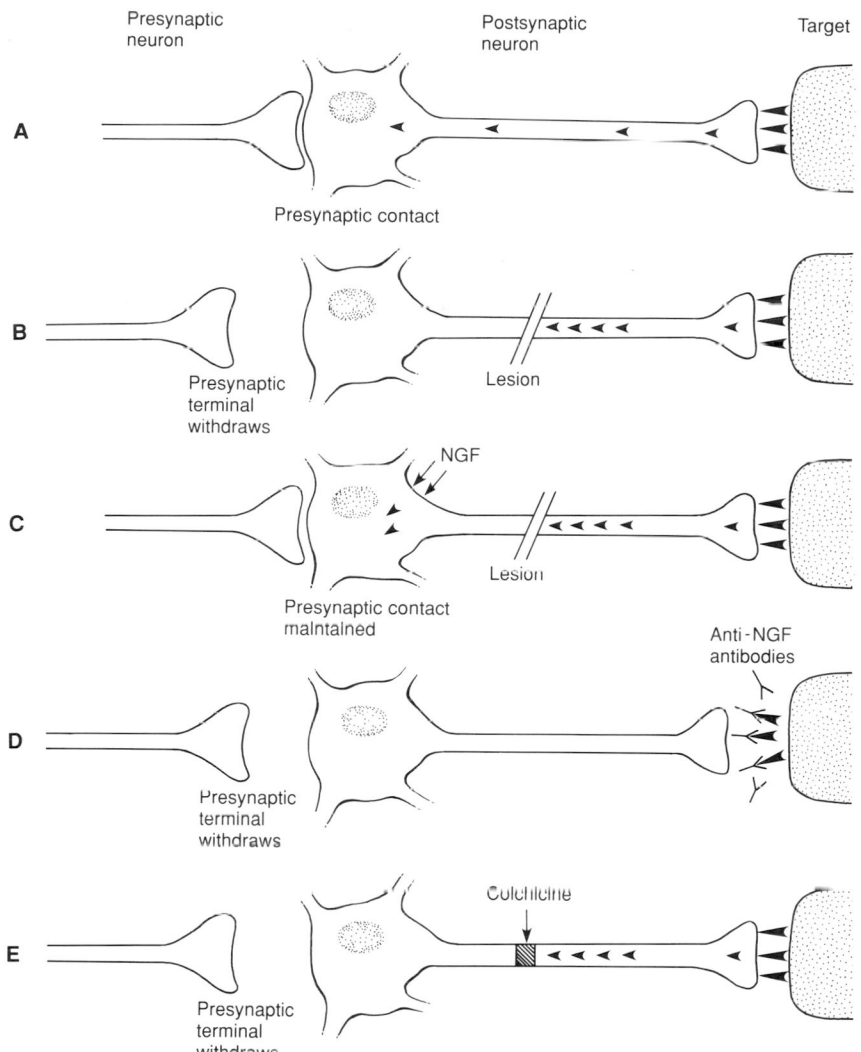

FIGURE 18–5

Schematic diagram showing the consequences of sectioning the axons of post ganglionic sympathetic neurons.

A. Normal contact made by a preganglionic terminal with a postganglionic neuron. The postganglionic neuron in turn contacts a peripheral target cell that releases nerve growth factor (NGF).

B. Sectioning the axons of postganglionic neurons causes preganglionic terminals to withdraw.

C. The withdrawal of presynaptic terminals after axonal section can be prevented by administration of NGF to the vicinity of the postganglionic sympathetic neuron.

D. Administration of anti-NGF antibodies, which prevent NGF released by the target cell from reaching the terminal of the postganglionic sympathetic neuron, also causes withdrawal of presynaptic terminals.

E. Blockade of retrograde axonal transport with drugs such as colchicine results in withdrawal of the presynaptic terminal. The retrograde transport of NGF itself or an intracellular messenger activated by NGF is required for maintenance of preganglionic axon terminals.

of NGF from the sympathetic target neurons. Injection of NGF into the vicinity of the nerve at the time the axon is cut prevents the withdrawal of many of the presynaptic terminals (Figure 18–5C). Conversely, injecting an animal with antibodies against NGF results in a marked withdrawal of presynaptic terminals, even though the axons of the postganglionic neurons have not been cut (Figure 18–5D). The loss of connections presumably results from the ability of the antibodies to inactivate NGF as it is secreted from the target cells, thus preventing the NGF from reaching the terminal of the postganglionic presynaptic neuron. The retrograde transport of NGF, or an intracellular messenger mobilized by activation of the NGF receptor, is thought to be essential to its trophic actions. Retrograde transport in intact axons can be abolished by application of drugs such as colchicine to the postganglionic nerve; under these conditions the presynaptic terminals withdraw, possibly because of the interruption of retrograde

flow of neurotrophic factors or second messengers (Figure 18–5E).

In addition to maintaining synaptic connections, NGF may also be required for the survival of mature neurons after injury. For example, NGF has a trophic influence on cholinergic neurons of the basal forebrain and septum in the central nervous system. Cholinergic neurons in the septum project to the hippocampus, a region of the limbic system with one of the highest concentrations of NGF in the central nervous system. Transection of the axons of septal cholinergic neurons causes the death of about half of these neurons. Intraventricular injection of NGF immediately after the transection substantially reduces the number of neurons that die. Neurons in the basal forebrain (nucleus basalis) degenerate markedly in Alzheimer's disease (as we shall see in Chapter 63). Administration of NGF prevents the death of these neurons in experimental animals. This raises the possibil-

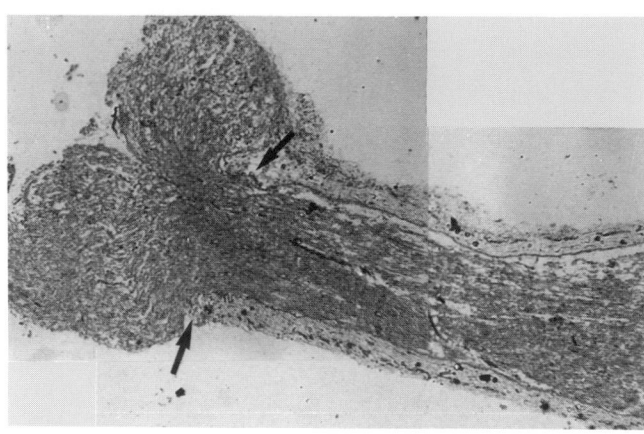

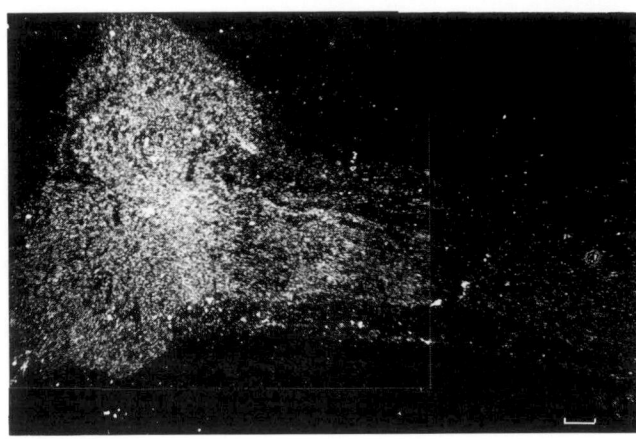

A

B

FIGURE 18–6

Nerve growth factor is synthesized by Schwann cells in response to crushing the sciatic nerve. This figure shows a longitudinal section of adult rat sciatic nerve four days after transection. (From Heumann et al., 1987.)

A. This micrograph of the sciatic nerve shows the site of crush (**arrows**).

B. Localization of NGF mRNA by *in situ* hybridization using radiolabeled nucleotide probes. In the micrograph the accumulation of silver grains (**bright dots**) reflects the high amounts of NGF mRNA in Schwann cells in the vicinity of the nerve cut. Scale bar = 40 μM.

ity that one contributing factor in the progression of Alzheimer's disease may be reduced amounts of NGF or other trophic factors in the central nervous system.

The mechanisms by which NGF prevents the death of adult neurons after axotomy are not yet understood. However, studies on sympathetic neurons grown in cell culture have demonstrated that neuronal degeneration induced by deprivation of NGF can be prevented, at least temporarily, by blocking RNA or protein synthesis. One interpretation of these findings is that NGF represses the synthesis of proteins that are toxic to the neuron, for example, proteases or other enzymes.

Support for the idea of gene products that control neuronal death comes from studies of cell death in other systems. For example, the hormonally induced death of lymphocytes and of some invertebrate neurons depends on RNA and protein synthesis. In the nematode worm, *Caenhorabditis elegans*, the death of certain neurons is developmentally programmed. Genes that regulate the survival of these and other neurons have been identified, although the structure and function of proteins encoded by these genes is still not known. It is conceivable that similar genes are activated in mammalian neurons after the supply of trophic factors from target cells is interrupted.

Schwann Cells Contribute to the Regeneration of Peripheral Axons

Some injuries, such as the crushing of a nerve, may transect peripheral axons but leave intact the sheath that surrounds it. In such injuries the sheath may act as a physical conduit that guides regenerating axons back to their targets. How does regeneration occur? One of the earliest

events after peripheral nerve damage is the recruitment of circulating macrophages to the site of the lesion. In addition to phagocytosing myelin debris, macrophages stimulate the proliferation of Schwann cells in the vicinity of the lesion, probably by secreting mitogenic growth factors. The proliferating Schwann cells secrete several extracellular proteins, in particular laminin, which promote axon extension. Adhesion molecules expressed on the surface of the Schwann cell may also promote the reextension of axons.

In sympathetic and sensory neurons, macrophages and Schwann cells interact in another way that contributes to the recovery of the axons. Macrophages that migrate to the site of the injury release a protein, interleukin 1, that mediates lymphocyte interactions in the immune system. Interleukin 1 evokes rapid and transient synthesis of NGF in Schwann cells near the site of the lesion (Figure 18–6). There is also increased synthesis of NGF in Schwann cells that surround the degenerating distal axonal segment. These Schwann cells may be a source of trophic factor to injured sympathetic and sensory neurons until they regain functional contact with their target cells. Normal Schwann cells surrounding intact axons do not synthesize NGF. Thus, the reestablishment of contact between regenerated axons and Schwann cells appears to suppress the synthesis of NGF by the Schwann cells.

Neurons in the Adult Central Nervous System Have Only Limited Capacity to Regenerate Their Axons

Unlike injuries to the peripheral nervous system, damage to the central nervous system is severe and irreversible, in part because of the failure of central neurons to regenerate

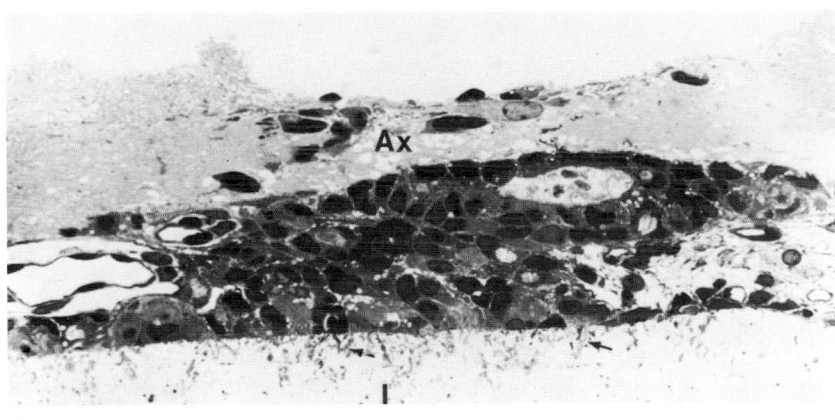

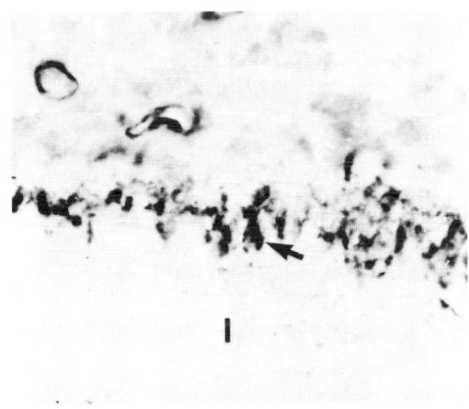

A

B

FIGURE 18–7
Central nervous system axons extend on substrates of immature astrocytes.

A. Frontal section through a nitrocellulose filter implanted into mice that have previously had their corpus callosum cut.

Axons (**Ax**) can be seen growing on a layer of astrocytes that cover the filter 72 hours after the transplant (× 4,400).

B. Immunocytochemical staining reveals the presence of laminin (**arrow**) in association with astrocytes covering the implant × 250. (From Smith et al., 1986.)

axons. Although the proximal stump of the damaged axon may sprout some short processes, in only very few cases is this local sprouting sufficient to restore functional connections. Why do central neurons lack this capacity, a feature that is so evident in peripheral neurons?

Early in neural development the extracellular matrix in both the central and peripheral nervous systems contains glycoproteins that are effective in promoting axon growth. Two such proteins, laminin and fibronectin, persist in the periphery but are virtually absent from the brain and spinal cord of adult mammals. Thus, the mature central nervous system lacks critical molecules in the extracellular matrix that may be needed for axons to regenerate. Developing axons also contain intracellular proteins associated with active growth. For example, one growth-associated protein with a molecular weight of about 43,000, called GAP-43, disappears from the axons of most adult central neurons but is expressed in neurons that have some capacity to sprout axons after injury, such as those in the hippocampus. In contrast, GAP-43 is present in many adult peripheral neurons. The function of GAP-43 is not yet known, but the inability of central neurons to continue synthesizing it and other similar proteins may contribute to the poor regrowth of axons in the mature central nervous system.

In addition to the lack of molecules that facilitate growth, the mature CNS may express molecules that actively inhibit the growth of axons. For example, when oligodendrocytes differentiate and begin to myelinate central axons, they synthesize glycoproteins that actively repress axon outgrowth. Moreover, in rats, antibodies against these molecules promote the regeneration of axons. These inhibitory glycoproteins are not present in the myelinating processes of Schwann cells around peripheral axons.

The formation of glial scars by astrocytes in the vicinity of the injury may also prevent regeneration of the axon. The formation of scars is a property associated with mature, but not embryonic or postnatal, astrocytes. This can be shown by cutting the corpus callosum of rats at different ages. In adult rats, axons fail to cross the midline at the site of the lesion and instead form a tangled knot. However, the growth of axons across the midline can be induced experimentally by surgically introducing a nitrocellulose filter coated with immature astrocytes (Figure 18–7). It is possible therefore that the loss of molecules that promote axon outgrowth and the appearance of inhibitory molecules during development may explain why central neurons gradually lose their capacity to regenerate.

Several Potential Manipulations Can Promote the Recovery of Function after Damage to the Central Nervous System

Peripheral Nerve Grafts Promote the Growth of Central Axons

As discussed above, the peripheral environment of autonomic sensory and motor axons supports axonal regeneration. This observation has prompted speculation that central axons might regenerate more effectively if they are exposed to a peripheral environment.

To test this idea, Albert Aguayo and his colleagues replaced central nervous tissue of the optic nerve of adult rats with segments of the peripheral sciatic nerve. The cut axons of ganglion neurons in the adult retina, which normally do not regenerate into the optic nerve, were able to regrow into the graft and reinnervate their targets in the superior colliculus (Figure 18–8). The regenerating retinal ganglion cell axons penetrated the superior colliculus for

A

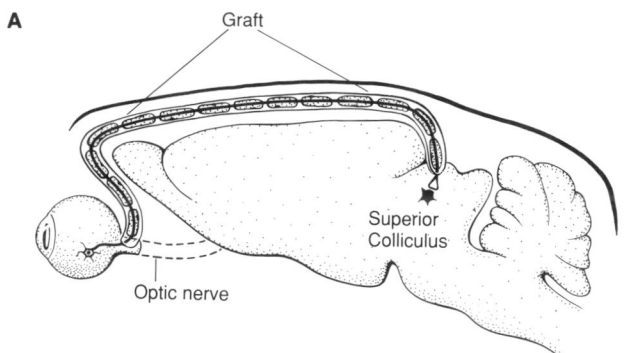

B

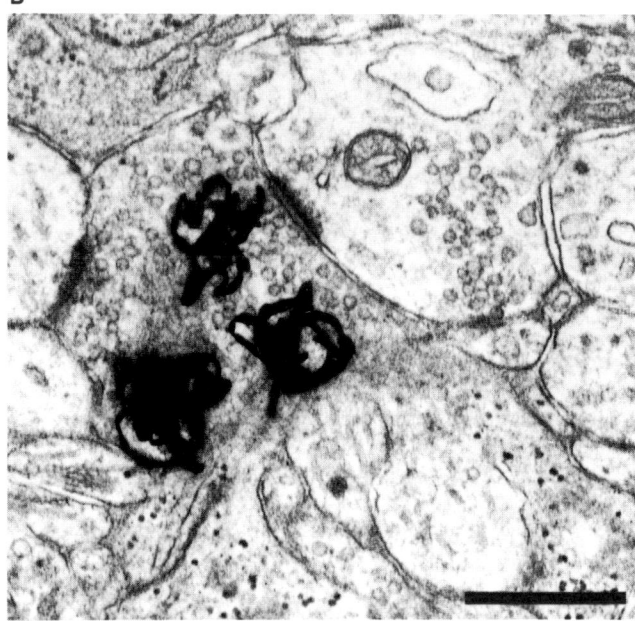

FIGURE 18–8

Grafting of peripheral nerve tissue in the central nervous system promotes the regeneration of the axons of adult central neurons. (Adapted from Bray et al., 1987.)

A. Diagram of an adult rat brain in sagittal section in which a peripheral sciatic nerve is grafted in place of the optic nerve, which has been transected near the eye. One end of the peripheral nerve is attached to the orbital stump of the optic nerve, the other end is inserted into the superior colliculus.

B. Micrograph of a regenerated retinal ganglion cell electron terminal in the superior colliculus of a rat 16 months after the retina and superior colliculus were connected by a peripheral nerve graft. The terminal, which contains pale mitochondria and spheroidal vesicles, and forms asymmetric contact with a dendritic shaft (**arrow**), is labeled with silver grains two days after the injection of [³H] leucine/proline into the eye. Scale bar = 0.5 μm.

distances of up to 500 μm and branched in the superficial layers that normally receive most retinal projections. Moreover, the ultrastructural features of the newly formed terminals resembled normal presynaptic structures. These findings demonstrate that regenerating axons can penetrate central nervous system tissue and form syn-

apses within the nearby gray matter. The regenerated synaptic contacts were detected in the superior colliculus for over a year, indicating that these connections are permanently restored.

Aguayo and his colleagues also assessed the function of synapses formed by regenerating retinal ganglion cell axons. In the region of the superior colliculus near the site of the graft insertion, cells were found that responded with either excitation or inhibition to flashes of light directed toward the retina (Figure 18–9). Because the formation and function of synaptic connections between regenerated retinal ganglion cell axons and the superior colliculus occurs in a context that is substantially different from that of the intact animal, it remains unclear to what extent synaptic transmission is translated into behavioral function and whether any retinotopic order is reestablished.

Nevertheless, these studies demonstrate that if regenerating axons are able to reach the general vicinity of their target cells they are capable of forming functional synaptic connections. The precision with which many injured neurons in the brain and spinal cord of lower vertebrates reestablish damaged axonal projections suggests that a similar accuracy might be achieved in the mammalian central nervous system if the extension of axons can be induced.

Transplantation of Embryonic Neurons into Adult Brain Promotes Recovery of Function after Damage

A different approach to repairing damage to brain tissue in the central nervous system, developed by Anders Björklund and others, involves the transplantation of cells from fetal or neonatal animals into the adult brain. Fetal neurons from a variety of brain regions can be successfully incorporated into the adult brain and subsequently identified by the neurotransmitter substances they produce (Figure 18–10). Such grafts can alleviate experimentally induced behavioral deficits in rats. For example, movement disorders induced by lesions of dopaminergic projections to the basal ganglia can be prevented by grafts of embryonic dopaminergic neurons. Complex cognitive functions that are impaired after lesions of the neocortex, such as maze learning, can also be partially restored by grafts of embryonic cortical cells.

The mechanisms of action of such neural grafts may be complex. Some transplanted cells may simply release transmitter onto distant target cells, much as transplanted endocrine cells do. For example, transplanted dopaminergic cells may release dopamine that diffuses from the site of the transplanted cells and interacts with nearby receptors. Transplanted embryonic cells may also release factors that exert a neurotrophic influence on cells in the damaged brain. Some transplanted neurons may actually form synaptic connections with neurons of the host animal. The embryonic surface adhesion molecules of the grafted cells could also provide a permissive environment through which damaged host neurons can reconnect with their targets.

A   Flash   B   Electrical stimulation

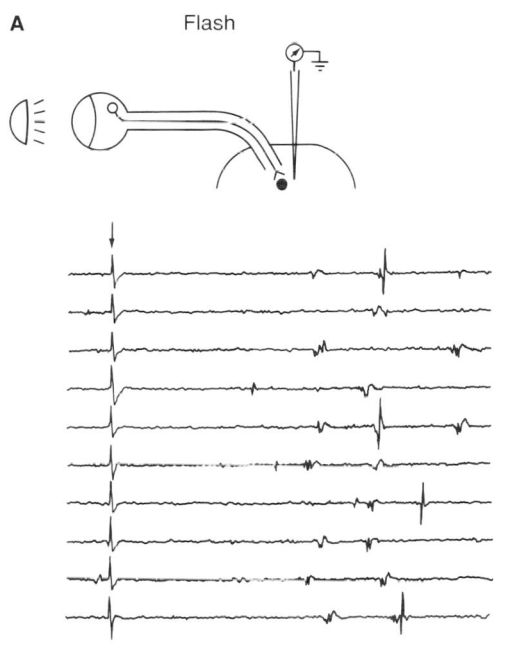

20 msec

FIGURE 18–9

Regenerating retinal axons can form functional connections with target neurons in the brain. Recordings are from the superior colliculus of a hamster with a peripheral nerve graft directed from the eye to the superior colliculus.

A. A single unit 250 μm below the surface of the superior colliculus responds to light flashes to the eye (**arrow**) with a single spike in 4 of 10 successive trials.

B. The same unit responds erratically with inconstant latency to a single electrical stimulus (**arrow**) delivered to the peripheral nerve graft (**trace 1**), but responds with a more constant latency, often with multiple spikes, to paired electrical stimuli (**arrows**) of the same intensity (**trace 2**). This pattern of response, reflecting postsynaptic summation of subthreshold EPSPs, is inconsistent with that expected from a retinal ganglion cell axon and thus identifies this unit as a superior colliculus neuron. (From Keirstead et al., 1989.)

FIGURE 18–10

Fetal neurons form synaptic connections after transplantation into the adult brain. (From Freund et al., 1985.)

A. Transplanted dopaminergic neurons (**arrows**) can be visualized in the light microscope by labeling with antibodies to tyrosine hydroxylase. Scale bar = 20 μM.

B. Tyrosine hydroxylase is seen in this electron micrograph of a nerve terminal formed by a grafted embryonic neuron. The terminal makes synaptic contact with the dendrite of an adult striatal neuron (**ds**, dendrite shaft; **s**, spine). Scale bar = 0.2 μM.

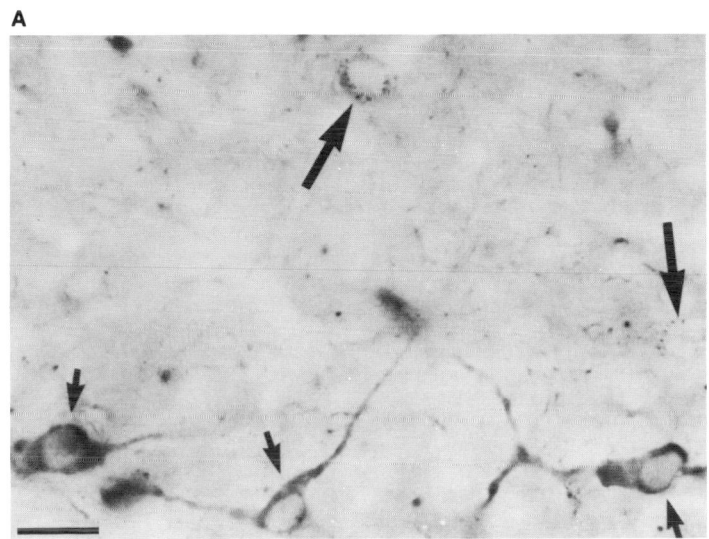

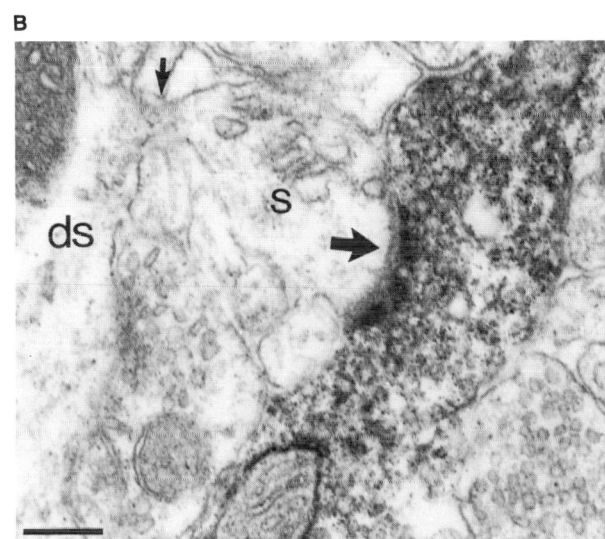

In Some Animals New Neurons Can Be Generated in the Adult Brain

Neurogenesis ceases early in the development of the mammalian brain, but persists into adulthood in some vertebrates, such as fish and birds. For example, Fernando Nottebohm and his colleagues found that the number of neurons in certain nuclei in the brains of adult songbirds changes cyclically on a seasonal basis. Studies using [^{3}H]thymidine as a marker of DNA synthesis have revealed that in the adult new neurons are born in the ventricular zone of the telencephalon and then migrate through the adult brain over considerable distances; moreover, these neurons generate action potentials and display normal synaptic potentials, raising the possibility that they may be integrated into neuronal circuits. Hormonal factors probably regulate the differentiation of these late-developing neurons. Elucidation of the detailed mechanisms that regulate the appearance and migration of new neurons in the adult brain may enable us to find out whether a similar capacity exists in the brain of adult mammals and, if so, whether cells can be induced to differentiate into neurons and rebuild functional neuronal circuits.

An Overall View

Considerable information on the contributions of particular neurons and groups of neurons to behavior has been gathered from analyses of both accidental and experimental lesions in the nervous system. The information gained in this way illustrates again a fundamental principle of the nervous system—that the behavioral role of a nerve cell is determined by its location in the brain and by its connections. Similar injuries have very different behavioral consequences depending on which neurons they affect.

The reactions of neurons to injury vary dramatically. A neuron may survive if it is able to restore functional connections after its axon is cut. If its connections with target cells are not restored, it will atrophy and die. The capacity of mammalian central neurons to regenerate axons after damage decreases dramatically in early postnatal stages of development, after which it is poor or nonexistent.

In the past decade there has been progress in four different areas of research directed at ameliorating the devastating loss of function in adult central nervous systems following damage. First, studies on the mechanisms underlying initial axonal overgrowth have characterized many cell-surface and extracellular molecules that promote axon growth. These molecules, such as laminin and fibronectin, are usually absent from the mature central nervous system. Inducing reexpression of these molecules in the environment of damaged central axons may be one way of promoting axon regeneration.

Second, it is becoming apparent that trophic factors produced by target cells are important in maintaining neurons. Deprivation of these factors contributes to the degeneration of neurons after injury. One such factor, NGF, has been well characterized, and other factors are likely to serve similar functions. Third, it is possible to promote

recovery of function in experimental animals by transplantation of peripheral nerve tissue, immature central nervous system glial cells, or embryonic neurons.

Finally, neurons can be generated from undifferentiated progenitor cells in the brain of some adult nonmammalian vertebrates. The underlying mechanisms of such differentiation are not understood well enough to determine whether cells in the adult mammalian central nervous system have a similar potential. Further exploration of this question may provide insights into both neuronal differentiation and regeneration.

Selected Readings

Aguayo, A. J., Bray, G. M., Rasminsky, M., Zwimpfer, T., Carter, D., and Vidal-Sanz, M. 1991. Synaptic connections made by axons regenerating in the CNS of adult mammals. J. Exp. Biol. In press.

Bray, G. M., Villegas-Pérez, M. P., Vidal-Sanz, M., and Aguayo, A. J. 1987. The use of peripheral nerve grafts to enhance neuronal survival, promote growth and permit terminal reconnections in the central nervous system of adults rats. J. Exp. Biol. 132: 5–19.

Dunnett, S. B., and Björklund, A. 1987. Mechanisms of function of neural grafts in the adult mammalian brain. J. Exp. Biol. 132:265–289.

Gage, F. H., and Fisher, L. J. 1991. Intracerebral grafting: A tool for the neurobiologist. Neuron 6:1–12.

Grafstein, B. 1983. Chromatolysis reconsidered: A new view of the reaction of the nerve cell body to axon injury. In F. J. Seil (ed.), Nerve, Organ, and Tissue Regeneration: Research Perspectives. New York: Academic Press, pp. 37–50.

Johnson, E. M., Jr., Taniuchi, M., and DiStefano, P. S. 1988. Expression and possible function of nerve growth factor receptors on Schwann cells. Trends Neurosci. 11:299–304.

Lieberman, A. R. 1971. The axon reaction: A review of the principal features of perikaryal responses to axon injury. Int. Rev. Neurobiol. 14:49–124.

Mendell, L. M., Munson, J. B., and Scott, J. G. 1976. Alterations of synapses on axotomized motoneurones. J. Physiol. (Lond.) 255:67–79.

Paton, J. A., and Nottebohm, F. N. 1984. Neurons generated in the adult brain are recruited into functional circuits. Science 225:1046–1048.

Perry, V. H. and Gordon, S. 1988. Macrophages and microglia in the nervous system. Trends Neurosci. 11:273–277.

Schwab, M. E. 1990. Myelin-associated inhibitors of neurite growth. Exp. Neurol. 109:2–5.

References

Alvarez-Buylla, A., and Nottebohm, F. 1988. Migration of young neurons in adult avian brain. Nature 335:353–354.

Freund, T. F., Bolam, J. P., Björklund, A., Stenevi, U., Dunnett, S. B., Powell, J. F., and Smith, A. D. 1985. Efferent synaptic connections of grafted dopaminergic neurons reinnervating the host neostriatum: A tyrosine hydroxylase immunocytochemical study. J. Neurosci. 5:603–616.

Hefti, F. 1986. Nerve growth factor promotes survival of septal cholinergic neurons after fimbrial transections. J. Neurosci. 6:2155–2162.

Heumann, R., Korsching, S., Bandtlow, C., and Thoenen, H. 1987. Changes of nerve growth factor synthesis in nonneuronal cells in response to sciatic nerve transection. J. Cell Biol. 104:1623–1631.

Kalil, K., and Skene, J. H. P. 1986. Elevated synthesis of an axonally transported protein correlates with axon outgrowth in normal and injured pyramidal tracts. J. Neurosci 6:2563–2570.

Keirstead, S. A., Rasminsky, M., Fukuda, Y., Carter, D. A., Aguayo, A. J., and Vidal-Sanz, M. 1989. Electrophysiologic responses in hamster superior colliculus evoked by regenerating retinal axons. Science 246:255–257.

Le Gros Clark, W. E., and Penman, G. G. 1934. The projection of the retina in the lateral geniculate body. Proc. R. Soc. Lond. [Biol.] 114:291–313.

Lindholm, D., Heumann, R., Meyer, M., and Thoenen, H. 1987. Interleukin-1 regulates synthesis of nerve growth factor in non-neuronal cells of rat sciatic nerve. Nature 330:658–659.

Martin, D. P., Schmidt, R. E., DiStefano, P. S., Lowry, O. H., Carter, J. G., and Johnson, E. M., Jr. 1988. Inhibitors of protein synthesis and RNA synthesis prevent neuronal death caused by nerve growth factor deprivation. J. Cell. Biol. 106:829–844.

Matthews, M. R., and Nelson, V. H. 1975. Detachment of structurally intact nerve endings from chromatolytic neurones of rat superior cervical ganglion during the depression of synaptic transmission induced by post-ganglionic axotomy. J. Physiol. (Lond.) 245:91–135.

Meiri, K. F., Pfenninger, K. H., and Willard, M. B. 1986. Growth-associated protein, GAP-43, a polypeptide that is induced when neurons extend axons, is a component of growth cones and corresponds to pp46, a major polypeptide of a subcellular fraction enriched in growth cones. Proc. Natl. Acad. Sci. U.S.A. 83:3537–3541.

Njå, A., and Purves, D. 1978. The effects of nerve growth factor and its antiserum on synapses in the superior cervical ganglion of the guinea-pig. J. Physiol (Lond.) 277:53–75.

Perry, V. H., Brown, M. C., and Gordon, S. 1987. The macrophage response to central and peripheral nerve injury: A possible role for macrophages in regeneration. J. Exp. Med. 165:1218–1223.

Rich, K. M., Luszczynski, J. R., Osborne, P. A., and Johnson, E. M., Jr. 1987. Nerve growth factor protects adult sensory neurons from cell death and atrophy caused by nerve injury. J. Neurocytol. 16:261–268.

Schnell, L., and Schwab, M. E. 1990. Axonal regeneration in the rat spinal cord produced by an antibody against myelin-associated neurite growth inhibitors. Nature 343:269–272.

Smith, G. M., Miller, R. H., and Silver, J. 1986. Changing role of forebrain astrocytes during development, regenerative failure, and induced regeneration upon transplantation. J. Comp. Neurol. 251:23–43.

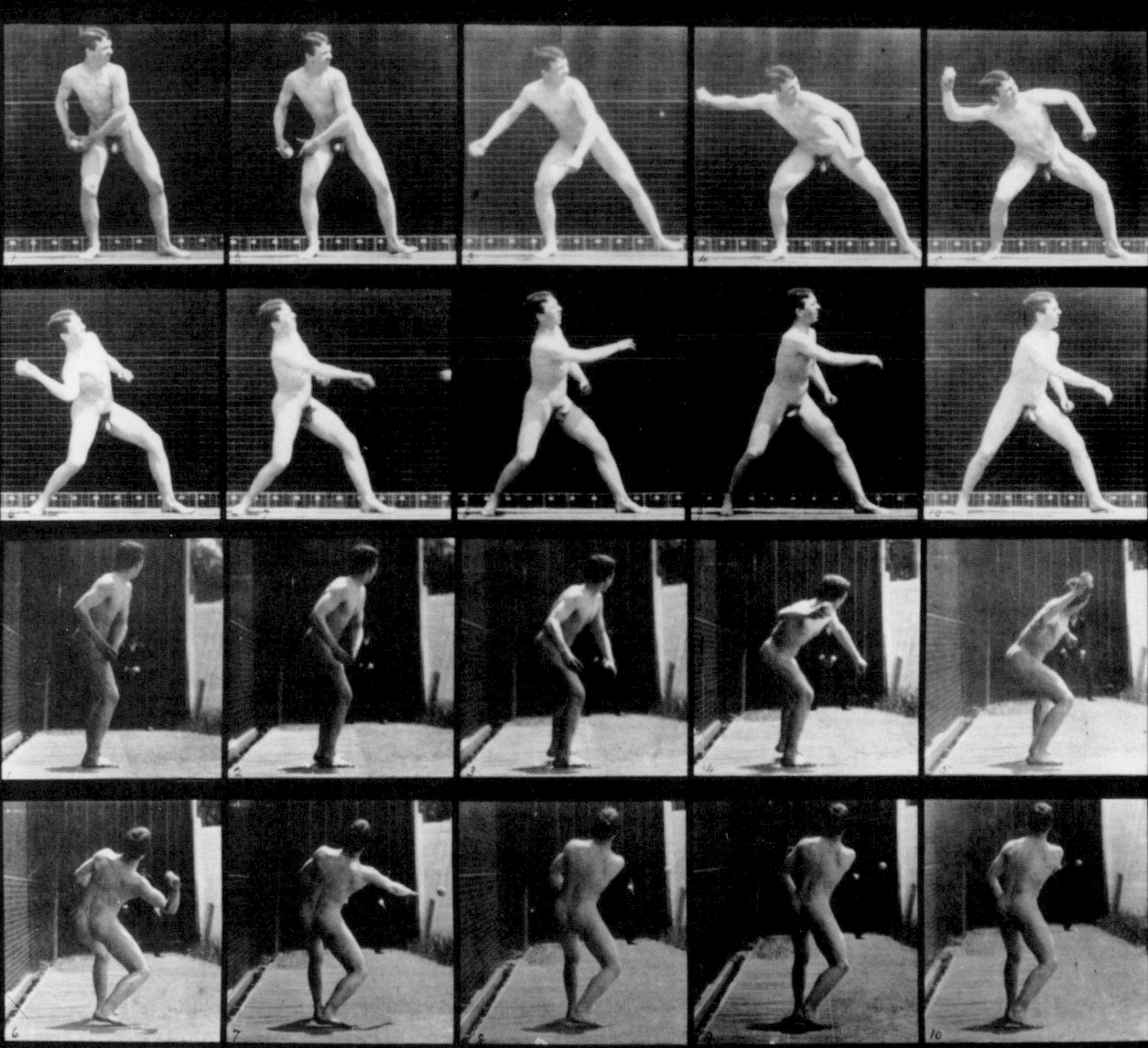

IV

Functional Anatomy of the Central Nervous System

In the same way that the detailed structure of proteins reveals important principles of protein function, knowledge of neuroanatomy, seemingly a static science, can provide profound insight into how the nervous system functions. Many of the prevailing ideas about the dynamic mechanisms involved in the development of connectivity in the nervous system were forecast a century ago by Ramón y Cajal on the basis of Golgi images of neurons in histological specimens. Today, much of our understanding of higher brain function depends on refined mapping of neuronal circuits with new anatomical and imaging techniques.

Indeed, many of the established properties of neuronal connectivity were first discovered by classical anatomy methods. Golgi staining first showed the existence of two major classes of nerve cells in the brain: projection neurons, whose axons connect the major regions of the nervous system, and local interneurons, which integrate information within specific nuclei of the brain. Next, trac-

ing techniques demonstrated the considerable convergence and divergence of projections between brain regions. Convergent pathways permit a given region of the brain to integrate the input it receives for different sensory systems. Divergent pathways permit small groups of cells to exert widespread influence on many different brain regions.

The introduction of electron microscopic methods to neuroanatomy in the 1950s revealed the structure of synapses, and illustrated that different classes of neurons form synapses with quite different features. Some synaptic terminals are located on dendrites, others on axon terminals, and still others on the soma of the postsynaptic cell. The location of the synapse on the neuronal surface affects the function of the cell in almost as critical a way as the organization of neuronal connections.

Modern neuroanatomical labeling techniques have also defined the principles by which neural circuits are organized. For example, the topographic organization of pro-

In 1872 Eadweard Muybridge, the photographer, was engaged by the University of Pennsylvania to study how people and animals move. This research, conducted in an open-air studio in the courtyard of the Veterinary Hall and Hospital, was supported by subscription to the resulting publication, *Animal Locomotion: An Electro-Photographic Investigation of Consecutive Phases of Animal Movements*. This work was published

in 1887 in 11 volumes and contained 781 collotype plates. These photographs show a man throwing a ball. Muybridge set up cameras at several different locations in order to catch multiple, simultaneous aspects of the moving subject. These images influenced many modern artists, dancers, and writers. (Original print courtesy of International Museum of Photography at George Eastman House, Rochester, New York.)

jections from one brain region to the next—maintaining the spatial relationship of inputs from the periphery in neighboring groups of neurons in the brain—ensures efficient coding of spatial information within the brain.

Modern imaging techniques have revolutionized the study of higher brain functions and placed neurology and psychiatry within reach of the methods of cell biology. The introduction of positron emission tomography (PET) and magnetic resonance imaging (MRI) has made the functional neuroanatomy of the living human brain accessible during behavioral experiments. As a consequence we now have a much clearer idea of the brain regions involved in many complex cognitive functions.

In this section we first examine the anatomical organization of the three functional systems within the nervous system: sensory, motor, and motivational. We then take a closer look at the structural organization of the central nervous system by following the flow of sensory information from the periphery into the spinal cord and brain, its transformation into a motor command, and the course of that command to the effector organ. In later sections of the book we shall explore each functional system of the brain in detail, examining how its specific structure and interconnections determine its particular function.

Because the three-dimensional structure of the brain has become important for accurate diagnosis of neurological and psychiatric disorders, we also examine how the brain develops. In the last chapter in this section we describe modern brain imaging techniques that reveal function in the living brain. These imaging techniques also are important diagnostic tools for diseases of the central nervous system.

PART IV

Chapter 19: Anatomical Organization of the Nervous System
Chapter 20: The Neural Basis of Perception and Movement
Chapter 21: Development as a Guide to the Regional Anatomy of the Brain
Chapter 22: Imaging the Living Brain

James P. Kelly
Jane Dodd

19

Anatomical Organization of the Nervous System

The Nervous System Has Peripheral and Central Components
The Peripheral Nervous System
The Central Nervous System

The Central Nervous System Consists of Six Main Regions

The Cerebral Cortex Is Divided into Four Lobes Concerned with Different Functions

The Motivational System Influences Behavior by Acting on the Somatic and Autonomic Motor Systems

Even Simple Behavior Involves the Activity of the Sensory, Motor, and Motivational Systems

Four Principles Govern the Organization of the Major Functional Systems
Each System Contains Synaptic Relays
Each System Is Composed of Several Distinct Pathways
Each Pathway Is Topographically Organized
Most Pathways Cross the Midline

An Overall View

To understand behavior it is necessary to appreciate how the nervous system is organized functionally and anatomically. The architecture of the nervous system, although complex, is governed by a relatively simple set of functional, organizational, and developmental principles. Taken together, these principles bring order to the myriad details of brain anatomy. In this chapter we shall first review the major parts of the peripheral and central nervous systems and then consider how the *functional systems* for perception, motor coordination, and motivation interact during a simple behavioral act. We shall then discuss four general principles that underlie the *anatomical organization* of these systems. In Chapter 21 we shall examine the *developmental principles* that underlie the structure of the brain.

The Nervous System Has Peripheral and Central Components

The nervous system has two components: the *central nervous system*, which is composed of the brain and the spinal cord, and the *peripheral nervous system*, which is composed of ganglia and peripheral nerves that lie outside the brain and spinal cord. The central and peripheral nervous systems are separated anatomically. Functionally they are interconnected and interactive.

The Peripheral Nervous System

The peripheral nervous system has two divisions, *somatic* and *autonomic*. The somatic division includes sensory neurons of the dorsal root and cranial ganglia that innervate the skin, muscles, and joints and provide sensory information to the central nervous system about muscle and limb position and about the environment outside the body. The axons of somatic motor neurons that innervate skeletal muscle and which project to the periphery are often considered part of the somatic division, even though their cell bodies are part of the central nervous system.

The autonomic division of the peripheral nervous system is the motor system for the viscera, the smooth muscles of the body, and exocrine glands. It consists of three spatially segregated subdivisions: the *sympathetic* system, the *parasympathetic* system, and the *enteric* nervous system. The sympathetic system participates in the response of the body to stress, whereas the parasympathetic system acts to conserve the body's resources and restore homeostasis. The enteric nervous system controls the function of smooth muscle of the gut. The organization and function of these three components of the autonomic nervous system are described in detail in Chapter 49.

The Central Nervous System

The central nervous system is organized along two major axes that are established early in development—a longitudinal rostral-to-caudal axis and a dorsal-to-ventral axis. In lower vertebrates the orientation of both axes is maintained into adult life, whereas in primates the longitudinal axis of the nervous system flexes during development (Figure 19–1). Because of this flexure several different terms are used to describe the orientation of structures in the mature human brain. In the spinal cord *rostral* means toward the head, *caudal* means toward the coccyx (Latin *cauda*, tail), *ventral* toward the belly, and *dorsal* toward the back. Above the flexure, in the brain, *rostral* means toward the nose, *caudal* toward the back of the head, *ventral* toward the jaw, and *dorsal* toward the top of the

FIGURE 19–1
The long axis of the nervous system bends as a result of flexure in the rostral brain stem.

A. 1. In lower vertebrates the central nervous system is organized along a straight line. **2.** In humans the central nervous system has a flexure at the junction between the midbrain and the diencephalon. Thus, in the cerebral hemisphere and upper brain stem the directions denoted by the terms *rostral, caudal, dorsal,* and *ventral* are different from those denoted in the spinal cord. Above

the diencephalon *rostral* means toward the nose, *caudal* toward the back of the head, *ventral* toward the jaw, and *dorsal* toward the top of the skull. At all levels of the nervous system the neuraxis is the longitudinal (rostral to caudal) axis.

B. In embryogenesis the neural tube forms the spinal cord and the brain vesicles that give rise to the mature brain. The brain vesicles are illustrated in a straightened-out view of the neural tube (**1**), and the flexures are illustrated in a side view (**2**).

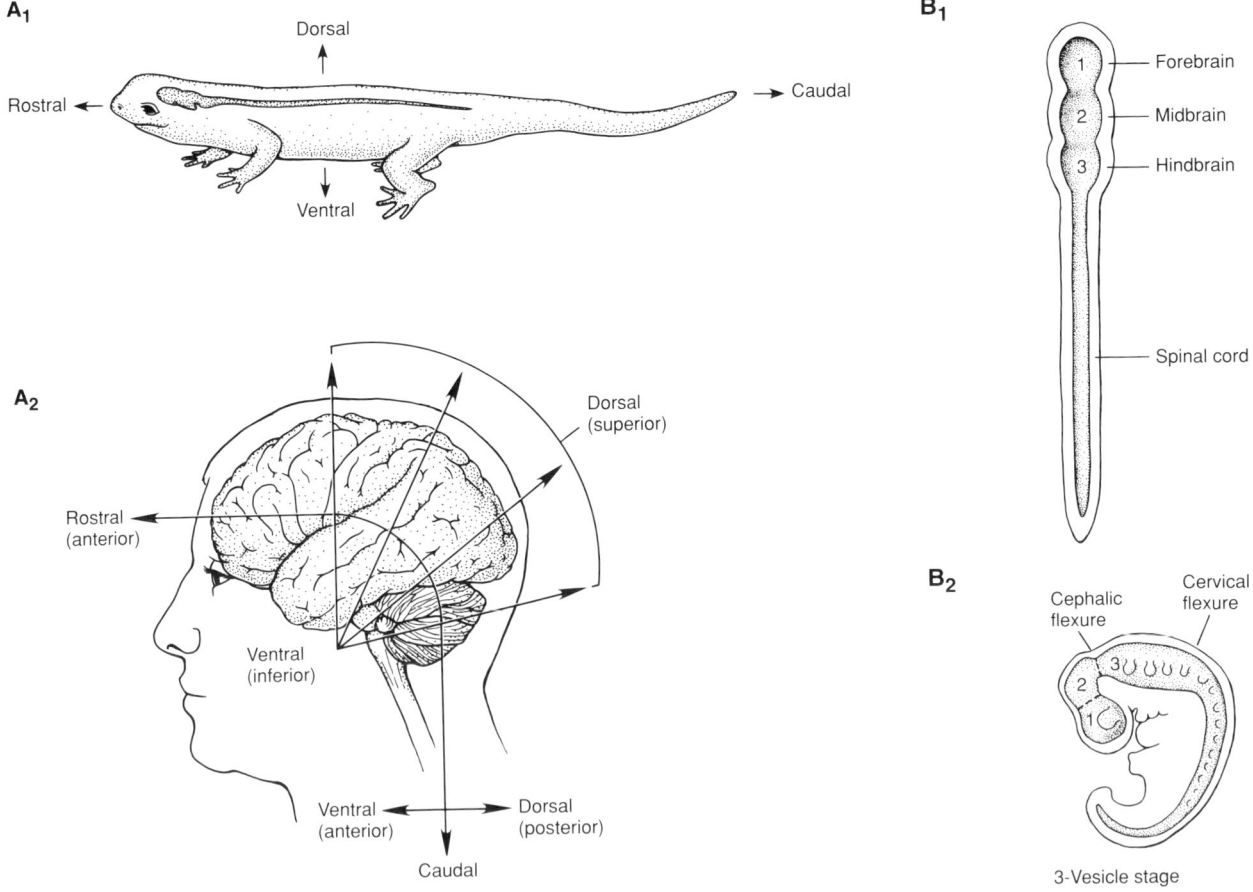

A₁

Dorsal

Rostral   Caudal

Ventral

A₂

Dorsal (superior)

Rostral (anterior)

Ventral (inferior)

Ventral (anterior)   Dorsal (posterior)

Caudal

B₁

1 — Forebrain
2 — Midbrain
3 — Hindbrain

Spinal cord

B₂

Cephalic flexure   Cervical flexure

3-Vesicle stage

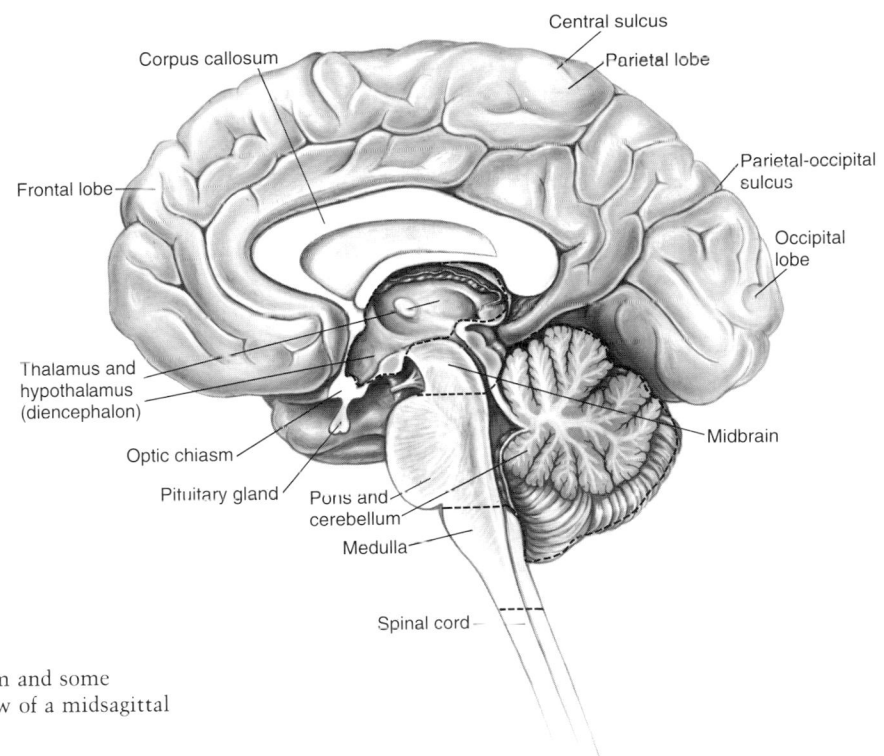

Corpus callosum

Central sulcus

Parietal lobe

Parietal-occipital sulcus

Occipital lobe

Frontal lobe

Thalamus and hypothalamus (diencephalon)

Midbrain

Optic chiasm

Pituitary gland

Pons and cerebellum

Medulla

Spinal cord

FIGURE 19–2
The major parts of the central nervous system and some important landmarks as seen in a medial view of a midsagittal section.

head. The terms *superior* (instead of *dorsal*) and *inferior* (instead of *ventral*) are also used to describe the relative positions of structures.

The Central Nervous System Consists of Six Main Regions

As described in Chapter 1, the adult central nervous system can be divided into six anatomical regions, each of which develops from a distinct division of the neural tube (Chapter 21). The six major divisions are: (1) the spinal cord; (2) the medulla; (3) the pons and cerebellum; (4) the midbrain; (5) the diencephalon; and (6) the cerebral hemispheres (Figure 19–2). Each of the six divisions is bilaterally paired.

1. The *spinal cord*, the simplest and most caudal part of the central nervous system, resembles the embryonic neural tube. It extends from the base of the skull through the first lumbar vertebra, and thus does not run the entire length of the *vertebral column*. The spinal cord receives sensory information from the skin, joints, and muscles of the trunk and limbs, and in turn contains the motor neurons responsible for both voluntary and reflex movements. It also receives sensory information from the internal organs and has clusters of neurons that control many visceral functions.

The spinal cord has a clear external segmentation evidenced in humans by 31 pairs of *spinal nerves*. The spinal nerves are peripheral nerves formed by the joining of the dorsal and ventral roots. The *dorsal roots* carry sensory information into the spinal cord from the muscles, skin, and viscera. The *ventral roots* carry outgoing motor axons that innervate muscles and preganglionic sympathetic and parasympathetic axons. Within the spinal cord there is an orderly arrangement of sensory cell groups that receive input from the periphery and motor cell groups that control specific muscle groups. In addition to these cell groups, the spinal cord contains ascending pathways through which sensory information reaches the brain and descending pathways that relay motor commands from the brain to motor neurons.

The next three divisions of the central nervous system—the medulla, the pons and cerebellum, and the midbrain—are collectively termed the *brain stem*. The brain stem is located rostral to the spinal cord. The sensory input and motor output of the brain stem is carried by *cranial nerves*, which are functionally analogous to spinal nerves. Whereas the spinal cord mediates sensation and motor control of the trunk and limbs, the brain stem is concerned with sensation from skin and joints in the head, neck, and face, as well as with specialized senses, such as hearing, taste, and balance. Motor neurons in the brain stem control the muscles of the head and neck. The brain stem also contains ascending and descending pathways that carry sensory and motor information to and from higher brain regions. In addition, a network of neurons in the brain stem, extending through the medulla, pons, and midbrain and known as the *reticular formation*, mediates aspects of arousal.

2. The *medulla* is the direct rostral extension of the spinal cord and resembles the spinal cord in both organization and function. Together with the pons it participates in regulating blood pressure and respiration.

3. The *pons* lies rostral to the medulla and appears as a protuberance from the ventral surface of the brain stem. It contains a large number of neurons that relay information from the cerebral hemispheres to the *cerebellum*. The cerebellum is not generally considered part of the brain stem. However, because many of the motor functions of the pons and cerebellum are closely related, and the cerebellum arises during development from the dorsal aspect of the hindbrain, it is discussed here with the brain stem.

The cerebellum lies dorsal to the pons and the medulla and extends laterally, wrapping around the brain stem. It has a characteristic foliated surface and is divided into several functionally independent lobes separated by distinctive fissures. The cerebellum receives somatosensory input from the spinal cord, motor information from the cerebral cortex, and input about balance from the vestibular organs of the inner ear. Integration of this information in the cerebellum coordinates the planning, timing, and patterning of skeletal muscle contractions during movement. The cerebellum also plays a role in the maintenance of posture and in the coordination of head and eye movements.

4. The *midbrain*, the smallest brain stem component, lies rostral to the pons. Several regions of the midbrain play a dominant role in the direct control of eye movements, whereas others are involved in motor control of skeletal muscles. The midbrain also contains essential relay nuclei of the auditory and visual systems.

5. The thalamus and the hypothalamus together form the *diencephalon*, or *between-brain*, so called because they lie between the cerebral hemispheres and the midbrain. The *thalamus* processes and distributes almost all sensory and motor information going to the cerebral cortex. It is also thought to regulate levels of awareness and emotional aspects of sensory experiences through a wide variety of effects on the cortex. The *hypothalamus* lies ventral to the thalamus and regulates the autonomic nervous system and the hormonal secretion by the pituitary gland. The hypothalamus has extensive afferent and efferent connections with the thalamus, the midbrain, and some cortical areas that receive information from the autonomic nervous system.

6. The *cerebral hemispheres* form by far the largest region of the brain. They consist of the cerebral cortex, the underlying white matter, and three deep-lying nuclei: the basal ganglia, the hippocampal formation, and the amygdala. The cerebral hemispheres are divided by the interhemispheric fissure and are concerned with perceptual, cognitive, and higher motor functions as well as emotion and memory.

The Cerebral Cortex Is Divided into Four Lobes Concerned with Different Functions

The cerebral cortex is the highly convoluted surface of the cerebral hemisphere. Its shape arose during evolution of the primate brain as the volume of the cerebral cortex increased more rapidly than the volume of the cranium. This disparity has resulted both in the convolutions of the cortical surface and in the folding of the structure as a whole (Figure 19–3). These evolutionary changes will be described in the next chapter.

The surface convolutions consist of grooves or *sulci* that separate elevated regions or *gyri*. Certain sulci have a consistent position in all human brains, and thus are used as landmarks to divide the cortex into four lobes. These lobes are named after the overlying cranial bones: *frontal, parietal, temporal,* and *occipital* (Figure 19–4).

Two other areas of cortex represent subdivisions that are comparable to lobes. The *insular cortex* is not visible on the surface of the brain; it occupies the medial wall of the lateral sulcus. The *limbic lobe* consists of the medial portions of the frontal, parietal, and temporal lobes that form a continuous band of cortex overlying the rostral brain stem and diencephalon. The limbic lobe is sometimes termed the *limbic system* because its neurons form complex circuits that collectively play an important role in learning, memory, and emotions.

Many areas of the cerebral cortex process sensory information or integrate cortical output that is important for the control of movement. Some cortical regions are more directly involved than others with sensory information (relayed from the thalamus) or with control of motor neurons (in the brain stem and spinal cord). These areas are known as *primary, secondary,* and *tertiary* sensory or motor areas. For example, the *primary motor cortex,* which lies within the precentral gyrus, contains neurons that project directly to the spinal cord; it mediates voluntary movements of the limbs and trunk because it contains neurons that project directly to the spinal cord to activate motor neurons. The *primary sensory areas* (the visual, auditory, somatic sensory, and gustatory areas) receive information from peripheral receptors with only a few synapses interposed. The *primary visual cortex* is located at the caudal pole of the occipital lobe, predominantly on its medial aspect. The *primary auditory cortex* lies in the temporal lobe, where it makes up a portion of the lower bank of the lateral sulcus. The *primary somatic sensory cortex* lies on the postcentral gyrus.

Surrounding the primary areas are the higher-order (secondary and tertiary) sensory and motor areas. These areas process complex aspects of a single sensory modality or information related to motor function. Higher-order sensory areas integrate information coming from the primary sensory areas. In contrast, higher-order motor areas send complex information required for a motor act to the primary motor cortex. The higher-order areas also include a portion of the posterior parietal lobe called the *posterior parietal cortex*. This region coordinates somatic sensation

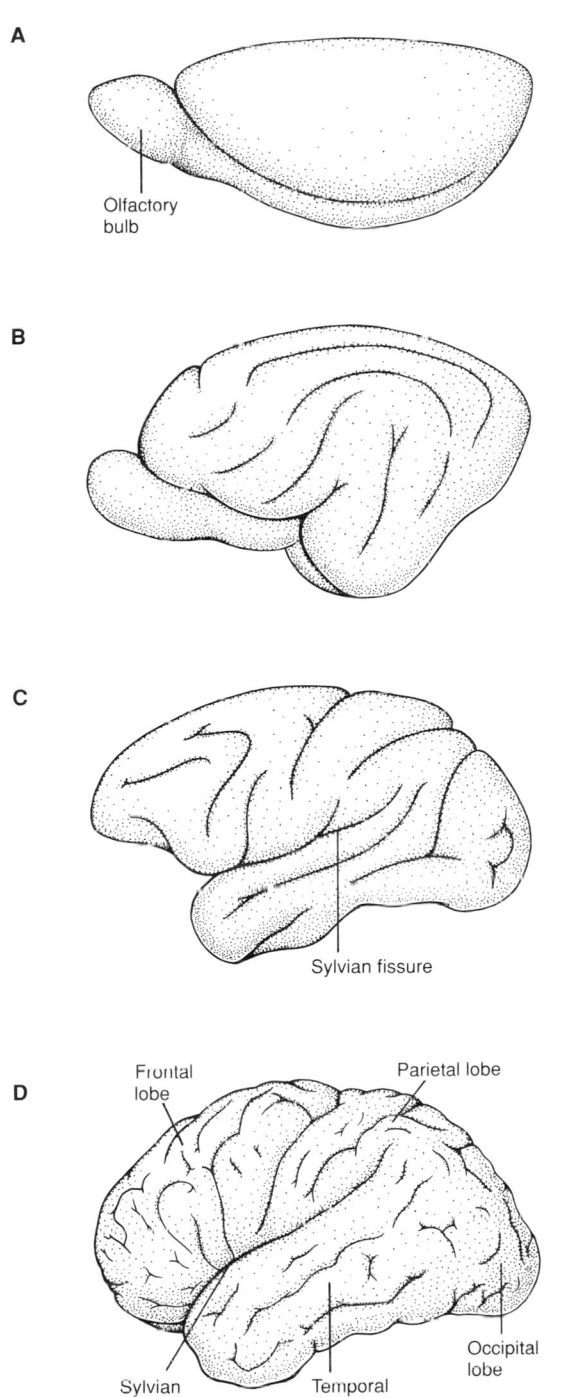

A

Olfactory
bulb

B

C

Sylvian fissure

D

Frontal
lobe

Parietal lobe

Sylvian
fissure

Temporal
lobe

Occipital
lobe

FIGURE 19–3
In the evolution of vertebrates the cerebral hemisphere has folded
into a horseshoe shape, resulting in emergence of the temporal
lobes. In the rat (**A**) the cerebral hemisphere is not folded. In the
cat (**B**) the folding is more evident; the caudal end of the cerebral
hemisphere extends slightly downward. In the monkey (**C**) and
man (**D**) the folding is pronounced: the cerebral hemisphere
curves from the frontal lobe into the temporal lobe, which reaches
forward around the brain stem. (From Nauta and Feirtag, 1986.)

and vision, and integrates aspects of these sensory perceptions with movement.

Three other large regions of cortex, called *association*
areas, lie outside the primary, secondary, and tertiary areas. In primates the association areas constitute by far the
largest area of cortex. Their function is mainly to integrate
diverse information for purposeful action, and they are
involved to different degrees in the control of three major
brain functions: perception, movement, and motivation.
The *parietal–temporal–occipital association cortex* occupies the interface between the three lobes for which it is
named (Figure 19–4B). It is concerned with higher perceptual functions related to somatic sensation, hearing, and
vision, the primary sensory inputs to these lobes. Information from these different sensory modalities is combined in the association cortex to form complex
perceptions. The *prefrontal association cortex* occupies
most of the rostral part of the frontal lobe; one important
function of this area is the planning of voluntary movement. The *limbic association cortex* is located on the medial and inferior surfaces of the cerebral hemispheres, in
portions of the parietal, frontal, and temporal lobes; it is
devoted mainly to motivation, emotion, and memory. The
organization of the association areas of the cortex is considered in greater detail in Chapter 53.

To summarize, the primary sensory areas of the cerebral cortex are devoted to the reception and initial cortical
processing of sensory information. The primary areas project to higher-order sensory areas that further elaborate
and process sensory input. The higher-order areas connect
to the association areas; these provide the link between
sensation and action by making connections with the
higher-order motor areas. The higher-order motor areas, in
turn, project to the primary motor cortex, which exerts
direct control over motor neurons.

Finally, three other, deep-lying structures are part of
the cerebral hemispheres: the basal ganglia, the hippocampus, and the amygdala. All three lie deep within the
cerebral cortex and its underlying white matter. The major components of the *basal ganglia* are the caudate nucleus and the putamen (together known as the corpus
striatum) and the globus pallidus. The basal ganglia have
an important role in the regulation of movement and also
contribute to cognition. They receive input from all four
lobes of the cerebral cortex but have efferent projections
only to the frontal cortex, via the thalamus.

The *hippocampus* and *amygdala* are part of the limbic
system. The hippocampus is involved in memory storage.
The amygdala coordinates the actions of the autonomic
and endocrine systems and is involved in emotions. While
the pathways that control the emotional quality of sensation or motor behavior are not understood completely, the
limbic system and the autonomic nervous system are
thought to participate in emotion because damage to these
areas affects emotional expression. By means of direct connections with the hypothalamus, the limbic system modulates the activity of the autonomic nervous system,
coordinating visceral responses (such as blood pressure,

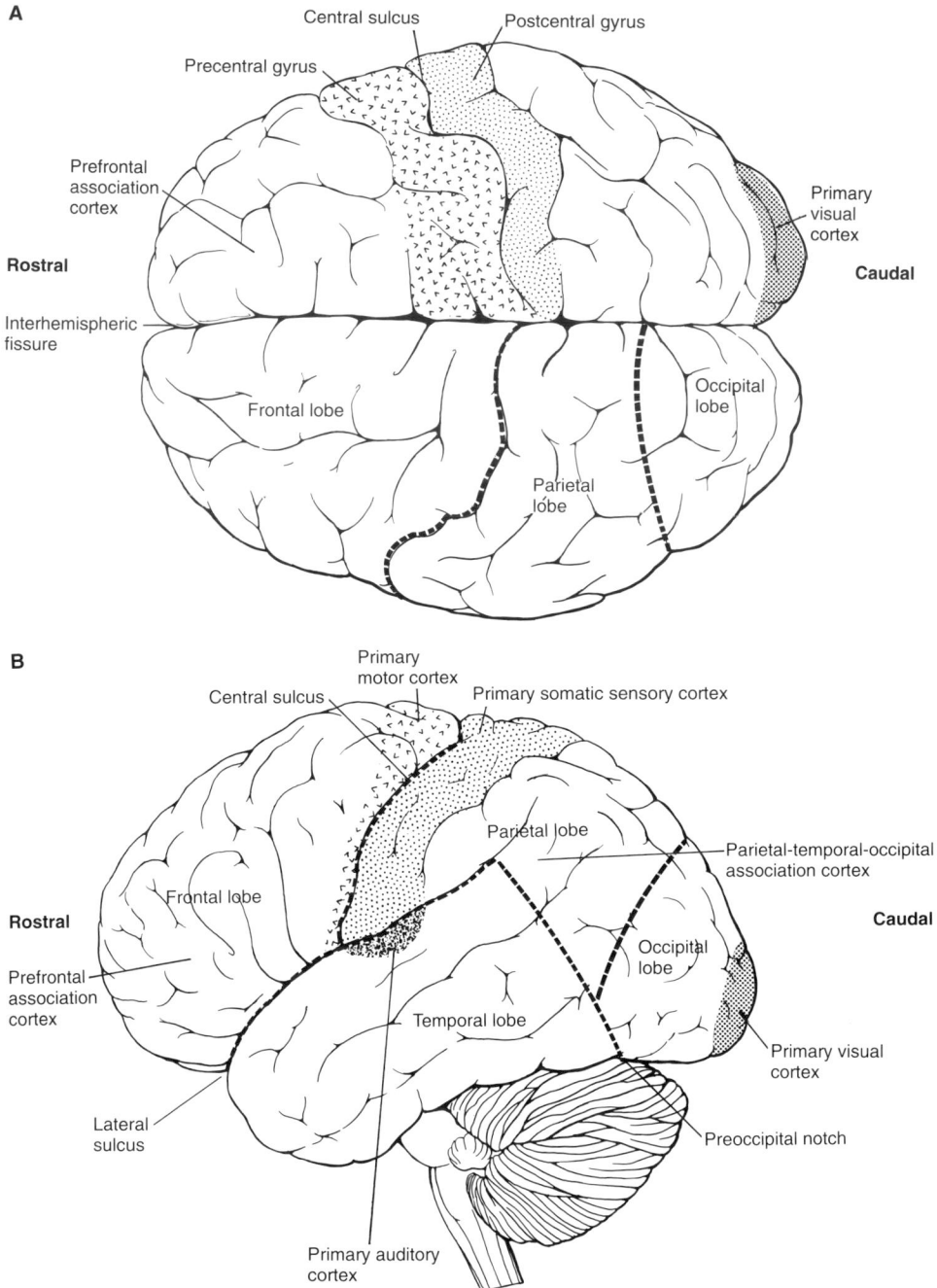

A

Central sulcus

Postcentral gyrus

Precentral gyrus

Prefrontal association cortex

Primary visual cortex

Rostral

Caudal

Interhemispheric fissure

Frontal lobe

Occipital lobe

Parietal lobe

B

Primary motor cortex

Central sulcus

Primary somatic sensory cortex

Parietal lobe

Parietal-temporal-occipital association cortex

Frontal lobe

Rostral

Caudal

Prefrontal association cortex

Occipital lobe

Temporal lobe

Primary visual cortex

Lateral sulcus

Preoccipital notch

Primary auditory cortex

FIGURE 19–4

The major divisions of the human cerebral cortex. The four lobes of the cerebral cortex take their names from the overlying bones of the skull: frontal, parietal, occipital, and temporal. The cortex of each lobe is thrown into folds, or *gyri*, separated by grooves called *sulci*. The boundaries between the lobes are defined somewhat arbitrarily along the lines of certain of the major sulci.

A. This dorsal view of the brain shows the separation of the cerebral hemispheres by the interhemispheric fissure. The central sulcus defines the border between the frontal and parietal lobes. The precentral gyrus, which contains the motor cortex, lies in the frontal lobe; the postcentral gyrus, which contains the somatic sensory cortex, lies in the parietal lobe. The occipital lobe, at the

caudal end of the hemisphere, contains the visual cortex. The temporal lobe, which lies ventrally, is not visible in this view of the brain.

B. A lateral view of the left hemisphere shows the locations of the primary sensory and motor areas and the various association areas of the four lobes. The primary auditory cortex, near the junction of the temporal and parietal lobes, lies within the Sylvian fissure and is hidden from view. Two large association areas are visible: the prefrontal association cortex and the parietal–temporal–occipital association cortex. The most prominent cleft visible in a lateral view of the brain is the Sylvian fissure, which separates the temporal lobe from the frontal and parietal lobes.

heart rate, and pupillary size) with motivational state. Because it regulates the release of hypothalamic hormones, the limbic system also exercises a major control over the endocrine systems of the body.

The Motivational System Influences Behavior by Acting on the Somatic and Autonomic Motor Systems

Voluntary movement is controlled by complex neural circuits in the brain interconnecting the sensory and motor systems. Although all voluntary movement is controlled directly by the motor system, the decision to initiate a voluntary movement is regulated by the motivational system. We reach for a glass of water if we are thirsty or a piece of fruit if we are hungry. The motivational system influences voluntary movement by acting on the somatic motor system in the brain. In addition, it influences behavior through its action on the *autonomic nervous system*, which innervates the exocrine glands, the viscera, and smooth muscles in all organs of the body. As we have seen, the autonomic nervous system has three major divisions: *sympathetic*, *parasympathetic*, and *enteric*. The sympathetic and parasympathetic divisions, which regulate the body's basic physiology, also mediate motivational and emotional states.

The main control center for the autonomic motor system is the hypothalamus, which is also critically involved in the regulation of endocrine hormone release. The hypothalamus sends out descending fibers that regulate sympathetic and parasympathetic nuclei in the spinal cord and brain stem. It receives information from many other structures, including the cerebral cortex and the reticular formation of the brain stem. The activity of the hypothalamus is also influenced by the blood concentrations of insulin and glucose. Thus, in its role as central governor of the autonomic motor system the hypothalamus directly regulates autonomic output and endocrine function and is responsive to a broad spectrum of behaviorally important stimuli.

Even Simple Behavior Involves the Activity of the Sensory, Motor, and Motivational Systems

To see how the sensory, motor, and motivational systems interact to produce purposeful behavior, let us examine the simple behavior of catching a ball. For this task several modalities of sensation processed by *sensory systems* are called into play: visual information about the motion of the ball, tactile information about the impact of the ball in the hand, and proprioceptive information about the position of the arms, legs, and trunk in space. Sensory information is fed to association areas of the cortex, where the movement is planned. From there, information is transmitted to the *motor system*, which generates commands for movements involved in anticipating, catching, and

holding the ball. These motor commands from the brain must be targeted to the correct muscles in the back, shoulder, arm, and hand. They must also be timed so that contraction and relaxation of appropriate muscle groups are coordinated, and they must regulate body posture as a whole. Finally, the motor systems are able to regulate motor performance based on continuous sensory information from the muscles about changes in muscular tension.

Whereas the sensory and motor systems are important in actually catching the ball, the stimulus to initiate and complete the behavior is provided by the *motivational system*. The motivational or limbic system modulates the motor output to skeletal muscles. How well the ball is caught may depend on whether the catcher is excited, bored, or distracted. The motivational system also coordinates the activities of the somatic and the autonomic motor systems. Thus, the same motivational system that modulates the activity of the skeletal motor system also controls the physiological signs of excitement, such as sweating and an increase in heart rate.

The major motor and sensory systems in the brain and spinal cord that process sensory information from the arm and control arm muscles are indicated in Figure 19–5. The interactions of these systems with the motivational system are summarized in Figure 19–6. In later chapters we shall see how separate neural pathways in the three major systems work together to produce appropriate motor responses to sensory stimuli.

Four Principles Govern the Organization of the Major Functional Systems

Each System Contains Synaptic Relays

The sensory, motor, and motivational systems are interrupted, usually at several points, by synaptic relays. These relays are not simple one-to-one connections between presynaptic and postsynaptic neurons within a system. Rather, neural information is modified by synaptic interactions between neurons in the relay nucleus itself and by synaptic inputs from higher centers in the system that converge on the relay nucleus to regulate the flow of information through it.

Relay nuclei typically contain several types of neurons, two of which are particularly important. (1) *Local inter neurons* have axons that are confined to the area of the relay nucleus itself. They mediate local excitatory and inhibitory synaptic interactions. (2) *Projection* (or *principal*) *interneurons* transmit the output of the nucleus. These neurons have long axons that leave the nucleus to synapse upon cells in other nuclei or in the cortex.

Synaptic relays are found throughout the spinal cord and brain, but perhaps the most prominent relay structure is the thalamus. The thalamus is actually a collection of many functionally distinct nuclei, most of which relay information about sensory input or motor performance to the cerebral cortex. Indeed, almost all of the sensory in-

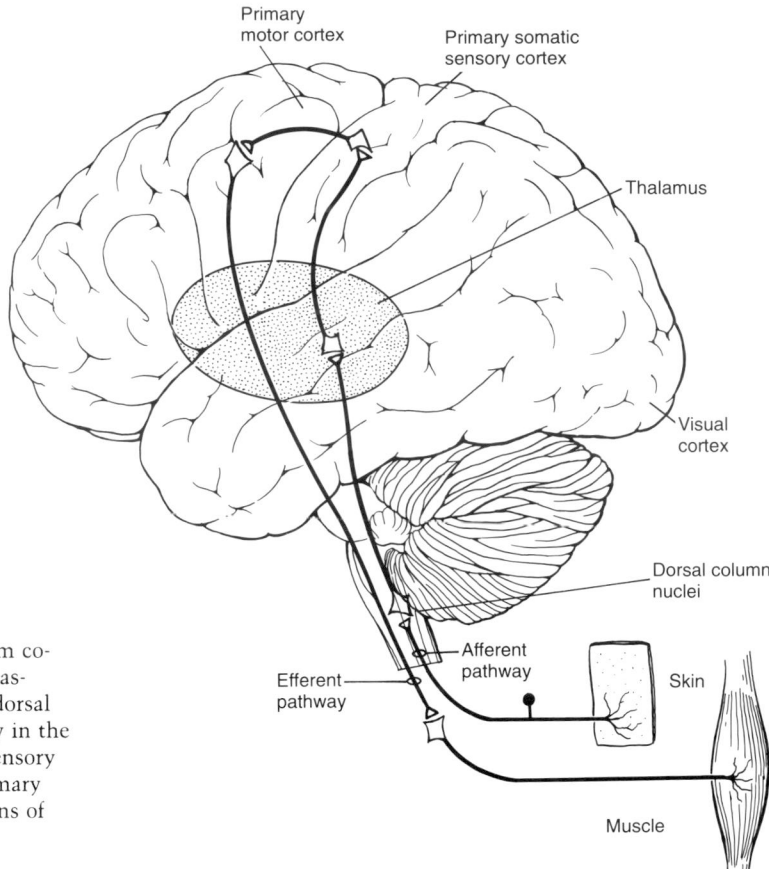

FIGURE 19–5

The major somatic sensory systems and the motor system co-operate to carry out most behavioral acts. Sensory input ascends through the spinal cord to a synaptic relay in the dorsal column nuclei of the brain stem, then to a synaptic relay in the thalamus, and eventually reaches the primary somatic sensory cortex. The direct motor pathway descends from the primary motor cortex through the brain stem to the motor neurons of the spinal cord, and from there to the muscle.

formation that reaches the cerebral cortex is first processed in the thalamus. The cerebral cortex, in turn, sends recurrent axons back to the thalamus.

Each System Is Composed of Several Distinct Pathways

The sensory, motor, and motivational systems each have anatomically and functionally distinct subsystems that perform specialized tasks. For example, each sensory modality (hearing, vision, touch, etc.) is mediated by a separate system. These specialized systems are divided into even more specialized pathways. The visual system, for example, has separate pathways for perceiving stationary objects and tracking moving objects. These pathways work together in the perception of moving objects. Similarly, anatomically separate somatic sensory pathways, such as those for touch and pain, relay information to the cerebral cortex from different receptors in the skin.

The motor system, too, consists of separate specialized pathways, running from the highest centers of information processing in the brain to the spinal cord. For example, the pyramidal tract controls accurate voluntary movements of the fingers and hand, while other motor pathways control overall body posture and regulate spinal reflexes.

Each Pathway Is Topographically Organized

The most striking feature of the sensory systems is that spatial relationships in the peripheral receptive surface—the retina of the eye, the cochlea of the inner ear, or the skin—are preserved throughout the central nervous system. For example, neighboring groups of cells in the retina project upon neighboring groups of cells in the thalamus, which in turn project upon neighboring regions of the visual cortex. In this way a *visuotopic* neural map, an orderly map of the visual field, is retained at each successive level in the brain. Not all parts of the visual field are represented equally in this visuotopic map. The central region of the retina, the area of greatest visual acuity, is represented by a disproportionately large cortical area because of the large number of neurons and synaptic connections involved. Similarly, the body surface is represented by a *somatotopic* neural map in the somatosensory cortex. This map, too, is not a one-to-one representation of receptors in the skin of the body. Regions that are particularly important for sensory discrimination, such as finger tips and lips, have more massive connections in the cortex and thus occupy the largest areas of the cortical map of the body. At each level of the auditory pathway neural codes for particular frequencies of sound excite distinct regions of the relay nuclei, so that the en-

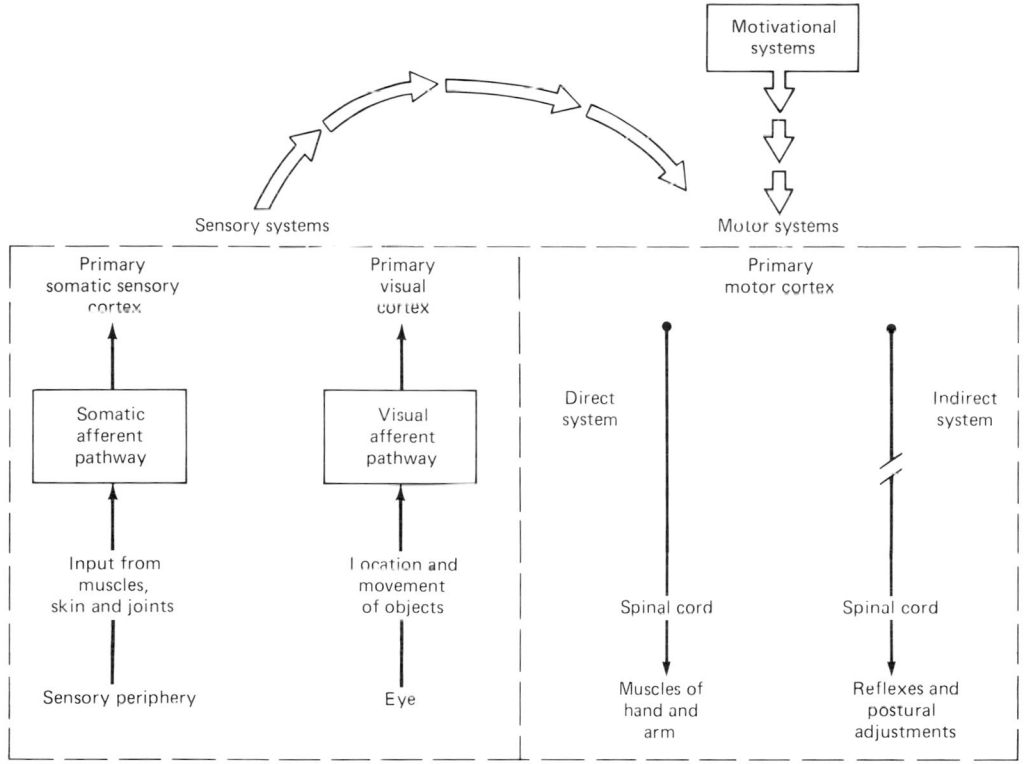

FIGURE 19–6

Most behavioral acts involve all three major functional systems of the brain—the sensory, motor, and motivational systems. In catching a ball, for example, information about the movement of the ball and its eventual impact in the hand is relayed to the primary sensory areas in the cerebral cortex. These areas provide input to the primary motor cortex through cortical connections, and through multisynaptic pathways involving the basal ganglia, the cerebellum, and the thalamus. The motivational system, which includes a portion of the limbic system of the brain, also sends information to the motor cortex. Direct and indirect motor pathways emerge from the motor cortex. The direct system regulates the activity of motor neurons that innervate the muscles of the hand and arm involved in the fine control of movement. The indirect system plays an important role in the overall regulation of body posture. The indirect motor system includes synaptic relays (represented by the break in the arrow). Different behaviors involve different relays.

tire sound spectrum to which the ear is sensitive is represented in a *tonotopic* neural map.

In the motor pathways neurons that regulate particular body parts are clustered together to form a *motor* map, which is particularly distinct in the primary motor cortex. The motor map, like the sensory maps, is not uniform, since the extent of central representation reflects the fineness of control of the movement of individual body parts.

These central sensory and motor maps are clinically important because damage to a particular subdivision of a pathway will produce characteristic deficits in motor or sensory function. Familiarity with the maps permits the neurologist to localize lesions in the central nervous system with precision.

Most Pathways Cross the Midline

An important but as yet unexplained aspect of the organization of the central nervous system is that most neural pathways are bilaterally symmetrical and cross over to the opposite (contralateral) side of the brain or spinal cord. As a result, sensory and motor events on one side of the body are relayed to and controlled by the cerebral hemisphere on the opposite side. Pathways cross at different anatomical levels in different systems. For example, the pathway for pain sensation crosses in the spinal cord, whereas the direct motor pathway from the motor cortex to the spinal cord crosses in the medulla. Crossings of this kind within the brain stem and spinal cord are called *decussations* (Latin, *decussare*, to cross in the shape of an X).

Structures that contain only decussating axons are termed *commissures*. Commissures in the brain contain fibers from functionally related areas in each half. By far the largest commissure, and indeed the largest fiber bundle in the brain, is the *corpus callosum*, which connects the two cerebral hemispheres (see Figure 19–2).

Crossing in the human visual system is slightly more complicated. About half of the axons from each retina cross to the opposite side of the brain, while the remaining axons terminate on the same side. The crossing of axons from the retina takes place in the optic chiasm, where the left and right optic nerves meet. Axons are redistributed in the chiasm so that each half of the brain receives all the fibers that mediate sight from the opposite half of the visual field, just as somatic sensation on one side of the body is represented in the opposite half of the brain.

An Overall View

The nervous system may be divided into the central nervous system, composed of the brain and the spinal cord, and the peripheral nervous system, composed of ganglia and peripheral nerves. The peripheral nervous system, which has somatic and autonomic components, relays information to the central nervous system and executes motor commands generated in the brain and spinal cord. Even a simple act involves the integrated activity of multiple sensory, motor, and motivational systems in the central nervous system. Each of these systems contains synaptic relays and each is composed of several distinct subdivisions. In addition, most pathways are ordered topographically based on function, and many pathways cross from one side of the nervous system to the other. These basic principles govern the organization of the nervous system from the level of the spinal cord, through the brain stem, to the highest levels of the cerebral cortex.

Selected Readings

Barr, M. L., and Kiernan, J. A. 1988. The Human Nervous System: An Anatomical Viewpoint, 5th ed. Philadelphia: Lippincott.

Brodal, A. 1981. Neurological Anatomy in Relation to Clinical Medicine, 3rd ed. New York: Oxford University Press.

Heimer, L. 1983. The Human Brain and Spinal Cord: Functional Neuroanatomy and Dissection Guide. New York: Springer.

Martin, J. H. 1989. Neuroanatomy: Text and Atlas. New York: Elsevier.

Nauta, W. J. H., and Feirtag, M. 1986. Fundamental Neuroanatomy. New York: Freeman.

References

Appenzeller, O. 1990. The Autonomic Nervous System: An Introduction to Basic and Clinical Concepts, 4th rev. and enl. ed. New York: Elsevier.

Noback, C. R., and Demarest, R. J. 1981. The Human Nervous System: Basic Principles of Neurobiology, 3rd ed. New York: McGraw-Hill.

Schmidt, R. F., and Thews, G. (eds.) 1989. Human Physiology. 2nd compl. rev. ed. M. A. Biederman-Thorson (trans.) Berlin: Springer.

20

James P. Kelly

The Neural Basis of Perception and Movement

The Spinal Cord Provides Sensory and Motor Innervation to the Trunk and Limbs

The Internal Structure of the Spinal Cord Varies at Different Levels

Sensory Axons Innervating the Trunk and Limbs Originate in the Dorsal Root Ganglia

Central Axons of Dorsal Root Ganglion Neurons Are Arranged Somatotopically in the Dorsal Column

The Dorsal Column–Medial Lemniscal System Is the Principal Pathway for Somatosensory Perception

The Thalamus Is the Principal Synaptic Relay for Information Reaching the Cerebral Cortex

The Highest Level of Information Processing Occurs in the Cerebral Cortex

The Corticospinal Tract Is a Direct Pathway for Voluntary Movement

Voluntary Movements Recruit the Actions of the Entire Motor System

Although the central nervous system is made up of about 100 billion neurons, the task of studying the connections between such a large number of cells is simplified by three considerations. First, individual neurons are not unique; for example, each of the many thousands of spinal motor neurons and hippocampal pyramidal cells serves a similar function. Second, different types of neurons are not randomly distributed but are clustered into *layers* or into discrete cellular groups called *nuclei*, which are connected to form the sensory, motor, and motivational systems. Thus, to understand the organization of the human central nervous system, we need only understand the major nuclear groups within the various sensory and motor systems and appreciate their relationships to each other and to the motivational system of the brain. Third, we now have a clearer idea of the functional importance of many key nuclear groups. As a result, brain anatomy can be studied in a more interesting and behaviorally relevant way than was possible in the past.

As we examine the organization of the central nervous system in this chapter, we shall be guided by these three considerations. To simplify our survey, we shall focus primarily on the somatic sensory and the motor systems and examine how information from the body surface ascends through the relays of the nervous system, is processed and transformed into a motor command, and descends again to the spinal cord to produce adaptive behaviors.

The Spinal Cord Provides Sensory and Motor Innervation to the Trunk and Limbs

The spinal cord is composed of *gray matter*, which contains the cell bodies and dendrites of neurons and glial cells, and *white matter*, which consists mainly of axons grouped into tracts (Figure 20–1).

FIGURE 20–1

This cross section of the spinal cord shows the bilaterally symmetrical divisions of white matter and gray matter. The white matter is organized into three columns (dorsal, lateral, and ventral) running parallel to the long axis of the cord. The central gray matter is divided into the dorsal horn, which comprises cells concerned with receiving afferent input, and the ventral horn, which contains the cells that generate the motor output of the cord. The intermediate zone, between the dorsal and ventral horns, contains neurons whose axons terminate in the spinal cord and brain stem. In the thoracic and part of the lumbosacral cord the intermediate zone (the lateral horn) contains the preganglionic neurons of the sympathetic and sacral parasympathetic systems.

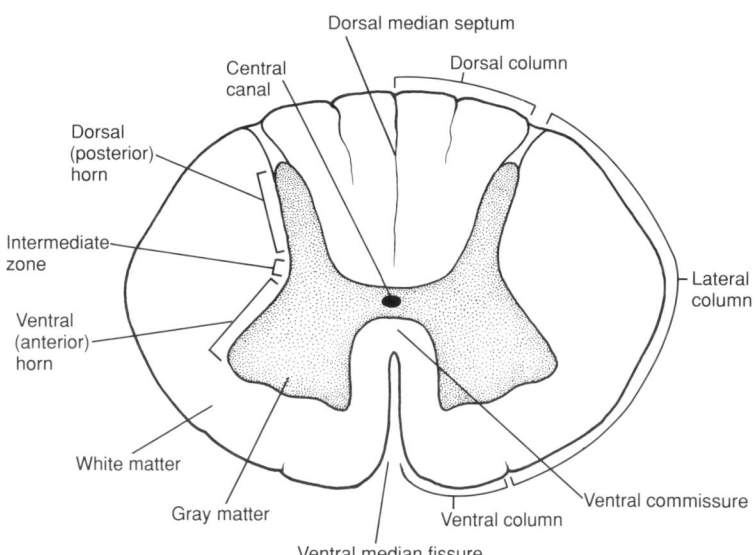

The gray matter of the spinal cord is shaped like the outline of a butterfly, and each half on either side of the midline may be subdivided into a *dorsal* (or *posterior*) and *ventral* (or *anterior*) horn. The dorsal horn contains sensory nuclei that are relay sites for somatosensory information entering the spinal cord. From here, ascending projection neurons transmit sensory information to the brain stem and thalamus. The ventral horn contains motor nuclei that innervate skeletal muscles. Interneurons in the gray matter modulate information flow from the dorsal horn (or from higher centers) to motor neurons, or from one group of motor neurons to another. The *intermediate zone*, between the dorsal and ventral horns, contains neurons whose axons terminate either in the ventral horn or in the brain stem and cerebellum. In the thoracic and upper lumbar segments, this zone also contains the preganglionic sympathetic neurons of the autonomic motor system (see below and Chapter 49), which are collected into a discrete longitudinal column called the intermediolateral cell column. The gray matter on the two sides of the spinal cord is connected by the gray matter that surrounds the *central canal*.

The white matter of the spinal cord surrounds the gray matter, and is divided into three large bilaterally paired bundles of axons arranged longitudinally—the dorsal, lateral, and ventral columns (Figure 20–1). The *dorsal columns* are composed of primary afferent axons that carry somatic sensory information to the brain stem. The *lateral columns* include axons that ascend to higher levels of the central nervous system as well as axons that project from nuclei in the brain stem and cortex upon motor neurons and interneurons in the gray matter of the spinal cord. The *ventral columns* include axons that relay information about pain and thermal sensation to higher levels of the central nervous system as well as descending motor axons that control axial muscles and posture. The *ventral commissure*, which is located ventral to the central canal, contains axons that cross from one side of the spinal cord

to the other side. This commissure contains axons that transmit information about pain and axons that control posture.

The Internal Structure of the Spinal Cord Varies at Different Levels

The spinal cord is divided into four major regions, each of which contains numerous segments. There are eight cervical segments, twelve thoracic segments, five lumbar segments, and five sacral segments (Figure 20–2). The organization of the spinal cord is determined by two important features. First, axons that project from the periphery to the spinal cord are added successively from the lower sacral region to the progressively higher lumbar, thoracic, and cervical levels. Similarly, the long descending axons originating in the brain terminate at various levels of the cord, so that fewer are left at each succeeding lower level, and only a small number remain in the sacral spinal cord. Thus, the sacral cord has very little white matter relative to gray matter (Figure 20–2, sacral 3 and 4), whereas the cervical cord, which contains many ascending and descending axons, has more white matter than gray matter (Figure 20–2, cervical 1). Second, the regions of the spinal cord that innervate the limbs have larger ventral and dorsal horns (known as the lumbosacral and cervical enlargements, respectively) than does the thoracic region, which innervates only the trunk. This is because more ascending

▷

FIGURE 20–2

Organization of the spinal cord at different levels.

A. The cross-sectional appearance of the spinal cord differs at each level. In the lumbar and sacral regions the ratio of gray to white matter is high because these regions contain the cell bodies of the motor neurons and interneurons that innervate the lower limbs and trunk. By contrast, most of the descending axons

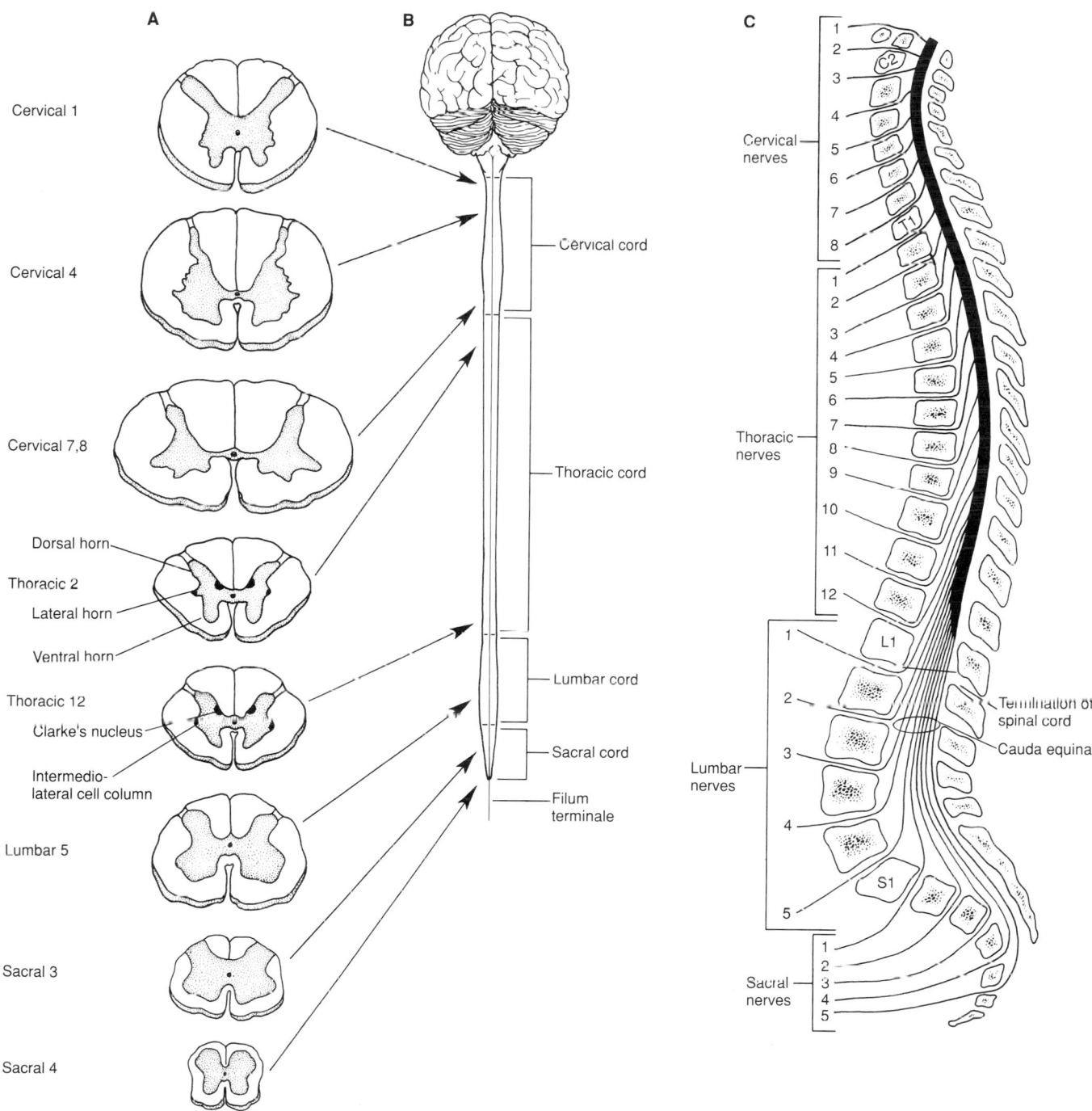

A

Cervical 1

Cervical 4

Cervical 7,8

Dorsal horn
Thoracic 2
Lateral horn
Ventral horn

Thoracic 12
Clarke's nucleus

Intermedio-
lateral cell column

Lumbar 5

Sacral 3

Sacral 4

B

Cervical cord

Thoracic cord

Lumbar cord

Sacral cord

Filum
terminale

C

Cervical
nerves

Thoracic
nerves

Lumbar
nerves

Sacral
nerves

C2

T1

L1

Termination of
spinal cord

Cauda equina

S1

terminate at higher levels of the cord. The cord is narrowest in the thoracic region and thickest in the so-called cervical enlargement, which contains numerous fibers innervating the upper limbs as well as ascending and descending fiber tracts. In the thoracic and parts of the lumbar spinal cord the intermediate zone bulges into the lateral column (the lateral horn).

B. Dorsal view of the brain and spinal cord. The *cervical cord* lies closest to the junction with the brain and contains the cervical enlargement. The *thoracic cord* is the longest division. The *lumbar* and the *sacral cord* together form the lumbosacral enlargement.

C. The individual spinal nerves are related to the four levels of the cord. There are eight cervical spinal nerves, even though there are only seven cervical vertebrae, because the first cervical spinal nerve emerges rostral to the first cervical vertebra. In the other spinal segments each spinal nerve is numbered after the vertebra rostral to the space through which the nerve exits. There are 12 thoracic nerves, five lumbar nerves, and five sacral nerves. The adult spinal cord does not run the whole length of the vertebral column but terminates at the border of the L1 vertebra. Therefore, the dorsal and ventral roots of lumbar and sacral nerves run some distance before exiting from the vertebral column. These rootlets are collectively termed the *cauda equina*.

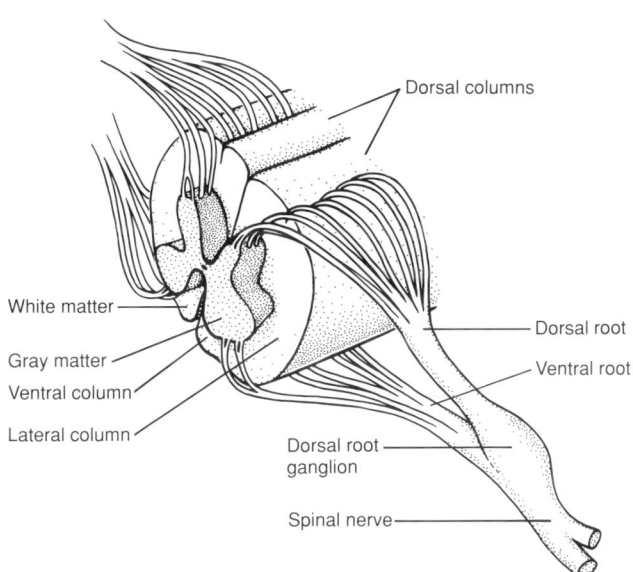

FIGURE 20–3

Each spinal nerve has a dorsal and ventral root. The dorsal root comprises the central branches of the dorsal root ganglion cells. These processes emerge from the nerve in small bundles before entering the spinal cord. Motor axons emerging from the cord join to form the ventral root.

sensory neurons, motor neurons, and interneurons are required to innervate the arms and legs.

In addition to variations in the dorsal and ventral horns, specific nuclei are present in the intermediate zone at some levels but not at others. For example, two important nuclei present only in the thoracic and upper lumbar segments are the intermediolateral cell column and the cells of Clarke's nucleus (Figure 20–2). The intermediolateral cell column contains the preganglionic sympathetic neurons of the autonomic motor system. These neurons project from the ventral root to neurons in the autonomic ganglia (see Figure 19–5). The interomediolateral cell column bulges laterally, distorting the outline of the gray matter into a *lateral horn* (Figure 20–2). The cells of Clarke's nucleus relay information about the position and movement of the leg and lower trunk directly to the cerebellum.

Sensory Axons Innervating the Trunk and Limbs Originate in the Dorsal Root Ganglia

Information from the skin, muscles, and joints of the limbs and trunk is relayed to the spinal cord by sensory cells located in the *dorsal root ganglia* that lie within the vertebral column immediately adjacent to the spinal cord (Figure 20–3). Dorsal root ganglion neurons are pseudounipolar neurons that have a central and a peripheral branch (Figure 20–4). The peripheral branch terminates in

skin, muscle, or other tissue as a free nerve ending or in association with specialized connective tissue or epithelial cells that contribute to the process in which stimulus energy is converted into neural events. Somatosensory information from the head and the neck is carried by the peripheral branches of neurons located in *cranial sensory ganglia*. Here we consider in detail only dorsal root ganglion neurons and their connections; the same general organization applies to the cranial sensory neurons.

The central processes of dorsal root ganglion neurons enter the spinal cord at the dorsal tip of the dorsal horn. Upon entry to the spinal cord the axons branch extensively and project to nuclei in the spinal gray matter and brain stem that process information about specific somatic sensory modalities, such as touch, pain, and temperature (Figure 20–5). In addition, the type of connection made by a central branch of a dorsal root ganglion neuron determines how the cell's sensory signal is used:

1. Connections with interneurons and motor neurons of the spinal cord mediate information for *reflex activity*.
2. Connections with neurons in the spinal cord whose output ascends through synaptic relays to the thalamus and then to the cerebral cortex mediate information for *perception* of sensory stimuli, such as touch or pain.
3. Connections with neurons of the reticular formation in the brain stem mediate information for *behavioral arousal* and *awareness*.

FIGURE 20–4

Neurons in the dorsal root ganglia have a single process that divides into two functionally distinct branches. The peripheral branch receives input from a receptor in the periphery, while the central branch relays input to the spinal cord or brain stem.

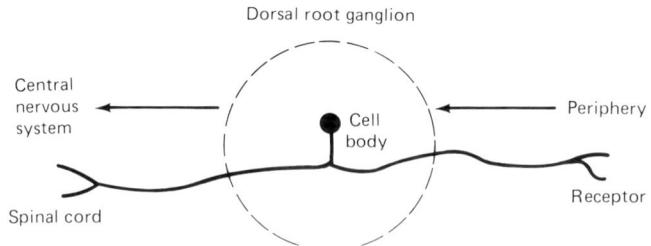

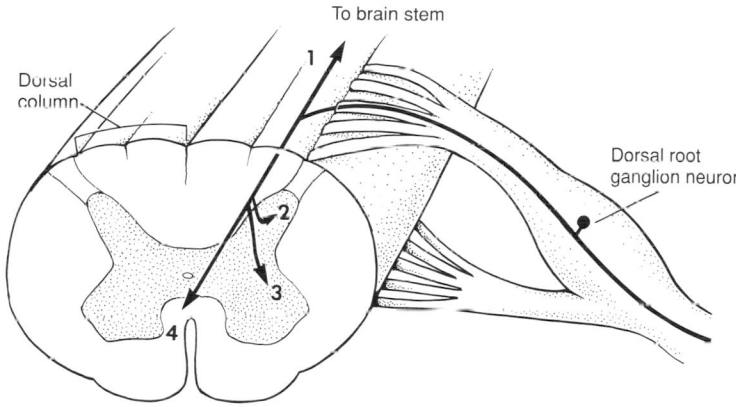

FIGURE 20–5
The axon of an individual dorsal root ganglion neuron that mediates pressure, touch, or proprioception has numerous branches in the spinal cord. The principal branch ascends in the dorsal column to the brain stem (**1**). Other branches terminate locally in the spinal cord (**2, 3**) or descend a few segments (**4**). Branches 2, 3, and 4 participate in local spinal reflexes or in sensory processing within the dorsal horn.

In this chapter we shall obtain an overall view of the brain pathways involved in the perception of touch and in movements of the limbs. We shall then examine these pathways in detail in Chapters 23 through 26. The reflex function of the various types of dorsal root fibers is examined in connection with the motor systems (Chapter 35), and arousal is discussed in the context of the brain stem (Chapter 44).

Central Axons of Dorsal Root Ganglion Neurons Are Arranged Somatotopically in the Dorsal Column

Neurons involved in tactile sensation project their central axons into the spinal cord, where the principal branch of the axon ascends rostrally in the dorsal columns. Axons that enter the cord in the sacral region are found near the midline; axons that enter the cord at successively higher levels are added in progressively more lateral positions. As a result, in the cervical cord sensory information from the region of the sacrum is carried medially, the leg and trunk more laterally, next the arm and shoulder, and finally, most laterally, the neck. This orderly representation of the axons relaying input from receptors in the skin and joints is termed the *somatotopic representation* of the body surface, and is maintained throughout the entire ascending somatosensory pathway, through the thalamus, to the somatosensory areas in the postcentral gyrus of the cerebral cortex.

The Dorsal Column–Medial Lemniscal System Is the Principal Pathway for Somatosensory Perception

The primary afferent fibers that carry somatosensory information enter the ipsilateral dorsal column and remain on the same side during their ascent to the medulla, where they synapse on cells in the *dorsal column nuclei*. The axons of the postsynaptic neurons in the dorsal column nuclei cross to the other side of the brain in an arc-shaped route as they emerge from the nuclei and ascend to the thalamus in a fiber bundle called the *medial lemniscus* (Figure 20–6B). As in the dorsal columns of the spinal cord, the fibers of the *medial lemniscus* are arranged somatotopically. Because of the crossing of the fibers, the right side of the brain receives sensory input from the limbs and trunk on the left side of the body, and vice versa. Other nuclei in the brain stem process inputs from the cranial nerves that innervate the head and neck and also generate the motor output of these nerves. We shall see in Chapter 44 that the brain stem contains 10 of the 12 cranial nerves. Some cranial nerves are sensory, some are motor, and some have mixed sensory and motor functions.

As we follow the medial lemniscus from the medulla upward through the brain stem, the next region encountered is the pons. The pons contains clusters of neurons (the *pontine nuclei*) whose axons cross the midline and run to the contralateral half of the cerebellum (Figure 20–6B2). These axons participate in the cerebellar control of movement and posture. The pons also contains the longitudinally oriented fibers that descend from the cerebral cortex to control muscles of the head, limbs, and trunk (corticospinal tract).

Finally, the medial lemniscus terminates in the thalamus, where several specialized nuclei process all somatosensory inputs to the central nervous system. The course of the medial lemniscus from the medulla to the thalamus is summarized in Figure 20–7.

The Thalamus Is the Principal Synaptic Relay for Information Reaching the Cerebral Cortex

The thalamus relays sensory input to the primary sensory areas of the cerebral cortex, as well as information about motor behavior to the motor areas of the cortex. Because of its central role in sensation and motor control, we shall consider this part of the brain in detail.

The thalamus is composed in part of distinct sensory nuclei that receive input about different sensory modalities, including somatic sensation, audition, and vision.

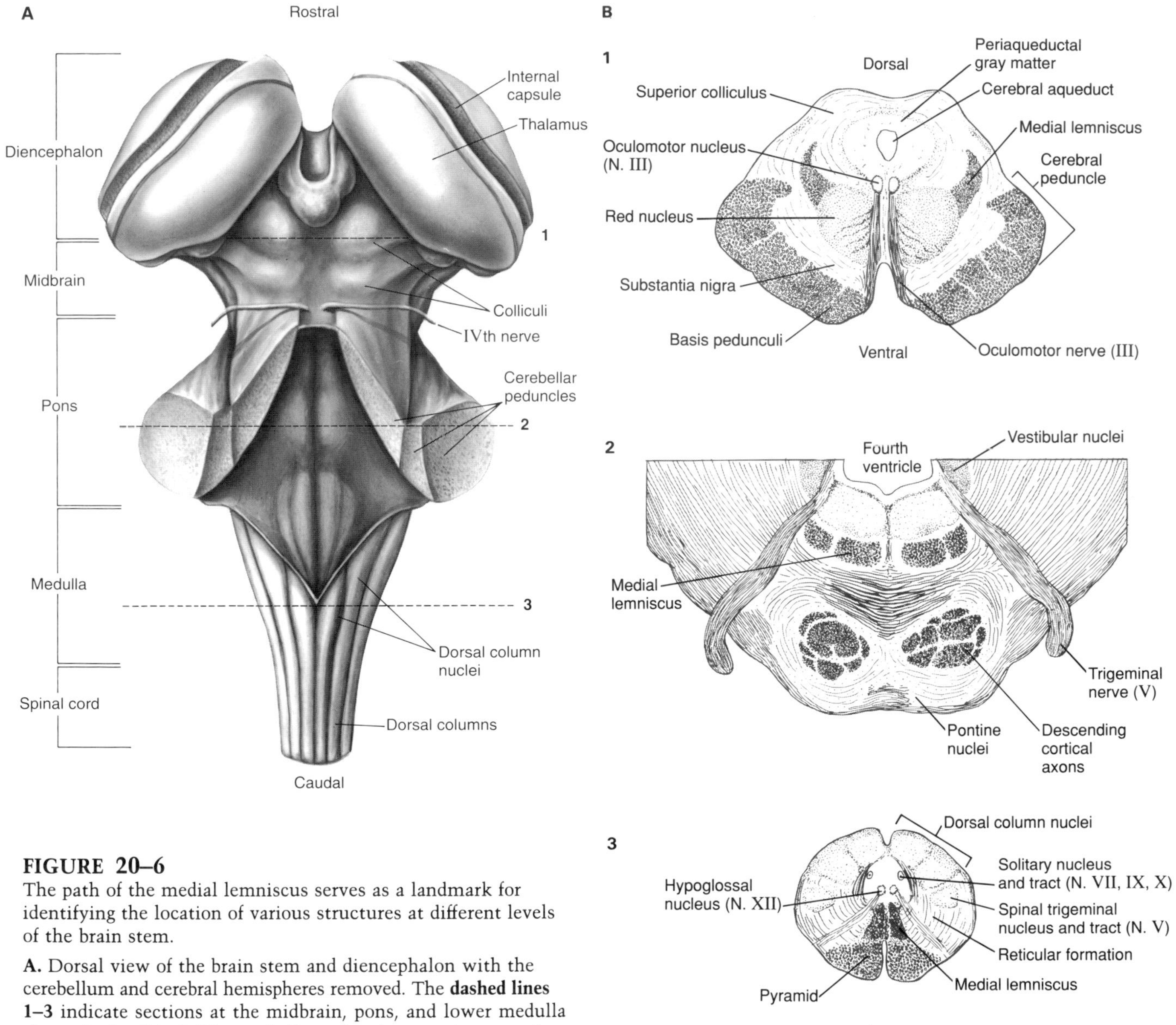

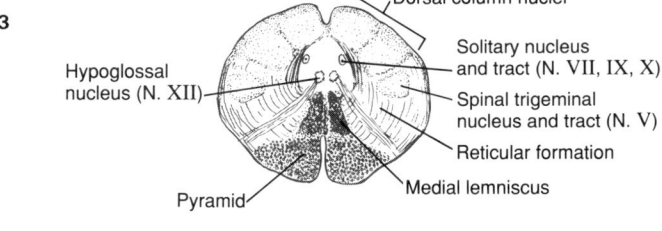

A. Dorsal view of the brain stem and diencephalon with the cerebellum and cerebral hemispheres removed.

Labels in A (top to bottom): Rostral; Internal capsule; Thalamus; 1; Colliculi; IVth nerve; Cerebellar peduncles; 2; Diencephalon; Midbrain; Pons; Medulla; Spinal cord; 3; Dorsal column nuclei; Dorsal columns; Caudal

Labels in B1: Dorsal; Periaqueductal gray matter; Superior colliculus; Cerebral aqueduct; Medial lemniscus; Oculomotor nucleus (N. III); Cerebral peduncle; Red nucleus; Substantia nigra; Basis pedunculi; Ventral; Oculomotor nerve (III)

Labels in B2: Fourth ventricle; Vestibular nuclei; Medial lemniscus; Trigeminal nerve (V); Pontine nuclei; Descending cortical axons

Labels in B3: Dorsal column nuclei; Solitary nucleus and tract (N. VII, IX, X); Hypoglossal nucleus (N. XII); Spinal trigeminal nucleus and tract (N. V); Reticular formation; Medial lemniscus; Pyramid

FIGURE 20–6

The path of the medial lemniscus serves as a landmark for identifying the location of various structures at different levels of the brain stem.

A. Dorsal view of the brain stem and diencephalon with the cerebellum and cerebral hemispheres removed. The **dashed lines 1–3** indicate sections at the midbrain, pons, and lower medulla shown in detail in B. The cerebellar peduncles contain axons that interconnect the cerebellum with the brain stem and spinal cord.

B. Cross sections made through the brain stem at the levels indicated in A. **1.** Section through the midbrain. The cerebral aqueduct connects the ventricular system in the diencephalon with the fourth ventricle in the pons and medulla. It is surrounded by the periaqueductal gray matter. The red nucleus is also a significant component of the midbrain. It gives rise to the rubrospinal tract, which descends to the spinal cord and regulates motor function. The substantia nigra and the basis pedunculi together constitute the cerebral peduncle. **2.** Section through the pons. At this level axons arise from the pontine nuclei and project to the cerebellum. These nuclei relay information from the cerebral cortex to the cerebellum on the opposite side. The vestibular nuclei lie beneath the floor of the fourth ventricle. **3.** Section through the lower medulla. The dorsal column nuclei and the medial lemniscus are evident at this level. Also seen are the nuclei of cranial nerves XII (hypoglossal) and V (trigeminal). The solitary nucleus and tract are important landmarks for identifying sections through the medulla. The pyramids, which carry the axons of the corticospinal (pyramidal) tract, make up the ventral surface of the medulla. The paired medial lemniscus tracts, shaped roughly like a triangle, lie dorsal to the pyramids and adjacent to the midline.

The thalamus also mediates motor functions by transmitting information from the cerebellum and basal ganglia to the motor regions of the frontal lobe—the primary motor cortex and higher-order motor areas. In addition, the thalamus is involved in autonomic reactions and the maintenance of consciousness. Almost all the thalamic nuclei project to and receive input from the cerebral cortex. Thalamocortical connections are made through the *internal capsule*, a large fiber bundle that carries most of the axons running to and from the cerebral hemisphere (Figure

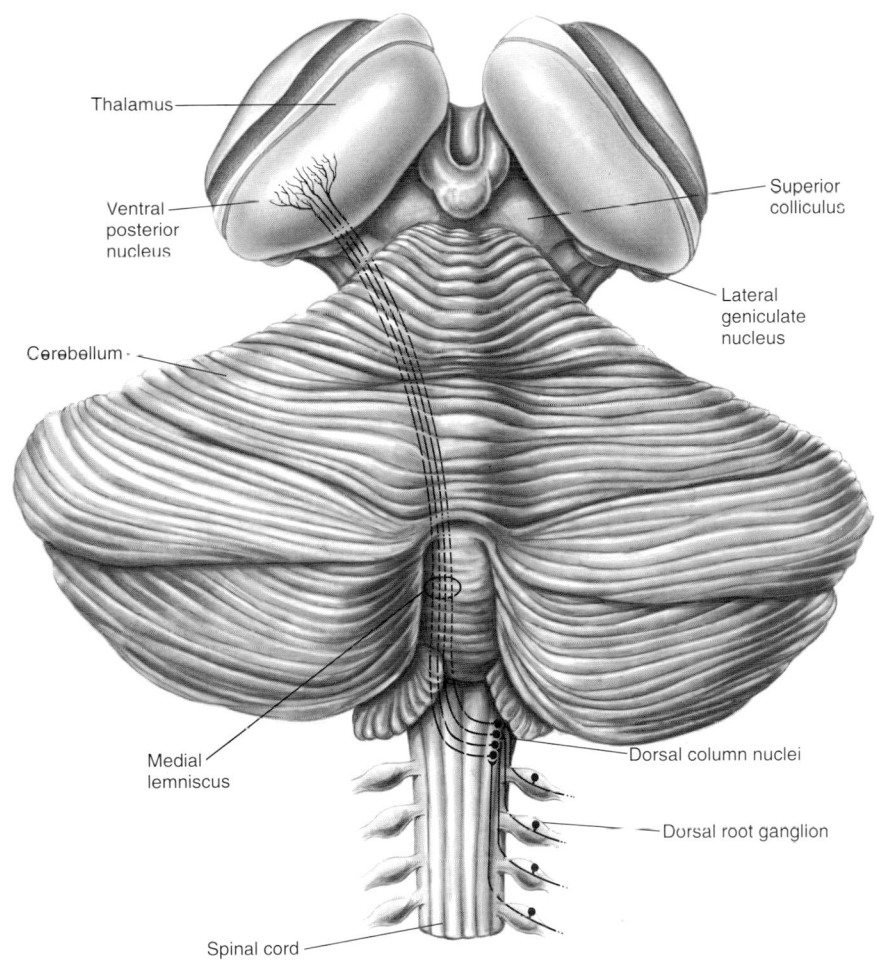

FIGURE 20–7

The course of the medial lemniscus from the medulla to the thalamus. (In this drawing the cerebral hemispheres have been removed. The cerebellum covers the dorsal surface of the brain stem). The medial lemniscus is composed of axons arising from the dorsal column nuclei. The axons, which cross the midline as they emerge from the nuclei, ascend close to the midline throughout the brain stem. Beginning in the pons they gradually veer away from the midline and terminate in the ventral posterior nucleus of the thalamus. (Adapted from Niewenhuys, Voogd, and van Huijzen, 1981.)

20–8). The internal capsule contains not only the rostral continuation of the somatic afferent pathway and the projection fibers from the various nuclei of the thalamus, but also the fibers descending from the cortex to the brain stem and spinal cord. We shall first consider a functional classification of the thalamic nuclei that relates them to the sensory and motor systems they serve. We shall then examine the regional classification of these nuclei.

Thalamic nuclei are classified into two functional groups: *relay nuclei* and *diffuse-projection nuclei* (Table 20–1).

Relay nuclei are characterized by three features: (1) each processes either a single sensory modality or an input from a distinct part of the motor system; (2) each projects to a specific local region of the cerebral cortex; and (3) each receives recurrent input from the region of the cerebral cortex to which it projects. These recurrent connections presumably allow the cortex to modulate the input it receives according to ongoing activity.

Diffuse-projection nuclei have more widespread connections than do the relay nuclei, and they influence the activity of cells not only in the cerebral cortex but also in the thalamus itself. The diffuse-projection nuclei are part of a system believed to govern the level of arousal of the brain (discussed in Chapter 48).

Each of the major functional divisions of the cerebral cortex that we considered in Chapter 19—sensory, motor, associative, and motivational—receives the axons of a particular type of thalamic relay nucleus. Thalamic sensory nuclei relay information about a particular sensory modality to local regions of the cerebral cortex. This information is the initial step in generating a sensory

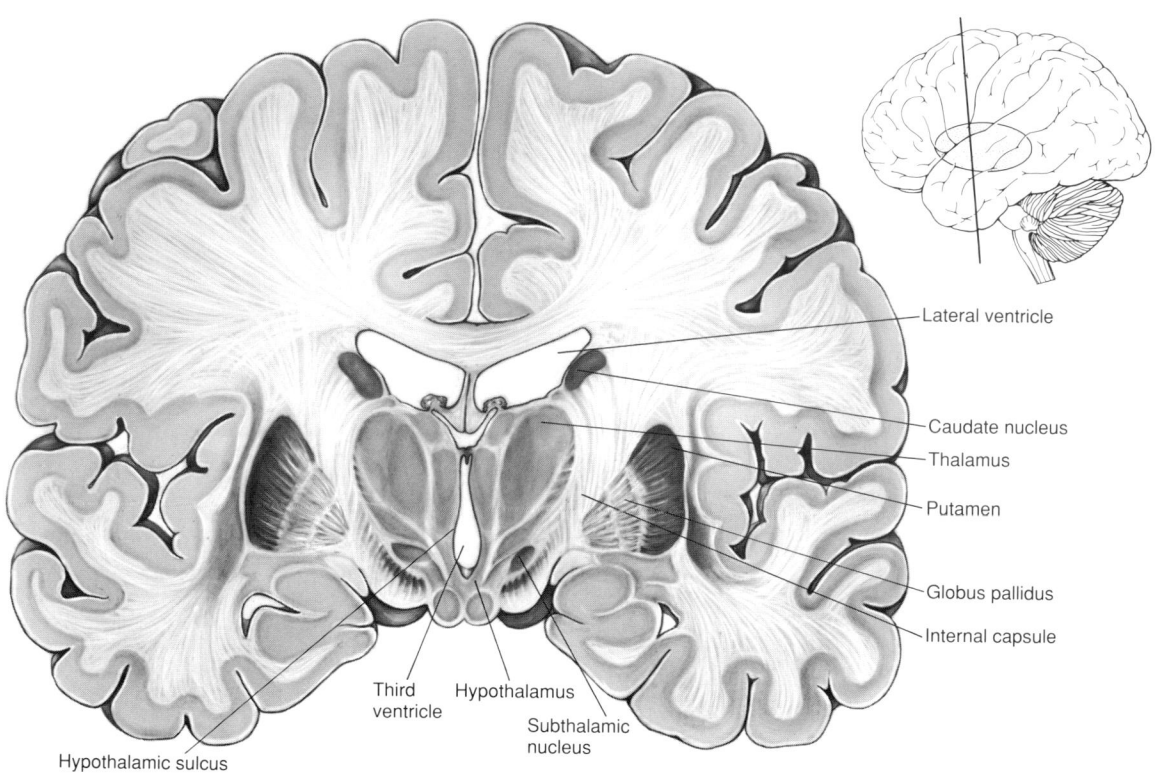

FIGURE 20–8
The thalamus is clearly visible in this coronal section through the diencephalon (the **inset** shows the plane of the section). The thalamus lies dorsal to the hypothalamus and forms the walls of the third ventricle. (Adapted from Nieuwenhuys, Voogd, and van Huijzen, 1981.)

perception. Other sensory nuclei send information to the association areas of the cortex, where inputs from several sensory systems are integrated to initiate behaviors. The thalamic motor nuclei send information to the motor cortex about activity in other regions of the brain that are involved in the control of motor output, such as the cerebellum. The motivational system also receives direct input from thalamic relay nuclei. In addition, all functional divisions of the cortex receive input from diffuse-projection nuclei. A single diffuse-projection nucleus may send its axons to different functional divisions of the cortex, where it is thought to regulate the overall level of excitability.

We shall return to the functional anatomy of the thalamus again in Chapters 25, 30, and 33 when we consider specific brain systems.

A Y-shaped sheet of fibers called the *internal medullary lamina* separates the thalamic nuclei into six groups:

Lateral (ventral and dorsal tiers)
Medial
Anterior
Intralaminar
Midline
Reticular

The lateral, medial, and anterior groups of nuclei are named according to their positions relative to the internal medullary lamina (Figure 20–9).

Each *lateral nucleus* receives restricted sensory or motor input and projects to and receives input from a specific region of sensory, motor, or association cortex (Table 20–1). The lateral nuclei are relay nuclei that are divided into two tiers, ventral and dorsal. The nuclei of the ventral tier are named according to their position within the tier: The ventral anterior and ventral lateral nuclei are important for motor control; the ventral posterior nucleus is important for somatic sensation. The medial and lateral geniculate nuclei, which are formed near the posterior part of the thalamus, are often included with the nuclei of the ventral tier. The medial geniculate nucleus mediates information about hearing, and the lateral geniculate information about vision. The three nuclei of the dorsal tier are the lateral dorsal, the lateral posterior, and the pulvinar (Figure 20–9).

The pulvinar, the largest of the thalamic nuclei, projects to the parietal–temporal–occipital association cortex, which includes Wernicke's speech area (described in Chapter 1). The pulvinar contains numerous subdivisions and forms the most posterior part of the thalamus (Figure 20–9). The pulvinar receives inputs from the superior colliculus of the midbrain, from the parietal–temporal–occipital association cortex (to which it also projects), and from the primary visual cortex. These diverse connections suggest that the pulvinar integrates sensory information.

TABLE **20–1.** Connections and Functions of Thalamic Nuclei

Nuclei	Principal afferent inputs	Major projection sites	Function
Relay nuclei			
Anterior nuclear group	Mammillary body of hypothalamus	Cingulate gyrus	Limbic
Ventral anterior	Globus pallidus	Premotor cortex (area 6)*	Motor
Ventral lateral	Dentate nucleus of cerebellum through brachium conjunctivum (superior cerebellar peduncle)	Motor and premotor	Motor
Ventral posterior			
Lateral portion	Dorsal column–medial lemniscal pathways and spinothalamic pathways	Somatic sensory cortex of parietal lobe	Somatic sensation (body)
Medial portion	Sensory nuclei of trigeminal nerve (V)	Somatic sensory cortex of parietal lobe	Somatic sensation (face)
Medial geniculate	Inferior colliculus through brachium of inferior colliculus	Auditory cortex of temporal lobe (areas 41 and 42)*	Hearing
Lateral geniculate	Retinal ganglion cells through optic nerve and optic tract	Visual cortex (area 17)*	Vision
Lateral dorsal	Cingulate gyrus	Cingulate gyrus	Emotional expression
Lateral posterior	Parietal lobe	Parietal lobe	Integration of sensory information
Pulvinar	Superior colliculus, temporal, parietal, and occipital lobes	Temporal, parietal, and occipital lobes	Integration of sensory information
Medial dorsal	Amygdaloid nuclear complex, olfactory, and hypothalamus	Prefrontal cortex	Limbic
Diffuse-projection nuclei			
Midline nuclei	Reticular formation and hypothalamus	Basal forebrain	Limbic
Intralaminar, centro-median, and centro-lateral nuclei	Reticular formation, spinothalamic tract, globus pallidus, and cortical areas	Basal ganglia and cortex	
Reticular nucleus	Cerebral cortex and thalamic nuclei, brain stem	Thalamic nuclei	Modulation of thalamic activity

*See Figure 20–11 for map of Brodmann's areas.

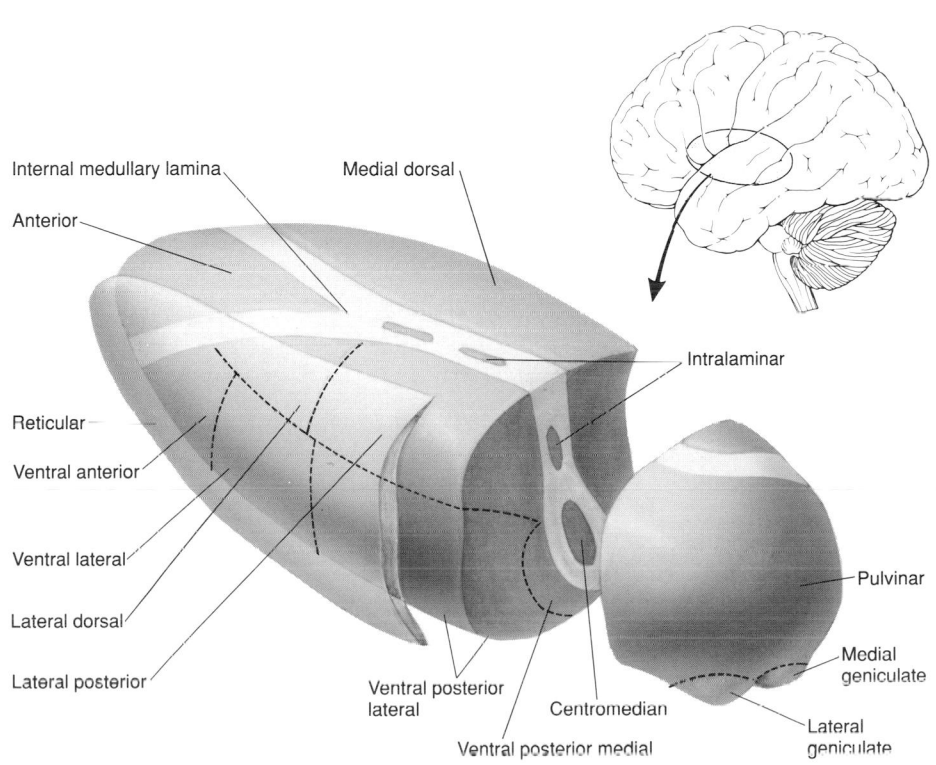

FIGURE 20–9
The major nuclei of the thalamus as seen on the left side of the brain. The internal medullary lamina divides the thalamus into the anterior, lateral, and medial nuclei. The lateral group is divided into dorsal and ventral tiers. The ventral tier is composed of the ventral anterior, ventral lateral, and ventral posterior nuclei; some anatomists include the lateral and medial geniculate nuclei. The dorsal tier includes the lateral dorsal and lateral posterior nuclei and the pulvinar. The medial dorsal nucleus is the largest of the medial group. Each nucleus in the ventral tier relays a specific sensory modality or motor information, while nuclei in the dorsal tier and the medial group have associational functions and project to the association cortex. The intralaminar nuclei lie within the internal medullary lamina, while the reticular nucleus caps the lateral aspect of the thalamus.

The *medial nuclei* are also relay nuclei. The largest component of the medial group is the medial dorsal nucleus.

The *anterior nuclei* participate in emotion by relaying information from the hypothalamus to the cingulate gyrus, a portion of the limbic system in the cerebral cortex.

The *intralaminar*, *reticular*, and *midline* nuclei are diffuse-projection nuclei (Table 20–1). The intralaminar nuclei lie within the internal medullary lamina; the largest of these cell groups is the centromedian nucleus (Figure 20–9). Cells in this nucleus have axons that terminate in several cortical areas in the frontal lobe and in two major components of the basal ganglia, the caudate nucleus and putamen. The reticular nucleus caps the entire lateral aspect of the thalamus and is separated from the lateral nuclei by another sheet of fibers, the *external medullary lamina*. Cells in the reticular nucleus receive input from a particular relay nucleus and in turn project back to that nucleus. The reticular nucleus is the only thalamic nucleus with an inhibitory output, and the only one that does not project to the cerebral cortex. The midline nuclei are diffuse-projection nuclei located in the dorsal half of the wall of the third ventricle.

The Highest Level of Information Processing Occurs in the Cerebral Cortex

The cerebral cortex is a folded sheet of cells that varies from 2 to 4 mm in thickness. The cortex that is visible on the external surface of the brain is called the *neocortex* because it is the part of the cortex most recently acquired in evolution. The neocortex is by far the largest component of the human brain. The most striking morphological feature of the neocortex is that its neurons are arranged in several well-defined layers. The other parts of the cortex arose earlier in vertebrate evolution and are called *allocortex* (Greek, *allos*, other). The allocortex lies deep within the temporal lobe near the zone where olfactory input reaches the cerebral cortex.

The cell bodies of cortical neurons have a variety of shapes, but in general two main types can be distinguished in all areas of the cortex: *pyramidal cells* and several types of *nonpyramidal* cells. Each of these classes can be further divided on the basis of the dendritic branching pattern. These distinctions based on cell configuration are not rigid, however.

Pyramidal cells are so called because they have a cell body shaped like a pyramid, with the apex pointing toward the surface of the brain. The apex gives rise to a dendrite (the apical dendrite) that runs toward the outermost layer of the cortex, intersecting the overlying layers roughly at right angles. The base of the cell body, which may be 30 μm across, gives rise to several dendrites (the basal dendrites) that course laterally within the layer containing the cell body. The nonpyramidal cells, in contrast, usually have round, smaller cell bodies, often stellate in shape, seldom measuring more than 10 μm in diameter. Their dendrites may arise from all aspects of the cell body (Figure 20–10).

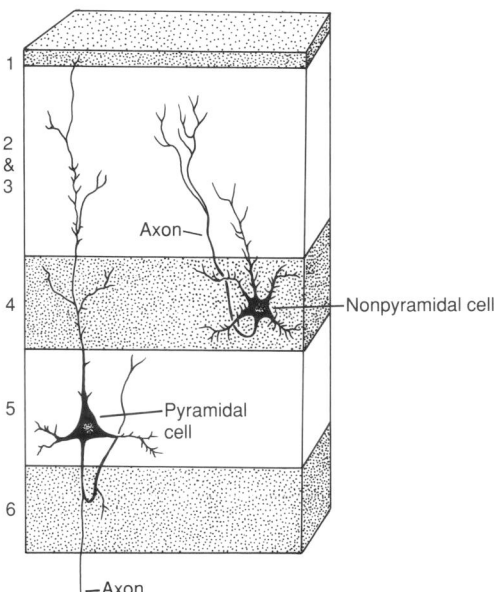

FIGURE 20–10
The cerebral cortex is organized into six distinct layers. Layer 1, the outermost layer, lies just below the pia mater; layer 6 lies just above the white matter. Layer 1 is made up mostly of glial cells and axons that run laterally through the layer and contains few cell bodies. Layers 2–6 contain different proportions of the two main classes of cortical neurons, pyramidal and nonpyramidal cells. Pyramidal cells send long axons down the spinal cord and are the major output neurons. They also have axonal branches that terminate in the local area. The axons of most nonpyramidal cells terminate locally.

The axons of pyramidal and nonpyramidal cells also differ. Although the axon of a pyramidal cell may have several collateral branches that terminate near the cell body, the main trunk of the axon enters the white matter and terminates either in another area of the cortex or at a more distant site in the central nervous system. In contrast, the axon of a nonpyramidal cell branches profusely in the region near the cell body and rarely extends beyond this region. Because of these differences, pyramidal cells are projection interneurons. They carry the output from a cortical area, although they also influence local processing through their collateral branches. Nonpyramidal cells are involved primarily in receiving input to the cortex and in the local processing of information.

Individual layers of the cortex do not contain equal proportions of pyramidal and nonpyramidal cells, and the type of cell that predominates in a layer provides an important clue about the function of that layer. For example, layers rich in pyramidal cells are predominantly output layers, whereas layers with many nonpyramidal cells are the principal sites of termination for thalamic and other afferent inputs.

The neocortex is divided into six layers, numbered sequentially from the surface next to the pia mater to the white matter underlying the cortex (Figure 20–10). Layer 1 contains only a few neuron bodies. It is composed largely of axons that run laterally through the layer (parallel to the pial surface) and glial cells (similar to those found in all cortical layers). The axons that run through layer 1 synapse on the apical dendrites of cells lying in deeper layers and presumably interconnect local cortical areas. Layer 2, which contains mostly small pyramidal neurons, and layer 3, which contains larger pyramidal cells, provide much of the output to other cortical regions. Layer 4 is rich in nonpyramidal cells and receives most of the afferent input from the thalamus. Layer 5 has the largest pyramidal cells; these cells give rise to long axons that leave the cortex and descend to the basal ganglia, the brain stem, and the spinal cord. Layer 6 also contains pyramidal cells, many of which project back to the thalamus. The white matter just below layer 6 carries axons to and from the cortex.

Although this six-layer structure is characteristic of the entire neocortex, the thickness of individual layers varies in different functional regions of the cortex. This variation in structure arises from two factors. First, layer 4 with its many nonpyramidal cells is usually expanded in primary sensory areas because these areas receive many inputs from sensory relay nuclei in the thalamus. A good example is the primary visual cortex, where layer 4 is greatly expanded and can be subdivided into three distinct sublayers. Second, in motor areas, which give rise to long descending pathways, layer 5 with its large pyramidal cells is prominent while layer 4 is much reduced. In association areas the pattern of layers is intermediate between those of the sensory and motor cortices.

The characteristic pattern of layering in different cortical areas was clearly shown at the turn of the century by Korbinian Brodmann, who examined the organization of the cells and fibers in the cortex using the Nissl stain for cell bodies and myelin stains for axons. Brodmann divided the human cerebral cortex into about 50 cytoarchitectural areas according to cell size, cell density, the number of layers in each region, and the density of myelinated axons. He assigned a number to each structural area, most of which have discrete functions (Figure 20–11). For example, the primary visual cortex, the area that receives direct input from the lateral geniculate nucleus, corresponds to Brodmann's area 17. He also correctly identified the boundaries of the primary motor and somatosensory areas and suggested that there may be many separate functional zones within individual association areas. Recent research has shown that there are, in fact, more functional zones in the association cortex than even Brodmann recognized.

The Corticospinal Tract Is a Direct Pathway for Voluntary Movement

The primary motor cortex of the frontal lobe is organized somatotopically, in a manner similar to the somatic sensory cortex. Specific regions in the motor cortex influence the activity of specific muscle groups in the periphery, just as each region in the somatic sensory cortex is related to specific portions of the sensory periphery. Axons from the primary motor cortex project directly to motor neurons in

Lateral view

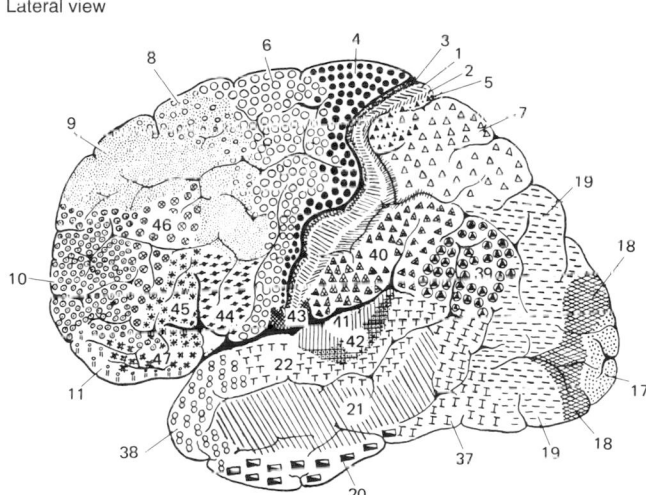

Medial view

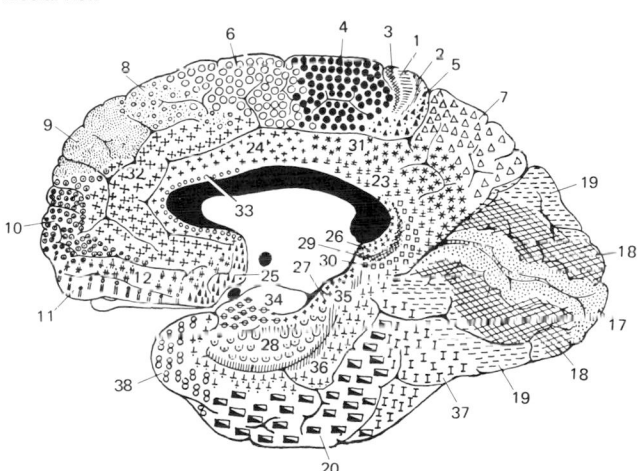

FIGURE 20–11

The human cerebral cortex was divided into about 50 discrete cytoarchitectonic areas more than 80 years ago by Korbinian Brodmann. Distinct areas are represented by different symbols and numbered as shown (there is no rationale for the numbering of the different fields). Brodmann's areas have consistently been found to correspond to distinctive functional fields, each of which has a characteristic pattern of connections. Area 4, the primary motor cortex, occupies most of the precentral gyrus. The primary somatic sensory cortex includes areas 1, 2, and 3 in the postcentral gyrus. Area 17 is the primary visual cortex. Areas 41 and 42 comprise the primary auditory cortex. The prefrontal association cortex and the parietal–temporal–occipital association cortex are also composed of a number of distinct cytoarchitectonic areas.

the spinal cord via the *corticospinal tract*. The fibers that synapse directly on motor neurons of the spinal cord arise from layer 5 of the primary motor cortex. The axons from the cortex descend through the white matter, the internal capsule, and the basis pedunculi, the fiber bundle that forms the base of the midbrain (Figure 20–12). The corticospinal tract accounts for only about 5% of the fibers in the basis pedunculi. It is bounded laterally and medially

A

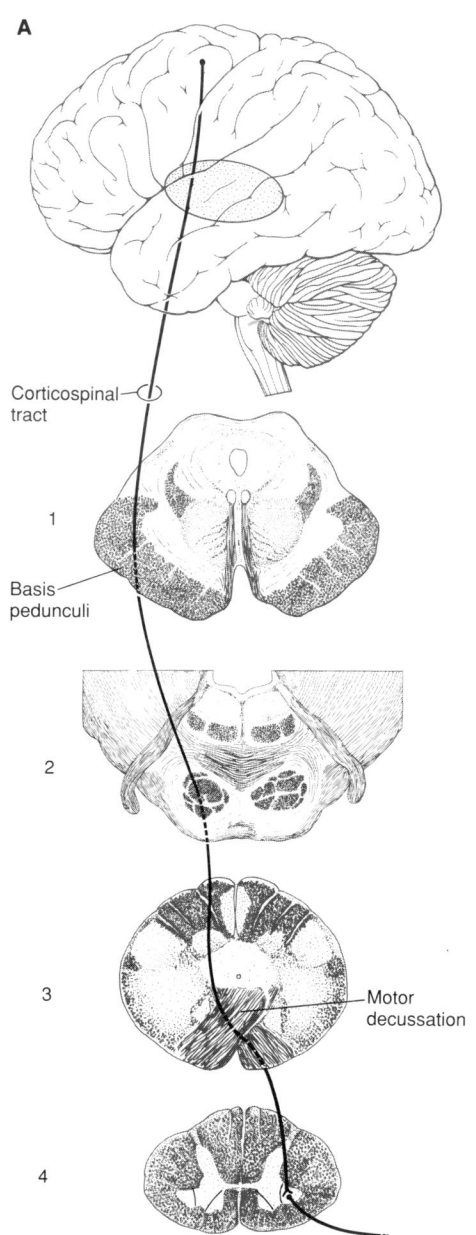

Corticospinal
tract

1

Basis
pedunculi

2

3

Motor
decussation

4

B

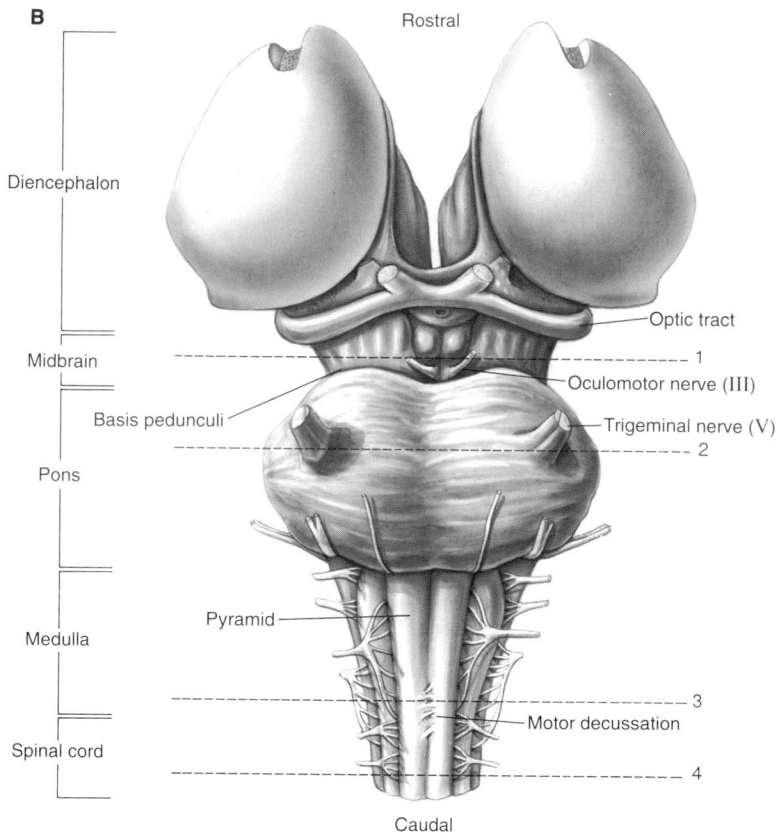

Rostral

Diencephalon

Optic tract

1

Midbrain

Oculomotor nerve (III)

Basis pedunculi

Trigeminal nerve (V)

Pons

2

Pyramid

Medulla

Spinal cord

3

Motor decussation

4

Caudal

FIGURE 20–12

Summary of the origin and course of the component of the corticospinal tract that originates in the motor cortex. **A** illustrates the location of the motor cortex in the frontal lobe and course of the corticospinal tract through the brain stem and the spinal cord, which is indicated in the four cross sections. **B**. The levels of the four cross sections illustrated in A are shown in B_1 to B_4: **1** midbrain; **2** pons; **3** medulla; **4** spinal cord. The corticospinal fibers descend through the basis pedunculi in the midbrain and cross to the other side at the medulla in the motor decussation. Individual fibers travel to different levels of the spinal cord and terminate directly upon motor neurons in the ventral horn.

by the *corticopontine fibers*, which terminate in the pons, and *corticobulbar fibers*, which terminate in the medulla (the *bulb* is an archaic term for the medulla). Fibers of the corticospinal tract descend into the medullary pyramids and therefore are sometimes called the *pyramidal tract*.

Like the ascending sensory system, the descending corticospinal tract on each side of the brain stem crosses to the opposite side of the spinal cord. Most of the corticospinal fibers cross the midline in the medulla, just caudal to the dorsal column nuclei (Figures 20–12A and B3). About 10% of the fibers continue on the same side until they reach their terminus in the spinal cord, where they then cross over the midline. Corticospinal axons terminate on groups of motor neurons in the spinal cord that innervate specific limb muscles, and on interneurons as-

sociated with the motor neurons. The corticospinal tract is primarily concerned with controlling distal muscles that are important for precise movements, such as those of the hand. Other motor pathways, which originate in brain stem nuclei, mediate the postural adjustments necessary during movement.

Voluntary Movements Recruit the Actions of the Entire Motor System

For voluntary movements to be well timed and accurate, they require coordinated tactile, visual, and proprioceptive information about the movement in progress. Voluntary movements thus depend on integration of the motor and the sensory systems. The cerebellum and the basal ganglia have an important role in motor integration; they receive sensory input and modulate the timing and trajectory of movements. These structures are essential for accurately aimed and smoothly executed movements.

Like the cerebral hemisphere, the cerebellum has a cortex that overlies white matter and deep nuclei. Whereas much of the input to the cerebral cortex passes through relay nuclei in the thalamus, input to the cerebellum excites both the three deep cerebellar nuclei (fastigial, interposed, and dentate) and the cerebellar cortex. In turn, the cerebellar cortex also influences activity in the deep cerebellar nuclei. It is, in fact, in the deep nuclei that most of the output axons of the cerebellum arise. The cerebellum is involved in the initiation and timing of movements.

The basal ganglia consist of three main components: the caudate nucleus, the putamen, and the globus pallidus. The caudate nucleus and putamen together are termed the corpus striatum and are involved in regulating the speed of movements. The control of movement by the cerebellum and basal ganglia is mediated by brain stem and thalamic motor nuclei. This is in contrast to the motor cortex, which controls movement directly through projections to motor neurons.

Lesions of the cerebellum or the basal ganglia cause characteristic disorders of movement. Damage to the cerebellum delays the onset of movements and affects the timing and trajectory of movements, so that even a simple movement such as touching the two index fingers together is difficult. Damage to the basal ganglia slows voluntary movement and frequently results in uncontrolled, involuntary movements.

Selected Readings

Brodal, A. 1981. Neurological Anatomy In Relation to Clinical Medicine, 3rd ed. New York: Oxford University Press.

References

Brodmann, K. 1909. Vergleichende Lokalisationslehre der Grosshirnrinde in ihren Prinzipien dargestellt auf Grund des Zellenbaues. Leipzig: Barth.

Martin, J. H. 1989. Neuroanatomy: Text and Atlas. New York: Elsevier.

Nieuwenhuys, R., Voogd, J., and van Huijzen, Chr. 1988. The Human Central Nervous System: A Synopsis and Atlas, 3rd rev. ed. Berlin: Springer.

John H. Martin
Thomas M. Jessell

21

Development as a Guide to the Regional Anatomy of the Brain

The Neural Tube Is the Embryonic Precursor of the Six Brain Regions

The Neural Tube Develops from the Neural Plate

The Neural Epithelium Gives Rise to the Entire Nervous System

The Spinal Cord and Brain Stem Follow Similar Developmental Plans

The Brain and Spinal Cord Become Segmented by Different Mechanisms

The Cavities of the Brain Vesicles Become the Ventricular System of the Brain

The Ventricular System Provides a Guide to Understanding the Regional Anatomy of the Diencephalon and Cerebral Hemispheres

The Caudate Nucleus Becomes C-Shaped Like the Lateral Ventricles

The Major Components of the Limbic System Also Develop into a C Shape

An Overall View

The subdivision of the brain into six regions may seem arbitrary and its regional anatomy forbidding. However, there is a logic to brain anatomy that becomes clearer when we understand how the brain develops. Early in development, the regional anatomy of the nervous system is simple but it subsequently becomes distorted by the folding and differentiation of neural cells. As a consequence, structures belonging to functionally unrelated systems often come to lie next to one another. Because of this, local injuries to the nervous system, whether from trauma, a tumor, or vascular disturbance, indiscriminately affect all functional systems within a given area. Our understanding of the spatial relationships between neighboring structures has been greatly facilitated by modern imaging techniques that allow regional anatomy to be visualized in the living brain (Chapter 22).

In this chapter we shall consider some general features of the development of the brain that help to explain its regional anatomy. We discuss the early development of the nervous system at the cellular and molecular levels in Chapters 57, 58, and 59.

The Neural Tube Is the Embryonic Precursor of the Six Brain Regions

There are three principal layers of cells in the mammalian embryo: *endoderm*, the innermost layer that gives rise to the gut, lungs, and liver; *mesoderm*, the middle layer that gives rise to connective tissues, muscle, and the vascular system; and *ectoderm*, the outermost layer that gives rise to all the major tissues of the central and peripheral nervous systems as well as the epidermis. The neurons and glial cells of the central nervous system derive from a specialized region of the ectoderm, the *neural plate*, which lies along the dorsal midline of the embryo (Figure 21–1A). This region becomes committed to the formation of the nervous system by a process called *neural induction*. As we shall see in Chapter 57, the molecular mechanisms responsible for neural induction remain elusive, but involve signals sent to the dorsal ectoderm from the mesoderm, including from a specific part of the mesoderm, the notochord.

The Neural Tube Develops from the Neural Plate

Soon after neural induction, the neural plate begins to fold at its lateral edges to form the neural groove, which then fuses at its dorsal-most extreme to form a hollow structure called the *neural tube* (Figure 21–1). This entire process is called *neurulation*. This change in shape of the neural ectoderm results in part from local cell rearrangement within the neural plate, but is also affected by adjacent mesodermal tissues, in particular the somites, which later give rise to the axial skeleton, limb musculature, and notochord.

In certain pathological conditions, the neural plate fails to close during development. When the caudal portion of the neural tube fails to close, a crippling developmental abnormality known as *spina bifida* results. In this condition the functions of the lumbar and sacral segments of the spinal cord are disrupted. Animal models indicate that in some instances, spina bifida may result from alterations in the rate of proliferation of neural cells, or from the failure of these cells to differentiate properly in the neural plate and neural tube. Other instances are thought to result from changes in mesodermal cells that indirectly affect the folding and closure of the neural plate. The neural tube can also fail to close at rostral levels. This leads to *anencephaly*, a condition in which the overall structure of the brain is grossly disturbed.

The Neural Epithelium Gives Rise to the Entire Nervous System

The cavity of the neural tube gives rise to the ventricular system of the central nervous system, while the epithelial cells that line the walls of the neural tube (the *neuroepithelium*) generate all the neurons and glial cells of the central nervous system. During these early stages of neural development, cells are dividing at an extremely rapid rate. However, the extent of cell proliferation is not uniform along the length of the neural tube; individual regions within the neuroepithelium expand differentially to give rise to the various specialized regions of the mature central nervous system.

The cells of the early neuroepithelium generate neuroblasts that remain within the central nervous system and differentiate into neurons of the brain and spinal cord. In addition, cells within the neuroepithelium also give rise to a specialized group of migratory cells, the *neural crest*. Neural crest cells emerge from the dorsal region of the neural tube soon after it has closed. After emerging, they

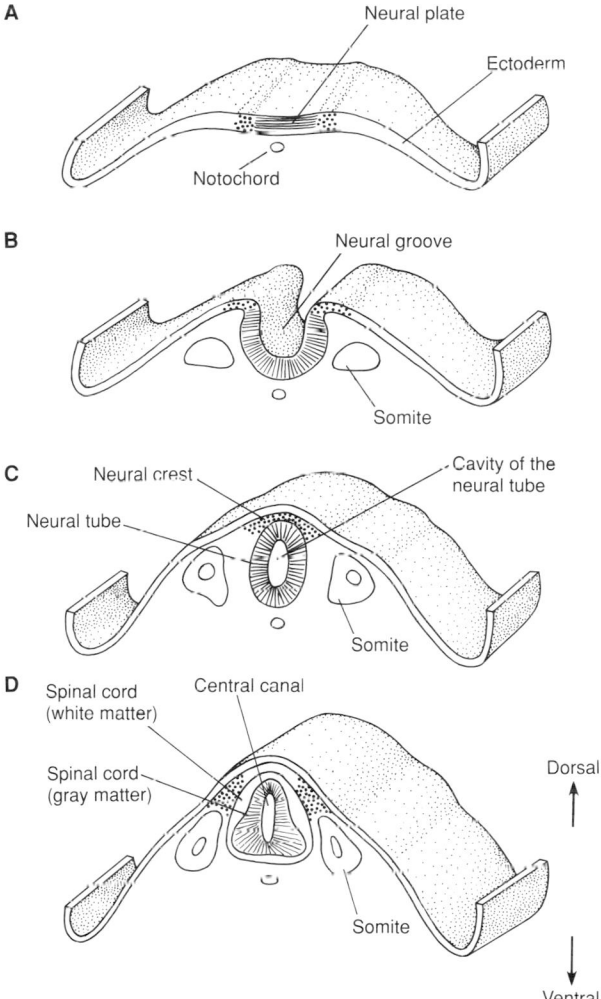

FIGURE 21–1

The embryonic neural tube is formed from the ectoderm during the third and fourth weeks of development. Its development is shown in sections through the dorsal surface of the embryo. (Adapted from Cowan, 1979.)

A. The neural plate is induced by adjacent mesoderm.

B. The neural plate folds to form the neural groove.

C. Opposing lips of the neural groove close to form the neural tube, and the neural crest develops.

D. The spinal cord begins to develop in the neural tube, as do other structures of the central nervous system.

migrate away from the neural tube to form a wide variety of peripheral tissues, including sensory and autonomic neurons in peripheral ganglia, melanocytes in the skin, and connective tissues of the face. One group of neural crest cells remains within the central nervous system to form the trigeminal mesencephalic nucleus, which contains sensory neurons that convey proprioceptive signals from jaw muscles.

The regional specialization that occurs in the early central nervous system is imposed, in part, by the underlying mesoderm at the time of neural induction. The caudal part

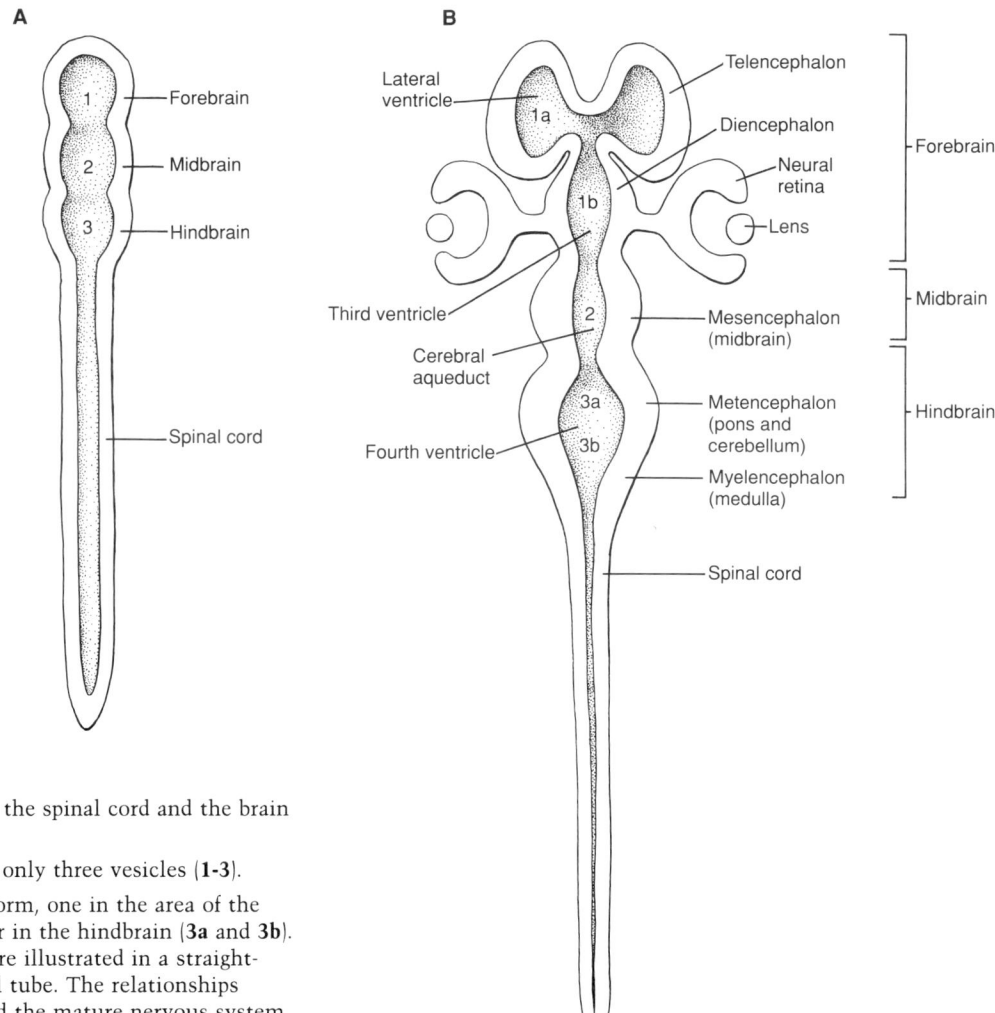

FIGURE 21–2

The embryonic neural tube forms the spinal cord and the brain vesicles.

A. In early development there are only three vesicles (**1-3**).

B. Later, two additional vesicles form, one in the area of the forebrain (**1a** and **1b**) and the other in the hindbrain (**3a** and **3b**). The vesicles at these two stages are illustrated in a straightened-out dorsal view of the neural tube. The relationships between these early structures and the mature nervous system are summarized in Table 21–1.

of the neural tube gives rise to the spinal cord (Figure 21–2). The rostral neural tube gives rise to the brain. It initially forms three brain vesicles called the *forebrain, midbrain,* and *hindbrain* (Figure 21–2A). At this early stage of development (the three-vesicle stage) the brain bends twice: at the *cervical flexure,* the junction of the spinal cord and hindbrain, and at the *cephalic flexure,* the junction of the hindbrain and midbrain (Figure 21–3A). A third flexure, the *pontine flexure,* forms later in development (Figure 21–3B). Both the cervical and pontine flexures eventually straighten out. The cephalic flexure, however, remains prominent throughout development and at maturity. Because of this flexure the longitudinal axis of the forebrain is different from that of the brain stem and spinal cord (Figure 20–3C) (see Chapter 19).

Next, two of the three primary embryonic vesicles, the forebrain and hindbrain, each subdivide; the midbrain

does not. As a result, these subdivisions, together with the spinal cord, make up the six major regions of the mature central nervous system (Figure 21–2B and Table 21–1). The primitive forebrain gives rise to: (1) the *telencephalon* (or endbrain), which gives rise to the constituents of the cerebral hemispheres, including the cerebral cortex, the basal ganglia, the hippocampal formation, and the amygdala; and (2) the *diencephalon* (or betweenbrain), lying between the cerebral hemispheres, which is composed principally of the thalamus, subthalamus, and hypothalamus. The diencephalon also gives rise to the optic cup, which later becomes the retina. (3) The *mesencephalon* (or midbrain) remains undivided during development and forms the midbrain in the mature central nervous system. The hindbrain gives rise to (4) the *metencephalon* (or afterbrain), consisting of the pons and cerebellum; and (5) the *myelencephalon* forms the medulla. The caudal

A Three-vesicle stage

Cephalic
flexure

Cervical
flexure

B Five-vesicle stage

Pontine
flexure

Cephalic flexure

Cervical
flexure

C Mature central nervous system

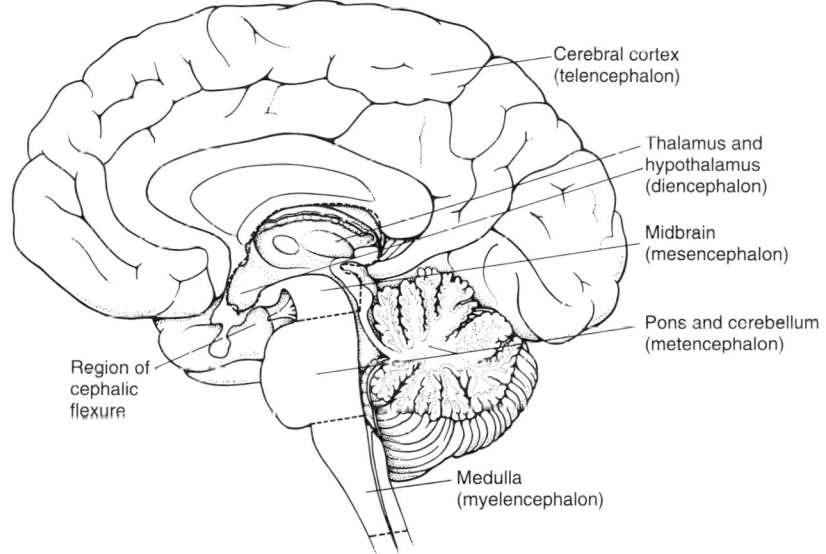

Cerebral cortex
(telencephalon)

Thalamus and
hypothalamus
(diencephalon)

Midbrain
(mesencephalon)

Pons and cerebellum
(metencephalon)

Region of
cephalic
flexure

Medulla
(myelencephalon)

FIGURE 21–3

The long axis of the central nervous system undergoes flexure at three points during development.

A. Lateral view of the three-vesicle stage (3–4 weeks).

B. Lateral view of the five-vesicle stage (5 weeks).

C. Midsagittal view of the mature central nervous system.

part of the neural tube remains undivided and becomes (6) the *spinal cord*. The diencephalon, basal ganglia, and cerebral cortex eventually develop more extensively than the more caudal portions of the central nervous system.

The cerebral hemispheres ultimately grow to cover most of the diencephalon and midbrain. The dorsal portion of the metencephalon, the cerebellum, is a second region of external growth (Figure 21-3C).

TABLE **21–1.** The Main Subdivisions of the Embryonic Central Nervous System and Mature Adult Forms

Three-vesicle stage	Five-vesicle stage	Major mature derivatives	Related cavity
1. Forebrain (prosencephalon)	1a. Telencephalon (endbrain)	1. Cerebral cortex, basal ganglia, hippocampal formation, amygdala, olfactory bulb	Lateral ventricles
	1b. Diencephalon	2. Thalamus, hypothalamus, subthalamus, epithalamus, retinae optic nerves and tracts	Third ventricle
2. Midbrain (mesencephalon)	2. Mesencephalon (midbrain)	3. Midbrain	Cerebral aqueduct
3. Hindbrain (rhombencephalon)	3a. Metencephalon (afterbrain)	4. Pons and cerebellum	Fourth ventricle
	3b. Myelencephalon (medullary brain)	5. Medulla oblongata	Fourth ventricle
4. Caudal part of neural tube	4. Caudal part of neural tube	6. Spinal cord	Central canal

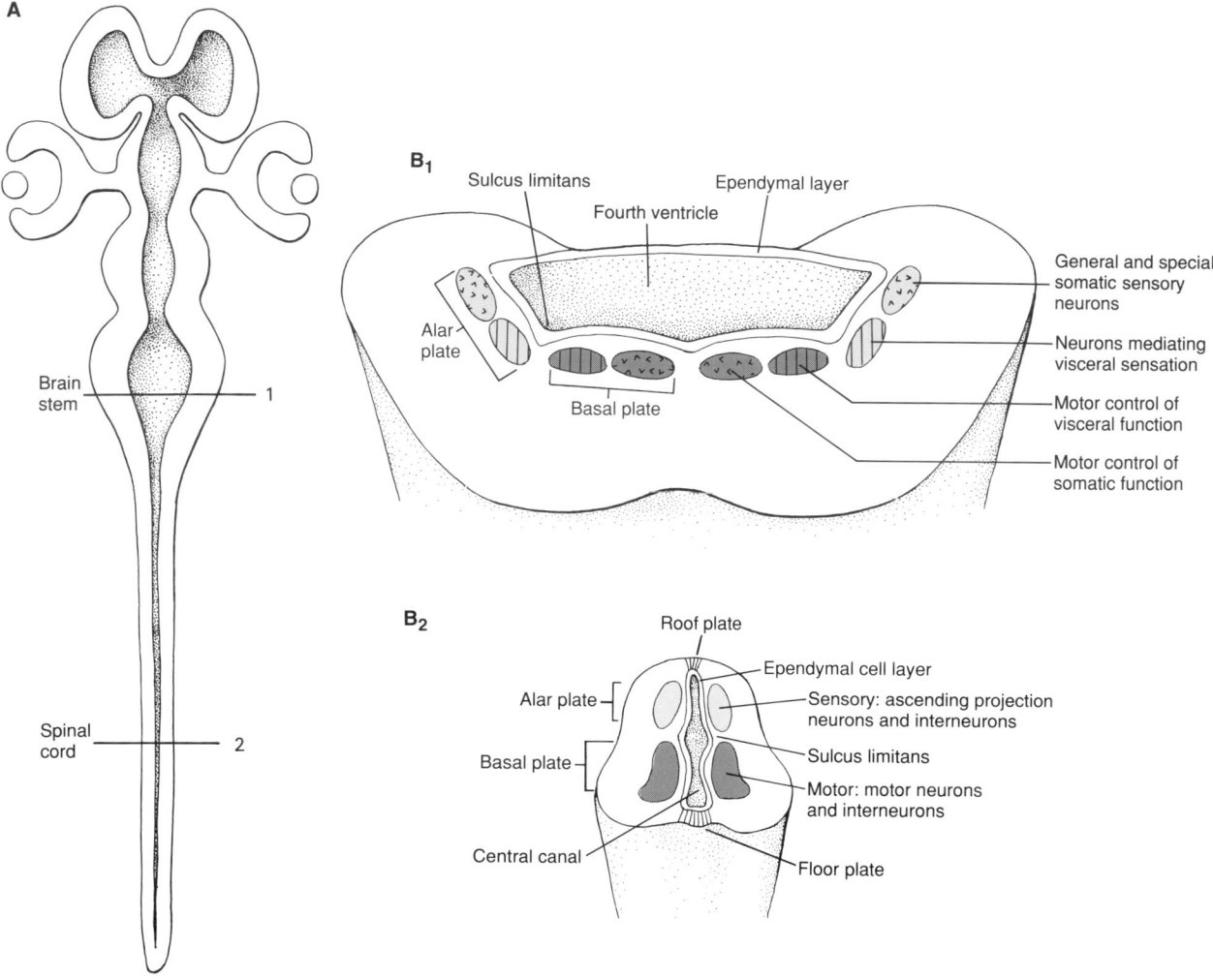

FIGURE 21–4

The spinal cord and brain stem follow similar developmental plans. During the development of each there is a region that serves sensory functions (the alar plate) and a motor region (the basal plate). In the spinal cord the alar plate is dorsal to the basal plate, whereas in the brain stem it is lateral to the basal plate.

A. Dorsal view of neural tube (see Figure 21–2).

B. Transverse sections of the brain stem (**1**) and spinal cord (**2**) at the levels indicated in **A.**

The Spinal Cord and Brain Stem Follow Similar Developmental Plans

The mature spinal cord is similar in organization to the embryonic form. In the developing spinal cord there are two major zones of proliferating cells: the *alar plate* in the dorsal portion of the neural tube wall and the *basal plate* in the ventral portion. These zones are organized as longitudinal columns of cells and are separated by a shallow groove, the *sulcus limitans* (Figure 21–4B). Alar plate cells become ascending projection neurons and interneurons of the dorsal spinal cord (the *dorsal horn*), which mediate body sensations such as touch and pain. Basal plate cells differentiate into the motor neurons and interneurons of the ventral spinal cord (the *ventral horn*). Precursor cells in the basal plate of the developing thoracic and lumbar spinal segments differentiate into autonomic neurons that become part of the *sympathetic division*, whereas those in the sacral spinal cord, together with others in the brain stem, become part of the *parasympathetic division*. The columnar organization of cells in the alar and basal plates is maintained after neuronal differentiation.

The developing central nervous system also contains a specialized ventromedial region termed the *floor plate* and a dorsomedial region termed the *roof plate*. In the spinal cord and brain stem the floor plate is the future site of the commissures, where the axons of somatic sensory relay neurons decussate.

In the mature central nervous system the spinal cord remains divided into a dorsal region, which is primarily involved in sensory processing, and a ventral region, which is involved in motor output. Ultimately, dorsal horn neurons become organized into thin sheets, whereas those of the ventral horn remain organized as columns that run rostrocaudally in the spinal cord.

During development there is a major change in the relationship of the size of the spinal cord to that of the vertebral column that surrounds it. Early in development the spinal cord runs the entire length of the vertebral column, but as development progresses the vertebral column lengthens more than the spinal cord. At birth the caudal end of the spinal cord lies at the level of the third lumbar vertebra (Figure 21–5). In adults the spinal cord extends only to the caudal margin of the first lumbar vertebra. Because of this difference the spinal roots projecting to and

from the lumbar and sacral segments must travel long distances within the vertebral canal. Like the spinal cord, these spinal roots, or *cauda equina*, are covered by the meninges. The space around the cauda equina, part of the subarachnoid space that surrounds the entire central nervous system, is called the *lumbar cistern* (Figure 21–5). Here cerebrospinal fluid can be tapped for clinical examination without damaging the spinal cord (Figure 21–6).

The caudal brain stem follows a developmental plan much like that of the spinal cord, resulting in a similar functional organization. It too has an alar and basal plate separated by the sulcus limitans (Figure 21–4B). As in the spinal cord, cells in the alar and basal plates are organized

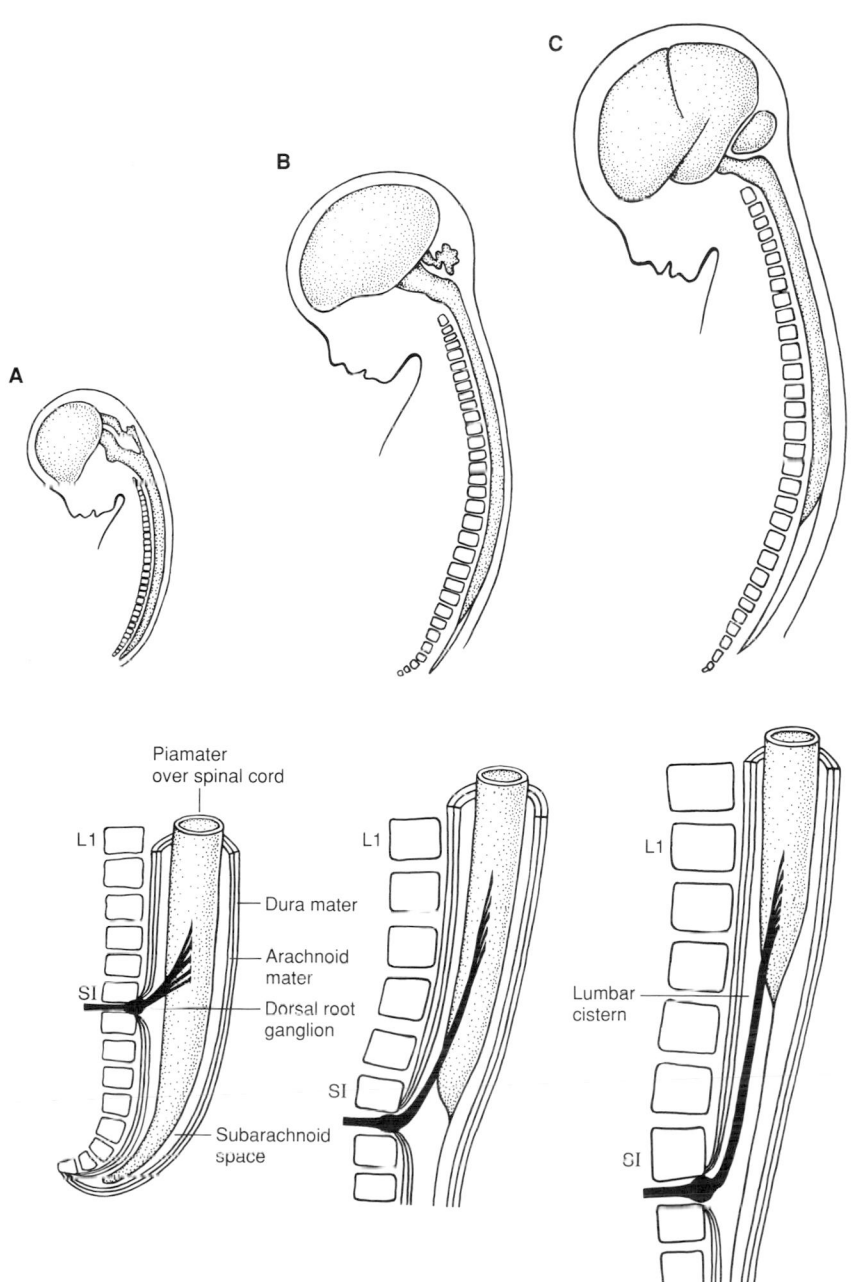

FIGURE 21–5

The vertebral column grows longer than the spinal cord. A side view and the detailed organization of the lumbosacral spinal cord and vertebral column are shown at three stages of development. (Adapted from Pansky, 1982.)

A. Fetus at 3 months.

B. Fetus at the end of 5 months.

C. Newborn. The lumbar cistern is the subarachnoid space around the caudal end of the vertebral canal. Spinal roots to and from the lumbar and sacral segments travel within this space before joining the spinal cord.

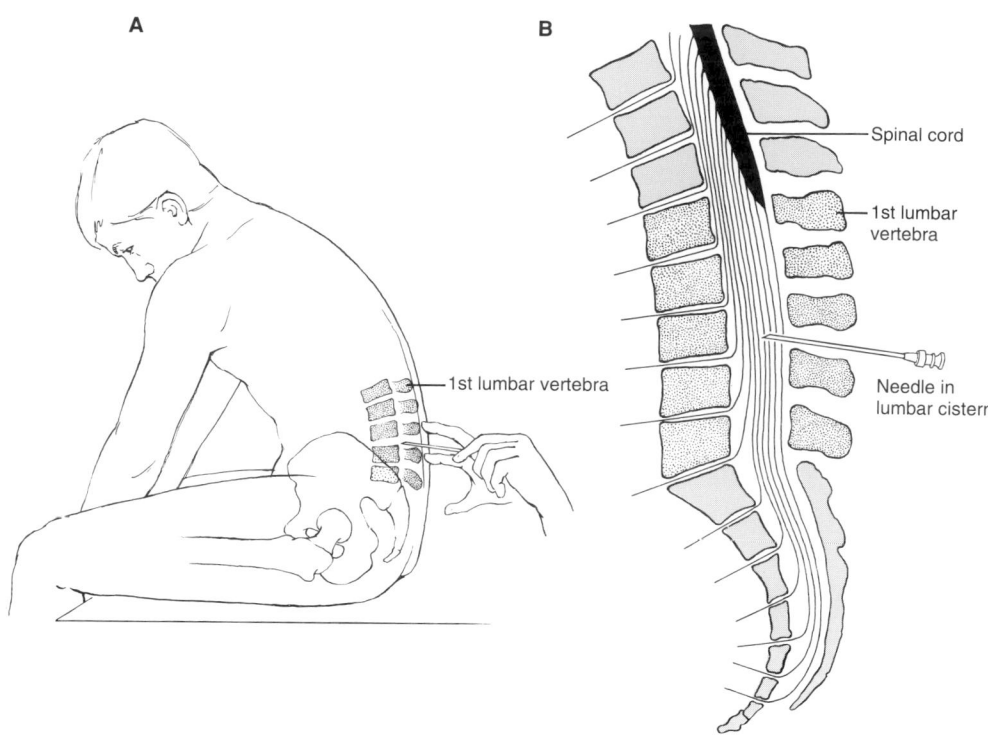

FIGURE 21-6
Cerebrospinal fluid is drawn from the lumbar cistern in a spinal tap. (Adapted from House, Pansky, and Siegel, 1979.)

A. The needle is inserted into the subarachnoid space of the lumbar cistern.

B. Because the spinal cord ends rostral to the injection site, it remains undamaged during the spinal tap. In this drawing of the caudal portion of the vertebral column and spinal cord the meninges have been omitted to better show the spinal rootlets in the lumbar cistern.

in columns. Cells in the alar plate in the brain stem differentiate into sensory neurons that mediate taste, hearing, balance, visceral sensation, and somatic sensation from the face. Some cells of the basal plate differentiate to become the motor neurons for the muscles of the eyes, head, and neck; others become parasympathetic preganglionic neurons that give rise to the cranial autonomic outflow. Neurons mediating sensation and motor control of the viscera are arranged in columns that are clearly separated from those for somatic sensation and innervation of somatic muscles. Rostral to the brain stem the separation of cells that derive from the alar and basal plates is less complete.

Unlike their counterparts in the spinal cord, the alar and basal plates of the brain stem give rise to some additional structures that are not strictly sensory or motor. For example, some cells of the basal plate differentiate into neurons of the reticular formation, which are involved in modulation of spinal reflexes, visceral functions, and behavioral arousal.

The Brain and Spinal Cord Become Segmented by Different Mechanisms

One striking feature of the anatomy of the mature nervous system is the segmental organization of the spinal cord. The axons of sensory and motor neurons enter and leave the spinal cord at regular intervals as the dorsal and ventral roots. The dorsal root ganglia and sympathetic ganglia also are arranged in a segmental order. Segmentation is also a property of the developing hindbrain but not of the midbrain.

Although segmentation is a common feature of both the spinal cord and the hindbrain, the events that lead to segmentation in these two regions differ in fundamental ways. In higher vertebrates the segmental organization of sensory and motor axons in the spinal cord is imposed by the segmented nature of the adjacent mesodermal tissues. The initial event in establishing segmentation in the spinal cord is the breakup of the paraxial mesoderm into segmented blocks called somites (Figure 21–1). The axons of motor neurons project into the anterior half of each somite and in this way initiate the segmental organization of motor nerves. Some neural crest cells also migrate into the anterior half of each somite after emerging from the neural tube. Here they coalesce to form the dorsal root ganglia, which appear at regular intervals on both sides of the developing spinal cord. The axons of sensory neurons that project from the newly formed dorsal root ganglia grow along the motor nerves, which explains why the patterns of sensory and motor projections in the periphery are similar.

In contrast, segmentation of the hindbrain is thought to result from processes intrinsic to the neural tube. The

A

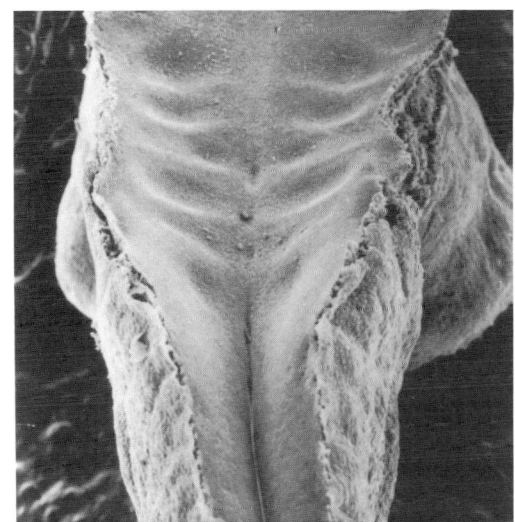

B

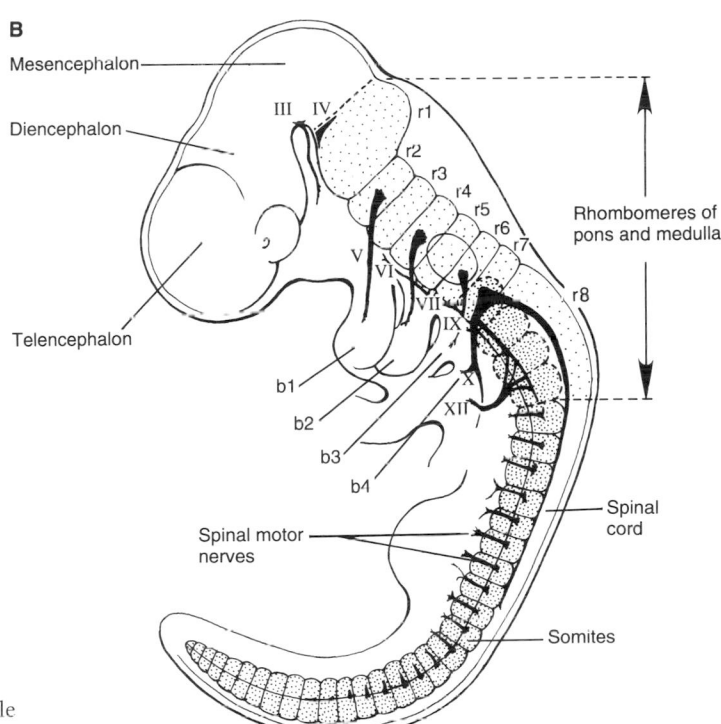

FIGURE 21–7

The segregation of cells into rhombomeres may be responsible for segmental organization of the hindbrain. (From Lumsden and Keynes, 1989.)

A. This scanning electron micrograph of an embryonic chick hindbrain at day 3 shows the dorsal surface of the basal and alar plates on either side of the midline floor plate. These rhombomeres are present in the hindbrain but not in the spinal cord. Scale bar = 300 μm.

B. This diagram of a stage 18 chick embryo shows the hindbrain and its rhombomeres (**r1–r8, light shading**), the cranial motor nerves (**III–XII**), and branchial arches (**b1–b4**). The somites (**dark shading**) and spinal motor nerves are also shown; somites alongside r7 and r8 are dispersed (**broken lines**). The

sensory ganglia have been omitted. The nuclei of nerves V, VII, and IX occupy serially adjacent positions along the anterior–posterior axis, and later form a continuous column of branchial and visceral efferent cell bodies. In contrast, the nuclei of the somatic motor system originate in discontinuous segments and retain this organization in maturity. The neurons of nerve IV originate in rhombomere r1; those of nerve VI arise en bloc between r4 and r7. Finally, the nucleus of nerve XII lies in the region of the medulla adjacent to the occipital somites (r8).

segmental form of the developing hindbrain can easily be observed in the conspicuous dorsal swellings termed *rhombomeres* (Figure 21–7). The segregation of cells into rhombomeres may be responsible for the segmental organization of individual cranial motor nerve nuclei and other developing hindbrain neurons. Segmentation of the hindbrain may also contribute to the patterning of nonneural tissues in the periphery. In contrast, in the spinal cord, the nonneural tissues contribute to the segmentation of the central nervous system.

The Cavities of the Brain Vesicles Become the Ventricular System of the Brain

The tubular structure of the developing central nervous system persists as the embryonic brain matures. The large cavities within the cerebral vesicles develop into the ventricular system of the brain, and the remaining caudal cavity becomes the central canal of the spinal cord. Later the cavity in the forebrain differentiates into the two *lateral*

ventricles (formerly called the first and second ventricles) and the *third ventricle*, located on the midline. The third ventricle extends to the *lamina terminalis*, the rostral end of the neural tube, and is interconnected with the lateral ventricles by the *interventricular foramen* (or foramen of Monro) (Figure 21–8).

As the dorsal region (or tectum) of the midbrain develops, the cavity within the midbrain narrows to become the *cerebral aqueduct* (or aqueduct of Sylvius). The cerebral aqueduct, located dorsal to the pons and medulla, is the conduit for the flow of cerebrospinal fluid to the *fourth ventricle* (Figure 21–8).

The cerebrospinal fluid cushions the brain and spinal cord within the skull and vertebral column (see Appendix C). It is produced mainly by the choroid plexus, a group of secretory cells in the ventricles. Cerebrospinal fluid in the ventricles bathes the interior of the brain while fluid within the subarachnoid space bathes the surface of the brain. The cerebrospinal fluid escapes into the subarachnoid space from the ventricles through three small open-

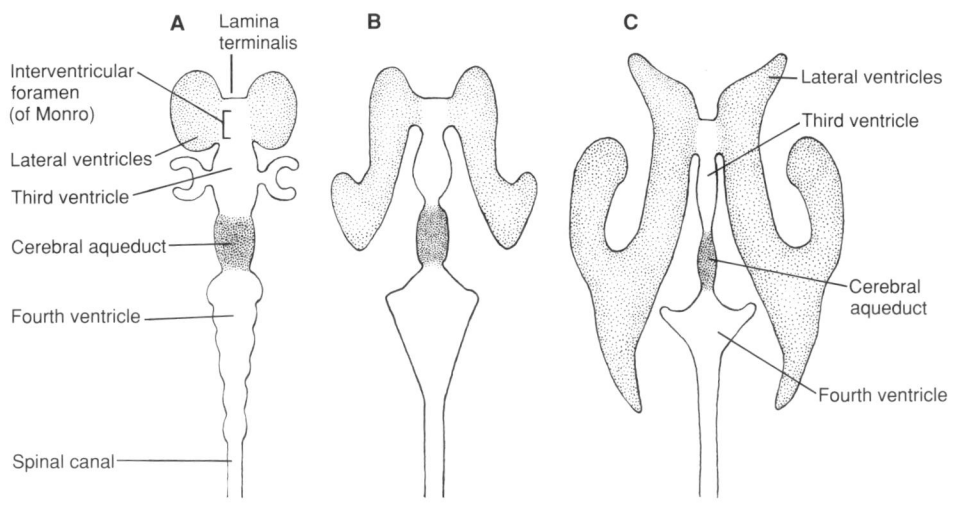

FIGURE 21–8

All of the major components of the ventricular systems are present at early developmental stages.

A. At 2 months the lateral ventricles are spherical in shape and lie close to the midline.

B. Later in development (5 months on this diagram) the lateral ventricles grow as the cerebral hemispheres enlarge. Portions of the lateral ventricle remain close to the midline, but others expand laterally.

C. Ventricular system of a newborn.

ings in the roof of the fourth ventricle: two situated laterally, the *foramina of Lushka*, and one in the midline, the *foramen of Magendie*.

The subarachnoid space is formed between two of the membranes (meninges) that cover the brain and spinal cord. The meninges (Greek *meninx*, covering) serve as a protective covering throughout life and consist of the dura mater, the arachnoid mater, and the pia mater (Figure 21–9). The *dura mater* is the thickest and most external of these membranes. The *arachnoid mater* adjoins but is not tightly bound to the dura mater, so that a potential space exists between them. This space is called the subdural

FIGURE 21–9

The central nervous system is covered by three membranes or meninges. The dura mater is the thickest and most external, and presumably evolved to protect the central nervous system. The arachnoid mater lies below the dura mater. The internal layer is the pia mater, which tightly adheres to the surface of the brain and spinal cord.

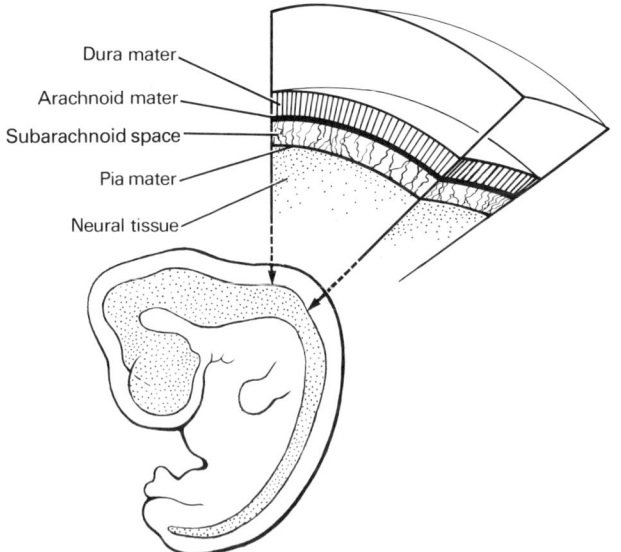

space. The *pia mater* follows the surface contours (gyri and sulci) of the brain.

During development cerebrospinal fluid produced by the choroid plexus in the lateral and third ventricles, along with that produced in the fourth ventricle, flows into the spinal cord through the central canal. Later in development the central canal closes. Obstruction of the cerebral aqueduct during pre- and postnatal development results in *hydrocephalus* (see Appendix A). In this condition cerebrospinal fluid produced in the lateral and third ventricles cannot pass freely to more caudal parts of the ventricular system and subarachnoid space. As a consequence, pressure within the lateral and third ventricles increases and eventually compresses the cerebral hemispheres and enlarges the cranium (which in the fetus and infant is still free to enlarge, since the bones of the skull have not yet fused). If untreated, this disorder can result in mental retardation.

The Ventricular System Provides a Guide to Understanding the Regional Anatomy of the Diencephalon and Cerebral Hemispheres

When the five-vesicle stage is first reached early in development, the cerebral hemispheres and lateral ventricles are spherical and lie lateral to the diencephalon and third ventricle (Figure 21–8). Later, the cells of the cerebral hemispheres undergo an enormous proliferation. As they proliferate the cerebral cortex first expands rostrally to form the frontal lobes, then dorsally to form the parietal lobes, and finally posteriorly and inferiorly to form the temporal and occipital lobes (Figure 21–10). This posterior and inferior expansion forces the cortex into a C shape. As a result, many of the underlying structures in the hemisphere, including the lateral ventricles, are also forced into a C shape. As the cerebral hemispheres develop, a part of the cortex becomes buried. This region, called the *insular cortex*, is covered by the opercular regions of the frontal, parietal, and temporal lobes.

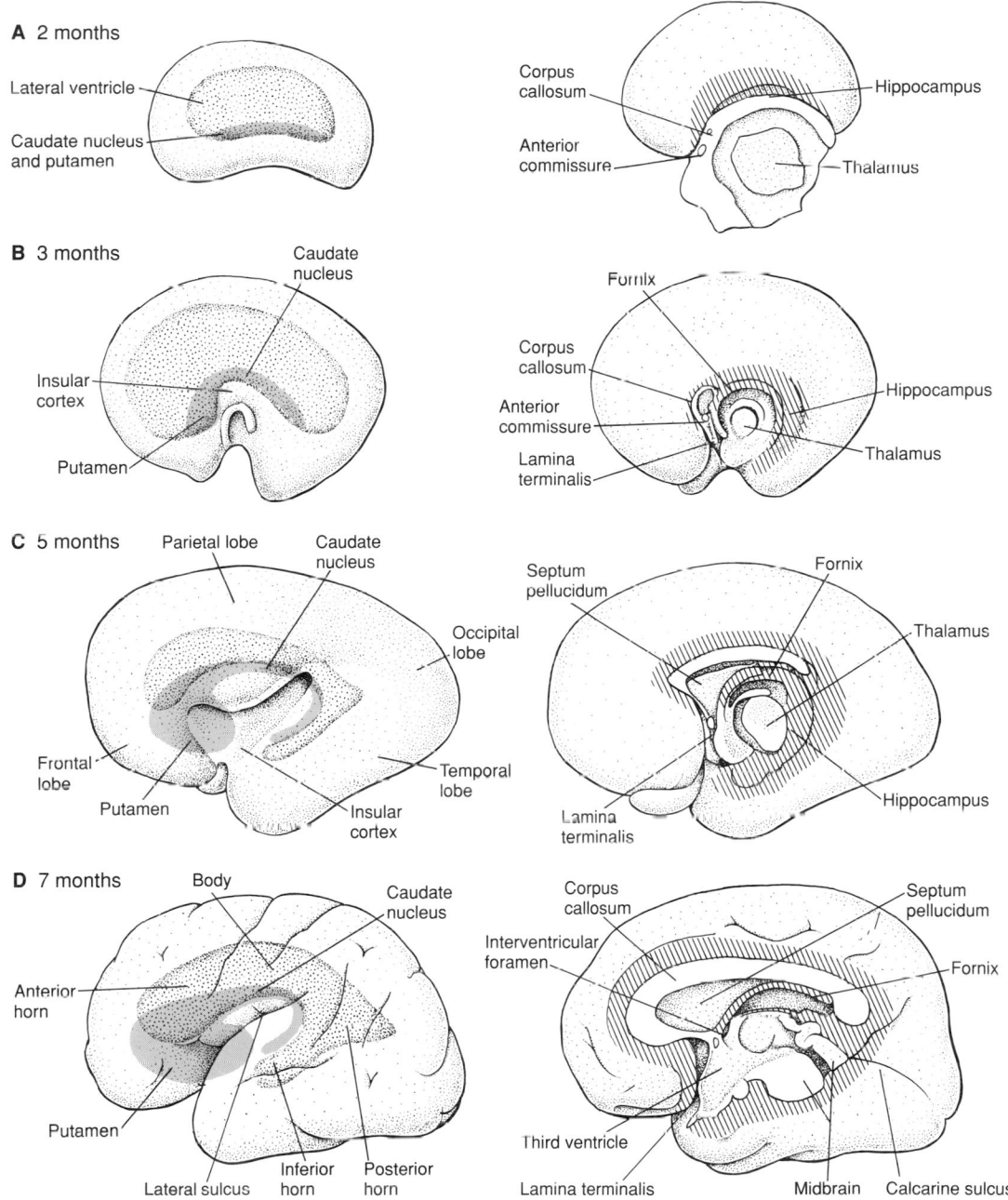

FIGURE 21–10

During development the lateral ventricle, caudate nucleus, and cortical limbic areas become C-shaped. The lateral view of the developing brain (**left**) shows the lateral ventricle (**stippled**) and the caudate nucleus (**shaded**), the medial view (**right**) shows the cortical limbic areas (**hatched**). At 2 months the caudate nucleus and putamen, which form a functional unit, are located on the floor of the lateral ventricle. As development of the brain proceeds, only the caudate nucleus and lateral ventricles become C shaped. (Adapted from Keibel and Mall, 1910–1912.)

The lateral ventricles are useful landmarks for understanding the regional anatomy of the cerebral hemispheres. The early development of the lateral ventricles is shown in Figure 21–10. In later developmental stages the four parts of the lateral ventricle become distinct: the *anterior* (frontal) *horn*, the *body*, the *posterior* (occipital) *horn*, and the *inferior* (temporal) *horn* (Figure 21–11). The medial wall of the anterior horn and body of the lateral ventricles is the septum pellucidum (Figure 21–10C). In addition to extending caudally and inferiorly, portions of the lateral ventricles expand laterally (Figure 21–8C).

The lateral ventricles are related anatomically to three structures that also have a characteristic C shape: the caudate nucleus of the basal ganglia, the hippocampal forma-

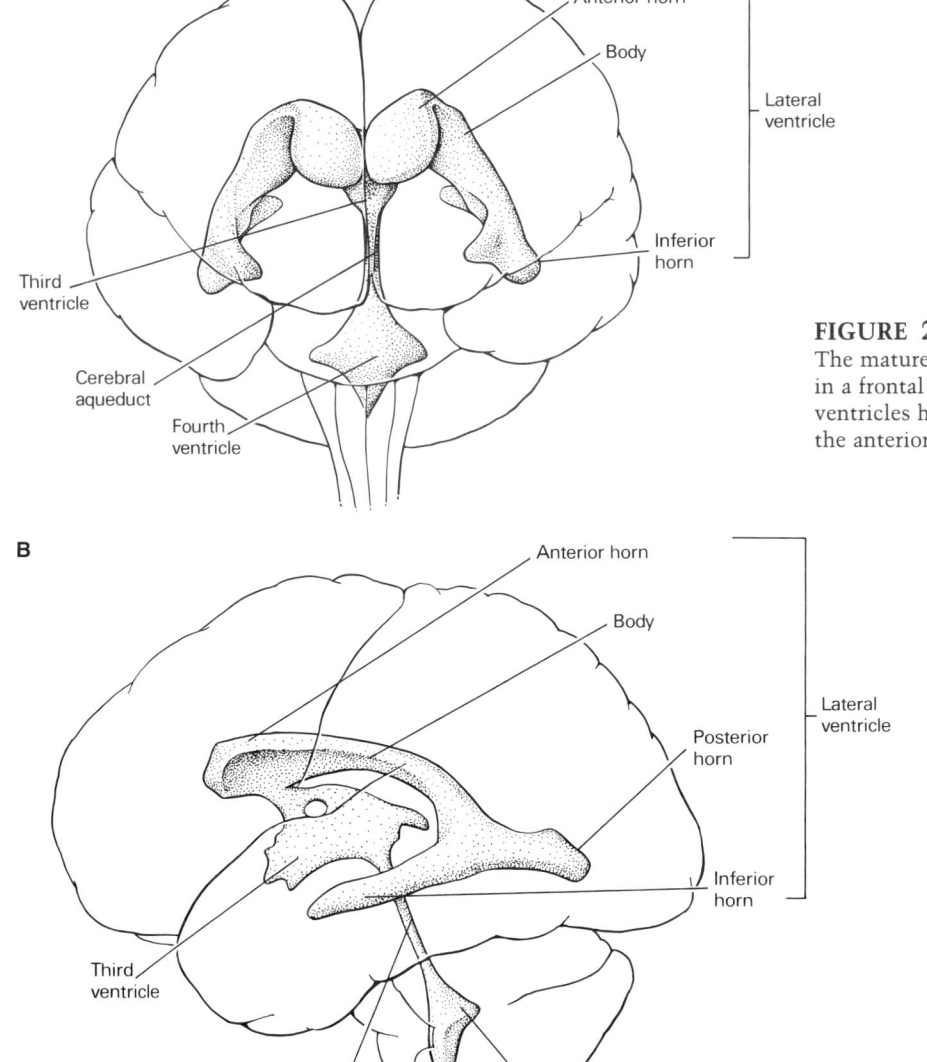

FIGURE 21–11
The mature ventricular system in the brain is shown in a frontal view (**A**) and lateral view (**B**). The lateral ventricles have four distinctive regions: the body and the anterior, posterior, and inferior horns.

tion of the limbic system, and the neocortical gyri of the limbic system (the cingulate and parahippocampal gyri). We shall next consider the development of each of these structures.

The Caudate Nucleus Becomes C-Shaped Like the Lateral Ventricles

The caudate nucleus, along with the putamen and the globus pallidus, are the three main parts of the basal ganglia and are important for controlling movement. Only the caudate nucleus is C-shaped; it roughly parallels the shape of the lateral ventricle (Figures 21–10C and 21–12). The mature caudate nucleus has a complex three-dimensional shape. Its most rostral portion or head forms the lateral

wall of the anterior horn of the lateral ventricle in the frontal lobe. The body of the caudate nucleus then runs along the lateral wall of the body of the lateral ventricle; it then curves inferiorly and forms part of the roof of the inferior horn of the lateral ventricle. This entire course describes a C shape. The caudate nucleus is only incompletely separated from the putamen by the *internal capsule*, a fan-like mass of afferent and efferent axons of the cortex. At the tip of the inferior horn of the lateral ventricle, near the end of the caudate nucleus, lies the *amygdala*, which is a part of the limbic system (Figure 21–12).

The most rostral part of the caudate nucleus is an important anatomical landmark in studying both the normal brain and certain neurological disorders. For example, in Huntington's chorea, a hereditary neurological disease, the caudate nucleus undergoes extensive cell death in

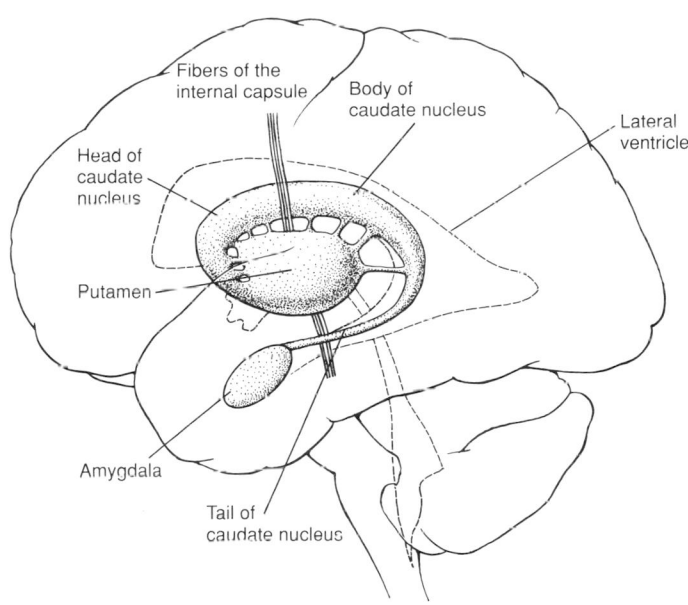

FIGURE 21–12
The shape of the caudate nucleus parallels that of the lateral ventricle. The head of the caudate forms part of the lateral wall of the anterior horn of the lateral ventricle; the body of the caudate forms part of the lateral wall of the body of the ventricle; and the tail of the caudate forms part of the roof of the inferior horn. The caudate nucleus and putamen (collectively called the *corpus striatum*) are separated by the internal capsule, a series of fiber tracts consisting of afferent and efferent axons of the cortex.

adulthood and diminishes in size. The caudate nucleus normally bulges into the anterior horn of the lateral ventricle, and thus can easily be visualized with computerized X-ray tomography and other imaging techniques. As we shall see in Chapter 42, in Huntington's disease the shrinkage in the caudate nucleus is reflected as a dramatic change in the contour of the anterior horn of the lateral ventricle.

The Major Components of the Limbic System Also Develop into a C Shape

The limbic system mediates emotions and aspects of learning and memory. It has four major components that form two C-shaped structures. The *hippocampus* and the *fornix* form one C shaped structure (Figure 21–13); the *cingulate* and *parahippocampal gyri* and their connections form the second (Figure 21–14). Early in development the hippocampal formation and cingulate gyrus are adjacent to one another. As development proceeds, however, they are pushed farther apart by axons that course through the *corpus callosum*, the large commissure that interconnects the cerebral cortices of the two hemispheres (Figures 21–10 and 21–13). Given the proximity of the hippocampal formation, cingulate gyrus, and parahippocampal gyrus in early development, it is easy to understand why these principal constituents of the limbic system are so closely interconnected.

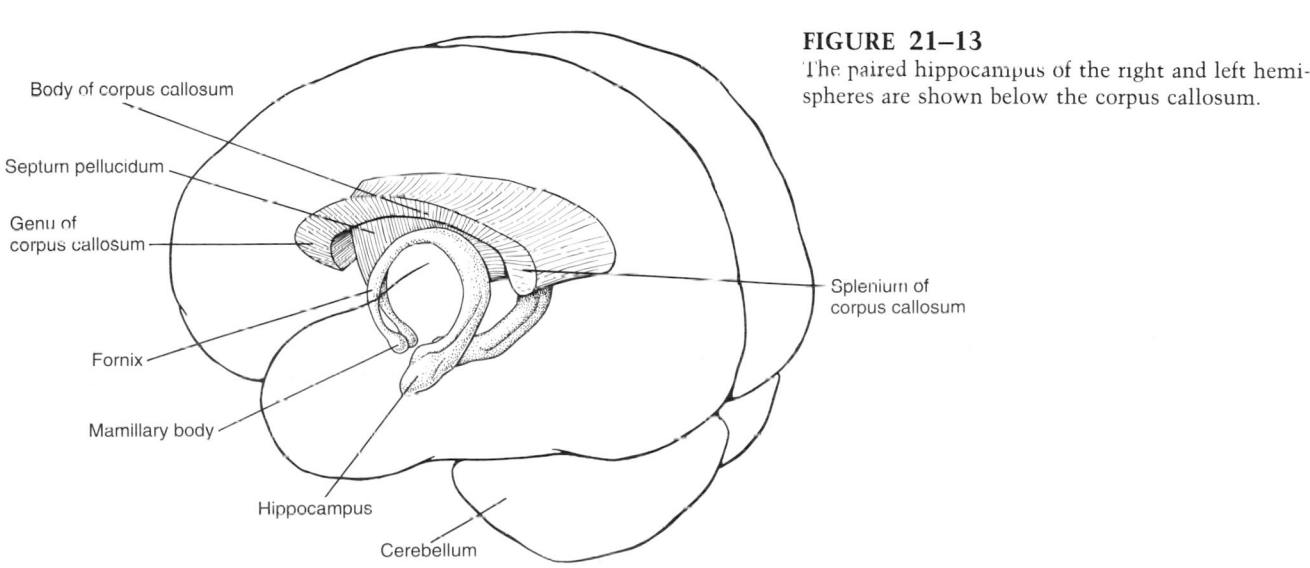

FIGURE 21–13
The paired hippocampus of the right and left hemispheres are shown below the corpus callosum.

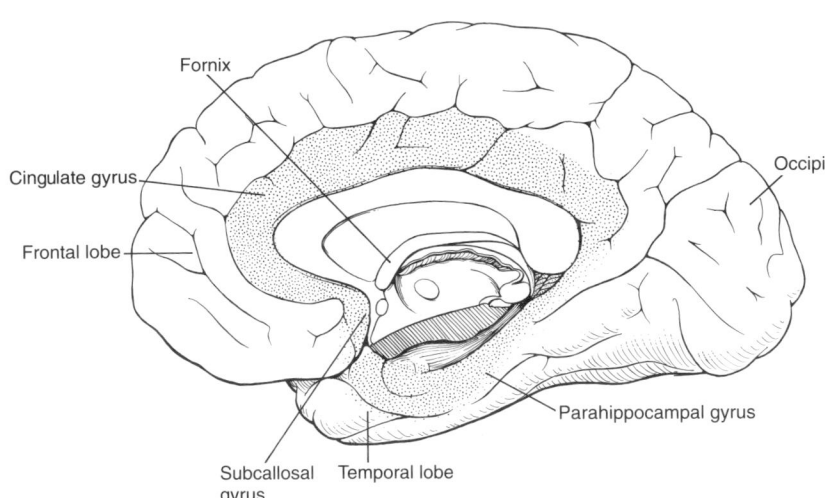

Fornix

Cingulate gyrus

Frontal lobe

Occipital lobe

Subcallosal gyrus   Temporal lobe

Parahippocampal gyrus

FIGURE 21–14
The cingulate gyrus and the parahippocampal gyrus (**stippled area**) are two components of the limbic system present on the medial surface of the cerebral hemisphere. The brain stem and a portion of the diencephalon have been removed to expose the parahippocampal gyrus.

An Overall View

The form of the central nervous system is not the result of the development of nervous tissue alone. A complex interplay between the neural ectoderm and surrounding mesodermal tissues is critical in shaping and regulating the differentiation of both germ layers. Many of these two-way interactions take the form of local tissue inductions that start at the onset of gastrulation and proceed throughout embryonic development. The cellular and molecular mechanisms that underlie neural differentiation are discussed in Chapters 57, 58, and 59.

The anatomy of the brain stem and spinal cord is relatively simple compared to the complex anatomy of the cerebral hemispheres. The proliferation of neurons in the cerebral hemispheres is also much greater than in other regions of the central nervous system. A more precise understanding of the relationship between the regional anatomy and localized function of the central nervous system is gradually emerging through the use of novel imaging techniques. These techniques, which are described in the next chapter, permit one to map the activity of populations of neurons in the living brain in a behavioral context.

Selected Readings

Cowan, W. M. 1979. The development of the brain. Sci. Am. 241(3):112–133.

Heimer, L. 1983. The Human Brain and Spinal Cord: Functional Neuroanatomy and Dissection Guide. New York: Springer.

Martin, J. H. 1989. Neuroanatomy: Text and Atlas. New York: Elsevier.

Nieuwenhuys, R., Voogd, J., and van Huijzen, Chr. 1988. The Human Central Nervous System: A Synopsis and Atlas, 3rd rev. ed. Berlin: Springer.

Purves, D., and Lichtman, J. W. 1985. Principles of Neural Development. Sunderland, Mass.: Sinauer.

Schoenwolf, G. C., and Smith, J. L. 1990. Mechanisms of neurulation: Traditional viewpoint and recent advances. Development 109: 243–270.

References

Copp, A. J., Crolla, J. A., and Brook, F. A. 1988. Prevention of spinal neural tube defects in the mouse embryo by growth retardation during neurulation. Development 104:297–303.

Hamburger, V., and Hamilton, H. L. 1951. A series of normal stages in the development of the chick embryo. J. Morphol. 88:49–92.

House, E. L., Pansky, B., and Siegel, A. 1979. A Systematic Approach to Neuroscience, 3rd ed. New York: McGraw-Hill.

Keibel, F., and Mall, F. P. (eds.) 1910–1912. Manual of Human Embryology. 2 vols. Philadelphia: Lippincott.

Keynes, R., and Lumsden, A. 1990. Segmentation and the origin of regional diversity in the vertebrate central nervous system. Neuron 4:1–9.

Keynes, R. J., and Stern, C. D. 1988. Mechanisms of vertebrate segmentation. Development 103:413–429.

Lumsden, A., and Keynes, R. 1989. Segmental patterns of neuronal development in the chick hindbrain. Nature 337:424–428.

Pansky, B. 1982. Review of Medical Embryology. New York: Macmillan.

John H. Martin
John C. M. Brust
Sadek Hilal

22

Imaging the Living Brain

**Imaging the Brain with X-Rays Depict Structures
with Large Differences in Absorbency of Radiation**

Brain Asymmetry Is Revealed on
Conventional Radiographs

Computerized Tomography Has Improved the
Depiction of Brain Structures within the Skull

**Positron Emission Tomography Localizes
Biochemical Processes in the Three-Dimensional
Living Brain**

**Magnetic Resonance Imaging Reveals the
Structure and the Functional State of the
Central Nervous System**

Proton Images Show Structural Lesions in
the Brain

The Paramagnetic Effects of Iron Allow Imaging
of Specific Neural Systems

Sodium and Phosphorus Scans Reveal Cerebral
Infarcts, Neoplastic Changes, and Metabolism

An Overall View

The study of the regional anatomy of the living brain has been revolutionized by the development of two imaging techniques: positron emission tomography (PET) and magnetic resonance imaging (MRI). These methods depict both brain structure and aspects of brain function. As a result, clinicians can now localize lesions of the brain with remarkable accuracy without invasive procedures that interfere with normal function and even endanger life. Moreover, a neuroscientist can examine the brain while people think, perceive, and initiate voluntary actions.

In this chapter we shall examine the principles underlying the major advances in imaging techniques that allow a new approach to the study of regional and functional neuroanatomy in the living brain. We shall focus on those brain structures that are behaviorally interesting and clinically important. Then we shall examine how PET is used to probe neuronal activity associated with different functional states, to locate neurons that contain particular receptors on their cell membranes, and to examine other aspects of the dynamic operation of different regions of the brain.

Imaging the Brain with X-Rays Depicts Structures with Large Differences in Absorbency of Radiation

Until recently only three radiological techniques were available to obtain images of the living brain: *conventional radiography*, still used for examining the skull; *pneumoencephalography*, replaced by newer imaging techniques; and *angiography*, still the best method for studying brain vasculature. Each of these methods relies on transmission of X-rays through the tissue and consequently cannot image neural structures.

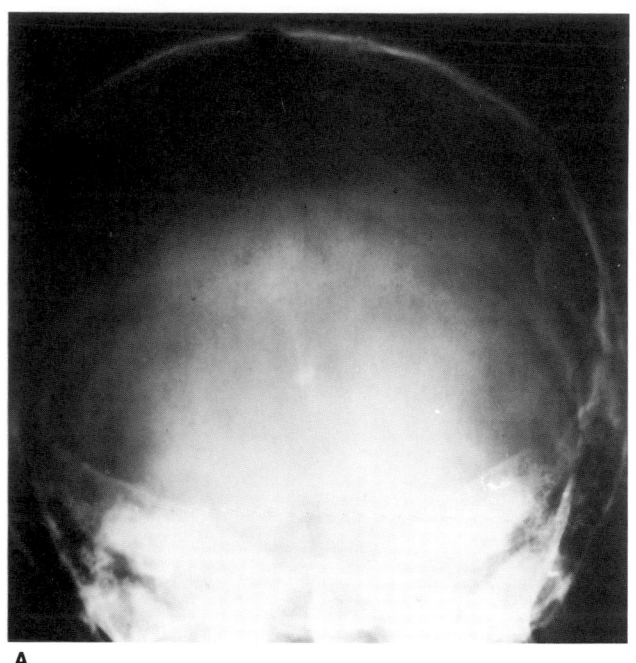

A

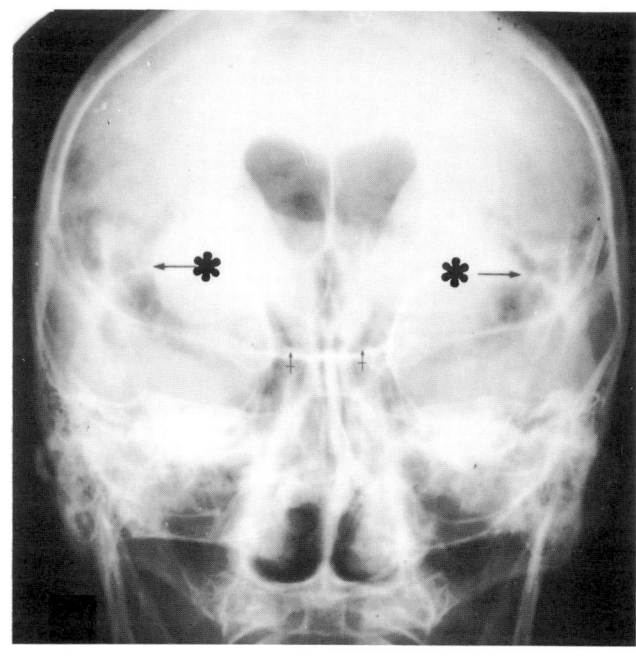

B

FIGURE 22–1

Traditional imaging methods: radiography, pneumoencephalography, and angiography.

A. In a radiograph of the skull, the bones and calcium-accumulating tissues absorb X-rays and appear light on the X-ray film.

B. In a pneumoencephalogram air replacing cerebrospinal fluid in the ventricles appears dark on the X-ray films. **Vertical arrows** (center) indicate air in basal subarachnoid cisterns; **arrows with asterisks** indicate air in lateral sulcus (Sylvian fissure). (Courtesy of Dr. Robert McMasters.)

C. In an angiogram a radiopaque material reveals the cerebral vasculature (frontal projection).

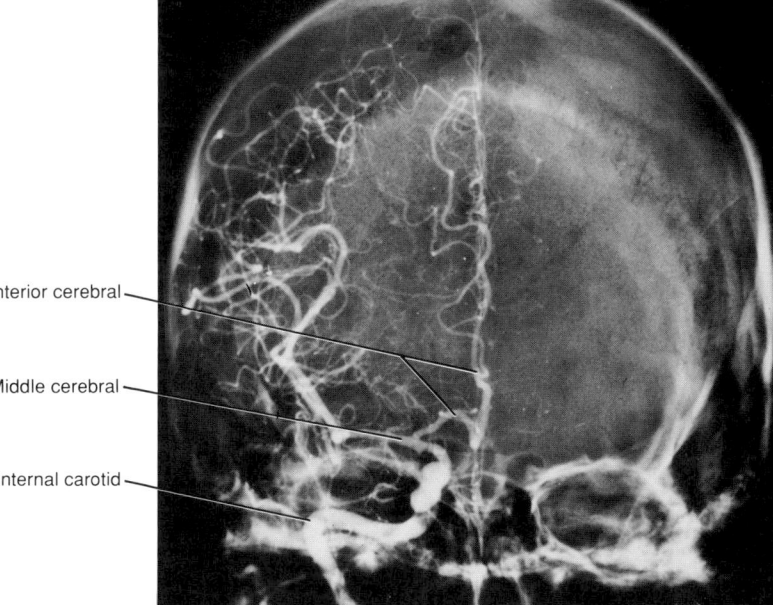

Anterior cerebral

Middle cerebral

Internal carotid

C

Brain Asymmetry Is Revealed on Conventional Radiographs

A conventional radiograph of the head is a picture of the skull and its contents. To produce a radiograph, a broad beam of X-rays is passed through the skull toward an X-ray film. The lucency of different tissues appears on X-ray films in inverse proportion to their absorption of X-rays. A radiograph is thus a two-dimensional representation of a three-dimensional object, a major limitation in studying the brain (Figure 22–1A). Another major limitation of con-

ventional radiographs of the head is that only those structures with large differences in X-ray absorbency are distinguished. For example, a conventional radiograph shows the detailed structure of the skull and any fractures or tumors involving the bones of the cranium. It cannot detect the gray matter or white matter, nor distinguish between them.

The advantage of a conventional radiograph is that it has high spatial resolution, on the order of 0.05 mm. Radiographs are therefore suitable for studying the skull and for detecting the distribution of radio-opaque compounds that enhance the contrast between intracranial structures, such as those used in angiography to image the arteries and veins of the brain. In addition, certain brain tissues that accumulate calcium with age, such as the pineal gland, also absorb X-rays and can often be recognized in conventional radiographs of the skull. The pineal gland is an unpaired structure in the diencephalon. It is normally located in the midline and is therefore a reliable landmark for brain symmetry. Lesions of the brain that occupy space, such as a hemorrhage or a tumor, often displace the pineal gland to one side or the other.

Unlike bone and other calcified tissue, air absorbs very little radiation and appears dark in radiographs. This fact has been exploited by neuroradiologists for imaging the ventricular system of the brain by a method called *pneumoencephalography* (Figure 22–1B). To obtain a pneumoencephalogram, a small amount of cerebrospinal fluid is removed from the subarachnoid space by spinal tap and replaced with air. Studying the path by which air enters the ventricles enables one to review the organization of the ventricular system. When the patient is erect the air travels up the subarachnoid space surrounding the spinal cord and brain. Some air passes through the three apertures in the roof of the fourth ventricle and enters the fourth ventricle, located in the medulla and pons. Air then travels through the cerebral aqueduct in the midbrain to the third ventricle, and then to the lateral ventricles through the interventricular foramen. Although pneumoencephalography is informative, it is also painful and

sometimes dangerous. It is therefore rarely used now having been superseded by computerized tomography and magnetic resonance imaging (MRI).

Angiography provides a wealth of information on the anatomy of the cerebral vasculature and the speed of circulation of blood in the brain in normal and diseased regions (see Appendix B). In angiography the patient receives an intravascular injection of a radio-opaque material (contrast medium). This results in the precise definition of blood vessels that contain the circulating radio-opaque material (Figure 22–1C). Angiography can identify aneurysms, vascular malformations, occlusive strokes, and vascular tumors, and is the optimal procedure for diagnosing lesions of the intracranial vascular system. Its drawback is that it is invasive; it involves intravascular injection of radio-opaque material, which can cause neurological complications. Recent advances in MRI allow intracranial vessels to be imaged through a noninvasive technique, magnetic resonance angiography (see below). Although magnetic resonance angiography has poor resolution compared to conventional angiography, with further technical advances it should supplant invasive angiography.

Computerized Tomography Has Improved the Depiction of Brain Structures within the Skull

X-ray *computerized tomography* (CT) allows us to explore the regional anatomy of the brain in normal subjects and in patients suffering from neurological disease. In contrast

---

Computerized Tomography   BOX 22–1

In computerized tomography (CT) a series of narrow, highly resricted beams of radiation are projected from the X-ray tube onto scintillation crystals, which are more sensitive than X-ray film. An X-ray source is rotated 180° around one side of the skull while the X-ray detectors are rotated around the opposite side. At each degree of rotation a series of transmission measurements is made (up to several hundred, depending on the model). The radiodensity of a single region of tissue is calculated by summing the readings of all beams passing through that region. The spatial resolution of CT scans is determined by the distance between these intersection points. The result for each section of brain is a matrix of *attenuation coefficients* computed from thousands of radiation intensity measurements and visually displayed as dark and light areas.

Computer-analyzed X-ray transmission profiles are able to resolve gray and white matter, blood, and cerebrospinal fluid, despite very small differences in radiodensity (less than 2%). Currently available CT equipment can produce scans with a resolution of less than 1 mm in soft tissue.

Intravenous injection of iodinated radiopaque material further enhances the contrast between tissue constituents in regions that have either increased

vasculature or impaired blood-brain barrier functions. By this means, blood vessels, tumors, or abscesses can be effectively visualized.

FIGURE 22–2
In CT scanning the transmission of X-rays through tissue is measured at each point of beam intersection. In the CT scan, dark areas correspond to regions of high X-ray transmittance and light areas correspond to low X-ray transmittance.

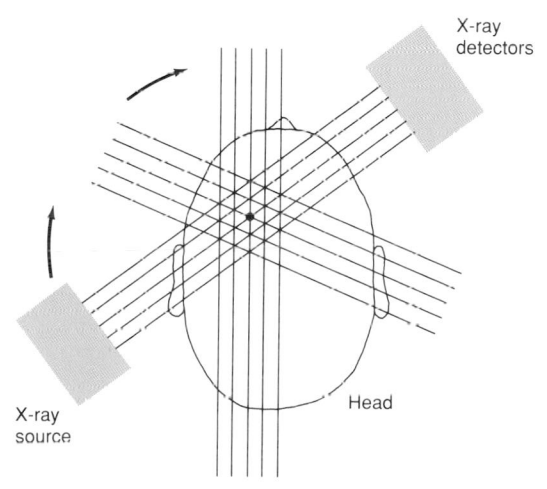

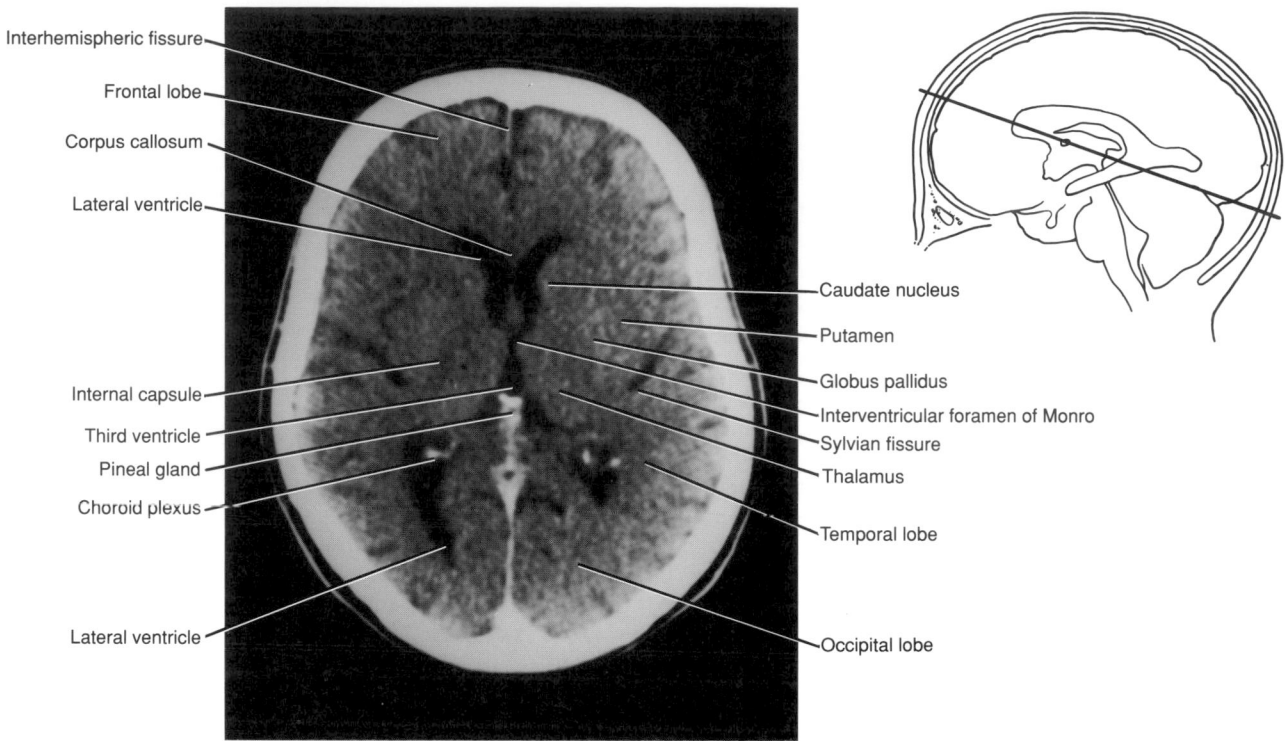

FIGURE 22–3

X-ray computerized tomography distinguishes gray and white matter in the brain. In this CT scan through the cerebral hemisphere and diencephalon the imaging plane is parallel to the line between the eye and the ear canal (canthomeateal line), which is an oblique plane between the transverse and horizontal planes.

to conventional radiography, the CT scan distinguishes gray and white matter. Computerized tomography is similar to conventional radiography in that the image is produced by the differential absorbtion of X-rays, but is much more sensitive (Box 22–1). The CT scan is an image of a single plane or section of tissue, hence the term tomography (Greek *tomos*, cut). A section of a tomogram is a true two-dimensional representation of a two-dimensional object (the thin plane), in contrast to a conventional radiograph, which represents a three-dimensional object in two dimensions.

X-ray computerized tomography provides images of bone, brain tissue, and cerebrospinal fluid (Figure 22–3). Even structures within the brain can be distinguished: the thalamus, basal ganglia, the gray and white matter of the cerebral cortex, and the ventricles. Because it reveals anatomical detail, computerized tomography has greatly expanded the clinician's capacity for diagnosis. Nevertheless, the views of the brain produced by computerized tomography are *static*—CT scans allow one to explore the structure but not the function of the brain. To produce images of the *dynamics* of the living brain, other techniques have been combined with CT.

Positron Emission Tomography Yields Images of Biochemical Processes of the Living Brain

Positron emission tomography (PET) provides images of brain function and has revolutionized the study of human cognitive processes and of psychiatric and neurological disease. Positron emission tomography combines the principles of computerized tomography and radioisotope imaging. In computerized tomography the X-ray source and detector are rotated around the head and the image is generated by differences in radiodensity. Emission tomography is based on similar principles but the image reflects the distribution in the tissue of an injected or inhaled isotope that *emits* radiation (Box 22–2).

A powerful application of PET scanning is the mapping of the glucose metabolism of neurons, a method introduced by Louis Sokoloff and his collaborators that reveals active nerve cells. Activity in a nerve cell is related to utilization of glucose. An analog of glucose, *2-deoxyglucose*, is taken up by neurons and phosphorylated by hexokinase in the same manner as glucose. Unlike glucose 6-phosphate, however, phosphorylated deoxyglucose cannot be further metabolized. Because it cannot cross the

Positron Emission Tomography

BOX 22–2

Nuclear imaging of neurophysiological processes requires isotopes of elements with low atomic numbers (e.g., hydrogen, carbon, nitrogen, and oxygen) that are constituents of biologically important compounds. However, these elements have few isotopes that emit gamma rays and their very short half-lives (seconds) make their clinical use impractical. Moreover, when gamma-emitting atoms are substituted, the activity of these compounds is usually altered. More useful are isotopes of elements that decay after longer half-lives (minutes to hours), and emit positrons (positively charged electrons). Radioactive isotopes of carbon (^{11}C), nitrogen (^{13}N), or oxygen (^{15}O) can be substituted in the structure of any of the compounds to be investigated; fluorine (^{18}F) can be substituted for hydrogen. Biological activity is preserved when a radioactive atom that decays by positron emission substitutes for a similar atom of low atomic number.

By binding positron-emitting isotopes to components of biological interest, a variety of biochemical processes can be examined. For example, brain metabolism can be probed by using a radioactive glucose analog, and the distribution and density of trans-mitter receptors can be studied by administering radiolabeled neurotransmitters. Position emission tomography is an extraordinarily sensitive analytical tool; it can detect picomolar changes in appropriately labeled chemical compounds.

Useful positron-emitting isotopes can be made in a cyclotron by accelerating protons into the nuclei of nitrogen, oxygen, carbon, and fluorine. Normally, these nuclei contain protons and neutrons in equal numbers. Incorporation of an extra proton into the nucleus produces an unstable isotope. For stability to be regained, the proton is broken down into two particles: (1) a neutron, which remains within the nucleus because a stable nucleus can contain extra neutrons; and (2) a positron, an unstable particle, which travels away from the site of generation, dissipating energy as it goes. The positron eventually collides with an electron, and the collision leads to their mutual annihilation and the emission of two gamma rays at precisely 180° from one another.

The two gamma rays emitted by the annihilation of a positron and electron ultimately reach a pair of detectors that will record an event when, and only when, two simultaneous detections are made. This method of coincident detection permits precise localization of the site of gamma emission. The resolution of PET is between 4 and 8 mm, greater than that of electroencephalograms and event-related electric potentials, the other major available methods for probing the dynamics of human brain activity (see Box 50–1).

FIGURE 22–4A

Gamma rays are detected by an array of crystal photomultipliers that surround the head. (Adapted from Oldendorf, 1980.)

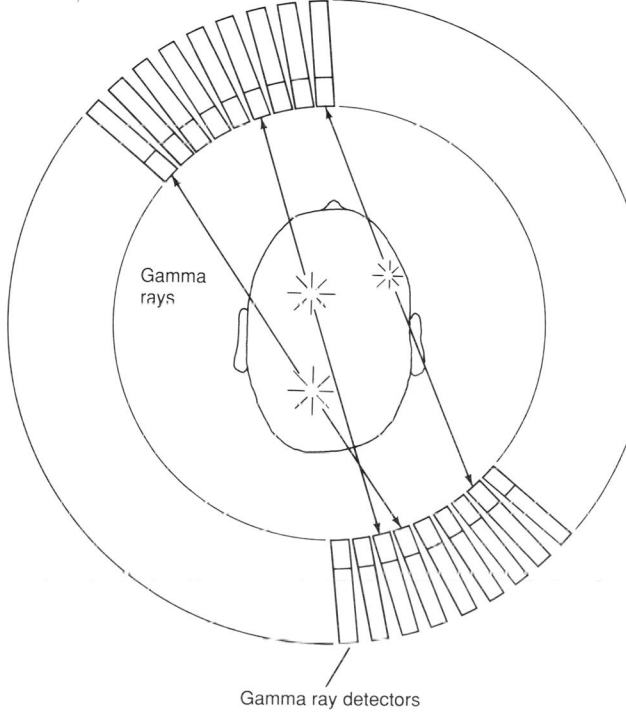

Gamma rays

Gamma ray detectors

FIGURE 22–4B

The site of positron annihilation that is imaged may be several millimeters from the site of origin. For example, the distance between sites of origin and annihilation is 2 mm for ^{18}F and 8 mm for ^{15}O. Because of this difference, ^{18}F scans can have greater resolution than ^{15}O scans.

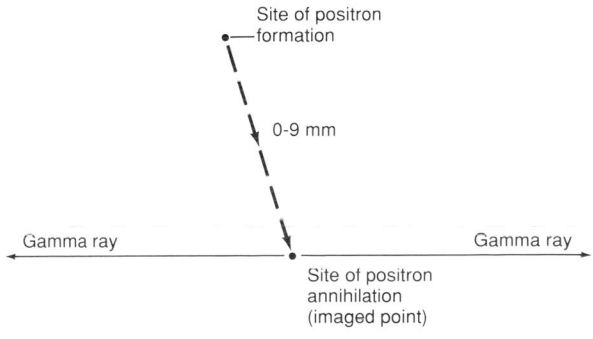

Site of positron formation

0-9 mm

Gamma ray   Gamma ray

Site of positron annihilation (imaged point)

cell membrane nor be metabolized further, deoxyglucose 6-phosphate accumulates within the active brain cells. By covalently bonding the positron-emitting isotope of fluorine-18 to deoxyglucose to make ^{18}F-labeled deoxyglucose, it is possible to assess glucose utilization in small regions of the brain.

The PET scans in Figures 22–5 through 22–7 show the degree of glucose metabolism in the brain of a person at rest and during perception. Figure 22–5 shows PET scans of 14 sections through the brain of a normal person at rest. The metabolic activity of various cortical gyri and sulci and subcortical nuclei is evident in these scans. Among the subcortical nuclei, we can see activity within the thalamus, caudate nucleus, putamen, and globus pallidus. Also visible are the posterior and anterior limbs of the internal capsule, brain stem, cerebellar hemispheres and vermis. Although these images illustrate functioning components, they also reflect the underlying nervous structure because all neural structures use glucose. White matter uses much less glucose than gray matter; moreover, different regions of gray matter have distinctive patterns of glucose metabolism.

Figure 22–6 shows PET scans of glucose metabolism in a normal person during visual stimulation. Transverse sections are shown with the eyes closed, open, and looking at a complex scene. With the eyes open, glucose metabolism increases in the primary visual cortex. When the subject views a complex scene, it increases further, and higher-order visual cortical areas become active as well. Figure 22–7 shows PET scans before and during auditory stimulation, which consisted of listening to a Sherlock Holmes adventure. This led to increased metabolism in the primary auditory cortex (Heschl's gyrus). Since the subject was instructed to remember key phrases of the story, activation of the hippocampus may be a consequence of the verbal memory task.

Transmitters or their precursors can also be labeled, as can receptor ligand molecules. A ligand that preferentially binds to dopamine receptors, [^{11}C]N-methylspiperone, can be used to map dopamine receptor location in the living human brain (Figure 22–8). Many dopamine receptors labeled in this manner are located in the caudate nucleus and putamen. Most of the dopamine in these structures comes from the nigrostriatal pathway, which originates in the substantia nigra, a midbrain nucleus, and terminates in the striatum.

Magnetic Resonance Imaging Reveals the Structure and the Functional State of the Central Nervous System

Like positron emission tomography, *magnetic resonance imaging* (MRI) is based on computerized tomography and can be used to explore function as well as structure, but with much better spatial resolution. Magnetic resonance technology was first developed in the early 1950s to measure the atomic constituents of chemical samples. Later it

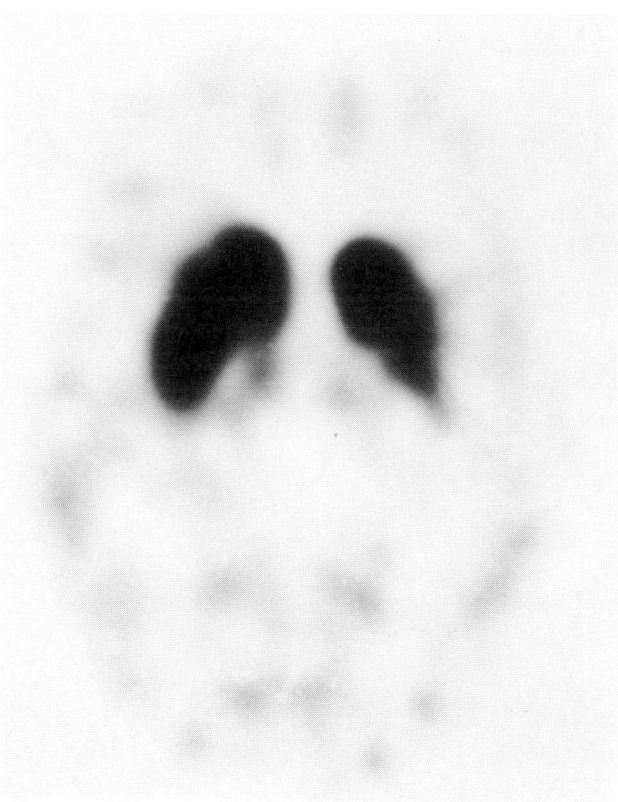

FIGURE 22–8

Dopamine receptors in the living brain are imaged in this PET scan. The ligand [^{11}C]N-methylspiperone, which binds to dopamine receptors, was injected intravenously 70–130 min before this PET scan was made. In this scan in the horizontal plane the isotope has accumulated in the caudate and putamen of the basal ganglia. (Courtesy of Dr. Henry. N. Wagner, Jr.)

was combined with computerized tomography to provide images that localize atomic nuclei. This combination resulted in a powerful imaging technique that can distinguish different body tissues because of their individual chemical compositions (Box 22–3). For example, gray matter can be strikingly differentiated from white matter, more so than by computerized tomography. As a result, the spatial resolution of MRI is comparable to that of fixed and sectioned anatomical material. Many of the key anatomical structures that were discussed in the previous three chapters can be clearly seen in MRI sections of the living brain.

The medial brain section (Figure 22–10) reveals all six major divisions of the central nervous system: the spinal cord, medulla, pons and cerebellum, midbrain, diencephalon, and cerebral hemispheres. Many of the components of the ventricular system can also be seen. MRI scans of the central nervous system in two other planes are illustrated in Figures 22–11 and 22–12.

Normal resting pattern

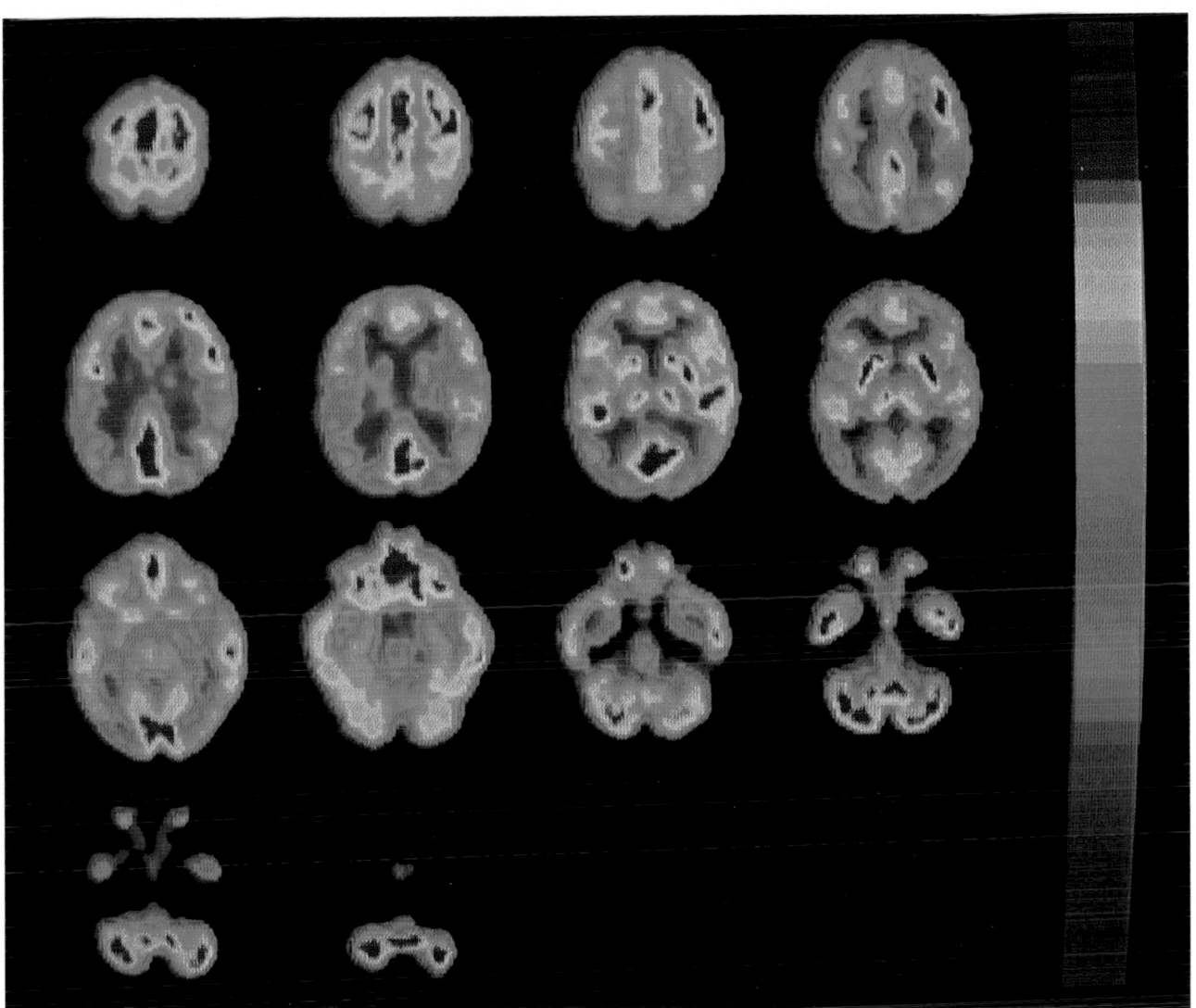

FIGURE 22–5

Positron emission tomography uses radioisotopes to reveal details of the functional organization of the brain. This series of PET scans used ^{18}F-labeled deoxyglucose to disclose the patterns of local utilization of glucose by the brain of a normal person at rest. **Red** represents the highest metabolic rate. The 14 consecutive sections of the brain are each 8 mm apart, from dorsal (**top**) to ventral (**bottom**) levels. Gray matter, which contains the cell bodies and dendrites of neurons as well as the regions of synaptic contact, is metabolically more active than white matter, which contains the myelinated axons. The areas of gray matter that are especially active are in the cerebral cortex, cerebellum, basal ganglia, and thalamus. (Courtesy of Drs. Michael E. Phelps and John C. Mazziotta.)

Visual stimulation

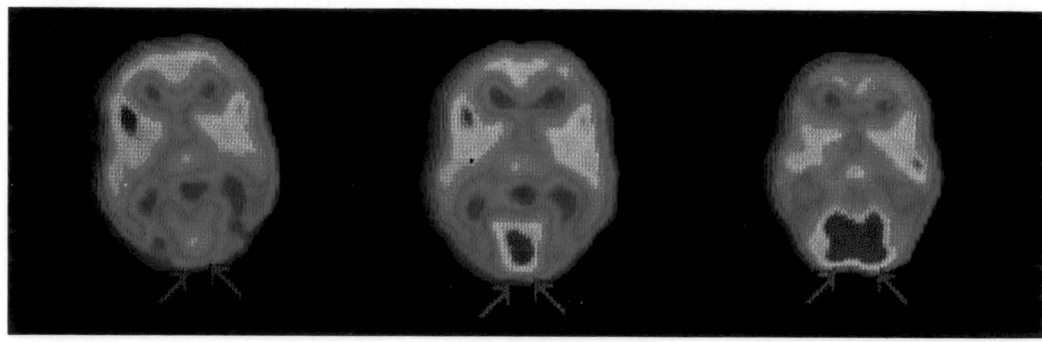

| Eyes closed | White light | Complex scene |

FIGURE 22–6

These PET scans show that different brain regions are activated by visual stimuli of different complexity. Even simple white-light illumination (**center**) causes the primary visual cortex (area 17) to be active. This can be seen by comparing the activity in this area when the eyes are open with activity when they are closed (**left**). However, higher-order visual cortices (such as area 18) become active only when the subject views a complex scene (**right.**) **Arrows** point to the occipital lobes. (Courtesy of Drs. Michael E. Phelps and John C. Mazziotta.)

Auditory stimulation

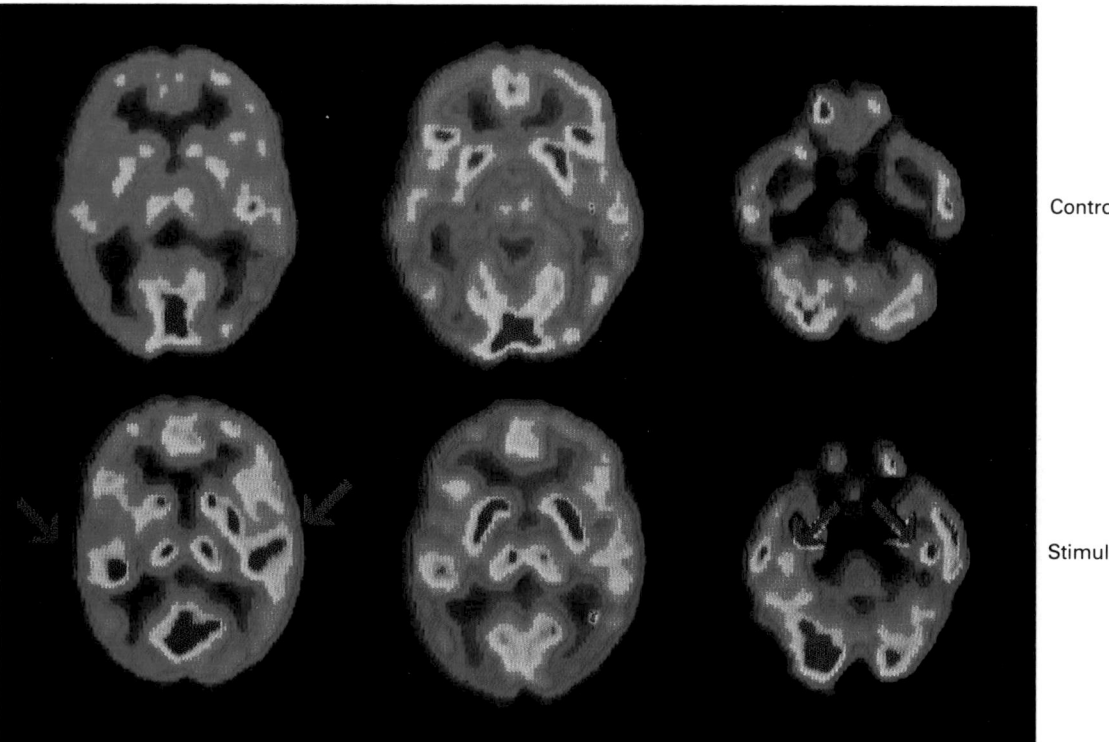

Control

Stimulation

FIGURE 22–7

These PET scans show how auditory stimulation alters the pattern of activity at three different levels of the brain. The bottom images are from an experimental subject who was read a story and told to remember specific phrases. The **top images** are from a control subject who was not read the story. Listening to the story increases metabolic activity in the experimental subject's primary and higher-order auditory cortices (**arrows, bottom left scan**), as well as in the hippocampus (**arrows, bottom right scan**), a structure important for memory. (Courtesy of Drs. Michael E. Phelps and John C. Mazziotta.)

When elements with an odd atomic weight, such as hydrogen, are exposed to a strong static homogeneous magnetic field, the nuclei behave as spinning magnets and develop a net alignment of their spin axes along the direction of the applied field (Figure 22–9A, large arrow). The atomic nuclei give rise to the magnetic resonance imaging (MRI) signal in the following way. The alignment of the spin axes can be perturbed by a brief pulse of radio waves, which serves to tip the spinning nuclei away from their parallel orientation with the strong magnetic field and provides energy for their subsequent gyroscope-like motions, called precession.

When the pulse is turned off, the nuclei tend to return to their original orientation, and in doing so release energy in the form of radio waves. The frequency of the radio wave given off is distinct for different atomic species as well as for a given atomic nucleus in different chemical or physical environments. The resonating nuclei thus become radio wave transmitters with characteristic frequencies and reveal their presence by their signals.

Different nuclear species absorb energy from radio waves of a particular frequency. The ability of the atomic nuclei to absorb energy from radio waves is called nuclear magnetic resonance. The atomic nuclei, having absorbed energy from the externally applied radio waves, then release it as a signal as they return to a lower-energy state.

The rate at which nuclei return to a lower-energy state is called *relaxation* and is usually described by its time constant (T). There are two types of relaxation of importance in MRI at present: spin-lattice relaxation (T_1) and spin–spin relaxation (T_2). For a particular atom, these relaxation times vary from compound to compound. For example, hydrogen has a much shorter relaxation time in fat than it has in water. Relaxation times also vary according to the local tissue conditions, such as water in the cerebrospinal fluid and water in the brain parenchyma. (Dense bone, which contains little water, is invisible on such images.) Since relaxation times are influenced by local tissue conditions, by emphasizing one or the other relaxation time an image can either discriminate between normal tissues of various composition or define pathological processes. For example, the difference between gray and white matter is best visualized by images emphasizing T_1, whereas cerebrospinal fluid is greatly enhanced on images emphasizing T_2.

Images can be generated that depict either the distribution of a particular relaxation time in a cross section of tissue or the actual concentration of a particular atomic nucleus. In MRI the greatest contrast is obtained when images represent tissue relaxation times rather than proton concentration. For example, the differences between the relaxation times of gray and white matter or white matter and cerebrospinal fluid are much greater than the differences between their proton concentrations.

FIGURE 22–9A

The alignment of atomic nuclei (**thick arrow**) with the direction of the applied magnetic field (**thin arrows**) is shown on the left; precession of atomic nuclei is shown on the right.

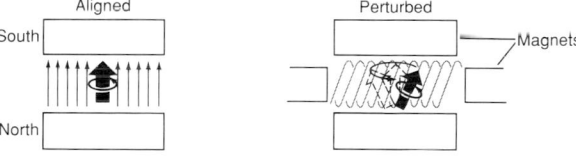

FIGURE 22–9B

The frequency of the radiowave emitted by an atomic nucleus depends directly upon the strength of the surrounding magnetic field. For a homogeneous sample of the nuclei in a homogeneous magnetic field, the resultant signal is at a single frequency. For the same sample exposed to two different strength fields simultaneously, the signal is split, the frequency of the signal emitted by the nuclei positioned in the weaker magnetic field is lower than that of nuclei positioned in the stronger field. If the strength of the applied magnetic field changes more often across the sample, each point on the frequency axis corresponds to a different spatial location within the sample.

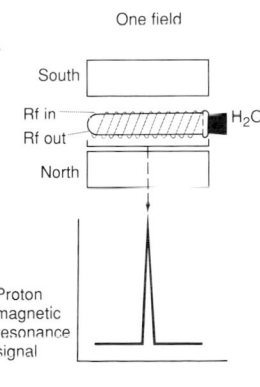
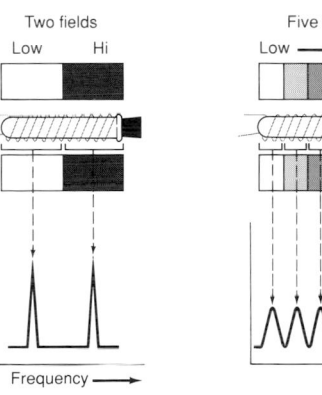

FIGURE 22–9C

Using the principle demonstrated in Figure 22–9B, one can translate signals coming from the brain into images by adding a small magnetic gradient onto the static homogeneous magnetic field. The frequency of the signal transmitted by nuclei in the higher end of the field is higher than that of nuclei in the lower end. The frequency of a given signal is therefore the indicator of spatial location. By changing the orientation of the applied magnetic gradient, one can obtain a large series of profiles of the brain (or any other part of the body). Using computer techniques similar to those applied in CT and PET, one can reconstruct an entire cross section of the brain from the information in the MRI profiles.

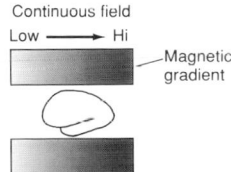
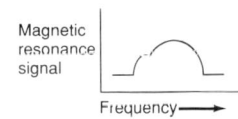

318

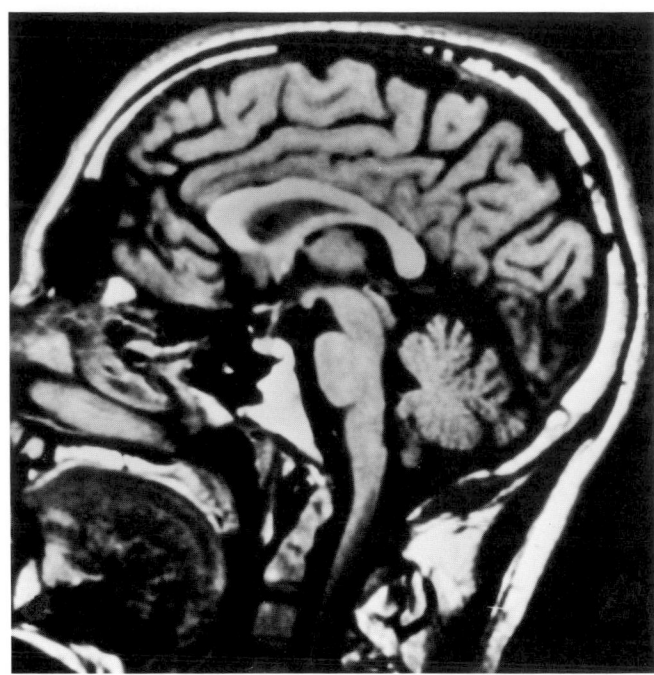

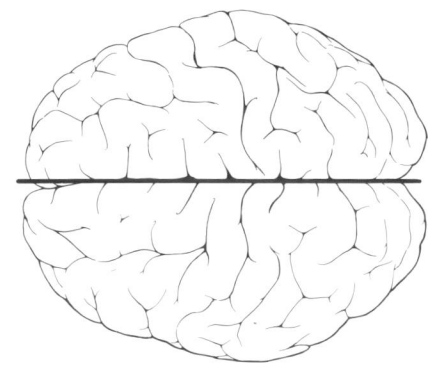

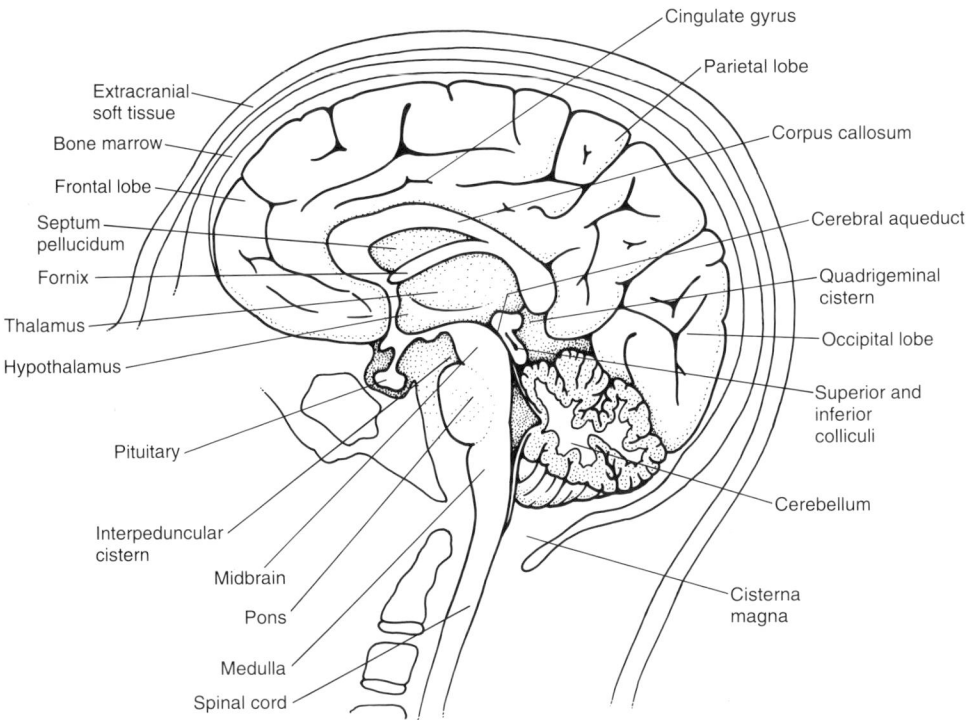

FIGURE 22–10

This MRI scan of a midsagittal section through the cerebral hemispheres, corpus callosum, brain stem, and spinal cord reveals all major regions of the central nervous system as well as components of the ventricular system. Whereas dense bone is not seen on MRI, marrow is. The diagram shows the detail visible in the MRI scan. The cingulate gyrus, a prominent gyrus on the medial surface, overlies the corpus callosum and fornix. These three structures each have a C shape. The cingulate gyrus and fornix are both part of the limbic system. The corpus callosum contains the axons of neurons that interconnect the two halves of

the cerebral cortex. The fornix can be seen to curve around the dorsal part of the thalamus, a major constituent of the diencephalon. The other major component of the diencephalon, the hypothalamus, can be seen ventral to the thalamus. The two lobes of the pituitary gland are also clearly revealed. The posterior lobe is distinguished from the anterior lobe by the presence of antidiuretic hormone in the terminals of neurosecretory cells, which produces an intense signal on MRI. The imaging plane in the scan cuts through the third ventricle. The cerebral aqueduct can be seen connecting the third and fourth ventricles.

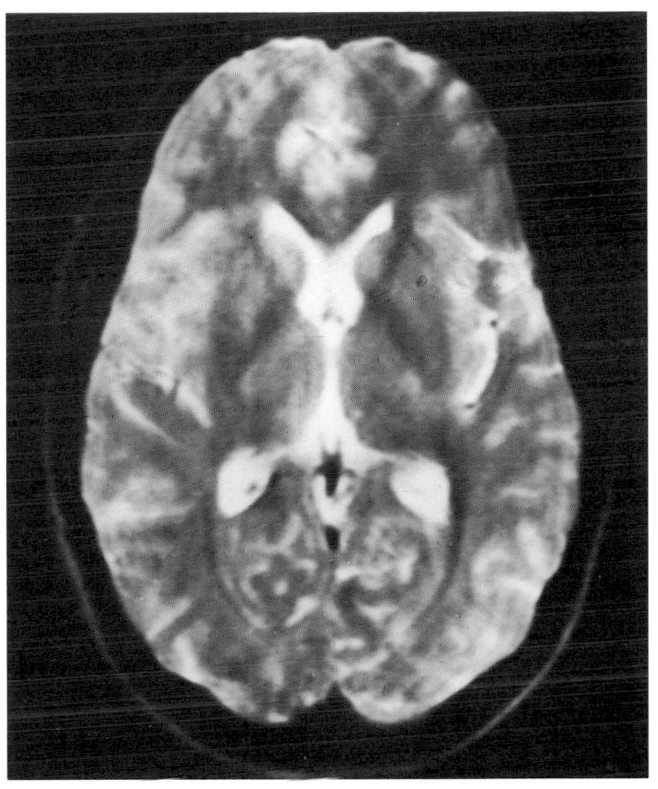

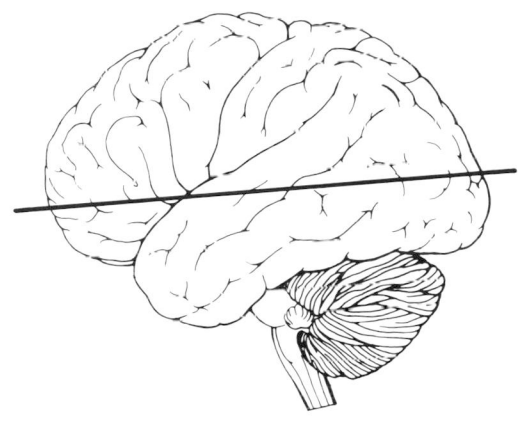

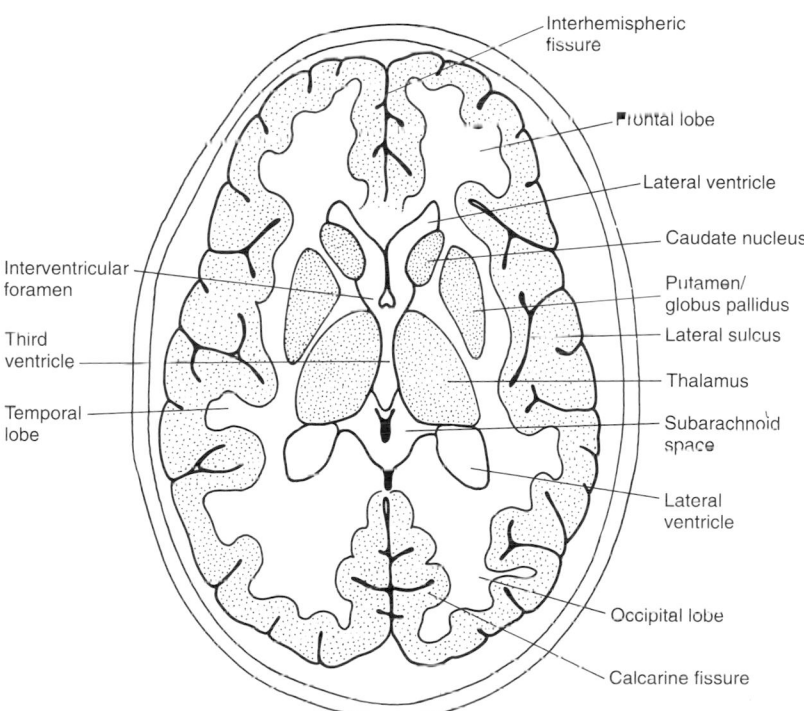

Interhemispheric fissure

Frontal lobe

Lateral ventricle

Caudate nucleus

Putamen/ globus pallidus

Lateral sulcus

Thalamus

Subarachnoid space

Lateral ventricle

Occipital lobe

Calcarine fissure

Interventricular foramen

Third ventricle

Temporal lobe

FIGURE 22–11

An MRI scan of a horizontal section through the cerebral hemisphere and diencephalon. The diagram shows the detail visible in the MRI scan. Some aspects of the nuclear organization of the thalamus can be seen. The caudate nucleus and putamen, the two major components of the basal ganglia, are clearly seen, as are components of the ventricular system. While the caudate nucleus is a C-shaped structure, only the head is visible; the body is above the plane of the section and the tail is too small to be seen on MR images. The calcarine fissure—the site of the primary visual cortex—can also be seen in the occipital lobe.

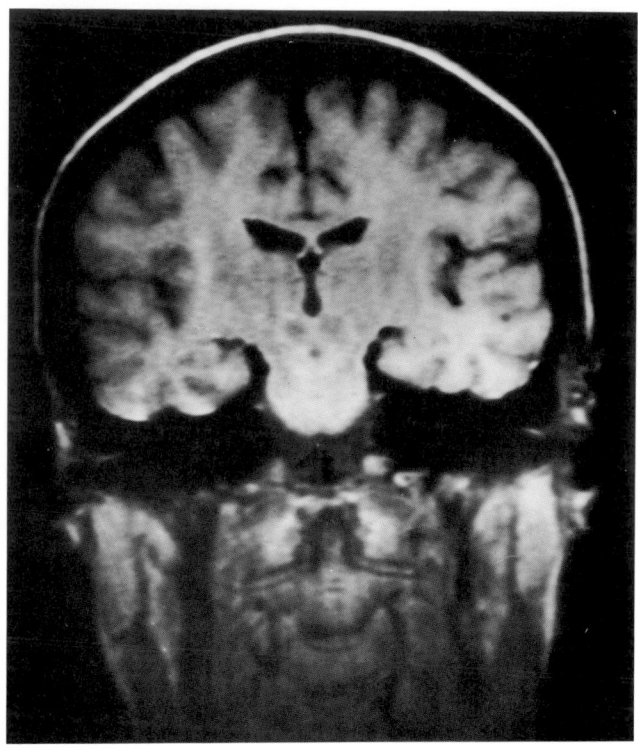

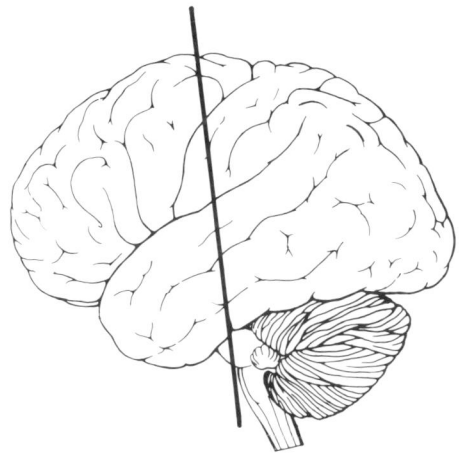

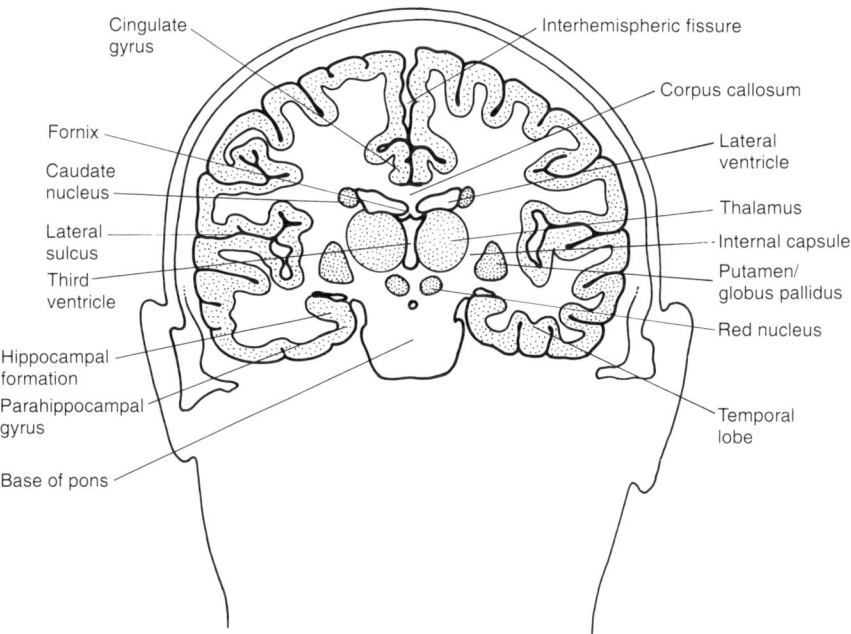

Cingulate gyrus

Interhemispheric fissure

Fornix

Corpus callosum

Caudate nucleus

Lateral ventricle

Lateral sulcus

Thalamus

Third ventricle

Internal capsule

Hippocampal formation

Putamen/ globus pallidus

Parahippocampal gyrus

Red nucleus

Base of pons

Temporal lobe

FIGURE 22–12

An MRI scan of a coronal section through the cerebral hemisphere and diencephalon. The diagram shows the detail visible in the MRI scan. The coronal section shows many of the structures that appear in the horizontal section in Figure 22–11. In addition, the hippocampal formation, a common site of epileptic seizures, can be seen. Two other key features of the internal structure of the brain are revealed in this section and Figure 22–11: the *third ventricle*, which separates the two halves of the thalamus, and the *internal capsule*, which separates the thalamus from components of the basal ganglia. In horizontal section the internal capsule

appears as an arrowhead, with its point, the genu, flanked by the anterior and posterior limbs. The internal capsule is particularly important clinically. Damage to this region is often devastating because axons descending from the motor regions of the cortex form a relatively compact bundle of fibers in this area. Occlusion of the vascular supply of the internal capsule, a common form of stroke, can result in paralysis of the opposite side of the body. The ascending sensory and descending motor axons course in the posterior limb of the internal capsule.

Magnetic resonance imaging can also detect the motion of water molecules. A technique called *magnetic resonance angiography* (MRA) selectively images the blood vessels (Figure 22–13). These techniques are promising because they are noninvasive, unlike conventional cerebral angiography, and can show the entire vascular system from many angles. Thus, MRA makes possible an accurate evaluation of the morphology of vessels and the detection of small atherosclerotic plaques. With MRA it is also possible to measure brain perfusion.

Proton Images Show Structural Lesions in the Brain

An MRI image of the brain based on the proton relaxation time (T_2) can reveal minute differences in tissue water concentration and is therefore a sensitive technique for the detection of brain lesions (see Box 22–3). This is because most structural disease processes expand the extracellular space. (The brain has the smallest extracellular space of all organs, approximately 20% of volume.) Extracellular water usually increases during brain swelling, for example, as a consequence of tumors or inflammatory processes. The advantages of MRI over computerized tomography for diagnosis is evident in Figure 22–14.

The Paramagnetic Effects of Iron Allow Imaging of Specific Neural Systems

Besides showing the water content of gray and white matter, MRI can show the distribution of naturally occurring elements with paramagnetic properties or artificially introduced substances. For example, under normal conditions the nuclei of the extrapyramidal system, a compo-

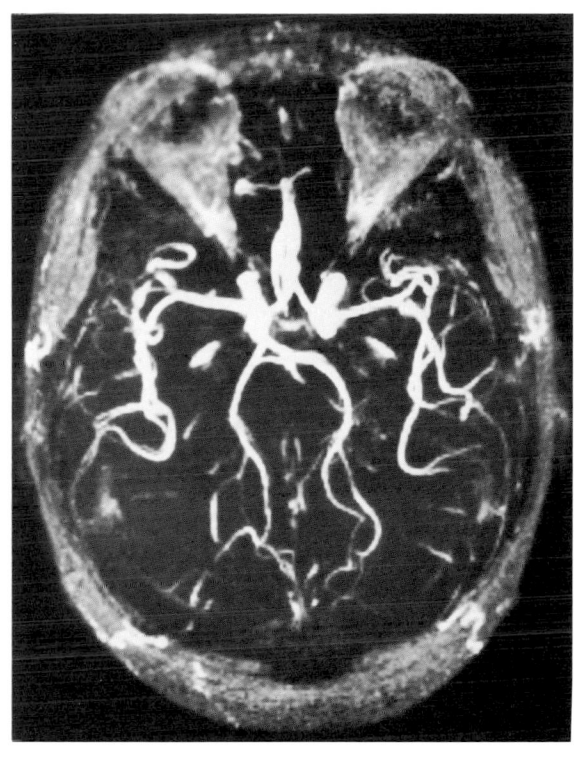

FIGURE 22–13
Magnetic resonance angiography (MRA) images blood vessels noninvasively. This image of the circulation of the cerebral hemispheres was reconstructed from MR images obtained at numerous levels. The three-dimensional organization of the cerebral arterial vasculature is projected into this two-dimensional image. The anterior, middle, and posterior cerebral arteries are clearly shown, as are the internal carotid arteries. Note that the posterior communicating artery is absent on the right side.

MRI

CT

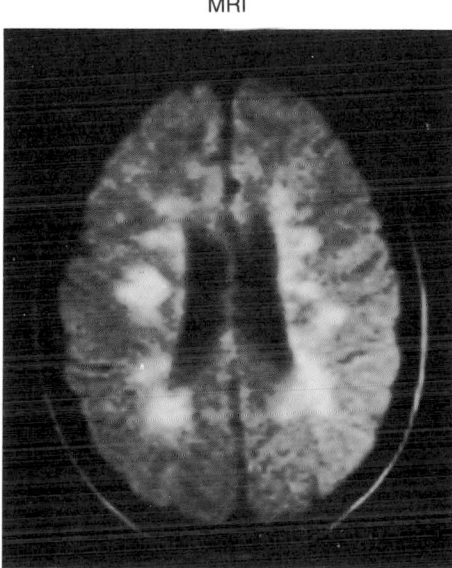
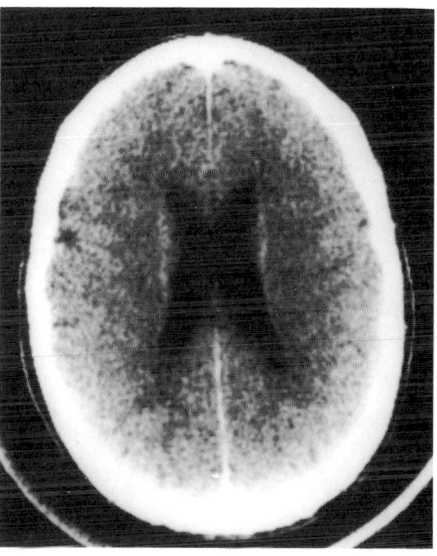

FIGURE 22–14
The diagnostic advantage of MRI over CT is shown in horizontal sections through the cerebral cortex and underlying white matter of a patient with multiple sclerosis. Demyelination of white matter is more clearly visible in the MRI scan. (Courtesy of Dr. Michael Aminoff.)

nent of the motor system, contain more iron than is found in other brain regions. Most of this iron is in ferritin. Because of the presence of iron, the magnetic field of the surrounding water is distorted; the signal from the water molecules is suppressed. These changes are most obvious with spin-spin relaxation (T_2) images. In a normal individual two components of the basal ganglia, the globus pallidus (Figure 22–11) and the substantia nigra as well as the red nucleus in the midbrain (Figure 22–12), appear darker than the rest of the brain because the signals from these tissues are reduced by the presence of ferritin. Movement disorders that result from diseases affecting the extrapyramidal system, like parkinsonism and dystonia, alter the distribution of iron and therefore the T_2 signal. Iron also plays an important role in imaging intracranial hemorrhage. Blood and its breakdown products also alter the signal on magnetic resonance images because of their iron content. As a result, MRI is the most sensitive way to detect a small hemorrhage in an area of stroke.

Paramagnetic substances, such as organic compounds synthesized with gadolinium, also alter the magnetic environment of water and therefore its relaxation properties. Intravascular injection of gadolinium compounds will outline brain vasculature and intracranial structures that have no blood–brain barrier, such as the meningeal membranes, the choroid plexus, the pineal gland, the pituitary stalk, and the pituitary gland. When the blood–

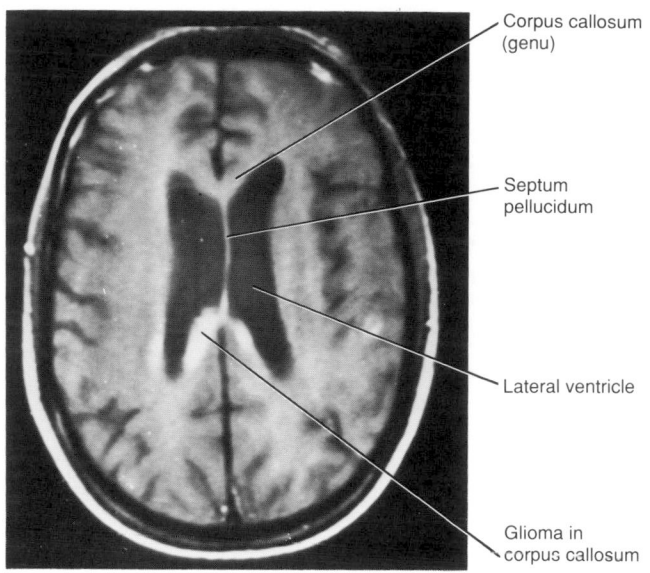

Corpus callosum (genu)

Septum pellucidum

Lateral ventricle

Glioma in corpus callosum

FIGURE 22–15

This MRI scan in the horizontal plane demonstrates a diffuse periventricular brain tumor (a glioma proven at autopsy). The T_1 image was obtained after intravascular injection of gadolinium. Multiple small areas of T_1 signal enhancement can be seen between the lateral ventricles and around the posterior portion of the corpus callosum.

FIGURE 22–16

These MRI scans show the distribution of Na^+ in a normal person. Scans from top left to lower right pass through successively more inferior levels of the cerebral hemispheres and brain stem. Note the prominent Na^+ signal from cerebrospinal fluid in the lateral ventricles (second and third rows), the subarachnoid space (third row), and vitreous fluid of the eyes (lower row).

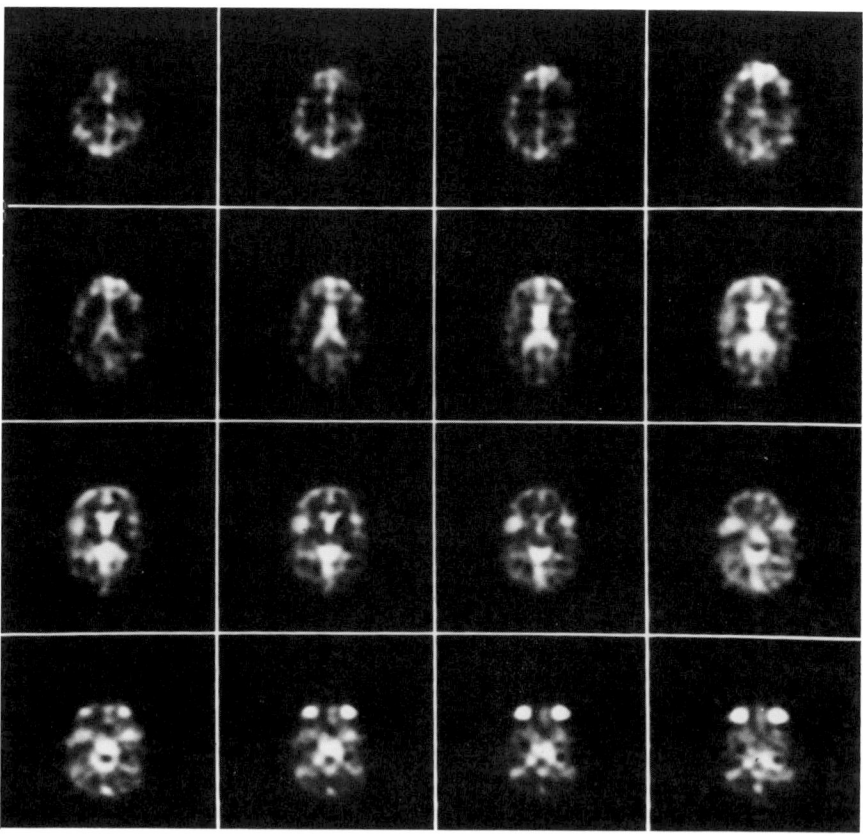

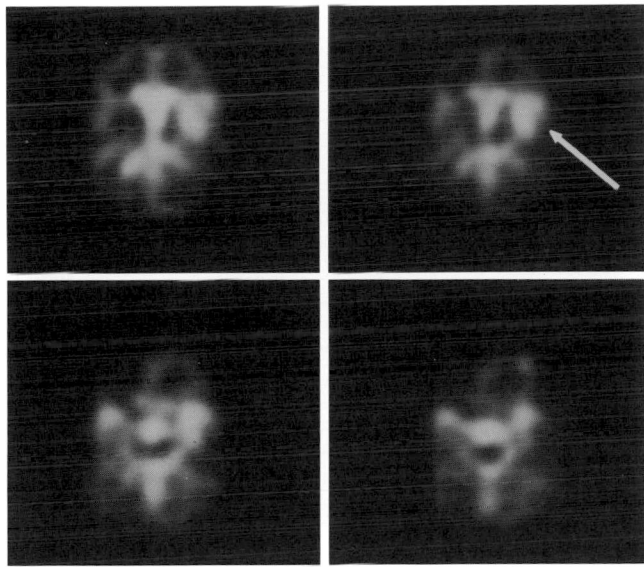

FIGURE 22–17
The increase in Na$^+$ at the site of a cerebral infarct is visible in this MRI scan (right frontal lobe, **arrow**). Slices are through superior (**upper left**) and inferior (**lower right**) cerebral hemispheres.

brain barrier is altered in abnormal conditions, such as tumors and stroke, leakage of the paramagnetic contrast agents makes lesions conspicuous (Figure 22–15).

Sodium and Phosphorus Scans Reveal Cerebral Infarcts, Neoplastic Changes, and Metabolism

Magnetic resonance imaging scanners image other atomic nuclei of biological importance. After hydrogen, Na$^+$ is the second most abundant element in the body and has been imaged in humans. After occlusive stroke, the concentration of Na$^+$ rises more rapidly than that of water, so that Na$^+$ imaging may reveal pathology earlier than proton imaging can. Magnetic resonance imaging scans of

normal persons show little or no Na$^+$ signal from the brain parenchyma but a large Na$^+$ signal from cerebrospinal fluid in the ventricles and subarachnoid space, as well as from the vitreous fluid of the eye because Na$^+$ is present primarily in the extracellular compartment (Figure 22–16). In patients with cerebral infarcts there is a remarkable increase in Na$^+$ at the site of the lesion (Figure 22–17).

Sodium is also an important indicator of neoplastic change. Under normal conditions the concentration of Na$^+$ within the cell is approximately 20 mM, while in the extracellular environment it is 140 mM. The Na$^+$ gradient between the intra- and extracellular space is maintained by the Na$^+$–K$^+$ pump in the cell membrane. Intracellular Na$^+$ concentration increases in neoplasms and in normal cells undergoing mitosis. In highly malignant cells it may increase to around 80 or 90 mM, whereas in lower-grade tumors it increases to between 40 and 60 mM. Thus, Na$^+$ imaging is a particularly good way to reveal precisely the size and extent of a tumor (Figure 22–18).

Magnetic resonance imaging can also show the distribution of phosphorus. It is possible to discriminate among the various compounds of phosphorus involved in energy production, including phosphocreatine and ATP. By providing an *in vivo* chemical analysis, MRI can detect metabolic processes, but PET is currently more sensitive than MRI for detecting small concentrations of a labeled compound.

An Overall View

The high-resolution techniques now available allow both the structural and the functional organization of the human brain to be imaged. A key to these techniques is the ability to reconstruct two- and three-dimensional spatial information from simple radiographic or biochemical measurements. Thus, computerized X-ray tomography has allowed us to evaluate the gross characteristics of brain structure. With the greater sensitivity of magnetic resonance imaging, the precise structure of the brain has been revealed with resolution that approaches that of low-magnification microscopic sections. Finally, with positron emission tomography, the biochemical composi-

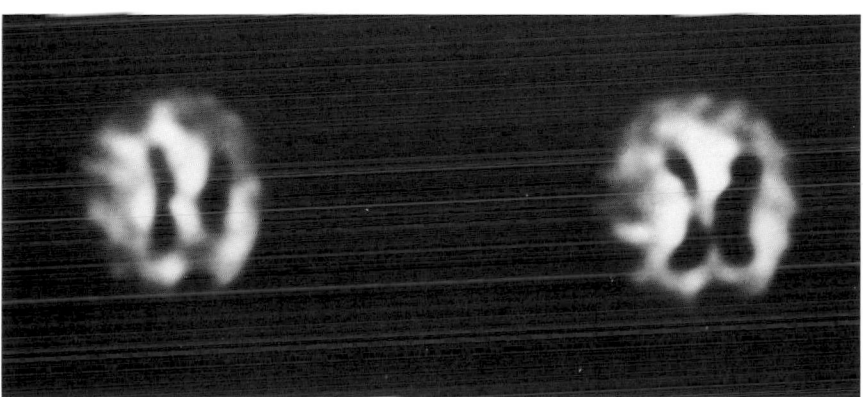

FIGURE 22–18
These derived images of intracellular Na$^+$ concentration show a remarkable increase in concentration (70 mM) within a neoplasm located around the body of the left lateral ventricle and crossing the midline to the opposite hemisphere. Unlike markers of blood–brain barrier description, Na$^+$ imaging can reveal the precise size and location of a neoplasm.

tion of neural tissue can be monitored. Thus, the biochemical function of local neural circuits can be studied during perception, movement, and thought. By combining PET and MRI we have obtained new insights into behavior by seeing how it is represented in the functional architecture of the human brain. These techniques have enabled us to localize more precisely disease processes and traumatic lesions in the brain, and develop therapies to deal with them.

Selected Readings

Andreasen, N. C. 1988. Brain Imaging: Applications in psychiatry. Science 239:1381–1388.

Brownell, G. L., Budinger, T. F., Lauterbur, P. C., and McGeer, P. L. 1982. Positron tomography and nuclear magnetic resonance imaging. Science 215:619–626.

Edelman, R. R. 1990. Magnetic resonance imaging of the nervous system. Discuss. Neurosci. 7:11–63.

Martin, J. H. 1989. Neuroanatomy: Text and Atlas. New York: Elsevier.

Moonen, C. T. W., van Zijl, P. C. M., Frank, J. A., Le Bihan, D., and Becker, E. D. 1990. Functional magnetic resonance imaging in medicine and physiology. Science 250:53–61.

Oldendorf, W., and Oldendorf, W., Jr. 1991. MRI Primer. New York: Raven Press.

Oldendorf, W. H. 1980. The Quest for an Image of Brain: Computerized Tomography in the Perspective of Past and Future Imaging Methods. New York: Raven Press.

Posner, M. I., Petersen, S. E., Fox, P. T., and Raichle, M. E. 1988. Localization of cognitive operations in the human brain. Science 240:1627–1631.

Pykett, I. L. 1982. NMR imaging in medicine. Sci. Am. 246(5): 78–88.

Raichle, M. E. 1987. Circulatory and metabolic correlates of brain function in normal humans. In F. Plum (ed.), Handbook of Physiology, Section 1: The Nervous System, Vol. V. Higher Functions of the Brain, Part 2. Bethesda, Md.: American Physiological Society, pp. 643–674.

Valk, J., and van der Knaap, M. S. 1989. Magnetic Resonance of Myelin, Myelination, and Myelin Disorders. Berlin: Springer.

References

Cormack, A. M. 1973. Reconstruction of densities from their projections, with applications in radiological physics. Phys. Med. Biol. 18:195–207.

Hilal, S. K., Ra, J. B., Oh, C. H., Mun, I. K., Einstein, S. G., and Roschmann, P. 1988. Sodium imaging. In D. D. Stark and W. G. Bradley, Jr. (eds.), Magnetic Resonance Imaging. St. Louis: Mosby, pp. 715–731.

Hounsfield, G. N. 1973. Computerized transverse axial scanning (tomography): Part 1. Description of system. Br. J. Radiol. 46: 1016–1022.

Lauterbur, P. C. 1973. Image formation by induced local interactions. Examples employing nuclear magnetic resonance. Nature 242:190–191.

Lukes, S. A., Crooks, L. E., Aminoff, M. J., Kaufman, L., Panitch, H. S., Mills, C., and Norman, D. 1983. Nuclear magnetic resonance imaging in multiple sclerosis. Ann. Neurol. 13:592–601.

Phelps, M. E., Mazziotta, J. C., and Huang, S.-C. 1982. Study of cerebral function with positron computed tomography. J. Cereb. Blood Flow Metab. 2:113–162.

Rutledge, J. N., Hilal, S. K., Silver, A. J., Defendini, R., and Fahn, S. 1987. Study of movement disorders and brain iron by MR. Am. J. Neuroradiol. 8:397–411.

Sokoloff, L. 1984. Modeling metabolic processes in the brain in vivo. Ann. Neurol. [Suppl] 15:S1–S11.

Wagner, H. N., Jr., Burns, H. D., Dannals, R. F., Wong, D. F., Langström, B., Duelfer, T., Frost, J. J., Ravert, H. T., Links, J. M., Rosenbloom, S. B., Lukas, S. E., Kramer, A. V., and Kuhar, M. J. 1984. Assessment of dopamine receptor densities in the human brain with carbon-11-labeled N-methylspiperone. Ann. Neurol. [Suppl.] 15:S79–S84.

I left the well-house

eager to l(ea)r n .   Ever y th ing

h a d   a   n a m e ,   and   e a ch

n a m e   g a v e   b i r th   to   a

n e w   th ou gh t .   A s   we

r e t u r n ed   to the   h ou s e ,

ever y   o b j e c t   I   t ou ch ed

s e e m ed   to q u i v er with   l i f e .

V

Sensory Systems of the Brain: Sensation and Perception

S ight, sound, touch, pain, smell, taste, and the sensation of bodily movements all originate in sensory systems. These perceptions, in turn, form the basis of our knowledge about the world. Perception begins in receptor cells that are sensitive to one or another kind of stimuli. Most sensory inputs are perceived as a sensation identified with a stimulus. Thus, short wavelength light falling on the eye is perceived as blue, and sugar on the tongue is perceived as sweet.

Psychophysics attempts to correlate quantitative aspects of physical stimuli with the sensations that they evoke. Important information about perception can be obtained from studying the various sensory receptors and the stimuli to which they respond, and the major sensory pathways that carry information from these receptors to the cerebral cortex. Psychophysical analysis is the basis for our understanding of how various stimuli alter the activity of the brain and generate specific perceptions.

Specific neurons in the sensory system, both peripheral receptors and central cells, encode some of the critical attributes of sensations: the location of the stimulus and its properties. Other attributes of sensation are encoded by the *pattern* of activity in a population of sensory neurons.

A major task of current research in sensory physiology is to determine the extent to which receptor specificity and patterns of activity are used in different sensory pathways. We know, for example, that receptor specificity is important for taste. In contrast, the pitch of an auditory stimulus depends, in large part, on pattern coding. Many other sensory systems involve combinations of sensory neuron specificity and response patterns.

Sensory pathways include neurons that link the receptor at the periphery with the spinal cord, brain stem, thalamus, and cerebral cortex. We feel a tactile stimulus on the hand when a population of appropriately connected touch receptors causes a discharge of action potentials in a population of afferent fibers, causing certain cells to discharge in the dorsal column nuclei of the thalamus and in several sequential areas in the cortex. The illusion of sensation in the hand can be elicited by electrical stimulation of the area of cortex that represents the hand, albeit a slightly blunted one. Therefore, it is important to learn

---

"... my teacher placed my hand under the spout. As the cool stream gushed over one hand, she spelled into the other the word water ... I knew then that 'w-a-t-e-r' meant the wonderful cool something that was flowing over my hand." Blind and deaf, in 1887 Helen Keller, then seven years old, learned the meaning of words as symbols through an unusual sensory modality, touch. She described how she began to understand language in *The Story of My Life* (1906, Garden City, N.Y., Doubleday & Company, Inc.), written as an undergraduate at Radcliffe College. A sentence from her autobiography is shown here in braille, a system of printing devised for reading words through touch. (Braille setting courtesy of Michael Helmers, The Associated Blind, New York.)

how sensation is analyzed by each component of a given sensory system. The most striking feature of the organization of sensory systems is that the inputs from the peripheral receptor sheet (the body surface, the cochlea, or the retina) are systematically mapped onto structures of the brain. These maps do not correspond point for point with the size and shape of the periphery but reflect the relative importance to perception of a particular part of the receptive sheet. Thus, the tips of our fingers have a large representation in the brain, whereas the skin on our back has a small representation.

Aspects of perception—of a visual object, a tactile sensation, or a melody—are carried and processed in parallel by different components of the sensory system processing that perception. Each system first analyzes and deconstructs the sensory information at the receptor level. It then abstracts the perception and represents it in the brain in different pathways and central regions through feature detection and pattern of firing. The central regions then interact to reconstruct the components into a unified conscious perception.

PART V

Chapter 23:   **Coding and Processing of Sensory Information**
Chapter 24:   **Modality Coding in the Somatic Sensory System**
Chapter 25:   **Anatomy of the Somatic Sensory System**
Chapter 26:   **Touch**
Chapter 27:   **Pain and Analgesia**
Chapter 28:   **Phototransduction and Information Processing in the Retina**
Chapter 29:   **Central Visual Pathways**
Chapter 30:   **Perception of Motion, Depth, and Form**
Chapter 31:   **Color Vision**
Chapter 32:   **Hearing**
Chapter 33:   **The Sense of Balance**
Chapter 34:   **Smell and Taste: The Chemical Senses**

23

John H. Martin

Coding and Processing of Sensory Information

Sensory Information Underlies Motor Control and Arousal As Well As Sensation

Sensory Systems Mediate Four Attributes of a Stimulus That Can Be Quantitatively Correlated with a Sensation

Modality

Intensity

Duration

Location

Sensory Systems Have a Common Plan

Sensory Receptors and Sensory Neurons in the Central Nervous System Have a Receptive Field

Sensory Information Is Processed by the Thalamus and Transmitted to the Cerebral Cortex

Sensory Systems Are Organized in Both a Hierarchical and Parallel Fashion

Sensory Systems Are Topographically Organized

Sensory Receptors Translate Stimulus Features into Neural Codes

Stimulus Intensity Is Encoded by Frequency and Population Codes

Stimulus Duration Is Encoded in the Discharge Patterns of Rapidly and Slowly Adapting Receptors

Modality Is Encoded by a Labeled Line Code

Stimulus Information Is Transmitted to the Central Nervous System by Conducted Action Potentials

An Overall View

We now turn to sensation and perception, historically the starting point for the scientific study of mental processes. The modern origins of this field date to the first third of the nineteenth century when the French philosopher Auguste Comte defined a new philosophy, which he called *positivism*, concerned with applying the empirical methods of natural science to the study of human behavior. Comte argued that the study of behavior should become a branch of the biological sciences, and that the laws governing the mind should be derived from objective observation. In this line of thought Comte was influenced by the British empiricists John Locke, George Berkeley, and David Hume, who maintained that all knowledge comes through sensory experience—what can be seen, heard, felt, tasted, or smelled. Locke proposed that at birth the human mind is blank, a *tabula rasa*, upon which experience leaves its marks.

Let us then suppose the Mind to be, as we say, white Paper void of all Characters without any Ideas: How comes it to be furnished? Whence comes it by that vast store, which the busie and boundless Fancy of Man has painted on it with an almost endless variety? Whence has it all the materials of Reason and Knowledge? To this I answer, in one word, From *Experience*. In that all of our Knowledge is founded; and from that it ultimately derives itself.

The empiricist view led to the emergence of psychology as a distinct academic discipline. Separate from philosophy, psychology developed as a discipline concerned with the experimental study of mental processes, emphasizing, in its early years, sensation as the key to the mind. Thus the founders of experimental psychology, Ernst Weber, Gustav Fechner, Hermann Helmholtz, and Wilhelm Wundt, were concerned with questions about the sequence of events by which a stimulus leads to a subjective experience.

They soon found that although the details of sensory reception differed for each of the senses, three steps were common to all senses: (1) a physical stimulus, (2) a set of events by which the stimulus is transduced into a message of nerve impulses, and (3) a response to the message, often in the perception or conscious experience of sensations. This sequence lent itself to two modes of analysis, giving rise to the fields of *psychophysics* and *sensory physiology*. Psychophysics focused on the relationship between the physical characteristics of a stimulus and the attributes of the sensory experience. Sensory physiology examined the neural consequences of a stimulus—how the stimulus is transduced by sensory receptors and processed in the brain. Much of the current excitement in the neurobiology of perception comes from the recent merging of these two approaches in experiments on animal and human subjects.

The early findings in psychophysics and sensory physiology soon revealed a weakness in the empiricist argument. The studies revealed that our mind is not blank nor is our perceptual world formed simply from a direct encounter of a naive brain with the physical properties of a stimulus. In fact, our perceptions differ qualitatively from the physical properties of stimuli because the nervous system only extracts certain information from a stimulus and then interprets this information in the context of its earlier experience. We experience electromagnetic waves of different frequencies not as waves but as actual colors that we see: red, blue, or green. We experience objects vibrating at different frequencies as different sounds that we hear. We experience chemical compounds dissolved in air or water as specific smells and tastes. Colors, tones, smells, and tastes are mental constructions created by the brain out of sensory experience. They do not exist, as such, outside of the brain. Thus, we can answer the traditional question raised by philosophers: Does a sound exist when a tree falls in the forest, if no one is near enough to hear it? We now believe that the fall causes vibration in the air but not sound. Sound only occurs when pressure waves from the falling tree reach and are perceived by a living being.

Even though sensory experience is a construction of the brain, such constructions seem not to be arbitrary. Although our perceptions of the size, shape, and color of objects are different from the images formed on our retinas, our perceptions appear to correspond to the physical properties of objects. Can we be sure of this? We cannot. Nevertheless, in most instances we can show that our perceptions of a shape, for example, the shape of a right triangle, is an accurate prediction of inferred reality because we can measure what we *see*. We can demonstrate, by measurement, that the square of its hypotenuse is equal to the sum of the squares of its sides. Perception therefore can be shown to be an accurate *organization* of the essential properties of an object that allows us to *manipulate* the objects successfully.

Thus, our perceptions are not direct records of the world around us but are constructed internally, at least in part, according to innate rules and constraints imposed by the capabilities of the nervous system. The philosopher Imanuel Kant referred to these inherent constraints as *preknowledge*. In opposition to empiricism, Kant argued that the mind is not a passive receiver of sense impressions, but is constructed to conform with ideal or objective preexisting categories, such as space, time, and causality, that exist independent of physical stimulation from outside the body. Knowledge, according to Kant, is based not only on sensory experience but also on the preknowledge that organizes sensory experience.

In subsequent chapters we shall see that the philosophical dialectic between Kant's idealism and Comte's empirical positivism continues to influence studies of perception. As we shall see in Chapter 30, Kant's emphasis on the preknowledge influenced the emergence of *Gestalt psychology*, which holds that aspects of perception reflect an inborn capability of the brain to order simple sensations in characteristic ways. Similarly, positivism influenced the emergence of *behaviorist psychology*, which focuses on the observable indices of behavior, the properties of the eliciting stimulus, and the subject's motor response.

In this chapter we introduce the study of perception by tracing the path followed by the early students of sensation. We first consider the psychophysical studies that allow us to evaluate the several functions of sensory information in behavior. Next, we examine the organizational features common to all sensory systems. Specifically, we shall consider how stimulus information is transduced by sensory receptors and encoded into neural signals. In later chapters we shall examine how the various sensory systems—for touch, pain, vision, hearing, balance, taste, and smell—allow us to perceive the physical world in which we live.

Sensory Information Underlies Motor Control and Arousal As Well As Sensation

Sensory systems receive information from the environment through receptors at the periphery of the body and transmit this information to the central nervous system. There the information is used for three main functions: sensation, control of movement, and maintaining arousal. Sensation is a conscious experience. Not all sensory information is perceived, however. For example, much of the sensory information used to control movement is not perceived. Consider the withdrawal of the hand after touching a hot surface—the sensory information drives the motor response automatically before we perceive the surface as hot.

In addition to stimulation from the external world, we also receive sensory information from within the body: from blood vessels, the viscera, and from the actions of skeletal muscles on joints. This information is used to regulate temperature, blood pressure, heart rate, respiratory rate, and reflex movements. Regulation of these essential body functions usually does not reach consciousness. We shall consider the important role that sensory information plays in the control of autonomic function and of movement in Chapter 49.

Sensory Systems Mediate Four Attributes of a Stimulus That Can Be Correlated Quantitatively with a Sensation

The modern study of sensation began in the nineteenth century with the work of Weber and Fechner, who pioneered sensory psychophysics. They discovered that the sensory systems extract four elementary attributes of a stimulus—modality (quality), intensity, duration, and location—that are combined in sensation. Here we shall examine each attribute and how it can be used to correlate specific features of behavior with the properties of sensory neurons.

Modality

Different forms of energy are transformed by the nervous system into different sensations or *sensory modalities*. Five major sensory modalities have been recognized since ancient times: vision, hearing, touch, taste, and smell. Each modality has many constituent qualities or *submodalities*. For example, taste can be sweet, sour, salty, or bitter; color and movement detection are submodalities of vision. In 1826 Johannes Müller advanced his "laws of specific sense energies." He proposed that modality is a property of the sensory nerve fiber. Each nerve fiber is activated by a certain type of stimulus because different stimuli activate different nerve fibers. In turn, the nerve fibers make specific connections within the nervous system, and it is these specific connections that are responsible for specific sensations. The unique stimulus that activates a specific receptor and therefore a particular nerve fiber was called an *adequate stimulus* by Charles Sherrington.

As we shall see later, the sensitivity of a sensory nerve fiber to a particular type of stimulus is not absolute; if a stimulus is strong enough, it can activate several kinds of nerve fibers. Nevertheless, under normal circumstances each nerve is primarily sensitive to one type of stimulus. For example, the retina is relatively insensitive to mechanical stimulation but very sensitive to light. A blow to the eye can nevertheless produce a flash of light (termed a phosphene), even though no light enters the eye. Müller's laws of specific sense energies are the basis of an important mechanism for neural coding of stimulus modality as well as the constituent qualities within a modality.

Intensity

Intensity or amount of a sensation depends on the strength of the stimulus. The lowest stimulus intensity a subject can detect is termed the *sensory threshold* and is determined statistically. A subject is presented a series of stimuli of progressively greater intensity, and the percentage of times the subject reports detecting the stimulus is plotted as a function of stimulus intensity. This relation is called the *psychometric function* (Figure 23–1). By convention, threshold is defined as the stimulus intensity detected in half of the trials.

Early in the study of psychophysics it became clear that sensory thresholds are not invariant and can be elevated or

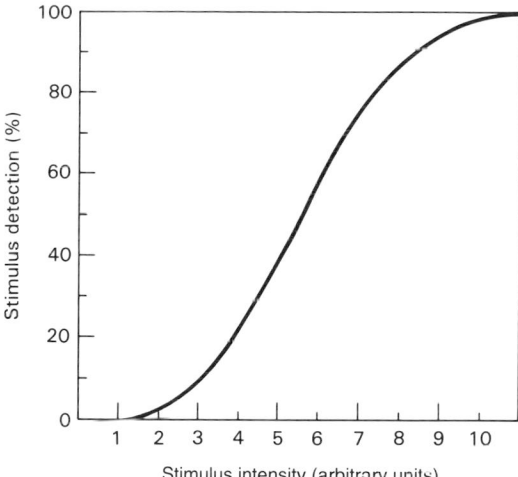

FIGURE 23–1
The percentage of stimuli (arbitrary units) detected as a function of stimulus intensity is called the psychometric function.

reduced. Threshold can be influenced by practice, fatigue, and the context in which the stimulus is presented. The threshold of a given stimulus also differs slightly depending on whether the intensity is increasing or decreasing. Modification of sensory thresholds by contextual cues is particularly intriguing and indicates that the perceptual thresholds are relative, not absolute. The threshold for pain is often heightened during competitive sports or in childbirth, as reflected in a shift in the psychometric function to higher stimulus intensities (Figure 23–2, curve c). Similarly, sensory thresholds can be lowered. Consider a runner at the starting line prepared to respond to the starter's shot. The excitement of the race manifests itself as a shift in the psychometric function, so that the runner now responds to a lower stimulus intensity, which would have been ignored previously (Figure 23–2, curve a).

FIGURE 23–2
The absolute sensory threshold (curve **b**) is an idealized relationship between stimulus intensity and the probability of stimulus detection. If the sensory system's ability to detect the stimulus is increased or the response criterion decreased, curve **a** would be observed; curve **c** illustrates the converse.

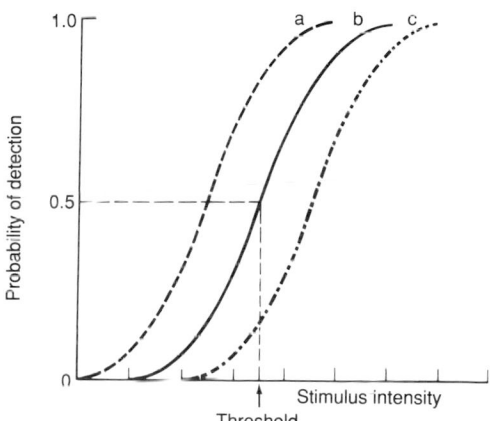

As we shall learn later in this chapter, these changes in sensory threshold do not result from changes in the threshold of the receptor in the periphery, but rather from changes of neurons in the central nervous system. These effects are produced not only by neurons in the sensory systems but also by neurons of the limbic system, which mediate the affective aspects of sensation.

The modifiability of sensory thresholds can be understood by considering two aspects of sensation: (1) the absolute *detectability* of the stimulus and (2) the *criterion* the subject uses to evaluate whether a stimulus is present. Detectability is a measure of the capacity of a sensory system to process a stimulus, whereas the response criterion reflects an attitude or bias of the subject toward the sensory experience. In the 1950s Wilson Tanner and John Swets developed the *signal detection theory* to explain the common observation that subjects often report a sensory experience (i.e., detection of a stimulus) when no stimulus is actually presented, a *false alarm*. In some situations (for example, the runner at the starting block), it is advantageous to respond as rapidly as possible. A consequence of this decrease in response criterion (or bias) is that a subject is more likely to report the presence of a stimulus when it is actually absent. The opposite condition, the reluctance to report the occurrence of a stimulus, is also common. In our culture men have a higher threshold for reporting pain than women.

The separate measures of stimulus detectability and response criterion can be combined with the concept of *threshold* to explain the mechanisms of drug action. For example, morphine, a potent analgesic, elevates pain threshold both by reducing the detectability of a painful stimulus and by elevating the criterion the subject uses to determine whether a stimulus is painful or not. Marijuana also increases pain thresholds, but by increasing response criterion, not decreasing stimulus detectability—the stimulus is just as painful but the subject is more tolerant.

The capacity of sensory systems to extract information about the intensity of the stimulus is important for two related discriminations: (1) for distinguishing between stimuli that differ only in intensity (as opposed to those that differ by modality or location), and (2) for evaluating stimulus intensity over a range of values, for example from weak to strong. The attribute of intensity includes the detection process (sensory threshold) as well as intensity discriminations and evaluations.

Historically, quantification of the intensity of a sensory experience evolved from considering how two stimuli with different intensities are distinguished. The sensitivity of the sensory system to differences depends on the strength of the stimuli. For example, we easily perceive that 1 kg is different from 2 kg, but it is difficult to distinguish between 50 and 51 kg. Yet both sets differ by 1 kg! This phenomenon was examined in 1834 by Weber, who proposed a quantitative relationship between stimulus intensity and discrimination, now known as Weber's law:

$$\Delta S = K \times S$$

where ΔS is the minimal difference in strength between a reference stimulus S and a second stimulus such that a

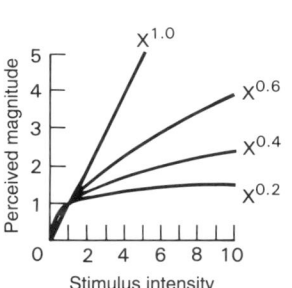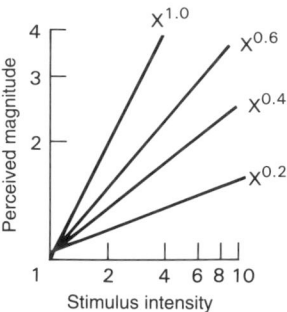

FIGURE 23–3

This figure illustrates idealized relations between stimulus intensity and the perceived magnitude of the stimulus described by power functions of different exponential values. Psychophysical measurements of different stimuli result in curves with distinctly different exponents. For example, the relationship between the perceived duration of a stimulus and the actual duration has an exponent close to one, whereas the relationship between perceived and actual brightness has an exponent close to 0.4. An extremely steep relationship is obtained for the perceived intensity of an electric shock, with an exponent of 3.5. In addition to enabling comparison between different modalities by quantifying the data in this manner, direct comparisons can be made between psychophysical and neurophysiological measurements to determine whether the properties of a particular component of the nervous system can explain sensory capacity. The relations shown in the left graph are plotted on linear scales; the relations in the right graph are plotted on logarithmic scales, which result in straight-line graphs.

difference can be perceived, and K is a constant. This is termed the *just noticeable difference* or JND. It follows that the difference in magnitude necessary to discriminate between a reference stimulus and a second stimulus increases with the intensity of the reference stimulus.

Fechner extended Weber's law in 1860 to describe the relationship between stimulus intensity and the intensity of the sensation experienced by a subject,

$$I = K \log \frac{S}{S_0}$$

where I is the subjectively experienced intensity, S_0 is the threshold, S is the suprathreshold stimulus used to estimate stimulus magnitude, and K is a constant. In 1953 Stanley Stevens noted that subjective experience is proportional not to the logarithm, as Fechner described, but to the nth power of the intensity of the suprathreshold stimulus (Figure 23–3). Over a limited range of intensity the power function may be similar to the log function. However, over an extended range of intensity subjective experience is best described by a power rather than by a logarithmic relationship:

$$I = K(S - S_0)^n.$$

This is important because natural stimuli vary greatly in intensity. For example, we experience a range of sounds, from a whisper to a shout.

As we shall see later in this chapter when we examine the physiological properties of peripheral receptors, an increase in stimulus intensity is paralleled by an increase in the discharge rate of sensory neurons. This relationship between the increase in sensory neuron discharge and perceived intensity is an important mechanism for encoding stimulus intensity.

Duration

The duration of sensation is defined by the relationship between the stimulus intensity and the perceived intensity. Typically, if a stimulus persists for a long time, the intensity diminishes. This decrease is called *adaptation*. Later we shall examine how sensory receptors adapt. Often the perceived stimulus intensity becomes subthreshold with time and the sensation is lost. For example, if a finger is immersed in warm water, the sense of warmth fades. This example raises a second important issue. Warmth fades over most of the finger but remains in the part of the finger at the interface between the cool air and the warm water. This perception is sharpest at regions of great contrast.

Location

There are two important measures of the awareness of the spatial aspects of sensory experience: (1) the ability to locate the site of stimulation and (2) the ability to distinguish two closely spaced stimuli. The ability to perceive two nearby stimuli as distinct is quantified by determining the minimum distance between two detectable stimuli, a measurement that Weber called the *two-point threshold*. As we shall see in the next chapter, the two-point threshold is small at the finger tip and increases markedly for more proximal parts of the body. As the two-point threshold increases from the finger tip to the arm, there is a corresponding decrease in the accuracy with which we are able to locate the site of stimulation.

Insights into the neural mechanisms for fine spatial discriminations on the finger tips have come from the work of Åke Vallbo and his colleagues, who have systematically studied mechanoreceptors that innervate the hairless (glabrous) skin of the human hand. They found that the density of receptor innervation is four times greater on the finger tips than on the palm. Similar principles apply to vision. One reason why the fovea of the retina has heightened visual acuity is because of its greater density of photoreceptors.

Sensory Systems Have a Common Plan

Despite their diversity, all sensory systems extract the same basic information from stimuli—modality, intensity, duration, and location. This may be one reason why the sensory systems are organized similarly (Figure 23–4). In each sensory system the initial contact with the external world occurs through specialized neural structures called *sensory receptors* (Figure 23–5). Each receptor is sensitive to a form of physical energy—mechanical, thermal, chemical, or electromagnetic (Table 23–1). The receptor transforms the stimulus energy into electrochemical energy, thereby establishing a common language for all sensory systems. This conversion process is called

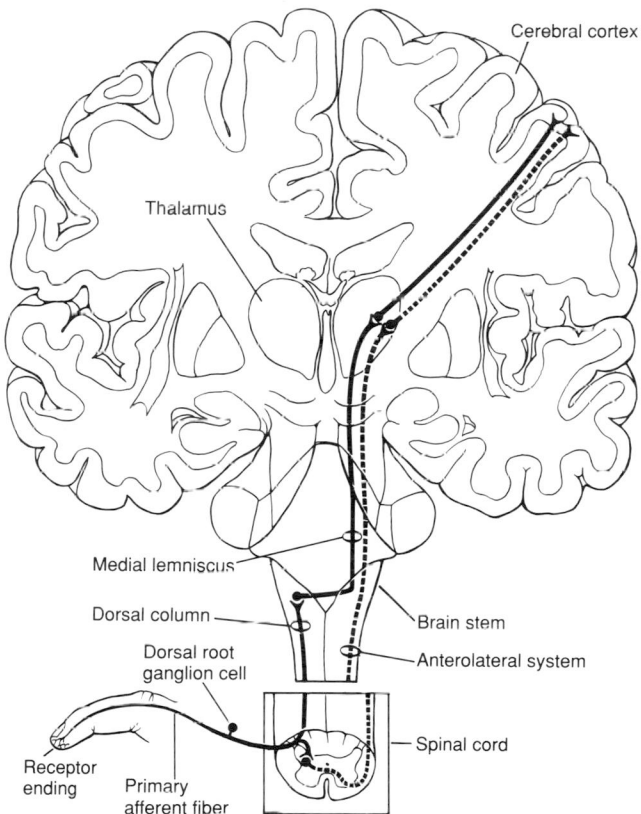

FIGURE 23–4

The hierarchical and parallel organization of sensory systems is demonstrated by two ascending parallel somatosensory pathways. The dorsal column–medial lemniscal system (**solid line**) is the main pathway for tactile information. The anterolateral system (**broken line**) mediates pain and, to a much lesser extent, tactile sensations. Only when the dorsal column–medial lemniscal pathway becomes damaged, as in certain degenerative neurological disorders, does the anterolateral pathway assume an important role in mediating tactile sensations.

FIGURE 23–5

Various sensory receptors have different morphologies and organization. (Adapted from Martin, 1989.)

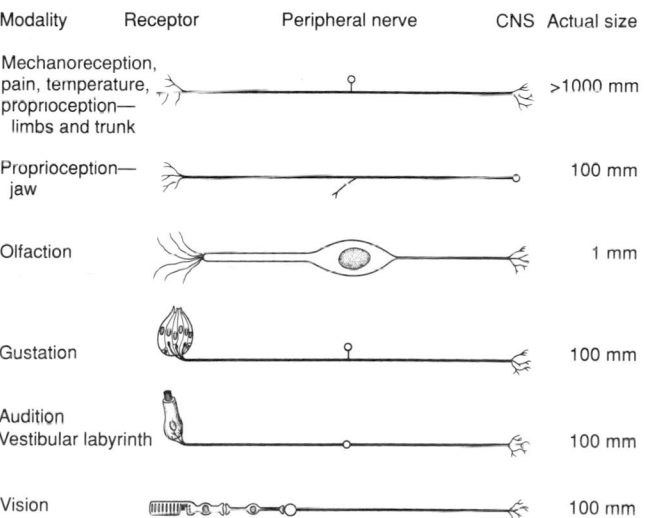

Modality	Receptor	Peripheral nerve	CNS	Actual size
Mechanoreception, pain, temperature, proprioception— limbs and trunk				>1000 mm
Proprioception— jaw				100 mm
Olfaction				1 mm
Gustation				100 mm
Audition Vestibular labyrinth				100 mm
Vision				100 mm

TABLE 23–1. Sensory Systems

Modality	Stimulus	Receptor types	Receptors
Vision	Light	Photoreceptor	Rods, cones
Audition	Sound	Mechanoreceptor	Hair cells (cochlear)
Balance	Head motion	Mechanoreceptor	Hair cells (semicircular canals)
Somatic	Mechanical, thermal, noxious (chemical)	Mechanoreceptor, thermoreceptor, nociceptor, chemoreceptor	Dorsal root ganglion neurons
Taste	Chemical	Chemoreceptor	Taste buds
Smell	Chemical	Chemoreceptor	Olfactory sensory neurons

stimulus transduction. (The transduction of stimulus energy is discussed later in this chapter.)

Stimulus information is then represented in a series of action potentials by a process called *neural encoding.* The four fundamental attributes of sensory information—modality, intensity, duration, and location—are each related to a separate stimulus feature, and codes exist for each. As we shall see in this and later chapters, there are only a limited number of mechanisms for encoding stimulus information. Neural codes may be the product of activity in single neurons, such as the mean impulse activity of the receptor and the time interval between impulses, or in populations of neurons. Because a stimulus activates many receptors, the distribution of activated receptors in the receptor population is itself a type of information provided to the sensory system and is a simple example of a population code.

The sensory receptor is the first neuron in each sensory pathway. Each sensory system handles the initial processing of stimulus information in somewhat different ways. In the somatic sensory and olfactory systems the receptor cell is a neuron whose axons generate action potentials. The somatic and olfactory receptors have two functions: stimulus transduction and neural encoding. In the gustatory, visual, auditory, and vestibular systems, however, these functions are carried out by separate cells (Figure 23–5). Whereas the different sensory systems share a common organization, the specific circuitry of each system reflects the particular demands imposed by the functions of the particular sensory information.

Sensory Receptors and Sensory Neurons in the Central Nervous System Have a Receptive Field

All sensory receptors have a *receptive field,* the space within the receptive sheet in which the sensory receptor is located and in which it transduces stimuli. The receptive field has a distinct structural basis. For example, the receptive field of a somatic sensory mechanoreceptor (for touch) is the portion of the skin directly innervated by the receptor terminals. The receptive field also includes the adjacent tissue through which a tactile stimulus can be conducted to reach the terminals. The receptive field of a photoreceptor is that portion of the retina in which the receptor is located.

Receptor neurons converge onto second-order neurons, which are often located in the central nervous system, and then to third- and higher-order neurons. At subcortical levels sensory information is passed from lower-order to higher-order neurons in particular *relay nuclei.* Neurons in each sensory relay nucleus also have a receptive field because they receive input directly or indirectly from sensory receptors (Figure 23–6A). However, the receptive fields of second-order and other higher-order sensory neurons are larger and more complex than those of receptor neurons. They are larger because they receive convergent input from many hundreds of receptors, each with a slightly different but overlapping receptive field (Figure 23–6A). They are more complex because they can be sensitive to specific stimulus features, such as movement in a particular direction in the visual field. Unlike the simple excitatory receptive field of the sensory receptor, the receptive field of higher-order sensory neurons commonly has both excitatory and inhibitory regions. Inhibitory components of receptive fields are produced by input from receptors that is relayed to the central neuron by inhibitory interneurons (Figure 23–6B). The addition of an inhibitory region in a receptive field is an important mechanism for increasing the contrast between stimuli and thus gives the sensory systems additional spatial resolving power.

Not all receptor neurons are concerned directly with spatial location. For example, auditory receptors are sensitive to the frequency of a sound and not to the location from which it originates; spatial location is a property of central auditory neurons. Whereas stimulus frequency is a feature of neurons in peripheral auditory structures, gustatory and olfactory receptors have chemospecificity.

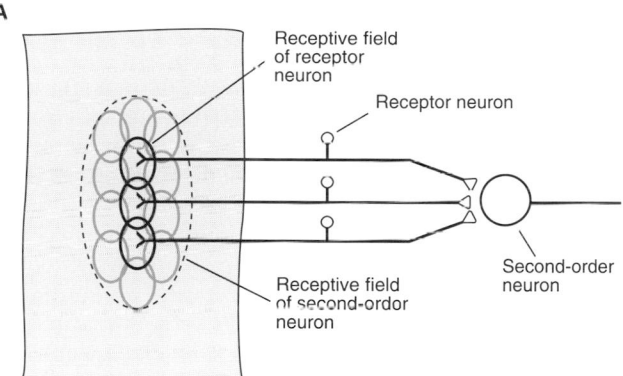

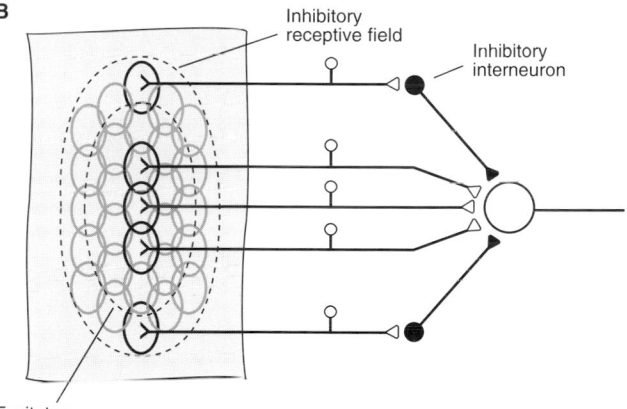

FIGURE 23–6

Receptive field structure.

A. Many peripheral receptors converge onto a single sensory neuron in the central nervous system. As a consequence, the receptive field for a central neuron is much larger.

B. The receptive field of a central sensory neuron may have a central excitatory receptive field surrounded by an inhibitory region.

Sensory Information Is Processed by the Thalamus and Transmitted to the Cerebral Cortex

The thalamus is an essential relay point in sensory processing. Virtually all pathways transmitting sensory information to the cerebral cortex make connections in the thalamus. In turn, the thalamic neurons of each sensory system project to a specific primary sensory area of the cerebral cortex. The only exception is the olfactory system, which transmits sensory information from the periphery directly to the primitive cortex of the medial temporal lobe.

The sensory regions of the cerebral cortex play a critical role in perception. This is most evident for the primary visual cortex. when it is damaged, a person becomes blind. Interestingly, damage to the primary visual cortex reveals that remaining regions do have a limited perceptual capacity. Under a variety of experimental conditions these blind patients can use visual information to guide some motor behaviors and identify a variety of visual stimulus features despite any visual awareness. The patient is unaware of this perceptual capacity and must be encouraged to guess. Even when the stimulus feature is perceived correctly (i.e., in better than 50% of the trials), the patient still does not acknowledge any visual capacity. The presence of residual visual capacity after lesions of the visual cortex has been named *blind sight* by its discoverer Lawrence Weiskrantz, and suggests that visual areas other than the primary visual cortex contribute to the perception of visual stimuli.

Sensory Systems Are Organized in Both a Hierarchical and Parallel Fashion

Sensory systems have a serial organization: Receptors project on first-order neurons in the central nervous system, which in turn project on second- and higher-order neurons. This sequence of connections gives rise to a *hierarchical organization* in which individual components can be assigned to distinct functional levels with respect to one another. For example, primary afferent fibers, which represent the lowest level in the hierarchy, determine the sensory properties of neurons of the next higher level. However, most sensory modalities are carried by more than one serial pathway. In the somatic sensory system, for example, two separate paths transmit information about shape and surface texture. Information about texture (obtained through mechanoreceptors in the skin of our fingertips) and about shape (obtained by activation of mechanoreceptors in the skin as well as those in subcutaneous tissue, muscle, and joints) is conveyed to the cerebral cortex in the same anatomical tract (the dorsal column–medial lemniscal system, Figure 23–4), but in functionally separate *parallel pathways*. Finally, additional tactile information, thought to be related to simple stationary contact and not motion of the fingers over the object, is carried by an anatomically separate path (the anterolateral system, Figure 23–4).

Thus, different features of a complex stimulus are processed separately by different paths that each transmit information to the brain. The visual system has parallel pathways from the retina to the cortex that separately carry information about the form, color, or movement of an object. The existence of parallel sensory pathways is often important clinically because there is actually some overlap in their functions. After damage to one sensory pathway, the remaining pathways may be able to mediate aspects of sensation originally served by the damaged pathway.

Sensory Systems Are Topographically Organized

The various portions of the peripheral receptive sheet are represented in the central nervous system in an orderly manner such that neighborhood relations in the periphery are preserved in the central nervous system. Receptors in adjacent portions of the peripheral receptive sheet ultimately project to neurons in adjacent portions of the

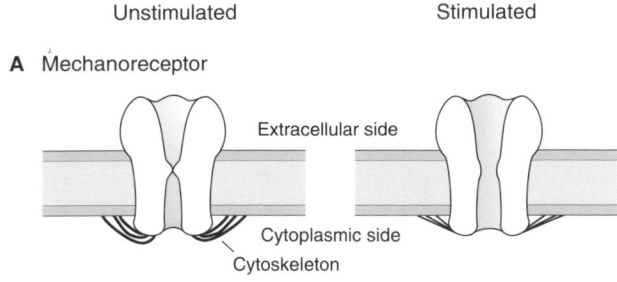

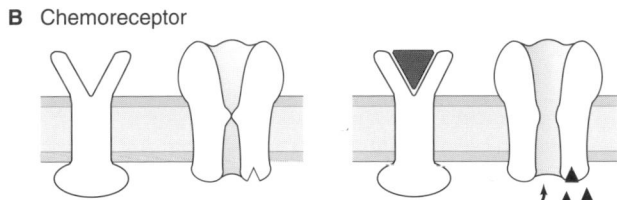

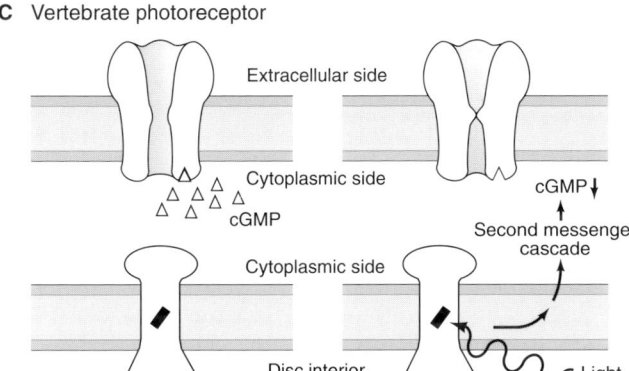

FIGURE 23–7

Transduction of different types of stimulus energies into neural activity. (Adapted from Shepherd, 1983.)

A. Mechanoelectric transduction is produced by direct mechanical interaction of the stimulus with the membrane channel. Few channels are open in the unstimulated membrane, whereas mechanical stimulation deforms the membrane and causes channels to open. Influx of Na^+ and K^+ causes the receptor terminal to depolarize locally producing the receptor potential.

B. Chemoelectric transduction is similar to mechanoelectric transduction except that a receptor–ligand interaction produces channel opening. A second messenger mediates channel opening in olfactory receptors and certain gustatory receptors.

C. Photoelectric transduction involves the absorption of light by photoreceptors. A photon–photopigment interaction on intracellular membranes produces a three-dimensional change in the photopigment. The resulting change in membrane permeability also involves a second-messenger system.

central nervous system. In the somatic sensory system, this organization is termed *somatotopy*. In visual and auditory systems the organization is called *retinotopy* and *tonotopy*, respectively.

Sensory Receptors Translate Stimulus Features into Neural Codes

How does the sensory receptor transduce natural stimulus energy into neural activity? The key to understanding sensory transduction lies in the analysis of the *receptor* (or *generator) potential*, a local potential that propagates electrotonically and is restricted to the receptive membrane. The receptor potential is often but not invariably depolarizing. The depolarizing potential is produced by an opening of cation channels selective for Na^+ and K^+, similar to those produced by the excitatory synaptic potential (see Chapter 10). The transduction process for three classes of receptors is shown schematically in Figure 23–7. When the stimulus is not present, only a few channels in a mechanoreceptor are open. Mechanical stimulation deforms the membrane, causing a change in its physical characteristics. As a result, more channels open and more Na^+ and K^+ ions flow through the membrane (Figure 23–7A). The mechanisms by which deformation of the membrane triggers the opening of channels is not known, but is thought to involve physical interactions between the channel protein and the structural components in the sensory ending (see Chapter 32).

Sensory transduction in other systems is similar to mechanoelectric transduction in the somatic sensory system. For example, inward current flow during stimulation of a chemoreceptor, such as an olfactory receptor, also causes a depolarizing inward current. However, for olfactory receptors and certain gustatory receptors, a specific receptor–ligand interaction leads to generation of a second messenger that opens the channel, thereby increasing the inward current (Figure 23–7B). Phototransduction in the retina is accomplished somewhat differently. In the dark there is a continuous flow of an inward current in photoreceptors. The channels close in response to light, thereby reducing the inward current (Figure 23–7C). In vision, as in smell, stimulation activates a second-messenger system that regulates channel gating.

When stimulus energy is transduced by the receptor into neural activity, specific features of the stimulus, such as intensity and duration, are represented in the resultant pattern of action potentials, or *neural code*. Numerous codes have been identified. The most common are based on the frequency and timing of action potentials in individual nerve fibers and on the overall distribution of activity in a population of fibers.

Stimulus Intensity Is Encoded by Frequency and Population Codes

In the 1920s Edgar Adrian first noted that the discharge frequency of an afferent fiber increases with increasing stimulus intensity. The *intensity function* of the primary afferent fiber describes the relationship between stimulus intensity and the rate or number of evoked action potentials. Suprathreshold stimuli lead to receptor potentials with faster rates of rise and greater amplitude, and these receptor potentials in turn evoke trains of action poten-

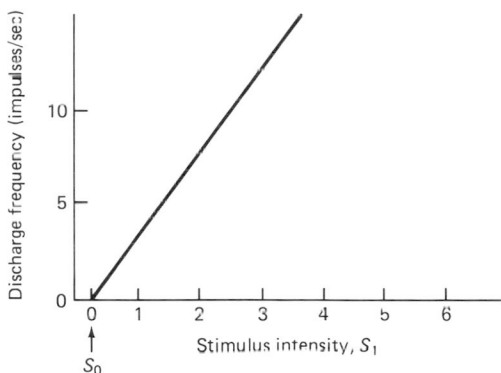

FIGURE 23–8

The frequency of discharge of a sensory neuron (recorded from the myelinated portion of the axon a few millimeters from the ending) is a function of the stimulus intensity. Afferent fibers begin discharging action potentials when the stimulus amplitude reaches S_0 (the absolute physiological threshold). At lesser amplitudes only passively propagated receptor potentials are generated. The absolute physiological threshold is important because stimulus information reaches the central nervous system only when action potentials are generated.

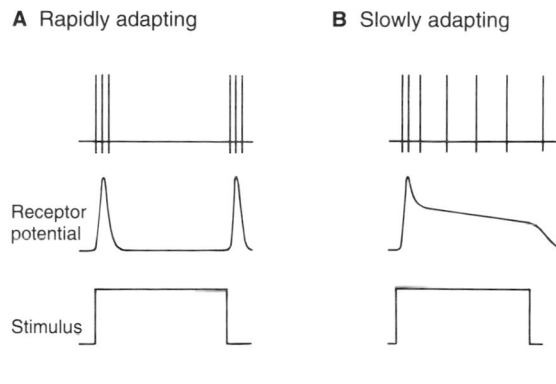

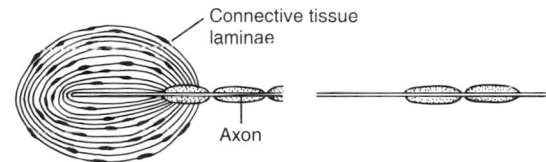

FIGURE 23–9

The response of a sensory receptor to sustained or constant stimulation diminishes over time.

A. The generator potential of a rapidly adapting receptor decreases rapidly to zero. Rapidly adapting receptors respond only at the beginning and end of the stimulus.

B. The generator potential of a slowly adapting receptor has an initial phase that adapts to a stable and maintained level of stimulus energy. Because of the properties of their generator potentials, slowly adapting receptors respond continually, albeit with decreased frequency, to an enduring stimulus.

C. The pacinian corpuscle is a rapidly adapting receptor. A cross section of this receptor (**left**) reveals concentrically arranged layers of connective tissue surrounding the sensory nerve terminal. An intact pacinian corpuscle responds with a receptor potential to the onset and termination of a mechanical stimulus but not during the intervening period. If the connective tissue laminae are removed (**right**), the receptor slowly adapts to the same mechanical stimulus. (Adapted from Loewenstein and Mendelson, 1965.)

tials with higher frequencies. This property of sensory neurons underlies the *frequency code* for stimulus intensity—stronger stimuli evoke larger receptor potentials, which cause both a greater number and a higher frequency of action potentials (Figure 23–8). The relationship between discharge frequency and stimulus intensity resembles the relationship between a subject's estimate of the magnitude of a stimulus and its intensity—both are monotonically increasing functions (see Figure 23–3).

In addition to increasing the frequency of firing, stronger stimuli also activate a greater number of receptors, so that the intensity of a stimulus is also encoded in the *size* of the responding receptor population. The activity of a population of responding receptors is called a *population* code. An increase in size of the responding neural population is a simple example of a population code. Thus, increases in stimulus intensity are encoded in two ways: (1) individual afferent fibers conduct a greater number of action potentials and (2) more fibers are activated. As we shall see in Part VI, these principles also apply to the motor systems. Here an increase in both the size of the population of active neurons and their frequency of firing determine the strength of muscle contraction.

Stimulus Duration Is Encoded in the Discharge Patterns of Rapidly and Slowly Adapting Receptors

An important feature of all sensory receptors is that they adapt to constant stimulation: The receptor potential invariably decreases in amplitude in response to a sustained stimulus. Receptor adaptation is thought to be an important component of perceptual adaptation. The response of a receptor can adapt rapidly or slowly. The pacinian corpuscle, which is located in subcutaneous tissue, is an example of a *rapidly adapting mechanoreceptor*. It responds transiently only at the onset of the stimulus and at the end of a step change in stimulus position. The duration of a maintained stimulus is therefore defined by the onset and termination of the stimulus, each of which causes a discharge in a rapidly adapting receptor (Figure 23–9A). The Merkel receptor, which is located in the skin and is sensitive to skin indentation, is an example of a *slowly adapting mechanoreceptor*. Stimulus duration may also be signaled by the persistent response of a slowly adapting receptor (Figure 23–9B).

Adaptation often results from characteristic response properties of the excitability of the membrane of the sensory neuron, such as inactivation of a Na^+ and Ca^{2+} channel or activation of a Ca^{2+}-dependent K^+ channel. Adaptation may also depend on the nonneural accessory

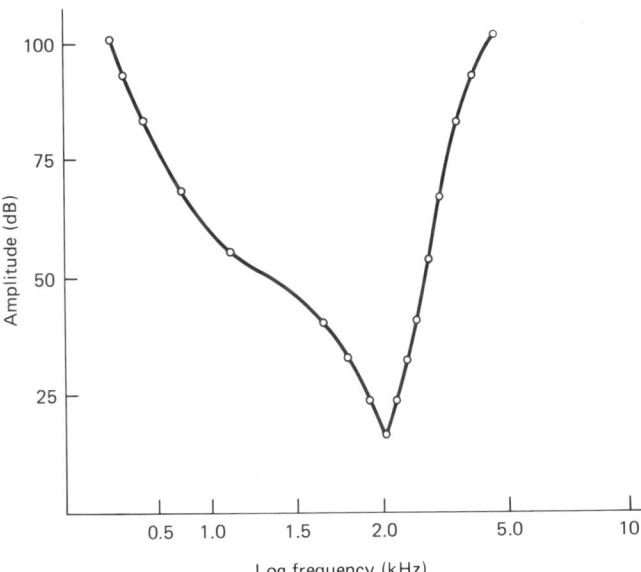

FIGURE 23–10

Each sensory receptor responds to a narrow range of intensities of a single type of energy. Physiological experiments can establish this range and enable the investigator to construct a tuning curve for individual receptors. The tuning curve shown here is for an auditory receptor most sensitive to sound at 2.0 kHz.

structure that surrounds the axon terminal. In the pacinian corpuscle, for example, this accessory structure consists of concentric layers of connective tissue surrounding an afferent nerve fiber terminal (Figure 23–9C). When a constant and persistent stimulus first impinges on the pacinian corpuscle, the outermost connective tissue layer and all deeper layers are deformed. This results in a coupled deformation of the axon membrane and leads to the response to stimulus onset. Gradually during the period of constant stimulation, the layers of the accessory structure slide between one another, so that the effective stimulus reaching the axon is mechanically dampened. In this way the accessory structure functions as a *filter*, eliminating steady or slow components of mechanical stimuli. As a result, the receptor responds only to rapid changes in pressure. Removal of the accessory structure transforms the pacinian corpuscle from a rapidly adapting into a slowly adapting receptor. Rapid adaptation in the pacinian corpuscle is an example of *feature extraction*, the selective detection and accentuation by sensory neurons of certain features of a stimulus.

Modality Is Encoded by a Labeled Line Code

As we saw earlier, specificity of function in committed neural pathways was first proposed by Müller in 1826. We now know that most sensory receptors are maximally sensitive to a single stimulus energy, a property sometimes termed *receptor specificity*. Specificity is a key property of a receptor and underlies the most important coding mech-

anism for stimulus modality, the *labeled line code*. The axons of the receptors function as modality-specific lines of communication between the periphery and the central nervous system carrying information about a specific modality. Whether pain or touch is perceived depends on the central connections of the receptors—different types of receptors have different sets of connections in the central nervous system. Thus, excitation of a particular receptor, whether by a natural stimulus or artificially by direct electrical stimulation, always elicits the same sensation. For example, electrical stimulation of the cochlear nerve can be used to signal tones of different frequencies in patients with deafness due to inner ear damage.

Not all sensory information is transmitted by labeled line codes. A relatively uncommitted receptor (or neural pathway) can signal different modalities by using different patterns of firing, called a *pattern code*. Certain types of chemoreceptors lack specificity to a single stimulus. It is thought that different modalities of chemical stimulation—for example, different aspects of taste—are elicited by different discharge patterns of chemoreceptors.

There are five specialized receptors in animals: chemoreceptors, mechanoreceptors, thermoreceptors, photoreceptors, and nociceptors (see Table 23–1). Other more specialized receptor classes have been identified in certain animals, such as infrared detectors in snakes. The type of stimulus energy to which the receptor is sensitive is called the *adequate stimulus*. Each receptor is sensitive to a narrow *range* of energy. For example, individual photoreceptors are not sensitive to all light but only to a small part of the spectrum. Thus, receptors are *tuned* to an adequate stimulus, and in physiological experiments we can generate a *tuning curve* (Figure 23–10). The tuning curve shows the maximal sensitivity of the receptor, the minimum stimulus intensity at which the receptor is activated. At greater or lesser values, stimulus intensity must be substantially increased to excite the receptor. For example, the auditory receptor shown in Figure 23–10 is most sensitive to a 2-kHz stimulus, but responds to a 1-kHz stimulus when the intensity is increased thirty times.

Stimulus Information Is Transmitted to the Central Nervous System by Conducted Action Potentials

Because the receptor potential propagates passively in the sensory receptor, the response of a sensory cell to stimulation is a purely local event. However, sensory information must be transmitted to the central nervous system for the stimulus to be perceived. In the somatic sensory and olfactory systems, the functions of sensory transduction and transmission of encoded information to the central nervous system are performed in specialized regions of the same receptor neuron (see Figure 23–5). The cell responds to an appropriate stimulus with a receptor potential that is a graded response similar to an excitatory postsynaptic potential (Figure 23–11). When the amplitude of the re-

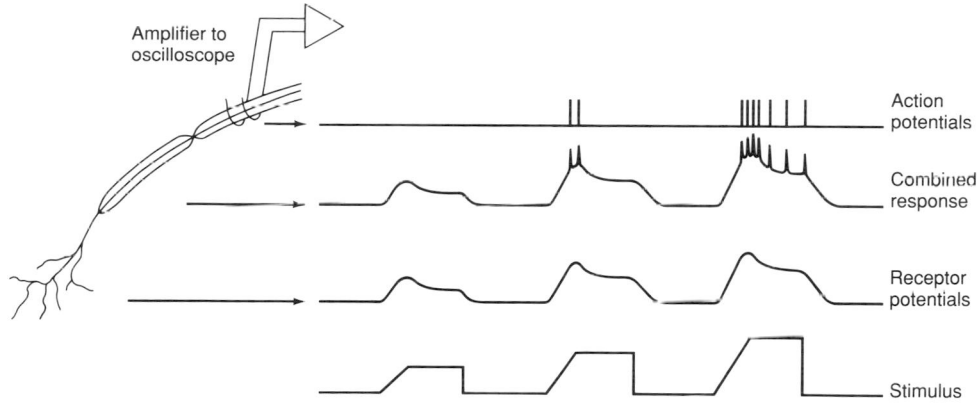

FIGURE 23–11

Different parts of a primary afferent fiber sensitive to skin stretch have different physiological characteristics. Receptor potentials are produced in the receptive membrane of the axon terminal in response to stimulation. The receptor potentials interact with the spike-generating membrane at the trigger zone, and action potentials are produced at the first node of Ranvier. Because the trigger zone is close to the receptive membrane, the potential across the trigger zone membrane reflects the sum of the receptor potential and action potentials. Further from the receptive membrane and trigger zone only action potentials are recorded.

ceptor potential reaches the threshold of the cell's trigger zone, an action potential is generated (see Chapter 10). The action potentials, which encode stimulus information, are then transmitted over distance to the central nervous system. In the visual, vestibular, auditory, and gustatory systems, these functions are performed by two different cells. Receptor cells only transduce the stimulus energy. The encoded information is conducted to the central nervous system by projection neurons.

An Overall View

Sensory experiences occur when stimulus energies excite receptors. Sensory receptors are sensitive transducers of energy—a single photon or micrometer of mechanical displacement is sufficient to excite photoreceptors or mechanoreceptors. Receptors report certain stimulus features selectively to the central nervous system. Individual receptors are tuned to one or several stimulus features. Sensory neurons in the central nervous system are also tuned to certain stimulus features because sensory receptors provide the major input to the next and subsequent neurons in the sensory pathway, albeit with modification.

The intensity of a sensation, which appears to be proportional to the strength of a stimulus, is mediated by two peripheral coding mechanisms for intensity. Stimuli of increasing intensity evoke progressively more activity in a receptor and recruit additional receptors with higher thresholds of activation. Localization of a sensation is a function of the receptive field of the receptor and central sensory neurons. The duration of a sensation is related both to the duration of the stimulus and the perceived intensity. Sensory systems are not only our means for perceiving the external world, but are also essential for maintaining arousal, forming our body image, and regulating movement.

Selected Readings

Hudspeth, A. J. 1989. How the ear's works work. Nature 341: 397–404.

Miller, G. A. 1962. Psychology: The Science of Mental Life. New York: Harper & Row.

Mountcastle, V. B. 1975. The view from within: Pathways to the study of perception. Johns Hopkins Med. J. 136:109–131.

Mountcastle, V. B. 1980. Sensory receptors and neural encoding: Introduction to sensory processes. In V. B. Mountcastle (ed.), Medical Physiology, 14th ed., Vol. 1. St. Louis: Mosby, pp. 327–347.

Stevens, S. S. 1961. The psychophysics of sensory function. In W. A. Rosenblith (ed.), Sensory Communication. Cambridge, Mass.: MIT Press, pp. 1–33.

Stevens, S. S. 1975. Psychophysics: Introduction to Its Perceptual, Neural, and Social Prospects. New York: Wiley.

Weiskrantz, L. 1986. Blindsight: A Case Study and Implications. Oxford: Clarendon Press.

References

Adrian, E. D., and Zotterman, Y. 1926. The impulses produced by sensory nerve-endings. Part 2. The response of a single end-organ. J. Physiol. (Lond.) 61:151–171.

Boring, E. G. 1942. Sensation and Perception in the History of Experimental Psychology. New York: Appleton-Century.

Clark, W. C., and Clark, S. B. 1980. Pain responses in Nepalese porters. Science 209:410–412.

Fechner, G. 1860. In D. H. Howes and E. G. Boring (eds.), Elements of Psychophysics, Vol. 1. H. E. Adler (trans.) New York: Holt, Rinehart and Winston, 1966.

Humphrey, N. K., and Weiskrantz, L., 1967. Vision in monkeys after removal of the striate cortex. Nature 215:595–597.

Locke, J. 1690. An Essay Concerning Human Understanding: In Four Books. London, Bk II, chap 1.

Loewenstein, W. R., and Mendelson, M. 1965. Components of receptor adaptation in a Pacinian corpuscle. J. Physiol. (Lond.) 177:377–397.

Martin, J. H. 1989. Neuroanatomy: Text and Atlas. New York: Elsevier.

Morawski, J. G. (ed.) 1988. The Rise of Experimentation in American Psychology. New Haven: Yale University Press.

Müller, J. 1833–40. Handbuch der Physiologie des Menschen für Vorlesungen, 2 vols. Coblenz: Hölscher.

Savage, C. W. 1970. The Measurement of Sensation: A Critique of Perceptual Psychophysics. Berkeley: University of California Press.

Shepherd, G. M. 1988. Neurobiology, 2nd ed. New York: Oxford University Press.

Sherrington, C. 1947. The Integrative Action of the Nervous System, 2nd ed. New Haven: Yale University Press.

Somjen, G. 1972. Sensory Coding in the Mammalian Nervous System. New York: Appleton-Century-Crofts.

Stevens, S. S. 1953. On the brightness of lights and the loudness of sounds. Science 118:576.

Tanner, W. P., Jr., and Swets, J. A. 1954. A decision-making theory of visual detection. Psychol. Rev. 61:401–409.

Vallbo, Å. B., Hagbarth, K.-E., Torebjörk, H. E., and Wallin, B. G. 1979. Somatosensory, proprioceptive, and sympathetic activity in human peripheral nerves. Physiol. Rev. 59:919–957.

Weber, E. H. 1846. Der Tastsinn und das Gemeingefühl. In R. Wagner (ed.), Handwörterbuch der Physiologie, Vol. III, Abt. 2. Braunschweig: Vieweg, pp. 481–588.

Weiskrantz, L., Warrington, E. K., Sanders, M. D., and Marshall, J. 1974. Visual capacity in the hemianopic field following a restricted occipital ablation. Brain 97:709–728.

Yang, J. C., Clark, W. C., Ngai, S. H., Berkowitz, B. A., and Spector, S. 1979. Analgesic action and pharmacokinetics of morphine and diazepam in man: An evaluation by sensory decision theory. Anesthesiology 51:495–502.

John H. Martin
Thomas M. Jessell

24

Modality Coding in the Somatic Sensory System

The Dorsal Root Ganglion Neuron Is the Sensory Receptor in the Somatic Sensory System

Different Sensory Receptors Have Distinguishing Anatomical Features

Pain Is Mediated by Nociceptors

Warmth and Cold Are Mediated by Thermal Receptors

Touch Is Mediated by Mechanoreceptors in the Skin

Glabrous and Hairy Skin Have Different Types of Mechanoreceptors

Mechanoreceptors Differ in Their Ability to Resolve Spatial and Temporal Features of Stimuli

Limb Proprioception Is Mediated by Muscle Afferent Fibers

Afferent Fibers of Different Diameters Conduct Action Potentials at Different Rates

An Overall View

In this and the next four chapters we shall consider the somatic sensory system, and examine how it receives and processes information from the body surface, from deep tissues, and from viscera. The somatic sensory system is distinctive for two reasons. First, the receptors for somatic sensation are distributed throughout the body, whereas those for other sensory systems are restricted to small, specialized organs. For this reason the somatic sensibilities are called the *skin senses* or *body senses*. Second, the somatic sensory system processes many kinds of stimuli and the sensations it mediates are diverse, whereas other sensory systems convey a single modality. There are four distinct somatic modalities:

1. *Touch*, elicited by mechanical stimulation of the body surface.
2. *Proprioceptive sensations*, elicited by mechanical displacements of the muscles and joints.
3. *Pain*, elicited by noxious (tissue damaging) stimuli.
4. *Thermal sensations*, elicited by cool and warm stimuli.

In addition to these elementary modalities, there are many *submodalities*. For example, we can distinguish several forms of tactile sensation, such as superficial touch and deep touch (pressure), and two forms of limb proprioception: static (position sense) and dynamic (kinesthesia). There are also *compound sensations*, such as wetness, that are achieved by combining elementary modalities and submodalities in different ways.

In this chapter we analyze the somatosensory receptor neurons of the dorsal root ganglia. We shall first examine the morphology and physiology of the receptor neurons. We then discuss the receptors that mediate the four modalities of somatic sensation. In the next chapter we turn to the two anatomical pathways that carry information from these receptors at the body surface to the cerebral cortex: (1) the *dorsal column–medial lemniscal system*, concerned with touch and limb proprioception, and (2) the *anterolateral system*, concerned with pain and temperature. In Chapters 26 and 27 we shall examine the processing of information by each of these two systems, using the perception of touch as an illustrative example of the functions of the dorsal column–medial lemniscal system (Chapter 26) and the perception of pain as an example of the functioning of the anterolateral system (Chapter 27).

The Dorsal Root Ganglion Neuron Is the Sensory Receptor in the Somatic Sensory System

Until the latter half of the twentieth century there was much debate as to how somatic sensory neurons encode the variety of somatosensory modalities. One view was that individual receptors respond selectively to one type of stimulus—the labeled line code. The other view was that different temporal patterns of activity in a single class of relatively nonspecialized receptors served as neural codes for different modalities—the pattern code. It is now clear that almost all modality coding by receptors is done by labeled line codes, described in Chapter 23. As we shall see below, however, pattern codes do have a role in some aspects of somatic sensation.

Each somatosensory modality—touch, limb proprioception, temperature sensation, and pain—is mediated by a separate class of receptors (Table 24–1). But irrespective of modality, all somatosensory information from the body is conveyed by *dorsal root ganglion neurons*. The dorsal root ganglion neurons have a complex morphology that is well suited to its two principal functions: stimulus transduction and transmission of encoded stimulus information to the central nervous system (Figure 24–1). The terminal of the peripheral branch of the axon is the only portion of the dorsal root ganglion cell that is sensitive to stimulus energy. The remainder of the peripheral branch together with the central branch are called the *primary afferent fiber*, and transmit the encoded stimulus information to the central nervous system. The central branch enters the dorsal root and terminates in the spinal cord or brain stem.

Different Sensory Receptors Have Distinguishing Anatomical Features

Dorsal root ganglion neurons differ in a variety of ways that reflect their distinct roles in sensation. Each cell can

TABLE 24–1. Receptor Types Active in Various Sensations

Receptor type	Fiber group	Quality
Nociceptors		Pain
Mechanical	Aδ	Sharp, pricking pain
Thermal and mechano-thermal	Aδ	Sharp, pricking pain
Thermal and mechano-thermal	C	Slow, burning pain
Polymodal	C	Slow, burning pain
Cutaneous and subcutaneous mechanoreceptors		
Meissner's corpuscle	Aβ	Touch
Pacinian corpuscle[1]	Aβ	Flutter
Ruffini corpuscle	Aβ	Vibration
Merkel's receptor	Aβ	Steady skin indentation
Hair-guard, hair-tylotrich	Aβ	Steady skin indentation
Hair-down	Aβ	Flutter
Muscle and skeletal mechanoreceptors		
Muscle spindle primary	Aα	Limb proprioception
Muscle spindle secondary	Aβ	
Golgi tendon organ	Aα	
Joint capsule mechanoreceptors	Aβ	

[1]Pacinian corpuscles are also located in the mesentery, between layers of muscle and on interosseous membranes.

be distinguished by (1) the morphology of its peripheral terminal, (2) its sensitivity to a stimulus energy, (3) the diameter of its axon and cell body, and (4) the presence (or absence) of a myelin sheath.

The peripheral terminal of dorsal root ganglion neurons, which is sensitive to stimulus energy, is either a bare nerve ending or an end organ consisting of a nonneural capsule surrounding the axon terminal (Figure 24–2). Nociceptors and thermoreceptors are all bare nerve endings. The selectivity of a bare nerve ending for a particular stimulus is presumably determined by the ending's membrane properties.

Virtually all mechanoreceptors have specialized endings (Table 24–1). Although the mechanoreceptor's sensitivity to stimuli is a property of the terminal membrane, its *dynamic response* is shaped by the specialized ending. As we saw in the previous chapter, removal of the connective tissue lamellae of the pacinian corpuscle trans-

FIGURE 24–1

The morphology of a dorsal root ganglion cell. The cell body lies in a ganglion on the dorsal root of a spinal nerve. The axon has two branches, one projecting to the periphery, where its specialized terminal is sensitive to a particular form of stimulus energy, and one projecting to the central nervous system.

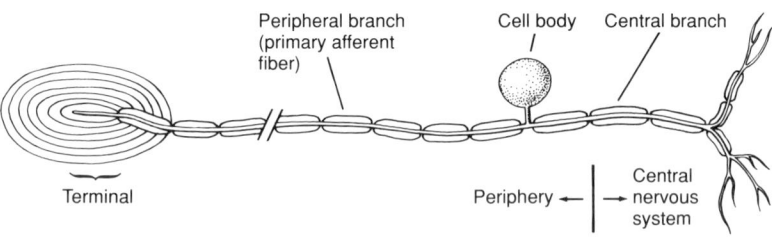

Terminal

Peripheral branch (primary afferent fiber)

Cell body

Central branch

Periphery ← | → Central nervous system

FIGURE 24-2

The location of various receptors in hairy and hairless (glabrous) skin of primates. Receptors are located in the superficial skin, at the junction of the dermis and epidermis, and more deeply in the dermis and in subcutaneous tissue. The receptors of the glabrous skin are: Meissner's corpuscles, located in the dermal papillae, Merkel's receptors, also located in the dermal papillae, and bare nerve endings. The receptors of the hairy skin are: hair receptors, Merkel's receptors (having a slightly different organization than their counterparts in the glabrous skin), and bare nerve endings. Subcutaneous receptors, beneath both glabrous and hairy skin, include pacinian and Ruffini's corpuscles. (Adapted from Light and Perl, 1984.)

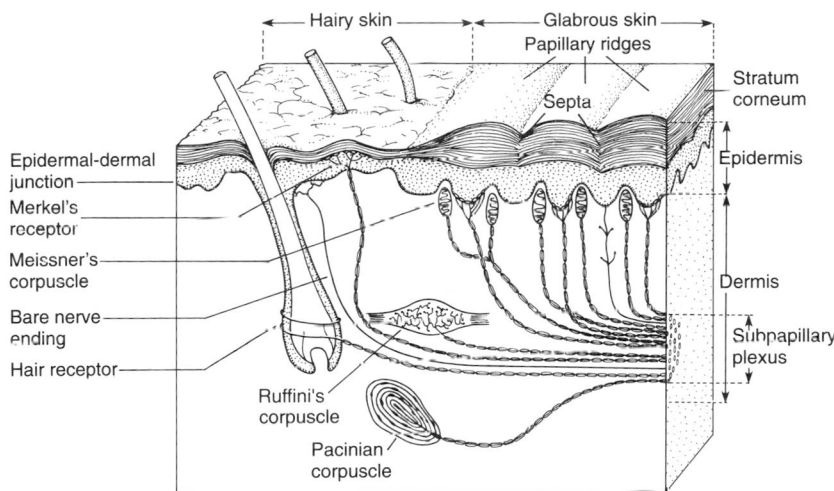

forms the cell's receptor potential from rapidly to slowly adapting. We now turn to consider the individual types of receptors. Later we shall examine the relationship between the diameter of their axons and their conduction velocity.

Pain Is Mediated by Nociceptors

The receptors that respond selectively to stimuli that can damage tissue are called *nociceptors* (Latin *nocere*, to injure). They respond directly to some noxious stimuli and indirectly to others by means of one or more chemical intermediaries released from cells in the traumatized tissue. Three types of nociceptors can be distinguished on the basis of the stimulus. (1) *Mechanical nociceptors* are activated only by strong mechanical stimulation, most effectively by sharp objects (Figure 24-3). (2) *Thermal nociceptors* respond selectively to heat or cold. Heat nociceptors in humans respond when the temperature of their receptive field exceeds 45°C, the heat pain threshold; cold nociceptors respond to noxious cold stimuli. (3) *Polymodal nociceptors* respond to several different kinds of noxious stimuli—mechanical, heat, and chemical.

Warmth and Cold Are Mediated by Thermal Receptors

Thermal sensations consist of the separate senses of warmth and cold. Temperature sensitivity is punctate: There are separate spots on the skin (each approximately 1 mm in diameter) where thermal stimulation elicits the sensation of either warmth or cold. The threshold for eliciting a thermal sensation at these spots is considerably lower than in surrounding regions of the skin.

Cold and warmth spots correspond to discrete zones of

FIGURE 24-3

A single mechanical nociceptor with a myelinated afferent fiber responds differently to different types of stimuli. Probing the cell's receptive field on the skin with a blunt tip (2 mm) elicits no response (**A**), but the tip of a needle produces a clear response (**B**). The **bottom traces** in parts A and B are the output of a force transducer coupled to the stimulator. Pinching the skin with serrated forceps (**C**), which is more traumatic than a pin prick, produces a brisk response. (Adapted from Perl, 1968.)

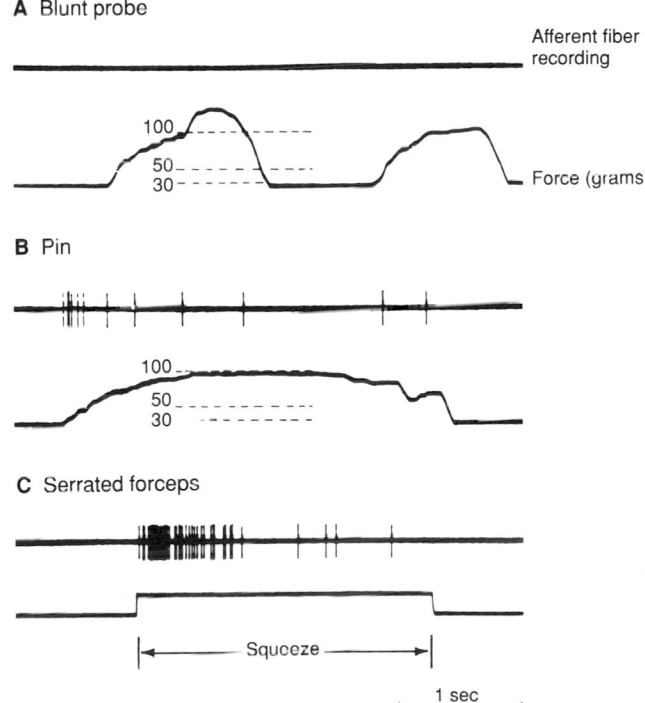

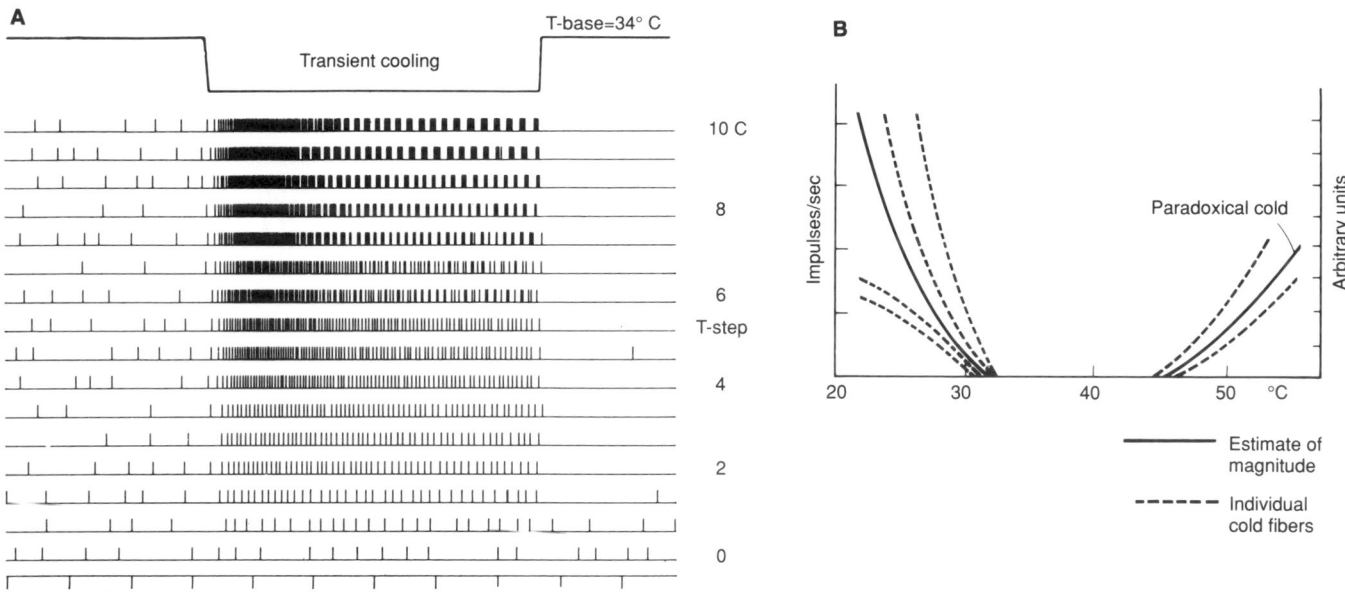

FIGURE 24-4

Cold receptors discharge when the skin is cooled below 34°C.

A. The frequency of discharge of a single cold fiber of a monkey increases with progressively greater cooling. (Adapted from Darian-Smith et al., 1973.)

B. When cold stimuli are applied to cold receptors in a monkey (**left plot**), the rate of discharge of individual fibers (**broken lines**) parallels human verbal estimations of the magnitude (**solid lines**) of cold stimuli of comparable intensities and duration. When heat (45°C) is applied to a cold receptor (**right plot**) the receptor still responds. A human subject reports the sensation as cold, a phenomenon called paradoxical cold.

innervation by cold and warmth receptors. Cold receptors discharge intensely when a cold stimulus is delivered to the receptive field, and the frequency of firing is proportional to the rate and degree at which temperature is lowered (Figure 24-4A). For example, cutaneous cold receptors are activated from approximately 1° to 20° below normal skin temperature (34°C). Over this range they are able to respond to very small changes in skin temperature. In addition, a curious sensory illusion called *paradoxical cold* occurs when a heat stimulus of 45°C is applied selectively to a cold spot on the skin (Figure 24-4B). This stimulus, which excites cold receptors, is ordinarily painful when applied diffusely to skin, but when applied to a single cold spot it is experienced by the subject as cold, not hot. Paradoxical cold is an example of labeled line coding—regardless of the stimulus, activity in the cold fiber population elicits the sensation of cold.

Warmth is mediated by a separate population of thermal receptors that are selectively activated by a range of temperatures between approximately 32°C and 45°C. With progressively warmer stimuli, warmth receptors discharge at a greater rate (Figure 24-5). Discharge rate and perceived magnitude of warmth increase in parallel (Figure 24-5). At temperatures greater than approximately 45°C warmth is not perceived but rather heat pain. In this range of painful thermal stimuli—the range over which thermal nociceptors are active—the discharge of warmth receptors is actually reduced. Thus, warmth is mediated by thermal receptors and heat pain is mediated by nociceptors.

FIGURE 24-5

The rate of discharge of individual warmth receptors in a monkey (**broken lines**) and the human estimation of the magnitude of heat stimuli (**solid line**) differ when the temperature exceeds 45°C and activates heat nociceptors instead.

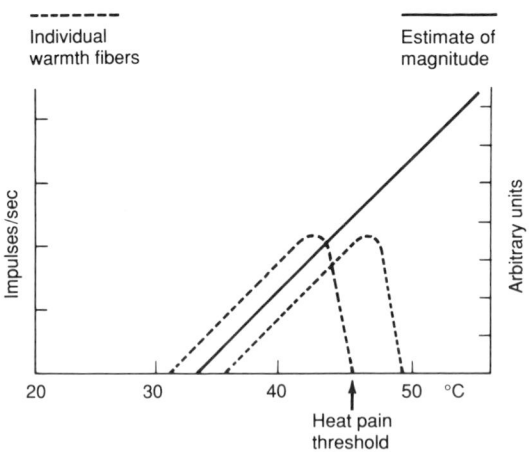

Touch Is Mediated by Mechanoreceptors in the Skin

The mechanoreceptors that mediate the sensation of touch can be divided into two major functional groups according to the way they respond to constant and enduring stimuli. *Slowly adapting* mechanoreceptors respond continuously to a persistent stimulus, whereas *rapidly adapting* mechanoreceptors respond at the onset, and often also at the termination, but not throughout the duration of the stimulus.

The relation between touch sensations and mechanoreceptor properties can be investigated directly in humans by recording from single primary afferent fibers in awake human subjects using the technique of *transdermal microneurography*. This technique was first used by Karl-Erik Hagbarth and Åke Vallbo to investigate the peripheral mechanisms underlying touch sensations. By comparing the subject's appraisal of a stimulus with the activity of individual afferent fibers, Vallbo and his colleagues sometimes found that the sensory threshold coincides with the receptive threshold of just one afferent fiber! Usually the minimum psychophysical threshold is higher than the receptive threshold of a single fiber, however.

Glabrous and Hairy Skin Have Different Types of Mechanoreceptors

The principal mechanoreceptor of the hairy skin, which covers most of the body, is the hair follicle receptor (Figure 24–2). In certain species three separate classes of receptors (down, guard, and tylotrich; see Table 24–1) innervate different types of hair follicles.

Glabrous (hairless) skin is a remarkably discriminating organ, and this sensitivity is most developed at the tips of the fingers. The two principal types of mechanoreceptors in the superficial glabrous skin are a rapidly adapting receptor, the Meissner's corpuscle, and a slowly adapting receptor, Merkel's receptor (Figure 24–2). Both have specialized accessory structures that are thought to be mechanical filters that confer the dynamic or static response specificity. Meissner's corpuscle is mechanically coupled to the surrounding tissue by thin strands of connective tissue. The Merkel's receptor is an unusual skin receptor. Electron microscopic studies suggest that a synapse is interposed between epithelial cells and the afferent fiber terminals. It is thought that an epithelial cell transduces a mechanical stimulus and forms a synaptic contact with the peripheral terminal of the dorsal root ganglion neuron. Whether this structure functions as a synapse physiologically is unclear, however. The size of the receptive field of Meissner's and Merkel's receptors is small, on average 2–4 mm (Figure 24–6).

Subcutaneous tissue beneath both hairy and glabrous skin contains two types of mechanoreceptors: the pacinian corpuscle, a rapidly adapting receptor, and Ruffini's corpuscle, a slowly adapting receptor. In contrast to the small receptive field size of Meissner's corpuscles and Merkel's receptors in superficial skin, the receptive fields of pacinian and Ruffini's corpuscles are large (Figure 24–6).

The size of the receptive fields of a population of receptors delimits the capacity of the receptors to resolve spatial detail of objects. The receptive field corresponds to

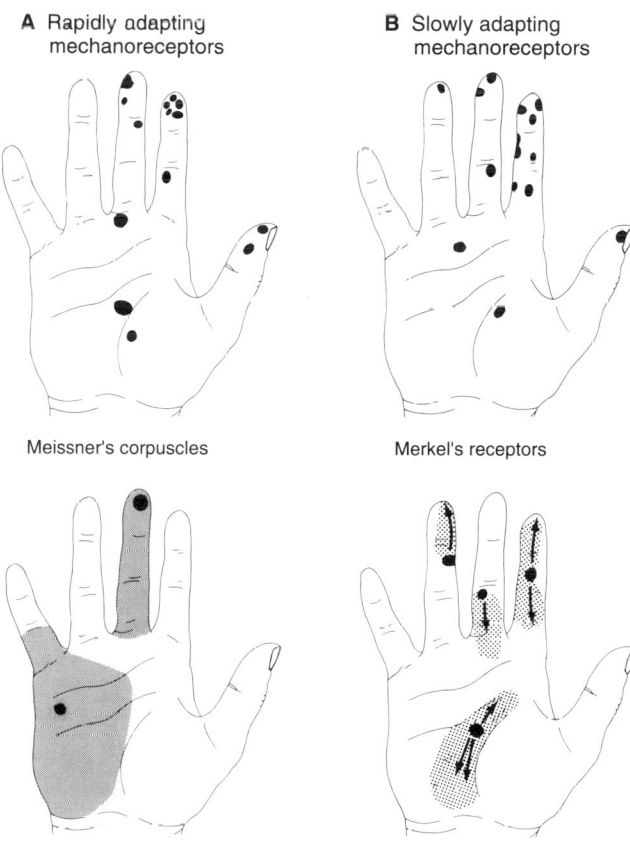

A Rapidly adapting mechanoreceptors

B Slowly adapting mechanoreceptors

Meissner's corpuscles

Merkel's receptors

Pacinian corpuscles

Ruffini's corpuscles

FIGURE 24–6

Mechanoreceptors in hairless skin vary both in the size of their receptive field and their rate of adaptation to stimuli. (Adapted from Johansson and Vallbo, 1983.)

A. The two rapidly adapting receptors are Meissner's corpuscle in the superficial skin and the subcutaneous pacinian corpuscle. The large receptive fields of pacinian corpuscles (**shaded areas**) have an inner zone of maximal sensitivity (**dark dot**). In contrast, the receptive field of Meissner's corpuscle is limited to a small area.

B. The two slowly adapting receptors are Merkel's corpuscle (superficial skin) and Ruffini's corpuscle (subcutaneous). Again, the receptor in the superficial skin has a highly localized receptive field, whereas the subcutaneous receptor has a large field (**stippled area**). Depending on their location, individual Ruffini's corpuscles are excited by stretch of the skin in different directions, indicated by **arrows**.

the region of tissue innervated by the terminals of the receptor and the area of the surrounding tissue through which the stimulus energy is conducted to the receptor's terminals. Meissner's corpuscle and Merkel's corpuscle, receptors with small receptive fields, can resolve fine spatial differences, whereas pacinian corpuscles and Ruffini's corpuscle, which have large receptive fields, can only resolve coarse spatial differences (see Figure 24–6).

As we saw in the previous chapter, spatial discrimination can be quantified psychophysically by the two-point

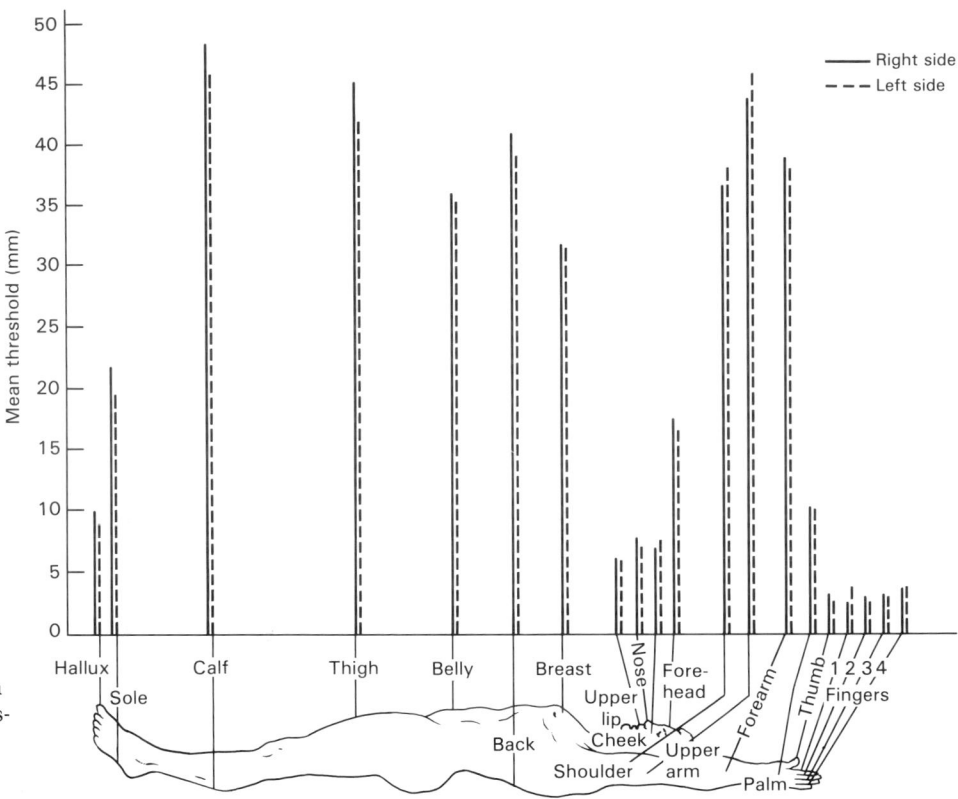

FIGURE 24–7
Two-point discrimination varies with location on body surface. Greatest discriminative capacity is present in the finger tips, lips, and tongue. (Adapted from Weinstein, 1968.)

threshold. The two-point threshold varies for different body regions (Figure 24–7); it is about 2 mm on the finger tip but increases to about 10 mm on the palm and 40 mm on the arm. This threshold variation has been examined in detail for the palmar surface of the hand, revealing a correlation between discriminative capacity and the innervation density of peripheral mechanoreceptors.

Mechanoreceptors Differ in Their Ability to Resolve Spatial and Temporal Features of Stimuli

A simple way to activate both rapidly and slowly adapting mechanoreceptors is to present a long-lasting stimulus, such as a steady skin indentation. This stimulus first evokes the sensation of contact or tap, which may be mediated by both rapidly and slowly adapting receptors. After several hundred milliseconds, however, only slowly adapting receptors remain active, and only then a steady skin indentation is felt (Figure 24–8A).

The sensitivities of the two types of rapidly adapting mechanoreceptors in the skin are best distinguished by their responses to mechanical stimuli that oscillate in a sinusoidal manner (Figure 24–8B). This can be illustrated by plotting the responses of the receptors to stimuli of different intensity and frequency. Meissner's corpuscles, located in the superficial glabrous skin, are most sensitive to low-frequency sinusoidal mechanical stimuli, whereas pacinian corpuscles, located in subcutaneous tissue, are most sensitive to high-frequency stimuli (Figure 24–9).

The excitation of Meissner's corpuscles is felt as a gentle fluttering in the skin. This sensation is well localized, reflecting the small size of the receptive field of Meissner's corpuscle. In contrast, the excitation of pacinian corpuscles evokes a diffuse, humming sensation in the deeper tissue. This vibration sense is poorly localized because of the large size of the receptive field of pacinian corpuscles.

These pure sensory experiences evoked by a tap or a sinusoidal mechanical stimulus are quite different from the tactile sensations evoked by the complex natural stimuli that we usually encounter. Natural stimuli rarely activate a single type of receptor; rather they activate different combinations of mechanoreceptors. Textures are a good example of complex stimuli that activate several mechanoreceptors.

To study texture discrimination, Kenneth Johnson and Graham Lamb compared the spatial discrimination of three classes of glabrous skin mechanoreceptors in the hands of monkeys. They examined the response of different types of mechanoreceptors to a braille dot pattern (Figure 24–10). Their findings suggest that different aspects of stimulus information are transmitted by rapidly and slowly adapting receptors. The discharge of the slowly adapting mechanoreceptors (Merkel's receptors) best encoded the spatial characteristics of the stimuli. The rapidly adapting receptors may provide timing information essential to the analysis of tactile information obtained under active conditions, as the finger tip is moved over a surface.

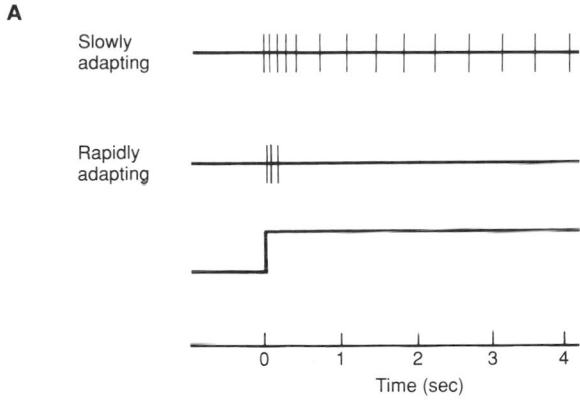

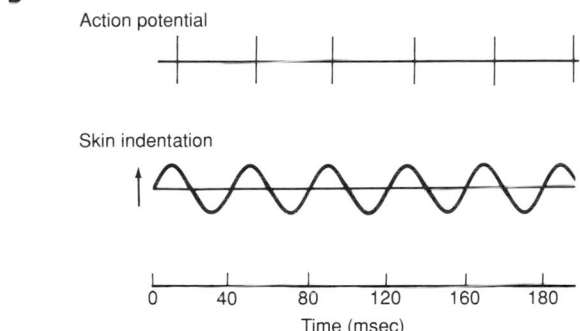

FIGURE 24–8

Slowly adapting mechanoreceptors continue responding to a steady stimulus, whereas rapidly adapting mechanoreceptors respond only at the beginning of the stimulus.

A. Responses of slowly and rapidly adapting mechanoreceptors to a step indentation of the skin.

B. A rapidly adapting mechanoreceptor responds to sinusoidal mechanical stimuli with a single action potential for each phase of the stimulus.

Limb Proprioception Is Mediated by Muscle Afferent Fibers

Limb proprioception is the sense of position and movement of the limbs. There are two submodalities of limb proprioception: the sense of stationary position of the limbs (*limb position sense*) and the sense of limb movement (*kinesthesia*). These sensations are important for maintaining balance, controlling limb movements, and for evaluating the shape of a grasped object.

Proprioceptive sensations of the limbs generally occur as a consequence of voluntary (or reflexive) movement. For this reason, it was long thought that limb proprioception depends not on signals from peripheral receptors, but rather on signals from brain regions controlling limb movement. Thus, limb proprioception was thought to differ from other somatosensory modalities, which are mediated by peripheral receptors. This view derives from the work of Herman Helmholtz, who over a century ago first

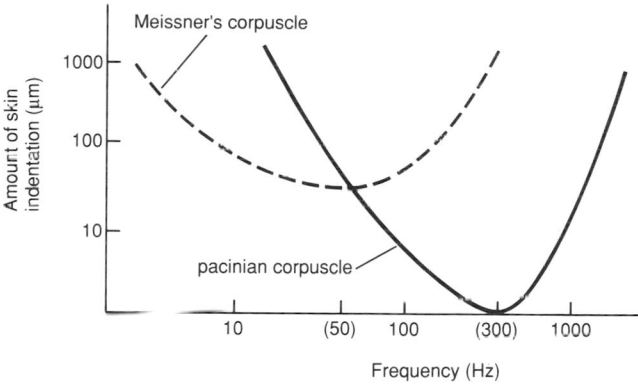

FIGURE 24–9

Meissner's corpuscles are more sensitive to low-frequency sinusoidal mechanical stimuli, whereas pacinian corpuscles are more sensitive to high-frequency stimuli. The ordinate indicates the magnitude of the threshold stimulus. The threshold of a mechanoreceptor corresponds to the lowest stimulus intensity that evokes one action potential per cycle of the sinusoidal stimulus (see Figure 24–8B).

called attention to the importance of motor centers in evoking sensation. According to this view, parts of the brain controlling movement transmit signals both to motor neurons—commanding skeletal muscle to contract—and to other parts of the central nervous system—informing them about the details of the planned movement.

One way to test whether corollary discharges are involved in proprioception is to produce a disparity between what the brain commands the muscles to do and what actually happens. This can be done by occluding circulation in a limb with a blood pressure cuff inflated above systolic pressure, thus altering the effectiveness of the neural signals responsible for muscle contraction in the limb. Distal to the cuff the nerves become anoxic. Peter Matthews and his colleagues found that the ability to move the limb and to perceive its movement are differentially affected under these conditions: The perception of voluntary movement diminishes before the movement itself because conduction of action potentials in the afferent nerves is blocked before conduction in efferent nerves to skeletal muscles.

Another way of assessing whether proprioceptive sensations are mediated by receptors or by corollary discharges is to compare the sensations of changes in limb position when the limbs are moved passively and actively. Studies using this method have shown that limb position sense and kinesthesia are well developed in the absence of voluntary muscle contraction. For example, at rest, the angle of the knee joint can be evaluated to within 0.5°. Thus, perception of limb position and movement is mediated by peripheral receptors.

Three main types of peripheral receptors signal the stationary position of the limb and the speed and direction of limb movement: (1) mechanoreceptors located in joint

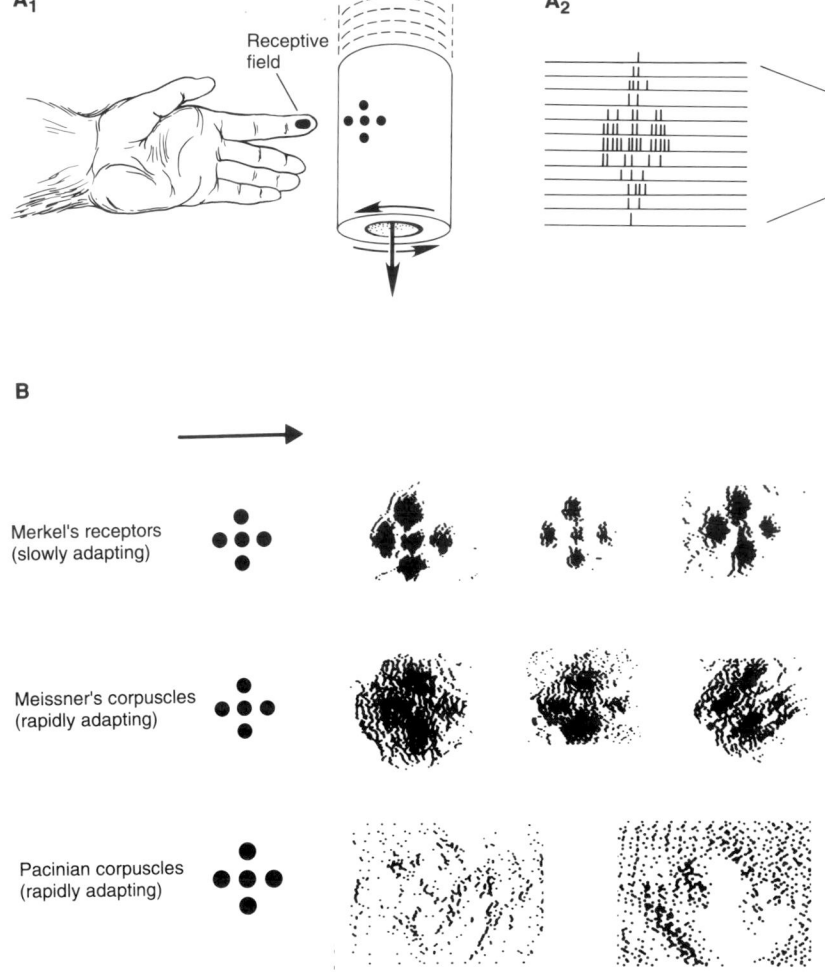

FIGURE 24–10

Complex stimuli activate more than one mechanoreceptor.

A. 1. The receptive field on a monkey's finger is stimulated with an embossed dot array on a drum. The array is swept across the skin at a given location in the receptive field by rotating the drum and then moved 200 μm within the receptive field and swept again. **2.** Action potentials discharged by the receptor during each sweep are recorded **(left)**. The recordings are ordered (from top to bottom) according to the sequence of stimulus presentation within the receptive field, as shown in part 1. To construct a *spatial event plot* **(right)**, each action potential shown at the left is represented by a dot. The locations of the dots are compressed vertically and horizontally to resemble the stimulus.

B. Representative examples of spatial event plots of three types of mechanoreceptors: slowly adapting Merkel's corpuscles **(top)**, rapidly adapting Meissner's corpuscles **(middle)**, and rapidly adapting pacinian corpuscles **(bottom)**. Stimuli are shown at the **left**. (Adapted from Johnson and Lamb, 1981.)

capsules, (2) muscle spindle receptors, mechanoreceptors in muscle that are specialized to transduce stretch of the muscle, and (3) cutaneous mechanoreceptors.

Richard Burgess and his colleagues carried out systematic psychophysical studies of limb position sense in humans. In separate experiments they examined the physiological properties of afferent fibers innervating the knee joint in cats to determine whether such receptors could signal joint angles. They found that the knee joint afferents are not sensitive to intermediate joint angles when the knee is bent halfway to full flexion; this is the range over which static position sense in humans is well developed. Rather, knee joint afferents are sensitive to extremes of joint angles. Moreover, patients with artificial joints can still have a good sense of static position. This evidence suggests that joint afferents may not play a dominant role in sensing position of the limb at rest. They do, however, participate in aspects of limb proprioception. Patients who have undergone total hip replacement are able to detect the direction of passive limb movement despite the lack of joint innervation; however, the threshold for detection is higher than before surgery.

Matthews, Burgess, and their colleagues found that joint angle is judged predominantly from information about muscle length provided by the muscle spindle receptors, slowly adapting mechanoreceptors that are entwined around a specialized muscle fiber (Figure 24–11). Muscle spindle receptors are sensitive to minute changes in muscle length. Matthews produced illusions of limb position and movement by applying a vibratory stimulus to the muscles of the forearm. Strong vibration causes the length of the muscle to vary by a small amount; these vibrations powerfully excite muscle spindle receptors. Vibration also excites pacinian corpuscles but their activity does not affect perceived limb position. When the muscle is vibrated, subjects report a disparity between the actual limb position and the perceived position (Figure 24–12A). For example, when the biceps is vibrated there is an illusion that the arm is more extended. During vibration, muscle spindles in the biceps discharge at higher rates. Normally, this higher discharge is produced by stretch of the biceps, i.e., limb extension. Even though the biceps does not increase in length, the higher discharge is perceived as limb extension. As we shall see in Chapter 37, muscle spindle recep-

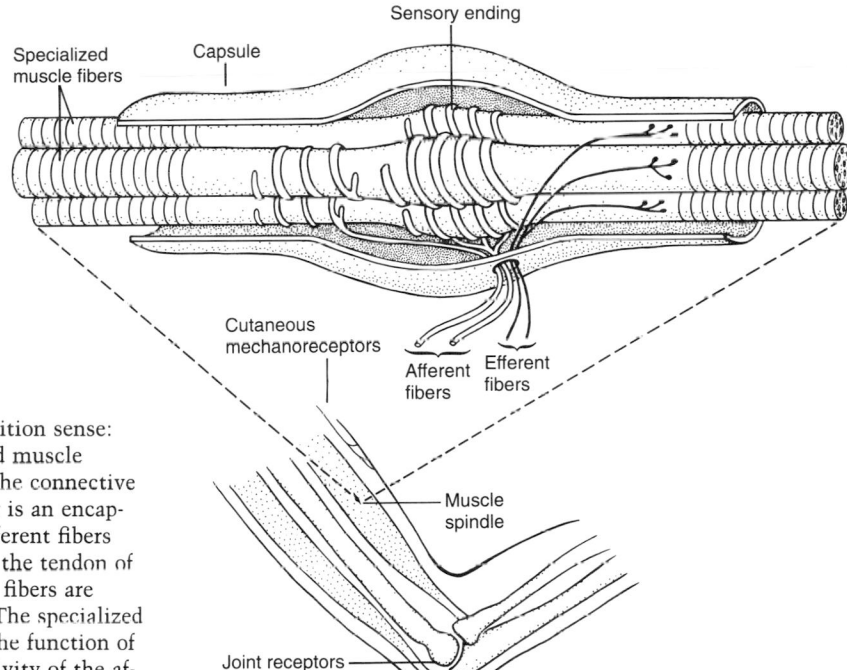

FIGURE 24–11

Three classes of receptors contribute to limb position sense: joint receptors, cutaneous mechanoreceptors, and muscle spindle receptors. The joint receptors innervate the connective tissue joint capsule. The muscle spindle receptor is an encapsulated stretch receptor (see **inset**) in muscle. Afferent fibers entwine around specialized muscle fibers. When the tendon of the muscle is stretched these specialized muscle fibers are stretched, thereby activating the afferent fibers. The specialized muscle fibers are innervated by efferent fibers. The function of this efferent innervation is to regulate the sensitivity of the afferent fibers during active muscle contractions (see Chapter 37).

tors have complex properties that are also controlled by efferent signals from the central nervous system.

Whereas the contribution of muscle spindle receptors to limb proprioception is clearly important, full proprioceptive sensitivity depends on the combined actions of muscle receptors, joint receptors, and cutaneous mechanoreceptors. Simon Gandevia and David McCloskey and their colleagues took advantage of the fact that the flexor and extensor muscles effectively become disengaged from the distal interphalangeal joint when it is held in a particular posture (Figure 24–12B). By manipulating finger position to eliminate the contribution of muscle receptors and administering local anesthetics to block cutaneous and joint afferent input, they studied proprioceptive acuity under three conditions: (1) with afferent input from muscles, joints, and skin intact, (2) with muscles disengaged, leaving only joint and skin input, and (3) with muscle afferents intact but input from joint and skin blocked by anesthesia. They found that performance deteriorated when only joint and cutaneous afferents provided joint angle information or when only muscle receptors provided information.

Afferent Fibers of Different Diameters Conduct Action Potentials at Different Rates

We have seen that the different qualities of somatic sensation—touch, proprioception, pain, and temperature sense—are mediated by the terminals of dorsal root ganglion cells that have different stimulus sensitivities and morphology. The axons of these different dorsal root ganglion cells conduct action potentials to the central nervous system at different rates. The speed at which an afferent fiber conducts action potentials also is related to the diameter of the fiber (see Chapter 7). In large myelinated fibers the conduction velocity (in meters per second) is approximately six times the axon diameter (in micrometers). The factor for converting axon diameter to conduction velocity is smaller for thinly myelinated fibers (approximately 5) and still smaller for unmyelinated fibers (1.5–2.5). Here we shall examine the relationship between action potential conduction velocity and receptor type.

To investigate the relationship of axonal diameter and conduction velocity of afferent fibers in peripheral nerves it is essential to eliminate the activity of efferent fibers. This can be done in experimental animals by cutting both the ventral roots (which contain the axons of the somatic motor neurons) and the nerve trunks that contain the postganglionic visceral motor supply (the gray rami). To ensure that the motor fibers distal to the transection degenerate, the animals are then allowed to recover for about four months before the nerves, now containing *only* afferent fibers, are examined histologically. The afferent fibers in the nerve then are counted, their diameters measured, and a frequency distribution plot of fiber diameter is constructed.

These graphs show that afferent fibers innervating muscle differ from those innervating the skin. The histogram of the distribution of these nerves in muscle has four peaks, corresponding to the four types of axons: large myelinated (I), small myelinated (II), smaller myelinated (III), and unmyelinated (IV) fibers (Figure 24–13A). Another nomenclature, Aα, Aβ, Aδ, C, is also used. Both nomen-

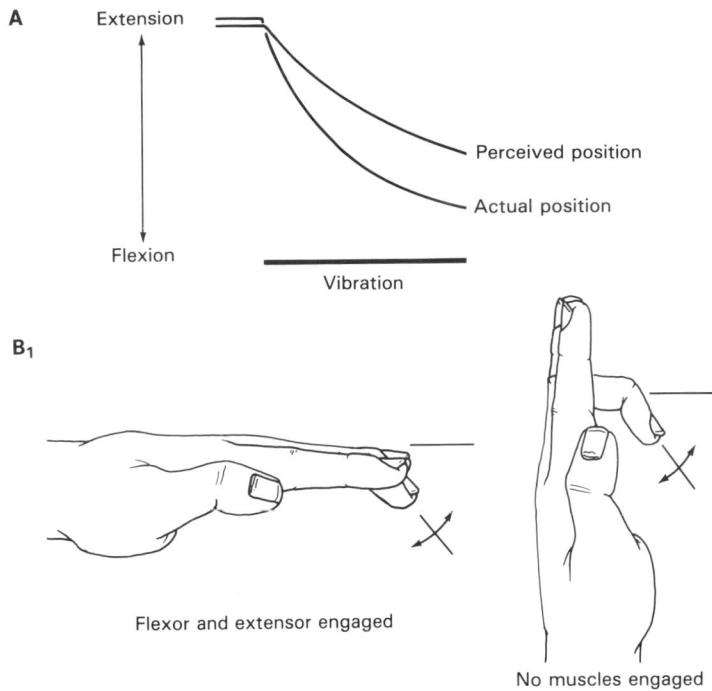

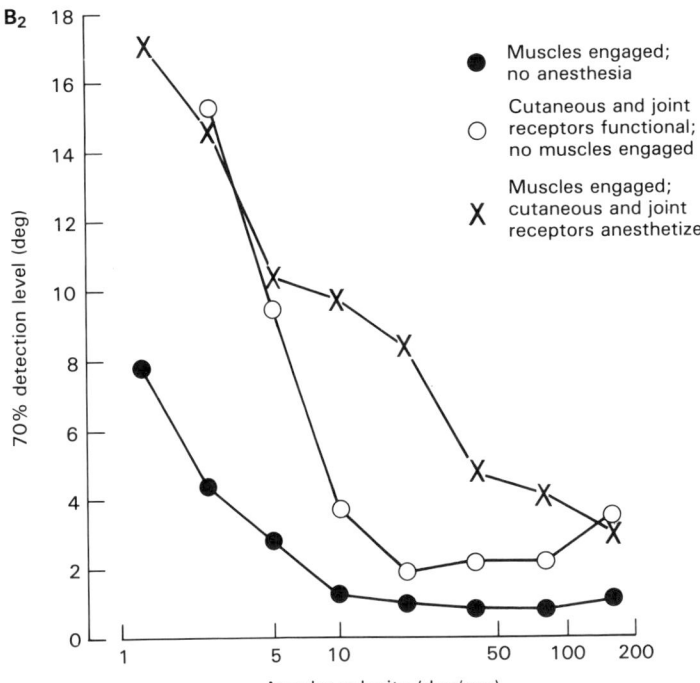

FIGURE 24–12

A. Vibration of muscle produces an illusion of limb position. Since the muscle spindles contain stretch receptors that excite the motor neurons innervating the muscle, vibrating a muscle is similar to tapping the tendon of a muscle: The stimulus causes the muscle to contract and the limb to move. Upon vibration of the biceps tendon the subject perceives his forearm to be somewhat more extended than the actual position. Note that the illusion of the limb movement is in the direction of limb extension.

B. Muscle receptors, joint receptors, and cutaneous receptors are required for complete proprioceptive acuity. The contribution of different receptors to limb position sense can be examined experimentally in human subjects. The joint and cutaneous receptors in the fingers are anesthetized by occluding local circulation. Under these conditions flexing the metacarpal–proximal phalangeal joint disengages the muscles of the distal phalanx. Thus, passive movement of the distal phalanx does not change muscle length and therefore does not activate muscle receptors.

clatures are based on conduction velocity (or axonal diameter). The numerical classification typically is used for muscle afferents, while the alphabetical scheme is used for cutaneous nerves. The fiber diameters and conduction velocities for the four types of axons are listed in Table 24–2. The distribution of cutaneous nerves has only three peaks because the group I (or Aα) afferents are absent in cutaneous nerves. The physiological properties of these group I afferents will be considered in detail in Chapter 37. Virtually all mechanoreceptors are Aβ and Aα fibers, whereas thermoreceptors and nociceptors belong to the Aδ and C fiber groups (Table 24–1).

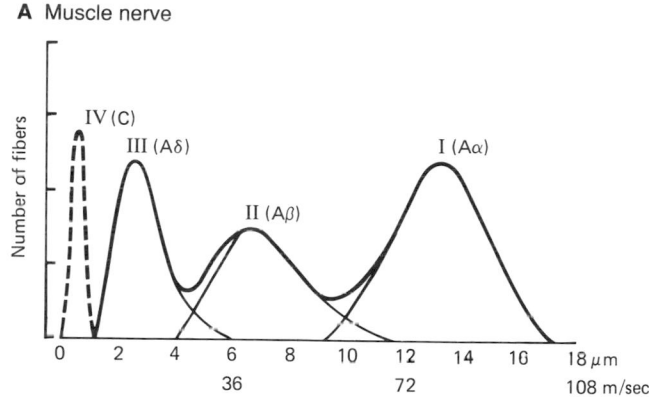

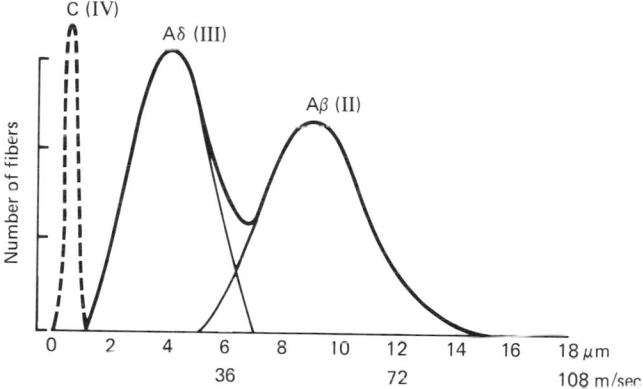

FIGURE 24–13

The distribution of different types of afferent fibers in muscle and cutaneous tissue. Axonal diameters are given in micrometers and conduction velocities are given in meters per second. (Adapted from Boyd and Davey, 1968.)

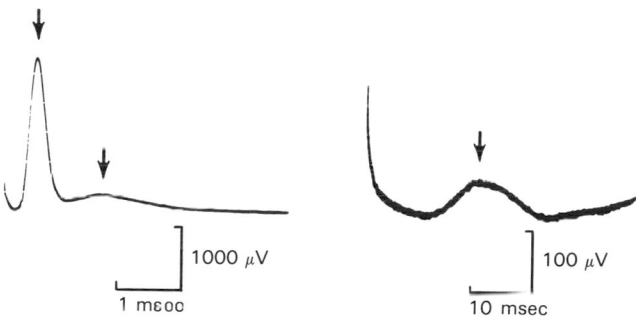

FIGURE 24–14

The compound action potential has three distinct peaks corresponding to Aα, Aδ, and C fibers. The compound action potential shown here was recorded *in vitro* since potentials from C fibers cannot be recorded *in vivo*. The nerve, from an 11-year-old boy whose leg had been amputated above the knee, was placed in a specialized recording chamber. The recording on the **left** shows peaks produced by Aα (left arrow) and Aδ (right arrow) fibers. The trace on the **right** is a high-gain, slow time scale recording of a C-fiber peak. (From Kimura, 1983.)

The conduction velocity of a fiber is important. The faster a fiber conducts action potentials, the quicker the central nervous system receives the information, and the sooner the central nervous system can act on the information. In an average adult a stimulus delivered to a finger tip activates receptors that are located about 1 meter from the spinal cord. An Aδ fiber, conducting at 25 ms, conveys information to the central nervous system in 0.04 s. In contrast, a C fiber, conducting at the rate of 0.5 ms, takes 2 s or more to convey information to the central nervous

system. If a stimulus is noxious and triggers reflex withdrawal, for example touching a hot surface, the appropriate muscle should contract as soon as possible. If the stimulus were carried only by the slow-conducting C fibers, damage to the finger tip could begin before the central nervous system receives the information.

The clinician takes advantage of the known distributions of conduction velocities of afferent fibers in peripheral nerves to diagnose diseases that result in sensory fiber degeneration. The *compound action potential* is produced by electrical stimulation of a peripheral nerve, at an intensity to activate all sensory fibers. This potential is the summation of action potentials of all sensory nerve fibers. It has two major deflections corresponding to action potentials conducted by large and small myelinated fibers (Figure 24–14). Action potentials of unmyelinated nerves are conducted slowly and produce a small late peak that typically cannot be recorded *in vivo*. In certain conditions there is a selective loss of axons; in diabetes, for example, large sensory fibers degenerate (large-fiber neuropathy). Such selective loss is reflected in a reduction in the appropriate peak of the compound action potential and a corresponding diminution of sensory capacity.

TABLE 24–2. Afferent Fiber Groups

	Muscle nerve	Cutaneous nerve	Fiber diameter (μm)	Conduction velocity (ms)
Myelinated				
Large	I	A–C	13–20	80–120
Small	II	Aβ	6–12	35–75
Smallest	III	Aδ	1–5	5–30
Unmyelinated	IV	C	0.2–1.5	0.5–2

An Overall View

There is a large variety of morphologically distinct somatic sensory receptors with different physiological characteristics. As we shall see in the next chapter, these different types of receptors also have different patterns of termination in the spinal cord dorsal horn. Thus, morphological specialization in the periphery sets the stage not only for the coding characteristics of the receptor, but also for the anatomical projections in the central nervous system and the role of the receptor in perception.

The relationship between somatic sensory modalities and the receptors mediating them is well understood. Discriminative mechanoreception and limb proprioception depend upon encapsulated receptors and axons with fast conduction velocities. In contrast, the sensations of pain and temperature are mediated by bare nerve endings and axons with slower conduction velocities. Each type of sensory receptor is tuned to a different quality of the stimulus. Mechanoreceptors are sensitive to a steady indentation or to low- or high-frequency vibration; thermal receptors are sensitive to cold or warmth. Nociceptors are sensitive to noxious stimuli.

The somatic sensory stimuli we encounter in everyday life are complex and often consist of multiple qualities. When all receptors in a given patch of skin are exposed to a complex stimulus, each type of receptor is selectively activated by a distinct component of the stimulus. The various types of receptors thus transmit selective information about the stimulus to the central nervous system. This information is analyzed and combined by subsequent processing stages in the central nervous system to produce perception.

Selected Readings

Boivie, J. J. G., and Perl, E. R. 1975. Neural substrates of somatic sensation. In C. C. Hunt (ed.), MTP International Review of Science. Physiology, Series 1: Neurophysiology, Vol. 3. Baltimore: University Park Press, pp. 303–411.

Burgess, P. R., and Perl, E. R. 1973. Cutaneous mechanoreceptors and nociceptors. In A. Iggo (ed.), Handbook of Sensory Physiology, Vol. 2: Somatosensory System. New York: Springer, pp. 29–78.

Burgess, P. R., Wei, J. Y., Clark, F. J., and Simon, J. 1982. Signaling of kinesthetic information by peripheral sensory receptors. Annu. Rev. Neurosci. 5:171–187.

Goodwin, G. M., McCloskey, D. I., and Matthews, P. B. C. 1972. The contribution of muscle afferents to kinaesthesia shown by vibration induced illusions of movement and by the effects of paralysing joint afferents. Brain 95:705–748.

Iggo, A., and Andres, K. H. 1982. Morphology of cutaneous receptors. Annu. Rev. Neurosci. 5:1–31.

Kass, J. H. 1990. Somatosensory system. In G. Paxinos (ed.), The Human Nervous System. San Diego: Academic Press, pp. 813–844.

McCloskey, D. I. 1978. Kinesthetic sensibility. Physiol. Rev. 58: 763–820.

Sathian, K. 1989. Tactile sensing of surface features. Trends Neurosci. 12:513–519.

Vallbo, Å. B., Hagbarth, K.-E., Torebjörk, H. E., and Wallin, B. G. 1979. Somatosensory, proprioceptive, and sympathetic activity in human peripheral nerves. Physiol. Rev. 59:919–957.

Willis, W. D., and Coggeshall, R. E. 1978. Sensory Mechanisms of the Spinal Cord. New York: Plenum Press.

References

Boyd, I. A., and Davey, M. R. 1968. Composition of Peripheral Nerves. Edinburgh: Livingstone.

Coggeshall, R. E., Applebaum, M. L., Fazen, M., Stubbs, T. B., III, and Sykes, M. T. 1975. Unmyelinated axons in human ventral roots, a possible explanation for the failure of dorsal rhizotomy to relieve pain. Brain 98:157–166.

Darian-Smith, I. 1984a. The sense of touch: Performance and peripheral neural processes. In I. Darian-Smith (ed.), Handbook of Physiology, Section 1: The Nervous System, Vol. III. Sensory Processes, Part 2. Bethesda, Md.: American Physiological Society, pp. 739–788.

Darian-Smith, I. 1984b. Thermal sensibility. In I. Darian-Smith (ed.), Handbook of Physiology, Section 1: The Nervous System, Vol. III. Sensory Processes, Part 2. Bethesda, Md.: American Physiological Society, pp. 879–913.

Darian-Smith, I., Johnson, K. O., and Dykes, R. 1973. "Cold" fiber population innervating palmar and digital skin of the monkey: Responses to cooling pulses. J. Neurophysiol. 36:325–346.

Gandevia, S. C., Hall, L. A., McCloskey, D. I., and Potter, E. K. 1983. Proprioceptive sensation at the terminal joint of the middle finger. J. Physiol. (Lond.) 335:507–517.

Johansson, R. S., and Vallbo, Å. B. 1983. Tactile sensory coding in the glabrous skin of the human hand. Trends Neurosci. 6:27–32.

Johnson, K. O., and Lamb, G. D. 1981. Neural mechanisms of spatial tactile discrimination: Neural patterns evoked by Braille-like dot patterns in the monkey. J. Physiol. (Lond.) 310: 117–144.

Kimura, J. 1989. Electrodiagnosis in Diseases of Nerve and Muscle: Principles and Practice, 2nd ed. Philadelphia: F. A. Davis.

Knibestol, M., and Vallbo, Å. B. 1976. Stimulus-response functions of primary afferents and psychophysical intensity estimation on mechanical skin stimulation in the human hand. In Y. Zotterman (ed.), Sensory Functions of the Skin in Primates with Special Reference to Man. Oxford: Pergamon Press, pp. 201–213.

Light, A. R., and Perl, E. R. 1984. Peripheral sensory systems. In P. J. Dyck, P. K. Thomas, E. H. Lambert and R. Burge (eds.), Peripheral Neuropathy, 2nd ed. Vol. 1. Philadelphia: Saunders, pp. 210–230.

Perl, E. R. 1968. Myelinated afferent fibres innervating the primate skin and their response to noxious stimuli. J. Physiol. (Lond.) 197:593–615.

Sherrington, C. S. 1900. The muscular sense. In E. A. Schäfer (ed.), Text-Book of Physiology, Vol. 2. Edinburgh: Pentland, pp. 1002–1025.

Weinstein, S. 1968. Intensive and extensive aspects of tactile sensitivity as a function of body part, sex, and laterality. In D. R. Kenshalo (ed.), The Skin Senses. Springfield, Ill.: Thomas, pp. 195–222.

25

John H. Martin
Thomas M. Jessell

Anatomy of the Somatic Sensory System

Afferent Fibers Enter the Spinal Cord Through the Dorsal Roots

The Spinal Cord Is the First Relay Point for Somatic Sensory Information

Spinal Gray Matter Contains Nerve Cell Bodies

Spinal White Matter Contains Myelinated Axons

Dorsal Root Fibers Branch In the White Matter and Terminate in the Gray Matter

Afferents Conveying Different Somatic Sensory Modalities Have Distinct Terminal Projections

Two Major Ascending Systems Convey Somatic Sensory Information to the Cerebral Cortex

The Dorsal Column-Medial Lemniscal System Mediates Tactile Sense and Arm Proprioception

The Anterolateral System Mediates Pain and Temperature Sense

The Primary Somatic Sensory Cortex Is Divided into Four Functional Areas

Pyramidal Cells in Layers 2, 3, 5, and 6 Are the Output Cells of the Primary Somatic Sensory Cortex

An Overall View

In the last chapter we saw that different sensory receptors respond to different stimulus qualities. In this chapter we shall examine the anatomical pathways whereby somatic modalities are conveyed from the various types of receptors in the periphery to different sites in the spinal cord and brain stem. Somatic sensory information is relayed next to the thalamus and then to the cerebral cortex by means of the two major somatosensory ascending pathways: the dorsal column–medial lemniscal pathway and the anterolateral pathway. Each of these ascending pathways mediates different sensory modalities, whose physiological properties we shall discuss in the next two chapters.

Here we examine only the somatic sensory representation of the body (arms, legs, and trunk). The innervation of the face, mediated by the trigeminal nerve, is considered separately in Chapter 45 because the trigeminal system illustrates several important features of the organization of the brain stem.

Afferent Fibers Enter the Spinal Cord Through the Dorsal Roots

Sensory information from the periphery is conveyed to the spinal cord by afferent nerve fibers bundled together in *peripheral nerves*. Individual peripheral nerves contain both the afferent and efferent nerve fibers for the same general part of the body. At various points between the periphery and the spinal cord the fibers in one peripheral nerve join fibers from other peripheral nerves. As they approach the spinal cord, peripheral nerves join together to form *spinal nerves*.

Near the spinal cord the afferent fibers separate dorsally from the efferent fibers and enter the spinal cord through

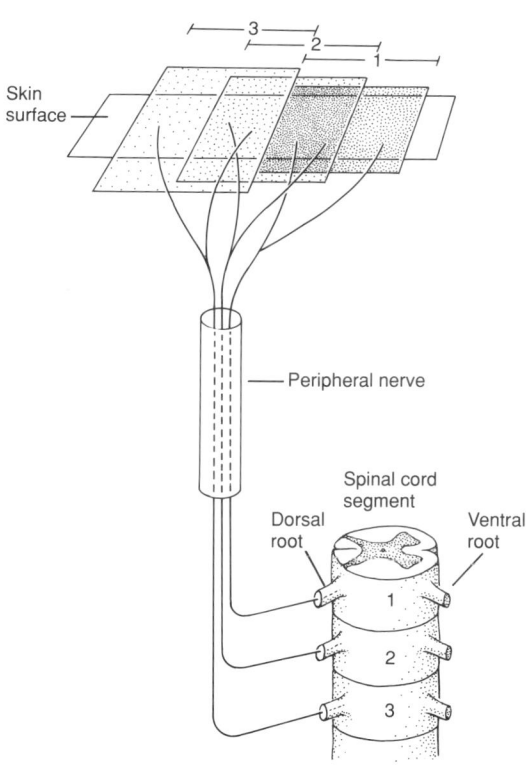

FIGURE 25–1
Afferent nerve fibers from one part of the skin are gathered in the peripheral nerves and then redistributed among the dorsal roots. The area of skin innervated by a single dorsal root is called a dermatome (areas **1, 2,** and **3**). The dermatomal boundaries overlap, because of the mixing of fibers from several dorsal roots in the peripheral nerve.

the *dorsal roots.* The area of skin innervated by a dorsal root is called a *dermatome.* Adjacent dermatomes overlap. As a result, the area innervated by an individual dorsal root is larger than the area innervated by a single peripheral nerve (Figure 25–1). This difference has important clinical consequences. Damage to a spinal nerve or dorsal root often results in only a small sensory deficit throughout the broad area innervated by these nerves. In contrast, cutting the distal portion of a peripheral cutaneous nerve results in a complete loss of sensory receptors in the circumscribed area innervated by the nerve. The distribution of dermatomes for all spinal segments have been mapped by studying sensation and reflex responsiveness that remain after injury to dorsal roots (Box 25–1).

Like the spinal cord, the dorsal and ventral roots are organized segmentally. The segmental organization of the dorsal roots in the spinal cord is preserved in the various ascending systems, reflecting one of the important principles of sensory organization: There is a topological relationship between adjacent regions of the receptive surface and many of the sites in the nervous system that receive sensory projections. This relationship in the somatic sensory system is considered in detail in Chapter 26.

The Spinal Cord Is the First Relay Point for Somatic Sensory Information

Sensory information conveyed to the brain from the limbs and trunk is first relayed through the spinal cord. As we saw in Chapter 20, the spinal cord has a butterfly-shaped

central gray area that contains the cell bodies of spinal neurons and a surrounding region of white matter that contains axons that ascend to and descend from the brain, most of which are myelinated (Figure 25–3B).

Spinal Gray Matter Contains Nerve Cell Bodies

The gray matter of the spinal cord is divided into three functionally distinct regions: the dorsal horn, the intermediate zone, and the ventral horn (Figure 24–3A).

1. The gray matter of the dorsal horn contains interneurons and ascending projection neurons that relay incoming sensory information to sites higher in the nervous system.
2. The gray matter of the ventral horn contains interneurons and motor neurons that control muscles of the trunk and the limbs.
3. The gray matter of the intermediate zone contains the autonomic preganglionic neurons and mediates a variety of visceral control functions as well as neurons that transmit afferent information to the cerebellum.

A scheme for subdividing the gray matter of the spinal cord into 10 layers (laminae), based on neuronal cytoarchitecture, was proposed in 1952 by Bror Rexed. This classification (Figures 25–4B) has endured because neurons in different laminae were later found to be functionally distinct and to have different patterns of projections. Laminae I–VI correspond to the dorsal horn, lamina VII is roughly equivalent to the intermediate zone, and laminae

Mapping the Innervation of the Dorsal Roots

BOX 25-1

The area of skin innervated by a single dorsal root, known as a *dermatome*, can be identified by probing the skin with different stimuli and observing the response of the fibers within the root. In experimental animals the response of each dorsal root in each modality (tactile, limb proprioceptive, pain, and temperature sense) can be systematically tested and the boundaries of individual dermatomes can be mapped across the skin. The boundaries overlap because of overlapping innervation by adjacent dorsal roots. The overlap varies depending on the modality. Pain dermatomes mapped with a pinprick overlap less than tactile dermatomes mapped with light mechanical stimuli. Because of this difference, injury to a single dorsal root is more easily identified by examining for pain than for touch. A method of determining the

area of innervation of dorsal root fibers in humans is to examine the spatial distribution of the skin lesions in shingles, a painful inflammation of dorsal root ganglia produced by infection with the virus herpes zoster.

Different testing methods produce somewhat different dermatomal maps, and even the same mapping technique can result in variation among subjects. Despite this variability, dermatomal maps are an important diagnostic tool for locating the site of injury to the spinal cord and dorsal roots. For example, on the basis of the dermatomal map for the human forearm, we know that sensory changes limited to the distal forearm and the fourth and fifth fingers are likely to result from injury to the spinal cord at levels C8 and T1.

FIGURE 25–2

The dermatomes follow a highly regular pattern on the body (**S**, sacral; **L**, lumbar; **T**, thoracic; **C**, cervical). In actuality,

the boundaries of the dermatomes are less distinct than shown here because of overlapping innervation.

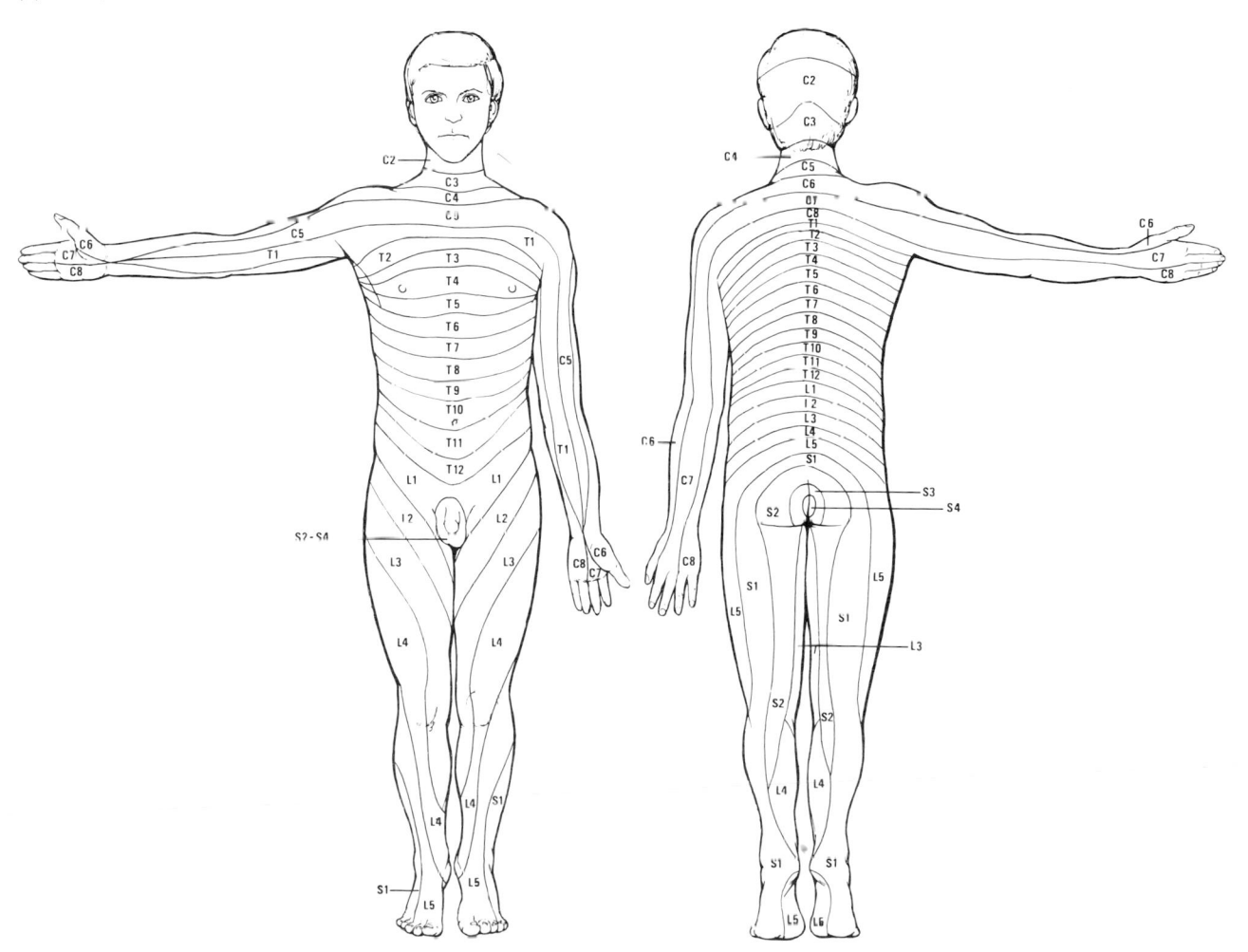

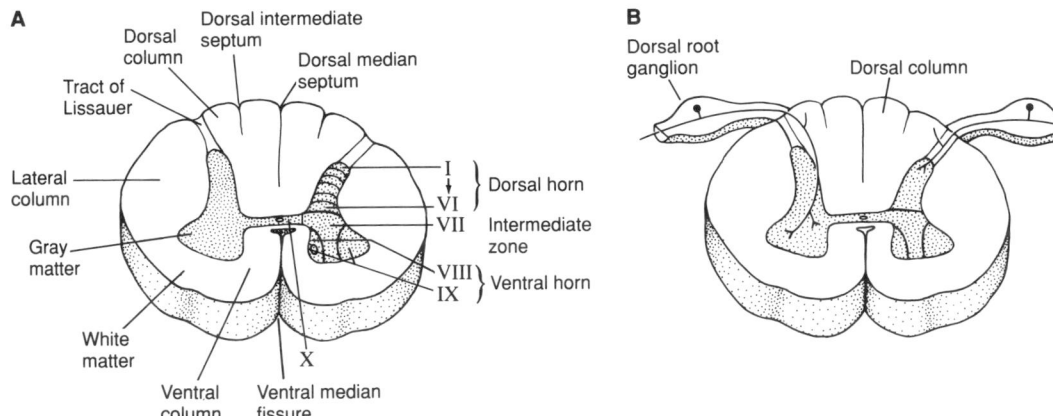

FIGURE 25–3

The white matter of the spinal cord contains afferent and efferent axons running in columns, and the gray matter is divided into layers of functionally distinct nuclei.

A. The columnar organization of the white matter is shown in this section. The spinal gray matter is divided into ten layers (I–X) comprising three major zones—the dorsal and ventral horns and the intermediate zone. Each layer includes functionally distinct groups of nerve cells (see Figure 25–4).

B. The termination pattern of large-diameter (left) and small-diameter (right) afferent fibers are illustrated. Large-diameter fibers terminate in the deeper portion of the gray matter, whereas the small-diameter fibers terminate superficially. Branches of the small-diameter fibers ascend and descend for a few segments in the tract of Lissauer.

VIII and IX comprise the ventral horn. Lamina X consists of the gray matter surrounding the central canal (Figure 25–4A). The functions of the spinal cord laminae (and corresponding nuclei) are as follows.

Lamina I, the *marginal zone*, is located in the most superficial region of the dorsal horn and is an important sensory relay for pain and temperature.

Lamina II, the *substantia gelatinosa*, receives afferent information from nonmyelinated fibers and integrates this information with that of thinly myelinated afferent fibers that project to lamina I.

Laminae III, IV, V, and VI contain the *nucleus proprius*, which integrates sensory input with information that descends from the brain and the region of the base of the dorsal horn where many of the neurons that project to the brain stem are located.

Lamina VII contains *Clarke's nucleus* or *cell column*, which is present in the thoracic and upper lumbar segments only and relays information about limb position and movement to the cerebellum. The *intermediolateral nucleus* or *cell column*, which is also located in the thoracic and upper lumbar segments, contains autonomic preganglionic neurons.

Lamina VIII contains interneurons that are important in regulating skeletal muscle contraction.

Lamina IX, the motor nuclei of the ventral horn, contains motor neurons innervating skeletal muscles.

Lamina X surrounds the central canal and receives afferent input similar to that of laminae I and II.

Spinal White Matter Contains Myelinated Axons

The white matter is divided into three bilaterally paired columns, or funiculi (Figure 24–3A).

1. The *dorsal columns*, medial to the dorsal horns, consist primarily of axons that relay somatic sensory information to the medulla.
2. The *lateral columns*, lateral to the gray matter, contain axons from sensory, motor, and autonomic control centers in the brain as well as somatic sensory pathways ascending to the brain.
3. The *ventral columns*, medial to the ventral horns, primarily contain axons descending from the brain that control axial musculature.

In addition to the major ascending (sensory) and descending (motor) tracts that make up these columns, the spinal cord contains two additional regions in which axons are located. The tract of Lissauer contains the central branches of small-diameter fibers. The *fasciculus proprius*, which contains the axons of propriospinal neurons that interconnect different regions of the spinal cord, is located along the margin of the gray matter and white matter.

Dorsal Root Fibers Branch in the White Matter and Terminate in the Gray Matter

The fibers that make up the dorsal roots project from cell bodies in the dorsal root ganglion and enter the spinal cord at its dorsolateral margin. As we have seen in Chapter 24, large-diameter fibers mediate touch and limb proprioception, whereas small-diameter fibers mediate pain and temperature sense. Although there is not a precise correlation between the diameter of the sensory neuron cell body and the diameter of the axon, most of the largest neurons have large myelinated axons, up to 20 µm in diameter. Neurons with intermediate- and small-diameter cell bodies have thinner myelinated and unmyelinated axons.

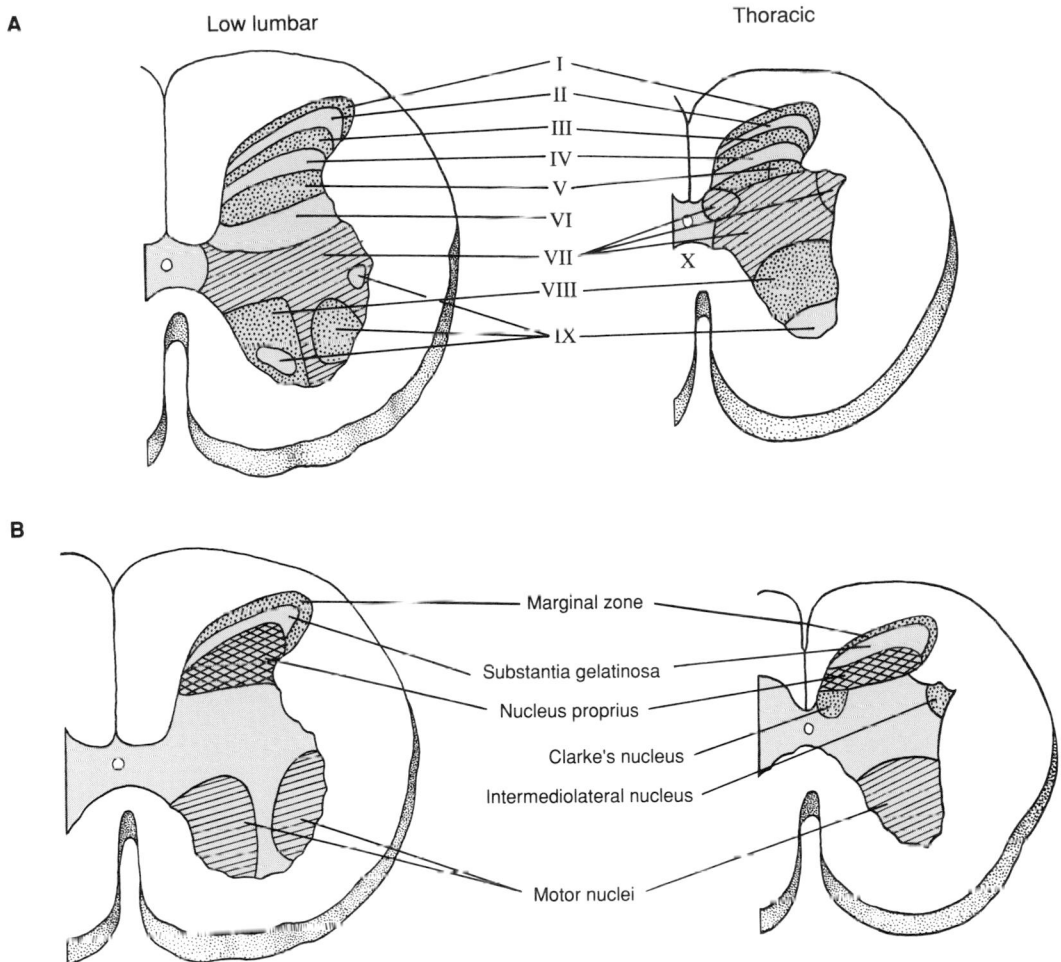

FIGURE 25–4

Detailed anatomy of the spinal gray matter in low lumbar and thoracic segments.

A. The laminae according to Rexed's classification. The lumbar (and sacral) segments, which innervate the lower limb, have a larger area of gray matter than thoracic segments. Note also that lamina VI is not ordinarily present in thoracic segments.

B. The important nuclei in the lumbar and thoracic segments.

After entering the spinal cord the primary afferent fibers branch in the white matter. In addition, afferent fibers give off collaterals that terminate in the gray matter. The axons from large and small cells, which mediate different somatic modalities, have different distributions in the gray and white matter (Figure 25–3B). Collaterals of small-diameter fibers, which mediate pain and temperature sense, do not enter the gray matter immediately. Instead they pass into the *tract of Lissauer* (Figure 25–3), where they bifurcate into branches that ascend and descend one to two segments before terminating in the superficial portion of the dorsal horn (Rexed's laminae I and II). Collaterals of large-diameter fibers, which mediate tactile sense and limb proprioception, enter the lateral aspect of the dorsal columns, where they ascend to the medulla. Large-diameter fibers also give off collaterals that enter the dorsal horn from its medial aspect (Figure 25–3B) and terminate in the deeper laminae of the gray matter.

In addition to their role in perception, afferent fibers also mediate reflex responses. Some large-diameter fibers terminate in motor nuclei (lamina IX) and mediate stretch reflexes. Two types of reflexes can be distinguished by the pattern of termination. *Intrasegmental reflexes* are generated by collaterals of afferent fibers that terminate in the gray matter of the same and adjacent segments. The knee jerk reflex is an example of an intrasegmental reflex. *Intersegmental reflexes* are mediated by collaterals of ascending and descending branches of the afferent fibers. The scratch reflex seen in cats and dogs and postural reflexes following a perturbation in body position are examples of intersegmental reflexes.

Afferents Conveying Different Somatic Sensory Modalities Have Distinct Terminal Projections

The different classes of primary afferent fibers that convey somatosensory modalities take specific routes and end in different regions of the spinal cord. By this means,

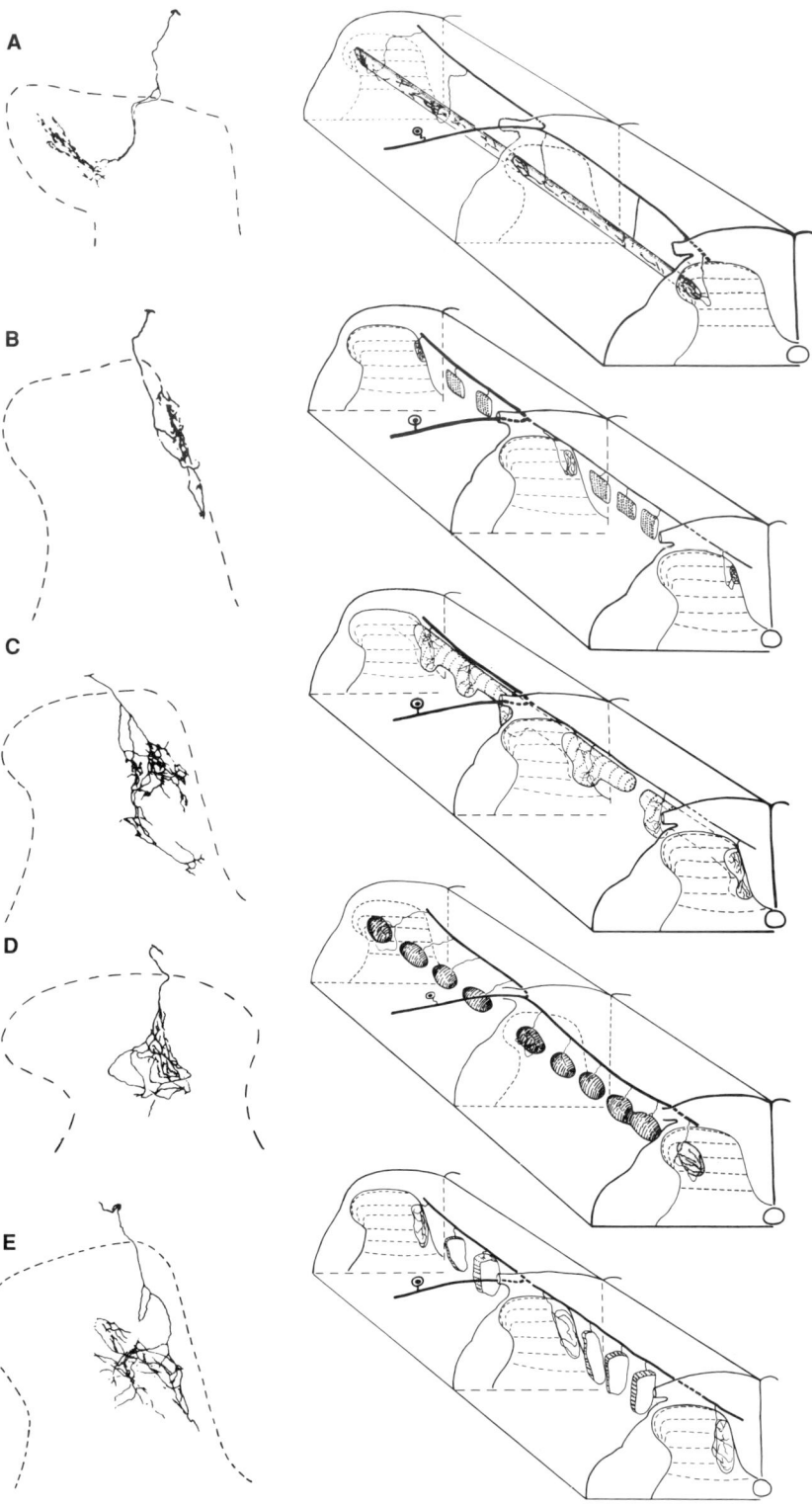

FIGURE 25–5

The anatomy of axon collaterals from identified cutaneous afferent fibers in the cat. Each pair of figures shows a typical collateral as seen in reconstructions from transverse sections (**left**) and a summary diagram of the three-dimensional organization of the axon and its collaterals (**right**).

A. Hair follicle afferent fibers. (Adapted from Brown et al., 1977.)

B. Rapidly adapting mechanoreceptive afferent fibers.

C. Pacinian corpuscle afferent fibers. (Adapted from Brown et al., 1980a.)

D. Slowly adapting type I afferent fibers. (Adapted from Brown et al., 1978.)

E. Slowly adapting type II afferent fibers.

the specific sensory information established by particular mechanoreceptors in the skin is maintained within the central nervous system. Each class of afferent fibers has a distinctive, and sometimes unique, central terminal projection (Figure 25–5). This specificity also extends to the fine details of their arborization pattern, the spacing of the collateral branches, and the arrangement of boutons on the axon terminals.

Two Major Ascending Systems Convey Somatic Sensory Information to the Cerebral Cortex

Somatic sensory signals are conveyed along two major ascending systems in the spinal cord: the dorsal column–medial lemniscal system and the anterolateral system (Figure 25–6). The *dorsal column–medial lemniscal system* relays information about tactile sensation—including touch and vibration sense—and limb proprioception. The system originates from both the ascending axons of large-diameter primary afferent fibers and, to a lesser extent, the axons of neurons in laminae III and IV of the dorsal horn. Initially, this pathway runs ipsilaterally in the spinal cord. The axons of the dorsal columns ascend to the caudal medulla, where they synapse on the cells of the *dorsal column nuclei*. From there, the tract decussates and projects to the thalamus as the *medial lemniscus*, a brain stem pathway, and then to the anterior parietal cortex through the *internal capsule*. Proprioceptive information

from the contralateral arm ascends in the dorsal column, whereas information from the contralateral leg ascends in the dorsal part of the lateral column, a region termed the dorsolateral column. We shall return to the medial lemniscal system in Chapter 26, where we describe the central pathways for touch.

The *anterolateral system* carries information chiefly about pain and temperature. It originates predominantly from neurons in lamina I and in deep laminae of the dorsal horn. These neurons send their axons to the contralateral side of the spinal cord and ascend in the anterolateral portion of the lateral column. Most of the axons of the anterolateral system terminate in three brain regions: the reticular formation of the pons and medulla, the midbrain, and the thalamus. In addition to pain and temperature, the anterolateral system also relays some tactile information. Because of this functional overlap with the dorsal columns, patients with a lesion of the dorsal columns retain some crude tactile sensibility. We shall consider the

FIGURE 25–6

Summary diagram of the major ascending somatic sensory systems. The dorsal column–medial lemniscal system mediates tactile sensations and arm proprioception; the anterolateral system mediates pain and temperature sensations, and, to a much lesser extent, tactile sensation. A general understanding of the organization of these two ascending systems reveals key principles underlying the organization of sensory systems of the brain

and provides a basis for localizing sites of injury following trauma. Both systems relay sensory information to the contralateral brain; however, decussation occurs at different levels. In the dorsal column–medial lemniscal system the axons of second-order neurons cross the midline in the medulla. In contrast, the anterolateral system decussates in the spinal cord. The organization within each pathway is both serial and parallel.

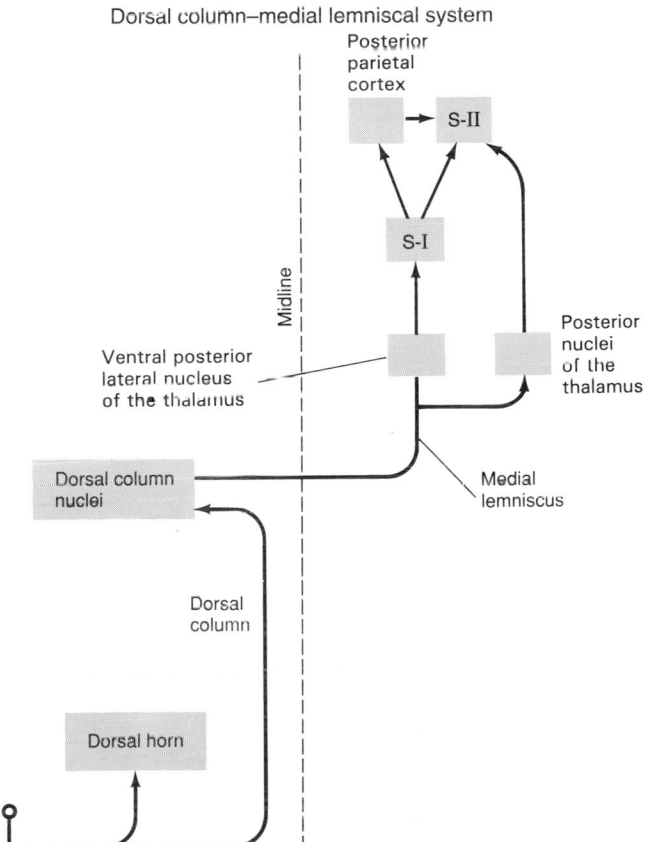

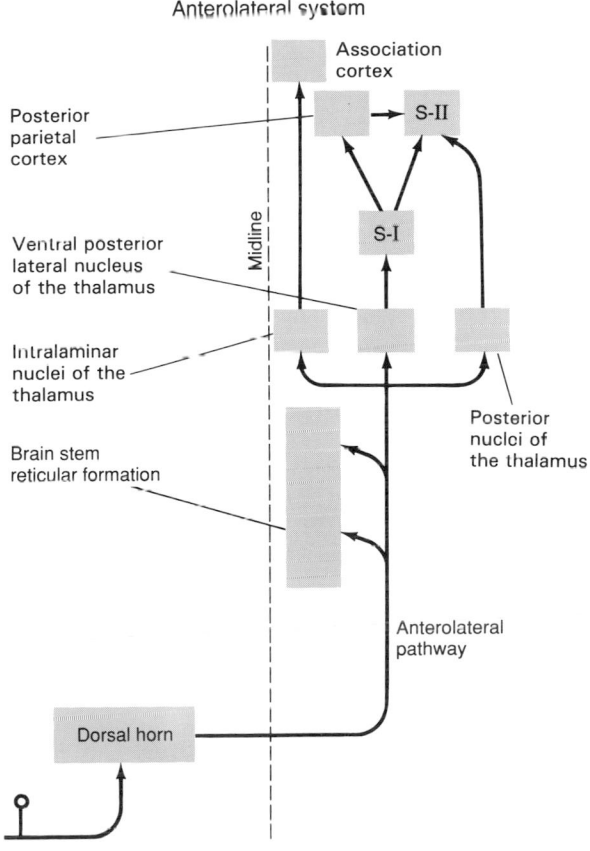

nociceptive pathways of the anterolateral system in Chapter 27.

As we saw in Chapter 23, the two ascending systems in the spinal cord are examples of parallel pathways. Even though each serves somewhat different functions, there is a degree of redundancy. Parallel pathways are advantageous for two reasons. They add subtlety and richness to a perceptual experience by allowing the same information to be handled in different ways. They also offer a measure of insurance—if one pathway is damaged, the others can provide residual perceptual capability.

The dorsal column–medial lemniscal system and components of the anterolateral system play an important role in perception. Other ascending somatic sensory pathways do not play a major role in perception, but participate in regulating movement, maintaining arousal, and visceral functions. It is therefore useful to distinguish between *sensory pathways*, which carry information that contributes to sensation, and *afferent pathways*, which carry information into the nervous system that does not enter conciousness. Proprioceptive information from the limbs provides an example of the different uses of information from peripheral receptors for perception and the regulation of movement. Proprioceptive information that is used for the perception of limb position is relayed to the somatic sensory cortex; proprioceptive information that is used in reflex control of movement is processed by local spinal cord circuits; and information used in regulating reflexes and voluntary movement ascends to the cerebellum, various brain stem nuclei, and the motor cortex. (Because the cerebellum does not participate in perception, the spinocerebellar pathways are considered in Chapter 41 in the context of motor control by the cerebellum.)

The Dorsal Column–Medial Lemniscal System Mediates Tactile Sense and Arm Proprioception

The dorsal columns are composed primarily of the central branches of dorsal root ganglion cells (primary afferent fibers) that ascend to the medulla, where they make synaptic connections. Many fibers in the dorsal columns (up to half by some measurements) are ascending axons of second-order neurons in the dorsal horn. At upper spinal levels the dorsal columns can be divided into two bundles (fascicles) of axons: the *gracile fascicle* and the *cuneate fascicle*. The gracile fascicle ascends medially and contains fibers from the ipsilateral sacral, lumbar, and lower thoracic segments, while the cuneate fascicle ascends laterally and includes fibers from the upper thoracic and cervical segments (Figure 25–7). The two bundles terminate in the lower medulla in the *gracile nucleus* and *cuneate nucleus*, respectively (Figure 25–8). The cuneate and gracile nuclei are located at about the same level in the caudal medulla and together are referred to as the *dorsal column nuclei*.

The pathways for proprioceptive information from the arms and legs to the medulla are somewhat different. The pathway for proprioceptive information from the arm is similar to that for tactile information: Axons in the cu-

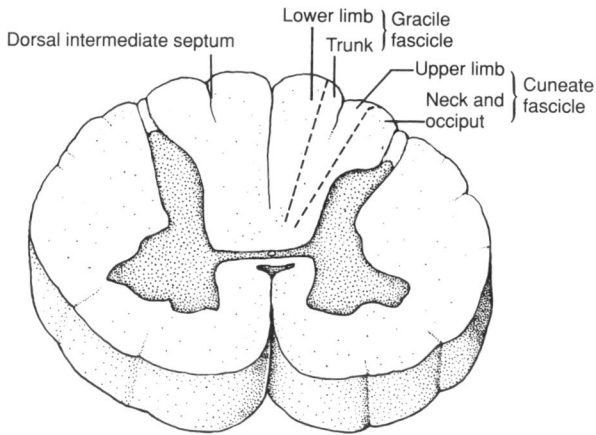

FIGURE 25–7
The organization of somatic sensory fibers in the dorsal column is illustrated in this cross section high in the cervical spinal cord.

neate fascicle synapse on neurons in a portion of the cuneate nucleus, whose axons project in the contralateral medial lemniscus. Proprioceptive information from the leg is relayed in the lateral column by the axons of neurons in Clarke's nucleus (see Chapter 20); in the caudal medulla these axons synapse on neurons that join the contralateral medial lemniscus. Information from the *trigeminal nerve*, which carries sensory information from the face, is transmitted to neurons in the pons whose axons also join the medial lemniscus. The organization of the ascending trigeminal pathways is discussed in Chapter 45.

In the medulla the fibers from the dorsal column nuclei arch across the midline, and for this reason are called the *internal arcuate fibers*. After they cross the midline they form the medial lemniscus and ascend to the thalamus (Figure 25–8). In the medulla the medial lemniscus lies dorsal to the medullary pyramids, at the approximate center of the reticular formation (see Figure 25–10). Like the dorsal columns, the medial lemniscus is somatotopically organized. However, this organization changes as the medial lemniscus ascends from the medulla. In the medulla, sensory fibers from the leg are located in the most ventral portion, and those from the arm are in the dorsal portion. Above the medulla the medial lemniscus assumes a more lateral position within the reticular formation. In the pons the sensory tract carrying information from the arm is medial to the tract from the leg. In the midbrain the medial lemniscus occupies an even more lateral position.

The fibers of the medial lemniscus synapse on neurons in the thalamus. The thalamus plays a key role in transforming sensory information that will eventually reach the cerebral cortex. With the exception of the olfactory system, all sensory pathways projecting to the cerebral cortex do so through specific relay nuclei in the lateral thalamus. Somatic sensation is mediated by the *ventral posterior nucleus*. Input from the trunk and limbs terminates on cells in the lateral division of the nucleus, or *ventral posterior lateral nucleus*; input from the face projects to the medial division, or *ventral posterior medial*

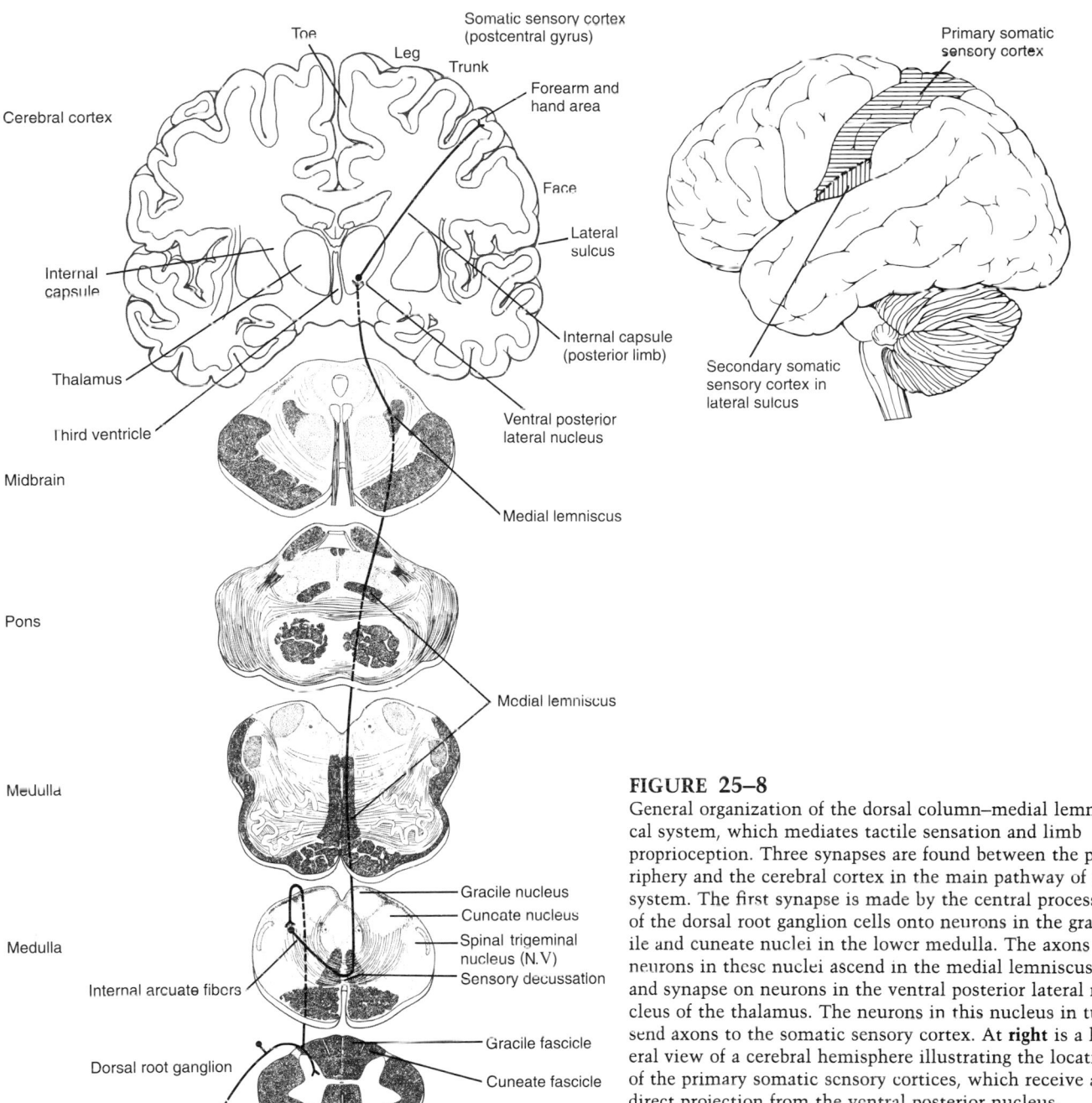

FIGURE 25–8

General organization of the dorsal column–medial lemniscal system, which mediates tactile sensation and limb proprioception. Three synapses are found between the periphery and the cerebral cortex in the main pathway of the system. The first synapse is made by the central processes of the dorsal root ganglion cells onto neurons in the gracile and cuneate nuclei in the lower medulla. The axons of neurons in these nuclei ascend in the medial lemniscus and synapse on neurons in the ventral posterior lateral nucleus of the thalamus. The neurons in this nucleus in turn send axons to the somatic sensory cortex. **At right** is a lateral view of a cerebral hemisphere illustrating the location of the primary somatic sensory cortices, which receive a direct projection from the ventral posterior nucleus. (Adapted from Carpenter and Sutin, 1983.)

nucleus (Figure 25–9). (This latter nucleus is discussed in Chapter 45 together with the ascending trigeminal pathways.)

Neurons in the ventral posterior nucleus, in turn, project through the posterior limb of the *internal capsule* to the *primary somatic sensory cortex*, which constitutes the major portion of the postcentral gyrus. Neurons in the medial and lateral divisions of the ventral posterior nucleus project to different parts of the primary somatic sensory cortex (Figures 25–8 and 25–9), preserving somatotopy in this portion of the cerebral cortex. In the primary somatic sensory cortex the axons from the thalamus terminate on pyramidal cells and excite them strongly. They also terminate on interneurons whose axons are oriented perpendicular to the surface and parallel to the apical dendrites of the pyramidal cells.

Sensory information about a particular modality from one part of the body is processed at each level in the dorsal column-medial lemniscal system by collections of neurons that form discrete functional units. As the medial

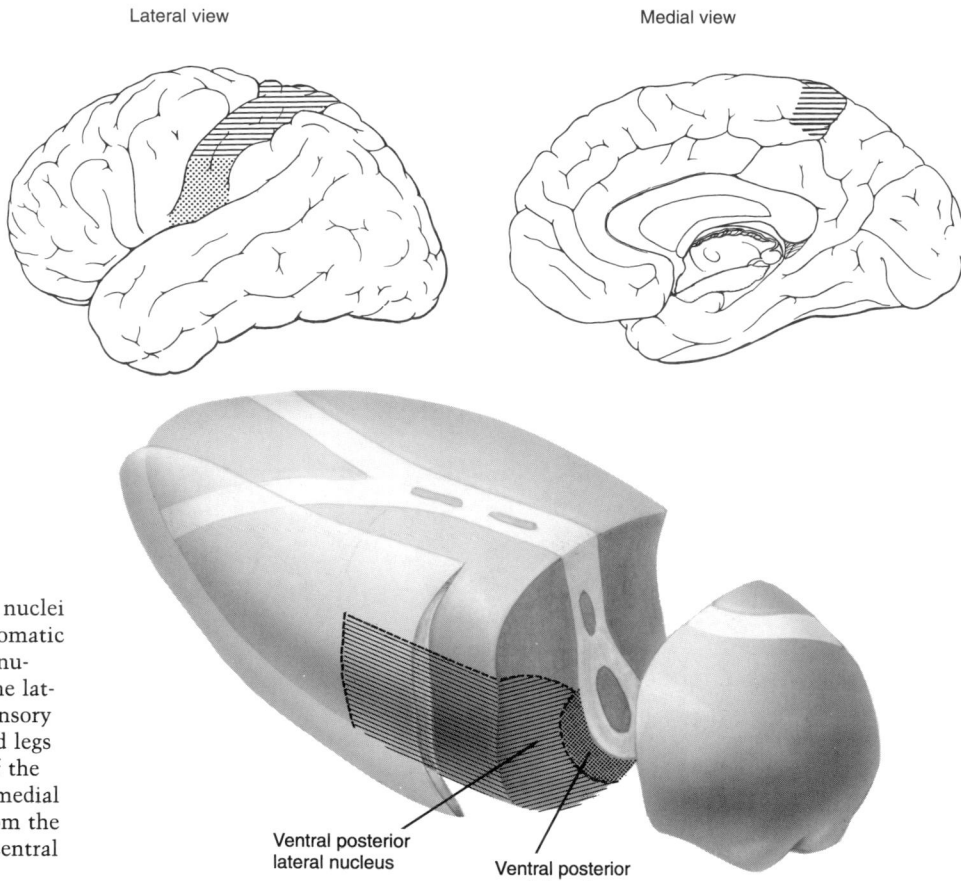

Lateral view   Medial view

FIGURE 25–9

Location of somatic sensory thalamic nuclei and their projections to the primary somatic sensory cortex. The ventral posterior nucleus contains two major divisions: the lateral division, which relays somatic sensory information from the arms, trunk, and legs to the medial and superior portions of the postcentral gyrus (**hatching**), and the medial division, which relays information from the face to the lateral portion of the postcentral gyrus (**stippled**).

Ventral posterior lateral nucleus

Ventral posterior medial nucleus

lemniscus enters the thalamus, this unit consists of a bundle of lemniscal axons that synapse on a group of cells that form a cylinder in the ventral posterior lateral nucleus. The axons of these thalamic neurons receiving this information terminate on cortical neurons with axons or dendrites oriented in columns. This columnar organization helps to limit the horizontal spread of afferent input to the cortex. This important feature of the organization of the cortex is discussed in the next chapter.

The Anterolateral System Mediates Pain and Temperature Sense

The anterolateral system is the second major ascending system that mediates somatic sensation. It is composed of three ascending pathways that together play a dominant role in pain and temperature sense and a minor role in tactile sense and limb proprioception. This system differs from the dorsal column–medial lemniscal system in four respects. (1) The cells of origin of the anterolateral system are located primarily in the dorsal horn and therefore are postsynaptic to the primary afferent fibers. In contrast, most axons in the dorsal columns are not from dorsal horn neurons but rather collaterals of primary afferent fibers. (2) The anterolateral system crosses in the spinal cord,

whereas the dorsal column–medial lemniscal system crosses in the medulla. (3) While most axons in the medial lemniscus terminate in the thalamus, anterolateral fibers terminate much more widely in the brain stem and hypothalamus as well as in the thalamus. (4) Whereas both the dorsal column-medial lemniscal and anterolateral systems transmit sensory information predominantly to the contralateral thalamus and cortex, the anterolateral system also projects ipsilaterally.

The three major pathways of the anterolateral system are the spinothalamic, spinoreticular, and spinomesencephalic tracts (Figure 25–10). The spinothalamic and spinoreticular tracts mediate noxious and thermal sensations, relayed from the periphery to the spinal cord by Aδ and C fibers. Axons in the spinoreticular tract end on neurons in the reticular formation of the medulla and pons, which relay information to the thalamus and other structures in the diencephalon. The spinomesencephalic (or spinotectal) tract terminates primarily in the tectum (roof) of the midbrain (in the superior colliculus). The spinomesencephalic tract also projects to the *mesencephalic periaqueductal gray*, the region surrounding the cerebral aqueduct. This area contains neurons that are part of a descending pathway that regulates pain transmission (Chapter 27).

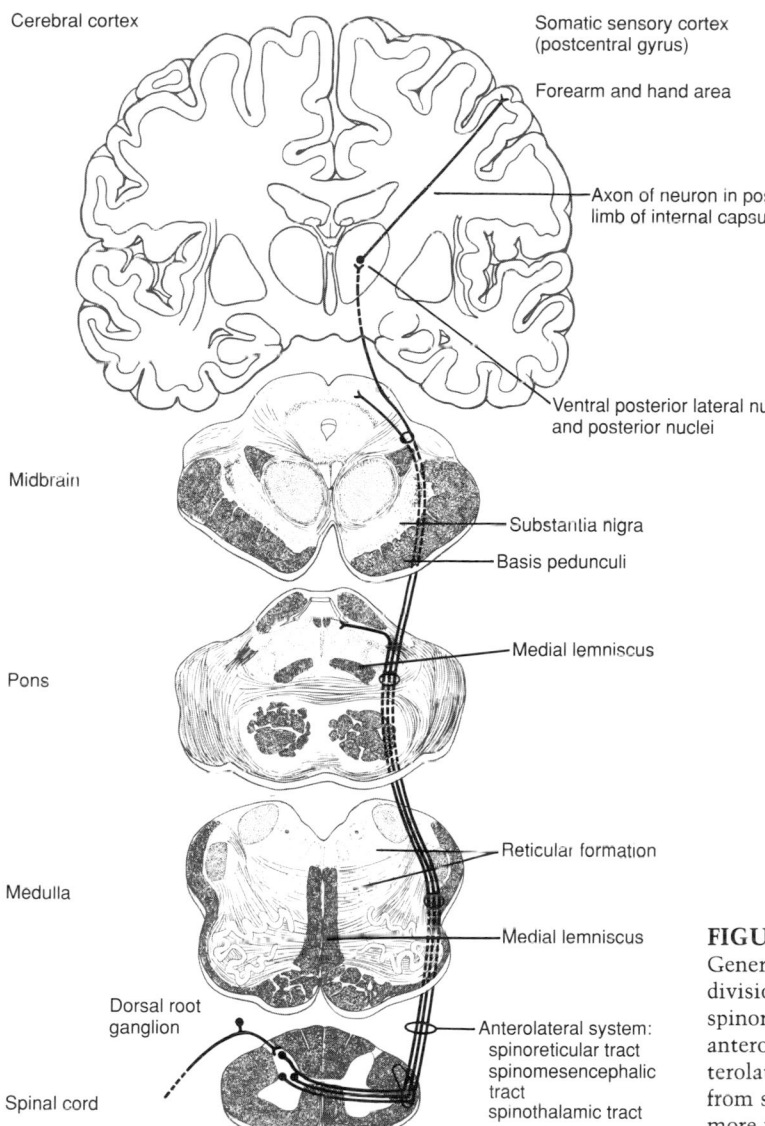

Cerebral cortex

Somatic sensory cortex
(postcentral gyrus)

Forearm and hand area

Axon of neuron in posterior
limb of internal capsule

Ventral posterior lateral nucleus
and posterior nuclei

Midbrain

Substantia nigra

Basis pedunculi

Medial lemniscus

Pons

Reticular formation

Medulla

Medial lemniscus

Dorsal root
ganglion

Anterolateral system:
spinoreticular tract
spinomesencephalic
tract
spinothalamic tract

Spinal cord

FIGURE 25–10

General organization of the anterolateral system. The three
divisions of the anterolateral system—the spinothalamic,
spinoreticular, and spinomesencephalic tracts—ascend in the
anterolateral portions of the spinal cord white matter. The anterolateral system is somatotopically organized. Sensory fibers
from successive spinal cord segments are added in progressively
more ventral and medial positions. (Adapted from Carpenter
and Sutin, 1983.)

In the medulla the fibers of the anterolateral system are
located on the lateral margin and separated from the medial lemniscus, which lies on the midline (Figures 25–8
and 25–10). In the pons the anterolateral system and
medial lemniscus move closer together, and in the midbrain the two systems are apposed in a more lateral position. At the level of the midbrain the anterolateral system
contains mostly spinothalamic fibers.

Whereas the medial lemniscus terminates chiefly in
the ventral posterior nucleus of the thalamus, fibers of the
anterolateral system synapse on neurons in three thalamic
regions: the ventral posterior lateral nucleus, the intralaminar nuclei, and the posterior nuclei. Neurons of
the ventral posterior lateral nucleus project only to the
somatic sensory cortical areas. The intralaminar nuclei
project more widely to areas of the cortex and to the basal

ganglia. The posterior nuclei project to regions of the parietal lobe outside the primary somatic sensory area.

The differences in functional organization of the anterolateral and dorsal column–medial lemniscal systems
are demonstrated most dramatically by considering the
effects of hemisection of the spinal cord on somatic sensation as might happen after a serious automobile accident. For example, tactile sense and limb proprioception,
which are relayed by the dorsal columns, are lost in the
ipsilateral arm and leg, whereas pain and temperature
sense, which are relayed by the anterolateral system, are
lost in the contralateral arm and leg. This loss of pain and
temperature sense begins a few segments below the level
of the lesion because decussation occurs over a few segments. The key features of the anterolateral and dorsal
column–medial lemniscal systems are compared in Table
25–1.

TABLE 25–1. Comparison of the Anterolateral and Dorsal Column–Medial Lemniscal Systems

	Anterolateral	Dorsal column–medial lemniscal
Modalities	Pain Temperature sense Crude touch	Tactile Proprioception (of arm only)
Location in spinal cord	Anterolateral column	Dorsal column
Level of decussation	Spinal cord	Medulla
Brain stem terminations	Brain stem reticular formation Midbrain tectal region Ventral posterior lateral nucleus, posterior nuclear group of thalamus, intralaminar nuclei	Ventral posterior lateral nucleus and posterior nuclear group of thalamus
Cortical terminations	Primary and secondary somatic sensory cortices and posterior parietal cortex	Primary and secondary somatic sensory cortices and posterior parietal cortex

The Primary Somatic Sensory Cortex Is Divided into Four Functional Areas

The somatic sensory cortex plays an important role in processing all of the somatic sensory submodalities. The somatic sensory cortex consists of several cytoarchitecturally distinct regions in the anterior part of the parietal lobe (Figure 25–11). The *primary somatic sensory cortex* (S-I) is located in the postcentral gyrus and in the depths of the central sulcus. It consists of four functional areas: Brodmann's areas 1, 2, 3a, and 3b, each of which has a somewhat different role in somatic sensation. Projections from the thalamus to S-I arise chiefly from the ventral posterior nucleus, are somatotopically organized, and transmit information from the contralateral body. Lateral and somewhat posterior to the primary somatic cortex is the *secondary somatic sensory cortex* (S-II), lying in the upper bank of the lateral sulcus. Deep within the lateral sulcus, in the insular region, are other sites that receive somatic sensory information. The secondary somatic sensory cortex receives input primarily from S-I and in turn projects to the somatic sensory fields in the insular region.

In addition to the primary and secondary somatic sensory cortical areas, the posterior parietal lobe also receives somatic inputs. This region is a higher-order sensory cortex similar in function to an association cortex; it relates sensory and motor processing and is concerned with integrating the different somatic sensory modalities necessary for perception.

Pyramidal Cells in Layers 2, 3, 5, and 6 Are the Output Cells of the Primary Somatic Sensory Cortex

There are two major classes of neurons within the somatosensory cortex: the pyramidal cells, which are the output cells of the cortex, and the nonpyramidal cells, which interconnect local regions of the cortex. Many subclasses of pyramidal neurons can be distinguished by their loca-

FIGURE 25–11

Sites of somatosensory processing in the cortex.

A. This lateral view of the cerebral hemisphere shows the locations of the primary (S-I) and secondary (S-II) somatic sensory cortices and the posterior parietal cortex.

B. This cross section (at level B in part A) shows the several cytoarchitecturally distinct areas of the region: S-I (Brodmann's areas 3a, 3b, 1, 2), part of the motor cortex (area 4), and part of the posterior parietal cortex (areas 5 and 7).

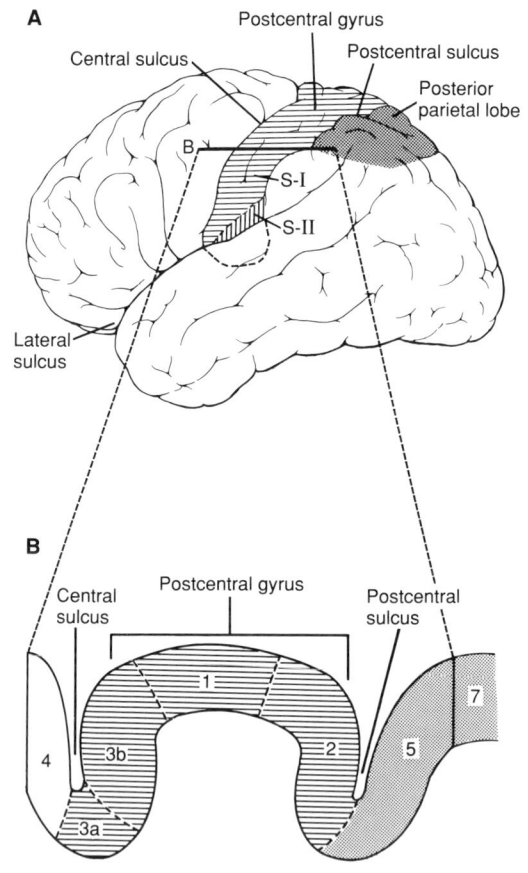

tion and projection targets. Pyramidal neurons in cortical layers 2 and 3 project to different cortical areas, whereas many pyramidal neurons in layers 5 and 6 send their axons to other subcortical areas and back to the thalamus. The axons of pyramidal neurons have a recurrent branch that excites neurons, both nonpyramidal and other pyramidal neurons locally. Nonpyramidal neurons also can be classified into several types; many have elaborate axonal ramifications and ornate names (double bouquet cells, chandelier cells, and spiderweb cells). Many of these neurons, which also receive direct input from thalamic afferents, are inhibitory and use γ-aminobutyric acid (GABA) as their neurotransmitter. This is in contrast to pyramidal cells, which are excitatory and use glutamate or aspartate as their neurotransmitters.

Pyramidal neurons in the somatic sensory cortex, which receive thalamic input, make three types of connections: association, callosal, and subcortical (or descending projections).

Association connections, made by neurons in layers 2 and 3, interconnect neurons in different cortical regions on the same side. There are association connections among the four areas of S-I (Brodmann's areas 1, 2, 3a, and 3b) and from S-I to the posterior parietal cortex (Brodmann's areas 5 and 7). Reciprocal association connections also exist between S-I and S-II and between these two somatic cortices and the motor cortex (in the precentral gyrus, Brodmann's area 4).

Callosal connections, which are also made by neurons in layers 2 and 3, interconnect symmetrical areas of the two hemispheres. Although most cortical areas of each cerebral hemisphere are connected through the *corpus callosum*, some are not. For example, bilateral cortical regions that receive inputs from the distal limbs are not connected through the corpus callosum.

Projection connections are characteristic of cortical neurons that send their axons to subcortical structures. The primary somatic sensory cortex has four major targets of descending projections: the basal ganglia, the ventral posterior nucleus of the thalamus, the dorsal column nuclei, and the dorsal horn of the spinal cord. Neurons that make descending projections are located in layers 5 and 6. The descending projections to the thalamus (from pyramidal cells in layer 6) and spinal cord (from pyramidal cells in layer 5) control the inflow of sensory information to the brain, an important feature of all sensory systems.

The projections of the cells of different layers of the cerebral cortex are summarized in Figure 25–12.

An Overall View

Sensory information from the body surface enters the central nervous system in the spinal cord, where the different modalities are conveyed to the brain in anatomically separate pathways. The two major ascending systems for somatic sensory input are the dorsal column–medial lemniscal system, which mediates touch and arm proprioception, and the anterolateral pathway, which mediates pain and temperature sense. These two systems follow separate pathways until they converge at the thalamus in the ventral posterior lateral nucleus. Even in the thalamus the different systems remain distinct, synapsing on separate populations of neurons.

Although information from the different somatic submodalities remains segregated in the spinal cord, brain stem, and thalamus, at each successive central relay site there is a convergence of spatial information. It is not until information reaches the somatic sensory areas in the cortex that input from the various submodalities interacts.

FIGURE 25–12

Neurons in the different layers of the primary somatic sensory cortex (S-I) project to different sites. Pyramidal cells in layers 2 and 3 project to other areas of the cortex, while those in layers 5 and 6 project to subcortical structures. Layer 1 contains few neurons; it consists mostly of dendrites of neurons that lie in deeper layers of S-I and axons from neurons in other parts of the cortex and brain stem. Layer 4 contains interneurons that connect with other cortical layers.

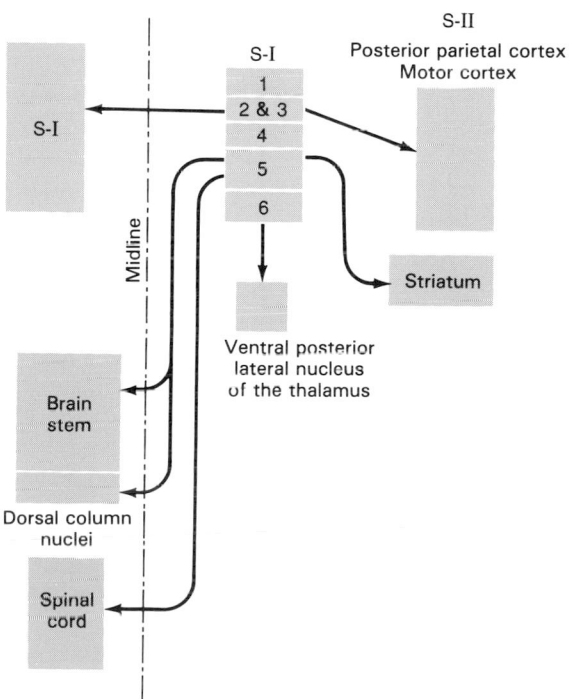

Selected Readings

Brodal, A. 1981. Neurological Anatomy in Relation to Clinical Medicine, 3rd ed. New York: Oxford University Press.

Brown, A. G. 1981. Organization in the Spinal Cord: The Anatomy and Physiology of Identified Neurones. New York: Springer.

Jones, E. G., and Powell, T. P. S. 1973. Anatomical organization of the somatosensory cortex. In A. Iggo (ed.), Handbook of Sensory Physiology, Vol. 2: Somatosensory System. New York: Springer, pp. 579–620.

Martin, J. H. 1989. Neuroanatomy: Text and Atlas. New York: Elsevier.

Rustioni, A., and Weinberg, R. J. 1989. The somatosensory system. In A. Björklund, T. Hökfelt, and L. W. Swanson (eds.), Handbook of Chemical Neuroanatomy, Vol. 7: Integrated Systems of the CNS, Part II. Central Visual, Auditory, Somatosensory, Gustatory. Amsterdam: Elsevier, pp. 219–321.

References

Brodmann, K. 1909. Vergleichende Lokalisationslehre der Grosshirnrinde in ihren Prinzipien dargestellt auf Grund des Zellenbaues. Leipzig: Barth.

Carpenter, M. B., and Sutin, J. 1983. Human Neuroanatomy, 8th ed. Baltimore: Williams & Wilkins.

Jones, E. G., and Wise, S. P. 1977. Size, laminar and columnar distribution of efferent cells in the sensory-motor cortex of monkeys. J. Comp. Neurol. 175:391–437.

Jones, E. G., Friedman, D. P., and Hendry, S. H. C. 1982. Thalamic basis of place- and modality-specific columns in monkey somatosensory cortex: A correlative anatomical and physiological study. J. Neurophysiol. 48:545–568.

Kuypers, H. G. J. M. 1973. The anatomical organization of the descending pathways and their contributions to motor control especially in primates. In J. E. Desmedt (ed.), New Developments in Electromyography and Clinical Neurophysiology, Vol. 3. Basel: Karger, pp. 38–68.

Light, A. R., and Perl, E. R. 1979. Reexamination of the dorsal root projection to the spinal dorsal horn including observations on the differential termination of coarse and fine fibers. J. Comp. Neurol. 186:117–131.

Rexed, B. 1952. The cytoarchitectonic organization of the spinal cord in the cat. J. Comp. Neurol. 96:415–495.

26

Eric R. Kandel
Thomas M. Jessell

Touch

Sensory Information About Touch Is Processed by a Series of Relay Nuclei

The Body Surface Is Represented in the Brain in an Orderly Fashion

Somatic Sensations Are Localized to Specific Regions of Cortex

Electrophysiological Studies Have Correlated Body Areas and Cortical Areas

Each Central Neuron Has a Specific Receptive Field

Sizes of Receptive Fields Vary in Different Areas of the Skin

Receptive Fields of Central Neurons Have Inhibitory and Excitatory Components

Lateral Inhibition Can Aid in Two-Point Discrimination

Inputs to the Somatic Sensory Cortex Are Organized into Columns by Submodality

Detailed Features of a Stimulus Are Communicated to the Brain

In the Early Stages of Cortical Processing the Dynamic Properties of Central Neurons and Receptors Are Similar

In the Later Stages of Cortical Processing the Central Nerve Cells Have Complex Feature-Detecting Properties and Integrate Various Sensory Inputs

An Overall View

The somatic sensory system is concerned with four major modalities: *discriminative touch* (required to recognize the size, shape and texture of objects and their movement across the skin), *proprioception* (the sense of static position and movement of limbs and body), *nociception* (the signaling of tissue damage, often perceived as pain), and *temperature sense* (warmth and cold). These modalities reach the brain through two major pathways. Most aspects of touch, as well as proprioception, are carried by the *dorsal column–medial lemniscal system*, with which we shall here be concerned. Sensations of pain and temperature are carried by the *anterolateral system*, which is discussed in the next chapter.

In this chapter we shall examine how neuronal activity within the dorsal column–medial lemniscal system gives rise to perception, using discriminative touch as an illustrative example. The sense of touch is most discriminating in the finger tips. Information transmitted to the brain from mechanoreceptors in the fingers enables us to feel the shape and texture of objects so we can read braille or play a musical instrument. Here we shall learn how we perceive the surface features of objects and why fingertips are better suited to the task than our toes or the skin of the back. Next we examine the degree to which the various somatic modalities are segregated functionally in the central nervous system and how they are combined for coherent perception. Since this chapter is the first in which we discuss the central projections of a sensory system, we also introduce the question: How does the cerebral cortex transform sensory information coming from the periphery?

Sensory Information About Touch Is Processed by a Series of Relay Nuclei

We have already considered the anatomical plan of touch sensation in Chapters 24 and 25 (see for example, Figure 25–8). The skin and underlying tissue contain four types

A

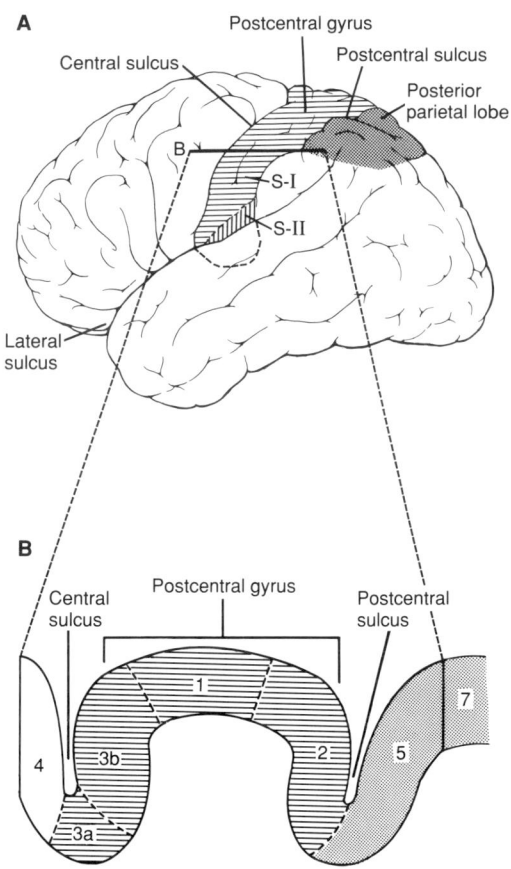

B

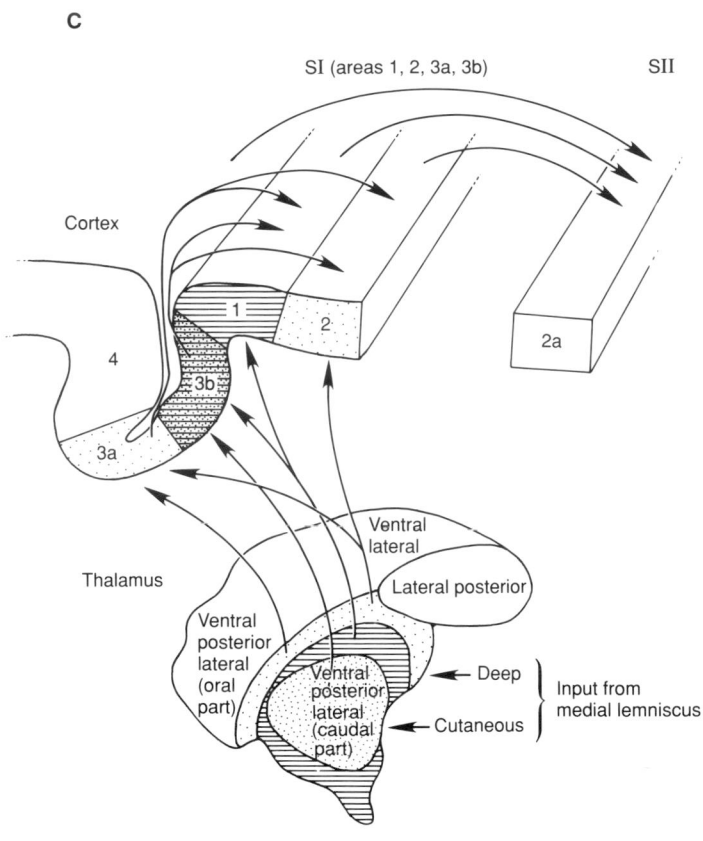

C

FIGURE 26–1

The somatic sensory cortex, located in the parietal lobe, has three major divisions: the primary (S-I) and secondary (S-II) somatosensory cortices and the posterior parietal cortex.

A. The relationship of S-I to S-II and to the posterior parietal cortex (Brodmann's areas 5 and 7) is seen best from a lateral perspective of the surface of the cerebral cortex.

B. The primary somatic cortex (S-I) is subdivided into four distinct cytoarchitectonic regions. This sagittal section shows these four regions (Brodmann's areas 3a, 3b, 1, and 2)

and illustrates their spatial relationship to area 4 of the motor cortex and area 5 and 7 of the posterior parietal cortex.

C. Fibers in the medial lemniscus project to the ventral posterior lateral nucleus of the thalamus. Neurons in this nucleus project to all areas in the primary somatic sensory cortex (S-I), primarily Brodmann's areas 3a and 3b but also to areas 1 and 2. In turn, neurons in areas 3a and 3b project to areas 1 and 2, and all of these project to the secondary somatic sensory cortex (S-II). (Adapted from Jones and Friedman, 1982).

of receptors. The superficial skin has rapidly adapting Meissner's corpuscles and slowly adapting Merkel's cells, both of which respond to touch. Deeper tissue contains the rapidly adapting pacinian corpuscles, which respond to vibration, and the slowly adapting Ruffini's corpuscles, which respond to rapid indentation of the skin. These four types of receptors are innervated by peripheral axons of nerve cells in the dorsal root ganglia; their central branches ascend in the dorsal columns and synapse with second-order neurons in the dorsal column nuclei. Axons of neurons in the dorsal column nuclei cross the midline in the medulla and ascend through the brain stem on the contralateral side as the medial lemniscus. In the thalamus they synapse on third-order cells in the ventral posterior medial and ventral posterior lateral nuclei.

The third-order neurons in the thalamus send axons to the *primary somatic sensory cortex* (S-I), located in the postcentral gyrus of the parietal lobe. This area is subdi-

vided into four cytoarchitectural areas: Brodmann's areas 1, 2, 3a, and 3b (Figure 26–1). Most thalamic fibers terminate in areas 3a and 3b. The cells in areas 3a and 3b then project to Brodmann's areas 1 and 2. Thalamic neurons also send a sparse projection directly to Brodmann's areas 1 and 2 and to the adjacent secondary somatic sensory cortex (S-II). In addition, S-II is innervated by neurons from each of the four areas of S-I (Figure 26–1C). Mortimer Mishkin and his colleagues found that the projections from S-I are required for the perceptual function of S-II. Removal of the neural connections in S-I that represent a particular part of the body, for example the hand area, completely prevents stimuli applied to the skin of the hand from activating neurons in S-II. In contrast, removal of parts of S-II has no effect on the response of neurons in S-I. Finally, some thalamic neurons project to the posterior parietal cortex (Brodmann's areas 5 and 7), which also receives input from S-I.

The anatomical plan of the somatic sensory system reflects an organizational principle common to all sensory systems: sensory information is processed in a series of relay regions within the brain. To understand the serial processing characteristic of sensory systems it is necessary to examine how incoming information is transformed within each relay nucleus.

Relay nuclei are composed of *projection* (or *relay*) *neurons* that send their axons to the next relay nucleus in the ascending pathway of sensory information. Each projection neuron receives synaptic input from many afferent axons. Nevertheless, in the dorsal column nuclei, for example, the synaptic actions of some afferent fibers are so effective that activity in a single afferent fiber can discharge a relay cell. When such a limited number of afferent fibers can activate a cell, information can be transmitted with high fidelity. As a result, in some nuclei (as in the lateral geniculate nucleus, the major relay nucleus for afferent signals from the retina) the afferent message is relayed to the next level without modification.

More commonly, however, sensory input to relay cells follows a pattern of extensive convergence and divergence, as shown in Figure 26–2. In addition to activating relay cells, afferent fibers also activate interneurons, both excitatory and inhibitory. These interneurons can contribute to the processing of incoming sensory information. In these relay nuclei the firing pattern of the projection neurons leaving the nucleus differs from that of the afferent fibers, reflecting transformation of the signal by the cells of the nucleus.

The processing of neural information at a sensory relay nucleus follows the same principles found in the motor relay nuclei that we examined in general in Chapter 2. In addition to the convergence and divergence of excitatory synaptic input, there are three types of inhibitory pathways: feed-forward, feedback, and distal inhibition (Figure 26–2).

Feed-forward (or *reciprocal*) *inhibition* allows activity in one group of neurons to inhibit a different group of neurons. Feed-forward inhibition permits what Sherrington called a *singleness of action*, a winner-take-all strategy, which ensures that only one of two or more competing responses is expressed. In contrast, *feedback* (or *recurrent*) *inhibition* allows the most active neurons to limit the activity of all adjacent elements that are less active, irrespective of their function, thereby enhancing the contrast in firing pattern between the actively firing cells and the surrounding less active neurons. Both types of inhibition create zones of contrasting activity within the central nervous system: a central zone of active neurons surrounded by a ring of less active neurons. As we shall see in Chapter 30, by enhancing or amplifying the contrast between highly active cells and their neighbors these cellular interactions contribute to *selective perception*, by which we attend to one stimulus and not another.

Inhibitory interactions are quite general in sensory systems. Although there is no inhibition of the peripheral receptor in the somatic sensory system, inhibitory actions are common in all subsequent relay nuclei. For example, both feed-forward and feedback inhibition are present in

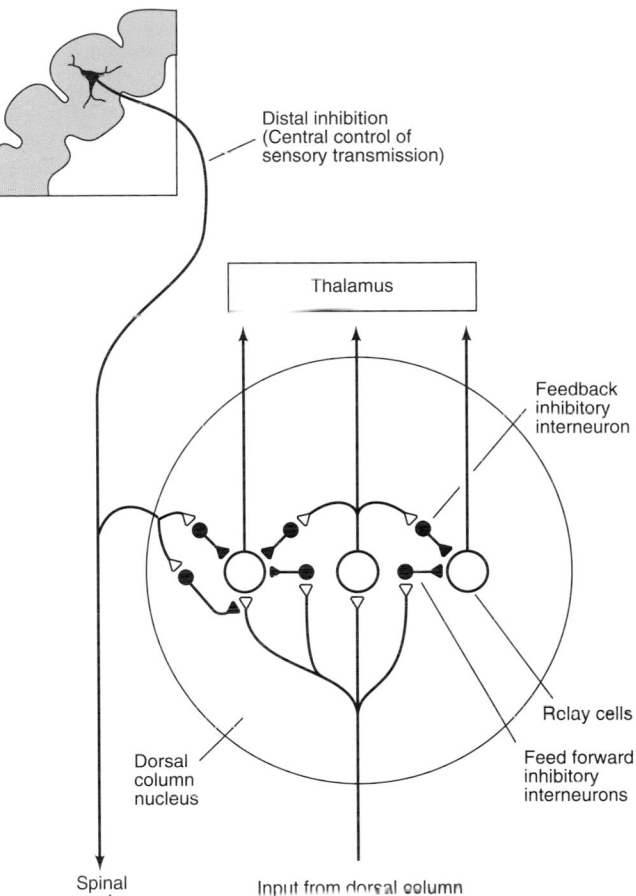

FIGURE 26–2
Cells in a sensory relay nucleus have complex inputs from both primary afferent fibers and local interneurons. This illustration is based on a dorsal column nucleus. The relay (or projection) cells of this nucleus receive convergent and divergent excitatory input from afferent fibers traveling in the dorsal columns. The afferent fibers also end on inhibitory interneurons that make feed-forward inhibitory connections onto adjacent relay cells. In addition, the activity in the relay cells inhibits the surrounding cells by means of feedback inhibition. Finally, neurons in the cerebral cortex modulate by distal inhibition the firing of relay cells, acting both pre- and postsynaptically. The relay cells in this nucleus project their axons to the thalamus. (In this, as in subsequent figures, excitatory synapses are indicated by **open triangles**, inhibitory synapses by **filled triangles**.)

the dorsal column nuclei, the first relay point in the somatic sensory system. The afferent fibers inhibit the activity of cells in the dorsal column nuclei that surround the cells they excite (feed-forward inhibition). In addition, the active cells in a nucleus inhibit the less active cells nearby by means of recurrent collateral fibers (feedback inhibition), thereby sharpening further the contrast between the active cells and their neighbors.

Feed-forward and feedback are local inhibitory mechanisms that operate within a relay nucleus. But neurons from more distant sites, such as the motor cortex and the brain stem, can also inhibit and thereby control the flow of information into relay nuclei. This mechanism is called *distal inhibition*. In the dorsal column nuclei distal inhibition operates mostly on presynaptic terminals. Distal inhibition illustrates still another principle of organization in the sensory system: Higher areas of the brain are able to control the sensory inflow from the peripheral receptors into relay nuclei.

The Body Surface Is Represented in the Brain in an Orderly Fashion

Our knowledge of how tactile information is represented in the central nervous system comes from two types of studies—clinical observations of humans and physiological studies in experimental animals.

Somatic Sensations Are Localized to Specific Regions of Cortex

The earliest information about the function of the somatic sensory system came from the analysis of disease states and traumatic injuries of the spinal cord. For example, one of the late consequences of syphilitic infection in the nervous system is a syndrome called *tabes dorsalis*, which destroys the large-diameter neurons in the dorsal root ganglia, causing the degeneration of myelinated afferent fibers in the dorsal columns. Patients with *tabes dorsalis* have severe deficits in touch and position sense but often little loss of temperature perception and of nociception. Additional information about the somatic afferent system comes from transection of the dorsal columns in experimental animals or as a result of trauma in humans. This type of injury results in a chronic deficit in certain tactile discriminations, such as detecting the direction of movement across the skin, the relative position of two cutaneous stimuli, and two-point discrimination. The deficit is ipsilateral to the lesion and occurs at levels below the lesion.

Experimental studies of the various somatic areas of the cortex have also provided valuable information about the function of different Brodmann's areas concerned with somatic sensibility. Total removal of S-I (areas 3b, 3a, 1, and 2) produces deficits in position sense and the ability to discriminate size, texture, and shape. Thermal and pain sensibilities usually are not abolished, but are altered. Small lesions in the cortical representation of the hand in Brodmann's area 3b produce deficits in the discrimination of the texture of objects as well as their size and shape. Lesions in area 1 produce a defect in the assessment of the texture of objects, whereas lesions in area 2 alter only the ability to differentiate the size and shape of objects. This is consistent with the idea that area 3b, which (together with 3a) is the principal target for the afferent projections from the ventral posterior lateral nucleus of the thalamus, receives information about texture as well as size and shape. Area 3b projects to both areas 1 and 2. The projection to area 1 is concerned primarily with texture, whereas the projection to area 2 is concerned with size and shape.

Because S-II receives inputs from all areas of S-I, removal of S-II causes severe impairment in the discrimination of both shape and texture and prevents monkeys from learning new tactile discriminations based on the shape of an object. Finally, damage to the posterior parietal cortex (the higher-order sensory cortex concerned with tactile perceptions) produces complex abnormalities in attending to the sensations from the contralateral half of the body.

Electrophysiological Studies Have Correlated Body Areas and Cortical Areas

Electrophysiological techniques were first used to study the cortical representation of the somatic sensory system in the late 1930s. This important series of experiments began with a chance observation made by Wade Marshall while studying the electrical activity of the cerebral cortex in the cat and monkey. Marshall found that by touching a specific part of the animal's body surface he could produce an *evoked potential* in the cortex over an area of several

FIGURE 26–3

A map of evoked potentials can be obtained in a monkey from the surface of the left postcentral gyrus of the cerebral cortex by applying stimuli to the body surface on the opposite side. This figure shows the responses of one large group of cells in the left postcentral gyrus to a light tactile stimulus applied to different points on the right palm. These cells respond much more effectively to tactile stimuli applied to the thumb and forefinger (**points 15, 16, 17, 20, 21, and 23**) than to those applied to the middle or the small finger (**points 1, 2, 3, 12, and 13**). (Adapted from Marshall, Woolsey, and Bard, 1941.)

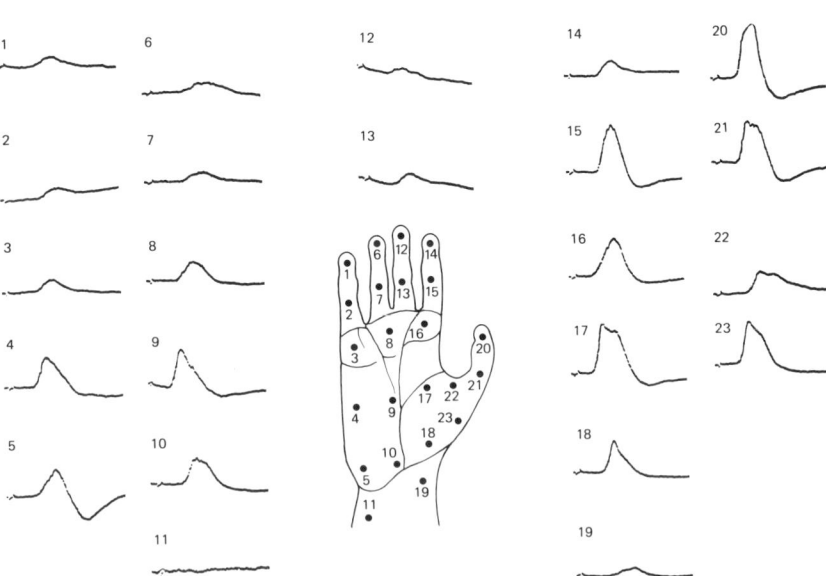

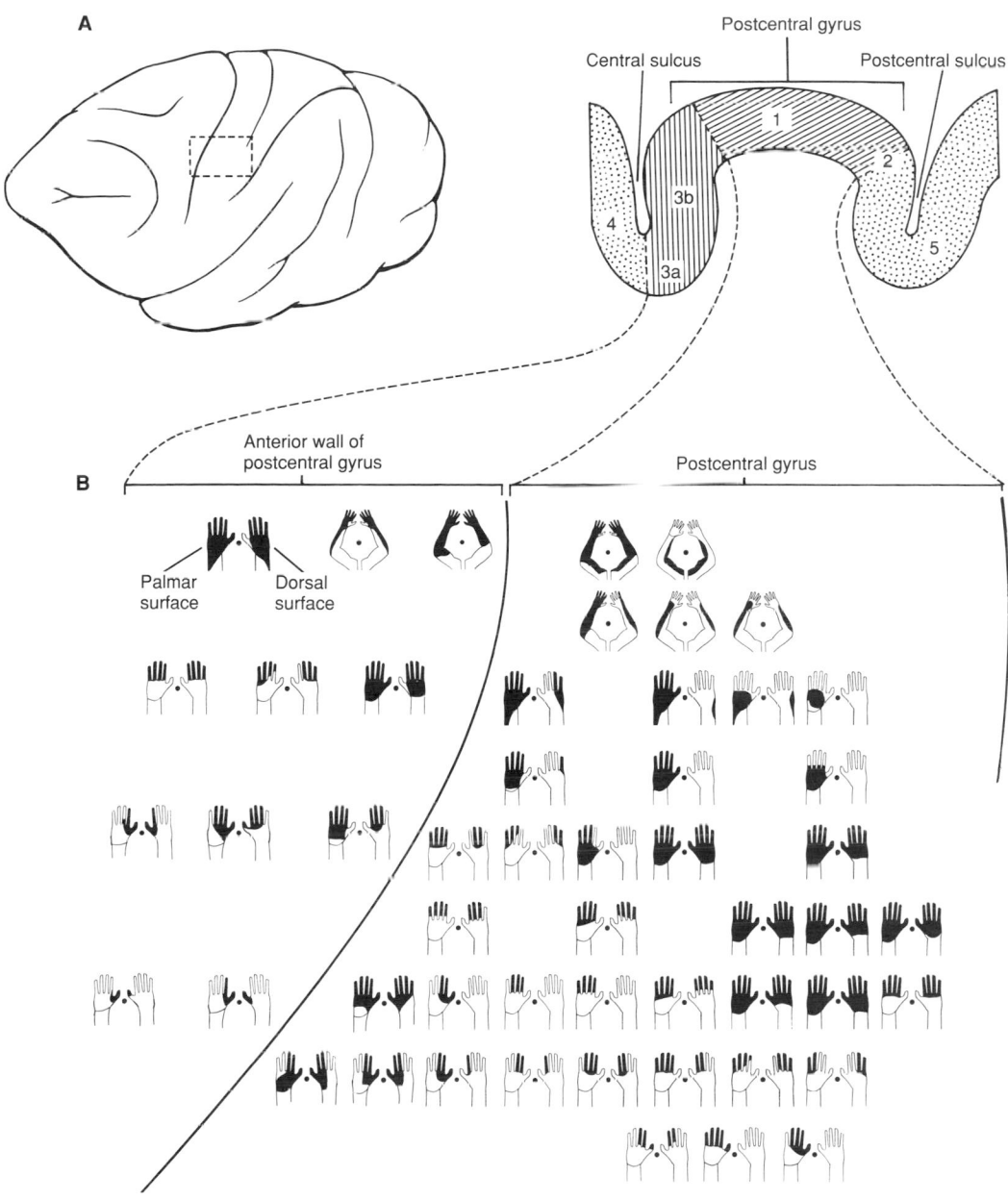

FIGURE 26–4

An early map of cortical responses to tactile stimulation in monkeys. (Adapted from Marshall, Woolsey, and Bard, 1941.)

A. Recordings were made in the primary somatic sensory cortex (S-I). The lateral view of the brain (**left**) shows the recording site. A sagittal view of S-I (**right**) shows Brodmann's subdivisions.

B. The maps reflect the responses evoked in different points of Brodmann's areas 3b and 1 by stimulation of the palmar and dorsal surfaces of the right hand. **Black dots** indicate sites in S-I that respond to stimulation of dorsal or palmar areas of the right hand. The sites on the **left side** of the figure are in the anterior wall of the postcentral gyrus, corresponding roughly to areas 3b and 3a in S-I. The sites on the **right side** of the figure are on the dorsal surface of the postcentral gyrus, corresponding roughly to area 1 in S-I.

millimeters. Evoked potentials are recorded electrical signals that represent the summed activity of thousands of cells and are obtained by using large, tipped metal electrodes or electrolyte-filled glass capillaries (Figure 26–3).

This evoked response method was later used by Marshall, Clinton Woolsey, and Philip Bard to map the representation of the body surface in Brodmann's area 1 of the postcentral gyrus in monkeys. The map was constructed by relating a point on the body surface to a point of maximal electrical activity in the cortex (Figures 26–4). Because each area in the map is involved in both convergent and divergent relationships, a coherent map of the body surface emerges only if one considers the points of maximal response. In later experiments the body surface and deep tissue were found to be represented in the thalamus and dorsal column nuclei as well.

A Sensory homunculus

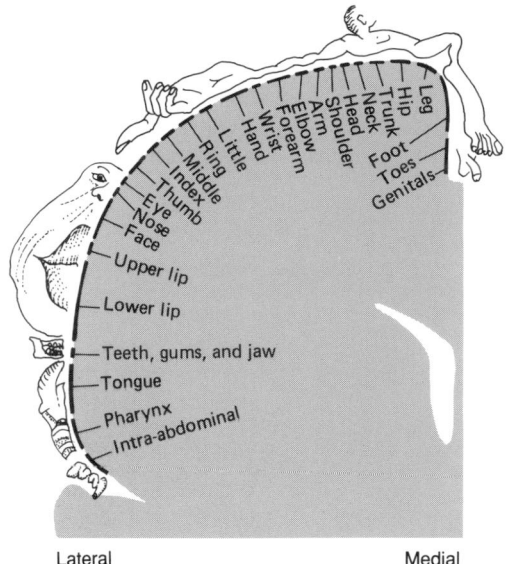

Lateral   Medial

B Motor homunculus

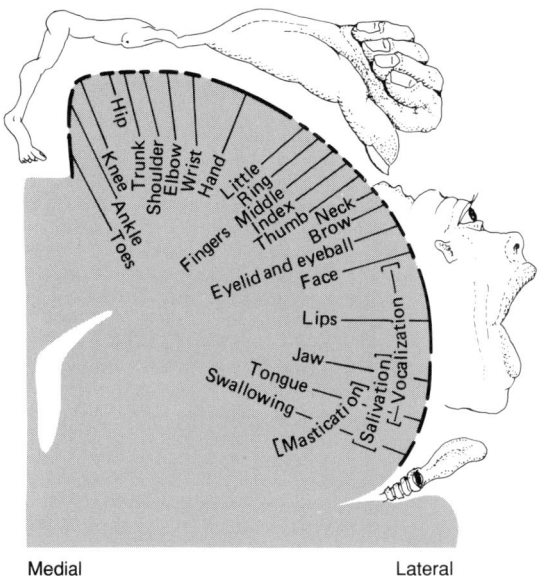

Medial   Lateral

FIGURE 26–5
Somatic sensory and motor projections from and to the body surface and muscle are arranged in the cortex in somatotopic order.

A. Sensory information from the body surface is received by the postcentral gyrus of the parietal cortex (areas 3a and 3b, and 1 and 2). Here the map for area 1 is illustrated. Areas of the body that are important for tactile discrimination, such as the tip of the tongue, the fingers, and the hand, have a disproportionately larger representation, reflecting their more extensive innervation. (Adapted from Penfield and Rasmussen, 1950.)

B. The analogous motor map exists for the motor cortex.

A similar organization was found in the human cortex by the neurosurgeon Wilder Penfield during operations for epilepsy and other brain disorders. Working with locally anesthetized patients, Penfield stimulated the surface of

the postcentral gyrus at various points in the area of S-I and asked the patients what they felt. (This procedure was necessary to ascertain the focus of the epilepsy and therefore to avoid unnecessary damage during surgery.) Penfield found that stimulation of points in the postcentral gyrus produced tactile sensations—paresthesias (numbness, tingling) and pressure—in discrete parts of the opposite side of the body. From these studies Penfield was able to construct a map of the neural representation of the body in the somatic sensory cortex.

As shown in Figure 26–5A, the leg is represented most medially, followed by the trunk, arms, face, and finally, most laterally, the teeth, tongue, and esophagus. Note that in Figure 26–5A, each part of the body is represented in the brain in proportion to its relative importance in sensory perception. The face is large compared with the back of the head; the index finger is gigantic compared with the big toe. As we shall see later, this distortion reflects differences in innervation density in different areas of the body. Similar distortion is seen in other species. In rabbits, for example, the face and snout have the largest representation because they are the animal's primary means of exploring its environment (Figure 26–6).

These cortical maps of the body surface and the parallel motor maps (Figure 26–5B) are important and explain why neurology has always been a precise diagnostic discipline, even though for many decades its practice relied on only the simplest tools—a wad of cotton, a safety pin, a tuning fork, and a reflex hammer. Disturbances within the somatic sensory system can be localized clinically because there is a direct relationship between the anatomical organization of the brain and specific perceptual and motor functions.

A particularly dramatic example of this relationship is the Jacksonian seizure, a characteristic sensory epileptic attack described by the neurologist John Hughlings Jackson. An early feature of the Jacksonian seizure is progression of numbness and paresthesia that begins in one place and spreads throughout the body. For example, numbness might begin at the fingertips, spread to the hand, up the arm, across the shoulder, into the back, and down the ipsilateral leg. The progress of this kind of sensory seizure is explained by the arrangement of the sensory projections in the brain (Figure 26–5A). In this example the seizure is initiated laterally, in the hand area, and propagates medially.

As we shall see in Chapter 50, potentials from the somatic sensory cortex can be recorded in humans in a completely noninvasive manner. Computers are used to obtain an average of many evoked signals so that the response can be distinguished from background electrical activity. Computer-averaged potentials provide clinical information that may not be detected in a routine neurological examination, about the somatic sensory cortex, and the ascending pathways in the spinal cord, brain stem, and thalamus. For example, the evoked potentials in the cortex can reveal a slowing of conduction in the spinal cord and brain stem due to demyelinating disease. This is useful in diagnosing *multiple sclerosis*, a common cause of demyelination in the central nervous system, since con-

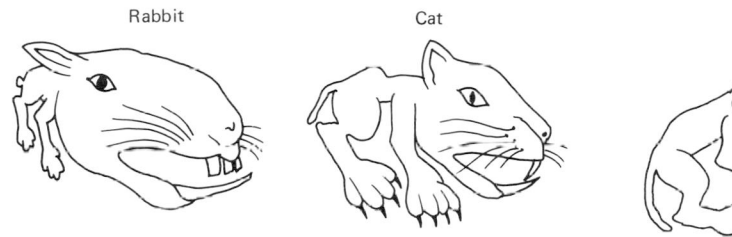
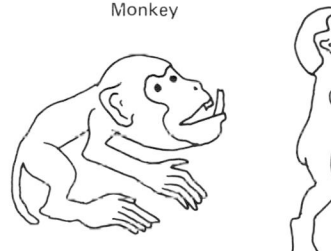
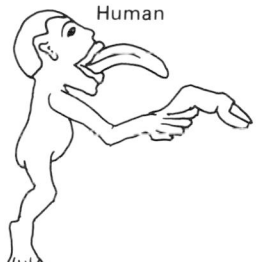

Rabbit   Cat   Monkey   Human

FIGURE 26–6

The relative importance of body regions in the somatic sensibilities of different species are shown in these drawings, which were based on studies of evoked potentials in the thalamus and cortex.

duction can be slowed at an early stage of the disease when sensation is still normal.

The first neural maps of the body surface—those developed by Marshall, Woolsey and Bard, and by Penfield—used gross recording electrodes that sampled more than 1 mm of cortex and probed primarily the convex region of the post central gyrus (Brodmann's area 1). Fine-resolution maps obtained more recently by Jon Kaas, Michael Merzenich, and their colleagues, using microelectrodes instead of gross recording electrodes, have revealed that

there are actually four independent and fairly complete maps in each Brodmann's area of the primary somatic sensory cortex (S-I): areas 3a, 3b, 1, and 2. The secondary somatic sensory cortex (S-II) has still another map. Each of the four areas in S-I has its own somatosensory input and most areas are interconnected. As illustrated in Figure 26–7, the somatosensory maps in Brodmann's areas 3b and 1 lie parallel to one another and correspond in their medial-to-lateral representation of the body surface. This explains why earlier studies, which probed a limited area of

FIGURE 26–7

Each of the four subregions of the primary somatic sensory cortex (Brodmann's areas 3a, 3b, 1, and 2) has its own complete representation of the body surface. This figure illustrates the representation for the hand and the foot in areas 3b and 1. (Adapted from Kaas et al., 1983.)

A. Somatosensory maps in areas 3b and 1 are shown in this dorsolateral view of the brain of an owl monkey. The two maps are roughly mirror images. The digits of the hand and foot are numbered D_1 to D_5.

B. 1. A more detailed illustration of the representation of the glabrous pads of the palm in areas 3b and 1. These include the palmar pads (numbered in order, P_4 to P_1), two insular pads (**I**), two hypothenar pads (**H**), and two thenar pads (**T**). **2.** An idealized map of the hands based on studies of a large number of monkeys. The distorted representations of the palm and digits reflect the extent of innervation of each palmar area in the cortex. The five digital pads (D_1 to D_5) include distal, middle, and proximal segments (**d, m, p**).

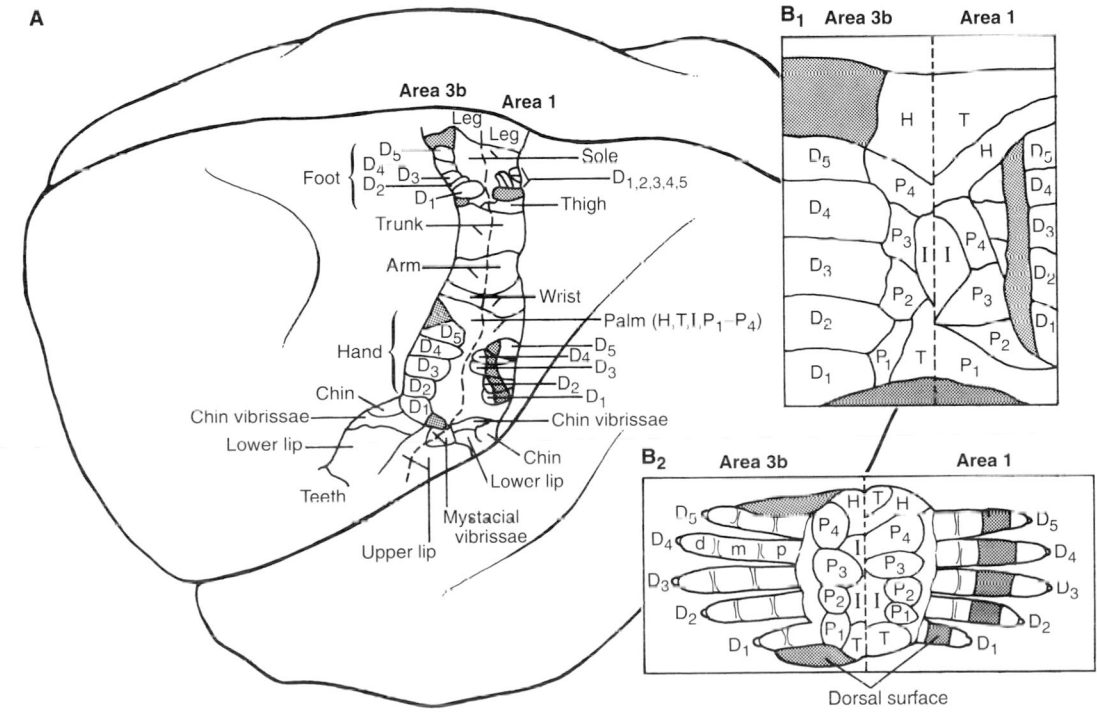

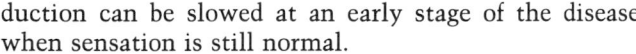

the postcentral gyrus and used techniques with poorer resolution, led to the inference that there was only a *single* large representation of the body surface in the cortex.

Each Central Neuron Has a Specific Receptive Field

When the first cortical maps of the body surface appeared in the 1930s they presented two puzzles. The contours of the map of each region of the body, like the hand area illustrated in Figure 26–4, are not sharply defined, and there is much overlap in the representation of parts of the body. This apparently inexact representation seemed inconsistent with the precise tactile sensibilities of humans. In addition, the various submodalities appeared to project to roughly the same area of cortex. Since superficial sensations can be discriminated from deep ones, and touch and position sense are distinct, the fact that there is only one map was puzzling.

To solve these problems, Vernon Mountcastle, Jerzy Rose, and their colleagues began in the late 1940s to examine the somatic sensory system at the cellular level. Using extracellular microelectrodes (which had just become available), they recorded the electrical responses of individual neurons. Extracellular recordings reveal only the action potentials of the cell; thus, they do not show synaptic activity except under certain circumstances. (It is more difficult to record intracellularly than extracellularly in the intact brain because the neurons are small and the brain pulsates, making it difficult to maintain intracellular penetrations.) Nevertheless, through extracellular recording a great deal has been learned about how sensory stimuli modulate the firing patterns of single cells.

Mountcastle and his colleagues found that cortical neurons in the somatic sensory system are mostly silent, with little or no spontaneous activity. Moreover, each cell responds only to stimulation of a specific area of the skin; that is, like the sensory receptors, central neurons have receptive fields. Any point on the skin is represented in the cortex by a population of cells connected to the afferent fibers that innervate that point on the skin. All of these cells will have similar receptive fields. When a point on the skin is touched the population of cortical neurons connected to that point on the skin will be excited. Stimulation of another point on the skin activates another population of cortical neurons. Thus, we perceive that a particular point on the skin is being stimulated because a specific population of neurons in the brain is activated. Conversely, as Penfield illustrated, when a point on the cortex is stimulated electrically, we experience tactile sensations on a specific part of the skin.

There are four other important features of receptive fields: their size and distribution on the body surface, modifiability, and fine structure.

Sizes of Receptive Fields Vary in Different Areas of the Skin

In the areas of the skin that are most sensitive to touch—the tongue and the tips of the fingers—the number of receptors per unit area of skin is large and the receptive field of each receptor is proportionally small. The finger tips of humans have the highest density of receptors: about 2500 per square centimeter! Of these, 1500 are Meissner's corpuscles, 750 are Merkel's cells, and about 75 are pacinian and Ruffini's corpuscles. These receptors are innervated by 300 myelinated axons per square centimeter. For example, each afferent fiber connects to about 20 Meissner's corpuscles and each corpuscle receives about two to five afferent fibers. The receptive fields for most of these receptors (the Meissner's corpuscles and Merkel's cells) are about 3 to 4 mm in diameter.

Moving up the arm, the receptive fields become larger, reflecting the density of innervation and thus the fineness of the tactile discrimination (Figure 26–8). In the trunk the receptive fields of sensory receptors are about 100 times larger than those in the finger tips. Conversely, the cortical magnification unit area of cortex per unit area of body surface is about 100 times greater for the fingers than for the trunk. Thus, receptive field size and cortical magnification are inversely related.

A remarkable feature of receptive fields in the somatic sensory system, and especially in the cerebral cortex, is that the size of the receptive field is not fixed. Although size stays approximately the same under normal conditions, it can be modified greatly by experience or injury. We shall consider this feature in Chapter 65 when we examine the neural mechanisms of learning.

Receptive Fields of Central Neurons Have Inhibitory and Excitatory Components

The discharge of a receptor cell is greatest when a stimulus is applied to the center of the receptive field, and weakest at the perimeter. This gradient of excitatory activity within the receptive field is maintained in the central nervous system at each relay point, including the cortex. In addition, there is a gradient of inhibition, which is largely masked by the more powerful excitation. The inhibition is also greatest at the center of the field and decreases with distance from the center. Since the inhibition is delayed, it gives rise to a sequence of synaptic actions—excitation followed by inhibition—at the center of the receptive field. Inhibition sometimes extends beyond the perimeter of the excitatory zone of the receptive field, giving rise to an inhibitory surround. Thus, at each relay point in the somatic afferent system a stimulus in the excitatory center of the receptive field produces a peak of excitation among the responding population of cells, which is surrounded by a population of inactive (inhibited) cells, and this spatial distribution of activity serves to sharpen the peak of activity within the brain (Figure 26–9).

Lateral Inhibition Can Aid in Two-Point Discrimination

Fine tactile discrimination, such as reading braille, involves perceiving textures. We can understand how this is accomplished by considering the simplest example of spatial discrimination: the ability to distinguish two closely placed point stimuli as two rather than as one. Mountcastle pro-

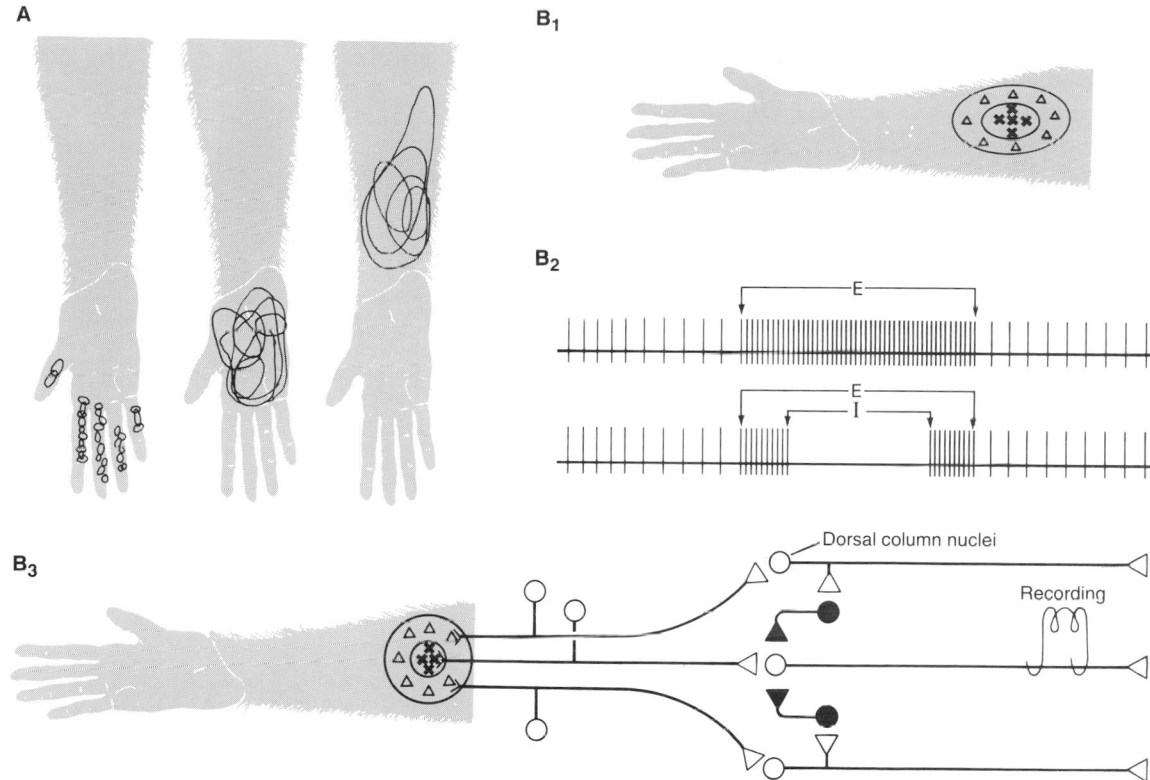

FIGURE 26–8

Fine structure of the receptive field of mechanoreceptors.

A. The size of the receptive fields of mechanoreceptors varies throughout the body. The fields are small in the distal finger tips; they become larger in the hand and even larger in the forearm.

B. 1. Idealized relationship of the excitatory (x) and inhibitory (Δ) zones of the receptive field of a neuron in the postcentral gyrus. In this example a larger zone of inhibition surrounds the excitatory zone. **2.** Extracellular recordings from a single cell in the cortex illustrate the dynamics of the excitatory (**E**) and inhibitory (**I**) zones of the receptive field. A stimulus applied steadily to the excitatory part of the receptive field elicits a steady firing in the cell (**trace 1**). When the inhibitory region on

the skin is stimulated along with the excitatory part, the excitation is inhibited. When the inhibitory stimulus is removed, the excitatory stimulus is again effective (**trace 2**). **3.** Simplified model of the input connections for a cell in the dorsal column nucleus (electrode) with a receptive field that has an excitatory region and inhibitory surround. A stimulus applied on the skin to the center of the receptive field activates receptors that excite one group of cells in the nucleus (the excited region or discharge zone). Stimulation of surrounding skin activates other receptors that end on inhibitory interneurons and suppress the firing of the cells activated by the excitatory center of the receptive field.

posed a model for two-point discrimination by reconstructing the neural events in the postcentral gyrus of the cortex produced by a light tactile stimulus on the skin. The model was derived from studies using a method called *reciprocal interpretation*. In this method a stimulus is moved systematically across the receptive field of a single nerve cell and the response of the cell is used to obtain an idea about how activity is distributed across a population of neurons. Reciprocal interpretation is based on the following argument. At each relay the stimulus activates a population of neurons with similar properties, whose responses are assumed to be uniformly distributed on the surface of the skin. Thus, moving the stimulus across the skin and examining the firing pattern of a single cell is equivalent to keeping the position of the stimulus constant and moving the recording electrode from one cell to the next in the relay nucleus receiving input from that piece of skin.

Consider first a single-point stimulus. This stimulus activates several touch receptors within a circumscribed

area around the stimulus, producing short trains of impulses in each receptor. These impulses then discharge a group of cells in a dorsal column nucleus, and those cells activate another group of cells in the ventral posterior nucleus of the thalamus, which in turn discharge a group of cells in the primary somatic sensory cortex. At each relay in the central nervous system the population of cells that discharges is limited by two factors: (1) the afferent pathway activated by the stimulus connects anatomically only to a limited number of central cells, the *responding population*, and (2) the population of neurons directly excited by the afferent signals at each relay also engages inhibitory interneurons that restrict, by means of recurrent inhibition, the firing of the responding population (Figure 26–9). This inhibition is not present at the level of the receptor but comes in at the dorsal column nuclei and is found at each subsequent relay step.

The *location* of a single stimulus on the body surface is thus signaled in the nervous system by the firing of specific populations of neurons activated by the stim-

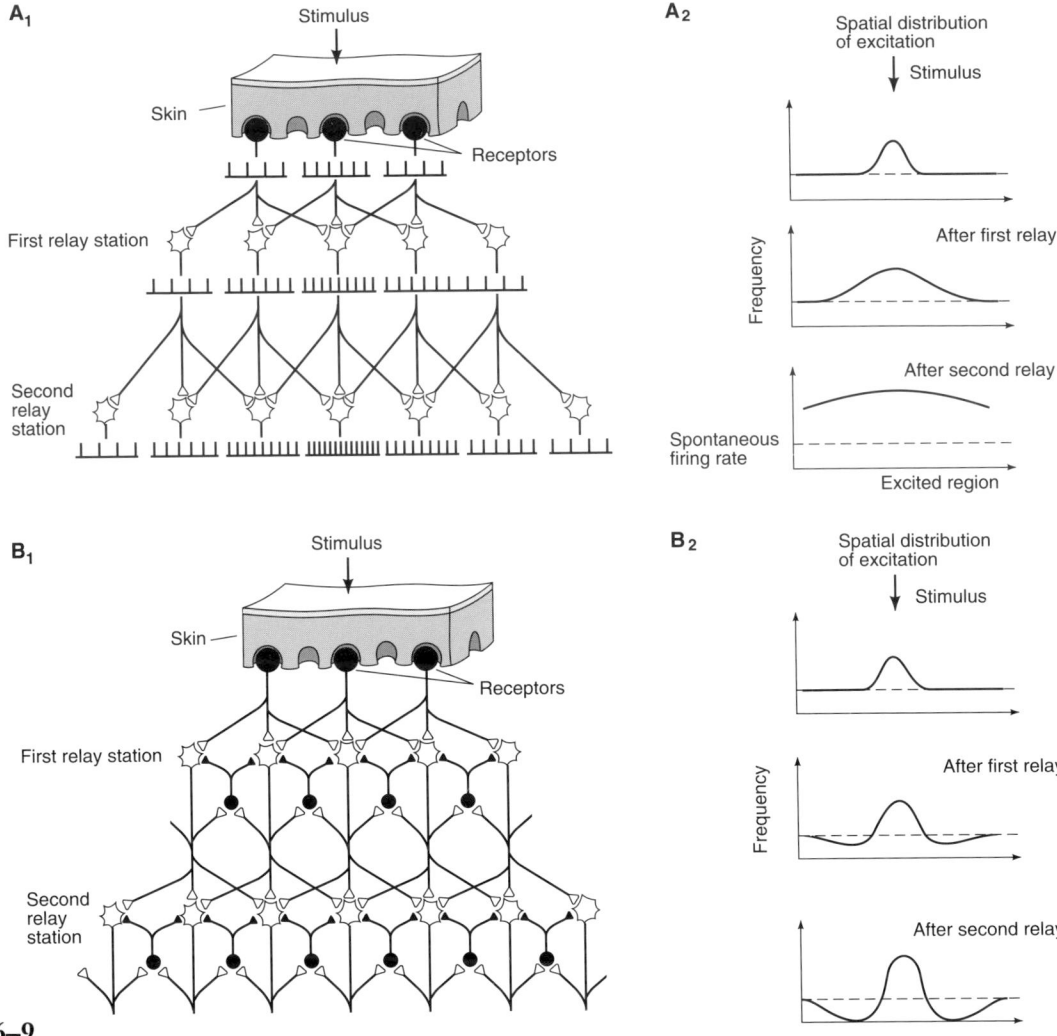

FIGURE 26–9

Effect of feedback inhibition. (Adapted from Dudel, 1983.)

A. 1. Diagram of the excitatory synaptic connections among three receptors and the interneurons at the next two relays in the absence and presence of inhibitory interneurons. The **inset** over each axon shows its relative rate of discharge during stimulation. **2.** In the absence of inhibitory interneurons, there is a large discharge zone (the *excitatory region* or *discharge zone*) at

each of the relays in response to a stimulus in the excitatory region of the receptive field.

B. The addition of inhibitory interneurons **(black)** narrows the discharge zone. On either side of the excitatory region the discharge rate is driven below the resting level by feedback inhibition.

ulus. Those populations are located at specific points in each relay nucleus as well as in the cerebral cortex. The *intensity* of the stimulus is signaled by the frequency of firing of the specific populations and by the size of the active populations, because a strong stimulus to the skin produces a higher frequency of firing and activates a larger population of cells than does a weak stimulus. Not all cells in this population respond in an identical manner. Cells at the center, which have the most powerful connections to the area being stimulated, discharge most effectively and with the shortest latency. Cells just off the center have a lower probability of firing and discharge fewer impulses with longer latency.

According to Mountcastle's model for two-point discrimination, two stimuli applied to different positions on

the skin set up excitatory gradients of activity in two cell populations at every relay point in the somatic sensory system. The activity in each population of cells has its own maximal region of activity, or peak, and the perception of two points rather than one occurs because two distinct populations are active. Neurons in each population have a receptive field with a central excitatory zone surrounded by a weaker excitatory zone, which is further depressed by the inhibitory surround. The inhibitory surround sharpens each peak and further enhances the distinction between the two peaks. When two stimuli are brought close together, the activity in the two populations tends to overlap so that the distinction between the two peaks could become blurred. However, as the stimuli are brought together, the inhibition produced by each summates. As a result of this more effective inhibition, the peaks of activity in the two responding populations become sharpened and the two active populations become more effectively separated spatially. This sculpturing role of the inhibition allows two distinct peaks of activity to continue to be registered at the cortical level, thus preserving the spatial separation of the two stimulus sites (Figure 26–10). At each level of the nervous system recurrent inhibition enhances contrast between stimuli. It is easy to see how this feature of neural organization can lead to the ability to recognize patterns and contours.

When two stimuli occur within a single large receptive field, as in the forearm, the separation of the two stimuli is encoded in the signals of a *single* population of receptors. Ian Darian-Smith, Esther Gardner, and their colleagues found that in such cases the spacing between two stimuli is encoded by the firing frequency of the individual afferent fibers. When the stimuli are widely separated they elicit high frequencies from the afferents responding to each stimulus. As the separation narrows, the frequencies decrease and the *duration* of their firing decreases so markedly that rapidly adapting receptors can distinguish spacing between stimulus probes as small as about 1 mm.

Inputs to the Somatic Sensory Cortex Are Organized into Columns by Submodality

Most nerve cells in the somatic sensory system are responsive to only one modality: touch, pressure, temperature, or pain. Neurons mediating touch are responsive to superficial tactile stimuli and not to deep pressure.

Neurons responsive to superficial stimuli are even more specialized. Some are responsive to movement of hairs while others respond to a steady indentation of skin. Throughout the somatosensory system, cells responding to one submodality tend to be grouped together.

A remarkable example of this feature is evident in the cerebral cortex. In a series of pioneering studies Mountcastle examined the distribution of the input from various receptors to the somatic sensory cortex. Because the cortex consists of six major cellular layers (see Chapter 20), he first looked for a correlation between cell layer and receptor type. He found none. Instead, he discovered that in all six layers neurons within a column or slab of cortex running from the cortical surface to the white matter respond to a single class of receptors. Some columns of cells are activated by rapidly adapting cutaneous receptors of the Meissner type, some by slowly adapting cutaneous receptors of the Merkel type, others by movement of hairs, and still others by subcutaneous rapidly adapting pacinian receptors. All neurons in a column also receive inputs from the same local area of skin. Neurons lying within a column therefore comprise an elementary functional module of the cortex. We shall see in later chapters that columnar organization is a basic structural principle of the cerebral cortex.

Although each of the four areas of the primary somatic sensory cortex (3a, 3b, 1, and 2) receives input from all areas of the body surface, Merzenich, Kaas, and their colleagues found that one modality tends to dominate in each area. In area 3a the dominant input is from muscle stretch receptors; in area 3b it is input from cutaneous receptors; in area 2, deep pressure receptors; and in area 1, rapidly adapting cutaneous receptors.

FIGURE 26–10
Two-point discrimination depends on separation of signals. (Adapted from Mountcastle and Darian-Smith, 1968.)

A. Stimulation of a single point of the skin activates one population of cells in the cortex with maximal activity in the center of the population.

B. Stimulation of two adjacent points activates two populations of cells, each with a peak of activity. In one population lateral

(recurrent) inhibition is shown. Here the active neurons excite inhibitory interneurons that in turn inhibit neighboring, less active cells. In the other population there is no lateral inhibition. Therefore, each active population has a broader representation in the cortex so that the two active peaks of activity readily merge into one another.

A One-point stimulus

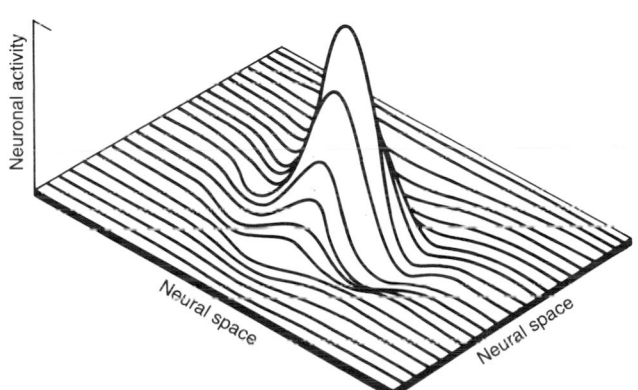

B Two-point stimulus

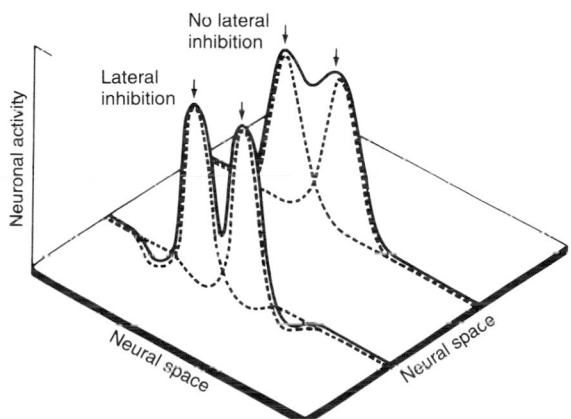

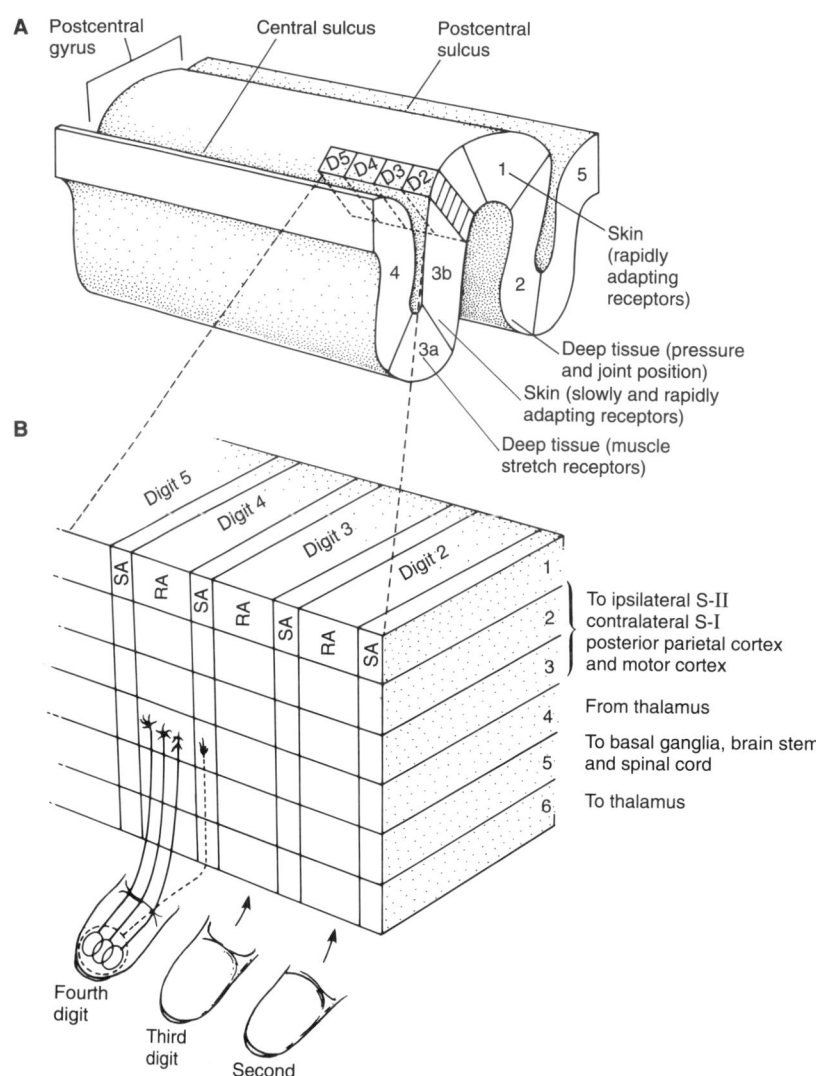

A Postcentral gyrus   Central sulcus   Postcentral sulcus

D5 D4 D3 D2   1   5

4   3b   2   Skin (rapidly adapting receptors)

3a

Deep tissue (pressure and joint position)

Skin (slowly and rapidly adapting receptors)

Deep tissue (muscle stretch receptors)

B

Digit 5   Digit 4   Digit 3   Digit 2

SA RA SA RA SA RA SA

1

2   To ipsilateral S-II contralateral S-I posterior parietal cortex and motor cortex

3

4   From thalamus

5   To basal ganglia, brain stem and spinal cord

6   To thalamus

Fourth digit

Third digit

Second digit

FIGURE 26–11

Inputs of individual modalities to the somatic sensory cortex are organized in columns. (Adapted from Kaas et al., 1979.)

A. Inputs to each region of the somatic sensory cortex—Brodmann's areas 3a, 3b, 1, and 2—are primarily from one type of receptor in the skin (indicated in the figure). Inputs from specific parts of the body are organized in columns of neurons that run from the surface to the white matter. This schematic drawing shows the columnar arrangement of inputs from digits 2, 3, 4, and 5.

B. This detail of columns for digits 2, 3, 4, and 5 in part A shows the arrangement of inputs in a portion of Brodmann's area 3b that receives inputs from rapidly adapting (**RA**) and slowly adapting (**SA**) cutaneous receptors of tactile stimuli.

In addition to being organized by modality, S-1 is further subdivided into submodalities. For example, in Brodmann's area 3b, the neural map of cutaneous receptors for each finger is divided into two columns, one each for inputs from rapidly adapting and slowly adapting receptors (Figure 26–11). Thus, within each of the four areas of S-I there are several interrelated modality-specific maps of the body surface.

How does the layering of the cortex participate in the modality-specific organization of the cortex? As described in Chapter 20, each layer of cells has connections with different parts of the brain: layer 6 projects back to the thalamus, layer 5 to subcortical structures, layer 4 *receives* input from the thalamus, and layers 2 and 3 project to other cortical regions. As a result, the modality-specific output from each column is conveyed to different regions of the brain. As we shall see in a later chapter, the visual cortex is also organized by submodalities.

Detailed Features of a Stimulus Are Communicated to the Brain

In Early Stages of Cortical Processing the Dynamic Properties of Central Neurons and Receptors Are Similar

Throughout the nervous system the various somatosensory submodalities are conveyed by anatomically separate pathways. Sensory receptors and primary sensory neurons responsive to one submodality are connected to clusters of cells in the dorsal column nuclei and thalamus that receive inputs only for that submodality. These relay neurons in turn project to modality-specific cells in the cortex. The cells that make up these anatomically distinct mechanoreceptor pathways have distinctive response properties. For example, as we saw in Chapters 23 and 24, some receptor cells in both the skin and deep tissue adapt rapidly to a stimulus and others adapt slowly. Psycho-

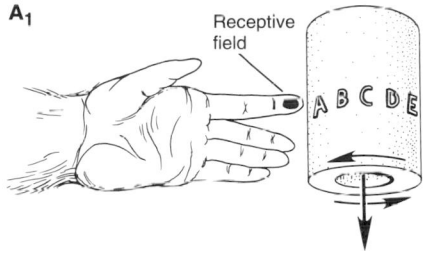

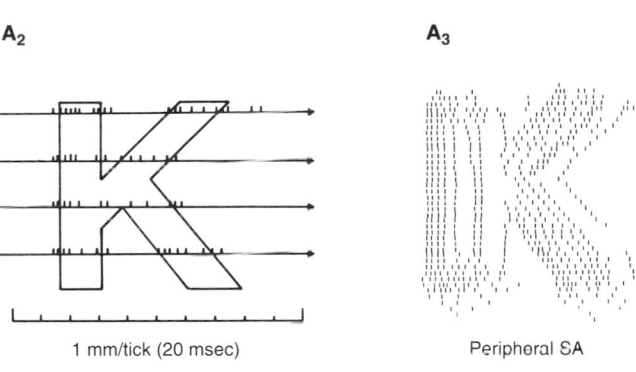

1 mm/tick (20 msec)

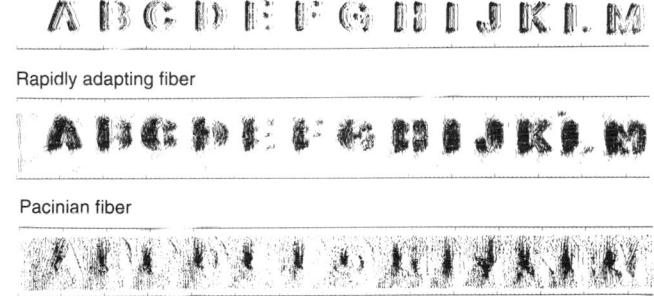

Peripheral SA

FIGURE 26–12

The spatial characteristics of embossed letters are represented in the discharge of cutaneous mechanoreceptors and neurons in primary somatic sensory cortex. (Adapted from Phillips et al., 1988.)

A. 1. Embossed letters on a cylindrical drum are used to study the spatial pattern of neuronal activity in mechanoreceptors innervating the finger tip and, in separate experiments, in cortical neurons in Brodmann's areas 3b and 1. Letters of the alphabet are repeatedly swept across a receptive field in the finger tip of a monkey by rotating the drum. The action potentials evoked by each letter in single afferent fibers (or cortical neurons) are plotted in *spatial event plots*. **2.** Spatial event plots are constructed as follows. Embossed letters (about 6.0 mm high and 500 μm in relief) are swept (50 times at 50 mm/s) across a given location within the receptive field of a single neuron innervating the finger pad, thereby producing action potentials. The drum is rotated and the stimulus is moved across the receptive field from proximal to distal (vertical bar of the K entered the receptive field first on each sweep). After each sweep, the drum is then shifted vertically within the receptive field by 200 μm and swept again. The time of occurrence of each action potential relative to adjacent stimulus position markers is recorded and ordered from top to bottom so as to assign a spatial location relative to the stimulus surface. **3.** In an actual spatial event plot for the letter K, each action potential in **A₂** is presented as a dot.

B. 1. Spatial event plots reconstructed from three types of afferent fibers in a monkey: slowly adapting (**top**), rapidly adapting (**middle**), and pacinian corpuscle (**bottom**). **2.** Spatial event plots reconstructed from five slowly adapting neurons in area 3b of an awake monkey.

B₁ Afferent fibers

Slowly adapting fiber

Rapidly adapting fiber

Pacinian fiber

B₂ Brodmann's area 3b: slowly adapting neurons

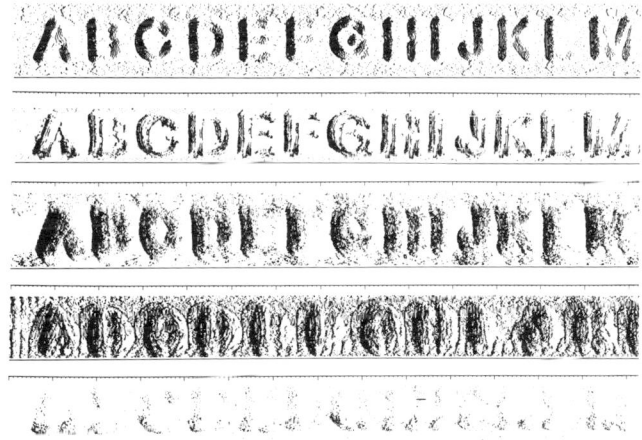

physical studies on flutter and vibration that we considered in Chapter 24 show that several types of human tactile perceptions are determined by the response properties of the receptors.

Mountcastle and his colleagues examined how these response property features are communicated to neurons in the brain and found that the dynamic properties of the receptors are matched by those of the central neurons to which they are connected. Rapidly adapting skin receptors connect to rapidly adapting neurons in the thalamus that connect to similar neurons in areas 3b and 3a in the primary somatosensory cortex (S-I). Likewise, slowly adapting receptors connect to neurons in the thalamus and 3b and 3a that also adapt slowly. Thus, the second- and third-order cells do not merely repeat the firing pattern of the primary afferent fibers but actually have adaptation properties similar to those of the receptors themselves. As a result, Mountcastle argued that the signal received by the input to the cortex faithfully reproduces the stimulus features encoded by the receptor in the skin.

How far does this fidelity extend? Kenneth Johnson and his colleagues addressed this question by examining the neural representation of the surface texture of objects. They examined the responses of single afferent fibers and cortical neurons in areas 3b and 1 when the fingers of awake monkeys were stimulated with embossed letters, the sort of stimulus used in pattern recognition experiments with humans. In separate experiments a single letter was repeatedly swept across the skin of the monkey's finger and the action potentials evoked in single receptor neurons and cortical neurons were plotted. Johnson and his colleagues found that both slowly and rapidly adapting receptors in the skin (Merkel's cells and Meissner's corpuscles) transmit a faithful neural image of the letters, while the pacinian receptors in deep tissue do not (Figure 26–12). As we have seen in considering two-point discrimination, the responses of a single neuron to a stimulus moved systematically across its receptive field can be assumed to represent the responses of a *population* of neurons with similar response properties.

Are these initial representations of the stimulus maintained at higher levels within the brain? In area 3b, the first stage of processing in the somatic sensory cortex, the projections from skin receptors give rise to relatively sharp images. In later stages, however, for example in area 1, the responses are more abstract. Since certain cutaneous peripheral afferents but not all cortical neurons represent letter stimuli faithfully, it should be possible to determine the steps by which the initial representation becomes abstracted.

In the Later Stages of Cortical Processing the Central Nerve Cells Have Complex Feature-Detecting Properties and Integrate Various Sensory Inputs

To sense the texture, form, and motion of an object the nervous system must integrate information from many different mechanoreceptors sensitive to superficial touch, deep pressure, and the position of the fingers and hand. How is this integration accomplished? At least four factors are involved: (1) the response properties of neurons at successive levels of sensory processing become more complex; (2) the submodalities converge on one common cell; (3) the size of the receptive field becomes larger at each level of processing; and (4) the profile of activity in the responding population changes.

The increasing complexity of response properties in somatic sensory systems was discovered by Gerhard Werner and his colleagues. They found cells in the hand region of the somatic sensory cortex that respond briskly to three-dimensional objects placed within the receptive fields, and particularly to movement of the object across the skin. These same cells, however, do not respond well to punctate stimuli, although cells located at earlier relay points are easily excited by such stimuli.

Studies by Juhani Hyvärinen and Antti Poranen, as well as by Yoshiaki Iwamura and by Gardner, revealed that neurons involved in the input to the cortex (areas 3b and 3a) respond to relatively simple punctate stimuli, whereas the neurons involved in subsequent cortical processing stations (areas 1 and 2) have complex response properties. For example, at least three types of neurons respond to movement across the skin in areas 1 and 2. *Motion-sensitive* neurons respond well to movement in all directions but do not respond selectively to movement in any one direction. *Direction-sensitive* neurons respond much better to movement in one direction than in another. *Orientation-sensitive* neurons respond best to movement along a specific axis of the receptive field (Figure 26–13).

Detection of movement and other features of the stimulus is a property of higher cortical neurons. These properties are not apparent in dorsal column nuclei, in the thalamus, or even in areas 3a and 3b. Feature-detecting neurons sensitive to stimulus direction and orientation are first found in area 1 and even more extensively in area 2, the areas concerned with *stereognosis* (the perception of the three-dimensional shape of objects) and with discriminating the direction of movement of objects on the skin. Thus, these complex stimulus properties arise not from thalamic input but from cortical processing of more elementary inputs. The convergent projections from areas 3a and 3b onto areas 1 and 2 also permit neurons in areas 1 and 2 to respond to other complex features, such as edge orientation. Whereas neurons in 3b and 1 respond only to touch, and neurons in areas 3a respond only to position sense, certain neurons in area 2 have both inputs. These neurons respond best when an object is grasped by the hand. As we shall see below, this information is thought to provide the necessary tactile clues for skilled movement of the fingers.

Neurons involved in the later stages of cortical processing also have larger receptive fields. For example, neurons in areas 3a and 3b, the sites of initial input of S-I, have quite small receptive fields that usually encompass one or two phalanges on a finger. In contrast, neurons in areas 1 and 2, which receive inputs from areas 3a and 3b, have receptive fields that include several fingers (Figure 26–14). Thus, the receptive fields and response properties of neurons in areas 1 and 2 reflect convergent input from different regions of the hand and fingers, areas that are separately represented in areas 3a and 3b (see Figure 26–11). Inputs for the finger areas are commonly adjacent to one another and the cells respond most effectively when adjacent fingers are stimulated, as when the hand is used to hold and manipulate an object. These complex cells in areas 1 and 2 become active during movements of the hand around an object, and seem to have a role in stereognosis, the tactile discrimination of three-dimensional shapes.

This increase in the complexity of neuronal response is important not only for perception but also for the execution of skilled movements. Indeed, area 2 sends somatosensory inputs from the entire body surface to the primary motor cortex. Moreover, reversible inhibition of neural

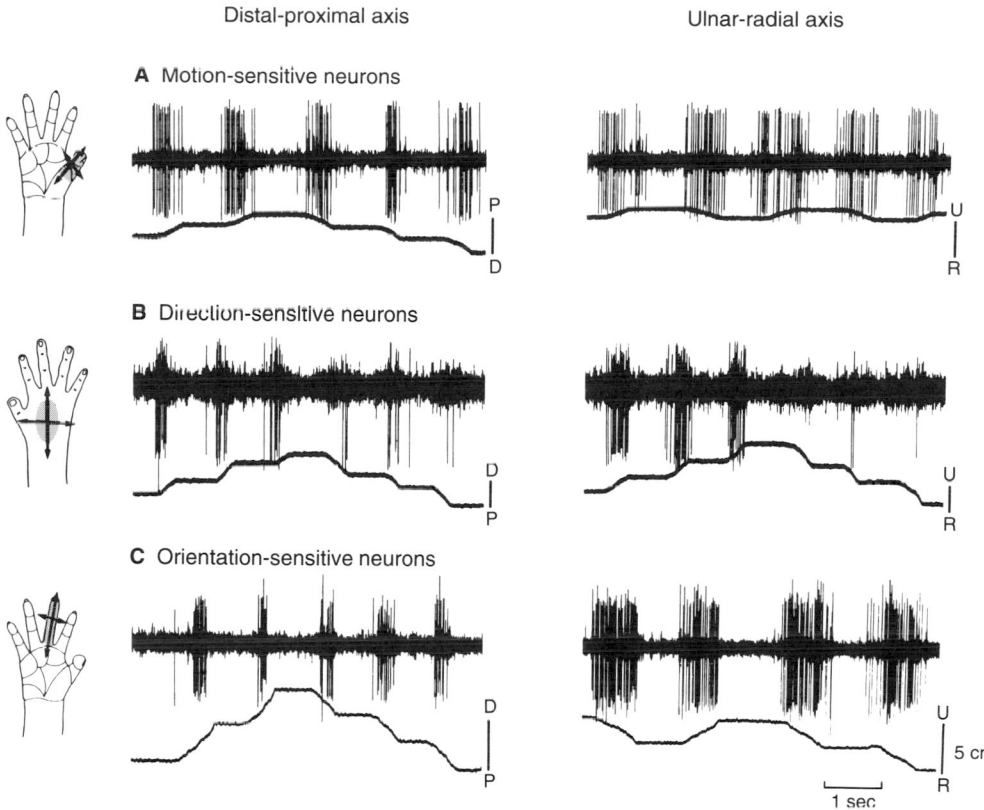

Distal-proximal axis   **Ulnar-radial axis**

A Motion-sensitive neurons

B Direction-sensitive neurons

C Orientation-sensitive neurons

5 cm

1 sec

FIGURE 26–13

Typical responses of three types of S-I cortical neurons to a grating wheel rolled across the hand of a monkey. The drawings of the hand at left show the locations of the receptive fields of the neurons tested and the directions of movement of the wheel across the skin. The recordings on the right show the responses of each type of neuron to movement of the wheel in four directions: longitudinally along a distal–proximal axis and transversely along an ulnar–radial axis. The trace below each cell record shows the output of a potentiometer measuring wheel rotation. Upward or downward deflections in the potentiometer indicate one complete sweep of the grating wheel across the receptive field in the indicated direction. During flat portions of the potentiometer recordings the grating was being lifted from the skin and repositioned for a new stimulus. (Adapted from Warren, Hamalainen, and Gardner, 1986.)

A. Motion-sensitive neurons respond to wheel motion in all directions. (Distance of wheel movement, 2.4 mm.)

B. Direction-sensitive neurons respond better to movement in one direction than another. Strongest responses are to motion in the ulnar direction; weakest responses are to the radial direction. Responses to distal movement are more vigorous than to proximal movement. (Distance of wheel movement, 1.2 mm.)

C. Orientation-sensitive neurons respond more vigorously to transverse than to longitudinal motion, but responses to motion in opposite directions are about the same. (Distance of wheel movement, 1.6 mm.)

activity in area 2 produced pharmacologically (using a GABA agonist that inhibits cortical cells) leads to an inability to assume functional postures of the hand and to coordinate the fingers for picking up small objects (Figure 26–15). In addition to projecting to the motor cortex for movement, the somatic sensory areas project to the posterior parietal cortex (Brodmann's areas 5 and 7), the cells of which have very complex properties, receive inputs from several modalities, and are often related to movement. There the information for tactile discrimination and position sense is integrated with visual information and with the neural systems in the brain stem, thalamus, and temporal lobe concerned with attention.

An Overall View

Examination of the receptive properties of neurons in the somatosensory cortex has revealed a precise representation of the external body surface onto the cortical surface. However, the somatosensory map or homunculus is not an exact representation of the body surface but is distorted. The finger tips, for example, are allotted a much greater cortical area than regions like the back. Receptive field sizes of cortical neurons are inversely related to the density of innervation. Somatotopy, the orderly projection of the sensory sheet in the brain, permits orderly intracortical connections.

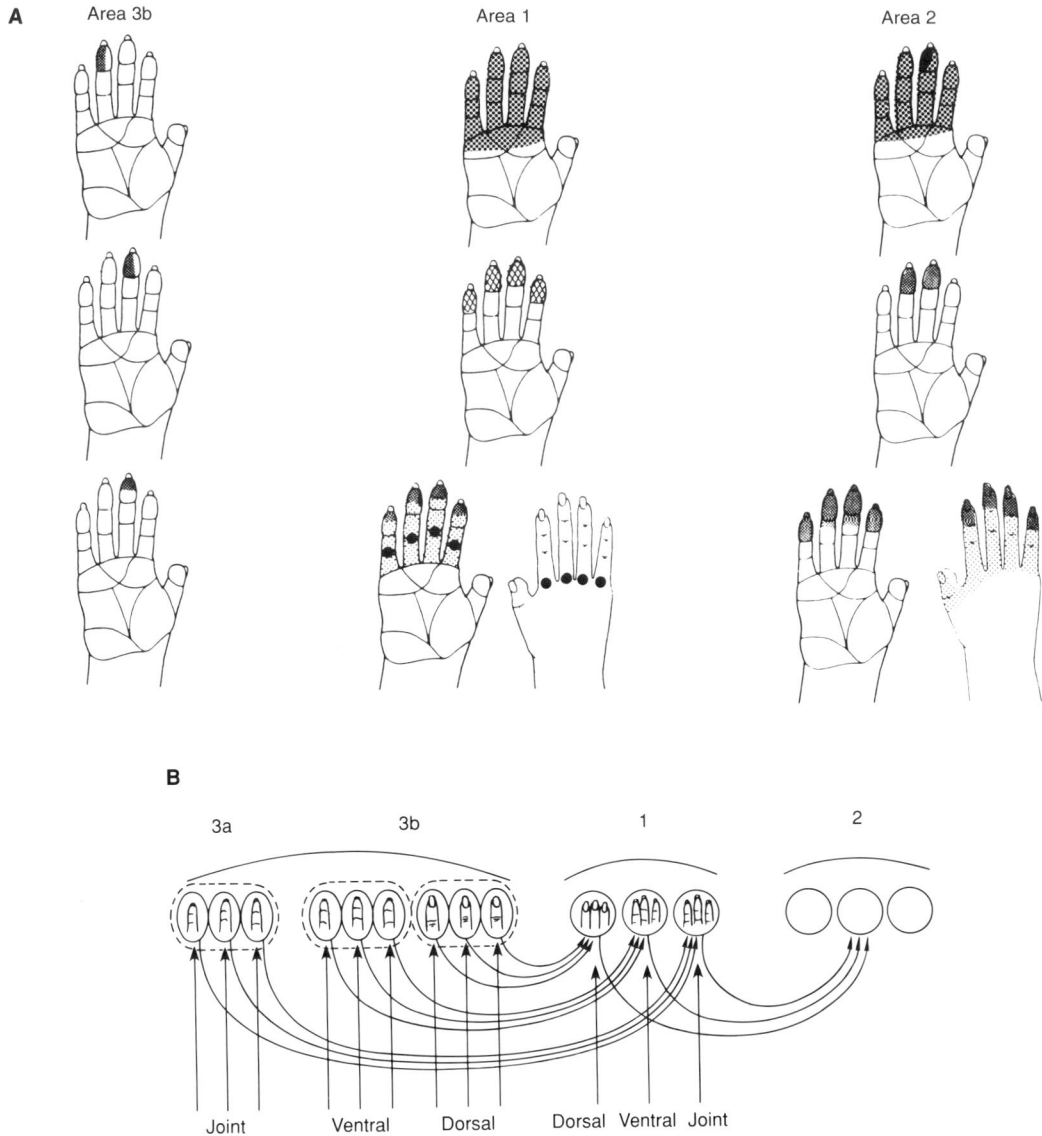

FIGURE 26–14

Neurons that participate in later stages of cortical processing (Brodmann's areas 1 and 2) have larger receptive fields.

A. These drawings illustrate the receptive fields of cells in areas 3b, 1, and 2 based on recordings made during a single electrode penetration close to the central sulcus. The neurons in

area 2 were all directionally sensitive. (Adapted from Gardner, 1988.)

B. Model showing how connections in S-I allow convergence of location and modality information onto single neurons in areas 1 and 2. (Adapted from Iwamura et al., 1985a,b.)

Like all sensory and motor modalities, tactile information from the periphery reaches the cortex by several pathways, each carrying both redundant and unique information. As a result, lesions of the medial lemniscus, which carry information from the dorsal column to the thalamus, do not completely abolish tactile perception. Patients with these lesions retain sensibility of crude touch through pathways that ascend in the anterolateral column.

In addition to parallel ascending pathways, many path-

ways project to more than one cortical area. Thus, there are five representations of the body surface in the parietal cortex, one in S-II and four in S-I. Why are there so many representations of the body surface? Somatic sensation involves the parallel analysis of different stimulus attributes in different cortical areas. Parallel processing in the brain is a form of processing that we shall encounter again. It is designed not to achieve multiplication of identical circuitry, but to allow different neuronal pathways and brain relays to deal with the same sensory information in

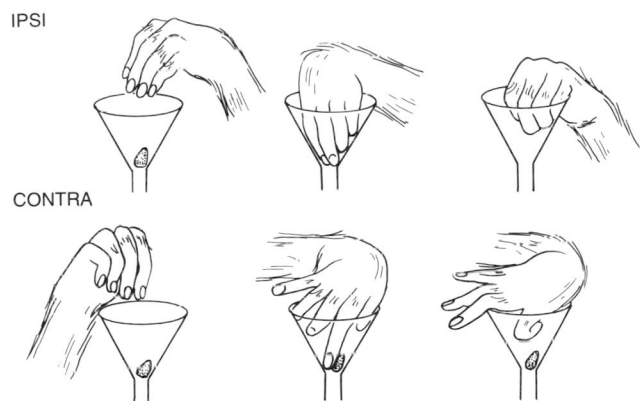

IPSI

CONTRA

FIGURE 26–15
A monkey's finger coordination is disrupted following the injection of muscimol, a GABA agonist that inhibits synaptic transmission in the somatic sensory cortex. The left hand **(ipsi)** is able to pick up an apple piece from a funnel. Two hours following the injection of muscimol into Brodmann's area 2 on the left side, the finger coordination of the right hand **(contra)** is severely disorganized. (Adapted from Hikosaka et al., 1985.)

slightly different ways. Because of parallel processing, simple neuronal transformations of signals based on synaptic excitation, synaptic inhibition, and action potentials are able to endow our perceptions with richness.

In the cortex sensory submodalities are arranged in columns, so that all six layers in any column represent the same modality. For example, layer 4 receives input from the thalamus, whereas other layers project out to other areas of the cortex and subcortex. Each of the four subregions in the somatosensory cortex contains its own map of the body surface, specific to a particular somatic sensory modality. Thus, area 3a primarily receives input from muscle stretch receptors, area 3b receives cutaneous receptor input, area 1 receives input from rapidly adapting receptors, and area 2 contains a map of deep pressure receptors. As a result, these different regions are involved in slightly different aspects of somatic sensation. Area 1 is involved in sensing the texture of objects, while area 2 is responsible for sensing the size and shape of objects.

Neurons in areas 2 and 1 are involved in the later-stages of somatosensory processing, have more complex feature-detecting properties, receive convergent input from a number of submodalities, and have larger receptive fields than first-order cortical neurons. At least three types of higher-order somatosensory cells have been found: motion-sensitive, orientation-sensitive, and direction-sensitive neurons. Even more complicated processing seems to be carried out by neurons activated when the hand is manipulating an object; these neurons project to the motor cortex for sensory–motor integration. Finally, the somatosensory cortex also sends outputs to the posterior parietal cortex, where integration with other senses takes place, and where an overall picture of the body is formed.

Selected Readings

Darian-Smith, I. 1982. Touch in primates. Annu. Rev. Psychol. 33:155–194.

Gardner, E. P., Hamalainen, H. A., Palmer, C. I., and Warren, S. 1989. Touching the outside world: Representation of motion and direction within primary somatosensory cortex. In J. S. Lund (ed.), Sensory Processing in the Mammalian Brain: Neural Substrates and Experimental Strategies. New York: Oxford University Press, pp. 49–66.

Hyvärinen, J., and Poranen, A. 1978. Movement-sensitive and direction and orientation-selective cutaneous receptive fields in the hand area of the post-central gyrus in monkeys. J. Physiol. (Lond.) 283:523–537.

Kaas, J. H., Nelson, R. J., Sur, M., Lin, C.-S., and Merzenich, M. M. 1979. Multiple representations of the body within the primary somatosensory cortex of primates. Science 204:521–523.

Kaas, J. H., Nelson, R. J., Sur, M., and Merzenich, M. M. 1981. Organization of somatosensory cortex in primates. In F. O. Schmitt, F. G. Worden, G. Adelman, and S. G. Dennis (eds.), The Organization of the Cerebral Cortex: Proceedings of a Neurosciences Research Program Colloquium. Cambridge, Mass.: MIT Press, pp. 237–261.

Mountcastle, V. B. 1984. Central nervous mechanisms in mechanoreceptive sensibility. In I. Darian-Smith (ed.), Handbook of Physiology, Section 1: The Nervous System, Vol. III. Sensory Processes, Part 2. Bethesda, Md.: American Physiological Society, pp. 789–878.

Pons, T. P., Garraghty, P. E., Friedman, D. P., and Mishkin, M. 1987. Physiological evidence for serial processing in somatosensory cortex. Science 237:417–420.

Vallbo, Å. B., Olsson, K. Å., Westberg, K.-G., and Clark, F. J. 1984. Microstimulation of single tactile afferents from the human hand: Sensory attributes related to unit type and properties of receptive fields. Brain 107:727–749.

References

Adrian, E. D., and Zotterman, Y. 1926. The impulses produced by sensory nerve-endings. Part 2. The response of a single end-organ. J. Physiol. (Lond.) 61:151–171.

Bard, P. 1938. Studies on the cortical representation of somatic sensibility. Harvey Lect. 33:143–169.

Costanzo, R. M., and Gardner, E. P. 1980. A quantitative analysis of responses of direction-sensitive neurons in somatosensory cortex of awake monkeys. J. Neurophysiol. 43:1319–1341.

Cracco, R. Q., and Bodis-Wollner, I. (eds.) 1986. Evoked Potentials. New York: Liss.

Dudel, J. 1983. General sensory physiology. In R. F. Schmidt and G. Thews (eds.), Human Physiology. M. A. Biederman-Thorson (trans.) Berlin: Springer, pp. 177–192.

Dykes, R. W. 1983. Parallel processing of somatosensory information: A theory. Brain Res. Rev. 6:47–115.

Gardner, E. P. 1988. Somatosensory cortical mechanisms of feature detection in tactile and kinesthetic discrimination. Can. J. Physiol. Pharmacol. 66:439–454.

Hikosaka, O., Tanaka, M., Sakamoto, M., and Iwamura, Y. 1985. Deficits in manipulative behaviors induced by local injections of muscimol in the first somatosensory cortex of the conscious monkey. Brain Res. 325:375–380.

Iwamura, Y., Tanaka, M., Sakamoto, M., and Hikosaka, O. 1983. Converging patterns of finger representation and complex response properties of neurons in area 1 of the first somatosensory cortex of the conscious monkey. Exp. Brain Res. 51:327–337.

Iwamura, Y., Tanaka, M., Sakamoto, M., and Hikosaka, O. 1985. Comparison of the hand and finger representation in areas 3, 1, and 2 of the monkey somatosensory cortex. In M. Rowe and W. D. Willis, Jr. (eds.), Development, Organization, and Processing in Somatosensory Pathways. New York: Liss, pp. 239–245.

Iwamura, Y., Tanaka, M., Sakamoto, M., and Hikosaka, O. 1985. Vertical neuronal arrays in the postcentral gyrus signaling active touch: A receptive field study in the conscious monkey. Exp. Brain Res. 58:412–420.

Jackson, J. H. 1931–1932. Selected Writings of John Hughlings Jackson. 2 vols. J. Taylor (ed.) London: Hodder and Stoughton.

Jones, E. G., and Friedman, D. P. 1982. Projection pattern of functional components of thalamic ventrobasal complex on monkey somatosensory cortex. J. Neurophysiol. 48:521–544.

Kaas, J. H., Merzenich, M. M., and Killackey, H. P. 1983. The reorganization of somatosensory cortex following peripheral nerve damage in adult and developing mammals. Annu. Rev. Neurosci. 6:325–356.

Marshall, W. H., Woolsey, C. N., and Bard, P. 1941. Observations on cortical somatic sensory mechanisms of cat and monkey. J. Neurophysiol. 4:1–24.

Mountcastle, V. B. 1957. Modality and topographic properties of single neurons of cat's somatic sensory cortex. J. Neurophysiol. 20:408–434.

Mountcastle, V. B., and Darian-Smith, I. 1968. Neural mechanisms in somesthesia. In V. B. Mountcastle (ed.), Medical Physiology, 12th ed., Vol. II. St. Louis: Mosby, pp. 1372–1423.

Norrsell, U. 1980. Behavioral studies of the somatosensory system. Physiol. Rev. 60:327–354.

Penfield, W., and Rasmussen, T. 1950. The Cerebral Cortex of Man: A Clinical Study of Localization of Function. New York: Macmillan.

Phillips, J. R., Johnson, K. O., and Hsiao, S. S. 1988. Spatial pattern representation and transformation in monkey somatosensory cortex. Proc. Natl. Acad. Sci. U.S.A. 85:1317–1321.

Randolph, M., and Semmes, J. 1974. Behavioral consequences of selective subtotal ablations in the postcentral gyrus of Macaca mulatta. Brain Res. 70:55–70.

Sherrington, C. 1947. The Integrative Action of the Nervous System, 2nd ed. New Haven: Yale University Press.

Warren, S., Hamalainen, H. A., and Gardner, E. P. 1986. Objective classification of motion- and direction-sensitive neurons in primary somatosensory cortex of awake monkeys. J. Neurophysiol. 56:598–622.

Werner, G., and Whitsel, B. L. 1973. Functional organization of the somatosensory cortex. In A. Iggo (ed.), Handbook of Sensory Physiology, Vol. 2: Somatosensory System. New York: Springer, pp. 621–700.

Woolsey, C. N. 1958. Organization of somatic sensory and motor areas of the cerebral cortex. In H. F. Harlow and C. N. Woolsey (eds.), Biological and Biochemical Bases of Behavior. Madison: University of Wisconsin Press, pp. 63–81.

27

Thomas M. Jessell
Dennis D. Kelly

Pain and Analgesia

Noxious Insults to the Body Activate Nociceptors

Nociceptors Are Activated by Mechanical,
Thermal, or Chemical Stimuli

Tissue Damage Can Sensitize Nociceptors

Local Pain Can Be Sensed Even When
Nociceptive Pathways Are Damaged

Pain Syndromes Can Result from Surgery
Intended to Alleviate Pain

**Primary Afferent Fibers Synapse with Dorsal
Horn Neurons**

**Primary Afferent Fibers Use Amino Acids and
Peptides As Transmitters**

**Nociceptive Information Is Conveyed to the Brain
Along Several Ascending Pathways**

**Pain Can Be Modulated by the Balance of Activity
Between Nociceptive and Other Afferent Inputs**

Pain Can Be Controlled by Central Mechanisms

Direct Electrical Stimulation of the Brain
Produces Analgesia

Nociceptive Control Pathways Descend to the
Spinal Cord

Opiate Analgesia Involves the Same Pathways
As Stimulation-Produced Analgesia

Endogenous Opioid Peptides and Their Receptors Are
Located at Key Points in the Pain Modulatory System

Supraspinal and Spinal Networks Coordinately
Modulate Nociceptive Transmission

Local Dorsal Horn Circuits Modulate Afferent
Nociceptive Input

**Behavioral Stress Can Induce Analgesia Through
Both Opioid and Nonopioid Mechanisms**

An Overall View

The sensations that we call pain—pricking, burning, aching, stinging, and soreness—have an urgent and primitive quality. Yet pain, like other sensations, can be modulated by a wide range of behavioral experiences—the joy of childbirth can suppress pain, whereas fear of the dentist can intensify otherwise innocuous sensations. The variability of human pain suggests that there are neural mechanisms that modulate transmission in pain pathways and modify the organism's emotional reaction to pain. As we shall see, both types of modulatory activity occur in the central nervous system.

A distinction needs to be made between pain and *nociception*. Nociception refers to the reception of signals in the central nervous system evoked by activation of specialized sensory receptors (nociceptors) that provide information about tissue damage. Not all noxious stimuli that activate nociceptors are necessarily experienced as pain. Pain is the *perception* of an aversive or unpleasant sensation that originates from a specific region of the body. The relationship between the perception of pain and the activation of nociceptors is a good example of the principle that we have encountered in earlier chapters: All perception involves an abstraction and elaboration of sensory inputs. The highly subjective nature of pain is one of the factors that makes it difficult to define and to treat clinically.

Pain is more than a conspicuous sensory experience that warns of danger. Chronic pain represents a massive economic problem—in the United States alone more than two million people are incapacitated by pain at any given time.

In this chapter we consider the mechanisms involved in signaling and modulating nociceptive stimuli. We also discuss how the activation of nociceptive pathways can lead to the perception of pain.

Noxious Insults to the Body Activate Nociceptors

Nociceptors Are Activated by Mechanical, Thermal, or Chemical Stimuli

Harmful stimuli applied to the skin or to subcutaneous tissue, such as joints or muscle, activate nociceptors, the peripheral endings of primary sensory neurons whose cell bodies are located in the dorsal root and trigeminal ganglia. Nociceptors are the least differentiated of the sensory receptors in the skin. Unlike the specialized receptors that convey other somatic sensory modalities, nociceptors exist as free nerve endings that do not have peripheral structures that transduce and filter peripheral stimuli.

Pain in humans is mediated by several different classes of nociceptive afferent fibers. *Thermal* or *mechanical nociceptors* have small-diameter, thinly myelinated Aδ fibers that conduct at about 5–30 m/s. Activation of these nociceptors is associated with sensations of sharp, pricking pain. *Polymodal nociceptors* are activated by a variety of high-intensity mechanical, chemical, and hot (greater than 45°C) or cold stimuli and have small-diameter, unmyelinated C fibers that conduct slowly at 0.5–2 m/s. Both Aδ and C fibers are widely distributed in skin as well as in deep tissues.

A noxious stimulus activates the nociceptor by depolarizing the membrane of the sensory ending. The mechanisms by which diverse chemical, thermal, and mechanical noxious stimuli depolarize free sensory endings and trigger an action potential are not known. It is believed that the transduction mechanism for each type of noxious stimulus is distinct since the threshold response of polymodal receptors to one type of stimulus can be changed without altering the threshold to others.

Tissue Damage Can Sensitize Nociceptors

When peripheral tissues are damaged, the sensation of pain in response to subsequent stimuli is enhanced. This phenomenon, termed *hyperalgesia,* may involve a lowering of threshold of the nociceptors or an increase in the magnitude of pain evoked by suprathreshold stimuli. Hyperalgesia can occur both at the site of tissue damage (primary hyperalgesia) and in the surrounding undamaged areas (secondary hyperalgesia).

What is responsible for primary hyperalgesia? Robert La Motte, James Campbell, and their colleagues have found that primary hyperalgesia can result from changes in the sensitivity of nociceptors. For example, repeated heating of the skin decreases the threshold of C and Aδ nociceptors (Figure 27–1). In contrast, repeated applications of noxious mechanical stimuli do not decrease the threshold of nociceptors, although they can sensitize nearby nociceptors that were previously nonresponsive to mechanical stimuli. Mechanical hyperalgesia may also result from changes in synaptic efficacy at the central terminals of primary afferent neurons in the spinal cord or brain.

The basis of secondary hyperalgesia is less clear. The spread of hyperalgesia in the periphery may occur through

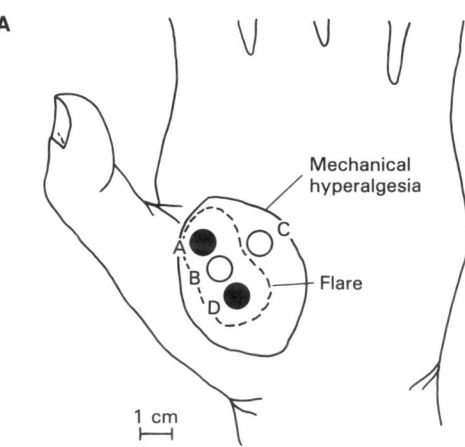

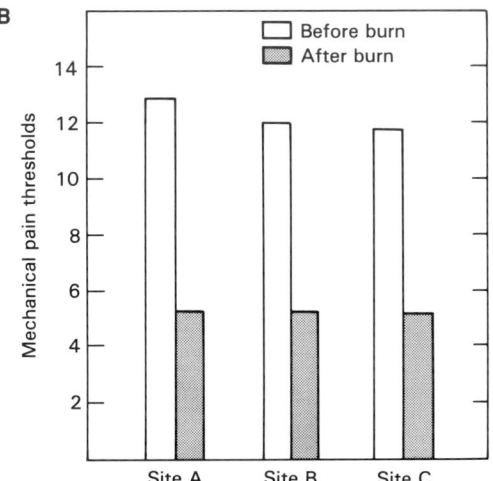

FIGURE 27–1

Burns to the glabrous skin of the hand produce both primary and secondary hyperalgesia to mechanical stimuli but only primary hyperalgesia to heat stimuli. (Reproduced with permission from Raja et al., 1989.)

A. Mechanical thresholds for pain were recorded at sites **A, B,** and **C** before and after burns at sites **A** and **D**. The burns consisted of a 53°C stimulus for 30 sec at both sites. The areas of reddening (flare) and mechanical hyperalgesia following the burns in one subject are also shown. In all subjects the area of mechanical hyperalgesia was larger than the area of flare. Mechanical hyperalgesia was present even after the flare disappeared.

B. Mean mechanical thresholds for pain before and after burns for seven subjects. The mechanical threshold for pain was significantly decreased following the burn.

the sensitization of nociceptors with diffuse collateral branches, one of which innervates the site of injury. This mechanism is similar to that proposed for the spread of vasodilation in the vicinity of a localized region of cutaneous injury, a phenomenon termed the *axon reflex*. Secondary hyperalgesia may also result from sensitization of central nociceptor neurons as a result of sustained activation.

TABLE 27–1. Some of the Naturally Occurring Agents that Activate or Sensitize Nociceptors

Substance	Source	Enzyme involved in synthesis	Effect on primary afferent fibers
Potassium	Damaged cells		Activation
Serotonin	Platelets	Tryptophan hydroxylase	Activation
Bradykinin	Plasma kininogen	Kallikrein	Activation
Histamine	Mast cells		Activation
Prostaglandins	Arachidonic acid-damaged cells	Cyclo-oxygenase	Sensitization
Leukotrienes	Arachidonic acid-damaged cells	5-Lipoxygenase	Sensitization
Substance P	Primary afferent		Sensitization

(Modified from Fields, 1987.)

The sensitization of nociceptors after injury or inflammation results from local tissue damage and the release of a variety of chemical mediators (Table 27–1). These agents have different cellular origins, but they all act to decrease the threshold and sometimes activate nociceptors (Figure 27–2). For example, histamine is released from damaged cells in response to tissue injury and excites polymodal nociceptors. In contrast, ATP, acetylcholine, and serotonin, which are also released from damaged cells, can act alone or in combination to sensitize nociceptors to other agents. Prostaglandin E2, a cyclo-oxygenase metabolite of arachidonic acid, is released from damaged cells and produces hyperalgesia and sensitizes nociceptors. Indeed, the reason why aspirin and other nonsteroidal anti-inflammatory analgesics are effective in controlling pain is because they inhibit the cyclo-oxygenase enzyme, preventing the synthesis of prostaglandin. The peptide bradykinin is one of the most active pain producing agents liberated during tissue damage. It activates both Aδ and C nociceptors and also increases the synthesis and release of prostaglandins from nearby cells.

The nociceptors themselves release peptides whose actions sensitize sensory endings. For example, substance P contributes to the spread of edema and hyperalgesia by vasodilation and by releasing histamine from mast cells, which then acts directly on the sensory ending.

Local Pain Can Be Sensed Even When Nociceptive Pathways Are Damaged

Although damage or loss of peripheral neurons that transmit noxious stimuli often impairs pain sensation, pain can arise spontaneously in the absence of activity in nociceptors. Pain due to injury of peripheral nerves is a major clinical problem that has several different causes. One is deafferentation; the loss of afferent input from the periphery to the spinal cord. This can occur when, for example, the dorsal roots over several segments are pulled away from the spinal cord (brachial plexus avulsion), a frequent result of motorcycle injuries. Patients feel a burning or electric pain in the dermatomes corresponding to the denervated, anesthetic area. The pain is thought to arise because of hyperactivity of dorsal horn neurons in the deafferented region of the spinal cord. In some cases it can be reduced by surgical ablation of the superficial dorsal horn in the deafferented region. Similarly, amputees often have the sensation of pain emanating from a missing limb, a phenomenon termed *phantom pain*. In this case, too, chronic overactivity of dorsal horn neurons may convey the illusion that the pain derives from the distal regions of a limb that no longer exists.

Activity of efferent fibers of the sympathetic nervous system following peripheral nerve injury can also trigger

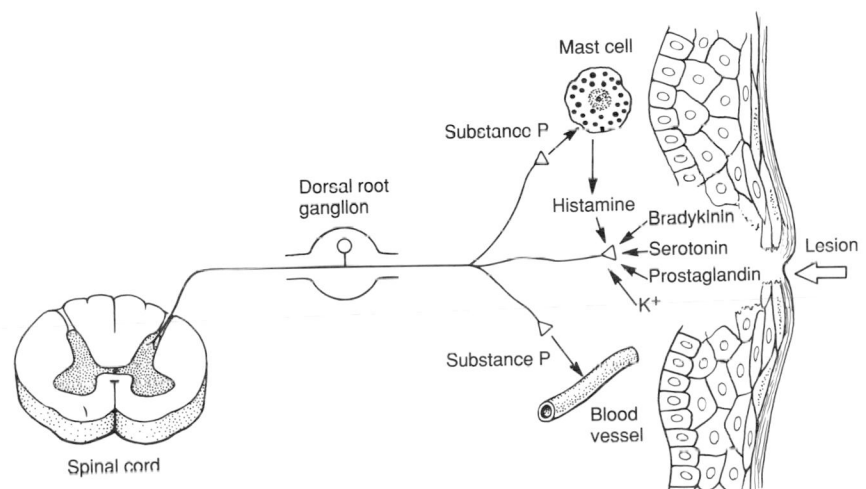

FIGURE 27–2
Chemical mediators can sensitize and sometimes activate the peripheral endings of nociceptors. Injury or tissue damage releases bradykinin (**BK**) and prostaglandins (**PG**), both of which activate and sensitize nociceptors. Activation of nociceptors leads to the release of substance P (**SP**) and other peptides. Substance P acts on mast cells in the vicinity of sensory endings to evoke degranulation and the release of histamine, which directly excites nociceptors. Substance P also produces dilation of peripheral blood vessels, and the resultant edema causes a further liberation of bradykinin. (See Table 27–1 for a list of chemicals that act on nociceptors.) (Adapted from Lembeck and Gamse, 1982, and Fields, 1987.)

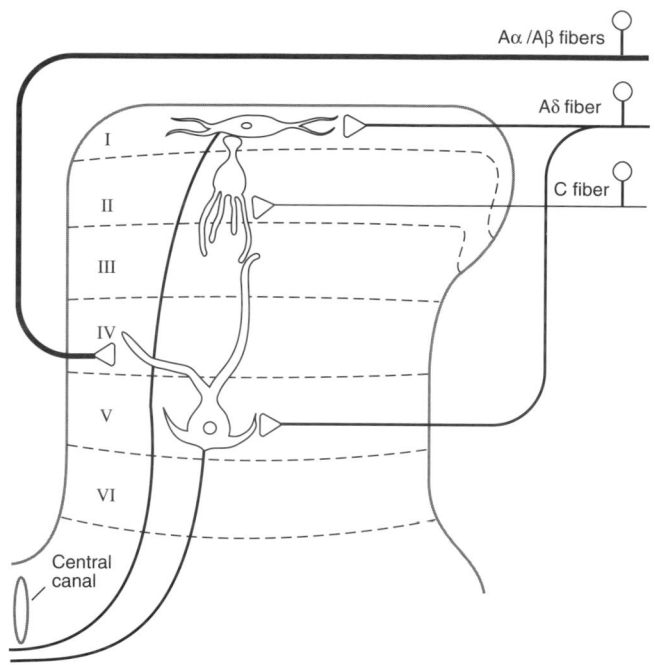

FIGURE 27–3

The afferent fibers of nociceptors terminate on projection neurons in the dorsal horn of the spinal cord. Projection neurons in lamina I receive direct input from myelinated (Aδ fiber) nociceptors and indirect input from unmyelinated (C fiber) nociceptors via stalk cell interneurons in lamina II. Lamina V neurons are predominately of the wide dynamic range type. They receive low-threshold input from large-diameter myelinated fibers (Aα) of mechanoreceptors as well as both direct and indirect input from nociceptive afferents (Aδ and C). In this figure the lamina V neuron sends a dendrite up through lamina IV, where it is contacted by the terminal of an Aα primary afferent. A lamina V cell dendrite in lamina III is contacted by the axon terminal of a lamina II interneuron. (Adapted from Fields, 1987.)

burning pain. This condition is called *causalgia* or *reflex sympathetic dystrophy syndrome*. In contrast to deafferentation pain, causalgic pain can be relieved by blocking sympathetic activity or depleting catecholamines from sympathetic nerve terminals. Sympathetic efferent activity is thought to cause pain by direct activation of damaged nociceptive afferents or by nonsynaptic electrical cross-talk (ephaptic transmission).

Pain Syndromes Can Result From Surgery Intended to Alleviate Pain

Over the years surgical intervention to treat pain has been attempted at every level of the nervous system, from the primary afferent fiber to the cortex. These surgical procedures are not very successful. Even when surgery is initially successful, the pain can return. The new sensations are unpleasant, often unlike anything the patients had ever felt before: spontaneous aching and shooting pain, numbness, cold, heaviness, burning, and other unsettling sensations that even the most articulate patients find difficult to describe. Central pain syndromes often cause more distress than the pain the operation was intended to relieve.

Many instances of chronic pain result from spontaneous lesions to central sites in nociceptive pathways. In 1906 Joseph Dejerine and Gustave Roussy described several cases of intractable pain resulting from vascular damage to the central nervous system. Autopsy revealed lesions in multiple regions of the thalamus, in particular the ventrobasal complex. As a consequence, they described this pain condition as the *thalamic syndrome*. Central pain syndromes are most commonly caused by lesions in the thalamus, but lesions can occur elsewhere in the ascending nociceptive pathway.

FIGURE 27–4

Signals from nociceptors in the viscera can be felt as pain elsewhere in the body. The source of the pain can be readily predicted from the site of referred pain.

A. Areas of deep referred pain in myocardial infarction and angina. (From Teodori and Galletti, 1962.)

B. Convergence of visceral and somatic afferents may account for referred pain. According to this hypothesis, afferent fibers from nociceptors in the viscera and afferents from specific areas of the periphery converge on the same projection neurons in the dorsal horn. The brain has no way of knowing the actual source of the noxious stimulus and mistakenly identifies the sensation with the peripheral structure. (Adapted from Fields, 1987.)

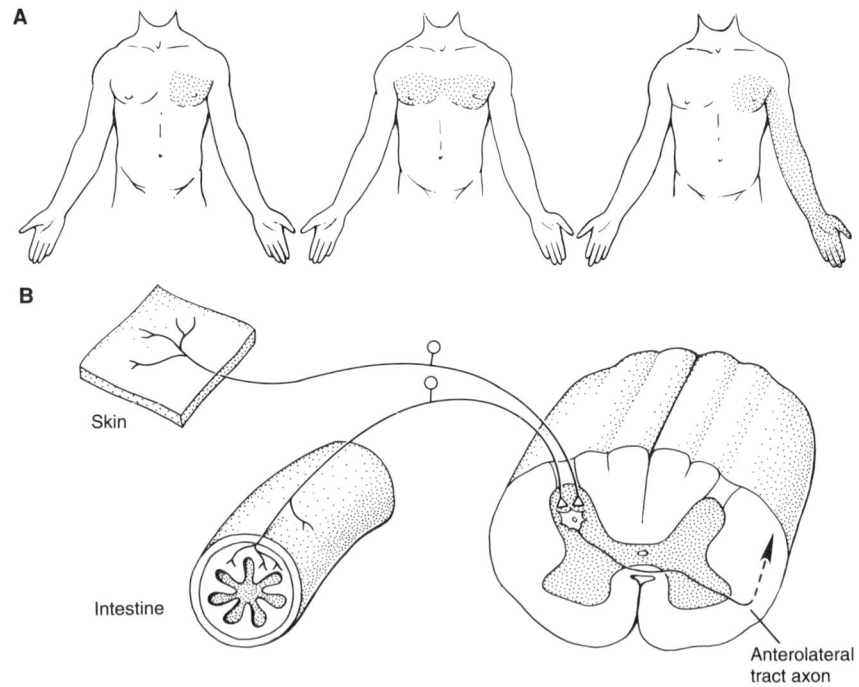

Primary Afferent Fibers Synapse with Dorsal Horn Neurons

Both Aδ and C nociceptive fibers bifurcate upon entering the spinal cord. Branches of these axons ascend and descend for a few segments as part of the tract of Lissauer, while axon collaterals synapse with neurons in the dorsal horn. Nociceptive fibers terminate primarily in the superficial dorsal horn, which comprises the marginal zone (lamina I) and the substantia gelatinosa (lamina II). Some Aδ nociceptive fibers also project more deeply and terminate in lamina V (Figure 27–3).

Nociceptive afferents form direct or indirect connections with three major classes of neurons in the dorsal horn: (1) projection neurons that relay incoming sensory information to higher centers in the brain; (2) local excitatory interneurons that relay sensory input to projection neurons; and (3) inhibitory interneurons that regulate the flow of nociceptive information to higher centers.

Lamina I of the dorsal horn contains a high density of projection neurons that process nociceptive information (Figure 27–3). One class is excited solely by nociceptors (both Aδ and C fibers) and is termed *nociceptive specific*. Other projection neurons in lamina I receive input from low-threshold mechanoreceptors in addition to those from nociceptors. These cells are termed *wide dynamic range* neurons. A second major population of wide dynamic range projection neurons is located in lamina V–VI.

Understanding the organization of afferent input to dorsal horn neurons is important in interpreting many clinical pain syndromes. For example, the organization of the cutaneous and visceral somatic sensory systems helps explain *referred pain*, pain that arises from nociceptors in deep visceral structures but is felt at sites on the body surface. The displacement of the pain to certain areas of the body is quite stereotyped. For example, patients with myocardial infarction frequently report pain not only from the chest but also from the left arm (Figure 27–4).

One possible mechanism of referred pain is the convergence of visceral and cutaneous nociceptors onto the same dorsal horn projection neurons, as first shown by Alden Spencer and Michael Seltzer. Since a single projection neuron receives both inputs, higher centers cannot distinguish the source of the input and incorrectly attribute the pain to the skin, perhaps because the cutaneous input normally predominates. The branching pattern of peripheral sensory neurons may account for some instances of referred pain, since one branch innervates visceral structures and the other a remote cutaneous site.

Primary Afferent Fibers Use Amino Acids and Peptides As Transmitters

Since nociceptive signals in the dorsal horn are transmitted by chemical means, identifying the chemical transmitters helps to understand how nociceptive information is transmitted to the brain. Indeed, if the transmitter used by nociceptors were distinct from transmitters used by other classes of sensory afferents, we might be able to design selective pharmacological blockades for specific

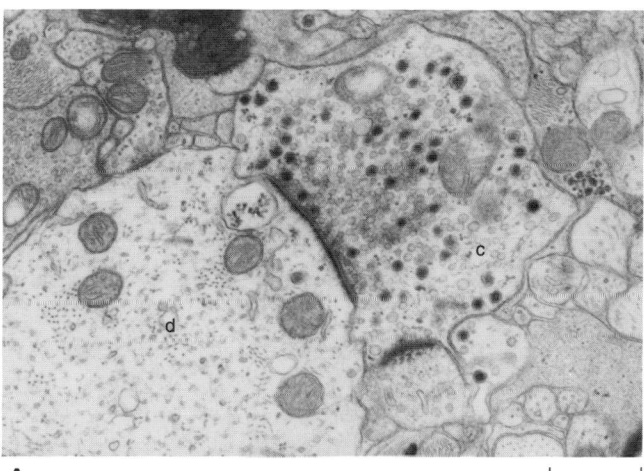

A   0.5 μm

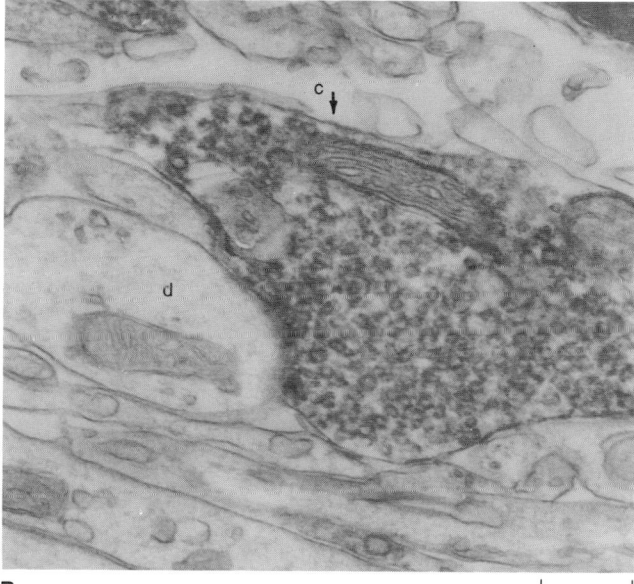

B   0.5 μm

FIGURE 27–5

Electron micrographs of synapses formed by nociceptive afferent neurons with substantia gelatinosa neurons in the dorsal horn of the spinal cord.

A. Synapse of an afferent C fiber terminal on the dendrite (**d**) of a dorsal horn neuron. Two classes of synaptic vesicles in the primary afferent terminal contain different transmitters. Small electron-translucent vesicles contain glutamate, while large dense-core vesicles contain neuropeptides. (Courtesy of H. J. Ralston, III.)

B. Localization of substance P in a C fiber afferent terminal in the dorsal horn. The electron-dense immunoreaction product is confined to large dense-core vesicles. (Courtesy of J. Priestley.)

pain syndromes. Ultrastructural studies of nociceptor terminals suggest that several different neurotransmitters are released by nociceptors. The terminals of Aδ nociceptive afferents include small electron-translucent synaptic vesicles that are thought to contain excitatory amino acids,

A Substance P

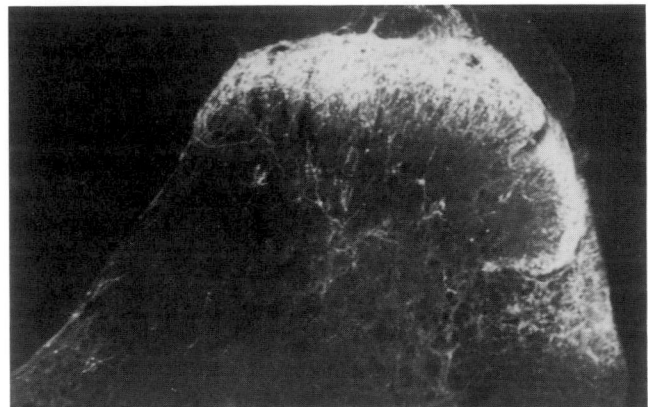

B Enkephalin

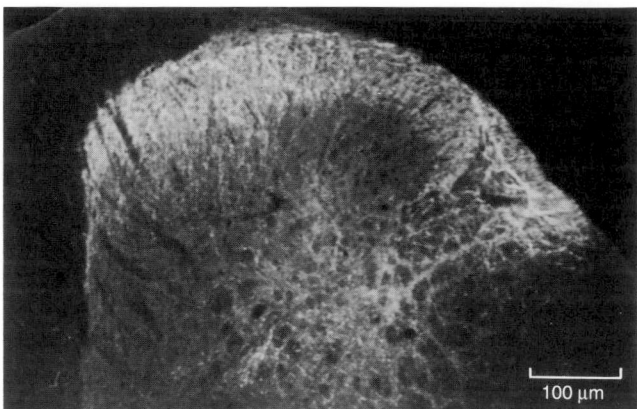

100 µm

FIGURE 27–6

Localization of peptides to the superficial dorsal horn of the spinal cord. (Courtesy of S. P. Hunt and J. Priestly.)

A. Substance P is concentrated in primary afferent terminals located in the superficial dorsal horn.

B. Enkephalin is localized in interneurons concentrated in the superficial dorsal horn, in the same region as afferent terminals containing substance P.

whereas the terminals of C fibers contain, in addition to the small clear vesicles, large dense-core vesicles known to store peptides (Figure 27–5).

Electrophysiological studies reveal that both Aδ and C fibers release an excitatory transmitter that evokes fast synaptic potentials in superficial dorsal horn neurons. The most likely candidate for this transmitter is glutamate. Pharmacological studies show that synaptic transmission is blocked by antagonists of excitatory amino acid receptors. Since glutamate also appears to be the transmitter at Ia afferent synapses with motor neurons, the same transmitter may be released from primary afferents conveying quite different sensory modalities.

Nociceptive afferents also elicit slow excitatory postsynaptic potentials through the release of a second class of transmitter, most likely peptides. C fibers and possibly Aδ fibers release a large variety of neuropeptides (Figure 27–6). Of these, the actions of substance P have been studied in most detail. Application of substance P to dorsal horn neurons evokes slow synaptic potentials that mimic those produced by high-intensity stimulation of primary afferents. Therefore, more than one type of transmitter may be released from the central terminals of nociceptors, in particular C fibers. This in turn may account for the existence of fast and slow excitatory postsynaptic potentials in dorsal horn neurons.

Nociceptive Information Is Conveyed to the Brain Along Several Ascending Pathways

Nociceptive input to the dorsal horn is relayed to higher centers in the brain by projection neurons. William Willis and others have shown that in primates nociceptive information is carried by five major ascending pathways that originate in different laminae of the dorsal horn.

1. The *spinothalamic tract* is the most prominent ascending nociceptive pathway in the spinal cord and originates from neurons in laminae I and V–VII. It is composed of the axons of nociceptive-specific and wide-dynamic-range neurons that terminate in the thalamus. It crosses the midline and ascends in the anterolateral white matter on the contralateral side (Figure 27–7).

2. The axons of nociceptive neurons in laminae VII and VIII make up the *spinoreticular tract*, which also ascends in the anterolateral quadrant of the spinal cord (Figure 27–7). In contrast to the spinothalamic tract, all the fibers of which cross the midline, some spinoreticular fibers form uncrossed projections. Some axons in this tract send branches that terminate in both the reticular formation and the thalamus.

3. Nociceptive neurons in laminae I and V project in the *spinomesencephalic tract* to the mesencephalic reticular formation, the lateral part of the periaqueductal gray region, and other midbrain sites (Figure 27–7). The periaqueductal gray region has reciprocal connections with the limbic system through the hypothalamus.

4. Most neurons in laminae III or IV of the dorsal horn respond solely to tactile stimuli, but some are also activated by noxious stimuli. Neurons in these two laminae project through the *spinocervical tract*, which runs in the dorsolateral spinal cord to the lateral cervical nucleus, a small cluster of neurons lateral to the dorsal horn in the upper cervical segments of the spinal cord. Axons from this nucleus cross the midline and ascend in the medial lemniscus in the brain stem to midbrain nuclei and to the thalamus (ventroposterior lateral and posterior medial nuclei).

5. Finally, some of the nociceptive neurons in laminae III and IV project their axons in the dorsal column of the spinal cord, along with the axon collaterals of large-diameter myelinated primary afferent fibers, to the cuneate and gracile nuclei in the medulla.

Spinothalamic   Spinoreticular   Spinomesencephalic

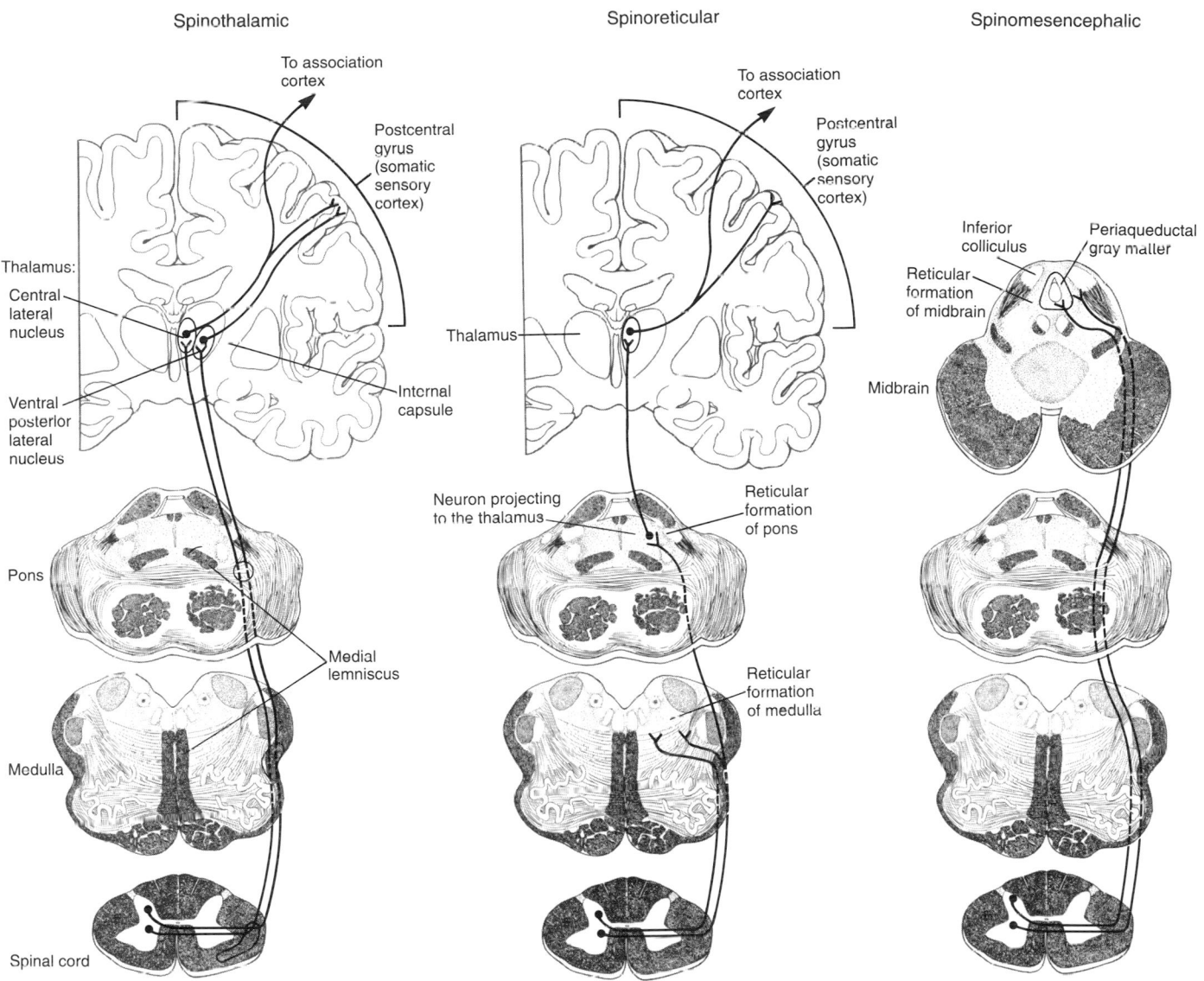

FIGURE 27–7
Three major ascending pathways transmit nociceptive information from the dorsal horn of the spinal cord to higher centers. (Adapted from Willis, 1985.)

Of these five tracts the spinothalamic has been studied in most detail, in part because of clinical evidence that lesions of this tract result in marked deficits in pain sensation, and also because electrical stimulation of the tract results in pain. Two major subdivisions of thalamic nuclei receive nociceptive input from spinal projection neurons. The *medial nuclear group*, which includes the central lateral nucleus and the intralaminar complex, receives its major input from neurons in laminae VI–VIII, which have large complex receptive fields. The *lateral nuclear group*, which includes the ventrobasal nucleus and the posterior nuclei, receives input primarily from nociceptive-specific and wide-dynamic-range neurons in laminae I and V. In

addition, the medial thalamus receives major somatosensory input from neurons in laminae VI–VIII by way of the reticular formation. This indirect pathway is bilateral and includes the spinoreticular tract that terminates in the medullary reticular formation and the subsequent reticular projection to the medial thalamus.

The response properties of neurons in the two major subdivisions of the thalamus that receive nociceptive input are similar to those of the spinothalamic neurons that synapse on them. Thus, some neurons in the ventrobasal complex in the lateral thalamus respond exclusively to noxious peripheral stimuli, and others respond to a wide range of somatosensory stimuli. Although many neurons in the medial thalamus respond optimally to noxious stimuli, the widespread projections of these neurons (to the basal ganglia and many different cortical areas) indicate that this region is not exclusively concerned with processing nociceptive information, but is part of a non-specific arousal system.

In vertebrate evolution, the indirect spinoreticular pathway appeared before the direct spinothalamic projection. The pathway to the medial thalamus was the first direct spinothalamic projection to appear and thus is also known as the *paleo*spinothalamic tract. The lateral thalamic projection to the ventrobasal nucleus, also known as the *neo*spinothalamic tract, is most developed in primates. Neurons in the medial intralaminar thalamus project diffusely to several regions of the ipsilateral cortex, whereas neurons in the lateral thalamic nuclei project directly to the primary somatosensory cortex, suggesting that there may be several pathways that process nociceptive information from the thalamus to the cortex.

Although we know a lot about the cortical processing of tactile, auditory, and visual information, there is still uncertainty about how the cortex processes pain. Two classes of neurons in the somatosensory cortex respond to noxious peripheral stimuli through inputs relayed through the thalamus. One class has a small contralateral receptive field and receives input from the ventrobasal bilateral nucleus in the lateral thalamus. The other class has a much more diffuse and bilaterally located receptive field and probably receives input from medial (intralaminar) thalamic nuclei. However, no orderly arrangement has been detected for nociceptive inputs to the cortex similar to the maps of tactile inputs. Moreover, clinical studies indicate that damage to large areas of the somatosensory cortex does not result in impaired responses to noxious stimuli or loss of pain. One difficulty in mapping nociceptive inputs to the cortex is that the thalamic nuclei that receive input from spinal nociceptive neurons project to different regions of the somatosensory cortex. Thus, as with other sensory modalities, there may be parallel or distributed processing of nociceptive information in the cortex.

Pain Can Be Modulated by the Balance of Activity Between Nociceptive and Other Afferent Inputs

Thus far, we have discussed the anatomical pathways involved in the transmission of nociceptive information from the periphery to the central nervous system. The variable nature of pain responses, however, suggests that there must be modulatory systems within the central nervous system that regulate pain. The activity of neurons in the spinal cord that receive input from nociceptive fibers may be modified by inputs from other nonnociceptive afferents.

In the early 1960s neurophysiological studies provided evidence that stimulation of low-threshold myelinated primary afferent fibers decreases the response of dorsal horn neurons to unmyelinated nociceptors, whereas blockade of conduction in myelinated fibers enhances the response of dorsal horn neurons. The firing of certain spinal cord neurons may therefore not simply be regarded by the level of activity in nociceptive afferent input but by the balance of activity between the unmyelinated nociceptors and the myelinated afferents not directly concerned with pain. This idea was introduced by Patrick Wall and Ronald Melzack as the *gate control theory*.

According to this theory, the neurons involved in modifying the output of dorsal horn neurons comprise low-threshold Aα/Aβ myelinated and unmyelinated C fibers, the dorsal horn projection neuron that relays incoming signals to the brain, and an inhibitory interneuron that inhibits the projection neuron. The projection neuron is directly activated by both the low-threshold myelinated and unmyelinated fibers. The crucial difference in the inputs from these two classes of afferents is that the myelinated fibers also activate the inhibitory interneuron, whereas the unmyelinated inputs suppress its activity (Figure 27–8). Thus, when low-threshold myelinated fibers are activated, the activity of the projection neuron (and thus the perception of pain) is reduced.

When the gate control theory was first introduced it provided a rational interpretation of previously confusing clinical observations. Moreover, some of its predictions

FIGURE 27–8
One explanation for the modulation of pain is the gate control hypothesis. This hypothesis focuses upon interactions of four classes of neurons in the dorsal horn of the spinal cord: (1) unmyelinated nociceptive afferents (C fiber), (2) myelinated non-nociceptive afferents (Aα/Aβ), (3) projection neurons, whose activity results in the sensation of pain, and (4) inhibitory interneurons. The inhibitory interneuron is spontaneously active and normally inhibits the projection neuron, thus reducing the intensity of pain. It is excited by the myelinated nonnociceptive afferent but inhibited by the unmyelinated nociceptor. The nociceptor thus has both direct and indirect effects on the projection neuron.

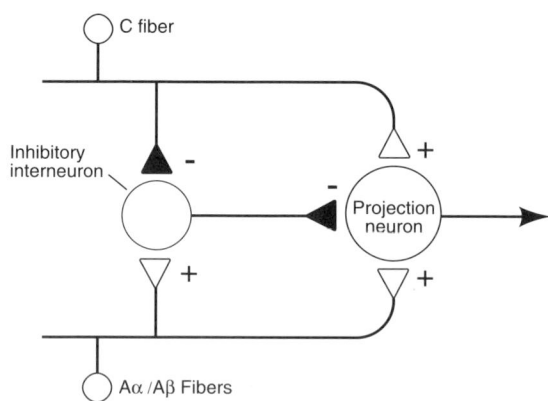

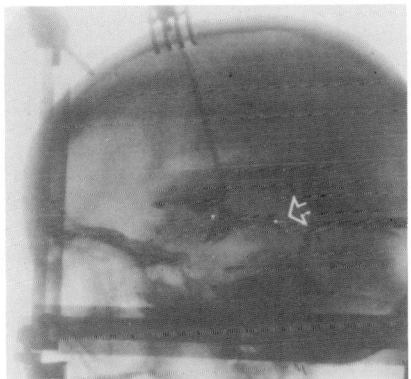

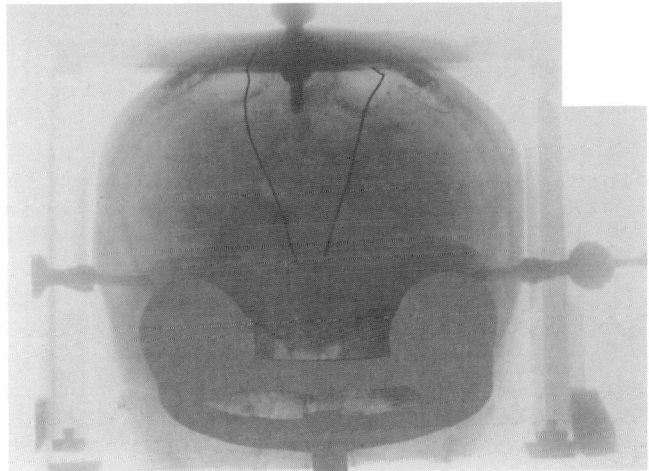

FIGURE 27–9
Stereotaxic method of electrode implantation in a human subject with chronic pain. The **top** radiograph shows a lateral view of a patient's cranium in the stereotaxic frame. Radiopaque medium is used to reveal the ventricular system. The target for placement of the electrodes is lateral to the point where the cerebral aqueduct meets the caudal end of the third ventricle **(arrow)**. The **bottom** radiograph, an anterior–posterior view of the same patient, shows the electrodes in place. (Courtesy of J. E. Adams, as shown in Fields, 1987.)

have led to effective clinical therapies. For example, the hypothesis that stimulation of the myelinated dorsal column fibers suppresses the pain transmission cell led to the successful practice of stimulating axons in the dorsal column and peripheral nerves transcutaneously as a way of relieving pain.

Pain Can Be Controlled by Central Mechanisms

The gate control theory introduced the idea that pain perception is sensitive to levels of activity in both nociceptive and nonnociceptive afferent fibers. It is also important to realize that nociceptive signals can also be modulated at successive synaptic relays along the central pathway. An additional advance has been the characterization of major pain control pathways that descend to the spinal cord from the brain. Here we outline five convergent lines of research that provide new information about these central mechanisms of pain control: (1) the finding that direct brain stimulation can suppress nociception; (2) the mapping of descending nociceptive control pathways; (3) the localization of morphine-sensitive sites in the brain; (4) the characterization of opiate receptors; and (5) the discovery of endogenous opioid peptides.

Direct Electrical Stimulation of the Brain Produces Analgesia

Damage to many regions of the central nervous system can result in increases in the firing rate of neurons and the perception of pain. However, in experimental animals stimulation of the gray matter that surrounds the third ventricle, cerebral aqueduct, and fourth ventricle can instead result in profound analgesia. In human patients stimulating electrodes placed for therapeutic reasons in the periventricular gray region, the ventrobasal complex of the thalamus, or the internal capsule reduce the severity of pain (Figure 27–9). This type of stimulation produces a profound suppression of activity in nociceptive pathways (analgesia). These subjects do not lose tactile sensibility—they still respond to touch, pressure, and temperature within the body area in which they are analgesic—but they feel less pain.

Nociceptive Control Pathways Descend to the Spinal Cord

Soon after stimulation-produced analgesia was discovered, the neural pathway that mediates this effect was defined. Two findings pointed to the existence of a descending inhibitory pathway that terminates on nociceptive neurons in the spinal cord. First, brain stem stimulation was found to inhibit nociceptive neurons in the dorsal horn of the spinal cord. Second, lesions of the dorsolateral funiculus abolished the suppression of pain responses evoked by brain stem stimulation.

The descending pathway modulating pain has three major components (Figure 27–10).

1. Neurons in the periventricular and periaqueductal gray matter in the midbrain make excitatory connections in the rostroventral medulla, a region that includes the serotonergic nucleus raphe magnus and the adjacent nucleus reticularis paragigantocellularis.
2. Neurons in the rostroventral medulla make inhibitory connections in laminae I, II, and V of the dorsal horn; these laminae are also the site of termination of nociceptive afferent neurons. Stimulation of these rostroventral medullary neurons inhibits dorsal horn neurons, including spinothalamic tract neurons that respond to noxious stimulation. Other descending fiber systems that originate in the medulla and pons also terminate in the superficial dorsal horn and suppress activity in nociceptive dorsal horn neurons.
3. Local circuits in the dorsal horn mediate the modulatory actions of the descending pathways. The organization of these local circuits is considered later in the chapter.

Opiate Analgesia Involves the Same Pathways As Stimulation-Produced Analgesia

Administration of low doses of opiates directly into specific regions of the rodent brain produces a powerful analgesia. The analgesic effects of systematically administered opiates are mediated not by acting on pain receptors in the periphery, but by direct actions on the central nervous system. The sites in the brain at which morphine is effective overlap with those used to evoke stimulation-produced analgesia. Thus, both the periaqueductal gray region and rostroventral medulla are highly sensitive to morphine (Figure 27–10). Moreover, administration of the narcotic antagonist naloxone into the periaqueductal gray region or rostroventral medulla blocks the analgesia produced by systemic administration of morphine. These observations suggested that opiates produce analgesia by activating the descending pain modulatory pathways.

Endogenous Opioid Peptides and Their Receptors Are Located at Key Points in the Pain Modulatory System

Two advances have greatly increased our understanding of the role of opioid systems in the modulation of nociception and pain perception. First was the demonstration by Solomon Snyder and Candace Pert, and independently by Lars Terenius and by Eric Simon, that morphine and related alkaloids exert their physiological actions by binding to specific membrane receptors. Second, John Hughes and

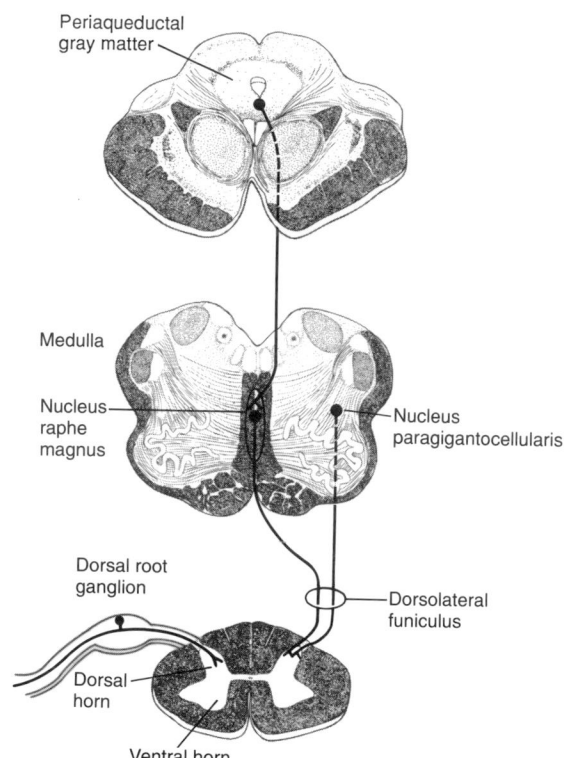

FIGURE 27–10
Interconnections of neural structures that contribute to control of nociceptive relay neurons in the spinal cord. The network includes connections from the midbrain periaqueductal gray region to the medullary nucleus raphe magnus and other serotonergic nuclei (not shown) via the dorsolateral funiculus, to the dorsal horn of the spinal cord. Additional spinal projections arise from the nucleus paragigantocellularis, which also receives input from the periaqueductal gray region, and the noradrenergic pontine and medullary cell groups. In the spinal cord these descending pathways inhibit nociceptive projection neurons through direct connections as well as through interneurons in the superficial layers of the dorsal horn. There is evidence that endorphin-containing interneurons in the periaqueductal gray region and the dorsal horn play an active role in pain modulation.

Hans Kosterlitz found that the brain contains endogenous opioid peptides.

There are three classes of endogenous opioid peptides. The first, identified by Hughes and Kosterlitz, is the enkephalins, two small peptides isolated from pig brain. The second class, discovered by Derek Smythe and Chao Ho Li, belongs to the proopiomelanocortin (POMC) family. The POMC precursor is expressed in the pituitary, and its peptide products are released into the blood stream in response to stress. The third class, discovered by Avram Goldstein and colleagues, belongs to the dynorphin family. Many other peptides with opioid activity have now been discovered, virtually all of which contain the sequence Tyr-Gly-Gly-Phe (Table 27–2).

Each of the endogenous opioids derives from one of three genes that encode the large polyprotein precursors of

TABLE 27–2. Amino Acid Sequences of Endogenous Opioid Peptides

Name	Amino acid sequence
Leucine-enkephalin	*Tyr-Gly-Gly-Phe*-Leu-OH
Methioine-enkephalin	*Tyr-Gly-Gly-Phe*-Met-OH
β-Endorphin	*Tyr-Gly-Gly Phe*-Met Thr-Ser-Glu-Lys-Ser-Gln-Thr-Pro-Leu-Val-Thr-Leu-Phe-Lys-Asn-Ala-Ile-Val-Lys-Asn-Ala-His-Lys Gly-Gln-OH
Dynorphin	*Tyr-Gly-Gly-Phe*-Leu-Arg-Arg-Ile-Arg-Pro-Lys-Leu-Lys-Trp-Asp-Asn-Gln-OH
α-Neoendorphin	*Tyr-Gly-Gly-Phe*-Leu-Arg-Lys-Tyr-Pro-Lys

(From Fields, 1987.)

the physiologically active peptides. These three genes are the POMC proenkephalin, and prodynorphin genes (Figure 27-11). Each of the five opioid peptides listed in Table 27–2 causes analgesia, although the enkephalins and β-endorphin are more potent than dynorphin.

Although the anatomical distributions of the peptides encoded by the three opioid genes differ, members of each family are located at sites associated with the processing or modulation of nociception. Enkephalin- and dynorphin-containing neuronal cell bodies and nerve terminals are found in the periaqueductal gray matter and rostroventral medulla and in the dorsal horn of the spinal cord, in particular in laminae I and II. In contrast, β-endorphin has a more restricted distribution and is confined primarily to neurons in the hypothalamus that send projections to the periaqueductal gray region and to noradrenergic nuclei in the brain stem.

Morphine and the opioid peptides bind to distinct subclasses of opiate receptors that have been defined on the basis of their ligand binding properties. There are three major classes of opiate receptors: *mu, delta,* and *kappa.* Opiate alkaloids, such as morphine, are potent agonists of the *mu* receptor. The endogenous enkephalins are active at both *mu* and *delta* receptors, and dynorphin is an agonist of the *kappa* receptor. Each of the three receptors is widely distributed throughout the central nervous system, suggesting that endogenous opioid systems are involved in physiological functions other than pain modulation. High levels of *mu* receptors are found in the periaqueductal gray region and in the superficial dorsal horn of the spinal cord,

FIGURE 27–11

The three families of endogenous opioid peptides. Each of the precursor molecules gives rise to multiple biologically active peptide fragments, about half of which are shown in this diagram.

A. Proopiomelanocortin (POMC) is so named because it gives rise to β-endorphin (β-endo), melanocyte-stimulating hormone (MSH), adrenocorticotropic hormone (ACTH), and corticotropin-like intermediate lobe peptide (CLIP).

B. Proenkephalin (pro-enk) gives rise to multiple copies of met-enkephalin (ME), a leucine-enkephalin (LE), and several extended enkephalins including ME-Arg-Gly-Leu (ME-RGL), ME-Arg-Phe (ME-RF), and peptides E, F, and B. Peptide E is further broken down into a family of large enkephalins that appear to be the most potent analgesic fragments derived from proenkephalin.

C. Prodynorphin (pro-dyn) gives rise to dynorphin (dyno), which contains the LE sequence, and neoendorphin (α-neo endo). (From Fields, 1987.)

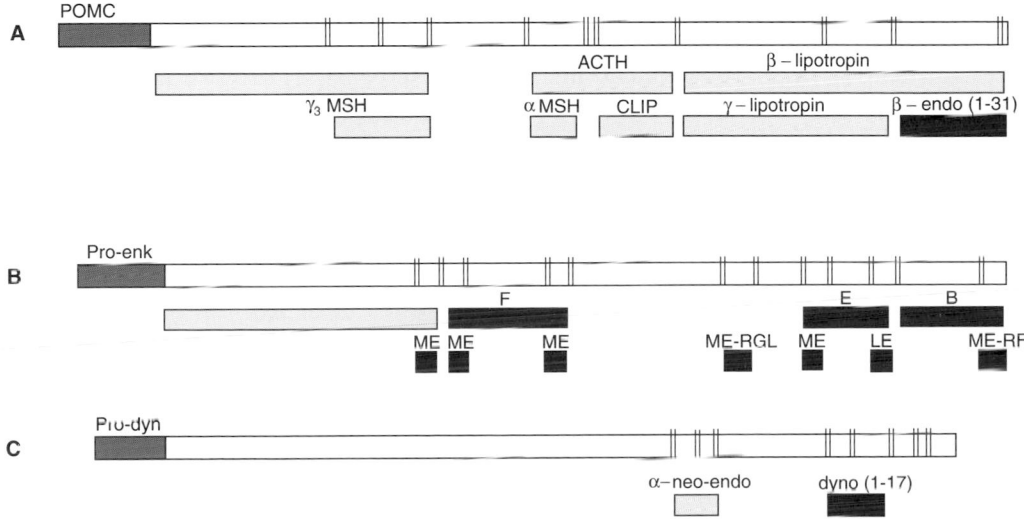

coincident with the distribution of enkephalin-containing neurons. Functional opioid systems are located in several regions of the brain involved in modulating nociception.

Opiate antagonists that are used clinically, such as naloxone, are structural analogs of morphine and consequently are most effective in antagonizing opiate actions at *mu* receptors. There is a good correlation between analgesic potency and agonist affinity at the *mu* receptor. This is not surprising since the *mu* receptor was originally defined by its affinity for analgesic compounds. In experimental studies *kappa* agonists suppress nociceptive responses after noxious mechanical stimulation, whereas *mu* agonists are most effective in analgesic tests that use noxious thermal stimuli. Different classes of opiate receptors may therefore be involved in modulating the activity of different classes of nociceptive afferent inputs.

Supraspinal and Spinal Networks Coordinately Modulate Nociceptive Transmission

Considerable progress in identifying the neurotransmitter systems involved in the modulation of nociception has also been made in the last decade. Many of the rostroventral medullary neurons that project to the spinal cord use serotonin as a transmitter. A second major descending pathway from the pons uses norepinephrine. The descending serotonergic pathway and noradrenergic pathways are a crucial link in the supraspinal modulation of nociceptive transmission. Destroying these neurons with neurotoxins or electrolytic lesions reduces or blocks the analgesic actions of systemically administered opiates. Similarly, the analgesia elicited by supraspinal administration of morphine can be reduced by applying serotonin receptor antagonists to the spinal cord. In addition, direct application of serotonin or norepinephrine to the spinal cord produces analgesia. These studies establish that the supraspinal analgesic actions of opiates are mediated in part through a descending monoaminergic projection to the spinal cord.

As discussed above, there is overlap between the supraspinal sites at which morphine is effective in eliciting analgesia and the locations at which stimulation-produced analgesia is effective. These findings indicate that morphine activates descending pathways that control nociceptive inputs. The activation of these pathways by morphine is thought to suppress the activity of an interneuron that releases γ-aminobutyric acid (GABA) and normally inhibits the activity of the descending pathways. In this way opiates activate descending projection neurons by a disinhibitory mechanism.

Opiates also exert a direct analgesic action on the spinal cord. For example, morphine can inhibit the firing of dorsal horn neurons in animals with spinal transections. Analgesia can also be produced by intrathecal injection of opiates into the subarachnoid space surrounding the spinal cord. Intrathecal opiate injection is used in certain pain states, for example to relieve labor pain. Intrathecal application of opiates reduces the incidence of respiratory

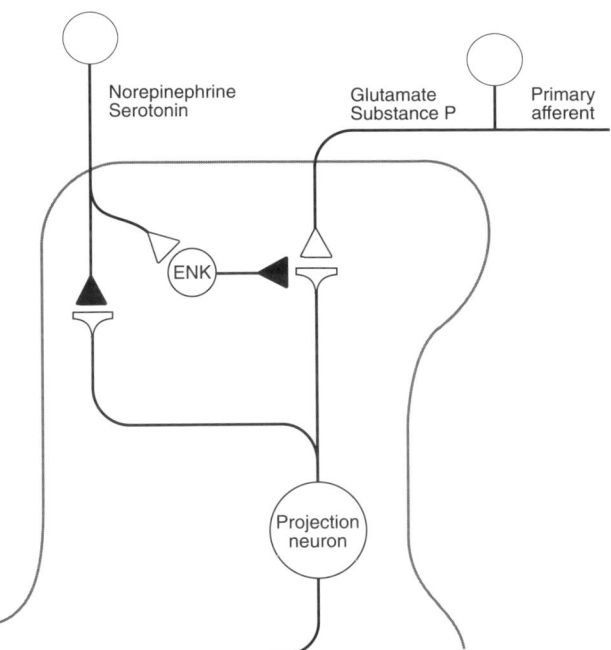

FIGURE 27–12

Possible interactions between primary afferents, local interneurons, and descending neurons in the dorsal horn of the spinal cord. Primary afferent fibers terminate on second-order spinothalamic projection neurons. Local enkephalin-containing interneurons (**ENK**) exert both presynaptic and postsynaptic inhibitory actions at primary afferent synapses. Descending brain stem neurons release serotonin, which activates local opioid interneurons and also suppresses the activity of spinothalamic tract neurons.

depression and other side effects of the actions of opiates in the brain stem.

These functional studies reinforce the idea derived from mapping the distribution of opioid peptides and opiate receptors that the analgesic actions of opiates is widespread in the central nervous system. The final output of these networks is the spinal cord, and we will now consider how the descending pathways interconnect with local spinal circuits to modulate incoming nociceptive sensory signals.

Local Dorsal Horn Circuits Modulate Afferent Nociceptive Input

Local circuits in the dorsal horn of the spinal cord play a critical role in processing nociceptive afferent input and in mediating the actions of descending pain modulating systems. The descending axons of serotonergic and noradrenergic neurons contact the dendrites of spinothalamic tract neurons and also local enkephalin-containing inhibitory interneurons in the superficial dorsal horn (Figure 27–12). Thus, the descending inhibition of spinothalamic tract neurons is likely to be mediated in part by the activation of enkephalin interneurons in the dorsal horn.

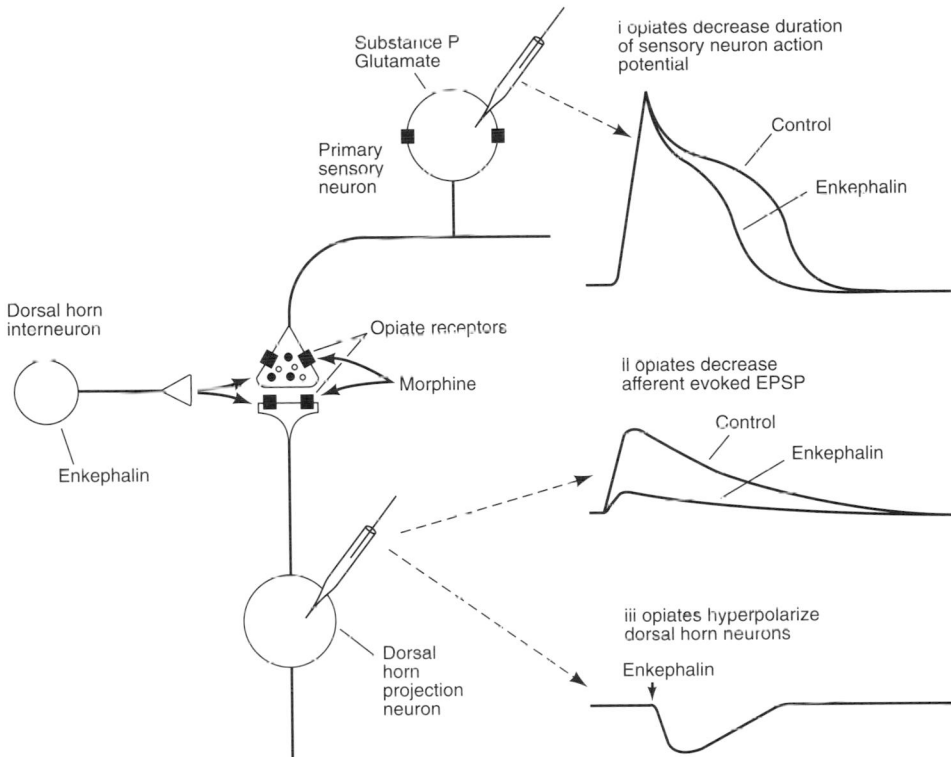

FIGURE 27–13

Electrophysiological analysis of the actions of opiates on sensory and dorsal horn neurons. A primary afferent neuron makes contact with a postsynaptic dorsal horn neuron. Opiates decrease the duration of the sensory neuron action potential, probably by decreased Ca^{2+} influx. Opiates may have a similar action at the terminals of the sensory neuron. Opiates hyperpolarize the membrane of dorsal horn neurons by activating a K^+ conductance. Stimulation of the sensory neuron normally produces a fast excitatory postsynaptic potential in the dorsal horn neuron, opiates decrease the amplitude of the postsynaptic potential.

How do endogenous opioid circuits and exogenous opiates regulate nociceptive transmission in the dorsal horn? The superficial dorsal horn contains a high density of enkephalin- and dynorphin-containing interneurons close to the terminals of nociceptive afferents and to the dendrites of the dorsal horn neurons that receive nociceptive afferent input. *Mu* opiate receptors are located both on the terminals of nociceptive afferents and on the dendrites of postsynaptic neurons. Pharmacological studies indicate that opiates and opioid peptides regulate nociceptive transmission in part by inhibiting the release of glutamate, substance P, and other transmitters from the sensory neurons. Transmitter release is suppressed by activation of opiate receptors on the sensory neurons, which decreases Ca^{2+} entry into the sensory terminal, either indirectly by activating K^+ conductances or directly by decreasing Ca^{2+} conductance (Figure 27–13).

Opiates also act postsynaptically at afferent synapses to suppress the activity of nociceptive dorsal horn neurons. Since most enkephalin-containing nerve terminals in the superficial dorsal horn contact the dendrites of postsynaptic neurons, it is likely that opioid peptide circuits are involved in regulating nociceptive transmission, in part by means of a postsynaptic mechanism. However, as with other peptide transmitters, enkephalins may diffuse from

the site of their release to interact with opiate receptors located presynaptically on nociceptive terminals.

It therefore seems likely that opiate alkaloids and endogenous opioid peptides modulate nociceptive transmission at the level of the primary afferent synapse by a combination of presynaptic and postsynaptic actions (Figure 27–13). This again reinforces the idea that opiate analgesia results from actions at multiple distinct neural locations. Sensory, spinal, and descending neurons that converge in the dorsal horn of the spinal cord also contain a variety of other neurotransmitters that are undoubtedly involved in transmitting and modulating nociceptive information. The clinical studies on the opioid and monoaminergic systems, however, highlight the fundamental role played by these two transmitter systems.

Behavioral Stress Can Induce Analgesia Through Both Opioid and Nonopioid Mechanisms

An important part of an organism's response to an emergency is a reduction in responsivity to pain. In meeting the behavioral demands prompted by exposure to stressful situations, such as those involving predation, defense, dominance, or adaptation to an extreme environmental demand, an animal's normal reactions to pain could prove disadvantageous. Pain normally promotes a set of reflex withdrawals, escape, rest, and other recuperative behaviors. During stress these reactions to pain can be suppressed in favor of more adaptive behavior. For example, when a laboratory animal is exposed to a novel and severe adverse stimulus, such as an inescapable electric shock to the foot, its sensitivity to other painful stimuli is reduced. The time course of such stress-induced analgesia may range from minutes to hours, depending on the stimulus used, its severity, and the method selected to measure pain thresholds.

If an animal's natural response to emergency includes diminished sensitivity to pain, then it seems reasonable that the pain inhibitory system we have considered above, which utilizes opioid peptides, might be involved. In support of this, there is evidence that stress can stimulate both opioid- and nonopioid-induced analgesia. Some laboratory examples of stress-induced analgesia are sensitive to opiate receptor blockade by naloxone, but others are not. Naloxone given alone does not cause pain but can significantly enhance the perceived intensity of protracted clinical pain, for example in patients recovering from dental surgery.

There is anecdotal evidence for stress-induced analgesia in humans. Soldiers wounded in battle and athletes injured in sports events report that they do not feel pain. Indeed, a century ago David Livingstone, the Scottish missionary and explorer of Africa, reported a particularly dramatic personal example. On an early journey to find the source of the Nile, Livingstone was attacked by a lion that crushed his shoulder.

. . . I heard a shout. Starting, and looking half round, I saw the lion just in the act of springing upon me. I was upon a little height; he caught my shoulder as he sprang, and we both came to the ground below together. Growling horribly close to my ear, he shook me as a terrier does a rat. The shock produced a stupor similar to that which seems to be felt by a mouse after the first shake of the cat. It caused a sort of dreaminess in which there was no sense of pain nor feeling of terror, though quite conscious of all that was happening. It was like what patients partially under the influence of chloroform describe, who see all the operation, but feel not the knife. . . . The shake annihilated fear, and allowed no sense of horror in looking round at the beast. This peculiar state is probably produced in all animals killed by the carnivora; and if so, is a merciful provision by our benevolent creator for lessening the pain of death.

(David Livingstone, *Missionary Travels*, 1857)

An Overall View

Pain is a highly complex perception. More than any other modality it is influenced by emotions and the environment. Because it is so dependent on experience, and therefore varies from person to person, pain is a difficult clinical problem. Moreover, our current understanding of the anatomy and physiology of specific pain circuits is still fragmentary. Nevertheless, recent advances in understanding the basic physiology of pain mechanisms have led to some effective pain therapies.

First, the finding that the balance of activity in small and large fibers is important in pain transmission led to the use of dorsal column stimulation and transcutaneous electrical nerve stimulation for certain types of peripheral pain. Second, the experimental finding that stimulation of specific sites in the brain stem produces profound analgesia may eventually lead to better ways of controlling pain by activating endogenous pain modulatory systems. Third, the discovery that opiates applied directly to the spinal cord exert potent analgesic effects has led to the use of intrathecal and epidural administration of opiates for certain conditions. Finally, the unraveling of the neurotransmitter systems underlying endogenous pain control circuits may provide a more rational basis for drug therapies in a variety of pain syndromes.

Selected Readings

Akil, H., Watson, S. J., Young, E., Lewis, M. E., Khachaturian, H., and Walker, J. M. 1984. Endogenous opioids: Biology and function. Annu. Rev. Neurosci. 7:223–255.

Basbaum, A. I., and Fields, H. L. 1984. Endogenous pain control systems: Brainstem spinal pathways and endorphin circuitry. Annu. Rev. Neurosci. 7:309–338.

Cassinari, V., and Pagni, C. A. 1969. Central Pain: A Neurosurgical Survey. Cambridge, Mass.: Harvard University Press.

Dubner, R., and Bennett, G. J. 1983. Spinal and trigeminal mechanisms of nociception. Annu. Rev. Neurosci. 6:381–418.

Fields, H. L. 1987. Pain. New York: McGraw-Hill.

Herbert, E., Oates, E., Martens, G., Comb, M., Rosen, H., and Uhler, M. 1983. Generation of diversity and evolution of opioid peptides. Cold Spring Harbor Symp. Quant. Biol. 48:375–384.

Iggo, A., Iversen, L. L., and Cervero, F. (eds.) 1985. Nociception and Pain. London: The Royal Society.

Melzack, R., and Wall, P. D. 1983. The Challenge of Pain. New York: Basic Books.

Terman, G. W., Shavit, Y., Lewis, J. W., Cannon, J. T., and Liebeskind, J. C. 1984. Intrinsic mechanisms of pain inhibition: Activation by stress. Science 226:1270–1277.

Wall, P. D., and Melzack, R. (eds.) 1989. Textbook of Pain, 2nd ed. Edinburgh: Churchill Livingstone.

Willis, W. D., Jr. 1985. The Pain System: The Neural Basis of Nociceptive Transmission in the Mammalian Nervous System. Basel: Karger.

References

Akil, H., Mayer, D. J., and Liebeskind, J. C. 1976. Antagonism of stimulation-produced analgesia by naloxone, a narcotic antagonist. Science 191:961–962.

Bromage, P. R. 1985. Clinical aspects of intrathecal and epidural opiates. In H. L. Fields, R. Dubner, and F. Cervero (eds.), Advances in Pain Research and Therapy, Vol. 9. New York: Raven Press, pp. 733–748.

Campbell, J. N., Raja, S. N., Cohen, R. H., Manning, D. C., Khan, A. A., and Mayer, R. A. 1989. Peripheral neural mechanisms of nociception. In P. D. Wall and R. Melzack (eds.), Textbook of Pain, 2nd ed. Edinburgh: Churchill Livingstone, pp. 22–45.

Carlen, P. L., Wall, P. D., Nadvorna, H., and Steinbach, R. 1978. Phantom limbs and related phenomena in recent traumatic amputations. Neurology 28:211–217.

Cervero, F., and Iggo, A. 1980. The substantia gelatinosa of the spinal cord. A critical review. Brain 103:717–772.

Christensen, B. N., and Perl, E. R. 1970. Spinal neurons specifically excited by noxious or thermal stimuli: Marginal zone of the dorsal horn. J. Neurophysiol. 33:293–307.

Dejerine, J., and Roussy, G. 1906. Le syndrome thalamique. Rev. Neurol. 14:521–532.

Hökfelt, T., Kellerth, J. O., Nilsson, G., and Pernow, B. 1975. Substance P: Localization in the central nervous system and in some primary sensory neurons. Science 190:889–890.

Hosobuchi, Y. 1986. Subcortical electrical stimulation for control of intractable pain in humans: Report of 122 cases (1970–1984). J. Neurosurg. 64:543–553.

Jessell, T. M., and Iversen, L. L. 1977. Opiate analgesics inhibit substance P release from rat trigeminal nucleus. Nature 268: 549–551.

Kuhar, M. J., Pert, C. B., and Snyder, S. H. 1973. Regional distribution of opiate receptor binding in monkey and human brain. Nature 245:447–450.

La Motte, R. H. 1984. Can the sensitization of nociceptors account for hyperalgesia after skin injury? Human Neurobiol. 3:47–52.

Lembeck, F., and Gamse, R. 1982. Substance P in peripheral sensory processes. Ciba Foundation Symp. 91:35–54.

Light, A. R., and Perl, E. R. 1984. Peripheral sensory systems. In P. J. Dyck, P. K. Thomas, E. H. Lambert, and R. Bunge (eds.), Peripheral Neuropathy, 2nd ed, Vol. 1. Philadelphia: Saunders, pp. 210–230.

Melzack, R., and Wall, P. D. 1965. Pain mechanisms: A new theory. Science 150:971–979.

Milne, R. J., Foreman, R. D., Giesler, G. J., Jr., and Willis, W. D. 1981. Convergence of cutaneous and pelvic visceral nociceptive inputs onto primate spinothalamic neurons. Pain 11:163–183.

Mudge, A. W., Leeman, S. E., and Fischbach, G. D. 1979. Enkephalin inhibits release of substance P from sensory neurons in culture and decreases action potential duration. Proc. Natl. Acad. Sci. U.S.A. 76:526–530.

Nashold, B. S., Jr., and Ostdahl, R. H. 1979. Dorsal root entry zone lesions for pain relief. J. Neurosurg. 51:59–69.

Noordenbos, W., and Wall, P. D. 1976. Diverse sensory functions with an almost totally divided spinal cord. A case of spinal cord transection with preservation of part of one anterolateral quadrant. Pain 2:185–195.

Raja, S. N., Campbell, J. N., and Meyer, R. A. 1984. Evidence for different mechanisms of primary and secondary hyperalgesia following heat injury to the glabrous skin. Brain 107:1179–1188.

Roberts, W. J. 1986. A hypothesis on the physiological basis for causalgia and related pains. Pain 24:297–311.

Ruda, M. A., Bennett, G. J., and Dubner, R. 1986. Neurochemistry and neural circuitry in the dorsal horn. Prog. Brain Res. 66: 219–268.

Teodori, U., and Galletti, R. 1962. Il dolore nelle affezioni degli organi interni del torace. Rome: Pozzi.

White, J. C., and Sweet, W. H. 1969. Pain and the Neurosurgeon: A Forty-Year Experience. Springfield, Ill.: Thomas.

Yaksh, T. L., and Noueihed, R. 1985. The physiology and pharmacology of spinal opiates. Annu. Rev. Pharmacol. Toxicol. 25:433–462.

Yaksh, T. L., Jessell, T. M., Gamse, R., Mudge, A. W., and Leeman, S. E. 1980. Intrathecal morphine inhibits substance P release from mammalian spinal cord in vivo. Nature 286:155–157.

Yoshimura, M., and North, R. A. 1983. Substantia gelatinosa neurones hyperpolarized in vitro by enkephalin. Nature 305:529–530.

28

Marc Tessier-Lavigne

Phototransduction and Information Processing in the Retina

The Retina Contains the Eye's Receptor Sheet

There Are Two Types of Photoreceptors:
Rods and Cones

Light Is Absorbed by Visual Pigments in the
Outer Segments of Rods and Cones

**Phototransduction Results from a Cascade of
Biochemical Events in the Outer Segment
of Photoreceptors**

Light Activates Pigment Molecules
in Photoreceptors

Activated Pigment Molecules Affect the
Cytoplasmic Concentration of Cyclic GMP

Cyclic GMP Gates Specialized Ion Channels in
the Plasma Membrane of the Photoreceptor

Closing of Cyclic GMP-Gated Ion Channels
in the Outer Segment Hyperpolarizes
the Photoreceptor

Changes in Intracellular Calcium Underlie
Light Adaptation in Photoreceptors

**Ganglion Cells Are the Output Neurons of
the Retina**

Ganglion Cell Receptive Fields
Have a Center and
Antagonistic Surround

The Properties of Ganglion Cells Enhance the
Ability to Detect Weak Contrasts and
Rapid Changes in the Visual Image

Ganglion Cells Are Also Specialized for
Processing Specific Aspects of the Visual Image

**Bipolar Cells and Other Interneurons Relay Signals
from Photoreceptors to Ganglion Cells**

Cone Signals Are Conveyed to Ganglion Cells
Through Direct or Lateral Pathways

Bipolar Cells Also Have Center-Surround
Receptive Fields

Each Class of Bipolar Cells Has Excitatory
Connections with Ganglion Cells
of the Same Class

Different Pathways Convey Rod Signals to
Ganglion Cells in the Moderately and
Extremely Dark-Adapted Eye

Some Chemical Synapses in the Retina Have
Distinctive Morphologies

An Overall View

Visual perception occurs in two stages. Light entering the cornea is projected onto the back of the eye where it is converted into an electrical signal by a specialized sensory organ, the retina. These signals are then sent through the optic nerve to higher centers in the brain for further processing. In this chapter we shall analyze the neural processing of visual signals in the retina. The next three chapters will be devoted to the processing that occurs in higher centers in the brain.

The retina bears careful examination for several reasons. First, it is a useful model system for understanding sensory transduction. Light is converted into electrical signals by specialized retinal neurons called *photoreceptors*. These are perhaps the best understood sensory cells, not just in humans but in any eukaryotic organism. Second, unlike other sensory structures, such as the cochlea or somatic receptors in the skin, the retina is not a peripheral organ but part of the central nervous system. During development the retina is derived from the neural ectoderm, the specialized part of the ectoderm that gives rise to the brain. The synaptic organization of the retina is therefore characteristic of other central neural structures (for instance, the major transmitter substances are glutamate and other amino acids).

Compared to other brain regions, however, the retina is relatively simple. It contains only five major classes of neurons linked in an intricate pattern of connections, but with an orderly, layered anatomical arrangement. This combination of physiological diversity and relatively simple structural organization makes the retina useful for understanding how information is processed by complex neural circuits in the brain.

For these reasons we shall describe neural processing in the retina in some considerable detail. This chapter is divided into two parts. In the first part we describe how photoreceptors transduce light into an electrical signal. In the second part we consider how these signals are shaped by other retinal neurons before being sent to the brain, and how synaptic connections among the retinal neurons are organized to accomplish this processing. But before discussing phototransduction, we shall review the overall organization of the retina and the basic physiological properties of the photoreceptor cells.

The Retina Contains the Eye's Receptor Sheet

The eye is foremost an optical device designed to focus the visual image on the retina with minimal optical distortion. As illustrated in Figure 28–1, light is focused by the cornea and the lens, then traverses the vitreous humor that fills the eye cavity before being absorbed by the photoreceptor cells. The retina is apposed to the *pigment epithelium* that lines the back of the eye. Cells in the pigment epithelium are packed with the black pigment *melanin*, which absorbs any light not captured by the retina, thereby preventing it from being reflected off the back of the eye back to the retina (which would degrade the visual image).

FIGURE 28–1

Photoreceptors are located in the retina. The location of the retina within the eye is shown at **left**. Detail of the retina at the fovea is shown on the **right** (the diagram has been simplified by eliminating lateral connections mediated by horizontal and amacrine cells; see Figure 28–6). In most of the retina light must pass through layers of nerve cells and their processes before it reaches the photoreceptors. In the center of the fovea, or foveola, these proximal neural elements are shifted to the side so that light has a direct pathway to the photoreceptors. As a result, the visual image received at the foveola is the least distorted.

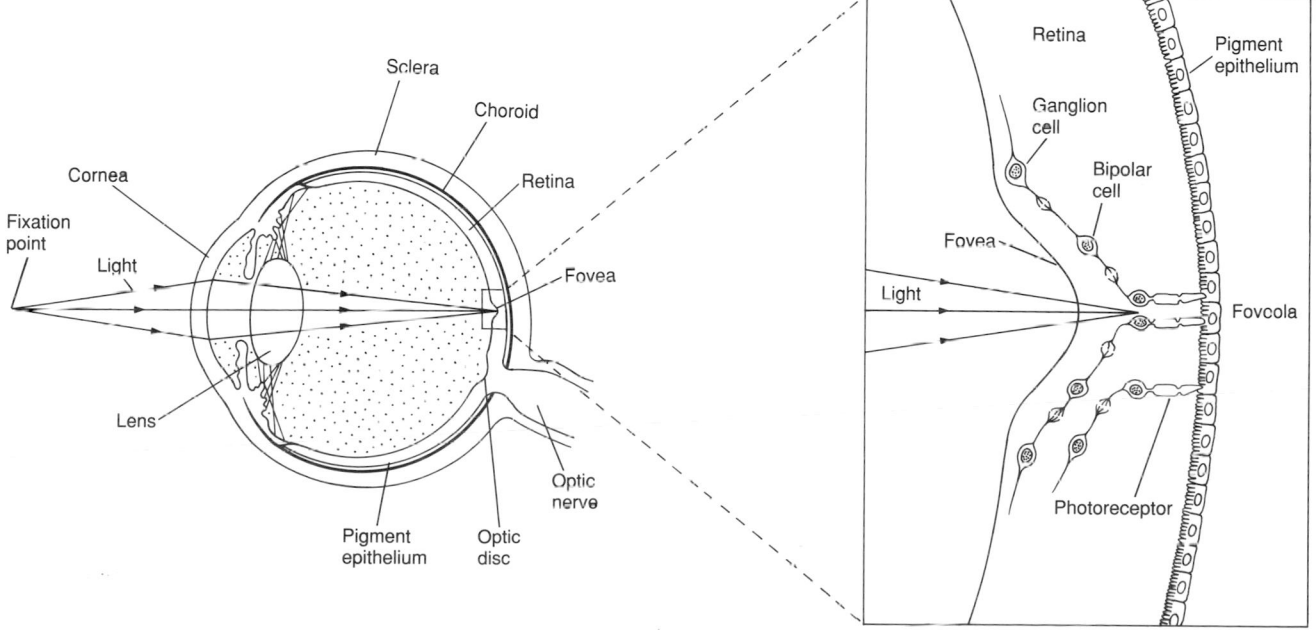

Pigment epithelial cells also assist photoreceptors with important aspects of their metabolism, in particular the resynthesis of the photosensitive visual pigments and, as we shall see later, the phagocytosis of outer segment tips. For this reason, photoreceptors directly contact the pigment epithelium, while the other retinal cells are closer to the lens (Figure 28–1). One remarkable consequence of this arrangement is that light must travel through all the other layers of retinal neurons before striking the photoreceptors. The proximal retinal neural layers are, however, unmyelinated and therefore relatively transparent, allowing light to reach the photoreceptors without being absorbed or greatly scattered (which would distort the visual image). In fact, in one region of the retina, the *fovea*, the cell bodies of the proximal retinal neurons have been shifted to the side, enabling the photoreceptors there to receive the visual image in its least distorted form (see Figure 28–1). This is most pronounced at the center of the fovea, the foveola. Humans therefore constantly move their eyes so that scenes of interest are projected onto their foveas. Nasal to the fovea is the optic disc where the optic nerve fibers leave the retina. This region has no photoreceptors and therefore creates a blind spot in the visual field (see Figure 29–5).

There Are Two Types of Photoreceptors: Rods and Cones

The human retina contains two types of photoreceptors, rods and cones. Cones are responsible for day vision; people who lose cone function are legally blind. Rods mediate night vision; they function in the dim light that is present at dusk or at night, when most stimuli are too weak to excite the cone system. Total loss of rods produces only night blindness.

Cones perform better than rods in all visual tasks except the detection of dim stimuli. Cone-mediated vision is of higher acuity than rod-mediated vision, and provides better resolution of rapid changes in the visual image (i.e., better *temporal resolution*). Cones also mediate color vision. The rod system is more sensitive than the cone system, but it is achromatic. These differences in performance are due partly to properties of the rods and cones themselves and partly to the connections they make with other neurons in the retina (the rod and cone systems). The most important factors that contribute to these differences are as follows.

Rods detect dim lights. Rods contain more photosensitive visual pigment than cones, enabling them to capture more light. Even more important, rods amplify light signals more than cones. As was first shown directly by Dennis Baylor and his colleagues, a single photon can evoke a detectable electrical response in a rod, whereas hundreds of photons must be absorbed by a cone to evoke a similar response. Conversely, fewer photons are required to evoke a maximal (or *saturating*) response in a rod. Only the rod response, not the cone, saturates in normal daylight.

Cones mediate color vision and provide greater spatial and temporal resolution. As we shall see in Chapter 31, the brain obtains information about color by comparing the responses of the three types of cones, each with a visual pigment that is more sensitive to a different part of the spectrum. In contrast, there is only one rod pigment so that all rods respond in the same way to different wavelengths. Rod vision is therefore achromatic.

Although rods outnumber cones by roughly 20 to 1, the cone system has better spatial resolution for two reasons. First, cones are concentrated in the fovea, especially in the foveola, where the visual image is least distorted. Second, the rod system is *convergent*: many rods synapse on the same target interneuron (a bipolar cell). The signals from these rods are pooled in the interneuron and reinforce one another, strengthening the response evoked by light in the interneuron and increasing the ability of the brain to detect dim lights. However, convergence in turn reduces the ability of the rod system to transmit spatial variations in the visual image because differences in the responses of neighboring rods are averaged out in the interneuron. In contrast, only a few cones converge on each bipolar cell, so that cones provide better spatial resolution. In fact, signals from cones in the foveola are not pooled at all.

Unlike most neurons, rods and cones do not fire action potentials. Instead, as we shall see below, they respond to light with graded changes in membrane potential. Rods respond slowly, so that the effects of photons absorbed during a 100 ms interval summate. This helps rods detect small amounts of light, but prevents them from resolving light flickering faster than about 12 Hz. The response of cones is much brisker, so that cones can detect flicker up to 55 Hz. Thus, cones also provide greater temporal resolution of the visual image. These differences are summarized in Table 28–1.

TABLE 28–1. Differences Between Rods and Cones and Between Their Neural Systems

Rods	Cones
High sensitivity, specialized for night vision:	Lower sensitivity, specialized for day vision:
More photopigment, capture more light	Less photopigment
High amplification, single photon detection	Less amplification
Saturate in daylight	Saturate only in intense light
Low temporal resolution: Slow response, long integration time	High temporal resolution: Fast response, short integration time
More sensitive to scattered light	Most sensitive to direct axial rays

Rod system	Cone system
Low acuity: highly convergent retinal pathways, not present in central fovea	High acuity: less convergent retinal pathways, concentrated in fovea
Achromatic: one type of rod pigment	Chromatic: three types of cones, each with a different pigment that is more sensitive to a different part of the visible spectrum

Light Is Absorbed by Visual Pigments in the Outer Segments of Rods and Cones

Rods and cones have similar functional regions: (1) a region specialized for phototransduction, called the *outer segment* (because it is located at the outer or distal surface of the retina); (2) a region containing the cell's nucleus and most of its biosynthetic machinery, called the *inner segment* (because it is located more proximally within the retina); and (3) a synaptic terminal that makes synaptic contact with the photoreceptor's target cells (Figure 28–2A). The outer segment is connected to the inner segment through a thin *stalk* or *cilium*, which contains microtubules organized in an array that is characteristic of other cilia (Figure 28–2).

The outer segments of rods and cones are effective light-catchers because they are densely packed with light-absorbing *visual pigments*. Each pigment molecule is a small light-absorbing molecule covalently attached to a large transmembrane protein. Rods and cones are capable of accommodating large numbers of these membrane proteins because they have evolved an elaborate system of stacked membranous *discs* in their outer segments that dramatically increase the surface area of the membrane in these cells (Figure 28–2B). These discs develop as a series of invaginations of the cell's plasma membrane. In cones they remain coextensive with the plasma membrane, while in rods they pinch off from the plasma membrane and become intracellular organelles. Each rod contains about 10^8 pigment molecules, each of which is oriented within the disc membrane to maximize the absorption of photons from a stream of light traversing the outer segment axially. The light-catching ability of rods and cones is further enhanced because the discs are stacked vertically, ensuring that light that escapes one disc is caught by the pigment in another.

Like other neurons, photoreceptors do not divide. Their outer segments are, however, being constantly renewed. In rods the discs are formed at the base of the outer segment and migrate outward to the tip. This process is rapid; every hour about three discs are synthesized. The discarded tips are removed by the phagocytotic activity of the pigment epithelial cells. Cones also undergo renewal and phagocytosis of the outer segment membranes, although it is not known how the renewal occurs.

Phototransduction Results from a Cascade of Biochemical Events in the Outer Segment of Photoreceptors

The absorption of light by visual pigments in rods and cones triggers a cascade of events that eventually leads to a change in ionic fluxes across the plasma membrane of these cells and a consequent change in membrane potential. In this section we shall examine in detail these biochemical steps and how they are controlled by light. A key intermediate in this cascade is the cyclic nucleotide 3'-5' cyclic *guanosine monophosphate*, or cGMP. It has long been recognized that phototransduction, at least in rods,

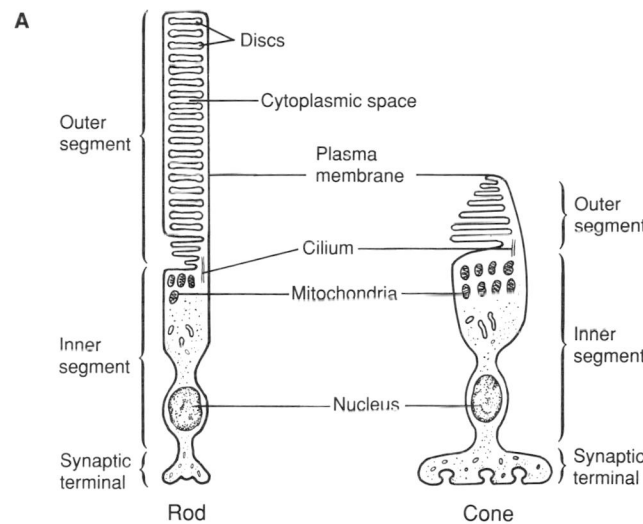

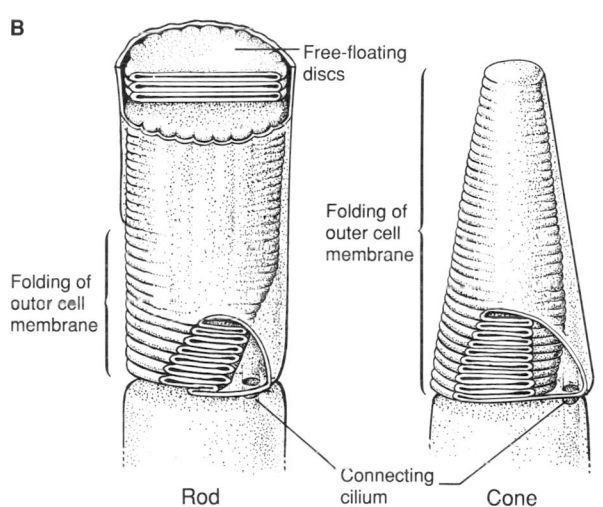

FIGURE 28–2

The two types of photoreceptors, rods and cones, have similar structures. (Adapted from O'Brien, 1982, and Young, 1970.)

A. Both rod and cone cells have inner and outer segments connected by a cilium. The inner segment contains the cell's nucleus and most of its biosynthetic machinery. The outer segment contains the light-transducing apparatus. The conical shape of the cone outer segment makes cones most sensitive to direct axial rays.

B. The outer segment consists of a stack of membranous discs, which contain the light-absorbing photopigments. In both types of cells these discs are formed by infolding of the plasma membrane. In rods, however, the folds pinch off so that the discs are free-floating within the outer segment.

must involve a cytoplasmic messenger that conveys information from the freely floating discs, where light is absorbed, to the cells' plasma membrane, where ionic fluxes are controlled. It is now known that this messenger is cGMP and that in both rods and cones cGMP controls

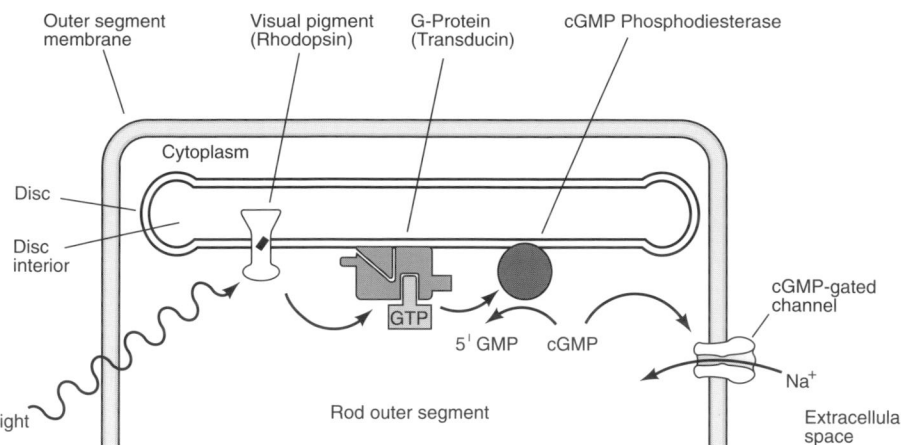

FIGURE 28–3

Phototransduction involves the closing of cation channels, illustrated here for rod photoreceptors. In the absence of light, cation channels in the outer segment membrane that conduct an inward current, carried largely by Na$^+$, are opened by intracellular cGMP. In the presence of light these channels are closed by a three-step process. (1) Light is absorbed by and activates pigment molecules (rhodopsin in rods) located in the disc membrane (the black rectangle in the rhodopsin molecule represents the light-absorbing chromophore, retinal). (2) The activated pigment stimulates a G-protein (transducin in rods), which in turn activates cGMP phosphodiesterase. This enzyme catalyzes the breakdown of cGMP to 5'-GMP. (3) As the cGMP concentration is lowered, these channels close, thereby reducing the inward current and causing the photoreceptor to hyperpolarize.

ionic fluxes across the plasma membrane by opening a specialized species of ion channel, the *cGMP-gated channel*. Recent experiments have shown that phototransduction occurs in three stages: (1) light activates visual pigments; (2) these activated molecules cause the stimulation of cGMP phosphodiesterase, an enzyme that reduces the cytoplasmic concentration of cGMP; (3) the reduction in cGMP concentration closes the cGMP-gated channels, thus hyperpolarizing the photoreceptor (Figure 28–3). We shall now examine each of these events step by step.

Light Activates Pigment Molecules in Photoreceptors

The visual pigment in rod cells, rhodopsin, has two parts. The protein portion, *opsin*, is embedded in the disc membrane and does not by itself absorb light (Figure 28–4A). The light-absorbing portion of the complex, *retinal*, is the aldehyde form of vitamin A and is covalently attached to opsin by a Schiff-base linkage at a specific site. Retinal can actually assume several different isomeric conformations, two of which are important in different phases of the visual cycle. In its nonactivated form rhodopsin contains the 11-*cis* isomer of retinal, which fits snugly into a binding site in the opsin molecule (Figure 28–4B).

The mechanism of activation of rhodopsin was discovered by George Wald and his colleagues, who found that the absorption of light causes retinal to change from the 11-*cis* to the all-*trans* configuration (Figure 28–4C). This reaction is the *only light-dependent step in vision*. As a result of this conformational change, retinal no longer fits into the binding site in opsin, so that opsin undergoes a conformational change. The rhodopsin molecule proceeds within a millisecond through a series of unstable intermediates to a semistable conformation called *metarhodopsin II*. This is the active form of rhodopsin that triggers the second step of phototransduction.

Metarhodopsin II is short-lived; within minutes the Schiff-base linkage between opsin and retinal hydrolyzes spontaneously, yielding opsin and all-*trans* retinal, which diffuses away. To be recycled for the synthesis of rhodopsin, all-*trans* retinal must be isomerized back to the 11-*cis* form, a reaction thought to take place in the neighboring pigment epithelium. Because retinal is not very water soluble, it is transported between rods and pigment epithelial cells by a special retinal-binding protein. All-*trans* retinal is reduced to all-*trans* retinol (vitamin A), the precursor for the synthesis of 11-*cis* retinal. Because all-*trans* retinol cannot be synthesized by humans, a nutritional deficiency in vitamin A can lead to night blindness and, if left untreated, to the deterioration of receptor outer segments and to total blindness.

As in rods, the visual pigments in cones are also composed of two parts: a protein called *cone opsin* and a light-absorbing molecule that, as in rods, appears to be 11-*cis* retinal. The excitation, breakdown, and regeneration of the cone pigments are believed to occur by mechanisms similar to those affecting rhodopsin. Each of the three types of cone cells in the retina of primates contains a different pigment designed to maximize absorption of light in a different part of the visible spectrum. This differentiation underlies normal human trivariant color vision (see Chapter 31). The three cone pigments contain different cone opsins, each of which interacts with 11-*cis* retinal in a different way, causing it to be more sensitive to

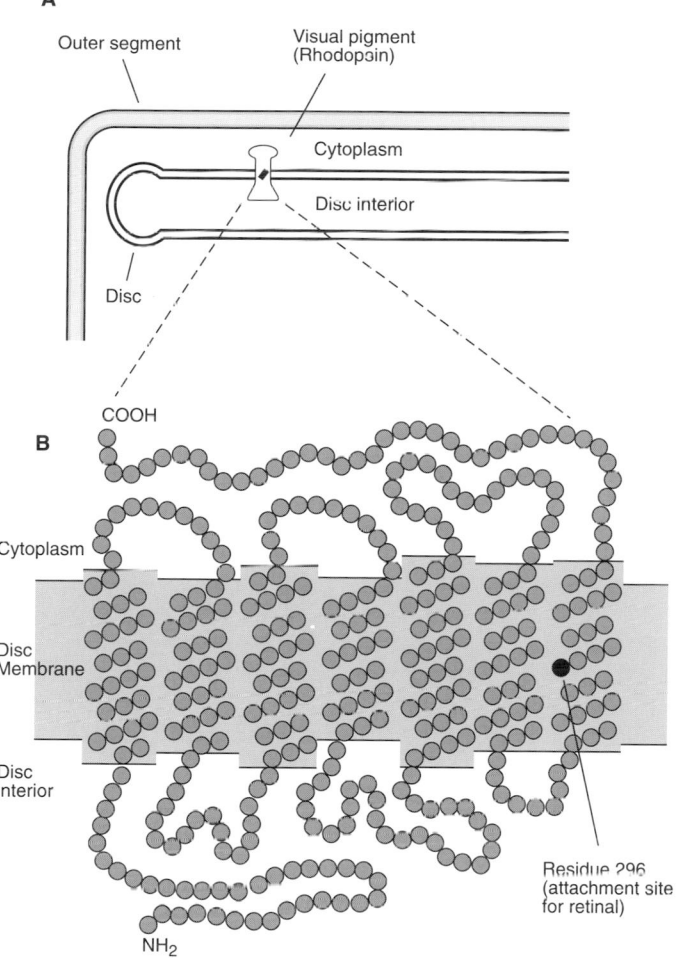

A

Outer segment

Visual pigment
(Rhodopsin)

Cytoplasm

Disc interior

Disc

B

COOH

Cytoplasm

Disc
Membrane

Disc
interior

NH₂

Residue 296
(attachment site
for retinal)

C

11-*cis* retinal
(M_r =268)

All-*trans* retinal

FIGURE 28–4

Location and structure of rhodopsin, the visual pigment in rod cells. Rhodopsin is the covalent complex of a large protein, *opsin*, and a small light-absorbing chromophore, *retinal*. Absorption of light by retinal causes a change in the three-dimensional structure of rhodopsin.

A. Location of rhodopsin in the disc membrane. The black rectangle represents the chromophore, retinal.

B. The structure of rhodopsin. Opsin has 348 amino acids and a molecular weight of about 40,000. It loops back and forth seven times across the membrane of the rod disc, with the N terminus lying in the intradiscal space and the C terminus on the cytoplasmic face of the membrane. Retinal is covalently attached to the side chain of a specific lysine residue in opsin, at residue 296 in the protein's seventh membrane-spanning region. The seven hydrophobic transmembrane segments are helical rods that appear to form a pocket enclosing the molecule of retinal. All other transmitter and hormone receptors that activate effector enzymes via a G-protein and whose structure has been determined show a high degree of structural similarity with rhodopsin. They also have seven distinct hydrophobic membrane-spanning regions that are connected by hydrophilic loops on the cytoplasmic and extracellular sides. (Adapted from Nathans and Hogness, 1984.)

C. In its nonactivated form rhodopsin contains the 11 *cis* isomer of retinal. The first event in visual transduction is the absorption of light by 11-*cis* retinal. This causes a rotation around the 11-*cis* double bond, allowing retinal to return to its more stable all-*trans* configuration. Because the all-*trans* isomer does not fit into the binding site in opsin, this causes a conformational change in the opsin portion of rhodopsin, which triggers the other events of visual transduction.

a particular part of the visible spectrum. Although the amino acid sequences of the rod opsin and the three cone opsins are known, it is not yet known which residues determine the spectral sensitivity of the 11-*cis* retinal.

Activated Pigment Molecules Affect the Cytoplasmic Concentration of Cyclic GMP

Activation of pigment molecules by light leads to a change in the cytoplasmic concentration of the second messenger cGMP. The concentration of cGMP is directly controlled by two enzymes. It is synthesized from GTP by guanylate cyclase, which is concentrated near the outer segment stalk, and it is hydrolyzed to 5'-GMP by cGMP phosphodiesterase, a protein peripherally associated with the disc membrane (Figure 28–3). The concentration of cGMP is affected by light because cGMP phosphodiesterase is itself controlled by the visual pigments. In darkness cGMP phosphodiesterase is only weakly active, and the concentration of cGMP is therefore relatively high, around 2 μM. Activation of pigment molecules by light leads to the activation of the phosphodiesterase, which breaks down cGMP and lowers its concentration.

This process shows a high degree of *amplification*: Photoactivation of a single rhodopsin molecule can lead to the hydrolysis of more than 10^5 molecules of cGMP in 1 second. This amplification is achieved through the regulatory protein *transducin*. One rhodopsin molecule can diffuse within the disc membrane and activate hundreds of transducin molecules, each of which stimulates a phosphodiesterase molecule. Each phosphodiesterase molecule in turn is capable of hydrolyzing over 10^3 molecules of cGMP per second.

The biochemical cascade initiated by the photoactivation of rhodopsin is similar to the signal transduction mechanism triggered by the binding of many hormones and neurotransmitters to their receptors. Indeed, the rod and cone opsins show a high degree of structural similarity with the family of hormone and transmitter receptors that activate effector enzymes (like adenylyl cyclase and phospholipase C) via *G-proteins*. Like these ligand-activated receptors, the rod and cone opsins have seven distinct hydrophobic membrane-spanning regions that are connected by hydrophilic loops (Figure 28–4B). (The opsins can actually be thought of as ligand-activated receptors, if the chromophore retinal is considered a light-sensitive ligand.) Moreover, transducin is a member of the family of G-proteins. Like other G-proteins, the activation of transducin involves a characteristic interaction with guanine nucleotides (see Chapter 12 and Figure 12–3). In its inactive form transducin binds a molecule of GDP tightly. Interaction with activated rhodopsin in the disc membrane causes transducin to exchange GDP for GTP. Once it has bound GTP, transducin can in turn stimulate the phosphodiesterase. Transducin becomes inactivated because it also has GTPase activity and eventually hydrolyzes the bound GTP molecule to GDP. This binding and subsequent hydrolysis of GTP is observed during activation of all G-proteins.

The mechanisms that terminate the light response are not as well understood as those that initiate it. As described, transducin inactivates itself by hydrolyzing bound GTP. The activated form of rhodopsin (metarhodopsin II) also breaks down spontaneously, but too slowly to explain the inactivation of the light response. It appears that activated rhodopsin becomes a target for phosphorylation by a specific protein kinase, opsin kinase, and that phosphorylated rhodopsin interacts with a specific regulatory protein called arrestin, leading to its rapid inactivation.

Cyclic GMP Gates Specialized Ion Channels in the Plasma Membrane of the Photoreceptor

The light-evoked decrease in cGMP causes a change in the photoreceptor's membrane potential because cGMP controls ion channels in the cell's plasma membrane, the cGMP-gated channels. How does cGMP open these channels? Evgeniy Fesenko and his colleagues, who discovered the cGMP-gated channels in rods, first provided evidence that cGMP produces its effect by binding directly to the cytoplasmic face of the channel and that channel activation occurs by the cooperative binding of at least three molecules of cGMP. This has recently been confirmed by Benjamin Kaupp and his colleagues, who have cloned the bovine rod cGMP-gated channel. The channel consists of a single type of polypeptide of molecular weight 63,000, which has several membrane-spanning regions and cytoplasmic domains. One particular cytoplasmic segment contains a region similar in amino acid sequence to the cGMP-binding domains of cGMP-dependent protein kinase and is believed therefore to bind cGMP. A functional channel is composed of three or more of these polypeptides (the exact number has not yet been determined).

The discovery that cGMP opens these channels directly came as a surprise. Before the discovery of the cGMP-gated channels, it was assumed that cGMP could not act directly on ion channels, but had to activate a cGMP-dependent protein kinase that would phosphorylate the channels. The cGMP-gated channel of photoreceptors was the first known example of an ion channel regulated by a cyclic nucleotide acting directly on the channel rather than through a protein kinase. Other channels directly gated by cyclic nucleotides have since been found in olfactory neurons (Chapter 34). Similar channels may also be present in some retinal bipolar cells (see below).

Closing of Cyclic GMP-Gated Ion Channels in the Outer Segment Hyperpolarizes the Photoreceptor

The change in the photoreceptor's membrane potential during illumination is determined both by the change in the current that flows through the cGMP-gated channels and by a current flowing across the photoreceptor membrane through K$^+$-selective, nongated (leakage) channels that are like those of other neurons. The K$^+$ channels tend to drive the photoreceptor's membrane potential to the equilibrium potential for K$^+$ (around -70 mV). In dark-

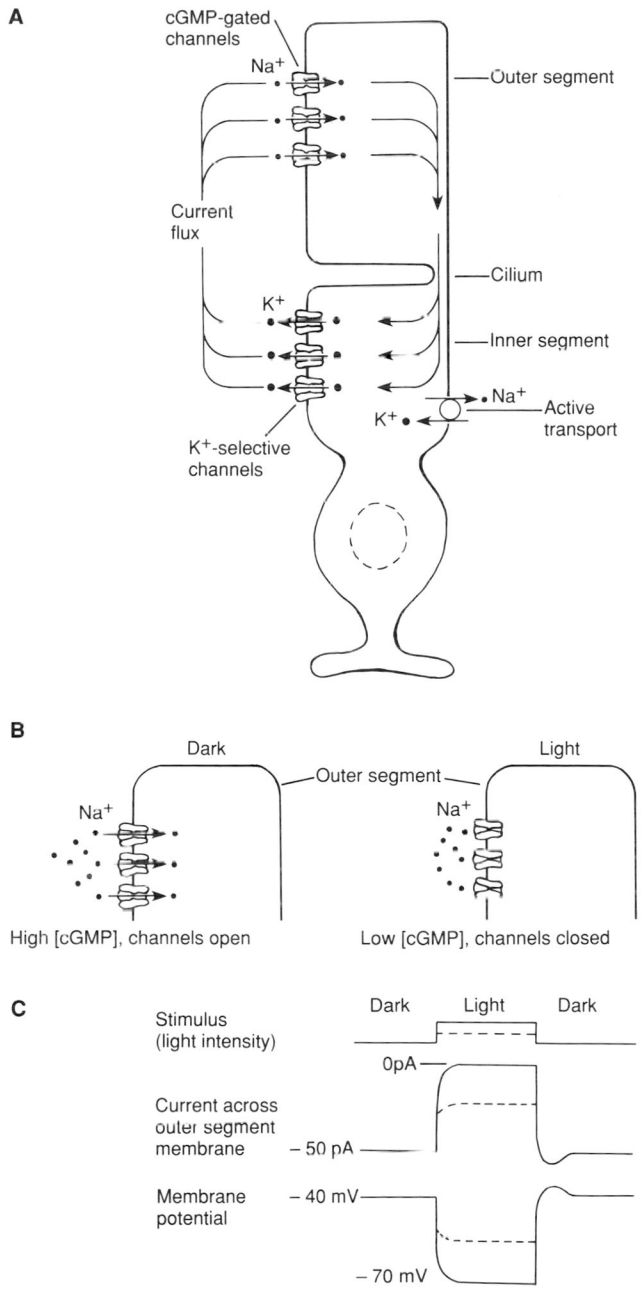

FIGURE 28-5

Closing of the cGMP-gated channels causes photoreceptors to hyperpolarize, as illustrated for a rod photoreceptor.

A. In darkness an inward current (the dark current), carried largely by Na⁺ ions, flows into the outer segment of photoreceptors through cGMP-gated channels. These channels are opened when cGMP binds to them on the cytoplasmic side of the outer segment membrane. The current flows out of the cell across the inner segment membrane, where it is carried largely by K⁺ ions flowing through K⁺-selective, nongated (leakage) channels. The current is driven by ion pumps in the inner segment that use metabolic energy to pump Na⁺ out and K⁺ in.

B. Absorption of light lowers the cytoplasmic concentration of cGMP in the outer segment, causing the closure of cGMP-gated channels and thus reducing the dark current partially or completely. This makes the photoreceptor hyperpolarize.

C. A bright (saturating) light (**solid line**) and a light of intermediate intensity (**dashed line**) have different effects on the inward current and the membrane potential of a cone photoreceptor. In the absence of light an inward current of 50 pA flows into the outer segment (because it is an inward current, it is shown as negative). A bright light suppresses this current completely by closing the cGMP-gated channels, thus hyperpolarizing the cell membrane from its resting level (−40 mV) to −70 mV, the equilibrium potential for K⁺. A light of intermediate intensity hyperpolarizes the cell to potentials between −40 and −70 mV.

ness, however, the high resting levels of cGMP in the cell keep the cGMP-gated channels open, allowing an inward current of about 50 pA, carried largely by Na⁺ ions, to flow into the cell. This steady inward current, called the *dark current*, maintains the photoreceptor membrane potential at around −40 mV. This resting potential is significantly more positive (or depolarized) than that of most other neurons, which is typically close to −70 mV (the K⁺ equilibrium potential).

As in other neurons, each type of ion channel in photoreceptors is found only in a certain region of the cell (Figure 28-5A). The cGMP-gated channels are confined to the outer segment, and in fact are the only species of ion channel there. In contrast, the K⁺ channels are confined to

the inner segment. In darkness, current flows through the photoreceptor, entering the outer segment through the cGMP-gated channels, where it is carried largely by Na⁺ ions, and flowing back out through the nongated K⁺ channels. (K⁺ flows out of these channels because the photoreceptors are depolarized with respect to the K⁺ equilibrium potential.) To maintain steady intracellular concentrations of Na⁺ and K⁺ in the face of these large fluxes, the photoreceptors have a high density of Na⁺-K⁺ pumps in the inner segment, which pump Na⁺ out and K⁺ in (Figure 28-5A).

When light reduces cGMP and the cGMP-gated channels close, the inward Na⁺ current that flows through these channels is reduced, thus hyperpolarizing the cell

(Figure 28–5B). A bright light can cause the closure of all the cGMP-gated ion channels. When this happens the large conductance produced by the nongated K^+ channels drives the photoreceptor's membrane potential to -70 mV. At intermediate light intensities the cGMP-gated channels are not all closed, and the photoreceptor hyperpolarizes to a potential between -40 mV and -70 mV (Figure 28–5C).

Changes in Intracellular Calcium Underlie Light Adaptation in Photoreceptors

The concentration of cGMP in the photoreceptor outer segments is modulated not only by light but also by the cytoplasmic concentration of Ca^{2+}. When Ca^{2+} is raised (as can be achieved experimentally by injecting Ca^{2+} ions into the outer segment), cGMP drops. In contrast to the effect of light on the level of cGMP, which is mediated by the activation of cGMP phosphodiesterase, the effect of Ca^{2+} is believed to be due largely to an inhibitory effect of Ca^{2+} on guanylate cyclase, the enzyme that synthesizes cGMP from GTP.

The modulatory effect of Ca^{2+} on cGMP is important in mediating *light adaptation*. Light adaptation is familiar to anyone who has stepped from a dark room into bright daylight. At first the light is blinding, but over a period of several seconds the eyes adapt. Adaptation involves many changes in the retina and eye (such as a contraction of the pupil to reduce the amount of light reaching the retina), but the most important change occurs in the cone photoreceptors. A very bright light closes all cGMP-gated channels, making the cones hyperpolarize from their resting potential (-40 mV) to -70 mV, the potential determined by the nongated K^+ channels. In this state the cones cannot respond to further increases in light intensity. However, if this background illumination is maintained, the cones slowly depolarize to a membrane potential between -70 and -40 mV, and are once again capable of hyperpolarizing in response to further increases in light intensity—the bright light is no longer blinding.

Light adaptation also involves a *desensitization* of the cone, a process that we shall not consider here. (The converse process of *dark adaptation*, the transition to dim light vision, occurs over a period of tens of minutes and involves several changes in rods that shall not be examined here either.)

The slow depolarization of the cone membrane potential that occurs during adaptation to maintained illumination is caused by a change in Ca^{2+} in the outer segment. The Ca^{2+} concentration is determined by two processes. Calcium constantly flows into the outer segment through the cGMP-gated channels because these channels are not selective for Na^+ ions (Ca^{2+} contributes about one-seventh of the current that flows through these channels). In darkness the Ca^{2+} concentration in the outer segment remains constant because the Ca^{2+} that enters is extruded by a specialized Ca^{2+} carrier in the outer segment membrane. During prolonged illumination the cGMP-gated channels

are closed, which reduces the influx of Ca^{2+}, causing a slow decrease in Ca^{2+} concentration (because the extrusion of Ca^{2+} continues). This relieves the inhibition of guanylate cyclase by Ca^{2+}, so that more cGMP is synthesized and the concentration of cGMP slowly increases. This results in the reopening of cGMP-gated channels and, consequently, slow depolarization of the cone.

The central role of Ca^{2+} in light adaptation was demonstrated by Trevor Lamb and King-Wai Yau and their colleagues, who succeeded in preventing changes in the Ca^{2+} concentration in photoreceptors by blocking the Ca^{2+} fluxes into and out of the outer segment. When the Ca^{2+} concentration is kept constant in this way, photoreceptors do not adapt during prolonged illumination.

Ganglion Cells Are the Output Neurons of the Retina

We now turn to the second topic of this chapter: How does the retina modify and process the signals evoked by light in photoreceptors before sending them to higher centers? The output neurons of the retina are the *ganglion cells*. Their axons form the optic nerve, which projects to the lateral geniculate nucleus and to the superior colliculus as well as to brain stem nuclei. Unlike photoreceptors, which respond to light with graded changes in membrane potential, ganglion cells transmit information as trains of action potentials. Sandwiched between the photoreceptors and the ganglion cells are three classes of interneurons: *bipolar*, *horizontal*, and *amacrine* cells (Figure 28–6). These cells transmit signals from the photoreceptors to the ganglion cells. They also combine signals from several photoreceptors, so that the electrical responses evoked in ganglion cells depend critically on the precise pattern of the light that stimulates the retina and how this pattern changes with time.

As ganglion cells are the output neurons of the retina, the simplest way of assessing how visual information is processed by the retina is to examine how ganglion cells respond to different patterns of light. There is a second reason for focusing on these cells. Much more is known about the responses of ganglion cells than of the three classes of retinal interneurons because ganglion cell activity can be measured relatively easily by recording from axons in the optic nerve with extracellular electrodes. Our knowledge of how the retinal interneurons respond to light is much more fragmentary because their activity can be monitored only by intracellular recording, which is especially difficult in the small cell bodies of interneurons in higher vertebrates. Accordingly, in this section we shall examine how ganglion cells respond to different patterns of light. In the final section we shall examine how the synaptic connections between the five classes of retinal neurons—the receptors, ganglion cells, and three classes of interposed interneurons (bipolar, horizontal, and amacrine cells)—appear to be organized to carry out the processing of the visual image.

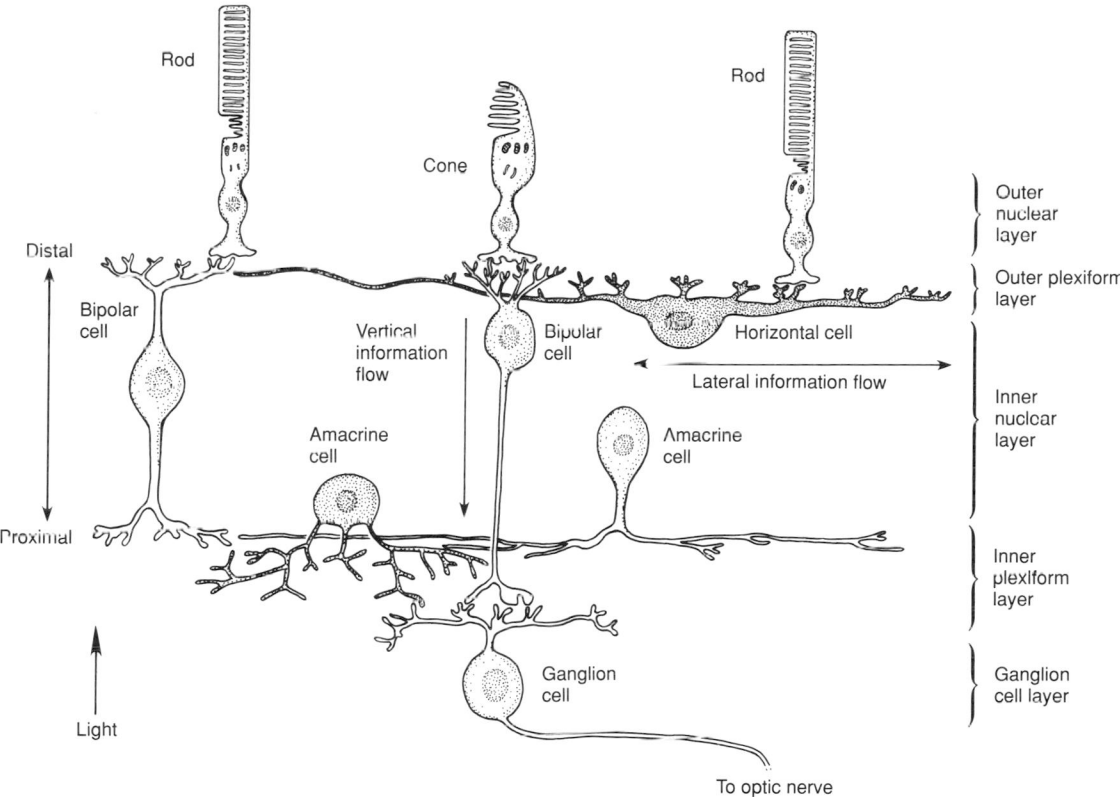

FIGURE 28–6

The retina has five major classes of neurons arranged into three nuclear layers: photoreceptors (rods and cones), bipolar cells, horizontal cells, amacrine cells, and ganglion cells. Photoreceptors, bipolar, and horizontal cells make synaptic connections with each other in the outer plexiform layer. The bipolar, amacrine, and ganglion cells make contact in the inner plexiform layer. Bipolar cells bridge the two layers. Details of these connections are illustrated in Figure 28–11. Information flows vertically from photoreceptors to bipolar cells to ganglion cells. Information also flows laterally, mediated by horizontal cells in the outer plexiform layer and amacrine cells in the inner plexiform layer. (Adapted from Dowling, 1979.)

Ganglion Cell Receptive Fields Have a Center and Antagonistic Surround

Modern studies of the retina began when Keffer Hartline, and subsequently Stephen Kuffler and Horace Barlow, recorded the pattern of action potentials fired by single ganglion cells in response to spots of light. They found that these cells are never silent, even in the dark, but that light modulates their spontaneous activity. (Of course, light does not directly affect the ganglion cells; it stimulates photoreceptors, which in turn send information to the ganglion cells.) Each ganglion cell responds to light directed to a specific area of the retina. This area is called the *receptive field* of the cell (see Chapter 23). The receptive field of a ganglion cell (or any other cell in the visual pathways) is that area of the retina where stimulation of photoreceptors with light causes either an increase or decrease of the ganglion cell's firing rate. In effect, it is the area of retina that the ganglion cell monitors. Ganglion cell receptive fields have three important features.

Ganglion cells have circular receptive fields. Using small spots of light to probe the properties of ganglion cell receptive fields, Kuffler found that these receptive fields are roughly circular, and that they vary in size across the retina. In the foveal region of the primate retina, where visual acuity is greatest, the receptive fields are small, with centers that are only a few minutes of arc (60 minutes = 1 degree). At the periphery of the retina, where acuity is low, the fields are larger, with centers of 3° to 5° (1° on the retina is equal to about 0.25 mm).

Ganglion cell receptive fields have a center and an antagonistic surround. The receptive field of most ganglion cells is not homogeneous but is divided into two parts: a circular zone at the center, called the *receptive field center*, and the remaining area of the field, called the *surround* (Figure 28–7).

Ganglion cells process visual information in two parallel pathways. Two classes of ganglion cells can be distinguished by their response to a small spot of light applied to the center of their receptive field. *On-center ganglion cells* fire few action potentials in darkness, and light directed to the center of their receptive field increases their firing rate (they are excited when light is turned on). Light applied to the surround inhibits the ef-

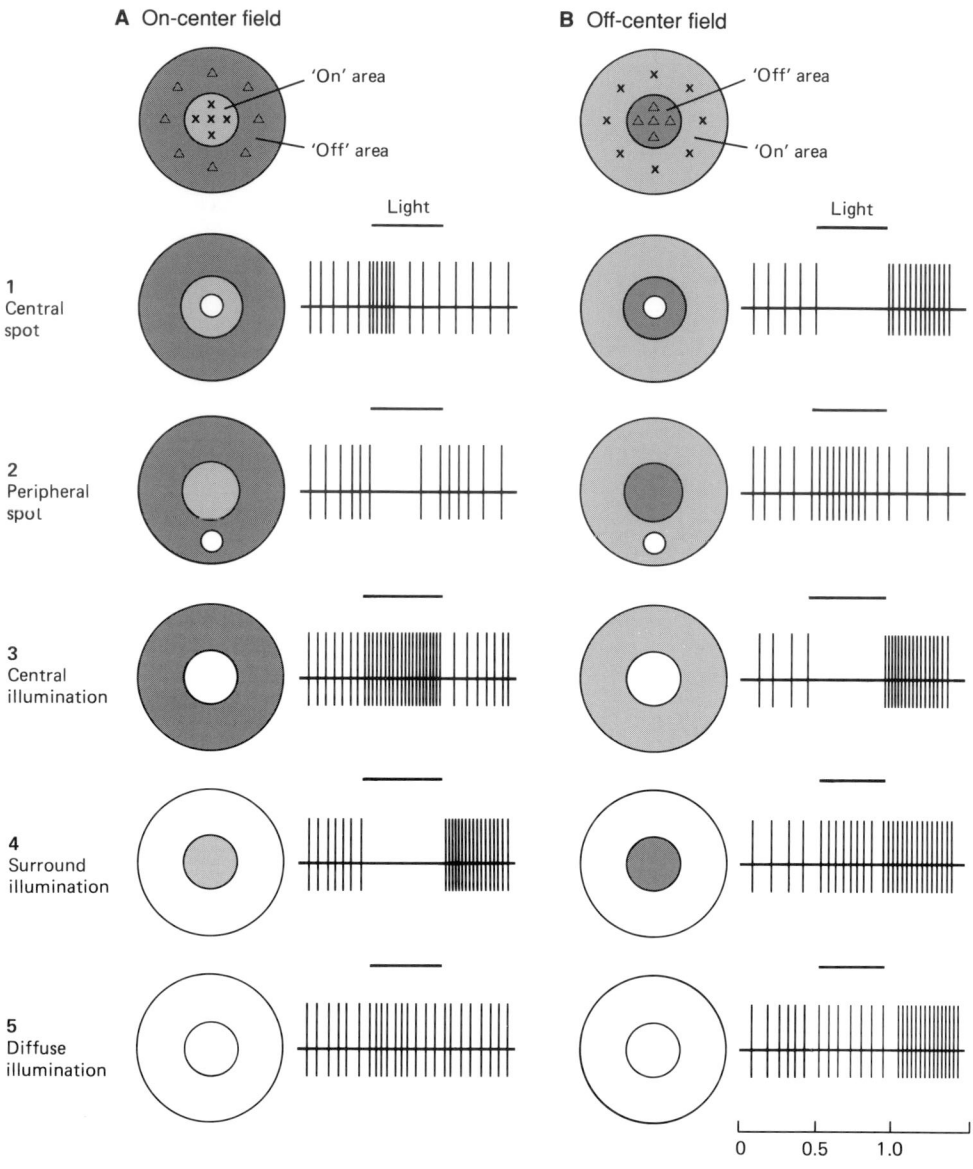

FIGURE 28–7

Retinal ganglion cells respond optimally to contrast in their receptive fields. Ganglion cells have circular receptive fields, divided into a center area and a surround. *On-center* cells are excited when stimulated in the center and inhibited when stimulated in the surround; *off-center* cells have the opposite responses. The figure shows the responses of both types of cells to five different light stimuli (the *white portion* of the receptive field represents the stimulated area). The pattern of action potentials fired by the ganglion cell in response to each stimulus is also shown in extracellular recordings. Duration of illumination is indicated by a bar above each record. (Adapted from Kuffler, 1953.)

A. On-center cells respond best when the entire central part of the receptive field is stimulated (**stimulus 3**). These cells also

respond well, but less vigorously, when only a portion of its central field is stimulated by a spot of light (**1**). Illumination of the surrounding area with a spot of light (**2**) or ring of light (**4**) reduces or suppresses the cell firing, which resumes more vigorously for a short period after the light is turned off. Diffuse illumination of the entire receptive field (**5**) elicits only a relatively weak discharge because the center and surround oppose each other's effects.

B. The spontaneous firing of off-center cells is suppressed when the central area is illuminated (**1,3**) but accelerates for a short period after the stimulus is turned off. Light shone onto the surround of an off-center receptive field excites the cell (**2,4**).

fect produced by illumination of the center; the most effective inhibitory stimulus is a ring of light on the entire surround. *Off-center ganglion cells* are inhibited by light applied to the center of their receptive field (Figure 28–7).

Their firing rate is highest for a short period of time after the light is removed (they are excited when the light is turned *off*). Light also excites an off-center ganglion cell when it is directed to the surround of the receptive field.

In both types of cells the response evoked by a ring of light on the entire surround cancels almost completely the response evoked by light in the center. For this reason, diffuse illumination of the entire receptive field evokes only a small response.

The receptive field properties of ganglion cells are invariant at most light intensities. However, after adaptation to extreme darkness or very dim light (e.g., starlight) for over an hour, these properties change so that illumination of the surround ceases to inhibit the response to illumination of the center. We shall examine the purpose and mechanism of this change later.

On- and off-center ganglion cells are present in roughly equal numbers and provide two *parallel pathways* for the processing of visual information. They are parallel in the sense that every photoreceptor sends outputs to both types of ganglion cells.

Not all ganglion cells have a center-surround receptive field organization. For example, a few ganglion cells respond to changes in the overall luminance of the visual field, and are important in controlling pupillary reflexes (Chapter 29).

The Properties of Ganglion Cells Enhance the Ability to Detect Weak Contrasts and Rapid Changes in the Visual Image

What is the purpose of the center-surround structure of ganglion cell receptive fields and why does the retina send visual information down parallel on-center and off-center pathways? As with many types of information processing in the brain it is difficult to determine all the advantages that are conferred on the visual system by these operations. But one function of this processing is probably to enhance the ability of higher centers to detect objects that contrast only weakly with their backgrounds as well as rapid changes in the visual image.

The fact that ganglion cells respond only weakly to uniform illumination (the center and surround inputs cancel each other), and respond best when the light intensities in the center and surround are quite different, reflects a key principle in the entire visual system: The cells in the visual system report principally on *contrast* in visual input rather than on its absolute intensity. The absolute amount of light reflected by objects is relatively uninformative because it is largely determined by the intensity of the light source. Doubling the ambient light intensity will double the amount of light reflected by objects, but will not alter contrasts between them. Thus, the information required to detect objects is contained mainly in *variations* in the light intensity across the visual scene.

As we shall see in Chapters 30 and 31, the brain also relies principally on information about contrast rather than the absolute amount of light in determining the brightness and color of objects. Thus, the *appearance* of an object is also influenced by the contrast between the object and its surrounding. For example, the same gray ring looks much lighter against a black background than against a white one (Figure 28–8).

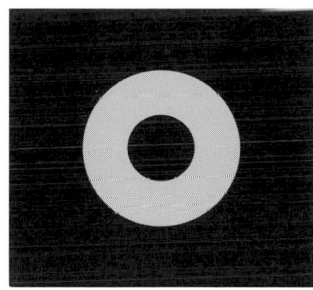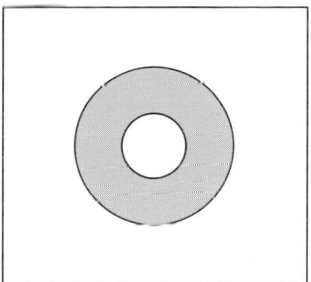

FIGURE 28–8
This visual illusion illustrates that the appearance of an object depends principally not on the intensity of the light source but on the contrast between the object and its surround. The two gray rings in the figures are identical in hue, but they appear to have different brightness because the different backgrounds produce different contrast. (From Brown and Herrnstein, 1975.)

Why does the detection of contrast start in the retina? Signals from photoreceptors could in principle be sent directly to higher centers for this processing. However, during transmission through several relay steps to the cortex, signals tend to be slightly distorted. If two photorecepors are illuminated by light of only slightly different intensity, so that their responses are only slightly different, errors in transmission could prevent higher centers from detecting the difference. One way of minimizing the effect of transmission errors is for the retina itself to measure the difference and to transmit a signal proportional to the difference. This, in effect, is what the ganglion cell does. The firing rate of a ganglion cell provides a measure of the difference in the intensities of light illuminating the center and surround. In this way information about small differences in intensities is directly transmitted to higher centers.

The segregation of information processing into parallel on-center and off-center pathways also enhances the performance of the visual system since the properties of each type of ganglion cell are best suited to signaling either a rapid increase or decrease in illumination. A rapid increase in the firing rate of on-center ganglion cells, which have a low rate of firing under dim illumination, signals rapid *increases* in light intensity. These same cells could not signal a rapid decrease in light intensity because they are already firing at a low rate. In contrast, a rapid increase in the firing rate of off-center ganglion cells, which have a low discharge rate in the light, signals rapid *decreases* in illumination. Peter Schiller and his colleagues have provided evidence that on-center ganglion cells are specialized for signaling rapid increases in illumination. They blocked the function of on-center ganglion cells in awake monkeys using a pharmacological agent, aminophosphonobutyrate (APB), which selectively blocks transmission from photoreceptors to on-center bipolar cells. Detection of rapid increases, but not decreases, in illumination was severely impaired in these animals.

Ganglion Cells Are Also Specialized for Processing Specific Aspects of the Visual Image

In addition to information on contrast and rapid change in illumination, the visual system also analyzes several other aspects of the visual image, such as color, form, and movement. In the visual cortex these features are processed by parallel pathways. Work by Christina Enroth-Cugell, John Robson, and others has shown that this parallel processing begins in the retina with parallel networks of ganglion cells.

Each region of the retina has several functionally distinct subsets of ganglion cells that serve the same photoreceptors in parallel. Most ganglion cells in the primate retina fall into two classes, M (or Pα) and P (or Pβ). Within each class there are both on-center and off-center cells. M cells have large cell bodies and a large dendritic arborization, while P cells have small cell bodies and small dendritic fields.

M cells have large receptive fields (reflecting their large dendritic arbors), and show a relatively transient response to sustained illumination. They respond to large objects and appear to be concerned with the analysis of gross features of a stimulus and its movement. The smaller P cells are more numerous, have small receptive fields, are for the most part wavelength-selective, and are involved in color vision. It is thought that P cells are responsible for the analysis of fine detail in the visual image, although some M cells may also be involved in this function. The primate retina also contains ganglion cells that do not fall into the P or M classes. The functions of these cells are largely unknown, although one type is known to report on the overall ambient light intensity.

Bipolar Cells and Other Interneurons Relay Signals from Photoreceptors to Ganglion Cells

How do the relatively simple responses of photoreceptors give rise to the complex responses of ganglion cells? Although the circuitry connecting the photoreceptors and ganglion cells appears complicated, on close examination it is relatively simple. Each type of interneuron in the retina (horizontal, bipolar, and amacrine cells) plays a specific role in shaping photoreceptor signals as they are transmitted through the retina. We will focus on the bipolar cells because they represent the most direct pathway between the receptors and ganglion cells.

Since vision in normal daylight relies on connections from cones to ganglion cells, we shall first describe the pathways that connect these cells and examine how different synaptic mechanisms shape signals as they are transferred from the receptors to the ganglion cells. We shall then briefly examine the pathways from rods to ganglion cells that convey visual information in dim light.

Cone Signals Are Conveyed to Ganglion Cells Through Direct or Lateral Pathways

Visual information is transferred from cones to ganglion cells along two types of pathways in the retina. Cones in the center of a ganglion cell's receptive field make direct synaptic contact with bipolar cells that in turn directly contact the ganglion cells (*direct* or *vertical pathways*). Signals from cones in the surround of the ganglion cell's receptive field are conveyed to the ganglion cell by means of horizontal and amacrine cells (*lateral pathways*). Horizontal cells transfer information from distant cones to nearby bipolar cells. Some types of amacrine cells transfer information from distant bipolar cells to the ganglion cells.

This orderly flow of information is reflected in the layered organization of the retina (Figure 28–6). The cell bodies of retinal neurons are organized into three *nuclear layers* (so-named because they contain the cells' nuclei): the *outer nuclear* layer, containing photoreceptors; the *inner nuclear* layer, containing bipolar, horizontal, and amacrine cells; and the *ganglion cell* layer. The processes of these cells are grouped in two plexiform layers where most synaptic contacts occur. The *outer plexiform* layer contains the processes of receptor, bipolar, and horizontal cells, while the *inner plexiform* layer contains the processes of bipolar, amacrine, and ganglion cells. This organization highlights the central position of bipolar cells, which bridge the two plexiform layers by having processes in both.

We have seen that photoreceptors respond to light with graded changes in membrane potential rather than by firing action potentials. The same is true of horizontal and bipolar cells. These cells lack voltage-gated Na$^+$ channels capable of generating action potentials, and instead transmit signals passively (Chapter 7). Because these small cells have short processes, signals are transmitted to their synaptic terminals without significant reduction. Passive signal transmission by cells with short processes occurs in many different parts of the brain. In contrast, the axons of ganglion cells project considerable distances to their targets in the brain, and, as we have seen, transfer information as trains of action potentials. Many types of amacrine cells also fire action potentials.

Bipolar Cells Also Have Center-Surround Receptive Fields

Bipolar cells are the key interneurons in the retina. As shown by Frank Werblin and John Dowling and by Akimichi Kaneko, bipolar cells have complex receptive field properties like those of ganglion cells: They have an antagonistic center-surround receptive field organization and are either on-center or off-center.

The cones in the receptive field center of a bipolar cell appear to be directly connected to the bipolar cell. On-center bipolar cells depolarize, while off-center bipolar cells hyperpolarize when light stimulates cones in the center of their receptive field (Figure 28–9A). In contrast, the inputs of cones in the bipolar cell's surround are relayed by horizontal cells, which can respond to inputs from distant sources because they have large dendritic trees and because they are electrically connected to other horizontal cells by gap junctions. When light stimulates cones in a bipolar cell's surround, it produces the opposite

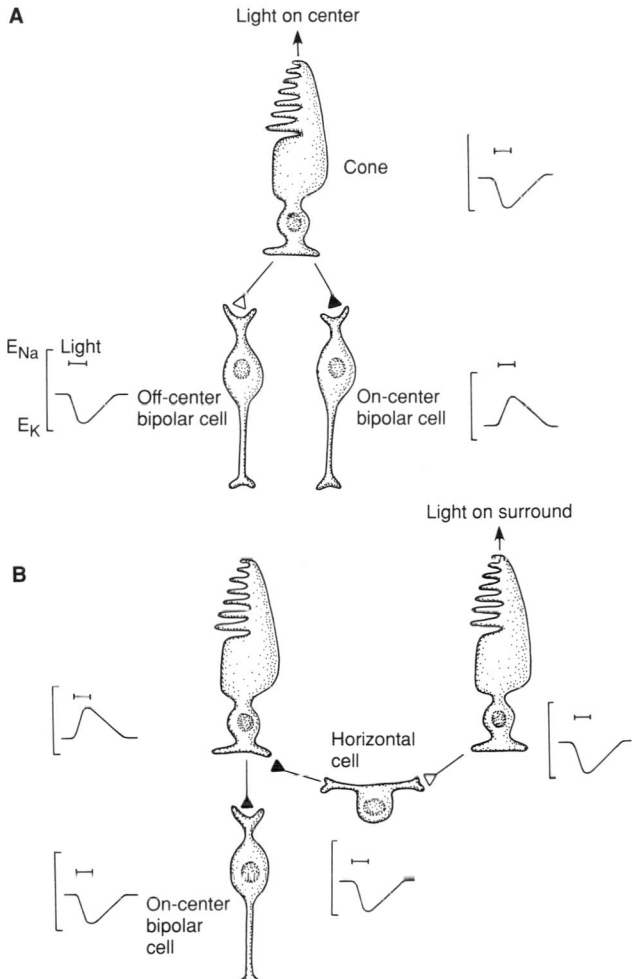

FIGURE 28–9
Bipolar cell responses are determined by inputs from photoreceptors and horizontal cells.

A. Visual information is segregated into on-center and off-center pathways. A single cone photoreceptor synapses on two bipolar cells. When the cone is hyperpolarized by light, the on-center bipolar cell is excited and the off-center bipolar cell is inhibited. These opposite actions are initiated by a transmitter substance (probably glutamate) released by the cone. In the dark the cone releases large amounts of transmitter because it is depolarized. Light, by hyperpolarizing the cone, causes a reduction in transmitter release. The same transmitter has different actions because the two types of bipolar cells have different postsynaptic receptors.

B. The response of a bipolar cell to stimulation of photoreceptors in the center of its receptive field is antagonized by stimulation of photoreceptors in the surround of its receptive field. This antagonistic interaction between neighboring retinal areas is mediated by the action of horizontal cells. Center-surround antagonism is illustrated here for a bipolar cell in the on-center pathway. In the dark, cones in the surround release glutamate steadily onto the horizontal cells, maintaining the cells in a slightly depolarized state (to -40 mV). In this state horizontal cells release an inhibitory transmitter that maintains cones in the center of the receptor field in a hyperpolarized state. Illumination of a cone in the bipolar cell's surround hyperpolarizes the cone, and this in turn results in the hyperpolarization of the horizontal cells connected to the cone. This causes a reduction in the amount of inhibitory transmitter released by the horizontal cell onto cones in the receptive field center, which results in the depolarization of these cones (the opposite effect of light absorption by center cones). This in turn hyperpolarizes the on-center bipolar cell, antagonizing the effect of illuminating the receptive field center.

response to that evoked by illumination of cones in the center (Figure 28–9B).

How does a cone depolarize the on-center bipolar cells and hyperpolarize the off-center bipolar cells with which it synapses? The cone releases a single neurotransmitter, thought to be glutamate, which has opposite actions on the two classes of bipolar cells. On-center bipolar cells are inhibited and off-center bipolar cells are excited. Recall, though, that the cone is depolarized in the dark (around -40 mV). This depolarization causes its synaptic terminals to release glutamate continuously, which maintains the on-center bipolar cells in a hyperpolarized state. When the cone is illuminated it hyperpolarizes, which causes a reduction in the amount of glutamate the cell releases, so that on-center bipolar cells depolarize. Conversely, glutamate released by the cone in the dark excites off-center bipolar cells, which therefore hyperpolarize when transmitter release is reduced by light (Figure 28–9A).

Glutamate produces different responses in the two classes of bipolar cells by gating different ion channels. It depolarizes off-center bipolar cells by opening cation channels that carry an inward, depolarizing Na$^+$ current into these cells. The mechanism by which it hyperpolarizes

on-center bipolar cells is unusual, and may be different for rod and cone cell synapses. At some synapses the transmitter appears to act by opening K$^+$-selective ion channels. At others it appears to close cation channels that are open and carry an inward Na$^+$ current in the absence of transmitter. Like the dark current in rods and cones, this sustained current maintains the cell in a depolarized state. Thus, when the channels are closed by transmitter, the cell hyperpolarizes. Scott Nawy and Craig Jahr have recently found that, like the dark current in photoreceptors, the sustained current in on-center bipolar cells flows through cGMP-gated channels that, in the absence of transmitter, are kept open by a high concentration of intracellular cGMP. Glutamate appears to cause the closure of these channels in precisely the same way as light causes the closure of cGMP-gated channels in photoreceptors — by activating a second messenger cascade that results in a lowering of the cytoplasmic concentration of cGMP. By analogy with photoreceptors, it is thought that the bipolar cells have a specific glutamate receptor that, like rhodopsin, activates a G-protein (perhaps transducin), which in turn activates cGMP phosphodiesterase.

How do horizontal cells mediate antagonistic inputs

from cones in the surround of the bipolar cell? It is believed that horizontal cells do not make direct synaptic contact with the bipolar cells. Instead, as was first shown by Dennis Baylor and his colleagues, the horizontal cells synapse onto *cones* in the center of the bipolar cell's receptive field. When the surround is illuminated, horizontal cells *depolarize* the cones in the center, the opposite effect of light absorption by these cones (Figure 28–9B). This mechanism can explain the antagonism between center and surround in bipolar cells; whether it accounts for the antagonism entirely is not yet known.

Each Class of Bipolar Cells Has Excitatory Connections with Ganglion Cells of the Same Class

The receptive field properties of a ganglion cell largely reflect those of the bipolar cells connected to it because each type of bipolar cell (on-center or off-center) makes *excitatory* synaptic connections with the corresponding type of ganglion cell. When on-center bipolar cells are depolarized by light, they depolarize on-center ganglion cells, which therefore fire more action potentials (Figure 28–10).

Although the responses of ganglion cells are largely determined by these direct inputs from bipolar cells, they are also shaped by amacrine cells, a group of interneurons with processes in the inner plexiform layer (Figure 28–6). There are over 20 morphologically distinguishable types of amacrine cells that use at least eight different neurotransmitters. Some amacrine cells have a similar function to horizontal cells: They mediate antagonistic inputs to ganglion cells from bipolar cells in the ganglion cell's surround. Others have been implicated in shaping the complex receptive field properties of specific classes of ganglion cells, such as the M-type ganglion cells that are orientation-selective.

Different Pathways Convey Rod Signals to Ganglion Cells in the Moderately and Extremely Dark-Adapted Eye

The pathways connecting cones to ganglion cells are used for vision in normal daylight. At lower light levels vision relies on rods. In the moderately dark-adapted eye (e.g., at dusk) rod signals are believed to be relayed to ganglion cells through cones. Rod signals can be transmitted directly to neighboring cones via gap junctions that connect these cells (Figure 28–11). The signals are then relayed by cones to ganglion cells through the pathways described in previous sections. For this reason, the receptive field properties of ganglion cells do not change as the eye becomes moderately dark-adapted.

During prolonged exposure to darkness or very dim light (such as starlight), the sensitivity of ganglion cells increases dramatically until these cells can detect the effects of individual photons absorbed by rods in their receptive field center. One factor that contributes to this extreme sensitivity is that ganglion cells are not inhibited

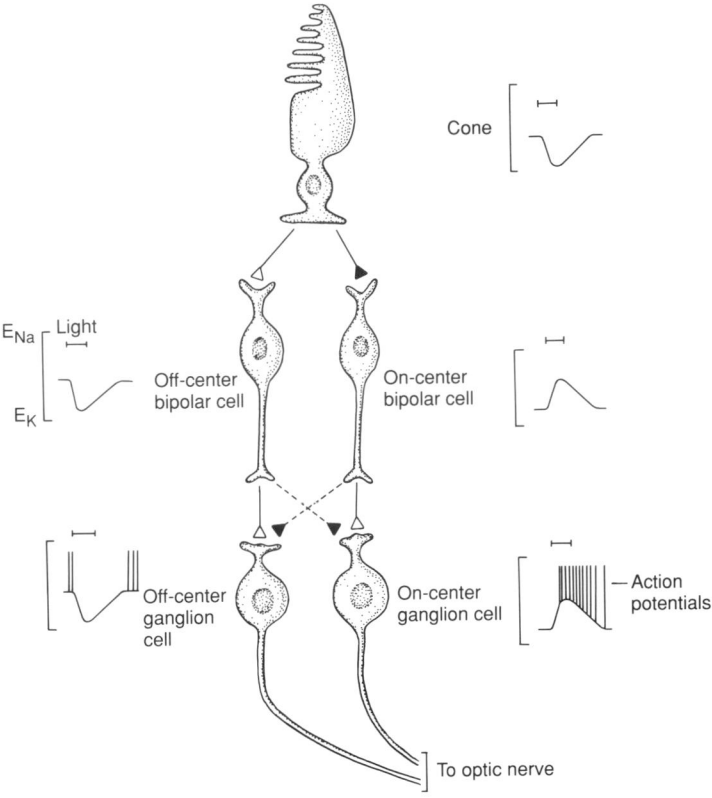

FIGURE 28–10

The responses of ganglion cells are largely determined by inputs from bipolar cells. Each type of bipolar cell makes excitatory connections with ganglion cells of the same class. Thus, an on-center bipolar cell depolarized by illumination of its receptive field center will depolarize the on-center ganglion cells connected to it. Peter Sterling and his colleagues have suggested that in mammals each type of bipolar cell also inhibits ganglion cells of the opposite class (**dashed connections**). For example, on-center bipolar cells excited by illumination of the center will hyperpolarize an off-center ganglion cell, thus reinforcing the hyperpolarization of the ganglion cell caused by the removal of excitatory inputs from off-center bipolar cells, which are inhibited by illumination of the center.

by illumination of their surround when the eye is fully dark-adapted. Under these conditions ganglion cells cease to be detectors of local contrast and instead become effective light detectors.

This change in receptive field properties is believed to result from a change in the pathways that convey rod signals to ganglion cells. During prolonged adaptation the gap junctions connecting rods and cones appear to close, preventing rod signals from being transferred through cones. Instead, the signals appear to be transferred to ganglion cells by *rod bipolar cells*, a specialized set of on-center bipolar cells that receive direct synaptic input only from rods. Unlike the cone bipolar cells, rod bipolar cells do not synapse directly onto ganglion cells. They send outputs to AII amacrine cells, which communicate di-

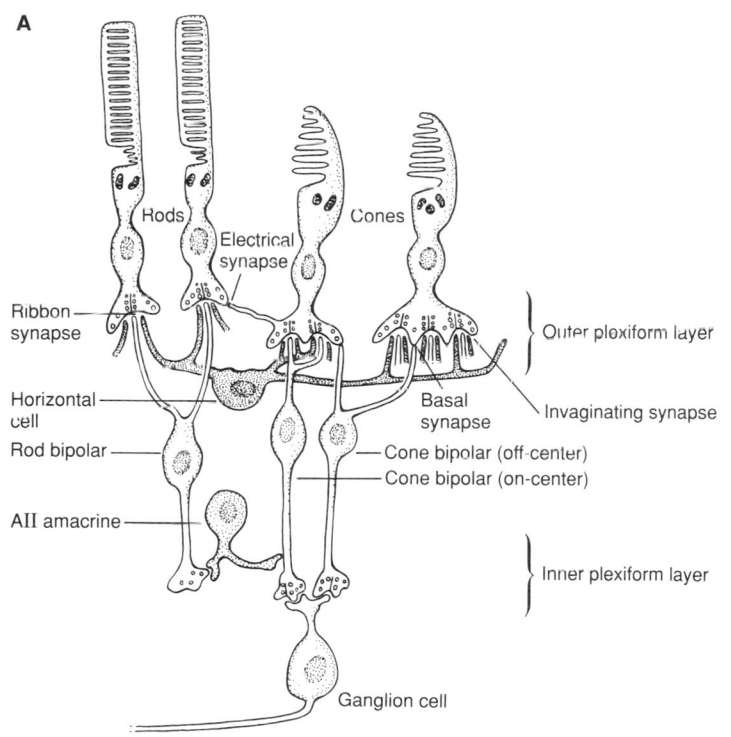

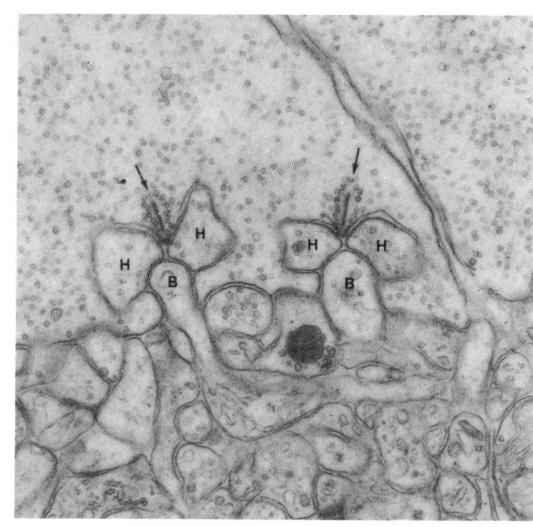

FIGURE 28–11

Rods and cones contact different populations of bipolar cells at synapses with distinctive morphologies.

A. In the outer plexiform layer the rods and cones synapse on bipolar and horizontal cells. Rods and cones each synapse on different bipolar cells, but these distinct pathways converge in the ganglion cell layer. However, the pathways prior to the ganglion cell connections are not independent because electrical synapses occur between cones and rods. Cones make contact with the two classes of bipolar cells at morphologically different synapses: They contact off-center bipolar cells at *basal* (flat) synapses, and on-center bipolar cells at *ribbon* synapses. The on-center bipolar cells send their dendrites into invaginations in the cone terminal (thus, these ribbon synapses are also called *invaginating* synapses). There they form the central element of three synapses, the other two being dendrites of horizontal cells. Horizontal cell processes are both post- and presynaptic at cone terminals (as illustrated in Figure 28–9B). Rods synapse on only one type of bipolar cell, which receives inputs only at ribbon synapses. These bipolar cells do not synapse directly on ganglion cells. Instead, they form synapses with type AII amacrine interneurons, which relay their inputs to ganglion cells by synapsing directly onto off-center ganglion cells (not illustrated) and onto bipolar cells that connect to on-center ganglion cells, as shown here.

B. Ribbon synapses at the photoreceptor terminal are characterized by an electron-dense ribbon (**arrows**) around which vesicles are clustered. One bipolar cell (**B**) and two horizontal cell (**H**) processes invaginate the presynaptic membrane. (From Dowling, 1979.)

rectly with off-center ganglion cells and indirectly with on-center ganglion cells by way of cone bipolar cells (Figure 28–11).

Some Chemical Synapses in the Retina Have Distinctive Morphologies

The retina contains both electrical synapses (gap junctions) and chemical synapses. Electrical synapses occur mainly between like neurons. As described in the last section, photoreceptors are connected to each other by gap junctions. Horizontal cells are also extensively interconnected electrically and can therefore mediate lateral information transfer over large distances. As in the rest of the brain, however, the predominant type of synapse in the retina is chemical. Many of these synapses are conventional chemical synapses that have a single presynaptic element that makes contact with a single postsynaptic element. The retina also contains two types of chemical synapses with distinctive morphologies: ribbon and basal synapses (Figure 28–11). They are the only synapses that photoreceptors make with horizontal and bipolar cells.

At *ribbon synapses* a single presynaptic specialization ends on more than one postsynaptic element, ensuring that transmitter is released simultaneously onto these elements. For example, photoreceptor ribbon synapses send input to three postsynaptic processes (called a *triad*). Typically, two horizontal cell processes occupy the two lateral positions and a single on-center bipolar cell process occupies the central position (Figure 28–11). Ribbon synapses are also found in connections between bipolar cells and postsynaptic amacrine and ganglion cells.

Basal synapses are unusual in that the presynaptic specialization does not contain synaptic vesicles. The main reason for believing that these contacts are synapses is that in higher vertebrates off-center bipolar cells receive inputs from cones only at these contacts (rods form only ribbon, not basal synapses, with bipolar cells). Because they lack synaptic vesicles, basal synapses could be specialized for a novel mechanism of transmitter release, *calcium-independent nonvesicular release*. Eric Schwartz has obtained evidence for this mechanism, although he has not yet determined whether it operates at basal synapses. He found that synaptic transmission from photoreceptors to some bipolar and horizontal cells can be maintained even when the extracellular Ca^{2+} concentration is drastically lowered and cobalt, a Ca^{2+} channel blocker, is added. Synaptic transmission at the neuromuscular junction is blocked under similar conditions because Ca^{2+} cannot enter the presynaptic terminal to trigger vesicle release. The specific mechanism of transmitter release at these retinal synapses is not known, but indirect evidence suggests that it results from the voltage-dependent transport of transmitter (glutamate) out of the cell by specific carrier proteins (similar to the carrier proteins that transport amino acids *into* cells).

An Overall View

The absorption of light and its transduction into electrical signals is carried out by the photoreceptors. Visual information is then transferred from the receptors to the ganglion cells via the bipolar cells. The ganglion cells in turn project to the brain: their axons form the optic nerve. Two types of interneurons (horizontal cells and amacrine cells) provide lateral inputs to bipolar cells and ganglion cells.

Recent studies have demonstrated the central role of the cyclic nucleotide cGMP in phototransduction. Absorption of light by the photosensitive visual pigments in the photoreceptor triggers a second-messenger cascade. The activated pigment molecules stimulate a G-protein, transducin, which in turn activates a phosphodiesterase that catalyzes the hydrolysis of cGMP. Light absorption therefore causes a reduction in the cytoplasmic concentration of cGMP. In darkness cGMP opens specialized ion channels that carry a depolarizing current into the cell, so that the reduction in cGMP makes the photoreceptor hyperpolarize.

As visual information is transferred from photoreceptors to ganglion cells, it is segregated into parallel on-center and off-center pathways. An on-center ganglion cell is excited when light stimulates the center of its receptive field and inhibited when light stimulates its surround. The opposite responses are observed in off-center ganglion cells. These transformations of the visual signal assist higher centers in detecting weak contrasts and rapid changes in light intensity. In addition, ganglion cells are specialized for processing different aspects of the visual image. Some are concerned with the general features of a stimulus and its movement. Others transmit information about fine spatial detail and color in the visual image.

The pattern of synaptic connections in the retina explains how the responses of ganglion cells arise. Bipolar cells, like ganglion cells, fall into two classes, on-center and off-center. The transmitter released by cones excites bipolar cells of one class and inhibits the others. Each cone makes contact with both cell types. Cones in the receptive field center of a ganglion cell synapse onto bipolar cells that make direct contact with the ganglion cell. Inputs from cones in the receptive field surround are relayed along lateral pathways by horizontal and amacrine cells.

As we shall see in later chapters, the segregation of information into parallel processing pathways, and the shaping of response properties by inhibitory lateral connections, are pervasive organizational principles in the visual system.

Selected Readings

Dowling, J. E. 1987. The Retina: An Approachable Part of the Brain. Cambridge, Mass.: Belknap Press of Harvard University Press.

Miller, R. F., and Slaughter, M. M. 1986. Excitatory amino acid receptors of the retina: Diversity of subtypes and conductance mechanisms. Trends Neurosci. 9:211–218.

Pugh, E., and Altman, J. 1988. A role for calcium in adaptation. Nature 334:16–17.

Rodieck, R. W. 1973. The Vertebrate Retina: Principles of Structure and Function. San Francisco: Freeman.

Schnapf, J. L., and Baylor, D. A. 1987. How photoreceptor cells respond to light. Sci. Am. 256(4):40–47.

Shapley, R., and Perry, V. H. 1986. Cat and monkey retinal ganglion cells and their visual functional roles. Trends Neurosci. 9:229–235.

Sterling, P. 1983. Microcircuitry of the cat retina. Annu. Rev. Neurosci. 6:149–185.

Stryer, L. 1986. Cyclic GMP cascade of vision. Annu. Rev. Neurosci. 9:87–119.

Stryer, L. 1987. The molecules of visual excitation. Sci. Am. 257(1):42–50.

Trends in Neurosciences. 1986. Special Issue: Information processing in the retina. Trends Neurosci. 9:181–240.

References

Barlow, H. B. 1953. Summation and inhibition in the frog's retina. J. Physiol. (Lond.) 119:69–88.

Baylor, D. A., Fuortes, M. G. F., and O'Bryan, P. M. 1971. Receptive fields of cones in the retina of the turtle. J. Physiol. (Lond.) 214:265–294.

Baylor, D. A., Lamb, T. D., and Yau, K.-W. 1979. Responses of retinal rods to single photons. J. Physiol. (Lond.) 288:613–634.

Brown, R., and Herrnstein, R. J. 1975. Psychology. Boston: Little, Brown.

Dowling, J. E. 1979. Information processing by local circuits: The vertebrate retina as a model system. In F. O. Schmitt and F. G. Worden (eds.), The Neurosciences: Fourth Study Program. Cambridge, Mass.: MIT Press, pp. 163–181.

Enroth-Cugell, C., and Robson, J. G. 1966. The contrast sensitivity of retinal ganglion cells of the cat. J. Physiol. (Lond.) 187:517–552.

Fesenko, E. E., Kolesnikov, S. S., and Lyubarsky, A. L. 1985. Induction by cyclic GMP of cationic conductance in plasma membrane of retinal rod outer segment. Nature 313:310–313.

Fung, B. K.-K., Hurley, J. B., and Stryer, L. 1981. Flow of information in the light-triggered cyclic nucleotide cascade of vision. Proc. Natl. Acad. Sci. U.S.A. 78:152–156.

Hartline, H. K. 1940. The receptive fields of optic nerve fibers. Am. J. Physiol. 130:690–699.

Kaneko, A. 1970. Physiological and morphological identification of horizontal, bipolar and amacrine cells in goldfish retina. J. Physiol. (Lond.) 207:623–633.

Kaupp, U. B., Niidome, T., Tanabe, T., Terada, S., Bönigk, W., Stühmer, W., Cook, N. J., Kangawa, K., Matsuo, H., Hirose, T., Miyata, T., and Numa, S. 1989. Primary structure and functional expression from complementary DNA of the rod photoreceptor cyclic GMP-gated channel. Nature 342:762–766.

Koch, K.-W., and Stryer, L. 1988. Highly cooperative feedback control of retinal rod guanylate cyclase by calcium ions. Nature 334:64–66.

Kuffler, S. W. 1953. Discharge patterns and functional organization of mammalian retina. J. Neurophysiol. 16: 37–68.

Matthews, H. R., Murphy, R. L. W., Fain, G. L., and Lamb, T. D. 1988. Photoreceptor light adaptation is mediated by cytoplasmic calcium concentration. Nature 334:67–69.

Matthews, H. R., Torre, V., and Lamb, T. D. 1985. Effects on the photoresponse of calcium buffers and cyclic GMP incorporated into the cytoplasm of retinal rods. Nature 313:582–585.

Nakatani, K., and Yau, K.-W. 1988. Calcium and light adaptation in retinal rods and cones. Nature 334:69–71.

Nathans, J., and Hogness, D. S. 1984. Isolation and nucleotide sequence of the gene encoding human rhodopsin. Proc. Natl. Acad. Sci. U.S.A. 81:4851–4855.

Nawy, S., and Jahr, C. E. 1990. Suppression by glutamate of cGMP-activated conductance in retinal bipolar cells. Nature 346:269–271.

O'Brien, D. F. 1982. The chemistry of vision. Science 218:961–966.

Saito, T., Kondo, H., and Toyoda, J. 1978. Rod and cone signals in the on-center bipolar cell: Their different ionic mechanisms. Vis. Res. 18:591–595.

Schiller, P. H., Sandell, J. H., and Maunsell, J. H. R. 1986. Functions of the ON and OFF channels of the visual system. Nature 322:824–825.

Schwartz, E. A. 1986. Synaptic transmission in amphibian retinae during conditions unfavourable for calcium entry into presynaptic terminals. J. Physiol. (Lond.) 376:411–428.

Schwartz, E. A. 1987. Depolarization without calcium can release γ-aminobutyric acid from a retinal neuron. Science 238:350–355.

Tomita, T. 1976. Electrophysiological studies of retinal cell function. Invest. Ophthalmol. 15:171–187.

Wald, G. 1968. Molecular basis of visual excitation. Science 162:230–239.

Werblin, F. S. 1972. Lateral interactions at inner plexiform layer of vertebrate retina: Antagonistic responses to change. Science 175:1008–1010.

Werblin, F. S., and Dowling, J. E. 1969. Organization of the retina of the mudpuppy, *Necturus maculosus*. II. Intracellular recording. J. Neurophysiol. 32:339–355.

Young, R. W. 1970. Visual cells. Sci. Am. 223(4):80–91.

Carol Mason
Eric R. Kandel

29

Central Visual Pathways

The Retinal Image Is an Inversion of the Visual Field

The Retina Projects to Three Subcortical Regions in the Brain

    The Pretectal Area of the Midbrain Controls Pupillary Reflexes

    The Superior Colliculus Controls Saccadic Eye Movements

    The Lateral Geniculate Nucleus Processes Visual Information

Neurons in the Lateral Geniculate Nucleus Have Concentric Receptive Fields

The Primary Visual Cortex Transforms Concentric Receptive Fields into Linear Segments and Boundaries

    Simple and Complex Cells Decompose the Outlines of a Visual Image into Short Line Segments of Various Orientation

    Some Feature Abstraction Can Be Accomplished by Progressive Convergence Within the Primary Visual Cortex

The Primary Visual Cortex Is Organized into Vertical Columns

Columnar Units Are Linked by Horizontal Connections

The Visual and Somatic Sensory Cortices Are Functionally Similar

Lesions in the Retino-Geniculate-Cortical Pathway Cause Predictable Changes in Vision

An Overall View

The whole organization of the lateral geniculate nucleus cries aloud that something is being segregated. The question before us is simply: What?

> G. L. Walls, *The Lateral Geniculate Nucleus and Visual Histophysiology,* 1953

The visual system is the most complex of all the sensory systems. The auditory nerve contains about 30,000 fibers, but the optic nerve contains one million, more than all the dorsal root fibers entering the entire spinal cord! Most of what we know about the functional organization of the visual system is derived from experiments that are similar to those used to investigate the somatic sensory system. The similarities of these systems allow us to identify general principles governing the transformation of sensory information in the brain and in the organization and functioning of the cerebral cortex.

In this chapter we examine the flow of visual information in two stages: first from the retina to the midbrain and thalamus, and then from the thalamus to the visual cortex. We shall begin by considering how the world is projected on the retina as visual fields, and describe the projection of the retina to three subcortical brain areas: the pretectal region, the superior colliculus of the midbrain, and the lateral geniculate nucleus of the thalamus. We shall then examine the pathways from the lateral geniculate nucleus to the cortex, focusing on the structure and function of the initial cortical relay in the primary visual cortex so as to elucidate the first steps in the cortical processing of visual information necessary for perception.

The Retinal Image Is an Inversion of the Visual Field

The regions of the visual field are defined with respect to the two retinas. The regions of the retina are named with reference to the midline: The *nasal hemiretina* lies medial to the fovea, and the *temporal hemiretina* is lateral to the fovea. Each half of the retina can also be divided into a *dorsal* and a *ventral* quadrant.

The visual field is the view seen by the two eyes without movement of the head. Imagine that the foveas of both eyes are fixed on a single point in space. It is then possible to define a *left* and a *right* half of the visual field. The *left hemifield*, or left half of the visual field, projects on the nasal hemiretina of the left eye and on the temporal hemiretina of the right eye. The *right hemifield* projects on the nasal hemiretina of the right eye and on the temporal hemiretina of the left eye. Light originating in the central region of the visual field enters *both* eyes; this area is called the *binocular zone*. In either half of the visual field there is also a *monocular zone*: Light from the temporal portion of the hemifield projects only onto the nasal hemiretina of the eye on the same side because the nose blocks this light from reaching the eye on the opposite side (Figure 29–1). This monocular portion of the visual field is also called the *temporal crescent* because it constitutes the crescent-shaped temporal extreme of each visual field. Since there is no binocular overlap in this region, vision is lost in the entire temporal crescent if this region of the retina is severely damaged.

FIGURE 29–1

The visual field has both binocular and monocular zones.

A. Light from the binocular zone (indicated in black) strikes both eyes, whereas light from the monocular zone strikes only the eye on the same side. The hemiretinas are defined with respect to the fovea, the region in the center of the retina with the highest acuity. The optic disc, the region where the ganglion cell axons leave the retina, is free of photoreceptors and therefore creates a gap, or blind spot in the visual field for each eye (see Figure 29–2).

B. Light from a monocular zone (temporal crescent) falls only on the ipsilateral nasal hemiretina and does not project upon the contralateral retina because it is blocked by the nose.

C. Each optic tract carries a complete representation of one half of the binocular zone in the visual field. Fibers from the nasal hemiretina of each eye cross to the opposite side at the optic chiasm, whereas fibers from the temporal hemiretina do not cross. In the illustration light from the right half of the binocular zone falls on the left temporal hemiretina and right nasal hemiretina. Axons from these hemiretinas thus contain a complete representation of the right hemifield of vision (see Figure 29–6).

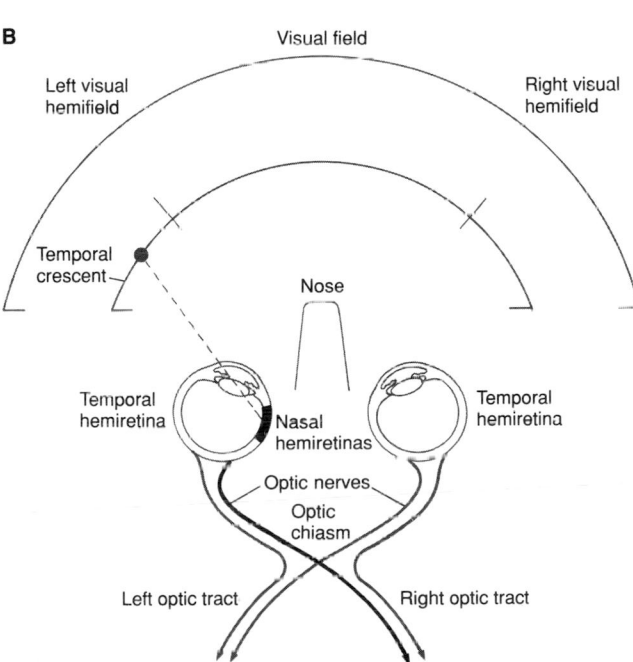

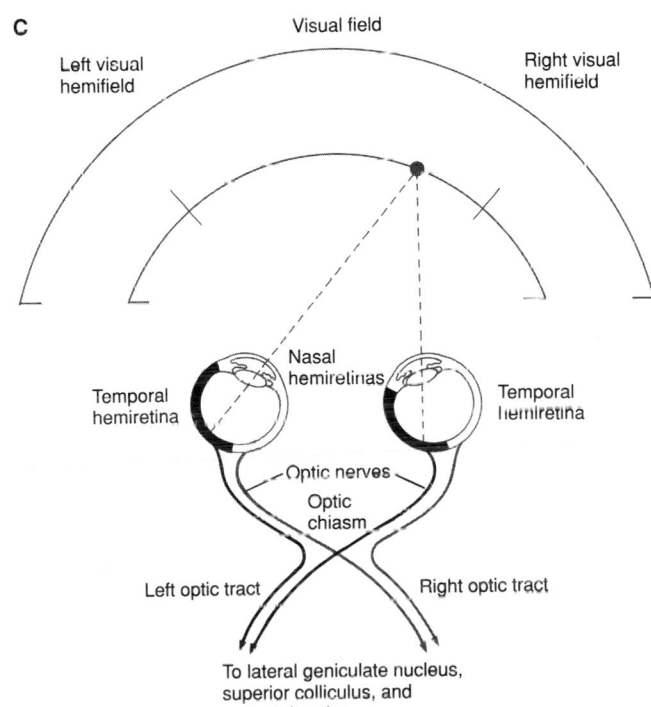

FIGURE 29–2

The blind spot in the left eye is located by shutting the right eye and fixating the upper cross with the left eye. If the book is held about 1.5 feet from the eye and is moved back and forth slightly, the circle on the left disappears since it is imaged on the blind spot. If the left eye fixates on the lower cross, the gap in the black line falls on the blind spot and the black line is seen as continuous because the gap is imaged on the blind spot. (Adapted from Hurvich, 1981.)

The optic disc, the region of the retina from which the ganglion cell axons exit, contains no photoreceptors and therefore is insensitive to light. Since the disc is medial to the fovea in both eyes (Figure 29–1A), light coming from a single point in the binocular zone never enters both optic discs, so that we are normally unaware of this blind spot. The blind spot of the left eye can be demonstrated by closing the right eye and looking at Figure 29–2 with the left eye. When the upper cross on the right of Figure 29–2 is viewed only with the fovea of the left eye at the appropriate distance (directly in front at about one and a half feet), the spot on the left disappears because it is projected medially from the left visual hemifield onto the optic disc of the left eye. This exercise demonstrates what blind peo-

FIGURE 29–3

The lens of the eye projects an inverted image on the retina in the same way as a camera. (Adapted from Groves and Schlesinger, 1979.)

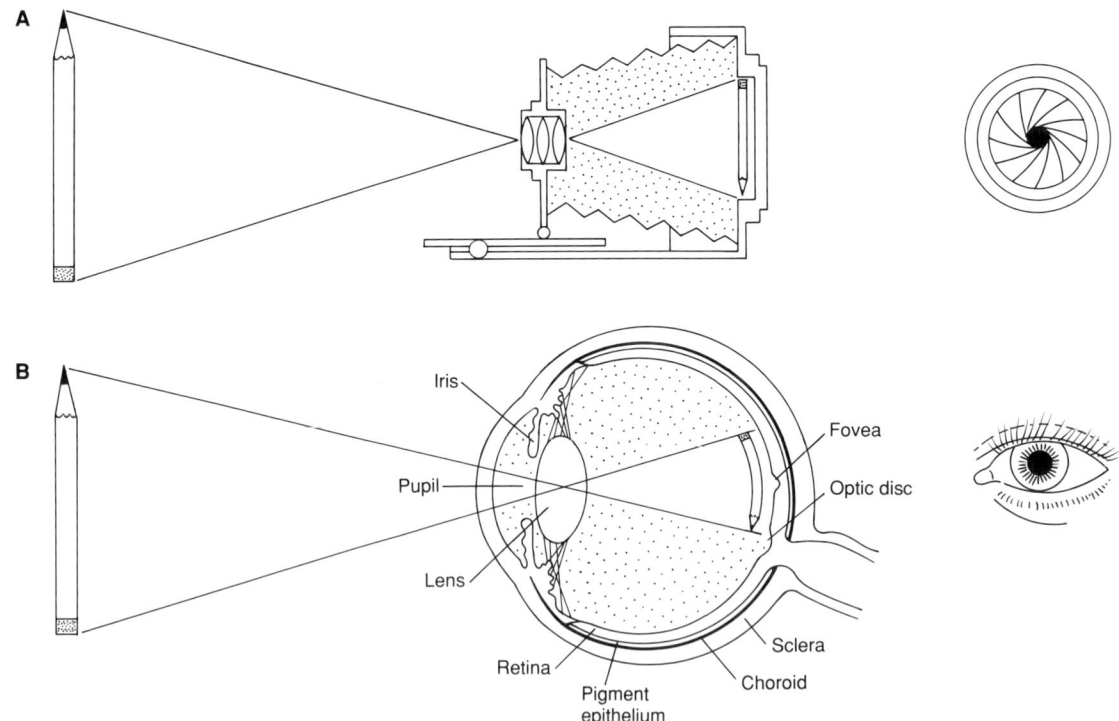

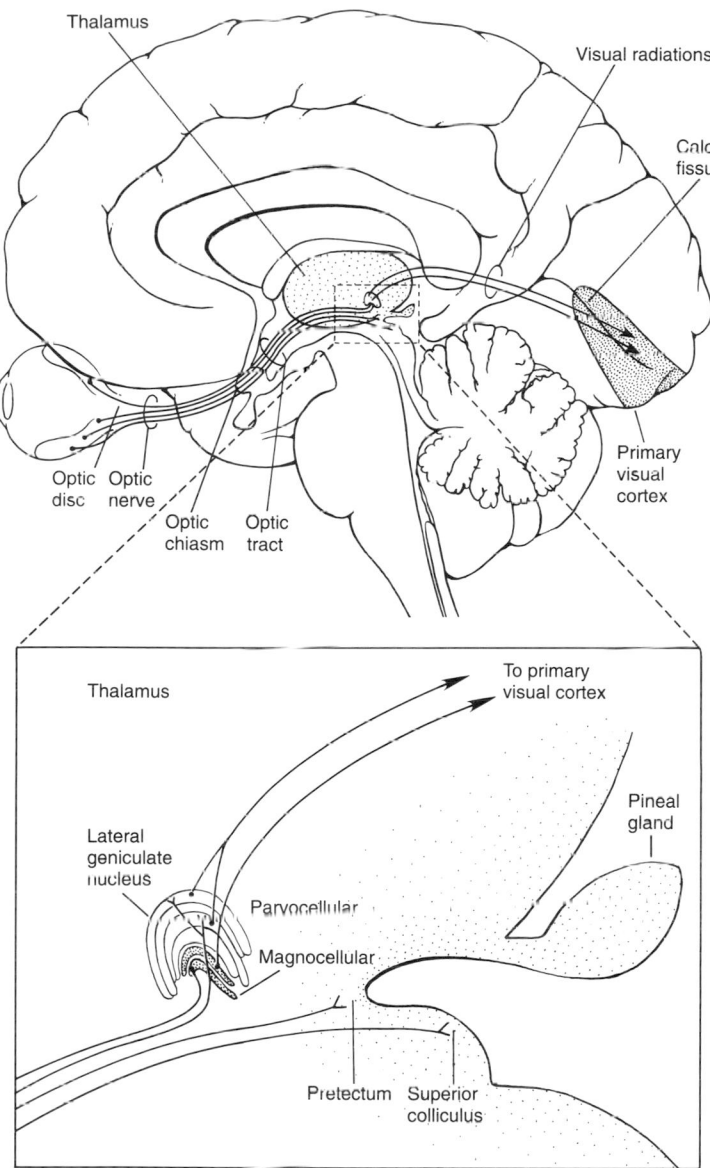

FIGURE 29–4

A simplified diagram of the projections from the retina to the various visual areas of the thalamus (lateral geniculate nucleus), midbrain (pretectum and superior colliculus), and area 17 of the cerebral cortex. The retinal projection to the pretectal area is important for pupillary reflexes and the projection to the superior colliculus mediates visually guided eye movements. The projection to the lateral geniculate nucleus and visual cortex processes visual information for perception.

ple experience—not blackness, but simply nothing. It also reveals why damage to large regions of the peripheral retina goes unnoticed. In these instances no large dark zone appears in the periphery, and it is usually by accidents, such as bumping into an unnoticed object, or by clinical testing of the visual fields, that the absence of sight is noticed.

It is important to keep in mind the correspondence between regions of the *visual field*, which is external, and the corresponding *retinal image.* First, the lens of the eye inverts the visual image upon the retina (Figure 29–3). The superior half of the visual field is projected onto the inferior (or ventral) half of the retina, and the inferior half of visual field is projected onto the superior (or dorsal) half of the retina. We see the world in its correct orientation because higher levels of the brain adjust this inversion. Thus, when an individual has sustained damage to the

inferior half of the retina of one eye, this causes a monocular deficit in the *superior half of the visual field.* Second, the binocular portion of each visual hemifield projects to different regions of the two retinas. For example, a point of light in the binocular half of the right visual hemifield falls upon the temporal hemiretina on the left eye and the nasal hemiretina of the right eye (Figure 29–1C).

The Retina Projects to Three Subcortical Regions in the Brain

The axons of all retinal ganglion cells stream toward the *optic disc,* where they become myelinated and together form the *optic nerve.* (Figure 29–4). The optic nerves from each eye join at the *optic chiasm.* There, fibers from each eye destined for one or the other side of the brain are sorted out. Retinal fibers from both eyes then enter each *optic tract*, which projects to three subcortical targets (Figure 29–4). Of the three subcortical regions receiving direct input from the retina, only one, the lateral geniculate nucleus, processes visual information that ultimately results in visual perception. The pretectal area of the midbrain uses inputs from the retina to produce pupillary reflexes, whereas the superior colliculus uses its input to generate eye movements.

The Pretectal Area of the Midbrain Controls Pupillary Reflexes

When light is shone upon one eye, it causes constriction of the pupil in that eye (the *direct response*) as well as in the other eye (the *consensual response*). Pupillary light reflexes are mediated by retinal ganglion neurons that respond to overall changes in brightness and project to the *pretectal area*, which lies just rostral to the superior colliculus where the midbrain fuses with the thalamus (Figure 29–5). The cells in the pretectal area project bilaterally to preganglionic parasympathetic neurons in the Edinger–Westphal (or accessory oculomotor) nucleus, which lies immediately adjacent to the neurons of the oculomotor (cranial nerve III) nucleus. Preganglionic neurons in the Edinger–Westphal nucleus send axons out of the brain stem in the oculomotor nerve to innervate the *ciliary ganglion*. This ganglion contains the postganglionic neurons that innervate the smooth muscle of the pupillary sphincter.

Pupillary reflexes are important clinically because they indicate the functional state of the afferent and efferent pathways mediating them. As an example, if light directed to the left eye of a patient elicits a consensual response in the right eye but not a direct one in the left eye, this response means that the afferent limb of the reflex, the optic nerve, is intact but the efferent limb to the left eye is damaged, possibly by a lesion of the oculomotor nerve. In contrast, if the optic nerve is lesioned unilaterally, light shone in the affected eye will cause no change in either pupil, but light shone in the normal eye will elicit both a direct and a consensual response. The absence of pupillary reflexes in an unconscious patient is a symptom of damage to the midbrain, the region from which the oculomotor nerve originates.

The Superior Colliculus Controls Saccadic Eye Movements

The superior colliculus coordinates visual, somatic, and auditory information, adjusting movements of the head and eyes toward a stimulus. Distributed within the seven layers of the colliculus are three sensory maps—a visual map, a map of the body surface, a map for sound in space— and a motor map. The most superficial layers receive both direct input from the retina and indirect input from the visual cortex. The deeper layers receive inputs primarily

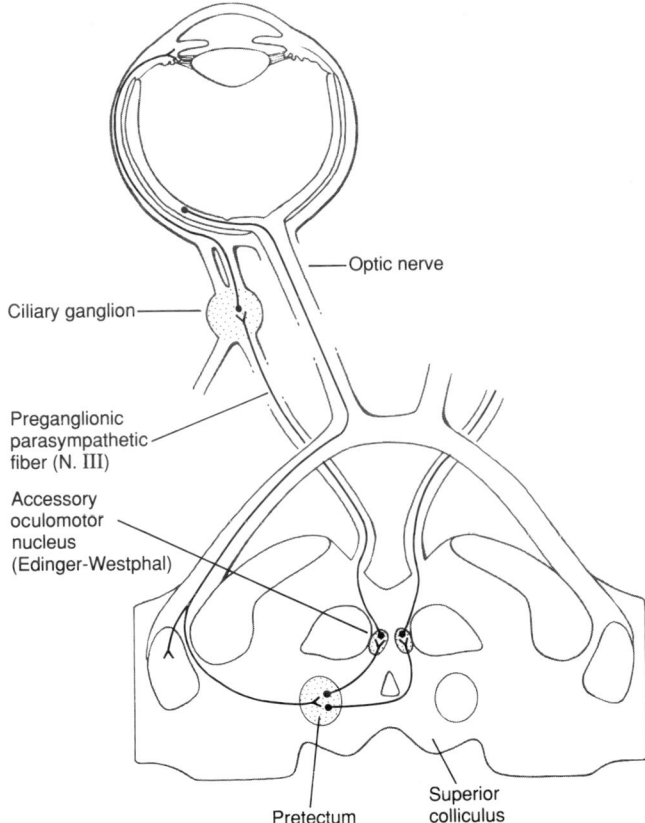

FIGURE 29–5
The reflex pathway mediating pupillary constriction. Light signals are relayed through the midbrain pretectum, to preganglionic parasympathetic neurons in the Edinger–Westphal nucleus, and out through the parasympathetic outflow of the oculomotor nerve to the ciliary ganglion. Postganglionic neurons then innervate the smooth muscle of the pupillary sphincter.

from the somatic sensory and auditory systems but also receive visual input through the upper layers. These deep cells are arranged according to the location of their respective somatic sensory or auditory receptive fields. These several sensory maps in the colliculus differ from those in the sensory cortical areas (Chapter 24). In the somatic sensory cortex the size of the central somatic representation of a peripheral structure (say, the hand) is determined by the importance of the structure as a tactile organ (reflected in the density of innervation of the structure). In contrast, the relative size of a somatic representation in the colliculus is determined by the visual map. Structures close to the eye, such as the nose and face, have greater representation than do structures located farther away, such as the finger tips.

As a result, a given location in the superior colliculus is thought to represent a given point in visual space around the animal and the organization of the different sensory maps reflect this function. The various sensory maps are aligned spatially with one another. For example, in the superficial visual map, neurons that receive information from the contralateral temporal visual field are located above neurons in the deeper auditory map that receive information from the same contralateral region of the animal's auditory space. Similarly, neurons in the corresponding portion of the somatosensory map receive information from cutaneous receptors on the contralateral parts of the body. In this way different sensory information about the location of a stimulus with respect to a particular part of the body is conveyed to a common region of the superior colliculus.

The three sensory maps in turn connect to a motor map located in the deeper layers of the superior colliculus. As a result, the colliculus can use the sensory information to control *saccadic* (high velocity) eye movements that orient the eye toward the stimulus, a function that the colliculus carries out together with a region of the frontal cortex called the *frontal eye fields* (to be considered in Chapter 42). Peter Schiller and his colleagues explored the roles of the superior colliculus and frontal eye fields in saccadic movements elicited by visual stimuli. They found that the colliculus receives information about three types of stimuli: those concerned with motion in the visual field, those concerned with visual attentiveness, and those concerned with identifying the broad outlines of objects. In contrast, the cortical frontal eye fields receive input from the primary visual cortex about fine visual discrimination and are concerned with generating saccadic movements to complex visual stimuli.

The superior colliculus projects to the regions of the brain stem that control eye movements. In addition, axons from the superior colliculus are also distributed in two descending tracts, the tectospinal and tectopontine tracts. The *tectospinal tract* is involved in the reflex control of head and neck movements; its axons cross the midline and descend to the upper spinal cord, where the neck motor neurons are located. The *tectopontine tract* relays visual input to the cerebellum for further coordination of eye and head movements.

The Lateral Geniculate Nucleus Processes Visual Information

The majority of retinal axons terminate in the lateral geniculate nucleus, the principal subcortical region that processes visual information for perception. Axons from the retina project through the optic chiasm, where the fibers from the nasal half of each retina cross to the opposite side of the brain. The axons from ganglion cells in the temporal hemiretina do not cross. Thus, the left optic tract contains axons from the right half of each retina—the temporal hemiretina of the left eye and the nasal hemiretina of the right eye. In other words, the left optic tract carries a complete representation of the right hemifield of vision (Figure 29–1C). Fibers from the right half of each retina (the nasal hemiretina of the left eye and the temporal hemiretina of

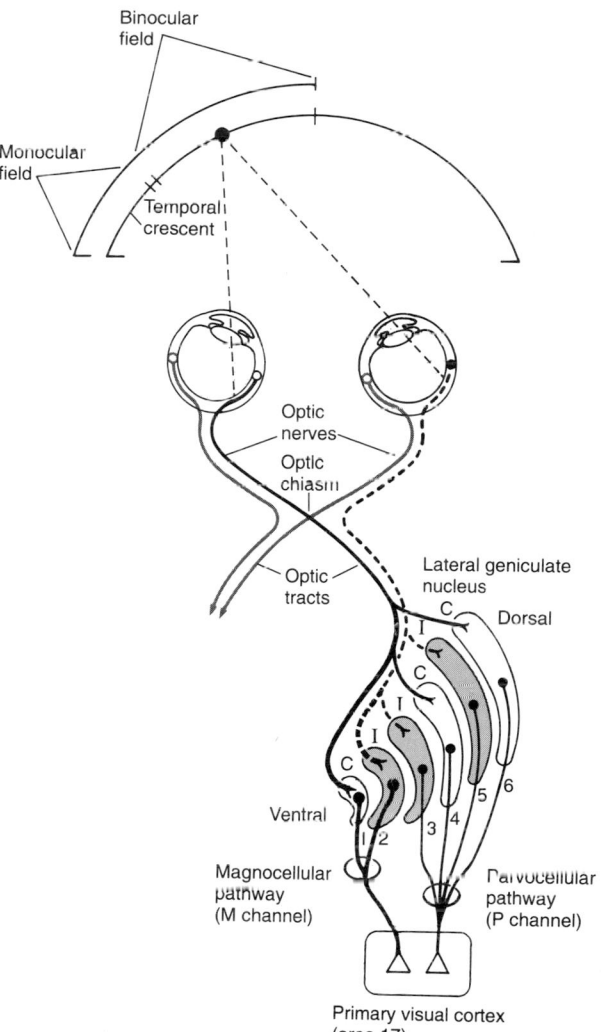

FIGURE 29–6

Inputs from the right hemiretina of each eye project to different layers of the right lateral geniculate nucleus to create a complete representation of the left visual hemifield. Similarly, fibers from the left hemiretina of each eye project to the left lateral geniculate nucleus. The temporal crescent is not represented in contralateral inputs (see Figure 29–1B). Layers 1 and 2 comprise the magnocellular layers; layers 4 through 6 comprise the parvocellular layers. All of these project to area 17, the primary visual cortex. There are major pathways from the retina through the lateral geniculate nucleus to area 17 of the cortex, which process, in parallel, different aspects of visual information. As we shall learn in the next chapter, three major parallel pathways have been identified: one magnocellular and two parvocellular pathways. The first is concerned primarily with movement and gross features of the stimulus; the second primarily carries information on detail and form; the third is concerned with color.

the right eye) project in the right optic tract to the right lateral geniculate nucleus (Figure 29–6). Similarly, fibers from the left hemiretina of each eye project in the left optic tract to the left lateral geniculate nucleus.

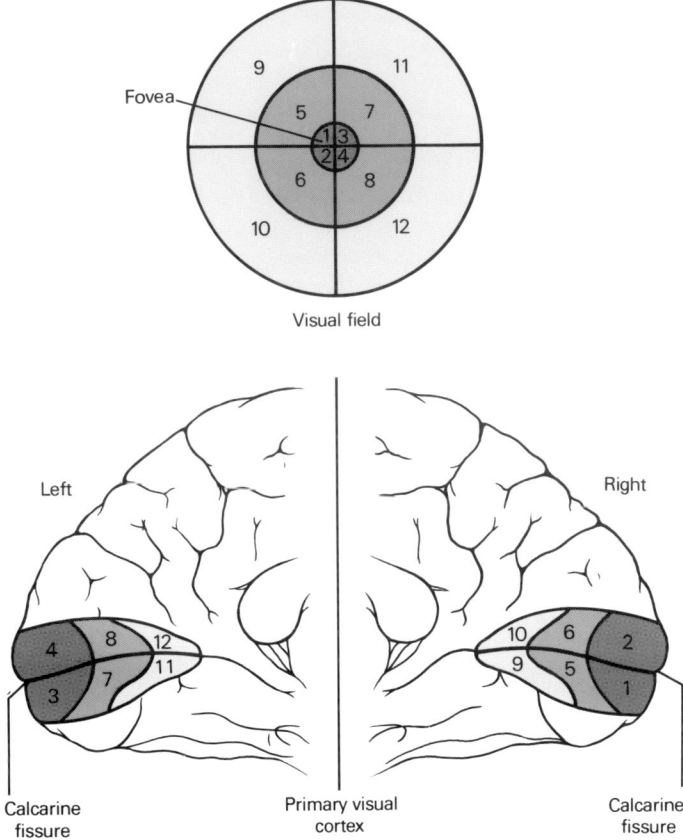

FIGURE 29–7

The primary visual cortex contains an orderly map of the visual field. In humans this cortex is located at the posterior pole of the cerebral hemisphere and lies almost exclusively on the me dial surface. (In some individuals it is shifted so that part of it extends onto the lateral surface.) Each half of the visual field is represented in the contralateral hemisphere. Areas in the primary visual cortex are devoted to specific parts of the visual field, as indicated by the corresponding numbers. The upper fields are mapped below the calcarine fissure, and the lower fields above it. The striking aspect of this map is that about half of the neural mass is devoted to representation of the fovea and the region just around it. This area has the greatest visual acuity.

Ganglion cells in the retina project in an orderly manner to points in the lateral geniculate nucleus, so that in each lateral geniculate nucleus there is a *visuotopic* representation of the contralateral half of the visual field. As in the somatosensory system, the surface of the retina is not represented isometrically in the lateral geniculate nucleus. The *fovea*, the area of the retina with greatest acuity, has the greatest density of ganglion cells and therefore has a much larger representation, proportionately, than does the periphery of the retina (Figure 29-1A). About half of the neural mass in the lateral geniculate nucleus (and in the primary visual cortex) represents the fovea and the region just around it (Figure 29–7). The much wider peripheral portions of the retina are less well represented.

The explanation for this disproportionate innervation can be found in the shape of the eye which is a globe designed to rotate in its socket. Because of this, the retina cannot have more area in the center than in the periphery. To compensate for this geometric constraint, the retinal ganglion cells in and near the fovea are densely packed. Since this physical limitation does not exist beyond the retina, neurons in the lateral geniculate nucleus and primary visual cortex are fairly evenly distributed. Thus, connections from the more numerous neurons in the fovea are distributed over a wide area. The ratio of the area in the lateral geniculate nucleus (or in the primary visual cortex) to the area in the retina representing one degree of the visual field is called the *magnification factor*.

The lateral geniculate nucleus of primates contains six layers of cell bodies separated by intervening layers of axons and dendrites. The layers are numbered from 1 to 6, ventral to dorsal (Figure 29–6). The two most ventral layers of the nucleus contain relatively large cells and are known as the *magnocellular layers*; their main retinal input is from Pα ganglion cells in the retina, also called M cells (after the layers in which they terminate). The four dorsal layers are known as *parvocellular layers* and receive input from Pβ ganglion cells in the retina, also called P cells. (Both types of ganglion cells are described in Chapter 28.) An individual layer in the nucleus receives input from one eye only: Fibers from the contralateral nasal hemiretina contact layers 1, 4, and 6; fibers from the ipsilateral temporal hemiretina contact layers 2, 3, and 5 (Figure 29–6).

Thus, each layer contains a representation of the contralateral *visual hemifield*. Since the layers of the nucleus are stacked on top of one another, the six maps of the contralateral hemifield are in precise vertical register. If an electrode were to pierce the layers, it would mark a single direction in visual space. The layers of the lateral geniculate nucleus that receive input from the nasal hemiretina in the contralateral eye contain a complete representation of the contralateral visual hemifield. In contrast, the layers that receive input from the temporal hemiretina in the ipsilateral eye contain only a 90% representation of the hemifield because they receive no input from the temporal crescent (Figure 29–1B).

Neurons in the Lateral Geniculate Nucleus Have Concentric Receptive Fields

Retinal ganglion cells have concentric receptive fields, with an antagonistic center-surround organization that allows them to measure the light intensity in their receptive field center relative to the surround (see Chapter 28).

How is the receptive field transformed in the lateral geniculate nucleus and in the cerebral cortex? These questions were first addressed in the early 1960s by David Hubel and Torsten Wiesel. They projected light patterns onto the retina of cats and monkeys by directing a light source to a screen in front of the subject. They found that receptive fields of neurons in the lateral geniculate nucleus are the same as those found in the retina: small concentric fields about 1° in diameter. As in the retina, the cells are either on-center or off-center. Like the retinal ganglion cells, cells in the lateral geniculate nucleus respond best to small spots of light within their receptive field center. Diffuse illumination of the whole receptive field produces only weak responses. This similarity of the receptive properties of cells in the lateral geniculate nucleus and those of retinal ganglion cells derives in part from the fact that each geniculate neuron receives its main retinal input from only a very few ganglion cell axons with very little transformation of the incoming information.

As in the retina, the on- and off-center pathways in the lateral geniculate nucleus are independent, and each of these pathways in turn is subdivided into *M* and *P pathways* or *M* and *P channels*. The M pathway seems to be concerned with the initial analysis of movement of the visual image, whereas the P pathways are concerned with the analysis of fine structure and color vision. Unlike the retina, however, the inputs of M and P cells in the lateral geniculate nucleus are segregated anatomically into different cellular layers. Thus, as we have seen, the M (Pα) cells from the retina project exclusively to the large-cell (magnocellular) layers 1 and 2, whereas the P (Pβ) cells project to the small-cell (parvocellular) layers 3–6 (Figure 29–6). The existence of these two pathways, each with on- and off-channels, is another example of *parallel processing*. Neurons at a single locus in the retina abstract different kinds of information from the visual world; the information from each locus is projected to different cells and even, as we shall learn, to different regions in the central nervous system.

Although we know a great deal about the cell types and circuitry of the lateral geniculate nucleus, and about the receptive field properties of different cell types, the actual function of the nucleus is not yet clear. In fact, only 10–20% of the presynaptic connections onto geniculate relay cells are from the retina! The majority of connections are from other regions, and many of these, particularly those from the reticular formation in the brain stem and from the cortex, are feedback connections. This input to the lateral geniculate nucleus may control the flow of information from the retina to the cortex.

The Primary Visual Cortex Transforms Concentric Receptive Fields into Linear Segments and Boundaries

The first relay point in visual processing where receptive field properties change significantly is the primary visual cortex (Brodmann's area 17), or visual area 1 (abbreviated as V1). It is also called the *striate cortex* because it contains a prominent stripe of white matter in layer 4, the *stripe of Gennari*, consisting of myelinated axons from the thalamus and other areas of the cortex. Like the lateral geniculate nucleus and superior colliculus, the primary visual cortex in each cerebral hemisphere receives information exclusively from the contralateral half of the

visual field (Figure 29–7), but the structure of the visual cortex is much more complex than that of the lateral geniculate nucleus.

The human visual cortex is about 2 mm thick and consists of six layers of cells (layers 1–6) between the pial surface and the underlying white matter. These layers are evident even on visual inspection because of differences in cell and fiber density. One of these, layer 4, the principal layer of inputs from the lateral geniculate nucleus, is further subdivided into four sublayers (sublaminae): 4A, 4B, 4Cα, and 4Cβ. By tracing resident cells and axonal inputs, Jennifer Lund and others have found that the M and P cells of the lateral geniculate nucleus terminate in different layers and even in different sublaminae (Figure 29–8A). The axons of M cells terminate principally in sublamina 4Cα; the axons of one group of P cells terminate principally in sublamina 4Cβ. Axons from a third group of cells, located in the interlaminar region of the lateral geniculate nucleus, terminate in layers 2 and 3, where they innervate patches of cells called blobs, a functional grouping that we shall discuss below.

As we have seen in Chapter 20, the cortex contains two basic classes of cells. *Pyramidal cells* are large and have long spiny dendrites; they are projection neurons whose axons project to other brain regions. *Nonpyramidal cells* are small, stellate in shape, and have dendrites that are either spiny (spiny stellate cells) or smooth (smooth stellates). They are local interneurons whose axons are confined to the primary visual cortex (Figure 29–8B). The pyramidal and spiny stellate cells are excitatory and many use glutamate or aspartate as their transmitters; the smooth stellate cells are inhibitory and many contain γ-aminobutyric acid (GABA).

Once afferents from the lateral geniculate nucleus enter the primary visual cortex, information flows systematically from one cortical layer to another, starting with the spiny stellate cells, which predominate in layer 4. These cells receive the direct input from the lateral geniculate nucleus and project up to layers 4B, 2, and 3. Cells in layers 2 and 3 project down to pyramidal cells in layer 5, which then feed via axon collaterals to pyramidal cells in layer 6. The pyramidal cells of layer 6 complete the local excitatory circuit by sending axon collaterals to layer 4 to excite the inhibitory smooth stellate cells. The inhibitory smooth stellate cells in turn contact and modulate the firing of the excitatory spiny stellate cells, completing an inhibitory feedback loop (Figure 29–8B,C). Thus, the spiny stellate cells distribute the input from the lateral geniculate nucleus to the cortex and the pyramidal cells feed axon collaterals upward and downward to integrate activity within the layers of V1.

How does the complexity of the circuitry in the cerebral cortex affect the response properties of cortical cells? Hubel, Wiesel and their colleagues found that most cells above and below layer 4 respond only to stimuli that are substantially more complex than those that excite cells in the retina and lateral geniculate nucleus. The most astonishing finding was that small spots of light—which are so

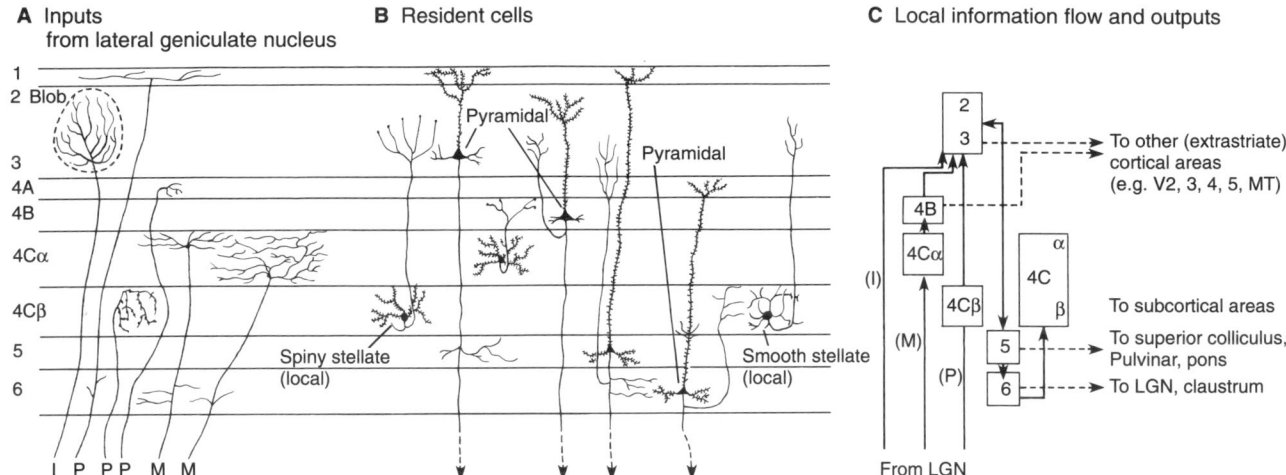

A Inputs
from lateral geniculate nucleus

B Resident cells

C Local information flow and outputs

FIGURE 29–8

The primary visual cortex has distinct anatomical layers, each with characteristic synaptic connections.

A. Most afferent fibers from the lateral geniculate nucleus terminate in layer 4. Axons of type P cells (in the parvocellular layers) terminate primarily in layer 4Cβ, with minor inputs to 4A and 1, while axons from type M cells (in the magnocellular layer) terminate primarily in layer 4Cα. Collaterals of both types of cells also terminate in layer 6. Cells of the intralaminar regions of the lateral geniculate nucleus terminate in layers 2 and 3.

B. Several types of resident neurons make up the primary visual cortex. Spiny stellate and pyramidal cells, both of which have spiny dendrites, are excitatory. Smooth stellate cells are inhibitory. Pyramidal cells project out of the cortex, whereas both types of stellate cells are local neurons.

C. Afferents from M and P cells in the lateral geniculate nucleus end on spiny stellate cells in layer 4C, and these cells project axons to layer 4B and the upper layers 2 and 3. Cells from the interlaminar zones (**I**) in the lateral geniculate nucleus project directly to layers 2 and 3. From there, pyramidal cells project axon collaterals to layer 5 pyramidal cells, whose axon collaterals project both to layer 6 pyramidal cells as well as back to cells in layers 2 and 3. Axon collaterals of layer 6 pyramidal cells then make a loop back to layer 4C onto smooth stellate cells. Each layer, except for 4C, has different outputs. The cells in layers 2, 3, and 4B project to higher visual cortical areas. Cells in layer 5 project to the superior colliculus, the pons, and the pulvinar. Cells in layer 6 project back to the lateral geniculate nucleus and the claustrum. (Adapted from Lund, 1988.)

effective in the retina, lateral geniculate nucleus, and in the input layer of the cortex 4C—are completely ineffective in all layers of the visual cortex except the blob regions in the superficial layers. Cells in all regions, except the blobs, do not have circular receptive fields. They respond only to stimuli that have linear properties, such as a line or bar (Figure 29–9). Hubel and Wiesel categorized the cells (in what we now know to be the regions outside the blobs) into two major groups, simple and complex, based on their responses to linear stimuli.

FIGURE 29–9

Comparison of the receptive fields of neurons in the retina and lateral geniculate nucleus with those of simple cells in the primary visual cortex. (Adapted from Hubel and Wiesel, 1962.)

A. Cells of the retina and lateral geniculate nucleus fall into two classes: on-center and off-center (×, excitatory; Δ, inhibitory).

B. Neurons of the primary visual cortex also fall into two major classes, simple and complex, but each of these classes has several subclasses. Several different types of simple cells, all with rectangular receptive fields, are illustrated here. Despite the variety, all simple cells are characterized by three features: (1) specific retinal position, (2) discrete excitatory and inhibitory zones, and (3) a specific axis of orientation. For simplicity, only receptive fields with a vertical axis of orientation (from 12 to 6 o'clock) are shown in this figure. In fact, all axes of orientation—vertical, horizontal, and various obliques—in each region of the retina are represented in the primary visual cortex.

A Concentric cells of retina and lateral geniculate nucleus

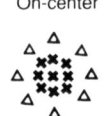
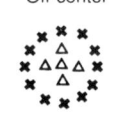

On-center   Off-center

B Simple cells of the cortex

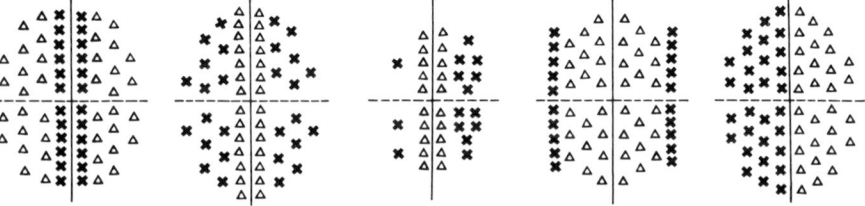

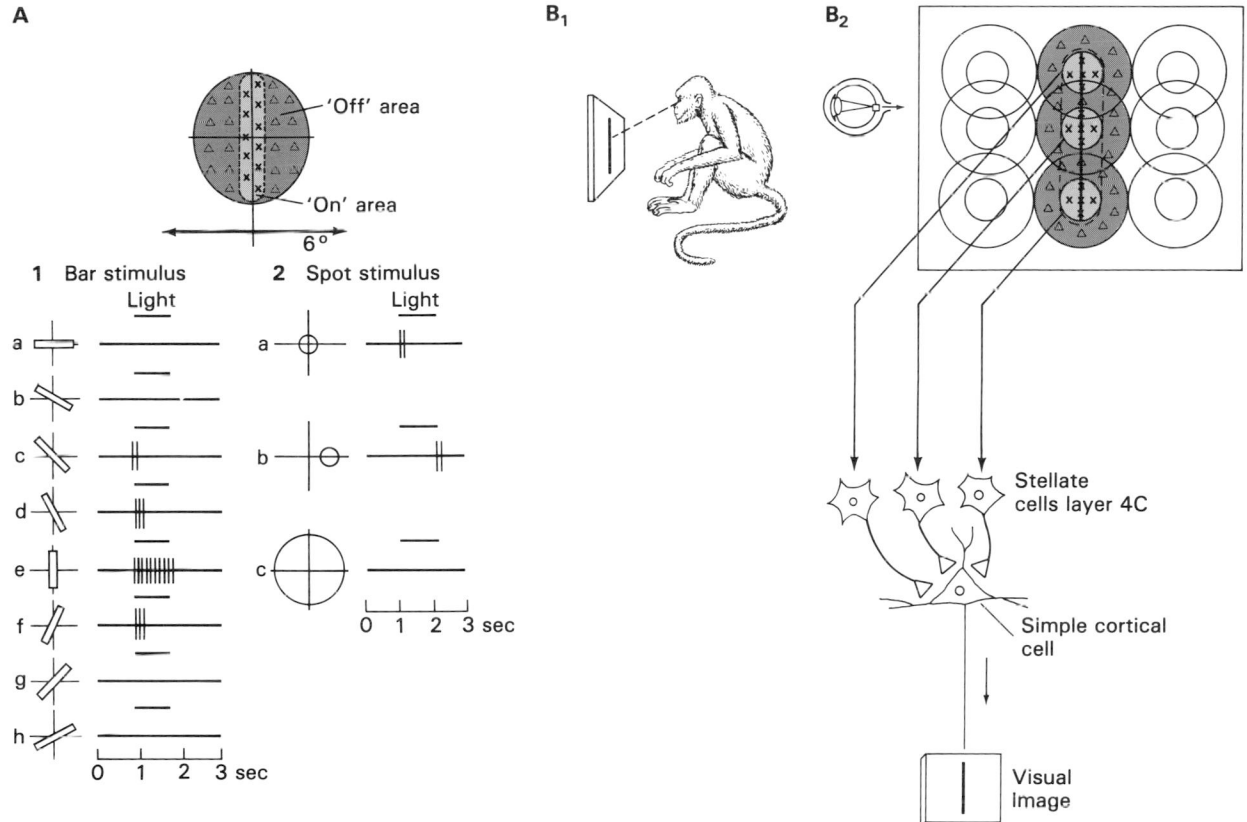

FIGURE 29–10

Receptive field of a simple cell in the primary visual cortex.

A. The receptive field has a narrow rectangular excitatory area (×) in the center flanked by symmetrical inhibitory areas (Δ). The patterns of action potentials fired by the cell in response to two types of stimuli are shown. **1.** The cell's response to a bar of light is strongest if the bar of light (1° × 8°) is vertically oriented in the center of its receptive field. Other orientations (rotated clockwise) are less effective or ineffective. Duration of illumination is indicated by a bar above each record. **2.** Spots of light consistently elicit weak responses or no response. A small spot in the excitatory center of the field (**a**) elicits only a weak excitatory response. A small spot in the inhibitory area (**b**) elicits a weak inhibitory response. Diffuse light (**c**) produces no response (Adapted from Hubel and Wiesel, 1959.)

B. Model for simple cells. **1.** Arrangement used by Hubel and Wiesel to study simple cells. A monkey faces a target screen on which bars with specific axes of orientation are projected. **2.** The exact process by which the circular receptive fields of geniculate cells are translated to the rectangular fields of simple cells in the visual cortex is not known. According to one idea, illustrated here, a simple cortical neuron in the primary visual cortex receives convergent excitatory connections from three or more stellate cells in layer 4C, each of which have a similar center-surround organization and which together represent light falling along a straight line in the retina. As a result, the receptive field of the simple cortical cell has an elongated excitatory region, indicated by the dashed outline in the receptive field diagram. (Adapted from Hubel and Wiesel, 1962.)

Simple cells resemble cells of the lateral geniculate nucleus, except that the on and off zones of their receptive fields are somewhat larger than those of geniculate cells. Moreover, unlike the circular fields of geniculate or retinal ganglion cells, these fields are rectangular with a specific axis of orientation. For example, a cell may have a rectangular *on* (excitatory) zone (with its long axis running from 12 to 6 o'clock) flanked on each side by rectangular *off* (inhibitory) zones (Figure 29–10A). The effective stimulus for the on zone of such a field must excite the specific segment of the retina, and have the correct linear properties (in this case a bar) and a specific axis of orientation (in this case vertical, running from 12 to 6 o'clock). The most effective stimulus is one that coincides with the bound-

aries of the subdivisions of the receptive field. For the cell described above, a stimulus with an orientation perpendicular or even oblique to the orientation of the cell's receptive field will be ineffective. Other cells in the cortex receiving impulses from the same point on the retina have similar receptive field shapes but their axes of orientation are horizontal or oblique. By this means, *every axis of rotation is represented for every retinal position.*

Hubel and Wiesel suggested that a rectilinear receptive field could be built up from many circular fields in appropriate connections with stellate cells in layer 4C in the primary visual cortex, the cells that receive direct input from the lateral geniculate nucleus (Figure 29–8B). This idea has received direct support from studies by Michael

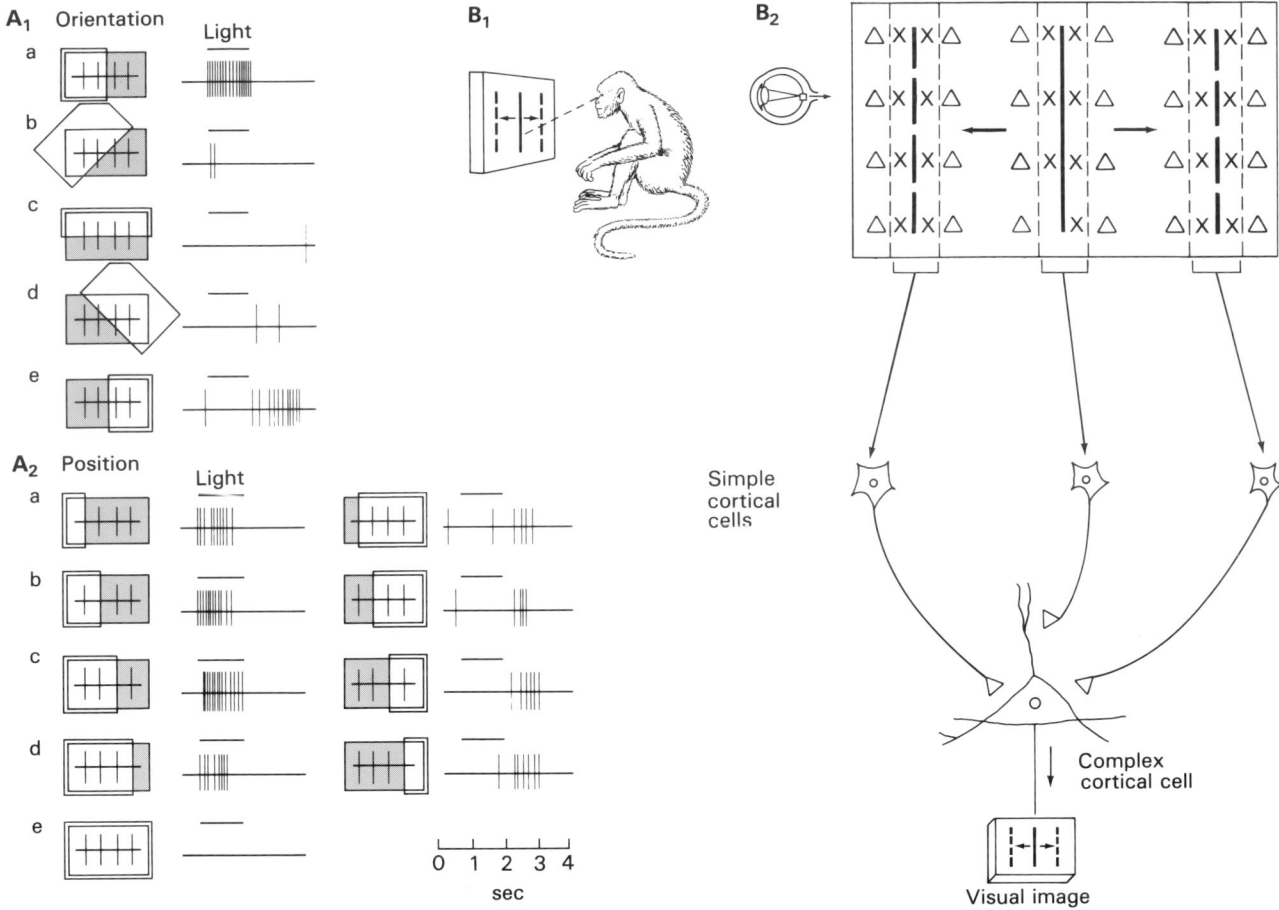

FIGURE 29–11

The receptive field of a complex cell in the primary visual cortex has no clearly distinct excitatory or inhibitory zones. Orientation of the light stimulus is important, but position within the receptive field is not. (Adapted from Hubel and Wiesel, 1962.)

A. In this example the cell responds best to a vertical edge.
1. Different orientations of the light stimulus produce different rates of firing in the cell. (The bar above each record indicates duration of illumination.) Light on the left and dark on the right produces a strong excitatory response (**a**). Light on the right produces an inhibitory response (**e**). Orientation other than vertical is less effective. **2.** The position of the border of the light within the field affects the type of response in the cell. If the edge of the light comes from any point on the right within the field, the stimulus produces an excitatory response. If the edge comes from the left, the stimulus produces an inhibitory response (**a–d**). Illumination of the entire receptive field produces no response (**e**).

B. Model for complex cells. **1.** Arrangement used to study complex cells as in Figure 29–10. **2.** According to Hubel and Wiesel, the properties of complex receptive fields may be explained by the pattern of input. A complex cortical neuron with a vertical orientation receives convergent excitatory input from several simple cortical cells, each of which has a vertical axis of orientation, a central excitation zone (×), and two flanking inhibitory regions (Δ), and thus represent light falling along a straight line in the retina. The receptive field of the complex cell is built up from the individual fields of the presynaptic cells.

Stryker, who found that the distribution of geniculate input onto simple cortical cells predicts its axes of orientation.

The receptive fields of *complex cells* are usually larger than those of simple cells. These fields also have a critical axis of orientation, but the precise position of the stimulus within the receptive field is less crucial because there are no clearly defined on or off zones (Figure 29–11). Movement across the receptive field is a particularly effective stimulus for certain complex cells. Although some complex cells have direct connections with cells of layer 4C, Hubel and Wiesel proposed that a significant input to complex cells comes from a family of simple cortical cells that have the same axis of orientation but slightly offset receptive field positions (Figure 29–11B).

Simple and Complex Cells Decompose the Outlines of a Visual Image into Short Line Segments of Various Orientation

What is the function of the simple and complex cells? Hubel and Wiesel suggest that these cells are important for analyzing the form of the visual image—its contours and boundaries—in terms of line segments. Moreover, the interaction between simple and complex cells may be important for perception of form independent of small head or eye movements. Consider a dark square on a light background in front of you. A vertical edge (or line) of the square excites a population of simple cells and a population of complex ones, each with the same vertical axis of orientation. If you now move your eye, or the square is moved against the background, a new population of simple cells will be excited, since these cells are sensitive to the exact position of the line in the receptive field. If the movement is small, however, the same population of complex cells will be excited, because these cells have large receptive fields without clearly delineated excitatory regions and are responsive to movement within the receptive field. This response to orientation over a range of positions seems to represent an elementary psychophysical mechanism for *positional invariance*, the ability to recognize the same feature anywhere in the visual field.

Another striking consequence of this analysis, which we have already encountered in considering the response properties of the retinal ganglion cells (Chapter 28, Figure 28–8), is that the cells of the visual system pay much more attention to the outlines of an object than to its interior. Each side of the dark square will activate simple and complex cells of the appropriate orientation. But, remarkably, in a way that is counter-intuitive, the interior of the dark square or the surface of the light background is largely ignored by the cells of the cortex because these monotonous surfaces contain no new visual information!

Some Feature Abstraction Can Be Accomplished by Progressive Convergence Within the Primary Visual Cortex

Hubel and Wiesel proposed that the convergent actions of cells in V1 are the initial steps in perception. In its simplest form, this scheme suggests that each complex cell surveys the activity of a group of simple cells. The simple cells survey the activity of a group of geniculate cells, which themselves survey the activity of a group of retinal ganglion cells. The ganglion cells survey the activity of bipolar cells that survey a group of receptors. *At each level, each cell has a greater capacity for abstraction than do the cells at the lower levels.*

Hubel and Wiesel postulated that the early visual pathways constitute a hierarchy of relay points, each of which is concerned with increasing visual abstraction. At the lowest level of the system, the level of the retinal ganglion and the geniculate cells, neurons respond primarily to contrast. This elementary information is repatterned by the simple and complex cells of the cortex into rectangular fields with relatively precise line segments and boundaries. Thus, the stimulus requirements necessary to activate a cell become more precise at each level of the afferent system. In the retina and lateral geniculate stimulus position is important. In simple cells, in addition to position, the axis of orientation is important. In complex cells, whose receptive fields are larger, the axis of orientation is also important, but these cells have an ability to detect orientation over a wide range of positions.

Moreover, both simple and complex cells in V1 receive input from two distinct functional pathways of the lateral geniculate nucleus, the magnocellular or parvocellular pathway. Cells receiving input from the magnocellular layers seem to be concerned more with movement and with the coarse outlines of the stimulus. In contrast, those cells that receive input primarily from the parvocellular layers are thought to be concerned more with color or texture and pattern. Both pathways could contribute to what the theoretical biologist David Marr called the *primal sketch*, the initial two-dimensional approximation of stimulus shape and contour.

The Primary Visual Cortex Is Organized into Vertical Columns

Like the somatic sensory cortex, the primary visual (or striate) cortex is organized into narrow columns, running from the pial surface to the white matter. Each column is about 30–100 μm wide and 2 mm deep, and each column contains cells in layer 4C with concentric receptive fields. Above and below there are simple cells with almost identical retinal positions and identical axes of orientation. For this reason these groupings are called *orientation columns*. Each orientation column also contains complex cells. The properties of these complex cells can most easily be explained by postulating that each complex cell receives direct connections from the simple cells in the column. Thus, in the visual system columns seem to be organized to allow local interconnection of cells, from which the cells are able to generate a new level of abstraction of visual information. For instance, the columns allow cortical cells to generate linear receptive field properties from the inputs of several cells in the lateral geniculate nucleus that respond best to small spots of light.

The discovery of columns in the various sensory systems was the most important advance in cortical physiology in the past several decades and immediately raised questions that have led to a family of new discoveries. For example, given that cells with the same axis of orientation tend to be grouped into columns, how are columns of cells with *different* axes of orientation organized in relation to one another? Detailed mapping of adjacent columns by Hubel and Wiesel, using tangential penetrations with microelectrodes, revealed a precise organization with an orderly shift in axis of orientation from one column to the next. Every 30–100 μm the electrode encounters a new column and a shift in axis of orientation of about 10 degrees.

The anatomical layout of the orientation columns was first demonstrated in electrophysiological experiments in which dyes were injected near the cells that are activated by stimuli at a given orientation. Later the anatomy was delineated by injecting 2-deoxyglucose, a glucose analog that can be radiolabeled and injected into the brain. Cells that are metabolically active take up the label and can then be detected in sections of cortex overlaid with X-ray film. Thus, when a stimulus of lines with a given orientation is presented, an orderly array of active and inactive stripes of cells is revealed (Figure 29–12A). A remarkable advance now allows the different orientation columns to be visualized directly in the living cortex. Using either a voltage-sensitive dye or inherent differences in the light

A

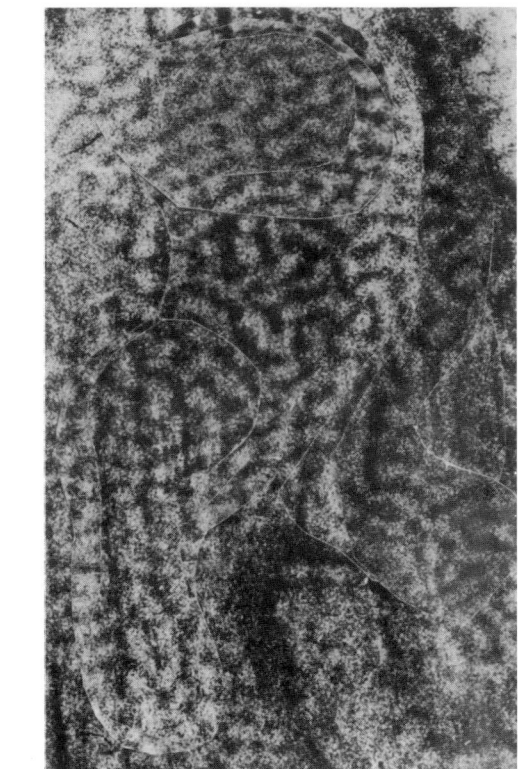

B

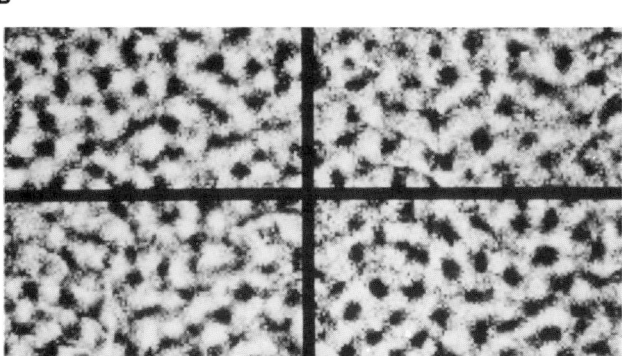

FIGURE 29–12

Orientation columns in the visual cortex.

A. A 2-deoxyglucose visualization of orientation columns in the visual cortex of a monkey binocularly stimulated with vertically oriented lines. Bright areas indicate those neurons responding to the stimulus. The cortex was sectioned tangentially. (From Hubel, Wiesel, and Stryker, 1978.)

B. Images of four different domains in the same cortical area of the primary visual cortex, imaged from the exposed surface of a living monkey brain with a sensitive camera. In each domain the constituent cells had the same axis of orientation. Differences in surface reflectance correspond to differences in the activity of cells. The darker areas correspond to regions of higher activity. Each view represents the pattern of activity occurring during the presentation of gratings having different orientations. (Courtesy of A. Grinvald, C. Gilbert, and R. Frostig.)

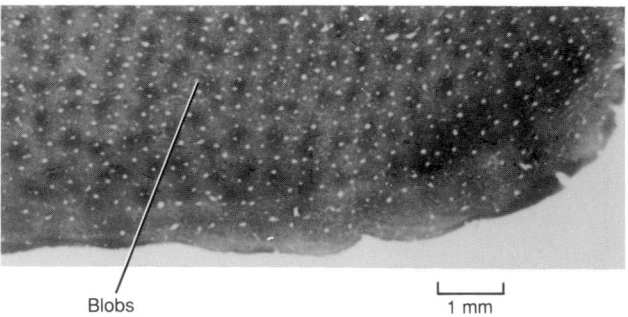

Blobs   1 mm

FIGURE 29–13

The distribution of the mitochondrial enzyme cytochrome oxidase in the superficial layers of the visual cortex, as seen in tangential sections of area 17 of the macaque monkey. The rows of dark patches or *blobs* represent areas of heightened enzymatic activity. This is thought to represent heightened neural activity in the blobs because of the lower response selectivity of these cells. (Courtesy of D. Ts'o, C. Gilbert, and T. Wiesel.)

scattering of active and inactive cells, a highly sensitive camera can detect the pattern of active and inactive orientation columns during presentation of a bar of light with a specific axis of orientation (Figure 29–12B).

The systematic shifts in axis of orientation from one column to another is occasionally interrupted by *blobs*, peg-shaped regions of cells in layers 2 and 3 of V1 first studied by Margaret Wong-Riley, Jonathan Horton, and Margaret Livingstone and Hubel (Figure 29–13). These cells in the blobs receive direct connections from the lateral geniculate nucleus (Figure 29–8). As we shall see in the next two chapters, the cells in the blobs are concerned with color and not with orientation.

In addition to columns devoted to axis of orientation and blobs related to color, a third alternating system of columns is devoted to the left or the right eye. These *ocular dominance columns* are important for binocular interaction. This set of columns is also arranged in an orderly manner in the primary visual cortex. The ocular dominance columns have been visualized using transynaptic transport of radiolabeled amino acids injected into one eye. In autoradiographs of sections of cortex cut perpendicular to the layers, patches in layer 4 that receive input from the injected eye are heavily labeled, and they alternate with unlabeled patches that mediate input from the uninjected eye (Figure 29–14A).

Hubel and Wiesel introduced the term *hypercolumn* to refer to a set of columns responsive to lines of all orientations from a particular region in space via *both* eyes. The relationship between the orientation columns, the independent ocular dominance columns, and the blobs within a hypercolumn is illustrated in Figure 29–15. (There are probably also columns for other aspects of vision.) A complete sequence of ocular dominance columns and orientation columns is repeated regularly and precisely over the surface of the primary visual cortex, each occupying a region of about 1 mm^2. This repeating organization illustrates nicely the modular organization characteristic of the cerebral cortex.

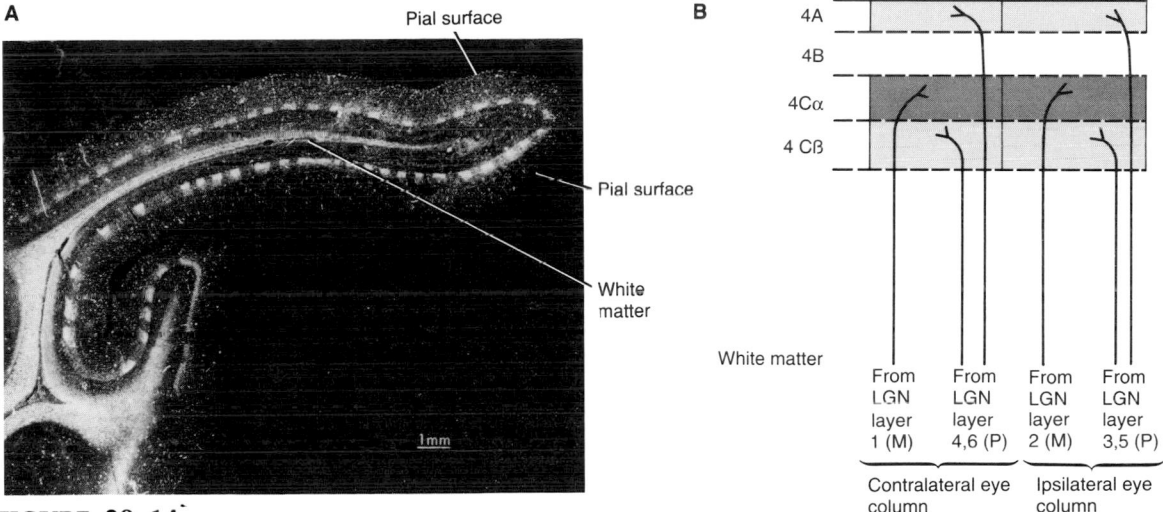

FIGURE 29-14

The ocular dominance columns.

A. This autoradiograph of the primary visual cortex in an adult monkey demonstrates the input from the lateral geniculate nucleus to the cortex. Labeling was achieved by injection of tritiated proline and fucose in the ipsilateral eye 2 weeks before. The label was transported to the lateral geniculate nucleus, then crossed synapses to the geniculocortical relay cells, whose axons terminate in layer 4 of the visual cortex. Areas that receive input from the injected eye are heavily labeled and appear white, and alternate with adjacent unlabeled patches that receive input from the uninjected eye. In all, some 56 columns can be counted in layer 4C. This section cuts through the gray matter of the cortex twice. Beginning at the pial surface (**top** of the figure) the section then goes through the gray matter and reaches layer 4, where the patches of label appear as bright bands. The section goes deeper through the gray matter to the underlying white matter, where labeled axons are evident. The section continues through the gray matter on the opposite side of the gyrus, through another band of columns in layer 4, and then reaches the pial surface. (From Hubel and Wiesel, 1979.)

B. Schematic representation of the projection from each eye through the lateral geniculate nucleus to the ocular dominance columns in subdivisions of layer 4 of the visual cortex. (See Figures 29-6 and 29-8.)

FIGURE 29-15

Small regions of the visual field are analyzed in the primary visual cortex by an array of complex cellular units called *hypercolumns*. A single hypercolumn represents the neural machinery necessary to analyze a discrete region of the visual field. Each contains a complete set of orientation columns, representing 360°, a set of left and right ocular dominance columns, and several blobs, regions of the cortex in which the cells are specific for color. Each ocular dominance column receives input from either the contralateral (**C**) or ipsilateral (**I**) eye via projections from cells in individual layers of the lateral geniculate nucleus that serve one or the other eye.

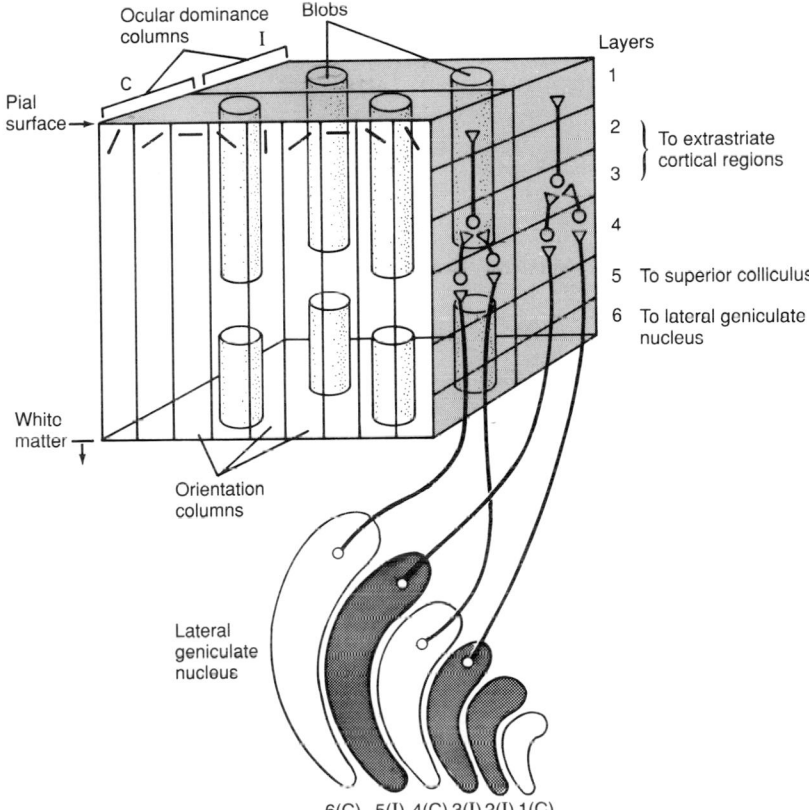

It is apparent from these findings that the primary visual cortex has at least three major functions: (1) it deconstructs the visual world into short line segments of various orientations, an early step in the process thought to be necessary for discrimination of form and movement; (2) it segregates information about color from that concerned with form and movement; and (3) it combines the input from the two eyes, a step in a sequence of transformations necessary for depth perception.

Besides being divided into columns, the cortex is also divided into six layers. What roles does the layered arrangement of cells have in the processing of visual information? Each layer in a column has slightly different inputs and outputs (Figure 29–8). The organization of the output connections from the primary visual cortex is similar to that of the somatic sensory cortex. There is output from all layers except 4C, and in each layer the principal output cells are the *pyramidal cells* (Figure 29–8). The cells in layers 2 and 3 make associational connections; they project to other higher visual cortical regions, such as Brodmann's area 18 (V2, V3, and V4). They also make connections via the corpus callosum to reciprocal cortical areas on the other side of the brain. Cells in layer 4B project to the medial temporal lobe (V5 or MT). Cells in layer 5 project to the superior colliculus, the pons, and the pulvinar. Cells in layer 6 project back to the lateral geniculate nucleus and to the claustrum. As we shall learn in Chapter 30, the claustrum and the pulvinar are thought to be important for visual attention.

Since each layer of the visual cortex performs a different task, the laminar position of a cell determines its functional properties. The morphology of the dendrites and collaterals of pyramidal cells varies according to the cells' efferent connections. Thus, superimposed on the hypercolumns—the columns of cells that together function as elementary computational devices—is a horizontal or layered organization. Hypercolumns receive a varied input, transform it, and send their output to a number of different regions of the brain. In this way the diverse synaptic circuits within each lamina and between laminae produce novel and more abstract levels of processing than those achieved in the retina or lateral geniculate nucleus.

Columnar Units Are Linked by Horizontal Connections

As we have seen, three major vertical units in the primary visual cortex have been delineated: (1) orientation columns, which contain the neurons that respond selectively to light bars with specific axes of orientation; (2) blobs, peg-shaped patches in upper layers (but not layer 4) that contain cells that respond to different color stimuli and whose receptive fields, like those of cells in the lateral geniculate nucleus, have no specific orientation; and (3) ocular dominance columns, which receive inputs from one or the other eye.

These regularly spaced columnar systems communicate with one another by means of horizontal connections that link cells within a layer. These connections have been delineated by Charles Gilbert and Wiesel, who injected horseradish peroxidase into individual pyramidal cells in layers 3 and 5 and found that the axon collaterals of these cells run long distances, parallel with the layers, and give rise to clusters of axon terminals in regular intervals that approximate the width of a hypercolumn (Figure 29–16A).

Independent evidence that a horizontal system interconnects columnar units came from Lund and Katherine Rockland. They injected horseradish peroxidase into restricted regions within superficial cortical layers (2–3) and found an elaborate honeycomb-like lattice of labeled cells and axons that formed walls around unlabeled patches about 500 μm in diameter. Hubel and Livingstone next found that injection of tracer into a site corresponding to a blob results in labeling of other blobs in a similar array. A honeycomb array also appears after labeling the non-blob cortex, suggesting that these lateral connections may allow communication between columns with similar function.

To examine this communication, Daniel Ts'o, Gilbert, and Wiesel recorded from cell pairs in superficial layers of cortex; each pair was separated by about 1 mm, the distance that typically separates the lattice arrays described above. They found that many cell pairs fire simultaneously in response to stimuli with a specific orientation and direction of movement (Figure 29–16B). They also established that color-selective cells in one blob are linked to cells with similar responses in other blobs.

Gilbert and Wiesel obtained additional evidence for horizontal communication when they examined cells that respond to a specific orientation. While presenting the stimulus, they injected radiolabeled 2-deoxyglucose and fluorescently labeled microbeads into the recording site. The beads are taken up by axon terminals at the injection site and transported back to the cell bodies. In sections tangential to the pia the overall pattern of cells labeled with the microbeads closely resembled the honeycomb-like lattice described above. In fact, the pattern labeled with 2-deoxyglucose could be superimposed on the pattern obtained with the microbeads. Thus, both anatomical and metabolic studies have established that cortical cells having receptive fields with the same orientation are connected by means of a horizontal network (Figure 28–16C). The visual cortex, then, is organized functionally into two sets of intersecting connections, one vertical, consisting of functional columns spanning the different cortical layers, and the other horizontal, connecting functional columns with the same response properties.

What is the functional importance of horizontal connections? Studies by Gilbert and Wiesel indicate that these connections integrate information over many millimeters of cortex. As a result, a cell can be influenced by stimuli *outside* its normal receptive field. Indeed, Gilbert and Wiesel find that a cell's axis of orientation is not completely invariant but is dependent on the context on which the feature is embedded. The psychophysical principle, called the *contextual effect*, whereby we evaluate objects in the context in which we see them, is thought to be mediated through horizontal connections.

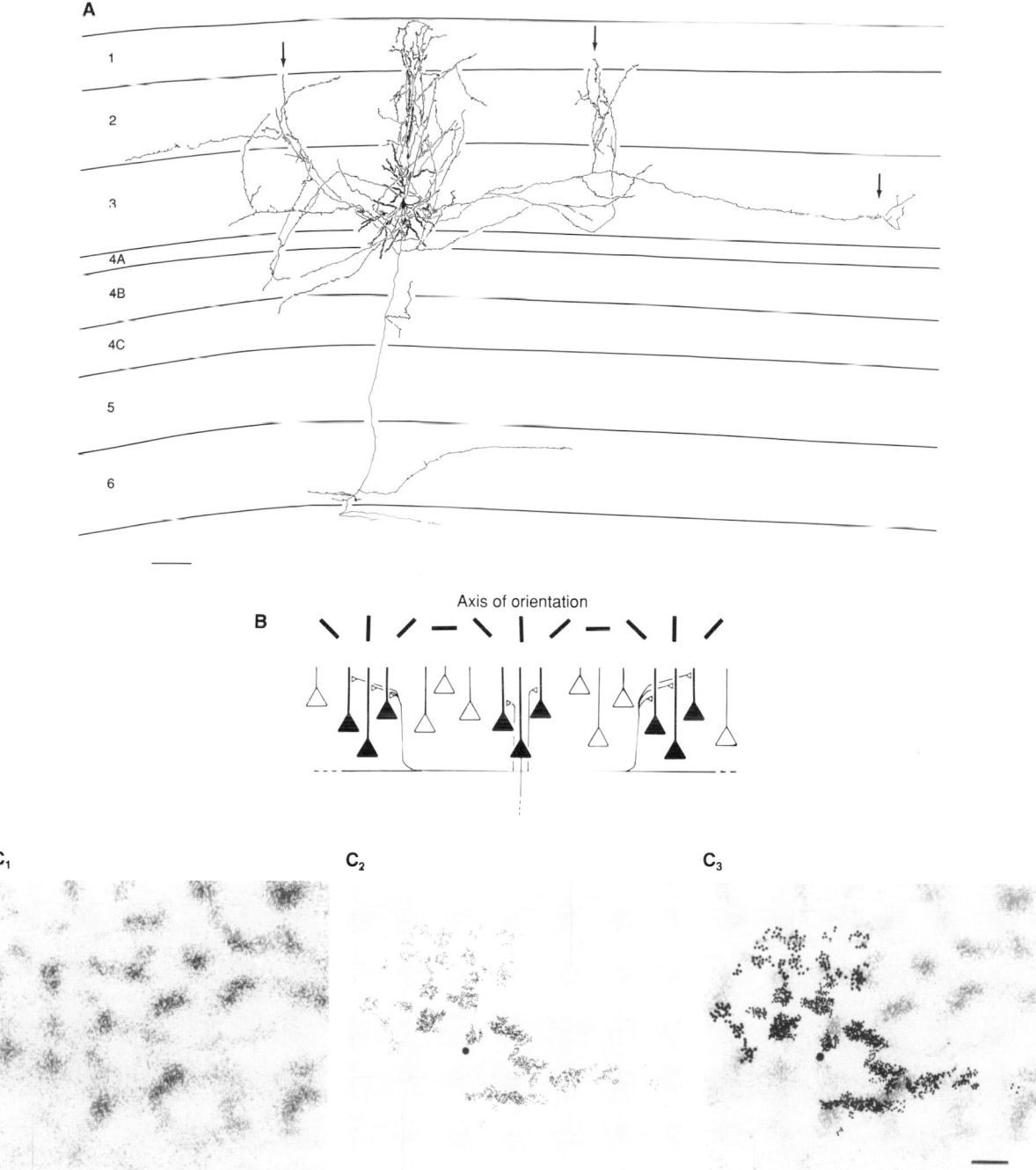

FIGURE 29–16

Columnar cell systems with similar function are linked through horizontal connections.

A. A camera lucida reconstruction of a pyramidal cell injected with horseradish peroxidase in layers 2–3 of V1 in a monkey. Several axon collaterals (**arrows**) branch off the descending axon and ramify near the dendritic tree and in three other clusters in layers 2 and 3. The clusters project horizontally and are given off at intervals, extending vertically into several layers. This collateral system is thought to interconnect cells in different cortical columns with similar functional properties. (From McGuire et al., 1990.)

B. The functional specificity of the long-range clustered horizontal connections, as demonstrated by cross-correlation analysis. The axon of one pyramidal cell, in the center of the diagram, synapses on other pyramidal cells in the immediate vicinity as

well as pyramidal cells some distance away. The axon makes connections only with cells with the same functional specificity. (Adapted from Ts'o, Gilbert, and Wiesel, 1986.)

C. Combined 2-deoxyglucose and fluorescent-bead labeling within area 17 demonstrate that cells in different columns responding to the stimulus of the same orientation are anatomically linked. **1.** A section of cortex labeled with 2-deoxyglucose shows a pattern of stripes after presentation of a stimulus with a particular orientation. **2.** Microbeads injected into the recording site are taken up by cell bodies through retrograde transport. Reconstruction of the distribution of bead-labeled cells in the same region is visualized in the same section. **3.** Superimposition of 1 and 2. The clusters of bead-labeled cells lie directly over the deoxyglucose-labeled areas, showing that groups of cells in different columns having the same axis of orientation are connected. Scale bar = 1 μm. (From Gilbert and Wiesel, 1989.)

The Visual and Somatic Sensory Cortices Are Functionally Similar

There are several striking similarities between the visual and somatic sensory cortices: both are modality specific, topographically organized, and have a modular organization. Both cortices are organized into layers, each concerned with distinct input and output functions. Finally, different submodalities are processed in anatomically distinct pathways that are topographically organized.

Based on these several similarities, Edward Jones suggested that the neuronal circuits for transforming somatic sensory and visual inputs follow a similar plan. This idea was tested by Douglas Frost and his colleagues. They surgically redirected the axons of the retinal ganglion cells of newborn hamsters and caused them to project to the ventrobasal nucleus, the thalamic nucleus of the somatic sensory system. The redirected retinal fibers formed a permanent retinotopic projection in the ventrobasal nucleus and in the somatosensory cortex. As a result, in adult animals the neurons in the somatic cortex responded to visual stimuli! The cells have distinct receptive fields and orientation specificity that are in several ways comparable to neurons in the primary visual cortex. Thus, although different cortical regions serve markedly different functions, the interesting possibility exists that they may all follow a common logic in transforming sensory information from peripheral receptors.

Lesions in the Retino-Geniculate-Cortical Pathway Cause Predictable Changes in Vision

Lesions of the visual system produce characteristic defects in vision that are best described in terms of the gaps they produce in the visual field, or the way in which the visual world is projected onto the retina (Figure 29–1).

As we have seen, the axons in the optic tract synapse in the lateral geniculate nucleus. From there, the axons sweep around the lateral ventricle in the *optic radiations* to the *primary visual cortex*. These fibers then radiate on the lateral surface of both the temporal and occipital horns of the lateral ventricle (Figure 29–17A). Fibers representing the inferior parts of the retina swing rostrally in a broad arc over the temporal horn of the ventricle and loop into the temporal lobe before turning caudally to reach the occipital pole. This group of fibers is called *Meyer's loop*. The geniculocortical fibers that relay input from the inferior half of the retina terminate in the inferior bank of the cortex lining a prominent sulcus called the calcarine fissure; the fibers relaying input from the superior half of the retina terminate in the superior bank (Figure 29–17B). Consequently, unilateral lesions in the temporal lobe affect vision in the *superior* quadrant of the contralateral visual hemifield because they disrupt Meyer's loop. A lesion in the *inferior* bank of the calcarine cortex causes a gap in the *superior* half of the contralateral visual field.

This arrangement illustrates a key principle: *At the initial stages of visual processing each half of the brain is concerned with the contralateral hemifield of vision.* This

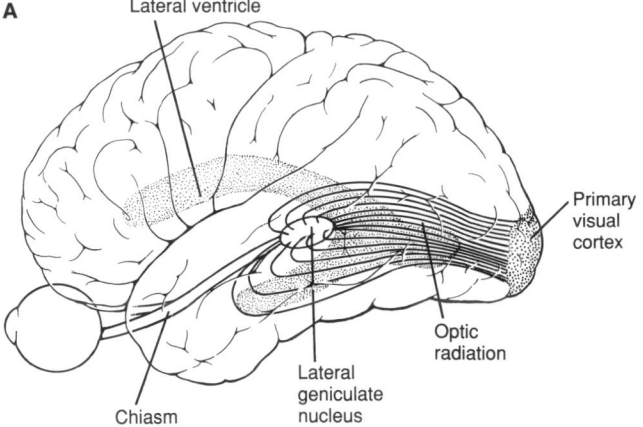

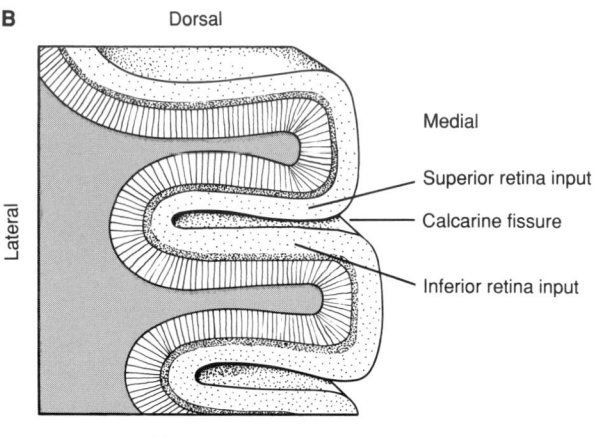

FIGURE 29–17

Projection of the retina and visual fields of the cortex.

A. Course of the fibers in the optic radiation as they sweep around the lateral ventricle to reach the primary visual cortex. Fibers that relay inputs from the inferior retina loop rostrally around the temporal horn of the lateral ventricle, forming Meyer's loop. (Adapted from Brodal, 1981.)

B. A cross section through the primary visual cortex in the occipital lobe. Fibers that relay input from the inferior half of the retina terminate in the inferior bank of the visual cortex; those that relay input from the superior half of the retina terminate in the superior bank.

pattern of organization begins with the segregation of axons in the optic chiasm, where fibers from the two eyes dealing with identical parts of the visual field are brought together (Figure 29–1C). In essence, this is similar to the somatic sensory system, in which each hemisphere mediates sensation on the contralateral side of the body.

To appreciate the projection of the visual world onto the primary visual cortex, let us consider the deficits produced by lesions at various levels leading up to the cortex. The visual field gaps caused by lesions at various levels of the visual pathway are summarized in Figure 29–18. After section of the optic nerve the visual field is seen monocularly by the eye on the intact side (Figure 29–18, 1). The

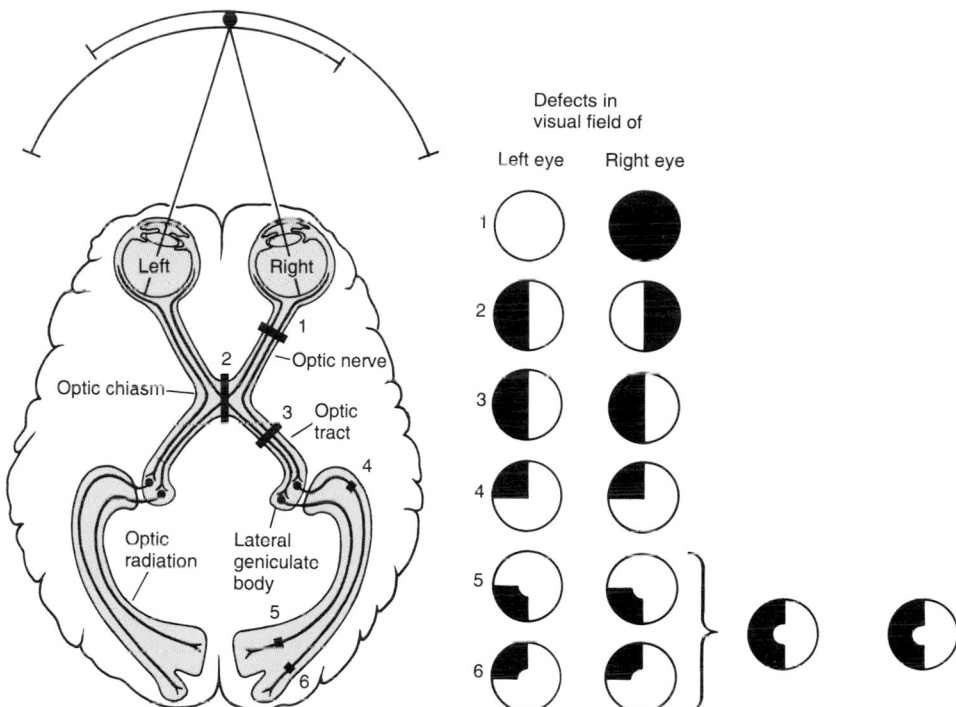

FIGURE 29–18

Visual deficits produced by lesions at various points in the visual pathway. The level of a lesion can be determined by the specific deficit in the visual field. In the diagram of the cortex the **numbers** along the visual pathway indicate the sites of lesions. The visual field deficits that result from lesions at each of these sites are shown in the visual field maps as **dark areas**. Deficits in the visual field of the left eye represent what an individual would see with the right eye closed, not deficits of the left visual hemifield.

1. A lesion of the right optic nerve causes a total loss of vision in the right eye.

2. A lesion of the optic chiasm causes a loss of vision in the temporal halves of both visual fields (bitemporal hemianopsia). Because the chiasm carries crossing fibers from both eyes, this is the only lesion in the visual system that causes a nonhomonymous deficit in vision, a deficit in two *different* parts of the visual field as a consequence of a single lesion.

3. A lesion of the optic tract causes a complete loss of vision in the opposite half of the visual field (contralateral hemianopsia).

4. After leaving the lateral geniculate nucleus the fibers representing both retinas mix in the optic radiation, although this is not indicated in the figure. A lesion of the optic radiation fibers that curve into the temporal lobe (Meyer's loop) causes a loss of vision in the upper quadrant of the opposite half of the visual field of both eyes (upper contralateral quadrantic anopsia).

5–6. Partial lesions of the visual cortex lead to partial field deficits on the opposite side. A lesion in the upper bank of the calcarine sulcus (**5**) causes a partial deficit in the inferior quadrant of the visual field on the opposite side. A lesion in the lower bank of the calcarine sulcus (**6**) causes a partial deficit in the superior quadrant of the visual field of both eyes on the opposite side. A more extensive lesion of the visual cortex, including parts of both banks of the calcarine cortex, would cause a more extensive loss of vision in the contralateral hemifield. The central area of vision, or macular area, is unaffected by cortical lesions (**5** and **6**), probably because the representation of the macula is so extensive that a single lesion is unlikely to destroy the entire representation. The representation of the periphery of the visual field is smaller and hence more easily destroyed by a single lesion.

temporal crescent is normally seen only by the nasal hemiretina on the same side. A person whose optic nerve is cut would therefore be blind in the temporal crescent on the lesioned side. Removal of binocular input in this way would also affect stereopsis, the perception of spatial depth.

Destruction of the fibers crossing in the optic chiasm would remove input from the temporal portions of both halves of the visual field. The deficit produced by this lesion is called *bitemporal hemianopsia* and occurs because fibers arising from the nasal half of each retina have been destroyed (Figure 29–18, 2). This kind of damage is

most commonly caused by a tumor of the pituitary gland that compresses the chiasm.

Destruction of one optic tract produces a *complete homonymous hemianopsia*: a loss of vision in the entire contralateral visual hemifield (Figure 29–18, 3). Destruction of the right tract causes *left homonymous hemianopsia*: loss of vision in the left nasal and right temporal hemiretinas (Figure 29–18, 4). Finally, a lesion of the optic radiation or of the visual cortex, where the fibers are more spread out, produces an *incomplete* or *quadrantic field defect* in the related part of the contralateral half of the visual field (Figure 29–18, 5,6).

An Overall View

Visual information important for perception flows from the retina to the lateral geniculate nucleus. In both structures cells respond to small circular stimuli. The primary visual cortex then transforms the concentric receptive fields in at least three ways. (1) Each part of the visual field is decomposed into short line segments of different orientation, through orientation columns. This is an early step in the process thought to be necessary for discrimination of form and movement. (2) Information about color is processed through regions called blobs, which lack orientation selectivity. (3) The input from the two eyes is combined through the ocular dominance columns; this is one step in a sequence of transformations thought to be necessary for fusion and depth perception.

To achieve this parallel processing, the central connections of the visual system are remarkably specific. Separate regions in the retina project to the lateral geniculate nucleus in the thalamus in such a way that a complete visual field for each eye is represented in the nucleus. Furthermore, different cell types in a single region of the retina project to different targets in the brain stem—some to the thalamus, some to the midbrain, others to both. Each geniculate axon terminates in the visual cortex, primarily in layer 4. Moreover, the cells in each layer have their own stereotyped patterns of connections with other subcortical regions.

In addition to the circuitry of the layers, cells in the visual cortex are arranged functionally into columnar systems: orientation-specific columns, ocular dominance columns, and blobs. Neurons within these columnar systems that have similar response properties are linked by horizontal connections. Information thus flows between different layers, in axes perpendicular to the pial surface, and horizontally through each layer. The columnar units seem to function as elementary computational modules—they receive varied inputs, transform them, and send their output to a number of different regions of the brain.

This kind of modular organization is present in all sensory cortices and may represent a basic plan of sensory representation that arises during development. Thus, if we were ever to understand completely the logic of one system, we might be well on the way toward understanding sensory processing in general.

Selected Readings

Gilbert, C. D., Hirsch, J. A., and Wiesel, T. N. 1990. Lateral interactions in the visual cortex. Cold Spring Harbor Symp. Quant. Biol. 55:663–677.

Hubel, D. H. 1988. Eye, Brain, and Vision. New York: Scientific American Library.

Hubel, D. H., and Wiesel, T. N. 1979. Brain mechanisms of vision. Sci. Am. 241(3):150–162.

Marr, D. 1982. Vision: A Computational Investigation into the Human Representation and Processing of Visual Information. San Francisco: Freeman.

Sherman, S. M. 1988. Functional organization of the cat's lateral geniculate nucleus. In M. Bentivoglio and R. Spreafico (eds.), Cellular Thalamic Mechanisms. New York: Excerpta Medica, pp. 163–183.

Stone, J., Dreher, B., and Leventhal, A. 1979. Hierarchical and parallel mechanisms in the organization of visual cortex. Brain Res. Rev. 1:345–394.

References

Boycott, B. B., and Wässle, H. 1974. The morphological types of ganglion cells of the domestic cat's retina. J. Physiol. (Lond.) 240:397–419.

Brodal, A. 1981. Neurological Anatomy in Relation to Clinical Medicine, 3rd ed. New York: Oxford University Press, chap. 8, "The Optic System".

Brown, R., and Herrnstein, R. J. 1975. Psychology. Boston: Little, Brown.

Gilbert, C. D., and Wiesel, T. N. 1979. Morphology and intracortical projections of functionally characterised neurones in the cat visual cortex. Nature 280:120–125.

Gilbert, C. D., and Wiesel, T. N. 1989. Columnar specificity of intrinsic horizontal and corticocortical connections in cat visual cortex. J. Neurosci. 9:2432–2442.

Grafstein, B., and Laureno, R. 1973. Transport of radioactivity from eye to visual cortex in the mouse. Exp. Neurol. 39:44–57.

Groves, P., and Schlesinger, K. 1979. Introduction to Biological Psychology. Dubuque, Iowa: W. C. Brown.

Guillery, R. W. 1982. The optic chiasm of the vertebrate brain. Contrib. Sens. Physiol. 7:39–73.

Horton, J. C., and Hubel, D. H. 1981. Regular patchy distribution of cytochrome oxidase staining in primary visual cortex of macaque monkey. Nature 292:762–764.

Hubel, D. H., and Wiesel, T. N. 1959. Receptive fields of single neurones in the cat's striate cortex. J. Physiol. (Lond.) 148:574–591.

Hubel, D. H., and Wiesel, T. N. 1962. Receptive fields, binocular interaction and functional architecture in the cat's visual cortex. J. Physiol. (Lond.) 160:106–154.

Hubel, D. H., and Wiesel, T. N. 1965. Binocular interaction in striate cortex of kittens reared with artificial squint. J. Neurophysiol. 28:1041–1059.

Hubel, D. H., and Wiesel, T. N. 1972. Laminar and columnar distribution of geniculo-cortical fibers in the macaque monkey. J. Comp. Neurol. 146:421–450.

Hubel., D. H., Wiesel, T. N., and Stryker, M. P. 1978. Anatomical demonstration of orientation columns in macaque monkey. J. Comp. Neurol. 177:361–379.

Hurvich, L. M. 1981. Color Vision. Sunderland, Mass.: Sinauer.

Jones, E. G. 1986. Neurotransmitters in the cerebral cortex. J. Neurosurg. 65:135–153.

Kaas, J. H., Guillery, R. W., and Allman, J. M. 1972. Some principles of organization in the dorsal lateral geniculate nucleus. Brain Behav. Evol. 6:253–299.

Katz, L. C. 1987. Local circuitry of identified projection neurons in cat visual cortex brain slices. J. Neurosci. 7:1223–1249.

Kisvarday, Z. F., Cowey, A., Smith, A. D., and Somogyi, P. 1989. Interlaminar and lateral excitatory amino acid connections in the striate cortex of monkey. J. Neurosci. 9:667–682.

LeVay, S., and Sherk, H. 1981. The visual claustrum of the cat. I. Structure and connections. J. Neurosci. 1:956–980.

Livingstone, M. S., and Hubel, D. H. 1984a. Anatomy and physiology of a color system in the primate visual cortex. J. Neurosci. 4:309–356.

Livingstone, M. S., and Hubel, D. H. 1984b. Specificity of intrinsic connections in primate primary visual cortex. J. Neurosci. 4:2830–2835.

Lund, J. S., 1988. Anatomical organization of macaque monkey striate visual cortex. Annu. Rev. Neurosci. 11:253–288.

Marshall, W. H., and Talbot, S. A. 1942. Recent evidence for neural mechanisms in vision leading to a general theory of sensory acuity. In H. Klüver (ed.), Visual Mechanisms. Lancaster, Pa.: Cattell, pp. 117–164.

Marshall, W. II., Woolsey, C. N., and Bard, P. 1941. Observations on cortical somatic sensory mechanisms of cat and monkey. J. Neurophysiol. 4:1–24.

Martin, K. A. C. 1988. The lateral geniculate nucleus strikes back. Trends Neurosci. 11:192–194.

McGuire, B. A., Gilbert, C. D., Rivlin, P. K., and Wiesel, T. N. 1991. Targets of horizontal connections in macaque primary visual cortex. J. Comp. Neurol. 305:370–392.

McGuire, B. A., Hornung, J.-P. Gilbert, C. D., and Wiesel, T. N. 1984. Patterns of synaptic input to layer 4 of cat striate cortex. J. Neurosci. 4:3021–3033.

Métin, C., and Frost, D. O. 1989. Visual responses of neurons in somatosensory cortex of hamsters with experimentally induced retinal projections to somatosensory thalamus. Proc. Natl. Acad. Sci. U.S.A. 86:357–361.

Mountcastle, V. B. 1976. The world around us: Neural command functions for selective attention. Neurosci. Res. Program Bull. 14 [Suppl.]

Rockland, K. S., and Lund, J. S. 1983. Intrinsic laminar lattice connections in primate visual cortex. J. Comp. Neurol. 216: 303–318.

Schiller, P. H. 1982. Central connections of the retinal ON and OFF pathways. Nature 297:580–583.

Schiller, P. H., Logothetis, N. K., and Charles, E. R. 1990. Functions of the colour-opponent and broad-band channels of the visual system. Nature 343:68–70.

Schiller, P. H., True, S. D., and Conway, J. L. 1980. Deficits in eye movements following frontal eye-field and superior colliculus ablations. J. Neurophysiol. 44:1175–1189.

Schmidt, R. F., and Thews, G. (eds.). 1989. Human Physiology, 2nd compl. rev. ed. M. A. Biederman-Thorson (trans.) Berlin: Springer.

Sherk, H., and LeVay, S. 1983. Contribution of the cortico-claustral loop to receptive field properties in area 17 of the cat. J. Neurosci. 3:2121–2127.

Sparks D. L., and Mays, L. E. 1990. Signal transformations required for the generation of saccadic eye movements. Annu. Rev. Neurosci 13:309–336.

Stryker, M. P., Chapman, B., Miller, K. D., and Zahs, K. R. 1990. Experimental and theoretical studies of the organization of afferents to single-orientation columns in visual cortex. Cold Spring Harbor Symp. Quant. Biol. 55:515–527.

Talbot, S. A., and Marshall, W. II. 1941. Physiological studies on neural mechanisms of visual localization and discrimination. Am. J. Ophthalmol. 24:1255–1264.

Ts'o, D. Y., Frostig, R. D., Lieke, E. E., and Grinvald, A. 1990. Functional organization of primate visual cortex revealed by high resolution optical imaging. Science 249:417–420.

Ts'o, D. Y., Gilbert, C. D., and Wiesel, T. N. 1986. Relationships between horizontal interactions and functional architecture in cat striate cortex as revealed by cross-correlation analysis. J. Neurosci. 6:1160–1170.

Walls, G. L. 1953. The Lateral Geniculate Nucleus and Visual Histophysiology. Berkeley: Univ. of California Press.

Wiesel, T. N., Hubel, D. H., and Lam, D. M. K. 1974. Autoradiographic demonstration of ocular-dominance columns in the monkey striate cortex by means of transneuronal transport. Brain Res. 79:273–279.

Wong-Riley, M. 1979. Changes in the visual system of monocularly sutured or enucleated cats demonstrable with cytochrome oxidase histochemistry. Brain Res. 171:11–28.

30

Eric R. Kandel

Perception of Motion, Depth, and Form

Visual Perception Is a Creative Process

Vision Is Thought to Be Mediated by Three Parallel Pathways That Process Information for Motion, Depth and Form, and Color

Psychological Evidence Supports the Idea That Separate Pathways Carry Different Visual Information

Clinical Evidence Is Also Consistent with Parallel Processing of Visual Information

Motion in the Visual Field Is Analyzed by a Special Neural System

Motion Is Represented in the Middle Temporal Area (V5) and Medial Superior Temporal Area (V5a)

Lesions of the Middle Temporal Area Selectively Impair the Ability to Analyze Motion

The Perceptual Judgment of Motion Direction Can Be Influenced by Microstimulation of Cells Within the Middle Temporal Area

Three-Dimensional Vision Depends on Monocular Depth Cues and Binocular Disparity

Monocular Cues Create Far-Field Depth Perception

Stereoscopic Cues Create Near-Field Depth Perception

Information from the Two Eyes Is First Combined in the Primary Visual Cortex

Recognition of Faces and Other Complex Forms Occurs in the Inferior Temporal Cortex

Visual Attention Focuses Perception by Facilitating Coordination Between Separate Visual Pathways

The Analysis of Visual Attention May Provide Important Clues Toward Understanding Conscious Awareness

An Overall View

We are so familiar with seeing, that it takes a leap of imagination to realize that there are problems to be solved. But consider it. We are given tiny distorted upside-down images in the eyes, and we see separate solid objects in surrounding space. From the patterns of stimulation on the retina we perceive the world of objects and this is nothing short of a miracle.

Richard L. Gregory, Eye and Brain, 1966

Most of our idea about the world and our memory of it is based on sight. How do we see? How do we perceive the movement of objects in space? How do we distinguish colors? Studies of artificial intelligence and of pattern recognition by computers have made us realize that the brain recognizes movement, form, and color using strategies that no existing computer begins to approach. Simply to look out into the world and recognize a face or enjoy a landscape entails an amazing computational achievement more difficult than that required for solving logic problems or playing chess.

How is this processing accomplished? A simple idea is that visual perception is achieved by a single hierarchical system of cells processing information from the retina to the striate and extrastriate cortex with receptive field properties that range from simple to complex and super-complex. In the previous chapter we saw that there is indeed a transformation of receptive field properties along a serial pathway. How far does this hierarchy reach? Is there a group of cells that receives input from the complex cells and makes us aware of the total image? Is there a special supercomplex cell group for each familiar object on top of the hierarchical processing?

There may be further elaboration of receptive field properties along a serial pathway as a result of higher-order cells in the occipital, inferotemporal, and posterior parietal areas abstracting the computational results of the striate cortex. But recent studies suggest that, in addition to serial processing, cells in *different* areas of the visual cortex respond to different perceptual attributes of objects—motion, form, or color. Each of these areas receives special information carried along separate pathways.

This chapter covers three areas. First we shall consider recent psychophysical and anatomical evidence for processing of motion, form, and color in three parallel pathways. Second, we shall examine the physiological mechanisms in two of these pathways. (In the next chapter we shall examine the processing of color). Finally, we shall examine how *visual attention* may bring these parallel transformations together into a single conscious image.

Visual Perception Is a Creative Process

Until recently, visual perception was often compared to the operation of a camera. Like the lens of a camera, the lens of the eye focuses an inverted image onto the retina. This analogy breaks down rapidly, however, because it does not capture what vision really does, which is to cre-

ate a three-dimensional perception of the world that is different from the two-dimensional images projected onto the retina. The comparison also fails to illustrate how our visual system can perceive an object under different conditions, conditions that cause the image on the retina to vary widely.

As we move about, or as the ambient illumination changes, the size, shape, and brightness of the images that an object projects onto the retina change. Yet under most conditions we do not perceive the object itself to be changing. As a friend walks toward you, you perceive the friend as coming closer; you do not perceive the friend as growing larger, even though the image on the retina does enlarge. As we move from a brightly lit garden into a dimly lit room, the intensity of light reaching the retina can vary 1000-fold. Yet in the dim light of a room, as in the bright light of the sun, we see a white shirt as white and a red tie as red. Our ability to perceive an object's size or color as unchanging illustrates clearly what is so remarkable about the visual system. It does not simply record images passively, like a camera. Instead, the visual system transforms transient light stimuli on the retina into mental constructs of a stable three-dimensional world.

The degree to which visual perception is transformational and therefore creative has only been fully appreciated recently. As we saw in the introduction to Chapter 23, earlier psychophysical thinking was greatly influenced by the British empiricist philosophers of the 17th and 18th centuries, notably John Locke and George Berkeley, who thought of perception as a simple process of assembling elementary sensations in an additive way, component by component. The modern view that perception is not atomistic but holistic, that it is an active and creative process that involves more than just the information provided by the retina was first emphasized in the early 20th century by the German psychologists Max Wertheimer, Kurt Koffka, and Wolfgang Köhle, who founded the school of *Gestalt psychology*.

The German term *Gestalt* means a configuration or image. The central idea of the Gestalt psychologists is that the act of perception creates a *Gestalt*—a figure or form that is not a property of an object observed but represents the *organization* of sensations by the brain. The Gestalt psychologists argued that the brain creates three-dimensional experiences from two-dimensional images by organizing sensations into stable patterns, or perceptual constancies. The visual system accomplishes this organization by following certain *rational principles* of shape, color, distance, and movement of objects in the visual field. That is, the brain makes certain assumptions about what is to be seen in the world, expectations that seem to derive in part from experience and in part from the built-in neural wiring for vision.

The Gestalt psychologists illustrated the brain's strategies with examples of visual illusions and perceptual constancies. Consider the array of dots in Figure 30–1A. The dots in the figure are equally spaced, yet the brain organizes them alternately into either rows or columns.

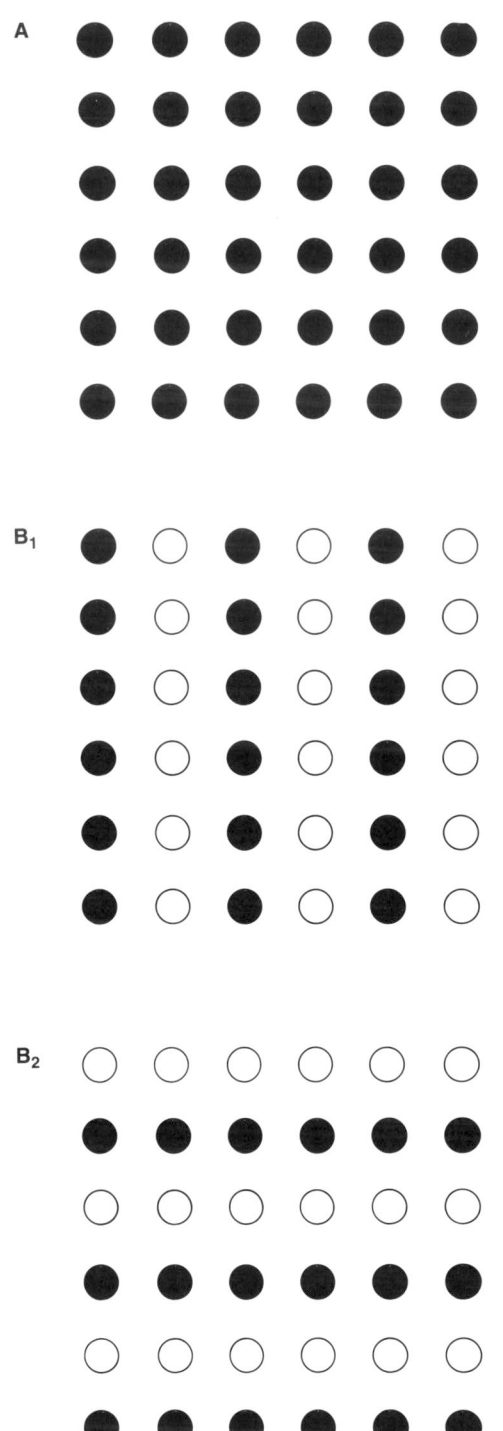

FIGURE 30–1
The array of dots in **A** can be seen as a pattern of either rows or columns. In the absence of additional clues, we alternatively see the pattern as either rows or columns of black dots. However, we can bias the way we organize the array by adding similarity and proximity clues. Thus, the two **lower figures** have the same spatial organization as A, but we see the cative image as a pattern of columns in **B₁** and rows in **B₂** because of the arrangement of black and white dots. (From Gleitman, 1981.)

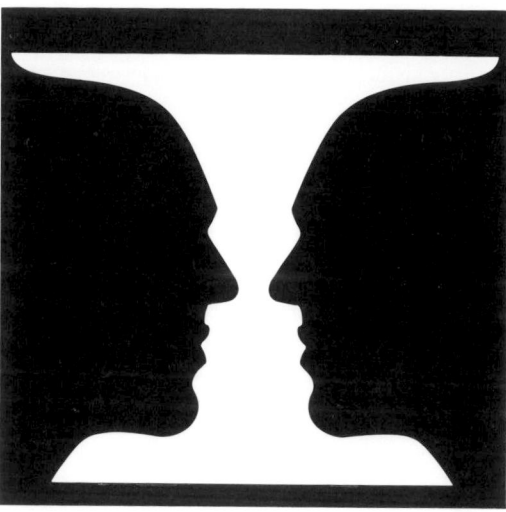

FIGURE 30–2
Figure–ground alternation. In this famous figure and ground by the Danish psychologist Edgar Rubin we sometimes see a pair of faces, sometimes a white vase. The perceptual decision of what is figure (or object) and what is ground is similar to the communication engineer's distinction between signal and noise. By focusing on one signal, the other becomes submerged into the background noise.

The tendency to see one pattern rather than another can be enhanced by adding clues such as *similarity* or *proximity*. For example, if some rows or columns of dots in Figure 30–1A appear similar, these dots will stand out as a group, so that we now perceive the *entire* image as a pattern of columns (Figure 30–1B, 1) or rows (Figure 30–1B, 2).

This process of organization is continuous and dynamic, as is evident in the well-known alternation of figures on a background, first illustrated in 1915 by the psychologist Edgar Rubin. Figure 30–2 can be seen as two faces in black against a white background or as a white vase against a black background, but it is difficult to see both images simultaneously. This organizational power of the visual system has been extensively exploited by the artists Kolomar Moser, Vassily Kandinsky, and Maurits Escher (Figure 30–3). Escher writes: "Our eyes are accustomed to fixing on specific objects. The moment this happens everything *around* is reduced to background . . . . The human eye and mind cannot be busy with two things at the same moment, so there must be a quick and continual jumping from one side to the other." The figure–ground dichotomy thus illustrates one principle of visual perception. In a *winner-take-all* perceptual strategy, similar to the singleness of action described by Sherrington for the motor system (Chapter 26), only part of the image can be selected as the focus of attention; the rest must become submerged into the background.

A

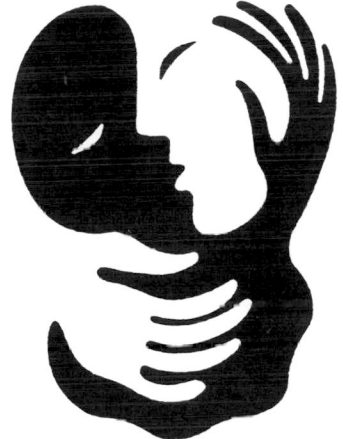

B

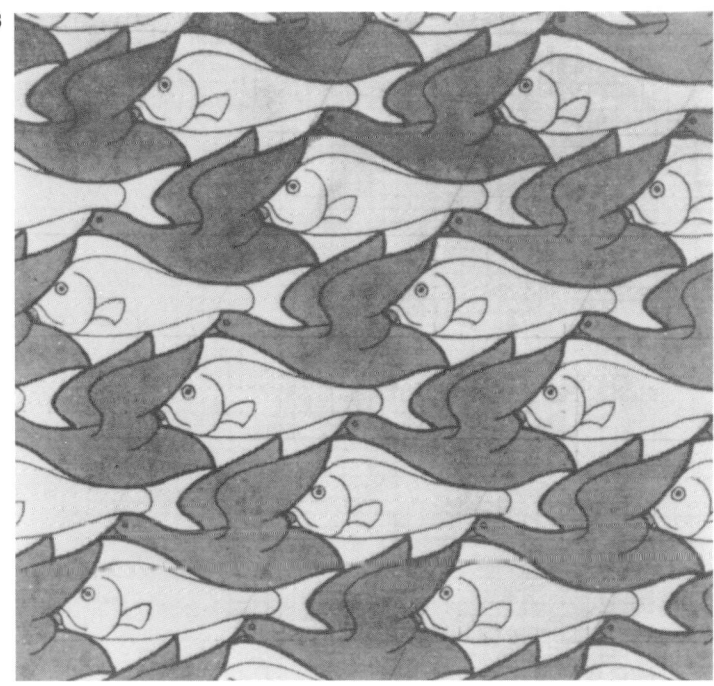

FIGURE 30–3
Figure–ground reversal has been used effectively by many graphic artists.

A. Here Victor Vasarely uses this technique to show two lovers embracing, one in black, the other in white. Either pattern can be seen as figure or ground. (From Gleitman, 1981.)

B. In this repeating pattern of fishes and birds by Maurits Escher, the same outline is shared by the two different figures. Normally, contours serve only to outline an object against its background.

The organizational mechanisms of vision—selection, distortion, filling in, and omissions—are best demonstrated by illusions. Illusions illustrate that perception is a creative construction based on unconscious conjecture about many of the assumptions the brain makes in interpreting visual data. In the classic Müller-Lyer illusion two lines of equal length appear to be unequal (Figure 30–4). As is characteristic of many illusions, learning does not prevent us from being taken in by this illusion. We consistently see the line with inwardly directed barbs as smaller than the line with outwardly directed barbs. We perceive them to be unequal because experience has taught us to use shape as an indicator of size.

In addition to previous knowledge, the context—the relationship of an object to the surrounding objects—also helps to interpret an image. Thus, we judge size by comparing objects to one another and to their immediate surroundings. For example, in the left photograph in Figure

FIGURE 30–4
Perceived length can differ from measured length, as illustrated by the classic Müller-Lyer illusion. The two horizontal lines are identical in length, but **line 1** appears shorter than **line 2**.

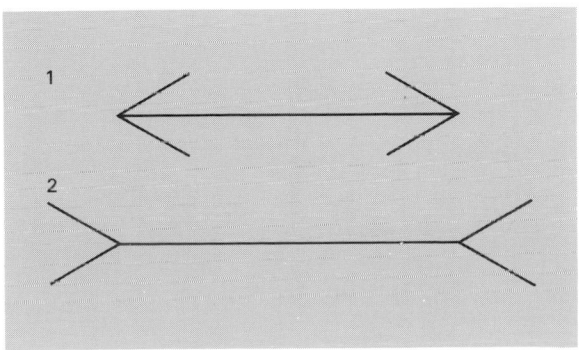

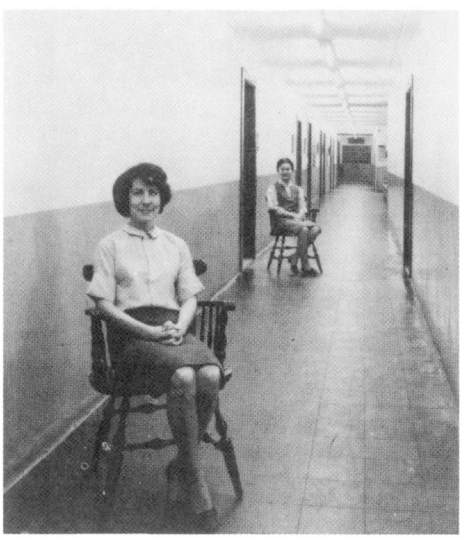
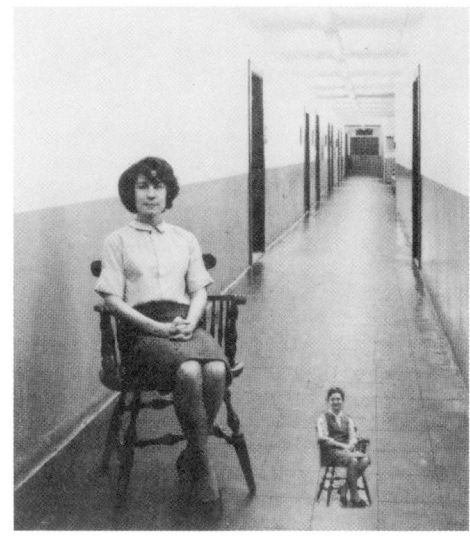

FIGURE 30–5

To judge size, we unconsciously compare the various objects in the visual field. In the picture on the **left** the nearer woman is 9 feet from the camera while the farther one is 27 feet away. Both appear to be the same size. The picture on the **right** was taken with the nearer woman in the same place but without the farther woman. The farther woman in the left picture was then cut out and pasted on the picture at right. To convince yourself that she is the same size as the one at left you will probably need to measure her. In the right picture she appears as small, not as being far away, because the corridor and tiles around her are not proportional, as they are in the left picture. (From Brown and Herrnstein, 1975.)

30–5 two women are at different distances from the camera. In that perspective they appear to be roughly equal in size. When viewed out of context, as in the photograph on the right, the size of the two women is seen to be quite different (Figure 30–5). Moving the distant woman next to the closer woman, where the corridor is wide and the tiles are larger, places her in a new perspective.

Some strategies used by the visual system seem to represent inferences built into the wiring of the brain by genetic and developmental processes. For example, the psychophysicist Vilyanur Ramachandran has explored the perception of shape from shadows, a phenomenon astronomers of the 19th century recognized as being based on the assumption that an image is illuminated by only one source of light. When a round shape is lit from above, it appears to be convex like the exterior of a sphere, whereas when it is lit from below it appears to be concave like the inside of a bowl (Figure 30–6A). The exact shape is ambiguous when the brain does not know the source of the light. With some conscious effort one can mentally shift the light source (assume it has a different direction) and change the apparent curvature of the object. In looking at an array of similar round shapes, our interpretation of one object will determine how we see the entire array.

Do the objects in the array appear all convex or all concave because we assume that similar objects in an array are identical? Or is our perception based on the assumption that there is only one source of light? To answer this question, Ramachandran created a display in which the objects in one column are the mirror images of those in the other column (Figure 30–6B). In this case we see one column of objects as concave and the other as convex. Again, the brain seems to assume that the entire visual image is illuminated by only one source of light. It does not assume that all the objects are facing one direction and that the different images are the result of different light sources. Ramachandran suggests that we make this assumption because we have evolved in a natural environ-

FIGURE 30–6

Spheres or cavities? The decision depends on where you assume the light source is.

A. You can reverse the depth of these objects by mentally shifting the light source from up to down.

B. In this array, once you see one column as convex the other column will appear concave. It is almost impossible to see both rows as simultaneously convex or concave. (Adapted from Ramachandran, 1987.)

A   B

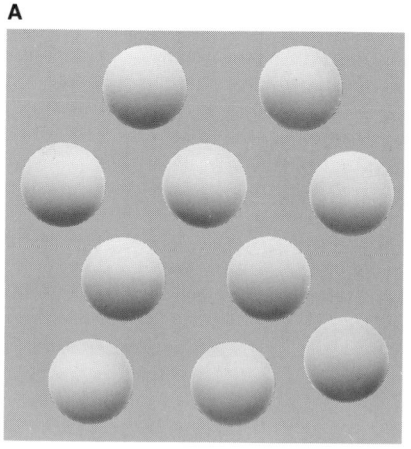
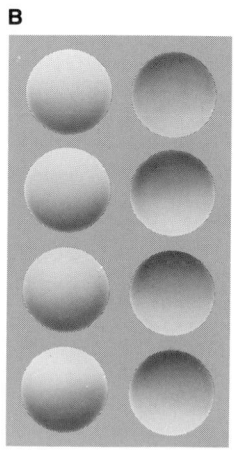

ment with only one source of light, the sun, and our brain assumes that the source of light is always above. Whether this particular explanation is correct, the finding supports the Gestaltist's contention that the derivation of shape from shading is not a strictly local operation restricted to a part of the image, but a global one that involves most, and perhaps all, of the visual field.

As a result of the influence of Gestalt theorists, most perceptual psychologists no longer ask the empiricist's question, "What are the basic components of this perception?" Rather, they—and we—are interested in the question, "What neural transformation produces this perception?" This question provides a common framework for the current attempts to merge psychological and neurobiological investigations of vision.

Vision Is Thought to Be Mediated by Three Parallel Pathways That Process Information for Motion, Depth and Form, and Color

In vision, as in the other mental operations, we experience the world as a whole. We saw above how the brain ana-

lyzes a visual image globally in interpreting shape from shading. Various otherwise unrelated attributes—movement, location, form, and color—are all coordinated in a visual image. This unity is achieved not by one hierarchical neural system concerned with vision but by at least three (and possibly more) parallel pathways in the brain. This view, first clearly enunciated by Semir Zeki, has become one of the major tenets of today's neurobiological study of vision.

At the beginning of the 20th century, the British neurologist Gordon Holmes inferred, based on clinical examination of patients with cortical lesions, that the spatial relationship of the photoreceptors in the retina was preserved in the striate cortex (Brodmann's area 17). This clinical impression was confirmed experimentally in 1941 when Wade Marshall and Samuel Talbot demonstrated that the striate cortex contains a complete *retinotopic map*. By 1985 Zeki, John Allman, Jon Kaas, and David Van Essen had found at least 20 other representations of the retina in the extrastriate cortex, the areas outside the striate cortex. Some of these representations are complete, others are only partial (Figure 30–7).

FIGURE 30–7

The striate and extrastriate visual areas.

A. 1. This lateral view of the right hemisphere shows exposed portions of visual areas V1, V2, and V4. (**Vertical line** indicates the location of the coronal section in 2.) **2.** An expanded view of the occipital lobe (anterolateral angle) shows areas V1, V2, V4, and V5. Area V5 lies in the buried MT area in the superior temporal sulcus at the rostral border of the occipital lobe.

B. This horizontal section through the occipital lobe at the location shown in A2 illustrates the approximate locations of known visual areas at this level.

C. A completely unfolded and flattened view of the right cerebral cortex shows the locations of different visual areas in relation to areas subserving other functions. In this flattened representation it is possible to see the relative dimensions of the different cortical areas. The visual cortex occupies the left posterior portion of the map and comprises roughly half of the surface area of cortex in monkeys. In humans it occupies somewhat less area. (Adapted from Maunsell and Newsome, 1987, and Movshon, 1989.)

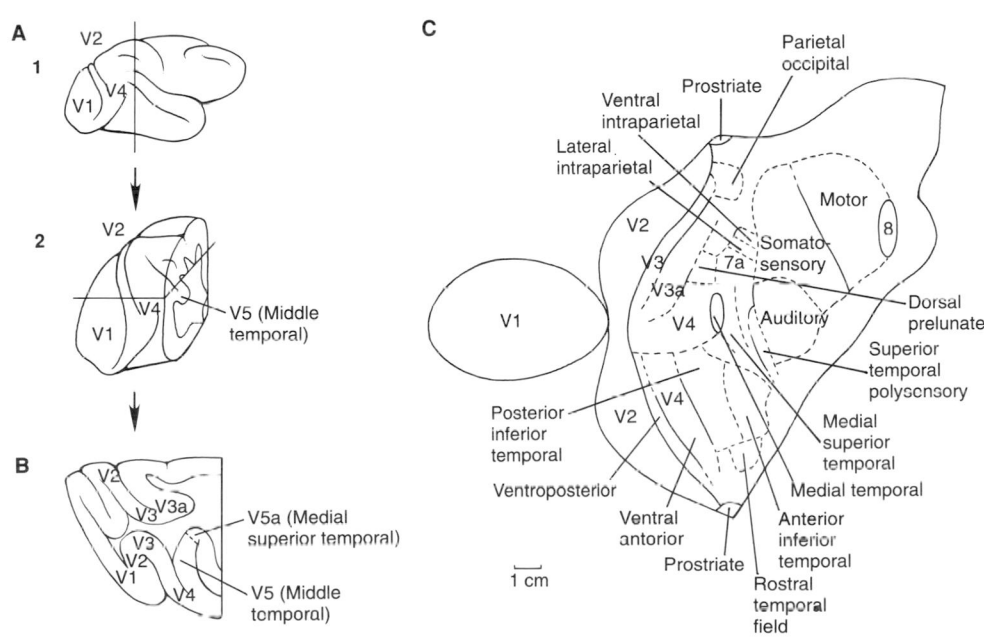

There are six retinotopic maps in the occipital lobe alone: one in area 17 (V1), two in area 18 (V2, V3), and three in area 19 (V3a, V4, and V5).[1] Area 5, or middle temporal area (MT),[2] lies on the posterior bank of the superior temporal sulcus; an adjacent parietal lobe visual area, V5a or medial superior temporal area (MST), lies on the anterior bank of the same sulcus. In addition, the posterior parietal cortex contains an area (7a) concerned with integrating somatic and visual sensations. All of these maps differ both in the precision with which the retina is represented topographically and in the features of stimuli to which the cells seem to respond. Thus the visual system, like the somatic sensory system, has several distinct representations of its receptive sheet, the retina, and these maps serve as the anatomical substrates for the parallel processing of different aspects of visual information. By recording from cells in various areas of the extrastriate cortex, Zeki identified the features of the visual image processed in each cortical area. For example, area V5 (MT) is primarily concerned with visual movement, while area V4 is much more concerned with color or the orientation of edges.

Later anatomical studies of the pathways, which we examined in the last two chapters, have independently led to the conclusion that visual processing involves parallel pathways from the retina to the lateral geniculate nucleus, to the striate, and finally to the extrastriate cortex.

As described in Chapter 28, the retina contains two types of ganglion cells, large cells called type M (or Pα) and small cells called type P (or Pβ). The large cells are not concerned with color. They do not treat the signals from the three types of color cones differently, but simply add them. These cells project to the magnocellular layers of the lateral geniculate nucleus. The small P ganglion cells, on the other hand, do distinguish among the three types of cones and therefore signal information about color. They project to the parvocellular layers of the lateral geniculate nucleus.

Margaret Wong-Riley, Jonathan Horton, Margaret Livingstone, and David Hubel provided a connecting link between the parvo- and magnocellular layers in the lateral geniculate nucleus and different retinotopic maps in the cortex. Wong-Riley and Horton stained the striate cortex (V1) for the mitochondrial enzyme cytochrome oxidase and found a precise and repeating pattern of dark, peg-like regions, about 0.2 mm in diameter. These so-called *blob regions*, that we encountered in Chapter 29, are especially

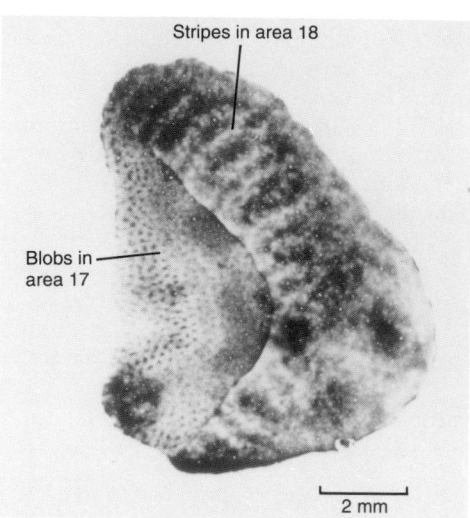

FIGURE 30–8
Section from the occipital lobe of a squirrel monkey at the border of areas 17 and 18 reacted with cytochrome oxidase. The cytochrome oxidase stains the blobs in area 17 and it stains the stripes (both thick and thin) in area 18. (Courtesy of M. Livingstone.)

prominent in the superficial layers 2 and 3, where they are separated by intervening regions that stain lighter, called *interblob regions*. Livingstone and Hubel extended these observations and delineated three pathways that project from cells in different layers of the lateral geniculate nucleus to the striate cortex. Two of these pathways end in the superficial layers, in either the blob or the interblob regions; the third pathway ends in the deeper layers.

Beyond the striate cortex (V1) lies V2 and the other visual representations of the extrastriate cortex (Figure 30–7). Roger Tootell next discovered cytochrome-rich patches in V2 that link the three pathways ending in V1 and the areas in the extrastriate cortex described by Zeki. In V2, instead of blobs the darkly stained cytochrome-rich patches take the form of alternating *thick* and *thin* stripes separated by *pale interstripes* (Figure 30–8). As proposed by Zeki, Van Essen, and Hubel and Livingstone, the striped regions of V2 are relay points for the three major pathways that course through V1 (Figure 30–9). These three pathways project to different extrastriate areas and form systems that appear to process distinct types of visual information.

The *magnocellular system* is specialized for motion and spatial relationships. It also contributes to stereopsis. This pathway extends from the large M-type ganglion cells in the retina to the magnocellular layers of the lateral geniculate nucleus. The pathway continues to layer 4Cα of V1 and then to layers 4B and 6. From there it leads to the thick stripes of V2, then to V3, and from V3 to MT (V5), the area found by Zeki to be concerned with depth and motion. MT projects to MST and other areas in the parietal cortex concerned with visuospatial function. Neurons throughout this system respond rapidly but only transiently. They are relatively insensitive to color and

---

[1]The abbreviations for the various visual areas (V1, V2, V3, V3a, V4) were originally based on the belief, no longer thought to be correct, that visual processing was strictly serial. In addition, some terms, such as 7a, 8, and TF, derive from old architectural maps of the cerebral cortex.

[2]The term MT, which is now generally used, may be confusing. It was originally used in reference to the owl monkey, where this region lies on the surface of the *middle temporal gyrus*. Today most work is done in macaque monkeys, where the homologous area lies in the *superior temporal sulcus*. Nevertheless, the term MT is still used, even in reference to the macaque monkey. In both the owl monkey and the macaque monkey, MT lies near the junction of the occipital, parietal, and temporal lobes.

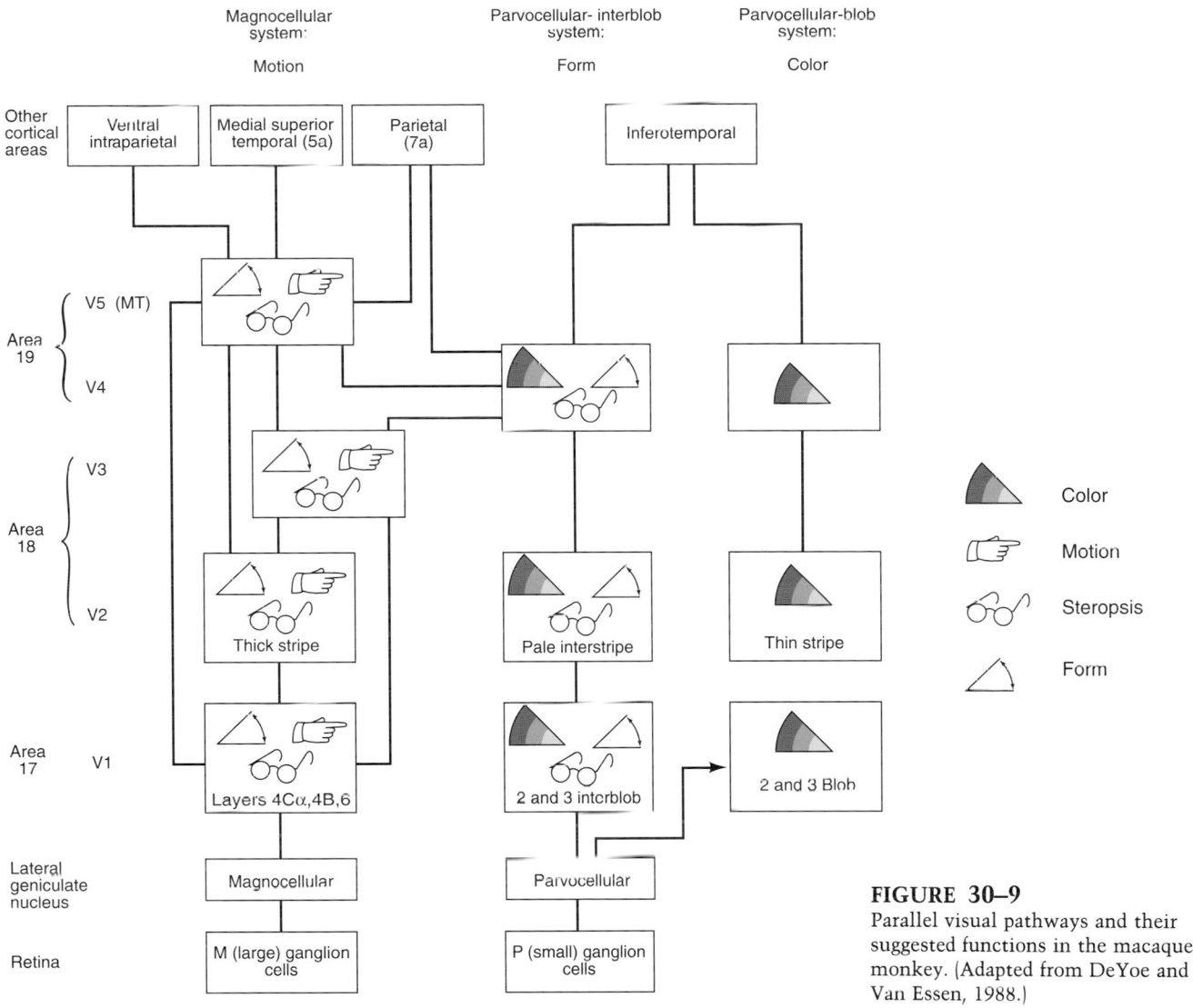

FIGURE 30–9
Parallel visual pathways and their suggested functions in the macaque monkey. (Adapted from DeYoe and Van Essen, 1988.)

therefore respond poorly to contours or borders discernible only on the basis of color contrast. The system is thought to be specialized for detecting the motion of objects and the three-dimensional organization of objects. Peter Schiller and his colleagues have found that this system also has a limited capability for depth perception. But the system is poor for analyzing stationary objects. It is concerned with seeing *where* as opposed to seeing *what*. As we shall see later, lesions in this pathway result in a selective deficit in motion perception and in eye movements directed toward moving targets.

The *parvocellular–interblob system* seems specialized for the detection of form (and to some degree color). This pathway projects from the small P-type ganglion cells in the retina to the parvocellular layers of the lateral geniculate nucleus. From there the pathway projects to layer 4Cβ, then to the interblobs of layers 2 and 3 in V1, then to the pale stripes of V2, to V4, and finally to the inferior temporal cortex. Neurons in this system are sensitive to

the orientation of edges. Because a great deal of the information about shape is derived from the borders, this system is important for perception of shape. These neurons are slowly adapting and capable of high resolution, which is probably important for seeing stationary objects in detail. Thus, this system is more concerned with seeing *what* than with seeing *where*. Lesions in the inferior temporal lobe produce deficits related to the recognition of objects and, in some regions, to the recognition of faces. The system is also important for depth perception.

The *parvocellular–blob system* is specialized for color. It also arises from the parvocellular subdivision of the lateral geniculate nucleus (and perhaps some additional cells in the interlaminal layer) and projects to the blobs of layers 2 and 3 in V1, then to the thin stripes of V2, and then to V4, the area described by Zeki as having many color-responsive cells. Like the parvocellular–interblob system, the parvocellular–blob system eventually terminates within the inferior temporal cortex.

These three pathways are interconnected at various levels. For example, both V4 and MT have some projections to the parietal cortex as well as their major projections to the inferior temporal cortex (Figure 30–9).

Psychological Evidence Supports the Idea That Separate Pathways Carry Different Visual Information

Can the perceptual strategies demonstrated by the Gestaltists be related specifically to the parallel pathways of the visual system? Can one experimentally relate components of global perception in humans to the specific pathways that run from the retina to the temporal or parietal cortex? How separable are movement and form, and either of these from color? This question has been addressed in two types of experiments.

First, Ramachandran and Richard Gregory attempted to reduce the contribution of what is now known as the magnocellular system by using *equiluminant stimuli*, stimuli that vary only in color but not in luminance (in ratio of brightness). A border between two equiluminant colors has color contrast but no brightness contrast. In a black-and-white photograph two equiluminant colors appear to be the same shade of gray. In theory, the magnocellular system is largely color blind. It therefore relies only on brightness clues and would not be able to distinguish borders between equiluminant red and green. Thus, equiluminant stimuli would reduce the contribution to perception of the magnocellular system. The color-sensitive cells of the parvocellular–blob system, however, should distinguish between red and green at any relative degree of brightness.

From their studies of human responses to equiluminant stimuli, Ramachandran and Gregory concluded that perception of motion disappears at equiluminance. Motion therefore seems to be processed independently of information about color—presumably by the magnocellular system and independent of the parvocellular system. Livingstone and Hubel have extended this approach to additional attributes of visual perception, including perspective, relative size of objects, depth perception, figure–ground relations, and visual illusions, and found that many of these relationships also disappear at equiluminance and therefore also seem to an important degree to be mediated by the magnocellular system.

Why are all of these relationships, and *these* relationships in particular, mediated by this one system? Following the arguments of the Gestalt psychologists and of Ann Treisman, whose ideas we shall learn more about later, Livingstone and Hubel proposed that to separate figure from ground we organize the components of a visual scene into coherent groups. Any object in the visual scene has a particular set of values of depth, brightness, and texture. In addition, when an object moves, a cluster of these elements will have a specific direction and velocity of motion. This moving cluster can also be used to separate that object from other objects. Moreover, unlike the analysis of form and color, which requires high-resolution vision, analysis of depth, brightness, and texture can be performed rapidly at low resolution. The ability to discriminate figure from ground, to link parts of a scene, and to perceive correct spatial relationships may all be mediated by the magnocellular–interblob system, which sees the whole image and its movements at low resolution. In contrast, the parvocellular–blob system is less concerned with movement and more concerned with the fine detail and with the color of a scene.

Although there is consensus that the visual system uses parallel processing, there is still controversy on how neatly the various functions are parceled out among the three pathways, and even exactly how many (two or three) key pathways there are. Part of the disagreement revolves around the question of whether equiluminant stimuli affect *only* the magnocellular pathway. Studies by Schiller and his colleagues suggest that equiluminant stimuli also *reduce* the activity of the parvocellular system. Indeed, there is now agreement that stereopsis, which also disappears at equiluminance and therefore should be restricted to the magnocellular pathway, nonetheless is mediated by the parvocellular systems to some degree. In psychophysical studies of monkeys with selective lesions of the parvocellular and magnocellular layers, Schiller found that, whereas only the magnocellular system is required for motion, both parvocellular systems are required for discrimination of stereopsis, as well as for aspects of color and form.

The findings from both types of studies, those examining human responses to equiluminant stimuli and those examining the responses of animals with damaged visual pathways, are consistent with the existence of three major parallel pathways—a magnocellular pathway concerned with motion and two parvocellular pathways, one more dedicated to color and the other to form. Stereopsis, however, seems to be mediated by both parvocellular pathways. Indeed, the psychophysical evidence on retinal disparity (which, as we shall see, is necessary for stereopsis) indicates that disparity is based on many visual clues, including color, boundaries, texture, and motion. These clues must involve all three parallel pathways to some degree.

Clinical Evidence Is Also Consistent with Parallel Processing of Visual Information

The idea that different aspects of visual perception may be localized to separate areas of the brain actually dates to the beginning of the twentieth century, when Sigmund Freud concluded that the inability of certain patients to recognize visual objects was due not to a peripheral sensory deficit but to a cortical defect that affects the ability to combine components of visual impressions into a complete pattern. These defects, which Freud called *agnosias*, can be quite specific depending on the area of the cortex damaged (Table 30–1). For example, *movement agnosia* occurs after bilateral damage in the cortex of MT or MST

TABLE 30–1. The Visual Agnosias

Type	Deficit	Most probable site of the lesion
Agnosia for form and pattern		
Object agnosia	Naming, using, recognition of real objects	Areas 18, 20, 21 on left and corpus callosum
Agnosia for drawings	Recognition of drawn objects	Areas 18, 20, 21 on right
Prosopagnosia	Recognition of faces	Areas 20, 21 bilaterally
Agnosia for color		
Color agnosia	Association of colors with objects	Area 18 on right
Color anomia	Naming colors	Speech zones or connections from areas 18, 37
Achromatopsia	Distinguishing hues	Areas 18, 37
Agnosia for depth and movement		
Visual spatial agnosia	Stereoscopic vision	Areas 18, 37 on right
Movement agnosia	Discerning movement of object	Bilateral medial temporal area (junction of occipital and temporal cortex)

(Modified from Kolb and Whishaw, 1980.)

and is manifest as a selective loss of movement perception without loss of any other perceptual capabilities. One well-studied patient with intact visual fields lost all perception of motion and could not distinguish between stationary and moving objects.

Some patients lose color vision (*achromatopsia*) because of localized damage to the temporal cortex, the area in humans that contains the homolog of V4. These patients, nonetheless, have reasonably good vision for form. Zeki and his colleagues have recently defined this color-processing area in the brain of living normal human subjects using PET scanning. In addition to movement agnosia and achromatopsia, there is an agnosia for form, which can be selective for inanimate or animate objects, or, as we shall see later, even for faces (*prosopagnosia*).

Visual agnosias rarely occur in pure form. Most patients with achromatopsia also have other deficits. This lack of complexity of the symptoms probably results from the fact that in humans lesions due to vascular accidents or tumors are not normally restricted to functionally discrete regions. In laboratory experiments, on the other hand, a region can be surgically removed with precision and without damage to adjacent areas so that one can locate the functional loss more clearly. Although the clinical evidence for the anatomical basis of visual agnosias is not always precise, it is nevertheless consistent with experimental findings that vision is mediated by interconnected parallel pathways.

How does this processing operate on the cellular level? To address this question we shall first examine the perceptual tasks involved in the analysis of motion, depth, and form. We shall next review the cellular evidence that motion and stereopsis are analyzed by the magnocellular system and that form is analyzed by the parvocellular-interblob system. Finally, to gain insight into the neuronal mechanisms responsible for the different types of perceptual processing, we shall consider the response properties of cells in these two pathways. The parvocellular–blob system, which is concerned with the assessment of color, will be considered in Chapter 31.

Motion in the Visual Field Is Analyzed by a Special Neural System

We usually move through the world we perceive. Appropriate behavior therefore requires that we receive accurate information about the motion of objects. Even when we or the objects that interest us do not move, the images these objects cast on the retina do move because the eyes and the head are never entirely still (Figure 30–10). The visual system has two ways of detecting motion: one related to the motion of the image, and the other (which we shall consider further in Chapter 43), related to the movement of the head and eyes (Figure 30–11).

Detection of motion of the image is so important to adaptive behavior in animals that only humans and other evolved primates can respond to objects that do not move. Simple vertebrate animals (such as frogs) cannot even see objects unless they are moving. In humans this limitation persists at the peripheral part of the retina. We are not able to identify an object at the sides of the visual field but will notice its motion. When the motion stops, our perception of the object also ceases. At the extreme periphery of the visual field, we cannot detect even motion. Instead, motion of an object at the extreme periphery triggers a reflex that rotates the eyes so as to bring the moving object into the central visual field.

Motion in the visual field is detected by comparing the position of images recorded at different times. Since most cells in the visual system are exquisitely sensitive to retinal position and can resolve events separated in time by a few tens of milliseconds, in principle, the visual system should be able to extract the necessary information from the position of the image on the retina by comparing the previous location of an object with its current location. What then is the evidence for a special neural subsystem specialized for motion?

The initial evidence for a special mechanism designed to detect motion independent of retinal position came from psychophysical observations on *apparent motion*, an illusion of motion such as occurs when lights separated in

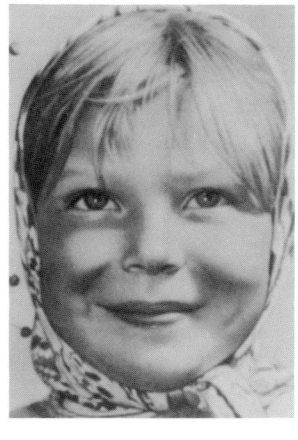
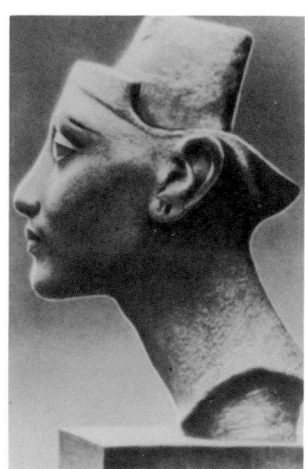
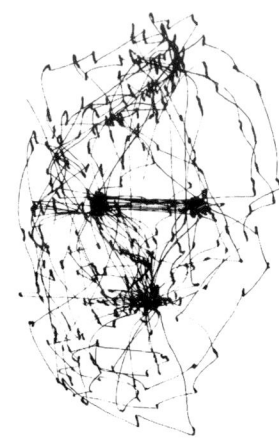
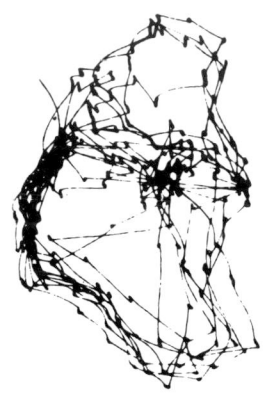

FIGURE 30–10

Our perception of an object in its entirety is built up from repeated scanning of areas of the object. The scanning consists of visually jumping back and forth between areas of interest. During these scanning movements, the image moves across the retina, yet we perceive the object as stationary. Below each photograph shown here is a record of the eye movements made during a two-minute examination of the photograph. (**Left,** photograph of "Girl from the Volga"; **right,** head of the statue of the Egyptian queen Nefertiti, about 1350 B.C.) (From Yarbus, 1967.)

space are alternately turned on and off at appropriate intervals (Figure 30–12). The perception of motion of objects that in fact have not changed position suggests that position and motion are signaled by separate pathways.

Motion Is Represented in the Middle Temporal Area (V5) and Medial Superior Temporal Area (V5a)

As we have seen, the motion pathway originates in the M-type retinal ganglion cells (Figure 30–9). Signals from these cells are relayed through the magnocellular layers of the lateral geniculate nucleus to layer 4Cα in V1, from there to layers 4b and 6, then to the thick stripes of V2, then to V3 and on to MT (V5). Signals from MT in turn are relayed to MST (V5a) and to the visual motor area of the parietal lobe. Although the type M cells in the retina have no special sensitivity to motion *per se*, they respond best to targets whose contrast varies with time. In V1, however, the information about motion—the temporal variation in contrast signaled by the type M cells—is transformed by neurons that respond to particular directions of motion. These signals are further elaborated in MT, where the firing pattern of neurons reflects the speed and direction of motion of visual targets. This information about motion is then extracted in MST and used for three different behavioral purposes, for visual perception, maintaining pursuit eye movements, and guiding bodily movement through the environment.

Neurons in both MT and MST project directly to the dorsolateral pontine nuclei in the brain stem. Cells in the pontine nuclei project to the contralateral cerebellar flocculus, where, as we shall learn in Chapter 43, cells discharge during pursuit eye movements, eye movements concerned with tracking a moving target. The flocculus, in turn, projects to the oculomotor area in the brain stem, which generates eye movement. Thus, the entire circuit of visual inputs to pursuit eye movements is known, at least in outline.

How is motion represented in the brain? When a simple

FIGURE 30–11

Movement in the visual field can be perceived in two ways.

A. When the eyes are held still, the image of a moving object traverses the retina. Information about movement is relayed to the brain through sequential firing of receptors in the retina.

B. When the eyes follow an object, the image of the moving object falls in one place on the retina and the information is conveyed to the brain by movement of the eyes or the head.

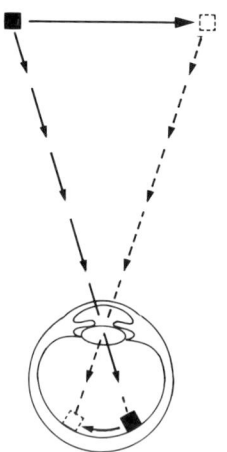
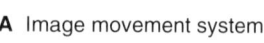
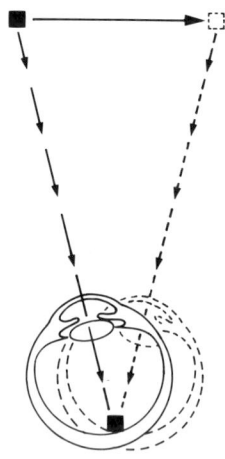

A Image movement system   B Eye-movement system

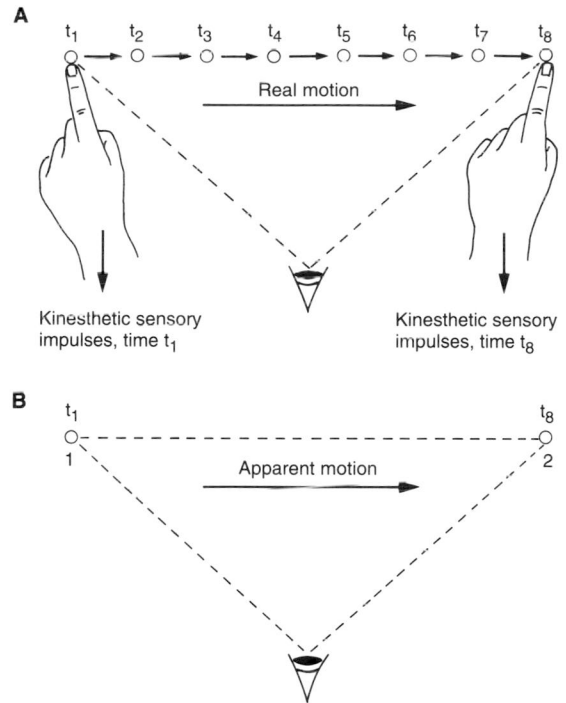

FIGURE 30–12

The perception of actual motion and apparent motion.

A. Actual motion is experienced as a sequence of visual sensations, each due to a different position on the retina (See Figure 30–11A). This can be documented, as illustrated here, by the memory of tactile sensations experienced when reaching out to grasp a moving object.

B. Apparent motion may actually be more convincing than actual movement illustrated in A, and is the perceptual basis for motion pictures. Thus when two lights at positions **1** and **2** are turned on and off at suitable intervals, we perceive a single light moving between the two points. This perceptual illusion cannot be explained by processing of information by means of different retinal positions, and is therefore evidence for the existence of a special visual system for the detection of motion. (From Hochberg, 1968.)

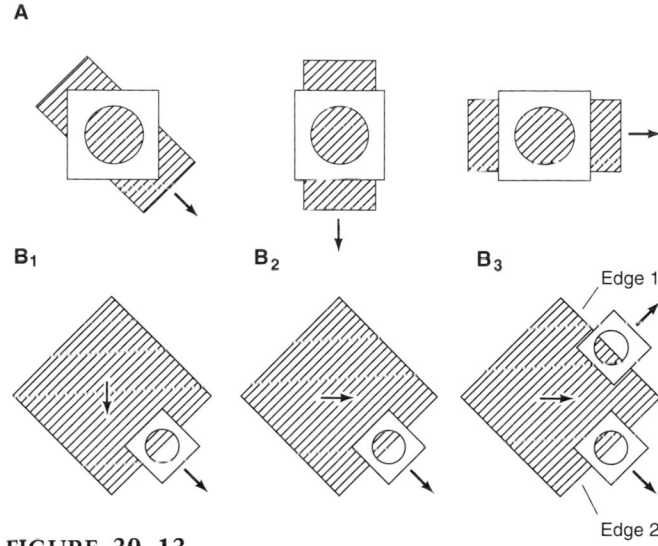

FIGURE 30–13

The aperture problem.

A. Motion in three different directions can produce the same physical stimulus and therefore can be perceived as motion in one direction. A simple grate is shown moving in three directions: obliquely right, directly down, and directly right. When seen through a small aperture, the grate appears in all three cases to move in the same direction: downward and to the right. This ambiguity is called the *aperture problem*. (Adapted from Movshon, 1985.)

B. The aperture problem is here illustrated with two diamonds, one moving downward (**1**) and one moving rightward (**2**). Again, locally measured motions (**circles**) do not reflect the motions of objects unambiguously. A formal solution to the aperture problem is presented in (**3**). According to this model, lower-order cells that respond to specific directions (perpendicular to their axis of orientation) obtain two or more local measurements to resolve the ambiguity inherent in single measurements of local movement. The several lower-order cells then project to higher-order cells that integrate the local movements encoded by the lower-order cells, thereby encoding the motion of the entire object. (Adapted from Movshon, 1990.)

one-dimensional object like an edge or a line is moved parallel to its own orientation, we perceive the direction of movement unambiguously. However, in our everyday experience we encounter complex two- and three-dimensional surfaces that readily give rise to ambiguities and illusions. Consider the example in Figure 30–13, which shows a large grating moving in three directions. When viewed through a small circular aperture, the direction of motion of a larger grating appears in all three cases to be the same. This example illustrates that when an observer examines only a limited area of the moving image—as is the case when looking through an aperture—the observer can only report the component of motion that is perpendicular to the orientation of the bars in the grating. This phenomenon has been called the *aperture problem*, and it illustrates a basic ambiguity of motion detection.

Most neurons in V1 have small receptive fields and are therefore subject to the aperture problem when confronted with a large moving object. Consider, for example, the response of a neuron in V1 whose receptive field is represented by the small aperture along the lower-right edge of the field of parallel lines in Figure 30–13B. The neuron will respond equally to motion of the field of lines downward or rightward because motion of the lines through the aperture will appear identical in both cases. Thus, neurons in V1 can only signal motion *perpendicular* to their axis of orientation (horizontal, vertical, or oblique). As a result, although the observer has no difficulty perceiving the direction, the responses of single neurons in V1 are ambiguous with respect to the direction of motion of the whole object. The cells in V1 cannot respond to, and therefore signal information about, the movement of the pattern as a whole. The global motion must therefore be computed subsequently by cells that receive information about the local analysis of motion carried out by a *number* of V1 neurons.

These considerations led David Marr and Shimon Ullman as well as Anthony Movshon and Edward Adelson to propose that information about motion in the visual field is extracted in two stages. The first stage is concerned with motion in one direction, that is, information about one-dimensional moving objects as well as measurement of the motion of the components of complex objects. In this initial stage, neurons that respond to a specific axis of orientation are primarily active and signal movement of components perpendicular to their axis of orientation. The second stage is concerned with establishing the motion of complex patterns. In this second stage, higher-order neurons combine and integrate the components of motion analyzed by several of the initial stage neurons. Thus, the analysis of the direction of motion of a pattern—a two-dimensional object—requires knowledge of the directions of motion of the components of the pattern.

Movshon, William Newsome, and Martin Gizzi tested this idea and found that the activation of different populations of motion-selective neurons corresponds to the two stages of motion processing. They simplified the aperture problem in their experiments by using plaid patterns, produced by superimposing two gratings (Figure 30–14A). The motion of these patterns creates visual ambiguities similar to those of a single grate viewed through an aperture. The motion of each component grating is perpendicular to the orientation of its bars. However, when the two gratings are superimposed to form a plaid, we perceive the motion as different from that of either component (obliquely upward and obliquely downward). For example, a rightward-moving grating and a downward-moving grating, when superimposed, produce a plaid stimulus that moves unambiguously to the right (Figure 30–14A).

Movshon and his colleagues found that the motion of each component is consistent with the properties of neurons in V1 as well as the majority of neurons in MT. They therefore called these neurons *component direction-selective neurons*. These cells respond only to motion perpendicular to their preferred orientation—vertical, horizontal, or oblique—and will signal the motion of component gratings that make up the plaid rather than the motion of the plaid itself (Figure 30–14B). These cells do not respond when the motion of the entire pattern is in the same direction as the axis of orientation for which the cell is selective. A second, smaller population of neurons in MT (about 20%) responds to the direction of motion of the entire pattern. These neurons, which Movshon and his colleagues called *pattern direction-selective neurons*, respond to the motion of the plaid. Pattern direction-selective neurons integrate information about motion, combining signals that report the motion of components in different directions. Pattern direction-selective neurons represent a level of abstraction not seen in V1. They carry information about motion that is independent of the orientation of the contours.

Lesions of the Middle Temporal Area Selectively Impair the Ability to Analyze Motion

These correlations raise the question: Is the activity of direction selective cells in MT causally related to the per-

ception of visual motion? The first approach to this question was taken by Robert Wurtz and his colleagues, who examined the smooth pursuit eye movements that allow the monkey to keep a moving target on its fovea, and used these eye movements as an indicator of the ability of the monkey to perceive motion. MT has a retinotopic map that conveys information about speed and direction of motion in the contralateral visual field to the system concerned with pursuit eye movement. Wurtz and his colleagues made discrete chemical lesions within different regions of the maps of MT using ibotenic acid, a neurotoxin that destroys neuronal cell bodies. They found that in the region of the visual field monitored by the damaged area the speed of the moving target could no longer be estimated correctly. In contrast, the lesions did not affect eye pursuit of targets in other regions of the visual field nor did it affect eye movements to stationary targets. Thus, visual processing in MT is *selective* for motion of the visual stimulus. Moreover, it is *necessary* for the analysis of motion.

The Perceptual Judgment of Motion Direction Can Be Influenced by Microstimulation of Cells Within the Middle Temporal Area

Like other cortical areas, MT is organized in a columnar fashion with neurons in a column having similar physiological properties. Within a single column, neurons fire action potentials in response to motion in a particular direction and show little or no response to motion in the opposite direction. The preferred direction of motion varies systematically from column to column, such that MT contains a complete representation of motion in all directions at each point in the visual field.

If cells in MT are directly involved in the analysis of motion, the firing patterns of neurons in these motion-selective columns presumably participate in forming the perceptual judgments about motion. How well does the firing pattern of these neurons actually correlate with behavior? To address this question, Newsome, Movshon, and Kenneth Britten recorded the activity of motion-selective neurons in MT in monkeys while the animals carried out a task designed to report the direction of motion in a random dot display. In this display some dots moved coherently while the rest moved randomly. The strength of the motion signal could be varied by varying the proportion of dots that moved coherently. At zero correlation the motion of all dots was random and at 100% correlation the motion of all dots was coherently in one direction. Using this method, Newsome and his colleagues found that the firing of most neurons on this task correlate extremely well with the performance of the monkey! Thus the directional information encoded by the neurons of a single column in MT is *sufficient* to account for the subject's judgment.

If this inference is correct then modifying the firing rates of the neurons that constitute a single column should alter the monkey's perception of motion. To test this idea, Newsome and his colleagues trained monkeys to report the direction of motion in the random dot display while

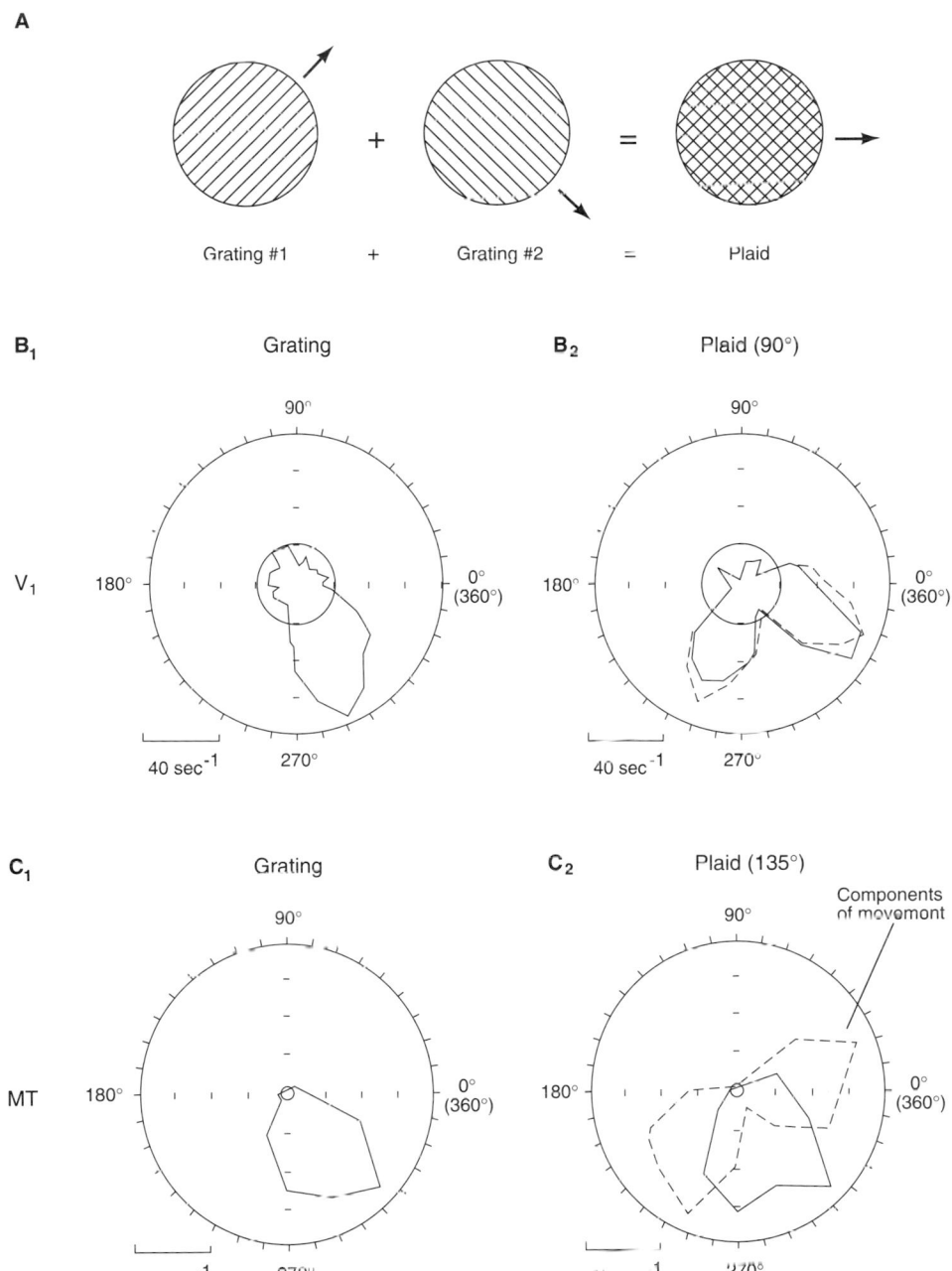

FIGURE 30–14

Plaid images simplify the study of the aperture problem and illustrate the direction selectivity of cortical neurons in the visual cortex.

A. Gratings 1 and 2 move at right angles to each other. When these two gratings are superimposed during movement, the resulting plaid pattern appears to move directly to the right.

B. These polar plots illustrate the motion signaled by lower order neurons in V1 (the striate cortex). The *direction* of stimulus motion is indicated by the angle of the plot (0° to 360°). The neuron's *maximal* response to the stimulus is indicated by the distance from the center to the point of the plot. The circle at the center indicates the neuron's activity when no stimulus is presented.
1. This neuron responds to movement of grating 2 in the direction parallel to its axis of orientation. 2. When presented with simultaneous motion of gratings 1 and 2, the neuron responds to the mo-

tion of both components (indicated by solid lines) but not to the unitary motion of the plaid. The dashed line indicates the expected response of the neuron to the plaid stimulus based on the response to individual gratings.

C. These polar plots illustrate the motion signaled by the higher-order neuron in MT. **1.** As is the case with the lower-order cell in V1, this cell in MT also responds to movement in a direction parallel to its axis of orientation. **2.** However, when presented with simultaneous motion of gratings 1 and 2, the neuron responds to the direction of the unitary motion of the resulting plaid pattern (**solid line**) and not to the component movements (indicated by the **dashed lines**). This indicates that the component signals of V1 have been processed in MT into a more accurate perception of the movement of the object. (From Movshon et al., 1986).

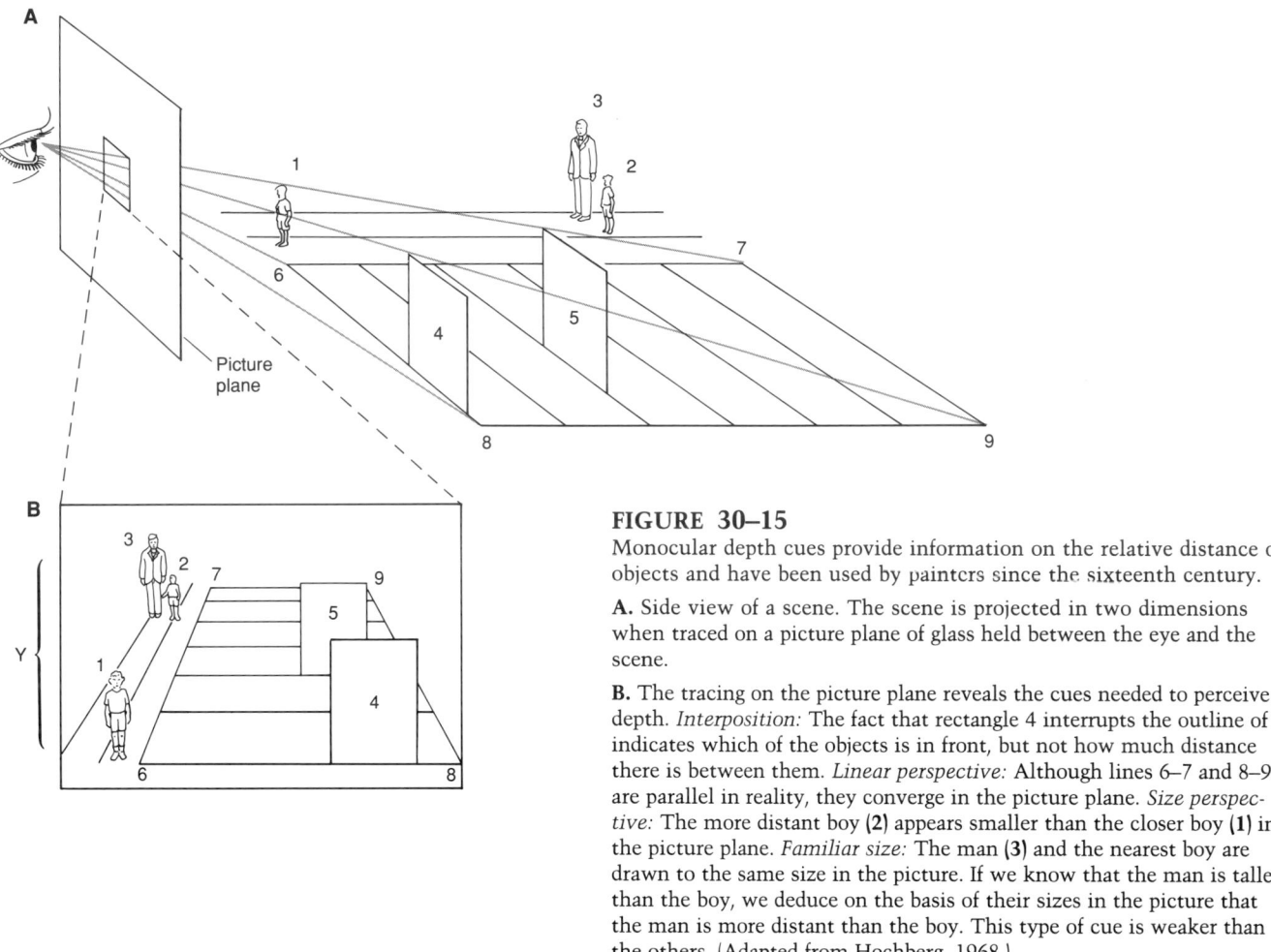

FIGURE 30–15

Monocular depth cues provide information on the relative distance of objects and have been used by painters since the sixteenth century.

A. Side view of a scene. The scene is projected in two dimensions when traced on a picture plane of glass held between the eye and the scene.

B. The tracing on the picture plane reveals the cues needed to perceive depth. *Interposition:* The fact that rectangle 4 interrupts the outline of 5 indicates which of the objects is in front, but not how much distance there is between them. *Linear perspective:* Although lines 6–7 and 8–9 are parallel in reality, they converge in the picture plane. *Size perspective:* The more distant boy (**2**) appears smaller than the closer boy (**1**) in the picture plane. *Familiar size:* The man (**3**) and the nearest boy are drawn to the same size in the picture. If we know that the man is taller than the boy, we deduce on the basis of their sizes in the picture that the man is more distant than the boy. This type of cue is weaker than the others. (Adapted from Hochberg, 1968.)

the experimenters stimulated clusters of directionally sensitive neurons in a single column with currents designed to increase the discharge rate of neurons. Stimulation, in fact, altered the animal's judgment, biasing it toward the particular direction of motion encoded by the neurons that were stimulated. Thus, the firing of a relatively small population of motion-sensitive neurons in MT, perhaps as few as 200 cells, directly contributes to perception. The relationship between functioning of the magnocellular pathway, the cells in the columns of MT, and the perception of motion is impressive.

Three-Dimensional Vision Depends on Monocular Depth Cues and Binocular Disparity

One of the major tasks of the visual system is to convert a two-dimensional retinal image into three dimensions. How is this transformation achieved? How do we tell how far one thing is from another? How do we estimate the relative depth of a three-dimensional object in the visual field? Psychophysical studies indicate that the convergence from two to three dimensions relies on two types of cues: cues for monocular depth and stereoscopic cues for binocular disparity.

*Monocular Cues Create Far-Field
Depth Perception*

At distances greater than about 100 feet, the retinal images seen by each eye are almost identical, so that looking at a distance we are essentially one-eyed. Nevertheless we can perceive depth with one eye by relying on a variety of *monocular depth cues*. There are at least five types of monocular depth cues (Figure 30–15). The first four of these were appreciated by the artists of antiquity, rediscovered during the Renaissance, and codified in the sixteenth century by Leonardo da Vinci.

1. *Previous familiarity.* If we know from experience something about the size of a person, we can judge the person's distance.

2. *Interposition.* If one person is partly hiding another person, we assume the person in front is closer.

3. *Linear* and *size perspectives.* Parallel lines, such as those of a railroad track, appear to converge with distance. The greater the convergence of lines, the greater the impression of distance. The visual system interprets the convergence as depth by assuming that parallel lines remain parallel.

4. *Distribution of shadows and illumination.* Patterns of light and dark can give the impression of depth. For example, brighter shades of colors tend to be seen as nearer. In painting this distribution of light and shadow is called *chiaroscuro.*

5. *Motion (or monocular movement) parallax,* perhaps the most important of these cues, is not a pictorial cue and therefore does not come to us from the study of painting. As we move our heads or bodies from side to side, the images projected by an object in the visual field moves across the retina. Nearby objects seem to move quickly and in the direction opposite to our own movement, whereas distant objects move more slowly.

Stereoscopic Cues Create Near-Field Depth Perception

Although monocular cues are important for depth perception at a distance, the perception of depth for near objects less than 100 feet away is also mediated by *stereoscopic vision.* This involves comparing the retinal images in the two eyes. When we fixate on a point, the image of this point falls upon the center of the retina in each eye. The convergence of the two eyes causes that point to fall on corresponding points on each central retina. The point of focus is called the *fixation point;* the parallel (vertical) plane of points on which it lies is called the *fixation plane.* The distance of an image from the center of the two eyes allows the visual system to calculate the distance of the object relative to the fixation point (Figure 30–16). Any point on the object that is nearer or farther than the fixation point will project an image at some distance from the center of the retina. Parts of the object that are closer to us will be farther apart on the retina in a horizontal direction. Parts of the object that are farther from us will project closer together on the retina.

Because the two eyes are about 6 cm apart, each eye views the world from a slightly different position. Thus, three-dimensional objects produce slightly different images on the two retinas. This can be clearly demonstrated by closing each eye in turn. As vision is switched from one to the other eye, any near object will appear to skip sideways. We adapt to this disparity by *sensory fusion,* by fixating both eyes on one point. By positioning the eyes so that the left and right images of the object fall on corresponding positions on the two retinas, we see one object. Fusion is not perfect, however, when we fix our gaze on a three-dimensional object. The two retinal images of the object do not fall on exactly corresponding positions. The difference in position, called *binocular disparity,* depends on the distance of the object from the fixation plane. Thus, points on the three-dimensional object just outside the fixation plane stimulate different points on each eye, and the multiple disparities provide cues for stereopsis, the perception of solid objects.

Surprisingly, not one of the great early students of optics—Euclid, Archimedes, Leonardo da Vinci, Newton, or Goethe—took notice of stereopsis, although each could readily have discovered it with the methods available to them. Stereoscopic vision was not discovered until 1838,

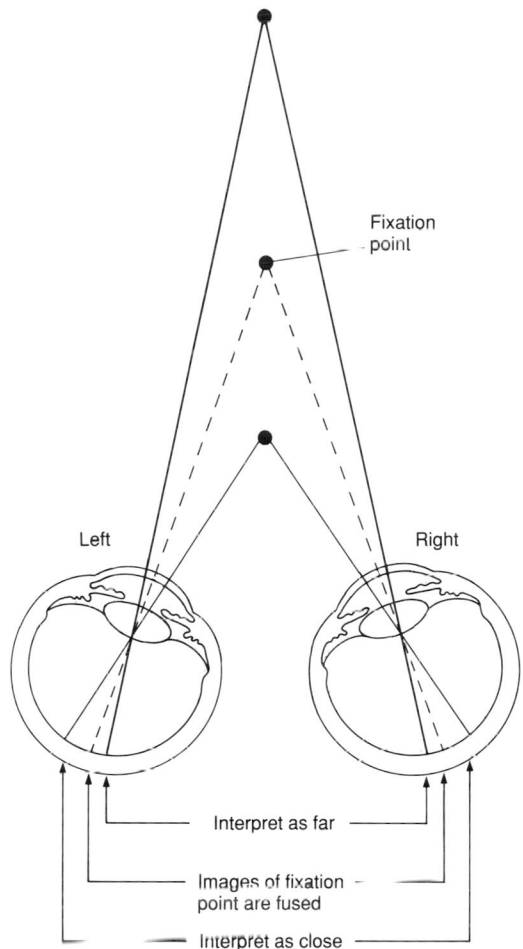

FIGURE 30–16
When we fix our eyes on a point on an object less than 100 feet away, the convergence of our eyes causes that point (the *fixation point*) to fall on identical portions of each retina. Cues for depth are provided by points just proximal or distal to the fixation point. These points produce *binocular disparity* by stimulating slightly different parts of the retina of each eye. When the lack of correspondence is in the horizontal direction only and is not greater than 0.6 mm or 2° of arc, the disparity is perceived as a single solid (3-D) spot. This phenomenon produces *stereopsis,* the perception of solidity or depth.

when the physicist Charles Wheatstone invented the *stereoscope.* Two photographs of a scene 60–65 mm apart, one from the position of each eye, are mounted into a binocular-like device such that the right eye sees only the picture taken from one position and the left eye sees only the other picture. Remarkably, this presentation produces a three-dimensional image.

How is stereopsis accomplished? Clearly the brain must somehow calculate the disparity between the images seen by the two eyes and then estimate distance based on simple geometric relations. But must the object first be recognized before the brain can match the corresponding points of the object in the two eyes? Until 1960 it was generally thought that this was so, and stereopsis

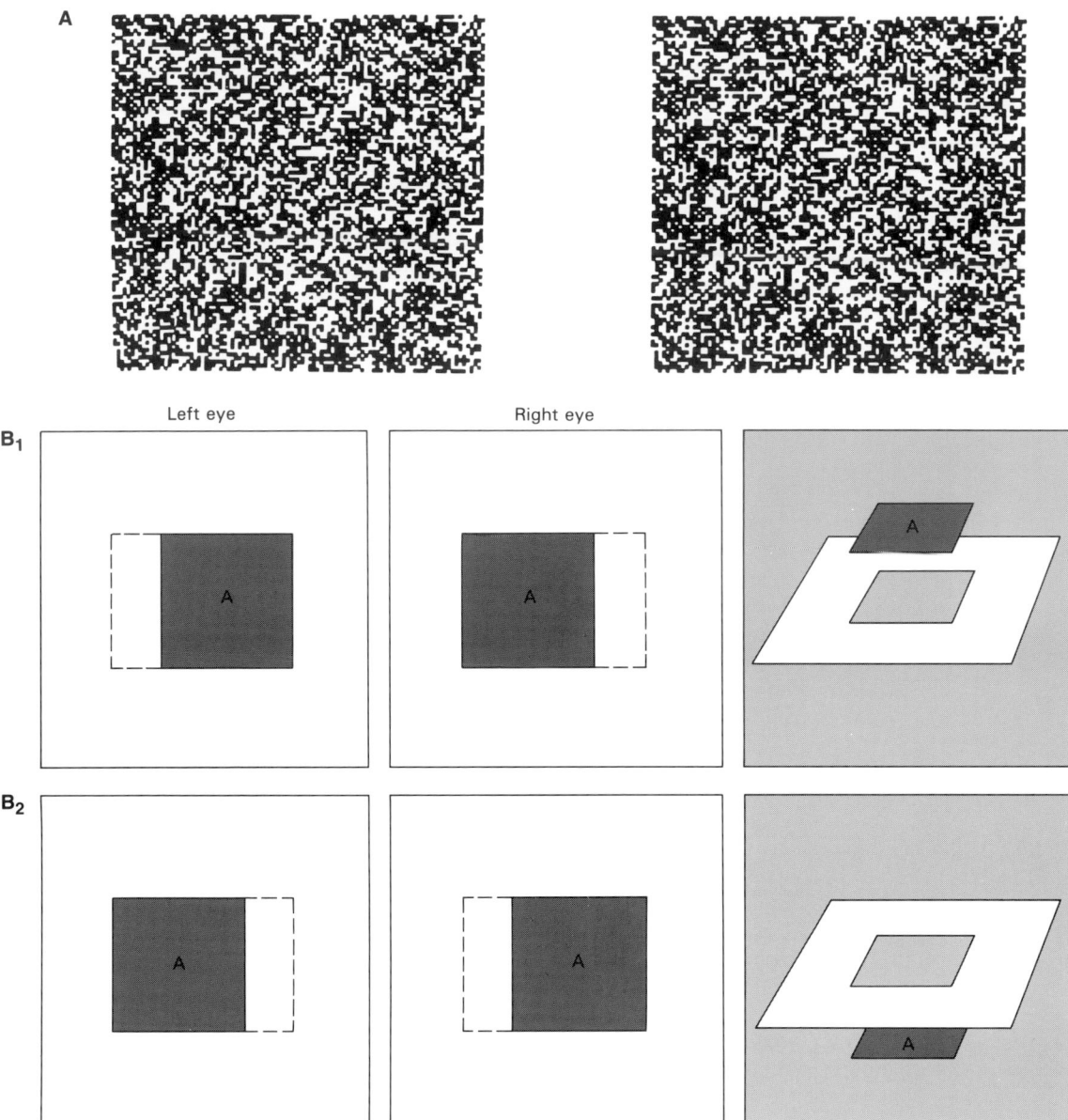

FIGURE 30–17

Stereopsis does not depend on form but can be produced by a random dot display.

A. These identical copies of a random array of dots have a central square that is not visible by looking at the image. Only when the two identical images are viewed in a stereoscope can the square be seen. This perception occurs only because of the ocular disparity of the two dot patterns, not because either eye recognizes the form of the square.

B. In the stereoscope each image is viewed through a rectangular frame in which the image can be shifted left or right. The central square is represented by the dark gray space labeled **A**. If the images are shifted so the left and right squares are closer together (**1**), the square is perceived in front of the dot array. If the images are shifted so that the two squares are further apart (**2**), the square appears to lie behind the dot image. (Adapted from Julesz, 1964.)

therefore was thought to be a late stage in visual processing.

In 1960 Bela Julesz proved that this view was wrong when he found that stereoscopic fusion and depth perception do not require monocular identification of form. The *only* clue necessary for stereopsis is retinal disparity. To demonstrate this remarkable fact, Julesz created a pattern composed entirely of random dots, in the middle of which are some dots arranged in a square. The square form is visible only when two identical copies of the pattern are viewed in a stereoscope. When the square in one of the copies is displaced slightly to one side, it appears in binocular view to lie in front of the rest of the pattern, and to be floating free of its background. If the displacement is in the opposite direction, the square appears to lie behind the rest of the pattern (Figure 30–17). By itself, each random dot pattern will not produce any clues. Only with stereoscopic vision can one see the square within the pattern.

With this method, Julesz demonstrated that humans can detect form and movement in depth from stereograms consisting only of randomly placed elements. Since all the dots are identical, it is remarkable that the visual system can discover which are the corresponding dots in the two pictures. Initially it was thought that this *correspondence problem* is solved by the cooperation of many sensors, each corresponding to a single point in the stereogram. It now seems more likely that the dots contain arrays of micropatterns or clusters so that the problem of correspondence is solved by matching a few of these with the input from the two eyes.

Julesz's experiments also showed that stereopsis does not have its origin in the retina or in the lateral geniculate nucleus, but occurs at the level of the striate cortex, or at an even higher level where the signals for the two eyes are combined. As a result, Julesz has called this kind of perception *cyclopean perception*, after the mythical Cyclops, who had only one eye in the middle of his forehead. Neither eye alone can make sense of the shapes or contours of the figures: Each receives only a meaningless assembly of random dots. Where then does fusion occur?

Information from the Two Eyes Is First Combined in the Primary Visual Cortex

Hubel and Wiesel first demonstrated that the initial opportunity for fusion occurs in V1. It is here that single cells in the visual system first receive input from the two eyes (Chapter 29). Stereopsis, however, requires that the inputs from the two eyes be slightly *different*—there must be a horizontal disparity in the two retinal images. The important finding that certain neurons in V1 are actually

FIGURE 30–18
Responses of cells to binocular disparity.

A. Responses of a cell that cannot distinguish disparity of retinal images. Both eyes were stimulated together by a vertical slit of light moving leftward. Three conditions were tested, illustrated in the panels on the left and representing different degrees of a disparity. In case **1** the slit is closer to the subject, in case **2** it is nearly in the plane of focus, and in case **3** it is farther from the subject. The cell is not tuned to disparity and responds to all three conditions with a similar brief burst of spikes. A graph (on the right) of the cell's responses to a range of disparity is nearly linear.

B. The responses of another cell to the same tests show this cell is tuned to fire only at zero disparity, when the slit of light is roughly in the plane of fixation. A graph of the cell's responses to a range of disparity shows the cell's selectivity for zero disparity. (Adapted from Hubel, 1988.)

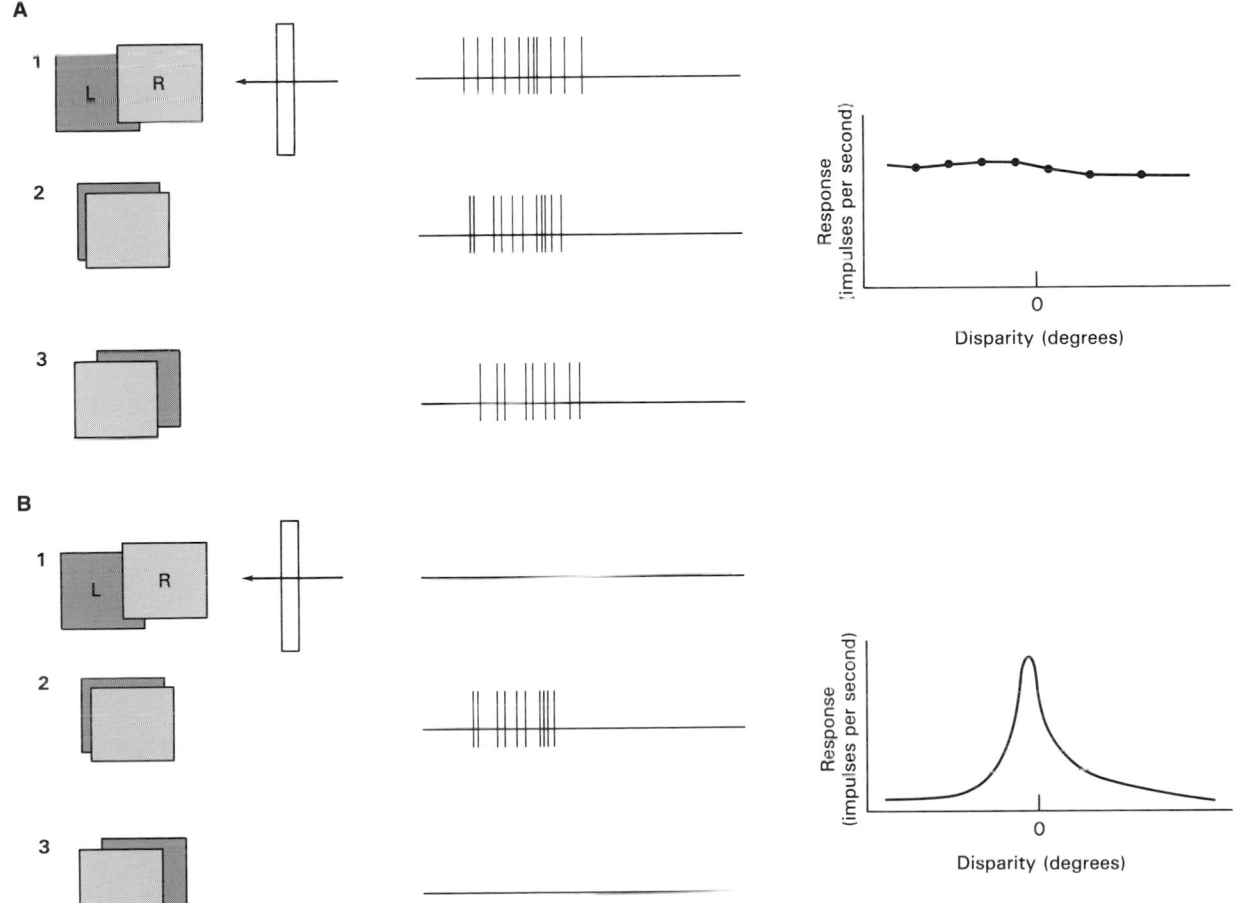

FIGURE 30–19

The response of a cell in area 17 to binocular disparity is the same whether the image is a solid figure or a random dot pattern. The monkey was trained to maintain a steady gaze while solid bars of selected size and orientation moved across the neuron's receptive field. The experiment illustrated the cell's similar response to on–off presentation of both solid figure and random dot patterns at a series of horizontal disparities centering around −20° to −15°. (Adapted from Poggio, 1986.)

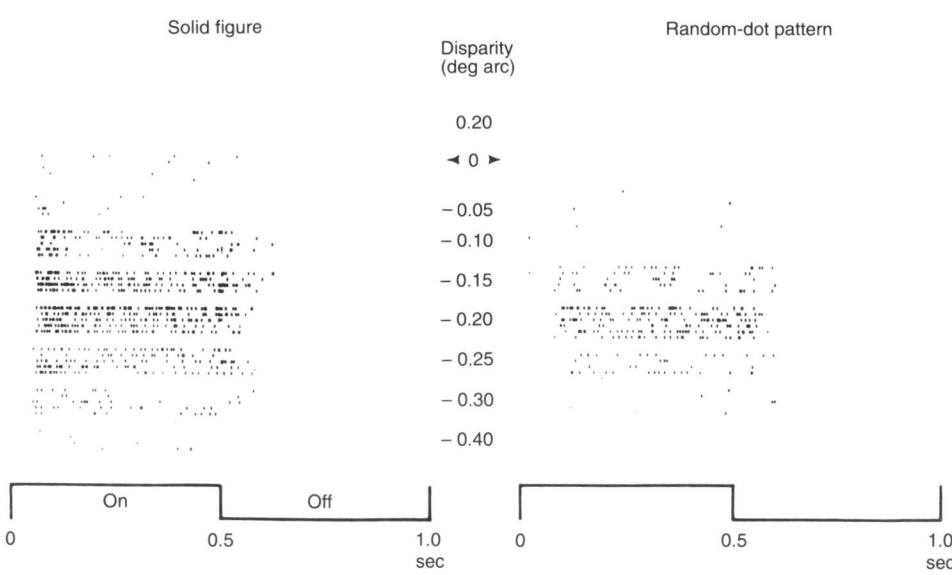

selective for horizontal disparity between the input from the two eyes was made in 1968 by Horace Barlow, Colin Blakemore, Peter Bishop, and Jack Pettigrew (Figure 30–18). Disparity-selective neurons have now been detected all along the magnocellular pathway: in V1, in the thick stripes of V2, and in MT.

Are these disparity-sensitive neurons important for stereopsis? This question has been addressed by Gian Poggio, who found that about 70% of both simple and complex cells in V1, V2, and V3 of alert monkeys respond to binocular disparity. Certain neurons are sensitive to stimuli nearer than the fixation plane, whereas others are sensitive to stimuli that are further away. As shown in Figure 30–16, stimuli nearer than the fixation plane are interpreted as close, and those further from the fixation plane are interpreted as far.

The existence of neurons sensitive to disparity raises the question: Do these neurons also respond to a stereogram that contains no depth clues except retinal disparity? To answer this, Poggio first located responsive cells using a solid (three-dimensional) bar as a stimulus. He then replaced the solid bar with a stereogram of a random-dot pattern. Many of the complex neurons that responded to the solid figure also responded to the random-dot stereogram (Figure 30–19). These analyses suggest that when a cell responds to a random-dot pattern it does so because the clusters of elements form a micropattern to which the cell responds effectively. When two such patterns are presented at the optimal disparity for the cell, the cell responds optimally. Thus the cell responds to the line pattern presented to each eye and the input to the two eyes yield summation.

Recognition of Faces and Other Complex Forms Occurs in the Inferior Temporal Cortex

We are capable of recognizing an almost infinite variety of shapes independent of their size or position on the retina.

Clinical work in humans and experimental studies in monkeys suggest that shape recognition is represented in the parvocellular–interblob system, extending from V1 to V2 and V4. From there, shape recognition is conveyed to the inferior temporal cortex. Perhaps the most dramatic evidence for this pathway comes from studies of the clinical syndrome called *prosopagnosia*, the impaired recognition of familiar faces. Patients with prosopagnosia can identify the parts of the face and even specific emotions expressed on the face. But they are unable to identify a *person* from the sight of their face. Patients with prosopagnosia often cannot recognize people whom they know well, such as members of the family, and may not even recognize their *own* faces in the mirror. However, it is not the identity of people that has been lost, but the *connection* between a particular face and a particular identity. To recognize even a close friend, patients must rely on the friend's voice or other nonvisual clues. In the purest form of prosopagnosia, which is very rare, only the recognition of faces is impaired; object recognition is not affected.

Lesions that cause prosopagnosia are always bilateral and are located on the inferior surface of both occipital lobes and extend forward to the inner surface of the temporal lobes. Norman Geschwind suggested that this region must be a critical part of the neural network specialized for the rapid and reliable recognition of faces. Studies of monkeys support this localization and show the inferior temporal cortex is necessary for normal visual learning and perception. Removal of the inferior temporal cortex impairs visual recognition of shapes and patterns without in any way disturbing other basic functions of visual perception, such as acuity or recognition of color and movement.

The inferior temporal cortex receives its input from V4, a retinotopically organized area that includes neurons sensitive to form and color. V4 receives information from V2 as well as from V3 and MT. Charles Gross, Edmund Rolls, and their collaborators have found that the response prop-

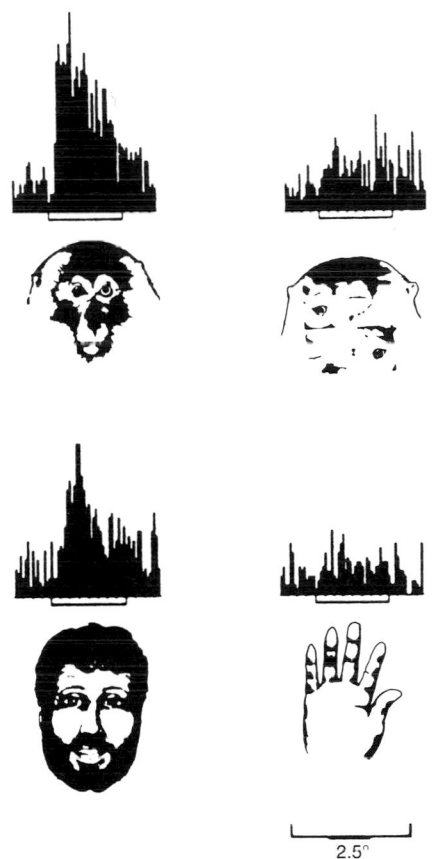

FIGURE 30–20
Response of a cell in the brain of a monkey to the face of a monkey and a man, as well as to degraded or different images. This cell in the inferior temporal cortex responds preferentially to faces. (From Gross et al., 1981.)

erties of cells in the inferotemporal cortex are those we might expect from an area involved in a later stage of pattern recognition.

For example, the receptive field of virtually every cell includes the foveal region, where fine discriminations are made. Unlike the striate cortex and most extrastriate visual areas, the cells in the inferotemporal area do not have a retinotopic organization. Also, unlike cells in the striate and extrastriate cortex, the receptive fields for most cells in the inferotemporal cortex are very large, on average 25° × 25°, and occasionally may include the entire visual field (both visual hemifields).

Most interesting is the finding that about 10% of these cells are selective for specific complex stimuli, such as the hand or face (Figure 30–20). For cells that respond to a hand, the individual fingers are a particularly critical visual feature; these cells do not respond when the spaces between the fingers are filled in. However, all orientations of the hand elicit similar responses. Among neurons selective for faces, the frontal view of the face is the most effective stimulus for some; for others it is the side view. Cells that respond to profiles or frontal views appear to

cluster separately, suggesting that they may be arranged systematically, perhaps in a columnar organization like orientation or motion-selective neurons. Moreover, whereas some neurons respond preferentially to faces, others respond preferentially to facial expressions. These groups, too, form separate clusters. Although the proportion of cells in the inferior temporal cortex responsive to hands or faces is small, their existence, together with the fact that lesions of this region lead to specific deficits in face recognition, indicate that the inferior temporal cortex is responsible for face recognition.

Visual Attention Focuses Perception by Facilitating Coordination Between Separate Visual Pathways

How is information about color, motion, depth, and form, which is carried by separate neuronal pathways, organized into cohesive perceptions? When we see a square purple box, we combine into one perception the sensations of color (purple), form (square), and solidity (box). We can equally well combine purple with a round box, a hat, or a coat. Clearly, the possible combinations are so great that the existence of distinct feature-detecting cells each responsive to only one set of combinations is improbable.

Instead, as we saw at the beginning of this chapter, complex visual images are typically built up at successively higher processing centers from the inputs of parallel pathways that process different features—movement, solidity, form, and color. To express the specific combination of properties in the visual field at any given moment, therefore, independent groups of cells, each of which processes a distinctive property, must be brought together in temporary association. There must be a mechanism whereby, for each percept, the brain associates the processing carried out independently in different cortical regions. This mechanism, as yet unspecified, is called *the binding problem.*

How does the nervous system achieve these associations? How does it solve the binding problem? In psychophysical studies Ann Treisman and her colleagues and Julesz have independently shown that formation of these associations requires *attention.* They began by trying to understand one of the problems addressed by the early Gestalt psychologists: How is attention focused on *one* object in the visual field? What features of the object make that object stand out from the background? Treisman and Julesz found that distinctive boundaries are created from *elementary properties*: brightness, color, and orientation of line. Consider, for example, Figure 30–21. Here a rectangle composed of small +'s within a field of large L's creates distinctive boundaries between the two. The rectangle easily stands out against its background.

Treisman and Julesz have found that when the boundaries are made up of elements that are clearly different the boundaries *pop out* almost automatically within 50 ms. In contrast, the detection of two similar but nonetheless different forms takes longer. Thus, in Figure 30–21 the square of +'s embedded in a background of L's emerges

A

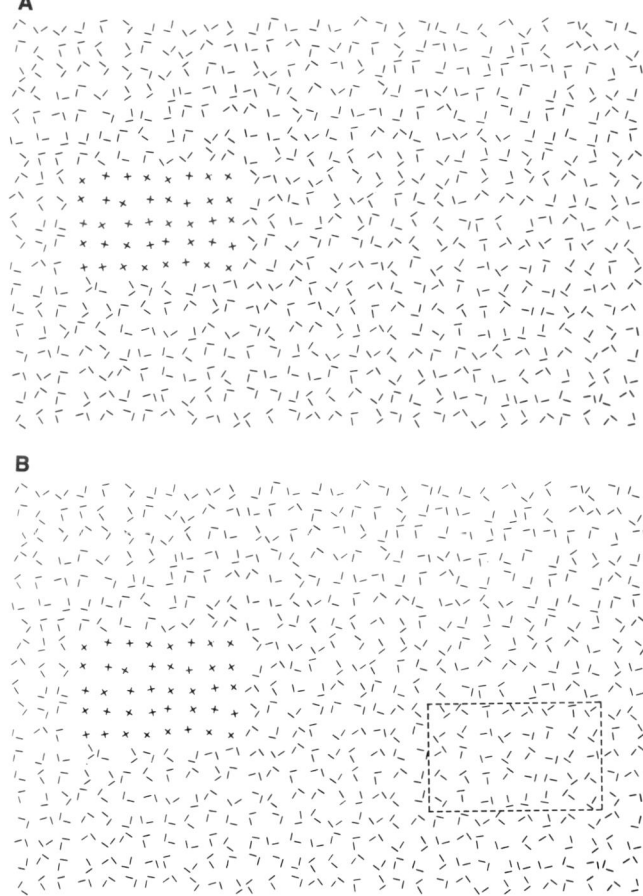

B

FIGURE 30–21

Some perceptions are produced by preattentive scanning; others require focal attention. (From Julesz and Bergen, 1983.)

A. In this figure the small rectangular area composed of +'s is effortlessly picked out from the surrounding area by simply looking at the figure. The figure also includes a rectangle composed of T's in contrast to the background. Can you find it? To do so, you must focus on each region of the figure.

B. The rectangular area of T's in A is outlined here.

effortlessly, whereas a second square of equal size but composed of T's can be found only after carefully scanning the figure because the T's are only subtly different from the background of L's.

Based on these observations, Treisman and Julesz suggest that there are two distinct processes in visual perception. An initial, *pre-attentive process* acts as a rapid scanning system and only is concerned with the detection of objects. This process rapidly scans the object's overall texture or features and encodes the useful elementary properties of the scene: color, orientation, size, or direction of movement. At this point, variation in a simple property may be discerned as a border or contour, but complex differences in combinations of properties are not detected. Treisman proposed that different properties are encoded in different *feature maps* in different brain regions. The later *attentive process* directs attention to spe-

cific features of an object, selecting and highlighting features that are initially segregated in the separate feature maps (Figure 30–22). This attentive process first described by the Gestaltists uses a *winner-take-all* strategy (perhaps similar to that achieved by feed-forward inhibition discussed in Chapter 26), whereby the salient features of the object are emphasized and attended to while other features and other objects are ignored.

The interaction of these two processes is illustrated in the perception of faces. Consider, for example, the two pictures in Figure 30–23. As we scan the two pictures initially (pre-attentive processing), we see that each picture shows the same face. However, when we turn the pictures rightside up and look at the individual features, we recognize, to our surprise, that one face is distorted. This recognition requires attention. Stated in neural terms, Treisman and Julesz argue that cells in different feature maps (maps for form, color, and movement) must be scanned, and associated with our memory of Leonardo da Vinci's painting of the Mona Lisa. To solve this binding problem, Treisman postulated that there may be a *master* or *saliency map* that codes only for key aspects of the image. This master map receives input from all feature maps but abstracts only those features in each map that distinguish the object of attention from its surround. Once these salient features have been selected, the information associated with this location in the master map is retrieved by referring back to the individual feature maps. In this way the master map selects the details in the feature map that are essential for attentive recognition. Recognition occurs when these salient locations in different feature maps are associated or bound together.

How does this binding occur? How is attention achieved in the visual system? Treisman speaks metaphorically of the *spotlight of attention*. Where is the switch for this spotlight located? What turns it on?

As may be appreciated from the evidence presented in this chapter, the neuronal mechanisms of attention and conscious awareness are now emerging as one of the great unresolved problems in perception and indeed in all of neurobiology. Based on the work of Wurtz, Patricia Goldman-Rakic, and others, Francis Crick and Christoff Koch suggest that visual attention may be mediated by one or more subcortical structures such as the pulvinar, claustrum, and superior colliculus, as well as perhaps by the prefrontal cortex. They argue that these structures may represent Treisman's saliency map and that bursts of action potentials in these structures may modulate the activity of the appropriate cells in the different feature maps.

In fact, three types of cellular studies of visual attention have illustrated that selective attention involves either enhanced firing of cells that respond to the object of interest or attenuated firing of cells that respond to objects that are being ignored. In the 1970s Wurtz, Michael Goldberg, and David Lee Robinson first explored the cellular basis of visual attention in the superior colliculus, in the striate cortex (V1), and in the posterior parietal cortex of awake primates. They examined the response of cells to a

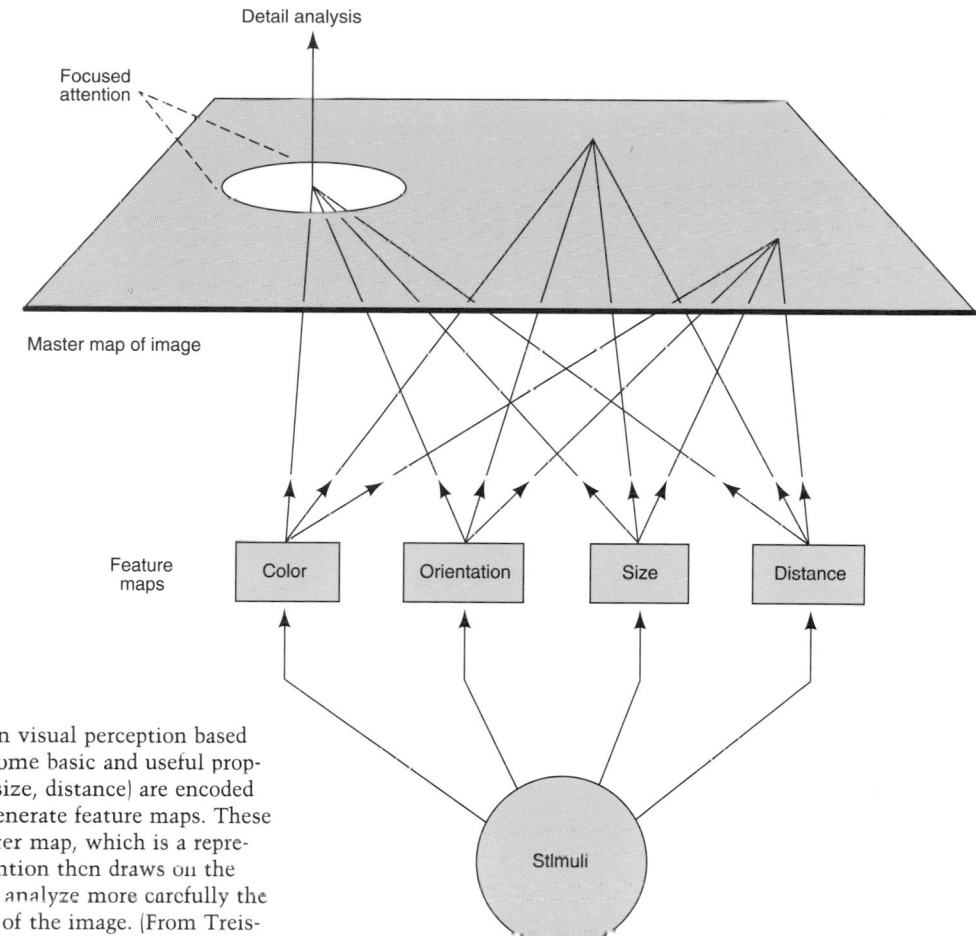

FIGURE 30–22

A hypothetical model of the stages in visual perception based on experiments by Ann Treisman. Some basic and useful properties of a scene (color, orientation, size, distance) are encoded in separate, parallel pathways that generate feature maps. These maps are then integrated into a master map, which is a representation of the image. Focused attention then draws on the information from the master map to analyze more carefully the features associated in a small region of the image. (From Treisman, 1988.)

spot of light under two conditions: when the animal looked elsewhere and did not attend to the spot, and when the animal was forced to fix its gaze on the spot by making saccadic eye movements to the spot of light. They found that the cells in the superior colliculus and in V1 responded more intensely when the animal attended to the spot than when it ignored it. However, the enhancement did not result from selective attention *per se*, but from changes in the general level of arousal and from the neural mechanisms involved in the initiation of eye movement. The enhancement did not occur when focused attention did not require eye movement. In contrast, in the posterior parietal cortex, a region known from clinical studies to be involved in attention to visual form, the enhancement is independent of eye movement or any other behavior of the animal in relation to the stimulus (Figure 30–24).

Based on these studies, Wurtz and his colleagues have proposed that when a subject attends visually to an object, cells in the posterior parietal cortex that respond to the object begin to discharge powerfully. As the subject moves its eyes toward the object to examine it further, cells in

FIGURE 30–23

These pictures appear similar at first glance because only our preattentive process is active. When the pictures are seen upright, the true detail in the two faces is revealed. (From Julesz, 1986, after an idea of Thompson, 1980.)

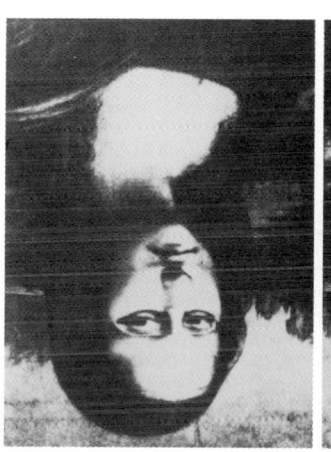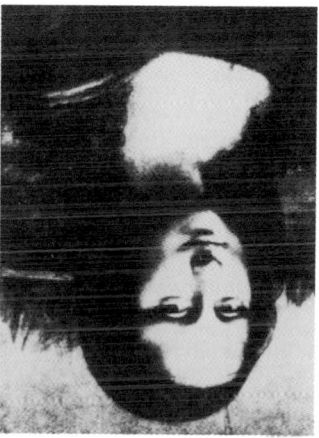

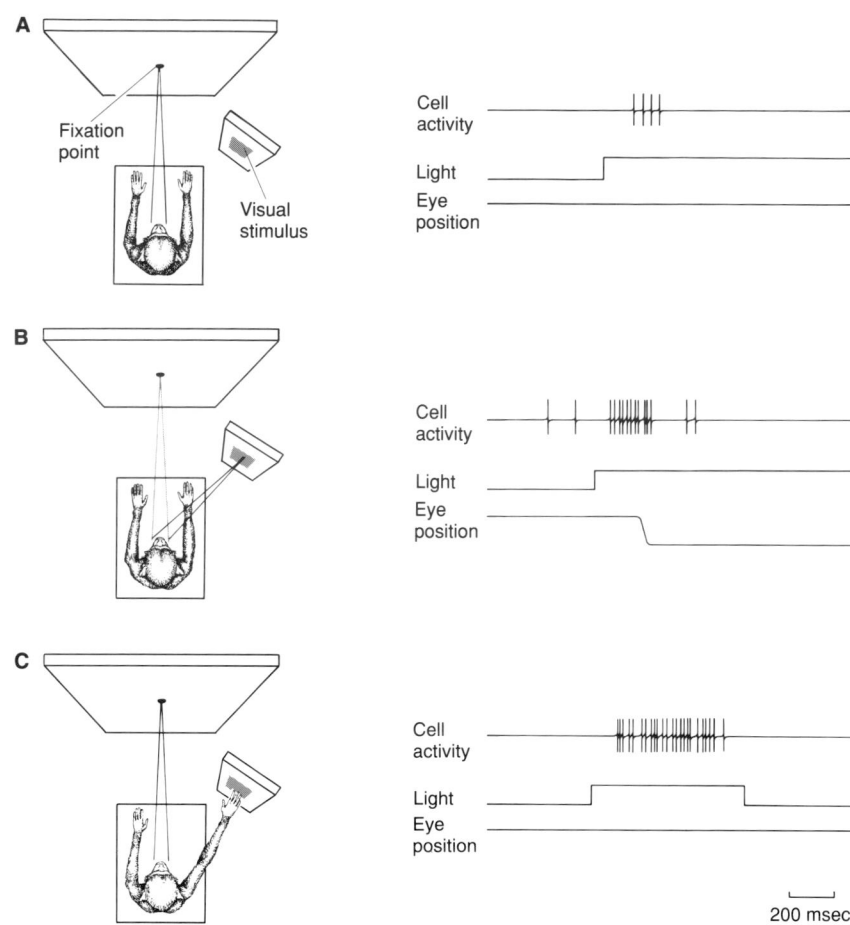

FIGURE 30–24

Neurons in the posterior parietal cortex of a monkey respond more effectively to stimuli that require attention. (From Wurtz and Goldberg, 1989.)

A. A spot of light elicits only a few action potentials in a cell.

B. The same cell's activity is enhanced when the spot is the target for a saccade.

C. The cell's activity is also enhanced when the monkey is required to touch the spot, but without moving his eyes. Neurons in the posterior parietal cortex differ from those in the superior colliculus (and also the striate cortex and the frontal eye field) in that their activity is enhanced by any mode of attention to the spot of light.

the superior colliculus and V1 also discharge more briskly. Thus, attention recruits the selective enhancement of the activity of cells in several visual regions of the cortex that respond to the object of interest.

This approach was extended to the inferior temporal cortex by Robert Desimone and his colleagues, who trained monkeys to attend selectively to a visual stimulus in one position of a neuron's receptive field while ignoring stimuli at another position. They found that while the activity of cells responding to the attended stimuli increased, the activity in cells responding to the unattended stimulus actually decreased.

A third insight into attention has come from Charles Gray and Wolfgang Singer, and Reinhold Eckhorn and his colleagues. They found that when a population of neurons in the visual cortex is activated by an object, the neurons activated tend to oscillate and fire in unison, at about 40 action potentials per second. In the most interesting case, two neurons 7 mm apart had receptive fields with similar axes of orientation. Each cell could be activated by a small bar of the correct orientation. When activated by small nonoverlapping bars, the two cells fire independently. When the bar was extended to cover both receptive fields, the neurons fire synchronously. Gray and Singer suggest that this synchrony might drive higher-order neurons more

effectively and thereby indicates to these higher-order cells that an object is being attended to (Figure 30–25). These findings raise the intriguing question whether synchrony also occurs among the extrastriate regions that analyze the color, motion, and forms of an object. Is synchrony a mechanism for binding, for integrating information from parallel pathways?

The Analysis of Visual Attention May Provide Important Clues Toward Understanding Conscious Awareness

The problem posed by selective attention was first defined in 1890 by William James in his *Principles of Psychology*:

Millions of items . . . are present to my senses which never properly enter my experience. Why? Because they have no *interest* for me. *My experience is what I agree to attend to.* . . . Everyone knows what attention is. It is the taking possession by the mind, in clear and vivid form, of one out of what seem several simultaneously possible objects of trains of thought. Focalization, concentration of consciousness are of its essence. It implies withdrawal from some things in order to deal effectively with others.

Thus, much of the sensory information received by the peripheral receptors in our body must eventually be fil-

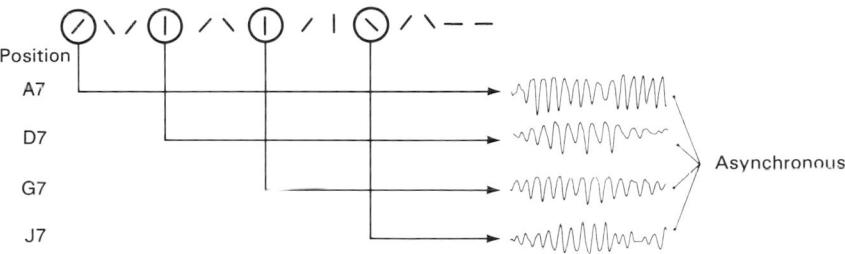

A₁ Figure–ground segregation

Ground

←Figure

Ground

A₂ Neuronal responses to contours in line 7

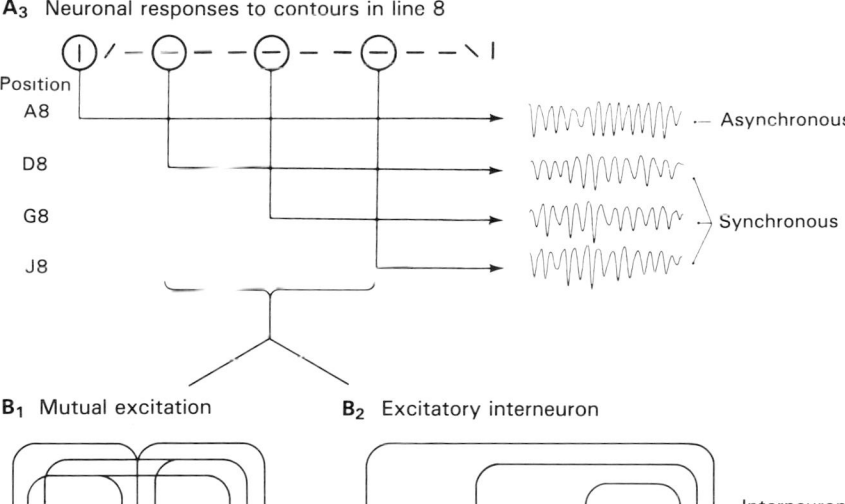

Position

A7

D7

G7

J7

Asynchronous

A₃ Neuronal responses to contours in line 8

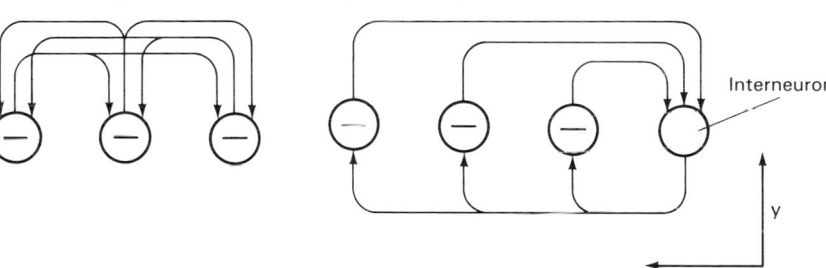

Position

A8

D8

G8

J8

Asynchronous

Synchronous

B₁ Mutual excitation   **B₂** Excitatory interneuron

Interneuron

y

x

FIGURE 30–25

Singer's speculative model of a neuronal assembly that segregates figure from ground by means of synchronous oscillations of the evoked response produced in small subpopulations of neurons whose receptive fields are activated in synchrony by the various components of the figure. (Adapted from Singer, 1990.)

A. 1. A *figure* is distinguished from the *background* by the contrast of the line segments within the image (the horizontal dashed line in **row 8**, running from **8C to 8L**), compared to all the other line segments in the total display (running as columns from **A to N** and as rows from **1 to 10**). The total display is assumed to indicate a complete set of cells representing all orientations. Each of the activated populations has a receptive field stimulated by part of the display. **2.** The neuronal responses encoded by the background. For any part of the background, such as **line 7**, the oscillatory responses evoked by each subpopulation do not have phase relationship to each other. For

example, the illustrated responses of neurons that contribute to the subpopulations at **A7, D7, G7,** and **J7** are out of synchrony and unrelated. **3.** Neuronal responses encoding the figure (**line 8**). In contrast to the background, the oscillatory responses of subpopulations of neurons encoding the figure (for example, **D8, G8** and **J8**) are synchronous. Thus, the figure running from **C8 to L8** is characterized by the coherent oscillatory responses of the subpopulations of cells whose receptive fields are activated by the figure. In contrast, all the subpopulations of cells activated by the background (**A to N; 1 to 10**) are out of phase in relation to one another and to the figure.

B. Two ways of coupling feature detectors that have similar preferences, so as to achieve a coherent oscillatory response. **1.** The corresponding sets of cells (feature detectors) are coupled by means of reciprocal excitatory connections. **2.** Feature detector cells with similar response properties drive common interneurons that feed back onto the corresponding feature detectors.

tered out and eliminated within the brain, much as we disregard the ground when we focus on the figure. Although the visual system contains extensive parallel pathways for processing different visual information, our ability to process different, simultaneous information is surprisingly limited by the mechanism of selective attention. As we saw in considering the figure–ground dichotomy, selective attention both filters out some features and sharpens our perception of others. In this winner-take-all strategy some stimuli stand out in consciousness while others recede into dim awareness.

It is attractive to think that exploration of visual attention will lead us to define the neural mechanisms of a specific instance of consciousness. Despite its central importance for a neurobiological understanding of mental processes, the problem of consciousness has so far eluded reductionist, cell biological approaches. But as this and later chapters illustrate, biological insights into any component of consciousness arc likely to give us at least a glimmer of understanding of some of the most complex components: of volition, intention, and self-awareness. If consciousness in its various forms is the product of a generalized set of neural mechanisms, then the study of visual attention could put us on the path to an understanding of self-awareness!

An Overall View

David Marr began his important book on the computational tasks of vision with the question: "What does it mean, to see?" Marr's answer was that vision is the process of discovering from images *what* is present in the visual world, and *where* it is.

Mortimer Mishkin and his colleagues first pointed out that these two tasks, identifying *what* and *where*, are carried by distinct anatomical pathways. The parvocellular–interblob system conveys information about form while the parvocellular–blob system reports color. These two pathways terminate in the inferior temporal cortex, the area identified by Mishkin as being important for the recognition of form. Location of the object in space is the task, in large part, of the magnocellular system. This pathway terminates in the posterior parietal cortex, the cortex identified by Mishkin as important for spatial organization.

The cells in each of these visual pathways show different selectivities. In view of the research on motion selectivity, it is attractive to think that the selectivities of particular classes of neurons are related to specific aspects of visual perception. Thus, orientation-selective neurons seem to provide information for the perception of shape and form, while disparity-selective neurons seem to provide information about the solidity of objects. Both types of cells could be important for perceiving *what*. Direction-selective neurons concerned with motion may tell us *where*.

Only recently has it become clear that visual processing involves parallel pathways rather than one serial pathway. But this important discovery has posed a new problem for the study of visual perception. Integration in a serial pathway is achieved *progressively*, in the transformation of information carried from one area to the next. In a system of parallel pathways, each with its own function, integration can be achieved only *interactively*.

How and where does this interaction occur in the visual system? David Van Essen and his colleagues argue that there are extensive interactions between the three pathways at almost all cortical levels. Each visual cue is handled in different ways by more than one pathway. In addition, the arguments of Treisman, Julesz, and Crick and Koch suggest we should look for inputs to visual areas from brain centers known to affect attention, such as the prefrontal cortex, the claustrum, or the pulvinar. These systems could serve to allow attention mechanisms to bind the visual process.

In this chapter we have focused on how we see. Obviously, vision is also important in guiding body movement. It is likely that much visual processing, particularly in the magnocellular pathway concerned with motion and spatial relationships, is essential for the control of our own movement. Simply moving about in the world requires complex analyses of visual stimuli, including the separation of figures from ground and the estimation of distance. We shall return to the visual guidance of movement later when considering the motor system.

Selected Readings

Bishop, P. O., and Pettigrew, J. D. 1986. Neural mechanisms of binocular vision. Vision Res. 26:1587–1600.

Crick, F., and Koch, C. 1990. Towards a neurobiological theory of consciousness. Sem. Neurosci. 2:263–275.

Gregory, R. L. 1978. Eye and Brain: The Psychology of Seeing, 2nd ed. New York: McGraw-Hill.

Hochberg, J. E. 1978. Perception, 2nd ed. Englewood Cliffs, N.J.: Prentice-Hall.

Hubel, D. H. 1988. Eye, Brain, and Vision. New York: Scientific American Library.

Lam, D. M.-K., and Gilbert, C. D. (eds.) 1989. Neural Mechanisms of Visual Perception. Proceedings of the Retina Research Foundation Symposia, Vol. 2. The Woodlands, Tex.: Portfolio Publishing.

Livingstone, M. S. 1988. Art, illusion and the visual system. Sci. Am. 258(1):78–85.

Marr, D. 1982. Vision: A Computational Investigation Into the Human Representation and Processing of Visual Information. San Francisco: Freeman.

Moran, J., and Desimone, R. 1985. Selective attention gates visual processing in extrastriate cortex. Science 229:782–784.

Rock, I., and Palmer, S. 1990. The legacy of Gestalt psychology. Sci. Am. 263(6):84–90.

Salzman, C. D., Britten, K. H., and Newsome, W. T. 1990. Cortical microstimulation influences perceptual judgements of motion direction. Nature 346:174–177.

Singer, W. 1990. Search for coherence: A basic principle of cortical self-organization. Concepts Neurosci. 1:1–26.

Stryker, M. P. 1989. Is grandmother an oscillation? Nature 338:297–298.

Teuber, M. L. 1974. Sources of ambiguity in the prints of Maurits C. Escher. Sci. Am. 231(1):90–104.

Treisman, A. 1986. Features and objects in visual processing. Sci. Am. 255(5):114B–125.

Wurtz, R. H., Goldberg, M. E., and Robinson, D. L. 1982. Brain mechanisms of visual attention. Sci. Am. 246(6):124–135.

Zeki, S. 1990. Colour vision and functional specialisation in the visual cortex. Discuss. Neurosci. 6(2):1–64.

Zeki, S., and Shipp, S. 1988. The functional logic of cortical connections. Nature 335:311–317.

References

Albright, T. D., Desimone, R., and Gross, C. G. 1984. Columnar organization of directionally selective cells in visual area MT of the macaque. J. Neurophysiol. 51:16–31.

Allman, J. M., and Kaas, J. H. 1971. Representation of the visual field in striate and adjoining cortex of the owl monkey (Aotus trivirgatus). Brain Res. 35:89–106.

Barlow, H. B., Blakemore, C., and Pettigrew, J. D. 1967. The neural mechanism of binocular depth discrimination. J. Physiol. (Lond.) 193:327–342.

Boycott, B. B., and Wässle, H. 1974. The morphological types of ganglion cells of the domestic cat's retina. J. Physiol. (Lond.) 240:397–419.

Brown, R., and Herrnstein, R. J. 1975. Psychology. Boston: Little, Brown.

Crick, F. 1984. Function of the thalamic reticular complex: The searchlight hypothesis. Proc. Natl. Acad. Sci. U.S.A. 81:4586–4590.

Desimone, R., Wessinger, M., Thomas, L., and Schneider, W. 1990. Attentional control of visual perception: Cortical and subcortical mechanisms. Cold Spring Harbor Symp. Quant. Biol. 55:963–971.

DeYoe, E. A., and Van Essen, D. C. 1988. Concurrent processing streams in monkey visual cortex. Trends Neurosci. 11:219–226.

Eckhorn, R., Bauer, R., Jordan, W., Brosch, M., Kruse, W., Munk, M., and Reitboeck, H. J. 1988. Coherent oscillations: A mechanism of feature linking in the visual cortex? Biol. Cybern. 60:121–130.

Escher, M. C. 1971. The Graphic Work of M. C. Escher. New Rev. and exp. ed. New York: Ballantine Books.

Geschwind, N. 1979. Specializations of the human brain. Sci. Am. 241(3):180–199.

Gleitman, H. 1986. Psychology: The Psychology of Seeing. 3rd ed. New York: Norton.

Goldman-Rakic, P. S. 1988. Topography of cognition: Parallel distributed networks in primate association cortex. Annu. Rev. Neurosci. 11:137–156.

Gray, C. M., and Singer, W. 1989. Stimulus-specific neuronal oscillations in orientation columns of cat visual cortex. Proc. Natl. Acad. Sci. U.S.A. 86:1698–1702.

Gray, C. M., König, P., Engel, A. K., and Singer, W. 1989. Oscillatory responses in cat visual cortex exhibit inter-columnar synchronization which reflects global stimulus properties. Nature 338:334–337.

Hasselmo, M. E., Rolls, E. T., and Baylis, G. C. 1989. The role of expression and identity in the face-selective responses of neurons in the temporal visual cortex of the monkey. Behav. Brain Res. 32:203–218.

Horton, J. C. 1984. Cytochrome oxidase patches: A new cytoarchitectonic feature of monkey visual cortex. Phil. Trans. R. Soc. London B 304:199–253.

Hurvich, L. M. 1981. Color Vision. Sunderland, Mass.: Sinauer.

James, W. 1890. The Principles of Psychology, The Works of William James, Vol. 1. Cambridge, Mass.: Harvard University Press, 1981.

Julesz, B. 1986. Stereoscopic vision. Vision Res. 26:1601–1612.

Julesz, B. 1984. Toward an axiomatic theory of preattentive vision. In G. M. Edelman, W. E. Gall, and W. M. Cowan (eds.), Dynamic Aspects of Neocortical Function. New York: Wiley, pp. 585–612.

Kaas, J. H. 1989. Changing concepts of visual cortex organization in primates. In J. W. Brown (ed.), Neuropsychology of Visual Perception. Hillsdale, N. J.: Erlbaum, pp. 3–32.

Kolb, B., and Whishaw, I. Q. 1985. Fundamentals of Human Neuropsychology, 2nd ed. New York: Freeman.

Livingstone, M. S., and Hubel, D. H. 1987. Psychophysical evidence for separate channels for the perception of form, color, movement, and depth. J. Neurosci. 7:3416–3468.

Lu, C., and Fender, D. H. 1972. The interaction of color and luminance in stereoscopic vision. Invest. Ophthalmol. 11:482–490.

Lueck, C. J., Zeki, S., Friston, K. J., Deiber, M.-P., Cope, P., Cunningham, V. J., Lammertsma, A. A., Kennard, C., and Frackowiak, R. S. J. 1989. The colour centre in the cerebral cortex of man. Nature 340:386–389.

Marshall, W. H., and Talbot, S. A. 1942. Recent evidence for neural mechanisms in vision leading to a general theory of sensory acuity. In H. Kluver (ed.), Visual Mechanisms. Lancaster, Pa.: Cattell, pp. 117–164.

Martin, K. A. C. 1988. From enzymes to visual perception: A bridge too far? Trends Neurosci. 11:380–387.

Maunsell, J. H. R., and Newsome, W. T. 1987. Visual processing in monkey extrastriate cortex. Annu. Rev. Neurosci. 10:363–401.

Movshon, A. 1990. Visual processing of moving images. In H. Barlow, C. Blakemore, and M. Weston-Smith (eds.), Images and Understanding: Thoughts About Images; Ideas About Understanding. New York: Cambridge University Press, pp. 122–137.

Movshon, J. A., Adelson, E. H., Gizzi, M. S., and Newsome, W. T. 1985. The analysis of moving visual patterns. In C. Chagas, R. Gattass, and C. Gross (eds.), Pattern Recognition Mechanisms. New York: Springer, pp. 117–151.

Newsome, W. T., Britten, K. H., and Movshon, J. A. 1989. Neuronal correlates of a perceptual decision. Nature 341:52–54.

Perrett, D. I., Mistlin, A. J., and Chitty, A. J. 1987. Visual neurones responsive to faces. Trends Neurosci. 10:358–364.

Perrett, D. I., Rolls, E. T., and Caan, W. 1979. Temporal lobe cells of the monkey with visual responses selective for faces. Neurosci. Lett. [Suppl. 3]:S358.

Poggio, G. F. 1984. Processing of stereoscopic information in primate visual cortex. In G. M. Edelman, W. E. Gall, and W. M. Cowan (eds.), Dynamic Aspects of Neocortical Function. New York: Wiley, pp. 613–635.

Poggio, G. F. 1990. Cortical neural mechanisms of stereopsis studied with dynamic random-dot stereograms. Cold Spring Harbor Symp. Quant. Biol. 55:749–758.

Ramachandran, V. S. 1987. Interaction between colour and motion in human vision. Nature. 328:645–647.

Ramachandran, V. S. 1988. Perceiving shape from shading. Sci. Am. 259(2):76–83.

Ramachandran, V. S., and Gregory, R. L. 1978. Does colour provide an input to human motion perception? Nature 275:55–56.

Rock, I. 1984. Perception. New York: Scientific American Books.

Schiller, P. H., True, S. D., and Conway, J. L. 1980. Deficits in eye movements following frontal eye-field and superior colliculus ablations. J. Neurophysiol. 44:1175–1189.

Talbot, S. A., and Marshall, W. H. 1941. Physiological studies on neural mechanisms of visual localization and discrimination. Am. J. Ophthalmol. 24:1255–1264.

Tootell, R. B., Hamilton, S. L., and Silverman, M. S. 1985. Topography of cytochrome oxidase activity in owl monkey cortex. J. Neurosci. 5:2786–2800.

Treisman, A. 1988. Features and objects: The Fourteenth Bartlett Memorial Lecture. J. Exp. Psychol. 40A(2):201–237.

Treisman, A., and Gormican, S. 1988. Feature analysis in early vision: Evidence from search asymmetries. Psychol. Rev. 95: 15–48.

Ullman, S. 1986. Artificial intelligence and the brain: Computational studies of the visual system. Annu. Rev. Neurosci. 9:1–26.

Ungerleider, L. G., and Mishkin, M. 1982. Two cortical visual systems. In D. J. Ingle, M. A. Goodale, and R. J. W. Mansfield (eds.), Analysis of Visual Behavior. Cambridge, Mass.: MIT Press, pp. 549–586.

Wong-Riley, M. T. T., and Carrol, E. W. 1984. Quantitative light and electron microscopic studies analysis of cytochrome oxidase-rich zones in VII prestriate cortex of the squirrel monkey. J. Comp. Neurol. 222:18–37.

Wurtz, R. H., and Goldberg, M. E. (eds.) 1989. The Neurobiology of Saccadic Eye Movements, Reviews of Oculomotor Research, Vol 3. Amsterdam: Elsevier.

Yarbus, A. L. 1967. Eye Movements and Vision. B. Haigh (trans.) New York: Plenum Press.

Zeki, S. M. 1976. The functional organization of projections from striate to prestriate visual cortex in the rhesus monkey. Cold Spring Harbor Symp. Quant. Biol. 40:591–600.

Zihl, J., Von Cramon, D., and Mai, N. 1983. Selective disturbance of movement vision after bilateral brain damage. Brain 106: 313–340.

31

Peter Gouras

Color Vision

Three Separate Cone Systems Respond Best to Different Parts of the Visible Spectrum

Color Discrimination Requires at Least Two Types of Photoreceptors with Different Spectral Sensitivities

Color Opponency, Simultaneous Color Contrast, and Color Constancy Are Key Features of Color Vision

In the Retina and Lateral Geniculate Nucleus Color Is Coded by Color Opponent Cells

In the Cortex Color Information Is Processed by Double-Opponent Cells in the Blob Zones

Double-Opponent Cells Help Explain Color Opponency, Color Contrast, and Color Constancy

Color Experience Is Based on Impressions of Hue, Saturation, and Brightness

Color Blindness Can Be Caused by Genetic Defects in Photoreceptors or by Retinal Disease

An Overall View

Perception of color greatly enriches our visual experience. But beyond this esthetic value, color vision is also important for detecting patterns and objects that would otherwise be elusive. Gradients of light energy are often small in natural scenes of everyday life. To distinguish an object against its background it is often helpful also to exploit the differences in wavelengths of the light reflected from the object and those reflected from the background. Think for a moment of a painting by a colorist such as Turner, Monet, or Renoir. In a black and white reproduction so many nuances of contrasting shapes evident in color are lost! Color perception thus serves to enhance contrast. It has evolved from simple brightness perception, which we considered in Chapters 28 and 29.

Color is a property of an object. However, the wavelength composition of the light reflected from the object is determined not only by its reflectance, but also by the wavelength composition of the light illuminating it. Since the composition of incident light varies, color vision compensates for this variation so that the object's color appears roughly the same. A lemon, for example, appears yellow whether seen in sunlight (which is whitish), under the light of a tungsten filament bulb (which is reddish), or by fluorescent (bluish) light. This property of color vision is known as *color constancy*. Color constancy is not entirely foolproof, however, as anyone can testify who has bought paint or a dress in artificial light and later was startled to see it appear as a different shade in daylight.

Color vision does not, therefore, simply record the physical parameters of the light reflected from the object's surface: Rather, it is a sophisticated abstracting process. What sort of abstraction is being performed? Clearly, the brain must somehow analyze the object in relation to its background. The importance of background is clear in experiments with a uniform field of color without pattern (a so-called *Ganzfeld*). Under these conditions the experience of color tends to disappear. In addition, different backgrounds can change the apparent color of an object illuminated by a constant light: A white object can appear pink or pale green against different backgrounds.

In this chapter we first describe how the visual system detects the wavelength composition of light using three different cone systems. We then examine how the nervous system processes this information in the retina and the visual cortex, and consider one explanation of how this processing analyzes objects in relation to their background. Finally, we shall discuss diseases that produce color blindness.

Three Separate Cone Systems Respond Best to Different Parts of the Visible Spectrum

The human eye is sensitive to wavelengths of light from 400 to 700 nm. Throughout this range the color of monochromatic light changes gradually from blue, through green, to red. People with normal color vision can readily match the color of any spectral composition of light by combining in an appropriate way three primary colors—blue, green, and red. This property of color vision called trivariancy results from three types of light-absorbing cone photoreceptors, each with a different visual pigment (see Chapter 28). These pigments have different but overlapping absorption spectra. As we shall see, the visual system extracts information on color by comparing the responses of the three classes of photoreceptors.

The idea that color vision is mediated by three classes of cone photoreceptors, each responsive to a primary color, was proposed at the beginning of the nineteenth century by Thomas Young. It was confirmed in 1964 when Edward MacNichol and his colleagues and George Wald and Paul Brown measured directly the absorption spectra

of visual pigments of single cones obtained from the retinas of humans. They found that individual cones contain only one of three pigments. One is primarily sensitive to short wavelengths in the visible spectrum, and makes a strong contribution to the perception of blue (it is called S, for *short*, or B, for *blue*). Another is selective for *middle* wavelengths and makes a strong contribution to the perception of *green* (it is called M or G). The third is responsive to *longer* wavelengths and makes a strong contribution to the perception of *red* (it is called L or R). Recent measurements show that B pigments absorb most strongly at 420 nm, G pigments at 531 nm, and R pigments at 558 nm (Figure 31–1).

Some people with genetic defects have only two cone pigments (dichromatopsia), while others have only one (monochromatopsia). It is possible to measure psychophysically the spectral sensitivity of the one cone system in individuals with monochromatopsia by ascertaining the subject's response to monochromatic light of different wavelengths. Data obtained in this way are consistent with direct measurements of the absorption spectra of cone pigments. By comparing results from monochromats with those obtained from dichromats and normal people, it is possible to estimate the relative sensitivities of the three cone systems at each wavelength (Figure 31–2). These sensitivities presumably reflect not only the relative sensitivities of the cone photoreceptors themselves, but also the relative numbers of the three types of cones in the retina, and how inputs from these three cone systems are weighted when they are combined in the brain.

Color Discrimination Requires at Least Two Types of Photoreceptors with Different Spectral Sensitivities

Individual cones do not transmit information about the wavelength of a light stimulus. When a cone absorbs a

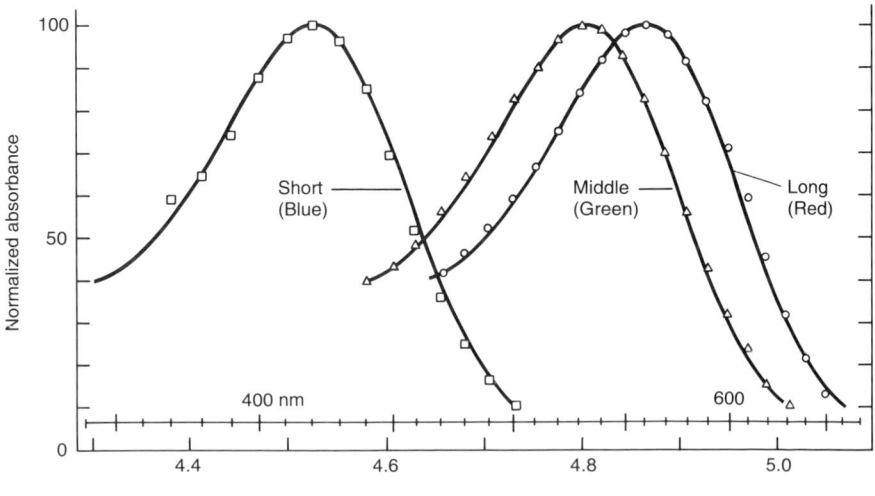

FIGURE 31–1

Each of the three types of human cones responds preferentially but not exclusively to short, middle, or long wavelengths as illustrated here by the absorption spectra of the outer segments of the cells. The short-wavelength cone contributes to the perception of blue, the middle to green, and the long to red. Note that the abscissa is the fourth root of wavelength, an empirically derived scale that makes the shapes of the three absorption spectra identical. (Adapted from Dartnall, Bowmaker, and Mollon, 1983.)

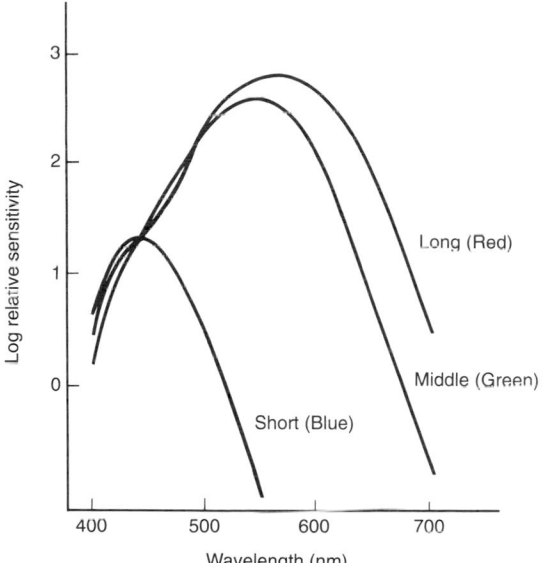

FIGURE 31–2
Spectral sensitivity curves of the three human cones can be obtained from psychophysical measurements of color-deficient subjects who have only one cone pigment. The different vertical positions of the three curves (which indicate the relative sensitivities of the three cone systems at each wavelength in a normal subject) reflect to a great extent the relative numbers of each class of photoreceptor in the normal retina. The ordinate scale is logarithmic rather than linear. (Adapted from Smith and Pokorny, 1975.)

photon, the electrical response that it generates is always the same, whatever the wavelength of the photon. This property, known as *univariance*, has been recognized by psychophysicists for many years but was only recently demonstrated directly by Dennis Baylor and his colleagues, who measured electrical responses of primate cones. Cones have this property because light absorption triggers the isomerization of the light-absorbing chromophore retinal from the 11-*cis* to the all-*trans* form (see Chapter 28). The all-or-none conformational change in the retinal molecule, and all the transduction events triggered by this change, is the same whatever the wavelength of the photon.

Although the wavelength of a photon does not shape the response of a cone, the number of photons absorbed by a cone does vary with wavelength. For example, an R-type cone is twice as likely to absorb a photon of 558 nm (its wavelength of peak sensitivity) as it is a photon of 490 nm (see Figure 31–1). An R-type cone will therefore absorb twice the number of photons from a 558 nm light as it will from a 490 nm light of the same intensity. By the same token, it will absorb the same number of photons from a 558 nm light as from a 490 nm light that is twice as intense: In either case the electrical response of the cone will be the same. In fact, a cell will respond equally to light of any wavelength as long as the intensity of the light

compensates for the cell's rate of absorbance at that wavelength! Thus, although individual cones respond preferentially to a particular color, the nervous system cannot determine from the response of, say, R-type cones whether the eye is being illuminated with red light or with much more intense blue light, or with a combination of lights of different wavelengths. Thus, people with only a single type of cone are unable to experience color (monochromatopsia).

Having a single-photoreceptor system results in vision similar to that experienced by normal people in dim light, which relies completely on rod vision. There is only one type of rod, with one visual pigment (rhodopsin); under these circumstances vision is achromatic, as we have all experienced at twilight. We can still distinguish an object if its *brightness* is stronger than that of the background, but we do not see it as colored. When an object in dim light appears colored (as when a full moon looks yellow), it is because its brightness is sufficient to excite cones.

Color vision requires at least two sets of photoreceptors with different spectral sensitivities. A two-receptor, or divariant, system would convey two values of brightness for each object. By comparing the two brightnesses, the brain would be able to distinguish colors (Figure 31–3B). If the object reflects primarily light of a long wavelength, the response in the longer wavelength cone system will be stronger than the response in the other system, and higher centers will interpret the object as being yellow. If the object reflects primarily shorter wavelengths, it will evoke a stronger response in the short-wavelength system and the object will be seen as blue. If the object reflects long and short wavelengths equally, it will be perceived as white, grey, or black, depending on the brightness of the background.

A divariant system may have been a first step in the evolution of color vision. Many color combinations of object and background are nevertheless invisible to a divariant system. An object that reflects light at both ends of the spectrum, and which appears against a background that reflects light in the midspectrum, will be invisible because both the object and the background produce the same response in both types of photoreceptors. These ambiguities are greatly reduced by a three-receptor or trivariant system (Figure 31–3C), but even this system does not eliminate all ambiguities.

Since color vision depends on a comparison of the outputs of different cones, it deteriorates when objects become so small that they stimulate only single cones. In addition, the optical resolution of the short-wavelength system is inherently limited because the optical image in this spectral region is more blurred, a phenomenon known as *chromatic aberration*. Consequently, the short-wavelength mechanism does not exist in the central fovea, where resolution of fine details is maximal (see Chapter 29). Thus, color vision in the central fovea is divariant. Because of these two limitations, color vision is not used to discriminate fine spatial detail, but rather to detect relatively large objects.

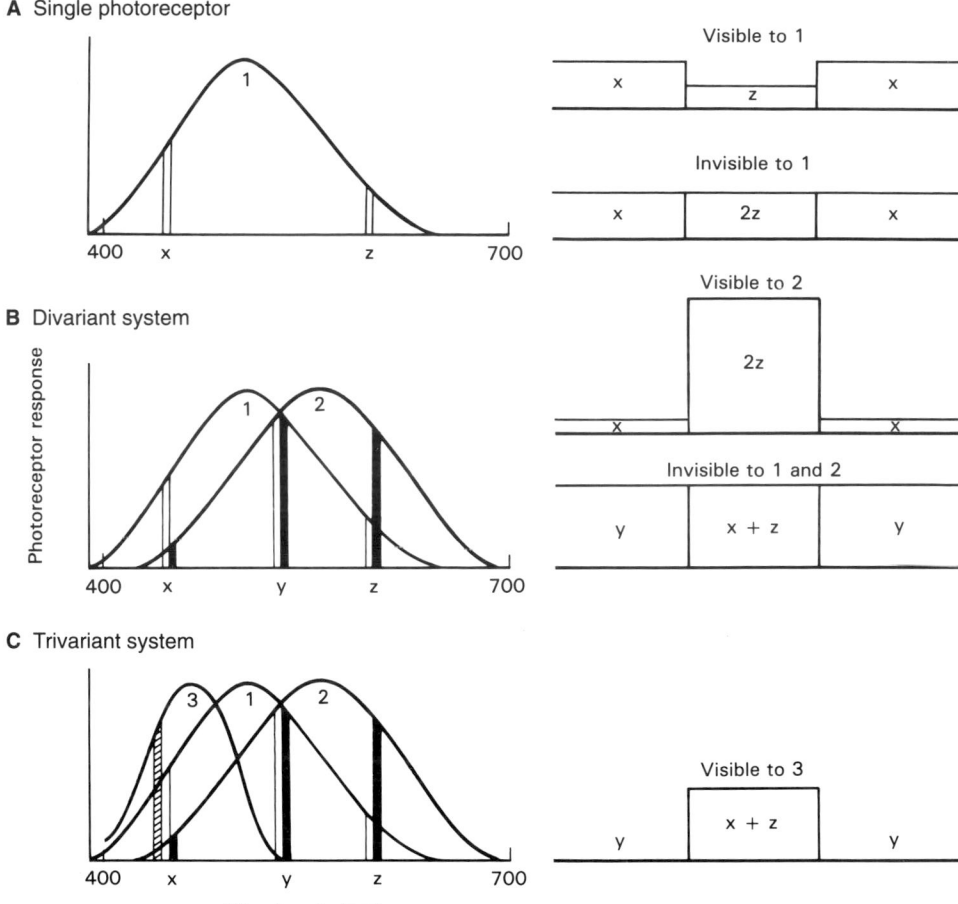

A Single photoreceptor

B Divariant system

C Trivariant system

Wavelength (nm)

Visible to 1

Invisible to 1

Visible to 2

Invisible to 1 and 2

Visible to 3

FIGURE 31–3

A trivariant system is clearly superior to monovariant or divariant systems for object discrimination. The curves on the left show the spectral response function of each type of photoreceptor system (400 nm = violet, 700 nm = deep red); the spectral characteristics of the reflectances from objects and backgrounds (**x**, **y**, and **z**) are also shown. The diagrams on the **right** illustrate the responses evoked in photoreceptors 1, 2, or 3 by an object (**middle region**) and its background (**flanking regions**).

A. In a single-photoreceptor system object **z** affects photoreceptor 1 about one-half as much as the background **x**; consequently if **x** and **z** reflect sunlight to the same extent, object **z** will appear dark in a bright background. However, if object **z** reflects sunlight about twice as much as the background (shown in the figure as **2z**), it will become invisible to photoreceptor 1 since the receptor response to the object will be about identical to the response generated by the background.

B. In a divariant system (two sets of photoreceptors, each with a different spectral response) objects invisible to a single-receptor system are usually visible. The object **2z** that is invisible to photoreceptor 1 when viewed against background **x** is strongly visible to photoreceptor 2. Some unusual, bispectrally reflectant objects, such as object (**x** + **z**), would stimulate photoreceptors 1 and 2 exactly the same as background **y** and consequently be invisible to both photoreceptors. One can work this out by showing that $x + z = y$ for both photoreceptors 1 and 2.

C. A trivariant system would be tougher to fool than the others, at least under natural light. The object (**x** + **z**) that is invisible to photoreceptors 1 and 2 when viewed against background **y** is visible to photoreceptor 3 because only **x** affects photoreceptor 3.

Color Opponency, Simultaneous Color Contrast, and Color Constancy Are Key Features of Color Vision

The theory of trivariant vision attributes color perception to the activity of three primary cone classes. This theory explains a large variety of data on color perception. For example, the combination of green and red is seen as yellow, and the combination of all three (what we perceive

individually as blue, green, and red) is seen as white. However, trivariancy alone fails to explain at least three important aspects of color perception.

The first is that certain colors cancel one another in such a way that they are never perceived in combination. For example, we cannot perceive reddish green or bluish yellow colors, even though we can readily see reddish blue (magenta), reddish yellow (orange), greenish yellow, or bluish green (cyan). Red and green lights can be mixed so

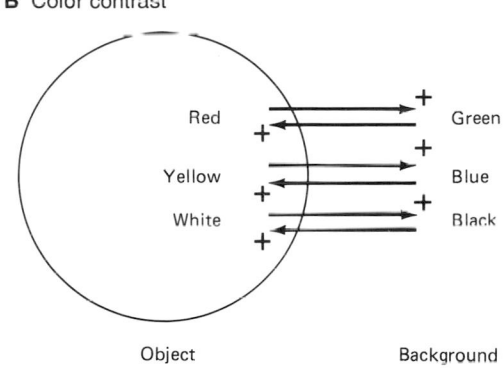

A Color opponency

Green → Red
Yellow → Blue
White → Black

Object

B Color contrast

Red → Green
Yellow → Blue
White → Black

Object   Background

FIGURE 31–4

Color opponency and color contrast are characteristic properties of human color vision.

A. Red and green, yellow and blue, and white and black antagonize each other in contributing to color perception when they emanate from the same point in space (e.g., when an object has both colors). The underlying physiological explanation is that, within the receptive fields of a single neuron, R cones and G cones are mutually antagonistic, as are B cones with G and R cones. Such opponent interactions are seen in the retina and the lateral geniculate nucleus of primates.

B. Red and green act synergistically *across* the boundaries of an object; similarly, yellow and blue as well as white and black enhance each other. The underlying physiological explanation for this phenomenon is the existence of so-called *double-opponent* cells. Thus, R cones on one side of an edge of contrast enhance the activity of G cones on the other side of the edge; likewise, B cones enhance R and G cone activity for yellow–blue contrasts. Double-opponent neurons have been found only in the visual cortex.

that all traces of the original redness or greenness are lost and a pure yellow is seen; yellow and blue lights can be mixed to produce white without any trace of the original blue or yellow.

This perceptual cancellation of colors led Ewald Hering to propose the *opponent process* theory. According to this theory the three primary colors have mutually antagonistic (or opponent) pairs: red–green, yellow–blue, and white–black. Hering postulated that these three color pairs are organized in the retina in three *color-opponent* neural channels. Accordingly, one channel responds in one direction (excitation or inhibition) to red and in the opposite direction to green. When properly balanced with the precise mixture of red and green, this channel produces no output. A second channel opposes the sensations of yellow and blue, a third opposes white and black (Figure 31–4A). As we shall see later in this chapter, the outputs from the three cone mechanisms are combined in opponent fashion, starting in the retina and lateral geniculate nucleus, and then in the cortex, in a way that can explain color opponency.

The color opponent theory explains why certain colors originating from the same point in space cancel one another. It does not, however, explain the phenomenon of *simultaneous color contrast*, which occurs *across* rather than within the boundaries of a perceived object. For example, a gray object seen in a background of red has a green tinge; in a background of green it has a red tinge. In these situations cone mechanisms appear to *facilitate* one another, rather than to cancel (Figure 31–4B). So-called *double opponent* cells in the visual cortex have properties

that can explain at least in part simultaneous color contrast.

Finally, a theory of color vision also needs to explain *color constancy*, which was described at the beginning of this chapter. We perceive the color of an object as relatively constant in the face of enormous changes in the spectral composition of the ambient light. We shall return to what is known about the constancy of color perception later.

In the Retina and Lateral Geniculate Nucleus Color Is Coded by Color Opponent Cells

Physiological evidence for the opponent process theory was obtained in the 1950s by Gunnar Svaetichin, who found that horizontal cells in the fish retina are hyperpolarized by one cone mechanism and depolarized by another. Svaetichin's discovery provided the first evidence for opponent interactions between cone cells. Later studies by Russell de Valois and by David Hubel and Torsten Wiesel identified similar cells in both the retina and lateral geniculate nucleus of primates.

Retinal ganglion cells and cells in the lateral geniculate nucleus of primates fall into several classes based on the way in which inputs from the three types of cones are combined (Figure 31–5). Most cells fall into two important classes: the concentric broad-band cells and the color-opponent cells.

The *concentric broad-band cells* have a concentric center-surround receptive field organization. A spot of white light on the receptive field center excites (or inhib-

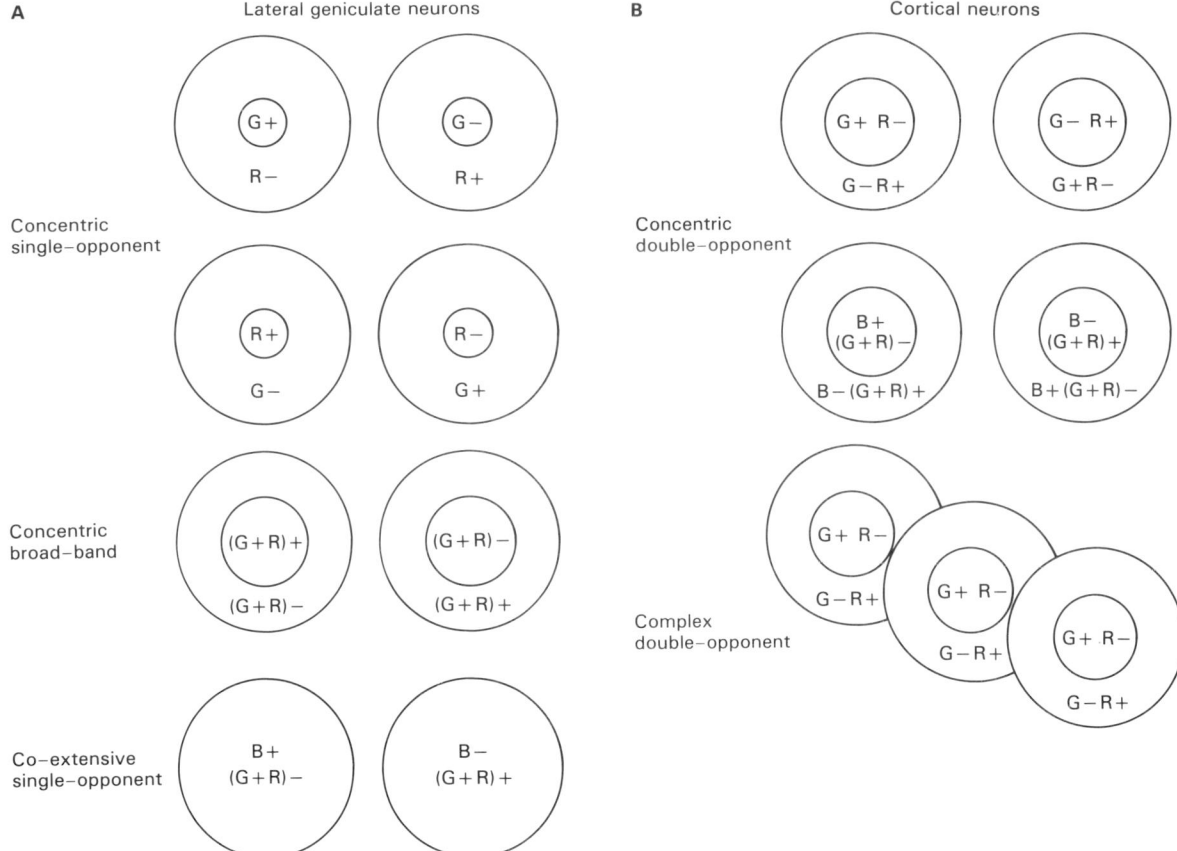

FIGURE 31–5

Retinal ganglion cells and geniculate neurons can be classified according to the way in which inputs from the three types of cones are combined.

A. The most common retinal ganglion cells and lateral geniculate neurons are *concentric single-opponent* cells: R and G cones act alone in either the center or surround of both on- and off-center cells and have opponent actions. The second most common are *concentric broad-band* cells: G and R cones act together in either the center or antagonistic surround. The least common are the *coextensive single-opponent* cells; within an un-

differentiated receptive field, the B cones are antagonized by the G and R cones acting together.

B. *Concentric double-opponent* cells are found in the visual cortex. The upper set respond preferentially to red–green contrasts, the lower set to yellow–blue contrasts. *Complex double-opponent* cells have similar properties to double-opponent cells, but spots do not have to appear in a precise spatial location within the visual field to elicit a response. Orientation-selective double-opponent cells have been found in striate cortex and complex double-opponent cells have been found in area 18.

its) the cell, whereas light applied to the surround elicits the opponent response. Diffuse light on these cells is thus a poor stimulus (see Figure 28–7). Although there is antagonism between center and surround, there is no antagonism between cone mechanisms in these cells. The center and the surround each combine inputs from both G and R cones. The broad-band cells therefore respond to the *brightness* of the center (compared to the brightness of the surround), and do not contribute to the perception of color. The B cones do not appear to contribute inputs to these cells. Presumably this reflects the fact that B cones are used only for color vision and not for detection of form, because chromatic aberration in the eye distorts images more at the blue (short wavelength) end of the spectrum.

Information about color is transmitted by *color-opponent cells* (Figure 31–5A). In most of these cells the

antagonism is between the R and G cones, and occurs within an antagonistic center-surround receptive field structure. Thus, the center receives inputs from R or G cones, and the larger antagonistic surround inputs from the other cones. These cells are called *single opponent* to distinguish them from double-opponent cells in the visual cortex (see below); because of the center-surround organization of their receptive fields they are called *concentric single-opponent* cells.

The responses of concentric single-opponent cells to different stimuli demonstrate that they transmit information about both color and achromatic brightness contrast. The responses of these cells to white or yellow light show the same center-surround antagonism as in broad-band cells because G and R cones absorb white or yellow light to similar degrees. When illuminated with white light

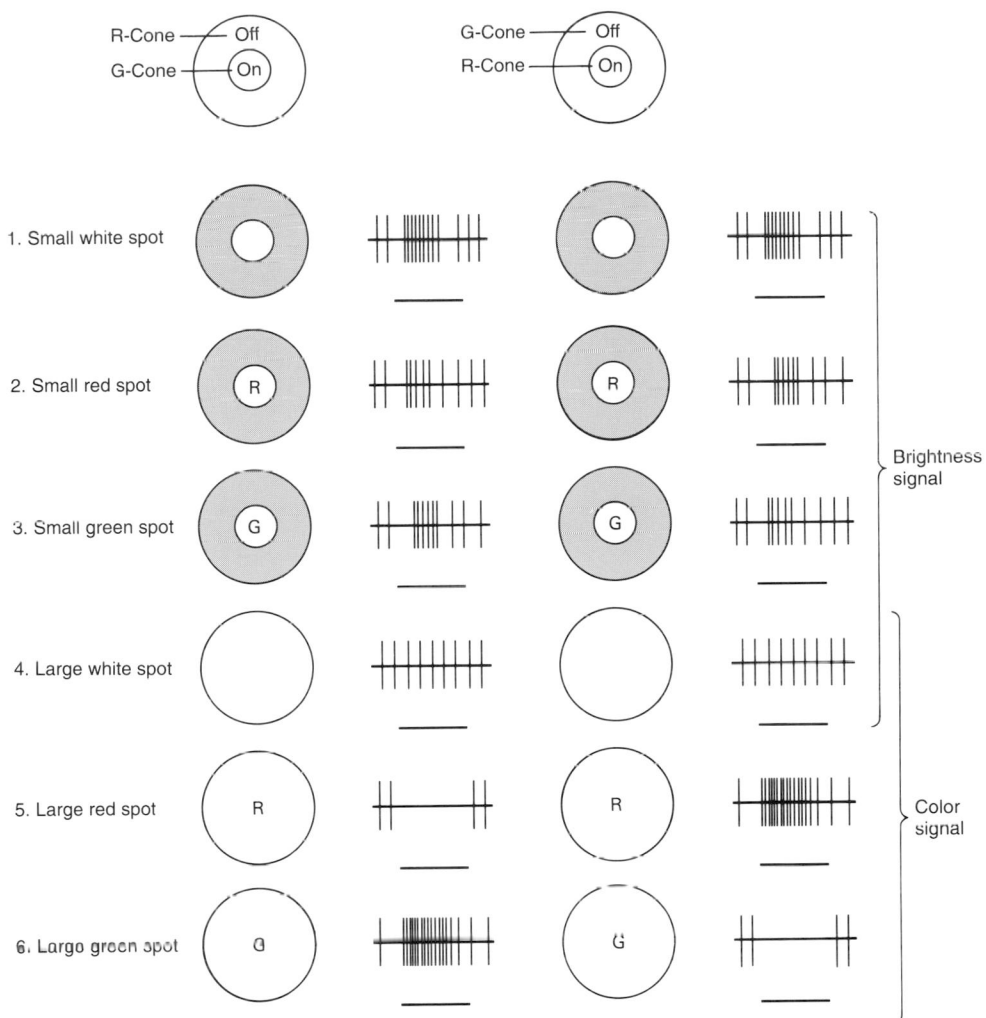

FIGURE 31-6

The receptive fields of concentric single-opponent cells in the retina of the cat are concentrically organized with a center and an antagonistic surround. The center and surround responses are mediated by *different* cone mechanisms. In the cell on the **left** the center (**inner circle**) is activated by the G cones and the surround (**outer ring**) by the R cones; the cell on the **right** has the reverse arrangement (R-center/G-surround). In the recordings excitation is indicated by an increased rate of firing. Both types of cells are excited by small, centered white spots (**1**) but are unresponsive to large white spots (**4**), because R and G cones have similar responses to white light so that the center and surround inputs cancel. Small centered red or green spots (**2, 3**) elicit a slightly weaker response than does a centered white spot (**R** and **G** indicate red and green spots, respectively). Large colored spots reveal the color selectivity of these cells. A large red spot (**5**) inhibits the cell on the left and excites the cell on the right; a large green spot (**6**) does exactly the opposite. The light stimulus is indicated by the bar below each recording.

they respond preferentially to small spots on either the center of their receptive field or the surround. At the same time these cells respond strongly to large spots of mono chromatic light of the appropriate wavelength. The R-center/G-surround cells respond best to red, while the G-center/R-surround cells respond best to green light (Figure 31–6).

Thus, these cells do not respond only to chromatic stimuli. It is impossible to know, for example, whether a strong excitatory response from an R-center/G-surround cell is due to a large red spot or a small bright spot of any color applied to the center of its receptive field (Figure 31–6). As we shall see in the next section, the visual cor-

tex has red–green opponent cells (the double-opponent cells) that do respond selectively to chromatic stimuli.

Finally, information from B cones is transmitted by a distinct class of single-opponent cells, the *coextensive single opponent* cells. These cells have a uniform receptive field in which inputs from B cones antagonize the combined inputs of R and G cones (Figure 31–5A).

In the Cortex Color Information Is Processed by Double-Opponent Cells in the Blob Zones

In preceding chapters we saw that many retinal ganglion cells fall into two general classes: the large M cells with

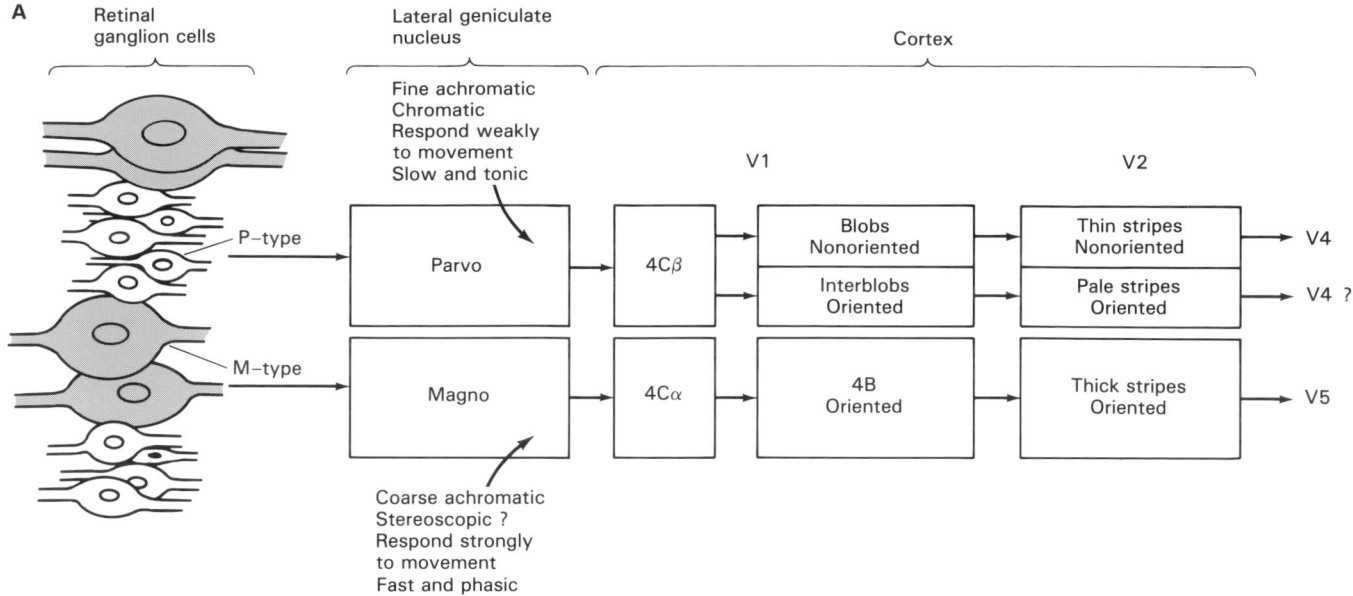

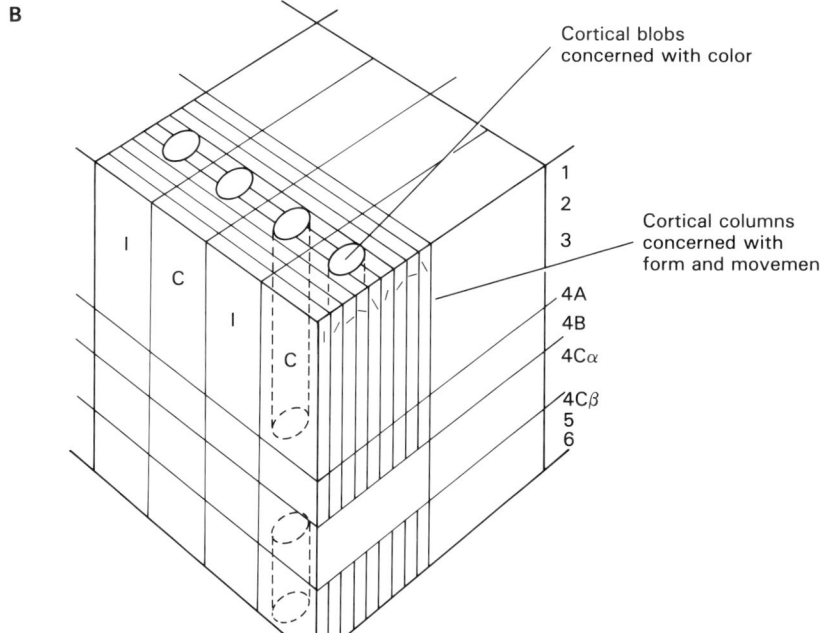

FIGURE 31–7

Color information is processed in the parvocellular–blob system. (Adapted from Livingstone and Hubel, 1984.)

A. Different aspects of the visual image are processed by separate pathways in the retina, lateral geniculate nucleus, and cortex.

B. Blobs in the primary visual cortex contain concentric double-opponent cells concerned with simultaneous color contrast (contrast across boundaries). The blobs are located in both the ipsilateral (**I**) and contralateral (**C**) ocular dominance columns and make up a system that is parallel to ocular dominance and orientation columns, whose cells are concerned with edges and contours.

fast conduction velocities, which project to the magnocellular layers of the lateral geniculate nucleus, and the smaller P cells, which project to the parvocellular layers. The broad-band ganglion cells described above can be either M-type or P-type, while single-opponent cells are exclusively P-type ganglion cells. Thus, the parvocellular layers relay all color information to the cortex in addition to information about achromatic contrast. The magnocellular layers are involved only in achromatic vision.

As we have seen in Chapters 29 and 30 and as illustrated again in Figure 31–7, the parvo- and magnocellular systems have different targets in the striate cortex. The parvocellular cells synapse in layer 4Cβ and this layer

projects in turn to layers 2 and 3. The color-sensitive cells in these layers are heavily concentrated in *blob* zones. These peg-like structures are centered within each ocular dominance column, extending from the upper to the lower layers (Figure 31–7B). The cells in the blobs are not selective for orientation, while most cells in the large interblob areas are selective for orientation but are not chromatic. It is thought that the same single-opponent parvocellular cells provide color contrast information to the cells in the blobs and achromatic brightness contrast information to cells in the interblob regions. Cells in the magnocellular layers project to layer 4Cα, which in turn projects to layer 4B. All the cells in these two layers are sensitive to ach-

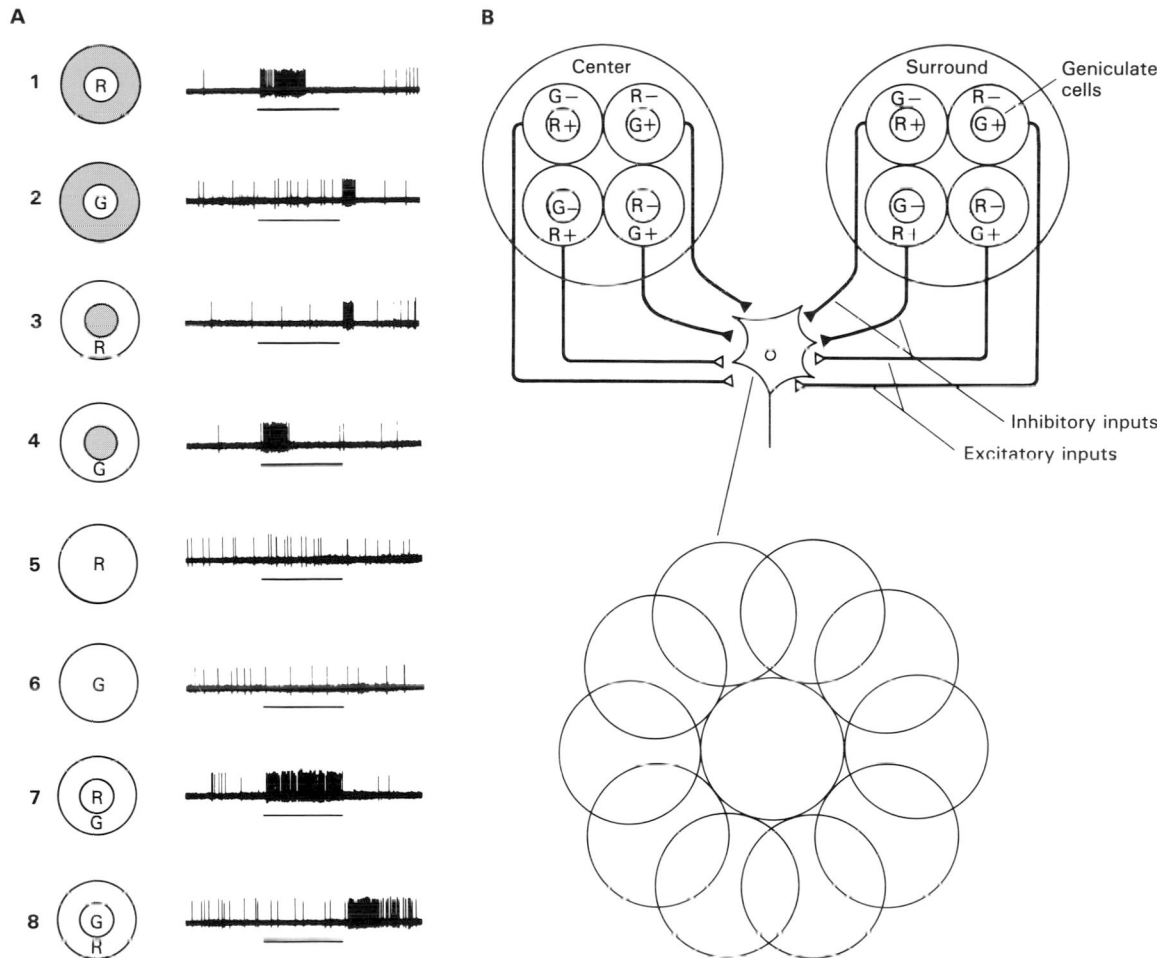

FIGURE 31–8

Concentric double-opponent red–green contrast cells in the cortex are highly sensitive to simultaneous color contrast.

A. The cell's responses to various red **(R)** and green **(G)** stimuli: Small spots of red and green light centered over the cell's receptive field **(1,2)**; red and green annuli **(3,4)**; large red and green spots **(5,6)**; and a red spot in a green background and the reverse **(7,8)**. The stimulus duration (1 sec) is indicated by the bar below each recording. This cell responds best to a red spot in a green background. (Adapted from Michael, 1978a.)

B. The concentric receptive field of the red–green contrast cell may be formed from the overlapping receptive fields of single-opponent cells in the lateral geniculate nucleus. Note that *both* on- and off-center single-opponent cells contribute to both the center and surround of double-opponent cells. The cell illustrated here responds best to a red spot in the center against a green background.

romatic contrast and show orientation selectivity. Thus, at the level of the cortex, chromatic and achromatic information is segregated into separate channels.

As we also have seen in Chapter 30, the parvocellular–interblob system appears to process information for the perception of form, the parvocellular–blob system codes for the perception of color, and the magnocellular system for stereopsis and the perception of movement. These three pathways project to separate interdigitating strips in V2. The magnocellular–interblob pathway then projects to V5, which contains cells sensitive to movement. The parvocellular–blob system projects to V4, the area described by Zeki in which color-selective cells predominate.

In the cortex, inputs from the single-opponent cells are combined to create so-called *double-opponent* cells, concentrated in the blob zones. These cells also have an antagonistic center-surround receptive field organization, but the cone organization of the receptive field is quite different from that of the single-opponent cells. Instead of one type of cone (e.g., G) operating in the center and another (R) in the surround, each type operates in all parts of the receptive field but has different actions in either the center or surround. For example, in some double-opponent cells, R cones excite in the center and inhibit in the surround. In these cells G cones have the opposite action: They inhibit in the center and excite in the surround (Figure 31–8B). These cells respond best to a red spot in the center against a green background, and they are more selective for chromatic stimuli than the concentric single-opponent cells (Figure 31–8A). They do not respond well to white light, whatever the size or the intensity of the stimulus, because the R and G cones absorb white light to similar extents and thus the two inputs cancel out each other's effect at all points in the receptive field.

There are three other classes of double-opponent cells: those that respond best to a green spot in a red background, and those that respond to a blue spot in a yellow background or vice versa (Figure 31–5B). Although these cells respond to some other contrasts, their maximum response is to these contrasts. Double-opponent cells have also been identified in higher processing centers. Some have orientation selectivity; others (in area 18), called complex double-opponent, respond only to spots of an appropriate size, but these spots do not have to appear in a precise spatial location within the visual field to elicit a response (Figure 31–5B). The neural circuitry that generates the receptive field of double-opponent cells from single-opponent cells has not yet been worked out, but the best candidate is illustrated in Figure 31–8B.

Double-Opponent Cells Help Explain Color Opponency, Color Contrast, and Color Constancy

Double-opponent cells were first discovered by Nigel Daw in studies of the retinal ganglion cells in goldfish. Although these cells are not present in the retina or geniculate of primates, they have been found in the cortex by Charles Michael and by Peter Gouras and Jurgen Kruger. Double-opponent cells clearly provide an explanation for the psychological phenomenon of color opponency, since different pairs of cone mechanisms oppose each other throughout the receptive fields of these cells (as postulated by Hering). In addition, their presence helps explain the phenomenon of simultaneous color contrast. For example, a double-opponent cell that is stimulated by red and inhibited by green in its center will respond the same to either a green light in its center or a red light in the surround. This may explain why a gray object seen against a background of green has a red tinge.

The organization of double-opponent cells may also contribute to the phenomenon of color constancy. An increase in the long-wavelength component of ambient light (such as occurs during a shift from fluorescent to incandescent illumination) has little effect on a double-opponent cell since the increase is the same for both the center and surround of the cell's receptive field. This helps explain why, in the example given at the beginning of this chapter, a lemon appears yellow under a variety of illumination conditions.

However, this compensation for changes in the ambient light does not explain why the lemon is perceived as *yellow* under all these conditions. In fact, a yellow lemon will not *always* be perceived as yellow. As first demonstrated by Edwin Land, the inventor of the Polaroid camera, objects reflecting identical wavelengths from their surfaces can appear to have totally different colors if they are set against different backgrounds. These experiments suggest that the visual system detects the color of objects by comparing all the objects in the visual scene.

The way in which the visual system does this is not understood. Nevertheless, Land has developed a quantitative method, the *retinex* (retina plus cortex) method, for predicting the colors of objects in any visual scene from the responses of the three cone mechanisms. The predicted colors are the same as the colors we perceive when observing the scene. The method correctly predicts that perceived colors remain roughly constant as the lighting conditions change, but that the perceived color of an object can change if its background is changed.

Land's method predicts color in three steps. For each type of cone, the brightness of each object in the scene is measured and this value is then normalized to the *brightest object in the scene*. In this way three numbers (one for each cone type) are assigned to each object. These numbers are then used to predict the color of all objects in the scene according to a rule devised by Land.

Does the cortex use this method to detect colors? Probably not in its simplest form. Indeed, it is unlikely that the cortex measures the brightness values of objects for each separate cone mechanism, since the inputs from the different cone mechanisms are combined in opponent fashion at a very early stage of visual processing. Land has shown, however, that his method works equally well if, instead of using brightness values for the three initial cone mechanisms, it uses values measured by the three color-opponent mechanisms (red–green, blue–yellow, and white–black). In this method each object is assigned a relative value of red–green brightness, blue–yellow brightness, and black–white brightness, and these three values are used to determine the object's color. It is certainly possible that the cortex uses the outputs of the different classes of double-opponent cells to determine colors in exactly the way that Land has suggested, although this has not been demonstrated.

Color Experience Is Based on Impressions of Hue, Saturation, and Brightness

The subjective perception of color can be broken down into three somewhat independent sensibilities: hue, saturation, and brightness.

Hue is what we ordinarily mean by color. This impression is determined by the proportion in which the three cones are activated by the object and its background. The brain must keep track of how much each of the three photoreceptor systems contributes to the detection of an object. Most of us have names for only a restricted number of hues, even though we are capable of discriminating 200 different ones.

Saturation, or richness of hue, indicates how much a hue has been diluted by grayness. This is determined by the degree to which all three cones are stimulated *to the same degree* by the object and by the background. At short and long wavelengths there are about 20 distinguishable steps of saturation for each hue. In the midspectral region

(530–590 nm) there are only about six distinguishable levels of saturation.

Brightness is the total effect of the object on all three cones (although, as we have seen, the short wavelength cone mechanism makes little or no contribution to the perception of brightness). It is the brightness factor that turns orange into brown, and gray into black or white. (Achromatic visual systems also distinguish brightness). There are 500 distinguishable steps of brightness. Thus, color vision has available about two million color gradations with which to detect the contours of objects in the external world (500 for brightness × 200 for hue × 20 for saturation).

Color Blindness Can Be Caused by Genetic Defects in Photoreceptors or by Retinal Disease

Color blindness can be inherited or acquired (Table 31–1). The most common causes of color blindness (red or green blindness) are recessive mutations located on the X chromosome. Thus, about 1% of men are red blind and 2% are green blind. In 1963 William Rushton used reflection densitometry to show that red or green blindness is a defect not in the neuronal circuitry mediating green or red color vision, but in the red or green cone pigments themselves. Since the defect was known to be X-linked, Rushton was able to infer that the genes for the red and green pigments are located on the X chromosomes.

Genetic variations in B-type cones (blue) also occur but very rarely. This form of color blindness is not X-linked but is an autosomal defect. The gene encoding the blue pigment has now been located on the seventh chromosome. The rhodopsin gene is on the third chromosome.

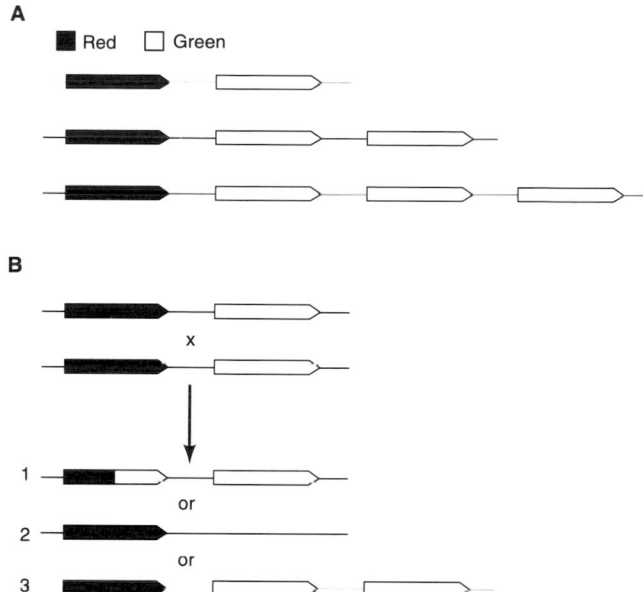

FIGURE 31–9

The arrangement of red and green pigment genes on the X chromosome may explain variations in these genes observed in both normal and color-blind males.

A. Arrangement of red and green pigment genes in color normal males. The base of each arrow corresponds to the 5'end of the gene and the tip corresponds to the 3'end. Color-normal males can have one, two, or three copies of the gene for the green pigment on each chromosome. (Adapted from Nathans et al., 1986.)

B. Because the genes for the green-absorbing and red-absorbing visual pigments of human cones are next to each other on a normal X chromosome, recombination between these genes can lead to the generation of a hybrid gene (**1**), the loss of a gene (**2**), or the duplication of a gene (**3**). (Adapted from Stryer, 1988.)

TABLE 31–1. Defects in Color Vision

Classification	Incidence (% males)
Congenital	
Anomalous	
Protanomaly (R-cone pigment abnormal)	1.3
Deuteranomaly (G-cone pigment abnormal)	5.0
Tritanomaly (B-cone pigment abnormal)	0.001
Dichromatopsia (two cones present)	
Protanopia (R-cone absent)	1.3
Deuteranopia (G-cone absent)	1.2
Tritanopia (B-cone absent)	0.001
Monochromatopsia (achromatic)	
Typical (all cones absent)	0.00001
Atypical (two cones absent)	0.000001
Acquired	
Tritanopia (outer retina layer disease)	
Protan-deuteran defects (inner retinal layer disease)	
Normal (three cones present)	91.2

The prefixes *protan-*, *deuteran-*, and *tritan-* refer to the long-, medium-, and short-wavelength mechanisms, respectively. The suffix *-opia* indicates a total absence of a cone; the suffix *-omaly* indicates an abnormality of function.

These chromosomal locations were confirmed with molecular techniques by Jeremy Nathans, who found a surprising variation in the genes that encode green pigment proteins in men with normal color vision. Each man was found to have a single copy of the gene for red pigment on the X chromosome and, located next to it, one, two, or even three copies of the gene for green pigment! How do these variations arise? Nathans suggested that if these genes are arranged in a tandem array, from head-to-tail, as illustrated in Figure 31–9, then variations in gene number could result from unequal homologous recombination. Since only the number of genes encoding the green pigment varies, Nathans has proposed that the red pigment lies at the beginning of this array.

Recombination between adjacent genes on the X chromosome could account not only for gene duplication but also for the loss of a gene or the generation of a hybrid gene, the pattern of gene rearrangement that occurs with red–green color blindness (Figure 31–9B). Thus, Nathans found that color variant males either lack the gene for

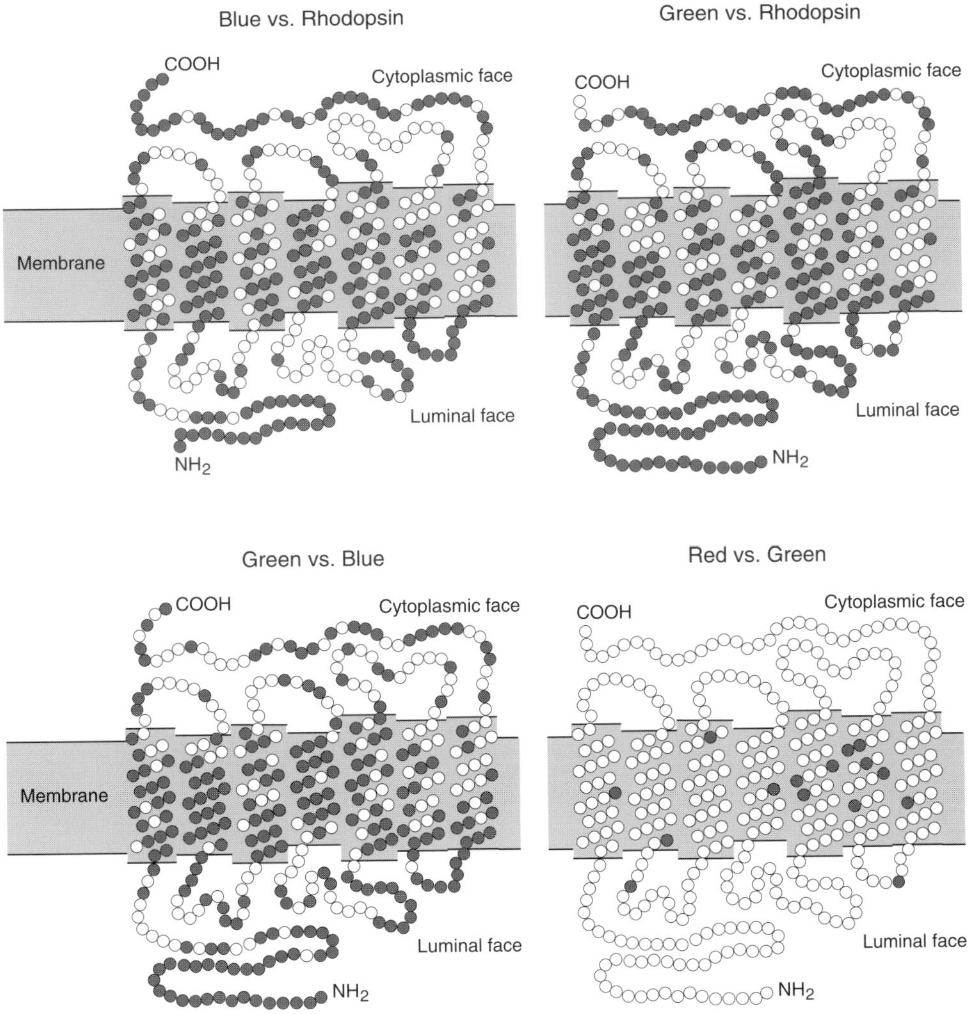

FIGURE 31–10

Pairwise comparisons of the amino acid sequences in the three visual pigments of cones (red, green, blue) and rods (rhodopsin). Each **dark circle** indicates an amino acid difference. (Adapted from Nathans et al., 1986.)

green pigment or have a hybrid gene that has intermediate spectral properties and is made up of segments from the green and red genes. With David Hogness, Nathans sequenced the gene for each of the three cone pigments and deduced their amino acid sequence. Each of the pigment genes encodes a transmembrane protein with seven inferred membrane-spanning regions, indicating that the proteins belong to the family of genes that also encodes rhodopsin, bacteriorhodopsins, and the invertebrate photopigments (Figure 31–10), as well as a variety of transmitter receptors that also interact with G-proteins (Chapter 12).

The three cone genes are quite similar to each other and to the rhodopsin gene, suggesting that all four evolved from a common ancestral rod gene by duplication and divergence. Comparison of amino acid sequences suggests that the blue cone pigment arose first from the rod gene. This short-wavelength gene then seems to have given rise to a single long-wavelength gene, a situation still found in contemporary New World monkeys, which have only two

color pigments. The long-wavelength gene then is thought to have duplicated and diverged to give rise to the red and green pigment genes only recently, about 30 million years ago, when Old World monkeys (which have all three pigments) separated from New World monkeys. Indeed, the red and green genes are closely related, with 90% identity in their amino acid sequences (Figure 31–10).

Although the number of extraretinal neurons involved in color vision is greater than retinal cells, most of the genetic defects involve only photoreceptors. This is undoubtedly because the genes that code for the cone pigments are more dedicated to color vision than are those that code for the neural circuitry that processes the information from photoreceptors. The genes involved in this neural circuitry must code for mechanisms common to much of the brain, and consequently mutations in them have a greater chance of being lethal.

Acquired defects of color vision are more complex. An old clinical rule, occasionally breached, states that diseases of the outer retinal layers tend to produce tritanopia (loss of the short-wavelength mechanism), whereas diseases of the inner layers and optic nerve produce protan–deutan defects (loss of the long- or medium-wavelength mechanisms). Finally, as we saw in Chapter 30, there are certain acquired forms of color blindness (prosopagnosia). These result from lesions that affect the areas V4 on both sides.

An Overall View

Individual cones do not transmit information about the wavelength of light. This is because the wavelength only affects the probability that the photon will be absorbed; it does not affect the electrical response of a cone. To detect color, the brain compares the responses of three types of cones, each most sensitive to a different part of the visible spectrum. This trivariancy of color vision explains why any color can be produced by appropriate combinations of red, blue, and green.

As information is transmitted to the brain, inputs from the three classes of cones are combined in a variety of ways. Many retinal ganglion cells, and cells in the lateral geniculate nucleus and cortex, are excited by one type of cone and inhibited by another. These opponent interactions of the three cone systems underlie the phenomena of color opponency (an object that is both red and green appears yellow since the red and green cancel each other out) and simultaneous color contrast (a gray object in a green background acquires a reddish tinge). The brain computes color perception of an object by comparing not only the responses of the cones stimulated by the object, but also the responses of all cones throughout the retina. In this way the brain is able to take into account changes in the spectral characteristics of ambient light so that an object's color appears roughly the same whatever the composition of the light, a phenomenon known as color constancy.

Color information is processed in a specialized pathway in the brain. The segregation of color information from information about form and movement starts in the retina. Information about color is processed by the parvocellular–blob system, which projects from the lateral geniculate nucleus to cortical area V4. As discussed in Chapter 30, we are just beginning to understand how information about color, form, and other aspects of the visual image is brought together in the brain.

Selected Readings

Boynton, R. M. 1979. Human Color Vision. New York: Holt, Rinehart and Winston.

Daw, N. W. 1984. The psychology and physiology of colour vision. Trends Neurosci. 7:330–335.

Gouras, P. 1984. Color vision. In N. N. Osborne and G. J. Chader (eds.), Progress in Retinal Research, Vol. 3. Oxford: Pergamon Press, pp. 227–261.

Hubel, D. H., and Wiesel, T. N. 1977. Ferrier Lecture: Functional architecture of macaque monkey visual cortex. Proc. R. Soc. Lond. [Biol.] 198:1–59.

Hurvich, L. M. 1972. Color vision deficiencies. In D. Jameson and L. M. Hurvich (eds.), Handbook of Sensory Physiology, Vol. 7, Part 4. Visual Psychophysics. Berlin: Springer, pp. 582–624.

Land, E. H. 1977. The retinex theory of color vision. Sci. Am. 237(6):108–128.

Livingstone, M., and Hubel, D. 1988. Segregation of form, color, movement, and depth: Anatomy, physiology and perception. Science 240:740–749.

Zeki, S. and Shipp, S. 1988. The functional logic of cortical connections. Nature 335:311–317.

References

Baylor, D. A., Nunn, B. J., and Schnapf, J. L. 1987. Spectral sensitivity of cones of the monkey Macaca fascicularis. J. Physiol. (Lond.) 390:145–160.

Brown, P. K., and Wald, G. 1963. Visual pigments in human and monkey retinas. Nature 200:37–43.

Damasio, A. R. 1985. Disorders of complex visual processing. Agnosias, achromatopsia, Baling's syndrome, and related difficulties of orientation and construction. In M.-M. Mesulam (ed.), Principles of Behavioral Neurology. Philadelphia: F. A. Davis, pp. 259–288.

Dartnall, H. J. A., Bowmaker, J. K., and Mollon, J. D. 1983. Microspectrophotometry of human photoreceptors. In J. D. Mollon and L. T. Sharpe (eds.), Colour Vision: Physiology and Psychophysics. New York: Academic Press, pp. 69–80.

Daw, N. W. 1968. Colour-coded ganglion cells in the goldfish retina: Extension of their receptive fields by means of new stimuli. J. Physiol. (Lond.) 197:567–592.

De Valois, R. L. 1960. Color vision mechanisms in the monkey. J. Gen. Physiol. 43[Suppl. 2]:115–128.

Gouras, P. 1991. The Perception of Colour. In Vision and Visual Dysfunction, Vol. VI London: Macmillan.

Gouras, P., and Krüger, J. 1979. Responses of cells in foveal visual cortex of the monkey to pure color contrast. J. Neurophysiol. 42:850–860.

Helmholtz, H. von. 1911. The Sensations of Vision. In J. P. C. Southall (ed. and trans.), Helmholtz's Treatise on Physiological Optics, Vol. 2. Wash., D. C.: Optical Society of America, 1924. Translated from the 3rd German edition.

Hering, E. 1964. Outlines of a Theory of the Light Sense. L. M. Herrick and D. Jameson (trans.) Cambridge, Mass.: Harvard University Press.

Hubel, D. H. 1988. Eye, Brain, and Vision. New York: Scientific American Library.

Hubel, D. H., and Livingstone, M. S. 1985. Complex-un-oriented cells in a subregion of primate area 18. Nature 315:325–327.

Kries, J. von. 1911. Appendix I. Normal and anomalous colour systems. In J. P. C. Southall (ed. and trans.), Helmholtz's Treatise on Physiological Optics, Vol. 2, pp. 395–425. Wash., D. C.: Optical Society of America, 1924. Translated from the 3rd German edition.

Livingstone, M. S., and Hubel, D. H. 1984. Anatomy and physiology of a color system in the primate visual cortex. J. Neurosci. 4:309–356.

Marks, W. B., Dobelle, W. H., and MacNichol, E. F., Jr. 1964. Visual pigments of single primate cones. Science 143:1181–1183.

Maxwell, J. C. 1890. The Scientific Papers of James Clerk Maxwell. 2 vols. W. D. Niven (ed.) Cambridge: The University Press.

Michael, C. R. 1978a. Color vision mechanisms in monkey striate cortex: Dual-opponent cells with concentric receptive fields. J. Neurophysiol. 41:572–588.

Michael, C. R. 1978b. Color vision mechanisms in monkey striate cortex: Simple cells with dual opponent-color receptive fields. J. Neurophysiol. 41:1233–1249.

Nathans, J. 1987. Molecular biology of visual pigments. Annu. Rev. Neurosci. 10:163–194.

Nathans, J., Piantanida, T. P., Eddy, R. L., Shows, T. B., and Hogness, D. S. 1986. Molecular genetics of inherited variation in human color vision. Science 232:203–210.

Nathans, J., Thomas, D., and Hogness, D. S. 1986. Molecular genetics of human color vision: The genes encoding blue, green, and red pigments. Science 232:193–202.

Nathans, J. 1987. Molecular biology of visual pigments. Annu. Rev. Neurosci. 10:163–194.

Pokorny, J., Smith, V. C., Verriest, G., and Pinckers, A. J. L. G. (eds.) 1979. Congenital and Acquired Color Vision Defects. New York: Grune & Stratton.

Rushton, W. A. H. 1963. A cone pigment in the protanope. J. Physiol. (Lond.) 168:345–359.

Sacks, O., Wasserman, R. L., Zeki, S., and Siegel, R. M. 1988. Sudden color-blindness of cerebral origin. Soc. Neurosci. Abstr. 14:1251.

Schiller, P. H., Logothetis, N. K., and Charles, E. R. 1988. The role of the color-opponent (C-O) and broad-band (B-B) channels in vision. Soc. Neurosci. Abstr. 14:456.

Smith, V. C., and Pokorny, J. 1975. Spectral sensitivity of the foveal cone photopigments between 400 and 500 nm. Vision Res. 15:161–171.

Stryer, L. 1988. Biochemistry, 3rd ed. New York: Freeman.

Svaetichin, G., and MacNichol, E. F., Jr. 1958. Retinal mechanisms for chromatic and achromatic vision. Ann. N. Y. Acad. Sci. 74:385–404.

Vollrath, D., Nathans, J., and Davis, R. W. 1988. Tandem array of human visual pigment genes at Xq 28. Science 240:1669–1672.

Young, T. 1802. The Bakerian Lecture. On the theory of light and colours. Phil. Trans. R. Soc. Lond., pp. 12–48.

James P. Kelly

32

Hearing

Sound Is Produced by Vibrations and Is Transmitted Through Air by Pressure Waves

Vibrations of the Conductive Apparatus Generate Fluid Waves in the Cochlea

Fluid Waves in the Cochlea Vibrate Hair Cells

Different Regions of the Cochlea Respond Selectively to Different Frequencies of Sound

Individual Hair Cells at Different Points Along the Cochlea Are Tuned to Different Frequencies of Vibration

Vibrations of Hair Cells Are Transformed into Electrical Signals in the Auditory Nerve

Central Auditory Neurons Are Specialized Physiologically to Preserve Time and Frequency Information

Bilateral Auditory Pathways Provide Cues to Localize Sound

The Auditory Cortex Is Composed of Separate Functional Areas

An Overall View

Over 100 years ago the physicist Georg Ohm proposed that the ear deconstructs complex sounds, like speech, into simple and discrete vibrations for subsequent analysis by the brain. Ohm suggested that the ear performs a type of spectral analysis, first described by the French mathematician Joseph Fourier, in which complex waveforms are simplified into the sum of many individual sine waves and cosine waves of appropriate frequencies, phases, and amplitudes. Modern research has confirmed Ohm's original idea. This chapter describes how sounds are transduced by the ear into neural signals and how these neural signals are processed by the brain.

We shall begin by considering the ear itself, which consists of three parts: the outer, the middle, and the inner ear. We shall then focus on the *cochlea* of the inner ear, a spiral bony canal that is filled with fluid and that contains the sensory transduction apparatus, the *organ of Corti*. Finally, we shall examine the organization and function of central neural pathways associated with hearing. The vestibular apparatus of the inner ear, which is important for the maintenance of body posture and the intergration of head and eye movements, will be considered in Chapter 33.

Sound Is Produced by Vibrations and Is Transmitted Through Air by Pressure Waves

Sound is produced by vibrations—for example the movement of speakers' diaphragms, piano strings or vocal cords—that result in the alternating compression and rarefaction (increased or decreased pressure) of the surrounding air. This disturbance radiates outward from the source as a pressure wave with alternating peaks and valleys of pressure (Figure 32–1). The *frequency* of the wave, or the

FIGURE 32–1

A sinusoidal sound wave propagating through space consists of alternating increases and decreases in the pressure of the ambient air. The pressure in this longitudinal wave is measured with a microphone probe at a fixed point. The speed of sound is a constant in air at standard temperature and pressure (approximately 340 m/s) and is related to both the wavelength (λ) and frequency (f) of the wave as shown in the equation in the figure. The tympanic membrane of the ear moves in response to the alternating compressions (peaks) and rarefactions (troughs) of the sound wave.

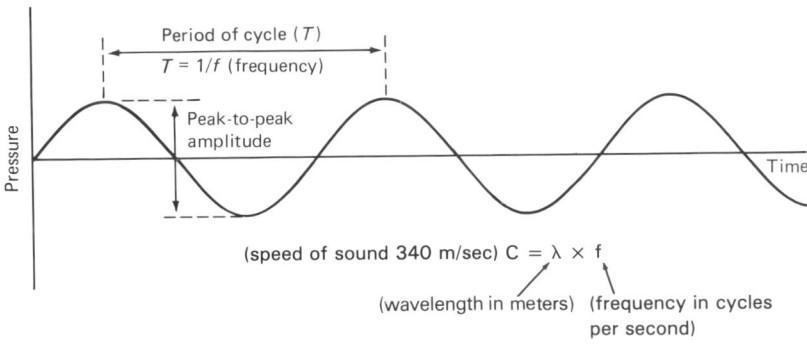

number of peaks that pass a given point per unit time, determines the *pitch* (highness or lowness) of the sound. Frequency is measured in cycles per second or Hz (hertz). For example, middle C on the piano has a frequency of 261 Hz. The human ear is sensitive to a wide range of frequencies from 20 to 20,000 Hz.

The *amplitude* of the wave is the maximum change in air pressure in either direction and is correlated with the *loudness* of the sound. The amplitude of pressure waves is measured with the decibel scale. The decibel (dB) is a logarithmic ratio defined as

$$\text{Sound pressure level (in decibels)} = 20 \log_{10} P_t/P_r$$
$$\text{(in newtons, N, per square meter)}$$

where P_t is the test pressure and P_r is the reference pressure (20 μN/m^2). This logarithmic scale was devised by Alexander Graham Bell, who found that the Weber–Fechner law (Chapter 23) applies to hearing. Incremental increases in subjective loudness correspond to equal increments of sound pressure level (SPL) regardless of the absolute value of the sound pressure level. In the equation above, P_r is the sound pressure required to make a sound between 1000 and 3000 Hz just audible to average listeners (human hearing is most acute in this range). A sound with test pressure 10 times greater than reference would have a loudness of 20 dB ($P_t/P_r = 10$, therefore 20 $\log_{10} 10$ = 20). Similarly, a test sound 100 times P_r would correspond to an SPL of 40 dB. For reference, conversational speech is about 65 dB.

The range of sound over which the ear responds is about 120 dB, so that the loudest sound that can be heard without discomfort has a million times greater pressure than the faintest sound the ear can detect. Sound pressures greater than 100 dB may damage the sensory apparatus of the cochlea. The extent of this damage depends on the intensity of the sounds, their frequency, and the duration of exposure.

Sounds reaching the ear travel through the external ear canal, or external auditory *meatus* (Latin, opening), and reach the middle ear, causing the *tympanic* (Latin, drum) *membrane* to vibrate. This vibration is then conveyed through the middle ear by a series of three small bones (ossicles), one of which, the *malleus* (Latin, hammer), is attached to the tympanic membrane. The vibration of the malleus is transmitted to an opening in the cochlea, the *oval window*, by the other two ossicles, the *incus* (Latin, anvil) and the *stapes* (Latin, stirrup) (Figure 32–2).

The major components of the middle ear—the tympanic membrane and ossicles—ensure that sounds from the air in the outer ear are transmitted efficiently to the fluid-filled cochlea of the inner ear. If the middle ear were absent, sounds would reach the fluid at the oval window directly. In that event, most of the sound energy would be reflected because fluid has a higher acoustic impedance than air and, as a result, the sound pressure required for hearing would be elevated.

Since the area of the tympanic membrane is greater than the area of the oval window, the total pressure (force per unit area) acting on the smaller oval window is increased. At frequencies near 1 kHz the ossicles also act as a system of levers to increase the pressure on the round window. This effect is reduced at both higher and lower frequencies because the tympanic membrane does not vibrate as a uniform plate, and therefore the ossicles cannot be viewed as a simple lever system. They are probably also arranged to reduce the inertial motion of the conductive apparatus resulting from head movements.

Vibrations of the Conductive Apparatus Generate Fluid Waves in the Cochlea

The cochlea spirals for two-and-a-half turns around a central pillar called the *modiolus* (Latin, pillar or hub). In Figure 32–2 the cochlea has been uncoiled for purposes of illustration. Here we can clearly see that the cochlea has three fluid-filled compartments or *scalae* (Italian, stairway). These are: (1) the *scala tympani*, which follows the outer contours of the cochlea; (2) the *scala vestibuli*, which follows the inner contours and is continuous with the scala tympani at the *helicotrema* (Greek, spiral hole); and, lying between these two, (3) the *scala media* (or cochlear duct), which extends finger-like into the cochlear channel and ends blindly near the apical end of the cochlea.

Sound entering the ear causes the stapes to oscillate, and these oscillations transmit energy to each of the three

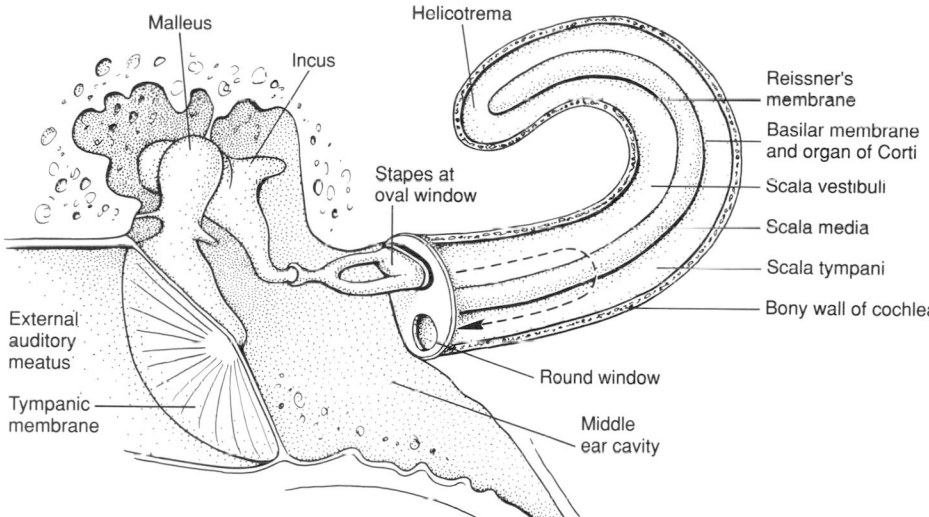

FIGURE 32–2

The major parts of the human ear consist of: (1) the external ear, including the pinna (not shown), the external auditory meatus, and the tympanic membrane; (2) the middle ear, which contains a series of three small bones or ossicles: the malleus, the incus, and the stapes; and (3) the internal ear, composed of the cochlea and the vestibular apparatus. Motion of the tympanic membrane, which is joined to the system of ossicles, causes motion of the stapes, which in turn initiates a propagated wave in the fluid-filled cochlea. The cochlea, a spiral bony canal, contains three compartments: the *scala tympani*, the *scala vestibuli*, and the *scala media*. The term *scala* was used by classical anatomists because of the fanciful resemblance between these compartments

and spiral stairways. (For purposes of illustration, the cochlea is shown here uncoiled.) The scala media is separated from the scala vestibuli by Reissner's membrane and from the scala tympani by the basilar membrane. The scala vestibuli and scala tympani communicate with each other at the helicotrema where the scala media ends, so that perilymph is continuous. The round window of the scala tympani is covered by a flexible membrane. Pushing the foot plate of the stapes at the oval window increases the fluid pressure in the cochlea, causing the round window membrane to bulge into the middle ear cavity. The flexible walls of the scala media are also set in motion by the pressure waves.

compartments. The transmission of pressure works as follows. When the stapes oscillates, it pushes into and out of the cochlea, putting varying pressure on the fluid in the scala vestibuli. Because fluid is not compressible, the pressure wave causes an alternating outward and inward movement of the round window membrane of the scala tympani. The pressure waves also cause oscillating movements of the scala media and of the basilar membrane (the floor of the scala media). The organ of Corti, the sensory transduction apparatus in the scala media, rests on the basilar membrane and is also stimulated by this movement (Figure 32–2).

Thus, the cochlear compartments are arranged to convert the differential pressure between the scala vestibuli and scala tympani into oscillating movements of the basilar membrane that excite and inhibit the sensory transducing cells in the organ of Corti.

Sounds can bypass the middle ear to reach the cochlea directly by *bone conduction*, that is, by vibration of the entire temporal bone, but this is an inefficient means of energy transfer and is important only as a part of audiological diagnosis. In the nineteenth century Heinrich Rinne developed a test to reveal the origin of hearing abnormalities by comparing a hearing-impaired patient's ability to detect air-conducted and bone-conducted sounds. In Rinne's test a tuning fork is struck and held near the patient's ear. When the patient can no longer hear the sound produced by the fork because the amplitude of

its vibration has decreased, the stem of the fork is placed behind the ear against the mastoid process of the temporal bone. If the patient once again hears the vibrations, this indicates that bone conduction is more sensitive than air conduction and implies some disruption of the air conductive apparatus.

Using Rinne's test it is possible to distinguish two broad classes of deafness: (1) conductive deafness, caused by damage to the middle ear, and (2) sensorineural deafness, caused by damage to the cochlea, the eighth nerve, or the central auditory pathway. In conductive deafness, as we have seen, air conduction is impaired. For example, in *otosclerosis* the footplate of the stapes becomes locked in place due to the growth of the bone around the annular ligament that binds the stapes to the oval window. In sensorineural deafness hearing by both bone and air conduction is impaired. The distinction is important clinically because many conductive defects can be repaired by surgery.

Fluid Waves in the Cochlea Vibrate Hair Cells

The sensory receptor cells of the inner ear, the *hair cells*, are contained within the organ of Corti. When the oscillating motion of the stapes causes changes in fluid pressure within the cochlea, motion is initiated in a particular portion of the basilar membrane and therefore in a particular set of hair cells.

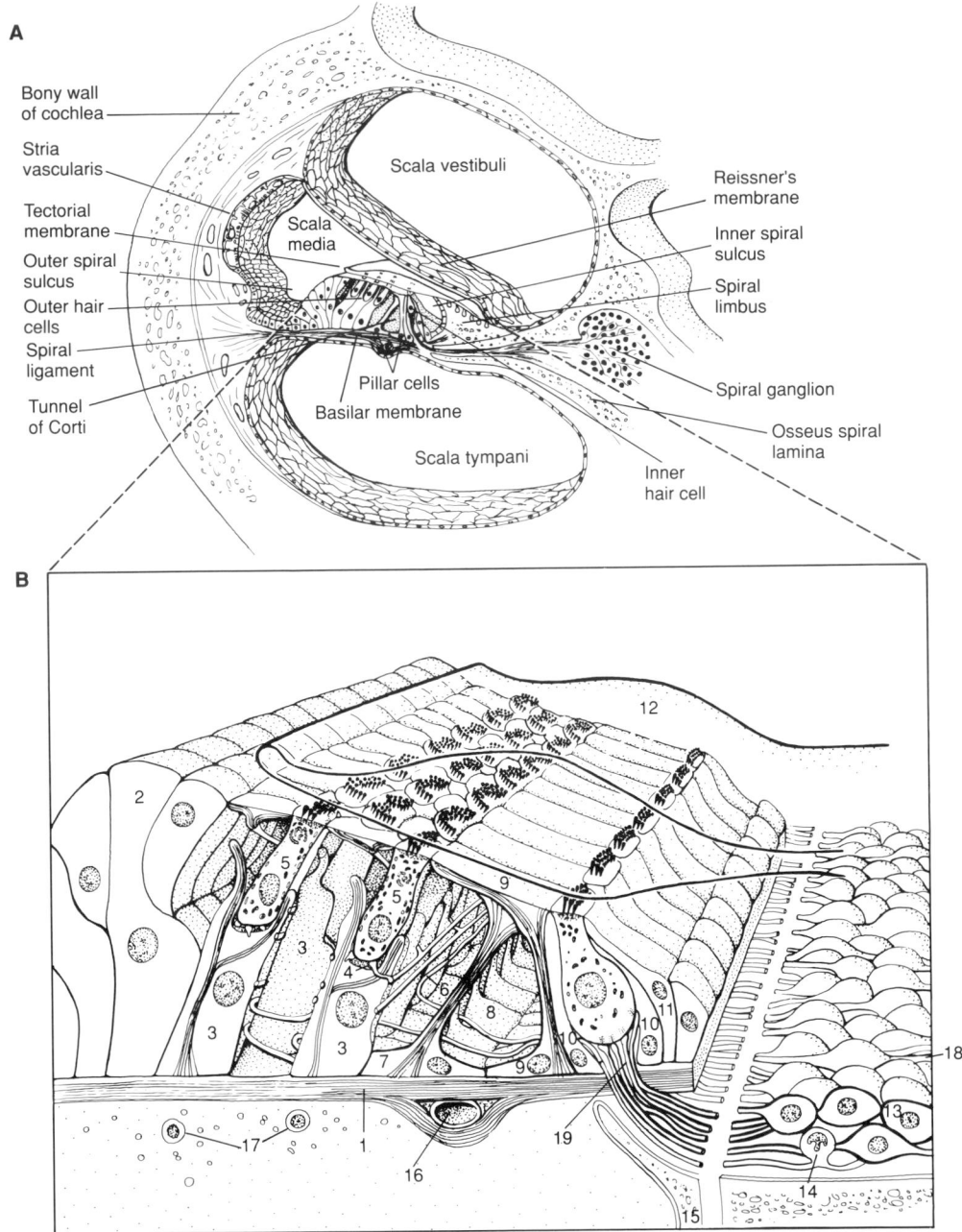

FIGURE 32-3

Organization of the scalae or compartments of the cochlea.

A. Two cavities in the osseous cochlea, the scala vestibuli and the scala tympani, contain *perilymph.* The central scala media or cochlear duct of the membranous cochlea contains *endolymph.* The floor of the scala media is the basilar membrane upon which rests the organ of Corti. The organ of Corti consists of receptor cells, the inner and outer hair cells, as well as a variety of supporting cells. The tectorial membrane extends from the vestibular lip of the spiral limbus over the internal spiral sulcus to cover the surfaces of the inner and outer hair cells. Reissner's membrane separates the scala vestibuli from the scala media. The lateral wall of the scala media consists in part of a region called the stria vascularis, which produces endolymph by selective pumping of ions. (Adapted from Bloom and Fawcett, 1975.)

B. Cellular architecture of the organ of Corti in the mammalian cochlea. There are differences among species, but the basic plan is similar for all mammals. The foreground represents the more

basal part of the cochlea. Here one hair cell is removed from the middle row of outer hair cells so that three-dimensional aspects of the relationship between supporting cells and hair cells can be seen. The diameter of an outer hair cell is approximately 7 μm. The most basal components are drawn so that some intracellular detail can be seen. Empty spaces at the bases of outer hair cells are occupied by efferent endings that have been omitted from the drawing. 1, Basilar membrane; 2, Hensen's cells; 3, Deiters's cells (outer phalangeal cells); 4, endings of spiral afferent fibers on outer hair cells; 5, outer hair cells; 6, outer spiral fibers; 7, outer pillar cells; 8, tunnel of Corti; 9, inner pillar cells; 10, inner phalangeal cells; 11, border cell; 12, tectorial membrane; 13, type I spiral ganglion cell (innervation for inner hair cells); 14, type II spiral ganglion cell (innervation for outer hair cells); 15, bony spiral lamina; 16, spiral blood vessel (found only in base of cochlea); 17, cells of the tympanic lamina; 18, axons of spiral ganglion cells (auditory nerve fibers); 19, radial fiber. (Adapted from Junqueira et al., 1977.)

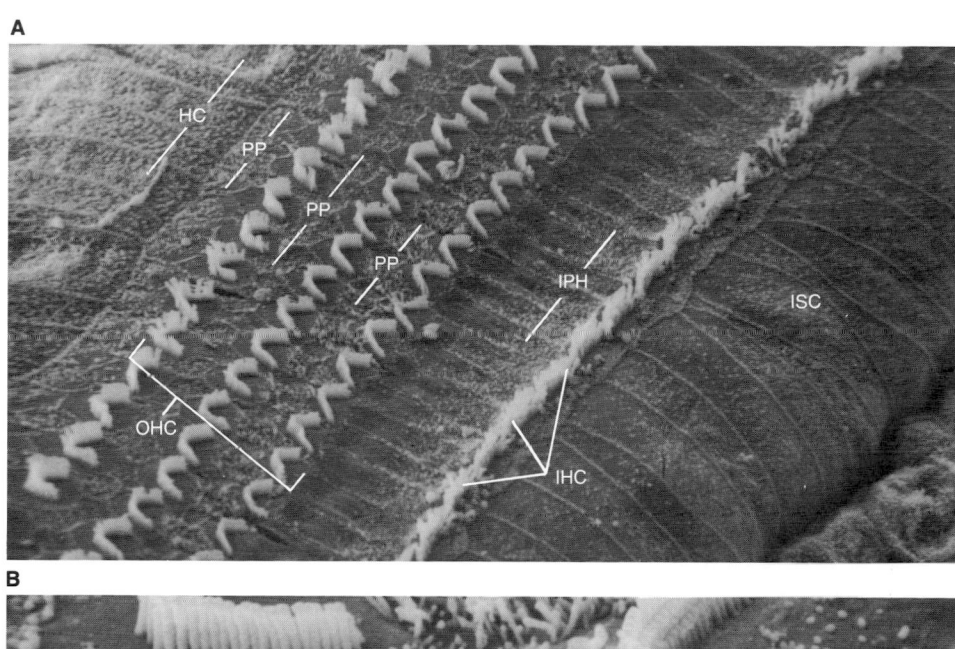

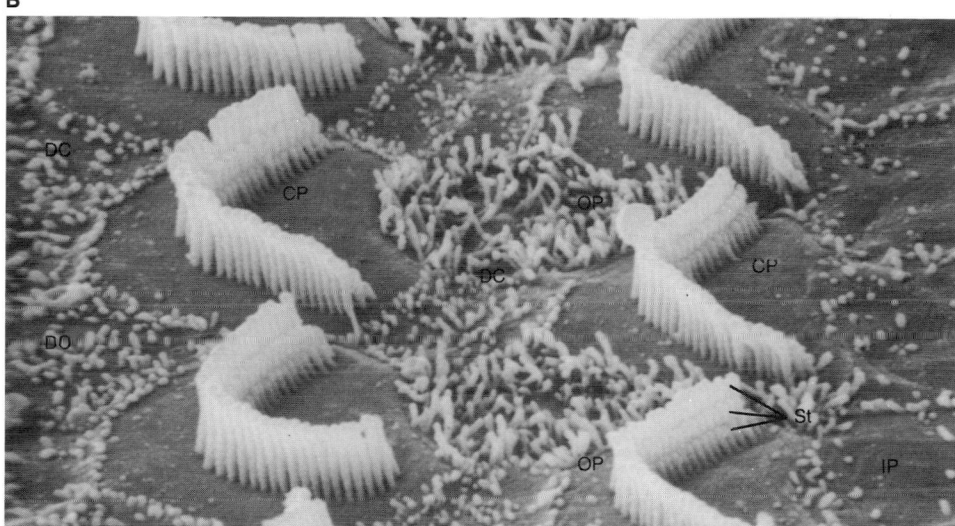

FIGURE 32–4

Scanning electron microscopy of the organ of Corti after removal of the tectorial membrane.

A. The single row of inner hair cells (**IHC**) contains stereocilia that are arranged linearly. In contrast, stereocilia associated with the three rows of outer hair cells (**OHC**) are arranged in a W configuration. It is also possible to distinguish the surfaces of a number of other cells within the organ of Corti in this figure. These include the inner spiral sulcus cells (**ISC**), the heads of the inner pillar cells (**IPH**), the phalangeal processes (**PP**) of Deiters's cells, and the surfaces of Hensen's cells (**HC**).

B. The W-shaped configuration of the stereocilia (**St**) of the first two rows of outer hair cells is shown at higher magnification in this scanning electron micrograph. The apical surfaces of the hair cells surrounding the stereocilia appear smooth and are termed cuticular plates (**CP**). The heads of the inner pillar (**IP**) cells form the roof of the tunnel of Corti. Extensions from the outer pillar heads (**OP**) run between the members of the first row of outer hair cells to separate the first row from the second. Deiters's cells (**DC**) form part of the separation between the rows of outer hair cells. The cuticular plates (**CP**) of the hair cells from which the stereocilia arise are smooth in comparison to the microvilli on the surfaces of supporting cells.

How do fluid waves produced by different sounds excite different hair cells at different points along the basilar membrane? A cross section of the cochlea shows the location of the hair cells in the organ of Corti (Figure 32–3). There are three rows of outer hair cells and one row of inner hair cells (the terms *inner* and *outer* refer to the relative proximity of the hair cells to the modiolus). On the apical surface of each hair cell is a bundle of *stereocilia* (Figure 32–4). They are stiff because they are filled with parallel arrays of cross-bridged actin filaments.

The stereocilia of the hair cells project into the overlying *tectorial membrane*. Because the tips of the stereocilia are embedded in this membrane and the bodies of the hair cells rest on the basilar membrane, the stereocilia will be displaced if the tectorial membrane and the basilar membrane move with respect to one another. Therefore, when

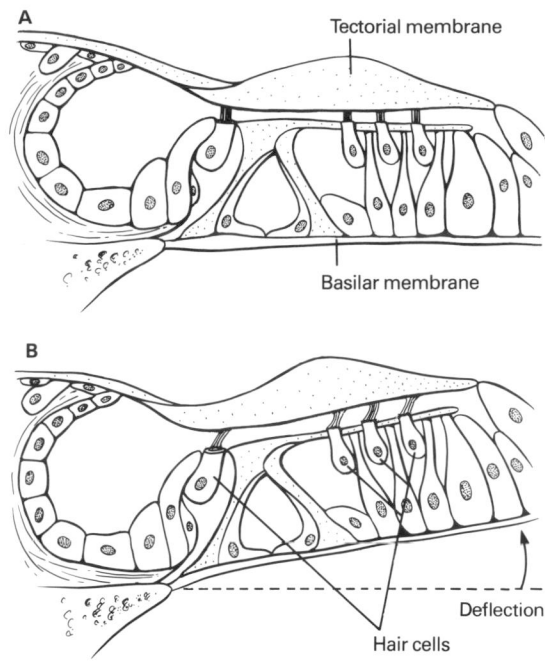

Tectorial membrane

Basilar membrane

Deflection

Hair cells

FIGURE 32–5

Vibration of the basilar membrane and the organ of Corti results in bending of hair cell stereocilia. Bending of the stereocilia causes a change in ionic conductance at the apical surface of the cell, a current flow, and resultant voltage change. (Adapted from Miller and Towe, 1979.)

A. Basilar membrane at rest.

B. Deflection of the basilar membrane results in angular displacement of stereocilia.

vibrations of the basilar membrane move the body of the hair cell, the stereocilia bend in relation to the hair cell body (Figure 32–5).

Motion of the stereocilia in one direction depolarizes the cell by opening ion channels that produce an inward current, carried by cations. Motion of the stereocilia in the opposite direction hyperpolarizes the cell. Thus, when a sound produces an oscillatory movement of the basilar membrane, the back-and-forth angular displacement of

the stereocilia results in sinusoidal (depolarizing-hyperpolarizing) potential changes at the frequency of the sound.

In addition to an input component at its apical end, the hair cell, like the photoreceptor of the retina, has specialized machinery for releasing chemical transmitter at its basal end (Figure 32–4). Here the cells are contacted by the peripheral branches of axons of bipolar neurons whose cell bodies lie in the spiral ganglion and whose central axons constitute the auditory nerve. Depolarization of the hair cell causes neurotransmitter to be released at the base of the cell. The transmitter excites the peripheral terminal of the sensory neuron, and this in turn initiates action potentials in the cell's central axon in the auditory nerve. Oscillatory changes in the potential of the hair cell therefore cause oscillatory release of transmitter and oscillatory firing of axons in the auditory nerve.

Different Regions of the Cochlea Respond Selectively to Different Frequencies of Sound

Given that hair cells respond to vibrations of their hair bundles, how are different frequencies of sound encoded into neural signals? This question was asked in the nineteenth century by Herman von Helmholtz, who discovered two interesting features about the organization of the cochlea. First, the basilar membrane has cross striations much like the strings of a piano. Second, the basilar membrane varies in width from the base to the apex of the cochlea. It is narrow (100 μm) and stiff near the oval window, and wider (500 μm) and more flexible near the apex of the cochlea (Figure 32–6). Helmholtz proposed that the cross striations of different portions of the basilar membrane resonate with different frequencies of sound, much as piano strings of different length and stiffness resonate with different frequencies. The cross striations of the stiff part of the basilar membrane at the base near the oval window would, in this view, resonate with high frequencies (about 15,000 Hz), while the striations in the flexible part of the membrane near the apex would resonate with low frequencies (about 100 Hz). Between these extreme frequencies there is a continuous spectrum of resonance. According to this *resonance theory*, different frequencies of sound affect different portions of the basilar membrane, which in turn affect different populations of hair cells.

FIGURE 32–6

The dimensions of the basilar membrane change along its length. In this surface diagram the human basilar membrane is shown as if it were uncoiled and stretched out flat.

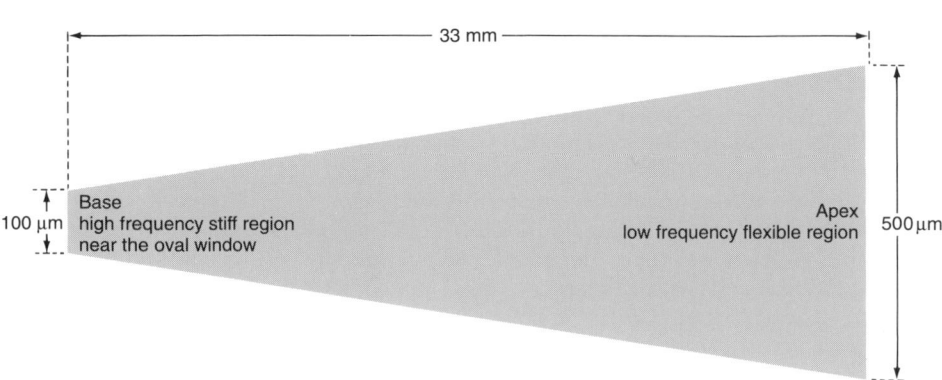

33 mm

100 μm   Base
high frequency stiff region
near the oval window

Apex
low frequency flexible region   500 μm

In the 1920s and 1930s Georg von Bekesy tested Helmholtz's idea directly by examining the pattern of mechanical vibrations in the cochlea. He sealed a microscope objective lens into the bony wall of the cochlea after spreading reflective crystals on the undersurface of the basilar membrane. In this way he could observe directly the motion of the basilar membrane in response to sound with minimal disruption of the normal fluid waves. In contradiction to the resonance hypothesis, Von Bekesy found that each sound does not lead to the resonance of only one narrow segment of the basilar membrane, but initiates a *traveling wave* along the length of the cochlea that starts at the oval window. The wave passes along the cochlea from the stapes to the helicotrema, much like snapping a rope tied at one end to a post causes a wave to pass along it from the snapped end to the fixed end.

Stimulation at a single frequency causes a very broad region of the basilar membrane to move (Figure 32–7). Different frequencies of sound produce different traveling waves with *peak* amplitudes at different points along the basilar membrane. This is possible because the mechanical properties of the basilar membrane vary along the length of the cochlea. At low frequencies the peak amplitude of the motion is near the apex of the cochlea, in the region of the helicotrema. As the frequency of the stimulus increases, the peak amplitude of motion occurs closer to the base of the cochlea. At any individual frequency, as the amplitude of the sound stimulation increases, the peak vibration increases in displacement and a broader region of the membrane vibrates. The representation of frequencies along the basilar membrane is logarithmic. The peak motion of the basilar membrane in response to sounds of different frequencies occurs at the points predicted by Helmholtz's resonance theory! Thus, although the wave travels along the membrane, the peak movement elicited in the organ of Corti by a given frequency of sound occurs at a particular position along the length of the cochlea. Different frequencies excite different hair cells at different positions in the cochlea, and the hair cells situated at the site where the oscillation is maximal are the most excited.

Individual Hair Cells at Different Points Along the Cochlea Are Tuned to Different Frequencies of Vibration

Until recently it was thought that frequency selectivity in the organ of Corti is determined only by variations in the mechanical properties of the basilar membrane, and not by differences in the properties of the hair cells. According to this view different hair cells respond not because of physiological differences, but because of their different positions along the basilar membrane.

Hair cells located within the organ of Corti at different points along the basilar membrane are not identical. They differ from one another in their electromechanical properties, and these variations may be the most important factors in determining frequency selectivity. At the base of the cochlea, where the basilar membrane is narrow and

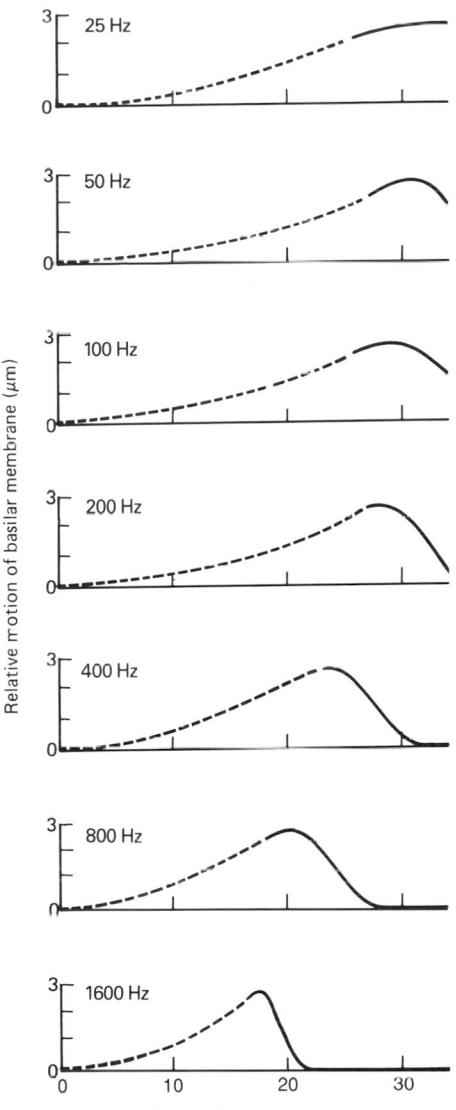

FIGURE 32–7

Plots of data from von Bekesy's experiments on the mechanics of the basilar membrane show that the peak amplitude of the traveling wave occurs at different points for sounds of different frequencies. The peak of wave motion moves progressively toward the base of the cochlea as sound frequency increases. Modern measurements show that these curves reflect only the overall envelope of motion of a more complex wave along the basilar membrane. The peak motion is now known to be sharp and restricted in distribution, although the exact waveform of the motion has not been established with certainty. (Adapted from von Bekesy, 1960.)

stiff, the outer hair cells and their stereocilia are short and stiff. In the apex, where the basilar membrane is more flexible, the hair cells and their stereocilia are more than twice as long and more flexible than those in the base. Because of this variation in physical structure, the hair cells are tuned mechanically—they have a *mechanical resonance.* Different sound waves activate different regions of the basilar membrane and in so doing may activate different populations of differently tuned hair cells.

In the 1980s two independent groups of scientists—Andrew Crawford and Robert Fettiplace, and Richard Lewis and Albert Hudspeth—discovered that the hair cells of certain lower vertebrates are also tuned electrically (*electrical resonance*). The hair cell membrane shows spontaneous oscillations in membrane potential. The frequencies of these oscillations vary in different hair cells according to their position along the basilar membrane. The characteristic frequency of the spontaneous electrical oscillation in each cell matches the frequency at which the cell is most responsive to mechanical stimuli (its mechanical resonance). As the mechanical activation opens and closes ion channels, the resulting potential changes in the hair cells amplify the spontaneous voltage oscillations. This can be shown experimentally by artificially passing depolarizing or hyperpolarizing currents into the hair cells.

How is this electrical resonance achieved? As the mechanical stimulus depolarizes and hyperpolarizes the cell, it increases and decreases the amplitude of the spontaneous oscillation of the Ca^{2+} and K^+ currents. Lewis and Hudspeth found that three different currents interact to produce the electrical resonance: a Ca^{2+} current, a Ca^{2+}-activated K^+ current, and a voltage-sensitive delayed K^+ current. The depolarizing phase is due to a depolarizing influx of Ca^{2+} near the apex of the cell. The influx of Ca^{2+} activates a Ca^{2+}-sensitive K^+ channel causing an outward K^+ current. The hyperpolarizing effect of the outward K^+ current is augmented by a voltage-sensitive delayed K^+ current. As Ca^{2+} is sequestered inside the cell, and the membrane potential returns to the resting state, both the Ca^{2+}-activated K^+ current and the voltage-sensitive K^+ current are reduced and the cell is ready for another cycle. The interaction of depolarizing and hyperpolarizing currents produces spontaneous voltage fluctuations around the resting potential. These currents have different kinetics for different hair cells, and hence different frequencies of oscillation (Figure 32–8).

The mechanical resonance of the hair cell (determined by the physical properties of the hair cell and its stereocilia) is coupled to its electrical resonance (determined by the electrical membrane characteristics of the cell). The interaction of these resonances tunes the hair cell to a particular frequency (Figure 32–8). Sound gives rise to traveling waves along the basilar membrane that excite the mechanical resonance of the hair cell. This excitation in turn amplifies the electrical resonance because in each cell both the electrical and mechanical oscillations are tuned to a narrow range of frequencies, and only these frequencies elicit large oscillatory changes in potential. Thus, the hair cell behaves like a tuned amplifier; the coupling of mechanical and electrical resonances optimizes the ability of the cell to transduce the mechanical stimuli of certain frequencies into electrical signals. Mechanical stimulation by frequencies different from the electrical resonance would cause a destructive interference between the mechanical and electrical signals. Inter-

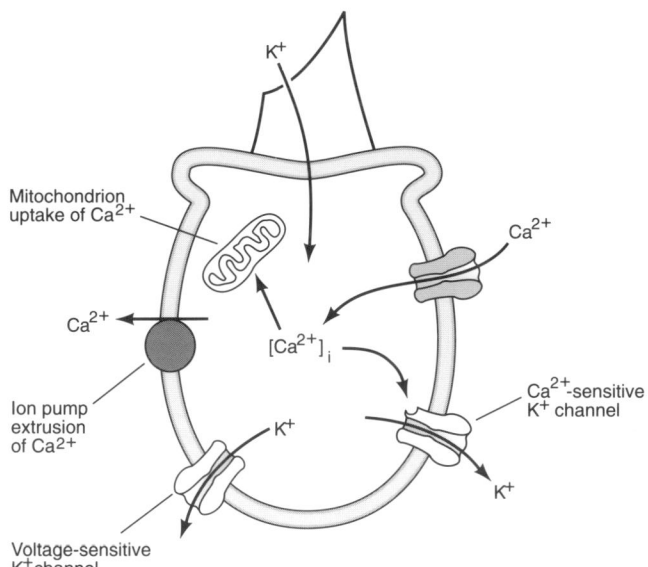

FIGURE 32–8

Individual hair cells have a characteristic electrical resonance due to spontaneous voltage fluctuations around the resting potential. Deflection of the stereocilia bundle mechanically opens ion transduction channels and positive ions enter the cell. Because the endolymph near the stereocilia of the cell has a concentration of K^+ that is greater than the intracellular concentration of K^+, there is an influx of K^+ in this region. The depolarization evoked by this current activates voltage-sensitive Ca^{2+} channels. As Ca^{2+} ions flow into the cell, they augment the depolarization. At the same time, however, the influx of Ca^{2+} raises the intracellular Ca^{2+} concentration, especially the local concentration just beneath the surface membrane. The high $[Ca^{2+}]_i$ brings into play the Ca^{2+}-sensitive K^+ channels, localized along the sides and the base of the cell. Since the fluid bathing this portion of the cell has a lower K^+ concentration, opening these channels causes efflux of K^+ from the cell. As K^+ exits through these pores, it begins to repolarize the membrane, thereby diminishing the activation of Ca^{2+} channels. A voltage-sensitive K^+ channel augments the hyperpolarization. By the time the membrane potential is somewhat more negative than its steady-state value, the intracellular Ca^{2+} concentration is reduced by its sequestration within mitochondria and by its extrusion through ion pumps. As the Ca^{2+}-sensitive K^+ channels close, the cell returns to approximately its initial condition, and another cycle of the electrical resonance commences. The stereocilia presumably have a mechanical resonance at the characteristic frequency of the cell. At this frequency, maximum displacement can be obtained with a minimal expenditure of energy, just as a child on a swing may be pushed almost effortlessly when the push is applied in phase with the oscillating swing. Maximal displacement would open more K^+ channels in the stereocilia, and the resultant receptor potential would be amplified by the oscillating sequence of Ca^{2+} entry and repolarization through Ca^{2+}-sensitive K^+ channels in the sides and bases of the cells. (Adapted from Hudspeth, 1985.)

ference of this kind may sharpen the tuning of hair cells to particular frequencies of mechanical stimulation.

Furthermore, the outer hair cells can alter their length and perhaps other mechanical characteristics, thus changing the tuning of the local region in the organ of Corti. William Brownell and his colleagues have shown that isolated outer hair cells maintained in culture can either increase or decrease the length of their cell bodies in response to transcellular alternating current stimulation. This change in length by the outer hair cells is an example of an active process that occurs within the organ of Corti in response to stimulation.

The whole transduction process can also work in reverse, so that the ear itself produces sounds, termed *otoacoustic emissions*. Hair cells may move, displacing cochlear endolymph and causing a fluid wave that displaces the foot plate of the stapes. This in turn leads to reverse transmission of vibration through the middle ear ossicles to the tympanic membrane. Emitted sounds produced by motion of the tympanic membrane may be recorded in the external ear canal and occur either as an echo in response to sound stimulation or spontaneously, probably as a consequence of spontaneous hair cell motility. Otoacoustic emissions, first described by David Kemp, may provide a simple clinical assay for the integrity of receptor cells and the active processes underlying transduction within the inner ear. *Tinnitus*, or ringing in the ear, may also be related to these emissions, although it is commonly caused by irritation of the auditory nerve.

Vibrations of Hair Cells Are Transformed into Electrical Signals in the Auditory Nerve

The hair cells are innervated by bipolar neurons of the *spiral ganglion* in the modiolus of the cochlea. The peripheral axons of the spiral ganglion cells are activated by transmitter released by the hair cells, and the central processes of these cells make up the auditory nerve. In the human cochlea there are about 33,000 spiral ganglion cells. Approximately 90% of the fibers innervate the inner hair cells; each inner hair cell (there are approximately 3000 in each cochlea) receives contacts from about 10 fibers and each fiber contacts only one inner hair cell. The remaining 10% of the fibers diverge to innervate many outer hair cells (Figure 32–3). Efferent fibers from the central nervous system also synapse on outer hair cells and on the afferent axons innervating inner hair cells.

As we have seen, the outer hair cells can contract the length of their cell bodies, and such changes may affect the mechanical properties of the organ of Corti and produce changes in sensitivity or in tuning. Since the outer hair cells are innervated by efferent fibers from the central nervous system, these changes in length may be under neural control. This system may change the mechanical sensitivity of the end-organ in a manner analogous to the γ efferents and the intrafusal muscle fibers of the muscle spindle that we shall learn about in Chapter 37. The inner hair cells are responsible for the detection of sound and the excitation of most afferent fibers in the auditory nerve. Selective modulation of the properties of outer hair cells, however, may alter the mechanical characteristic of the organ of Corti and provide the brain with a mechanism for tuning the ear to sounds of particular interest. The outer and inner hair cells are coupled through their common insertion into the tectorial membrane, so changes in the properties of outer hair cells may regulate the tuning of inner hair cells. In this way the entire dynamic function of the cochlea may be influenced by the brain.

Since most spiral ganglion cells innervate only a single hair cell, it is not surprising that individual auditory nerve fibers characteristically respond to a particular frequency of sound. By recording the response of a single auditory nerve fiber to brief pulses of sound at various frequencies and amplitudes, a *tuning curve* for the fiber can be established. Tuning curves are plots of the amplitude of sound required to produce detectable responses to various frequencies of sound and thus show the sensitivity of the fiber. Although an individual fiber responds to a range of frequencies (since a substantial portion of the basilar membrane moves in response to a single frequency of sound, even at moderate intensities), it is most sensitive to a particular frequency, its *characteristic frequency*. This tuning corresponds to the tuning of the hair cell that the fiber innervates; fibers innervating hair cells near the oval window at the base of the cochlea have high characteristic frequencies, whereas those innervating hair cells near the apex of the cochlea have low characteristic frequencies. A sample tuning curve for an auditory nerve fiber with a characteristic frequency of 2 kHz is shown in Figure 32–9.

Earlier in the chapter we described the responses of hair cells and afferent fibers in a somewhat simplified way: Coupled oscillations of the receptor potential in the hair cell release a transmitter that excites the afferent fibers. For several reasons the underlying mechanism of hearing is more complicated. First, nerve fibers cannot fire rapidly enough to follow high-frequency sounds by generating one

FIGURE 32–9

Every fiber of the auditory nerve has a characteristic frequency, corresponding to that of the hair cell it innervates. This tuning curve for a fiber with a characteristic frequency of 2 kHz shows its sensitivity to sounds. The fiber's response is just detectable when stimulated with a 2 kHz tone at about 15 dB. At another frequency, about 4 kHz, a much louder sound (nearly 80 dB) is required to elicit a just-detectable response.

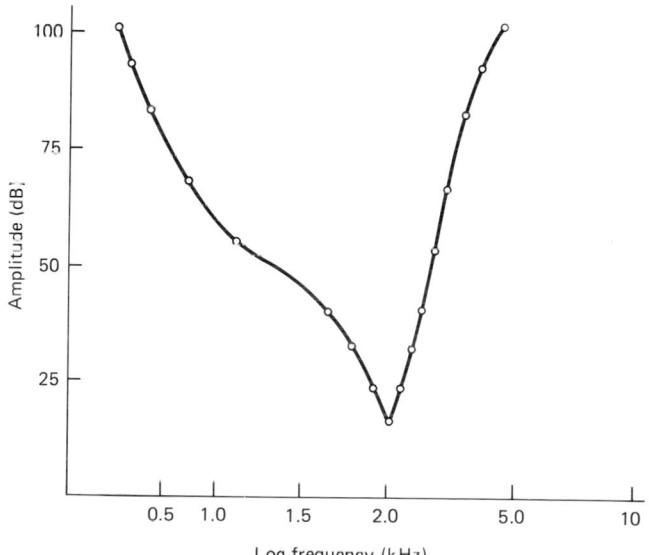

A Tone burst level (dB) above threshold

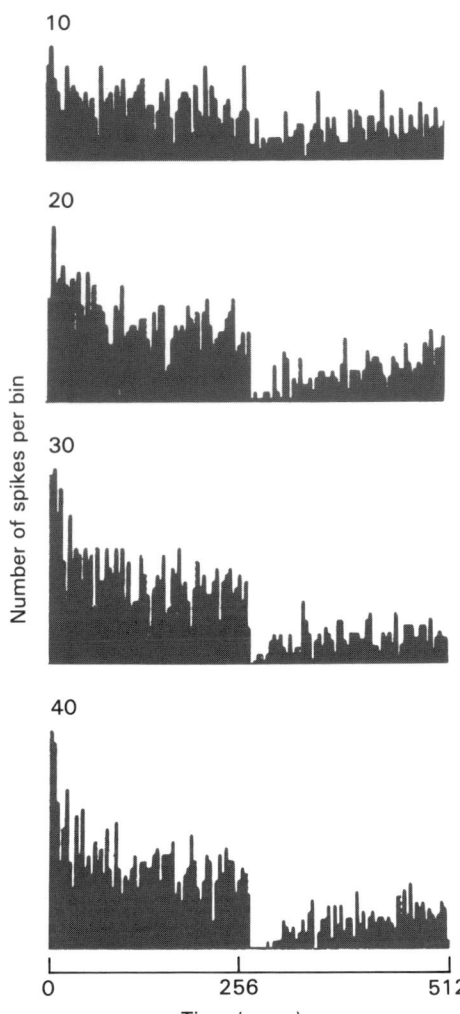

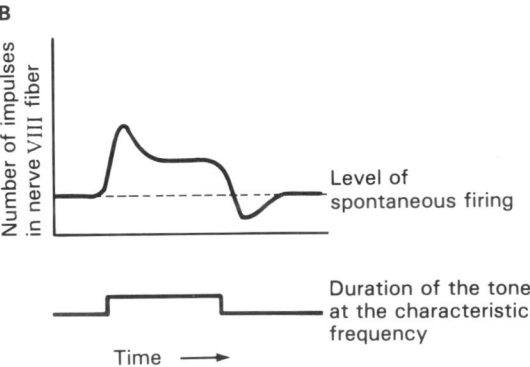

B

FIGURE 32–10

Post-stimulus time histograms show the average response patterns of an auditory nerve fiber to tone bursts as a function of stimulus level.

A. Zero time of each histogram is 2.5 ms before the onset of the electrical input to the earphone. The stimuli were tone bursts at about 5000 kHz (the characteristic frequency of the unit), lasting 250 ms, with a 2.5 ms rise-fall time. The stimulus was followed by a quiet period lasting 250 ms, then was repeated again, over a period of 2 min. The entire sample period is divided into a number of small time units, or bins, and the number of spikes occurring in each bin is measured. The four consecutive responses are averaged bin by bin. There is an initial phasic increase in firing correlated with the onset of the stimulus. A maintained discharge occurs during the course of the stimulus, and there is a decrease in activity following termination. This pattern is evident when the stimulus is >20 dB above threshold. There is a gradual return to baseline activity during the interstimulus interval. (Adapted from Kiang, 1965.)

B. An auditory nerve fiber responds to a pure tone at its characteristic frequency. At the initiation of the tone the firing rate increases above the plateau rate and remains there throughout the tone burst. When the tone ceases, there is a transient decrease to below the spontaneous firing level.

action potential for each cycle of the sound wave. The rate of firing in afferent fibers is limited to about 0.5 kHz because of the refractory period, which lasts approximately 1 ms. Consequently, even if the duration of both the action potential and the refractory period in auditory nerve fibers were reduced, it would still not be possible for the fibers to follow an input greater than 500 Hz with one action potential per cycle. Since the upper range of human hearing extends to frequencies near 20 kHz, some mechanism other than one-to-one firing must be operative. Second, the temporal pattern of the response to a brief tone burst, even at frequencies less than 500 Hz, is not an instantaneous response at the input frequency. The increase in the firing rate of a nerve fiber takes some time to build during the response to a tone, and the pattern of response from one stimulus presentation to the next is not the same. Third, most sounds that are biologically significant to humans, such as speech, contain amplitude-modulated (AM) and frequency-modulated (FM) components, so there should be some mechanism in the auditory system to demodulate these components in order to receive the input signal.

For these reasons an analysis of the responses of auditory nerve fibers requires information about both the average characteristics of the response and its time structure. Computer-based methods that provide this information were first applied to the auditory system by Nelson Kiang and his colleagues.

A *post-stimulus time histogram* is a plot of the average number of spikes recorded in an individual auditory nerve fiber in response to many identical stimuli. The number of spikes is plotted versus time relative to the beginning of the stimulus. Even though each response differs, it is possible to establish the average characteristics of the response using this approach. As illustrated in Figure 32–10, the time structure of the response becomes clearer as the stimulus intensity is increased.

The temporal pattern of the response to a brief tone burst at the characteristic frequency is similar from one auditory nerve fiber to the next. There is an initial phasic increase in firing rate above the spontaneous level, followed by a maintained tonic discharge that persists for the duration of the tone. When the tone is turned off, there is a transient decrease in firing rate below the spontaneous level before the fiber returns to its resting state. This pattern of response is shown schematically in Figure 32–10B.

A *period histogram* shows the probability of firing during a particular phase of the input sound wave. If, for example, a nerve fiber responded selectively to the peak in an input sound wave, there would be a peak at 90° in the period histogram. This preferential firing at a particular point of the sound wave is called *phase locking* and has been observed in auditory nerve fibers at frequencies as high as 8 kHz. Therefore, even though a nerve fiber may not fire in response to each cycle of the sound wave, a period histogram may show that the nerve fiber transmits information about the sound wave by locking its activity to a particular phase of the input waveform.

Since auditory nerve fibers may phase lock to high-frequency sounds without responding to each cycle, it is possible that several fibers firing during different cycles of the stimulus and converging on a central target could provide the brain with input about each cycle of a high-frequency sound. This idea, that auditory nerve fibers work in concert to signal high frequencies, is called the *volley principle*, a theory developed by Glen Weaver. Another theory put forward to explain our sensitivity to different frequencies of sound proposes that a nerve fiber is in some way identified by the site it innervates in the cochlea. This theory, termed the *place principle*, emphasizes the importance of ordered connections between the auditory nerve and the brain as the basis for our ability to detect a broad range of sound frequencies. If the fiber innervates a hair cell located near the base of the cochlea, where high frequencies of sound are transduced, then activity in the fiber would be interpreted by the brain as high-frequency input, while activity in fibers innervating the apex would signal low-frequency input. Fibers inner-

vating intermediate regions of the cochlea would provide a spectrum of input between the extremes of low and high frequency.

The detection of speech waves poses special problems for the ear. Speech sounds are generated by vibrations of the vocal cords, which excite resonances in the vocal tract, principally the mouth and tongue. In effect, the relatively slow vibrations of the mouth and tongue act to modulate the higher-frequency waves produced by the vocal cords. It would be difficult to detect directly the sound produced by vibrations of the mouth and tongue since they occur at about 10 Hz, less than the low-frequency limit of hearing. However, the ear can decode these modulated sounds. First, the sharp tuning of receptor cells and nerve fibers in the ear allows the system to act as a frequency analyzer so that speech *formants*, spectral peaks at particular frequencies that characterize different vowel sounds, are represented in specific temporal and spatial patterns of nerve fiber discharges. Second, an individual fiber may have spectral components in its firing pattern at both the frequency of vocal cord vibration and at the lower modulating frequency imposed on the speech sound by the resonances of mouth and tongue. In this way the ear functions like a demodulator in a radio to extract significant low-frequency information from a high frequency carrier wave.

Central Auditory Neurons Are Specialized Physiologically to Preserve Time and Frequency Information

Auditory fibers in the eighth nerve terminate in the *cochlear nucleus*, lying on the external aspect of the inferior cerebellar peduncle (Figure 32–11). The cochlear nucleus is divided into dorsal and ventral divisions. Auditory

FIGURE 32–11

This myelin-stained section through the lower pons shows the location of the cochlear nucleus on the external aspect of the inferior cerebellar peduncle. (Adapted from Ranson and Clark, 1953.)

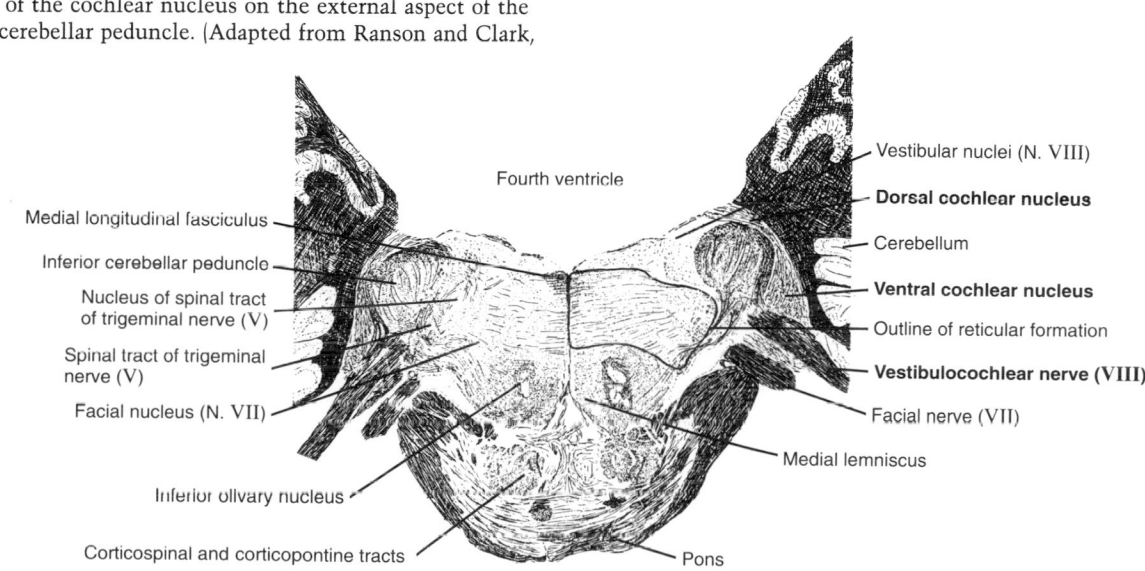

Medial longitudinal fasciculus
Inferior cerebellar peduncle
Nucleus of spinal tract of trigeminal nerve (V)
Spinal tract of trigeminal nerve (V)
Facial nucleus (N. VII)
Inferior olivary nucleus
Corticospinal and corticopontine tracts

Fourth ventricle

Vestibular nuclei (N. VIII)
Dorsal cochlear nucleus
Cerebellum
Ventral cochlear nucleus
Outline of reticular formation
Vestibulocochlear nerve (VIII)
Facial nerve (VII)
Medial lemniscus
Pons

nerve fibers enter the ventral division at about the middle of its rostrocaudal extent, thereby separating the ventral division into an *anteroventral* and a *posteroventral cochlear nucleus*. Each auditory nerve fiber branches as it enters the cochlear nucleus. An ascending branch innervates the anteroventral nucleus, and a descending branch innervates the posteroventral and dorsal cochlear nuclei.

The most important principle governing the topography of the cochlear nucleus is the *tonotopic organization* of its cells and fibers. Primary auditory fibers that innervate the base of the cochlea penetrate deeply into the nucleus before terminating in its three principal divisions. Primary axons that innervate the apex of the cochlea terminate at more superficial levels in the nucleus. Fibers that innervate the middle region of the cochlea terminate in an ordered array between these two extremes.

Donata Oertel and her colleagues have approached the study of this portion of the auditory system in a novel way by recording the electrical properties of cells in tissue slices cut from the cochlear nucleus and maintained in culture. The two main cell types of the ventral cochlear nucleus, stellate cells and bushy cells, could be identified by injecting them with dye while making intracellular recordings. When a stellate cell is depolarized by a steady current pulse, the cell generates a spaced series of action potentials at regular intervals, termed a *chopper response*. Therefore, stellate cells fire at a regular rate during sound stimulation in spite of any slight asynchrony in the inputs. Because the frequency of the chopper response varies from one stellate cell to the next, different sets of cells signal the different frequency components in the sound stimulus. In contrast, when bushy cells are stimulated with a steady depolarizing current pulse, they generate only one or two spikes at the beginning of the pulse. Therefore, bushy cells signal the onset of a sound, and are most concerned with timing information which, as we shall see, is important for the localization of the sound (Figure 32–12).

FIGURE 32–12

Comparison of the shapes of stellate cells and bushy cells in the ventral cochlear nucleus and their response to brief current pulses. (Adapted from Oertel et al., 1988.)

A. The stellate cells of the cochlear nucleus have several dendrites. Numerous small synaptic terminals establish contacts with the dendrites of each cell. The responses of a stellate cell to brief (less than 40 ms) depolarizing and hyperpolarizing current pulses (0.4 nA) are shown. Depolarizing pulses cause the cell to fire repetitively at a fixed frequency, the so-called *chopper response*.

B. Bushy cells have a single dendritic trunk and establish contact with a few very large terminals called end bulbs that surround the cell. Bushy cells respond to a depolarizing current pulse with a single action potential. These cells therefore signal the onset or timing of a sound. Bushy cells respond like stellate cells to hyperpolarizing currents.

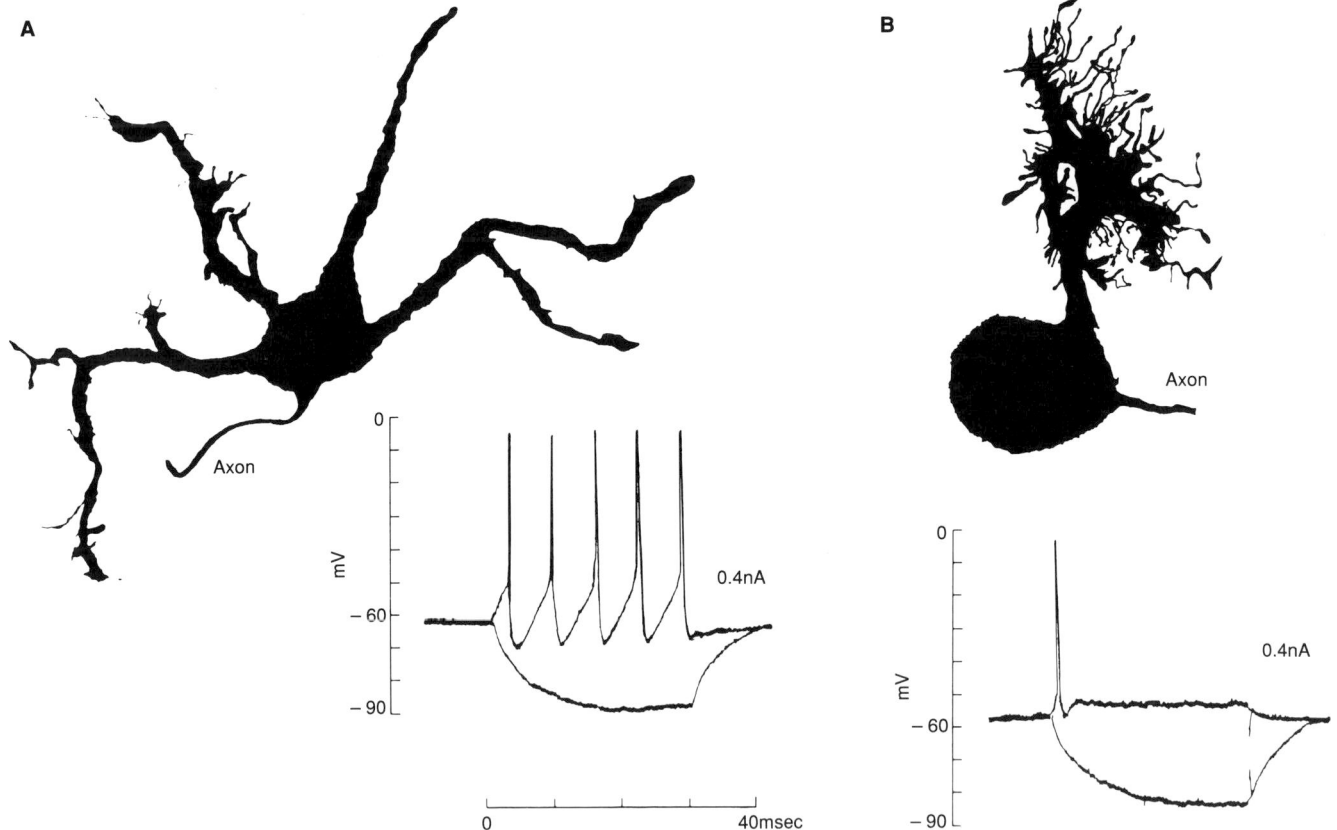

Bilateral Auditory Pathways Provide Cues to Localize Sound

To understand the organization of the projections that leave the cochlear nuclei and ascend to the auditory cortex, particularly the extensive crossing that occurs in these projections, it is necessary to consider the binaural interactions underlying sound localization. The localization of sounds in space is achieved in the brain by comparison of differences in the intensity and timing of sounds received in each ear. These two cues for localization, time and intensity, are related to the frequency of the sound to be localized. A *brief* sound, a click for example, originating on one side would strike the ear on that side first and then, after a delay, strike the ear on the opposite side. The duration of the delay is determined by the distance between the two ears, the speed of sound, and the location of the sound source. If the sound source were located along the midline, either in front or in back of the head, the sound would strike the two ears simultaneously and the delay would be zero. At 90° to the right or left the interaural delay would reach a maximal value of approximately 50 μs. At points between these extremes there is a spectrum of *interaural time difference*. For low frequencies of sound (<1400 Hz), a *continuous tone* can be localized on the basis of a phase difference that results from a difference in the time of the arrival of the sound wave at the two ears. At higher frequencies, where the wavelength of the sound is less than the distance between the ears, the phase or time difference of a continuous tone becomes ambiguous, because multiple cycles of the sound wave are possible between the ears and the brain cannot detect whether the phase difference is within one cycle or between multiple cycles. At these frequencies, however, the head acts as a sound shield, reflecting and absorbing the shorter wavelengths of sound to produce an *interaural intensity difference*.

Marc Konishi and his colleagues have analyzed the neural mechanisms underlying sound localization using the owl's brain as a model system. Neurons concerned with the detection of interaural timing differences are found in the laminar nucleus, a part of the central auditory pathway in the medulla of the bird's brain. This bilateral nucleus receives fibers from the cochlear nuclei on either side and is organized tonotopically into a number of isofrequency zones, where the neurons and fibers share the same characteristic frequency. When a recording electrode is advanced through each isofrequency zone to record the response of successive fibers to a sound stimulus, orderly shifts in the time of arrival of spikes phase-locked to the sound stimulus are observed. Neurons in the isofrequency zones act as coincidence detectors by integrating inputs from fibers at the same frequency but at different interaural delays. Therefore, frequency and time are mapped along orthogonal axes in the *timing pathway* of the brain (Figure 32–13).

Interaural differences in sound intensity are analyzed using excitatory and inhibitory interactions between in-

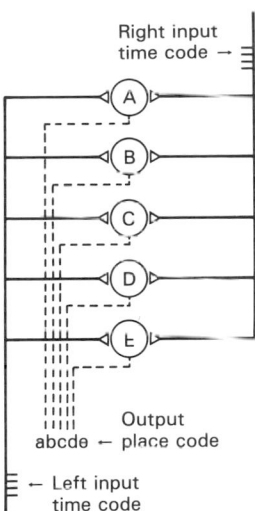

FIGURE 32–13

Model of neural circuits for measuring and encoding interaural time differences. The binaural neurons **A–E** fire maximally when signals from the two sources arrive simultaneously. Thus, the neurons serve as coincidence detectors. In the model, delays in signal transmission are a function of the variable lengths of the incoming axons. The axonal paths to the binaural neurons (**solid lines**) increase systematically along the array but in opposite directions for the left and right channels. This pattern of innervation creates left-right asymmetries in transmission delays. When binaural disparities in acoustic signals exactly compensate for these asymmetries, the neurons fire maximally. For example, if sound were to arrive at the two ears simultaneously, neuron C in the array would be excited by coincident inputs. If sound to the left ear were delayed, neurons D or E would be excited depending on the duration of the delay. The output axons (**dotted lines**) project to higher centers in the brain. Only the place of a neuron in the array determines the interaural time difference to which the neuron responds maximally. (Adapted from Konishi et al., 1988.)

puts from the two ears in the *intensity pathway* of the bird's brain. Neurons in the principal relay nucleus of this pathway are excited by contralateral stimulation and inhibited by ipsilateral stimulation of the ear. When both ears are stimulated equally, excitation and inhibition from the inputs balance, and there is little response in the postsynaptic cell. However, when sound amplitude is decreased in one ear, neurons in the intensity pathway on the same side respond, since excitatory input from the opposite side would remain the same while inhibition would be decreased (Figure 32–14). Neurons in this pathway are arranged according to the specific interaural intensity difference to which they are most responsive. At higher levels of the bird's brain the timing and intensity pathways converge upon neurons that are broadly tuned in frequency but specific in spatial localization of sound.

Similar time and intensity pathways exist in the mammalian brain. Axons from the cochlear nuclei project to several brain stem auditory nuclei and thus there are

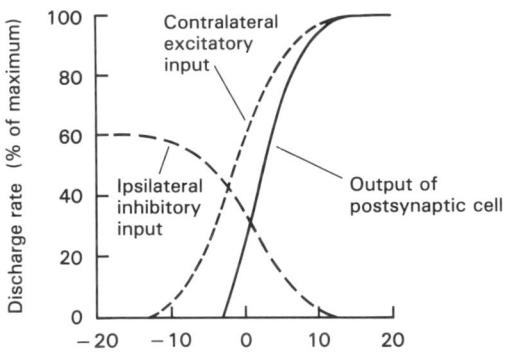

FIGURE 32–14

A neural model of excitatory and inhibitory interactions underlying sound localization through the detection of interaural differences in sound intensity. A difference of 0 dB between the stimuli to the two ears indicates the input to both ears is the same in amplitude and frequency. A negative interaural intensity difference means that the stimulus to the ipsilateral inhibitory ear is increased while the stimulus to the contralateral excitatory ear is decreased. For a −10 dB intensity difference, for example, the intensity to the ipsilateral ear is increased by 5 dB, while the stimulus to the contralateral ear is decreased by 5 dB, and the average intensity of the stimuli to the two ears remains constant. The dynamic range of the postsynaptic cell is approximately 20 dB. This means that the cell shows a pronounced change in firing rate if the interaural intensity difference is varied by approximately ±10 dB with respect to zero interaural difference. When the intensity difference is −20 dB, the cell shows no response because the stimulus is loudest in the ipsilateral ear, and inhibition dominates. As the stimulus to the excitatory ear is increased, and the stimulus to the inhibitory ear decreased, the cell begins to respond. The slope of the solid curve is greatest near 0 dB, indicating that the postsynaptic cell is most sensitive to slight differences in intensity between the two ears. (Adapted from Manley et al., 1988.)

many possibilities for interconnections among the relay nuclei.

The axons of cells in the cochlear nucleus stream out along three pathways: the *dorsal acoustic stria*, the *intermediate acoustic stria*, and the *trapezoid body* (Figure 32–15). The most important pathway is the trapezoid body. It contains fibers destined for the *superior olivary nuclei* on both sides of the brain stem. The *medial superior olive* is concerned with sound localization on the basis of interaural time differences. This nucleus is composed of spindle-shaped neurons with one medial and one lateral dendrite, which receive input from the contralateral and ipsilateral cochlear nuclei, respectively. The binaural cells in the medial superior olive are very sensitive to phase differences between continuous tones presented to the two ears. The *lateral superior olive* is concerned with interaural differences in sound intensity.

Axons arising from the superior olivary nuclei join the crossed and uncrossed axons from the cochlear nucleus to form the *lateral lemniscus*. Thus, from the outset there is

extensive bilateral auditory input in the central nervous system, so that lesions of the central auditory pathway do not cause monaural disability. The lateral lemniscus courses through the *nuclei of the lateral lemniscus*, where some fibers synapse. Here again there is extensive crossing between the two sides through *Probst's commissure*. All fibers in the lateral lemniscus eventually synapse in the *inferior colliculus*. The cells of the inferior colliculus receive binaural input and are arranged tonotopically. Most of the cells in the inferior colliculus send their axons to the *medial geniculate body* of the thalamus on the same side of the brain. The cells in the medial geniculate body send their axons to the ipsilateral *primary auditory cortex* in the superior temporal gyrus (Brodmann's areas 41 and 42).

The Auditory Cortex Is Composed of Separate Functional Areas

The primary auditory cortex contains several distinct tonotopic maps of the frequency spectrum, analogous to the multiple representations of the periphery in the somatic sensory and visual cortices. The different layers of the auditory cortex establish patterns of connections with other regions of the brain in a manner that also is similar to other primary cortical areas. Layer IV, for example, is the input layer, layer V projects back to the medial geniculate nucleus, and layer VI projects back to the inferior colliculus.

Several aspects of the organization of the primate auditory cortex, studied by John Brugge and his colleagues, are of particular interest. First, like the somatic sensory and visual cortices, the auditory cortex is functionally organized into columns. Binaural cells are found clustered into two alternating columnar groups, *summation columns* and *suppression columns*, running from the pial surface to the underlying white matter. Most cells within a column display similar binaural interactions. In summation columns the response of a cell to binaural input is greater than to monaural input. In suppression columns input from one ear is dominant; the response of a cell to input from the dominant ear is greater than to binaural input. Columns of this kind may be related to spatial maps of sound localization in the cortex.

Second, the auditory cortex has important callosal connections. Zones that receive callosal connections are interspersed with zones that do not receive them. The two types of zones, which branch and appear to join one another occasionally in a manner similar to the ocular dominance columns of the visual cortex (see Chapter 29), may be the anatomical subdivisions of binaural interaction columns.

Third, because of the extensive inputs from each ear in both hemispheres, unilateral lesions of the auditory cortex do not dramatically disrupt the perception of sound frequency, although they do affect the ability to localize sounds in space. Each hemisphere is concerned principally with localizing sounds on the contralateral side. To localize the position of a sound source, the auditory cortex uses

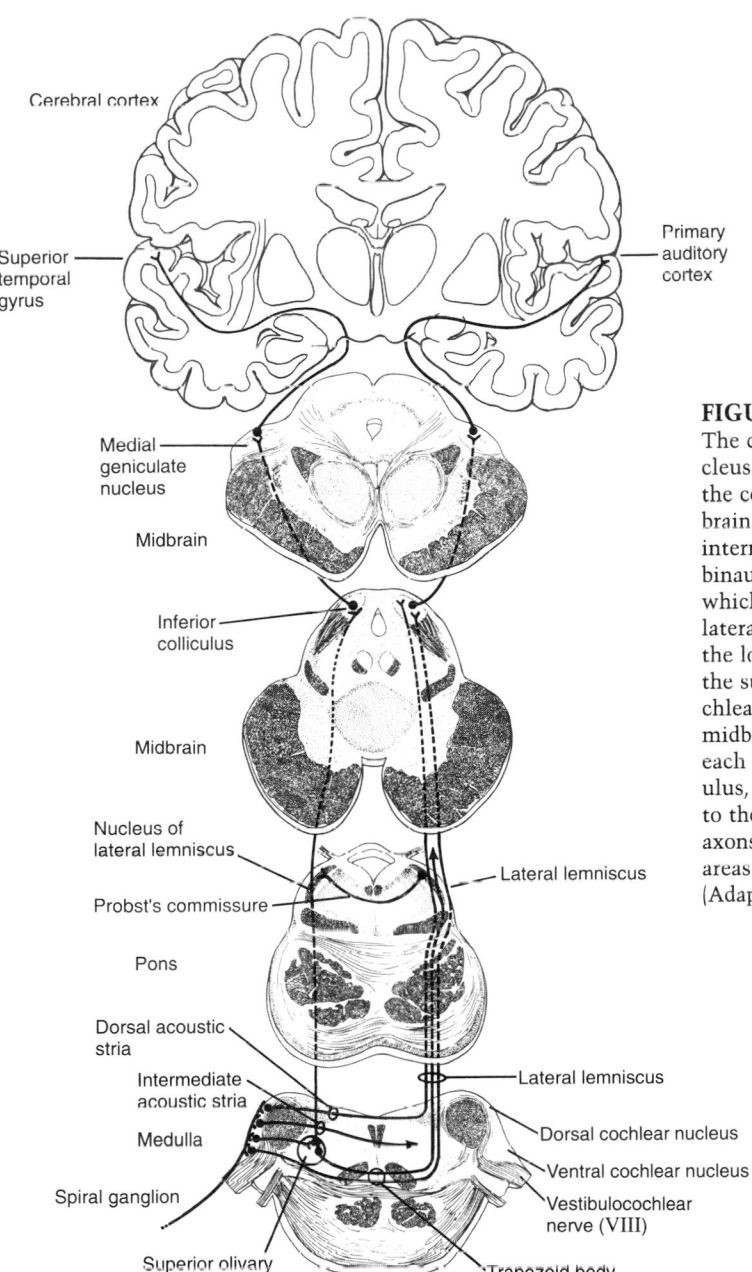

FIGURE 32–15

The central auditory pathways extend from the cochlear nucleus to the primary auditory cortex. Postsynaptic neurons in the cochlear nucleus send their axons to other centers in the brain via three main pathways: the dorsal acoustic stria, the intermediate acoustic stria, and the trapezoid body. The first binaural interactions occur in the superior olivary nucleus, which receives input via the trapezoid body. The medial and lateral divisions of the superior olivary nucleus are involved in the localization of sounds in space. Postsynaptic axons from the superior olivary nucleus, along with axons from the cochlear nuclei, form the lateral lemniscus, which ascends to the midbrain. Axons relaying input from both ears are found in each lateral lemniscus. The axons synapse in the inferior colliculus, and postsynaptic cells in the colliculus send their axons to the medial geniculate body of the thalamus. The geniculate axons terminate in the primary auditory cortex (Brodmann's areas 41 and 42), a part of the superior temporal gyrus. (Adapted from Brodal, 1981.)

the cues of interaural differences in intensity and time of arrival of sound. However, only large lesions of the auditory cortex affect this ability to any significant extent. In this way the auditory cortex differs from the primary visual cortex, where even small lesions produce noticeable deficits in vision.

In addition to cortical areas important for the representation of sound frequency and localization, the human cerebral cortex contains functional areas in the frontal and temporal lobes (Broca's area and Wernicke's area) related to the perception of speech sounds. Speech functions are unique to the human brain, and therefore it is not imme-

diately evident if an animal model is suitable for the study of neuronal interactions underlying speech perception. Oddly enough, the neural machinery in echolocating bats uses many of the same sound cues known to be important for speech.

Bats locate prey by emitting sounds and analyzing the echoes from these sounds. Nobuo Suga and his colleagues have made a thorough study of the central neural pathways involved in echolocation and found that the sounds emitted by echolocating bats have two principal components: (1) a *constant frequency component* similar to the formants in vowel sounds, and (2) a *frequency*

FIGURE 32–16

The mustached bat analyzes the echo of its own emitted sounds to determine the location and size of objects. (Adapted from Suga, 1988.)

A. Schematized sonogram of the mustached bat orientation sound (**solid lines**) and the Doppler-shifted echo (**dashed lines**). The orientation sound is also called a pulse. The four harmonics (**H**) of both the orientation sound and the echo each contain a long constant frequency component (**CF**) and a short frequency modulated component (**FM**). The relative amplitude of each harmonic in the orientation sound differs: H_2 is the strongest, followed by H_3 (6–12 dB weaker than H_2), H_4 (12–24 dB weaker than H_2), and H_1 (18–26 dB weaker than H_2).

B. As the mustached bat flies at a constant speed toward a stationary object, the frequency of the echo (**dashed line**) becomes higher than the frequency of the emitted sound (**solid line**). The difference in frequency between the two arrowheads indicates the extent of the Doppler shift, a measure of the bat's velocity during approach to a stationary target.

C. Target size is determined from both target range and subtended angle.

D. Relationship between echo properties and target properties. As noted in C, the Doppler shift provides a measure of the relative velocity of the bat with respect to the target. The amplitude of the echo is greater for the targets that subtend larger angles. The delay in the echo indicates the distance or range of the target from the bat. When both the subtended angle and the range are known, the absolute size of the target may be estimated. The amplitude spectrum or modulation of the echo indicates details about the surface contours of the target. Interaural time or amplitude differences in the echo are binaural cues that indicate the

azimuth or position of the target on the horizontal axis. Reflections of sound within the pinna and tragus are cues used to locate the target in the vertical axis.

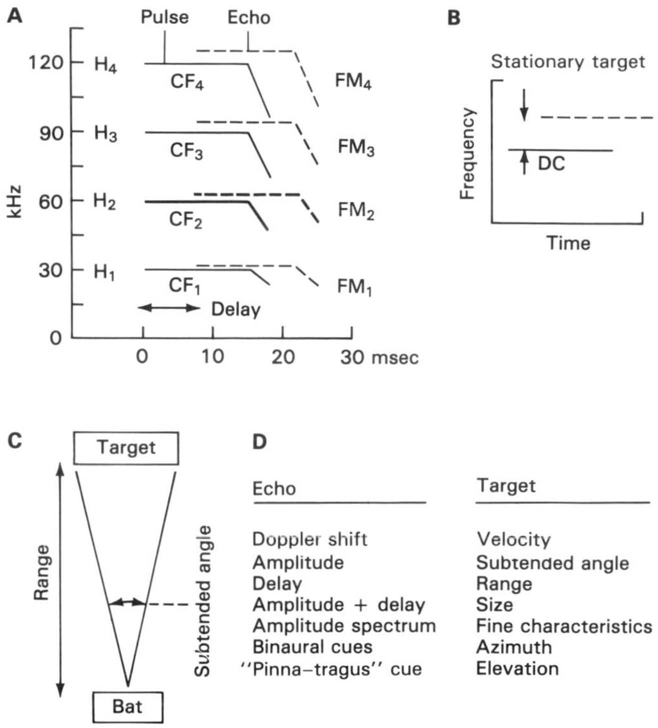

modulated component similar to the changing frequencies in consonants.

The frequency of a sound changes as a result of motion of either the source or receiver. This Doppler shift in frequency is experienced in everyday life as the increasing pitch of an automobile horn as it approaches and the decreasing pitch as it moves away. The bat uses the Doppler shift in the constant frequency component to determine the velocity of the prey. For example, if the prey is flying toward the bat, the constant frequency component in the emitted sound will be shifted to a slightly higher frequency in the reflected sound. The degree of shift is determined by the relative velocity of the bat and its prey. The bat uses the frequency-modulated component to estimate the range or distance of the prey by determining the time delay between emission and reflection. Each emitted sound has four constant frequency components that are harmonics or integral multiples of the lowest frequency, and four frequency-modulated components, one related to each of the constant frequencies (Figure 32–16). Between the emitted sound and the echo, therefore, the bat must distinguish 16 components to gauge the velocity and distance of the prey! This is qualitatively similar to the task of perceiving the subtleties in speech sounds.

The bat's cerebral cortex is composed of distinct areas that represent the constant frequency and frequency-modulated components of emitted sounds and their echoes (Figure 32–17). Neurons in the *constant frequency area* respond selectively to combinations of two frequencies: a constant frequency in the emitted sound and the Doppler-shifted echo. Neurons in this area are arranged in bands according to the frequency of the emitted component. Neurons within each band are excited by echo components that differ slightly in frequency and correspond to the differences in Doppler shift that would be produced by prey moving at different velocities. Neurons in the *frequency-modulation area* respond only to a pair of frequency-modulated sounds separated by a time delay between 0.4 and 18 ms. These neurons serve as range finders to detect the delay between the time of sound emission and reception of the echo.

Thus, as is the case with somatic sensation and vision, the brain has parallel pathways for processing auditory information, and these pathways project to areas in the cortex that process several aspects of sound. Some areas in the primate brain appear to receive information on both frequency and location of sound, both of which are critical to the perception of music. There is strong evidence that the bat's cerebral cortex includes areas where harmonic combinations of frequencies are represented. Although no

A

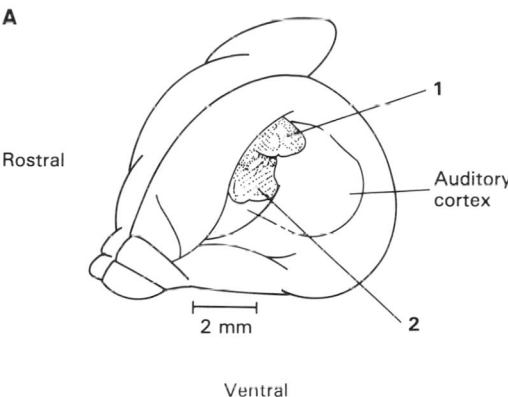

Rostral

1

Auditory cortex

2 mm

2

Ventral

B

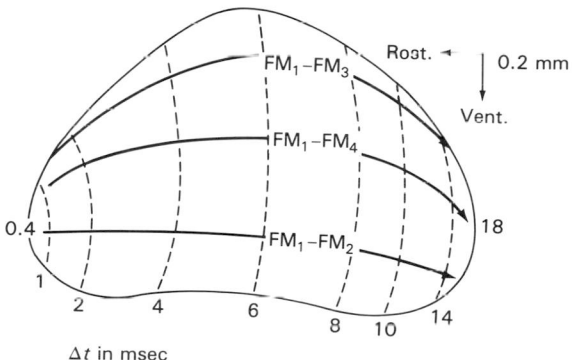

Rost.

0.2 mm

Vent.

FM₁–FM₃

FM₁–FM₄

FM₁–FM₂

0.4

1

2   4   6   8   10   14

18

Δt in msec

C₁   Tonotopic representation

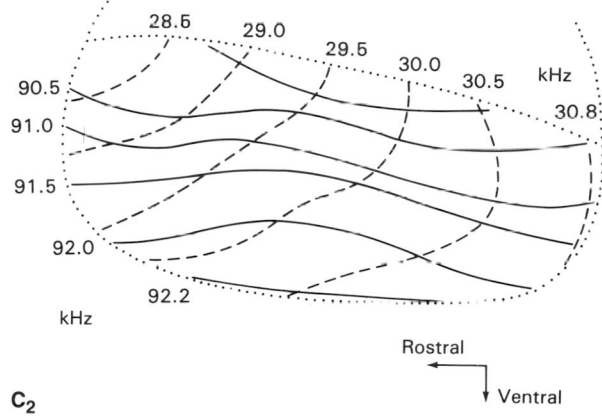

28.5   29.0   29.5   30.0   30.5   kHz

90.5
91.0
91.5
92.0
92.2

30.8

kHz

Rostral

Ventral

C₂

Iso–velocity contours

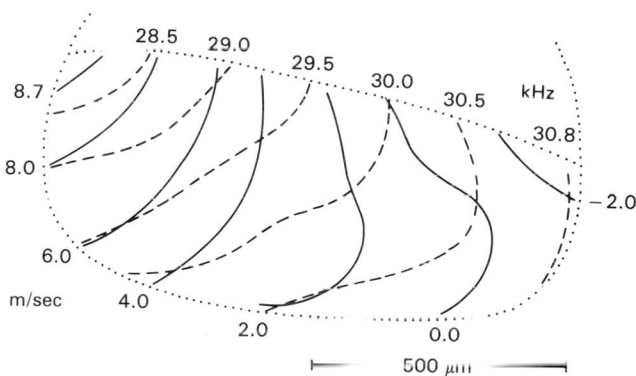

28.5   29.0   29.5   30.0   30.5   kHz

8.7
8.0
6.0
4.0
2.0   0.0

30.8

–2.0

m/sec

500 μm

FIGURE 32–17

The auditory cortex of the echolocating bat has several distinct functional areas for processing complex sounds. (Adapted from Suga, 1988.)

A. This view of the cerebral hemisphere of the mustached bat shows the auditory cortex and two functional areas within it: the frequency modulation area, where the range of a target is computed (**1**), and the constant frequency area, where the velocity of a target is computed (**2**).

B. The functional organization of the frequency modulation area. The differences in time between emitted sound and echo for three pairs of frequency modulation sweeps are represented in this area. Each pair is represented in a strip of cells running from rostral to caudal (**solid lines**). The difference in timing (Δt) between emission and echo is represented in cells along the orthogonal axis from dorsal to ventral (**dashed lines**). The range of timing differences is 0.4–18 ms, corresponding to a range in distance of 7–310 cm.

C. The functional organization of the constant frequency area. **1.** The tonotopic organization of the area. Cells respond best to combinations of two tones that are close, but not exact, pairs in a harmonic series. In a harmonic series ascending frequencies are integral multiples of a fundamental frequency, for example 30 kHz, 60 kHz, and 90 kHz. The cells in the constant frequency area respond best when the two tones from the harmonic series are mismatched in frequency. This shift corresponds to the Doppler shift or increase in frequency that would occur as the bat flies toward a target. Cells in this particular area respond best to an emitted tone of 28.5–30.8 kHz in combination with a second tone of 90.5–92.2 kHz corresponding to a Doppler-shifted echo. **2.** The Doppler shift in the echo can be converted to a map of target velocity. If the emitted sound and the echo have an exact harmonic relation, there is no velocity difference between the bat and its target. The cells in this area can detect velocities ranging from 0.0 to 8.7 meters per second.

such cells have yet been found in the human brain, they would be ideal detectors of the multiple frequencies in the speech sounds produced by the human voice.

In addition to parallel pathways, the auditory system has an extensive set of *feedback connections*. As we have seen, some cells in the auditory cortex send their axons back to the medial geniculate nucleus, and some back to

the inferior colliculus. The inferior colliculus in turn sends recurrent fibers to the cochlear nucleus. A cluster of cells near the superior olivary complex gives rise to the efferent *olivocochlear bundle*, which terminates either on the hair cells of the cochlea directly or on the afferent fibers innervating them. These connections may be important for regulating attention to particular sounds by modulating the transduction mechanism in the organ of Corti.

An Overall View

The auditory system, composed of the ear and the auditory pathways of the brain, enables us to detect the frequency composition of sound and to locate sound sources despite the fact that the energy in a sound wave, even a loud one, is exceedingly small and most sounds are composed of a multitude of different frequencies in the midst of a noisy environment. This remarkable signal analysis is accomplished by the sophisticated mechanoelectric transduction system of the inner ear working in conjunction with neural systems of the brain that compare signals from the two ears. No man-made technology currently available can match the human auditory system in sensitivity and dynamic range. Humans are capable of detecting sounds ranging from 20 to 20,000 Hz, over a million-fold range of intensities, with a spatial resolution as great as one degree of arc. This is a consequence of the mechanical design of the ear and the specificity of wiring in the brain.

The external ear and the middle ear form collectively a mechanical transmission system that converts sounds, or air pressure waves, into fluid waves in the inner ear. The receptors of the inner ear, the hair cells, act like miniature amplifiers, each tuned mechanically to provide a maximal electrical response when vibrated at a particular frequency by the fluid waves of the inner ear. The hair cells are a set of frequency filters ordered spatially within the cochlea; those with high-pass frequencies occupy the bass, and those with low-pass frequencies occupy the apex. Sensory transduction occurs in the organ of Corti, where the hair cells interact with supporting elements to convert fluid waves into the bending of the hair bundles and resultant ion influxes. The organ itself is under dynamic control from the brain, so it may be tuned to sounds of particular interest.

Signal coding occurs initially at the synapse between the hair cells and the fibers of the auditory nerve. Using only the digital code of action potentials, the nerve provides a profile of sound input, including the spectrum of frequencies, the phase or timing relations of different frequency components, and their relative amplitudes. Given the complexity of the information encoded, it is not surprising that this code is not understood completely. It seems clear, however, that there is a relationship between the site a nerve fiber innervates in the cochlea and the frequency characteristics of the fiber. Thus, each fiber responds best to a very narrow band of frequencies, although most fibers are excited to some extent by a wide range of frequencies.

In the brain, inputs from the two ears are combined by ascending pathways that cross the midline extensively. The pathways separate information about the *timing* and the *intensity* of signals, the binaural cues for sound localization. The information ascends in parallel to the auditory cortex where the timing, intensity, and frequency of the sound are mapped. The diversity of separate areas within the auditory cortex reflects the complexity of the task underlying perception of complex sounds. As in the visual cortex, where form, color, and stereopsis are processed in separate areas, in the auditory cortex separate functional regions deconstruct speech into components to generate a perception of location, loudness, and pitch.

Selected Readings

Black, H. S. 1953. Modulation Theory. New York: Van Nostrand.

Brodal, A. 1981. Neurological Anatomy in Relation to Clinical Medicine, 3rd ed. New York: Oxford University Press, chap. 9, "The Auditory System."

Goldstein, M. H., Jr. 1980. The auditory periphery. In V. B. Mountcastle (ed.), Medical Physiology, 14th ed., Vol. 1. St. Louis: Mosby, pp. 428–456.

Helmholtz, H. L. F. 1877. On the Sensations of Tone as a Physiological Basis for the Theory of Music. (2nd English ed.). New York: Dover, 1954.

Hudspeth, A. J. 1983. Transduction and tuning by vertebrate hair cells. Trends Neurosci. 6:366–369.

Imig, T. J., and Adrián, H. O. 1977. Binaural columns in the primary field (A1) of cat auditory cortex. Brain Res. 138:241–257.

Imig, T. J., and Brugge, J. F. 1978. Sources and terminations of callosal axons related to binaural and frequency maps in primary auditory cortex of the cat. J. Comp. Neurol. 182:637–660.

Khanna, S. M., and Leonard, D. G. B. 1982. Basilar membrane tuning in the cat cochlea. Science 215:305–306.

Kiang, N. Y.-S. 1965. Discharge Patterns of Single Fibers in the Cat's Auditory Nerve. Cambridge, Mass.: MIT Press.

Konishi, M., Takahashi, T. T., Wagner, H., Sullivan, W. E., and Carr, C. E., 1988. Neurophysiological and anatomical substrates of sound localization in the owl. In G. M. Edelman, W. E. Gall, and W. M. Cowan (eds.), Auditory Function: Neurobiological Bases of Hearing. New York: Wiley, pp. 721–745.

Lorente de Nó, R. 1933. Anatomy of the eighth nerve. III. General plan of structure of the primary cochlear nuclei. Laryngoscope 43:327–350.

Merzenich, M. M., and Reid, M. D. 1974. Representation of the cochlea within the inferior colliculus of the cat. Brain Res. 77:397–415.

Morest, D. K. 1964. The laminar structure of the inferior colliculus of the cat. Anat. Rec. 148:314.

Rhode, W. S. 1971. Observations of the vibration of the basilar membrane in squirrel monkeys using the Mössbauer technique. J. Acoust. Soc. Am. 49:1218–1231.

Suga, N. 1988. Auditory neuroethology and speech processing: Complex-sound processing by combination-sensitive neurons. In G. M. Edelman, W. E. Gall, and W. M. Cowan (eds.), Auditory Function: Neurobiological Bases of Hearing. New York: Wiley, pp. 679–720.

References

Art, J. J., Fettiplace, R., and Fuchs, P. A. 1984. Synaptic hyperpolarization and inhibition of turtle cochlear hair cells. J. Physiol. (Lond.) 356:525–550.

Bloom, W., and Fawcett, D. W. 1975. A Textbook of Histology, 10th ed. Philadelphia: Saunders.

Brawer, J. R., Morest, D. K., and Kane, E. C. 1974. The neuronal architecture of the cochlear nucleus of the cat. J. Comp. Neurol. 155:251–300.

Brownell, W. E., Bader, C. R., Bertrand, D., and de Ribaupierre, Y. 1985. Evoked mechanical responses of isolated cochlear outer hair cells. Science 227:194–196.

Brugge, J. F., and Merzenich, M. M. 1973. Responses of neurons in auditory cortex of the macaque monkey to monaural and binaural stimulation. J. Neurophysiol. 36:1138–1158.

Carr, C., and Konishi, M. 1988. Axonal delay lines for time measurement in the owl's brainstem. Proc. Natl. Acad. Sci. U.S.A. 85:8311–8315.

Crawford, A. C., and Fettiplace, R. 1981. An electrical tuning mechanism in turtle cochlear hair cells. J. Physiol. (Lond.) 312:377–412.

Goldberg, J. M., and Brown, P. B. 1969. Response of binaural neurons of dog superior olivary complex to dichotic tonal stimuli: Some physiological mechanisms of sound localization. J. Neurophysiol. 32:613–636.

Hudspeth, A. J. 1985. The cellular basis of hearing: The biophysics of hair cells. Science 230:745–752.

Hudspeth, A. J., and Lewis, R. S. 1988. Kinetic analysis of voltage- and ion-dependent conductances in saccular hair cells of the bull-frog, *Rana catesbeiana*. J. Physiol. (Lond.) 400:237–274.

Hudspeth, A. J., and Lewis, R. S. 1988. A model for electrical resonance and frequency tuning in saccular hair cells of the bull-frog, *Rana catesbeiana*. J. Physiol. (Lond.) 400:275–297.

Junqueira, L. C., Carneiro, J., and Contopoulos, A. N. 1977. Basic Histology, 2nd ed. Los Altos, Calif: Lange Medical Publications.

Kemp, D. T. 1978. Stimulated acoustic emissions from within the human auditory system. J. Acoust. Soc. Am. 64:1386–1391.

Lewis, R. S., and Hudspeth, A. J. 1983. Frequency tuning and ionic conductances in hair cells of the bullfrog's sacculus. In R. Klinke and R. Hartmann (eds.), Hearing—Physiological Bases and Psychophysics. Berlin: Springer, pp. 17–24.

Manley, G. A., Köppl, C., and Konishi, M. 1988. A neural map of interaural intensity differences in the brain stem of the barn owl. J. Neurosci. 8:2665–2676.

Miller, J. M., and Towe, A. L. 1979. Audition: Structural and acoustical properties. In T. Ruch and H. D. Patton (eds.), Physiology and Biophysics, Vol. 1. The Brain and Neural Function, 20th ed. Philadelphia: Saunders, pp. 339–375.

Oertel, D., Wu, S. H., and Hirsch, J. A. 1988. Electrical characteristics of cells and neuronal circuitry in the cochlear nuclei studied with intracellular recordings from brain slices. In G. M. Edelman, W. E. Gall, and W. M. Cowan (eds.), Auditory Function: Neurobiological Bases of Hearing. New York: Wiley, pp. 313–336.

Ranson, S. W., and Clark, S. L. 1953. The Anatomy of the Nervous System: Its Development and Function, 9th ed. Philadelphia: Saunders.

Stotler, W. A. 1953. An experimental study of the cells and connections of the superior olivary complex of the cat. J. Comp. Neurol. 98:401–431.

von Békésy, G. 1960. Experiments in Hearing. E. G. Wever (ed. and trans.) New York: McGraw-Hill.

Wersäll, J., Flock, Å., and Lundquist, P.-G. 1965. Structural basis for directional sensitivity in cochlear and vestibular sensory receptors. Cold Spring Harbor Symp. Quant. Biol. 30:115–132.

33

James P. Kelly

The Sense of Balance

The Organs of Balance Are Located in the Inner Ear

The Vestibular Labyrinth Is Filled with Endolymph

Specialized Regions of the Vestibular Labyrinth Contain Hair Cells

Vestibular Hair Cells Respond to Changes in Movement or Position of the Head

The Hair Cells Are Polarized Structurally and Functionally

The Semicircular Ducts Respond to Angular Acceleration in Specific Directions

The Utricle Responds to Linear Acceleration in All Directions

The Central Connections of the Vestibular Labyrinth Reflect Its Dynamic and Static Functions

The Lateral Vestibular Nucleus Participates in the Control of Posture

The Medial and Superior Vestibular Nuclei Mediate Vestibulo-Ocular Reflexes

The Inferior Vestibular Nucleus Integrates Inputs from the Vestibular Labyrinth and the Cerebellum

An Overall View

Unlike taste, smell, hearing, vision, and somesthesis, the sense of balance is not prominent in our consciousness. Nevertheless, this sensibility is essential for the coordination of motor responses, eye movement, and posture. Moreover, disruption of the sense of balance leads to dizziness and nausea—sensations that all too quickly impinge upon consciousness.

Proper balance and posture require continuous information about the position and motion of all body parts, including the head and eyes. Feedback information from the head and eyes must be independent of each other since the eyes can be fixed on a target even when the head is moving. In addition, the position and movement of the eyes must be based on nonvisual cues, since the eyes are capable of moving with respect to the body and the body can move with respect to the visual field.

The vestibular system of the brain and inner ear fulfills these requirements. The vestibular system is so named because the peripheral organs are found partially within the vestibule of the inner ear, a hollow expansion of the petrous bone near the region of the oval window.

In this chapter we shall first consider the structure of the two principal organs of equilibrium: the semicircular ducts and the otolith organs. We shall then examine how specialized receptor cells in these two organs, vestibular hair cells, are able to transduce mechanical displacement into neural signals. Finally, we shall discuss the central connections of the vestibular system. In later chapters we shall consider the role of the vestibular system in controlling postural reflexes (Chapter 39) and eye movements (Chapter 43).

The Organs of Balance Are Located in the Inner Ear

The inner ear, or labyrinth, is made up of two parts: the bony labyrinth and the membranous labyrinth. The *bony labyrinth* consists of several cavities in the petrous portion of the temporal bone that house both the vestibular and the auditory sense organs. Within these cavities is the *membranous labyrinth*, so called because it consists of fine membranes made up of a simple epithelium. In specialized regions the membranous labyrinth becomes elaborated into a sensory epithelium that serves as a transducing structure for both audition and balance. In the last chapter we considered the auditory division of the membranous labyrinth, which is specialized to form the organ of Corti. Here we shall consider the vestibular division.

The vestibular portion of the membranous labyrinth consists of two principal sets of structures: (1) a pair of saclike swellings—*the otolith organs*—called the *utricle* and the *saccule*; and (2) three directionally sensitive, more or less mutually perpendicular *semicircular ducts*. The organization of the membranous labyrinth is depicted in Figure 33–1. The two otolith organs lie in the vestibule (middle portion) of the inner ear. The saccule communicates directly with the cochlear duct and with the membranous semicircular ducts. These ducts lie in the bony *semicircular canals* and are separated from them by narrow sheaths of connective tissue.

The sensory receptor cells in each of these structures respond to accelerated movement of the head, or to changes in acceleration resulting from an altered position of the head. Different segments of the end organ respond to different types of acceleration. The three semicircular ducts lie in different planes that are perpendicular to one another. As a consequence of their arrangement in three-dimensional space, they detect angular acceleration of the head in any of these three directions. The otolith organs detect linear acceleration when the head moves and they are also important for determining the position of the head with respect to gravity.

Information from both components of the peripheral end-organ—the semicircular ducts and the otolith organs—is relayed by the vestibular portion of the eighth nerve to the vestibular nuclei in the brain stem and to the vestibular portion of the cerebellum (the flocculonodular lobe). Different subdivisions of the vestibular nuclear complex in turn connect in a highly specific manner with the motor nuclei of the extraocular muscles and with the spinal cord. The whole system functions to keep the body balanced, to coordinate head and body movements, and most remarkably to keep the eyes fixed on a point in space even when the head is moving.

The Vestibular Labyrinth Is Filled with Endolymph

The membranous labyrinth is filled with *endolymph*, an unusual extracellular fluid in that its ion composition is similar to that of intracellular fluid. The space surrounding the membranous labyrinth is filled with *perilymph*, which has an ionic composition similar to cerebrospinal fluid. The endolymph has a high K^+ concentration (≈150 mM) and a low Na^+ concentration (≈2 mM). Although these ion concentrations vary somewhat in different portions of the labyrinth, they never approach the normal ion balance found in other extracellular fluids. The unusual ion concentration of endolymph is produced by ionic pumps in the membranous labyrinth. These pumps generate a net potential difference between endolymph in the membranous labyrinth and the surrounding perilymph, so that the cochlear duct is about 80 mV positive with respect to the surrounding perilymph. The absolute value of this potential is somewhat smaller in the vestibular portion of the labyrinth.

The significance of these potentials is not completely understood, but they probably contribute to the ability of hair cells to transduce stimuli. The potential serves as a battery to set up a large extracellular driving force of 140 mV across the tops of the hair cells, since the extracellular space is +80 mV while the resting potential of the hair cell is −60 mV. This driving force causes ionic current flow through channels of the hair cells when they are opened by motion of the stereocilia. Reduction of the extracellular potential diminishes threshold responses of the hair cells.

Endolymph is probably produced by secretory cells in the transitional epithelium surrounding the sensory epithelia, and by the *stria vascularis*, the epithelium lining the upper part of the cochlear duct. It drains into the venous sinuses of the dura mater through the endolymphatic duct (Figure 33–1). Perilymph is thought to be secreted by arterioles in the periosteum surrounding the labyrinth; it drains into the subarachnoid space through the perilymphatic duct. If normal production or drainage of either fluid is disturbed, the function of the entire labyrinth is impaired. For example, the overproduction of endolymph may lead to a condition called Meniere's syndrome, in which both auditory and vestibular function are disturbed. Given the continuity between the cochlear duct and the vestibular labyrinth, it is not surprising that both hearing and balance are affected by excessive production of endolymph. The disease is characterized by transient attacks of dizziness or vertigo that are so severe that the afflicted individual cannot stand or walk. Nausea, vomiting, abnormal eye movements (nystagmus), and a sensorineural hearing loss also occur. The transient character of the symptoms may be a consequence of changes in fluid pressure within the labyrinth.

Specialized Regions of the Vestibular Labyrinth Contain Hair Cells

Both ends of each fluid-filled semicircular duct terminate in the utricle, although one limb of the superior duct fuses with the posterior duct before joining the utricle (Figure 33–1). One end of each duct dilates before joining the utricle. Within this dilatation, called the *ampulla*, the epithelium thickens in a region called the *ampullary crest*. This

A

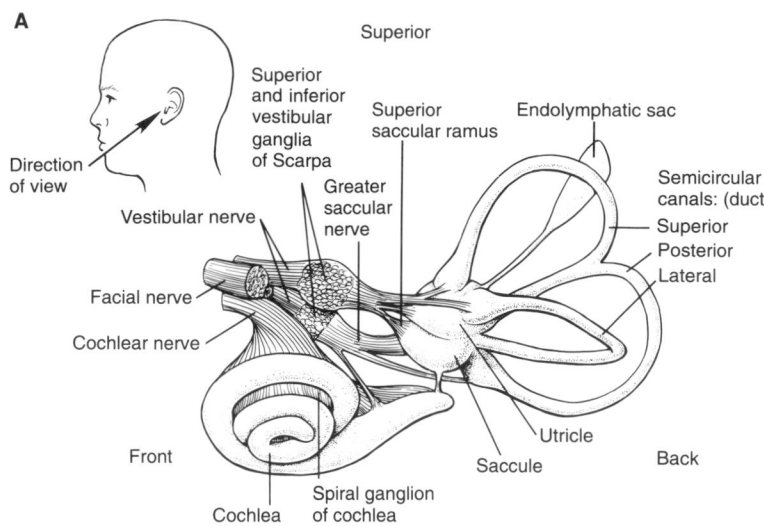

B

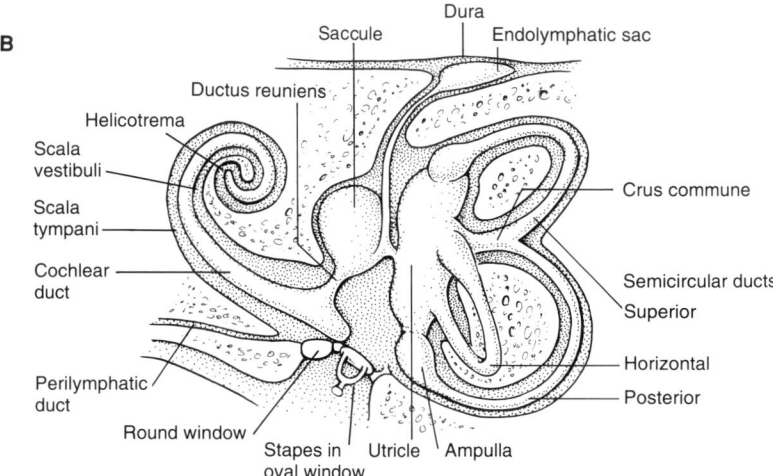

FIGURE 33–1

A. Location of vestibular and cochlear divisions of the inner ear with respect to the head.

B. The inner ear is divided into bony and membranous labyrinths. The bony labyrinth is bounded by the petrous portion of the temporal bone. Lying within this structure is the membranous labyrinth, a membrane-bound structure that contains the organs of hearing (the cochlear duct) and equilibrium (the utricle, saccule, and semicircular ducts). The space between bone and membrane is filled with perilymph, while the membranous labyrinth is filled with endolymph. Sensory cells in the utricle, saccule, and the ampullae of the semicircular ducts respond to motion of the head. (Adapted from Iurato, 1967.)

FIGURE 33–2

The organization of the ampulla of the semicircular duct.

A. A thickened zone of epithelium, the ampullary crest, contains the receptor cells. Stretching from the crest to the roof of the ampulla is a gelatinous material called the cupula.

B. The cupula is displaced by the flow of endolymph when the head moves. As a result, cilia extending from the receptor cells into the cupula are also displaced.

A

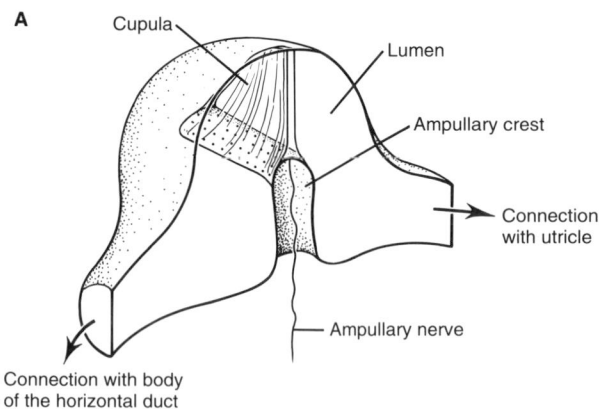

B

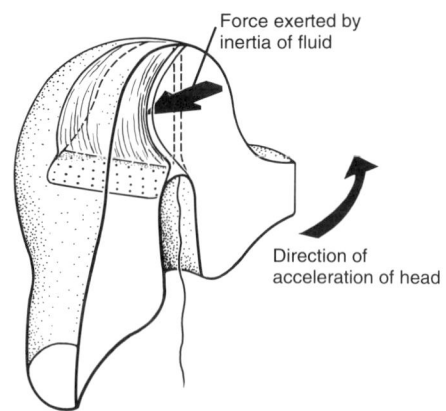

region of epithelium contains specialized receptor cells, the *vestibular hair cells*, which are innervated by peripheral processes of bipolar sensory neurons in the ampullary nerve.

The ampullary crest is covered by a gelatinous, diaphragm-like mass, the *cupula*, that stretches to the roof of the ampulla. When the head is rotated, the force exerted by the inertia of the fluid in the semicircular ducts acts against the cupula (Figure 33–2). This action produces a displacement of the sensory hairs on the receptor cells. As we shall see, the resulting distortion of the cupula elicits a receptor potential in the hair cells of the crest and eventually alters the level of activity in the nerve fibers innervating them.

The receptor system of the vestibular apparatus is so sensitive that it can respond to angular accelerations or decelerations as small as $0.1°/s^2$. The displacement of the cupula at the threshold of sensitivity is less than 10 nm, which is somewhat greater than the physical displacement of the basilar membrane produced by low-amplitude sounds in the auditory system. The displacement of the base of the cupula is greatest near the center of the ampullary crest, and therefore receptor cells near the center of the crest are sensitive to low amplitudes of fluid motion. Increasing acceleration recruits more and more receptor cells toward the periphery of the crest, since these cells are located near the edge of the diaphragm and are stimulated when this portion of the cupula is displaced. This anatomical relationship therefore leads to a graded response in the population of hair cells.

As in the ampullae of the semicircular ducts, a portion of the floor of the utricle is also thickened and contains hair cells. This zone of the utricle, the *macula* (Latin, spot), also contains the distal branches of vestibular ganglion cells. The macula is covered with a gelatinous substance in which are embedded crystals of calcium carbonate, called *otoliths* (Greek *lithos*, stone; (see Figure 33–10). The macula of the utricle lies roughly in the horizontal plane when the head is held erect, so that the otoliths rest directly upon it. If the head is tilted or undergoes linear acceleration, the otoliths deform the gelatinous mass, which in turn bends the hairs of the receptor cells.

A receptor-rich macula is also found in the saccule. In contrast to the macula of the utricle, the macula of the saccule is oriented vertically when the head is in its normal position. The macula of the saccule also detects the position of the head in space, but it responds selectively to vertically directed linear force.

Vestibular Hair Cells Respond to Changes in Movement or Position of the Head

The Hair Cells Are Polarized Structurally and Functionally

Hair cells in the vestibular apparatus are restricted to the ampullary crests of the semicircular ducts and the maculae of the saccule and utricle. They are separated from one another by supporting cells, to which they are joined

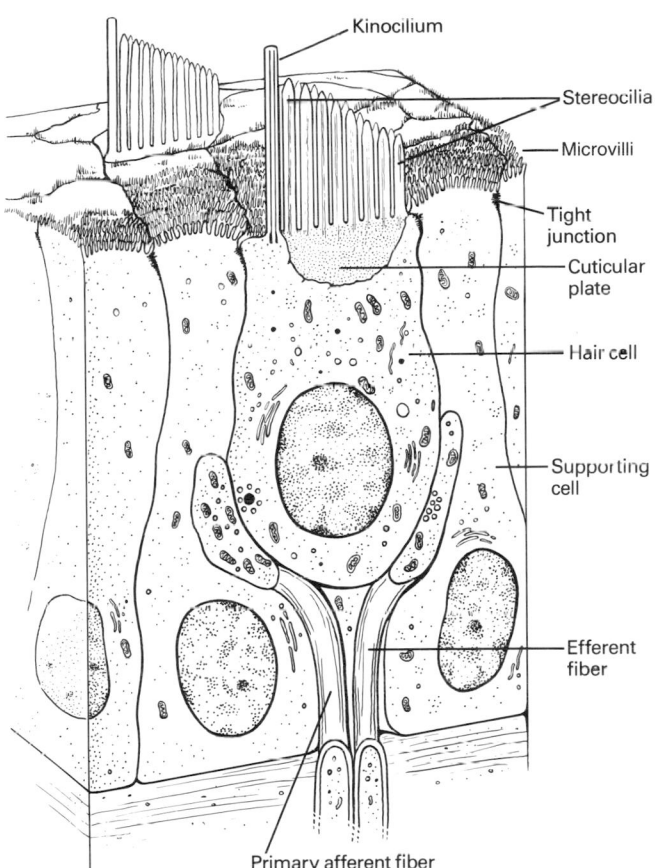

FIGURE 33–3

The hair cells of the vestibular sensory epithelium are surrounded by supporting cells, to which they are joined at their apex by tight junctions. The surfaces of the supporting cells are covered with microvilli. The hair cell is innervated at its base by the afferent process of a single vestibular ganglion cell, and by efferent terminals that arise from cells in the brain stem. The efferent processes provide a pathway for the brain to regulate directly the activity of vestibular receptor cells. The apical surface of the hair cell has several rows of stereocilia, which are packed with actin filaments, and a single kinocilium. Each stereocilium is anchored to the hair cell by a rootlet that extends into the underlying cuticular plate. The kinocilium arises from the cytoplasmic surface of the hair cell and is longer than the stereocilia. In the ampullae of the semicircular ducts the stereocilia extend into the overlying cupula. In the maculae of the utricle and saccule they extend into the overlying otolithic membrane.

by tight junctions. The free surface of each hair cell is differentiated into 40–70 stereocilia and a single motile *kinocilium*. Stereocilia vary in length, the longest being those next to the kinocilium, and tapering down with distance from the kinocilium (Figure 33–3). In the semicircular ducts, the stereocilia project into the overlying cupula. The kinocilium is always found on one side of the hair bundle. This gives each hair cell a *morphological axis of polarity*, running from the smallest stereocilium to the kinocilium.

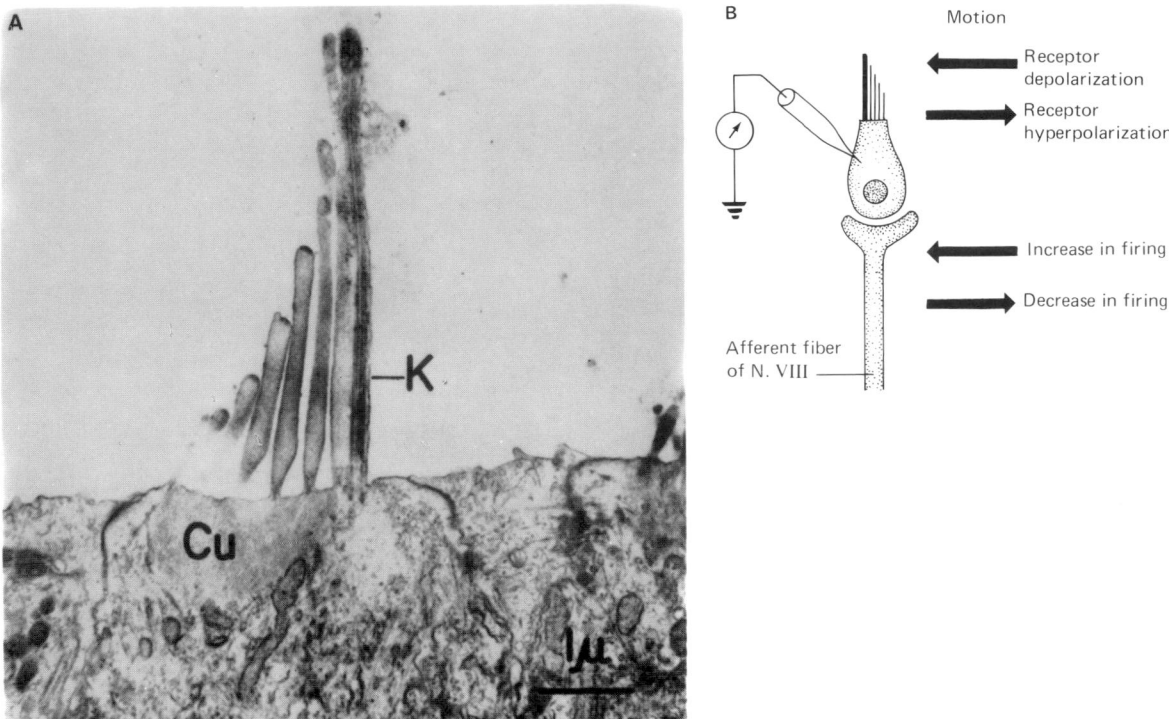

FIGURE 33–4

The arrangement of the stereocilia and the kinocilium on the surface of a vestibular hair cell determines the structural polarization of the cell.

A. A transmission electron micrograph shows that the stereocilia increase in length toward the kinocilium (**K**). The stereocilia are anchored to the cell by rootlets that extend into the cuticular plate (**Cu**).

Osmium tetroxide fixation, uranyl acetate stain. Magnification × 11,000. (From Flock, 1964.)

B. The direction in which the apical hairs bend (toward or away from the kinocilium) affects the membrane potential of the hair cell and the firing rate of the afferent fiber.

This structural arrangement is important because it allows hair cells to respond differently to bending of the hairs in different directions. The hair cells release transmitter tonically, even when the hair bundle is not bent. Bending of the hair bundle toward the kinocilium leads to depolarization of the hair cell, an increase in the release of transmitter, and an increase in the firing of the afferent fibers. Conversely, bending away from the kinocilium leads to hyperpolarization of the hair cell, a decrease in the release of transmitter, and decreased firing in the afferent fibers (Figure 33–4).

Variable tension in the linkage between adjacent stereocilia is probably the mechanical stimulus for transduction in hair cells. Rows of stereocilia parallel to the axis of polarity of the cell are connected by minute links at their tips. The links do not interconnect stereocilia within the same row (that is, in a direction perpendicular to the axis). These links may act as minute springs, opening the excitatory transduction channels as follows. During the resting state a fraction (about 10%) of the transduction channels may be open. When the hair bundle is displaced along the axis of polarization, tension on the elastic links or gating springs is increased, since they are stretched in a direction parallel to the morphological axis. This mechan-

ical event opens additional transduction channels, producing a receptor potential. Displacing the bundle in the opposite direction reduces tension on the links by relaxing the springs. This action decreases the number of open channels, produces a hyperpolarization of the membrane potential, and leads to a decrease in the firing rate of the afferent fibers. Displacements of the hair bundle perpendicular to the axis of polarity have little effect, since the links remain at their resting length. Finally, some additional mechanical element exists in series with the links, so that the whole bundle can adapt to maintained displacements and adjust the dynamic range of the transduction mechanism. Experimental evidence for this pattern of response to a mechanical stimulus, and a mechanical model of the hair bundle with elastic links, is presented in Figure 33–5.

The hair cells of the semicircular ducts are arranged in an orderly pattern. In the horizontal ducts the axis of polarization points toward the utricle, and therefore bending of the hairs in the direction of the utricle is excitatory (Figure 33–6). In the superior and posterior ducts the axis of polarization points away from the utricle, so that bending of the hairs in the direction away from the utricle is excitatory. The outcome of this morphological polarity can be

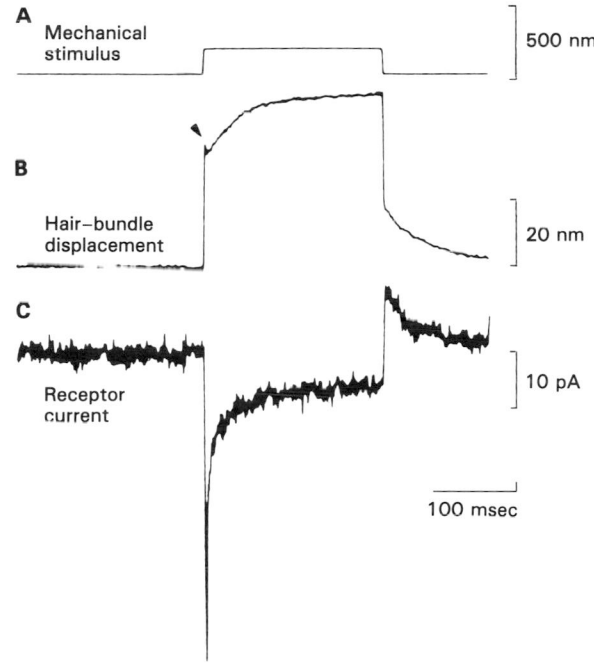

A Mechanical stimulus — 500 nm

B Hair–bundle displacement — 20 nm

C Receptor current — 10 pA

100 msec

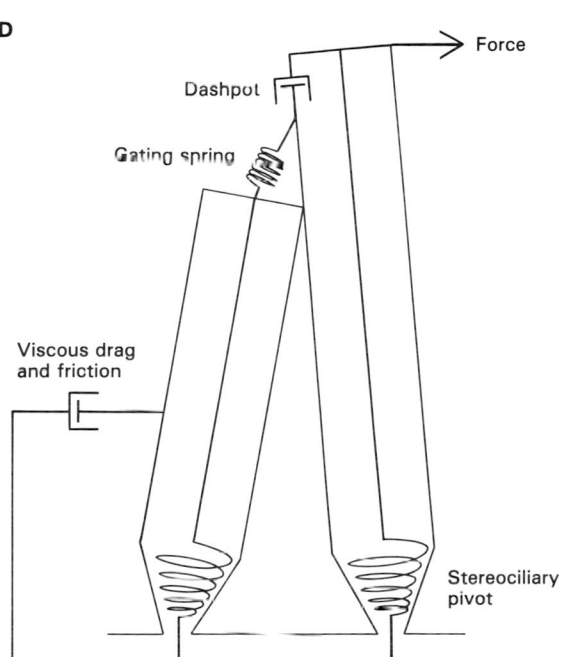

D

Force

Dashpot

Gating spring

Viscous drag and friction

Stereociliary pivot

◁ **FIGURE 33–5**

FIGURE 33–5

Simultaneous recording of hair bundle displacement and receptor current in a vestibular hair cell in response to an externally applied step of force.

A. A glass fiber used to move the hair bundle is displaced by 186 nm using a piezoelectric micromanipulator.

B. In response to the force, the hair bundle undergoes an abrupt initial displacement followed by a slow exponential adaptation. With cessation of stimulation there is another abrupt response followed by exponential relaxation.

C. The current measured simultaneously with a two-electrode voltage clamp has an initial fast, inward, transient component followed by a slower, adaptation component. An overshoot and slow adaptation occurs at the end of the step. The two components of adaptation in the receptor current (at the onset and end of the stimulus) have time courses similar to those of the mechanical responses. The cell's membrane potential is effectively clamped at −70 mV. The stiffness of the stimulating fiber is 340 μN/m.

D. A mechanical model of the vestibular hair bundle. The mechanical elements are only schematic analogies for cellular structure and function. A spring signifies mechanical stiffness, and a dashpot signifies viscous drag and fluid friction. Actin might contribute stiffness to the hair bundles, while the components of the cell membrane along with surrounding fluid might contribute drag. The transduction channels are thought to be at one or both ends of the gating spring and to be gated by tension in that spring. Note that when the hair bundle is deflected, the gating springs elongate but the pivotal springs bend.

FIGURE 33–6

The axis of polarity of all hair cells in the ampullary crest of the horizontal duct is toward the utricle.

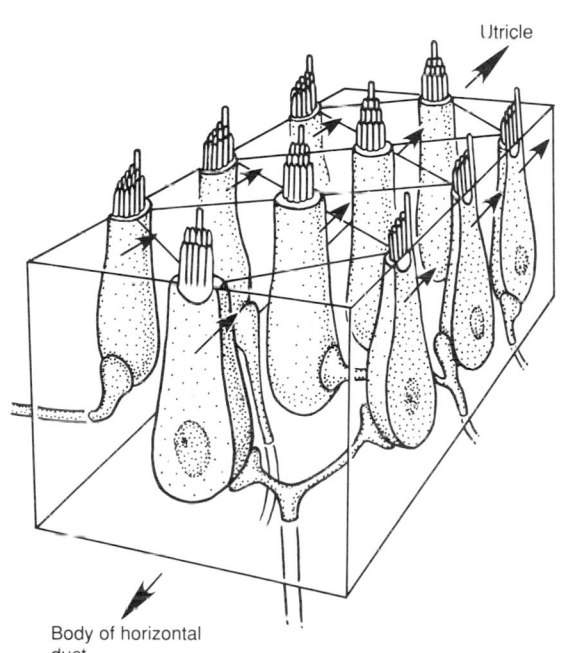

Utricle

Body of horizontal duct

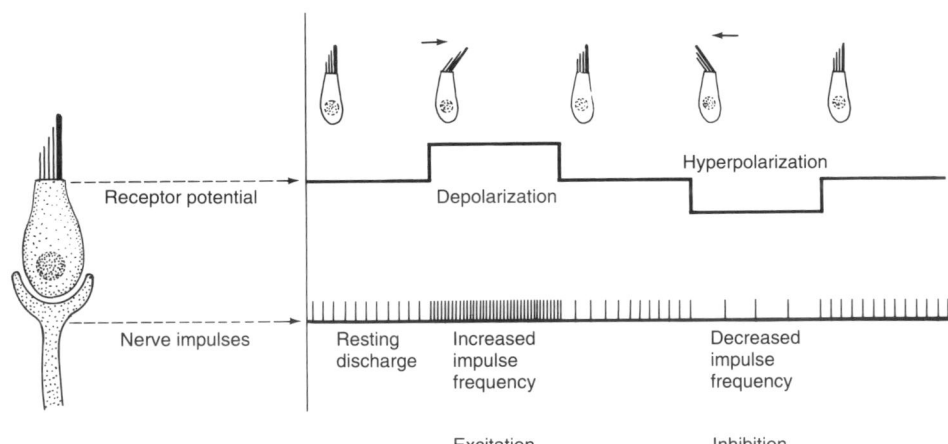

FIGURE 33–7
The firing of vestibular nerve fibers depends on the direction in which the hairs are bent. Bending toward the kinocilia causes hair cells to depolarize and produces an increased rate of firing in the afferent fibers. Bending away from the axis of polarity causes the hair cells to hyperpolarize and produces a decreased rate of firing in the afferent fibers. (Adapted from Flock, 1965.)

demonstrated by recording the activity of afferent fibers innervating the hair cells. At rest, the fibers discharge spontaneously at a rate of about 100 spikes per second. If the sensory hairs are bent in one direction, this rate is increased; if they are bent in the other, the rate is decreased (Figure 33–7). Therefore, in each duct the vestibular nerve fibers are excited by rotation in only one direction. Since there is a resting discharge, the fibers show a decrease in activity following rotation in the opposite direction.

The Semicircular Ducts Respond to Angular Acceleration in Specific Directions

To examine how paired ducts on either side of the head work together, imagine that we are looking down on the two horizontal ducts. The morphological axis of polarization of each hair cell in both horizontal ampullae points toward the utricle, to which the ducts are connected. As the head turns to the left, the fluid in the ducts lags behind the turning motion because of inertia. As a consequence, the fluid in the left duct deflects the hair bundles in the direction of their axes of polarity, while the fluid in the right duct deflects the hair bundles against their axes (Figure 33–8). The hair cells of the left ampulla therefore depolarize and release more transmitter to excite the afferent fibers innervating them. The hair cells of the right ampulla hyperpolarize, release less transmitter, and the firing rate of the afferent fibers innervating them decreases. The brain then receives two reports of this turning motion: an increase in the firing of nerve fibers on one side, and a decrease on the other.

The bilateral horizontal ducts can work together to detect motion because they lie in approximately the same plane. The situation is not as simple for the other ducts because of their orientation in the head. The *anterior duct* on one side lies approximately in the same plane as the *posterior duct* on the opposite side, so the anterior and posterior ducts of either side are functional pairs (Figure 33–9). Nevertheless, like the horizontal ducts, these duct pairs also provide a bilateral indication of head movement: Motion of fluid in the plane of these ducts causes

excitation of hair cells on one side and inhibition on the other.

The Utricle Responds to Linear Acceleration in All Directions

Hair cells in the macula of the utricle are also arranged in an orderly pattern, but their kinocilia do not face in a single direction. As a result, the utricle can respond to tilt or to linear acceleration in any one of several directions. The hair cells of the utricle are located in a specialized epithelium much like the crests of the ampulla. Their cilia project into the otolithic membrane, an overlying gelatinous matrix studded with otoliths (Figure 33–10).

FIGURE 33–8
View of the horizontal ducts from above shows how paired canals work together to provide a bilateral indication of head movement. Movement of the head to the left causes endolymph to move to the right because of inertia. This moves the stereocilia in the left duct in the direction of their axis of polarity, therefore exciting the afferent fibers to increase their firing rate. The opposite occurs on the right.

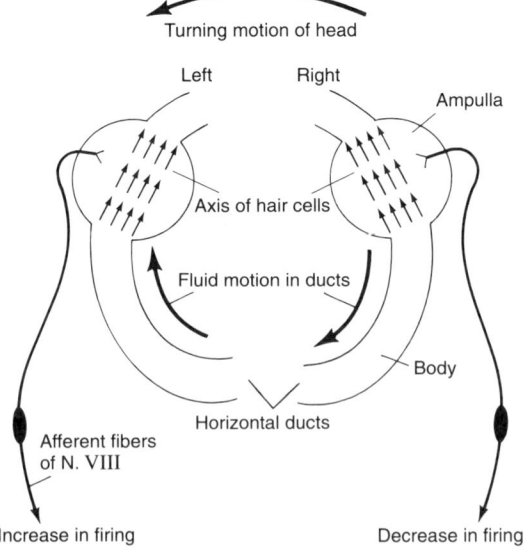

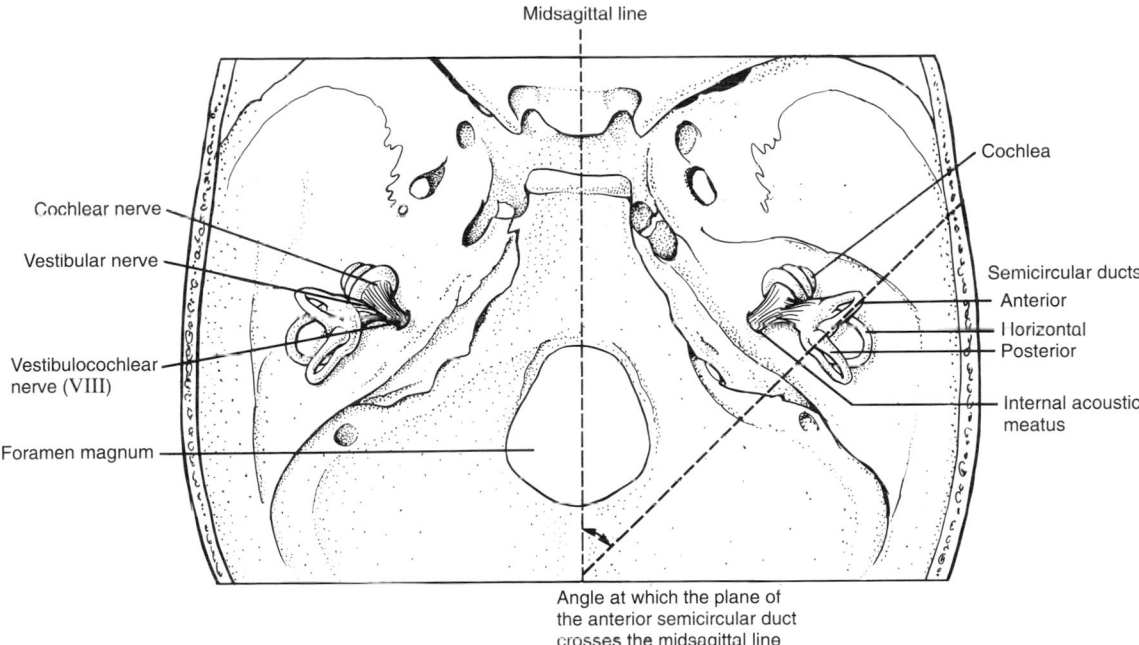

Midsagittal line

Cochlear nerve

Vestibular nerve

Vestibulocochlear nerve (VIII)

Foramen magnum

Cochlea

Semicircular ducts:
Anterior
Horizontal
Posterior

Internal acoustic meatus

Angle at which the plane of the anterior semicircular duct crosses the midsagittal line

FIGURE 33–9

The orientation of the semicircular ducts within the head. The horizontal ducts on both sides lie in the same plane and therefore are functional pairs. In contrast, the *anterior* duct on one side and the *posterior* duct on the opposite side lie in the same plane and are therefore functional pairs.

A

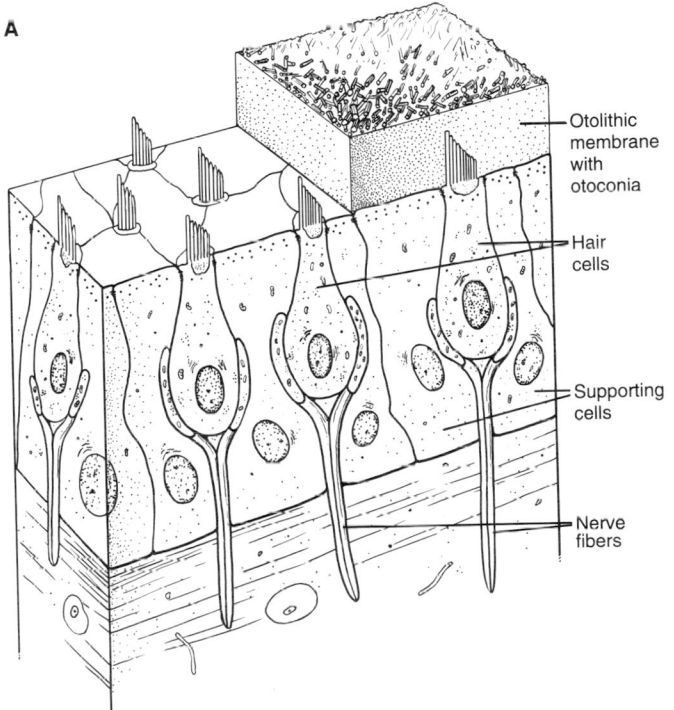

Otolithic membrane with otoconia

Hair cells

Supporting cells

Nerve fibers

FIGURE 33–10

The macula of the utricle is organized structurally to detect tilt of the head in any direction.

A. The hair bundles of hair cells in the macula of the utricle project into the otolithic membrane. This membrane is a gelatinous material in which calcium carbonate stones (otoliths) are embedded. The hair bundles are polarized with the kinocilium at one end, but not all cells are oriented in the same direction. (Adapted from Iurato, 1967.)

B. The response of an individual hair cell in the utricle to a tilt of the head depends upon the direction in which its hairs are bent by the gravitational force of the otoliths. The direction of gravitational force is constant. When the head is tilted in the direction of the axis of polarity for a particular cell, it depolarizes and excites the afferent fiber. When the head is tilted in the opposite direction, that cell hyperpolarizes and inhibits the afferent fiber.

B Gravitational force exerted by otoliths

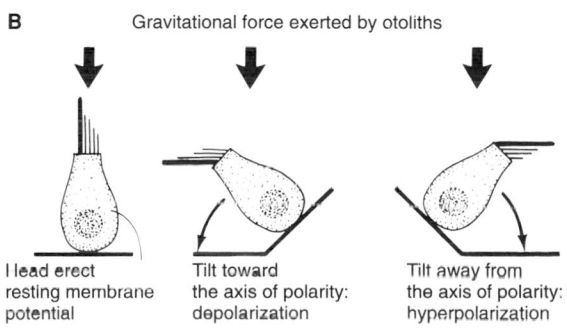

Head erect resting membrane potential

Tilt toward the axis of polarity: depolarization

Tilt away from the axis of polarity: hyperpolarization

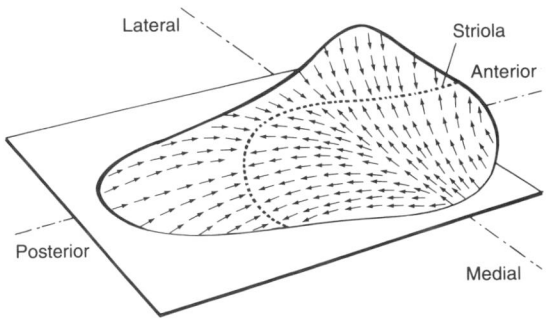

FIGURE 33–11
The axes of polarity (**arrows**) of all hair cells in the macula of the utricle are oriented toward the striola, a curved border running across the surface of the macula (**dotted line**). Therefore, tilt in any direction depolarizes some cells and hyperpolarizes others, while having no effect on a third group. (Adapted from Spoendlin, 1966.)

Individual utricular hair cells respond to the gravitational force exerted by the otoliths and the otolithic membrane as shown in Figure 33–10B. An intriguing structural feature of the hair cells in the utricle is that all cells are oriented toward a curving landmark, the *striola* (Figure 33–11). Thus, tilt in *any* direction depolarizes some utricular hair cells and hyperpolarizes others. This complex signal provides the brain with an accurate measure of head position.

The Central Connections of the Vestibular Labyrinth Reflect Its Dynamic and Static Functions

It should be clear by now that the vestibular labyrinth has two interrelated functions. The *dynamic* function, mediated principally by the semicircular ducts, enables us to track the rotation of the head in space and is important for the reflex control of eye movements. Since there are no steady-state angular forces that affect the head, the semicircular ducts serve a uniquely dynamic function. The *static* function, mediated principally by the utricle and saccule, enables us to monitor the absolute position of the head in space, and this plays a pivotal role in the control of posture. The utricle and saccule also detect linear accelerations, so in actuality they have both a static and dynamic function. We shall now consider the central connections of the ganglion cells that innervate the hair cells of the semicircular ducts and the utricle and saccule. As might be expected, the central connections of these two sets of ganglion cells differ in ways that reflect their distinctive physiological roles.

The cell bodies of the afferent fibers of the vestibular system lie in the vestibular ganglion (Scarpa's ganglion) near the internal auditory meatus. There are about 20,000 cells in each vestibular ganglion. These cells are bipolar: the peripheral axon innervates the hair cells and the central axon terminates in the brain stem. Like most of the cells in the spiral ganglion of the cochlea, both the axons

and the cell bodies of the neurons in the vestibular ganglion are myelinated, because action potentials propagate directly through the bipolar cell body from the peripheral to the central branches.

The vestibular ganglion is divided into two portions. The *superior division* innervates the macula of the utricle, the anterior part of the macula of the saccule, and the ampullae of the horizontal and anterior semicircular ducts. The *inferior division* innervates the posterior part of the macula of the saccule and the ampulla of the posterior duct. The centrally directed axons of cells in Scarpa's ganglion join with axons from the spiral ganglion of the cochlea in the vestibulocochlear nerve, the eighth cranial nerve. This nerve runs through the internal auditory meatus along with the facial nerve. After leaving the meatus, the eighth nerve runs through the cerebellopontine angle to reach the lateral aspect of the pons, where it enters the vestibular nuclei of the brain.

The vestibular nuclear complex occupies a substantial portion of the medulla beneath the floor of the fourth ventricle (Figure 33–12). This complex includes four distinct nuclei: the lateral vestibular nucleus, the medial vestibular nucleus, the superior vestibular nucleus, and the inferior, or descending, vestibular nucleus. Each nucleus can be distinguished on the basis of its architecture, and each has a distinctive set of connections with the periphery and with certain regions in the central nervous system, notably the spinal cord, the oculomotor nuclei (III, IV, and VI) of the brain stem, and the cerebellum.

The Lateral Vestibular Nucleus Participates in the Control of Posture

The lateral vestibular nucleus (also known as Deiters's nucleus) is diamond shaped when seen from a lateral view. The ventral portion receives primary vestibular input from the macula of the utricle and the semicircular ducts. Cells in this part of the nucleus contribute to vestibulo-ocular pathways. The dorsal portion of the nucleus receives input from the cerebellum and the spinal cord. Many of the cells in the dorsal part of the nucleus send their axons into the lateral vestibulospinal tract, which terminates ipsilaterally in the ventral horn of the spinal cord. The lateral vestibulospinal tract has a pronounced facilitatory effect on both alpha and gamma motor neurons that innervate muscles in the limbs. This tonic excitation of the extensors of the leg and the flexors of the arm enables us to maintain an upright body posture (Chapter 39).

Some neurons in Deiters's nucleus respond selectively to tilting of the head. These neurons have a resting discharge that increases in response to tilt in one direction and decreases in response to tilt in the opposite direction. The magnitude of the response increases with increasing angle of tilt. Other neurons respond whenever the angle of the head is changed. Both types of cells receive input from the macula of the utricle. The dorsocaudal part of the nucleus receives direct inhibitory input from Purkinje cells in the vermis of the cerebellum.

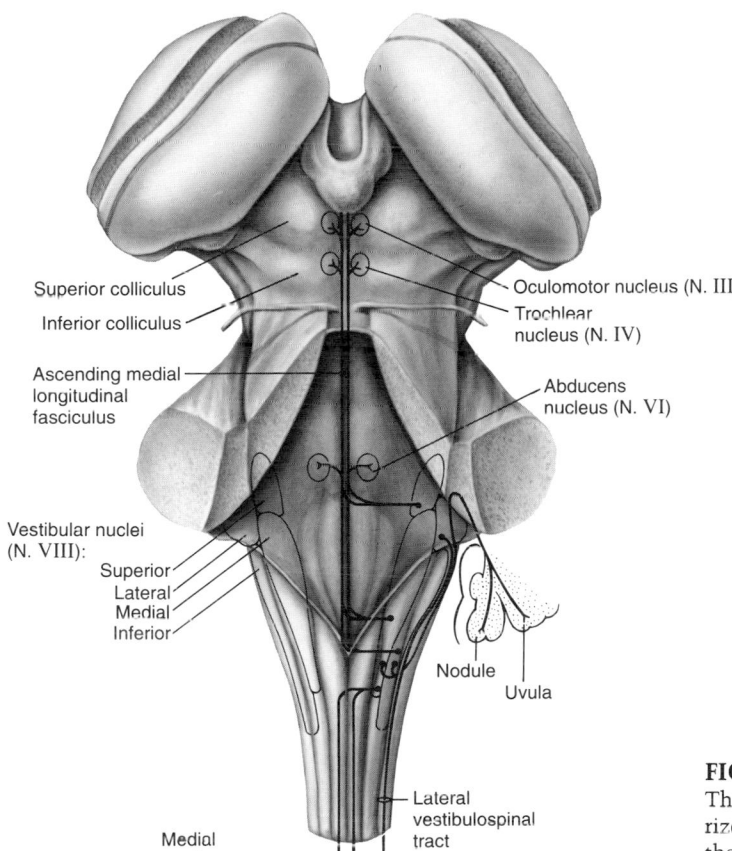

Superior colliculus

Inferior colliculus

Ascending medial
longitudinal
fasciculus

Oculomotor nucleus (N. III)

Trochlear
nucleus (N. IV)

Abducens
nucleus (N. VI)

Vestibular nuclei
(N. VIII):
Superior
Lateral
Medial
Inferior

Nodule

Uvula

Lateral
vestibulospinal
tract

Medial
vestibulospinal
tract

FIGURE 33–12
The central connections of the vestibular nuclei are summarized in this dorsal view of the brain stem. Each component of the vestibular complex has distinctive connections with the periphery and with regions of the brain and spinal cord.

Electrical stimulation of the anterior part of the cerebellar vermis reduces decerebrate rigidity, a condition of increased reflex tone in the flexors of the upper limb and the extensors of the lower limb resulting from transection of the brain stem above the level of the vestibular nuclei (Chapter 39). If the transection is caudal to the vestibular nuclei, the rigidity does not occur. Decerebrate rigidity is undoubtedly due to the unopposed excitatory effect of the lateral vestibulospinal tract and the reticulospinal pathway upon motor neurons supplying the antigravity muscles. If the portion of the cerebellum connected to Deiters's nucleus is removed, decerebrate rigidity is greatly exacerbated because the inhibitory action of the Purkinje cells on the giant cells of Deiters's nucleus is eliminated.

The Medial and Superior Vestibular Nuclei Mediate Vestibulo-Ocular Reflexes

The medial and superior vestibular nuclei receive input principally from the ampullae of the semicircular ducts. The medial vestibular nucleus gives rise to the medial vestibulospinal tract, which terminates bilaterally in the cervical region of the cord. The axons in this tract make monosynaptic connections with motor neurons innervat-

ing the neck muscles. This tract participates in the reflex control of neck movements so that the position of the head can be maintained accurately and is correlated with eye movements.

Cells in both the medial and superior vestibular nuclei participate in vestibulo-oculomotor reflexes. They send their axons into the *medial longitudinal fasciculus*, a tract running to rostral parts of the brain stem just beneath the midline of the fourth ventricle. The locations of these structures are indicated in Figure 33–13. The function of the medial and superior vestibular nuclei can be illustrated by examining an elementary vestibulo-oculomotor reflex arc. If the head is tilted to one side, the eyes rotate in the opposite direction, and this helps to maintain the visual field in the horizontal plane. The central pathways that mediate this reflex have not been traced completely, but the reflex is known to be dependent upon tonic input from the utricle. The motor pathways mediating vestibulo-ocular reflexes are described in Chapter 43, along with the disturbances of eye movements that result from the interruption of these pathways.

The coordination of the vestibulo-oculomotor reflexes was examined experimentally in the 1950s by Janos Szentagothai. He sealed a cannula in the left horizontal semicircular duct of an experimental animal and alter-

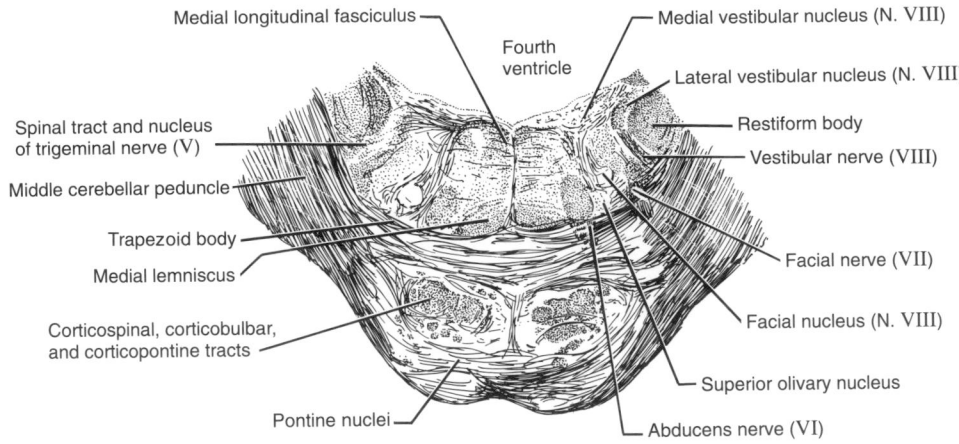

FIGURE 33–13
This transverse section of the lower pons stained for myelin shows the location of the medial longitudinal fasciculus in relation to the medial vestibular nucleus.

nately pushed and pulled the endolymph while recording the tension in each of the extraocular muscles. When the endolymph was pushed, simulating a rotational movement to the left, the medial rectus of the left eye and the lateral rectus of the right eye contracted, while the lateral rectus of the left eye and the medial rectus of the right eye showed reduced tension.

As we shall see in Chapter 43, the *voluntary* control of eye movements is independent of the vestibular system. The most important regions of the cerebral cortex involved in voluntary movements of the eyes are the frontal eye fields, located in the frontal lobes.

The Inferior Vestibular Nucleus Integrates Inputs from the Vestibular Labyrinth and the Cerebellum

The inferior vestibular nucleus appears to receive primary vestibular fibers from the semicircular ducts and from the utricle and saccule. Like Deiters's nucleus, this nucleus also receives afferents from the vermis of the cerebellum. The majority of efferent fibers contribute to the vestibulospinal and vestibuloreticular pathways. This nucleus integrates input from the vestibular labyrinth and the cerebellum, and affects centers at higher levels in the brain stem, perhaps in the thalamus.

A striking feature of the vestibulo-ocular system is the plasticity of its synaptic connections. Clinical insight to this plasticity is well documented, since individuals adapt in the long term to the vestibular disturbances brought about by unilateral damage to the vestibular division of the eighth nerve. This implies that some degree of plastic change must occur on the intact side to compensate for a unilateral deprivation of input. G. Melvill Jones and his colleagues studied changes in the pattern of the vestibulo-ocular reflexes by fitting individuals with prisms that re-

verse the direction (in the horizontal plane only) of movement perceived visually. When tested with stimuli involving rotation of the head, these individuals demonstrated eye movements in a direction opposite to normal. This change in the direction of the reflex eye movements occurred slowly, over a period of months, but was reversed somewhat more rapidly once the reversing prisms were removed.

An Overall View

The input to the vestibular system comes from a complex peripheral receptor, the vestibular hair cell, whose physiological properties are unique. Most peripheral receptors, for example the pacinian corpuscle, depolarize in response to an appropriate stimulus. Some, such as vertebrate photoreceptors, hyperpolarize. The vestibular hair cell, however, may either depolarize or hyperpolarize depending upon the direction of head movement or tilt. Furthermore, any motion of the head affects both sides, so there must be extensive interaction in the central nervous system between the inputs arising from both labyrinths. The bidirectional nature of the hair cell response, along with the coordination of inputs from the bilateral labyrinths, provides the central nervous system with multiple indications of head movement and position.

Selected Readings

Brodal, A. 1981. Neurological Anatomy in Relation to Clinical Medicine, 3rd ed. New York: Oxford University Press, pp. 470–495.

Corey, D. P., and Hudspeth, A. J. 1979. Ionic basis of the receptor potential in a vertebrate hair cell. Nature 281:675–677.

Eatock, R. A., Corey, D. P., and Hudspeth, A. J. 1987. Adaptation of mechanoelectrical transduction in hair cells of the bullfrog's sacculus. J. Neurosci. 7:2821–2836.

Flock, Å. 1964. Structure of the macula utriculi with special reference to directional interplay of sensory responses as revealed by morphological polarization. J. Cell Biol. 22:413–431.

Howard, J., and Hudspeth, A. J. 1988. Compliance of the hair bundle associated with gating of mechanoelectrical transduction channels in the bullfrog's saccular hair cell. Neuron 1:189–199.

Hudspeth, A. J., and Corey, D. P. 1977. Sensitivity, polarity, and conductance change in the response of vertebrate hair cells to controlled mechanical stimuli. Proc. Natl. Acad. Sci. U.S.A. 74:2407–2411.

Ohmori, H. 1987. Gating properties of the mechano-electrical transducer channel in the dissociated vestibular hair cell of the chick. J. Physiol. (Lond.) 387:589–609.

Wilson, V. J., and Melvill Jones, G. 1979. Mammalian Vestibular Physiology. New York: Plenum Press.

References

Crawford, A. C., and Fettiplace, R. 1981. An electrical tuning mechanism in turtle cochlear hair cells. J. Physiol. (Lond.) 312:377–412.

Crawford, A. C., and Fettiplace, R. 1981. Non-linearities in the responses of turtle hair cells. J. Physiol. (Lond.) 315:317–338.

Crawford, A. C., and Fettiplace, R. 1985. The mechanical properties of ciliary bundles of turtle cochlear hair cells. J. Physiol. (Lond.) 364:359–379.

Flock, Å. 1965. Transducing mechanisms in the lateral line canal organ receptors. Cold Spring Harbor Symp. Quant. Biol. 30: 133–145.

Iurato, S. 1967. Submicroscopic Structure of the Inner Ear. Oxford: Pergamon Press.

Melvill Jones, G., and Milsum, J. H. 1971. Frequency-response analysis of central vestibular unit activity resulting from rotational stimulation of the semicircular canals. J. Physiol. (Lond.) 219:191–215.

Spoendlin, H. 1966. Ultrastructure of the vestibular sense organ. In R. J. Wolfson (ed.), The Vestibular System and Its Diseases. Philadelphia: University of Pennsylvania Press, pp. 39–68.

Szentágothai, J. 1950. The elementary vestibulo-ocular reflex arc. J. Neurophysiol. 13:395–407.

Wersäll, J., and Flock, Å. 1965. Functional anatomy of the vestibular and lateral line organs. In W. D. Neff (ed.), Contributions to Sensory Physiology, Vol 1. New York: Academic Press, pp. 39–61.

Jane Dodd
Vincent F. Castellucci

34

Smell and Taste: The Chemical Senses

Smell and Taste Result from the Activation of Specific Receptors

The Sensation of Smell Is Transduced by Neurons Within the Olfactory Epithelium

Presentation of Odorants to the Receptor Cell May Involve an Olfactory Binding Protein

Olfactory Transduction Involves Second Messenger-Regulated Ion Channels

Individual Olfactory Neurons Respond to a Variety of Odorants

Olfactory Information Is First Encoded in the Paleocortex and Then Projects to the Neocortex via the Thalamus

Abnormalities of Olfaction Can Give Rise to Both Sensory Loss and Hallucination

The Sensation of Taste Is Transduced by Gustatory Receptor Cells

Taste Receptor Cells Are Innervated by Primary Afferent Neurons

Four or Five Basic Stimulus Qualities Can Be Distinguished

There Are Distinct Representations of Taste in the Thalamus and Cortex

Afferents from Taste Buds Project to the Gustatory Nucleus

Taste Sensations Are Encoded by Specific Pathways and by Patterns of Activity Across These Pathways

Both Inborn and Learned Taste Preferences Are Important for Behavior

An Overall View

And soon, mechanically, weary after a dull day with the prospect of a depressing morrow, I raised to my lips a spoonful of the tea in which I had soaked a morsel of the cake. No sooner had the warm liquid, and the crumbs with it, touched my palate than a shudder ran through my whole body, and I stopped, intent upon the extraordinary changes that were taking place. . . . I was conscious that it was connected with the taste of tea and cake, but that it infinitely transcended those savors, could not, indeed, be of the same nature of theirs.

. . . When from a long-distant past nothing subsists, after the people are dead, after the things are broken and scattered, still, alone, more fragile, but with more vitality, more unsubstantial, more persistent, more faithful, the smell and taste of things remain poised a long time, like souls, ready to remind us. . . .

Marcel Proust, *Remembrance of Things Past*

We are continuously bombarded by molecules released into our environment. Through the senses of smell and taste these molecules provide us with important information that we use constantly in our daily lives. They signal pleasure or danger and inform us about food and drink, or the presence of something to seek or avoid. Thus, like the other senses we have so far considered (somatic sensibility, vision, and hearing), smell and taste inform us about the external world. In addition, however, they also connect that perception with information about our internal environment, its needs, and its satisfactions: hunger, thirst, sex, and satiety.

Smell and taste are phylogenetically primitive sensibilities. The sense of smell, for example, is unique among the sensory systems in that its central connections first project to phylogenetically older portions of the cerebral cortex before reaching the thalamus and eventually the neocortex. Smell and taste also have access to neural circuits that controls both emotional states of the body and certain memories. As the passage from Proust illustrates, special memories come to mind in response to a particular taste or aroma.

The neural systems that convey smell and taste are remarkably sensitive, capable of detecting and discriminating stimuli at extremely low concentrations. Although served by anatomically and morphologically distinct systems, the sensations of smell and taste often function in concert. For example, wine tasters report that they can distinguish more than 100 different components of taste based on combinations of flavor and aroma.

Although the modalities of smell and taste have been studied intensively, the inaccessibility of the cells that serve as receptors for odorants and flavors and the difficulty of defining precisely the stimuli involved have made it difficult to study transduction processes for these senses on the cellular level. However, recent methodological advances have shown that smell and taste use mechanisms for transduction that are similar to those used by other sensory receptor cells. In this chapter we consider how chemical information is transduced and how this information reaches consciousness. In so doing we examine how the diversity of chemicals involved in taste and smell are coded by the nervous system. Finally, we consider the importance of the chemical senses to behavior.

Smell and Taste Result from the Activation of Specific Receptors

The neural systems for smell and taste can discriminate thousands of different odors and flavors. This selectivity is thought to be achieved through the activation of receptors that recognize discrete chemical structures. The most compelling evidence for specific receptors comes from studies of the response to stereoisomeric compounds. For example, D-carvone smells of spearmint whereas L-carvone smells of carraway. Similarly, the artificial sweetener aspartame is the L-isomer of aspartic acid-L-phenylalanine methyl ester; the D-aspartic acid form of the same molecule has no sweet taste.

The findings of genetic studies of human taste responses are also consistent with the existence of specific receptors. For example, phenylthiourea, an aromatic sulfur-containing compound, produces a bitter taste that results from the thiocarbonyl group of the molecule. Individuals can be classified as tasters or nontasters according to their ability to sense phenylthiourea as a bitter substance. Nontasters can perceive sweet, sour, salty, and all bitter substances except those containing the thiocarbonyl group. This difference in perception is thought to result from the presence or absence of a particular receptor protein for the thiocarbonyl structure on the surface of taste receptor cells. Sensitivity to phenylthiourea is a dominant trait, thus nontasters carry two recessive genes.

Genetic studies of this kind have been used to obtain an estimate of the number of receptor types. The ability of phenylthiourea nontasters to taste other bitter compounds, such as quinine, suggests that more than one receptor for bitter compounds must exist. In many genet-

ically determined diseases that result in a loss of the sense of smell (*anosmias*), several distinct sensory modalities are absent, suggesting the presence of many distinct receptor types. These receptors appear to be broadly tuned to a large group of compounds with similar chemical properties. This may have important functional consequences for the central processing of chemosensory information.

The Sensation of Smell Is Transduced by Neurons Within the Olfactory Epithelium

The discriminative capability of the olfactory system is extraordinary. Humans can distinguish thousands of odoriferous chemicals and can detect odorants at concentrations as low as a few parts per trillion.

The sense of smell (olfaction) is carried by receptors that lie deep within the nasal cavity. In humans these receptors are confined to a patch of specialized epithelium, the olfactory epithelium, covering roughly 5 cm^2 of the dorsal posterior recess of the nasal cavity and lying over the turbinate cartilage (Figure 34–1). This epithelium contains receptor cells, supporting cells, and basal cells (Figure 34–2).

The receptors are bipolar neurons that have a short peripheral process and a long central process. The short peripheral process extends to the surface of the mucosa, where it ends in an expanded *olfactory knob*. The knob gives rise to several cilia that are thought to be immobile in humans and that form a dense mat at the mucosal surface (Figure 34–2). The cilia are thought to interact with odorants within the layer of mucus that covers this surface. In frogs removal of the cilia and knobs results in the loss of olfactory responses. The longer central process, an

FIGURE 34–1

Olfactory receptors lie in the olfactory epithelium, located in the dorsal posterior recess of the nasal cavity (**striped area**). The olfactory bulb is a small, flattened, ovoid body that rests on the cribriform plate of the ethmoid bone.

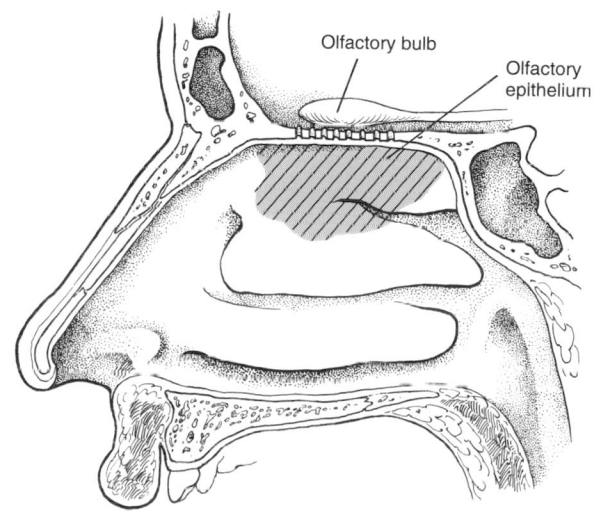

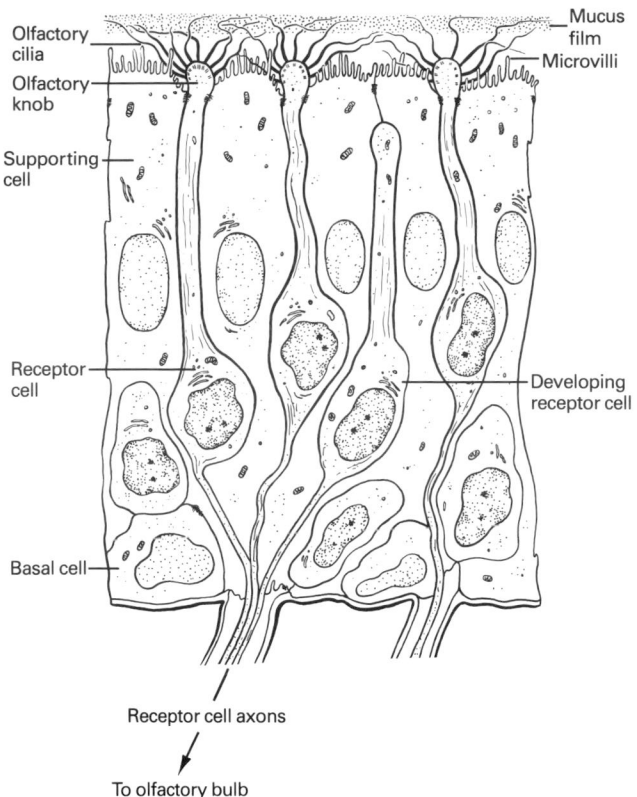

FIGURE 34–2

The vertebrate olfactory epithelium contains receptor, supporting, and basal cells. (Adapted from Andres, 1966.)

FIGURE 34–3

The olfactory receptors in the nasal cavity project to the olfactory bulbs, the first relay in the olfactory receptor system. Afferent terminals form glomerular complexes with mitral cell dendrites. Granule cells in the olfactory bulb act as local inter-

unmyelinated axon, joins between 10 and 100 others to form a bundle of axons, surrounded by Schwann cell processes, that projects through the cribriform plate to the ipsilateral *olfactory bulb* on the under surface of the frontal lobe (Figure 34–3).

Olfactory neurons differ from most other neurons in mammals in that they are generated throughout the life of the mature animal. New receptor cells are generated approximately every 60 days from precursor basal cells. This is remarkable because the olfactory neurons must extend their axons into the central nervous system and form synapses with target mitral cells in the olfactory bulb. The cells in the olfactory bulb like other cells of the central nervous system do not divide and therefore must accept new synapses continually.

Presentation of Odorants to the Receptor Cell May Involve an Olfactory Binding Protein

Odorants are first absorbed into the mucous layer overlying the receptor cell. It is thought that they then diffuse to the cilia of the receptor neurons or are presented attached to binding proteins present in the mucosa. A nasal tissue-specific protein, known as *olfactory binding protein*, has been identified. It is secreted at the tip of the nasal cavity by the lateral nasal gland, is soluble, and binds to a wide variety of structurally diverse odorants.

Olfactory binding protein belongs to a family of proteins that act as carriers for small lipophilic molecules. These include the retinol-binding proteins that transport retinol to the pigment epithelium and to the photorecep-

neurons, modifying olfactory input. The olfactory bulbs are connected to each other by the anterior commissure. (Adapted from Ottoson, 1983.)

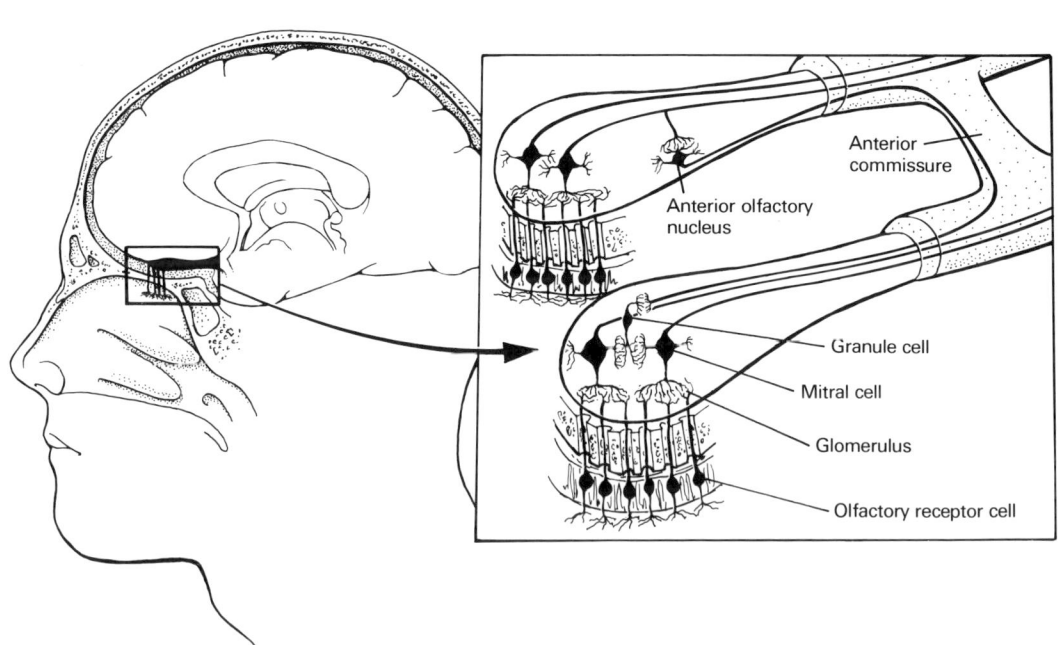

tors. By analogy with retinol-binding proteins and other members of this family, olfactory binding protein may trap odorants entering the nasal cavity and carry them to the nasal area, perhaps concentrating them at the receptor sites. Alternatively, olfactory binding protein may act as a sink or filter, protecting olfactory neurons from exposure to excessively high concentrations of odorants. A salivary gland protein called von Ebner's gland protein also belongs to this family and may concentrate and deliver molecules to gustatory receptors.

Olfactory Transduction Involves Second Messenger-Regulated Ion Channels

The application of odorants to olfactory neurons generates a depolarizing receptor potential that causes a graded increase in the frequency of action potentials (Figure 34-4). The receptor potential is thought to result from the opening of ion channels specific for Na^+. As with the receptor potential produced in photoreceptors, one mechanism of transduction of olfactory stimuli may involve cyclic nucleotide second messengers. A large number of odorants, though not all, increase the level of cAMP by enhancing the activity of an adenylyl cyclase in the olfactory epithelium. The rank order of potency of odorants in evoking firing of olfactory neurons parallels their ability to stimulate adenylyl cyclase. The greatest stimulation of the cyclase occurs with fruity, floral, and herbaceous agents, while putrid stimuli are much weaker. Consistent with the importance of the cAMP pathway in olfactory signal transduction, Randall Reed and his colleagues have cloned from the olfactory epithelium an olfactory-specific GTP-binding protein of the G_s family (called G_{olf}) and an olfactory-specific adenylyl cyclase. Both of these proteins are highly enriched in the cilia. Furthermore, Linda Buck and Richard Axel have discovered a large family of genes, also restricted in their expression to the olfactory epithelium, that encode receptor proteins with seven trans-membrane

spanning regions, suggesting that they are coupled to G-proteins (Chapter 12). It is likely that these genes encode olfactory receptors.

Like phototransduction in the visual system the increase in cAMP evoked by the binding of odorants to olfactory receptors opens a cation channel selective for Na^+. The olfactory channel has been cloned by Reed and his colleagues and found to be gated directly by cAMP and cGMP and to be highly homologous to the Na^+ channel involved in phototransduction.

Some odorants may interact with receptors that activate second messenger pathways other than cAMP. Support for this idea has come from comparative studies of olfaction in mammals and insects. Detection of odorants and pheromones in insects is mediated by receptors located on olfactory sensory cells that are clustered beneath the cuticle in structures called *sensilla*. The sensitivity of detection of odorants and pheromones in insects is similar to or greater than that of vertebrates. Odorant-induced changes in second messengers have been compared in isolated preparations of rat olfactory cilia and insect antennae. Application of a menthol analog to the rat olfactory cilia preparation resulted in a rapid and transient rise in cAMP, supporting the idea that cAMP mediates responses to some odorants in vertebrates. In contrast, application of an insect pheromone, periplanone B, to insect antenna produced a transient increase in inositol trisphosphate (IP_3) with no change in cAMP levels. Thus, different second messengers may be involved in olfactory transduction in different organisms, and perhaps in the same organisms in response to different odorants.

Individual Olfactory Neurons Respond to a Variety of Odorants

In color vision, three cone pigments are sufficient to convey the myriad hues that we can discriminate. The dis-

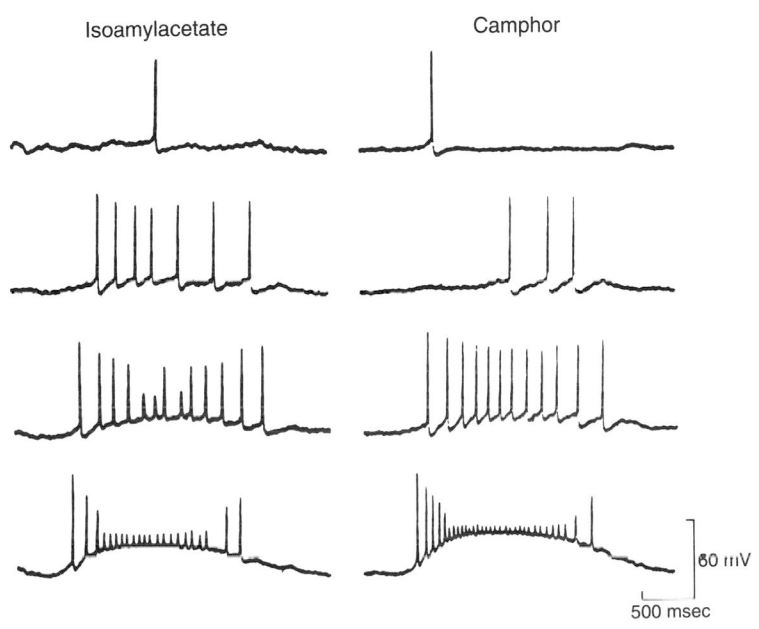

FIGURE 34-4
Intracellular recordings from an olfactory receptor showing the responses to isoamylacetate and camphor. The rate of impulse firing of the receptor increases with increasing concentration (**from top trace down**). (From Trotier and McLeod, 1983.)

covery of a large family of potential olfactory receptors suggests that hundreds of receptors, each recognizing a single or a few odorants, enable us to detect a wide range of odorants. It is not yet known whether individual olfactory neurons have multiple receptors, nor is it known how narrowly tuned a given receptor is to individual odorants. Electrophysiological studies indicate that single olfactory receptor cells can respond to several different odorants. Nevertheless, the size of the family suggests that individual neurons express only small numbers of distinct receptor molecules.

Although responses to specific odorants occur throughout the epithelium, measurement of olfactory responses in different regions of the epithelium combined with the use of 2-deoxyglucose mapping reveals areas of high sensitivity (hot spots) for individual odorants. For example, butanol best activates neurons in the anterior regions of the mucosa whereas limonene preferentially activates neurons in the posterior mucosa. When the stimulus intensity is increased, however, it is possible to activate pre-

viously silent olfactory receptors in and around the area of maximal sensitivity. Thus, increasing the concentration of odorant will activate additional receptor cells and change the overall firing pattern.

Olfactory Information Is First Encoded in the Paleocortex and Then Projects to the Neocortex via the Thalamus

The small unmyelinated axons of the olfactory neurons terminate in the olfactory bulb, the first relay in the olfactory system. Within the olfactory bulb are specialized synaptic areas called *glomeruli*. Here the primary axons synapse on the dendritic arbors of large mitral cells and on small tufted cells, the main output cells of the bulb (Figure 34–5).

The axons of mitral and tufted cells project in the olfactory tract to the secondary olfactory areas of the olfactory cortex. This region of cortex is divided into five parts:

FIGURE 34–5

The mammalian olfactory bulb is organized in layers of cells.

A. Olfactory receptors make contact with the dendrites of mitral cells and tufted cells in specialized areas, the glomeruli. The dendritic structure of the mitral cell is richly arborized with primary (1°) and secondary (2°) dendrites and recurrent axon collaterals. Periglomerular cells and granule cells are inhibitory interneurons. The bulb is divided into five layers according to the distribution of these elements. (Adapted from Shepherd, 1972.)

B. This circuit diagram shows the pervasive inhibitory actions of the periglomerular and granule cells. The primary olfactory

axons synapse with the mitral cells, the tufted cells, and the periglomerular cells. The dendrites of mitral cells are synaptically connected with the inhibiting periglomerular cells. Secondary dendrites of the mitral cells make and receive synaptic contacts with the dendrites of the inhibiting granule cells. The inhibitory interneurons provide a curtain of inhibition that must be penetrated by the peaks of excitation generated by odorant stimuli. The output of the bulb is carried by the mitral cells and the tufted cells. Various centrifugal fibers from the central nervous system act directly on the periglomerular and granule cells. (Adapted from Shepherd, 1972.)

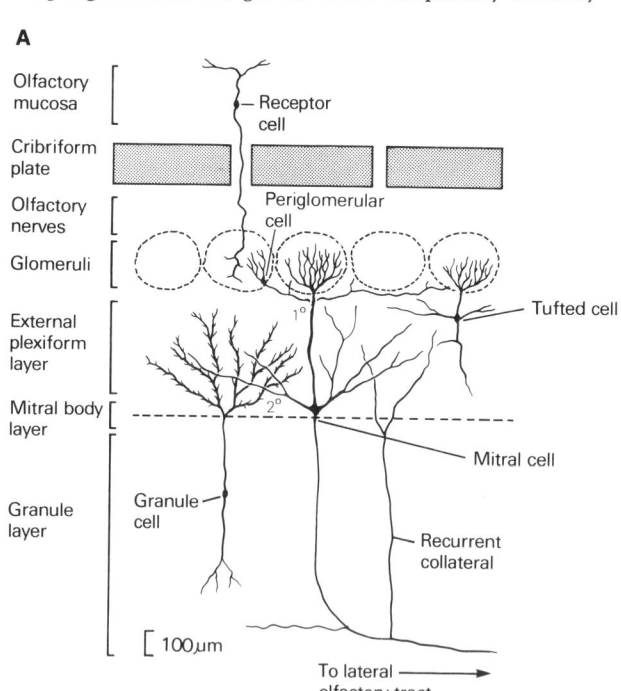

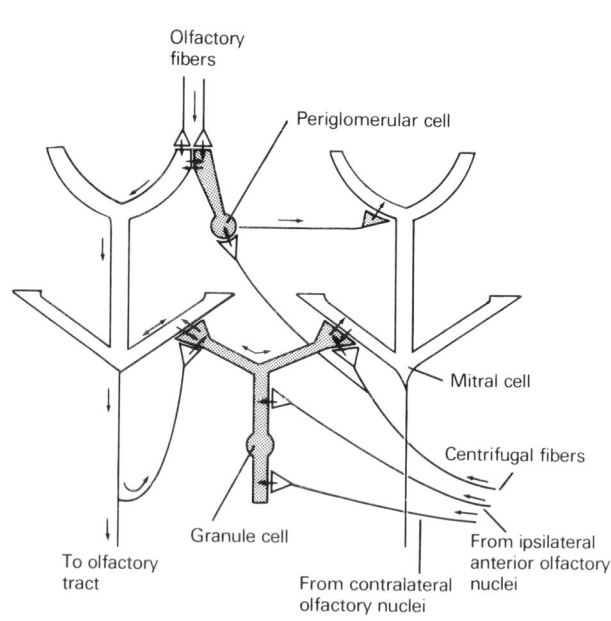

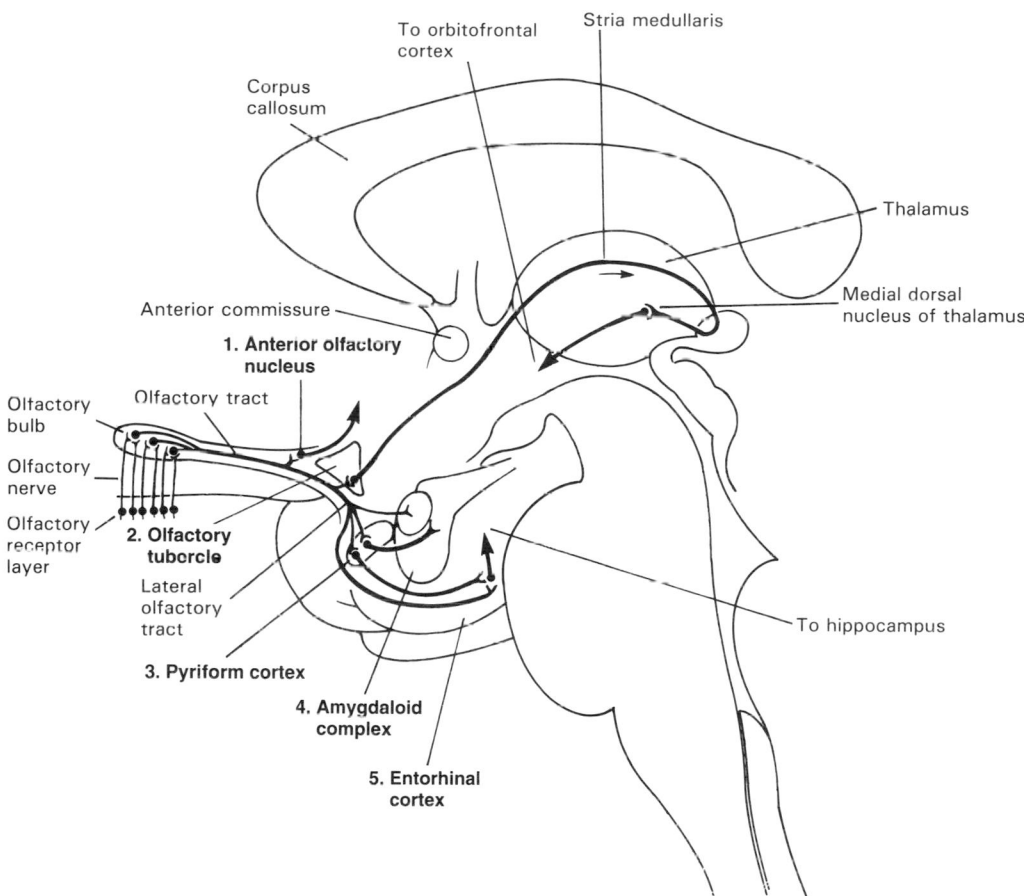

FIGURE 34-6

The axons of mitral and tufted cells project in the olfactory tract and synapse on neurons in five separate regions of the olfactory cortex. The anterior olfactory nucleus (1) projects via the anterior commissure to the contralateral olfactory bulb. The olfactory tubercle (2) and the pyriform cortex (3) project to other olfactory cortical regions and to the medial dorsal nucleus of the thalamus.

Together, these cortical and thalamic regions are thought to be involved in conscious perception of odors. The cortical nucleus of the amygdala (4) and the entorhinal area (5) are components of the limbic system and may be involved in the affective components of odors.

the anterior olfactory nucleus, which connects the two olfactory bulbs through a portion of the anterior commissure; the olfactory tubercle; the pyriform cortex, the main olfactory discrimination region; the cortical nucleus of the amygdala; and the entorhinal area, which in turn projects to the hippocampus (Figure 34-6).

Unlike the somatosensory and visual systems, where afferent input is organized in a rather precise topographic manner, there is no strict relationship between the arrangement of the projections of olfactory neurons in the olfactory bulb and the regions of mucosa from which they originate. Therefore, the olfactory bulb and higher centers must be able to interpret different signals from the same subregion as different odors.

Functional mapping of the topographic projections of olfactory neurons can be performed using 2-deoxyglucose autoradiography in awake animals after exposure to various odorants. This method shows that the activity of cells in specific glomeruli increases preferentially in response to certain odorants (Figure 34-7). As the concentration of an odorant is increased, additional glomeruli are activated, suggesting that groups of cells with higher thresholds are recruited. These distributed patterns of activity thus seem to carry the information about the odor molecule.

The local circuitry of the olfactory bulb plays an active role in processing incoming olfactory information before transmitting it to higher centers. Recordings from mitral or tufted cells show that the periglomerular and granule neurons constitute local inhibitory circuits. As with other sensory systems, olfactory information is ultimately relayed through the thalamus to the neocortex. The olfactory tubercle projects to the medial dorsal nucleus of the thalamus, which in turn projects to the orbitofrontal cortex, the region of cortex thought to be involved in the conscious perception of smell.

A Camphor summary

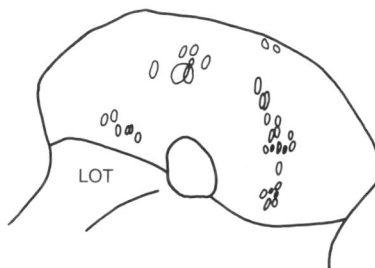

B Camphor and amylacetate

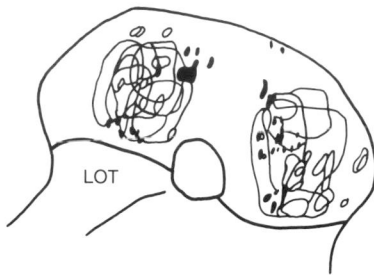

C Pure air

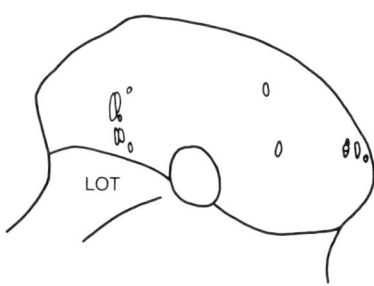

FIGURE 34–7
Different odors elicit different degrees of activity in different
regions of the glomerular layer of the olfactory bulb. (**LOT**,
lateral olfactory tract.) (Adapted from Stewart, Kauer, and
Shepherd, 1979.)

A. Summary map of six experiments using camphor as a stimulus.

B. Comparison of summary maps of camphor (**dark areas**) and
amylacetate.

C. Summary map of 12 experiments using filtered air as a stimulus.

In addition, there are olfactory pathways to the limbic
system (the amygdala and hippocampus). The amygdala
acts as a relay center that connects the olfactory cortex
with the hypothalamus and the tegmentum of the midbrain. This limbic pathway is thought to mediate the
affective component of odors. In contrast, the thalamus–
neocortex projection is thought to be involved in the conscious perception of smell. People with lesions of the
orbitofrontal cortex cannot discriminate odors.

Abnormalities of Olfaction Can Give Rise to Both Sensory Loss and Hallucination

Olfactory acuity varies enormously from person to person.
Sensitivity may vary as much as a thousandfold even
among people with no obvious abnormality. In the medical literature the term *hyposmia* (diminished sense of
smell) is favored for milder olfactory defects that are comparatively general in extent, such as occur during the
common head cold. General hyposmia occurs in conjunction with cystic fibrosis of the pancreas and Parkinson's
disease. Hyposmia is also found in patients with untreated
adrenal insufficiency.

Specific anosmia, a common olfactory abnormality, is a
lowered sensitivity to a single odorant or a few related
compounds, while perception of most other odors remains
normal. Total loss or an absence of the sense of smell is
known as *general anosmia* or simply *anosmia*. The olfactory nerve can become inoperative for one or another reason, such as mechanical blockage of the airway, infection,
chemical interference with olfactory receptors, or the
presence of a tumor. In addition, the sense of smell may
diminish during the later decades of life. For example, the
threshold for detecting various odors, including cherry,
grape, and lemon, is considerably higher in older people.

Olfactory hallucinations of repugnant smells (*cacosmia*) occur as part of uncinate epileptic seizures. This
symptom generally indicates a focal onset in the anterior
medial portion of the temporal lobe, where the pyriform
and entorhinal cortices are located.

The Sensation of Taste Is Transduced by Gustatory Receptor Cells

Taste receptor cells transduce soluble chemical stimuli
into electrical signals that can be transmitted to the brain.
The receptor cells are epithelial cells clustered in sensory
organs called *taste buds*, which are located primarily in
numerous projections (papillae) embedded in the epithelia
of the tongue (Figure 34–8), palate, and pharynx. Taste
buds are also found in the epiglottis and upper third of the
esophagus. In regions other than the tongue, the taste buds
are not usually found in papillae.

In humans there are three types of papillae: fungiform,
foliate, and circumvallate. Fungiform papillae look like
small blunt mushrooms; each contains between one and
five taste buds (Figure 34–8). There are several hundred
fungiform papillae, located on the anterior two-thirds of
the tongue. Foliate papillae form leaf-like folds on the posterior edge of the tongue. Circumvallate papillae appear as
large round structures surrounded by a groove and are located in the posterior third of the tongue. The foliate and
circumvallate papillae contain thousands of taste buds
(see Figure 34–10A).

In addition to containing between 50 and 150 receptor
cells, each taste bud has two other types of cell: basal cells
and supporting cells (Figure 34–9). Basal cells are round

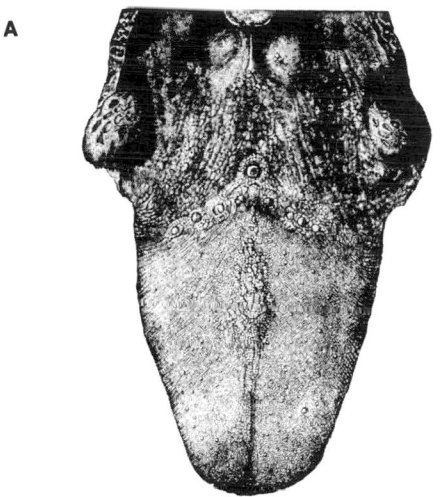

A

FIGURE 34–8
Taste sensitivity, cranial nerve innervation, and papilla type differ throughout the human tongue.

A. Surface of dorsum and root of human tongue. (From Bloom and Fawcett, 1962.)

B. Innervation pattern of the tongue. The taste buds of the anterior two-thirds of the tongue are innervated by the afferent fibers that travel in a branch of the facial nerve (VII) called the chorda tympani. The taste buds of the posterior third of the tongue are innervated by afferent fibers that travel in the lingual branch of the glossopharyngeal nerve (IX). (Adapted from Shepherd, 1983.)

C. Schematic cross sections of the main types of taste papillae. Each type predominates in specific areas of the tongue, indicated by the **arrows** from part B.

D. Regions of lowest threshold for sweet, salty, sour, and bitter tastes in the human tongue.

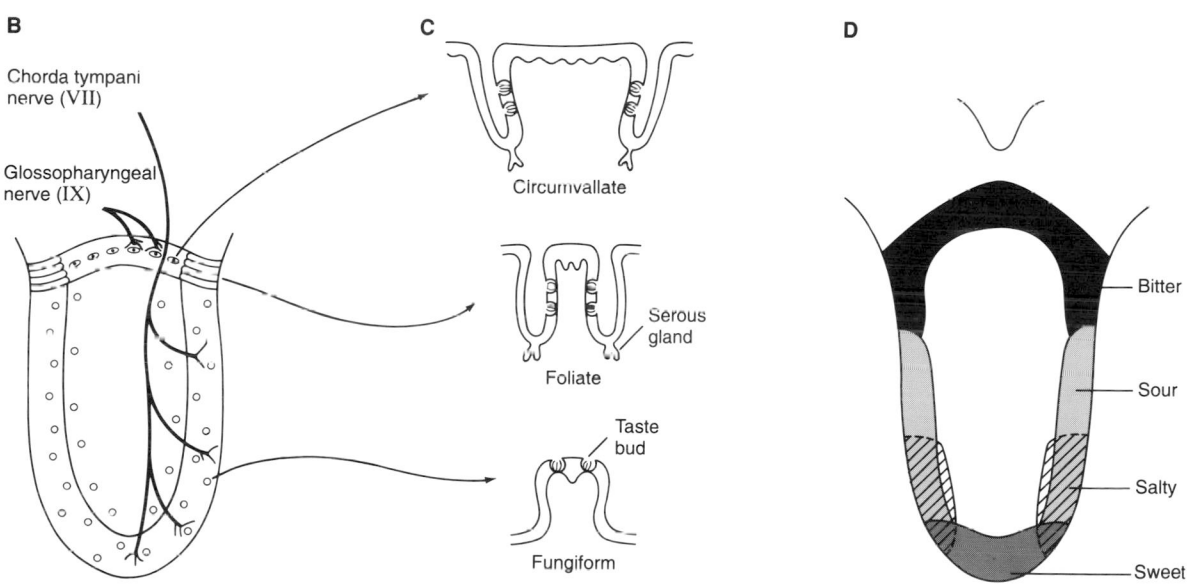

Taste Receptor Cells Are Innervated by Primary Afferent Neurons

cells located at the base of the taste bud. They may act as interneurons within the taste bud or as transitional cells, eventually differentiating to become new receptor cells. Supporting cells have glial-like properties and may provide structural or trophic support for the primary receptor cells.

Taste buds are embedded in the epithelium of the tongue and are connected to the surface of the tongue by an opening called the *taste pore*. Small processes (microvilli) extend from the apical surface of each receptor cell through the taste pore to the surface of the tongue (Figure 34–9). The microvilli are the only parts of the receptor cell exposed to compounds within the oral cavity, and are thought to be the sites at which sensory transduction takes place. The basolateral surface of receptor cells is occluded from the oral cavity by tight junctions that connect the receptor cells in their apical regions.

Each receptor cell is innervated at its base by the peripheral branch of a primary afferent fiber (Figure 34–10). Each afferent fiber branches many times, innervating several papillae and, within each taste bud, several receptor cells. Thus, the electrical activity recorded from a single afferent fiber represents the input of many receptor cells. The contacts between the receptor cell and the sensory fiber have the morphological characteristics of chemical synapses, suggesting that taste cells communicate with afferent nerve endings by synaptic transmission.

The taste buds in the anterior two-thirds of the tongue are innervated by afferents that travel in the chorda tympani, a branch of the facial nerve (cranial nerve VII), with cell bodies in the geniculate ganglion (see Figures 34–8

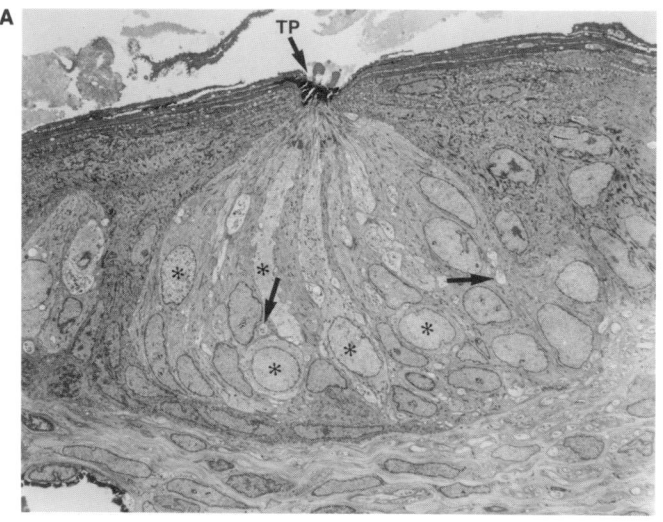

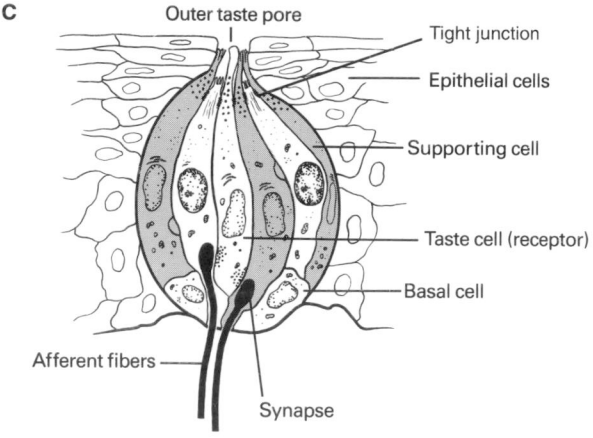

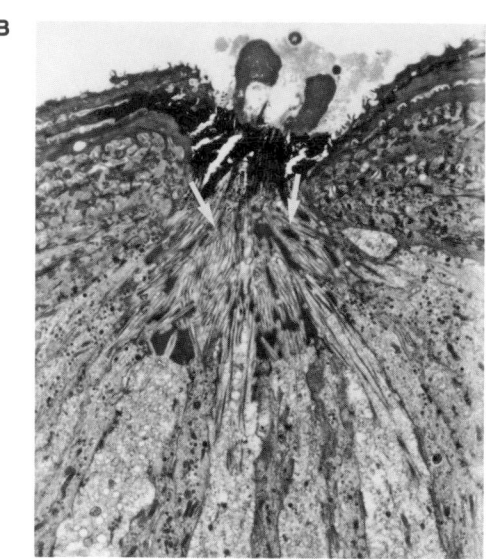

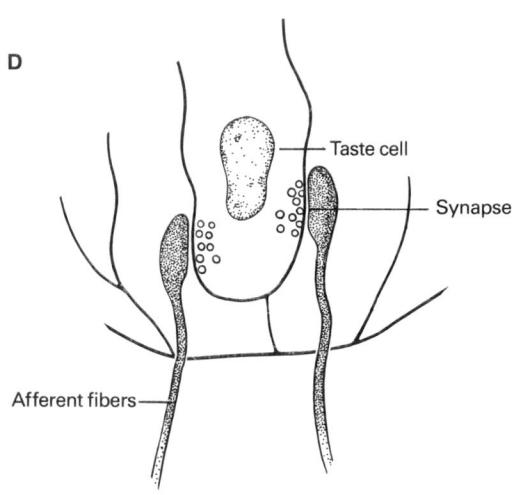

FIGURE 34–9

Taste receptor cells are contained in taste buds.

A-B. These transmission electron micrographs of longitudinal sections through a rabbit foliate taste bud show the microvilli **(arrows)** projecting into the taste pore **(TP)**. Nuclei and apical processes of taste receptor cells (labeled with **asterisks** in **A**) can be seen. Intragemmal nerve fibers are indicated by arrowheads. $\approx \times 860$. (A From Royer and Kinnamon, 1991. B Courtesy of Royer and Kinnamon.)

C. The taste bud contains three types of cells: basal, supporting, and receptor cells. Taste cells are innervated at their base.

D. The contact between the receptor cell and the afferent nerve has the characteristics of a chemical synapse: clustering of vesicles and parallel membranes at the zone of apposition. (C and D adapted from Murray, 1973.)

and 34–14). Taste buds in the posterior third of the tongue are innervated by the peripheral branches of sensory neurons that derive from the petrosal ganglion and travel in the lingual branch of the glossopharyngeal nerve (cranial nerve IX). The taste buds on the palate are innervated by the greater superficial petrosal branch of cranial nerve VII, and the buds on the epiglottis and esophagus by the superior laryngeal branch of cranial nerve X. Each of these nerves also carries somatosensory afferents that innervate regions of the tongue that surround the taste buds. The

presence of these somatosensory afferents makes it difficult to distinguish pure taste sensations carried by gustatory nerve fibers from somatosensory information carried by other classes of sensory fibers.

Vertebrate taste cells contain voltage-gated Na^+, K^+, and Ca^{2+} channels similar to those found in neurons. As a result, taste cells are electrically excitable and can generate action potentials in response to electrical and chemical stimulation. During normal physiological responses, however, the signals that are generated are thought to be

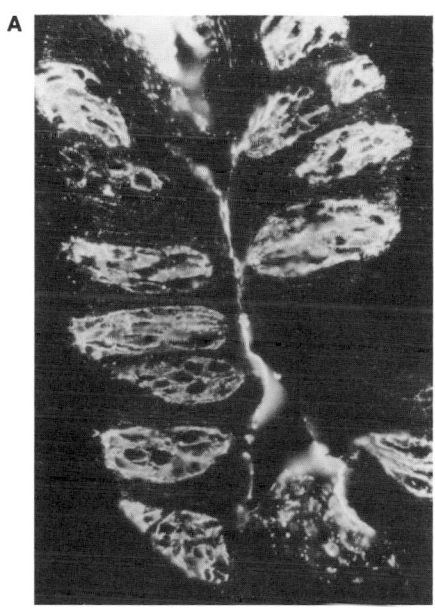

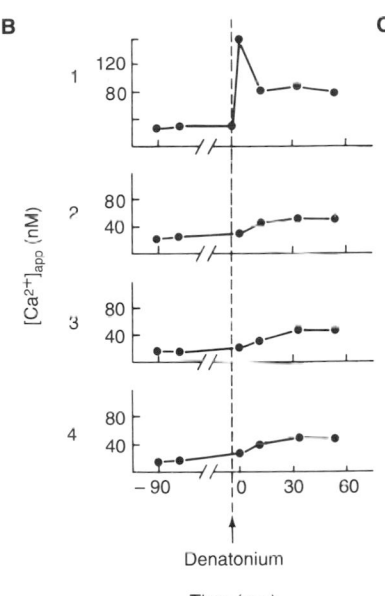

Denatonium

Time (sec)

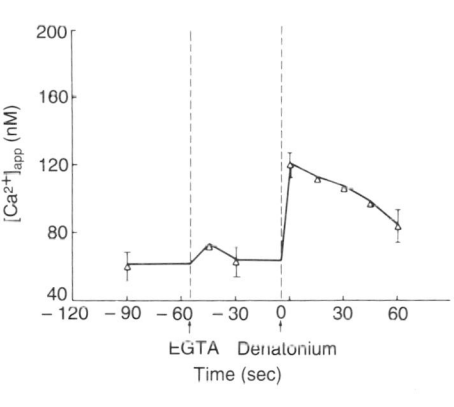

EGTA Denatonium

Time (sec)

FIGURE 34–10

Identification of taste buds *in vivo* and *in vitro* permits analysis of their responses to chemical stimuli.

A. Taste buds in a circumvallate papilla of the rat tongue labeled with a monoclonal antibody. Many taste cells are clustered in several buds lining the wall of the papilla. (From Akabas et al., 1988.)

B. Increases in intracellular Ca^{2+} concentration in a taste cell responsive to a bitter stimulus, denatonium chloride (**1**). Three adjacent nonreceptive cells (**2,3,4**) showed no change in intracellular Ca^{2+} concentration. The Ca^{2+} concentration was calculated using a Ca^{2+}-sensitive dye, Fura-2. (From Akabas et al., 1988.)

C. Increases in intracellular Ca^{2+} concentration in the taste cell derive from mobilization of intracellular stores. When taste cells isolated in culture were bathed in a Ca^{2+}-free medium, (EGTA) denatonium chloride remained an effective stimulus.

small and subthreshold, so that taste receptor cells generally do not produce action potentials. Information is thought to be processed primarily by graded receptor potentials that lead, possibly through increase in the level of intracellular Ca^{2+} and the consequent release of a chemical transmitter, to the generation of action potentials in the sensory afferents that innervate the taste buds.

Four or Five Basic Stimulus Qualities Can Be Distinguished

Like olfaction, the complexity of gustatory sensation probably results from the activation of many different classes of receptors. In 1927 Hans Henning suggested that the richness of a taste is due to the presence of specific receptors for four basic qualities: bitter, salty, sour, and sweet. The response to more complex taste stimuli may be due to the activation of specific combinations of receptors encoding the four basic taste modalities.

Although the basis by which complex stimuli are encoded is not well understood, there is general agreement that these four basic stimulus qualities are detected by distinct gustatory receptor cells. Monosodium glutamate may represent a fifth category, but this is controversial. There may be anatomical separation of distinct receptor types. For example, the tip of the tongue is responsive to all four basic qualities but is more sensitive to sweetness and saltiness, whereas the lateral part of the tongue is more responsive to sourness, and the back of the tongue to bitterness (Figure 34–8). The cellular mechanisms of transduction of these four basic stimuli by taste cells are discussed in the following section.

Bitterness. Bitterness, a taste that is often associated with harmful stimuli, is elicited by chemically heterogeneous compounds, although it is not known which chemical structures are responsible for the sensation. The transduction mechanism of bitter taste has been studied in single taste cells isolated from the circumvallate papillae of rodents (Figure 34–10). Here, bitter stimuli cause the release of Ca^{2+} from intracellular stores (Figure 34–10), which may be triggered either by IP_3 or by cAMP. The rise in intracellular Ca^{2+} is thought to cause the release of neurotransmitter from taste cells, thereby activating the sensory fiber.

Sweetness. The sweetest compounds known to humans are the proteins thaumatin and monellin, which are 100,000 times sweeter than sucrose and can be detected at concentrations of 10^{-8} M. Although the structures of these two proteins are quite different, they are likely to bind to the same receptor. Folding of each protein is

Monellin

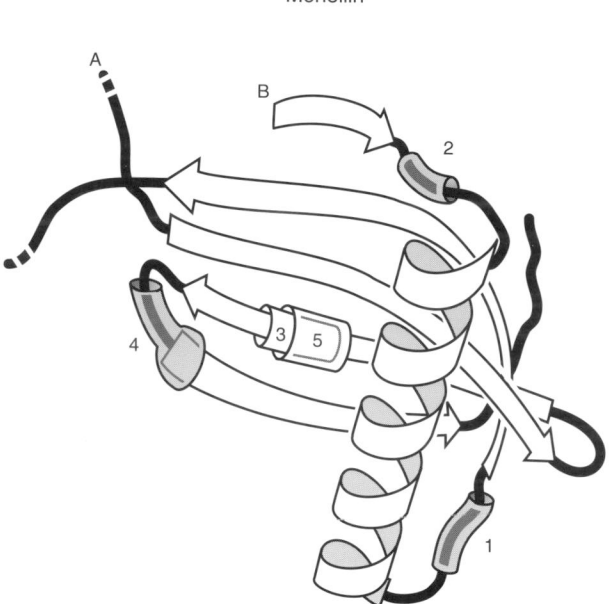

Thaumatin

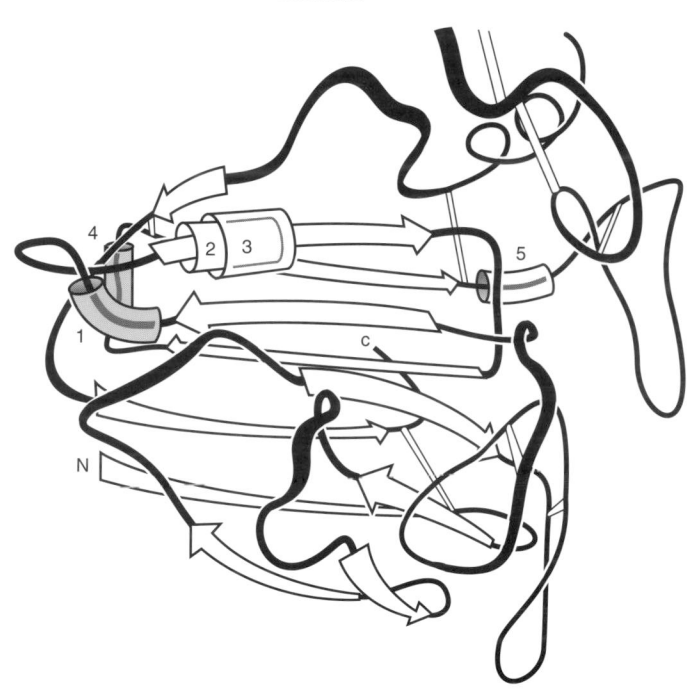

FIGURE 34–11

Molecular structure of two sweet-tasting compounds. Schematic drawings of the backbone structures of monellin and thaumatin. Although both proteins are active only in their native form, and despite the fact that they appear to interact with the same receptor, thaumatin and monellin bear no resemblance to each other in their amino acid sequence or their three-dimensional backbone structures, determined by X-ray crystallography. The two proteins are immunologically cross-reactive, however, and antibody–protein complexes do not elicit sweet taste. Other sweet compounds compete for the antibodies while nonsweet derivatives do not, suggesting that the antigenic site is also the receptor-binding site. Further examination of the amino acid sequence revealed several tripeptide sequences in the two proteins, which are not statistically homologous but which could combine to form an antigenic site. These regions are indicated by tube sections in the figure; homologous tripeptide pairs are identified by the same number. Any one tripeptide by itself is not large enough to be an antigenic site. However, two of these regions (1 and 4) in each molecule are located in looping, exposed parts of the folded proteins and share the same sequence and topology in each molecule. Thus, in their native conformations thaumatin and monellin may activate the sweet receptor through the juxtaposition of a pair of tripeptides. (Adapted from Ogata et al., 1987.)

thought to bring together two tripeptide sequences to form structurally similar local domains in the two proteins. These domains are thought to combine with the sweetness receptor (Figure 34–11).

Two mechanisms for the transduction of sweet taste have been proposed. The first mechanism uses a Na^+-selective, voltage-independent channel in the apical membrane of taste cells. Intracellular recordings show that sucrose evokes a depolarization that has a reversal potential near the Na^+ equilibrium potential. This depolarization is inhibited by amiloride, a compound that blocks cation channels in other epithelia. The second mechanism involves a membrane depolarization resulting from the closure of a voltage-dependent leakage K^+ channel, which is normally open at resting membrane potential. The channel, located in the basolateral membrane of the taste cells, is closed by elevations in cAMP. Consistent with this mechanism, sugar stimulates adenylyl cyclase activity in the lingual epithelial membranes. It is not clear whether both mechanisms operate in the same receptor cell or whether different cells have different transduction mechanisms.

Sourness. Acids elicit a sour taste. These compounds seem to penetrate the membrane of the taste cell directly, without the intervention of specific membrane receptors, and act to block voltage-dependent Na^+, Ca^{2+}, and K^+ channels. In amphibian taste cells the resting potential is dominated by K^+ channels, which are restricted to the apical membrane of the cell. The blockade of these K^+ channels by acidic compounds is likely to account for the depolarizing receptor potential (Figure 34–12). Voltage-gated Na^+ and Ca^{2+} channels are distributed throughout the membrane of the taste cells and most are therefore not accessible to sour compounds. Thus, after blockade of most or all of the K^+ channels, Na^+ and Ca^{2+} channels on the basolateral membrane are still able to carry the current required to generate the receptor potential.

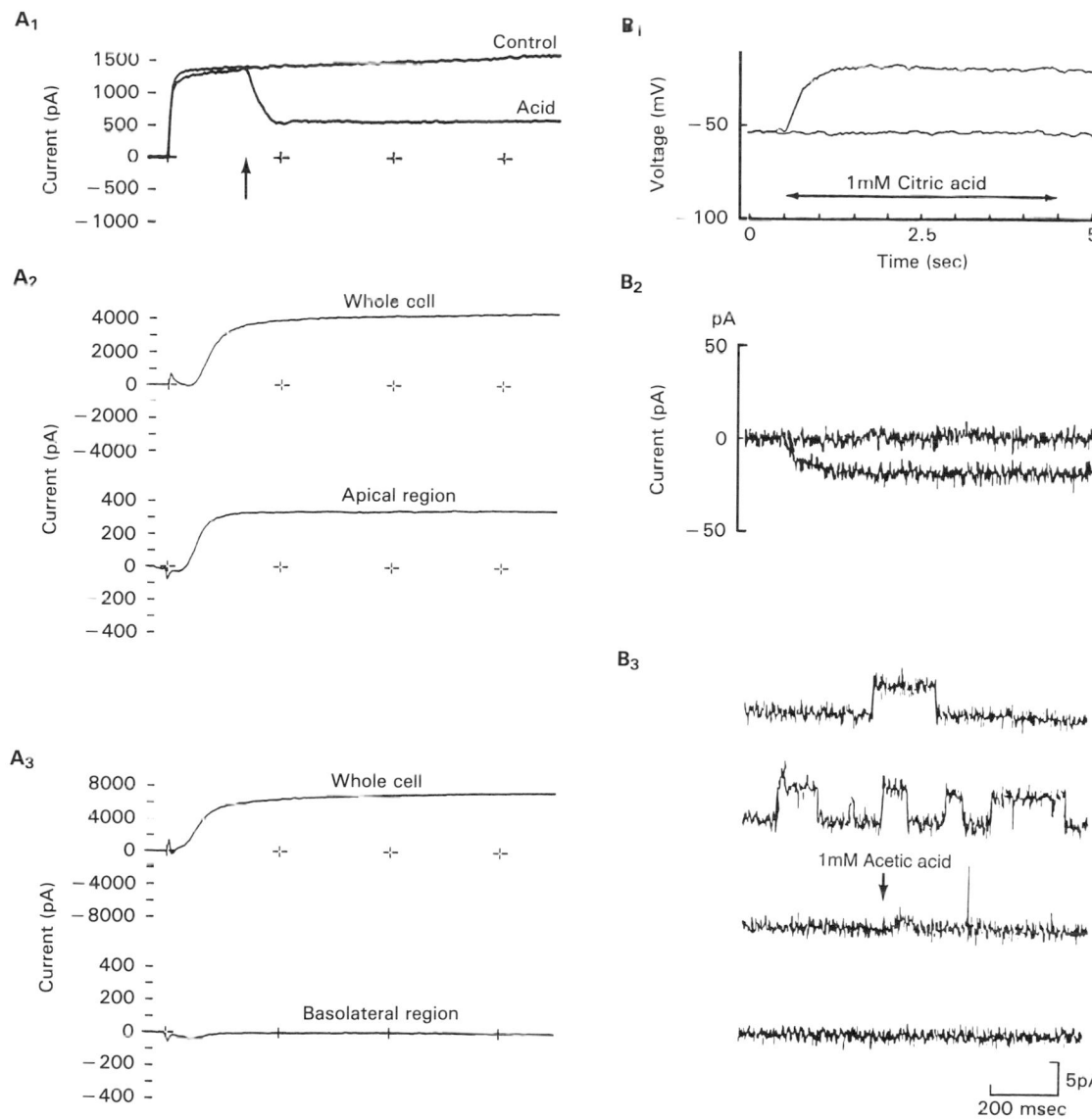

FIGURE 34–12

Sour taste transduction results from a cluster of ion channels.

A. Recordings from isolated mudpuppy taste cells. **1.** Focal application of citric acid to the taste cell reduces the whole-cell K$^+$ current. **2-3.** Approximately 10% of the whole-cell K$^+$ current was recorded near the apical region **(2)** but less than 0.5 near the basolateral region **(3)**. Potassium current was recorded in response to a 20 mV depolarization from −100 mV. (From Kinnamon, 1988.)

B. Responses of isolated salamander taste cells and cell-free patches to acids. **1.** Citric acid (1 mM) elicited a slow depolarization of the taste cell, which was associated with an increase in membrane resistance (not shown). **2.** Under voltage clamp, the acid-induced response was observed as a sustained inward current. **3.** This continuous recording of single K$^+$ channels in outside-out patches of taste cell membrane shows the channels rapidly (and reversibly) blocked by acetic acid. (From Teeter et al., 1989.)

Saltiness. Salt taste appears to result from passage of ions through voltage-independent cation channels in the apical membrane, altering directly the membrane potential of the receptor cells. This transduction mechanism does not seem to require the existence of specific membrane receptors. Rather, the active molecules are thought to be capable of binding to and acting on specific ion channels. Sodium influx through these voltage-independent and amiloride-sensitive cation channels is thought to mediate the transduction of salt taste. Support for this idea comes from the finding that amiloride can block the response of primary gustatory nerve fibers to salt. In addition, psychophysical studies in humans indicate that amiloride partially blocks the taste of Na$^+$ salts.

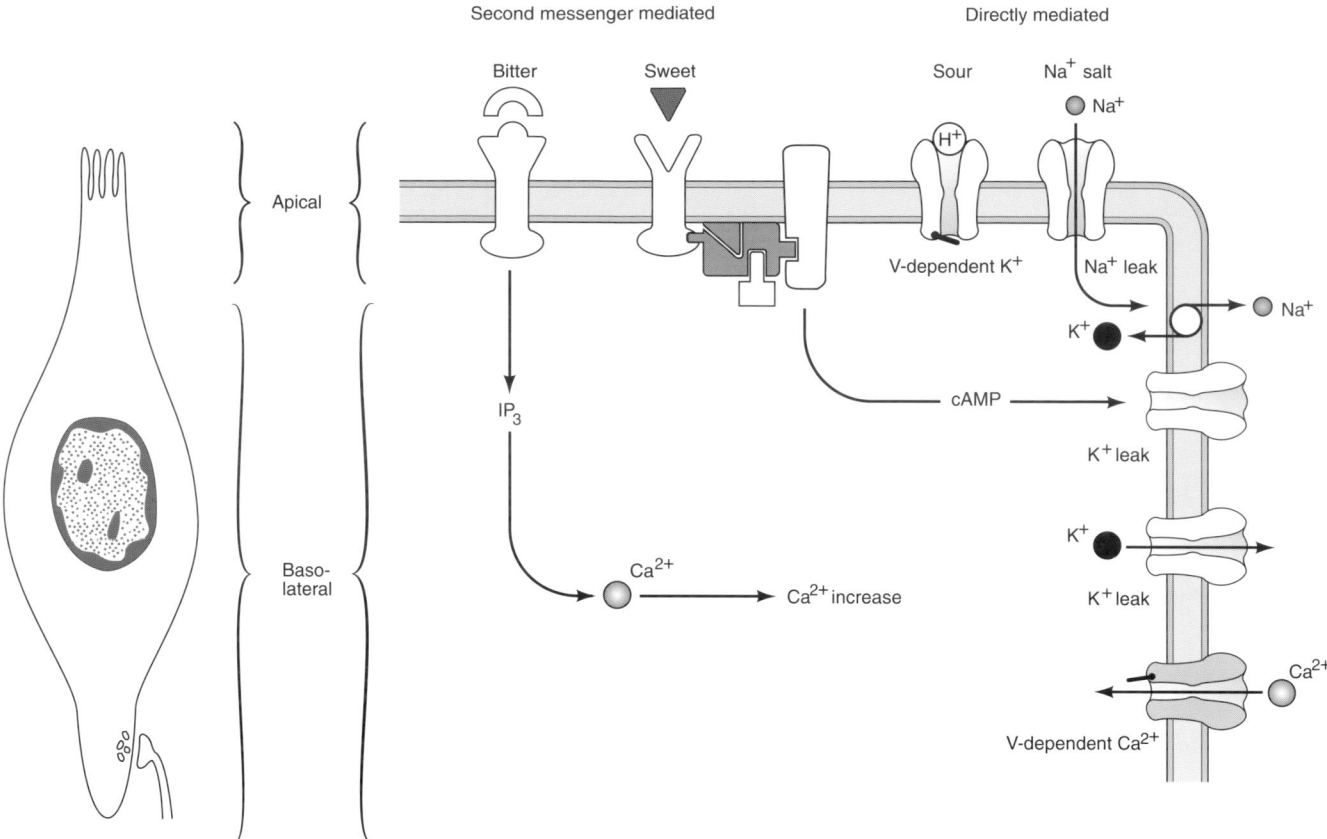

FIGURE 34–13

Diagrammatic representation of possible taste transduction mechanisms. Activation of receptors on the taste cell may lead to rises in intracellular cAMP and to the generation of IP_3 and Ca^{2+} release. Second messengers may activate ion channels in the cell membrane leading to membrane potential changes. (Adapted from Kinnamon, 1988.)

In summary, several different extracellular and intracellular events underlie the transduction of the four basic stimuli. These proposed mechanisms are shown in Figure 34–13. They fall into two general categories. Molecules that signal bitterness and sweetness use second messengers; molecules that signal sourness and saltiness act on channels directly. The saliva may also contain proteins that bind nonselectively to many bitter substances and other lipophilic compounds and play a role in delivering the stimulus to the receptor cell.

There Are Distinct Representations of Taste in the Thalamus and Cortex

Gustatory information is transmitted from the taste buds to the cerebral cortex. As with somatic, visual, and auditory information that enters conscious perception, gustatory information is relayed in the thalamus before reaching the cortex. Unlike the other sensory pathways, however, including the somatic sensory pathway from the tongue, the majority of gustatory fibers project to the thalamus in an uncrossed pathway.

Afferents from Taste Buds Project to the Gustatory Nucleus

The first synapse of the gustatory system is at the taste bud itself. There, individual receptor cells synapse on the terminals of the sensory afferent fibers (Figure 34–9). Each sensory afferent innervates many receptor cells and each receptor cell receives input from several afferent fibers. This results in complex and overlapping receptive fields. The sensory fibers that receive input from the taste cells run in cranial nerves VII, IX, and X and enter the solitary tract in the medulla (Figure 34–14). All the afferent fibers then synapse on neurons in a thin column in the rostral and lateral part of the solitary nuclear complex, called the *gustatory nucleus*. The solitary nuclear complex is an important visceral relay nucleus. Neurons in its ventral region relay afferent information from the gut, lungs, and cardiovascular system to more rostral brain stem nuclei.

Neurons in the gustatory nucleus project in the central tegmental tract to the thalamus, where they terminate in the small-cell (parvocellular) region of the ventral posterior medial nucleus. There the cells serving taste are grouped separately from neurons related to other sensory

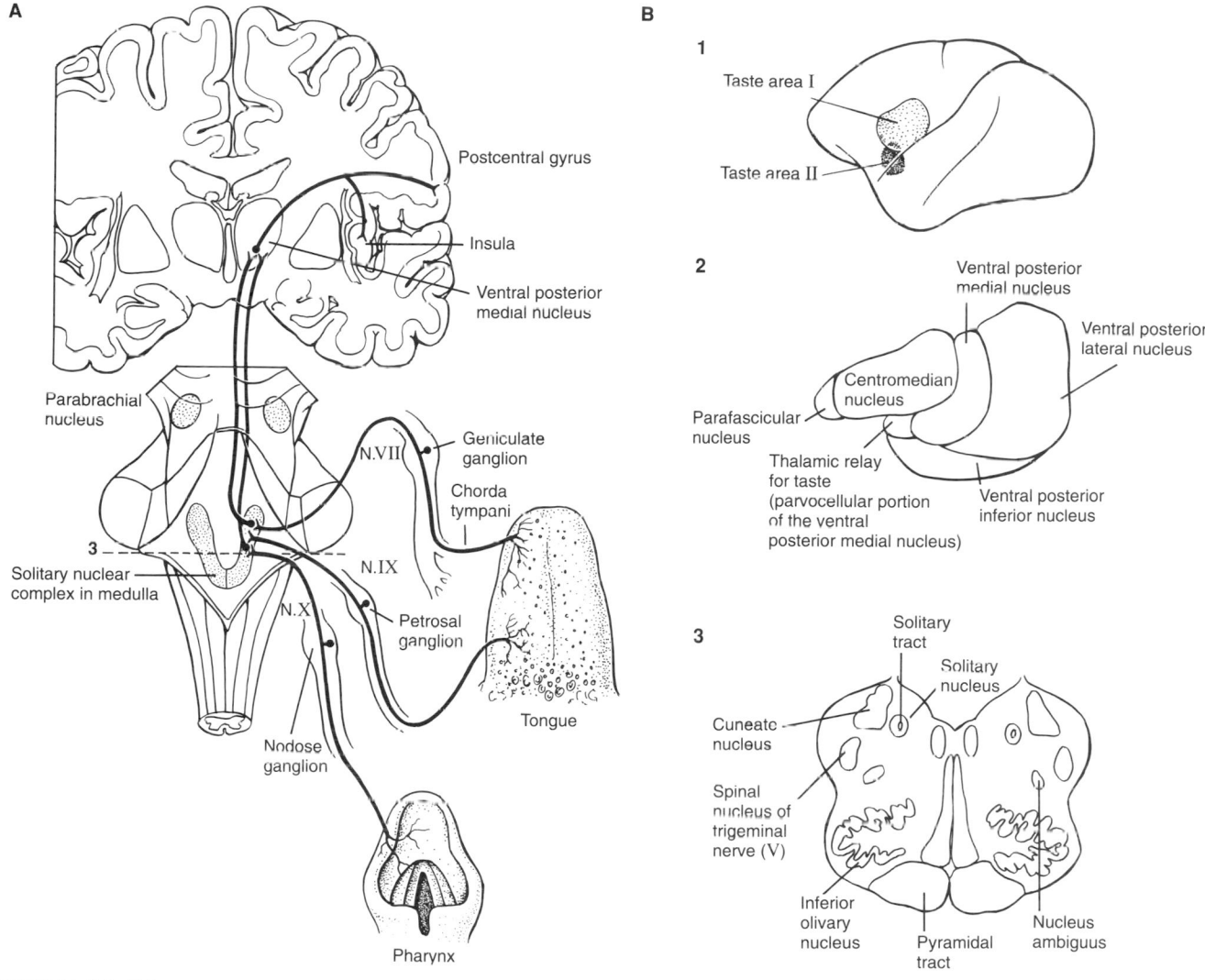

FIGURE 34–14

Taste information is transmitted from the taste buds in the tongue to the cerebral cortex via synapses in the brain stem and thalamus.

A. This diagram of tongue innervation and central pathways of the taste system is derived from studies in monkeys.

B. Cortical representation of taste. **1.** Areas in the somatosen-

sory cortex to which the chorda tympani and glossopharyngeal nerves project. Taste area II is in the insula shown in part A. **2.** The thalamic relay center for taste is shown in this coronal section. **3.** The solitary tract and solitary nucleus are visible in this cross section through the medulla. (Adapted from Burton and Benjamin, 1971.)

modalities of the tongue. Some neurons in the gustatory nucleus project to the pontine parabrachial nuclei, which may mediate autonomic reflexes to taste stimuli and the affective aspects of taste perception. However, in primates gustatory information is not relayed via the parabrachial nucleus but reaches the thalamus directly from the nucleus of the solitary tract.

The neurons of the parvocellular region project to two regions of cerebral cortex: the gustatory region of the postcentral gyrus (in Brodmann's area 3b) and the inner face of the frontal operculum and insula. The region of sensory cortex that receives gustatory input lies just ventral and rostral to the somatosensory representation of the tongue.

Taste Sensations Are Encoded by Specific Pathways and by Patterns of Activity Across These Pathways

A comprehensive scheme for the central coding of gustatory information must account for the discrimination of a variety of complex stimuli. This could be achieved by a labeled line system in which information about single taste qualities is transmitted in separate pathways through the medulla, thalamus, and cortex. Alternatively, the activity of all receptor cells across the lingual epithelium could be broadly tuned, with some receptors activated more strongly than others. Variations of receptor

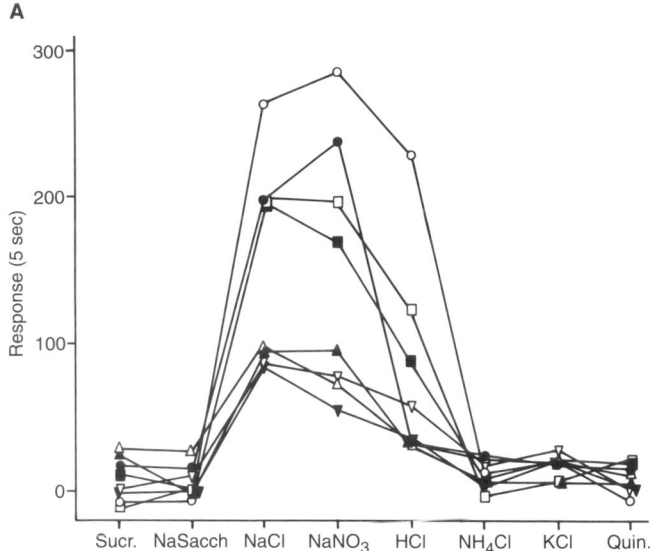

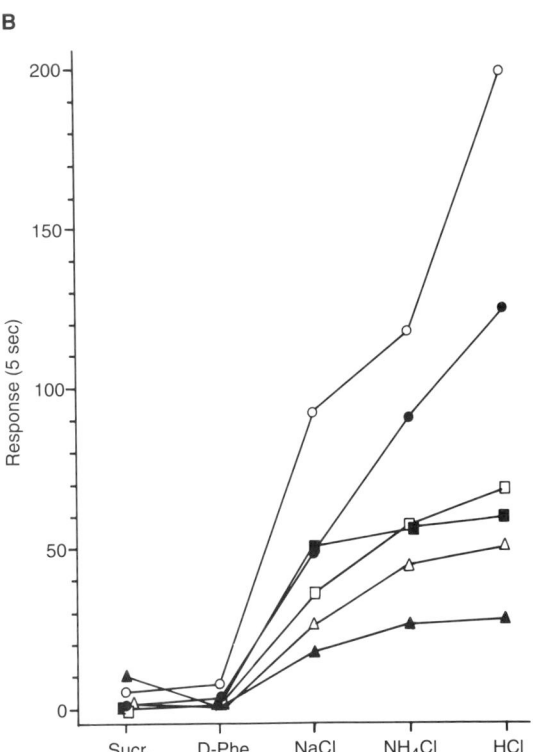

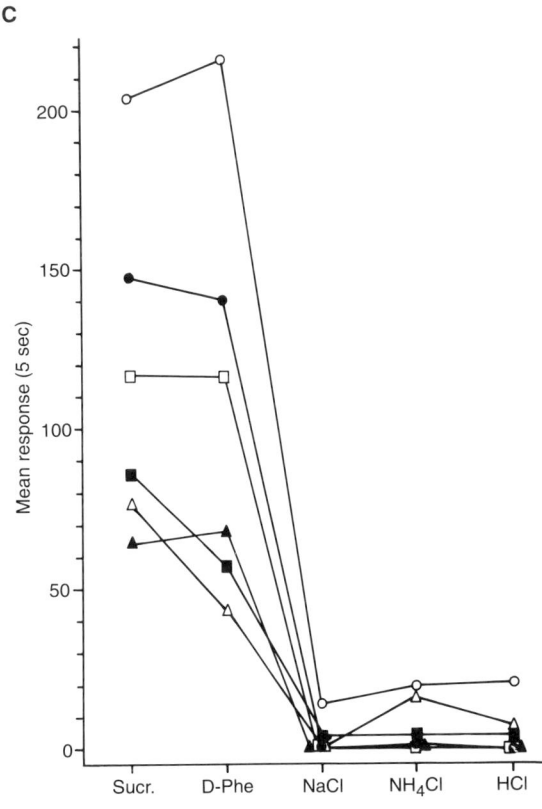

FIGURE 34–15

Response profiles of chorda tympani fibers of the hamster. (From Frank, 1985.)

A. Response profiles for eight fibers that responded more to two sodium salts than to HCl.

B. Profiles for six fibers that responded to HCl, NaCl and NH$_4$Cl.

C. Profiles for six fibers that responded rather specifically to sucrose and D-phenylalanine, which are both sweet.

activity would generate distinctive patterns of activity in the afferent nerve, with each pattern representing a signature for a given complex stimulus.

As already described, there is evidence for the existence of different types of receptors that respond to four basic categories of stimuli, each distributed differentially across the tongue and with distinct transduction mechanisms. The spatial segregation of receptor subtypes in the tongue is preserved in the gustatory nucleus, the thalamus, and the cortex. Thus, it would be possible to maintain independent processing of individual taste modalities at the level of both the peripheral receptors and their central projection sites.

Experiments on taste responses have led to two general theories to explain taste perception. One theory, the *specific pathway theory*, proposes that a single class of neurons may be able to signal one basic taste quality. For example, in the squirrel monkey small groups of gustatory axons respond preferentially to one sweet compound (sucrose), while the nerve as a whole exhibits a greater sensitivity to a different sweet compound (fructose). At the behavioral level, however, the animal's preference is for sucrose, suggesting that taste perception has an important labeled line component.

The other theory involves the principle of *across-fiber pattern coding*. According to this theory, central neurons compare inputs from a whole population of afferent fibers, each of which responds preferentially to a certain stimulus but which also has significant sensitivity to other stimulus types. It is not clear how many different receptors are expressed by individual taste cells. However, there is substantial divergence of innervation of taste cells by the afferent axons. Recordings from the hamster chorda tympani have revealed that single fibers respond to several stimuli of different qualities. For example, fibers that respond primarily to salt also respond to acid, and fibers that respond primarily to acid also respond to bitterness (Figure 34–15). Thus, each sensation is carried centrally by sets of fibers that respond to more than one modality. These results suggest that the perception of each taste results from the comparison of the pattern of activation of all fibers in a population.

Other experiments suggest that both theories are correct; central coding of a stimulus results from a comparison of the activity in a preferred line for that stimulus with the activity in lines for other taste qualities. Thus, the coding for taste resembles the coding in other sensory systems. In the visual system, cortical cells have a preferred axis of orientation but also respond to other orientations. In the auditory system, afferent fibers have a preferred frequency but also respond to other frequencies. Late steps in the processing of visual and auditory stimuli must involve a comparison of the activity of different cells with different preferred orientations and frequencies. The three different photopigments in the photoreceptors also are broadly tuned across the visual spectrum. Color discrimination derives from the central processing of the outputs of all three cone systems. Even the recognition of form in the absence of color depends on contrast. Thus, the mechanism of taste coding—comparison across fibers—represents a general principle of sensory processing.

Both Inborn and Learned Taste Preferences Are Important for Behavior

Smell and taste exert profound control over food and water intake. An observation that first called attention to this aspect of taste perception was the discovery of *specific hunger* by Curt Richter in 1940. Richter reported that animals have an inborn ability to compensate for deficiencies in their diet by selecting foods that contain the missing nutrient. Most dramatic was the discovery of an *innate hunger for salt*. He encountered this hunger in a child whose adrenal cortex had been destroyed by a tumor. As a result, the child had lost the ability to secrete adrenal cortical hormones that maintain normal salt balance in the body, and thus was constantly deprived of salt. Richter found that, given unlimited access to food, this child compensated for his salt deficiency by an extraordinary craving for salt. He found a similar craving in rats whose

adrenals were surgically removed. Robert Contreras extended these observations by showing that removal of the adrenal gland makes the salt receptors in the tongue less sensitive to salt.

Hunger for salt and for certain other foods is innate, but we also learn to prefer some foods and to avoid others. A particularly powerful demonstration of this phenomenon has come from the work of John Garcia. Garcia exposed rats to two stimuli: a specific taste and an auditory stimulus, a tone. He paired the two stimuli with a mild poison that produced nausea. Even though the poison was paired with both the taste and the tone, only the taste became aversive. From then on, the animal invariably avoided food with that particular taste. In a complementary experiment he gave rats the same two stimuli (taste of food and tone) but now paired them with a shock to the foot. Only the tone and not the taste became aversive.

This experiment illustrates that animals have evolved neural mechanisms that enable them to associate smell and taste (and not other sensory modalities) with nausea and stomach illness. The evolutionary advantage that this specific learning ability would provide is obvious; animals that are poisoned by a distinctively flavored food and survive do well not to eat it again. Food avoidance learning is not unique to lower animals but occurs commonly in our everyday life, as the psychologist Martin Seligman has described so vividly:

Sauce Bearnaise is an egg-thickened, tarragon-flavored concoction, and it used to be my favorite sauce. It now tastes awful to me. This happened several years ago, when I felt the effects of the stomach flu about six hours after eating filet mignon with sauce Bearnaise. I became violently ill and spent most of the night vomiting. The next time I had sauce Bearnaise, I couldn't bear the taste of it. At the time, I had no ready way to account for the change, although it seemed to fit a classical conditioning paradigm: conditioned stimulus (sauce) paired with unconditioned stimulus (illness) and unconditioned response (vomiting) yields conditioned response (nauseating taste). But if this was classical conditioning, it violated at least two Pavlovian laws: The delay between tasting the sauce and vomiting was about 6 hours, and classical conditioning isn't supposed to bridge time gaps like that. In addition, neither the filet mignon, nor the white plate off which I ate the sauce, nor *Tristan und Isolde*, the opera that I listened to in the interpolated time, nor my wife, Kerry, became aversive. Only the sauce Bearnaise did. Moreover, unlike much of classical conditioning, it could not be seen as a "cognitive" phenomenon, involving expectations. For I soon found out that the sauce had not caused the vomiting and that a stomach flu had.... Yet in spite of this knowledge, I could not later inhibit my aversion.

Martin Seligman, in *Biological Boundaries of Learning*

An Overall View

Smell and taste are fascinating because they are so vivid emotionally and perceptually and so important nutritionally for the regulation of bodily function. Smell and taste were for many years thought to be different from the other senses; however, modern studies suggest that this is not so. In both the olfactory and gustatory systems the transduction of sensory stimuli involves the activation of membrane receptors that trigger a variety of intracellular second messengers. These second messengers are probably similar to those used in other sensory cells. The ion channels expressed by olfactory and gustatory receptor cells are similar to those expressed by other sensory neurons. In addition, the same general rules for coding that we have encountered in the other senses—labeled line codes, analysis of contrast, and parallel processing—may also apply to smell and taste. Thus, all sensory systems rely on the same basic principles of processing and organization, not only in humans, but throughout much of phylogeny. The mechanisms of perception have therefore been remarkably conserved during evolution.

Selected Readings

Beidler, L. M. 1980. The chemical senses: Gustation and olfaction. In V. B. Mountcastle (ed.), Medical Physiology, 14th ed., Vol. 1. St. Louis: Mosby, pp. 586–602.

Brand, J. G., Teeter, J. H., Cagan, R. H., and Kare, M. R. (eds.) 1989. Chemical Senses, Vol. 1: Receptor Events and Transduction in Taste and Olfaction. New York: Marcel Dekker.

Carpenter, M. B., and Sutin, J. 1983. Human Neuroanatomy, 8th ed. Baltimore: Williams & Wilkins.

Finger, T. E., and Silver, W. L. (eds.) 1987. Neurobiology of Taste and Smell. New York: Wiley.

Kauer, J. S. 1987. Coding in the olfactory system. In T. E. Finger and W. L. Silver (eds.), Neurobiology of Taste and Smell. New York: Wiley, pp. 205–231.

Norgren, R. 1984. Central neural mechanisms of taste. In I. Darian-Smith (ed.), Handbook of Physiology, Section 1: The Nervous System, Vol. III. Sensory Processes, Part 2. Bethesda, Md.: American Physiological Society, pp. 1087–1128.

Pfaff, D. W. (ed.) 1985. Taste, Olfaction, and the Central Nervous System. New York: Rockefeller University Press.

Ramón y Cajal, S. 1909. Histologie du Système Nerveux de l'Homme & des Vertébrés, Vol. 1. L. Azoulay (trans.). Madrid: Instituto Ramón y Cajal, 1952.

Reed, R. R. 1990. How does the nose know? Cell 60:1–2.

Roper, S. D. 1989. The cell biology of vertebrate taste receptors. Annu. Rev. Neurosci. 12:329–353.

Shepherd, G. M. 1988. Neurobiology. 2nd ed. New York: Oxford University Press, chap. 11, "Chemical Senses."

References

Akabas, M. H., Dodd, J., and Al-Awqati, Q. 1988. A bitter substance induces a rise in intracellular calcium in a subpopulation of rat taste cells. Science 242:1047–1050.

Andres, K. H. 1966. Der Feinbau der Regio olfactoria von Makrosmatikern. Z. Zellforsch. 69:140–154.

Avenet, P., and Lindemann, B. 1989. Chemoreception of salt taste: The blockage of stationary sodium currents by amiloride in isolated receptor cells and excised membrane patches. In J. G. Brand, J. H. Tetter, R. H. Cagan, and M. R. Kare (eds.), Chemical Senses, Vol. 1.: Receptor Events and Transduction in Taste and Olfaction. New York: Marcel Dekker, pp. 171–182.

Bignetti, E., Cavaggioni, A., Pelosi, P., Persaud, K. C., Sorbi, R. T., and Tirindelli, R. 1985. Purification and characterisation of an odorant-binding protein from cow nasal tissue. Eur. J. Biochem. 149:227–231.

Bloom, W., and Fawcett, D. W. 1975. A Textbook of Histology, 10th ed. Philadelphia: Saunders, pp. 392–410.

Breer, H., Boekhoff, I., and Tareilus, E. 1990. Rapid kinetics of second messenger formation in olfactory transduction. Nature 345:65–68.

Buck, L., and Axel, R. 1991. A novel multigene family may encode odorant receptors: A molecular basis for odorant recognition. Cell 65:175–187.

Burton, H., and Benjamin, R. M. 1971. Central projections of the gustatory system. In L. M. Beidler (ed.), Handbook of Sensory Physiology, Vol. IV: Chemical Senses, Part 2, Taste. Berlin: Springer, pp. 148–164.

Contreras, R. J. 1977. Changes in gustatory nerve discharges with sodium deficiency: A single unit analysis. Brain Res. 121:373–378.

Dhallan, R. S., Yau, K.-W., Schrader, K. A., and Reed, R. R. 1990. Primary structure and functional expression of a cyclic nucleotide-activated channel from olfactory neurons. Nature. 347:184–187.

Erickson, R. P. 1968. Stimulus coding in topographic and non-topographic afferent modalities: On the significance of the activity of individual sensory neurons. Psychol. Rev. 75:447–465.

Frank, M. 1973. An analysis of hamster afferent taste nerve response functions. J. Gen. Physiol. 61:588–618.

Frank, M. E. 1985. On the neural code for sweet and salty tastes. In D. W. Pfaff (ed.), Taste, Olfaction and the Central Nervous System. New York: Rockefeller University Press, pp. 107–128.

Frank, M. E., Contreras, R. J., and Hettinger, T. P. 1983. Nerve fibers sensitive to ionic taste stimuli in chorda tympani of the rat. J. Neurophysiol. 50:941–960.

Frisch, D. 1967. Ultrastructure of mouse olfactory mucosa. Am. J. Anat. 121:87–119.

Garcia, J., Hankins, W. G., and Rusiniak, K. W. 1974. Behavioral regulation of the milieu interne in man and rat. Science 185:824–831.

Getchell, T. V. 1977. Analysis of intracellular recordings from salamander olfactory epithelium. Brain Res. 123:275–286.

Getchell, T. V., and Shepherd, G. M. 1978. Responses of olfactory receptor cells to step pulses of odour at different concentrations in the salamander. J. Physiol. (Lond.) 282:521–540.

Henning, H. 1922. Psychologische Studien am Geschmackssinn. Handbh. Biol. Arbeitsmeth. 6A:627–740.

Hwang, P. M., Verma, A., Bredt, D. S., and Snyder, S. H. 1990. Localization of phosphatidylinositol signaling components in rat taste cells: Role in bitter taste transduction. Proc. Natl. Acad. Sci. U.S.A. 87:7395–7399.

Jones, D. T., and Reed, R. R. 1989. G_{olf}: An olfactory neuron specific-G protein involved in odorant signal transduction. Science 244:790–795.

Kauer, J. S. 1988. Real-time imaging of evoked activity in local circuits of the salamander olfactory bulb. Nature 331:166–168.

Kimura, K., and Beidler, L. M. 1961. Microelectrode study of taste receptors of rat and hamster. J. Cell. Comp. Physiol. 58:131–139.

Kinnamon, J. C. 1987. Organization and innervation of taste buds. In T. E. Finger, and W. L. Silver (eds.), Neurobiology of Taste and Smell. New York: Wiley, pp. 277–297.

Kinnamon, S. C. 1988. Taste transduction: A diversity of mechanisms. Trends Neurosci. 11:491–496.

Kinnamon, S. C., Dionne, V. E., and Beam, K. G. 1988. Apical localization of K^+ channels in taste cells provides the basis for sour taste transduction. Proc. Natl. Acad. Sci. U.S.A. 85:7023–7027.

Krupinski, J., Coussen, F., Bakalyar, H. A., Tang. W.-J., Feinstein, P. G., Orth, K., Slaughter, C., Reed, R. R., and Gilman, A. G.

1989. Adenylyl cyclase amino acid sequence: Possible channel- or transporter-like structure. Science 244:1558–1564.

Mathews, D. F. 1972. Response patterns of single neurons in the tortoise olfactory epithelium and olfactory bulb. J. Gen. Physiol. 60:166–180.

Moulton, D. G. 1976. Spatial patterning of response to odors in the peripheral olfactory system. Physiol. Rev. 56:578–593.

Murray, R. G. 1973. The ultrastructure of taste buds. In I. Friedmann (ed.), The Ultrastructure of Sensory Organs. New York: American Elsevier, pp. 1–81.

Nakamura, T., and Gold, G. H. 1987. A cyclic nucleotide-gated conductance in olfactory receptor cilia. Nature 325:442–444.

Nieuwenhuys, R., Voogd, J., and van Huijzen, Chr. 1988. The Human Central Nervous System: A Synopsis and Atlas, 3rd rev. ed. Berlin: Springer.

Ogata, C., Hatada, M., Tomlinson, G., Shin, W.-C., and Kim, S.-H. 1987. Crystal structure of the intensely sweet protein monellin. Nature 328:739–742.

Ottoson, D. 1983. Physiology of the Nervous System. New York: Oxford University Press.

Ozeki, M., and Sato, M. 1972. Responses of gustatory cells in the tongue of rat to stimuli representing four taste qualities. Comp. Biochem. Physiol. 41A:391–407.

Pace, U., Hanski, E., Salomon, Y., and Lancet, D. 1985. Odorant-sensitive adenylate cyclase may mediate olfactory reception. Nature 316:255–258.

Pelosi, P., Baldaccini, N. E., and Pisanelli, A. M. 1982. Identification of a specific olfactory receptor for 2-isobutyl-3-methoxy pyrazine. Biochem. J. 201:245–248.

Pevsner, J., Hwang, P. M., Sklar, P. B., Venable, J. C., and Snyder, S. H. 1988. Odorant-binding protein and its mRNA are localized to lateral nasal gland implying a carrier function. Proc. Natl. Acad. Sci. U.S.A. 85:2383–2387.

Pevsner, J., Reed, R. R., Feinstein, P. G., and Snyder, S. H. 1988. Molecular cloning of odorant-binding protein: Member of a ligand carrier family. Science 241:336–339.

Pfaffmann, C. 1941. Gustatory afferent impulses. J. Cell. Comp. Physiol. 17:243–258.

Pfaffmann, C. 1955. Gustatory nerve impulses in rat, cat and rabbit. J. Neurophysiol. 18:429–440.

Pfeuffer, E., Mollner, S., Lancet, D., and Pfeuffer, T. 1989. Olfactory adenylyl cyclase. J. Biol. Chem. 264:18803–18807.

Richter, C. P. 1942. Total self regulatory functions in animals and human beings. Harvey Lect. 38:63–103.

Rolls, E. T. 1989. Information processing in the taste system of primates. J. Exp. Biol. 146:141–164.

Royer, S. M., and Kinnamon, J. C. 1991. HVEM serial-section analysis of rabbit foliate taste buds. I. Type III cells and their synapses. J. Comp. Neurol. 306:49–72.

Schiffman, S. S. 1983. Taste and smell in disease. N. Engl. J. Med. 308:1337–1343.

Schmale, H., Holtgreve-Grez, H., and Christiansen, H. 1990. Possible role for salivary gland protein in taste reception indicated by homology to lipophilic-ligand carrier proteins. Nature 343:366–369.

Scott, T. R., Jr., and Erickson, R. P. 1971. Synaptic processing of taste-quality information in thalamus of the rat. J. Neurophysiol. 34:868–884.

Seligman, M. E. P., and Hager, J. L. 1972. Biological Boundaries of Learning. Englewood Cliffs, N. J.: Prentice-Hall.

Shepherd, G. M. 1972. Synaptic organization of the mammalian olfactory bulb. Physiol. Rev. 52:864–917.

Sloan, H. E., Hughes, S. E., and Oakley, B. 1983. Chronic impairment of axonal transport eliminates taste responses and taste buds. J. Neurosci. 3:117–123.

Smith, D. V., Van Buskirk, R. L., Travers, J. B., and Bieber, S. L. 1983. Coding of taste stimuli by hamster brain stem neurons. J. Neurophysiol. 50:541–558.

Stewart, W. B., Kauer, J. S., and Shepherd, G. M. 1979. Functional organization of rat olfactory bulb analysed by the 2-deoxyglucose method. J. Comp. Neurol. 185:715–734.

Teeter, J. H., Sugimoto, K., and Brand, J. G. 1989. Ionic currents in taste cells and reconstituted taste epithelial membranes. In J. G. Brand, J. H. Teeter, R. H. Cagan, and M. R. Kare (eds.), Chemical Senses, Vol. 1.: Receptor Events and Transduction in Taste and Olfaction. New York: Marcel Dekker, pp. 151–170.

Trotier, D., and MacLeod, P. 1983. Intracellular recordings from salamander olfactory receptor cells. Brain Res. 268:225–237.

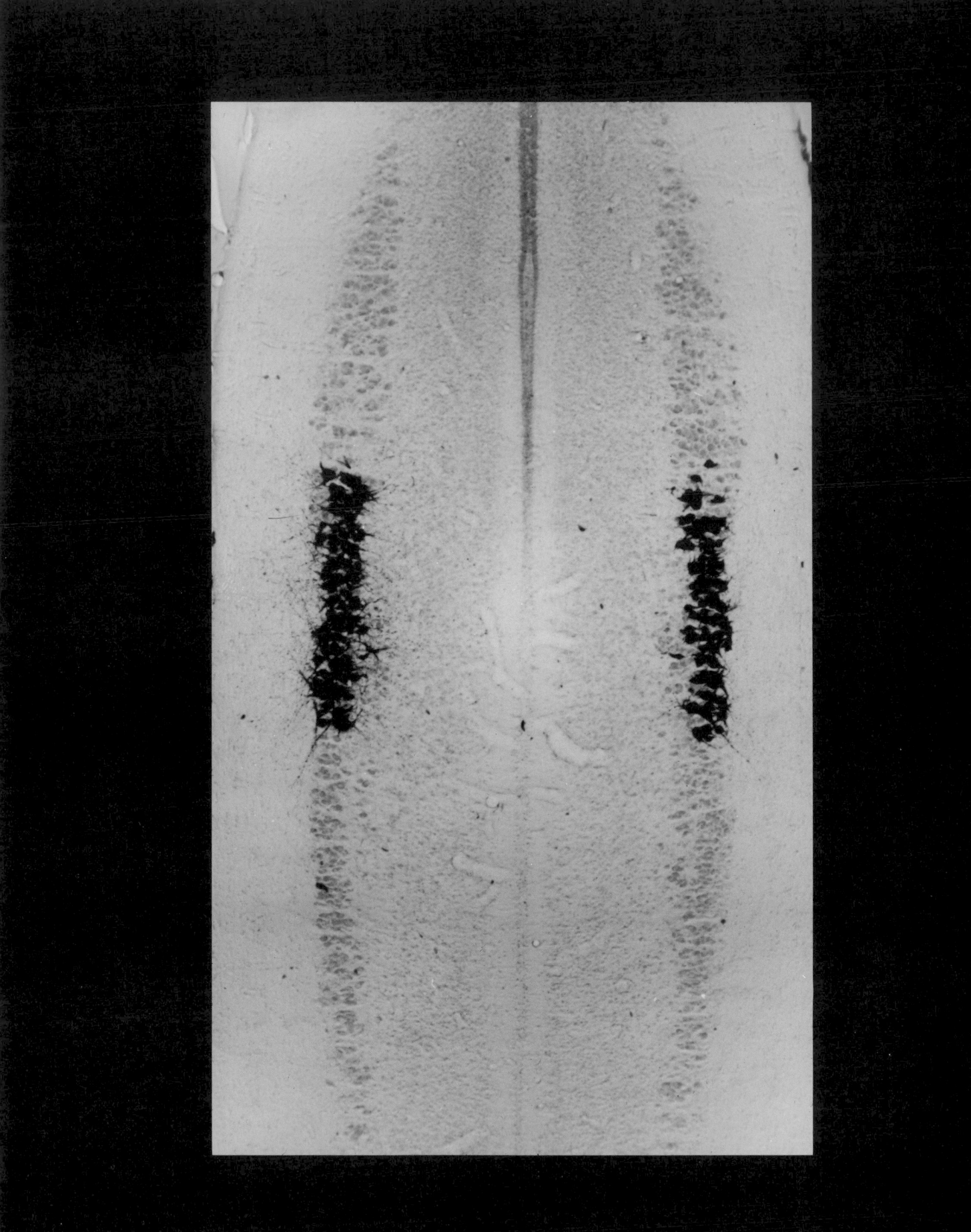

Motor Systems of the Brain: Reflex and Voluntary Control of Movement

Individuals select from the continuous, changing array of external stimuli and organize motor output to achieve a *particular* and *single goal*. Charles Sherrington, the English physiologist, referred to this purposeful behavior as the *integrative action* of the nervous system. Sherrington was interested in how various regions of the nervous system are coordinated to produce purposeful action even in the presence of conflicting stimuli. He correctly recognized that reflexes within the spinal cord are the simplest examples of a purposeful action. Indeed, spinal mechanisms are critical for the execution of all movements. Through motor neurons and their associated interneuronal circuits, the spinal cord is the final output for voluntary as well as reflex actions. In addition, as we saw in Part V, the spinal cord also is an important sensory structure.

The spinal cord is only the lowest level, however, in the hierarchy of structures that subserves motor function.

This hierarchy also includes the brain stem and cerebral cortex. Each of these higher levels contains several anatomically distinct areas that project in parallel to the spinal cord. A characteristic feature of most of these areas is that, like the sensory systems, they are organized in a somatotopic fashion—movements of adjacent body parts are controlled by neighboring parts of each area of the brain. Thus, the motor cortex contains a complete motor map of the body just as the nearby somatic sensory cortex contains a complete map of the body surface. Two associated structures, the cerebellum and basal ganglia, are not involved directly in producing movement. Rather, they modulate the corticospinal and the brain stem systems that control the motor neurons and related spinal interneurons.

Some functions of the motor systems and their disturbance by disease are now understood at the level of the biochemistry of specific transmitter systems. Information

Motor neurons are the final common pathway for all behavioral acts. These neurons form a column in the ventral horn that extends up through the spinal cord and into the brain stem. This photomicrograph shows a horizontal section through the brachial region of the frog's spinal cord. Here, the triceps motor neuron pools are identified by the retrograde accumulation of horseradish peroxidase transported from motor nerve endings after injection of the marker enzyme in the vicinity of target muscles. (Courtesy of Eric Frank, University of Pittsburgh.)

about transmitters in the basal ganglia and their deficits in Parkinsonism suggests that other neurological and psychiatric disorders also result from altered functioning of chemical transmitter systems—malfunction of synthesis, transport, release, and interaction with the postsynaptic receptor. We now know that in Huntington's disease a mutation can lead to premature death of nerve cells, which results in the symptoms of disease. With the identification of the genes and proteins important for motor function, we may soon understand the molecular mechanisms of the integrative action of the nervous system.

PART VI

Chapter 35: **The Control of Movement**
Chapter 36: **Muscles: Effectors of the Motor Systems**
Chapter 37: **Muscle Receptors and Spinal Reflexes: The Stretch Reflex**
Chapter 38: **Spinal Mechanisms of Motor Coordination**
Chapter 39: **Posture**
Chapter 40: **Voluntary Movement**
Chapter 41: **The Cerebellum**
Chapter 42: **The Basal Ganglia**
Chapter 43: **The Ocular Motor System**

Claude Ghez

The Control of Movement

Sensory Information Is Necessary for the Control of Movement

Sensory Information Is Used to Correct Errors Through Feedback and Feed-forward Mechanisms

Patients with Impaired Sensation in the Limbs Show Deficits in Both Feedback and Feed-forward Control of Movement

There Are Three Levels in the Hierarchy of Motor Control

The Spinal Cord, the Brain Stem, and Cortical Motor Areas Are Organized Hierarchically and in Parallel

The Cerebellum and Basal Ganglia Control the Cortical and Brain Stem Motor Systems

Motor Neurons in the Spinal Cord Are Subject to Afferent Input and Descending Control

Spinal Motor Neurons Are Topographically Organized into Medial and Lateral Groups That Innervate Proximal and Distal Muscles

The Terminations of Medial and Lateral Interneurons and Propriospinal Neurons Have Different Distributions

The Brain Stem Modulates Motor Neurons and Interneurons in the Spinal Cord Through Four Systems

Medial Pathways Control Axial and Proximal Muscles

Lateral Pathways Control Distal Muscles

Aminergic Pathways Modulate the Excitability of Spinal Neurons

The Motor Cortex Acts on Motor Neurons Directly via the Corticospinal Tract and Indirectly Through Brain Stem Pathways

The Corticospinal Tract Is the Largest Descending Fiber Tract from the Brain

Cortical Control of Movement Is Achieved Only Late in Phylogeny

Lesions of the Cortical Motor Areas and Their Projections Cause Characteristic Symptoms

Muscle Weakness May Result from Disturbances in Descending Motor Pathways or in the Spinal Motor Neurons Themselves

Parallel Control of Motor Neurons Allows Recovery of Function Following Lesions

An Overall View

The sensory systems provide an internal representation of the outside world. A major function of this representation is to extract the information necessary to guide the movements that make up our behavioral repertoire. These movements are controlled by a set of motor systems that allow us to maintain balance and posture, to move our body, limbs, and eyes, and to communicate through speech and gesture. In contrast to the sensory systems, which transform physical energy into neural information, the motor systems transform neural information into physical energy by issuing commands that are transmitted by the brain stem and spinal cord to skeletal muscles. The muscles translate this neural information into a contractile force that produces movements.

As our perceptual skills are a reflection of the capabilities of the sensory systems to detect, analyze, and estimate the significance of physical stimuli, so our agility and dexterity are reflections of the capabilities of the motor systems to plan, coordinate, and execute movements. The beautifully executed pirouette of a ballet dancer, the powered backhand of a tennis player, the fingering technique of a pianist, and the coordinated eye movements of a reader all require a remarkable degree of motor skill that no robot approaches. Yet once trained, the motor systems execute the motor program for each of these skills with ease, almost automatically.

The movements of which our motor systems are capable can be divided into three broad, overlapping classes: voluntary movements, reflex responses, and rhythmic motor patterns. These movements differ in their complexity and degree of voluntary control.

Voluntary movements, reading, manipulating an object, or playing the piano, represent the most complex actions. These movements are characterized by several features. First, they are purposeful. They may be initiated in response to a specific, external stimulus or to the will. Second, voluntary movements are goal directed. Finally, movements are largely learned and their performance improves greatly with practice. As these skilled movements are mastered with practice, they require less or ultimately no conscious participation. Thus, once you have learned to drive a car you do not think through the actions of shifting gears or stepping on the brake before performing them.

Reflex responses, the knee jerk, the withdrawal of a hand from a hot object, or coughing are the simplest motor behaviors and are least affected by voluntary controls. Reflexes are rapid, somewhat stereotyped, and involuntary responses that are usually controlled in a graded way by the eliciting stimulus.

Rhythmic motor patterns, walking, running, chewing, combine features of voluntary and reflex acts. Typically only the initiation and termination of the sequence are voluntary. Once initiated, the sequence of relatively stereotyped, repetitive movements may continue almost automatically in reflex-like fashion.

Muscles relax and contract in each of these classes of movements. Most movements occur at joints, where two or more bones form a lubricated contact point with low friction. Since individual muscles can only pull (they cannot push), separate sets of muscles are required at the opposite side of the joint, and use it as a fulcrum (Figure 36–15). Each movement at a joint thus brings into play two opposing sets of muscles: *Agonists*, the prime movers, are counterbalanced by the *antagonists*, which help to decelerate the moving limb.

Beyond simply contracting and relaxing, the motor systems need to carry out three additional tasks. First, the motor systems must convey accurately timed commands not only to *one* muscle group but to *many* groups, since even a simple movement, such as raising the arm, involves many different joints: the wrist, the elbow, as well as the shoulder. Second, the motor systems must consider the distribution of body mass and make postural adjustments appropriate for the particular movements to be executed. For example, while standing, our leg muscles must contract before we raise an arm, otherwise the arm movement would shift our center of gravity, causing us to fall. Finally, the motor systems must take into account the *motor plant*: the mechanical arrangement of the muscles, bones, and joints. With each movement the motor systems must adjust their commands to compensate for the inertia of the limbs and the mechanical arrangement of the muscles, bones, and joints being moved.

To integrate these three features into voluntary and reflex acts, the motor systems rely on two important and interrelated organizational features. One, the motor systems have available to them a continuous flow of sensory information about events in the environment, the position and orientation of the body and limbs, and the degree of contraction of the muscles. The motor systems use this information to select the response that is appropriate and to make adjustments in ongoing movement. Two, the components of the motor systems are organized as a hierarchy of control levels and each level is provided with that sensory information that is relevant for the functions it controls. Thus, higher levels concerned with strategic issues, such as the selection of a response appropriate to a specific goal, need not monitor the moment-to-moment sensory details of the response. This detailed sensory monitoring goes on at a lower level of the motor hierarchy.

In this chapter we introduce the study of movement by observing how different classes of movement are governed by these two organizational features—the flow of sensory information and the hierarchy of control levels. In later chapters we shall examine in detail the individual components of the motor systems and the pathways through which they act on motor neurons and muscles to produce purposeful motor activity. In addition, we shall also see how the motor systems function cooperatively to control the major classes of movements.

Sensory Information Is Necessary for the Control of Movement

The functioning of the motor systems is intimately related to that of the sensory systems. Experiments conducted in the 1950s by Richard Held and Allan Hein showed that when young kittens were passively moved about and not allowed to actively interact with their environment, they failed to develop the capacity to discriminate important visual cues. The proper moment-to-moment functioning of motor systems depends on a continuous inflow of sensory information. First, vision, hearing, and receptors on the body surface inform us about where objects are in space and our own position relative to them. Second, proprioceptors in the muscle, joints, and the vestibular apparatus inform the motor systems about the length and tension of muscles, the angles of the joints, and the position of the body in space. Both types of information are essential for planning movements and refining those that are in progress.

Sensory Information Is Used to Correct Errors Through Feedback and Feed-forward Mechanisms

When we reach for an object, the arm may initially be off course, but we can correct the end of its trajectory by a feedback process. Many man-made devices, such as thermostats and power steering, use similar feedback processes. How do these feedback mechanisms work? Both natural and man-made systems that use feedback mechanisms have sensors that monitor the output. These sensors provide a *feedback signal*, which is compared to a *reference signal* that indicates the desired output value (Figure 35–1A). With *negative feedback* the feedback signal is subtracted from the reference signal by a device called a *comparator*, and the resultant error signal acts on a device called a *controller* to increase or decrease the output of the controlled system. Thus, in reaching for an object the controlled system is the arm and the difference between the actual position of the hand (feedback signal) and the position we intend for it (reference signal) should be brought to zero. If we do not reach the target, perhaps because an obstacle unexpectedly deflects the hand (disturbance), an error signal is sent to the controller, which issues another command to continue further in the same direction. If we overshoot, a command is emitted to move in the opposite direction.

Feedback can be used either to maintain or to modulate a variable such as position or force. When the variable is to be maintained around a set value, the reference signal remains constant, a process termed *regulation*. An example of regulation is the continued maintenance of a standing posture on a moving boat. Here motion of the support surface (the deck of the boat) is sensed in the feet and ankles and is used by postural mechanisms to maintain the body in a vertical position. In the nervous system feedback is limited to slow movements and to the control of sequential acts because the time taken to process sensory inputs is relatively long. For example, it may take several hundred milliseconds to respond to a visual cue (see Chapter 40) while a quick movement itself may last only 150–200 ms. It is therefore impossible to rely on feedback to

catch a ball, or to reach for a rapidly moving object. In addition, when the effect of a feedback loop is very powerful—a condition referred to as a *high gain*—and there are long time delays. The system can readily be driven into an undesirable state of oscillation. This phenomenon is discussed in Chapter 37 in the context of spasticity.

Sensory events can often control motor action more effectively by providing *advance* rather than feedback information. Advance information can then be used to adjust the controlled variables before events occur that would influence them. This *feed-forward control* is essential in a wide variety of movements (Figure 35–1B). Consider the task of catching a ball. To catch the ball it is necessary to predict its trajectory and to place the hand at a point that will intercept its path. As is apparent in the example of catching a ball, the feed-forward control system must interpret visual cues correctly to tense the muscles in anticipation of impact and to set the position feedback correctly. This requires dynamic representations or *internal models* of both the ball's trajectory and the properties of the musculoskeletal system. (See Chapter 30).

These representations are updated by information from additional sensors that monitor changes in the state of the controlled system (labeled as state variables in Figure 35–1B). Proprioceptors in muscles and joints, which sense the length and tension of muscles and the angles of joints, are critical in providing state information to the motor system. However, vision and vestibular inputs are also quite important.

Although the same sensors may provide information for both feedback and feed-forward control, the way in which the information is processed is quite different. With feedback, error signals are computed continuously and control the ongoing response from moment to moment. As a result of the long conduction delay of neural impulses, biological feedback processes generally operate relatively slowly and are therefore used primarily to maintain posture and regulate slow movements. In catching a ball even the most rapid feedback responses would not prevent us from dropping it if we have incorrectly estimated the force of impact. On the other hand, such feedback is crucial for stabilizing the hand once the ball has been caught. In contrast, feed-forward systems, which are not affected by loop delays, operate more quickly. In contrast to feedback control, which operates continuously, feed-forward control is often triggered intermittently, and the resulting state is then reevaluated after the response is completed.

Patients with Impaired Sensation in the Limbs Show Deficits in Both Feedback and Feed-forward Control of Movement

The importance of proprioceptive inputs in the feedback and feed-forward control of posture and movement can be demonstrated dramatically by the motor deficits of patients with impaired proprioception. This occurs in a condition known as *large-fiber sensory neuropathy* in which

A Feedback control

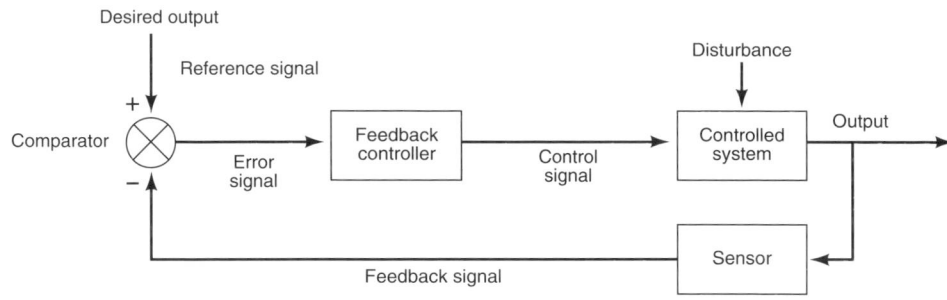

B Feed-forward control

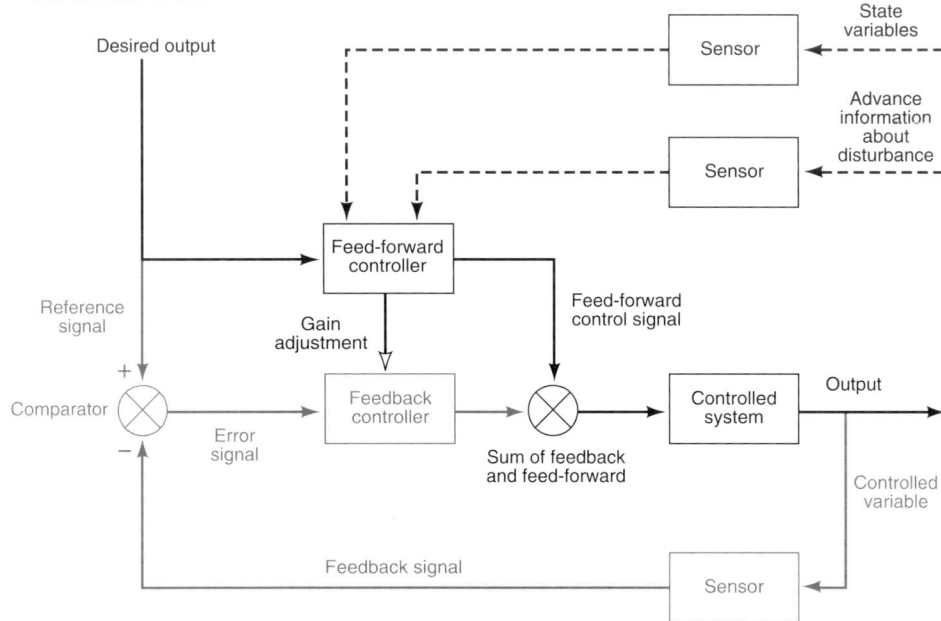

FIGURE 35–1

Feedback and feed-forward control circuits.

A. In a feedback system a feedback signal is compared to a reference signal by a comparator. In reaching slowly for an object, the arm is the controlled system and the intended position of the arm is the reference. The difference between the position of the hand and the reference should be brought to zero to execute the action properly. If the hand is unexpectedly disturbed, an error signal is sent to the controller and a command to continue in the direction of the target is issued. In a feedback system, error signals are sent continuously to control the action from moment to moment. Feedback control is usually used for slow movements and to maintain posture.

B. Feed-forward control is essential for rapid movements and relies on advance information to adjust controlled variables. In catching a ball, advance information on the ball's trajectory and possible placement of the hand are advance information received by sensors and fed forward by the controller. Feedback control comes into play to position the hand properly after the ball is caught. Feed-forward control also monitors the system to deal with changes that take place over time, such as fatigue, through the mechanism of the adaptive controller.

the large afferent fibers that carry proprioceptive and tactile inputs degenerate. Unless they can see their limbs these patients cannot sense their position nor can they detect motion of their joints, because these sensations are mediated primarily by receptors in muscles and joints supplied by large-diameter fibers. Tendon reflexes are also absent because information from muscle spindles that

triggers these reflexes does not reach the spinal cord. Finally, tactile sensation is impaired. Tactile feedback allows one to estimate contact with objects more precisely than does visual monitoring of the hand. When this feedback system does not function, manual dexterity is severely impaired even in such habitually performed tasks as writing or buttoning clothes. On the other hand, pain and temperature sensation are preserved since these modalities are carried by small-diameter afferent fibers.

Without proprioceptive feedback, patients can maintain their limbs in a steady position only when they can see them. When the patient attempts to hold the arm outstretched while closing the eyes, the arm starts to drift randomly after a few seconds (this is termed *pseudo-athetosis*). Similarly, if large axons are affected in the sensory nerves of the legs, the patient is unsteady when walking and falls if the eyes are closed (*Romberg's sign*). Proprioceptive feedback from the ankles is crucial for the control and maintenance of a standing posture (see Chapter 39).

Because loss of proprioceptive inputs provides the state information (including the angle and orientation of the joints) needed for feed-forward control, rapid movements to targets in space are profoundly inaccurate. Whereas normal subjects move their hands straight to a target even if they are prevented from monitoring the movement visually, patients with large fiber neuropathy make large errors in both the direction and amplitudes of their movements. In addition, at the end of movement their hands do not stop in a stable position; their hands drift away even though the patients believe them to be stationary (Figure 35–2).

Vision can compensate for the loss of proprioceptive sensation through feed-forward as well as through feedback mechanisms. Thus, if the patient is allowed to see the limb *before* making the movement, the errors in direction and extent are much reduced, even when the patient is then prevented from seeing the limb *during* the movement itself. This inaccuracy therefore reflects defective feed-forward control. The errors in direction arise because the motor systems lack a precise representation of the state of the limb (its position in space and the tension of the different muscles) and its current properties. As a result they cannot select the muscles that are appropriate to move the limb in the desired direction.

The defects in feedback and feed-forward regulation also impair the ability to use vision effectively, even to control slow movement of the limbs. While normal subjects can make deliberate movements at a slow speed, stopping precisely at the desired end point, patients with large-fiber sensory neuropathy cannot (Figure 35–2C). These patients are unable to sense the resistance of the surface on which their hand is moving or the tension that is being developed by their muscles, and thus their movements are jerky. Errors in direction are improperly corrected because by the time visual feedback occurs the hand is in a new and unexpected position.

These deficits can be explained by means of the model illustrated in Figure 35–1B. In the deafferented patient the adaptive controller receives incomplete information about the state of the limb and fails to receive proprioceptive feedback. The adaptive mechanism therefore cannot construct an accurate internal model of the limb and cannot set the characteristics of either the feed-forward or the feedback controller. This results in errors in both the feed-forward control of direction, as a result of an incorrect selection of the muscles to be activated, and in the initial

acceleration of movement. Once movement is in progress, errors in proprioceptive feedback produce oscillations and irregular movements.

There Are Three Levels in the Hierarchy of Motor Control

The Spinal Cord, the Brain Stem, and Cortical Motor Areas Are Organized Hierarchically and in Parallel

How do the motor systems integrate motor commands with ongoing sensory information so as to control the complicated mechanical machinery of musculoskeletal systems? This is achieved by distributing feedback, feed-forward, and adaptive mechanisms among three levels of motor control: the spinal cord, the descending systems of the brain stem, and the motor areas of the cerebral cortex (Figure 35–3). These different levels of the motor systems are organized both hierarchically and in parallel. By their hierarchical organization the lower levels have the capacity to generate complex spatiotemporal patterns of muscle activation in the form of reflexes. This enables higher centers to give relatively general commands without having to specify the details of the motor action.

By means of their parallel organization motor systems can issue commands that can act directly on the lowest level of the chain to adjust the operation of reflex circuits. For example, the corticospinal tract controls pathways descending from the brain stem but, in addition, it also controls spinal interneurons and motor neurons directly. The combination of parallel and hierarchical mechanisms results in an overlap of different functional components of the motor systems, similar to that which we encountered in the sensory systems. This overlap is also important in the recovery of function after local lesions.

The lowest level of the hierarchy, the *spinal cord*, contains neuronal circuits that mediate a variety of automatic and stereotyped reflexes. These reflexes can function even when the cord is disconnected from the rest of the brain. At the beginning of this century Sherrington demonstrated that virtually all reflexes involve the integrated activation and inhibition of activity in different muscle groups. He suggested that many of these actions are coordinated by spinal interneurons. For example, both reflex withdrawal from noxious stimuli and the alternating activity in flexors and extensors during locomotion are organized by networks of spinal interneurons. Even simple descending commands can produce complex effects through these interneurons. It is now known that the same networks of interneurons that organize reflex behavior are also involved in voluntary movements. Ultimately, however, all interneuronal controls converge on the motor neurons that innervate the skeletal muscles. To stress the importance of this convergence, Sherrington called the motor neurons the *final common path*.

The next level of the motor hierarchy, the *brain stem*, contains three neuronal systems (medial, lateral, and

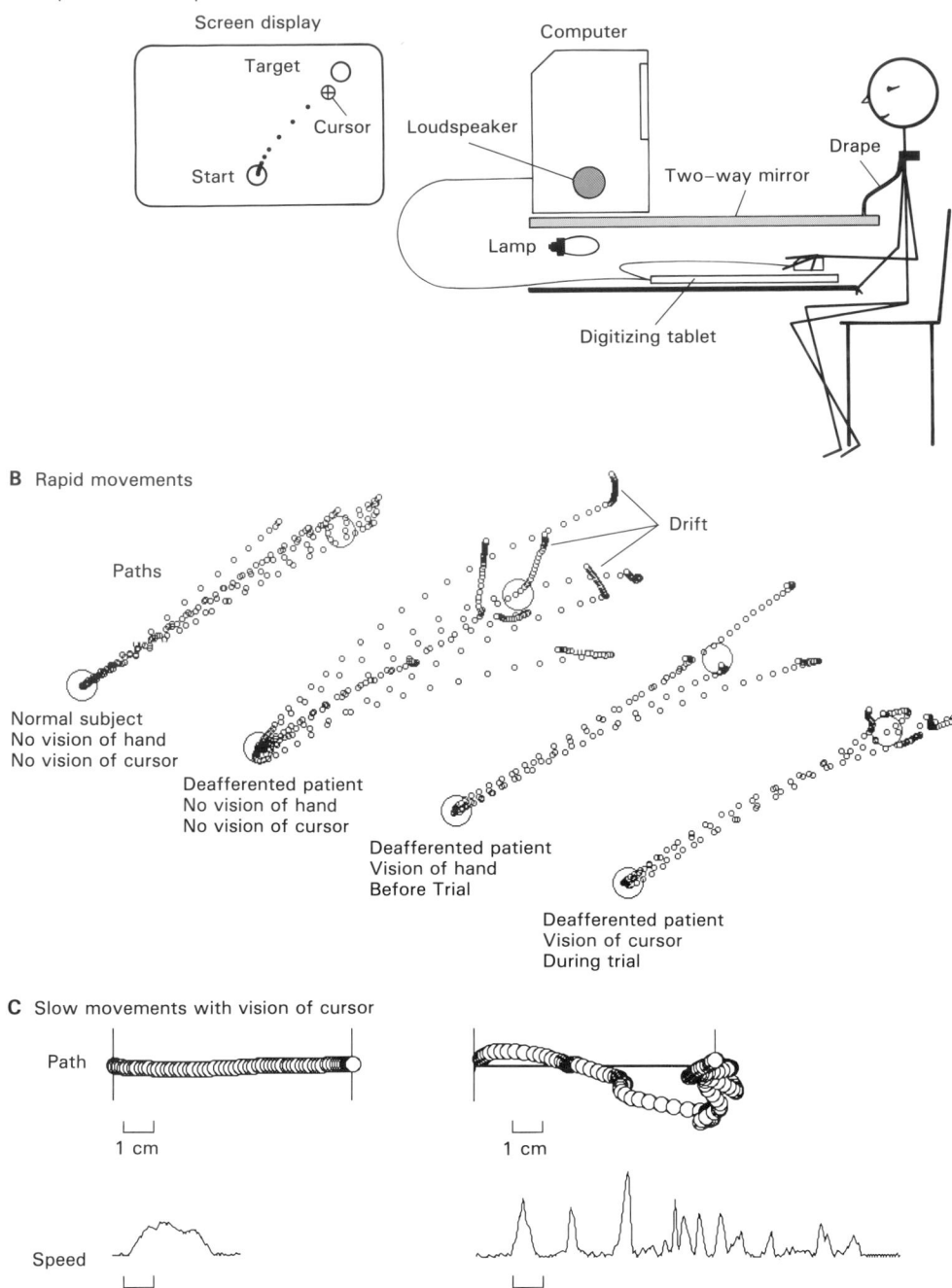

FIGURE 35–2

Patients with large-fiber sensory neuropathy make large errors in aiming and controlling their movements unless they can see their hands.

A. The subject is seated facing a computer screen and moves a hand-held cursor on a digitizing tablet. The position of the cursor on the tablet is displayed on the computer screen as a cross hair. Circular targets or lines to be traced are also displayed on the screen. Vision of the arm is made possible by turning on a lamp under the two-way mirror.

B. Accuracy of rapid arm movement made without visual feedback in a normal subject and deafferented patient. The subject is told to move the cursor rapidly from a start circle to a target, both shown on the screen. The screen cursor is blanked just before the subject's movement and shown again at the end of movement. Although target locations were varied randomly, movements to only one location are illustrated here. The small circles indicate successive positions of the hand every 20 ms. The normal subject

correctly aims and carries out each movement without either viewing the screen cursor or his hand and maintains a stable position at the end of movement. The sensory-impaired patient shows marked variation in movement direction and extent and his hand drifts at the end of the movement. The directional errors and drifts are reduced if the patient can see the hand between trials. A similar degree of reduction occurs when the screen cursor remains visible.

C. Slow movements with visual feedback in normal and deafferented patient. The subjects are told to move the cursor slowly and regularly along a straight horizontal line on the screen (between the two parallel lines) while viewing the cross hair on the screen. The subject with intact sensation makes a slow movement and maintains his speed close to a steady value, whereas movements made by the deafferented patient are jerky, indicating multiple adjustments to errors in direction.

aminergic) whose axons project to and regulate the segmental networks of the spinal cord. The brain stem systems integrate visual and vestibular information with somatosensory inputs and play an important role in modulating spinal motor circuits in the control of posture (Chapter 39). In addition, brain stem nuclei control eye and head movements (Chapter 44).

The highest level of motor control consists of three areas of cerebral cortex: the *primary motor cortex*, the *lateral premotor area* (or premotor cortex), and the *supplementary motor area*. Each area projects directly to the spinal cord through the corticospinal tract as well as indirectly through the brain stem motor systems. The premotor and supplementary motor areas also project to the primary motor cortex. The lateral premotor and supplementary motor areas are important for coordinating and planning complex sequences of movement. Both areas receive information from the posterior parietal and prefrontal association cortices. We shall consider these areas in Chapters 40 and 53.

Three organizational features of the motor hierarchy are important. First, each component of the motor system contains somatotopic maps—spatial relations are preserved so that neurons that influence adjacent body parts are adjacent to each other. Moreover, this organization is important in the interconnections between different levels. Thus, regions of primary motor cortex that control the arm receive input from arm-control areas in the premotor cortex and, in turn, influence corresponding arm-control areas of the descending brain stem pathways. Second, each level of control receives information from the periphery, so that sensory input can modify the action of descending commands. Third, higher levels can control the information that reaches them by facilitating or suppressing the transmission of afferent input in sensory relay nuclei.

The Cerebellum and Basal Ganglia Control the Cortical and Brain Stem Motor Systems

In addition to the three hierarchical levels—spinal cord, brain stem, and cortex—two other parts of the brain also regulate motor function—the cerebellum and basal ganglia. The cerebellum improves the accuracy of movement by comparing descending motor commands with information about the resulting motor action. The cerebellum does this by acting on the brain stem and on the cortical motor areas that project directly to the spinal cord, monitoring both their activity and the sensory feedback signals they receive from the periphery. We shall examine this further in Chapter 43.

The basal ganglia receive inputs from all cortical areas and project principally to areas of frontal cortex that are concerned with motor planning. Diseases of the basal ganglia produce a range of motor abnormalities including loss of spontaneous movements, abnormal involuntary movements, and disturbances in posture. We shall discuss the physiology and diseases that affect the basal ganglia in Chapter 42.

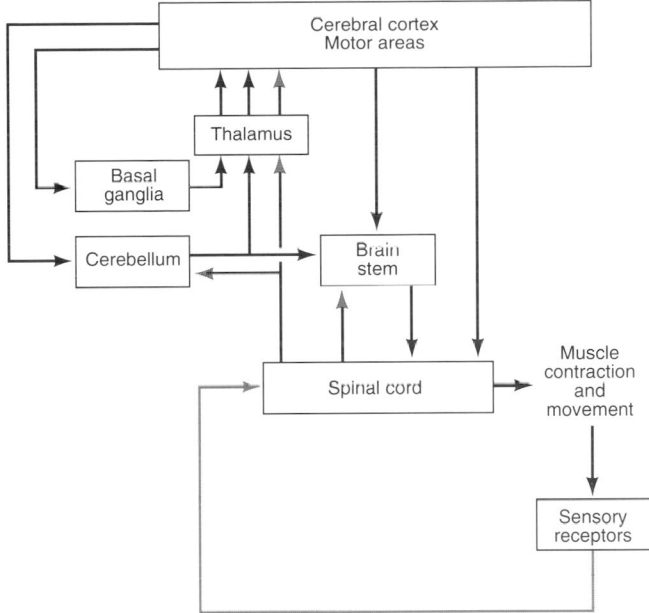

FIGURE 35-3
The motor system consists of three levels of control organized both hierarchically and in parallel. Thus, the motor areas of the cerebral cortex can influence the spinal cord both directly and through the brain stem descending systems. All three levels of the motor systems receive sensory inputs and are also under the influence of two independent subcortical systems: the basal ganglia and the cerebellum. Both the basal ganglia and cerebellum act on the cerebral cortex through relay nuclei in the thalamus.

We now turn to consider each of the three levels of the motor hierarchy.

Motor Neurons in the Spinal Cord Are Subject to Afferent Input and Descending Control

Spinal Motor Neurons Are Topographically Organized into Medial and Lateral Groups That Innervate Proximal and Distal Muscles

The cell bodies of motor neurons that innervate individual muscles are clustered in *motor nuclei*, or *motor neuron pools*, which form longitudinal columns extending one to four spinal segments. The spatial organization of the different motor nuclei follows two important anatomical and functional rules: a *proximal–distal rule* and a *flexor–extensor rule*.

According to the proximal–distal rule the motor neurons innervating the most proximal muscles are located most medially, while those innervating more distal muscles are located progressively more laterally. The motor nuclei of axial muscles, innervating muscles of the neck and back, form a distinct group in the most medial part of the ventral horn that extends throughout the entire length of the spinal cord. In the lower cervical and lumbosacral spinal cord segments there is also a larger cluster of motor

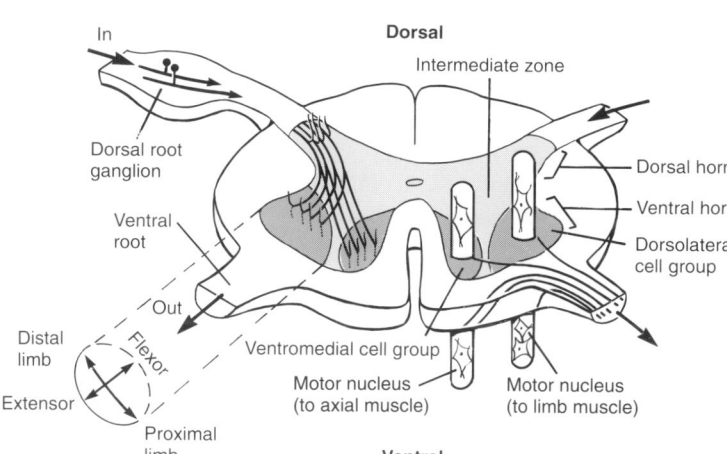

FIGURE 35–4
The motor nuclei of the spinal cord are grouped functionally in distinct medial and lateral positions. The
medial group contains the motor neurons innervating
axial muscles of the neck and back. Within the lateral
group, the most medial motor neurons innervate
proximal muscles while the most lateral innervate
distal muscles. Ventrally located motor neurons innervate extensors while dorsal ones innervate flexors.

nuclei in the lateral part of the ventral horn. Within these
groups, motor neurons innervating the proximal girdle
muscles (the shoulder and pelvis) are medial, while those
innervating the distal hand and foot muscle are lateral.

According to the flexor–extensor rule, motor neurons
that innervate extensor muscles lie ventral to those innervating flexor muscles (Figure 35–4). These anatomical
relationships account for an important functional distinction: Proximal muscles (especially the extensor muscles
of the legs) are predominantly used to maintain equilibrium and posture, whereas distal muscles (especially those
of the upper extremity) are used for fine manipulatory activities. We will now see that the medial and lateral motor
neurons are controlled by separate populations of local
interneurons, propriospinal neurons, and descending pathways.

The Terminations of Medial and Lateral Interneurons and Propriospinal Neurons Have Different Distributions

The fact that the most medial motor neurons innervate
the proximal muscles and the most lateral motor neurons
the distal muscles is also reflected in the organization of
local interneurons and propriospinal neurons that terminate in more than one segment. The local interneurons in
the most medial parts of the intermediate zone project to
the medial motor nuclei that control axial muscles on
both sides of the body, both ipsilaterally and contralaterally. More laterally located interneurons project only ipsilaterally to the motor neurons innervating girdle muscles,
while the most lateral ones synapse on motor neurons
that innervate the most distal ipsilateral muscles (Figure
35–5).

The axons of propriospinal neurons run up and down
the white matter of the spinal cord and terminate both on

interneurons and on motor neurons located several segments away from the cell bodies (Figure 35–5).[1] Axons of
medial propriospinal neurons run in the ventral and medial columns, are longer, and may even extend the entire
length of the spinal cord; more laterally placed propriospinal neurons interconnect a smaller number of segments and are topographically less diffuse. This pattern of
organization allows the axial muscles, which are innervated from many spinal segments, to be coordinated during postural adjustment. In contrast, distal limb muscles,
which tend to be used independently, are controlled by the
more highly focused lateral propriospinal systems.

The Brain Stem Modulates Motor Neurons and Interneurons in the Spinal Cord Through Four Systems

Many groups of neurons in the brain stem project to the
spinal gray matter. Based on their location and distribution in the spinal cord, Hans Kuypers classified these projections into two main pathways (see Figure 35–6). The
medial pathways terminate in the ventromedial part of
the spinal gray matter and thus influence motor neurons
that innervate axial and proximal muscles. The *lateral
pathways* terminate in the dorsolateral part of the spinal
gray matter and influence motor neurons that control distal muscles of the extremities. A third system made up of
the *aminergic pathways*, originates in nuclei in the brain
stem and branches diffusely throughout the spinal cord.

---

[1]The term *interneuron* is used here to indicate a spinal neuron whose
main branches are confined to the same or adjacent spinal segment. Propriospinal neurons are spinal neurons whose main axon branches terminate in distant spinal segments. Some propriospinal neurons have branches
that ascend outside of the spinal cord like the projection neurons of sensory
and spinocerebellar tracts.

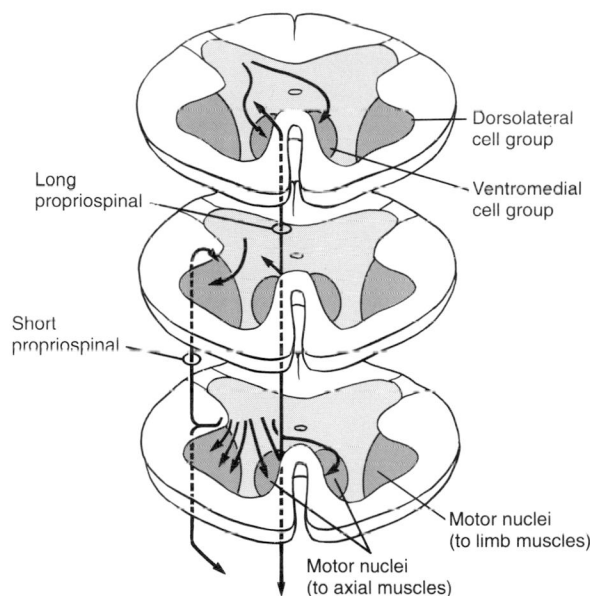

FIGURE 35–5
Medial motor nuclei are interconnected by long propriospinal neurons whereas lateral motor nuclei are interconnected by short propriospinal neurons.

Medial Pathways Control Axial and Proximal Muscles

The medial system has three major components: the vestibulospinal tracts (medial and lateral), the reticulospinal tracts (medial and lateral), and the tectospinal tract. These pathways descend in the ipsilateral ventral columns of the spinal cord and terminate predominantly on interneurons and long propriospinal neurons in the ventromedial part of the intermediate zone. They also terminate directly on some motor neurons, particularly those of the medial cell group, which innervate axial muscles (Figure 35–6A).

The medial and lateral *vestibulospinal tracts* originate in the vestibular nuclei and carry information for the reflex control of balance and posture from the vestibular labyrinth (see Chapter 40).

The medial and lateral *reticulospinal tracts* originate from several nuclei located primarily in the reticular formation of the pons and medulla (see Chapter 40). These systems have both excitatory and inhibitory connections with spinal interneurons and motor neurons. The reticulospinal systems are important for the maintenance of posture. They integrate information from a variety of inputs, notably the vestibular nuclei and cerebral cortex. Axons originating from the primary motor and premotor cortex synapse with reticulospinal neurons to form a *cortico-reticulospinal pathway*. This pathway is particularly important for the suppression of spinal reflexes and activity by motor cortical areas (see Chapter 39).

The *tectospinal tract* originates in the superior colliculus of the midbrain and is the only medial brain stem pathway to project contralaterally. However, it does not project lower than the cervical segments of the spinal cord. This system is important in coordinating head and eye movements and can be controlled from the cerebral cortex by means of a *cortico-tectospinal pathway*.

Lateral Pathways Control Distal Muscles

The column of fibers descending in the lateral quadrant of the spinal cord terminates in the lateral portion of the intermediate zone and among the dorsolateral groups of motor neurons innervating more distal limb muscles (Figure 35–6B). The main lateral descending pathway from the brain stem is the *rubrospinal tract*, which originates in the magnocellular portion of the red nucleus in the midbrain. Rubrospinal fibers descend through the medulla to the dorsal part of the lateral column of the spinal cord.

The difference in the distributions of the lateral and medial systems corresponds to their fundamentally different roles in motor function. The medial system is phylogenetically the oldest component of the descending motor systems. It is important in maintaining balance and posture, both of which rely on proximal and axial muscles. The wide area of termination of individual axons is important in distributing control to a variety of different motor nuclei that are functionally related. The medial pathways provide the basic postural control system upon which the cortical motor areas can organize more highly differentiated movements. The lateral pathways function in more varied ways by controlling distal muscles used in a variety of fine movements, such as reaching and manipulating objects with the fingers and hand. In anthropoid apes and humans, where the rubrospinal system is small and vestigial, this function is largely assumed by the corticospinal system.

Aminergic Pathways Modulate the Excitability of Spinal Neurons

Two sets of aminergic pathways send axons to the entire spinal cord. One, the *ceruleospinal system*, is noradrenergic. It originates in the locus ceruleus and from some neurons in the pontomedullary reticular formation and descends in the ventrolateral part of the lateral column. The other, the *raphe–spinal system*, is serotonergic. It originates from nuclei in the raphe of the brain stem and projects through both lateral and ventral columns (Chapter 44). Axons of both systems terminate in the intermediate zone and on motor nuclei throughout the spinal cord. Individual neurons send collaterals to many, and perhaps all, segments. The raphe–spinal system also projects to the outer layers of the dorsal horn, where it modulates the transmission of painful stimuli to projection neurons and spinal interneurons.

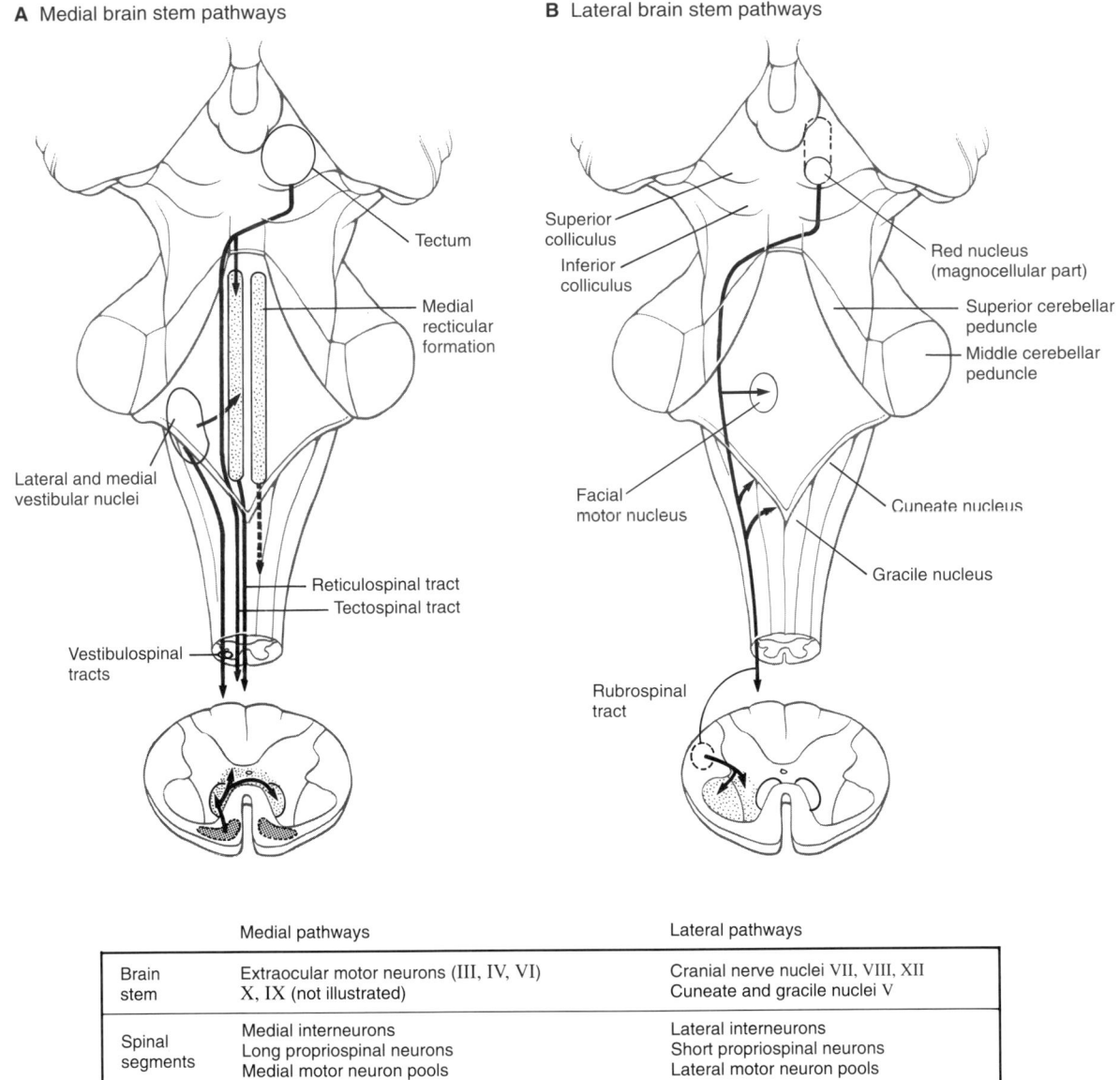

A Medial brain stem pathways

Tectum

Medial recticular formation

Lateral and medial vestibular nuclei

Reticulospinal tract
Tectospinal tract

Vestibulospinal tracts

B Lateral brain stem pathways

Superior colliculus
Inferior colliculus

Red nucleus (magnocellular part)

Superior cerebellar peduncle

Middle cerebellar peduncle

Facial motor nucleus

Cuneate nucleus

Gracile nucleus

Rubrospinal tract

	Medial pathways	Lateral pathways
Brain stem	Extraocular motor neurons (III, IV, VI) X, IX (not illustrated)	Cranial nerve nuclei VII, VIII, XII Cuneate and gracile nuclei V
Spinal segments	Medial interneurons Long propriospinal neurons Medial motor neuron pools	Lateral interneurons Short propriospinal neurons Lateral motor neuron pools
Muscles	Proximal ≫ Distal Extensors ≫ Flexors	Distal ≫ Proximal Flexors ≫ Extensors

FIGURE 35–6

Two groups of descending brain stem pathways control different groups of neurons and different groups of muscles.

A. The main components of the medial pathways are the reticulospinal, the medial and lateral vestibulospinal, and the tectospinal tracts that descend in the ventral column. These terminate in the shaded portions of the gray spinal matter.

B. The main lateral pathway is the rubrospinal tract, which originates in the caudal, magnocellular portion of the red nucleus. The rubrospinal tract descends in the contralateral dorsolateral column terminating in the shaded area of the spinal gray matter.

The Motor Cortex Acts on Motor Neurons Directly Via the Corticospinal Tract and Indirectly Through Brain Stem Pathways

The ability to organize complex motor acts and to execute fine movements with precision depends on control signals transmitted from the motor areas in the cerebral cortex through the corticobulbar and corticospinal tracts. The *corticobulbar fibers* control the cranial motor nerve nuclei, and thus the facial muscles, while the *corticospinal fibers* control the motor neurons innervating the spinal segments. Corticospinal axons act directly on motor neurons and interneurons. They also influence motor activity indirectly through the descending brain stem pathways, notably through cortico-reticulospinal and cortico-rubrospinal projections and other corticobulbar projections.

The Corticospinal Tract Is the Largest Descending Fiber Tract from the Brain

The corticospinal tract is a massive bundle of fibers containing about one million axons. About a third of these originate from the primary motor cortex located in the precentral gyrus of the frontal lobe (Brodmann's area 4). Electrical stimulation of the primary motor cortex evokes movements of different contralateral muscle groups. Another third of the corticospinal fibers originate from the premotor motor areas (area 6), a larger zone that lies rostral to area 4 in the frontal lobe. The remaining third originate in areas 3, 2, and 1 in the somatic sensory cortex and regulate the transmission of afferent input to control structures.

The corticospinal fibers course through the posterior limb of the internal capsule together with corticobulbar fibers to reach the ventral portion of the midbrain. As they descend through the pons the corticospinal fibers separate into small bundles of fibers that course between the pontine nuclei. The fibers regroup in the medulla to form the *medullary pyramid*, a conspicuous landmark on the ventral surface of the medulla. Because of this regrouping, the corticospinal tract is sometimes referred to as the pyramidal tract. This usage is incorrect, however, because some fibers leave the medullary pyramids to terminate in brain stem nuclei, such as the dorsal column nuclei.)

At the junction of the medulla and the spinal cord about three-quarters of the corticospinal fibers cross the midline in the *pyramidal decussation*. The crossed fibers descend in the dorsal part of the lateral columns (dorsolateral column) of the spinal cord, forming the *lateral corticospinal tracts*. The uncrossed fibers descend in the ventral columns as the ventral corticospinal tracts (Figure 35–7).

The lateral and ventral corticospinal tracts terminate in approximately the same regions of spinal gray matter as do the lateral and medial descending brain stem systems (Figure 35–7). The lateral corticospinal tract projects primarily to the motor nuclei of the lateral part of the ventral horn and to interneurons in the intermediate zone. The ventral corticospinal tract projects bilaterally to the ventromedial cell column, which contains the motor neurons that innervate the axial muscles and to adjoining portions of the intermediate zones.

The corticobulbar fibers that control muscles of the head and face terminate in both motor and sensory cranial nerve nuclei in the brain stem. In humans there are monosynaptic connections between corticobulbar fibers and motor neurons in the trigeminal, facial, and hypoglossal nuclei. The projections to the trigeminal motor nucleus are bilateral and approximately equal in size. Although the projection to the facial nucleus is also bilateral, the

motor neurons innervating muscles of the lower face receive predominantly contralateral fibers. As a result, unilateral damage to corticobulbar fibers on one side produces weakness only of the muscles of the contralateral lower part of the face.

Cortical Control of Movement Is Achieved Only Late in Phylogeny

Phylogenetically, the corticospinal and corticobulbar pathways first appear in mammals. In the most primitive mammals the motor outflow from the cortex first appears as a mechanism that controls and adjusts sensory inflow to spinal interneurons and projection neurons. In the hedgehog the corticospinal tracts are located in the dorsal columns and terminate exclusively in the dorsal horn. Moreover, in hedgehogs and other primitive mammals the somatic sensory representations of the body surface in the cerebral cortex overlap with the motor representation.

Higher mammals have distinct sensory and motor representations of the body in the cortex and have additional corticospinal terminations within the intermediate zone of the spinal cord. With still further phylogenetic development, there is a gradual increase in the number of corticospinal fibers distributed to more ventral regions of the spinal cord, so that corticospinal neurons make direct connections to motor neurons in the lateral motor nuclei that control distal limb muscles and later, phylogenetically, also in medial motor nuclei. Thus, in the phylogeny of primates the number of corticospinal axon terminals ending on spinal motor neurons increases progressively from prosimians to monkeys, anthropoid apes, and finally to humans. In the more primitive primates direct connections are present only in the most dorsolateral cell groups innervating the most distal muscles, but in monkeys the entire lateral group of motor nuclei receives corticospinal input; in higher apes and humans the medial motor nuclei also receive dense corticospinal terminations. In most carnivores corticospinal fibers terminate exclusively in the dorsal horn and dorsolateral parts of the intermediate zone and do not make any direct connections with motor neurons (Figure 35–8).

Lesions of the Cortical Motor Areas and Their Projections Cause Characteristic Symptoms

Lesions of cortical-motor areas or their projections are especially common in neurological practice. This is easy to understand because of the large size of these areas and because corticospinal axons extend from the cerebral cortex through the brain stem to the spinal cord, and can be damaged by lesions at any of these locations. The most common cause of the lesions is vascular occlusion producing *cerebral infarction*, neuronal cell death. The blood supply of the brain is discussed in Appendix B. Especially common are occlusion of the *middle cerebral artery* (whose branches supply the lateral surface of the cortex and the internal capsule) or of the *vertebrobasilar system*

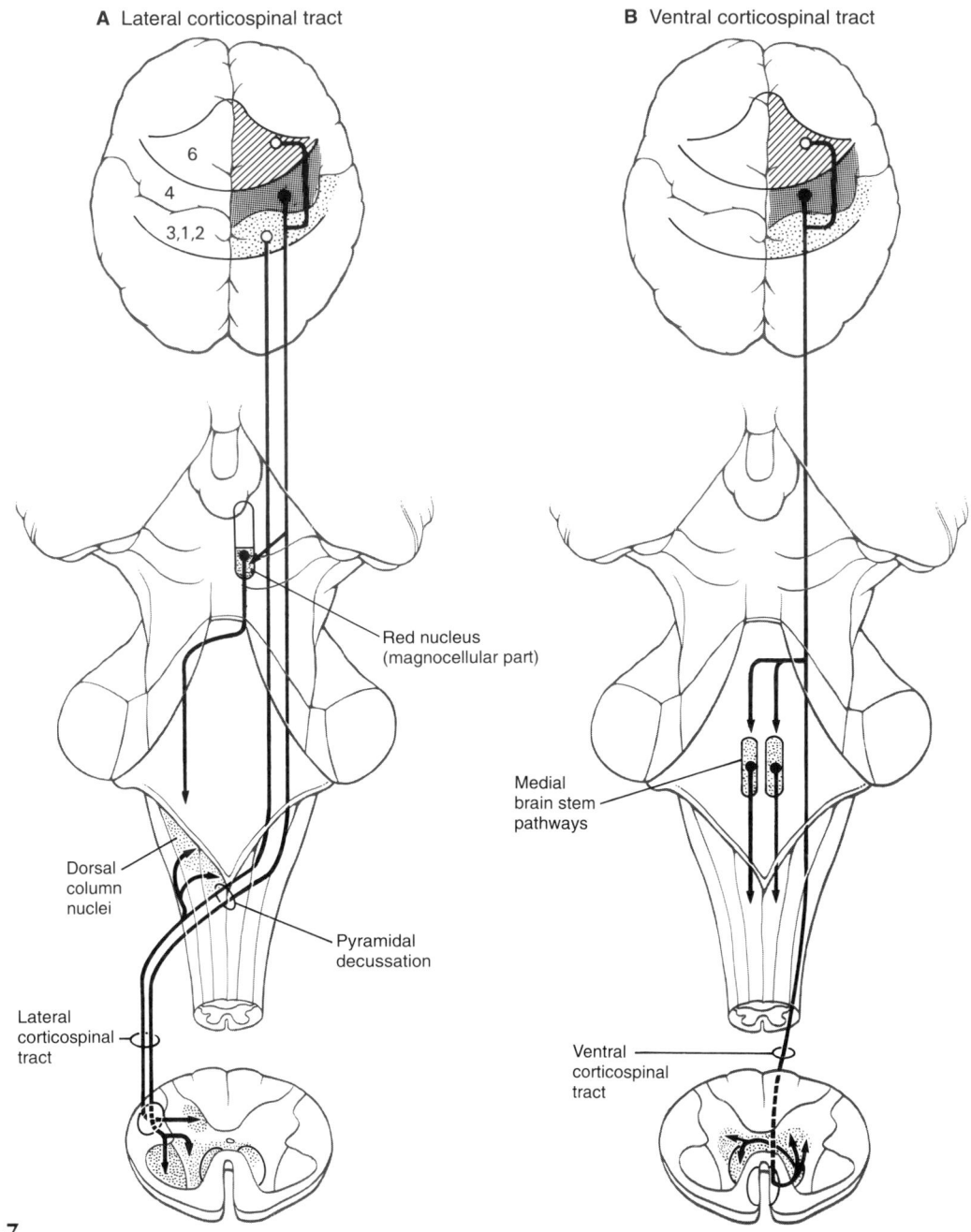

A Lateral corticospinal tract

B Ventral corticospinal tract

6
4
3,1,2

Red nucleus
(magnocellular part)

Medial
brain stem
pathways

Dorsal
column
nuclei

Pyramidal
decussation

Lateral
corticospinal
tract

Ventral
corticospinal
tract

FIGURE 35–7

The descending cortical pathways to the spinal segments.

A. The crossed lateral corticospinal tract originates from Brodmann's areas 4 and 6, and sensory areas 3, 2, and 1. The tract then crosses at the pyramidal decussation, descends in the dorsolateral column, and terminates in the shaded area of spinal gray matter. Corticorubral neurons are mainly located in area 6. The principal area of termination of the corticospinal

neurons originating from the sensory cortex is the medial portion of the dorsal horn. Collaterals project to dorsal column nuclei.

B. Uncrossed pathways (ventral corticospinal tract) originate principally in Brodmann's area 6 and in zones controlling the neck and trunk in area 4. Terminations are bilateral and collaterals project to the medial brain stem pathways.

(supplying the brain stem). Tumor, trauma, and demyelinating diseases are other common causes of damage to the corticospinal system.

John Hughlings Jackson first recognized that lesions of the nervous system give rise to two kinds of abnormal function, which he defined as *negative* and *positive*. Neg-

ative signs reflect the loss of particular capacities normally controlled by the damaged system, for example, weakness or loss of strength. Positive signs represent stereotyped abnormal responses that may emerge after the lesion. These *release phenomena* are explained by the withdrawal of inhibitory influences on normal interneu-

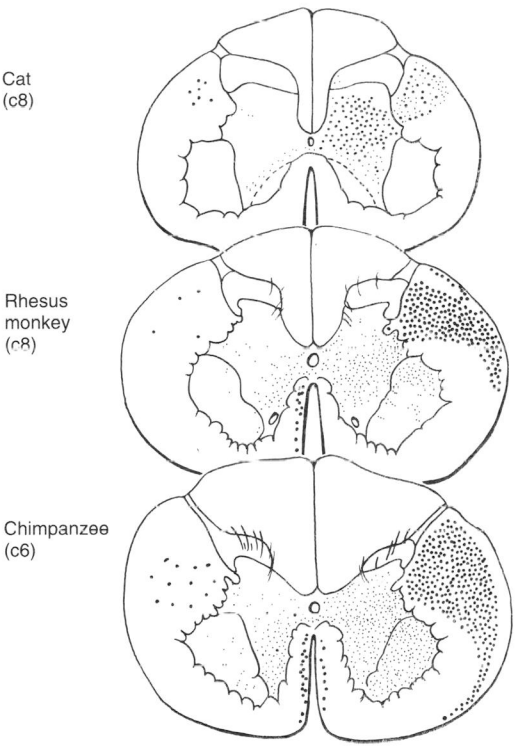

FIGURE 35–8

Cortical motor neurons in different species have different patterns of termination in the spinal cord. In the cat the corticospinal fibers terminate principally on neurons in the ventral parts of the dorsal horn and in the spinal intermediate zone. In lower primates, such as the rhesus monkey, most terminations remain in the intermediate zone but a small number also reach the motor neurons. In the more highly evolved primates, such as the chimpanzee and humans, where lateral brain stem pathways recede, there are extensive terminations throughout the contralateral intermediate zone and both medial and lateral motor neuron groups. A substantial ipsilateral fiber tract is also present and terminates primarily on proximal muscles important for postural control. (Adapted from Kuypers, 1985.)

ronal networks that mediate the responses. Examples of positive signs are the pathological reflexes seen with lesions of descending pathways or the involuntary movements that occur with certain lesions affecting the basal ganglia.

The extensor plantar reflex is an important positive sign of corticospinal damage and is widely used in clinical neurology. The sign was discovered in 1896 by the neurologist Joseph Babinski, then in charge of a ward of syphilitic patients at the Pitié Hospital in Paris. A form of this disease, meningovascular syphilis, produces vascular lesions of the brain that often affect the corticospinal tract. Babinski noted that the reflex response, elicited by stroking the lateral aspect of the foot with a sharp object, was different in patients with lesions of the corticospinal tract than in patients without such lesions. This stimulus normally produces flexion of all the toes, including the large one. In affected patients, however, there is a reflex extension of the big toe, which may be accompanied by fanning of the others (Figure 35–9).

William Landau and others have demonstrated that the extensor plantar response is actually an enhanced withdrawal reflex and is part of a larger family of responses to noxious stimuli that are released by pyramidal lesions. The appearance under pathological conditions of a reflex response that is normally absent illustrates clearly that central lesions can lead to both negative and positive signs: to the loss of some specific functions and to the release of others that are otherwise inhibited.

Muscle Weakness May Result from Disturbances in Descending Motor Pathways or in the Spinal Motor Neurons Themselves

Some pathological processes affecting motor nerves and central motor systems can cause muscle weakness by interfering with the output of spinal motor neurons. When diagnosing the cause of weakness clinicians must first determine whether the disturbance is at the level of the motor neuron or whether it reflects an abnormality in the balance of excitatory and inhibitory inputs to motor neurons, as may arise with lesions of descending pathways. As we have seen in Chapter 17, in clinical literature the motor neurons in the spinal cord and brain stem that innervate skeletal muscles of the body and head are often called *lower motor neurons*. The signs of direct damage to motor neurons (the *lower motor neuron syndrome*) differ from those produced by damage to descending pathways that clinicians call *upper motor neuron* syndrome.

The lower motor neuron syndrome results from dis-

FIGURE 35–9

The Babinski sign is diagnostic of a lesion of the corticospinal tract. When the sole of the foot is stroked firmly along the path indicated, the normal response is flexion of the foot and toes. The Babinski sign is extension of the big toe and fanning of the others.

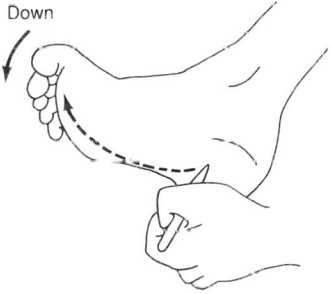

Normal plantar response

Down

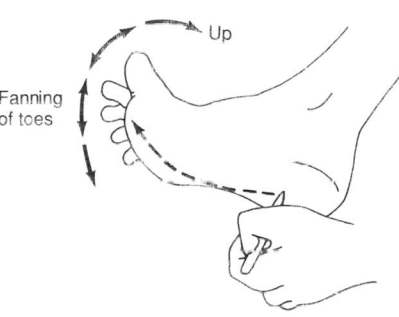

Extensor plantar response (Babinski sign)

Up

Fanning of toes

eases or lesions affecting the motor neuron at the level of the cell body or its axon. An example is poliomyelitis, a viral disease that attacks motor neurons in localized areas of spinal cord, causing weakness of small groups of muscles while nearby muscles may remain normal. Affected muscles often exhibit fasciculation (twitches of muscle fascicles under the skin) and atrophy (loss of muscle volume). The affected muscles always show decreased tone, and tendon reflexes are reduced or absent (see Chapter 18).

In the upper motor neuron syndrome there is damage or interference with the central excitatory drive to the motor neurons. Typically, the disturbance results from dysfunction of descending motor systems other than the corticospinal tract (see Chapter 40). In the upper motor neuron syndrome groups of muscles (synergists) are invariably all affected, atrophy is rare, and there are no fasciculations. In addition there is *spasticity*, a condition in which muscle tone and deep tendon reflexes are both increased (see Chapter 39).

Parallel Control of Motor Neurons Allows Recovery of Function Following Lesions

In primates the corticospinal system provides the only direct descending control over distal limb motor neurons. These connections endow higher primates with the ability to control individual muscles independently, a capacity known as *fractionation of movement*. This ability is completely and irretrievably lost following lesions of the corticospinal fibers in the medullary pyramid. Monkeys whose corticospinal tracts have been interrupted cannot grasp small objects between two fingers (the so-called precision grip) or make isolated movements of the wrist or elbow. When attempting to grasp a small object, the animal uses its hand as a shovel or contracts all the digits simultaneously around the object. These animals are able to maintain balance and can control axial and girdle muscles, however; therefore, they can walk and climb without difficulty.

The fact that several levels of control (segmental interneurons, brain stem, cortex) act on motor neurons contributes to the recovery of function that may occur after lesions of one or another component of the descending motor systems. For example, in monkeys, section of the medullary pyramids is immediately followed by severe weakness. With time, strength recovers; however, the animals are unable to move as rapidly as before. The weakness is much more severe if, in addition to damage of the primary motor area, the outflow from the premotor areas to the brain stem and spinal cord is also damaged.

Younger patients typically recover more muscle strength than do older ones. Several factors contribute to the amount of strength recovered, including the transfer of some of the functions of the corticospinal system to descending brain stem pathways, as well as the sprouting of other axons into the synaptic areas vacated by the degenerating corticospinal axons. If the connections from the primary motor cortex to lateral brain stem pathways are spared, the cerebral cortex can control limb muscles through cortico-rubrospinal and cortico-reticulospinal pathways. This anatomical reorganization is also much greater in neonatal and young animals than in adults. In higher primates the number of axons in the rubrospinal tract decreases substantially relative to that of monkeys and other species, and the degree of functional recovery following cortical lesions is correspondingly smaller.

An Overall View

Behavior involves the contraction of muscles and is controlled by motor systems. These systems are hierarchically organized, so that spinal circuits for automatic reflex behaviors are subject to control from the brain stem and motor cortex. These three components—spinal cord, brain stem, and cortex—also function in parallel, so that any one set of controls can to some extent control movement independently of the other two.

Different parts of the motor system carry out distinct but interrelated functions. Thus, while the spinal cord and brain stem mediate reflexive and simple automatized voluntary responses, the cortical motor areas initiate more complex voluntary movements. The prefrontal motor cortex and basal ganglia are thought to be involved in the planning of movement and in large-scale coordination between body parts. The cerebellum is responsible for coordinating precisely timed activity by integrating intended motor output with ongoing sensory feedback.

Sensory information influences motor output in many ways and at all levels of the motor system. Sensory input to the spinal cord directly triggers reflex responses. It is also essential for determining the parameters of programmed voluntary responses. Finally, sensory input, especially proprioceptive information, is integral to both feedback and feed-forward mechanisms, which provide flexibility in the control of motor output.

Three distinct groups of pathways from the brain stem descend in the medial spinal cord to influence the activity of spinal motor circuits: the vestibulospinal, reticulospinal, and tectospinal pathways. The first two originate in the vestibular nuclei and reticular formation, respectively, and are involved in the control of posture and balance, which are mediated by motor neurons of axial muscles. The tectospinal pathway descends only as far as the cervical spinal cord and coordinates head and eye movements.

The corticospinal tract originates in the frontal, prefrontal, and parietal cortex. Pathways from the motor and premotor cortex and red nucleus descend in the lateral spinal cord to control the motor neurons that innervate distal muscles that are used in fine independent movements. These fibers pass through the internal capsule and make their way to the medullary decussation, where three-fourths cross the midline and become the lateral corticospinal tracts, while the remaining one-fourth becomes the ipsilateral medial corticospinal tract. The lateral tracts innervate distal motor neurons, while the fewer medial fibers innervate axial motor neurons.

Parallel descending motor pathways offer the advantage that if one pathway is lesioned, the remaining ones can to some extent take over its functions. For example, lesions in the corticospinal tract produce both negative signs (loss of function) and positive signs (release of function). Some of the deficits can, with time, be recovered by the remaining cortico-rubrospinal and cortico-reticulospinal tracts.

Selected Readings

Alexander, G. E., and DeLong, M. R. 1986. Organization of supraspinal motor systems. In A. K. Asbury, G. M. McKhann, and W. I. McDonald (eds.), Diseases of the Nervous System, Vol. I. Clinical Neurobiology. Philadelphia: Saunders, pp. 352–369.

Bernstein, N. 1967. The Co-ordination and Regulation of Movements. Oxford: Pergamon Press.

Houk, J. C., and Rymer, W. Z. 1981. Neural control of muscle length and tension. In V. B. Brooks (ed.), Handbook of Physiology, Section 1: The Nervous System, Vol. II. Motor Control, Part 1. Bethesda, Md.: American Physiological Society, pp. 257–323.

Jackson, J. H. 1932. Selected Writings of John Hughlings Jackson, Vol. II. J. Taylor (ed.) London: Hodder and Stoughton.

Kuypers, H. G. J. M. 1981. Anatomy of the descending pathways. In V. B. Brooks (ed.), Handbook of Physiology, Section 1: The Nervous System, Vol. II. Motor Control, Part 1. Bethesda, Md.: American Physiological Society, pp. 597–666.

Kuypers, H. G. J. M. 1985. The anatomical and functional organization of the motor system. In M. Swash, and C. Kennard (eds.), Scientific Basis of Clinical Neurology. New York: Churchill Livingstone, pp. 3–18.

Lundberg, A. 1979. Integration in a propriospinal motor centre controlling the forelimb in the cat. In H. Asanuma and V. J. Wilson (eds.), Integration in the Nervous System. Tokyo: Igaku-Shoin, pp. 47–64.

Marsden, C. D., Rothwell, J. C., and Day, B. L. 1984. The use of peripheral feedback in the control of movement. Trends Neurosci. 7:253–257.

Miles, F. A., and Evarts, E. 1979. Concepts of motor organization. Annu. Rev. Psychol. 30:327–362.

Sherrington, C. 1947. The Integrative Action of the Nervous System, 2nd ed. New Haven: Yale University Press.

Tower, S. S. 1940. Pyramidal lesion in the monkey. Brain 63:36–90.

References

Babinski, J. 1896. Sur le réflexe cutané plantaire dans certaines affections organiques du système nerveux central. C. R. Soc. Biol. (Paris) 48:207–208.

Ghez, C., Gordon, J., Ghilardi, M. F., Christakos, C. N., and Cooper, S. E. 1990. Roles of proprioceptive input in the programming of arm trajectories. Cold Spring Harbor Symp. Quant. Biol. 55:837–847.

Held, R., and Hein, A. 1963. Movement-produced stimulation in the development of visually guided behavior. J. Comp. Physiol. Psychol. 56:872–876.

Landau, W. M., and Clare, M. H. 1959. The plantar reflex in man, with special reference to some conditions where the extensor response is unexpectedly absent. Brain 82:321–355.

Rothwell, J. C., Traub, M. M., Day, B. L., Obeso, J. A., Thomas, P. K., and Marsden, C. D. 1982. Manual motor performance in a deafferented man. Brain 105:515–542.

Sanes, J. N., Mauritz, K. H., Dalakas, M. C., and Evarts, E. V. 1985. Motor control in humans with large-fiber sensory neuropathy. Human Neurobiol. 4:101–114.

36

Claude Ghez

Muscles: Effectors of the Motor Systems

Movement and Force Are Produced by the Contraction of Sarcomeres

Contraction Results from the Sliding of Filamentous Proteins within the Muscle Fiber

The Force of Contraction Depends on the Length of the Muscle

The Force of Contraction Also Depends on the Relative Rates of Movement of the Thick and Thin Filaments

Muscles Contract Slowly and the Force Generated by a Train of Impulses Summates

Repeated Activation of Muscles Causes Fatigue

A Single Motor Neuron and the Muscle Fibers It Innervates Constitute a Motor Unit

Three Types of Motor Units Are Distinguished by the Properties of Their Muscle Fibers

The Properties of Motor Neurons Are Closely Matched to Muscle Fibers

The Nervous System Grades the Force of Muscle Contraction in Two Ways

Motor Units Are Recruited in a Fixed Order from Weakest to Strongest

Increases in Firing Rate of Motor Units Produce Increasing Force Output

Muscle Properties Limit the Strategies Available to Control Movement

Several Strategies Can Produce a Given Joint Angle

Skeletal Muscles Are Low-Pass Filters of Neural Input

An Overall View

. . . .To move things is all that mankind can do; . . . for such the sole executant is muscle, whether in whispering a syllable or in felling a forest.

Charles Sherrington, 1924

The major output of the elaborate information processing that takes place in our brain is the generation of contractile force in our skeletal muscles. The controlled contraction of muscle allows us to move our limbs, maintain posture, and perform a variety of tasks with great precision.

In this chapter we shall first review the structure of skeletal muscles and the mechanisms by which neural signals produce mechanical forces. We shall see how the amount of force generated by muscles depends on the length of the muscle fibers and on the rate of change in length, and then consider the mechanisms by which the motor systems produce finely graded forces and movements of different speeds. Finally, we shall see how limitations in the mechanical properties of muscles and in their speed of contraction determine specific strategies by the nervous system for controlling movement.

Movement and Force Are Produced by the Contraction of Sarcomeres

Contraction Results from the Sliding of Filamentous Proteins within the Muscle Fiber

Skeletal muscles are composed of groups of elongated multinucleated cells called *muscle fibers*. These fibers contain longitudinal bundles of *myofibrils* that contract in response to neural or electrical stimuli. Under the light microscope the myofibrils appear as alternating light and dark bands whose widths change during contraction. Un-

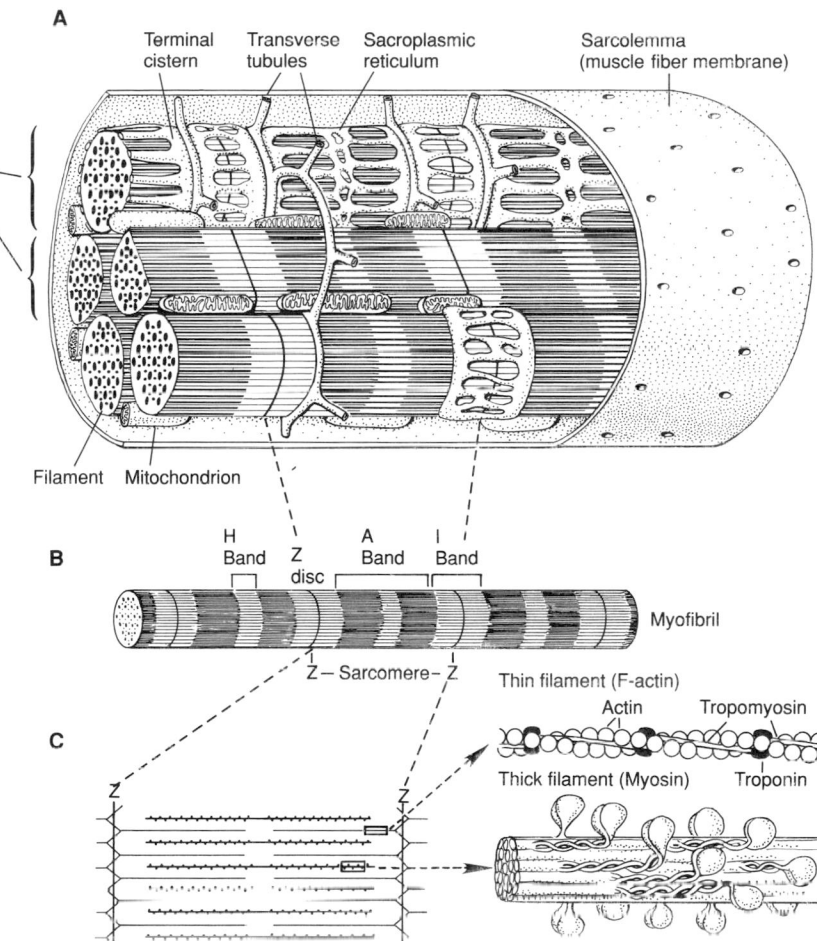

A.

Terminal cistern   Transverse tubules   Sacroplasmic reticulum   Sarcolemma (muscle fiber membrane)

Myofibrils

Filament   Mitochondrion

B.

H Band   Z disc   A Band   I Band

Myofibril

Z — Sarcomere — Z

C.

Thin filament (F-actin)
Actin   Tropomyosin

Thick filament (Myosin)   Troponin

FIGURE 36–1

Alternating light and dark bands within the myofibrils give skeletal muscle its characteristic striated appearance. (Adapted from Bloom and Fawcett, 1970; Loeb and Gans, 1986.)

A. Three-dimensional reconstruction of a sector of muscle fiber showing the relationships of the membrane and tubular system to the myofibrils.

B. Individual myofibril showing light and dark bands. Individual sarcomeres are separated by thin Z disks. The dark bands correspond to regions of overlap of thin and thick filaments.

C. Schematic cross section of an individual sarcomere. The thin filaments are composed principally of polymerized actin whereas the thick filaments are made up of arrays of myosin molecules. The myosin molecule includes a stem and a globular double-head that protrudes from the stem.

der the electron microscope the myofibrils can be seen to consist of repeated cylindrical units, called *sarcomeres*, separated by thin Z disks (Figure 36–1). The myofibrils are enveloped by a flattened bag-like structure called the sarcoplasmic reticulum, which is sealed off from the intracellular space containing the myofibrils. Another space, interweaving among the myofibrils, is the transverse tubule (T-tubule) system formed by minute invaginations of the muscle membrane. The T-tubule is sealed off from both the cytoplasm and the sarcoplasmic reticulum but communicates directly with the extracellular space.

The sarcomere represents the smallest contractile unit. It is composed of two distinct fibrillar proteins, the thin and the thick filaments. The *thin filaments* are discontinuous and attach to the Z disk on one end or the other, while the *thick filaments* lie in the center of the sarcomere, interdigitated among the thin filaments. Motion of the thin filaments relative to the thick filaments occurs during contraction and produces the changes in the widths of the striations seen under the microscope. The main

constituents of the thin filaments are pairs of polymerized actin monomers arranged as a helix. The thin filament also contains two other proteins, tropomyosin (a long filamentous protein that lies in the grooves formed by the paired strands of actin) and troponin (small molecular complexes that are attached to the tropomyosin filament at discrete intervals). The thick filaments are made up of about 250 myosin molecules. Each myosin molecule has two entwined tails about 150 nm long and a double globular head (Figure 36–1C). The myosin heads are powerful ATPases.

Until the early 1950s it was believed that muscle contraction resulted from the contraction of a protein molecule within the myofibrils. In 1954, however, on the basis of ultrastructural and biophysical studies of contracting muscle, Hugh Huxley and Andrew Huxley proposed the *sliding filament theory*, according to which contraction arises from cyclical interactions between the thin (actin) and thick (myosin) filaments. During contraction the globular heads of the myosin molecules attach themselves to receptor sites on the actin molecules, forming *cross bridges* between the thick and thin filaments. The myosin heads then undergo a conformational change that exerts a pulling force on the actin filaments. Finally, the myosin heads detach themselves and the cycle starts over. The access of the myosin heads to the attachment sites on the actin molecules is regulated by the tropomyosin and troponin molecules in the thin filament and is dependent on ATP and Ca^{2+}. The muscle shortens because the myosin molecules slide over the actin molecules, not because either molecule changes its length.

Contraction is set off by the depolarization of the muscle fiber. When an action potential in a motor axon reaches the neuromuscular junction it generates an endplate potential, which in turn triggers an action potential in the muscle fiber. This action potential is propagated rapidly over the surface of the fiber and conducted into the muscle fiber by means of the system of T-tubules (Figure 36–1A). The T-tubule system insures that the contraction that follows a single action potential, termed a *twitch*, spreads throughout the entire fiber. Without such a mechanism, contracting segments of the myofibrils would stretch the slack ones and force would not be transmitted to the ends of the fibers.

A key aspect of the electromechanical mechanism by which the action potential triggers mechanical contraction, a process termed *excitation–contraction coupling*, is a sudden increase in intracellular Ca^{2+}. The spreading depolarization causes Ca^{2+} to be released from the sarcoplasmic reticulum, where Ca^{2+} is normally sequestered into the intracellular space of the muscle fiber, which contains the actin and myosin filaments. The depolarization of the T-tubule system acts on specialized voltage-sensitive channels in the terminal cisterns located in apposing regions of the sarcoplasmic reticulum membrane. By mechanisms that are not fully understood, these local voltage-sensitive channels cause the release of Ca^{2+} throughout the membrane of the sarcoplasmic reticulum. Later, when the muscle relaxes, Ca^{2+} is actively and efficiently pumped out of the intracellular space and back into the sarcoplasmic reticulum (Figure 36–1A).

The interaction between myosin and actin is made possible because some of the Ca^{2+} binds to troponin, producing a conformational change in the actin molecule that exposes a receptor site for the myosin head. Adjacent sites on the myosin head then bind successively to a series of adjacent sites on the actin molecule and this rotates the myosin head. The rotation exerts a force that pulls the thin filaments over the thick filaments and toward the center of the sarcomere (Figure 36–2). After the myosin head has fully rotated, it dissociates from the actin filament and returns to its original relaxed position.

The detachment cocks the myosin head, preparing it for attachment and rotation on an adjacent actin monomer. This detachment is an active process that uses energy derived from the hydrolysis of ATP. When the myosin head is attached to the actin molecule it has a potent ATPase activity that catalyzes the breakdown of

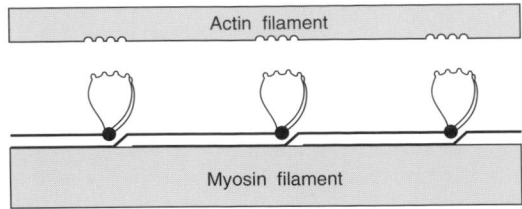

Relaxed

Actin filament

Myosin filament

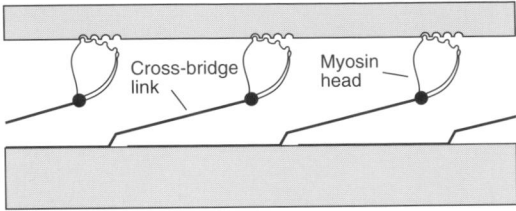

Attached

Cross-bridge link   Myosin head

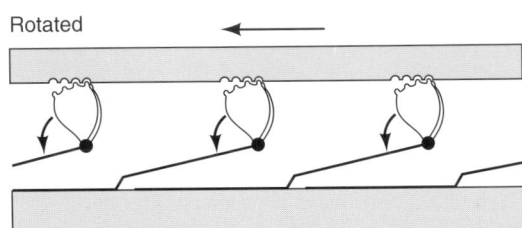

Rotated

FIGURE 36–2

Muscle contraction occurs when the sarcomere shortens. The heads of individual myosin molecules project from the myosin filament toward the actin filament. By an active process, the myosin heads or cross bridges attach themselves to the actin filament in a manner that draws the actin filament toward the center of the A-band. (Adapted from Huxley, 1969.)

A. Relaxed state.

B. Attachment of myosin heads to actin.

C. Successive attachment of sites on each myosin head pulls the actin filament toward the center of the A-band (see Figure 36–1C).

ATP into ADP and P_i, which remain bound to the myosin molecule. This process is, however, also dependent on the Ca^{2+} released from the sarcoplasmic reticulum. The process of attachment, rotation, and detachment continues as long as Ca^{2+} and ATP are present in the myofibril in sufficient amounts. During a single twitch an individual cross bridge attaches and detaches many times. When depolarization ends, Ca^{2+} is pumped back into the sarcoplasmic reticulum and relaxation occurs because cross bridges can no longer form. Both the association and the detachment of the cross bridges require ATP. When ATP is no longer regenerated from ADP, as happens after death, the muscle becomes rigid, a state termed *rigor mortis*.

The Force of Contraction Depends on the Length of the Muscle

The amount of contractile force that a muscle can produce depends markedly on its initial length. Andrew Huxley stimulated small groups of frog muscle fibers while he maintained them at a fixed length during contraction, and found that the relationship of force to length consists of a series of linear segments with different slopes (Figure 36–3). The finding of discrete linear segments is consistent with the sliding filament theory, which predicts that the contractile force should be linearly proportional to the number of cross bridges. Each linear segment of the force-length relationship corresponds to a different pattern of overlap of thick and thin filaments. In each region small increments in length result in different relative changes in the number of cross bridges.

These mechanical events in individual sarcomeres are reflected in the muscle as a whole. However, when the whole muscle is stimulated a smoother curve is produced. This is because the sarcomeres themselves cannot be maintained at a constant length. Some of the force they generate is taken up by the tissues through which they are attached to bone and by deformation of the cross bridges, all of which act like springs (see Box 36–1). Thus, some

degree of stretch of elastic elements of the muscle is inevitable as the activated sarcomeres develop force.

Like a spring, muscles generate a restoring force when they are stretched beyond their resting length. After this resting length is exceeded, each increment in length produces additional increments in restoring force (Figure 36–4B). When the muscle is stimulated, the contractile elements shorten and the muscle starts to develop tension at a much shorter length than it does in the passive state (Figure 36–4B, dotted lines). This is equivalent to taking up the slack of a rubber band by excising a portion of it. Stiffness also increases during contraction (as shown by the increased slope of the lines in Figure 36–4B) because of the active stiffness contributed by the cross bridges. As the rate of stimulation increases, the steep portion of the length–force relationship occurs at progressively shorter muscle lengths.

If a weight were attached directly to the muscle, the weight would be pulled up progressively as the rate of stimulation increases until its restoring force precisely matches the weight. The length at which the muscle comes to rest is called the *equilibrium point*. At the end of this chapter we will see that a fundamental task for the motor systems is to produce neural signals that are precisely calibrated to the loads imposed on the muscles, so that the equilibrium points of the muscles match their desired lengths.

FIGURE 36–3

The amount of active tension developed during contraction depends upon the degree of overlap of thick and thin filaments. When the sarcomere is stretched beyond the length at which the thick and thin filaments overlap (length **a**), no active tension develops because cross bridges cannot form. As the filaments overlap (lengths **a** to **b**), the tension that can develop increases linearly as length decreases because of the progressive increase in the number of sites available for cross bridges to form. Around the muscle's resting length (lengths **b** to **c**), the level of tension remains constant because the central portion of the thick filaments is devoid of myosin heads. Additional sites gained at

either end of the thin filament are matched by losses in the center. With further reductions in length (lengths **c** to **d**) additional binding sites at the ends of the thick filaments are matched by losses in the center because the progressive overlap of thin filaments occludes potential attachment sites and the tension begins to fall. Once the thick filaments abut the Z disks the continued cross-bridge cycling deforms the filaments (lengths **d** to **e**), further reducing the number of myosin heads that can find attachment sites and causing the force to drop at a higher rate. (Adapted from Gordon et al., 1966.)

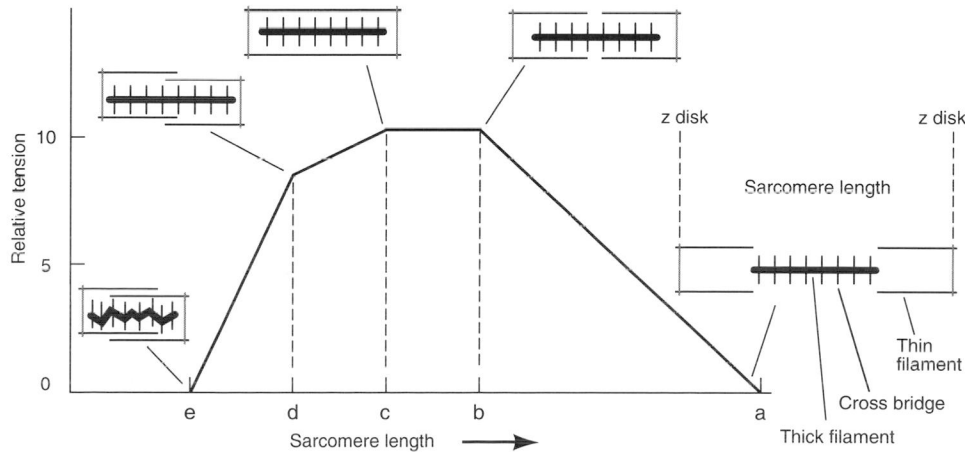

Mechanics of Muscle Contraction

BOX 36–1

A spring is a mechanical device that responds to an increase in length by generating a *restoring force* that is proportional to the change in length. However, this force is developed only when the length exceeds a threshold known as the *set point* or *resting length* (L_0). Until L_0 is exceeded, the spring is slack. Once the length is increased beyond L_0, tension increases linearly.

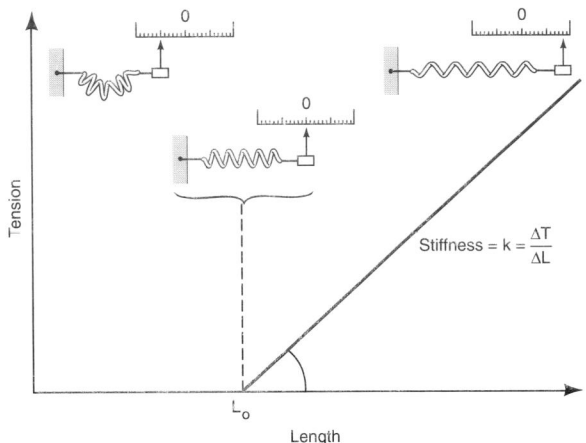

The slope of the line shown in the figure, the incremental force (ΔF) corresponding to a unit change in length (ΔL), represents the spring constant k, also known as the stiffness.

$$k = \Delta F / \Delta L$$

Thus, the tension or force produced by the spring can be described by the simple equation

$$F = k(L - L_0)$$

In muscles the sarcomeres have spring-like properties because they shorten when activated. Thus, muscles can be represented by two elements connected in series: a contractile element (depicted below as a rack and pinion), and an elastic element (depicted by the spring).

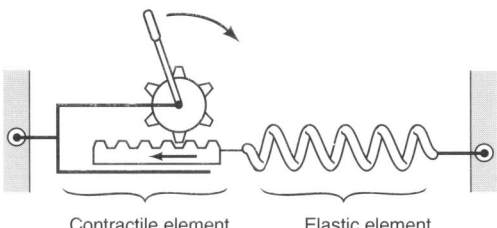

Contractile element   Elastic element

The elastic element includes a passive and an active component. The tendon and connective tissue elements through which the sarcomeres exert force on the bone are the passive component. The cross bridges themselves, where external forces can counteract the rotation at the necks of the myosin heads, are the active component. A more complete model of the muscle would include two other components. First, an elastic element, representing elastic proteins between myofibrils and connective tissue between muscle fibers, acts in parallel with the serially connected contractile and elastic elements. Second, a viscous element provides resistance to stretch; this resistance increases with the speed of stretch. For simplicity, these elements are not included here.

The Force of Contraction Also Depends on the Relative Rates of Movement of the Thick and Thin Filaments

So far we have considered the contractile forces produced by muscles only when their length is held fixed, a condition termed *isometric*. Under natural conditions, however, the length of muscles varies during contraction. As we shall see, the change in length itself influences the time it takes cross bridges to form in the sarcomeres, the amount of force they develop, and the speed of shortening.

The speed of shortening is, of course, greatest when there is no external load. When the load imposed on the muscle matches the force generated by cross-bridge cycling, no net movement occurs and velocity is zero. In this condition there is as much forward as backward sliding of cross bridges. When the load is greater than the forces produced by cross-bridge cycling, the thin filaments will slide backward relative to the thick filaments, and the contracting muscle will actually lengthen. Substantially more force is needed to stretch the contracting muscle—a *lengthening contraction*—than to maintain the muscle at a fixed length, because cross bridges need to be broken to stretch the muscle, and the stiffness of the cross-bridges in the muscle is quite high. About twice as much tension can be produced during lengthening contractions as under isometric conditions. The motor systems regularly exploit this capacity for greater force production. For example, when stepping down stairs, the gastrocnemius contracts to plantar flex the ankle well before the ball of the foot touches the ground. As we move our weight to the foot, the ankle dorsiflexes, thus lengthening the contracting gastrocnemius, which can then provide the force needed to cushion the impact of the body weight.

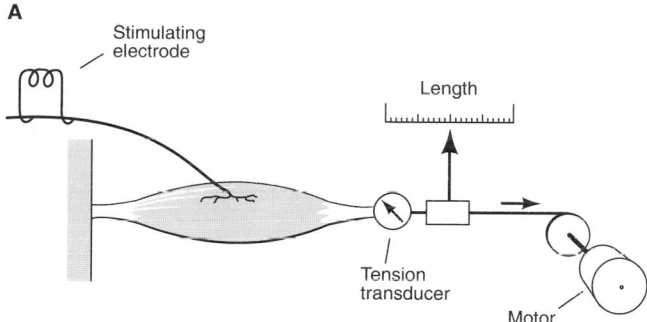

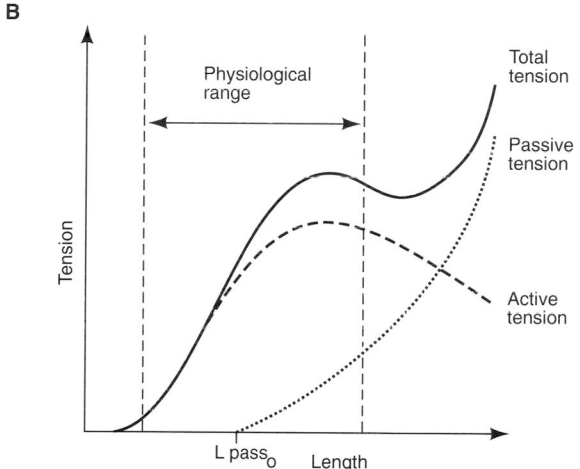

FIGURE 36–4

Tension developed during contraction in whole muscle depends upon its length.

A. Measurements of tension are taken at a series of fixed muscle lengths while stimulating the muscle nerve at different frequencies. The motor serves to pull the muscle and maintain it at a series of set lengths, where a long train of stimuli is applied to the muscle nerve. The steady tension at each of these lengths is recorded by the tension transducer (strain gauge).

B. Length–tension relationship in stimulated muscle. The **dotted line** is the passive stiffness of the muscle. The **solid line** is the length–tension curve for the same muscle when it is stimulated to produce maximal tetanic tension. The amount of tension increases as the muscle is stretched. For lengths greater than $Lpass_0$ the total tension (**solid line**) is the sum of the active (**dashed line**) and passive components (**dotted line**).

When the muscle is maximally activated, detached cross bridges find new attachment sites rapidly. However, when muscle activation is submaximal and the external force is applied very quickly, many cross bridges break abruptly at the same time and the myosin heads need more time to find new attachment sites. This time can be relatively long if a large number of heads are simultaneously trying to find attachment sites. When this occurs, the elastic restoring force of the muscle transiently collapses (Figure 36–5) and the muscle yields, giving way much like chewing gum when it is rapidly stretched. This

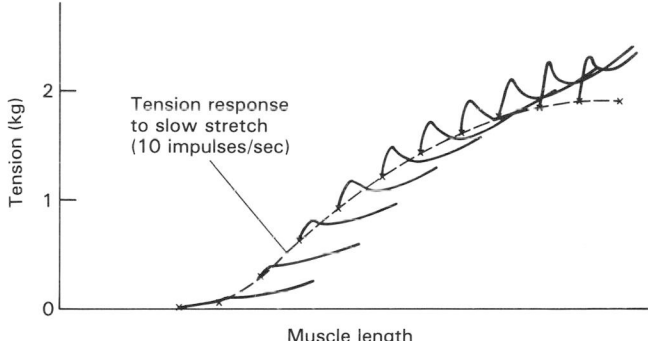

FIGURE 36–5

The length–tension relationship breaks down when muscle is subjected to rapid stretch. The interrupted curve is the length–tension relationship of a muscle when its nerve is stimulated at a rate of 10 impulses per second. The several solid curves are the force–length trajectories that result from stretching the muscle at a constant velocity at different initial muscle lengths while the muscle nerve is being stimulated. (Adapted from Joyce et al., 1969.)

response, which is readily demonstrated in isolated nerve–muscle preparations, would be disastrous if it were to occur during natural behaviors, causing us for example to fall when going down stairs. However, muscle yielding is prevented from occurring because very small amounts of stretch are detected by specialized receptors, the muscle spindles, and this information is rapidly transmitted to motor neurons that quickly increase their level of activation, compensating for the yield. This compensatory mechanism, which acts through the stretch reflex, will be discussed in greater detail in Chapter 37.

Muscles Contract Slowly and the Force Generated by a Train of Impulses Summates

In comparison with the brief time course of a single nerve or muscle action potential (1–3 ms), the time required for a twitch, the contraction and relaxation of a muscle fiber, is very long (10–100 ms). This is, in part, because it takes time for Ca^{2+} that controls cross-bridge cycling to be pumped back into the sarcoplasmic reticulum (Figure 36–6). Thus, successive action potentials may activate the muscle fiber before it has fully relaxed. The forces produced by each twitch will then summate until a plateau of force, or *tetanus*, is reached.

When the rate of stimulation is relatively low, successive stimuli activate the muscle after the peak force of the twitch, and tension is recorded as a characteristic ripple (Figure 36–6C). This is termed an *unfused tetanus* because individual twitches can still be detected. As the stimulation rate increases, the average force increases progressively to a maximum value and the record of the tension becomes smooth. This is called a *fused tetanus* because

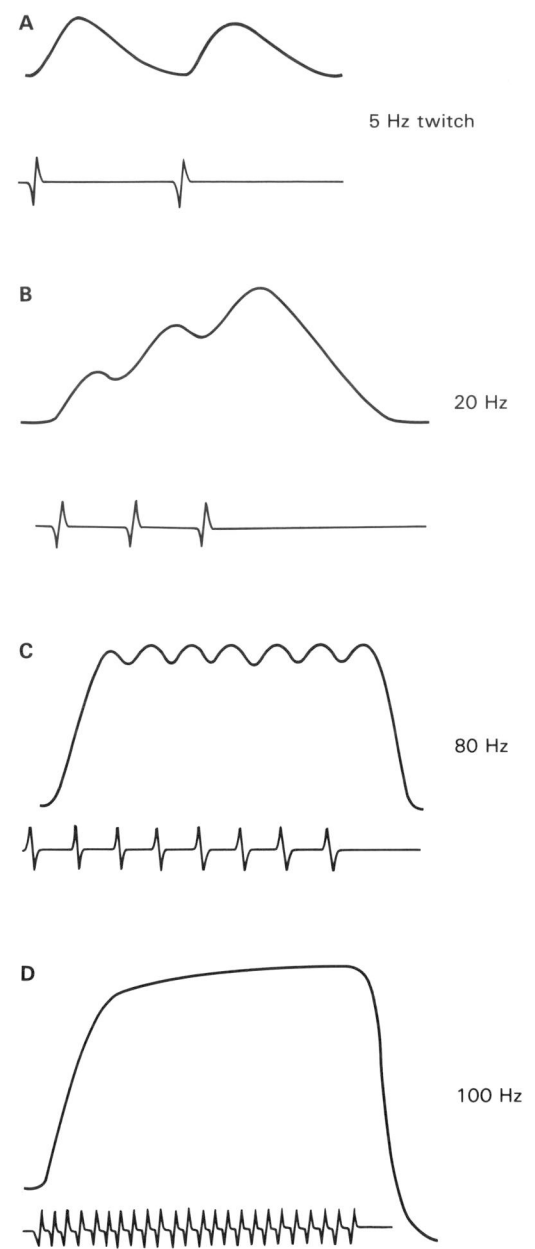

FIGURE 36–6

Active tension varies with the rate of stimulation. Twitch and tetanic contractions elicited by stimulating muscle nerve.

A. Successive isometric force twitches evoked at 5 Hz.

B. Summation of successive twitch contractions.

C. Unfused tetanus.

D. Fused tetanus.

individual twitches can no longer be distinguished (Figure 36–6D). We shall see later that muscle fibers differ in the amount of and time course of their twitch tension and in the frequency that produces fusion. Under conditions of steady contraction, however, muscles are never activated at rates high enough to result in a fused tetanus.

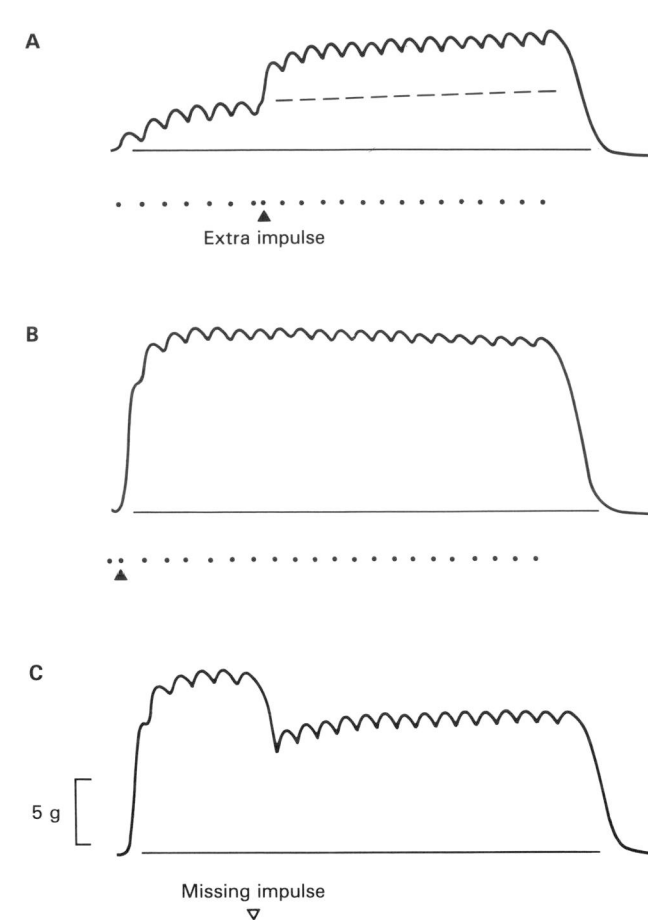

FIGURE 36–7

Active tension depends upon the pattern of stimulation.

A. Unfused tetanus produced by a train of 12 Hz stimuli. Inserting an extra impulse during the train (**arrow**) produces a long-lasting increase in the tension.

B. Adding an impulse at the beginning of a train significantly increases the force and rate of change of force.

C. A missing impulse within a train produces a significant and long-lasting step in tension. (Adapted from Burke et al., 1970.)

The amount of force produced by muscle fibers depends not only on the average rate at which they are stimulated but also on the pattern of stimulation of impulses in the stimulus train. Robert Burke and his colleagues have found that the insertion of a single extra action potential in a low-frequency train of action potentials profoundly enhances the tension (Figure 36–7). The cause of this property is not known. Since following an extra impulse the muscles can be transiently activated at a higher rate than that required for the maintenance of a steady level of force, the motor systems use this non-linear increase in force to make quick movements.

Repeated Activation of Muscles Causes Fatigue

When muscle fibers are repeatedly activated, energy supplies are depleted and the muscles fatigue, producing less force. Muscle fibers also take longer to relax because relaxation is an active process that requires ATP. The prolongation in the mechanical relaxation time has the paradoxical effect of allowing the force produced by successive nerve impulses to summate at lower frequencies (with longer interspike intervals) than when the muscle is rested. As a result, early during fatigue the force produced by unfused tetanic stimulation decreases less than that produced during individual twitches. Brenda Bigland-Ritchie found that during fatigue the firing frequency of motor neurons automatically decreases to compensate for the increased summation of force. In the next chapter we shall see how receptors in the muscles can perform this compensation through reflex actions on motor neurons.

A Single Motor Neuron and the Muscle Fibers It Innervates Constitute a Motor Unit

Each muscle fiber is innervated by only one motor neuron, although each motor neuron innervates a number of skeletal muscle fibers. Since all muscle fibers innervated by one motor neuron contract in response to an action potential in the motor axon, Edward Liddell and Sherrington introduced the term *motor unit* in 1925 to indicate that this combination of elements—the motor neuron and all the muscle fibers it innervates—represents the smallest functional unit controlled by the motor systems.

The number of muscle fibers innervated by one motor neuron is called the *innervation ratio*. Although the innervation ratio varies considerably from one muscle to another, it is roughly proportional to the size of the muscle. In human extraocular muscles, which are very small, the ratio is about 10; in the hand muscles, which are somewhat larger, it is about 100, and in the still larger gastrocnemius muscle it is about 2000. A low innervation ratio indicates a greater capacity for finely grading the muscle's total force, much as small receptive fields allow greater spatial resolution in the somatic sensory and visual systems.

Three Types of Motor Units Are Distinguished by the Properties of Their Muscle Fibers

Some skeletal muscles have a pale color while others are dark red. When electrically stimulated, the pale muscles contract more rapidly than the red and are called *fast muscles*, whereas the dark red muscles are called *slow muscles*. The differences in contraction time reflect differences in the contractile and biochemical characteristics of the muscle fibers in the different motor units. All the muscle fibers belonging to a motor unit have similar physiological properties and are always of the same biochemical type. Motor units are classified physiologically into three basic classes according to the time the fibers take to achieve the peak force during a twitch and the degree to which they fatigue (Figure 36–8).

The first group, called *fast fatigable*, contracts and relaxes rapidly, but fatigues rapidly when stimulated repeatedly. These units generate the largest force during a twitch or tetanic contraction. The second group, termed *slow fatigable*, has a much longer contraction time and is highly resistant to fatigue. These units, however, can only generate 1–10% of the force of the fast fatigable units. The third group, called *fast fatigue-resistant*, has properties that are intermediate between the other two; their contraction time is only slightly slower than fast fatigable units but such units are almost as resistant to fatigue as are the slow units, which produce about twice as much force (Figure 36–9).

The muscle fibers in these three types of motor units also differ in their histochemical and biochemical profiles. Fast fatigable fibers have fewer mitochondria and rely on glycolysis, using the anaerobic breakdown of glycogen for their energy requirements. These fibers have high levels of glycogen and glycolytic enzymes, such as phosphorylase. During contraction these fibers build up an oxygen debt that is restored during relaxation. The rapid contraction and relaxation times correlate with high levels of myosin ATPase and phosphorylase. In contrast, muscle fibers of the slow units are more dependent on oxidative metabolism and have many more mitochondria as well as high levels of oxidative enzymes, such as succinic dehydrogenase. The large number of mitochondria and the low rate of utilization of ATP account for the low fatigability of these fibers. Slow fibers also contain large amounts of myoglobin, which is a heme protein with an oxygen storage capacity. Leg muscles in fowl, for example, owe their dark red color to the predominance of slow fibers. The fast fatigue-resistant fibers, whose properties are intermediate between the slow and fast fatigable, have high quantities of myosin ATPase and phosphorylase, as well as large numbers of mitochondria and oxidative enzymes.

The three types of units vary substantially in the force they generate. Fast fatigable units produce 100 times more force than slow units. The differences in force are due to two major factors: (1) the innervation ratio is greatest and (2) the cross-sectional areas of individual muscle fibers are largest in fast fatigable and least in the slow fibers. In addition, there are intrinsic differences in the myosin molecules and the force generation capacity of the cross bridges in the three groups of fibers.

Individual muscles contain varying proportions of the different motor unit types and the muscle fibers belonging to a given motor unit are widely distributed within each muscle (Figure 36–10). Typically, however, the slow units, which are by far the most numerous and require the most metabolic support, are located more deeply within muscles. Fast fatigable units, which rely on glycolysis, are often closer to the surface, where vascularization is less. Some muscles, such as the soleus, have a preponderance of slow motor units while others, such as extraocular muscles, have primarily fast motor units. These differences correspond well to the functional demands of the different muscles.

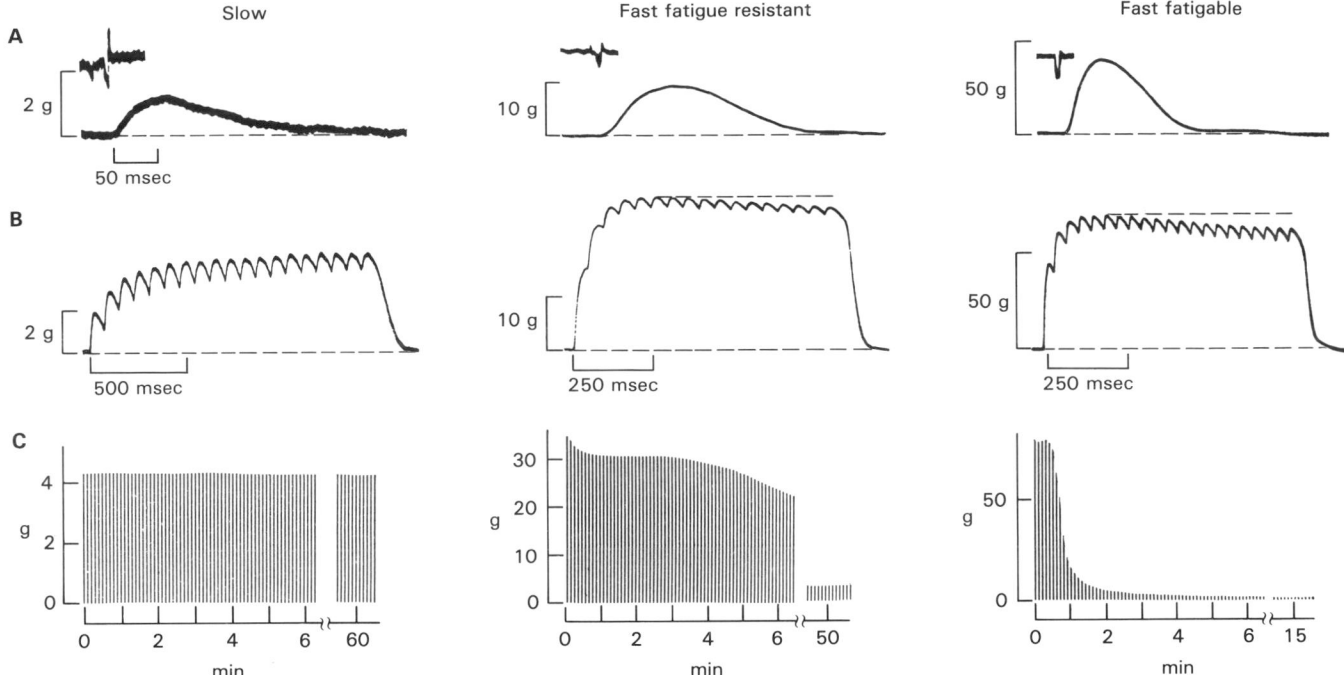

FIGURE 36–8

Twitch tetanic force and fatigability vary in different types of motor units. Slow, fast fatigue-resistant, and fast fatigable motor units were activated by stimulating motor neurons intracellularly. The traces in **A** show the twitches of the three motor units, and in **B** the tetanic tensions produced by a train of 12 Hz stimuli. Note the markedly increased twitch and tetanic forces produced by fast fatigue-resistant and fast fatigable units relative to slow units. In **C**, the muscle is activated by tetanic stimuli lasting

330 seconds and repeated every second. The force produced by each tetanus, recorded at slow speed, appears as a single vertical line. In the slow type unit, the force remains essentially constant for over an hour of repeated stimulation, whereas in the fast fatigable unit the force drops abruptly after only a minute. The fast fatigue-resistant unit shows substantial resistance to fatigue and the force declines slowly over many minutes; some residual force remains after 50 minutes. (From Burke et al., 1974.)

The Properties of Motor Neurons Are Closely Matched to Muscle Fibers

In a motor unit the properties of the neuron and muscle fibers are closely correlated. First, the diameter and conduction velocities of axons supplying fast-fatigable fibers are greater than those of axons supplying fast fatigue-resistant and slow fibers. As a result, the speed of the contraction of the muscle fiber is correlated with the speed of conduction along the axon. Second, motor neurons of slow motor units only fire at low frequencies because each action potential is followed by a large hyperpolarizing afterpotential, which prevents another impulse from occurring immediately (Figure 36–11).

The Nervous System Grades the Force of Muscle Contraction in Two Ways

Motor Units Are Recruited in a Fixed Order from Weakest to Strongest

In the 1960s Elwood Henneman and his colleagues observed that motor neurons are recruited by synaptic action

in a fixed order determined by the conduction velocity and therefore the diameter of their axons. Since the size of the cell body varies with the diameter of its axon, Henneman proposed that when a motor neuron pool is activated the smallest cell bodies are recruited first and by the weakest inputs because they have the lowest threshold for synaptic activation. As the synaptic input increases in strength, progressively larger motor neurons are recruited. This ranking of recruitment is called the *size principle*.

The finding that motor units are recruited according to a stereotyped order has been confirmed under a wide variety of conditions in both experimental animals and in human subjects. This recruitment occurs during both reflex and voluntary contraction. The weakest inputs recruit the slow units, which generate the smallest force and are most resistant to fatigue (Box 36–2 and Figure 36–13). The fast fatigue-resistant units are recruited next, followed by the fast fatigable units. This stereotyped order of recruitment has three important functional consequences.

First, orderly recruitment simplifies the task of modulating force. Higher centers need only determine the overall level of synaptic drive to the motor neuron pool as a whole and do not have to select specific combinations of

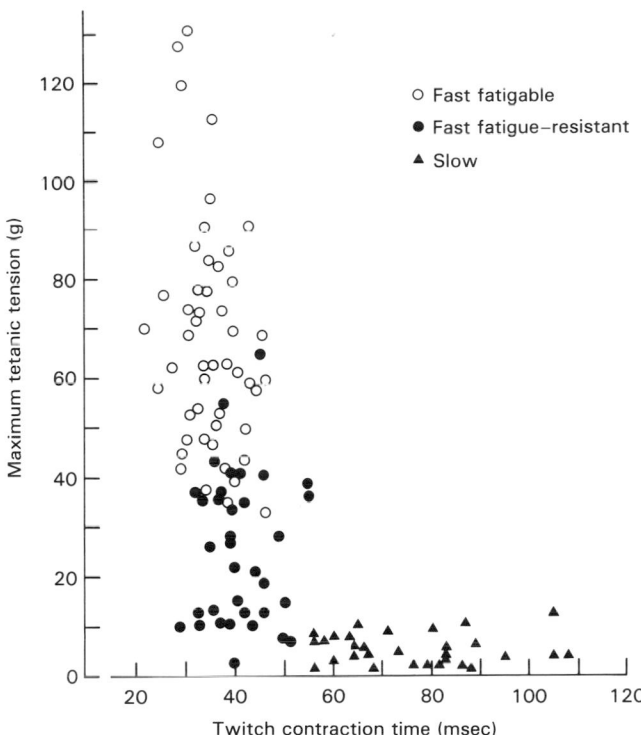

FIGURE 36–9

Physiological profiles of a population of motor units in the gastrocnemius muscle of the cat show three distinct groupings. The fast fatigable units produce larger tension than the fast fatigue-resistant units. The slow units have very long twitch contraction times and generate very low force. (From Burke et al., 1974.)

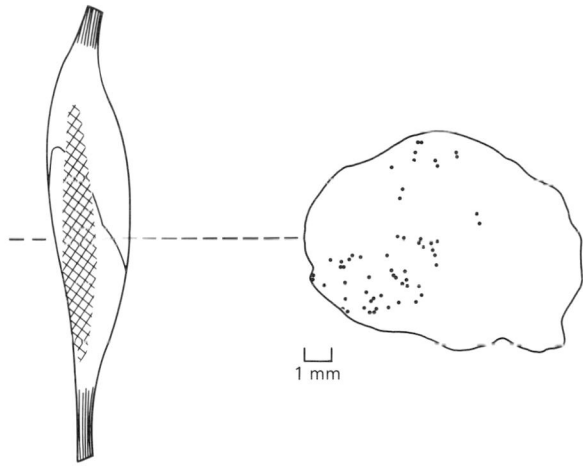

FIGURE 36–10

A single motor neuron innervates many muscle fibers, and these muscle fibers are typically distributed quite widely, as shown by this example in the soleus muscle. The **hatched** area is the approximate size of the motor unit territory projected onto the muscle surface. The location of individual muscle fibers making up the motor unit was determined by stimulation of a single motor neuron for a prolonged period of time; this caused all the muscle fibers to which that motor neuron connected to contract and deplete their stores of glycogen. The fibers were then identified histochemically with a stain selective for glycogen. On the right is a schematic cross section of the muscle at the level indicated by the **broken line**; each **dot** represents a single muscle fiber. (Adapted from Burke et al., 1974.)

motor units to produce the desired amount of force. Second, orderly recruitment assures that the increments of force generated by successively activated motor units increases the synaptic drive in proportion to the force threshold at which they are recruited. Since there may be

fluctuation in the descending synaptic drive during a sequence of movements, the precision of control (i.e., the relative variability of successive responses) remains nearly the same at all levels of force. This consequence of orderly recruitment is formally similar to Weber's law of sensory

FIGURE 36–11

Motor neurons innervating fast muscle fibers show a progressive drop in firing rate. Changes in firing rate and force are shown here for two motor neurons innervating fast and slow muscle fibers, respectively. The cells were impaled with microelectrodes and a steady depolarizing current was applied. The motor neuron connected to the slow-type muscle fiber maintained a steady firing rate during the depolarization, whereas the firing rate of the motor neuron connected to the fast fatigable muscle fiber decreased rapidly over 30 seconds. This reduction in firing rate results in still further reduction in the force produced over the time interval. (From Kernell and Monster, 1982.)

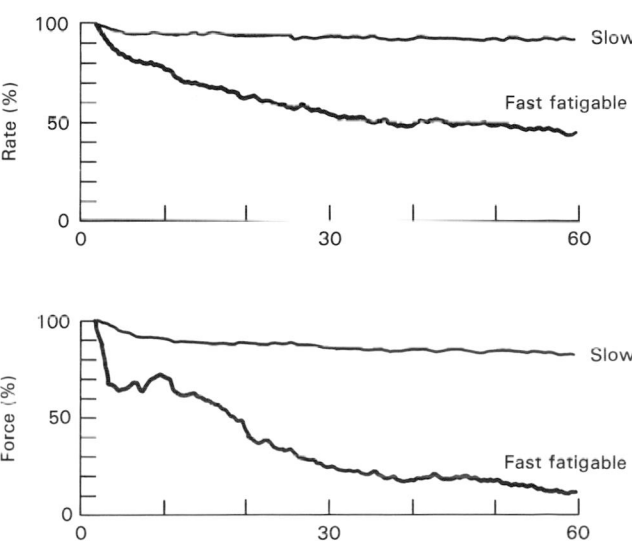

Measurement of Twitch Contraction Time

BOX 36–2

In sensory or motor physiology it is often important to characterize the effect of stimulating a particular neural pathway on a physiological response and to determine the time course of the effect. For example, one commonly needs to ascertain the influence of a neuronal action potential on the force exerted by a particular muscle group.

One approach to this problem is to stimulate the pathway and to record its effect. Unfortunately, stimuli can coactivate nearby pathways or structures that may also affect the structure or variable of interest. In 1968 Lorne Mendell and Elwood Henneman introduced an ingenious computer averaging technique, called *spike-triggered averaging*, that overcame these limitations and made it possible to identify even minute effects of single nerve or muscle action potentials.

Richard Stein and his collaborators used this approach to measure the twitch force of single motor units in awake volunteers. The action potentials from a muscle fiber are recorded with small intramuscular electrodes inserted into a muscle such as the first dorsal interosseous, and muscle force is measured with a strain gauge.

The force generated after a single action potential during the steady contraction of a muscle is not normally recognizable as a clear deflection. This is because the twitch force of a single motor unit is small and because other motor units firing around the same time are also causing the force record to fluctuate. It is, however, possible to isolate the force produced by a series of consecutive spikes in the same unit. This is done by taking advantage of the fact that the change in force it produces remains time locked to the action potential, while the twitches of asynchronously firing motor units is not. Since the action potential associated with a particular unit has a constant size and shape, it can be recognized by a device called a *discriminator*. This device is used to trigger an averaging computer, which then samples the force for a predetermined period of time. With successive action potentials, the changes in tension that are not correlated with the recorded action potential will cancel each other out, while the forces that result specifically from the action potential are time locked with it and become progressively more distinct. Thus, with enough occurrences of the action potentials, typically several hundred, the time course of the twitch becomes more and more evident (Figure 36–12).

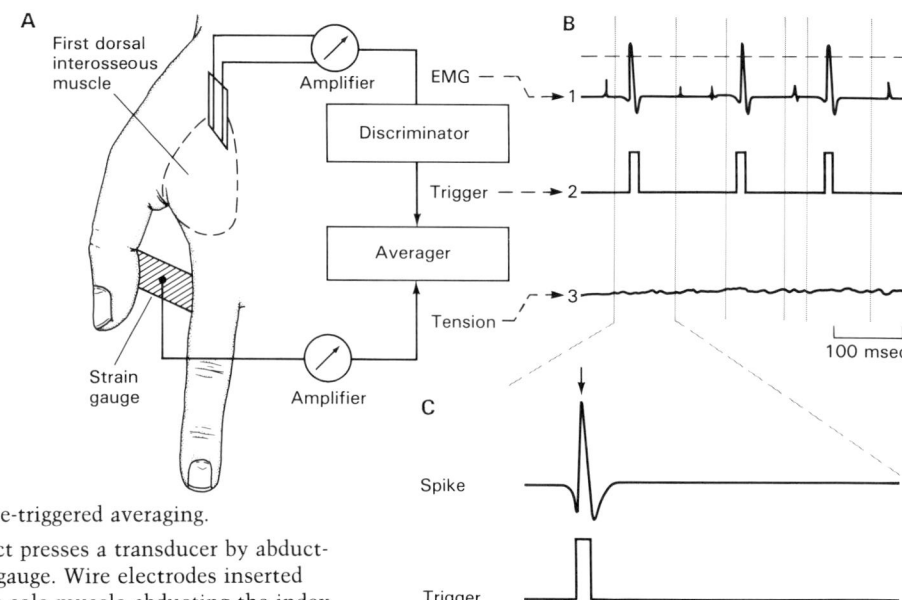

FIGURE 36–12

Twitch tension estimated using spike-triggered averaging.

A. Experimental arrangement. Subject presses a transducer by abducting the index finger against a strain gauge. Wire electrodes inserted into the first dorsal interosseous, the sole muscle abducting the index finger, records action potentials from motor neurons near the bared tip of the electrode. (Adapted from McComas, 1977.)

B. Sample records of a number of single motor units, each with a different size or shape (**1**). Horizontal dotted line shows the level set by the discriminator, which produces a standard pulse (**2**) with each occurrence of large action potentials. The simultaneously recorded force (**3**) does not show obvious inflections corresponding to action potentials.

C. Spike, discriminator pulse, and averaged tensions produced by one, 10, 100, and 500 spikes. Note that with more than 10 spikes a systematic deflection in force becomes evident and the signal to noise ratio increases with increased numbers of traces forming the average.

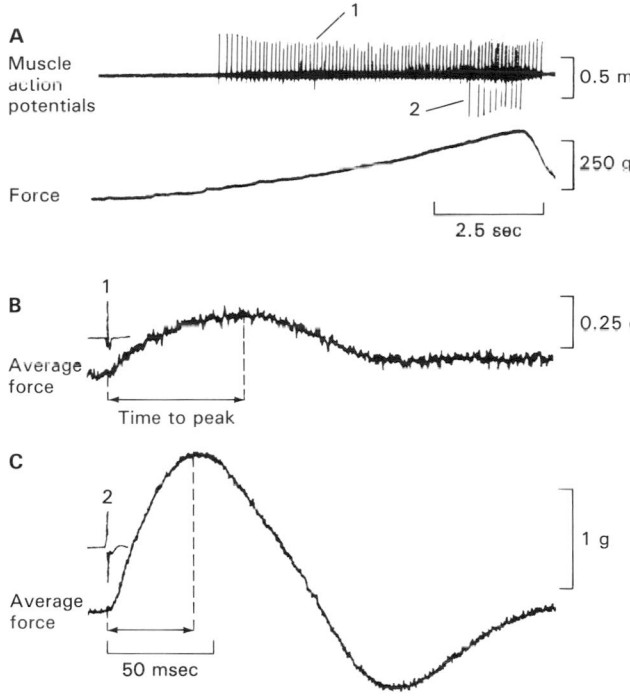

FIGURE 36–13

Motor units producing a low force are recruited before motor units producing large force. Two single motor units were recorded from the first dorsal interosseous of a human subject through the same electrode, which produced a slowly rising force (**A**). Spike-triggered averaging (see Box 36–2) shows that the unit recruited first produces a lower twitch force and has a longer twitch contraction time (**B**) than does the second (**C**). (Adapted from Desmedt and Godaux, 1977.)

discrimination, which states that the smallest difference (jnd) that can be detected between two stimuli (reflecting the precision of perception) is a constant proportion of the reference stimulus (Chapter 23).

Third, the more numerous slower motor units are the most heavily used and must be provided with the greatest metabolic support. Burke and his colleagues found that half the motor units in the hind limb of the cat are slow and are used for standing and walking, activities that require only about 20% of the total force of the muscle. The remaining half of the units, the fast fatigable units, generate the greatest forces but are used only occasionally, for such strenuous activities as running and jumping. Thus, although half of the body's muscle mass is active only rarely, the metabolic cost to have this reserve capacity available is relatively low since the fast fatigable units depend primarily on anaerobic metabolism.

The mechanism underlying the stereotyped recruitment order of motor neurons is not completely understood. Three factors appear to be important. First, as Henneman initially proposed, recruitment order depends on the size of the nerve cell body. This is reasonable since the size of the synaptic potential produced by a standard input varies with the input resistance of the motor neuron. From Ohm's law $(E = IR)$ we know that the size of an excitatory synaptic potential depends on the product of the synaptic current and the input resistance of the neuron. There is an inverse relationship between a neuron's surface area and its input resistance: The smaller the neuron, the larger its passive input resistance. Thus, the same synaptic current would produce a larger synaptic potential in a small neuron than in a larger one. Second, intracellular studies of motor neurons have revealed that the density of synaptic current increases progressively from slow to fast fatigue-resistant to fast fatigable motor units. Third, intrinsic differences in the excitability of motor neurons correlate with the twitch tension of the muscle fibers. Thus, while the idea of size initially referred to the physical dimensions of the neuronal cell bodies, axons, muscle fibers, and the innervation ratio, the most clear basis of orderly recruitment is instead the motor unit force.

There are some notable exceptions to the orderly recruitment of motor units from low- to high-force units. For example, the recruitment of motor neurons innervating muscles with multiple mechanical actions is orderly only if the direction of movement is the same. For example, the first dorsal interosseous can produce both flexion and abduction of the index finger. For voluntary contraction of this muscle, recruitment is orderly (from low to high force units) only for a single direction of movement. Another exception arises when synaptic inputs to motor neuron pools act selectively on specific types of motor units. For example, polysynaptic inputs from cutaneous receptors preferentially inhibit slow motor units while exciting fast ones. Such cutaneous receptors can be activated during manipulatory movements, when the preferential recruitment of fast, high-force motor units might compensate for frictional forces.

Increases in Firing Rate of Motor Units Produce Increasing Force Output

In addition to modulating muscular force by orderly recruitment, the nervous system can vary force by modulating the rate of firing of motor neurons (*rate modulation*). Increases in force with increased firing frequency occurs because successive twitches can then summate. Under normal conditions, however, firing rates stay within a relatively narrow range. For steady voluntary muscle contractions the lowest firing rate of motor units is about 8 Hz; frequencies are rarely higher than 25 Hz during even the most intensely maintained contractions (Figure 36–14). Although these firing rates produce unfused tetanic contractions, movements are smoothly executed because the different motor units are activated asynchronously. In this way the peaks and troughs of motor unit twitches average out. Higher rates of firing that would produce a fused tetanus occur only transiently during the early phase of rapid contraction.

Recruitment and rate modulation are not mutually exclusive. For motor tasks that require a slowly increasing force, single motor units are recruited one at a time in an orderly fashion and their rate is modulated as the force increases.

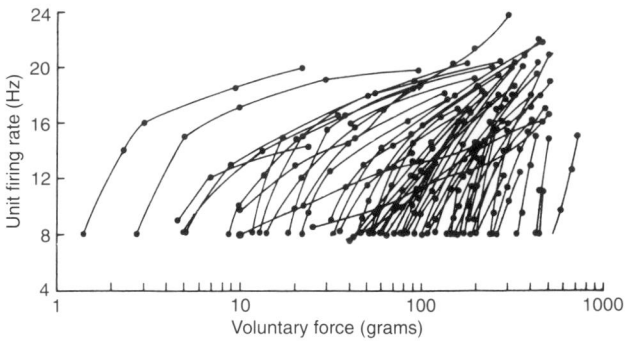

FIGURE 36–14
During slow rising forces different motor units are recruited and their firing frequency increases progressively. Motor units recorded in the extensor digitorum communis of a human subject produce gradually rising forces. Units fire at about 8 Hz when they are recruited and their firing rate increases progressively as the subject produces more force. (Adapted from Monster and Chan, 1977.)

Muscle Properties Limit the Strategies Available to Control Movement

Several Strategies Can Produce a Given Joint Angle

The large number of muscles acting at each joint provide the motor systems with a variety of means for controlling

the position and trajectory of the body and limbs. However, the properties of muscles also impose limitations. For example, neither the force of muscle contraction nor the length of muscle can be determined directly by the amount of neural activity. Instead, since muscles behave like springs, the motor systems control their stiffness and set point. How the motor systems take advantage of the spring-like property of muscle can be illustrated by an example of purposeful motor action: flexing the arm a few degrees. Let us assume that this flexion is produced by contracting the biceps muscle and that the triceps exerts no opposing force. The biceps can be represented as contractile and elastic elements arranged in series, as shown in Figure 36–15. Neural activity shortens the contractile element, shown in the figure as the clockwise rotation of the gear in contact with the rack. The shortening of the contractile element pulls on the spring, which in turn moves the forearm to the equilibrium point, where the forces generated balance the weight of the forearm.

In reality, however, the triceps muscle opposes the biceps, so that its state of contraction also needs to be controlled. Emilio Bizzi and his colleagues proposed that this control of opposing muscles allows the central nervous system to produce a given change in joint angle in several different ways. Two of these—reciprocal innervation and co-contraction—are illustrated schematically in Figure 36–16.

Each of these two has a benefit and a cost. Reciprocal innervation is more energy efficient, but it requires that loads be accurately known by central processes involved

A

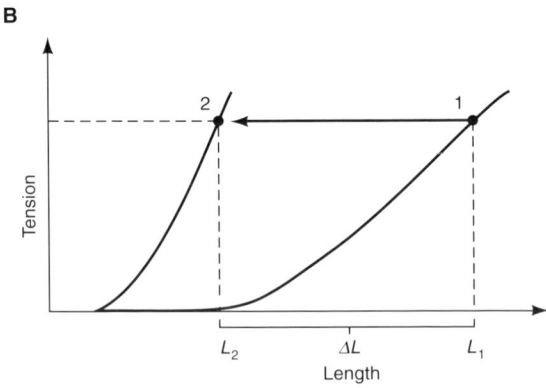

FIGURE 36–15
Changes in limb position result from changes in stiffness and set point of muscle.

A. The mechanical action of the elbow flexor muscle (biceps) is shown here as a rack and pinion gear (contractile element) and a spring (elastic element). Clockwise rotation of the gear resulting from increased neural activity pulls on the spring, which flexes the forearm.

B. The change in length–tension relationships under different conditions. In **1** the set point (**L1**) is longer and the stiffness (slope) is less than in **2**. The change in length (**ΔL**) occurs because the opposing force (the mass of the arm) remains the same in the two positions.

in planning the movement. Co-contraction uses more energy but does not require that loads be known precisely. This co-contraction provides greater adaptability to unanticipated changes in external forces or loads. Because the joint is stiffer with co-contraction, a difference between the actual and expected load will have only a smaller effect on the final limb position than if reciprocal activation were used. As we learn to anticipate loads during the development of motor skill, the motor system switches from a strategy of co-contraction to that of reciprocal innervation.

Skeletal Muscles Are Low-Pass Filters of Neural Input

The nervous system does not control skeletal muscles through a simple one-to-one relationship of trains of action potentials and changes of muscle length or tension.

Rather, changes in muscle tension represent a transformation of the frequency of neural impulses. This type of signal transformation can be demonstrated by applying sinusoidally varying trains of stimuli to the muscle nerve and examining the resulting changes in muscle tension. This method allows one to determine how faithfully a signal reaching a processing element, such as a neuronal synapse or nerve–muscle synapse, is represented in the output of the system, or whether the amplitude and time course of the signal has been systematically distorted. This method has also been used extensively to characterize the properties of sensory transduction, and was first applied to muscle by Lloyd Partridge.

At low frequencies sinusoidal trains of stimuli produce oscillations in muscle tension that are also sinusoidal but that lag behind the fluctuations in impulse frequency (Figure 36–17A). When the frequency of the sinusoidal train is increased, however, the magnitude of the change in ten-

FIGURE 36–16

The same change in equilibrium point or joint angle can be produced by reciprocal innervation or by co-contraction. Contractions of biceps (agonist) and triceps (antagonist) muscles are again shown as rotations of rack-and-pinion gears operating on springs. Rotation of the gears changes the set points of the springs (muscles).

A. The elbow is flexed by reciprocal innervation. The set point of the excited biceps is lowered and the muscle shortens while the inhibited triceps relaxes. The activation of the biceps increases its stiffness and decreases its set point length, whereas the relaxation of the triceps brings about a decrease in stiffness and a corre-

sponding increase in set point length in this muscle as well. The concomitant changes in both muscles specify a new equilibrium position of the limb, and the elbow is flexed to the new joint angle.

B. The elbow is flexed by co-contraction. The biceps must contract enough to overcome the force of the contracting antagonist triceps. The decrease in set point and stiffness of both muscles results in an overall increase in the stiffness of the joint itself. Thus, with the contraction of two opposing muscles, the central nervous system can independently vary both the angle and the stiffness of the joint.

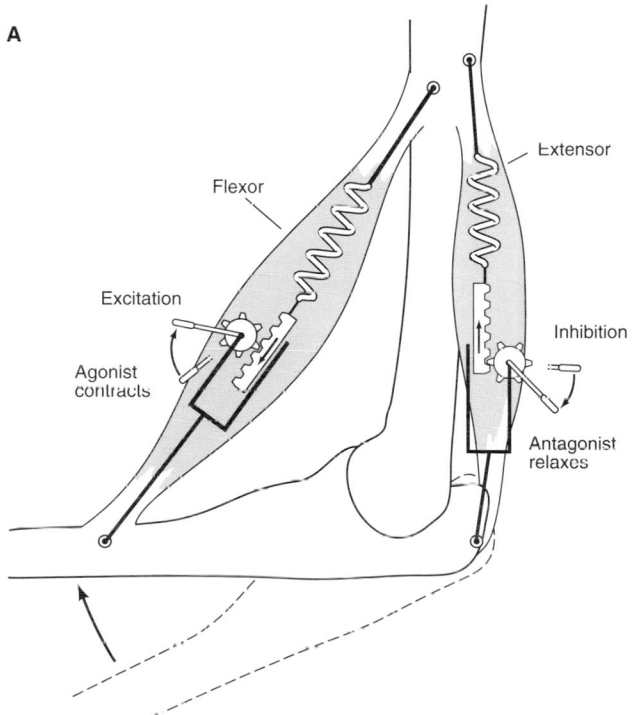

A

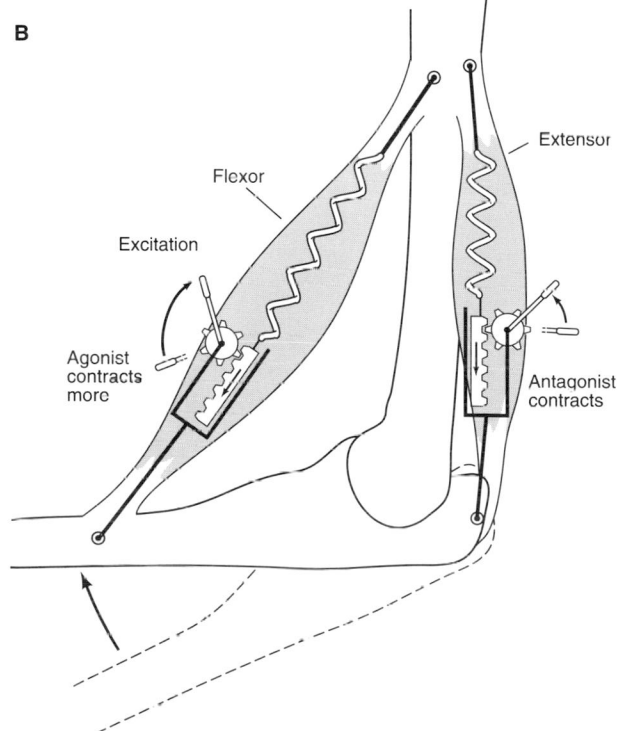

B

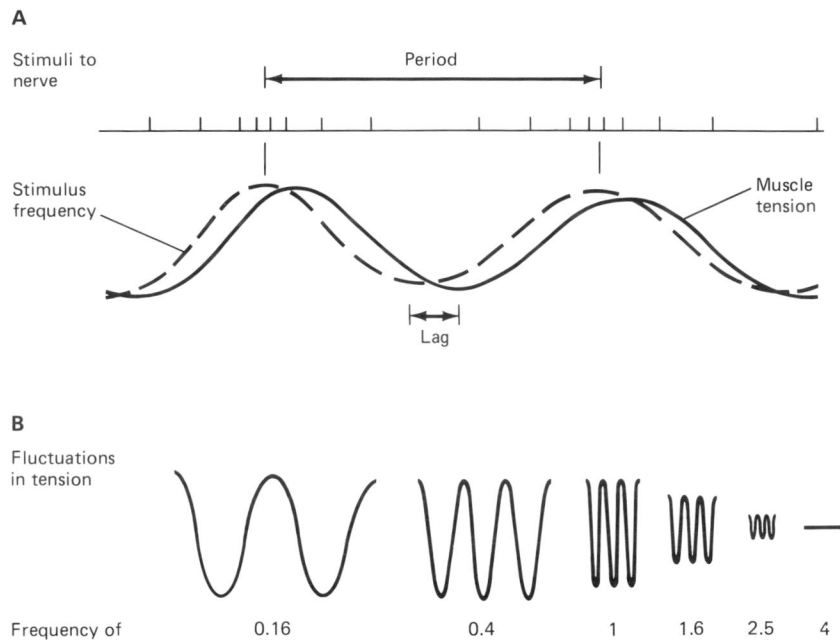

FIGURE 36–17

Muscle mechanics filter the information contained in a train of neural impulses.

A. The stimuli are applied to the muscle nerve with a sinusoidal frequency (**broken line** in lower trace). The oscillation in the muscle tension (**solid line** in lower trace) lags behind the changes in stimulus frequency.

B. Changes in the frequency of the sinusoidal stimulation cause changes in the frequency and amplitude of muscle tension. When the sinusoidal train is delivered at high frequency, muscle tension remains at a fixed level and no longer reflects the change in sinusoidal stimulus rate. (Adapted from Partridge, 1966.)

sion decreases and the change in tension lags progressively more. From 0.16 Hz the magnitude decreases 50% to 1.6 Hz; by 4 Hz almost no fluctuation in muscle tension is present (Figure 36–17B).

From these observations Partridge concluded that muscles are low-pass filters; they are unable to transform high frequencies in the modulation of neural impulses into fluctuations in force. This important property of muscle derives from the fact that the time course of a muscle twitch produced by a single action potential is longer (by several hundred milliseconds) than that of the action potential itself. In controlling movement the motor systems take into account this feature of muscles—that they only reproduce faithfully, slowly varying trains of impulses. The motor systems produce a fast-rising force by activating the agonist muscle to a greater degree and more quickly than normal. When this occurs the motor system must then activate the antagonist muscle to truncate the force at the desired level. If the antagonist were not activated, the level of force, corresponding to the maximal rate of rise, would be excessive. In rapid movements this sequential activation gives rise to a characteristic triphasic pattern of activation of the opposing muscles (Figure 36–18). The late contractions, first in the antagonist and then in the agonist, decelerate the movement and smooth late oscillations at the end of movement (Figure 36–18).

An Overall View

Precision in the control of movement is complicated by two properties of muscles: their spring-like quality and their slow response to neural activation.

First, like a spring, the tension exerted by a muscle

varies with the muscle's length. Changes in muscle length depend not only on neural drive but also on the initial length of the muscle and on the external loads. The muscle's mechanical response to rapid stretching is consider-

FIGURE 36–18

Rapid voluntary limb movements are associated with a triphasic pattern of muscle contraction. First, the agonist muscle shows a burst of activation (**arrow**) forming the first agonist burst. As the limb reaches maximal velocity, agonist activity is transiently silenced and the antagonist is activated to decelerate the movement (reciprocal antagonist burst [**arrow**]). Later, agonist activation resumes, frequently with an initial phasic activation, the second agonist burst (**arrow**). (Courtesy of C. Ghez and J. I. Martin.)

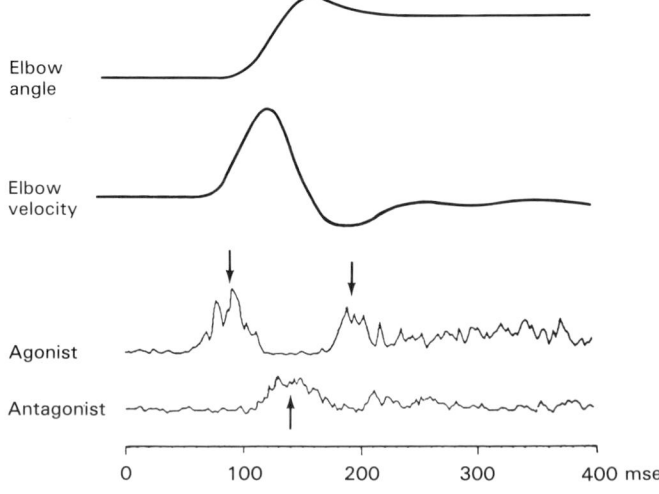

ably more complex than a spring. In the next chapter we shall see that the regulation of muscle length and tension by the brain is also controlled by spinal mechanisms, which compensate for some of the more complex properties of muscles. The complex properties of muscles and the loads to which they are ultimately attached also require that motor commands be calibrated on the basis of experience. Skilled motor performance is therefore highly dependent on learning.

Second, because the mechanical response of muscles to neural activity is slow, changes in muscle tension do not represent a simple one-to-one correspondence to the firing patterns of motor neurons. Rather, the temporal pattern of the incoming train of action potentials is modified by the muscles themselves. Because of this filtering action, muscles faithfully reproduce only those signals that vary slowly. To produce rapid changes in tension, the motor systems must alternate contraction in opposing muscles.

Selected Readings

Bizzi, E., and Abend, W. 1983. Posture control and trajectory formation in single- and multi-joint arm movements. In J. E. Desmedt (ed.), Motor Control Mechanisms in Health and Disease. Advances in Neurology, Vol. 39. New York: Raven Press, pp. 31–45.

Desmedt, J. E. 1985. Patterns of motor commands during various types of voluntary movement in man. In E. V. Evarts , S. P. Wise, and D. Bousfield (eds.), The Motor System in Neurobiology. New York: Elsevier, pp. 133–139.

Eckert, R. 1988. Animal Physiology: Mechanisms and Adaptations, 3rd ed. New York: Freeman, Chap. 10, "Muscle and movement."

Freund, H.-J. 1983. Motor unit and muscle activity in voluntary motor control. Physiol. Rev. 63:387–436.

Huxley, A. F. 1974. Review lecture: Muscular contraction. J. Physiol. (Lond.) 243:1–43.

Partridge, L. D., and Benton, L. A. 1981. Muscle, the motor. In V. B. Brooks (ed.), Handbook of Physiology, Section 1: The Nervous System, Vol. II, Motor Control. Part 1. Bethesda, Md.: American Physiological Society, pp. 43–106.

Polit, A., and Bizzi, E. 1978. Processes controlling arm movements in monkeys. Science 201:1235–1237.

Stuart, D. G., and Enoka, R. M. 1983. Motoneurons, motor units and the size principle. In R. N. Rosenberg (ed.), The Clinical Neurosciences, Vol. 5. Neurobiology. New York: Churchill Livingstone, pp. 471–517.

References

Bigland-Ritchie, B., Johansson, R., Lippold, O. C. J., Smith, S., and Woods, J. J. 1983. Changes in motoneurone firing rates during sustained maximal voluntary contractions. J. Physiol. (Lond.) 340:335–346.

Bizzi, E., Accornero, N., Chapple, W., and Hogan, N. 1982. Arm trajectory formation in monkeys. Exp. Brain Res. 46:139–143.

Bloom, W., and Fawcett, D. W. 1975. A Textbook of Histology, 10th ed. Philadelphia: W. B. Saunders.

Buchtal, F. 1942. The mechanical properties of the single striated muscle fibre at rest and during contraction and their structural interpretation. Dan. Biol. Medd. 17(2).

Burke, R. E., Levine, D. N., Salcman, M., and Tsairis, P. 1974. Motor units in cat soleus muscle: Physiological, histochemical and morphological characteristics. J. Physiol. (Lond.) 238:503–514.

Burke, R. E., Rudomin, P., and Zajac, F. E., III. 1970. Catch property in single mammalian motor units. Science 168:122–124.

Burke, R. E., Rudomin, P., and Zajac, F. E. III. 1976. The effect of activation history on tension production by individual muscle units. Brain Res. 109:515–529.

Desmedt, J. E., and Godaux, E. 1977. Fast motor units are not preferentially activated in rapid voluntary contractions in man. Nature 267:717–719.

Garnett, R., and Stephens, J. A. 1981. Changes in the recruitment threshold of motor units produced by cutaneous stimulation in man. J. Physiol. (Lond.) 311:463–473.

Gordon, A. M., Huxley, A. F., and Julian, F. J. 1966. The variation in isometric tension with sarcomere length in vertebrate muscle fibres. J. Physiol. (Lond.) 184:170–192.

Henneman, E., Somjen, G., and Carpenter, D. O. 1965. Functional significance of cell size in spinal motoneurons. J. Neurophysiol. 28:560–580.

Huxley, A. F., and Niedergerke, R. 1954. Structural changes in muscle during contraction. Interference microscopy of living muscle fibres. Nature 173:971–973.

Huxley, H. E. 1969. The mechanism of muscular contraction. Science 164:1356–1366.

Huxley, H., and Hanson, J. 1954. Changes in the cross-striations of muscle during contraction and stretch and their structural interpretation. Nature 173:973–976.

Joyce, G. C., Rack, P. M. H., and Westbury, D. R. 1969. The mechanical properties of cat soleus muscle during controlled lengthening and shortening movements. J. Physiol. (Lond.) 204:461–474.

Kernell, D., and Monster, A. W. 1982. Motoneurone properties and motor fatigue: An intracellular study of gastrocnemius motoneurones of the cat. Exp. Brain Res. 46:197–204.

Liddell, E. G. T., and Sherrington, C. S. 1925. Recruitment and some other features of reflex inhibition. Proc. R. Soc. Lond. [Biol.] 97:488–518.

Loeb, G. E., and Gans, C. 1986. Electromyography for Experimentalists. Chicago: University of Chicago Press.

McComas, A. J. 1977. Neuromuscular Function and Disorders. London: Butterworths.

Mendell, L. M., and Henneman, E. 1968. Terminals of single Ia fibers: Distribution within a pool of 300 homonymous motor neurons. Science 160:96–98.

Milner-Brown, H. S., Stein, R. B., and Yemm, R. 1973. The contractile properties of human motor units during voluntary isometric contractions. J. Physiol. (Lond.) 228:285–306.

Monster, A. W., and Chan, H. 1977. Isometric force production by motor units of extensor digitorum communis muscle in man. J. Neurophysiol. 40:1432–1443.

Partridge, L. D. 1966. Signal-handling characteristics of load-moving skeletal muscle. Am. J. Physiol. 210:1178–1191.

Stein, R. B., French, A. S., Mannard, A., and Yemm, R. 1972. New methods for analysing motor function in man and animals. Brain Res. 40:187–192.

James Gordon
Claude Ghez

37

Muscle Receptors and Spinal Reflexes: The Stretch Reflex

Muscles Contain Specialized Receptors That Sense Different Features of the State of the Muscle

Muscle Spindles Respond to Stretch of Specialized Muscle Fibers

Golgi Tendon Organs Are Sensitive to Changes in Tension

Functional Differences Between Spindles and Tendon Organs Derive from Their Different Anatomical Arrangements within Muscle

Muscle Spindles Are Sensitive to Muscle Stretch

The Primary and Secondary Endings of Spindle Afferents Respond Differently to Phasic Changes in Length

Two Types of Gamma Motor Neurons Alter the Responsiveness of Spindles

Spindle Afferents and Efferents Innervate Different Types of Intrafusal Fibers

The Central Nervous System Can Control Sensitivity of the Muscle Spindles Through the Gamma Motor Neurons

The Fusimotor System Maintains Spindle Sensitivity During Muscle Contraction

Fusimotor Output Can Be Adjusted Independently of Motor Output

Discharge of Muscle Spindle Afferents Produces Stretch Reflexes

The Stretch Reflex Has Phasic and Tonic Components

Group Ia Afferents Make Monosynaptic Connections to Motor Neurons

The Main Connections of Group II and Group Ib Afferents to Motor Neurons Are Polysynaptic

Stretch Reflexes Contribute to Muscle Tone

Stretch Reflexes Regulate Muscle Tone Through Negative Feedback

Stretch Reflexes Allow Muscles to Respond Smoothly to Stretch and Release

An Overall View

In the previous chapter we considered how the nervous system modulates the contraction of skeletal muscles through motor neurons, the final common pathway for motor processing. The force produced in the contracting muscle and the resulting change in its length are dependent on three factors: the initial length of the muscle, the velocity of length change, and the external loads acting to oppose movement. For effective control of muscle the central nervous system therefore needs information about the lengths of the muscles and the forces they are generating. This proprioceptive information is transmitted to the central nervous system by two types of muscle receptors: muscle spindles and Golgi tendon organs.

Muscle spindles and tendon organs convey complementary information about the state of the muscle: The muscle spindles signal changes in length, while the tendon organs signal changes in tension. In the first part of this chapter we shall examine the different structures and anatomical arrangements within muscles of these two receptors. Muscle spindles are of particular interest because they are innervated by efferent axons that allow the nervous system to adjust the sensitivity of the sensory endings. Thus, muscle spindles provide a particularly well-studied example of how the central nervous system can control its own sensory inflow.

Information from muscle spindles and tendon organs reaches all levels of the nervous system. At the highest levels, such as the cerebral cortex, this proprioceptive information is used for the perception of limb position and for planning movements. At lower levels muscle receptors control motor behavior through *reflexes*, the simplest of behaviors.

A reflex is an involuntary and relatively stereotyped response to a specific sensory stimulus. Two features of the sensory stimulus are particularly important in shaping the reflex response. First, the *locus* of the stimulus determines in a fixed way the particular muscles that contract to produce the reflex response. Second, the strength of the stimulus determines the amplitude of the response. Reflexes therefore are typically graded.

Spinal reflexes are reflexes in which the sensory stimuli arise from receptors in muscles, joints, and skin, and in which the neural circuitry responsible for the motor response is entirely contained within the spinal cord. Although the neuronal circuits that mediate spinal reflexes are relatively simple, descending influences from higher brain centers often use these spinal circuits to generate more complex behavior. Therefore, an understanding of the organizational principles of spinal reflexes is essential for understanding more complex motor sequences. Spinal reflexes also are valuable for clinical diagnosis. They can be used to assess the integrity of both afferent and motor connections as well as the general excitability of the spinal cord. Brain stem reflexes, such as gagging and the vestibulo-ocular reflex, follow basically similar rules.

In this chapter we shall examine the neural circuitry of one spinal reflex: the stretch reflex. This is the simplest of reflexes; it depends only on the monosynaptic connections between primary afferent fibers from muscle spindles and motor neurons innervating the same muscle. In other spinal reflexes, such as those produced by cutaneous stimuli, one or more interneurons may be interposed between the primary afferent fibers and the motor neurons. In the next chapter we shall consider the more complex circuitry of other spinal reflexes and we shall examine the role of these reflexes in posture, locomotion, and other complex motor acts.

Muscles Contain Specialized Receptors That Sense Different Features of the State of the Muscle

Skeletal muscles are richly supplied with a variety of receptors. Two receptors are particularly important for motor control: the *muscle spindles* and the *Golgi tendon organs*. Both receptors are distributed extensively throughout most skeletal muscles. Muscle spindles are elongated structures within the fleshy portions of muscles; they are parallel to the skeletal muscle fibers (Figure 37–1). Golgi tendon organs are located at the junction between muscle fibers and tendon; they are therefore connected in series to a group of skeletal muscle fibers.

Muscle spindles are innervated by group I (large myelinated) and group II (small myclinated) afferent fibers; Golgi tendon organs are innervated only by group I afferent fibers. The group I afferents innervating muscle

FIGURE 37–1

Muscle spindles and Golgi tendon organs are encapsulated structures found in skeletal muscle. The main skeletal muscle fibers, or extrafusal fibers, are innervated by large-diameter alpha motor axons. The muscle spindle has a fusiform shape and is arranged in parallel with extrafusal fibers. It is innervated by both afferent and efferent fibers. The Golgi tendon organ is found at the junction between a group of extrafusal fibers and the tendon; it is therefore in series with extrafusal fibers. Each tendon organ is innervated by a single afferent axon. (Adapted from Houk et al., 1980.)

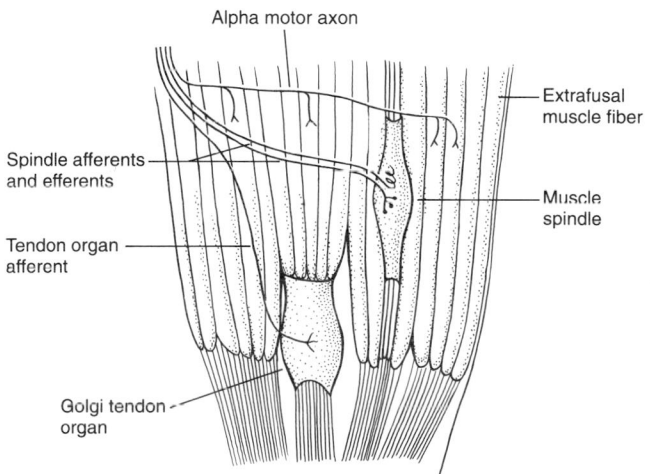

Alpha motor axon

Extrafusal muscle fiber

Spindle afferents and efferents

Muscle spindle

Tendon organ afferent

Golgi tendon organ

Tendon

spindles are called *group Ia* afferents whereas those innervating tendon organs have slightly smaller diameters and are referred to as *group Ib* afferents. Almost all of the group I afferents arising in muscle innervate either spindles or tendon organs. Most group II afferents from muscle terminate on spindles but a few terminate as free nerve endings or in other types of receptors.

Many other small-diameter afferent fibers in muscle nerves arise from receptors other than muscle spindles and tendon organs. Most have unmyelinated axons (group IV), terminate as free nerve endings, and probably serve nociceptive and thermoregulatory functions. Some of these afferents play an important role in regulating the response of the body to exercise, such as increasing blood pressure and respiration.

Muscle Spindles Respond to Stretch of Specialized Muscle Fibers

Muscle spindles are encapsulated structures, ranging from 4 to 10 mm in length. Each spindle has three main components: a group of specialized muscle fibers, sensory axons that terminate on the muscle fibers, and motor axons that regulate the sensitivity of the spindle (Figure 37–2). The center of the spindle is enclosed by a connective tissue capsule filled with a gelatinous fluid that facilitates sliding of the muscle fibers within it. Thus, the spindle is slightly swollen in the center, and the ends are tapered, giving it a fusiform or spindle-like shape.

The specialized muscle fibers of the muscle spindle are called *intrafusal fibers* to distinguish them from ordinary skeletal muscle fibers, the *extrafusal fibers*. Intrafusal fibers are smaller than extrafusal muscle fibers and do not contribute significant force to muscle contraction. Their central regions have very few myofibrils and are essentially noncontractile; only the polar regions actively contract. Three types of intrafusal muscle fiber can be distinguished: one type of nuclear chain and two types of nuclear bag fibers. *Nuclear chain fibers* are short and slender; their nuclei lie in single file within the fiber. *Nuclear bag fibers* are thicker in diameter and have nuclei clustered in their central regions, which thus appear slightly swollen. Physiological studies have further distinguished two types of nuclear bag fibers, dynamic and static. A typical mammalian muscle spindle contains two nuclear bag fibers, one of each type, and a variable number of nuclear chain fibers, usually about five. As we shall see, the different properties of the three types of intrafusal fibers play a major role in determining the firing characteristics of the sensory endings of the spindle.

The myelinated sensory axons enter the capsule in its central part and terminate on or near the central portions of the intrafusal fibers. Most afferent endings spiral around individual intrafusal fibers (Figure 37–2). When the fibers

FIGURE 37–2
The main components of the muscle spindle are intrafusal fibers, sensory endings, and motor axons.

A. The intrafusal fibers are specialized muscle fibers; their central regions are not contractile. The sensory endings spiral around the central regions of the intrafusal fibers and are responsive to stretch of these fibers. Gamma motor neurons innervate the contractile polar regions of the intrafusal fibers. Contraction of the intrafusal fibers pulls on the central regions from both ends and increases the sensitivity of the sensory endings to stretch. (Adapted from Hullinger, 1984.)

B. The muscle spindle contains three types of intrafusal fibers: dynamic nuclear bag, static nuclear bag, and nuclear chain fibers. A single group Ia afferent fiber innervates all three types of intrafusal fiber, forming a primary ending. A group II afferent fiber innervates chain and static bag fibers, forming a secondary ending. Two types of efferent axon innervate different intrafusal fibers. Dynamic gamma motor axons innervate only dynamic bag fibers; static gamma motor axons innervate various combinations of chain and static bag fibers. (Adapted from Boyd, 1980.)

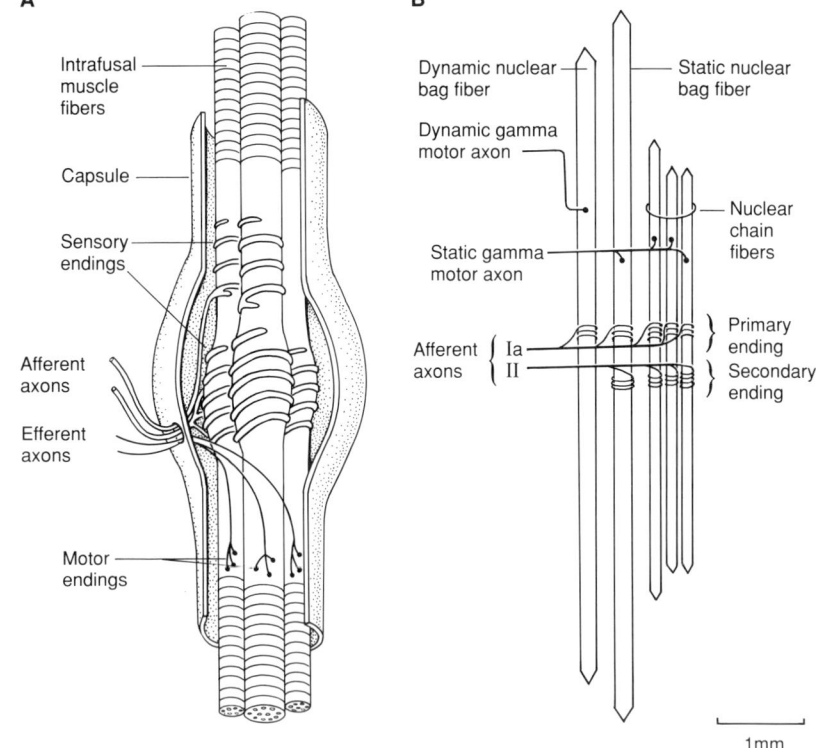

A.

Intrafusal muscle fibers

Capsule

Sensory endings

Afferent axons

Efferent axons

Motor endings

B.

Dynamic nuclear bag fiber

Dynamic gamma motor axon

Static gamma motor axon

Afferent axons { Ia / II

Static nuclear bag fiber

Nuclear chain fibers

Primary ending

Secondary ending

1mm

are stretched, often referred to as *loading* the spindle, the endings increase their firing rate. This happens because stretching of the spindle lengthens the central region of the intrafusal fibers around which the afferent endings are entwined. The resulting elongation of the afferent endings activates stretch-sensitive channels that depolarize the membrane and generates action potentials. When the stretch is released, referred to as *unloading*, the intrafusal fibers slacken and the firing rate in the afferent endings decreases.

There are two types of sensory endings in muscle spindles: primary and secondary. There is usually just one *primary ending* in each spindle, consisting of all the branches of a single *group Ia* afferent axon. Group Ia afferents terminate on all three types of intrafusal fibers. There is also usually one *secondary ending* in a spindle consisting of the terminations of a single *group II* afferent. The group II fibers terminate only on chain fibers and static bag fibers. The primary and secondary endings have different signaling characteristics. Primary endings are much more sensitive to the rate of change of length than secondary endings. We will consider the functional differences between the two types of ending and the reasons for them in a later section.

The motor axons that regulate the sensitivity of the muscle spindle terminate on the polar regions of the intrafusal fibers. In amphibians and other lower vertebrates, the motor axons are collaterals of the motor axons innervating the extrafusal fibers. In mammals, however, the motor innervation of intrafusal and extrafusal fibers is generally separate. This was first demonstrated in 1945 by Lars Leksell, who established that the intrafusal fibers are innervated by small *gamma motor neurons*, while the extrafusal fibers are innervated by larger *alpha motor neurons*. Leksell used pressure to block conduction in the large motor axons in ventral roots, so that stimulation of the ventral roots excited only the small-diameter motor axons. The excitation produced no significant increase in muscle tension, but did increase the discharge rate of spindle afferents. Thus, the gamma motor neurons can modulate the discharge of spindle afferents.

The gamma motor neurons that innervate muscle spindles are often referred to as the *fusimotor system*, while the alpha motor neurons that innervate extrafusal fibers are referred to as the *skeletomotor system*. Recent studies have shown that some collaterals from alpha motor neurons innervate intrafusal fibers. These are referred to as *skeletofusimotor* or beta efferents. A significant though still unquantified degree of skeletofusimotor innervation has been found in both cat and human muscle spindles.

How does stimulation of gamma efferents modulate the discharge rate of spindle afferents? Whereas the sensory afferents terminate in the central region of intrafusal fibers, the gamma fibers innervate the polar regions, where the contractile elements are located (Figure 37–2). Activation of a gamma efferent causes contraction and shortening of the polar regions of the intrafusal fibers, which in turn stretches the non-contractile central region

from both ends, leading to an increase in firing rate of the sensory endings. Contraction of the intrafusal fibers also changes the sensitivity of the spindle afferent endings to stretch. How the central nervous system uses the fusimotor system to control the information coming from the spindles is discussed later in this chapter.

Golgi Tendon Organs Are Sensitive to Changes in Tension

Golgi tendon organs are slender encapsulated structures about 1 mm long and 0.1 mm in diameter. They are typically located at the junction of muscle and tendon, where collagen fibers arising from the tendon attach to the ends of groups of extrafusal muscle fibers (Figure 37–3). Collagen bundles within the capsule of the tendon organ divide into fine fascicles that form a braided structure.

Each tendon organ is innervated by a single group Ib axon that loses its myelination after it enters the capsule and branches into many fine endings, each of which in-

FIGURE 37–3
Golgi tendon organs are specialized structures found at the junctions between muscle and tendon. Collagen fibers in the tendon organ attach to the muscle fibers. A single Ib afferent axon enters the capsule and branches into many unmyelinated endings that wrap around and between the collagen fibers. When the tendon organ is stretched (usually because of contraction of the muscle), the afferent axon is compressed by the collagen fibers (see insert at lower right) and increases its rate of firing. (Adapted from Schmidt, 1983; inset adapted from Swett and Schoultz, 1975.)

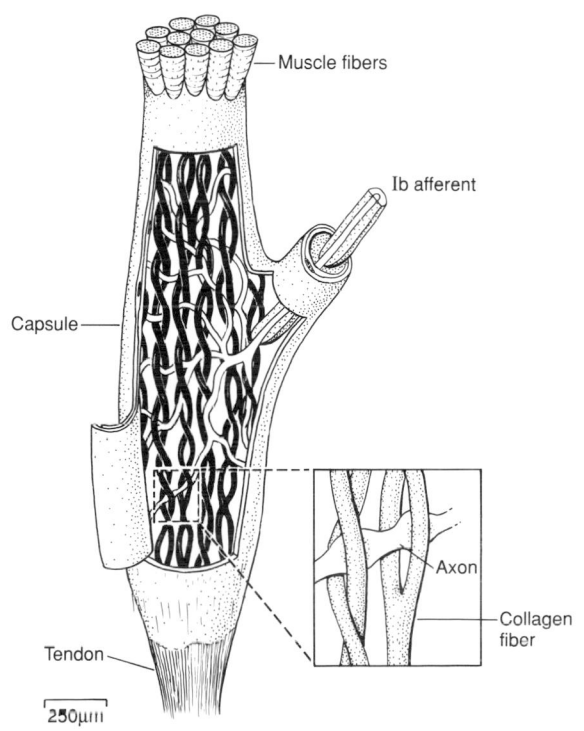

Muscle fibers

Ib afferent

Capsule

Axon

Collagen fiber

Tendon

250μm

tertwines among the braided collagen fascicles. Stretching of the tendon organ straightens the collagen fibers. This compresses and elongates the nerve endings and causes them to fire. Because the free nerve endings intertwine among the collagen fiber bundles, even very small stretches of the tendon organ can deform the nerve endings. The firing rate of tendon organs is very sensitive to changes in tension of the muscle. Tendon organs stretch most easily when the muscle tension increases due to contraction. James Houk and Elwood Henneman found that a twitch contraction of a single motor unit is sufficient to increase the firing rate of a tendon organ afferent.

Functional Differences Between Spindles and Tendon Organs Derive from Their Different Anatomical Arrangements within Muscle

In 1933 Bryan Matthews obtained the first recordings from axons of muscle afferents and discovered that muscle spindles and Golgi tendon organs convey different information (Figure 37–4). When he stretched the muscle, the spindle afferents showed a brisk increase in their rate of discharge, while tendon organs showed only a slight and inconsistent increase. On the other hand, when the muscle contracted

after stimulating its motor nerve, the firing rate of the tendon organ increased markedly, but the firing rate of the spindle decreased or ceased altogether.

Matthews reasoned that this difference in response results from the different anatomical relationships of the two types of receptors to the extrafusal muscle fibers. The spindles are arranged *in parallel* with extrafusal fibers, whereas the Golgi tendon organs are arranged *in series*. Stretching of the muscle elongates the intrafusal fibers stretching the sensory endings in the spindle and leading to increased firing. In tendon organs, however, the collagen fibers from the tendon are stiffer than the muscle fibers with which they are in series. Therefore, most of the stretch is taken up by the more compliant muscle fibers; little direct mechanical deformation of the tendon organ takes place. When the muscle contracts, however, the muscle fibers themselves pull directly on the collagen fibers and transmit the stretch to the tendon organ more effectively. As a result, tendon organs always respond more robustly to contraction than to stretch of the muscle. Spindles, in contrast, decrease their firing rate when the muscle contracts because, as the extrafusal fibers shorten with contraction, the parallel intrafusal fibers also shorten.

FIGURE 37–4

The two types of muscle stretch receptors, the spindle afferent and the Golgi tendon organ, have different responses to muscle stretch and to muscle contraction. Both afferents discharge to stretch of the muscle (**A**), the Golgi tendon organ much less than the spindle. However, when the muscle is made to contract by stimulation of its motor neuron (**B**), the spindle is unloaded and therefore goes silent, whereas the Golgi tendon organ firing rate increases. (Adapted from Patton, 1965.)

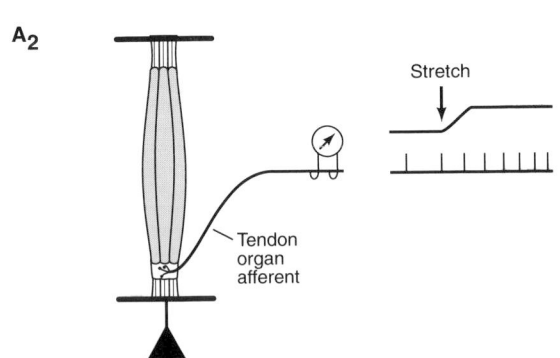

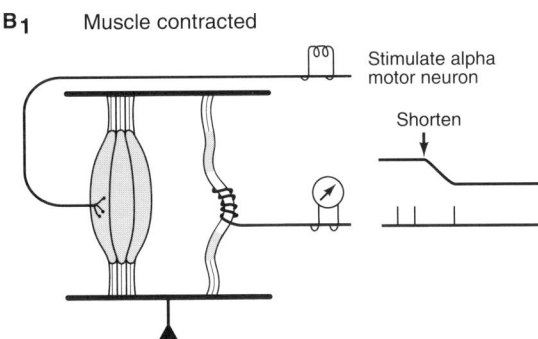

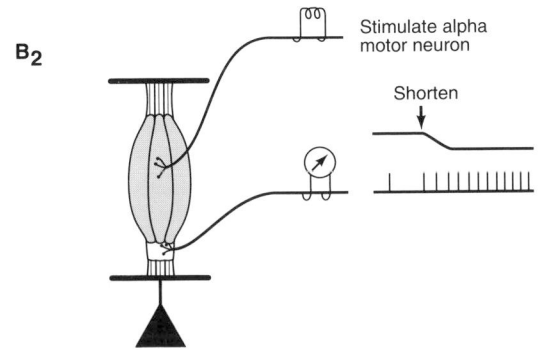

Spindles and tendon organs provide complementary information about the mechanical state of the muscle. Because the length of a muscle varies with the angle of the joint it acts upon, the sensory input from the spindles is used by the brain to determine the relative positions of the limb segments. Sensory input from Golgi tendon organs about the tension produced by muscles is useful for a variety of motor acts, such as maintaining a steady grip on an object or compensating for the effects of fatigue (when a steady neural drive to the muscle would produce decreasing levels of tension).

We shall return to Golgi tendon organs in the next chapter, where we discuss the function of spinal reflexes in motor control. In the rest of this chapter we shall focus on muscle spindles. First, we shall see that the spindles are capable of transmitting information not only about the absolute change in length but also about the velocity of the length change. Next, we shall consider the functional role of the gamma motor axons in regulating the sensitivity of the spindle. Finally, we shall examine the spinal connections of spindle afferents and their role in stretch reflexes.

Muscle Spindles Are Sensitive to Muscle Stretch

The Primary and Secondary Endings of Spindle Afferents Respond Differently to Phasic Changes in Length

When muscle is stretched or released from stretch, there are two phases of the change in length: a dynamic phase, the period during which length is changing, and a static or steady-state phase, when the muscle has stabilized at a new length. In 1961 Sybil Cooper recorded from the primary and secondary endings of muscle spindles and found that they respond quite differently during the dynamic phase of a change in muscle length (Figure 37–5A). When a muscle is lengthened, both endings increase their firing rates to a higher steady-state rate. When a muscle is shortened and released from stretch, both endings decrease their firing to a lower rate. During the dynamic phase of the stretch, however, the primary ending fires at a much higher rate than during the later steady-state phase. The firing of the secondary ending increases only gradually, and is not much higher during the dynamic phase than during the steady-state phase.

The primary endings of the muscle spindle are highly sensitive to the rate of change of muscle length, a property referred to as *velocity sensitivity* (Figure 35–5B). The increase in firing rate in primary endings during stretch reflects the rate of change in muscle length—higher rates occur during faster stretches. Velocity sensitivity is also seen when the muscle shortens: during a rapid shortening primary endings pause in firing, then resume firing at a lower rate when shortening stops. Because of their high degree of dynamic sensitivity, primary endings respond with bursts of firing to transient stimuli, such as brief taps or vibration of the muscle (Figure 37–5A). Secondary endings, in contrast, are relatively unaffected by such phasic

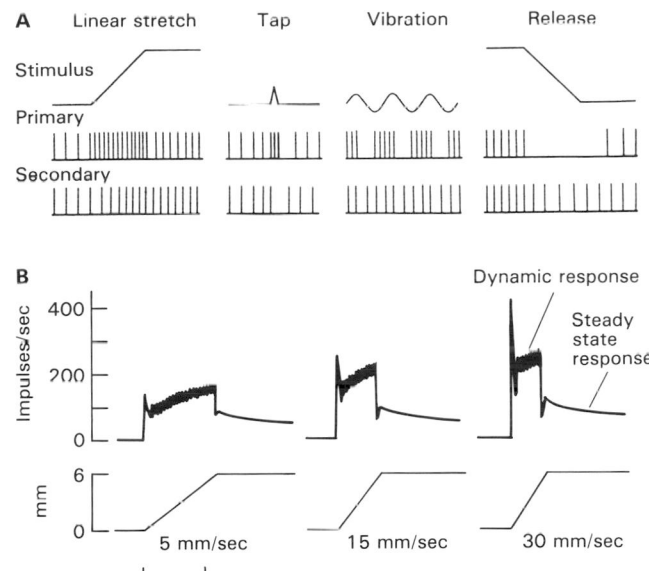

FIGURE 37–5

Primary and secondary ending in muscle spindles have different firing properties.

A. When the muscle is stretched or released, both endings reach a steady-state firing rate that reflects the new muscle length. In addition, the primary ending shows a burst of firing during the dynamic phase of stretch and a transient silence during release. Primary endings are therefore very sensitive to transient or changing stimuli, such as taps or vibration of the muscle. (Adapted from Matthews, 1964.)

B. The primary ending is highly sensitive to the velocity of stretch. Its firing rate during the dynamic phase reaches higher levels with faster stretches. Primary endings are particularly sensitive to very small stretches; this is reflected in the transient increase in the firing rate at the very beginning of the stretch. (Adapted from Matthews, 1972.)

stimuli because the changes in muscle length occur too quickly to be reflected in the steady-state discharge of these endings.

Since primary endings encode not only the length of a muscle but also the rate of length change, they provide information about the speed of movements as well as the static positions of joints. Two important factors also affect the firing rate of primary endings. First, primary endings are most sensitive to small changes in muscle length (less than 0.1 mm). This sensitivity is often reflected in a transient increase in firing rate at the beginning of a stretch (Figure 37–5B). The dynamic sensitivity of primary endings decreases dramatically with large changes in length. Second, primary endings are able to reset their responsiveness to very small stretches after they come to a new length. Consequently, they are able to sense small changes in length regardless of the steady-state length of the muscle. Thus, the relationship between the rate of spindle firing and rate of change in length is not linear and depends in complex ways on other factors, most notably the initial length and the recent history of spindle firing.

Two Types of Gamma Motor Neurons Alter the Responsiveness of Spindles

Two types of gamma motor neurons selectively alter the static and dynamic responsiveness of spindle afferents. In 1964 Peter Matthews recorded from isolated Ia afferent fibers and stretched the muscle at a controlled rate, while at the same time stimulating the axons of individual gamma motor neurons. Stimulation of different neurons produced two different effects. Stimulation of some gamma axons markedly enhanced the steady-state discharge from the primary afferent during the static phase, with little effect on its dynamic responsiveness during stretch. These afferents are thus classified as *static* gamma motor neurons. They have a similar effect on the output of secondary endings. Stimulation of other gamma axons markedly enhanced the high-frequency burst during the dynamic phase of stretch. These are classified as *dynamic* gamma motor neurons (Figure 37–6).

Selectively increasing the steady-state discharge of spindle afferents reduces the differences between the dynamic response and the steady-state (Figure 37–6B). Thus, when static gamma motor neurons are activated the information from spindles primarily reflects the actual length of the muscle, whereas with activation of dynamic gamma motor neurons the overall spindle input becomes more *phasic*, thus communicating information about small and quick fluctuations in length.

Spindle Afferents and Efferents Innervate Different Types of Intrafusal Fibers

The different firing properties of primary and secondary afferents as well as the different actions of the two types of gamma motor neurons probably do not derive from major intrinsic differences in the properties of the neurons themselves. Rather, these properties differ primarily because the neurons innervate different types of intrafusal fibers, each of which has distinct mechanical and contractile properties. Primary spindle endings terminate on all the intrafusal fibers within a spindle: dynamic bag fibers, static bag fibers, and nuclear chain fibers (Figure 37–2B). Therefore, the firing pattern of primary endings derives from the combined properties of all three types of intrafusal fiber. Secondary endings on the other hand innervate chain fibers and static bag fibers. Their firing patterns thus reflect the properties of these types of intrafusal fibers. The two types of gamma motor neurons also innervate different types of intrafusal fibers. Dynamic gamma motor neurons innervate only the dynamic nuclear bag fibers. Static gamma motor neurons innervate both nuclear chain fibers and static bag fibers.

The functional consequences of this differential innervation have been demonstrated by Ian Boyd, who observed the operation of spindles under the microscope while stimulating alpha and gamma motor neurons. Boyd found that the high degree of dynamic sensitivity of primary afferent fibers derives from the peculiar mechanical behavior of the dynamic nuclear bag fibers (Figure 37–7A).

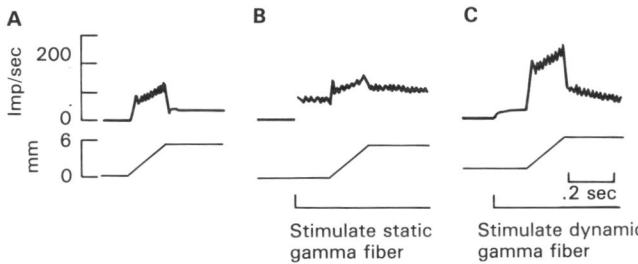

FIGURE 37–6

Selective stimulation of the two types of gamma motor neurons has different effects on the firing of spindle endings. (Adapted from Brown and Matthews, 1966.)

A. With no gamma stimulation the primary ending shows a small dynamic response to stretch and a modest increase in steady-state firing.

B. With stimulation of a static gamma motor neuron the steady-state response of the ending increases but there is no change in the dynamic response. Because the difference between the dynamic and steady-state response has decreased, the spindle shows *less* dynamic sensitivity.

C. With stimulation of a dynamic gamma motor neuron, the dynamic response of the ending is markedly enhanced but the steady-state response gradually returns to its original level. Because the difference between the dynamic and steady-state response has increased, the spindle shows *greater* dynamic sensitivity.

These intrafusal fibers have nonuniform characteristics along their length. The central region acts much like a spring, while the polar regions exhibit viscous resistance to the stretch; that is, resistance is low when the stretch is slow but increases as the rate of change of length increases. When the dynamic bag fiber is stretched quickly, the central region lengthens immediately, whereas the polar regions lengthen only gradually (Figure 37–7B). As the polar regions slowly lengthen, the lengthened central region creeps back to a slightly shorter length. Boyd called this behavior *intrafusal creep*. The sensory ending on these fibers responds to stretch with a burst of firing, which then diminishes as the central region creeps back to a shorter length. Nuclear chain fibers and static bag fibers, on the other hand, are more uniformly stiff along their length, and therefore the central region does not creep back to a shorter length at the end of a quick stretch.

The different effects of dynamic and static gamma efferents can also be explained by the different properties of the intrafusal fibers they innervate. Boyd showed that activation of dynamic bag fibers by dynamic gamma motor neurons prior to muscle stretch produces little actual shortening of the polar contractile portions of the intrafusal fiber (Figure 37–7C). Instead, the polar regions stiffen and their viscous resistance to stretch increases. This has the effect of enhancing stretch of the central sensory region, and thus the dynamic sensitivity of the primary ending. Nuclear chain fibers and static bag fibers, on the other hand, behave much more like extrafusal muscle fibers. When stimulated, the contractile regions shorten

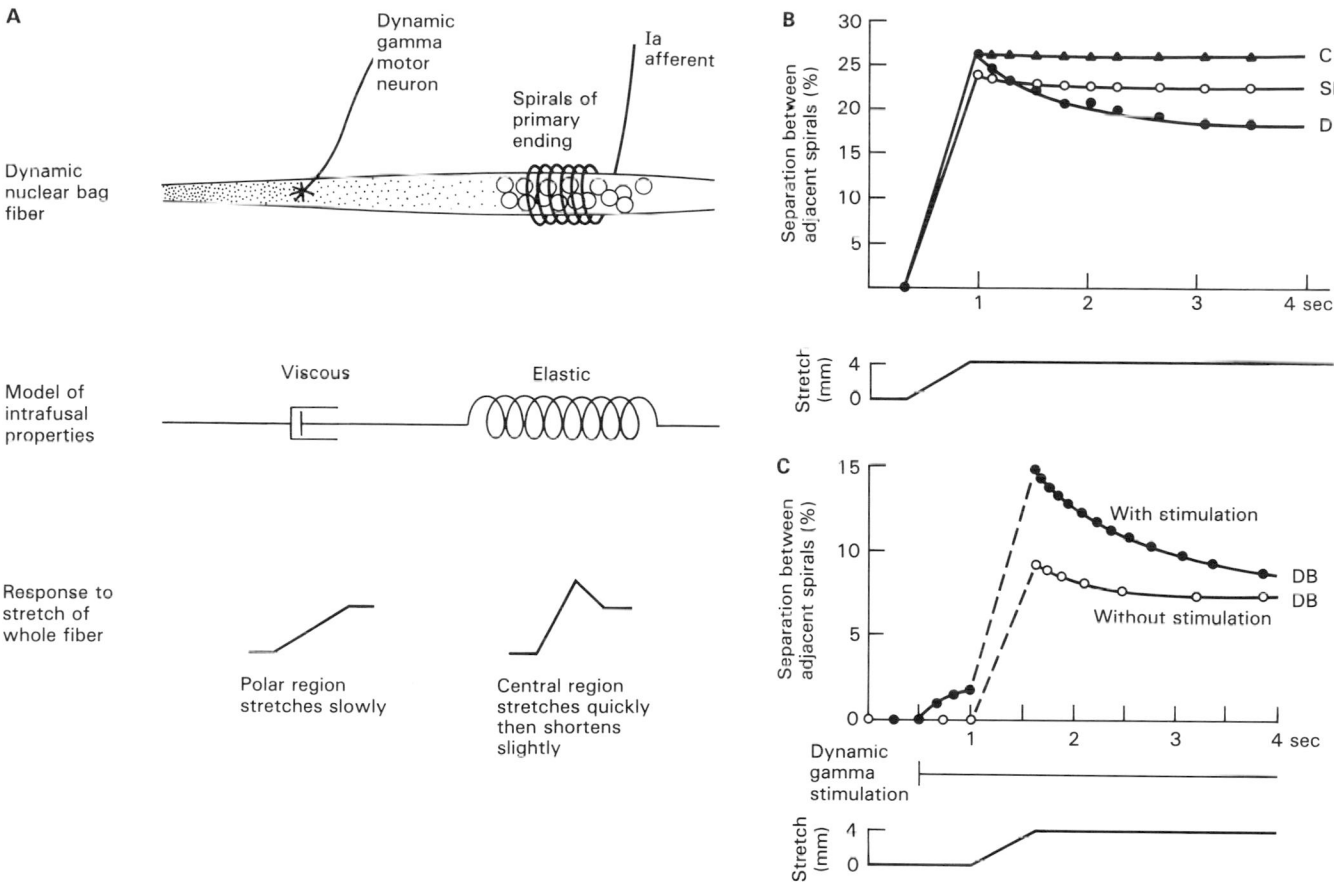

FIGURE 37–7

The dynamic sensitivity of primary endings results from unusual mechanical properties of the dynamic nuclear bag fibers of the muscle spindle.

A. The dynamic bag fiber has an elastic response to stretch in its central region and a viscous response in its polar regions. When the fiber is stretched the central region lengthens quickly but then "creeps" back to a shorter length because of the slower response of the polar regions.

B. The effect of muscle stretch on intrafusal fibers is assessed by measuring the distance between adjacent spirals of the sensory endings. Spirals around the dynamic nuclear bag fiber (**DB**) spread quickly and then creep back. This accounts for the burst of firing in the primary endings. Spirals around nuclear chain (**C**) and static nuclear bag (**SB**) fibers remain separated during the stretch. (Adapted from Boyd and Smith, 1984.)

C. Stimulation of a dynamic gamma motor neuron enhances intrafusal creep but has little effect on the steady-state response of the dynamic nuclear bag fiber.

rapidly, stretching the sensory regions. Thus, activation of these fibers by gamma static efferents increases the steady-state discharge rate of both primary and secondary endings even in the absence of muscle stretch.

The Central Nervous System Can Control Sensitivity of the Muscle Spindles Through the Gamma Motor Neurons

The Fusimotor System Maintains Spindle Sensitivity During Muscle Contraction

The parallel arrangement of muscle spindles relative to extrafusal fibers raises an interesting problem. Because intrafusal fibers slacken when a muscle shortens, the spindle discharge should cease when the muscle shortens.

Were this to occur, however, the spindle would fail to transmit information about changes in length at the very time when that information is most critical—when the contracting muscle is shortening. How then does the central nervous system ensure that it will receive information on changes in muscle length during contraction? In the early 1950s Carlton Hunt and Stephen Kuffler found that the central nervous system activates gamma motor neurons during contraction to maintain the tension of the intrafusal fibers of the muscle spindle.

Hunt and Kuffler examined the activity of isolated spindle afferents and stimulated gamma efferents innervating the same muscle spindles as well as alpha motor neurons supplying the extrafusal fibers (Figure 37–8). To accomplish this task they dissected and identified single axons in the dorsal and ventral roots of anesthetized cats.

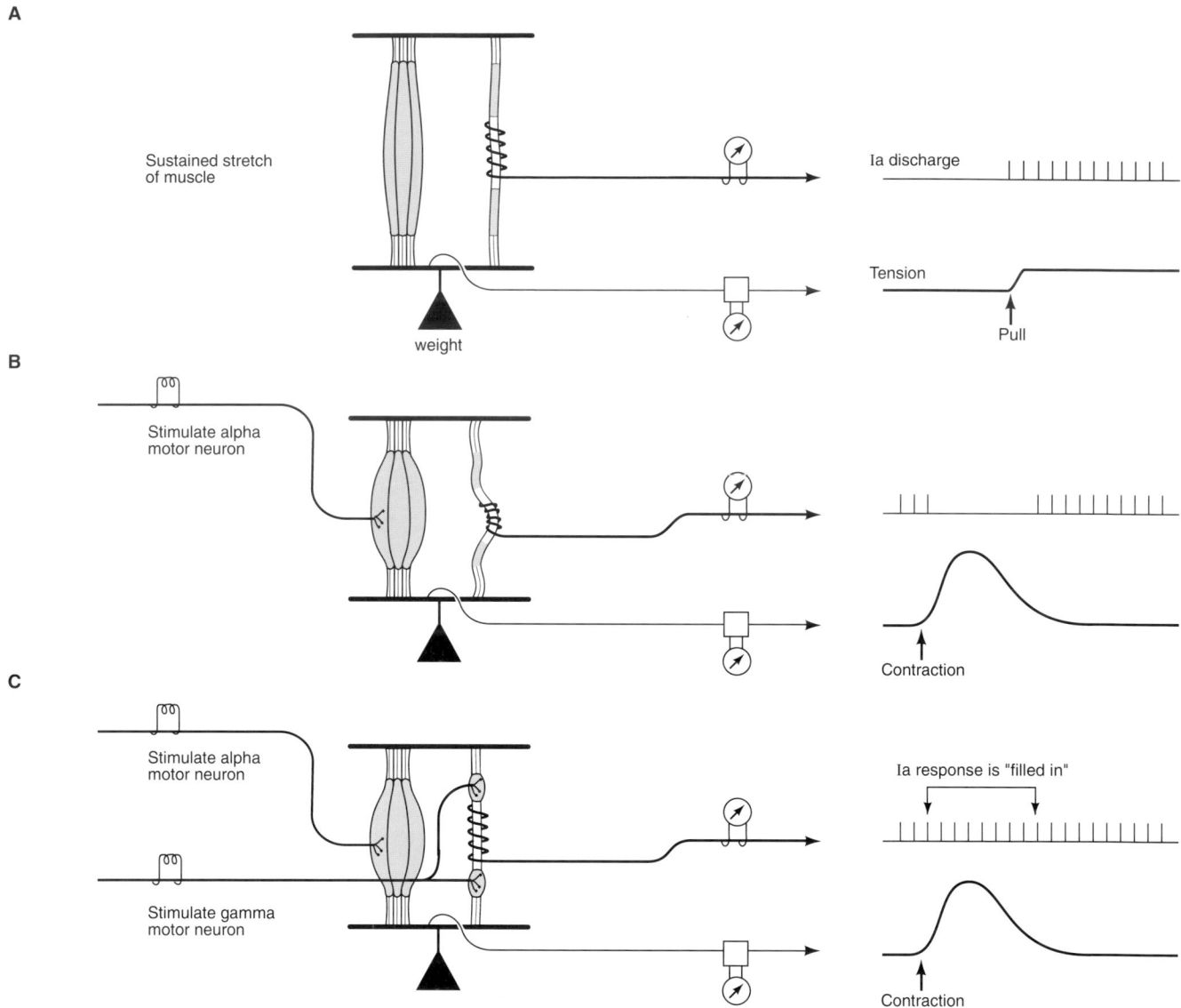

FIGURE 37–8

During active muscle contractions the ability of the spindles to sense length changes is maintained by activation of gamma motor neurons. (Adapted from Hunt and Kuffler, 1951.)

A. Sustained tension elicits steady firing of the Ia afferent.

B. A characteristic pause occurs in ongoing Ia discharge when the muscle is caused to contract by stimulation of its alpha motor neuron alone. The Ia fiber stops firing because the spindle is unloaded by the contraction.

C. If during a comparable contraction a gamma motor neuron to the spindle is also stimulated, the spindle is not unloaded during the contraction and the pause in Ia discharge is "filled in."

When they stimulated alpha motor neurons alone there was a pause in firing of the afferents during contraction, because the muscle shortened and therefore unloaded the spindle. When, however, a gamma motor neuron supplying the spindle was stimulated at the same time as the alpha motor neurons, the pause in afferent discharge did not occur. This is because the fusimotor system counteracts the slackening of the intrafusal fibers when the muscle shortens. In later experiments Ragnar Granit found that electrical stimulation of the motor cortex and other higher centers typically leads to simultaneous activation

of alpha and gamma motor neurons. He called this pattern *alpha–gamma coactivation.*

The experiments of Hunt and Kuffler and Granit were carried out with electrical stimulation in anesthetized animals. Testing of the hypothesis that alpha–gamma coactivation occurs during natural movements required techniques for recording from spindle afferents in unanesthetized animals and human subjects. In the late 1960s Åke Vallbo and Karl-Erik Hagbarth developed a technique known as microneurography to record from the larger afferent neurons in the peripheral nerves of awake human subjects. By this method the activity of spindle afferents can be directly measured during voluntary movement. However, since gamma motor neurons are too small to isolate and identify, activity in these neurons must be inferred from changes in the activity of the Ia afferents during voluntary contractions. The activity of alpha motor neurons can be estimated from recordings of electromyographic activity.

How can the patterns of activation of gamma motor neurons be inferred from recordings of the discharge of spindle afferents? Vallbo showed that in slow movements, Ia afferent fibers often increase their rate of discharge even when the muscle shortens as it contracts. The gamma motor neurons must therefore have been activated in synchrony with the alpha motor neurons. If there were no gamma activation, spindle discharge would decrease or pause during a shortening contraction, as Hunt and Kuffler demonstrated, because of slackening of the intrafusal fibers. Vallbo thus confirmed that during voluntary contraction alpha-gamma coactivation can maintain spindle firing.

Vallbo also explored how the maintenance of spindle sensitivity by alpha–gamma coactivation can be useful to the nervous system. He recorded the discharge rate of a Ia afferent from a finger flexor in a subject attempting to make a slow flexion movement at a constant velocity (Figure 37–9). The trajectory of the movement showed small deviations from a constant velocity—at times the muscle shortened quickly and at other times more slowly. The firing of the Ia afferent mirrored the irregularities in the trajectory. When the velocity of flexion increased transiently, Ia discharge decreased in rate because the muscle was shortening more rapidly, thus exerting less tension on the intrafusal fibers. When the velocity decreased, Ia discharge increased because the muscle was shortening more slowly, and therefore relative tension on the intrafusal fibers increased.

Thus, in this movement the Ia afferent's discharge rate is very sensitive to variations in the *rate of change* of muscle length. These findings illustrate the functional importance of a property of the primary spindle endings that we discussed earlier: Primary endings are most sensitive to very small changes in length. This information can be used by the nervous system to compensate for the irregularities in the movement trajectory. Since the muscle is shortening throughout the movement, the sensitivity of the Ia discharge to small changes in velocity clearly depends upon alpha-gamma coactivation. If the gamma motor neurons supplying the intrafusal fibers of this spindle were not firing, the afferent discharge would steadily decrease as the muscle shortens, and it would eventually stop.

Fusimotor Output Can Be Adjusted Independently of Motor Output

As we have noted, in lower vertebrates collaterals from alpha motor neurons are the only axons innervating intrafusal fibers and provide the equivalent of alpha–gamma

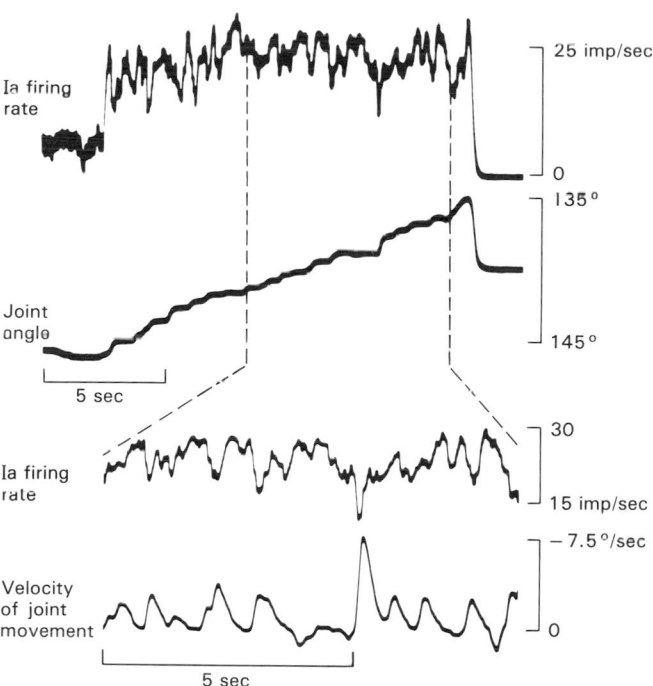

FIGURE 37–9

Gamma motor neurons are coactivated during voluntary movements. Recordings from a spindle afferent during a slow flexion of a finger show that the spindle's firing mirrors irregularities in the movement velocity, shown below. These changes in spindle firing can be used by the nervous system to compensate for the irregularities and thus smooth the movement. The ability of the spindle to signal these irregularities depends on alpha-gamma coactivation. If the gamma motor neurons were not active the spindle would slacken as the muscle shortened. (Adapted from Vallbo, 1981.)

coactivation. When these neurons are activated, unloading of the spindle by contraction of extrafusal fibers is at least partially compensated by contraction of intrafusal fibers. In mammals the gamma motor neurons have evolved as an *independent* system, thus uncoupling the control of muscle spindles from the control of the muscles. As we will now see, this provides greater flexibility in the control of spindle output in different functional contexts.

Under what circumstances does the nervous system modulate the contraction of intrafusal fibers independently of extrafusal fibers? Arthur Prochazka and Manuel Hulliger have found that, in natural movements of cats, there is more to gamma control than an invariant linkage of alpha and gamma activation. Rather, the amount and type of gamma activation (static or dynamic) is preset at a fairly steady level, which varies according to the specific task or context. Prochazka and Hulliger refer to this type of control as *fusimotor set*. In general, both static and dynamic gamma motor neurons are set at higher levels as the speed and difficulty of the movement increase (Figure 37–10). Unpredictable conditions, as when a cat is picked

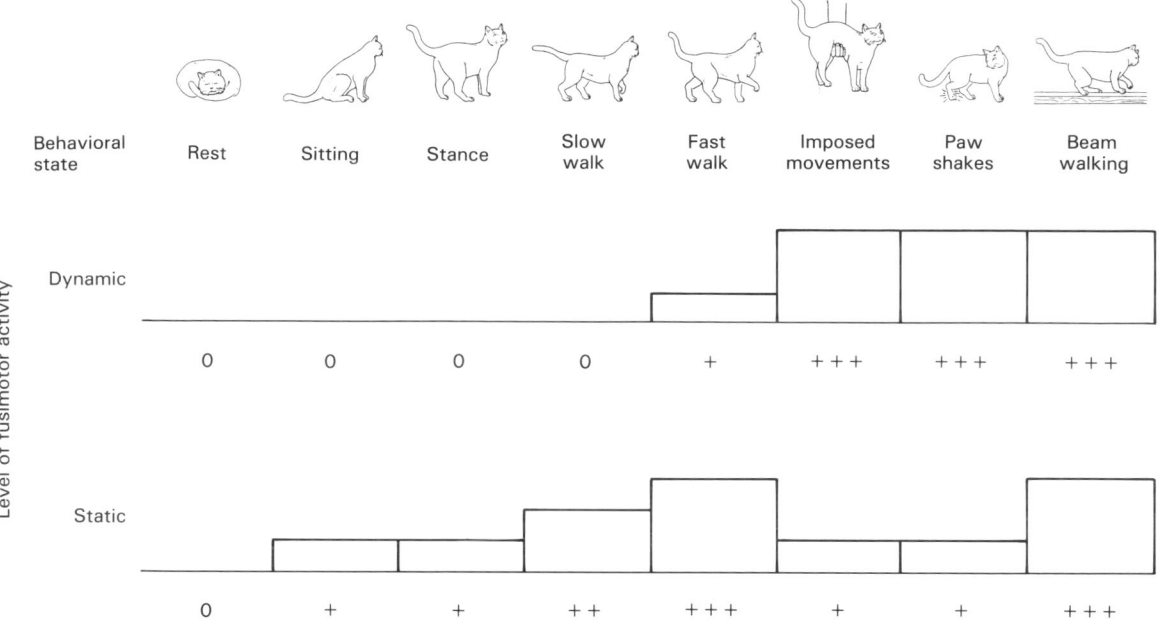

Behavioral state	Rest	Sitting	Stance	Slow walk	Fast walk	Imposed movements	Paw shakes	Beam walking
Dynamic	0	0	0	0	+	+++	+++	+++
Static	0	+	+	++	+++	+	+	+++

FIGURE 37–10

Fusiform (gamma) activity is set at different levels for different types of behavior. During activities in which muscle length changes slowly and in a predictable fashion, only static gamma neurons are active. Dynamic gamma neurons are activated during behaviors in which muscle length may change rapidly and unpredictably. (Adapted from Prochazka et al., 1988.)

up or handled, lead to marked increases in dynamic gamma activity reflected in greatly increased spindle responsiveness. When the animal is performing a difficult task, such as walking across a narrow beam, high levels of both static and dynamic gamma activation are present. Thus, by adjusting the balance between activation of static and dynamic gamma motor neurons, the nervous system uses the fusimotor system to fine-tune the spindles, so that the ensemble output of the muscle spindles provides information most appropriate for the specific task.

Discharge of Muscle Spindle Afferents Produces Stretch Reflexes

So far we have considered the muscle spindles and tendon organs as sensory receptors—as transducers of changes in muscle length and tension. How is this information used by the nervous system to regulate motor output? As we saw in Chapter 20, afferent axons from muscle spindles, tendon organs, and other somatosensory receptors ascend to the brain stem and cerebral cortex through various pathways and relay nuclei. These pathways convey information about the muscles to centers of the brain that participate in planning and controlling motor behavior. In addition muscle spindles and tendon organs also influence motor neurons directly through spinal reflex circuits.

Perhaps the most important, certainly the most stud-

ied, spinal reflex is the stretch reflex. Stretch reflexes are contractions of muscle that occur when the muscle is lengthened. They were once thought to result from intrinsic properties of muscles themselves. But at the turn of the century Charles Sherrington discovered that stretch reflexes could be abolished by cutting either the dorsal or the ventral roots, thereby establishing that these reflexes require both sensory input from the muscle to the spinal cord and a return path to the muscles. The receptor that senses the change of length is the muscle spindle. The afferent axons from this receptor make direct excitatory connections to motor neurons.

The Stretch Reflex Has Phasic and Tonic Components

To study the central circuits that mediate spinal reflexes in their simplest form, Sherrington transected the brain stem at the level of the midbrain, between the superior and inferior colliculi. In this *decerebrate preparation* the cerebrum is disconnected from the spinal cord, blocking sensations of pain as well as normal modulation of reflexes by higher brain centers. Many spinal reflexes are heightened and more stereotyped, making it easier to examine the factors controlling their expression. Decerebrate animals also show a dramatic increase in extensor muscle tone, sometimes sufficient to support the animal in the standing position.

When Sherrington attempted to flex passively the rigidly extended hindlimb of a decerebrate cat, he encountered increased contraction of the muscles being stretched. He called this the *stretch* or *myotatic reflex* and found that it has two components: (1) a brisk but short-lasting *phasic* contraction, which is triggered by the dynamic change in muscle length; and (2) a weaker but longer-lasting *tonic* contraction, determined by the static stretching of the muscles at the new longer length. He also discovered that stretching a muscle caused the antagonist muscles to relax. Sherrington concluded that stretch caused excitation of some motor neurons in the spinal cord and inhibition of others. He referred to this dual action as *reciprocal innervation.*

Stretch reflexes are weaker and considerably more variable in intact animals than in decerebrate animals. In decerebrate animals brain stem pathways powerfully facilitate the reflex circuits involved in stretch reflexes. In contrast, in intact animals there is a balance between facilitation and inhibition of reflex circuits; descending pathways from the cerebral cortex and other higher centers of the brain continuously modulate the strength of stretch reflexes according to changing tasks.

The tonic component of stretch reflexes is not apparent in intact animals unless the stretched muscle is already contracting. This is because the steady-state discharge of muscle spindles is not strong enough to raise the resting potential of motor neurons above threshold for firing, even when the muscle is stretched to its longest possible length. When the motor neurons are already firing, however, even small increases in length modulate the firing rate of motor neurons and thus increase the strength of the contraction. In decerebrate animals extensor muscles fire tonically and thus, as Sherrington found, the tonic component of the stretch reflex is readily elicited in these muscles and, along with the phasic component, is greatly exaggerated.

Group Ia Afferents Make Monosynaptic Connections to Motor Neurons

After Sherrington's analysis of the effects of muscle stretch, other investigators began to analyze the neural circuits responsible for the stretch reflex. In the 1940s David Lloyd measured the latency of the stretch reflex to determine how many different synapses intervene between the spindle afferent and motor neuron. Because a nerve fiber's threshold to electrical stimulation is inversely proportional to the diameter of its axon, Lloyd was able to activate selectively Ia afferent axons from muscle spindles, the largest of the sensory axons, with weak electrical stimuli. He stimulated the Ia afferent fibers in the dorsal roots and recorded a large potential in the ventral root after a latency of less than 1 ms. Birdsey Renshaw, working in the laboratory next door to Lloyd, had just discovered that the delay introduced by a single synapse is between 0.5 and 0.9 ms. With this information Lloyd concluded correctly that the stretch reflex is produced by a

two-neuron circuit consisting of a single synaptic connection between the Ia afferent and the alpha motor neurons. Lloyd then demonstrated that the Ia afferent from a muscle excites not only the motor neurons innervating the same (homonymous) muscle, but also those innervating synergist muscles. Synergist muscles are those that control the same joint and have a similar mechanical action. At the ankle joint, for example, the soleus muscle is a synergist of the gastrocnemius.

The monosynaptic connection between motor neurons and Ia afferents was confirmed in the 1950s by Eccles through intracellular recordings from motor neurons. In addition, Eccles discovered that the discharge of Ia afferent fibers produces inhibitory synaptic potentials in motor neurons innervating the antagonist muscles. Eccles determined that a single spinal interneuron was interposed in this pathway. This set of connections accounts for the reciprocal innervation described by Sherrington.

How extensive are the connections between a single Ia afferent fiber and motor neurons? Using computerized averaging techniques (see Box 36–2), Lorne Mendell and Elwood Henneman found that each Ia afferent in the medial gastrocnemius motor neurons of the cat makes excitatory connections with *all* motor neurons innervating the homonymous muscle. They also found that Ia axons provide excitatory inputs to many of the motor neurons supplying synergists (up to 60% for some synergists).

The structure of the spinal circuit responsible for stretch reflexes that has emerged from these studies is illustrated in Figure 37–11A. Group Ia afferent fibers enter the spinal cord through the dorsal roots. Within the dorsal horn they separate into numerous branches. Some branches make direct excitatory connections with motor neurons that innervate the same muscle, some with motor neurons innervating synergists. Still other branches make excitatory connections with interneurons that inhibit antagonist motor neurons.

How does this spinal circuitry produce the stretch reflex? A simple stretch reflex in flexor muscles is illustrated in Figure 37–11B and C. A brisk passive extension of the limb lengthens the flexor muscles, causing an increase in the discharge rate of Ia fibers arising from these muscles. The discharge of the Ia afferents excites motor neurons to both homonymous and synergist muscles, causing a contraction that opposes the lengthening. Because the discharge of the Ia afferent also inhibits antagonist motor neurons, the antagonist muscles tend to relax, an action that indirectly assists the reflex resistance to the stretch.

It is usually necessary to stretch the muscle briskly to elicit an observable reflex because the primary endings in muscle spindle receptors are most sensitive to the dynamic phase of a change in length. A sharp tap on a tendon, for example, produces a brief stretch of most or all of the spindles in a muscle. The ensuing volley of action potentials from many Ia afferents reaches the homonymous and synergist motor neurons at the same time, and the result is a powerful temporal summation of excitatory

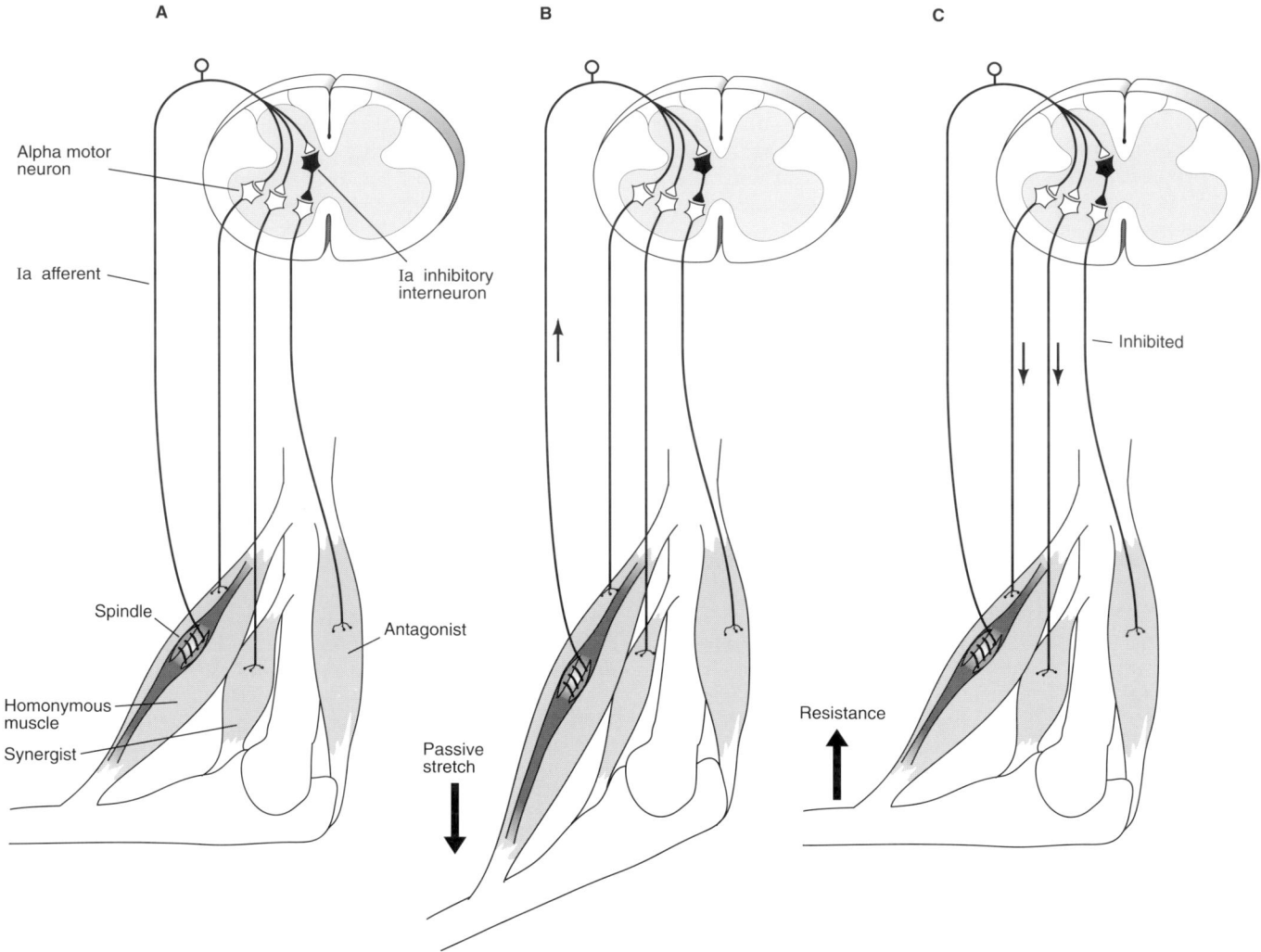

FIGURE 37-11

Excitation of muscle spindles is responsible for the stretch reflex.

A. Ia afferent fibers make monosynaptic excitatory connections to alpha motor neurons innervating the same (homonymous) muscle from which they arise and motor neurons innervating synergist muscles. They also inhibit motor neurons to antagonist muscles through an inhibitory interneuron.

B. When a muscle is stretched the Ia afferents increase their firing rate.

C. This leads to contraction of the same muscle and its synergists and relaxation of the antagonist. The reflex therefore tends to counteract the stretch, enhancing the spring-like properties of the muscles.

potentials in the motor neurons. This leads to a brisk phasic contraction in the stretched muscles, sometimes called a tendon jerk.

Because of the relative simplicity of the neural circuits responsible for the stretch reflex, testing the strength of tendon jerks is useful in clinical diagnosis. Absent or weak (hypoactive) tendon jerks often indicate a disorder of one or more components of the reflex circuit: sensory or motor axons, the cell bodies of motor neurons, or the muscle itself. Hypoactive stretch reflexes can also result from lesions of the central nervous system, because the excitability of motor neurons is dependent on both excitatory and inhibitory descending influences. Hyperactive stretch reflexes result from central lesions that lead to a net increase in the excitatory input to motor neurons. They are often associated with disorders of tone, such as spasticity and rigidity. These will be discussed in more detail later in this chapter and in Chapter 39.

The Main Connections of Group II and Group Ib Afferents to Motor Neurons Are Polysynaptic

Although group II spindle afferents have monosynaptic excitatory connections with homonymous motor neurons, this connection is relatively weak. The main connections of group II afferents to motor neurons are polysynaptic, involving several classes of interneurons. Because the group II endings in the spindles are most sensitive to steady-state length, these connections with motor neurons primarily affect the tonic component of the stretch reflex.

Group Ib afferents from Golgi tendon organs also make polysynaptic connections to motor neurons. Stimulation of tendon organ afferents inhibits homonymous motor neurons and excites antagonist motor neurons. However, because interneurons mediate these effects, the function of these connections is complex. These circuits will be discussed in the next chapter.

Stretch Reflexes Contribute to Muscle Tone

The term muscle tone refers to the force with which a muscle resists being lengthened, that is, its stiffness. It is assessed clinically by passively extending and flexing the patient's limbs and feeling the resistance offered by the muscles. As we saw in the previous chapter, one component of muscle tone derives from the intrinsic elasticity of the muscles themselves. Muscles have elastic elements which resist lengthening. A muscle behaves like a spring. In addition to this intrinsic stiffness, however, there is a neural component of muscle tone. As we have seen, the stretch reflex also acts to resist lengthening of the muscle. Thus, stretch reflexes enhance the spring-like quality of muscles.

Normal muscle tone serves several important functions. First, the tone of muscles assists in maintaining posture. For example, as we sway back and forth while standing, the muscles resist being stretched, preventing the amount of sway from becoming too large. Second, muscles, like springs, can store energy and release it later. This is particularly important in walking and running. As weight is accepted on a limb, the muscles stretch and store mechanical energy. When the leg pushes off, some of this energy is released and assists the active contraction of muscles; less active contraction of muscles is required to propel the leg forward. Thus, the elasticity of muscles makes locomotion more efficient. Finally, the spring-like qualities of muscles help to smooth movements. If muscles acted simply like the motors that control a robot's limbs, movements would be jerky, with sudden starts and stops. The elasticity of muscle smooths out these jerks, because like a spring the muscle achieves an equilibrium length more gradually.

Stretch Reflexes Regulate Muscle Tone Through Negative Feedback

To understand how the stretch reflex contributes to tone, it is useful to view the reflex circuit as a negative feedback loop in which the regulated variable is muscle length (Figure 37–12). A negative feedback system counteracts deviations of the regulated variable from a desired value (see Chapter 35). The desired value of muscle length is determined by the sum of the descending excitatory and inhibitory influences on the motor neuron. Deviations from the desired muscle length are sensed by the muscle spindles and "fed back" to the motor neurons. The motor neurons in turn signal the level of force needed by the muscle to change its length to the desired value. If an external disturbance, such as an increase in load, lengthens the muscle, the discharge rate of the spindle afferents increases. This causes the muscle to contract, counteracting the stretch produced by the load. If the external load is decreased and the muscle shortens, spindle firing decreases, leading to less muscle force and a consequent lengthening of the muscle to its desired length. Thus, the stretch reflex loop acts continuously to keep muscle length close to a set value.

Two crucial determinants of the behavior of a feedback system are its *gain* and its *loop delay*. The *gain* of a feedback system refers to its strength or effectiveness. The larger the gain of the stretch reflex, the greater will be the muscle force that results from an imposed change in length. The gain of the stretch reflex can be modulated by the central nervous system in three ways: (1) by adjusting the level of fusimotor activity, (2) by presynaptic modulation (Chapter 13) that modulates the effectiveness of synaptic inputs to the motor neurons, and (3) by direct synaptic inputs to the alpha motor neurons. Thus, the spinal circuits responsible for the stretch reflex provide the central nervous system with a mechanism for adjusting muscle tone, according to the behavioral task. For example, when maintaining a standing position in a moving bus, the gain of stretch reflexes can be increased to compensate for the large disturbances. Similarly, during walking or running the gain of stretch reflexes in extensor muscles is increased during the periods when weight is being accepted on a limb.

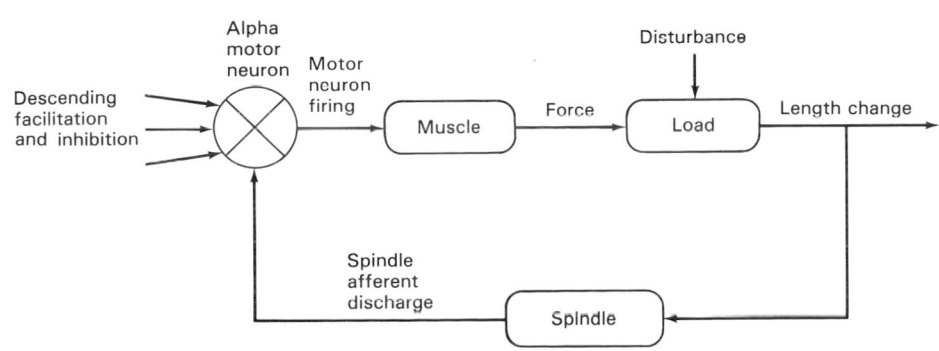

FIGURE 37–12
The stretch reflex acts like a negative feedback loop. The controlled variable is muscle length. The desired value is determined by descending signals to the motor neuron. If a disturbance causes muscle length to increase, the spindle increases its firing rate, causing the motor neuron to fire and the muscle to shorten. Decreases in muscle length produce the opposite effect. This system therefore corrects for deviations from the desired muscle length.

The *loop delay* in a feedback system is the time between a disturbance and the compensatory response. For the stretch reflex, the total loop delay is the sum of the sensory and motor conduction times, synaptic delays, and the time required for excitation-contraction coupling. The slow mechanical response of the muscle adds significant delay to the compensation for a disturbance. Such delays are obviously undesirable if a disturbance is to be counteracted rapidly. Muscle spindles, by virtue of their velocity sensitivity, enhance the responsiveness of the feedback system by contributing a measure of the rate of change of the disturbance to the feedback. This makes the feedback signal larger and more effective when the regulated variable changes rapidly.

The gain of stretch reflexes is normally kept quite low, except for transient increases. When feedback gain is high and a delay is present in the loop, a disturbance may lead to oscillations of the regulated variable. Oscillations occur because with high gain a disturbance will produce large corrections which, because of the delay, are not terminated early enough and thus overshoot the desired value of the regulated variable. Subsequent corrections, also delayed and therefore excessive, then swing back and forth around the desired value. Certain lesions of the central nervous system that interrupt descending motor pathways lead to abnormally high gain of stretch reflexes, resulting in an increase in muscle stiffness, or *hypertonus*. The most common form of hypertonus is *spasticity*, a condition in which muscles show abnormally high resistance to rapid stretch (Chapter 39). Spasticity is often associated with *clonus*, in which rapid oscillations of contraction and relaxation occur in response to stretch. For example, clonus of ankle extensors in spastic patients is elicited by an abrupt and steadily applied dorsiflexion of the foot by the examiner. This leads to a series of rhythmic contractions of the ankle extensors at about 4 Hz, which may continue as long as the foot is dorsiflexed.

Stretch Reflexes Allow Muscles to Respond Smoothly to Stretch and Release

A characteristic aspect of muscle tone is that the tension produced by the muscle increases approximately in proportion to the amount of stretch. Moreover, when muscle is released from a stretch the tension decreases progressively to its resting level. This symmetrical response is present whether the muscle is stretched slowly or abruptly. It derives from a combination of the mechanical properties of muscle and the neural component provided by the stretch reflex. In slowly imposed stretches this spring-like behavior occurs because of the intrinsic length–tension properties of muscle. In rapid stretches, however, the intrinsic mechanical response is an initial increase in tension followed by a transient collapse even as the muscle continues to be stretched. As we saw in the last chapter, this yielding occurs because of rupture of the myosin cross bridges (see Figure 36–6).

Recent studies by T. Richard Nichols and James Houk have shown that the stretch reflex compensates for this irregularity and also assures the consistent and symmetrical response of muscles to rapid stretch and release. Nichols and Houk measured the tensions produced by controlled stretches and releases of the soleus muscle in decerebrate cats before and after cutting the dorsal roots (Figure 37–13A). With the dorsal roots sectioned, which eliminates the stretch reflex, the mechanical response to rapid stretch showed the expected initial stiffness and transient yield. Moreover, at the end of the stretch, even though the muscle was maintained at a longer length, the tension transiently dropped again and the steady-state tension was only slightly higher than before the stretch was imposed. Releasing the muscle by the same amount produced a drop in tension that was much greater than the corresponding increase during stretch. This shows that the intrinsic mechanical response of the muscle to rapid stretch and release is markedly asymmetric. In contrast, when the dorsal roots were intact and thus the stretch reflex was allowed to function, Nichols and Houk found that the responses of the muscle to stretch and release were smoother and much more symmetric. The muscle did not yield during stretch and the tension continued to build up while stretch continued. Although there was still a small drop in tension at the onset of the steady stretch, the steady tension produced during the maintained stretch was much larger than when the stretch reflex was blocked by dorsal root section.

In later studies, Houk, Patrick Crago, and W. Zev Rymer showed that the high sensitivity of the muscle spindles to small changes in length is responsible for the reflex responses that rapidly counteracts the yield of the muscles shortly after the onset of stretch. Records of the patterns of discharge of muscle spindle primaries during these changes in length also showed that the asymmetry in the tension changes produced by stretch and release of the deafferented muscle are matched by a corresponding opposite asymmetry in the spindle discharge (Figure 37–13B). Thus, the transducer characteristics of the muscle spindle are well adapted, perhaps by evolutionary processes, to compensate for the apparent irregularities and asymmetries in muscle properties. Houk has suggested that this compensation simplifies the control of movement by the brain because the mechanical consequences of external disturbances and self-generated movements are more regular and therefore easier to predict.

An Overall View

The muscle spindle is a remarkable sensory organ whose elegant design and operation have intrigued physiologists for over a century. It contains specialized elements that sense muscle length and velocity of length change. In conjunction with the Golgi tendon organ, which senses muscle tension, it provides the central nervous system with continuous information about the mechanical state of the muscle. Innervation of the muscle spindle by an indepen-

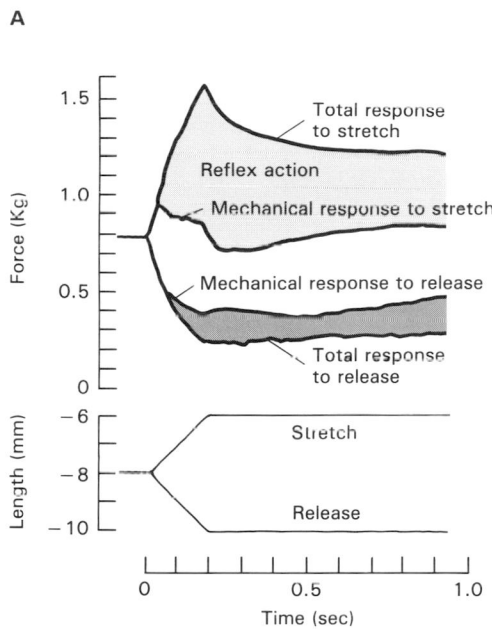

A

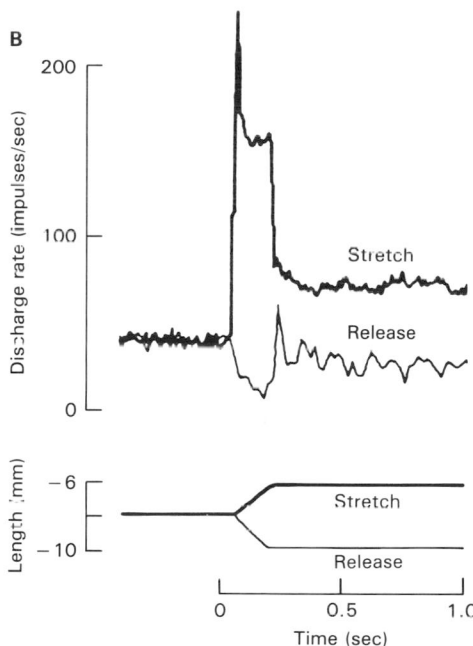

B

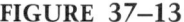

FIGURE 37–13

Reflex action compensates for the nonlinear properties of muscle. (Adapted from Houk and Rymer, 1981.)

A. The force produced by a rapid stretch and a release from stretch is shown under two conditions: when the stretch reflex is eliminated by deafferentation (mechanical response alone) and when the stretch reflex is intact. The purely mechanical response of a muscle to stretch is asymmetric and nonlinear. In particular, the muscle yields abruptly when it is stretched rapidly. When the

reflex is intact, the force responses are symmetric and yielding does not occur.

B. The asymmetry in mechanical response of the muscle is matched by an opposite asymmetry in the firing rate of the primary afferent of the muscle spindle. Thus, the stretch reflex makes the response to stretch and release more symmetric and consistent.

dent system of gamma motor neurons allows the central nervous system to adjust the sensitivity of the spindle and thus to fine tune the information it receives. In this sense the muscle spindle is like the eye, in which the motor innervation of the lens and extraocular muscles allows the nervous system to control how light impinges on the retina.

However, the finer control conferred by this motor innervation has a cost in the added complexity of perceptual processing by higher centers. Since the firing rate of muscle spindles depends on both muscle length and the level of gamma activation of the intrafusal fibers, the nervous system, in interpreting the signals from muscle spindles, must also monitor and take into account the fusimotor drive. This illustrates the close relationship between sensory and motor processing. In virtually all higher-order perceptual processes, sensory input must be correlated with motor output to get an accurate picture of external events.

The stretch reflex presents us with a model of sensory-motor integration. Although relatively simple, it embodies many of the principles that we shall see in more complex reflex pathways in the next chapter. The stretch reflex is the only known monosynaptic reflex in the mammalian nervous system. Because the participating afferent

and efferent axons have large diameters and are among the most rapidly conducting neurons in the nervous system, the stretch reflex pathway is adapted for speed of operation. The economy of the neural circuit for the stretch reflex allows muscle tone to be regulated quickly and efficiently without direct intervention by higher centers. Descending control signals adjust the gain of the reflex loops, adapting them to the requirements of specific motor acts.

Selected Readings

Boyd, I. A. 1980. The isolated mammalian muscle spindle. Trends Neurosci. 3:258–265.

Hasan, Z., and Stuart, D. G. 1984. Mammalian muscle receptors. In R. A. Davidoff (ed.), Handbook of the Spinal Cord. Vols. 2 & 3: Anatomy and Physiology. New York: Marcel Dekker, pp. 559–607.

Houk, J. C., and Rymer, W. Z. 1981. Neural control of muscle length and tension. In V. B. Brooks (ed.), Handbook of Physiology, Section 1: The Nervous System, Vol. II. Motor Control, Part 1. Bethesda, Md.: American Physiological Society, pp. 257–323.

Hulliger, M. 1984. The mammalian muscle spindle and its central control. Rev. Physiol. Biochem. Pharmacol. 101:1–110

Matthews, P. B. C. 1981. Evolving views on the internal operation and functional role of the muscle spindle. J. Physiol. (Lond.) 320:1–30.

Prochazka, A., and Hulliger, M. 1983. Muscle afferent function and its significance for motor control mechanisms during voluntary movements in cat, monkey, and man. In J. E. Desmedt (ed.), Motor Control Mechanisms in Health and Disease. Advances in Neurology, Vol. 39. New York: Raven Press, pp. 93–132.

References

Boyd, I. A., and Smith, R. S. 1984. The muscle spindle. In P. J. Dyck, P. K. Thomas, E. H. Lambert, and R. Bunge (eds.), Peripheral Neuropathy, Vol. 1. Philadelphia: Saunders, pp. 171–202.

Boyd, I. A., and Ward, J. 1975. Motor control of nuclear bag and nuclear chain intrafusal fibres in isolated living muscle spindles from the cat. J. Physiol. (Lond.) 244:83–112.

Brown, M. C., and Matthews, P. B. C. 1966. On the sub-division of the efferent fibres to muscle spindles into static and dynamic fusimotor fibres. In B. L. Andrew (ed.), Control and Innervation of Skeletal Muscle. Dundee: University of St. Andrews, pp. 18–31.

Cooper, S. 1961. The responses of the primary and secondary endings of muscle spindles with intact motor innervation during applied stretch. Q. J. Exp. Physiol. 46:389–398.

Crowe, A., and Matthews, P. B. C. 1964. The effects of stimulation of static and dynamic fusimotor fibres on the response to stretching of the primary endings of muscle spindles. J. Physiol. (Lond.) 174:109–131.

Eccles, J. C. 1964. The Physiology of Synapses. Berlin: Springer.

Eccles, J. C., Fatt, P., and Koketsu, K. 1954. Cholinergic and inhibitory synapses in a pathway from motor-axon collaterals to motoneurones. J. Physiol. (Lond.) 126:524–562.

Granit, R. 1970. The Basis of Motor Control. London: Academic Press.

Houk, J. C., Crago, P. E., and Rymer, W. Z. 1981. Function of the spindle dynamic response in stiffness regulation—a predictive mechanism provided by non-linear feedback. In A. Taylor and A. Prochazka (eds.), Muscle Receptors and Movement. London: Macmillan, pp. 299–309.

Houk, J. C., Crago, P. E., and Rymer, W. Z. 1980. Functional properties of the Golgi tendon organs. In J. E. Desmedt (ed.), Spinal and Supraspinal Mechanisms of Voluntary Motor Control and Locomotion, Vol. 8. Progress in Clinical Neurophysiology. Basel: Karger, pp. 33–43.

Houk, J., and Henneman, E. 1967. Responses of Golgi tendon organs to active contractions of the soleus muscle of the cat. J. Neurophysiol. 30:466–481.

Hunt, C. C., and Kuffler, S. W. 1951. Stretch receptor discharges during muscle contraction. J. Physiol. (Lond.) 113:298–315.

Leksell, L. 1945. The action potential and excitatory effects of the small ventral root fibres to skeletal muscle. Acta Physiol. Scand. 10 (Suppl. 31):1–84.

Liddell, E. G. T., and Sherrington, C. 1924. Reflexes in response to stretch (myotatic reflexes). Proc. R. Soc. Lond. [Biol.] 96:212–242.

Lloyd, D. P. C. 1943. Conduction and synaptic transmission of the reflex response to stretch in spinal cats. J. Neurophysiol. 6:317–326.

Loeb, G. E. 1984. The control and responses of mammalian muscle spindles during normally executed motor tasks. Exer. Sport Sci. Rev. 12:157–204.

Matthews, B. H. C. 1933. Nerve endings in mammalian muscle. J. Physiol. (Lond.) 78:1–53.

Matthews, P. B. C. 1964. Muscle spindles and their motor control. Physiol. Rev. 44:219–288.

Matthews, P. B. C. 1972. Mammalian Muscle Receptors and Their Central Actions. London: Arnold.

Mendell, L. M., and Henneman, E. 1971. Terminals of single Ia fibers: Location, density, and distribution within a pool of 300 homonymous motoneurons. J. Neurophysiol. 34:171–187.

Nichols, T. R., and Houk, J. C. 1976. Improvement in linearity and regulation of stiffness that results from actions of stretch reflex. J. Neurophysiol. 39:119–142.

Patton, H. D. 1965. Reflex regulation of movement and posture. In T. C. Ruch and H. D. Patton (eds.), Physiology and Biophysics, 19th ed. Philadelphia: Saunders, pp. 181–206.

Prochazka, A., Hulliger, M., Trend, P., and Dürmüller, N. 1988. Dynamic and static fusimotor set in various behavioural contexts. In P. Hník, T. Soukup, R. Vejsada, and J. Zelena (eds.), Mechanoreceptors: Development, Structure, and Function. New York: Plenum Press, pp. 417–430.

Prochazka, A., Hulliger, M., Zangger, P., and Appenteng, K. 1985. 'Fusimotor Set': New evidence for α-independent control of γ-motoneurones during movement in the awake cat. Brain Res. 339:136–140.

Prochazka, A., and Wand, P. 1981. Independence of fusimotor and skeletomotor systems during voluntary movement. In A. Taylor and A. Prochazka (eds.), Muscle Receptors and Movement. London: Macmillan, pp. 229–243.

Renshaw, B. 1940. Activity in the simplest spinal reflex pathways. J. Neurophysiol. 3:373–387.

Schmidt, R. F. 1983. Motor systems. In R. F. Schmidt and G. Thews (eds.), Human Physiology. M. A. Biederman-Thorson (trans.) Berlin: Springer, pp. 81–110.

Stein, R. B., and Capaday, C. 1988. The modulation of human reflexes during functional motor tasks. Trends Neurosci. 11:328–332.

Swett, J. E., and Schoultz, T. W. 1975. Mechanical transduction in the Golgi tendon organ: A hypothesis. Arch. Ital. Biol. 113:374–382.

Vallbo, Å. B. 1970. Discharge patterns in human muscle spindle afferents during isometric voluntary contractions. Acta Physiol. Scand. 80:552–566.

Vallbo, Å. B. 1981. Basic patterns of muscle spindle discharge in man. In A. Taylor and A. Prochazka (eds.), Muscle receptors and Movement. London: Macmillan, pp. 219–228, 263–275.

Vallbo, Å. B., Hagbarth, K.-E., Torebjörk, H. E., and Wallin, B. G. 1979. Somatosensory, proprioceptive, and sympathetic activity in human peripheral nerves. Physiol. Rev. 59:919–957.

James Gordon

38

Spinal Mechanisms of Motor Coordination

Interneurons Are the Building Blocks of Spinal Reflexes

Convergent and Divergent Connections Are the Basis of Reflex Pathways

Networks of Interneurons Coordinate the Timing of Reflex Components

Inhibitory Interneurons Coordinate Muscle Action Around a Joint

Group Ia Inhibitory Interneurons Coordinate Opposing Muscles

Renshaw Cells Are Part of a Negative Feedback Loop to Motor Neurons

Group Ib Inhibitory Interneurons Receive Convergent Input from Several Types of Receptors

Cutaneous Stimuli Elicit Complex Reflexes That Serve Protective and Postural Functions

Cutaneous Stimuli Modulate the Excitability of Specific Motor Neuron Pools

Flexion Reflex Pathways Coordinate Whole Limb Movements

Certain Reflexes Consist of Rhythmic Movements

Certain Reflexes Adapt to Different Body Postures

Spinal Circuits Generate Rhythmic Locomotor Patterns

Tonic Descending Signals from the Brain Stem Activate the Spinal Circuits Responsible for Locomotion

NMDA Receptors Are Involved in Generating the Locomotor Pattern

Goal-Directed Locomotion Requires Intact Supraspinal Systems

Afferent Information Modifies the Rhythmic Locomotor Pattern

An Overall View

Purposeful motor behavior requires the coordinated action of many muscles. Even a relatively simple act—reaching to pick up a glass of water—requires contraction of dozens of muscles to move the hand to the glass and to grasp it, and contraction of many muscles in the trunk and legs to maintain stability of the body. Motor coordination is the process of linking the contractions of many independent muscles so that they act together and can be controlled as a single unit.

Neural circuits in the spinal cord play an essential role in motor coordination. Spinal reflexes provide the nervous system with a set of elementary patterns of coordination that can be activated either by sensory stimuli or by descending signals from the brain stem and cerebral cortex. In the last chapter we examined the stretch reflex, which involves a relatively simple circuit in the spinal cord—primary afferent fibers from muscle spindles excite motor neurons to the same muscle through monosynaptic connections. Most spinal reflexes, however, have more complex circuits. First, although a few reflexes have primarily local actions on single muscles, most coordinate the actions of groups of muscles; the afferent inputs are distributed widely, sometimes spanning several joints. Second, most reflex pathways are polysynaptic—one or more *interneurons* are interposed between the sensory and motor neurons. This feature allows descending signals as well as other afferent inputs to modify the expression of the reflex.

In this chapter we shall first consider the different roles that interneurons play in reflex circuits. We shall then analyze the pathways responsible for two general types of spinal reflexes: those elicited by signals arising in muscle and those elicited by cutaneous stimuli. We shall see that reflex circuitry is hierarchical, with three main levels of control: (1) control of individual muscles, (2) coordination of muscle action around a joint, and (3) coordination of muscles at several joints. Finally, we shall consider the neural control of locomotion, a complex behavior in which spinal circuits play an important role.

Interneurons Are the Building Blocks of Spinal Reflexes

Reflex pathways consist of primary afferent neurons, motor neurons, and one or more interneurons. Spinal interneurons are neurons that are restricted to the spinal cord and influence other nearby neurons. They are distinct from primary afferent neurons that carry incoming sensory information from the periphery, from motor neurons (the final common pathway of motor output), and from neurons that project in the long tracts of the spinal cord. Interneurons form spinal networks that mediate between input and output elements and produce varied reflex behaviors. Here we shall consider the elementary types of connections between neurons in the spinal cord.

Convergent and Divergent Connections Are the Basis of Reflex Pathways

As we first learned in chapter 2, the most basic mechanisms of neural integration are divergence and conver-gence. *Divergence* refers to the distribution of the output of a single neuron to a number of target neurons by branching of the axon (Figure 38–1A). Virtually all spinal neurons, including afferent neurons, interneurons, and motor neurons, show some degree of divergence. For example, Ia afferent fibers from the muscle spindle branch extensively in the spinal cord, terminating on most homonymous motor neurons (that innervate the same muscle), many synergist motor neurons, and interneurons that inhibit antagonist motor neurons. Reflexes in which a focal stimulus leads to coordinated contractions of many muscles depend on the divergent connections of afferent neurons and interneurons to distribute excitation and inhibition to the appropriate motor neurons.

Convergence refers to the processing of input from several neurons onto one neuron. All motor neurons and interneurons receive convergent input and thus their activity at any given time reflects the summation of excitatory and inhibitory postsynaptic potentials from several sources (Figure 38–1B). The convergent inputs onto a single neuron may include sensory inputs from the periphery, descending signals from supraspinal regions, and signals from interneurons.

Convergence of descending signals onto interneurons that also receive input from peripheral receptors is an important mechanism by which higher centers can control the expression of reflex behavior. By exciting or inhibiting spinal interneurons, descending signals can enhance or suppress specific reflex actions. For example, when a slippery object is gripped with one's fingers, descending signals can enhance the excitatory and inhibitory effects of cutaneous signals from the finger tips on motor neurons innervating finger muscles to allow for quick reactions to slips. Moreover, some interneurons act as *gates* that control whether a peripheral input reaches motor neurons (Figure 38–1C). Gating allows higher centers to preselect which of several possible responses will follow a stimulus. This enables the organism to react more quickly to certain stimuli, since higher centers do not have to process the afferent information to decide on a response. Gating can also be achieved directly by descending fibers on the terminals of afferent fibers acting through presynaptic connections (Figure 38–1D).

Networks of Interneurons Coordinate the Timing of Reflex Components

Divergent and convergent connections in reflex pathways play an important role in the *spatial* organization of reflex behaviors, determining which sensory inputs are enhanced or suppressed and which muscles contract or relax. Other types of connections determine the *temporal* organization of reflexes. For example, *reverberating circuits*, closed circuits of interneurons that re-excite themselves, are responsible for some reflexes that outlast the stimulus (Figure 38–1E). More complex temporal patterns are produced by networks of interneurons called *central pattern generators*.

A hypothetical model of a central pattern generator that produces rhythmic alternation in opposing muscles

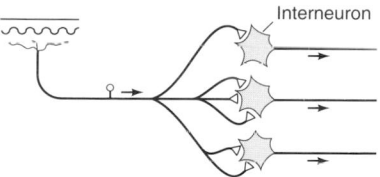

A Divergence

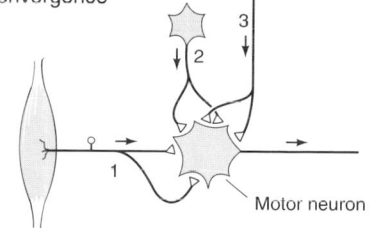

B Convergence

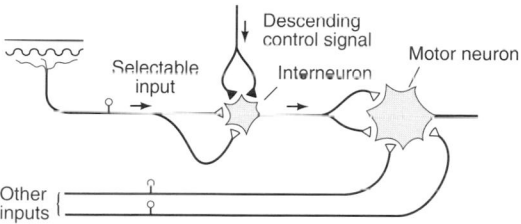

C Gating by interneurons

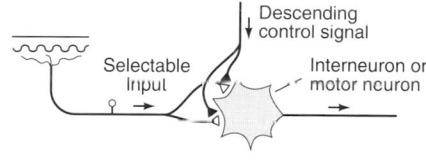

D Gating by presynaptic inhibition

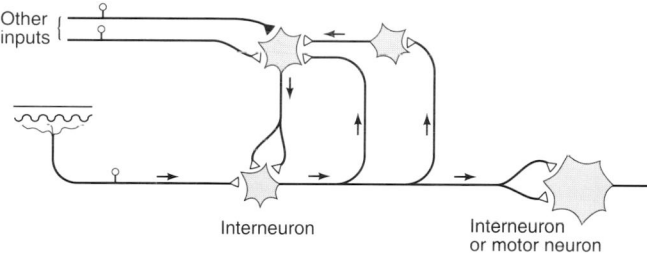

E Reverberating circuit

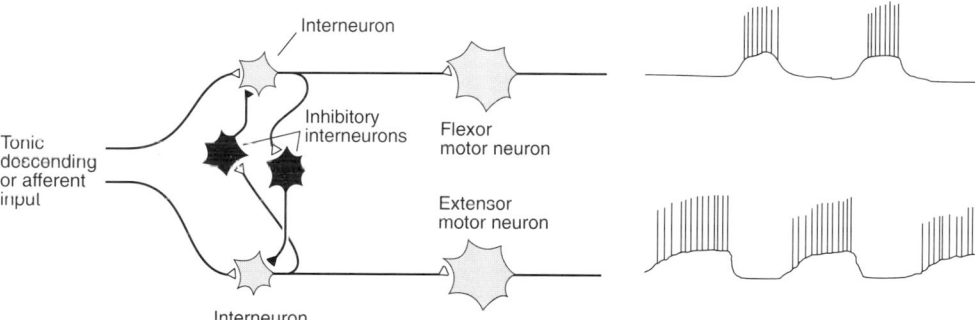

F Rhythmic alternating activity

FIGURE 38–1

Several types of interneuronal circuits act on motor neurons.

A. Divergence. Collaterals of a single neuron synapse on several target neurons.

B. Convergence. The activity of a single neuron, such as the motor neuron shown here, depends on the sum of inputs from afferent fibers (**1**), interneurons (**2**), and descending fibers from supraspinal regions (**3**).

C. Gating by interneurons. An inhibitory command can prevent peripheral input from discharging an interneuron that acts on a motor neuron.

D. Gating by presynaptic inhibition. A descending command can turn afferent input on or off by acting on presynaptic terminals of afferent fibers.

E. Reverberating circuits. Axon collaterals re-excite the same neuron through excitatory interneurons, thus prolonging a reflex response.

F. Half-center model of rhythmic alternating activity in the flexor and extensor motor neurons. Flexor and extensor motor neurons, together with their associated interneurons, each constitute a half-center. The two half-centers are assumed to mutually inhibit each other, so that when one is active, the other is inactive. Tonic input causes both interneurons to fire, but because of random fluctuations in excitability or other inputs, one half-center dominates and inhibits the other at any one time. For rhythmic activity to be generated, some mechanism is needed to switch the activity from one half-center to the other. One possible switching mechanism would be an intrinsic limit to the duration of inhibition by the active half-center, which would have the effect of lessening the inhibition of the other half-center, enabling it to become active. (Adapted from Pearson, 1976.)

in response to a tonic input is called the half-center model (Figure 38–1F). The simplest form of this model proposes that interneurons controlling flexor and extensor motor neurons have reciprocal inhibitory connections. The model assumes that the duration of reciprocal inhibition is limited by some intrinsic factor. Graham Brown, who proposed the half-center model, hypothesized that a limiting factor could be *fatigue* of the inhibitory synapses, which causes the strength of synaptic transmission to decline with time. Other possible intrinsic processes, now considered more plausible, are *adaptation*, in which a neuron responds to constant excitatory input with a declining rate of output, and *post-inhibitory rebound*, in which the threshold for excitation of a neuron decreases transiently as a result of past inhibition.

The tonic input to the network initiates firing in both interneurons, but fluctuations in excitability cause one of the interneurons to fire more strongly at first. Thus, if the interneurons to flexor motor neurons fire more strongly, they inhibit the firing of extensor muscles. However, the inhibition of extensor interneurons decreases with time, because of the intrinsic limit to the duration of inhibition. As a result, the extensor interneurons eventually become sufficiently depolarized to fire, and then they in turn inhibit the flexor motor neurons. As long as a tonic synaptic drive is present, this network of neurons will produce alternating flexion and extension.

Inhibitory Interneurons Coordinate Muscle Action Around a Joint

In the previous chapter we considered the monosynaptic connections of group Ia fibers with homonymous motor neurons that give rise to the stretch reflex. There we emphasized the functional role of the stretch reflex in controlling the tone of individual muscles. In addition, spindle afferents also make direct connections to motor neurons innervating synergist muscles and to interneurons that inhibit motor neurons innervating the antagonist muscles. These divergent connections of spindle afferents establish strong neural linkages between muscles acting around a joint, so that the muscles do not act independently of each other. Lloyd referred to this system of reflex pathways as the *myotatic unit*. Inputs from Golgi tendon organs and the secondary endings of muscle spindles also contribute to the myotatic unit through interneurons.

The myotatic unit coordinates the actions of individual synergist and antagonist muscles so that they act as a unit to regulate the mechanical properties of the joint. Most joints are not simple hinges, but rather allow movement in two or three planes. The muscles that surround these joints act in different combinations and with different relative forces depending on the particular direction of movement. When a stretch stimulus is applied to such a joint, the divergent connections of spindle afferents ensure that the appropriate combination of synergists will be activated and the appropriate combination of antagonist muscles

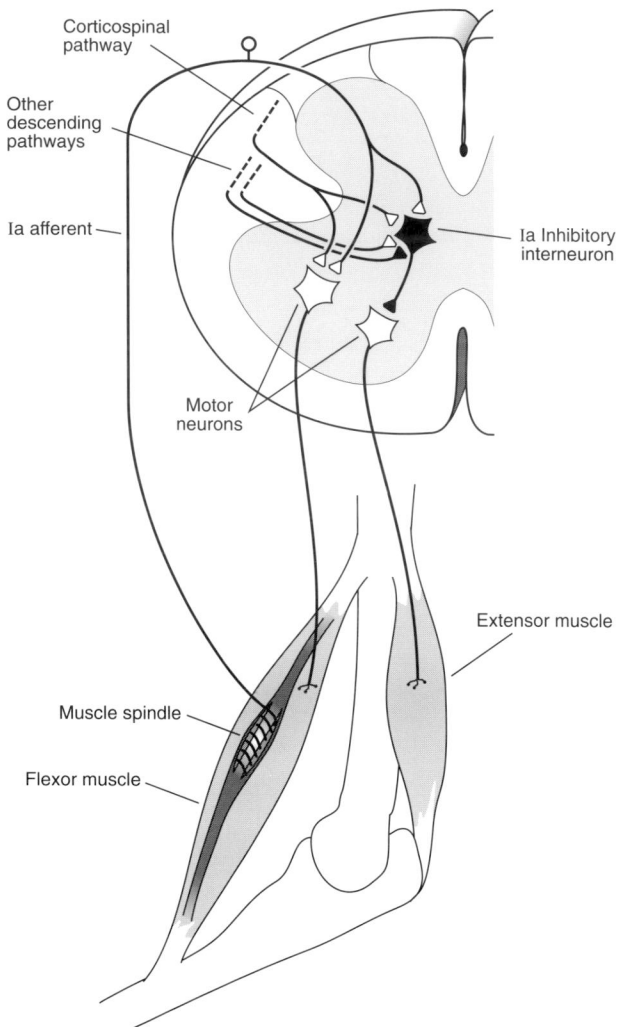

FIGURE 38–2

The Ia inhibitory interneuron allows higher centers to coordinate opposing muscles at a joint through a single command. This inhibitory interneuron mediates reciprocal innervation in stretch reflex circuits. In addition, it receives inputs from corticospinal descending axons, so that a descending signal to activate one set of muscles automatically leads to relaxation of the antagonists. Other descending pathways make excitatory and inhibitory connections to this interneuron. When the balance of inputs is shifted to greater inhibition, reciprocal inhibition will be decreased, and co-contraction of opposing muscles will occur. (Only a few of the many inputs to the Ia interneuron and motor neurons are shown in this highly simplified diagram.)

inhibited. Thus, the myotatic unit regulates the stiffness of the whole joint.

Different interneurons play specific roles in the coordination of reflex action around a joint. For instance, inhibitory interneurons play a special role in reflex pathways by reversing the sign of the reflex effect from excitatory to inhibitory. In this section we shall examine three types of inhibitory interneurons, each of which acts directly on motor neurons.

Group Ia Inhibitory Interneurons Coordinate Opposing Muscles

The most intensively studied of the inhibitory interneurons involved in reflex pathways is the Ia inhibitory interneuron. In the stretch reflex this interneuron mediates the reciprocal inhibition (through excitatory inputs from muscle spindle afferents) that coordinates the actions of opposing muscles; as one muscle contracts, the other relaxes (see Figure 37–11). This mode of coordination is useful not just in stretch reflexes but also in voluntary movements. Relaxation of the antagonist muscle during movement enhances speed and efficiency because the muscles that act as prime movers are not working against the contraction of opposing muscles. In addition to its role in the stretch reflex, the Ia inhibitory interneuron also allows higher centers to control opposing muscles at a joint in a reciprocal fashion. Elzbieta Jankowska has found that descending axons from the motor cortex, which make direct excitatory connections to spinal motor neurons, also send collaterals to Ia inhibitory interneurons. This *reciprocal innervation* means that higher centers do not have to send separate commands to the opposing muscles (Figure 38–2).

Reciprocal innervation of opposing muscles is not the only useful mode of coordination. Sometimes it is advantageous to contract the prime mover and the antagonist muscles simultaneously. This *co-contraction* has the effect of stiffening the joint and is most useful when precision and joint stabilization are critical (see Figure 36–16). The Ia inhibitory interneuron receives both excitatory and inhibitory signals from all of the major descending pathways (Figure 38–2). The pattern of connections to the Ia inhibitory interneuron allow the nervous system to shift from reciprocal coordination to co-contraction. By changing the balance of excitatory and inhibitory inputs onto this interneuron, supraspinal centers can control the relative amount of joint stiffness to meet the requirements of a motor act.

Renshaw Cells Are Part of a Negative Feedback Loop to Motor Neurons

A second class of inhibitory interneurons is the *Renshaw cell*, named by John Eccles for Birdsey Renshaw, who described it in 1941. Histological studies had shown that motor neurons send collaterals to small interneurons in the ventral horn. These interneurons make synaptic connections with several populations of motor neurons, including the motor neurons that send collaterals to the same interneurons (Figure 38–3). Renshaw found that motor neurons in the ventral horn became *less* excitable when their axons were stimulated electrically. Because electrical stimulation of axons produces action potentials that travel in both directions, he suggested that impulses traveling in the antidromic direction (opposite to the normal physiological direction) invaded the recurrent collaterals and caused the firing of a population of inhibitory interneurons. He therefore referred to the action of the interneurons on the presynaptic motor neurons as *recur-*

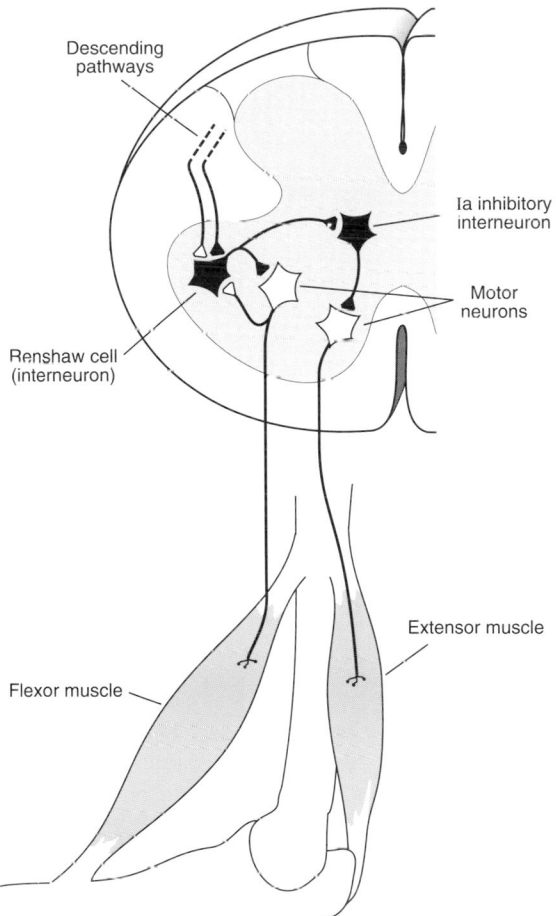

FIGURE 38–3
Renshaw cells produce recurrent inhibition of motor neurons. These spinal interneurons are excited by collaterals from motor neurons and then inhibit the same motor neurons. This negative feedback system regulates motor neuron excitability and stabilizes firing rates. Renshaw cells also send collaterals to synergist motor neurons (not shown) and to Ia inhibitory interneurons. Thus, descending inputs that modulate the excitability of the Renshaw cell adjust the excitability of all the motor neurons around a joint.

rent inhibition. Later, Eccles confirmed Renshaw's hypothesis by recording intracellularly from these interneurons.

The connections of Renshaw cells to presynaptic motor neurons form a negative feedback system, which regulates the firing rate of the motor neurons. If the firing rate of the motor neuron increases, recurrent inhibition of the motor neuron increases, thus limiting the change in firing rate. Decreases in motor neuron firing rate lead to less inhibition and thus increase the net excitability of the motor neuron. Recurrent inhibition thus stabilizes motor neuron firing rates by counteracting large transient changes.

Renshaw cells also make inhibitory connections with the Ia inhibitory interneurons that act on antagonist motor neurons (Figure 38–3). Thus, when they fire, they not only inhibit certain motor neurons, they also *disinhibit* antagonist motor neurons. Renshaw cells also inhibit motor neurons innervating synergist muscles. Therefore, the effect of recurrent inhibition on motor neuron excitability is distributed to muscles around a joint, in much the same way that stretch reflex effects are distributed to synergists and antagonists.

Renshaw cells receive significant synaptic input from descending pathways. By changing the excitability of these cells, higher centers can adjust the sensitivity of motor neurons to other descending inputs or to afferent inputs. Because Renshaw cells make divergent connections to motor neurons affecting the whole joint, the input from descending pathways modifies the excitability of the myotatic unit as a whole.

Group Ib Inhibitory Interneurons Receive Convergent Input from Several Types of Receptors

Golgi tendon organs, which are responsive to the tension in a muscle, influence homonymous motor neurons indirectly by way of a third type of inhibitory interneuron, the *Ib inhibitory interneuron* (Figure 38–4). Tendon organ input provides a negative feedback mechanism for regulating muscle tension, parallel to the negative feedback from muscle spindles that regulates muscle length. This system tends to counteract small changes in muscle tension by increasing or decreasing the inhibition to the motor neurons.

The influence of the Ib inhibitory interneuron on motor neuron excitability depends on the combined input from many sources, both central and peripheral. Anders Lundberg and his colleagues found that, in addition to input from tendon organs, the Ib inhibitory interneuron receives convergent input from Ia afferents from muscle spindles, low-threshold cutaneous afferents, and joint afferents, as well as both excitatory and inhibitory input from various descending pathways (Figure 38–4). These connections have important functional implications. For example, they provide a spinal mechanism for the fine control of exploratory movements, such as active touch. When the hand first contacts a physical object, muscle force will be strongly inhibited by combined activation of tendon organs and cutaneous afferents, allowing an immediate reduction in muscle force to soften the contact. Because descending pathways also modulate the Ib inhibitory interneuron, the strength of this inhibitory effect can be tuned up, as it is when the object is fragile, or tuned down, as when a more forceful push is desired.

Cutaneous Stimuli Elicit Complex Reflexes That Serve Protective and Postural Functions

Cutaneous Stimuli Modulate the Excitability of Specific Motor Neuron Pools

Tactile stimulation of many areas of skin causes reflex contraction of specific muscles, usually those underlying the area of stimulation. For example, stroking the abdomen (usually done from lateral to medial) causes reflex

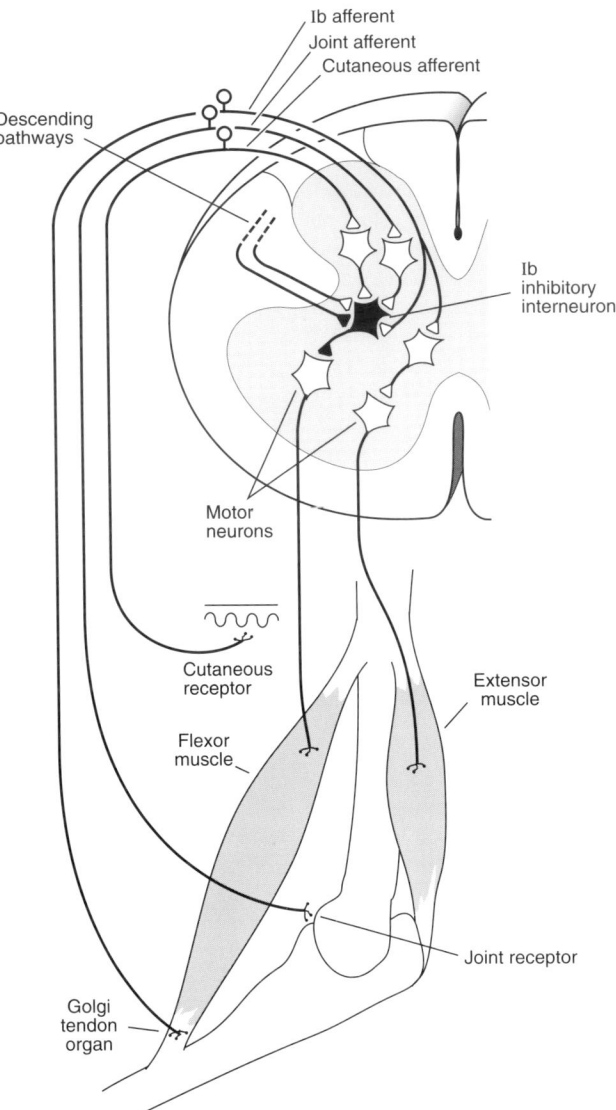

FIGURE 38–4

Ib afferent fibers from Golgi tendon organs provide a negative feedback system for regulating muscle tension. Ib afferents inhibit homonymous and synergist motor neurons (not shown) through the Ib inhibitory interneuron. They also excite antagonist motor neurons through an excitatory interneuron. Thus, the reflex effect of stimulating tendon organs is opposite to that of stimulating muscle spindles. The Ib inhibitory interneurons receive convergent input from joint and cutaneous receptors and from descending pathways, and thus mediate control of movements in which integration of different sensory modalities is important, as in touch.

contraction of abdominal muscles, often visible as a deviation of the umbilicus toward the side of stimulation. Stroking the upper abdomen causes contraction of upper abdominal muscles, whereas stimulation of the lower abdomen causes contraction of lower abdominal muscles. This fixed spatial relationship between the locus of the stimulus and the particular muscles that contract is called *local sign*.

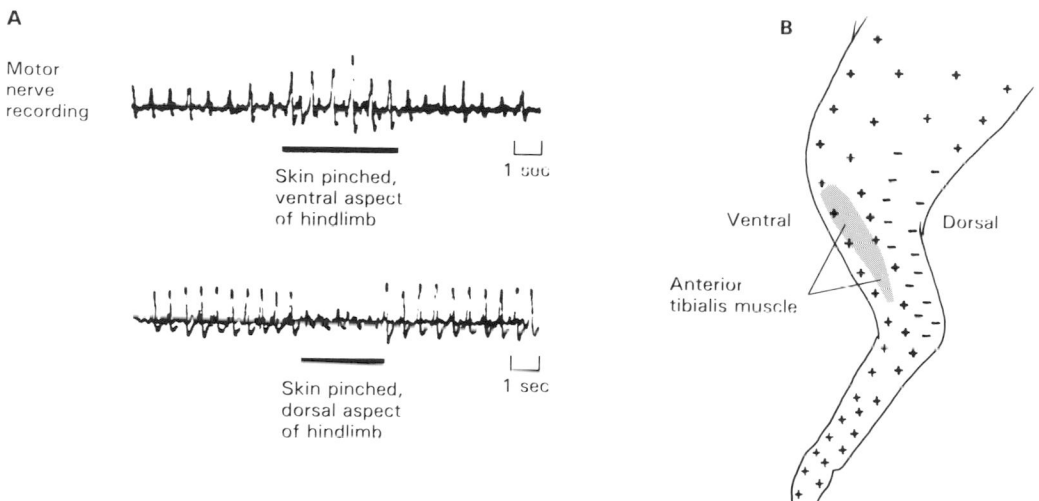

FIGURE 38-5

Cutaneous stimuli modify the excitability of specific motor neurons in a reciprocal fashion. (Adapted from Hagbarth, 1952.)

A. Tonic stimulation of Ia afferents from the tibialis anterior muscle in a spinal cat elicits a monosynaptic reflex contraction of the muscle. The strength of this contraction is then used experimentally to monitor the effects of cutaneous stimuli in different areas of skin on the excitability of the motor neurons. Pinching the skin over the muscle increases the strength of the

contraction, indicating that the motor neurons have been facilitated by the stimulus. Pinching the skin over the antagonist muscle diminishes muscle contraction, indicating that the motor neurons have been reciprocally inhibited.

B. Diagram of the cat hindlimb shows the excitatory (+) and inhibitory (−) stimulus areas of skin for the tibialis anterior muscle.

Although they may not always produce an observable response, cutaneous stimuli usually have subthreshold effects on motor neuron excitability. An example of such a cutaneous reflex effect was demonstrated by Karl-Erik Hagbarth in 1952. Using low-intensity electrical stimulation, Hagbarth selectively activated large spindle afferents of a motor nerve in cats, thereby producing a contraction of the muscle through the monosynaptic stretch reflex pathway. Mild pinching of wide areas of the skin overlying the contracting muscle increased the strength of the electrically evoked reflex contraction, while pinching the skin over the antagonist muscle inhibited it (Figure 38–5). Thus, the effects of cutaneous stimuli on motor neuron excitability are both spatially specific and reciprocal; they cause excitation of specific motor neurons and inhibition of motor neurons to the corresponding antagonist muscles.

The reflex effect of cutaneous stimulation often depends on the quality of the stimulus. For example, stroking the plantar surface of the foot in normal individuals (usually from heel to toe) leads to plantar flexion of the toes, and in some cases the whole foot. This is referred to as a *plantar reflex*. In contrast, light pressure on the plantar surface leads to a generalized extensor response in the whole leg, referred to as *extensor thrust*. This reflex is usually subliminal in normal individuals; it probably enhances support during standing and walking. In contrast, it is often exaggerated after certain neurological lesions and in some patients can interfere with standing and walking. Finally, a painful stimulus such as a pinch or pin prick applied to the same area produces *flexion withdrawal*

of the limb from the stimulus, caused by contraction of all flexor muscles of the limb.

Flexion Reflex Pathways Coordinate Whole Limb Movements

Flexion withdrawal from a noxious stimulus is a protective reflex involving coordinated muscle contractions at multiple joints through polysynaptic reflex pathways (Figure 38–6). Flexion reflexes, like stretch reflexes, involve reciprocal innervation: Flexor muscles of the stimulated limb are contracted at the same time the extensor muscles of the limb are inhibited. Along with flexion of the stimulated limb, the reflex produces an opposite effect in the contralateral limb: Extensor muscles are excited and flexor muscles are inhibited. This *crossed extension reflex* serves to enhance postural support during withdrawal from a painful stimulus. Thus, flexion withdrawal is a complete, albeit simple, motor act.

Although the flexion reflex is a relatively stereotyped response to a variety of painful stimuli, both the size and strength of muscle contraction reflect stimulus intensity. Touching a warm stove may produce moderately fast withdrawal only at the wrist and elbow, while touching a hot stove invariably leads to a forceful contraction at all joints and rapid withdrawal of the entire limb. Moreover, the contractions produced in a flexion reflex always outlast the stimulus, and duration of the reflex usually increases with stimulus intensity. Thus, like most reflexes, flexion reflexes are not simply stereotyped movement patterns, but are modulated in different ways according to the properties of the stimulus.

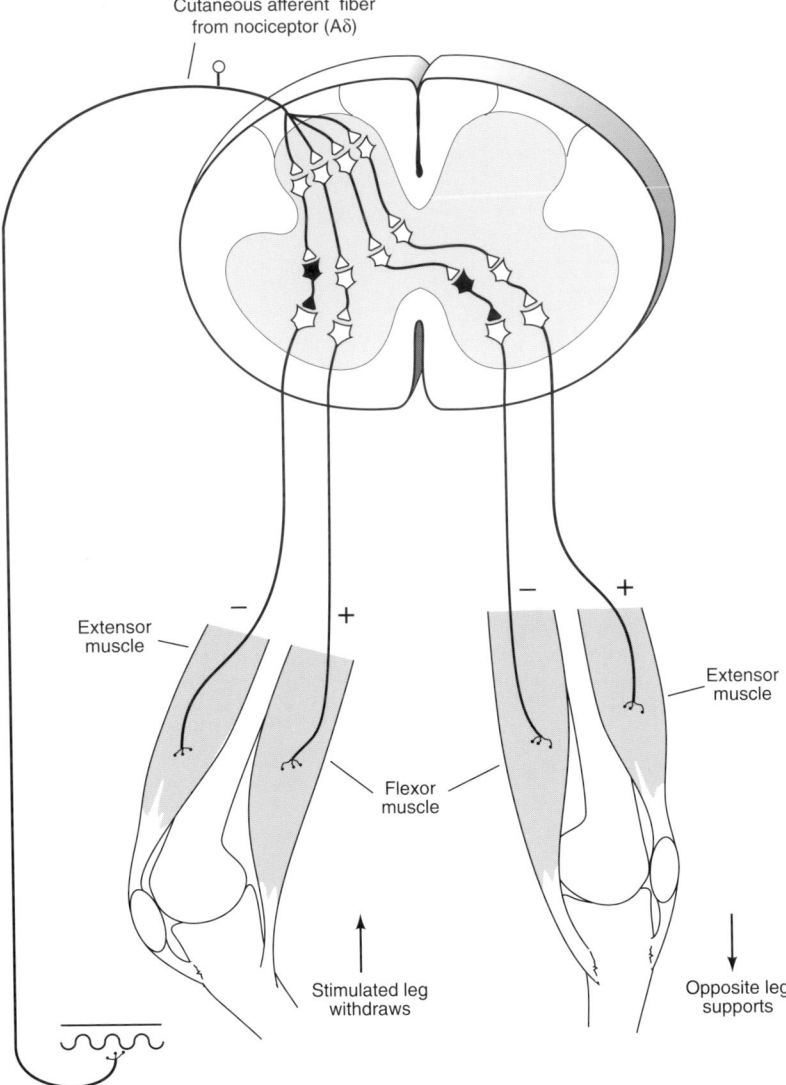

Cutaneous afferent fiber from nociceptor (Aδ)

Extensor muscle

Extensor muscle

Flexor muscle

Stimulated leg withdraws

Opposite leg supports

FIGURE 38–6

The flexion withdrawal reflex produces flexion of the stimulated limb and extension of the opposite limb. Stimulation of cutaneous afferents, such as an Aδ fiber from a nociceptor, produces excitation of ipsilateral flexor muscles and inhibition of ipsilateral extensor muscles, while producing the opposite response in the contralateral limb (the crossed extensor reflex). The cutaneous input is distributed over many spinal segments, so that the full reflex involves contraction of muscles at all joints of both limbs. The pathways are schematically illustrated here for one spinal segment only. (Adapted from Schmidt, 1983.)

The spinal circuits responsible for flexion withdrawal and crossed extension do more than mediate protective reflexes—they also serve to coordinate limb movements in voluntary movements. Lundberg and his colleagues have found that interneurons in these pathways receive convergent inputs from different types of afferent fibers, not just nociceptive ones, and from descending pathways. Thus, many receptors, in addition to having spatially specific actions on motor neurons (such as those illustrated in Figure 38–5), send collaterals to interneurons in the flexion reflex pathways. Under certain circumstances stimulation of these afferents can evoke a generalized flexion reflex. Such *flexor reflex afferents* include group II and group III afferents from skin, joints, and muscles, and the group II afferents from the secondary endings of muscle spindles.

Why should there be so much multisensory convergence onto the same interneurons? This convergence would seem to mix together inputs from many different sources, resulting in the loss of specificity of sensory processing. However, if these same interneurons mediate de-

scending commands for voluntary movements, as Lundberg has proposed, this convergence makes sense. Most active movements lead to excitation not just of muscle receptors but also of cutaneous and joint receptors. This proprioceptive and cutaneous input therefore facilitates and reinforces the spinal circuits that activate the movement. This provides the nervous system with a local spinal mechanism for regulating the movement—its strength and duration will depend in part on the direct inputs of somatosensory receptors.

Flexor reflex afferent, despite its name, does not always lead to excitation of ipsilateral flexor motor neurons and contralateral extensors. Under certain conditions the opposite effect can be evoked. Thus, distinct flexor reflex afferent pathways mediate different movement patterns within a limb, generally classified as either flexion or extension patterns. The different flexor reflex afferent pathways appear to be mutually inhibitory—when one pathway is active, others are inhibited. The mutual inhibition between flexor reflex afferent pathways is reminiscent of the half-center hypothesis discussed earlier.

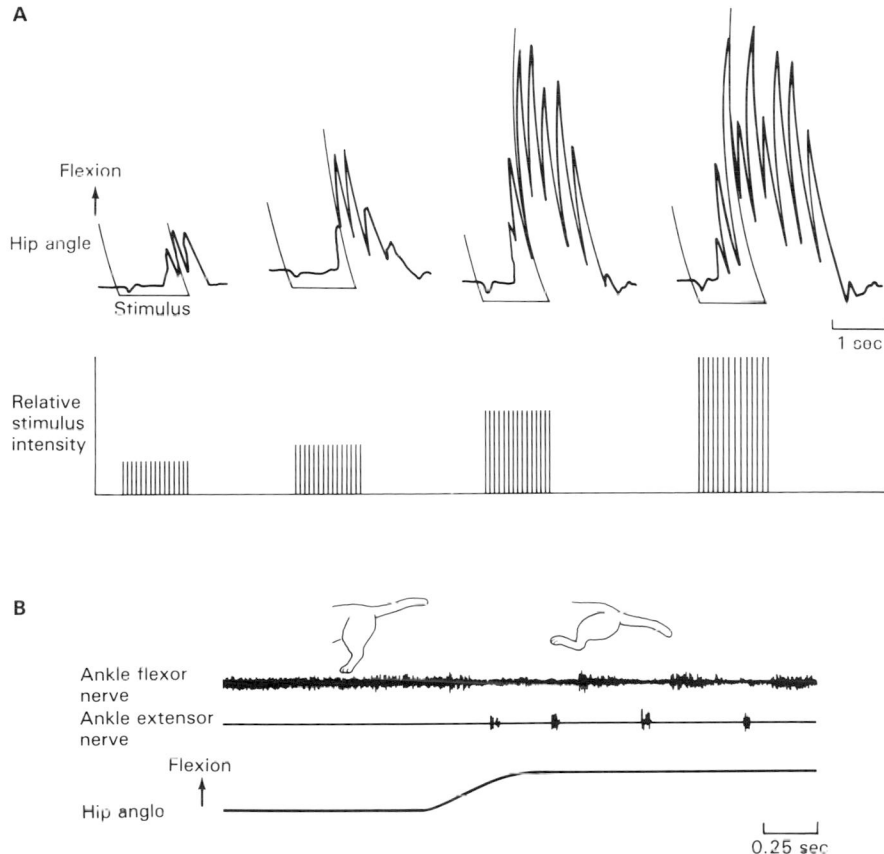

FIGURE 38–7

FIGURE 38–7

The spinal cord generates a rhythmic movement in the scratch reflex without a rhythmic stimulus.

A. Records from Sherrington's experiments with spinal dogs early in the century show the effect of increasing stimulus strength on the scratch reflex. The tracings show movement of the hindlimb in response to a mild electrical stimulus. As the intensity of the stimulus is increased, the amplitude of movement and duration of the reflex increase but the rhythm remains constant. (Adapted from Sherrington, 1947.)

B. When the muscles to the limb are paralyzed with curare, the motor nerves will respond to cutaneous stimulation, but no movement can occur. Under these conditions the motor neurons will not begin firing in alternating bursts until the hip is passively flexed. Thus, afferent signals from the hindlimb play a gating role: They enable rhythmic motor activity when the limb is in the proper position. (Adapted from Deliagina et al., 1975.)

Indeed, Lundberg has proposed that flexor reflex afferent pathways producing flexion and extension are elements of central pattern generators that control muscle activity in locomotion and other rhythmic behaviors. He and his colleagues have shown that after administration of L-dihydroxyphenylalanine (L-DOPA) in the acute spinal cat, stimulation of flexor reflex afferents sometimes produces rhythmically alternating contractions in flexor and extensor muscles. Apparently, L-DOPA releases the flexor reflex afferent pathways from tonic inhibitory control. As we shall see later, L-DOPA has a similar effect in activating locomotor behavior in spinal cats.

Certain Reflexes Consist of Rhythmic Movements

The ability of isolated spinal circuits to generate rhythmically alternating movements was appreciated quite early in motor physiology. Sherrington was one of the first to study this phenomenon systematically in the *scratch reflex* of dogs. The scratch reflex is a rhythmic movement, most often observed in furry animals, that removes an annoying stimulus such as a flea. Like the flexion withdrawal reflex, it is a complex behavior with a clear purpose. The reflex begins with movement of the hindlimb into a position close to the location of the stimulus; rhyth-

mic scratching occurs only after the limb has been brought to the correct starting position. Crossed extensor reflexes maintain the standing posture of the animal. The end result is that the animal is able to execute a well-coordinated series of scratches appropriately directed to the irritated area of skin.

Sherrington evoked the scratch reflex by applying a mild electrical stimulus to the flank or back of dogs in which the cervical spinal cord had been transected (Figure 38–7A). He found that the scratch reflex is intact in spinal animals and that, like flexion reflexes, many of the properties of the reflex are dependent on the intensity and duration of the stimulus. Thus, with increasing intensity of stimulation, the latency of the reflex decreases while the strength of muscle contractions and the number of repetitions increase. The most salient feature of this reflex, however, is that the rhythm of the reflex is independent of features of the stimulus. In fact, Sherrington found that the rhythmic reflex output typically outlasts the stimulus. A rhythmic output occurs without a rhythmic input, and the same rate of alternation of flexion and extension is maintained even as the force and duration of the output change.

Although Sherrington's findings demonstrated that a sustained rhythmic alternation of movements does not depend on supraspinal inputs, the possibility remained that such movements might require rhythmic input from muscle receptors in the moving limb. To exclude this input, Sherrington cut the dorsal roots carrying sensory input from the hindlimb. Even after this deafferentation, cutaneous stimulation in spinal animals elicited rhythmic scratching movements, although they were less well-coordinated and not as effective in reaching the site of the stimulus. Thus, the circuits responsible for alternation of flexion and extension are intrinsic to the spinal cord and do not require input either from supraspinal centers or from the periphery.

Although not necessary for the generation of rhythmic scratching, afferent input from the moving limb does influence the behavior. The nature of this influence has been investigated using *d*-tubocurare, a competitive inhibitor of acetylcholine, which blocks synaptic transmission at the neuromuscular junction (Chapter 10). When an irritative stimulus is applied after administration of tubocurare, the motor nerves to flexor and extensor muscles fire alternately, but no scratching movements actually occur. Since no movement takes place, the signals carried by afferent nerves from the limb cannot be responsible for the rhythm of the neural output. Such *fictive reflexes* have been used to analyze the central neural circuits underlying several types of spinal reflexes, as well as locomotor behaviors. In the fictive scratch reflex, rhythmic activity in the motor nerves does not begin unless the hindlimb is raised by flexing the hip (Figure 38–7B). Thus, while it is not responsible for the rhythmic alternation itself, tonic afferent input from the hindlimb nonetheless plays a gating role in that it enables the alternation to occur.

Certain Reflexes Adapt to Different Body Postures

Although reflexes are usually thought of as stereotyped patterns of neural output, all reflexes have some degree of adaptability to circumstances. The high degree of adaptability of some spinal reflexes was demonstrated by Anatol Feldman and his colleagues in a study of the wiping reflex of frogs. Like the scratch reflex, the purpose of the wiping reflex is removal of an irritative stimulus. To elicit the reflex a small blotter dipped in a mild acid solution was placed on the forelimb of spinal frogs. A frog with a high cervical transection of the spinal cord will make one or more quick wiping movements of the hindlimb directed at the source of irritation. If the position of the forelimb is changed but the irritant is applied to the same spot, the pattern of hindlimb wiping changes markedly so that the wipe is again directed to the site of the stimulus (Figure 38–8). Thus, the specific pattern of the reflex is determined by the position of the joints at the time of stimulation.

FIGURE 38–8

A frog with a transection of the cervical spinal cord varies its reflex movements to take into account the relative position of its limbs. Wiping movements of the hindlimb were elicited by placing an irritant on a specific part of the forelimb. In **A** the forelimb is placed forward; in **B** the forelimb is held back. In both cases the stimulated area of skin is the same, but because the initial position of the forelimb is different, the movement directed to the stimulus is different, as can be seen in the movement trajectories of the tip of the hindlimb (traced from film recordings). (Adapted from Berkinblit et al., 1986.)

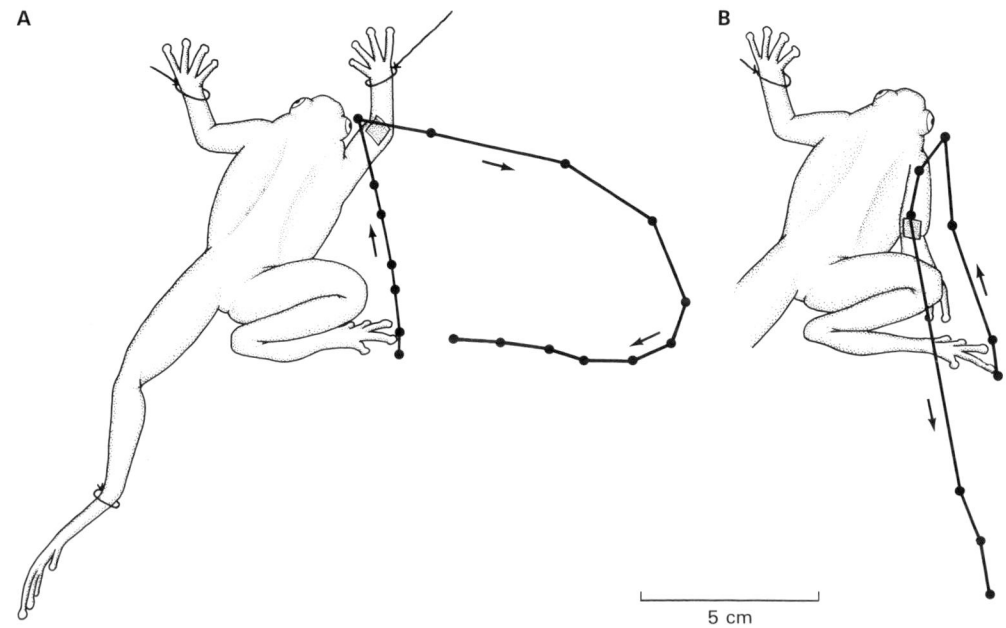

5 cm

Spinal Circuits Generate Rhythmic Locomotor Patterns

Locomotion is one of the most automatic of voluntary actions. When we walk we barely notice the alternating stepping movements of our legs that propel our body forward, and we superimpose upon these movements all manner of purposeful actions, such as carrying a suitcase, throwing a ball, speaking to a friend, even reading a book. To a large extent, the automaticity, and hence the ease, of normal locomotion can be attributed to intrinsic spinal circuits that take care of the details of the complex coordination of muscle contractions needed to generate rhythmic stepping movements of the legs.

In 1914 Brown demonstrated that spinal animals are capable of rhythmic stepping after transection of the dorsal roots, indicating that spinal circuits alone generate sustained rhythmic output, without requiring rhythmic input from either supraspinal structures or sensory receptors. He further proposed that a half-center organization of interneurons in the spinal cord (which we considered earlier) could account for the rhythmic stepping.

Sten Grillner and his colleagues have confirmed that spinal circuits act as central pattern generators, producing a well-differentiated and functional motor output for stepping. To analyze this phenomenon they transected the lower thoracic spinal cord of a cat, isolating the part of the spinal cord that controls the hindlimbs from descending signals (Figure 38–9A). Under these conditions the spinal cat will walk on a moving treadmill with a near normal stepping pattern, although the cat does require external support for balance (Figure 38–9B).

The overall stepping pattern consists of a rhythmic alternation between contractions of flexor and extensor muscles. The step cycle during locomotion has two phases: the swing phase (when the foot is off the ground and flexing forward) and the stance phase (when the foot is planted and the leg is extending relative to the body). The swing phase is generally controlled by contraction of flexor muscles, the stance phase by contraction of extensors. However, the pattern of muscle activation in the limbs of the spinal cat is not simply stereotyped flexion and extension, but rather consists of a differentially timed and spatially distributed *synergy* of muscle contractions, similar in form to that of normal cats. Similar observations have been made on cats whose spinal cords were transected at 1–2 weeks of age. Thus, the central pattern generators are innate, built into the architecture of the spinal circuitry.

Grillner showed that there are individual pattern generators for each limb. If one hind limb is prevented from moving on the treadmill, the other limb continues stepping normally. He observed that the one limb is frozen in midcycle, while the other continues to cycle rhythmically. Thus, the pattern generator for each limb can act independently of the other generators. In normal locomotion, however, the pattern generators for each limb are coupled to one another. When a cat walks on a treadmill,

for example, the movements of the left and right hindlimb are exactly out of phase with each other, so that while one is flexing the other is extending (Figure 38–9C). Increasing the treadmill speed dramatically shifts the temporal coupling between the limbs, as the animal changes from walking to trotting to galloping. In galloping the hindlimbs are in phase with each other; that is, they flex and extend together. Thus, independent but connected pattern generators provide for flexibility in interlimb coordination.

As noted above, passive movements of the limbs produced by the moving treadmill activate peripheral sensory receptors, and these stimuli are usually sufficient to initiate locomotion even in spinal cats. In spinal cats injected with tubocurare or in deafferented cats, however, these stimuli do not reach the spinal cord. Grillner found that intravenous administration of L-DOPA in such animals is sufficient to induce locomotion. This finding lends support to Lundberg's proposal that flexor reflex afferent pathways are part of the central pattern generators for locomotion, since the flexor reflex afferent pathways also show rhythmic alternating activity in the presence of L-DOPA. The neural circuits that constitute the central pattern generators for locomotion are probably not dedicated to this one function, but rather share interneurons with spinal circuits that generate other behaviors, such as flexion and scratch reflexes.

Tonic Descending Signals from the Brain Stem Activate the Spinal Circuits Responsible for Locomotion

L-DOPA stimulates synthesis and release of transmitters, such as norepinephrine, from presynaptic terminals of monoaminergic neurons in the spinal cord, and virtually all of these originate in the brain stem. The experiments with spinal cats are done soon after transection of the spinal cord, before there is sufficient time for descending fibers to degenerate. Thus, the fact that L-DOPA stimulates locomotion in these cats suggests that descending monoaminergic pathways from the brain stem activate the spinal circuits responsible for locomotion.

Further insight into how the brain stem controls locomotion has come from experiments by Mark Shik and Grigori Orlovsky, who found that tonic electrical stimulation of the *mesencephalic locomotor region* in decerebrate cats caused the animals to walk normally when placed on a treadmill. The rhythm of the locomotor pattern was unrelated to the pattern of electrical stimulation, and depended only on its intensity. Weak stimulation produced a walking gait that increased in speed as the intensity increased; progressively stronger stimulation produced trotting and finally galloping (Figure 38–9C). Thus, a relatively simple control signal from the brain stem, modulated only in intensity, can activate locomotion and cause changes in speed. The details of the loco-

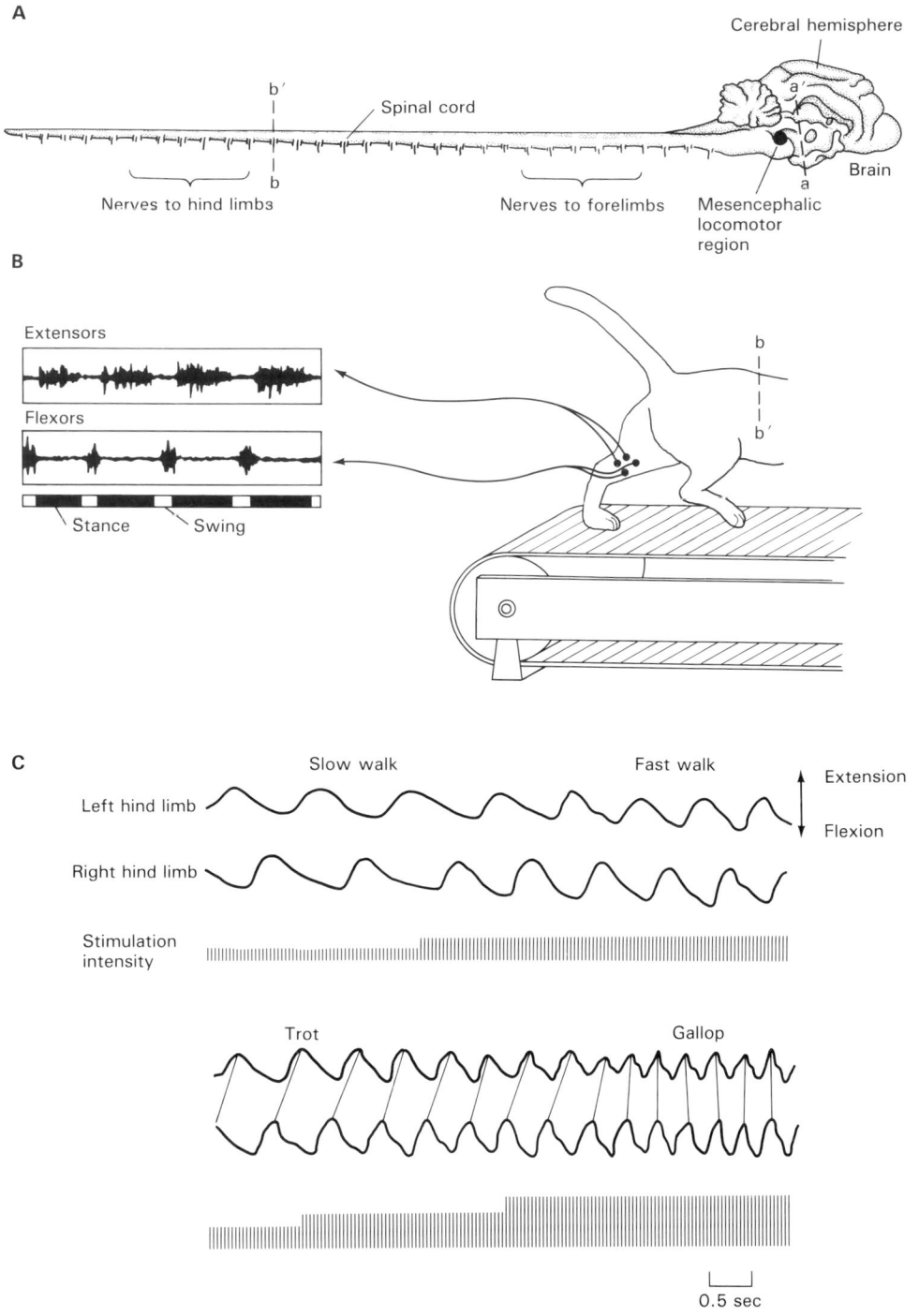

FIGURE 38–9

In mammals rhythmic locomotor patterns are generated by intrinsic spinal cord circuits that are activated by descending signals from the brain stem. (Adapted from Pearson, 1976.)

A. Transection of the spinal cord of a cat at the level of **b'-b** isolates the hindlimb segments of the cord. The hindlimbs are still able to walk on a treadmill after recovery from surgery. Transection at the level **a'-a** isolates the spinal cord and lower brain stem of the cat from the cerebral hemispheres. Locomotion can be produced in the animal by electrical stimulation of the mesencephalic locomotor region.

B. Locomotion of a cat transected at **b'-b** as demonstrated on a motorized treadmill. Reciprocal bursts of electrical activity can be recorded from flexors during the swing phase and from extensors during the stance phase of walking.

C. Locomotion of a cat transected at **a'-a** as demonstrated on a freely moving treadmill. The mesencephalic locomotor region is stimulated with increasing intensity. Bottom traces show movements of left and right hindlimbs and stimulus intensity. As the stimulus intensity increases, the gait becomes faster. As the cat progresses from trotting to galloping, the hindlimbs shift from alternating to simultaneous flexion and extension.

motor synergy are handled by intrinsic circuits in the spinal cord.

The mesencephalic locomotor region stimulated by Shik and Orlovsky is a rather circumscribed part of the midbrain. Axons from this region descend to the spinal cord through monoaminergic pathways. In later studies Grillner and Shik found that low intensities of electrical stimulation of this region, below the threshold for producing locomotion, modify flexor reflexes in ways similar to the effect of L-DOPA in the acute spinal cat. Several other regions of the brain stem can produce locomotion when stimulated, in particular a *subthalamic locomotor region* in the rostral brain stem and a *pontine locomotor region*. How these different brain stem regions interact in normal control of locomotion is still not known.

NMDA Receptors Are Involved in Generating the Locomotor Pattern

The generation of locomotor patterns relies heavily on *N*-methyl-D-aspartate (NMDA) receptors. Grillner and his colleagues, working on the lamprey, and Nicholas Dale and Alan Roberts working on amphibian embryos, found that NMDA can evoke a pattern of activity in the isolated spinal cord appropriate to the control of swimming. In addition, NMDA antagonists block the activation of swimming reflexes in response to natural stimulation. Moreover, application of NMDA to the isolated spinal cord of the lamprey evokes pacemaker oscillations of the membrane potential of motor neurons and many interneurons that participate in the locomotor pattern generator. These oscillations have a cycle similar to that of swimming and probably contribute to the generation of the swimming pattern by reinforcing the ability of the spinal network to generate a rhythmic motor output.

These pacemaker oscillations depend importantly on the unique properties of the NMDA receptor-channel, which we considered in Chapter 11, namely the channel's permeability to Ca^{2+} and its voltage-dependent blockade by Mg^{2+}. Depolarization leads to an unblocking of the NMDA channel by Mg^{2+}, allowing Ca^{2+} influx. The Ca^{2+} influx activates a Ca^{2+}-dependent K^+ current that repolarizes the membrane and restores the blockade of the channel by Mg^{2+}. The channel blockade in turn reduces the inward current through the NMDA channel. The continued inward leakage current depolarizes the membrane again, thereby repeating the cycle of pacemaker oscillations.

The involvement of NMDA receptors in both the lamprey and the amphibian embryo, as well as in mammals, suggests that these receptors may play an important role in the control of locomotion in all vertebrates. This idea is supported by Norio Kudo and Toshiya Yamada, who found that application of NMDA to the isolated spinal cord of the neonatal rat causes a pattern of ventral root activation appropriate for coordinated walking movements in the hindlimb.

Goal-Directed Locomotion Requires Intact Supraspinal Systems

Normal locomotion requires multiple levels of neural control. To support the body against gravity and to propel it forward the nervous system must coordinate muscle contractions at many joints. This is accomplished by the spinal circuits, which are activated by tonic signals from brain stem nuclei. Other descending systems, including reticulospinal, rubrospinal, and corticospinal pathways, are phasically active during locomotion and appear to be important for modulating the strength of the muscle contractions. At the same time, the nervous system must exert active control to maintain balance of the moving body, and it must adapt the locomotor pattern to the environment and to the overall behavioral goals. Although a spinal cat can produce relatively normal stepping patterns, it is not capable of maintaining balance. Adequate balance depends on parallel descending signals from other brain stem structures, especially from the vestibular system (Chapter 39). Adaptation of the locomotor pattern is partially accomplished by spinal reflex pathways and brain stem structures, but successful goal-directed locomotion requires the participation of cortical and subcortical structures, including the motor cortex (Chapter 40), basal ganglia (Chapter 42), and cerebellum (Chapter 41).

Afferent Information Modifies the Rhythmic Locomotor Pattern

Although sensory input is not necessary for the generation of a rhythmic locomotor pattern, the speed of walking is slowed and the locomotor synergy is less well-coordinated in the absence of peripheral input. Grillner and his colleagues Hans Forssberg and Serge Rossignol have demonstrated how afferent information interacts with the locomotor pattern. First, afferent input assists in switching the pattern from one phase of the step cycle to another. Preventing extension during the stance phase of one hind limb in a spinal cat inhibits the swing phase of that limb, so that extensor muscle activity in the limb persists. When the limb is slowly extended, the extensor activity suddenly ceases at a critical point, and flexion promptly occurs. Thus, during a critical part of the stance phase afferent input allows the central pattern generator to switch to the swing phase. In normal locomotion this mechanism ensures that the limb will not be lifted until adequate extension has occurred.

Afferent input also compensates for external disturbances. If the limb of a walking cat contacts an obstacle as it swings forward, a brisk flexion allows the limb to clear the obstacle. A weak electrical stimulus to the dorsum of the foot produces exactly the same reflex. This *stumble corrective reaction* appears to be elicited by tactile stimuli, since it can be abolished by cutaneous anesthesia. Grillner examined this reflex in spinal cats during locomotion on a treadmill. They found that electrical stimulation of the top of the foot during the swing phase enhances flexion of the limb, while the same stimulation during the stance phase enhances extension. The effect of the stimulus is channeled, through interneurons, to flexors during the flexion phase of walking and to extensors during the extensor phase.

This *reflex reversal* is functionally important because a particular reflex may not be appropriate at certain times. For example, the stumble corrective reflex is appropriate for stepping over an obstacle and thus is adaptive during the swing phase. However, if the same flexion reflex were produced during the stance phase, when the animal's weight is being supported by the limb, the animal might collapse.

An Overall View

In the chapters that follow we shall examine control of movement by higher centers of the brain. We shall see that most descending axons influence motor neurons indirectly through interneurons. Interneurons in spinal circuits are not merely relay neurons that carry messages from sensory neurons to higher centers and from higher centers to motor neurons. Rather, they constitute a powerful neural machinery that has the capacity to link muscles together into functional units.

We get a glimpse of this organization in the spinal reflexes, which are really fragments of more complex behaviors. Reflex circuits provide the higher centers with a set of elementary patterns of coordination, from relatively simple combinations, like reciprocal innervation at a single joint, to more complex spatial patterns of movement, such as flexion reflexes, and temporal patterns, as in the scratch reflex. Although they are relatively stereotyped, these wired-in movement patterns are nevertheless remarkably adaptable to current conditions, as when the frog's wiping reflex adjusts to different positions of the part of the body being stimulated. Thus, reflexes are not entirely stereotyped but rather are adapted to the initial position of the body segments and the external loads acting to oppose movement. Because this information reaches the lower levels directly, higher centers can activate these reflex circuits to produce voluntary movements and need not be concerned with the details of shaping the movement patterns to current circumstances.

Locomotion provides an excellent example of how the spinal circuits responsible for simple reflexes simplify the control of voluntary movement. The spinal circuits that generate the locomotor synergy allow higher centers to control a very complex movement pattern with relatively simple descending signals.

Our understanding of the neural mechanisms involved in locomotion has come almost exclusively from experiments on animals. How relevant are these experiments to human voluntary movement? Indirect evidence indicates they are most likely of great importance. Although humans with complete transections of the spinal cord are incapable of rhythmic stepping like those observed in spinal cats, developmental studies indicate that human infants are born with innate reflex circuits capable of rhythmic pattern generation. Newborn infants exhibit rhythmic stepping when placed on a moving treadmill, and there is evidence that this reflex pattern is a forerunner of the mature locomotor synergy. Human locomotion differs from most animal locomotion in that it is bipedal, placing greater demands on descending systems that control posture during walking. Therefore, the spinal networks that contribute to human locomotion are probably more dependent on supraspinal centers.

A large body of experimental work on such different types of locomotion as swimming, flying, and walking, in both vertebrates and invertebrates, indicates that all forms of locomotion rely on the same general principles of neuronal organization—intrinsic oscillatory networks are activated and modulated by afferent input and by higher motor centers in the brain stem and cortex. Thus, evolutionary processes have led to the development of similar strategies in a variety of species, and there is no reason to believe that humans are fundamentally different.

Selected Readings

Baldissera, F., Hultborn, H., and Illert, M. 1981. Integration in spinal neuronal systems. In V. B. Brooks (ed.), Handbook of Physiology, Section 1: The Nervous System, Vol. II. Motor Control. Part 1. Bethesda, Md.: American Physiological Society, pp. 509–595.

Grillner, S., and Wallén, P. 1985. Central pattern generators for locomotion, with special reference to vertebrates. Annu. Rev. Neurosci. 8:233–261.

Grillner, S., Wallén, P., and Viana di Prisco, G. 1990. Cellular network underlying locomotion as revealed in a lower vertebrate model: Transmitters, membrane properties, circuitry, and simulation. Cold Spring Harbor Symp. Quant. Biol. 55:779–789.

Lundberg, A. 1975. Control of spinal mechanisms from the brain. In D. B. Tower (ed.), The Nervous System, Vol. 1: The Basic Neurosciences. New York: Raven Press, pp. 253–265.

Pearson, K. 1976. The control of walking. Sci. Am. 235(6):72–86.

Sherrington, C. 1947. The integrative Action of the Nervous System, 2nd ed. New Haven: Yale University Press.

References

Adams, R. D., and Victor, M. 1989. Principles of Neurology, 4th ed. New York: McGraw-Hill.

Armstrong, D. M. 1988. Review lecture: The supraspinal control of mammalian locomotion. J. Physiol. (Lond.) 405:1–37.

Berkinblit, M. B., Feldman, A. G., and Fukson, O. I. 1986. Adaptability of innate motor patterns and motor control mechanisms. Behav. Brain Sci. 9:585–638.

Brown, T. G. 1911. The intrinsic factors in the act of progression in the mammal. Proc. R. Soc. Lond. [Biol.] 84:308–319.

Dale, N., and Roberts, A. 1985. Dual-component amino-acid-mediated synaptic potentials: Excitatory drive for swimming in Xenopus embryos. J. Physiol. (Lond.) 363:35–59.

Deliagina, T. G., Feldman, A. G., Gelfand, I. M., and Orlovsky, G. N. 1975. On the role of central program and afferent inflow in the control of scratching movements in the cat. Brain Res. 100:297–313.

Easton, T. A. 1972. On the normal use of reflexes. Am. Sci. 60:591–599.

Eccles, J. C. 1964. The Physiology of Synapses. Berlin: Springer.

Eccles, J. C., Fatt. P., and Koketsu, K. 1954. Cholinergic and inhibitory synapses in a pathway from motor-axon collaterals to motoneurones. J. Physiol. (Lond.) 126:524–562.

Forssberg, H. 1982. Spinal locomotor functions and descending control. In B. Sjölund and A. Björklund (eds.), Brain Stem Control of Spinal Mechanisms. Amsterdam: Elsevier, pp. 253–271.

Forssberg, H. 1985. Ontogeny of human locomotor control. I. Infant stepping, supported locomotion and transition to independent locomotion. Exp. Brain. Res. 57:480–493.

Friesen, W. O., and Stent, G. S. 1978. Neural circuits for generating rhythmic movements. Annu. Rev. Biophys. Bioeng. 7:37–61.

Gelfand, I. M., Orlovsky, G. N., and Shik, M. L. 1988. Locomotion and scratching in tetrapods. In A. H. Cohen, S. Rossignol, and S. Grillner (eds.), Neural Control of Rhythmic Movements in Vertebrates. New York: Wiley, pp. 167–199.

Grillner, S., and Shik, M. L. 1973. On the descending control of the lumbosacral spinal cord from the "mesencephalic locomotor region." Acta Physiol. Scand. 87:320–333.

Hagbarth, K.-E. 1952. Excitatory and inhibitory skin areas for flexor and extensor motoneurones. Acta Physiol. Scand. 26 (Suppl. 94):1–58.

Jankowska, E., Padel, Y., and Tanaka, R. 1976. Disynaptic inhibition of spinal motoneurones from the motor cortex in the monkey. J. Physiol. (Lond.) 258:467–487.

Kudo, N., and Yamada, T. 1987. N-methyl-D,L-aspartate-induced locomotor activity in a spinal cord-hindlimb muscles preparation of the newborn rat studied in vitro. Neurosci. Lett. 75:43–48.

Lloyd, D. P. C. 1946. Integrative pattern of excitation and inhibition in two-neuron reflex arcs. J. Neurophysiol. 9:439–444.

Lundberg, A., Malmgren, K., and Schomburg, E. D. 1975. Convergence from Ib, cutaneous and joint afferents in reflex pathways to motorneurones. Brain Res. 87:81–84.

Nichols, T. R. 1989. The organization of heterogenic reflexes among muscles crossing the ankle joint in the decerebrate cat. J. Physiol. (Lond.) 410:463–477.

Renshaw, B. 1941. Influence of discharge of motoneurons upon excitation of neighboring motoneurons. J. Neurophysiol. 4:167–183.

Renshaw, B. 1946. Central effects of centripetal impulses in axons of spinal ventral roots. J. Neurophysiol. 9:191–204.

Rossignol, S., Lund, J. P., and Drew, T. 1988. The role of sensory inputs in regulating patterns of rhythmical movements in higher vertebrates: A comparison between locomotion, respiration, and mastication. In A. H. Cohen, S. Rossignol, and S. Grillner (eds.), Neural Control of Rhythmic Movements in Vertebrates. New York: Wiley, pp. 201–283.

Schmidt, R. F. 1983. Motor systems. In R. F. Schmidt and G. Thews (eds.), Human Physiology. M. A. Biederman-Thorson (trans.) Berlin: Springer, pp. 81–110.

Shik, M. L., and Orlovsky, G. N. 1976. Neurophysiology of locomotor automatism. Physiol. Rev. 56:465–501.

Wallén, P., and Grillner, S. 1987. N-methyl-D-aspartate receptor-induced, inherent oscillatory activity in neurons active during fictive locomotion in the lamprey. J. Neurosci. 7:2745–2755.

Claude Ghez

Posture

Postural Stability During Standing and Walking Is Maintained by Both Feedforward Control and Rapid Feedback Compensatory Corrections

Three Classes of Sensory Input Are Important for Triggering Postural Responses but Are Normally Used in Different Ways

The Topography of Rapid Postural Responses Is Dependent on Context

Postural Responses Are Triggered Centrally Before Voluntary Movements

Vestibular and Neck Reflexes Stabilize the Head and Eyes

Vestibulocollic and Vestibulospinal Reflexes Maintain the Head Vertical with Respect to Gravity

Neck and Vestibular Reflexes Are Synergistic in the Neck but Antagonistic in the Limbs: Cervicocollic and Cervicospinal Reflexes

Vestibular and Neck Afferents Converge on the Vestibular Nuclei and Propriospinal Neurons

Brain Stem and Spinal Mechanisms Play a Major Role in the Control of Posture

The Pontine Reticular Nuclei Facilitate Motor Neurons Whereas Medullary Reticular Nuclei Produce Both Facilitation and Inhibition

Section of the Brain Stem above the Vestibular Nuclei Produces Decerebrate Rigidity

Lesions of the Cerebellum Modify Vestibular and Reticular Influences on Posture

Spasticity Is a Common Manifestation of Supraspinal Lesions in Humans

An Overall View

Posture represents the overall position of the body and limbs relative to one another and their orientation in space. Postural adjustments are necessary for all motor tasks and need to be integrated with voluntary movements. A boxer who fails to adjust his posture while throwing a punch would topple to the ground. Runners jogging over uneven terrain encounter other challenges to postural control: Their center of gravity is continuously advancing and the legs must move forward at the right moment to support the body. To maintain a stable position and stand erect while keeping the parts of the body aligned—the head upright on the neck and the torso upright on the pelvis—a family of adjustments is needed. These adjustments serve three behavioral functions. First, they support the head and body against gravity and other external forces. Second, they maintain the center of the body's mass aligned and balanced over the base of support on the ground. Third, they stabilize supporting parts of the body while others are being moved.

Postural adjustments are achieved by means of two major mechanisms. First, there are *anticipatory* or *feedforward mechanisms* that predict disturbances and produce preprogrammed responses that maintain stability. These anticipatory responses are modified by experience and their effectiveness improves with practice. A key role of anticipatory responses is to generate postural adjustments before voluntary movements occur. In their absence the body would become destabilized and fall. Second, *compensatory* or *feedback responses* are evoked by sensory events following loss of balance. These automatic postural adjustments, typically produced by body sway, are extremely rapid and, like reflexes, they have relatively stereotyped spatiotemporal organization. Unlike reflexes, however, these postural responses are appropriately scaled to achieve the goal of stable posture. If the system fails in one situation, adjustments are made on subsequent attempts to prevent falling. Also, unlike reflexes, postural adjustments are refined continuously by practice and learning, much like skilled voluntary movements.

These postural mechanisms are recruited by information coming from a variety of sensory receptors: cutaneous, proprioceptive, and visual. Cutaneous receptors signal the shearing forces on the skin of the feet from the ground. Proprioceptors signal changes in the position of the limbs and alterations in the orientation of the head relative to the body. Visual detection of movement in the surrounding world signals orientation relative to the horizon. Sensory inputs from these various modalities trigger anticipatory and compensatory responses that are automatic and contribute to posture without our awareness.

To integrate posture and voluntary movements postural responses make use of cortical circuits as well as spinal and brain stem reflexes. In this chapter we first examine how postural stability is maintained by the coordination of reflex and voluntary movements. We next consider the brain stem and spinal mechanisms that stabilize the head and eyes and that align the head and body. Finally, we shall describe the neural circuits of the brain stem that mediate posture and the disorders in posture that are produced by lesions of the brain stem.

Postural Stability During Standing and Walking Is Maintained by Both Feedforward Control and Rapid Feedback Compensatory Corrections

In quadrupeds the mechanics of standing are relatively simple and extensor rigidity can maintain a decerebrate animal erect, provided the ground or support surface remains immobile. In bipeds on the other hand, the standing position is unstable and reflexes alone cannot maintain an upright posture. Maintenance of balance during walking or running is even more demanding. When the body is progressing forward it can readily be destabilized by variations in the terrain and foot placement may need to be visually guided to avoid obstacles. The mechanisms that maintain postural stability in natural conditions requires the participation of cortical and other supraspinal mechanisms. We begin by considering how vertical posture is maintained when ground support is unsteady and during voluntary movements.

Three Classes of Sensory Input Are Important for Triggering Postural Responses but Are Normally Used in Different Ways

To analyze how humans adjust their balance while standing, Lewis Nashner and his colleagues studied postural control of subjects standing on a movable platform that made them sway forward (by moving the platform backward), or backward (by moving the platform forward). Nashner found that the swaying movements induced by moving the platform in either direction elicited rapid and highly stereotyped postural responses in many muscles that maintain the center of body mass over the center of

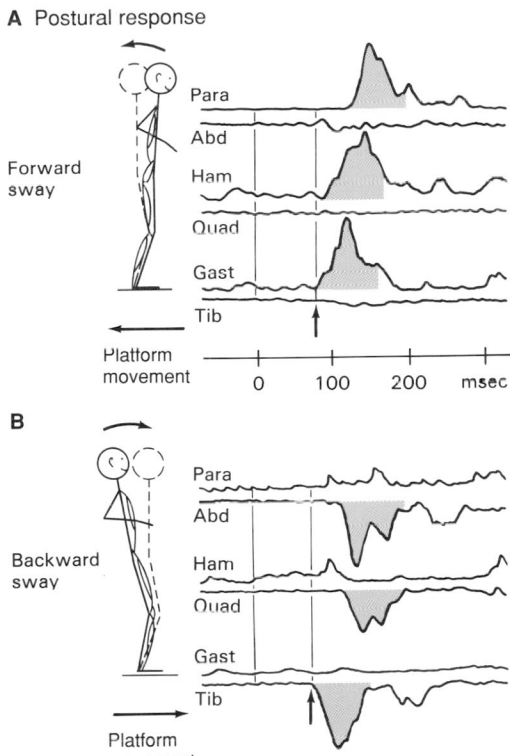

A Postural response

B

FIGURE 39–1

A movable platform is used to perturb stance in various ways. (Adapted from Horak and Nashner, 1986.)

Backward movement of the platform makes the subject sway forward (**A**). This elicits a compensatory response organized in the distal to proximal sequence (first the gastrocnemius, then the hamstrings and lumbar paraspinal muscles).

This distal to proximal pattern of postural responses, however, can become reorganized when the conditions of support change, for example, if the platform is very narrow. Then, the ball of the foot is no longer in contact with the ground and ankle motion cannot counteract body sway. In that case (**B**), the postural response to a forward sway begins with the abdominal and hip muscles acting on the pelvis to bend the body forward at the hip. Traces are electromyograms (EMGs) of: **Para**, paraspinal muscles (rectified and integrated); **Abd**, abdominal muscles; **Ham**, hamstring muscles; **Quad**, quadriceps; **Gast**, gastrocnemius; **Tib**, anterior tibial muscles.

foot support. Moreover, the contraction of different muscles that make up the postural responses occur in a highly characteristic distal-to-proximal sequence: The first muscles to contract are those that are closest to the base of support. During forward sway, the ankle extensors (such as the gastrocnemius) contract first. During backward sway, the tibialis anterior (an ankle flexor) contracts first (this muscle is stretched during backward sway). Only after these distal muscles contract do the thigh and then the trunk muscles contract (Figure 39–1).

Postural responses are triggered by three types of sensory inputs: (1) *muscle proprioceptors* that sense changes in length or tension in ankle muscles; (2) *vestibular receptors* that sense sway through head motion; and (3)

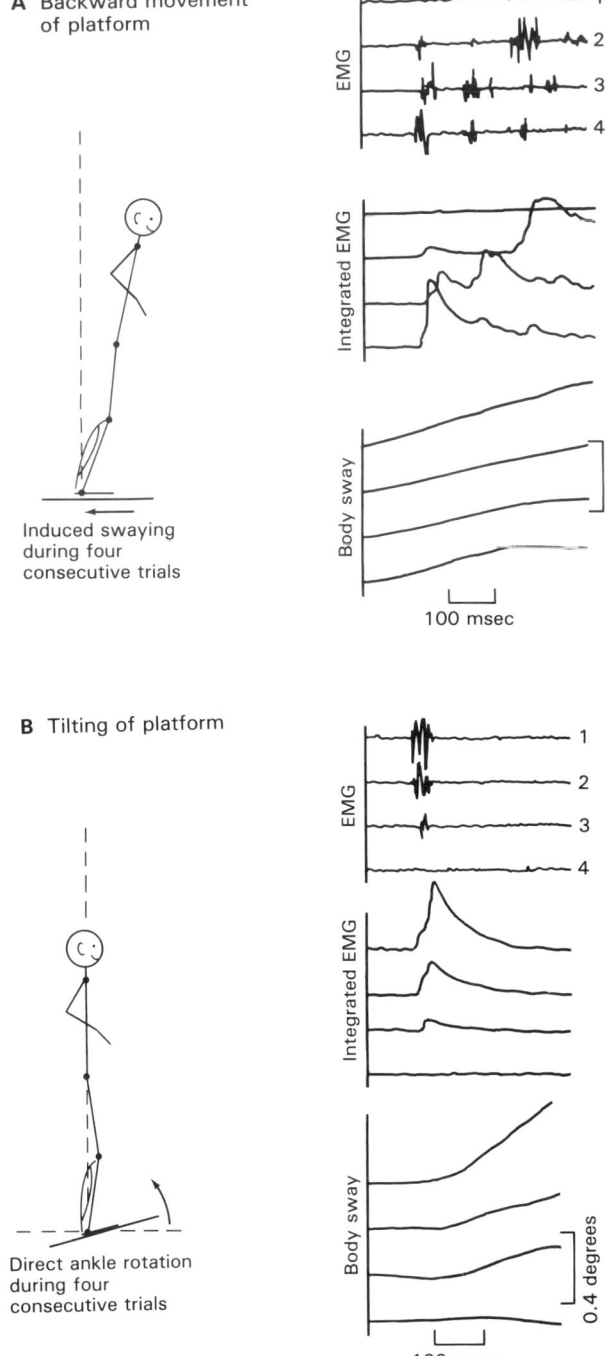

A Backward movement of platform

EMG

Integrated EMG

Body sway

0.4 degrees

Induced swaying during four consecutive trials

100 msec

B Tilting of platform

EMG

Integrated EMG

Body sway

0.4 degrees

Direct ankle rotation during four consecutive trials

100 msec

FIGURE 39–2

The muscles that contract during body sway are adapted to counteract the disturbance. (Adapted from Nashner, 1976.)

A. Sway induced by unexpected backward movement of the platform triggers a rapid postural response in the gastrocnemius muscle that occurs progressively earlier with repeated trials. (Numbers opposite EMG traces refer to consecutive trials.)

B. When the ankle is unexpectedly tilted in the toes up direction, the large contraction of gastrocnemius on the first trial initially destabilizes posture and induces large body sway. However, this response is attenuated after a few trials and sway is reduced.

visual inputs that detect motion in the visual field. By varying the sensory input available to the subject, Nashner discovered that each modality plays a different role (Figure 39–1). Postural responses elicited by muscle receptors that sense muscle stretch have the shortest latencies and can be triggered at 70 to 100 ms.[1] Responses based exclusively on either vestibular or visual inputs are almost twice as slow. Visual and proprioceptive information alone do not allow the central nervous system to distinguish whether the head or the external environment is in motion. To accomplish this task, information from both modalities need to be correlated with each other and with concurrent vestibular inputs.

The Topography of Rapid Postural Responses Is Dependent on Context

Despite the reflex-like stereotypy of postural responses to body sway, the pattern of contraction elicited by a particular stimulus depends on the subject's prior experience and expectations. This was discovered by Nashner when he next compared the responses of subjects standing on the moving platform to types of motion: backward translation and upward rotation. Both motions produce the same ankle rotation and therefore act as the same stimulus; however, the response that is appropriate to maintain the body upright is quite different. By sliding the platform backward, Nashner induced forward sway and, as we saw earlier, subjects maintained balance by contracting the ankle extensors, the gastrocnemius muscle. When the platform instead was suddenly tilted upward, bringing the toes up, Nashner induced backward sway. Subjects initially responded the same way they did to forward sway; they contracted the gastrocnemius. This is because in both forward sway (produced by sliding the platform) and backward sway (produced by tilting the platform) the gastrocnemius muscle is stretched by the movement, triggering a stretch-evoked response that extends the ankle joint. However, the consequences of active ankle extension produced by contraction of the gastrocnemius are quite different for the two movements. In induced forward swaying, ankle extension *opposes* sway and therefore serves to maintain normal posture. In the backward sway produced by tilting the platform upward, ankle extension *increases* sway, a movement that is inappropriate. Within a few trials, however, the subjects learn to stabilize posture by contracting at the same latency an ankle flexor, the tibialis anterior muscle, instead of the ankle extensors (Figure 39–2). Moreover, a response that stabilizes posture becomes facilitated progressively with repeated trials. In contrast, a response that destabilizes posture adapts and becomes progressively weaker (Figure 39–2B). As a result the same effective stimulus, stretch of the ankle extensors, ultimately evokes contraction of one group of muscles in one condition and of its antagonist in another.

These results illustrate an essential feature of postural

---

[1]For purposes of comparison, segmental stretch reflexes in the lower extremities require only about 50 ms.

control. An individual's postural response to a perturbing stimulus is shaped by experience, and the form of the response is adjusted so that balance is maintained. In one context a stimulus can produce a short-latency feedback response in one muscle group, yet in another context the same stimulus can produce contraction of a different muscle group. The responses are powerful enough in both conditions, to stabilize the body, and in both conditions a feedforward or anticipatory mechanism predicts the disturbance and preprograms the stabilizing response. Nashner used the term *postural set* to describe the preparatory state in which a specific postural response is selected in advance of the stimulus so that it is then executed automatically.

FIGURE 39–3

The contraction of arm and leg muscles are coordinated during voluntary arm movements.

A. The subject pulls on the handle as soon as possible after an auditory stimulus (**arrow**), however, muscle contraction starts in the leg muscles.

B. The subject is leaning against a support while grasping the handle. When the handle is suddenly displaced forward, the subject's arm is extended. This evokes a stretch reflex in the biceps at very short latency, which blends in with later, more tonic activation. No activity is evoked in the leg muscles.

C. If the subject is not supported and the handle is jerked forward, extending the subject's arm as in B and moving the subject's center of mass forward as in A, the initial stretch reflex in the biceps is largely suppressed and arm muscle response is coordinated with a response in the gastrocnemius, as in A.

Postural Responses Are Triggered Centrally Before Voluntary Movements

Lifting or pulling a heavy object can have the same destabilizing effect as movements of the surface of support, because the force exerted will pull the body toward the object. In lifting or pulling, postural muscles contract to maintain equilibrium *before* destabilizing movements are executed. Paul Cordo and Nashner found that when subjects pull in response to a cue they contract the gastrocnemius and hamstrings before the biceps (Figure 39–3A). If the subject's body is braced by a support that prevents the pulling action of the biceps from moving the body forward, the biceps is contracted at the time the gastrocne-

D. The biceps can also be incorporated into a rapid postural response at a latency only slightly longer than the stretch reflex when the standing subject grasps the handle and the platform moves forward. This moves the subject's center of mass backwards. A modest stretch-evoked response occurs in the leg muscles. However, movement of the platform now extends the elbow, because the subject is grasping the handle, and evokes a large response in the biceps. (Adapted from Nashner, 1982.)

E. Posture and movement are integrated using feedforward and feedback. Commands triggering movement of a limb are coordinated with feedforward triggering of postural adjustment, and in this way the destabilizing effect of the movement is anticipated. The postural control system is also prepared to respond quickly and appropriately to feedback on disturbances in the event that feedforward control does not produce complete stabilization. (Adapted from Gahery and Massion, 1981.)

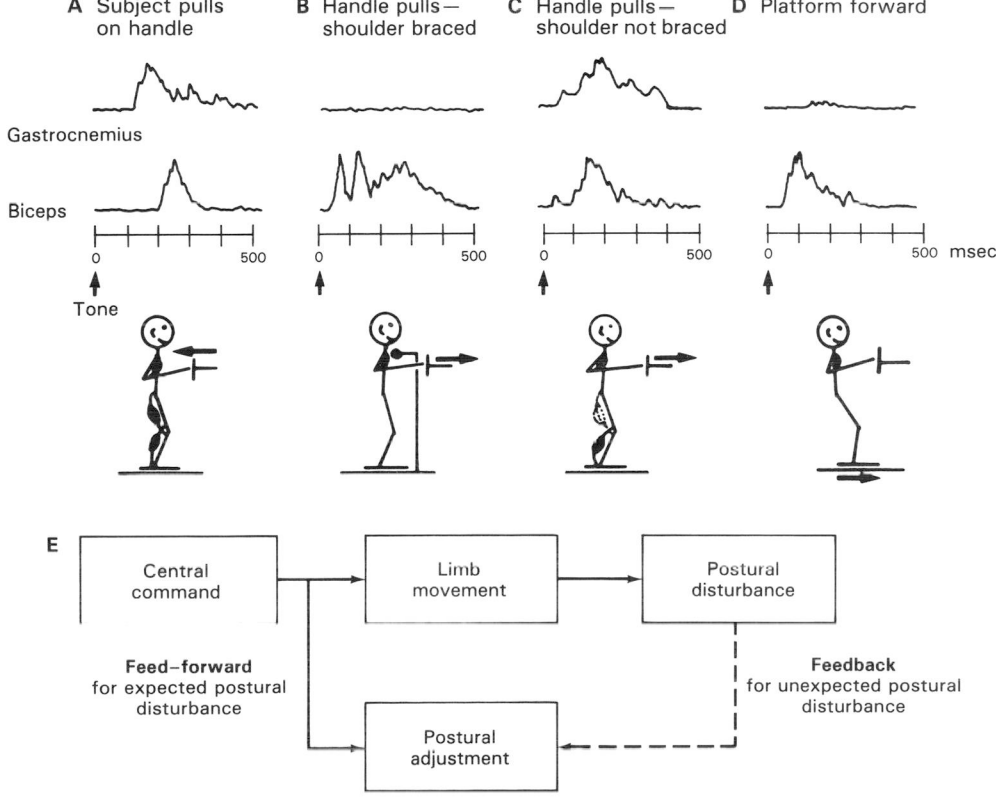

A Subject pulls on handle   B Handle pulls— shoulder braced   C Handle pulls— shoulder not braced   D Platform forward

Gastrocnemius

Biceps

0   500   0   500   0   500   0   500 msec

Tone

E Central command → Limb movement → Postural disturbance

Feed–forward for expected postural disturbance

Feedback for unexpected postural disturbance

Postural adjustment

mius would have contracted. In the unsupported condition the arm movement is normally delayed until the execution of a postural response that anticipates movement of the center of the body's mass. Thus, the planning of movement involves the coordination of commands to both the limb muscles and to a wide variety of postural muscles. In the next chapter we shall see that the supplementary motor area is important in this process.

Spinal reflexes are also modulated in accordance with the conditions of postural support. Cordo and Nashner asked subjects to grasp a handle mounted on a motor that suddenly pulled on the arm and stretched the biceps. If subjects were braced so that the arm pull could not displace their body and they were then told to counteract the pull, a large stretch reflex response occurred in the biceps of the arm. This response merged with later tonic activation of voluntary origin (Figure 39–3B). If, however, subjects had to maintain their balance without being braced, the short-latency reflex response in the biceps to the handle pull was markedly decreased, while a large response occurred in the gastrocnemius. Substantial activation in the biceps occurred only after this postural response was well under way (Figure 39–3C). Thus, the gain or strength of the stretch reflex in the biceps was profoundly reduced because it would destabilize the subject. Similarly, when the subjects were asked to steady themselves by holding onto the handle and the platform then was moved forward the expected response in the gastrocnemius was markedly attenuated, and instead a brisk response in the biceps was evident (Figure 39–3D). These results illustrate an essential point: *descending influences* generated by postural set can act on spinal neurons to gate and modulate reflex circuits (see Chapter 38).

These examples illustrate two key principles that govern posture. First, as we have seen before, postural adjustments anticipate the occurrence of disturbances that would cause the loss of balance. This feedforward control is essential for coordinating posture with voluntary movement. Feedforward control also is evident in postural adjustment during walking: For example, when stepping down stairs the plantar flexors of the ankle are contracted before the foot reaches the next step.

Second, when disturbances actually occur, feedback mechanisms produce rapid corrective responses. When we can predict the nature of a disturbance but not its exact timing, higher motor centers enhance or reduce the strength of short-latency pathways that operate automatically (Figure 39–3E).

While we do not yet know all the circuits that mediate automatic postural adjustments, a short-latency transcortical pathway is important for the most rapid responses to proprioceptive inputs. Afferent information that triggers these responses ascends through the dorsal column–medial lemniscal system and is relayed through the thalamus, where neurons project both directly to the primary motor cortex and indirectly through the somatic sensory cortex (Chapter 40).

Vestibular and Neck Reflexes Stabilize the Head and Eyes

In the preceding section we focused on responses evoked by perturbations of the support surface. The consequent responses maintain our body upright. We now discuss mechanisms that align our head and body with respect to gravity. These mechanisms require vestibular and neck reflexes. *Vestibular reflexes* are evoked by changes in the position of the head, whereas *neck reflexes* are triggered by tilting (bending) or turning the neck. Both reflexes produce coordinated effects on muscles of the arms, legs, and neck. Movement of the head also evokes vestibulo-ocular reflexes that stabilize visual images on the retina. (We shall consider these later in Chapter 43.)

The vestibular and neck reflexes were identified at the beginning of this century by Rudolph Magnus. These reflexes are mediated principally by neural circuits in the brain stem and spinal cord and are most pronounced when the spinal circuits are released from cortical inhibition, much like certain spinal reflexes described in the preceding chapter. Magnus stimulated the vestibular end organs selectively by placing human subjects on an examining table that allowed the neck and body to be tilted together without bending the neck. He also studied patients with damage to the vestibular end organs and was thereby able to examine neck reflexes in the absence of concurrent vestibular reflexes.

Vestibulocollic and Vestibulospinal Reflexes Maintain the Head Vertical with Respect to Gravity

Vestibular reflexes act on the neck (the *vestibulocollic reflexes*) and on the limbs (the *vestibulospinal reflexes*); they are evoked principally by sensory input from the otolith organs: the utricle and the saccule in the vestibule of the inner ear. These organs give rise to signals that inform the brain about the direction of gravity and the acceleration produced during head movement in the horizontal and sagittal planes (see Chapter 33). The semicircular canals have weaker influences on the spinal circuits and serve predominantly to control extraocular muscles and coordinate head and eye movements.

Vestibulocollic and vestibulospinal reflexes are primarily static and are elicited by positioning the head in different orientations relative to gravity. The *vestibulocollic reflexes* counteract head movements keeping the head stable. For example, when the head is tilted forward without bending the neck (as when the body is pitched forward with the head straight), the vestibulocollic reflexes return the head to the vertical by contracting dorsal neck muscles. The *vestibulospinal reflexes* contract the limb muscles and prepare the subject for landing during falls. Tilting the head *forward* produces extension of arms (or upper limbs) and flexion of the lower ones, a combination of movements that reduces the impact of a fall.

FIGURE 39–4

The actions of neck reflexes on the limb muscles of standing humans. (Adapted from Tokizane et al., 1951.)

A. Normal posture.

B. Bending the neck backward produces extension of arms and legs, while bending the neck forward produces flexion of arms and legs. It should be noted that in animals, bending the neck backward produces extension of the forelimbs and flexion of the hindlimbs. The reverse occurs with bending the neck forward.

C. Rotating the head to the right or bending it to the right produces extension of the right arm (*extension of the chin limbs*) and leg and flexion of the left (contralateral) limbs.

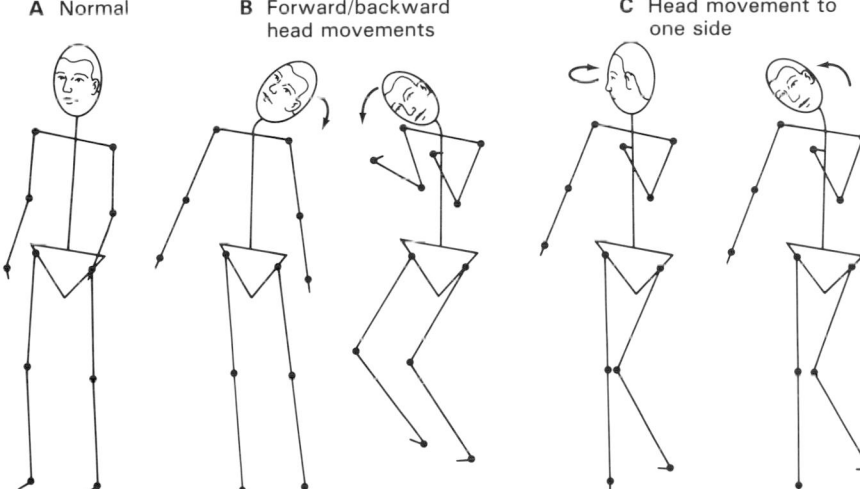

A Normal   B Forward/backward head movements   C Head movement to one side

Neck and Vestibular Reflexes Are Synergistic in the Neck but Antagonistic in the Limbs: Cervicocollic and Cervicospinal Reflexes

Bending the neck and turning the head relative to the body also evokes reflexes in both neck muscles (*cervicocollic reflexes*) and limb muscles (*cervicospinal reflexes*) (Figure 39–4). Spindles in neck muscles and receptors in the joints of the upper cervical vertebrae are the receptors responsible for these actions. They have both phasic and tonic components.

Cervicocollic reflexes contract neck muscles that are stretched. A movement of the head (for example, by an externally imposed force) in one direction will stretch the neck muscles on the opposite side and cause them to contract. This will act to realign the head. Cervicocollic reflexes are therefore synergistic with the vestibulocollic reflexes produced by the same head movements. In contrast, the actions of cervicospinal reflexes on the limb muscles oppose those of vestibulospinal reflexes. For example, bending the neck forward elicits flexion of the upper extremities (Figure 39–4), but tilting the head (together with the body to avoid stretching neck muscles) produces extension of the upper extremities. The opposite actions

FIGURE 39–5

Vestibular and neck reflexes have opposing actions on limb muscles. To distinguish the effects of vestibular and neck reflexes, the dorsal roots innervating the first two cervical vertebrae were sectioned in a decerebrate cat. Vestibular reflexes were then elicited by tilting the head. Neck reflexes were produced by turning the second cervical vertebra, thus activating afferents at levels below C2. This procedure has the same effect as would occur when the intact animal rotates the head, but without stimulating the otoliths. The upper panels of the figure show how vestibular reflexes are elicited by tilting the head with the vertebrae fixed in the normal orientation. The circle with vertical line represents the orientation of the vertebrae and spinous process. The lower panels show how neck reflexes are evoked by rotation of the axis (see the reorientation of the spinous process). (Adapted from Roberts, 1978.)

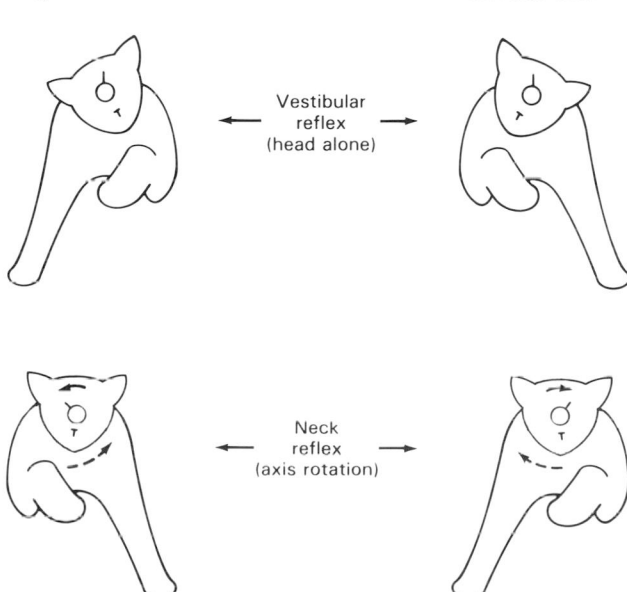

Right side down   Left side down

Vestibular reflex (head alone)

Neck reflex (axis rotation)

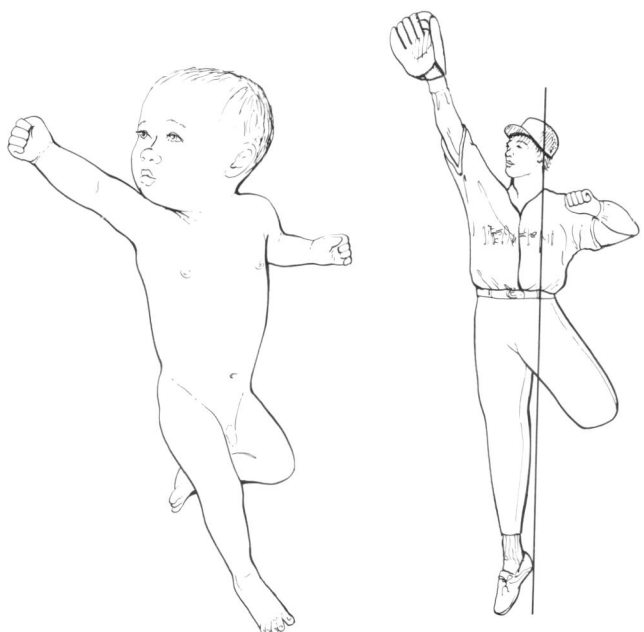

FIGURE 39–6
Neck reflexes are readily elicited in newborns and are expressed in adults when posture requires optimal control. (Adapted from Fukuda, 1961.)

of vestibular and neck receptors on limb muscles were clearly demonstrated by Tristam Roberts for side to side motions in an experiment illustrated in Figure 39–5. Since most voluntary and imposed movements of the head are accompanied by bending or twisting of the neck, the reflexes are generally combined and tend to cancel out.

Vestibular and neck reflexes are readily elicited in newborns and in patients with major cerebral lesions by tilting the head (and body) or by bending the neck. In normal adults, however, these effects are unusual. For example, neck reflexes are seen in the movements of athletes and dancers (Figure 39–6). Passive bending or turning of the neck produces only small changes in muscle activation that are detectable only by electromyographic recordings. However, if the vestibular apparatus is damaged (as may occur in certain diseases or following treatment with some antibiotics) neck reflexes on neck, limb, and even eye muscles become prominent.

Vestibular and Neck Afferents Converge on the Vestibular Nuclei and Propriospinal Neurons

In contrast to the simpler reflexes we examined in earlier chapters, the vestibular and neck reflexes produce complex patterns of facilitation and inhibition in motor neurons innervating widely distributed muscles. Inputs from the otolith organs and proprioceptive inputs from neck afferents are relayed in the vestibular nuclei. Vestibular neurons project to the spinal cord through two vestibulospinal tracts and influence spinal circuits indirectly

through connections with the pontine and medullary reticular formation. Reticular neurons in turn project to the spinal cord in two reticulospinal tracts. Both the vestibulospinal and reticulospinal tracts excite interneurons and long propriospinal neurons responsible for distributing the patterns of excitation and inhibition widely to many groups of motor neurons (see Chapter 35). Both descending systems also make monosynaptic connections (both excitatory and inhibitory) on spinal motor neurons innervating axial muscles of the neck and back. We shall first review the major connections of the vestibulospinal system and, in the next section, examine how vestibular and neck inputs are further integrated by the reticulospinal system.

Inputs to neck motor neurons from the semicircular canals and otolith organs are mediated by neurons in the *medial* and *inferior vestibular nuclei*. The axons of these neurons project bilaterally down the medial vestibulospinal tract to cervical and thoracic segments, where they terminate on the medial motor neuron groups that innervate neck and back muscles and on nearby interneurons and propriospinal neurons (Figure 39–7). Some of these axons make direct excitatory connections with ipsilateral neck motor neurons, others have direct inhibitory connections with contralateral neck motor neurons.

Inputs to limb motor neurons from the otolith organs are mediated by neurons in the *lateral vestibular nucleus* (Deiters's nucleus), which project ipsilaterally to all segments of the spinal cord in the lateral vestibulospinal tract. Axons in this tract primarily facilitate extensor motor neurons and inhibit flexor motor neurons of both the upper and lower extremities through interneurons and propriospinal neurons.

Even though muscle spindles are abundant in neck muscles, direct monosynaptic connections between these muscle afferents and the homonymous motor neurons are very weak. Instead, excitation of homonymous motor neurons produced by stretch of these muscles is mediated by local interneurons. Vestibular and neck afferent signals are integrated at several levels, beginning in the vestibular nuclei, where input from neck muscle spindles strongly modulates the discharge of neurons projecting down both the medial and lateral vestibulospinal tracts. They are also integrated by neurons in the pontine and medullary reticular formation.

Brain Stem and Spinal Mechanisms Play a Major Role in the Control of Posture

The Pontine Reticular Nuclei Facilitate Motor Neurons Whereas Medullary Reticular Nuclei Produce Both Facilitation and Inhibition

The brain stem contains the discrete sensory and motor nuclei of the different cranial nerves and a central core, of more diffusely organized nuclei, called the *reticular formation*. In 1946 Horace Magoun and Ruth Rhines identified two groups of nuclei in the reticular formation of the pons and the medulla that were involved in the control of

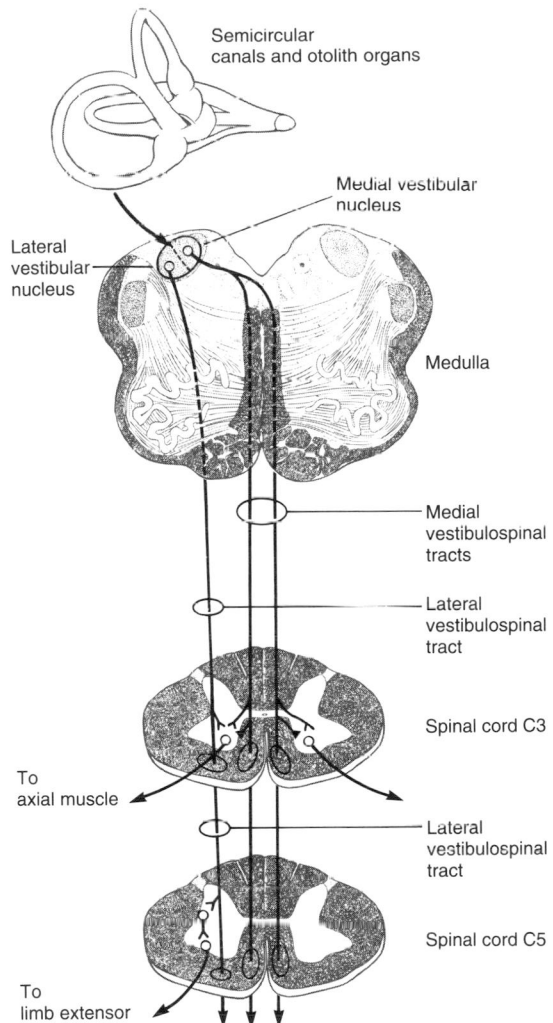

FIGURE 39–7
Vestibulospinal projections to axial and limb motor neurons.

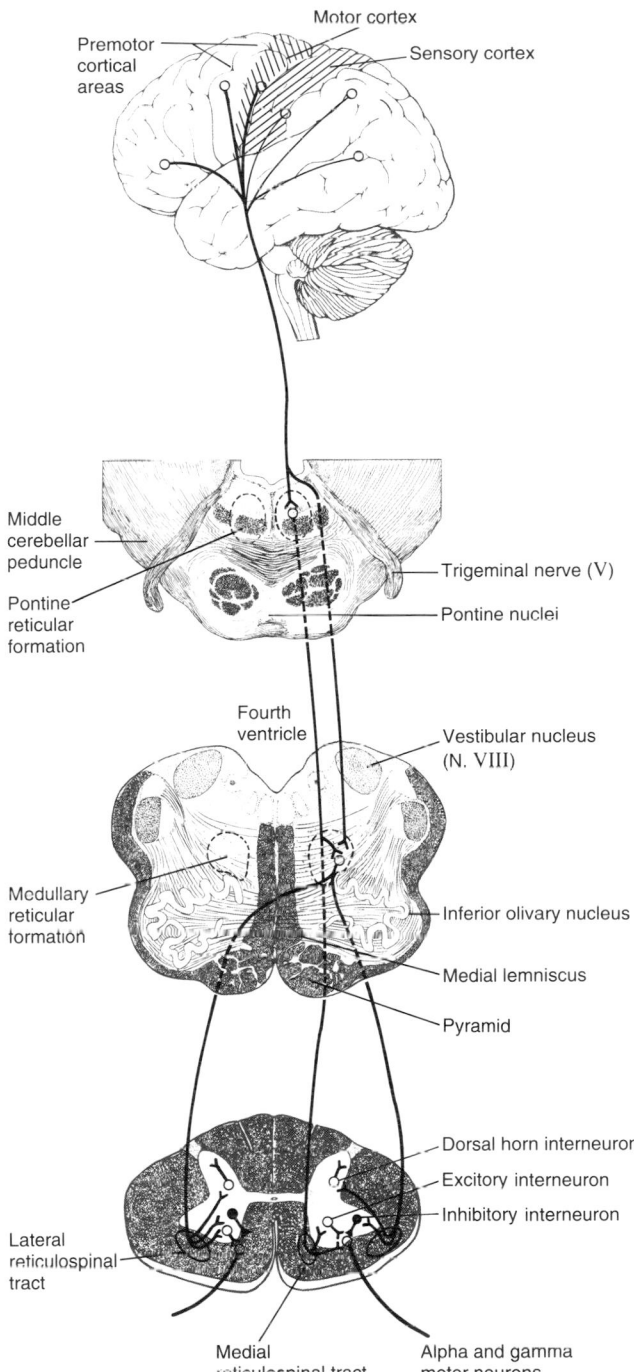

FIGURE 39–8
Reticulospinal and corticoreticular pathways.

posture. Electrical stimulation of nuclei located in the pons *facilitated* spinal reflexes. Stimulation of nuclei located in the medulla *inhibited* spinal reflexes. These nuclei project through the medial and lateral reticulospinal tracts to all levels of the spinal cord (Figure 39–8).

The *pontine reticular formation* consists mainly of the nucleus reticularis pontis oralis and caudalis, and projects ipsilaterally to the spinal cord by way of the *medial reticulospinal tract* in the ventral columns. Most of the axons of this tract terminate on and facilitate motor neurons that innervate axial muscles and extensors of the limbs. The *medullary reticular formation* consists mainly of the gigantocellular nucleus and gives rise to the *lateral reticulospinal tract* that projects bilaterally down the ventral part of the lateral columns. The lateral reticulospinal tract produces monosynaptic inhibition of neck and back motor neurons, much like the medial vestibulospinal tract. The lateral re-

ticulospinal pathway also makes widespread polysynaptic inhibitory connections with extensor motor neurons and excitatory connections with flexor motor neurons (Figure 39–8). In addition to the inhibitory actions suggested by Magoun and Rhines, some axons of the lateral tract also excite motor neurons innervating extensor muscles and inhibit flexors.

Both the medial and the lateral reticulospinal fibers also modulate reflex action during ongoing movements and produce different effects, depending on the movement in progress at the time the stimulus is applied. Thus, Trevor Drew and Serge Rossignol found that in freely moving animals stimulation of a small group of reticular neurons produces extension during the stance phase of locomotion; during the swing phase the same stimulus produces flexion.

The reticulospinal system coordinates posture and movement by integrating vestibular and other sensory inputs with commands from the cerebral cortex (Figure 39–8). The importance of the reticular formation in coordinating the posture and movement of cats has been demonstrated by Gahéry and his colleagues. Whenever a standing cat lifts its forepaw to reach for an object, a stereotyped postural adjustment is set in motion. This consists of a shift in body weight from an even distribution over all four feet to a diagonal pattern, where the weight is borne principally by the nonreaching forelimb and the hindlimb ipsilateral to the movement. This shift balances the animal during the limb movement. The same shift can also be induced in an alert cat by electrically stimulating the forelimb area of the cerebral cortex with implanted electrodes. However, if the medullary reticular formation is pharmacologically inactivated, the anticipatory postural adjustments do not occur during the limb movement. Instead, the cat loses balance transiently and relies on a rapid feedback to correct its balance. This shows that even though the corticospinal pathway causes the limb to contract the postural adjustment is governed indirectly through the corticoreticulospinal system.

Section of the Brain Stem above the Vestibular Nuclei Produces Decerebrate Rigidity

In humans and many other animals, transection of the brain stem above the level of the vestibular nuclei but below the red nucleus produces *decerebrate rigidity*. In quadrupeds, where it was first described by Sherrington in 1896, all four limbs become tonically extended: The animal stands unsupported in a posture that Sherrington called exaggerated standing. Believing this to be a useful model for understanding normal posture, Sherrington analyzed the processes that control muscle tone in the decerebrate state. Even though these studies revealed important principles of neural integration and first demonstrated the role of afferent input in the maintenance of posture, decerebrate animals cannot regulate posture when the support surface is unstable.

When decerebration occurs in primates, or when it occurs in patients as a result of cerebral hemorrhage or large tumors, it produces a less pronounced increase in extensor tone. Typically, the classical extensor posture is intermittent or seen only if a noxious peripheral stimulus is ap-

plied to a bony pressure point, such as the sternum or forehead. Eliciting decerebrate posture and other brain stem reflexes (such as vestibulo-ocular reflexes; see Chapter 43) is helpful in diagnosing the condition of a patient in coma by indicating the approximate level of residual function within the nervous system.

Decerebrate posture results from the combined effects of tonic activity in the vestibulospinal and pontine reticulospinal neurons, whose dominant action is to activate both alpha and gamma motor neurons that innervate extensor muscles (Figure 39–9). As a result, stretch reflexes of extensor muscles are hyperactive and muscle tone in these muscles is increased. As we saw in Chapter 38, Sherrington found that the tonic muscle contraction of the decerebrate limb disappears when the dorsal roots are cut. This interrupts the stretch reflex, preventing spindle endings from providing tonic facilitation to motor neurons. The profound effect of cutting the dorsal root on decerebrate rigidity provides an indication of the importance of stretch reflexes in maintaining muscle tone. Other factors also contribute to extensor rigidity following decerebration. For example, tonic activity in reticulospinal and aminergic brain stem fibers also inhibits polysynaptic flexion reflex pathways of the spinal cord.

Lesions of the Cerebellum Modify Vestibular and Reticular Influences on Posture

Since activity of neurons in the vestibular and reticular nuclei is maintained by tonic input from the otolith organs, cutting the vestibular nerves reduces decerebrate rigidity. The activity of these vestibular and reticular neurons is modulated by the cerebellum, which can thus influence muscle tone throughout the body. Sherrington found that stimulation of the anterior lobe of the cerebellar cortex reduces decerebrate rigidity; destruction of this region increases contraction of tonic extensors and produces hyperextension of the neck. As we shall see in Chapter 41, the output neurons of the cerebellar cortex, the Purkinje neurons, inhibit their target neurons, which include the cells of the lateral vestibular nucleus. Therefore when this part of the cerebellum is destroyed, neurons that give rise to the lateral vestibulospinal tract are released from inhibition and then facilitate extensor motor neurons.

Stereotyped decerebrate posture no longer occurs when the brain stem is transected above the level of the red nucleus. Then, posture is regulated by rubrospinal and other tonically active midbrain neurons that project to the spinal cord. Activity in these pathways opposes that of the vestibulo- and reticulospinal systems of the lower brain stem. After the transection, postural ability differs considerably among species, depending on the size and distribution of rubrospinal fibers and on the degree of control exerted by the cerebral cortex on postural mechanisms. In cats and monkeys, which have a substantial rubrospinal pathway, tonic activity in this system, which pre-

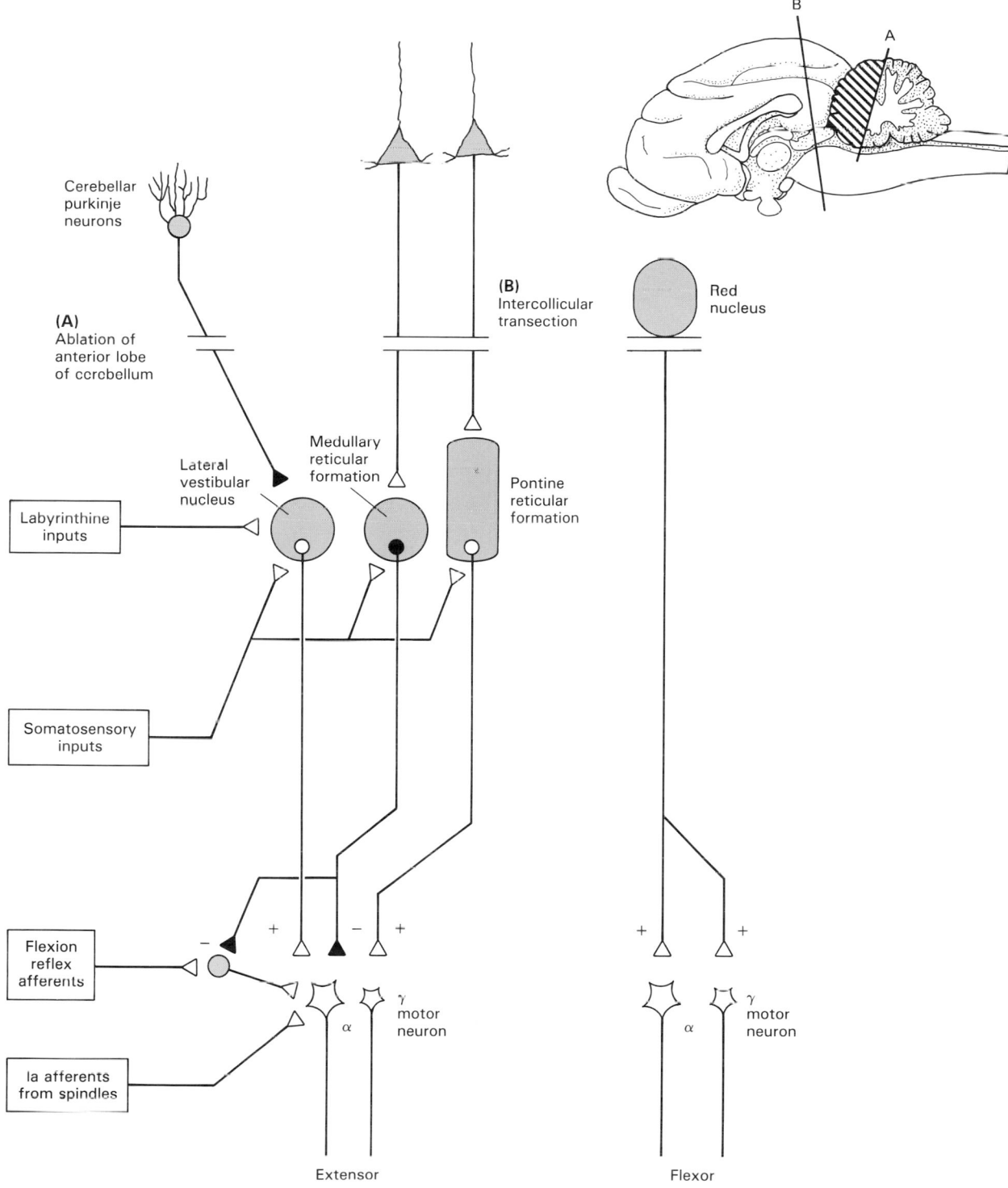

FIGURE 39–9

Decerebrate rigidity is mediated primarily by the vestibulospinal and reticulospinal pathways, which are tonically active when disconnected from cerebral control. Decerebrate rigidity is modulated by the cerebellum and is enhanced following removal of the anterior lobe of the cerebellum because a major inhibitory input to the lateral vestibular nucleus, the Purkinje neurons, is then moved. Excitatory and inhibitory reticulospinal influences on extensor motor neurons tend to cancel each other; however, reticulospinal inhibition of interneurons mediating flexion reflexes adds to the overall extensor bias.

dominantly facilitates flexors and inhibits extensors (see Chapter 35), counteracts the actions of vestibulo- and reticulospinal neurons. The so-called midbrain cat is able to right itself and exhibits a varied repertory of postural responses. These responses are more limited in monkeys, in which behavioral control and balance are dependent to a greater degree on the cerebral cortex.

Humans with severe lesions of the cerebral hemispheres but whose brain stem circuitry is still intact exhibit a postural state known as *decorticate rigidity*. In this condition the extensors of the legs and the flexors of the arm contract steadily. One reason for this is that the rubrospinal tract in humans only projects as far as the cervical cord and may counteract vestibulospinal facilitation of arm but not leg extensors.

Spasticity Is a Common Manifestation of Supraspinal Lesions in Humans

Lesions of the premotor areas or their outflow produce *spasticity*, a form of increased muscle tone. In patients the extensor muscles in the legs and flexors in the arms typically show the greatest increase in tone, much as in decorticate rigidity. Spasticity is associated with hyperactive stretch reflexes and tendon jerks: When a limb is moved passively the measured resistance varies with the speed of the movement. A movement rapidly imposed meets greater resistance than a slow one and may elicit clonus. The reduced threshold of the stretch reflex results from increased excitability of the monosynaptic pathway itself, and the weakness of these patients results in part from abnormalities in the recruitment of motor units.

In spastic patients, when passive movements are imposed slowly on the limb segment, measured resistance may abruptly melt away (a response called the *clasp knife phenomenon*). This sudden drop in muscle force depends on joint angle and muscle length. This length-dependent inhibition results from the activation of afferents in the muscle that are distinct from those in muscle spindles. In experimental animals this reflex is released by lesioning reticulospinal axons.

In clinical practice it is important to distinguish *spasticity* from *rigidity*, which also involves increased resistance to passive movement of the limb and which occurs in diseases of the basal ganglia, notably in Parkinson's disease (see Chapter 41).[2] The increased tone in Parkinsonian and other forms of rigidity has a more plastic character. Once the limb segment has been rotated it tends to remain at the same angle when the examiner releases it. In contrast to spasticity, this increase in tone is evenly distributed to flexors and extensors. While in rigidity there is no increase in monosynaptic reflexes or tendon jerks,

long-latency polysynaptic effects also produced by muscle stretch appear to be markedly increased. This increase is thought to result from the activity in pathways involving the primary motor cortex (see Chapter 40).

An Overall View

A characteristic feature of voluntary movements is that subjects respond more quickly to a stimulus if they know in advance the response required. The latency of voluntary responses is longer when the subject must choose which response to make, using information from the stimulus. This is not so for postural responses: Subjects make the correct responses at the same latency to body sway whether they expect to be moved in one way or another. For this reason postural responses are thought to be governed by organized motor programs that are merely triggered by external perturbations.

While postural set probably involves the gating of short-latency feedback pathways through the cortex, postural set also prepares lower level feedback mechanisms to respond appropriately to disturbances. Thus the stretch reflex itself can be enhanced or reduced according to the needs for postural stabilization during rapid voluntary movements. Similar graded adjustments in stretch reflex occur during locomotion.

A rich variety of reflex circuits coordinate the muscle contractions needed to maintain the head vertical and aligned with the body. Inputs from the vestibular labyrinth maintain the head in a vertical orientation and neck reflexes maintain the head aligned with the body. Vestibular and neck reflexes also act on limb muscles to cushion falls and to stabilize the body in relation to the support surface. Much of the neuronal circuitry that coordinates movements is located in the brain stem and spinal cord and integrates information from the labyrinth and neck receptors. The patterns of coordinated activity that they generate are used in a variety of automatic postural tasks but are normally under powerful descending control. Lesions of the brain stem and spinal cord give rise to alterations in posture and to stereotyped stimuli, and are important to characterize abnormal clinical conditions.

Selected Readings

Brodal, A. 1981. Neurological Anatomy in Relation to Clinical Medicine, 3rd ed. New York: Oxford University Press.

Gahéry, Y., and Massion, J. 1981. Co-ordination between posture and movement. Trends Neurosci. 4:199–202.

Magnus, R. 1926. Physiology of posture. Part I. Local static reactions. Lancet ii:531–536.

Magnus, R. 1926. Physiology of posture. Part II. General static reactions of the mid-brain animal. Lancet ii:585–588.

Nashner, L. M. 1982. Adaptation of human movement to altered environments. Trends. Neurosci. 5:358–361.

Nashner, L. M. 1983. Analysis of movement control in man using the movable platform. In J. E. Desmedt (ed.), Motor Control Mechanisms in Health and Disease. Advances in Neurology, Vol. 39. New York: Raven Press, pp. 607–619.

---

[2]By convention the term *rigidity* is used clinically to refer to the alteration in tone in diseases of the basal ganglia. It should not be confused with the conditions of decerebrate or decorticate rigidity. Physiologically, these are more closely related to spasticity.

Peterson, B. W., and Richmond, F. J. (eds.) 1988. Control of Head Movement. New York: Oxford University Press.

Plum, F., and Posner, J. B. 1980. The Diagnosis of Stupor and Coma. Philadelphia: F. A. Davis.

Roberts, T. D. M. 1979. Neurophysiology of Postural Mechanisms. London: Butterworths.

Wilson, V. J., and Peterson, B. W. 1981. Vestibulospinal and reticulospinal systems. In V. B. Brooks (ed.), Handbook of Physiology, Section 1: The Nervous System, Vol. II. Motor Control, Part 1. Bethesda: American Physiological Society, pp. 667–702.

References

Andrews, C., Knowles, L., and Lance, J. W. 1973. Corticoreticulospinal control of the tonic vibration reflex in the cat. J. Neurol. Sci. 18:207–216.

Beloozerova, I. N., and Sirota, M. G. 1988. Role of motor cortex in control of locomotion. In V. S. Gurfinkel, M. E. Ioffe, J. Massion, and J. P. Roll (eds.), Stance and Motion: Facts and Concepts. New York: Plenum Press, pp. 163–176.

Bjursten, L.-M., Norrsell, K., and Norrsell, U. 1976. Behavioural repertory of cats without cerebral cortex from infancy. Exp. Brain Res. 25:115–130.

Brink, E. E., Suzuki, I., Timerick, S. J. B., and Wilson, V. J. 1985. Tonic neck reflex of the decerebrate cat: A role for propriospinal neurons. J. Neurophysiol. 54:978–987.

Cordo, P. J., and Nashner, L. M. 1982. Properties of postural adjustments associated with rapid arm movements. J. Neurophysiol. 47:287–302.

Dichgans, J., Bizzi, E., Morasso, P., and Taghasco, V. 1973. Mechanisms underlying recovery of eye-head coordination following bilateral labyrinthectomy in monkeys. Exp. Brain Res. 18:548–562.

Drew, T., and Rossignol, S. 1984. Phase-dependent responses evoked in limb muscles by stimulation of medullary reticular formation during locomotion in thalamic cats. J. Neurophysiol. 52:653–675.

Drew, T., and Rossignol, S. 1990. Functional organization within the medullary reticular formation of intact unanesthetized cat. I. Movements evoked by microstimulation. J. Neurophysiol. 64:767–781.

Drew, T., and Rossignol, S. 1990. Functional organization within the medullary reticular formation of intact unanesthetized cat. II. Electromyographic activity evoked by microstimulation. J. Neurophysiol. 64:782–795.

Feldman, M. H. 1971. The decerebrate state in the primate. I. Studies in monkeys. Arch. Neurol. 25:501–516.

Feldman, M. H., and Sahrmann, S. 1971. The decerebrate state in the primate. II. Studies in man. Arch. Neurol. 25:517–525.

Fukuda, T. 1961. Studies on human dynamic postures from the viewpoint of postural reflexes. Acta. Oto-Laryngol. Suppl. 161:1–52.

Gillies, J. D., Burke, D. J., and Lance, J. W. 1971. Supraspinal control of tonic vibration reflex. J. Neurophysiol. 34.302–309.

Gurfinkel, V. S., and Shik, M. L. 1973. The control of posture and locomotion. In A. A. Gydikov, N. T. Tankov, and D. S. Kosarov (eds.), Motor Control. New York: Plenum Press, pp. 217–234.

Horak, F. B, and Nashner, L. M. 1986. Central programming of postural movements: Adaptation to altered support-surface configurations. J. Neurophysiol. 55:1369–1381.

Lacquaniti, F., and Maioli, C. 1989. The role of preparation in tuning anticipatory and reflex responses during catching. J. Neurosci. 9:134–148.

Lindsay, K. W., Roberts, T. D. M., and Rosenberg, J. R. 1976. Asymmetric tonic labyrinth reflexes and their interaction with neck reflexes in the decerebrate cat. J. Physiol. (Lond.) 261:583–601.

Luccarini, P., Gahery, Y., and Pompeiano, O. 1990. Cholinoceptive pontine reticular structures modify the postural adjustements during the limb movements induced by cortical stimulation. Arch. Ital. Biol. 128:19–45.

Magoun, H. W. 1963. The Waking Brain, 2nd ed. Springfield, Ill.: Thomas, chap. 2, "Reticulo-spinal influences and postural regulation." Springfield, Ill.: Thomas, pp. 23–38.

Magoun, H. W., and Rhines, R. 1946. An inhibitory mechanism in the bulbar reticular formation. J. Neurophysiol 9:165–171.

Mott, F. W., and Sherrington, C. S. 1895. Experiments upon the influence of sensory nerves upon movement and nutrition of the limbs. Preliminary communication. Proc. R. Soc. Lond. 57:481–488.

Nashner, L. M. 1976. Adapting reflexes controlling the human posture. Exp. Brain Res. 26:59–72.

Pal'tsev, Ye. I., and El'ner, A. M. 1967. Preparatory and compensatory period during voluntary movement in patients with involvement of the brain of different localization. Biophysics 12:161–168.

Rademaker, G. G. J. 1924. The significance of the red nuclei and the other parts of the mesencephalon for muscle tonus for normal attitudes and for labyrinthine reflexes. Brain 47:390–393.

Sherrington, C. S. 1898. Decerebrate rigidity, and reflex coordination of movements. J. Physiol. (Lond.) 22.319–332.

Stein, R. B., and Capaday, C. 1988. The modulation of human reflexes during functional motor tasks. Trends Neurosci. 11:328–332.

Tokizane T., Murao, M., Ogata, T., and Kondo, T. 1951. Electromyographic studies on tonic neck, lumbar and labyrinthine reflexes in normal persons. Jap. J. Physiol. 2:130–146.

Wilson, V. J., Schor, R. H., Suzuki, I., and Park, B. R. 1986. Spatial organization of neck and vestibular reflexes acting on the forelimbs of the decerebrate cat. J. Neurophysiol. 55:514–526.

40

Claude Ghez

Voluntary Movement

The Motor Areas of the Cerebral Cortex Are Organized Somatotopically

The Primary Motor, Supplementary Motor, and Premotor Areas Contribute the Majority of Axons in the Corticospinal Tract

Inputs to Motor Areas from the Periphery, Cerebellum, and Basal Ganglia Are Mediated by Other Areas of Cortex and the Thalamus

Corticospinal Axons Influence Segmental Motor Neurons Through Direct and Indirect Connections

Neurons of the Primary Motor Cortex Encode the Direction of the Force Exerted

Individual Corticospinal Neurons Control Small Groups of Muscles

Neurons in the Primary Motor Cortex Encode the Amount of Force to Be Exerted

Movement Direction Is Encoded by Populations of Neurons, Not by Single Cells

Neurons in the Motor Cortex Are Informed of the Consequences of Movements

Premotor Cortical Areas Prepare the Motor Systems for Movement

Motor Preparation Time Is Longer Than the Response Time to Stimuli

Lesions of the Premotor Cortex, Supplementary Motor, and Posterior Parietal Areas Impair the Ability to Execute Purposeful Movements

The Supplementary Motor Area Is Important in Programming Motor Sequences and in the Coordination of Bilateral Movements

The Premotor Cortex Controls the Proximal Movements that Project the Arm to Targets

The Posterior Parietal Lobe Plays a Critical Role in Providing the Visual Information for Targeted Movements

An Overall View

Voluntary movements differ from reflex movements in several important ways. First, voluntary movements are purposeful. The motor systems can use different strategies in different circumstances to achieve the same end. For example, when writing on a piece of paper we use primarily the fingers and wrist, but writing on a blackboard we use the arm and shoulder. Donald Hebb called this flexibility of strategy *motor equivalence*. Second, the effectiveness of voluntary movements improves with experience and learning. Thus, the precision of a reach or a throw increases and its variability decreases with practice. The muscle contractions of successive responses become more efficient as co-contraction and movement time decrease. Third, although voluntary movements may be evoked by sensory stimuli as are reflexes, an external stimulus need not precede them. Thus, the trajectory of our hand is the same when we reach for a real target or to its remembered or imagined location. The higher levels of our motor systems can therefore dissociate the information content of a stimulus—which tells us *where* or *how* to move—from its capacity to trigger movement—which tells us *when* to move. Moreover, many movements are initiated by thoughts or emotions as acts of will.

The neural events leading even to a simple voluntary movement, such as reaching for a glass of water, involve three complex processes: identification and localization of the target, a plan of action, and execution of the movement. First, the glass is identified and its position located in space. Second, a plan of action is selected that will bring the glass to the mouth. To specify which body parts are needed and in what direction they are to be moved, the location of the glass must be assessed in relation to the position of the hand and body. This information allows the motor systems to determine the hand's trajectory. Finally, the response is executed. Commands are conveyed by the cortical and brain stem descending pathways to the final common pathway, the motor neurons. These commands specify the temporal sequence of muscle activation, the forces to be developed, and the changes in joint angles. In addition, while reaching, the hand and fingers are oriented to fit the contours of the glass, coordinating movements of the shoulder and arm with those at the wrist and digits so that the glass will be grasped on contact without delay.

These three phases, target identification, plan of action, and execution are governed by distinct regions of the cerebral cortex: the posterior parietal cortex, the premotor areas of the frontal cortex, and the primary motor cortex. We shall begin by considering the organization of these three cortical areas. There are distinct somatotopic motor maps within each of these motor areas. Then we examine how the primary motor cortex encodes the features of movements and how the premotor and association areas participate in planning movement and programming its various components.

The Motor Areas of the Cerebral Cortex Are Organized Somatotopically

In 1870 Gustav Fritsch and Eduard Hitzig provided the first direct evidence that distinct areas of the brain control movement on the contralateral side of the body. They discovered that electrical stimulation of different parts of the cortex of dogs produces contractions of different contralateral muscles. These observations were soon extended to monkeys by David Ferrier, who elicited movements of contralateral limbs by stimulating the precentral and postcentral gyri and movements of the eyes by stimulating the posterior parietal cortex. Alfred Leyton and Sherrington next discovered that in primates motor effects are elicited most readily from the precentral gyrus. This region corresponds to Brodmann's area 4 and is now called the *primary motor cortex.*

The discovery that different areas of cerebral cortex control movements of different parts of the body had immediate clinical relevance. It explained why damage of different areas of the contralateral frontal lobe results in weakness of the face, arm, or leg. It also enabled clinicians to understand the mechanism of focal motor seizures. For example, the Jacksonian seizure, described by Hughlings Jackson, typically begins with a series of tonic and clonic (abrupt, intense, and repetitive) involuntary contractions of muscles on one side, commonly the finger flexors. The contractions then gradually spread proximally to the wrist, then to the elbow, shoulder, trunk, and other muscles. The abrupt, intense muscle jerks that occur during the seizure resemble those elicited by cortical stimulation. Jackson correctly surmised that the sequential activation of different muscle groups during the seizure results from the progressive spread of abnormal motor activity from a site in the cortex controlling distal extremity muscles to ones that control more proximal ones. Frequently, these focal seizures are triggered by tumors, scars, or other abnormalities in nearby areas of the brain. The neurosurgeon Wilder Penfield used cortical stimulation, a technique he learned from Sherrington, in patients undergoing brain surgery to identify functional areas that had to be spared when excising abnormal tissue in the brain.

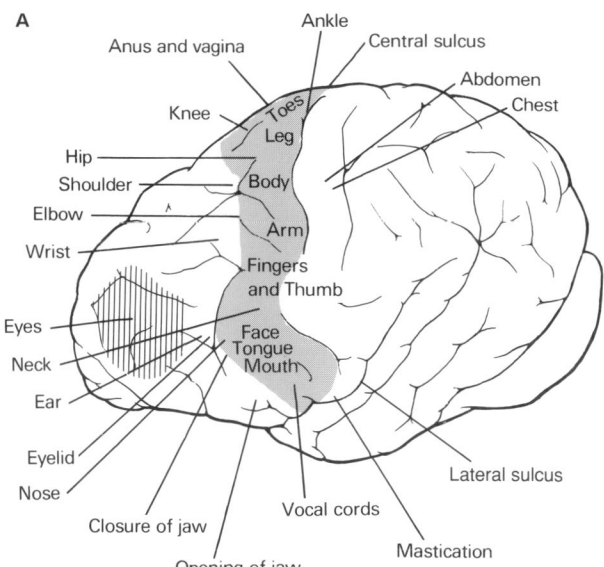

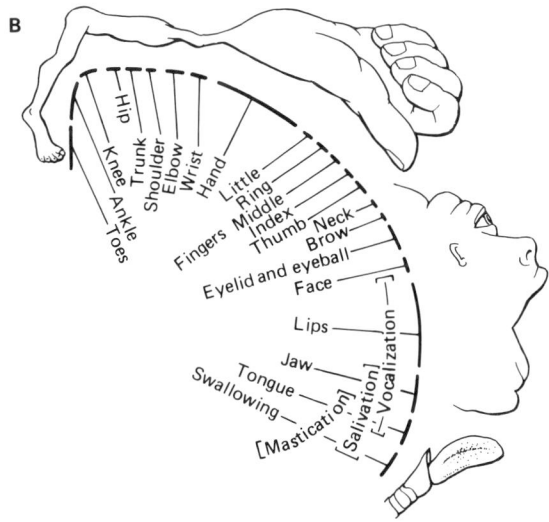

FIGURE 40–1

Comparison of the somatotopic representation in the primary motor cortex in chimpanzees (**A**) and humans (**B**). This sequence of representation is similar, with the ankles being medial, and the face, mouth, and muscles of mastication lateral. But the human motor cortex has a much larger representation of the face and digits. (Part A from Leyton and Sherrington, 1917; part B adapted from Penfield and Rasmussen, 1950.)

Penfield's work in patients and similar studies by Clinton Woolsey in monkeys showed that the primary motor cortex contains a *motor map* of the body. The head is represented close to the lateral sulcus; above it are representations of the arms, trunk, and legs (Figure 40–1A). As with the sensory maps, not all body parts are represented equally in the motor map. The parts of the body used in tasks requiring precision and fine control, such as the face and hands, have a disproportionately large representation in the motor map (Figure 40–1B).

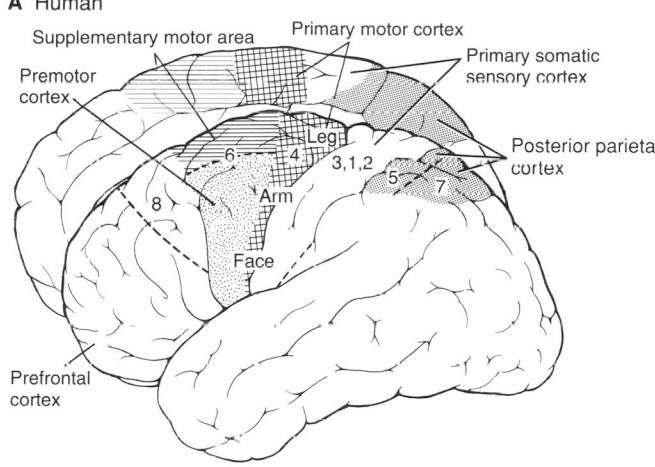

A Human

Supplementary motor area

Primary motor cortex

Premotor cortex

Primary somatic sensory cortex

Posterior parietal cortex

Leg

6   4

3,1,2

5   7

Arm

8

Face

Prefrontal cortex

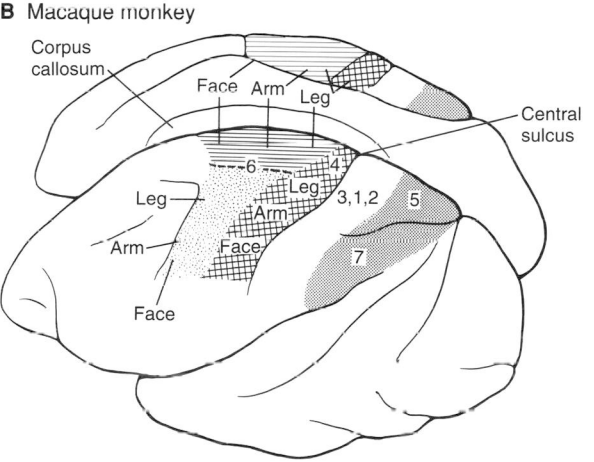

B Macaque monkey

Corpus callosum

Face Arm Leg

Central sulcus

6   4

Leg

Leg   3,1,2   5

Arm

Arm   Face

7

Face

FIGURE 40–2

Locations of the primary and premotor cortical areas in humans (**A**) and the macaque monkey (**B**). Behind the primary motor areas lies the somatic sensory cortex, Brodmann's areas 3, 1, 2, and the posterior parietal cortex, areas 5 and 7.

The studies by Penfield and Woolsey also revealed that stimulation in Brodmann's area 6, anterior to the primary motor cortex, could also produce motor effects. These areas are called the *premotor areas*. The axons of neurons in the premotor areas project to the primary motor cortex, as well as to subcortical structures and to the spinal cord. While the size of the primary motor cortex remains constant across primate phylogeny in proportion to body weight, the premotor areas increase in size sixfold from the macaque monkey to humans. There are two principal premotor areas: the *supplementary motor area* (sometimes referred to as the *secondary motor cortex*, or MII), located on the superior and medial aspects of the hemisphere, and the *premotor cortex*, located on the lateral surface of the hemisphere (Figure 40–2). Movements produced by stimulation of the supplementary motor or premotor areas are more complex and require larger stimulus currents than those produced by stimulation of

the primary motor cortex. Stimulation of the premotor areas typically evokes coordinated contractions of muscles at more than one joint and, in the case of the supplementary motor area, on both sides of the body as well. The supplementary motor and premotor areas are also organized somatotopically. Anatomical studies have identified additional premotor areas, notably one located within the cingulate gyrus (area 24), which may be important in allowing motivation to influence motor planning directly.

The Primary Motor, Supplementary Motor, and Premotor Areas Contribute the Majority of Axons in the Corticospinal Tract

The cytoarchitecture of the three cortical motor areas differs from that of the sensory areas behind them and the prefrontal areas in front. Layer 4, the major input layer for sensory cortices, is absent in the motor areas. Since layer 4 is called the *internal granular layer*, these motor areas are referred to as *agranular cortex* (Figure 40–3A). Layer 5 in the primary motor cortex contains a distinctive population of giant (50–80 mm in diameter) pyramidal neurons, the Betz cells, named after their discoverer Vladimir Betz. The axons of these cells run in the corticospinal tract. The 30,000 Betz cells represent only one of several populations of nerve cells contributing to the one million axons that make up the corticospinal tract. The tract originates from neurons of all sizes in layer 5 (Figure 40–3B). About half of the axons in the tract come from the primary motor cortex (Brodmann's area 4). Most of the others come from cells in area 6, mainly from the supplementary motor area; a smaller proportion arises from the lateral premotor area and somatic sensory cortex (areas 3, 2, and 1). As noted in Chapter 35, axons of the corticospinal tract originating from the motor cortex terminate in the intermediate and the ventral zones of the spinal cord, while those from the somatic sensory cortex terminate primarily in the dorsal horn.

Inputs to Motor Areas from the Periphery, Cerebellum, and Basal Ganglia Are Mediated by Other Areas of Cortex and the Thalamus

The motor areas of the cerebral cortex receive input from three sources. First, they receive information from the periphery. This input is transmitted either directly to the primary motor cortex from the thalamus (nucleus VPLo) and the primary somatosensory cortex, or indirectly to the premotor areas from the sensory association areas. Second, the motor areas receive input from the cerebellum. This input is principally distributed to the primary and premotor cortex by way of the thalamus (the oral part of the ventral posterolateral nucleus, VPLo, the caudal part of the ventrolateral nucleus VLc, and a recently identified subdivision of the thalamus referred to as area X). The third source of input is the globus pallidus of the basal ganglia. This input is also relayed through the thalamus, however, from an area situated more anteriorly (the oral part of the ventrolateral nucleus VLo, and the ventral anterior nucleus VA) than the cerebellar relay (Figure 40–4A).

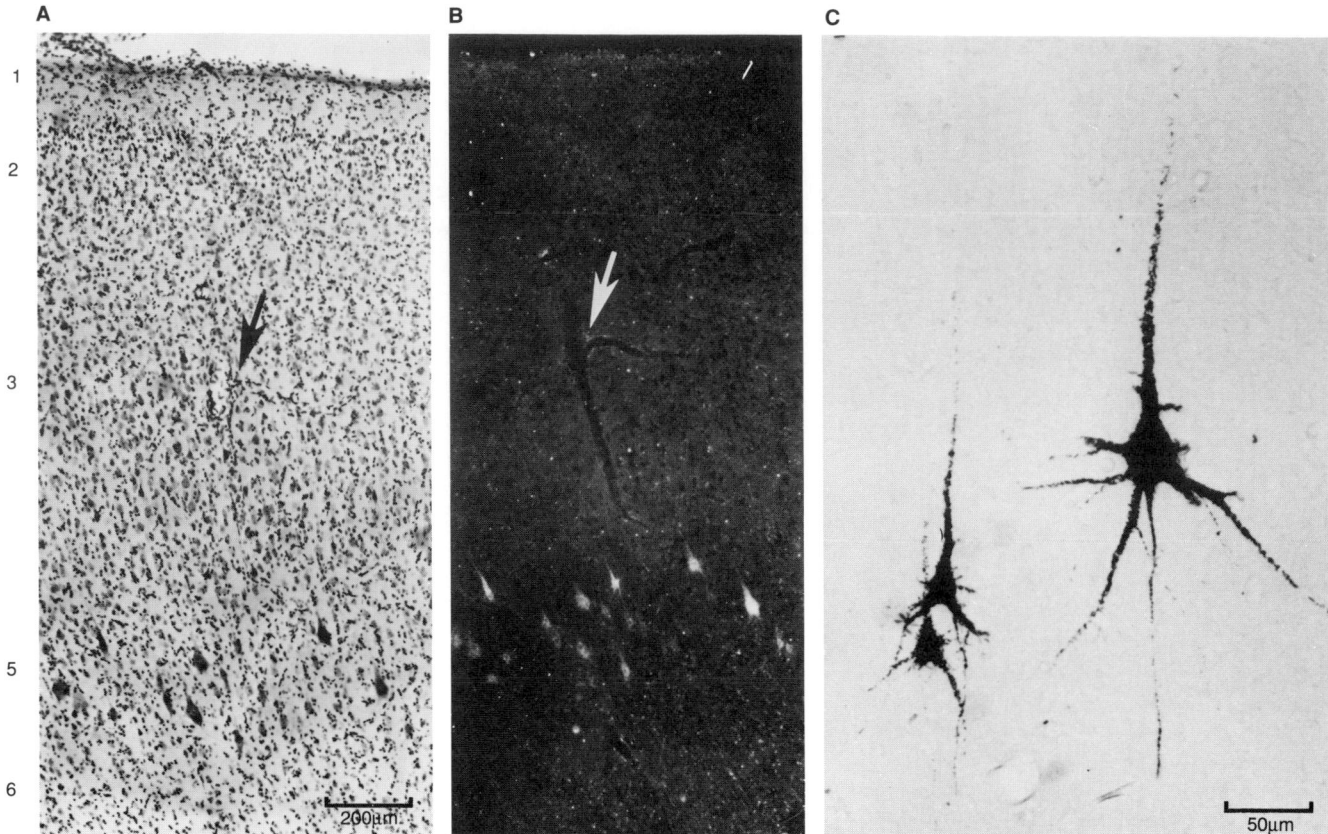

FIGURE 40–3

In the primary motor cortex, layer 4 (also called the *internal granular layer*) is reduced or absent, and layer 5 contains large and small pyramidal neurons. As a result, the motor cortex is called the *agranular cortex*. (From Murray and Coulter, 1981.) Bright-field (**A**) and dark-field (**B**) photomicrographs of Nissl-stained monkey primary motor cortex with corticospinal neurons retrogradely labeled following horseradish peroxidase injection into the contralateral lumbar spinal cord. The labeled neurons are better visualized under dark-field illumination (**B**). In both photographs arrows point to the same branch of the blood vessel. A cluster of three corticospinal neurons of different sizes are located in layer 5 (**C**). These neurons were retrogradely labeled from the contralateral spinal cord.

The motor cortical areas also receive important input from the sensory cortex and sensory association areas. In the monkey there are significant connections to the primary motor cortex from the primary somatic sensory cortices, Brodmann's area 2, and the posterior parietal somatic association area, Brodmann's area 5. These connections are organized in a homotopic fashion. Moreover, areas of motor cortex representing a given body part receive sensory input from the portion of sensory cortex representing the same body part. In addition, intracortical input to the primary motor cortex arises in the lateral and supplementary motor areas, which are in turn influenced by primary input from posterior parietal and prefrontal association cortices (Figure 40–4).

Corticospinal Axons Influence Segmental Motor Neurons Through Direct and Indirect Connections

How do corticospinal neurons act on the spinal motor neurons? By stimulating the primary motor cortex and recording synaptic potentials in spinal motor neurons,

James Preston and Charles Phillips separately discovered that corticospinal neurons in primates make powerful and direct excitatory connections with alpha motor neurons. Corticospinal axons also excite gamma motor neurons through polysynaptic pathways. As we have seen, this coactivation of alpha and gamma motor neurons allows muscle spindles to sense changes in muscle length, even when limb movement produces muscle shortening (see Chapter 37).

Besides direct connections, corticospinal neurons influence motor neurons indirectly. Anders Lundberg and his co-workers have found that one important indirect pathway to the motor neurons innervating the muscles of the arm involves propriospinal neurons in the upper cervical segments of the spinal cord that project to motor nuclei located two or more segments below. A second indirect path involves the Ia inhibitory interneuron that mediates the disynaptic corticospinal inhibition of motor neurons.

Although the corticospinal tract projects to motor nuclei controlling proximal and distal muscles, the role of the corticospinal tract is to control the distal muscles of

A

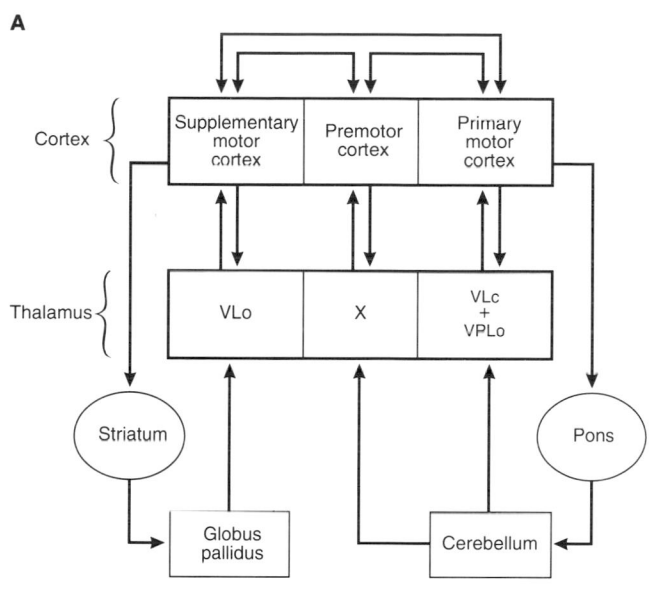

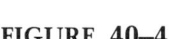

B

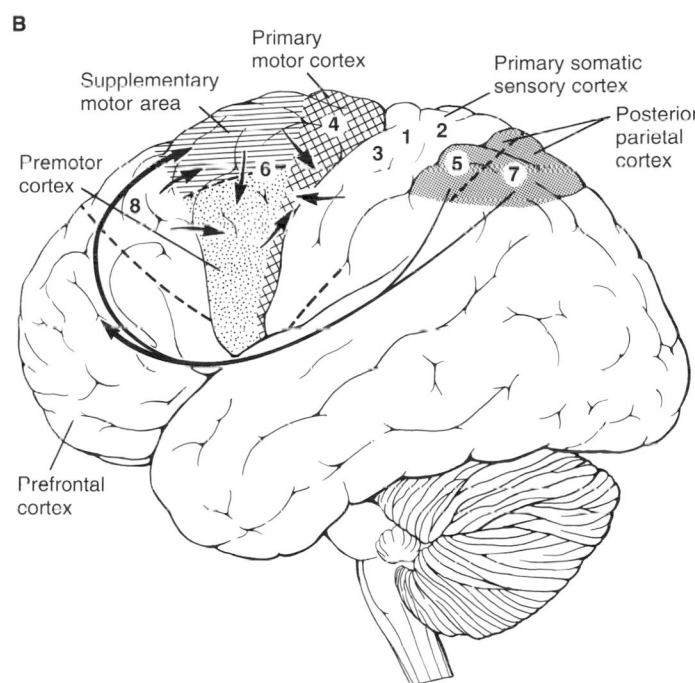

FIGURE 40–4

The motor areas receive both subcortical and corticocortical input.

A. Subcortical input from thalamic nuclei. **VLo** and **VLc** are, respectively, the oral (rostral) and caudal portions of the ventro-

lateral nucleus and thalamus. **VPLo** is the oral portion of the ventral posterolateral nucleus and **X** represents nucleus X.

B. Corticocortical connections. Although the arrows are unidirectional, the interconnecting pathways are reciprocal.

the fingers. Indeed, the synaptic potentials produced by cortical stimuli are largest in motor neurons innervating distal muscle. Destruction of the primary motor cortex abolishes not only all effects on distal muscles that normally result from stimulation of the motor cortex, but also abolishes the distal effects produced by stimulation of premotor and supplementary motor areas. Thus, both the supplementary motor area and the premotor cortex act on distal muscles principally through their projections to the primary motor cortex.

The motor cortical areas also exert indirect control over spinal motor neurons through parallel projections to brain stem neurons. For example, neurons in the primary motor cortex and premotor and supplementary motor areas terminate on reticulospinal and other brain stem neurons that project to the spinal cord. These various polysynaptic connections allow motor cortical areas to control complex patterns of muscle activation whose details are organized either in the spinal cord or brain stem.

Neurons of the Primary Motor Cortex Encode the Direction of the Force Exerted

Individual Corticospinal Neurons Control Small Groups of Muscles

The discovery of a somatotopic motor map in the primary motor cortex led Hiroshi Asanuma and his colleagues in

the 1960s to ask: How finely detailed is this map? Asanuma inserted microelectrodes into the motor cortex and stimulated small groups of neurons. Using low-current stimuli that activate only a dozen neurons, he was able to produce the isolated contraction of individual muscles. Asanuma next discovered that the sites where stimulation produces contraction of a given muscle are arranged in radial arrays, similar to the columns of neurons found in the somatic sensory and visual cortices.

Despite this fine localization, detailed mapping studies with microelectrodes have shown that certain muscles, notably distal muscles, are represented at more than one site. Conversely, cortical stimuli that activate a given muscle frequently also influence several other muscles. More importantly, Eberhard Fetz and Paul Cheney discovered that individual corticospinal axons frequently diverge to influence monosynaptically the motor neurons that innervate several muscles. However, this divergence is small for the most distal muscles of the fingers. This divergence has now been confirmed anatomically (Figure 40–5).

Neurons in the Primary Motor Cortex Encode the Amount of Force to Be Exerted

While ablation and stimulation studies show that specific cortical motor areas control movements of contralateral body parts, they provide no clues as to how these areas

FIGURE 40–5

Corticospinal axons have multiple branches within the spinal cord. A single axon identified physiologically was injected with horseradish peroxidase and its course was reconstructed.

A. Longitudinal view showing branches terminating at several levels.

B. Transverse view showing terminations in four different motor nuclei. (From Shinoda et al., 1981.)

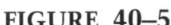
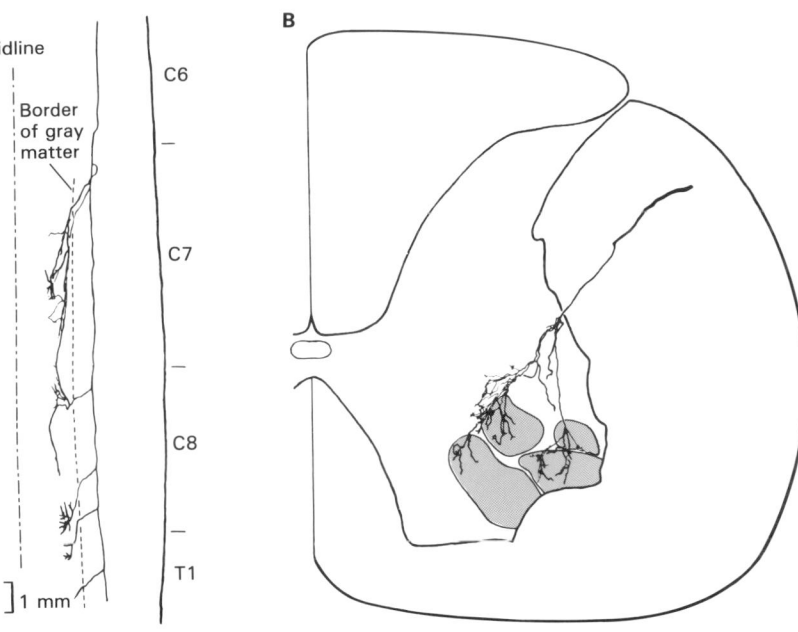

A

Midline

Border of gray matter

C6

C7

C8

T1

] 1 mm

B

might participate in its initiation or control. In order to address this question we would have to know how neuronal discharge is modulated during the performance of a motor task itself. Edward Evarts was the first to investigate this issue by recording from single neurons in the primary motor cortex of monkeys trained to perform various simple tasks. He studied how cortical neurons in the wrist area of primary motor cortex are modulated during flexion and extension of the wrist (Figure 40–6B). He found that different populations of neurons were active during flexion and during extension and that the modulation in their activity typically occurred *before* the contraction of the relevant muscles. This provided direct evidence that the primary motor cortex actually participates in the initiation or triggering of movement.

What aspect of movement is controlled by the activity of individual corticospinal tract neurons? Is it the extent of the limb movement (that is, a change in position) or the degree of force exerted by the muscles of the limb? If these neurons encode an intended change in position, without regard to force, then their discharge should have the same firing pattern for the same movement against different loads. But, if the cells encode the force exerted, neuronal activity should change with the load and not be affected by the change in position.

Evarts determined that the discharge frequency of corticospinal tract neurons encodes the amount of force used to move the limb rather than the change in the position of the limb. For example, the firing rate of a neuron that becomes active during wrist flexion increases with the flexor load. When the weight is shifted to assist flexion and oppose extension, flexion occurs passively by the relaxation of the antagonist (extensor) muscles and the neuron no longer fires (Figure 40–6B).

In addition to neurons that encode the amount of force exerted, some neurons in the primary motor cortex encode the rate of change of force. These neurons are likely to control the speed of movement. They are assisted by neurons in the rubrospinal system, whose activity is principally related to the dynamics of force and to limb velocity (Figure 40–7).

Movement Direction Is Encoded by Populations of Neurons, Not By Single Cells

The observation that flexion and extension of wrist or elbow are associated with the firing of different populations of cortical neurons fit with the idea of a muscle-like map in primary motor cortex. However, since individual neurons in primary motor cortex can influence multiple muscles, the question arises of how the direction of typical multijoint arm movements might be encoded by cortical neurons. This question was addressed by Apostolos Georgopoulos and his colleagues by studying how neuronal activity varied when monkeys move a handle to one of several targets arranged around a central starting position. They found that activity of individual neurons did indeed vary with the direction of the movement: they fired most briskly for movements in a preferred direction and fell silent during movements in the opposite direction. Moreover, the preferred directions of neurons located within a column of cortex were quite similar. The directional tuning of all recorded neurons was, however, surprisingly broad. Individual neurons contribute predominantly to movements in a preferred direction but also to lesser degrees to movements in other directions (Figure 40–8).

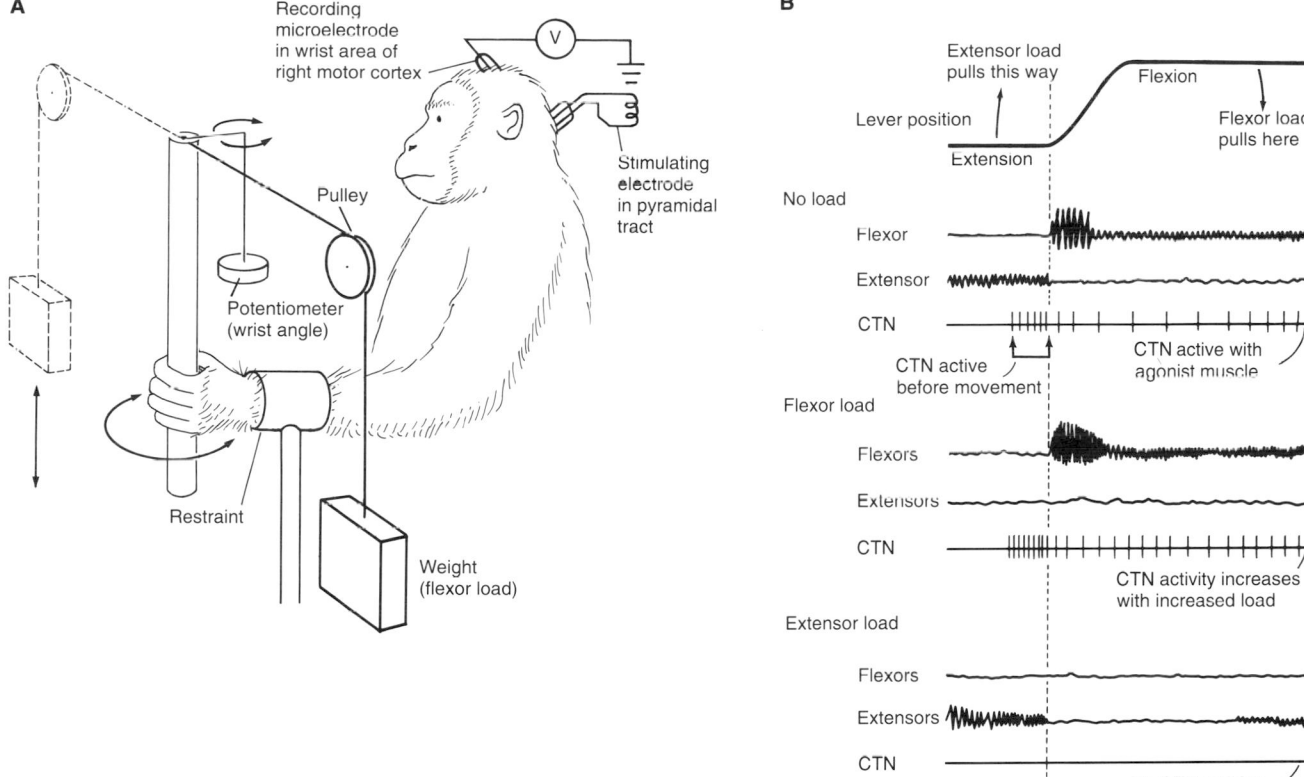

FIGURE 40–6

The activity of motor cortical neurons codes the direction of force exerted. (Adapted from Evarts, 1968.)

A. Setup for recording specific corticospinal tract neurons in the motor cortex of an awake monkey. The apparatus permits the animal alternately to flex and extend its wrist. To ascertain that the neuron being recorded projects through the corticospinal tract, corticospinal fibers are stimulated through a separate electrode implanted in the ipsilateral medullary pyramid to produce antidromic action potentials, thus activating output neurons in the motor cortex at a short and consistent latency.

B. Records of a corticospinal tract neuron (**CTN**) that increases its activity with flexion of the wrist. Note that the cell starts firing before movement. Electromyograms of flexor and extensor muscles and discharge records of a corticospinal tract neuron are shown under different load conditions. Absence of neuronal activity with extensor load indicates that the neuron codes for force rather than displacement.

FIGURE 40–7

Dynamic, static, and mixed neurons have distinctive patterns of firing during voluntary isometric contraction in the cat. dF/dt = rate of change of force. **Broken line** denotes onset of movement. (Adapted from Ghez and Vicario, 1978; and Vicario, Martin, and Ghez, 1983.)

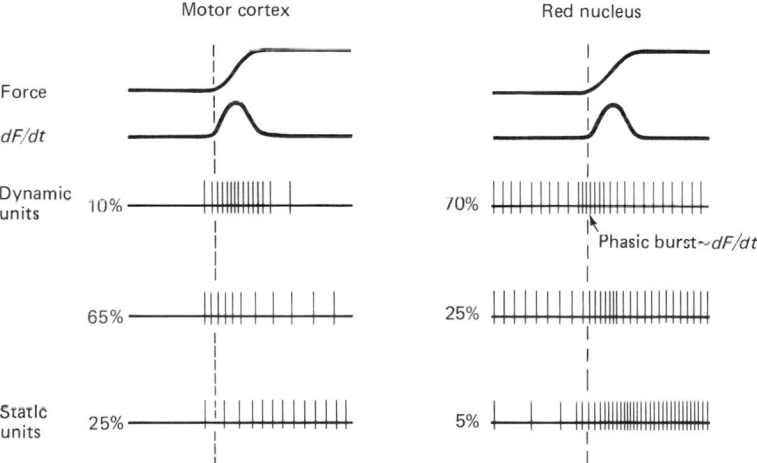

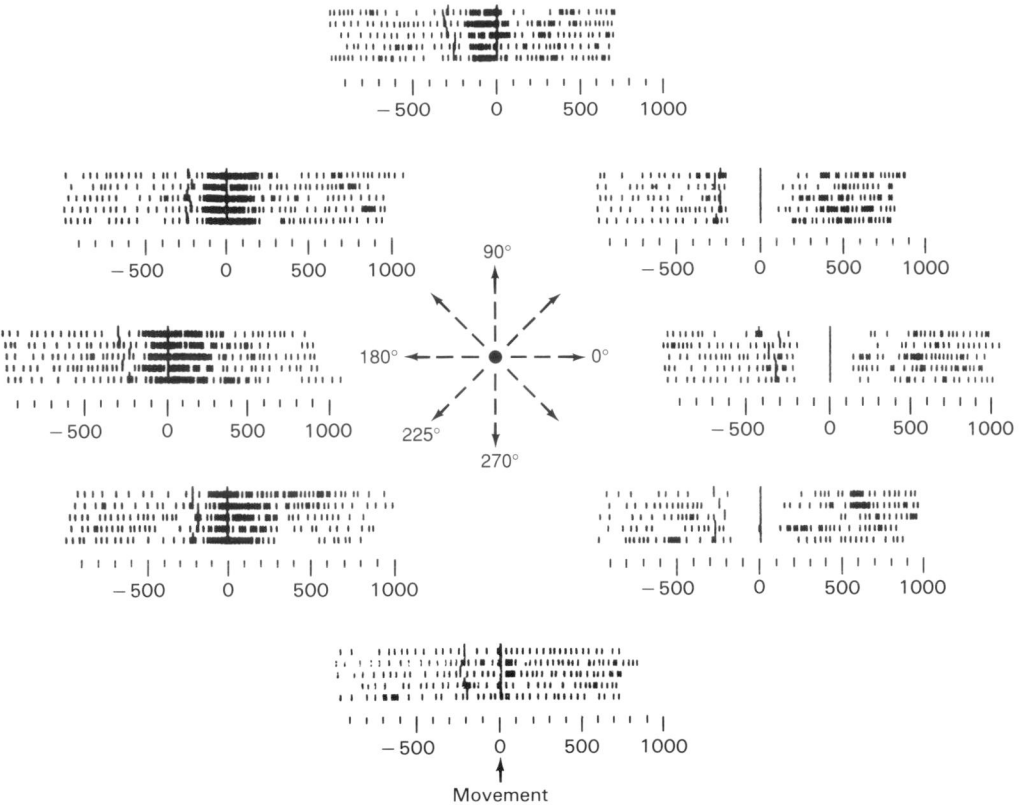

FIGURE 40–8

Individual cortical neurons are broadly tuned to the direction of movement. Raster plots show the firing pattern of a single neuron during movement in eight directions. A monkey was trained to move a handle to eight different locations, represented by light-emitting diodes, arranged radially in one plane around a central starting position. Each row of tics in each raster plot represents activity in a single trial. The rows are aligned at zero time (the onset of movement). The center diagram shows the directions of the eight movements. It can be seen that the cell fires at relatively high rates during movements made in a range of directions from 90° to 225°. (From Georgopoulos et al., 1982.)

How can movement direction be coded precisely by neurons that are so broadly tuned? Georgopoulos proposed that movement in a particular direction is determined not by the action of single neurons but by the net action of a broad population of neurons. Furthermore, he suggested that the contributions of each neuron to movement in a particular direction could be represented as a vector whose length depended on the degree of activity during movements in that particular direction. The contributions of individual cells could then be added vectorally to produce a *population vector*. Georgopoulos has proposed that the direction of the population vector would determine the direction of movement.

To test this idea and to determine the relationship between the direction of the population vector and the ensuing movement, Georgopoulos analyzed the activity of neurons in monkeys reaching toward targets in different directions and found that the directions of the computed population vectors closely match the directions of movement (Figure 40–9). This finding is evidence for the idea that this voluntary behavior is determined by the activity of a population of neurons and cannot be predicted from the discharge patterns of any one neuron. This situation contrasts with that in motion detection where small populations of cells seem to be critically important for perception.

Although neurons in the primary motor cortex encode direction and force exerted during movement, their contribution is not invariant and depends on the nature of the task being performed. For example, Roger Lemon found that neurons that fire when a monkey squeezes a small transducer precisely between the thumb and index finger may remain silent when the monkey exerts the same force by grasping a rod with all fingers together. Similarly, while neurons in the motor cortex may govern an arm movement performed to reach an object, a similar arm movement made during an outburst of anger or an emotional upset may occur without a change in the activity of neurons in the motor cortex. As still another example, cortical neurons in the face area that are active during the jaw movement of a trained biting response have been shown to remain silent when the animal uses the same muscles for chewing, which is a more automatic response.

Neurons in the Motor Cortex Are Informed of the Consequences of Movements

Neurons in the primary motor cortex are kept informed about the position and speed of movement through sen-

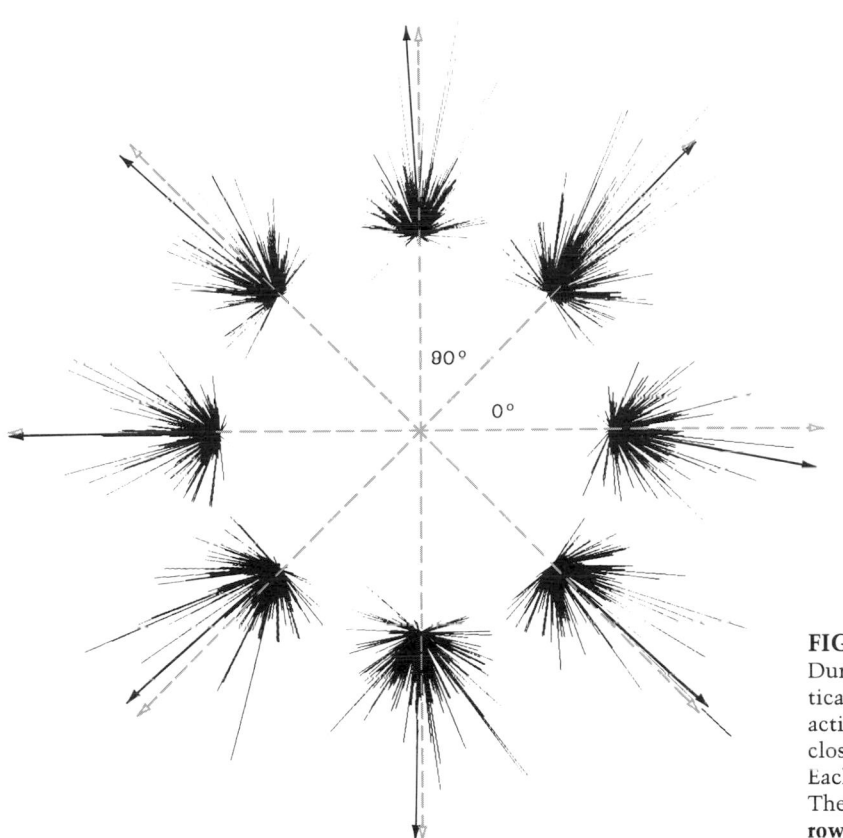

FIGURE 40–9
During movements in any given direction various cortical neurons with different preferred directions are active but the direction of the population vector closely matches that of the direction of movement. Each cluster represents the activity of one population. The directions of the population vectors (**dashed arrows**) closely match the direction of the targets.

sory input. Like neurons in the somatic sensory cortex, neurons in the motor cortex have receptive fields in the periphery. Some respond to tactile stimuli, others to movements of the hands, and still others to stretch of individual muscles or rotation of joints.

What is the relationship between the location of these receptive fields on the body and the muscle groups controlled by local sectors of motor cortex? Asanuma and his colleagues found that some neurons in the motor cortex receive proprioceptive input from the muscle to which they project, while others receive input from regions of skin that tend to be contacted during contraction of that same muscle (Figure 40–10). This sensory input is transmitted to the motor cortex by both corticocortical fibers from the somatic sensory cortex, and by direct pathways from the thalamus.

The correspondence between the muscle receptors providing proprioceptive input to cortical neurons and the target muscles of these same neurons is similar to that of muscle afferents and homonymous motor neurons in the spinal cord. Phillips suggested that the motor cortex might therefore function in parallel with the spinal stretch reflex. He envisioned that transcortical circuits convey afferent information from muscles and control contraction of muscles by a long loop pathway through the motor cortex (Figure 40–10). This feedback would provide assistance, supplementing the stretch reflex, when

FIGURE 40–10
Input-output organization of the cortical neurons controlling a flexor of a digit. The neurons are activated by either stretch of the muscle or stimulation of the skin. A parallel mechanism, the spinal loop, is also shown. (Adapted from Asanuma, 1973.)

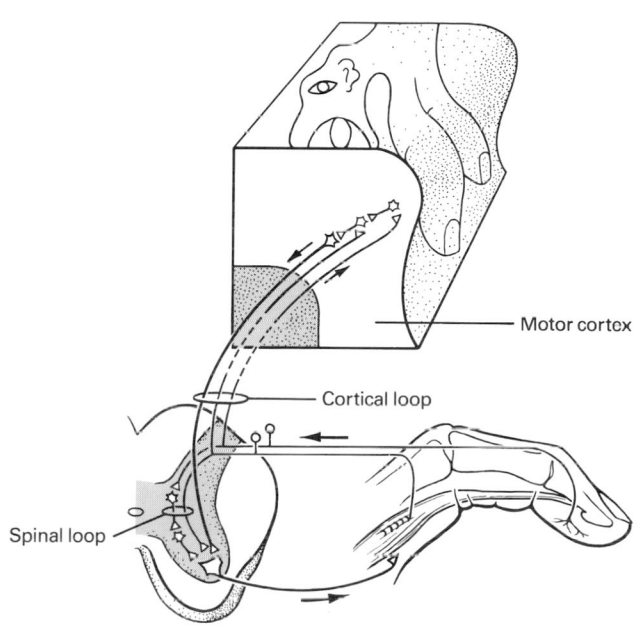

the moving limb encountered an unexpected obstacle: If the movement were appreciably slowed, misalignment would occur between the length of the muscle and its spindles, causing the primary spindle afferents to fire. This input would then boost the cortical output as well as act directly on motor neurons through the stretch reflex arc. A similar process might be set in motion from cutaneous receptors that also influence motor cortical neurons.

Phillips's suggestion that the transcortical pathway mediates kinesthetic inputs is supported by experiments of Vernon Brooks, who trained monkeys to move a handle between two target zones, flexing and extending the forearm. Through a motor attached to the handle, a force opposing the movement could be introduced at any time during the movement, so that the monkey would unexpectedly have to use more force to bring the handle into the target zone. The sudden occurrence of an additional load produced a marked change in the pattern of cortical discharge. First, there was a burst of activity in response to the additional load, and later a more prolonged response during which the monkey repositioned the lever in the target zone (Figure 40–11). The early, short-latency burst of cortical activity indicates that the motor cortex responds to muscle stretch in the same way as the alpha motor neurons in the spinal cord, consistent with Phillips's hypothesis. The effect of the boost in cortical response compensates only for relatively small disturbances. Large disturbances trigger new voluntary responses based

FIGURE 40–11

An unexpected load increases the activity of neurons in the motor cortex. The monkey is trained to move a handle from an extension to a flexion target. On random trials a load is introduced just after movement begins. From **top to bottom**: position of the arm, electromyograms of the triceps and biceps, typical records of neuronal discharge during a single trial, and histograms of neuronal activity over 20 trials. (Adapted from Conrad et al., 1974.)

A. Control movement (flexion) of the arm between two target zones (**hatched rectangles**).

B. Movement opposed by a transient increase in opposing force (at **arrow**). The two periods of increased neuronal activity following the application of the load reflect, first, the activation of the neuron's receptive field and then the execution of a second motor command to overcome the load.

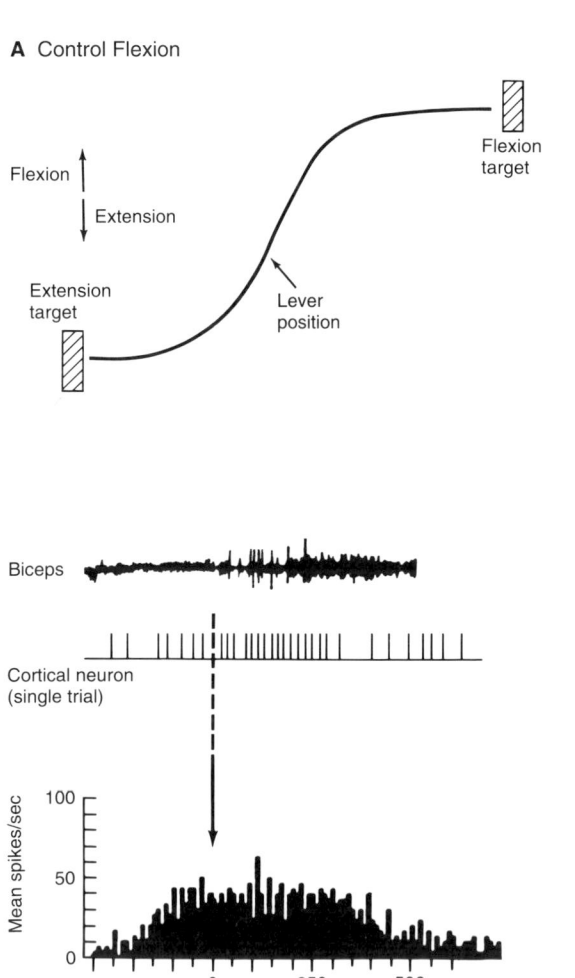

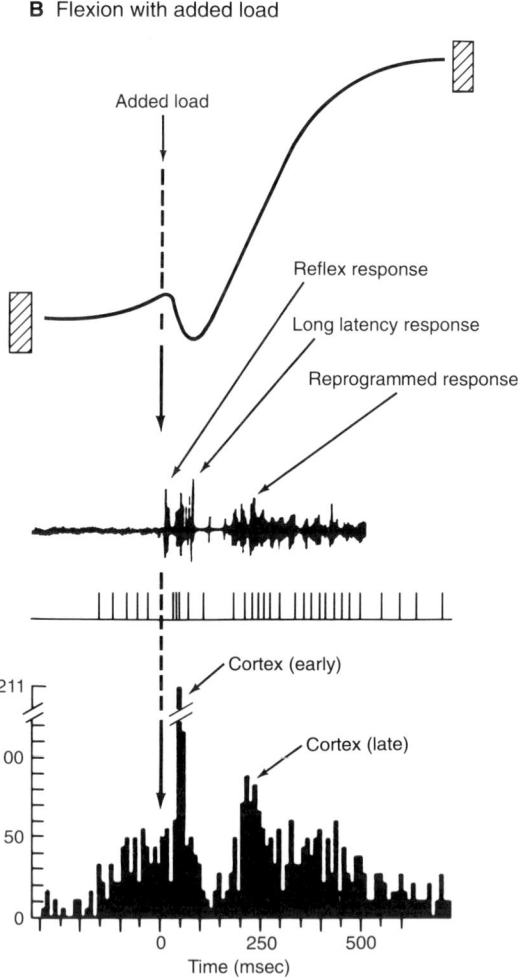

on an updated computation of the new load opposing the movement (Figure 40–11).

Premotor Cortical Areas Prepare the Motor Systems for Movement

Motor Preparation Time Is Longer Than the Response Time to Stimuli

Under optimal conditions of attention, we can respond to a sensory stimulus in 120 to 150 ms (the shortest time is for proprioceptive or auditory stimuli, the longest for visual stimuli, because of extra retinal synapses). In contrast, the time needed to prepare for a spontaneous movement may take several hundred milliseconds (Figure 40–12). This preparation time increases with the anticipated complexity of the response and the degree of precision required for the task. It also depends on the amount of processing needed to decide which response is appropriate to a particular stimulus. The latency is shortest when the subject knows in advance which stimulus will occur and which response to make (*simple reaction time*). Reaction time is longer when the subject must anticipate several different stimuli, each requiring a different response (*choice reaction time*). Choice reaction time increases linearly with the number of alternative responses that are available, a relationship that reflects the added processing needed to select and program the appropriate response.

Lesions of the Premotor Cortex, Supplementary Motor, and Posterior Parietal Areas Impair the Ability to Execute Purposeful Movements

Lesions of the lateral premotor, supplementary motor, and posterior parietal areas cause more complex movement disorders than do lesions of the primary motor cortex. While lesions of the primary motor cortex cause weakness, lesions of premotor areas impair the ability to develop an appropriate strategy for movement. When monkeys with lesions of these areas are presented with food behind a transparent shield with an opening to the side of the food, they do not reach through the opening but instead aim directly for the food, bumping their hands into the shield.

These symptoms in monkeys are similar to *apraxias* that occur in humans with lesions of the frontal association or posterior parietal cortices. Patients with apraxia show neither weakness nor sensory loss and are able to make simple movements accurately, but they are unable to perform complex acts requiring sequences of muscle contractions or a planned strategy such as combing their hair or brushing their teeth (Figure 40–13).

The Supplementary Motor Area Is Important in Programming Motor Sequences and in the Coordination of Bilateral Movements

The supplementary motor area plays an important role in programming complex sequences of movement. Movements elicited by stimulating the supplementary motor area require more intense and longer-lasting trains of pulses than do movements evoked from the primary motor cortex. These include such complex patterns of movement as orienting the body or opening or closing the hand. Many of the movements are bilateral. Movements involving proximal muscles can be mediated through direct projections from the supplementary motor area to the spinal cord. Those involving distal muscles appear to be mediated indirectly through connections to the motor cortex, since they are abolished by lesions of the motor cortex.

The role of the supplementary motor area in programming rather than executing complex movement sequences was discovered by Per Roland and his co-workers while studying local cerebral blood flow in humans performing motor tasks of increasing complexity. During

FIGURE 40–12
Neurons in the lateral premotor area begin firing about 800 ms before a voluntary finger movement. Traces are based on recordings from the human scalp over the frontal cortex. (Adapted from Deeke et al., 1969.)

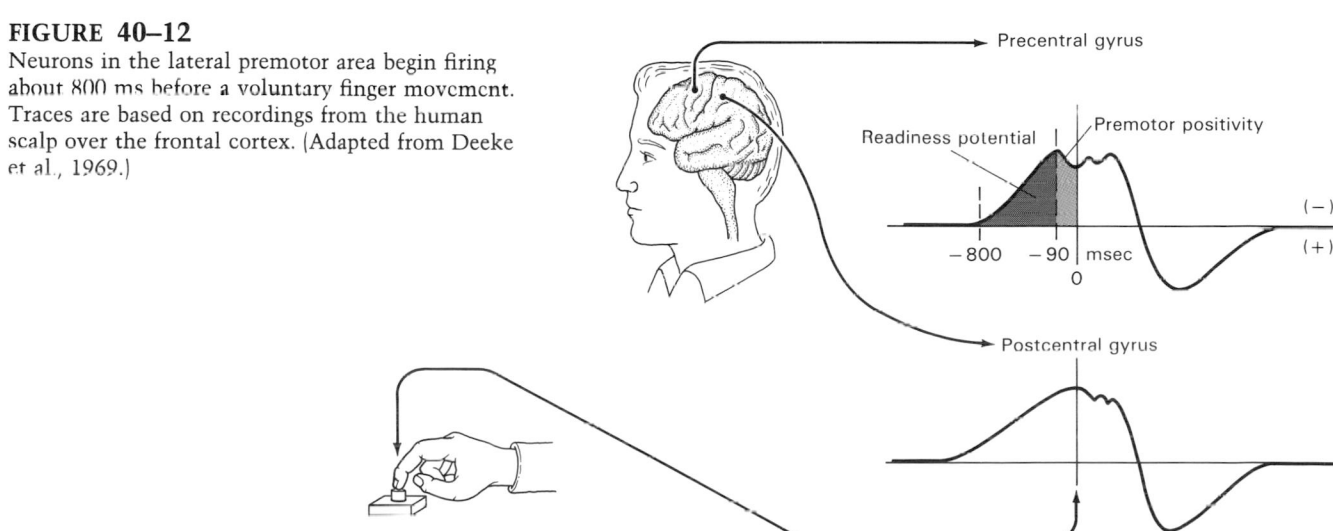

Precentral gyrus

Readiness potential

Premotor positivity

−800 −90 | msec
0

(−)
(+)

Postcentral gyrus

A Normal   **B** Apraxic

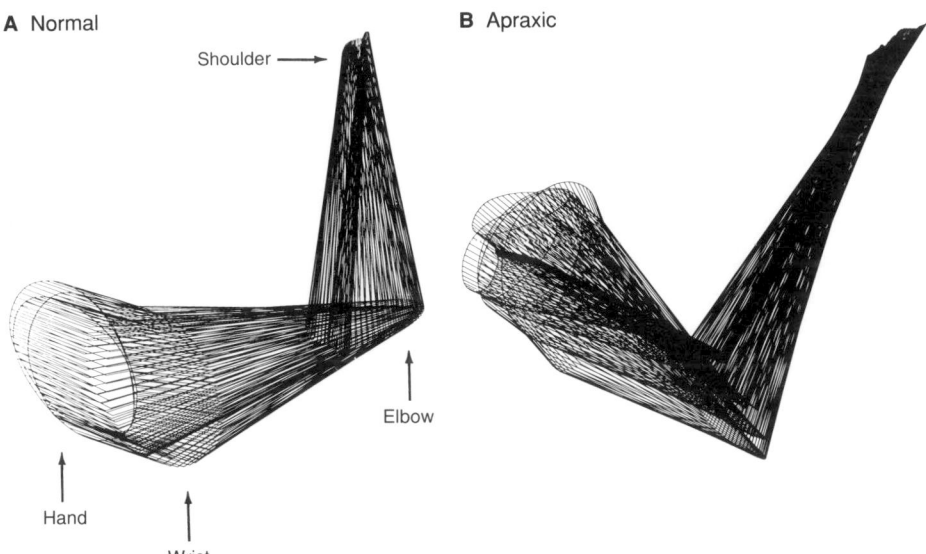

FIGURE 40–13
Three-dimensional reconstruction of the motions of the hand and arm of a normal subject (**A**) and apraxic subject (**B**) performing the gesture of winding a window. The normal subject makes repeated circular motions of the hand, whereas the movements made by the apraxic are tentative and irregular. (From Poizner, 1990.)

simple tasks blood flow increased dramatically within the contralateral hand areas of both the primary motor and somatic sensory cortices but did not increase significantly over lateral premotor areas (Figure 40–14C). During a complex sequence of movements involving all of the digits, the increase in cerebral blood flow extended to the supplementary motor area. When subjects were told to rehearse the sequence of finger movements mentally but not to perform the sequence, blood flow increased *only* in the supplementary motor area (Figure 40–14C).

Cobie Brinkman found two major motor deficits following lesions of the supplementary motor area. These findings also are consistent with the role of this area in programming and coordinating complex movements. First, monkeys are unable to orient their hands and digits appropriately while reaching for a peanut in a small well; rather, the hand assumes awkward positions as it approaches the peanut. Second, monkeys are severely impaired in their ability to use both hands to retrieve a morsel of food stuck into a hole drilled in a transparent plastic plate (Figure 40–15).

The supplementary motor area also plays an important role in coordinating posture and voluntary movement. Jean Massion and his colleagues asked subjects to maintain flexion of the elbow when a weight placed on their wrists was suddenly removed. The ability to perform this task depended on whether the weight was removed actively (by the subject) or passively (by the experimenter). When subjects removed the weight with their free hands, the biceps of the supporting arm relaxed concurrently and without delay as the weight was removed. But if the examiner removed the weight, the subjects could not maintain flexion of the arm, even though they anticipated the removal. Similarly, flexion could not be maintained when the weight was removed passively with an electromechan-

ical device operated by the subject. The biceps relaxed only after a delay, corresponding to a brief simple reaction time following removal of the weight (Figure 40–16).

Patients with unilateral lesions of the supplementary motor area are unable to coordinate muscle contractions of their arms when the weight was placed on the affected (contralateral) arm. Subjects invariably responded with a delay to both active and passive removal of the weight. Task performance was normal, however, if the weight was placed on the unaffected (ipsilateral) limb. This result supports the idea that during the performance of a voluntary movement, two relatively independent but coordinated motor programs operate. One initiates the limb movement; the other program generates a coordinated postural response. This second program requires the integrity of the supplementary motor area.

The Premotor Cortex Controls the Proximal Movements that Project the Arm to Targets

Although the lateral premotor cortex is the most poorly understood of the cortical regions that project to the motor cortex, some preliminary insights into its functions emerge from studies correlating anatomy, single-cell recording, and behavior. The premotor cortex receives its principal input from the posterior parietal cortex. It sends abundant projections to regions of the brain stem that contribute to the medial descending systems (notably the reticulospinal system) and to the region of the spinal cord that controls proximal and axial muscles. These connections led Hans Kuypers to suggest that the premotor cortex plays a primary role in the control of proximal and axial muscles as well as in the initial phases of orienting the body and arm to a target. Many neurons in the premo-

A Simple finger flexion (performance)

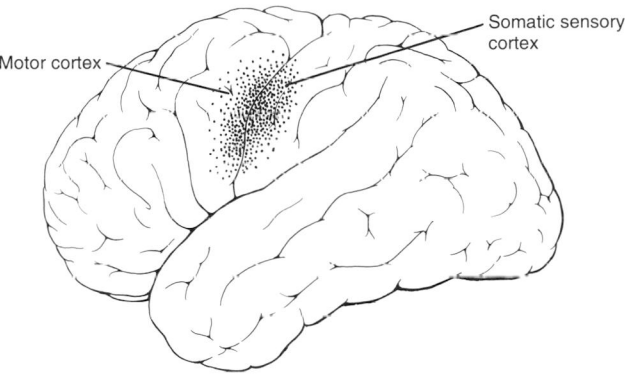

Motor cortex
Somatic sensory cortex

B Finger movement sequence (performance)

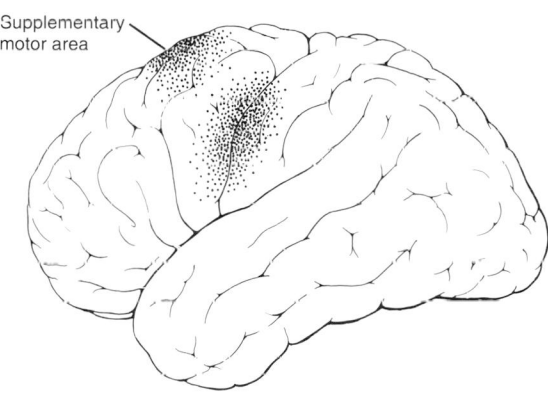

Supplementary motor area

FIGURE 40–14

Local increases in cerebral blood flow during a behavior indicate which areas of motor cortex are involved in the behavior. (Adapted from Roland et al., 1980.)

A. When a finger is pressed against a spring, increased blood flow is detected in the hand areas of the primary motor and sensory cortices. The increase in the motor area was related to the execution of the response whereas the increase in the sensory area reflected the activation of peripheral receptors.

B. During a complex sequence of finger movements, the increase in blood flow extends to the supplementary motor area.

C. During mental rehearsal of the same sequence illustrated in B, blood flow increases only in the supplementary motor area. Blood flow was measured by intravenously injecting radioactive xenon dissolved in a saline solution and measuring the radioactivity over different parts of cortex using arrays of detectors placed over the scalp. Since local tissue perfusion varies with neural activity, the measured radioactivity provides a good index of regional activity in the surface of the brain.

C Finger movement sequence (mental rehearsal)

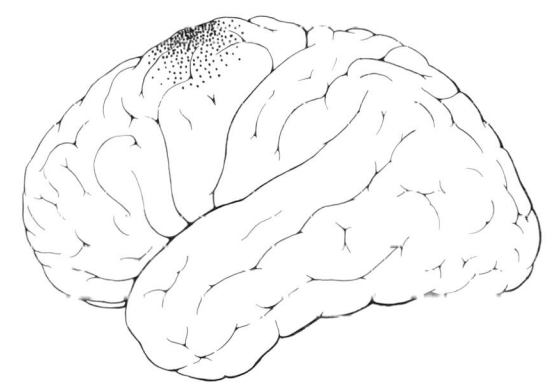

FIGURE 40–15

A unilateral lesion of the supplementary motor area results in a deficit in bimanual coordination. A normal monkey pushes food through the hole with one hand and catches it with the other. The lesioned animal uses both index fingers to push the food from top and bottom. (Adapted from Brinkman, 1984.)

Normal animal

5 months after right SMA lesion

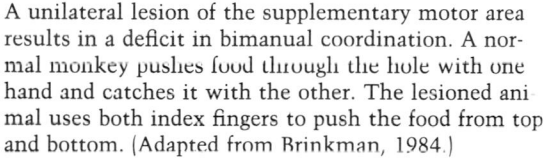
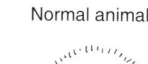
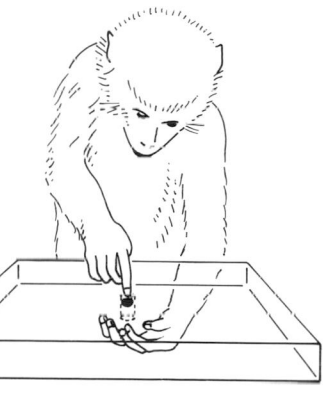
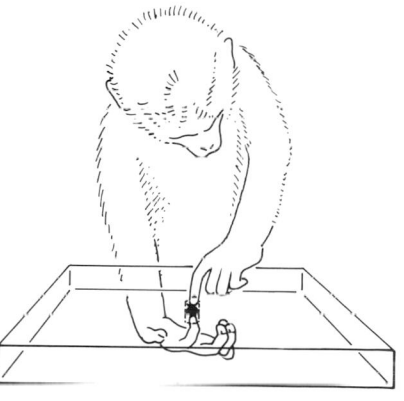

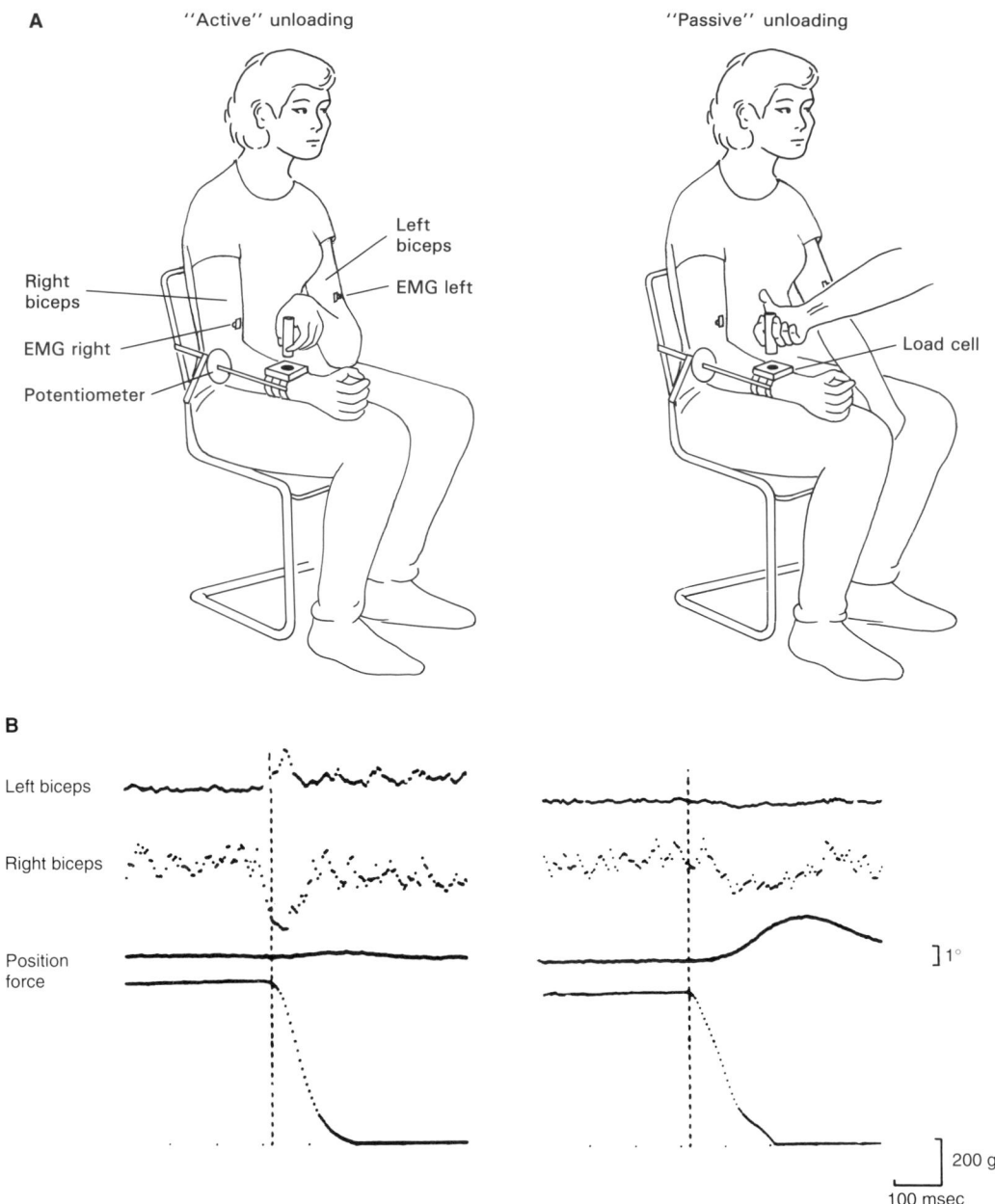

FIGURE 40–16

The dependence of certain postural reflexes on voluntary movement is demonstrated in this experiment. A weight is placed on a force transducer resting on the right arm and a potentiometer measures the elbow angle. The weight is removed by the subject with the left hand (active unloading) or by the experimenter (passive unloading). The records show recordings of force, joint position of the elbow, and rectified and integrated myograms of the left and right biceps. Mean value of 15 trials. Active and passive unloading result in different postural adjustments. At the onset of active unloading the elbow joint does not change position and activity in the biceps is inhibited. In contrast, with passive unloading the supporting biceps is not inhibited and the arm rises. (From Hugon et al., 1982.)

tor cortex fire when the animal receives an instruction telling it to move to a particular location in response to a subsequent go-signal (Figure 40–17). Such neurons are termed *set-related* to indicate that their activity reflects what the animal is preparing to do and indicate a role for the lateral premotor area in the preparatory process itself.

The Posterior Parietal Lobe Plays a Critical Role in Providing the Visual Information for Targeted Movements

An important step in preparing for movement is the focusing of attention on salient stimuli, such as the spatial relationships among objects. Information about the exter-

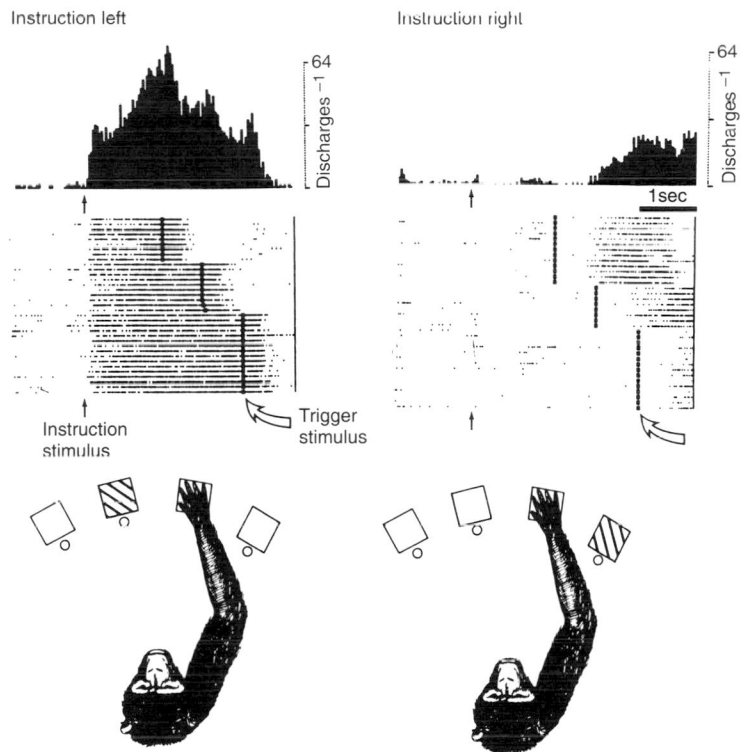

FIGURE 40–17

A set-related neuron in the lateral premotor area becomes active while the animal prepares itself to make a movement to the left. An instruction signal, illumination of one of the four panels, tells the animal which panel it will have to depress when the trigger signal, illumination of the nearby light-emitting diode, is presented. Each dot on each line represents a spike in the recorded neuron. Each line is one trial, and successive trials are aligned on the onset of the instruction signal. The delay between the instruction and trigger signals varied randomly among three values. In the figure the responses made with each delay time are grouped to show that the discharge of the neuron coincides with the instruction signal (**IS**) and lasts until the response is made after the trigger signal (**TS**).

nal world conveyed through the various sensory modalities needs to be correlated with information about the position of our body and limbs and our motivational state. There is now clear anatomical and physiological evidence that the posterior parietal cortex plays a role in these processes (see also Chapter 52).

In monkeys the posterior parietal cortex comprises areas 5 and 7 (Figure 40–2). In humans it also includes the supramarginal gyrus (area 39) and the angular gyrus (area 40), which show a strong hemispheric specialization: The left posterior parietal cortex is specialized for processing linguistic information and the right posterior parietal cortex is specialized for processing spatial information. Patients with lesions in these areas have severe attentional disturbances, referred to as neglect, of tactile or visual stimuli on one side of their body. They also make peculiar errors in locating objects in space, and their ability to recognize or perform complex gestures is defective (see Chapter 53). Although sensation may be entirely normal, these patients are unable to recognize complex objects placed in the hand or to draw three-dimensional objects. They typically do not make use of any information from either the contralateral side of the body or the contralateral visual field. They synthesize their spatial coordinates incorrectly and their movements are not in accord with the coordinates of the object in space. For example, when drawing a clock, a patient with a posterior parietal lesion puts all the numbers on one side and does not notice that the drawing is inaccurate.

Area 5 receives its main input from the somatic sensory cortex, Brodmann's areas 3, 1, and 2 and relates this somatosensory input to limb position. Area 5 is also informed by the vestibular system about the orientation of the head in space, by the premotor areas about motor plans, and by inputs from limbic cingulate cortices about motivational state. Area 5 in turn projects both posteriorly to area 7 and anteriorly to the premotor areas. Area 7 is involved primarily in the processing of visual information that relates to the location of objects in space (as opposed to information about the features of the visual scene. In area 7 visual information is integrated with somatosensory inputs from area 5 and auditory inputs from area 22. Area 7 directs movement by its projections to the premotor areas and to the lateral cerebellum (see Chapter 41).

Major insights into the roles of posterior parietal association areas in motor control have been obtained by Vernon Mountcastle and his colleagues studying neuronal activity in these regions during natural behaviors. They found that the discharge of neurons in these areas is modulated by states of attention. Two classes of neurons in area 5 are of further interest for their possible role in the initiation of movement. The first, called *arm projection neurons*, fire only when a monkey reaches for a desired object (food or reward-related stimuli) within its immediate surroundings. These neurons were otherwise unresponsive to sensory stimulation and do not fire when the animal moves its limb to the same region of space as when the object of interest was absent. The second class of neurons, in area 5, called *hand manipulation neurons*, became active only when the animal manually explored objects of interest. Neurons with similar movement-dependent properties are found in area 7.

Thus, neurons in the posterior parietal cortex can be driven by sensory stimuli, but only in the context of specific behavioral motor responses. By integrating information about the state of the animal with that of potential targets, the posterior parietal areas are thought to create a context or frame of reference for directing movement.

An Overall View

The discovery that the motor areas of the cerebral cortex are electrically excitable and organized somatotopically has had important implications for understanding neurological diseases. However, these motor areas are not simple distribution centers as was long believed. Rather, three advances have given us new insight into the cortical mechanisms subserving voluntary movement. First, the motor areas have a modular organization. In the primary motor cortex, local modules in the form of columnar arrays of neurons control the direction of limb movements. However, individual cortical neurons control direction by acting on single muscles for the most distal movements such as those of the digits. For movements of more proximal body parts, the directional signal is distributed both through axon collaterals and spinal interneurons to produce facilitation and inhibition in multiple motor neurons. It seems likely that this branching provides the elements of a fundamental motor vocabulary.

Second, the firing of individual cortical neurons encodes simple movement parameters such as the amount of force or the rate of change of force that needs to be developed. This intensity coding is nevertheless continuously modulated by feedback from the periphery. Thus, the distinction between sensory and motor processes is somewhat blurred by the tight interactions that continuously take place between these processes.

Finally, studies of premotor and parietal association areas provide new and deep insights into how intention is translated into action. In premotor and parietal association areas, neuronal activity does not simply result from external stimulation, but also reflects the subject's intentions. Neurons in these areas do not encode the fine detail of actions to be executed; instead they are concerned with more global aspects of motor tasks—the coordination of posture and movements, particularly those performed by different body parts. Premotor and parietal areas appear to participate in a fundamental event necessary to purposeful movement—the translation of sensory inputs into the motor coordinates needed to specify precise movements.

Selected Readings

Georgopoulos, A. P. 1986. On reaching. Annu. Rev. Neurosci. 9:147–170.

Hepp-Reymond, M. C. 1988. Functional organization of motor cortex and its participation in voluntary movements. In H. D. Steklis and J. Irwin (eds.), Comparative Primate Biology, Vol. 4. Neurosciences. New York: Liss, pp. 501–624.

Humphrey, D. R. 1979. On the cortical control of visually directed reaching: Contributions by nonprecentral motor areas. In R. E. Talbott and D. R. Humphrey (eds.), Posture and Movement. New York: Raven Press, pp. 51–112.

Wise, S. P. 1985. The primate premotor cortex: Past, present, and preparatory. Annu. Rev. Neurosci. 8:1–19.

Wise, S. P., and Strick, P. L. 1984. Anatomical and physiological organization of the non-primary motor cortex. Trends Neurosci. 7:442–446.

References

Asanuma, H., and Rosén, I. 1972. Topographical organization of cortical efferent zones projecting to distal forelimb muscles in the monkey. Exp. Brain Res. 14:243–256.

Betz, V. 1874. Anatomischer Nachweis zweier Gehirncentra. Centralbl. Med. Wiss. 12:578–580, 595–599.

Brinkman, C. 1984. Supplementary motor area of the monkey's cerebral cortex: Short- and long-term deficits after unilateral ablation and the effects of subsequent callosal section. J. Neurosci. 4:918–929.

Buys, E. J., Lemon, R. N., Mantel, G. W. H., and Muir, R. B. 1986. Selective facilitation of different hand muscles by single corticospinal neurones in the conscious monkey. J. Physiol. (Lond.) 381:529–549.

Cheney, P. D., and Fetz, E. E. 1980. Functional classes of primate corticomotoneuronal cells and their relation to active force. J. Neurophysiol. 44:773–791.

Conrad, B., Matsunami, K., Meyer-Lohmann, J., Wiesendanger, M., and Brooks, V. B. 1974. Cortical load compensation during voluntary elbow movements. Brain Res. 71:507–514.

Deecke, L., Scheid, P., and Kornhuber, H. H. 1969. Distribution of readiness potential, pre-motion positivity, and motor potential of the human cerebral cortex preceding voluntary finger movements. Exp. Brain Res. 7:158–168.

Evarts, E. V. 1966. Pyramidal tract activity associated with a conditioned hand movement in the monkey. J. Neurophysiol. 29:1011–1027.

Evarts, E. V. 1968. Relation of pyramidal tract activity to force exerted during voluntary movement. J. Neurophysiol. 31:14–27.

Evarts, E. V., and Tanji, J. 1976. Reflex and intended responses in motor cortex pyramidal tract neurons of monkey. J. Neurophysiol. 39:1069–1080.

Ferrier, D. 1875. Experiments on the brain of monkeys–No. 1. Proc. R. Soc. Lond. 23:409–430.

Fetz, E. E., Cheney, P. D., and German, D. C. 1976. Corticomotoneuronal connections of precentral cells detected by post-spike averages of EMG activity in behaving monkeys. Brain Res. 114:505–510.

Fritsch, G., and Hitzig, E. 1870. Ueber die elektrische Erregbarkeit des Grosshirns. Arch. Anat. Physiol. Wiss. Med., pp. 300–332.

Fulton, J. F., and Keller, A. D. 1932. The Sign of Babinski: A Study of the Evolution of Cortical Dominance in Primates. Springfield, Ill.: Thomas.

Georgopoulos, A. P., Kalaska, J. F., Caminiti, R., and Massey, J. T. 1982. On the relations between the direction of two-dimensional arm movements and cell discharge in primate motor cortex. J. Neurosci. 2:1527–1537.

Ghez, C., and Vicario, D. 1978. Discharge of red nucleus neurons during voluntary muscle contraction: Activity patterns and correlations with isometric force. J. Physiol. (Paris) 74:283–285.

Hebb, D. O., and Donderi, D. C. 1987. Textbook of Psychology, 4th ed. Hillsdale, N.J.: Lawrence Erlbaum.

Hoffman, D. S., and Luschei, E. S. 1980. Responses of monkey precentral cortical cells during a controlled jaw bite task. J. Neurophysiol. 44:333–348.

Hugon, M., Massion, J., and Wiesendanger, M. 1982. Anticipatory postural changes induced by active unloading and comparison with passive unloading in man. Pflügers Arch. 393:292–296.

Jackson, J. H. 1931. Selected Writings of John Hughlings Jackson, Vol. I. J. Taylor (ed.) London: Hodder and Stoughton.

Jane, J. A., Yashon, D., DeMyer, W., and Bucy, P. C. 1967. The contribution of the precentral gyrus to the pyramidal tract of man. J. Neurosurg. 26:244–248.

Jankowska, E., Padel, Y., and Tanaka, R. 1976. Disynaptic inhibition of spinal motoneurones from the motor cortex in the monkey. J. Physiol. (Lond.) 258:467–487.

Jones, E. G. 1981. Anatomy of cerebral cortex: Columnar input-output organization. In F. O. Schmitt, F. G. Worden, G. Adelman, and S. G. Dennis (eds.), The Organization of Cerebral Cortex: Proceedings of a Neuroscience Research Program Colloquium. Cambridge, Mass.: MIT Press, pp. 199–235.

Kohlerman, N. J., Gibson, A. R., and Houk, J. C. 1982. Velocity signals related to hand movements recorded from red nucleus neurons in monkeys. Science 217:857–860.

Kubota, K., and Hamada, I. 1978. Visual tracking and neuron activity in the post-arcuate area in monkeys. J. Physiol. (Paris) 74:297–312.

Leyton, A. S. F., and Sherrington, C. S. 1917. Observations on the excitable cortex of the chimpanzee, orang-utan, and gorilla. Q. J. Exp. Physiol. 11:135–222.

Lynch, J. C., Mountcastle, V. B., Talbot, W. H., and Yin, T. C. T. 1977. Parietal lobe mechanisms for directed visual attention. J. Neurophysiol. 40:362–389.

Massion, J., Viallet, F., Massarino, R., and Khalil, R. 1989. La région de l'aire motrice supplémentaire est impliquée dans la coordination entre posture et mouvement chez l'homme. C. R. Acad. Sci. 308:417–423.

Merton, P. A., and Morton, H. B. 1980. Stimulation of the cerebral cortex in the intact human subject. Nature 285:227.

Moll, L., and Kuypers, H. G. J. M. 1977. Premotor cortical ablations in monkeys: Contralateral changes in visually guided reaching behavior. Science 198:317–319.

Mountcastle, V. B. 1978. An organizing principle for cerebral function: The unit module and the distributed system. In G. M. Edelman and V. B. Mountcastle, The Mindful Brain. Cambridge, Mass.: MIT Press, pp. 7–50.

Mountcastle, V. B., Lynch, J. C., Georgopoulos, A., Sakata, H., and Acuna, C. 1975. Posterior parietal association cortex of the monkey: Command functions for operations within extrapersonal space. J. Neurophysiol. 38:871–908.

Muir, R. B., and Lemon, R. N. 1983. Corticospinal neurons with a special role in precision grip. Brain Res. 261:312–316.

Murray, E. A., and Coulter, J. D. 1981. Organization of corticospinal neurons in the monkey. J. Comp. Neurol. 195:339–365.

Penfield, W., and Rasmussen, T. 1950. The Cerebral Cortex of Man: A Clinical Study of Localization of Function. New York: Macmillan.

Poizner, H., Mack, L., Verfaellie, M., Rothi, L. J. G., and Heilman, K. M. 1990. Three-dimensional computergraphic analysis of apraxia. Neural representations of learned movement. Brain 113:85–101.

Preston, J. B., and Whitlock, D. G. 1961. Intracellular potentials recorded from motoneurons following precentral gyrus stimulation in primate. J. Neurophysiol. 24:91–100.

Roland, P. E., Larsen, B., Lassen, N. A., and Skinhøf, E. 1980. Supplementary motor area and other cortical areas in organization of voluntary movements in man. J. Neurophysiol. 43:118–136.

Rothwell, J. C., Thompson, P. D., Day, B. L., Boyd, S., and Marsden, C. D. 1991. Stimulation of the human motor cortex through the scalp. Exp. Physiol. 76:159–200.

Schell, G. R., and Strick, P. L. 1984. The origin of thalamic inputs to the arcuate premotor and supplementary motor areas. J. Neurosci. 4:539–560.

Sherrington, C. 1947. The Integrative Action of the Nervous System, 2nd ed. New Haven: Yale University Press.

Shinoda, Y., Yokota, J.-I., and Futami, T. 1981. Divergent projection of individual corticospinal axons to motoneurons of multiple muscles in the monkey. Neurosci. Lett. 23:7–12.

Smith, A. M., Hepp-Reymond, M.-C., and Wyss, U. R. 1975. Relation of activity in precentral cortical neurons to force and rate of force change during isometric contractions of finger muscles. Exp. Brain Res. 23:315–332.

Vicario, D. S., Martin, J. H., and Ghez, C. 1983. Specialized subregions in the cat motor cortex: A single unit analysis in the behaving animal. Exp. Brain Res. 51:351–367.

Weinrich, M., and Wise, S. P. 1982. The premotor cortex of the monkey. J. Neurosci. 2:1329–1345.

Woolsey, C. N. 1958. Organization of somatic sensory and motor areas of the cerebral cortex. In H. F. Harlow and C. N. Woolsey (eds.), Biological and Biochemical Bases of Behavior. Madison: University of Wisconsin Press, pp. 63–81.

Claude Ghez

41

The Cerebellum

The Regional Organization of the Cerebellum Reflects Its Different Functions

The Cerebellum Is Divided into Three Lobes

Two Longitudinal Furrows Divide the Cerebellum into Medial and Lateral Regions

The Cellular Organization of the Cerebellum Is Highly Regular

The Cerebellar Cortex Is Divided into Three Distinct Layers

The Purkinje Cells Provide the Output of the Cerebral Cortex and Receive Excitatory Input from Three Fiber Systems

Purkinje Cells Are Inhibited by Local Interneurons

The Cerebellum Has Three Functional Divisions

The Vestibulocerebellum Controls Balance and Eye Movements

The Vestibulocerebellum Receives Input Directly from the Vestibular Nuclei

Diseases of the Vestibulocerebellum Cause Disorders in the Control of Eye Movements and Disturbances of Equilibrium

The Spinocerebellum Adjusts Ongoing Movements

The Spinocerebellum Contains Complete Somatosensory Maps of the Body

Somatic Sensory Information Reaches the Spinocerebellum Mainly Through Direct and Indirect Mossy Fiber Pathways

Efferent Spinocerebellar Projections Control the Medial and Lateral Descending Systems in the Brain Stem and Cerebral Cortex

The Spinocerebellum Uses Sensory Feedback to Control Muscle Tone and the Execution of Movement

The Cerebrocerebellum Coordinates the Planning of Limb Movements

The Cerebrocerebellum Is the Center of a Complex Feedback Circuit that Modulates Cortical Motor Commands

Lesions of the Cerebrocerebellum Produce Delays in Movement Initiation and in Coordination of Limb Movement

The Cerebellum Participates in Motor Learning

Cerebellar Diseases Have Distinctive Symptoms and Signs

An Overall View

The cerebellum (Latin, little brain) constitutes only 10% of the total volume of the brain, yet it contains more than half of all the neurons. These neurons are arranged in a highly regular manner that results from repetition of the same basic circuit module. Despite its structural regularity the cerebellum is divided into several distinct regions, each of which makes connections with different areas of the brain. These features suggest that all areas of the cerebellum perform similar functions but that each area performs that function on a different set of inputs. What are these functions? The cerebellum is not necessary for perception or for the movement of muscle. Even though the cerebellum contains both sensory and motor components, its complete removal does not impair either sensory perception or muscle strength. Rather, the cerebellum regulates movement and posture *indirectly* by adjusting the output of the major descending motor systems of the brain. Lesions of the cerebellum disrupt coordination of limb and eye movements, impair balance, and decrease muscle tone. The signs of cerebellar damage thus differ dramatically from those of damage to the motor cortex (upper motor neuron signs), which reduces the strength and speed of movement and causes a patient to lose the ability to contract individual muscles.

How does the cerebellum adjust the output of the motor systems? The most attractive idea is that it acts as a *comparator* that compensates for errors in movement by comparing intention with performance. Three features of its organization are important for this function:

1. The cerebellum receives information about plans for movement from brain structures concerned with the programming and execution of movement. This type of feedback information is called *corollary discharge* or *internal feedback*. For example, neurons in the motor and premotor cortex project their axons to different regions of the cerebellum (the corticopontocerebellar system). The cerebellum also monitors control signals to spinal motor neurons from collaterals of propriospinal neurons and from collaterals of interneurons that integrate descending and peripheral information in the spinal cord (for example the ventral spinocerebellar tract).

2. The cerebellum receives information about motor performance from sensory feedback arising in the periphery during the course of movement. This type of information is called *reafference* or *external feedback*.

   These internal and external feedback signals allow the cerebellum to compare central information (corresponding either to the intended goal or to a desired trajectory) with the actual motor response.

3. The cerebellum projects to the descending motor systems of the brain.

Through comparisons of external and internal feedback signals, the cerebellum is able to correct ongoing movements when they deviate from their intended course and modify central motor programs so that subsequent movements can fulfill their goal. In part, these corrections depend on the capacity of certain classes of inputs to modify cerebellar circuits for long periods of time. The function of the cerebellum is changed by experience. It thus plays an important role in the learning of motor tasks.

In this chapter we first consider how the cerebellum is organized and how this organization reflects the various functions of the cerebellum. We then examine its wiring diagram to see how this structure is represented on the cellular level. Finally, we shall review disorders of cerebellar function.

The Regional Organization of the Cerebellum Reflects Its Different Functions

The cerebellum occupies most of the posterior cranial fossa. It is composed of an outer mantle of gray matter (the *cerebellar cortex*), internal white matter, and three pairs of *deep nuclei*, which project out of the cerebellum: the *fastigial*, the *interposed* (itself composed of two nuclei, the *globose* and *emboliform*), and the *dentate* nuclei (Figure 41-1A).

The cerebellum receives input from the periphery and from all levels of the central nervous system. Afferent pathways synapse on neurons in both the deep nuclei and the cerebellar cortex. The outflow from most regions of the cerebellar cortex projects first to the deep nuclei, rather than directly out of the cerebellum. The phylogenetically oldest parts of the cerebellar cortex project directly to the vestibular nuclei in the brain stem, which are functionally analogous to the deep cerebellar nuclei. Together, the deep cerebellar nuclei and the vestibular nuclei transmit the entire output of the cerebellum. This output is focused on the motor regions of the cerebral cortex and the brain stem.

The input and output connections of the cerebellum run through three symmetrical pairs of tracts that connect to the brain stem. These tracts, called the *cerebellar peduncles*, consist of the inferior cerebellar peduncle (or restiform body), the middle cerebellar peduncle (or brachium pontis), and the superior cerebellar peduncle (or brachium conjunctivum) (Figure 41-1).

The Cerebellum Is Divided into Three Lobes

A striking feature of the cerebellar surface is the many parallel transverse convolutions that run from one side to the other. Two deep transverse fissures divide the cerebellum into three major lobes. The primary fissure, located on the upper surface, divides the cerebellum into *anterior* and *posterior lobes*. The posterolateral fissure on the underside of the cerebellum separates the large posterior lobe from the small *flocculonodular lobe*. Shallower fissures subdivide the anterior and posterior lobes into several *lobules*. In a sagittal section (Figure 41-1C) the lobes and lobules have the appearance of branches on a common trunk of white matter (Figure 43-1C). Many small offshoots, called *folia* (Latin, leaves), spring from each branch and represent the cut sections of the fine convolutions that run from side to side.

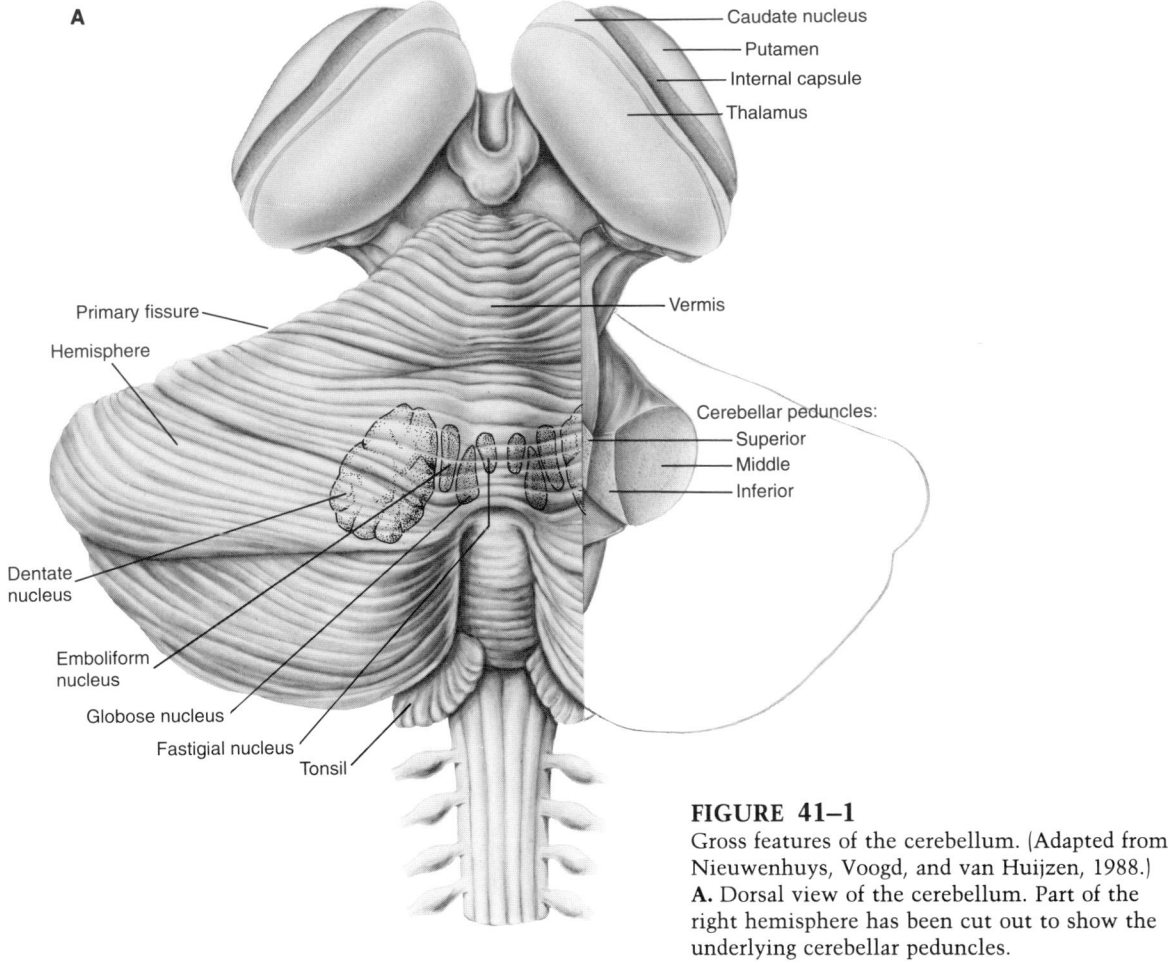

A

Caudate nucleus
Putamen
Internal capsule
Thalamus

Primary fissure
Hemisphere

Vermis

Cerebellar peduncles:
Superior
Middle
Inferior

Dentate
nucleus

Emboliform
nucleus

Globose nucleus

Fastigial nucleus

Tonsil

FIGURE 41–1
Gross features of the cerebellum. (Adapted from
Nieuwenhuys, Voogd, and van Huijzen, 1988.)
A. Dorsal view of the cerebellum. Part of the
right hemisphere has been cut out to show the
underlying cerebellar peduncles.

Anatomists have identified 10 different lobules (Figure
41–2). Although their names need not be learned, one set
of lobules is clinically important. These are the *cerebellar
tonsils*, situated on the undersurface of the cerebellum
(Figures 41–1A and 41–2B). The tonsils are often injured
when a mass in a cerebral hemisphere (for example, a tumor or hemorrhage) displaces the brain stem and cerebellum downward through the *foramen magnum* (tonsillar
herniation).

Two Longitudinal Furrows Divide the Cerebellum into Medial and Lateral Regions

Two longitudinal furrows, most prominent on the undersurface of the cerebellum's posterior lobe, separate three
areas: a thin longitudinal strip in the midline, known as
the *vermis* (Latin, worm), and the left and right cerebellar
hemispheres on either side (Figures 41–1 and 41–2). Each
hemisphere is composed of an *intermediate* and *lateral*
part (Figure 41–2B).

Jan Jansen and Alf Brodal discovered that these parts
represent distinct functional subdivisions that have distinct connections. The vermis and the two parts of each
hemisphere are connected to different deep nuclei and to
different components of the descending systems. The ver-

FIGURE 41–2
The cerebellum is divided into anatomically distinct lobes.

A. The cerebellum is unfolded to reveal the lobes normally hidden from view.

B. The main body of the cerebellum is divided by the primary
fissure into anterior and posterior lobes. The posterolateral fissure separates the flocculonodular lobe. Shallower fissures divide the anterior and posterior lobes into nine lobules
(anatomists consider the flocculonodular lobe as the tenth lobule). The cerebellum has three functional regions: the central
vermis and the lateral and intermediate zones in each hemisphere.

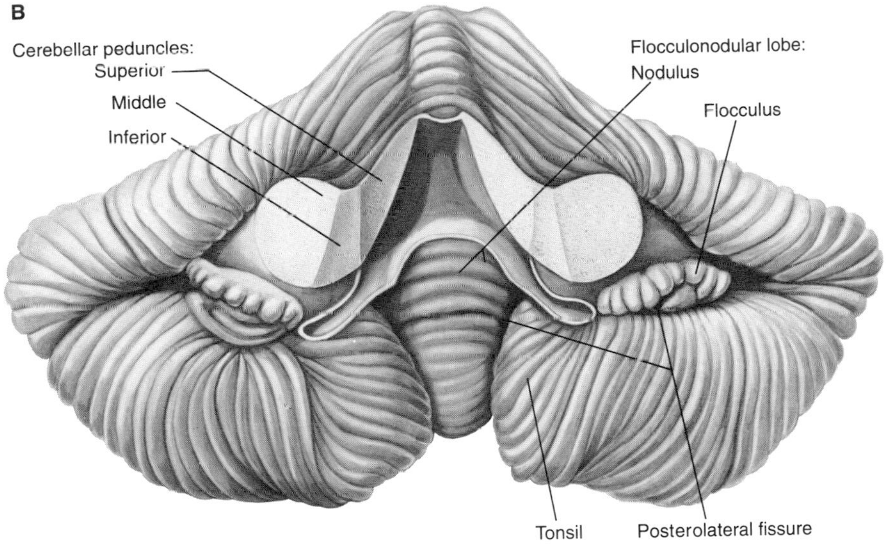

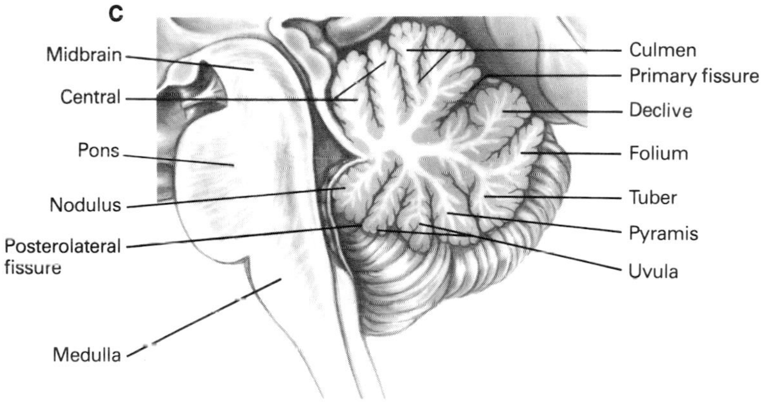

B

Cerebellar peduncles:
Superior
Middle
Inferior

Flocculonodular lobe:
Nodulus
Flocculus

Tonsil
Posterolateral fissure

C

Midbrain
Central
Pons
Nodulus
Posterolateral fissure
Medulla

Culmen
Primary fissure
Declive
Folium
Tuber
Pyramis
Uvula

B. Ventral view of the cerebellum detached from the brain stem.

C. Midsagittal section through the brain stem and cerebellum, showing the branching structures of the cerebellum.

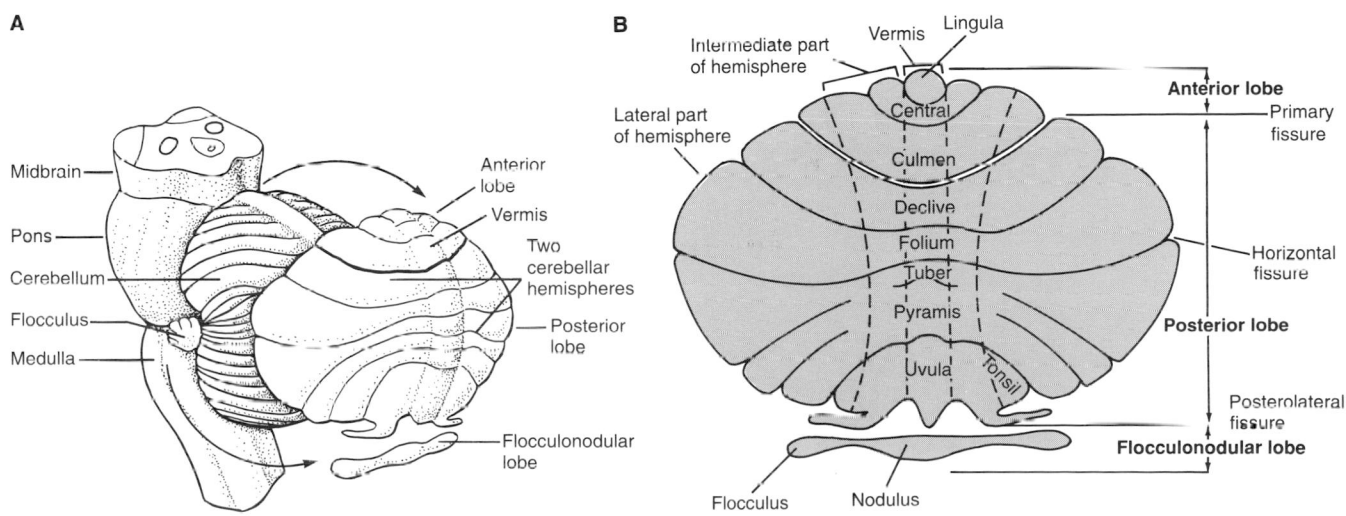

A

Midbrain
Pons
Cerebellum
Flocculus
Medulla

Anterior lobe
Vermis
Two cerebellar hemispheres
Posterior lobe
Flocculonodular lobe

B

Intermediate part of hemisphere
Lateral part of hemisphere
Vermis
Lingula
Central
Culmen
Declive
Folium
Tuber
Pyramis
Uvula
Tonsil
Flocculus
Nodulus

Anterior lobe
Primary fissure
Horizontal fissure
Posterior lobe
Posterolateral fissure
Flocculonodular lobe

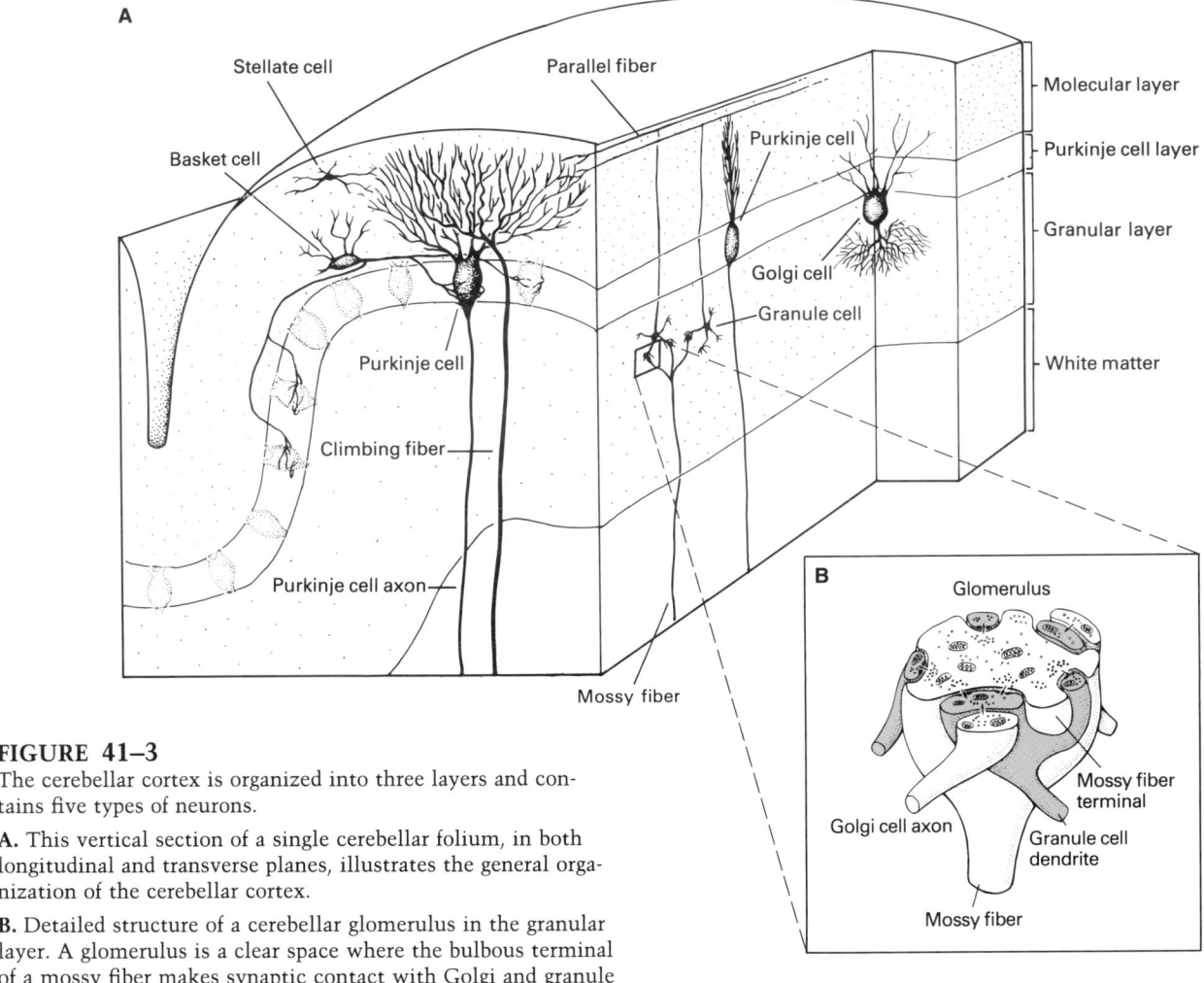

FIGURE 41–3

The cerebellar cortex is organized into three layers and contains five types of neurons.

A. This vertical section of a single cerebellar folium, in both longitudinal and transverse planes, illustrates the general organization of the cerebellar cortex.

B. Detailed structure of a cerebellar glomerulus in the granular layer. A glomerulus is a clear space where the bulbous terminal of a mossy fiber makes synaptic contact with Golgi and granule cell axons.

mis projects by way of the fastigial nucleus to cortical and brain stem regions that give rise to the medial descending systems, controlling proximal muscles. The intermediate zone projects via the interposed nucleus to the cortical and brain stem regions that give rise to the lateral descending systems, through which distal limb muscles are controlled. The lateral zone projects to the dentate nucleus, which connects primarily with motor and premotor regions of the cerebral cortex; these regions are involved in the planning of voluntary movements.

The Cellular Organization of the Cerebellum Is Highly Regular

The Cerebellar Cortex Is Divided into Three Distinct Layers

The cerebellar cortex is a simple structure consisting of three layers that contain only five types of neurons: stellate, basket, Purkinje, Golgi, and granule cells (Figure 41–3).

The outermost or *molecular layer* is composed primarily of the axons of granule cells, known as *parallel fibers*, that run parallel to the long axis of a folium. It also contains scattered stellate and basket cells, which function as interneurons, as well as the dendrites of the underlying Purkinje neurons.

Beneath the molecular layer is the *Purkinje cell layer*. It contains the large (50–80 μm) cell bodies of the Purkinje neurons that are arranged side by side in a single layer. The Purkinje neurons have extensive dendritic trees that extend up into the molecular layer in a single plane perpendicular to the main axis of a folium. The Purkinje neurons send their axons down into the underlying white matter. They are the sole output of the cerebellar cortex. Masao Ito discovered that all Purkinje neurons are inhibitory and that they use γ-aminobutyric acid (GABA) as their neurotransmitter.

The innermost or *granular layer* contains a vast number of densely packed small neurons, mostly small granule cells. Their number, about 10^{11}, exceeds the total in the cerebral cortex! A few larger Golgi cells are found at the outer border. The granular layer contains small clear spaces called *cerebellar glomeruli*, where cells in the granular layer form complex synaptic contacts with the bulbous expansions of afferent (mossy) fibers (see Figure 41–3B).

The Purkinje Cells Provide the Output of the Cerebral Cortex and Receive Excitatory Input from Three Fiber Systems

Information flowing from the cerebellum acts initially on the deep nuclei, which together with the vestibular nuclei transmit all output from the cerebellum. The activity of the Purkinje cells, the only output from the cerebellar cortex, is determined by two excitatory afferent inputs: *mossy fibers* and *climbing fibers* (Figure 41–3).

Mossy and climbing fibers arise from different sources (as we shall see below), terminate in different ways in the cerebellum, and have different functional roles. Both send collateral axon branches to the deep cerebellar nuclei. These collateral pathways, given off by the mossy and climbing fibers to activate neurons in deep nuclei, form the primary cerebellar circuit. This primary circuit is then modulated by the inhibitory action of the cerebellar cortex (mediated by the Purkinje neurons), which is driven by the same inputs (Figure 41–4).

The *mossy fibers* constitute the major afferent input. They originate from a variety of brain stem nuclei and from neurons in the spinal cord that give rise to the spinocerebellar tracts. Mossy fibers influence Purkinje neurons indirectly through synapses with the granule cells, which are excitatory interneurons in cerebellar glomeruli (Figure 41–3B). The mossy fiber pathway activated by peripheral stimuli typically activates local clusters of granule cells. Granule cell axons ascend into the molecular layer and, along the way, make powerful excitatory connections with nearby Purkinje cells. In the molecular layer the axons of the granule cell bifurcate and give rise to fibers called parallel fibers, which extend several millimeters along the long axis of the cerebellar folia. The parallel fibers intersect the dendrites of a row of Purkinje cells, all of which are oriented perpendicular to the parallel fibers. Each Purkinje cell receives converging input from approximately 200,000 parallel fibers from granule cells and each granule cell collects input from many mossy fibers.

The *climbing fibers*, the other excitatory input, originate in a single site in the medulla, the inferior olivary nucleus. Climbing fibers are so named because of the morphology of their terminations on the Purkinje neurons. Their axons enter the cortex and wrap around the soma and dendrites of Purkinje neurons, where they make numerous synaptic contacts, primarily on the proximal portions of the dendrites. Their synapses are all excitatory. Each climbing fiber contacts only 1–10 Purkinje neurons, and each Purkinje neuron receives synaptic input from only a single climbing fiber.

The synaptic connection made by climbing fibers on Purkinje neurons is one of the most powerful in the nervous system. A single action potential in a climbing fiber

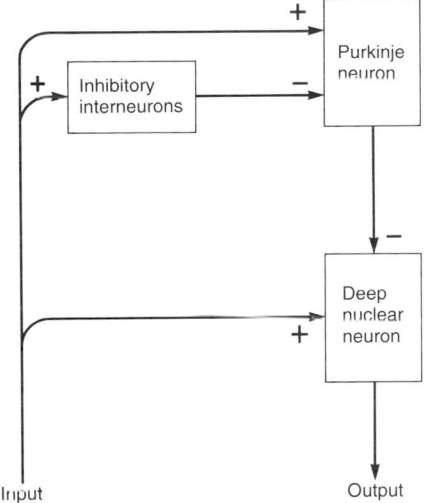

FIGURE 41–4
The excitatory input of the cerebellum can be modulated by inhibitory interneurons.

elicits very large excitatory postsynaptic potentials in both the soma and dendrites of the Purkinje cells that trigger a large action potential followed by a high-frequency burst of smaller action potentials. This characteristic grouping is called a *complex spike* and is associated with a large Ca^{2+} influx into the Purkinje neuron. Mossy fiber input results in smaller excitatory postsynaptic potentials. Spatial and temporal summation of these smaller postsynaptic potentials is required for the Purkinje cell to produce a single action potential, called a *simple spike* (Figure 41–5).

Mossy and climbing fiber inputs are each modulated quite differently in response to sensory stimulation and during motor acts. The neurons that give rise to the mossy fibers and the granule cells both fire spontaneously at high rates, producing 50–100 spikes per second in Purkinje neurons. Sensory stimuli or voluntary movements acting through mossy fibers can modulate this firing and control

FIGURE 41–5
Responses of a Purkinje neuron to excitatory input from a climbing fiber (**left**) and a mossy fiber (**right**).

Complex spike   Simple spike

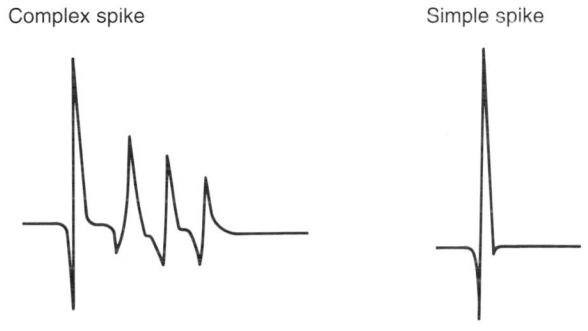

the moment-to-moment firing rate of the Purkinje cell. In contrast, the neurons in the inferior olivary nucleus that give rise to the climbing fibers fire spontaneously at low rates, producing on average one complex spike per second in the Purkinje cell. Sensory stimuli or movement elicit only one or two complex spikes. Since temporal and spatial summation are normally required to produce significant effects in postsynaptic neurons, the low firing frequency resulting from variations in climbing fiber activity is unlikely to have a major influence on the target neurons of the Purkinje cells. However, climbing fiber input to the Purkinje cells is important in modulating the effect of mossy fibers upon Purkinje cells and occurs in two distinct ways. Through mechanisms that are not fully understood, the climbing fibers can transiently enhance the effect of mossy fiber inputs on Purkinje cells. The climbing fibers also can produce a *long-lasting depression* of the efficacy of selected mossy fiber inputs through a heterosynaptic action responsible for some forms of motor learning discussed later in the chapter.

The cerebellar cortex also receives diffuse afferents from *aminergic fibers* arising in two groups of brain stem nuclei, the *raphe nuclei* and the *locus ceruleus*. The projection from the raphe nuclei is serotonergic and terminates in both the granular and the molecular layers. The projection from the locus ceruleus is noradrenergic and terminates as a plexus in all three layers of the cerebellar cortex. Both inputs have widespread modulatory actions.

Purkinje Cells Are Inhibited by Local Interneurons

The activity of the Purkinje neurons is modulated by three types of inhibitory interneurons: the stellate and basket cells in the molecular layer and Golgi cells in the granular layer (Figure 43–3). Like the Purkinje cells, stellate and basket cells receive excitatory connections from the parallel fibers (granule cell axons). Stellate cells have short axons that contact nearby dendrites of Purkinje cells in the molecular layer, while basket cell axons run perpendicular to the parallel fibers and contact the cell bodies of more distant Purkinje cells. As a result, when a group of parallel fibers excites a row of Purkinje neurons and neighboring basket cells, the excited basket cells inhibit the Purkinje neurons outside the beam of excitation (Figure 41–6). This results in a field of activity that resembles the center-surround antagonism that we have encountered in sensory neurons.

The third inhibitory interneuron, the Golgi cell located in the granular layer, has an elaborate dendritic tree in the molecular layer, where it receives its principal input (excitatory) from the parallel fibers. In the granular layer the terminals of the Golgi cells are distributed to the granule cells as axodendritic synapses within the glomeruli (Figure 41–3B). Thus, the Golgi neurons suppress the excitation of the granule cells to mossy fiber input and curtail the duration of the excitation, ultimately reaching the Purkinje cell through the parallel fibers. GABA appears to be the neurotransmitter used by Golgi neurons.

The Cerebellum Has Three Functional Divisions

The cerebellum is organized into three functional regions, each with distinct anatomical connections to the brain and spinal cord: the vestibulocerebellum, the spinocerebellum, and the cerebrocerebellum. These three regions correspond roughly to anatomical subdivisions that have evolved successively in phylogeny. Each region receives its main inputs from a different source and sends its outputs to a different part of the brain (Figure 41–7). Lesions of each of the three regions give rise to distinctive characteristic clinical syndromes.

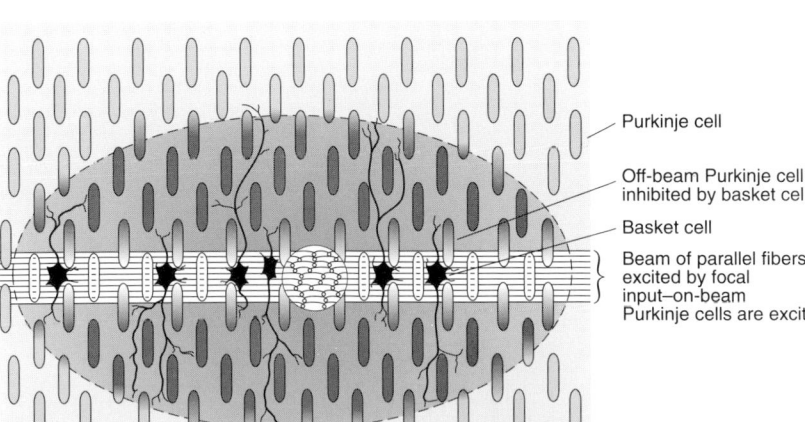

Purkinje cell

Off-beam Purkinje cell inhibited by basket cell

Basket cell

Beam of parallel fibers excited by focal input–on-beam Purkinje cells are excited

FIGURE 41–6

Excitation of a beam of parallel fibers by focal mossy fiber input leads to excitation of a central (on-beam) region of Purkinje cells and inhibition of surrounding (off-beam) Purkinje cells (via excitation of inhibitory basket cells). In this schematic view of the surface of the cerebellar folium the dark area surrounding the excited beam of parallel fibers indicates inhibitory effects. (Adapted from Eccles, Ito, and Szentagothai, 1967.)

A Outputs

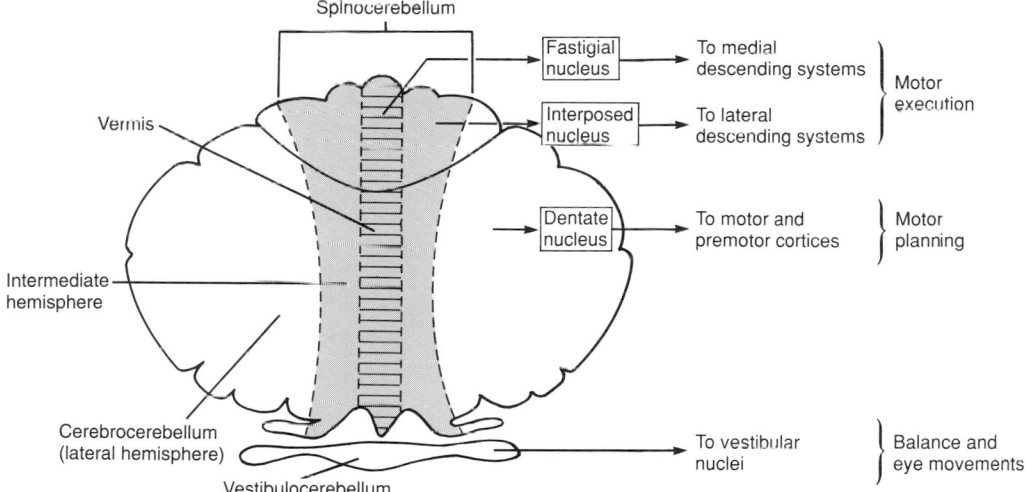

B Inputs

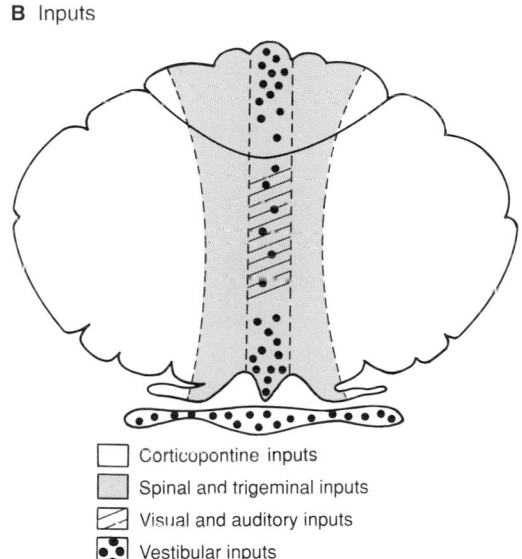

☐ Corticopontine inputs
▨ Spinal and trigeminal inputs
▨ Visual and auditory inputs
▨ Vestibular inputs

FIGURE 41–7

The cerebellum has three functional components with different outputs (**A**) and inputs (**B**).

The *vestibulocerebellum* is coextensive with the flocculonodular lobe. This region receives its input from the vestibular nuclei in the medulla and projects directly back to them, hence its name. This part of the cerebellum appeared first in vertebrate evolution. Through its afferent and efferent connections with the vestibular nuclei, the vestibulocerebellum of humans governs eye movements and body equilibrium during stance and gait.

Two functionally distinct areas form the body of the cerebellum: the spinocerebellum and the cerebrocerebellum. The *spinocerebellum* extends rostrocaudally through the central part of both the anterior and posterior lobes and includes two sagittally oriented regions: the vermis at the midline and the intermediate part of the hemispheres. These two regions receive sensory information from the periphery. The spinocerebellum is so named because a major source of its input arises in the spinal cord. Purkinje neurons in the vermis project to the fastigial nuclei, and those in the intermediate zone project to the interposed nuclei. Through these two deep nuclei the spinocerebellum controls the medial and lateral components of the descending motor systems and thus plays a major role in controlling the ongoing execution of limb movement.

The *cerebrocerebellum* is the lateral part of the cerebellar hemisphere and forms a third sagittal region in the main body of the cerebellum. Its inputs originate exclusively in pontine nuclei that relay information from the cerebral cortex, and its output is conveyed by the dentate nucleus to the thalamus and from there to the motor and premotor cortices. In conjunction with the motor and pre-

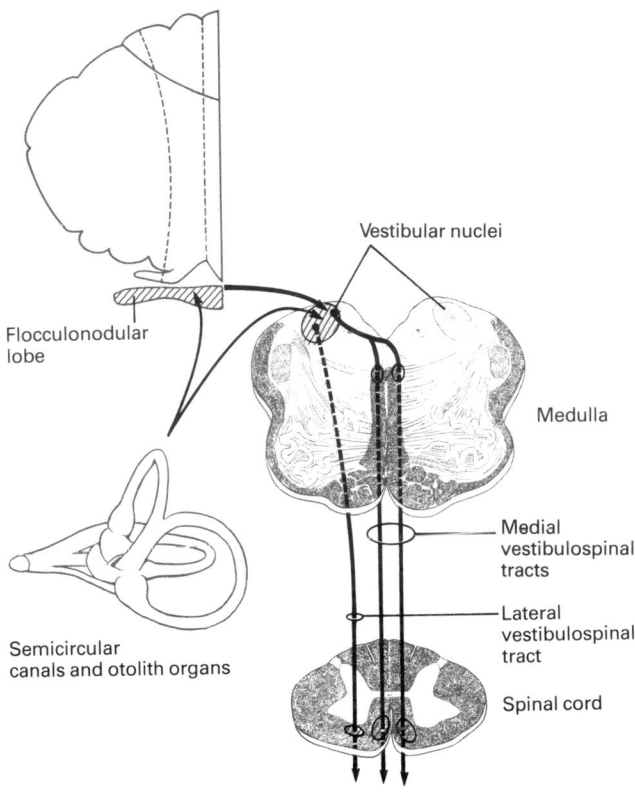

FIGURE 41-8
The vestibulocerebellum (flocculonodular lobe) receives input from the vestibular labyrinth and projects directly to the vestibular nuclei. (Oculomotor connections of the vestibular nuclei are omitted for clarity.)

motor regions of cerebral cortex with which it is connected, the cerebrocerebellum is thought to play a special role in the planning and initiation of movement.

The principal input and output pathways of the cerebellum are summarized in Table 41–1.

The Vestibulocerebellum Controls Balance and Eye Movements

The Vestibulocerebellum Receives Input Directly from the Vestibular Nuclei

The dominant afferent inputs to the vestibulocerebellum come from two sources: (1) the semicircular canals (which signal changes in head position); and (2) the otolith organs, (which signal the orientation of the head with respect to gravity) (See Chapter 33). These two types of primary vestibular afferents are the only afferents that reach the cerebellar cortex directly from ganglion cells in the periphery without an intervening relay. Secondary afferents arise from the vestibular nuclei (Figure 41–8). The vestibulocerebellum also receives visual information from the lateral geniculate nucleus, superior colliculi, and stri-

ate cortex, most of which is relayed through the pontine nuclei.

The output of the vestibulocerebellum is projected back to the vestibular nuclei. By its action on the vestibular nuclei, the vestibulocerebellum is important for equilibrium and the control of the axial muscles that are used to maintain balance. The vestibulocerebellum also controls eye movement and coordinates movements of the head and eyes (Chapter 43).

Diseases of the Vestibulocerebellum Cause Disorders in the Control of Eye Movements and Disturbances of Equilibrium

Because of the connections of the vestibular system with the flocculonodular lobe, diseases of the flocculonodular lobe cause disturbances of equilibrium, including ataxic gait, a compensatory wide-based standing position, and nystagmus. Patients with lesions of the flocculonodular lobe lack the ability to use vestibular information to coordinate movements of either body or eyes. However, when the patient moves while lying down no deficits are seen.

The Spinocerebellum Adjusts Ongoing Movements

The Spinocerebellum Contains Complete Somatosensory Maps of the Body

The principal input to the spinocerebellum is somatosensory information from the spinal cord through the spinocerebellar tracts. The spinocerebellum also receives information from the auditory, visual, and vestibular systems. As first shown by Edgar Adrian and Ray Snider, these afferent projections are organized somatotopically.

FIGURE 41-9
Two regions of the cerebellar surface each contain somatotopic maps of the entire body. In both maps the head and trunk are located medially in the vermis. This region also receives input from labyrinthine, visual, and auditory receptors. The limb representations are located on either side of the midline, in the intermediate part of the cerebellar hemispheres.

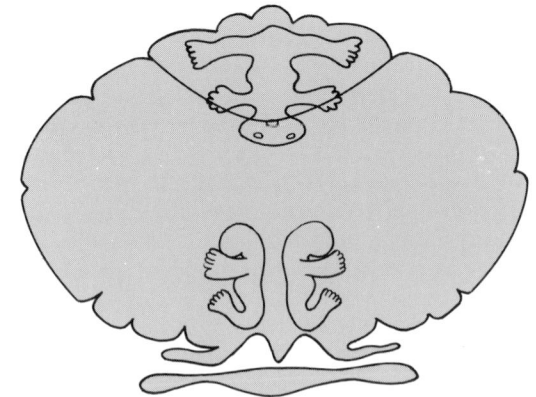

TABLE **41–1.** Principal Input and Output Pathways of the Cerebellum

Functional region	Anatomical region	Principal input	Deep nucleus	Principal destination	Function
Vestibulocerebellum	Flocculonodular lobe	Vestibular labyrinth	Lateral vestibular	Medial systems: axial motor neurons	Axial control and vestibular reflexes
Spinocerebellum	Vermis	Vestibular labyrinth, proximal body parts; facial, visual, and auditory inputs to posterior lobe only	Fastigial	Medial systems: vestibular nucleus, reticular formation, and motor cortex	Axial and proximal motor control; ongoing execution of movement
Spinocerebellum	Intermediate part of hemisphere	Spinal afferents (distal body parts)	Interposed	Lateral systems: red nucleus (magnocellular part) and distal regions of motor cortex	Distal motor control; ongoing execution
Cerebrocerebellum	Lateral part of hemisphere	Cortical afferents	Dentate	Integration areas: red nucleus (parvocellular part) and premotor cortex (area 6)	Initiation, planning, and timing

The body is mapped in two different areas of the spinocerebellar cortex, one in the anterior lobe and the other in the posterior (Figure 41–9). These two maps are inverted relative to one another: The body map in the anterior lobe has the feet oriented forward while the face extends backward into the first lobule of the posterior lobe. The body map in the posterior lobe is oriented head forward and is located in the vermis and intermediate part of the hemisphere.

More refined studies using single-cell recordings have complicated this simple view. First, mossy fiber input from circumscribed peripheral sites diverges to influence several discrete patches of granule cells, each of which excites a small array of Purkinje neurons. This is dramatically seen in the detailed maps of mossy fiber inputs to granule cells in the rat obtained by Georgia Shambes and her colleagues (Figure 41–10). Even though input from a given peripheral site activates a small, sharply demarcated area, adjacent regions may receive information from distant body parts—an arrangement that has been called a *fractured somatotopy.* Recordings of surface potentials for a particular region of cerebellar cortex thus reflect only the predominant input and do not give a full picture of the somatotopic connections. The spinocerebellum also receives topographically organized projections from the primary motor and somatic sensory cortex. This input is in register with that from the periphery.

Somatic Sensory Information Reaches the Spinocerebellum Mainly Through Direct and Indirect Mossy Fiber Pathways

Information from the spinal cord is conveyed to the cerebellum by numerous pathways terminating in the vermis and the intermediate zone. Four pathways carry somatic

sensory information to the cerebellar cortex directly from the spinal cord. The dorsal and ventral spinocerebellar tracts are the direct pathways from the trunk and legs and the cuneo- and rostral spinocerebellar tracts are the direct pathways from the arms and neck.

Anders Lundberg, Olov Oscarsson, and their colleagues suggested that the dorsal and ventral spinocerebellar tracts convey fundamentally different information. Signals in the dorsal spinocerebellar tract faithfully reflect sensory events in the periphery and provide the cerebellum with information about evolving movements. Signals running in the ventral spinocerebellar tract reflect the activity of segmental interneurons that integrate both descending and peripheral inputs. The ventral spinocerebellar neurons are principally driven by central commands that regulate the locomotor cycle. This internal feedback allows the cerebellum to monitor the operation of spinal circuits.

Efferent Spinocerebellar Projections Control the Medial and Lateral Descending Systems in the Brain Stem and Cerebral Cortex

As we saw earlier, the Purkinje neurons in the cerebellar vermis and the adjacent intermediate part of the hemisphere project to different deep nuclei. These nuclei in turn control different components of the descending motor pathways.

Fastigial nuclei receive somatotopically organized projections from the vermis in the anterior and posterior lobes and project bilaterally to the brain stem reticular formation and to the lateral vestibular nuclei. Both the vestibular nuclei and the reticular formation give rise to fibers that descend to the spinal cord. The fastigial nuclei also have crossed ascending projections that reach the

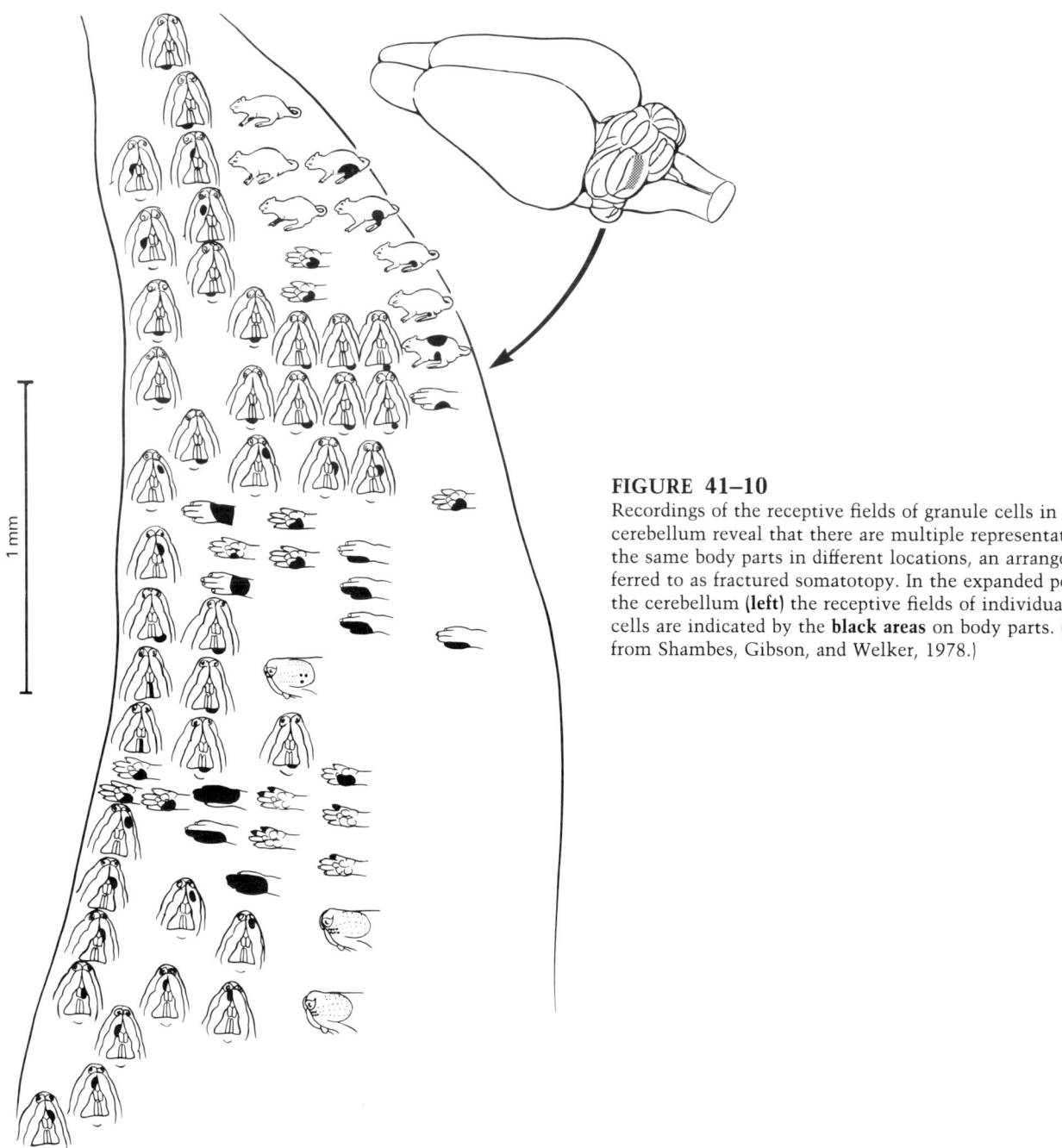

FIGURE 41–10
Recordings of the receptive fields of granule cells in the rat cerebellum reveal that there are multiple representations of the same body parts in different locations, an arrangement referred to as fractured somatotopy. In the expanded portion of the cerebellum **(left)** the receptive fields of individual granule cells are indicated by the **black areas** on body parts. (Adapted from Shambes, Gibson, and Welker, 1978.)

ventrolateral nucleus of the thalamus. From there information is relayed to the primary motor cortex. Through both its ascending and descending projections, the medial region of the cerebellum controls mainly the cortical and brain stem components of the medial descending systems. This region of the cerebellum regulates axial and proximal musculature (Figure 41–11A).

The cortex of the intermediate part of the cerebellar hemisphere projects to the interposed nuclei, which modulate cortical commands for movement through their connections to the brain stem and cortical components of the lateral descending systems: the rubrospinal and lateral

corticospinal tracts. The interposed nuclei project to the contralateral magnocellular portion of the red nucleus (Figure 41–11B) in the brain stem via the superior cerebellar peduncle. Many of these fibers continue rostrally to the ventral lateral nucleus of the thalamus, where they end on neurons projecting to the limb areas of motor cortex. (The region of the ventral lateral nucleus also receives projections from the globus pallidus; the pallidal and cerebellar projections terminate on separate populations of neurons.)

By acting on the cells of origin of the rubrospinal and corticospinal systems, the intermediate zone and the interposed nuclei focus their action on distal limb muscles.

Because these cerebellar projections that project to the contralateral rubrospinal and corticospinal systems cross in the decussation of the superior cerebellar peduncle, and these latter two pathways cross before terminating in the spinal cord, the deficits produced by lesions of the intermediate zone affect limbs on the same side as the lesion (Figure 41–11B).

The Spinocerebellum Uses Sensory Feedback to Control Muscle Tone and the Execution of Movement

The spinocerebellum controls the execution of movement and regulates muscle tone. It carries out these functions by regulating the peripheral muscular apparatus to compensate for small variations in loads encountered during movement and to smooth out small oscillations (physiological tremor). This control is thought to be dependent both on information that the spinocerebellum receives from cortical motor areas about the intended motor command and on feedback from the spinal cord and periphery, which provides details about the evolving movement. These inputs allow the spinocerebellum to correct for deviations from the intended movement.

The importance of the spinocerebellum in maintaining muscle tone was first recognized by Gordon Holmes, who described patients with cerebellar lesions causing a decrease in tonic muscle tension, or *hypotonia*. Similar defects are also seen in monkeys following lesions of the interposed or fastigial nuclei. Sid Gilman discovered that the activity of gamma motor neurons is profoundly reduced. This drop in the fusimotor drive to muscle spindles produces a decrease in the steady background of spindle afferent activity and a reduction in the input to motor neurons during motion of the limb.

Because they receive dual inputs from the periphery and from primary sensory and motor cortices, the nucleus interpositus neurons are modulated by peripheral inputs and by central commands triggering movement. This modulation is especially pronounced in response to imposed mechanical oscillations of the limbs. They are also modulated shortly before self-paced voluntary movements.

The Cerebrocerebellum Coordinates the Planning of Limb Movements

The Cerebrocerebellum Is the Center of a Complex Feedback Circuit That Modulates Cortical Motor Commands

The cerebrocerebellum receives most of its input from sensory and motor cortices and from premotor and posterior parietal cortices (Figure 41–12). These regions do not project directly to the cerebellum but rather to the pontine nuclei, which then distribute cortical information to the contralateral cerebellar hemisphere through the middle cerebellar peduncle.

The lateral zone of the cerebellar cortex projects to the dentate nucleus, which sends fibers through the superior cerebellar peduncle to the ventral lateral nucleus of the thalamus. From the ventral lateral nucleus, the dentate nucleus influences motor and premotor regions of the cerebral cortex. The dentate nucleus also projects to the parvocellular component of the red nucleus. This portion of the red nucleus does not contribute to the rubrospinal tract but is part of a complex feedback circuit that sends information back to the cerebellum, primarily through the ipsilateral inferior olivary nucleus.

Lesions of the Cerebrocerebellum Produce Delays in Movement Initiation and in Coordination of Limb Movement

The lateral parts of the cerebellar hemispheres are largely devoted to achieving precision in the control of rapid limb movements and in tasks requiring fine dexterity. Lesions on either side of the dentate nuclei or the overlying cortex produce four kinds of disturbances: (1) delays in initiating and terminating movement; (2) terminal tremor at the end of movement; (3) disorders in the temporal coordination of movements involving multiple joints; (4) disorders in the spatial coordination of hand and finger muscles.

Two mechanisms have been proposed to account for the delay in the initiation of movement. First, the dentate nuclei might provide background facilitation to either cortical or subcortical neurons so that, after dentate lesions, commands to initiate movement could bring the motor neurons to fire only after an increased period of summation. Alternatively, the dentate nucleus might participate in, or indeed convey, the commands initiating movement.

In an attempt to distinguish between these two alternatives, Vernon Brooks and his colleagues recorded the patterns of activity of neurons in the motor cortex of monkeys while the animals performed prompt movements to a visual cue, and then compared these patterns before and after the dentate nucleus was reversibly inactivated. Inactivation was achieved by a cooling probe inserted into the deep cerebellar nuclei. If the dentate merely provides background excitation to subcortical structures, the change in activity of neurons in motor cortex should occur at the normal time, but more time would have elapsed before the onset of movement. This, however, was not found. When the dentate nucleus was cooled, both the discharge of motor cortex neurons associated with the movement and the onset of the movement itself were delayed. These results suggest that the dentate nucleus provides important information capable of triggering activity in the primary motor cortex. However, since movement does eventually occur, it is likely that activity in the lateral cerebellum participates together with the premotor cortical areas in this process.

Comparisons of the modulations of dentate and interposed neurons during performance of different tasks emphasize their dissimilar roles. These differences support the idea that the cerebrocerebellum contributes to the preparation of movement while the spinocerebellum is

638

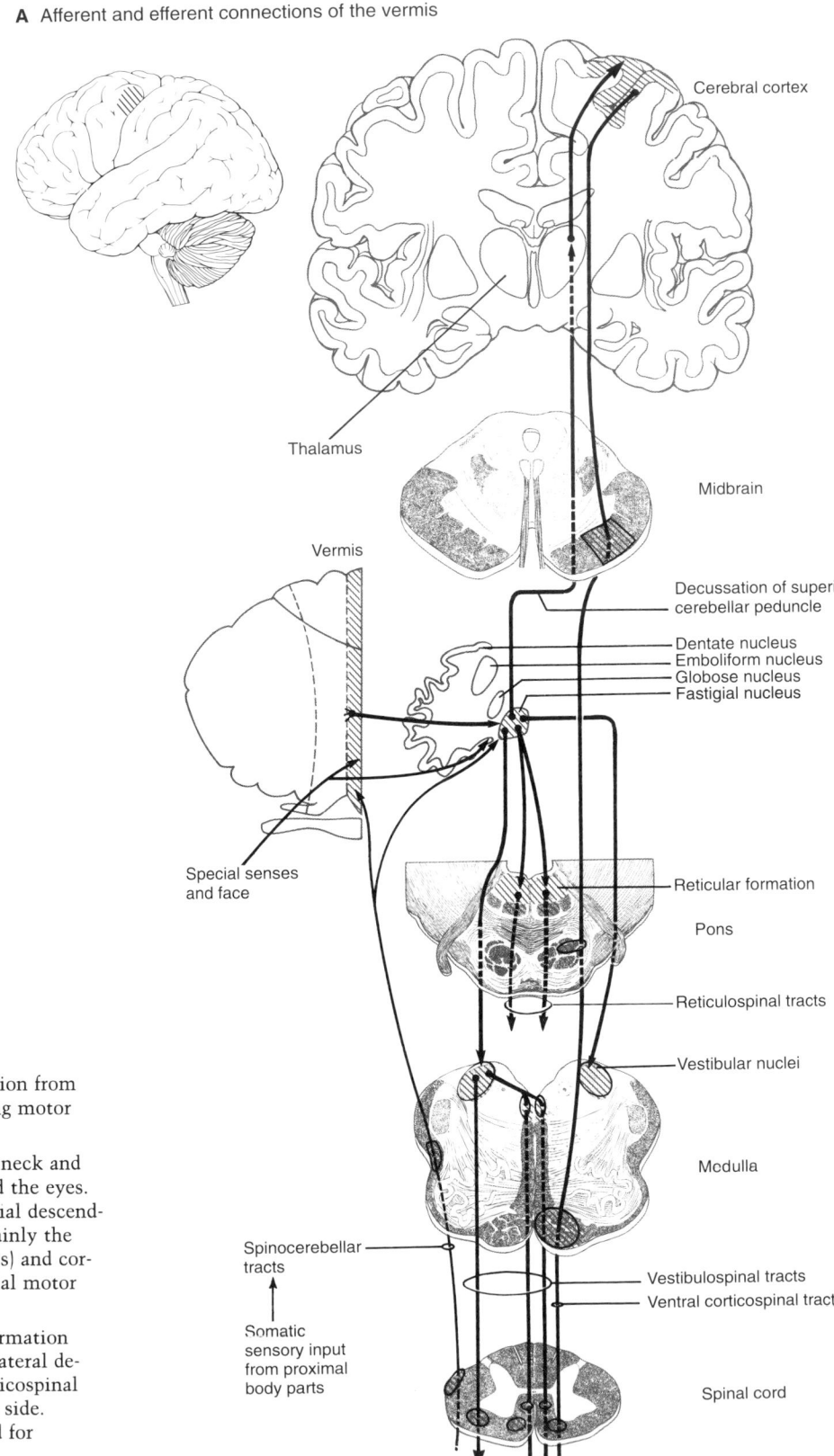

A Afferent and efferent connections of the vermis

Cerebral cortex

Thalamus

Midbrain

Vermis

Decussation of superior
cerebellar peduncle

Dentate nucleus
Emboliform nucleus
Globose nucleus
Fastigial nucleus

Special senses
and face

Reticular formation

Pons

Reticulospinal tracts

Vestibular nuclei

Medulla

Spinocerebellar
tracts

Vestibulospinal tracts
Ventral corticospinal tract

Somatic
sensory input
from proximal
body parts

Spinal cord

FIGURE 41–11

The spinocerebellum receives information from
the periphery and projects to descending motor
systems.

A. The vermis receives input from the neck and
trunk as well as from the labyrinth and the eyes.
Its output is focused on the ventromedial descending systems of both the brain stem (mainly the
reticulospinal and vestibulospinal tracts) and cortex (corticospinal fibers acting on medial motor
neurons).

B. The intermediate zone receives information
from the limbs and controls the dorsolateral descending systems (rubrospinal and corticospinal
tracts) acting on the limbs of the same side.
(Climbing fiber input has been omitted for
simplicity.)

B Afferent and efferent connections of the intermediate hemisphere

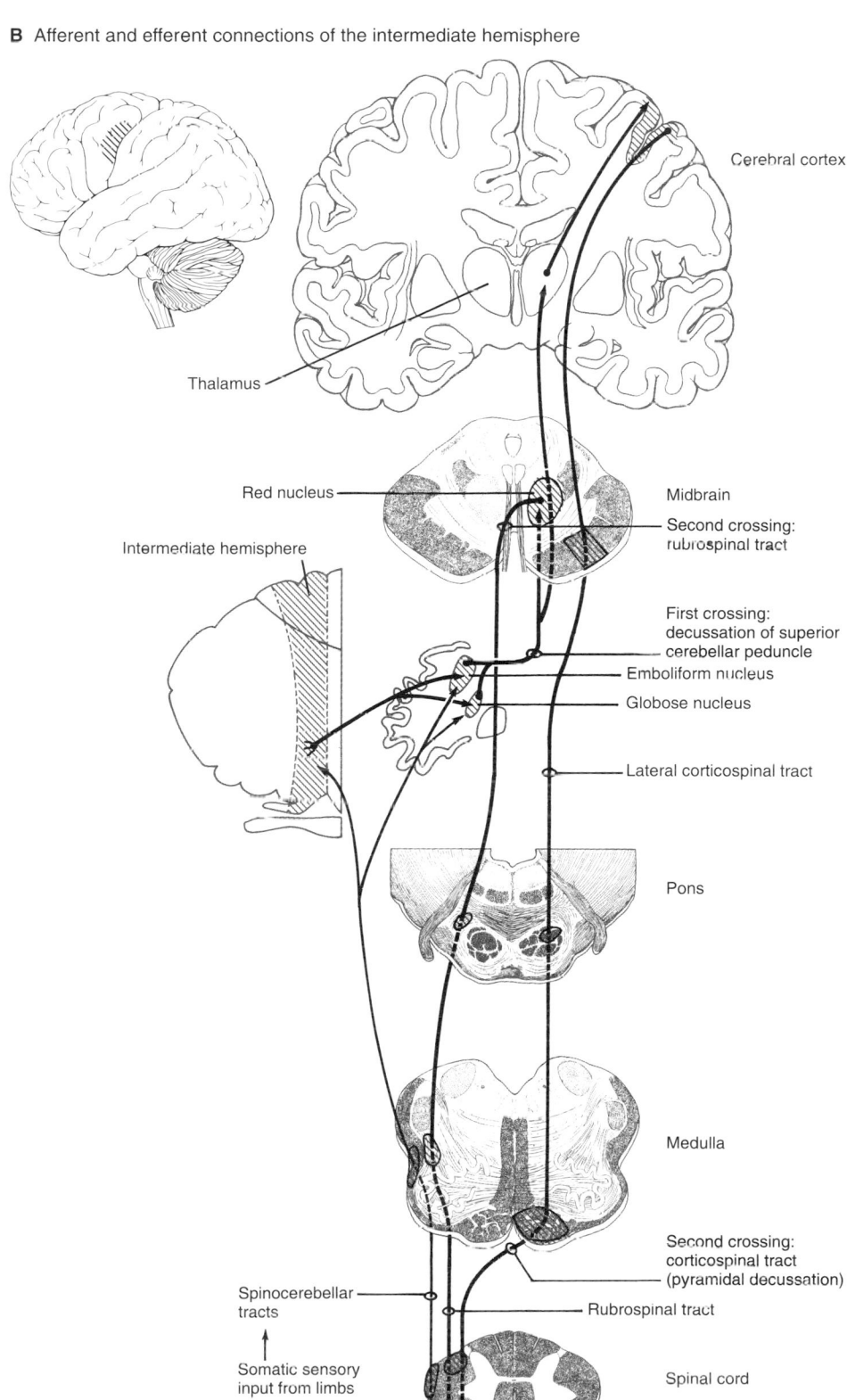

Cerebral cortex

Thalamus

Red nucleus

Midbrain

Second crossing:
rubrospinal tract

Intermediate hemisphere

First crossing:
decussation of superior
cerebellar peduncle

Emboliform nucleus

Globose nucleus

Lateral corticospinal tract

Pons

Medulla

Second crossing:
corticospinal tract
(pyramidal decussation)

Spinocerebellar
tracts

Rubrospinal tract

Somatic sensory
input from limbs

Spinal cord

640

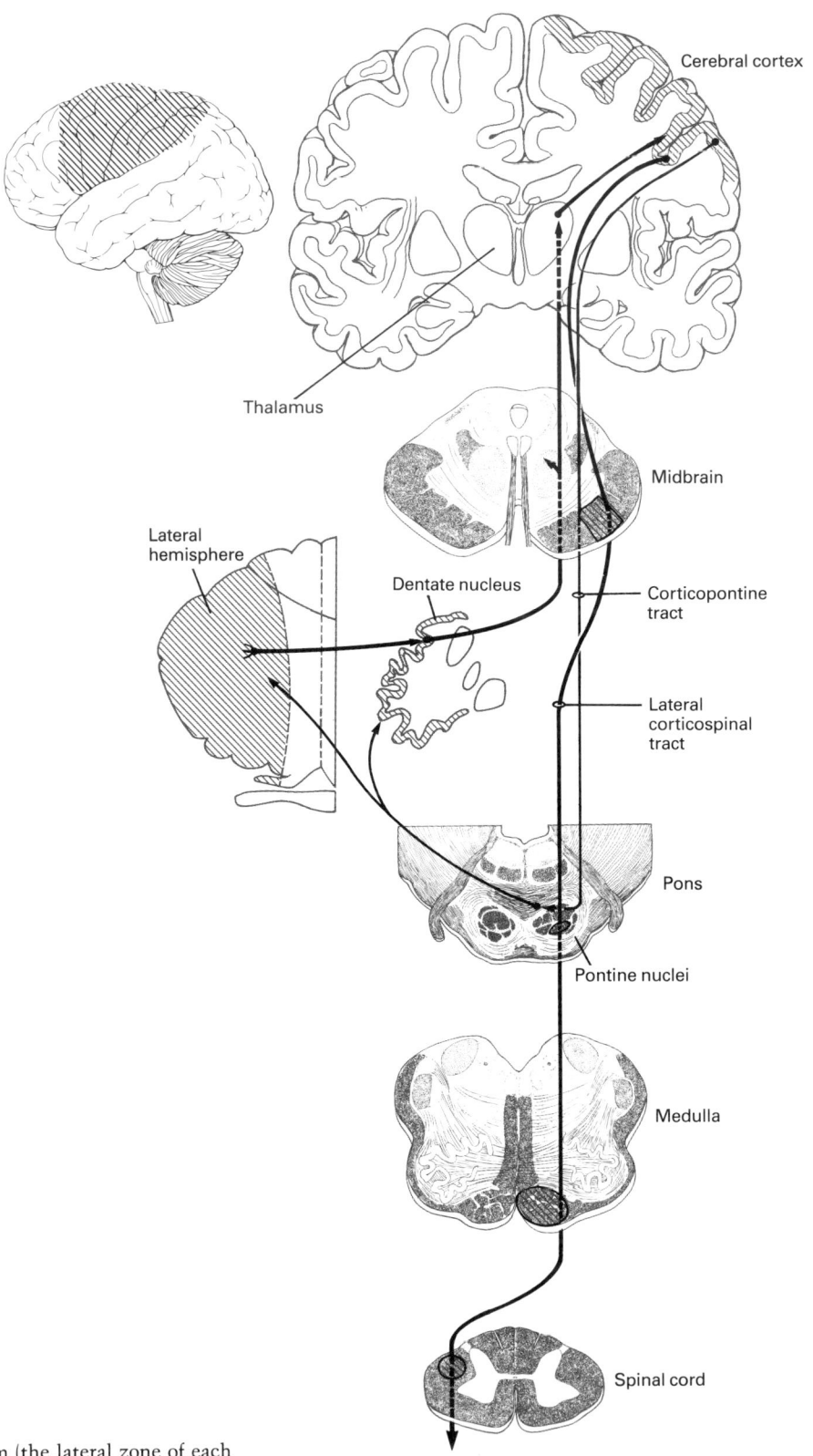

Cerebral cortex

Thalamus

Midbrain

Lateral
hemisphere

Dentate nucleus

Corticopontine
tract

Lateral
corticospinal
tract

Pons

Pontine nuclei

Medulla

Spinal cord

FIGURE 41–12
The cerebrocerebellum (the lateral zone of each
hemisphere) receives cortical input via the pontine
nuclei and influences the motor and premotor
cortices via the ventral lateral nucleus of the
thalamus.

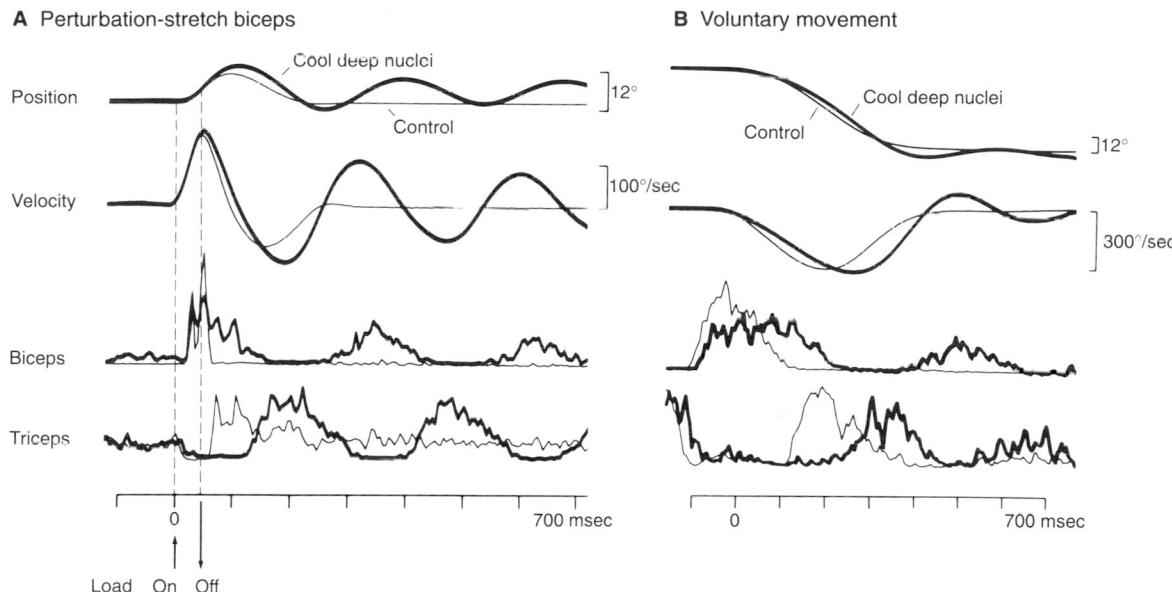

A Perturbation-stretch biceps

Position

Cool deep nuclei

Control

]12°

Velocity

]100°/sec

Biceps

Triceps

0   700 msec

Load On Off

B Voluntary movement

Cool deep nuclei

Control

]12°

]300°/sec

0   700 msec

FIGURE 41–13

Oscillations in limb position occur when the interposed and dentate nuclei are inactivated by cooling. (Courtesy of Jonathan Hore.)

A. Effects of cooling on responses to transient passive displacement of the limb. Position, acceleration, and electromyographic responses in biceps and triceps following a torque–pulse perturbation applied to the limb maintained in a stationary position by a trained monkey. Prior to cooling the limb returns to its original

position upon termination of the external torque; only minimal overshooting is evident on the acceleration trace. During cooling the limb returns with marked overshoot; sequential corrections produce oscillations. (From Vilis and Hore, 1977.)

B. Effects of cooling on movement trajectories. As in the case of passive movement, cooling of deep nuclei during voluntary movement produces oscillations in the trajectory.

more concerned with movement execution and feedback adjustments. The role played by the cerebrocerebellum in programming movement is particularly critical for multijoint (as opposed to single-joint) movements, and in those requiring fractionated digit movements. These movements are the ones that are most impaired following lesions or reversible inactivation of the dentate nucleus.

To study the contribution of the lateral cerebellum to movement, Jonathan Hore and his colleagues analyzed motor responses of monkeys during reversible inactivation of the dentate nuclei produced by local cooling with a chronically implanted probe. They found that cooling disrupted the precisely timed sequence of agonist and antagonist activation that occurs with normal rapid movements (Chapter 36). Agonist activation becomes slower and more prolonged while activation of the antagonist, which is needed to stop the movement at the right moment, is delayed and prolonged. As a result, rapid movements are characteristically overshot (*hypermetria*) as they are in patients with cerebellar lesions. This delayed deceleration results in an unintended movement in the opposite direction, constituting a new error that needs to be corrected. This correction gave rise to further errors and a period of terminal instability called *terminal tremor*. The same tremor occurs in patients with cerebellar lesions when the limb is passively displaced, or in monkeys

whose deep cerebellar nuclei are disrupted by cooling (Figure 41–13).

The lateral cerebellum may also perform a more general timing function that affects cognitive as well as motor performance. Richard Ivry and Steven Keele have found that cerebellar lesions interfere with the ability of patients to produce a sequence of simple but precisely timed tapping movements. They next asked: Does the irregularity shown by patients with cerebellar lesions reflect a disturbance in a central timing mechanism or a disturbance in the timing of movement execution. They found that, whereas medial cerebellar lesions interfered with the accurate execution of the response, lateral lesions interfered with the cognitive ability to set up a central clock-like mechanism. Patients with lateral lesions not only showed motor deficits in timing but their ability to judge elapsed time in purely perceptual tasks was severely disturbed. For example, they could not assess whether a tone of a given duration was longer or shorter than another, nor could they judge the speed of moving stimuli.

These current views of the role of the intermediate and lateral cerebellum are consistent with a model first proposed in the 1970s by Gary Allen and Nakaakira Tsukahara (Figure 41–14). According to this model the basal ganglia and lateral cerebellum process information originating in the sensory association cortex. This processing

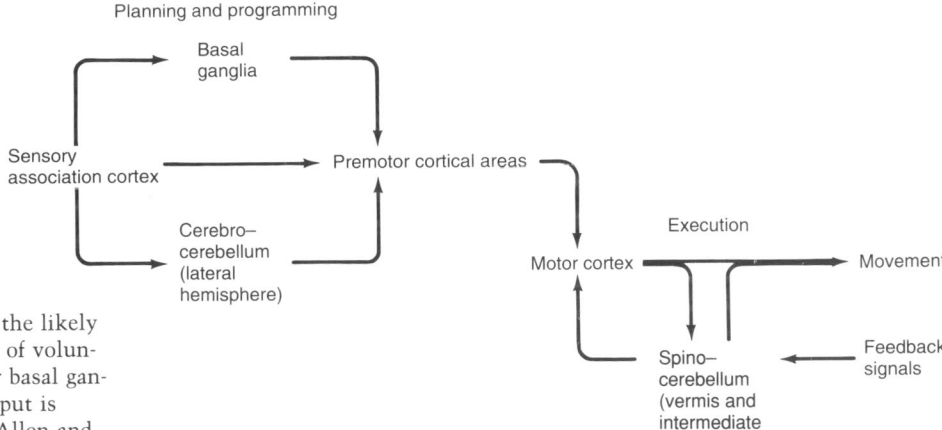

Planning and programming

FIGURE 41–14
This hypothetical flow diagram shows the likely role of the cerebellum in the initiation of voluntary movement. The thalamic relay for basal ganglia, cerebellar, and somatic sensory input is omitted for simplicity. (Adapted from Allen and Tsukahara, 1974.)

is critical for planning movement and preparing the motor systems to act. Eventually, the processed information forms the commands for movement issued by the lateral cerebellum and the basal ganglia to the premotor and motor cortical areas (and to subcortical centers that are not shown in Figure 41–14). These motor areas execute movement and inform the spinocerebellum of the ongoing commands. In turn the spinocerebellum then corrects for errors that have occurred or compensates for impending errors in the commands for movement.

The Cerebellum Participates in Motor Learning

On the basis of functional modeling of the cerebellum's circuitry during the early 1970s, first David Marr and later James Albus suggested that the cerebellum is necessary for the learning of motor skills. Both investigators proposed that the function of the climbing fiber input is to modify the response of Purkinje neurons to mossy fiber inputs for prolonged periods of time. Ito had already suggested that the information coming in to the cerebellum is processed in the deep nuclei, and that this processing is regulated by changing levels of Purkinje inhibition. In the context of Ito's idea, Marr suggested that the climbing fiber input on specific Purkinje cells acts to increase the effectiveness of mossy fiber synapses on any one Purkinje neuron. Albus then suggested that the climbing fiber input decreases the effectiveness of the mossy fibers and thereby acts to correct mismatches between intended and actual movement.

Several lines of evidence now support the idea that cerebellar circuits are modified by experience and that these changes are important for motor learning. Much of this work has focused on the vestibulo-ocular reflex, which maintains the orientation of the eyes on a fixed target when the head is rotated. In this reflex, motion of the head in one direction is sensed by the vestibular labyrinth which initates eye movements in the opposite direction to maintain the image on the retina (see Chapter 43). When

humans and experimental animals wear prismatic lenses that reverse the left and right visual fields, the vestibulo-ocular reflex is initially maladaptive. This is because the resulting eye movement accentuates motion of the visual field on the retina. However, as was discovered by Aaron Gonshor and Geoffrey Melville Jones and his colleagues, with time the direction of the reflex gradually becomes reversed. This learning is prevented by lesions of the vestibulocerebellum. This same kind of adaptation occurs in experimental animals such as the cat, and these adaptations also are prevented by lesions of the vestibulocerebellum.

To examine the neural mechanisms whereby the cerebellum participates in the learning of motor skills, Peter Gilbert and Thomas Thatch examined the activity of climbing fibers in monkeys who were trained to grasp a movable handle and then had to learn to maintain the handle in a new location using the flexors or extensors of the wrist. By connecting the handle to a motor, Gilbert and Thatch could introduce loads that unexpectedly displaced the handle. When the load was kept constant the trained animal returned the level rapidly and smoothly to the required position from trial to trial. However, when the load was changed unexpectedly the animal's response became inaccurate for many trials, until gradually it learned to counteract the load with the correct force (Figure 41–15).

Gilbert and Thatch now asked: What happens to the climbing fibers and to the mossy fibers during this learning task? They found that when the load was constant and predictable, each movement was accompanied by stereotyped fluctuations in simple spikes from mossy fiber, with an occasional interspersed complex spike from the climbing fibers (as we saw earlier, complex spikes only fire about once per second). When the load was changed suddenly, the pattern of firing of complex spikes increased dramatically and this increase was paralleled by a gradual decrease in firing frequency of simple spikes. As the animals learned the task and its performance became

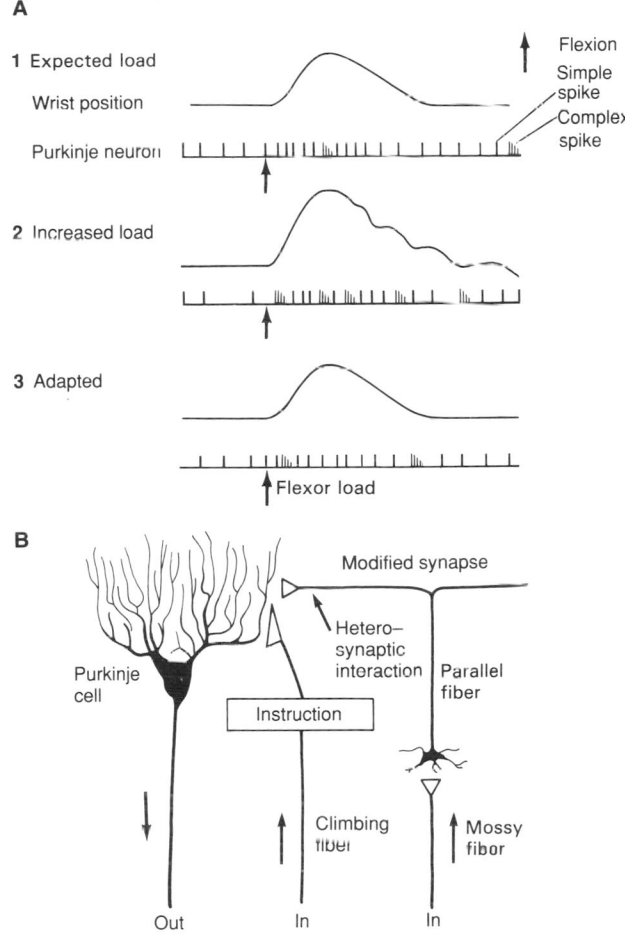

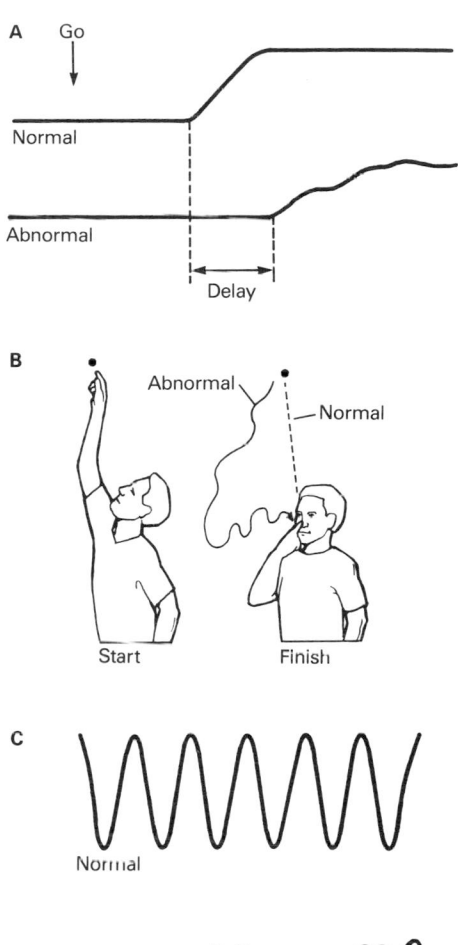

FIGURE 41–15

Cerebellar circuits are modified during learning.

A. Changes in simple and complex spike activity in the Purkinje neuron take place as a monkey learns to adapt to an increased load on wrist flexion. **1.** A control response is produced with only occasional complex spikes. **2.** In the trial immediately following application of an increased load, the neuron fires numerous complex spikes. **3.** After practice with the new load, activity in the neuron returns to the control frequency of complex spikes while the frequency of simple spikes has decreased. (Adapted from Gilbert & Thach, 1972.)

B. Simplified neural circuit showing the convergence of the two major inputs, the mossy fibers and climbing fibers, onto the cerebellum. The changes that occur in the cerebellum following the learning of a novel motor task result from the ability of the climbing fibers to depress the actions of the parallel fibers on the Purkinje cells. According to this view, the climbing fibers instruct or modulate the action of the mossy fibers. (Adapted from Ito, 1984.)

FIGURE 41–16

Typical defects observed in cerebellar diseases.

A. A lesion in the right cerebellar hemisphere causes a delay in the initiation of movement. The patient is told to flex both arms at the same time on a "go" signal. The left arm is flexed later than the right, as evident in the recordings of elbow position.

B. A patient moving his arm from a raised position to touch the tip of his nose exhibits dysmetria (inaccuracy in range and direction) and unsmooth movement with increased tremor on approaching the nose.

C. Dysdiadochokinesia, an irregular pattern of alternating movements, can be seen in the abnormal position trace.

smooth, the firing frequency of the complex spikes gradually returned to control levels. However, the firing of simple spikes remained decreased, as if firing of the mossy fibers had been modified so as to be adjusted to the new load. These findings demonstrate that the activity of the climbing fiber is modulated during motor learning, and

suggests that this modulation might serve to reduce, by heterosynaptic inhibition, the strength of the mossy fiber input to the Purkinje neurons. The reduction of mossy fiber input following the perturbing stimulus would in turn lead to a decrease in firing of the Purkinje cells and to an increase in the output (due to disinhibition) of the neurons in the deep nuclei. Consistent with the idea that these cellular changes actually mediate learned changes in behavioral response, Thatch and his colleagues have found that pharmacological inactivation of the cerebellar cortex prevents behavioral adaptation from occurring. The results agree with Albus's idea that the climbing fibers can decrease the activity of the mossy fibers, and that this heterosynaptic inhibition is designed to correct any mismatch between the intended movement and the results achieved.

The cerebellum's contribution to motor adaptation may reflect its more general role in forms of classical or Pavlovian conditioning (see Chapter 64). Richard Thompson and others have found that lesions of the cerebellum in the rabbit prevent the acquisition and disrupt the retention of a conditioned eyeblink reflex. The unconditioned stimulus is conveyed to the cerebellar Purkinje cells via the climbing fibers while mossy fibers relay the conditioned stimulus. After repeated pairing of conditioned and unconditioned stimuli, the conditioned stimulus lowers the firing rate of the Purkinje cells, as suggested by Albus. This in turn would cause an increase in firing of the nuclear cell and thereby produce a conditioned response. Thus, the cerebellum appears to have functions that go beyond the control of movement. Its role in motor learning is required because even normal motor behavior requires constant adaptation as circumstances change.

Cerebellar Diseases Have Distinctive Symptoms and Signs

Disorders of the cerebellum result in distinctive symptoms and signs first described in the 1920s and 1930s by Gordon Holmes. From his studies of patients who sustained gunshot wounds to the cerebellum in the first World War, Holmes described three principal deficits.

The first consists of *hypotonia*, and is manifest as a diminished resistance to passive limb displacements and in a delay in the response to such rapid imposed movements. This latter sign, also called *lack of check*, reflects the patient's inability to stop the limb rapidly so that the limb overshoots and may rebound excessively. It also is manifest in the *pendular reflexes*.

Second, Holmes described a variety of abnormalities in the execution of voluntary movements which can be globally referred to as *ataxia* (Figure 41–16). These abnormalities include several distinctive defects: a delay in initiating responses with the affected limb, errors in the range and force of movement or *dysmetria* (i.e., errors in the metrics of movement), and errors in the rate and regularity of movements. This last deficit is most readily demonstrated when the patient attempts to perform rapid alternating movements, such as tapping one hand with the other, alternating between the back and the palm of the hand. Patients cannot sustain a regular rhythm nor produce an even amount of force, a sign referred to as *dysdiadochokinesia*. Holmes also noted that patients made errors in the relative timing of the components of complex multijoint movements (*decomposition of movement*) and frequently failed to brace proximal joints against the forces generated by movement of more distal joints.

Third, patients may show a specific form of tremor called *action tremor* or *intention tremor*, although it is the act of moving rather than the intention to move that causes the tremor. A characteristic of cerebellar tremor is that it becomes most marked at the end of movement, when the patient attempts to achieve the greatest precision.

Several anatomical and physiological principles can guide the effort to localize disease processes to the cerebellum. One, lesions in the cerebellum produce disorders in the limbs ipsilateral to the lesion. This occurs because the output pathways of the cerebellum course through the superior cerebellar peduncle, which is crossed, and disturb mainly the action of the corticospinal and rubrospinal systems, which are also crossed.

Two, because of the somatotopic organization of the spinocerebellum, lesions of the midline vermis and fastigial nuclei principally produce disturbances in axial and truncal control. This may be manifest as *titubation*, a tremor in the trunk during standing or sitting, or as the drunken sailor's gait, an ataxia of gait in which stance is wide and balance is unsteady. Such patients may even have difficulties sitting erect, if unsupported. Because facial control is also localized to the vermis, there also may be a disorder in articulating speech (dysarthria) with slurring and slowing of speech with a characteristic singsong quality known as scanning-speech.

A restricted form of cerebellar cortical degeneration involves the anterior lobes (vermis and leg areas) and is common in alcoholic patients. The cardinal features of disease in this part of the cerebellum are involvement of the legs and impaired gait; the arms are relatively unaffected. The heel–shin test, which consists of sliding the heel of one foot slowly down the shin of the opposite leg, shows abnormal movements (*asynergia*). Gait is wide-based and ataxic. In contrast to the ataxia of gait following lesions of the flocculonodular lobe, the ataxia that accompanies disease of the anterior lobe vermis is not improved when the patient initiates walking while lying down. Thus, it is a more general deficit than an inability to control leg movements according to gravity.

More lateral lesions that impinge either on the intermediate cerebellum or the interposed nuclei produce ataxia of limb movements and action tremor. The disorders produced by lesions of the lateral cerebellar hemispheres, the cerebrocerebellum, consist principally in delays in initiating movement and decomposition of multijoint movements. This is especially manifest in movements of the distal joints with inability to flex single fingers while fixing the others.

Three, the most severe disturbances are produced by lesions of the superior cerebellar peduncle and the deep nuclei.

Four, the symptoms of cerebellar disease tend, however, to improve gradually with time if the underlying disease process does not itself progress. Recovery can be impressive when the lesions occur in childhood and, indeed, developmental anomalies in which the cerebellum is absent produce remarkably few signs. However, second cerebral lesions sustained at a later time may again reveal previously compensated cerebellar signs, suggesting that in young people cerebellar functions may be taken over by other parts of the brain.

An Overall View

Whereas lesions of other motor structures produce paralysis or involuntary movements, lesions of the cerebellum produce errors in the planning and execution of movements. How do these errors occur? The inputs and outputs of the subregions of the cerebellum indicate that it is able to compare internal feedback signals that reflect the *intended* movement with external feedback signals that reflect the *actual* movement. To generate corrective signals, the cerebellum computes errors. The corrective adjustments take the form of feedback and feed-forward controls that operate on the descending motor systems of the brain stem and cortex. The oscillations and the tremor that occur following lesions of the cerebellum are due to failure to correct movement properly or to defective use of sensory inputs in feedback correction.

The cerebellum also plays a role in motor learning. As we have seen in Chapter 35, most motor actions need to be initiated in an open loop way and to be planned in advance. Because of variations in the musculo-skeletal system, this feed-forward control requires calibration and adaptive adjustments of motor programs. The cerebellum is crucial to learned movement because even normal motor behavior requires constant adaptation as circumstances change. In addition, the Marr Albus model provides a framework for understanding the role played by the climbing fibers. Because of their low firing frequencies, these powerful inputs have a very modest capacity for transmitting moment-to-moment changes in sensory information. This would be a serious problem for feedback control but not for a mechanism that would adaptively adjust the operation of the system for a subsequent response. Finally, the cerebellum seems to participate in perception.

Nevertheless, it is instructive to recall a comment made by a patient of Gordon Holmes who had a lesion of his right cerebellar hemisphere: "The movements of my left arm are done subconsciously, but I have to think out each movement of the right (affected) arm. I come to a dead stop in turning and have to think before I start again." John Eccles proposed that the cerebellum spares us this mental task: A general movement command from higher brain centers leaves the details of the execution of the movement to subcortical, notably cerebellar, control mechanisms.

Selected Readings

Adams, R. D., and Victor, M. 1989. Principles of Neurology, 4th ed. New York: McGraw-Hill.

Asanuma, C., Thach, W. T., and Jones, E. G. 1983. Anatomical evidence for segregated focal groupings of efferent cells and their terminal ramifications in the cerebellothalamic pathway of the monkey. Brain Res. Rev. 5:267–297.

Brooks, V. B., and Thach, W. T. 1981. Cerebellar control of posture and movement. In V. B. Brooks (ed.), Handbook of Physiology, Section 1: The Nervous System, Vol. II. Motor Control, Part 2. Bethesda, Md.: American Physiological Society, pp. 877–946.

Gilman, S. 1985. The cerebellum: Its role in posture and movement. In M. Swash and C. Kennard (eds), Scientific Basis of Clinical Neurology. New York: Churchill Livingstone.

Glickstein, M., and Yeo, C. 1990. The cerebellum and motor learning. J. Cogn. Neurosci. 2:69–80.

Holmes, G. 1939. The cerebellum of man. Brain 62:1–30.

Ito, M. 1984. The Cerebellum and Neural Control. New York: Raven Press.

Keele, S. W., and Ivry, R. 1990. Does the cerebellum provide a common computation for diverse tasks? A Timing Hypothesis. Ann. N.Y. Acad. Sci. 608:179–211.

Llinás, R. 1981. Electrophysiology of the cerebellar networks. In V. B. Brooks (ed.), Handbook of Physiology, Section 1: The Nervous System, Vol. II. Motor Control, Part 2. Bethesda, Md.: American Physiological Society, pp. 831–876.

Thach, W. T., Kane, S. A., et al., (eds.) 1991. Cerebellar Output: Multiple Maps and Modes of Control in Movement Coordination, Ramon-y Cajal Centenary. Berlin: Springer. In press.

References

Adrian, E. D. 1943. Afferent areas in the cerebellum connected with the limbs. Brain 66:289–315.

Albus, J. S. 1971. A theory of cerebellar function. Math. Biosci. 10:25–61.

Allen, G. I., and Tsukahara, N. 1974. Cerebrocerebellar communication systems. Physiol. Rev. 54:957–1006.

Arshavsky, Yu. I., Berkenblit, M. B., Fukson, O. I., Gelfand, I. M., and Orlovsky, G. N. 1972. Recordings of neurones of the dorsal spinocerebellar tract during evoked locomotion. Brain Res. 43:272–275.

Arshavsky, Yu. I., Berkenblit, M. B., Fukson, O. I., Gelfand, I. M., and Orlovsky, G. N. 1972. Origin of modulation in neurones of the ventral spinocerebellar tract during locomotion. Brain Res. 43:276–279.

Botterell, E. H., and Fulton, J. F. 1938. Functional localization in the cerebellum of primates. II. Lesions of midline structures (vermis) and deep nuclei. J. Comp. Neurol. 69:47–62.

Botterell, E. H., and Fulton, J. F. 1938. Functional localization in the cerebellum of primates. III. Lesions of hemispheres (neocerebellum). J. Comp. Neurol. 69:63–87.

Chan-Palay, V., and Palay, S. L. 1984. Cerebellar Purkinje cells have glutamic acid decarboxylase, motilin, and cysteine sulfinic acid decarboxylase immunoreactivity: Existence and coexistence of GABA, motilin, and taurine. In V. Chan-Palay and S. L. Palay (eds.), Coexistence of Neuroactive Substances in Neurons. New York: Wiley, pp. 1–22.

Eccles, J. C., Ito, M., and Szentágothai, J. 1967. The Cerebellum as a Neuronal Machine. New York: Springer.

Flament, D., and Hore, J. 1986. Movement and electromyographic disorders associated with cerebellar dysmetria. J. Neurophys. 55:1221–1233.

Flament, D., and Hore, J. 1988. Comparison of cerebellar intention tremor under isotonic and isometric conditions. Brain Res. 439:179–186.

Flament, D., Vilis, T., and Hore J. 1984. Dependence of cerebellar tremor on proprioceptive but not visual feedback. Exp. Neurol. 84:314–325.

Gibson, A. R., Robinson, F. R., Alam, J., and Houk, J. C. 1987. Somatotopic alignment between climbing fiber input and nuclear output of the cat intermediate cerebellum. J. Comp. Neurol. 260:362–377.

Gilbert, P. F. C., and Thach, W. T. 1977. Purkinje cell activity during motor learning. Brain Res. 128:309–328.

Gilman, S. 1969. The mechanism of cerebellar hypotonia. An experimental study in the monkey. Brain 92:621–638.

Gilman, S., Carr, D., and Hollenberg, J. 1976. Kinematic effects of deafferentation and cerebellar ablation. Brain 99:311–330.

Gonshor, A., and Melvill Jones, G. 1976. Short-term adaptive changes in the human vestibulo-ocular reflex arc. J. Physiol. (Lond.) 256:361–379.

Gravel, C., and Hawkes, R. 1990. Parasagittal organization of the rat cerebellar cortex: Direct comparison of Purkinje cell compartments and the organization of the spinocerebellar projection. J. Comp. Neurol. 291:79–102.

Groenewegen, H. J., and Voogd, J. 1977. The parasagittal zonation within the olivocerebellar projection. I. Climbing fiber distribution in the vermis of cat cerebellum. J. Comp. Neurol. 174:417–488.

Groenewegen, H. J., Voogd, J., and Freedman, S. L. 1979. The parasagittal zonation within the olivocerebellar projection. II. Climbing fiber distribution in the intermediate and hemispheric parts of cat cerebellum. J. Comp. Neurol. 183:551–601.

Hore, J., and Flament, D. 1986. Evidence that a disordered servo-like mechanism contributes to tremor in movements during cerebellar dysfunction. J. Neurophysiol. 56:123–136.

Hore, J., and Vilis, T. 1984. Loss of set in muscle responses to limb perturbations during cerebellar dysfunction. J. Neurophysiol. 51:1137–1148.

Ivry, R. B., and Keele, S. W. 1989. Timing functions of the cerebellum. J. Cogn. Neurosci. 1:136–152.

Ivry, R. B., Keele, S. W., and Diener, H. C. 1988. Dissociation of the lateral and medial cerebellum in movement timing and movement execution. Exp. Brain Res. 73:167–180.

Jansen, J., and Brodal, A. (eds.) 1954. Aspects of Cerebellar Anatomy. Oslo: Grundt Tanum.

Keating, J. G., and Thach, W. T. 1990. Cerebellar motor learning: Quantitation of movement adaptation and performance in rhesus monkeys and humans implicates cortex as the site of adaptation. Soc. Neurosci. Abstr. 16:762.

Llinás, R. 1985. Functional significance of the basic cerebellar circuit in motor coordination. In J. R. Bloedel, J. Dichgans, and W. Precht (eds.), Cerebellar Functions. Berlin: Springer, pp. 170–185.

Lundberg, A., and Weight, F. 1971. Functional organization of connexions to the ventral spinocerebellar tract. Exp. Brain Res. 12:295–316.

Marr, D. 1969. A theory of cerebellar cortex. J. Physiol. (Lond.) 202:437–470.

McCormick, D. A., and Thompson, R. F. 1984. Cerebellum: Essential involvement in the classically conditioned eyelid response. Science 223:296–299.

Meyer-Lohmann, J., Conrad, B., Matsunami, K., and Brooks, V. B. 1975. Effects of dentate cooling on precentral unit activity following torque pulse injections into elbow movements. Brain. Res. 94:237–251.

Meyer-Lohmann, J., Hore, J., and Brooks, V. B. 1977. Cerebellar participation in generation of prompt arm movements. J. Neurophysiol. 40:1038–1050.

Miall, R. C., Weir, D. J. and Stein, J. F. 1987. Visuo-motor tracking during reversible inactivation of the cerebellum. Exp. Brain Res. 65:455–464.

Nieuwenhuys, T., Voogd, J., and van Huijzen, Chr. 1988. The Human Central Nervous System: A Synopsis and Atlas, 3rd rev. ed. Berlin: Springer.

Oscarsson, O. 1973. Functional organization of spinocerebellar paths. In A. Iggo (ed.), Handbook of Sensory Physiology, Vol. 2: Somatosensory System. New York: Springer, pp. 339–380.

Robinson, D. A. 1976. Adaptive gain control of vestibuloocular reflex by the cerebellum. J. Neurophysiol. 39:954–969.

Shambes, G. M., Gibson, J. M., and Welker, W. 1978. Fractured somatotopy in granule cell tactile areas of rat cerebellar hemispheres revealed by micromapping. Brain Behav. Evol. 15:94–140.

Snider, R. S., and Stowell, A. 1944. Receiving areas of the tactile, auditory, and visual systems in the cerebellum. J. Neurophysiol. 7:331–357.

Yeo, C. H., Hardiman, M. J., and Glickstein, M. 1984. Discrete lesions of the cerebellar cortex abolish classically conditioned nictitating membrane response of the rabbit. Behav. Brain Res. 13:261–266.

Soechting, J. F., Ranish, N. A., Palminteri, R., and Terzuolo, C. A. 1976. Changes in a motor pattern following cerebellar and olivary lesions in the squirrel monkey. Brain Res. 105:21–44.

Strick, P. L. 1983. The influence of motor preparation on the response of cerebellar neurons to limb displacements. J. Neurosci. 3:2007–2020.

Thach, W. T. 1978. Correlation of neural discharge with pattern and force of muscular activity, joint position, and direction of intended next movement in motor cortex and cerebellum. J. Neurophysiol. 41:654–676.

Vilis, T., and Hore, J. 1977. Effects of changes in mechanical state of limb on cerebellar intention tremor. J. Neurophysiol. 40:1214–1224.

Vilis, T., and Hore, J. 1980. Central neural mechanisms contributing to cerebellar tremor produced by limb perturbations. J. Neurophysiol. 43:279–291.

Voogd, J., and Bigaré, F. 1980. Topographical distribution of olivary and cortico nuclear fibers in the cerebellum: A review. In J. Courville, C. de Montigny, and Y. Lamarre (eds.), The Inferior Olivary Nucleus: Anatomy and Physiology. New York: Raven Press. pp. 207–234.

Yeo, C. H., Hardiman, M. J., and Glickstein, M. 1984. Discrete lesions of the cerebellar cortex abolish the classically conditioned nictitating membrane response of the rabbit. Behav. Brain Res. 13:261–266.

Lucien Côté
Michael D. Crutcher

42

The Basal Ganglia

The Basal Ganglia Consist of Five Nuclei

The Basal Ganglia Receive Input from and Project to the Cortex By Way of the Thalamus

> Internuclear Connections in the Basal Ganglia Are Topographically Organized

> The Basal Ganglia Project to Nuclei in the Thalamus

The Neostriatum Is Organized into Modules Called Striosomes and Matrix

The Motor Portion of the Basal Ganglia Is Somatotopically Organized and Involved in Higher-Order Aspects of Movement

The Basal Ganglia Are Linked to Cortex for Behavioral Functions Unrelated to Voluntary Movements

The Circuits within the Basal Ganglia Use Different Neurotransmitters

Diseases of the Basal Ganglia Have Characteristic Disorders in Transmitter Metabolism

> Loss of Dopaminergic Cells Leads to Parkinson's Disease

> The Neurotoxin MPTP Produces a Parkinsonian Syndrome

> Huntington's Disease Results from the Loss of Striatal Neurons

> There Are Now Genetic Markers for Huntington's Disease

> Tardive Dyskinesia Is a Response to Long-Term Treatment with Antipsychotic Drugs

Glutamate-Induced Neuronal Cell Death Contributes to Huntington's Disease

An Overall View

The basal ganglia consist of five large subcortical nuclei that participate in the control of movement. Unlike most other components of the motor system, the basal ganglia do not make either direct input or direct output connections with the spinal cord. Their primary input is from the cerebral cortex and their output is directed through the thalamus back to the prefrontal, premotor, and motor cortices. The motor functions of the basal ganglia are therefore mediated by the frontal cortex.

That the basal ganglia are involved in controlling movement first emerged from clinical observations. Postmortem examination of patients with Parkinson's disease, Huntington's disease, and hemiballismus revealed pathological changes in the basal ganglia. These diseases produce three characteristic types of motor disturbances: (1) tremor and other involuntary movements; (2) changes in posture and muscle tone; and (3) poverty and slowness of movement without paralysis. Primarily because of these clinical findings the basal ganglia were believed to be the major components of the so-called *extrapyramidal motor system*, which was thought to control movement in parallel with and independent of the *pyramidal* (or *corticospinal*) *motor system*. Thus, two different motor syndromes were distinguished: the *pyramidal tract syndrome*, characterized by spasticity and paralysis, and the *extrapyramidal syndrome*, characterized by involuntary movements, muscular rigidity, and immobility without paralysis.

There are several reasons why this simple dichotomy is no longer satisfactory. First, we now know that in addition to the extrapyramidal (basal ganglia) and pyramidal (corticospinal) systems, other parts of the brain participate in voluntary movement. Thus, disorders of the motor nuclei of the brain stem, red nucleus, or cerebellum also result in disturbances of movement. Second, the extrapyramidal and pyramidal systems are not independent, but are extensively interconnected and cooperate in the control of movement. Indeed, the motor actions of the basal ganglia

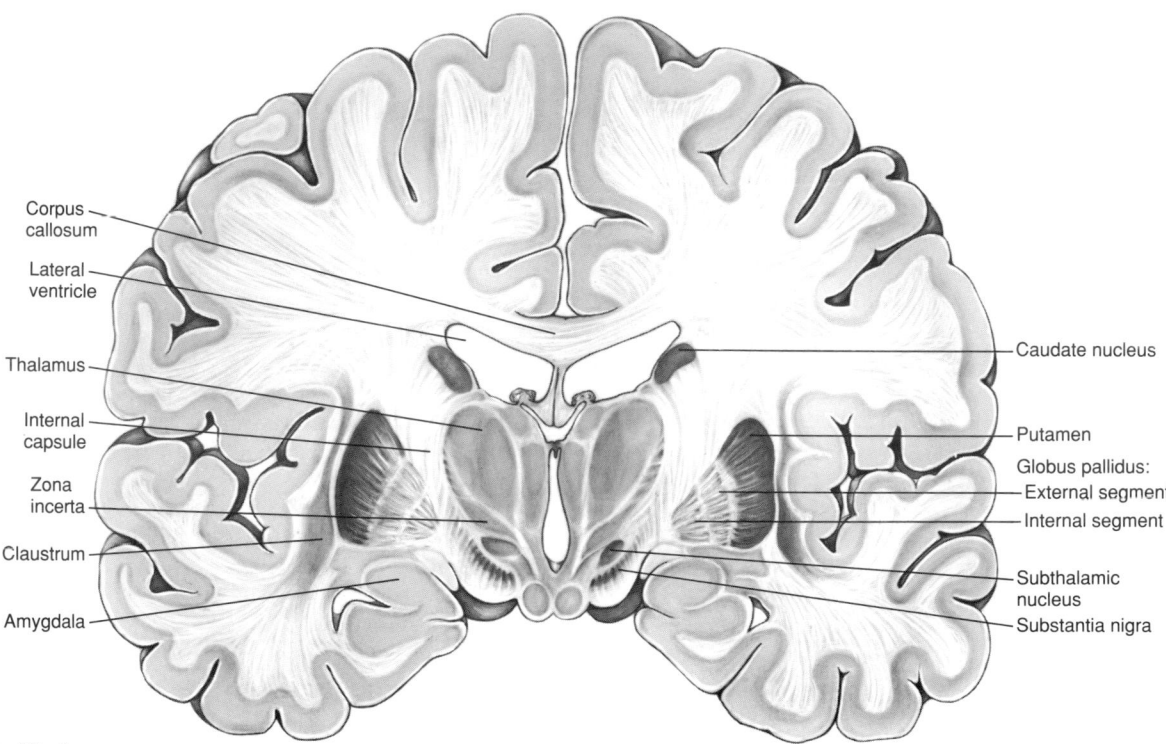

FIGURE 42–1
This coronal section shows the basal ganglia in relation to surrounding structures. (Adapted from Nieuwenhuys, Voogd, and van Huijzen, 1981.)

are mediated in part through the pyramidal system. Finally, the basal ganglia are involved in behaviors unrelated to movement. The basal ganglia have a role in cognitive function, which was first recognized in the characteristic cognitive disturbances of Huntington's disease. In addition, patients with Parkinson's disease have disturbances of affective as well as cognitive function. For these reasons, the concept of the extrapyramidal motor system, while historically important, is no longer adequate.

Diseases of the basal ganglia have always been important in clinical neurology because they are so common. In addition, Parkinson's disease was the first disease of the nervous system to be identified as a *molecular disease*. Here a specific defect in transmitter metabolism was shown to have a causal role. Therefore, in addition to providing important information about motor control, the study of diseased basal ganglia has also provided a paradigm for studying the relationship of transmitter molecules to disorders of mood and thought, a theme we shall consider again in Chapters 55 and 56.

The Basal Ganglia Consist of Five Nuclei

The basal ganglia consist of five extensively interconnected subcortical nuclei: the caudate nucleus, putamen, globus pallidus, subthalamic nucleus, and substantia nigra (Figure 42–1). The *caudate nucleus* and *putamen* develop from the same telencephalic structure; as a result, they are composed throughout of identical cell types and are fused anteriorly. Together the two nuclei are called the *neostri-*

atum (or *striatum*). They serve as the input nuclei for the basal ganglia.

The *globus pallidus* (or *pallidum*) is derived from the diencephalon and lies medial to the putamen and lateral to the internal capsule (Figure 42–1). It is divided into internal and external segments. The *subthalamic nucleus* lies below the thalamus at its junction with the midbrain. The *substantia nigra* lies in the midbrain and has two zones. A ventral pale zone, the *pars reticulata*, resembles the globus pallidus cytologically. A dorsal, darkly pigmented zone, the *pars compacta*, is comprised of dopaminergic neurons whose cell bodies contain neuromelanin. This dark pigment, a polymer derived from dopamine, gives the substantia nigra its name (Latin, black substance), because in humans this part of the brain appears black in cut sections. Because of the striking similarities in cytology, connectivity, and function of the internal segment of the globus pallidus and the substantia nigra pars reticulata, these two nuclei can be considered as a single structure arbitrarily divided by the internal capsule, much like the caudate and putamen. The globus pallidus and the substantia nigra pars reticulata constitute the major output nuclei of the basal ganglia.

The Basal Ganglia Receive Input from and Project to the Cortex By Way of the Thalamus

Almost all afferent connections to the basal ganglia terminate in the neostriatum. The neostriatum receives input from two major sources outside the basal ganglia: the

A Afferent connections

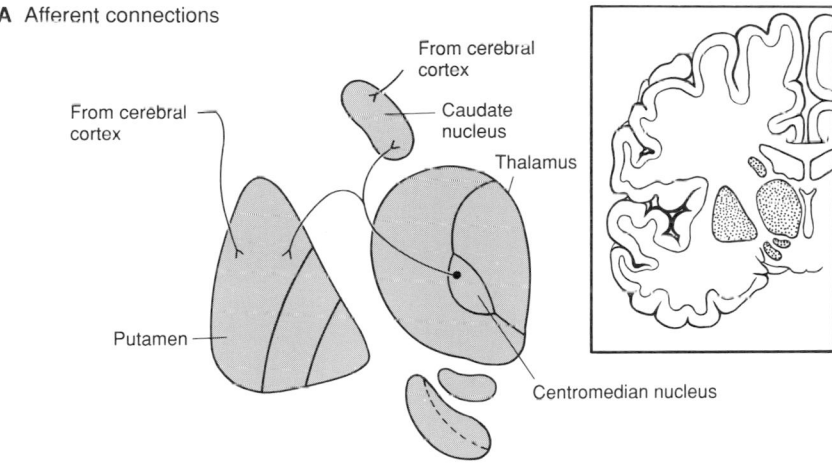

B Connections among basal ganglia

C Efferent connections

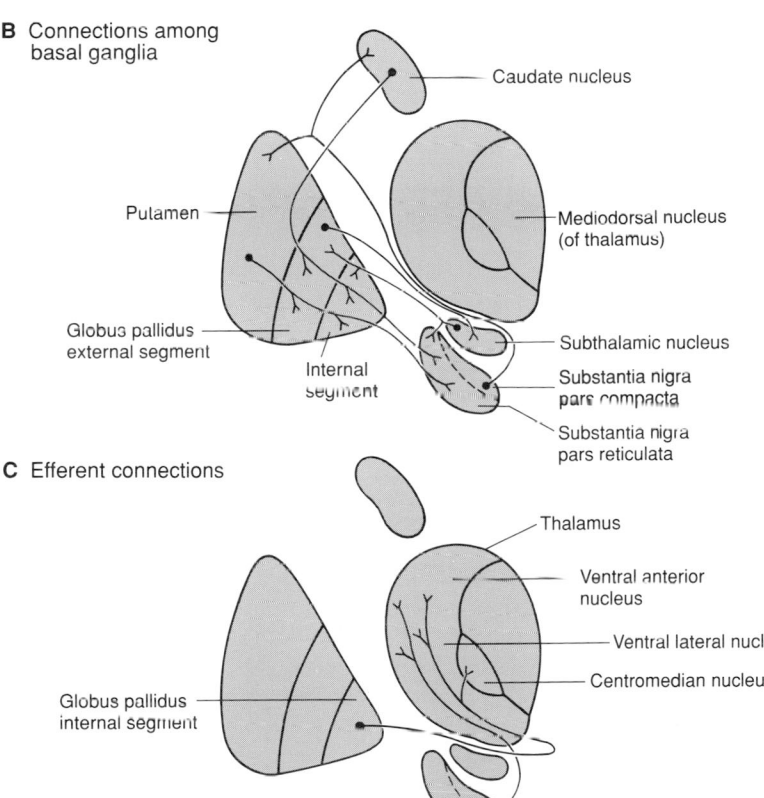

FIGURE 42–2

Major anatomical connections of the basal ganglia.

A. The caudate nucleus and putamen receive almost all afferent input to the basal ganglia.

B. The internuclear connections include topographically organized connections between all of the nuclei of the basal ganglia.

C. The principal target of efferent connections from the basal ganglia is the thalamus.

cerebral cortex and the intralaminar nuclei of the thalamus (Figure 42–2A). The most important input, the *corticostriate projection*, arises from the cerebral cortex. This pathway contains fibers from the entire cerebral cortex, including motor, sensory, association, and limbic areas. This projection is topographically organized; specific areas of the cortex project to different parts of the neostriatum, which therefore have specific behavioral functions. For example, the putamen is primarily concerned with motor control, the caudate is involved in the control of

eye movements and with certain cognitive functions, and the ventral striatum is related to limbic functions.

The input to the neostriatum from the intralaminar nuclei of the thalamus also is topographically organized. An important component of that input arises from the centromedian nucleus and terminates in the putamen. Because the centromedian nucleus receives input from the motor cortex, its projection to the neostriatum is an additional pathway by which the motor cortex can influence the basal ganglia.

Internuclear Connections in the Basal Ganglia Are Topographically Organized

The input cells of the neostriatum (the caudate and putamen) project to the globus pallidus (the *striatopallidal pathway*) and to the substantia nigra (the *striatonigral pathway*) (Figure 42–2B). These projections are organized so that each part of the neostriatum projects to specific parts of the globus pallidus and substantia nigra. Because the corticostriatal, the striatopallidal, and striatonigral pathways are all topographically organized, specific parts of the cortex act through the neostriatum on specific parts of the globus pallidus and substantia nigra.

The subthalamic nucleus receives the output of the external segment of the globus pallidus and has topographically organized projections to both segments of the globus pallidus and to the substantia nigra pars reticulata. The subthalamic nucleus also receives direct, topographically organized inputs from the motor and premotor cortices, providing the motor cortex another means for modulating the output of the basal ganglia. Finally, the neostriatum receives an important dopaminergic projection from the substantia nigra pars compacta.

The Basal Ganglia Project to Nuclei in the Thalamus

The major output pathways of the basal ganglia arise from the internal segment of the globus pallidus and the pars reticulata of the substantia nigra and project to three nuclei in the thalamus: the *ventral lateral*, *ventral anterior*, and *mediodorsal nuclei* (Figure 42–2C). The internal segment of the globus pallidus has an additional projection to the centromedian nucleus of the thalamus. The portions of the thalamus that receive input from the basal ganglia project to the prefrontal cortex, the premotor cortex, the supplementary motor area, and the motor cortex. Through this projection the basal ganglia influence other descending systems, such as the corticospinal and the corticobulbar systems. In addition to influencing movements of the body and limbs, the basal ganglia also influence eye movements by means of an additional projection from the substantia nigra pars reticulata to the superior colliculus.

The basal ganglia and cerebellum are the major constituents of two important subcortical loops of the motor system. Both receive major projections from the cerebral cortex and both project back to the cortex via the thalamus (Figure 42–3). There are three important differences, however, between the connections of the basal ganglia and those of the cerebellum. First, the basal ganglia receive inputs from the entire cerebral cortex. In contrast, the cerebellum receives input only from that part of the cortex that is directly related to sensorimotor functions. Second, the output of the cerebellum is directed back to the premotor and motor cortex, whereas the output of the basal ganglia is directed not only to the premotor and motor cortex but also to the prefrontal association cortex. Finally, the cerebellum receives somatic sensory informa-

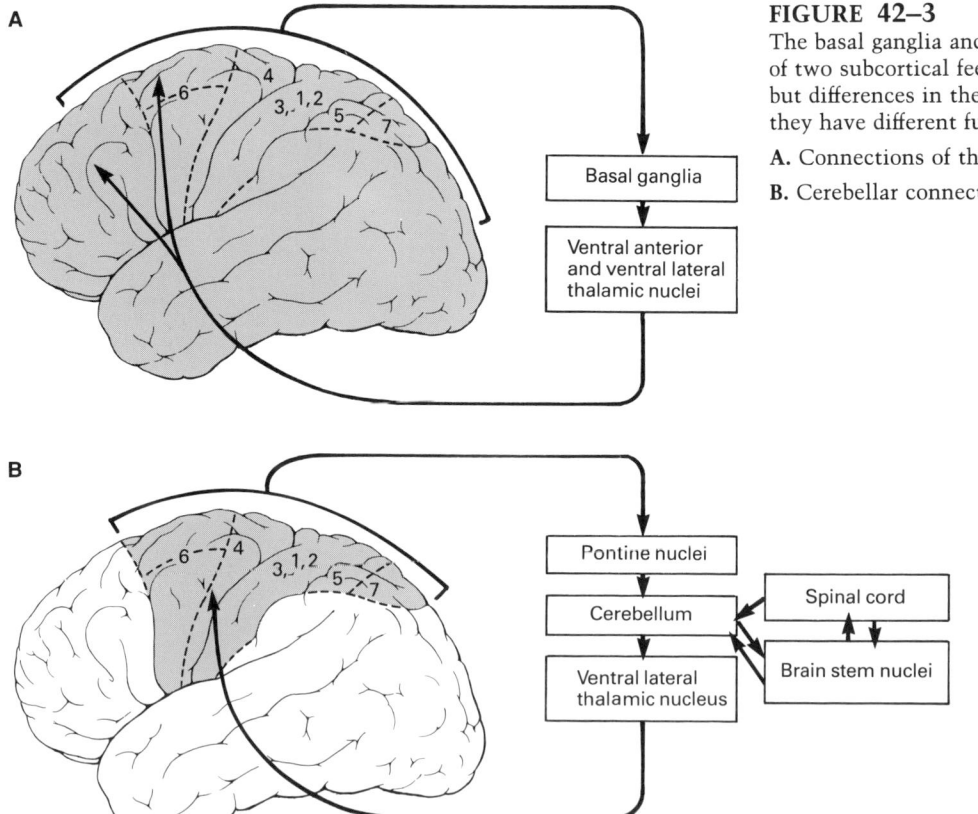

FIGURE 42–3

The basal ganglia and cerebellum are major components of two subcortical feedback loops of the motor system, but differences in their anatomical connections suggest they have different functions.

A. Connections of the basal ganglia.

B. Cerebellar connections.

tion directly from the spinal cord and has major afferent and efferent connections with many brain stem nuclei that are directly connected with the spinal cord. In contrast, the basal ganglia have relatively few connections to the brain stem and no direct connections at all to the spinal cord.

These differences suggest that the cerebellum directly regulates execution of movement, whereas the basal ganglia are involved in higher-order, cognitive aspects of motor control: the planning and execution of complex motor strategies. In addition, because of their extensive connections with association cortex and limbic structures, the basal ganglia unlike the cerebellum are involved in many functions other than motor control.

The Neostriatum Is Organized into Modules Called Striosomes and Matrix

Using a variety of techniques Ann Graybiel and Patricia Goldman-Rakic found that inputs to the striatum from cortex and thalamus end in patches or modules that appear to be analogous to the columns of the cortex. These modules have also been identified by the patchy distribution of markers for various neurotransmitters and neuropeptides, including dopamine, enkephalin, and substance P. The smaller of these neurochemically specialized compartments are called *striosomes*. These are in turn embedded in a larger compartment called the *matrix*.

The majority of cortical projections to the striatum concerned with sensation and movement terminate in the *matrix compartment*. This compartment projects to the pallidum and substantia nigra pars reticulata and is thought to mediate information critical for motor or cognitive behavior. The limbic projections terminate in the striosomes which project to the dopaminergic neurons of the substantia nigra. Thus the striosome compartment may modulate the dopaminergic pathway.

Further evidence for the modular organization of the striatum comes from electrophysiological studies of the activity of single cells during movement. These studies reveal that during passive movements of a single joint the cells in certain compartments become active, whereas during active movements of the same joint, cells of other compartments become active. Thus, these compartments in the neostriatum represent functionally distinct modules much like the functional columns of the cortex.

The Motor Portion of the Basal Ganglia Is Somatotopically Organized and Involved in Higher-Order Aspects of Movement

The anatomical basis for the motor functions of the basal ganglia is illustrated in Figure 42–4. Those portions of the cerebral cortex most closely related to the control of movement (supplementary motor area, premotor cortex,

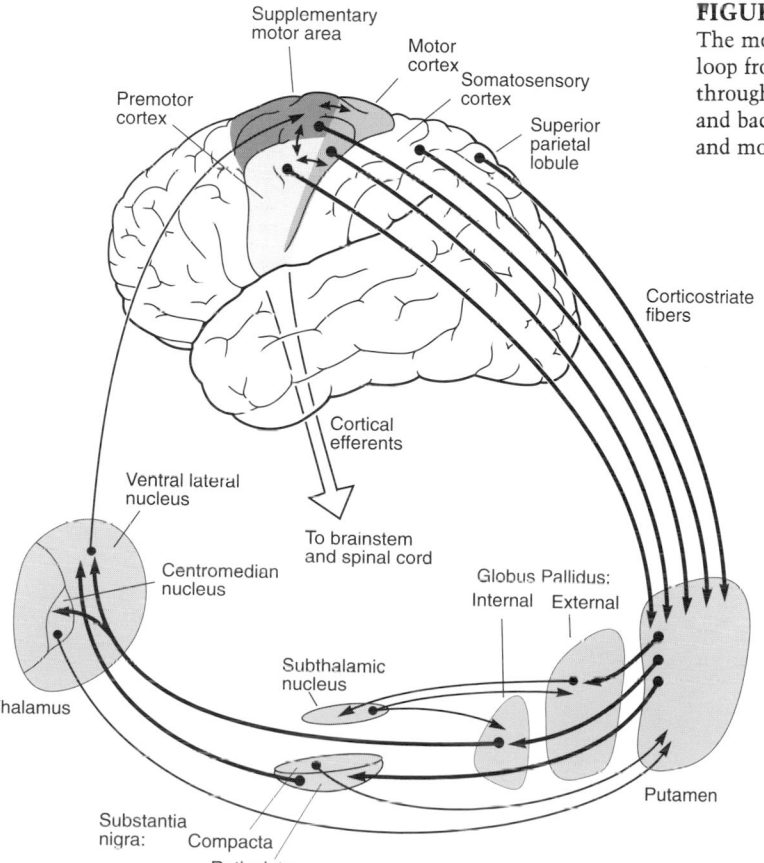

FIGURE 42–4
The motor circuit of the basal ganglia is a subcortical feedback loop from the motor and somatosensory areas of the cortex, through restricted portions of the basal ganglia and thalamus, and back to the premotor cortex, supplementary motor area, and motor cortex.

motor cortex, somatosensory cortex, and the superior parietal lobule) make dense, topographically organized projections to the motor portion of the putamen. The output of this pathway, termed the *motor circuit* of the basal ganglia, is directed primarily back to the supplementary motor area and premotor cortex. These areas are reciprocally interconnected with each other and with the motor cortex and all have direct descending projections to brain stem motor centers and the spinal cord. Thus, the motor functions of the basal ganglia are not mediated directly but by means of these three cortical motor areas and their descending projections.

The activity of some neurons in the basal ganglia resembles the activity of cells in the motor and supplementary motor area. The activity is related to discrete and directionally selective passive and active movements of individual parts of the body, usually movements of a single joint. Despite this resemblance, the activity of neurons in the putamen differs from that of neurons in the cortex and supplementary motor area in several interesting ways.

First, in response to visually guided tracking tasks the cells in the basal ganglia that are selective for movement fire later than cells in the cortical motor areas. Second, neurons in the putamen are more likely to be selective for the direction of limb movement than for the activation of specific muscles. These findings indicate that the basal ganglia do not play a significant role in the initiation of stimulus-triggered movements and do not specify directly the muscular forces necessary for the execution of movement.

What do the basal ganglia do? Why, for example, do lesions of the basal ganglia and the motor cortex or cerebellum result in distinctly different motor disturbances? Perhaps the basal ganglia selectively facilitate some movements and suppress others, analogous to the inhibitory surround characteristic of receptive fields in the sensory systems. This idea is attractive because it can explain many of the diverse symptoms characteristic of diseases of the basal ganglia. Alternatively, the basal ganglia may compare commands for movement from the precentral motor fields with proprioceptive feedback from the evolving movement. This might be useful for regulating a movement or for monitoring its consequences. Finally, the basal ganglia may be involved in the initiation of internally generated movements. This possibility is consistent with the striking inability to initiate movement (akinesia) exhibited by patients with Parkinson's disease.

The Basal Ganglia Are Linked to Cortex for Behavioral Functions Unrelated to Voluntary Movements

In addition to the motor circuit of the basal ganglia (the pathway from the cortical motor areas to the putamen to the globus pallidus and substantia nigra and back to the supplementary motor and premotor areas), there are at least three other circuits that connect the basal ganglia to the thalamus and cortex.

(1) *The Oculomotor Circuit.* The frontal eye fields and several other cortical areas project to the body of the caudate. The caudate then projects to both the superior colliculus and the frontal eye fields via the thalamus. The circuit is involved in the control of saccadic eye movements.

(2) *The Dorsolateral Prefrontal Circuit.* The dorsolateral prefrontal cortex and several other areas of association cortex project to the dorsolateral head of the caudate nucleus, which in turn projects back to the dorsolateral prefrontal cortex via the thalamus. This circuit is probably involved in aspects of memory concerned with orientation in space.

(3) *The Lateral Orbitofrontal Circuit.* This circuit links the lateral orbitofrontal cortex with the ventromedial caudate. It is thought to be involved in the ability to change behavioral set.

Thus the basal ganglia subserve many functions, perhaps all of the functions served by the cortex itself!

The Circuits within the Basal Ganglia Use Different Neurotransmitters

Figure 42–5 shows a model of the circuitry of the basal ganglia. The cortical inputs to the neostriatum are excitatory and mediated by glutamatergic neurons. There are two major pathways through the basal ganglia. The *direct pathway* is the striatal projection to the internal segment of the globus pallidus and substantia nigra pars reticulata (the output nuclei of the basal ganglia), which then project to the thalamus. The *indirect pathway* is the circuit from the neostriatum to the external segment of the globus pallidus, which projects to the subthalamic nucleus. The subthalamic nucleus in turn projects back to both pallidal segments and the substantia nigra.

The direct pathway from the striatum to the output nuclei is mediated by GABA and substance P. This pathway is inhibitory as is the pathway from the output nuclei to the thalamus, mediated by GABA. Movement results when the thalamic cells are released from tonic inhibition. This occurs when corticostriate inputs excite striatal neurons, which results in phasic disinhibition, an inhibition of inhibitory cells in the basal ganglia output nuclei. The resulting activation of thalamocortical neurons is thought to facilitate movement by exciting premotor and supplementary motor areas and thus activating their projections to the motor cortex, the brain stem, and the spinal cord.

The indirect pathway of the basal ganglia operates differently (Figure 42–5). Corticostriatal excitation results in inhibition of the external segment of the pallidum, mediated by GABA and enkephalin, and disinhibition of the subthalamic nucleus, mediated by GABA, which excites the output nuclei, mediated by glutamate. This inhibits the thalamus and decreases the excitation of the supplementary motor area.

The dopaminergic projection from the substantia nigra has several effects on neurons in the neostriatum. Dopamine excites the direct pathway, the striatal neurons that send GABA and substance P projections to the output nu-

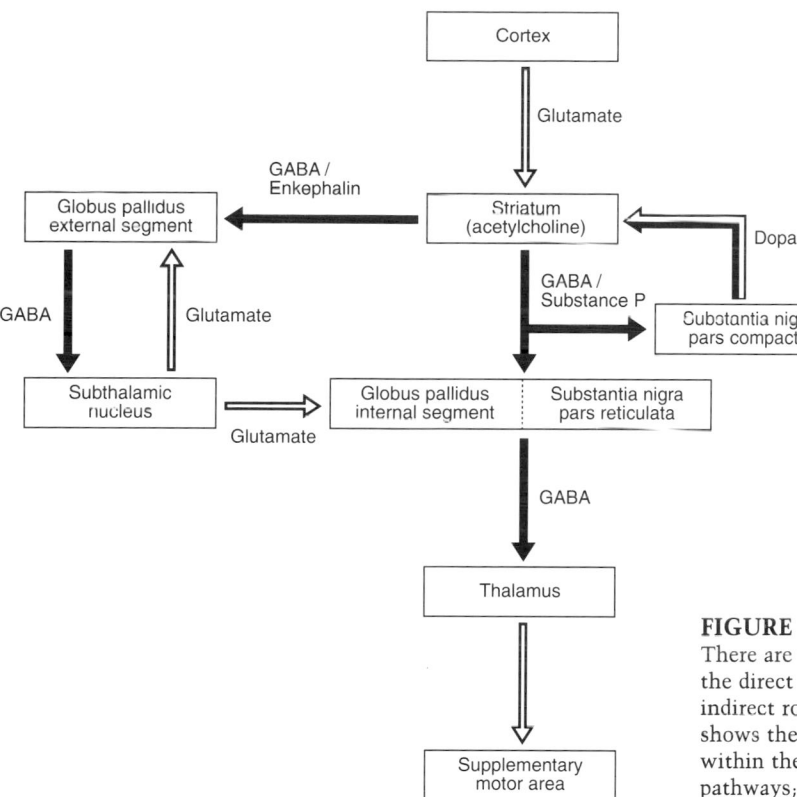

FIGURE 42–5

There are two different pathways through the basal ganglia: the direct route from the striatum to the output nuclei and the indirect route through the subthalamic nucleus. This figure shows the possible interactions of different neurotransmitters within the basal ganglia. (**Black arrows** represent inhibitory pathways; **white arrows** represent excitatory projections.)

clei. In contrast, dopamine inhibits the indirect pathway, the striatal neurons that send GABA and enkephalin projections to the external segment of the pallidum. Since the direct pathway appears to facilitate movement by exciting the supplementary motor area while the indirect pathway has the opposite effect, dopamine appears to facilitate movement by acting on both pathways.

These two pathways seem to counterbalance one another. Activation of the striatum can have opposite effects on the output nuclei (and thus on the thalamus and cortex). Disturbances in the activity of different portions of these two interrelated pathways, either as a result of diseases of transmitter metabolism, as in Parkinson's disease, or following lesions, as in hemiballismus, can disrupt this balance. Depending on the site of the disturbance, this can lead either to the production of involuntary movements or to such impairments of movement as lack of movement (akinesia), slowness of movement (bradykinesia), and the shuffling gait of Parkinson's disease.

We now turn to the specific alterations in basal ganglia output responsible for these clinically different disorders.

Diseases of the Basal Ganglia Have Characteristic Disorders in Transmitter Metabolism

Diseases of the basal ganglia characteristically produce involuntary movements. These include *tremors* (rhythmic, involuntary, oscillatory movements), *athetosis* (slow, writhing movements of the fingers and hands, and some-

times of the toes), *chorea* (abrupt movements of the limbs and facial muscles), *ballism* (violent, flailing movements), and *dystonia* (a persistent posture of a body part which can result in grotesque movements and distorted positions of the body). These symptoms often occur together and may have a common basis.

As we have seen in Chapter 35, Hughlings Jackson divided all motor disorders into two classes: negative signs attributed to the loss of function of specific neurons, and positive signs (or *release phenomena*) caused by the emergence of an abnormal pattern of action in neurons when their controlling input (usually their inhibitory input) is impaired. The abnormal movements that occur in basal ganglia disease are thought to belong to the second category. The major disorders of movement are summarized in Table 42–1.

Aspects of basal ganglia disease can be simulated by manipulating specific transmitter systems. For example, akinesia (difficulty in initiating a movement), often associated with rigidity and postural abnormalities, results from destruction or blockade of the ascending dopamine pathways. These symptoms, which resemble those of Parkinson's disease, can be produced in experimental animals more easily by altering specific transmitter systems, which causes an abnormal output from the basal ganglia, than by lesions in the basal ganglia, which eliminate the output. Therefore it is likely that the underlying pathology of disorders of the basal ganglia in humans is a disruption of transmitter metabolism.

TABLE 42–1. Disorders of the Basal Ganglia

Disorder	Pathophysiology	Chemical changes	Clinical manifestations	Treatment
Parkinson's disease	Degeneration of the nigrostriatal pathway, raphe nuclei, locus ceruleus, and motor nucleus of vagus	Reduction in dopamine, serotonin, and norepinephrine	Slowly progressive; third most common neurological disease (affects 500,000 Americans); about 15% of patients have a first-degree relative with the disease; mean age of onset is 58 years; findings are tremor at rest (3–6 beats/s), cogwheel rigidity, akinesia, bradykinesia, and postural reflex impairment	L-DOPA with or without peripheral DOPA decarboxylase inhibitor; anticholinergic agents: trihexyphenidyl or benztropine
Huntington's disease	Degeneration of intrastriatal and cortical cholinergic neurons and GABA-ergic neurons	Reduction in choline acetyltransferase, glutamic acid, decarboxylase, and GABA	Progressive disease with associated dementia and death within 10–15 years; about 10,000 cases in the United States; autosomal dominant; onset at any age, but usually in adulthood; findings are chorea, decreased tone (may occur), and dementia	No specific therapy; dopamine antagonists phenothiazines and butyrophenones, useful in controlling chorea
Ballism	Damage to one subthalamic nucleus, often due to acute vascular accident		Most severe form of involuntary movement disorder known; tends to clear up slowly	Neuroleptics (butyrophenones)
Tardive dyskinesia	Alteration in dopaminergic receptors causes hypersensitivity to dopamine and its agonists		Iatrogenic disorder due to long-term treatment with phenothiazines or butyrophenones; abnormal involuntary movements especially of the face and tongue; usually temporary but can be permanent	Stop offending drug

Loss of Dopaminergic Cells Leads to Parkinson's Disease

In 1817 James Parkinson, a physician working in London, described the motor disorder that now bears his name:

. . . involuntary tremulous motion, with lessened muscular power, in parts not in action and even when supported; with a propensity to bend the trunk forwards, and to pass from a walking to a running pace, the senses and intellects being uninjured.

Parkinson's disease (paralysis agitans) is one of the best characterized diseases of the basal ganglia. Its symptoms are (1) a rhythmical tremor at rest, (2) a unique increase in muscle tone or rigidity that often has a cogwheel- or ratchet-like characteristic, (3) difficulty in the initiation of movement and paucity of spontaneous movements (akinesia), and (4) slowness in the execution of movement (bradykinesia). This slowness is often most evident in the way the patient gets up from a bed or chair and in the characteristic shuffling gait. In Parkinson's disease there is a marked decrease in the dopaminergic projection from the substantia nigra.

Several advances in our understanding of diseases of the basal ganglia were made in the late 1950s, when Arvid Carlsson observed that 80% of the dopamine in the brain is localized in the basal ganglia—an area that makes up less than 0.5% of the total weight of the brain! Soon afterwards, Oleh Hornykiewicz, studying brains obtained at postmortem examination, found that in patients with Parkinson's disease the content of dopamine, norepinephrine, and serotonin was low. He next observed that, of the three biogenic amines, dopamine was most drastically reduced. Parkinson's disease therefore became the first example of a disease of the brain associated with a deficiency in a specific neurotransmitter. This discovery stimulated a thorough search for alterations in neurotransmitters in other disorders of the brain, including depression, schizophrenia, and dementia.

In addition to a reduction of dopamine the brains of patients with Parkinson's disease also have loss of nerve cells and depigmentation in the two pigmented nuclei of the brain stem: the substantia nigra and the locus ceruleus. The severity of changes in the substantia nigra parallels the reduction of dopamine in the striatum. Because the pars compacta of the substantia nigra contains many of the dopaminergic nerve cell bodies in the brain, these observations suggest that the dopaminergic pathway from the substantia nigra to the striatum is disturbed in Parkinson's disease.

Walter Birkmayer and Hornykiewicz reasoned that patients with Parkinson's disease might be helped if the amount of dopamine in the brain were restored to normal. They therefore gave L-3,4-hydroxyphenylalanine (L-DOPA) intravenously to patients with Parkinson's disease. This amino acid is the immediate precursor of dopamine but, unlike dopamine, it crosses the blood-brain barrier. Birkmayer and Hornykiewicz observed a remarkable but brief remission in their patients' symptoms and thus suggested a new approach to the treatment of Parkinson's disease.

How L-DOPA ameliorates the symptoms of Parkinson's disease is still unclear. Dopamine is synthesized in the neostriatum, in the nerve endings of dopaminergic neurons whose cell bodies lie in the substantia nigra. At these nerve endings the transmitter is taken up into vesicles and released in the synaptic cleft when the cell fires. In Parkinson's disease as many as 90% of the dopaminergic neurons degenerate. What then is the fate of L-DOPA in patients with Parkinson's disease? Presumably the L-DOPA is taken up and converted into dopamine (see Chapter 14) by the remaining dopaminergic nerve cells. The few healthy dopaminergic neurons and those that have partially degenerated may be able to compensate by carrying out the entire function of the nigrostriatal system once tyrosine hydroxylase, the rate-limiting enzyme for the synthesis of dopamine, is bypassed with the large amounts of L-DOPA. Another possibility is that DOPA decarboxylase, which is not specific to dopaminergic neurons, can synthesize dopamine from the orally administered L-DOPA in nondopaminergic cells—for example, in serotonergic neurons or other neurons, or perhaps even in glial cells. This exogenously formed dopamine might then be generated in amounts large enough to act on appropriate target cells.

In addition to the dopaminergic projection to the neostriatum, there are also dopaminergic projections to parts of the limbic system and the frontal neocortex. The akinesia seen in patients with Parkinson's disease may be due partly to dopamine depletion in the limbic system, especially in the nucleus accumbens. Some of the specific cognitive deficits of the disease may also be due to loss of dopamine from nerve endings in the cortex.

Although recent evidence suggests that the loss of striatal dopamine alone accounts for most of the symptoms, in Parkinson's disease there are also losses of noradrenergic neurons in the locus ceruleus and serotonergic neurons in the raphe nuclei.

The Neurotoxin MPTP Produces a Parkinsonian Syndrome

In 1982 seven drug abusers in northern California tried intravenous forms of a synthetic heroin derivative. As a result they all developed the signs and symptoms of Parkinson's disease: rigidity, akinesia, bradykinesia, tremor, and bent posture. It was soon discovered that the drug contained a toxic contaminant 1-methyl-4-phenyl-1,2,3,6-tetrahydropyridine (MPTP). When MPTP is injected into experimental animals, the animals also develop the same clinical symptoms. These findings led to an important advance: an animal model of Parkinson's disease. In the animal model there is a significant reduction in dopamine levels in the brain, resulting from loss of dopaminergic cells in the substantia nigra pars compacta and the ventral tegmental area.

The discovery that MPTP is highly toxic to the dopaminergic neurons of the substantia nigra suggested that an environmental toxin may play a role in the development of Parkinson's disease. No toxic agent that has this action has yet been discovered in humans. Research on the mechanisms by which MPTP produces its effects revealed that the toxin needs to be converted to MPP^+ (1-methyl-4-phenylpyridinium) by monoamine oxidase. This suggested the possibility that inhibitors of monoamine oxidase might block the progression of Parkinson's disease. Recent evidence suggests that L-deprenyl, a selective inhibitor of monoamine oxidase B, slows the progression of Parkinson's disease and raises the level of dopamine in the brains of parkinsonian patients. (The latter effect occurs presumably because monoamine oxidase also catalyzes the degradation of dopamine.) Consequently, L-deprenyl is now used effectively together with L-DOPA to treat patients with Parkinson's disease.

Although L-DOPA therapy has been hailed as the most significant advance in the treatment of Parkinson's disease, it has not been the panacea hoped for when it was first introduced. At that time it was hoped that L-DOPA might not only ameliorate the symptoms of Parkinson's disease, but also arrest it and even reverse some of the degenerative changes seen in the substantia nigra. This does not happen. L-DOPA only controls some of the symptoms; it does not alter the course of the disease. In addition, many patients become refractory or suffer side effects after treatment with L-DOPA for several years.

Two approaches have been used to overcome the limitations of L-DOPA therapy. First, fetal dopamine cells have been transplanted into the striatum (see also Chapter 18). The clinical usefulness of these transplants is still being debated. Second, thalamotomy has been found to reduce the tremor and rigidity, but does not improve the bradykinesia or gait impairment.

Huntington's Disease Results from the Loss of Striatal Neurons

In 1872 George Huntington, a physician living on Long Island in New York, described a disease that he, his father, and his grandfather had observed in several generations of their patients. The disease was characterized by four features: heritability, chorea (Greek, dance), dementia, and death 15 or 20 years after onset. This disease, now called Huntington's disease, affects men and women with equal frequency, about 5 per 100,000 population. In most patients the onset of the disease occurs in the fourth to fifth decade of life. Thus, the disease strikes after most individuals have married and had children. Each child of an affected parent has a 50% chance of inheriting the disease. One of the tragic aspects of the disease in the past was that no test was available to make the diagnosis before the symptoms become apparent. As a result, the children of a patient lived for decades in the fear that they, too, may have inherited the gene for the disease.

The first signs of the disorder are subtle: absentmindedness, irritability, and depression, accompanied by fidgeting, clumsiness, or sudden falls. Uncontrolled movements, a prominent feature of the disease, gradually increase until the patient is confined to bed or to a wheelchair. Speech is slurred at first, then incomprehensible, and finally stops altogether as facial expressions become distorted and grotesque. Cognitive functions also deteriorate, and eventually the ability to reason disappears. No treatment is available. Once the disease has begun its inexorable course, the patient faces years of gradually decreasing capacity, followed by total disability and certain death.

Huntington's disease results from the loss of specific sets of cholinergic and GABA-ergic neurons in the striatum. Nerve cell death (up to 90%) in the striatum is thought to cause the chorea. The impaired cognitive functions and eventual dementia may be due either to the concomitant loss of cortical neurons or to the disruption of normal activity in the cognitive portions of the basal ganglia, namely the dorsolateral prefrontal and lateral orbitofrontal circuits described previously. It is now possible to demonstrate selective loss of neurons in the caudate nucleus of a patient with Huntington's disease while the individual is still alive, using imaging techniques described in Chapter 22.

Normally a balance is maintained among the activities of three biochemically distinct but functionally interrelated systems: (1) the nigrostriatal dopaminergic system; (2) the intrastriatal cholinergic neurons; and (3) the GABA-ergic system, which projects from the striatum to the globus pallidus and substantia nigra (Figure 42–5). In Parkinson's disease reduction of the dopaminergic system causes an increase in the output of the basal ganglia to the thalamus, leading to tremor, rigidity, and bradykinesia. In Huntington's disease, on the other hand, the intrastriatal cholinergic and GABA-ergic neurons are destroyed.

The loss of striatal neurons in Huntington's disease is at first selective, involving the population of GABA-ergic neurons projecting to the external segment of the pallidum. This loss releases the inhibition of the external pallidum and thus suppresses subthalamic activity as a result of the increased GABA-ergic input. Lesions of the subthalamic nucleus, both in humans with strokes and in experimental animals, result in involuntary movement of the limbs on one side of the body (hemiballismus). The chorea characteristic of Huntington's disease may also be due to a reduction in activity in the subthalamic nucleus.

Thus, Huntington's disease and Parkinson's disease, which clinically are present with opposite types of symptoms (one hyperkinetic and hypotonic, the other hypokinetic and hypertonic), are associated with almost opposite alterations in basal ganglia output (decreased in Huntington's disease and increased in Parkinson's disease). Moreover, in both disorders the subthalamic nucleus is strongly implicated in mediating the abnormal basal ganglia output.

Both choline acetyltransferase, the enzyme required for the formation of acetylcholine, and glutamic acid decarboxylase, the enzyme required to synthesize GABA, are markedly decreased in the striatum of patients with Huntington's disease. These enzyme deficits are consistent with the clinical observation that choreic movements worsen in patients with Huntington's disease following administration of L-DOPA. Conversely, a parkinsonian patient given too much L-DOPA develops involuntary movements such as chorea, athetosis, and dystonia. Thus, an imbalance anywhere in the dopamine, acetylcholine, or GABA systems can cause involuntary movements.

There Are Now Genetic Markers for Huntington's Disease

The genetic transmission of Huntington's disease became evident when it was discovered that practically all patients with this disease on the east coast of the United States were descendants of two ancestors who were born in Suffolk, England, and who emigrated to Salem, Massachusetts in 1630. In all likelihood, several of the apparently deranged women in Salem who were executed as witches were actually exhibiting symptoms of the disease. The familial pattern is impressive; traced through 12 generations (over 300 years), the disease has been expressed in each generation.

Huntington's disease is inherited as a highly penetrant, autosomal dominant disorder. As we have seen in Chapter

17, the normal human complement of chromosomes consists of 22 pairs of autosomes (nonsex chromosomes) and one pair of sex chromosomes. Using a technique to map gene restriction fragment length polymorphisms (see Box 17-1), James Gusella and his colleagues located the region on chromosome 4 that contains the mutated gene responsible for Huntington's disease. For this purpose, they screened DNA samples from a group of Venezuelans known to carry the gene by epidemiological studies. These people all were descended from a woman who lived near Lake Maracaibo at the beginning of the nineteenth century and who suffered from Huntington's disease most likely because her father, an English sailor, carried the gene. Most of this woman's descendants married and remained near Lake Maracaibo, and she now has more than 3,000 living descendants, 100 of them with Huntington's disease. In addition, there are 1,100 children, each with a 50% chance of inheriting the disease. Gusella, Nancy Wexler, and their colleagues found a consistent correlation between Huntington's disease and a restriction enzyme DNA fragment estimated to be several million base pairs from the end of the short arm of chromosome 4, the site of the mutation (Figure 42–6). Another marker was found recently that is only within one million base pairs of the genetic defect.

Although the locus of the Huntington's disease gene has not yet been identified, the localization that has been obtained has two important consequences. First, it may allow the disease to be diagnosed before symptoms develop or even prenatally. Second, this localization will eventually allow the defective gene to be cloned, a prerequisite for identifying the gene product and ultimately determining how a mutation of this gene causes the disease.

Tardive Dyskinesia Is a Response to Long-Term Treatment with Antipsychotic Drugs

Tardive dyskinesia is another clinical disorder that may involve the basal ganglia; its symptoms are involuntary movements, especially of the face and tongue. It is a medically induced (iatrogenic) disorder caused by long-term treatment with antipsychotic agents that decrease the function of dopaminergic cells—the phenothiazines (e.g., chlorpromazine, perphenazine) and the butyrophenones (e.g., haloperidol). These drugs appear to block dopaminergic transmission and may eventually make dopaminergic receptors hypersensitive to dopamine. The balance between the dopaminergic, intrastriatal cholinergic, and GABA-ergic systems is thus altered, and involuntary movements appear as a consequence.

Glutamate-Induced Neuronal Cell Death Contributes to Huntington's Disease

Cells die for a number of reasons. Which of these contribute to diseases of the basal ganglia? One cause of cell

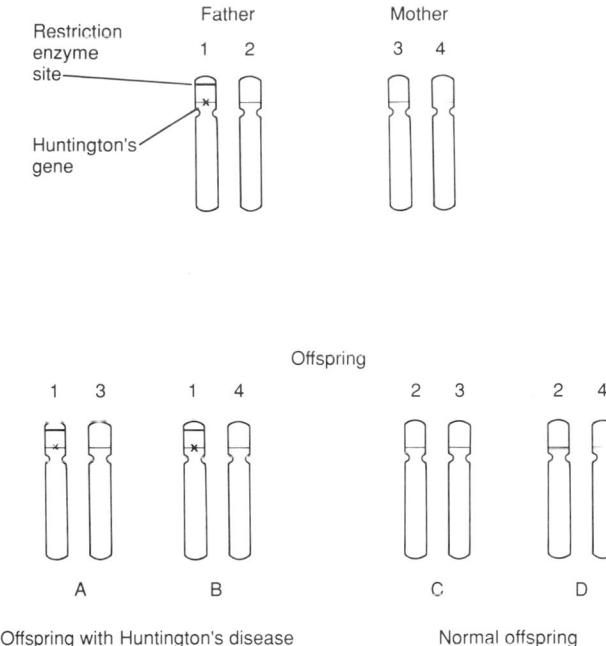

FIGURE 42–6
The inheritance of the gene responsible for Huntington's disease can be traced by following the inheritance of restriction fragment polymorphisms for chromosome 4.

death, observed in the nematode worm *Caenorhabditis elegans*, is genetically programmed and occurs during development (Chapter 18). A second kind of cell death, found during development in the vertebrate nervous system, involves an overproduction of neurons followed by death of a subset of these neurons. This type of cell death is thought to result from the failure of some outgrowing neurons to compete successfully for a limited amount of growth factor (as discussed in Chapter 59). Many studies now indicate that a third and common cause of pathological cell death occurs in the mature nervous system as a result of the transformation of normal transmitter signaling mechanisms into a mechanism for cell destruction (see Chapter 11).

Glutamate is the principal excitatory transmitter in the central nervous system. It excites virtually all central neurons and is present in the nerve terminals in extremely high concentrations (10^{-3} M). In normal synaptic transmission the level of glutamate rises in the synaptic cleft only transiently and this rise is restricted to the synaptic cleft. In contrast, sustained and diffuse increases in glutamate kills neurons. This mechanism of cell death occurs primarily by the persistent action of glutamate on the N-methyl-D-aspartate (NMDA) type of glutamate receptors and the resulting excessive influx of Ca^{2+} (Chapter 11). Excess Ca^{2+} has several damaging consequences leading to cytoxicity and death. First, it can mobilize active Ca^{2+}-dependent proteases. Second, Ca^{2+} activates phos-

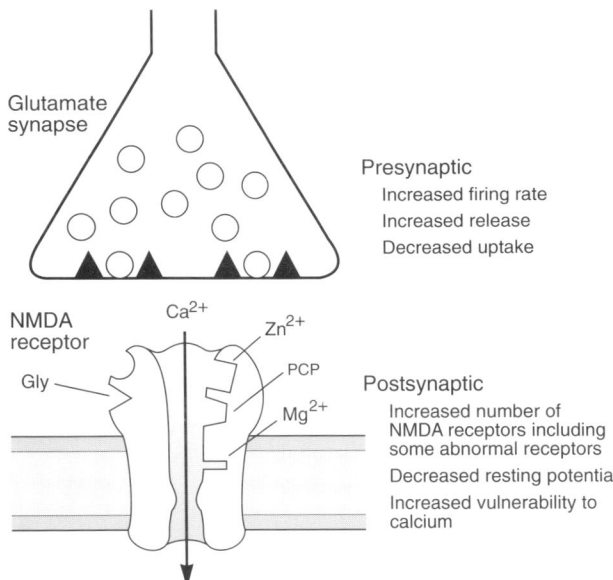

Presynaptic
- Increased firing rate
- Increased release
- Decreased uptake

Postsynaptic
- Increased number of NMDA receptors including some abnormal receptors
- Decreased resting potential
- Increased vulnerability to calcium

FIGURE 42–7

Possible presynaptic and postsynaptic mechanisms of N-methyl-D-aspartate (NMDA) receptor-mediated toxicity in Huntington's disease. Different presynaptic and postsynaptic abnormalities affecting glutamate synapses could produce NMDA receptor-mediated neurotoxicity in Huntington's disease. Presynaptically, there might be excessive neuronal activity, excessive glutamate release, or reduced glutamate uptake (into nerve terminals or glia). Postsynaptically, an abnormally large number of NMDA receptors, altered NMDA receptor-channel complexes (e.g., with increased mean channel open time), reduced average resting potential (leading to decreased Mg^{2+} block), or increased vulnerability to Ca^{2+}-mediated damage (e.g., due to reduced Ca^{2+} buffering capability). All could underlie NMDA receptor-mediated injury. In addition, NMDA receptor-mediated toxicity could also be produced by abnormalities in modulatory factors, reduced synaptic Zn^{2+}, excess synaptic glycine (Gly), or an abnormal amount of a modifying NMDA agonist (like quinolinate). If NMDA receptor-activated channels are normally partially blocked by an endogenous ligand for the phencyclidine (PCP) site, reduced levels of such a ligand would be another possibility. (From Choi, 1988.)

pholipase A_2, which liberates arachidonic acid, leading to the production of substances causing inflammation and possibly free radicals can trigger still other destructive events.

Toxic changes produced by glutamate, called *glutamate excitotoxicity*, are thought to cause cell damage and death following acute brain injury such as stroke or excessive convulsions. In addition, excitotoxicity may contribute to chronic degenerative diseases of the brain, such as Huntington's disease. Joseph Korland, Patrick McGeer, and their colleagues have found that injection of NMDA agonists into the rat striatum reproduces the pattern of neuronal cell loss characteristic of Huntington's disease. Thus, it is possible that the abnormal gene on chromosome 4 produces an abnormality that leads to excessive activation of NMDA receptors (Figure 42–7).

An Overall View

In 1949 Linus Pauling revolutionized medical thinking by introducing the concept of a molecular disease. He and his collaborators observed a change in the electrophoretic mobility of hemoglobin S and reasoned that sickle cell anemia, a disease known to be genetic, could be explained by a mutation of a gene for a specific protein. A decade later Vernon Ingram showed that this alteration in charge occurs in the amino acid sequence of hemoglobin S, where a glutamic acid residue is replaced by a valine. This change from a single negatively charged residue in normal hemoglobin to a neutral one explains the altered molecular properties of hemoglobin S, and these in turn account for the intermolecular and cellular differences observed in sickled red cells. Thus, the molecular change is fundamental to understanding the patient's pathology, symptoms, and prognosis.

While the explanation for other diseases may not be as simple, it is a fundamental principle of modern medicine that each disorder has a molecular basis. Parkinson's disease and myasthenia gravis are disorders that historically have made the medical community realize that specific molecular components of chemical synapses are likely to be targets for disease. In myasthenia gravis the molecular target is the acetylcholine receptor. In the disorders of the basal ganglia some components of the synthesis, packaging, or turnover of dopamine and serotonin are altered. What causes the pathological alterations at these loci, whether genetic, infectious, toxic or degenerative, is not yet known. Although we may soon be in a position to identify the mutant gene for Huntington's disease, as yet we have no idea about the molecule(s) affected by the disorder. Rational treatment for diseases of transmitter metabolism requires a good understanding of synaptic transmission in the affected pathways. The diseases of the basal ganglia are a powerful motive for expanding our insight into synaptic physiology and motor behavior.

Selected Readings

Albin, R. L., Young, A. B., and Penney, J. B. 1989. The functional anatomy of basal ganglia disorders. Trends Neurosci. 12:366–375.

Alexander, G. E., and Crutcher, M. D. 1990. Functional architecture of basal ganglia circuits: Neural substrates of parallel processing. Trends Neurosci. 13:266–271.

Alexander, G. E., DeLong, M. R., and Strick, P. L. 1986. Parallel organization of functionally segregated circuits linking basal ganglia and cortex. Annu. Rev. Neurosci. 9:357–381.

Barden, H. 1981. The biology and chemistry of neuromelanin. In R. S. Sohal (ed.), Age Pigments. Amsterdam: Elsevier North-Holland Biomedical Press, pp. 155–180.

Botstein, D., White, R. L., Skolnick, M., and Davis, R. W. 1980. Construction of a genetic linkage map in man using restriction fragment length polymorphisms. Am. J. Hum. Genet. 32:314–331.

DeLong, M. R. 1990. Primate models of movement disorders of basal ganglia origin. Trends Neurosci. 13:281–285.

DeLong, M. R., and Georgopoulos, A. P. 1981. Motor functions of the basal ganglia. In V. B. Brooks (eds.), Handbook of Physiology, Section 1: The Nervous System, Vol. II. Motor Control, Part 2. Bethesda, Md.: American Physiological Society, pp. 1017–1061.

DiFiglia, M. 1990. Excitototoxic injury of the neostriatum: A model for Huntington's disease. Trends Neurosci. 13:286–289.

Harper, P. S. 1984. Localization of the gene for Huntington's chorea. Trends Neurosci. 7:1–2.

Kopin, I. J., and Markey, S. P. 1988. MPTP toxicity: Implications for research in Parkinson's disease. Annu. Rev. Neurosci. 11: 81–96.

Langston, J. W., and Irwin, I. 1986. MPTP: Current concepts and controversies. Clin. Neuropharmacol. 9:485–507.

Martin, J. B. 1984. Huntington's disease: New approaches to an old problem. Neurology 34:1059–1072.

Yurek, D. M., and Sladek, J. R., Jr. 1990. Dopamine cell replacement: Parkinson's disease. Annu. Rev. Neurosci 13:415–440

References

Bertler, Å., and Rosengren, E. 1959. Occurrence and distribution of dopamine in brain and other tissues. Experientia 15:10–11.

Birkmayer, W., and Hornykiewicz, O. (eds.) 1976. Advances in Parkinsonism: Biochemistry, Physiology, Treatment. Fifth International Symposium on Parkinson's Disease (Vienna). Basel: Roche.

Carlsson, A. 1959. The occurrence, distribution and physiological role of catecholamines in the nervous system. Pharmacol. Rev. 11:490–493.

Choi, D. W. 1988. Glutamate neurotoxicity and diseases of the nervous system. Neuron 1:623–634.

Crutcher, M. D., and DeLong, M. R. 1984. Single cell studies of the primate putamen. I. Functional organization. Exp. Brain Res. 53:233–243.

Goldman, P. S., and Nauta, W. J. H. 1977. An intricately patterned prefronto-caudate projection in the rhesus monkey. J. Comp. Neurol. 171:369–385.

Graybiel, A. M. 1984. Neurochemically specified subsystems in the basal ganglia. In D. Evered and M. O'Connor (eds.), Functions of the Basal Ganglia. Ciba Foundation Symposium 107. London: Pitman, pp. 114–149.

Gusella, J. F., Wexler, N. S., Conneally, P. M., Naylor, S. L., Anderson, M. A., Tanzi, R. E., Watkins, P. C., Ottina, K., Wallace, M. R., Sakaguchi, A. Y., Young, A. B., Shoulson, I., Bonilla, E., and Martin, J. B. 1983. A polymorphic DNA marker genetically linked to Huntington's disease. Nature 306:234–238.

Hikosaka, O., and Wurtz, R. H. 1983. Visual and oculomotor functions of monkey substantia nigra pars reticulata. I. Relation of visual and auditory responses to saccades. J. Neurophysiol. 49:1230–1253.

Hikosaka, O., and Wurtz, R. H. 1983. Visual and oculomotor functions of monkey substantia nigra pars reticulata. II. Visual responses related to fixation of gaze. J. Neurophysiol. 49: 1254–1267.

Hikosaka, O., and Wurtz, R. H. 1983. Visual and oculomotor functions of monkey substantia nigra pars reticulata. III. Memory-contingent visual and saccade responses. J. Neurophysiol. 49:1268–1284.

Hikosaka, O., and Wurtz, R. H. 1983. Visual and oculomotor functions of monkey substantia nigra pars reticulata. IV. Relation of substantia nigra to superior colliculus. J. Neurophysiol. 49:1285–1301.

Hikosaka, O., and Wurtz, R. H. 1985. Modification of saccadic eye movements by GABA-related substances. I. Effect of muscimol and bicuculline in monkey superior colliculus. J. Neurophysiol. 53:266–291.

Hikosaka, O., and Wurtz, R. H. 1985. Modification of saccadic eye movements by GABA-related substances. II. Effects of muscimol in monkey substantia pars reticulata. J. Neurophysiol. 53:292–308.

Hornykiewicz, O. 1966. Metabolism of brain dopamine in human parkinsonism: Neurochemical and clinical aspects. In E. Costa, L. J. Côté, and M. D. Yahr (eds.), Biochemistry and Pharmacology of the Basal Ganglia. New York: Raven Press, pp. 171–185.

Housman, D., and Gusella, J. 1982. Molecular genetic approaches to neural degenerative disorders. In F. O. Schmitt, S. J. Bird, and F. E. Bloom (eds.), Molecular Genetic Neuroscience. New York: Raven Press, pp. 415–422.

Huntington, G. 1872. On chorea. Med. Surg. Reporter 26:317–321.

Ingram, V. M. 1957. Gene mutations in human haemoglobin: The chemical difference between normal and sickle cell haemoglobin. Nature 180:326–328.

Jackson, J. H. 1932. Selected Writings of John Hughlings Jackson, Vol. 2. J. Taylor (ed.) London: Hodder & Stoughton.

Johnson, T. N., and Rosvold, H. E. 1971. Topographic projections on the globus pallidus and the substantia nigra of selectively placed lesions in the precommissural caudate nucleus and putamen in the monkey. Exp. Neurol. 33:584–596.

Landau, W. M. 1990. Clinical neuromythology VII - Artificial intelligence: The brain transplant cure for parkinsonism. Neurology 40:733–740.

Lee, T., Seeman, P., Rajput, A., Farley, I. J., and Hornykiewicz, O. 1978. Receptor basis for dopaminergic supersensitivity in Parkinson's disease. Nature 273:59–61.

McGeer, P. L., Eccles, J. C., and McGeer, E. G. 1987. Molecular Neurobiology of the Mammalian Brain, 2nd ed. New York: Plenum Press.

Nieuwenhuys, R., Voogd, J., and van Huijzen, Chr. 1981. The Human Central Nervous System: A Synopsis and Atlas, 2nd ed. Berlin: Springer.

Parkinson, J. 1817. An Essay on the Shaking Palsy. London.

Pauling, L., Itano, H. A., Singer, S. J., and Wells, I. C. 1949. Sickle cell anemia: A molecular disease. Science 110:543–548.

Ungerstedt, U., Ljungberg, T., Hoffer, B., and Siggins, G. 1975. Dopaminergic supersensitivity in the striatum. In D. Calne, T. N. Chase, and A. Barbeau (eds.), Dopaminergic Mechanisms. Advances in Neurology, Vol. 9. New York: Raven Press, pp. 57–65.

Watson, J. D., Tooze, J., and Kurtz, D. 1983. Recombinant DNA: A Short Course. New York: Scientific American Books.

Michael E. Goldberg
Howard M. Eggers
Peter Gouras

43

The Ocular Motor System

Five Neuronal Control Systems Keep the Fovea on Target

The Vestibulo-ocular and Optokinetic Reflexes Compensate for Head Movement

The Smooth Pursuit System Keeps Moving Targets in the Fovea

The Saccadic System Points the Fovea Toward Objects of Interest

The Vergence Movement System Aligns the Eyes to Look at Targets with Different Depths

The Eye Is Moved by Three Complementary Pairs of Muscles

Eye Position and Velocity Are Signaled by Extraocular Motor Neurons

The Vestibulo-ocular Reflex Is Coordinated in the Brain Stem

The Semicircular Canals Send an Eye Velocity Signal to Brain Stem Oculomotor Centers

Disease of the Vestibular System Causes Nystagmus

A Brain Stem Network Coordinates the Horizontal Vestibulo-ocular Reflex

A Neural Integrator Maintains Eye Position After the Head Has Stopped Moving

Modulation of the Vestibulo-ocular Reflex Requires the Cerebellum

Subcortical and Cortical Structures Contribute to the Optokinetic Reflex

Saccades and Smooth Pursuit Are Organized in Pontine and Mesencephalic Reticular Centers

Horizontal Saccades Are Generated in the Pontine Reticular Formation

Vertical Saccades Are Generated in the Mesencephalic Reticular Formation

Modulation of the Saccadic System by Experience Requires the Cerebellum

Smooth Pursuit Requires the Cerebral Cortex, Cerebellum, and Pons

Vergence Is Organized in the Midbrain

Patients with Brain Stem Lesions Have Characteristic Deficits in Eye Movements

The Saccade Generator in the Brain Stem Is Controlled in the Cerebral Cortex

The Superior Colliculus Transmits Cortical Oculomotor Signals to the Brain Stem

The Frontal Eye Field Sends a Specific Movement Signal to the Superior Colliculus

An Overall View

In the last several chapters we learned about the motor systems that control the head and body. In this chapter we consider the ocular motor system, the motor system that controls the position of the eyes. The neural control of eye movements is simpler than that for limb movement. The repertoire of eye movements is small, consisting of only five types of movements, and each eye has only six muscles. This simplicity has made the oculomotor system attractive for neural scientists interested in the neurobiology of behavior.

Although we detect objects over a large visual angle of about 200°, we see objects best with the fovea, the central 1° of the visual field, which is less than 1 mm in diameter. Thus, when we look around in an exploratory manner we have to move the fovea quickly from one object to another to make the search efficient. Once we find something, however, we want to stabilize its image on the retina so we can see it clearly, even when the head moves. The oculomotor system, then, has two major functions: (1) to bring targets onto the fovea, and (2) to keep them there. We shall examine here the five different types of eye movements, the anatomy of the muscles that move the eyes, and the neural systems that produce and modify eye movements.

Five Neuronal Control Systems Keep the Fovea on Target

Although Hermann von Helmholz and the psychophysicists of the nineteenth century who studied vision also were interested in eye movement, they did not appreciate that there is more than one kind of eye movement. Only in 1890 did Edmund Landolt discover that the eyes do not move smoothly along the line in reading a page of print but make little jerky movements, each followed by a little pause. By 1902 Raymond Dodge was able to outline five separate movement systems that put the fovea on a target and keep it there. Each of these movement systems shares the same effector pathway—the three bilateral groups of ocular motor neurons in the brain stem.

The five systems can be divided into two that stabilize the eye during head movement, and three that keep the fovea on a visual target (Table 43–1): (1) *vestibulo-ocular movements* hold images stable on the retina during brief head movements; (2) *optokinetic movements* hold images during sustained head rotation; (3) *saccadic eye movements* shift the fovea rapidly to a target spotted at the periphery; (4) *pursuit movements* keep the image of a moving target on the fovea; (5) *vergence movements* move the eyes in opposite directions so that the image is positioned on both foveae. The first four of these movements are conjugate: Each eye moves the same amount in the same direction. The fifth is disconjugate: The eyes move in different directions and sometimes by different amounts.

The Vestibulo-ocular and Optokinetic Reflexes Compensate for Head Movement

The vestibulo-ocular and optokinetic reflexes are the earliest eye movements, to appear phylogenetically, and it is useful to consider them first. During head movements in any direction the semicircular canals of the vestibular labyrinth signal how fast the head is rotating, and the oculomotor system responds to this signal by rotating the eyes at an equal and opposite velocity (Figure 43–1). This stabilizes the eyes relative to the external world and keeps visual images fixed on the retina.

The vestibulo-ocular reflex is active almost all the time. For example, as you look at this book, turn your head to the left. As you turn your head to the left, your eyes compensate by rotating to the right at the same speed. Were that not to happen the image of the page would slip on the retina and reading would be impossible. Thus, the vestibulo-ocular reflex allows us to see clearly even as we are moving.

The value of stabilizing gaze in space can be appreciated by seeing what happens when hair cells in the semicircular canals are damaged. This was described by a physician whose vestibular system was destroyed by a toxic reaction to the antibiotic streptomycin. Immediately following the onset of streptomycin toxicity, he could not

TABLE **43–1.** A Functional Classification of Eye Movement

Eye movement	Function
Movements that stabilize the eye when the head moves	
Vestibulo-ocular	Uses vestibular input to hold images stable on the retina during brief or rapid head rotation
Optokinetic	Uses visual input to hold images stable on the retina during sustained or slow head rotation
Movements that keep the fovea on a visual target	
Saccade	Brings new objects of interest onto the fovea
Smooth pursuit	Holds the image of a moving target on the fovea
Vergence	Adjusts the eyes for different viewing distances in depth

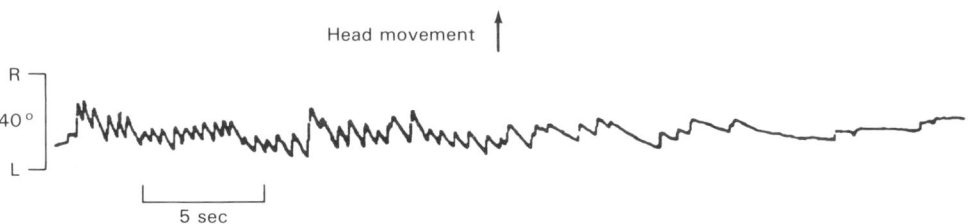

FIGURE 43–1

The vestibulo-ocular reflex. A human subject's horizontal eye position as he is rotated rightward in total darkness. Horizontal position is plotted against time. Eye position is always plotted as degrees of rotation. The subject begins to rotate at 50° per second and the eyes move leftward to hold the eyes still in space. Note that the eyes move in the direction *opposite* the head. When the eyes become too eccentric they move back toward the center of the orbit with a quick phase movement. The reflex gradually habituates and has disappeared by about 30 seconds. (From Leigh and Zee, 1991.)

read in bed without some means of steadying the head to keep it motionless. Even after recovery was partially complete, he still could not read street signs or recognize friends while walking in the street; he had to stop to see clearly.

Vestibular Nystagmus Resets Eye Position During Sustained Rotation. One would think that sustained rotation in any direction would drive the eyes to the edge of the orbit and keep them there. This does not occur because as the eyes slowly approach the edge of the orbit they rapidly reverse direction, moving back across the center of the gaze. This rapid reversal of the direction is called a *quick phase.* The combination of slow and quick phases results in a rhythmic oscillatory pattern, nystagmus (Greek, nod), so called because a nod has a slow phase as the head drops and a quick phase as the head snaps back to an erect position.

In the dark nystagmus does not continue forever, but gradually slows down as the semicircular canals adapt to the constant rotation. This habituation of the reflex (see Chapter 65) occurs because the semicircular canals adapt to repeated movement in the same direction: They habituate with a time constant of 5 seconds, and they also respond poorly to very slow movements. Brain stem circuitry extends the effective habituation time constant to 25 seconds, but during sustained or slow head movement the vestibular signal ultimately fails and the eyes begin to move in space.

The Optokinetic System Uses Visual Information to Complement the Vestibulo-ocular Reflex. Stabilization fails only when a subject is rotated in the dark. In the light, rotatory nystagmus continues as long as the subject rotates. This is because the optokinetic system compensates for the defects in the vestibular system by using the visual motion of head movement to drive the eyes.

As your eyes move in space, the stable aspects of the environment, for example the trees and buildings, move on the retina in a direction opposite to that of the head. The optokinetic system drives the eyes in the direction of this full-field motion, which is opposite the head move-

ment inducing that motion (Figure 43–2). The optokinetic reflex has a long latency and slow buildup that complements the short latency and slow decay of the vestibular system. Although the vestibular system is relatively insensitive to slow head movement, the optokinetic system responds well to the slow visual motion induced by slow head movement. In fact, the system interprets visual motion as head movement. A familiar example of this visual input to the vestibular system is the sudden sensation of backward motion you experience when you are stopped at a red light and the car next to you moves forward.

The functioning of the optokinetic system can be demonstrated by placing a subject inside a cylindrical drum covered with vertical stripes. As the drum begins to rotate the subject develops an optokinetic nystagmus that resembles the nystagmus he would have developed had the chair been rotating in the opposite direction, and he will report the sensation of actually being rotated.

The Vestibulo-ocular and Optokinetic Reflexes Are Under Adaptive Control. The efficiency or *gain* of a reflex is evaluated by comparing its actual response with the stimulus that elicits the response. Since the function of the vestibulo-ocular reflex is to stabilize the visual world

FIGURE 43–2

The optokinetic reflex. A human's horizontal eye position as he sits still inside a vertically striped drum rotating slowly to his right. Eye position is plotted against time. Note that during the slow phase the eyes move in the same direction as the striped drum so as to keep the drum still on the retina.

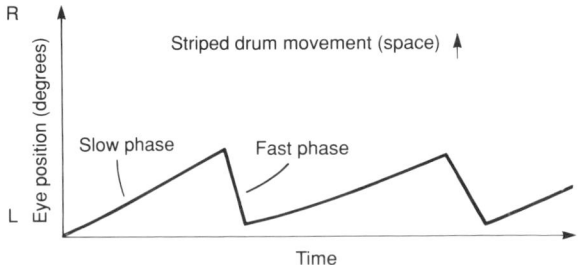

on the retina, the gain of the reflex must be close to unity or else the image will move.

As we saw in Chapter 35, a reflex can be controlled in either a feedback or *closed loop* manner, or a feed-forward or *open loop* manner. With closed loop control the output is fed back and compared with the input to regulate the gain of the *current* movement. With open loop control the result of the movement is used to set the gain so that the next movement will be more accurate. The input to the vestibulo-ocular reflex is head movement, and the output of the reflex is eye movement. The only way to measure the efficacy of that eye movement is to measure the movement of visual images on the retina. The latency of the vestibulo-ocular reflex is 14 ms from head movement to eye movement, but the latency of visual processing is much longer. It takes the retinal ganglion cells alone almost 20–30 ms to respond to light, and the latency of the cortical motion-sensitive cells is more than 60 ms. The reflex therefore cannot be regulated through closed loop control because it is over by the time the visual information can reach the controller. Instead it must be controlled in an open loop manner; visual information is used to calibrate the responsiveness of the system to head movement so that less image movement will occur during the next head movement.

The gain of the reflex can be adjusted by long-term adaptation. For example, if you are wearing eye glasses for myopia, the retinal image is smaller than that ordinarily projected by the lens in your eye. When you move your head, the image motion produced by that movement is less than it would be if you were not wearing glasses. To stabilize the image your eyes must move less than when you are without the glasses. This in fact happens, and the gain of the reflex is less than 1, since the open loop control system has used your visual experience to calibrate the gain. Similarly, magnifying spectacles increase movement of the retinal image with head rotation, and require an increase in the gain of the reflex. The reflex can even be reversed in direction in subjects who have worn reversing prisms for several days. In these subjects the eyes move in the same direction as the head, even in darkness.

In addition, the vestibulo-ocular reflex is capable of rapid modifications in gain that are independent of, and superimposed upon, the long-term adjustments. Sometimes the reflex is counterproductive. If you are looking at something that is moving with you, you want the eyes to travel with the head. Since the vestibulo-ocular reflex forces the eyes to remain in their original position in space, they would not remain focused on the moving target. Luckily, the reflex is suppressible and can be switched off voluntarily.

The Smooth Pursuit System Keeps Moving Targets in the Fovea

Whereas the optokinetic system stabilizes the eyes in space when head movement causes the entire retinal image to move, the smooth pursuit system *moves* the eyes in space to keep a single target on the fovea by calculating

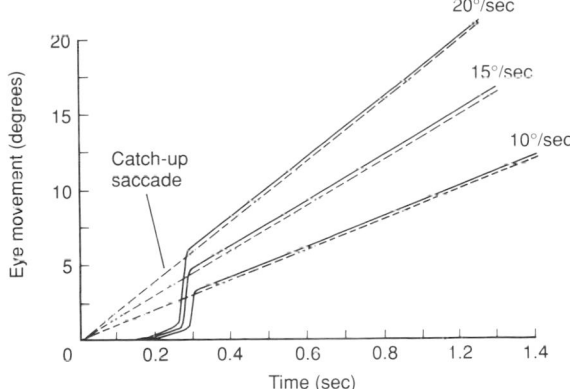

FIGURE 43–3
The smooth pursuit system. A monkey's eye position (**solid line**) plotted against time as he follows a target (**dotted line**) that begins to move at time 0. Note that the monkey makes a rapid movement (saccade) to catch up to the target and then follows it with an eye movement that has the same speed as the target. Pursuit is shown for three different target speeds. (Adapted from Fuchs, 1967.)

how fast the target is moving and moving the eyes accordingly. Smooth pursuit is a voluntary movement and requires a moving stimulus to calculate the proper eye velocity (Figure 43–3). You cannot make a smooth pursuit movement in response to a verbal command alone in the absence of a moving stimulus. Smooth pursuit requires that you attend to an object to pursue it, unlike optokinetic movement, which is involuntary. Smooth pursuit movements have a maximum velocity of about 100°/s. Drugs, fatigue, alcohol, and even distraction degrade the quality of smooth pursuit movements.

FIGURE 43–4
The saccadic system. A human's eye position as he looks at a spot of light that suddenly jumps to the right. Eye position (**solid line**) and target position (**dotted line**) plotted superimposed against time. Eye velocity is shown beneath. The eye stays still for about 200 ms and then moves rapidly to the new target position. The eye velocity rises and falls smoothly.

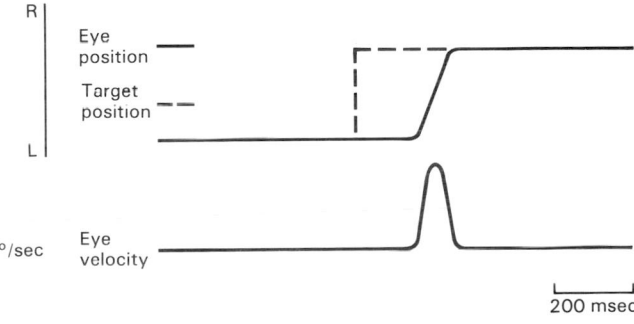

The Saccadic System Points the Fovea Toward Objects of Interest

If you look at a target whose image suddenly moves away from the fovea, your eyes maintain their position for about 200 ms, then move quickly to bring the target back onto the fovea. (Figure 43–4). This rapid eye movement is the *saccade*. It resembles the quick phase of vestibular nystagmus. Saccades are highly stereotyped; they have a standard waveform that reflects a single smooth increase and decrease of eye velocity. Unlike smooth pursuit, which requires a visual stimulus, accurate saccades can also be made in response to sounds, tactile stimuli, memories of locations in space, and even to verbal commands ("look left").

The velocity of saccadic eye movement is determined by the distance of the target from the fovea, whereas in smooth pursuit eye velocity is determined by target velocity. You can voluntarily change the amplitude and direction of saccades, but you cannot voluntarily change their velocities. Like smooth pursuit, only fatigue, drugs, or pathological states can slow saccades. Saccades are so fast, occurring within a fraction of a second, at speeds up to 900°/s, that ordinarily there is no time for visual feedback to modify the course of the saccade; corrections are made in small saccades after the primary one.

Like the vestibulo-ocular reflex, the saccadic system can adapt to changes in muscle function. When there is a weakness of one of the extraocular muscles, as occurs with a partial paralysis due to nerve damage, saccades will be weaker than normal (*hypometric*) and the eye will not move as far as the central nervous system expects. Since the innervation of each eye is equal, the signal will be inadequate for the weakened eye. However, if the strong eye is patched so it cannot see, the system must rely on the weak eye for visual input, and in a few days the output pattern will change to allow the weak eye to move more accurately, resulting in significant overshoot of the strong, patched eye.

The Vergence Movement System Aligns the Eyes to Look at Targets with Different Depths

All of the preceding systems move both eyes the same amount in the same direction. These movements are called *conjugate*. However, the eyes also move in opposite directions when they converge or diverge to focus on objects at different distances from the viewer. These *disconjugate* movements are generated by the vergence system. Thus, when we view an object that moves toward or away from us, each eye moves differently (disconjugately) to keep the image of the object aligned precisely on each fovea. If the object moves closer, the eyes must converge; if the object moves away, the eyes diverge.

The difference in retinal position of an object in one eye compared to its position in the other is referred to as *retinal disparity*. The range of retinal disparity that drives the vergence system is much larger than that responsible for stereopsis, which we considered in Chapter 30. Disparities used as cues for stereopsis can be a few tens of seconds of arc. In contrast, the retinal disparities that evoke vergence movements require a few minutes of arc. Vergence occurs whether or not stereopsis is present.

Targets approaching the eyes normally become blurred and are brought into focus by contraction of the ciliary muscle, which changes the radius of curvature of the crystalline lens in the eye. This process is called *accommodation*, and accommodation and vergence are linked together. Blur, the accommodative stimulus, can induce convergence as well as accommodation. Vergence can induce accommodation even when there is no blur.

The Eye Is Moved by Three Complementary Pairs of Muscles

To understand how the eye muscles move the eye to produce the five types of behavioral responses, it is necessary to understand the geometry of the eye and the functions of the eye muscles. The eye's orientation can be defined by three axes of rotation—horizontal, vertical, and torsional—that intersect at the center of the eyeball. To a good approximation, the eyeball rotates around a single point that is fixed in both the eye and orbit (Figure 43–5). The Y axis is the line of sight when the eye is in the primary position (looking straight ahead); the Z and X axes are mutually perpendicular to each other and to the Y axis, intersecting at the center of the globe. Eye movements are described as rotations around these axes. Abduction and adduction are the horizontal rotations (around the Z axis) away from and toward the nose respectively; elevation and depression are the vertical rotations (around the X axis); and intorsion and extorsion are the rotations of the top of the cornea toward and away from the nose (around the Y axis).

Although each eye has three degrees of freedom, it does not assume all possible torsional rotations. Perceptual stability of horizontal lines requires that the lines be perpendicular to the X axis in all positions of gaze; otherwise lines perceived as horizontal in some positions of gaze would be perceived to tilt in others. Torsional movements are necessary to minimize the tilt, and only become apparent when they are exaggerated by pathological processes.

Six muscles attach to each eye: four rectus muscles (superior, inferior, medial, and lateral) and the two oblique muscles (superior and inferior). The recti originate at the apex of the orbit and insert on the sclera, the outer coat of the eyeball, anterior to the equator of the eye (Figure 43–6). The obliques approach the eye from the anteromedial aspect and insert posterior to the equator.

The medial and lateral recti adduct and abduct the eye. The actions of the four remaining muscles are complicated by the fact that they do not pull the eye around the X and Y axes only. Each of these muscles also has some torsional component to its action, depending upon the and inferior obliques (depression–intorsion versus elevation–extorsion). For conjugate movements the two eyes are yoked together. To follow a target moving upward to the left, the left eye moves upward and away from the nose and the right eye moves upward and toward the nose. This requires that each pair of muscles in one eye has a functional complement in the other orbit that can rotate the eye in the same plane but the opposite direction. The medial and lateral recti complement each other, but the vertical muscles do not. Thus, the obliques on one side have roughly the same pulling planes as the superior and inferior recti on the other.

Eye Position and Velocity Are Signaled by Extraocular Motor Neurons

Extraocular muscles are innervated by three groups of motor neurons whose cell bodies form nuclei in the brain stem (Figure 43–8). The lateral rectus is innervated by the motor neurons of the *abducens nucleus* (cranial nerve nucleus VI) in the pons, in the floor of the fourth ventricle. The medial, inferior, and superior recti, and the inferior oblique muscles are innervated by the ocular motor neurons that form the *oculomotor nucleus* (cranial nerve nucleus III) in the midbrain at the level of the superior colliculus. The levator palpebrae, which elevates the eyelid, and the ciliary muscle, which constricts the pupil, are also innervated by fibers traveling in the oculomotor nerve. The superior oblique muscle is innervated by the *trochlear nucleus* (cranial nerve nucleus IV), located in the midbrain at the level of the inferior colliculus.

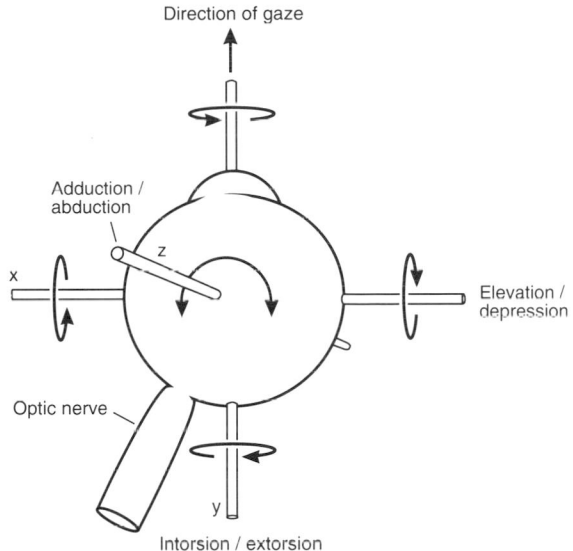

FIGURE 43–5
The three principal axes of eye rotation. Horizontal rotation occurs about the vertical axis (**Z**), vertical rotation about the transverse axis (**X**), and torsion about the anterior-posterior axis (**Y**). Note that the Y axis goes through the center of gaze but is medial to the optic nerve, which defines the central axis of the orbit.

horizontal position of the eye in the orbit (Figure 43–7, Table 43–2).

Thus, three pairs of muscles have complementary actions: the medial and lateral recti (adduction versus abduction), the inferior and superior recti (depression–extorsion versus elevation–intorsion), and the superior

FIGURE 43–6
The origins and insertions of the extraocular muscles.

A. Lateral view with orbital wall cut away. Note that the recti insert in front of the equator of the globe and contraction rotates the cornea *toward* the insertion. The obliques insert behind the equator, and contraction rotates the cornea away from the

insertion. The superior oblique muscle passes through a pulley of bone, the trochlea, before it inserts.

B. Superior view with roof of orbit cut away.

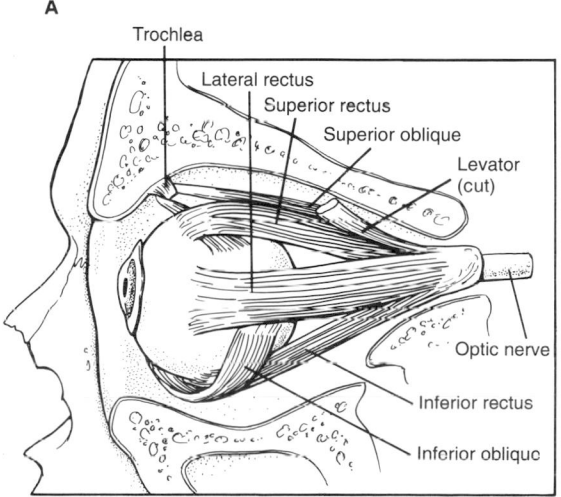

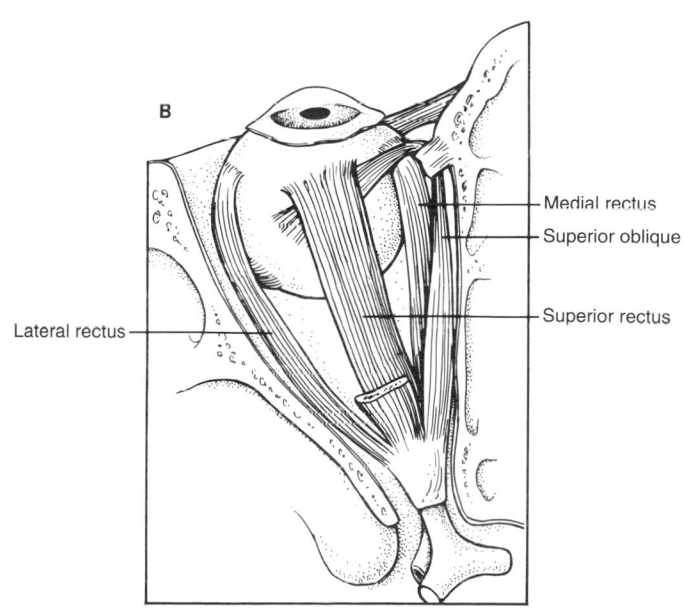

A Right superior rectus

B Right superior oblique

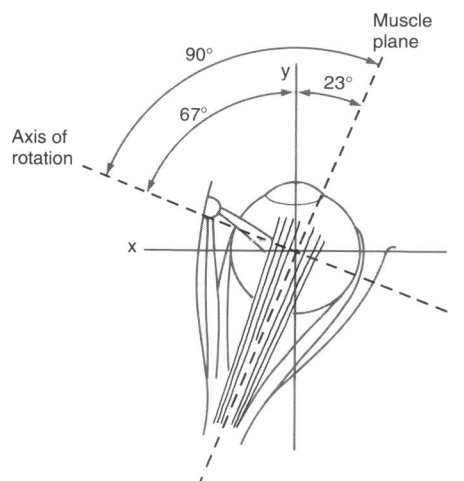
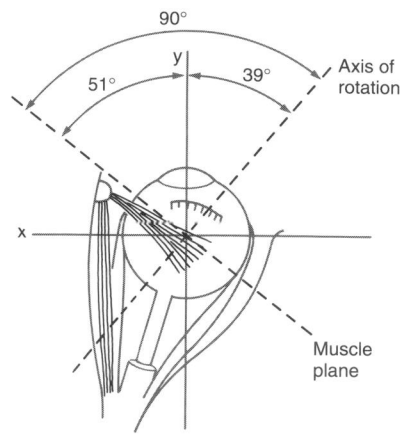

FIGURE 43–7

The directions of action of the superior vertical muscles of the right eye. (From Von Noorden as reproduced in Leigh and Zee, 1991.)

A. When the eye is abducted 23° from its primary position (the Y axis) the right superior rectus muscle is a pure elevator of the globe. When the eye is fully adducted, the action of the superior rectus is principally intorsional. Thus, the superior rectus muscle

acts as a pure elevator of the eye only when the eye is 23° or more lateral to the primary position; it has a significant intorsional component when the eye is more medial.

B. Right superior oblique muscle. When the eye is abducted 39° from the Y axis its action is pure intorsion. When the eye is fully adducted its main action is depression of the globe.

The discharge frequency of each extraocular motor neuron is directly proportional to the position of the eye and to its velocity (Figure 43–9B). Since the saccade has a very high velocity, the bulk of activity during the saccade is proportional to eye velocity, and has been described as a *pulse* of activity, a rapid increase in the firing rate of the neuron. The pulse serves to drive the eyes as rapidly as possible, and to overcome the viscous drag of the eye in the orbit. Once the eye has achieved its new position, it is held there by a steady contraction of the extraocular muscles. The difference between the initial and final discharge levels is described as a *step* in activity. Thus, the control signal to the ocular motor neurons for a saccade has the form of a *pulse-step* (Figure 43–9B). The height of the step determines the amplitude of the saccade, while the duration of the pulse determines the duration of the saccade.

The greater the amplitude of the pulse, the faster the saccade. The longer the duration of the burst (pulse), the longer the saccade.

Oculomotor neurons differ from spinal motor neurons in several ways. First, all eye motor neurons participate equally in all five types of eye movements. There are no motor neurons specialized for saccades or for smooth pursuit. Second, unlike skeletal muscle, the eye motor neurons have a fixed sequence of recruitment regardless of the type of eye movement being made. Recruitment order is determined as a function of orbital position of the eye: Each neuron begins to discharge when the eye is beyond a certain position in the orbit. Third, the extraocular muscles never have to respond to unpredictably changing external loads. As a result, oculomotor neurons do not respond to muscle stretch, even though the muscles are rich in muscle spindles—the receptors that mediate the stretch reflex of skeletal muscle. Finally, there is no recurrent inhibition on oculomotor neurons, nor are there special fast-twitch and slow-twitch muscles.

Patients with lesions of the extraocular muscles or their nerves complain of *diplopia*, double vision. Each nerve has a characteristic syndrome. Thus, a lesion of the abducens nerve causes an inability of the eye to move lateral to the primary position, causing *diplopia on lateral gaze*. A deficit of the oculomotor nerve, prevents the eye from moving medially or upward from the mid position.

TABLE 43–2. Vertical Muscle Action in Adduction and Abduction

Muscle	Abduction	Adduction
Inferior rectus	Depression	Extorsion
Superior oblique	Intorsion	Depression
Inferior oblique	Extorsion	Elevation
Superior rectus	Elevation	Intorsion

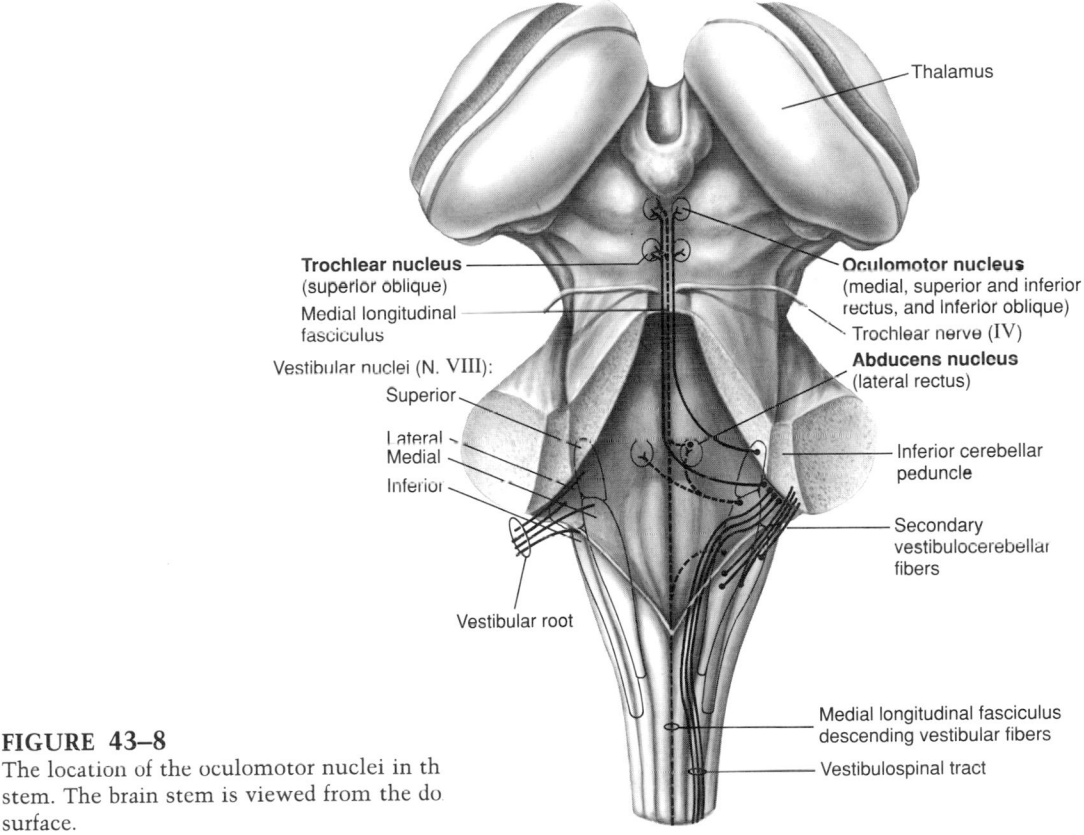

Thalamus

Trochlear nucleus
(superior oblique)

Medial longitudinal
fasciculus

Vestibular nuclei (N. VIII):

Superior

Lateral
Medial

Inferior

Vestibular root

Oculomotor nucleus
(medial, superior and inferior
rectus, and inferior oblique)

Trochlear nerve (IV)

Abducens nucleus
(lateral rectus)

Inferior cerebellar
peduncle

Secondary
vestibulocerebellar
fibers

Medial longitudinal fasciculus
descending vestibular fibers

Vestibulospinal tract

FIGURE 43–8
The location of the oculomotor nuclei in th
stem. The brain stem is viewed from the do
surface.

Downward movement is partial because the action of the superior oblique (innervated by the trochlear nerve) is intact but is not balanced by that of the inferior rectus muscle, so the eye intorts as it moves downward. Since nerve fibers to the levator palpebrae and pupilloconstrictor muscles also travel in the oculomotor nerve, damage to this nerve is also accompanied by drooping of the eyelid (*ptosis*) and pupillary dilatation (*mydriasis*).

An isolated lesion of the trochlear nerve results in an eye with deficits in intorsion and depression, which vary as a function of position of the eye in the orbit. This results in a *skew deviation* (eyes at different vertical positions in the orbit) and a torsional deficit. Patients with trochlear damage frequently keep their heads tilted toward the side of the weak muscle to minimize diplopia.

The Vestibulo-ocular Reflex Is Coordinated in the Brain Stem

Binocular eye movements require coordination among the 12 muscles and are always described in terms of gaze—where the eyes point. The best understood gaze process is the horizontal vestibulo-ocular reflex, which keeps the visual image still by compensating for head movement. This reflex coordinates the action of four muscles, the lateral and medial recti, so they can drive the eyes with a velocity equal to and opposite to that of the head.

The Semicircular Canals Send an Eye Velocity Signal to Brain Stem Oculomotor Centers

How does the vestibulo-ocular reflex work? The basic reflex involves only a three neuron arc that begins with afferent neurons innervating the hair cells in each semicircular canal. These neurons signal the *velocity* of head movement to interneurons in the vestibular nuclei, which then provide the ocular motor neurons with an appropriate eye velocity signal.

The vestibular sensory organ consists of the semicircular canals, which detect rotation of the head around the three axes of space, and the otolith organs, which sense linear movements of the head and the orientation of the head with respect to gravity. There are three pairs of canals organized roughly in three mutually perpendicular planes, each of which lies approximately in the pulling direction of two pairs of complementary extraocular muscles: (1) the left and right horizontal canals in the plane of the medial and lateral recti, (2) the left anterior and right

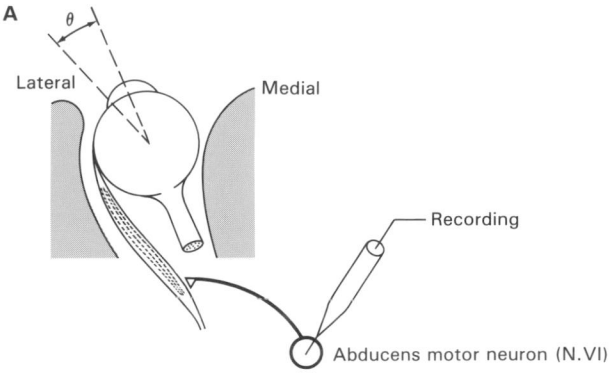

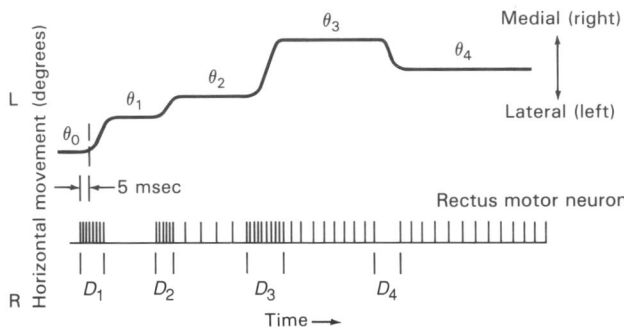

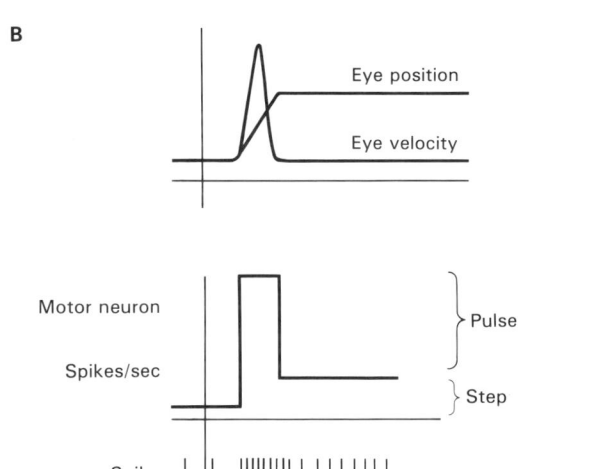

FIGURE 43–9

Action of a left abducens neuron in the monkey.

A. Relation of discharge rate to eye position and velocity. When the eye is in the right of the orbit the cell is silent (position θ_1 and θ_2), except during leftward saccades (D_1 and D_2). As the eye moves rightward the cell fires with a higher frequency at increasingly eccentric positions (θ_2 and θ_3). The cell does not fire during the rightward saccade (D_4) even though it fires when the eye is still at these positions.

B. Pulse and step of innervation during a saccade. A single saccade is shown in an extended time base, with motor neuron spikes/second compared with eye position and velocity. Note that the neuron bursts while the eye is moving (the **pulse**) and resumes a new stable discharge level (the **step**) after the saccade.

posterior canals in a plane close to that of the left superior and inferior recti and right superior and inferior obliques, and (3) the right anterior and left posterior canals near that of the right vertical recti and the left obliques (Figure 43–10).

Neurons in the vestibular nuclei project to the motor nuclei in such a way that the inputs from each canal excite and inhibit complementary muscles in both eyes. For example, the left horizontal canal excites the left medial rectus and right lateral rectus while inhibiting the left lateral rectus and right medial rectus. The individual canals and their associated eye muscles are listed in Table 43–3.

Disease of the Vestibular System Causes Nystagmus

Each canal transmits a tonic signal to the vestibular nerve even when the eyes are still. Head rotation in the canal's plane to the same side causes an increased signal; rotation away from the canal results in a decreased signal. The rightward head rotation in the horizontal plane excites the right and inhibits the left horizontal canal. The eyes remain still when the head is still because the various tonic discharges from all six canals to all 12 muscles are in balance. Any imbalance of this tonic signal causes a pathological nystagmus: Both eyes are driven in one direction by the imbalance, and jerked back by the quick-phase mechanism in the other. Nystagmus when the head is still is the hallmark of disease of the labyrinth and its central connections, and resembles normal nystagmus that occurs with head rotation.

A Brain Stem Network Coordinates the Horizontal Vestibulo-ocular Reflex

The best known neural pathways by which the vestibular signal is transformed into an eye movement are those for the horizontal vestibulo-ocular reflex. Leftward head movement causes rightward eye movement. The leftward head rotation increases activity in the nerve from the left horizontal canal and decreases activity in the right horizontal canal nerve. This change in activity is proportional to head velocity. The signal from the canals is distributed to the muscles by a network of interneurons (Figure 43–11). The lateral rectus motor neurons in the pons are driven directly by interneurons in the vestibular nucleus. The medial rectus motor neurons in the midbrain are driven by interneurons in the abducens nucleus, which receive the same signal as the motor neurons but project to the midbrain rather than to the muscle. This projection crosses the midline and ascends in the contralateral medial longitudinal fasciculus. This tract is critical for coordinating the medial rectus and lateral rectus for all horizontal gaze processes, and its length and vulnerability make it clinically important, as will be described later.

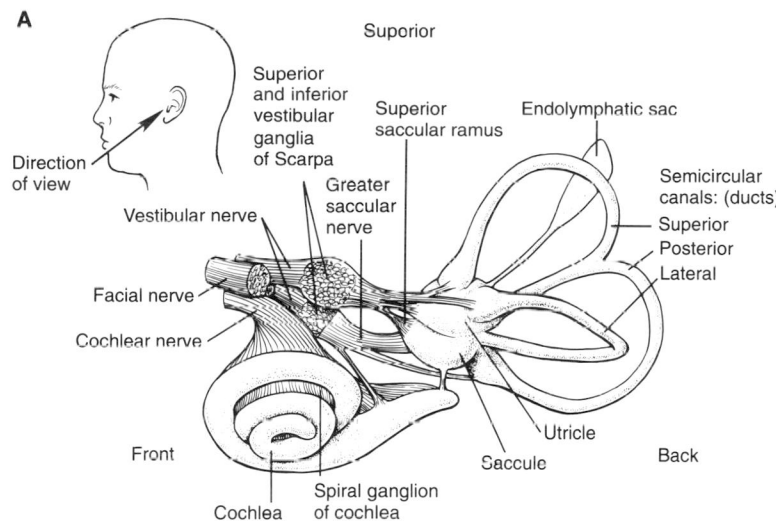

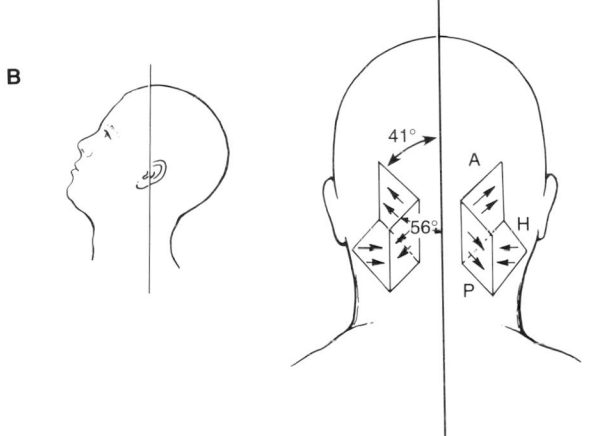

FIGURE 43–10

The vestibulo-oculomotor reflex is initiated in the membranous labyrinth of the inner ear (shown for the left ear).

A. Location and innervation of the vestibular end-organs in the human temporal bone. The vestibular nerve is composed of axons of bipolar cell bodies lying in the superior and inferior vestibular (Scarpa's) ganglia. Distal processes of bipolar cells divide into branches to innervate the three canals and the two otolith organs. The facial and cochlear divisions of nerve VIII are also shown. (From Hardy, 1934.)

B. Preferred stimulus direction for hair cells of the semicircular canal. (Adapted from Patton et al., 1989.)

A Neural Integrator Maintains Eye Position After the Head Has Stopped Moving

The vestibulo-ocular reflex circuit changes the head velocity signal into an eye velocity signal. However, as we have seen, the ocular motor neurons carry two signals, a velocity signal and a position signal. If the vestibular velocity signal were the only signal to reach the eyes as a result of head movement, the eyes would continue to move as long as the head moves; when the head stops, the eyes drift back to the starting position because there is no new position signal. David Robinson pointed out that a new position signal is necessary to hold the eyes in place after they have been moved by the vestibulo-ocular reflex, and that the generation of this signal is the neural equivalent of the mathematical process of integration of the velocity signal. (Velocity is the derivative of position, and position, the integral of velocity.) Neural integration of the vestibular velocity signal requires the cerebellar flocculus, the medial vestibular nucleus, and another brain

TABLE 43–3. Effects of Semicircular Canals on Eye Muscles

Canal	Excites	Inhibits
Horizontal	Ipsilateral medial rectus, contralateral lateral rectus	Ipsilateral lateral rectus, contralateral medial rectus
Posterior	Ipsilateral superior oblique, contralateral inferior rectus	Ipsilateral inferior oblique, contralateral superior rectus
Anterior	Ipsilateral superior rectus, contralateral inferior oblique	Ipsilateral inferior rectus, contralateral superior oblique

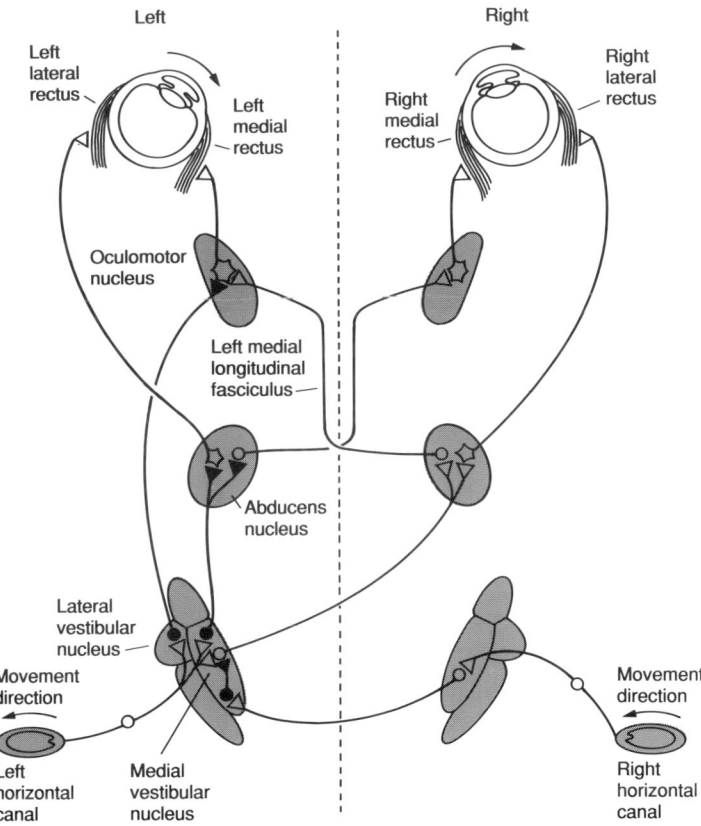

FIGURE 43–11
The pathways of the horizontal vestibulo-ocular reflex in the brain stem for leftward head movement. Inhibitory connections are shown as filled neurons, excitatory connections as unfilled neurons. For simplicity, only the projections from the left vestibular nuclei are shown. Leftward head movement stimulates the left horizontal canal and inhibits the right, resulting in increased discharge in the right lateral and left medial rectus and decreased discharge in the left lateral and right medial rectus. The leftward head rotation increases activity in the vestibular afferents innervating the left horizontal canal. These in turn excite excitatory and inhibitory interneurons in the left medial and lateral vestibular nuclei. These neurons have at least four functions: (1) medial vestibular excitatory axons cross to the right abducens nucleus and directly excite motor neurons, which excite the right lateral rectus muscles, and interneurons whose axons ascend in the left medial longitudinal fasciculus to excite the left medial rectus motor neurons; (2) medial vestibular inhibitory neurons suppress the activity of left abducens motor neurons and interneurons, thus decreasing activity in the left lateral rectus and right medial rectus muscles; (3) medial vestibular excitatory neurons cross to the right medial vestibular nucleus and excite interneurons that inhibit the right medial vestibular projection for the right abducens nucleus; and (4) left lateral vestibular neurons suppress activity in the left medial rectus motor neurons. The same head rotation decreases activity in the right horizontal canal afferents, resulting in activity reciprocal to that evoked by the left canal afferents. The sum of this activity is that both eyes move with a velocity equal and opposite to that of the head.

stem nucleus, the *nucleus prepositus hypoglossi*. Lesions of these regions affect the way the eyes hold position.

Modulation of the Vestibulo-ocular Reflex Requires the Cerebellum

Adjustments to the gain of the vestibuloocular reflex, either by short-term suppression or long-term adaptation, involve the cerebellar flocculus. Vestibular signals project directly to the flocculus, and floccular Purkinje cells project to and can inhibit vestibular interneurons, providing a control on the reflex. Cerebellar lesions prevent even short-term modification of the reflex.

The mechanism of long-term adaptation is uncertain. Frederick Miles and his colleagues found that floccular Purkinje cells in the monkey respond to the visual signal that arises from the mismatch of head velocity and eye velocity. The gain of the reflex is then altered to minimize this error (i.e., to eliminate motion of the visual world on the retina), presumably by changing the sensitivity of some interneurons to signals from the semicircular canals. In the primate, the Purkinje cells themselves do not show a gain change. Steven Lisberger demonstrated in the monkey that brain stem neurons that receive input from the flocculus and the semicircular canals are capable of such changes.

Subcortical and Cortical Structures Contribute to the Optokinetic Reflex

How does the optokinetic system provide the vestibular system with a visual signal? Retinal neurons project to the nucleus of the optic tract in the pretectum, which then projects to the medial vestibular nucleus. Thus, neurons in the vestibular nucleus that receive signals from vestibular afferents also receive visual signals. Cells in the nucleus of the optic tract respond preferentially to stimuli moving in a temporal-to-nasal direction, and to stimuli moving with low velocity.

In primates the subcortical reflex is supplemented by a cortical component that responds to stimuli moving with higher velocities or in a nasal-to-temporal direction. This cortical system includes the visual motion pathway outlined in Chapter 30: the magnocellular layers of the lateral geniculate nucleus, the striate cortex (area 17), the middle temporal area, and the medial superior temporal area. Patients with lesions of this region have defective optokinetic nystagmus to visual stimuli moving toward the side of the lesion.

Saccades and Smooth Pursuit Are Organized in Pontine and Mesencephalic Reticular Centers

As we have seen, the activity of ocular motor neurons describes the velocity and position of the eye at any given time. Interneurons in the brain stem reticular formation provide the velocity and step signals to the motor neurons for saccades and smooth pursuit. The horizontal component of these movements is organized in the paramedian pontine reticular formation. The vertical component of these movements is organized in the mesencephalic reticular formation.

Horizontal Saccades Are Generated in the Pontine Reticular Formation

All conjugate gaze movements are paralyzed in the direction of the side of the lesion in patients with pontine lesions. Bernard Cohen and his colleagues found that electrical stimulation in this area drives the eyes in the ipsilateral direction, and cells here drive ipsilateral horizontal saccades and smooth pursuit. Klaus Hepp and Volker Henn showed that chemical lesions destroying the cells in this region eliminate saccades and smooth pursuit without affecting the vestibuloocular reflex. There are four types of neurons in this region related to horizontal saccades: burst cells, tonic cells, burst-tonic cells, and pause cells. We shall consider each of these cells in turn (Figure 43–12).

The command to the motor neurons for a saccade has the form of a pulse-step. The neurons that give rise to the pulse component are called *burst cells*. The burst neurons for horizontal saccades lie within the paramedian pontine reticular formation. The burst cells discharge at a high frequency just before and during saccades of the ipsilateral eye, and their activity resembles the pulse component of motor neuron discharge but without the step.

There are a variety of burst cells. *Medium-lead burst cells* make direct excitatory connections to motor neurons and interneurons in the ipsilateral abducens. *Long-lead burst neurons* drive the medium-lead burst cells and receive excitatory input from higher centers. *Inhibitory burst neurons* located more caudally suppress neurons in the contralateral abducens nucleus.

Where does the signal for the step component arise? We have seen that when the eyes are moved to a new position by the vestibular velocity signal, the signal must be integrated in order for the eyes to remain in the new position. The same mechanism holds for the saccadic system. The velocity pulse from the burst neurons must be integrated to provide the signal that enables the eye to hold the new position; the difference in firing before and after the saccade is the step. Lesions in the nucleus prepositus hypoglossi destroy the integrator. Monkeys with such lesions can make accurate saccades but cannot keep looking at the target. Instead of maintaining gaze, the eyes drift back to the mid position with an exponential waveform; repeated efforts to fixate an eccentric target result in nystagmus.

This integrated eye position signal is carried by *tonic* neurons in the paramedian pontine reticular formation. These cells fire at a steady rate during eye fixation, but the firing rate increases linearly with increasing horizontal movement of the eye, thus signaling the position of the eye in the orbit. During saccades their activity changes from the steady presaccadic level to the faster postsaccadic level.

Burst-tonic neurons carry both the step and pulse signals, much like oculomotor neurons. The tonic discharge of these cells is related to eye position; they fire in a velocity-related burst during ipsilaterally directed saccades and pause during contralaterally directed saccades.

Pause cells are located in the nucleus of the dorsal raphe, on the midline just behind and below the abducens nucleus. They project to contralateral pontine and mesencephalic burst neurons and fire at all times except during saccades. The pause in firing precedes the saccade by approximately 16 ms and ends with or slightly before the end of the saccade. Electrical stimulation of pause neurons during a saccade stops the saccade, which resumes when the stimulation stops. It is therefore thought that the pause neurons inhibit the burst neurons, and that the pause in their firing allows burst cells to initiate a saccade.

These neurons are connected together as a network to generate saccades. The long-lead burst cells receive excitatory input from higher structures that specifies how far the eye should move, and this signal also turns off the pause cells, enabling the long-lead burst cells to excite the medium-lead burst cells. This activates both classes of neurons in the ipsilateral abducens nucleus. The motor neurons drive the ipsilateral lateral rectus muscle, and interneurons excite the contralateral medial rectus motor neurons by way of the median longitudinal fasciculus. The eyes move conjugately and rapidly in an ipsilateral direction. The inhibitory burst neurons inhibit the motor neurons of the antagonist muscles and also the pause neurons. When the eye is on target, the burst neurons stop

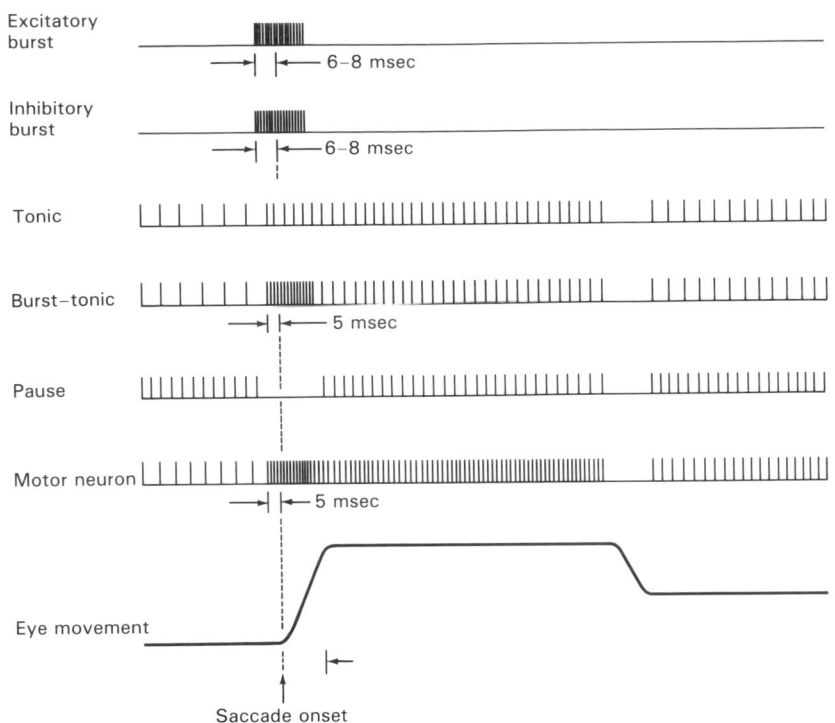

Excitatory burst

6–8 msec

Inhibitory burst

6–8 msec

Tonic

Burst–tonic

5 msec

Pause

Motor neuron

5 msec

Eye movement

Saccade onset

FIGURE 43–12
Saccade-related neurons in the pontine reticular formation. Spike discharge patterns of burst, burst-tonic, tonic, and pause neurons are shown compared with a motor neuron and eye position. Note that the pause occurs first, followed by bursts in the burst, burst-tonic, and finally motor neurons. The tonic neuron fires through the saccade but has no burst. During a saccade in the opposite direction all neurons are silent.

firing, thus turning off the inhibitory input to the pause neurons. The neural integrator integrates the burst signal and sends the eye position signal to the tonic neurons.

Vertical Saccades Are Generated in the Mesencephalic Reticular Formation

Only horizontal saccades are organized in the paramedian pontine reticular formation. The burst, tonic, and burst-tonic neurons for vertical saccades lie in the *rostral interstitial nucleus of the medial longitudinal fasciculus* in the mesencephalic reticular formation. The pontine pause cells control the mesencephalic burst neurons as well as those in the pons. Both the pontine and mesencephalic systems participate in the generation of oblique saccades, which have both horizontal and vertical components. Purely vertical saccades require activity on both sides of the mesencephalic reticular formation, and communication between the two sides traverses the posterior commissure.

Modulation of the Saccadic System by Experience Requires the Cerebellum

The gain of the saccadic system, like that of the vestibuloocular reflex, can be modulated by experience, for example to compensate for the weakness of a muscle. This adaptation to partial paralysis is produced by two mechanisms: (1) a change in the duration of the innervation pulse, and (2) a change in the height of the step size relative to the pulse size (see Figure 43–9B). Guntram Kommerell and his colleagues described these adaptive processes in patients who

preferentially used one eye with weak muscles because vision in the eye with normal muscles was poor. When a patch is placed over the eye with normal muscles, the gain of the system increases so that the eye with weak muscles is able to make adequate saccades. However, this results in too intensive innervation to the eye with normal muscles, and since this eye is patched, no visual information tells the system of the errors. Thus, the saccades made by the normal eye are larger than normal (*hypermetric*). Because the burst is too large for the step, the integrated signal is too small and the eye drifts back toward the original target (*postsaccadic drift*).

Damage to the cerebellum prevents both of these adaptive changes. Lesions of the dorsal cerebellar vermis and fastigial nuclei prevent changes only in the pulse size. Lesions of the flocculus prevent only the matching of saccadic step size to the pulse size. Thus, the flocculus maintains the pulse-step match and the dorsal vermis and fastigial nuclei maintain accurate pulse size.

Smooth Pursuit Requires the Cerebral Cortex, Cerebellum, and Pons

Rolf Eckmiller showed that neurons in the paramedian pontine reticular formation carry velocity signals for smooth pursuit but not for the vestibulo-ocular reflex. This area receives input from the flocculus of the cerebellum, where neurons also have a velocity signal that drives smooth pursuit (Figure 43–13). The gaze velocity signal must also be integrated for eye position to be maintained.

The smooth pursuit pathway uses the same cortical motion pathway that processes visual signals for the opto-

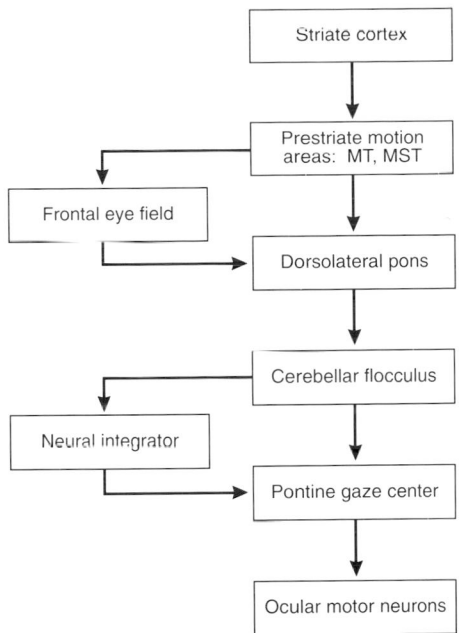

FIGURE 43–13

Smooth pursuit pathways. The cerebral cortex processes visual motion information and sends it to the pontine gaze center via the dorsolateral pons and the cerebellar flocculus, where a gaze velocity signal is generated.

kinetic reflex: the striate cortex and the motion-sensitive region in the superior temporal sulcus and the middle temporal and medial superior temporal areas (Figure 43–14). Robert Wurtz and his colleagues found that lesions of the middle temporal areas disrupt the ability to respond to targets moving in regions of the visual field represented in the damaged cortical area. Lesions of the medial superior temporal area results in similar defects in eye movements, together with difficulty in pursuit movements toward the side of the lesion. The output of these cortical areas is directed to the dorsolateral pons and thence to the flocculus, and this cortical activity tells the system how fast the visual target is moving.

Vergence Is Organized in the Midbrain

Looking at a near object requires simultaneous adduction of both eyes, which is accomplished by increasing medial rectus tone and decreasing lateral rectus tone. Looking at a distant object requires simultaneous abduction of both eyes, accomplished by increasing lateral rectus tone and decreasing medial rectus tone bilaterally. Accommodation and vergence are controlled by neurons in the midbrain in the region of the oculomotor nucleus.

Patients with Brain Stem Lesions Have Characteristic Deficits in Eye Movements

We can now understand how different hindbrain lesions can cause different, characteristic syndromes. Lesions that include the pontine gaze centers result in paralysis of ipsilateral horizontal gaze, but pure upward gaze can be intact. Conversely, lesions that include the midbrain vertical gaze centers will cause paralysis of vertical gaze. Lesions of the median longitudinal fasciculus will cause disconnection of the medial rectus motor neurons from the abducens interneurons. The medial rectus will be unable to contract in horizontal saccades or pursuit, but it will function perfectly well in vergence. This medial rectus deficit in lateral gaze with normal vergence is called internuclear ophthalmoplegia and is often seen in patients with multiple sclerosis.

Patients with cerebellar lesions cannot adjust the accuracy of their eye movements, so their saccades tend to

FIGURE 43–14

Cortical areas active in movements. Visual motion processing important for optokinetic and smooth pursuit eye movements occurs in striate cortex, medial temporal, and medial superior temporal areas. The posterior parietal cortex (Brodmann's area 7) is important in visual attentional processing for saccades. The frontal eye fields, the supplementary eye fields, and the dorsolateral prefrontal cortex are all important in the generation of saccades.

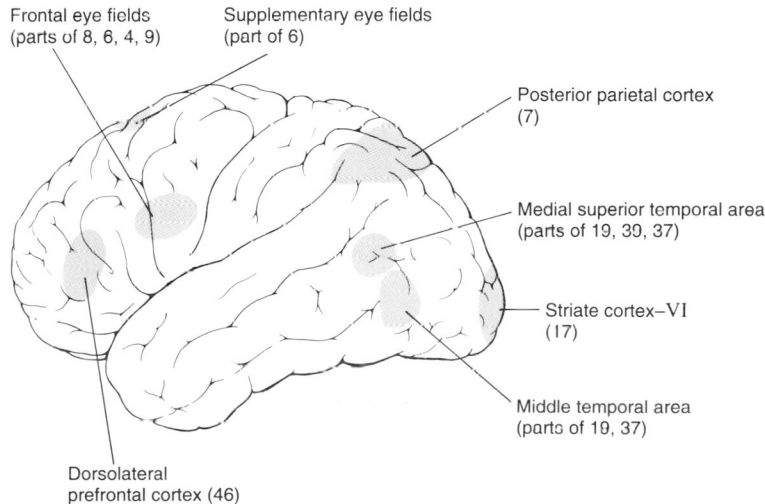

be inaccurate. If the lesions are in the vestibulocerebellum, the patient will have nystagmus and be incapable of smooth pursuit. Moving targets, no matter how slow, are tracked by a series of saccades. Finally, such patients cannot suppress the vestibulo-ocular reflex when necessary.

The Saccade Generator in the Brain Stem Is Controlled in the Cerebral Cortex

Humans make an average of three saccades a second. You make saccades whether you are doing something that requires moving your fovea, like reading this book, or doing something for which vision is irrelevant, like doing mental arithmetic in darkness. All saccades are organized by the pontine and mesencephalic burst circuits, usually under the control of the *superior colliculus*. The saccades that are important for visual behavior are under the control of the cerebral cortex, which can act through the superior colliculus and also independently (Figure 43–15).

The Superior Colliculus Transmits Cortical Oculomotor Signals to the Brain Stem

The superior colliculus can be divided into two regions: the superficial layers and the intermediate and deep layers.

The three superficial layers of the superior colliculus receive both direct input from the retina and a projection from striate cortex for the entire contralateral visual hemifield. Neurons in the superficial superior colliculus have specific visual receptive fields: Half of the neurons have a higher frequency discharge in response to a visual stimulus when a monkey is going to make a saccade to that stimulus. If the monkey attends to the stimulus without making a saccade to it, for example by making a hand

movement in response to a brightness change, these neurons do not give an enhanced response.

Cells in the two intermediate and deep layers are primarily related to the oculomotor system. These cells receive visual inputs from prestriate, middle temporal, and parietal cortices, and motor input from the frontal eye field. In addition, there is also representation of the body surface and of the locations of sound in space. As we have seen in Chapter 29, these maps are in register with the visual maps. Thus, if the image of a bird excites a visual neuron, the bird's chirp will excite a nearby auditory neuron, and both stimuli will excite a bimodal neuron.

Recordings from awake animals reveal that the majority of neurons in the intermediate layers fire before contralateral saccades of specific size and direction. This motor output drives the long-lead burst cells of the paramedian pontine reticular formation that specify how far the eye should move. These cells have *movement fields* analogous to the receptive fields of sensory neurons. The movement field is that part of the visual field to which the eye moves in response to activity in the cell. Peter Schiller and Michael Stryker found that electrical stimulation of the superior colliculus evokes saccades into the movement field of the stimulated neurons. The movement fields are in register with the visual and auditory receptive fields, so that neurons that drive eye movements to a certain target are found in the same region as the cells excited by the sounds and image of that target.

The movement fields are large, so that each cell fires before a wide range of saccades but most intensely before those of one optimal direction and amplitude. Therefore a large population of broadly tuned cells is active before each saccade. David Sparks and his colleagues found that the actual eye movement is coded by the entire ensemble of activated cells, and is the average of the optimal direction for each cell weighted by the intensity of the cell's

FIGURE 43–15

Higher control of saccadic eye movements. The brain stem saccade generator receives a motor command from the superior colliculus. The colliculus receives direct excitatory projections from the frontal eye field and the posterior parietal cortex, and an inhibitory projection from the substantia nigra. Nigral inhibition can be suppressed by the caudate nucleus, which in turn receives a motor command from the frontal eye field.

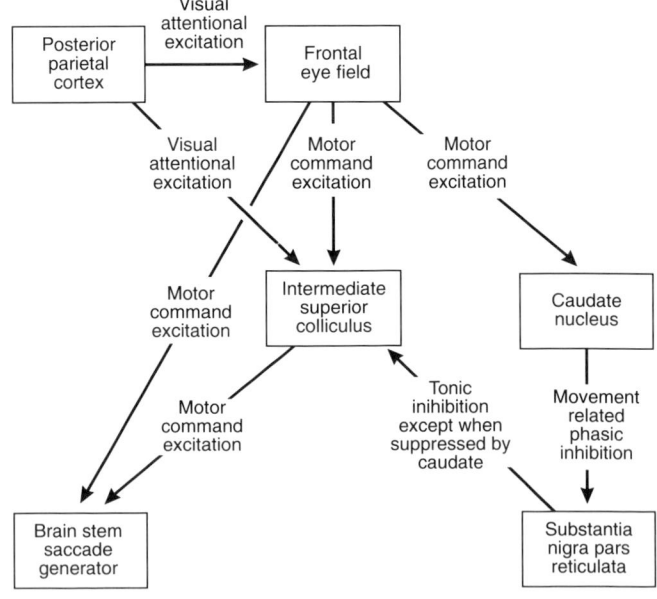

discharge before the movement. Since each cell makes only a small contribution to the direction and amplitude of a movement, any variability or noise in the discharge of a given cell is minimized. Similar population coding is found for voluntary movement (Chapter 40) and for the sense of smell (Chapter 34).

In each of two sets of layers in the superior colliculus—the superficial and deep—activity can occur independently of the other. Thus, sensory activity in the superficial layers need not lead to motor output from the intermediate layers, and output can occur without sensory activity in the superficial layers. In fact, neurons in the superficial layers do not project directly to the intermediate layers. Instead, they send their fibers to the pulvinar and lateral posterior nuclei of the thalamus, from there the signals are relayed to the cortical regions that project back to the intermediate layers. Lesions of a small part of the colliculus transiently affect the latency, accuracy, and velocity of saccades; lesions of the entire colliculus transiently render a monkey unable to make any contralateral saccades, but this quickly recovers. The monkey at first makes saccades that are slower, less accurate, and have a longer reaction time than before the lesion, but ultimately even these recover almost entirely.

The Frontal Eye Field Sends a Specific Movement Signal to the Superior Colliculus

In monkeys roughly half of the neurons in the frontal eye field respond to visual stimuli, and half of these visual neurons have enhanced responses to stimuli that become targets for saccadic eye movements. Unlike neurons in the parietal cortex, they do not have enhanced responses when the animal attends to the stimulus without making a saccade to it. These neurons require visual stimuli.

A second class of cells discharge before both visually guided and memory-guided saccades, and do not respond to visual stimuli that are not the targets for saccades. Unlike the movement cells in the superior colliculus that discharge before all saccades, these cells discharge only before saccades that are relevant to the monkey's behavior. This class, and not the visual neurons, project to the superior colliculus. Electrical stimulation of the frontal eye field evokes saccades to the movement fields of the stimulated cells. Bilateral stimulation of the frontal eye field evokes vertical saccades.

The frontal eye field controls the superior colliculus in two ways: (1) the movement neurons project directly to the intermediate layers of the superior colliculus, exciting the movement neuron ensembles; and (2) neurons from the same layer of the frontal eye field project to the caudate and excite those neurons that inhibit the substantia nigra. Movement activity in the frontal eye field presents a saccadic signal, simultaneously exciting the superior colliculus and releasing it from the inhibition from the substantia nigra by way of the caudate nucleus. The frontal eye field also projects to the pontine and mesencephalic reticular formations, although not directly to the burst-cell regions.

In monkeys lesions of the frontal eye field cause a transient contralateral neglect and paresis of contralateral gaze that rapidly recover. The residual deficits are more subtle. Animals have no trouble making visually guided saccades but have great difficulty learning to make memory-guided saccades. They cannot make predictive saccades. As compared with these subtle deficits, bilateral lesions of both the frontal eye fields and the superior colliculus render monkeys unable to make saccades at all, as if there were no higher control on the brain stem mechanisms.

Two other cortical regions are thought to be important in the control of saccades: both the dorsolateral prefrontal cortex and the supplementary eye field at the most rostral part of the supplementary motor area. Neurons in these areas project to the frontal eye field. In addition, the supplementary eye field projects directly to subcortical areas.

We can now understand the effects of lesions of these regions on the generation of saccades. Collicular lesions in the monkey produce transient damage to the saccadic system because the frontal brain stem projection is intact. With parietal damage the system can function normally after the neglect period because the frontal signals are sufficient to suppress the nigra and stimulate the colliculus.

Frontal damage causes more subtle deficits. Transient gaze paralysis may be related to the fact that in the absence of inputs from the frontal eye field there is no adequate control on the substantia nigra, which then will not permit the colliculus to generate any saccades. Eventually the system must adapt so that the colliculus can respond to a parietal signal. However, this parietal signal is an undifferentiated attentional signal rather than a carefully crafted movement command, so the system tends to generate more stimulus-bound saccades than in the normal case. Thus, Daniel Guitton and his colleagues found that patients with frontal lesions made accurate saccades to the target but had difficulty making saccades away from targets without first looking at the targets. We would expect this if the superior colliculus responded to a parietal signal without the attendant frontal-nigral control.

An Overall View

The oculomotor system provides an advantageously placed window into the nervous system, for both the clinician and the scientist. Patients with oculomotor deficits experience diplopia, and this alarming symptom sends them quickly to seek medical help. A physician with a thorough knowledge of the oculomotor system can describe and diagnose most oculomotor deficits at the bedside, and can localize precisely the site of the lesion because so much is known about the neuroanatomy and the neurophysiology of eye movements. Our understanding of neural processes has been greatly enriched by using the oculomotor system as a model of motor control.

Yet at every level of the oculomotor system important questions remain unanswered. For example, we know precisely the signal of each oculomotor neuron in terms of eye position and velocity. But since different orbital positions require different forces for equilibrium, the ultimate factor in muscular control must be the differential recruitment of neurons, and we have no idea how recruitment is controlled.

We know that the eye muscles have as many spindle stretch receptors as skeletal muscles, and that the number of spindles increases from the carnivore to the non-human primate to man. Nonetheless, the extraocular muscles have no stretch reflexes; we have no idea how the spindles function.

We know that oculomotor processes are under adaptive control, and that this adaptive control requires the cerebellum. Adaptive control must require a permanent modification of synaptic sensitivity, so that a given visual or vestibular input will have a different effect on a premotor neuron. But the location of these modifiable synapses is not clearly known.

We have a general idea of how the brain stem organizes saccades and, for example, that this organization must involve feeding back a signal to the burst and pause neurons. But we do not know the signals that are fed back or the anatomical location of the feedback loops.

We know that we explore the world with saccadic eye movements and that the cerebral cortex chooses the objects for our exploration. But we do not know the processes underlying that choice. Perhaps if we understood these processes we would have a better understanding of all motor control.

Selected Readings

Becker, W. 1989. Metrics. In R. H. Wurtz and M. E. Goldberg (eds.), The Neurobiology of Saccadic Eye Movements, Reviews of Oculomotor Research, Vol. 3. Amsterdam: Elsevier, pp. 13–67.

Fuchs, A. F. 1989. The vestibular system. In H. D. Patton, A. F. Fuchs, B. Hille, A. M. Scher, and R. Steiner (eds.), Textbook of Physiology, 21st ed. Excitable Cells and Neurophysiology, Vol. 1. Philadelphia: Saunders, pp. 582–607.

Fuchs, A. F., Kaneko, C. R. S., and Scudder, C. A. 1985. Brainstem control of saccadic eye movements. Annu. Rev. Neurosci. 8:307–337.

Goldberg, M. E., and Colby, C. L. 1989. The neurophysiology of spatial vision. In F. Boller and J. Grafman (eds.), Handbook of Neuropsychology, Vol. 2. Amsterdam: Elsevier Science Publishers, pp. 301–315.

Hikosaka, O., and Wurtz, R. H. 1989. The basal ganglia. In R. H. Wurtz and M. E. Goldberg (eds.), The Neurobiology of Saccadic Eye Movements, Reviews of Oculomotor Research, Vol. 3. Amsterdam: Elsevier, pp. 257–281.

Lisberger, S. G., Morris, E. J., and Tychsen, L. 1987. Visual motion processing and sensory-motor integration for smooth pursuit eye movements. Annu. Rev. Neurosci. 10:97–129.

Raphan, T., and Cohen, B. 1978. Brainstem mechanisms for rapid and slow eye movements. Annu. Rev. Physiol. 40:527–552.

Robinson, D. A. 1981. Control of eye movements. In V. B. Brooks (ed.), Handbook of Physiology, Section 1: The Nervous System, Vol. II. Motor Control, Part 2. Bethesda, Md.: American Physiological Society, pp. 1275–1320.

Sparks, D. L. 1986. Translation of sensory signals into commands for control of saccadic eye movements: Role of primate superior colliculus. Physiol. Rev. 66:118–171.

Wurtz, R. H., Komatsu, H., Dürsteler, M. R., and Yamasaki, D. S. 1990. Motion to Movement: Cerebral cortical visual processing for pursuit eye movements. In G. M. Edelman, W. E. Gall, and W. M. Cowan (eds.), Signal and Sense: Local and Global Order in Perceptual Maps. New York: Wiley-Liss, pp. 233–260.

Zee, D. S., and Optican, L. M. 1985. Studies of adaptation in human oculomotor disorders. In A. Berthoz, and G. Melvill Jones (eds.), Adaptive Mechanisms in Gaze Control: Facts and Theories. Amsterdam: Elsevier, pp. 165–176.

References

Becker, W., and Jürgens, R. 1979. An analysis of the saccadic system by means of double step stimuli. Vision Res. 19:967–983.

Bruce, C. J., and Goldberg, M. E. 1985. Primate frontal eye fields: I. Single neurons discharging before saccades. J. Neurophysiol. 53:603–635.

Büttner-Ennever, J. A., Büttner, U., Cohen, B., and Baumgartner, G. 1982. Vertical gaze paralysis and the rostral interstitial nucleus of the medial longitudinal fasciculus. Brain 105:125–149.

Carpenter, R. H. S. 1988. Movements of the Eyes, 2nd ed. rev. enl. London: Pion.

Cohen, B., Matsuo, V., and Raphan, T. 1977. Quantitative analysis of the velocity characteristics of optokinetic nystagmus and optokinetic after-nystagmus. J. Physiol. (Lond) 270:321–344.

Cumming, B. G., and Judge, S. J. 1986. Disparity-induced and blur-induced convergence eye movement and accommodation in the monkey. J. Neurophysiol. 55:896–914.

Dodge, R. 1903. Five types of eye movement in the horizontal meridian plane of the field of regard. Am. J. Physiol. 8:307–329.

Dufossé, M., Ito, M., Jastreboff, P. J., and Miyashita, Y. 1978. A neuronal correlate in rabbit's cerebellum to adaptive modification of the vestibulo-ocular reflex. Brain Res. 150:611–616.

Dürsteler, M. R., and Wurtz, R. H. 1988. Pursuit and optokinetic deficits following chemical lesions of cortical areas MT and MST. J. Neurophysiol. 60:940–965.

Eckmiller, R. 1987. Neural control of pursuit eye movements. Physiol. Rev. 67:797–857.

Fuchs, A. F. 1967. Saccadic and smooth pursuit eye movements in the monkey. J. Physiol. (Lond.) 191:609–631.

Gonshor, A., and Melvill Jones, G. 1976. Short-term adaptive changes in the human vestibulo-ocular reflex arc. J. Physiol. (Lond) 256:361–379.

Gordon, B. 1973. Receptive fields in deep layers of cat superior colliculus. J. Neurophysiol. 36:157–178.

Guitton, D., Buchtel, H. A., and Douglas, R. M. 1985. Frontal lobe lesions in man cause difficulties in suppressing reflexive glances and in generating goal-directed saccades. Exp. Brain Res. 58:455–472.

Hardy, M. 1934. Observations on the innervation of the macula sacculi in man. Anat. Rec. 59:403–418.

Helmholtz, H. von. 1911. The Sensations of Vision. In J. P. C. Southall (ed. and trans.), Helmholtz's Treatise on Physiological Optics, Vol. 2. Wash., D. C.: Optical Society of America, 1924. Translated from the 3rd German edition.

Henn, V., Lang, W., Hepp, K., and Reisine, H. 1984. Experimental gaze palsies in monkeys and their relation to human pathology. Brain 107:619–636.

Hikosaka, O., and Wurtz, R. H. 1983. Visual and oculomotor functions of monkey substantia nigra pars reticulata. I. Relation of visual and auditory responses to saccades. J. Neurophysiol. 49:1230–1253.

Hikosaka, O., and Wurtz, R. H. 1983. Visual and oculomotor functions of monkey substantia nigra pars reticulata. III. Memory-contingent visual and saccade responses. J. Neurophysiol. 49:1268–1284.

Judge, S. J., and Cumming, B. G. 1986. Neurons in the monkey midbrain with activity related to vergence eye movement and accommodation. J. Neurophysiol. 55:915–930.

Keller, E. L., and Robinson, D. A. 1971. Absence of a stretch reflex in extraocular muscles of the monkey. J. Neurophysiol. 34:908–919.

Kommerell, G., Olivier, D., and Theopold, H. 1976. Adaptive programming of phasic and tonic components in saccadic eye movements. Investigations in patients with abducens palsy. Invest. Ophthalmol. 15:657–660.

Landolt, E., and von Helmholtz, H. 1928. Handbook of physiological optics, 3rd ed. (J. P. C. Southall, trans.) Arch. Ophthalmol. (Paris) 11:385–395.

Leigh, R. J., and Zee, D. S. 1991. The Neurology of Eye Movements, 2nd ed. Philadelphia: F.A. Davis.

Lynch, J. C., and McLaren, J. W. 1989. Deficits of visual attention and saccadic eye movements after lesions of parietooccipital cortex in monkeys. J. Neurophysiol 61:74–90.

Lynch, J. C., Mountcastle, V. B., Talbot, W. H., and Yin, T. C. T. 1977. Parietal lobe mechanisms for directed visual attention J. Neurophysiol. 40:362–389.

Miles, F. A., and Lisberger, S. G. 1981. Plasticity in the vestibulo-ocular reflex: A new hypothesis. Annu. Rev. Neurosci. 4:273–299.

Mountcastle, V. B., Lynch, J. C., Georgopoulos, A., Sakata, H., and Acuna, C. 1975. Posterior parietal association cortex of the monkey: Command functions for operations within extrapersonal space. J. Neurophysiol. 38:871–908.

Optican, L. M., and Robinson, D. A. 1980. Cerebellar-dependent adaptive control of primate saccadic system. J. Neurophysiol. 44:1058–1076.

Patton, H. D. 1989. The autonomic nervous system. In H. D. Patton, A. F. Fuchs, B. Hille, A. M. Scher, and R. Steiner (eds.), Textbook of Physiology: Excitable Cells and Neurophysiology, 21st ed., Vol. 1, Section VII: Emotive Responses and Internal Milieu. Philadelphia: Saunders, pp. 737–758.

Robinson, D. A. 1970. Oculomotor unit behavior in the monkey. J. Neurophysiol. 33:393–404.

Schiller, P. H., and Stryker, M. 1972. Single-unit recording and stimulation in superior colliculus of the alert rhesus monkey. J. Neurophysiol. 35:915–924.

Schlag, J., and Schlag-Rey, M. 1987. Evidence for a supplementary eye field. J. Neurophysiol. 57:179–200.

Schwarz, U., Busettini, C., and Miles, F. A. 1989. Ocular responses to linear motion are inversely proportional to viewing distance. Science 245:1394–1396.

Westheimer, G. 1954. Eye movement responses to a horizontally moving visual stimulus. Arch. Ophthalmol. 52:932–941.

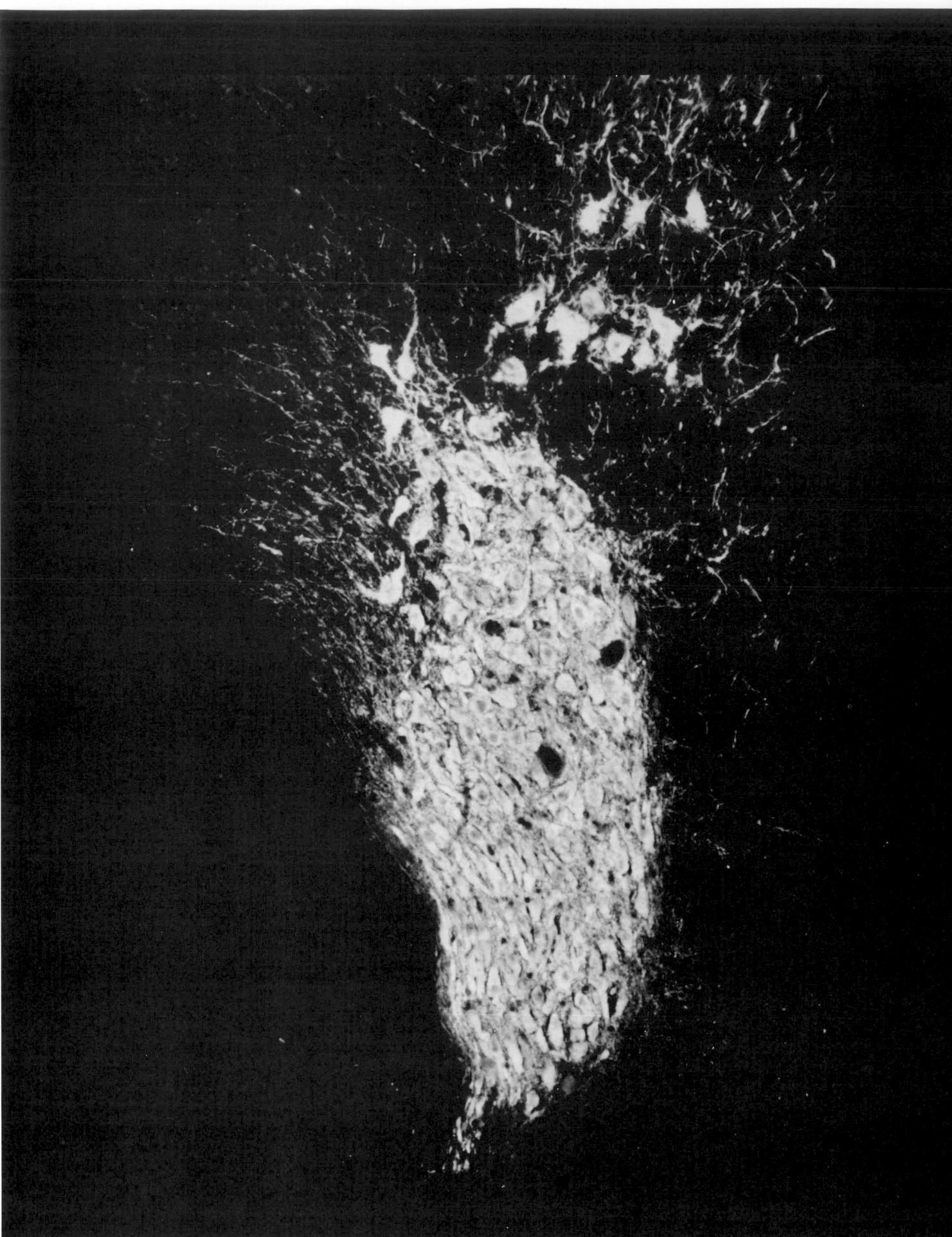

VII

The Brain Stem and Reticular Core: Integration of Sensory and Motor Systems

The brain stem—the small region of the central nervous system between the spinal cord and the diencephalon—has a clinical significance that is far out of proportion to its size. Damage to the brain stem can profoundly affect motor and sensory processes as well as consciousness.

The brain stem contains three types of structures: nuclear groups, long tracts (both motor and sensory), and the components of the reticular formation, a loosely organized collection of cells concerned with modulating awareness and behavioral performance. Most of the cranial nerves arise from nuclear groups in the brain stem and innervate structures of the head and neck. The general principles underlying the organization of the cranial nerves are similar to those of the spinal nerves, but the nerves innervating the head are anatomically more complex. Some cranial nerves are concerned with sight, hearing, taste, and smell.

Neurological syndromes that result from damage to the brain stem often consist of many symptoms that seem unrelated. These confusing syndromes occur because long ascending and descending tracts run near different nuclear groups. Despite this proximity, however, the long tracts and the nuclei are concerned with different functions. A single lesion can therefore affect neurons that mediate quite different aspects of sensation and motor function. Nevertheless, the organization of the brain stem is sufficiently well defined that knowledge of the location of even a small lesion can be used to predict its clinical consequences. For this reason, the clinical symptoms can indicate the precise location of damage within the brain stem.

In many ways the brain stem can be considered a rostral continuation of the spinal cord. Relatively small in volume, it contains all of the tracts that bring sensory information from the body and that deliver commands from the brain, as well as centers that control vital functions, like respiration and heart beat. The brain stem also contains a center thought to be crucial for attention, and therefore to higher mental functions: the *locus ceruleus*. Half of the noradrenergic neurons of the brain are clustered together in this small nucleus in the reticular formation of the brain stem. This nucleus is visualized here in the rat by immunofluorescence histochemical localization of tyrosine hydroxylase, the rate-limiting enzyme in the synthesis of noradrenaline. Intense immunofluorescence delineates the noradrenergic cell bodies and their initial axonal projections. (Courtesy of Thomas Hökfelt, Karolinska Institute.)

PART VII

Chapter 44:   **The Brain Stem: Cranial Nerve Nuclei and the Monoaminergic Systems**

Chapter 45:   **Trigeminal System**

Chapter 46:   **Clinical Syndromes of the Spinal Cord and Brain Stem**

Lorna W. Role
James P. Kelly

The Brain Stem: Cranial Nerve Nuclei and the Monoaminergic Systems

Most Cranial Nerves Are Located in the Brain Stem

Cranial Nerves Contain Motor, Visceral, and Somatic Afferent Fibers

There Are Three Classes of Motor Neurons in the Brain Stem

There Are Four Classes of Sensory Neurons

The Cranial Nerve Nuclei Are Organized into Columns

The Motor Nuclei

The Sensory Nuclei

Several Principles Govern the Organization of the Brain Stem

Most Motor Nuclei in the Brain Stem Project to Their Targets Through a Single Cranial Nerve

The Sensory Nuclei in the Brain Stem Receive Input from Several Cranial Nerves

Somatic Sensory and Motor Tracts Traverse the Brain Stem

Cranial Nerve Fiber Types May Intermingle in the Periphery

Nuclei in the Reticular Formation Form Widespread Networks

There Are Three Major Monoaminergic Systems in the Brain Stem

The Noradrenergic System Originates in Two Nuclear Groups: The Locus Ceruleus and the Lateral Tegmental Nucleus

The Dopaminergic System Originates in the Midbrain and Projects to the Striatum, Limbic System, and Neocortex

The Serotonergic System Originates in the Raphe Nuclei

An Overall View

The brain stem is a relatively small region between the spinal cord and the diencephalon, yet its functional significance is far out of proportion to its size. It regulates both motor and sensory processes and it is required for consciousness; a small lesion causes coma. As the rostral extension of the spinal cord, the brain stem follows the organizing principles evident in the cord.

The brain stem includes three major regions—the medulla, pons, and midbrain—which contain somatic and visceral sensory and motor fibers, as well as the nuclei of the cranial nerves. Embedded around the major tracts and nuclei of the brain stem are the nerve cells of the reticular formation. These have an important modulatory effect on the spinal cord as well as on the cerebral cortex. Neurons in the reticular formation are arranged in distinctive functional groups on the basis of their connections and the biochemical nature of their transmitter. Thus, the distinct neuronal groups in the brain stem are the major source of noradrenergic, dopaminergic, and serotonergic inputs to most parts of the brain.

In this chapter we first describe the anatomical organization of the cranial nerves in relation to the three regions of the brain stem. We then discuss the division of brain stem neurons into longitudinal columns. Appreciating this columnar organization is important for understanding the functional organization of the cranial nerves and the brain stem. Finally, we examine the nuclei of the reticular formation, their afferent and efferent connections, their physiological properties, and their role in modulating or controlling a variety of behaviors.

Most Cranial Nerves Are Located in the Brain Stem

The cranial nerves have three main functions: (1) they provide the motor and general sensory innervation of the skin, muscles, and joints in the head and neck; (2) they mediate vision, hearing, olfaction, and taste; and (3) they

TABLE **44–1.** Functions of the Cranial Nerves

Cranial nerve	Type of nerve	Functions
Olfactory (**I**)	Sensory	Smell
Optic (**II**)	Sensory	Sight
Oculomotor (**III**)	Motor	Eye movements: innervates all extraocular muscles except the superior oblique and lateral rectus muscles (see N. IV and VI); innervates the striated muscle of the eyelid; mediates pupillary constriction and accommodation of the lens for near vision
Trochlear (**IV**)	Motor	Eye movements: innervates superior oblique muscle
Trigeminal (**V**)	Mixed	Sensory: mediates cutaneous and proprioceptive sensations from skin, muscles, and joints in the face and mouth, and sensory innervation of the teeth Motor: innervates muscles of mastication
Abducens (**VI**)	Motor	Eye movements: innervates lateral rectus muscle
Facial and intermediate (**VII**)	Mixed	Motor: innervates muscles of facial expression, lacrimal glands, salivary glands Sensory: mediates taste sensation from the anterior two-thirds of the tongue, and sensation from skin of external ear
Vestibulocochlear (**VIII**)	Sensory	Hearing, balance, postural reflexes, and orientation of the head in space
Glossopharyngeal (**IX**)	Mixed	Autonomic fibers innervate the parotid gland Swallowing: mediates visceral sensations from the palate and posterior one-third of the tongue Innervates the carotid body Innervates taste buds in posterior third of the tongue
Vagus (**X**)	Mixed	Autonomic fibers innervate smooth muscle in the heart, blood vessels, trachea, bronchi, esophagus, stomach, and intestine Innervates striated muscles in the larynx and pharynx and controls speech Mediates visceral sensation from the pharynx, larynx, thorax, and abdomen Innervates taste buds in the epiglottis
Spinal accessory (**XI**)	Motor	Motor innervation of the trapezius and sternocleidomastoid muscles
Hypoglossal (**XII**)	Motor	Motor innervation of the intrinsic muscles of the tongue

carry the parasympathetic innervation of autonomic ganglia that control visceral functions, such as breathing, heart rate, blood pressure, coughing, and swallowing.

The 12 pairs of cranial nerves are numbered in rostrocaudal sequence. Some of them are purely motor, others purely sensory, and the rest are mixed (Table 44–1). Assessment of the function of these nerves is important in neurological examinations because functional abnormalities of one or more of the cranial nerves often reflect lesions of the brain stem. Since these nerves originate in different regions in the brain stem, dysfunction of specific nerves can provide valuable information about the site of a lesion in the brain stem.

The origins of most cranial nerves can be seen in a ventral view of the brain stem with the cerebral hemispheres and cerebellum removed (Figure 44–1). The remaining cranial nerves are best seen in a lateral view (Figure 44–2). Three purely motor nerves (nerves III, VI, and XII) exit from the brain stem close to the midline. Ontogenetically and phylogenetically, these three cranial nerves belong to a common class (the somatic motor nerves), and the neurons that give rise to them are found adjacent to the midline. The oculomotor nerve (III) lies most rostrally and emerges at the caudal border of the midbrain. The abducens (VI) lies below it, at the caudal border of the pons. The hypoglossal (XII) lies still further below and emerges from the medulla just lateral to the

medullary pyramids. The oculomotor and abducens nerves innervate extraocular muscles; the hypoglossal nerve innervates the intrinsic muscles of the tongue. Only one cranial nerve, the trochlear (IV), exits from the dorsal aspect of the brain stem. The trochlear nerve is purely motor. It exits from the midbrain just caudal to the inferior colliculus near the midline and innervates the superior oblique muscle of the eye (Figure 44–2).

The trigeminal nerve (V) enters the pons; this mixed sensory–motor nerve mediates sensation from the face and innervates the muscles of the jaw. The facial (VII) and vestibulocochlear (VIII) nerves originate at the junction between the pons and the medulla. The glossopharyngeal (IX), vagus (X), and accessory (XI) nerves arise as a series of fine rootlets just dorsal to the inferior olive. Two cranial nerves do not terminate in the brain stem: the optic (II) terminates in the thalamus and midbrain, and the olfactory (I) nerve in the olfactory bulb. They are described in relation to vision (Chapter 29) and olfaction (Chapter 34).

Cranial Nerves Contain Motor, Visceral, and Somatic Afferent Fibers

As we have seen in Chapter 21, the development of the motor and sensory cranial nerve nuclei of the brain stem follows a pattern similar to that of the spinal cord. The

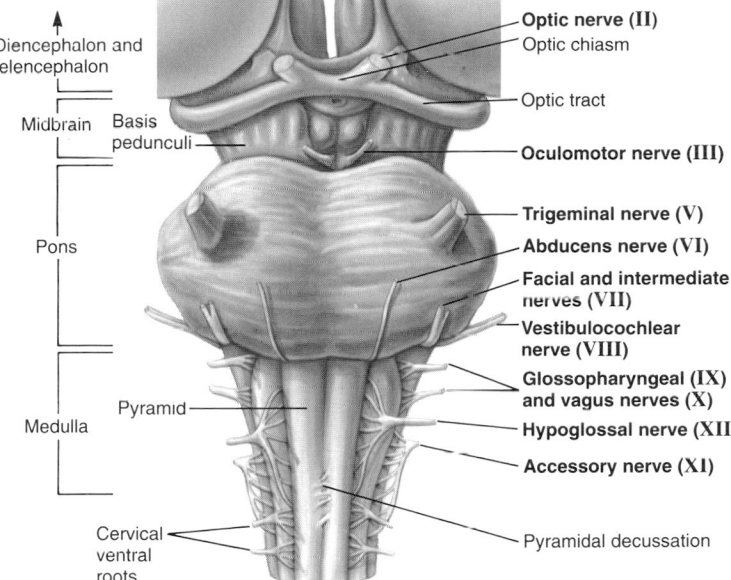

Diencephalon and telencephalon

Midbrain

Basis pedunculi

Pons

Medulla

Pyramid

Cervical ventral roots

Optic nerve (II)
Optic chiasm
Optic tract

Oculomotor nerve (III)

Trigeminal nerve (V)
Abducens nerve (VI)
Facial and intermediate nerves (VII)
Vestibulocochlear nerve (VIII)
Glossopharyngeal (IX) and vagus nerves (X)
Hypoglossal nerve (XII)
Accessory nerve (XI)

Pyramidal decussation

FIGURE 44–1

The origins of most of the cranial nerves are evident in a ventral view of the brain stem.

FIGURE 44–2

A lateral view of the brain stem illustrates the emergence of the cranial nerves in rostrocaudal sequence. The trochlear (IV) nerve, the only cranial nerve that exits from the dorsal aspect of the brain stem, as well as the origins of the facial (VII) and vestibulocochlear (VIII) nerves are best seen in this lateral view of the brain stem.

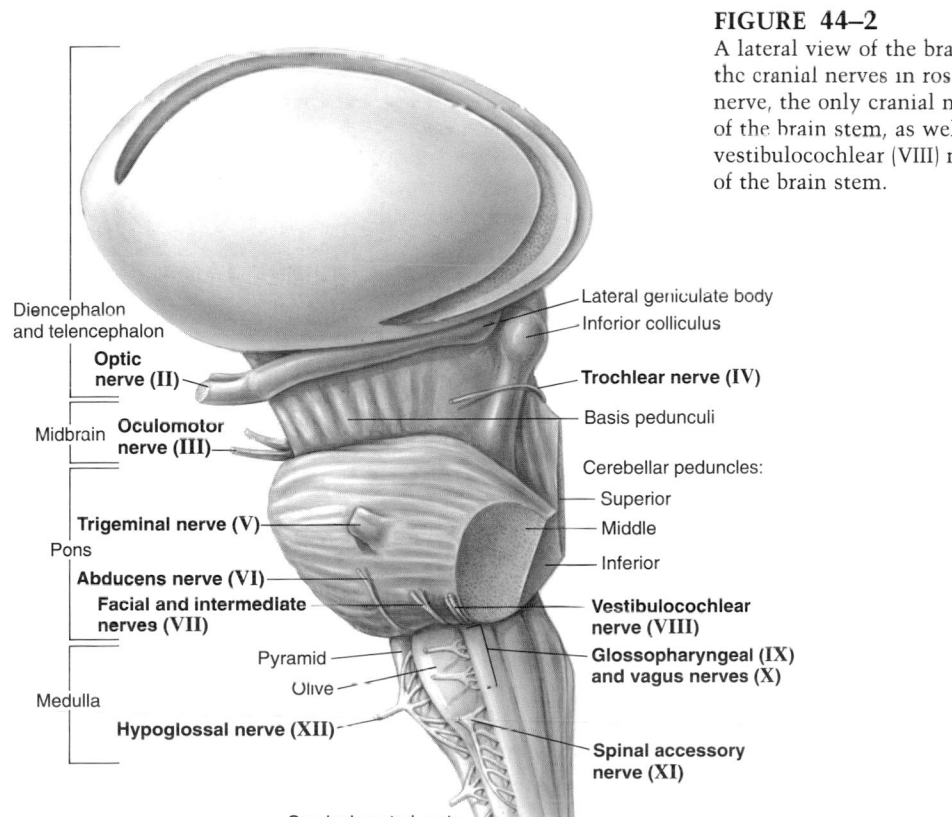

Diencephalon and telencephalon

Optic nerve (II)

Midbrain

Oculomotor nerve (III)

Trigeminal nerve (V)

Pons

Abducens nerve (VI)
Facial and intermediate nerves (VII)

Pyramid
Olive

Medulla

Hypoglossal nerve (XII)

Cervical ventral roots

Lateral geniculate body
Inferior colliculus

Trochlear nerve (IV)

Basis pedunculi

Cerebellar peduncles:
Superior
Middle
Inferior

Vestibulocochlear nerve (VIII)

Glossopharyngeal (IX) and vagus nerves (X)

Spinal accessory nerve (XI)

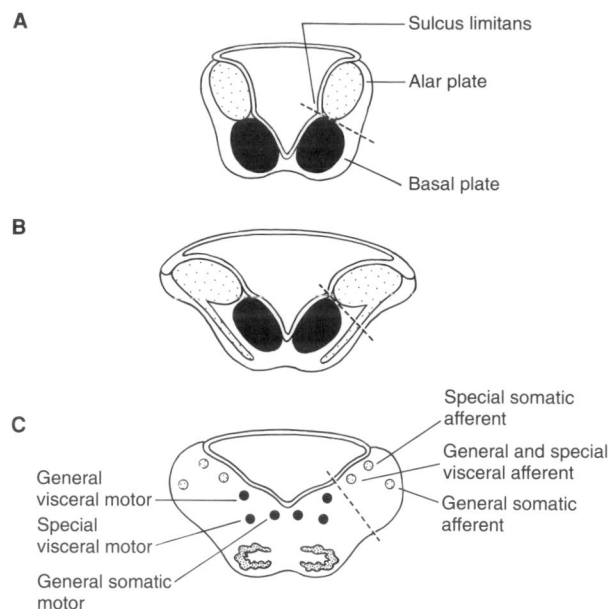

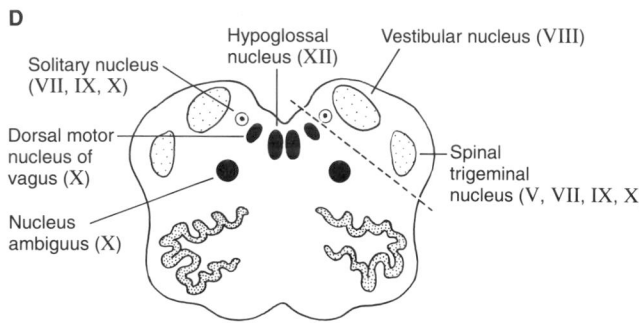

FIGURE 44–3

The sensory and motor nuclei of the cranial nerves develop from the alar and basal plates.

A–C. Drawings of transverse sections through the medulla show three stages of development. Cranial nerve sensory nuclei arise from the alar plate, whereas the motor nuclei develop from the basal plate.

D. Drawing of a myelin-stained section of the mature medulla shows some of the sensory and motor cranial nuclei relative to the approximate position of the sulcus limitans at earlier stages.

developing brain stem is comprised of separate alar and basal plates (Figure 44–3). Neurons that arise from the alar plate of the brain stem become sensory (or afferent) neurons; those arising from the basal plate develop into motor (or efferent) neurons. As in the spinal cord, the alar and basal plates of the brain stem are divided by the *sulcus limitans*, which separates the sensory and motor nuclei (Figure 44–3).

There are two classes of motor neurons in the spinal cord. *Somatic motor neurons* innervate the muscle of the trunk and limbs. *Visceral (autonomic) motor neurons* innervate the ganglion cells of the autonomic nervous system. These ganglion cells innervate blood vessels, glands,

and the viscera of the body cavity. There are also two classes of sensory neurons that project to the spinal cord: *somatic afferent neurons* and *visceral (autonomic) afferent neurons*. Both classes of afferent neurons have their cell bodies outside the spinal cord in the dorsal root ganglia. Somatic afferent neurons innervate the skin, muscles, and joints of the trunk and limbs, and mediate touch as well as proprioception. Visceral afferent fibers innervate the viscera of the body cavity and mediate autonomic reflexes.

The functional organization of the cranial nerves is similar to that of the spinal nerves. As in the spinal cord, the cell bodies of motor and sensory fibers in the cranial nerves are found in different locations. The cell bodies of motor neurons whose axons run in the cranial nerves are located within the brain stem, whereas those of the afferent fibers lie outside the brain stem, either in ganglia analogous to the dorsal root ganglia or in specialized end-organs such as the eye. We next describe the functional classes of motor and sensory neurons associated with the cranial nerves.

There Are Three Classes of Motor Neurons in the Brain Stem

Whereas the spinal cord contains only two classes of motor neurons (*somatic* and *visceral*), the brain stem contains three: one class of somatic motor neurons and two classes of visceral motor neurons (*special* and *general*). All three classes of motor neurons are located in the cranial motor nuclei of the brain stem. Like spinal motor neurons, cranial motor neurons are lower motor neurons (see Chapter 35). Although the somatic and special visceral motor neurons innervate skeletal muscles of the head and neck, they innervate distinct sets of striated muscle of different developmental origins (Table 44–2).

The *somatic motor neurons* innervate the extraocular muscles and the intrinsic muscles of the tongue (through nerves III, IV, VI, and XII). These muscles develop from the myotomes of the embryo and their development is similar to that of other striated muscles in the body. The somatic motor neurons resemble the large motor neurons of the ventral horn of the spinal cord. The *special visceral motor neurons* innervate striated muscles that control chewing, facial expression, the larynx, and the pharynx (through nerves V, VII, IX, X, and XI). These muscles develop from the branchial arches of the embryo. Special visceral motor neurons are found lateral to the somatic motor neurons. The *general visceral motor neurons* are parasympathetic preganglionic neurons. They regulate the activity of ganglionic neurons that innervate glands, blood vessels, and smooth muscle (through nerves III, VII, IX, and X).

Sympathetic neurons that innervate structures in the head have their cell bodies in the superior cervical ganglion, the most rostral of the sympathetic ganglia (Chapter 49). Axons of these sympathetic neurons run along the internal carotid artery for part of their course and eventually join one of the cranial nerve branches to reach the appropriate end-organ.

TABLE **44–2.** Functional Classes of Cranial Nerves

Classification	Functions	Structures innervated	Cranial nerves
Afferent fibers			
General somatic	Touch, pain, temperature, and proprioception	Skin, skeletal muscles of head and neck, mucous membrane of mouth, and teeth	V, VII, IX, X
Special somatic[a]	Hearing, vision, balance	Cochlea, vestibular organ	II, VIII
General visceral	Mechanical, pain, temperature, and proprioception	Pharynx, larynx, gut	V, VII, IX, X
Special visceral	Olfaction, taste	Taste buds, olfactory epithelium	I, VII, IX, X
Motor fibers			
General somatic	Skeletal muscle control (somites)	Extraocular and tongue muscles	III, IV, VI, XII
General visceral	Autonomic control	Tear glands, sweat glands, gut	III, VII, IX, X
Special visceral	Skeletal muscle control (branchiomeric)	Muscles of facial expression, jaw, neck, larynx, and pharynx	V, VII, IX, X, XI

[a]The optic nerve (II) is considered part of the special somatic afferent class, but is not included here because it does not contain the axons of primary sensory neurons but rather those of third-order neurons in the visual pathway.

There Are Four Classes of Sensory Neurons

The sensory nuclei in the brain stem are composed of second-order neurons that receive input from the primary afferent fibers that originate in sensory ganglia outside the brain stem. Because of the presence of special sensory organs in the head as well as the mixed embryological origin of muscle in the facial region, the cranial nerves include specialized types of afferent fibers that are not present in spinal nerves. As a result, the two classes of afferent neurons (somatic and visceral) in the cranial nerves may be further subdivided.

General somatic afferent fibers innervate the skin of the face and the mucous membranes of the mouth. *Special somatic afferent* fibers arise from the cochlea and vestibular apparatus, the sensory organs of the inner ear. *General visceral afferent* fibers provide sensory innervation to internal organs, and to the larynx and pharynx. *Special visceral afferent* fibers innervate the taste buds and mediate the sense of taste. The general functions and sites of innervation of all four classes of afferent fibers are summarized in Table 44–2.

The Cranial Nerve Nuclei Are Organized into Columns

The cranial nerve nuclei are organized into seven longitudinal columns within the brain stem (Figure 44–4). These columns represent the division of neurons on the basis of embryological origin from either the alar or basal plate (sensory versus motor), and the nature of the structure innervated. Neurons innervating structures that develop from somites are segregated from neurons innervating structures that develop from branchial arches. Neurons mediating special senses are also segregated in particular columns. The cell columns run roughly parallel to the longitudinal axis of the brain stem, but they are not always continuous. At any level of the brain stem, however, a particular functional group or column is located medially or laterally, depending on whether it is motor or sensory and somatic or visceral.

The functional significance of this columnar organization is twofold. First, neurons with similar functions are brought into proximity by this pattern of organization. For example, neurons processing afferent information pertaining to taste are found in the same location relative to the midline, even though they may receive input from several different cranial nerves. The functional organization of neurons into columns here and elsewhere in the nervous system has the net effect of economizing neural connections. Second, because of this functional organization, different functions are affected by local damage in the brain stem, depending on whether the damage is restricted to regions near the midline or to lateral regions. Therefore, when discussing neurological deficits in the brain stem, the site of damage is often described with respect to the midline (for example, see the discussion of lateral medullary syndrome in Chapter 46).

In the following sections we describe the motor and sensory nuclei associated with individual cranial nerves and the locations of these nuclei within functional columns. The location of the nuclei with respect to the major landmarks of the brain stem are shown in Figures 44–4 and 44–5.

The Motor Nuclei

Neurons that innervate the somatic muscles of the head that are derived from the myotomes form the *somatic motor column*. They are situated adjacent to the midline, immediately ventral to the floor of the fourth ventricle. Motor neurons that innervate the branchiomeric muscles that are derived from the branchial arches form the *special visceral motor column*. They are displaced ventrally and laterally from the somatic motor column. The parasympathetic neurons of the *general visceral motor column* are found immediately lateral to the somatic motor column.

The Somatic Motor Column. The somatic motor column, the most medial of the motor columns, consists of four nuclear groups: the oculomotor (III), trochlear (IV), abducens (VI), and hypoglossal (XII) nuclei (Figure 44–4B).

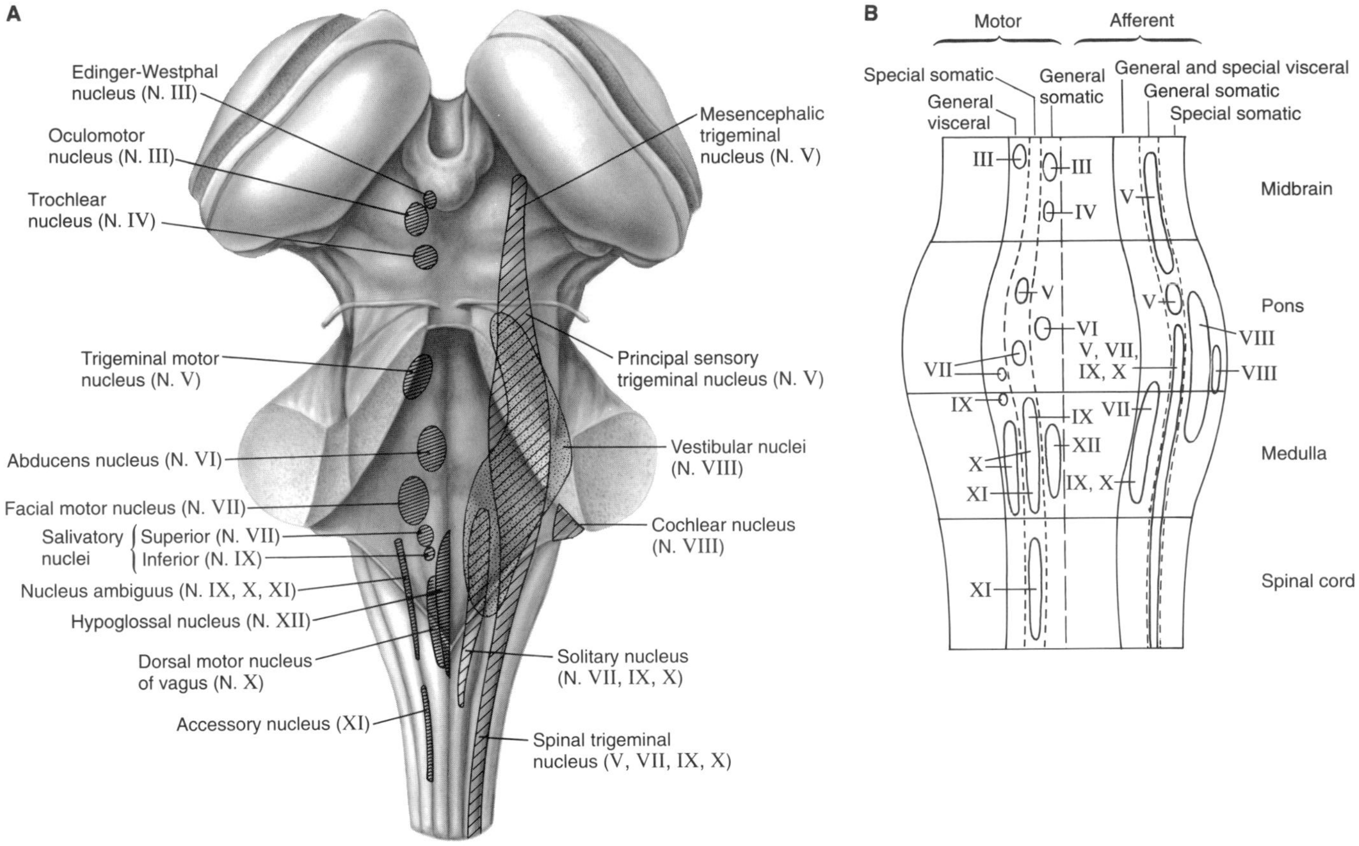

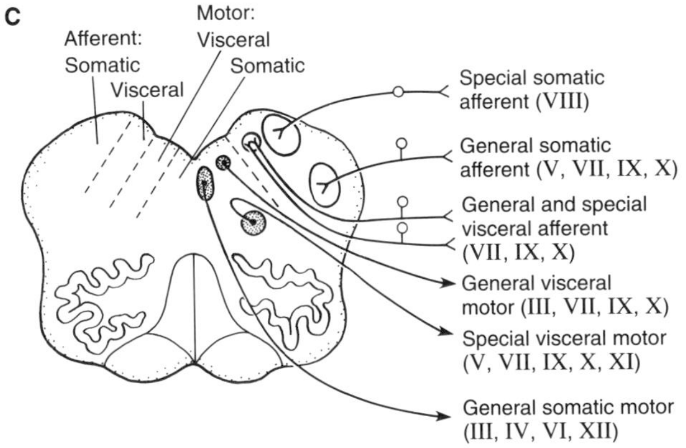

A

Edinger-Westphal
nucleus (N. III)

Oculomotor
nucleus (N. III)

Trochlear
nucleus (N. IV)

Trigeminal motor
nucleus (N. V)

Abducens nucleus (N. VI)

Facial motor nucleus (N. VII)

Salivatory { Superior (N. VII)
nuclei   { Inferior (N. IX)

Nucleus ambiguus (N. IX, X, XI)

Hypoglossal nucleus (N. XII)

Dorsal motor nucleus
of vagus (N. X)

Accessory nucleus (XI)

Mesencephalic
trigeminal
nucleus (N. V)

Principal sensory
trigeminal nucleus (N. V)

Vestibular nuclei
(N. VIII)

Cochlear nucleus
(N. VIII)

Solitary nucleus
(N. VII, IX, X)

Spinal trigeminal
nucleus (V, VII, IX, X)

B

Motor   Afferent

Special somatic.   General   General and special visceral
General somatic   somatic   General somatic
General   Special somatic
visceral

III   V   Midbrain

IV

v   v   Pons

VI   VIII
VII   V, VII,   VIII
IX, X

IX   IX VII   Medulla
XII
X   IX, X

XI

XI   Spinal cord

C

Motor:
Visceral
Afferent: Somatic
Somatic
Visceral

Special somatic
afferent (VIII)

General somatic
afferent (V, VII, IX, X)

General and special
visceral afferent
(VII, IX, X)

General visceral
motor (III, VII, IX, X)

Special visceral motor
(V, VII, IX, X, XI)

General somatic motor
(III, IV, VI, XII)

FIGURE 44–4

Cranial nerve nuclei are functionally organized in columns.

A. This dorsal view of the brain stem illustrates the columnar organization of the cranial nerve nuclei. The motor (efferent) nuclei are shown on the **left** and the sensory (afferent) nuclei are shown on the **right**.

B. This horizontal dorsal view of the columnar organization of the afferent and efferent nuclei shows the rostrocaudal positions of the nuclei.

C. The positions of the motor and afferent nuclei with respect to each other are shown in this cross section through the medulla.

These nuclei are not continuous along the rostrocaudal extent of the motor column, but each is found in the same relative position, just ventral to the floor of the ventricular system near the midline. The *oculomotor* (III) *nucleus* lies in the rostral part of the midbrain at the level of the superior colliculus (Figure 44–5). The *trochlear* (IV) *nucleus* lies more caudally in the midbrain at the level of the inferior colliculus. Both of these nuclei lie ventral to the cerebral aqueduct. The *abducens* (VI) *nucleus* is within the midpons region, and the *hypoglossal* (XII) *nucleus* is within the rostral medulla. Both of these nuclei lie ventral to the floor of the fourth ventricle.

The Special Visceral Motor Column. The motor neurons of the special visceral motor column are also clustered in four nuclei, displaced ventrally and laterally from the somatic motor column (Figure 44–4B). The most rostral component of the special visceral motor column, the motor nucleus of the *trigeminal nerve* (V), lies in the rostral pons (Figure 44–5) and contains the motor neurons that innervate the muscles of mastication. The motor component of the *facial* (VII) *nucleus* lies caudal to the motor nucleus of the trigeminal nerve in the pons (Figure 44–5) and contains the neurons that innervate the muscles of facial expression.

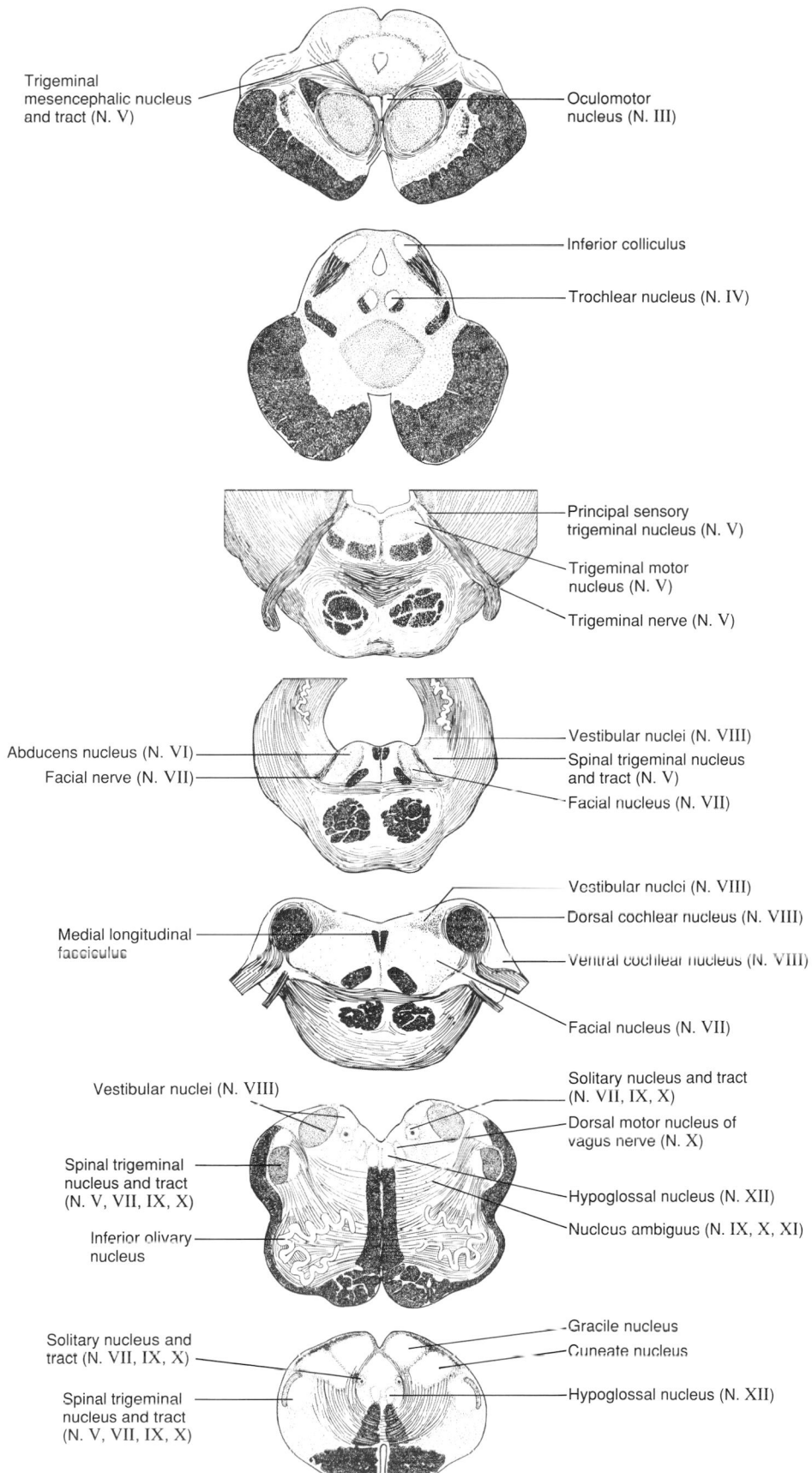

FIGURE 44–5

Transverse sections of the brain stem stained for myelin show the cranial nerve nuclei at various levels of the brain stem.

The motor neurons contributing to the glossopharyngeal (IX), vagus (X), and spinal accessory (XI) nerves lie in the medulla (Figure 44–4B). The motor neurons of the glossopharyngeal and vagus nerves are clustered in a single group, the *nucleus ambiguus*, in the rostral medulla (Figure 44–5). This nucleus innervates striated muscles in the larynx and pharynx that control both speech and swallowing. The most caudal nucleus in this column, the *spinal accessory (XI) nucleus*, stretches into the cervical region of the spinal cord and innervates the sternocleidomastoid and trapezius muscles.

The General Visceral Motor Column.   The general visceral motor column has four principal nuclei that lie just lateral to the somatic motor column (Figure 44–4B). The most rostral of these is the *Edinger–Westphal nucleus* (Figure 44–5). It lies adjacent to the oculomotor (III) nucleus and contains some, but not all, of the parasympathetic preganglionic neurons whose axons run in nerve III. These axons terminate in the ciliary ganglion, the cells of which innervate the pupillary constrictor and ciliary muscles of the eye. The parasympathetic innervation of the eye is balanced by the sympathetic innervation from the superior cervical ganglion, the cells of which innervate three smooth muscles in the orbit.

The *superior* and *inferior salivatory nuclei* lie in the rostral part of the medulla, but the borders of these nuclei are difficult to delineate. Axons of neurons in the superior salivatory nucleus run in the root of the intermediate branch of the facial nerve (VII), while those from the inferior salivatory nucleus run in the glossopharyngeal nerve (IX). The visceral motor axons in both of these nerves leave the nerve trunk to synapse in autonomic ganglia in the head that innervate salivary glands, mucous glands, and blood vessels. The inferior salivatory nucleus innervates the parotid gland through the otic ganglion. The superior salivatory nucleus innervates the sublingual and submandibular glands through the submandibular ganglion, and the lacrimal glands through the pterygopalatine ganglion.

The last component of the general visceral motor column, the *dorsal motor nucleus of the vagus* (X), lies adjacent to the hypoglossal (XII) nucleus in the rostral medulla (Figure 44–5). Axons of neurons in this nucleus run in the various branches of the vagus nerve to innervate the heart, lungs, and gut. Vagal stimulation decreases heart rate, whereas sympathetic stimulation increases it. In the gut the vagus nerve promotes peristalsis, while sympathetic fibers decrease intestinal motility (see Chapter 49).

Just lateral to the general visceral motor column there is the sulcus limitans. As described above, this cleft marks the division between sensory and motor regions in the developing neural tube (Figure 44–3). In the adult brain stem it marks the division between the afferent and efferent cell columns. The motor neurons described above are medial to the sulcus limitans, whereas the afferent cell columns (described next) lie lateral to it.

The Sensory Nuclei

The General and Special Visceral Afferent Column. The visceral afferent column is adjacent to the general visceral motor column and contains a single nucleus in the medulla called the *solitary nucleus* (Figure 44–4A). Neurons in this nucleus receive afferent fibers mediating the sense of taste, as well as fibers from the carotid body, the larynx and pharynx, the heart, lungs, and gut. The solitary nucleus has two parts. The rostral part is a relay for taste, whereas the caudal part receives input from the carotid body, which monitors carbon dioxide in the blood and is important for cardiovascular control. Other neurons in the caudal part of the nucleus receive afferent input from the lungs and bronchi.

The cell bodies of fibers conveying afferent input to the solitary nucleus lie in sensory ganglia outside the brain stem as part of the facial (VII), glossopharyngeal (IX), and vagus (X) nerves. Their central axons run into the brain stem and join the *solitary tract*, which terminates in the solitary nucleus. Fibers from the solitary nucleus that mediate taste sensation synapse in the thalamus. Thalamic neurons, in turn, relay information about taste to the cerebral cortex. The other regions of the nucleus, which deal with cardiovascular function, have local connections with the reticular formation and indirect connections with the limbic system of the forebrain.

The Special Somatic Afferent Column.   The special somatic afferent column lies lateral to the visceral afferent column (Figure 44–4B). It contains the two nuclei that receive the fibers of the vestibulocochlear nerve (VIII). The *cochlear nucleus* lies in the rostral medulla and the caudal pons and receives input from neurons in the spiral ganglion, whose central axons run in the cochlear division of nerve VIII. The *vestibular nucleus* extends from the mid pons to the rostral medulla and receives input from the vestibular division of nerve VIII. Both of these nuclei lie near the lateral recess of the fourth ventricle (Figure 44–5).

The General Somatic Afferent Column.   The general somatic afferent column is ventral and lateral to the other afferent columns and includes the three separate divisions of the trigeminal sensory nucleus nerve (Figure 44–4B). General somatic afferent input is primarily conveyed by the trigeminal nerve and, to a lesser extent, by branches of the facial glossopharyngeal and vagus nerves. The most rostral nucleus, the mesencephalic trigeminal nucleus, lies principally in the mesencephalon and mediates jaw proprioception. The main trigeminal sensory nucleus lies in the rostral pons, while the spinal trigeminal nuclei run the entire length of the medulla and extend into the spinal cord. These nuclei receive afferent input from the teeth, the skin of the face, and the mucous membranes of the mouth. This sensory input is conveyed to the thalamus and then to the cerebral cortex. The organization of the trigeminal nuclei is discussed in detail in Chapter 45.

Several Principles Govern the Organization of the Brain Stem

Most Motor Nuclei in the Brain Stem Project to Their Targets Through a Single Cranial Nerve

The oculomotor nucleus has its own nerve (III), as do the trochlear (IV), abducens (VI), and hypoglossal nuclei (XII). The neurons of the hypoglossal nucleus are analogous to lower motor neurons in the spinal cord. They receive input from the motor area of the cerebral cortex and send their axons to muscles in the periphery. The same principle applies to the motor nuclei of the trigeminal (V), facial (VII), and spinal accessory (XI) nerves.

The Sensory Nuclei in the Brain Stem Receive Input from Several Cranial Nerves

In contrast to the motor nuclei, sensory nuclei in the brain stem receive input from several cranial nerves. Sensory information of a particular type is forwarded to a single nucleus regardless of which cranial nerve pathway this information takes. The solitary nucleus, for example, receives information pertaining to taste from the facial, glossopharyngeal, and vagus nerves. This principle was considered before in our discussions of sensory systems: *Afferent fibers conveying similar sensory modalities of input usually terminate within the same region in the brain* (see Chapters 23 and 25).

Somatic Sensory and Motor Tracts Traverse the Brain Stem

It is important to stress that *all descending cortical* projections (i.e., corticospinal and corticobulbar tracts) as well as *all somatic afferent* projections (i.e., the medial lemniscal and spinothalamic tracts) traverse the brain stem. These tracts are compactly arranged within the brain stem along with the afferent and efferent projections of the cranial nerve nuclei, the fibers of the reticular formation, and the projections of the various amine-containing nuclei described below.

Cranial Nerve Fiber Types May Intermingle in the Periphery

Even though the motor neurons of the cranial nerves and their associated sensory nuclei lie in distinct regions of the brain, there is considerable mixing of different fiber types in the periphery. The peripheral course of the facial nerve (VII) illustrates this principle (Figure 44–6). As the facial and vestibulocochlear nerves leave the brain stem they are joined by the intermediate branch of the facial nerve, which carries both sensory and visceral efferent fibers. The facial nerve and its intermediate branch run to-

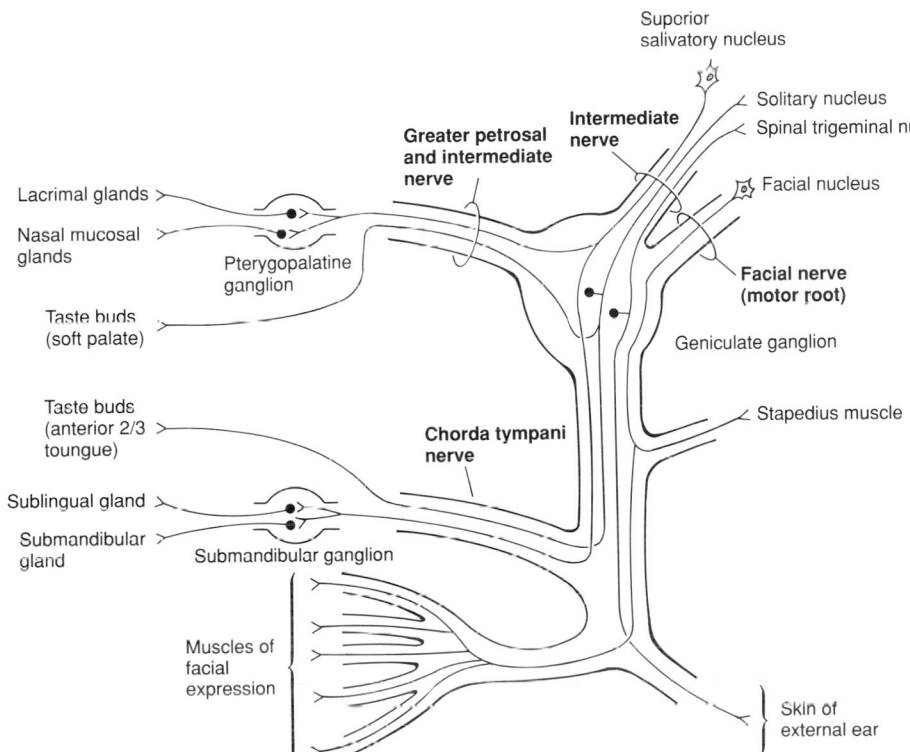

FIGURE 44–6
The peripheral course of the facial nerve illustrates how cranial nerve fiber types can intermingle. The facial nerve and its intermediate branch as well as the petrosal and a branch of the trigeminal nerve (not shown) course together in the periphery.

gether until the nerve courses through the facial canal. There some of the motor axons of the facial nerve leave the main trunk to innervate muscles of the middle ear, while others branch widely in the periphery to innervate certain facial muscles. The intermediate branch joins the greater petrosal nerve, which contains sympathetic axons arising from the sympathetic chain ganglia. These two nerves eventually reach the pterygopalatine ganglion. The postganglionic fibers of this parasympathetic ganglion innervate the lacrimal glands, joined along their course by a branch of the trigeminal nerve (V).

This example underscores the functional consequences of the mixing of cranial nerve fiber types in the periphery. This lesion of the facial nerve, as it exits from the brain stem in association with the intermediate nerve, disturbs secretion of tears and results in altered perception of sound as well as paralysis of the muscles of facial expression.

Nuclei in the Reticular Formation Form Widespread Networks

The reticular formation is composed of neurons that are outside the major nuclear groups of the brain stem. It represents the rostral extension of the interneuronal network of the spinal cord but is considerably more extensive. The reticular formation is distributed throughout the medulla, pons, and midbrain and is most conveniently divided into nuclear groups along a medial-to-lateral axis (Figure 44–7). Lying in the midline are the *raphe nuclei*, so named because of their proximity to the midline seam or raphe.

Adjacent to the raphe is the large-cell region of the reticular formation; more laterally is the small-cell region.

The unique feature of reticular neurons is that they distribute their axons widely, often in both rostral and caudal directions from the brain stem. An example of the axonal plexus established by a single gigantocellular reticular neuron is shown in Figure 44–8. The axon not only descends to the dorsal column nuclei and the spinal cord, but also ascends to the thalamus and hypothalamus. Although not all reticular neurons branch as broadly as this one, their widespread connections give them extensive influence over many neurons.

The reticular formation was originally thought to be a diffuse activating system that regulated alertness. This view came from the work of Giuseppe Moruzzi and Horace Magoun in the late 1940s, in which stimulation of the reticular formation of deeply anesthetized animals produced changes in the overall electrical activity of the brain, transforming the electroencephalogram pattern from a state resembling sleep to the awake state. Subsequent anatomical studies have shown that the reticular formation is not diffusely organized, but instead is composed of many morphologically and biochemically defined groups of neurons.

Activation of the brain for behavioral arousal and for different levels of awareness is only one physiological role of reticular neurons. At least three other functions are associated with the reticular formation. First, the reticular formation modulates segmental stretch reflexes and muscle tone by means of the pontine and medullary reticulospinal tracts. The reticulospinal axons originate

FIGURE 44–7
The locations of some major reticular cell groups are shown in a brain section cut through the medulla at the level of the cochlear nuclei. (Adapted from Nieuwenhuys, Voogd, and Huizen, 1981.)

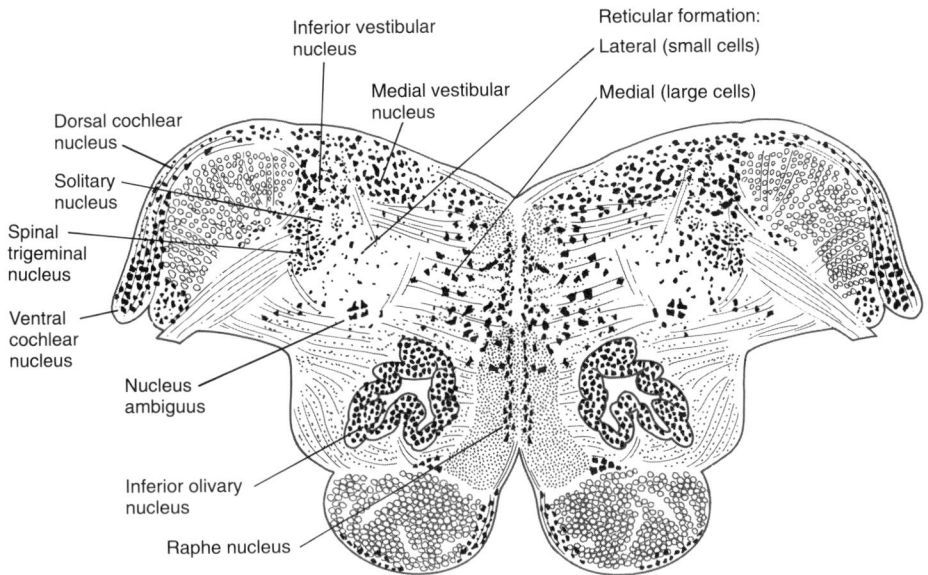

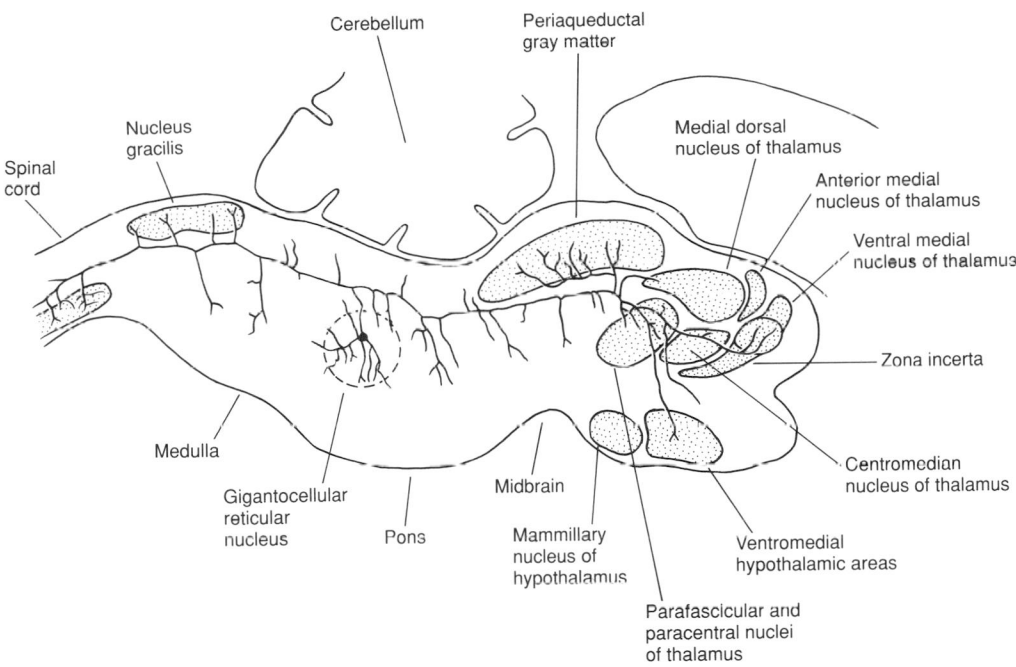

FIGURE 44–8

The axonal plexus established by an individual gigantocellular neuron of the reticular formation is widespread, as shown by this example in a two-day-old rat. It projects an axon that bifurcates into an ascending and a descending branch. The latter gives off collaterals to the adjacent gigantocellular reticular nucleus, the gracile nucleus, and the ventral horn in the spinal cord. The ascending branch gives off collaterals to the reticular formation and the periaqueductal gray and appears to supply several thalamic nuclei (the parafascicular, paracentral, and others), the hypothalamus, and the zona incerta. (Adapted from Scheibel and Scheibel, 1958.)

principally in the medial regions of the pons and medulla, where large reticular neurons are found. The *pontine reticulospinal tract* terminates near the motor nuclei of the ventral horn. Activity of these reticulospinal neurons enhances extensor muscle tone. The *medullary reticulospinal tract* arises from the gigantocellular reticular nucleus and terminates widely in the intermediate zone of the ventral horn from cervical to lumbar levels of the spinal cord. Activity in this tract exerts an inhibitory influence on extensor muscle tone. The antagonistic activity of these two tracts is important for the control of motor function (discussed in Chapter 38).

Second, the reticular formation is involved in the control of breathing and cardiac function. Many reticular neurons that regulate respiration send their axons to the spinal cord, where they control the activity of motor neurons innervating the muscles for inhalation and expiration. Reticular neurons important for cardiovascular functions receive input from a wide variety of peripheral receptors, including the carotid body, through a relay in the solitary tract. The activity of these neurons is also influenced from higher areas in the hypothalamus and prefrontal association cortex. These neurons regulate the output of preganglionic neurons associated with the vagus nerve and of preganglionic sympathetic neurons in the intermediolateral cell column of the spinal cord. The function of these neurons is to accelerate or depress the heart rate in response to an appropriate stimulus (see Chapter 49).

Finally, reticulospinal pathways modulate the sense of pain by influencing the flow of information through the dorsal horn of the spinal cord (Chapter 27). These four principal functions of the reticular formation—behavioral arousal, regulation of muscle reflexes, coordination of autonomic functions, and modulation of pain sensation—are carried out by distinct groups of neurons that make more extensive connections than those made by neurons in the major sensory and motor systems. Embedded within the reticular formation of the brain stem are major nuclear groups for the noradrenergic, adrenergic, dopaminergic, and serotonergic neurons of the brain. We now turn to consider these groups.

There Are Three Major Monoaminergic Systems in the Brain Stem

Formaldehyde-induced fluorescence to visualize noradrenergic, dopaminergic, and serotonergic pathways revolutionized the mapping of brain stem neuronal projections and revealed previously unknown connections within the reticular formation (Figure 44–9). These histochemical techniques reveal three major aminergic cell groups in the brain stem. These groups are distinguished by their trans-

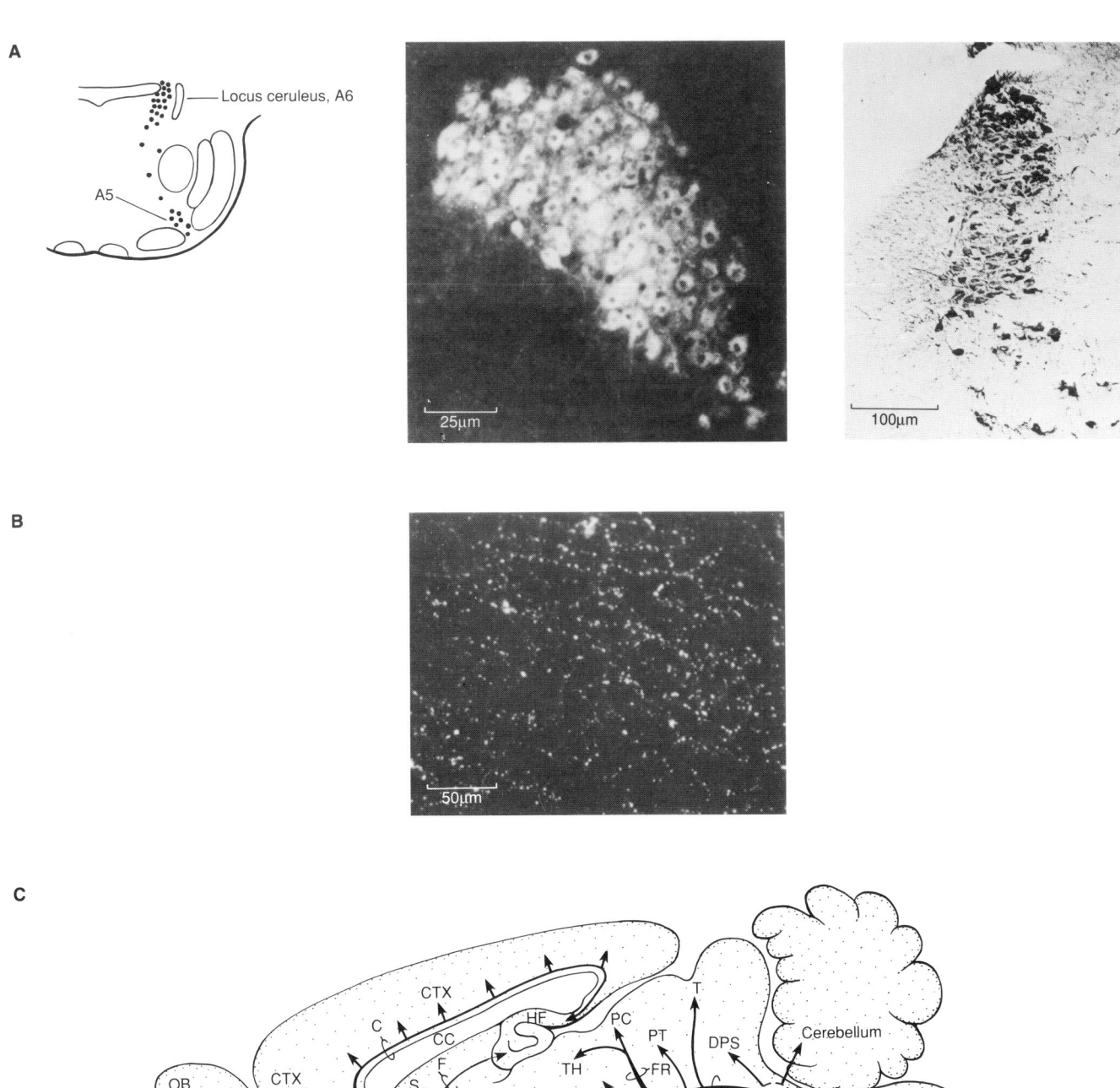

FIGURE 44–9

Noradrenergic cell groups of the locus ceruleus. (From Moore and Bloom, 1979.)

A. Neurons of the locus ceruleus visualized with histofluorescent (middle panel) and immunocytochemical (right panel) techniques.

B. An example of the terminal arborization of these noradrenergic cells in the hippocampus.

C. Summary diagram of the projections of the locus ceruleus (sagittal plane). **AP-VAB,** ansa peduncularis–ventral amygaloid bundle system; **BS,** brain stem; **C,** cingulum; **CC,** corpus callo-

sum; **CER,** cerebellum; **CTT,** central tegmental tract; **CTX,** cerebral cortex; **DPS,** dorsal periventricular system; **DTB,** dorsal tegmental bundle; **EC,** external capsule; **F,** fornix; **FR,** fasciculus retroflexus; **H,** hypothalamus; **HF,** hippocampal formation; **LC,** locus ceruleus; **ML,** medial lemniscus; **MT,** mammilothalamic tract; **OB,** olfactory bulb; **PC,** posterior commissure; **PT,** pretectal area; **RF,** reticular formation; **S,** septal area; **SC,** spinal cord; **SM,** stria medullaris; **ST,** stria terminalis; **T,** tectum; **TH,** thalamus.

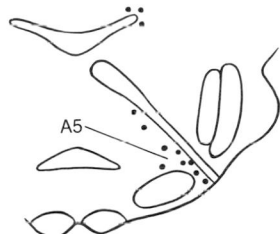

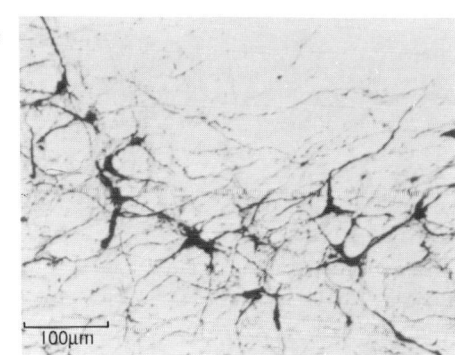

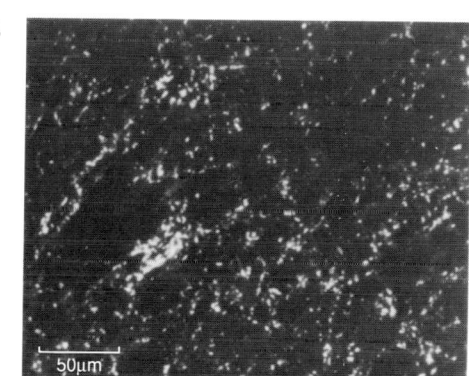

FIGURE 44–10

Noradrenergic cell groups of the lateral tegmentum. (From Moore and Bloom, 1979.)

A. Neurons of the lateral tegmental group (A5). **1.** Schematic indicating position of the A5 neurons within the brain stem. **2.** A5 neurons visualized with peroxidase-antiperoxidase immunohistochemistry, using an antibody to tyrosine hydroxylase.

B. Terminal arborization within the motor trigeminal nucleus visualized by flourescent histochemical techniques.

C. Location and projections of noradrenergic lateral tegmental neurons as viewed in the horizontal plane.

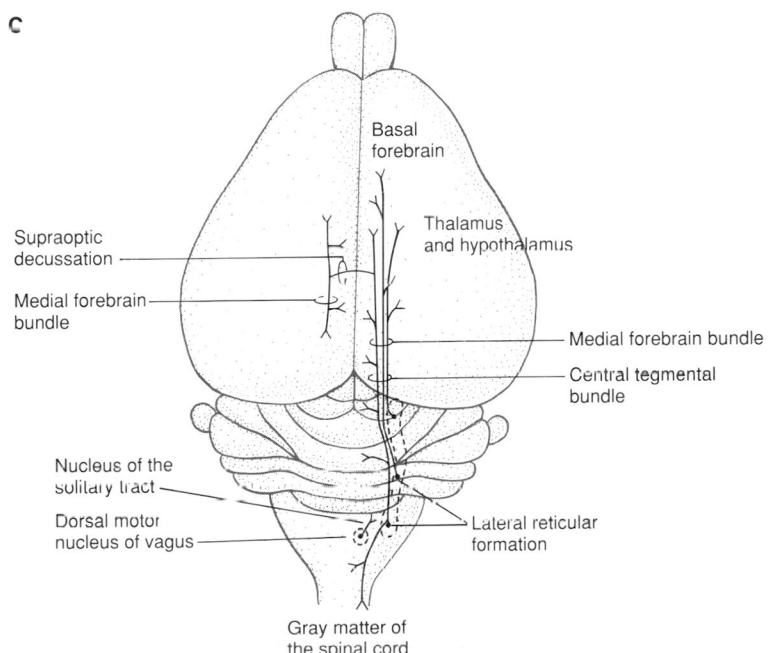

mitter: norepinephrine (noradrenaline), dopamine, and serotonin. Another important aminergic group of neurons in the dorsal and lateral tegmental area contain epinephrine (adrenaline); these cells project to the spinal cord, brain stem, hypothalamus, and thalamus, but we shall not consider them here.

The Noradrenergic System Originates in Two Nuclear Groups: The Locus Ceruleus and the Lateral Tegmental Nucleus

Two principal nuclei in the brain stem contain noradrenergic neurons. These are (1) the *locus ceruleus* (so named because of the slightly bluish appearance of this nucleus in fresh human tissue), located in the rostral pontine central gray region, and (2) the *lateral tegmental neurons*, which are more scattered in the *medullary lateral pontine tegmentum.*

The neurons of the locus ceruleus have both descending and ascending axonal branches. The descending branches go to the spinal cord (predominantly to the ventral horn) and to the brain stem itself (primarily to sensory nuclei). Ascending projections terminate in the diencephalon (largely in the dorsal thalamus, with a smaller projection terminating in the hypothalamus), in the cerebellum, the basal forebrain (including the hippocampus), and the neocortex (Figure 44–9). The locus ceruleus receives only two major inputs. These come from two brain stem nuclei: the nucleus paragigantocellularis and the nucleus hypoglossi prepositus. Thus, the locus ceruleus receives restricted afferent input yet makes very broad efferent projections.

The locus ceruleus only contains half of the total number of noradrenergic neurons in the brain stem. The rest are distributed diffusely throughout the ventral lateral tegmentum. An example of this group are the lateral tegmental neurons (Figure 44–10A). Like the neurons of the locus ceruleus, the axons of the lateral tegmental neurons have extensive collaterals and dense terminal arborizations. The axons project to three major sites: (1) the spinal cord, (2) the brain stem and (3) the thalamus and cerebellar and cerebral cortices (where the input is minor compared to that of the locus ceruleus).

In general neurons of the lateral tegmental region do not overlap their targets with those of the locus ceruleus. Thus, whereas the neurons of the locus ceruleus provide the principal noradrenergic input to the neocortex, the lateral tegmental neurons provide the major noradrenergic input to the brain stem and spinal cord. The physiological significance of these divergent noradrenergic projections is illustrated by the extensive behavioral effects produced by drugs that alter central norepinephrine action.

When neurons of the locus ceruleus are activated by novel sensory input, they respond as a group with an increased burst of activity. This coordinate response to a change in sensory input suggests that these neurons have a role in orienting and attending to sudden contrasting, or aversive sensory input.

How does this noradrenergic system modulate neural activity? To examine this question Roger Nicoll and his colleagues studied the response of hippocampal neurons, one of the targets of the locus ceruleus, and found that norepinephrine increases the excitability of these cells. Norepinephrine activates β-adrenergic receptors on hippocampal neurons, which activate the cAMP-dependent protein kinase, leading to inhibition of a Ca^{2+}-activated K^+ conductance. In other cortical neurons Floyd Bloom and his colleagues found that norepinephrine activates α-adrenergic receptors, producing the opposite effect on cellular excitability. In these cells norepinephrine causes a slow

TABLE **44–3.** Organization of the Mesencephalic Dopaminergic Cell Groups

System	Cells of origin	Projections
Mesostriatal		
Dorsal part	Substantia nigra (area A9)	Striatal areas, including caudate–putamen, globus pallidus, subthalamic nucleus, neocortex
Ventral part	Ventral tegmentum (area A10)	Nucleus accumbens, olfactory tubercle, nuclei of stria terminalis, neocortex
	Retrorubral nucleus (area A8)	Ventral striatum
Mesolimbic and mesocortical	Area A10 (some area A9)	Limbic and cortical areas, including cingulate cortex, habenula and limbic brain stem regions, septum, amygdala, pyriform and entorhinal cortices, locus ceruleus

(From Björklund and Lindvall, 1984.)

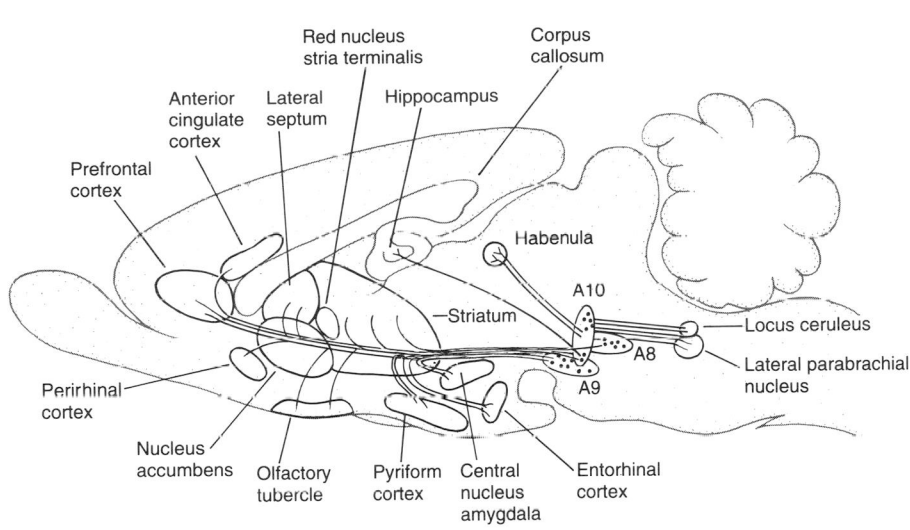

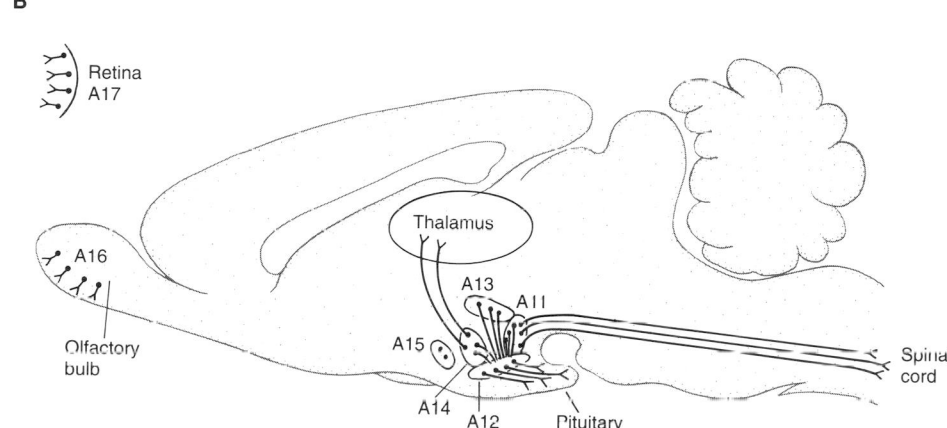

FIGURE 44–11

Dopaminergic cell groups within the brain stem.

A. The two major dopaminergic cell groups in the midbrain. The mesostriatal and mesolimbocortical systems are located in **A8** (retrorubral nucleus), **A9** (substantia nigra), and **A10** (ventral tegmentum).

B. Other dopaminergic cell groups of the central nervous system. Areas **A11–A14** are the diencephalic dopaminergic cell groups, in-cluding the tuberohypophyseal incertohypothalamic and medullary periventricular neurons; area **A15** includes cells in the dorsal and ventrolateral preoptic areas and the hypothalamus; area **A16** contains olfactory bulb and **A17**, the retinal dopaminergic neurons. (Adapted from Cooper, Bloom, and Roth, 1986.)

hyperpolarization and a decrease in the rate of spontaneous firing.

Neurons of the lateral tegmental noradrenergic system contribute to the integration of autonomic function in brain stem and spinal cord nuclei through projections to sympathetic preganglionic neurons in the intermediolateral cell column as well as to the nucleus of the solitary tract and the dorsal motor nucleus of the vagus nerve. Direct activation of lateral tegmental neurons leads to a profound decrease in mean arterial pressure, heart rate, and blood pressure (see Chapter 50).

The Dopaminergic System Originates in the Midbrain and Projects to the Striatum, Limbic System, and Neocortex

There are about three to four times as many dopaminergic neurons as noradrenergic neurons in the brain. In contrast to the diffuse projections of the noradrenergic system, the dopaminergic system is highly organized topographically. On the basis of their efferent projections, dopaminergic cell groups have been broadly classified into two groups: (1) the mesostriatal system, and (2) the mesolimbic and mesocortical systems.

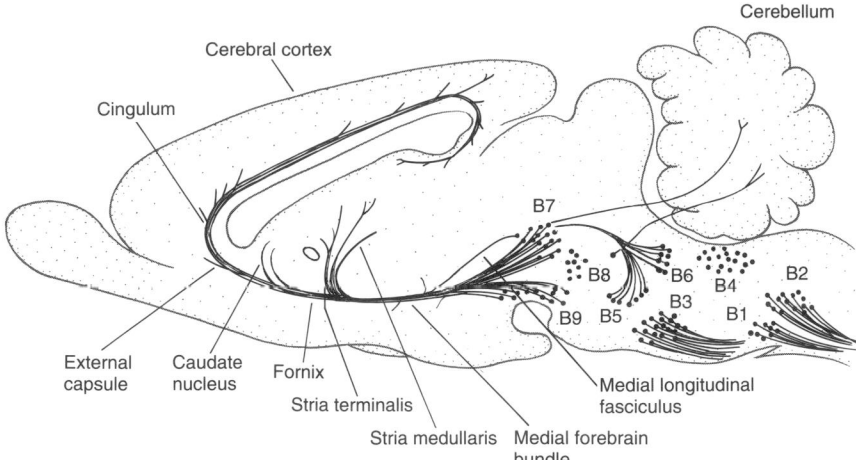

FIGURE 44–12
Serotonergic cell groups within the brain stem. **B1**, nucleus raphe pallidus; **B2**, nucleus raphe obscurus; **B3**, nucleus paragigantocellularis; **B4**, nucleus raphe magnus; **B5**, nucleus raphe pontis; **B6** and **B7**, nucleus raphe dorsalis; **B8**, nucleus centralis superior; **B9**, nucleus tegmenti reticularis pontis and adjacent tegmentum.

The *mesostriatal system* projects from the substantia nigra and the ventral tegmentum to several striatal areas. This system is critically involved in the control of voluntary movement (Chapter 40). Selective destruction or degeneration of the mesostriatal dopaminergic system results in the motor disorders of Parkinson's disease.

The *mesolimbic* and *mesocortical systems* project from the ventral tegmentum to limbic and cortical areas. The function of these projections are not known, but they are thought to participate in cognition. As we shall learn in Chapter 56, the dopaminergic system is considered the primary site of action of many stimulants (e.g., amphetamines) as well as antipsychotic drugs.

The projections of these two groups are summarized in Table 44–3 and Figure 44–11A. Dopaminergic neurons are also found in other regions of the central nervous system (Figure 44–11B).

The Serotonergic System Originates in the Raphe Nuclei

The most extensive monoaminergic system in the brain stem is the serotonergic system, whose neurons outnumber the noradrenergic and dopaminergic cells of the brain stem. The vast majority of serotonergic neurons are located within the raphe nuclei and adjacent nuclear groups (Figure 44–12). The three most caudal serotonergic groups (the *nucleus raphe magnus, pallidus,* and *obscurus*) provide the principal descending serotonergic projections to the spinal cord. The descending projections of the raphe nuclei modulate spinal sensory and motor neurons. Application of serotonin results in increased excitability of motor neurons, presumably through 5-HT$_{1b}$-type receptors. There are also dense projections from serotonergic cells to the superficial zone of the dorsal horn of the spinal cord (laminae I and II). As we saw in Chapter 27, these fibers depress afferent nociceptive input.

The raphe nuclei of the midbrain and upper pons project primarily in the medial forebrain bundle to an array of rostral sites, including the cerebral cortex, striatum, limbic structures, olfactory tubercle, hippocampus, and the diencephalon. All parts of the forebrain receive overlapping but differential input from the dorsal versus median raphe nucleus and the B9 cell group. The dorsal raphe nucleus projects most strongly to the frontal cortex and the striatum; the median raphe nucleus projects primarily to the septum and the hippocampus. The cerebellum receives relatively few serotonergic fibers, primarily from area B4 (Figure 44–12). Areas within the brain stem with quite dense serotonergic projections include the raphe nuclei, the substantia nigra, and the oculomotor and facial motor nuclei.

The excitatory effects of serotonin have been best characterized in the projections of the raphe nuclei to the facial motor nucleus. Here, George Aghajanian and his collegues have found that 5-HT activates 5-HT$_2$ receptors, which results in closure of K$^+$ channels and a slow depolarization. Serotonin produces similar actions on pyramidal neurons in the cerebral cortex.

Serotonin acting through other receptors also can inhibit neuronal discharge. Thus, Menahem Segal and his colleagues have found that in the hippocampus, serotonin causes inhibition by opening a K$^+$ channel and producing a hyperpolarization of these neurons. A similar inhibitory action occurs in the cerebral cortex and the neostriatum.

An Overall View

A knowledge of the anatomy of the nuclear groups of the brain stem and their relationship to the afferent and efferent tracts of the cranial nuclei is essential to clinical neurology, since lesions in this region typically affect several contiguous structures. The localization of function is due to the clustering of neurons with similar physiological roles into longitudinal columns early in development.

The reticular neurons of the brain stem have many functions. Recent anatomical techniques have changed our understanding of the arrangement of the reticular formation, revealing a large number of morphologically and biochemically discrete groups of cells. In addition to having an integrative function, such as mediating a general state of arousal, these neurons regulate muscle reflexes, coordinate autonomic function, and modulate the perception of pain.

Selected Readings

Aghajanian, G. K., and Vandermaelen, C. P. 1986. Specific systems of the reticular core: Serotonin. In F. E. Bloom (ed.), Handbook of Physiology, Section 1: The Nervous System, Vol. IV. Intrinsic Regulatory Systems of the Brain. Bethesda, Md.: American Physiological Society, pp. 237–256.

Björklund, A., and Hökfelt, T. (eds.) 1984. Handbook of Chemical Neuroanatomy, Vol. 2: Classical Transmitters in the CNS. Part I. Amsterdam: Elsevier.

Björklund, A., and Lindvall, O. 1986. Catecholaminergic brain stem regulatory systems. In F. E. Bloom (ed.), Handbook of Physiology, Section 1: The Nervous System, Vol. IV. Bethesda, Md.: American Physiological Society, pp. 155–235.

Brodal, A. 1981. Neurological Anatomy in Relation to Clinical Medicine, 3rd ed. New York: Oxford University Press, chap. 7, The Cranial Nerves.

Cooper, J. R., Bloom, F. E., and Roth, R. H. 1991. The Biochemical Basis of Neuropharmacology, 6th ed. New York: Oxford University Press.

Dahlström, A., and Fuxe, K. 1964. Evidence for the existence of monoamine-containing neurons in the central nervous system. Acta Physiol. Scand. Suppl. 232:1–55.

Foote, S. L., and Morrison, J. H. 1987. Extrathalamic modulation of cortical function. Annu. Rev. Neurosci. 10:67–95.

Molliver, M. E. 1987. Serotonergic neuronal systems: What their anatomic organization tells us about function. J. Clin. Psychopharmacol. 7[suppl. 6]:3S–23S.

Moore, R. Y., and Bloom, F. E. 1979. Central catecholamine neuron systems: Anatomy and physiology of the norepinephrine and epinephrine systems. Annu. Rev. Neurosci. 2:113–168.

Nicoll, R. A. 1988. The coupling of neurotransmitter receptors to ion channels in the brain. Science 241:545–551.

Nieuwenhuys, R. 1985. Chemoarchitecture of the Brain. Berlin: Springer.

References

Aston-Jones, G., Foote, S. L., and Bloom, F. E. 1984. Anatomy and physiology of the locus coeruleus neurons: Functional implications. In M. G. Ziegler and C. R. Lake (eds.), Norepinephrine. Frontiers of Clinical Neuroscience, Vol. 2. Baltimore: Williams & Wilkins, pp. 92–116.

Björklund, A., and Lindvall, O. 1984. Dopamine-containing systems in the CNS. In A. Björklund and T. Hökfelt (eds.), Handbook of Chemical Neuroanatomy, Vol. 2.: Classical Transmitters in the CNS, Part 1. Amsterdam: Elsevier, pp. 55–122.

Bowker, R. M., Westlund, K. N., Sullivan, M. C., Wilber, J. F., and Coulter, J. D. 1983. Descending serotonergic, peptidergic and cholinergic pathways from the raphe nuclei: A multiple transmitter complex. Brain Res. 288:33–48.

Chan-Palay, V. 1979. Combined immunocytochemistry and autoradiography after in vivo injections of monoclonal antibody to substance P and ^{3}H-serotonin: Coexistence of two putative transmitters in single raphe cells and fiber plexuses. Anat. Embryol. 156:241–254.

Clark, R. G. 1975. Manter and Gatz's Essentials of Clinical Neuroanatomy and Neurophysiology, 5th ed. Philadelphia: F. A. Davis.

DeArmond, S. J., Fusco, M. M., and Dewey, M. M. 1989. Structure of the Human Brain: A Photographic Atlas, 3rd ed. New York: Oxford University Press.

Falck, B., Hillarp, N.-Å., Thieme, G., and Torp. A. 1962. Fluorescence of catechol amines and related compounds condensed with formaldehyde. J. Histochem. Cytochem. 10:348–354.

Hökfelt, T., Lundberg, J. M., Schultzberg, M., Johansson, O., Ljungdahl, Å., and Rehfeld, J. 1980. Coexistence of peptides and putative transmitters in neurons. In E. Costa and M. Trabucchi (eds.), Neural Peptides and Neuronal Communication. New York: Raven Press, pp. 1–23.

Jacobs, B. L., and Gelperin, A. (eds.) 1981. Serotonin Neurotransmission and Behavior. Cambridge, Mass.: MIT Press.

Molliver, M. E., Grzanna, R., Lidov, H. G. W., Morrison, J. H., and Olschowka, J. A. 1982. Monoamine systems in the cerebral cortex. In Chan-Palay, V., and Palay, S. L. (eds.), Neurology and Neurobiology, Vol. 1: Cytochemical Methods in Neuroanatomy. New York: Liss, pp. 255–277.

Moruzzi, G., and Magoun, H. W. 1949. Brain stem reticular formation and activation of the EEG. Electroencephalogr. Clin. Neurophysiol. 1:455–473.

Nicoll R. A. 1982. Neurotransmitters can say more than just "yes" or "no." Trends Neurosci. 5:369–374.

Ranson, S. W., and Clark, S. L. 1953. The Anatomy of the Nervous System: Its Development and Function, 9th ed. Philadelphia: Saunders.

Roberts, P. J., Woodruff, G. N., and Iversen, L. L. (eds.) 1978. Dopamine: Advances in Biochemical Psychopharmacology, Vol. 19. New York: Raven Press.

Scheibel, M. E., and Scheibel, A. B. 1958. Structural substrates for integrative patterns in the brain stem reticular core. In H. H. Jasper, L. D. Proctor, et al. (eds.), Reticular Formation of the Brain (Henry Ford Hospital International Symposium). Boston: Little, Brown, pp. 31–55.

Segal, M. 1981. The action of serotonin in the rat hippocampus. Adv. Exptl. Med. Biol. 133:375–390.

45

Jane Dodd
James P. Kelly

Trigeminal System

**The Trigeminal Nerve Has Three Major Branches
That Innervate the Face, Oral Cavity, and
Dura Mater**

**Trigeminal Nerve Fibers Ascend to the
Principal Sensory Nucleus and Descend
to the Spinal Nucleus**

Tactile Sensation from the Face Is Mediated by
the Principal Sensory Nucleus

Pain and Temperature Sensation Are Mediated
by the Spinal Nucleus

Lesions of the Trigeminal Sensory System Have
Elucidated the Functional Organization of the
Spinal Nucleus

Proprioceptive Responses from the Jaw Muscles
Are Mediated by the Mesencephalic Nucleus

**The Trigeminal Motor Nucleus Controls the
Activity of the Jaw Muscles**

**Trigeminal Sensory Information Is Mapped
Somatotopically in the Cortex**

**Whiskers Are Represented in the Unique Modular
Organization in the Cortex**

An Overall View

The trigeminal or fifth cranial nerve conveys most of
the sensory information from the face, conjunctiva,
oral cavity, and dura mater, as well as the motor innervation of the muscles responsible for mastication. We consider the trigeminal nerve separately from the other
cranial nerves because somatic sensation in the face, lips,
and mouth is so important in everyday life. As a result, the
representation of the face, and especially of the lips, in the
primary somatosensory cortex is especially large compared to the rest of the body surface.

The trigeminal system illustrates two important points
about the organization of the brain stem. First, the trigeminal system allows us to see how the sensory and motor
nuclei of the brain stem are the direct, rostral extension of
the sensory and motor systems in the spinal cord. Second,
the trigeminal system also illustrates how fibers within a
single nerve can carry different modalities of sensation
and project that information to distinct nuclei within the
brain stem.

The Trigeminal Nerve Has Three Major Branches
That Innervate the Face, Oral Cavity, and
Dura Mater

The fifth nerve is named *trigeminal* because it branches
peripherally into three major nerves: the ophthalmic, the
maxillary, and the mandibular. The ophthalmic and maxillary branches are pure sensory nerves, while the mandibular branch carries both sensory and motor fibers. The
three divisions exit from the skull through three separate
openings: the superior orbital fissure, the foramen rotun-
dum, and the foramen ovale. The trigeminal is thus a
mixed nerve that is functionally equivalent to a peripheral
spinal nerve. As in the spinal system, the central branches

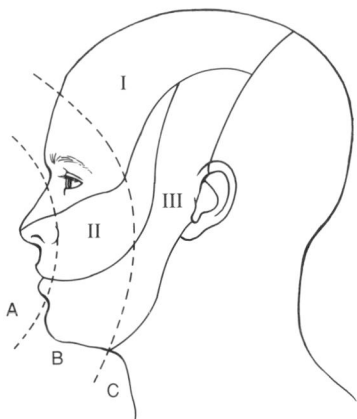

FIGURE 45–1
Different areas of the facial skin are innervated by the three branches of the trigeminal nerve: the ophthalmic (I), maxillary (II), and mandibular (III). The dashed concentric lines separate the regions of the face as represented in the nucleus caudalis. The perioral region (**A**) is represented in the rostral part of the nucleus. Areas **B** and **C** are represented progressively more caudally. (Adapted from Brodal, 1981.)

of the sensory and motor axons enter and exit the brain separately as the sensory (afferent) and motor (efferent) trigeminal roots.

The cell bodies of most of the trigeminal sensory fibers are clustered in ganglia in the periphery, the bilateral *trigeminal ganglia* (also called the semilunar or Gasserian ganglia). Each trigeminal ganglion lies within a cavity of the skull ventral to the pons. In a departure from this anatomical organization the cell bodies of one functional class of trigeminal sensory neurons, the proprioceptive neurons, are located centrally in the *mesencephalic trigeminal nucleus*. This is the only central nervous system site in which primary sensory neuron cell bodies that derive from the neural crest have been found. The cell bodies of the motor fibers form the *trigeminal motor nucleus* in the pons.

The peripheral axons of trigeminal ganglion neurons run in all three branches of the trigeminal nerve. The area of facial skin innervated by each branch is shown in Figure 45–1. In the perioral region there is bilateral innervation, so that unilateral destruction of the fifth nerve does not completely deprive this region of sensation on the affected side. The skin of the face has three physiological classes of receptors that transmit information via the trigeminal nerve: mechanoreceptors, thermoreceptors, and nociceptors. In addition, certain animals, most notably rodents, have whiskers called *mystacial vibrissae* that are used to explore the environment around the animal's head.

The trigeminal nerve also carries the sensory innervation of most of the oral mucosa, the anterior two-thirds of the tongue, and the dura mater of the anterior and middle cranial fossae. It also innervates the tooth pulp and surrounding gingiva and the periodontal membrane.

Trigeminal Nerve Fibers Ascend to the Principal Sensory Nucleus and Descend to the Spinal Nucleus

The trigeminal sensory nucleus consists of three nuclei that comprise the general somatic afferent column and extend from the rostral spinal cord to the midbrain. These nuclei are the *spinal*, *principal* (or *main*), and *mesencephalic trigeminal nuclei*. The central branches of neurons in the trigeminal ganglion enter the ventral pons. Like dorsal root fibers, many entering axons bifurcate into ascending and descending branches that project to discrete regions within the principal and spinal nuclei of the trigeminal nerve (Figure 45–2). The locations of the trigeminal nuclei are illustrated in Figure 45–3.

Tactile Sensation from the Face Is Mediated by the Principal Sensory Nucleus

The afferent fibers that carry tactile information from the face are large-diameter axons that branch to two nuclei. A short ascending branch projects to the ipsilateral principal nucleus and a longer descending branch runs within the spinal trigeminal tract to the ipsilateral spinal nucleus. The second-order sensory neurons in the principal nucleus project to the thalamus. Most fibers arising from the principal nucleus travel to the contralateral ventral posterior nucleus of the thalamus through the trigeminal lemniscus (Figure 45–2A), a decussating pathway that joins the ascending spinal dorsal column medial lemniscus. Some neurons in the dorsomedial region of the principal nucleus are thought to give rise to a minor ipsilateral pathway that terminates in the ipsilateral ventral posterior nucleus of the thalamus.

The principal nucleus and its major thalamic projection are analogous both functionally and anatomically to the dorsal column–medial lemniscal system of the spinal cord. In addition, second-order neurons in the spinal trigeminal nucleus that receive tactile input are analogous to dorsal horn neurons that receive tactile input and project within the dorsal columns to the posterior nucleus of the thalamus.

Pain and Temperature Sensation Are Mediated by the Spinal Nucleus

Trigeminal afferents that carry the sensations of pain and temperature are small-diameter, thinly myelinated and unmyelinated axons. They descend in the spinal trigeminal tract and terminate in the spinal trigeminal nucleus; they do not appear to project rostrally to the principal nucleus (Figure 45–2).

Primary trigeminal fibers descending in the tract are somatotopically organized. Sensory fibers from the ophthalmic division of the nerve are found ventrolaterally in the tract; fibers from the mandibular division are found dorsomedially; and fibers from the maxillary division lie in between. Thus, there is an inverted representation of

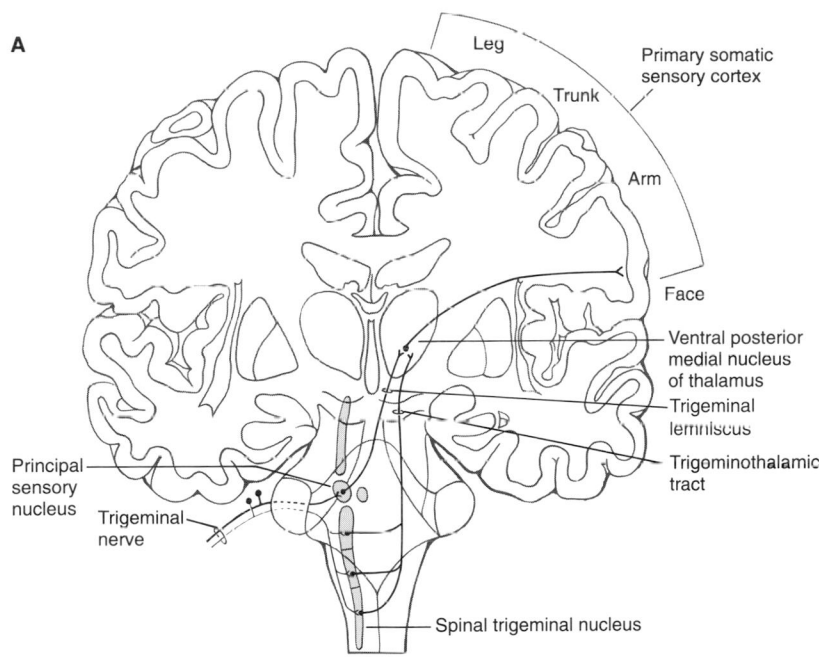

A

Leg

Trunk

Arm

Primary somatic
sensory cortex

Face

Ventral posterior
medial nucleus
of thalamus

Trigeminal
lemniscus

Trigeminothalamic
tract

Principal
sensory
nucleus

Trigeminal
nerve

Spinal trigeminal nucleus

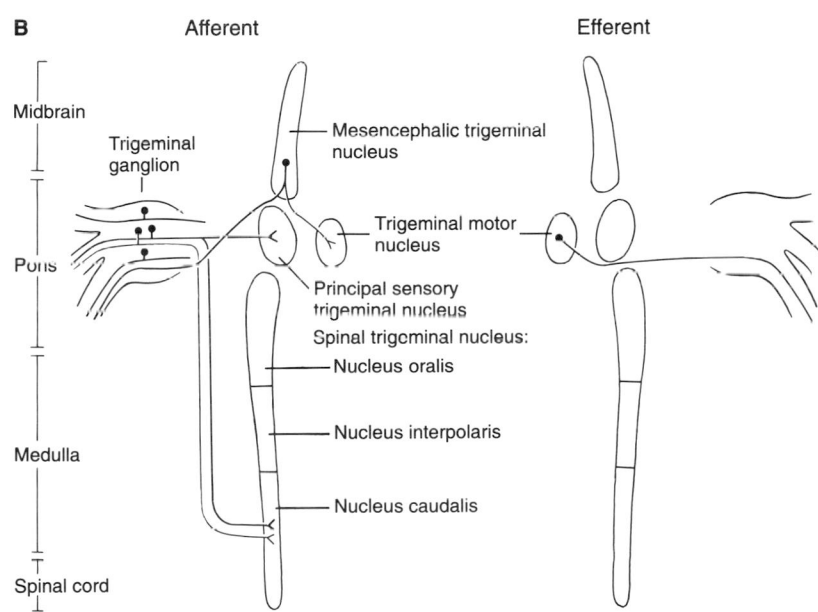

B   Afferent   Efferent

Midbrain

Trigeminal
ganglion

Mesencephalic trigeminal
nucleus

Trigeminal motor
nucleus

Pons

Principal sensory
trigeminal nucleus

Spinal trigeminal nucleus:

Nucleus oralis

Nucleus interpolaris

Medulla

Nucleus caudalis

Spinal cord

FIGURE 45–2
The location of the afferent and efferent components of the trigeminal system. (Adapted from Brodal, 1981.)

A. The major central pathways of the afferent limb of the trigeminal system.

B. The distribution of the sensory (afferent) and motor (efferent) nuclei is shown. For clarity, the sensory component is shown on the left and the motor component on the right. However, both components are bilaterally symmetrical.

the ipsilateral face in the spinal tract of the trigeminal nerve. Primary sensory fibers from other cranial nerves (VII, IX, and X) also enter the descending tract of nerve V; these fibers carry input from the skin of the external ear, and the mucous membranes of the larynx and the pharynx. Near their point of termination, trigeminal fibers in the descending tract turn abruptly inward and ramify in the underlying spinal trigeminal nucleus (Figure 45–3C). This nucleus is contiguous rostrally with the principal nucleus and extends caudally through the medulla into the spinal cord, to the level of C2.

The spinal nucleus has three morphologically distinct

subdivisions along its rostrocaudal extent, each of which has a different function, considered below. The *nucleus caudalis* is the most caudal of the three and is continuous with and resembles the dorsal horn of the cervical spinal cord. It consists of a dorsal marginal zone overlying the substantia gelatinosa, and the subnucleus magnocellularis, a deeper region composed of large neurons. The latter may be equivalent to the nucleus proprius of the dorsal horn of the spinal cord, while the spinal trigeminal tract overlying the marginal zone of the nucleus caudalis is the functional equivalent of Lissauer's tract in the spinal cord.

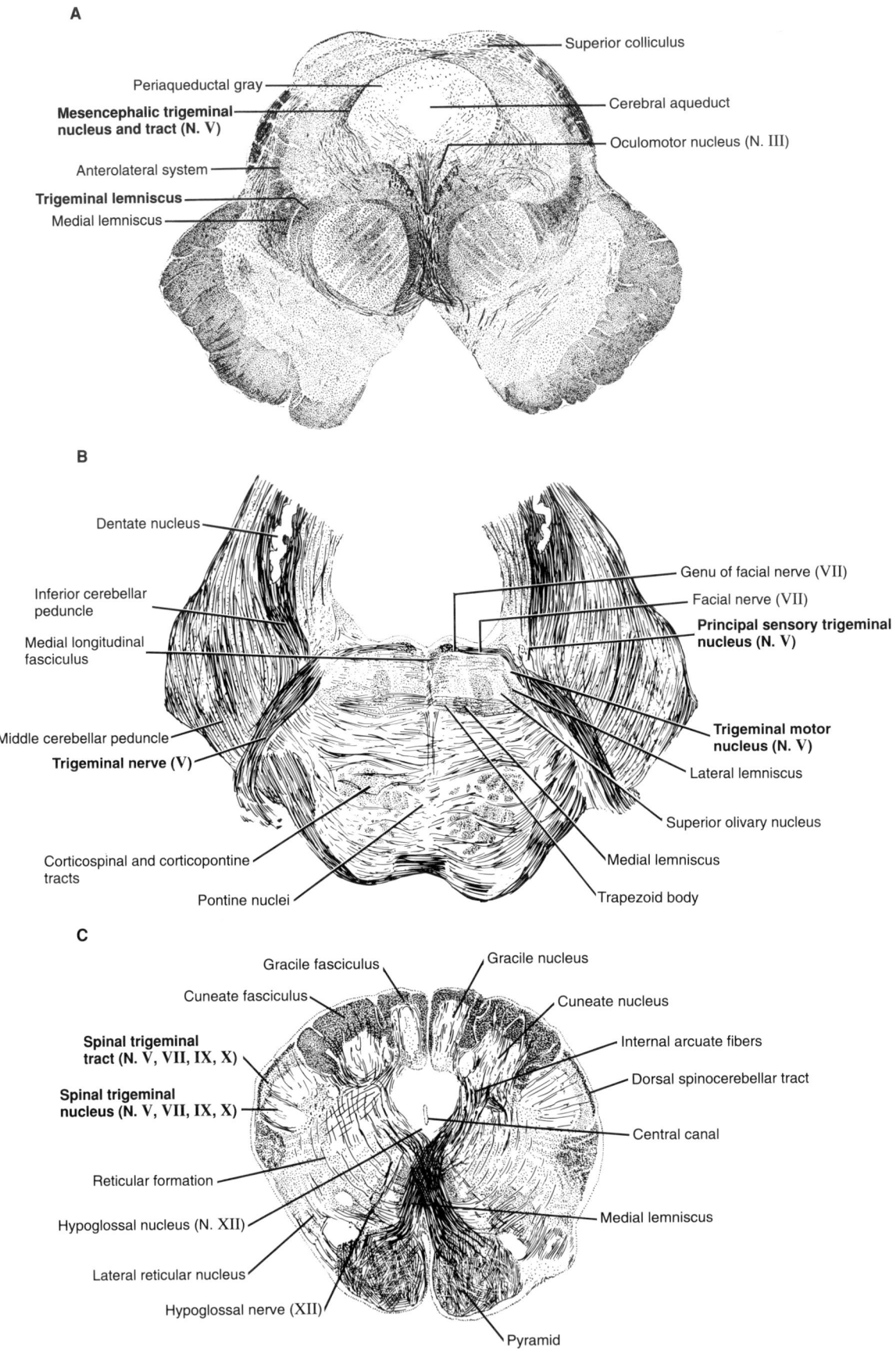

A

Superior colliculus

Periaqueductal gray

Mesencephalic trigeminal nucleus and tract (N. V)

Cerebral aqueduct

Oculomotor nucleus (N. III)

Anterolateral system

Trigeminal lemniscus

Medial lemniscus

B

Dentate nucleus

Inferior cerebellar peduncle

Medial longitudinal fasciculus

Middle cerebellar peduncle

Trigeminal nerve (V)

Corticospinal and corticopontine tracts

Pontine nuclei

Genu of facial nerve (VII)

Facial nerve (VII)

Principal sensory trigeminal nucleus (N. V)

Trigeminal motor nucleus (N. V)

Lateral lemniscus

Superior olivary nucleus

Medial lemniscus

Trapezoid body

C

Gracile fasciculus

Cuneate fasciculus

Spinal trigeminal tract (N. V, VII, IX, X)

Spinal trigeminal nucleus (N. V, VII, IX, X)

Reticular formation

Hypoglossal nucleus (N. XII)

Lateral reticular nucleus

Hypoglossal nerve (XII)

Gracile nucleus

Cuneate nucleus

Internal arcuate fibers

Dorsal spinocerebellar tract

Central canal

Medial lemniscus

Pyramid

FIGURE 45-3

Locations of the trigeminal nuclei. (Adapted from Ranson and Clark, 1953.)

A. The mesencephalic trigeminal nucleus and tract are shown in a transverse section through the midbrain.

B. The principal trigeminal sensory nucleus and the trigeminal motor nucleus are shown in a section through the pons. The trigeminal nerve can be seen entering the pons ventrally.

C. The spinal trigeminal nucleus and tract are shown in a transverse section through the medulla.

More rostrally, near the obex, the cytoarchitecture of the spinal nucleus changes and is composed predominantly of scattered small cells. This change marks the boundary with the *nucleus interpolaris* (Figure 45–2). More rostral still and extending to the principal sensory nucleus is the *nucleus oralis*, which consists of gray matter with tightly packed neurons.

Neurons of the spinal nucleus project to the ventral posterior medial and intralaminar nuclei of the thalamus. These axons also send collaterals to the reticular formation. The majority of ascending axons decussate and travel with the contralateral anterolateral system that mediates the sensations of pain and temperature from the body. A small number of fibers ascend in the ipsilateral anterolateral system. Within the ventral posterior medial nucleus of the thalamus there is a somatotopic representation of the contralateral face, with the lower jaw represented in the ventral region and the mouth represented closest to the midline (Figure 45–4). The ascending trigeminal axons and the anterolateral system have complementary termination sites in the thalamus such that sensory input from the face is in appropriate anatomical register with the projections of the body and limbs in the adjacent ventral posterior lateral nucleus (Figure 45–4).

Lesions of the Trigeminal Sensory System Have Elucidated the Functional Organization of the Spinal Nucleus

Trigeminal neuralgia is a condition characterized by severe facial pain in the absence of any local damage to the skin or skull. One treatment for this ailment is to sever the fifth nerve root, thereby depriving the face of its sensory innervation. This procedure offers relief in many patients with trigeminal neuralgia, but has deleterious side effects. Cutting the fifth nerve interrupts the afferent limb of the blinking reflex by making the cornea anesthetic, so that keratitis (a drying out and thickening of the cornea) often develops.

During the 1930s Olof Sjöqvist found that the smallest-diameter fibers of the trigeminal root terminate selectively in the nucleus caudalis. He therefore suggested that cutting the spinal trigeminal tract just before it enters the nucleus caudalis might remove the pain fibers selectively, leaving other aspects of facial sensation intact. The oper-

ation is possible because the spinal tract and the trigeminal nucleus bulge out of the lateral medulla (Figure 45–3C) and can be visualized directly. The operation, called the trigeminal tractotomy of Sjöqvist, often alleviates trigeminal neuralgia without totally eliminating facial sensation.

The success of the Sjöqvist procedure prompted others to look for specific nociceptive neurons in the nucleus caudalis. The responses of cells in deep regions of the nucleus caudalis to mechanical stimuli delivered to the face were examined in cats under general anesthesia. The neurons responded to both noxious and innocuous input, not selectively to noxious stimuli. These neurons may therefore correspond to the wide dynamic range nociceptive neurons found in the dorsal horn of the spinal cord. Later experiments showed that cells in the substantia gelatinosa of the nucleus caudalis respond selectively to strong mechanical stimuli that evoke pain reactions in awake cats. Specific nociceptors therefore appear to be confined to the substantia gelatinosa of the nucleus caudalis. Thermoreceptors are also confined to the substantia gelatinosa of the nucleus caudalis.

Trigeminal tractotomy has also revealed aspects of the somatotopic organization of the nucleus caudalis. The spinal trigeminal tract can be severed at different rostrocaudal levels and facial sensitivity to pain and temperature tested later. Transection of the tract at the rostral border of the nucleus caudalis results in disruption of nociception and thermoreception throughout the face. Tractotomy at more caudal levels results in loss of sensation in more discrete regions of the face; thus, perioral and nasal skin (areas A and B in Figure 45–1) are spared after caudal lesions. As lesions are placed more rostrally, the spared region becomes progressively smaller and more central, indicating that the area of the face that is most caudal and continuous with the cervical spinal cord is represented in the caudal portion of the nucleus caudalis, adjacent to the cervical spinal cord representation. Neurons that innervate the perioral region project most rostrally in the nucleus caudalis.

The nucleus interpolaris plays an important role in mediating sensation from the teeth. In rats when the tooth pulp is removed from all the mandibular teeth on one side of the jaw and the peripheral branch of the trigeminal nerve innervating the tooth pulp is severed, the trigeminal neurons degenerate. The degenerating terminals of neurons in such experimental animals have been found principally in the nucleus interpolaris and in the substantia gelatinosa of the rostral nucleus caudalis.

Proprioceptive Responses from the Jaw Muscles Are Mediated by the Mesencephalic Nucleus

The mesencephalic trigeminal nucleus extends from the rostral end of the principal nucleus to the superior colliculus in the midbrain (Figures 45–2 and 45–3A). It consists of a column of primary sensory neurons that develop from the neural crest and can therefore be considered equivalent to a peripheral sensory ganglion.

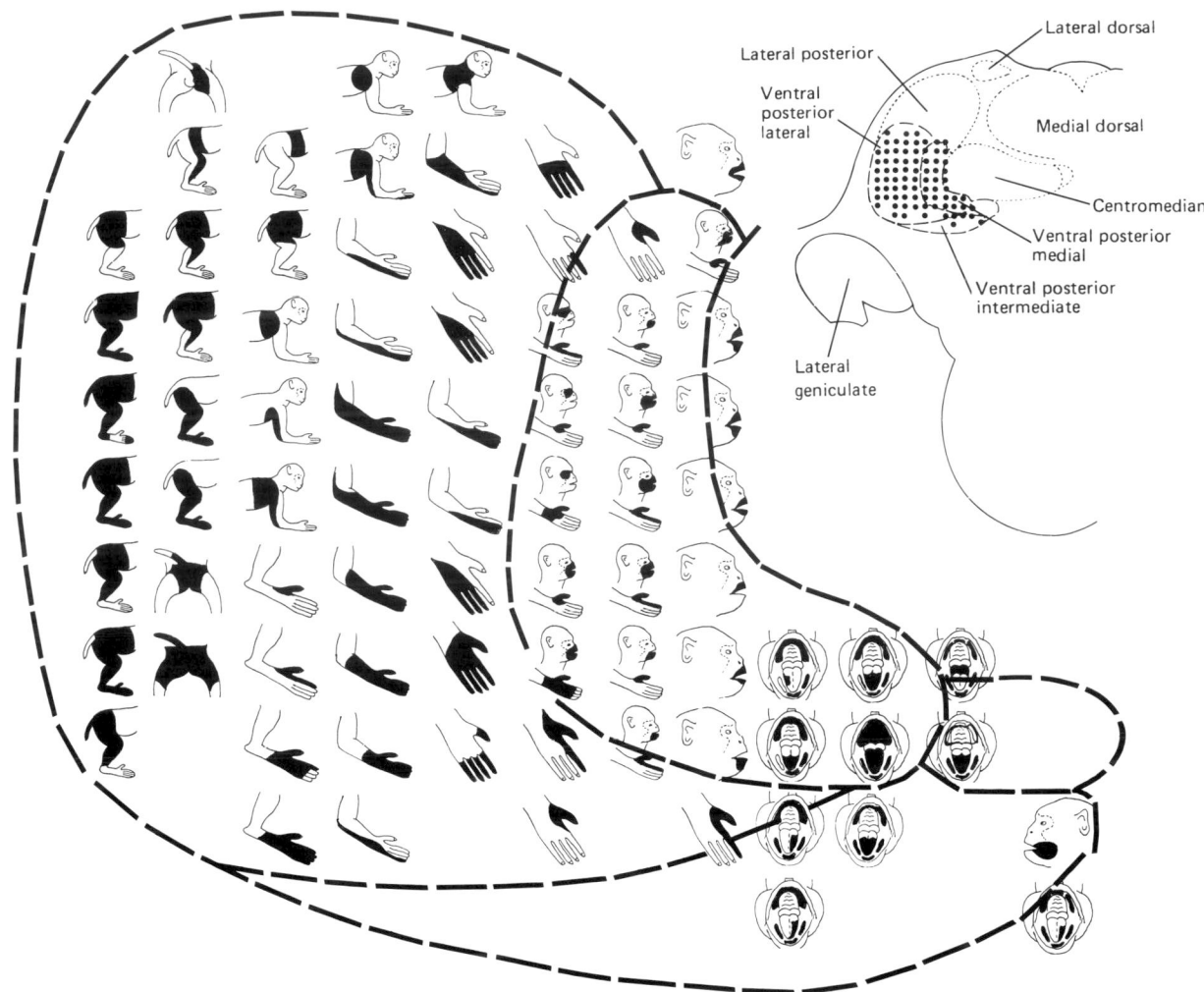

FIGURE 45–4

The somatotopic organization of sensory input in the ventral posterior lateral and medial nuclei of the thalamus in the monkey. The map was determined by the evoked potential technique. The drawing of the thalamus was prepared from a frontal section of the brain in the plane of electrode penetrations. Tactile stimulation of the skin of the black areas in the figurines evoked responses at the points (**dots**) indicated in the drawing of the thalamus. (The arrangement of figurines is identical to that of the dots.) With the exception of ipsilateral intraoral and perioral regions, all responses were obtained from stimulation of only the contralateral side of the body and head. (Adapted from Mountcastle and Henneman, 1952.)

The peripheral branches of mesencephalic neurons innervate stretch receptors in the jaw muscles and mechanoreceptors in the periodontal membrane. The majority of peripheral fibers of the mesencephalic nucleus appear to travel with the mandibular branch of the trigeminal nerve. A collateral branch, analogous to the central branch of a spinal proprioceptive primary neuron, projects directly in the mesencephalic trigeminal tract to the trigeminal motor nucleus (Figure 45–2A). This arrangement provides a monosynaptic reflex arc to the motor neurons similar to the stretch reflex arc mediated by the Ia afferents in the spinal cord. This trigeminal reflex, known as the jaw reflex, consists of a contraction of the muscles of mastication in response to pressure on the mandibular teeth and depression of the lower jaw.

The Trigeminal Motor Nucleus Controls the Activity of the Jaw Muscles

The motor nucleus of the trigeminal nerve is the most rostral nucleus in the column of special visceral efferent nuclei. Its position in the pons, medial to the principal sensory nucleus, can be seen in Figures 45–2B and 45–3B. It contains large neurons that resemble motor neurons found in the spinal cord and midbrain. Motor axons leave the nucleus, projecting out of the ventral pons through a motor root that is medial to and much smaller than the sensory trigeminal root. The motor fibers pass ventral to the ganglion before joining the mandibular division of the peripheral nerve. Trigeminal motor neurons principally innervate the muscles of mastication, the masseter, temporalis, and pterygoid muscles, as well as the tensor tympani.

The trigeminal motor neurons receive input from the proprioceptive neurons of the mesencephalic nucleus and form the effector limb of the jaw reflex. In addition, neurons in the motor nucleus receive input from corticobulbar fibers, either directly or indirectly through interneurons in the reticular formation.

Trigeminal Sensory Information Is Mapped Somatotopically in the Cortex

Trigeminal sensory information is carried centrally via the ventral posterior medial nucleus of the thalamus to the primary somatosensory cortex. The ventral posterior medial nucleus projects via the posterior limb of the internal capsule to the lateral region of the postcentral gyrus (Figure 45–5A) where there is a complete representation of the contralateral face and bilateral representation of the perioral region. Somatosensory information from the arms, trunk, and legs also projects to the postcentral gyrus. The cortical representation of the face is ventral and lateral to that of the arms, trunk, and legs. The representation of the perioral region is disproportionately large in humans, reflecting the important role of sensory information from this region of the face in human behavior (Figure 45–5B).

The projection from the ventral posterior medial nucleus terminates principally in the primary somatosensory cortex (S-I) but some trigeminal input ascends directly to the secondary somatosensory cortex (S-II) from the posterior thalamic nuclei.

Whiskers Are Represented in the Unique Modular Organization in the Cortex

The mechanisms by which somatotopic organization is achieved can be studied in animals in which the cortical representation of the face is particularly clear. In rodents, whose whiskers are the principal tactile receptors, the region surrounding the mouth is more extensively represented in the cortex than are the paws. Each whisker is innervated by a separate vibrissal nerve containing about 100 myelinated fibers, which are activated by movements of the whiskers. The central terminals of vibrissal fibers are in the principal trigeminal nucleus and the nucleus oralis of the spinal nucleus. As we have seen, these nuclei project to the ventral posterior medial nucleus of the thalamus and to S-I.

In 1970 Thomas Woolsey and Hendrick van der Loos showed that animals with mystacial vibrissae have a unique arrangement of cells in the portion of S-I representing the face. In layer 4 of the somatosensory cortex, where the fibers from the ventral posterior medial nucleus terminate, the neurons are arranged in discrete functional units called barrels (Figure 45–6). A single barrel contains about 2500 neurons arranged in a cylindrical array around a hollow center. Each barrel processes tactile input derived from a single whisker. The number of barrels is the same as the number of vibrissae on the contralateral side of the face and the barrels are arranged in a pattern that corresponds to the topography of the whiskers. This organization of the central representation of whisker stimuli is similar in principle to the columnar representation of the

FIGURE 45–5
Somatosensory representation in the cortex. (Adapted from Penfield and Rasmussen, 1950.)

A. A lateral view of the cerebral hemisphere showing the representation of the limbs, trunk, and face in the postcentral gyrus.

B. Somatotopic organization of the postcentral gyrus.

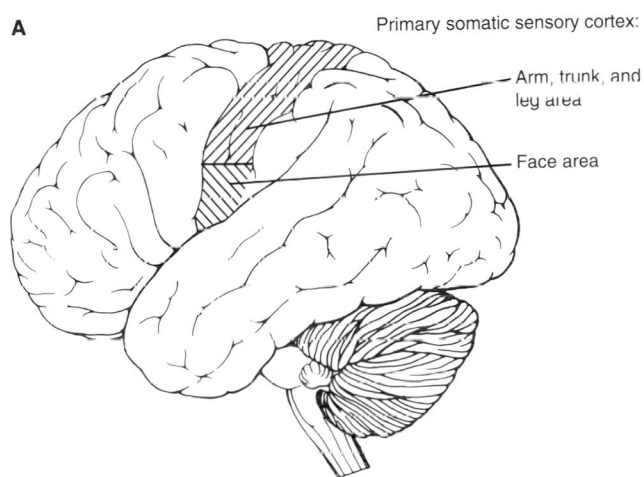

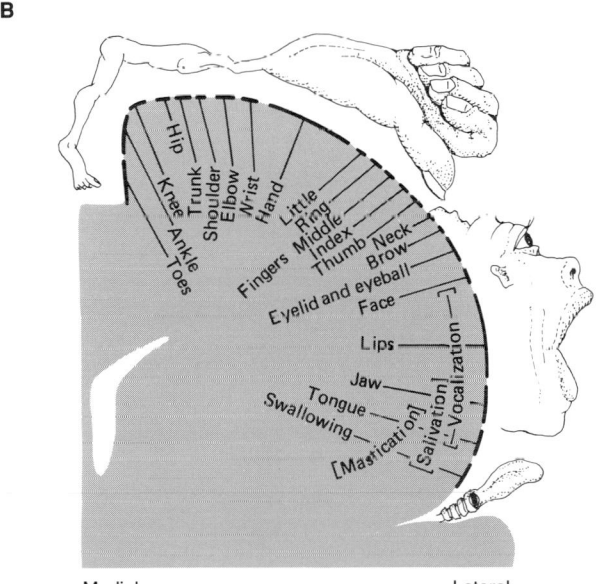

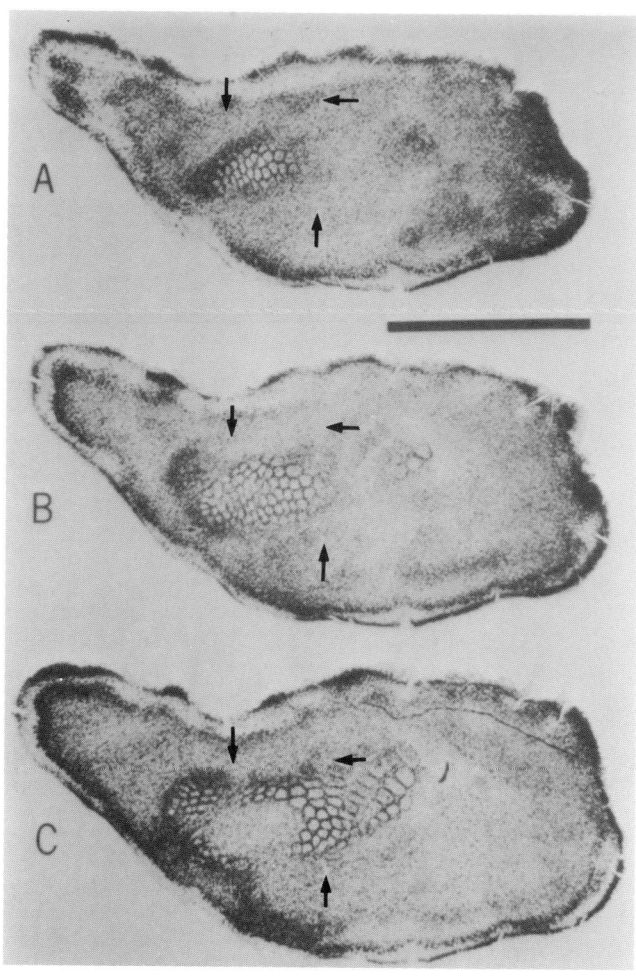

FIGURE 45–6

The barrel arrangement of somatosensory cortex. Photomicrographs of three serial tangential sections of the somatosensory cortex of the mouse show neurons that receive projections from mystacial vibrissae arranged in discrete units, or barrels, in layer 4. The **top** section is the most superficial, the **bottom** section the deepest. Orientation: anterior, **left**; posterior, **right**; medial, **up**; lateral, **down**. Some of the vessels commonly used to relate serially cut sections spatially to one another are marked by **arrows**. Bar=2 mm. (Adapted from Woolsey and van der Loos, 1970.)

somatosensory system (Chapter 26) and the visual system (Chapter 29).

The pattern of barrels in S-I is a faithful one-to-one representation of the spatial organization of the vibrissae. This was demonstrated by van der Loos and his colleagues, who compared the barrel fields of strains of mice that were bred to differ from each other only in the number or pattern of mystacial vibrissae. Mice with extra whiskers developed the same number of extra barrels, the position of which relative to other barrels, reflected the topological relationship of the extra whiskers to the other whiskers. Figure 45–7 illustrates the precise correspondence of number and position between extra vibrissae and extra barrels in S-I. The innervation of the whole barrel field is also altered, such that the extra barrels are innervated at the expense of neighboring barrels, which receive fewer axons per barrel area. No changes in the number of axons innervating each normal vibrissal follicle were found. These observations led Welker and van der Loos to suggest that during the formation of the barrel field map there must be competition for cortical space.

Removal of vibrissae or vibrassal follicles also results in alterations in the cortical map. Within the barrels corresponding to the ablated vibrissae, cytochemical and morphological changes in neurons are accompanied by a loss of activity. Thus, although features of the central representation, such as the size of the overall barrel field in S-I and its orientation and location within the cortex, may be determined centrally, modifications of neuronal activity in the periphery regulate the dynamic organization of the cortex during both development and maintenance of the map. Presumably, plasticity of the central representation of the whisker field exists also at other central nervous system sites between the periphery and the cortex, such as the trigeminal nucleus. The mechanisms by which the periphery exerts its influence are unclear.

An Overall View

Functionally and anatomically the trigeminal system resembles the spinal sensory and motor systems. The underlying plan of organization is that distinct modalities of sensory information are processed independently. This

FIGURE 45–7

The pattern of barrels in the cortex reflects that of the whiskers on the snout. Photomicrographs of whisker pads are paired with drawings of corresponding barrel fields for each of six strains of mouse bred to have different numbers of patterns of whiskers.

NOR mice were bred for the absence of supernumerary whiskers. These mice possess the standard set of whisker follicles (and barrel fields), distributed over the whisker pad in five horizontal rows of four follicles (**A–E**) and one vertical row of four follicles (α, β, γ, and δ).

A/A mice were bred for the presence of one supernumerary whisker at the rostral end of the A row, called A5.

H/H mice have two supernumerary whiskers representing fifth elements of the A and the B rows.

MAP mice were bred for the presence of many extra whiskers in a strip of skin medial to the A row, called the A′ whiskers, as well as an A5 whisker.

MCP mice have several extra whiskers between the B and C rows, called C′, as well as extra A5 and B5 whiskers.

M/M mice were bred for maximal numbers of whiskers regardless of position. In the case illustrated, A5, B5, A′, and C′ were present. In all cases extra barrel fields were present (indicated by **hatched arrow**) that corresponded in position to the supernumerary whisker follicles. (From Welker and van der Loos, 1986.)

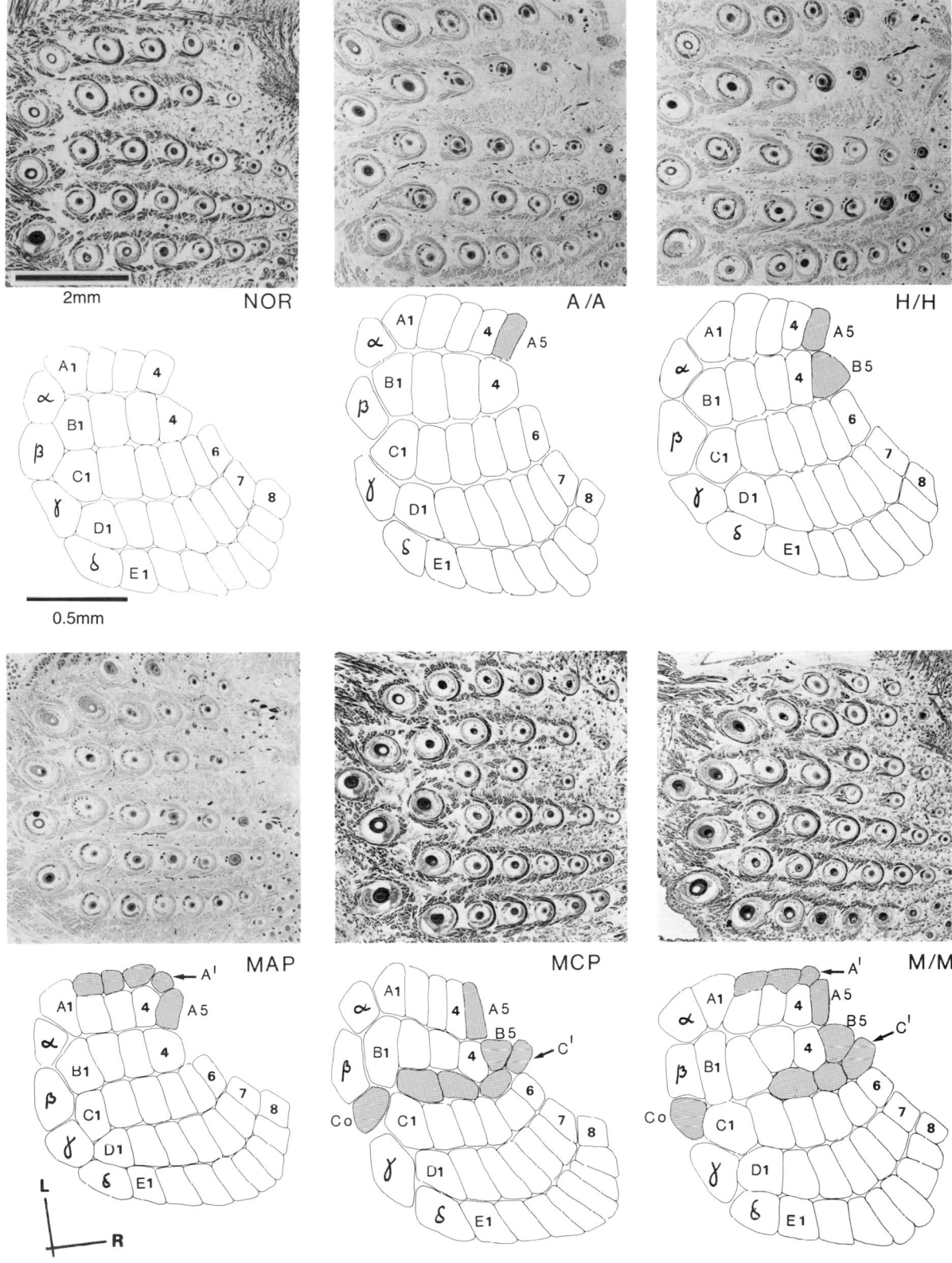

principle holds for both primary sensory neurons and the central representation of somatosensory information. Thus, the principal sensory nucleus mediates tactile information while the spinal trigeminal nucleus is mainly involved in processing pain and temperature sensation. At all levels of the trigeminal central projection, a topographic map of the face is maintained and its position relative to the sensory representation of the body is faithful.

Selected Readings

Brodal, A. 1981. Neurological Anatomy in Relation to Clinical Medicine, 3rd ed. New York: Oxford University Press, pp. 508–532.

Dubner, R., and Bennett, G. J. 1983. Spinal and trigeminal mechanisms of nociception. Annu. Rev. Neurosci. 6:381–418.

References

Carpenter, M. B. 1985. Core Text of Neuroanatomy, 3rd ed. Baltimore: Williams & Wilkins.

Gobel, S., and Binck, J. M. 1977. Degenerative changes in primary trigeminal axons and in neurons in nucleus caudalis following tooth pulp extirpations in the cat. Brain Res. 132:347–354.

Hayashi, H., Sumino, R., and Sessle, B. J. 1984. Functional organization of trigeminal subnucleus interpolaris: Nociceptive and innocuous afferent inputs, projections to thalamus, cerebellum, and spinal cord, and descending modulation from periaqueductal gray. J. Neurophysiol. 51:890–905.

Henry, M. A., Westrum, L. E., and Johnson, L. R. 1986. Light- and electron-microscopic localization of primary dental afferents to medullary dorsal horn (pars caudalis). Somatosens. Res. 3:291–307.

Martin, J. H. 1989. Neuroanatomy: Text and Atlas. New York: Elsevier.

Mosso, J. A., and Kruger, L. 1973. Receptor-categories represented in spinal trigeminal nucleus caudalis. J. Neurophysiol. 36: 472–488.

Mountcastle, V. B., and Henneman, E. 1952. The representation of tactile sensibility in the thalamus of the monkey. J. Comp. Neurol. 97:409–439.

Penfield, W., and Rasmussen, T. 1950. The Cerebral Cortex of Man: A Clinical Study of Localization of Function. New York: Macmillan.

Sjöqvist, O. 1938. Studies on pain conduction in the trigeminal nerve. Acta Psychiatr. Neurol. [Suppl.] 17:1–139.

Wall, P. D., and Taub, A. 1962. Four aspects of trigeminal nucleus and a paradox. J. Neurophysiol. 25:110–126.

Welker, E., Soriano, E., and Van der Loos, H. 1989. Plasticity in the barrel cortex of the adult mouse: Effects of peripheral deprivation on GAD-immunoreactivity. Exp. Brain Res. 74:441–452.

Welker, E., and van der Loos, H. 1986. Quantitative correlation between barrel-field size and the sensory innervation of the whiskerpad: A comparative study in six strains of mice bred for different patterns of mystacial vibrissae. J. Neurosci. 6:3355–3373.

Westrum, L. E., Canfield, R. C., and Black, R. G. 1976. Transganglionic degeneration in the spinal trigeminal nucleus following removal of tooth pulps in adult cats. Brain Res. 101:137–140.

Woolsey, T. A., and van der Loos, H. 1970. The structural organization of layer IV in the somatosensory region (S I) of mouse cerebral cortex. The description of a cortical field composed of discrete cytoarchitectonic units. Brain Res. 17:205–242.

46

Lewis P. Rowland

Clinical Syndromes of the Spinal Cord and Brain Stem

The Clinically Important Anatomy of the Spinal Cord Involves Four Descending or Ascending Tracts

Somatotopic Organization of the Spinothalamic Tract Is an Aid to Diagnosis and Treatment of Chronic Pain

Function Is Lost Below a Transverse Spinal Lesion

  The Site of a Spinal Cord Lesion May be Indicated by Focal Weakness (the Motor Level)

  The Site of a Spinal Cord Lesion Is More Often Indicated by the Pattern of Sensory Loss (the Sensory Level)

It Is Important to Distinguish Intra-Axial from Extra-Axial Spinal Lesions

Lesions of the Spinal Cord Often Give Rise to Characteristic Syndromes

  Complete Transection

  Partial Transection

  Hemisection (Brown-Séquard Syndrome)

  Multiple Sclerosis

  Syringomyelia

  Subacute Combined Degeneration

  Friedreich's Ataxia

The Brain Stem Is the Site of A Number of Essential Functions

Extra-Axial Lesions of the Brain Stem Are Illustrated by the Acoustic Neuroma and Other Tumors of the Cerebellopontine Angle

Intra-Axial Lesions of the Brain Stem Often Cause Gaze Palsies and Internuclear Ophthalmoplegia

  Gaze Palsies

  Syndrome of the Median Longitudinal Fasciculus: Internuclear Ophthalmoplegia

Vascular Lesions of the Brain Stem and Midbrain May Cause Characteristic Syndromes

  Medial Syndromes of the Medulla and Pons

  Lateral Syndromes of the Medulla and Pons

  Midbrain Syndromes

  Coma and the Locked-In Syndrome

An Overall View

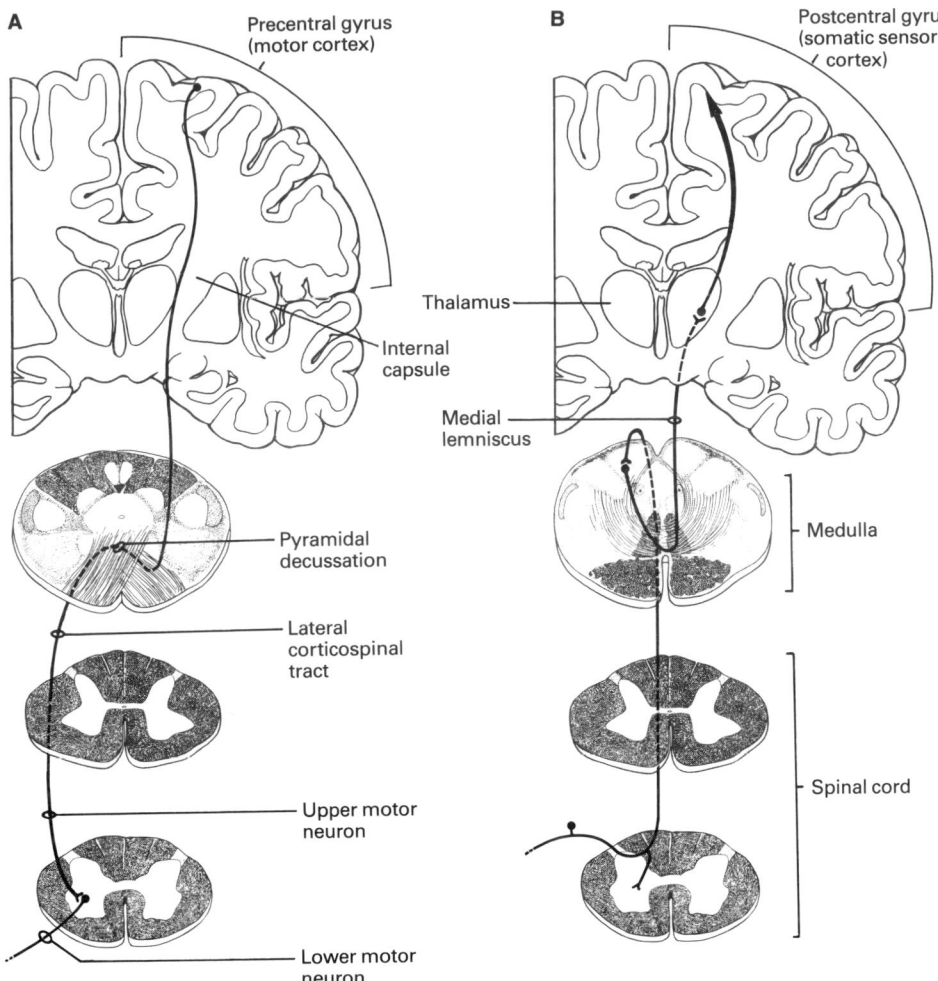

FIGURE 46–1

Clinically important ascending and descending tracts.

A. The corticospinal tract is the major descending pathway in which lesions lead to clinically detectable changes.

B. The dorsal column–medial lemniscal system conveys sensations of light touch, vibration, and joint position.

C. The lateral spinothalamic tracts carry sensations of pain, temperature, and crude touch from the other side of the body. These fibers ascend two to three segments and cross in the anterior commissure to join the medial fibers of the contralateral spinothalamic tract.

D. The spinocerebellar tracts convey unconscious proprioception.

I n this chapter we review the neurological disorders of the spinal cord and brain stem. To localize diseases to these structures and to identify their nature, one must know the detailed anatomy and physiology of the spinal cord and brain stem. For example, in the spinal cord, the specific transverse level of the sensory or motor impairment helps specify the level of the lesion. Similarly in the brain stem, abnormalities in the function of specific cranial nerves can localize the lesion to a particular horizontal level, such as the medulla or pons. In addition, at any given level the signs caused by lesions of the long tracts, such as the corticospinal tract (medially) or the spinothalamic tract (laterally), can further localize the lesion to the medial or lateral segment of the spinal cord and brain stem.

The Clinically Important Anatomy of the Spinal Cord Involves Four Descending or Ascending Tracts

The only descending tract of major clinical importance is the corticospinal tract in the lateral columns of the spinal cord (Figure 46–1A). Other descending pathways, such as the rubrospinal tract, also function in the control of posture and movement, but only lesions of the corticospinal tract have clinically evident effects. In contrast, three ascending tracts are important clinically:

1. The dorsal column–medial lemniscal system carries sensations of discriminative touch, vibration, and joint position. The axons run ipsilateral to the roots of entry

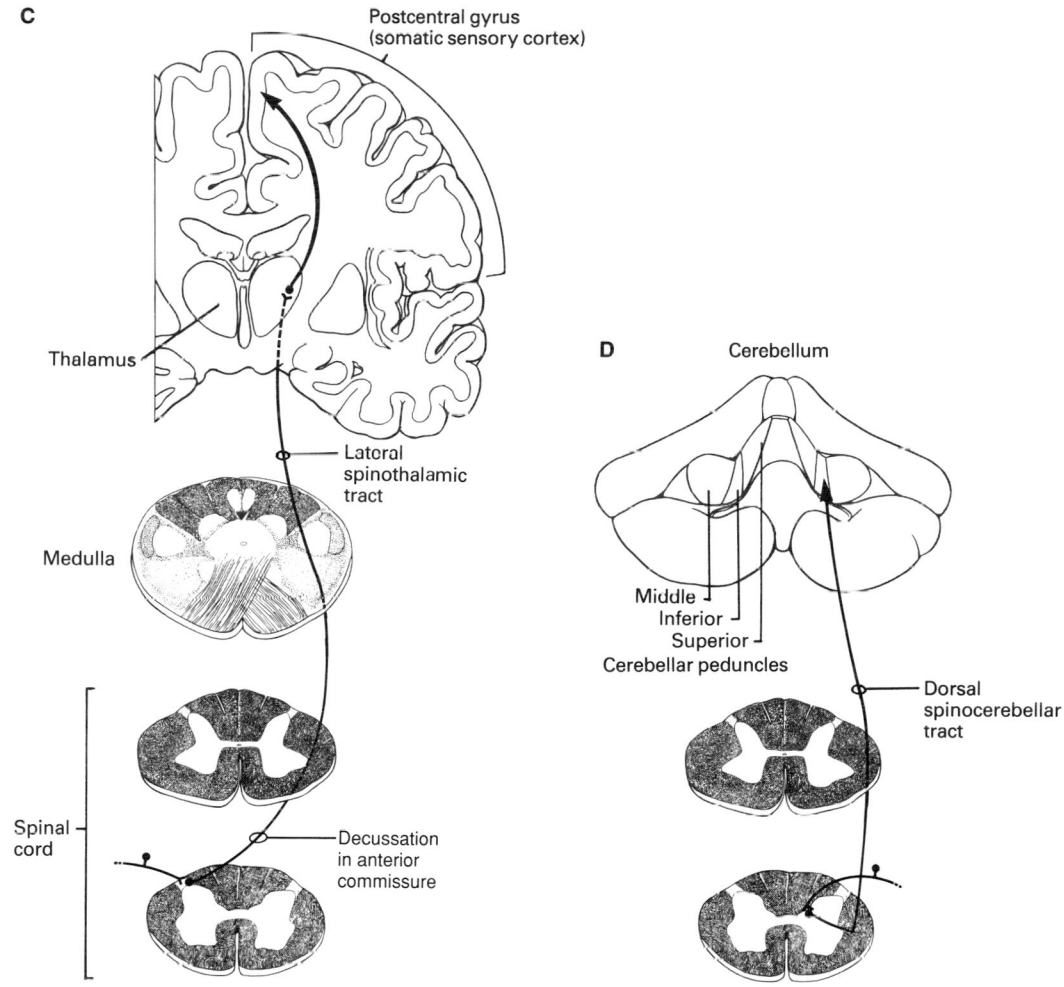

FIGURE 46–1 C and D

and cross to the other side above the spinal cord, in the medulla, after synapsing in the dorsal column nuclei (Figure 46–1B).

2. The lateral spinothalamic tract conveys sensations of pain, temperature, and crude touch from the contralateral side of the body (Figure 46–1C).

3. The spinocerebellar tract provides information about the position of the body in space and about the position of body segments relative to one another (Figure 46–1D). This tract is affected in some hereditary ataxias (Chapter 43) but is not the source of symptoms in other spinal cord diseases.

Somatotopic Organization of the Spinothalamic Tract Is an Aid to Diagnosis and Treatment of Chronic Pain

The fibers in the corticospinal tract, posterior columns, and spinothalamic tract are somatotopically organized.

This organization is clinically important in two conditions, both of which affect the spinothalamic tract: (1) lesions of the central parts of the cervical or thoracic cord, and (2) surgical procedures designed to relieve pain.

In the thoracic and cervical cord, fibers originating in the lowermost (sacral) region are pushed laterally by fibers entering from successively higher levels. Therefore, when lesions, such as tumors, arise in the innermost portion of the thoracic or cervical cord, a phenomenon called *sacral sparing* may result. As these lesions extend outward, they first compress the most medial fibers from higher segments but they may not affect the most lateral sacral fibers. In such cases all cutaneous sensation may be abolished below the level of the lesion but the sacral segments (perineum, scrotum, and saddle area) are spared (Figure 46–2F).

Neurosurgeons take advantage of the somatotopic organization of these tracts in the operation called *cordotomy*, which is sometimes performed to control

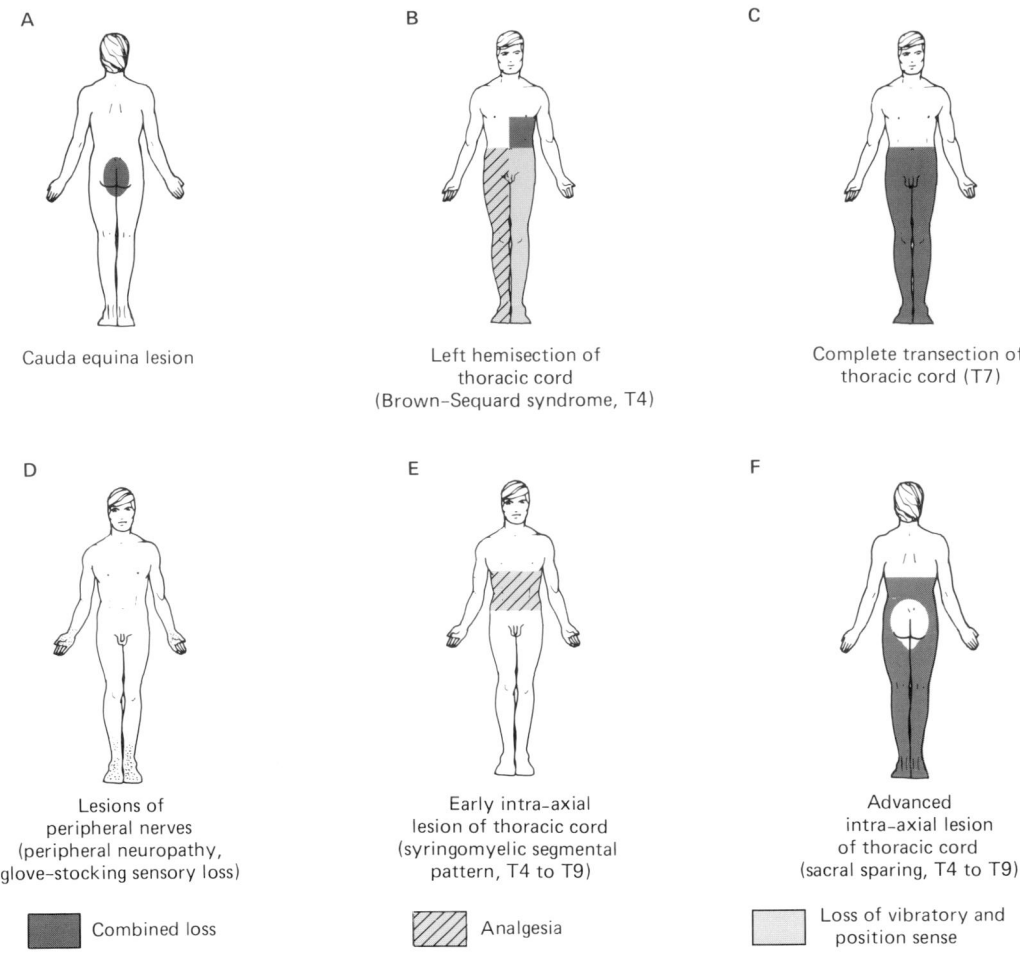

A
Cauda equina lesion

B
Left hemisection of
thoracic cord
(Brown–Sequard syndrome, T4)

C
Complete transection of
thoracic cord (T7)

D
Lesions of
peripheral nerves
(peripheral neuropathy,
glove-stocking sensory loss)

E
Early intra-axial
lesion of thoracic cord
(syringomyelic segmental
pattern, T4 to T9)

F
Advanced
intra-axial lesion
of thoracic cord
(sacral sparing, T4 to T9)

Combined loss   Analgesia   Loss of vibratory and
position sense

FIGURE 46–2
The sensory deficit is correlated with the anatomical level of
the lesion. (Adapted from Collins, 1962.)

intractable pain in the pelvis or legs. Because pain is not experienced in the spinal cord itself, it is possible to section the spinothalamic tract selectively under local anesthesia. When the scalpel enters the outer aspect of the spinal cord and spinothalamic tract, it encounters the sacral fibers first. As the knife goes deeper, the level at which sensation is lost rises. Because the patient is awake and cooperative, the extent of sensory loss can be ascertained continuously during the procedure to ensure that only the desired level is attained.

Cordotomy, however, is not always successful. The procedure may be open, requiring a laminectomy to reach the cord, or it may be percutaneous, a less extensive procedure but one that has to be done under radiological guidance for proper placement of the lesion. In either method the pain may not be relieved completely, or relief may be only temporary. Moreover, cervical cordotomy is not without risk. If the pain is in the midline, as in pelvic

tumors, bilateral cordotomies are needed, increasing the likelihood that there will be injury to the corticospinal tract, descending autonomic fibers, or respiratory fibers. Bladder control is impaired in up to 50% of cases after bilateral procedures. Weakness, incoordination of the legs, and respiratory insufficiency are less common risks.

Function Is Lost Below a Transverse Spinal Lesion

Lesions of the spinal cord give rise to motor or sensory symptoms that are often related to a particular sensory or motor segmental level of the spinal cord. Identification of the appropriate level of the motor or sensory loss (called a *motor* or *sensory level*) is crucial for recognizing focal lesions within the spinal cord or external compressive lesions that interrupt functions below the lesion.

TABLE 46–1. Indicators of Motor Level Lesions

Root	Major muscles affected	Reflex loss
C3–5	Diaphragm	—
C5	Deltoid, biceps	Biceps
C7	Triceps, extensors of wrist and fingers	Triceps
C8	Interossei, abductor of fifth finger	—
L2–4	Quadriceps	Knee jerk
L5	Long extensor of great toe, anterior tibial	—
S1	Plantar flexors, gastrocnemius	Ankle jerk

The Site of a Spinal Cord Lesion May be Indicated by Focal Weakness (the Motor Level)

When motor roots are involved, or when motor neurons are affected focally, clinical findings may indicate the spinal level of injury. The clinical evidence would include the typical lower motor neuron signs: weakness, wasting, fasciculation, and loss of tendon reflexes. The muscles and tendon reflexes that serve as landmarks for locating motor level lesions are listed in Table 46–1. However, because it is clinically difficult to relate the innervation of muscles of the trunk and thorax to specific spinal segments, the motor level may not be evident. For instance, a lesion anywhere above the first lumbar segment may cause signs of upper motor neuron disease in the legs. Under these circumstances sensory abnormalities are more valuable in localizing the lesion.

The Site of a Spinal Cord Lesion Is More Often Indicated by the Pattern of Sensory Loss (the Sensory Level)

The characteristic pattern of sensory loss after a transverse spinal cord lesion is loss of cutaneous sensation below the level of the lesion (Figure 46–2C); if the lesion is unilateral, the loss is contralateral (Figure 46–2B). The sensory level is often more evident than the motor level. However, sensory loss due to spinal lesions must be differentiated from the pattern of sensory loss caused by lesions of peripheral nerves or isolated nerve roots. When multiple peripheral nerves are affected by disease (polyneuropathy), there is a glove-and-stocking pattern of impaired perception of pain and temperature. This pattern is attributed to impaired axonal transport, or dying back (see Chapter 17). The parts of the axons most severely affected are those most distant from the sensory neuron cell bodies in the dorsal root ganglia. When single peripheral nerves are injured, the distribution of sensory loss is more restricted and can be recognized by reference to sensory charts that were originally generated by studies of the long-term effects of traumatic injuries incurred during war.

Nerve root or segmental sensory loss and spinal sensory levels can be identified by the dermatomes typically affected (Figure 46–3 and Box 25–1). The landmarks for the major sensory levels are listed in Table 46–2. The spinal cord ends at the level of the base of the second lumbar (L2) vertebra. Below this level the spinal canal is occupied by the lower nerve roots (cauda equina).

It Is Important to Distinguish Intra-Axial from Extra-Axial Spinal Lesions

In practical terms it is important to know whether a lesion arises within the spinal cord (whether it is intra-axial or intramedullary), or whether the spinal cord is being compressed by an external mass (whether it is extra-axial or extramedullary). Clinical evidence may give some clues that are helpful in making the distinction. For instance, pain is more common in extra-axial lesions because a compressing lesion (such as a tumor) may affect the dura, posterior nerve roots, or blood vessels that are innervated by sensory neurons mediating pain. In contrast, because there are no pain receptors within the spinal cord itself (or the brain), intra-axial lesions may be painless. Intra-axial lesions may be marked by sacral sparing of sensation (Figure 46–2F) or may cause a segmental pattern of sensory loss (Figure 46–2E), as in syringomyelia (described below). In addition, bladder function is affected earlier in intra-axial than in extra-axial disease.

None of these characteristics is absolutely reliable, however; definite diagnosis depends on radiographic contrast procedures, the most important of which is myelography. In this procedure a radio-opaque material is introduced into the subarachnoid space to outline the spinal cord, the nerve roots, and the bony margins of the canal, permitting assessment of compressive lesions or those that distort the cord from within. Vascular lesions can be assessed by spinal angiography, in which spinal blood vessels are selectively catheterized and injected with radio-opaque dyes.

To provide more detailed views of the contents of the spinal canal, computerized tomography is combined with injection of contrast material (metrizamide) into the subarachnoid space. As we saw in Chapter 22, magnetic resonance imaging may soon provide this information without the discomfort, expense, and hazards of injection into the subarachnoid space (Figure 46–4).

It is also possible to evaluate conduction in the human dorsal column–medial lemniscal system by measuring

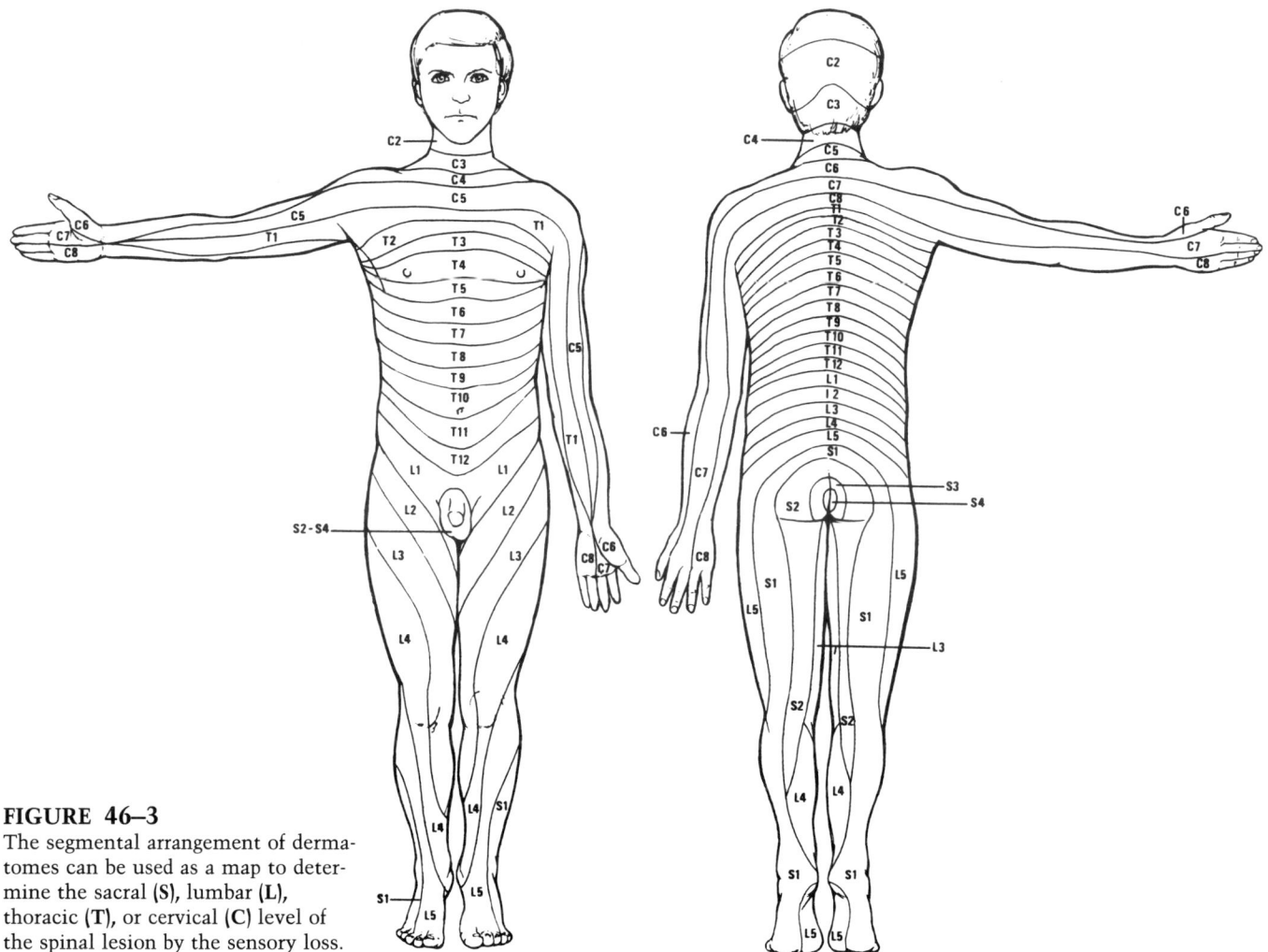

FIGURE 46–3

The segmental arrangement of dermatomes can be used as a map to determine the sacral (**S**), lumbar (**L**),
thoracic (**T**), or cervical (**C**) level of
the spinal lesion by the sensory loss.

TABLE 46–2. Indicators of Sensory Level Lesions

Root	Major sensory areas affected
C4	Clavicle
C8	Fifth finger
T4	Nipples
T10	Umbilicus
L1	Inguinal ligament
L3	Anterior surface of the thigh
L5	Great toe
S1	Lateral aspect of the foot
S3–5	Perineum

somatic sensory evoked potentials, a series of waves that
are recorded at the scalp or over the spine in response to a
sensory stimulus. (For a discussion of somatic sensory
evoked potentials see Chapters 24, 27, and Box 50–1.)

Evoked potentials are a measure of central conduction,
and the test is of greatest use in evaluating patients with
suspected multiple sclerosis or other demyelinating diseases (in which conduction within myelinated fiber tracts
may be slowed or blocked altogether). Because of the lesion, one or more peaks of the somatic sensory evoked
potential may be absent or delayed. Evoked potentials are
valuable because they may reveal lesions that are not detectable clinically, and they aid in interpreting a clinically
equivocal symptom or sign. Somatic sensory evoked
potentials may also be abnormal with compressive or in-
filtrative lesions, but the type of abnormality does not
vary with etiology. In addition, these evoked potentials
are used in the operating room to prevent spinal cord injury during surgical procedures on the spine or cord itself.

Lesions of the Spinal Cord Often Give Rise to Characteristic Syndromes

Spinal cord injuries are most often caused by trauma, especially automobile accidents. The resulting syndrome
depends on the extent of direct injury of the cord or compression of the cord by displaced vertebrae or blood clots.
In extreme cases trauma may lead to complete or partial
transection of the spinal cord.

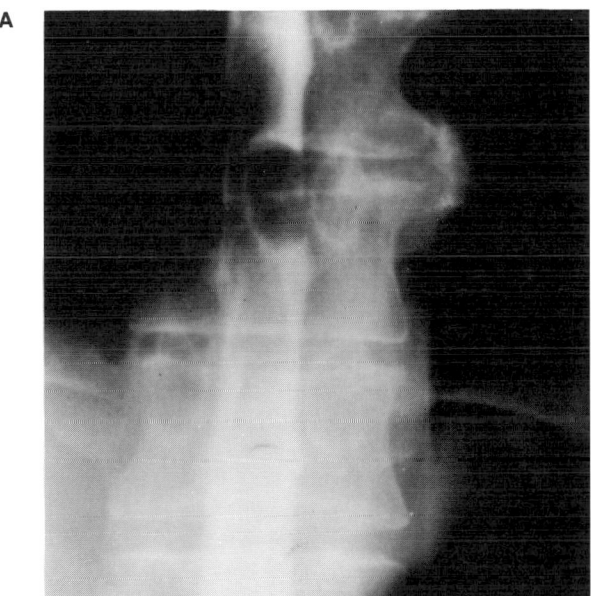

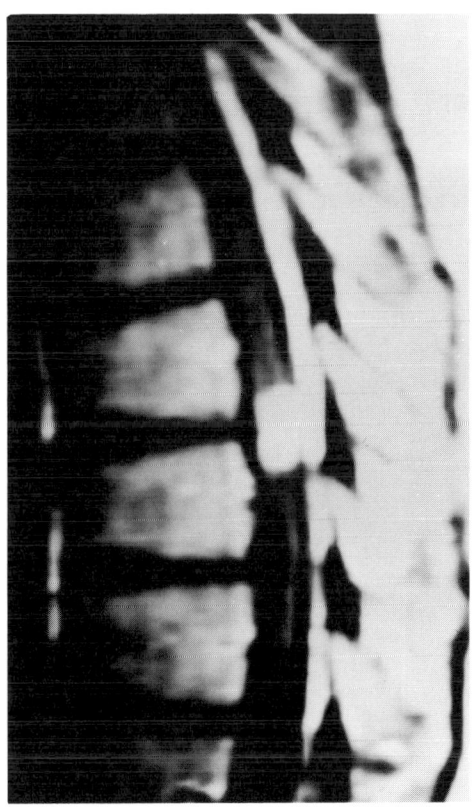

FIGURE 46–4

Magnetic resonance imaging often provides information without the hazards and discomfort of a myelogram, but both techniques were useful in demonstrating this thoracic schwannoma, an extradural tumor. (Courtesy of A. J. Silver and S. K. Hilal.)

A. A frontal view myelogram using the contrast agent iohexol. The contrast agent fills the subarachnoid space (white columns) on either side of the spinal cord, which appears as the dark central column. Several features indicate that the mass is extramedullary not intradural: the contours of the mass are cup-like; the mass indents the subarachnoid space; there is widening of the subarachnoid space above and below the mass; and there is lateral displacement of the overtly compressed spinal cord.

B. A lateral sagittal view magnetic resonance image of the same patient as in A. The mass is evident as a white, well-defined nodule that enhances after intravenous administration of the contrast agent gadolinium, which enters the lesion because the blood—CNS barrier is defective in the area of the mass. Without other views such as those in A, it would be impossible to determine whether this lesion is intramedullary or, as it appears in A, extramedullary. But the lateral sagittal view shows the extent of the mass and reveals that it is solid, not cystic.

Complete Transection

The spinal cord may be completely severed in fracture-dislocations of vertebrae or by knife or bullet wounds. Acute transection of the cord may also result from an inflammatory condition called *transverse myelitis* or from compression due to a tumor, especially metastatic tumors. Symptoms of acute transection resulting from myelitis or tumors evolve in days or weeks.

Traumatic section of the cord, however, results in immediate loss of all sensation (Figure 46–2C) and all voluntary movement below the lesion. Bladder and bowel control are also lost. If the lesion is above C3, breathing may be affected. Although upper motor neuron signs might be expected, tendon reflexes are usually absent—a condition of spinal shock that persists for several weeks. After a while, reflex activity returns at levels below the lesion. Hyperactive reflexes, *clonus* (rapid and repeated contraction and relaxation of passively stretched muscle), and Babinski signs then appear as signs of damage to the corticospinal tract. The legs become spastic; this condition is often preceded by intermittent hypertonia and flexor spasms that occur spontaneously or may be provoked by cutaneous stimuli. Later, flexor and extensor spasms may alternate, and the ultimately fixed posture may be either flexion or extension of the knees and hips. Bladder and bowel function may become automatic, with emptying in response to moderate filling. Automatic bladder emptying may be retarded by severe distension of the bladder or infection in the acute stage, or by damage to lumbar or sacral cord segments.

Partial Transection

In partial transection of the spinal cord, some ascending or descending tracts may be spared. In slowly progressing lesions, as in compression by an extramedullary tumor, the same tracts may be affected but less severely. Partial function is retained, but specific motor and sensory signs are evident.

Hemisection (Brown-Séquard Syndrome)

Because of spinal cord anatomy, hemisection of the right side of the cervical spinal cord (at C4, for example) has four main clinical consequences.

1. Ipsilateral (right) signs of a lesion in the corticospinal tract. There is weakness of the right arm and leg, with more active tendon reflexes in the right arm and leg. In addition, several abnormal reflexes appear. The Babinski sign, abnormal extension of the great toe, instead of the normal downward (flexor) plantar reflex, in response to a moving tactile stimulus on the lateral border of the sole of the foot, reliably indicates a disorder of the corticospinal tract on that side of the spinal cord. Another abnormal reflex is the Hoffmann sign, an abnormal flexor reflex of the thumb and other fingers induced by stretching the flexors of the middle finger by flicking the distal phalanx of that finger. Finally, there may be *clonus*, which is best detected at the ankle when the examiner abruptly moves the patient's foot upward (stretching the gastrocnemius). Sometimes clonus is so easily evoked that it occurs vigorously in response to a simple tap on the Achilles tendon or when the patient places the foot on the floor. The reaction can be stopped promptly by passively moving the foot down or plantarflexing the foot, relieving the stretched position of the gastrocnemius.
2. Ipsilateral signs of a lesion in the posterior columns and dorsospinocervical tract are indicated by loss of position sense and vibratory sensation.
3. Contralateral loss of pain and temperature perception to the level of C4 follows interruption of the right spinothalamic tract.
4. Loss of autonomic function results in Horner's syndrome—constricted pupil (*miosis*) and lid-drop (*ptosis*) —on the same side.

Multiple Sclerosis

The two most common nontraumatic disorders of the spinal cord are probably amyotrophic lateral sclerosis (described in Chapter 18) and multiple sclerosis. Upper motor neuron signs and proprioceptive sensory loss are almost always present in advanced cases of multiple sclerosis, although there may be no signs referable to a lesion of the spinal cord. Nonetheless, when patients who have had these signs come to autopsy, there are usually many small lesions throughout the spinal cord. Some combinations of signs are almost diagnostic of multiple sclerosis: for instance, the combination of proprioceptive sensory loss and signs of upper motor neuron disease together with evidence of either cerebellar dysfunction—ataxia, tremor of the arms, disorders of eye movement (nystagmus), difficulty speaking (dysarthria)—or a history of optic neuritis. In addition to signs of disorder elsewhere in the nervous system, there is often a clinical episode of transverse myelitis with corresponding motor and sensory levels.

Syringomyelia

Syringomyelia is a condition defined by formation of cysts within the spinal cord. The cause is unknown, but the lesion affects the central portion of the cord first and then spreads peripherally. Intramedullary tumors may also cause the same clinical syndrome. The clinical picture of syringomyelia is characterized by two unusual patterns of segmental dysfunction (involving cutaneous sensation and motor neurons) as well as interruption of ascending or descending tracts. Because the lesion starts centrally, the first fibers to be affected are those carrying pain and temperature sensations as they cross in the anterior commissure (Figure 46–5). This usually causes bilateral loss of cutaneous sensation, restricted to the segments involved and resulting in a shawl or cuirass (French, breastplate) pattern, affecting a few cervical or thoracic segments and sparing sensation below (Figure 46–2E). Sometimes the segmental sensory loss is unilateral. The lesion is chronic and the loss of sensation may lead to painless injuries of the digits or painless burns. Because touch perception is conveyed in posterior columns as well as in the spinothalamic tract, there may be dissociated sensory loss, sparing touch as well as position and vibration sense (Figure 46–5). If motor neurons in the diseased segment are affected, lower motor neuron signs, such as weakness, wasting, and

FIGURE 46–5

Syringomyelia may disrupt pain sensation, not proprioception. The cavity **(hatched area)** within the spinal cord interrupts transmission of information about painful stimuli to the brain stem and thalamus. Sensory loss is seen only in the segments affected (as in Figure 47–2). In contrast, tactile sensation and limb proprioception remain undisturbed because the cavity does not encroach upon the posterior columns. Large cavities may extend into the anterior horn to disrupt motor neuron function in the affected segments. (Adapted from Collins, 1962.)

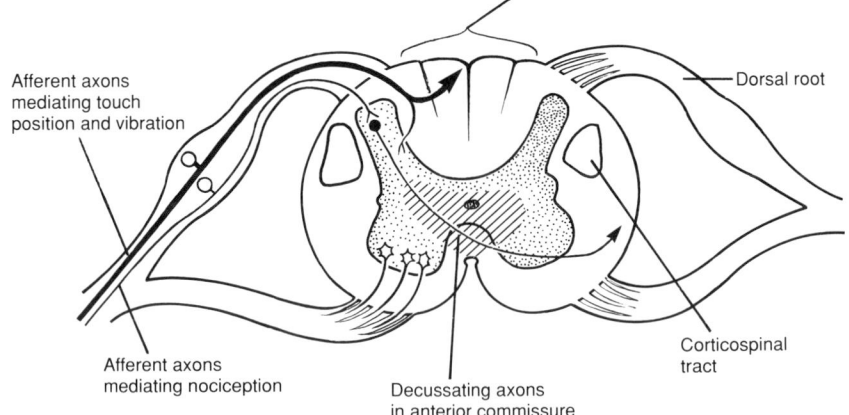

loss of reflexes, are present in the appropriate area. If the lesion extends laterally, the corticospinal tract is affected and upper motor neuron signs may be present in the legs.

Subacute Combined Degeneration

Degeneration of the spinal cord that affects both the corticospinal tracts and the posterior columns (often called combined degeneration) is usually the result of vitamin B_{12} deficiency. This disorder is most commonly due to loss of gastric intrinsic factor, resulting in macrocytic anemia (pernicious anemia). As a consequence of the combined degeneration there is a gait disorder, with upper motor neuron signs and loss of position and vibratory perception in the legs. The loss of position sense may be so severe that the patients are uncertain where their feet are. The unsteady gait is therefore due to sensory loss rather than motor incoordination, a disorder called *sensory ataxia*. Because the spinothalamic tract is not involved primarily, loss of cutaneous sensation would not be expected but almost always occurs and is attributed to concomitant degeneration of peripheral nerves. The peripheral neuropathy may also abolish tendon reflexes, modifying or masking the expected upper motor neuron signs. Because this is a system degeneration rather than a focal cord lesion, there is no motor or sensory level.

The clinical pattern of combined degeneration is also seen in the vacuolar myelopathy of patients with acquired immunodeficiency syndrome (AIDS). The pathogenesis of this lesion is uncertain and may be due to direct effects of the human immunodeficiency virus (HIV), secondary infection with other viruses, or interference with the metabolism of vitamin B_{12}. Another viral infection, tropical spastic paraparesis, can cause a similar pattern of cord disease and is due to infection by human lymphotropic virus type I (HTLV-I). The disease is common in subtropical areas around the globe and is seen in the United States in immigrants from Caribbean countries or from Central or South America. In this condition the dominant signs are due to lesions in the corticospinal tract, causing the paraparesis.

Friedreich's Ataxia

Friedreich's ataxia is a genetic condition in which the distribution of spinal cord lesions is similar to that of combined system disease. In addition, the spinocerebellar tract is affected. As a result, the first symptoms, occurring in adolescence, are usually unsteadiness or ataxia in walking. There may be spastic weakness of the legs and loss of proprioception. The combination of lesions results in the incongruous appearance of Babinski signs, although knee and ankle jerks are lost. Other signs of cerebellar disease (nystagmus and tremor of the arms) may appear later. (It is not clear why tendon reflexes are lost; there is no cutaneous sensory loss to imply peripheral neuropathy. Perhaps cerebellar influences on reflexes are important.)

Thus the spinal cord may be affected by three types of diseases: traumatic, inherited, and acquired. The damage resulting in the spinal cord in each of these three types of disease may be segmental or longitudinal. The pattern of motor and sensory signs, and the severity of the resulting disorder, depend on the extent of the lesion.

The Brain Stem Is the Site of a Number of Essential Functions

As we have seen in Chapter 44, the spinal cord continues rostrally as the brain stem (Figure 46–6). No other region of the central nervous system compares to the brain stem in being as densely packed with vital structures. Crowded into the small space of the brain stem are the nuclear groups and nerve fibers of the cranial nerves, the long sensory tracts ascending from the spinal cord to the thalamus and cortex, and the motor pathways descending from the cortex and the subcortical nuclei to the brain stem and spinal cord. In addition, the brain stem contains the reticular formation, with autonomic centers that control respiration, blood pressure, and gastrointestinal functions as well as centers that mediate arousal and wakefulness. Finally, the brain stem surrounds a narrow passage for the circulation of cerebrospinal fluid; that channel, the aqueduct of Sylvius, is susceptible to occlusion. It is therefore not surprising that a small lesion in the brain stem can have disastrous results.

To localize lesions within the brain stem, it is useful to delineate structures along two planes, the longitudinal and the cross-sectional. Along the longitudinal plane, areas of the brain stem that lie in the direction of the cerebral hemispheres are called *upper*, *superior*, or *rostral*; areas that lie in the direction of the spinal cord are called *lower*, *inferior*, or *caudal* (Figures 46–5 and 46–6). In cross section the lowermost structures are called *ventral*, the upper structures are called *dorsal* or *tegmental*.

As with spinal cord disease, it is critical to determine whether the site of a lesion lies within or outside the brain stem proper. A lesion that directly affects the tissue of the brain stem is called *intra-axial*, *intramedullary*, or *parenchymal*. A lesion outside the brain stem, such as one affecting the peripheral course of a cranial nerve, is called *extra-axial*.

Because of the anatomical arrangement, unilateral lesions within the brain stem tend to cause crossed syndromes, in which some signs are ipsilateral and others are contralateral to the lesion. Extra-axial lesions may affect only specific groups of cranial nerves, but extra-axial tumors may also compress the brain stem so that ascending and descending tracts are compromised, making it difficult to distinguish between intra- and extra-axial lesions on clinical grounds.

Extra-Axial Lesions of the Brain Stem Are Illustrated by the Acoustic Neuroma and Other Tumors of the Cerebellopontine Angle

Small extra-axial lesions affecting the brain stem often begin by compressing and interfering with the function of

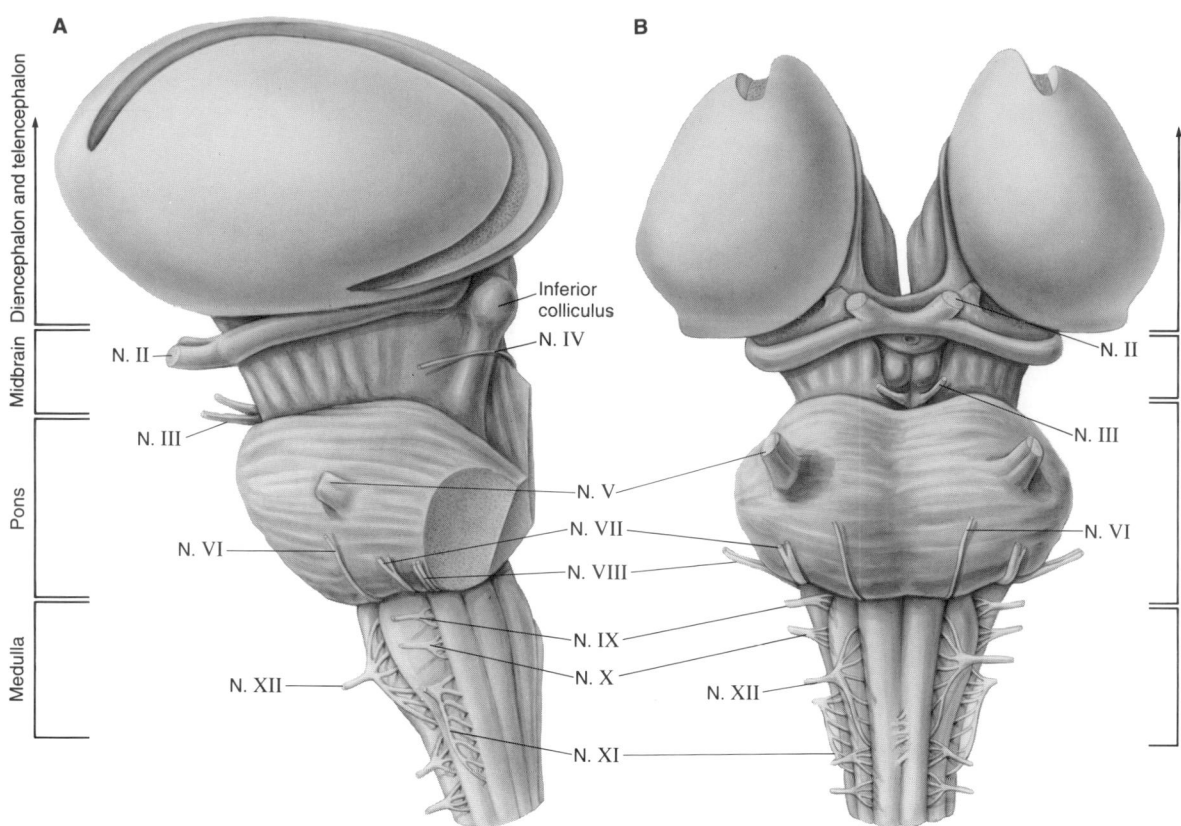

FIGURE 46-6
Two views of the brain stem show the location of the cranial nerves: lateral view (**A**) and ventral view (**B**).

individual cranial nerves. Neighboring structures within the brain stem may then be affected, causing long tract signs. Isolated cranial nerve disorders, however, are more likely to be due to peripheral lesions, affecting the nerves as they exit through the foramina of the skull. Intracranial tumors outside the brain stem may also begin by compressing cranial nerves.

As an example of a common extra-axial lesion we shall consider the acoustic neuroma. This extramedullary tumor originates from Schwann cells of the sheath of the acoustic nerve (VIII) within the acoustic canal and grows in the angle between the cerebellum and the pons (the cerebellopontine angle). The acoustic neuroma first compresses the cochlear nerve, causing ringing in the ear (tinnitus), loss of hearing, and ultimately deafness. The distance from the internal auditory meatus to neighboring nerves and the brain stem is short (Figure 46–7). As the tumor grows into the angle between the cerebellum and the pons, the corneal reflex (the reflex blink on touching the cornea) may be lost, signifying compression of afferent fibers of the trigeminal nerve (V). Later, other trigeminal motor and sensory functions may also be lost.

The next signs may involve the facial nerve (VII) or the ipsilateral cerebellar hemisphere. When the facial nerve is affected, there is a lower motor neuron type of paralysis on the same side of the face. If the cerebellar hemisphere is compressed, there is ipsilateral limb ataxia and intention tremor (a tremor that is intensified by voluntary movement), or nystagmus (rhythmical oscillation of the eyes, with a fast movement in one direction and a slow movement in the other) (Figure 46–8). The brain stem ultimately becomes compressed, causing corticospinal tract signs or narrowing the aqueduct to cause hydrocephalus (enlargement of the ventricular system) and symptoms of increased intracranial pressure (as explained in Appendix C). The tumor is now usually detected by computerized tomography or magnetic resonance imaging before the condition progresses to hydrocephalus. Acoustic neuromas are benign and accessible tumors that can be removed surgically.

Intra-Axial Lesions of the Brain Stem Often Cause Gaze Palsies and Internuclear Ophthalmoplegia

Gaze Palsies

Many lesions of the brain stem cause abnormalities of gaze (conjugate movements of both eyes) or nystagmus. It

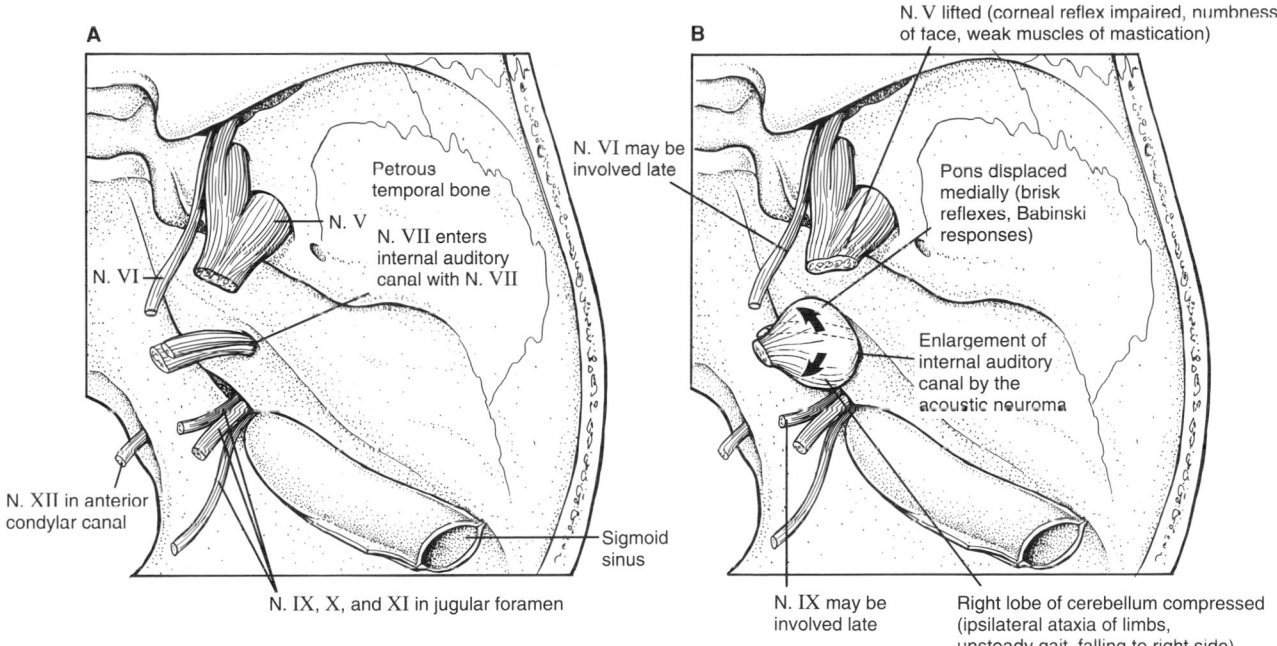

FIGURE 46–7

The acoustic neuroma grows in the cerebellopontine angle and causes a characteristic syndrome. (Adapted from Patten, 1977.)

A. A view of the inner surface of the cranium with the brain stem and cerebellum removed showing the normal cerebellopontine angle.

B. Changes caused by an acoustic neuroma.

is therefore useful to review the relationship between two of the centers controlling eye movements that we considered in Chapter 42—the occipital and frontal eyefields and the pontine gaze center (Figure 46–8).

Discharging epileptic foci or electrical stimulation of frontal or occipital eye fields on one side causes both eyes to move conjugately to the opposite side, called an adversive movement of the eyes (Figure 46–9A). Conversely, destructive lesions of the frontal cortical area may result in impaired gaze toward the side opposite the lesion. A patient with a lesion in the right frontal lobe, for example, cannot move the eyes conjugately to the left, and the eyes therefore tend to drift to the right (right gaze preference). If a lesion in the right hemisphere also causes a left hemiplegia, the eyes look away from the hemiplegia (Figure 46–9B).

The fibers descending from the cortical eye fields cross the midline to the contralateral gaze center in the pontine reticular formation, near the sixth-nerve nucleus (Figure 46–8A). Lesions in or near the pontine gaze centers impair gaze toward the side of the lesion. For instance, a destructive lesion on the right side of the pons impairs gaze to the right, and the eyes tend to drift to the left. If corticospinal fibers are also involved, the right-sided lesion is above the decussation of the descending fibers and a left hemiplegia

results. In this case the eyes look toward the side of the hemiplegia (Figure 46–9C).

Syndrome of the Median Longitudinal Fasciculus: Internuclear Ophthalmoplegia

Gaze to the right requires the coordinated activity of the right lateral rectus muscle (innervated by the sixth nerve) and the left medial rectus (innervated by the third nerve). This integration depends upon functions of the pontine gaze center (or paramedian pontine reticular formation). This structure sends fibers to the ipsilateral abducens nucleus and the contralateral oculomotor nucleus (Figure 46–8A). These fibers travel with vestibular and other fibers in the medial longitudinal fasciculus. Lesions in the medial longitudinal fasciculus cause a characteristic combination of signs called *internuclear ophthalmoplegia*. In young adults the most common cause of internuclear ophthalmoplegia is multiple sclerosis. Later in life the syndrome is most often caused by occlusion of the basilar artery (described below) or paramedian branches of that artery.

If the lesion is unilateral, adduction of the eye on that side is impaired or paralyzed (Figure 46–9). By convention,

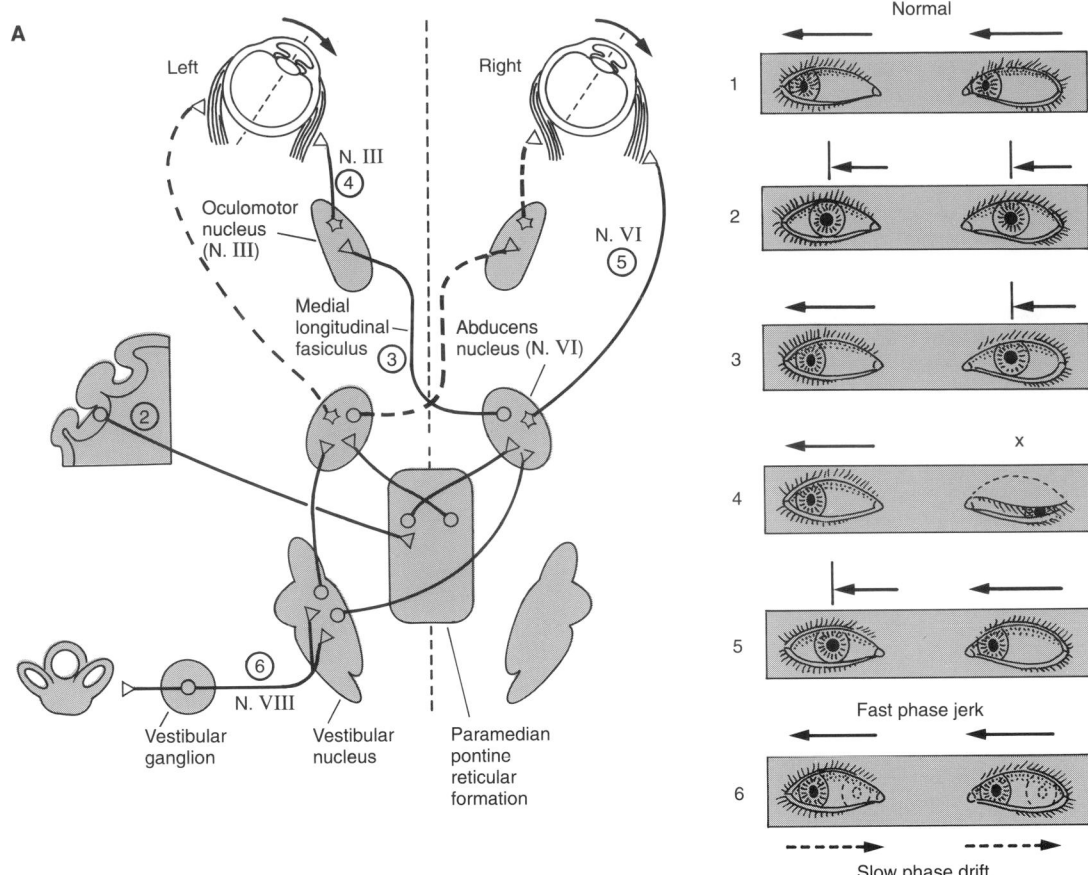

FIGURE 46–8

Lesions of the neural pathways mediating horizontal gaze lead to specific effects. (Adapted from Sears and Franklin, 1980.)

A. Pathways for horizontal gaze. Numbers indicate sites of lesions.

B. Abnormalities of eye movements on attempted gaze to the right correspond to the numbered lesions in the horizontal gaze system shown in part A. **1.** Normal right gaze. **2.** Left cortical

lesion (gaze to the right is impaired). **3.** Left medial longitudinal fasciculus lesion (impaired adduction of the left eye; nystagmus of abducting right eye). **4.** Left oculomotor nerve lesion (impaired adduction of left eye plus other manifestations of third-nerve palsy, including the ptosis illustrated). **5.** Right abducens nerve lesion, with isolated paralysis of lateral rectus. **6.** Left vestibular nerve lesion (jerk nystagmus).

lesions within the medial longitudinal fasciculus—as opposed to those in the paramedian pontine reticular formation—are named for the side of the affected medial rectus. The supranuclear nature of the impaired adduction on attempted gaze can be deduced because the function of the medial rectus is preserved in the reflex responses of convergence for near vision.

In internuclear ophthalmoplegia there is often nystagmus of the abducting eye when the patient tries to look toward that side. The abducting nystagmus is characterized by an adducting drift of the eye (a slow medial movement) followed by a corrective abducting saccade (a rapid lateral movement). The pathophysiology is not known and several theories have been advanced. For instance, the nystagmus affects the eye contralateral to the affected medial rectus, and the medial drift has been attributed to failure of inhibition of the normal medial rectus in the

abducting eye. Alternatively, there may be an abnormal state of persistent convergence; that is, the patient uses the only possible eye movement mechanism (convergence) to adduct the paretic medial rectus. Convergence, however, involves both eyes and the abducting eye therefore adducts momentarily. To resume its proper position, the abducting eye makes a quick movement to refixate on the laterally placed target, and this appears as nystagmus.

Vascular Lesions of the Brain Stem and Midbrain May Cause Characteristic Syndromes

Vascular lesions of the brain stem often affect functions other than movement of the eyes. It is therefore important to understand the principles of the vascular anatomy of this area. The medulla is supplied by branches of the ver-

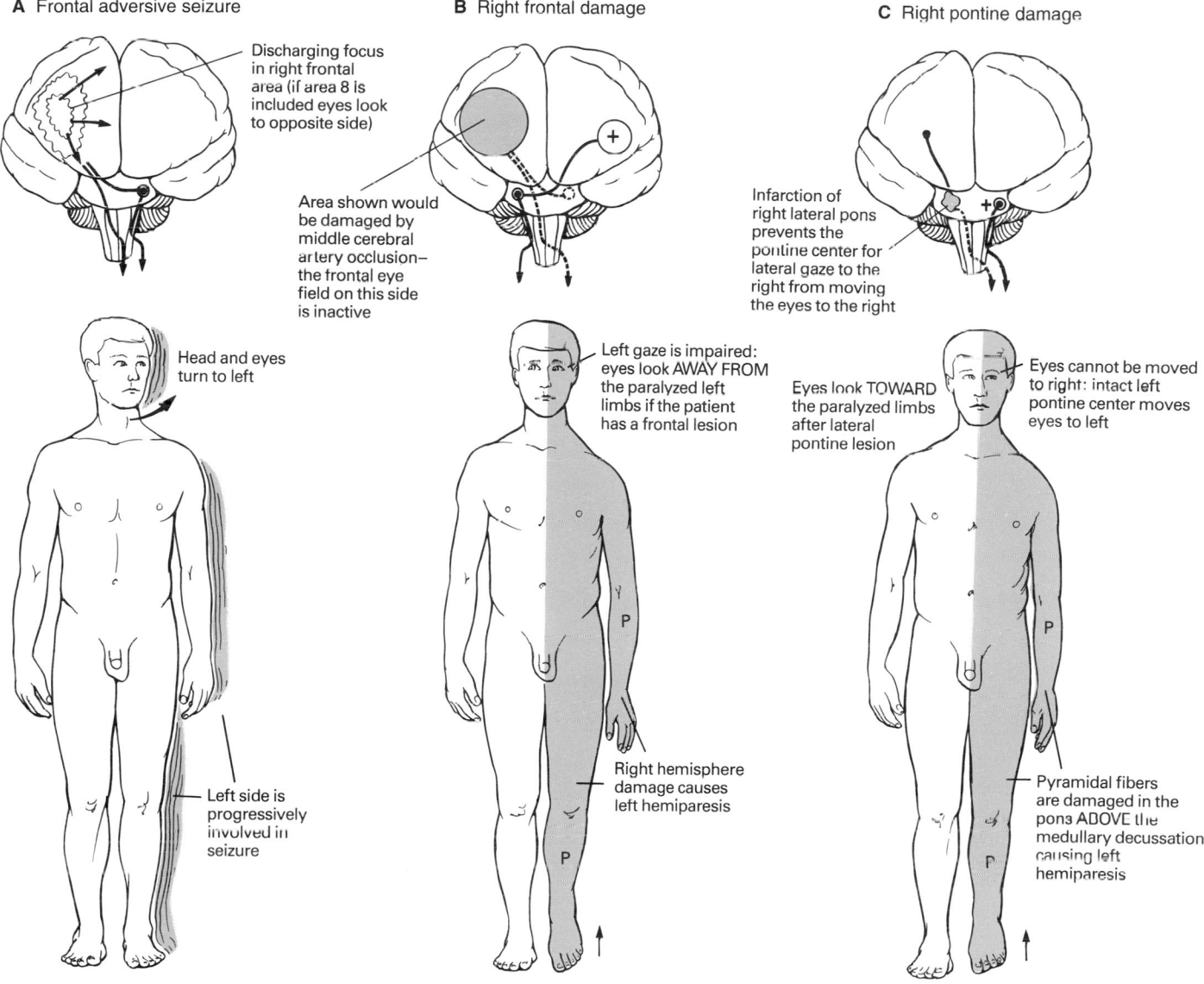

A Frontal adversive seizure

Discharging focus in right frontal area (if area 8 is included eyes look to opposite side)

Head and eyes turn to left

Left side is progressively involved in seizure

B Right frontal damage

Area shown would be damaged by middle cerebral artery occlusion—the frontal eye field on this side is inactive

Left gaze is impaired: eyes look AWAY FROM the paralyzed left limbs if the patient has a frontal lesion

Right hemisphere damage causes left hemiparesis

C Right pontine damage

Infarction of right lateral pons prevents the pontine center for lateral gaze to the right from moving the eyes to the right

Eyes look TOWARD the paralyzed limbs after lateral pontine lesion

Eyes cannot be moved to right: intact left pontine center moves eyes to left

Pyramidal fibers are damaged in the pons ABOVE the medullary decussation causing left hemiparesis

FIGURE 46–9

Disorders of gaze in relation to other impairments can indicate the nature of the lesion. Direction of gaze (see eyes), functioning gaze center (+), paretic limbs (**P**), and the presence of the Babinski sign (↑) are indicated. (Adapted from Patten, 1977.)

A. Effects of discharging epileptic lesions in the right frontal lobe.

B. Right frontal damage.

C. Right pontine damage.

tebral artery (Figure 46–10), including the posterior inferior cerebellar artery (Figure 46–11). The two vertebral arteries of each side join to form the basilar artery, which runs along the base of the pons and produces three sets of branches: (1) paramedian branches, which supply midline structures of the pons; (2) short circumferential branches, which supply the lateral aspect of the pons and the middle and superior cerebellar peduncles; and (3) long circumferential arteries, the inferior and superior cerebellar arteries, which also supply lateral portions of the brain stem and

run around the pons to reach the cerebellar hemispheres. (The basilar artery terminates by dividing into the two posterior cerebral arteries. These vessels are then linked to the corresponding carotid arteries by the posterior communicating arteries, completing the posterior portion of the circle of Willis.)

Sometimes only a branch of the basilar artery is occluded, resulting in a restricted lesion in the brain and often a characteristic syndrome. More often either the vertebral or the basilar artery itself is occluded, giving rise

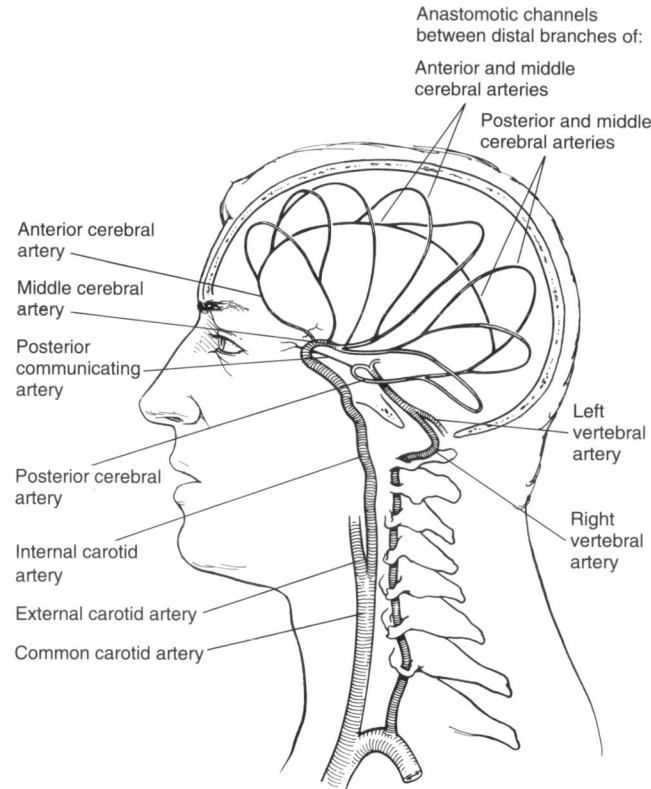

Anastomotic channels
between distal branches of:

Anterior and middle
cerebral arteries

Posterior and middle
cerebral arteries

Anterior cerebral
artery

Middle cerebral
artery

Posterior
communicating
artery

Posterior cerebral
artery

Internal carotid
artery

External carotid artery

Common carotid artery

Left
vertebral
artery

Right
vertebral
artery

FIGURE 46–10
Course of the major cerebral arteries over the lateral and medial cortical surfaces. Anastomotic channels between the middle and anterior cerebral arteries, which is one site for collateral circulation, are depicted. (Adapted from Fisher, 1975, and Martin, 1989.)

to a more extensive lesion, which may be unilateral or bilateral. Bilateral lesions cause signs of more than one of the characteristic syndromes that occur when only a single branch is occluded. Here we shall consider the simple case of a single occluded branch vessel giving rise to a single syndrome. In actual clinical situations, however, the occlusion often leads to mixtures of the individual syndromes.

The longitudinal continuity of ascending and descending pathways places the different tracts in relatively constant medial or lateral positions that are maintained in cross sections at different levels. Because the location of tracts and cranial nerve nuclei are fixed, specific combinations of signs reliably indicate the site of the lesion. Analysis of disorders of the brain stem is therefore greatly simplified by answers to two questions:

1. Is the lesion medial or lateral? At levels below the midbrain, lesions in long ascending and descending tracts lead to clinical signs that indicate whether the damage is medial or lateral (Table 46–3).
2. What is the level of the lesion? Specific cranial nerve signs delineate the actual level of the lesion (Table 46–4).

These signs, which localize the lesion in both the longitudinal and horizontal extent of the brain stem, can be best understood by referring to the figures that accompany the following descriptions of the lesions.

Medial Syndromes of the Medulla and Pons

Medial lesions arise from occlusion of the paramedian branches of the basilar artery. A unilateral medial lesion in either the pons or upper medulla affects the corticospinal tract and medial lemniscus, with corresponding signs on the other side of the body: contralateral hemiparesis and contralateral loss of position and vibratory sensation (Table 46–3 and Figure 46–12). The spinothalamic tracts are spared, so cutaneous sensation is preserved.

Medial syndromes of the medulla and pons can be differentiated by cranial nerve signs (Table 46–4 and Figure 46–12). In the medial syndrome of the medulla the emerging fibers of the hypoglossal nerve (XII) are involved (Figure 46–12A), causing ipsilateral weakness and later wasting of that half of the tongue. In the medial syndrome of the pons the lateral rectus muscle may be paralyzed if the lesion is rostral and extends dorsally to affect the nucleus of the abducens nerve (VI) or the emerging fibers of the nerve (Figures 46–12B and Fig 46–13). Lesions involving the nucleus of nerve VI are likely to cause ipsilateral gaze palsy rather than isolated paralysis of the abducens because of the proximity of the paramedian pontine reticular formation (Figure 46–8). Nystagmus may also be present if the lesion involves vestibular or cerebellar connections or the medial longitudinal fasciculus.

725

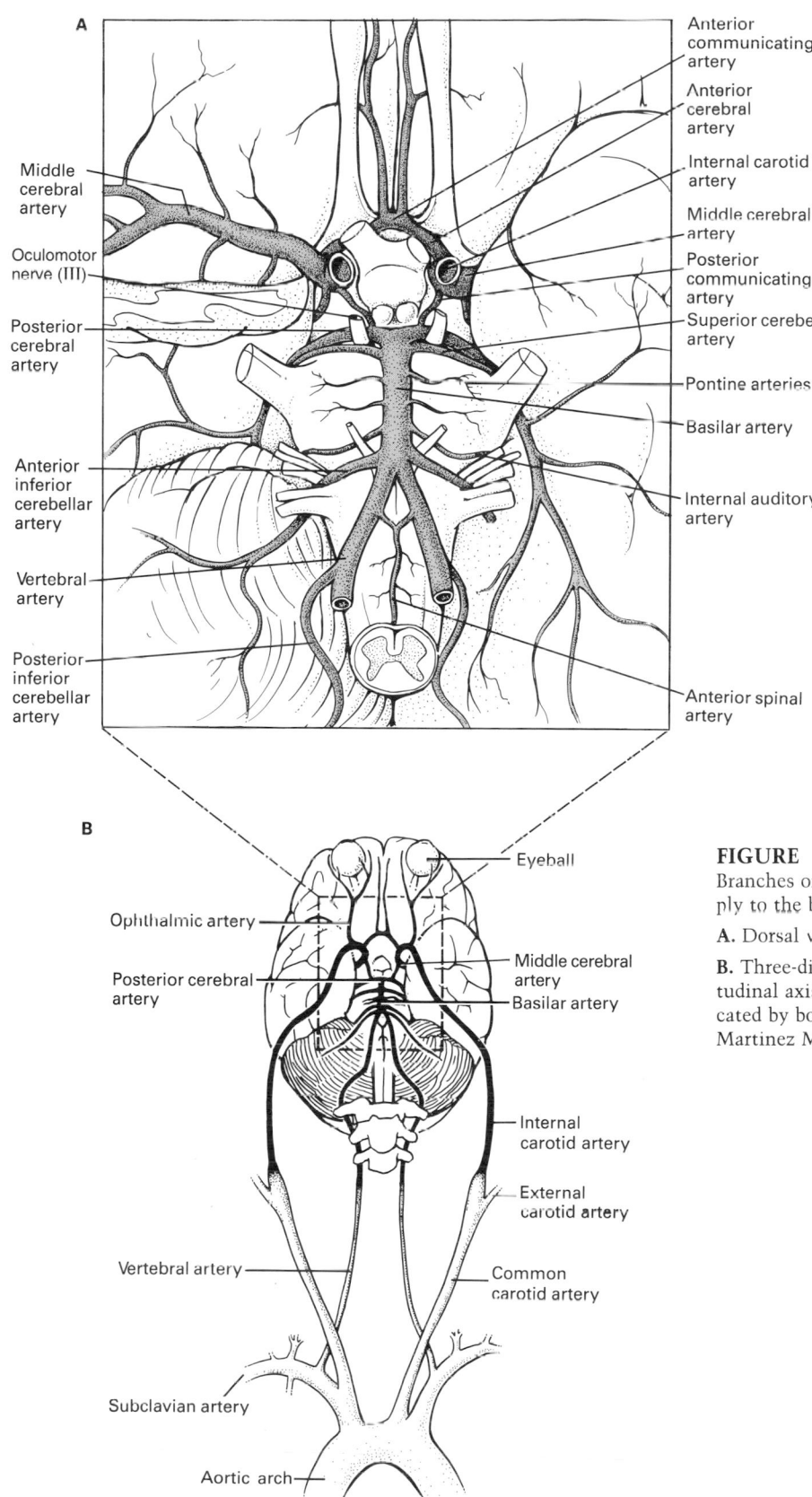

A

Middle cerebral artery

Oculomotor nerve (III)

Posterior cerebral artery

Anterior inferior cerebellar artery

Vertebral artery

Posterior inferior cerebellar artery

Anterior communicating artery

Anterior cerebral artery

Internal carotid artery

Middle cerebral artery

Posterior communicating artery

Superior cerebellar artery

Pontine arteries

Basilar artery

Internal auditory artery

Anterior spinal artery

B

Ophthalmic artery

Posterior cerebral artery

Vertebral artery

Subclavian artery

Aortic arch

Eyeball

Middle cerebral artery

Basilar artery

Internal carotid artery

External carotid artery

Common carotid artery

FIGURE 46–11

Branches of the vertebral arteries carry the blood supply to the brain stem.

A. Dorsal view. (Adapted from Patten, 1977.)

B. Three-dimensional blown-up view along the longitudinal axis of the brain stem. Details of area indicated by box are illustrated in part A. (Adapted from Martinez Martinez, 1982.)

TABLE 46–3. Features Common to Medial and Lateral Syndromes at Any Level of the Medulla or Pons

Syndromes	Structure involved	Signs
Medial	Corticospinal tract	Hemiparesis (contralateral)
	Medial lemniscus	Loss of position and vibration sense (contralateral)
	Cerebellar connections (pons)	Limb ataxia or nystagmus (ipsilateral)
Lateral	Cerebellar connections	Limb ataxia (ipsilateral)
	Sensory nucleus or descending sensory tract of trigeminal nerve	Loss of cutaneous sensation on face (ipsilateral)
	Descending autonomic fibers	Horner syndrome: miosis, ptosis, impaired sweating (ipsilateral)
	Spinothalamic tract	Loss of pain and temperature sensation (contralateral)
	Vestibular nuclei and connections	Nystagmus, nausea, vomiting
	Uncertain	Hiccup

Lateral Syndromes of the Medulla and Pons

Lateral lesions arise from occlusion of the posterior inferior cerebellar artery or the anterior inferior cerebellar artery. The resulting lesions affect lateral structures (not those affected in medial lesions). Lateral lesions involve the spinothalamic tract, descending autonomic fibers, the nucleus or descending sensory tract of the trigeminal nerve, vestibular nuclei, and cerebellar connections.

All lateral lesions involve a set of six common manifestations that may appear together or in different combinations (Table 46–3): (1) contralateral loss of pain and temperature sensation of the limbs and trunk due to damage in the spinothalamic tract; (2) ipsilateral Horner syndrome with miosis (small pupil with normal reaction to light), ptosis of the eyelid, and decreased sweating on the ipsilateral side of the face due to interruption of descending autonomic fibers; (3) ipsilateral loss of cutaneous sensation on the face from involvement of the sensory trigeminal nucleus or descending tract; (4) nystagmus and nausea attributed to involvement of vestibular connections; (5) ataxia of the ipsilateral limbs due to interruption of cerebellar connections (the restiform body in the medulla, and the middle and superior peduncles in the pons); and for reasons not known (6) hiccup. Lateral lesions do not cause hemiparesis or loss of proprioception.

Vascular lesions affect the brain stem at several levels, producing a variety of syndromes. Involvement of specific cranial nerves distinguishes the actual level of the syndrome.

TABLE 46–4. Specific Syndromes Produced at Different Levels by Vascular Lesions of the Brain Stem

Syndromes	Artery affected	Structure involved	Specific manifestations
Medullary			
Medial	Paramedian branches	Emerging fibers of nerve XII	Ipsilateral hemiparalysis of tongue
Lateral	Posterior inferior cerebellar	Emerging fibers of nerves IX and X	Dysphagia, hoarseness, ipsilateral paralysis of vocal cord; ipsilateral loss of pharyngeal reflex
		Solitary nucleus and tract	Loss of taste on tongue
Inferior pontine			
Medial	Paramedian branches	Pontine gaze center, near nucleus of nerve XI	Paralysis of gaze to side of lesion
		Vestibular nucleus or connections, or medial longitudinal fasciculus	Gaze-evoked nystagmus
		Nucleus or emerging fibers of nerve VI	Paralysis of ipsilateral lateral rectus
Lateral	Anterior inferior cerebellar	Emerging fibers of nerve VII	Ipsilateral facial paralysis
		Pontine gaze center	Paralysis of gaze to side of lesion
		Nerve VIII or cochlear nucleus	Deafness, tinnitus
Superior pontine			
Medial	Paramedian branches	Medial longitudinal fasciculus	Internuclear ophthalmoplegia
		Uncertain	Palatal myoclonus

A Medulla

Nucleus of N. XII
Medial lemniscus
Tractus solitarius with nucleus
Vestibular nucleus
Medial longitudinal fasciculus
Interior cerebellar peduncle
Olivocerebellar fibers
Nucleus ambiguus (motor nucleus of N. IX and X)
Descending tract of N. V
Descending sympathetic tract
Dorsal spinocerebellar tract
N. X
Ventral spinocerebellar tract
Spinothalamic tract
Lateral medullary syndrome (posterior inferior cerebellar artery)
Inferior olive
Pyramid   N.XII
Medial medullary syndrome (parmedian branches of basilar artery)

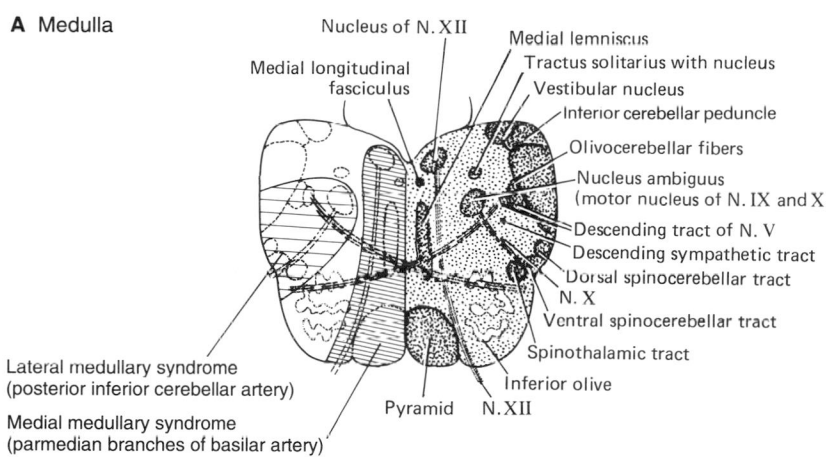

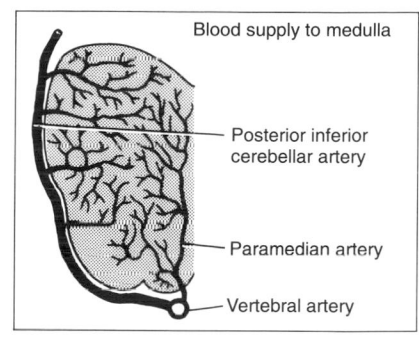

Blood supply to medulla
Posterior inferior cerebellar artery
Paramedian artery
Vertebral artery

B Lower pons

Medial longitudinal fasciculus
Nucleus of N.VI
Vestibular nucleus
Inferior cerebellar peduncle
Nucleus of N.VII
Dorsal cochlear nucleus
Spinal tract and nucleus of N. V
N.VIII
N.VII
Spinothalamic tract
Middle cerebellar peduncle
N. VI
Medial lemniscus
Lateral inferior pontine syndrome (anterior inferior cerebellar artery)
Corticospinal and corticobulbar tracts
Medial inferior pontine syndrome (paramedian branches of basilar artery)
Pontine nuclei and pontocerebellar fibers

C Upper pons

Medial longitudinal fasciculus
Superior cerebellar peduncle
Spinothalamic tract
Lateral lemniscus
Central tegmental bundle
Medial lemniscus
Pontine nuclei and pontocerebellar fibers
Corticospinal tract
Lateral superior pontine syndrome (superior cerebellar artery)
Medial superior pontine syndrome (paramedian branches of basilar artery)

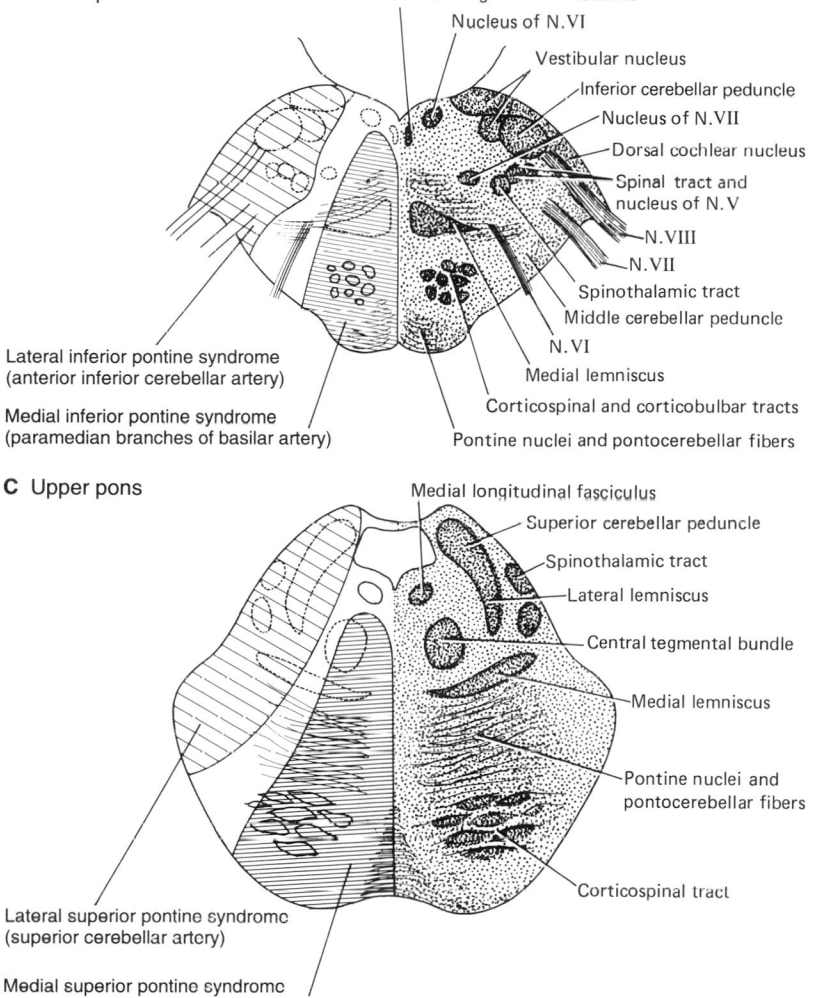

FIGURE 46–12

Syndromes of brain stem vascular lesions, indicated on the left in each figure. (Adapted from Adams and Victor, 1977.)

The lateral medullary syndrome (Wallenberg syndrome) is caused by an infarction in the distribution of the posterior inferior cerebellar artery (Figure 46–12A). Often, however, the actual occlusion is found in the parent vessel, the vertebral artery. The damaged area includes the dorsal portion of the lateral medulla, the lateral medullary tegmentum. In addition to the six common characteristics listed above, glossopharyngeal (IX) and vagal (X) nerves may be involved, causing difficulty in swallowing (dysphagia), hoarseness of the voice because of paralysis of the ipsilateral vocal cord, and loss of the ipsilateral pharyngeal reflex (Table 46–4). The solitary nucleus may also be destroyed, leading to loss of taste on the ipsilateral half of the tongue.

The lateral syndrome of the lower pons results from occlusion of the anterior inferior cerebellar artery (Figure 46–12B). It includes the six common manifestations noted above and three additional specific signs that arise from damage of the facial (VII) and auditory (VIII) nuclei: (1) ipsilateral facial paralysis of the lower motor neuron type because the lesion involves either the facial nucleus or the emerging fibers of the seventh nerve; (2) deafness and tinnitus; and (3) ipsilateral gaze paralysis if the lesion extends medially to affect the pontine gaze center.

Lateral lesions of the midpons result from occlusion of a short circumferential artery and cause a syndrome identical to that of lateral lesions in the lower pons, except that nerves VII and VIII are spared and there is no abnormality of facial movement or hearing. Instead, trigeminal motor functions are implicated: Bilateral lesions cause difficulty in chewing while unilateral lesions cause deviation of the jaw toward the side of the lesion when the mouth is opened. Lateral lesions of the superior pons (Figure 46–12C) arise from occlusion of the superior cerebellar artery;

there are no specific cranial signs. In other words, facial paralysis and hearing loss imply a lateral lesion of the lower pons; impaired trigeminal functions imply a lesion of the midpons; and none of these cranial nerves is affected by lesions of the upper pons.

Midbrain Syndromes

The clinical anatomy of the mesencephalon is less complicated than that of the medulla and pons, but even in this small area three separate syndromes are recognized (Figure 46–14). In the ventral syndrome (Weber syndrome) a lesion of the cerebral peduncle causes (1) contralateral hemiparesis, including supranuclear facial paresis due to damage of the corticospinal and corticobulbar tracts, and (2) ipsilateral oculomotor nerve palsy from damage of the emerging third-nerve fibers.

In the central or tegmental syndrome oculomotor nerve palsy is again seen because of a lesion in either a nucleus or emerging fibers, but there is also a tremor or involuntary movement of the contralateral limbs. This condition, called *hemichorea*, is attributed to a lesion in the red nucleus. In addition, there is contralateral hemianesthesia that affects both primary forms of sensation: cutaneous sensation (carried by the spinothalamic tract) and proprioception (carried in the medial lemniscus). The corticospinal tract is spared if the lesion is limited, as in Figure 46–14.

The dorsal midbrain or collicular syndrome (Parinaud syndrome) is usually caused by an extra-axial lesion, most often a tumor of the pineal gland (pinealoma) that compresses the superior colliculi and pretectal structures. This compression causes paralysis of upward gaze but does not affect other eye movements.

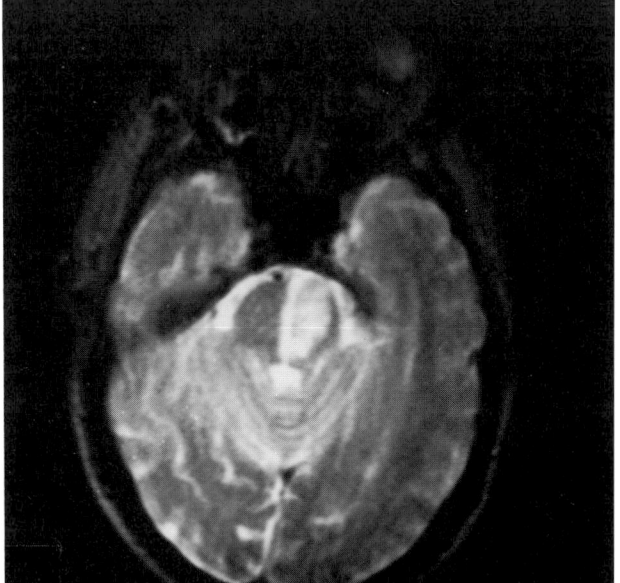

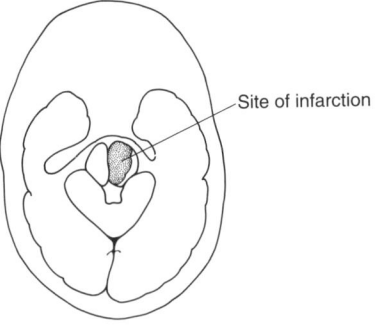

FIGURE 46–13
Magnetic resonance imaging shows a white highlight in the ventral portion of the left half of the pons. The lesion stops abruptly at the midline, suggesting unilateral occlusion of one or more paramedian vessels. (Note that the various observed parts of the brain are different in imaging and anatomic sections. In this figure, the ventral portion of the brain stem is uppermost, and the left side of the brain is on the right.)

Site of infarction

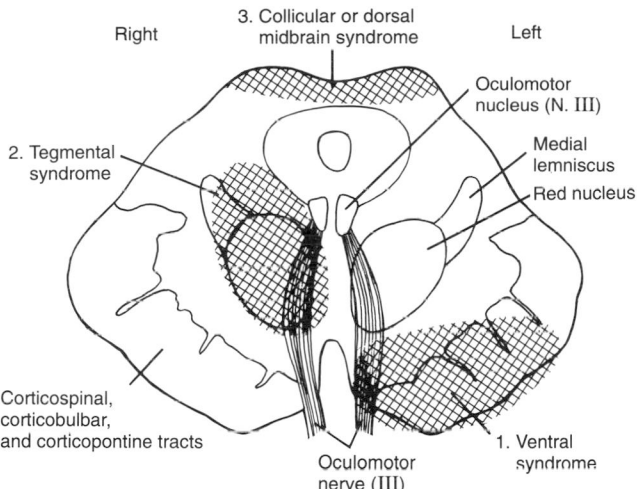

FIGURE 46–14
The three midbrain syndromes. (Adapted from Gatz, 1966.)

Coma and the Locked-In Syndrome

Because brain stem mechanisms are so important in maintaining alertness, lesions in this area often cause coma. It is therefore important to recognize brain stem signs in the examination of a comatose patient (see Chapter 52) or patients with space-occupying lesions, such as tumors, that are likely to cause brain stem signs due to downward tentorial herniation or herniation of the cerebellum through the foramen magnum.

Bilateral lesions of the ventral pons, usually due to occlusion of the basilar artery, may interrupt the corticobulbar and corticospinal tracts on both sides. As a result, the patient is quadriplegic, unable to speak, and incapable of facial movement. This state may resemble coma, but the eyes are open and move, and the patient is fully conscious and able to communicate by movement of the eyelids or eyes, although otherwise completely immobile or locked in.

An Overall View

The spinal cord may be affected by three types of diseases: traumatic, inherited, and acquired. The damage resulting in the spinal cord in each of these three types of disease may be segmental or longitudinal. The pattern of motor and sensory signs and the severity of the resulting disorder depend on the extent of the lesion.

Segmental lesions result most commonly from trauma or from tumors. There is characteristically a spinal level of disability below which motor or sensory functions are impaired. The pattern and severity of the resulting disorder depend on the extent of the lesion. For instance, traumatic transection of the cord may be complete or partial, and this difference is expressed in different patterns of neurological abnormality. Some segmental lesions pose diag-

nostic problems, however. For instance, syringomyelia and intramedullary tumors may be impossible to differentiate clinically because either lesion may cause segmental loss of cutaneous sensation or segmental loss of motor neuron function, with or without long tract signs. Another difficult distinction is that between intramedullary tumors and extramedullary compressive lesions. Myelography, angiography, computerized tomography, or magnetic resonance imaging are then necessary to determine the precise nature of the lesion.

Longitudinal disorders are those that involve particular ascending or descending tracts, whereas segmental disorders are caused by focal lesions. Longitudinal disorders are usually the result of heritable or metabolic conditions that selectively affect particular sets of nerve cells and their axons in the spinal cord (system degeneration). Sometimes, as in multiple sclerosis, there are clinical signs of both segmental and longitudinal lesions. The clinical syndromes that result from either segmental or longitudinal disorders are important diagnostically. They also provide insight into the organization of cells and tracts in the spinal cord.

In contrast to disorders of the spinal cord, syndromes of the brain stem are recognized because specific cranial nerve functions are affected. The cranial nerves are sometimes affected on one side and long tracts on the other, resulting in characteristic crossed syndromes that identify a brain stem lesion. In addition to stroke, multiple sclerosis and brain tumors are among the conditions that often affect brain stem nuclei and the tracts that ascend or descend. Knowledge of neuroanatomy often makes it possible to localize the lesion, even without the aid of elaborate technology, but modern imaging has made diagnosis of brain stem lesions much more precise. Analysis of brain stem syndromes tells us how the brain stem is organized and how it functions.

Selected Readings

Adams, R. D., and Victor, M. 1989. Principles of Neurology, 4th ed. New York: McGraw-Hill.

Ash, P. R., and Keltner, J. L. 1979. Neuro-ophthalmic signs in pontine lesions. Medicine (Baltimore) 58:304–320.

Bauer, G., Gerstenbrand, F., and Rumpl, E. 1979. Varieties of the locked-in syndrome. J. Neurol. 221:77–91.

Bilaniuk, L. T., Zimmerman, R. A., Littman, P., Gallo, E., Rorke, L. B., Bruce, D. A., and Schut, L. 1980. Computed tomography of brain stem gliomas in children. Radiology 134:89–95.

Caplan, L. R. 1980. "Top of the basilar" syndrome. Neurology 30:72–79.

Daniels, D. L., Williams, A. L., and Haughton, V. M. 1982. Computed tomography of the medulla. Radiology 145:63–69.

Fields, H. L. 1987. Pain. New York: McGraw-Hill.

Fields, H. L. (ed.) 1990. Pain Syndromes in Neurology. London: Butterworths.

Glaser, J. S. 1978. Neuro-ophthalmology. Hagerstown, Md.: Harper & Row.

Martin, J. H. 1989. Neuroanatomy: Text and Atlas. New York: Elsevier.

Plum, F., and Posner, J. B. 1980. The Diagnosis of Stupor and Coma, 3rd ed. Philadelphia: F. A. Davis.

References

Baloh, R. W., Furman, J. M., and Yee, R. D. 1985. Dorsal midbrain syndrome: Clinical and oculographic findings. Neurology 35: 54–60.

Barkhof, F., and Valk, J. 1988. "Top of the basilar" syndrome: A comparison of clinical and MR findings. Neuroradiology 30: 293–298.

Beal, M. F. 1990. (Editorial). Multiple cranial-nerve palsies: A diagnostic challenge. N. Engl. J. Med. 322:461–463.

Bydder, G. M., Steiner, R. E., Thomas, D. J., Marshall, J., Gilderdale, D. J., and Young, I. R. 1983. Nuclear magnetic resonance imaging of the posterior fossa: 50 cases. Clin. Radiol. 34:173–188.

Chiappa, K. H., and Ropper, A. H. 1982. Evoked potentials in clinical medicine. N. Engl. J. Med. 306:1205–1211.

Collins, R. D. 1962. Illustrated Manual of Neurologic Diagnosis. Philadelphia: Lippincott.

Cook, A. W., Nathan P. W., and Smith, M. C. 1984. Sensory consequences of commissural myelotomy. A challenge to traditional anatomical concepts. Brain 107:547–568.

Emerson, R. G., and Pedley, T. A. 1986. Effect of cervical spinal cord lesions on early components of the median nerve somatosensory evoked potential. Neurology 36:20–26.

Fisher, C. M. 1975. The anatomy and pathology of the cerebral vasculature. In J. S. Meyer (ed.), Modern Concepts of Cerebrovascular Disease. New York: Spectrum Publications.

Flannigan, B. D., Bradley, W. G., Jr., Mazziotta, J. C., Rauschning, W., Bentson, J. R., Lufkin, R. B., and Hieshima, G. B. 1985. Magnetic resonance imaging of the brainstem: Normal structure and basic functional anatomy. Radiology 154:375–383.

Freddo, L., Sacco R. L., Bello, J. A., Mohr, J. P., Tatemichi, T., and Petty, G. W. 1989. Lateral medullary syndrome: Clinicoanatomical features studied by magnetic resonance and vascular imaging. Ann. Neurol. 26:157.

Gatz, A. J. 1966. Manter's Essentials of Clinical Neuroanatomy and Neurophysiology, 3rd ed. Philadelphia: Davis.

Gildenberg, P. L., and Hirshberg, R. M. 1984. Limited myelotomy for the treatment of intractable cancer pain. J. Neurol. Neurosurg. Psychiatry 47:94–96.

Harner, S. G., and Laws, E. R., Jr. 1981. Diagnosis of acoustic neurinoma. Neurosurgery 9:373–379.

Ho, K.-L., and Meyer, K. R. 1981. The medial medullary syndrome. Arch. Neurol. 38:385–387.

Ischia, S., Luzzani, A., Ischia, A., and Maffezzoli, G. 1984. Bilateral percutaneous cervical cordotomy: Immediate and longterm results in 36 patients with neoplastic disease. J. Neurol. Neurosurg. Psychiatry 47:141–147.

Jagiella, W. M., and Sung, J. H. 1989. Bilateral infarction of the medullary pyramids in humans. Neurology 39:21–24.

Kalovidouris, A., Mancuso, A. A., and Dillon, W. 1984. A CT-clinical approach to patients with symptoms related to the V, VII, IX–XII cranial nerves and cervical sympathetics. Radiology 151:671–676.

Knepper, L., Biller, J., Adams, H. P. Jr., Yuh, W., Ryals, T., and Godersky, J. 1990. MR imaging of basilar artery occlusion. J. Comput. Assist. Tomogr. 14:32–36.

Levin, B. E., and Margolis, G. 1977. Acute failure of automatic respirations secondary to a unilateral brainstem infarct. Ann. Neurol. 1:583–586.

Lindenbaum, J., Healton, E. B., Savage, D. G., Brust, J. C. M., Garrett, T. J., Podell, E. R., Marcell, P. D., Stabler, S. P., and Allen, R. H. 1988. Neuropsychiatric disorders caused by cobalamin deficiency in the absence of anemia or macrocytosis. N. Engl. J. Med. 318:1720–1728.

Markand, O. N., Farlow, M. R., Stevens, J. C., and Edwards, M. K. 1989. Brain-stem auditory evoked potential abnormalities with unilateral brain-stem lesions demonstrated by magnetic resonance imaging. Arch. Neurol. 46:295–299.

Martinez Martinez, P. F. A. 1982. Neuroanatomy: Development and Structure of the Central Nervous System. Philadelphia: Saunders.

Masamitsu, A., Kjellberg, R. N., and Adams, R. D. 1989. Clinical presentations of vascular malformations of the brain stem: Comparison of angiographically positive and negative types. J. Neurol. Neurosurg. Psychiatry 52:167–175.

Mawad, M. E., Silver, A. J., Hilal, S. K., and Ganti, S. R. 1983. Computed tomography of the brain stem with intrathecal metrizamide. Part I: The normal brain stem. Am. J. Neuroradiology 4:1–11.

Patten, J. 1977. Neurological Differential Diagnosis. New York: Springer.

Pryse-Phillips, W. 1989. Infarction of the medulla and cervical cord after fitness exercises. Stroke 20:292–294.

Reznik, M. 1983. Neuropathology in seven cases of locked-in syndrome. J. Neurol. Sci. 60:67–78.

Schwaighofer, B. W., Klein, M. V., Lyden, P. D., and Hesselink, J. R. 1990. MR imaging of vertebro basilar disease. J. Comput. Assist. Tomogr. 14:895–904.

Seales, D. M., Torkelson, R. D., Shuman, R. M., Rossiter, V. S., and Spencer, J. D. 1981. Abnormal brainstem auditory evoked potentials and neuropathology in "locked-in" syndrome. Neurology 31:893–896.

Sears, E. S., and Franklin, G. M. 1980. Diseases of the cranial nerves. In R. N. Rosenberg (ed.), The Science and Practice of Clinical Medicine, Vol. 5: Neurology. New York: Grune & Stratton, pp. 471–494.

Sever, J. L., and Gibbs, C. J. Jr. (eds.) 1988. Retroviruses in the nervous system. Ann. Neurol. Suppl. 23:S1–S217.

Uppington, J., and Warfield, C. A. 1988. Chronic pain in the perineum, groin, and genitalia. Hosp. Prac. 23:37–52.

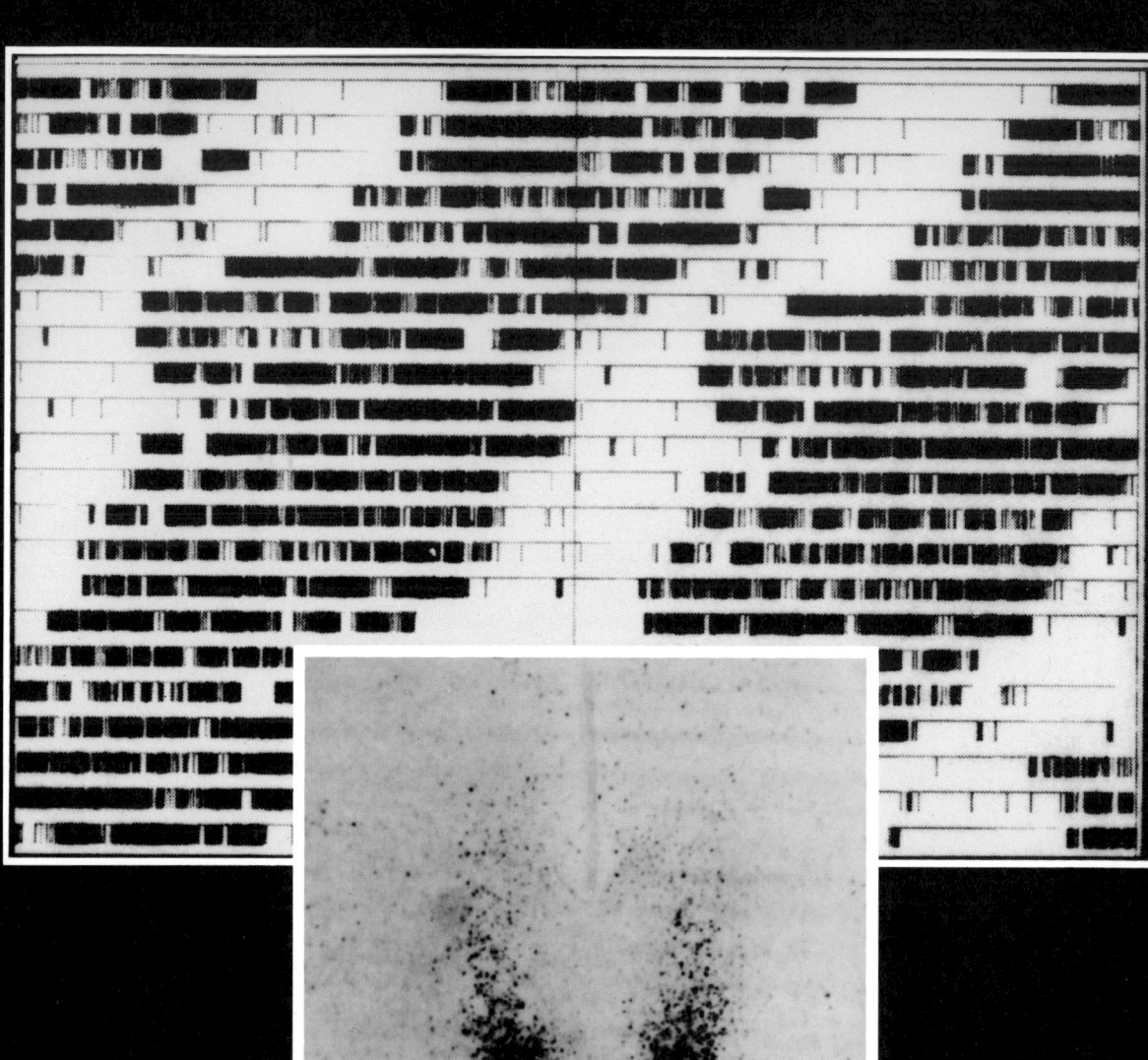

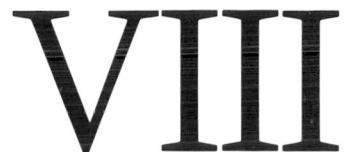

Hypothalamus, Limbic System, and Cerebral Cortex: Homeostasis and Arousal

O ne function of the nervous system is to maintain the constancy of the internal environment. These regulatory processes have intrigued many of the founders of modern physiology, Claude Bernard, Walter Cannon, and Walter Hess. Although virtually the whole brain is involved in homeostasis, neurons controlling the internal environment are concentrated in the hypothalamus, a small area of the diencephalon that comprises less than 1% of the total volume of the brain.

The hypothalamus and closely linked structures in the limbic system keep the internal environment constant by regulating endocrine secretion, the autonomic nervous system, and emotions and drives. Through its control of the endocrine system and autonomic nervous system, the

hypothalamus acts *directly* on the internal environment to maintain homeostasis. Through its control of emotions and motivated behavior, the hypothalamus acts *indirectly* in maintaining homeostasis by motivating animals and human beings to act on their environment. In regulating emotional expression, the hypothalamus functions in conjunction with higher control systems in the limbic system and neocortex.

In addition to regulating specific motivated behaviors, the hypothalamus and the cerebral cortex are involved in arousal—the maintenance of a general state of awareness. The level of arousal varies from different degrees of excitement to drowsiness, sleep, and coma.

Our lives are governed by daily fluctuations in many physiological activities. A prominent example is sleep and wakefulness. These cyclic behaviors are mediated by complex neuronal circuits, several of which have now been identified. Through phylogeny, these mechanisms were shaped by the earth's daily rotation around the sun, which results in night and day. The behavioral cycles are therefore called circadian rhythms. In vertebrates the neurons that mediate circadian rhythms are located in the suprachiasmic nucleus. The top panel shows activity traces, obtained in humans, without time cues. The periods of activity become longer than 24 hours. (Courtesy of

J. Zimmerman, reproduced from Moore-Ede, Sulzman, and Fuller, *The Clocks That Time Us*, Harvard University Press, 1982.) One of the cellular mechanisms involved in circadia behaviors is altered gene expression. The bottom panel shows that circadian rhythm is reflected in the expression of the *fos* oncoprotein in neurons of the suprachiasmatic nucleus of a hamster after exposure to light. The protein is detected immunohistochemically with anti-*fos* antibodies. In animals deprived of light, *fos* cannot be detected in these neurons. (Courtesy of Benjamin Rusak, Dalhousie University, Canada.)

PART VIII

Chapter 47: **Hypothalamus and Limbic System: Peptidergic Neurons, Homeostasis, and Emotional Behavior**
Chapter 48: **Hypothalamus and Limbic System: Motivation**
Chapter 49: **The Autonomic Nervous System**
Chapter 50: **The Collective Electrical Behavior of Cortical Neurons: The Electroencephalogram and the Mechanisms of Epilepsy**
Chapter 51: **Sleep and Dreaming**
Chapter 52: **Disorders of Sleep and Consciousness**

47

Irving Kupfermann

Hypothalamus and Limbic System: Peptidergic Neurons, Homeostasis, and Emotional Behavior

The Anatomy of the Hypothalamus and Limbic System Reflects Their Interrelated Functions

Higher Cortical Centers Communicate with the Hypothalamus via the Limbic System

The Structure of the Hypothalamus Reflects Its Diverse Functions

The Hypothalamus Contains Various Classes of Peptidergic Neuroendocrine Cells

Peptidergic Neurons Control Endocrine Function

Magnocellular Neurons Secrete Oxytocin and Vasopressin

Parvocellular Neurons Secrete Inhibiting and Releasing Hormones

Both Magnocellular and Parvocellular Neurons Contain Multiple Peptides that Are Found Throughout the Nervous System

Hypothalamic Neurons Participate in Four Classes of Reflexes

Milk Ejection and Uterine Contraction Are Regulated by Neural Input and Humoral Output

Urine Flow Is Regulated by Humoral Input and Output

Feedback Loops Involve Humoral Input and Output

Central Effects of Hormones on Behavior Involve Humoral Input and Neural Output

Neurons in the Hypothalamus Undergo Structural and Biochemical Changes in Response to Behavioral Demands

The Hypothalamus Helps Regulate the Autonomic Nervous System and Is Involved in Emotional Behavior

An Overall View

The living organism does not really exist in the *milieu exterieur*—the atmosphere it breathes, salt or fresh water if that is its element—but in the liquid *milieu interieur* formed by the circulatory organic liquid which surrounds and bathes all the tissue elements; this is the lymph and the plasma. . . . The *milieu interieur* surrounding the organs, the tissue and their element never varies. . . . Here we have an organism which has enclosed itself in a kind of hot house. The peripheral changes of external conditions cannot reach it; it is not subject to them, but is free and independent. . . . All the vital mechanisms, however varied they may be, have only one object, that of preserving constant the conditions of life in the internal environment.

> Claude Bernard, *Leçons sur les phénomènes de la vie communs aux animaux et aux végétaux*, 1878–1879

Constancy in the internal environment of the body is the result of a system of control mechanisms that limit the variability of body states. The tendency toward stability in the body is called *homeostasis*, a concept introduced by the physiologist Walter Cannon in 1932. The key neuronal mechanisms related to maintaining homeostasis are located in the hypothalamus, which acts on three major systems: the endocrine system, autonomic nervous system, and an ill-defined neural system concerned with motivation.

The hypothalamus and related structures in the limbic system receive information directly from the internal environment and act directly on the internal environment. Other parts of the brain affect the internal environment largely indirectly, through action on the external environment. The indirect and direct ways of regulating the internal environment often function in parallel. For example, if a room is cold, body temperature can be kept constant directly by peripheral vasoconstriction, or indirectly by closing the window or turning up the heat.

In this chapter we shall first briefly examine the anatomy of the hypothalamus and limbic system. We shall then consider the role of the hypothalamus in organizing

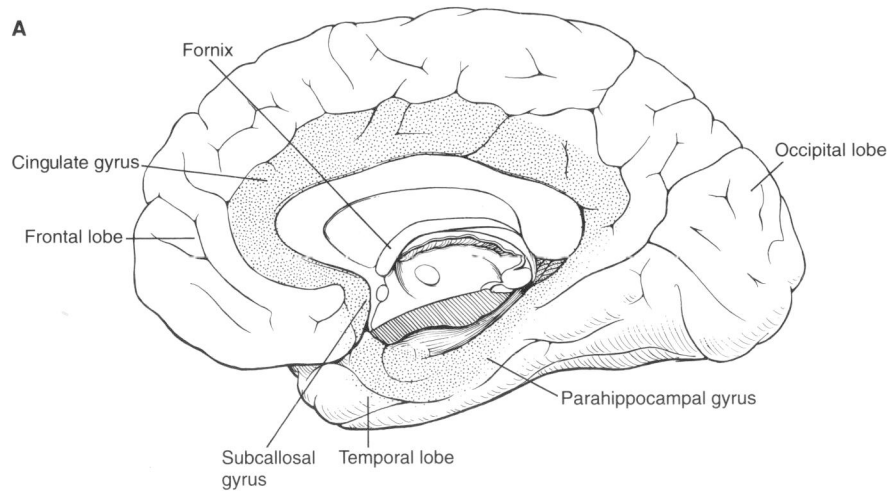

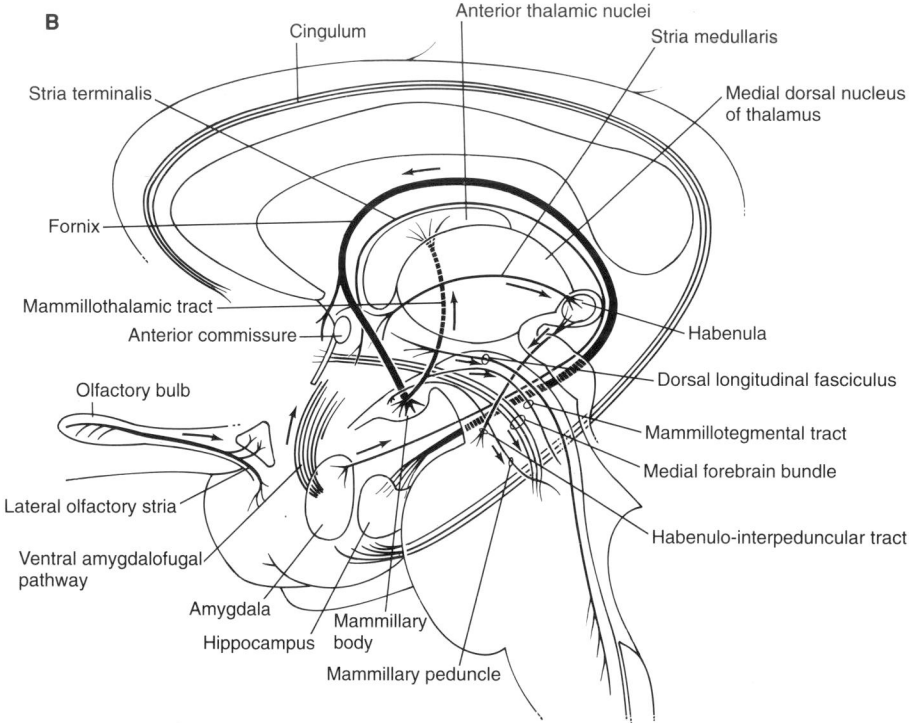

FIGURE 47–1

The limbic system consists of the limbic lobe and deep-lying structures. (Adapted from Nieuwenhuys, Voodg, and van Huijzen, 1981.)

A. This medial view of the brain shows the limbic lobe, which consists of primitive cortical tissue (**stippled area**) that encircles the upper brain stem. Also included in the limbic lobe are the underlying cortical structures (hippocampus and dentate gyrus).

B. Interconnections of the deep-lying structures included in the limbic system. The predominant direction of flow of neural activity in each tract is indicated by an arrow, but the designated tracts typically have bidirectional activity.

endocrine and autonomic functions. Although the hypothalamus constitutes less than 1% of the total volume of the human brain, it contains a large number of neuronal circuits that regulate vital functions: temperature, heart rate, blood pressure, blood osmolarity, and water and food intake. In the next chapter we shall focus on the role of motivational states in homeostatic regulation. In Chapter 49 we shall consider the primary role of the autonomic nervous system in feedback-regulated control of the internal environment.

Hypothalamic and limbic structures are also important in regulating emotional behavior and reproduction. We shall therefore examine in this chapter the role of the

hypothalamus in organizing motor and endocrine responses that constitute adaptive emotional behavior. Emotions are further considered in Chapter 56 and sexual behavior is discussed in Chapter 61.

The Anatomy of the Hypothalamus and Limbic System Reflects Their Interrelated Functions

The hypothalamus is extensively interconnected with a ring of cortical structures that are part of the limbic system. We shall first consider the structure and interconnections of the components of the limbic system, and then the hypothalamus.

Higher Cortical Centers Communicate with the Hypothalamus via the Limbic System

The concept of the limbic system derives from the idea of a limbic lobe (Latin, *limbus* border), a term introduced by Paul Broca to characterize gyri that form a ring around the brain stem and consist of what is considered to be phylogenetically primitive cortex. The limbic lobe includes the parahippocampal gyrus, the cingulate gyrus, and the subcallosal gyrus, which is the anterior and inferior continuation of the cingulate gyrus (Figure 47–1A). It also includes the underlying cortex of the hippocampal formation, which is morphologically more simple than the overlying cortex. The hippocampal formation includes the hippocampus proper, the dentate gyrus, and the subiculum.

In 1937 James Papez suggested that the limbic lobe formed a neural circuit that provides the anatomical substratum for emotions. Based on experiments suggesting that the hypothalamus has a critical role in the expression of emotion (see later section), Papez argued that, since emotions reach consciousness and thought and conversely, higher cognitive functions affect emotions, the hypothalamus must communicate reciprocally with higher cortical centers. He proposed that the cortex influences the hypothalamus through connections of the cingulate gyrus to the hippocampal formation. According to this idea, the hippocampal formation would process this information and project it to the mammillary bodies of the hypothalamus by way of the fornix (a distinct fiber bundle, see Figures 47–1B and 47–3B, C). The hypothalamus would in turn provide information to the cingulate gyrus by a pathway from the mammillary bodies to the anterior thalamic nuclei (through the mammillothalamic tract) and from the anterior thalamic nuclei to the cingulate gyrus (Figure 47–2, thick lines).

The concept of the limbic system was later expanded by Paul MacLean to include other structures functionally and anatomically related to those described by Papez. MacLean included in the limbic system parts of the hypothalamus, the septal area, the nucleus accumbens (a part of the striatum), neocortical areas such as the orbitofrontal cortex, and the amygdala. The amygdala is a subcortical structure located at the dorsomedial tip of the temporal lobe and continuous with the uncus of the parahippocampal gyrus.

Modern anatomical studies have supported Papez's outline of the limbic system, and have demonstrated extensive and direct connections between neocortical areas, the hippocampal formation, and the amygdala (Figure 47–2, connections indicated in thin lines). These studies have shown that the hippocampus receives its major input from the entorhinal cortex by way of the *perforant path*. The entorhinal cortex in turn receives its input from areas of the association cortex and thereby provides a link between the neocortex and the limbic system. Fibers from the entorhinal cortex that reach the hippocampus by means of the perforant pathway pass through the subiculum, an area of cortex that receives major output from the

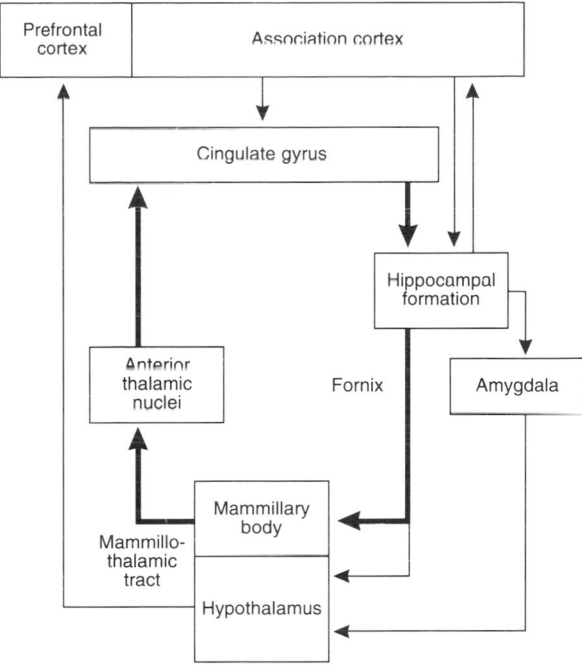

FIGURE 47–2
A proposed neural circuit for emotion. The circuit originally proposed by James Papez is indicated by **thick lines;** more recently described connections are shown by **fine lines**. Known projections of the fornix to hypothalamic regions (mammillary bodies and other hypothalamic areas) and of the hypothalamus to the prefrontal cortex are indicated. A pathway interconnecting the amygdala to limbic structures is shown. Finally, reciprocal connections between the hippocampal formation and the association cortex are indicated. The hippocampal formation includes the hippocampus proper and surrounding structures, including entorhinal cortex and the subicular complex.

hippocampus and has extensive reciprocal connections with many areas of the brain, including several areas of the neocortex. The subiculum (and pre- and parasubiculum) is the origin of those fibers in the fornix that innervate the hypothalamus. The fornix also contains axons of hippocampal pyramidal cells that innervate nonhypothalamic structures. It is significant that the relative size of the subiculum increases in phylogeny and is largest in humans.

The amygdala is composed of many nuclei that are reciprocally connected to the hypothalamus, hippocampal formation, neocortex, and thalamus. It gives rise to two major efferent (descending) projections: the stria terminalis and the ventral amygdalofugal pathway (Figure 47–1B). The *stria terminalis* innervates the bed nucleus of the stria terminalis, the nucleus accumbens, and the hypothalamus. The *ventral amygdalofugal pathway* provides input to the hypothalamus, dorsal medial nucleus of the thalamus, and rostral cingulate gyrus. The amygdala in turn receives an important afferent input from the olfactory system and also inputs from the other afferent systems.

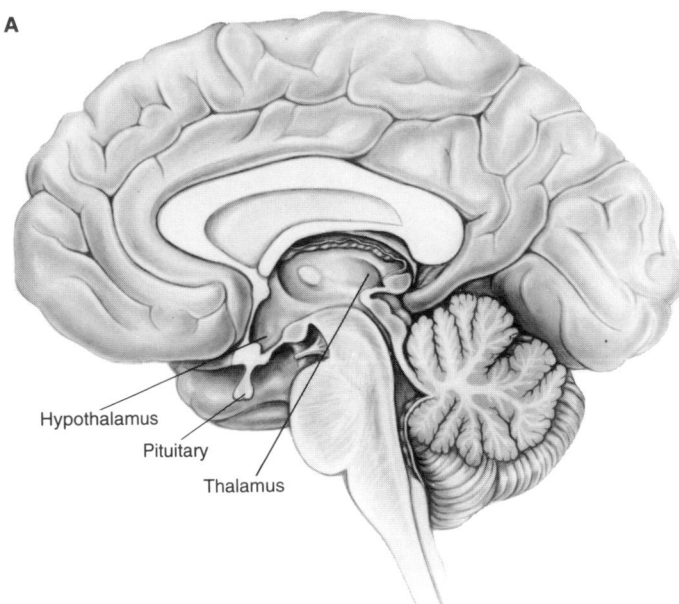

A

Hypothalamus

Pituitary

Thalamus

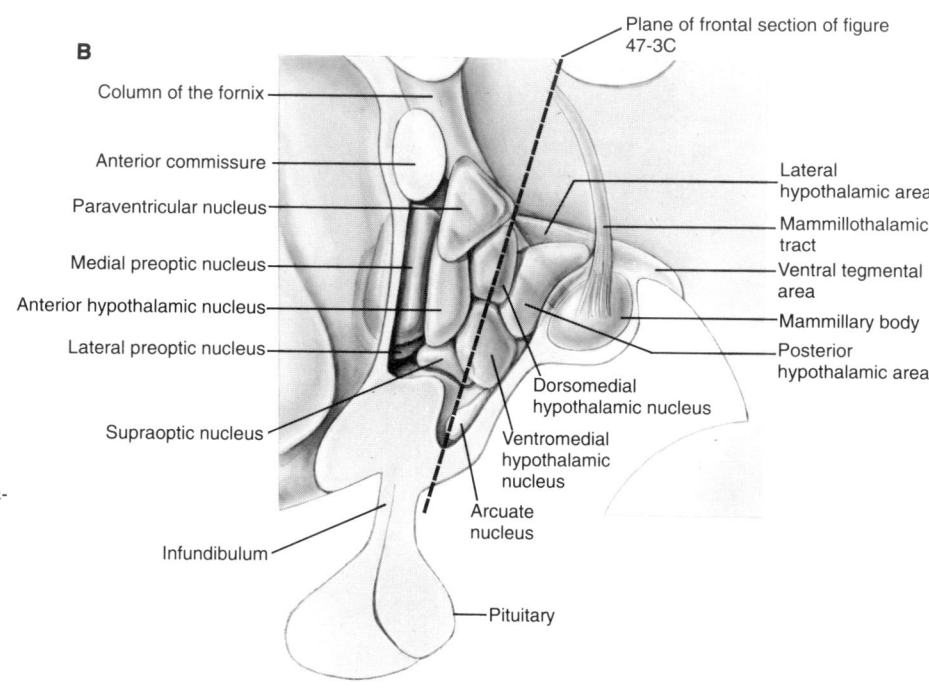

B

Plane of frontal section of figure 47-3C

Column of the fornix

Anterior commissure

Paraventricular nucleus

Medial preoptic nucleus

Anterior hypothalamic nucleus

Lateral preoptic nucleus

Supraoptic nucleus

Infundibulum

Lateral hypothalamic area

Mammillothalamic tract

Ventral tegmental area

Mammillary body

Posterior hypothalamic area

Dorsomedial hypothalamic nucleus

Ventromedial hypothalamic nucleus

Arcuate nucleus

Pituitary

FIGURE 47–3

The location and structure of the hypothalamus. (Adapted from Nieuwenhuys, Voodg, and van Huijzen, 1981.)

A. Medial view showing the relationship of the hypothalamus to the pituitary and thalamus.

B. Medial view showing positions of the main hypothalamic nuclei. Some nuclei are visible only in the frontal view in part C.

C. Frontal view of the hypothalamus (section along plane shown in part A).

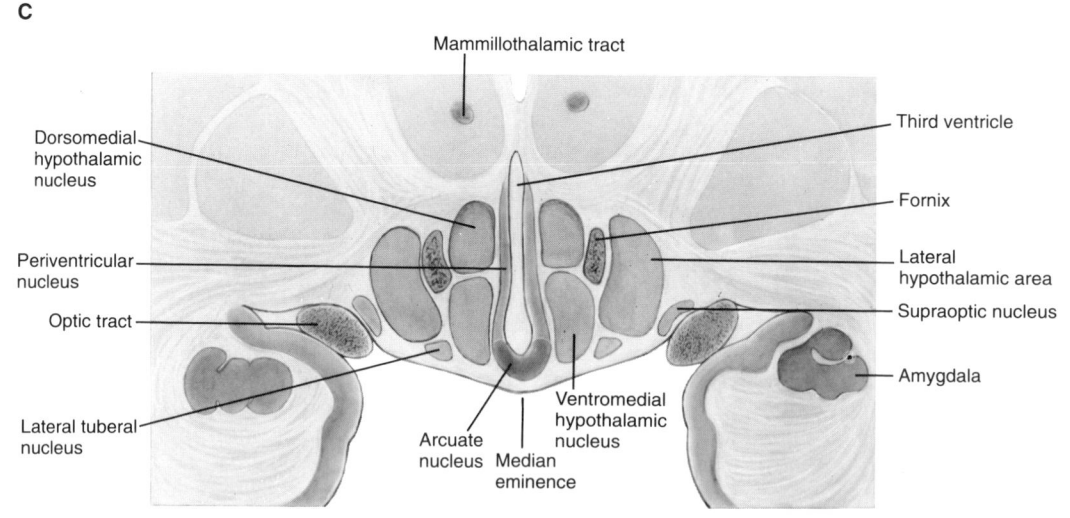

C

Mammillothalamic tract

Dorsomedial hypothalamic nucleus

Periventricular nucleus

Optic tract

Lateral tuberal nucleus

Arcuate nucleus

Median eminence

Ventromedial hypothalamic nucleus

Third ventricle

Fornix

Lateral hypothalamic area

Supraoptic nucleus

Amygdala

Despite its extensive olfactory input, the amygdala is not essential for olfactory discrimination. Lesions and electrical stimulation of the amygdala produce a variety of effects on autonomic responses, emotional behaviors, and feeding. These effects are often similar to those associated with stimulation and lesioning of the lateral or medial regions of the hypothalamus (discussed below and in Chapter 48). Finally, the amygdala has been implicated in the process of learning, particularly those tasks that require coordination of information from different sensory modalities, or the association of a stimulus and an affective (emotional) response.

In 1937, the same year that Papez described the limbic circuit, Heinrich Klüver and Paul Bucy reported their finding that bilateral destruction of the temporal lobe, which includes several limbic structures, such as the hippocampus and amygdala, produced dramatic changes in the emotional behavior of monkeys. Papez, Klüver, and Bucy provided the background for many later theoretical and experimental approaches to the neurobiology of emotions.

The Structure of the Hypothalamus Reflects Its Diverse Functions

One of the prime functions of the hypothalamus is to control the pituitary gland, to which it is attached by a stalk called the *infundibulum* (Figure 47–3B). The posterior extent of the hypothalamus is delimited by the mammillary bodies. The anterior extent is delimited by the optic chiasm, preoptic area, and lamina terminalis.

The hypothalamus can be grossly divided in the lateral-medial direction into lateral, medial, and periventricular regions. It can also be divided in the anterior-posterior direction into anterior, middle, and posterior regions. The *lateral region* has long fibers that project to the spinal cord and cortex, and also has extensive short-fiber, multisynaptic ascending and descending pathways. Most prominent of these fiber systems is the medial forebrain bundle, a major tract that runs through the lateral hypothalamus and continues rostrally to end in the telencephalon. Many aminergic neurons originating in the brain stem project to neocortical regions by way of fibers in the medial forebrain bundle and its rostral continuation in the cingulum bundle. The *medial region* of the hypothalamus is separated from the lateral region by the descending columns of the fornix. It contains most of the well-delineated nuclei of the hypothalamus, including (1) the preoptic nuclei and suprachiasmatic nuclei in the anterior region; (2) the dorsomedial, ventromedial, and paraventricular nuclei in the middle region; and (3) the posterior nucleus and mammillary bodies in the posterior region (Figure 47–3B and C). The *periventricular region* consists of those parts of the hypothalamus immediately bordering the third ventricle. The basal portion of the medial region and the periventricular region contain many of the small (parvicellular) hypothalamic neurons that secrete the substances that control the release of anterior pituitary hormones (discussed later in the section on peptidergic neurons). Within the basal region are the tuberal nuclei, found in primates, and the arcuate nucleus, found in lower animals.

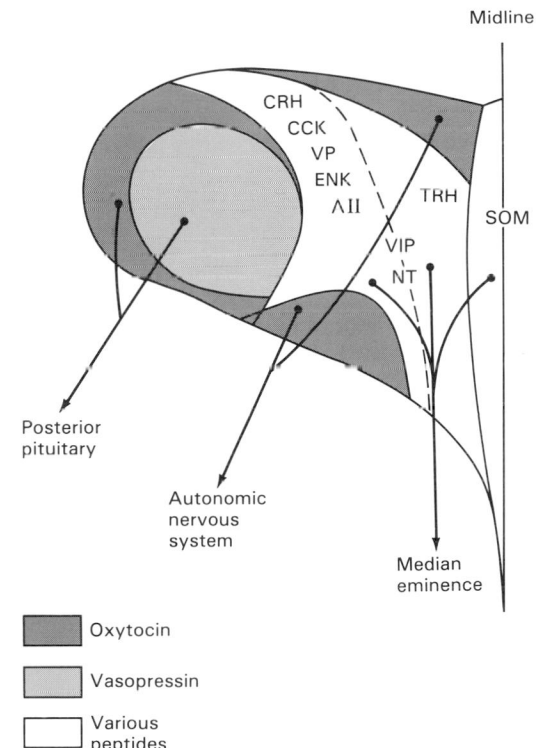

FIGURE 47–4

The paraventricular nucleus of the hypothalamus (frontal section, see Figure 47–3). This schematic representation shows some of the major peptides as well as the projection sites of neurons in different subregions of the nucleus. Abbreviations: **AII**, angiotensin II; **CRH**, corticotropin-releasing hormone; **CCK**, cholecystokinin; **ENK**, enkephalin peptides; **NT**, neurotensin; **SOM**, somatostatin; **TRH**, thyrotropin-releasing hormone; **VIP**, vasoactive intestinal peptide; **VP**, vasopressin. (Adapted from Kiss, 1988, and Swanson and Sawchenko, 1983.)

Each nucleus of the hypothalamus typically subserves a variety of functions. This is most clearly seen in the paraventricular nucleus (PVN), a highly differentiated structure that contains anatomically discrete regions of neurons containing specific peptides and combinations of peptides (Figure 47–4). The neurons can be classified into three groups: those that project to the posterior pituitary, those that project to the median eminence, and those associated with the autonomic nervous system.

Most fiber systems of the hypothalamus are bidirectional. Projections to and from areas caudal to the hypothalamus are carried in the medial forebrain bundle, the mammillotegmental tract, and the dorsal longitudinal fasciculus. Rostral structures are interconnected to the hypothalamus by means of the mammillothalamic tract, fornix, and stria terminalis. There are two important exceptions to the rule that fibers are bidirectional in the hypothalamus. The hypothalamohypophyseal tract contains only descending axons of paraventricular and supraoptic neurons, which terminate primarily in the posterior pituitary. The hypothalamus also receives one-way afferent connections directly from the retina. These fibers terminate primarily in the suprachiasmatic nucleus, which is involved in generating light-dark cycles (circadian rhythms, see Chapters 48 and 51).

The Hypothalamus Contains Various Classes of Peptidergic Neuroendocrine Cells

Many neurons in the hypothalamus are specialized for the synthesis and secretion of peptides, and individual neurons typically release more than one peptide. Some of the neurons release their peptides into a synaptic cleft where these peptides act locally as neurotransmitters. Others release their peptides into the circulation and these peptides act as hormones on distant cells. The actions of peptides tend to be enduring and to serve modulating functions, controlling neuron excitability and synaptic effectiveness (see Chapter 12). These long-lasting actions are thought to be important for a variety of behavioral functions, including mood, motivational state, and learning.

Peptidergic Neurons Control Endocrine Function

One of the main functions of the hypothalamus is the control of the endocrine system. This is accomplished in two ways: (1) *directly*, by secretion of neuroendocrine products into the general circulation through the vasculature of the *posterior pituitary* (neural lobe or neurohy-

pophysis), and (2) *indirectly*, by secretion of regulating hormones into the local portal plexus (within the median eminence), which drains into the blood vessels of the *anterior pituitary* (adenohypophysis). The hypothalamic regulating hormones, which can be either releasing or inhibiting, control the synthesis and release of anterior pituitary hormones into the general circulation.

Our current understanding of the endocrine function of the hypothalamus is based on the analysis of the direct and indirect types of control by Ernst and Berta Scharrer and Geoffrey Harris. The Scharrers developed the concept of *neurosecretion*, the idea that certain neurons function in two roles: as nerve cells that receive and transmit electrical information, and as endocrine cells that release their secretory products into the blood stream (Figure 47–5). They function as neuroendocrine transducers that convert neural information into hormonal information. Harris recognized the importance of the blood supply that connects the pituitary to the hypothalamus—the pituitary–hypophyseal–portal system—and showed that this vascular link carries hormonal information from the hypothalamus to the pituitary (Figure 47–6). These ideas are the basis of modern neuroendocrinology and our current understanding of the hypothalamic control of endocrine activity.

Each type of endocrine control (direct and indirect) is mediated by a distinct class of peptidergic neuroendocrine neurons. In both classes of neurons the neurohormone or

FIGURE 47–5

In contrast to conventional autonomic neurons, hypothalamic neuroendocrine cells release secretory products into the blood stream. (Adapted from Reichlin, 1978.)

A. Conventional autonomic neurons.
1. Exocrine glands are innervated by postganglionic neurons that stimulate secretion through synaptic action of acetylcholine (ACh). **2.** The adrenal medulla is innervated by sympathetic preganglionic neurons.

B. In hypothalamic neuroendocrine cells, the neurohormone or precursor peptide is synthesized in the cell body and transported by axoplasmic flow to release sites. **1.** In the *neurohypophyseal system* the secretions (vasopressin or oxytocin) are transported to the nerve terminals in the neural lobe of the pituitary. Activity of the neuron leads to the release of the hormone into the general circulation. **2.** In the *adenohypophyseal system* the secretions (releasing or regulating hormones) are transported to nerve terminals in the median eminence (and in some species, the pituitary stalk). Activity of these neurons leads to secretion of the regulating hormones into the hypophyseal-portal circulation and the release or inhibition of release of hormones from the anterior pituitary.

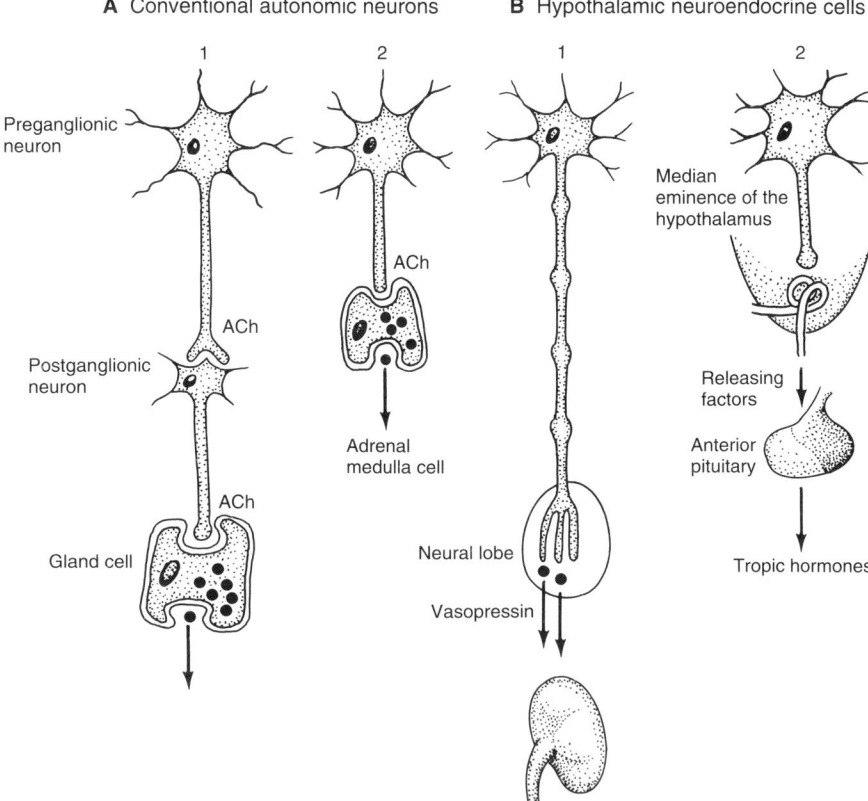

A Conventional autonomic neurons

B Hypothalamic neuroendocrine cells

FIGURE 47–6

Various functional elements participate in the control of the pituitary by the hypothalamus. Peptidergic neurons (5) release oxcytocin or vasopressin into the general circulation via the posterior pituitary. Two general types of neurons are involved in regulation of the anterior pituitary. Peptidergic neurons (3,4) form the releasing hormones that enter the capillary plexus of the hypophyseal–portal vessels. The second type of neuron is the link between the rest of the brain and the peptidergic neuron. These neurons, some of which are monoaminergic, are believed to end on the cell body of the peptidergic neuron in a conventional manner (1), or to end on the axon terminal of the peptidergic neuron (2) by means of axo-axonic synapses. (Adapted from Reichlin, 1978, Gay, 1972.)

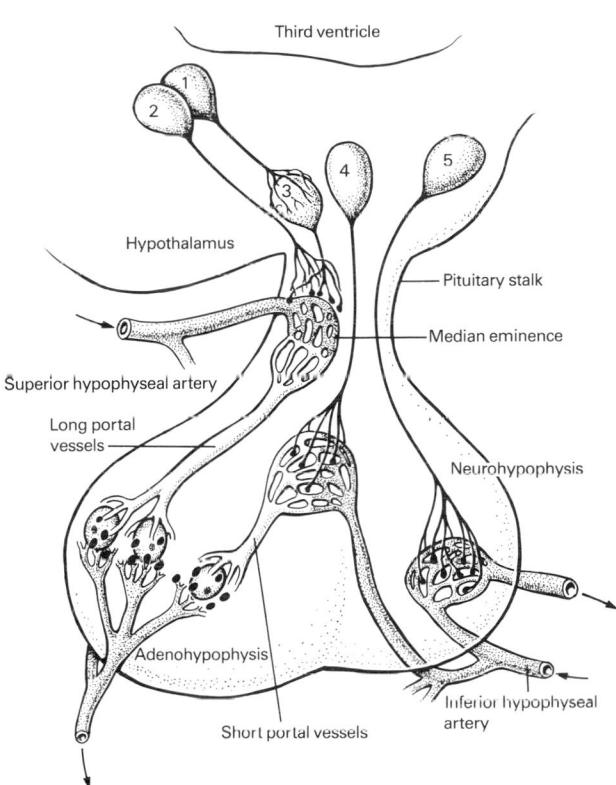

precursor peptide is synthesized in the cell body and packaged in neurosecretory vesicles that are transported down the axon to the terminal, where they are stored and released by secretion when the neuron is stimulated. The *magnocellular* (large) neuroendocrine neurons are located in the paraventricular and supraoptic nuclei. Some of the cells release the neurohypophyseal hormone *oxytocin*, and others release *vasopressin* into the general circulation by way of the posterior pituitary. The *parvocellular* (small) neuroendocrine neurons are located in several hypothalamic regions: the medial basal region, the arcuate and tuberal nuclei, the periventricular region, and the preoptic and paraventricular nuclei. The parvocellular neurons secrete peptides into the portal vasculature to stimulate or inhibit secretions from the anterior pituitary gland. The capillaries of the posterior pituitary and median eminence are highly fenestrated (perforated), facilitating the entry of the magnocellular hormones into the general circulation (through the posterior pituitary) or of the parvocellular hormones into the portal plexus (from the median eminence).

Magnocellular Neurons Secrete Oxytocin and Vasopressin

In 1950 Vincent du Vigneaud determined the amino acid sequence of oxytocin. Four years later he worked out the sequence of vasopressin, thereby providing the first evidence that these hormonal functions of the brain are mediated by peptides. Vasopressin and oxytocin contain nine amino acid residues each (Table 47–1). As with most peptide hormones, both vasopressin and oxytocin are cleaved from a larger prohormone. The prohormones for vasopressin and oxytocin are synthesized in the cell bodies of the magnocellular neurons, and are cleaved within the vesicles during their transport down the axons. The peptide *neurophysin* is a cleavage product of the processing of both vasopressin and oxytocin; however, the neurophysin formed in neurons that release vasopressin differs somewhat from that produced in neurons that release oxytocin. Each neurophysin is released along with its hormone at the terminals in the posterior pituitary.

TABLE 47–1. Neurohypophyseal Hormones

Name	Structure	Function
Vasopressin	H-Cys-Tyr-Phe-Gln-Asn-Cys-Pro-Arg-Gly-NH$_2$ └─────────S–S─────┘	Vasoconstriction, water resorption by the kidney
Oxytocin	H-Cys-Tyr-Ile-Glu-Asn-Cys-Pro-Leu-Gly-NH$_2$ └─────────S–S─────┘	Uterine contraction and milk ejection

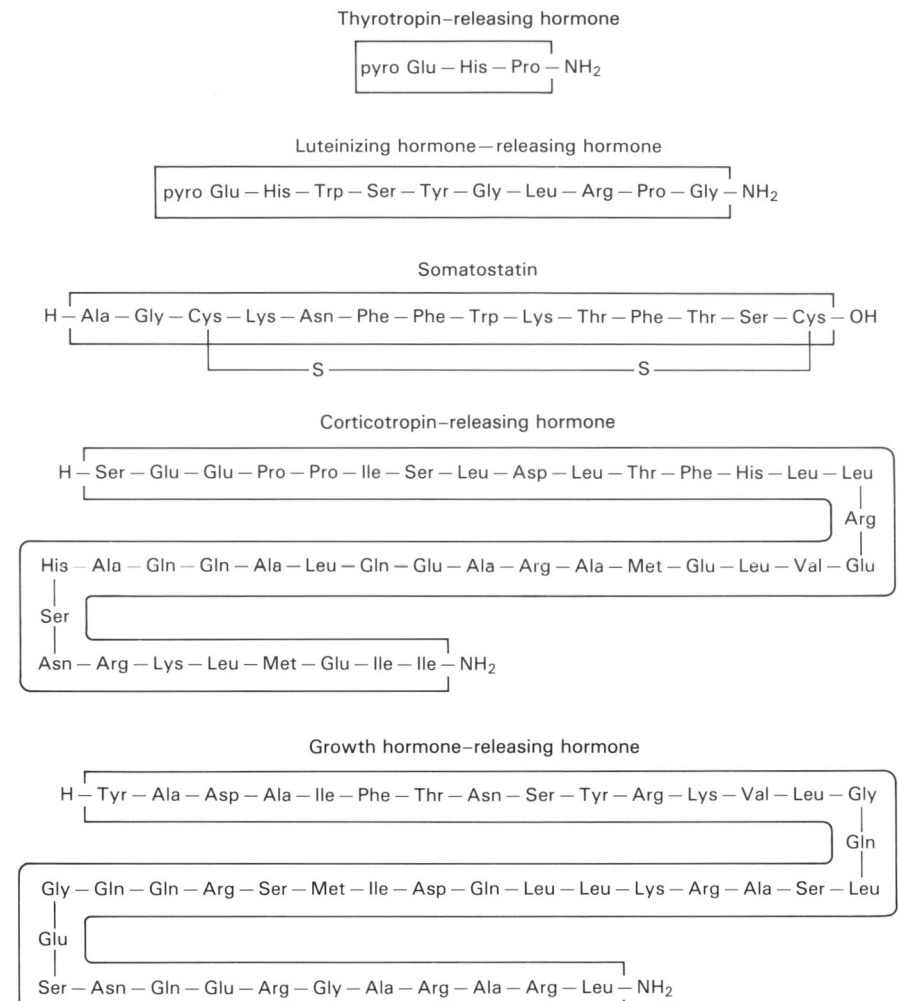

FIGURE 47–7

Structures of some hypothalamic releasing and inhibiting hormones.

Parvocellular Neurons Secrete Inhibiting and Releasing Hormones

Most hormones of the anterior pituitary are controlled by peptide neurohormones synthesized by small neurons that release their product into the capillaries of the median eminence. The determination of the structure of oxytocin and vasopressin and the work of Harris on the neural control of the anterior pituitary inspired Roger Guillemin, Andrew Schally, and their colleagues to isolate and characterize the structure of hormones that regulate the anterior pituitary. After 12 years of intense work on several tons of hypothalamic fragments, the laboratories of Guillemin and Schally independently characterized the structure of *thyrotropin-releasing hormone* (Figure 47–7). In 1971 Schally characterized *luteinizing hormone-releasing* hormone, and in 1973 Guillemin characterized somatostatin (Figure 47–7). More recently, *corticotropin-releasing hormone* (CRH, also called corticotropin-releasing factor, CRF) and *growth hormone-releasing hormone* (GRH) have been sequenced. CRH is found in

several regions of the hypothalamus. The CRH that is released in the median eminence to act on the pituitary appears to originate in parvocellular neurons in the paraventricular nucleus (Figure 47–4).

The release of the hormones of the anterior pituitary is regulated by antagonistic enhancing and inhibiting substances. For example, the release of growth hormone is stimulated by growth hormone-releasing hormone and inhibited by somatostatin. There is evidence that at least one inhibiting hormone is not a peptide: Prolactin release is inhibited by dopamine released from the median eminence. In many instances a single releasing hormone affects more than one pituitary hormone. The known hypothalamic releasing and inhibiting hormones are listed in Table 47–2 along with their most common abbreviations and the anterior pituitary hormones they affect.

Systematic electrical recordings from identified groups of neurons secreting releasing factors have not been made, but there is reason to believe that many of the parvocellular neurons discharge in bursts of action potentials. This inference is based on the observation that hormonal se-

TABLE 47–2. Hypothalamic Substances That Release or Inhibit the Release of Anterior Pituitary Hormones

Hypothalamic substance	Anterior pituitary hormone
Releasing	
Thyrotropin-releasing hormone (TRH)	Thyrotropin, prolactin
Corticotropin-releasing hormone (CRH)	Adrenocorticotropin, β-lipotropin
Gonadotropin-releasing hormone (GnRH)	LH, FSH
Growth hormone releasing hormone (GHRH or GRH)	GH
Prolactin-releasing factor (PRF)	Prolactin
Melanocyte-stimulating hormone-releasing factor (MRF)	MSH, β-endorphin
Inhibiting	
Prolactin release-inhibiting hormone (PIH), dopamine	Prolactin
Growth hormone release-inhibiting hormone (GIH or GHRIH; somatostatin)	GH, thyrotropin
Melanocyte-stimulating hormone release-inhibiting factor (MIF)	MSH

cretion is typically pulsatile: Blood concentrations of hormones show periodic surges throughout the day. This pattern is seen even for hormones, such as growth hormone, that regulate presumably nonepisodic physiological functions. Episodic firing may have evolved because this pattern is particularly effective for the release of peptides. In addition, periodic stimulation of receptors may limit receptor inactivation (down regulation).

Both Magnocellular and Parvocellular Neurons Contain Multiple Peptides that Are Found Throughout the Nervous System

Vasopressin, oxytocin, and the regulating hormones are not the only peptides of neurobiological interest in the hypothalamus. The opioid peptides, β-endorphin, and the enkephalins (see Chapter 27) are also found here, as are angiotensin II, substance P, neurotensin, cholecystokinin, and a host of other peptides. Almost every type of peptidergic neuron that has been carefully studied, including both parvocellular and magnocellular hypothalamic neurons, has been found to contain more than one peptide. For example, some parvocellular neurons in the paraventricular nucleus that contain corticotropin-releasing factor (CRH) also contain vasopressin, which is released together with CRH from the median eminence. Interestingly, the action of CRH in releasing ACTH from the pituitary is greatly potentiated by vasopressin, indicating that the two substances act synergistically.

Peptides released by the hypothalamic magnocellular and parvocellular neurons are not unique to these cells and have also been found in other regions of the nervous system. Some of these peptides are present in the terminals of parvocellular hypothalamic neurons that project to

regions of the brain and spinal cord, but others are synthesized in cell bodies outside of the hypothalamus.

CRH, for example, is widely distributed within as well as outside of the hypothalamus, especially in neurons of the limbic structures and nuclei related to the autonomic nervous system. This is also the case for other hypothalamic peptides. Thus, neurons in the arcuate nucleus that contain adrenocorticotropin, β-endorphin, and related peptides project to the thalamus, periaqueductal gray matter, limbic structures (nucleus accumbens, bed nucleus of the stria terminalis, and amygdala), and to major catecholamine-containing nuclei of the brain. The paraventricular nucleus, in addition to its magnocellular peptidergic projections to the posterior pituitary, sends axons of parvocellular oxytocin- or vasopressin-containing neurons to the locus ceruleus, solitary nucleus, dorsal vagal complex, and intermediolateral cell column of the spinal cord (see Figure 47–4). These peptidergic projections are well suited for coordinating neuroendocrine and autonomic responses. For example, regulatory peptides released at brain sites other than the median eminence may modulate behavior by actions independent of the release of pituitary hormones. The behavioral effects of regulatory peptides are thematically related to the types of endocrine effects produced by the same peptide acting on the pituitary. For example, injection of gonadotropin-releasing hormone into the medial preoptic area and arcuate nucleus of the hypothalamus of estrogen-treated female rats increases mating behavior as measured by lordosis (the stereotyped receptive behavior of the female). The action of this releasing hormone does not appear to be mediated through the ovaries, since the effect is not abolished by hypophysectomy or ovariectomy as long as estrogen is provided. A final example of a regulatory peptide that has central actions is CRH, which acts on the pituitary in response to stress. When injected intraventricularly, CRH evokes many of the behavioral and autonomic reactions normally seen in response to stress.

Hypothalamic Neurons Participate in Four Classes of Reflexes

Since the hypothalamus has both neural and humoral outputs and inputs it participates in four classes of reflexes: (1) conventional reflexes involving neural input and neural output; (2) reflexes in which the input to the hypothalamus is neural and the output is humoral; (3) reflexes in which the input is humoral and the output is neural; and (4) reflexes in which both the input and output are humoral. We shall consider simple examples of these four types of reflexes, keeping in mind that normal behavior typically involves more than one of these hypothalamic reflex modes.

Milk Ejection and Uterine Contraction Are Regulated by Neural Input and Humoral Output

The paraventricular and supraoptic nuclei contain magnocellular neurons that release oxytocin, which induces contraction of the myoepithelial cells of the mammary gland. Oxytocin also increases the amplitude of contraction of uterine smooth muscle if the muscle is appropriately primed by estrogens. This action of the hormone facilitates expulsion of the baby during delivery. The properties of hypothalamic magnocellular neurons resemble conventional neurons in many respects. They have resting potentials, fire action potentials, and receive excitatory and inhibitory synaptic input. Electrical stimulation of the posterior pituitary results in antidromic action potentials in these neurons, demonstrating that they send axons to the posterior pituitary.

In 1974 Dennis Lincoln and J. Wakerley succeeded in recording from identified neuroendocrine cells in female rats while they were suckling their pups, a natural stimulus for oxytocin release. Milk ejection was simultaneously measured by recording intramammary pressure. Lincoln and Wakerley found that a continuous suckling stimulus produced periodic bursts of action potentials in many of the identified neuroendocrine cells. Approximately 13 seconds after each burst there was an increase in intramammary pressure, indicating the arrival of a pulse of oxytocin to the mammary glands (Figure 47–8). Thus, the oxytocin cells participate in a relatively simple reflex in which the afferent pathway is neural and the efferent pathway is humoral.

As appears to be true for all hypothalamic neurosecretory products, the release of oxytocin can be regulated by higher brain structures. For example, the sight or sound of her child can trigger milk ejection in a lactating mother. Presumably, excitatory cortical influences project to oxytocin-containing cells in the hypothalamus. Inhibitory cortical influences may also affect these cells since anxiety and worry can inhibit the milk ejection reflex.

Urine Flow Is Regulated by Humoral Input and Output

The paraventricular and supraoptic nuclei also contain neurons that release the hormone vasopressin. Vasopressin alters the membrane permeability of the collecting ducts and convoluted tubules of the kidneys so that their membranes become more permeable to water. As a result, the recovery of water after filtration is facilitated, urinary volume decreases, and body water is conserved. For this reason vasopressin is also called antidiuretic hormone.

In contrast to the neurons that release oxytocin, which tend to fire in a single burst of activity, the neurons that release vasopressin are spontaneously active and provide a constant, basal concentration of the hormone in the blood. This concentration is decreased or increased according to physiological demand. When the animal is deprived of water, vasopressin-releasing neurons fire more rapidly and in a burst pattern. They fire less rapidly when the animal is well hydrated. The vasopressin system therefore functions analogously to that of graded neural reflexes, whereas the oxytocin system functions more like that of fixed-action pattern responses (to be considered in Chapter 65).

The hypothalamic neurons involved in the release of vasopressin respond directly to the state of the internal environment (specifically, the blood), although they can also be influenced through afferent neuronal pathways. Direct response to humoral factors, first suggested by E. B. Verney in 1947, is strongly supported by the observation made by John Sundsten and Charles Sawyer in 1961 that animals can regulate release of vasopressin even when the hypothalamus is disconnected from all structures except the pituitary. Vasopressin-producing cells as well as other hypothalamic cells and circumventricular neurons (located in structures in which the blood–brain barrier is weak, such as the subfornical organ) respond directly to osmotic stimuli or to changes in the blood concentration of Na^+ (see the next chapter). Other humorally mediated stimuli can affect vasopressin release directly or indirectly. For example, anesthetic agents and circulating hormones (such as angiotensin II) increase the release of vasopressin, while ethanol decreases its release.

The release of vasopressin is also controlled by neural inputs from blood volume receptors in blood vessels: Decreased blood volume enhances vasopressin release, while increased volume inhibits release. Temperature receptors in the skin may also affect vasopressin release; cold inhibits the release of vasopressin, while warmth enhances its release, perhaps to conserve water because of increased water loss due to sweating. Finally, vomiting is associated with a strong release of vasopressin.

Feedback Loops Involve Humoral Input and Output

A hormone produced in a peripheral endocrine gland (typically steroid hormones that readily cross the blood–brain barrier) can limit its own production by directly inhibiting

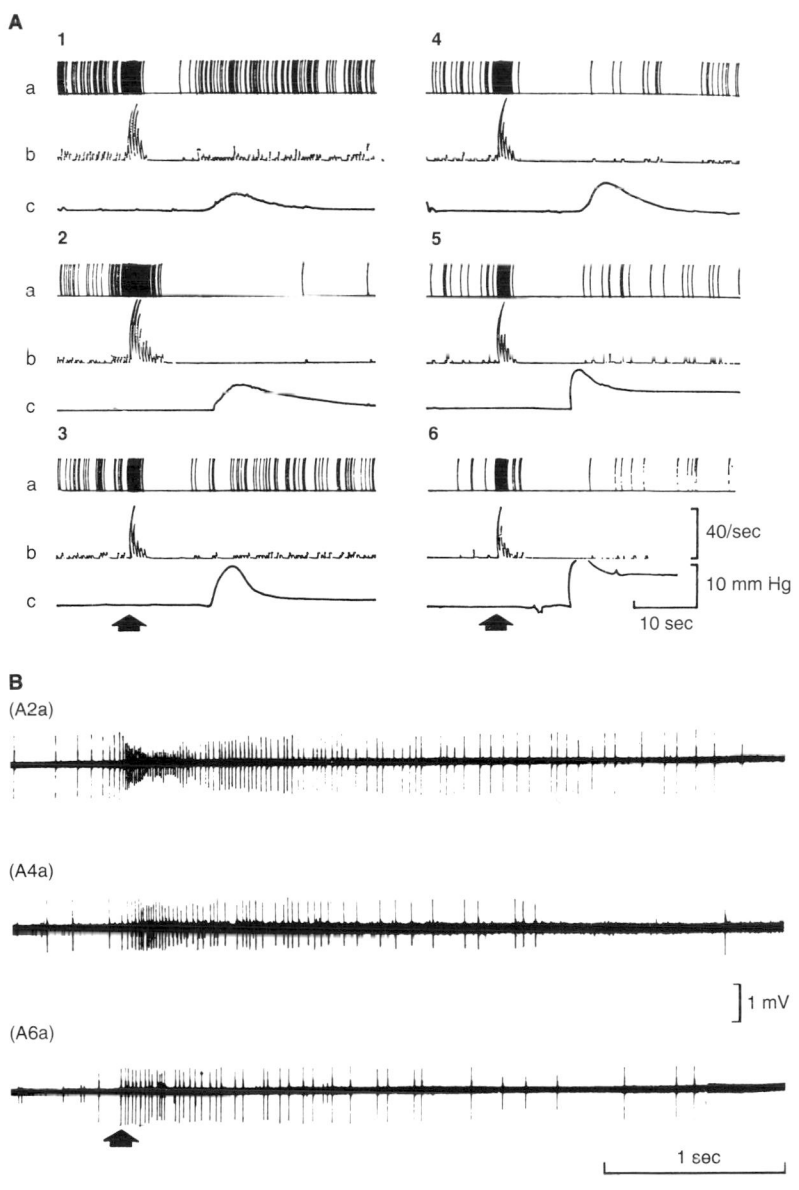

FIGURE 47–8

Recordings from oxytocin releasing neuroendocrine cells in the female rat during suckling of pups illustrate the correlation of spike activity with milk ejection. **Arrows** indicate onset of neurosecretory response. (Adapted from Lincoln and Wakerley, 1974.)

A. Polygraph records of six responsive supraoptic neurons (**1–6**). For each cell, approximately 40 s of spike activity, spanning one milk ejection, is shown. **Trace a** shows unit activity, in which each vertical deflection corresponds to a single action potential. **Trace b** is an integration of the unit recording in which the height of the trace is proportional to frequency. **Trace c** is a record of intramammary pressure. Note the difference in the background activity of the six units, the dramatic and stereotyped acceleration in spike activity about 13 s before milk ejection, the peak rates of spike discharge (30–50 spikes per s), the duration of the response, and the period of after-inhibition.

B. Records on a greatly expanded time scale show the spike trains in three of the units (2, 4, 6) illustrated in A.

the brain or the anterior pituitary. This is achieved through long feedback loops involving neurons in the limbic system and hypothalamus that have receptors for the hormone. This control of hormone production is an example of a reflex in which both input and output are humoral.

Central Effects of Hormones on Behavior Involve Humoral Input and Neural Output

Although certain hormones circulate widely through the brain, only a subset of neurons possess receptors to a specific hormone. Therefore, the action of circulating hormones can be quite specific, and a given hormone that can cross the blood–brain barrier or be released into the extracellular space or cerebrospinal fluid will activate or inhibit only a restricted population of neurons. Hormonal effects on central nerve cells (sometimes referred to as modulatory effects) are slow and thus suited to long-term regulation of excitability or synaptic effectiveness. These hormonal actions are thought to be involved in modifying mood and behavioral states or in triggering complex motor patterns in which the details are dependent upon conventional transmitter actions.

The action of steroid and thyroid hormones on the hypothalamus and elsewhere typically involves binding to intracellular steroid receptors that act as factors that regulate transcription. During development these hormones alter the differentiated state and connections of neurons (see Chapter 61). In the adult brain the same hormones reversibly alter the expression of neuropeptides, neuroreceptors, enzymes, and structural proteins.

Neurons in the Hypothalamus Undergo Structural and Biochemical Changes in Response to Behavioral Demands

The hypothalamus is involved in many stereotypic and automatic responses. Nevertheless, its functioning is hardly static, and many hypothalamic neurons exhibit dramatic forms of plasticity in response to prolonged demands placed on the system. Many hypothalamic neurons that control the release of circulating endocrine hormones are affected by these very same hormones. These feedback effects are both short term as well as long term. For example, glucocorticoids that are injected into an animal or are released from the adrenal glands following stress act rapidly on neurons that release CRH. This results in a short-term suppression of the response of these neurons to stressful stimuli, which in turn reduces the release of adrenal glucocorticoids to additional stress. Long-term exposure (over days or weeks) to glucocorticoids inhibits the transcription of the gene for CRH and, particularly, for vasopressin in parvocellular neurons. In contrast, adrenalectomy, by stimulating CRH release, produces a dramatic increase in the synthesis of CRH and vasopressin, such that vasopressin becomes expressed in CRH neurons that normally have little or no vasopressin.

As mentioned previously, CRH and vasopressin can act synergistically in releasing ACTH. Stress, pain, and anxiety, which increase vasopressin release, also increase the release of adrenocorticotropin, and prolonged stress may alter the expression of CRH and vasopressin or oxytocin. In addition, studies by Robert Sapolsky and his colleagues indicate that severe stress or a chronic increase of glucocorticoids can result in damage to hippocampal pyramidal neurons. In contrast, Robert Sloviter and colleagues found that other neurons, such as hippocampal granule cells, may degenerate when circulating glucocorticoids are eliminated by adrenalectomy. The variety of effects of glucocorticoids on the hippocampus was explained by Bruce McEwen, who found that the hippocampus contains an unusually high concentration of glucocorticoid receptors, and that chronic alterations of glucocorticoid levels in the blood produces complex biphasic responses that result in either enhancement or depression of hippocampal function. The nature of the response is a function of the duration of exposure, age, and various other unidentified factors.

Lactation, parturition, and severe dehydration result in dramatic structural changes in magnocellular neurons as well as in the glia associated with the cell bodies and the posterior pituitary terminals of the neurons. The structural changes, such as increased cell size, promote the functioning of the system during increased demand.

The Hypothalamus Helps Regulate the Autonomic Nervous System and Is Involved in Emotional Behavior

Although the hypothalamus has important hormonal inputs and outputs, it also mediates conventional reflexes involving neural inputs and neural outputs. In this role the hypothalamus functions as the so-called head ganglion of the autonomic nervous system. Much of what we know about the autonomic function of the hypothalamus stems from a long series of experiments, starting in the early 1930s, by Stephen Ranson and Walter Hess. Ranson took advantage of the stereotaxic method developed by Horsley and Clark, which permits the precise and reproducible placement of electrodes in the deep structures of the brains of experimental animals by means of a triple-coordinate system that locates each subcortical nucleus uniquely. (This technique was later refined to permit neurosurgeons to make therapeutic lesions deep within the brain.) In previous attempts to stimulate the hypothalamus, investigators had used drastic surgical procedures to visualize the appropriate structures. Ranson systematically stimulated different regions of the hypothalamus and evoked almost every conceivable autonomic reaction, including alterations in heart rate, blood pressure, and gastrointestinal motility, as well as erection of hairs and bladder contraction. The most prominent responses involved the sympathetic nervous system, and these effects tended to occur with stimulation of the lateral and posterior hypothalamus.

Most of Ranson's experiments were done on anesthetized animals. Hess extended Ranson's approach by implanting electrodes and permanently fixing them to the skull of the animal. By attaching a long flexible cable to the implanted electrode, he could observe the effects of brain stimulation in awake and completely unrestrained animals. Hess found that stimulation of different parts of the hypothalamus produced characteristic constellations of responses that appeared to be organized behavior. For example, electrical stimulation of the lateral hypothalamus in cats elicited autonomic and somatic responses characteristic of anger: increased blood pressure, raising of the body hair, pupillary constriction, arching of the back, and raising of the tail.

These observations provided the basis for the important conclusion that the hypothalamus is not a motor nucleus for the autonomic nervous system, but rather is a coordinating center that integrates various inputs to ensure a well-organized, coherent, and appropriate set of autonomic and somatic responses. Since many of these responses resemble those seen during various types of emotional behaviors, Hess suggested that the hypothalamus integrates and coordinates the behavioral expression of emotional states. This idea is supported by lesion studies that associate different hypothalamic structures with a wide range of emotional states. Whereas stimulation of the lateral hypothalamus elicits anger, lesions of the same area result in placidity. In contrast, animals with lesions of the medial hypothalamus become highly excitable and are easily triggered into aggressive responses.

Similar irritability is also produced by decortication. Decorticated cats exhibit lashing of the tail, vigorous arching of the back, jerking of the limbs, clawing, attempts to bite, and such autonomic responses as erection of the tail hairs, sweating (of the toe pads), urination, defecation, and increased blood pressure. There is also an increase in adrenal secretions, including epinephrine and corticosteroids. In 1925 Walter Cannon and S. W. Britton termed this constellation of responses *sham rage*, because it appeared to lack elements of conscious experience that are characteristic of naturally occurring rage. Sham rage reactions also differ from genuine rage in that responses can occur spontaneously or be triggered by very mild tactile and other stimuli. Even when elicited by strong stimuli, the sham rage subsides very quickly when the stimulus is removed. Finally, the aggressive responses are undirected, and the animals sometimes even bite themselves.

In 1928 Philip Bard further analyzed sham rage by means of progressive transections down the neuraxis (Figure 47–9). When the hypothalamus was included in the ablation, the sham rage disappeared. Although some expression of emotional responses could be obtained in animals in which the hypothalamus and all rostral forebrain structures had been removed, very strong stimuli were required to elicit the responses, and they were much less coordinated than those seen when the ablation did not include the hypothalamus. Such responses were first described by Robert Woodworth and Sherrington in 1904, who called them *pseudo-affective reflexes*.

Sham rage was originally described as resulting from total decortication. Bard and Vernon Mountcastle, however, found that large portions of the neocortex could be removed without producing sham rage. Sham rage phenomena were seen when the ablation included structures of the limbic system (for example, the cingulate cortex).

In 1937 Klüver and Bucy reported that bilateral removal of the temporal lobe in the monkey—including the amygdala and the hippocampal formation as well as the nonlimbic temporal cortex—produced a dramatic behavioral syndrome. The animals, formerly quite wild, became tame, showed a flattening of emotions, and exhibited remarkable oral tendencies (they put all manner of objects into their mouths). They also exhibited an enormous increase in sexual behavior, including mounting of inappropriate objects and species. Finally, the animals showed a compulsive tendency to take note of and react to every visual stimulus, hypermetamorphosis, but failed to recognize familiar objects. Some of the features of the Klüver-Bucy syndrome tend to be the opposite of those encountered in patients with temporal lobe epilepsy, who, as we saw in Chapter 1, show decreased sexuality and heightened emotionality.

What structures account for the individual symptoms of the Klüver-Bucy syndrome? Damage to the amygdala is particularly important in producing the oral tendencies, hypersexuality, and tameness; and damage to the visual association areas of the temporal cortex contributes to the visual deficits. In addition, these animals presumably have defects in certain memory functions because of the removal of the hippocampus (see Chapter 64).

Thus, our current models of the neural basis of emotional behavior are built on ideas that James Papez proposed more than 50 years ago. We think of the hypothalamus as integrating the motor and endocrine re-

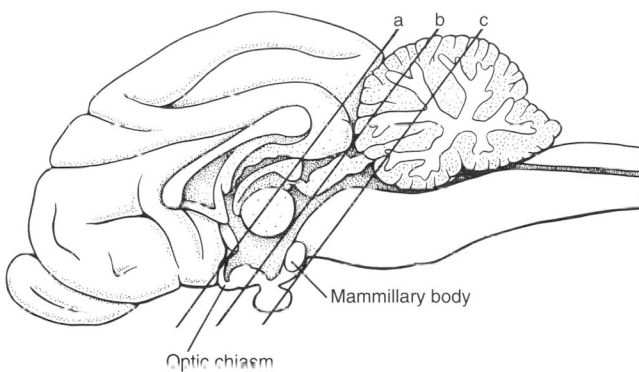

FIGURE 47–9
This midsagittal section of the cat brain shows the level of brain transections used to study sham rage. Transection of the forebrain (at level **a**) causes an animal to exhibit sham rage. Transection at the level of the hypothalamus (**b**) also produces sham rage. If the posterior hypothalamus is included (**c**), only isolated elements of a rage response can be elicited.

sponses that produce appropriate emotional behavior, and we think of the telencephalon suppressing emotional responses to trivial and inconsequential stimuli. The telencephalon connects the hypothalamus to the outer world in a manner that allows appropriate autonomic and endocrine concomitants of emotions to be expressed in response to external conditions. Telencephalic structures also provide the neural mechanisms needed to direct skeletomotor responses to external events, so that, for example, an object is appropriately approached or avoided. Finally, the neocortex seems to be crucial for the conscious experience of emotions.

Current thinking has deemphasized the role of the mammillary bodies and anterior thalamic nuclei in emotions; these structures appear to be more closely related to the process of memory storage. On the other hand, the amygdala, which Papez did not include in his circuit, appears to play an important role in emotions by conveying higher cognitive information to hypothalamic structures other than the mammillary bodies. The amygdala not only receives information from cortical structures, including the hippocampus, but also receives direct afferent input from the thalamus. Joseph LeDoux suggests that this direct thalamic input may mediate short-latency primitive emotional responses and prepare the amygdala for the reception of more sophisticated information from higher centers. The output of the amygdala, as well as afferent input that is triggered as a consequence of the activity of autonomic effectors, feeds back to cortical structures, such as the prefrontal cortex, and results in a conscious emotional experience.

An Overall View

The interplay between the neural activity of the hypothalamus and the activity of higher centers results in emotional experiences that we describe as fear, anger, pleasure, and contentment. The behavior of patients in whom the prefrontal cortex or cingulate gyrus (parts of which are related to the limbic system) has been removed supports this idea. These patients are no longer bothered by chronic pain. When they do perceive pain and exhibit appropriate autonomic reactions, the perception is no longer associated with a powerful emotional experience (see Chapters 27 and 53).

Thus, noxious or pleasurable stimuli have dual effects. First, these stimuli trigger autonomic and endocrine responses that are integrated by the hypothalamus and that alter the internal state, thus preparing the organism for attack, flight, sexual experience, or other adaptive behaviors. These internal reactions are relatively simple to execute and require no conscious control. Once the animal interacts with its external environment, however, a second set of mechanisms come into play. These involve the telencephalon and modulate the animal's behavior much as proprioceptive feedback from an uneven terrain modulates the central program for locomotion. Perhaps consciousness evolved to deal with the enormous complexity of the external environment. Compared to our internal environment, the external environment is far less predictable and provides a much richer variety of stimuli. Furthermore, in dealing with the external environment we often have the luxury of delaying our responses, thus permitting actions to be guided by plans and strategies.

Selected Readings

Carithers, J. R., and Johnson, A. K. 1988. Fine structural studies of the effects of AV3V lesions on the hypothalamo-neurohypophyseal neurosecretory system. In A. W. Cowley, Jr., J.-F. Liard, and D. A. Ausiello (eds.), Vasopressin: Cellular and Integrative Functions. New York: Raven Press, pp. 301–319.

Gainer, H., 1988. Mechanisms of neuropeptide precursor processing. Implications for neuropharmacology. In M. Avoli, T. A. Reader, R. W. Dykes, and P. Gloor (eds.), Neurotransmitters and Cortical Function: From Molecules to Mind. New York: Plenum Press, pp. 527–546.

Guillemin, R. 1978. Control of adenohypophysial functions by peptides of the central nervous system. Harvey Lect. 71:71–131.

Hess, W. R. 1954. Diencephalon: Autonomic and Extrapyramidal Functions. New York: Grune & Stratton.

Isaacson, R. L. 1982. The Limbic System, 2nd ed. New York: Plenum Press.

Koizumi, K., Kollai, M., Oomura, Y., Yamashita, H., and Wayner, M. J. (eds.) 1988. The hypothalamus: Selected topics. Brain Res. Bull. 20:651–902.

McEwen, B. S. 1989. Steroid hormone receptors and the brain: Linking the genome with the environment in health and disease. In Neural Control of Reproductive Function. New York: Liss, pp. 5–31.

Meyerson, B. J. 1979. Hypothalamic hormones and behaviour. Med. Biol. (Helsinki) 57:69–83.

Ranson, S. W. 1934. The hypothalamus: Its significance for visceral innervation and emotional expression. Trans. Coll. Physicians Phila. 2:222–242.

Renaud, L. P. 1981. A neurophysiological approach to the identification, connections and pharmacology of the hypothalamic tuberoinfundibular system. Neuroendocrinology 33:186–191.

Silverman, A.-J., and Zimmerman, E. A. 1983. Magnocellular neurosecretory system. Annu. Rev. Neurosci. 6:357–380.

Swanson, L. W., and Sawchenko, P. E. 1983. Hypothalamic integration: Organization of the paraventricular and supraoptic nuclei. Annu. Rev. Neurosci. 6:269–324.

References

Bard, P. 1928. A diencephalic mechanism for the expression of rage with special reference to the sympathetic nervous system. Am. J. Physiol. 84:490–515.

Bard, P., and Mountcastle, V. B. 1948. Some forebrain mechanisms involved in expression of rage with special reference to suppression of angry behavior. Res. Publ. Assoc. Res. Nerv. Ment. Dis. 27:362–404.

Bernard, C. 1878–1879. Leçons sur les phénomènes de la vie communs aux animaux et aux végétaux, 2 Vols. Paris: Baillière.

Broca, P. 1878. Anatomie comparée de circonvolutions cérébrales. Le grand lobe limbique et la scissure limbique dans la série des mammifères. Rev. Anthropol. 1:385–498.

Cannon, W. B., and Britton, S. W. 1925. Studies on the conditions of activity in endocrine glands. XV. Pseudoaffective medulliadrenal secretion. Am. J. Physiol. 72:283–294.

Du Vigneaud, V. 1956. Hormones of the posterior pituitary gland: Oxytocin and vasopressin. Harvey Lect. 50:1–26.

Gay, V. L. 1972. The hypothalamus: Physiology and clinical use of releasing factors. Fertil. Steril. 23:50–63.

Harris, G. W. 1955. Neural Control of the Pituitary Gland. Monograph No. 3 of The Physiological Society. London: Arnold.

Kandel, E. R. 1964. Electrical properties of the hypothalamic neuroendocrine cells. J. Gen. Physiol. 47:691–717.

Kiss, J. Z. 1988. Dynamism of chemoarchitecture in the hypothalamic paraventricular nucleus. Brain Res. Bull. 20:699–708.

Klüver, H., and Bucy, P. C. 1939. Preliminary analysis of functions of the temporal lobes in monkeys. Arch. Neurol. Psychiatry 42:979–1000.

LeDoux, J. E. 1989. Cognitive-emotional interactions in the brain. Cognition Emotion 3:267–289.

Lincoln, D. W., and Wakerley, J. B. 1974. Electrophysiological evidence for the activation of supraoptic neurones during the release of oxytocin. J. Physiol. (Lond.) 242:533–554.

MacLean, P. D. 1955. The limbic system ("visceral brain") and emotional behavior. Arch. Neurol. Psychiatry 73:130–134.

Nieuwenhuys, R., Voogd, J., and van Huijzen, Chr. 1981. The Human Central Nervous System: A Synopsis and Atlas, 2nd rev. ed. Berlin: Springer.

Papez, J. W. 1937. A proposed mechanism of emotion. Arch. Neurol. Psychiatry 38:725–743.

Reichlin, S. 1978. Introduction. In S. Reichlin, R. J. Baldessarini, and J. B. Martin (eds.), The Hypothalamus. Res. Publ. Assoc. Res. Nerv. Ment. Dis. 56:1–14.

Sawchenko, P. E., and Swanson, L. W. 1985. Localization, colocalization, and plasticity of corticotropin-releasing factor immunoreactivity in rat brain. Fed. Proc. 44:221–227.

Schally, A. V. 1978. Aspects of hypothalamic regulation of the pituitary gland: Its implications for the control of reproductive processes. Science 202:18–28.

Scharrer, E., and Scharrer, B. 1954. Hormones produced by neurosecretory cells. Recent Prog. Horm. Res. 10:183–232.

Sloviter, R. S., Valiquette, G., Abrams, G. M., Ronk, E. C., Sollas, A. L., Paul, L. A., and Neubort, S. 1989. Selective loss of hippocampal granule cells in the mature rat brain after adrenalectomy. Science 243:535–538.

Sundsten, J. W., and Sawyer, C. H. 1961. Osmotic activation of neurohypophysial hormone release in rabbits with hypothalamic islands. Exp. Neurol. 4:548–561.

Uno, H., Tarara, R., Else, J. G., Suleman, M. A., and Sapolsky, R. M. 1989. Hippocampal damage associated with prolonged and fatal stress in primates. J. Neurosci. 9:1705–1711.

Vale, W., Spiess, J., Rivier, C., and Rivier, J. 1981. Characterization of a 41-residue ovine hypothalamic peptide that stimulates secretion of corticotropin and β-endorphin. Science 213: 1394–1397.

Verney, E. B. 1947. The antidiuretic hormone and the factors which determine its release. Proc. R. Soc. Lond. [Biol.] 135: 25–106.

Woodworth, R. S., and Sherrington, C. S. 1904. A pseudaffective reflex and its spinal path. J. Physiol. (Lond.) 31:234–243.

48

Irving Kupfermann

Hypothalamus and Limbic System: Motivation

Motivation Is an Inferred Internal State Postulated to Explain Variability of Behavioral Responses

Homeostatic Processes Such as Temperature Regulation, Feeding, and Thirst Correspond to Motivational States

Temperature Regulation Involves Integration of Autonomic, Endocrine, and Skeletomotor Responses

Feeding Behavior Is Regulated by a Great Variety of Mechanisms

Body Weight Is Regulated Around a Set Point

Dual Controlling Elements Are Involved in the Control of Food Intake

Chemical Stimulation of the Hypothalamus Alters Feeding Behavior

Thirst Is Regulated by Tissue Osmolality and Vascular Volume

Motivational States Can Be Regulated by Factors Other Than Tissue Needs

Ecological Constraints

Anticipatory Mechanisms

Hedonic Factors

Intracranial Stimulation Can Simulate Motivational States and Reinforce Behavior

An Overall View

The internal environment of the body is regulated by three classes of mechanisms: neuroendocrine, autonomic, and motivational. In the last chapter we examined the role of the limbic system and the hypothalamus in the neuroendocrine and autonomic regulation of homeostasis. In this chapter we shall consider the control of homeostasis by motivational states, the internal conditions that arouse and direct voluntary behavior. These motivated behavioral responses typically occur in parallel to the autonomic and neuroendocrine responses. We shall first consider how the study of motivation has become more amenable to biological experimentation by use of control systems analysis. We shall next examine how motivated behaviors are regulated by factors other than simple tissue deficits. Finally, we shall discuss systems of the brain concerned with a specific component of motivation: reward and reinforcement.

Motivation Is an Inferred Internal State Postulated to Explain Variability of Behavioral Responses

Specific motivational states, or *drives*, represent urges or impulses based upon bodily needs that impel humans and other animals into action. For example, a temperature-regulating drive is said to control behaviors that directly affect body temperature, such as shivering or rubbing the hands together. Other conditions that control behavior but which do not appear to be based on any well-defined physiological deprivation, such as curiosity and sexual arousal, are also referred to as drives because, like classical homeostatic drives, they also involve arousal and satiation.

Drives or motivational states are inferred mechanisms postulated to explain the intensity and direction of a variety of complex behaviors, such as temperature regulation, feeding, thirst, and sex. Behavioral scientists posit these internal states because observable stimuli in the external environment are not sufficient to predict all aspects of these behaviors. In simple reflexes—for example, the pupillary response—the properties of the stimulus appear to account in large part for the properties of the behavior. On the other hand, more complex activities are not consistently correlated with external stimulus conditions. For example, at certain times food might stimulate vigorous feeding. At other times it produces no response or even rejection. The motivational states of hunger and satiety are inferred to explain the loose correlation between the food stimulus and the feeding response at different times.

Homeostatic Processes Such as Temperature Regulation, Feeding, and Thirst Correspond to Motivational States

Neurobiologists are now beginning to define the actual physiological states that correspond to the motivational states inferred by psychologists. In some instances it has been possible to approach motivational states as examples of interaction between external and internal stimuli. The problem of motivation thus can be reduced to that of a complex reflex under the excitatory and inhibitory control of multiple stimuli, some of them internal. This approach has worked particularly well with temperature regulation. In contrast, the relevant internal stimuli for hunger, thirst, and sexual behavior have been exceedingly difficult to identify or to manipulate. Nevertheless, even for these behaviors the concept of drive state remains useful for behavioral scientists. As more is learned about the actual physiology of hypothetical drive states, the need for invoking these states to explain behavior may ultimately disappear, to be replaced by more precise concepts derived from physiology and systems theory.

Homeostatic mechanisms can be understood in terms of the types of control systems, or *servomechanisms*, that regulate machines. While the existence of specific physiological control systems regulating homeostatic variables has never been demonstrated, this approach has provided a convenient and precise language to describe both concepts and experimental results. It permits us to organize our thinking about highly complex systems. Furthermore, the servomechanism concept makes it possible to define the problem of physiological control experimentally. This approach has been most successfully applied to temperature regulation. The approach has been less successful when applied to more complex regulatory behaviors, such as feeding and thirst, but it is probably still the best approach to the analysis of these poorly understood functions.

Control systems regulate a *controlled variable* that is maintained within a certain range. As we saw in Chapter 35, the controlled variable can be a movement. However, homeostatic variables such as body temperature also can be regulated by similar control mechanisms. One way of regulating the controlled variable is to measure it by means of a *feedback detector* and to compare it with a desired value or *set point*. This is accomplished by an *integrator* or *error detector* that generates an *error signal* when the measurement of the controlled variable does not match the set point signal. The error signal then drives *controlling elements* that adjust the controlled system in the desired direction. The error signal is not only controlled by internal feedback stimuli but also is affected by external stimuli. External stimuli (e.g., the sight or smell of food) that are capable of driving behavior are termed *incentive stimuli*. All examples of physiological control seem to involve dual effects, inhibitory and excitatory, which function together to adjust the control system (Figure 48–1). The control system used to heat a home

FIGURE 48–1

Homeostatic processes can be analyzed in terms of control systems.

A. A system using a set point to turn behavior on or off can be used to regulate motivated behaviors. When a feedback signal indicates the level of the controlled variable is below or above the set point, an error signal is generated; this signal serves to turn on (or facilitate) appropriate behaviors and physiological responses, and to turn off (or suppress) incompatible responses. A drive signal also can be generated by external incentive stimuli.

B. A negative feedback system without a set point controls fat stores. (Based on data of Di Girolamo and Rudman, 1968.)

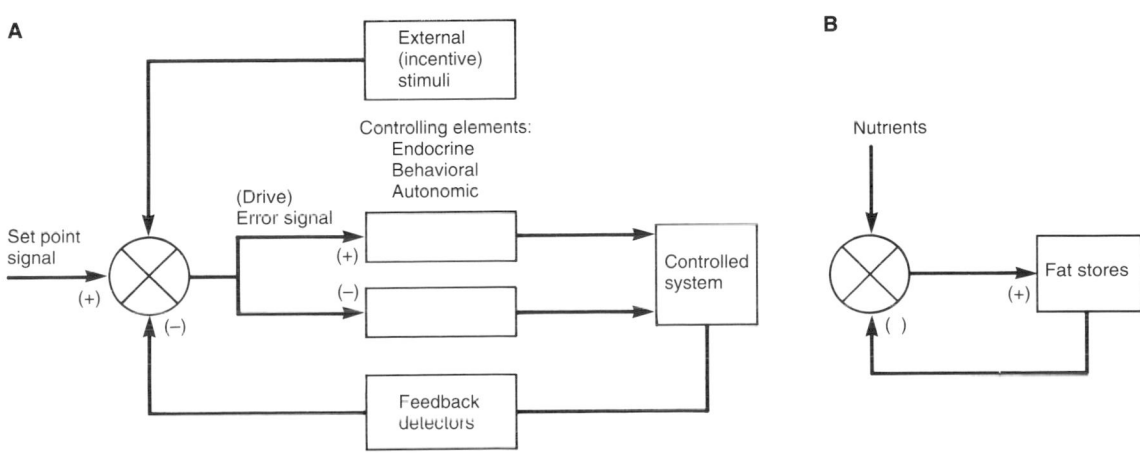

illustrates these principles. The furnace system is the controlling element. The room temperature is the controlled variable. The home thermostat is the error detector. The setting on the thermostat is the set point. Finally, the output of the thermostat that turns the controlling element on or off is the error signal.

Temperature Regulation Involves Integration of Autonomic, Endocrine, and Skeletomotor Responses

In the system of temperature regulation, the integrator and many controlling elements appear to be located in the hypothalamus. Temperature regulation nicely fits the model of a servocontrol system (or several systems), and normal body temperature is the set point. The feedback detector appears to collect information about body temperature from two main sources: peripheral temperature receptors located throughout the body (in the skin, spinal cord, and viscera) and central temperature receptors concentrated in the hypothalamus. Although both anterior and posterior hypothalamic areas are involved in temperature regulation, detectors of temperature, both low and high, are located only in the anterior hypothalamus. The hypothalamic receptors are probably neurons whose firing rate is highly dependent on local temperature, which in turn is determined primarily by the temperature of the blood.

Because temperature regulation requires integrated autonomic, endocrine, and skeletomotor responses, the anatomical connections of the hypothalamus make this structure well suited for this task. Electrical stimulation of the hypothalamus indicates that it includes dual mechanisms that control, respectively, increases and decreases in body temperature. Electrical stimulation of the anterior hypothalamus in unanesthetized animals causes dilation of blood vessels in the skin and a suppression of shivering, responses that result in a drop in body temperature. Electrical stimulation of the posterior hypothalamus produces a set of opposite responses that function to generate or conserve heat (Figure 48–2). As with fear responses evoked by electrical stimulation of the hypothalamus (see Chapter 47), electrically induced temperature regulation also includes appropriate responses involving the skeletomotor system. For example, anterior hypothalamic (preoptic area) stimulation produces panting, while posterior stimulation produces shivering.

The results of ablation experiments corroborate the critical role of the hypothalamus in regulating temperature. Lesions of the anterior hypothalamus result in chronic hyperthermia and eliminate the major responses that normally dissipate excess heat. Lesions in the posterior hypothalamus have relatively little effect if the animal is maintained at room temperature (approximately 22°C). If the animal is exposed to cold, however, it quickly becomes hypothermic because of failure of the homeostatic mechanisms that generate and conserve heat.

The hypothalamus also controls endocrine responses to temperature challenges. Thus, long-term exposure to cold can enhance an animal's release of thyroxine and thereby increase body heat by increasing tissue metabolism.

The error signal of the temperature control system, in addition to driving appropriate autonomic, endocrine, and nonvoluntary skeletal responses, can also provide a signal to drive voluntary behavior that moves the controlled system in the direction that minimizes the error signal. For example, a rat can be taught to press a button to re-

FIGURE 48–2
The hypothalamic regions concerned with heat conservation and heat dissipation are shown in a sagittal section of the human brain.

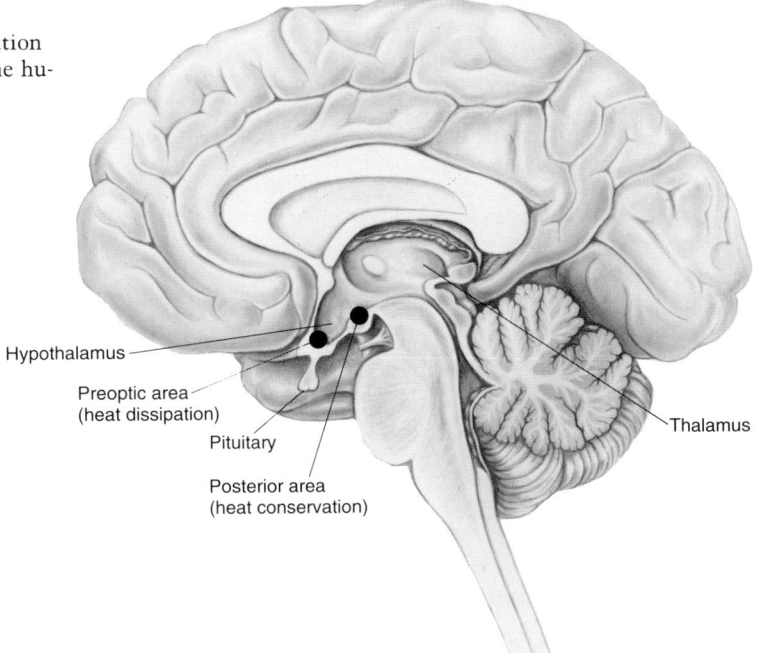

Hypothalamus

Preoptic area
(heat dissipation)

Pituitary

Posterior area
(heat conservation)

Thalamus

ceive a puff of cool air in a hot environment. When placed in a room at normal temperature, the rat will not press the cool-air button. If the anterior hypothalamus is locally warmed by perfusing warm water through a hollow probe, the rat will run to the cool-air button and press it. Summation of peripheral and central input to the hypothalamus in the same rat can be demonstrated by heating the environment and concurrently cooling or heating the hypothalamus (Figure 48–3). When both the environment and hypothalamus are heated, the rat presses faster than when either one is heated alone (see points c and d in Figure 48–3). Button pressing for cool air in a hot environ ment can be suppressed completely by directly cooling the hypothalamus (see point e in Figure 48–3).

Recordings from neurons in the preoptic area and anterior hypothalamus by Tetsuro Hori, Jack Boulant, and their colleagues support the idea that the hypothalamus integrates peripheral and central information relevant to temperature regulation. Units in this region, called *warm-sensitive neurons*, increase their firing when the local hypothalamic tissue is warmed. Other neurons, called *cold-sensitive neurons*, respond to local cooling. The warm-sensitive neurons, in addition to responding to local brain warming, are generally excited by warming of the skin or spinal cord and are inhibited by cooling of the skin or spinal cord. The cold-sensitive neurons exhibit the opposite behavior. Thus, these neurons could serve to integrate thermal information from the periphery with that from the brain. Furthermore, many temperature-sensitive neurons also respond to nonthermal stimuli, such as osmolarity, glucose, sex steroids, and blood pressure.

Although the temperature set point mechanism ordinarily maintains body temperature within close limits, the set point can be altered by pathological states, most notably by the action of pyrogens, which induce fever. Systemic pyrogens, such as the macrophage product interleukin-1, appear to enter the brain at regions in which the blood–brain barrier is incomplete, and act on the preoptic area. This results in an increase of the temperature set point, and body temperature rises until that new point is reached. Experiments by Norman Kasting and collaborators have found that the brain also has an antipyretic area, which appears to be activated during fever, and which functions to limit the magnitude of the fever response. The antipyretic area includes the septal nuclei, which are located anteriorly to the preoptic area, near the anterior commissure. Substantial evidence indicates that the antipyretic area is activated by inputs that use the peptide vasopressin. Injection of vasopressin into the septal area counteracts fever in a manner similar to that of antipyretic drugs, suggesting that some of the effects of these drugs may be mediated by the central release of vasopressin. The antipyretic action of nonsteroidal anti-inflammatory drugs such as indomethacin is blocked by injection of a vasopressin antagonist into the septal nuclei. Finally, there is evidence that convulsions brought on by high fevers may in part be evoked by the peptide vasopressin that is released in the brain as part of an antipyretic response.

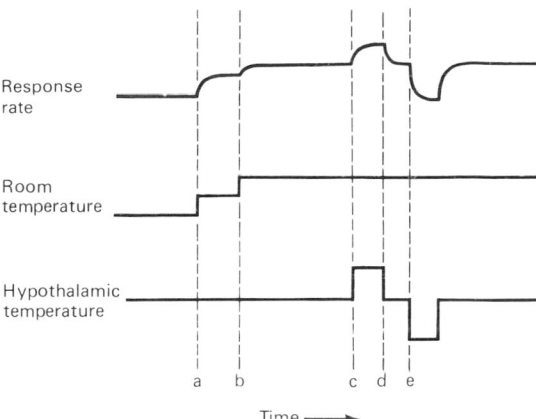

FIGURE 48–3
Peripheral and central information on temperature is summated in the hypothalamus. Changes in room temperature or hypothalamic temperature alter the response rate of rats trained to press a button to receive a brief burst of cool air. When the room temperature is increased, thus presumably increasing skin temperature, the response rate increases roughly in proportion to the temperature increase (points **a** and **b**). If the hypothalamic temperature is also increased, the response rate reflects a summation of the skin temperature and hypothalamic temperature inputs (points **c** and **d**). If skin temperature remains high but the hypothalamus is cooled, the response rate decreases or is suppressed altogether (point **e**). (From Corbit, 1973, and Satinoff, 1964.)

The control of body temperature is a clear example of the integrative function of the hypothalamus in autonomic, endocrine, and drive-state control, and illustrates how the hypothalamus operates directly on the internal environment or provides signals (derived from the internal environment) to control higher neural systems.

Feeding Behavior Is Regulated by a Great Variety of Mechanisms

The analysis of feeding behavior can also be approached in terms of a control system in much the same fashion as temperature regulation, although at every level of analysis the understanding of feeding is less complete.

Body Weight Is Regulated Around a Set Point

One reason it appears that control theory can be applied to feeding behavior is that body weight seems to be controlled by some type of set point system. Humans often maintain the same body weight over a period of many years. Since even a small excess or deficit of daily caloric intake could result in a substantial change of body weight over a long period of time, in some way the body must provide feedback signals that control nutrient intake and metabolism. Control of nutrient intake can be clearly seen

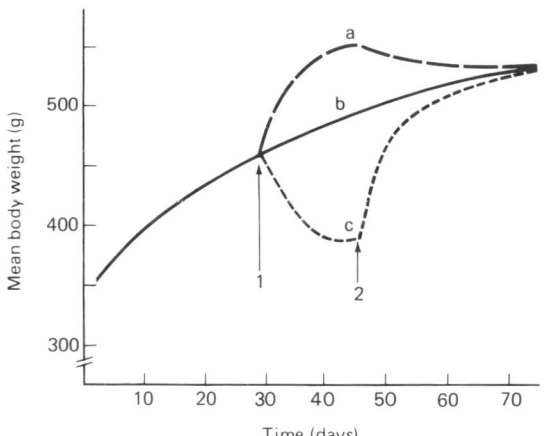

FIGURE 48–4

Animals tend to adjust their food intake to achieve a normal body weight. The plots show a schematized growth curve for a group of rats. At arrow **1** one-third of the animals were maintained on their normal diet (curve **b**), one-third were force-fed (curve **a**), and one-third were placed on a restricted diet (curve **c**). At arrow **2** all rats were placed on a normal (*ad libitum*) diet. The force-fed animals lost weight and the starved animals gained weight until the mean weight of the two groups approached that of the normal growth curve (**b**). (Adapted from Keesey et al., 1976.)

in animal studies in which body weight is altered from the set point either by food deprivation or by force-feeding. In both instances animals adjust their subsequent food intake (either up or down) until they regain a body weight appropriate for their age (Figure 48–4). Animals are said to defend their body weight against perturbations.

Regulation of body weight, however, is different from regulation of body temperature. Whereas body temperature is remarkably similar from individual to individual, body weight has an equally remarkable dissimilarity from individual to individual. Furthermore, the apparent set point of an individual can vary as a function of stress, palatability of the food, exercise, and many other environmental and genetic factors. One possible explanation for these observations is that the set point itself can change on the basis of different factors. Another possibility is that feeding behavior is regulated by some control systems that have no formal set point mechanisms, but which function as if there were set points. Feedback systems of this type do exist in the body. A negative feedback system for the regulation of fat stores in cells is shown in Figure 48–1B. Apparently, the more fat stored in the cell, the less conversion there is of nutrients to fat. Thus, fat stores may directly or indirectly exert a negative feedback that is proportional to the amount of fat. Because of this feedback mechanism, fat stores tend to be stable in the face of varying nutrient input. If nutrient input is increased, however, the system will seek a new set point that is above the former value. In this system the fat stores cannot increase the negative feedback signal (to meet the demands of higher nutrient input), unless the fat stores are first increased somewhat. Automatic physiological feedback sys-

tems of this type appear to play an important role in regulating body weight.

Although body weight varies from animal to animal across and within species, there is a remarkable constancy of the daily expenditure of energy (kcal) expressed per metabolic mass, i.e., body weight (g) raised to the 0.75 power, when animals are permitted to eat freely. The ratio is approximately 70. This relationship (sometimes called Kleiber's rule) holds true for freely feeding animals of different species (Figure 48–5A) as well as for animals within a species (Figure 48–5B). Animals can be driven way above their normal weight by force-feeding or being fed an unusually palatable diet. They can be driven below their normal weight by calorie restriction. Under these circumstances the ratio of energy expenditure to body weight gradually changes: Underweight animals require fewer calories to maintain their weight, whereas overweight animals require more calories to maintain their weight. For the underweight rat, the ratio falls below what would be expected for the new lower weight, and vice versa for the overweight rat (see arrows in Figure 48–5B). Thus, these self-regulating mechanisms tend to return the animal to a weight at which the ratio of energy expenditure to body weight$^{0.75}$ is close to 70.

An important conclusion from these considerations is that the individual's body weight set point can be thought of as that weight at which the ratio of energy expenditure to body weight$^{0.75}$ is close to 70. There is evidence that if the organism is repeatedly subjected to weight loss (as in human dieting patterns), long-term changes may occur; fewer calories will be needed to maintain a given weight, which has the effect of increasing the body weight set point or increasing the person's weight at which the ratio of energy expenditure to body weight$^{0.75}$ is close to 70. Some previously obese individuals who have maintained lower weight for years have abnormally low metabolic rates, and thus can maintain their weight loss only by restricting their caloric intake well below other individuals at the same weight.

Dual Controlling Elements Are Involved in the Control of Food Intake

Food intake is thought to be under the control of two centers in the hypothalamus. In 1942 A. Hetherington and Stephen Ranson reported that destruction in the region of the ventromedial hypothalamic nuclei (see Figure 48–4) and surrounding tissue produces hyperphagia, which results in severe obesity. In contrast, B. K. Anand and John Brobeck found in 1951 that bilateral lesions of the lateral hypothalamus produce the opposite effect—a severe aphagia in which the animal dies unless force-fed and hydrated. Electrical stimulation produces the opposite effects: Lateral stimulation elicits feeding, whereas medial stimulation suppresses feeding. These observations were originally interpreted to mean that the lateral hypothalamus contains a feeding center, and the medial hypothalamus a satiety center. This conceptually attractive conclusion is faulty, however, since the brain is not orga-

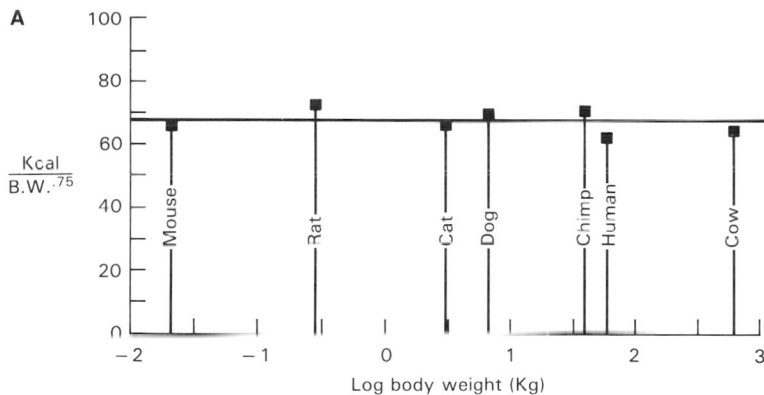

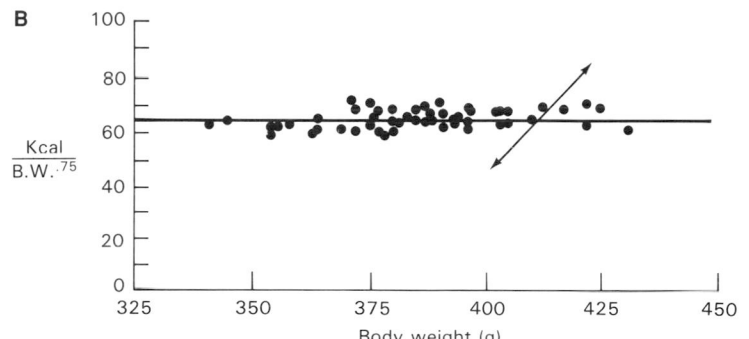

FIGURE 48–5

Daily energy expenditure (kcal) is relatively constant when expressed per metabolic body size (body weight$^{0.75}$). (Adapted from Keesey, 1989, and Kleiber, 1947.)

A. Body weight and daily energy expenditure of various species of mammals.

B. Relative constancy of daily energy expenditure (kcal), expressed per metabolic body size (body weight$^{0.75}$), of individual male rats of the same strain and age at the body weight each spontaneously maintains. If rats are forced to increase or decrease their weight they become, respectively, hyper- or hypometabolic (**arrows**). (Example is for two rats normally weighing 410 grams.)

nized into discrete centers that control specific functions in isolation. Rather, individual functions are performed by neural circuits distributed among several structures in the brain.

The observed results of lateral or medial hypothalamic lesions on feeding are thought to be due to several factors, including (1) alteration of sensory information, (2) alteration of set point, (3) alteration of hormonal balance, and (4) effects on fibers of passage and interference with behavioral arousal. We shall discuss each of these factors, drawing primarily from experiments done on animals, although one or more of them may be seen in patients who have sustained damage to the hypothalamus from vascular disease or a tumor.

Sensory and Motor Deficits. Lateral hypothalamic lesions sometimes result in a lesion of fibers of the trigeminal system, and the resultant sensory loss can contribute to the aphagia. Sectioning of peripheral trigeminal input can also disturb feeding behavior. Sensory or motor deficits might contribute to the phenomenon of sensory neglect seen after lateral hypothalamic lesions. Sensory neglect is most easily studied after unilateral lesions of the lateral hypothalamus. Orienting responses to visual, olfactory, and somatic sensory stimuli presented contralateral to the lesion are greatly reduced; feeding responses to food presented contralaterally are also diminished. It is not clear whether this phenomenon is due to disruption of sensory systems or to interference with motor systems directing responses contralateral to the lesion.

Altered sensory responses are also seen in animals with hyperphagia due to lesions in the region of the ventromedial nucleus. The responsiveness of these animals to the aversive or attractive properties of food and other stimuli is heightened. On a normal diet they eat more than nonlesioned animals, but if the food is adulterated with a bitter substance, they eat less than normal animals. This effect is similar to that seen in normal animals that are made obese by force feeding. Therefore, the altered sensory responsiveness to food of animals with ventromedial hypothalamic lesions probably is, at least in part, a consequence rather than a cause of the obesity. This interpretation is supported by the finding of Stanley Schachter that some obese humans with no evidence of damage to the region of the ventromedial hypothalamus are also unusually responsive to the taste of food.

Alterations of Set Point. Several experiments have indicated that hypothalamic lesions may alter the set point for regulating body weight. In some experiments animals were starved to reduce their weight before a relatively small lateral hypothalamic lesion was made. When the animals resumed eating, ordinarily at a reduced level of intake, they ate more than normally and gained weight, whereas the controls (nonstarved) lost weight (Figure 48–6). The prestarvation apparently brings the weight of these animals below the set point determined by the lateral lesion. Conversely, animals given ventromedial hypothalamic lesions do not overeat, as they ordinarily do, if their weight before the lesion is first increased by force-feeding.

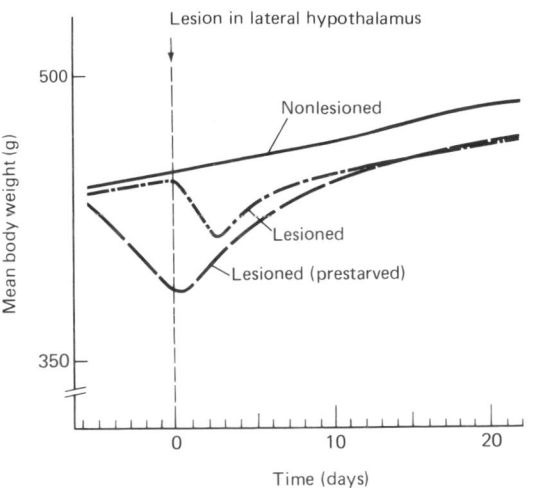

FIGURE 48–6

The set point for body weight appears to be altered by lateral hypothalamic lesions. Three groups of rats were used in this experiment. The control group was maintained on a normal diet. On day zero the animals of the other two groups received small lesions of the lateral hypothalamus. One of these groups had been maintained on a normal diet; the other group had been starved before the lesion and consequently had lost body weight. Following the lesion, all animals were given free access to food. The lesioned animals that had not been prestarved initially decreased their food intake and lost body weight, while those that were prestarved at normal levels rapidly gained weight until they reached the level of the other lesioned animals. (Adapted from Keesey et al., 1976.)

Alteration of Hormonal Balance. Feeding behavior is affected by many hormones, including sex steroids, glucagon, insulin, and growth hormone. Large lesions of the hypothalamus invariably affect many of these hormonal control systems. For example, lesions of the medial hypothalamus result in a greatly increased release of insulin when animals eat. This response may explain, at least in part, the hyperphagia and weight gain seen after medial lesions, since a large amount of insulin in the blood can elicit feeding responses and also promotes the conversion of nutrients into fat. Interestingly, animals with medial hypothalamic lesions show a relative increase in body fat even when their overeating is controlled by limiting their caloric intake to normal levels.

Hypothalamic Lesions and Fibers of Passage. Lesions of the lateral hypothalamus have been found to damage dopamine-containing fibers coursing from the substantia nigra to the striatum. Such lesions may also disrupt dopaminergic fibers that emanate from the ventral tegmental area (the mesolimbic projections) and extensively innervate structures associated with the limbic system, such as the prefrontal cortex and nucleus accumbens (see Chapter 41). In addition, if the dopaminergic fibers themselves are sectioned outside of the hypothalamus, animals exhibit a hypoarousal state and aphagia similar to that observed after lateral hypothalamic lesions. The aphagia following lateral hypothalamic lesions, however, can be more profound and differs in detail.

The possibility that the effects of lateral hypothalamic lesions may be due to interruption of fibers of passage have led investigators to question whether the hypothalamus itself has any role in feeding behavior. This issue has been clarified by the use of chemical lesioning of the hypothalamus. In this technique the lateral hypothalamus is injected locally with kainic or ibotenic acid, glutamate analogs that destroy neuronal cell bodies without affecting fibers of passage. This technique produces aphagia and certain other aspects of a lateral hypothalamic syndrome. Furthermore, Edmund Rolls and his collaborators have found that the hypothalamus contains many neurons that respond to the sight or taste of food and that the cells only respond when the animal is hungry.

Chemical Stimulation of the Hypothalamus Alters Feeding Behavior

Some of the strongest evidence implicating the hypothalamus in the control of feeding comes from studies by Sarah Leibowitz and several other investigators who have shown that chemical stimulation of the hypothalamus by a wide spectrum of transmitters produces profound alterations of feeding behavior. Studies of the paraventricular nucleus (PVN) and the lateral hypothalamic area clearly illustrate that feeding behavior consists of many different components and that different brain systems are involved in the control of specific aspects of feeding. For example, when animals feed, they differentially regulate the type of nutrient ingested, and different transmitters appear to be concerned with the regulation of different nutrients. For example, application of norepinephrine to the paraventricular nucleus greatly stimulates feeding behavior, but animals given a choice of carbohydrate, protein, or fat eat more of the carbohydrate food. Application of the peptide galanin selectively increases ingestion of fat, whereas opiates can enhance consumption of protein.

Although we have emphasized the importance of the hypothalamus in a variety of regulatory mechanisms in this and the preceding chapter, other structures in the nervous system also contribute to homeostatic regulation. Indeed, a limited degree of homeostatic regulation of food intake continues even after the hypothalamus and structures rostral to it are removed. For example, a rat with this type of lesion will eat if food is placed in its mouth and will reject food (satiate) after an appropriate amount of food has been eaten.

A great deal of research has been devoted to analyzing the cues the organism uses to regulate feeding. There are two main sets of regulatory cues for hunger: *short-term cues* regulate the size of individual meals, and *long-term cues* regulate overall body weight. Short-term cues consist primarily of chemical properties of the food that act in the mouth to stimulate feeding behavior and in the gastrointestinal system and liver to inhibit feeding. The short-term satiety signals impinge on the hypothalamus through visceral afferent pathways communicating primarily with lateral hypothalamic regions. The effectiveness of short-term cues is modulated by some long-term signal reflecting body weight (perhaps related to total fat stores). By this means, body weight is kept reasonably constant over a broad range of activity and diet. Body weight, however, is also maintained at a relatively set level by means of self-regulating feedback mechanisms that appropriately adjust metabolic rate when the organism drifts away from its characteristic set point. Thus, if an animal is put on a reduced-calorie diet, its metabolic rate decreases, so that it needs less food to maintain its weight. If the organism is repeatedly subjected to weight loss, a long-term reduction of metabolic rate may occur, such that even when the weight returns to normal, the normal weight will be maintained only if fewer than normal calories are consumed.

Several humoral signals are thought to be important for regulating feeding behavior. The hypothalamus has glucoreceptors that respond to blood glucose levels. This system, however, probably stimulates feeding behavior (in contrast to autonomic responses related to blood glucose) only in pathological emergency states in which blood glucose falls drastically. Other humoral signals that may control feeding include gut hormones that are released during a meal and may contribute to satiety. The best evidence is for a role of the peptide cholecystokinin. Cholecystokinin is released from the duodenum and upper intestine when amino acids and fatty acids are present in the tract. Moreover, systemic injection of cholecystokinin can inhibit feeding behavior by actions that involve peripheral receptors. Cholecystokinin also appears to be released by neurons of the brain (see Chapter 13). Injection of small quantities of cholecystokinin and several other peptides (including neurotensin, calcitonin, and glucagon) into the ventricles or specifically the paraventricular nucleus also inhibits feeding. Therefore, cholecystokinin released in the brain may also inhibit feeding, independently of its release from the gut.

Cholecystokinin is an example of a hormone or neuromodulator that appears to have independent central and peripheral actions that are functionally related. Other examples include luteinizing hormone-releasing hormone (sexual behavior), adrenocorticotropin (stress and avoidance behavior), and angiotensin (responses to hemorrhage; see the section on thirst). The use of the same transmitter for related central and peripheral functions is a widespread phenomenon. In invertebrates, for example, serotonin enhances feeding responses by acting directly on muscles that are involved in consuming food, but also promotes behavioral arousal by acting on the central motor neurons that innervate these muscles.

Thirst Is Regulated by Tissue Osmolality and Vascular Volume

As discussed in Chapter 47, the hypothalamus regulates water balance by direct physiological actions. The hypothalamus also regulates behavioral aspects of drinking. Unlike feeding, as long as a sufficient amount of water is ingested, the precise amount of water taken in is relatively unimportant. Within broad limits, excess intake is readily eliminated. Nevertheless, a set point or ideal amount of

water intake appears to exist, since too much or too little drinking represents inefficient behavior. If an animal takes in too little liquid at one time, it must soon interrupt other activities and resume its liquid intake to avoid underhydration. Drinking a large amount at one time results in unneeded time spent drinking, as well as urinating to eliminate the excess fluid.

Drinking is controlled by two main physiological variables: *tissue osmolality* and *vascular (fluid) volume*. These variables appear to be handled by separate but interrelated mechanisms. Drinking also can be controlled by dryness of the tongue, and by hyperthermia, detected at least in part by thermosensitive neurons in the anterior hypothalamus.

The feedback signals for water regulation derive from many sources. Osmotic stimuli can act directly on osmoreceptor (or sodium-level receptor) cells (probably neurons) in the hypothalamus. The feedback signals for vascular volume are located in the low-pressure side of the circulation—the right atrium and adjacent walls of the great veins. Large volume changes may also affect arterial baroreceptors in the aortic arch and carotid sinus, and signals from these sources can initiate drinking. Low blood volume (as well as other conditions that decrease body sodium) also results in an increase of renin secreted from the kidney. Renin, a proteolytic enzyme, cleaves plasma angiotensinogen into angiotensin I, which is then hydrolyzed to the highly active octapeptide angiotensin II. Angiotensin II elicits drinking as well as three other physiological actions that compensate for water loss: (1) vasoconstriction, (2) increased release of aldosterone, and (3) increased release of vasopressin.

Alan Johnson has begun to unravel the mode of action of angiotensin and baroreceptor afferents in regulating drinking. It was long suspected that for blood-borne angiotensin to affect behavior it was likely to stimulate those regions of the brain that permitted substances to pass the blood–brain barrier. Studies by Alan Epstein and collaborators showed that angiotensin operates at one such region—the subfornical organ. This organ is a small neuronal structure that extends into the third ventricle and has fenestrated capillaries that readily permit the passage of blood-borne molecules. As previously discussed (Chapter 47), the subfornical organ responds to very low concentrations of angiotensin II in the blood. A neural pathway between the subfornical organ and the preoptic area conveys this information to the hypothalamus. This pathway uses an angiotensin-like molecule as a transmitter. Thus, the same molecule regulates drinking by functioning as a hormone and also as a neurotransmitter. The preoptic area also receives information from baroreceptors throughout the body. This information is integrated and then conveyed to various brain structures that activate the animal to seek water and to drink. Information from baroreceptors is also sent to structures such as the paraventricular nucleus, which mediates the release of vasopressin (see Chapter 47), which in turn regulates water retention.

The signals that terminate drinking are less well understood than those that initiate drinking. It is clear, however, that the termination signal is not always merely the absence of the initiating signal. This principle holds for many examples of physiological and behavioral regulation, including feeding. Thus, for example, drinking initiated by low vascular fluid volume (e.g., after severe hemorrhage) terminates well before the deficit is rectified. This is highly adaptive since it prevents water intoxication due to excessive dilution of extracellular fluids. It also seems to prevent overhydration that could result from absorption of fluid in the alimentary system long after the cessation of drinking.

Motivational States Can Be Regulated by Factors Other Than Tissue Needs

We have so far dealt with the role of tissue needs in signaling the nervous system to initiate appropriate behavioral and physiological responses to minimize or eliminate deficits. A thorough understanding of motivated behaviors, however, requires knowledge of many factors not related to tissue deficit. For example, sexual responses and curiosity do not appear to be controlled by the lack of specific substances in the body. Even homeostatic responses, such as drinking and feeding, are regulated by innate and learned mechanisms that modulate the effects of the feedback signals that indicate tissue deficits. In humans, in particular, learned habits and subjective feelings of pleasure can override interoceptive feedback signals. For example, people often choose to go hungry rather than eat food they have learned to avoid. Here we shall briefly describe three factors that regulate motivated behaviors: the particular ecological requirements of the organism, anticipatory mechanisms, and hedonic (pleasure) factors.

Ecological Constraints

The details of particular behavior patterns are determined by evolutionary selection, which shapes responses so that they are appropriate for the ecology of the particular animal. One means of analyzing motivated behaviors in an ecological context is to do cost-benefit analyses similar to those done by economists. For feeding behavior, costs include the time and effort to search for and procure food. The benefit consists of nutrient intake that will ultimately support a given level of reproductive success. The spacing and duration of meals can be considered to reflect the operation of brain mechanisms that have evolved to maximize gain and minimize costs. According to this type of analysis, carnivores may eat very rapidly not because they have exceptionally powerful feedback signals indicating severe deprivation, but because they have evolved mechanisms that help ensure that their kill will not have to be shared with other animals. Ecological considerations need not preclude consideration of homeostatic mechanisms, since homeostatic mechanisms also have evolved to assist the organism in adapting to its particular environmental conditions.

Anticipatory Mechanisms

Homeostatic regulation often is anticipatory and can be initiated before any physiological deficit occurs. Clock mechanisms turn physiological behavioral responses on and off before the occurrence of tissue deficit or need. One such common mechanism is a daily rhythm with a free-running period typically close to 24 hours, called a *circadian rhythm* (Latin *circa*, around, and *dies*, a day). In the presence of a repeated 24-hour signal (typically light–dark cycles) the circadian rhythm runs exactly 24 hours. However, circadian rhythms are autogenous—they continue under constant dark, although in periods of somewhat more or less than 24 hours.

Circadian rhythms exist for virtually every homeostatic function of the body. Since many of the rhythms are coordinated, the hypothalamus would seem to be the ideal location for a major clock mechanism that would drive them, or at least coordinate independent clock mechanisms located throughout the brain. The results of lesion studies of the suprachiasmatic nucleus of the rat support this suggestion (Figure 48–7). Animals with these lesions lose 24-hour rhythmicity of corticosteroid release, feeding, drinking, locomotor activity, and several other responses. Furthermore, Benjamin Rusak and his colleagues have found that exposure of animals to light pulses just at the phases of the circadian rhythm during which light can shift the rhythm leads to an increase in the products of immediate-early genes, such as *c-fos*, in neurons in the suprachiasmatic nucleus. The immediate-early gene products may alter DNA transcription and thereby play a role in regulating the circadian pacemaker. (See also Chapter 51.)

In primates, including humans, there appear to be two primary oscillators that are linked during normal light–dark cycles but that run free with independent cycles under conditions of constant light. One oscillator controls

FIGURE 48–7

Lesions of the suprachiasmatic nucleus affect the daily activity rhythm of the rat. Normal animals exhibit 24-hour rhythms during periods of light and dark (**white** and **hatched areas**, respectively) and approximately 24-hour rhythms in constant dark. Animals with lesions of the suprachiasmatic nucleus completely lose the 24-hour rhythm.

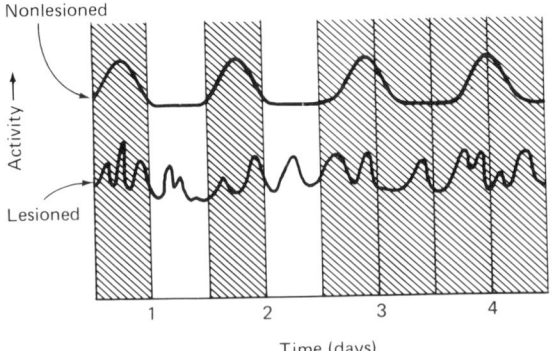

such functions as slow-wave sleep, plasma growth hormone, skin temperature, and calcium excretion and appears to be driven by the suprachiasmatic nucleus. Direct retinal projections to this nucleus may provide the cyclical light–dark signals. The suprachiasmatic nucleus provides a means of regulating the rhythm of many different systems with a minimal amount of wiring, and it illustrates the advantage of clustering related functions into an anatomically discrete structure. The second oscillator controls rapid eye movement (REM) sleep, plasma corticosteroids, body core temperature, and potassium excretion.

Hedonic Factors

Unquestionably, pleasure is a factor in the control of motivated behaviors of humans. Humans will sometimes even subject themselves to deprivation in order to heighten the pleasure obtained when the deprivation is relieved (e.g., skipping lunch in order to enjoy dinner more), or to obtain pleasure by satisfying some other need (e.g., dieting to look attractive). Since pleasure is subjective, it is difficult to study in animals, but there are reasons to believe that a similar variable may control motivated animal behavior. For example, in 1976 Anthony Sclafani found that rats given a very palatable diet containing a variety of junk foods (chocolate chip cookies, salami) eat much more than when they are given a bland and comparably nutritious diet of rat chow. The neural bases of pleasure are poorly understood, but it seems reasonable to hypothesize that these mechanisms overlap or even coincide with brain mechanisms (including those in the hypothalamus) that are concerned with reward and the reinforcement of learned behavior.

Intracranial Stimulation Can Simulate Motivational States and Reinforce Behavior

One of the most influential discoveries related to mechanisms of drive was the finding by James Olds and Peter Milner in 1954 that intracranial electrical stimulation of the hypothalamus and associated structures can act as reinforcement in operant conditioning of animals (see Chapter 62 for a discussion of operant conditioning). In many respects brain stimulation appears to act like ordinary reinforcing stimuli, such as food, but with one important difference. Ordinary stimuli are effective only if the animal is in a particular drive state; for example, food serves as a reinforcing stimulus only in hungry animals. In contrast, brain stimulation seems to work regardless of the drive state of the animal. These considerations led Anthony Deutsch and C. Howarth in 1963 to postulate that brain stimulation produces reinforcement in two ways: (1) it evokes a drive state, and (2) it activates systems that are normally activated by a reinforcing stimulus. Support for this idea has come from subsequent observations that many of the points in the brain that are effective in producing reward also stimulate complex behavioral patterns such as feeding and drinking.

Although stimulation has been found to be reinforcing at many different sites in the brain, hypothalamic sites are particularly effective. Very effective sites are found along the medial forebrain bundle and the structures it innervates. Stimulation of the nucleus accumbens is also reinforcing. In fact, addictive drugs such as cocaine may induce euphoria by enhancing the action of dopamine at the nucleus accumbens, which receives substantial dopaminergic input.

There have been many attempts to relate reinforcing brain stimulation to pathways that use specific neurotransmitters, usually one or another biogenic amine. The available evidence indicates that dopaminergic pathways may be involved in some way, although it is unlikely that a complex behavioral phenomenon like reinforcement involves only a single transmitter.

An Overall View

The hypothalamus is concerned with the regulation of various behaviors that are directed toward homeostatic goals such as food, water, or sexual gratification. The hypothalamus contributes to these behaviors by receiving information from both external incentive stimuli and internal stimuli that report on the homeostatic state of the animal. Many functions of the hypothalamus can be understood in terms of servocontrol systems.

Although other structures in the nervous system participate in regulatory functions, the hypothalamus, because of its intimate relationship with both the autonomic system and the endocrine system, appears to play a central role in regulating the complex behaviors of higher organisms.

Selected Readings

Bligh, J. 1973. Temperature Regulation in Mammals and Other Vertebrates. Amsterdam: North-Holland.

Booth, D. A., Toates, F. M., and Platt, S. V. 1976. Control system for hunger and its implications in animals and man. In D. Novin, W. Wyrwicka, and G. A. Bray (eds.), Hunger: Basic Mechanisms and Clinical Implications. New York: Raven Press, pp. 127–143.

Boulant, J. A. 1981. Hypothalamic mechanisms in thermoregulation. Fed. Proc. 40:2843–2850.

Friedman, M. I., and Stricker, E. M. 1976. The physiological psychology of hunger: A physiological perspective. Psychol. Rev. 83:409–431.

Keesey, R. E. 1989. Physiological regulation of body weight and the issue of obesity. Med. Clinics N. Am. 73:15–27.

Kissileff, H. R., and Van Itallie, T. B. 1982. Physiology of the control of food intake. Annu. Rev. Nutr. 2:371–418.

Moore-Ede, M. C. 1983. The circadian timing system in mammals: Two pacemakers preside over many secondary oscillators. Fed. Proc. 42:2802–2808.

Rolls, B. J., and Rolls, E. T. 1982. Thirst. Cambridge, England: Cambridge University Press.

Rolls, E. T. 1981. Central nervous mechanisms related to feeding and appetite. Br. Med. Bull. 37:131–134.

Schoener, T. W. 1971. Theory of feeding strategies. Annu. Rev. Ecol. Syst. 2:369–404.

Toates, F. 1986. Motivational Systems. Cambridge, England: Cambridge University Press.

Weiss, K. R., Koch, U. T., Koester, J., Rosen, S. C., and Kupfermann, I. 1982. The role of arousal in modulating feeding behavior of *Aplysia*: Neural and behavioral studies. In B. G. Hoebel and D. Novin (eds.), The Neural Basis of Feeding and Reward. Brunswick, Me.: Haer Institute, pp. 25–57.

References

Anand, B. K., and Brobeck, J. R. 1951. Localization of a "feeding center" in the hypothalamus of the rat. Proc. Soc. Exp. Biol. Med. 77:323–324.

Boulant, J. A., and Silva, N. L. 1988. Neuronal sensitivities in preoptic tissue slices: Interactions among homeostatic systems. Brain Res. Bull. 20:871–878.

Corbit, J. D. 1973. Voluntary control of hypothalamic temperature. J. Comp. Physiol. Psychol. 83:394–411.

Deutsch, J. A., and Howarth, C. I. 1963. Some tests of a theory of intracranial self-stimulation. Psychol. Rev. 70:444–460.

Di Girolamo, M., and Rudman, D. 1968. Variations in glucose metabolism and sensitivity to insulin of the rat's adipose tissue, in relation to age and body weight. Endocrinology 82: 1133–1141.

Epstein, A. N., Fitzsimons, J. T., and Rolls, B. J. 1970. Drinking induced by injection of angiotensin into the brain of the rat. J. Physiol. (Lond.) 210:457–474.

Hetherington, A. W., and Ranson, S. W. 1942. The spontaneous activity and food intake of rats with hypothalamic lesions. Am. J. Physiol. 136:609–617.

Hori, T., Nakashima, T., Koga, H., Kiyohara, T., and Inoue, T. 1988. Convergence of thermal, osmotic and cardiovascular signals on preoptic and anterior hypothalmic neurons in the rat. Brain Res. Bull. 20:879–885.

Johnson, A. K., and Cunningham, J. T. 1987. Brain mechanisms and drinking: The role of lamina terminalis-associated systems in extracellular thirst. Kidney Int. 32[Suppl 21]:S-35–S-42.

Jonsson, G. 1980. Chemical neurotoxins as denervation tools in neurobiology. Annu. Rev. Neurosci. 3:169–187.

Kleiber, M. 1947. Body size and metabolic rate. Physiol. Rev. 27:511–541.

Kasting, N. W. 1989. Criteria for establishing a physiological role for brain peptides. A case in point: The role of vasopressin in thermoregulation during fever and antipyresis. Brain Res. Rev. 14:143–153.

Keesey, R. E., Boyle, P. C., Kemnitz, J. W., and Mitchel, J. S. 1976. The role of the lateral hypothalamus in determining the body weight set point. In D. Novin, W. Wyrwicka, and G. A. Bray (eds.), Hunger: Basic Mechanisms and Clinical Implications. New York: Raven Press, pp. 243–255.

Leibowitz, S. F., and Stanley, B. G. 1986. Brain peptides and the control of eating behavior. In T. W. Moody (ed.), Neural and Endocrine Peptides and Receptors. New York: Plenum Press, pp. 333–352.

Moore, R. Y., and Lenn, N. J. 1972. A retinohypothalamic projection in the rat. J. Comp. Neurol. 146:1–14.

Olds, J., and Milner, P. 1954. Positive reinforcement produced by electrical stimulation of septal area and other regions of rat brain. J. Comp. Physiol. Psychol. 47:419–427.

Rolls, E. T., Sanghera, M. K., and Roper-Hall, A. 1979. The latency of activation of neurones in the lateral hypothalamus and substantia innominata during feeding in the monkey. Brain Res. 164:121–135.

Rusak, B., Robertson, H. A., Wisden, W., and Hunt, S. P. 1990. Light pulses that shift rhythms induce gene expression in the suprachiasmatic nucleus. Science. 248:1237–1240.

Satinoff, E. 1964. Behavioral thermoregulation in response to local cooling of the rat brain. Am. J. Physiol. 206:1389–1394.

Schachter, S. 1971. Some extraordinary facts about obese humans and rats. Am. Psychol. 26:129–144.

Sclafani, A. 1976. Appetite and hunger in experimental obesity syndromes. In D. Novin, W. Wyrwicka, and G. A. Bray (eds.), Hunger: Basic Mechanisms and Clinical Implications. New York: Raven Press, pp. 281–295.

Stellar, J. R., and Stellar, E. 1985. The Neurobiology of Motivation and Reward. New York: Springer.

Jane Dodd
Lorna W. Role

49

The Autonomic Nervous System

The Autonomic Nervous System Is a Visceral and Largely Involuntary Motor System

The Autonomic Nervous System Is Organized into Three Divisions

The Sympathetic (Thoracolumbar) Division

The Parasympathetic (Craniosacral) Division

The Enteric Division

The Hypothalamus and the Nucleus of the Solitary Tract Play a Major Role in Controlling the Output of the Autonomic Nervous System

The Autonomic Nervous System Has Been Studied at the Cellular Level

Synaptic Transmission in Autonomic Ganglia Is Predominantly Cholinergic

Autonomic Targets Are Regulated by Both Cholinergic and Noradrenergic Input

Autonomic Control of Target Function Is Coordinately Regulated

An Overall View

T he concept that body states are regulated toward a steady state (homeostasis) was proposed by Walter Cannon in 1932. At the same time, Cannon introduced the idea of *negative feedback regulation*.

If a state remains steady, it does so because any tendency for change is automatically met by increased effectiveness of the factor or factors which resist the change. As examples, I may cite thirst when there is need of water; the discharge of adrenaline which liberates sugar from the liver, when the concentration of sugar in the blood falls below a critical point; and the increased breathing which reduces carbonic acid when the blood tends to shift toward acidity.

Cannon further proposed that an important part of this feedback-regulated control is mediated by the autonomic nervous system through the hypothalamus.

The autonomic nervous system has three major divisions: sympathetic, parasympathetic, and enteric. Cannon suggested that two of these, the sympathetic and the parasympathetic divisions, have a primary role in regulating the internal environment. The sympathetic division governs the *fight and flight* reaction, whereas the parasympathetic system is responsible for *rest and digest*. In emergency situations the body is called on to cope with a sudden change in its external or internal environment—combat, athletic competition, severe change in temperature, blood loss. To respond rapidly to the external environment, the hypothalamus activates the sympathetic nervous system. This results in increased sympathetic outflow to the heart and other viscera, peripheral vasculature, sweat glands, as well as the piloerector and ocular muscles. The increased cardiac output, altered body temperature and blood glucose, and pupillary dilation permit rapid responses to potentially disturbing external conditions. In contrast, the parasympathetic system maintains basal heart rate, respiration, and metabolism under normal conditions.

Cannon demonstrated that without a sympathetic nervous system an animal can survive when it is sheltered, kept warm, and not stressed. A sympathectomized animal cannot carry out strenuous work or fend for itself. In these animals blood sugar is not mobilized on demand from the liver, red blood cells do not increase in the circulation in response to exercise, and normal reactions to cold do not occur; there is no vasoconstriction or elevation of hairs. In short, the animal cannot survive in a harsh environment. The autonomic nervous system is not only recruited for emergency or restorative purposes, however. Many sympathetic and parasympathetic pathways are tonically active and operate in conjunction with the somatic motor system to regulate normal behavior and to maintain a steady internal environment in the face of changing external conditions.

The Autonomic Nervous System Is a Visceral and Largely Involuntary Motor System

The autonomic nervous system is primarily an effector system. It controls smooth muscle, heart muscle, and exocrine glands. As a result, it often is referred to as the *autonomic* (or *visceral*) *motor system*, in contrast to the *somatic motor system*. The anatomical principles underlying the organization of both motor systems are similar and the two systems function in parallel to adjust the body to environmental changes. Nevertheless, the two systems differ in important ways.

First, most movements initiated by the somatic motor system are under voluntary control, whereas most autonomic adjustments are automatic—they are not subject to significant voluntary control nor are they accessible to conscious inspection. The autonomic nervous system is therefore also called the *involuntary motor system*, in contrast to the *voluntary (somatic) motor system*. However, the differences in voluntary control between the two motor systems is relative and not absolute. Certain movements, particularly reflex responses, are involuntary. At the same time, certain autonomic adjustments, for example those involved in blood pressure regulation, can be brought under partial voluntary control with practice.

Second, all somatic motor neurons are located within the central nervous system, either within cranial motor nuclei or in the ventral horn of the spinal cord (Chapters 35 and 45). Moreover, the efferent pathway to skeletal muscle is *monosynaptic*—the central motor neurons project directly to skeletal muscle. In contrast, all autonomic motor neurons are located peripherally within autonomic ganglia that lie outside the central nervous system (Figures 49–1 and 49–2). These autonomic motor neurons

FIGURE 49–1

Schematic representations of the anatomical organization of somatic motor and autonomic motor systems.

A. Somatic motor neurons project directly to their target skeletal muscles from the central nervous system.

B. Autonomic preganglionic motor neurons project to autonomic postganglionic motor neurons, which in turn synapse on their visceral targets.

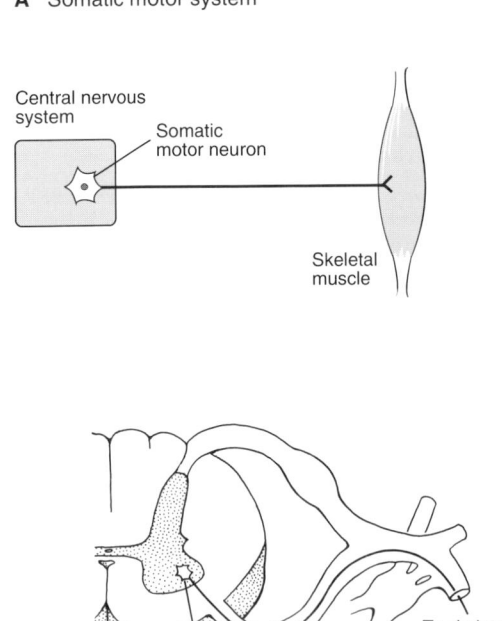

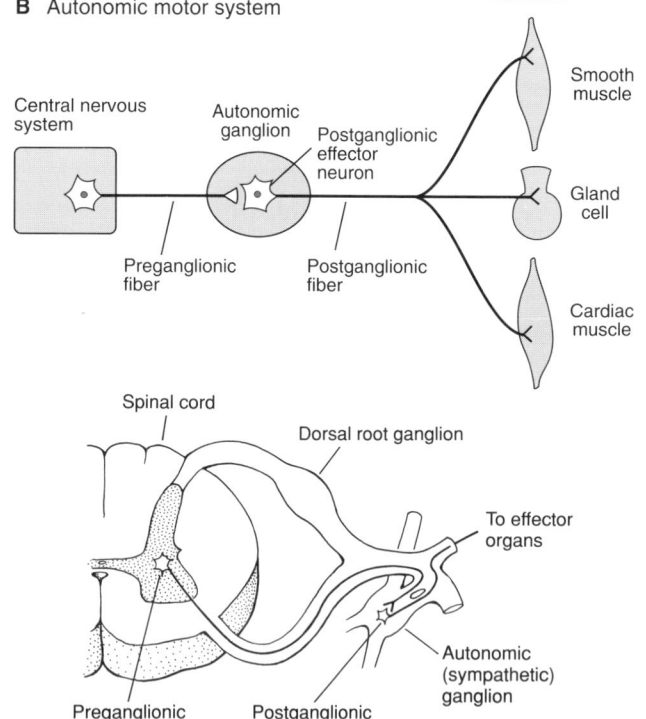

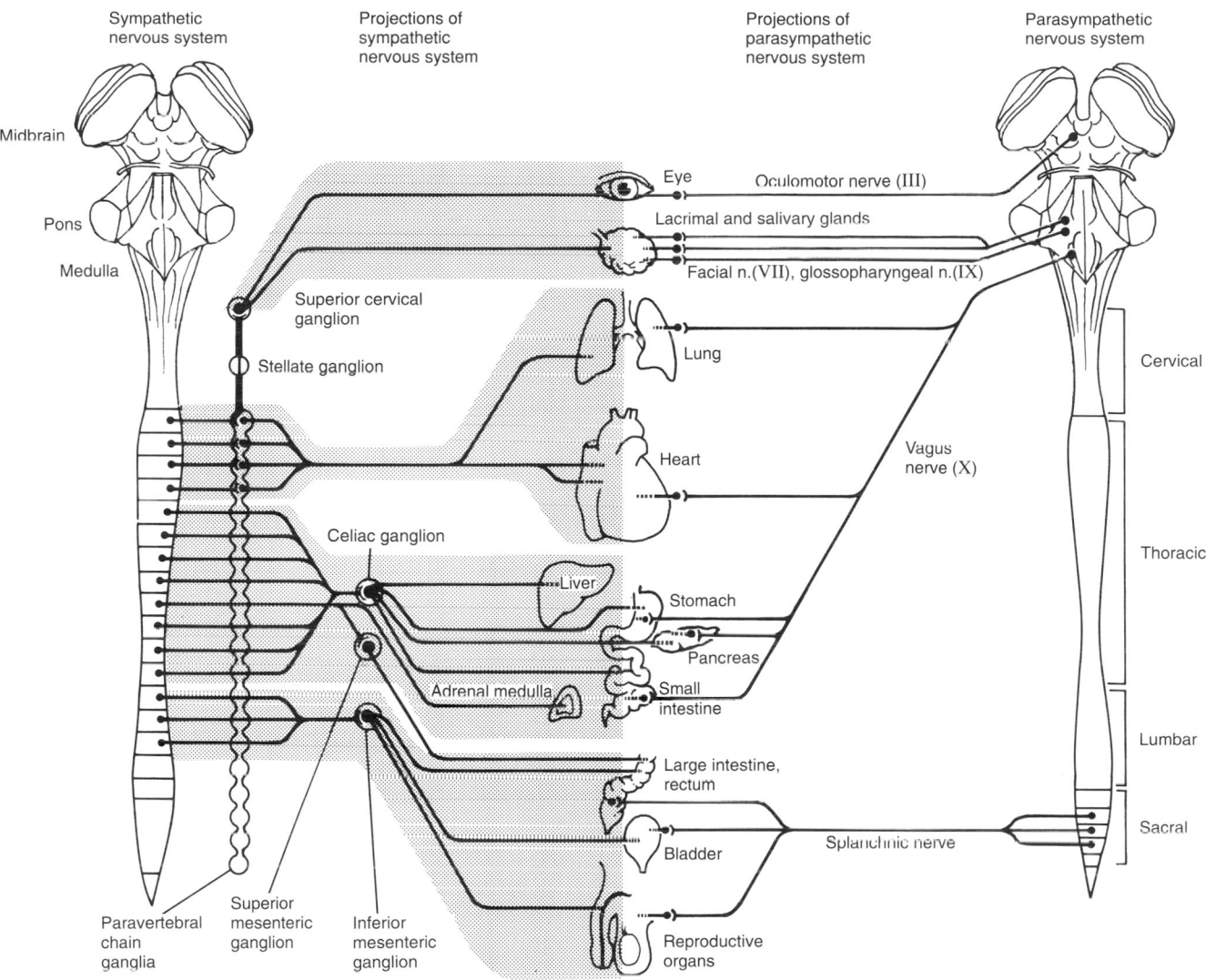

FIGURE 49–2

Sympathetic and parasympathetic divisions of the autonomic nervous system. Preganglionic neurons of the sympathetic division extend from the first thoracic spinal segment to lower lumbar segments. Parasympathetic preganglionic neurons are located within the brain stem and in segments S2 to S4 of the spinal cord. This figure also illustrates the coordinate innervation of a subset of targets by these two divisions of the autonomic nervous system.

(also called *postganglionic neurons*) are activated by columns of *preganglionic neurons* within brain stem nuclei and the spinal cord. Thus, in the visceral motor system the efferent pathway to the target is *disynaptic*: A synapse in a peripheral autonomic ganglion is interposed between the efferent neuron in the central nervous system and the target organ in the periphery.

Third, the somatic and autonomic motor systems differ in the mechanisms by which motor output is inhibited. All somatic motor neurons are excitatory; inhibition is exerted centrally onto the motor neuron. Thus, relaxation of skeletal muscle is achieved not by inhibiting the muscle directly but by inhibiting the motor neurons in the spinal cord that excite the muscle. In contrast, autonomic targets typically receive direct inhibitory inputs. The abil-

ity of the autonomic nervous system to excite and inhibit targets directly, combined with the anatomical arrangement of effector neurons in the interconnected autonomic ganglia, permits the system to respond to environmental demands in a concerted fashion (Figure 49–2).

The Autonomic Nervous System Is Organized into Three Divisions

The autonomic nervous system has three principal divisions: the sympathetic (or thoracolumbar), the parasympathetic (or craniosacral), and the enteric. Anatomically, the three differ in the positions of the preganglionic neurons and in the organization of postganglionic neurons. We shall consider each in turn.

The Sympathetic (Thoracolumbar) Division

Preganglionic cells of the sympathetic division extend from the first thoracic spinal segment to lower lumbar segments. The cell bodies of the preganglionic neurons are found within the spinal cord primarily within the intermediolateral gray matter (Figure 49–2 and 49–3). Axons of preganglionic neurons emerge from the spinal cord through the ventral root, enter the spinal nerve, and then separate from the somatic motor axons to project through the white rami communicantes (communicating branches, which are white because fibers in them are myelinated) to the *paravertebral chain ganglia*. Preganglionic fibers exit the spinal cord at the segmental level at which their cell bodies are located; they may innervate sympathetic ganglia at the same spinal level or ganglia more rostral or caudal to it by traveling within the ganglionic connective (or trunk) (Figure 49–3). Each preganglionic fiber synapses with many postganglionic neurons that are often distributed among different paravertebral ganglia. This divergence permits coordinated activation of sympathetic neurons at several spinal levels.

The axons of postganglionic neurons within the paravertebral ganglia exit through the gray rami communicantes, and those that innervate structures in the head travel along branches of the carotid arteries to their targets. Those innervating the rest of the body travel in the spinal peripheral nerves to their autonomic targets. Some neurons of the cervical and upper thoracic ganglia innervate cranial and peripheral vessels, sweat glands, and hair follicles while others innervate visceral organs and glands of the head and chest, including lacrimal and salivary glands, as well as the heart, lungs, and vascular smooth muscle (Figure 49–2). Lower thoracic and lumbar paravertebral ganglia innervate peripheral blood vessels, sweat glands, and pilomotor smooth muscle.

Some preganglionic fibers pass without interruption through the paravertebral sympathetic ganglia and branches of the splanchnic nerves to synapse on neurons of the *prevertebral* (or collateral) *ganglia*, which include the coeliac ganglion and the superior and inferior mesenteric ganglia (Figures 49–2 and 49–3). The prevertebral sympathetic ganglia innervate the gastrointestinal system and the accessory gastrointestinal organs, including the

FIGURE 49–3

Organization of the sympathetic division of the autonomic nervous system. (From Loewy and Spyer, 1990.)

A. Anatomical organization of the projection path of sympathetic preganglionic and postganglionic axons.

B. 1. General organization of sympathetic innervation.
2. Specific projections of sympathetic preganglionic and postganglionic axons.

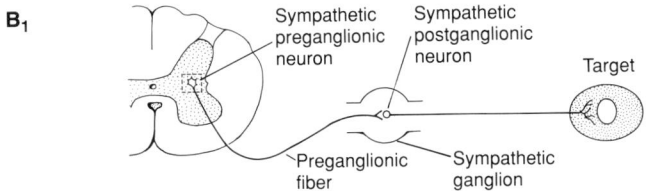

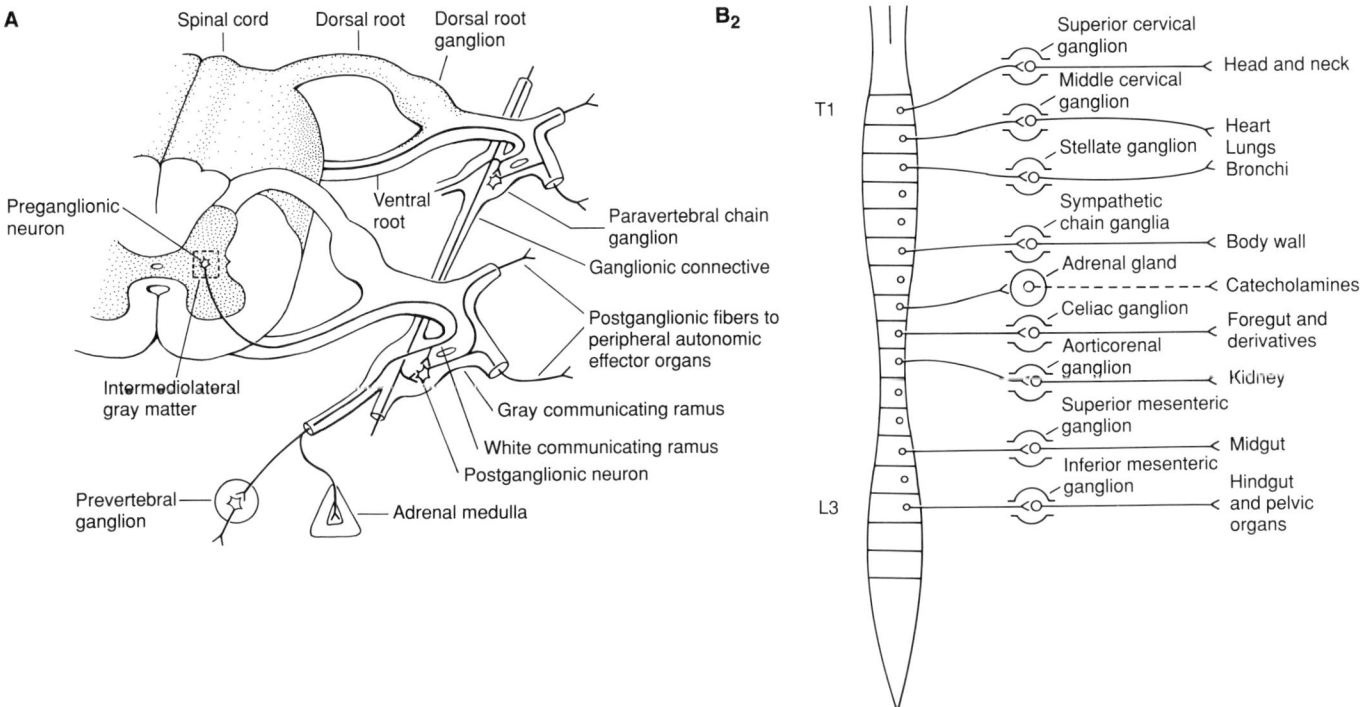

A General organization of parasympathetic innervation

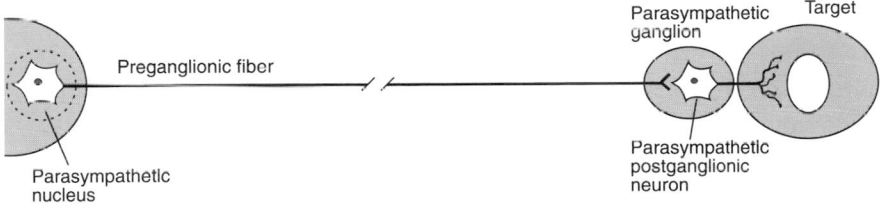

B 1 Midbrain

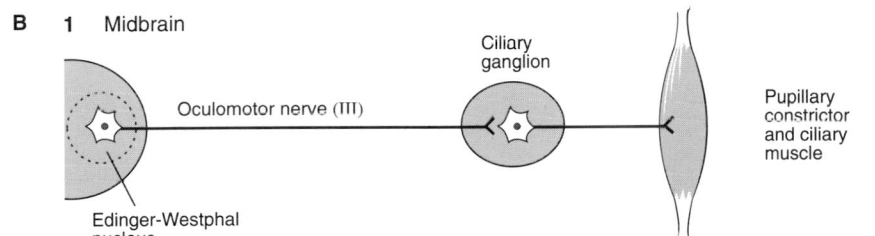

2 Pons

3 Medulla

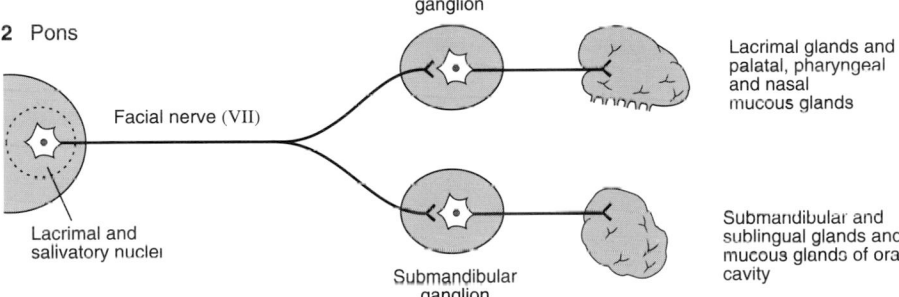

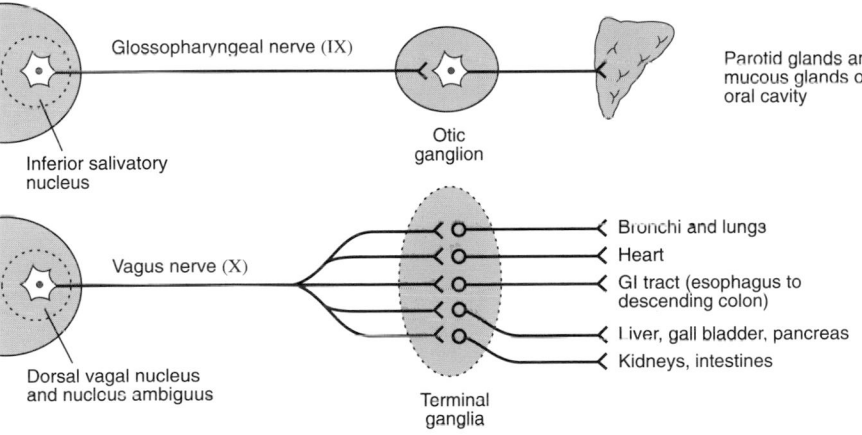

4 Sacral spinal cord

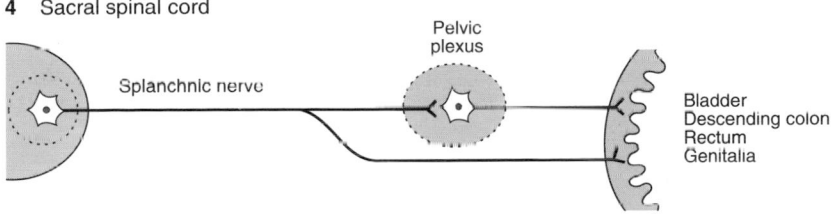

FIGURE 49–4

Organization of the parasympathetic division of the autonomic nervous system.

A. General scheme of the projection path of parasympathetic preganglionic and postganglionic axons.

B. Specific projections of parasympathetic preganglionic and postganglionic axons.

kidneys, pancreas, and liver, and also provide the major sympathetic innervation of the bladder and external genitalia. Another group of preganglionic fibers runs with the thoracic splanchnic nerve into the abdomen and innervates cells of the adrenal medulla. The adrenal medullary cells are developmentally and functionally related to postganglionic sympathetic neurons (see below).

A major difference between the sympathetic and parasympathetic systems is the extent of their divergence. In the sympathetic system the ratio of preganglionic to postganglionic fibers is approximately 1 : 10. In contrast, the peripheral projections of the parasympathetic system are less diffuse, with a ratio of preganglionic to postganglionic fibers of approximately 1 : 3. These differences are paralleled in the diffuse adrenergic transmitter actions characteristic of the sympathetic postganglionic neurons and the more specific cholinergic actions of the parasympathetic postganglionic neurons (to be described later).

The Parasympathetic (Craniosacral) Division

The cell bodies of the preganglionic neurons of the parasympathetic division are located within the brain stem in several nuclei and in segments S2–S4 of the spinal cord (Figures 49–2 and 49–4). Characteristically, axons of parasympathetic preganglionic neurons are considerably longer than those of postganglionic neurons (see Figure 49–4). Thus, parasympathetic preganglionic neurons within both the brain stem and the spinal cord project to postganglionic neurons in ganglia that are close to visceral targets or actually embedded in them. In contrast, sympathetic ganglia within the para- or prevertebral chains are distant from their targets.

Parasympathetic preganglionic nuclei in the brain stem include the Edinger–Westphal nucleus (associated with cranial nerve III), the superior and inferior salivatory nuclei (associated with cranial nerves VII and IX, respectively), and the dorsal vagal nucleus and the nucleus ambiguus (both associated with cranial nerve X). Preganglionic axons leave the brain stem through their respective cranial nerves and project to postganglionic neurons in the ciliary, pterygopalatine, submandibular, and otic ganglia (Figure 49–4). Parasympathetic preganglionic fibers such as the vagus innervate parasympathetic ganglion neurons, which in turn innervate the target tissues. The axons of motor neurons in the dorsal vagal nucleus project in the vagus nerve to postganglionic neurons embedded in thoracic and abdominal targets—the lungs, esophagus, stomach, liver, gall bladder, pancreas, and upper intestinal tract (see Figures 49–3 and 49–4). Neurons of the ventrolateral nucleus ambiguus provide the principal parasympathetic innervation of the cardiac ganglion, which innervates the heart. Neurons in or very close to the nucleus ambiguus also project to the esophagus.

The parasympathetic preganglionic cell bodies in the sacral spinal cord occupy an intermediolateral position but do not form a column as distinct as that of sympathetic preganglionic neurons within the thoracic and lumbar cord. The axons of spinal parasympathetic pre-

ganglionic neurons leave the spinal cord via the ventral roots and project in the pelvic nerve to parasympathetic postganglionic neurons in the pelvic ganglion plexus. Pelvic ganglion neurons innervate the descending colon, bladder, and external genitalia (Figures 49–3, 49–4, and 49–11).

The Enteric Division

The enteric nervous system innervates the gastrointestinal tract, the pancreas, and the gall bladder. It is composed of local sensory neurons that register alterations in the tension of the gut walls and the chemical environment, as well as interneurons and motor neurons that control the muscles of the gut wall and vasculature and the secretory activity of the mucosa. Thus, the enteric nervous system can function autonomously, though its activity is normally regulated by central nervous system reflexes. By its control of gastrointestinal blood vessel tone, motility, gastric secretion, and fluid transport, the enteric nervous system plays a major role in homeostasis.

The neurons of the enteric nervous system are arranged in interconnected plexuses—complex meshworks of ganglia and interconnecting nerve fibers. The plexuses are situated between the various layers of muscle and endothelium (Figure 49–5). The two major intrinsic plexuses are the myenteric (or Auerbach's) and the submucous (or Meissner's) plexuses. The myenteric plexus lies between the external longitudinal and circular smooth muscle layers while the submucosal plexus lies within the connective tissue of the submucosa between the circular muscle and the mucosa.

The enteric nervous system is regulated by an extrinsic innervation that is supplied by the parasympathetic and sympathetic systems. Parasympathetic preganglionic neurons project directly to enteric ganglia of the stomach, colon, and rectum through the vagus and the pelvic splanchnic nerves. The sympathetic innervation is primarily postganglionic from prevertebral sympathetic ganglia, with some innervation from the cervical paravertebral chain. These ganglia project to plexuses in the wall of the stomach, the small intestine, and the colon. The innervation of the gut by the sympathetic and parasympathetic fibers of the autonomic nervous system provides a second level of control of motility and secretion, but also can override intrinsic enteric activity in situations of emergency or stress.

The Hypothalamus and the Nucleus of the Solitary Tract Play a Major Role in Controlling the Output of the Autonomic Nervous System

The output of the autonomic nervous system is influenced by many regions of the brain: the cerebral cortex, the hippocampus, the entorhinal cortex, parts of the thalamus, basal ganglia, cerebellum, and the reticular formation. Most of these regions produce their actions by way of the hypothalamus. The hypothalamus in turn integrates

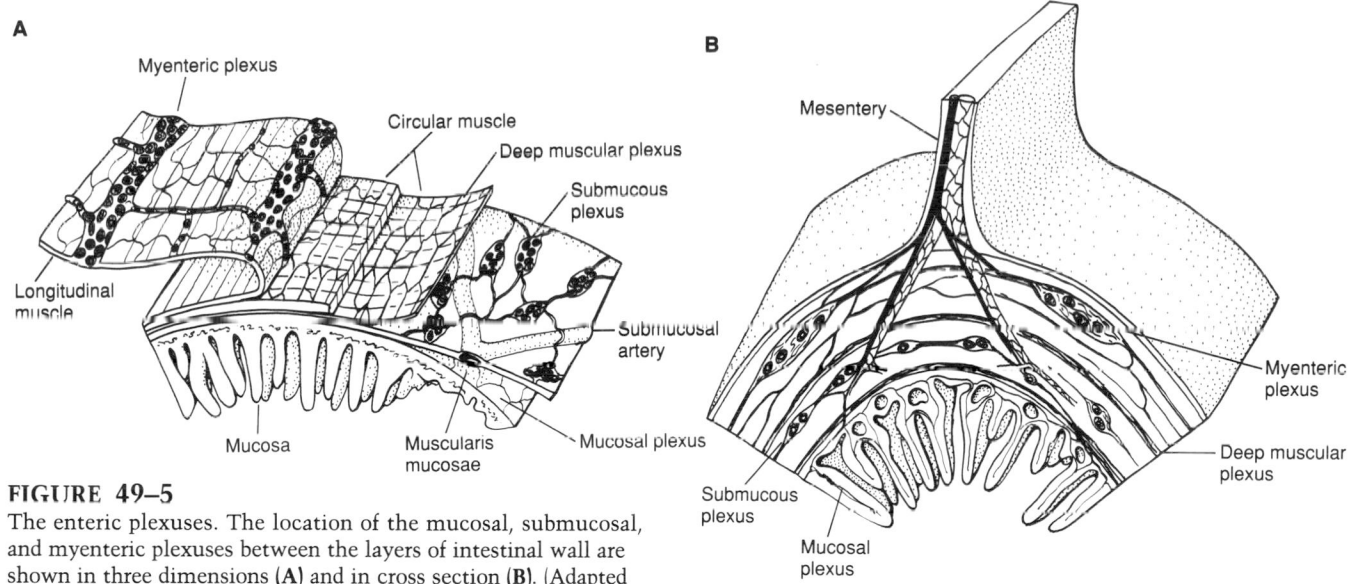

FIGURE 49–5

The enteric plexuses. The location of the mucosal, submucosal, and myenteric plexuses between the layers of intestinal wall are shown in three dimensions (**A**) and in cross section (**B**). (Adapted from Furness and Costa, 1980.)

the information it receives from these structures into a coherent pattern of autonomic response. As we learned in Chapter 47, the hypothalamus regulates the autonomic nervous system in two ways. First, it projects to nuclei in the brain stem and the spinal cord that act on preganglionic autonomic neurons to control temperature, heart rate, blood pressure, and respiration. Thus, stimulation of the lateral hypothalamus leads to general sympathetic activation—piloerection, increase in blood pressure and heart rate, sweating, and dilatation of the pupils. Second, the hypothalamus acts on the endocrine system to release hormones that influence autonomic function.

Although the hypothalamus exerts a major overall control over the autonomic nervous system (so that it is called the *head ganglion* of the autonomic nervous system), many autonomic functions do not require continuous monitoring by the hypothalamus. Indeed, transection of the brain stem above the pons leaves regulation of cardiovascular and respiratory functions intact, indicating that nuclei in the brain stem can also coordinate autonomic functions. The major coordinating center for autonomic function in the brain stem is the *nucleus of the solitary tract* (Figure 49–6). This nucleus receives sensory information from most major organs of the body, and then

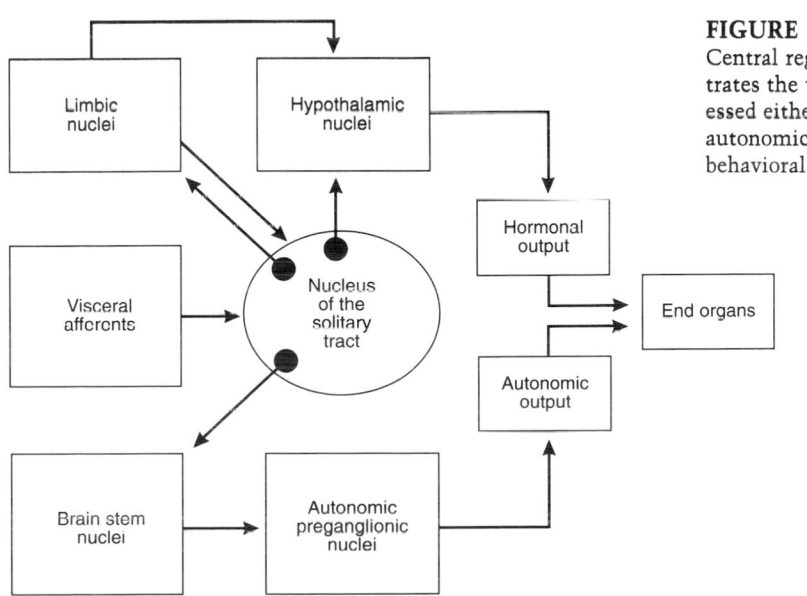

FIGURE 49–6

Central regulation of autonomic output. The drawing illustrates the ways in which visceral afferent information is processed either for reflex responses or as a part of a central autonomic circuit that can affect autonomic, hormonal, and behavioral activities. (Adapted from Loewy and Spyer, 1990.)

uses this information to modulate autonomic function in two ways.

First, the nucleus controls simple autonomic function by means of a set of reflex circuits. Sensory (visceral afferent) fibers from the heart, lungs, and gastrointestinal tract project to specific subnuclei within the nucleus of the solitary tract in a viscerotopic manner. These neurons project to lower brain stem nuclei that connect to autonomic motor neurons controlling effectors.

Second, the nucleus coordinates elaborate homeostatic adjustments by transmitting information from autonomic targets to both higher and lower brain regions. These regions then relay integrated information required for more complex autonomic control back to the nucleus of the solitary tract. In particular, visceral afferents from an array of autonomic targets terminate in a common region of the nucleus of the solitary tract called the *commissural nucleus*, which in turn projects to a wide range of brain stem and forebrain nuclei, including the amygdala, the paraventricular hypothalamic nucleus, and the bed nucleus of the stria terminalis. These nuclei then project back to the nucleus of the solitary tract, as well as to other lower brain stem nuclei. In addition, these brain stem nuclei project directly to the autonomic output nuclei for the gastrointestinal system, in particular the dorsal vagal nucleus and sympathetic preganglionic nuclei.

The Autonomic Nervous System Has Been Studied at the Cellular Level

Synaptic Transmission in Autonomic Ganglia Is Predominantly Cholinergic

Autonomic ganglia integrate information from the central nervous system and relay it to peripheral effector organs. The principal neurons within each preganglionic, sympathetic and parasympathetic ganglion receive and combine convergent inputs from several sources. The postganglionic neurons, in turn, act on their targets by means of the transmitter acetylcholine (ACh) and one or more peptide neurotransmitters. For example, the prevertebral ganglion combine input from the intestinal wall, the stellate ganglion from the lungs and aorta, and the superior cervical ganglion from the carotid sinus.[1]

Presynaptic stimulation of fibers to an autonomic ganglion evokes a variety of postsynaptic potentials that depend on the particular receptors expressed by the principal neurons. In all cases the release of ACh evokes a fast excitatory synaptic potential (EPSP) that is mediated by nicotinic ACh receptors. This fast EPSP is often large enough to generate an action potential in the postganglionic neuron, and is thus regarded as the principal synaptic pathway

---

[1]Sympathetic ganglia also contain small cells that are chromaffin-like and are usually clustered close to blood vessels. These cells, called small intensely fluorescent (or SIF) cells, contain dopamine, epinephrine, or norepinephrine that can be visualized by histofluorescence techniques. The function of SIF cells is not yet known.

A

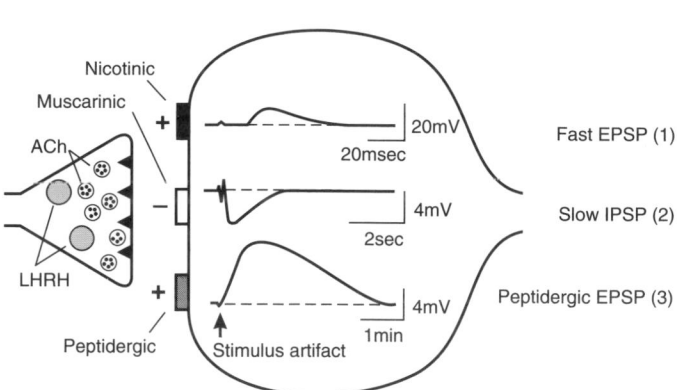

B

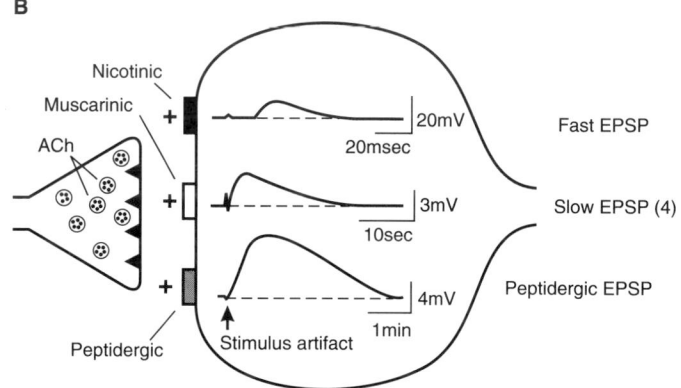

FIGURE 49–7

Nicotinic, muscarinic, and peptidergic synapses in the sympathetic chain ganglia in the bullfrog. Presynaptic terminals release both ACh and LHRH-like peptide stored in large vesicles (**A**) or stored in small vesicles (**B**). These two transmitters produce four types of postsynaptic potentials (**1–4**) in different postganglionic neurons. (From Jan and Jan, 1983).

A. A single presynaptic stimulus evokes a fast nicotinic EPSP (**1**). Repetitive stimulation evokes, in addition, a slow muscarinic IPSP (**2**) and a slow peptidergic EPSP (**3**).

B. In another class of postganglionic neurons, a single presynaptic stimulus also evokes a fast nicotinic EPSP. Repetitive stimulation now leads to a muscarinic EPSP (**4**). This class of neurons also evokes the slow peptidergic EPSP, but only in response to stimulation of the preganglionic fibers shown in A. The peptide diffuses from these remote terminals to distant receptors.

---

in both sympathetic and parasympathetic ganglia. Drugs that selectively block nicotinic ACh receptors, such as hexamethonium or curare, completely block ganglionic output. The nicotinic receptors on ganglionic neurons are related to the nicotinic receptors at the neuromuscular junction that we considered in Chapter 10. However, unlike the ACh receptors of skeletal muscle, Stephen

Heinemann and others have found that neuronal ACh receptors contain only two types of subunits, termed α and β. Expression of different combinations of one of the several neuronal α-subunits with any of the different β-subunits results in ACh receptor-channels with distinct conductance, kinetics, and pharmacology.

In addition to the fast nicotinic excitation all sympathetic and some parasympathetic ganglia exhibit slow synaptic potentials that can modulate the firing of the principal neurons. There is a slow EPSP and a slow IPSP mediated by ACh, as well as a slow EPSP mediated by peptides (Figure 49–7).

The slow EPSP is produced by muscarinic receptors opening Na^+ and Ca^{2+} channels while closing K^+ channels. The K^+ channel that is closed is called the *M channel* (because it was first demonstrated using the muscarinic agonist muscarine). It is active at the resting membrane potential; closure of the channel depolarizes the membrane (Chapter 12).

The slow IPSP is produced in some postganglionic neurons. It is mediated by activation of muscarinic receptors, which open K^+ channels. This in turn causes the cell to hyperpolarize and reduces its ability to fire action potentials. The inhibition has interesting properties. It does not suppress action potentials elicited by fast nicotinic EPSPs but inhibits repetitive firing initiated by the slow peptidergic EPSP (Figure 49–8). Thus, a single suprathreshold nicotinic EPSP will *always* give rise to a postsynaptic action potential, but repetitive firing can be modulated by subsequent presynaptic stimuli that generate the IPSP. The dual expression of slow inhibitory and excitatory mechanisms in a single postsynaptic neuron thus allows complex transformation between convergent presynaptic and patterned postsynaptic activity.

A variety of peptides are present in preganglionic fibers (Table 49–1) and are thought to be co-released with ACh. One peptide is a luteinizing hormone-releasing hormone-like (LHRH-like) peptide. Lily Jan, Yuh-Nung Jan, and Stephen Kuffler demonstrated its co-localization with ACh in sympathetic ganglia of the bullfrog (Figure 49–7). The peptide can diffuse considerable distances within the ganglion. High-frequency stimulation of preganglionic fibers releases the peptide, producing a long-latency, slow depolarization in all postganglionic neurons (Figure 49–7). As described in Chapter 12, the late slow peptidergic EPSP, like the slow muscarinic EPSP, results in the closure of the $M—K^+$ channel and concomitant opening of both Na^+ and Ca^{2+} channels.

Peptides appear often to be modulatory in action: They affect the efficacy of cholinergic transmission rather than produce direct excitatory or inhibitory responses on postganglionic neurons. The effects of LHRH and other peptides are slow, lasting up to several minutes. This contrasts with the nicotinic EPSP, which has a considerably faster time course. Interaction of subthreshold nicotinic EPSPs with the slow peptidergic EPSP results in repetitive firing of action potentials. Thus, one major function of peptides in autonomic ganglia is to alter neu-

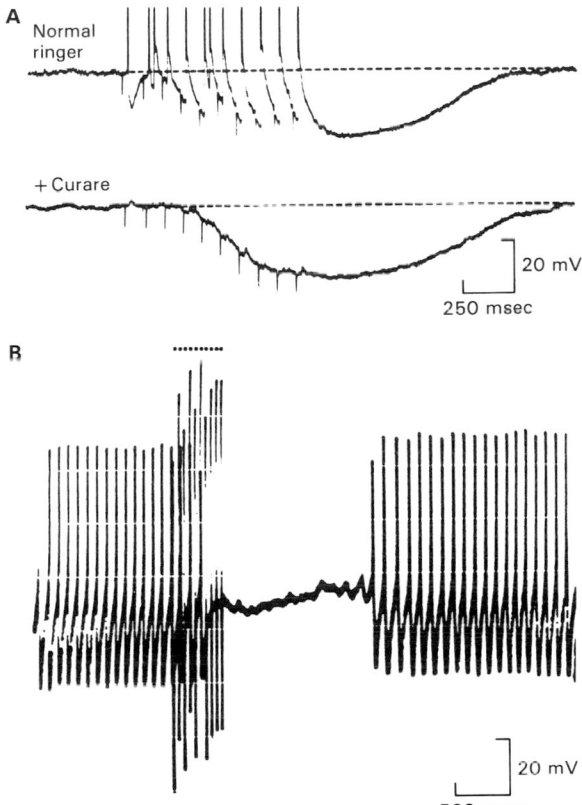

FIGURE 49–8

Synaptic integration in a bullfrog sympathetic neuron. The IPSP does not inhibit nicotinic excitation. (From Horn and Dodd, 1983.)

A. A train of 10 presynaptic stimuli produces 12 suprathreshold nicotinic EPSPs followed by the IPSP **(top trace).** Curare blocks the nicotinic EPSPs. It now becomes clear that the IPSP starts as early as the fourth stimulus and is almost fully developed by the tenth. Comparison of the two records demonstrates that the IPSP, even as it approaches its maximum amplitude, does not inhibit nicotinic EPSPs from initiating action potentials.

B. The IPSP inhibits repetitive firing of bullfrog sympathetic neurons. A train of presynaptic stimuli, applied at the times indicated by the dots above the trace, produced an IPSP. As the IPSP developed, the repetitive firing was inhibited. As the IPSP subsided, the membrane potential began to oscillate and repetitive firing recommenced.

ronal excitability and thereby modulate the effectiveness of cholinergic synaptic transmission.

Autonomic Targets Are Regulated by Both Cholinergic and Noradrenergic Input

The stimulation of sympathetic or parasympathetic postganglionic axons leads to the release of norepinephrine or ACh, respectively, at target sites. In addition, autonomic

TABLE 49–1. Some Peptides in Sympathetic Neurons

Peptide[a]	Localization	Sympathetic ganglia[b]	Species
BOM	Preganglionic fibers	CMG	Rat
CCK	Preganglionic fibers	IMG, CMG	Guinea pig
DYN	Postganglionic neurons	CMG	Guinea pig, rat
ENK	Preganglionic fibers	IMG, CMG, SCG, SCG	Rat, guinea pig
GRH	Preganglionic fibers	CMG, paravertebral	Human, rat, guinea pig
LHRH	Preganglionic fibers	Paravertebral	Bullfrog
NPY	Postganglionic neurons	IMG, CMG, SCG, STG	Human, rat, cat, guinea pig
	Peripheral terminals		Human, rat, cat, guinea pig, pig
NT	Preganglionic fibers	SMG, IMG, CMG	Guinea pig
SOM	Postganglionic neurons	SCG, IMG, CMG	Guinea pig, rat
	Preganglionic fibers	IMG	Cat
SP	Preganglionic fibers	IMG, CMG, SCG	Guinea pig, cat
		SCG	Rat
VIP	Preganglionic fibers	IMG, CMG, SCG	Human, guinea pig, rat
	Postganglionic fibers	IMG, CMG, paravertebral	Human, guinea pig
	Peripheral terminals		Human, rat, cat, dog, guinea pig

[a]BOM, bombesin; CCK, cholecystokinin; DYN, dynorphin; ENK, enkephalin; GRH, gastrin-releasing hormone; LHRH, luteinizing hormone-releasing hormone; NPY, neuropeptide Y; NT, neurotensin; SOM, somatostatin; SP, substance P; VIP, vasoactive intestinal peptide.

[b]CMG, coeliac mesenteric ganglion; SMG, superior mesenteric ganglion; IMG, inferior mesenteric ganglion; SCG, superior cervical ganglion; STG, stellate ganglion.

(Adapted from Karczmar et al., 1986.)

postganglionic axons also contain and probably release a variety of peptides that may regulate target activity (Table 49–1).

The effects of acetylcholine are usually discrete and limited to the site of release in the autonomic neuron. In contrast, the actions of catecholamines are more diffuse, typically extending beyond an individual target. Some norepinephrine released from nerve terminals escapes re-uptake and enters the circulation. In addition, the adrenal medulla releases epinephrine and norepinephrine into the circulation. This diffuse release of catecholamines, along with the divergent anatomical organization of sympathetic preganglionic axons, underlies the ability of the sympathetic nervous system to achieve a concerted hormone-like activation of sympathetic targets in situations of stress.

Although some autonomic targets—sweat glands, liver, and spleen—receive input from only one division of the autonomic nervous system, most targets are controlled by coordinated and reciprocal sympathetic and parasympathetic innervation. For example, cholinergic output from the parasympathetic division promotes absorption of food and digestion by enhancing salivary, gastric, intestinal, and pancreatic secretions by increasing motility of the gut and by relaxing pyloric and intestinal sphincters. In contrast, the catecholaminergic output of the sympathetic division decreases the motility and secretory activity of the gastrointestinal system. Although sympathetic control of the gastrointestinal tract comes into play only in response to stress, the reciprocal control of other organs by both autonomic divisions is coordinated and necessary for normal function. A good example of this is the autonomic regulation of blood pressure. The degree of control

is so fine that alteration in heart rate can occur within a single beat following activation of neural input. We now turn to consider this and other examples of reciprocal control.

Autonomic Control of Target Function Is Coordinately Regulated

Cardiovascular Function. Changes in blood pressure are sensed by afferents innervating the carotid sinus and aortic baroreceptors. These receptors detect changes in stretch, but, because their firing rate is increased at the onset of a pressure pulse, they are referred to as pressoreceptors or baroreceptors. The neural pathways mediating the response to a rise in arterial pressure are indicated in Figure 49–9. A rise in blood pressure that activates baroreceptor afferents results in both direct and indirect activation of the parasympathetic vagal innervation of the heart, thereby decreasing heart rate (see below and Figures 49–9 and 49–10).

Both sympathetic and parasympathetic fibers innervating the heart are tonically active. A rise in blood pressure, detected by carotid baroreceptors, activates the afferent and central autonomic pathways that project to sympathetic preganglionic neurons and inhibit their tonic activity (Figure 49–9). This is accompanied by increased vagal output, which causes a further decrease in heart rate and cardiac output. The sympathetic and parasympathetic neurotransmitters have opposite effects on cardiac function. Norepinephrine and epinephrine increase cardiac output; acetylcholine decreases it. These effects are achieved through modulation of both the electrical and the mechanical activity of the heart.

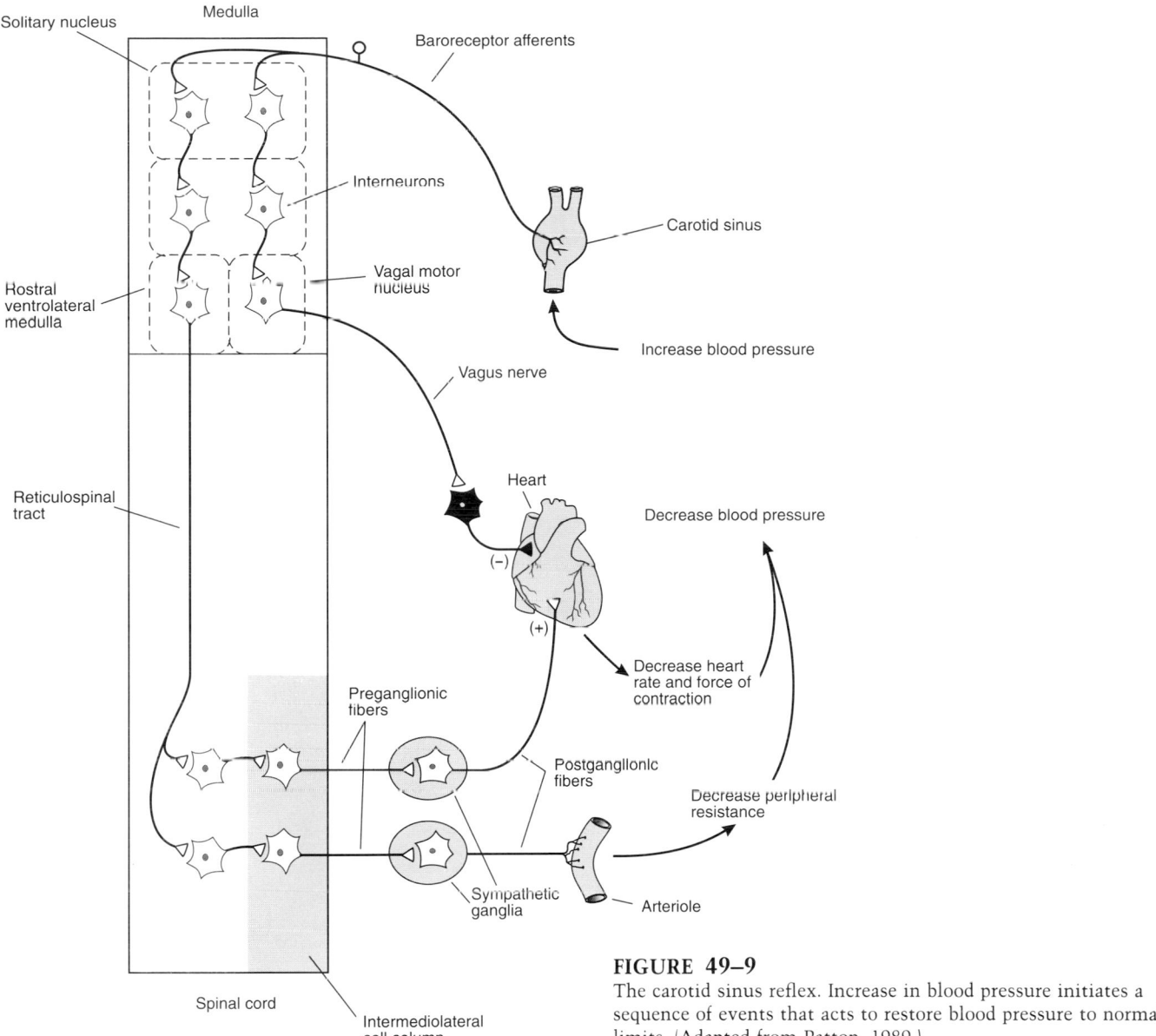

FIGURE 49–9

The carotid sinus reflex. Increase in blood pressure initiates a sequence of events that acts to restore blood pressure to normal limits. (Adapted from Patton, 1989.)

Sympathetic Regulation of Cardiovascular Function. Norepinephrine released from sympathetic postganglionic neurons acts on cardiac muscle to stimulate heart rate and contractility. Neurally released and circulating catecholamines act primarily through β-adrenergic receptors to modulate several ionic currents. The long-lasting (or L type) Ca^{2+} current of heart muscle cells is enhanced by norepinephrine, contributing to an increase in the net force of contraction (Figure 49–10). In the early 1970s several investigators discovered that enhancement of the long-lasting Ca^{2+} current by β-adrenergic agonists was mediated by cAMP. This was the first demonstration that neurotransmitter modulation of an ionic conductance occurred through a second messenger.

In addition to the modulation of Ca^{2+} current, activation of β-adrenergic receptors has two other effects. First, it increases a K^+ current of the delayed rectifier-type (Chapter 8). Enhancement of this K^+ current counteracts the increase in the inward Ca^{2+} current. Although the increase in the L current would tend to broaden the action potential, the concomitant effect of norepinephrine to increase the K^+ current keeps the action potential duration constant. Second, activation of the β receptors decreases the threshold for the pacemaker current (I_f), and thereby increases heart rate. It is now appreciated that the other actions of norepinephrine on β-adrenergic receptors are mediated by the cAMP-dependent protein kinase (Chapter 12). Finally, all of the effects of neurally released norepinephrine on cardiac function are potently reinforced by circulating epinephrine from the adrenal medulla.

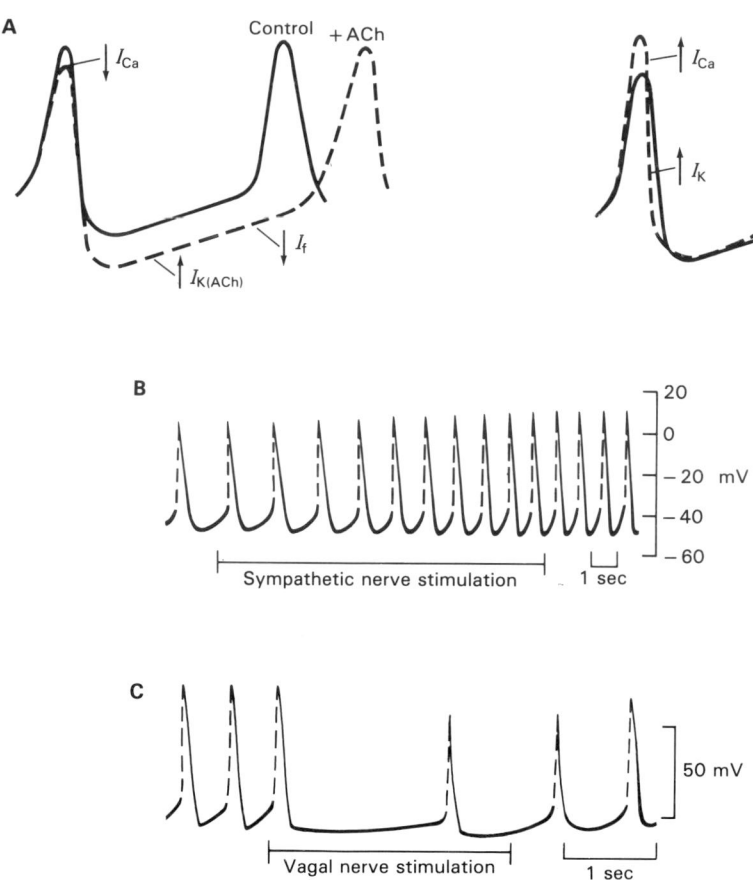

FIGURE 49–10

Action of sympathetic and vagal transmitters on electrical activity of cardiocytes from the sinoatrial node.

A. Ionic currents in the heart are differentially regulated by ACh and norepinephrine (NE), as indicated by the **arrows**.

B. Acceleratory effect of sympathetic nerve stimulation of the frog sinus venosus. Nerve stimulation increased firing rate. (Adapted from Hutter and Trautwein, 1956.)

C. Effect of vagal nerve stimulation on cardiocytes from the sinotrial node. Nerve stimulation slows firing and shortens the amplitude of the action potential. (Adapted from Toda and West, 1967.)

Neurally released norepinephrine also acts on α-adrenergic receptors to increase peripheral vascular resistance, therefore increasing venous return, and increasing blood pressure. When baroreceptors detect an increase in blood pressure, the vasomotor brain centers cause net inhibition of the sympathetic preganglionic neurons, decreasing sympathetic vasomotor tone, thereby decreasing peripheral vascular resistance. There is not a corresponding parasympathetic control of vascular resistance. Thus, the regulation of blood pressure in the periphery is an important example of the way in which autonomic control can be mediated largely through inhibition of tonically active autonomic neurons.

Parasympathetic Regulation of Cardiovascular Function. Activation of neurons of the vagal motor nucleus profoundly decreases heart rate and cardiac contractility, resulting in a net decrease in cardiac output. These inotropic effects are mediated by vagal activation of parasympathetic preganglionic neurons that innervate cholinergic ganglion neurons in the heart (see Box 49–1).

Acetylcholine slows the heart rate by acting on muscarinic receptors in the cardiocytes of the sinoatrial and atrioventricular nodes or atrial muscle, and increasing a resting K^+ conductance called $I_{K(ACh)}$ (Figure 49–10). Activation of $I_{K(ACh)}$ hyperpolarizes sinoatrial cells and slows

conduction through the atrioventricular node. The activation of $I_{K(ACh)}$ by acetylcholine apparently involves direct gating of the K^+ channel by a G-protein (see Chapter 13).

Acetylcholine also decreases heart rate by shifting the pacemaker current (I_f) in a manner opposite to that of norepinephrine, thereby increasing its threshold for activation and decreasing heart rate. Finally, acetylcholine decreases the sustained (L-type) Ca^{2+} current, primarily by antagonizing the effects of the cAMP-dependent modulation of L current. Acetylcholine decreases L current by reducing the synthesis of cAMP and by activating a cAMP phosphodiesterase. This latter action is achieved through the production by acetylcholine of another second messenger, cGMP. Acetylcholine also decreases cardiac output by causing a decrease in Ca^{2+} influx. This is due to both a decrease in Ca^{2+} current and an increase in resting K^+ current, which shortens the duration of the action potential.

Autonomic Control of the Eye: The Pupillary Light Reflex. The diameter of the pupils is controlled jointly by parasympathetic and sympathetic innervation of the two muscles of the iris. Parasympathetic postganglionic fibers from the ciliary ganglion innervate the pupillary sphincter muscle, which constricts the pupil. Sympathetic fibers from the superior cervical ganglion innervate the pupillary

---

First Isolation of a Chemical Transmitter   **BOX 49–1**

Although John Langley and Henry Dale and their students had postulated the existence of chemical messengers on the basis of their pharmacological studies dating from the beginning of the century, convincing evidence for a neurotransmitter was provided by Otto Loewi in 1920 in a simple but decisive experiment examining the autonomic innervation of two isolated, beating frog hearts. In his own words,

> The night before Easter Sunday of that year I awoke, turned on the light, and jotted down a few notes on a tiny slip of paper. Then I fell asleep again. It occurred to me at six o'clock in the morning that during the night I had written down something most important, but I was unable to decipher the scrawl. The next night, at three o'clock, the idea returned. It was the design of an experiment to determine whether or not the hypothesis of chemical transmission that I had uttered seventeen years ago was correct. I got up immediately, went to the laboratory, and performed a simple experiment on a frog heart according to the nocturnal design. I have to describe briefly this experiment since its results became the foundation of the theory of chemical transmission of the nervous impulse.

The hearts of two frogs were isolated, the first with its nerves, the second without. Both hearts were attached to Straub cannulas filled with a little Ringer solution. The vagus nerve of the first heart was stimulated for a few minutes. Then the Ringer solution that had been in the first heart during the stimulation of the vagus was transferred to the second heart. It slowed and its beat diminished just as if its vagus had been stimulated. Similarly, when the accelerator nerve was stimulated and the Ringer from this period transferred, the second heart speeded up and its beat increased. These results unequivocally proved that the nerves do not influence the heart directly but liberate from their terminals specific chemical substances which, in their turn, cause the well-known modifications of the function of the heart characteristic of the stimulation of its nerves.

Loewi called this substance *Vagusstoff* (vagus substance). Soon after, *Vagusstoff* was identified chemically as acetylcholine.

---

dilator muscle to enhance dilation of the pupil. During the pupillary light reflex, in response to a bright light, the parasympathetic input is activated and the sympathetic dilator system is inhibited, causing a net decrease in pupillary diameter. Pupillary dilation results from increasing tonic activity in sympathetic neurons and decreasing activity in parasympathetic neurons. Thus, the mechanism underlying the control of ciliary muscle is analogous to the antagonism involved in flexion and extension of a limb. The parasympathetic fibers innervate the circular constrictor muscle and the sympathetic fibers innervate the antagonistic radial dilator muscle.

Autonomic Control of Salivary Glands. Control of salivary secretion differs from that of other autonomic targets because the inputs do not exert opposing effects on all aspects of salivary gland function. Activity in both sympathetic and parasympathetic fibers that directly innervate salivary gland cells evoke a maximal increase in secretion. However, the two pathways trigger release of different fluids. Activation of sympathetic neurons produces a more viscous secretion with a high amylase content; parasympathetic stimulation produces watery saliva.

The effects of the two autonomic systems on the blood vessels in the salivary gland are antagonistic. Sympathetic activation causes vasoconstriction, decreasing blood flow and salivary output; parasympathetic fibers dilate the vessels increasing secretion. Thus, the composition and volume of the final output of the gland reflect the balance between sympathetic and parasympathetic activity.

Autonomic Control of the Bladder. Bladder filling and urination are controlled by the interplay not only of sympathetic and parasympathetic neurons but also of somatic motor neurons. All three systems are activated by reflexes that are regulated at both spinal and supraspinal levels.

The excitatory input to the bladder wall that causes contraction and promotes emptying is parasympathetic. Cholinergic axons originating in the intermediolateral region of the sacral spinal cord travel in the pelvic nerve to the pelvic ganglion plexus, whose neurons are dispersed near to and within the bladder wall (Figure 49–11). Pelvic ganglion neurons activate the muscles of the bladder wall by releasing ACh, which acts on muscarinic receptors. The parasympathetic neurons are quiescent during initial bladder filling. However, bladder distension initiates impulses in visceral afferents that travel in the pelvic nerve to the sacral spinal cord and activate parasympathetic preganglionic neurons.

The activity of the parasympathetic system is counteracted and also controlled directly by the sympathetic input. In humans the sympathetic innervation of the bladder originates in the thoracic and upper lumbar spinal cord. Preganglionic neurons project to the inferior mesenteric ganglion. Postganglionic fibers travel from the inferior mesenteric ganglion in the hypogastric nerve to the pelvic ganglion, the bladder wall, and the internal urethral sphincter muscle (Figure 49–11). Sympathetic preganglionic neurons are activated by low levels of activity in sensory afferents that respond to tension in the bladder walls. Stimulation of the sympathetic innervation results

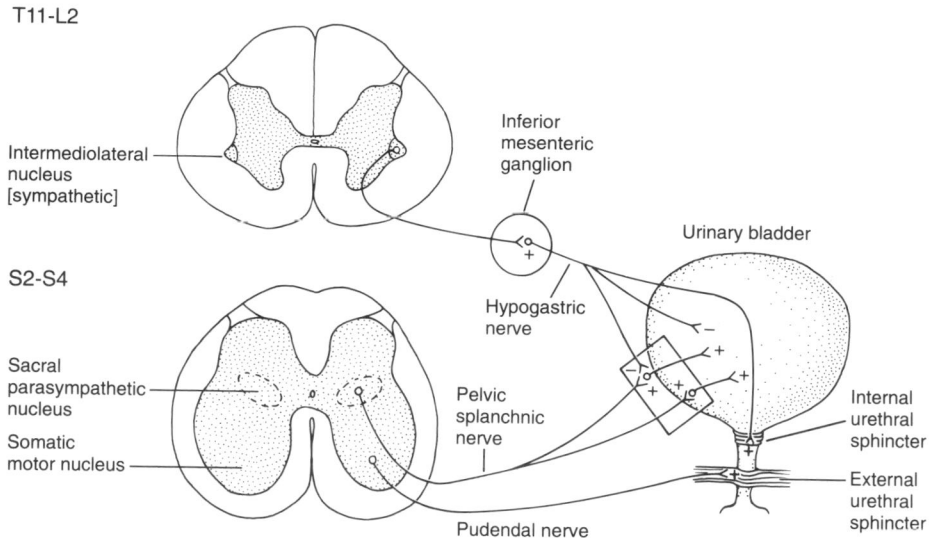

FIGURE 49–11
Somatic and autonomic motor innervation of the urinary bladder.

in an α-adrenergic inhibition of parasympathetic activity in the pelvic ganglion, relaxation of the muscles of the bladder wall (mediated by β-adrenergic receptors) and excitation of the internal sphincter muscle. Thus, during bladder filling the activity of the sympathetic innervation promotes bladder wall relaxation directly and also indirectly through inhibition of parasympathetic activity, and causes closure of the internal sphincter.

Regulation of bladder function also involves the somatic motor system. Motor neurons in the ventral horn of the sacral spinal cord innervate the external sphincter and cause contraction (Figure 49–11). These motor neurons are stimulated by activity in visceral afferents that respond to low levels of bladder distension. At high levels of distension supraspinal neurons that inhibit the firing of both the sympathetic and the somatic motor neurons are activated so that the sympathetic depression of parasympathetic activity is released and both sphincters relax, permitting bladder contraction and urine flow.

Although control of bladder function operates through the interaction of the parasympathetic, sympathetic, and somatic systems at the spinal reflex level in very young, anesthetized, or paraplegic subjects, under normal circumstances the voluntary control of bladder function operates through the supraspinal regulation of all three reflexes.

An Overall View

The three divisions of the autonomic nervous system comprise an integrated motor system that acts in parallel with the somatic motor system and is responsible for homeostasis. Essential to the functioning of the system, in addition to motor outflow, are the visceral sensory afferents, the hypothalamus, and several brain stem nuclei such as the nucleus of the solitary tract. Afferent information about peripheral organs is integrated and relayed through the brain stem nucleus of the solitary tract back to autonomic nuclei to regulate autonomic outflow.

Several features of the autonomic nervous system permit rapid integrated responses to changes in the environment. The activity of effector organs is finely controlled by coordinated and balanced excitatory and inhibitory inputs from tonically active postganglionic neurons. Moreover, the sympathetic system is tremendously divergent, permitting the entire body to respond to extreme conditions (the fight or flight reaction).

In addition to the classically defined neurotransmitters—ACh, adrenaline, and noradrenaline—a wide variety of peptides and other neurotransmitters are thought to be released by autonomic neurons either onto postganglionic cells or their targets. Many of these transmitters act in a modulatory capacity, altering the efficacy of cholinergic or adrenergic transmission and providing a further level of control of target organ activity.

Selected Readings

Bacq, Z. M. 1975. Chemical Transmission of Nerve Impulses: A Historical Sketch. Oxford, England: Pergamon Press.

Brown, A. M., and Birnbaumer, L. 1990. Ionic channels and their regulation by G protein subunits. Annu. Rev. Physiol. 52:197–213.

Cannon, W. B. 1932. The Wisdom of the Body. New York: Norton.

Ciriello, J., Calaresu, F. R., Renaud, L. P., and Polosa, C. (eds.) 1987. Organization of the Autonomic Nervous System: Central and Peripheral Mechanisms. New York: Liss.

Furness, J. B., and Costa, M. 1987. The Enteric Nervous System. Edinburgh: Churchill Livingstone.

Gershon, M. D. 1981. The enteric nervous system. Annu. Rev. Neurosci. 4:227–272.

Langley, J. N. 1921. The Autonomic Nervous System. Cambridge, England: Heffer & Sons.

Loewy, A. D., and Spyer, K. M. (eds.) 1990. Central Regulation of Autonomic Functions. New York: Oxford University Press.

Randall, W. C.,(ed.) 1984. Nervous Control of Cardiovascular Function. New York: Oxford University Press.

Reuter, H., and Scholz, H. 1977. The regulation of the calcium conductance of cardiac muscle by adrenaline. J. Physiol. (Lond.) 264:49–62.

Tseng, G.-N., and Siegelbaum, S.A., 1990. Molecular biological approach to drug-receptor interactions: Structure-function relationship of ion channels. In M. R. Rosen, M. J. Janse, and A. L. Wit (eds.), Cardiac Electrophysiology: A Textbook. Mt. Kisco, N.Y.: Futura Publishing, pp. 969–993.

References

Brown, D. A., and Adams, P. R. 1980. Muscarinic suppression of a novel voltage-sensitive K⁺ current in a vertebrate neurone. Nature 283:673–676.

Deneris, E. S., Boulter, J., Connolly, J., Wada, E., Wada, K., Goldman, D., Swanson, L. W., Patrick, J., and Heinemann, S. 1989. Genes encoding neuronal nicotinic acetylcholine receptors. Clin. Chem. 35:731–737.

Dodd, J., and Horn, J. P. 1983. Muscarinic inhibition of sympathetic C neurones in the bullfrog. J. Physiol. (Lond.) 334:271–291.

Furness, J. B., and Costa, M. 1980. Types of nerves in the enteric nervous system. Neuroscience 5:1–20.

Horn, J. P., and Dodd, J. 1983. Inhibitory cholinergic synapses in autonomic ganglia. Trends Neurosci. 6:180–184.

Hutter, O. F., and Trautwein, W. 1956. Vagal and sympathetic effects on the pacemaker fibers in the sinus venosus of thed heart. J. Gen. Physiol. 39:715–733.

Jan, L. Y., and Jan, Y. N. 1982. Peptidergic transmission in sympathetic ganglia of the frog. J. Physiol. (Lond.) 327:219–246.

Jan, Y. N., and Jan, L. Y. 1983. A LHRH-like peptidergic neurotransmitter capable of 'action at a distance' in autonomic ganglia. Trends Neurosci. 6:320–325.

Karczmar, A. G., Koketsu, K., and Nishi, S. (eds.) 1986. Autonomic and Enteric Ganglia: Transmission and Its Pharmacology. New York: Plenum Press.

Langley, J. N. 1905. On the reaction of nerve cells and nerve endings to certain poisons chiefly as regards the reaction of striated muscle to nicotine and to curari. J. Physiol. (Lond.) 33:374–473.

Loewi, O. 1921. Über humorale Übertragbarkeit der Herzenvenwirkung. Pflügers Arch. 189:239–242. (English translation "On the humoral propagation of cardiac nerve action." In I. Cooke and M. Lipkin, Jr., (eds.), 1972. Cellular Neurophysiology: A Source Book. New York: Holt, Rinehart, and Winston, pp. 460–466.

Patton, H. D. 1989. The autonomic nervous system. In H. D. Patton, A. F. Fuchs, B. Hille, A. M. Scher, and R. Steiner (eds.), Textbook of Physiology: Excitable Cells and Neurophysiology, Vol. 1, Section VII: Emotive Responses and Internal Milieu. Philadelphia: Saunders, pp. 737–758.

Pfaffinger, P. J., Martin, J. M., Hunter, D. D., Nathanson, N. M., and Hille, B. 1985. GTP-binding proteins couple cardiac muscarinic receptors to a K channel. Nature 317:536–538.

Toda, N., and West, T. C. 1967. Interactions of K, Na, and vagal stimulation in the S-A node of the rabbit. Am. J. Physiol. 212:416–423.

50

John H. Martin

The Collective Electrical Behavior of Cortical Neurons: The Electroencephalogram and the Mechanisms of Epilepsy

The Collective Behavior of Neurons Can Be Studied Noninvasively in Humans with Macroelectrodes

The Cellular Mechanisms Underlying Electroencephalography

The EEG Is Generated in the Cortex by the Flow of Synaptic Currents Through the Extracellular Space

The EEG Reflects Primarily Synaptic Potentials in Pyramidal Cells

Epilepsy Interrupts Normal Brain Function

Partial and Generalized Seizures Have Different Clinical and EEG Features

Large Populations of Neurons Are Activated Synchronously During an Epileptic Seizure

A Depolarization Shift Underlies Focal Seizures

Excitatory Connections Between Cortical Neurons Synchronize Discharges in an Epileptic Focus

Synaptic Inhibition May Limit Seizure Spread

Generalized Epilepsy Can Be Produced Experimentally

An Overall View

The enormous growth of the human cerebral cortex differentiates it from the cortex of other mammals. One of the challenges for neurobiology is to understand how the cerebral cortex is organized and how this organization relates to the special perceptual, motor, and linguistic competence of humans.

The various parts of the cerebral cortex have many distinguishing features; they also have features in common. For example, individual cortical areas subserving the various sensory, motor, and cognitive functions are distinguished from one another by their input and output connections. Nevertheless, despite differences in input and output, almost all sensory and motor cortices are similarly organized into vertical columns that run from the pial surface to the white matter. Within each column the cells have similar receptive field positions and response properties. Moreover, the inputs and outputs of different cortices, although distinctive, are distributed in much the same way. For example, the major input to all sensory cortices comes from the thalamus and terminates predominantly in layer 4. Neurons of layer 4 in turn distribute the information to neurons within the same column. The output functions are served by neurons in layers 2, 3, 5, and 6.

In earlier chapters we focused on the distinctive features of cortical regions as expressed in their patterns of interconnections and their role in behavior. In this chapter we shall examine these features of organization common throughout the cortex and consider how these contribute to collective or ensemble properties characteristic of the cerebral cortex. These ensemble properties are particularly evident in certain normal behavioral states, such as sleep, wakefulness, and arousal, as well as in certain disease states, such as epilepsy—when neurons throughout the cortex may be recruited in synchronous activity—and coma.

The ensemble properties of the cerebral cortex are best studied with techniques that record the activity of many cortical neurons simultaneously. One such technique is the electroencephalogram (or EEG), which we shall consider in detail. Unlike intracellular recordings of individual neurons, the EEG records the activity of many hundreds of thousands of neurons through electrodes placed on the scalp. Because it is noninvasive, the EEG is important in the clinical assessment of cortical function. It provides important indices for studying arousal, wakefulness, sleep, and dreaming, and for diagnosing epilepsy and coma.

The Collective Behavior of Neurons Can Be Studied Noninvasively in Humans with Macroelectrodes

The functioning of a cortical column depends on the operations of neuronal ensembles rather than on the actions of any single neuron. The behavior of a neuronal ensemble can be estimated by probing the responses of the individual cells with microelectrodes. This approach is time-consuming, however, and ethically can be done only in experimental animals. Another approach is to use macroelectrodes (similar to those used initially by investigators to map responses in the somatic sensory cortex) to record the summated activity of large groups of neurons. Recordings of electrical responses of neuronal ensembles can be obtained in humans when the cortical surface is exposed during surgery (*electrocorticogram*, ECoG), or noninvasively from the surface of the scalp (*electroencephalogram*, EEG).

An EEG is a record of the fluctuations of the electrical activity of large ensembles of neurons in the brain (Figure 50–1). Specifically, it is a measure of the extracellular current flow associated with the summed activity of many individual neurons. As we shall see later, surface recorded potentials reflect predominantly the activity of cortical neurons in the area underlying the EEG electrode, and postsynaptic potentials rather than action potentials.

To record the EEG at least two electrodes are used. An *active electrode* is placed over a site of neuronal activity, and an *indifferent electrode* is placed at some distance from this site. In clinical EEG recordings numerous active electrodes are situated over different parts of the head. (All recordings, however, measure the potential difference between two electrodes, either between the active and indifferent electrode or between two active electrodes.) The recording electrodes are usually placed over the frontal, parietal, occipital, and temporal lobes according to a conventional scheme (Figure 50–2). In special circumstances placement of nasopharyngeal or sphenoidal electrodes enhances detection of activity in the medial temporal lobes. This type of recording is particularly important in patients suspected of having seizures originating in structures of the limbic system, such as the hippocampus.

The EEG is a record of the electrical activity of the brain while the subject is sitting quietly or sleeping. The EEG is also recorded during specific sensory stimulation,

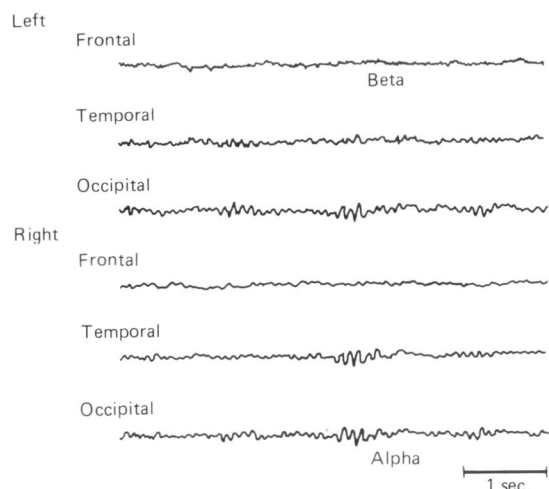

FIGURE 50–1

The EEG recorded in a human subject at rest from the scalp surface at various points over the left and right hemispheres. Three pairs of EEG electrodes are positioned so as to overlie the frontal, temporal, and occipital lobes. (See Figure 50–2 for the standardized placement of EEG electrodes.) *Beta* activity is recorded over the frontal lobes. This is the EEG activity with the highest frequency and lowest amplitude. *Alpha* activity is recorded in the occipital and temporal lobes. This is a signature of a brain in a relaxed and wakeful state. The presence of alpha activity in the occipital lobe suggests that the subject's eyes were closed.

such as presentation of a flash of light or a tone. The component of the EEG related specifically to a significant stimulus is called a *sensory evoked potential* or *event related potential* (see Box 50–1). Electroencephalograms are analyzed in the temporal (i.e., frequency) and spatial domains. Analysis of the frequency components of the EEG is usually based on principles developed by the mathematician Jean Baptiste Fourier, who found that any function of a variable, in this case voltage with respect to time, can be expanded into a series of sine wave harmonics. Different combinations of electronic filtering can be used alone or in combination with Fourier algorithms to analyze the EEG.

The frequencies of the potentials recorded from the surface of the scalp of a normal human typically vary from 1–30 Hz, and the amplitudes typically range from 20–100 μV. The amplitude of the EEG is attenuated by the meninges and cerebrospinal fluid, as well as by the skull and scalp. Although the frequency characteristics of the EEG potential are extremely complex and the amplitude may vary considerably even within a relatively short time interval, a few dominant frequency bands and amplitudes are typically observed. They are called alpha (8–13 Hz), beta (13–30 Hz), delta (0.5–4 Hz), and theta (4–7 Hz).

Alpha waves are generally associated with a state of relaxed wakefulness; they are recorded best over the parietal and occipital lobes (Figure 50–1). Alpha waves are sometimes called *Berger rhythm* after Hans Berger, who pioneered the study of the EEG. *Beta waves* are normally

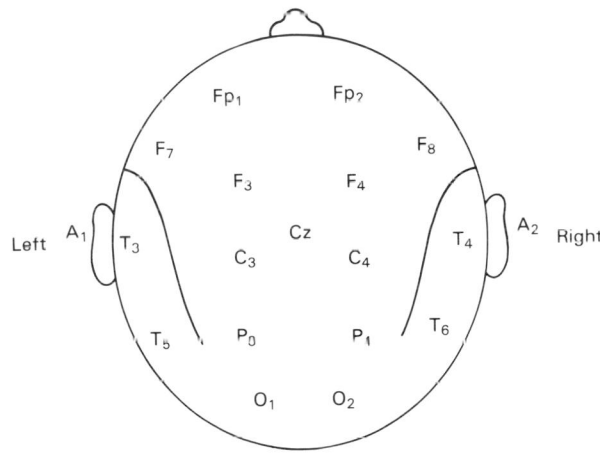

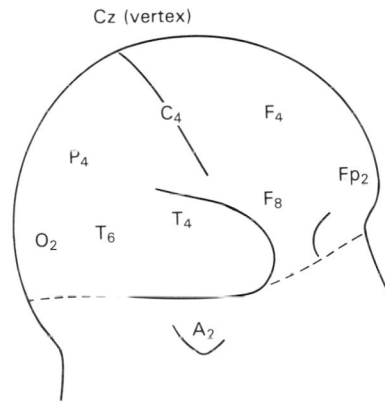

FIGURE 50–2
The standard placement of EEG recording electrodes at the top and side of the head. Abbreviations for multiple electrode placements are: **A**, auricle; **C**, central; **Cz**, vertex F, frontal; **FP**, frontal pole; **O**, occipital; **P**, parietal; **T**, temporal. The multiple electrodes placements overlying a given area (eg., temporal) are indicated by numerical subscripts. Placement **C₄** overlies the region of the central sulcus.

seen over the frontal regions and over other regions during intense mental activity. Beta waves have the smallest amplitudes of recorded EEG activity (Figure 50–1). *Delta* and *theta waves*, which are associated with sleep in the normal adult, have the largest amplitudes of EEG activity.

A new and radically different technique called *optical imaging* has been developed recently to examine the ensemble properties of neurons. Optical imaging permits a high-resolution spatial record of activity in a neural population by using *voltage-sensitive dyes*, which respond to changes in membrane potential by changing their fluorescence or absorption. The dynamic properties of neural ensembles can then be examined by following changes in the optical characteristics of the tissue that occur with time. More recently, neurons have been found to emit activity-dependent signals based on their *intrinsic fluorescence*, even in the absence of voltage-sensitive dyes. Optical im-

aging based on voltage-sensitive dyes or intrinsic fluorescence is invasive; it requires direct visualization of the cortical surface. It is currently being used only in studies of experimental animals. This method of imaging neural populations might one day be applied to the human cortex, much like positron emission tomography (PET) or magnetic resonance imaging (MRI).

The Cellular Mechanisms Underlying Electroencephalography

To appreciate the physiological mechanisms underlying the EEG we must briefly review aspects of cortical morphology that are considered in Chapter 20. As we have seen in Chapter 20 the cerebral cortex contains several different types of nerve cells that fall into two major classes, pyramidal and nonpyramidal, based on morphology, laminar distribution, and neurotransmitter content (Figure 50–5). The *pyramidal cells* project their axons to other areas of the brain and to the spinal cord. They are excitatory neurons; their transmitter is thought to be glutamate. Pyramidal cells are the major projection neurons of the cerebral cortex. In addition to their projections from a local region of cortex, pyramidal cells also have recurrent axon collaterals that project locally. Some axon collaterals may extend many millimeters in a plane parallel to the cortical layers. Connections made by axon collaterals play an important role in the collective electrical activity of cortical neuron ensembles and in the establishment and spread of seizure activity during epilepsy.

The dendritic organization of pyramidal cells facilitates the integration of a variety of inputs. The apical dendrites of pyramidal cells often cross several layers and are always oriented perpendicular to the surface of the brain. This allows input from the different cortical layers to impinge at different points along the dendritic tree. In addition, the dendrites contain local regions capable of generating action potentials that amplify synaptic currents, thereby making distant synaptic sites much more effective than would be possible based on the passive properties of dendrite membranes (Chapter 7 and below). The electrical activity of pyramidal cells is the principal source of EEG potentials.

Nonpyramidal cells of the cerebral cortex have oval-shaped cell bodies. Their axons typically do not leave the cortex but terminate on nearby neurons. Most cortical interneurons are nonpyramidal cells and are morphologically heterogeneous. *Stellate cells* form a dominant group of nonpyramidal cells. One class of stellate cells has axons that are oriented vertically in the plane of the cortical columns. These cells receive information directly from thalamic neurons, which they convey to other interneurons or to pyramidal cells in the same column. An example of this kind of stellate interneuron is the spiny stellate cell of the visual cortex, whose dendrites are covered with small spines.

Some nonpyramidal cells have axons that are oriented horizontally in the plane of the cortical layers. An important example is the *basket cell*, which forms dense

Sensory Evoked Potentials Measure Activity in Specific Sensory Pathways   BOX 50–1

The sensory evoked potential is a specific change in the ongoing EEG resulting from stimulation of a sensory pathway. Sensory evoked potentials are distinguished from event-related potentials, which are dependent on the context in which the stimulus is presented, such as whether the stimulus is expected or a surprise.

The sensory evoked potential is extracted from the EEG using computer averaging techniques (Figure 50–3). The EEG is recorded during repetitive natural stimulation, such as a tap on the skin, presentation of a tone, or a flash of light, which activates sensory receptors. A computer samples the EEG for a brief period before and after the stimulus and the sampled data are averaged to enhance the signal-to-noise ratio.

Sensory evoked potentials consist of multiple components related to various aspects of subcortical and cortical processing. Although the recordings made from scalp electrodes predominantly reflect cortical processing in the immediate environment of the electrode, earlier components reflecting subcortical processing also can be distinguished.

Because the sensory-evoked potentials reflect the processing of the physical characteristics of the stimulus, they are clinically useful for assessing the function of sensory systems or evaluating demyelinating diseases, such as multiple sclerosis. Since destruction of the myelin sheath causes conduction velocity to decrease, the latencies of the evoked potentials are longer than normal. Later components of the sensory evoked potential are important in clinically assessing higher brain functions.

Of the various sensory systems, the components of the auditory evoked potential have been most extensively studied. The auditory evoked potential consists of two sets of deflections generated by different components of the auditory system. The *brain stem evoked potentials* are the first set of deflections. The first brain stem evoked potential is produced by the auditory apparatus in the inner ear, immediately followed by potentials produced by each of the major auditory relay nuclei in the pons and midbrain, as well as transmission in the ascending auditory pathway (Figure 50–4). These early components of the evoked potential recorded from the scalp are sometimes termed *far-field potentials* because they originate from distant sites. The second set of deflections have longer latencies than the brain stem potentials and are generated by the thalamic auditory relay nucleus and neurons in the auditory cortex.

Auditory event-related potentials, which are believed to be mediated by higher-order auditory areas and portions of the association cortex, have longer latencies than the sensory evoked potentials. The amplitude of the event-related potentials changes depending on the context in which the stimulus is presented.

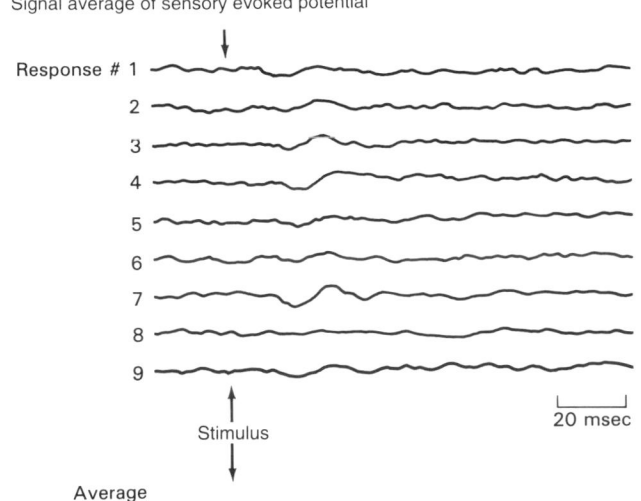

FIGURE 50–3

These tracings show nine separate records of the ensemble activity of cortical neurons during which a stimulus, for example a flash of light or a tap, was presented. The evoked potential occurs at a predictable interval following the stimulus. Since the size of the response in an individual record is small in relation to the amplitude of the fluctuations of the EEG, numerous records must be averaged using a computer to reveal the characteristic evoked potential. In this procedure the randomly occurring fluctuations in the EEG cancel each other out, leaving a record of an average sensory evoked potential that clearly illustrates the time course and waveform of the sensory activity.

FIGURE 50–4

The auditory evoked potential has separate components corresponding to electrical activity at each relay and the cortex. Components I to VI are generated by successive structures in the auditory pathway, from the cochlea to the medial geniculate nucleus. Sources for later negative components (N_0, N_a, N_b, and N_2) and positive components (P_0, P_a, P_1, P_2) include thalamic nuclei other than the medial geniculate nucleus, the auditory cortex, and association cortices. The potentials are plotted on logarithmic scales. (Adapted from Picton et al., 1974.)

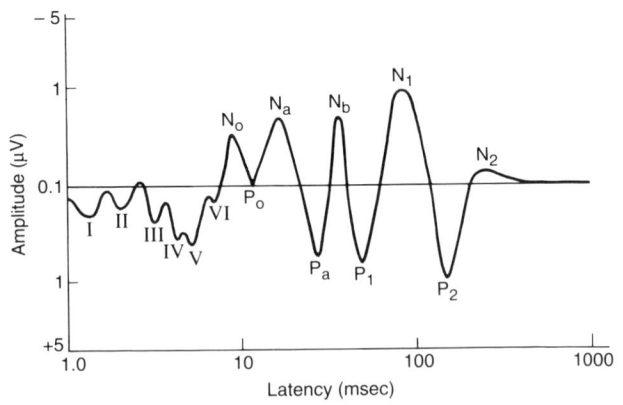

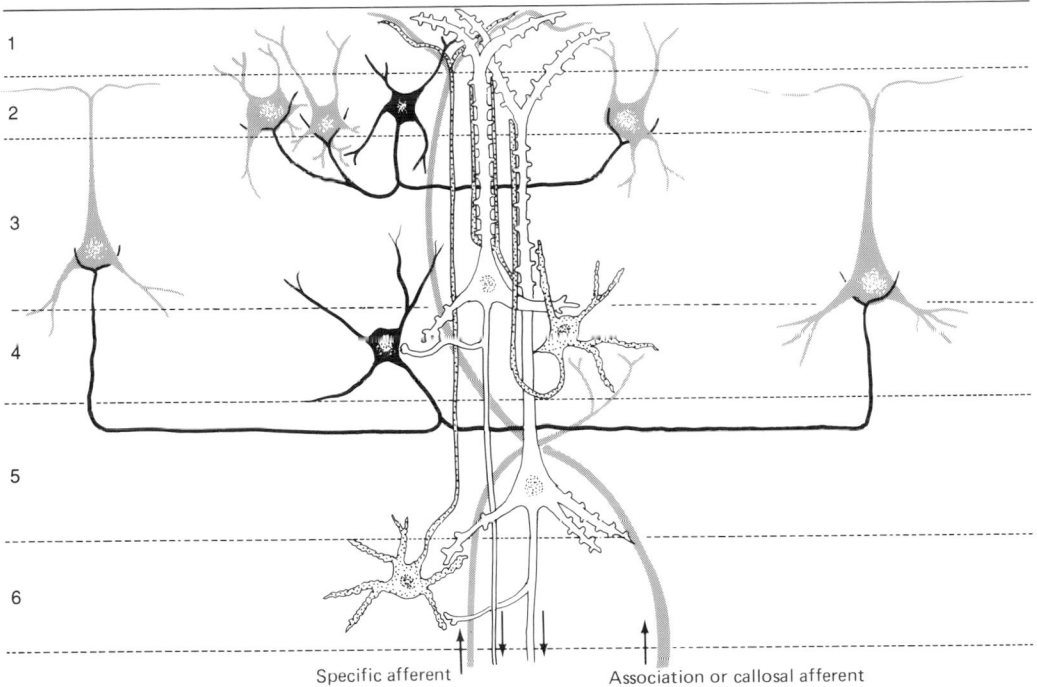

FIGURE 50–5

The principal neuron types and their interconnections are similar in the various regions of the cerebral cortex. Note that the two large pyramidal cells **(white)** in layers 3 and 5 receive multiple synaptic contacts from the star-shaped interneuron (stellate cell, **stippled**) in layer 4. The inhibitory action of the basket cells **(black)** is directed to the cell bodies of cortical neurons **(gray)**.

Major input to the cortex derives from specific thalamic relay nuclei (specific afferents) and is directed mostly to layer 4; association and callosal input (association and callosal afferents) is, in large part, directed to more superficial layers. (Adapted from Szentágothai, 1969.)

synaptic connections that envelop the soma of the postsynaptic neuron (hence the name basket). The terminals of basket cells contain large amounts of the enzyme glutamic acid decarboxylase, which catalyzes the synthesis of the inhibitory neurotransmitter γ-aminobutyric acid (GABA) (Box 50–2). The basket cell is thought to produce surround or pericolumnar inhibition (See Chapter 26), which enables neurons in a given cortical column to function in relative isolation from neighboring columns. These and other nonpyramidal cells that use GABA as their neurotransmitter are considered further in Box 50–2.

The EEG Is Generated in the Cortex by the Flow of Synaptic Currents Through the Extracellular Space

The EEG is an extracellular recording obtained by using macroelectrodes rather than microelectrodes. Macroelectrode recording from cortex is similar in principle to electrocardiography. Recordings are made at sites distant from the source of the electrical activity. Both the EEG and ECG are based on the theory of *volume conduction*, which describes the flow of ionic current generated by nerve cells or cardiac muscle through the extracellular space.

Potential changes recorded from the scalp are generated by the summed ionic currents of the many thousands of neurons located under the recording electrode. The net ionic current is recorded as a voltage across the resistance of the extracellular space. To elucidate the EEG we shall first review the response of a single neuron to an excitatory input as detected in intracellular recordings. Next we shall examine that neuron's response, and those of its neighbors, as detected with a microelectrode positioned just outside the cell. Finally, we shall examine the summed responses of the neurons of the entire ensemble recorded by a macroelectrode located on the scalp.

Let us first consider the flow of current produced by an excitatory synaptic potential on the apical dendrite of a cortical pyramidal cell (Figure 50–8A). The excitatory postsynaptic potential (EPSP) is produced by a current, I_{EPSP}, flowing inward through the synaptic membrane and outward along the large expanse of the extrasynaptic membrane (Chapters 10 and 11). The intracellular record is the measured voltage, V_m, across both the membrane resistance, R_m, and extracellular resistance, R_{ex} (Figure 50–8B). Because the extracellular resistance is so small compared with the large resistance of the membrane, the voltage is effectively equal to the current multiplied by the membrane resistance ($I_{EPSP} \times R_m$).

Synaptic Inhibition in the Cerebral Cortex

BOX 50–2

Inhibition in the cerebral cortex is mediated principally by GABA. GABA or its synthesizing enzyme glutamic acid decarboxylase can be found in a variety of nonpyramidal cells using immunological staining techniques. These nonpyramidal cells are largely devoid of dendritic spines and hence are termed *nonspiny neurons* (Figure 50–6). Neurons that contain GABA (or glutamic acid decarboxylase) project locally. (An interesting exception is the Purkinje cell of the cerebral cortex, a GABAergic projection neuron.) A large percentage of cortical neurons that are immunoreactive for GABA are also immunoreactive for many of the known neuropeptides (see Chapter 14). Inhibition in the cortex, as well as other supraspinal structures, is powerful and may do more than simply

cancel the effect of excitation. In the cortex inhibitory synapses generally are located close to the cell body, whereas excitatory synapses are located primarily on the dendrites. For example, *basket cells* (Figure 50–6) are inhibitory interneurons that synapse on the cell bodies of pyramidal cells. Therefore they have a direct inhibitory influence on action potential generation at the initial axon segment of the pyramidal cell. Not only are inhibitory synapses on cortical neurons strategically placed for influencing signaling, but their action endures. Cortical inhibitory presynaptic potentials are much larger and last 10–20 times longer than the inhibitory actions exerted on spinal motor neurons (Figure 50–7).

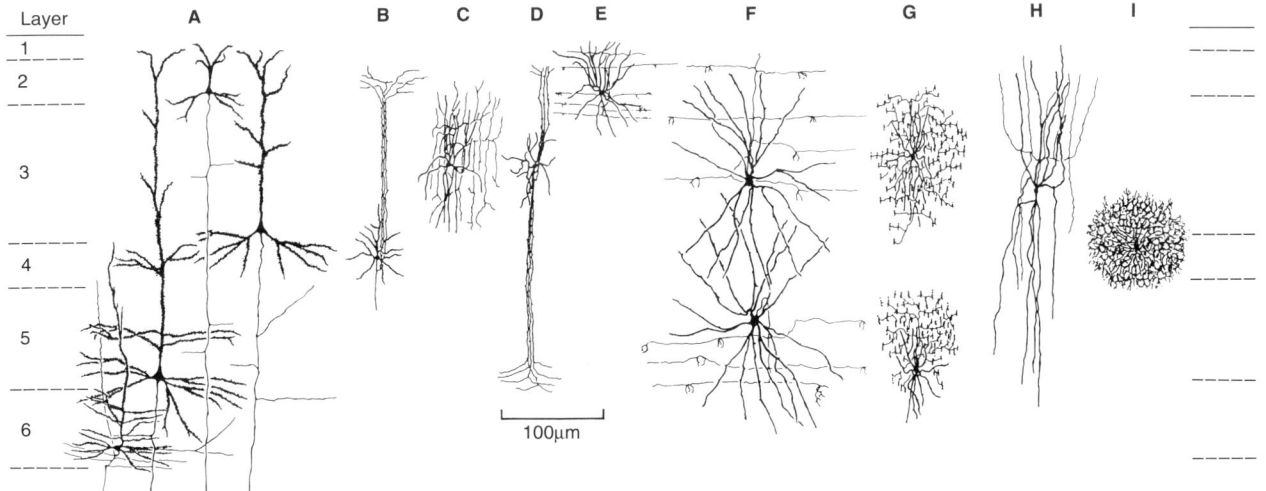

FIGURE 50–6

Morphological types of cells identifiable in monkey cerebral cortex, based on studies of the primary somatic sensory and motor cortex. Pyramidal cells (**A**) contain dendritic spines and are the only output neurons on the cortex. They are likely to use glutamate as a neurotransmitter and therefore are excitatory neurons, as is the interneuron (**B**). Most

nonpyramidal cells are thought to use GABA, and in some cases neuropeptides, as a transmitter. These neurons do not have dendritic spines. **C.** Cell with axonal "arcades". **D.** Double bouquet cell. **E** and **F.** Basket cells. **G.** Chandelier cells. **H.** Long, stringy cells (contain neuropeptides or acetylcholine). **I.** Neurogliaform cell. (Adapted from Jones, 1987.)

FIGURE 50–7

The inhibitory postsynaptic potential recorded from a hippocampal pyramidal cell is much greater than that recorded from a spinal motor neuron. (From Spencer and Kandel, 1968.)

Large cortical inhibitory postsynaptic potentials have a powerful influence on the activity of a population of cells. For example, in normal tissue recurrent inhibition may limit the size of a neuronal population that responds to a stimulus and thereby serve as a mechanism for enhancing the contrast between active and inactive cells in the population (see Chapter 26).

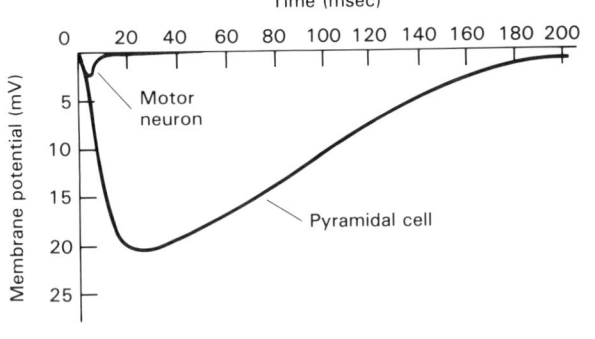

A

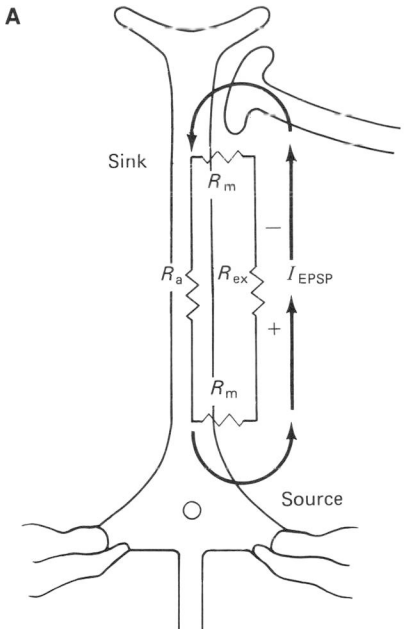

B

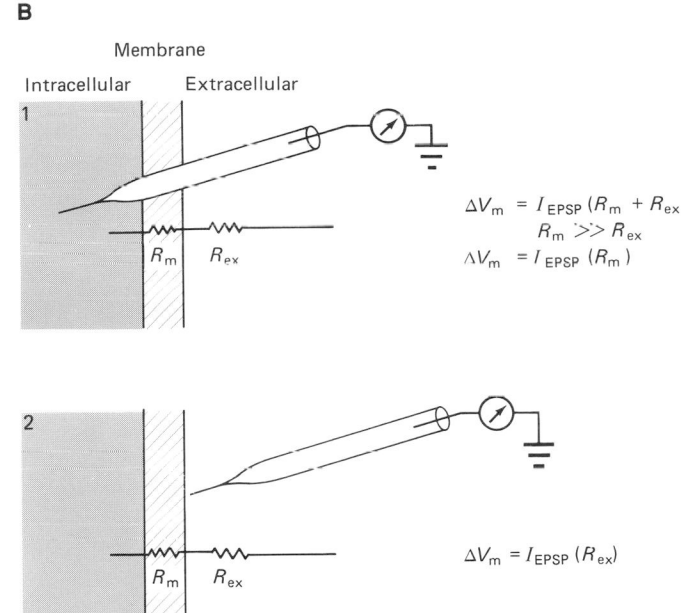

FIGURE 50–8
Intracellular potentials are recorded primarily across the membrane resistance, whereas extracellular potentials are recorded across the extracellular resistance.

A. Current flow (I_{EPSP}) in and around a cortical pyramidal cell. (R_{ex} extracellular resistance; R_m membrane resistance; R_a axoplasmic resistance.)

B. Comparison of intracellular (**1**) and extracellular (**2**) recording configurations. Intracellular recordings measure the voltage drop principally across R_m; extracellular recordings are measurements across R_{ex}. Because R_m is much greater than R_{ex}, an electrical event recorded from within a cell is larger than the same event recorded outside the cell.

To understand extracellular potentials, we must now focus on this small extracellular resistance. As shown in Figure 50–8B, a recording is made across only the extracellular resistance. A given current (I_{EPSP}) flowing across the large membrane resistance (R_m) causes a much greater change in potential across the membrane, ΔV_m, than does the same current (I_{EPSP}) flowing across the small extracellular resistance (R_{ex}). This is one reason that intracellular potentials are large (in the range of millivolts) and extracellular potentials are small (in the range of microvolts). As a first approximation, we can use Ohm's law to calculate the voltage difference between potentials recorded intracellularly and extracellularly. The current resulting from the EPSP is the same throughout the circuit, and flows across the membrane resistance (R_m) and the extracellular resistance (R_{ex}). Therefore, if we assume an intracellularly recorded EPSP of 5 mV, the extracellular signal measured just outside the cell would be about 2.5 μV:

$$\frac{\Delta V_m}{R_m} = \frac{\Delta V_{ex}}{R_{ex}} = \frac{5 \times 10^{-3}\,V}{1 \times 10^5\,\Omega} = \frac{\Delta V_{ex}}{5 \times 10^1 \Omega}$$

$$\Delta V_{ex} = \frac{(5 \times 10^{-3})\,V}{(1 \times 10^5)\,\Omega} = 2.5\ \mu V.$$

To interpret the polarity of the recorded potential it is important to distinguish the sites of inward and outward current. The site of inward current is called the *sink* because this is where the current flows into the cell. The site of outward current is called the *source*. (For simplicity, in Figure 50–8A only one path of inward and outward current is shown.) The sink is on the negative side of the extracellular potential; the source is on the positive side.

At the site of generation of an EPSP the extracellular recording has a negative sign because the tip of the recording electrode is close to the site of inward current (the sink). When the tip is close to the site of outward current (the source), a positive potential is recorded (Figure 50–9). In contrast, when the electrode tip is inside the cell, EPSPs are always recorded as depolarizing potentials produced by the influx of positively charged ions, irrespective of the recording site.

We have illustrated extracellular recordings with a signal from one cell, but in fact an extracellular microelectrode records signals from many cells. The recorded signal comes principally from neurons near the tip of the electrode and only to a small extent from more distant neurons. As the electrode is moved from the site of generation of activity, the recorded amplitude of the signal decreases rapidly by the square root of the distance. In addition to the small value of the extracellular resistance, the rapid drop of potential with distance also contributes to the small size of the recorded extracellular potentials.

The small size of potentials recorded extracellularly poses a serious problem when the electrode is far from the

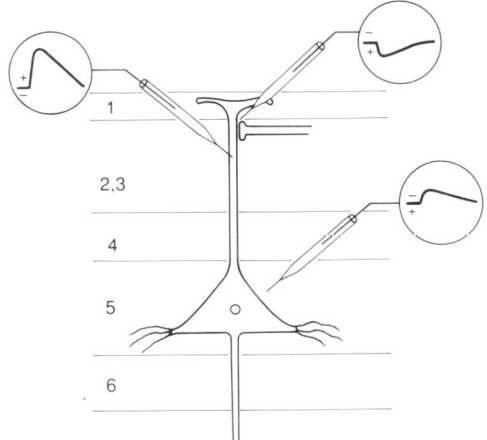

FIGURE 50-9

The polarity of extracellular recordings depends on whether the electrode is near the site of inward or outward current flow. Two extracellular recordings are shown on the **right** in response to an EPSP in the superficial portion of layer 2. The **top right** recording is near the site of inward current flow (sink) and the one **below** is near the site of outward current flow (source). An intracellular recording is shown on the **left.**

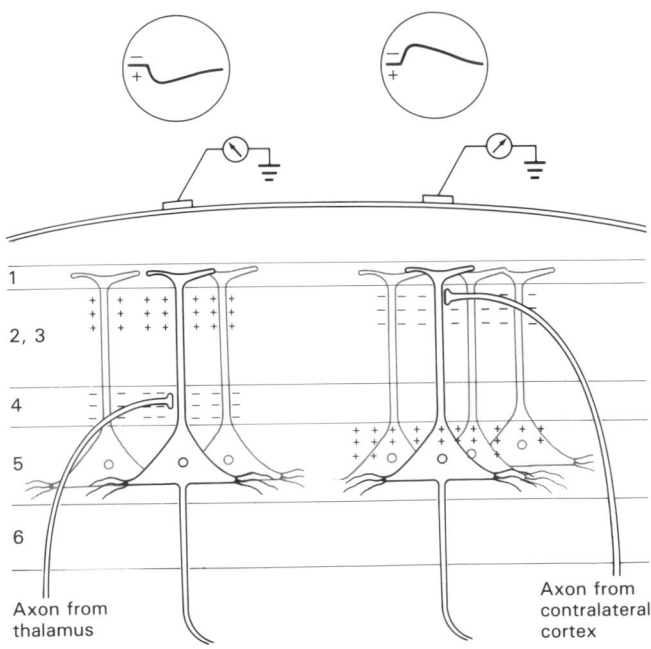

FIGURE 50-10

Scalp recordings depend on the depth of synaptic activity in the cortex. The convention adopted for the polarity of *extra*cellular recording is that upward deflections represent negative potentials when recording near the synapse, where the current flow is inward. In deeper cortical layers, away from the synapse, these same excitatory synaptic potentials are observed as a downward deflection on an EEG. (In *intra*cellular recordings upward deflections represent positive potentials.)

Left: A potential recorded from a scalp electrode following activation of thalamic inputs. The terminals of thalamocortical neurons make excitatory connections on cortical neurons predominantly in layer 4. Thus, the site of inward current flow (sink) is in layer 4 and the site of outward current flow (source) is in the superficial cortical layers. Since the recording electrode on the scalp is closer to the site of outward current flow, it records a positive potential.

Right: A potential recorded from excitatory inputs from callosal neurons in the contralateral cortex. The axons of callosal neurons terminate in the superficial cortical layers. A negative potential (upward deflection) is recorded because the electrode is closer to the site of inward current flow than that of the outward flow.

active neurons, as in recording from the scalp with a macroelectrode. The activity of single neurons cannot be recorded from the scalp because the amplitude of their potentials is too small and macroelectrodes are insufficiently selective to distinguish this activity from that of its neighbors. Fortunately, the scalp recording is the summed activity of large numbers of neurons.

Thalamic input activates thousands of cortical neurons synchronously. The initial cortical response to thalamic input is the formation of a sink in deeper layers (where the excitatory synapses are located) and a source in superficial layers (Figure 50–10, left). A recording electrode on the surface of the scalp is therefore closer to the source than to the sink. With further intracortical processing the configuration of sinks and sources may change. The sign of the electrical signal will differ depending on where in the cortex the excitatory synapses are located (whether in the superficial or in deep layers). The right half of Figure 50–10 shows the scalp-recorded potential in response to excitation by callosal neurons, whose axons terminate in layers 2 and 3. The sink is closer to the recording electrode and the recording is an upward deflection. During inhibition the relationship between synaptic location and recording polarity is reversed (see Table 50–1).

Thus, cortical synaptic events cannot be unambiguously determined from surface recording alone. For example, a positive wave recorded from the surface of the scalp may correspond to either superficial excitation or deep inhibition. Additional information about the anatomical organization of cortical synapses is needed to define the synaptic mechanisms underlying surface-recorded potentials. The directions of deflection of recorded potentials in response to excitation and inhibition are summarized in Table 50–1.

The EEG Reflects Primarily Synaptic Potentials in Pyramidal Cells

Although it might seem that the most obvious source for the extracellular potentials recorded in the EEG is the action potential—the largest signal generated by neurons—action potentials actually contribute little to surface potentials except possibly when there are synchronous action potentials in large numbers of neurons. Most potentials recorded from the scalp are the result of extracellular current flow associated with summated synaptic potentials in the activated pyramidal cells.

TABLE 50–1. Directions of Deflection in Recordings of Excitatory and Inhibitory Potentials

Postsynaptic potential	Cellular response	Intracellular recording	Extracellular surface recording	
			Synapse in superficial layer	Synapse in deeper layer
Excitatory	Depolarization	Upward	Upward	Downward
Inhibitory	Hyperpolarization	Downward	Downward	Upward

The reason why pyramidal cell activity contributes more to the EEG than nonpyramidal cell activity is that pyramidal cells are oriented parallel to one another, and their dendrites are oriented perpendicular to the surface of the cortex. Therefore, a synaptic potential generated on the dendrites is recorded with little attenuation because the sources and sinks are all oriented perpendicular to the cortical surface. In contrast, most nonpyramidal cells and individual glial cells are not oriented in any particular fashion relative to one another or to the pyramidal cells; their contribution to the EEG is probably insignificant. Synaptic potentials contribute more to the EEG because they are slower than action potentials, and thus can summate.

Epilepsy Interrupts Normal Brain Function

The extensive neuronal interconnections within a local area of cortex and between distant areas underlie the extensive serial and parallel processing of sensory and motor information. However, such connections—many of which are excitatory—result in an abnormal synchrony of discharge in large ensembles of neurons. During such synchronous interactions, an epileptic seizure that has serious behavioral consequences will occur. Synchronous discharge produces stereotyped and involuntary paroxysmal alterations in behavior: jerking movements, transient loss of awareness, and even massive convulsions and loss of consciousness. These behavioral changes profoundly alter the life of epileptic patients. Abnormal cellular discharge may be caused by many factors: trauma, oxygen deprivation, tumors, infection, and toxic states. In about half of the patients, however, no specific causative factors are found. Next to strokes, epilepsy is the most common neurological disease: About 0.5 to 1% of the population suffers from epilepsy.

Partial and Generalized Seizures Have Different Clinical and EEG Features

Epileptic seizures can be either partial or generalized. *Partial* (or *focal*) epilepsy is a form of seizure that begins in a restricted brain region and either remains localized or spreads to adjacent cortex. Partial seizures do not necessarily disrupt consciousness. The clinical manifestations of a partial seizure reflect the region of the brain involved (Figure 50–11A). For example, an epileptic focus in the motor cortex results in involuntary contractions of individual or small groups of striated muscles of the body.

In some partial seizures of the motor cortex there is sequential activation of different muscle groups as the abnormal electrical activity spreads from the focus to neighboring motor cortical tissue. In these seizures the motor activity may involve first the fingers, followed by the wrist, elbow, shoulder, and eventually the face and leg. As we saw in Chapter 1, Hughlings Jackson first described the somatotopic organization of the motor cortex from observations made in patients with this type of seizure. These attacks are therefore called *Jacksonian motor seizures*. A patient experiencing a Jacksonian seizure remains conscious if the abnormal activity is restricted to one hemisphere. If epileptic activity spreads to the other hemisphere, consciousness may be lost.

Complex partial seizures, sometimes referred to as *psychomotor* seizures, are characterized by complicated illusory phenomena and semipurposeful complicated motor acts. Psychomotor seizures involve limbic system structures within the temporal lobe and orbital frontal cortex.

The electrophysiological consequences of focal seizures can be recorded in a noninvasive manner with scalp electrodes. The signature of a focal seizure is a brief pointed wave, often called an *EEG spike* (Figure 50–11A). As we shall see below, this signal corresponds to the synchronous discharge of cortical neurons beneath the electrode. EEG spikes occur with high frequency during a seizure but can also be seen between attacks.

Generalized (or *nonfocal*) *epilepsy* involves large parts of the brain from the outset (Figure 50–11B) and invariably loss of consciousness. The difference in the spatial distribution of abnormal electrical activity recorded during generalized and focal seizures is significant. Like focal seizures, generalized seizures also result in EEG spikes; unlike focal seizures, generalized seizure activity is present on EEG traces all over the skull simultaneously. There are several forms of generalized seizures. Two of the more prominent are petit mal and grand mal. *Petit mal seizures*, which begin during childhood, are accompanied by a transient loss of consciousness (absence seizure). The EEG during petit mal seizures shows a three-cycle-per-second generalized spike-wave discharge. Petit mal seizures interrupt perception, cognition, and memory, but such functions return almost immediately when the seizure stops. Muscle tone is maintained so that patients rarely fall. *Grand mal seizures* occur as a startling and

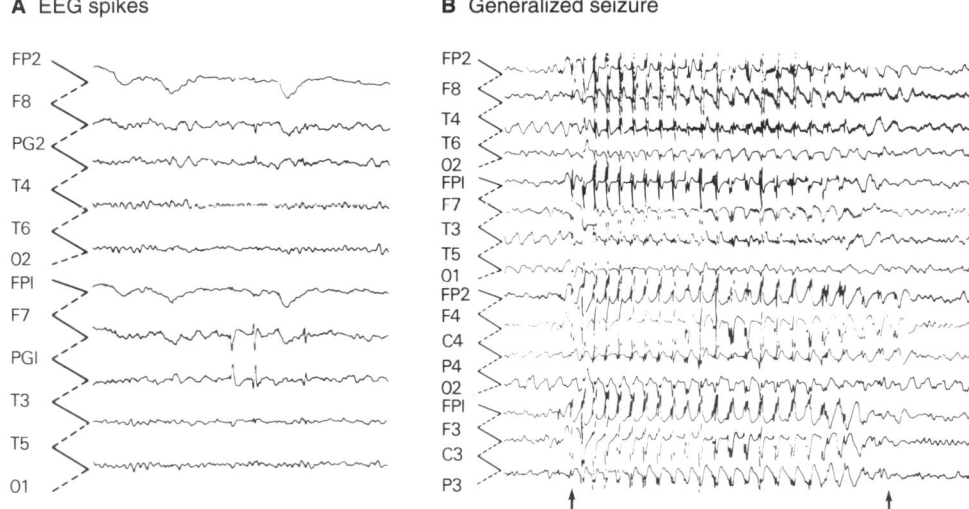

FIGURE 50–11

Scalp recordings during a focal epileptic seizure and a generalized seizure. Various scalp electrodes record ongoing electrical activity over different cortical regions. The location and nomenclature of the electrodes conform to an international convention (see Figure 50–2). (Adapted from Merritt, 1979.)

A. In this record of a focal seizure, sharp deflections (so-called EEG spikes) are recorded between electrodes F7 and PG1 and between PG1 and T3.

B. The beginning and end of this generalized seizure are indicated by the **arrows**. During a generalized seizure abnormal electrical activity is recorded by electrodes. In contrast, focal seizures are characterized by abnormal electrical activity from only a subset of electrodes.

abrupt loss of consciousness and postural control. The patient falls to the ground and suffers tonic–clonic movements, i.e., periods of increased muscle tone (the tonic phase) alternating with periods consisting of jerky movements (the clonic phase). In contrast to petit mal seizures, the loss of consciousness and other behavioral changes of the grand mal seizure may persist after the seizure.

Large Populations of Neurons Are Activated Synchronously During an Epileptic Seizure

Large-amplitude waves on the normal EEG occur when the activity of groups of neurons is synchronized. This occurs during some high-voltage alpha waves and during theta and delta activity. Synchronous neuronal activation also characterizes the EEG spike and the spike and wave complex recorded during partial and generalized seizures. Our understanding of the cellular mechanisms of epilepsy is most detailed for focal epilepsy. Focal epilepsy has been studied most widely because it is prevalent and is easy to produce in experimental animals.

Experimental focal epilepsy can be established by a variety of physical and chemical insults applied to a small neuronal ensemble. One way is to apply *convulsant drugs* transiently to the surface of the cortex of an experimental animal. For example, direct application of large doses of penicillin blocks the action of the inhibitory neurotransmitter GABA. As we shall see below, reducing the amount of inhibition in a cortical region has a major impact on the behavior of neuronal ensembles. Application of a convul-

sant drug produces an acute focal epilepsy without morphological changes in cells. In contrast, topical application of alumina cream can produce chronic focal epilepsy accompanied by morphological changes, such as a reduction in the number of dendritic spines, reduced dendritic branching, or a reduction in the number of inhibitory synapses.

Repeated electrical stimulation can also produce electrophysiological, and perhaps even morphological, changes in the local tissue. It has been known since the early 1960s that stimulus-produced seizure activity can be progressively intensified by repeated high-frequency stimulation of certain components of the limbic system at intervals ranging from minutes to days. This phenomenon is termed *kindling*, by analogy to starting a fire. Kindling involves a long-lasting change in the properties of neurons. Months after stimulation, an intense seizure can be elicited by relatively few electrical stimuli. Kindling induced in experimental animals (by stimulating the amygdala, for example) shares many features with human psychomotor epilepsy (similar EEG changes, changes in behavior patterns during the seizure, and responsiveness of the seizures to anticonvulsant drug therapy). This similarity raises the very interesting possibility that certain forms of human epilepsy may be produced by a relatively brief event that triggers a series of changes in the properties of neural circuits. The mechanisms underlying kindling may be similar to long-term potentiation, in which a brief period of intense activity gives rise to a persistent change in synaptic strength.

There are also experimental models for the study of generalized seizures. One important model also relies on the use of penicillin at toxic doses administered systemically rather than locally. There are also genetic models for generalized epilepsy in which animals show the characteristic spike–wave discharges and even convulsions when perturbed in specific ways. We shall next consider three important questions that have been examined in experimental epilepsies: (1) the cellular mechanisms producing focal seizures, (2) the mechanisms by which a focal seizure becomes generalized, and (3) the mechanisms of generalized seizure. Because much of modern research on epilepsy has focused on the properties of cortical neurons and the circuitry involved in the generation of seizures, we shall examine the electrophysiological properties of normal cortical neurons and compare them with those of cortex made epileptic through experimental manipulations.

A Depolarization Shift Underlies Focal Seizures

The electrical activity recorded from the surface of the brain during a focal seizure produced by penicillin application is similar to that recorded from epileptic foci in humans. The first abnormal electrical event of the activated focal seizure is the appearance of intermittent high-voltage negative waves on the EEG (Figure 50–12). These are called *interictal spikes* because they resemble the spikes seen on the EEG of humans between seizures. As the interictal spikes become more frequent, they become associated with a slower negative wave. Collectively, the fast (spike-like) and slow components may also be associated with low-voltage fast waves riding on the crest. When a full-blown seizure occurs, it typically arises from these low-voltage components.

The interictal spike is recorded with a surface electrode. Intracellular recordings from neurons within the experimental epileptic focus show a characteristic abrupt depolarizing potential, termed a *depolarization shift*, during the initial component of the interictal spike. A burst of action potentials is often concurrent with and superimposed on this potential (Figure 50–12). The depolarization shift is thought to be generated by an excitatory postsynaptic potential that is enhanced and subsequently amplified by intrinsic (voltage-dependent) membrane responses.

This enhancement may be due to a variety of mechanisms, including reduction in synaptic inhibition. The amplification is also thought to involve several processes. One is the production of regenerative *dendritic* action potentials. In contrast to axonal action potentials, there are two kinds of dendritic action potentials: small fast ones and large slow ones. The fast action potentials were identified in 1961 with intrasomatic recordings from pyramidal cells of the hippocampus by Alden Spencer and Eric Kandel. They suggested that the fast spikes (termed fast prepotentials) are active responses in the dendrites that are detected remotely in the cell body.

David Prince and his colleagues later showed with in-

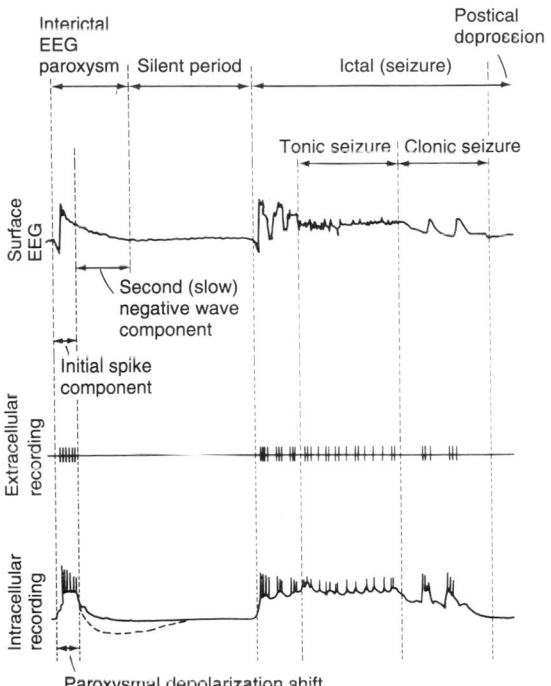

FIGURE 50–12

Relationship between surface-recorded EEG discharges and intracellular and extracellular activity in a cortical epileptic focus in an experimental animal. Application of penicillin to the cortical surface produces an epileptic focus. Within the focus, and restricted to it, a characteristic sequence of events occurs. Before the occurrence of the focal seizure there are fast spike-like potentials in the EEG. These potentials correspond to the interictal EEG paroxysms and are thought to be produced by an abrupt depolarization of the underlying cortical neurons, called the *paroxysmal depolarization shift*. The slow wave that follows the EEG spike occurs during the period when the cortical neurons are hyperpolarized. (The **dashed line** on the bottom trace corresponds to the afterhyperpolarization.) As the experimental epileptic focus develops, the frequency of occurrence of the interictal EEG paroxysms increases until a generalized projected seizure occurs. After the seizure there is a decrease in neuronal excitability. (Adapted from Ayala et al., 1973).

tradendritic recordings in hippocampal slices (see Box 50–3) that the fast action potentials can be blocked by tetrodotoxin (a Na^+ channel blocker), indicating that they are Na^+ spikes. In contrast, the larger dendritic action potentials are insensitive to tetrodotoxin and are inhibited by Mg^{2+}, which blocks Ca^{2+} channels. Dendritic trigger zones are believed to function as booster zones under normal conditions so that synaptic currents that are remote from the spike initiation zone at the axon hillock may result in generation of action potentials. During epilepsy the normal balance of excitation and inhibition is altered, favoring excitation. An excitatory postsynaptic potential may trigger a burst of dendritic action potentials, especially Ca^{2+} spikes, which summate to produce a large and prolonged depolarization (Figure 50–15).

Mammalian Brain Slice Preparation

BOX 50–3

The tissue slice technique has revolutionized the study of the electrophysiological properties of mammalian neurons. Brain slices, which range from 70–400 µM thick, are prepared by quickly removing the brain and immersing it into chilled saline and then sectioning the tissue with a special type of microtome. This technique preserves the basic circuitry of

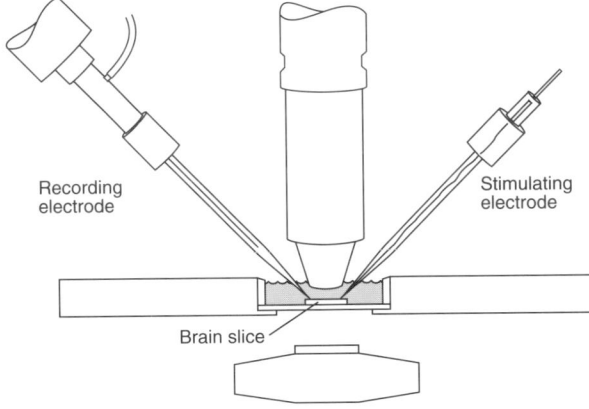

Recording electrode

Stimulating electrode

Brain slice

FIGURE 50–13
Set-up for recording from neurons in a brain slice. The slice is mounted in a chamber to the X-Y stage of a microscope. A water-immersion objective allows visualization of the slice at high power through the saline solution. Separate stimulation and recording electrodes can be placed in the tissue under direct visualization through a microscope. (Adapted from Konnerth, 1990.)

FIGURE 50–14
Photograph of a rat hippocampal slice. (Courtesy of Dr. A. Konnerth.)

A. Nomarski image from the cut surface of the slice revealing the pyramidal cell layer in the CA1 region of the hippocampus.

neurons in the slice. The slice is placed in a recording chamber (Figure 50–13) through which oxygenated saline solution is circulated.

There are two principal advantages to recording from neurons in tissue slices. First, more stable electrophysiological recordings can be made because there are no mechanical pulsations due to respiration or the pumping of blood. This allows recording from very fine neuronal processes, such as dendrites. Second, the tissue is visualized under a microscope. When the microscope is equipped with special optics, for example Nomarski optics, individual neurons actually can be seen (Figure 50–14). Direct visualization of neurons allows them to be identified from their morphology or from their efferent projections (by retrogradely filling a neuron's cell body with a fluorescent compound before the slice is removed from the brain). In addition, direct visualization facilitates patch clamping of individual neurons.

Recording from brain slices has been used to investigate various aspects of the function of mammalian neurons, including the response of neurons to different neurotransmitters and neuromodulators and the properties of single channels. Through the use of tissue slice techniques, cell and molecular biological approaches can be applied to virtually any part of the mammalian brain. Information obtained from recordings made in brain slices has provided important insights into such problems as synaptic plasticity, the mechanisms of epilepsy, and the actions of drugs on the brain.

B. A single pyramidal cell is filled with the fluorescent dye Lucifer yellow. The upside-down configuration of the hippocampus results in the large apical dendrite projecting toward the bottom of the photograph, and the basilar dendrites toward the top. The large neuronal cell body can be seen at the tip of the dye-containing pipette.

A

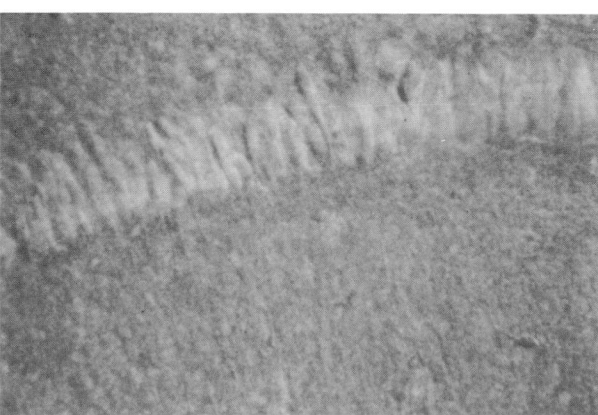

B

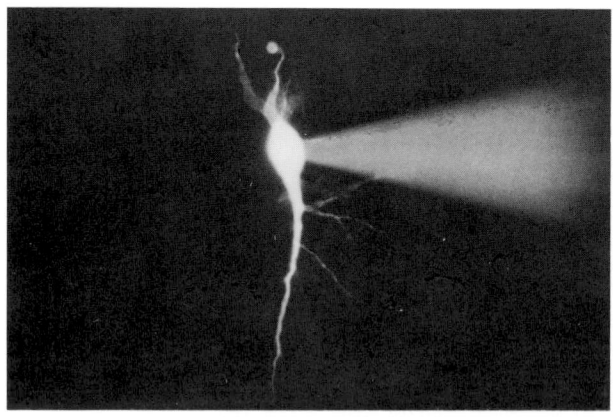

Excitatory Connections Between Cortical Neurons Synchronize Discharges in an Epileptic Focus

The interictal spike reflects the synchronous activity of a large neuronal ensemble. In fact, because a large spike is recorded from the cortical surface, we know that many hundreds or thousands of neurons must be firing in synchrony. How is the activity of the neuronal ensemble synchronized? Normally, communication between neurons in an ensemble is highly constrained, because inhibition in the cortex is very strong (see Box 50–2). One mechanism for synchronizing large ensembles in focal epilepsy may be a decrease in postsynaptic inhibition.

With a decrease in cortical GABAergic inhibition, cells fire bursts of action potentials and strongly excite their postsynaptic targets. Richard Miles and Robert Wong found that during periods of reduced GABAergic inhibition, produced by application of the GABA antagonist picrotoxin, a pyramidal cell in a hippocampal tissue slice excites its target neurons strongly, but also excites the neurons that normally are excited by the target neurons. Before GABA blockade, a given neuron has only a 5% chance of exciting a nearby neuron; this increases to 30% when GABA inhibition is antagonized. Inhibition of GABA's action can thus begin a cascade of excitation that results in the synchronous activation of a neuronal ensemble.

The axon of a pyramidal cell has many postsynaptic targets. A neuron that fires a single action potential may not activate postsynaptic neurons because the excitatory postsynaptic potential may be subthreshold. A burst of action potentials is much more likely to excite the postsynaptic cells because of temporal summation (see Chapter 11). Any modification that increases neuronal excitability and therefore favors burst production will presumably lead to recruitment and synchronization of neurons in the ensemble. In addition to synaptic inhibition, extracellular events may play an important role in synchronizing neuronal activity. For example, when large neuronal ensembles discharge, summation of extracellular currents can alter the excitability of neurons. Also, certain changes in the ionic environment (for example, accumulation of K^+ ions in the extracellular space) can increase neuronal excitability.

Synaptic Inhibition May Limit Seizure Spread

Interictal spikes and focal seizures are often limited in their spread; the entire cerebral cortex does not become affected. This limitation occurs because the depolarization shift (and associated burst of action potentials), thought to underlie the interictal spike, is followed by a period of hyperpolarization during which neuronal excitability is reduced.

One important mechanism contributing to the hyperpolarization, and thus limiting the spread of the seizure, is the very potent synaptic inhibition in the cortex (see Box 50–2). A second mechanism thought to be important in the afterhyperpolarization (and therefore a factor limiting seizure spread) is the turning on of both voltage-sensitive and Ca^{2+}-dependent K^+ channels.

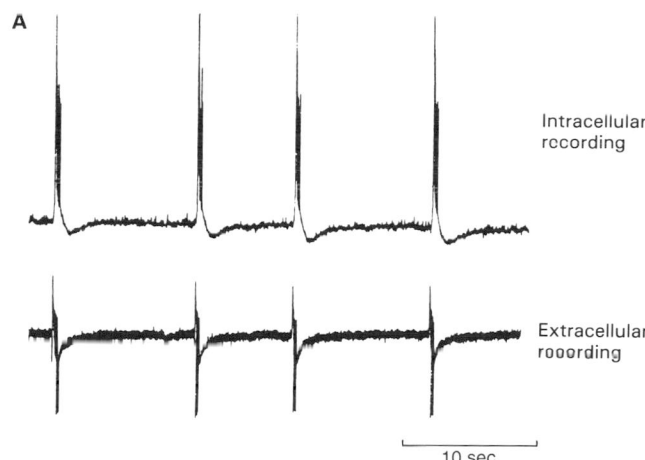

A

Intracellular recording

Extracellular recording

10 sec

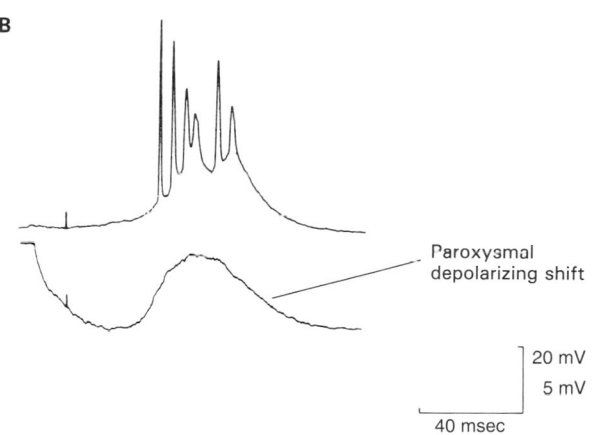

B

Paroxysmal depolarizing shift

20 mV
5 mV
40 msec

FIGURE 50–15

Interictal discharges occur spontaneously in the *in vitro* hippocampus when the GABA blocking agent bicuculline is applied to the fluid bathing the tissue slice. (Adapted from Wong et al., 1984.)

A. Rhythmic epileptiform discharges can be seen in the intracellular recording from a hippocampal pyramidal cell (top trace). Large neuronal ensembles are discharging in synchrony and their summed activity is recorded extracellularly (bottom trace).

B. Large-amplitude action potentials from the cell body and the dendrites (top trace) are superimposed upon the paroxymal depolarization shift, a slow depolarization that is revealed when the neuron is hyperpolarized (bottom trace).

Generalized Epilepsy Can Be Produced Experimentally

The signature of generalized epilepsy in the EEG is a characteristic spike-wave discharge that is present simultaneously over the entire brain. These electroencephalographic features can be produced in animal models of generalized epilepsy. The neurological signs of experimental epilepsy are also similar to those observed in human epilepsy. Generalized spike-wave discharge and convulsions can be elicited in certain baboons by presenting a flickering light. While some insights into the cellular mechanisms of generalized epilepsy have been obtained in baboons, other animals are better suited to a physiological analysis. For example, systemic administration of high doses of penicillin to cats produces a state that is similar to petit mal epilepsy. Bilaterally synchronous bursts of spike-wave discharges occur in the EEG, during which time the cat is behaviorally unresponsive. Pierre Gloor and his co-workers have found that the EEG oscillations are critically dependent on thalamic as well as cortical circuitry.

The phasing of the discharges in generalized epilepsy produced by high doses of penicillin may result from the strong recurrent inhibitory connections within the cortex. During focal seizures a reduction in GABA-mediated inhibition seems to be critical to the establishment and spread of the seizure. But during generalized seizures in this experimental model, GABA is needed to antagonize neuronal activity. Indeed, the concentration of penicillin in the brain of animals with generalized seizures is one to two orders of magnitude lower than when penicillin is applied locally to produce a focal seizure. Gloor and his colleagues have suggested that the long-lasting intracortical inhibition (see Figure 50–7 in Box 50–2) restricts excitatory influences to the brief interval between inhibitory postsynaptic potentials (IPSPs). This mechanism is similar to that proposed for the rhythmic alpha-wave activity observed in the EEG during slow-wave sleep.

While epilepsy produced by penicillin may help explain some of the temporal features of generalized epilepsy, it does not help us understand the generalized nature of the discharges. This may derive from a combination of factors such as an impingement on a hyperexcitable cortex of a diffuse input from the brain stem reticular formation, transmitted by way of midline thalamic nuclei. Recently, attention has focused on the ascending biogenic amine and cholinergic systems (Chapter 44).

An Overall View

The collective properties of the cerebral cortex are clearest in behavioral states such as sleep, arousal, and convulsive activity. These states can be examined noninvasively with scalp electrodes to record the EEG. The EEG reflects the activity of large ensembles of neurons, primarily that of cortical pyramidal cells. The apical dendrites of pyramidal cells are parallel to each other, an orientation that produces summation of extracellular current flow. The EEG also records the activity of other brain regions but only under special circumstances; the amplitude of these potentials are so small that computer averaging techniques are needed to extract the signal from the EEG. Distant neural signals as well as signals originating from neurons directly beneath the recording electrode are detected because the recording is based on volume conduction (i.e., extracellular currents are recorded across the resistance of the extracellular space).

While the EEG has been used successfully to examine fundamental questions in the neural mechanisms of cognition and perception, it is most commonly used clini-

cally to diagnose neurological disease, especially epilepsy. The two major forms of epilepsy, focal and generalized, produce distinctive EEG patterns. Changes in the EEG during focal epilepsy are initially restricted to a circumscribed portion of the cortex, but may spread. In contrast, changes in the EEG during generalized epilepsy are evident over the entire brain at seizure onset.

These distinctive patterns have encouraged the development of experimental models of human epilepsy. We are beginning to understand aspects of focal epilepsy in terms of the electrophysiological properties and connections of cortical neurons. Thus, the establishment of focal epilepsy is thought to involve a reduction in cortical inhibition mediated by GABA combined with divergent excitation, probably mediated by glutamate.

Since epilepsy is a disease that is reflected in the collective electrical behavior of the brain, research in epilepsy is unique in illustrating the effective use of cellular electrophysiology in elucidating the defects underlying a disease of the nervous system.

Selected Readings

Ayala, G. F., Dichter, M., Gumnit, R. J., Matsumoto, H., and Spencer, W. A. 1973. Genesis of epileptic interictal spikes. New knowledge of cortical feedback systems suggests a neurophysiological explanation of brief paroxysms. Brain Res. 52: 1–17.

Dichter, M. A., and Ayala, G. F. 1987. Cellular mechanisms of epilepsy: A status report. Science 237:157–164.

Duffy, F. H. (ed.) 1986. Topographic mapping of Brain Electrical Activity. Boston: Butterworths.

Fischer, R. S. 1989. Animal models of the epilepsies. Brain Res. Rev. 14:245–278.

Gloor, P. 1975. Contributions of electroencephalography and electrocorticography to the neurosurgical treatment of the epilepsies. In D. P. Purpura, J. K. Penry, and R. D. Walter (eds.), Neurosurgical Management of the Epilepsies. Advances in Neurology, Vol. 8. New York: Raven Press, pp. 59–105.

Hounsgaard, J., and Midtgaard, J. 1989. Dendrite processing in more ways than one. Trends Neurosci. 12:313–315.

Knowles, W. D., Traub, R. D., Wong, R. K. S., and Miles, R. 1985. Properties of neural networks: Experimentation and modeling of the epileptic hippocampal slice. Trends Neurosci. 8:73–79.

Konnerth, A. 1990. Patch-clamping in slices of mammalian CNS. Trends Neurosci. 13:321–323.

McCormick, D. A. 1989. Cholinergic and noradrenergic modulation of thalamocortical processing. Trends Neurosci. 12:215–221.

McNamara, J. O. 1986. Kindling model of epilepsy. In A. V. Delgado-Escueta, A. A. Ward, Jr., D. M. Woodbury, and R. J. Porter (eds.), Basic Mechanisms of the Epilepsies: Molecular and Cellular Approaches. Advances in Neurology, Vol 44. New York: Raven Press, pp. 303–318.

Møller, A. R., and Jannetta, P. J. 1986. Simultaneous surface and direct brainstem recordings of brainstem auditory evoked potentials (BAEP) in man. In R. Q. Cracco and I. Bodis-Wollner (eds.), Evoked Potentials, Frontiers of Clinical Neuroscience, Vol. 3. New York: Liss, pp. 227–234.

Pedley, T. A., and Traub, R. D. 1990. Physiological basis of the EEG. In D. D. Daly and T. A. Pedley (eds.), Current Practice of Clinical Electroencephalography, 2nd ed. New York: Raven Press, pp. 107–137.

Prince, D. A. 1978. Neurophysiology of epilepsy. Annu. Rev. Neurosci. 1:395–415.

Schwartzkroin, P. A., and Wyler, A. R. 1980. Mechanisms underlying epileptiform burst discharge. Ann. Neurol. 7:95–107.

References

Glaser, G. H. 1979. Convulsive disorders (epilepsy). In H. H. Merritt (ed.), A Textbook of Neurology, 6th ed. Philadelphia: Lea & Febiger, pp. 843–883.

Goddard, G. V. 1967. Development of epileptic seizures through brain stimulation at low intensity. Nature 214:1020–1021.

Hubel, D. H., and Wiesel, T. N. 1977. Ferrier Lecture: Functional architecture of macaque monkey visual cortex. Proc. R. Soc. Lond. [Biol.] 198:1–59.

Jones, E. G. 1984. Identification and classification of intrinsic circuit elements in the neocortex. In G. M. Edelman, W. E. Gall, and W. M. Cowan (eds.), Dynamic Aspects of Neocortical Function. New York: Wiley, pp. 7–40.

Jones, E. G. 1987. GABA-peptide neurons of the primate cerebral cortex. J. Mind Behav. 8:519–536.

Llinás, R., and Nicholson, C. 1971. Electrophysiological properties of dendrites and somata in alligator Purkinje cells. J. Neurophysiol. 34:532–551.

Marshall, W. H., Woolsey, C. N., and Bard, P. 1941. Observations on cortical somatic sensory mechanisms of cat and monkey. J. Neurophysiol. 4:1–24.

McCormick, D. A. 1989. GABA as an inhibitory neurotransmitter in human cerebral cortex. J. Neurophysiol. 62:1018–1027.

Miles, R., and Wong, R. K. S. 1987. Inhibitory control of local excitatory circuits in the guinea-pig hippocampus. J. Physiol. (Lond.) 388:611–629.

Mountcastle, V. B. 1978. An organizing principle for cerebral function: The unit module and the distributed system. In G. M. Edelman and V. B. Mountcastle, The Mindful Brain. Cambridge, Mass.: MIT Press, pp. 7–50.

Orbach, H. S., Cohen, L. B., and Grinvald, A. 1985. Optical mapping of electrical activity in rat somatosensory and visual cortex. J. Neurosci. 5:1886–1895.

Picton, T. W., Hillyard, S. A., Krausz, H. I., and Galambos, R. 1974. Human auditory evoked potentials. I: Evaluation of components. Electroencephalogr. Clin. Neurophysiol. 36:179–190.

Rowland, L. P. (ed.) 1984. Merritt's Textbook of Neurology, 7th ed. Philadelphia: Lea & Febiger.

Spencer, W. A. 1977. The physiology of supraspinal neurons in mammals. In E. R. Kandel (ed.), Handbook of Physiology, Section 1: The Nervous System, Vol. I. Cellular Biology of Neurons. Part 2. Bethesda, Md.: American Physiological Society, pp. 969–1021.

Spencer, W. A., and Kandel, E. R. 1961. Electrophysiology of hippocampal neurons. IV. Fast prepotentials. J. Neurophysiol. 24:272–285.

Spencer, W. A., and Kandel, E. R. 1968. Cellular and integrative properties of the hippocampal pyramidal cell and the comparative electrophysiology of cortical neurons. Int. J. Neurol. 6:266–296.

Szentágothai, J. 1969. Architecture of the cerebral cortex. In H. H. Jasper, A. A. Ward, Jr., and A. Pope (eds.), Basic Mechanisms of the Epilepsies. Boston: Little, Brown, pp. 13–28.

Ts'o, D. Y., Frostig, R. D., Lieke, E. E., and Grinvald, A. 1990. Functional organization of primate visual cortex revealed by high resolution optical imaging. Science 249:417–420.

Wong, R. K. S., Miles, R., and Traub, R. D. 1984. Local circuit interactions in synchronization of cortical neurones. J. Exp. Biol. 112:169–178.

Wong, R. K. S., Prince, D. A., and Basbaum, A. I. 1979. Intradendritic recordings from hippocampal neurons. Proc. Natl. Acad. Sci. U.S.A. 76:986–990.

51

Dennis D. Kelly

Sleep and Dreaming

Sleep Is an Active and Rhythmic Neural Process

Normal Sleep Is Composed of a Recurring Succession of Identifiable Stages

Slow-Wave Sleep Stages Are Distinguished Principally by Electroencephalographic Criteria

An Active Sleep Stage Can Be Distinguished by Rapid Eye Movements (REM Sleep)

Sleep Architecture Refers to the Pattern of Sleep Stages Throughout the Night

There Are Several Clues to the Biological Importance of REM Sleep

Selective Deprivation of REM Sleep Results in a REM Rebound

The Need for REM Sleep Steadily Declines During Early Development

The Need for REM Sleep Differs Markedly Across Species

REM Sleep Can Occur Without Atonia Following Damage to the Pons

The Mental Content of Dreams Is Linked to the Physiology of Sleep

Several Neural Mechanisms May Be Responsible for the Sleep–Wake Cycle

Sleep Factors Interact with the Immune System

Early Concepts of the Reticular Activating System Cast Sleep as a Passive Process

Active Sleep-Inducing Neurons Reside in the Brain Stem

The Suprachiasmatic Nucleus Serves as the Biological Clock for the Sleep–Wake Cycle

Distinct Regions of the Brain Stem May Trigger REM Sleep

An Overall View

Ideas about sleep and dreaming have always been central to man's concepts of mind and consciousness. Thinking about sleep has followed two lines. One characterizes sleep as an analog of death during which mental function ceases—Hesiod called sleep "the brother of death." The other view holds that sleep, like wakefulness, is a special form of mental activity. Like Shakespeare's Hamlet, many have viewed sleep less as a suspension of life than as a chance to dream, a chance to engage in a special form of mental activity. In 1900 Sigmund Freud significantly expanded the latter view. In *The Interpretation of Dreams* Freud proposed that dreaming might represent a unique avenue by which unconscious motivation could be explored. When waking consciousness is periodically interrupted by sleep, he argued, mental activity is not simply laid to rest; rather, the mental experience of waking is replaced with the even more intense mental experience of dreaming.

Given the special importance of sleep as an expression of brain activity, how are we to define it? In a book published in 1913 that was to influence sleep research for several decades, Henri Pieron defined three features of sleep: (1) it is periodically necessary, (2) it has a rhythm relatively independent of external conditions, and (3) it is characterized by complete interruptions of the sensory and motor functions that link the brain with the environment. We now know that the third part of Pieron's definition is not correct. Isolation from the environment is far from complete even in the deepest stages of sleep. Sensory impulses from the periphery penetrate cortical areas even during sleep, and, conversely, cortical motor commands reach alpha motor neurons in the spinal cord during specific sleep stages, although the output of the motor neurons is actively inhibited. Nevertheless, Pieron's definition remains interesting today, for it focuses our attention on two unsolved questions: How and why does the brain regularly undergo such a profound change in its activity?

In this chapter we shall weigh the current theories and evidence as to how and why we sleep. The various stages of sleep will be described physiologically, including one strongly coupled with dreaming. The need for sleep will then be explored in different species and at different times within the lifespan. We shall conclude with an examination of the neural mechanisms responsible for behavioral sleep and dreams.

Sleep Is an Active and Rhythmic Neural Process

There is a strict periodicity to sleep throughout the life cycle: from the polyphasic sleep–wake cycle of the newborn, to the biphasic pattern of the child who naps in the afternoon, and to the monophasic, circadian cycle of the adult. The sleep–wake cycle is one of the endogenous rhythms of the body that become entrained to the day–night cycle. If a person is completely isolated from the diurnal changes of light and temperature, from social cues, and especially from the knowledge of time, his sleep–wake rhythm will gradually drift from a strict 24-hour cycle to one of approximately 25 hours. This represents the length of the endogenous sleep–wake rhythm for three-quarters of the adult population. In the rest, the period between successive awakenings under isolated, free-running conditions is even longer.

An example of a person whose free-running sleep–wake cycle lengthened to an average of 33 hours is shown in Figure 51–1. These data illustrate that there is no single biological clock that regulates all of the body's circadian rhythms. Under free-running conditions, the various rhythmic functions, such as maintenance of temperature, formation of urine, and secretion of cortisol, may become desynchronized with each other and with the sleep–wake cycle. Body temperature, for example, normally varies in a circadian pattern from a high in the late afternoon to a low

in the early morning hours during sleep. Under normal conditions the sleep–wake and body temperature rhythms are linked. Under free-running conditions, however, most vegetative functions cannot follow cycles longer than 25 hours (Figure 51–1). Therefore, when the sleep–wake cycle lengthens beyond this value, the rhythms become desynchronized and run free with different periodicities.

Until the late 1950s sleep research was dominated by a passive theory of sleep, which held that the brain lapses into sleep when there is insufficient sensory stimulation to keep it awake. Because sleep was viewed as a lapse in the waking state, the central problem for neurophysiology was reduced to specifying those neural systems that maintained wakefulness—the primary, active state. We shall encounter this view in the next chapter in relation to the study of coma.

Compared with the simple notion of sleep as an idling state somewhere near the low end of a continuum of vigilance, the concept of sleep that emerged during the 1950s and 1960s was revolutionary. Sleep was recognized as an active process characterized by a cyclic succession of different psychophysiological phenomena. The stages of sleep are programmed in a relatively predictable sequence each night, and they appear to be controlled by different, but linked, neurochemical systems.

Normal Sleep Is Composed of a Recurring Succession of Identifiable Stages

Slow-Wave Sleep Stages Are Distinguished Principally by Electroencephalographic Criteria

The primary method for monitoring the stages of human sleep is the electroencephalogram (EEG), described in Chapter 50. Stages 1–4 of slow-wave sleep are characterized by progressively slower frequencies and higher volt-

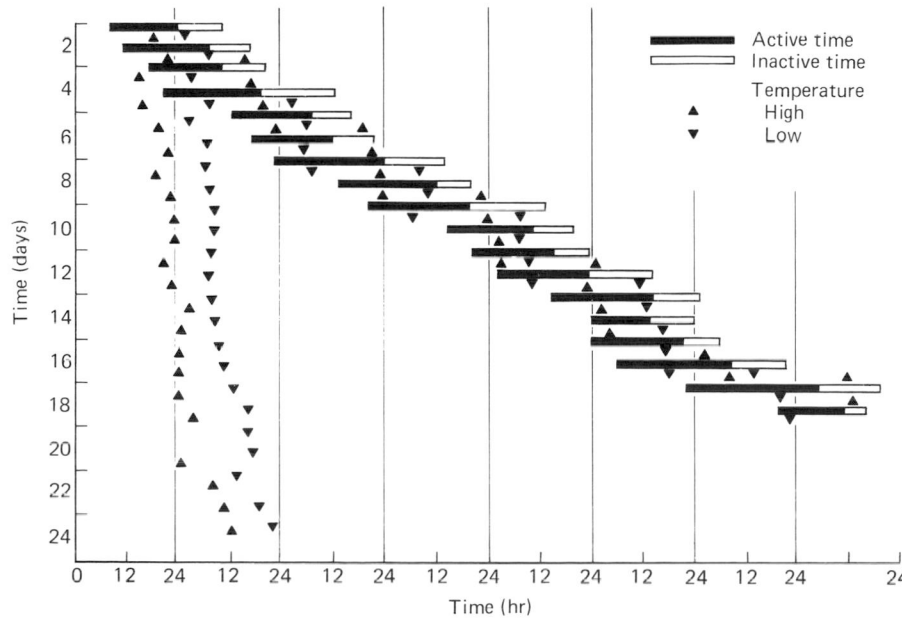

Active time
Inactive time
Temperature
▲ High
▼ Low

FIGURE 51–1

Body rhythms that are synchronized under normal conditions can become desynchronized under isolated, free-running conditions. In this subject the free-running sleep-wake cycle lengthened to an average of 33 hours, as evidenced by the drift to the right in the bars showing cycles of activity (**black**) and rest (**white**). The drift in the activity-rest plot is caused by the subject awakening (the beginning of the line) several hours later each day. Thus, the subject experienced only 18 sleep-wake cycles in 24 days. Rectal temperature (**triangles** plotted separately to the **left**) maintained a 24.8-hour rhythm. Thus, when superimposed on the activity-rest plot, temperature shows more than one maximum or minimum per 33-hour cycle. (Adapted from Aschoff, 1969.)

Time (days)

Time (hr)

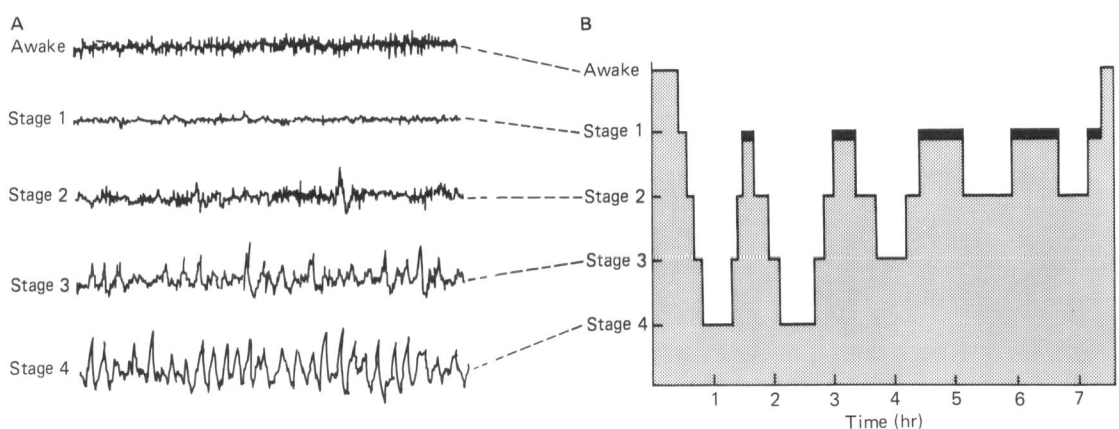

FIGURE 51–2

Stages of sleep form a cyclical pattern.

A. EEG recordings during different stages of wakefulness and sleep. Each record spans 30 s. The **top recording** of low-voltage, fast activity is that of an awake brain; the **next four** represent successively deeper stages of slow-wave sleep. Note that the stage 2 recording contains several characteristic bursts of waxing and waning waves (sleep spindles) lasting 1–2 s. Stage 1 rapid eye movement (REM) sleep can be distinguished from stage 1 non-REM sleep only by additional electrooculographic and electromyographic criteria.

B. A typical night's pattern of sleep in a young adult. The time spent in REM sleep is represented by a **black bar.** The first REM period is usually short (5–10 min), but tends to lengthen in successive cycles. Conversely, stages 3 and 4, which together are often referred to as "delta sleep," dominate the slow-wave sleep periods in the first third of the night, but are often completely absent during the later, early morning cycles. The amount of stage 2 slow-wave sleep increases progressively until it completely occupies the slow-wave periods toward the end of the night. Note that in this example, because the morning awakening interrupted the last REM period, the likelihood of a dream recall is good. If, instead, the REM period had been completed and the sleeper had been awakened by an alarm clock from the next stage 2 slow-wave sleep, the chance of a dream being recalled would be greatly reduced.

age activities and correspond to successively deeper states of sleep (Figure 51–2A). As a person initially falls asleep, the EEG progresses through all four stages of slow-wave sleep over a period of 30–45 minutes, and then retraces the same stages in reverse order during a similar time span (Figure 51–2B). During slow-wave sleep the muscles are relaxed, but somatic activity is not absent. The normal sleeper makes a major postural adjustment on the average of once every 20 minutes, and some sleepers do so every 5 minutes. During slow-wave sleep, parasympathetic activity predominates. Heart rate and blood pressure decline; gastrointestinal motility increases. The threshold for arousal in slow-wave sleep varies inversely with EEG frequency; therefore the delta-wave sleep of stage 4 is the most difficult to interrupt.

An Active Sleep Stage Can Be Distinguished by Rapid Eye Movements (REM Sleep)

About 90 minutes after the onset of sleep, several abrupt physiological changes occur. The EEG becomes desynchronized, showing a low-voltage, fast activity pattern similar, but not identical, to that of the waking state. As a result, this sleep state has been variously called paradoxical sleep, active sleep, and desynchronized sleep. Recordings from deep electrodes in animals reveal that, although cortical activity is desynchronized, the hippocampal EEG is highly synchronized at 4–10 Hz (theta wave). Neuronal generators for the theta rhythm are located in the pyrami-

dal cell layers of the CA1 field, of the dentate gyrus, and of the entorhinal cortex. A hippocampal theta rhythm is also observed in the waking state, particularly when the neocortical EEG is maximally desynchronized.

This elaborate, active brain pattern is coupled with profound loss of muscle tone throughout the body. Only those skeletal muscles controlling the movements of the eyes, the middle ear ossicles, and respiration escape the generalized paralysis. The sleeper suddenly loses the ability to regulate body temperature, which begins to change in the direction of the ambient temperature. This is one reflection of a broad suppression of sympathetic activity; another is severe pupillary contraction (miosis). Reduced homeostasis is both a dramatic and fundamental property of this sleep stage.

In 1957 William Dement and Nathaniel Kleitman described the association of rapid eye movements (REM) during sleep with the desynchronized EEG. This active sleep stage has consequently been called *REM sleep*, the term we shall use. Actually, most of the eye movements during REM sleep are slow and rolling; discrete bursts of rapid eye movements are superimposed upon this background of slow eye movements. These rapid eye movements, as well as phasically active middle ear muscles, appear to be driven by phasic bursts of electrical activity that can be recorded in animals from a variety of structures in the brain stem (the dorsolateral pons, motor nuclei of the oculomotor, trigeminal, and facial nerves), in the thalamus (lateral geniculate nuclei), and in the visual and auditory cortex. These monophasic sharp waves propagate rostrally from the pons and are referred to as pontine–geniculate–occipital (PGO) spikes. The conclusion that they represent a primary triggering process for phasic ocular movements is supported by the finding that in cats the first derivative of the electrooculogram during episodes of REM is perfectly correlated with PGO spike activity. In fact, pontine-generated phasic activity is thought to be a pacemaker that drives many of the phasic events of REM sleep, including middle-ear muscle activity, muscle twitches, changes in respiration, and surges in heart rate and coronary blood flow, in addition to eye movements.

During REM sleep the threshold for arousal by environmental stimuli is increased; so, by the criterion of external arousability, REM is the deepest stage of sleep. At the same time, a sleeping rat, cat, or human is also more likely to awake spontaneously from REM sleep than from any other stage. By the criterion of internal arousability, REM is the lightest stage of sleep. In contrast, these two measures of arousability covary closely across the stages of slow-wave sleep. Clearly, depth of sleep is not a unitary parameter.

Finally, most sleepers awakened from REM sleep readily recall dreaming (74–95%), whereas less than half of those awakened from slow-wave sleep (0–51%) report any mental activity. The range in these values depends principally on the definition of dreaming adopted by different investigators as reflected in their method of questioning, such as whether recall of a storyline is required to score as a dream or merely recall of a thought.

Sleep Architecture Refers to the Pattern of Sleep Stages Throughout the Night

During a typical night's sleep, the normal adult alternates between periods of REM and slow-wave sleep, with REM stages recurring at regular intervals four to six times each night (Figure 51–2B). After the first REM period, the intervals between successive REM periods *decrease* throughout the night, while the length of each REM episode tends to *increase*. In all, REM sleep occupies approximately 20–25% of the sleep time of young adults. Stage 2 slow-wave sleep occupies about one-half of total sleep time, and stage 3 and stage 4 slow-wave sleep about 15%.

The deeper stages of slow-wave sleep (stages 3 and 4) occur primarily in the first half of the sleep period. The lighter stages of slow-wave sleep and longer REM periods occur preferentially in the second half, and thus the early morning hours are normally associated with more frequent awakenings.

Stage 4 slow-wave sleep and REM sleep have distinctive characteristics. As we shall see in the next section, they have markedly different developmental patterns over the life span of the individual. Stage 4 slow-wave sleep is highly influenced by the amount of prior wakefulness, whereas REM sleep is much less so. REM and stage 4 slow-wave sleep are also differentially affected by certain drugs. Many psychoactive agents, particularly alcohol and the barbiturates, suppress REM sleep, whereas stage 4

slow-wave sleep is less responsive to these drugs but does respond selectively to others. For instance, stage 4 slow-wave sleep is reduced by the benzodiazepines to a much greater extent than REM sleep. We shall return to this important point in the next chapter when we consider the treatment of insomnia.

There Are Several Clues to the Biological Importance of REM Sleep

Selective Deprivation of REM Sleep Results in a REM Rebound

By arousing subjects as they pass into REM sleep, REM sleep time can be drastically reduced without curtailing slow-wave sleep. The initial interest in selective REM deprivation was the possible consequence for subsequent waking behavior. However, even total REM deprivation does not lead to psychosis, bizarre behavior, anxiety, or irritability, as once was feared. Subjects deprived of REM sleep for as long as 16 days show no signs of serious psychological disturbance.

The most important effect of REM deprivation is a dramatic shift in subsequent sleep patterns when the subject is allowed to sleep without interruption. Curtailment of REM sleep for several nights is followed by earlier initiation, marked lengthening, and increased frequency of REM periods. The longer the deprivation the larger and longer the REM rebound. The existence of an active compensatory mechanism for the recovery of lost or suppressed REM sleep suggests that REM sleep is physiologically necessary. It also affirms the common belief that dreaming serves some important need. In 1900 Freud proposed that dreams may permit the sleeper to discharge during sleep psychologically upsetting stimuli that might arise from the environment, from concerns of the previous day, and from unsatisfied repressed impulses that might otherwise disturb sleep: "The dream-process allows the result of such a combination to discharge itself through the channel of a harmless hallucinatory experience, and thus insures the continuity of sleep." On the assumption, widely held, that the content of dreams represents thoughts that are deeply repressed and hence unavailable to consciousness, many psychoanalysts make use of the interpretation of dreams in therapy. The purpose of dreaming remains largely unexplained. Thus, chronic medication with monoamine oxidase inhibitors can virtually extinguish REM sleep and dreaming for years without apparent deleterious psychological consequences.

The Need for REM Sleep Steadily Declines During Early Development

Thus far we have considered only the sleep pattern of the mature human brain. There are also dramatic ontogenetic and phylogenetic determinants of sleep. In humans the daily sleep requirement declines steadily throughout childhood and adolescence, levels off during the middle

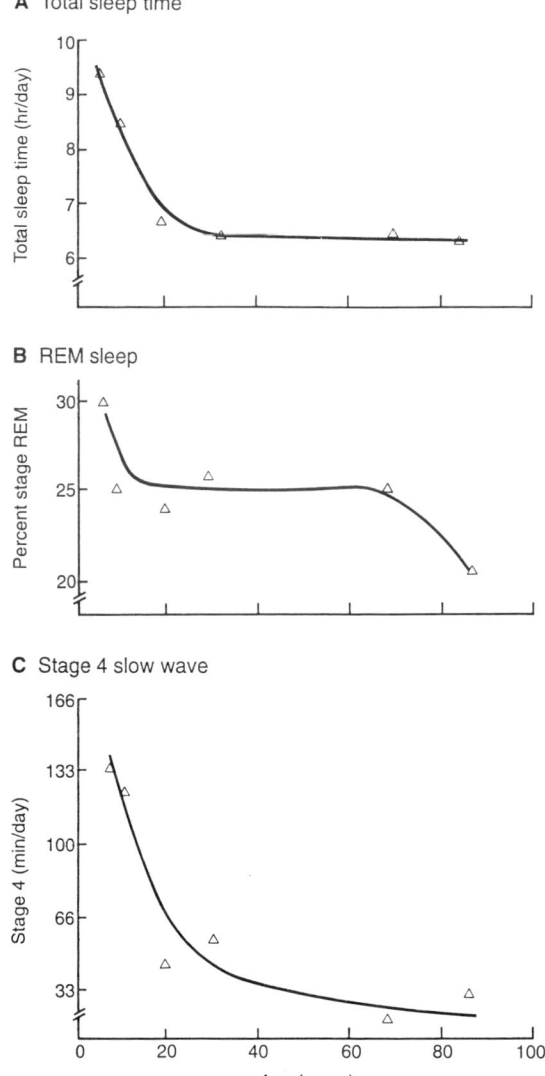

FIGURE 51–3

The human sleep pattern changes with age. Each plot shows data points for the ages of 6, 10, 21, 30, 69, and 84 years. (Adapted from Feinberg, 1969.)

years, and then often declines further with old age (Figure 51–3). The inevitability and significance of disturbed sleep in the elderly is not yet clear. Whereas those with dementia show dramatic sleep changes, healthy individuals show much less of a decline in sleep time as they age.

The most striking maturational changes in the pattern of human sleep involve the amount of stage REM and stage 4 slow-wave sleep (Figure 51–3B and C). The need for REM sleep begins *in utero*. REM sleep fills approximately 80% of the total sleep time of infants born 10 weeks prematurely, and 60–65% of the sleep time of those born 2–4 weeks prematurely. In full-term neonates REM sleep fills one-half of the normal 16-hour total daily sleep time. REM sleep declines sharply to 30–35% of sleep time by age 2

and stabilizes at about 25% by 10 years of age, after which it shows little change until the seventh or eighth decade. Thus, the absolute amount of REM sleep per day declines sharply from about 8 hours at birth to 1.5–1.75 hours by the onset of puberty. Stage 4 slow-wave sleep, on the other hand, declines exponentially throughout the developing and middle years, and often disappears after 60 years of age. This decline in stage 4 slow-wave sleep in the elderly is correlated with an increase in the number of normal spontaneous awakenings and ultimately with a return to a biphasic circadian pattern of sleep (that is, a nap in the afternoon).

What is the developmental importance of these striking and systematic changes in REM sleep? Because the ontogenetic pattern of REM sleep roughly parallels cerebral myelinization, in 1966 Howard Roffwarg suggested that REM sleep plays a role in the developing nervous system analogous to that of physical exercise in the development of muscles. This early theory took into account that REM sleep causes intense activation of neuronal circuits; indeed, the brain consumes more oxygen during REM sleep than during either intense physical or mental exercise in the waking state. Thus, REM sleep was postulated to be a potent source of internal stimulation necessary for proper maturation of the brain. However, this theory does not explain why dreaming continues after the brain has fully developed.

The Need for REM Sleep Differs Markedly Across Species

Throughout phylogeny, the pattern of sleep, like that of dietary habits, is partly determined by ecological adaptation. A lion sleeps by day and hunts at night, while the giraffe takes short daytime naps and then spends the night relaxed, but awake and vigilant. Dement suggested that the human pattern of a single extended period of sleep through the night may have evolved as a protective measure—in primitive conditions it would be safer to sleep at night huddled in a cave than to hunt or graze when nocturnal carnivores are searching for prey.

In the early 1970s Michel Jouvet developed a novel theory to account for the phylogeny of REM sleep. EEG recordings show that sleep stages in nonhuman primates are similar to those of humans. However, the sleep of rodents, smaller mammals, and birds is characterized by only two distinct stages: a slow-wave sleep similar to human stage 4, and activated sleep equivalent to REM sleep in humans. On the other hand, sleep associated with EEG desynchronization has not been clearly established in reptiles or amphibians, although EEG criteria may be useless for establishing the homology of sleep patterns in species that possess no neocortex. Because REM sleep is recognizable in mammals and birds but not in snakes or other reptiles, Jouvet suggested that REM may be a later phylogenetic process related to warm-blooded animals. REM sleep occupies between 15–20% of the existence of most placental mammals. Because advanced animals spend more time in REM sleep than in many other activities essential for survival, we must ask: What is the selective advantage conveyed by the REM state? Unfortunately, most research is directed at understanding *how* we sleep, not *why* we sleep.

REM Sleep Can Occur Without Atonia Following Damage to the Pons

In 1965 Jouvet discovered that the paralysis that occurs during REM sleep could be selectively eliminated by lesions in the pons, specifically in the locus ceruleus. Interruption of the strong motor inhibition of the REM state revealed the unparalyzed behavior of cats during REM sleep. The behaviors most often observed were such species-typical patterns as predatory attack, rage, flight, grooming, and exploration. The movements exhibited during this striking REM state were strongly linked to bursts of PGO spikes during REM sleep. Jouvet assumed that, by analogy with the human REM state, these cats appeared to be acting out dreams.

These observations led Jouvet to suggest that the REM dreams of lower mammals may be a vehicle for programming species-typical behaviors, a means of practicing vital behavioral patterns before the eliciting situation is actually encountered in waking life. This is why, Jouvet argued, instinctive acts are executed flawlessly the very first time they are required in nature—they have been rehearsed during REM sleep. By extension, the REM sleep of all animals may be genetically programmed. That is, the neuronal circuits controlling instinctive behavioral sequences may be organized during REM sleep according to a genetic blueprint and in this way added to the repertoire of the maturing brain. The reason why cold-blooded animals may not require REM sleep, Jouvet hypothesized, is that this developmental process may be completed *in ovo* before birth. Hence, in precocial species (aptly derived from the Latin word for *precooked*), there may be no need for the REM state after parturition. Only one mammal has been found to lack REM sleep—an egg-laying monotreme, the spiny anteater.

Despite the attractiveness of this comprehensive phylogenetic theory, we must acknowledge that there are many opportunities other than REM sleep for practicing instinctive behaviors. In particular, instinctive motor patterns emerge in the play behavior of young animals during the waking state. We also know, through Adrian Morrison's studies of REM sleep without atonia, that the range of motor behaviors unveiled during REM sleep depends upon the site and size of the experimental lesion in the brain stem. Progressively larger lesions of the pontine reticular formation result in progressively more elaborate behavioral displays during REM sleep. In fact, the predictability of this relationship suggests to Morrison that these cats are not acting out their dreams. As an example, aggressive behavior was observed during REM only when lesions extended rostroventrally into the midbrain. On the other hand, the same animals were also chronically aggressive in their waking state, which might suggest that aggressiveness was elevated nonspecifically, be it during waking or REM sleep.

In summary, the paralysis that normally accompanies the REM state may be neither a necessary nor an essential aspect of this sleep stage. Still it clearly serves a useful protective function for the sleeper, an important fact to which we shall return in the next chapter when we discuss an equally dramatic human sleep syndrome, REM sleep behavior disorder.

The Mental Content of Dreams Is Linked to the Physiology of Sleep

The discovery of a strong correlation between REM sleep and visual dreaming in humans has reversed many commonly held notions about dreams. Whereas it was previously believed that dreaming is rare, modern physiological studies have shown that everyone dreams in regular cycles several times every night. The reason that dreams were thought to be infrequent is that they are not well remembered. The probability of recall in a dream falls to zero during slow-wave levels within 8 minutes after REM sleep. As a result, we usually remember only morning dreams, which also turn out to be those with the oldest and most emotional psychological content.

During a single night's sleep, the physiological intensity of successive REM periods intensifies, as measured by the frequency of phasic events (PGO spikes, rapid eye movements, middle ear muscle contractions, cardiorespiratory irregularities, or muscular twitching). There is also a parallel increase through successive REM periods in the intensity of emotional tone and the activity of visual imagery in the content of the recalled dream. In this limited sense, eye movements appear to be related to dream imagery: Eventful dreams are associated with more frequent REM than inactive dreams. It is a matter of dispute whether a more detailed, or even causal, correspondence exists—whether, for example, the eyes are scanning or looking at the dream. Some investigators find occasional correlations between specific eye movements and shifts of gaze in dream imagery; others find that eye movements are driven in the same frequency pattern as other phasic phenomena. Rather than being guided by subjective dream content, eye movements are most likely phasically activated by the same neuronal spiking mechanism that generates dream imagery. Hence the two tend to be synchronized.

Finally, penile erection is a common physiological correlate of REM sleep. Erections slightly precede, then accompany, virtually every REM epoch in males. They usually bear little relationship to dream content, and they rarely correlate with overtly sensual dreaming, although there may be modulation of tumescence and even ejaculation at appropriate moments in a dream story. The ability to attain a normal erection during REM sleep is used by sex therapists to distinguish between physical and psychogenic causes of impotence.

From ancient times dreams have been regarded as important and often believed to provide insight into the future. Because of their presumed predictive value, dreams were extensively catalogued in antiquity. The most famous dream book was written by Artemidorus of Daldis in the second century. The dreams recorded are remarkably similar to contemporary ones.

Many normal dreams are unpleasant. Calvin Hall catalogued over 10,000 dreams from normal people and found that approximately 64% were associated with sadness, apprehension, or anger. Only 18% were happy or exciting. Hostile acts by or against the dreamer, such as murder, attack, or denunciation, outnumbered friendly acts by more than two to one. Only 1% of dreams involve sexual feelings or acts, and very few of these involve sexual intercourse. Dreams are primarily visual, although perhaps no more so than the perceptions experienced in the waking state. The congenitally blind have auditory dreams, and those who lose their sight gradually lose their ability to dream visually.

Despite many popular anecdotes to the contrary, the passage of time in dreams is not compressed. On the assumption that it would take more words to describe a long dream than a short one, Dement counted the number of words in dream reports and compared these to the length of the REM episodes. The length of dream narratives showed a highly positive correlation with the duration of REM sleep. In another experiment in the same series, Dement awakened subjects either 5 or 15 minutes after the onset of REM sleep and asked them to specify whether they had dreamt a short or long time based upon the apparent duration of whatever dream material they could recall. A correct choice was made in 83% of instances.

Although vivid dreaming occurs primarily in REM sleep, mental activity also occurs during slow-wave sleep. In general, mentation during slow-wave sleep is more poorly recalled, less vivid and visual, more conceptual and plausible, under greater volitional control, less emotional,

and more pleasant (Table 51–1). An important exception is that most episodes of sleep terror nightmares occur during stages 3 and 4 of slow-wave sleep, a point to which we shall return in Chapter 52. The essential symptoms of these latter slow-wave sleep nightmares are respiratory oppression, paralysis, and anxiety. However, as is typical of mental activity during slow-wave sleep, such episodes are not accompanied by full dream narratives; rather, a single oppressive situation is recalled, such as being locked up in a tomb.

Several Neural Mechanisms May Be Responsible for the Sleep–Wake Cycle

Sleep Factors Interact with the Immune System

In 1913 Henri Pieron suggested that physical or mental activity during the day may produce some chemical that induces sleep and that during sleep the chemical is destroyed. Pieron siphoned cerebrospinal fluid from dogs kept awake for several days and injected it into the ventricular system of recipient dogs, who as a result slept for 2–6 hours.

In the past 15 years, improved biochemical techniques have led to the discovery and characterization of many potential sleep-promoting factors. The list includes: muramyl peptides, lipopolysaccharides, prostaglandins, interleukin-1, interferon-α_2, tumor necrosis factor, delta sleep-inducing peptide, vasoactive intestinal peptide, and serotonin. Besides enhancing sleep, all also exert effects upon body temperature and upon the immune response. Because so many substances that lead to immune responses can also induce sleep and are found in the brain, one theory is that an important ancillary function of the

TABLE 51–1. Characteristics of Mental Activity During REM and Slow-Wave Sleep Reported by Subjects

	Sleep stage		
	Slow-wave 3 and 4	Ascending 2	REM
Features present (percent positive responses)			
Dreaming content	51%	51%	82%
Thinking content	19%	23%	5%
Emotion felt by self	28%	29%	50%
Visual	73%	62%	90%
Physical movement of self	33%	38%	67%
Only one other character	62%	50%	34%
Shift in scene	28%	38%	63%
Recall makes sense to dreamer in terms of recent experience[a]	69%	75%	48%
Median reported duration of mental experience	5 min	5 min	5 min
Mean self-rating of dream characteristic[b]			
Anxiety	0.71	1.00	1.19
Violence/hostility	0.12	0.59	0.71
Distortion	1.12	0.41	1.68

[a]Question asked on postsleep questionnaire rather than during nocturnal interview.
[b]Scale runs from 0 (low) to 5 (high).
(Adapted from Foulkes, 1966.)

sleep state may be to optimize the processes that counter infections.

As examples of potential sleep factors, we shall consider only two peptides from the list, one originally isolated from blood, the other from cerebrospinal fluid. In 1977 Guido Schoenenberger and Marcel Monnier isolated a nonapeptide from the blood of rabbits in which the thalamus had been electrically stimulated to induce sleep. Because administration of this peptide (Trp–Ala–Gly–Gly–Asp–Ala–Ser–Gly–Glu) into the cerebral ventricles enhanced EEG delta waves typical of slow-wave sleep and reduced general locomotor activity, it has been named *delta sleep-inducing peptide*. However, in most studies this peptide has proven to be a mild hypnotic and, like other peptides, its normal passage across the blood–brain barrier is difficult and slow.

Another sleep-promoting substance was concentrated by means of selective filtration from the cerebrospinal fluid of sleep-deprived goats by John Pappenheimer and Manfred Karnofsky. This factor, with a molecular weight of less than 500, acts by increasing the duration of slow-wave sleep (but not REM sleep) and by decreasing locomotor activity in recipient subjects. Chemical analysis showed this factor to be a peptidoglycan with a muramic acid residue. This type of compound had previously been thought to occur only in bacteria, where muramyl peptides are the monomeric building blocks of bacterial cell wall peptidoglycans. The origin of muramyl peptides in mammalian tissue remains controversial, and may involve bacteria present in the gastrointestinal tract. The muramyl peptides have even been likened to vitamins in that they are required but cannot be synthesized by the host. The biological activity of muramyl peptides may be regulated through structural changes caused by enzymes in the mammalian brain. Every muramyl peptide with somnogenic properties has also proven to be pyrogenic and immunoactive.

The effects of murayml peptides upon sleep may involve the serotonergic system. Sleep-promoting doses increase serotonin turnover. Administration of parachlorophenylalanine (PCPA), which blocks synthesis of serotonin, inhibits sleep, a fact to which we shall return later; this effect is completely antagonized by muramyl peptide. There is also direct evidence that serotonin and muramyl peptides compete for common binding sites both on macrophages and in the brain. This competitive (agonist) relationship between a neurotransmitter and an immunomodulator is all the more interesting in light of the discovery that serotonin (5-HT$_2$) receptor affinity is markedly altered by sleep deprivation.

Early Concepts of the Reticular Activating System Cast Sleep as a Passive Process

Whether sleep is induced by a factor present in blood, brain, or cerebrospinal fluid, or none of these, it is now certain that the onset of sleep is actively induced. This has been widely accepted only in the past 30 years, largely through the efforts of Giuseppe Moruzzi. The earlier theory that sleep was a passive function of the brain took root in the mid-1930s because of the experiments of the neurophysiologist Frederic Bremer.

Bremer was interested in whether the isolated forebrain, disconnected from the caudal brain stem and thus deprived of almost all sensory input, would continue to cycle between sleep and wakefulness. When Bremer completely transected the midbrain of a cat at a level between the superior and inferior colliculi (a *cerveau isolé* preparation), the isolated forebrain displayed a continuous EEG pattern typical of sleep, although only high-voltage slow-wave activity and permanently constricted pupils were evident. However, when the transection was made lower in the brain stem between the caudal medulla and the spinal cord (an *encephale isolé* preparation), normal cycles of sleep and waking were recorded in the forebrain.

Bremer reasoned that the isolated forebrain of the cerveau isolé preparation slept incessantly because there was insufficient sensory input to arouse it. In contrast, transection between the medulla and spinal cord preserved the sensory input of the cranial nerves, particularly the fifth (trigeminal) and eighth (vestibulocochlear), and this input in turn preserved normal sleep–wake cycling. To support this interpretation, Bremer showed that if the brain stem cranial sensory nerves were cut in an encephale isolé preparation, a state of continuous forebrain sleep resulted similar to that with the cerveau isolé.

Bremer's assumption was that the stimulation that normally aroused the forebrain is carried rostrally by means of the normal sensory pathways. However, in 1949 Moruzzi and Horace Magoun significantly qualified Bremer's theory by making partial lesions rather than complete brain stem transections at the midbrain level of the cat. They found that lateral tegmental lesions, which severed the direct ascending sensory pathways, did not significantly alter the balance between sleep and wakefulness. However, midline lesions that cut the rostral projections of the reticular formation resulted in a behavioral stupor and a continuous EEG delta pattern that resembled sleep. Moruzzi and Magoun concluded that the ascending projections of a tonically active reticular formation (fed by collaterals from the specific sensory systems) activate the cortex and keep the forebrain awake, and that a reduction in this activity results in sleep. This passive view of sleep as a functional deafferentation regulated by an ascending reticular activating system dominated sleep research for many years.

Active Sleep-Inducing Neurons Reside in the Brain Stem

In the late 1950s Moruzzi and his colleagues began to question the unitary view of the nonspecific reticular activating system. They found that when brain stem transections were performed at the midpontine level, only a few millimeters caudal to the midbrain cuts of Bremer, cats could not sleep. This suggested that the rostral reticular formation contains a population of neurons whose activity is required for wakefulness and, conversely, that the caudal brain stem contains neurons that are necessary for sleep. As Moruzzi demonstrated in 1959, these neurons are part of the reticular formation.

In brief, Moruzzi showed that when injections of a barbiturate anesthetic were restricted to the rostral pons and cerebrum (by selectively tying off various cerebral arteries), awake cats were put to sleep, as might be expected. However, when only the caudal brain stem was anesthetized, sleeping cats wakened, and synchronous EEG activity was replaced by desynchronous EEG activity. Thus, these experiments demonstrate that somewhere in the caudal brain stem are neurons, either clustered or dispersed, whose *activity* is needed to induce sleep. Because these experiments are relevant to understanding coma that follows lower brain stem lesions, we will consider them more fully in Chapter 52.

Early studies suggested that the sleep-inducing region in the brain stem might be either the raphe nucleus, a collection of serotonergic cells that lie together in the midline of the medulla, or the nucleus of the solitary tract. Although few hold to this conclusion today, it is instructive to review the evidence that led to this long-held belief, for the quest for the *sleep center* guides much sleep research even today.

Raphe Nuclei. Jouvet found that intracerebral injections of serotonin induced sleep and that destruction of 80–90% of raphe cells produced complete insomnia in cats for 3–4 days. Slow-wave sleep, but not REM sleep, gradually returned but never exceeded 2 hours per day (cats normally sleep 14.5 hours per day). Smaller raphe lesions resulted in greater recovery, but REM sleep never reappeared until slow-wave sleep totaled at least 3.5 hours per day. All of which seemed very convincing.

The critical difficulty with the serotonin hypothesis of sleep, however, was first revealed by experiments with PCPA, which inhibits the synthesis of serotonin. When PCPA is administered chronically, it leads initially to insomnia, as expected. But after only one week of daily injections both REM and slow-wave sleep return to within 70% of normal, despite continued and complete suppression of brain serotonin levels (Figure 51–4). In the same subjects, however, REM phasic activity is no longer confined to REM sleep periods, but emerges in all sleep stages, and even in the waking state. It is now known that in normal individuals serotonergic cells decrease their firing rate from the waking state to slow-wave sleep, and become completely silent during REM sleep. Thus, these cells inhibit phasic REM sleep events; the reason why raphe lesions initially prevent sleep is because waking stimuli cannot be shut off.

Nucleus of the Solitary Tract. A secondary medullary system, located in the vicinity of the nucleus of the solitary tract, may also be involved in inducing sleep. Since activation of this area promotes sleep but damaging it does not result in insomnia, it may produce its effects upon sleep by modulating the arousal properties of the reticular

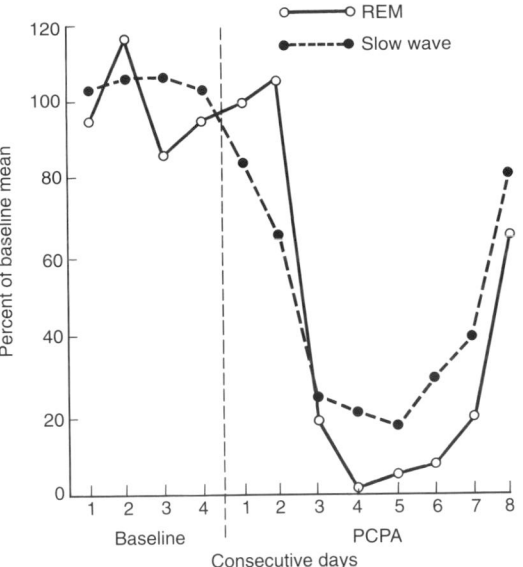

FIGURE 51–4

Serotonin may not be the crucial factor for the normal production of either REM or slow-wave sleep. Although parachlorophenylalanine (PCPA) inhibits the synthesis of serotonin, it produces only a short-term effect on REM and slow-wave sleep. In this experiment PCPA was administered to a cat for 8 consecutive days, and its effects on REM and slow-wave sleep were compared with the cat's normal sleep as measured for 4 days before treatment (baseline). Shortly after treatment began both types of sleep diminished sharply, but by the eighth day both approach their normal level. In contrast, serotonin levels remained at approximately zero during the entire course of treatment. (Adapted from Dement, 1965.)

formation (see Chapter 44). Electrical stimulation of the nucleus of the solitary tract has a synchronizing effect upon forebrain EEG activity that long outlasts the stimulation. This portion of the medulla is involved in autonomic regulation and receives taste and visceral afferent input principally from the vagus (tenth) nerve (Chapter 49). Stimulation of afferent fibers in the vagus nerve also produces EEG synchrony, as does mild low-frequency (3–8 Hz) stimulation of certain cutaneous nerves. Perhaps this frequency-sensitive mechanism calms the gently rocked baby.

The Suprachiasmatic Nucleus Serves as the Biological Clock for the Sleep–Wake Cycle

At least two areas in the hypothalamus and adjacent basal forebrain are also essential for the induction of normal sleep—the preoptic area and the suprachiasmatic nucleus. Direct application of serotonin to the *preoptic area* can induce slow-wave sleep, as can certain patterns of electrical stimulation. Both effects can be attenuated by prior treatment with PCPA. Destruction of the preoptic area results in abrupt insomnia in rats.

As we saw earlier in reference to Figure 51–1, the sleep–wake cycle is one of the endogenous rhythms of the

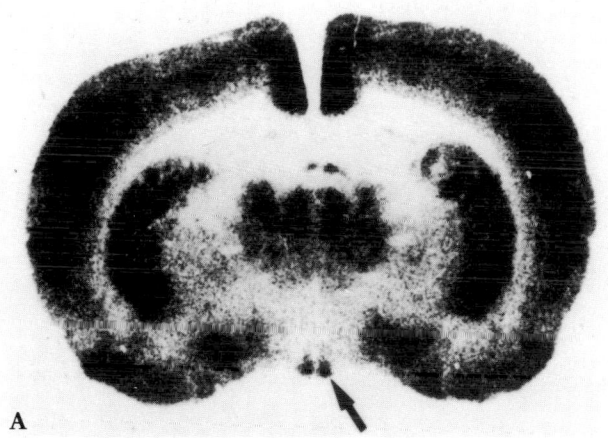 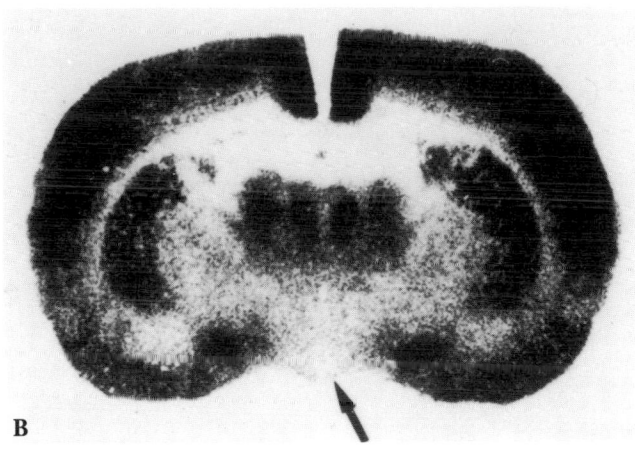

FIGURE 51–5

The metabolic activity of the suprachiasmatic nucleus becomes entrained to the circadian light–dark cycles. These two autoradiographs of transverse sections through the rat brain were made after injections of radioactive 2-deoxyglucose. (From Schwartz and Gainer, 1977.)

A. Metabolic activity in the suprachiasmatic nucleus increased when the injections took place during the light phase.

B. Glucose injections during the dark phase did not produce evidence of metabolic activity at this site.

body that normally become entrained to the day–night cycle. Light serves as a *Zeitgeber*, literally a time giver, a stimulus that entrains an endogenous rhythm to the circadian clock. However, when both the primary optic tracts and the accessory optic system are severed caudal to the optic chiasm, light continues to entrain the sleep–wake cycle of animals. This unexpected result prompted the hypothesis that a direct retinohypothalamic pathway conveyed information about light to the internal circadian pacemaker. There is now evidence that, at least in experimental animals, the primary biological clock is located in the *suprachiasmatic nucleus.*

This hypothalamic nucleus receives direct input from retinal fibers. (In some species there are also retinal fibers that terminate in the preoptic area.) The suprachiasmatic nucleus is also remarkable for the density of dendrodendritic synapses that link its cells together and thus bias them toward synchronous activity. In 1972 Robert Moore and Irving Zucker independently discovered that destruction of the suprachiasmatic nucleus not only prevents entrainment of rhythms by light, but also disrupts various endogenous behavioral and hormonal circadian rhythms, including the sleep–wake cycle. Therefore, the suprachiasmatic nucleus may house self-contained circadian oscillators, and the retinohypothalamic pathway may serve to couple the mammalian circadian system to the external light–dark cycle.

A remarkable demonstration of the circadian activity patterns of the suprachiasmatic nucleus can be found in Figure 51–5. William Schwartz and Harold Gainer injected rats entrained on a strict light–dark cycle with radiolabeled 2-deoxyglucose. As we have seen, this metabolically inert analog of glucose is taken up by cells and terminals in proportion to their activity, for glucose is the normal energy source for neurons. When animals were prepared and observed during the light phase, the suprachiasmatic

nucleus became heavily labeled (Figure 51–5A), a consequence of the high metabolic activity in this nucleus when the retinal hypothalamic tract is stimulated. When animals were prepared and observed in the dark phase of their normal circadian cycle, the nucleus was not labeled. However, the metabolic activity of the suprachiasmatic nucleus was not due solely to the presence of light; the nucleus displayed an entrained endogenous rhythm. When rats were sacrificed in the dark, but during hours corresponding to their habitual light phase, the entrained nucleus was metabolically active. The mechanism by which the sun's rise and fall synchronize the endogenous clock to local time also involves cells in the suprachiasmatic nucleus (Figure 51–6). In the next chapter we shall see how light stimulation at appropriate times in the circadian cycle can be used to reset the human body clock.

Distinct Regions of the Brain Stem May Trigger REM Sleep

In addition to the postulated involvement of brain stem nuclei in slow-wave sleep, there is thought to be a special subset of anatomically and biochemically distinct regions that may trigger REM sleep. Most serotonergic neurons in the dorsal raphe nucleus in the midbrain periaqueductal gray matter fire maximally during waking and drastically reduce their firing rate during REM sleep. This pattern fits with the suggestion that they may normally suppress PGO waves. In the transition from slow-wave sleep to REM, most raphe neurons specifically cease firing prior to PGO spikes, and subsequently they remain silent throughout REM episodes. Jouvet suggested that these neurons normally inhibit phasic REM events and that their silence during REM sleep indicates a termination of this inhibition.

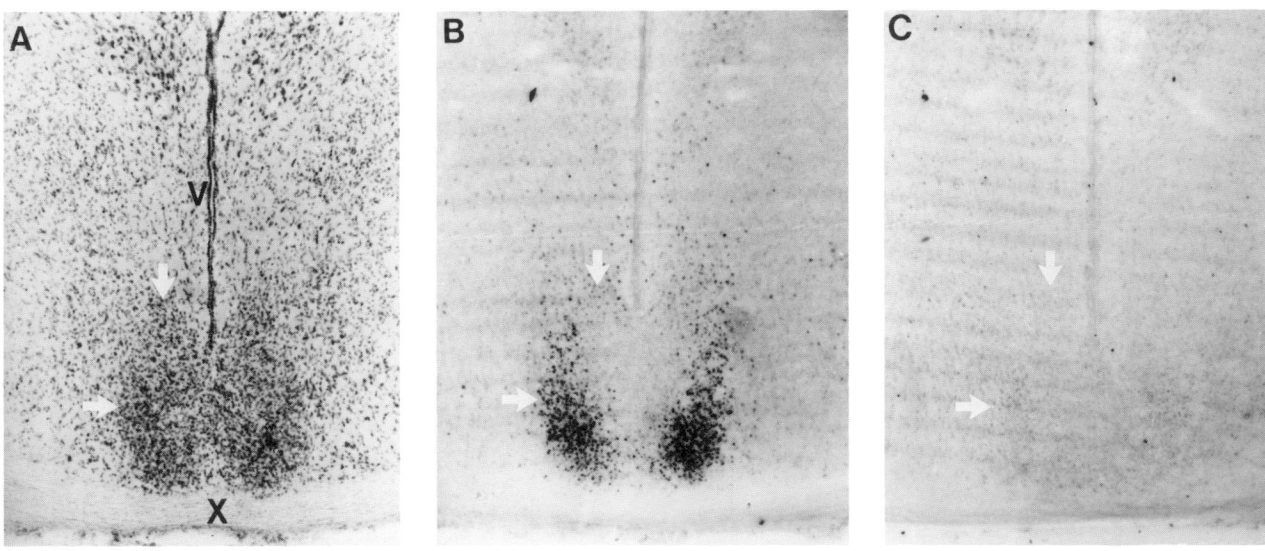

FIGURE 51–6

Light exposures synchronize circadian rhythms by altering the activity of cells in the suprachiasmatic nucleus (SCN). (Adapted from Rusak et al., 1990.)

A. The hypothalamus of a hamster stained with cresyl violet shows the location of the SCN. The **white arrows** show the approximate dorsal and lateral borders of the left suprachiasmatic nucleus. (**V**, third ventricle; **X**, optic chiasm.)

B. The same region stained for Fos immunoreactivity in a hamster exposed to light for 1 hour during the normally dark phase

of the daily light–dark cycle. There is nuclear staining of SCN cells.

C. Fos immunoreactivity is negligible in a hamster not exposed to light during the dark phase. In hamsters kept in the dark for 2 extra days and then exposed to light during the hours corresponding to their normal light cycle, Fos staining is also absent. Thus the increase in c-*fos* gene expression after light exposure is specific to the time of day during which light can phase shift rhythms.

Another population of brain stem cells that may be involved in the induction or maintenance of REM sleep either secretes or is sensitive to acetylcholine (ACh). Microinjection of cholinergic agonists into the pontine tegmentum results in prolonged REM sleep in cats. Although these trigger sites for REM sleep have no cholinergic neurons, input to these areas has been mapped by James Quattrochi, Allan Hobson, and their colleagues. Carbachol, a mixed muscarinic-nicotinic cholinergic agonist, is effective in eliciting REM sleep. By conjugating carbachol to fluorescent microspheres, the same pharmacologically active probe caused a behavioral state change from waking to REM and also labeled anatomically defined neurons projecting into the injection site. Retrograde labeling was found in a widely distributed brain stem network, including some nuclei known to contain cholinergic neurons and some not. Prominent among the latter were the aminergic cell clusters of the dorsal raphe and locus ceruleus. These findings are consistent with the view that REM sleep is the result of activation of various neuronal groups using different transmitters.

Hobson and Robert McCarley have called attention to the possible reciprocal roles of ACh in REM sleep and the monoamines in slow-wave sleep. They found two interconnected populations of neurons that either fire or are inhibited during REM sleep. One population, cholinoceptive cells in the gigantocellular tegmental field, fires rap-

idly and in a phasic manner throughout REM sleep and is correlated with PGO spikes, rapid eye movements, and muscle twitches (see Figure 44–7). The second population, monoaminergic cells in the locus ceruleus and the raphe nuclei, are slowed down in their firing during REM sleep. This led Hobson and McCarley to propose that an intrinsic pattern of alternating activity between cholinergic and noradrenergic cells might account for the cyclicity of REM and slow-wave sleep. Later, however, Jerome Siegel and Dennis McGinty found that the discharge of giant tegmental cells is also highly correlated with movements in alert, awake animals, and thus appears not to be selective for REM sleep but for motor activation per se.

An Overall View

What is the function of sleep? Why does the brain require periodic episodes of sleep to function effectively in wakefulness? Why do we dream? What are the mechanisms that underlie the alternation from wakefulness to sleep, and from slow-wave sleep to REM sleep? These are some of the central questions that guide sleep research. Most still lack convincing scientific answers. Indeed, in light of the discouraging findings regarding the aminergic and cholinergic models of sleep, it may now seem as if we actually know less about the neurobiology of sleep than was presumed only 25 years ago, when the amine hypothesis was first framed by Jouvet and before the experiments that challanged it were carried out.

But scientific progress need not be measured in terms of the durability of its models. In this chapter we have noted several true advances in the recent understanding of basic sleep mechanisms. As primary examples, we can cite the cholinergic mediation of REM sleep and the parallel finding that during REM sleep the aminergic cells of the raphe nucleus and the locus cerulcus are shut down. These remarkable discoveries, however, do not exhaust the potential mechanisms that control REM sleep. For example, glutamate can also induce a REM-like state when injected into the pons. Moreover, two or more transmitters (one often a peptide) can be colocalized in the majority of brain stem neurons. It is not yet established whether the coexpressed chemical messengers might be competitive or synergistic, short term or long, and whether such circadian or behavioral events as sleep deprivation might regulate the blend of neurosecretory products expressed in these cells.

Since Pieron and before, each generation has sought the presumed hypnogenic substance in the brain and experienced disappointment. Others have sought *the* sleep center. Perhaps the format of the single neurochemical or single regional models of sleep needs to be reexamined. As we have seen, sleep is not a unitary process, but rather a complex, repeating sequence of biological and mental phenomena. A convincing scientific explanation of sleep is likely to be no less complex.

Selected Readings

Borbély, A., and Valatx, J.-L. (eds.) 1984. Sleep Mechanisms. Exp. Brain Res. Suppl. 8. Berlin: Springer.

Gaillard, J.-M. 1983. Biochemical pharmacology of paradoxical sleep. Br. J. Clin. Pharmacol. 16:205S–230S.

Hastings, J. W., Rusak, B., and Boulos, Z. 1991. Circadian rhythms: The physiology of biological timing. In C. L. Prosser (ed.), Neural and Integrative Animal Physiology, Comparative Animal Physiology, 4th ed. New York: Wiley-Liss, pp. 435–546.

Hobson, J. A. 1988. The Dreaming Brain. New York: Basic Books.

Hobson, J. A., and Steriade, M. 1986. Neuronal basis of behavioral state control. In F. E. Bloom (ed.) Section 1: The Nervous System, Vol. IV. Intrinsic Regulatory Systems of the Brain. Bethesda, Md.: American Physiological Society, pp. 701–823.

Kryger, M. H., Roth, T., and Dement, W. C. (eds.) 1989. Principles and Practice of Sleep Medicine. Philadelphia: Saunders.

McGinty, D., and Szymusiak, R. 1990. Keeping cool: A hypothesis about the mechanisms and functions of slow-wave sleep. Trends Neurosci. 13:480–487.

Rosenwasser, A. M. 1988. Behavioral neurobiology of circadian pacemakers: A comparative perspective. Prog. Psychobiol. Physiol. Psychol. 13:155–226.

Steriade, M., and McCarley, R. W. 1990. Brainstem Control of Wakefulness and Sleep. New York: Plenum Press.

References

Allison, T., and Cicchetti, D. V. 1976. Sleep in mammals: Ecological and consitutional correlates. Science 194:732–734.

Artemidorus Daldianus. ca. 140–180 A.D. The Interpretation of Dreams (Oneirocritica). R. J. White (trans.) Park Ridge, N. J.: Noyes Press, 1975.

Aschoff, J. 1969. Desynchronization and resynchronization of human circadian rhythms. Aerosp. Med. 40:844–849.

Batini, C., Moruzzi, G., Palestini, M., Rossi. G. F., and Zanchetti, A. 1958. Persistent patterns of wakefulness in the pretrigeminal midpontine preparation. Science 128:30–32.

Bremer, F. 1936. Nouvelles recherches sur le mécanisme du sommeil. C. R. Seances Soc. Biol. Fil. (Paris) 122:460–464.

Campbell, S. S., and Tobler, I. 1984. Animal sleep: A review of sleep duration across phylogeny. Neurosci. Biobehav. Rev. 8:269–300.

Curran, T., and Franza, B. R., Jr. 1988. Fos and Jun: The AP-1 connection. Cell 55:395–397.

Dement, W., and Kleitman, N. 1957. Cyclic variations in EEG during sleep and their relations to eye movements, body motility, and dreaming. Electroencephalogr. Clin. Neurophysiol. 9:673–690.

Dement, W. C. 1965. An essay on dreams: The role of physiology in understanding their nature. In New Directions in Psychology II. New York: Holt, Rinehart and Winston, pp. 135–257.

Feinberg, I. 1969. Effects of age on human sleep patterns. In A. Kales (ed.), Sleep: Physiology & Pathology. Philadelphia: Lippincott, pp. 39–52.

Foulkes, D. 1966. The Psychology of Sleep. New York: Scribner's.

Freud, S. 1900–1901. The Interpretation of Dreams, Vols. IV and V. J. Strachey (trans.) London: Hogarth Press and The Institute of Psycho-Analysis, 1953.

Freud, S. 1933. New Introductory Lectures on Psycho-Analysis. W. J. H. Sprott (trans.) London: Hogarth Press and The Institute of Psycho-Analysis, 1949.

Hall, C. S., and Van de Castle, R. L. 1966. The Content Analysis of Dreams. New York: Appleton-Century-Crofts.

Hobson, J. A., McCarley, R. W., and Wyzinski, P. W. 1975. Sleep cycle oscillation: Reciprocal discharge by two brainstem neuronal groups. Science 189:55–58.

Jouvet, M., and Delorme, F. 1965. Locus coeruleus et sommeil paradoxal. C. R. Seances Soc. Biol. Fil. [Paris] 159:895–899.

Kirby, D. A., and Verrier, R. L. 1989. Differential effects of sleep stage on coronary hemodynamic function. Am. J. Physiol. 256: H1378–H1383.

Krueger, J. M., and Karnovsky, M. L. 1987. Sleep and the immune response. In B. D. Janković, B. M. Marković, and N. H. Spector (eds.), Neuroimmune Interactions. Proceedings of the Second International Workshop on Neuroimmunomodulation. Ann. N.Y. Acad. Sci. 496:510–516.

Lai, Y. Y., and Siegel, J. M. 1988. Medullary regions mediating atonia. J. Neurosci. 8:4790–4796.

Moore, R. Y., and Eichler, V. B. 1972. Loss of a circadian adrenal corticosterone rhythm following suprachiasmatic lesions in the rat. Brain Res. 42:201–206.

Morrison, A. R. 1988. Paradoxical sleep without atonia. Arch. Ital. Biol., 126:275–289.

Moruzzi, G., and Magoun, H. W. 1949. Brain stem reticular formation and activation of the EEG. Electroencephalogr. Clin. Neurophysiol. 1:455–473.

Pappenheimer, J. R., Koski, G., Fencl, V., Karnovsky, M. L., and Krueger, J. 1975. Extraction of sleep-promoting factor S from cerebrospinal fluid and from brains of sleep-deprived animals. J. Neurophysiol. 38:1299–1311.

Piéron, H. 1913. Le Problème Physiologique du Sommeil. Paris: Masson.

Quattrochi, J. J., Mamelak, A. N., Madison, R. D., Macklis, J. D., and Hobson, J. A. 1989. Mapping neuronal inputs to REM sleep induction sites with carbachol-fluorescent microspheres. Science 245:984–986.

Roffwarg, H. P., Muzio, J. N., and Dement, W. C. 1966. Ontogenetic development of the human sleep-dream cycle. Science 152:604–619.

Rusak, B., Robertson, H. A., Wisden, W., and Hunt, S. P. 1990. Light pulses that shift rhythms induce gene expression in the suprachiasmatic nucleus. Science 248:1237–1240.

Sastre, J.-P., and Jouvet, M. 1979. Le comportement onirique du chat. Physiol. Behav. 22:979–989.

Schoenenberger, G. A., and Monnier, M. 1977. Characterization

of a delta-electroencephalogram(-sleep)-inducing peptide. Proc. Natl. Acad. Sci. U.S.A. 74:1282–1286.

Schwartz, W. J., and Gainer, H. 1977. Suprachiasmatic nucleus: Use of ^{14}C-labeled deoxyglucose uptake as a functional marker. Science 197:1089–1091.

Siegel, J. M., and McGinty, D. J. 1977. Pontine reticular formation neurons: Relationship of discharge to motor activity. Science 196:678–680.

Stephan, F. K., and Zucker, I. 1972. Circadian rhythms in drinking behavior and locomotor activity of rats are eliminated by hypothalamic lesions. Proc. Natl. Acad. Sci. U.S.A. 69:1583–1586.

52

Dennis D. Kelly

Disorders of Sleep and Consciousness

Insomnia Is a Symptom with Many Causes, Not a Unitary Disease

   The Sleep of Insomniacs Differs Physiologically from That of Normal Sleepers

   Anticipation of Insomnia May Cause Insomnia

   Psychopathology Is Often Mirrored in Disturbed Sleep

   Temporary Insomnia Is a Natural Consequence of Altered Circadian Rhythms

   Sleep Problems Are Magnified in the Elderly

   The Barbiturates: Earlier Sleep Medications Initially Helped, Then Harmed Sleep

   The Benzodiazepines: Subjective Benefits to Insomniacs May Exceed Objective Improvements in Sleep Measures

Parasomnias Are Behavioral Dysfunctions Associated with Sleep, Sleep Stages, or Partial Arousals

   Nocturnal Enuresis Is Not Caused by Dreaming

   Sleepwalking Is Triggered by Arousal from Slow-Wave Sleep

   REM Behavior Disorder: REM Sleep Without Atonia Causes Violent Episodes in Human Sleepers

   Night Terrors, Nightmares, and Terrifying Dreams Occur in Different Stages of Sleep

Sleep Apnea: Persistent Nocturnal Arousals Can Result from Lapses in Breathing

Narcolepsy: Irresistible Sleep Attacks Are Accompanied by Several REM-Related Symptoms

Loss of Consciousness: Coma Is Not Deep Sleep

   Transient Losses of Consciousness Can Result from Decreased Cerebral Blood Flow

   Coma Has Many Causes

   The Determination of Cerebral Death Constitutes a Medical, Legal, and Social Decision

The inability to sleep, or to stay awake, is a hardship that can disrupt a life with extraordinary thoroughness. By conservative estimates, about 15% of people living in industrialized countries have serious or *chronic* sleep problems. An additional 20% complain of occasional insomnia. Among certain populations, such as institutionalized mental patients, the incidence is much higher still: In a survey of 700 patients at St. Elizabeth's Hospital in Washington, D. C., 70% had initially sought medical help because of a sleep problem.

In 1979 the Association of Sleep Disorders Centers published the first comprehensive classification of the disorders of sleep and arousal. This classification scheme included four main categories: (1) disorders of initiating and maintaining sleep, or insomnias; (2) disorders of excessive somnolence, or the hypersomnias, such as sleep apnea and narcolepsy; (3) disorders of the sleep–wake schedule, essentially rhythm disruptions; and (4) the parasomnias, behavioral dysfunctions associated with sleep, sleep stages, or partial arousals.

In this chapter we shall consider only the most important sleep disorders, and a few that illuminate the neural mechanisms of sleep outlined in Chapter 51. A consideration of sleep disorders should not only deepen our understanding of normal sleep but also demonstrate that sleep is not an isolated behavioral event. Its disturbance may be linked to other changes in mood and performance, which in turn can exert far-reaching effects upon one's life. We will conclude with an analysis of the special states of *un*consciousness encountered in comatose patients.

Insomnia Is a Symptom with Many Causes, Not a Unitary Disease

Insomnia is a complaint, like a pain in the abdomen. W. C. Fields once remarked that the only thing wrong with insomniacs is that they don't get enough sleep. As we shall see, even this need not be so. Insomnia is a symptom of many disorders, most still poorly understood.

A widely accepted definition of insomnia is the chronic inability to obtain the amount or quality of sleep necessary to maintain adequate daytime behavior. Thirty percent of all sleep clinic applicants complain of insomnia. Because this initial complaint depends upon the self-evaluation of the patient, the perception of insomnia can be independent of the actual number of hours the person sleeps.

To place an insomniac's complaint in an appropriate context, some understanding of the range of normal sleep habits is necessary. Few people adhere literally to Alfred the Great's formula of eight hours for work, eight hours for play, and eight hours for sleep. Young adults do sleep on average 7–8 hours each day, yet the normal range extends from 4–10 hours. Brief sleepers spend proportionately less time than do others in the lighter stages 1 and 2 of slow-wave sleep, and more time in REM and in the deepest stage 4 of slow-wave sleep, a potentially important fact for the diagnosis of certain insomnias.

Patients with insomnia usually underestimate actual sleep compared to polygraph recordings (*polysomnograms*) throughout the night. Some self-professed insomniacs have been found to sleep and dream normally in the laboratory, but their subjective report in the morning is of poor quality, unrefreshing sleep. In an early study William Dement examined 127 sleepers who complained of insomnia and observed a mean sleep onset time of 15 minutes and sleep duration of 7 hours. An estimated 10–12% of all self-defined insomniacs have normal physiological sleep. Theirs is known formally as the *sleep misperception syndrome* or as *pseudoinsomnia*.

Another 30% of insomniacs are kept awake by physiological events of which they are unaware. Most common are periodic stereotyped leg twitches known as *nocturnal myoclonus*. A related condition occurs in fewer patients who, while awake and relaxed before sleep, have an irresistible urge to keep the limbs in motion (restless leg syndrome), which can delay sleep onset. Due to the prevalence of these movement syndromes and of pseudoinsomnia, it should be evident that an objective finding of insomnia cannot be made solely through interview in a physician's office without the benefit of a sleep clinic evaluation. The reason is nearly half of all "insomniacs" either sleep normally or are disturbed by physical events of which they are not aware.

The Sleep of Insomniacs Differs Physiologically from That of Normal Sleepers

Polysomnographic studies of chronic insomniacs indicate relatively small irregularities in sleep patterns. Some studies find shorter sleep time, more intermittent awakenings, and lower sleep efficiency; but these aggregate deviations are usually mild compared to the severity of the patient's perception of the disturbance. Thus, continuity, particularly during slow-wave stages, may be a more important determinant of sleep quality than how much total time is spent sleeping. However, some insomniacs clearly do show decreased delta sleep, the deepest stage of slow-wave sleep. Using quantitative electroencephalogram (EEG) criteria, J. Christian Gillin has successfully distinguished these insomniacs from depressed patients, whose disturbed sleep pattern we shall consider later.

Perhaps the most dependable physiological alteration in the sleep of chronic insomniacs can be measured with a rectal thermometer. People who report poor sleep maintain higher core body temperatures throughout sleep than do good sleepers (Figure 52–1). This is not due to a phase shift in the temperature rhythm (as was observed in the free-cycling subject in Figure 51–1), nor is it attributable to more frequent awakenings. One possibility is that the insomniac suffers a form of autonomic hyperarousal that may be associated with the perception of poor sleep. Another is that the lack of temperature decline normally associated with sleep onset results in the decreased deep slow-wave sleep in insomniacs.

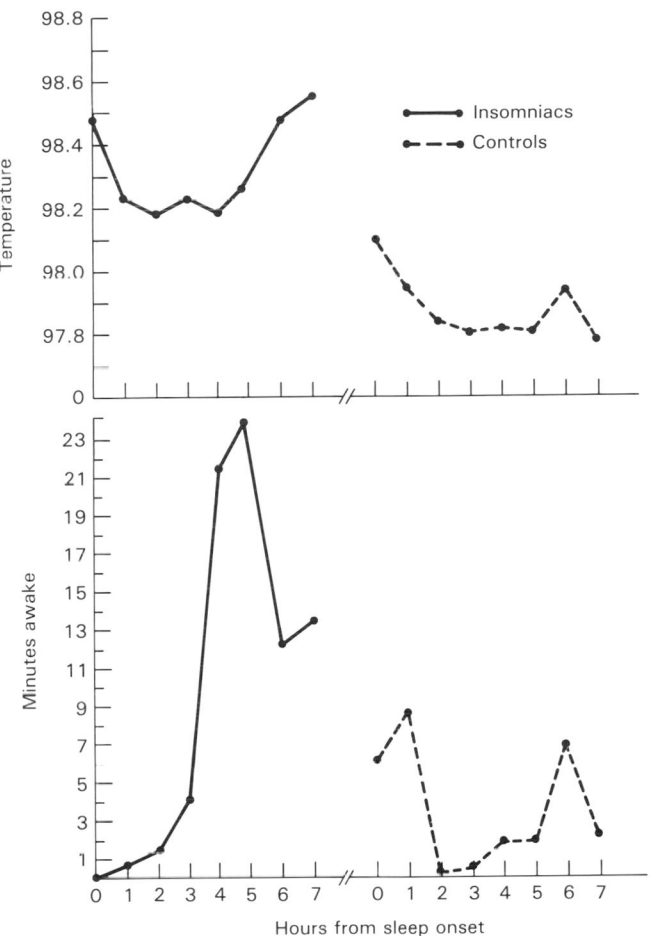

FIGURE 52–1

Insomniacs maintain higher than normal rectal temperature throughout sleep. The plots show core temperature and waking time after sleep onset in 10 insomniacs and age- and sex-matched controls. (Adapted from Mendelson et al., 1984.)

Anticipation of Insomnia May Cause Insomnia

Learning and anticipation play a major role in at least 15% of insomnia cases, which are classified as *psychophysiological insomnia*. These apprehensive patients fear *not* being able to sleep and associate their customary sleep environment and habits with not sleeping. After repeated self-fulfilling pairings of negative expectations and subsequent sleep problems, a measurable exaggeration of muscle tone develops as bedtime approaches. One consequence of this form of conditioned insomnia is that, in contrast to normal sleepers, these patients often sleep *better* in a hotel or sleep laboratory.

Psychopathology Is Often Mirrored in Disturbed Sleep

Perhaps the most common cause of insomnia is emotional disturbance, estimated to account for 35% of insomnias.

Anxiety tends to be correlated with difficulty falling asleep, depression with early awakenings. At times the underlying psychological problem can be hidden, so that the sleep disturbance is presented as the primary complaint. What is more, psychopathology and poor sleep can potentiate each other; and drugs that affect one usually affect the other, although not always in the desired manner. In one study the likely cause in 70% of patients with insomnia was an emotional problem, with depression heading the list. However, most of these depressed patients had initially been treated symptomatically with sleeping pills because their presenting complaint was lack of sleep, not depression.

There are some consistent quantitative differences in the sleep of depressed patients. They obtain less delta sleep (combined stages 3 and 4 slow-wave). Although total rapid eye movement (REM) sleep is not curtailed, David Kupfer and Gordon Foster found that seriously depressed persons consistently enter REM sleep shortly after the onset of sleep. Some depressed patients enter REM sleep within 5–15 minutes after sleep onset. However, most depressed patients have REM latencies that are about 25–35 minutes below the normal REM latency of 80–90 minutes. Compared with depressed or even severely anxious persons, chronic schizophrenic patients sleep well.

Temporary Insomnia Is a Natural Consequence of Altered Circadian Rhythms

In modern society some transient encounters with insomnia are normal, if not always anticipated. These will result from disruptions, usually intentional, of our normal circadian rhythms or of their entrainment. Normal circadian rhythms are commonly disrupted by travel (jet lag) as well as such behavioral changes as late-afternoon naps during vacations, altered meal times, and so on. As we saw in Chapter 51, the body's endogenous sleep–wake rhythm is entrained to the diurnal cycle: The stimuli that entrain internal circadian rhythms to the 24-hour day, or *Zeitgebers*, include not only the sun, but also clocks, regular work or meal habits, rhythmic noise or silence (e.g., traffic), or even regularly occurring behavioral interactions imposed by another person's activity–rest cycle. Changes in any of these can result in a phase shift of the circadian cycle and, in turn, in a disturbance of sleep, because the altered clock times of the phase shifts conflict with the customary times of sleeping and waking in the society (Figure 52–2).

Just as circadian rhythms can be disrupted as a by-product of behavioral change, they can also be deliberately manipulated. For example, phase shifts to a more appropriate sleep cycle can be established by forcing persistent arousal at a specified time each day. Similarly, people who stay in bed too long on one day may have insomnia the next night. Sunday night insomnia after long weekend mornings in bed is common.

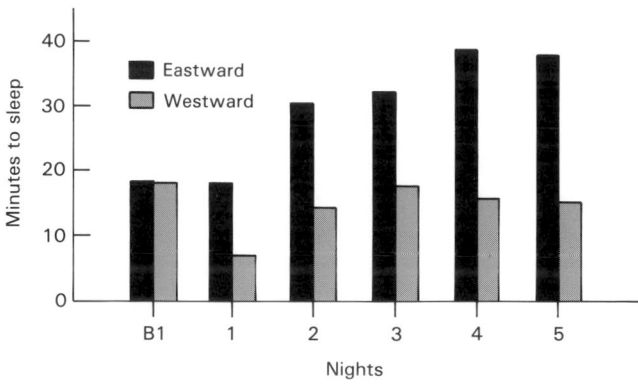

FIGURE 52–2

The symptoms experienced after rapid time zone transitions (jet lag) are more severe following eastward flights, and reentrainment of the sleep–wake cycle takes longer. In this study subjects flew from London to Detroit and back (a 5-hour shift). Following eastward travel to London, it took longer once in bed to fall asleep (sleep latency). Night B1 is a baseline night's sleep before the flight. In both scheduled shifts (eastward and westward) there was increased sleepiness and reduced performance during waking periods. (Adapted from Nicholson et al., 1986.)

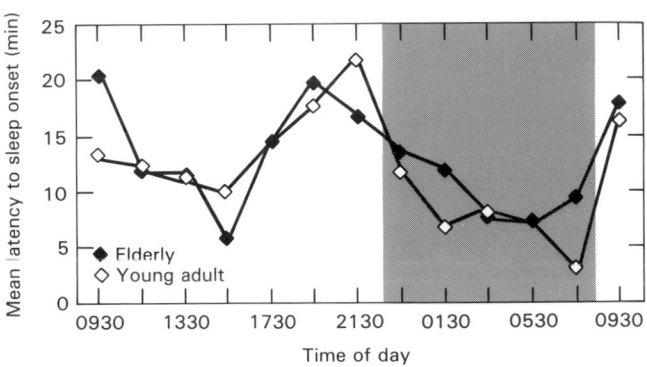

FIGURE 52–3

The circadian rhythm pattern of sleepiness is biphasic. Healthy normal young adult and elderly subjects were tested every 2 hours throughout the 24-hour day. During the sleep period (shaded, 2330–0800 hours) sleep latency testing was accomplished by awakening subjects for 15 minutes and then allowing them to return to sleep. Two troughs of sleepiness occurred in the afternoon (1400–1800) and early morning nocturnal hours (0200–0600). (Adapted from Carskadon and Dement, 1987.)

The human body clock can also be reset predictably and with precision by exposure to light, a recent finding of potential importance to both jet-lagged travelers and those whose sleep pattern is disrupted by sleeping late or odd shifts. Charles Czeisler and Richard Kronauer found that the body rhythms for temperature, urine formation, and several hormones could be reset by exposing young men to 5 hours of bright light at the time when their body temperature was lowest. The first daily exposure made the circadian variations irregular, the second markedly reduced them, and the third restarted the clock as if it were daytime, regardless of the actual time. The magnitude and direction of the rhythm change were also affected by the interim exposure of the subjects to low levels of illumination, as from normal room lights. The implication here is that insomniacs who turn on a reading light when they cannot sleep may compound their problem by altering their biological clocks.

Sleep Problems Are Magnified in the Elderly

As we saw in Chapter 51, one of the most significant determinants of a person's normal sleep pattern is age. The amount of stage 4 slow-wave sleep declines with age and in many people is virtually eliminated by the seventh decade. As a consequence, older people spend proportionately more time in the lighter stages of slow-wave sleep, from which they awaken more often. Noise that will awaken an older sleeper may produce only a temporary shift toward lighter sleep in an EEG of a young adult. In our society most adults learn to sleep in one extended period at night. However, the circadian rhythm of sleepiness is actually

biphasic, and normal afternoon drowsiness is more pronounced in the elderly (Figure 52–3). Furthermore, for reasons not wholly understood, the older one grows the more difficult it is to reset one's biological clock rapidly. Thus, travel across time zones more seriously upsets the normal sleep patterns of the elderly.

Despite the age-dependent reorganization in sleep staging toward a pattern of lighter sleep, serious insomnia is not an inevitable consequence of aging. Many aged individuals still sleep 8 hours per day. Markedly shortened sleep time relative to prior habits is often secondary to other health problems in the elderly. Because they are more susceptible to such problems, surveys of sleep habits in the elderly have often underestimated their normal sleep requirements. Patients with Alzheimer's-type dementia, common among the elderly, sleep often during the day, show fragmented sleep at night, and display other circadian rhythm disruptions.

The Barbiturates: Earlier Sleep Medications Initially Helped, Then Harmed Sleep

Until the mid-1970s barbiturates were the hypnotic drugs most commonly prescribed to treat insomnia. Although initially helpful, they became ineffective within 2 weeks. This unfortunate history is worth reviewing because it both illuminates certain principles of normal sleep physiology and illustrates the possible public health consequences of a uniform, collective pattern of drug prescription. Most patients showed rebound insomnia when withdrawn from hypnotics. The repeated administration of barbiturates, such as secobarbital, gradually led

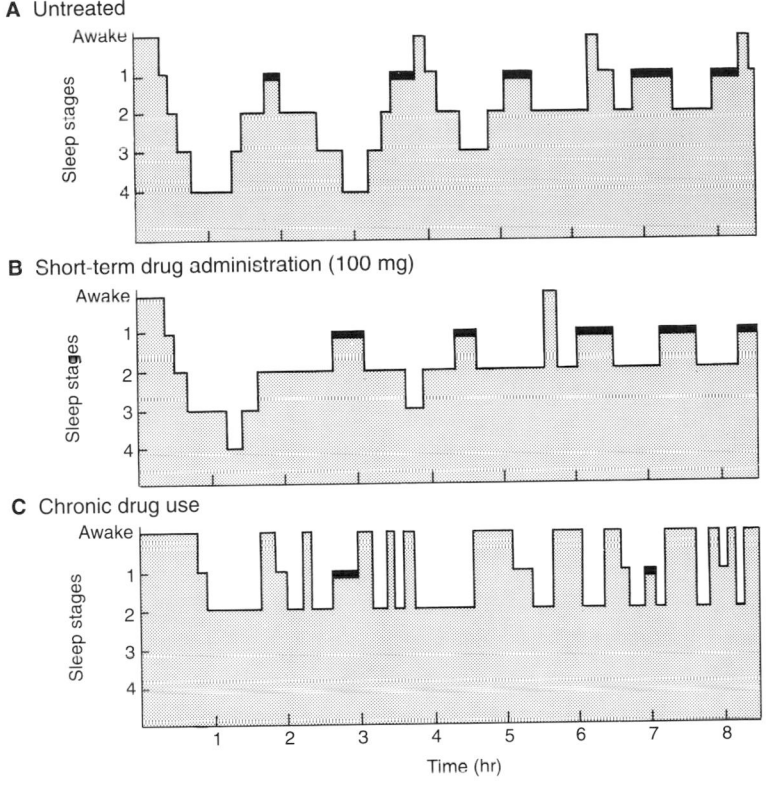

FIGURE 52–4

Effect of pentobarbital treatment on sleep staging in a young adult. Time spent in REM sleep is indicated by the **black bars.** (Adapted from Kales and Kales, 1973.)

A. Untreated patient complained of early morning awakenings.

B. Administration of 100 mg of pentobarbital initially lengthened the latency to the first REM period and decreased spontaneous awakenings.

C. With chronic nightly use of pentobarbital and an increased dose reflecting tolerance, the patient took almost 1 hour to fall asleep and there were 12 awakenings during the night. Note also that both REM sleep and stages 3 and 4 slow-wave sleep are suppressed.

to an increase in the liver enzymes responsible for degrading these drugs. As a result, their pharmacological action progressively diminished with prolonged use (Figure 52–4). Moreover, since these enzymes tend to be relatively nonspecific, a broad cross-tolerance to other hypnotics developed at the same time. Barbiturate hypnotics severely suppressed REM sleep, and drug withdrawal was associated with a profound REM rebound (Figure 52–5). Because of these properties, the administration of barbiturates longer than several days actually aggravated the sleep problems of insomniacs. For these reasons there has been a virtually complete shift away from the use of barbiturates as sleeping pills and toward the use of benzodiazepines.

The Benzodiazepines: Subjective Benefits to Insomniacs May Exceed Objective Improvements in Sleep Measures

Approximately 20 million prescriptions for benzodiazepine hypnotics, including flurazepam and triazolam, are written each year. One peculiar aspect of the benzodiazepines is that they enhance the subjective quality of sleep and yet are potent suppressors of deep slow-wave sleep, which has long been considered the most restful stage. This unusual blend of properties makes these drugs effective in treating both certain insomnias and certain delta sleep disorders, like night terrors, as we shall see later. Another puzzling result from polysomnographic

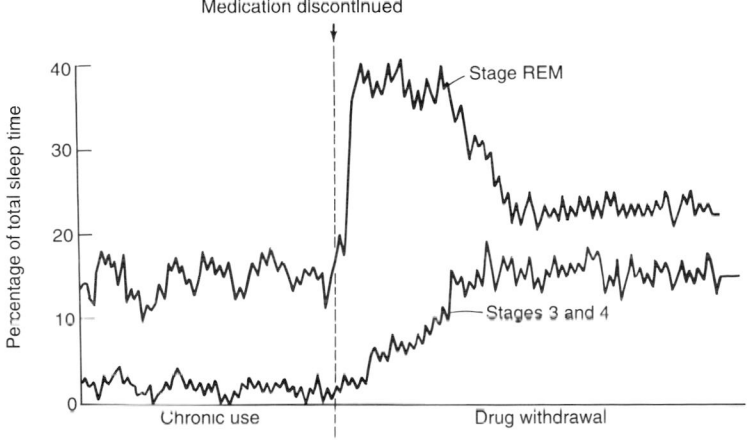

FIGURE 52–5

Abrupt withdrawal of hypnotic drugs causes a marked increase in previously suppressed REM sleep, as well as the frequency and intensity of dreaming. Stages 3 and 4 slow-wave sleep also recover to normal levels, but they do so gradually, displaying no overshoot or rebound phenomena. (Adapted from Kales and Kales, 1973.)

studies was that the quantitative improvement caused by these hypnotic drugs in total sleep time (e.g., 6–8% in a 1-month trial of 30 mg flurazepam) and in sleep onset latencies seemed very modest relative to the subjective benefits reported by insomniacs. Moreover, most improvement in insomniacs taking flurazepam is limited to an increase in stage 2 slow-wave sleep.

It now seems that conventional sleep stage scoring may not be the best gauge of the sleep protecting effects of benzodiazepines. Recent experiments have found that the benzodiazepines sharply curtail the number of micro-wakes, which, lasting but a few seconds each, severely diminish the restorative dimension of sleep. Benzodiazepine drugs may therefore help people sleep more continuously, if not much longer.

It is probably significant that benzodiazepines lower core temperature, because insomniacs typically have higher body temperatures throughout sleep. Since slow-wave sleep is sensitive to body temperature, perhaps the salutary changes in sleep induced by benzodiazepines result in part from the effect of these drugs on body temperature, as might their efficacy in treating insomnia. Even though safer than barbiturates, benzodiazepines are habit forming. Their abrupt withdrawal causes extremely distressing symptoms.

There is evidence that the mechanism of flurazepam's sleep-inducing properties involves the neuronal benzodiazepine receptor, which in turn may be involved in the physiological regulation of normal sleep (see Chapter 51). Wallace Mendelson and his colleagues found that in rats a benzodiazepine receptor antagonist (3-hydroxymethyl-β-carboline) induces a dose-dependent increase in sleep latency, a reduction in slow-wave (but not active REM) sleep, and a state of persistent wakefulness, without causing any major changes in motor activity. Furthermore, at a low dose that by itself did not affect sleep, the same drug blocked induction of sleep by large doses of flurazepam. Because this β-carboline drug also antagonizes the anxiolytic actions of the benzodiazepines, the previously noted relation between insomnia and anxiety states may be traced to actions at a common neuronal receptor.

Most drugs that are used to prevent or reduce sleep, such as amphetamine, also cause profound alterations in motor activity and other behaviors. If a compound like β-carboline were found to act more directly upon a normal sleep mechanism and thus reduce sleep without eliciting other major changes in motor behavior, it could be defined as a somnolytic, a drug class that sleep researchers have long sought to develop. Such compounds might be useful in the treatment of sleep disorders that are characterized by excessive somnolence. We shall consider these disorders later in the chapter.

Parasomnias Are Behavioral Dysfunctions Associated with Sleep, Sleep Stages, or Partial Arousals

The *parasomnias* are a broad set of normally undesirable behaviors that either occur exclusively during sleep or are exaggerated by sleep. We shall focus upon those that are associated with specific sleep stages and that illuminate certain mechanisms of normal sleep biology.

Nocturnal Enuresis Is Not Caused by Dreaming

Nocturnal enuresis, or bed-wetting, was once considered a dream-related disorder, as were sleepwalking and night terrors. However, as a result of laboratory studies made possible by the physiological discoveries outlined in Chapter 51, these common disturbances of sleep in the young have all been found to occur independently of normal REM stage dream periods.

Bed-wetting is common in children, especially boys, and young adults. Its incidence has been estimated at 3–6% for the general population, 15% for psychologically disturbed children, and 30% for institutionalized children. Idiopathic or essential enuresis (that is, enuresis whose cause is not known) is correlated with decreased bladder capacity and is now widely believed to be related to a maturational lag in neurological control, despite lack of experimental proof. Occasionally bed-wetting may be due to urinary tract anomalies, cystitis, diabetes mellitus, diabetes insipidus, or epilepsy.

In a typical enuretic episode, the sleeper awakes to find himself in soaked bedclothes, and can report little else. On the other hand, an observer can usually note a preceding period of agitated sleep, including gross body movements, succeeded by several seconds of tranquility and apparent continuation of sleep, followed in turn by enuresis. Immediately after the incident, it is difficult to waken the sleeper; when finally awakened, the patient is confused, even to the extent of denying that the bed is wet, and unable to recall any dreams.

Laboratory studies have confirmed that few enuretic episodes (3 of 22 in one study) are related to REM sleep. The trigger of an enuretic episode (the initial body movements) is most often associated with EEG patterns of stage 4 slow-wave sleep, and this is followed by a rapid emergence from the deeper stages of slow-wave sleep. Micturition occurs in slow-wave stages 4, 3, 2, or stage 1 REM, depending upon the length of the period of calm intervening between the initial body movements and enuresis. The dreams often reported by patients to explain the enuresis are recounted in the laboratory only if the subject is allowed to sleep into the next REM episode, during which the sensations arising from the wet bedclothes become incorporated into the dream.

Sleepwalking Is Triggered by Arousal from Slow-Wave Sleep

In the typical sleepwalking episode (somnambulism) the sleeper sits up quietly, gets out of bed, and walks about, rather unsteadily at first, with eyes open and with a blank expression. Soon the somnambulist's behavior becomes more coordinated and complex—avoiding objects, dusting tables, or going to the bathroom, and occasionally mumbling or speaking incoherently. It is difficult to attract the sleepwalker's attention. There may be monosyllabic replies to questions. If left alone, the sleeper usually goes back to bed and upon awakening acknowledges little

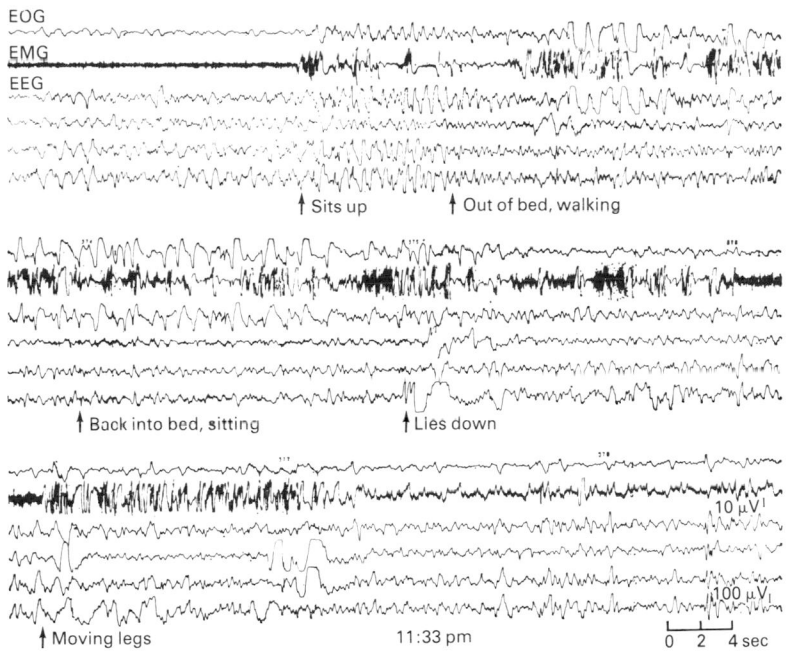

EOG
EMG
EEG

↑ Sits up   ↑ Out of bed, walking

↑ Back into bed, sitting   ↑ Lies down

10 μV

100 μV

↑ Moving legs   11:33 pm   0 2 4 sec

FIGURE 52–6

Electrooculogram (EOG), electromyogram (EMG), and EEG records of a sleepwalking incident observed under laboratory conditions. A high-voltage slow-wave EEG pattern commences as the sleepwalker sits up in bed, and slow wave sleep patterns are maintained throughout the episode. (Adapted from Jacobson et al., 1965.)

recollection of the night's activities or of dreaming. Until recently somnambulism was almost universally interpreted as acting out dream material.

In the laboratory sleepwalking occurs almost always in stage 3 or 4 slow-wave sleep. In an early study in which 25 sleepwalkers were observed for five nights each, 41 incidents occurred, all initiated during the deepest stages of slow-wave sleep. Given the intense descending inhibition of spinal motor neurons and consequent paralysis during REM sleep, it would seem reasonable that slow-paced somnambulistic episodes are unrelated to REM episodes.

Later studies have confirmed that sleepwalking occurs exclusively during slow-wave sleep, most frequently in the first third of the night when stages 3 and 4 predominate. In a remarkable study by Allan Jacobson and coworkers, all night EEG records revealed that high-voltage, slow-wave patterns often *commenced* as the sleeper began the nocturnal ramblings (Figure 52–6).

Both enuresis and somnambulism originate in slow-wave sleep. They are not under the sleeper's control. Both disorders run in the same families. One-third of the military recruits who had enuresis also had a personal history of sleepwalking, while another one-fourth said that someone in their family sleepwalked. As with enuresis, somnambulism is more common in children than adults; its decline with age parallels the normal decrease in the proportion of sleep time spent in stage 4 slow-wave sleep.

REM Behavior Disorder: REM Sleep Without Atonia Causes Violent Episodes in Human Sleepers

In Chapter 51 we noted that cats with certain brain stem lesions are able to enter and maintain REM sleep without the normally attendant paralysis. A similar state under-

lies the fascinating syndrome known as *REM behavior disorder*. Whereas most parasomnias, like bed-wetting and sleepwalking are harmless, the violent moving nightmares of this state are often as menacing to sleep partners as they are dangerous to the dreaming sleeper. In one study 85% of the violent sleepers had injured themselves, and 44% had injured their bed partners, sometimes seriously. Although some REM behavior disorder patients have identifiable brain stem lesions or other neurological problems ("soft" signs), between 50 and 60% are without obvious deficits in the waking state. In fact, most violent sleepers are not aggressive when awake—but then few of us dream as we think when awake.

In REM behavior disorder the normal paralysis of REM sleep is lost, and the person literally jumps out of bed and enacts the dream he experiences. One sleeper, a 67-year-old grocer, woke up with a gash on his head. He had been dreaming that he was a football player in full pads charging at an opponent in uniform. In reality he was wearing pajamas and had slammed into his bedroom dresser. His wife of 40 years said, "That's enough," and took him to a sleep clinic. Fortunately these patients respond well to drugs with strong anticonvulsant activity, in particular clonazepam, a benzodiazepine, and carbamazepine, an iminostilbene related to tricyclic antidepressants.

Night Terrors, Nightmares, and Terrifying Dreams Occur in Different Stages of Sleep

Upsetting dreams may occur during either REM or slow-wave sleep. Moreover, they possess, often to an exaggerated degree, the physiological and psychological characteristics of normal dreams as outlined in Chapter 51. Bad dreams, during both REM and slow-wave sleep, may occur in either children or, less frequently, adults.

The *night terror* (*pavor nocturnus*) attack in children is perhaps the best characterized. Usually within 30 minutes of falling asleep, the child abruptly sits up in bed, screams, and appears to be staring wide-eyed at some imaginary object. His face is covered with perspiration, and breathing is labored. In the same manner that sleepwalkers appear to be oblivious to external stimuli, consoling stimuli have no effect on the terrorized child. After the attack, which may last 1 or 2 minutes, dream recall is rare and usually fragmentary. The next morning there is no recollection of the episode. This fragmented pattern of recall resembles mentation during slow-wave sleep. Thus, it was not surprising that when Henri Gastaut observed night terror episodes in seven children in his laboratory, all attacks occurred during a sudden arousal from stages 3 or 4 slow-wave (delta) sleep. There is recent evidence that diazepam may suppress night terrors, coincident with a measurable decline in the amount of stage 4 (delta-wave) slow-wave sleep.

A related slow-wave sleep parasomnia is also seen in adults, although less frequently. The core symptoms of these attacks are respiratory oppression, partial paralysis, and anxiety—usually in that sequence. The anxiety is intense, accompanied by sweating, a fixed facial expression, dilated pupils, and difficulty in breathing. Dream activity is rarely well structured; it consists not of a story but of a poor recollection of a single oppressive situation, such as having rocks piled on the chest. Like night terror attacks in children, the patient usually has little memory of the attack the next morning. These patients also show greater than normal daytime anxiety. The name of these slow-wave sleep attacks in the adult is *incubus*, which, given the Latin root *incubare* (to lie upon), is an appropriate term for a phenomenon characterized by respiratory oppression. It also seems likely that the word *nightmare* may have originally described the anxiety and difficult breathing of slow-wave sleep attacks. From the Middle Ages and before it was believed that nightmares were caused by a nocturnal demon pressing upon the sleeper's chest. The German word *Nachtmar* and the French word *cauchemar* both contain the ancient Teutonic root *mar*, which means devil. *Cauchemar* also derives from *caucher*, an old French verb meaning to press, thus literally referring to a pressing devil.

In contrast to the night terrors and nightmares of delta sleep are the more common frightening dreams that occur during normal REM periods in sleepers of all ages. As would be expected from the study of normal REM events, these terrifying dreams contain complex imagery, have a story line, are vividly recalled, and are not accompanied by depressed respiration, but rather by an exaggerated increase in all the phasic activity that normally characterizes REM sleep, probably including pontine–geniculate–occipital spikes, although these cannot be measured directly in humans. Because REM sleep becomes more extensive and more physiologically intense as sleep continues, most terrifying REM dreams occur in the early morning hours. Often these terrifying REM episodes are also referred to as nightmares.

Whatever the nomenclature, it is clinically useful to distinguish the high-anxiety dream phenomena that occur during REM from those that occur during slow-wave stages of sleep. Like other slow-wave disturbances such as enuresis and somnambulism, night terrors decline with age along with delta sleep, and they can be alleviated by drugs, such as the benzodiazepines, that selectively reduce delta sleep. In contrast, REM sleep time does not change appreciably after childhood, nor is it suppressed by the same drugs. Hence, the prognosis for childhood slow-wave sleep disturbances differs from terrifying REM dreams, and the two should be treated differently.

Sleep Apnea: Persistent Nocturnal Arousals Can Result from Lapses in Breathing

Another remarkable disturbance of sleep is characterized by frequent, periodic breathing pauses, called *sleep apnea*. Both the causes of sleep apnea and the presenting complaints of patients suffering from this disorder are extremely broad. It is unlikely that sleep apnea represents a single disorder. In some cases of sleep apnea, the shift from wakefulness to sleep is assumed to be associated with a suppression of activity in the medullary respiratory center. This causes the diaphragm and the intercostal muscles to become immobile. In this phase of apnea, which lasts for 15–30 seconds, blood oxygen falls and carbon dioxide rises, eventually stimulating the respiratory center and causing the respiratory muscles to function again. Often, however, the lungs do not fill with air because the throat has collapsed, perhaps a reflection of the relaxed state of most body muscles during slow-wave sleep. The extreme changes in the concentrations of oxygen and carbon dioxide in the blood that develop after one minute or more without air rouse the sleeper. Muscle tone returns to the throat, and a few noisy, choking gasps refill the lungs. Arousal may last for only a few seconds until the blood gases return to normal. Then the person returns immediately to sleep and the cycle can be repeated—as many as 500 times during the night!

Different types of sleep apneas can sometimes be distinguished operationally in the sleep laboratory. *Central sleep apnea* can be defined by an absence of respiratory effort; although the upper airway remains open, the diaphragm stops moving and there is no exchange of air. *Obstructive sleep apnea*, the more common type, is defined by a collapse of the upper airway and a lack of air flow, despite persistent respiratory efforts. Whether the apnea involves central nervous system dysfunction or upper airway obstruction, or a combination of both (*mixed apnea*), these patients all literally stop breathing and begin to suffocate repeatedly during their sleep (Figure 52–7).

Some sleep apnea patients are apparently oblivious of their persistent nocturnal arousals and may actually complain of too much sleep. These patients were first described by Gastaut in 1965, who called their disorder *hypersomnolent apnea syndrome*. Later, Dement described another group of patients with a similarly disturbed sleep pattern who complained instead of insomnia. Apparently these patients do not habituate to the frequent nocturnal arousals or do not return to sleep immediately after the apnea. Approximately one out of 10 patients with

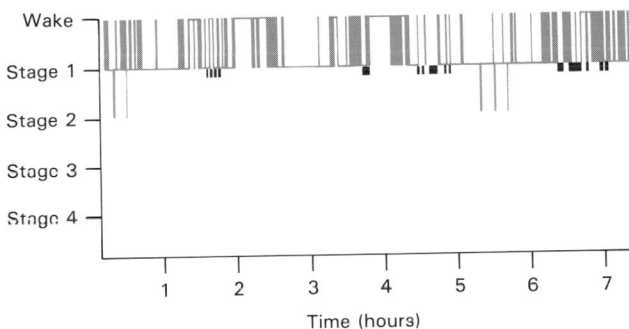

FIGURE 52–7
The sleep of a 64-year-old male patient with obstructive sleep apnea is interrupted by frequent awakenings. Slow-wave sleep (stages 3 and 4) is absent. The REM portion of sleep is only 10%. The person spends most of the night in active EEG stage 1 sleep without accompanying REM signs, a light stage of sleep only rarely observed in normal sleepers. (Adapted from data supplied by G. Nino-Murcia to Carskadon and Dement, 1989.)

sleep apnea complains of insomnia and the rest of hypersomnia.

Sleep apnea affects all ages and both sexes. It has been proposed as one of the factors in sudden infant death syndrome, or crib death, and there is a high prevalence of sleep apnea in the elderly. One laboratory study found that 30% of people over the age of 65 have some form of sleep apnea, although most are otherwise asymptomatic and noncomplaining. In almost all diagnosed cases of serious sleep apnea, a critical factor is a report from a sleep partner that the patient snored loudly. Affected people tend to be obese, but about one-third are not. Weight loss is the first therapeutic step—it works, but why is not clear. No drugs have yet proven effective in treating sleep apnea, although many are under investigation. In those cases in which the cause is some form of upper airway obstruction, a mechanical approach can be taken. A new treatment, continuous positive airway pressure, is like a pneumatic splint of the airway; a tight-fitting mask delivers high-pressure air that keeps the throat expanded between breaths. Surgery to enlarge the upper airway by cutting away the uvula and trimming away mucous and lymphoid tissue is also successful in 50–60% of serious cases.

Narcolepsy: Irresistible Sleep Attacks Are Accompanied by Several REM-Related Symptoms

The principal symptom of narcolepsy is irresistible *sleep attacks* lasting 5–30 minutes during the day. These attacks occasionally occur without warning and at inappropriate moments. More often the narcoleptic feels an overwhelming drowsiness preceding the attack and attempts to fight it off. If the patient naps, he awakes refreshed; 15 minutes is usually sufficient. One serious danger posed by narcolepsy is accidental death, and automobile accidents are a more frequent occurrence with narcolepsy than with epilepsy. In one study 40% of the narcoleptic patients questioned admitted that they had fallen asleep while driving.

In the late 1950s Robert Yoss and David Daly described an idiosyncratic set of symptoms that characterized narcoleptics from all walks of life and virtually all personality types. They discovered that, in addition to sleep attacks, the narcoleptic patient often exhibits an abrupt loss of muscle tone, a swoonlike reaction termed *cataplexy*. In a typical attack the jaw sags, the head falls forward, the arms drop to the side, and the knees buckle. Cataplexy is usually triggered by emotion, for example, laughter, anger, or even sexual excitement. A classic example is an angry parent who wants to spank a child but who instead collapses to the floor, fully conscious, yet unable to control muscle movement.

A third symptom of narcolepsy is *sleep paralysis*. These reversible episodes of muscle inhibition occur while the person is lying in bed and drifting into or out of sleep. Conscious, but unable to move or speak, the patient often experiences shallow breathing. A fourth symptom is *hypnagogic hallucinations*, which may be auditory or visual. These occur only at sleep onset, whether daytime naps or nocturnal sleep. Sleep paralysis and hallucinations occur in only a minority of narcoleptics.

These four symptoms reflect the intrusion of the normally inhibited properties of REM sleep into the waking state (sleep attacks and cataplexy) or into the transitions between wakefulness and sleep (sleep paralysis and hallucinations). In fact, narcoleptic patients can enter into REM sleep almost directly from the waking state (Figure 52–8). In approximately 50% of sleep recordings REM sleep appears in narcoleptics within 10 minutes of sleep onset. As a result, *sleep-onset REM*, a fifth defining symptom is now considered diagnostic of narcolepsy.

A sixth sign of narcolepsy is *decreased voluntary sleep latency*. When tested every 2 hours throughout the day while lying in bed, narcoleptics can usually fall asleep upon request within 2 minutes, whereas normal subjects take an average of 15 minutes to get to sleep. Interestingly, the narcoleptic's need for sleep is apparently satiated at a normal rate. Yasuo Hishikawa and his colleagues found that, despite excessive daytime drowsiness, when narcoleptics were asked to sleep as long as possible, they slept no longer than normal.

The cataplexy and sleep paralysis of narcolepsy may have a common cause. Both may be related to the activation of those brain stem neurons responsible for the massive descending inhibition of spinal motor neurons during stage REM sleep. A state resembling the cataplexy of the awake narcoleptic can be induced in animals by direct injection of carbachol, a cholinergic agonist, into the dorsal pontine reticular formation. The effective region for inducing this state of atonia without REM sleep corresponds very well with the pontine area whose destruction results in REM sleep without atonia described in Chapter 51.

As we also observed in Chapter 51, the loss of muscle tonus during REM sleep does not extend to the eye and middle ear muscles. During a cataplectic attack the narcoleptic remains capable of moving his eyes, and can even do so voluntarily in response to questions. During sleep paralysis patients can also move the eyes. Some narcolep-

FIGURE 52–8

Narcoleptic patients can enter into REM sleep almost directly from the waking state. (Adapted from Dement, Guilleminault, and Zarcone, 1975.)

A. Sleep onset in the normal person is typified by a gradual change from a waking EEG dominated by alpha activity (10 Hz) to mixed lower-frequency patterns coupled with the development of slow, rolling eye movements in the electrooculogram (EOG) and little change in the electromyographic (EMG) recording of muscle tonus.

B. In narcoleptics sleep onset is preceded by several seconds of markedly reduced EMG activity (indicated by **brackets** on EMG trace) and then accompanied by conjugate (both traces) rapid eye movements. Sleep-onset REM usually lasts 10–20 minutes, after which, if the narcoleptic remains asleep, there follows a typical progression through stages 1–4 of slow-wave sleep.

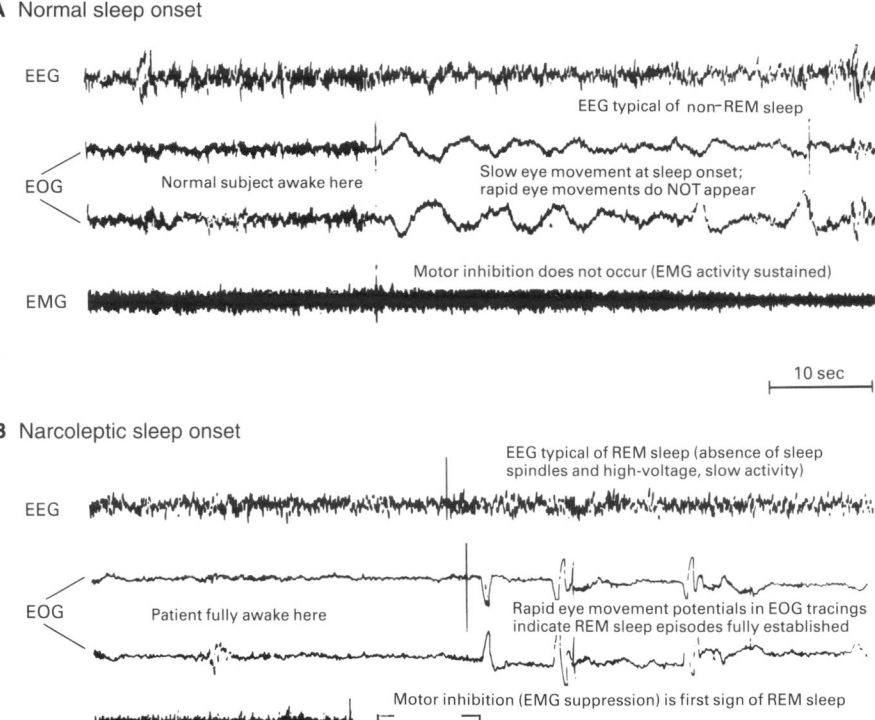

A Normal sleep onset

EEG
EEG typical of non-REM sleep

EOG
Normal subject awake here
Slow eye movement at sleep onset; rapid eye movements do NOT appear

EMG
Motor inhibition does not occur (EMG activity sustained)

10 sec

B Narcoleptic sleep onset

EEG typical of REM sleep (absence of sleep spindles and high-voltage, slow activity)

EEG

EOG
Patient fully awake here
Rapid eye movement potentials in EOG tracings indicate REM sleep episodes fully established

Motor inhibition (EMG suppression) is first sign of REM sleep
EMG

tics have learned to terminate paralysis by first vigorously moving the eyes, then fluttering the eyelids, and then by moving facial muscles. In this way they establish a gradual spread of voluntary control using the unparalyzed movements of the eye as an initial base. (Sleep paralysis can also be reversed immediately by the touch of another person.) Like the narcoleptic human, a cat made cataplectic by pontine injections of carabachol can also blink its eyes and visually track a moving object, despite the suppression of all other somatic reflexes.

In spite of the ability to fall asleep quickly and to enter the first REM period rapidly, narcoleptics generally show significantly less total REM time than normal and a disturbed sleep architecture. Polysomnographic records on narcoleptics show excessive shifting among sleep stages, especially from REM sleep to stage 1 slow-wave sleep. As a result, REM sleep is frequently interrupted, a narcoleptic sign known as *REM sleep fragmentation*. For these reasons, one early hypothesis suggested that the irresistible and recuperative sleep attacks during the daytime reflect increased pressure to obtain REM sleep. Because stimulant drugs were commonly administered to control the sleep attacks, this proposal was somewhat unsettling. These drugs suppress REM sleep, and thus it was feared that the treatment might contribute to the illness rather than its cure. However, it now seems that narcolepsy is more complex than a simple state of REM deprivation. Moreover, as outlined in Chapter 51, the consequences of experimental REM deprivation are largely restricted to subsequent sleep periods and intrude very little upon waking behavior.

Drugs that enhance transmission at central catecholaminergic synapses affect the various symptoms of narcolepsy differently. The stimulants methylphenidate and *d*-amphetamine, by enhancing the release of newly synthesized transmitter at nerve terminals (and, to a lesser extent, attenuating reuptake), aid in the control of sleep attacks and drowsiness, but have no effect on the other symptoms of narcolepsy. The tricyclic antidepressants, which block reuptake of both norepinephrine and serotonin by presynaptic terminals, prevent cataplexy but have no effect on sleep attacks. As a rule, any medication effective in treating sleep attacks has only a slight effect on cataplexy and vice versa. This suggests that the symptoms of narcolepsy, like the physiological components of REM sleep, reflect the activities of separate neuronal populations.

There is a strong inherited component to narcolepsy, even though onset is usually delayed, often until the second decade. Narcolepsy is not rare, ranging in incidence between 0.04 and 0.09% of the population. Because many of these cases are not diagnosed, narcoleptics may be subject to unwarranted disapproval for apparent laziness.

A promising advance in our understanding of the molecular genetic basis of narcolepsy is the discovery by Yutaka Honda and colleagues of the association of narcolepsy with the inheritance of a class II antigen (known as DR2) of the major histocompatibility complex. The major histocompatibility complex, or MHC, is a cluster of genes that encode surface molecules involved in antigen recognition and cell interactions in the immune system. Each gene has several allelic forms, which means that every member of the species has the gene, but different members have different forms of the gene. Class II genes of the MHC encode a series of molecules, called Ia antigens, that are expressed primarily on lymphocytes. Class II genes also control the level of the immune response to some antigens, hence they are also called the immune response genes. Honda discovered that all Japanese narcoleptics were DR2 positive, as compared to only 25% of the general population. The association between DR2 and narcolepsy is important because of the relation of the MHC gene complex to autoimmune diseases. Several other diseases, including multiple sclerosis, have been associated with the DR2 locus, and all are associated with immune dysfunction.

Loss of Consciousness: Coma Is Not Deep Sleep

At one time it was commonly held in both the clinical and basic neural sciences that a continuum of consciousness existed that ranged in graded levels from attention, alertness, relaxation, and drowsiness to sleep, stupor, and coma. It was generally believed that the level of excitation in the ascending reticular activating system determined the level of consciousness. Sensory impulses entering the reticular formation from the different modalities were assumed to merge and lose their specificity within this network of neurons. The reticular formation, in turn, acted as an energizer and exerted a broad facilitatory influence on the rest of the nervous system. A reduction in the amount of impulses from the reticular formation would reduce the overall activity of the brain and consequently result in sleep.

With the discovery of the extraordinary neural activity that characterizes sleep, the idea of a neurophysiological continuum from quiescence to excitation was abandoned. Moreover, activity of the reticular formation alone does not account for variations in levels of consciousness. Nevertheless, the brain stem reticular core plays a role in many clinical disorders of consciousness.

Transient Losses of Consciousness Can Result from Decreased Cerebral Blood Flow

Fainting, or syncope, most often results from a general reduction in cerebral blood flow, which compromises the ability of the brain to extract oxygen and needed nutrients. This involves a failure of the autoregulatory reflexes of the cerebral vessels, which normally maintain a constant blood flow over a wide range of perfusion pressures. Autoregulation may fail if perfusion pressure falls below 60 mm Hg; too precipitous a fall can result from decreased cardiac output or, more frequently, from decreased peripheral resistance, or both. One type of syncope, termed *vasovagal*, is reflexive in origin and is almost always related to pain, fear, or other emotional stress. In vasovagal syncope, stimulation of the autonomic nervous system usually precedes the drop in blood pressure and the patient is usually aware of light-headedness and impending fainting.

Coma Has Many Causes

Sleep and coma differ behaviorally in their arousal threshold, or relative reversibility. They can also be easily distinguished physiologically. Sleep is a highly active neurophysiological state during which cerebral oxygen uptake does not decline from normal waking levels. In fact, Seymour Kety found that cerebral oxygen uptake increases above normal during REM episodes. In contrast, oxygen uptake falls below the normal resting level in every studied example of coma. Thus, *coma* may be defined by exclusion as a nonsleep loss of consciousness that, unlike syncope, lasts for an extended period. Within the range of this definition, different levels of unconsciousness, including lethargy, loss of sensation, stupor, and coma, have been distinguished clinically by the degree of indifference of the patient to such common stimuli as talking, shouting, shaking, or noxious prodding. *Stupor* is a state in which someone is responsive only to shaking, shouting, or noxious stimuli, whereas *coma* refers to total unresponsiveness.

Two general types of pathological processes may impair consciousness. One consists of a set of conditions that can cause widespread functional depression of the cerebral hemispheres; the other includes more specific conditions that depress or destroy critical brain stem areas. In 1982 Fred Plum and Jerome Posner suggested that diseases causing stupor or coma must either affect the brain widely or encroach upon deep central structures. They classified these diseases into three categories, using as a reference the conventional landmark, the tentorium of the cerebellum (a taut extension of the inner dura mater located between the occipital lobe and the cerebellum): (1) sub- or infratentorial mass or destructive lesions (such as pontine hemorrhage) that directly damage the central core of the brain stem; (2) supratentorial mass lesions (such as may result from subdural hematomas) that indirectly compress deep diencephalic structures; and (3) metabolic disorders (such as hypoglycemia) that widely depress or interrupt brain functions. Some of the clinical causes of coma in these three categories are listed (Table 52–1) along with their relative frequencies.

The first question that usually arises for the physician confronted with a patient in coma is: Where is the lesion and what is the cause? Another question that is often of diagnostic importance is: In what direction is the process evolving? In coma the sequence of signs is likely to be as important in revealing the source as the full clinical picture at any given moment. The answers to these questions can often place the disease in one of the above categories and thus reduce the number of inferences required to specify the nature of the disorder.

Infratentorial Lesions. A pathological process that affects the brain stem reticular formation will probably never be restricted to the reticular formation alone. A tu-

TABLE 52–1. Final Diagnosis in 386 Patients with Coma of Unknown Etiology

Diagnosis	Number	Percent of subtype	Percent of total
Supratentorial mass lesions			
Epidural hematoma	2	2.8	
Subdural hematoma	21	30.4	
Intracerebral hematoma	33	47.8	
Cerebral infarct	5	7.3	
Brain tumor	5	7.3	
Brain abscess	3	4.4	
Subtotal	69		17.9
Subtentorial lesions			
Brain stem infarct	37	71.2	
Brain stem tumor	2	3.9	
Brain stem hemorrhage	7	13.5	
Cerebellar hemorrhage	4	7.7	
Cerebral abscess	2	3.9	
Subtotal	52		13.5
Metabolic and diffuse cerebral disorders			
Anoxia or ischemia	51	19.5	
Concussion and postictal states	9	3.5	
Infection (meningitis and encephalitis)	11	4.2	
Subarachnoid hemorrhage	10	3.8	
Exogenous toxins	99	37.9	
Endogenous toxins and deficiencies	81	31.0	
Subtotal	261		67.6
Psychiatric disorders	4		1.0

(Adapted from Plum and Posner, 1982.)

mor, vascular disorder, or infection is likely to involve other structures as well, with resulting signs and symptoms that involve cranial nerves, long ascending and descending pathways, and various nuclei (see Chapters 44 and 46). Tumors involving the midbrain and diencephalon may be followed by a loss of consciousness that lasts for months. The EEG in these patients may show synchronization, suggesting that this type of coma might actually involve normal sleep mechanisms. If these EEG signs are present, the clinical state of stupor might more appropriately be referred to as *hypersomnia*. This often reversible condition may also occur with tumors below the floor of the third ventricle. If the tumor is cystic and is emptied by aspiration, the stupor may disappear promptly. However, in other cases of tumors in the upper midbrain and diencephalon, decerebrate rigidity may be present in addition to loss of consciousness. This pattern may also be seen after occlusion of the basilar artery. Thus, in broad terms these clinical and EEG patterns are compatible with the view that the upper brain stem and diencephalic regions are concerned with the general activation of the brain, or what is clinically called crude consciousness.

The role of the lower brain stem in consciousness is less clear. Because the medulla and lower pons regulate respiration and cardiovascular functions, lesions of the lower brain stem are apt to be rapidly fatal. Unconsciousness in these cases is often accompanied by disturbances in breathing, lowered blood pressure, and other brain stem signs (tetraplegia, Babinski signs due to corticospinal tract

damage, pinpoint but reactive pupils after disruption of descending sympathetic pathways, and absence of ocular movements). Pontine hemorrhage results in these clinical signs before there are disorders of blood pressure and respiration.

On those rare occasions when patients with extensive lesions of the pons and medulla survive for long periods, the EEG may have a desynchronized pattern, as in the waking state (*alpha coma*). These clinical findings in humans corroborate the classic experiments performed on cats in 1959 by Moruzzi, Alberto Zanchetti, and their colleagues. They were the first to provide evidence for a region in the caudal brain stem that actively puts the brain to sleep. They tied off cerebral blood vessels so that the arterial supply to the medulla and lower pons was isolated from that of the upper pons, midbrain, and cerebrum (Figure 52–9). Injections of the barbiturate anesthetic thiopental into the rostral brain stem and forebrain anesthetized the cat, as might be expected. However, when only the caudal brain stem was anesthetized, the cat awakened as if it had been sleeping. The synchronous EEG of slow-wave sleep was replaced by a desynchronized waking EEG. Among the structures in the lower pons and medulla that might be responsible for the active induction of slow-wave sleep are the midline raphe nuclei and the nucleus of the solitary tract. The solitary nucleus is a pontine structure that receives both taste and visceral information, but it also causes a synchronizing of the cortical EEG when stimulated with low-frequency current.

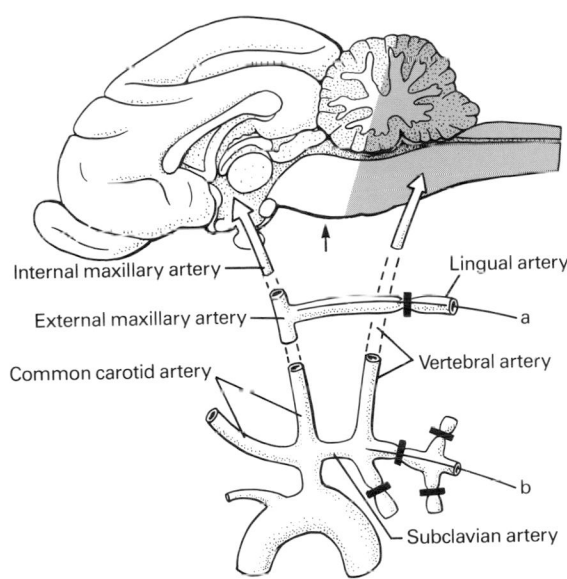

FIGURE 52–9

Procedure for establishing separate perfusion in a cat's brain of the medulla, caudal pons, and posterior cerebellum (**shaded**) served by the vertebral artery, and of the anterior cerebellum, rostral pons, midbrain, and forebrain (**unshaded**) served by the internal carotid. **Black arrow** indicates where the basilar artery is clamped to prevent mixing of vertebral and carotid blood. Injections are made through plastic tubes at **a** and **b**. (Adapted from Magni et al., 1959.)

Both clinical observations of coma due to infratentorial lesions and experimental studies of limited brain stem dysfunction suggest that the subset of reticular neurons responsible for activation of the cerebrum is not distributed evenly throughout the brain stem, but only in the most rostral part.

Supratentorial Lesions. Supratentorial structural lesions usually cause coma in one of two ways, either by destroying a critical amount of cerebral cortex bilaterally, or by compressing the brain stem and diencephalic structures that lie below the tentorium. If the lesion is unilateral, it may cause transtentorial downward herniation of either the medial temporal lobe (*uncal herniation*) or more medial diencephalic structures (*central herniation*). As a result of the asymmetry of the lesion, there may be asymmetry of limb movements or tendon reflexes due to involvement of the corticospinal tract. There may also be decerebrate posturing (arms and legs extended) in response to noxious stimuli. This may be due to the compromised function of the rubrospinal and corticospinal systems, which normally exert a net facilitatory effect on flexor muscles, and the consequent release of the vestibulospinal system, which facilitates extensor muscle groups.

The pupillary response to light is decreased or absent. In uncal herniation the most sensitive sign is that the ipsilateral pupil is dilated because the third cranial nerve is compressed as it passes through the tentorium, leaving sympathetic influence on the pupil unopposed. In central herniation one or both pupils tend to be in midposition

because the pressure on the midbrain disrupts both parasympathetic and sympathetic pupillary influences. With continuing, long-term compression of the brain stem, eye movements cease, including reflex responses to head rotation and to ice water applied to the tympanic membrane. (The normal response is a forced deviation of the eyes to the opposite side, away from the stimulus.) As brain stem compression moves caudally, a sequence of abnormal respiratory patterns ensues: Cheyne-Stokes breathing, characterized by rhythmic waxing and waning of the depth of respiration, with regularly recurring periods of apnea; prolonged periods of hyperventilation; intermittent bouts of irregular or ataxic breathing; and, finally, apnea.

Cerebral infarctions do not often cause coma unless massive and accompanied by considerable brain swelling. In fact, the loss of extensive amounts of cerebral tissue (even hemispherectomy) may be sustained without impaired alertness. More important as a cause of coma is brain swelling. Therefore, cerebral hemorrhage is more likely to cause coma than infarction, and it is often accompanied by the typical signs of rostral–caudal transtentorial herniation outlined above. Other supratentorial lesions that commonly cause coma are subdural hematoma, cerebral tumor, or cerebral abscess.

Metabolic Coma. Metabolically caused coma is usually preceded by gradual changes in cognition. However, in some conditions, such as hypoglycemia, the onset of coma may be abrupt. For obvious reasons, asymmetrical changes in tendon reflexes or other focal signs are less likely in metabolic states than with structural lesions. Common symptoms in metabolic comas are tremor, *asterixis* (rapid loss of postural tone, most easily demonstrated by asking the patient, if sufficiently awake, to extend the wrists), and *myoclonus* (sudden, nonrhythmic jerks of limbs). The respiratory changes in metabolic coma vary with the cause. For instance, opiate drug overdose depresses respiration, while hepatic coma is characterized by hyperventilation. As a rule (which is useful in diagnosis), ocular movements are only rarely affected in metabolic coma, unless the coma is quite severe. The pupillary reflex to light is also normally preserved until death, except in comas caused by anoxia or ischemia or by certain toxins, such as atropine.

The causes of metabolic coma are extremely varied and difficult to systematize. They include diffuse brain anoxia or ischemia, hypo- or hyperglycemia, thiamine deficiency, poisons (including ethanol, opiates, barbiturates, heavy metals, and aspirin), acid–base derangements, hyper- or hypocalcemia, pulmonary disease (carbon dioxide narcosis), uremia, liver failure, hypo- or hyperthermia, and meningitis.

The Determination of Cerebral Death Constitutes a Medical, Legal, and Social Decision

Despite improved techniques for resuscitation, some comas are not reversible. Because the brain is particularly susceptible to acute anoxia, it is likely to suffer irreparable

TABLE 52–2. Criteria for Cerebral Death (Brain Death)

Prerequisite: All appropriate diagnostic and therapeutic procedures have been performed
Criteria (to be present for 30 minutes at least 6 hours after the onset of coma and apnea):
  1. Coma with cerebral unresponsivity (see definition 1)
  2. Apnea (see definition 2)
  3. Dilated pupils
  4. Absent cephalic reflexes (see definition 3)
  5. Electrocerebral silence (see definition 4)
Confirmatory test: Absence of cerebral blood flow

Definitions
  1. Cerebral unresponsivity—a state in which the patient does not respond purposively to externally applied stimuli, obeys no commands, and does not utter sounds spontaneously or in response to a painful stimulus.
  2. Apnea—the absence of spontaneous respiration, manifested by the need for controlled ventilation (that is, the patient makes no effort to override the respirator) for at least 15 minutes.
  3. Cephalic reflexes—pupillary, corneal, oculoauditory, oculovestibular, oculocephalic, ciliospinal, snout, pharyngeal, cough, and swallowing.
  4. Electrocerebral silence—an EEG with an absence of electrical potentials of cerebral origin over 2 μV from symmetrically placed electrode pairs over 10 cm apart and with interelectrode resistance between 100 and 10,000 Ω.

(Adapted from A Collaborative Study by Ninos, NIH, 1977.)

damage while resuscitative measures may be restoring vitality to less vulnerable organs. The resulting dilemma is that of a dead brain in an otherwise living body—a condition beyond deep coma. Under the law, physicians determine whether a patient is alive or dead. In medical practice the signs of brain death are irreversible coma and lack of spontaneous respiration, although the specific criteria used to diagnose brain death differ in different hospitals. The development of equipment that mechanically maintains respiration and other vital functions and the need of modern transplant surgery for access to viable organs have focused ethical and legal attention on the desirability of agreeing on the medical criteria of cerebral death. One set of criteria was suggested by a task force organized by the National Institute of Neurological and Communicative Diseases and Stroke (Table 52–2).

Because cerebral death usually results from a severe anoxic condition that affects the brain diffusely, the cardinal clinical symptoms (1-4 in Table 52–2) reflect a complete absence of centrally mediated behavioral responses and reflexes, including respiration. However, the criteria were drafted particularly to guard against the false terminal diagnosis of patients made comatose and apneic by reversible drug intoxication or by other lesions that occasionally can mimic cerebral death. One serious and common problem is that persons with self-induced metabolic coma have often taken several drugs, including alcohol, that together may have synergistic effects and may make

the identification of drugs in the blood difficult—hence the need for stringent laboratory testing of brain viability.

The most widely used indication of brain death is an isoelectric EEG, or *electrocerebral silence*. This hybrid term is operationally defined as an EEG record with no biological activity greater than 2 μV between scalp or referential electrode pairs 10 cm or more apart with interelectrode resistance of 100–10,000 Ω (with needle electrodes, 100–100,000 Ω). While the EEG offers the most significant laboratory information concerning cerebral death, an isoelectric EEG does not indicate the location of the lesion. Electrocerebral silence occurs in about the same percentage of patients with brain stem, or infratentorial, lesions (63%) as those with diffuse cerebral lesions (60%) or focal cortical lesions (62%).

In many European countries brain death is equated with total cerebral infarction, and the absence of cerebral blood flow is the principal legal sign. Unfortunately, angiography and most other techniques for determining cerebral blood flow are currently too invasive for routine use in patients hovering between life and death. However, in more chronic cases the demonstration of intracranial circulatory arrest for 30 minutes should reasonably eliminate the possibility of cerebral viability even if blood flow can then be reestablished. Of 2650 patients surveyed who displayed coma, apnea, and an isoelectric EEG in the absence of drug intoxication and hypothermia, none survived. Thus, empirically, these criteria are conservative. However, judgments about life and death are always applied in a social context. In addition to being clinically acceptable, it is also important that the criteria not offend society's notion of what constitutes reasonable assurance of death.

Selected Readings

Black, P. McL. 1978. Brain death (two parts). N. Engl. J. Med. 299:338–344 and 393–401.

Honda, Y., and Juji, T. (eds.) 1988. HLA in Narcolepsy. Heidelberg: Springer.

Kryger, M. H., Roth, T., and Dement, W. C. (eds.) 1989. Principles and Practice of Sleep Medicine. Philadelphia: Saunders.

Lydic, R., and Biebuyck, J. F. (eds.) 1988. Clinical Physiology of Sleep. Bethesda, Md.: American Physiological Society.

Mendelson, W. B. 1987. Human Sleep: Research and Clinical Care. New York: Plenum Medical Book Co.

Plum, F., and Posner, J. B. 1980. The Diagnosis of Stupor and Coma, 3rd ed. Philadelphia: F. A. Davis.

Solomon, F., White, C. C., Parron, D. L., and Mendelson, W. B. 1979. Sleeping pills, insomnia, and medical practice (summary of report of the Institute of Medicine, National Academy of Sciences). N. Engl. J. Med. 300:803–808.

References

Association of Sleep Disorders Centers and the Association for the Psychophysiological Study of Sleep. 1979. Diagnostic classification of sleep and arousal disorders. Sleep 2:1–137.

Billiard, M., and Seignalet, J. 1985. Extraordinary association between HLA-DR2 and narcolepsy. Lancet 1: 226–227.

Brodal, A. 1981. Neurological Anatomy in Relation to Clinical

Medicine, 3rd ed. New York: Oxford University Press, chap. 6, "The Reticular Formation and Some Related Nuclei."

Carskadon, M. A., and Dement, W. C. 1987. Daytime sleepiness: Quantification of a behavioral state. Neurosci. Biobehav. Rev. 11:307–317.

Carskadon, M. A., and Dement, W. C. 1989. Normal human sleep: An overview. In M. H. Kryger, T. Roth, and W. C. Dement (eds.), Principles and Practice of Sleep Medicine. Philadelphia: Saunders, pp. 3–13.

Collaborative Study by NINDS, NIH. 1977. An appraisal of the criteria of cerebral death. A summary statement. J.A.M.A. 237:982–986.

Czeisler, C. A., Kronauer, R. E., Allan, J. S., Duffy, J. F., Jewett, M. E., Brown, E. N., and Ronda, J. M. 1989. Bright light induction of strong (Type 0) resetting of the human circadian pace maker. Science 244:1328–1333.

Dement, W., Guilleminault, C., and Zarcone, V. 1975. The pathologies of sleep: A case series approach. In D. B. Tower (ed.), The Nervous System, Vol. 2: The Clinical Neurosciences. New York: Raven Press, pp. 501–518.

Gastaut, H., Tassinari, C. A., and Duron, B. 1965. Étude polygraphique des manifestations épisodiques (hypniques et respiratoires), diurnes et nocturnes, du syndrome de Pickwick. Rev. Neurol. (Paris) 112:568–579.

Hishikawa, Y., Wakamatsu, H., Furuya, E., Sugita, Y., Masaoka, S., Kaneda, H., Sato, M., Nan'no, H., and Kaneko, Z. 1976. Sleep satiation in narcoleptic patients. Electroencephalogr. Clin. Neurophysiol. 41:1–18.

Honda, Y., Doi, Y., Juji, T., and Satake, M. 1985. Positive HLA-DR2 finding as a prerequisite for the development of narcolepsy. Folia Psychiatrica Neurol. Japon. 39:203–204.

Horne, J. A., Moore, V. J., Reid, A. J., and Shackell, B. S. 1985. Waking body temperature manipulation and subsequent sleep (SWS). Sleep Res. 14:15.

Jacobson, A., Kales, A., Lehmann, D., and Zweizig, J. R. 1965. Somnambulism: All-night electroencephalographic studies. Science 148:975–977.

Kales, A., and Kales, J. 1973. Recent advances in the diagnosis and treatment of sleep disorders. In G. Usdin (ed.), Sleep Research and Clinical Practice. New York: Brunner/Mazel, pp. 59–94.

Karacen, I., Thornby, J. I., Anch., M., Holzer, C. E., Warheit, G. J., Schwab, J. J., and Williams, R. L. 1976. Prevalence of sleep disturbance in a primarily urban Florida County. Soc. Sci. Med. 10:239–244.

Kety, S. S. 1960. Sleep and the energy metabolism of the brain. In G. E. W. Wolstenholme and M. O'Connor (eds.), The Nature of Sleep. Boston: Little, Brown, pp. 375–381.

Kupfer, D. J., and Foster, F. G. 1972. Interval between onset of sleep and rapid-eye-movement sleep as an indicator of depression. Lancet 2:684–686.

Magni, F., Moruzzi, G., Rossi, G. F., and Zanchetti, A. 1959. EEG arousal following inactivation of the lower brain stem by selective injection of barbiturate into the vertebral circulation. Arch. Ital. Biol. 97:33–46.

Mahowald, M. W., and Schenck, C. H. 1989. REM Behavior Disorder. In M. H. Kryger, T. Roth, and W. C. Dement (eds.), Principles and Practice of Sleep Medicine. Philadelphia: Saunders, pp. 389–401.

Mendelson, W. B., Cain, M., Cook, J. M., Paul, S. M., and Skolnick, P. 1983. A benzodiazepine receptor antagonist decreases sleep and reverses the hypnotic actions of flurazepam. Science 219:414–416.

Mendelson, W. B., Garnett, D., Gillin, J. C., and Weingartner, H. 1984. The experience of insomnia and daytime and nighttime functioning. Psychiatry Res. 12:235–250.

Mendelson, W. B., Weingartner, H., Greenblatt, D. J., Garnett, D., and Gillin, J. C. 1982. A clinical study of flurazepam. Sleep 5:350–360.

Mitler, M. M., and Dement, W. C. 1974. Cataplectic-like behavior in cats after micro-injections of carbachol in pontine reticular formation. Brain Res. 68:335–343.

Nicholson, A. N., Pascoe, P. A., Spencer, M. B., Stone, B. M., Roehrs, T., and Roth, T. 1986. Sleep after transmeridian flights. Lancet 2:1205–1208.

Sewitch, D. E. 1984. NREM sleep continuity and the sense of having slept in normal sleepers. Sleep. 7:147–154.

Sewitch, D. E. 1987. Slow wave sleep deficiency insomnia: A problem in thermo-downregulation at sleep onset. Psychophysiology 24:200–215.

Yoss, R. E., and Daly, D. D. 1957. Criteria for the diagnosis of the narcoleptic syndrome. Proc. Staff Meet. Mayo Clin. 32:320–328.

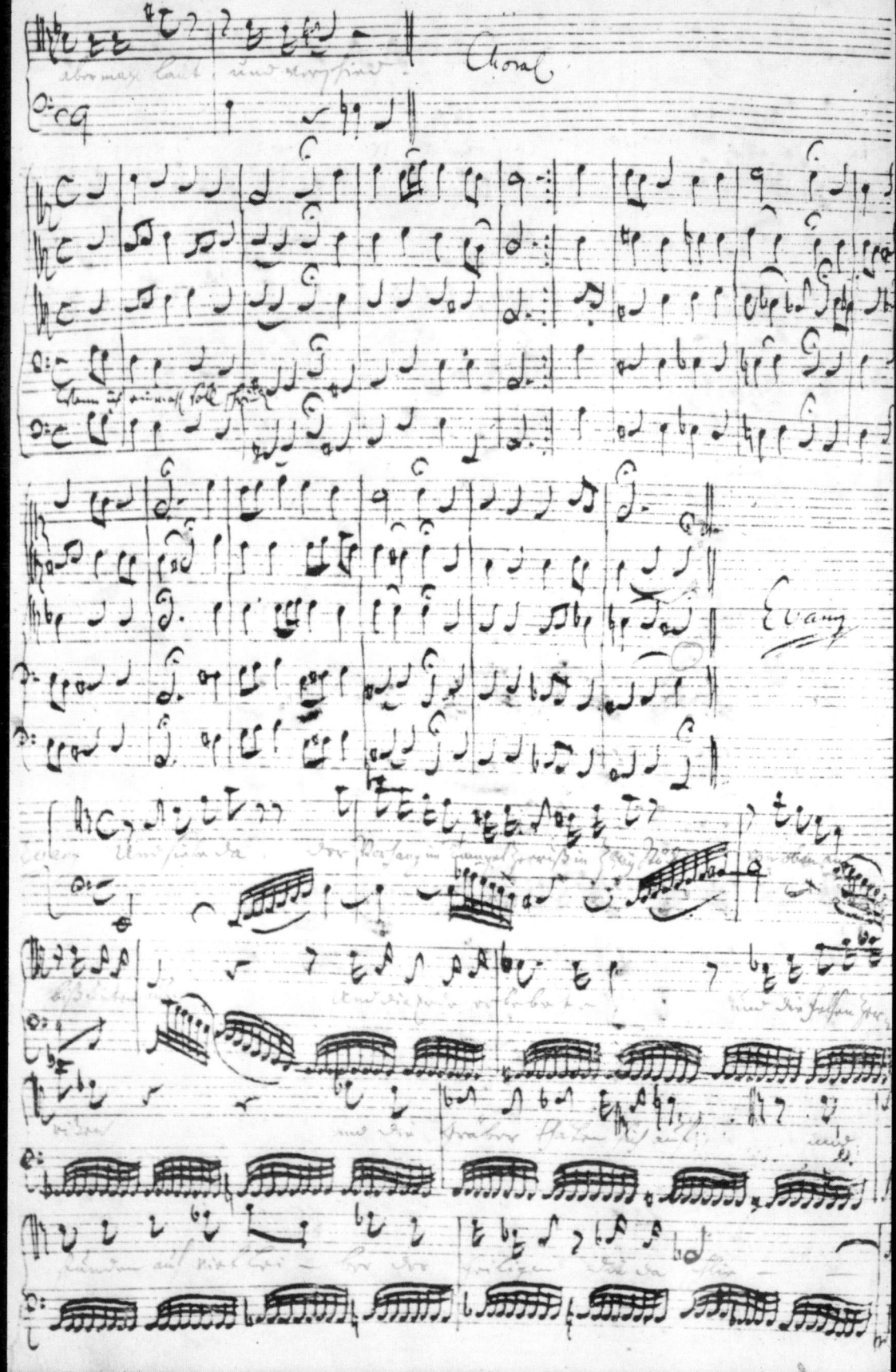

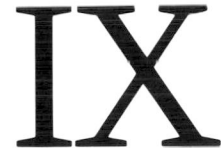

Localization of Higher Functions and the Disorders of Language, Thought, and Affect

The attempt to localize function in the cerebral cortex dates from the discovery of two types of motor control in specific areas of the frontal lobe: control of speech by Pierre Paul Broca in 1862, and control of voluntary movement by Gustav Fritsch and Eduard Hitzig in 1870. Next came the elucidation of the various primary sensory cortices—for vision, audition, somatic sensation, and taste—in the occipital, parietal, and temporal lobes. These motor and sensory cortices, however, account for less than one-half of the cerebral cortex in humans. The remaining areas, called the *association cortices*, coordinate events arising in areas dedicated to motor and sensory processes. The association cortices can be divided into three major regions: the prefrontal, which is concerned with motor functions, the parietal–temporal–occipital, which is important in sensory function, and the limbic, which is important for motivation. These areas are involved in planning, thinking, and feeling: in perception, speech, memory, and skilled movements.

Most of the early evidence relating higher cognitive functions to regions of association cortex came from clinical studies of brain damage. Study of patients with lesions of these areas, and more recently study of experimental animals, provide new insight into neural mechanisms that underlie higher mental functions. For example, the study of language and its disorders is now yielding important information about how human mental processes are distributed in the two hemispheres of the brain. In this section we shall examine the evidence that specific higher functions are related to cortical regions and that each higher mental function is controlled by several cortical regions that work together.

Music is especially suited to represent higher cognitive functions. Usually abstract, it nevertheless conforms to complex rules, requires the operation of many parts of the brain, and clearly involves both thought and affect. Another important feature is that musical talent may have a strong genetic component. This autograph copy of a page from Johann Sebastian Bach's *St. Matthew Passion* (Part II, number 72 and 73), now in the Deutsche Staatsbibliothek in der Stiftung Preussischer Kulturbesitz, Berlin-Musikabteilung (Mus. ms. Bach P 25), represents these features: The passion is complex, has strong emotional impact, and was written by a composer who had many children, five of whom are known to have been distinguished musicians and composers. In addition, his only grandson was a composer and harpsichordist to the Court of Prussia. In 1730, Bach proudly wrote that he was able to "put on a vocal and instrumental concert with my own family."

PART IX

Chapter 53: Localization of Higher Cognitive and Affective Functions: The Association Cortices
Chapter 54: Disorders of Language: The Aphasias
Chapter 55: Disorders of Thought: Schizophrenia
Chapter 56: Disorders of Mood: Depression, Mania, and Anxiety Disorders

Irving Kupfermann

Localization of Higher Cognitive and Affective Functions: The Association Cortices

The Three Association Areas Are Involved in Different Higher Functions

The Association Areas of the Frontal Region Are Thought to Be Involved in Cognitive Behavior and Motor Planning

Lesions of the Principal Sulcus in Monkeys Interfere with Specific Motor Tasks

Lesions of the Inferior Prefrontal Convexity Interfere with Appropriate Motor Responses

The Association Areas of the Limbic Cortex Are Involved in Memory and in Aspects of Emotional Behavior

The Orbitofrontal Cortex and Cingulate Gyrus Are Concerned with Emotional Behavior

The Temporal Lobe Portion of the Limbic Association Cortex Is Thought to Be Concerned with Memory Functions

The Association Areas of the Parietal Lobes Are Involved in Higher Sensory Functions and Language

The Two Hemispheres Are Not Fully Symmetrical and Differ in Their Capabilities

Split-Brain Experiments Reveal Important Asymmetries and Show That Consciousness and Self-Awareness Are Not Unitary

Why Is Function Lateralized to One Hemisphere?

Cognitive Functions Can Be Simulated by Connectionist Networks Capable of Parallel Distributed Processing

An Overall View

More than a century ago Franz Joseph Gall and his student Johann Spurzheim developed a new approach to mental function, called phrenology. Phrenologists believed that the size of specific bumps on the surface of the head reflected the size and degree of function of the underlying brain tissue. Although the experimental evidence for phrenology was eventually rejected, the idea that specific higher functions are associated with distinct cortical regions received strong support from the studies of the aphasias by Pierre Paul Broca, Karl Wernicke, and other clinical neurologists (see Chapter 1). Despite these findings, many clinical and experimental neurologists still favored the idea that the brain, and particularly the cerebral cortex, acts as a whole.

The holistic view was expounded most forcefully by Karl Lashley, who believed that with certain types of higher functions, such as learning, virtually any part of the cortex could substitute for any other. Nevertheless the proponents of the holistic view admitted that specific sensory and motor functions could be associated with well-defined anatomical loci. Later evidence, which we shall consider in this chapter, revealed that even highly complex brain functions can be associated with the operation of specific brain areas. Localization does not imply that any specific function is mediated exclusively by one region of the brain. Most functions require the integrated action of neurons in different regions. Rather, *localization of function* means that certain areas of the brain are more concerned with one kind of function than with others.

Some of the most compelling evidence for localization of higher functions has come from studies of the *association areas* of the cerebral cortex. The association areas are

TABLE 53–1. Major Sensory, Association, and Motor Cortices

Functional designation	Lobe	Location in lobe	Brodmann's area
Primary sensory cortex			
Somatic sensory	Parietal	Postcentral gyrus	1,2,3
Visual	Occipital	Calcarine fissure	17
Auditory	Temporal	Heschl's gyrus	41,42
Higher-order sensory cortex			
Somatic sensory II	Parietal	Dorsal bank of Sylvian fissure	2 (opercular portion)
Visual II	Occipital	Occipital gyri	18
Visual III, IIIa, IV, V	Occipital, temporal	Occipital gyri and superior temporal sulcus	19 and area rostral to 19
Visual Inferotemporal area	Temporal	Anterior and inferior temporal cortex	21,20
Posterior parietal cortex (somatic sensation, vision)	Parietal	Superior parietal lobule	5 (somatic) 7 (visual)
Auditory	Temporal	Superior temporal gyrus	22
Association cortex			
Parietal–temporal–occipital (polymodal sensory, language)	Parietal, temporal, and occipital	Junction between lobes	39,40 and portions of 19,21,22,37
Prefrontal (cognitive behavior and motor planning)	Frontal	Rostral portion of dorsal and lateral surface	Area rostral to 6
Limbic (emotion and memory)	Temporal, parietal, and frontal	Cingulate and parahippocampal gyri, temporal pole, and orbital surface of frontal lobe	23,24,38,28,11
Higher-order motor cortex			
Premotor (including supplementary motor area)	Frontal	Rostral to postcentral gyrus	6,8
Primary motor cortex	Frontal	Precentral gyrus	4

concerned with the integration of more than one sensory modality and with the planning of movement. They were once considered more extensive than is now believed. As our understanding of sensory and motor processes has increased, some areas that were thought to be association cortex have proved instead to be secondary or tertiary processing centers for sensory or motor information. Table 53–1 summarizes the major primary and higher-order sensory and motor areas and association areas of the cerebral cortex. In this chapter we shall focus primarily, but not exclusively, on the functions of true association areas, which are located in three regions: prefrontal association cortex, limbic association cortex, and parietal–temporal–occipital association cortex.

Because the association cortices produce few or no obvious motor or sensory effects when electrically stimulated, they were at one time called silent areas. They were believed to have two main functions: to integrate the activity of the various primary sensory cortices, and to link the sensory cortices to the motor cortices. On the basis of these roles, the association cortices were thought to be the anatomical substrates for the highest brain functions—thought and perception. Modern evidence supports this idea. Not surprisingly, the relative extent of the association cortices increases throughout phylogeny, and they reach their greatest size in humans (Figure 53–1).

FIGURE 53–1

Drawings (approximately to scale) of the cerebral hemispheres of four mammals. Note the increase both in size and relative amount of higher-order sensory, motor, and association cortices.

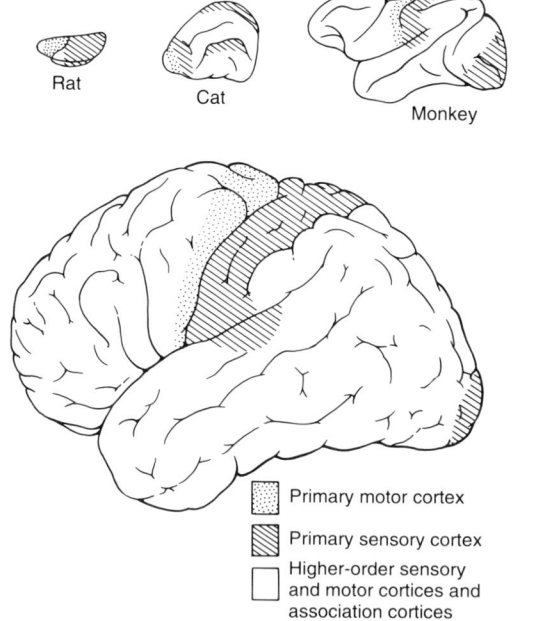

Rat   Cat   Monkey

▨ Primary motor cortex

▨ Primary sensory cortex

☐ Higher-order sensory and motor cortices and association cortices

Much of what we know about the function of association areas has come from the study of two types of patients—those with damage to the cortex (due to trauma, cerebrovascular disease, or tumors), and those who have undergone brain surgery for a behavioral or neurological disorder. Evidence from the second group of patients has been particularly instructive because each patient has had a relatively well-defined surgical lesion. In some instances, insight obtained from clinical studies has been extended by experiments on animals, in which it is possible to make localized lesions and to obtain detailed behavioral and electrophysiological information. Most recently, brain imaging techniques have begun to provide information on localization of function in normal humans.

In this chapter we shall first consider the structures and functions of the three association areas. We shall then focus on the discovery that the human brain, which has many symmetrical features, is actually not perfectly symmetrical. The left and right hemispheres each have their own special capabilities and limitations, and consequently the association areas of the cerebral cortex are not symmetrical either.

The Three Association Areas Are Involved in Different Higher Functions

How does information reach an association area of the cerebral cortex? As we have seen in Chapter 20, each primary sensory area of cortex is adjacent to and connects with a series of higher-order sensory processing centers. For example, Brodmann's area 17, the primary visual cortex, is adjacent to and interconnects with the higher-order visual cortex in area 18. These higher-order areas are concerned with more detailed analysis of sensation. Unlike primary sensory areas, the higher-order sensory cortices do not always contain maps of the peripheral receptive sheet. Higher-order sensory areas project to one or another, or to all three of the major association cortices (Figure 53–2).

Together, the association cortices are involved in many aspects of higher functions, including voluntary movement, sensory perception, cognition, emotional behavior, memory, and language. Nevertheless, a given association cortex appears to specialize in only one or another of these functions. The prefrontal cortex is concerned with complex motor actions, the parietal–temporal–occipital area with integration of sensory functions and language, and the limbic area with memory and emotional and motivational aspects of behavior. First, we briefly consider the intracortical connections of these association cortices.

The *parietal–temporal–occipital association cortex* consists of several functional areas that are intercalated between higher-order somatic, visual, and auditory areas and that receive projections from them. The parietal–temporal–occipital association cortex is therefore thought to link information from several sensory modalities, a step important in the processing of sensory information for perception and language.

The portion of the frontal lobe that is anterior to the primary motor area has traditionally been divided into two regions: premotor areas (the supplementary motor area and *premotor area*), which lie just anterior to the precentral gyrus, and the *prefrontal association cortex*, which lies anterior to the premotor area (Figure 53–2). As noted in Chapter 40, the premotor area is important in the initiation of movement. The prefrontal cortex, as we shall see later, is important for the planning of responses.

The prefrontal and premotor areas receive input from various regions of higher-order sensory cortex. Those portions of higher-order sensory cortex that are more closely connected with primary sensory areas project to the premotor cortex (which in turn projects to the motor cortex). Those areas of higher-order sensory cortex that are less directly connected to primary sensory areas project to the prefrontal cortex (which projects to the premotor cortex)

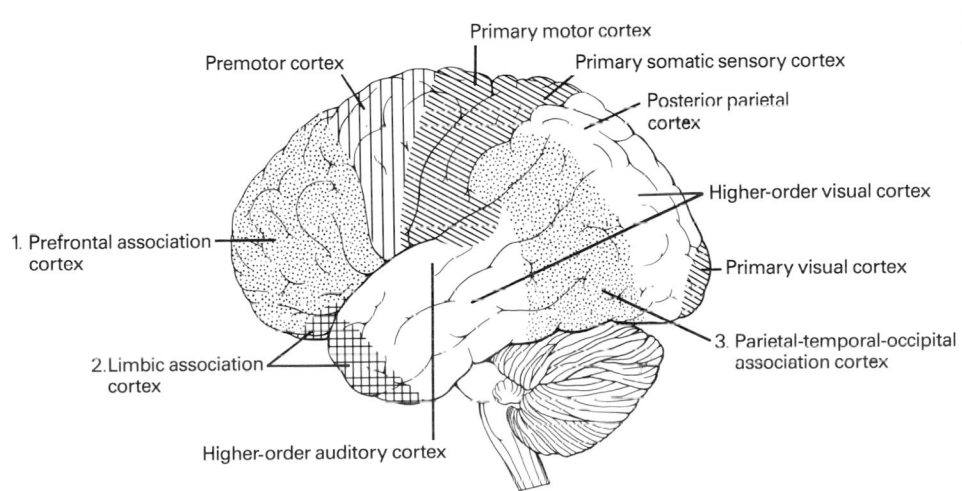

FIGURE 53–2
This schematic drawing of the lateral surface of the human brain shows the regions of the primary sensory and motor cortices, the higher-order motor and sensory cortices, and the three association cortices.

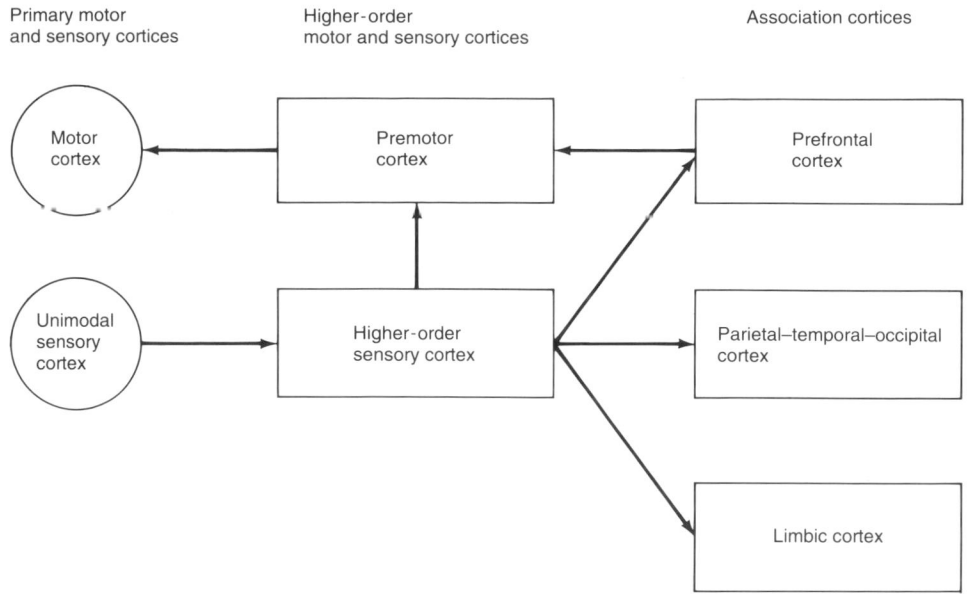

FIGURE 53-3

The intercortical connections of primary motor and sensory cortices, higher-order motor and sensory cortices, and association cortices are shown here in a simplified form. The same general pattern is repeated for each of the main primary sensory cortices (for vision, somesthesis, and hearing). For simplicity, a number of pathways, such as those interconnecting the three association cortices, have been omitted.

(Figure 53–3). These differential patterns of connections permit the more precise representation of sensory information to influence the execution of movement (by way of successive projections to the premotor and then to the motor cortex). Concomitantly, the more abstract representations of sensory information can influence the planning of movement (by way of successive projections to the prefrontal cortex, the premotor cortex, and then the motor cortex).

The *limbic association cortex* is located in the medial and ventral surfaces of the frontal lobe, the medial surface of the parietal lobe, and the anterior tip of the temporal lobe (called the *temporal pole*) (Figure 53–2). The limbic association cortex includes the orbitofrontal cortex, the cingulate region, and the parahippocampal area. It receives projections from the higher-order sensory areas and sends projections to other cortical regions, including the prefrontal cortex. This provides one pathway by which emotions can affect motor planning.

Even though the association areas are concerned with higher mental functions, they all share organizational principles with the primary sensory and motor cortices. This discovery emerged from the work of Patricia Goldman-Rakic and Walle Nauta, who found that in monkeys the pattern of termination of intercortical connections between regions of association cortex of the parietal lobe and the frontal lobe is organized into distinct, vertically oriented columns. These columns are 200–500 μm wide and extend across all layers of cortex. Thus, columnar organization is not unique to sensory or motor cortices, but is a general feature of all neocortex.

The Association Areas of the Frontal Region Are Thought to Be Involved in Cognitive Behavior and Motor Planning

The association functions of the various regions of the frontal cortex are too diverse to be easily summarized. One important function of the frontal lobes is thought to be related to the capacity of the organism to weigh the consequences of future actions and to plan accordingly. The frontal lobes integrate the interoceptive and exteroceptive information that they receive so as to select the appropriate motor response from the many available.

Functional and anatomical studies on monkeys suggest that the prefrontal association area can be divided into numerous subregions, but there are two main regions: the prefrontal association cortex proper, located on the dorsolateral surface of the frontal lobes, and the *orbitofrontal cortex*, located on the medial and ventral surface of the brain. These two regions assume prodigious proportions in nonhuman primates and humans (Figure 53–4). Both regions receive a prominent afferent input from the medial dorsal thalamic nucleus and have a prominent input layer, the granule cell layer (4). Both regions therefore are sometimes referred to as *frontal granular cortex*, in distinction to the agranular cortex of the motor and premotor areas. The orbitofrontal cortex is part of the limbic association cortex, having direct connections with limbic structures, such as the amygdala. We shall first consider the prefrontal cortex, which in the monkey has three subdivisions: principal sulcus, superior prefrontal convexity, and inferior prefrontal convexity (Figure 53–5).

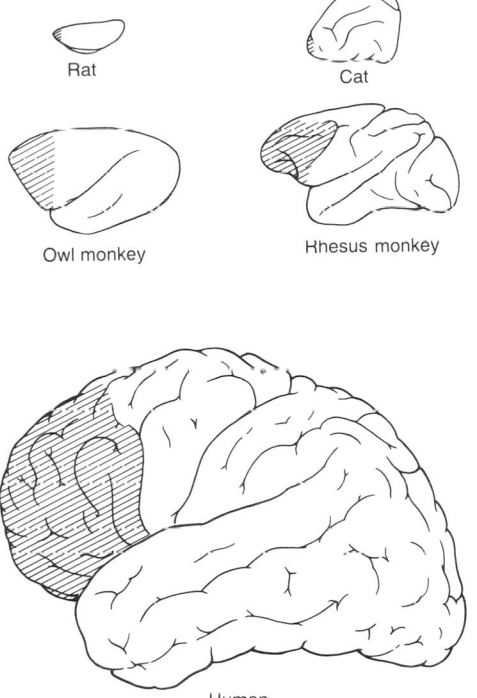

FIGURE 53–4
Proportion of the brain taken up by the frontal association cortex (**hatched area**) in five species. (Drawings not to scale.)

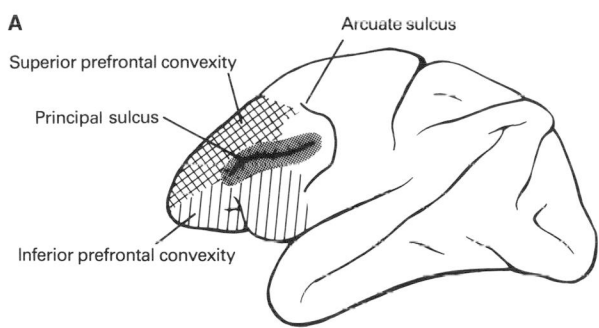

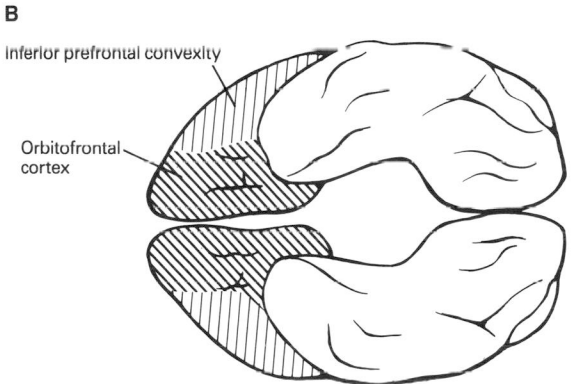

FIGURE 53–5
Simplified scheme of the basic subdivisions of the frontal association cortex of the monkey, as shown in two views. (Data from Rosenkilde, 1979.)

A. The lateral view illustrates the dorsoventral surface of the prefrontal lobe, the region of the prefrontal association cortex.

B. This ventral view illustrates the orbitofrontal cortex, a subdivision of the limbic association cortex.

Lesions of the Principal Sulcus in Monkeys Interfere with Specific Motor Tasks

The principal sulcus is concerned with the strategic planning for higher motor actions, including cognitive tasks. The first evidence leading to our understanding of the cognitive role of the principal sulcus came from a dramatic experiment in the 1930s by Carlyle Jacobsen, who studied two chimpanzees and discovered that bilateral removal of the frontal association cortex, an area that includes the principal sulcus, impairs the ability to perform a task involving delayed spatial response. In this experiment a hungry animal is shown a piece of food and, while the animal watches, the food is placed randomly under one or the other of two identical opaque containers, one on the left, one on the right. After a delay of 5 seconds or longer, the monkey is permitted to select one of the containers. Normal animals quickly learn to select the container covering the food, whereas animals with frontal damage do poorly on this task. The lesioned animals perform well only if there is no delay after the experimenter covers the food. Jacobsen therefore thought that the prefrontal region might be involved in short-term memory. Specifically, he proposed that the frontal association areas are needed for the execution of complex motor tasks in which the essential cues are not available at the time of responding but must be recalled by a short-term memory process.

Later research suggested that this interpretation is correct but that the lesions do not produce a generalized deficit involving all short-term memory. Rather, the deficit is specific for *working-memory*, a temporary storing of information used to guide a future action. Moreover, the deficit of working memory is specific to certain types of tasks. Experiments involving limited lesions of the frontal association cortex have revealed that this region is functionally heterogeneous. Functional heterogeneity has been most thoroughly studied using a type of delayed spatial response task, in which monkeys must choose alternately between two containers, one on the right and one on the left, with a delay interposed between each choice (Figure 53–6). A relatively small lesion around the principal sulcus is sufficient to produce a deficit in this task. This deficit is highly specific to this type of problem and is evident only if the task involves both a delay and a spatial aspect. Animals with lesions in the principal sulcus have no difficulty with discrimination problems in-

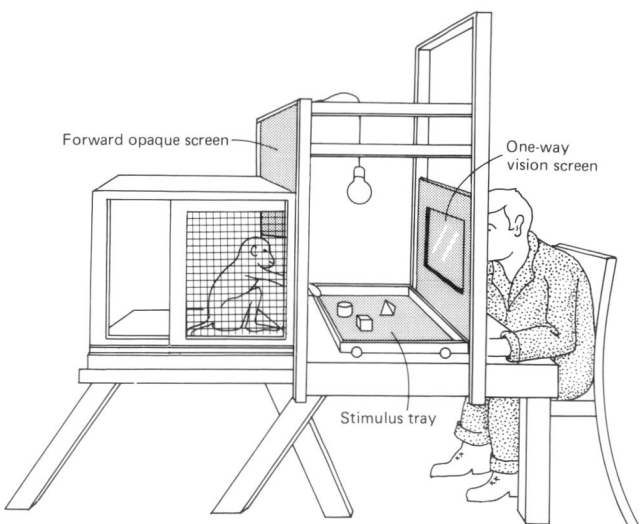

FIGURE 53–6
The Wisconsin General Testing Apparatus is used to test monkeys in a variety of discrimination and learning problems. (Adapted from Harlow, 1958.)

volving no delay or with tasks for which spatial cues are not important. For example, lesioned animals can be trained so that when shown several objects, they will correctly select that object which was shown on the previous trial. This task requires a response after a delay but does not have any spatial aspects, such as responding to the left or right cue.

The idea that the principal sulcus of the prefrontal association cortex is involved in delayed response tasks is also supported by cellular studies. Joaquin Fuster found that many neurons in this region increase their firing when a cue is presented and continue to fire throughout the delay period even when the cue is no longer there. Shintaro Funahashi, Charles Bruce, and Goldman-Rakic found that during the delay some neurons in the principal sulcus fire, whereas others are inhibited. Furthermore, during the delay period individual neurons respond only to stimuli at a particular position in the visual field, usually in the contralateral hemifield. This pattern of cellular response suggests that the prefrontal region contains a complete map of the contralateral visual field that can be used for the purpose of working memory. The adjacent frontal eye field (posterior to the principal sulcus) has a similar map, but this area appears to be specific for directing eye movements in space, whereas the principal sulcus is involved in both eye and hand movements in space.

Anatomical studies suggest that the dorsolateral prefrontal association cortex works closely with the posterior parietal association cortex; the two regions are the most densely interconnected areas of association cortex and they both project to numerous common cortical and subcortical structures (Figure 53–7). James Gnadt and Richard Andersen have found posterior parietal neurons that, like

prefrontal neurons, are active during a time period when the animal has to remember the position of a visual target to which eye movement will be made. Thus, the activity of the units may represent the intent to make an eye movement of a specific direction and amplitude.

Other lines of evidence also implicate the principal sulcus in mediating delayed response tasks. For example, Lawrence Weiskrantz and collaborators found that electrical stimulation of the prefrontal sulcus, which disrupts normal function, interferes with delayed spatial response tasks. Furthermore, Goldman-Rakic and Harold Rosvold found that a delayed response is severely disrupted when dopamine is depleted from the principal sulcus by means of localized cortical injection of 6-hydroxydopamine,

FIGURE 53–7
Common projections of parietal and prefrontal association areas. The diagram shows third-party connections of the posterior parietal and caudal principal sulcus based on double-label studies in which one anterograde tracer was injected into the prefrontal cortex and another into the parietal cortex of the same animal. Superimposition of adjacent sections shows these areas projecting to different target areas. Major targets of prefrontal and parietal projections are limbic areas on the medial surface and opercular and superior temporal cortices on the lateral surface. **Stippling**, intraparietal sulcus and principal sulcus. (From Goldman-Rakic, 1987.)

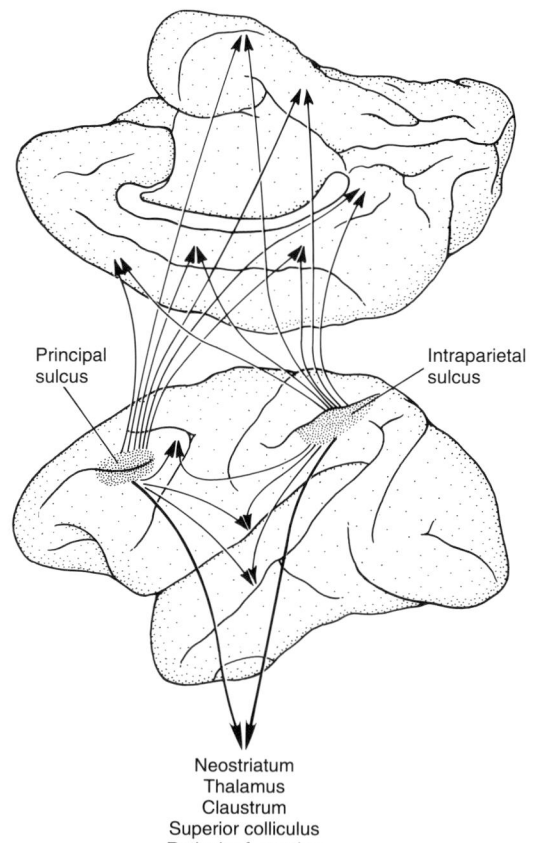

which selectively destroys terminals that use catecholamines as their transmitter.

These findings are interesting clinically. Delayed response involves several conceptual skills: visual discrimination, short-term memory, and planning and execution of a visual motor task. Since the prefrontal cortex is essential for tasks of this complexity, it is likely that it participates in a variety of related cognitive skills. In addition, the prefrontal area of primates and other animals has a particularly prominent dopaminergic innervation; since depletion of dopamine from this area produces effects similar to those of lesions, disturbances of this system may contribute to human cognitive disorders, such as schizophrenia, that are thought to involve alterations in dopaminergic transmission in the brain (see Chapter 55).

Imaging studies of the brains of schizophrenic patients support this idea. The frontal lobe tends to be smaller in schizophrenics than in normal individuals. Furthermore, when challenged by a task that engages prefrontal functions, such as the Wisconsin Card Sort Test (described later in the chapter), blood flow into the prefrontal areas of normal people increases, whereas no such increase is seen in many people with schizophrenia. In normal, nonmoving, unstimulated persons, the blood flow and metabolism of the frontal lobes is considerably higher than that of postcentral regions. This hyperfrontal pattern has been interpreted to reflect cognitive activity of the frontal lobes, even when the brain is otherwise at rest. These regional differences are less marked or are absent in sleep or coma.

Lesions of the Inferior Prefrontal Convexity Interfere with Appropriate Motor Responses

In contrast to lesions of the principal sulcus, lesions of the inferior prefrontal convexity affect the ability of an animal to perform any type of delayed response whether or not it has a spatial element. These lesions appear to interfere with tasks that require the animal to inhibit certain motor responses at appropriate times. Lesions of the arcuate concavity, which is adjacent to the principal sulcus, do not disturb delayed response, however, they diminish the animal's ability to choose among various types of motor responses in response to different sensory cues. For example, animals have difficulty learning a task in which they must move to the left when an auditory cue comes from above the cage, or move to the right when the cue comes from below the cage.

The Association Areas of the Limbic Cortex Are Involved in Memory and in Aspects of Emotional Behavior

The limbic association cortex consists of several major subareas located in different lobes: the orbitofrontal cortex, the cingulate gyrus, and portions of the temporal lobe. We shall first consider the orbitofrontal cortex and cingulate gyrus.

The Orbitofrontal Cortex and Cingulate Gyrus Are Concerned with Emotional Behavior

Jacobsen and later investigators found that if lesions of the frontal cortex encompass regions of the frontal limbic cortex, which includes orbitofrontal or anterior cingulate cortex, the result is an alteration of the emotional responsiveness of animals, in addition to deficits of delayed responses. For example, lesioned animals sometimes fail to exhibit signs of rage and anger when they do not receive expected rewards in a training task. If damage is limited to the orbitofrontal cortex, the normal aggressiveness and emotional responsiveness of primates is reduced. Furthermore, electrical stimulation of the orbitofrontal cortex produces many autonomic responses (increases in arterial blood pressure, dilation of the pupils, salivation, and inhibition of gastrointestinal contractions), suggesting that this area may be involved in a generalized arousal reaction. This interpretation is supported by the observation that orbitofrontal stimulation induces a generalized desynchronization of the cortical electroencephalogram (see Chapter 50) and increases plasma cortisol. Finally, lesions that include limbic association cortex also reduce chronic intractable pain, suggesting still another effect of the limbic cortex on emotional behavior (see Chapter 47).

In 1935 John Fulton and Jacobsen reported their observations of the calming effect of frontal cortical lesions (lobotomy) in chimpanzees. Egas Moniz, a Portuguese neuropsychiatrist, attended this meeting and suggested that severance of the frontal–limbic association connections in humans might serve as a treatment for severe mental illness. Moniz assembled a surgical team and performed the first prefrontal lobotomies in humans within a few months of Fulton and Jacobsen's report.

These early attempts were soon followed by extensive application of various procedures that involved either ablation of frontal association areas or interruption of the fiber tracts that connect the frontal lobes with subcortical structures or other areas of cortex. These tracts include the cingulum, a bundle of axons in the cingulate gyrus that contains aminergic fibers from the brain stem as well as fibers that connect the frontal and parietal lobes with the parahippocampal gyrus and adjacent temporal cortex. A second major surgical procedure (capsulotomy) involves sectioning the anterior limb of the internal capsule, which contains axons that connect the medial dorsal nucleus of the thalamus with the prefrontal cortex.

The early results of frontal lobotomy appeared favorable. Many patients seemed to show a reduction in anxiety. The results from later, more controlled studies were equivocal. Furthermore, lobotomy was associated with a high incidence of complications, including the development of epilepsy and abnormal personality changes, such as a lack of inhibition or a lack of initiative and drive. However, intellectual capability as measured on conventional tests of intelligence was little affected, even though large lesions were made. This was surprising since the huge frontal lobes in humans were thought to be related to higher mental functions, such as abstract thought and reasoning.

Although global intelligence is not greatly affected by frontal lesions (which include prefrontal cortex and premotor cortex), lobotomized patients do show deficits in certain specific tasks. Brenda Milner found that patients with frontal lesions experience difficulty in changing strategies when required to do so. For example, they do poorly on the Wisconsin Card Sort Test. This task requires that the individual sort picture cards on the basis of some criterion (such as similar colors or shapes). When the patient solves the problem, the solution is changed, and the patient must select on the basis of a different criterion. The patients with frontal lesions persist with their previously successful solution; they fail to alter their choices, even when informed that their choices are no longer correct. Perseverance and failure to inhibit inappropriate responses are frequently observed in monkeys with frontal lesions, particularly of the inferior frontal convexity. Patients with frontal lesions also show difficulty in rapid verbal naming from memory and in performing certain types of pencil-and-paper maze tasks. In addition, studies by Bryan Kolb and his colleagues suggest that these patients may exhibit a generalized decrease in spontaneity of behavior.

After several studies failed to show clear benefits from prefrontal psychosurgery, the use of these operations dwindled in the 1950s. In recent years there has been increased interest in modified forms of psychosurgery based on attempts to make highly localized lesions that might reduce anxiety without producing unfavorable side effects. Several studies suggest that a small lesion limited to the cingulum produces favorable results. Despite the relatively high percentage of patients who show improvement, it is not possible to conclude unequivocally that the improvement is due to lesion of a specific structure rather than to a placebo effect or to spontaneous recovery. In drug studies the drug can be administered and withdrawn, thus allowing an accurate assessment of the drug's effectiveness. The effects of brain surgery, however, are irreversible. These studies therefore require a matched sample of untreated control patients, and this requirement is rarely fulfilled. Despite the fact that frontal lobe surgery for the treatment of behavioral disorders has been practiced for over a half century, the formidable ethical and scientific questions regarding this procedure are not settled (see for example *The Psychosurgery Debate*, edited by Elliot Valenstein).

The Temporal Lobe Portion of the Limbic Association Cortex Is Thought to Be Concerned with Memory Functions

In monkeys, lesions of the inferior temporal region, a higher-order visual region, result in deficits in the rate of learning of visual tasks. The deficits, which are not due to blindness, are most dramatic when the visual task is com-plex. For example, inferior temporal lesions interfere with the ability of an animal to improve performance progressively (to develop a learning set) when a long series of related visual problems is presented. In addition to interfering with the *acquisition* of a learned visual task, these lesions interfere with the *retention* or *memory* of visual tasks. Similarly, damage to the superior temporal cortex of animals does not produce deafness, but impairs learning of auditory patterns (such as discriminating dah, dit, dah, from dit, dah, dit).

As we saw in Chapter 1, major insights into the functions of the human temporal lobes have come from the work of the neurosurgeon Wilder Penfield. Penfield stimulated various points on the temporal lobe electrically in awake patients before he removed diseased epileptic tissue. As expected, stimulation of the primary auditory areas produced crude auditory sensations. In contrast, stimulation of the superior temporal gyrus produced alterations in the perception of sounds, and auditory illusions and hallucinations. The hallucinations had a rather startling feature. The patients reported that the experience was remarkably real, almost as if they were actually re-experiencing a past event. The evocation of complex experiential phenomena after stimulation of the temporal lobes appears to occur only in patients with epilepsy in the temporal lobe; such experiences are relatively specific to the temporal lobe and are not reported when other cortical areas are stimulated.

Many of the patients studied by Penfield and others had a temporal lobe subsequently removed for the treatment of epilepsy. The lesion did not include Wernicke's speech area, but did typically include portions of the hippocampus. The capacities of these patients have been thoroughly studied by Milner. In the few patients in whom both the left and the right temporal lobes were removed, there was a profound and irreversible impairment of the capacity to form certain types of long-term memories (see Chapter 64).

Milner also found some interference with memory after unilateral damage of a temporal lobe, although the deficit was mild compared with the bilateral lesions. Furthermore, the degree of impairment depended on the side of the brain that had the lesion and on the type of material to be memorized. Patients whose left temporal lobes had been lesioned had difficulty remembering verbal material, such as a list of nouns. Patients with a right-sided lesion had normal verbal memory but were impaired in their ability to remember patterns of sensory input. When presented with a series of pictures of human faces, some of which were repeated, patients in whom the right temporal lobe had been removed had difficulty remembering whether they had previously seen a given face. These patients had no difficulty with geometric figures, but had problems with irregular patterns of line drawings.

One explanation for these observations may be the existence of neurons in the temporal cortex that specifically respond to images of faces, since such cells have been identified in nonhuman primates (see Chapter 30). An additional factor is that geometric patterns can easily be named and then stored as verbal data (square, triangle, etc.), but faces and irregular patterns cannot be readily encoded verbally. Studies of brain-damaged patients have repeatedly demonstrated that left-hemisphere lesions impair the processing of verbal material, while right-hemisphere lesions interfere with the processing of nonverbal information.

Stimulation (or ablation) of the temporal portion of the limbic association cortex alters emotions. For example, Penfield reported that stimulation of the anterior and medial temporal cortex could produce emotional feelings, particularly fear. The role of the temporal lobes in emotional behavior is also supported by the finding of a so-called temporal lobe personality in patients with temporal-lobe epilepsy. As described in Chapter 1, these patients tend to have an overall deepening of emotional responses. They also have a variety of other personality characteristics that suggest altered emotional responses. Finally, as we shall see in Chapter 56, brain-imaging studies by Eric Reiman and Marcus Raichle and their associates have revealed that the anterior poles of the temporal lobes may be activated during emotional experiences, such as anticipating an electric shock or during (and even before) panic attacks.

The Association Areas of the Parietal Lobes Are Involved in Higher Sensory Functions and Language

The anterior parietal lobe contains the primary somatic sensory cortex, whereas the more posterior region contains higher-order sensory areas (the posterior parietal association area) and an association area of extensive polymodal convergence. Studies of the posterior parietal cortex (Brodmann's areas 5 and 7) of animals and humans have revealed that lesions in this area produce subtle deficits in the learning of tasks requiring knowledge of the body in space.

Studies of single cells in the parietal cortex of monkeys by Vernon Mountcastle and his colleagues and by David Robinson, Michael Goldberg, and their colleagues reveal that certain cells respond to visual stimuli or to visually guided movements. Unlike cells in the visual cortex, the intensity of the response of these cells to a series of identical stimuli is remarkably variable. In particular, the activity of the cells is enhanced when the animal pays attention to the stimulus. These results are consistent with the notion that the parietal cortex is involved with attention to the spatial aspects of sensation and perhaps with the manipulation of objects in space. This interpretation is also supported by the anatomical finding that the parietal and prefrontal cortex regions that are involved in spatial aspects of sensory processing, are interconnected and project to common targets.

Patients with damage to the parietal lobes often show striking deficits, including abnormalities in body image

and perception of spatial relations. In addition, damage to the dominant (usually left) parietal lobe tends to produce *aphasia* (disorders of language, see Chapter 54), and *agnosia* (the inability to perceive objects through otherwise normally functioning sensory channels). A particularly dramatic agnosia after damage to the parietal cortex is *astereognosia*, an inability to recognize the form of objects by touch even though there is no pronounced loss of somatosensory sensitivity.

A historically important syndrome associated with damage to the inferior regions of the left parietal cortex is known as *Gerstmann's syndrome*. Patients with Gerstmann's syndrome are characterized by (1) *left–right confusion*, an inability to distinguish between left and right, (2) *finger agnosia*, difficulty in naming fingers when a specific finger is touched, despite the absence of major deficits of finger sensations, (3) *dysgraphia*, a writing disability, despite the absence of motor or sensory deficits of the upper extremities, and (4) *dyscalculia*, an inability to carry out mathematical calculations. Not all the symptoms are seen in every patient with inferior parietal lobe damage, even in those with large lesions, and consequently this tetrad of symptoms may be of limited diagnostic utility.

Balint's syndrome is also instructive for understanding the function of posterior parietal cortex. This syndrome is seen following bilateral damage to the parieto-occipital regions and consists of (1) an inability to make voluntary eye movements to a point in space, although spontaneous eye movements are unaffected, (2) a deficit in using visual guidance to grasp an object (*optic ataxia*), and (3) difficulty in attending to visual stimuli.

Lesions of the nondominant (usually right) parietal lobe do not cause obvious disturbances of language. Instead, patients with right parietal lobe damage demonstrate a lack of appreciation of the spatial aspects of all sensory input from the left side of the body as well as of external space. Although somatic sensations are relatively intact, patients sometimes completely ignore half of the body (*neglect syndrome*) and may fail to dress, undress, and wash the affected side. The patients may deny that their arm or leg belongs to them when the limb is passively brought into their field of vision. They may also deny the existence of associated hemiplegia and may attempt to leave the hospital prematurely since they feel there is nothing wrong with them. Disturbance of the appreciation of external space is seen as neglect of visual stimuli on that side of the body. These patients sometimes also exhibit a severe disturbance in their ability to copy drawn figures (*constructional apraxia*). In some patients this deficit may be so severe that the patient may draw a figure in which one-half of the body is completely left out.

Patients with a neglect syndrome due to an inferior right parietal lesion can show a deficit in the processing of the nonsyntactic component of language. Kenneth Heilman found that patients with lesions in the inferior right parietal lobe fail to appreciate those aspects of a verbal message that are conveyed by the tone, loudness, and timing of the words (e.g., emotional tone) as opposed to the literal sense of the words. The patients also have difficulty in modulating the sound of their speech and convey poorly the affective aspects of language. As we shall see again in Chapter 54, these observations suggest that the right homolog of Wernicke's area may also be concerned with language and, specifically, with intonation and other nonsyntactic aspects of language.

The Two Hemispheres Are Not Fully Symmetrical and Differ in Their Capabilities

As recently as 1968 it was widely believed that there was no gross anatomical asymmetry in the human brain. At that time Norman Geschwind and Walter Levitsky published the results of a simple experiment. They studied the gross dimensions of 100 human brains, using a camera and a ruler to make measurements of the *planum temporale*, a region on the upper surface of the temporal lobe that includes the classical speech area of Wernicke. The results were clear-cut (Figure 53–8). The left planum was larger in 65% of the brains; the right planum was larger in only 11% of the brains; and in 24% of the brains the left and right sides were approximately equal in size. Later work with a variety of techniques, including computerized tomography, confirmed these results and established that similar asymmetries are present even in the human fetus. These observations suggest that an inherent anatomical asymmetry may initially favor the left hemisphere for the development of language functions. Once one hemisphere begins to specialize, it may excel at that function, which could in turn prompt its further development.

In addition to being asymmetrical, the two hemispheres differ in their capabilities—an important discovery in the study of cortical localization. Several techniques have illustrated this in patients without brain damage. One procedure of great clinical importance is the *sodium amytal test*, which was developed to determine the dominant hemisphere for speech functions in order to avoid neurosurgical procedures that might destroy language ability. In this test the patient is instructed to count aloud or speak. Meanwhile, sodium amytal, a fast-acting barbiturate, is injected into the left or right internal carotid artery. The drug is preferentially carried to the hemisphere on the same side as it is injected and produces a brief period of dysfunction of that hemisphere. When the hemisphere dominant for speech is affected, the patient stops speaking and does not respond to a command to continue.

The relationship between handedness and lateralization of speech functions was one of the first problems explored with the sodium amytal test. Do left-handed individuals have left-hemisphere speech, as do right-handed people, or do they have right-hemisphere speech? The test has revealed that almost all right-handed people have left-hemisphere speech. Surprisingly, the majority of left-handed people also have left-hemisphere speech, but a

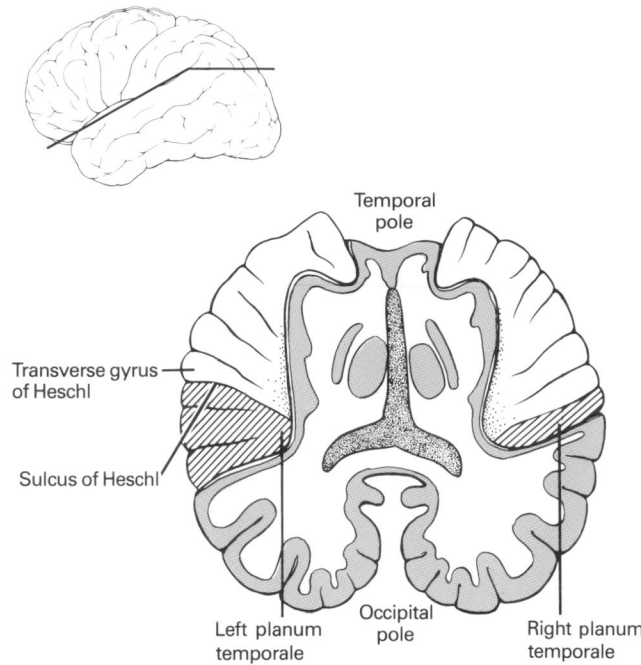

FIGURE 53–8
The planum temporale is larger in the left hemisphere than in the right in the majority of human brains (horizontal section in the plane of the Sylvian fissure). (Adapted from Geschwind and Levitsky, 1968.)

significant number (15%) have right-hemisphere speech. Furthermore, some left-handed people have control of speech in both the right and left hemispheres (Table 53–2). In these patients neither right nor left injections of sodium amytal suppress speech function. Thus, the restriction of language to one hemisphere is largely or completely absent in some left-handed people.

The sodium amytal test has yielded another unexpected result. Unilateral injection of the drug affects not only speech, but also mood. Some studies indicate that the effect on mood is related to the side of injection: left injections tend to produce a brief depression, and right injections, euphoria. The effects occur at doses smaller than those needed to block speech. These results suggest that functions related to mood may also be lateralized in the human brain to some degree. This is consistent with the clinical observation that some patients with damage to the left hemisphere are exceptionally upset about their

TABLE 53–2. Linguistic Dominance and Handedness

Handedness	Dominant hemisphere (%)		
	Left	Right	Both
Left or mixed handed	70	15	15
Right handed	96	4	0

(Data from Rasmussen and Milner, 1977.)

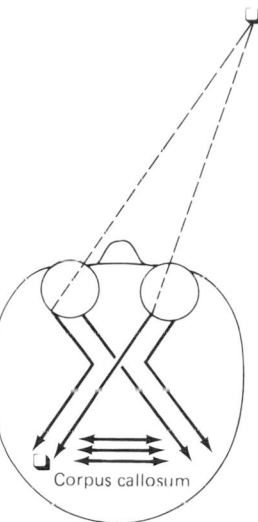

FIGURE 53–9
An image in the right visual field stimulates the left temporal retina and right nasal retina. Because projections from the nasal retina project contralaterally, whereas those from the temporal retina project ipsilaterally (shown in a superior view of the brain), the information projects to the left hemisphere, although it can secondarily reach the right hemisphere if the corpus callosum is intact.(Adapted from Sperry, 1968.)

symptoms. In contrast, some patients with damage to the right hemisphere exhibit a pathological indifference to their disability.

Results from several indirect, noninvasive methods correlate well with those from the sodium amytal test. In one test a tachistoscope is used. This device presents very brief visual stimuli to the right or left visual hemifield. Subjects are given tasks that engage either visuospatial processes (e.g., recognizing a face) or verbal processes (e.g., recognizing a word). Because of the crossing of the visual pathways, the image of a visual stimulus restricted to one visual field is projected first to the opposite hemisphere (Figure 53–9). The information is then transmitted, presumably in a slightly degraded form, to the other hemisphere via the corpus callosum. On verbal tasks, right-handed subjects typically perform slightly better when the stimuli are presented to the right visual field, which is contralateral to the speech hemisphere. In contrast, spatial tasks are performed better when stimuli are presented to the left visual field. Left-handed subjects show greater variability with regard to the visual field superior for the task.

Similar results are obtained with the *dichotic auditory task*, in which hemispheric lateralization is assessed by simultaneously presenting different auditory stimuli to both ears and determining which ear is better at recognizing the auditory inputs. In right-handed subjects the left ear tends to be better for nonverbal auditory tasks (e.g., recognition of music), whereas the right ear is better for

verbal material. The results of this test suggest that the crossed auditory pathways are more important for perception than the uncrossed pathways.

Split-Brain Experiments Reveal Important Asymmetries and Show That Consciousness and Self-Awareness Are Not Unitary

Perhaps the most dramatic evidence for the localization of function to one rather than another hemisphere comes from research on epileptic patients in whom the corpus callosum and anterior commissure (the major fiber pathways interconnecting the two hemispheres) have been cut in an attempt to prevent the spread of epileptic activity from one side of the brain to the other. Studies of these patients show that each hemisphere is capable of functioning independently when isolated from its companion. Although the right hemisphere is generally mute and cannot communicate about its experience verbally, it can do many of the things that the verbal hemisphere is capable of doing. Such basic processes as sensory analysis, memory, learning, and calculation can be performed by either hemisphere. The ability of the right hemisphere is very limited, however, when the task involves complex reasoning or analysis.

Intuitively, it seems obvious that the corpus callosum and other commissures integrate the functions of the two hemispheres. Yet it is difficult to tell from casual observation that there is anything wrong with patients with sectioned hemispheric commissures. Indeed, early investigators failed to find any deficiencies. By 1940 Warren McCulloch concluded with irony that the only certain role of the corpus callosum was "to aid in the transmission of epileptic seizures from one to the other side of the body." As recently as 1950 Lashley facetiously reiterated his feeling that the purpose of the corpus callosum "must be mainly mechanical . . . to keep the hemispheres from sagging."

The functional role of the hemispheric commissures first became apparent in split-brain studies of animals by Ronald Myers and Roger Sperry. In addition to sectioning the corpus callosum, Myers and Sperry limited visual input to one hemisphere by cutting the optic chiasm and thereby destroying the crossed visual fibers. The split-brain animals were trained in complex visual discriminations using one eye; unlike normal animals, when tested with the untrained eye, they behaved as if they were completely naive. The effects of the training experience were limited to the hemisphere receiving the visual input.

Later, in a classic series of studies, Sperry, Michael Gazzaniga, and Joseph Bogen examined the function of the corpus callosum in humans by carefully studying a group of epileptic patients whose corpus callosum had been sectioned. Sperry and his colleagues not only confirmed the earlier studies on animals, but also demonstrated that under certain experimental conditions these patients were severely limited in the ability to perform tasks that required one hemisphere to work independently of the other.

One reason these patients do so well in real-life situations, despite the absence of direct interhemispheric communication, is that ordinarily both hemispheres independently obtain similar information that allows integration of function. For example, each hemisphere ordinarily receives a complete representation of the world. Since the optic chiasm is intact in these patients, portions of the same visual images are projected to each hemisphere. However, Sperry and Gazzaniga could arrange the experimental situation so that these cross-cues were eliminated. One simple way to accomplish this is to present visual stimuli with a tachistoscope to either the right or left visual field. Such visual stimuli project only to the opposite hemisphere, for in the absence of callosal fibers the briefly presented visual information is unable to gain access to the ipsilateral hemisphere (Figure 53–9).

A simple experiment using this technique immediately revealed the deficit. When a subject was presented with an apple in the right visual field and questioned about what he saw, he said—not surprisingly—"apple." If, however, the apple was presented to the left visual field the patient denied having seen anything, or if prompted to give an answer, guessed or confabulated. This is not because the right hemisphere is blind or is unable to remember a simple stimulus. The patient could readily identify the object if he could point to it or, using tactile cues, could pick it out from several others presented under a cover (Figure 53–10). Thus, when visual stimuli were limited to the right hemisphere, the patient could not *name* what he saw but was able to identify the object by nonverbal means. This suggests that although the right hemisphere cannot talk, it indeed can perceive, learn, remember, and issue commands for motor tasks.

Furthermore, the right hemisphere may be capable of primitive understanding of language. For example, many words projected to the right hemisphere can be read and understood. If the letters D-O-G were flashed to the right hemisphere (the left visual field), the patient selected a model of a dog with his left hand. More complicated verbal input to the right hemisphere, such as commands, were comprehended poorly. The right hemisphere appears to be almost totally incapable of language *output* but is able to process very simple linguistic inputs.

The right hemisphere is not merely a copy of the left hemisphere without verbal capacity, however. In fact, on certain perceptual tasks the right hemisphere performs better than the left. For example, in a task involving fitting together pieces of colored wooden blocks to make a coherent pattern, patients performed better with the left hand than with the right. Thus, as indicated earlier, the nonspeech hemisphere is superior on spatial-perceptual problems.

There is some indication that in commissurotomized patients the two hemispheres not only can function independently, but even interfere with each other's function. In block design tasks performed with the nondominant hand (the hand ipsilateral to the verbal hemisphere), the

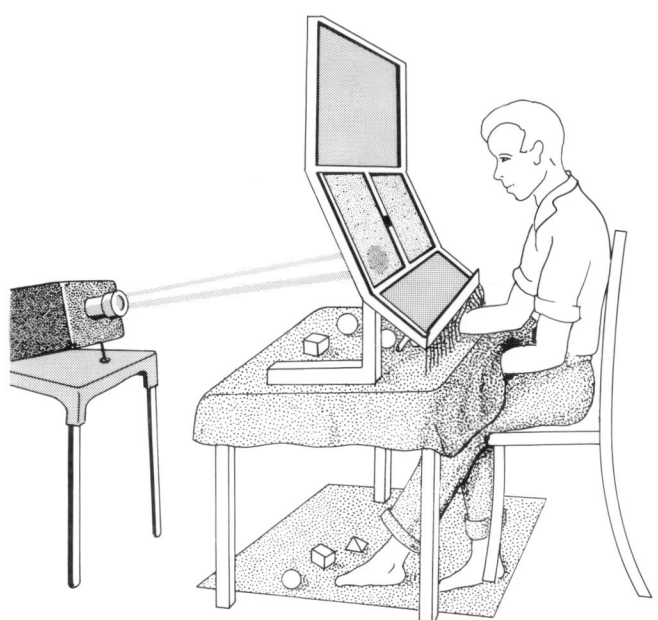

FIGURE 53–10

In this experimental setup a commissurotomized subject's gaze is fixed between the two screens. Words or images of objects can be briefly flashed on the translucent screens in either the left or right visual field of the subject. The subject can identify the stimuli either verbally or nonverbally by touching and then pointing to objects hidden behind the screen. (Adapted from Sperry, 1968.)

dominant hand sometimes attempts to interfere, usually impeding the successful solution of the problem. In addition, the dominant hemisphere sometimes initiates verbal comments about the performance of the nondominant hemisphere, frequently exhibiting a false sense of confidence on problems in which it cannot know the solution, since the information was projected exclusively to the nondominant hemisphere.

Studies of patients in which the corpus callosum has been sectioned have led to the notion that these individuals function with two independent minds, the left under the control of consciousness, the right largely functioning unconsciously and automatically. In these patients either hemisphere is capable of directing behavior. Which hemisphere gains control seems to depend on which hemisphere is best suited for the type of task to be performed. This is seen clearly in experiments with chimeric figures, for example, a face in which the right half is male and the left half is female (Figure 53–11). When shown this chimeric figure, commissurotomized patients report that the face is that of a man; but if asked to select the face from a series of whole faces, they point to a female face. Presumably, either hemisphere is capable of pointing; nevertheless, in this task the more competent right hemisphere is in control. When the task requires a verbal answer, of which the right hemisphere is incapable, the left hemisphere controls the task.

Each isolated hemisphere has its own strengths and weaknesses with regard to a given task. Certain tasks are best performed in an analytic mode, in which the problem

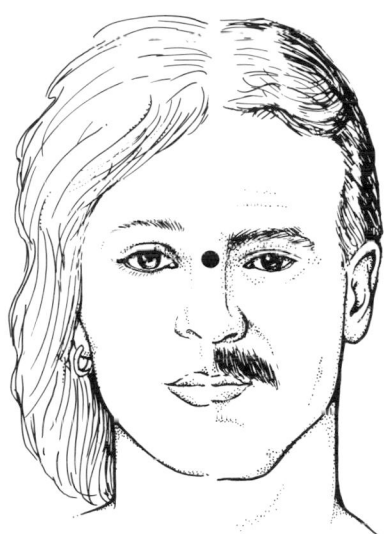

FIGURE 53–11

Hybrid (chimeric) figures, like this face, are used in experiments with commissurotomized patients to clarify the circumstances under which each hemisphere exerts dominant control. After fixating on the dot in the center of the figure, the patient is asked to describe verbally what he sees or to point to a face that matches the one he sees. When a verbal response is required, the left hemisphere predominates; since the left hemisphere receives its input from the right visual field, the patient reports seeing the face of a man. In the pointing task the right hemisphere (which receives input from the left visual field) exerts dominant control, and the patient responds by pointing to the face of a woman.

is broken down into logical elements. This type of task is well suited to verbalization and verbal encoding. Other tasks may be best performed not by sequential analysis but by some type of simultaneous processing of the whole input. For example, we ordinarily recognize a familiar face not by serially determining that it has or does not have given features, say a mustache, glasses, and small nose, but rather by some process by which all these elements are simultaneously integrated into a single perception. The face simply looks familiar or not familiar. If we had to verbalize how we recognize a face, we would find it difficult and time-consuming.

It is sometimes said that we may think of our brains as consisting of a left hemisphere that excels in intellectual, rational, verbal, and analytical thinking, and a right hemisphere that excels in perceiving and in emotional, nonverbal, and intuitive thinking. Current research, however, emphasizes that in the normal brain with extensive commissural connections the interaction of the two hemispheres is such that it is not likely we shall ever be able to dissociate clearly the specialized functions of the two hemispheres. In fact, there is now evidence that the capacity of one hemisphere to perform a particular task may deteriorate following commissurotomy. For example, Gazzaniga has described a patient who could perform a tactile task (discrimination of the detailed shapes of wire

figures) with either hand before split-brain surgery. After the surgery the subject could not perform the task with either hand, suggesting that interaction between the hemispheres for this task is needed, even though other evidence indicates that this task may primarily be mediated by the right hemisphere. Thus, despite the dramatic differences in capacities of the isolated hemispheres, when they are interconnected they seem to aid one another in a variety of tasks, both verbal and nonverbal.

Why Is Function Lateralized to One Hemisphere?

The question as to why lateralization of function exists in the human brain involves two major issues. First, how does lateralization develop within the life span of the individual? Second, what functional advantages, if any, does lateralization confer? We shall consider each of these questions in turn.

Analysis of verbal deficits in children who have sustained left- or right-hemisphere damage suggests that left dominance is already present when language is first expressed. Nevertheless, in sharp contrast to adults, children who sustain damage to the left hemisphere, even substantial damage, usually recover language capability in later life because the right hemisphere can perform language functions if the left hemisphere is nonfunctional.

If either hemisphere can attain linguistic competence in the developing individual, why does the left hemisphere become dominant in most people? It is likely that, at least in part, dominance develops in the left hemisphere because of an inherent anatomical asymmetry in the human brain, which is present even in the human fetus. As mentioned earlier, this asymmetry may initially favor the left hemisphere for language functions. Specialization of function in turn prompts further development in that area. It has been suggested that functions that require extensive intracortical connectivity may become lateralized. The number of fibers within the corpus callosum, which provides connections between the hemispheres, is far less than the number of intracortical fibers within a hemisphere. In fact, if the corpus callosum provided a richness of connections comparable to that of the intracortical connections, it would have to be as big as the brain. Thus, within the limited size of the cranial cavity, it may be computationally advantageous to locate highly complex functions, such as language, primarily to one hemisphere.

One would expect some insight into the possible advantages or disadvantages of lateralization of function to emerge from studies of the capacities of left-handed individuals, since a relatively high proportion of them appear to lack distinct lateralization. Nevertheless, careful studies of populations of normal individuals have not revealed any deficits in left-handed people. Curiously, a number of studies have indicated that in various clinical populations with behavioral problems there is a slightly greater incidence of individuals who are left-handed or who exhibit incomplete lateralization. An above normal incidence of left-handedness has been reported among patients with epilepsy, cerebral palsy, stuttering, mental retardation, and dyslexia. One possible reason for this is that the incidence of brain damage may be slightly higher in left-handed individuals than in right-handed individuals. When (and if) early brain damage produces a switch of handedness, it results in a greater number of right to left switches than left to right, simply because there is a much greater incidence of right handedness. Of course, the overwhelming majority of left-handed individuals do not have brain damage. Although on theoretical grounds cerebral lateralization should provide for more efficient function, as yet there is no conclusive evidence establishing this point.

Whatever factors promote lateralization of function, they are not limited to humans. Anatomical asymmetry of the brain has been demonstrated in the great apes, monkeys, cats, rats, and birds. This is particularly well documented in birds that learn their song by listening to other birds. There are also interesting sex differences in hemispheric dominance in birds as there are in human beings (Chapter 61). Fernando Nottebohm found that centers for vocal control are larger in male birds, which learn to sing, than in females, which normally do not sing. Several of the song control areas in the left hemisphere contain neurons that bind testosterone. In the canary the presence or absence of circulating testosterone modulates the amount of singing during the life span of the bird.

Cognitive Functions Can Be Simulated by Connectionist Networks Capable of Parallel Distributed Processing

In recent years it has become possible to model cognitive processes using neuron-like elements that are linked into circuits. For many years cognitive scientists attempted to model cognitive processes, using computer programs in which each operation was performed in sequence. These serial models were very slow in processing information, and were not very successful in simulating actual thought processes. We now recognize that the brain does not operate exclusively by serial processing, and that parallel processing is an important component. The development of parallel computer devices that perform relatively sophisticated operations in an architecture reminiscent of brain networks has generated some excitement among neuroscientists.

Parallel distributed processing (so-called PDP) models consist of elements that are interconnected in circuits. Each element is influenced in positive or negative ways by other elements. The effect of the activity of one element on another is the product of its output level and its connection strength. An element summates the effects of its various inputs and produces an output that is a linear or nonlinear function of the inputs. The elements of PDP models can be considered to be analogous to neurons, but they can also represent higher-order elements such as words, percepts, or ideas. One of the most powerful and interesting PDP models is the *layered network* pioneered by David Rummelhardt and John McClelland. This consists of a set of input neuron-like elements connected to a

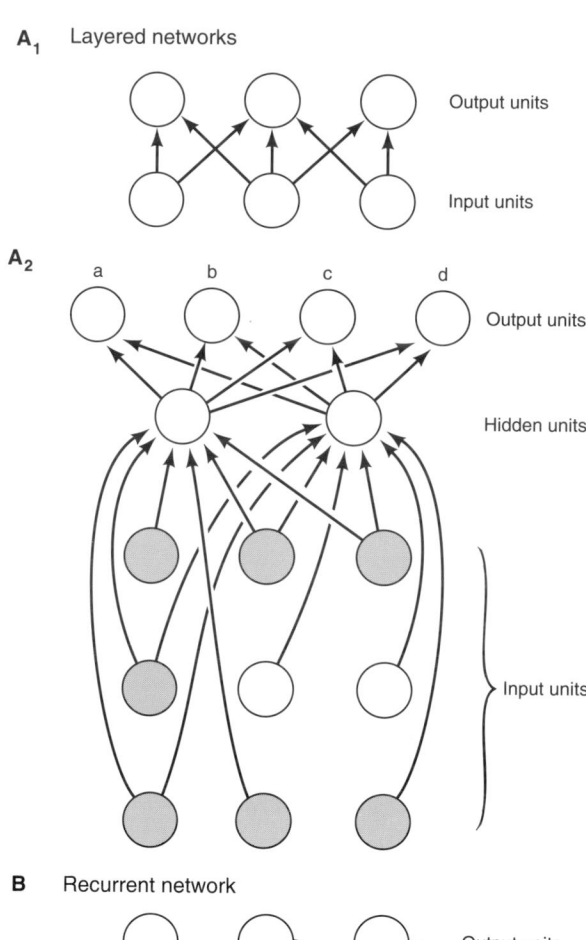

FIGURE 53–12
Certain cognitive functions can be simulated by networks capable of parallel distributed processing.

A. In layered networks the input units are connected directly to the output units (**arrows**). Each connection strength can be different. For a given trial the input units are each provided with a level of activation (a value from 0 to 1). Each output unit then becomes activated as a function of the sum of the activations from its input units. The degree of activation provided by an input unit is a function of the product of the level of activation of the input unit times the magnitude of the connection strength to the output unit. **1.** A layered network consisting of an input and output layer. **2.** A layered network containing a hidden layer. The input layer in this example is a two-dimensional array, such as a retina. It has been stimulated with the letter C. The output layer has four choices: a, b, c, or d. By training the network, the connection strength between units can be adjusted such that presentation of each letter primarily activates the corresponding output unit. For simplicity, not all connections typically present in connectionist models have been indicated in these examples.

B. In recurrent network the output units provide feedback (indicated by **curved arrows**) to earlier units in the circuit.

set of output elements (Figure 53–12A,1). This network is capable of performing a variety of computations, particularly if the input layer does not directly connect to the output layer, but rather connects through one or more intermediate (so called hidden) layers (Figure 53–12A,2).

The level of performance of the network is dependent on the strength and pattern of the connections between the elements. The power of the PDP models comes from the fact that the connection strengths required to perform a given calculation can be discovered through successive applications of algorithms that calculate the appropriate strength for each connection. The most popular and powerful technique is *back propagation*, so-called because it involves a series of calculations that start at the last (output) layer of the network and proceed back through successive layers until the first (input) layer is reached. In simplified terms, this procedure involves the following steps. A computational problem is defined. For example, one output element may be asked to output a value of one if the number of input elements is even, while another may be asked to output a value equal to the total number of input elements. An initial network is set up with random connection strengths between elements of one layer to the next. Different sets of inputs are provided and each time the resulting output of each output unit is compared by the system to the desired output. An error is calculated by the system for each output unit based on the difference between the desired and actual activity of the output unit.

Next, the connection strengths of units connecting to that output unit are slightly modified by the model system in proportion to the extent that they contributed to the error. The error terms of the output units are then used as a measure of the error signal of the units in the layer before, and the connection strengths of the inputs to this penultimate layer are adjusted proportional to these errors. Over many iterations of training this self-correcting network typically improves in performance until it solves or comes close to solving the problem. This procedure has been used to perform a variety of sensory tasks. For example, it has been used to classify visual stimuli, such as letters presented through a two-dimensional array of input elements (see Figure 53–12A,2). The procedure has also performed motor computations, such as calculating the correct joint angles to move an artificial limb to a particular point in space. Back-propagation is one of many techniques used to optimize connections so that networks can solve interesting problems. One recently developed technique simulates the evolutionary forces that may have originally determined the connections during phylogenesis. These *genetic algorithms* appear to be capable of finding optimum sets of connections, even when other algorithms fail.

A second type of network that has been studied is the *recurrent network* (Figure 53–12B). In these networks there is feedback between the output and input elements. Therefore, unlike nonrecurrent layered networks, recurrent networks sometimes have no stable state; once presented with an input they continue to cycle interminably from one mode to another. Algorithms have been developed, however, that allow connection strengths to be set,

such that the networks will assume one of several steady states. The network then has the property that if only a portion or a distorted replica of one of the stable states is presented, the network assumes the complete stable state. Thus, these networks form associative memories in which a part of a stimulus evokes a larger related memory.

The reason the PDP models have generated interest is not because they are likely to be replicas of actual processing in the nervous system. Rather, they illustrate the types of operations that can be performed by networks of interconnected units. The similarity between these circuits and real brains is the extensive parallel processing that occurs in both. A second similarity is that the operations of PDP networks are not dependent upon any single unit. They exhibit graceful degradation, which means removal of a modest number of units in the circuit results in only minimal computational dysfunction. Furthermore, the PDP models can generalize, so that the correct output can be calculated from an incomplete or distorted input. Current thinking is that some areas of cortex may be specialized for given computations, but that in other areas PDP-like processing may occur, in which the action of specific units is not critical to the functioning of the area. Thus, both strictly localized as well as nonlocalized processes may occur in cortical functioning.

An Overall View

Analysis of behavior indicates that even the most complex functions of the brain are localized to some extent. This has great clinical importance and explains why certain syndromes are characteristic of disease in specific regions of the brain. Nevertheless, assigning functions to specific regions presents a problem, since no part of the nervous system functions in the same way alone as it does in concert with other parts. When a part of the brain is removed in a lesion study, the behavior of the animal is more a reflection of the adjusted capacities of the remaining brain than of the part of the brain that was removed. It is unlikely, therefore, that any complex behavior—especially higher functions such as thought, perception, and language—are localized in only one region of the brain without considering the relationship of that region to other regions.

Furthermore, although failure of a lesion to disrupt a particular task is informative, it does not mean that the lesioned area of brain is not involved in that task. First, the brain can reorganize, sometimes very quickly, sometimes more slowly, so that other areas take over the function. Second, and perhaps more important, is the possibility that some individual units or small groups of units, and perhaps even large ensembles of units, can be removed without dramatically altering the function of the system because of the parallel organization of brain circuits. This is a general property of parallel computers in which the computations are in effect distributed throughout the network.

Finally, modern imaging techniques have revealed that multiple areas of cortex are typically activated even by the performance of simple tasks.

Nevertheless, the current approach to the nervous system, reducing its activities into anatomically discrete units, is clinically useful and gives us clues about the contribution of individual parts to the functioning of the whole.

Selected Readings

Andersen, R. A. 1987. Inferior parietal lobule function in spatial perception and visuomotor integration. In F. Plum (ed.), Handbook of Physiology, Section 1: The Nervous System, Vol. VI. Higher Functions of the Brain, Part 2. Bethesda, Md.: American Physiological Society, pp. 483–518.

Andreasen, N. C. 1988. Brain imaging: Applications in psychiatry. Science 239:1381–1388.

Fulton, J. F. 1951. Frontal Lobotomy and Affective Behavior: A Neurophysiological Analysis. New York: Norton.

Fuster, J. M. 1989. The Prefrontal Cortex: Anatomy, Physiology, and Neuropsychology of the Frontal Lobe, 2nd ed. New York: Raven Press.

Geschwind, N. 1979. Specializations of the human brain. Sci. Am. 241(3):180–199.

Goldberg, D. E. 1989. Genetic Algorithms in Search, Optimization, and Machine Learning. Reading, Mass.: Addison-Wesley.

Goldman-Rakic, P. S. 1987. Circuitry of primate prefrontal cortex and regulation of behavior by representational memory. In F. Plum and V. B. Mountcastle (eds.), Handbook of Physiology, Section 1: The Nervous System, Vol. V. Higher Functions of the Brain, Part 1. Bethesda, Md.: American Physiological Society, pp. 373–417.

Hardyck, C., and Petrinovich, L. F. 1977. Left-handedness. Psychol. Bull. 84:385–404.

Kolb, B., and Whishaw, I. Q. 1990. Fundamentals of Human Neuropsychology, 3rd ed. New York: Freeman.

Milner, B. 1974. Hemispheric specialization: Scope and limits. In F. O. Schmitt and F. G. Worden (eds.), The Neurosciences: Third Study Program. Cambridge, Mass.: MIT Press, pp. 75–89.

Pandya, D. N., and Seltzer, B. 1982. Association areas of the cerebral cortex. Trends Neurosci. 5:386–390.

Rumelhart, D. E., and McClelland, J. L. (eds.) 1986. Parallel Distributed Processing, Explorations in the Microstructure of Cognition, Vol. 1: Foundations. Cambridge, Mass.: MIT Press.

Valenstein, E. S. (ed.) 1980. The Psychosurgery Debate: Scientific Legal, and Ethical Perspectives. San Francisco: Freeman.

References

Brozoski, T. J., Brown, R. M., Rosvold, H. E., and Goldman, P. S. 1979. Cognitive deficit caused by regional depletion of dopamine in prefrontal cortex of rhesus monkey. Science 205:929–932.

Funahashi, S., Bruce, C. J., and Goldman-Rakic, P. S. 1989. Mnemonic coding of visual space in the monkey's dorsolateral prefrontal cortex. J. Neurophysiol. 61:331–349.

Gazzaniga, M. S. 1989. Organization of the human brain. Science 245:947–952.

Geschwind, N., and Levitsky, W. 1968. Human brain: Left-right asymmetries in temporal speech region. Science 161:186–187.

Gnadt, J. W., and Andersen, R. A. 1988. Memory related motor-planning activity in posterior parietal cortex of macaque. Exp. Brain Res. 70:216–220.

Goldman, P. S., and Nauta, W. J. H. 1977. Columnar distribution of cortico-cortical fibers in the frontal association, limbic, and motor cortex of the developing rhesus monkey. Brain Res. 122:393–413.

Harlow, H. F. 1958. Behavioral contributions to interdisciplinary research. In H. F. Harlow and C. N. Woolsey (eds.), Biological and Biochemical Bases of Behavior. Madison: University of Wisconsin Press, pp. 3–23.

Jacobsen, C. F. 1935. Functions of frontal association area in primates. Arch. Neurol. Psychiatry 33:558–569.

Lashley, K. S. 1950. In search of the engram. Symp. Soc. Exp. Biol. 4:454–482.

Levy, J., Trevarthen, C., and Sperry, R. W. 1972. Perception of bilateral chimeric figures following hemispheric deconnexion. Brain 95:61–78.

Milner, B. 1968. Visual recognition and recall after right temporal-lobe excision in man. Neuropsychologia 6:191–209.

Moniz, E. 1936. Tentatives Operatoires dans le Traitement de Certaines Psychoses. Paris: Masson.

Mountcastle, V. B., Lynch, J. C., Georgopoulos, A., Sakata, H., and Acuna, C. 1975. Posterior parietal association cortex of the monkey: Command functions for operations within extrapersonal space. J. Neurophysiol. 38:871–908.

Myers, R. E. 1955. Interocular transfer of pattern discrimination in cats following section of crossed optic fibers. J. Comp. Physiol. Psychol. 48:470–473.

Nottebohm, F. 1979. Origins and mechanisms in the establishment of cerebral dominance. In M. S. Gazzaniga (ed.), Handbook of Behavioral Neurobiology, Vol. 2: Neuropsychology. New York: Plenum Press, pp. 295–344.

Penfield, W. 1958. Functional localization in temporal and deep Sylvian areas. Res. Publ. Assoc. Res. Nerv. Ment. Dis. 36:210–226.

Rasmussen, T., and Milner, B. 1977. The role of early left-brain injury in determining lateralization of cerebral speech functions. Ann. N.Y. Acad. Sci. 299:355–369.

Reiman, E. M., Fusselman, M. J., Fox, P. T., and Raichle, M. E. 1989. Neuroanatomical correlates of anticipatory anxiety. Science 243:1071–1074.

Robinson, D. L., Goldberg, M. E., and Stanton, G. B. 1978. Parietal association cortex in the primate: Sensory mechanisms and behavioral modulations. J. Neurophysiol. 41:910–932.

Rosenkilde, C. E. 1979. Functional heterogeneity of the prefrontal cortex in the monkey: A review. Behav. Neural Biol. 25:301–345.

Sperry, R. W. 1964. The great cerebral commissure. Sci. Am. 210(1):42–52.

Sperry, R. W. 1968. Mental unity following surgical disconnection of the cerebral hemispheres. Harvey Lect. 62:293–323.

Tucker, D. M., Watson, R. T., and Heilman, K. M. 1977. Discrimination and evocation of affectively intoned speech in patients with right parietal disease. Neurology 27:947–950.

Weiskrantz, L., Mihailović Lj. and Gross, C. G. 1962. Effects of stimulation of frontal cortex and hippocampus on behaviour in the monkey. Brain 85:487–504.

Richard Mayeux
Eric R. Kandel

54

Disorders of Language: The Aphasias

Language Is Distinctive from Other Forms of Communication

Animal Models of Human Language Have Been Largely Unsatisfactory

What Is the Origin of Human Language?

Is the Capability for Language an Innate Skill or Learned?

Aphasias Are Disorders of Language that Also Interfere with Other Cognitive Functions

The Wernicke–Geschwind Model for Language Is a Useful Clinical Model for Distinguishing Damage to the Two Major Language Regions of the Brain

Recent Cognitive and Imaging Studies of Normal Subjects and Aphasic Patients Have Clarified the Interconnections of the Two Language Regions

Seven Types of Aphasia Can Be Distinguished and Related to Different Anatomical Systems

Wernicke's Aphasia

Broca's Aphasia

Conduction Aphasia

Anomic Aphasia

Global Aphasia

Transcortical Aphasias

Subcortical Aphasia

Certain Affective Components of Language Are Affected by Damage to the Right Hemisphere

Some Disorders of Reading and Writing Can Be Localized

Alexias and Agraphias Are Acquired Disorders of Reading and Writing

Dyslexia and Hyperlexia Are Developmental Disorders of Reading

An Overall View

Language is particularly interesting from a neurobiological point of view because its specific and localized organization has given us the keenest insight into the functional architecture of the dominant hemisphere of the brain. The study of language also represents a striking example of how neurobiology, in collaboration with disciplines ranging from anthropology and linguistics to developmental and clinical neurology, might help us understand even the most complex of human behaviors.

Language Is Distinctive from Other Forms of Communication

Language is distinguished from other kinds of human communication by its creativity, form, content, and use.

Creativity. Just as vision is not simply an assembly of sensations but the outcome of a transformational or creative processing of physical stimuli by the brain, so is speech creative and transformational. We do not learn a language by repeating memorized stock sentences, but by understanding the rules for creating meaningful utterances. With every new thought we speak we create original sentences. Listening is also creative. We readily interpret the sentence spoken by others.

Form. Language is formed from arrangements of a limited set of sounds in predictable sequences that signal content. Each of the world's languages is based on a small fraction of the sounds humans are capable of making, and not all languages use the same set of sounds. The sounds that make up a language are called *phonemes.* These are the smallest differences in sound that distinguish different contents, for example, the difference between the sounds *d* and *t*.

Content. In natural language two further levels of structure can be distinguished: (1) the combination of phonemes to form words (morphology), and (2) the combination of words to form phrases and sentences (grammar). Unlike simple sign systems, in which meaning is tied to highly specific situations, language provides a means of shaping and communicating abstractions whose meanings are independent of the immediate situation. Language is rooted in the ability to give a single name to various appearances under different conditions. In addition, language has an emotional content that is supported by such extralinguistic means as gesture, tone of voice (flatness, whining, whispering, loudness), facial expression, and posture. Specific languages have different content structures.

Use. Language is fundamentally a means for social communication. Language is not merely a neutral medium of exchange of facts and observations about the world. Whenever we speak or write we have a social purpose. Through language we organize our sensory experience and express our thoughts, feelings, and expectations.

Certain diseases interfere more with one than with another of these features. Form can be affected by disease of the cerebellum, resulting in dysarthria (the inability to articulate words clearly), or by lesions of the cerebral cortex, resulting in Broca's aphasia. Content is disturbed in Wernicke's aphasia, in conduction aphasia, and in schizophrenia. Use is affected in the aprosodias, and in some psychiatric illnesses, such as schizophrenia.

In this chapter we shall consider the distinctive features of human language and examine why animal research has increased understanding of human language only modestly. In contrast, much has been learned about language from two sources: from the study of language acquisition in children and from neurological disorders of language. Therefore, we shall review the major findings regarding the development of language and then examine in some detail the clinical disorders of speech, reading, writing, and gesture. This family of disorders can now be understood with a model of language developed by Karl Wernicke in the nineteenth century and expanded first by Norman Geschwind, and more recently by Antonio Damasio, Michael Posner, and Marcus Raichle.

In 1984 Damasio and Geschwind summarized the progress in our understanding of the biological basis of language:

As late as the mid 1960s, the standard view regarding cerebral dominance for language stated that [language] had no anatomical correlates, that it did not exist in other species, and that its evolution in humans could not be studied. . . . But the discoveries of the past 15 years have proven that each of these standard views was false and have opened up entirely new avenues of study.

It is these avenues that we shall pursue here.

Animal Models of Human Language Have Been Largely Unsatisfactory

Approaches to a neural analysis of cognitive and other behavioral functions have often depended on animal models. Considerable effort therefore has been expended in developing animal models of language. Animals as simple as crickets and bees have an elementary form of communication, a sort of natural language. The song of birds is even more elaborate (see Chapter 61). Nevertheless, these forms of communication cannot be considered interpersonal—they are at best inter*individual*—and their form, content, use, and creativity are highly stereotyped.

What about our closest relatives, the nonhuman primates? Do they have creative language? Can they be used to study human speech? In the past few decades opinion on this question has swung back and forth several times. In the 1930s it was generally thought that chimpanzees could learn to speak if they were raised in a human home as human children are. With this idea in mind, William and Lorna Kellogg raised a chimpanzee, Gua, with their own child. The chimpanzee adopted many human behaviors, understood a few spoken commands, and mastered a few hand gestures, but never learned to speak. By the early 1960s chimpanzees were thought to lack the intellectual capacity for language. Noam Chomsky, a linguist, wrote in 1968: "Anyone concerned with the study of human nature and human capacity must somehow come to grips with the fact that all normal humans acquire spoken language whereas acquisition of even the barest rudiments is quite beyond the capacity of an otherwise intelligent ape."

Shortly thereafter it was discovered that the vocal apparatus of chimpanzees is unable to produce the full range of human sounds. The possibility remained, however, that chimpanzees might show a capacity for language if they did not have to produce speech sounds. Allen and Beatrice Gardner circumvented the need for sound production by training a female chimpanzee named Washoe to use signs borrowed from American Sign Language, the language of the American deaf. Within four years Washoe achieved a vocabulary of 160 words, including signs for objects (bird, hand), attributes (blue, green, different), and modifiers (more, less). Although these results demonstrate that chimpanzees can learn words and use symbols, the vocabulary they acquire is much smaller than that of a human infant. A child of four has a vocabulary of more than 3000 words, as compared with Washoe's 160.

To explore whether chimpanzees understand relationships, David Premack trained a chimpanzee, Sarah, to communicate with plastic chips that had different signs inscribed on them. In this training Premack tried to preserve many features that are universal in natural languages. He taught Sarah to interpret commands contained in an arrangement of the signs on different chips and to construct her own sentences. Sarah eventually learned the concepts of negation, similarity, and difference, the expression "is the name of," compound sentences, if–then statements, and how to ask questions. Most interesting were experiments in which Premack showed Sarah pairs of objects in which the second was a transformed version of the first (an apple and an apple cut into pieces; a dry towel and a wet towel). Sarah was then asked to select one of several other objects that would explain the correlation (for example, a knife and a bowl of water) and insert it between these pairs. She made the appropriate choice about 80% of the time. Sarah appeared to be able to express in symbols her understanding of the causal relationship between physical events.

Thus, chimpanzees (and probably gorillas as well) are able to communicate through symbols in a rudimentary fashion. It is not certain, however, if they can go beyond that. For example, there is no evidence as yet that chimpanzees can understand syntax, the rules that organize words into sentences, so that they can creatively recombine words and express different ideas with them. Thus, Washoe can use the words *Washoe*, *me*, and *banana*, but most students of language think that she cannot distinguish "me give Washoe banana" from "Washoe give me banana." Indeed, most linguists are struck by the *noncreative*, imitative, and mechanical nature of the language acquired by chimpanzees.

Although the analogy between the use of human language forms by chimpanzees and the fluent and creative language of humans seems weak, this work does show that apes (and even much simpler animals, as we now have good reason to believe) share with humans certain cognitive capabilities such as knowledge of causality. Whether these capabilities are crucial to linguistic competence, however, remains unclear. It is hard to know, for example, whether animals do not express propositions because their communication abilities are insufficient or because they do not think.

Because animal models have proven to be of limited usefulness in the study of human language, students of language rely primarily on anthropological, developmental, and clinical studies.

What Is the Origin of Human Language?

Although it is difficult to pinpoint the time or way in which language evolved, some cerebral structures that are prerequisite for language appear to have arisen early in human evolution. This conclusion has come from the work of Marjorie LeMay, who examined endocranial casts of human fossils. In most individuals the left hemisphere is dominant for language and the cortical speech area of the temporal lobe (the planum temporale) is larger in the left than in the right hemisphere. Since important gyri and sulci often leave an impression upon the skull, LeMay searched the fossil record for the morphological asymmetries associated with speech in modern humans and found them in Neanderthal man (dating back 30,000 to 50,000 years) and in Peking man (dating back 300,000 to 500,000 years). The left hemisphere is also dominant for the recognition of species-specific cries in Japanese macaque monkeys, and asymmetries similar to those of humans are present in brains of modern-day great apes, such as the chimpanzee. Whether these anatomical and functional asymmetries originally evolved for language, for other forms of communication, or for an entirely different function, is not known.

Although the anatomical structures that are prerequisites for language may have arisen early (perhaps as many as 500,000 years ago), many linguists believe that language *per se* emerged rather late in the prehistoric period of human existence (about 100,000 years ago) and that perhaps it arose only *once*. According to this view, all human languages are thought to have arisen together with the evolution of animals from a single language first spoken in Africa.

Did human language evolve from ape-like communication? Since human evolution is itself not understood, and since apes, as we have seen, have only rudimentary language capabilities, these questions are speculative. Two hypotheses about the origin of language have been advanced: gestural and vocal.

Gestural theories propose that language evolved from a system of gestures that emerged when certain apes assumed an erect posture, freeing the hands for social communication. Subsequently, vocal communication may have arisen to free the hands for purposes other than communication. *Vocal theories* contend that language evolved from an extensive group of instinctive calls that were expressive of emotional states, such as distress, elation, and sexual arousal. About 100,000 years ago changes in the structure of the mouth, jaw, and vocal tract made it possible to control the production of different sounds reliably and consciously. As a result, sounds could at least in principle be used creatively in different combinations. When these ancestors of modern humans dispersed into separate colonies, geographical isolation allowed for the development of different sound systems. The possibility that language emerged *once* in history might explain why all human languages have so many features in common.

Alternatively, language may have emerged from the co-evolution of gesture and vocalization. This possibility might account for the still inexplicable correlation of verbal language and hand dominance (gesture), both localized to the left hemisphere.

Is the Capability for Language an Innate Skill or Learned?

Although the acquisition of language clearly involves learning, studies of the anatomical localization of language and of language development in children suggest that a large part of the process is innate. First, as we saw in Chapter 53, both natural and sign language functions are localized; language is predominantly represented in the left hemisphere.

Second, the localization of language in the left hemisphere seems to be related to anatomical differences between the two hemispheres. For example, the planum temporale, the area of the temporal lobe specialized for speech, is larger in the left hemisphere in most right-handed people (Chapter 53). Third, this anatomical asymmetry in the planum temporale is present early in development (by the thirty-first week of gestation), suggesting that this asymmetry does not develop in response to experience but is innate.

Fourth, infants at birth are sensitive to distinctions in a broad range of sounds, an ability that is crucial for the comprehension of any human language. Indeed, some of this sensitivity is lost later, when a specific language is acquired. For example, most adult Japanese cannot perceive the difference between the sounds of *r* and *l*. Japanese infants can distinguish these sounds, however, and only lose this ability when they mature. Peter Eimas has suggested that the neural basis of this decline in perceptual discrimination is similar to that underlying the loss of visual acuity in kittens raised in a restricted visual environment (see Chapter 60).

Finally, there are universal regularities in the acquisition of language. Children progress from babbling to one-word speech, to two-word speech with syntax, to complex speech (Table 54–1). Some children progress through these stages faster than others, but the average age for each stage is the same in all cultures. Moreover, language capacity (as measured by the ability to acquire a new language) is reduced dramatically after puberty. These several findings suggest that there is a critical period during development when language, whether verbal or signed, is acquired effortlessly. Presumably, this period of development corresponds to the maturation of the human brain, although studies have not yet attempted to correlate language acquisition with maturation of specific areas related to language. During this period children learn the rules of language by simply listening to the speech around them. These rules, the grammar of the language, are clearly understood by the time the child begins to form sentences. Although a specific language must be learned through experience, Noam Chomsky argues that humans have some innate program that prepares them to learn language in general. According to Chomsky, an infant learns a language by testing the specifics of the language heard daily against a genetically determined system of rules or

TABLE 54–1. Stages of Development in the Acquisition of Language

Average age	Language ability
6 months	Beginning of distinct babbling.
1 year	Beginning of language understanding; one-word utterances.
1½ years	Words used singly; child uses 30–50 words (simple nouns, adjectives, and action words) one at a time but cannot link them to make phrases; does not use functors (the, and, can, be) necessary for syntax.
2 years	Two-word (telegraphic) speaker; 50 to several hundred words in the vocabulary; much use of two-word phrases that are ordered according to syntactic rules; child understands propositional rules.
2½ years	Three or more words in many combinations; functors begin to appear; many grammatical errors and idiosyncratic expressions; good understanding of language.
3 years	Full sentences; few errors; vocabulary of around 1000 words.
4 years	Close to adult speech competence.

(Based on E. H. Lenneberg, 1967.)

generative grammar. These rules reflect innately determined neural mechanisms that limit the possible characteristics of a natural language. That is, children have an innate ability to recognize the *universals* that characterize a natural language in the environment. When exposed to a language with these universals, a child learns it avidly. Chomsky argues that a language that violated these universals would be unlearnable.

In summary, linguists and psychologists now believe that the mechanisms for the universal aspects of language acquisition are determined by the structure of the human brain. According to this view, the human brain is prepared as a result of development to learn and use speech. The particular language spoken and the dialect and accent are determined by the social environment.

The question now being debated by linguists is whether linguistic universals derive from the neural structures specifically related to language acquisition or from cognitive universals that are more general. Chomsky argues that there are neural constraints specific to language acquisition, but many psychologists disagree. Children are able to understand abstract rules before they learn to speak. They can, for example, distinguish between causative and noncausative actions.

The challenge for the neurobiological approach to cognition and language is to address these problems. One avenue of investigation has come from the study of aphasia. Researchers working with aphasic patients are asking two sorts of questions. First, are disorders of language isolated cognitive disorders, or are they related to more general disturbances of cognitive processes? Second, what are the neural structures that underlie the innate universal rules of grammar?

Aphasias Are Disorders of Language that Also Interfere with Other Cognitive Functions

The aphasias are disturbances of language caused by insult (vascular damage, trauma, or tumor) to specific regions of the brain—usually, but not invariably, to regions of the cerebral cortex. Damage of the cerebral cortex does not result in an overall reduction in language ability; rather, lesions in different parts of the cerebral cortex cause selective disturbances. Furthermore, these disorders involve more than a breakdown in the production and comprehension of spoken language: The damage to the brain often affects other cognitive and intellectual skills to some degree. For example, as we shall see later, some aphasic patients have difficulty comprehending both speech and writing (Wernicke's aphasia). Others have difficulty expressing thoughts in either written or spoken language (Broca's aphasia).

Such selective disruptions of cortical function afford unusual insight into how the brain is organized for language. One of the most impressive insights has been provided by Ursula Bellugi and her colleagues in their study of sign language. Unlike speech, signing is expressed by hand gestures rather than by sounds, and is perceived by visual rather than auditory pathways. Nonetheless, signing, which has the same structural complexities characteristic of spoken languages, is also localized to the left hemisphere. Thus, following lesions in the left hemisphere, deaf individuals become aphasic for sign language. Lesions in the right hemisphere do not produce these defects in signing. Moreover, defects in signing following left hemisphere damage can be quite specific, involving either sign comprehension and grammar or signing fluency.

This illustrates three points. First, the left hemisphere contains the cognitive capability for language and this capacity is independent of the sensory or motor modalities used for processing language. Second, speech and hearing are not a prerequisite for the emergence of language capabilities in the left hemisphere. Third, spoken language represents only one of a family of cognitive skills mediated by the left hemisphere.

The aphasias are distinguished from other disorders of speech, such as *dysarthria*, a disturbance in articulation, and *dysphonia*, a disturbance in vocalization. These disorders result from weakness or incoordination of the muscles controlling the vocal apparatus and are simply disorders of the mechanical process of speech. They do not basically affect language comprehension or the central processes of expression. Patients with cerebellar disorders who are dysarthric, or those with Parkinson's disease who are dysphonic, retain their language ability despite severe speech impairment. In contrast, the hallmark of aphasia is a disturbance in language ability, either in comprehension or production, or both, that is not attributable to a mechanical impediment.

The most common cause of aphasia is head trauma, which produces 200,000 cases in the United States each year. The next most frequent cause is stroke: 40% of major vascular events in the cerebral hemispheres produce language disorders. In the United States stroke leads to 100,000 cases of aphasia each year. Studies of patients with discrete vascular lesions have increased our understanding of aphasia because these lesions do not progress and the anatomy of the damaged region often directly relates to the distribution of critical blood vessels.

The Wernicke–Geschwind Model for Language Is a Useful Clinical Model for Distinguishing Damage to the Two Major Language Regions of the Brain

There is no universally accepted classification for the aphasias. A useful classification was developed by Geschwind and Damasio as an elaboration of the Wernicke–Geschwind model of language and gesture, and we shall use that scheme here (Figure 54–1).

This model for language can best be illustrated by considering the simple task of repeating a word that has been heard. According to the original Wernicke–Geschwind

FIGURE 54–1

Primary language areas of the brain.

A. The classical nomenclature of gyri and sulci are indicated in this lateral view of the exterior surface of the left hemisphere. Broca's area, the motor-speech area, is adjacent to the region of the motor cortex (precentral gyrus) that controls the movements of facial expression, articulation, and phonation. Wernicke's area lies in the posterior superior temporal lobe near the primary auditory cortex (superior temporal gyrus) and includes the auditory comprehension center. Wernicke's and Broca's areas are joined by a fiber tract called the *arcuate fasciculus*. In the figure Broca's and Wernicke's areas are referred to as *regions* to indicate their status as part of complex networks rather than independent language *centers*.

B. The cytoarchitectonic areas (Broadmann's classification) are illustrated in this lateral view of the left hemisphere. Area 4 is the primary motor cortex; area 41 is the primary auditory cortex; area 22 is Wernicke's region; and area 45 is Broca's region.

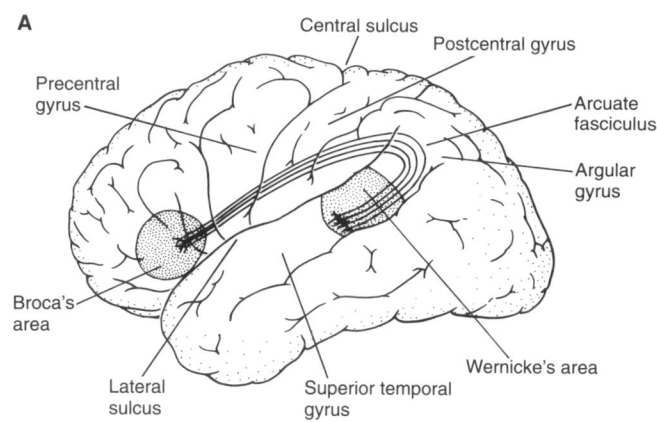

Lateral surface of the left hemisphere

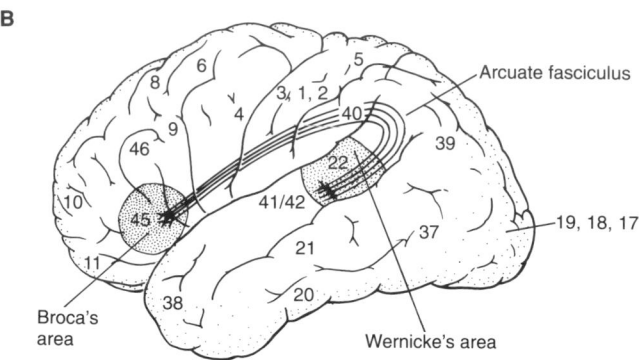

model, this task involves transfer of information from the basilar membrane of the auditory apparatus to the auditory nerve and medial geniculate nucleus. The information then flows first to the primary auditory cortex (Brodmann's area 41), then to the higher-order auditory cortex (Brodmann's area 42), before it is conveyed to a specific region of the parietal–temporal–occipital association cortex, the *angular gyrus* (Brodmann's area 39), which is thought to be concerned with the association of incoming auditory, visual, and tactile information. From here the information is projected to Wernicke's area and then, by means of the arcuate fasciculus, to Broca's area, where the perception of language is translated into the grammatical structure of a phrase and where the memory for word articulation is stored. This information about the sound pattern of the phrase is then conveyed to the facial area of the motor cortex that controls articulation so that the word can be spoken.

A similar pathway was thought by Wernicke and Geschwind to be involved in naming an object that has been visually recognized (Figure 54–2). According to their model visual information is transferred from the retina to the lateral geniculate nucleus, and from there to the primary visual cortex (Brodmann's area 17). The information then travels to a higher-order center (area 18), where it is

conveyed first to the angular gyrus of the parietal–temporal–occipital association cortex, and then to Wernicke's area, where the visual information is transformed into a phonetic (auditory) representation of the word. The phonetic pattern is formed and then conveyed to Broca's area by means of the arcuate fasciculus.

The original Wernicke–Geschwind model made several interesting predictions that are useful clinically. First, it predicted the outcome of a lesion in Wernicke's area. Words reaching the auditory cortex fail to activate Wernicke's area and thus fail to be comprehended. If the lesion extends posteriorly and inferiorly beyond Wernicke's area, it will also affect the pathway concerned with the processing of visual input to language. As a result, the patient will be incapable of understanding either the spoken or the written word. Second, the model correctly predicts that a lesion in Broca's area will not affect the comprehension of written and spoken language, but will cause a major disruption of speech and verbal production because the pattern for sounds and for the structure of language are not passed on to the motor cortex. Third, the model predicts that a lesion in the arcuate fasciculus, by disconnecting Wernicke's area from Broca's, will disrupt verbal production because the auditory input is not conveyed to the part of the brain involved with production of language.

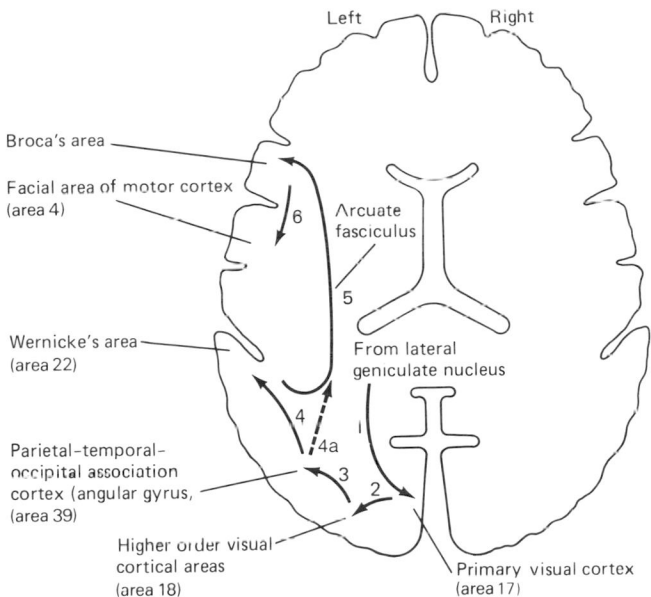

Left   Right

Broca's area

Facial area of motor cortex
(area 4)

Arcuate
fasciculus

6

5

Wernicke's area
(area 22)

From lateral
geniculate nucleus

4

4a

Parietal-temporal-
occipital association
cortex (angular gyrus,
(area 39)

3

2

Higher order visual
cortical areas
(area 18)

Primary visual cortex
(area 17)

FIGURE 54–2

The neural pathways involved in naming a visual object according to the Wernicke–Geschwind model of cortical processing. The diagram here shows a schematic drawing of a horizontal section of the human brain at the level of the corpus callosum. The naming begins with input from the retina through the optic nerve. Recent evidence suggests that the actual flow of information is almost identical to the sequence shown here, except that, following step 3, a component of the arcuate fasciculus (4a) conveys information directly from the association cortex to Broca's area, bypassing Wernicke's area. (Adapted from Patton, Sundsten, Crill, and Swanson, 1976.)

Recent Cognitive and Imaging Studies of Normal Subjects and Aphasic Patients Have Clarified the Interconnections of the Two Language Regions

Even though the modified Wernicke–Geschwind model continues to be useful clinically, recent cognitive and imaging studies comparing the uses of language by normal and aphasic patients by Damasio, Raichle, Posner, and their colleagues indicate that the Wernicke–Geschwind model may be oversimplified in several ways. First, the emphasis in the Wernicke–Geschwind model on the importance of Broca's and Wernicke's areas for expression and reception was based on lesions that actually affected much larger regions. When lesions are restricted to the areas originally identified by Broca and Wernicke, they usually do not give rise to the full symptoms characteristic of Wernicke's or Broca's aphasia. The typical symptoms are usually the result of damage to the surrounding regions as well.

Second, the Wernicke–Geschwind model emphasizes the importance of cortical regions (and interconnecting pathways running through subcortical white matter). There now is evidence that subcortical structures, specifically the left thalamus, the left caudate nucleus, and adjacent white matter, also are important for language. For example, lesions in the left caudate lead to a defect in auditory comprehension presumably by interrupting the auditory–motor integration required for linguistic processing.

Third, as we saw in Chapter 1, an auditory input—a spoken word—is indeed projected from the auditory cortex to the angular gyrus and then to Wernicke's area before being conveyed to Broca's area (Figure 54–3). However, visual information, such as a written word, is not con-

veyed to Wernicke's areas, but goes from the visual association cortex directly to Broca's area. Words that are read are therefore *not* transformed into an auditory representation. Rather, visual and auditory perceptions of a word are processed independently by modality-specific pathways that have independent access to Broca's area and to the higher-order regions concerned with the meaning and expression of language.

Finally, cognitive studies of language disagree with the Wernicke–Geschwind model on more than the pathway for processing auditory information. For example, there is good evidence that not all auditory input is processed in the same way. Nonsense sounds—words without meaning—are processed independently from conventional, meaningful words. Thus, there are thought to be separate pathways for *sounds*, the *phonological* aspects of language, and for *meaning*, the semantic aspects of language. Similarly, although Broca's area is the common output for both spoken and written words that have meaning, there may be an independent output for nonsense words. Finally, a number of studies by psycholinguists indicate that patients with both Broca's and Wernicke's aphasia not only have language deficits but also have deficits in one or another aspect of cognitive processing. These difficulties muddy the simple distinction between impairment of reception or expression. In actuality, therefore, language deficits are never as pure as the Wernicke–Geschwind model would predict.

These and related findings indicate that language involves a larger number of areas and a more complex set of interconnections than just the serial interconnection of Wernicke's area to Broca's area. A more realistic scheme illustrating the neural processing of language is shown in Figure 54–3.

FIGURE 54–3

Recent models of the neural processing of language are more complex than the Wernicke-Geschwind model but nonetheless are built on its basic ideas. The particular model illustrated in this figure represents a fairly simple circuit and shows the relationship between various anatomical structures and functional components of language. Other networks are plausible. At each point in the circuit the anatomical structure is indicated in italics. The function of the structure is shown below the structure name and the specific language skill is shown above the name. Both visual and auditory inputs as well as spoken and written expression are illustrated. (From Petersen et al., 1988.)

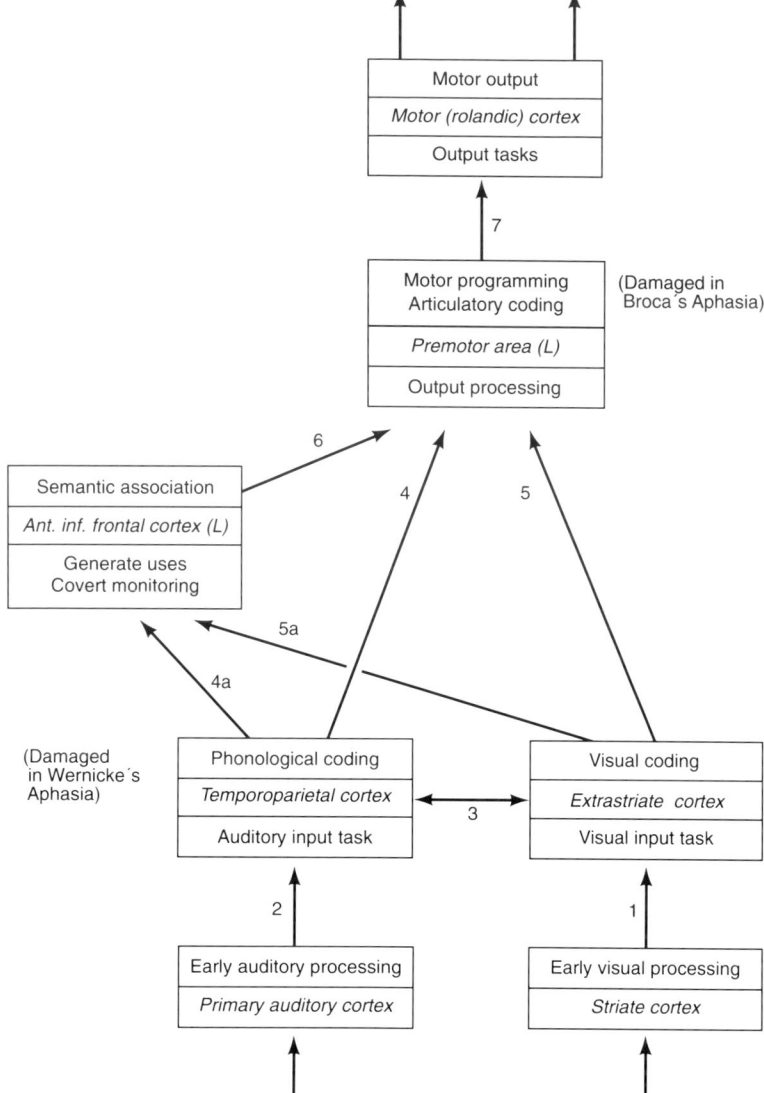

Seven Types of Aphasia Can Be Distinguished and Related to Different Anatomical Systems

We now turn to the major clinical syndromes of aphasia. In practice, the symptoms of a patient may not always fall simply into one category or another because lesions producing cortical damage are not always coextensive with a functional site (Table 54–2).

Wernicke's Aphasia

Wernicke's aphasia is characterized by a prominent deficit in comprehension. The lesion primarily affects Wernicke's area—the left posterior portion of the temporal lobe, or Brodmann's area 22—although it often extends to the superior portions of the temporal lobe (areas 40 and 39) and inferiorly to area 37. When the lesion is extensive, comprehension of both visual and auditory language input is severely impaired. In contrast, speech is fluent. Language is normal in rate, rhythm, and melody, although patients may use the wrong word or combination of words (*paraphasia*). These patients tend to add additional syllables to words and additional words to phrases. They may make up new words, called *neologisms*. The neologistic or paraphasic distortions most frequently involve key lexical items (nouns, verbs, adjectives, adverbs), especially nouns.

Language may be excessive (*logorrhea*); this phenomenon has been called *press of speech*. Because of the abundance of words, their speech often conveys little meaning,

TABLE 54–2. Clinical Characteristics of Cortical Aphasias

Type	Verbal output	Repetition	Compre-hension	Naming	Associated signs	Lesions
Broca's	Nonfluent	Impaired	Normal	Marginally impaired	RHP and RHH apraxia of the left limbs and face	Left posterior inferior frontal
Wernicke's	Fluent	Impaired	Impaired	Impaired		Left posterior superior temporal
Conduction	Fluent	Impaired	Normal	Impaired (paraphasic)	± RHS, apraxia of all limbs and face	Left parietal
Global	Nonfluent	Impaired	Impaired	Impaired	RHP, RHS, RHH	Left frontal temporal parietal
Anomic	Fluent	Normal (anomic)	Normal	Impaired	None	Left posterior inferior temporal, or tempo-ral-occipital region
Transcortical motor	Nonfluent	Normal	Normal	Impaired	RHP	Left medial frontal or anterior border zone
Sensory	Fluent	Normal	Impaired	Impaired	± RHH	Left medial parietal or posterior border zone
Mixed	Nonfluent	Normal	Impaired	Impaired	RHP, RHS	Left medial frontal pari-etal or complete bor-der zone

RHP, right hemiparesis; RHH, right homonomous hemianopsis; RHS, right hemisensory defect.

however. For example, when asked where he lived, a patient with Wernicke's aphasia replied, "I came there before here and returned there." Patients with Wernicke's aphasia fail to convey the ideas they have in mind, an impairment called *empty speech*. They generally are unaware of this failure, probably because language comprehension is impaired. The ability to repeat words and phrases is also impaired because comprehension is severely disturbed. In addition, patients with Wernicke's aphasia have severe reading and writing disabilities. Except for these symptoms of aphasia, other neurological signs may be absent, but occasionally a right visual field defect is encountered.

Broca's Aphasia

In Broca's aphasia comprehension is usually preserved, at least in part, but language production is not fluent. Patients have damage to the motor association cortex in the frontal lobe, usually extending to the posterior portion of the third frontal gyrus (Brodmann's areas 44 and 45) which forms part of the frontal operculum (Broca's area). In severe cases there is also damage to the surrounding premotor and prefrontal regions (areas 6, 8, 9, 10, and 46). The deficit in language production ranges from almost complete muteness to a slowed, deliberate speech constructed from very simple grammatical structures. Patients with Broca's aphasia use only key words. They usually express nouns in the singular, verbs in the infinitive or participle, and often eliminate articles, adjectives, and adverbs altogether. For example, instead of saying "the large gray cat," a patient with Broca's aphasia may say "gray cat."

These omissions are even more dramatic in more complex sentences. Here we can see the second characteristic of this defect: a breakdown in the construction and coordination of several constituent phrases within a sentence. Consider the sentence: "The ladies and gentlemen are now all invited into the dining room." A patient with Broca's aphasia may only be able to say "Ladies, men, room." When asked his occupation, a mailman with Broca's aphasia said "Mail . . . Mail . . . M . . . ." In addition to such telegraphic or nongrammatical speech, repetition is always impaired, and naming ability may be slightly to moderately impaired. Unlike Wernicke's aphasia, patients with Broca's aphasia are generally aware of these errors.

Although production of language is severely disturbed, comprehension of both spoken and written language is less disturbed, because Wernicke's area is not damaged. However, patients with Broca's aphasia have difficulty reading aloud, and writing (like speech) is abnormal. Work by Rita Berndt and Alfonso Caramazza suggests that Broca's aphasics may also have some difficulty comprehending those aspects of syntax that they have difficulty producing.

Because Broca's area is located near the motor cortex and the underlying internal capsule, a right hemiparesis and homonymous hemianopsia (loss of vision) is almost always present in this type of aphasia.

Conduction Aphasia

As pointed out in Chapter 1, conduction aphasia was predicted by Wernicke. He proposed that an area in the temporal lobe, concerned with the comprehension of language, projected to Broca's area by means of a pathway that connected the two regions. He therefore inferred that a lesion could leave both Broca's and Wernicke's areas intact but disconnect the two. Clinical studies verified this prediction. Lesions in the arcuate fasciculus, which runs in the white matter and connects Wernicke's and Broca's areas, lead to a conduction aphasia. Damage to the fasciculus occurs with injury of the supramarginal gyrus of the parietal lobe, or, less frequently, injury of the posterior and superior aspect of the left temporal lobe (Figure 54–1). Thus, the lesion is not restricted to white matter but also involves the cortex.

Like patients with Wernicke's aphasia, patients with conduction aphasia are fluent but have many paraphasic errors, errors in which incorrect words or sounds are substituted for correct ones. The degree of fluency may be somewhat less than that seen in Wernicke's aphasia, but comprehension is good. However, damage to the pathways from Wernicke's area to Broca's area greatly impairs the ability to repeat. Other characteristics of conduction aphasia are also consistent with a functional separation of Broca's and Wernicke's areas. Naming is severely impaired. Reading aloud is abnormal, but patients can read silently with good comprehension. Writing may also be disturbed; spelling is poor, with omissions, reversals, and even substitutions of letters.

Many patients with conduction aphasia have some degree of impairment of voluntary movement.

Anomic Aphasia

In anomic aphasia the only disturbance is a difficulty in finding the correct words. This is an unusual form of aphasia that typically follows lesions in the posterior aspect of the left inferior temporal lobe, near the temporal–occipital border. Occasionally, patients with anomic aphasia also have a defect in the right superior quadrant visual field.

Global Aphasia

Patients with global aphasia are unable to speak or comprehend language; they cannot read, write, repeat, or name objects. Lesions that cause global or total aphasia usually include the entire perisylvian region, thereby compromising both Broca's and Wernicke's areas and the arcuate fasciculus. Symptoms also include a complete right hemiplegia, right hemisensory defect, and usually a right homonymous hemianopsia.

Transcortical Aphasias

Transcortical aphasias have two important characteristics: (1) the patients have the ability to repeat spoken language, and (2) their lesion lies outside the perisylvian language centers. These aphasias most often result from vascular damage at the junction between the middle, anterior, and posterior cerebral arteries, a region known as the *border zone* or *watershed area*. This border zone includes association areas that are important for memory of the meaning of words and the supplementary motor cortex, which is important for skilled motor acts.

Transcortical motor aphasia results from a lesion that disconnects Broca's area from the supplementary motor cortex. The lesion is usually in the frontal lobe anterior to Broca's area. The lesion gives rise to a nonfluent aphasia in which the patient cannot produce creative speech. The patient will attempt conversation but can utter only a few syllables. In striking contrast, these patients are able to repeat words and phrases well. Comprehension of language is less disturbed, as is reading (both silently and aloud), but writing may be impaired seriously.

Transcortical sensory aphasia follows disconnection of Wernicke's area from the posterior parietal temporal association area. This gives rise to a fluent aphasia with defective comprehension, to a defect in thinking about or remembering the meaning of signs or words. The patient cannot read or write and has marked difficulty in finding words, but is able to repeat spoken language easily and fluently. This type of aphasia usually results from a lesion in the parietal–temporal–occipital junction.

A combination of transcortical motor and transcortical sensory aphasias produces *mixed transcortical aphasia* or *isolation of the speech area*. This is an extremely rare disorder. The patient is unable to speak unless spoken to, and responses are usually a direct echo of the examiner's words, a behavior called *echolalia*. The patient is not competent in any other language function.

Subcortical Aphasia

We have so far considered some aphasia due to *cortical* damage. Lesions that do not affect the cerebral cortex, typically vascular lesions in the basal ganglia and thalamus, can also result in aphasia.

Lesions in the left caudate nucleus or putamen cause a fluent aphasia with neologistic language. The language deficit is characteristically transient, however. Lesions in the thalamus can produce an aphasia that is often similar to that observed in the transcortical aphasias. The most frequent signs are a combination of paraphasia, poor comprehension of spoken language, and an intact ability to repeat. These disorders are typically transient; many patients fully recover.

Hypometabolism in the corresponding left temporoparietal area has been observed in patients with impaired comprehension following a subcortical aphasia. This also supports the concept that normal language is dependent not only on cortical–cortical but also on subcortical connections.

Certain Affective Components of Language Are Affected by Damage to the Right Hemisphere

We have so far considered only the cognitive components of language. Human language, and more generally human communication, has important affective components as well. These components include musical intonation (*prosody*) and emotional gesturing.

Elliott Ross found that certain affective components of language rely on specialized processes of the right hemisphere. Disturbances in affective components of language associated with damage to the right hemisphere are called *aprosodia*. The organization for prosody in the right hemisphere seems to mirror the anatomical organization for the cognitive aspects of language in the left hemisphere. Thus, patients with lesions in the anterior portion of the right hemisphere have a flat tone of voice whether they are happy or sad. Patients with posterior lesions do not comprehend the affective content of other people's language.

Some Disorders of Reading and Writing Can Be Localized

Reading disorders are either congenital (called the *dyslexias*) or acquired (called *acquired dyslexias* or *alexias*). We shall first focus on the alexias because they are particularly instructive for understanding language and illustrate interesting extensions of the Wernicke–Geschwind model of language.

Alexias and Agraphias Are Acquired Disorders of Reading and Writing

Alexia (disruption of the ability to read) and agraphia (disruption of the ability to write) are quite remarkable because they demonstrate that small lesions of the brain in an adult can selectively destroy the ability to read or write, or both, without interfering with speech or other cognitive functions. This discovery was made by the French neurologist Jules Dejerine, who described word blindness in two papers published in 1891 and in 1892. In the first, Dejerine described a patient with a disorder of both reading and writing (alexia with agraphia). The second patient had a pure word blindness (alexia without agraphia).

Word Blindness Accompanied by Writing Impairment (Alexia with Agraphia). The first patient described by Dejerine could speak and understand spoken language, but had ceased to be able to read or write. Autopsy of this and later cases revealed that alexia with agraphia is usually associated with lesions of the angular or supramarginal gyrus of the parietal–temporal–occipital association cortex. As we saw in Chapter 53, this association cortex is concerned with the integration of visual, auditory, and tactile information. Once integrated, the information is conveyed to the speech areas of the temporal lobe and then to those of the frontal lobe. When the association cortex of the angular or the supramarginal gyrus is damaged, patients cannot read or write because they cannot connect visual symbols (letters) with the sounds they represent. Similarly, these patients cannot recognize words spelled out loud, nor can they spell. They also are unable to recognize embossed letters by feeling the letters because the angular and supramarginal gyri mediate the transfer of cutaneous sensory information into language areas.

Pure Word Blindness: Alexia without Agraphia. Dejerine's second patient could speak. An intelligent and highly articulate man, he suddenly observed that he could not read. The patient was able, however, to derive meaning from words spelled aloud and was able to spell correctly. Even though he could not comprehend written words, he could copy them correctly and could recognize and understand them after writing the individual letters.

The patient was blind in the right visual field (indicating damage to the left visual cortex) but otherwise had normal visual acuity. Postmortem examination of this and other patients revealed damage to the left occipital (visual) cortex and the splenium (the posterior portion of the corpus callosum), which carries visual information between the two hemispheres by interconnecting area 18 of the occipital cortex of one hemisphere with that of the other. Although the visual information from the left visual field could still be processed by the right hemisphere, damage to the splenium prevented its transfer to the angular gyrus and to language areas of the left hemisphere.

As might be predicted from the location of the lesion, many patients have selective deficits in visual perception due to damage in the visual portion of Brodmann's area 18 (see Chapter 29). For example, 50% of patients with pure alexia have either a *color agnosia* (they are capable of matching colors but cannot name them) or an *achromatopsia* (they cannot perceive color and therefore see objects only as shades of gray).

John Trescher and Frank Ford extended Dejerine's findings by noticing that surgical disruption of the splenium (the posterior portion of the corpus callosum) results in the loss of reading ability in the left but not the right visual field. In contrast, section of the anterior portion of the corpus callosum (which does not transmit visual information) does not interfere with reading. However, patients in whom the anterior portion of the corpus callosum has been transected cannot write with their left hands (controlled by the right hemisphere), because the right hemisphere no longer has access to the left hemisphere language centers. The patients also cannot name objects held in the left hand because the somatic sensory information does not reach the language areas in the left hemisphere.

Phonetic Symbols and Ideographs Are Localized to Different Regions of the Cerebral Cortex. An interesting disturbance in reading and writing occurs among the Japanese. There are two distinct systems of writing Japanese. One, *kata kana*, is phonetic: words are represented by a series of phonetic symbols (graphemes). There are 71 graphemes in the *kana* system. The other writing system, *kanji*, is in good part ideographic: root words are represented by one or more ideograms derived from Chinese. There are over 40,000 *kanji* ideograms to which are added affixes for phonemic reference. *Kana* words are comprehended syllable by syllable and, unlike Western words, are not easily identified at a glance. In contrast, the *kanji* system represents both sound and meaning; it has both phonetic and morphemic reference.

Because these two writing systems rely on phonemic processing to differing degrees, one might expect that certain focal lesions might affect reading or writing in one system but not the other. This is in fact the case. Both systems rely on language centers in the left hemisphere but each is processed by a different intrahemispheric mechanism. Lesions of the angular gyrus of the parietal–temporal–occipital association cortex severely disrupt reading of *kana* (syllabic) writing, but leave comprehension of *kanji* (ideographic) writing largely intact. Such lesions can disrupt reading of *kanji* to some degree, but the disruption entails primarily phonemic processing; patients may be unable to read the *kanji* word aloud but can accurately explain its meaning. In contrast, these patients are unable to understand the same idea expressed in *kana*.

These observations support the conclusion from brain imaging studies that the angular gyrus of the left hemisphere, concerned with auditory representation, is not involved with the processing of the visual representation of words. Other dissociations between the processing of *kana* and *kanji* scripts also occur and have provided further insight into the mechanisms of information processing in the production and comprehension of language.

Dyslexia and Hyperlexia Are Developmental Disorders of Reading

Dyslexia is an inability to read effortlessly or with understanding. Except for the reading impairment, the cognitive and intellectual capacities of these children are often normal and may even be superior. Children with dyslexia seem particularly impaired in phonemic processing—the ability to associate letters with the sounds they represent. However, they can usually understand other signs or symbols of communication, such as traffic signs or words that have a unique visual appearance (such as the Coca-Cola trademark). Indeed, Paul Rozin and his colleagues have found that American dyslexic children can easily learn to read English when entire words are represented by single characters rather than a sequence of characters. The specificity of this disorder and the parallels to alexic disorders caused by strokes have led to the suggestion that dyslexia might result from abnormalities in connections between visual and language areas.

Some dyslexic children also exhibit a strong tendency to read a word from right to left (confusing words like "was" and "saw") and have particular difficulty distinguishing between letters that have the same configuration but in different orientations (for example, p and q, or b and d). These mistakes occur in both reading and writing. These errors and the disproportionate percentage of left-handers among dyslexics led Samuel Orton to suggest that dyslexia might involve a deficit in the development of dominance by the left hemisphere. Albert Galaburda and Thomas Kemper have provided evidence supporting this hypothesis. They found that the normal hemispheric discrepancy in the size of the planum temporale was much reduced in dyslexic males. In addition, the left planum temporale exhibited striking cytoarchitectonic abnormalities, including an incomplete segregation of cell layers. In contrast, the right hemisphere appeared normal. These observations suggest that normal migration of neurons to the left cortex during development is slowed in dyslexic patients.

An Overall View

Language is a uniquely human ability. In both its written and spoken forms it represents meaningful interpersonal interaction, not just in the present but also across time. The study of language therefore presents problems of common interest to biology and the humanities. Given this special opportunity we may well ask, What can neurobiologists say to psychologists and humanists that would shed light on the biological process of human cognition?

The first and most important insight is that language abilities can be localized to one of the two cerebral hemispheres. The hemispheric asymmetry that ultimately gave rise to language emerged early in human evolution, perhaps as early as 300,000 years ago. The capability for language seems to be present at birth, and universal features of language are thought to derive in part from the structure of the cortical regions concerned with language in the left hemisphere.

From a biological standpoint, language is not a single capability but a family of capabilities, two of which, comprehension and expression, can be separated by distinctive functional sites in the brain. As first suggested by Wernicke, profound aphasia can result from simply disconnecting these two sites. Success in correlating major components of language with different anatomical regions led to the development of a simple model of language, the Wernicke–Geschwind model, which can account for a family of language-related disorders. This model, although clinically helpful, is overly simple and incorrect in detail.

Despite some notable insights, the neurobiological understanding of language is very rudimentary. The Wernicke–Geschwind model, although modified since its introduction, is only a beginning in the localization of cognitive functioning. It has, however, provided an important bridge between the analysis of language and its disorders by psycholinguists and the neuroanatomical localization of language function by neural scientists.

Selected Readings

Bellugi, U., Poizner, H., and Klima, E. S. 1989. Language, modality and the brain. Trends Neurosci. 12:380–388.

Caplan, D. 1987. Neurolinguistics and Linguistic Aphasiology: An Introduction. Cambridge, England: Cambridge University Press.

Chomsky, N. 1968. Language and the mind. Psychol. Today 1(9):48–68.

Damasio, A. R., and Geschwind, N. 1984. The neural basis of language. Annu. Rev. Neurosci. 7:127–147.

Gardner, R. A., and Gardner, B. T. 1969. Teaching sign language to a chimpanzee. Science 165:664–672.

Geschwind, N. 1965. Disconnexion syndromes in animals and man. Brain 88:237–294, 585–644.

Gleitman, L. R., and Gleitman, H. 1981. Language. In H. Gleitman (ed.), Psychology. New York: Norton, chap. 10.

LeMay, M. 1976. Morphological cerebral asymmetries of modern man, fossil man, and nonhuman primate. Ann. N.Y. Acad. Sci. 280:349–366.

Miller, G. A. 1981. Language and Speech. San Francisco: Freeman.

Petersen, S. E., Fox, P. T., Posner, M. I., Mintun, M., and Raichle, M. E. 1989. Positron emission tomographic studies of the processing of single words. J. Cognt. Neurosci. 1:153–170.

Premack, D. 1976. Intelligence in Ape and Man. Hillsdale, N.J.: Erlbaum.

References

Benson, D. F. 1979. Aphasia, Alexia, and Agraphia. New York: Churchill Livingstone.

Berndt, R. S., and Caramazza, A. 1980. A redefinition of the syndrome of Broca's aphasia: Implications for a neuropsychological model of language. Appl. Psycholinguistics 1:225–278.

Brown, R. 1973. A First Language: The Early Stages. Cambridge, Mass.: Harvard University Press.

Bruner, J. 1983. Child's Talk: Learning to Use Language. New York: Norton.

Brunner, R. J., Kornhuber, H. H., Seemuller, E., Suger, G., and Wallesch, C.-W. 1982. Basal ganglia participation in language pathology. Brain Language 16:281–299.

Chomsky, N. 1972. Language and Mind, 2nd ed. New York: Harcourt Brace Jovanovich.

Coltheart, M. 1985. Cognitive neuropsychology and the study of reading. In M. I. Posner and O. S. M. Marin (eds.), Attention and Performance XI. Hillsdale, N. J.: Erlbaum, pp. 3–37.

Damasio, H., and Damasio, A. R. 1980. The anatomical basis of conduction aphasia. Brain 103:337–350.

Damasio, A. R., and Geschwind, N. 1984. The neural basis of language. Annu. Rev. Neurosci. 7:127–148.

Dejerine, J. 1891. Sur un cas de cécité verbale avec agraphie, suivi d'autopsie. C. R. Seances Mem. Soc. Biol. 43:197–201.

Dejerine, J. 1892. Contribution a l'étude anatomo-pathologique et clinique des différentes variétés de cécité verbale. C. R. Seances Mem. Soc. Biol. 44:61–90.

Eimas, P. D. 1985. The perception of speech in early infancy. Sci. Am. 252(1):46–52.

Galaburda, A. M. 1988. The pathogenesis of childhood dyslexia. In F. Plum (ed.), Language, Communication, and the Brain. New York: Raven Press, pp. 127–137.

Galaburda, A. M., and Kemper, T. L. 1979. Cytoarchitectonic abnormalities in developmental dyslexia: A case study. Ann. Neurol. 6:94–100.

Geschwind, N. 1967. The varieties of naming errors. Cortex 3:97–112.

Geschwind, N. 1975. The apraxias: Neural mechanisms of disorders of learned movement. Am. Sci. 63:188–195.

Geschwind, N., Quadfasel, F. A., and Segarra, J. M. 1968. Isolation of the speech area. Neuropsychologia 6:327–340.

Heilman, K. M., and Scholes, R. J. 1976. The nature of comprehension errors in Broca's, conduction and Wernicke's aphasics. Cortex 12:258–265.

Iwata, M. 1984. Kanji versus Kana: Neuropsychological correlates of the Japanese writing system. Trends Neurosci. 77:290–293.

Karbe, H., Herholz, K., Szelies, B., Pawlik, G., Weinhard, K., and Heiss, W.-D. 1989. Regional metabolic correlates of Token test results in cortical and subcortical left hemispheric infarction. Neurology 39:1083–1088.

Kaufmann, W. E., and Galaburda, A. M. 1989. Cerebrocortical microdysgenesis in neurologically normal subjects: A histopathologic study. Neurology 39:238–244.

Kellogg, W. N. 1968. Communication and language in home-raised chimpanzee. Science 162:423–427.

Lenneberg, E. H. 1967. Biological Foundations of Language. New York: Wiley.

Liepmann, H. 1914. Bemerkungen zu v. Monakows Kapitel "Die Lokalisation der Apraxie." Monatsschr. Psychiatr. Neurol. 35: 490–516.

Metter E. J., Kempler, D., Jackson, C., Hanson, W. R., Mazziotta, J. C., and Phelps, M. E. 1989. Cerebral glucose metabolism in Wernicke's, Broca's and conduction aphasia. Arch. Neurol. 46: 27–34.

Naeser, M. A., Alexander, M. P., Helm-Estabrooks, N., Levine, H. L., Laughlin, S. A., and Geschwind, N. 1982. Aphasia with predominantly subcortical lesion sites. Arch. Neurol. 39:2–14.

Ojemann, G. A. 1983. Brain organization for language from the perspective of electrical stimulation mapping. Behav. Brain Sci. 6:189–230.

Orton, S. T. 1937. Reading, Writing and Speech Problems in Children. New York: Norton.

Patton, H. D., Sundsten, J. W., Crill, W. E., and Swanson, P. D. 1976. Introduction to Basic Neurology. Philadelphia: Saunders.

Petersen, S. E., Fox, P. T., Posner, M. I., Minton, M., and Raichle, M. E. 1988. Positron emission tomographic studies of the cortical anatomy of single-word processing. Nature 331: 585–589.

Ross, E. D. 1981. The aprosodias: Functional-anatomic organization of the affective components of language in the right hemisphere. Arch. Neurol. 38:561–569.

Rozin, P., Poritsky, S., and Sotsky, R. 1971. American children with reading problems can easily learn to read English represented by Chinese characters. Science 171:1264–1267.

Saffran, E. M. 1982. Neuropsychological approaches to the study of language. Br. J. Psychol. 73:317–337.

Schwartz, M. F. 1985. Classification of language disorders from a psycholinguistic viewpoint. In J. Oxbury, R. Whurr, M. Coltheart, and M. Wyke (eds.), Aphasia. London: Butterworth.

Skinner, B. F. 1957. Verbal Behavior. Advances in Neurology, Vol. 42. New York: Appleton-Century-Crofts.

Vignolo, L. A. 1984. Aphasias associated with computed tomography scan lesions outside Broca's and Wernicke's areas. In F. C. Rose (ed.), Progress in Aphasiology. Advances in Neurology, Vol. 42. New York: Raven Press, pp. 91–98.

55

Eric R. Kandel

Disorders of Thought: Schizophrenia

**Defining a Psychiatric Syndrome Poses
Unusual Difficulties**

There Are Now Reliable Clinical Criteria for
Classifying Mental Illnesses

Schizophrenia Has Been Studied Extensively
to Improve Classification and Diagnosis
of the Illness

**Schizophrenia Is Characterized by Psychotic
Episodes Preceded by Prodromal Signs and
Followed by Residual Symptoms**

**Schizophrenia Has an Important
Genetic Predisposition**

**Some People with Schizophrenia Have Prominent
Anatomical Changes in the Brain**

**Antipsychotic Drugs Are Effective in the
Treatment of Schizophrenia**

Antipsychotic Drugs Block Dopamine Receptors

Excess Dopaminergic Transmission
May Contribute to the Development
of Schizophrenia

Schizophrenic Symptoms Have Been Associated
with Distinct Anatomical Components Within
the Dopaminergic System

Abnormalities in Dopaminergic Transmission
Do Not Account for All Aspects
of Schizophrenia

An Overall View

Neurobiological advances in the analysis of language and its disorders have inspired biological investigations into the disturbances of thinking and mood. In this and the next chapter we shall examine the four most serious mental illnesses, schizophrenia, depression, mania, and the anxiety states. These disorders involve disturbances in thought, self-awareness, perception, affect, and social interaction.

Understanding mental illness is not only challenging to science, but is also of great social importance. In the United States mental illness accounts for about 20% of *all* hospitalizations. Before the advent of psychopharmacological agents, schizophrenia and the affective disorders alone accounted for 50% of all hospital bed occupancy!

Defining a Psychiatric Syndrome Poses Unusual Difficulties

As we have seen in earlier chapters on diseases of nerve and muscle, the study of any illness requires that there be good criteria for diagnosis. Ultimately, diagnosis should be based on *causes*, on whether the illness results from a genetic defect, a viral or bacterial infection, toxins, or stress. Unfortunately, the causes for most psychiatric illnesses are not known. As a result, psychiatric disorders are still grouped, as they were at the end of the nineteenth century, according to which of the four major mental faculties are affected: (1) disorders of thinking and cognition (schizophrenia and delirium); (2) disorders of mood (affective disorders and anxiety); (3) disorders of social behavior (character defects and personality disorders); and (4) disorders of learning, memory, and intelligence (mental retardation and dementia). This classification paralleled the system of classification adopted slightly earlier for inter nal medicine, where disorders were classified according to the primary target organ (disorders of the heart, lung, kidney, and stomach). The mental faculties—thinking, mood, social competence, intelligence—were similarly thought to reflect the functioning of different mental organs.

The first to emphasize the importance of objective description and classification in psychiatry was Emil Kraepelin, who at the turn of the century directed The Psychiatry Clinic in Heidelberg. Prior to Kraepelin, psychiatrists had arranged symptoms along arbitrary lines that had no medical significance. Kraepelin, following the lead of Rudolf Virchow and Julius Cohn Levin, the pioneers of cellular pathology, began to study psychiatric disorders as *disease processes* whose specific signs and symptoms emerged at specific points and evolved over time. He therefore focused on three features: (1) the signs that the disease presented, (2) the course of the disease, and (3) its outcome. Although our understanding of the brain has increased significantly since then, the delineation of the major mental illnesses in terms of signs, course, and outcome still constitutes the basis of the current classification of psychiatric illnesses.

There Are Now Reliable Clinical Criteria for Classifying Mental Illnesses

Following Kraepelin, the search for a reliable means of classifying mental illnesses has led to the development of three criteria for establishing a *diagnostic category*. These are: (1) that a group of *signs* (what the examiner sees) and *symptoms* (what the patient reports) be identified so that they can be reliably assessed; (2) that in certain patients, these signs and symptoms be shown to cluster together forming a *syndrome* that effectively distinguishes the group from normal people or people with other syndromes; (3) that the proposed syndrome be validated by one or more of three independent measures. The three independent measures commonly used are the following.

1. *Natural history (clinical course and outcome).* As Kraeplin first pointed out, a syndrome may occur at a characteristic age or be associated with a specific precipitant. It may also follow a characteristic clinical course. For example, there is a characteristic progressive and unremitting deterioration in schizophrenia, whereas in the major affective disorders there are cycles of recovery and relapse.
2. *Response to specific treatment.* A syndrome may respond specifically to one class of drugs and not to another. For example, manic-depressive illness, but not other mental illnesses, responds to lithium (Li$^+$).
3. *Causality (etiology and pathogenesis).* Definition of a syndrome does not imply that it has a specific cause, and therefore is not a specific disease. The ultimate validation of a syndrome is therefore finding a specific pathology, an anatomical or molecular defect, and a specific cause. Once a distinct cause has been identified, diagnosis of a specific *disease entity* can be made.

Traditionally, *demonstrable pathology*, the defining of a structural abnormality in the brain, has helped characterize specific diseases. Thus, a lesion in the head of the caudate nucleus helps define Huntington's disease. Even more informative about causality in this disease is the finding of a disproportionately higher incidence of Huntington's disease in blood relatives or twins of patients than in the population at large. This knowledge about pedigree and genetic predisposition led to the identification of a locus on chromosome 4 responsible for the disease. The most powerful insight into cause is the discovery of a specific molecular abnormality, as is the case with the gene that encodes for dystrophin in Duchenne's muscular dystrophy. This membrane-associated protein is always absent or abnormal in the disease.

There are, unfortunately, only a few psychiatric disorders in which the clinical manifestations can be correlated with a demonstrable pathology, as in Huntington's disease. The defects underlying most psychiatric disorders presumably involve more subtle structural and molecular changes, and these changes have so far remained elusive. The elusiveness of anatomical pathology distinguishes diseases of the mind from those of other areas of medicine, including neurology. Diseases of the heart, lung, kidney, and intestines, and even most traditional neurological diseases, can be validated by objective tissue pathology and, in addition, by quantitative examination of specific organ function, independent of the physical signs and symptoms. In contrast, diseases of the mental faculties can usually only be evaluated in terms of altered thinking, mood, and social behavior, and these clinical features can be difficult to ascertain and even more difficult to quantify. Psychiatric diagnosis therefore must rely heavily on the individual patient's history and the patient's response to treatment. These limitations have made it difficult in the past to achieve consensus in the evaluation of psychiatric symptoms and to investigate psychiatric illness scientifically. Nonetheless, substantial progress has been made recently in diagnosing mental illness, and there is reason to hope that a genuine neuropathology of mental illness might emerge soon.

Schizophrenia Has Been Studied Extensively to Improve Classification and Diagnosis of the Illness

Schizophrenia is perhaps the most devastating disorder of humankind. A fairly common disorder, schizophrenia affects both sexes equally and strikes about 1% of the population worldwide. Another 2–3% have *schizotypal personality disorder*, a milder form of the disease. Because of its prevalence and severity, schizophrenia has been studied extensively in an effort to develop better criteria for diagnosing the illness. Yet improved criteria have emerged only recently, after decades of research that began in the early part of the twentieth century with the clinical observations of Kraepelin and Eugene Bleuler in Switzerland.

Based on the long-term outcomes of hundreds of patients, Kraepelin distinguished two major mental illnesses. He called one illness *dementia praecox* (early deterioration of the intellect) because of its early age of onset, typically in adolescence, and his observation that the disease usually followed a progressive course without remission, leading ultimately to a dramatic deterioration of intellect. Kraepelin called the second illness the *manic depressive psychosis*. This condition usually has different symptoms, but most important it has a very different course: The onset is characteristically later, followed by remissions and relapses without progressive deterioration.

Bleuler objected to the term *dementia praecox* because he saw patients in whom the condition began in adulthood, while others occasionally experienced remission. He concluded that the symptoms described by Kraepelin reflected not a single entity but a group of closely related illnesses characterized by disorder of thought rather than dementia. He proposed that the thought disorder reflected the splitting of the cognitive side of the personality from the affective or emotional side and therefore called this group of diseases *schizophrenia*, a splitting of the mind. (This is not to be confused with multiple or split personalities, a rare disease in which a person alternately assumes two or more *identities*.) A patient with schizophrenia may show inappropriate affect (emotion) by laughing while recounting a tragic event, or may show no emotion (a flat affect) while describing a joyous occasion. Alternatively, he may experience a fragmentation of self by experiencing hallucinations; for instance, internal voices may tell him he is a terrible person who smells intolerably.

As is true for most other severe mental disturbances, schizophrenia is characterized by *psychotic episodes*—discrete, often reversible, mental states in which the patient loses the ability to *test reality*. During a psychotic episode patients are unable to examine their beliefs and perceptions realistically, and to compare them to what actually is happening in the world. Loss of *reality testing* is accompanied by other disturbances of higher mental functioning, especially *hallucinations* (abnormal perceptions), *delusions* (aberrant beliefs), incoherent thinking, disordered memory, and sometimes confusion.

Psychotic episodes are not specific to schizophrenia, however, and often occur in affective disorders and in states of toxic delirium. By using the validating methods described above, psychiatrists following Kraepelin and Bleuler were eventually able to differentiate schizophrenia more clearly from psychotic disorders with similar features which were often lumped with schizophrenia into a common diagnostic category. These included certain psychoses associated with drug intoxication (for example, psychosis due to phencyclidine or angel dust, which we shall learn about later), forms of manic depressive illness, brief reactive psychoses, and paranoid states.

Recent advances in the classification of mental disease, reflected in the revised third edition of the *Diagnostic and Statistical Manual of the American Psychiatric Association* (DSM-III-R), have led to the development of objective and rigorous descriptive criteria (as opposed to theoretical ones). These include both the features that are required to make the diagnosis (*inclusive criteria*) and those that would cause one to reject it (*exclusive criteria*). Moreover, each criterion in DSM-III-R has been demonstrated to be useful for making a diagnosis since independent observers agree on their meaning in actual clinical contexts.

Schizophrenia Is Characterized by Psychotic Episodes Preceded by Prodromal Signs and Followed by Residual Symptoms

The first psychotic episode of schizophrenia often is preceded by *prodromal signs*. These include social isolation and withdrawal, impairment in role function, odd behavior and ideas, neglect of personal hygiene, and blunted affect. The prodromal period is then followed by one or more psychotic episodes, separated by long periods in which the patient is not overtly psychotic, but nonetheless behaves eccentrically, is socially isolated, has poverty of speech, a poor attention span, a flat affect, and a lack of motivation.

These symptoms of the nonpsychotic period are called *residual* or *negative symptoms* because they reflect the *absence* of normal social and interpersonal function. These negative symptoms contrast with the abnormalities of a psychotic episode called the *positive symptoms* because they reflect the *presence* of distinctive behaviors, such as delusions, hallucinations, and markedly bizarre or disorganized behavior. Because they persist, these negative symptoms are the most unmanageable part of the illness.

The modern criteria for the diagnosis of schizophrenia require that a patient be continuously ill for at least six months, and that there be at least one psychotic phase followed by a residual phase. During the psychotic phase one or more of the following three groups of psychotic symptoms must be present:

1. Bizarre delusions (for example, of being persecuted or of having one's feelings, thoughts, and actions controlled by God or an outside force).
2. Prominent hallucinations, usually auditory (for example, hearing voices commenting on one's actions).
3. Disordered thoughts, incoherence, loss of the normal association between ideas, or marked poverty of speech accompanied by a loss of emotional content (flattening of affect).

During the psychotic phase schizophrenic patients may also exhibit bizarre behavior, unusual postures, mannerisms, or rigidity. On the basis of these criteria and other differences, schizophrenia is often divided into two or more subtypes, including *catatonic schizophrenia*, in which mutism and abnormal posture dominate, and *paranoid schizophrenia*, in which delusions of persecution predominate.

In diagnosing schizophrenia it is important to exclude a

disorder of mood, especially manic-depressive illness or a drug-induced psychosis, such as those due to amphetamine or phencyclidine, which we shall later consider. The prognosis for schizophrenia is generally (but not always) poor; there are frequent relapses into psychotic behavior. After each relapse social functioning may deteriorate progressively as the years go by.

Most students of schizophrenia view the purely psychotic episodes (or positive symptoms) and the residual (or negative) symptoms as different phases of the same disease, with the residual symptoms commonly representing the long-term outcome of positive symptoms. Some students of schizophrenia, however, have emphasized the distinctiveness of the two types of symptoms and believe that cases in which negative symptoms predominate represent a more severe disease, one in which the outcome is poorer.

Schizophrenia Has an Important Genetic Predisposition

Identifying the causes of schizophrenia is now one of the most challenging goals of psychiatric research. Recent studies indicate that schizophrenia is, at least in part, a genetic abnormality. For many years clinicians argued that social and environmental factors, particularly poor parenting, are important factors in the genesis of schizophrenia. For example, mothers of schizophrenic patients often manifest disturbed patterns of thinking and communication. The investigators in these earlier studies probably mistook the signs of a hereditary disorder for a poor social *interaction* between parent and child.

Franz Kallmann provided the earliest direct evidence that genetic endowment is important to the development of schizophrenia. Kallmann was impressed with the fact that approximately 1% of the general population suffers from schizophrenia. This rate is fairly uniform throughout the world, even though the social and environmental factors vary. Kallmann found, however, that the incidence of schizophrenia among parents, children, and siblings of patients with the disease is 15%, strong evidence that the disease runs in families. A genetic basis for schizophrenia cannot simply be inferred from the increased incidence in families, however. Not all conditions that run in families are necessarily genetic—wealth and poverty, habits and values run in families, and in earlier times even the nutritional deficiency pellagra ran in families.

To distinguish genetic from environmental factors, Kallmann and other investigators developed several research strategies. One strategy was to compare the rates of illness in monozygotic (identical) and dizygotic (fraternal) twins. Monozygotic twins have essentially identical genomes, whereas dizygotic twins share only half of their genetic material and are genetically equivalent to siblings. Therefore, monozygotic twins should be more or less identical in their tendency to develop schizophrenia if the disease is caused entirely by genetic factors. Even if genetic factors were necessary but not sufficient for the development of schizophrenia, because additional environmental factors are involved, a monozygotic twin of a patient with schizophrenia should be at significantly higher risk than a dizygotic twin. The tendency for twins to have the same illness is called *concordance*.

Studies on twins have established that the concordance for schizophrenia in monozygotic twins is about 30–50%. In contrast, it is only about 15% in dizygotic twins, about the same as for siblings, and 1% in the population at large. If schizophrenia were caused entirely by the genetic abnormalities, then the concordance rate of monozygotic twins would be nearly 100%. The 30–50% rate clearly indicates that genetic factors are not the only cause. However, these data do indicate that genetic factors must be critical because the risk for schizophrenia in a monozygotic twin is two to four times greater than that for dizygotic twins, and 30–50 times the risk in the general population!

Some critics argue that the high concordance in identical twins might be explained by the psychological trauma of having an identical twin who has schizophrenia. It has been argued that monozygotic twins might be prone to higher rates of perinatal trauma than dizygotic twins. To address these issues, and to disentangle further the effects of nature and nurture, Leonard Heston studied patients in the United States and David Rosenthal, Paul Wender, and Seymour Kety studied patients in Denmark. Heston compared the incidence of schizophrenia in adopted children whose biological parents suffered from schizophrenia with those of adopted children born of normal parents. Rosenthal and their colleagues compared the rate of illness in the biological relatives of schizophrenic adoptees with the rate among relatives of nonschizophrenic adoptees. All of the children were adopted at an early age by parents free of the illness, so that social factors were well controlled. In both sets of studies, the rate

TABLE 55–1. Evidence for the Importance of Genetic Factors in Schizophrenia

	Biological relatives		Adoptive relatives	
	With Schizophrenia	Control	With Schizophrenia	Control
Chronic schizophrenia	2.9% *	0%	1.4%	1.1%
Latent schizophrenia	3.5	1.7	0	1.1
Schizophrenia, uncertain subtype	7.5 *	1.7	1.4	3.3
Total	14.0 *	3.4	2.7	5.5

*Statistically significant.
(Adapted from Kety et al., 1975.)

of schizophrenia was higher among adopted children whose biological parents were schizophrenic than among adopted children with normal biological parents. The difference in rate—about 10–15%—was the same observed earlier by Kallman (Table 55–1).

In addition to documenting the importance of genetic factors in schizophrenia, studies of adoptees who develop schizophrenia show that rearing plays only a minor role in the disease. These studies also reveal that even when not overtly suffering from schizophrenia, some of the children of patients with schizophrenia are odd; they are socially isolated, have poor rapport with people, ramble in their speech, tend to be suspicious, have eccentric beliefs, and engage in magical thinking. This group of symptoms, which has been called the *schizotypal personality disorder*, may be a mild form of the disease, a nonpsychotic condition related to schizophrenia.

The view that schizophrenia is inherited is now beginning to be analyzed with the techniques of molecular genetics. Major advances in the study of genetic linkages have been achieved using a new technique to identify human DNA polymorphisms, places in the genome in which humans differ. As we have seen in our discussion of Duchenne's muscular dystrophy (Chapter 17), in the past, genetic markers were derived primarily from variations in gene products, such as enzymes or antigens from the histocompatibility complex blood groups. However, this method mapped only the coding sequences, or about 20% of the total human genome. It is now possible to saturate the human genome with restriction fragment length polymorphisms, genetic markers that are based on common variations in DNA sequences, including noncoding as well as coding sequences (see Chapter 17, Box 17–1).

Linkage studies using restriction fragment length polymorphism have recently been applied to families of patients with schizophrenia. By examining a few British and Icelandic families that contain many family members with schizophrenia, Robin Sherrington and his colleagues discovered a linkage between schizophrenia and two DNA polymorphisms on the long arm of chromosome 5. A similar chromosomal location was discovered by Anne Bassett and her colleagues in two related patients with schizophrenia, both of whom had a partial trisomy of chromosome 5. Cytogenetic studies of Bassett's patients revealed that an identical extrachromosomal segment of the long arm of chromosome 5 had been inserted into the long arm of chromosome 1.

This locus on chromosome 5 probably is only one of several (perhaps many) genetic loci for schizophrenia. In fact, most populations that show a genetic predisposition to schizophrenia do not show this particular defect, suggesting that schizophrenia may arise from a number of genetic abnormalities, both major and minor. The data of Sherrington and of Bassett indicate that there are probably a few *major* genes in the population, the alteration of any one of which can cause schizophrenia. These major genes, however, seem to account for only a small percentage of the genetic determinants of schizophrenia. More commonly, schizophrenia probably results from the concerted actions of many genes, each of which makes only a small contribution. This is consistent with evidence from other areas of behavioral genetics, which suggests that the normal range of a given behavioral variation usually reflects the combined actions of *many* genes, each with only a small effect. When acting alone, most of these alleles presumably alter behavior only subtly.

Moreover, the consistent finding that only 30–50% of monozygotic twins of schizophrenics have schizophrenia indicates that nongenetic factors also are important. Thus, most forms of schizophrenia differ dramatically from Duchenne's muscular dystrophy and Huntington's disease, two genetic diseases of the nervous system we considered earlier (Chapters 17 and 41), in which there is transmission of a *dominant* gene. The penetrance of these two diseases (the frequency with which the diseases are manifested by individuals carrying the conditioning genes) approaches 100%, and there are only minor nongenetic influences in their expression. Also, the transmission pattern of schizophrenia differs from such simple *recessive* diseases as phenylketonuria. Here neither parent may have the phenotype but one in four children will have the disease. For diseases that show classical dominant or recessive Mendelian inheritance, such as Huntington's, Duchenne's, and phenylketonuria, relatively routine studies of pedigrees are sufficient to pinpoint the mode of transmission.

The pattern of inheritance manifest in most forms of schizophrenia is more complex. As is the case with other multifactorial, polygenic diseases, such as diabetes and hypertension, most forms of schizophrenia are thought to require the accumulation of several genetic defects as well as environmental factors. Thus, to understand schizophrenia it will be essential to learn how several genes combine to predispose an individual to the disease and to determine how the environment influences the penetrance of these genes. Environmental influences include not only parenting and other early social interactions but also, and perhaps particularly important, perinatal injury and infections of childhood. Moreover, Sherrington's finding that in certain families a single allele can be linked with various subtypes of the illness (paranoid, catatonic, and even schizotypal personality) indicates that, under the influence of environmental factors, the genetic defect may be expressed in a range of phenotypes rather than only one phenotype.

Some People with Schizophrenia Have Prominent Anatomical Changes in the Brain

In addition to a genetic abnormality, a second important clue about the biology of schizophrenia has come from anatomical studies of patients with the disease. Computerized tomography and magnetic resonance imaging studies have shown that *some* patients with schizophrenia have three major anatomical abnormalities: (1) enlarged lateral ventricles; (2) enlarged third ventricles; and (3) widening of sulci, reflecting a reduction of cortical tissue, especially in the frontal lobe.

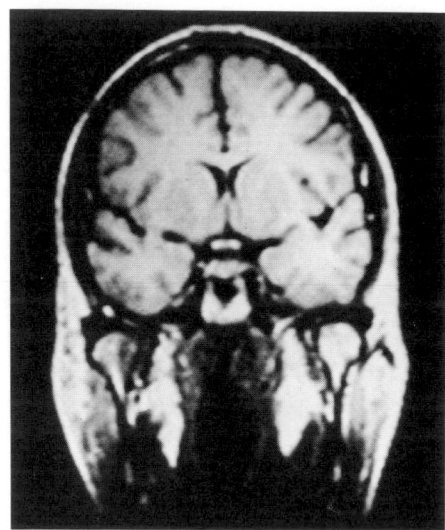
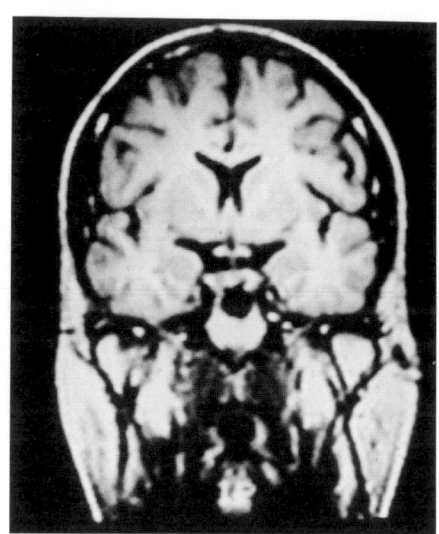

Unaffected twin   Schizophrenic twin

FIGURE 55–1
Comparison of MRI scans of monozygotic twins, only one of which is affected with schizophrenia. The affected twin on the right shows marked lateral ventricular enlargement. This has been found to correlate strongly with the presence of the disease. (Adapted from Suddath et al., 1989.)

Patients with ventricular enlargement often have a history of a prominent prodromal period with poor social functioning before the onset of psychotic symptoms, suggesting that the disease starts early in life. Ventricular enlargement is not specific to this disease, however; this abnormality also occurs in patients with dementia of the Alzheimer's type. Nonetheless, brain imaging techniques have had an important impact on the study of schizophrenia by providing clear evidence that many patients with schizophrenia have atrophy of the brain, particularly of the prefrontal region, and enlargement of the ventricles. This point is clearly made in Figure 55–1, which shows magnetic resonance image scans from a pair of monozygotic twins. The twin with schizophrenia has enlarged ventricles, while the normal twin has normal ventricles. Daniel Weinberger and his colleagues have now examined 15 twin pairs. In 12 pairs the twin with schizophrenia had enlarged ventricles that could be diagnosed from simply inspecting the image. This difference in monozygotic twins suggests the intriguing possibility that the structural change is nongenetic, resulting perhaps from perinatal injury or other developmental disturbance.

Antipsychotic Drugs Are Effective in the Treatment of Schizophrenia

The evidence for a genetic component of schizophrenia was soon followed by evidence of possible physiological mechanisms. Until the 1950s there were no treatments specifically effective for schizophrenia. During the 1950s, however, antipsychotic drugs were found that dramatically improved the treatment of the psychotic phase of the illness. The first of these drugs was reserpine. This was followed by a group of drugs now called the *typical antipsychotics*, which include the phenothiazines (beginning with chlorpromazine), the butyrophenones (haloperidol), and the thioxanthenes (Figure 55–2). More recently a new group of drugs called the *atypical antipsychotics* (clozapine) have proven useful in schizophrenia.

These antipsychotic drugs were originally thought to act as tranquilizers, calming patients without sedating them unduly. Acutely agitated, aggressive patients are calmed within hours. However, by 1964 the drugs were found to have an even more powerful long-term therapeutic effect that was specific to the psychotic symptoms of schizophrenia. When taken over several weeks the drugs mitigate or abolish delusions, hallucinations, and some types of disordered thinking (Table 55–2). Maintaining remitted patients on antipsychotic medication also reduces the rate of relapse.

TABLE 55–2. Response of Schizophrenic Symptoms to Phenothiazines

Symptoms	Response to phenothiazines*
Schizophrenic symptoms	
Thought disorder	+++
Blunted affect	+++
Withdrawal	+++
Autistic behavior	+++
Hallucinations	++
Paranoid ideation	+
Grandiosity	+
Hostility, belligerence	0
Nonschizophrenic symptoms	
Anxiety, tension, agitation	0
Guilt, depression	0

*0, no response; +++, best response.
(Adapted from Klein and Davis, 1969.)

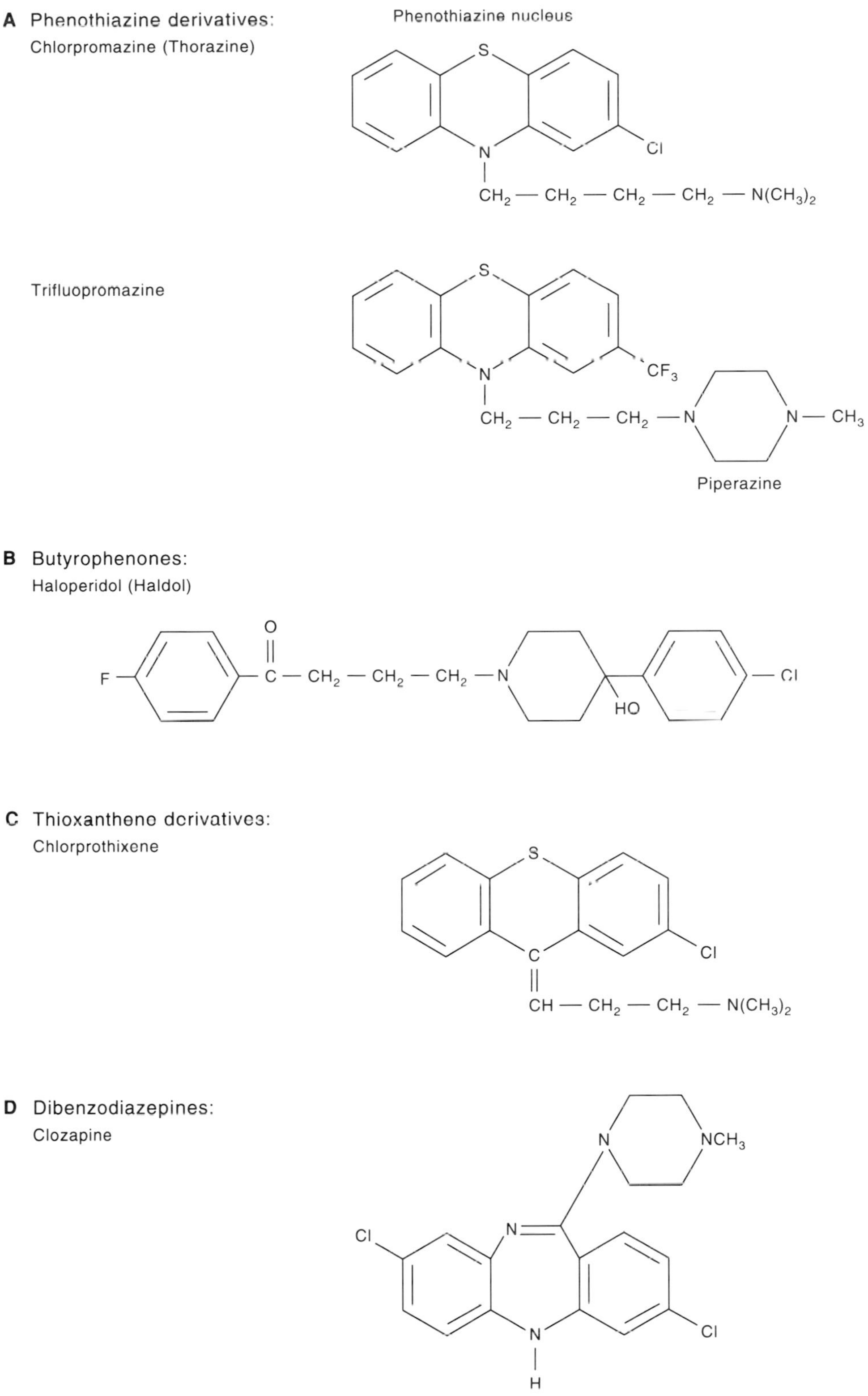

FIGURE 55–2

Chemical structures of the four major groups of antipsychotic drugs used to treat schizophrenia. The *typical antipsychotic* drugs, the phenothiazincs (**A**), butyrophenones (**B**), and thioxanthenes (**C**) bind to D_2 receptors. These typical antipsychotic drugs give rise to extrapyramidal side effects (**D**). The *atypical antipsychotic* drugs—such as the dibenzodiazepine, clozapine—bind to D_3 and D_4 receptors, and these do not give rise to the extrapyramidal side effects.

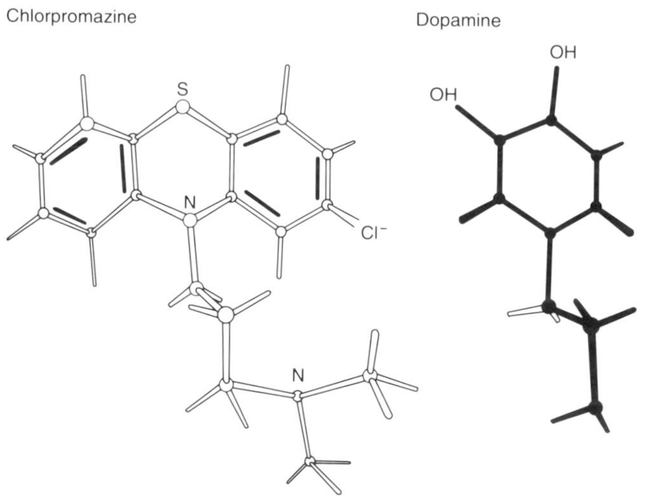

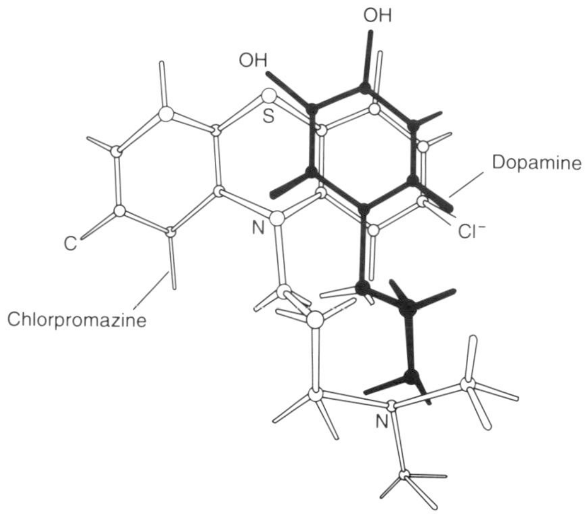

FIGURE 55–3
A comparison of the molecular structure of dopamine and chlorpromazine demonstrates why the latter acts on dopamine receptors. It has a similar shape and therefore fits the receptor. However, because of differences in structure, chlorpromazine simply binds to the receptor without triggering a response. (Adapted from Snyder, 1986.)

Antipsychotic Drugs Block Dopamine Receptors

The first clue to the cellular action of antipsychotic drugs came from an analysis of their major side effects. The drugs often produce a syndrome resembling parkinsonism. Like parkinsonism, which involves a deficiency in dopaminergic transmission (see Chapter 41), this drug-induced syndrome is reversed by anticholinergic agents. Following a suggestion by Avid Carlsson, a number of studies found that, despite differences in their chemical structure, many effective antipsychotic agents block dopamine receptors (Figure 55–3). It was therefore thought that an excess of dopamine transmission could be an important part of the pathogenesis of schizophrenia.

To localize the pathology further it was important to identify the receptor sites at which the drugs exert their effect. There are now at least six major types of dopamine receptors (D_1, D_{2a}, D_{2b}, D_3, D_4, and D_5). Isoforms of each of these receptors have been cloned by Olivier Civelli, Marc Caron, J.-C. Schwartz, Philip Seeman, and their colleagues. As expected of G-protein-coupled receptors, the amino acid sequences of each of these receptor subtypes has the characteristic seven membrane-spanning regions (Table 55–3).

The D_1 and D_5 dopamine receptors are coupled to a G-protein (G_S) that activates adenylyl cyclase, the enzyme that converts ATP to cAMP (Chapter 13). These receptors are expressed in neurons of the cortex and hippocampus and have a low affinity for most types of antipsychotic drugs.

The D_2 dopamine receptors are expressed in neurons of the caudate and the limbic systems, specifically in the nucleus accumbens, the amygdala, the hippocampus, and parts of the cerebral cortex. There are at least two subtypes. One (D_{2a}) is linked to an inhibitory G-protein (G_i) that inhibits adenylyl cyclase. A second subtype (D_{2b}) is linked through another G-protein that increases phosphoinositide turnover (Figure 55–5). The D_2 receptors have a high affinity for typical antipsychotic drugs (of the phenothiazine, butyrophenone, and thioxanthene variety) and are therefore thought to be one of the major sites of the therapeutic action of these drugs. Indeed, the clinical potency of these antipsychotic agents in patients with schizophrenia is closely correlated with their affinity for the D_2 receptors (Figure 55–4). Since D_2 receptors are expressed in the caudate, they presumably contribute to extrapyramidal side effects of the antipsychotic drugs. The D_{2a} receptors are of further interest because they are present on dopaminergic neurons themselves, on both the cell body and on the terminals. Here they act as *inhibitory autoreceptors* to control both the rate of firing of the neuron and the release of dopamine by the action potential at the terminal (Figure 55–5). The conventional antipsychotic drugs are thought to exert some of their actions at the D_{2a} autoreceptors.

The D_3 and D_4 dopamine receptors are restricted in

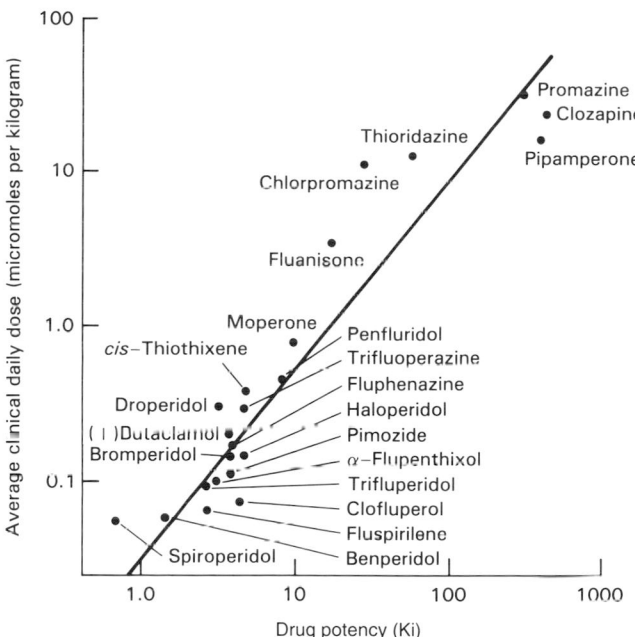

FIGURE 55-4
There is a strong correlation between the clinical potencies of antipsychotic drugs and the ability of the drugs to block dopamine D_2 receptors. On the **vertical axis** is the average daily dose required to achieve the same clinical effect. On the **horizontal axis** is the concentration of drug required to bind half the receptors. The higher the concentration required, the lower the affinity for the receptor. (Based on Seeman et al., 1976.)

their expression to the limbic system and cortex; they are only weakly expressed in the basal ganglia. This selective distribution may explain why atypical antipsychotic agents, such as clozapine that bind effectively to D_3 and D_4 receptors, do not give rise to extrapyramidal side effects.

Excess Dopaminergic Transmission May Contribute to the Development of Schizophrenia

The finding that antipsychotic drugs block certain dopamine receptors has led to the suggestion that an excess of dopaminergic transmission underlies at least some aspects of the pathogenesis of schizophrenia. This idea has received additional support from two discoveries in humans. First, drugs that increase the level of dopamine—such as L-dihydroxyphenylalanine (L-DOPA), cocaine, and amphetamine—cause a psychosis that resembles the paranoid subtype of schizophrenia (Figure 55–6). Some of these drugs, such as amphetamine, also cause bizarre repetitive, stereotyped behavioral acts in monkeys. Antipsychotic drugs reverse not only the amphetamine psychosis in humans, but also the bizarre behavioral syndrome in monkeys. Second, the brains of schizophrenic patients studied at autopsy contain an increased number of D_2 receptors in the caudate nucleus, nucleus accumbens (ventral striatum), and olfactory tubercule. This increase is particularly

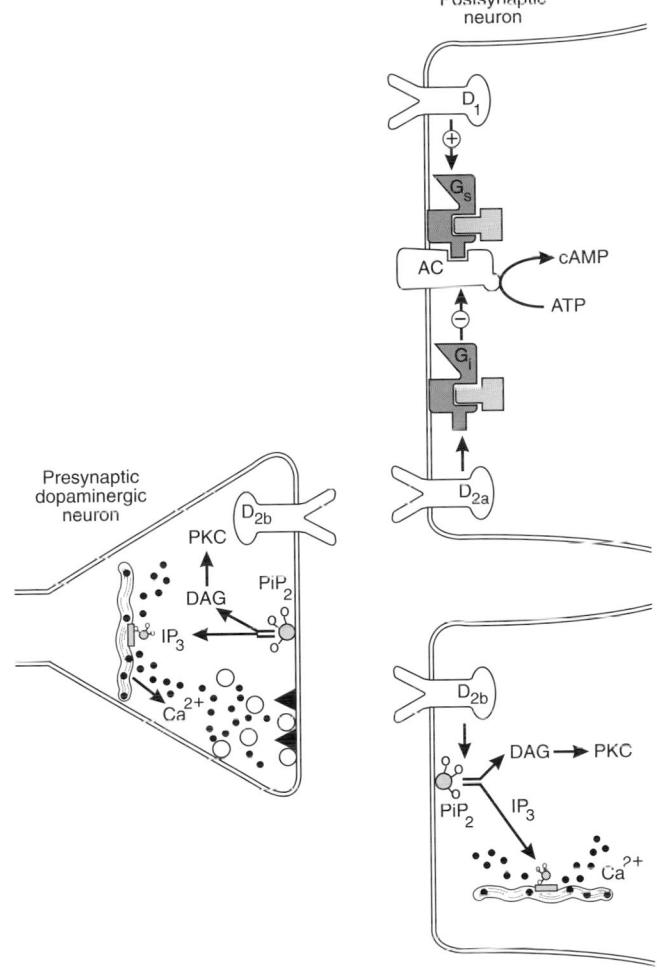

FIGURE 55-5
There are at least six types of dopamine receptors, three of which are illustrated here. The postsynaptic receptor D_{2a} inhibits adenylyl cyclase by an inhibitory G-protein (G_i). The presynaptic inhibitory autoreceptor D_{2b} regulates, via a phosphoinositide second-messenger system, the amount of dopamine released in response to an action potential. (PiP_2, phosphoinositide diphosphate; IP_3, inositol triphosphate; **DAG**, diacylglycerol; **PKC**, protein kinase C.) The presynaptic receptor D_{2b}, and the postsynaptic receptor D_{2a} have a high affinity for the typical antipsychotic drugs of the phenothiazine, butyrophenone, and thioxanthene classes, and are thought to be key targets for their therapeutic actions. There are, in addition, four other dopamine receptors. D_1 and D_5 stimulate adenylyl cyclase (**AC**) by a stimulatory G-protein (G_s). These have a low affinity for antipsychotic drugs and are therefore not thought to be involved in mediating the effects of these drugs on schizophrenic symptoms. The receptors D_3 and D_4 bind the atypical antipsychotic drugs.

prominent in patients with positive symptoms and has now been demonstrated in positron emission tomography (PET) scans of living patients who have never been treated with antipsychotic medication, so that the finding appears not to be a secondary effect of treatment with drugs.

These changes in D_2 receptors need not be the primary

TABLE 55–3. Six Types of Postsynaptic Dopamine Receptors

	D_1 and D_5	D_{2a}	D_{2b}	D_3 and D_4
Molecular structure	Seven membrane-spanning regions	Seven membrane-spanning regions	Seven membrane-spanning regions	Seven membrane-spanning regions
Effect on cyclic AMP	Increases	Decreases	Increases phospho-inositide turnover	?
Agonists				
Dopamine	Full agonist (weak)	Full agonist (potent)		
Apomorphine	Partial agonist (weak)	Full agonist (potent)		
Antagonists				
Phenothiazines	Potent	Potent		
Thioxanthenes	Potent	Potent		
Butyrophenones	Weak	Potent		
Clozapine	Inactive	Weak	Weak	Potent

FIGURE 55–6

The key steps in the synthesis and degradation of dopamine (DA) and the sites of action of various psychoactive substances at the dopaminergic synapse. (Adapted from Cooper, Bloom, and Roth, 1986.)

1. *Enzymatic synthesis.* The conversion of tyrosine to DOPA (dihydroxyphenylalanine) by tyrosine hydroxylase is stimulated by L-DOPA and is blocked by the competitive inhibitor α-methyl-tyrosine.

2. *Storage.* Reserpine and tetrabenazine interfere with the uptake and storage of dopamine by the storage granules. Reserpine is an effective antipsychotic drug; the depletion of dopamine by reserpine is long-lasting and the storage granules appear to be irreversibly damaged. Tetrabenazine also interferes with the uptake and storage mechanism of the granules, but only transiently.

3. *Release.* Cocaine releases dopamine from dopaminergic neurons by blocking reuptake.

4. *Receptor interaction.* Typical antipsychotics such as perphenazine and haloperidol are particularly effective in blocking the D_2 and the postsynaptic autoreceptors.

5. *Reuptake.* Dopamine activity is terminated when dopamine is taken up into the presynaptic terminal. Amphetamine, as well as the anticholinergic drug benzotropine, is a potent inhibitor of this reuptake mechanism. Amphetamine induces a psychosis that is reversed by antipsychotic drugs.

6. *Degradation.* Dopamine present in a free state within the presynaptic terminal can be degraded by the enzyme monoamine oxidase (MAO). Pargyline is an effective inhibitor of MAO. Some MAO is also present outside the dopaminergic neuron. Dopamine also can be inactivated by the enzyme catechol-O-methyltransferase (COMT), which is believed to be localized outside the neuron in the postsynaptic cell.

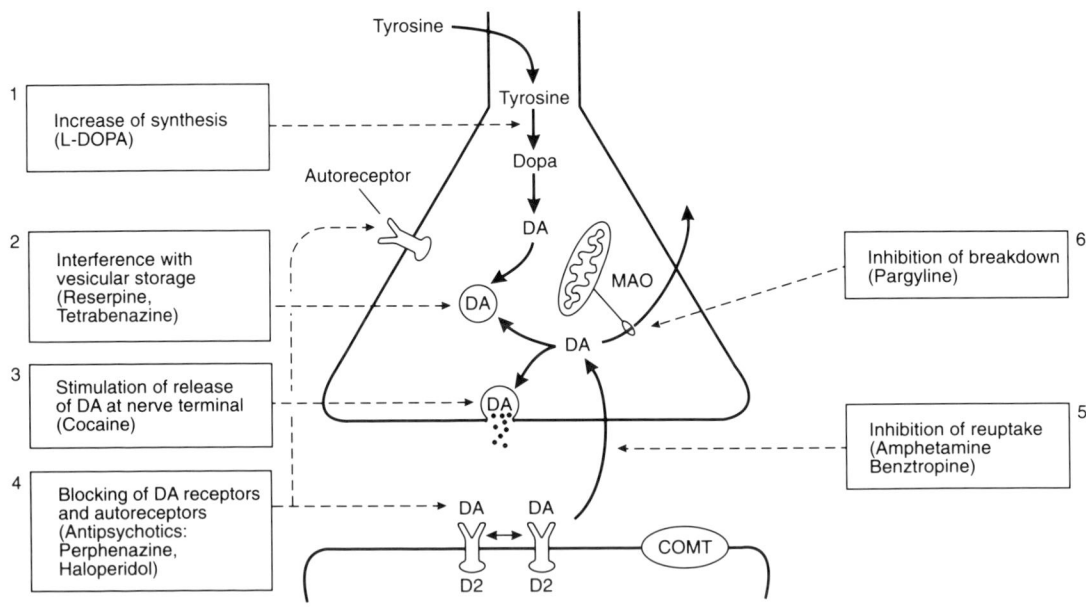

defect, however; they might be secondary to disturbances elsewhere in the brain that are mediated by dopamine receptor mechanisms.

Moreover, there is still no direct evidence that the excessive activity of dopaminergic cells implied by the PET studies actually contributes to the defect underlying schizophrenia. The challenge in schizophrenia (as in the depressive disorders, which we shall consider in Chapter 56) is to advance from an initial set of pharmacological clues to more precise anatomical insights. To explore the roles of dopaminergic transmission in schizophrenia further, we therefore need to know which component of the dopamine system is involved in the disease.

Schizophrenic Symptoms Have Been Associated with Distinct Anatomical Components Within the Dopaminergic System

As discussed in Chapter 44, dopamine neurons are not randomly distributed in the brain but are organized into four major subsystems: the tuberoinfundibular, nigrostriatal, mesolimbic, and mesocortical systems (Figure 55–7). These systems have been revealed through the use of formaldehyde-induced histofluorescence microscopy (described in Chapter 14).

The *tuberoinfundibular dopaminergic system* originates in cell bodies of the arcuate nucleus of the hypothalamus and projects to the pituitary stalk. This system is important for prolactin regulation and may contribute to some of the secondary neuroendocrine abnormalities in schizophrenia.

The *nigrostriatal dopaminergic system* originates in the substantia nigra and projects primarily to the putamen and caudate nucleus. As pointed out in Chapter 41, partial degeneration of this system contributes to the symptoms of Parkinson's disease. This system may also be involved in the short-term extrapyramidal side effects of antipsychotics, such as hand tremor and rigidity of muscles, as well as the long-term side effect known as *tardive dyskinesia*. When the caudate degenerates in Huntington's disease, it causes movement disorders similar to that seen with tardive dyskinesia.

The *mesolimbic dopaminergic system* has its origin in cell bodies in the ventral tegmental area, which is medial and superior to the substantia nigra. These cells project to the *mesial* component of the limbic system, the nucleus accumbens, the nuclei of the stria terminalis, parts of the amygdala and hippocampus, to the lateral septal nuclei, and the mesial frontal, anterior cingulate, and entorhinal cortex. The role of the mesolimbic system in emotions and memory (see Chapters 48 and 64), and the similarity between schizophrenia and certain types of psychomotor (limbic system) epilepsy in which disturbances of thought and perception are prominent (see Chapter 1), led Arvid Carlsson to propose that the positive symptoms of schizophrenia result from overactivity of the mesolimbic components of the dopaminergic system. Among the projections of the mesolimbic system, those to the nucleus accumbens are thought to be particularly important. This nucleus is a convergence site for input from the amygdala,

hippocampus, entorhinal area, anterior cingulate area, and parts of the temporal lobe. The mesolimbic dopaminergic projection is thought to modulate this convergent flow of neural activity and thereby transform the information conveyed by the nucleus accumbens to the septum, hypothalamus, anterior cingulate area, and frontal lobes. All of these areas, as we shall see later, are thought to be disturbed in schizophrenia. Overactive modulation of the output to these areas from the nucleus accumbens could contribute to positive symptoms.

The *mesocortical dopaminergic system* originates in the ventral tegmental area and projects to the neocortex, and most densely to the prefrontal cortex. As we have seen in Chapter 53, the prefrontal cortex is involved in motivation and planning, the temporal organization of behavior, attention, and social behavior. This component may be important in the negative symptoms of schizophrenia. Whereas the positive symptoms of schizophrenia might involve increased activity in the mesolimbic dopaminergic system, the negative symptoms of schizophrenia bear some resemblance to the defects seen following surgical disconnection of the frontal lobes, especially the dorsal prefrontal cortex (Chapter 53). After loss of the dorsal prefrontal cortex patients are poorly motivated, plan poorly, and have a flat affect.

Consistent with this idea, David Ingvar has found that in patients with schizophrenia the blood flow in the frontal lobe is reduced and is not further enhanced during intellectual tasks as it is in normal subjects. Moreover, Goldman-Rakic and her colleagues found that the modulatory pathway from the mesocortical dopaminergic system is essential for the normal function of the dorsolateral prefrontal cortex: for motivation, planning, and aspects of cognition. Depletion of dopamine in the prefrontal cortex (using the toxin 6-hydroxydopamine) impairs the performance of monkeys in cognitive tasks, similar to the effect of ablating the prefrontal cortex. This cognitive deficit can be reversed by giving the dopamine precursor L-DOPA or the agonist apomorphine. In fact, patients with Parkinson's disease, who have lost dopaminergic neurons, suffer not only from a motor disorder (reflecting the deficit in the nigrostriatal dopaminergic system), but also lack motivation and have flat affect and reduced spontaneity, defects that may reflect a decrease in transmission in the mesocortical dopaminergic pathways. Similarly, lesions that destroy the ventral tegmental area, which gives rise to the mesolimbic dopaminergic system, cause dementia and psychotic episodes.

These several findings have led Weinberger to suggest that there are two different disturbances in dopaminergic transmission in schizophrenia: (1) an *increase* in activity in the mesolimbic component of the dopaminergic system (perhaps mediated primarily through D_2, D_3, and D_4 receptors), which accounts for the positive symptoms and responds to antipsychotic drugs often quite dramatically, and (2) a *decrease* in activity of the prefrontal area, which accounts for the negative symptoms and does not respond as effectively to antipsychotic drugs. Weinberger stresses an imbalance between cortical and subcortical dopaminergic transmission in the genesis of schizophrenia. He pro-

864

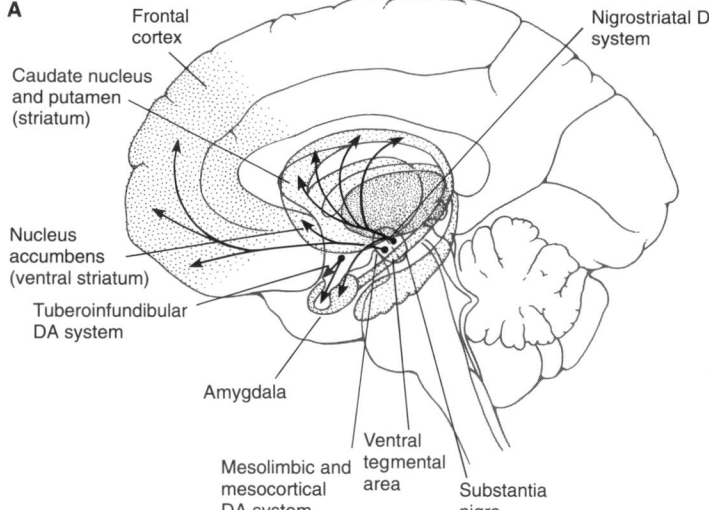

A

Frontal cortex

Caudate nucleus and putamen (striatum)

Nigrostriatal DA system

Nucleus accumbens (ventral striatum)

Tuberoinfundibular DA system

Amygdala

Mesolimbic and mesocortical DA system

Ventral tegmental area

Substantia nigra

FIGURE 55–7

There are four major dopaminergic tracts in the brain: (1) the nigrostriatal, from the substantia nigra to the putamen and caudate; (2) the tuberoinfundibular, from the arcuate nucleus of the hypothalamus to the pituitary stalk; (3) the mesolimbic, from the ventral tegmental area to many components of the limbic system; and (4) the mesocortical, from the ventral tegmental area to the neocortex, especially prefrontal areas. The mesolimbic system may be involved in the positive symptoms of schizophrenia and the mesocortical system in the negative symptoms.

A. A midsagittal section shows the approximate anatomical routes of the four tracts.

B. A coronal section shows the sites of origin and the targets of all four tracts.

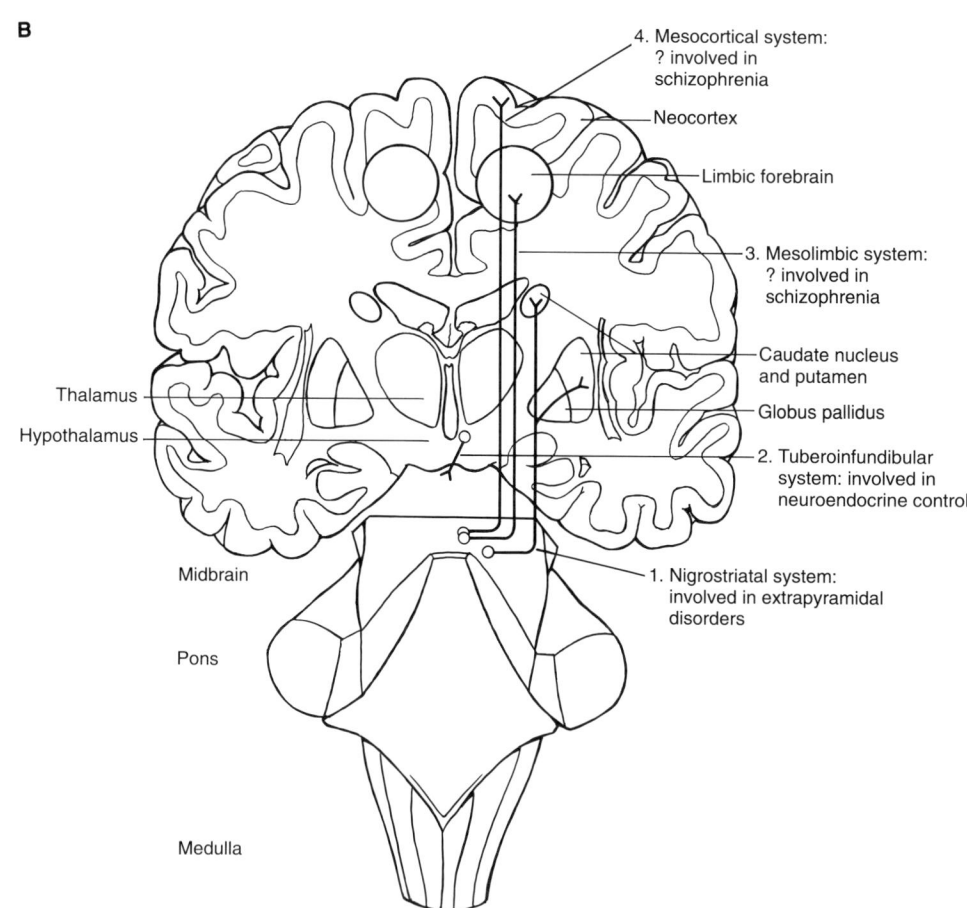

B

4. Mesocortical system: ? involved in schizophrenia

Neocortex

Limbic forebrain

3. Mesolimbic system: ? involved in schizophrenia

Caudate nucleus and putamen

Globus pallidus

2. Tuberoinfundibular system: involved in neuroendocrine control

1. Nigrostriatal system: involved in extrapyramidal disorders

Thalamus

Hypothalamus

Midbrain

Pons

Medulla

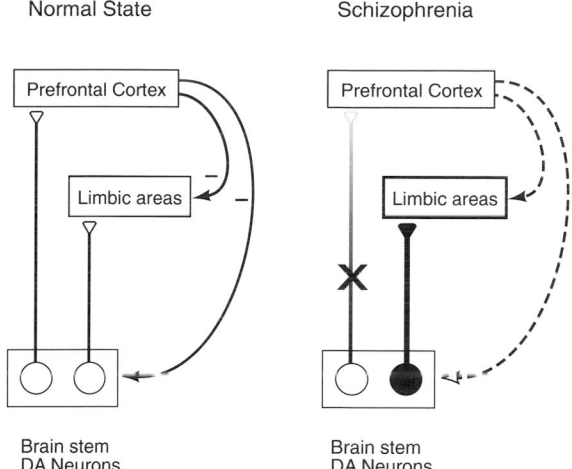

FIGURE 55–8

A neuro-anatomical model of schizophrenia. According to this view, the mesocortical pathway and prefrontal areas normally inhibit by feedback inhibition the activity of the limbic areas and the mesolimbic pathway. A primary defect in schizophrenia may be depressed activity in the mesocortical dopaminergic projection to the frontal lobe. This could lead to loss of inhibitory feedback and a consequent hyperactivity of the dopaminergic mesolimbic pathway. (Adapted from Weinberger, 1987.)

poses that activity in the mesocortical pathway to the prefrontal cortex normally inhibits the limbic components by feedback inhibition, and that the primary defect in schizophrenia is a reduction in prefrontal activation by the mesocortical pathway, which leads to disinhibition and overactivity in the mesolimbic pathway (Figure 55–8).

Although Weinberger's scheme is still untested, there is evidence for an interaction between the mesolimbic and mesocortical components in experimental animals. Christopher Pycock and his colleagues found that lesioning of the mesocortical pathway in experimental animals with 6-hydroxydopamine induces enhanced synaptic responsiveness in the mesolimbic pathways, specifically in its terminations in the nucleus accumbens. It is not known how loss of dopaminergic terminals in the prefrontal cortex leads to increased activity of the mesolimbic pathway in the nucleus accumbens. However, Pycock and his collaborators suggest that reduced activity in one pathway may result in compensatory neuronal growth in the other. Weinberger has further argued that the mesocortical system is important in the normal response to stress. If so, reduced function in this system, perhaps due to a number of gene defects, may make a person particularly vulnerable to the stresses of adolescence and thus contribute to the onset and progression of schizophrenia.

Abnormalities in Dopaminergic Transmission Do Not Account for All Aspects of Schizophrenia

As these interesting but still speculative arguments illustrate, we are far from understanding the role of dopaminergic transmission in normal mental function and in schizophrenia. Moreover, even if our preliminary ideas about the role of dopamine in mental function were correct in outline, it is still unlikely that schizophrenia results only from a defect in dopaminergic transmission. First, the major argument for the involvement of dopaminergic pathways in schizophrenia comes from the analysis of the mechanisms of action of the antipsychotic drugs. It is difficult, in principle, to extrapolate from the mechanisms of action of a therapeutic agent to the causal mechanisms of a disease. Pharmacological manipulation may produce changes that compensate for the disease without directly affecting the disordered mechanism itself. For example, the primary defect in Parkinson's disease is a decrease in dopamine levels, but as we have seen in Chapter 42, the symptoms can be alleviated by drugs that *block* cholinergic transmission.

This issue can be further illustrated by referring to the

FIGURE 55–9

This scheme shows how an antischizophrenic drug blocking a dopamine receptor could ameliorate symptoms without directly acting on the neurons that are responsible for the disease. Here it is assumed that schizophrenia is due to an imbalance of synaptic input as a result of overactivity of an inhibitory neuron. Blocking the effectiveness of a parallel dopaminergic inhibitory neuron acting at the same postsynaptic cell could ameliorate the disease by reducing the net inhibition converging on the postsynaptic cell. However, it would be incorrect to assume that because the block partially restored the balance and thereby improved the patient's behavior, these dopaminergic neurons were the site of pathology. (Adapted from R. Zigmond, personal communication.)

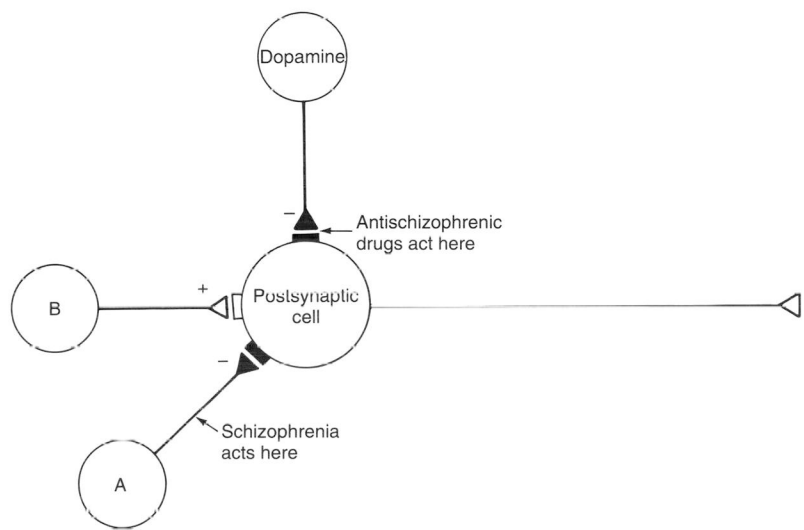

simple model illustrated in Figure 55–9. Consider the hypothetical situation of three presynaptic neurons converging on a postsynaptic neuron, with each presynaptic neuron releasing a different transmitter (transmitters A, B, and dopamine). Transmitter A and dopamine reduce the excitability of the postsynaptic cell, whereas transmitter B directly excites it. If schizophrenia resulted from a defect in neuron A or its transmitter, causing an excess of this modulatory transmitter to act on the postsynaptic cell, one might improve the symptoms by simply blocking the action of dopamine, the other modulatory transmitter, because this intervention would reduce net inhibition onto the postsynaptic cell. However, this model could easily prove inadequate for determining the best treatment. For instance, the dopaminergic neuron and neuron A might have very different inputs converging on them. If so, inhibiting dopaminergic transmission might cause an imbalance in the inputs and therefore inappropriate signals in the postsynaptic neuron. Even this simple example illustrates that a correlation between excess dopamine and schizophrenia, however strong, is not sufficient to allow a conclusion about the underlying cause of the disease.

In addition, there are some reasons to question whether the affinity of antipsychotic agents for D_2 (as well as D_3 and D_4) receptors is the only basis of the clinical efficacy of these drugs. Although antipsychotic drugs occupy dopamine receptors very quickly following administration, there often is a delay of 1–2 weeks in the appearance of maximal therapeutic (antipsychotic) effects. This seems to indicate that the blockade of dopaminergic transmission as demonstrated in these binding assays is not related to the therapeutic effect. The antipsychotic action may be secondary to other consequences in the brain that evolve over a period of several weeks. For example, some neuronal circuitry may need to adjust to a new level of modulation. In addition, the drugs might produce alterations in gene expression in cells responding to dopamine, the consequences of which may not become manifest for one or more weeks.

One late consequence of long-term dopamine blockade, which may well involve gene induction, is an increase in the number of dopamine receptors, resulting in receptor supersensitivity. A second possible late consequence, supported by electrophysiological data, is a decrease in the activity of dopaminergic neurons. Finally, as we have seen in Figure 55–9, the delayed actions might reflect adjustments of other interacting neuronal systems. For example, most antipsychotic agents also act on a class of serotonin receptors, the 5-HT$_2$ receptors (see Chapters 44 and 56). These receptors also are the site of action of LSD and other psychedelic hallucinogens. Long-term administration of antipsychotic agents leads to a down regulation of 5-HT$_2$ receptors that parallels in time course the therapeutic action of the antipsychotic drugs. Finally, many antipsychotic agents also bind, although with low affinity, to the D_1 receptor, and this may enhance the action of dopamine at the D_2 site.

Perhaps one of the reasons we do not understand better to what degree a defect in dopamine transmission contributes to schizophrenia is that we are just beginning to de-

lineate the full extent of the dopaminergic receptor family. For example, it has long been known that at least 20% of schizophrenic patients do not improve following treatment with dopaminergic blockers that act on D_2 receptors. Studies by John Kane and his colleagues indicate that patients who do not respond to conventional antipsychotic agents often respond to clozapine (a dibenzodiazepine), which is only a weak blocker of D_2 receptors. Clozapine has the additional interesting property that it produces few, if any, parkinsonian (extrapyramidal) side effects, which characteristically occur with blockade of D_2 receptors. It now turns out that clozapine binds effectively to D_3, and even better to D_4, two newly discovered species of dopamine receptors that are limited in their distribution to the limbic system. However, as is the case with the typical antipsychotic agents, clozapine is not limited in its action to the dopamine system. It also blocks the serotonin 5-HT$_2$ receptor, as well as α_1-adrenergic and H$_1$ histamine receptors. It is therefore likely that just as schizophrenia is a multifactorial disease and perhaps affects more than one set of pathways in the brain (mesolimbic and mesocortical), so the actions of antipsychotic drugs are exerted on more than one molecular target.

Further evidence that disorders in transmitter systems other than dopamine might also contribute to schizophrenia comes from the finding that the addictive drug phencyclidine (PCP), known as angel dust, produces a psychosis that resembles the psychosis in schizophrenia. Normal subjects given intravenous PCP experience depersonalization and feel disconnected from their environment. They also suffer delusions of being controlled by external agents and have auditory and visual hallucinations. PCP binds to two identified molecular targets in the brain: (1) the N-methyl-D-aspartate (NMDA) class of glutamate receptors and (2) certain classes of K$^+$ channels at higher concentrations. Most of the behavioral effects of PCP are due to its blocking of the NMDA receptor-channels. Indeed, specific drugs developed to block NMDA receptors selectively (and used for the treatment of NMDA-induced neurotoxicity following stroke or prolonged seizure activity) have the undesirable side effect of producing psychosis. Why blockade of the NMDA receptor should lead to psychotic behavior is not at all clear, however.

The existence of drugs that produce psychotic behavior by binding to the NMDA receptor illustrates that psychotic behavior can probably be produced by interfering with several transmitter systems other than dopamine, either alone or in combination.

An Overall View

In considering the biological defect in schizophrenia we have focused on current insights into the molecular mechanisms of the disease and not on the social and psychological factors that act on an individual before, during, and even after they have the disease. In this context it is useful to be reminded of two common misconceptions.

First, it is sometimes thought that in classifying mental disorders we are classifying *people*; in reality, we are classifying *disorders* that people have. People are not schizophrenic, they *have* schizophrenia. Second, even though all the people who have a given mental illness are similar in ways that are important and all of these people will, by definition, share the *defining* features of the disease, the individuals suffering from the disease will likely differ in quite fundamental ways that may influence both the course and the outcome of the disease.

In addition to social factors, further research on schizophrenia needs to build on four established aspects of the disease: (1) there is an important genetic component, (2) the disease often becomes clinically apparent in late adolescence and early adulthood, (3) blockers of dopamine D_2, D_3, and D_4 receptors are often effective clinically, and (4) the disease can lead to enlarged lateral ventricles and widening of cortical sulci, especially in the frontal lobes in some cases. The hypothesis emerged from the finding that dopaminergic agonists are capable of producing psychosis and that the potency of antischizophrenic drugs that bind to dopamine D_2 receptors is directly correlated with their clinical potency in alleviating psychotic symptoms. Postmortem studies have indeed found increases in the number of dopamine receptors in these limbic areas.

In addition, almost all patients with schizophrenia show attentional and motivational deficits similar to patients with deficits in prefrontal cortex function. These considerations suggest that a second defect in schizophrenia may be found in the prefrontal cortex or its connections. How this prefrontal defect relates to the defect in the mesolimbic projection is unclear, and how either is related to the structural changes in the brain remains the great challenge of this disease. Initial clues to the answers for these questions should come from cloning genes involved in schizophrenia.

Selected Readings

Andreasen, N. C., Olsen, S. A., Dennert, J. W., and Smith, M. R. 1982. Ventricular enlargement in schizophrenia: Relationship to positive and negative symptoms. Am. J. Psychiatry 139: 297–302.

Creese, I., Sibley, D. R., Hamblin, M. W., and Leff, S. E. 1983. The classification of dopamine receptors: Relationship to radioligand binding. Annu. Rev. Neurosci. 6:43–71.

Crow, T. J. 1980. Molecular pathology of schizophrenia: More than one disease process? Br. Med. J. 280.66–68.

Early, T. S., Posner, M. I., Reiman, E. M., and Raichle, M. E. 1989. Left strio-pallidal hyperactivity in schizophrenia. Part II: Phenomenology and thought disorder. Psychiatric Dev. 2:109–121.

Goodwin, D. W., and Guze, S. B. 1989. Psychiatric Diagnosis, 4th ed. New York: Oxford University Press.

Hart, B. 1962. The Psychology of Insanity. Cambridge, England: Cambridge University Press.

Havens, L. L. 1973. Approaches to the Mind: Movement of the Psychiatric Schools from Sects Toward Science. Boston: Little Brown.

Klein, D. F., Gittelman, R., Quitkin, F., and Rifkin, A. 1980. Diagnosis and Drug Treatment of Psychiatric Disorders: Adults and Children, 2nd ed. Baltimore: Williams & Wilkins.

Lander, E. S. 1988. Splitting schizophrenia. Nature 336:105–106.

Plomin, R. 1990. The role of inheritance in behavior. Science 248:183 188.

Sherrington, R., Brynjolfsson, J., Petursson, H., Potter, M., Dudleston, K., Barraclough, B., Wasmuth, J., Dobbs, M., and Gurling, H. 1988. Localization of a susceptibility locus for schizophrenia on chromosome 5. Nature 336:164–167.

Snyder, S. H. 1986. Drugs and the Brain. New York: Scientific American Books.

Suddath, R. L., Christison, G. W., Torrey, E. F., Casanova, M. F., and Weinberger, D. R. 1990. Anatomical abnormalities in the brains of monozygotic twins discordant for schizophrenia. New Engl. J. Med. 322:789–794.

Touchette, N. 1990. A new dopamine receptor: The gain falls mainly in the brain. J. NIH Res. 2:59–62.

Wong, D. F., Wagner, H. N., Jr., Tune, L. E., Dannals, R. F., Pearlson, G. D., Links, J. M., Tamminga, C. A., Broussolle, E. P., Ravert, H. T., Wilson, A. A., Toung, J. K. T., Malat, J., Williams, J. A., O'Tuama, L. A., Snyder, S. H., Kuhar, M. J., and Gjedde, A. 1986. Positron emission tomography reveals elevated D_2 dopamine receptors in drug-naive schizophrenics. Science 234:1558–1563.

References

Bassett, A. S. 1989. Chromosome 5 and schizophrenia: Implications for genetic linkage studies. Schizophrenia Bull. 15:393–402.

Benes, F. M., Davidson, J., and Bird, E. D. 1986. Quantitative cytoarchitectural studies of the cerebral cortex of schizophrenics. Arch. Gen. Psychiatry 43:31–35.

Bleuler, E. 1911. Dementia Praecox or the Group of Schizophrenias. J. Zinkin (trans.) New York: International Universities Press, 1950.

Brozoski, T. J., Brown, R. M., Rosvold, H. E., and Goldman, P. S. 1979. Cognitive deficit caused by regional depletion of dopamine in prefrontal cortex of rhesus monkey. Science 205:929–932.

Bunzow, J. R., Van Tol, H. H. M., Grandy, D. K., Albert, P., Salon, J., Christie, M., Machida, C. A., Neve, K. A., and Civelli, O. 1988. Cloning and expression of a rat D_2 dopamine receptor cDNA. Nature 336:783–787.

Carlsson, A. 1974. Antipsychotic drugs and catecholamine synapses. J. Psychiatr. Res. 11:57–64.

Cooper, J. R., Bloom, F. E., and Roth, R. H. 1991. The Biochemical Basis of Neuropharmacology, 6th ed. New York: Oxford University Press.

Creese, I. 1982. Dopamine receptors explained. Trends Neurosci. 5:40–43.

Davis, J. M., and Garver, D. L. 1978. Neuroleptics: Clinical use in psychiatry. In L. L. Iversen, S. D. Iversen, and S. H. Snyder (eds.), Handbook of Psychopharmacology, Vol. 10: Neuroleptics and Schizophrenia. New York: Plenum Press, pp. 129–164.

Dearry, A., Gingrich, J. A., Falardeau, P., Fremeau, R. T., Jr., Bates, M. D., and Caron, M. G. 1990. Molecular cloning and expression of the gene for a human D_1 dopamine receptor. Nature 347:72–76.

Havens, L. L. 1965. Emil Kraepelin. J. Nerv. Ment. Dis. 141:16–28.

Heston, L. L. 1970. The genetics of schizophrenic and schizoid disease. Science 167:249–256.

Ingvar, D. H. 1987. Evidence for frontal/prefrontal cortical dysfunction in chronic schizophrenia: The phenomenon of "hypofrontality" reconsidered. In H. Helmchen and F. A. Henn (eds.), Biological Perspectives of Schizophrenia. Chichester, England: Wiley, pp. 201–211.

Kallmann, F. J. 1938. The Genetics of schizophrenia. New York: Augustin.

Kane, J. M. 1987. Treatment of schizophrenia. Schizophrenia Bull. 13:133–156.

Kennedy, J. L., Giuffra, L. A., Moises, H. W., Cavalli-Sforza, L. L.,

Pakstis, A. J., Kidd, J. R., Castiglione, C. M., Sjogren, B., Wetterberg, L., and Kidd, K. K. 1988. Evidence against linkage of schizophrenia to markers on chromosome 5 in a northern Swedish pedigree. Nature 336:167–170.

Kety, S. S., Rosenthal, D., Wender, P. H., Schulsinger, F., and Jacobsen, B. 1975. Mental illness in the biological and adoptive families of adopted individuals who have become schizophrenic: A preliminary report based on psychiatric interviews. In R. R. Fieve, D. Rosenthal, and H. Brill (eds.), Genetic Research in Psychiatry. Baltimore: Johns Hopkins University Press, pp. 147–165.

Kirch, D. G., and Weinberger, D. R. 1986. Anatomical neuropathology in schizophrenia: Post-mortem findings. In H. A. Nasrallah and D. R. Weinberger (eds.), The Neurology of Schizophrenia. Amsterdam: Elsevier Science Publishers., pp. 325–348.

Klein, D. F., and Davis, J. M. 1969. Diagnosis and Drug Treatment of Psychiatric Disorders. Baltimore: Williams & Wilkins.

Kraepelin, E. 1909. Dementia Praecox and Paraphrenia. From Kraepelin's Text-Book of Psychiatry, 8th ed. R. M. Barclay (trans.) Edinburgh: Livingstone, 1919.

Nauta, W. J. H., Smith, G. P., Faull, R. L. M., and Domesick, V. B. 1978. Efferent connections and nigral afferents of the nucleus accumbens septi in the rat. Neuroscience 3:385–401.

Olney, J. W., Labruyere, J., and Price, M. T. 1989. Pathological changes induced in cerebrocortical neurons by phencyclidine and related drugs. Science 244:1360–1362.

Posner, M. I., Early, T. S., Reiman, E., Pardo, J. P., and Dhawan, M. 1988. Asymmetries in hemispheric control of attention in schizophrenia. Arch. Gen. Psychiatry 45:814–821.

Pycock, C. J., Kerwin, R. W., and Carter, C. J. 1980. Effect of lesion of cortical dopamine terminals on subcortical dopamine receptors in rats. Nature 286:74–77.

Reveley, A. M., Reveley, M. A., Clifford, C. A., and Murray, R. M. 1982. Cerebral ventricular size in twins discordant for schizophrenia. Lancet 1:540–541.

Roberts, P. J., Woodruff, G. N., and Iversen, L. L. (eds.) 1978. Advances in Biochemical Psychopharmacology, Vol. 19: Dopamine. New York: Raven Press.

Seeman, P., and Lee, T. 1975. Antipsychotic drugs: Direct correlation between clinical potency and presynaptic action on dopamine neurons. Science 188:1217–1219.

Seeman, P., Lee, T., Chau-Wong, M., and Wong, K. 1976. Antipsychotic drug doses and neuroleptic/dopamine receptors. Nature 261:717–719.

Seeman, P., Ulpian, C., Bergeron, C., Riederer, P., Jellinger, K., Gabriel, E., Reynolds, G. P., and Tourtellotte, W. W. 1984. Bimodal distribution of dopamine receptor densities in brains of schizophrenics. Science 225:728–731.

Shelton, R. C., and Weinberger, D. R. 1986. X-ray computerized tomography studies in schizophrenia: A review and synthesis. In H. A. Nasrallah and D. R. Weinberger (eds.), The Neurology of Schizophrenia. Amsterdam: Elsevier Science Publishers, pp. 207–250.

Slater, E., and Roth, M. 1969. Mayer-Gross Slater and Roth Clinical Psychiatry, 3rd ed. Baltimore: Williams and Wilkins.

Snyder, S. H., and Largent, B. L. 1989. Receptor mechanisms in antipsychotic drug action: Focus on sigma receptors. J. Neuropsychiatr. Clin. Neurosci. 1:7–15.

Sokoloff, P., Giros, B., Martres, M.-P., Bouthenet, M.-L., and Schwartz, J.-C. 1990. Molecular cloning and characterization of a novel dopamine receptor (D_3) as a target for neuroleptics. Nature 347:146–151.

Sunahara, R. K., Guan, H.-C., O'Dowd, B. F., Seeman, P., Laurier, L. G., Ng, G., George, S. R., Torchia, J., Van Tol, H. H. M., and Niznik, H. B. 1991. Cloning of the gene for a human dopamine D_5 receptor with higher affinity for dopamine than D_1. Nature 350:614–619.

Torack, R. M., and Morris, J. C. 1988. The association of ventral tegmental area histopathology with adult dementia. Arch. Neurol. 45:497–501.

Van Tol, H. H. M., Bunzow, J. R., Guan, H.-C., Sunahara, R. K., Seeman, P., Niznik, H. B., and Civelli, O. 1991. Cloning of the gene for a human dopamine D_4 receptor with high affinity for the antipsychotic clozapine. Nature 350:610–614.

Weinberger, D. R. 1987. Implications of normal brain development for the pathogenesis of schizophrenia. Arch. Gen Psychiatry 44:660–669.

56

Eric R. Kandel

Disorders of Mood: Depression, Mania, and Anxiety Disorders

The Major Affective Disorders Can Be Either Unipolar or Bipolar

> Unipolar Depression Is Most Likely Several Disorders
>
> Bipolar Depressive (Manic-Depressive) Disorders Give Rise to Euphoria and Depression

There Is a Strong Genetic Predisposition for Affective Disorders

Depressive and Manic-Depressive Disorders Can Now Be Treated Effectively

> Drugs Effective in Depression Act on Serotonergic and Noradrenergic Pathways
>
> An Abnormality in Biogenic Amine Transmission May Contribute to the Affective Disorders

Depression May Involve Disturbances of Neuroendocrine Function

There Are Two Major Types of Anxiety Disorders

> Panic Attacks Are Brief Episodes of Terror
>
> Generalized Anxiety Disorder Is Long-Lasting

An Overall View

E mil Kraepelin, who developed the first modern classification of mental illness, was careful to distinguish dementia praecox, the progressive illness now known as schizophrenia, from the recurrent and more benign *manic-depressive illness* (a term Kraepelin coined) and from neurotic processes such as the anxiety syndromes. By so doing he drew a distinction between disturbance of a person's cognitive faculties (*disorders of thought*) and disturbance of emotional life (*disorders of mood*).

In clinical descriptions of an individual's emotions the term *mood* refers to a sustained emotional state. A person's immediate or momentary emotional state is called *affect* or *affective response*. In practice, mood is a symptom; it is what patients tell you they feel. Affect is a sign; it is what can be observed. Normal affective responses range from euphoria to elation, pleasure, surprise, anger, anxiety, disappointment, sadness, grief, despair, and even depression. Three of these normal affective responses can become so sustained and dominant as to constitute a disorder. These three are euphoria (which in its sustained form becomes mania), depression, and anxiety.

We shall consider all three and examine the biological insights into the nature of these diseases. All three are disorders of mood. By tradition, however, depression, mania, and anxiety are referred to as disorders of affect. To avoid confusion, we shall preserve the older terminology here as we first consider depression and mania. We shall then go on to examine the anxiety states. Throughout we shall emphasize important interrelationships between the three mood disorders.

The Major Affective Disorders Can Be Either Unipolar or Bipolar

The most common affective disorder, unipolar depression, was described in the fifth century B.C. in the Hippocratic writings. In the Hippocratic view, moods were thought to depend upon the balance of four humors—blood, phlegm, yellow bile, and black bile—an excess of which was believed to cause depression. In fact, the ancient Greek term for depression, *melancholia*, means black bile. Though this explanation for the etiology of depression seems fanciful today, the underlying view that psychological disorders reflect physical processes is correct.

Efforts to update the Hippocratic formulation were hindered by an inability to classify affective disorders precisely. In 1917, in a paper entitled *Mourning and Melancholia*, Sigmund Freud wrote: "Even in descriptive psychiatry the definition of melancholia is uncertain; it takes on various clinical forms (some of them suggesting somatic rather than psychogenic affections) that do not seem definitely to warrant reduction to a unity." Only in the past two decades have relatively precise criteria for classifying affective syndromes been developed in parallel with those for cognitive disorders (see Chapter 55). We shall describe here the two major affective syndromes: unipolar depression (major depression) and bipolar depression (manic-depressive illness).

Unipolar Depression Is Most Likely Several Disorders

The clinical features of unipolar, major depression can be summarized readily. In Hamlet's words, "How weary, stale, flat, and unprofitable seem to me all the uses of this world!" Untreated, the usual episode of depression lasts 4–12 months and is characterized by a pervasive unpleasant (dysphoric) mood that is present most of the day, day-in and day-out. This is accompanied by intense mental pain, by an inability to experience pleasure (anhedonia), and by a generalized loss of interest. The diagnosis also requires at least three of the following symptoms to be present: disturbed sleep, usually insomnia with early morning awakening (but sometimes, as we shall see, oversleeping or hypersomnia), diminished appetite and loss of weight (but sometimes overeating), loss of energy, decreased sex drive, restlessness (psychomotor agitation), or slowing down of thoughts and actions (retardation), difficulty in concentrating, indecisiveness, feelings of worthlessness, guilt, pessimistic thoughts, and thoughts about dying and suicide. Although not required for diagnosis, other common symptoms are constipation, decreased salivation, and diurnal variation in the severity of symptoms, which are usually worse in the morning.

In addition to the inclusion criteria there are exclusion criteria; for example, schizophrenia or other neurological diseases need to be excluded. There also should be no ev-idence of recent death in the family, since, as we shall see later, some of the symptoms of depression are also normal expressions of personal loss and mourning.

When the syndrome is defined in this manner, about 5% of the world's population suffer from major depression. In the United States 8,000,000 people at any given time are affected. Severe depression can be profoundly debilitating. In extreme cases patients stop eating or maintaining basic personal cleanliness. The average age of onset is about 30, but the first episode can occur at almost any age. Indeed, depression is common among young children and adolescents but often is not recognized. Depression also occurs in the elderly, but usually older people who become depressed have had an earlier episode. It is rare to have the first episode after the age of 60. Women are affected about two to three times more often than men. Although some people suffer only a single episode, usually the illness is recurrent. About 70% of patients who suffer one major depressive episode will have at least one other.

Major depression is most likely not a single illness but a group of disorders. However, the attempt to distinguish subtypes has been only partially successful so far. For example, some clinicians subdivide the major depressions into two subgroups, *endogenous* and *reactive*, based on the absence or presence of a precipitating social stress.

Endogenous depression (also called depression of the *melancholic type*) represents the clearest subtype among the major depressions and accounts for 40–60% of people hospitalized for depression. In endogenous depression there often is no obvious external precipitating cause—no loss or rejection or obvious change in external conditions. The disease is characterized by five symptoms: (1) depression with diurnal variations in mood (worse in the morning), (2) insomnia with early morning wakening, (3) anorexia with significant weight loss, (4) psychomotor agitation and mental pain, and (5) loss of interest in almost all activity and lack of response to pleasurable stimuli (anhedonia).

Patients with melancholic depression often have a history of one or more previous episodes of major depression with recovery. In addition, many patients show characteristic abnormalities in sleep pattern as measured by electroencephalography. These abnormalities occur primarily during the first half of the night, when the rapid eye movement (REM) phase of sleep is shortened. In more than half of melancholic-type patients there is also some frequent awakening. Unlike other types of depression, melancholic depression does not lead to emotional or intellectual underactivity (retardation). On the contrary, there is a rather painful state of arousal and an active and persistent preoccupation with perceived deficiencies and inadequacies of one's character.

Reactive depression (also called *nonmelancholic*) is thought to be the result of a specific stress, such as the loss of a family member, rejection, loss of job, loss of health, or transient loss of self-esteem. Seen in this way, reactive depression is an extension or intensification of normal responses to distressing circumstances. According to this view, stress transiently overwhelms the individual's ability to cope with loss and disappointment. Reactive depression tends to occur in people who previously have exhibited neurotic behavior and have a predisposition to depressive behavior. Patients frequently do not manifest any of the five features that characterize endogenous depression. They also tend to be younger than melancholic patients and to respond less well to antidepressant drugs.

Although the distinction between endogenous and reactive depression is sometimes useful, it is not firm. For example, the contribution of genetic factors is identical in both categories. In addition, when patients with endogenous depression are carefully examined, over 80% report a psychosocial or somatic stress that preceded their depression. Nevertheless, in such cases the psychosocial factors are thought to act on a biological predisposition for major depressive illness. Thus, rather than being distinct entities, endogenous and reactive depression may represent extreme points on a continuum of melancholic depressive illness.

There is, however, reason to believe that melancholic depression can be distinguished from another depressive disorder called *atypical depression*. This disorder accounts for about 15% of patients hospitalized for major depressive disorders. The disease is called atypical because the patients show symptoms that are the opposite of those with melancholic depression. The patients do not have loss of appetite and weight loss but instead overeat and gain weight; they do not report insomnia but rather tend to have prolonged periods of sleep, and their depression is worse, not better, in the evening. The patients also have prominent symptoms of anxiety.

It is important to remember that we normally experience grief or despondency following loss of a family member (or following a major illness). In such cases people may show any of the individual symptoms of atypical or melancholic depression. However, they have fewer suicidal thoughts and, more important, they have lower rates of suicide than patients with atypical or melancholic depression. Most helpful in making the diagnosis, however, is the finding of *reactive affect*. Unlike the situation in a major depression, the depression normally experienced following a personal loss is not unrelenting and pervasive—it does not persist *every day, all day*. Most people are able to experience and *react to* moments of pleasure and contentment that relieve the sadness in a way that a person with a major depression cannot.

Bipolar Depressive (Manic-Depressive) Disorders Give Rise to Euphoria and Depression

About 25% of patients with major depression (or 2 million people in the United States) will also experience a manic episode, if only a mild one, sometime later in life. Patients who experience both depressive and manic episodes suffer from a distinct disorder called bipolar depressive illness. The illness affects men and women equally, and the average age of onset is a decade younger than that of unipolar depression (the onset usually occurs at age 20 rather than 30).

Episodes of depression in bipolar disorders are clinically similar to those of the unipolar type. The manic episodes are characterized by an elevated, expansive, or irritable mood lasting at least one week, together with several of the following symptoms: overactivity, overtalkativeness (pressure of speech), social intrusiveness, increased energy and libido, pressure of ideas, grandiosity, distractibility, decreased need for sleep, and reckless involvements. In severe cases patients are delusional and have hallucinations. Most episodes have no detectable psychosocial precipitant. Bipolar disorder is also a recurrent illness; following the initial episode of euphoria, episodes (of either depression or euphoria) occur about twice as often as in unipolar disease. One of the most amazing aspects of bipolar illness is that a patient may switch from depression to euphoria or vice versa quite rapidly, sometimes in a matter of minutes.

There Is a Strong Genetic Predisposition for Affective Disorders

As in schizophrenia, genetic factors are important in both unipolar and bipolar affective disorders. The morbidity rate of depression is much higher in first-degree relatives (parents, siblings, and children) of patients with depressive illness than in the general population. As with schizophrenia, the overall concordance rate for monozygotic twin pairs is approximately 50%; the rate for dizygotic twins is approximately 10% (the same as for siblings).

Seymour Kety, Paul Wender, and David Rosenthal extended their studies of the relative contributions of genetic and environmental factors to schizophrenia in adoptees (Chapter 55) to those with manic-depressive disorders. They found that among adoptees who developed depressive or manic-depressive illness the rate of affective illness in the biological parents was higher than in the adoptive parents (or than in the biological and adoptive parents of mentally healthy adoptees). Particularly impressive was the finding that the incidence of suicide among biological relatives of adoptees who suffered from depression was 6–10 times higher than among the biological relatives of normal adoptees (Figure 56–1). Furthermore, monozygotic twins reared apart have a concordance rate of 40–60%, similar to the concordance of those reared together.

Molecular genetic studies have supported the idea that a genetic defect contributes to the pathogenesis of affective disorders. However, as with schizophrenia, the major depressive disorders have a variety of different etiologies. Transmission does not follow a classic single-gene Men-

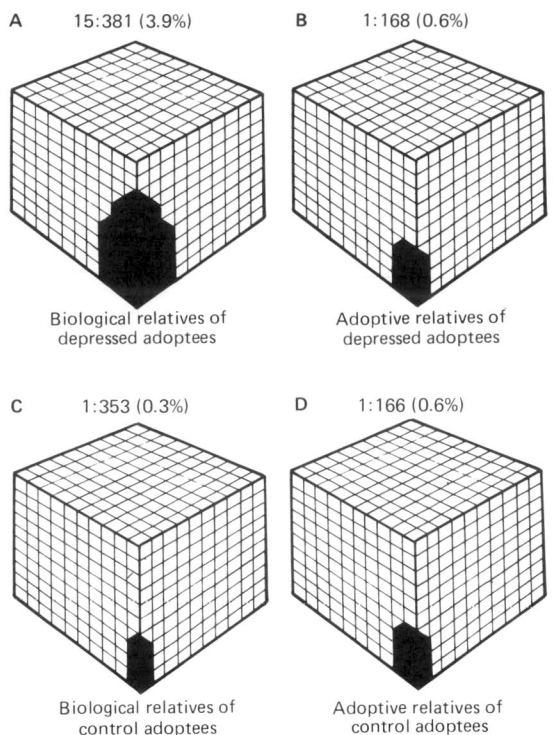

A 15:381 (3.9%)   **B** 1:168 (0.6%)

Biological relatives of
depressed adoptees

Adoptive relatives of
depressed adoptees

C 1:353 (0.3%)   **D** 1:166 (0.6%)

Biological relatives of
control adoptees

Adoptive relatives of
control adoptees

FIGURE 56–1
Incidence of suicides among biological and adoptive relatives of
depressed patients. There is a higher incidence of suicide
among biological relatives of adoptees who suffered from bipolar depression (**A**) than among their adoptive relatives (**B**). The
rates in the adoptive relatives of depressed patients are similar
to those of both the biological (**C**) and adoptive (**D**) relatives of
mentally healthy adoptees. Each ratio shows the number of relatives who committed suicide with respect to the total number
of relatives. (Adapted from Kety, 1979.)

delian pattern. Instead, different genetic defects can result
in affective illness. For example, Miron Baron and his
colleagues have found evidence that bipolar illness in
Ashkenazi Jews from northern Europe is linked to a dominant X chromosome locus, whereas other populations do
not show this linkage. In addition to an occasional major
single gene defect, in many individuals depression will
most likely involve the action of many genes, each with a
small effect. Moreover, as with schizophrenia, the discor-
dance for monozygotic twin pairs indicates that nongenetic factors influence whether an affective disorder
will be expressed.

The importance of nongenetic factors in depression is
also supported by two important *secular trends* in depression over the past 50 years. Since 1940 the age of onset has
become younger (28 rather than 35) and the incidence of
depression in the families of patients has increased. Perhaps people vulnerable to depression and exposed to
stressful environments are now more likely to become
depressed than they were half a century ago.

Depressive and Manic-Depressive Disorders Can Now Be Treated Effectively

There are three effective treatments for major depressive
and bipolar illness: electroconvulsive therapy (ECT), antidepressant drugs, and lithium. Of the three, electroconvulsive therapy has been used for the longest period of
time, over 50 years. Although antidepressants are generally used first in the treatment of major depression, electroconvulsive therapy is very effective. It produces full
remission or marked improvement in about 90% of patients with well-defined major depression. It is therefore
often useful for patients with heart conditions in which
some antidepressant drugs can have undesirable effects.

The critical therapeutic factor in electroconvulsive
therapy is the induction of a generalized brain seizure. The
motor component of the seizure is not necessary for therapeutic results, and modern electroconvulsive therapy is
given under anesthesia with complete muscle relaxation.
On the average, 6 to 8 treatments given at two-day intervals over a period of 2 to 4 weeks usually suffice to produce a complete remission of symptoms. As might be
predicted from our knowledge of seizure activity (Chapter
50), electroconvulsive therapy creates many temporary
changes in brain functions. Although the mechanism of
its therapeutic action is not understood, it may be related
to changes in aminergic receptor sensitivity, as we shall
see below.

The most widely used antidepressant drugs fall into
three major classes: (1) the *monoamine oxidase inhibitors*, such as phenelzine (Figure 56–2A), (2) the *tricyclic
compounds*, such as imipramine, so named for their
three-ring molecular structure (Figure 56–2B), and (3) the
serotonin uptake blockers, fluoxetine and trazodone. The
monoamine oxidase inhibitors and the tricyclic antidepressants produce remission or marked improvement in
about 70% of patients with major depressions. When high
doses are given (and blood drug levels are monitored so as
to achieve and maintain an adequate therapeutic concentration), the success rate with tricyclic drugs and the specific serotonin uptake inhibitors may reach 85%, almost
as effective as electroconvulsive therapy. Patients with bipolar depression occasionally become manic during treatment with either class of antidepressant. Although a few
patients begin to improve immediately, there usually is a
lag of 1–3 weeks before the symptoms of depression begin
to improve, and 4 to 6 weeks are generally required for full
response.

Lithium salts, first introduced in the psychiatric treatment of manic-depressive illness in 1949 by John Cade,
are effective in terminating manic episodes. Moreover,
maintenance lithium therapy, first used by Mogens
Schou, is an effective prophylactic and prevents or atten-
uates recurrent manic and, to a lesser extent, depressive
episodes. Lithium is not used to treat major depression,
however. Antipsychotic drugs (see Chapter 55) also are
quite effective in terminating manic episodes. Antipsychotic drugs are also used frequently in combination with

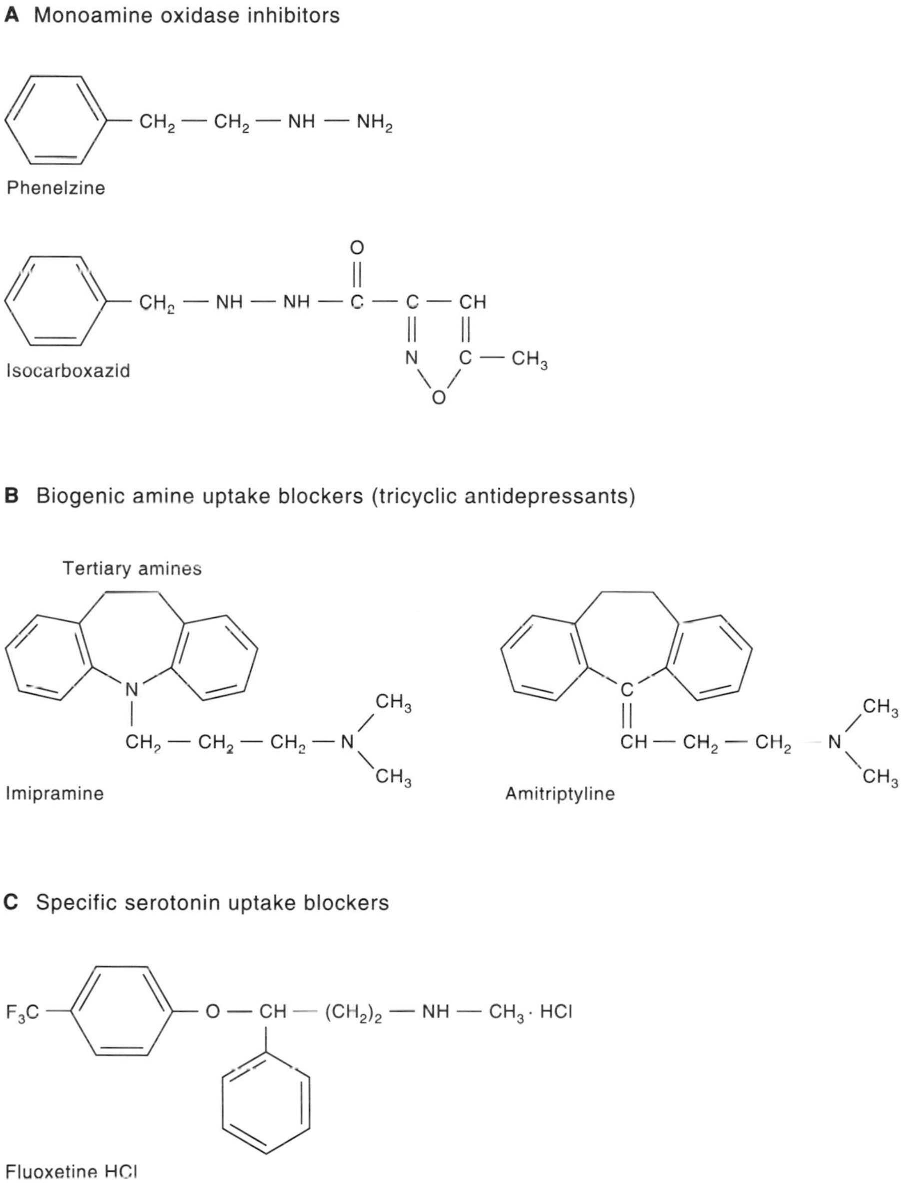

A Monoamine oxidase inhibitors

Phenelzine

Isocarboxazid

B Biogenic amine uptake blockers (tricyclic antidepressants)

Tertiary amines

Imipramine

Amitriptyline

C Specific serotonin uptake blockers

F_3C — ⟨ ⟩ — O — CH — $(CH_2)_2$ — NH — $CH_3 \cdot$ HCl

Fluoxetine HCl

FIGURE 56–2

Representative drugs from the three types of antidepressants: monoamine oxidase (MAO) inhibitors, biogenic amine uptake blockers (tricyclics), and serotonin uptake blockers.

A. Clinically useful MAO inhibitors are chemically diverse. It is thought that these drugs act by decreasing the breakdown of biogenic amines in the brain, thereby making more neurotransmitter available for release at aminergic synapses. The antidepressant effects of the drugs take several weeks to fully develop.

B. Tricyclic drugs are modifications of phenothiazine (see Figure 55–2). They have immediate and long-term effects: Blockage of the reuptake of biogenic amine neurotransmitters from the synapse is evident soon after administration. The therapeutic action of antidepressants usually begins 4 days to 3 weeks after starting the medication.

C. Serotonin uptake blockers are now considered the most effective antidepressants.

A Serotonergic pathway

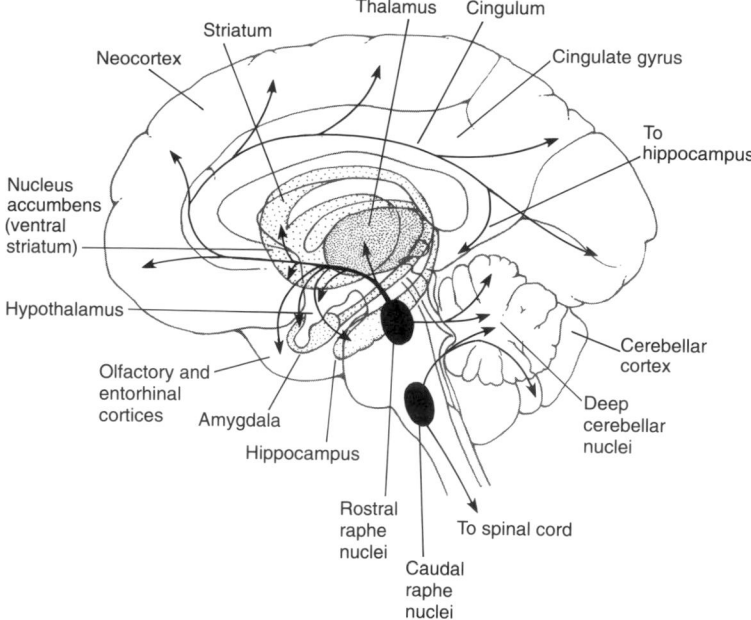

FIGURE 56–3

Serotonergic pathways.

A. Lateral view of the brain. Although the raphe nuclei form a fairly continuous collection of cell groups close to the midline throughout the brain stem, they are illustrated here in a distinct rostral and caudal group for the sake of simplicity. The rostral raphe nuclei project to a large number of forebrain structures. In this highly schematic drawing the fibers projecting laterally through the internal and external capsules to neocortex are not indicated.

B. Coronal view of the serotonergic projections from the rostral raphe nuclei. This schematic drawing demonstrates some of the major targets of the raphe nuclei neurons. (Adapted from Heimer, 1983.)

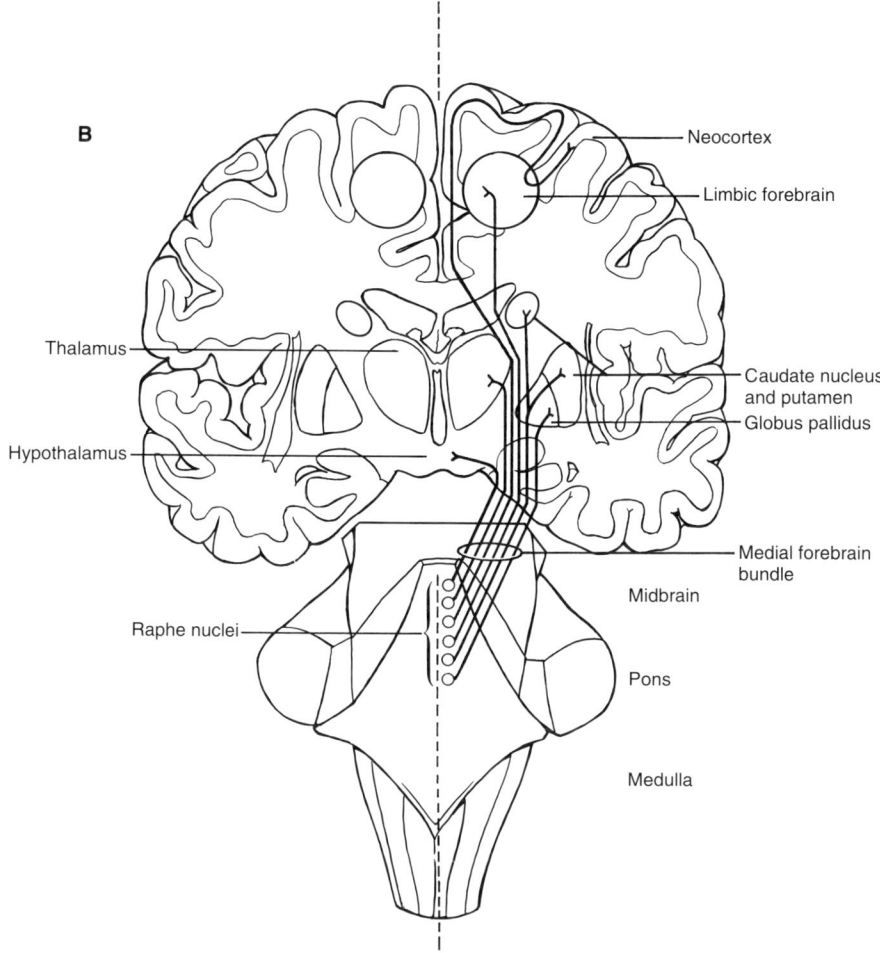

tricyclic drugs when depression is accompanied by psychosis with delusions and hallucinations.

Drugs Effective in Depression Act on Serotonergic and Noradrenergic Pathways

Drugs effective in treating depression act on the serotonergic and noradrenergic systems of the brain. The action of these drugs, therefore, provides the first clues to a neurochemical basis of depressive disorders. The serotonergic pathways have their major origin in the raphe nuclei of the brain stem (Figure 56–3). Cells from the rostral parts of these nuclei project diffusely to the forebrain. The branches of even a single neuron can project to hundreds of target cells, thus covering a large target area. The cells of the caudal part of the raphe nuclei project to the spinal cord.

The serotonergic receptors on the postsynaptic membrane have been classified traditionally into four groups: 5-HT$_1$, 5-HT$_2$, 5-HT$_3$, and 5-HT$_4$ (Table 56–1). Now that several serotonin receptors have been cloned, a classification based on receptor mechanisms is emerging based on the second-messenger system to which the receptor is coupled. Some receptors (such as 5-HT$_{1A}$ and 5-HT$_4$) are coupled negatively or positively to adenylyl cyclase, others (such as 5-HT$_2$) are coupled to phosphotidylinositide turnover, and still others (such as 5-HT$_3$) are directly coupled to an ion channel.

The noradrenergic pathways originate in the locus ceruleus (Figure 56–4). The ascending axons of locus ceruleus neurons innervate the hypothalamus and all regions of the cerebral cortex, including the hippocampus. The descending axons of the locus ceruleus reach the dorsal and ventral horns of the spinal cord. As is the case with serotonergic cells, noradrenergic neurons also innervate targets that have a variety of receptors in their transmitters (Table 56–2).

As we learned in Chapter 44, electrical stimulation of the locus ceruleus produces a state of heightened arousal. Whereas certain components of the noradrenergic system appear to be involved with arousal and anxiety, other components are involved with positive motivation and the perception of pleasure (Chapter 48). The pervasive anxiety and the loss of pleasure in melancholic and atypically depressed patients might therefore be related to disregulation of these two components of the locus ceruleus system. Consistent with these findings, monoamine oxidase inhibitors and tricyclic agents effective in depression decrease the firing of neurons in the locus ceruleus of experimental animals.

An Abnormality in Biogenic Amine Transmission May Contribute to the Affective Disorders

Although drugs that are clinically effective in affective disorders act on the receptors for 5-HT and norepinephrine, the primary disorder could be anywhere in the brain activated by the noradrenergic or serotonergic systems. As discussed in Chapters 14 and 15, norepinephrine is synthesized from tyrosine, and serotonin from tryptophan. When the neuron is stimulated the transmitters are packaged in synaptic vesicles that are released into the synaptic cleft by means of exocytosis. Both norepinephrine and serotonin interact with specific postsynaptic receptors and this activity is curtailed by active uptake of the released transmitter into the presynaptic terminals as well as into glial cells and even the postsynaptic cell. Inside the presynaptic terminals they are packaged again in vesicles or catabolized primarily by the mitochondrial enzyme monoamine oxidase.

Until recently the consensus view, expressed in the form of the *catecholamine hypothesis*, was that depression represented a decreased availability of either norepinephrine or serotonin or of both amines. Euphoria was believed to result from the overactivity of noradrenergic systems. This hypothesis was derived from studies of the effects of various drugs on the serotonergic and noradrenergic systems of the brain. The initial idea for this hypothesis came from the observation in 1950 that reserpine, a Rauwolfia alkaloid then used extensively in the treatment of hypertension, precipitated depressive syndromes in about 15% of treated patients. This finding had a parallel in animal studies in which reserpine produced a

TABLE 56–1. Classification of Serotonin Receptors

Receptors	Gene family
Receptors linked to second-messenger systems	
5-HT$_1$	
5-HT$_{1A}$ (linked to inhibition of adenylyl cyclase)	
5-HT$_{1B}$ (linked to inhibition of adenylyl cyclase)	
5-HT$_{1C}$ (linked to stimulation of PI turnover)	Superfamily of receptors with 7 transmembrane
5-HT$_{1D}$ (linked to inhibition of adenylyl cyclase)	regions that are coupled to G-proteins
5-HT$_2$ (linked to phospholipase and PI turnover)	
5-HT$_4$ (linked to stimulation of adenylyl cyclase)	
Receptors linked to an ion channel	Superfamily of ligand-gated ion channels
5-HT$_3$	

876

A Noradenergic pathway

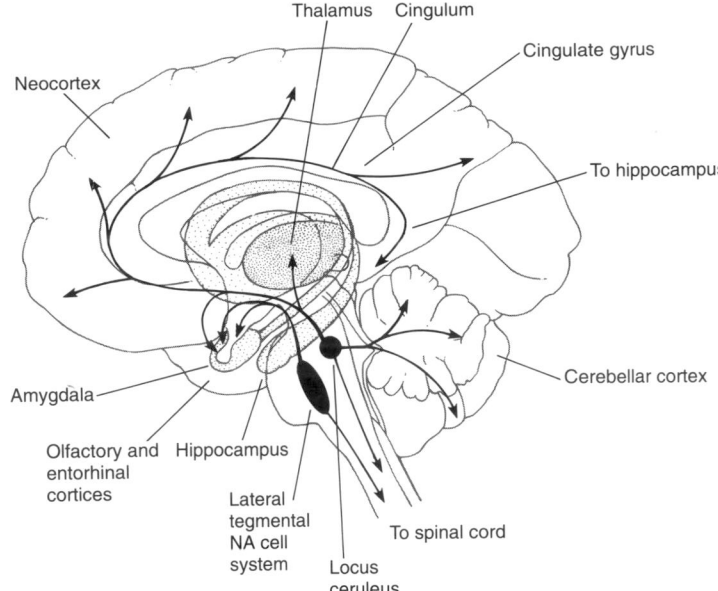

Thalamus Cingulum

Cingulate gyrus

Neocortex

To hippocampus

Amygdala

Cerebellar cortex

Olfactory and entorhinal cortices

Hippocampus

Lateral tegmental NA cell system

To spinal cord

Locus ceruleus

FIGURE 56–4

Noradrenergic pathways. The locus ceruleus, located immediately beneath the floor of the fourth ventricle in the rostrolateral pons, is the best understood noradrenergic nucleus in the brain. Its projections reach many areas in the forebrain, cerebellum, and spinal cord. Noradrenergic neurons in the lateral brain stem tegmentum innervate several structures in the basal forebrain including the hypothalamus and the amygdaloid body.

A. A lateral view of a midsagittal cut demonstrates the course of the major noradrenergic pathways emanating from the locus ceruleus and from the lateral brain stem tegmentum.

B. A coronal section shows schematically the major targets of neurons from the locus ceruleus. (Adapted from Heimer, 1983.)

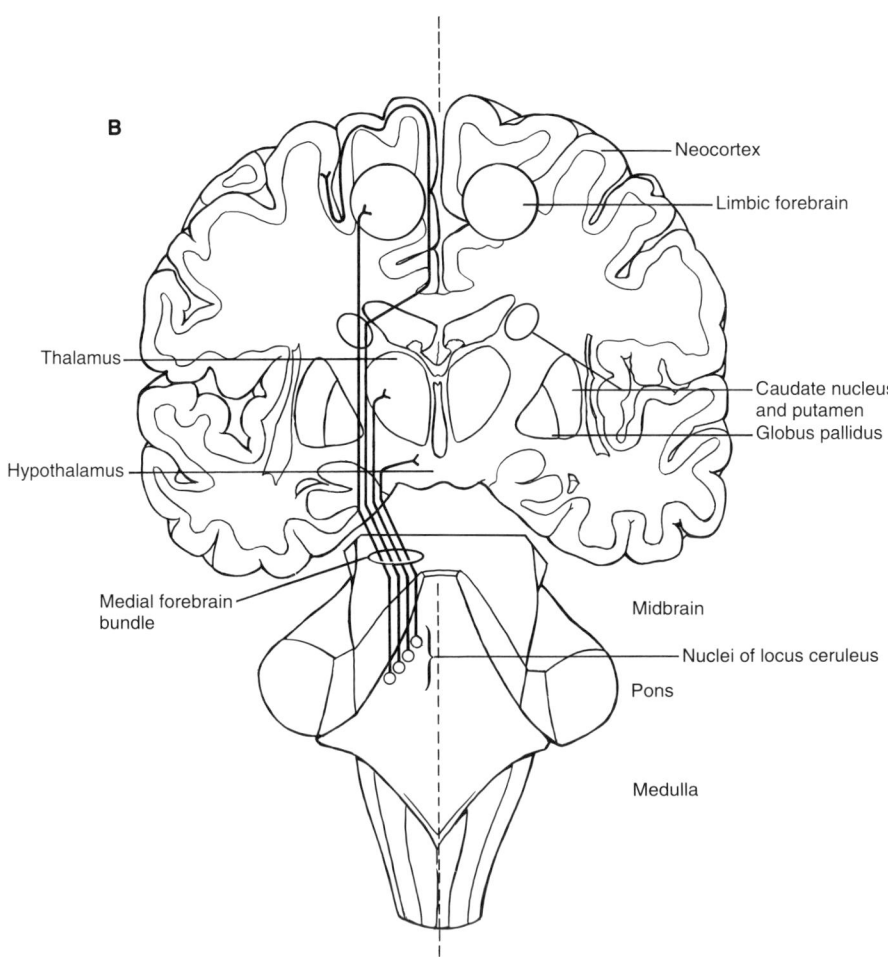

B

Neocortex

Limbic forebrain

Thalamus

Caudate nucleus and putamen
Globus pallidus

Hypothalamus

Medial forebrain bundle

Midbrain

Nuclei of locus ceruleus

Pons

Medulla

TABLE 56–2. Classification of Noradrenergic Receptors Linked to Second-Messenger Systems

Type	Second-messenger system	Gene family	Location
β_1	Linked to stimulation of adenylyl cyclase	Superfamily of receptors with 7 transmembrane regions that are coupled to G proteins	Cerebral cortex, cerebellum
β_2	Linked to stimulation of adenylyl cyclase		Cerebral cortex, cerebellum
α_1	Linked to inhibition of adenylyl cyclase in peripheral tissues		Brain, blood vessels, spleen
α_2	Phospholipase C mobilization of intracellular Ca^{2+}		Presynaptic nerve terminals throughout the brain

depression-like syndrome with motor retardation and sedation. Bernard Brodie and his colleagues found that reserpine depletes the brain of serotonin and norepinephrine (as well as other biogenic amines) by causing the transmitter vesicles to release these neurotransmitters into the cytoplasm prior to exocytosis. Once released from their intracellular stores, the transmitters undergo degradation by monoamine oxidase in the cytoplasm (Figure 56–5).

Inhibitors of monoamine oxidase, such as iproniazid, were later found to be effective antidepressants. Iproniazid was initially developed in the 1980s to treat tuberculosis. In the course of clinical trials it was noted that some depressed tuberculosis patients experienced elevations in mood when treated with the drug. Iproniazid was next tried in depressed nontubercular patients and found to be effective. Monoamine oxidase inhibitors increase the concentration of serotonin and norepinephrine in the brain by decreasing the degradation of these transmitters by monoamine oxidase (Figure 56–5). In experimental animals, monoamine oxidase inhibitors prevent reserpine's sedative effects on behavior as well as its degradation of the amines released into the cytoplasm.

Further support for the view that monoamine oxidase inhibitors exercise their therapeutic action by increasing the availability of serotonin and biogenic amines came with the discovery of a second class of effective antidepressants, the tricyclic compounds. These agents block the active reuptake of transmitter released by serotonergic and noradrenergic neurons, thereby prolonging the period during which serotonin or norepinephrine persist and act in the synaptic cleft (Figure 56–5). Thus, both major classes of antidepressants affect uptake or accumulation of norepinephrine and serotonin.

Other studies focused on measuring the metabolites of serotonin and norepinephrine in depressed patients and controls (as an index of transmitter metabolism in the brain). Because some of the metabolites of these transmitters do not cross the blood-brain barrier, the concentrations are measured in body fluids, such as the cerebrospinal fluid. Marie Åsberg found that the major metabolite of serotonin, 5-hydroxyindole acetic acid (5-HIAA), is reduced in the spinal fluid of about half of all severely depressed patients studied, particularly in those who had committed suicide. A similar association has now been found with aggressive and impulsive patients.

All of these observations, however, provide only circumstantial support for the idea that aminergic transmission is altered in depression. Moreover, the catecholamine hypothesis fails to account for a number of important clinical phenomena. For example, the onset of the clinical response to monoamine oxidase inhibitors and tricyclics is about the same, even though the biochemical action of some monoamine oxidase inhibitors is slow, while the tricyclic agents rapidly block the high-affinity reuptake systems for serotonin and norepinephrine as soon as they are given. In addition, the tricyclic drugs vary widely in their relative abilities to block serotonin or norepinephrine reuptake, yet their clinical efficacies in depressed patients are all about the same, particularly when doses are adjusted to achieve comparable blood concentrations. Moreover, in some depressed patients the onset of the illness is associated not with decrease but an *increase* in the level of norepinephrine in spinal fluid and plasma, and treatment leads to reduction to a normal level.

Some clues are emerging that might resolve at least some of these discrepancies. For example, it is now clear that antidepressant agents affect processes other than uptake and accumulation. These findings might explain the lack of correlation between the slow time course of the clinical action of tricyclic drugs and the rapid effect on uptake mechanisms. The evidence is perhaps most instructive for serotonin. In addition to their rapid biochemical effects on uptake, both monoamine oxidase inhibitors and tricyclic antidepressants produce a delayed but long-term increase in the sensitivity of receptors to serotonin. Conversely, a new class of uptake blockers highly selective for serotonin (fluoxetine) produces a delayed decrease in the sensitivity of an inhibitory presynaptic serotonin autoreceptor, leading to increased release of serotonin. Both of these actions lead to a slowly developing increase in the effectiveness of serotonergic synapses.

Similarly, electroconvulsive therapy, as well as antidepressants, produce a delayed down-regulation of presynaptic β-adrenergic autoreceptors, which normally inhibit release of norepinephrine. Inhibition of these autoreceptors also enhances release of norepinephrine. In addition, long-term antidepressant treatments lead to an up-regulation of the α_1 receptor. Perhaps most interesting is the finding by Fridolin Sulser that the serotonergic and noradrenergic systems interact. For example, destruction of the serotonergic systems prevents down-regulation of

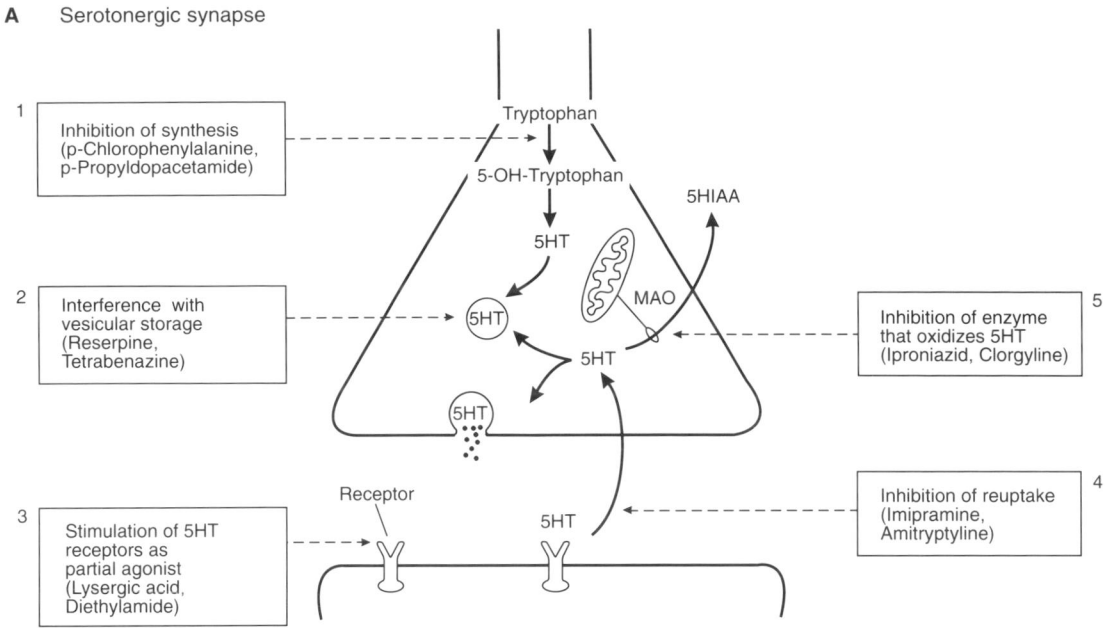

A   Serotonergic synapse

FIGURE 56–5

Key steps in serotonergic and noradrenergic transmission.

A. Five possible sites where antidepressant drugs act on central serotonergic neurons.

1. *Enzymatic synthesis.* Tryptophan, the precursor of serotonin, is converted to 5-hydroxytryptophan (5-OH-tryptophan) by the enzyme tryptophan hydroxylase. This enzyme can be effectively inhibited by *p*-chlorophenylalanine and *p*-propyldopacetamide.

2. *Storage.* Reserpine and tetrabenazine interfere with the uptake–storage mechanism of the amine granules, causing a marked depletion of serotonin.

3. *Receptor interaction.* Lysergic acid diethylamide (LSD) acts as a partial agonist at postsynaptic serotonergic receptors in the central nervous system. A number of specific compounds have now been suggested to act as receptor-blocking agents at various serotonergic synapses.

4. *Reuptake.* The action of serotonin is terminated by being taken up into the presynaptic terminal. Tricyclic drugs with a tertiary nitrogen, such as imipramine and amitryptyline, appear to be potent inhibitors of this uptake mechanism and thus increase the efficacy of transmission.

5. *Degradation by monoamine oxidase (MAO).* Serotonin present in a free state within the presynaptic terminal can be degraded by the enzyme MAO, which is localized in the outer membrane of mitochondria. Iproniazid and clorgyline are effective inhibitors of MAO.

B. Seven possible sites of antidepressant drug action in central noradrenergic neurons.

1. *Enzymatic synthesis.* **(a)** The reaction catalyzed by tyrosine hydroxylase is blocked by the competitive inhibitor, α-methyl-tyrosine. **(b)** The reaction catalyzed by dopamine β-hydroxylase, converting DOPA to dopamine (DA), is blocked by a dithiocarbamate derivative, FLA 63.

---

the β-adrenergic receptors by long-term antidepressant treatment.

Given these contradictory findings, where does the catecholamine hypothesis stand? There seems to be general consensus that the catecholamine hypothesis is no longer valid in its initial simple form—that reduction of catecholamines leads to depression, and elevation to euphoria. There probably is no simple relationship between catecholamines and depression. Indeed, there are important instances of depression where norepinephrine levels are not decreased but became elevated. If a relationship exists at all, which seems likely, it is complicated by three factors. First, depression is most likely a single disorder not a group of illnesses with several underlying pathologies. Second, disturbances in one of several transmitter systems can lead to depression. Finally, the transmitter systems do not function independently of one another but interact.

Specifically, there is cross talk between second messengers activated by these transmitters.

For example, the cholinergic and GABAergic systems are known sites of action of antidepressant drugs. Cholinergic neurons excite the noradrenergic cells of the locus ceruleus through muscarinic receptors, and cholinergic agonists can induce depression. Indeed, patients with a history of depression tend to be hyper-responsive to cholinergic agonists, even when they are normal.

Since most serotonergic and adrenergic receptors activate or inhibit adenylyl cyclase or stimulate phosphoinositide turnover, it is perhaps not surprising that drugs acting directly on these second-messenger pathways are now being developed. For example, Rolpram, an inhibitor of cAMP phosphodiesterase (one of several enzymes that degrades cAMP), is effective in certain forms of depression. Moreover, lithium salts, which are highly effective

B   Noradrenergic synapse

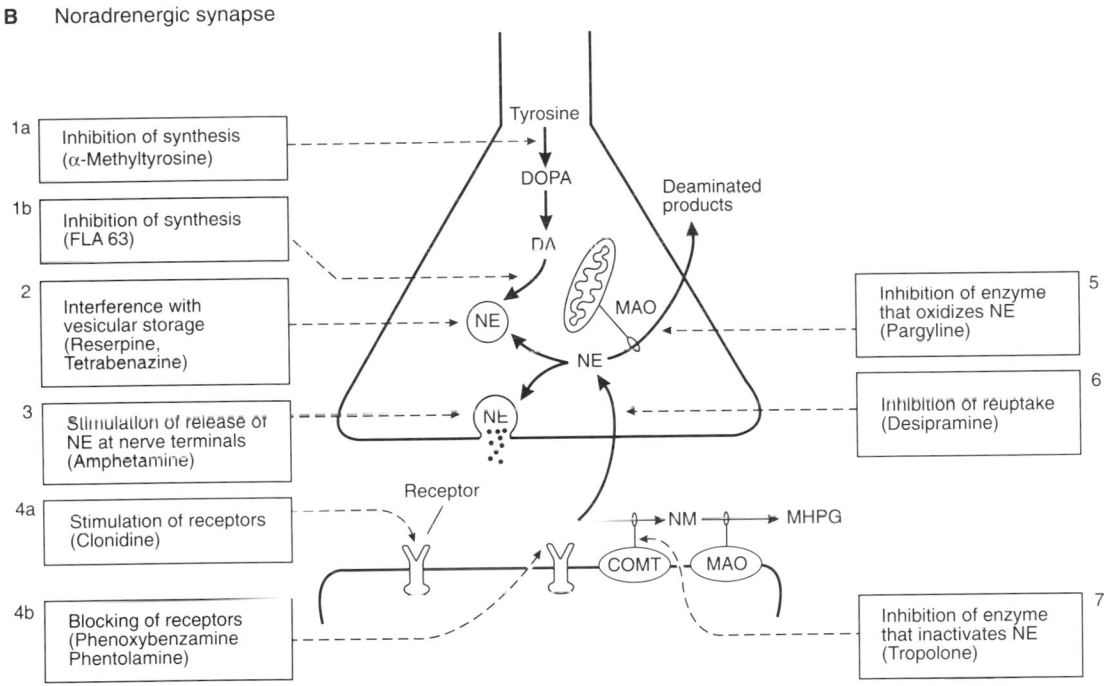

2. *Storage.* Reserpine and tetrabenazine interfere with the uptake–storage mechanism of the amine granules. The depletion of norepinephrine (NE) by reserpine is long-lasting and the storage granules are irreversibly damaged, causing permanent depletion of NE available for release transmission. Tetrabenazine also interferes with the uptake of free cytoplasmic NE into the granules.

3. *Release.* Amphetamine appears to cause an increase in the net release of norepinephrine, most likely due to its ability to block the reuptake.

4. *Receptor interaction.* **a.** Clonidine is a very potent β-receptor-agonist. **b.** Phenoxybenzamine and phentolamine are effective α-receptor blocking agents. Recent experiments have indicated that these drugs also have a presynaptic site of action.

5. *Degradation by monoamine oxidase (MAO).* Norepinephrine present in a free state within the presynaptic terminal can be degraded by the enzyme MAO, which appears to be localized in the outer membrane of mitochondria. Pargyline is an effective inhibitor of MAO.

6. *Reuptake.* The action of norepinephrine is terminated by uptake into the presynaptic terminal. The tricyclic drug desipramine is a potent inhibitor of this uptake mechanism. Norepinephrine thus remains in the synapse longer and has a greater postsynaptic effect.

7. *Degradation by catechol-O-methyltransferase (COMT).* Norepinephrine can be inactivated by the enzyme COMT, which is believed to be localized outside the postsynaptic neuron. Tropolone is an inhibitor of COMT.

---

in mania and in bipolar depression, block the enzyme inositol-1-phosphatase, which recycles inositol phosphate back to inositol, thus resulting in a buildup of inositol phosphate (IP₃), which is known to be active in Ca²⁺ metabolism (Figure 56–6). Inhibition of this enzyme is thought to reduce the responsiveness of those neurons in which transmitter receptors are coupled to the IP₃ pathway. This could be a means by which lithium acts therapeutically, perhaps by dampening excessive neural activity in the manic phase of illness.

Depression May Involve Disturbances of Neuroendocrine Function

There are many clinical signs of hypothalamic disturbance in depression, suggesting that hypothalamic modulation of neuroendocrine activity might also be affected.

The best-established neuroendocrine disturbance in severe depression is a hypersecretion of cortisol from the adrenal cortex in response to excessive secretion of adrenocorticotropin (ACTH) by the pituitary. Excessive secretion of cortisol occurs in 40–60% of depressed patients. In normal people the secretion of cortisol follows a circadian rhythm in which secretion peaks at 8:00 a.m. and is relatively lower in the evening and early morning hours. In contrast, about one-half of depressed patients secrete excessive amounts of cortisol, primarily during the afternoon and evening (Figure 56–7). This disturbance of cortisol secretion in depression is not dependent on stress, and it is not found in other psychiatric disorders. Cortical secretion returns to normal with recovery.

Philip Gold and his colleagues have found that the increased secretion of cortisol results from hypersecretion of corticotropin-releasing hormone (CTRH) from the hypo-

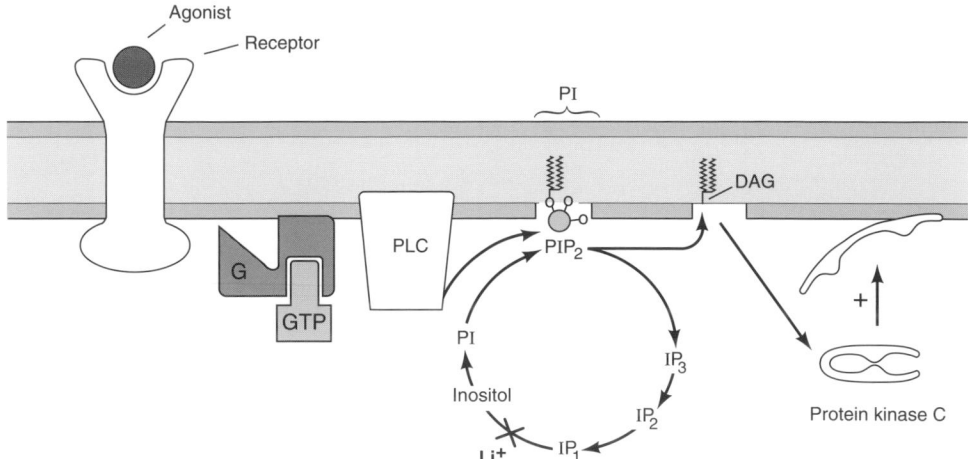

FIGURE 56–6

The exact mechanism of action for lithium, used to treat bipolar depression, is unknown. However, lithium has recently been shown to affect the phosphoinositide second-messenger system. As illustrated in this figure many synaptic receptors act through a G-protein to mediate the conversion of phosphoinositol diphosphate (**PIP₂**), a membrane lipid, into diacylglyc-

erol (**DAG**) and inositol triphosphate (**IP₃**). IP₃ is further broken down to inositol phosphate (**IP**), which is then converted to free inositol by the enzyme inositol-1-phosphatase. Lithium blocks this enzyme and therefore causes IP₃ to accumulate in the cytoplasm. The role of IP₃ and protein kinase C in cellular function is discussed in Chapter 13.

thalamus. The level of CTRH correlates positively with depression. Of interest is the finding that CTRH induces anxiety in experimental animals. Release of CTRH is stimulated by norepinephrine and acetylcholine and inhibited by GABA. Thus, Gold and his colleagues have suggested that CTRH and the noradrenergic system may reinforce one another.

The hypersecretion of cortisol in the evening by depressed patients is sometimes also resistant to normal feedback suppression by the potent synthetic corticosteroid dexamethasone, which acts to depress adrenocorticotropin. This *dexamethasone suppression test* has been used to diagnose depression because at least 40% of rigorously diagnosed depressed patients show abnormalities of this test. The test is not specific, however. Dexamethasone suppression is also abnormal in patients suffering

from dementia, anorexia nervosa, bulimia, alcohol withdrawal, or weight loss.

There Are Two Major Types of Anxiety Disorders

The key feature of anxiety disorders is the frequent occurrence of symptoms of fear—arousal, restlessness, heightened responsiveness, sweating, racing heart, increased blood pressure, dry mouth, a desire to run or escape, and avoidance behavior. Just as grief is a normal response to personal loss, anxiety is a normal response to threatening situations. Sometimes the threats are active and direct, and sometimes they are indirect, such as the absence of people or objects that represent security. Anxiety is adaptive; it signals potential danger and can contribute to the

FIGURE 56–7

The mean hourly plasma cortisol concentration over a 24-hour period for seven patients with unipolar depression compared with the mean for 54 normal subjects. Each point represents the mean cortisol concentration every 60 minutes. Significant changes occur during the early morning and evening hours, resulting in a much weaker diurnal rhythm in the depressed patients.

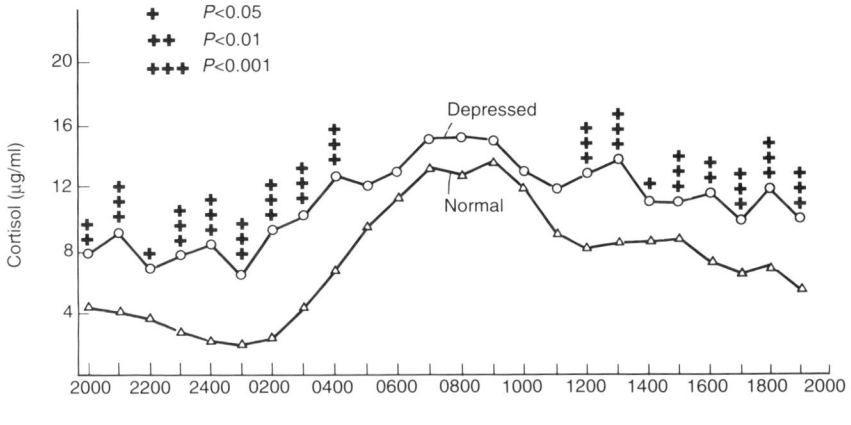

mastery of a difficult situation and thus to personal growth. Excessive anxiety, on the other hand, is maladaptive, either because it is too intense or because it is inappropriately provoked by events that present no real danger. Thus, anxiety is pathological when excessive and persistent, or when it no longer serves to signal danger.

Anxiety has subjective as well as objective manifestations. The subjective manifestations range from a heightened sense of awareness to a deep fear of impending disaster and death. Anxiety disorders are the most common psychiatric disorders, found in 10–30% of the general population. Anxiety can be subdivided into several types based on clinical characteristics and response to psychopharmacological agents. We shall focus only on panic attacks and general anxiety disorders.

Panic Attacks Are Brief Episodes of Terror

Panic attacks are brief, recurrent, spontaneous episodes of terror without a clearly identifiable cause. The attacks are usually brief, most commonly lasting 15 to 30 minutes; occasionally, but only rarely, they last hours. An essential feature of the attack is that at the onset of the disease the attacks are *unexpected*. They do not occur in situations that normally evoke fear or in which the patient is the focus of other people's attention. The attacks are characterized by a sense of impending disaster accompanied by an intense overactivity of the sympathetic nervous system (referred to as a *sympathetic crisis*). The heart races, there is shortness of breath, dizziness, trembling or shaking of the hands and legs, flushes or chills, chest pain, fear of dying or of going crazy or of doing something uncontrolled. The attacks first occur usually in the late 20s. They are recurrent over a period ranging from months to several years and are often experienced several times a week.

An interesting aspect of panic attacks is that they can be induced in some patients suffering from this disorder, but not in most normal subjects, by the infusion of sodium lactate into the blood or by the inhalation of carbon dioxide. Moreover, regular use of antidepressants that are effective for spontaneous panic will also prevent the panic induced by the infusion. Thus, sodium lactate infusion provides an approach for studying the mechanism underlying this disorder because the onset of an attack can be timed precisely. Using this approach, Eric Reiman and his colleagues have found a circumscribed bilateral abnormality in the temporal poles of patients suffering from panic attacks (see Chapter 1). This abnormality can also be activated by infusion of lactate. A unilateral abnormality in the right parahippocampal area is present in susceptible subjects, even when panic attacks are not actually occurring. Thus, a predisposition to this particular emotional disorder can be traced to a permanent and localized abnormality in an anatomically specific region of the brain. This region also participates in normal anxiety: When normal subjects experience anxiety, they show a transient increase in blood flow in the area.

A significant proportion of patients with panic disor-

ders—twice that of the normal population—have mitral valve prolapse. Moreover, the disease seems to have a strong genetic predisposition. Sixty percent of patients have relatives who suffer from the disorder, and there is overlap in the transmission of panic disorder and depression. In fact, half the patients with panic attacks also have depression, a finding that has led to the suggestion that panic attacks are a variant of depressive illness. This is consistent with the initially surprising finding that this form of anxiety responds to antidepressants, both to tricyclics and to monoamine oxidase inhibitors. Now that more is known about the function of the locus ceruleus, this finding is perhaps less surprising. The noradrenergic cells in this nucleus respond most effectively to stimuli that produce intense fear in the animal.

Generalized Anxiety Disorder Is Long-Lasting

The key feature of generalized anxiety is unrealistic or excessive worry, lasting not minutes but six months or longer. The symptoms are *motor tension* (trembling, twitching, muscle aches, restlessness), *autonomic hyperactivity* (shortness of breath, palpitations, increased heart rate, sweating, cold hands), and *vigilance and scanning* (feeling on edge, exaggerated startle response, difficulty in concentrating). The disorder sometimes follows an episode of depression.

The drugs most effective in treating generalized anxiety disorders are the benzodiazepines, such as chlordiazepoxide (Librium) and its derivative diazepam (Valium). In 1978 John Tallman found that benzodiazepines produced their therapeutic effect by enhancing activity of the $GABA_A$ receptor. GABA, as we have seen in Chapter 11, is the major inhibitory transmitter in the brain. The $GABA_A$ receptor acts by opening Cl^- channels that initiate hyperpolarization and inhibition of target cells. Benzodiazepine increases the affinity of the receptor for GABA, thereby

FIGURE 56–8
Diazepam is an effective drug in treating generalized anxiety disorders. Electrical tracings compare the response of a mouse spinal cord neuron to GABA, the major inhibitory neurotransmitter in the brain, and GABA in the presence of diazepam.

A. When GABA is bound to a $GABA_A$ receptor, it opens Cl channels and thus hyperpolarizes the cell.

B. Diazepam increases the affinity of the receptor for GABA and thus increases the Cl^- conductance and the hyperpolarization.

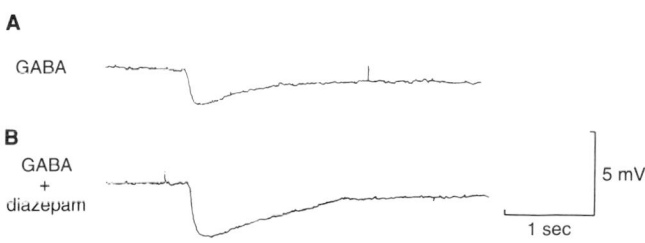

A

GABA

B

GABA
+
diazepam

5 mV

1 sec

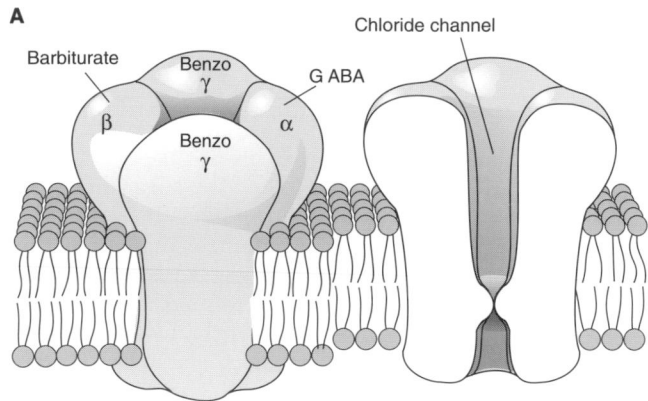

A

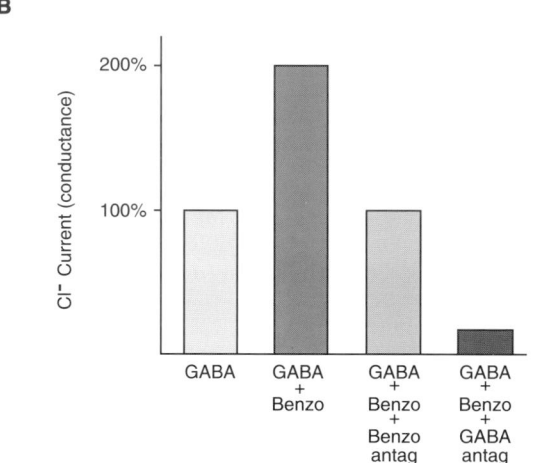

B

FIGURE 56–9

Structural model of the GABA_A chloride channel.

A. There are three different subunit types: α, β, γ. Benzodiazepines bind to the γ-subunits. GABA binds to the α-subunit, and barbiturates bind to the β-subunit. All the subunits contribute to forming the Cl⁻ channel.

B. Modulation of chloride flux through the GABA_A receptor channel by benzodiazepine. GABA enhances the influx of Cl⁻ into the nerve cell. Benzodiazepine enhances the effect of GABA, so that basal levels of GABA are more effective in gating the channel. Benzodiazepine antagonists prevent enhancement of GABA effects but do not reduce basal conductance of Cl⁻. GABA antagonists prevent gating of Cl⁻ channels in spite of the presence of benzodiazepines.

resulting in an increase in Cl⁻ influx through the Cl⁻ channel (Figure 56–8).

The GABA_A receptor has three functional domains: (1) a binding site for GABA, (2) a site for barbiturates, and (3) a site for benzodiazepines (Chapter 11). The protein is allosteric; binding of any one of the three ligands (GABA, benzodiazepine, or barbiturate) influences the binding of the other two and facilitates GABA's action. In particular, GABA will bind more tightly when a benzodiazepine also is bound to its site on the receptor. Nevertheless, all three sites are distinct from each other. Indeed, analysis of the

primary structure of the GABA receptor indicates that there are at least three subunits (alpha, beta, and gamma), with benzodiazepine binding only to the gamma subunit (Figure 56–9).

The calming effects of benzodiazepines are therefore best explained by an enhancement of certain of GABA's inhibitory effects. The GABA receptors to which benzodiazepines bind are concentrated in the limbic system, specifically in the amygdala, an area thought to be of central importance for emotional behavior.

An Overall View

Certain major depressive illnesses may be the result of genetically determined disorders of chemical transmission involving at least two major transmitter pathways of the brain: the serotonergic and the noradrenergic systems. Although the mechanisms that cause the defect remain obscure, rapid developments in this field in the last two decades provide great hope that aspects of the molecular basis of affective disorders will soon be elucidated.

Anxiety is less well understood. However, like major depression and schizophrenia, two types of anxiety, panic attacks and generalized anxiety disorder, seem to represent alterations in synaptic functioning. Since panic attacks respond well to antidepressants, they too may reflect an abnormality in the biogenic amine pathways of the brain. In contrast, generalized anxiety disorder seems to involve the GABA_A receptor system. Although the pathology underlying the anxiety disorders has not been localized precisely, PET scanning has shown that both normal anxiety and panic attacks involve the same anatomical site. This discovery is the first specific anatomical localization of a major psychiatric syndrome.

Selected Readings

Gold, P. W., Goodwin, F. K., and Chrousos, G. P. 1988. Clinical and biochemical manifestations of depression (parts I and II). New Engl. J. Med. 319:348–353 and 413–420.

Goodwin, D. W., and Guze, S. B. 1989. Psychiatric Diagnosis. New York: Oxford.

Goodwin, F. K., and Jamison, K. R. 1990. Manic-Depressive Illness. New York: Oxford University Press.

Jonowsky, A. and Sulser, A. 1987. Alpha and beta adrenergic receptor in brain. In H. T. Meltzer (ed.), Psychopharmacology, The Third Generation of Progress. New York: Raven Press, pp. 249–256.

Kety, S. S. 1979. Disorders of the human brain. Sci. Am. 241(3): 202–214.

Kleiman, E. 1983. The Scope of Depression. In J. Angst (ed.), The Origins of Depression: Current Concepts and Approaches. Dahlem Konferenzen. Heidelberg: Springer-Verlag.

References

Anden, N.-E., Dahlstrom, A., Fuxe, K., Larsson, K., Olson, L., and Ungerstedt, U. 1966. Ascending monoamine neurons to the telencephalon and diencephalon. Acta. Physiol. Scand. 67: 313–326.

Åsberg, M., Traskman, L., and Thoren, P. 1976. 5-HIAA in the cerebrospinal fluid. A biochemical suicide predictor? Arch. Gen. Psychiatry 33:1193–1197.

Baron, M. 1990. Genetic linkage in mental illness. Nature 346: 618.

Carroll, B. J., Feinberg, M., Greden, J. F., et al. 1981. A specific laboratory test for the diagnosis of melancholia. Arch. Gen. Psychiatry 38:15–22.

Cooper, J. R., Bloom, F. E., and Roth, R. H. 1986. The Biochemical Basis of Neuropharmacology, 5th ed. New York: Oxford University Press.

Davis, J. M., and Moss, J. W. (eds.). 1983. The Affective Disorders. Washington, D.C.: American Psychiatric Press.

Everett, G. M., and Toman, J. E. P. 1959. Mode of action of Rauwolfia alkaloids and motor activity. In J. H. Masserman (ed.), Biological Psychiatry. New York: Grune & Stratton, pp. 75–81.

Freud, S. 1917. Mourning and melancholia. In The Collected Papers, Vol. IV. New York: Basic Books, 1959, pp. 152–170.

Kety, S. S., Rosenthal, D., Wender, P. H., Schulsinger, F., and Jacobsen, B. 1975. Mental illness in the biological and adoptive families of adopted individuals who have become schizophrenic: A preliminary report based on psychiatric interviews. In R. R. Fieve, D. Rosenthal, and H. Brill (eds.), Genetic Research in Psychiatry. Baltimore: Johns Hopkins University Press, pp. 147–165.

Klein, D. F. 1974. Endogenomorphic depression: A conceptual and terminological revision. Arch. Gen. Psychiatry 31:447–454.

Kraepelin, E. 1909. Dementia Praecox and Paraphrenia. From Kraepelin's Textbook of Psychiatry, 8th ed. R. M. Barclay (trans.). Edinburgh: Livingstone, 1919.

Pletscher, A., Shore, P. A., and Brodie, B. B. 1956. Serotonin as a mediator of reserpine action in brain. J. Pharmacol. Exp. Ther. 116:84–89.

Posner, M. I., Early, T. S., Reiman, E., Pardo, J. P., and Dhawan, M. 1988. Asymmetries in hemispheric control of attention in schizophrenia. Arch. Gen. Psychiatry. 45:814–821.

Sachar, E. J., Asnis, G., Halbreich, U., Nathan, R. S., and Halpern, F. 1980. Recent studies in the neuroendocrinology of major depressive disorders. Psychiatr. Clin. North Am. 3:313–326.

Schou, M., Juel-Nielson, N., Stromgen, E., and Volotry, H. 1954. The treatment of manic psychosis by the administration of lithium salts. J. Neurol. Neurosurg. Psychiat. 17:250.

Styron, W. 1990. Darkness Visible: A Memoir of Madness. New York: Random House.

Tallman, J. F., and Gallagher, D. W. 1985. The GABA-ergic system: A locus of benzodiazepine action. Ann. Rev. Neurosci. 8:21.

Van Praag, H. M. 1982. Neurotransmitters in CNS disease. Lancet 2:1259–1263.

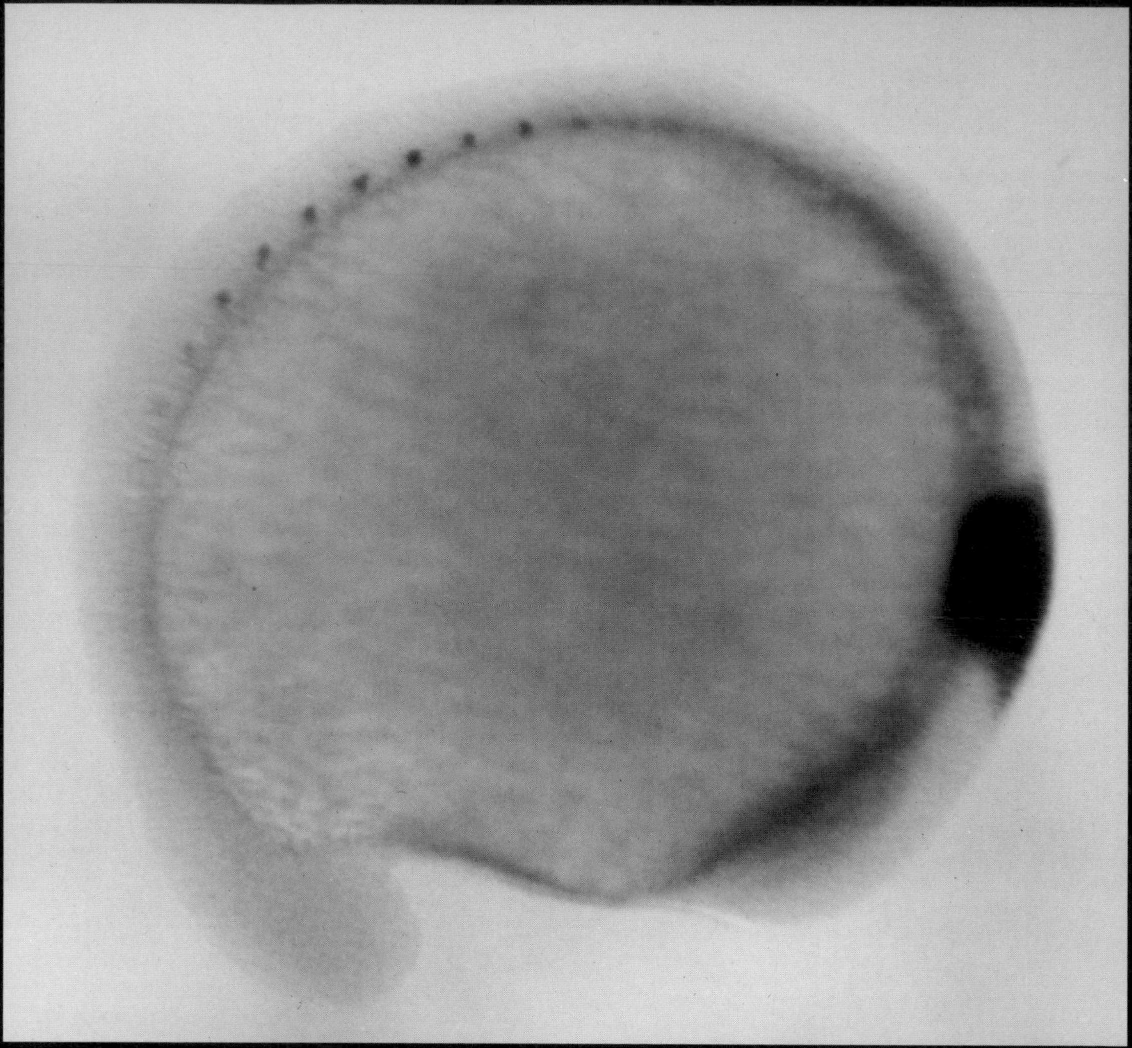

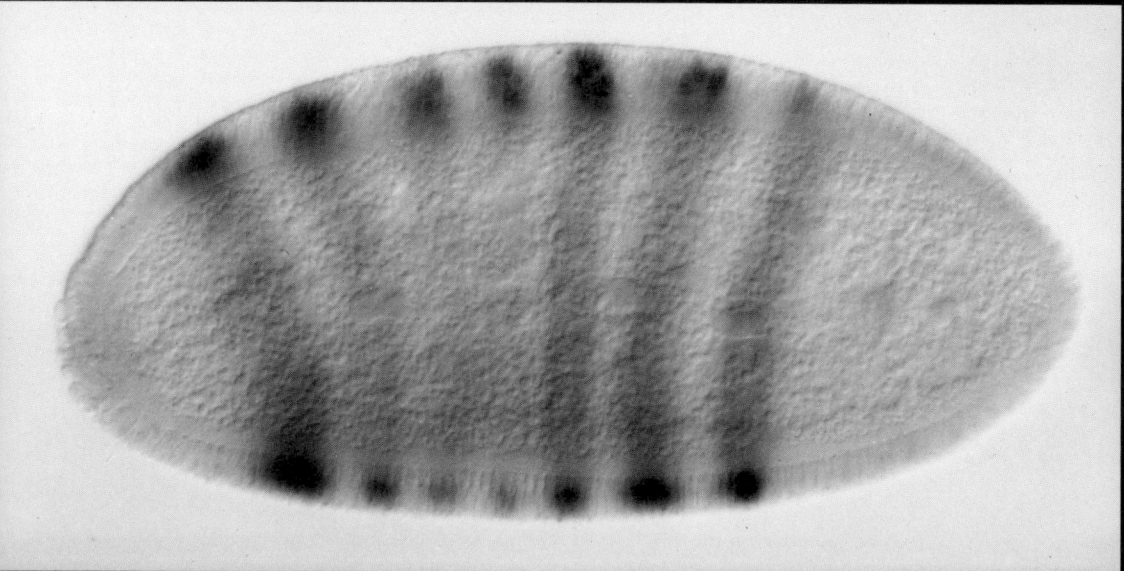

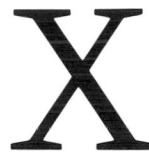

Development, Critical Periods, and the Emergence of Behavior

Our understanding of the adult nervous system and its control of behavior has been enhanced by research into the development of the brain. Behavior is dependent on individual classes of nerve cells with specialized functions and on the formation of specific interconnections between them. Studies of the development of the nervous system aim to elucidate how neural cells acquire specific identities and how patterns of neuronal connections are established and maintained. The nervous system develops in a series of ordered steps, with a precise temporal sequence that is characteristic of each neural structure. Moreover, each neuron connects with only a selected subset of potential target cells. In addition, the connections are formed only at specific regions of the target cell's surface membrane.

It is evident that the total genetic information available to an animal—perhaps 10^5 genes in mammals—is not sufficient to specify the total number of neuronal interconnections that are made—perhaps as many as 10^{15}. Thus, the development of the nervous system must also involve *epigenetic* processes that activate specific subsets of genes in a combinatorial manner at specific times during development.

Epigenetic influences that control neural cell differentiation originate from within the embryo and from the external environment. Influences that derive from the embryo involve intercellular signals that consist of many diffusible factors and surface molecules. The external environment provides nutritive factors, sensory and social experiences, and learning, which mediate their effects through changes in neural activity. Many internal and external factors impinge upon the developing cell. Thus, the appropriately timed actions of a complex array of distinct factors are critical for the proper differentiation of an individual neural cell.

In the next series of chapters, we consider successive stages in the development of the nervous system. In addition to examining the early stages of development that

Even though the body form of different animals is strikingly distinct, the developmental programs that govern animal form seem to be remarkably conserved throughout phylogeny. In each case development depends on a sequential program of gene expression. In many instances gene expression is governed by specific DNA-binding proteins, one class of which are termed homeobox genes. Homeobox genes are used to shape the development of both vertebrate and invertebrate embryos.

The top figure shows the segmentally repeated pattern of expression of the even-skipped homeobox protein in cells of the early *Drosophila* embryo. Proteins with similar homeobox domains are also found in vertebrate embryos. The bottom figure shows the segmentally repeated expression of the *engrailed* homeobox protein in cells of the zebrafish embryo. *Engrailed* gene homologs are found in many invertebrate and vertebrate species. (Courtesy of Corey S. Goodman and Nipam Patel.)

control neural cell identity, the guidance of axons and the formation of synaptic circuits, we look at how the interactions with the external world and the social and sensory environment modify and consolidate the connection formed early in development. Depriving an animal of its normal environment during an early critical period can have profound consequences for later maturation of the brain and for behavior. We also consider how internal factors, such as androgen hormones, continue to influence the structure of the brain during early postnatal development. Finally, we consider the aging of the brain.

PART X

Chapter 57:   **Control of Cell Identity**

Chapter 58:   **Cell Migration and Axon Guidance**

Chapter 59:   **Neuronal Survival and Synapse Formation**

Chapter 60:   **Early Experience and the Fine Tuning of Synaptic Connections**

Chapter 61:   **Sexual Differentiation of the Nervous System**

Chapter 62:   **Aging of the Brain: Dementia of the Alzheimer's Type**

Thomas M. Jessell
Samuel Schacher

57

Control of Cell Identity

Cell Lineage Can Control the Fate of Neural Cells

In Most Species the Fate of Neural Cells Is Not Determined by Cell Lineage

Neural and Epidermal Cell Fate Is Regulated by Local Cell Interactions

Induction of the Neural Plate from the Ectoderm Is Dependent on Interactions with the Adjacent Mesoderm

Regional Differentiation Within the Neural Plate Is Also Controlled by the Mesoderm

Studies of Invertebrate Embryos Have Identified Genes that Control the Fate of Ectodermal Cells

Diffusible Factors Control Glial Cell Differentiation in the Central Nervous System

Cell Position Controls the Identity of Photoreceptors in the *Drosophila* Eye

The Fate of Neural Crest Cells Is Controlled by the Local Environment

The Transmitter Choice of Peripheral Neurons Is Controlled by Signals from Neighboring Cells

An Overall View

The complex and diverse functions of the mature nervous system—perception, motor coordination, motivation, and memory—depend on the precise interconnections formed by many thousands of neural cell types. Establishment of the mature pattern of neuronal connections is a gradual process that can be considered to occur in six major stages. First, a uniform population of neural precursor cells is induced from undifferentiated ectoderm by signals from the mesoderm. Second, these neural cells begin to diversify, giving rise to glial cells and immature neurons. Third, immature neurons migrate from germinal zones to their final position. Fourth, neurons extend axons, which project to the vicinity of their eventual targets. Fifth, axons form synaptic connections with a selected subset of target cells. Finally, some of the synaptic contacts that are formed initially are modified to generate the mature pattern of neural connections.

Although these sequential steps lead to a greater variety of cell types within the nervous system than in any other organ of the body, the problems inherent in understanding the mechanisms underlying this diversification are simply an extension of the central question in development: How does a single cell, the fertilized egg, give rise to each of the many differentiated cell types in the entire organism? Modern insights into principles that control cellular differentiation began with the studies of Theodor Boveri and Edmund Wilson around the turn of the century, culminating in the work of Jacques Monod and Francois Jacob in the late 1950s. Monod and Jacob proposed that cell differentiation is achieved by the activation of specific sets of genes, with each distinct cell type expressing a different subset of genes. The differential activation of specific genes within individual cells is now known to be controlled, in a direct manner, by nuclear proteins that bind to DNA sequences, thereby regulating the transcription of specific genes (see Box 12–1). These transcriptional regulatory proteins are themselves controlled by other cellular signaling proteins. The mechanisms by which transcriptional regulatory proteins are controlled define two major programs of cell differentiation: cell lineage and cell-cell interactions.

The differentiated fate of some cells depends exclusively on lineage, on the program of division that the cell undergoes. Lineage-dependent programs of cell differentiation are controlled by cytoplasmic or nuclear proteins that are inherited asymmetrically by the progeny of a dividing precursor cell. As a result, different daughter cells inherit distinct differentiation signals. The differentiation of other cells depends on external signals from other cells in the environment. These local signals can be secreted or they can be cell surface molecules. Many of the receptors for these signaling molecules are membrane proteins that transduce signals across the plasma membrane, triggering intracellular second-messenger pathways that directly or indirectly regulate the activity of transcription factors. Other receptors for diffusible signals, for example, steroid hormones, are located within the nucleus and are themselves transcriptional regulatory proteins.

The different strategies of neural cell differentiation discussed in this chapter therefore depend on whether transcriptional regulatory proteins are regulated by signaling mechanisms that are intrinsic to the cell, and are therefore dependent on the lineage of the cell, or by extrinsic signals triggered from surrounding cells. But no single organism, vertebrate or invertebrate, has so far provided a complete picture of the signaling mechanisms underlying neural development. To illustrate the fundamental principles of neural cell differentiation we therefore have selected examples from different species. First, we discuss how the development of some neural cells can be controlled in an autonomous cell lineage-dependent manner by the program of division that a cell undergoes, using the nematode worm *Caenorhabditis elegans* as an example. However, unlike *C. elegans* the fate of most neural cells in invertebrate and vertebrate embryos is not cell autonomous but depends on external signals. We emphasize this point with four examples of cell-cell interactions that illustrate the way in which the fate of neural cells is restricted progressively during development. We first discuss the binary decision that is fundamental in determining whether embryonic ectodermal cells progress along a neural or an epidermal pathway of differentiation. Second, we examine the mechanisms that control glial cell diversification, highlighting how diffusible factors determine neural cell fate. Third, we discuss how cells that are already committed to a neural fate differentiate into specific classes of neurons. Finally, we discuss further refinements that occur once cells are committed to a specific neuronal or glial fate, illustrating how the choice of neurotransmitter that a cell uses also is controlled by environmental signals.

In Chapter 58 we discuss the next steps involved in neuronal differentiation: in particular, the growth of axons to their targets, a process that is critical to establishing neural circuits. Once axons reach the vicinity of their targets they need to establish functional synaptic con-

nections. The mechanisms involved in the survival of neurons and the formation of synaptic connections are described in Chapter 59. Axonal extension and synapse formation are not the only processes that determine the eventual pattern of neuronal connections, however. The stability of initial synaptic connections is dependent on subsequent neuronal experience. Thus neuronal activity plays a crucial role in selecting which synapses are stabilized and which exist only transiently. The role of neuronal activity in the rearrangement and stabilization of synapses during development is discussed in Chapter 60.

Cell Lineage Can Control the Fate of Neural Cells

Every cell in the nervous system has a developmental history that can in principle be depicted as a *fate map* that traces the ancestry of the cell from the fertilized egg through successive cell divisions. Identification of individual cells or groups of cells by direct visual inspection or by cell marking techniques has made it possible to follow the fate of certain cells for long periods of time, in some cases until they stop dividing. Fate maps for the precursors of neural cells have been obtained in several species, and with this information it is possible to determine whether the program of cell divisions—the *lineage* of the cell—is important in defining its eventual fate. Some invertebrate animals have highly stereotyped developmental programs that are reflected in invariant cell lineages. The best characterized animal that exhibits an invariant cell lineage is the nematode worm, *C. elegans*, first studied by Sydney Brenner and his colleagues in the early 1960s. The lineage of every somatic cell has been mapped in detail by John Sulston, Robert Horvitz, and their colleagues (Figure 57–1). Each animal has precisely 302 neurons and 56 glial support cells. The nervous system in *C. elegans* does not derive from a single precursor cell, but from precursors spaced out along the body of the worm (Figure 57–1). Each neuronal precursor in every animal exhibits the same sequence and pattern of cell divisions. The developmental history of each of these neurons can be traced back to the zygote.

The invariance of this program of neuronal development can be demonstrated by monitoring the fate of a single cell after deleting one or several of its neighbors. In *C. elegans* and some other invertebrate species-specific cells can be killed by focusing the beam of a laser at the nucleus of the cell. Laser ablation of single cells has been used to show that in many cases the fate of an individual cell that is destined to give rise to a neuron is not affected by the absence of its neighbor, or by the appearance of new neighbors. In some cases, however, deletion of a single cell does result in one of its neighbors changing its fate, sometimes even adopting the fate of the missing cell. Thus, even in animals such as *C. elegans*, whose cell lineage program is highly stereotyped, local cell interactions—signals from other cells—have a role in regulating cell fate.

The factors that determine cell fate in *C. elegans* can be studied effectively using genetics (Figure 57–2). Genetic analysis is simplified in *C. elegans* because the animal can

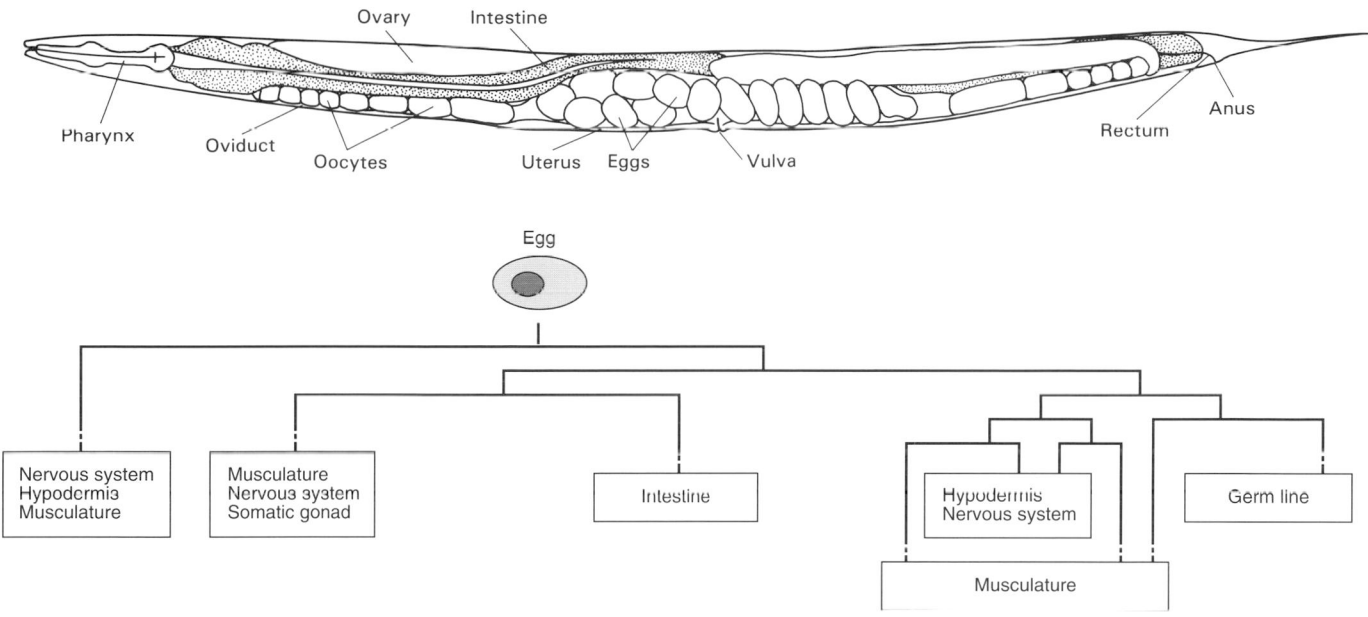

FIGURE 57–1

The nematode *Caenorhabditis elegans* has been used to study the relationship between cell lineage and differentiation. The top panel shows a schematic drawing of an adult *C. elegans* with the major tissues and organs labeled. The lower panel, a simplified lineage tree, depicts the major cell division pathways that give rise to these major tissues, including the nervous system. Like most other organs, cells of the nervous system do not derive from a single branch of the lineage tree. (From Sulston and Horvitz, 1977.)

FIGURE 57–2

Genes that control cell lineage in *Caenorhabditis elegans* are involved in cell-cell interactions.

A. A simplified lineage diagram illustrating some of the ways in which genetic mutations may affect cell lineage. In each cell division in *C. elegans* a progenitor cell with a particular fate (A) divides into cells with fates B and C. Mutations in which both progeny adopt fate B define genes whose normal function is to generate different fates in the two progeny. Mutations in which one of the cells adopts fate A define genes whose normal function is to make progeny different from the progenitor.

B. The gene *Lin-12* specifies the fate of cells. In wild-type *C. elegans* the left and right cellular homologs (defined by the prior pattern of cell division) give rise to different progeny (**top** diagram). Mutations that eliminate the function of the *lin-12* gene transform the pattern of cell division of the left homolog into the pattern characteristic of the right cell. Conversely, mutations that result in overproduction of the Lin-12 protein, or result in constitutive activity of this protein, transform the pattern of cell division of the right cell into the one characteristic of its left homolog. (Adapted from Horvitz et al., 1983.)

C. The protein product of the *lin-12* gene is a transmembrane protein with structural repeats in its extracellular domain similar to those of epidermal growth factor (**EGF**). Asterisks indicate the position of mutations in the *lin-12* gene that cause the gain-of- function phenotypes shown in part B. Each mutation results in a single amino acid change at the indicated position. (Adapted from Greenwald and Seydoux, 1990.)

A

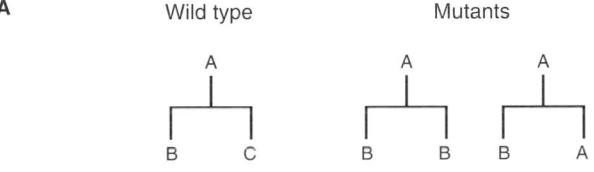

Wild type   Mutants

B

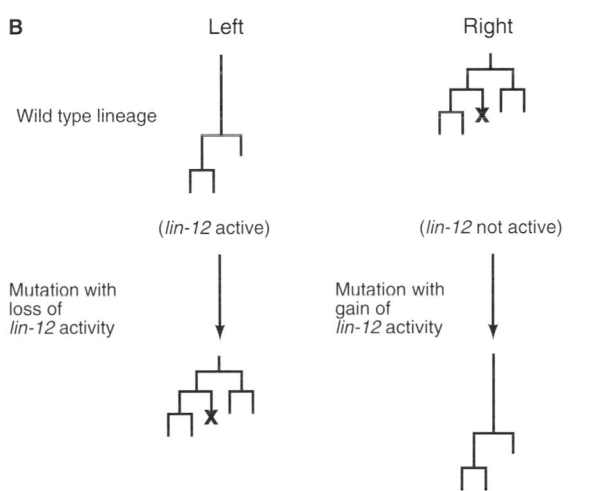

C   Structure of the Lin-12 protein

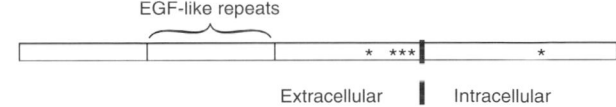

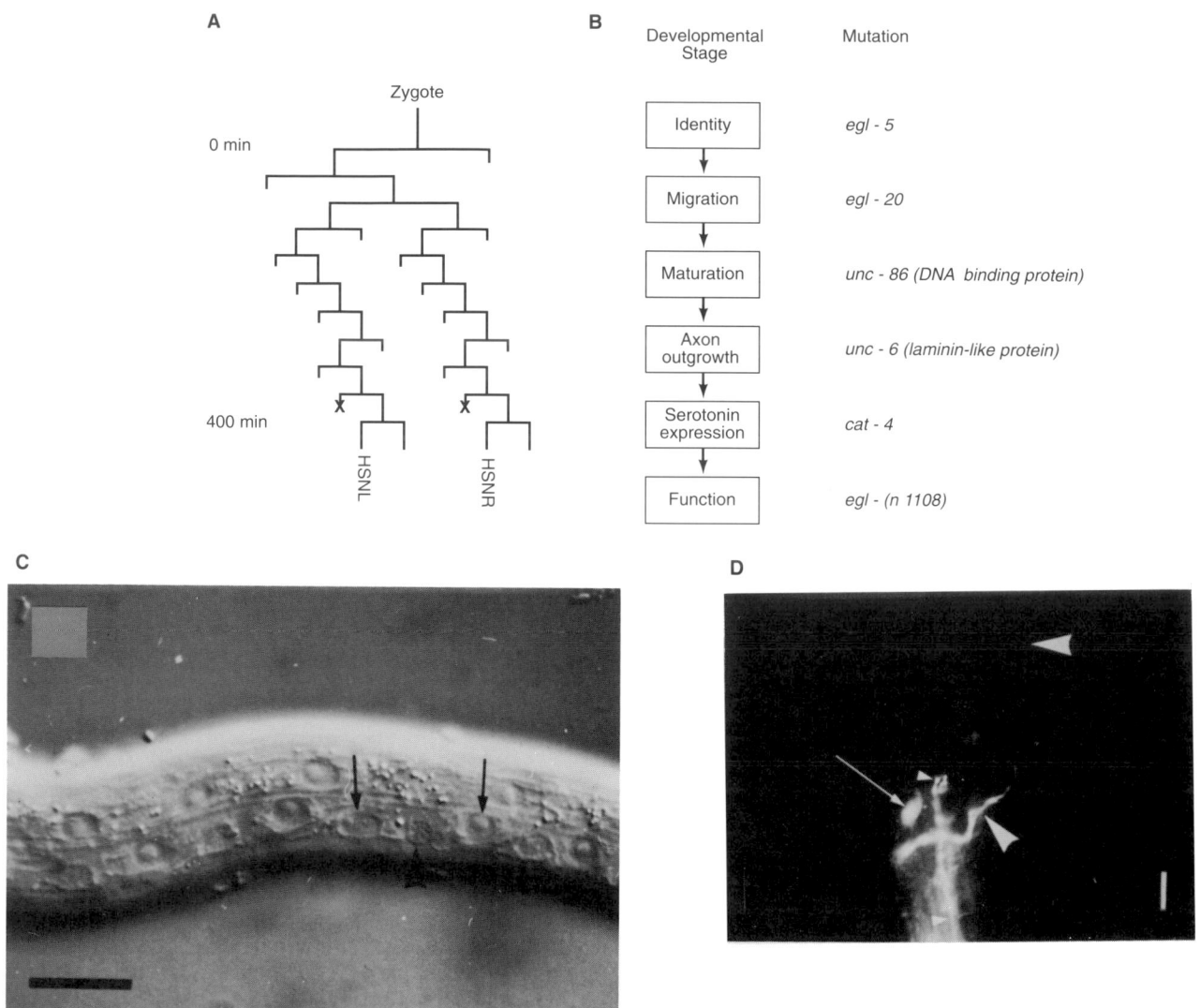

FIGURE 57–3

Genetics can be used to define sequential steps involved in the differentiation of identified neurons. In this example the development of the HSN motor neurons in *Caenorhabditis elegans* has been analyzed.

A. The entire lineage of the HSN motor neurons has been traced. Similar lineage diagrams can be drawn for all the other neurons and glial cells in the *C. elegans* nervous system.

B. The developmental stages responsible for the complete differentiation of the HSN motor neuron have been defined. Mutations that affect each successive stage have also been isolated, and the names of these mutations are shown next to the process that they

disrupt. The structure of some of these genes has now been determined. For example, the *unc-86* gene encodes a DNA-binding protein and the *unc-6* gene encodes a laminin-like extracellular matrix protein.

C. The HSN motor neuron can be identified in a recently hatched *C. elegans* larva simply by using interference contrast (Nomarski) microscopy.

D. The axon deriving from the HSN motor neuron expresses the neurotransmitter serotonin as revealed by immunocytochemistry. The acquisition of transmitter-specific properties is one of the final events in neuronal differentiation. (From Desai et al., 1988.)

exist either as a male or a self-fertilizing hermaphrodite, which makes propagation of stocks and cross breeding easy. Moreover, *C. elegans* has a rapid generation time and a program of cell divisions that is readily monitored by microscopic observation. Finally, a physical map of most of the *C. elegans* genome has been derived from cloned

DNA fragments. Because of these experimental advantages, many genes that affect the lineage of cells in the nervous system have been identified. One approach to the characterization of such genes is to examine the functional deficit that results when a specific neuron is killed by laser ablation, then to mutagenize animals and screen for mutants, which show the same deficit, and finally to analyze the development of those mutants to discriminate genes affecting development from those affecting function. Using this approach, Robert Horvitz and his colleagues have identified a hierarchy of genes that regulates the program of development of a single class of motor neurons from early cell divisions to the acquisition of neurotransmitter properties (Figure 57–3).

The structure of some of the genes that affect cell fate in early neural lineage in *C. elegans* is known. For example, the gene *unc-86* encodes a DNA binding protein that functions to regulate the transcription of other genes. Other genes, such as *lin-12*, encode membrane-spanning proteins that may function as ligands or receptors that participate in signaling with nearby cells (Figure 57–2).

In Most Species the Fate of Neural Cells Is Not Determined by Cell Lineage

The identity of individual neurons is, however, not achieved through any single developmental strategy. Some neurons depend critically on their lineage and develop independently of other cells, but the differentiation of other neurons, for example, those in the vertebrate retina, appears to be largely independent of any lineage relationship, depending exclusively on signals received from neighboring groups of cells.

As we have seen in Chapter 28, the vertebrate retina consists of a complex array of interconnected photoreceptors, bipolar cells, horizontal, amacrine, retinal ganglion cells, as well as supporting glial cells. A single precursor cell can give rise to different classes of cells, for example, to a glial cell and a photoreceptor, to a photoreceptor and an amacrine cell, or in fact to almost any combination of cell types (Figure 57–4). This finding has been demonstrated using two types of experimental techniques. Experiments with chick and frog embryos using direct intracellular injection of markers such as horseradish peroxidase or fluorescent dextran into single precursor cells have shown that there is no lineage restriction in the progeny of marked cells, regardless of the developmental stage at which the cell is injected. In mammals, where direct injection into brain cells is technically more difficult, another technique has been developed for tracing lineage. Dividing neural cells can be infected with a recombinant retrovirus. Part of the viral genome is replaced by the gene that codes for a protein marker that can be detected easily in single cells, usually the β-galactosidase enzyme of the bacterium *Escherichia coli*. The retrovirus is incapable of spreading from infected cells or their progeny because the genes required for packaging the viral genome have been deleted. Thus, if a single cell is infected with the virus, all the progeny of that cell will express the marker enzyme, providing a permanent and nondiluted lineage marker (see Figure 58–1).

Injection of fluorescent dye or retrovirus into the retina of newborn rats results in the labeling of precursor cells that give rise to virtually every combination of cell types.

Moreover, the progeny of single cells labeled by direct injection or retroviral infection are organized in columns within the retina. It appears therefore that cell lineage does not play a major role in determining the identity of individual cells in the vertebrate retina.

Neural and Epidermal Cell Fate Is Regulated by Local Cell Interactions

How is the decision of a cell to progress along a pathway that results in neural differentiation first reached? As we learned in Chapter 21, the vertebrate nervous system develops from a region of ectoderm that lies along the dorsal midline of the embryo. As neural ectodermal cells begin to differentiate, they elongate more than the remainder of the ectoderm, giving rise to a columnar epithelium known as the *neural plate*. The ectodermal cells lateral to the neural plate eventually give rise to epidermis. Soon after the neural plate forms it becomes regionally differentiated along its anteroposterior axis. Regional specialization of the neural plate occurs concomitantly with a series of changes in cell shape and the folding of the flat sheet of neural ectodermal cells into a tubular structure, the *neural tube*. During this process, called *neurulation*, cells in the anterior part of the neural plate begin to form the primitive forebrain and midbrain, whereas cells in the posterior part form the hindbrain and spinal cord.

To understand the mechanisms that give rise to the differentiation of distinct populations of cells, we need first to address two major questions. First, what controls the formation of the neural plate? Second, what defines the regional specification of the neural plate along its anteroposterior and dorsoventral axes? We discuss these two questions in turn.

Induction of the Neural Plate from the Ectoderm Is Dependent on Interactions with the Adjacent Mesoderm

Hans Spemann and Hilde Mangold discovered in 1924 that the differentiation of the neural plate from the uncommitted ectoderm is induced by adjacent mesodermal tissues. The role of the mesoderm in inducing the embryonic nervous system was demonstrated by transplanting tissues to new locations in amphibian embryos. First, Spemann and Mangold transplanted cells from a region of the embryo destined to form the dorsal mesoderm, called the dorsal lip of the blastopore, into or underneath the ventral ectoderm of a host embryo, a region that normally gives rise to ventral epidermal tissues (Figure 57–5). The transplanted cells were removed from a pigmented embryo and grafted into an unpigmented host, thus permitting the fate of the grafted cells to be assessed. The cells of the dorsal blastopore lip that were transplanted to this ventral site differentiated into axial mesoderm, consistent with their normal fate. Strikingly, these transplanted cells also re-

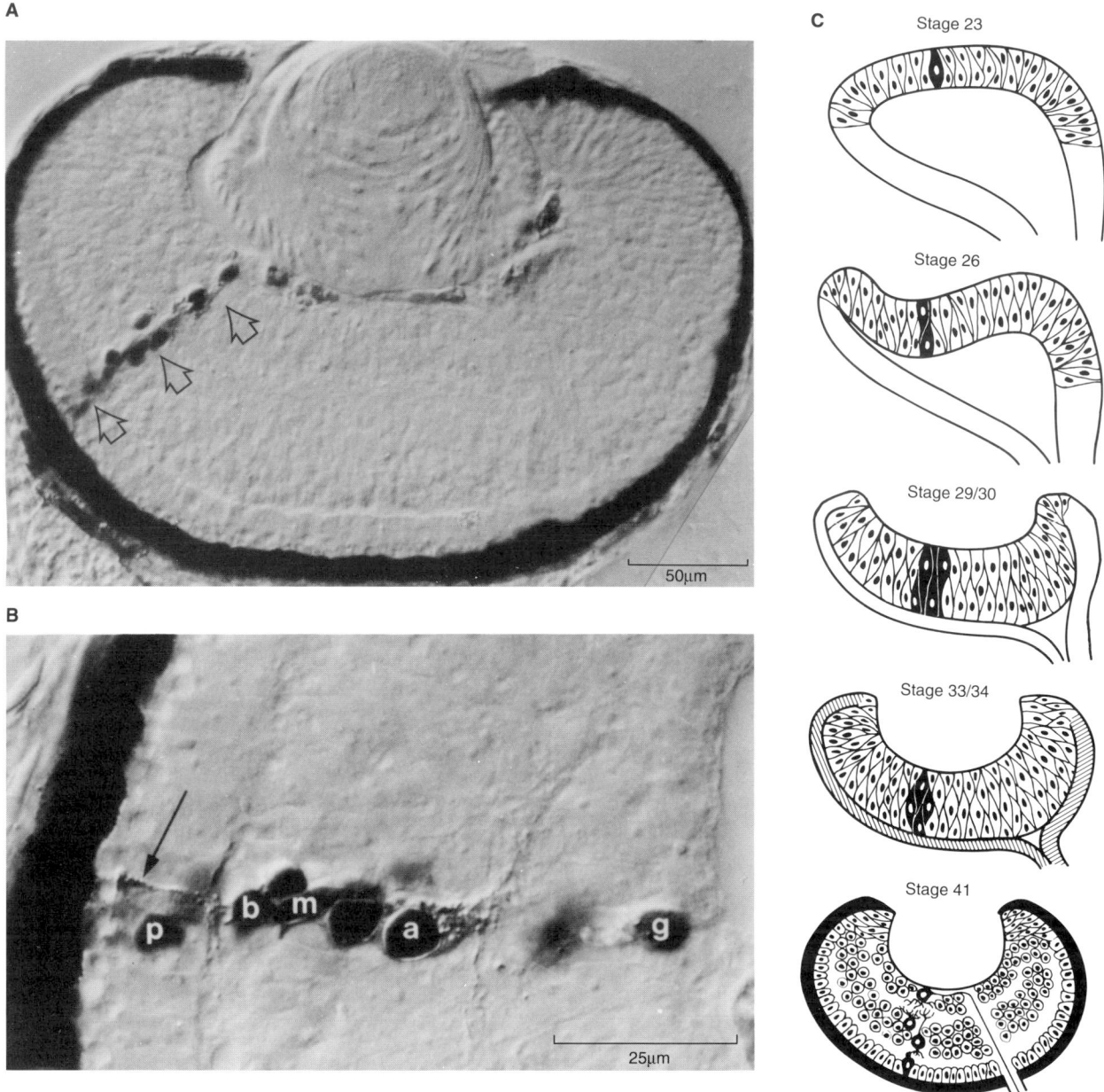

FIGURE 57–4

Lineage does not determine the developmental fate of cells that form the vertebrate retina.

A. Section through the eye of a *xenopus* embryo showing the dorsal location and radial alignment of this column of clonally related retinal cells, marked by injection of the marker enzyme horseradish peroxidase.

B. Same clone at a higher magnification with some of the identified cell types labeled (**p**, photoreceptors; **b**, bipolar; **m**, Müller; **a**, amacrine; and **g**, ganglion). The **arrow** points to a rod cell in partial focus.

C. Scheme for the generation of cell types in the frog (*Xenopus*) retina. A single cell at stage 23 may give rise by division to a contiguous collection of cells, all of which have left the cell cycle by stage 29/30 but may not yet be functionally committed. As the retina breaks up into layers (near stage 33/34), clonally related postmitotic cells distribute themselves radially and end up in different microenvironments. Local cell interactions in these different environments lead them to adopt distinct fates, which become obvious by stage 41. (From Holt et al., 1988.)

programmed the fate of host ectodermal cells, inducing them to form a second body axis that included a virtually complete nervous system. Other regions of the early gastrula transplanted to ectopic sites in the embryo lack the capacity of the dorsal blastopore lip to self-differentiate and induce a second body axis. This prompted Spemann to call this special region the *organizer*. Spemann and Mangold's finding suggested that during normal development the nervous system is induced by the adjacent mesoderm.

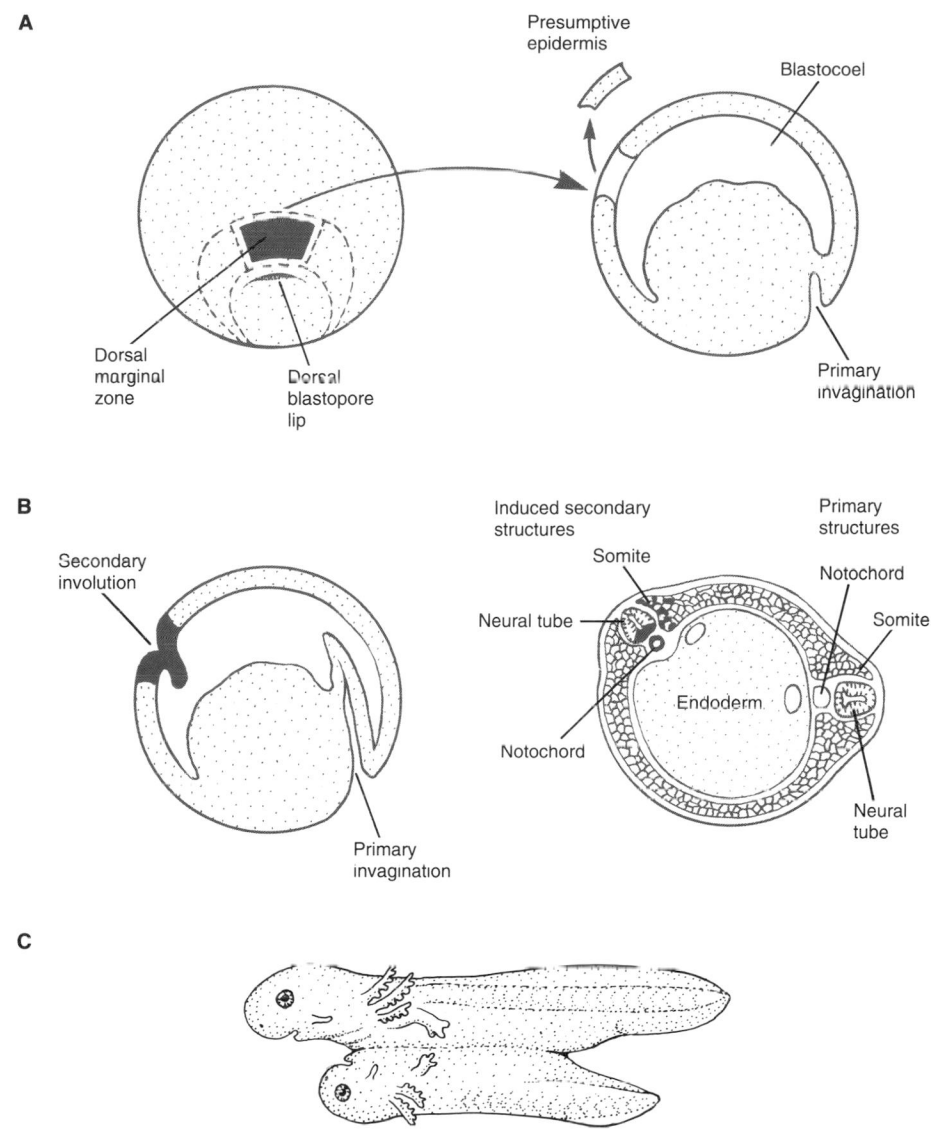

FIGURE 57–5

Transplantation of the dorsal lip of the blastosphere can induce a second embryonic axis in amphibian embryos. (Adapted from Gilbert, 1991.)

A. A dorsal blastopore lip from an early gastrula is transplanted into another early gastrula in the region that normally becomes the ventral epidermis.

B. The tissue invaginates and induces a second embryonic axis, including an entire nervous system. Both donor (**black**) and host (**white**) tissues are seen in the induced neural tube, notochord, and somites.

C. As the embryo matures, the high degree of differentiation of the secondary embryo becomes apparent.

A second set of experiments that reinforced this conclusion was carried out by Johannes Holtfreter in the early 1930s. By raising the isotonicity of the salt solution in which amphibian embryos develop, Holtfreter reversed the normal involution of the mesoderm during gastrulation. The mesoderm now moved outward and away from the ectoderm, forming a disordered embryo called an *exogastrula*. In exogastrulae the mesoderm is never located under the prospective neural ectoderm and in such embryos there was no histologically detectable neural ec-

toderm. These results strengthened the idea that proximity between the axial mesoderm and overlying ectoderm is essential for the differentiation of neural ectoderm.

Although these two sets of experiments suggested that induction of neural ectoderm is influenced by the underlying axial mesoderm, Spemann had considered earlier that induction occurred by a signal that spreads from the blastopore lip through the ectoderm before gastrulation. Recent experiments on neural induction by Christopher Kintner and others have provided evidence that the dorsal

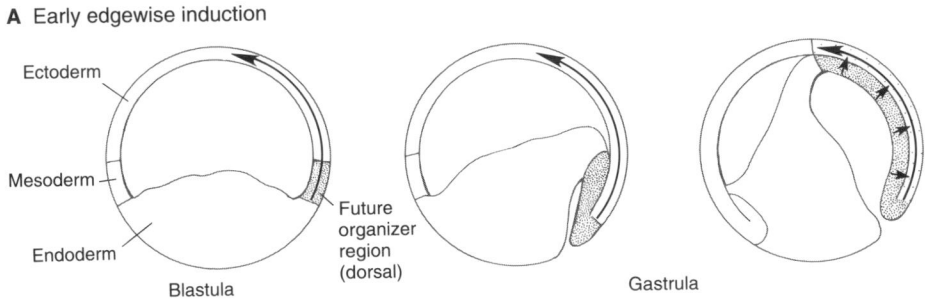

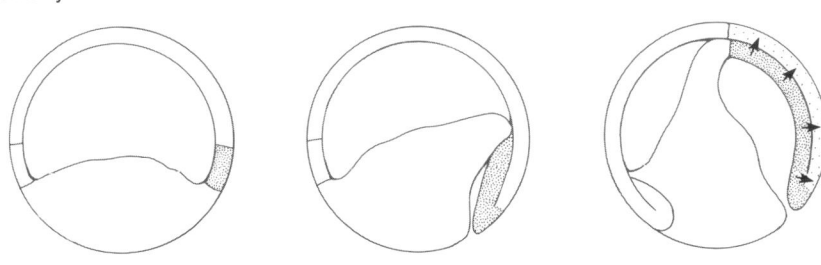

FIGURE 57-6

Two different models for the source of signals required for induction of neural ectoderm. (Adapted from Kintner and Dixon, 1989.)

A. The "organizer" region (dorsal lip of the blastopore) is the source of early inductive signals, which spread in an edgewise manner through the ectoderm. After involution, the dorsal mesoderm may provide (**hatched area**) additional inducing signals.

B. The major source of signals responsible for neural induction comes from the dorsal mesoderm after it has involuted. The induced neural plate is shown as the **stippled** area of ectoderm.

blastopore does begin to induce neural ectoderm before involution of the mesoderm, supporting Spemann's original suggestion. Neural induction may therefore occur in two steps. There may be partial induction of neural ectoderm before gastrulation movements begin. This initial signal may then be reinforced by signals from the mesoderm after it has extended under the ectoderm (Figure 57–6).

The molecular signals responsible for the initial differentiation of the neural plate are not known. However, several genes expressed by the neural ectoderm soon after its induction have been identified. Some of these genes encode cell-surface molecules such as the neural cell adhesion molecule NCAM and N-cadherin, both of which we shall consider in detail in Chapter 58. These adhesion molecules may play a role in organizing neural tissue as it begins to differentiate. Other genes expressed soon after neural induction encode DNA binding proteins that are similar in structure to proteins involved in pattern formation in early *Drosophila* embryos. Many of these proteins contain a conserved 60 amino acid sequence termed a "homeobox" (named because mutations in many of these genes cause *homeotic transformations*, the formation of a body part with characteristics normally found in a related part at another site in the body). This conserved region of the protein is directly involved in binding to DNA. As in

the case of *Drosophila* there is increasing evidence that homeobox genes have important roles in establishing regional differences early in the development of the vertebrate nervous system. Moreover, there are striking parallels in the structure, pattern of expression, and chromosomal organization of homeobox genes in *Drosophila* and vertebrates, suggesting that these genes have roles in organizing the body plan of highly divergent species (see Box 57–1).

Although these genes do not appear to be involved in the initial events of neural induction, their identification has permitted the design of quantitative and selective assays that will help to identify the signals responsible for neural induction (Figure 57–8). Attempts to characterize these signaling molecules have been further stimulated by the identification of molecules that mediate induction of the mesoderm. In early amphibian embryos the mesoderm that induces neural tissue is itself induced by endodermal cells located at the vegetal pole of the embryo. Mesoderm inducing factors belong to two large families of peptides originally identified as growth factors acting on mammalian cells: the fibroblast growth factor (FGF) and transforming growth factor β (TGFβ) families. The addition of FGF- and TGFβ-related molecules, in particular a TGFβ-like molecule called *activin*, to early amphibian ectoderm causes a potent induction of mesoderm, and suggests that

Genetic Control of the Body Plan During Development

BOX 57–1

Studies of early development in *Drosophila* have provided important insights into the mechanisms underlying the development of body form. In the early 1980s Christiane Nüsslein-Volhard and Eric Weischaus performed the first systematic screen for genes that affect the body pattern in the *Drosophila* embryo. They, and subsequently other groups, have identified dozens of genes that contribute to the establishment of the body plan. These genes can be ordered into a hierarchical series that control the organization of individual regions of the embryo in progressively finer detail.

Molecular cloning of these genes has revealed that many of them, particularly those expressed early in development of the *Drosophila* embryo, encode nuclear proteins that bind to DNA and activate the transcription of downstream genes, many of which are also transcriptional regulatory factors. Several of these *Drosophila* regulatory proteins contain a 60 amino acid sequence termed a *homeobox* domain.

This protein domain forms three alpha-helical regions, one of which is involved in binding to specific DNA target sequences. Other transcriptional regulatory proteins involved in the establishment of the *Drosophila* body plan contain different structural motifs. For example, proteins with zinc finger domains have peptide loops that are stabilized by the formation of complexes with heavy metal ions. These proteins also interact directly with target sequences in DNA (see Box 12–1).

In *Drosophila* many of the homeobox-containing proteins are clustered together in the genome, and the domains of expression of these genes in the developing embryo correspond to the linear arrangement of these genes on the chromosome. Several structurally related homeobox-containing genes have been identified in mammals. There is a remarkable conservation not only in the structure of these genes but also in the overall order and alignment of related genes in the *Drosophila* and mouse genome.

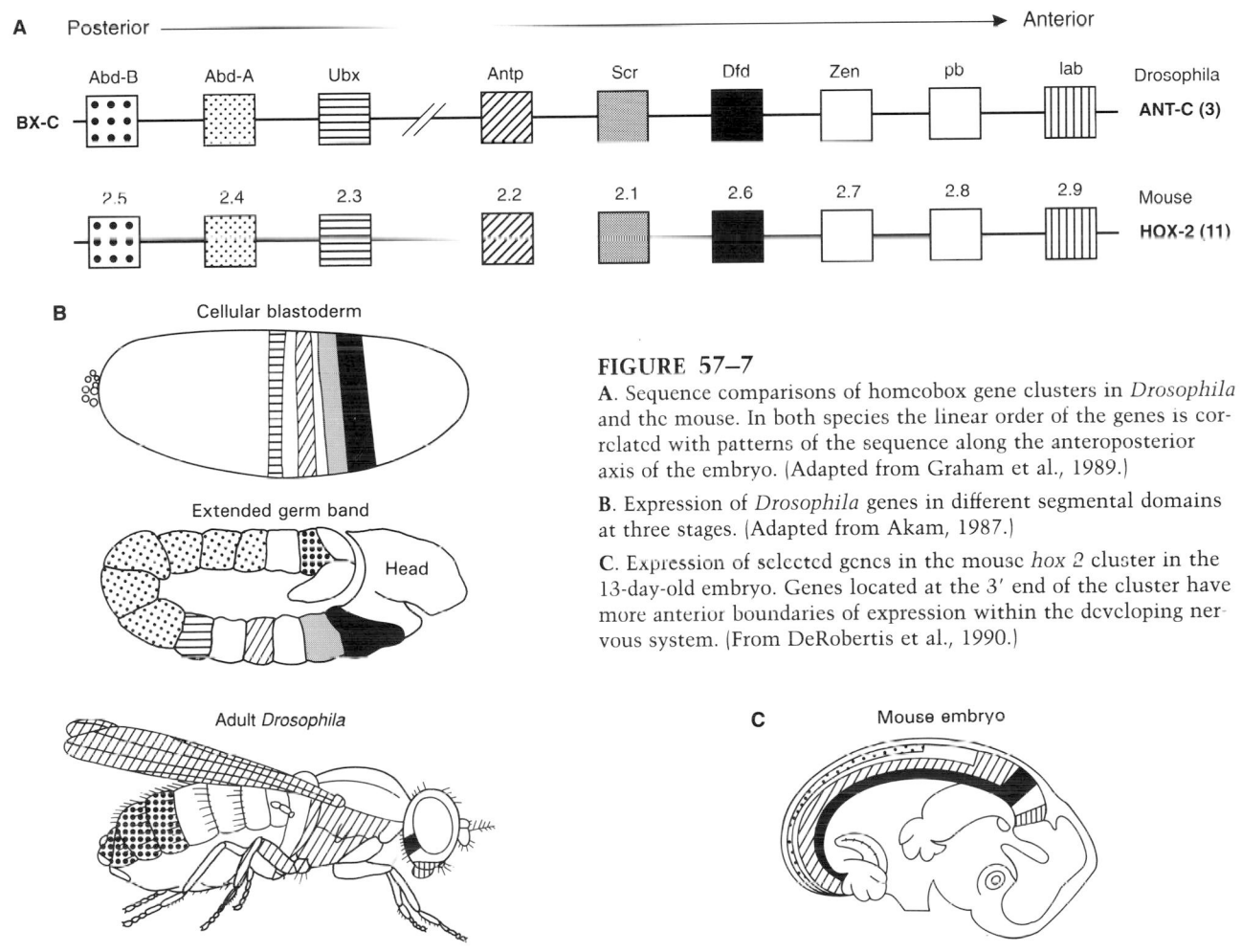

FIGURE 57–7

A. Sequence comparisons of homeobox gene clusters in *Drosophila* and the mouse. In both species the linear order of the genes is correlated with patterns of the sequence along the anteroposterior axis of the embryo. (Adapted from Graham et al., 1989.)

B. Expression of *Drosophila* genes in different segmental domains at three stages. (Adapted from Akam, 1987.)

C. Expression of selected genes in the mouse *hox 2* cluster in the 13-day-old embryo. Genes located at the 3' end of the cluster have more anterior boundaries of expression within the developing nervous system. (From DeRobertis et al., 1990.)

A

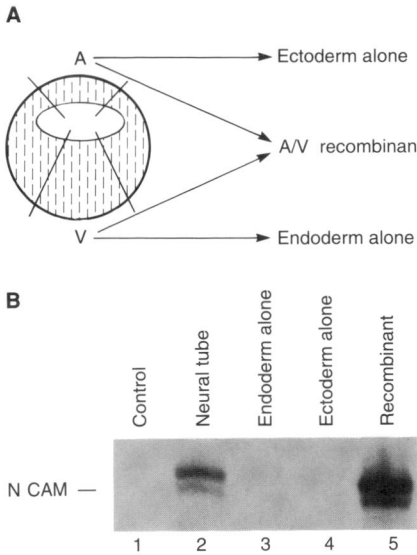

A ──────→ Ectoderm alone

A/V recombinant

V ──────→ Endoderm alone

B

N CAM —

Control / Neural tube / Endoderm alone / Ectoderm alone / Recombinant

1   2   3   4   5

FIGURE 57–8

Design of a quantitative assay to measure neural induction in frog (*Xenopus*) embryos.

A. Ectoderm can be removed from the animal pole and endoderm from the vegetal pole of the pregastrula *Xenopus* embryo. These tissue pieces can be maintained *in vitro* in isolation or in combination.

B. The neural cell adhesion molecule NCAM serves as a selective and sensitive marker for neural induction. The levels of NCAM mRNA can be measured autoradiographically using an RNAse protection assay. The intensity of the autoradiographic band indicates the level of mRNA. **Lane 1.** In the absence of added tissue (control) there is no detectable NCAM mRNA. **Lane 2.** The neural tube dissected from a neurula stage embryo expresses high levels of NCAM mRNA. **Lanes 3** and **4.** Ectoderm and endoderm tissue pieces maintained alone *in vitro* do not express NCAM mRNA. **Lane 5.** When ectoderm and endoderm are combined *in vitro*, high levels of NCAM mRNA are induced. The first step in this process is the induction of mesoderm. The mesoderm then acts on the remaining ectoderm to trigger the formation of neural ectoderm expressing NCAM. (From Kintner and Melton, 1987.)

neural induction may be triggered by similar types of molecules.

Regional Differentiation Within the Neural Plate Is Also Controlled by the Mesoderm

If neural induction is triggered by signals from the mesoderm, how can one explain the regional differentiation of the neural plate, which leads to the formation of structures as distinct as the forebrain, hindbrain, and spinal cord? Studies by Otto Mangold in 1933 demonstrated that the regional specificity of neural differentiation is influenced by the underlying mesoderm. Mangold removed axial mesoderm from different anteroposterior regions of amphibian embryos that had just completed gastrulation, and transplanted them individually into the ventral region of early gastrulae. The most anterior mesoderm induced

neural ectodermal structures with anterior character, such as eyes and brain vesicles, whereas mesoderm from more posterior regions induced neural structures with posterior character, such as hind brain and spinal cord (Figure 57–9). These findings suggest that the regional character of the neural ectoderm is dependent, at least in part, on regional differences in the properties of the underlying mesoderm. However, as discussed earlier, the differentiation of neural ectoderm into anterior or posterior structures may also be controlled by signals that spread anteriorly through the neural ectoderm from the blastopore lip.

Although the molecular basis of the regional differences along the anteroposterior axis of the mesoderm and neural plate is not known, several genes have been identified whose expression is restricted to specific regions along the anteroposterior axis of the mesoderm and neural ectoderm. Almost all these genes were isolated on the basis of their structural relationship to genes involved in organizing the segmental pattern of *Drosophila* embryos (see Box 57–1). In the frog one such gene, called *Xhox-3* (Xenopus homeobox), is expressed in a posterior-to-anterior gradient in the axial mesoderm. When this gradient is abolished by injecting *Xhox-3* RNA transcripts into an early frog embryo, resulting in uniformly high levels of Xhox-3 protein, anterior structures fail to develop and a headless embryo forms. Thus, the graded distribution of *Xhox-3* may be important in the patterning of mesoderm and, indirectly, of the neural ectoderm.

The differentiation of individual classes of neural cells along the dorsoventral axis of the neural tube also appears to be initiated by the mesoderm. Experiments in chick embryos show that the dorsoventral pattern of neural cell differentiation is regulated by signals derived from axial mesodermal cells of the notochord. The notochord induces a specialized group of cells at the ventral midline of the neural tube called the *floor plate*. Grafting an additional notochord or floor plate to ectopic positions adjacent to the neural tube induces new motor neurons. Inversely, removing the notochord and floor plate prevents the differentiation of motor neurons and other classes of neurons in the ventral region of the central nervous system. Thus, as in many other developing tissues, the pattern of cell differentiation in the neural tube appears to depend on the organizing properties of specialized cell groups—in this case the notochord and floor plate.

Studies of Invertebrate Embryos Have Identified Genes that Control the Fate of Ectodermal Cells

The principle first described by Spemann and Mangold that the nervous system arises by inducing a change in fate of ectodermal cells is also encountered in studies of neurogenesis in invertebrates such as *Drosophila*. Here we have been able to obtain information about the molecules that regulate the differentiation of ectodermal cells into either neural or epidermal cells. As in vertebrate embryos, a restricted region of the *Drosophila* ectoderm gives rise to neuronal precursor cells. This region of the ectoderm lies

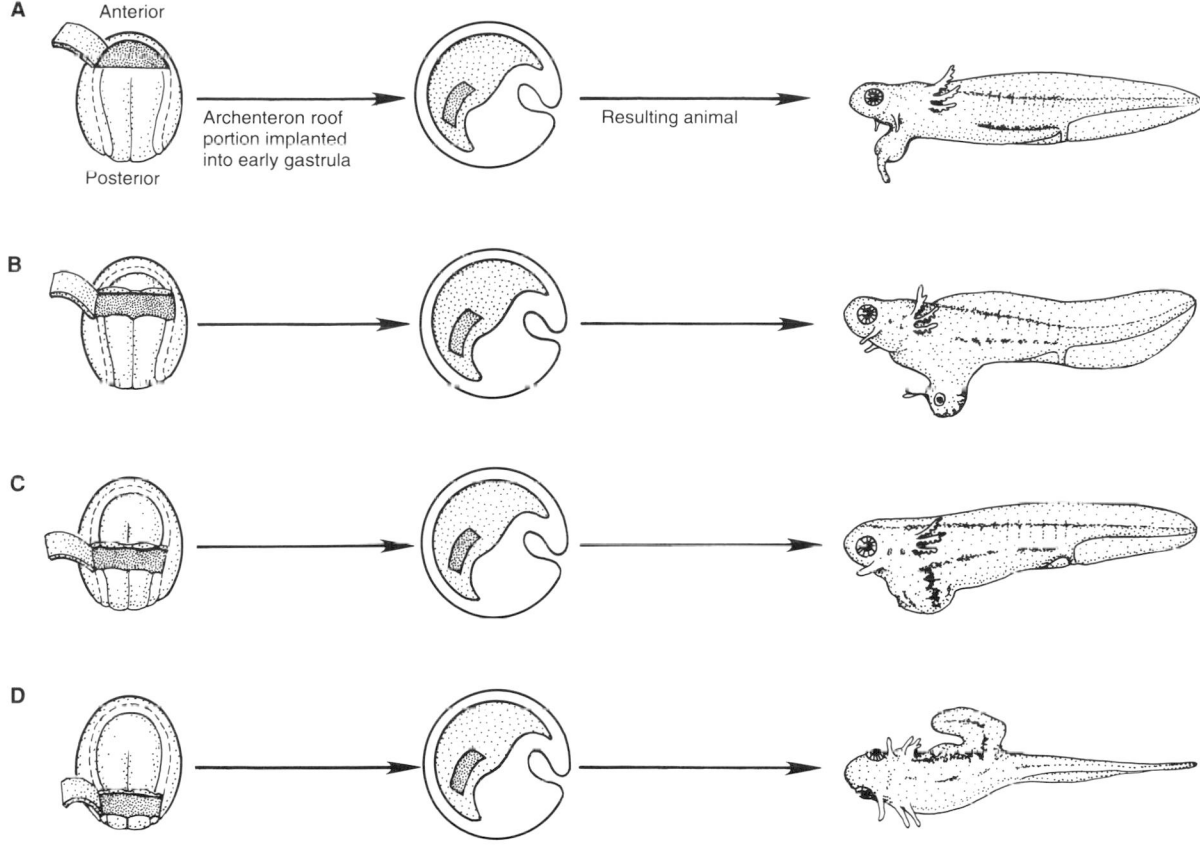

FIGURE 57–9

Dorsal mesoderm can control the regional differentiation of neural ectoderm along the anterior–posterior axis of the embryo. Implanting different regions of the mesoderm of an early newt embryo into the blastocoel cavity gives rise to secondary structures, the anterior–posterior character of which depends on the level from which the mesoderm was obtained. (Adapted from Mangold, 1933.)

A. A secondary head appears at an anterior position.

B. A secondary head with eyes and forebrain is formed.

C. The posterior part of a secondary head is induced.

D. A trunk–tail segment is induced in a posterior position.

alongside the ventral midline of the embryo and is termed the *neurogenic region*. About 25% of all cells in the neurogenic region become neuroblasts, and the remainder give rise to the ventral epidermis.

Cellular studies performed on the neurogenic region of the grasshopper, an arthropod related to *Drosophila*, have provided support for the involvement of local cell interactions in the control of neural cell fate. Christopher Doe and Corey Goodman found that neuroblasts arise from single cells that emerge from a local region of the ectodermal layer. All of the cells in the area immediately surrounding the newly formed neuroblast remain within the ectoderm and differentiate into epidermal cells. However, if the emerging neuroblast is killed by laser ablation one of the surrounding cells becomes a neuroblast and exhibits the full developmental potential of the original cell (Figure 57–10). This suggests that the newly emerged neuroblast transmits a signal to surrounding ectodermal cells that inhibits their differentiation along a neural pathway.

Genes that regulate the neural or epidermal fate of these ectodermal cells in *Drosophila* embryos have been identified by defining mutations that cause virtually all cells to progress along a neural pathway at the expense of the epidermal cells. The genes that affect the decision to differentiate along a neural or ectodermal pathway are called neurogenic genes, and the structure of several of these genes is known. Two of them, named *notch* and *delta*, have been shown by Spiros Artavanis-Tsakonas, Michael Young, Jose Campos-Ortega, and their colleagues to encode membrane-spanning proteins that have domains similar to those of the vertebrate epidermal growth factor receptor and the *lin-12* gene of *C. elegans* that we discussed earlier (Figure 57–10). These two genes may be involved in transmitting or receiving local signals that control cell fate in this region of the ectoderm.

Comparison of the initial steps of insect and vertebrate neural development has thus revealed that there are parallels in underlying strategies. First, local cell signaling

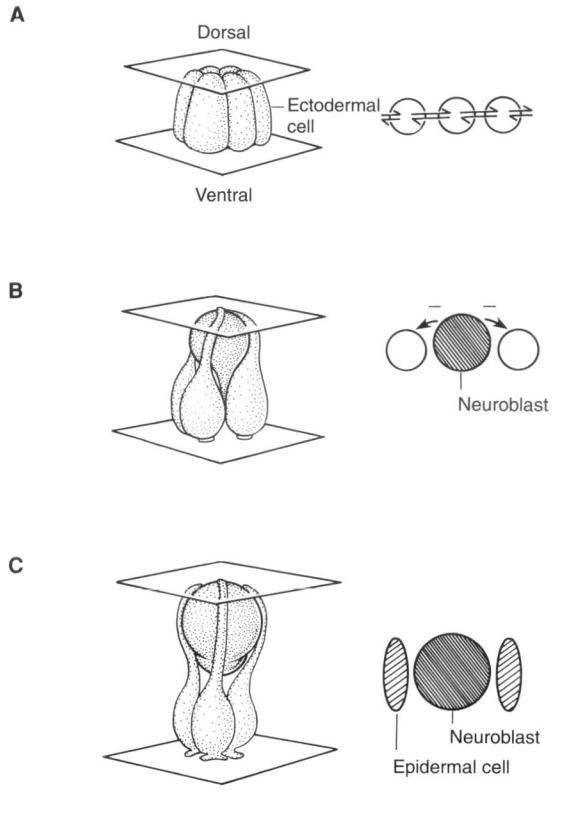

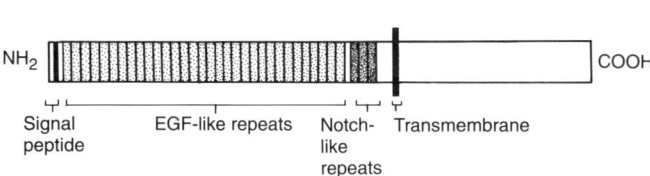

FIGURE 57–10

Local cell interactions control the differentiation of neuroblasts and epidermal cells in the neurogenic region of the grasshopper embryo. (Adapted from Doe et al., 1985.)

A. Initially, all ectodermal cells in the neurogenic region are equivalent and in contact with each other (**half-arrows**).

B. One ectodermal cell begins to differentiate into a neuroblast. The cytoplasm and nucleus of this cell shift dorsally and delaminate from the ventral surface of the embryo. The onset of differentiation of the neuroblast inhibits the adjacent cells from becoming neuroblasts (**arrows**). Neurogenic genes, such as *notch* and *delta*, are involved in this process, although their precise function is not known.

C. The new neuroblast has delaminated from the ventral surface. Adjacent cells differentiate into support cells. If a neuroblast is ablated, the adjacent cells are released from inhibition and one will enlarge to replace it.

D. The structure of the *notch* gene product. This gene has been implicated in cell–cell interactions that influence the decision of a cell to become a neuroblast or an epidermal cell. Like the Lin-12 protein, the *notch* gene product is a transmembrane protein that has EGF-like repeats in its extracellular domain.

appears to be important in determining neural and epidermal cell fate. Second, growth factors and their receptors are important in mediating these intercellular signals. Although the principles appear similar, there may be important differences in detail. In vertebrates an inducing signal may be necessary to trigger differentiation of ectodermal cells along a neural pathway; in its absence, differentiation into epidermis occurs. In insects cell-cell interactions are required for ectodermal cells to progress along an epidermal pathway of differentiation. In the absence of such signals all ectodermal cells differentiate into neurons.

Diffusible Factors Control Glial Cell Differentiation in the Central Nervous System

Once a cell becomes committed to a program of neural rather than epidermal differentiation, it has two basic choices: to become a neuron, or one of several different classes of supporting glial cell. Glial cell differentiation in the rat optic nerve is one of the better understood examples of cell interactions that define cell type in the vertebrate nervous system. As with mesodermal and perhaps neural induction, growth factors appear to play a crucial role in the diversification of glial cells in the rat optic nerve. There are three distinct classes of glial cells in cultures of optic nerve: oligodendrocytes and two types of astrocytes, termed type 1 and type 2 astrocytes. Each class of glial cell can be distinguished by its expression of specific intracellular and surface antigens. Because optic nerve cultures are relatively simple, for example, they do not contain neurons, the lineage and cellular interactions that control glial cell diversification can be readily analyzed. Oligodendrocytes (O) and type 2 astrocytes (2A) differentiate postnatally from a common precursor called the O-2A progenitor cell. Oligodendrocytes appear in the optic nerve soon after birth, whereas type 2 astrocytes do not appear for at least another week. Type 1 astrocytes differentiate during embryonic development from a distinct precursor cell.

Martin Raff and his colleagues have examined the cellular interactions that control the proliferation and pathway of differentiation of O-2A progenitor cells in culture. They found that the fate of O-2A progenitor cells is controlled by signals from type 1 astrocytes. When O-2A progenitor cells are cultured in the absence of type 1 astrocytes, they stop dividing and differentiate almost immediately; when grown in the presence of type 1 astrocytes, they continue to proliferate. Thus type 1 astrocytes secrete a mitogenic signal required for the proliferation of O-2A cells. One factor responsible for maintaining O-2A cell proliferation has been identified as *platelet-derived growth factor* (PDGF). After a set period of time and number of cell divisions, however, O-2A progenitor cells lose the ability to respond to PDGF and differentiate into either oligodendrocytes or type 2 astrocytes.

The decision to differentiate into type 2 astrocytes or oligodendrocytes is also regulated by type 1 astrocytes. When O-2A precursor cells are cultured alone in serum-free medium, they invariably differentiate into oligodendrocytes. However, optic nerve extracts or proteins

A

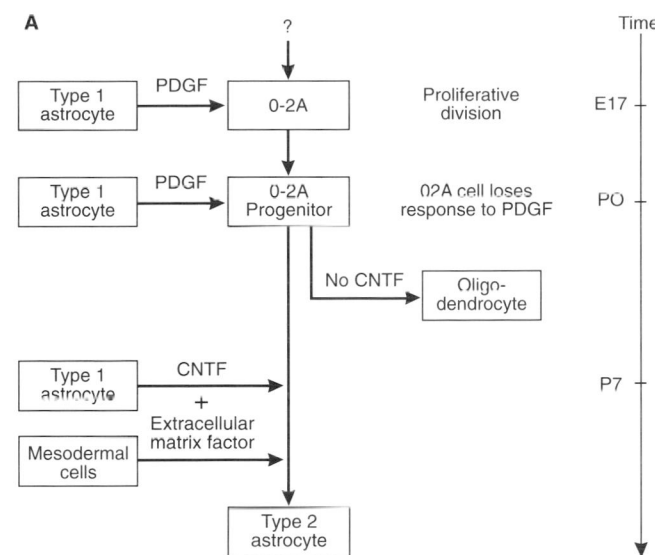

FIGURE 57–11
Growth factors control glial cell diversification in the rat optic nerve.

A. During embryogenesis platelet derived growth factor (PDGF) secreted by type 1 astrocytes maintains the proliferation of O-2A cells. Postnatally, O-2A cells begin to lose sensitivity to PDGF, even though it is still secreted by type 1 astrocytes, and cells begin to differentiate into oligodendrocytes. About 7 days after birth, type 1 astrocytes begin to secrete a CNTF-like molecule that promotes the differentiation of type 2 astrocytes from O-2A progenitors. The complete differentiation of type 2 astrocytes requires an unidentified factor that is associated with the extracellular matrix of mesodermal cells. (Adapted from Lillien and Raff, 1990.)

B.-D. Micrographs show the appearance of cultured O-2A progenitor cells (**B**), type 2 astrocytes labeled with an antibody against glial-fibrillary acidic protein (**C**), and oligodendrocytes labeled with an antibody against galactocerebroside (**D**).

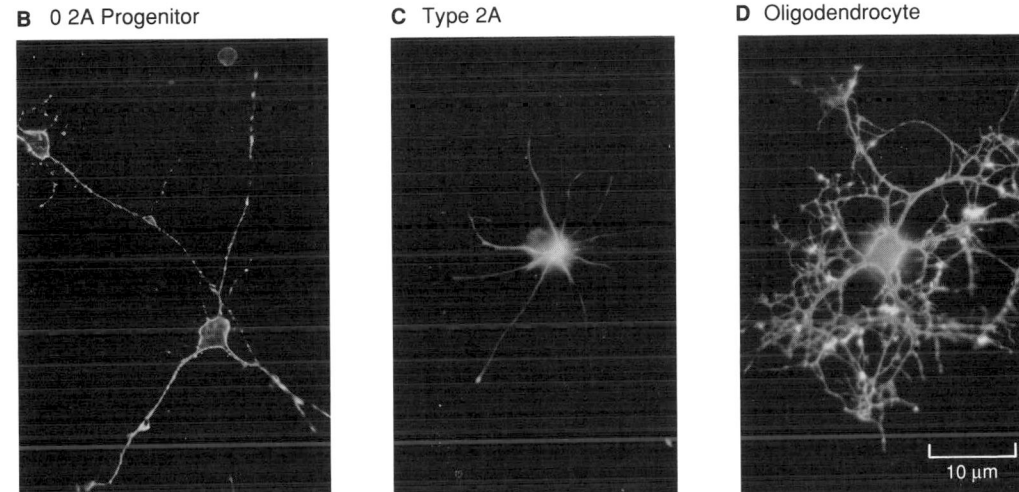

B 0 2A Progenitor   **C** Type 2A   **D** Oligodendrocyte

released by type 1 astrocytes induce the differentiation of O-2A progenitor cells into type 2 astrocytes. Raff and his colleagues have identified the protein that promotes type 2 astrocyte differentiation as *ciliary neurotrophic factor* (CNTF). Ciliary neurotrophic factor can initiate type 2 astrocyte differentiation but alone is insufficient to complete this process. Molecules that seem to be made by mesenchymal cells and are associated with the extracellular matrix collaborate with CNTF to complete type 2 astrocyte differentiation (Figure 57–11).

These findings suggest that the differentiation of astrocytes and oligodendrocytes in the developing central nervous system is controlled by local interactions between different classes of glial cells. In addition they illustrate how mechanisms that control the differentiation of specific cell types in the developing vertebrate nervous system can be defined in the absence of genetic tools. A crucial element in the success of this approach was the identification of cell specific markers, which permitted the lineage of each individual cell type to be defined and

the use of cell culture in which the developing system could be reconstituted and manipulated. As with all cell culture experiments, however, it will be important in the future to show that the same cellular and molecular mechanisms operate in the intact developing nervous system.

Cell Position Controls the Identity of Photoreceptors in the *Drosophila* Eye

The commitment of cells to a neural fate is followed by additional interactions that control the differentiation of these cells into specific classes of neurons. Some of the signals that control neuronal cell fate act over extremely short distances, influencing the decision of one cell but not its immediate neighbor. For example, studies of the compound eye of *Drosophila* by Seymour Benzer, Donald Ready, Andrew Tomlinson, Gerald Rubin, Lawrence Zipursky and their colleagues have provided evidence that the precise position a cell occupies in relation to its neighbors

A

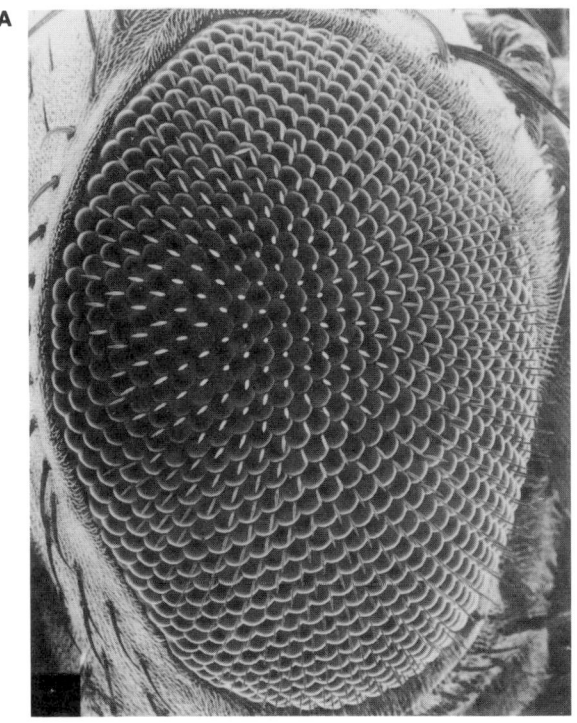

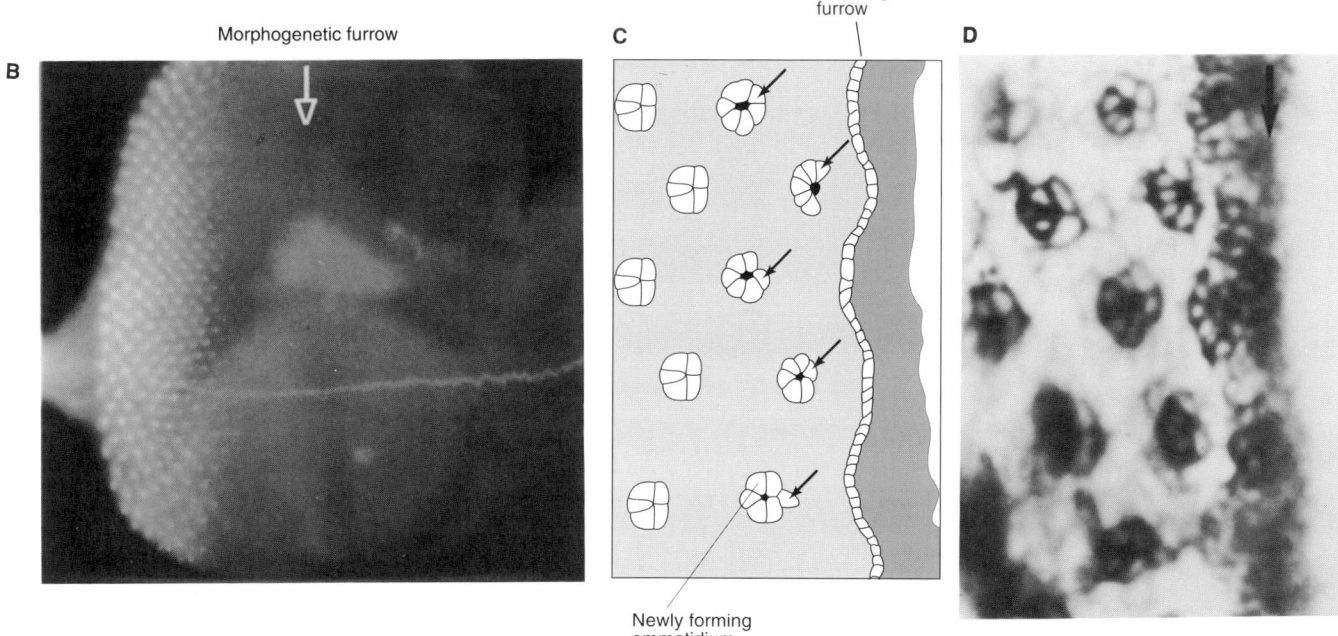

Morphogenetic furrow

B

C

Morphogenetic
furrow

D

Newly forming
ommatidium

FIGURE 57–12

Development of the compound eye in *Drosophila melanogaster*. (From Ready et al., 1976; Tomlinson, 1988; and Banerjee and Zipursky, 1990.)

A. A regular array of identical units (ommatidia) covers the surface of the adult eye. Each ommatidium consists of 20 cells.

B. During larval development a wave of cell division and cell rearrangement sweeps across the eye imaginal disc. This wave can be observed as a morphogenetic furrow (**arrow**), which represents the movement of cells in the epithelial sheet of the eye disc.

C. As the morphogenetic furrow passes across the eye disc, cells in the epithelial layer begin to form clusters in the wake of the furrow.

D. These clusters represent the beginning of each ommatidium and can be recognized by antibodies that label differentiating photoreceptor cells.

can have a critical role in determining the type of neuron it will become.

The compound eye consists of a highly ordered array of identical units called *ommatidia* (Figure 57–12). Each ommatidium consists of 20 cells, of which eight are specialized photoreceptor neurons. These photoreceptors, called R1-R8, can be classified into three distinct groups on the basis of the opsin pigments that they express and the projection pattern of their axons. Photoreceptors R1-R6 express a common opsin, which responds to light with

wavelength in the visible range. R8 expresses a distinct visible wavelength opsin and R7 an opsin that is activated by ultraviolet light.

How do each of these photoreceptor neurons acquire their unique differentiated characteristics? At first it was thought that the orderly and progressive assembly of each ommatidium must be controlled by cell lineage. However, it is now clear that the identity of developing photoreceptors results from local cell signaling.

The molecular analysis of this problem has focused pri-

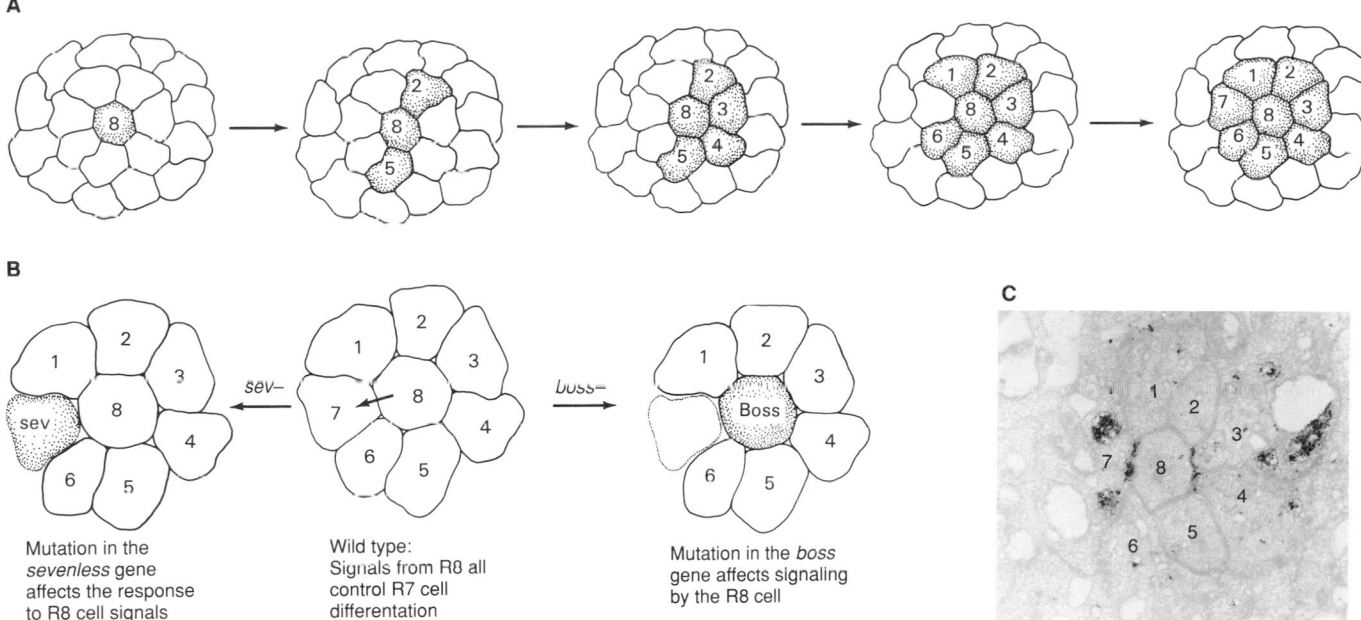

FIGURE 57–13

Differentiation of photoreceptor cells in *Drosophila*.

A. The first photoreceptor cell to express neuron-specific antigens is R8. This is followed by the simultaneous differentiation of cells R2 and R5. Shortly after, R3 and R4 begin to differentiate, followed by R1 and R6. The final cell to be added to the developing cluster is R7. (Adapted from Banerjee and Zipursky, 1990.)

B. Development of the R7 cell depends on local cell interactions, which are controlled by at least two genes: the *sevenless* gene in the R7 cell and the *boss* gene in the R8 cell. Mutations

in the *sevenless* gene block the ability of the prospective R7 cell to respond to signals from the R8 photoreceptor. The *boss* gene product may be a ligand for the Sevenless protein or may be required in the R8 cell for expression of the *sevenless* ligand. (Based on Banerjee and Zipursky, 1990; Tomlinson, 1988.)

C. Immunocytochemical localization of the Sevenless protein at the junction of the R7 and R8 cells. Even though the Sevenless protein is expressed in other photoreceptor types, only R7 depends on this gene for its development. (Provided by A. Tomlinson.)

---

marily on the last photoreceptor to develop, the R7 cell, which is responsible for the response of the fly to ultraviolet light. Genes involved in R7 cell development or physiology can be identified by screening for mutations that abolish the ability of the fly to move toward an ultraviolet light source. The first series of screens for mutants that cannot undergo phototaxis in response to ultraviolet light was carried out by William Harris and Seymour Benzer and generated one mutation (called *sevenless*) in which the R7 photoreceptor was missing, even though the other photoreceptors were normal. Detailed studies of the assembly of the ommatidium by Andrew Tomlinson and Donald Ready showed that mutation of the *sevenless* gene causes the cell destined to become the R7 photoreceptor to give rise instead to a supporting cell.

These findings suggested that the *sevenless* mutant defines a gene involved in the cellular signaling required for the differentiation of the R7 photoreceptor. By using X-rays to induce mitotic recombinations that result in small clones of genetically marked cells carrying the *sevenless* mutation, Benzer and his colleagues established that the function of this gene is required in the prospective R7 cell itself, and not the neighboring cells. These studies suggested that the *sevenless* gene is a receptor for a signal

transmitted by neighboring photoreceptor cells (Figure 57–13). Gerald Rubin and his colleagues, and independently Seymour Benzer and his colleagues, cloned the *sevenless* gene and found that the encoded protein spans the plasma membrane, has a large extracellular domain and an intracellular domain that functions as a tyrosine kinase. This structure is consistent with the idea that the Sevenless protein functions as a receptor for a localized inducing signal. The kinase function of the cytoplasmic domains is critical for signal transduction since mutations that destroy tyrosine kinase activity abolish the ability of the Sevenless protein to promote the differentiation of the R7 photoreceptor.

Once the receptor function of the Sevenless protein was established, it became important to know which cells send the signal that induces R7 differentiation. Lawrence Zipursky and colleagues, using genetic screens similar to those that identified the *sevenless* gene, identified another gene which, when mutated, leads to the loss of the R7 photoreceptor. However, in contrast to *sevenless*, this new gene, named *boss* (bride of sevenless), is required solely in the R8 photoreceptor. Since the phenotype of these two mutations is identical, it is probable that the R8 cell is involved in transmitting the signal necessary for

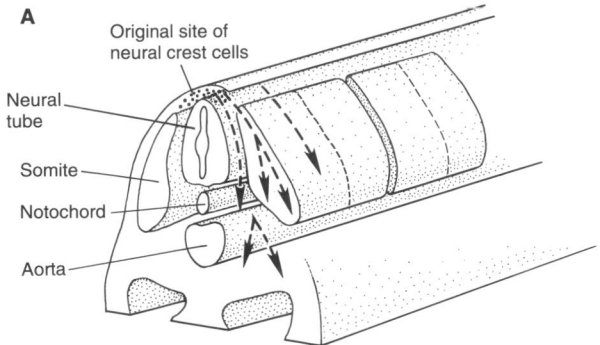

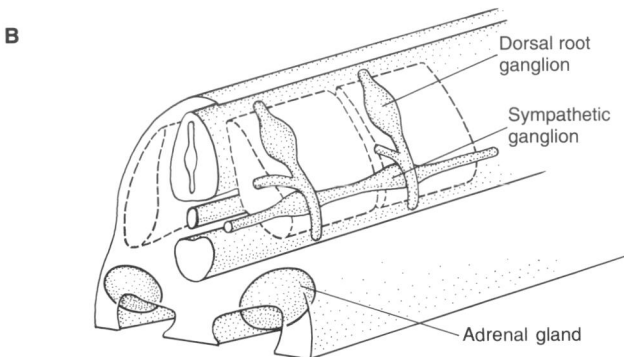

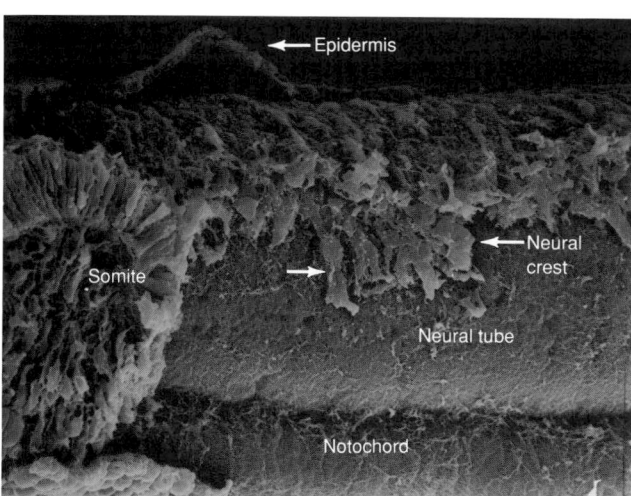

FIGURE 57–14

The main pathways of neural crest cell migration in a chick embryo. The diagram shows a cross section through the middle part of the trunk.

A. The cells that take the superficial pathway, just beneath the ectoderm, will form pigment cells of the skin. Those that take the deep pathway via the somites will form sensory ganglia, sympathetic ganglia, and parts of the adrenal gland.

B. The positions at which sympathetic and sensory ganglia are located after neural crest migration is complete.

C. Scanning electron micrograph showing neural crest cells migrating away from the dorsal surface of the neural tube of a chick embryo. (Provided by K. Tosney.)

differentiation of the R7 cell (Figure 57–13). This is consistent with the fact that the R8 cell touches the R7 cell at the time that the latter's fate is determined. The *boss* gene encodes a membrane protein with a large extracellular domain. This protein appears to act directly as the ligand for the *sevenless* receptor.

The genetic analysis of the development of the R7 photoreceptor provides a clear example of the way in which cell-specific inductive interactions can determine the identity of individual neurons. Together with studies of the neurogenic genes in *Drosophila* and of peptide growth factors in vertebrate embryos, these findings illustrate the importance of cell surface and diffusible molecules as signals in the determination of neural cell identity.

The Fate of Neural Crest Cells Is Controlled by the Local Environment

The evidence emerging from studies of *Drosophila* and vertebrate development, that the fate of neural cells is influenced by signals from neighboring cells and not by cell lineage, can be tested by changing the position of a cell in relationship to its neighbors. This is difficult to achieve with most vertebrate and invertebrate neural cells, because their entire program of differentiation occurs within a densely packed and relatively inaccessible environment in which undifferentiated precursor cells are intermingled with newly differentiated neurons and glial cells. However, one vertebrate system, the *neural crest*, has permitted comparison of the normal fate and developmental potential of neural precursor cells when moved to new positions in the embryo.

The neural crest is a transient and migratory group of cells that emerge from the dorsal region of the neural tube and rapidly disperse along different pathways (Figure 57–14). Their migration terminates at many peripheral locations, where they coalesce to form the neurons and Schwann cells of the sensory and autonomic nervous systems, the chromaffin cells of the adrenal medulla, the melanocytes of the skin, and mesenchymal tissues of the face and skull (Figure 57–15).

A major advance in analyzing the migration and fate of neural crest cells was introduced by Nicole Le Douarin in the late 1960s. Le Douarin made use of the difference in appearance of chromatin within the nuclei of chick and quail cells. In chick cells chromatin is diffusely distributed, whereas in quail cells it is tightly packed. Thus, it is possible to graft quail tissue into chick embryos and follow the fate of the grafted quail cells with a simple histological stain.

The extensive migration of neural crest cells has made it possible to follow the fate of neural crest cells located at different points along the neuraxis. These fate maps reveal that distinct cell types, for example neurons, melanocytes, and Schwann cells, derive from neural crest cells that occupy the same position along the neuraxis. Some neural crest descendants, for example the neurons in the enteric nervous system, originate from a restricted region of the neuraxis.

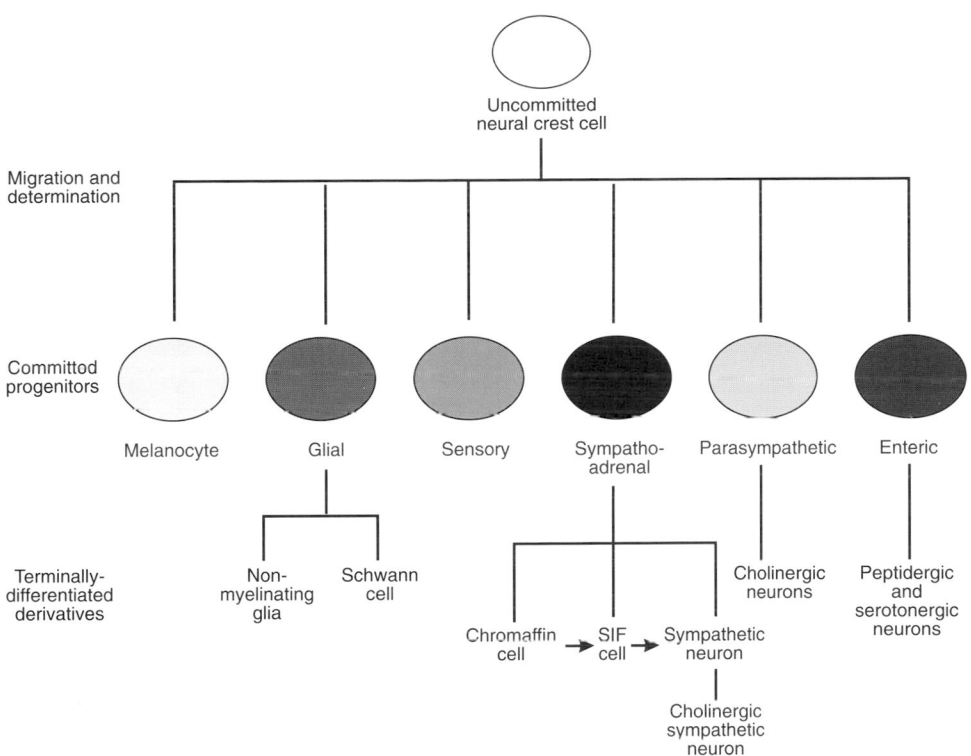

FIGURE 57–15
The different classes of committed progenitor cells that may derive from the earliest neural crest cells. No order of appearance is implied and the variety of differentiated cell types is not complete. (Adapted from Anderson, 1989.)

To test whether the number of distinct cell types a neural crest cell can give rise to is greater than the number actually observed in the embryo, Le Douarin and her colleagues, James Weston and others grafted neural crest cells into ectopic positions along the neuraxis. These experiments revealed that most neural crest cells can give rise to a far wider range of cell types than they do normally. Changing the position of neural crest cells may lead to the selection of different subpopulations of committed precursors. Alternatively, the different migratory paths taken by neural crest cells may control the fate of uncommitted precursors.

There is now considerable evidence that early neural crest cells have the potential to differentiate into a wide variety of cell types, and that the developmental fate of a cell is critically dependent on the signals it receives from the environment through which it migrates. The restriction in cell fate appears to occur during the process of cell migration. Transplantation of cells from newly formed sensory or autonomic ganglia back into the neural crest of younger host embryos has shown that by the time cells are located in sensory and autonomic ganglia their fate is in part restricted. The developmental options of neural crest cells therefore appear to be gradually restricted by changes in cellular environment as they migrate in the periphery.

The multipotentiality of many neural crest cells prior to migration has been confirmed by examining the range of cell types that derive from a single neural crest cell *in vitro*. In some experiments clones of up to 20,000 cells have been generated, with each clone producing a highly diverse array of differentiated cell types, including sensory neurons, melanocytes, and Schwann cells. Intracellular

injection of fluorescent tracers into neural crest cells *in vivo* has also revealed that single neural crest cells can give rise to many distinct cell types.

Some of the molecules that control the fate of a neural crest cell have been identified in the sublineage that gives rise to the sympathetic nervous system and adrenal medulla (the sympatho-adrenal lineage). This lineage comprises the major catecholaminergic descendants of the neural crest: sympathetic neurons, chromaffin cells, and cells in the sympathetic ganglia defined on the basis of intense catecholamine histofluorescence, called *small intensely fluorescent cells* (SIF). Precursors to these distinct cell classes can be isolated from the embryonic adrenal medulla or sympathetic ganglia. When grown in culture, it is possible to control the fate of these progenitor cells by varying the culture conditions (Figure 57–16).

The differentiation of adrenal progenitor cells into chromaffin cells is dependent on the presence of glucocorticoid hormones. Differentiation of chromaffin cells from neural crest precursors is probably triggered by the migration of these cells into the adrenal gland and are exposed to the high levels of glucocorticoids synthesized by the adrenal cortex. Glucocorticoids activate nuclear receptors that function directly as transcriptional regulatory proteins. Neural crest cells that form sympathetic ganglia follow one of two fates: They can become SIF cells or sympathetic neurons. As with chromaffin cells, the decision to become an SIF cell may also be dependent on glucocorticoids in the blood supply, since *in vitro* low concentrations of glucocorticoids promote the appearance of SIF cells.

The factors that promote the differentiation of neural

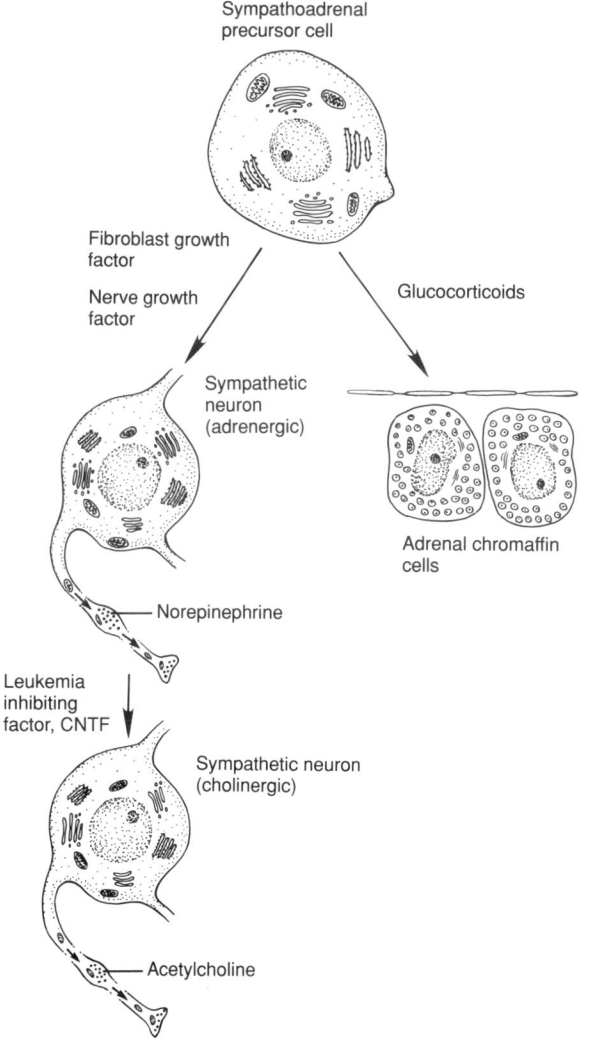

Sympathoadrenal
precursor cell

Fibroblast growth
factor

Nerve growth
factor

Glucocorticoids

Sympathetic
neuron
(adrenergic)

Adrenal chromaffin
cells

Norepinephrine

Leukemia
inhibiting
factor, CNTF

Sympathetic neuron
(cholinergic)

Acetylcholine

FIGURE 57–16

Summary of the developmental potential of an undifferentiated precursor cell in the sympatho-adrenal lineage. Glucocorticoids cause the precursor cell to differentiate into chromaffin cells, which have large (150–350 nm) dense-core granules. Fibroblast growth factor and nerve growth factor induce precursor cells to differentiate into sympathetic neurons, which possess 50 nm electron-dense vesicles and synthesize norepinephrine as transmitter. If these neurons are cultured in the presence of conditioned medium containing leukemia inhibiting factor, they acquire cholinergic properties, synthesize acetylcholine, and contain small (30–50 nm) electron-translucent vesicles. (Adapted from Doupe et al., 1985.)

crest precursors into neurons are less well established. However, fibroblast growth factor (FGF) has been shown to promote the differentiation of chromaffin cells into neurons. As discussed earlier in the chapter, FGF also induces the differentiation of mesoderm. Thus a single growth factor may have several roles in neural development, acting on distinct classes of neural cells at different

times. As neural crest cells begin to differentiate into sympathetic neurons they gradually lose sensitivity to glucocorticoids and acquire dependence on nerve growth factor for survival. Thus the responsiveness of developing nerve cells to environmental signals changes as they differentiate.

The Transmitter Choice of Peripheral Neurons Is Controlled by Signals from Neighboring Cells

We have discussed how a programmed cell lineage and signals from neighboring cells can generate the diverse neuronal and glial cell types found in the nervous system. However, differentiation does not stop when cells leave the cell cycle and adopt a neuronal or a glial fate. For a mature neuron to function as part of a neuronal circuit it must go on to express many highly specialized properties, including the transmitters that mediate chemical signaling with other neurons and the transmitter receptors that permit the cell to respond to incoming synaptic inputs. In vertebrate peripheral neurons the choice of transmitter is acquired at a comparatively late stage of neuronal development and can be modified by changing the environment of the neuron.

Paul Patterson, Story Landis, and their colleagues have studied the regulation of transmitter choice of neural crest descendants in the autonomic nervous system. Most sympathetic neurons in the autonomic nervous system use norepinephrine as their primary transmitter. However, one class of sympathetic neuron, which innervates the exocrine sweat glands in the foot pads, uses acetylcholine.

Studies by Landis and her colleagues have shown that newly differentiated sympathetic neurons that innervate sweat glands in the skin initially express many of the properties of adrenergic neurons. However, once the axons of these cells reach the sweat glands, these adrenergic properties disappear and are replaced by cholinergic properties. Landis and her colleagues demonstrated that the target sweat glands may be critical in inducing cholinergic properties in sympathetic neurons by transplanting the sweat glands from the foot pad of a newborn rat into a cutaneous site that normally is innervated by adrenergic sympathetic neurons. The sympathetic neurons that innervated the sweat glands acquired cholinergic transmitter properties. Thus, in at least one case the signal from the target can induce a change in the transmitter properties of developing sympathetic neurons.

Patterson and Linda Chun showed that when sympathetic neurons are grown *in vitro* in the absence of any other cell type, they express adrenergic transmitter properties. However, when grown in the presence of a variety of non-neuronal background cells, or in medium conditioned by these cells, these sympathetic neurons synthesize acetylcholine as their transmitter (Figure 57–17).

Edwin Furshpan, David Potter, and their colleagues also demonstrated the transition in transmitter choice by recording the response of cardiac muscle cells innervated by sympathetic neurons. Sympathetic neurons grown in

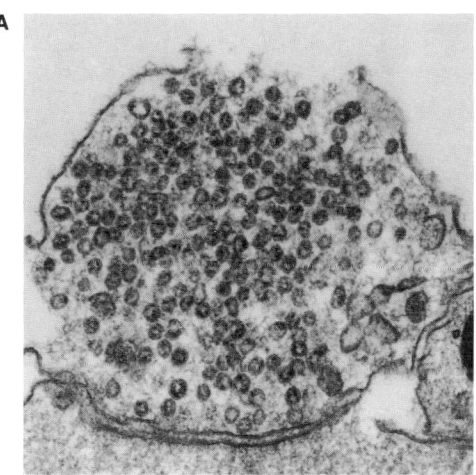

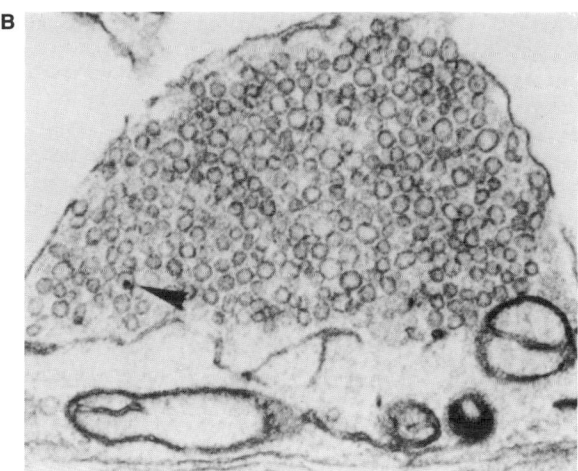

FIGURE 57–17

Morphology of synaptic vesicles in cultured sympathetic neurons grown in the absence or presence of cholinergic-inducing factor derived from heart cells. (Adapted from Landis, 1980.)

A. Sympathetic neuron grown under conditions in which adrenergic differentiation is maintained. An axonal varicosity forms a

synapse on an adjacent cell body. Most of the synaptic vesicles in this profile are dense-core vesicles. ×50,000.

B. Sympathetic neuron grown in culture in the presence of cholinergic-inducing factor. The terminal varicosity contains almost exclusively clear vesicles. ×38,000.

isolation release norepinephrine as their transmitter, which increases the rate of firing of cardiac muscle cells, whereas neurons grown in a medium conditioned by other cell types release acetylcholine, which decreases the rate of firing of the muscle cells. In physiological assays that tested the same neuron *in vitro* over a period of months Furshpan and Potter found that in the presence of conditioned medium a single neuron switches gradually from adrenergic to cholinergic properties, passing through a stage in which the neuron releases both norepinephrine and acetylcholine. Other properties of the sympathetic neuron are also changed. For example, in a conditioned medium that promotes cholinergic differentiation the neuron gradually changes its vesicle content from the large dense-core granules found in adrenergic neurons to the small electron-translucent vesicles typical of cholinergic neurons (Figure 57–17). These findings indicate that *in vitro*, and probably also *in vivo*, transmitter choice of sympathetic neurons is regulated by signals released from other cells in the environment.

Patterson and his colleagues have purified a glycoprotein of molecular weight 43,000 that is released by rat heart cells and promotes the cholinergic differentiation of sympathetic neurons. This factor is identical to leukemia inhibitory factor (LIF), a protein with actions in the immune system. CNTF, the molecule discussed above that promotes type 2 astrocyte differentiation, also promotes cholinergic differentiation in sympathetic neurons. These observations provide additional examples of growth and differentiation factors that exert quite distinct effects on different cell types in the developing embryo.

An Overall View

The early development of the nervous system is a continuation of cellular events initiated during gastrulation and involves a gradual restriction in the developmental potential of individual cells. In all developing nervous systems, cell differentiation depends on a series of signals that ultimately control the transcription of specific genes. When cells undergo cell-autonomous differentiation, these signals are initiated by inheritance of asymmetrically distributed cytoplasmic determinants and are perpetuated by an internal cascade of interactions between nuclear factors that regulate transcription. With cells whose fate is more plastic, the critical signals derive from the environment and they control indirectly the expression or activity of nuclear transcription factors. The relative contribution of these two basic programs of differentiation varies among species and between different types of cells in the same embryo. The development of the nematode *Caenorhabditis elegans* is based in part on autonomous cell development, whereas vertebrate embryos rely almost exclusively on local cell interactions to restrict developmental potential and to consolidate the differentiated properties of cells. Cell-to-cell interactions play a critical role in all stages of vertebrate neural development, from neural induction to the choice of neurotransmitter.

Some of the cellular and molecular mechanisms that underlie the cell autonomous and environmentally regulated programs have now been established. Not surprisingly, many of the genes that control the fate of invertebrate cells in a cell-autonomous manner are nuclear proteins that regulate the transcription of other genes. In contrast, local cell interactions in the nervous system, as in many nonneuronal tissues, involve diffusible signaling molecules and membrane receptors. Many of these signaling molecules are not restricted to the nervous system but have critical roles in the differentiation of other organs. Similarly, the receptors for these signaling molecules, for example transmembrane tyrosine kinases, are familiar proteins found in many different eukaryotic cell types. Thus, the molecules that control the differentiation and fate of cells in the nervous system are identical or closely related to the molecules that regulate other aspects of embryonic development. Insights into the early stages of neuronal development therefore continue to benefit from studies of the differentiation of other eukaryotic cells.

Once the identity of individual cells within the nervous system is established, axonal extension begins and complex but precise connections between these cells begin to form. How these neuronal circuits are established during development is discussed in the next chapter.

Selected Readings

Anderson, D. J. 1989. The neural crest cell lineage problem: Neuropoiesis? Neuron 3:1–12.

Doe, C. Q., Kuwada, J. Y., and Goodman, C. S. 1985. From epithelium to neuroblasts to neurons: The role of cell interactions and cell lineage during insect neurogenesis. Philos. Trans. R. Soc. Lond. [Biol.] 312:67–81.

Gilbert, S. F. 1991. Developmental Biology. 3rd ed. Sunderland, Mass.: Sinauer.

Greenwald, I. 1989. Cell-cell interactions that specify certain cell fates in C. elegans development. Trends Genet. 5:237–241.

Gurdon, J. B. 1987. Embryonic induction—molecular prospects. Development 99:285–306.

Hamburger, V. 1988. The Heritage of Experimental Embryology. Hans Spemann and the Organizer. New York: Oxford University Press.

Horvitz, H. R., Sternberg, P. W., Greenwald, I. S., Fixsen, W., and Ellis, H. M. 1983. Mutations that affect neural cell lineages and cell fates during the development of the nematode Caenorhabditis elegans. Cold Spring Harbor Symp. Quant. Biol. 48:453–463.

Jan, Y. N., and Jan, L. Y. 1990. Genes required for specifying cell fates in Drosophila embryonic sensory nervous system. Trends Neurosci. 13:493–498.

Le Douarin, N. M. 1986. Cell line segregation during peripheral nervous system ontogeny. Science 231:1515–1522.

Lillien, L. E., and Raff, M. C. 1990. Differentiation signals in the CNS: Type-2 astrocyte development in vitro as a model system. Neuron 5:111–119.

Rubin, G. M. 1989. Development of the Drosophila retina: Inductive events studied at single cell resolution. Cell 57:519–520.

Simpson, P. 1990. Notch and the choice of cell fate in Drosophila neuroepithelium. Trends Genet. 6:343–345.

Sternberg, P. W., and Horvitz, H. R. 1984. The genetic control of cell lineage during nematode development. Annu. Rev. Genet. 18:489–524.

Tomlinson, A. 1988. Cellular interactions in the developing Drosophila eye. Development 104:183–193.

References

Akam, M. 1987. The molecular basis for metameric pattern in the Drosophila embryo. Development 101:1–22.

Artavanis-Tsakonas, S. 1988. The molecular biology of the Notch locus and the fine tuning of differentiation in Drosophila. Trends Genet. 4:95–100.

Banerjee, U., and Zipursky, S. L. 1990. The role of cell-cell interaction in the development of the Drosophila visual system. Neuron 4:177–187.

Boveri, T. 1904. Ergebnisse über die Konstitution der chromatischen Substanz des Zellkerns. Jena: Fisher.

Brenner, S. 1974. The genetics of Caenorhabditis elegans. Genetics 77:71–94.

De Robertis, E. M., Oliver, G., and Wright, C. V. E. 1990. Homeobox genes and the vertebrate body plan. Sci. Am. 263 (1):46–52.

Desai, C., Garriga, G., McIntire, S. L., and Horvitz, H. R. 1988. A genetic pathway for the development of the Caenorhabditis elegans HSN motor neurons. Nature 336:638–646.

Dixon, J. E., and Kintner, C. R. 1989. Cellular contacts required for neural induction in Xenopus embryos: Evidence for two signals. Development 106:749–757.

Doupe, A. J., Landis, S. C., and Patterson, P. H. 1985. Environmental influences in the development of neural crest derivatives: Glucocorticoids, growth factors, and chromaffin cell plasticity. J. Neurosci. 5:2119–2142.

Furshpan, E. J., Potter, D. D., and Landis, S. C. 1982. On the transmitter repertoire of sympathetic neurons in culture. Harvey Lect. 76:149–191.

Graham, A., Papalopulu, N., and Krumlauf, R. 1989. The murine and Drosophila homeobox gene complexes have common features of organization and expression. Cell 57:367–378.

Greenwald, I. and Seydoux, G. 1990. Analysis of gain-of-function mutations of the lin-12 gene of Caenorhabditis elegans. Nature 346:197–199.

Hedgecock, E. M. 1985. Cell lineage mutants in the nematode Caenorhabditis elegans. Trends Neurosci. 8:288–293.

Holt, C. E., Bertsch, T. W., Ellis, H. M., and Harris, W. A. 1988. Cellular determination in the Xenopus retina is independent of lineage and birth date. Neuron. 1:15–26.

Holtfreter, J. 1933. Die totale Exogastrulation, eine Selbstablösung des Ektoderms vom Entomesoderm. Entwicklung und funktionelles Verhalten nervenloser organe. Wilhelm Roux's Arch. Entwicklungsmech. Org. 129:669–793.

Ingham, P. W. 1988. The molecular genetics of embryonic pattern formation in Drosophila. Nature 335:25–34.

Keynes, R., and Lumsden, A. 1990. Segmentation and the origin of regional diversity in the vertebrate central nervous system. Neuron 4:1–9.

Kidd, S., Kelley, M. R., and Young, M. W. 1986. Sequence of the Notch locus of Drosophila melanogaster: Relationship of the encoded protein to mammalian clotting and growth factors. Mol. Cell. Biol. 6:3094–3108.

Kintner, C. R., and Melton, D. A. 1987. Expression of Xenopus N-CAM RNA in ectoderm is an early response to neural induction. Development 99:311–325.

Landis, S. C. 1980. Developmental changes in the neurotransmitter properties of dissociated sympathetic neurons: A cytochemical study of the effects of medium. Dev. Biol. 77:349–361.

Mangold, O. 1933. Über die Induktionsfähigkeit der verschiedenen Bezirke der Neurula von Urodelen. Naturwissenschaften 21:761–766.

Monod, J., and Jacob, F. 1961. General conclusions: Teleonomic mechanism in cellular metabolism, growth, and differentiation. Cold Spring Harbor Symp. Quant. Biol. 26:389–401.

Nüsslein-Volhard, C., and Wieschaus, E. 1980. Mutations affecting segment number and polarity in *Drosophila*. Nature 287: 795–801.

Patterson, P. H., and Chun, L. L. Y. 1974. The influence of non-neuronal cells on catecholamine and acetylcholine synthesis and accumulation in cultures of dissociated sympathetic neurons. Proc. Natl. Acad. Sci. U.S.A. 71:3607–3610.

Ready, D. F., Hanson, T. E., and Benzer, S. 1976. Development of the *Drosophila* retina, a neurocrystalline lattice. Dev. Biol. 53:217–240.

Reinke, R., and Zipursky, S. L. 1988. Cell-cell interaction in the *Drosophila* retina: The bride of *sevenless* gene is required in photoreceptor cell R8 for R7 cell development. Cell 55:321–330.

Ruiz i Altaba, A., and Melton, D. A. 1989. Interaction between peptide growth factors and homeobox genes in the establishment of antero-posterior polarity in frog embryos. Nature 341: 33–38.

Schotzinger, R. J., and Landis, S. C. 1988. Cholinergic phenotype developed by noradrenergic sympathetic neurons after innervation of a novel cholinergic target *in vivo*. Nature 335:637–639.

Spemann, H., and Mangold, H. 1924. Über Induktion von Embryonalanlagen durch Implantation artfremder Organisatoren. Wilhelm Roux Arch. Entwicklungsmech. Org. 100:599–638.

Sulston, J. E., and Horvitz, H. R. 1977. Post-embryonic cell lineages of the nematode, *Caenorhabditis elegans*. Dev. Biol. 56: 110–156.

Turner, D. L., and Cepko, C. L. 1987. A common progenitor for neurons and glia persists in rat retina late in development. Nature 328:131–136.

Vassin, H., Bremer, K. A., Knust, E., and Campos-Ortega, J. A. 1987. The neurogenic gene Delta of *Drosophila melanogaster* is expressed in neurogenic territories and encodes a putative transmembrane protein with EGF-like repeats. EMBO J. 6:3431–3440.

Weston, J. A. 1963. A radioautographic analysis of the migration and localization of trunk neural crest cells in the chick. Dev. Biol. 6:279–310.

Wetts, R., and Fraser, S. E. 1988. Multipotent precursors can give rise to all major cell types of the frog retina. Science 239:1142–1145.

Wilson E. B. 1896. The Cell in Development and Inheritance. New York: Macmillan.

Yamada, T., Placzek, M., Tanaka, H., Dodd, J., and Jessell, T. M. 1991. Control of cell pattern in the developing nervous system: Polarizing activity of the floor plate and notochord. Cell 64:635–647.

Yamamori, T., Fukada, K., Aebersold, R., Korsching, S., Fann, M.-J. and Patterson, P. H. 1989. The cholinergic neuronal differentiation factor from heart cells is identical to leukemia inhibitory factor. Science 246:1412–1416.

58

Thomas M. Jessell

Cell Migration and Axon Guidance

The Migration Pattern of Neurons Establishes the Basic Plan of the Central Nervous System

The Birthday of a Neuron Defines Its Eventual Position and Properties

Immature Neurons in the Brain Migrate on a Scaffold of Radial Glial Cells

The Growth Cone Guides the Axon to Its Target

The Pathways of Developing Axons Are Accurate

Studies in Invertebrates Reveal the Precision of Axon Pathfinding and the Existence of Specific Cellular Cues

Guidance Cues Can Be Inhibitory

Some Growth Cones Are Guided by Chemotropic Molecules

Adhesion Molecules Are Involved in Axon Extension

Several Major Classes of Glycoproteins Are Involved in Neural Cell Adhesion

Many Glycoproteins Involved in Axon Fasciculation Are Members of the Immunoglobulin Superfamily

Axons Often Pause As They Project to Their Targets

Molecular Gradients May Help Axons Find Their Correct Location Within a Target Field

Pruning of Axons Focuses Their Projection to Targets

The Initial Formation of Synaptic Connections Is Often Accurate

An Overall View

E ach function of the mature nervous system, from a simple reflex response to a complex behavior, depends on the actions of distinct neuronal circuits. These circuits function correctly because their component neurons are connected appropriately to each other. A fundamental problem in neurobiology is to understand how this intricate pattern of neuronal connections is established during development. In the central nervous system of higher vertebrates the complexity of such circuits is intimidating. There are millions of nerve cells, many of which have axons that project widely throughout the brain, forming thousands of connections with different classes of target neurons. The diversity of connections formed by a single nerve cell is one of the key features that distinguishes neurons from cells in other tissues of the body.

To understand how the pattern of connections of a neuron is established, we need to know how the neuronal cell body comes to occupy its particular position in the nervous system and the signals that guide the course of its axon. In this chapter we discuss the principles and mechanisms underlying the migration of neural cells and the projection of axons to their targets. In the next two chapters we shall consider the processes of synapse formation and modification.

The Migration Pattern of Neurons Establishes the Basic Plan of the Central Nervous System

A characteristic feature of many neuronal precursors (neuroblasts) and neurons is that they migrate from the sites at which they begin to differentiate. For example, as we discussed in Chapter 57, neurons in the peripheral nervous system derive from neural crest cells that migrate extensively throughout the body before completing their differentiation into autonomic, sensory, and enteric neurons. Similarly, in the central nervous system the eventual position of many different classes of neurons is achieved by the migration of neuroblasts from the site of their proliferation in the ventricular zones of the neuroepithelium. Different classes of neuroblasts migrate at different stages; some migrate before and some after they have extended their axons. For example, motor neurons in the ventral horn of the spinal cord migrate from the ventricular zone of the neural tube to form the motor column before they send an axon out into the periphery. Other neurons, such as granule cells of the cerebellum, extend axons for considerable distances, and only at a relatively late stage in the maturation of the neuron does the cell body migrate from the external granular layer to its final settling place in the granule cell layer. The migration of neuronal precursors serves a dual function. First, it has a role in establishing the identity of some neurons. Second, it may define the functional properties and future connections of the neuron.

The Birthday of a Neuron Defines Its Eventual Position and Properties

Many regions of the central nervous system are notable for the orderly arrangement of neurons into layers. For example, as we have seen in Chapter 20, neurons in the cerebral cortex that have different morphologies and connections are organized into well-defined layers. Large pyramidal-shaped projection neurons are located in layer 5 and smaller stellate neurons are found in layer 4. Yet all of the different neurons that eventually populate the several layers of the cerebral cortex derive from neuroblasts that originate in the ventricular zone near the ventricles of the brain.

The layering of cortical neurons appears to be associated with the birthdays of these neurons. The term *birthday* is used to indicate the time at which a dividing precursor undergoes its final round of cell division to give rise to a postmitotic neuron. Neuronal birthdays can be determined by applying pulses of ^{3}H-thymidine to developing neuroblasts. Precursor neuroblasts that are in the S-phase of the cell cycle incorporate ^{3}H-thymidine. Postmitotic daughter cells that arise from the next mitotic division are heavily labeled but if cells continue to divide, the label is diluted. Thus, heavily labeled cells are those that are born a short time after the pulse of ^{3}H-thymidine. Using this technique it has been shown that neurons born at early stages of cortical development end up in the deepest cortical layers, while those born at later times end up in progressively more superficial layers. Neurons born at later times must therefore migrate past neurons that have already reached their final position in the cortex. Thus, the organization of cortical layers is achieved by an inside-out sequence of neuronal differentiation. Similar processes of cell migration are also seen in many other layered structures in the brain.

The mechanisms by which neurons in different cortical layers come to acquire different properties have not been resolved. The identity and function of a neuron could be defined by its birthday. Alternatively, interactions within the local environment could be more important. Studies of neuronal cell migration in the *reeler* mutant mouse have provided some evidence that cell birthday is important in defining the eventual properties and projections of neurons in the cerebral cortex. In *reeler* mice the normal inside-out layering of cortical neurons is inverted; neurons born at early times end up in the most superficial layers, whereas neurons born at later stages end up in deeper layers. Although these neurons are located in inappropriate positions, they still appear to acquire their normal morphology and connections, leading to an inversion in the functional arrangement of cortical neurons. These observations suggest that the position occupied by a neuron in the cortex is less critical in determining its final identity and connections than is its birthday or other events in its developmental history.

The time of commitment of cortical neurons has been examined in ferrets by Susan McConnell, who transplanted embryonic cortical neuronal precursors destined for layers 5 and 6 into the ventricular zone of newborn animals where the surrounding cells migrate to layers 2 and 3. Many of the transplanted neurons migrated to layers 5 and 6 and developed axonal projections appropriate for their birthday. The stage of the cell cycle affects the fate of these transplanted cells. Progenitor cells in S-phase are altered after transplantation into older hosts and these cells migrate to the host-specific layers 2 and 3. If, however, progenitors are transplanted late in the cell cycle or after the production of postmitotic daughters, those daughters are committed to their normal laminar fates, migrating to layer 6 and forming axonal connections appropriate for their birthday. Thus, commitment occurs prior to migration, and laminar fates are determined just before the neuron is born.

The principles of cortical cell development differ from those of neural crest cells discussed in the previous chapter, which showed that the migratory route and final location of crest cells are more important than cell birthday in determining their eventual fate.

Immature Neurons in the Brain Migrate on a Scaffold of Radial Glial Cells

The neural tube consists of a layer of epithelial cells that give rise both to neurons and glial cells. Soon after the neural tube forms, many of the epithelial cells near its lumenal surface begin to proliferate and give rise to neuroblasts. However, a distinct group of neural cells, the *radial glial cells*, retain contacts with both the lumenal and pial surfaces of the neural tube. In many regions of the developing brain the migration of neuroblasts and neurons is dependent on radial glial cells (Figure 58–1).

In the primate cortex the radial glial cells are extremely elongated, extending from the ventricular to the pial surface before neuronal migration has begun (Figure 58–2).

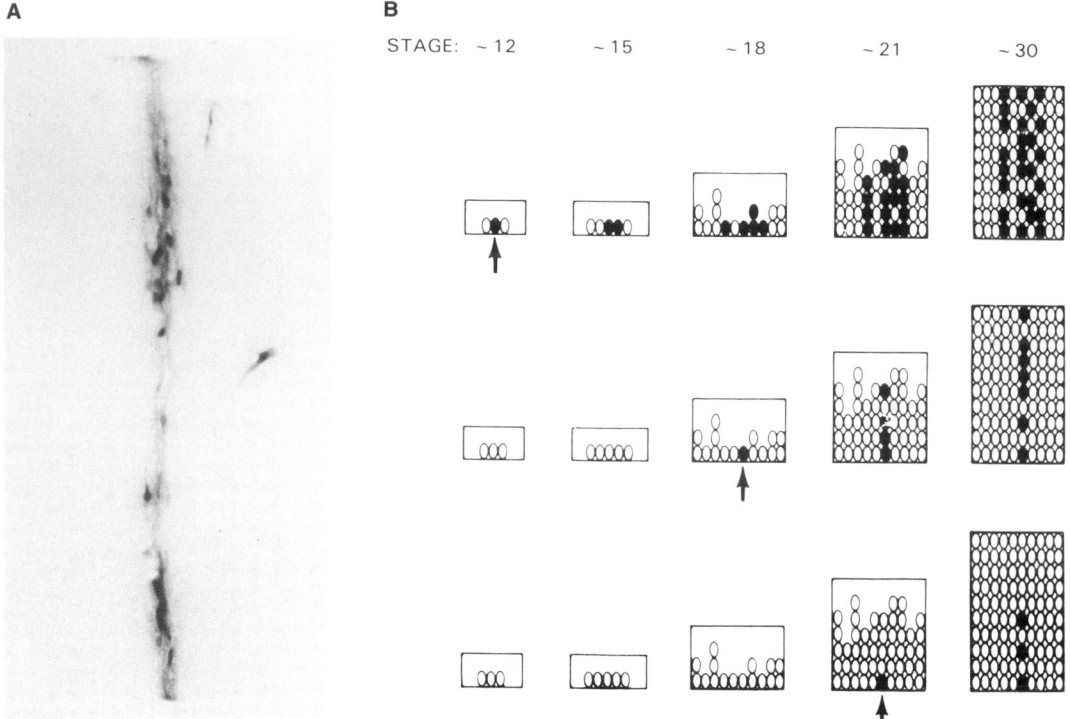

FIGURE 58–1

Retroviruses can be used to trace the migratory paths of cells in the vertebrate brain.

A. A clonally related group of cells in the chick optic tectum. The cells are identified by expression of the enzyme β-galactosidase after the developing brain is injected with a small number of retroviral particles, which can express the gene encoding this enzyme. The clone of cells migrates in strict radial order as the laminae of the optic tectum form.

B. The pattern of labeled cells changes with the age at which the retrovirus is injected. Injection at early stages of development results in a broad band of marked cells, suggesting that the founder cell gives rise to cells that spread laterally within the ventricular zone before migrating radially. With progressively later injection times (**arrows**), labeled cells give off progeny that migrate radially without first spreading in the ventricular zone. (Adapted from Sanes, 1989.)

From electron-microscopic reconstruction of embryonic primate cerebral cortex, Pasko Rakic and his colleagues observed that migrating neurons align themselves and form intimate contacts with the radial glial cells. Similarly, granule cells, a class of excitatory interneurons in the cerebellum, align with radial glial fibers as they migrate from the external granular layer to the internal granular layer, their final destination (Figure 58–2).

Additional evidence that radial glial fibers act as substrates for migrating neurons has come from studies of the *weaver* mutant mouse. In *weaver* embryos the radial glial cells are misaligned. The granule cells are unable to migrate to their correct location in the cerebellum and are arrested in more superficial layers (Figure 58–3). The correct orientation of radial glial fibers therefore appears to be critical for the normal migration of granule cells.

Daniel Goldowitz and Richard Mullen examined whether the genetic defect that leads to the aberrant migration of granule cells in the *weaver* mouse affects the function of the radial glial cell or that of the granule cell. They produced chimeric mice by mixing blastomeres

from a *weaver* mouse and implanting them into a genetically marked wild-type host embryo. In the chimeric mice that resulted, some cells in the cerebellum derived from the mutant *weaver* background and some from the wild-type strain. The origins of the different cells can be recognized by expression of high glucuronidase activity in the wild-type strain. The genetic background of radial glial and granule cells in local regions of the cerebellum was correlated with arrested granule cells. Goldowitz and Mullen found that arrested granule cells are always derived from *weaver* mice. Moreover, using cultured cerebellar cells, Mary Beth Hatten and Carol Mason found that granule cells from *weaver* embryos cannot migrate on radial glia from wild-type embryos, whereas wild-type granule cells migrate normally on glial cells of the *weaver* background (Figure 58–3B). These two lines of evidence indicate that the inability of granule cells to migrate along the surface of the radial glial cells in the *weaver* mutant results from a defect in the granule cell itself.

The normal organization of radial glia may be dependent on interactions with granule cells. Wild-type radial

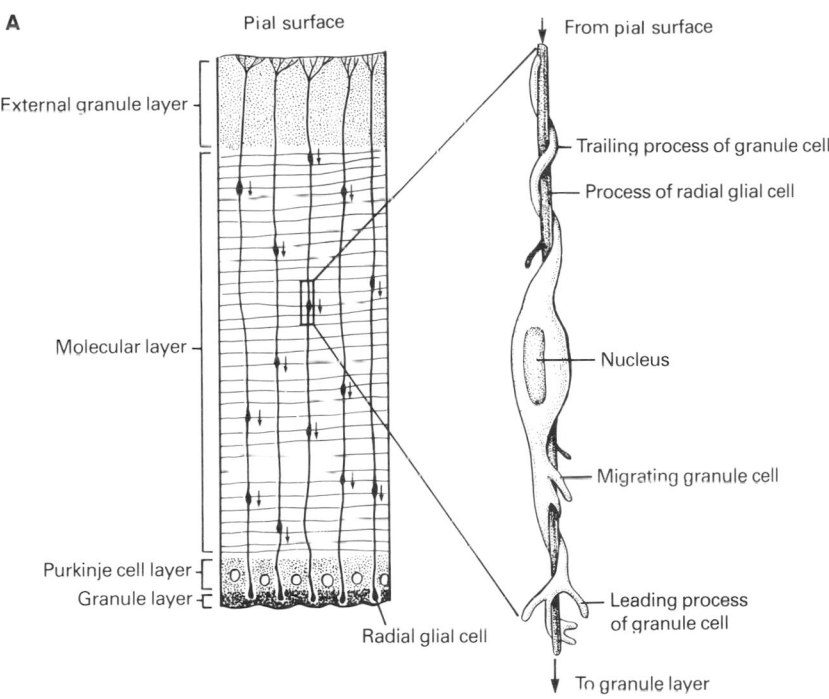

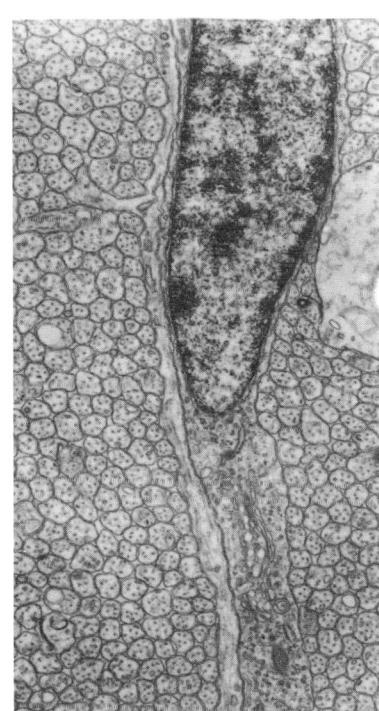

FIGURE 58–2

Neurons use radial glial cell fibers as scaffolds for migration.

A. Granule cells migrate through the molecular and Purkinje cell layers along processes of radial glial cells (Bergmann astrocytes), which extend from the granule layer to the pial surface. The cell bodies of the radial glial cells are located near the junction of the Purkinje and granule cell layers. (Adapted from Rakic, 1971.)

B. This electron micrograph shows the vertically oriented cell body of a migrating granule cell in the molecular layer. Note the abundance of cytoplasmic organelles in the leading process, particularly the elaborate reticulum and ribosomes. On the left side of the cell is an electron-lucent longitudinally oriented Bergmann glial fiber. The Bergmann process has a lateral protrusion (**arrow**) but the surface shared in common with the migrating granule cell is relatively smooth. The cytoplasm of the leading process close to the nucleus is rich in organelles, including mitochondria, free ribosomes, Golgi apparatus, and multivesicular bodies. × 16,500. (From Rakic, 1971.)

glia in the vicinity of *weaver* granule cells are disorganized, suggesting that the *weaver* mutation indirectly affects the properties of the radial glia. Hatten and her colleagues have identified a granule cell-surface protein, astrotactin, that may be involved in adhesive interactions between granule cells and radial glia.

Many neurons in the cerebral cortex also use radial glia to guide their migration from the ventricular zones to their final destinations. However, there must be other ways of guiding migrating cells since many neuroblasts migrate in regions of the central nervous system in which there are no radial glial fibers. Similarly, as discussed in Chapter 57, neural crest cells migrate in the absence of any organized glial structures. Extracellular matrix molecules, including laminin and fibronectin (see below), have been implicated in the migration of neural crest cells.

The Growth Cone Guides the Axon to Its Target

Once a neuron has migrated to its final position, and sometimes even before, it begins to extend an axon. The axon extends at its growing tip by means of a specialized structure called the *growth cone*. The possibility that growth cones are involved in axon pathfinding was first suggested by Ramón y Cajal in the 1890s. In 1909 Ross Harrison invented the technique of tissue culture for the purpose of determining whether the axon grows out from the cell body as Ramón y Cajal proposed. Harrison also observed living growth cones and deduced that the growth of axons occurs by extension of the growth cone.

Growth cones appear as an enlargement of the shaft of the axon. Several finger-like extensions, called *filopodia*, project from the growth cone. Filopodia are highly motile and continually extend and retract. In between the filopodia are thin membranes called *lamellipodia*, which are also motile and give the growth cone its characteristic ruffled appearance (Figure 58–4). In tissue culture, where many studies of growth cones have been performed, the leading process of the growth cone is flattened and has few organelles, whereas the body of the growth cone is packed with microtubules, mitochondria, and a variety of other organelles. The ultrastructural features of the growth cone

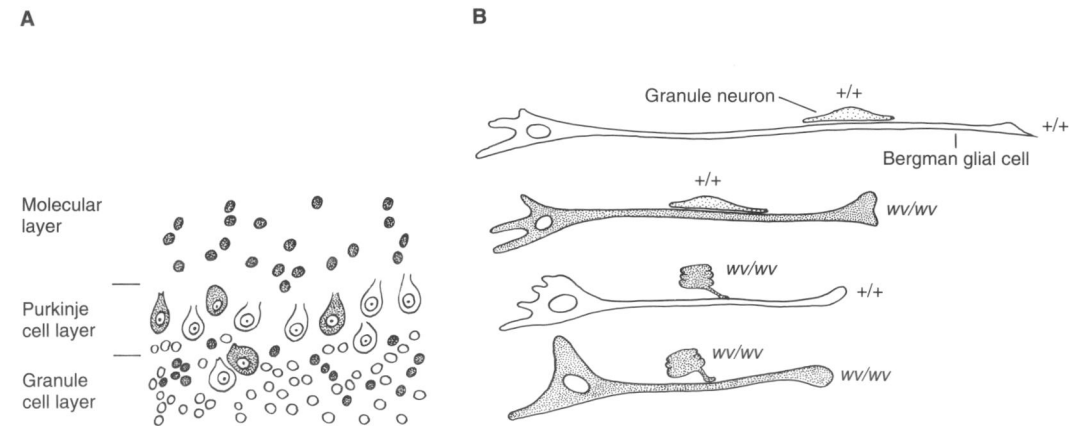

FIGURE 58–3

Granule cell migration is perturbed in the cerebellum of the *weaver* mutant mouse.

A. Schematic diagram of neurons in the cerebellum of a chimeric mouse created from embryonic cells from a wild-type and a heterozygous *weaver* mouse embryo. The wild-type cells are **white**, while the cells from the *weaver* embryo are shown in **black**. Arrested granule cells are located in the molecular layer and nearly all of them derive from the *weaver* embryo. (Adapted from Goldowitz, 1989.)

B. Abnormal cell interactions between *weaver* granule neurons and wild-type radial glial cells can be demonstrated *in vitro*. Diagram showing interactions of normal (**+/+**) and *weaver (wv/wv)* granule neurons with wild-type and *weaver* cerebellar glial cells. Normal granule neurons migrate on both wild-type (**clear**) and *weaver* (**black**) glial cells and induce morphological differentiation of both wild-type and mutant glia. In contrast, *weaver* granule neurons fail to make close contacts with either wild-type or *weaver* astroglial cells. Glial differentiation is poor in the presence of *weaver* neurons. (From Hatten et al., 1986.)

FIGURE 58–4

Growth cone morphology *in vivo* and *in vitro*.

A. Growth cone of a motor neuron observed *in situ* in a salamander embryo. The growth cone is viewed growing along the dorsal surface of a somite and has many filopodia. The bundle of axons (**arrow**) emerges from the spinal cord. (From Roberts and Patten, 1985.)

B. Whole-mount electron micrograph of a growth cone *in vitro*. Two distinct cytoplasmic domains are present. The approximate boundary between the two domains is shown by the dotted line. The central (**C**) domain contains microtubules (**mt**), mitochondria (**m**), and dense-core vescicles. The peripheral domain contains bundles of microfilaments (**arrows**) that form the core of the majority of filopodia. (From Bridgman and Dailey, 1989.)

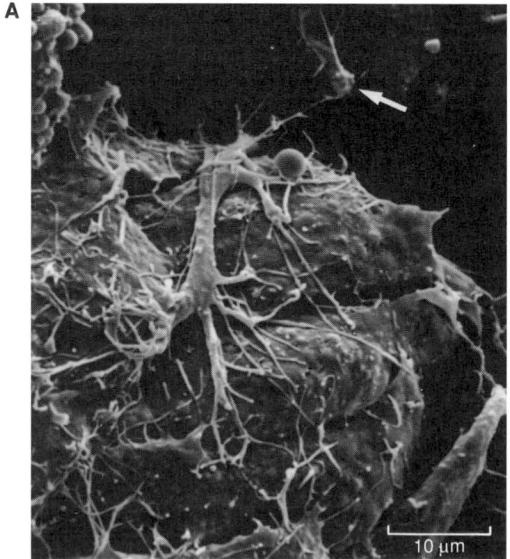

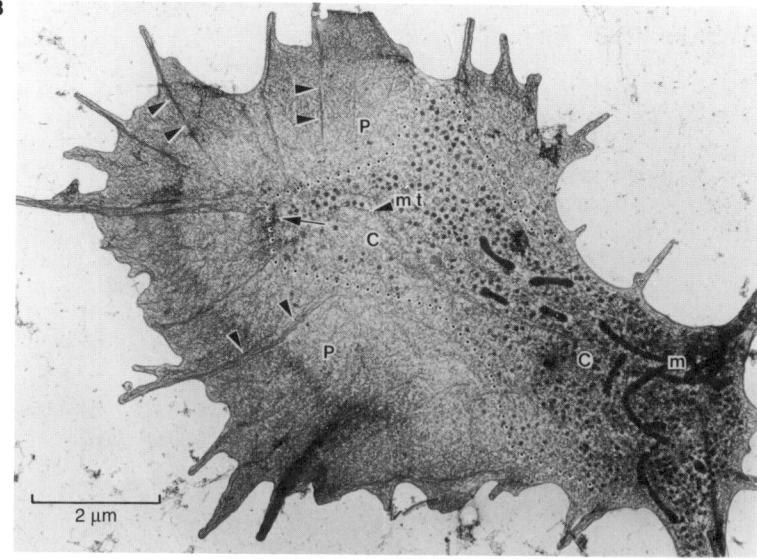

A

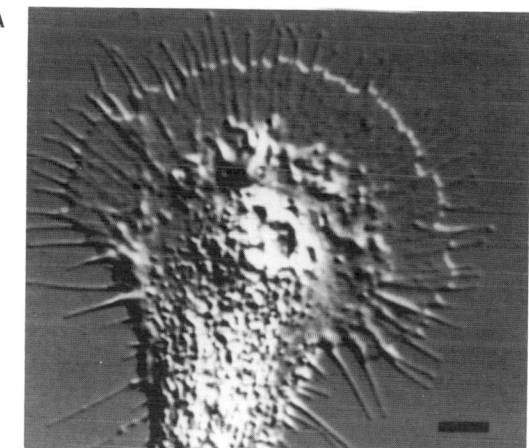

B

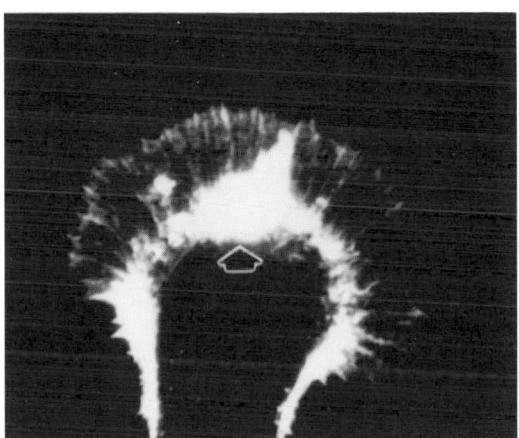

C

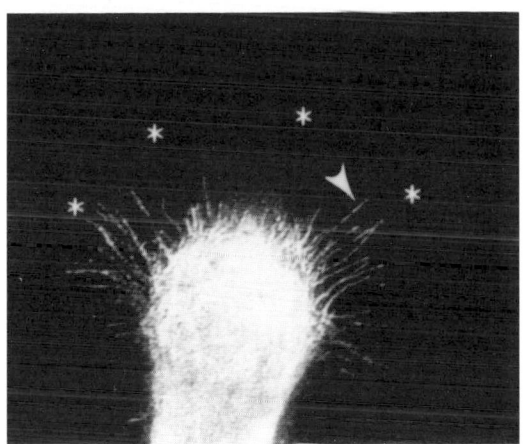

FIGURE 58–5

Actin and microtubule domains are localized in different regions of the growth cone. Scale bar = 5 μm. (From Forscher and Smith, 1988.)

A. A growth cone from a neuron isolated from the marine snail *Aplysia californica* viewed under differential interference contrast optics. Numerous filopodia extend from the growth cone.

B. The distribution of filamentous actin in the same growth cone shown in part A is revealed by labeling with fluorescent phalloidin. Most of the actin filaments are in the periphery of the growth cone.

C. The localization of microtubules in the same growth cone is revealed using an antibody to tubulin. Most of the microtubules are concentrated in the central core of the growth cone. **Asterisks** mark the border of the growth cone.

are similar to those of the leading process of fibroblasts and neutrophils. Thus, the basic mechanisms underlying the locomotion of neurons and other motile cells are probably similar.

The force that extends the axon derives from changes that occur within the growth cone. Both the lamellipodia and filopodia of the growth cone contain a high density of actin filaments (Figure 58–5). There is increasing evidence that the degree of actin polymerization regulates growth cone motility (Figure 58–6). One hypothesis suggests that actin subunits are assembled into filamentous polymers at the leading edge of the growth cone, then move in a retrograde direction to the shafts of the growth cone where depolymerization occurs. The actin monomers are then recycled to the leading edge of the growth cone, where they assemble into filaments (Figure 58–6). In this model the extension of the growth cone would result from actin filament assembly at the leading edge. Retraction of the growth cone would result from depolymerization of actin filaments.

Direct evidence for the involvement of actin filaments in growth cone motility has come from experiments using cytochalasins, fungal toxins that inhibit actin polymerization. When treated with these toxins, growth cones show little or no movement or extension. Other details of growth cone motility still require explanation. For example, we need to understand how the adhesion molecules on the surface of growth cones interact with the actin cytoskeleton and to identify proteins that regulate the cycle of actin polymerization within the growth cone.

Several different second-messenger pathways can be activated in growth cones by environmental signals and may regulate growth cone motility by modifying the structure or function of cytoskeletal and other proteins in the growth cone. For example, the binding of ligands to neurotransmitter receptors on growth cones can lead to changes in intracellular calcium concentration and result in marked effects on growth cone motility. As with many other motile cells the intracellular proteins that serve as substrates for these second-messenger and protein kinases are not well characterized. One protein, GAP-43, first characterized by Mark Willard, is expressed at high levels in active growth cones and growing axons but at lower levels in mature neurons. Biochemical studies have shown that GAP-43 is a substrate for calcium-dependent and phospholipid-dependent protein kinase C. Moreover, GAP-43 binds calmodulin at low calcium levels. Thus,

A

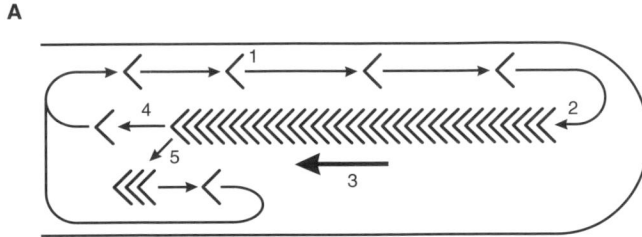

B₁

B₂

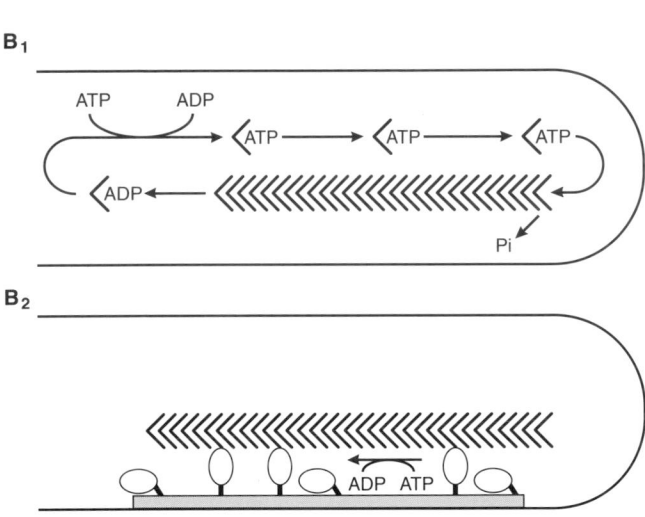

FIGURE 58–6

Schematic diagram of a growth cone, showing how actin may control the motility of growth cones. (See also Chapter 4.)

A. Actin subunits (**1**) diffuse to the tip of the filopodium (**2**), where they add to the barbed end of an actin filament (the end nearest the tip of the filopodium). The actin filament is translocated (**3**) toward the center of the cell, where it depolymerizes into monomers (**4**) or fragments into pieces by depolymerization (**5**).

B. Two possible ways of powering retrograde actin filament flow. **1.** Retrograde actin flow is powered by the insertion of actin subunits between the membrane and the barbed end of the actin filament and the simultaneous loss of subunits from the pointed end nearer to the center of the growth cones. This process can occur because the insertion of actin is coupled to ATP hydrolysis. The subunits adding to the tip have bound ATP, which is hydrolyzed soon after polymerization; hence the bulk of the polymer contains ADP actin. ADP actin disassembles from the pointed end before reassembly of the monomer. ATP is exchanged for ADP. **2.** In this model retrograde actin flow is powered by myosin, most probably myosin type 1, which is shown as **ellipses** anchored to an as yet undefined submembranous matrix. The force exerted by the myosin accompanying ATP hydrolysis drives the actin filaments to the left in the figure. The direction of movement is dictated by the polarity of the actin subunit and the properties of myosin. (Adapted from Smith, 1988.)

GAP-43 may represent one growth cone protein whose function is modified by second messengers.

As the axon extends, the surface area of the neuronal membrane increases. New membrane is synthesized in

the cell body, packaged into vesicles, and transported along microtubules that extend into the body of the growth cone. Once in the growth cone, these vesicles fuse and are incorporated into the surface membrane. Although the growth cone also recycles membrane via endocytosis, there is a net addition of new membrane.

Growth cones also orient growing axons. Orientation of the growth cone depends on two classes of interaction: (1) contacts made with other cell surfaces and with molecules in the extracellular matrix, and (2) diffusible molecules that bind to surface receptors on the growth cone and which transmit signals across the plasma membrane. The cellular and molecular mechanisms involved in guiding developing growth cones are discussed later in the chapter. First we discuss the evidence that growth cones project to their targets in a precise manner using specific guidance cues.

The Pathways of Developing Axons Are Accurate

For over a century neurobiologists have been intrigued by the way in which the axons of developing neurons reach their targets. Ramón y Cajal's early descriptions of developing axons left the impression that growth cones move in an ordered and directed manner. Direct observation of growth cone movement in tissue culture by Harrison and in living amphibian embryos by Carl Spiedel supported this idea. However, by the 1930s the idea that guided axonal growth contributed to the specificity of neuronal connection was still not widely accepted. Instead, the prevailing opinion was that initial outgrowth of axons occurred randomly and in an undirected manner. Paul Weiss, in particular, held the view that the specificity of connections was due solely to selective retention of those connections in which the pattern of electrical activity of the presynaptic neuron matched that of its target. This idea was known as the *resonance hypothesis*.

The demise of the resonance theory, and the reemergence of ideas of specificity in axonal pathfinding is largely attributable to Roger Sperry. In the 1940s and 1950s Sperry assessed the regenerative capacity of axons in the visual and somatosensory systems. In experiments on the visual system of the newt he examined how retinal neurons regenerate axons and reestablish connections with target cells in the optic tectum when the optic nerve is cut. Sperry cut the optic nerve and inverted the eye in its orbit by 180° before regeneration was allowed to occur. The animals subsequently behaved as if their visual world had been inverted. For example, visual stimuli presented above and to the left of the animal evoked a motor response directed to the lower right. Moreover, the behavioral response was not corrected by visual experience. The implication of this finding was that the axons of retinal ganglion neurons had grown back to their original targets in the optic tectum even though the regenerated connections were behaviorally inappropriate. Sperry later obtained anatomical evidence to support this proposal.

These and many similar experiments by Sperry on other neural systems provided evidence for a high degree

A Stages 15-16

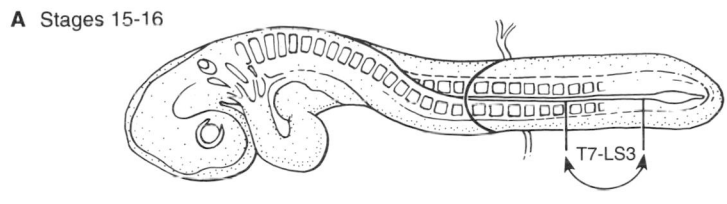

T7-LS3

B Stage 28½ control   Stage 28½ reversed

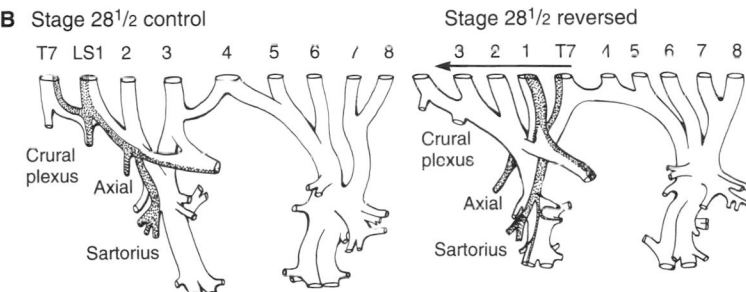

T7 LS1 2   3   4   5   6   7   8   3   2   1   T7   4   5   6   7   8

Crural
plexus
Axial

Sartorius

Crural
plexus

Axial

Sartorius

FIGURE 58-7

Axon pathfinding is directed to highly specific targets in early development. (Adapted from Lance-Jones and Landmesser, 1981.)

A. A length of spinal cord comprising several segments (T7–LS3) is reversed along the anterior–posterior axis at an early stage of development (stages 15–16) in the chick embryo.

B. Anterograde transport of horseradish peroxidase injected into one or two spinal cord segments (**black lines**) reveals the pattern of axon projection at a later stage (after about 6 days incubation; stage 28½). The normal projection pattern of segments T7 and LS1 is shown on the left. On the right is the pattern after the reversal operation shown in part A. Despite displacement of the motor neuron cell bodies, the axons of these neurons find their correct peripheral nerves and eventually innervate appropriate muscles.

of specificity in the formation of synaptic connections. He proposed that this specificity depends on selective chemical affinities that exist between individual neurons. The basic idea of this *chemoaffinity hypothesis* is that individual neurons acquire distinctive molecular markers early in development. The establishment of appropriate connections between two neurons would thus depend on the correct matching of molecules present on the pre- and postsynaptic neuron. More refined techniques have since been used to reexamine the development of neural connectivity in many of the systems that Sperry studied. Although some of the details of Sperry's studies have been revised, the basic idea that the selectivity of synaptic connections depends on the recognition of specific molecular cues in the vicinity of the target is now widely accepted.

These studies have also shown that the initial outgrowth of axons early in development is directed and that axons select particular pathways by recognizing cues in their environment. A good example of axon pathfinding in vertebrate embryos is the selection of peripheral pathways by the axons of developing motor neurons. Lynn Landmesser and her colleagues examined the development of pathways of different populations of motor axons in the chick embryo using an anatomical marker. As different classes of motor neurons project from the spinal cord, their axons are intermingled. However, when the axon bundle reaches the base of the developing limb, individual axons leave the bundle and reassemble to form new branches that contain only those motor axons destined for the same muscle target (Figure 58–7). This suggests that growth cones of different classes of motor neurons recognize specific cues within the limb. The sorting of motor axons occurs in a restricted region of the limb that Landmesser called a *decision region*. These guidance cues also appear to be effective in directing the correct projection of motor axons that have been experimentally forced to enter

the limb in an inappropriate position (Figure 58–7). Moreover, the fact that many distinct sets of motor axons segregate from a mixed bundle of fibers implies a high degree of selectivity in the recognition of these guidance cues.

Decision regions have been identified in the pathway of other classes of axons in the central and peripheral nervous systems. Growth cones change their appearance at these regions, become more expanded with a greater number of filopodia. These changes in morphology may indicate that a growth cone is actively searching for specific guidance cues or, alternatively, they may occur once the growth cone has successfully located its cue.

Studies in Invertebrates Reveal the Precision of Axon Pathfinding and the Existence of Specific Cellular Cues

In vertebrate embryos it is difficult to follow the path of an individual axon. In certain insect embryos, however, the trajectory of a single axon can be traced and thus the signals involved in growth cone migration can be detected more easily. For example, developing sensory neurons in the embryonic grasshopper limb are thought to extend over epithelial surfaces by following an adhesive substrate distributed in a graded fashion along the epithelium of the limb. At specific locations there are abrupt changes in the direction of extension of the growth cone. These changes occur as the filopodia of the growth cone contact specific cells. The cells that trigger the change in trajectory have been termed *guidepost cells*, which are often immature neurons (Figure 58–8). Direct experimental evidence that these cells guide the migration of growth cones has been obtained by killing the guidepost cells by laser ablation before they are contacted by the growth cone. In the absence of these cells the growth cone meanders, often veering off in an inappropriate direction. Cells with similar

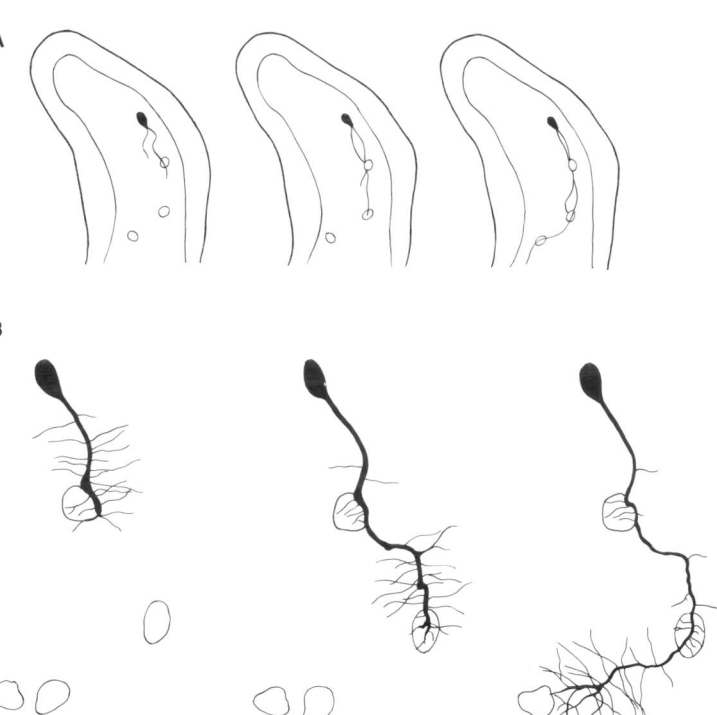

FIGURE 58–8

Specialized cells guide developing sensory neurons in the grasshopper embryo along precise pathways. (Adapted from Taghert et al., 1982.)

A. Diagram of developing sensory neurons (**black**) and their axons in whole-mounted grasshopper limbs at successive stages of development. The axons take a stereotyped route as they project centrally, contacting several cells along their path.

B. The growth cones of the sensory axons send out extensive filopodia, some of which adhere preferentially to another differentiating neuron (called a *guidepost cell*) and thus direct the growth of the axons toward the cell.

roles in axon guidance are thought to exist in other regions of invertebrate and vertebrate nervous systems.

The growth cones of invertebrate neurons also use the axons of other neurons as scaffolds upon which to extend. Corey Goodman and his colleagues found that in grasshopper embryos the growth cone of an identified neuron consistently migrates along the same axon bundles, even though several other bundles are within reach of the filopodia of the growth cone. When the preferred axon bundle was eliminated by killing the neurons that give rise to these axons, growth cones did not switch to neighboring axons. Instead, they frequently stopped in the vicinity of the missing bundle or wandered within the neuroepithelium without recognizing the remaining axons. Thus, there is a high degree of specificity in the ability of growth cones to recognize axon tracts.

There is increasing evidence for a similar specificity in growth cone guidance in the vertebrate nervous system. For example, Charles Kimmel, John Kuwada, and their colleagues have shown in zebra fish embryos that the axons of identified neurons follow the same trajectory in different embryos. Indeed, many of the major principles of axon guidance defined from studies in invertebrates—cell and substrate adhesion, guidepost cells that function as intermediate targets, and selective axon fasciculation— are likely to operate in the vertebrate nervous system.

Guidance Cues Can Be Inhibitory

Many growth cues for developing axons involve adhesive contacts between the growth cone and molecules on the surface of neighboring cells or in the extracellular matrix.

However, not all of the cues that guide axons necessarily involve adhesion. Neurons may also be guided by cell-surface molecules that repel growth cones. Support for this idea comes from *in vitro* studies on vertebrate neurons. For example, growth cones of central neurons retract when they contact the axons of peripheral neurons but are not affected when they contact the axons of other central neurons. Likewise, the growth cones of developing peripheral neurons collapse when they contact the axons of central neurons.

Oligodendrocytes, one of the major classes of glial cells in the central nervous system, also inhibit the extension of axons. Martin Schwab and his colleagues have found that the inhibitory properties of oligodendrocytes result from two cell-surface glycoproteins with molecular weights of 35,000 and 250,000. Antibodies to these proteins neutralize the inhibitory properties of the oligodendrocyte cell surface. These two proteins are first expressed in the brain postnatally as oligodendrocytes begin to synthesize myelin and persist in the adult central nervous system. As we saw in Chapter 18, Schwann cells, the myelinating cells of the peripheral axons, promote axon regeneration and do not express these two proteins. Thus, neuronal regeneration in the central, but not the peripheral, nervous system may be prevented by components of myelin with inhibitory properties.

Some Growth Cones Are Guided by Chemotropic Molecules

Developing axons may also be guided by gradients of diffusible factors that are released by restricted groups of tar-

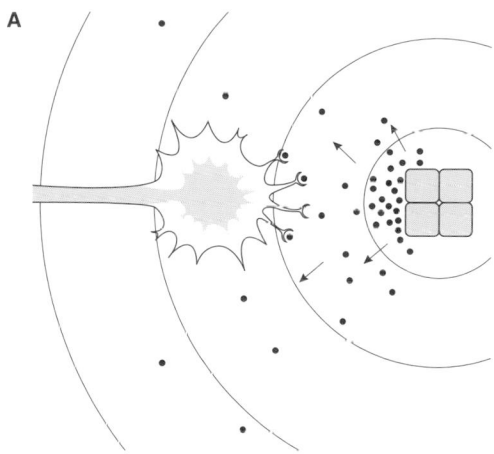

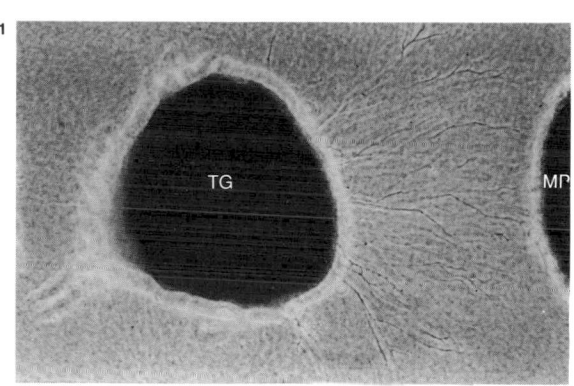

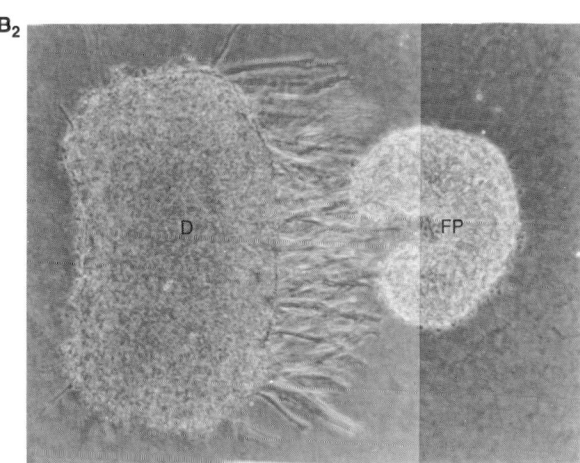

FIGURE 58–9

Chemotropic factors released from target cells guide axons in the developing mammalian nervous system.

A. A group of target cells releases a diffusible chemoattractant that is distributed in a graded manner in the path of a developing axon. Growth cones orient up a concentration gradient of this factor and grow toward the target.

B. Photomicrograph of explants of neuronal and target tissue cocultured *in vitro* in three-dimensional collagen gels. **1.** Neurites of sensory neurons emerge from the embryonic trigeminal ganglion (**TG**) and grow toward their peripheral target tissue, the epithelial cells of the maxillary process (**MP**). Scale bar = 200 μm. (Courtesy of A. Lumsden.) **2.** Commissural neurons in an embryonic rat dorsal spinal cord (**D**) extend bundles of axons toward the floor plate (**FP**), an intermediate target in their pathway. Scale bar = 100 μm. (Adapted from Tessier-Lavigne et al., 1988.)

get cells (Figure 58–9). Such oriented growth is termed *chemotropism* (or *chemotaxis*) and was first proposed as a mechanism of axon guidance by Ramón y Cajal after studying axon growth in the developing retina. Many other classes of cells in the body, in particular neutrophils and fibroblasts, exhibit chemotaxis, which can be assayed as the migration of cells toward local sources of diffusible factors. In the nervous system *in vitro* studies have provided evidence for chemotropic guidance of three different sets of neurons. First, sensory neurons in the trigeminal ganglion direct their axons toward the source of a factor secreted by the maxillary epithelium, one of the normal peripheral targets of these axons. Second, the axons of commissural neurons are directed toward the ventral midline of the central nervous system by a chemoattractant factor released by a group of cells called the *floor plate* (Figure 58–9). Third, some cortical neurons project collateral branches in response to a diffusible factor released from target cells in the pons. These chemotropic factors may be distinct from trophic molecules such as nerve growth factor (NGF), brain-derived neurotrophic factor (BDNF), and neurotrophin 3 (NT3), all of which support the survival of neurons (see Chapter 59).

Nonneural cells can detect differences as small as 1%

in the local concentration of the chemotactic factor, and it is likely that growth cones have similar discriminatory abilities. The mechanisms by which growth cones detect gradients of diffusible molecules is not clear, although it is likely that chemotropic factors bind to surface receptors and that these receptors transduce signals to the cytoplasm of the growth cone. Studies on chemotactic response of neutrophils and other cells have shown that second-messenger pathways involving intracellular Ca^{2+}, cAMP-dependent protein kinase, and protein kinase C are activated in response to chemotactic factors.

Adhesion Molecules Are Involved in Axon Extension

Some of the guidance molecules on the surface of the axon and on the substrate upon which the axon grows, have been identified over the past decade. Some of these molecules appear to mediate general adhesive interactions between the growth cone and its environment, while others may help growth cones choose cell surfaces upon which to extend (Figure 58–10). We next discuss the structure and function of some of these molecules.

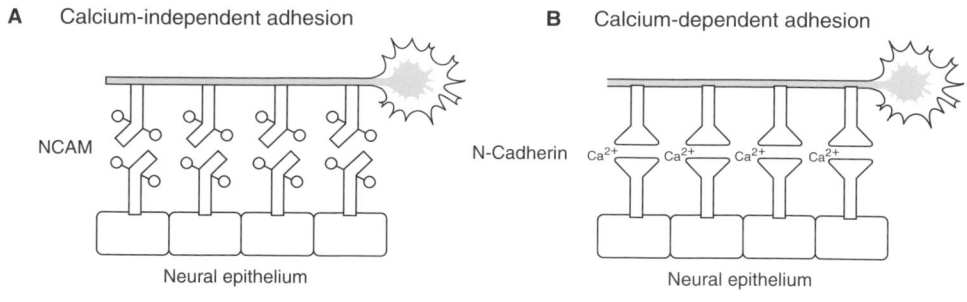

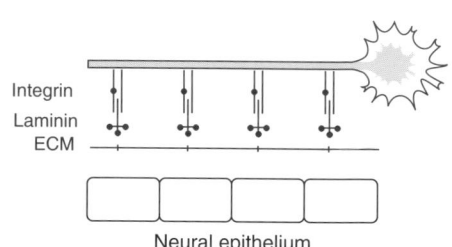

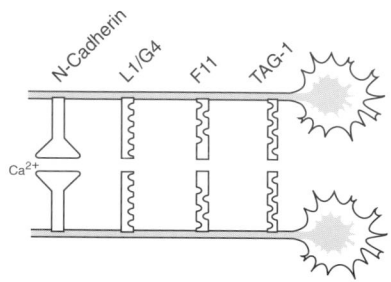

FIGURE 58–10

Some of the different molecular mechanisms thought to contribute to axonal growth. (Adapted from Dodd and Jessell, 1988.)

A. Growth cones extend in contact with neural epithelial cells. Homophilic binding of Ca²⁺-independent adhesion molecules on the surface of the axon and on the neural epithelial cell, such as NCAM, may promote axonal growth.

B. Growth cone extension on neural epithelial cells may also involve homophilic binding between Ca²⁺-dependent adhesion molecules, such as N-cadherin.

C. Growth cones may also extend on extracellular matrix (**ECM**) substrates. Glycoproteins in the ECM, such as laminin, promote axon growth by interacting with integrins on the axonal surface.

D. Later in development, when most neural epithelial cells have differentiated, growth cones extend on other axons. Many different types of molecules mediate interactions between axons, including N-cadherin and members of the immunoglobulin superfamily, such as L1/G4, F11, and TAG-1.

Several Major Classes of Glycoproteins Are Involved in Neural Cell Adhesion

Many of the glycoproteins involved in the adhesion of neural cells belong to one of three major structural families. The first is the immunoglobulin superfamily. The second family comprises a group of structurally related glycoproteins called cadherins, of which N-cadherin is a prominent member expressed within the nervous system. The third family consists of a large family of glycoproteins called integrins. The integrins mediate interactions between the cell surface and molecules in the extracellular matrix. Each integrin consists of two distinct subunits that together confer the binding properties of the molecule. Members of these three families of glycoproteins are expressed at high levels on neurons but are also expressed by nonneural cells. Thus, molecules that underlie adhesive properties of neurons may carry out similar functions on nonneural cells.

Neural cell adhesion molecule (NCAM) is one of the most abundant adhesion molecules on the surface of neural cells. NCAM was identified by Gerald Edelman and his colleagues in the 1970s. The protein was defined using antibodies that prevented the aggregation of retinal cells using *in vitro* assays, and the protein was identified biochemically by its ability to neutralize these antisera. NCAM is expressed on almost all neural cells from the time of neural induction and is likely to contribute to the general adhesive properties of neural cells.

NCAM derives from a single gene but exists in multiple protein forms derived from alternatively spliced RNAs and from extensive post-translational modification. Two of the major forms of NCAM are transmembrane glycoproteins; a third is attached to the membrane via a glycosyl-phosphatidylinositol linkage; and a fourth form is secreted. These four forms have a conserved extracellular region with five domains, which fold in a manner similar to that found in immunoglobulins (Figure 58–11). As we discuss below, this family now includes many other proteins. In addition to the immunoglobulin-like domains, NCAM also includes regions of homology with the glycoprotein fibronectin, an extracellular substrate adhesion molecule that we discuss later in the chapter. The different structural domains of NCAM may therefore have distinct adhesive functions.

The protein backbone of NCAM is modified exten-

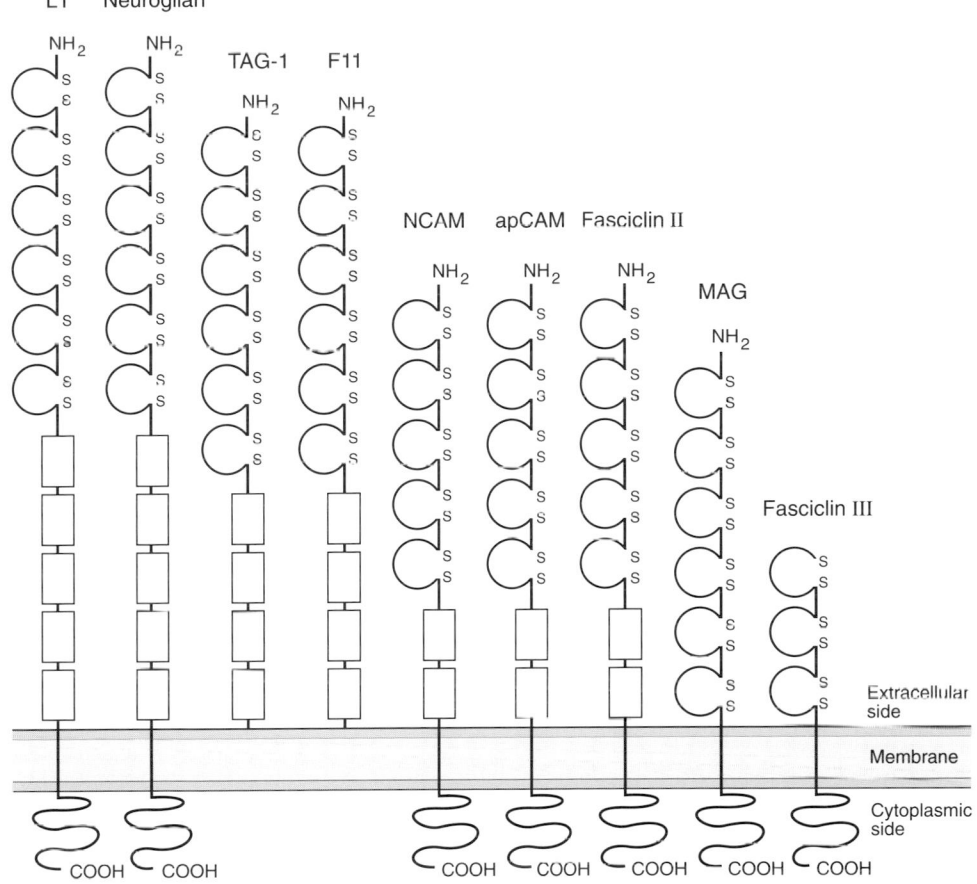

FIGURE 58-11

Structures of different members of the immunoglobulin family of neural adhesion molecules. The extracellular domain of these proteins is divided into two major structures: (1) an amino-terminal series of immunoglobulin-like repeats (**loops**), characterized by a regularly spaced disulfide linkage; and (2) repeats of about 100 amino acids in length (**boxes**), which share structural features with a sequence in the fibronectin molecule, called a type III repeat. The number of these repeats varies between molecules. In addition, the mode of attachment to the cell surface differs between molecules. L1, neuroglian, MAG, NCAM, fasciclin II, and fasciclin III exist in transmembrane forms and have cytoplasmic domains. In contrast, TAG-1, F11, and some forms of NCAM, neuroglian, fasciclin II, and apCAM are anchored to the cell surface by a glycosyl-phosphatidylinositol linkage.

sively by glycosylation. In particular, each of the protein forms of NCAM found in developing embryos have an extremely high sialic acid content amounting to approximately 30% of the mass of the protein. In contrast, NCAM found in the adult nervous system has a much lower (~10%) sialic acid content. The structure of this carbohydrate is unusual, consisting of long chains of 2,8-linked sialic acid. The degree of sialylation changes markedly during development. In embryos the major forms of NCAM express high amounts of the polysialic acid side group whereas in adults sialylation decreases considerably.

NCAM mediates the binding of cells by a *homophilic* mechanism, that is, an NCAM molecule on one cell binds to a counterpart NCAM molecule on an adjacent cell. Association between NCAM molecules is thought to occur through the amino terminal immunoglobulin-like domains of the protein. Differences in the structure of NCAM may affect its binding function. In particular, the regulation of NCAM sialylation may be important functionally since NCAM molecules with a high polysialic acid content have been found to bind at a lower affinity than NCAM molecules that have a low degree of sialylation. The mechanism by which polysialic acid reduces the rate of cell binding is not established but may involve a steric perturbation of the homophilic binding domain. The binding function of NCAM may also be regulated by interactions with heparan sulphate proteoglycans, large extracellular matrix proteins with a high degree of glycosylation.

The second major family of proteins involved in neural cell adhesion is the *cadherins*. Over ten cadherin molecules have been characterized in vertebrates, and there may be still other members of this family. Unlike NCAM, related cadherin molecules derive from different genes. A

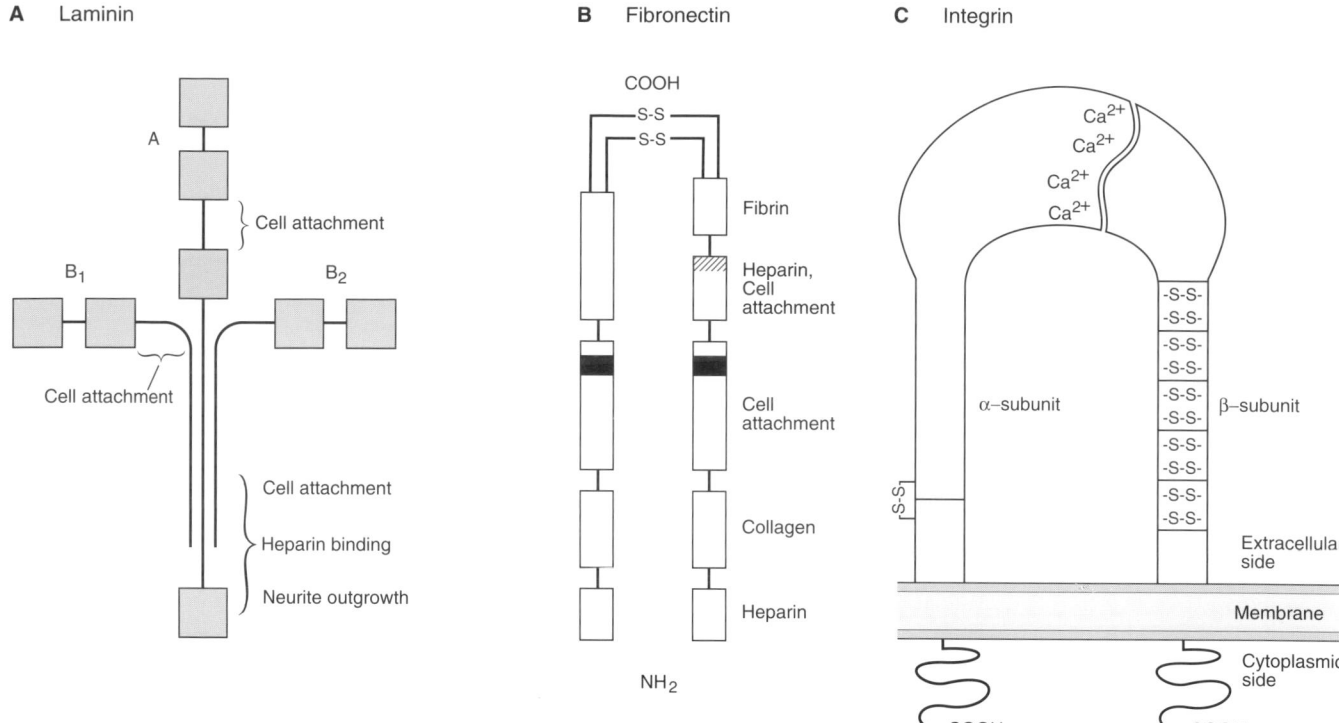

FIGURE 58–12

Some of the proteins that mediate cell substrate adhesion.

A. The extracellular matrix molecule *laminin* is composed of three subunits, termed A, B₁, and B₂. The diagram shows the domain that supports cell attachment, heparin binding, and neurite outgrowth.

B. The extracellular matrix glycoprotein *fibronectin* has multiple binding sites for cells, other extracellular matrix proteins, and proteoglycans. The approximate positions of these binding sites are shown.

C. Each *integrin* molecule consists of a heterodimer of one α- and one β-subunit. The β-subunit has extensive internal disulfide linkages (**-S-S**). The binding site for extracellular matrix glycoproteins is formed near the amino-terminal globular head of the protein. The binding of Ca^{2+} near the recognition site of each integrin is important for binding function. (Adapted from Nermut et al., 1988.)

major cadherin present within the nervous system is N-cadherin. N-cadherin, like NCAM, is expressed on most neural cells and mediates cell adhesion by homophilic binding. However, in contrast to NCAM, the binding function of the cadherins is critically dependent on the presence of Ca^{2+} in the extracellular environment. Calcium ions are thought to stabilize the cadherins by binding to a charged region in the extracellular domain of the protein. The cytoplasmic domain of cadherins is thought to bind to a family of proteins called catenins, which interact with the cytoskeleton. This association appears to be important for the adhesive properties of the molecule.

The cadherins appear to have a major role in the adhesion of neural cells. N-cadherin is expressed in the nervous system from the time of neural induction and is maintained by both neurons and glial cells after they differentiate. Adding N-cadherin antibodies to neural tissues causes them to disaggregate into single cells. Most neural cells express both of the major glycoproteins involved in cell-cell adhesion: NCAM, which mediates Ca^{2+}-independent cell adhesion, and N-cadherin, which is the predominant Ca^{2+}-dependent adhesion molecule.

The third major family of glycoproteins involved in neural cell adhesion are the integrins. Whereas NCAM and cadherins mediate adhesion between the surfaces of neural cells, the integrins mediate the adhesion of neural cells to glycoproteins in the extracellular matrix. The integrins consist of two noncovalently linked subunits, termed α and β (Figure 58–12C). Different α- and β-subunits are expressed by distinct cell types. The particular combination of subunits defines which set of extracellular and matrix proteins will be recognized by each integrin. Thus, in contrast to NCAM and N-cadherin, the integrins mediate adhesion between cells and their substrates through a heterophilic binding mechanism.

Fibronectin and laminin are the two most prominent extracellular matrix glycoproteins that interact with integrins and have roles in neural cell adhesion. Laminin is a large protein with a molecular weight of about 1,000,000 and is composed of three subunits designated A, B₁ and B₂ (Figure 58–12A). Two other laminin-like subunits have been identified, suggesting that there may be a family of laminin molecules. Laminin is a major component of the basement membrane in nonneural tissues and of the basal lamina in the peripheral nervous system. Fibronectin is composed of two disulfide-linked subunits, each of which has many distinct binding sites (Figure 58–12B). Fibronectin is secreted by fibroblasts and other mesenchymal cells and is also found in the peripheral nervous system, where it is involved in the migration of neural crest cells and possibly in the regeneration of damaged axons.

Many Glycoproteins Involved in Axon Fasciculation Are Members of the Immunoglobulin Superfamily

The biochemical and functional characterization of NCAM, the cadherins, the integrins, and extracellular matrix glycoproteins have provided insight into the mechanisms of neural cell adhesion. However, these molecules are expressed by virtually all neurons and there may be other molecules involved in the directed growth of axons. Surface molecules with more restricted distributions have been identified and may participate in more selective growth cone interactions with other axons. Many of these proteins also belong to the immunoglobulin superfamily (Figure 58–11).

Each of these immunoglobulin-like proteins has an overall structure that is similar to that of NCAM, with multiple immunoglobulin-like domains as well as sequences that resemble domains of the fibronectin molecule. Differences in the combinations of these glycoproteins expressed on different populations of neurons may be recognized by migrating growth cones and used to select the correct set of axons upon which to grow.

Axons Often Pause As They Project to Their Targets

The rate at which axons grow to their targets is not constant. Frequently the growth cone of an axon will grow for a brief period, then stop for as long as 24 hours before continuing. For example, the axons of chick motor neurons on their way to target muscles in the limb and the axons of thalamic neurons projecting to the cortex wait just before entering the target region. The reason why axons pause is not yet clear, but three suggestions have been advanced. First, the waiting period may permit cells in the target region to differentiate and acquire the molecular properties that enable the approaching axons to recognize appropriate target areas and synaptic partners. Second, the waiting period may reflect the time it takes growth cones to locate guidance cues in a complex environment. Third, waiting axons may form transient synapses whose function is important for subsequent development of neuronal circuitry.

Molecular Gradients May Help Axons Find Their Correct Location Within a Target Field

Once axons have arrived in the vicinity of their targets, they often arrange themselves in highly ordered connections within the target field. Sperry proposed that precise topography in axonal projections occurs because growth cones recognize molecules that are distributed in a graded manner within the target field. Experimental evidence to support this idea has come from studies of the projections of retinal ganglion neurons to their targets in the tectum.

As we saw in Chapter 28, the visual world is transmitted through the lens of the eye and projected as an inverted image onto the retina. The axons of retinal ganglion neurons themselves form an inverted map on the tectum. Thus, neurons in the dorsal region of the retina project to ventral regions of the tectum, while neurons in the ventral retina project to the dorsal tectum. Similarly, neurons in the nasal region of the retina project to the posterior region of the tectum, while neurons in the temporal retina project to anterior regions of the tectum.

Sperry and later Marcus Jacobson, Michael Gaze, and their collaborators studied the specificity of regenerating retinal axons that projected into the tectum after cutting the optic nerve and found that regenerating axons showed a high degree of specificity (Figure 58–13). However, since the tectum had previously been innervated by retinal axons, it was not clear whether the ability of retinal axons to regenerate the topographic map had any bearing on the events that occurred during the initial innervation of the tectum.

The precision of the initial projection of retinal axons has been examined in the frog, goldfish, and chick. In experiments on frogs using a variety of anatomical tracing techniques, Hajime Fujisawa, William Harris, Christine Holt, Scott Fraser, and their colleagues have found that the initial projection of retinal axons into the tectum is quite accurate along the dorsoventral axis, although it overlaps slightly along the anterior–posterior (nasal–temporal) axis. Similar studies in the developing chick show that the initial projection pattern is also reasonably accurate. As we shall see later in the chapter, axons that make errors in their projection and end up in inappropriate locations correct their initial projection or are eliminated.

How is the precision of the initial retinal projection onto the tectum achieved? Friedrich Bonhoeffer and his colleagues provided evidence that some retinal axons recognize a molecule that is distributed in a graded manner along the anterior–posterior axis of the tectum. When axons from the temporal (anterior) part of the retina are confronted in vitro with a substrate of alternating stripes of anterior or posterior membranes, the axons extend only on the anterior membrane stripes (Figure 58–14). Retinal axons choose anterior tectal membranes not because of some growth-promoting activity in the anterior tectum, but because the posterior membranes have a higher concentration of a repellent molecule. This repellent molecule is a protein of 33,000 molecular weight linked to the surface membrane by a glycosyl-phosphatidylinositol linkage of the type discussed in Chapter 4.

There is also evidence for an adhesive gradient along the dorsoventral axis of the retinotectal system. In addition, monoclonal antibodies have identified several molecules that have a graded distribution along the dorsoventral axis of the retina and tectum. One of these, a glycoprotein with a molecular weight of 47,000, named the

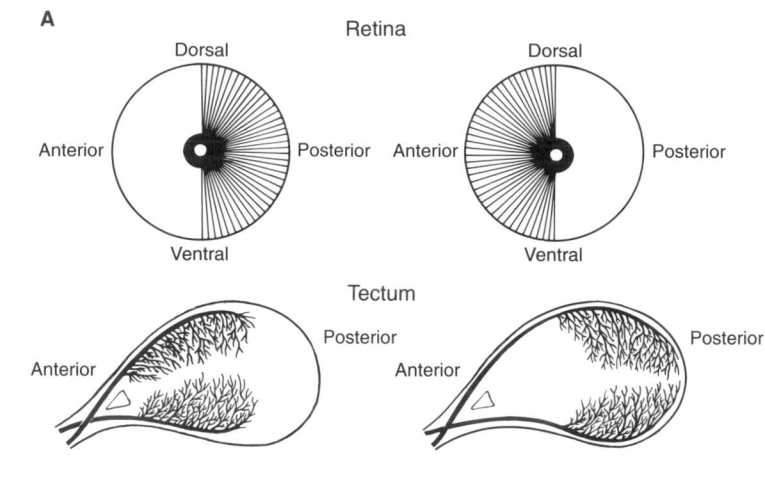

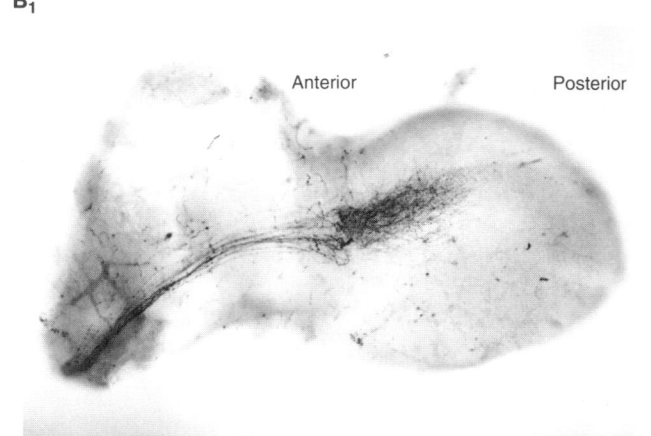

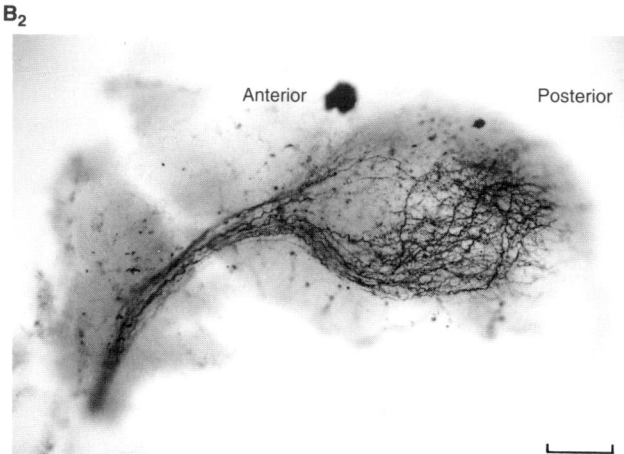

FIGURE 58-13

The axons of retinal ganglion neurons project to appropriate positions on the tectum during regeneration and early development.

A. In the adult goldfish the anterior or posterior half retinae were removed surgically and the optic nerve was cut. The course and termination of the regenerating axons were observed several weeks later using silver staining techniques to visualize retinal axons. Posterior retinal axons projected to the anterior tectum and anterior retinal axons to the posterior tectum. (From Sperry, 1963.)

B. Demonstration of the initial specificity of retinal ganglion axon projections to the tectum in the *Xenopus* embryos. Small regions of the retina were labeled with horseradish peroxidase, which is transported by retinal ganglion axons in the vicinity of the projection. Injections into the posterior retina (**1**) label axon terminals in the anterior tectum, while injections into the anterior retina (**2**) label terminals in the posterior tectum. Scale bar = 200 μm (From Fujisawa et al., 1982.)

TOP antigen, has its highest concentration in the dorsal retina and is also found in the ventral tectum (Figure 58-15). The TOP antigen is therefore a candidate for guiding axons along the dorsoventral axis of the tectum.

Molecular gradients therefore appear to guide axons to appropriate locations within the developing retinotectal system. The guidance of axons in this system can be controlled both by positive adhesive forces and by molecules that inhibit the growth of axons. Thus, the specificity of axon guidance may depend on a balance between the actions of these adhesive and repellent molecules.

Pruning of Axons Focuses Their Projection to Targets

We have seen that the migration of neuroblasts and the projection of axons to their targets can be quite precise and that molecules implicated in the guidance of growth cones have even been identified. Despite these guidance cues, however, some of the initial axonal projections are eventually eliminated. Maxwell Cowan, Giorgio Innocente, and their colleagues independently found that many neurons in the brain send axons to a much wider set of targets

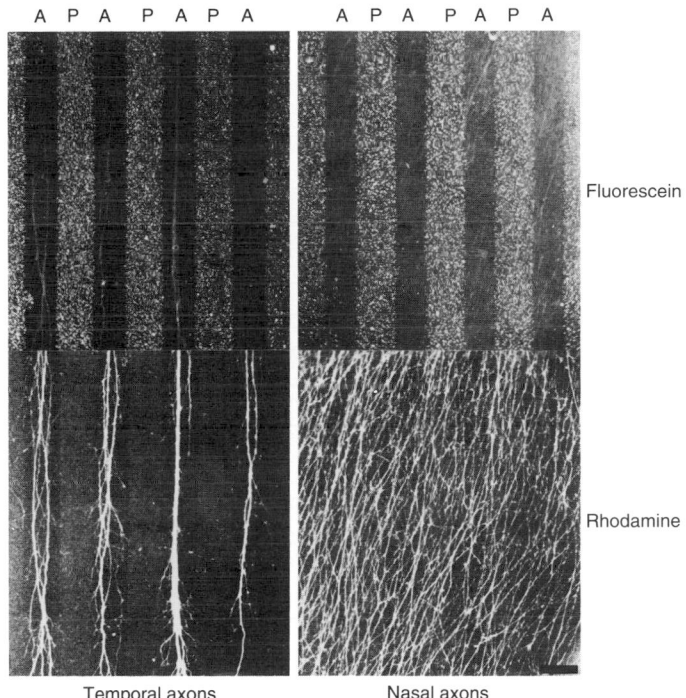

A P A P A P A   A P A P A P A

Fluorescein

Rhodamine

Temporal axons   Nasal axons

FIGURE 58–14

Retinal ganglion axons discriminate anterior and posterior tectal membranes *in vitro*. Membranes were prepared separately from anterior and posterior optic tectum from a chick and laid down on a suitable substrate in alternating, thin (90 μm wide) stripes. Fluorescent beads were added to the posterior membrane to visualize the stripes. The **top panels** show the alternating stripes of anterior and posterior tectal membrane viewed under fluorescent optics to visualize the beads in the lanes with posterior tectal membranes. Pieces of temporal and nasal retina labeled with a different colored fluorescent dye are then placed perpendicular to the stripes and allowed to extend axons. The **lower panels** show the growth pattern of temporal and nasal axons viewed under fluorescent optics. Temporal axons grow preferentially on anterior membranes and avoid the posterior membranes. In this assay nasal retinal axons do not discriminate between anterior and posterior tectal membranes. However, they will grow preferentially on posterior membranes that have been prepared in a different manner. (From Walter et al., 1987.)

than is eventually detected in the adult animal. For example, in young kittens axons that cross the midline in the corpus callosum project to virtually the entire visual cortex. Later in development these projections are focused to discrete areas of the cortex by elimination of many of the axons. The pruning of axons during development is a widely used mechanism for removing projections to inappropriate targets and for refining the specificity of axonal projections (Figure 58–16).

In many neurons the axon branches that are normally eliminated can be retained if other major axonal inputs to the same target area are removed experimentally. This finding suggests that there is competition between different classes of axons for particular targets. Competition between developing neurons regulates axonal branching patterns and also the formation of synapses and the survival of neurons. The role of competition in neuronal development is discussed more fully in the next two chapters.

The Initial Formation of Synaptic Connections Is Often Accurate

As we shall see in the next chapter, some synapses are eliminated or rearranged during later stages of development. There is evidence, however, that connections formed by developing axons can be specific from the outset and do not require subsequent rearrangement. The degree of specificity differs depending on the particular connection studied. One example of selectivity in the formation of connections between nerve and muscle has come from experiments by Sanes and Donald Wigston. They removed the superior cervical ganglion and transplanted intercostal muscles from different segments of the

FIGURE 58–15

Gradient of TOP antigen in the developing chick retina. Retinae from 14-day chick embryos were cut into pie slices, as shown in the top diagrams (the **black area** is the choroid fissure, which served as a reference point). The slices were then dissociated and incubated with a solution of radioactively labeled TOP antibody. The numbers within each slice correspond to the numbers on the abscissa of the graph. About 35 times more antigen was detected in the dorsal retina than in the ventral retina. (Adapted from Trisler et al., 1981.)

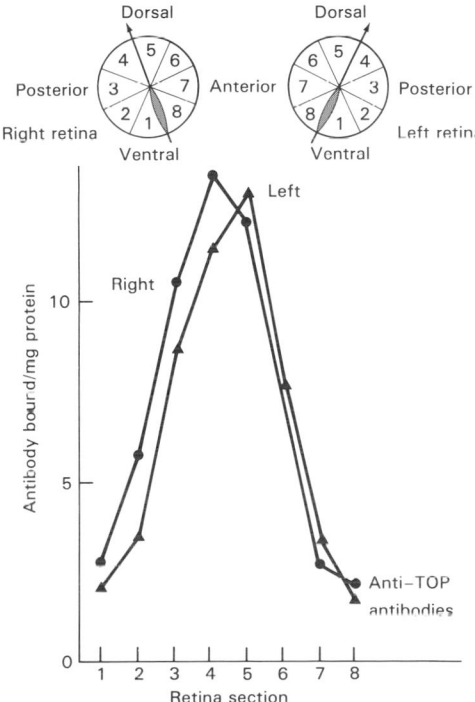

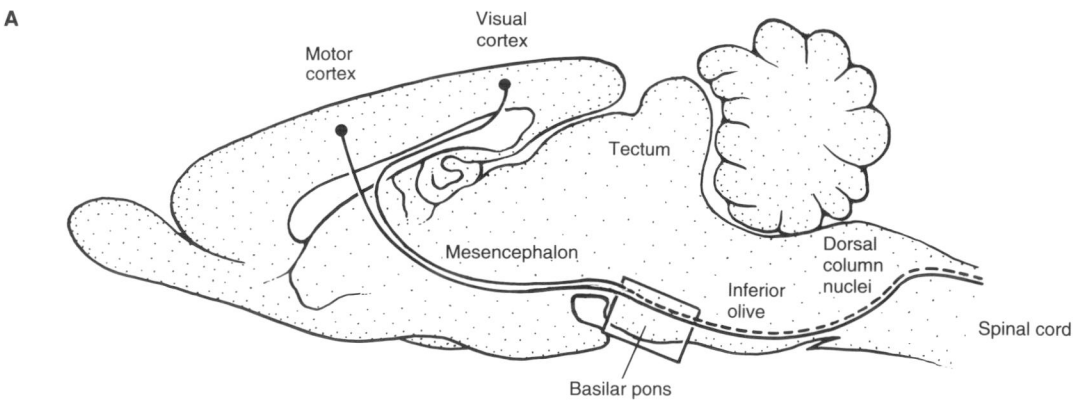

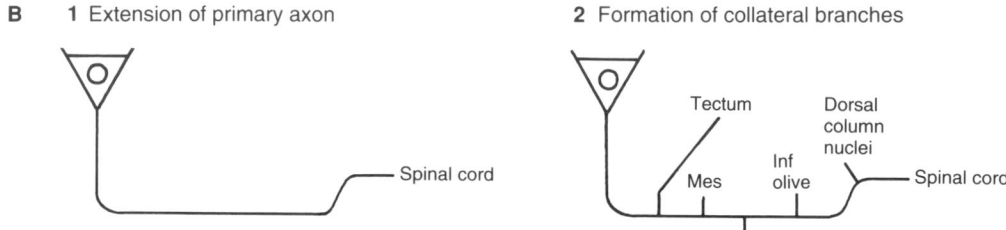

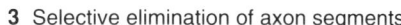

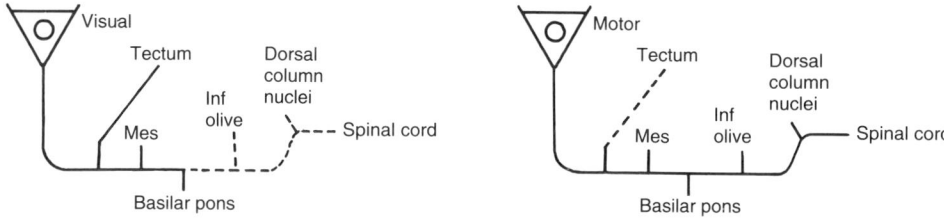

FIGURE 58–16

Branches of developing axons in the central nervous system are pruned during development.

A. Schematic, parasagittal view of the basic, subcortical trajectory of the parent axons that form the corticospinal and corticopontine projections. The pathway originating in the visual cortex is transient (the **dashed** part of trajectory) beyond the basilar pons.

B. Phases in the development of projections of layer 5 cortical neurons. **1.** The initial projection of the primary axon to the spinal cord is the same for neurons in both motor and visual cortex. **2.** The pattern of collateral branches from the primary axons is similar for neurons in motor and visual cortex. **3.** Neurons in the motor and visual cortex eliminate different branches, resulting in distinctive projection patterns at maturity. (Adapted from O'Leary and Terashima, 1988.)

body wall into the position of the ganglion. Presynaptic cholinergic axons at different segmental levels of the spinal cord were then stimulated and the number and strength of synaptic inputs to the target muscle assayed by intracellular recording. Presynaptic axons from a particular segmental level preferentially innervated the intercostal muscle from its appropriate segmental level rather than muscles from a different segmental level. This preference, however, was weak.

Additional evidence for selectivity in connections has been obtained at certain synapses between neurons, for example in the autonomic nervous system. Studies carried out by John Langley around 1900 demonstrated that sym-

pathetic preganglionic axons from different spinal segments would innervate postganglionic neurons in a positionally appropriate manner. The specificity of reinnervation was shown at a functional level by monitoring sympathetic responses to stimulation of individual ventral roots, which contain the preganglionic axons. For example, progressively more posterior regions of skin are activated by stimulation of progressively more posterior spinal cord segments. Moreover, when preganglionic sympathetic fibers reinnervate sympathetic ganglia after denervation, the resulting functional organization is reestablished, implying a high degree of selectivity in reinnervation.

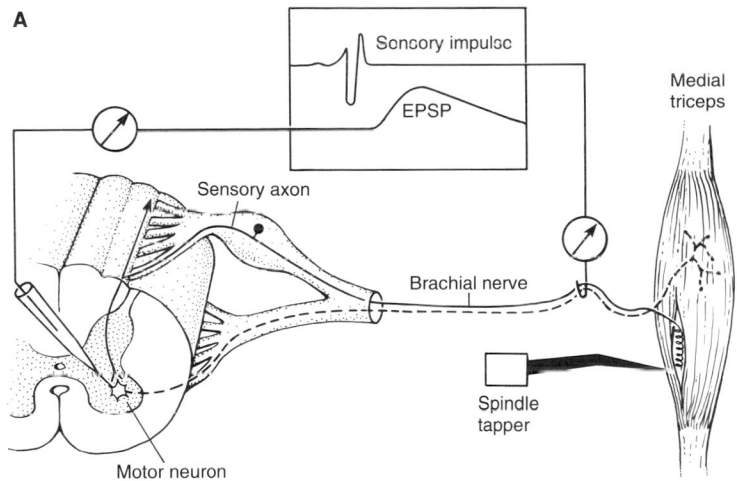

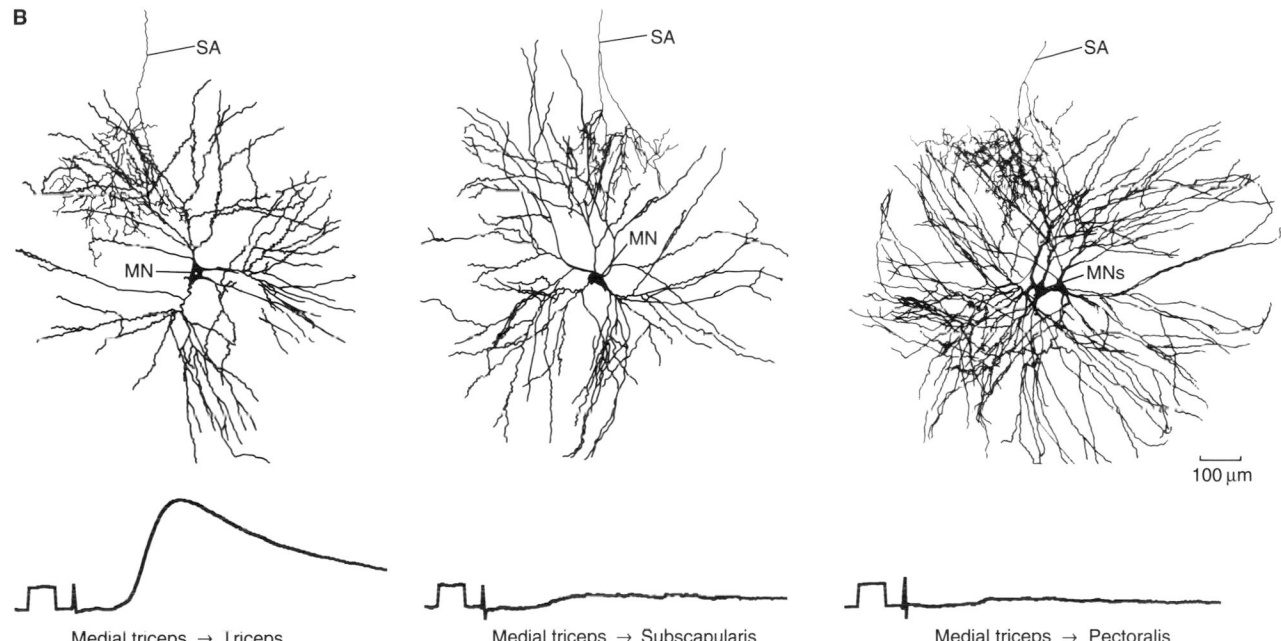

FIGURE 58–17

Developing muscle spindle afferents form specific connections with appropriate motor neurons. (Adapted from Frank et al., 1988.)

A. The preparation used to measure unitary excitatory postsynaptic potentials (EPSPs) in motor neurons is a hemisected frog spinal cord removed in continuity with the brachial nerve and the medial triceps muscle. Tapping a stretch-sensitive sensory ending in the muscle elicits an impulse that is detectable in the peripheral nerve. A simultaneous intracellular recording from a triceps motor neuron shows an EPSP elicited by the sensory impulse.

B. Reconstruction of labeled afferents and motor neuron dendrites. The terminal arbor of triceps sensory afferents (**SA**) overlap extensively with the dendrites of three different types of motor neurons (the triceps, subscapularis, and pectoralis). EPSPs elicited from medial or internal–external triceps sensory afferents are larger in synergistic triceps motor neurons than in subscapular or pectoralis motor neurons, even though all classes of neuron are located in the same region of the spinal cord. These results provide evidence that primary afferent fibers are able to select the appropriate subset of dendrites as synaptic partners.

Dale Purves and his colleagues have confirmed and extended Langley's original findings using intracellular recording methods. Purves's studies show that each neuron in the superior cervical ganglion is innervated by about a dozen different axons that arise from several adjacent spinal cord segments. However, each neuron receives its strongest input from one particular segment, and axons leaving the spinal cord at segments far removed from the dominant segment do not provide any inputs to the neuron. Moreover, when these preganglionic axons have been severed and reinnervate the ganglion the original pattern of connections is reformed. These regenerated connections are accurate from the outset. Similar studies have shown that the preganglionic innervation of other autonomic ganglia is also accurate from the time that initial contacts are made.

A similar specificity in synaptic connectivity can be found in the central nervous system. One synapse that has been studied intensively is the connection between the muscle spindle sensory afferent and the primary motor neuron. Eric Frank and his colleagues have found that in the bullfrog the muscle spindle afferents form the strongest connections with motor neurons that project back to the same muscle group from which the afferent derives. From the outset the developing muscle sensory afferent is able to form connections with appropriate target motor neurons amid a jumble of dendrites of inappropriate motor neurons (Figure 58–17). The specificity of connections made by sensory afferents with motor neurons in the spinal cord may be controlled by contacts already established between the peripheral end of the sensory fiber and the muscle.

An Overall View

The growth of developing vertebrate axons to their targets is dependent on guidance cues from cells and extracellular matrices with which the growth cones form contacts. The first clear evidence for this view emerged from the analysis of developing motor axons in the chick embryo. The demonstration that motor neuron growth cones recognize specific guidance cues refuted earlier proposals that axon outgrowth is a random process and at the same time marked a resurgence of interest in Sperry's concept of chemoaffinity. Studies of the retinotectal system have provided direct cellular evidence for selectivity in growth cone recognition. Through the use of *in vitro* assays, molecules that mediate neural adhesion and recognition have been isolated and characterized. Many of these proteins belong to multigene families, whose other members serve similar recognition and adhesive functions in nonneural cells. Chemotropism and contact-mediated inhibition have also been established as mechanisms of guidance.

Despite these advances, there are still deficiencies in our understanding of the mechanisms by which growth cones interact with their environment. Current approaches to defining adhesion and recognition molecules rely heavily on *in vitro* assays, and in most cases there is no clear evidence that these molecules operate in the same way *in vivo*. The molecular cloning of genes that encode neural adhesion molecules has, however, provided information on the function of these molecules *in vitro*, and in some cases has provided methods for assessing their role in developing embryos. It is also necessary to identify cell-surface and diffusible recognition molecules that at present are only inferred on the basis of cellular assays. Finally, we also need to gain a more detailed molecular understanding of interactions between adhesion molecules and to delineate signaling mechanisms in growth cones.

The existence of a variety of guidance cues does not,

however, prevent errors in axon navigation. Thus, in addition to molecular cues that actively guide the axon, there are mechanisms for eliminating axons that project to inappropriate targets.

Selected Readings

Bonhoeffer, F., and Gierer, A. 1984. How do retinal axons find their targets on the tectum? Trends Neurosci. 7:378–381.

Bray, D, and Hollenbeck, P. J. 1988. Growth cone motility and guidance. Annu. Rev. Cell Biol. 4:43–61.

Cowan, W. M., Fawcett, J. W., O'Leary, D. D. M., and Stanfield, B. B. 1984. Regressive events in neurogenesis. Science 225: 1258–1265.

Dodd, J., and Jessell, T. M. 1988. Axon guidance and the patterning of neuronal projections in vertebrates. Science 242:692–699.

Goodman, C. S., Bastiani, M. J., Doe, C. Q., du Lac, S., Helfand, S. L., Kuwada, J. Y., and Thomas, J. B. 1984. Cell recognition during neuronal development. Science 225:1271–1279.

Hunt, R. K., and Cowan, W. M. 1990. The chemoaffinity hypothesis: An appreciation of Roger W. Sperry's contributions to developmental biology. In C. Trevarthen (ed.), Brain Circuits and Functions of the Mind. Cambridge, England: Cambridge University Press, pp. 19–74.

Jessell, T. M. 1988. Adhesion molecules and the hierarchy of neural development. Neuron 1:3–13.

McConnell, S. K. 1989. The determination of neuronal fate in the cerebral cortex. Trends Neurosci. 12:342–349.

Mitchison, T., and Kirschner, M. 1988. Cytoskeletal dynamics and nerve growth. Neuron 1:761–772.

Patterson, P. H. 1988. On the importance of being inhibited, or saying no to growth cones. Neuron 1:263–267.

Purves, D., and Lichtman, J. W. 1985. Principles of Neural Development. Sunderland, Mass.: Sinauer.

Ramón y Cajal, S. 1911. Histologie du Système Nerveux de l'Homme & des Vertébrés, Vol. 2. L. Azoulay (trans.) Paris: Maloine. Republished in 1955. Madrid: Instituto Ramón y Cajal.

Reichardt, L. F., Bixby, J. L., Hall, D. E., Ignatius, M. J., Neugebauer, K. M., and Tomaselli, K. J. 1989. Integrins and cell adhesion molecules: Neuronal receptors that regulate axon growth on extracellular matrices and cell surfaces. Dev. Neurosci. 11:332–347.

Sanes, J. R. 1989. Extracellular matrix molecules that influence neural development. Annu. Rev. Neurosci. 12:491–516.

Smith, S. J. 1988. Neuronal cytomechanics: The actin-based motility of growth cones. Science 242:708–715.

Sperry, R. W. 1963. Chemoaffinity in the orderly growth of nerve fiber patterns and connections. Proc. Natl. Acad. Sci. U.S.A. 50:703–710.

Takeichi, M. 1987. Cadherins: A molecular family essential for selective cell-cell adhesion and animal morphogenesis. Trends Genet. 3:213–217.

Udin, S. B., and Fawcett, J. W. 1988. Formation of topographic maps. Annu. Rev. Neurosci. 11:289–327.

References

Bentley, D., and Caudy, M. 1983. Navigational substrates for peripheral pioneer growth cones: Limb-axis polarity cues, limb-segment boundaries, and guidepost neurons. Cold Spring Harbor Symp. Quant. Biol. 48:573–585.

Berlot, J., and Goodman, C. S. 1984. Guidance of peripheral pioneer neurons in the grasshopper: Adhesive hierarchy of epithelial and neuronal surfaces. Science 223:493–496.

Bridgman, P. C., and Dailey, M. E. 1989. The organization of myosin and actin in rapid frozen nerve growth cones. J. Cell Biol. 108:95–109.

Caroni, P., and Schwab, M. E. 1988. Two membrane protein fractions from rat central myelin with inhibitory properties for neurite growth and fibroblast spreading. J. Cell Biol. 106: 1281–1288.

Caroni, P., and Schwab, M. E. 1988. Antibody against myelin-associated inhibitor of neurite growth neutralizes nonpermissive substrate properties of CNS white matter. Neuron 1:85–96.

Caviness, V. S., Jr. 1982. Neocortical histogenesis in normal and reeler mice: A developmental study based upon [³H]thymidine autoradiography. Dev. Brain Res. 4:293–302.

Caviness, V. S., Jr., and Rakic, P. 1978. Mechanisms of cortical development: A view from mutations in mice. Annu. Rev. Neurosci. 1:297–326.

Chang, S., Rathjen, F. G., and Raper, J. A. 1987. Extension of neurites on axons is impaired by antibodies against specific neural cell surface glycoproteins. J. Cell Biol. 104:355–362.

Edelman, G. M. 1986. Cell adhesion molecules in the regulation of animal form and tissue pattern. Annu. Rev. Cell Biol. 2:81–116.

Edmondson, J. C., Liem, R. K. H., Kuster, J. E., and Hatten, M. E. 1988. Astrotactin: A novel neuronal cell surface antigen that mediates neuron-astroglial interactions in cerebellar microcultures. J. Cell Biol. 106:505–517.

Eisen, J. S., Pike, S. H., and Debu, B. 1989. The growth cones of identified motoneurons in embryonic zebrafish select appropriate pathways in the absence of specific cellular interactions. Neuron 2:1097–1104.

Forscher, P., and Smith, S. J. 1988. Actions of cytochalasins on the organization of actin filaments and microtubules in a neuronal growth cone. J. Cell Biol. 107:1505–1516.

Frank, E., and Mendelson, B. 1990. Specification of synaptic connections between sensory and motor neurons in the developing spinal cord. J. Neurobiol. 21:33–50.

Fujisawa, H., Tani, N., Watanabe, K., and Ibata, Y. 1982. Branching of regenerating retinal axons and preferential selection of appropriate branches for specific neuronal connections in the newt. Dev. Biol. 90:43–57.

Gaze, R. M., Keating, M. J., and Chung, S. H. 1974. The evolution of the retinotectal map during development in Xenopus. Proc. R. Soc. Lond. [Biol.] 185:301–330.

Goldowitz, D. 1989. The weaver phenotype is due to intrinsic action of the mutant locus in granule cells: Evidence from homozygous weaver chimeras. Neuron 2:1565–1575.

Goldowitz, D., and Mullen, R. J. 1982. Granule cell as a site of gene action in the weaver mouse cerebellum: Evidence from heterozygous mutant chimeras. J. Neurosci. 2:1474–1485.

Gundersen, R. W., and Barrett, J. N. 1979. Neuronal chemotaxis: Chick dorsal-root axons turn toward high concentrations of nerve growth factor. Science 206:1079–1080.

Harrison, R. G. 1910. The outgrowth of the nerve fiber as a mode of protoplasmic movement. J. Exp. Zool. 9:787–846.

Hatten, M. E., Liem, R. K. H., and Mason, C. A. 1986. Weaver mouse cerebellar granule neurons fail to migrate on wild-type astroglial processes in vitro. J. Neurosci. 6:2675–2683.

Heffner, C. D., Lumsden, A. G. S., and O'Leary, D. D. M. 1990. Target control of collateral extension and directional axon growth in the mammalian brain. Science 247:217–220.

Holt, C. E., and Harris, W. A. 1983. Order in the initial retinotectal map in Xenopus: A new technique for labelling growing nerve fibres. Nature 1:150–152.

Hunt, R. K., and Jacobson, M. 1974. Neuronal specificity revisited. Curr. Top. Dev. Biol. 8:203–259.

Innocenti, G. M. 1981. Growth and reshaping of axons in the establishment of visual callosal connections. Science 212: 824–827.

Kapfhammer, J. P., Grunewald, B. E., and Raper, J. A. 1986. The selective inhibition of growth cone extension by specific neurites in culture. J. Neurosci. 6:2527–2534.

Kuwada, J. Y. 1986. Cell recognition by neuronal growth cones in a simple vertebrate embryo. Science 233:740–746.

Lance-Jones, C., and Landmesser, L. 1981. Pathway selection by chick lumbosacral motoneurons during normal development. Proc. R. Soc. Lond. [Biol.] 214:1–18.

Lance-Jones, C., and Landmesser, L. 1981. Pathway selection by embryonic chick motoneurons in an experimentally altered environment. Proc. R. Soc. Lond. [Biol.] 214:19–52.

Langley, J. N. 1897. On the regeneration of pre-ganglionic and of postganglionic visceral nerve fibres. J. Physiol. (Lond.) 22:215–230.

Lankford, K., Cypher, C., and Letourneau, P. 1990. Nerve growth motility. Curr. Opin. Cell Biol. 2:80–85.

Lumsden, A. G. S., and Davies, A. M. 1983. Earliest sensory nerve fibres are guided to peripheral targets by attractants other than nerve growth factor. Nature 306:786–788.

McConnell, S. K. 1988. Development and decision-making in the mammalian cerebral cortex. Brain Res. Rev. 13:1–23.

Mendelson, B., and Kimmel, C. B. 1986. Identified vertebrate neurons that differ in axonal projection develop together. Dev. Biol. 118:309–313.

Nermut, M. V., Green, N. M., Eason, P., Yamada, S. S., and Yamada, K. M. 1988. Electron microscopy and structural model of human fibronectin receptor. EMBO J. 7:4093–4099.

O'Leary, D. D. M., and Terashima, T. 1988. Cortical axons branch to multiple subcortical targets by interstitial axons budding: Implications for target recognition and "waiting periods." Neuron 1:901–910.

O'Rourke, N. A., and Fraser, S. E. 1990. Dynamic changes in optic fiber terminal arbors lead to retinotopic map formation: An in vivo confocal microscopic study. Neuron 5:159–171.

Purves, D., and Lichtman, J. W. 1983. Specific connections between nerve cells. Annu. Rev. Physiol. 45:553–565.

Rakic, P. 1971. Neuron-glia relationship during granule cell migration in developing cerebellar cortex. A Golgi and electron-microscopic study in Macacus rhesus. J. Comp. Neurol. 141: 283–312.

Rakic, P. 1972. Mode of cell migration to the superficial layers of the fetal monkey neocortex. J. Comp. Neurol. 145:61–83.

Ramón y Cajal, S. 1892. Le rétine des vertébrés. La Cellule 9:121–246. In The Structure of the Retina. S. A. Thorpe and M. Glickstein (Comp. and Trans.). Springfield, Ill.: Thomas, 1972.

Raper, J. A., Bastiani, M. J., and Goodman, C. S. 1984. Pathfinding by neuronal growth cones in grasshopper embryos. IV. The effects of ablating the A and P axons upon the behavior of the G growth cone. J. Neurosci. 4:2329–2345.

Roberts A., and Patton, D. J. 1985. Growth cones and the formation of central and peripheral neurites by sensory neurons in amphibian embryos. J. Neurosci. Res. 13:23–38.

Rutishauser, U., Acheson, A., Hall, A. K., Mann, D. M., and Sunshine, J. 1988. The neural cell adhesion molecules (NCAM) as a regulator of cell-cell interactions. Science 240:53–57.

Sanes, J. R. 1989. Analysing cell lineage with a recombinant retrovirus. Trends Neurosci. 12:21–28.

Shatz, C. J., and Luskin, M. B. 1986. The relationship between the geniculocortical afferents and their cortical target cells during development of the cat's primary visual cortex. J. Neurosci. 6:3655–3668.

Speidel, C. C. 1941. Adjustments of nerve endings. Harvey Lect. 36:126–158.

Stuermer, C. A. O., and Raymond, P. A. 1989. Developing retinotectal projection in larval goldfish. J. Comp. Neurol. 281:630–640.

Taghert, P. H., Bastiani, M. J., Ho, R. K., and Goodman, C. S. 1982. Guidance of pioneer growth cones: Filopedial contacts and coupling revealed with an antibody to Lucifer Yellow. Dev. Biol. 94:391–399.

Tessier-Lavigne, M., Placzek, M., Lumsden, A. G. S., Dodd, J., and Jessell, T. M. 1988. Chemotropic guidance of developing axons in the mammalian central nervous system. Nature 336:775–778.

Tomaselli, K. J., Neugebauer, K. M., Bixby, J. L., Lilien, J., and Reichardt, L. F. 1988. N-cadherin and integrins: Two receptor systems that mediate neuronal process outgrowth on astrocyte surfaces. Neuron 1:33–43.

Trisler, D., and Collins, F. 1987. Corresponding spatial gradients of TOP molecules in the developing retina and optic tectum. Science 237:1208–1209.

Trisler, G. D., Schneider, M. D., and Nirenberg, M. 1981. A topographic gradient of molecules in retina can be used to identify neuron position. Proc. Natl. Acad. Sci. U.S.A. 78:2145–2149.

Walter, J., Henke-Fahle, S., and Bonhoeffer, F. 1987. Avoidance of posterior tectal membranes by temporal retinal axons. Development 101:909–913.

Walter, J., Kern-Veits, B., Huf, J., Stolze, B., and Bonhoeffer, F. 1987. Recognition of position-specific properties of tectal cell membranes by retinal axons in vitro. Development 101:685–696.

Weiss, P. 1941. Nerve patterns: The mechanics of nerve growth. Growth 5 (Suppl.):163–203.

59

Thomas M. Jessell

Neuronal Survival and Synapse Formation

The Survival of Neurons Is Regulated by Interactions with Their Targets

The Survival of Many Classes of Neurons Depends on Nerve Growth Factor

The Activity of Target Muscle Regulates the Survival of Motor Neurons

Synapse Formation Is a Gradual Process

The Presynaptic Nerve Terminal Triggers Biochemical and Morphological Changes in the Postsynaptic Membrane

The Distribution and Stability of Nicotinic Acetylcholine Receptors Change After Innervation of Skeletal Muscle

The Functional Properties of Nicotinic Acetylcholine Receptors in Muscle Change After Innervation

Other Components of the Nerve–Muscle Synapse Are Also Regulated by Innervation of Muscle

Innervation Changes the Contractile Properties of Muscle

Presynaptic Neurons Also Regulate the Development of Nicotinic Receptors in Neurons

The Postsynaptic Muscle Cell Regulates the Differentiation of the Motor Nerve Terminal

Some Synapses Are Eliminated During Development

An Overall View

The formation of contacts between developing axons and their targets is an essential step in the establishment of neuronal connections. Contact between a presynaptic neuron and its target is also important for the survival of the presynaptic neuron—if an axon does not reach its target the neuron often dies.

In the first part of this chapter we outline the evidence that the death of neurons is a widespread phenomenon during development and that the extent of cell death in a population of neurons can be increased by removing the target and prevented by providing additional targets. Neurons are dependent on their target because they require trophic factors that are supplied by the target tissue. Some of these trophic factors have been identified, and their role in neuronal survival has been analyzed. In this chapter we use the term *trophic factor* to indicate those factors that are essential for the survival of neurons as opposed to *growth factors* that promote cell division but which are not required for survival.

In the second part of this chapter we discuss the mechanisms involved in the formation and maintenance of synaptic connections in the nervous system. The contact of the axonal growth cone with its target cell triggers the formation of synaptic contacts. The maturation of these contacts involves the assembly of specialized structures in both pre- and postsynaptic cells. This process appears to be dependent on communication between the nerve terminal and its target.

The Survival of Neurons Is Regulated by Interactions with Their Targets

In invertebrates, such as the nematode *Caenorhabditis elegans*, the death of some neurons during development is genetically programmed and does not appear to depend on the environment of the neuron (see Chapter 57). However, in vertebrates the survival of neurons during development is critically dependent on interactions between the neuron and its target. Studies by Samuel Detwiler, Viktor Hamburger, and others in the 1920s and 1930s showed that the number of sensory neurons in the dorsal root ganglion of amphibian embryos can be increased by transplanting an additional limb bud. Conversely, the number of neurons could be decreased by removing the normal target. In these early experiments the difference in the final number of neurons was thought to result from an effect of the target on the proliferation and differentiation of sensory neuroblasts.

In the late 1940s this interpretation was revised when Rita Levi-Montalcini and Hamburger found that neuronal cell death occurred in normally developing embryos. An excess number of neurons is generated initially, and this number is eventually reduced by cell death so that the population of surviving neurons is matched in number to the size of the target. For example, more neurons survive in chick dorsal root ganglia that innervate a large target field such as a limb than in ganglia that innervate small targets such as the neck. Moreover, Levi-Montalcini and Hamburger showed that the extent of neuronal death was markedly enhanced when the target of the neurons was removed.

These studies were important for several reasons, but

their significance became appreciated only gradually. First, they established that the death of neurons is a normal and widespread occurrence during embryonic development, often resulting in the loss of up to half of the number of neurons initially generated. Second, they showed that alteration in the size of the neuronal target affects the survival of postmitotic neurons and not the division of neuronal precursor cells. This process of neuronal overproduction followed by death is now known to occur in almost all regions of the central and peripheral nervous systems and is usually referred to as *naturally occurring neuronal death*.

The Survival of Many Classes of Neurons Depends on Nerve Growth Factor

Shortly after Hamburger and Levi-Montalcini determined that target tissues have a role in regulating neuronal numbers, a former student of Hamburger, Elmer Bueker, performed experiments to determine whether implantation of various tumor tissues into mice might serve as a substitute for extra peripheral targets in supporting the survival of sensory neurons. Bueker found that the mouse sarcoma tissue evoked extensive growth of sensory fibers into the tumor. He also observed that dorsal root ganglia

FIGURE 59–1
Structure of nerve growth factor.

A. The prohormone (130,000 molecular weight) is cleaved into two α-, one β-, and two γ-subunits. (Courtesy of D. Ishii.)

B. The amino acid sequence of a monomer of the β-subunit, which is the active growth-promoting component of the larger protein precursor. (Based on Angeletti and Bradshaw, 1971; and Patterson and Purves, 1982.)

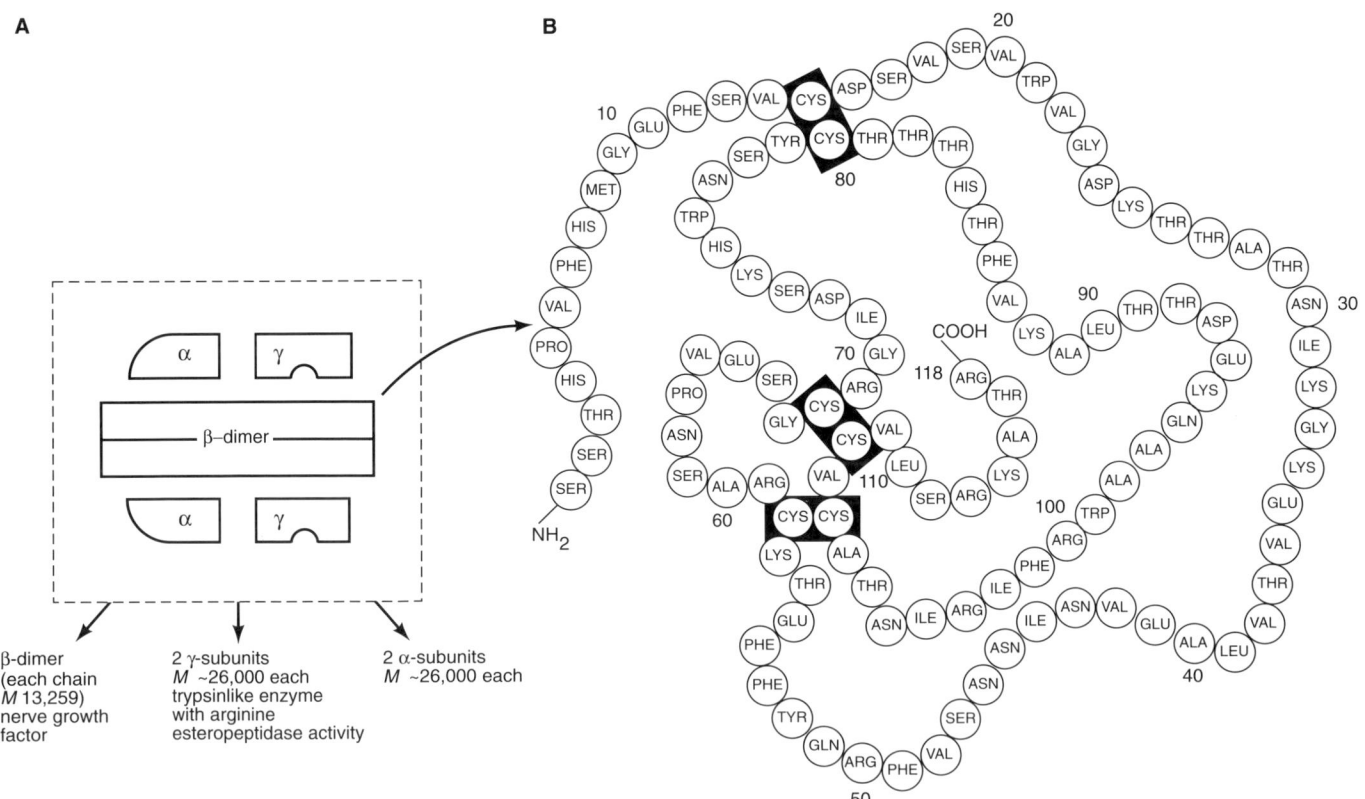

near the site of tumor implantation were significantly larger than the corresponding ganglia on the opposite side of the spinal cord. These experiments were extended by Levi-Montalcini and Hamburger, who noted a dramatic increase in the size of sympathetic ganglia in the vicinity of the sarcoma implants. Further studies showed that the effect of the sarcoma was caused by a diffusible factor. Levi-Montalcini developed quantitative *in vitro* assays to measure the effects of the tumor tissue on the survival and outgrowth of axons from sensory and sympathetic ganglia and together with Stanley Cohen started to purify the diffusible molecule, which by this time had been named *nerve growth factor* (NGF).

In a key experiment Cohen and Levi-Montalcini tried to rule out DNA or RNA as a source of the neurotrophic activity. They used a crude preparation of snake venom as a source of phosphodiesterase to degrade nucleic acids present in partially purified preparations of the factor. They found that the snake venom itself produced a far greater degree of axon extension than the NGF sample. Cohen then found that a mammalian counterpart of the snake venom gland, the male mouse submaxillary gland, contained a rich source of NGF. This fortuitous discovery provided an abundant source of NGF for purification and

protein sequencing. However the large amount of NGF in this gland is of unknown significance in neuronal development.

Purified native nerve growth factor exists as a complex of three subunits, α, β, and γ, in a stoichiometry of $\alpha_2\beta_2\gamma_2$, and a molecular weight of 130,000 (Figure 59–1). The active component is the 118 amino acid β-subunit, which exists as a homodimer in solution.

The membrane receptor for NGF appears to consists of two subunits. One subunit, termed p75, has a molecular weight of 75,000 and binds NGF with low affinity but does not transduce the biological actions of NGF. A second subunit, of molecular weight 130,000, is a transmembrane tyrosine kinase that was first identified as the *trk* oncogene. *Trk* also binds NGF directly and in a complex, and alone or with p75 may mediate the biological effects of NGF. The related proteins Trk_B and Trk_C appear to function as receptors for two other NGF-related neurotrophic factors, brain-derived neurotrophic factor (BDNF) and neurotrophin 3 (NT3), which are discussed later in the chapter.

Two key sets of experiments established the physiological role of NGF in the survival of sensory and sympathetic neurons. First, Cohen and Levi-Montalcini found

FIGURE 59–2

Nerve growth factor (NGF) antiserum treatment impairs the development of sympathetic ganglia in neonatal rodents. (From Levi-Montalcini, 1972.)

A. Cross section of a superior cervical ganglion from a normal 9-day-old mouse (**above**) compared to a similar section from a 9-day-old mouse injected daily since birth with NGF antiserum (**below**). The superior cervical ganglion of the treated mouse shows marked atrophy, with obvious loss of nerve cells.

B. Whole mounts of the stellate and thoracic sympathetic chain ganglia of control (**right**) and experimental (**left**) mice injected since birth with NGF antiserum and examined at 20 days of age. The sympathetic chain from the experimental mouse shows gross atrophy.

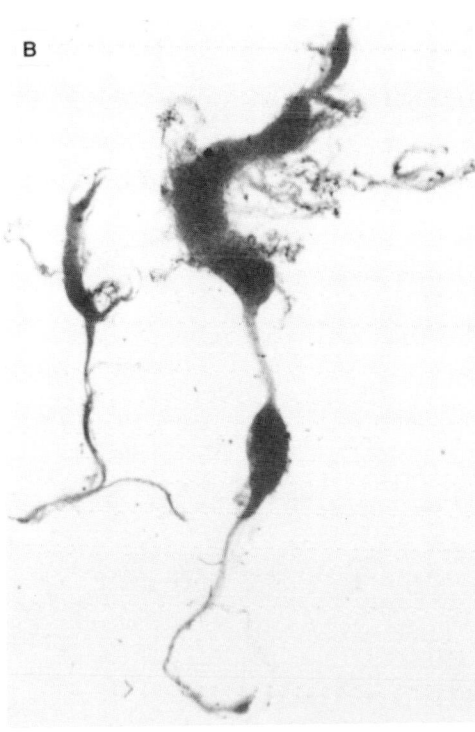

A

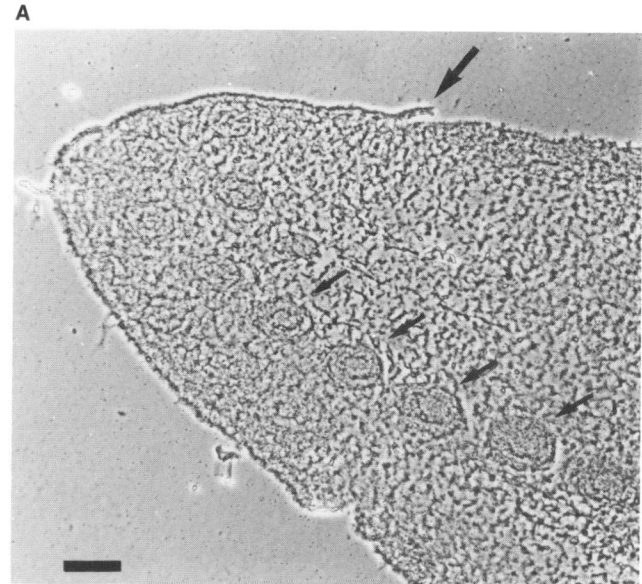

B

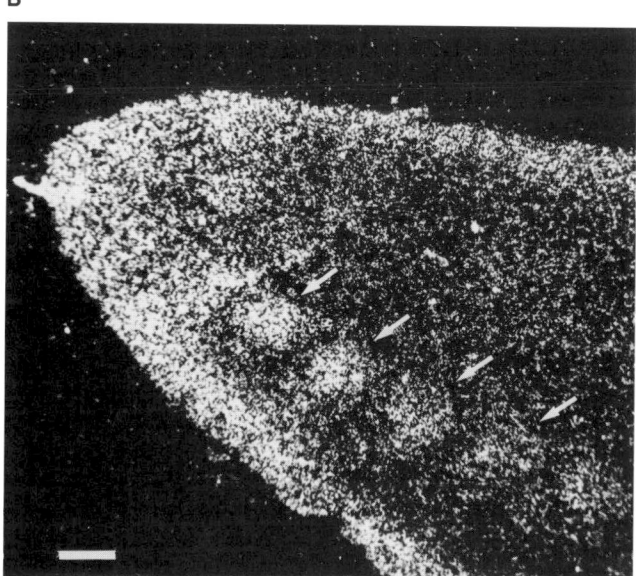

FIGURE 59–3

Nerve growth factor mRNA is localized in the whisker target field of the mouse embryo. *In situ* hybridization shows the distribution of mRNA. (From Bandtlow et al., 1987.)

A. This phase-contrast micrograph of a section is processed for autoradiography. High levels of mRNA are found near the sensory endings in the target field after the phase of neuronal death. Scale bar = 100 μm.

B. In this dark-field micrograph both the surface epithelium, the thickness of which can be seen by a small piece that has become detached **(large arrow)**, and the epithelial components of developing whisker follicles **(small arrows)** are densely labeled. The presumptive dermis, the mesenchyme just beneath the surface epithelium, is more densely labeled than the poorly innervated deep mesenchyme.

A

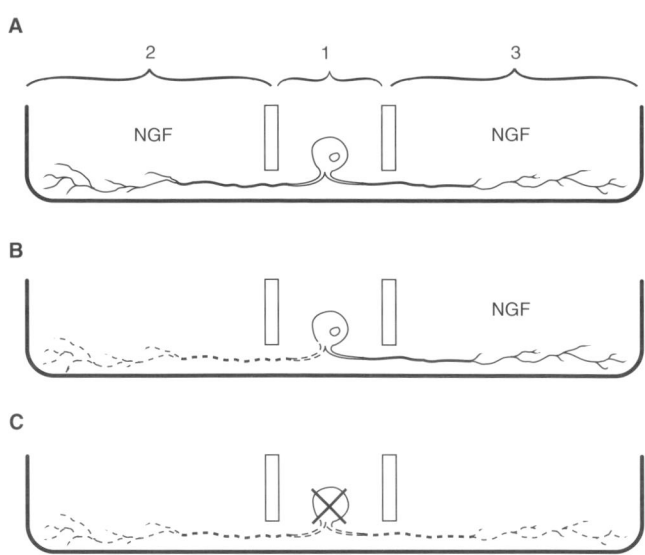

FIGURE 59–4

Nerve growth factor can influence the growth of neurites *in vitro* by a local action. Three sections of a culture dish are separated from one another by a Teflon divider, which is sealed to the bottom of the culture dish with grease. (Based on Campenot, 1981; and Purves, 1988.)

A. Isolated rat sympathetic ganglion cells plated in compartment 1 extend neurites along a collagen substrate, through the grease seal, and into compartments 2 and 3, both of which contain NGF.

B. Removal of NGF from compartment 2 causes local regression of neurites but does not affect the survival of neurons in compartment 2 or the growth of neurites in compartment 3.

C. Removal of NGF from all three compartments results in the death of neurons.

that when antibodies against NGF were injected into newborn mice and rats, the sympathetic ganglia almost completely disappeared (Figure 59–2). Nerve growth factor antibodies administered at earlier stages of development reduce the number of dorsal root ganglion neurons. Thus, both sympathetic and sensory neurons depend on this factor for their survival. Moreover, administration of large amounts of NGF to embryonic or newborn animals prevents the naturally occurring death of many sensory and sympathetic neurons.

The production of NGF by the targets of sensory and sympathetic neurons is critical to the survival of these neurons. Assays capable of detecting minute amounts of NGF protein and its mRNA have shown a correlation between the levels of NGF and the density of sympathetic innervation in target tissues. However, the total amount of NGF in even the most heavily innervated of these targets is very low (Figure 59–3), consistent with the idea that peripheral axons compete for a limited supply of trophic factor.

The binding of NGF to receptors on neuronal targets triggers various second-messenger pathways. As discussed in Chapter 17, NGF bound to receptors is taken up by nerve terminals (Figure 59–4) and transported back to the cell body. Interruption of retrograde transport blocks the effect of NGF and results in the death of neurons that are dependent on this factor. It is not clear which is crucial to neuronal survival: the transport of NGF itself or the second messengers that it activates.

Sensory and sympathetic neurons lose their dependence on NGF at later developmental stages, after target innervation has been stabilized. Although many adult neurons do not require NGF for their survival, they nevertheless remain sensitive to it. For example, NGF increases the synthesis of enzymes involved in neurotransmitter synthesis such as tyrosine hydroxylase in sympathetic neurons and the peptide transmitter substance P in adult sensory neurons.

Although NGF was originally purified on the basis of its trophic activity toward peripheral neurons, it has been found that certain neurons in the developing central nervous system are also dependent on this factor. In rats, for example, cholinergic neurons in the basal forebrain that project to the hippocampus and cortex die when they are separated from their cortical targets. In some cases the death of these neurons can be prevented by intraventricular injections of NGF. Moreover, many regions of the developing central nervous system, including the hippocampus, synthesize both NGF and its receptor. As discussed in Chapter 18, these findings may have clinical relevance, as the cholinergic forebrain neurons that respond to NGF in rats are similar to cholinergic neurons in humans that die in Alzheimer's disease.

Many neurons that appear to be dependent on their targets for survival are not supported by NGF. For example, NGF does not support the survival of parasympathetic neurons, spinal motor neurons, and sensory neurons that derive from ectodermal placodes rather than from the neural crest. Some sensory neurons that do not respond to NGF are instead supported by a factor named *brain-derived neurotrophic factor* (BDNF). Yves-Alan Barde and his colleagues purified brain-derived neurotrophic factor and found it to be a basic protein of molecular weight 12,300. A third member of this family, *neurotrophin 3*, (NT3) has also been identified by Barde and others. Neurotrophin 3 supports the survival of dorsal root ganglion neurons and proprioceptive neurons of the trigeminal mesencephalic nucleus. The primary structures of NGF, BDNF, and NT3 as determined by cloned cDNAs for these factors are very similar to one another. These findings suggest that the survival of diverse groups of neurons may be supported by different members of a multi-gene family encoding closely related but distinct polypeptides. Ciliary ganglion neurons in the parasympathetic nervous system are supported by a distinct factor with molecular weight 22,000 named *ciliary neuronotrophic factor* (CNTF) that bears no sequence similarity to NGF.

The Activity of Target Muscle Regulates the Survival of Motor Neurons

Many classes of neurons in the central nervous system also undergo naturally occurring cell death. The cellular interactions that regulate the death of central neurons

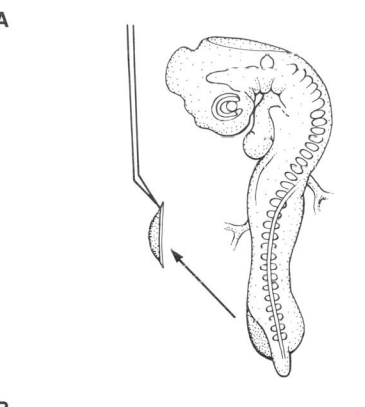

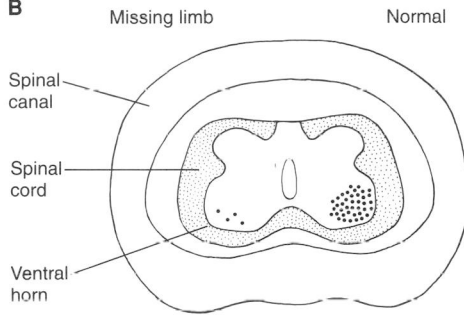

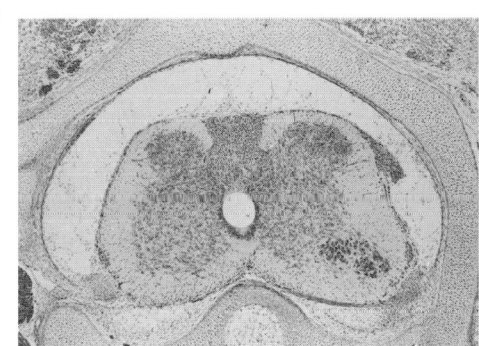

FIGURE 59–5

Removing a developing limb results in a marked decrease in the number of motor neurons. (Based on Hamburger, 1975; Purves, 1988.)

A. Limb bud amputation in a chick embryo at about 2.5 days.

B. Cross section of the lumbar spinal cord of an embryo 1 week following removal of a limb. Few motor neurons remain on the side of the spinal cord that normally innervates the hindlimb. The number of motor neurons on the contralateral side is normal.

C. Photomicrograph showing section through lumbar spinal cord of an embryo in which one hindlimb has been removed. A marked reduction in motor neurons is apparent on the operated (left) side.

have been best studied in the case of spinal motor neurons. Hamburger found that about 22,000 motor neurons are born during the development of the lumbar lateral motor column in the chick. Over the course of the next 5–7 days about 10,000 of these neurons die, after which the number of neurons remains constant. The role of the target in motor neuron cell death was first inferred from the finding that the onset of motor neuron cell death coin-

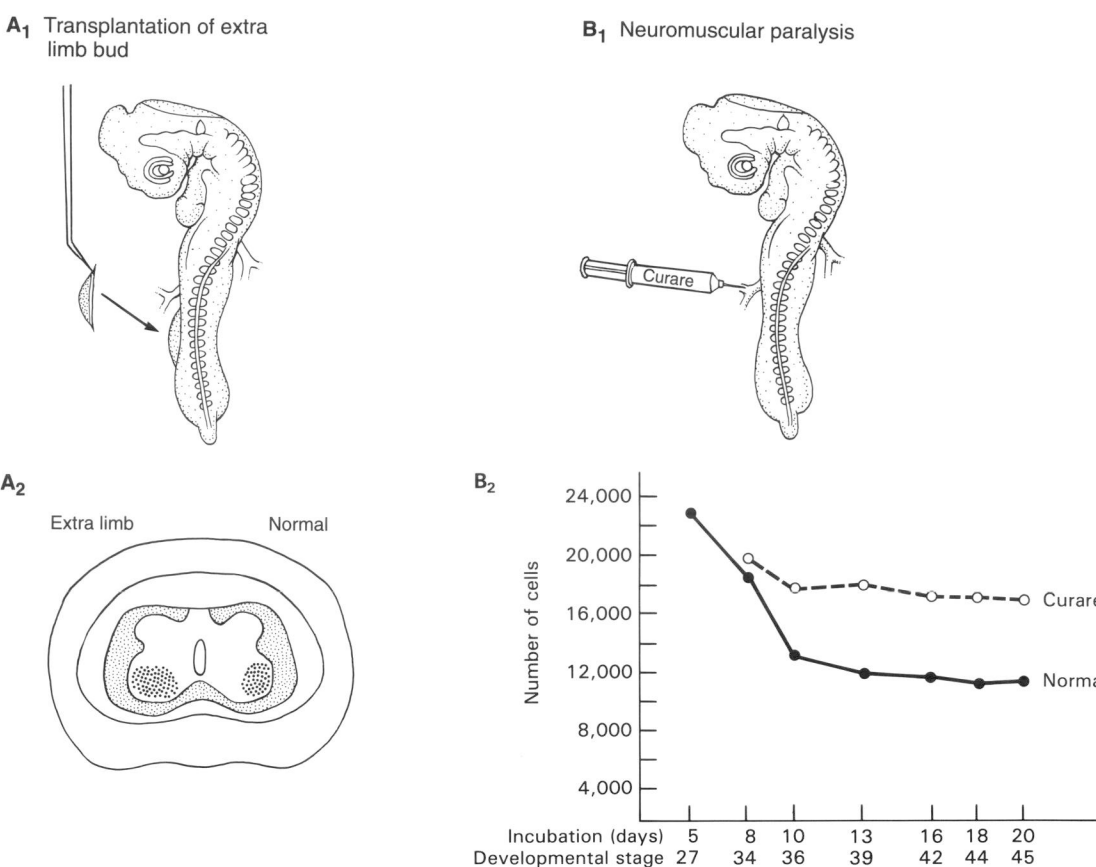

A₁ Transplantation of extra limb bud

A₂

Extra limb   Normal

B₁ Neuromuscular paralysis

Curare

B₂

FIGURE 59–6

Increasing the size of the target or preventing neuromuscular transmission reduces the extent of naturally occurring neuronal death during development.

A. 1. Transplantation of an extra limb bud prior to the normal period of cell death in a chick embryo. **2.** Cross section of the lumbar spinal cord in a late-stage embryo after limb transplantation, showing an increased number of limb motor neurons on the operated side. (Adapted from Purves, 1988.)

B. 1. Neuromuscular transmission can be blocked early in development by application of curare, a drug that blocks activation of acetylcholine receptors. **2.** Blockade of neuromuscular transmission with curare (day 6 to day 9 of development) reduces the extent of motor neuron loss. (Based on Purves, 1988; Oppenheim, 1981.)

cided with the time that axons reached their targets. Anatomical studies by Ronald Oppenheim and his colleagues have shown that nearly all motor neurons that die during development do so after reaching the vicinity of their target muscles. In addition, in experiments analogous to those on sensory ganglia Hamburger and his colleagues found that the number of motor neurons that died was increased by removal of the target and reduced by the presence of an additional limb (Figure 59–5 and 59–6). Thus, target muscle has a critical role in the survival of spinal motor neurons.

Why do some motor neurons die after reaching their targets? A widely accepted view is that motor nerve terminals compete with each other for a limited amount of an essential nutrient or trophic factor provided by the target muscle. Thus, eliminating the target eliminates the factor, and increasing the size of the target increases the supply. Although the identity of these factors is not known, there is considerable evidence to support the idea that trophic factors support the survival of spinal motor

neurons. For example, motor neurons removed from the embryonic spinal cord and grown in cell culture in standard medium die very rapidly, usually within 2–3 days. However, they can be kept alive in culture for weeks and sometimes months in the presence of muscle extracts or skeletal muscle cells.

These findings have focused attention on the mechanisms by which the supply of trophic factors to motor neurons is regulated. Oppenheim and his colleagues found that after initial synapses have formed the survival of motor neurons can be correlated with muscle activity. Blockade of neuromuscular transmission, with drugs such as curare, produces a dramatic increase in the number of motor neurons that survive (Figure 59–6). Conversely, direct stimulation of the muscle increases the death of motor neurons. There are two ways in which muscle activity may regulate survival of motor neurons. It could affect the production of the trophic factor by the muscle. That is, a blockade of activity would increase the production of the factor and an increase in activity would reduce production. If the supply of the trophic factor is normally limiting, further reduction will lead to a greater degree of motor neuron death. This view is derived largely by analogy with studies of the regulation of the supply of nerve growth factor, the best-characterized neurotrophic factor. Alternatively, activity may alter the ability of the motor nerve terminal to reach the source of the factor. The muscle-derived factors that promote the survival of motor neu-

rons have not been identified, although CNTF has been shown to rescue brain stem motor neurons deprived of their muscle targets.

Synapse Formation Is a Gradual Process

No matter how efficiently the processes of cell determination, neuronal differentiation, and axonal guidance are

A

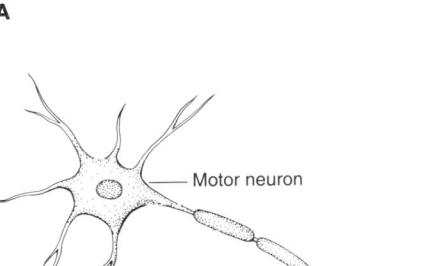

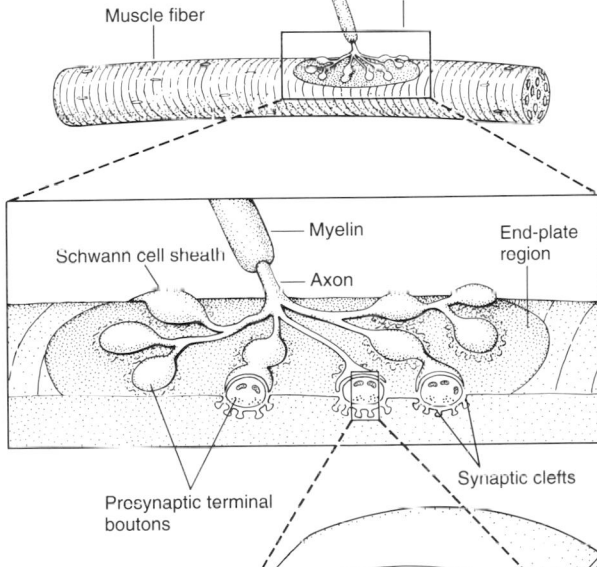

FIGURE 59–7
Organization of the mature vertebrate neuromuscular synapse.

A. Top panel shows the axon of a spinal motor neuron contacting a target muscle fiber. **Middle panel** shows the neuromuscular junction in greater detail. The axon terminal branches, giving rise to a complex terminal network consisting of numerous presynaptic terminal boutons ensheathed in Schwann cells. The **lower panel** shows a more detailed view of a presynaptic terminal bouton and the postsynaptic clefts. The presynaptic bouton contains clusters of synaptic vesicles concentrated around the active zones (**dark shading**) opposite the junctional folds.

B. Ultrastructure of the frog neuromuscular junction.
1. Electron micrograph of the presynaptic terminal (**top half** of photo) and the postsynaptic folds and contractile filaments of the muscle fiber (**bottom half**). The plane of section is the same as the lower panel in part A. × 29,400. **2.** A quick-frozen, fractured, and deep-etched image of a similar junction showing cytoskeletal elements and extracellular matrix material in the synaptic cleft and functional folds. × 42,000. (From Hirokawa and Heuser, 1982.)

B₁

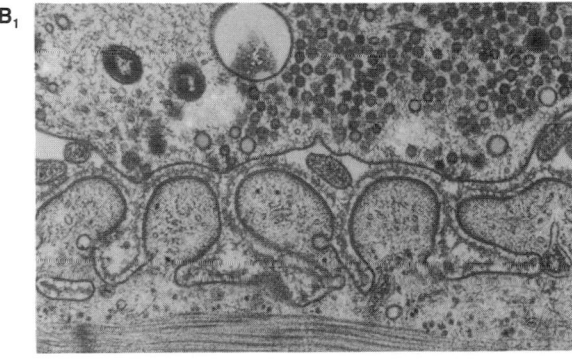

B₂

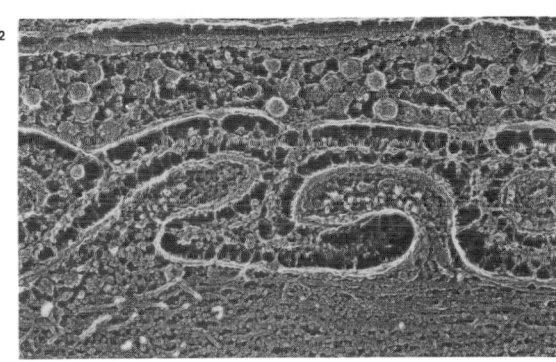

controlled, the nervous system cannot function effectively unless synaptic connections are formed with appropriate target neurons. For a synapse to function correctly, several key events must take place. First, the axon of a developing neuron must make contact with a postsynaptic partner, whether this is another neuron, a muscle cell, or a gland cell. Initial contacts between the growth cone of the neuron and its target cell must then be stabilized. This process of stabilization involves the assembly of specialized structures that permit the release of synaptic transmitter from the nerve terminal and its efficient reception by the target cell.

We shall first discuss the factors that control the functional organization of the synapse using the neuromuscular junction as a paradigm (Figure 59–7). We then discuss the evidence that some synapses exist only transiently and see how initial synaptic connections are modified and rearranged to give rise to the final connections of the nervous system.

Many of the steps in the formation, stabilization, and modification of synaptic connections are probably controlled in similar ways in different classes of neurons. Because not all synapses are equally accessible, however, our understanding of synapse formation is more advanced in the peripheral nervous system. For this reason, many of the details included in this chapter focus on the synapse between motor neurons and skeletal muscle—the best studied vertebrate synapse. Many of the features that have emerged from studies of the neuromuscular junction are likely to apply to synapses in the central nervous system.

When a developing motor axon first approaches a target skeletal muscle fiber, neither the axon nor the muscle cell is well equipped to participate in synaptic transmission. The axonal growth cone does not resemble a mature presynaptic nerve terminal, and the postsynaptic muscle mass has not yet cleaved to form individual muscles. Despite this, a primitive form of synaptic transmission exists from the moment the axon reaches the muscle target. This can be shown by recording intracellularly from embryonic muscle fibers. Spontaneous miniature end-plate potentials can be recorded from muscle fibers in frog embryos as soon as the motor neurons can be seen to project into the region of the muscle. The onset of synaptic transmission immediately after contact between the nerve and

muscle shows two important features of the early development of neuromuscular synapses. First, the presynaptic axon is capable of releasing its neurotransmitter, acetylcholine (ACh), before it makes contact with its postsynaptic target muscle. Second, the postsynaptic muscle membrane is capable of responding to ACh before it is contacted by the motor neuron. In support of this, ACh receptors have been shown to be present on muscle cell precursors that have not yet fused to form multinucleated myofibers.

The ability of growth cones to release ACh before they contact muscle has been demonstrated *in vitro*. By placing a patch-clamp pipette onto which is attached a small piece of muscle membrane rich in nicotinic ACh receptors near a motor neuron growth cone, it is possible to record the opening of individual receptor channels. These channels open when the patch approaches the growth cone, and the frequency of openings provides a sensitive measure of the spontaneous and evoked release of ACh from the growth cone (Figure 59–8). Thus, growth cones have the capacity to store and release transmitter before they contact muscle. The amount of transmitter released spontaneously and in response to an action potential in the growth cone is, however, very much less than that released by the mature motor neuron terminal.

Soon after initial contact between the motor neuron and muscle fiber, the amplitude of the end-plate potentials increases dramatically. This increase in transmission appears to involve changes in both the pre- and postsynaptic components of the synapse and occurs over a surprisingly protracted period of time—over three weeks in the rat. This process involves many different biochemical and morphological changes: the redistribution of ACh receptors, the appearance of acetylcholinesterase and a specialized basement membrane, a change in the metabolic stability and functional properties of ACh receptors, and changes in the number of nerve–muscle contacts.

The Presynaptic Nerve Terminal Triggers Biochemical and Morphological Changes in the Postsynaptic Membrane

The arrival of the motor nerve terminal triggers a dramatic series of changes in the properties of the postsynaptic

FIGURE 59–8
Motor neuron growth cones release ACh before they contact muscle. To demonstrate this an intracellular or extracellular electrode is used to stimulate the axon of a cholinergic neuron. The train of action potentials recorded from the neuron is shown in the trace on the **left**. A patch-clamp pipette containing a patch of skeletal muscle membrane is maneuvered close to the growth cone. The muscle membrane patch contains functional nicotinic ACh receptors. Acetylcholine released from the growth cone (either spontaneously or after electrical stimulation) interacts with the ACh receptors and opens channels, as shown in the trace on the **right**. (Based on Hume et al., 1983.)

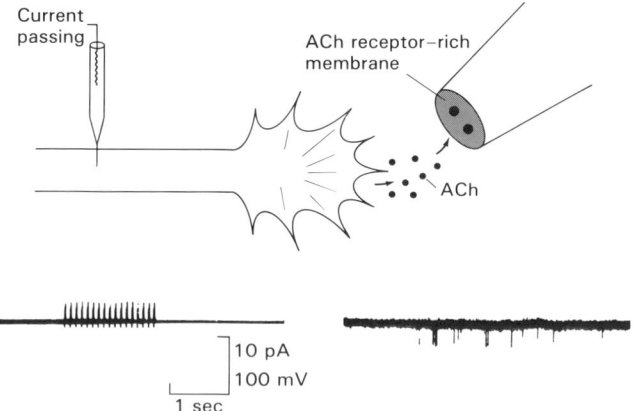

muscle cell. These changes enhance the efficiency and reliability of chemical transmission and the subsequent transduction of the end-plate potential into the contractile force of the muscle fiber. Here we discuss primarily those changes that affect chemical signaling between nerve and muscle.

The Distribution and Stability of Nicotinic Acetylcholine Receptors Change After Innervation of Skeletal Muscle

Before the arrival of the motor nerve, nicotinic ACh receptors are distributed relatively uniformly over the surface of muscle fibers. The distribution of receptors can be mapped physiologically by measuring the sensitivity of the muscle membrane to local ionophoretic applications of ACh with an intracellular recording electrode, or by measuring inward current flow with an extracellular electrode placed close to the muscle surface. The distribution of receptors can also be visualized using radiolabeled α-bungarotoxin, a snake venom protein that binds selectively and almost irreversibly to nicotinic receptors, or with monoclonal antibodies directed against extracellular regions of the receptor.

These labeling techniques reveal a dramatic change in the distribution of nicotinic ACh receptors after innervation of the muscle fiber. There is a large increase in the density of receptors at the site of innervation and a decrease in the density of receptors at extrasynaptic sites. By the time these changes are complete, the density of ACh receptors at the synaptic site is several thousandfold greater than at regions of the muscle membrane away from the synapse, approaching 20,000 molecules per μm².

In the past 15 years there has been considerable progress in understanding the molecular events that control ACh receptors in the postsynaptic membrane, in large part because of the establishment of tissue culture systems for studying the initial events of nerve–muscle synapse formation. Skeletal myotubes in culture can be innervated by spinal motor neurons and the resulting synapses recapitulate many of the events observed *in situ*. Using such culture systems, Gerald Fischbach, Monroe Cohen, and their colleagues found that a marked accumulation of ACh receptors on the muscle surface occurs precisely at sites of ACh release from the presynaptic motor axon.

By careful mapping of the distribution of ACh receptors on individual muscle fibers before and after innervation, Fischbach, Cohen, and their colleagues were able to show that synapses do not form at pre-existing clusters of ACh receptors. Instead, the nerve induces a new cluster of receptors at the site of ACh release (Figure 59–9). The accumulation of receptors at sites of transmitter release occurs by two mechanisms. First, there is a redistribution of pre-existing receptors that are already present in the muscle membrane. These receptors diffuse within the plane of the membrane and become immobilized at the synaptic site. Second, there is an increase in the synthesis of new receptors, which are inserted into the local muscle mem-

brane at or near to the synaptic site. These results indicate that the nerve terminal controls both the synthesis and distribution of receptors on the postsynaptic membrane.

The influence of the nerve on ACh receptor distribution is mediated by diffusible factors released by the presynaptic nerve terminal. Acetylcholine itself is not the molecule responsible for the clustering of ACh receptors—ACh receptors do not cluster in response to local application of ACh and receptor clustering can occur when all ACh receptors are blocked by drugs such as curare. Three molecules that are likely to contribute to the nerve-induced clustering of receptors at synaptic sites have now been identified. First, Fischbach and his col-

FIGURE 59–9

The presynaptic neuron induces clustering of ACh receptors on skeletal myotubes. (Adapted from Frank and Fischbach, 1979.)

A. A cholinergic axon approaches a skeletal muscle fiber that expresses ACh receptors. Most of the preexisting receptors are diffusely distributed but some already exist in clusters (not shown).

B. After the nerve contacts and grows along the muscle fiber, sites of transmitter release can be identified by focal extracellular recording of nerve evoked currents. The sites of transmitter release from the nerve do not coincide with the preexisting clusters of ACh receptors.

C. Some time after the nerve begins to release transmitter, ACh receptor clusters are localized to the site of transmitter release.

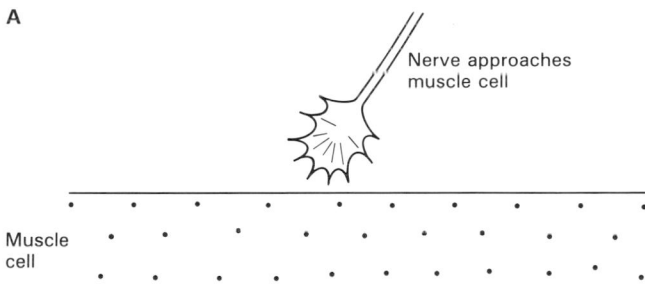

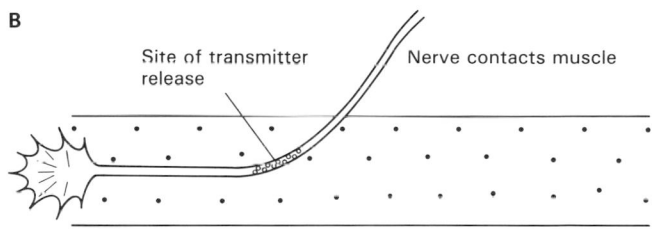

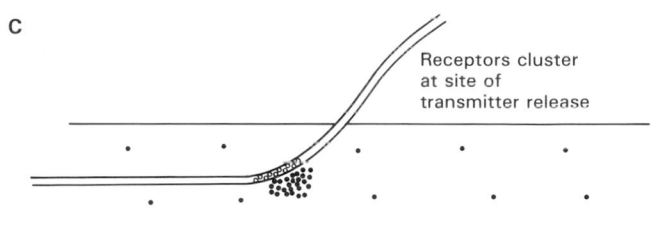

A

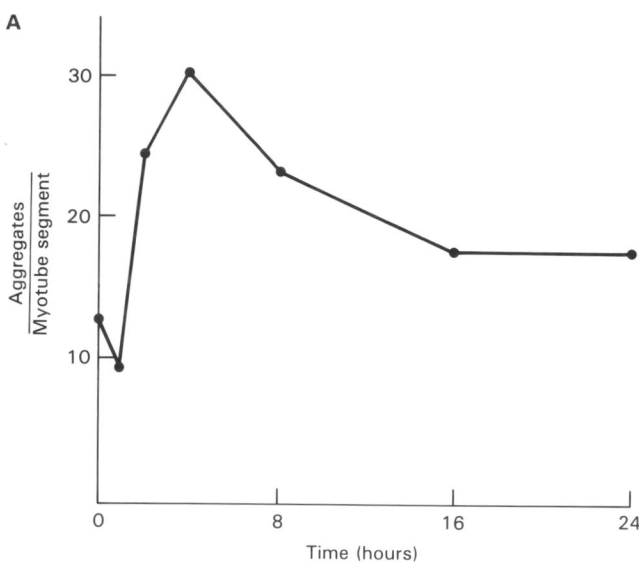

B₁

B₂

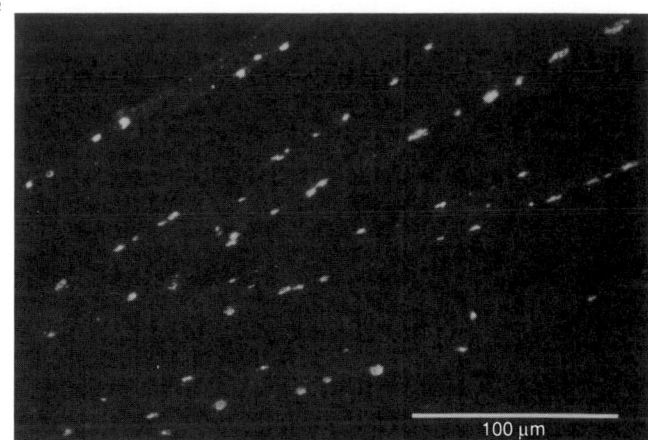

100 μm

FIGURE 59–10

The protein agrin induces the clustering of ACh receptors on the muscle membrane. (From McMahan and Wallace, 1989.)

A. Application of agrin causes the rapid formation of a large number of ACh receptor clusters; the number of aggregates declines to a plateau although the size of each aggregate increases. Receptors were identified using rhodamine–α-bungarotoxin and visualized by fluorescence microscopy.

B. Agrin-containing extracts of the electric organ of the *Torpedo* fish cause the formation of aggregates of ACh receptors on chick myotubes in culture. Fluorescence micrographs show the control culture (**1**) and the culture treated overnight with agrin-containing extracts (**2**).

leagues have purified a 43,000 molecular weight protein named ARIA (acetylcholine receptor inducing activity) that produces an increase in both the total number of ACh receptors on the muscle surface and the number of receptor clusters. Second, Jack McMahan and his colleagues have characterized a 200,000 molecular weight protein named agrin that is localized in the synaptic basal lamina and causes the clustering of pre-existing receptors. Agrin also causes the clustering of several other post-synaptic membrane components, including acetylcholinesterase, suggesting that it coordinately regulates the assembly of the motor end-plate (Figure 59–10). Third, calcitonin gene-related peptide (CGRP), a peptide that is synthesized by motor neurons, increases the number of ACh receptors on the muscle surface, apparently by activating cAMP within the muscle cell. Anatomical studies have shown that ARIA, agrin, and CGRP are expressed in motor neurons in the spinal cord (Figure 59–11). Thus, motor nerve terminals release several molecules that regulate ACh receptors on the muscle surface.

Concomitant with the appearance of ACh receptor clusters at the synapse, extrasynaptic receptors disappear. The loss of extrajunctional ACh receptors is controlled by a mechanism distinct from that responsible for the clustering of receptors at synaptic sites. Studies by several groups have shown that the expression of extrajunctional receptors during normal development is regulated by the level of electrical activity of the muscle. If mature muscle is denervated there is a gradual appearance of ACh receptors at extrajunctional sites. Terye Lømo and Jean Rosenthal found that the appearance of extrajunctional receptors after denervation can be suppressed if the muscle is activated by direct electrical stimulation at a frequency similar to that of innervated muscle. These and other experiments indicate that the loss of extrajunctional receptors during the initial innervation of muscle is due to an activity-dependent suppression in the synthesis of ACh receptors in extrajunctional regions.

This observation raises the question of how ACh receptor synthesis is controlled in different regions of the muscle fiber. Since there are many nuclei within a single muscle fiber, the synthesis of ACh receptor mRNA may be controlled independently by individual nuclei. In support of this, Jean Pierre Changeux, Walter Gilbert, and their colleagues have independently shown, by *in situ* hybridization histochemistry, that nuclei in synaptic regions synthesize higher levels of receptor subunit mRNA than nuclei in nonsynaptic areas.

The Functional Properties of Nicotinic Acetylcholine Receptors in Muscle Change After Innervation

The motor nerve terminal triggers many other changes in the properties of the postsynaptic receptor. First, ACh receptors at junctional sites lose their ability to diffuse in the plane of the membrane and gradually become fixed at the site of the synapse. Second, ACh receptors at junctional sites have a much longer half-life than extrajunctional receptors. Steven Burden found that receptors at newly formed end-plates in embryonic chicks have a half-life of about 24 hours, which is similar to that of extrajunctional receptors. With increasing time after synapse formation, junctional receptors become more stable, turning over with a half-life of about 120 hours, whereas extrajunctional receptors are not stabilized. The time at which the lateral mobility of junctional receptors decreases coincides with the onset of receptor stabilization.

There are also striking changes in the functional properties of nicotinic ACh receptors after skeletal muscle is innervated. Acetylcholine receptor channels in embryonic rat muscle have a relatively small conductance (about 30 pS) but remain open for long periods (about 5–10 ms) and have therefore been termed slow channels. In contrast, junctional receptors at mature end-plates have a significantly larger conductance (about 50 pS) but remain open for a much shorter period (usually only about 1 ms) and are called fast channels. By monitoring the fraction of these two classes of channels present during the development of end-plates in rat muscles, Bert Sakmann and his colleagues and Fischbach and Stephen Schuetze found that the number of embryonic channels decreases gradually after innervation. The appearance of fast channels can be prevented if muscle is denervated, indicating that the nerve is important in evoking this change in channel properties.

The change in channel properties of ACh receptors at embryonic and mature end-plates results from a change in the subunit composition of ACh receptor. Shosaku Numa and colleagues found that the subunit composition of embryonic receptors is α_2, β, γ, and δ. Numa and colleagues identified a novel ACh receptor subunit in bovine muscle, termed ε subunit, that closely resembles the γ-subunit. Acetylcholine receptors on embryonic muscle contain the γ-subunit, whereas ACh receptors in adult muscle contain

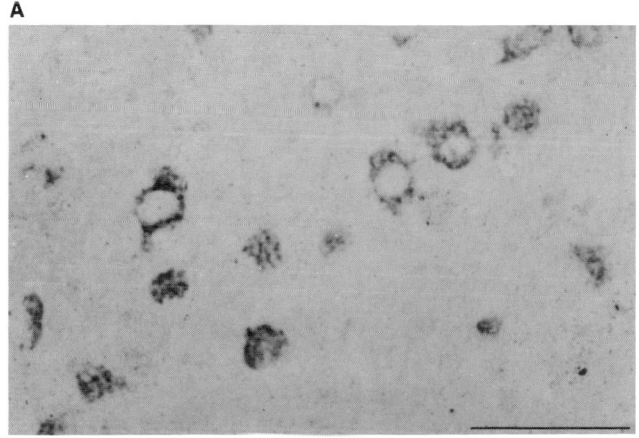

A

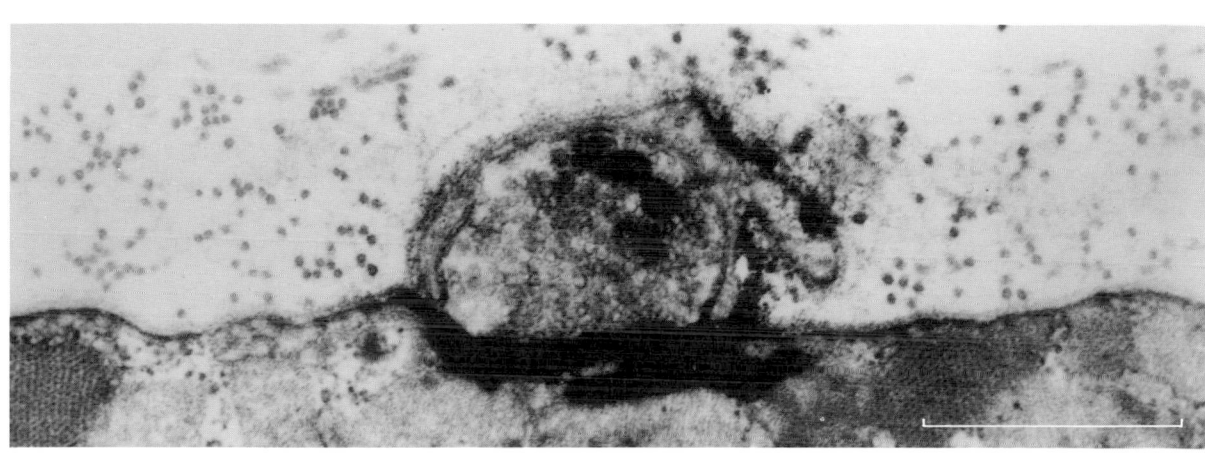

B

FIGURE 59–11

Localization of agrin in motor neurons and the synaptic cleft. (From McMahan and Wallace, 1989.)

A. The localization of agrin mRNA by *in situ* hybridization histochemistry in the cell bodies of frog motor neurons in the spinal cord is shown in this micrograph. Scale bar = 100 μm.

B. Agrin is present at high density in the synaptic cleft but not at extrasynaptic sites. The localization of agrin was determined by electron microscopic immunocytochemistry using anti-agrin antibodies. Scale bar = 1 μm.

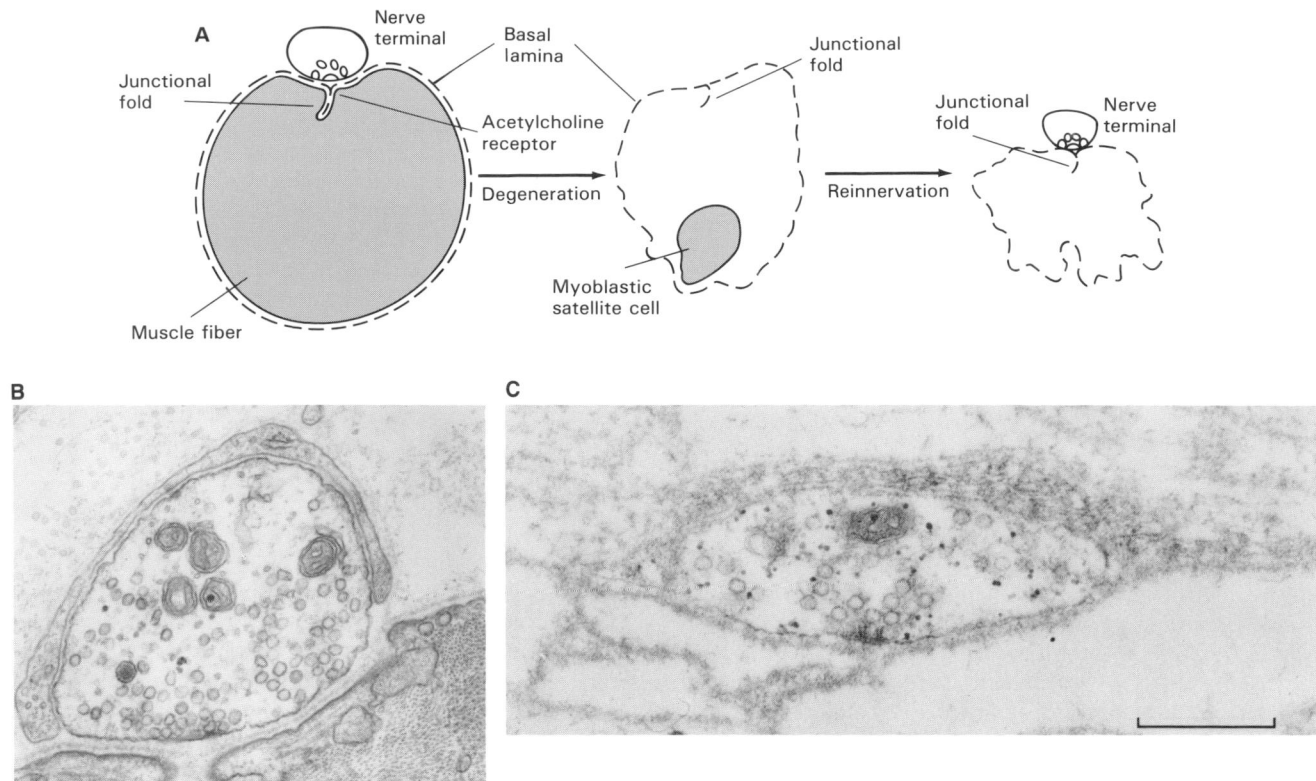

FIGURE 59–12

Reinnervation of damaged muscle occurs at the old synaptic site.

A. Synaptic basal lamina has a role in synaptic regeneration at the frog neuromuscular junction. Nerve terminals (**N**) and muscle fibers (**M**) degenerate when they are injured, but the basal lamina (**BL**) sheath of the muscle fiber persists. Myotubes regenerate from myoblast satellite cells (**Mb**) within the basal lamina but are prevented from doing so by x-irradiation. Axons that regenerate in the absence of myotubes contact the basal lamina at original synaptic sites and form active zones opposite tails of basal lamina that mark the sites where mouths of junctional folds (**F**) once were. (**R**, acetylcholine-receptor-rich postsynaptic membrane.) (From McMahan and Wallace, 1989.)

B. Terminal and preterminal portions of axons in frog muscle. Electron micrographs of a nerve terminal at a normal adult neuromuscular junction. An active zone in the terminal apposes a junctional fold in the postsynaptic membrane. (From Glicksman and Sanes, 1983.)

C. Electron micrograph of a nerve terminal reinnervating a muscle fiber basal lamina after the muscle was damaged and denervated. The regenerating axon has contacted the basal lamina sheath at an original synaptic site which is marked by the basal lamina tail that once lined the junctional fold. The presynaptic terminal contains synaptic vesicles and an active zone at this site. This provides evidence that the synaptic basal lamina may organize the presynaptic nerve terminal. (From McMahan and Wallace, 1989.)

the ε-subunit. When mixtures of α-, β-, γ-, and δ-subunit mRNAs are injected into *Xenopus* oocytes, the expressed channels have the properties of embryonic receptors. When transcripts encoding the ε-subunit are substituted for the γ-subunit, the resulting channels have the properties of adult receptors. This switch in subunit composition is likely to contribute in large part to the developmental change in end-plate channel properties.

The transition in channel properties during development may ensure that synaptic transmission works efficiently at all stages of maturation of the synapse. Soon after initial contact, the amount of transmitter released is low and the postsynaptic membrane is relatively unspecialized. The presence of channels with large open times results in a large current flow, sufficient to ensure muscle contraction. In contrast, at mature synapses the presence of channels with brief open times may help maintain the stimulus-response relationship between motor neuron firing and muscle contraction.

Other Components of the Nerve–Muscle Synapse Are Also Regulated by Innervation of Muscle

So far we have focused on the role of the motor neuron in regulating the distribution and properties of postsynaptic ACh receptors. However, for synapses to function effectively, many other features of the synapse need to be controlled in step with the development of ACh receptors. For example, the basal lamina, the extracellular matrix that is interposed between the presynaptic terminal and the muscle surface, is highly specialized at synaptic sites. It consists of a complex mixture of structural components, such as collagens and proteoglycans, which are present both in the region of the end plate and at extrajunctional regions.

The function of the synaptic basal lamina has been studied by McMahan and his colleagues. McMahan found that cut motor axons will regrow to their old synaptic sites and form new synapses precisely at the location of the original synapse (Figure 59–12). The ability of the motor axon to relocate the original synaptic site is independent of cues provided by the postsynaptic muscle fiber or by nearby Schwann cells. By elimination, the only guidance cue left for the ingrowing axon is the basal lamina at the old synaptic site.

Molecules associated with the synaptic basal lamina may play critical roles in guiding the regenerating motor axon back to its original location and in ensuring that ACh receptors remain at the site of the regenerating synapse. Recognition of the basal lamina by the ingrowing nerve terminal may depend on specific glycoproteins found primarily or exclusively at synaptic sites. Many of these extracellular glycoproteins are thought to be involved in the formation and operation of neuromuscular synapses.

One such molecule is a large polypeptide called s-laminin. This molecule was isolated and characterized by John Merlie and Joshua Sanes and shown to be a protein that is closely related to the B_1 chain of the extracellular matrix glycoprotein laminin discussed in the previous chapter. Although the structures of s-laminin and the laminin B_1 chain are closely related, these two proteins may have distinct functions. Fragments of s-laminin promote the adhesion of cholinergic neurons from the ciliary ganglion but, unlike laminin, do not promote the outgrowth of axons from these neurons. Thus, the restricted distribution of s-laminin at synaptic sites may act as a stop signal, instructing the incoming motor axon to adhere but not to extend further.

Innervation Changes the Contractile Properties of Muscle

Mammals have two classes of muscles that can be distinguished on the basis of color and speed of contraction: fast (pale) and slow (red). Fast muscles (also called twitch muscles) depend on glycolytic metabolism, whereas slow muscles, rich in myoglobin, depend on aerobic respiration. Fast muscles are involved in phasic contractions; slow muscles are involved in postural adjustment. John Eccles found that motor neurons and muscles have matching properties. Motor neurons that innervate fast muscles have a rapid conduction velocity and a brief hyperpolarizing afterpotential and can therefore fire rapidly, at 30–60 impulses per second. Motor neurons that innervate slow muscles conduct slowly and have a larger afterpotential and thus fire more slowly, at 10–20 impulses per second.

Newborn kittens have only slow muscles; their muscles differentiate into fast or slow over a period of weeks after birth. Arthur Buller, John Eccles, and Rosamond Eccles examined whether motor neurons determine the properties of the muscle, or whether the muscle determines the properties of the motor neuron. They found that when nerves and muscles were switched surgically, the neurons retained their properties. In contrast, the muscles changed their contractile properties when the innervating motor neuron was changed: A fast muscle was converted to slow muscle by a slow motor neuron, and slow muscles were converted to faster muscles by fast motor neurons (Figure 59–13). This transformation is notable for two rea-

sons. First, it shows that differentiation into fast or slow muscle is not an irreversible process. A change in innervation at any time will change the contractile properties of the muscle. Second, fast and slow muscles differ in their myosin light chains. Thus, the initial differentiation and subsequent changes in muscle properties involve an alteration in gene expression. Lømo and his colleagues found that differentiation of muscle is determined at least in part by the frequency of muscle contraction.

It is clear from these studies of the developing and regenerating neuromuscular junction that the motor nerve terminal plays a fundamental role in organizing both the postsynaptic muscle membrane and the extracellular matrix components involved in synapse formation and function, such as acetylcholinesterase and s-laminin.

Presynaptic Neurons Also Regulate the Development of Nicotinic Receptors in Neurons

Presynaptic neurons can also regulate the properties of nicotinic ACh receptors in postsynaptic neurons. Studies on nicotinic synapses in bullfrog lumbar sympathetic ganglia by Lawrence Marshall have shown that there are two classes of postsynaptic neurons in these ganglia, B and C cells. B cells receive input from presynaptic B fibers and C cells from presynaptic C fibers. Marshall has shown that the ACh receptors on postsynaptic B and C cells remain open for quite different durations: B cells remain open for about 5 ms, C cells for about 10 ms. When B cells are denervated they are reinnervated by the C fiber preganglionic input that normally projects to the C neurons. Under these conditions, the ACh receptors on the postsynaptic B neuron acquire the properties of those expressed by the C neuron; that is, they remain open for prolonged periods. The mechanisms that regulate development of postsynaptic receptors on peripheral neurons may be similar to those operating at neuromuscular synapses. It remains to be seen whether the properties of synaptic receptors in the brain are controlled in a similar way.

The Postsynaptic Muscle Cell Regulates the Differentiation of the Motor Nerve Terminal

As we discussed earlier, the presynaptic terminal is quite undifferentiated at the point of initial contact between nerve and muscle and only gradually acquires its characteristic specializations: the active zone, clusters of synaptic vesicles, and a high density of Ca^{2+} channels in the presynaptic neuron membrane. How does the progressive differentiation of the presynaptic terminal come about? From studies of regenerating motor axons, McMahan and colleagues have found that components in the basal lamina can organize the presynaptic nerve terminal. Even in the absence of the postsynaptic muscle, contact with the synaptic basal lamina is sufficient to organize the active zone and the clustering of synaptic vesicles in the region of the presynaptic terminal precisely opposite the original postjunctional fold. Thus, components of the synaptic basal lamina also appear to regulate the differentiation of the presynaptic nerve terminal, at least during regenera-

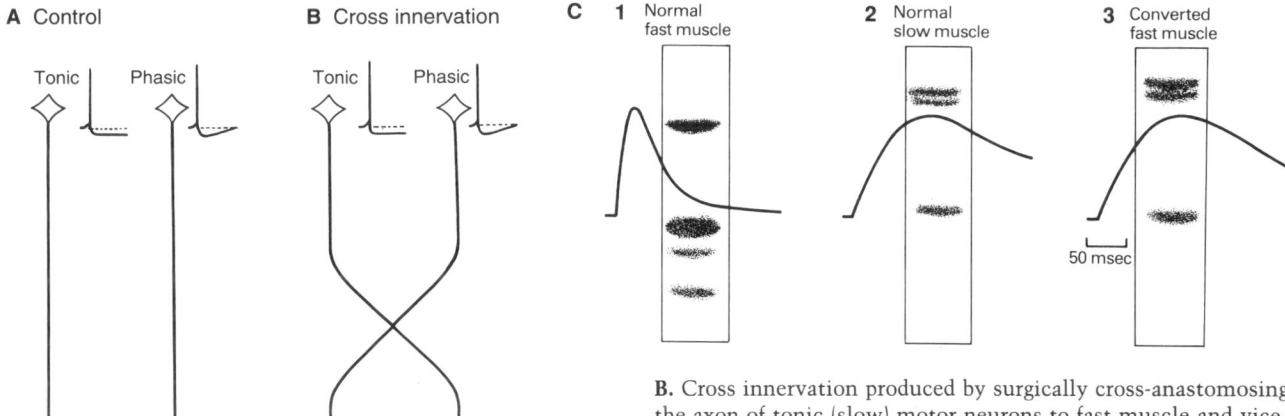

FIGURE 59–13
Switching motor axons between slow and fast muscles transforms the contractile properties of the muscles.

A. Normal innervation of fast and slow muscles by tonic and phasic motor neurons.

B. Cross innervation produced by surgically cross-anastomosing the axon of tonic (slow) motor neurons to fast muscle and vice versa. The unique characteristics of the two species of motor neurons do not change, but the contractile properties of the muscles are completely transformed. The fast muscles behave like slow muscles and slow muscles are changed into an intermediate form.

C. Changing the pattern of stimulation alters contractile proteins of muscle, as illustrated in SDS gels of the myosins from muscle. **1-2.** The gel pattern for myosin from normal fast and slow muscles. **3.** The gel for fast muscle that has been stimulated for 20 weeks at frequencies characteristic of a slow motor neuron. The myosin pattern, like the contractile response, now resembles that of a slow muscle. (Adapted from Salmons and Sréter, 1976.)

tion. Some of these components may conceivably play a role in the differentiation of the presynaptic terminal during the initial stages of synapse formation.

Some Synapses Are Eliminated During Development

We have discussed the mechanisms involved in the formation of a single synaptic connection, using the neuromuscular synapse as an example. The function of the neuromuscular system also depends on precise regulation of the number of motor nerve terminals on each muscle fiber. Most muscle fibers in adults are connected to a single motor axon; that is, there is one end-plate per muscle fiber. At earlier stages of neuromuscular development, however, this is not the case—single muscle fibers are innervated by several different motor axons.

This feature of neuromuscular development was first shown with anatomical techniques by J. F. Tello and later confirmed with electrophysiological recordings by Paul Redfern. Intracellular recordings from fast-twitch skeletal muscle fibers in neonatal animals have detected multiple postsynaptic responses that can be resolved into individual inputs by varying the intensity of stimulation of the motor nerve. During the first weeks after birth, the number of individual synaptic inputs that can be recorded from a single muscle fiber decreases, so that eventually a single muscle fiber is contacted by only one motor axon (Figure 59–14). The reduction in synaptic input cannot be accounted for by a decrease in the number of motor neurons or a developmental increase in the number of muscle fi-

bers. Synapses are thought to be eliminated by the withdrawal of the presynaptic branch into the motor axon. Although the number of distinct inputs to a skeletal muscle fiber decreases during development, the complexity of the one remaining presynaptic terminal increases over the same period; it acquires more synaptic boutons and release sites. Thus, the strength of synaptic input to the muscle fiber can actually increase during the period of synapse elimination.

Synapse elimination can also be observed during the development of many regions of the central and peripheral nervous systems. Elimination of neuronal synapses has been easiest to document in the autonomic ganglia of the peripheral nervous system. Here, as at the neuromuscular junction, there is a decrease in the number of presynaptic axons that contact a single postsynaptic neuron. For example, in the ciliary ganglion of the parasympathetic nervous system there is a twofold reduction in the number of preganglionic axons that innervate each ciliary postganglionic neuron (Figure 59–14). As with the neuromuscular junction, this decrease is not attributable to a change in the number of preganglionic neurons innervating the ganglion or of ciliary ganglion neurons, and must therefore reflect the elimination of connections. The number of synaptic contacts formed by each remaining axon increases during the period that preganglionic inputs are eliminated, increasing the overall strength of synaptic transmission.

Synapse elimination also occurs in the central nervous system. For example, each Purkinje neuron in the adult cerebellum is innervated by only a single climbing fiber

A Motor neuron innervation of skeletal muscle

Early: polyneuronal innervation

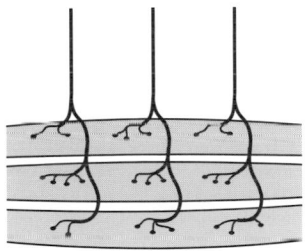

Late: single innervation

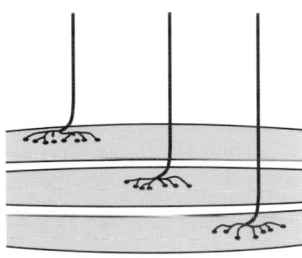

B Presynaptic innervation of autonomic ganglion neurons

Early: polyneuronal innervation

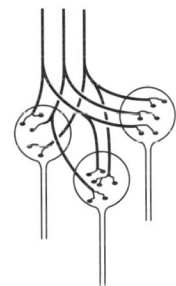

Late: single innervation

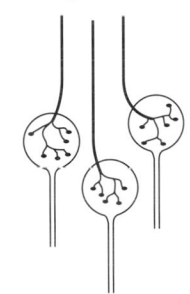

FIGURE 59–14

Rearrangement of synaptic connections in the peripheral nervous system of mammals during the first few weeks of postnatal life. In muscles (**A**) and ganglia comprising neurons without dendrites (**B**) each axon innervates more target cells at birth than in maturity. The number of neurons innervating each target cell decreases with development, but the size and complexity of the arbor of the remaining terminal increases with time. (Based on Purves and Lichtman, 1980; and Purves, 1988.)

axon from the inferior olive. However, during development each Purkinje neuron receives input from three or four different climbing fibers.

The elimination of synapses during development may involve competition between different axons that innervate the same target cell. Early in development several motor neurons innervate each muscle fiber, and a single motor axon innervates several distinct muscle fibers. With time, the number of muscle fibers innervated by a single motor neuron decreases, possibly because other motor axons have been more successful in maintaining input to many of the muscle fibers. In fact, when other competing motor axons are removed, the number of muscle fibers innervated by the remaining motor axon does not decrease. Motor axons may compete with each other for supply or access to trophic factors that maintain synaptic contacts. Thus, trophic factors may promote the survival of neurons and regulate the number of synaptic contacts made by the neuron.

These few examples illustrate that the formation of an initial synaptic contact is not the final event in neuronal connectivity. The elimination and rearrangement of synaptic connections plays an equally important role in

sculpting the circuitry of the nervous system. In effect, the process of synapse elimination and rearrangement is similar to the phenomenon of axon collateral elimination that we discussed in the previous chapter.

An Overall View

The ability of an axon to reach its appropriate target is essential for the survival of the neuron; if the target is absent, neurons often atrophy and die. There is now considerable evidence that target cells supply neurotrophic factors that maintain presynaptic neurons during the formation of functional synaptic connections. The matching of the number of presynaptic neurons with the size of the target organ may also be controlled by the availability of trophic factors.

Several neurotrophic factors have now been identified, in particular nerve growth factor, brain-derived neurotrophic factor, neurotrophin 3, and ciliary neurotrophic factor, each of which supports the survival of distinct groups of neurons.

The formation of synaptic contacts involves a complex series of interactions between the nerve terminal and its postsynaptic target. In many cases the presynaptic terminal plays a critical role in organizing the postsynaptic membrane to ensure that synaptic transmission functions efficiently. For example, the presynaptic terminal regulates the number and distribution of transmitter receptors and other molecules on the postsynaptic membrane. Conversely, the postsynaptic cell may also regulate the differentiation of the presynaptic terminal.

In some regions of the nervous system the initial synaptic contacts between cells are accurate and stable, providing evidence for a high degree of initial specificity in cell recognition. In other regions, however, initial contacts are dramatically rearranged and many synapses are eventually eliminated during development.

Selected Readings

Barde, Y.-A. 1989. Trophic factors and neuronal survival. Neuron 2:1525–1534.

Lømo, T., and Westgaard, R. H. 1976. Control of ACh sensitivity in rat muscle fibers. Cold Spring Harbor Symp. Quant. Biol. 40:263–274.

McMahan, U. J., and Wallace, B. G. 1989. Molecules in basal lamina that direct the formation of synaptic specializations at neuromuscular junctions. Dev. Neurosci. 11:227–247.

Purves, D., Snider, W. D., and Voyvodic, J. T. 1988. Trophic regulation of nerve cell morphology and innervation in the autonomic nervous system. Nature 336:123–128.

Scheutze, S. M., and Role, L. W. 1987. Developmental regulation of nicotinic acetylcholine receptors. Annu. Rev. Neurosci. 10: 403–457.

Thoenen, H., and Barde, Y.-A. 1980. Physiology of nerve growth factor. Physiol. Rev. 60:1284–1335.

References

Anderson, M. J., and Cohen, M. W. 1977. Nerve-induced and spontaneous redistribution of acetylcholine receptors on cultured muscle cells. J. Physiol. (Lond.) 268:757–773.

Angeletti, R. H., and Bradshaw, R. A. 1971. Nerve growth factor from mouse submaxillary gland: Amino acid sequence. Proc. Natl. Acad. Sci. U.S.A. 65:2417–2420.

Bandtlow, C. E., Heumann, R., Schwab, M. E., and Thoenen, H. 1987. Cellular localization of nerve growth factor synthesis by in situ hybridization. EMBO J. 6:891–899.

Brenner, H. R., and Sakmann, B. 1983. Neurotrophic control of channel properties at neuromuscular synapses of rat muscle. J. Physiol. (Lond.) 337:159–171.

Bueker, E. D. 1948. Implantation of tumors in the hind limb field of the embryonic chick and the developmental response of the lumbosacral nervous system. Anat. Rec. 102:369–389.

Buller, A. J., Eccles, J. C., and Eccles, R. M. 1960. Interactions between motoneurones and muscles in respect of the characteristic speeds of their responses. J. Physiol. (Lond.) 150:417–439.

Burden, S. 1977. Acetylcholine receptors at the neuromuscular junction: Developmental change in receptor turnover. Dev. Biol. 61:79–85.

Bursztajn, S., Berman, S. A., and Gilbert, W. 1989. Differential expression of acetylcholine receptor mRNA in nuclei of cultured muscle cells. Proc. Natl. Acad. Sci. U.S.A. 86:2928–2932.

Campenot, R. B. 1981. Regeneration of neurites in long-term cultures of sympathetic neurons deprived of nerve growth factor. Science 214:579–581.

Cohen, M. W., Anderson, M. J., Zorychta, E., and Weldon, P. R. 1979. Accumulation of acetylcholine receptors at nerve–muscle contacts in culture. Prog. Brain Res. 49:335–349.

Cohen, S. 1960. Purification of a nerve-growth promoting protein from the mouse salivary gland and its antiserum. Proc. Natl. Acad. Sci. U.S.A. 46:302–311.

Detwiler, S. R. 1936. Neuroembryology: An Experimental Study. New York: Macmillan.

Fischbach, G. D., and Schuetze, S. M. 1980. A post-natal decrease in acetylcholine channel open time at rat end-plates. J. Physiol. (Lond.) 303:125–137.

Fontaine B., and Changeux, J.-P. 1989. Localization of nicotinic acetylcholine receptor α-subunit transcripts during myogenesis and motor endplate development in the chick. J. Cell Biol. 108:1025–1037.

Frank, E., and Fischbach, G. D. 1979. Early events in neuromuscular junction formation in vitro: Induction of acetylcholine receptor clusters in the postsynaptic membrane and morphology of newly formed synapses. J. Cell Biol. 83:143–158.

Glicksman, M. A., and Sanes, J. R. 1983. Differentiation of motor nerve terminals formed in the absence of muscle fibres. J. Neurocytol. 12:661–671.

Hamburger, V. 1975. Cell death in the development of the lateral motor column of the chick embryo. J. Comp. Neurol. 160:535–546.

Hamburger, V., and Levi-Montalcini, R. 1949. Proliferation, differentiation and degeneration in the spinal ganglia of the chick embryo under normal and experimental conditions. J. Exp Zool. 111:457–501.

Hirokawa, N., and Heuser, J. E. 1982. Internal and external differentiations of the postsynaptic membrane at the neuromuscular junction. J. Neurocytol 11:487–510.

Hohn, A., Leibrock, J., Bailey, K., and Barde, Y.-A. 1990. Identification and characterization of a novel member of the nerve growth factor/brain–derived neurotrophic factor family. Nature 344:339–341.

Hume, R. I., Role, L. W., and Fischbach, G. D. 1983. Acetylcholine release from growth cones detected with patches of acetylcholine receptor-rich membranes. Nature 305:632–634.

Hunter, D. D., Shah, V., Merlie, J. P., and Sanes, J. R. 1989. A laminin-like adhesive protein concentrated in the synaptic cleft of the neuromuscular junction. Nature 338:229–234.

Kaplan, D. R., Hempstead, B. L., Martin-Zanca, D., Chao, M. V., and Parada, L. F. 1991. The trk proto-oncogene product: A signal transducing receptor for nerve growth factor. Science 252:554–558.

Klein, R., Jing, S., Nanduri, U., O'Rourke, E., and Barbacid, M. 1991. The trk proto-oncogene encodes a receptor for nerve growth factor. Cell 65:189–197.

Leibrock, J., Lottspeich, F., Hohn, A., Hofer, M., Hengerer, B., Masiakowski, P., Thoenen, H., and Barde, Y.-A. 1989. Molecular cloning and expression of brain-derived neurotrophic factor. Nature 341:149–152.

Levi-Montalcini, R. 1972. The morphological effects of immunosympathectomy. In G. Steiner and E. Schönbaum (eds.), Immunosympathectomy. Amsterdam: Elsevier, pp. 55–78.

Lømo, T., Westgaard, R. H., and Dahl, H. A. 1974. Contractile properties of muscle: Control by pattern of muscle activity in the rat. Proc. R. Soc. Lond. [Biol.] 187:99–103.

Lømo, T., and Rosenthal, J. 1972. Control of ACh sensitivity by muscle activity in the rat. J. Physiol. (Lond.) 221:493–513.

Marshall, L. M. 1986. Presynaptic control of synaptic channel kinetics in sympathetic neurones. Nature 317:621–623.

Nitkin, R. M., Smith, M. A., Magill, C., Fallon, J. R., Yao, Y.-M. M. Wallace, B. G., and McMahan, U. J. 1987. Identification of agrin, a synaptic organizing protein from Torpedo electric organ. J. Cell Biol. 105:2471–2478.

Oppenheim, R. W. 1981. Neuronal cell death and some related regressive phenomena during neurogenesis: A selective historical review and progress report. In W. M. Cowan (ed.), Studies in Developmental Neurobiology: Essays in Honor of Viktor Hamburger. New York: Oxford University Press, pp. 74–133.

Oppenheim, R. W. 1989. The neurotrophic theory and naturally occurring motoneuron death. Trends Neurosci. 12:252–255.

Patterson, P. H., and Purves, D. 1982. Readings in Developmental Neurobiology. Cold Spring Harbor, N.Y.: Cold Spring Harbor Laboratory.

Purves, D. 1988. Body and Brain. A Trophic Theory of Neural Connections. Cambridge, Mass.: Harvard University Press.

Purves, D., and Lichtman, J. W. 1980. Elimination of synapses in the developing nervous system. Science 210:153–157.

Redfern, P. A. 1970. Neuromuscular transmission in new-born rats. J. Physiol. (Lond.) 209:701–709.

Rupp, F., Payan, D. G., Magill-Sole, C., Cowan, W. M., and Scheller, R. 1991. Structure and expression of a rat agrin. Neuron 6:811–823.

Salmons, S., and Sréter, F. A. 1976. Significance of impulse activity in the transformation of skeletal muscle type. Nature 263:30–34.

Tello, J. F. 1917. Genesis de las terminaciones nerviosas motrices y sensitivas. Trav. Labs Invest. Biol. Univ. Madrid 15:101–199.

Usdin, T. B., and Fischbach, G. D. 1986. Purification and characterization of a polypeptide from chick brain that promotes the accumulation of acetylcholine receptors in chick myotubes. J. Cell Biol. 103:493–507.

Wigston, D. J., and Sanes, J. R. 1982. Selective reinnervation of adult mammalian muscle by axons from different segmental levels. Nature 29:464–467.

Young, S. H., and Poo, M.-M. 1983. Spontaneous release of transmitter from growth cones of embryonic neurones. Nature 305:634–637.

60

Eric R. Kandel
Thomas Jessell

Early Experience and the Fine Tuning of Synaptic Connections

Normal Development Depends on Sensory Experience and Social Interaction

There Is an Early Critical Period in the Development of Social and Perceptual Competence

Isolated Young Monkeys Do Not Develop Normal Social Behavior

Early Sensory Deprivation Alters Perceptual Development

Early Sensory Deprivation Alters the Development of Neural Circuits

The Development of Ocular Dominance Columns Is an Important Example for Understanding the Development of Behavior

Cooperation and Competition Are Important for Segregating Afferent Inputs into the Ocular Dominance Columns

Cooperation Requires Synchronous Activity

Different Regions of the Brain Have Different Critical Periods of Development

Studies of Development Are Important Clinically

An Overall View

The mature brain is precisely wired to process sensory information into coherent patterns of activity that form the basis of our perception, thoughts, and actions. This precise wiring is not fully developed at birth, however. The pattern of connections that emerges as a result of cell recognition events during prenatal development only roughly approximates the final wiring. This initially coarse pattern of connections is subsequently refined by activity-dependent mechanisms that match precisely the presynaptic neurons to their appropriate target cells. This activity-dependent matching can be modulated by normal or aberrant sensory experience.

As a result, at critical stages of postnatal development the integrative action of the brain, and at the cellular level the detailed wiring of the brain, is dependent upon specific interactions between the organism and its environment. This influence of the environment on the brain, and therefore on behavior, changes with age. Abnormal environmental experiences usually have more profound effects during early stages of postnatal development than in adulthood.

In previous chapters we examined the molecular events that underlie the prenatal development of the nervous system. Here we shall look at the postnatal development of functioning organisms, in particular the human infant. We shall focus on the development of vision because studies of the effects of experience on the developing visual system have been generally instructive in furthering our understanding of how experience shapes the developing neural circuitry of the brain. In Chapter 65 we shall consider how experience affects the adult brain.

Normal Development Depends on Sensory Experience and Social Interaction

There Is an Early Critical Period in the Development of Social and Perceptual Competence

As we have seen in Chapter 57, at certain irreversible decision points during development, nerve cells become committed to one or another pathway of differentiation. There are similar *critical periods* in the development of behavior, both in the acquisition of sexual identity (Chapter 61), and in the development of social and perceptual competence. During these critical periods the infant must interact with a normal environment if development is to proceed satisfactorily.

A particularly well-studied example of a critical period in the acquisition of a normal behavior is *imprinting*, a form of learning encountered in birds and examined in detail by the Austrian ethologist Konrad Lorenz. Just after birth, birds become attached to a prominent moving object in their environment, typically the mother. Imprinting is important for the protection of the hatchling; it is acquired rapidly, and once acquired the attachment generally persists. However, imprinting can be acquired only during a critical period (which in some species lasts a few hours) early in postnatal development. Imprinting therefore illustrates the close relationship between genetically programmed development and learning.

The clearest way to show that certain social or perceptual experiences are important for development is to deprive an infant of these stimuli and to examine the consequences on later perceptual or social competence. For ethical reasons deprivation experiments on human infants are not conducted by scientists. However, deprivation is sometimes imposed, often unintentionally, by parents or institutions. There are a few reliable histories of children who survived abandonment in the wild and who later were returned to civilization. There is also abundant anecdotal evidence on the fate of newborn infants left unattended during the major part of each day, being fed but not otherwise cared for. As might be expected, severely deprived children are socially maladjusted, usually in an irreversible way. The social behavior of these abandoned children is abnormal, and they are often mute and incapable of learning language.

The first compelling evidence that early social interaction with other humans is essential for normal development came from studies in the 1940s by the psychoanalyst René Spitz. Spitz compared the development of infants raised in a foundling home for abandoned children with the development of infants raised in a nursing home attached to a woman's prison. Both institutions were clean, and provided adequate food and medical care. The babies in the nursing home were all cared for by their mothers, who, because they were in prison and away from their families, tended to shower affection on their infants in the limited time allotted to them each day. In contrast, infants in the foundling home were cared for by nurses, each of whom was responsible for seven babies. As a result,

children in the foundling home had much less contact with other humans than those in the prison's nursing home.

The two institutions also differed in another respect. In the nursing home the cribs were open, so that the infants could readily watch the activity in the ward; they could see other babies play and observe their mothers and the staff go about their business. In the foundling home the bars of the cribs were covered by sheets that prevented the infants from seeing outside. This dramatically reduced the infants' environment. In short, the babies in the foundling home lived under conditions of relative sensory and social deprivation.

Spitz followed a group of newborn infants at each of the two institutions throughout their early years. At the end of the first four months the infants in the foundling home scored better than those in the nursing home on several developmental tests. This suggested to Spitz that genetic factors did not favor the infants in the nursing home. However, eight months later, at the end of the first year, the motor and intellectual performance of the children in the foundling home had fallen far below that of children in the nursing home, and many had developed a syndrome that Spitz called *hospitalism* (now often called *anaclitic depression*). These children were withdrawn, showed little curiosity or gaiety, and were prone to infection.

By their second and third years, children in the nursing home were similar to children raised in normal families at home: They walked well and talked actively. In contrast, the development of the children in the foundling home was delayed. Only two of 26 children in the foundling home were able to walk and speak, and even they could say only a few words. Normal children at this age are agile, have a vocabulary of hundreds of words, and speak in sentences. Thus, severe social and sensory deprivation in early childhood can have catastrophic consequences for later development. In contrast, isolation later in life (although often unpleasant) is much better tolerated.

Isolated Young Monkeys Do Not Develop Normal Social Behavior

Spitz's work was carried one important step further in the 1960s when Harry and Margaret Harlow studied monkeys reared in isolation. They found that newborn monkeys isolated for six months to one year were physically healthy but behaviorally devastated. These monkeys crouched in a corner of their cages and rocked back and forth like severely disturbed (autistic) children. They did not interact with other monkeys, nor did they fight, play, or show any sexual interest. A six-month period of social isolation during the first one and a half years of life produces persistent and serious alterations in behavior. By comparison, isolation of an older animal for a comparable period was innocuous. Thus, in monkeys, as in humans, there is a critical period for social development.

The Harlows next sought to determine the factors that need to be introduced into the isolation experience to prevent the development of the isolation syndrome. They found that the syndrome could be partially reversed by giving an isolated monkey a surrogate mother—a cloth-covered wooden dummy. This elicited clinging behavior in the isolated monkey but was insufficient for the development of fully normal social behavior. Social development would occur normally only if, in addition to a surrogate mother, the isolated animal had contact for a few hours each day with a normal infant monkey who spent the rest of the day in the monkey colony. Subsequently, Stephen Suomi and the Harlows found that the isolation syndrome can sometimes be reversed fully by contact with certain monkeys with special personality traits, such as unflagging gregariousness. These monkeys (who might be considered monkey psychotherapists) persistently engage the isolate in social and aggressive behavior until the isolate begins to respond.

Early Sensory Deprivation Alters Perceptual Development

Early deprivation does not have to be so all-encompassing as social isolation to have behavioral consequences. For example, there is also a critical period in the development of normal perception. Even restricted sensory deprivation may have dire consequences. For example, in 1932 Marius von Senden reviewed the world literature on cataracts in the newborn. Cataracts are opacities of the lens that interfere with the optics of the eye but not with the nervous system; they can be fully corrected surgically in the infant. Von Senden discovered several children who were born with binocular cataracts that were removed much later in life (from ages 10 to 20). The presence of these cataracts in early childhood resulted later in a permanent impairment of the ability to perceive form. Even after the cataracts were removed these patients could recognize colors but had difficulty recognizing shapes and patterns.

The idea that normal sensory experience is required for perceptual development was supported by the work of Austin Riesen, who raised newborn monkeys in the dark for the first 3–6 months of their lives. When these monkeys were later introduced to a normal visual world, they could not discriminate even simple shapes. It took weeks or even months of training to teach them to distinguish a circle from a square, whereas normal monkeys learn such discrimination in days. Thus, the development of normal perception requires exposure to patterned visual stimulation early in development.

Early Sensory Deprivation Alters the Development of Neural Circuits

An important step toward understanding the role of patterned visual stimulation in the development of perception was made by Torsten Wiesel and David Hubel in studies on newborn kittens and monkeys. In particular, Wiesel and Hubel examined the effects of visual deprivation on cellular responses in area 17 of the visual (striate) cortex.

As we have seen in Chapters 29 and 30, Wiesel and Hubel had earlier recorded from single cells at various

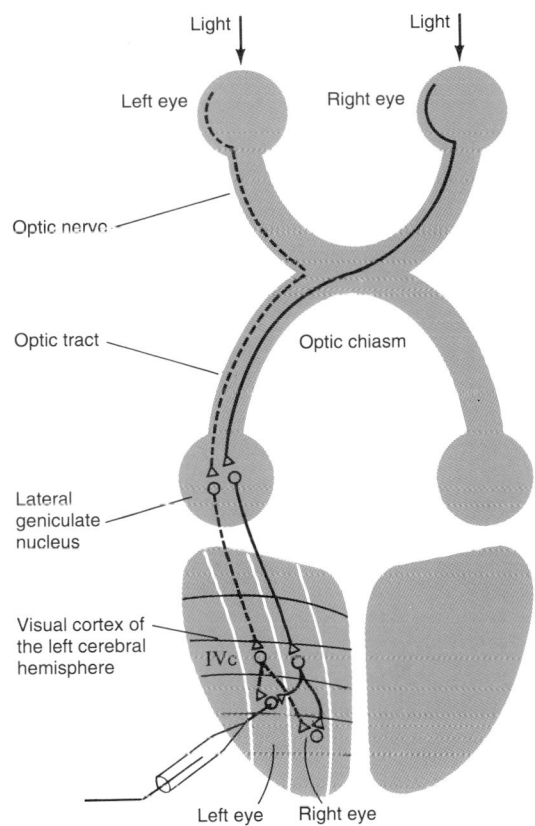

FIGURE 60–1
The input from the two eyes is segregated up to the level of the visual cortex. The retinal ganglion cells of each eye project to separate layers of the lateral geniculate nucleus. The axons of cells in the lateral geniculate nucleus form synaptic connections with neurons in layer 4c of area 17, the primary visual cortex. Neurons in layer 4c are organized in two sets of ocular dominance columns that each receives input from only one eye. The axons of the cells in layer 4c go to the adjacent columns as well as the upper and lower layers in the same column. As a result of these connections, the input becomes mixed so that most cells in the upper and lower layers of the cortex receive information from both eyes.

points in the visual pathway to determine where the fusion of visual images begins. They found that cells in the retina, the lateral geniculate nucleus, and layer 4c of the striate cortex respond only to input from one or the other eye. In the monkey, binocular interaction (convergence of input from the two eyes on a common target cell) first occurs in the cells above and below layer 4c (Figure 60–1). Thus in the monkey most cells above and below layer 4c respond to an appropriate stimulus presented to either eye; only a small proportion of cells, those in layer 4c, responds exclusively to the left or the right eye (Figure 60–2A and B).

However, if a monkey is raised from birth up to six months of age with one eyelid sutured shut, the animal permanently loses useful vision in that eye after the occluding sutures are removed. Electrical recordings from the retinal ganglion cells in the deprived eye and from

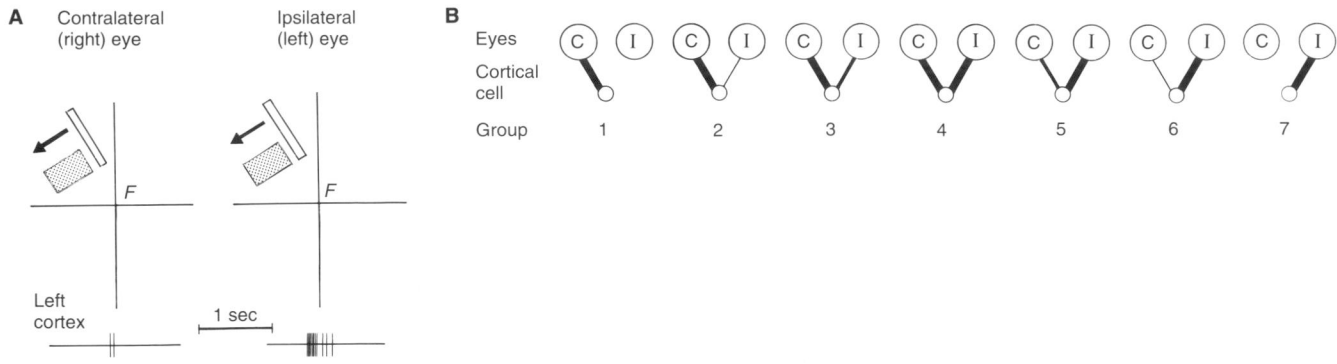

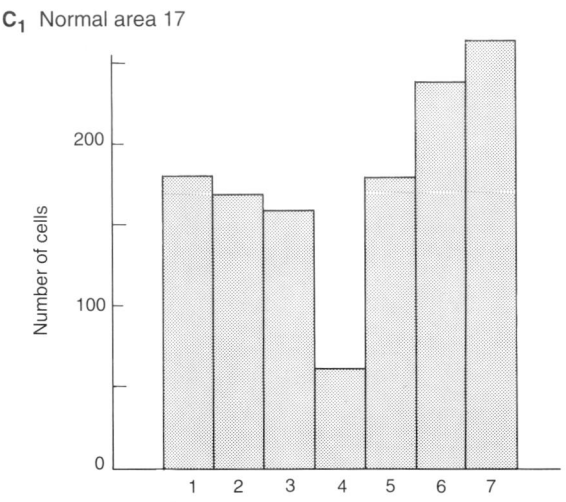

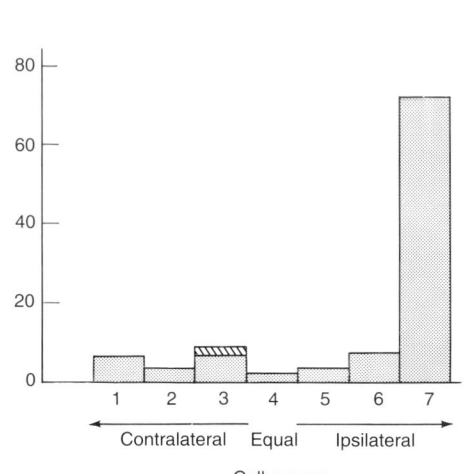

C₁ Normal area 17

C₂ Area 17 after monocular closure of contralateral eye

FIGURE 60–2

Binocular interaction and plasticity in area 17 of the monkey's visual cortex. (Adapted from Hubel and Wiesel, 1977.)

A. The response of a typical neuron in the visual cortex of the left hemisphere to a diagonal bar of light moving to the left across the cell's receptive field (**shaded rectangle**). The receptive fields are shown with respect to the location of the foveal region (**F**), the region of greatest visual acuity. The visual fields as seen by the right and the left eyes are drawn separately for clarity, although in normal vision the two visual fields are superimposed. The fields in the two eyes are similar in orientation, position, shape, and size and respond to the same form of stimulus. The action potential recordings below show that the cortical cell responds more effectively when the stimulus is presented to the ipsilateral eye than to the contralateral eye.

B. On the basis of the responses of the sort illustrated in part A, Hubel and Wiesel divided the response properties of cortical neurons into seven ocular dominance groups. Cells receiving input

only from the contralateral eye (**C**) fall into group 1. Cells that receive input only from the ipsilateral eye (**I**) fall into group 7. In other cells one eye may influence the cell much more than the other (groups 2 and 6), or the differences may be slight (groups 3 and 5). According to these criteria, the cell shown in part A would fall into group 6.

C. Histograms of the responsiveness of cells to stimulation of one eye or the other in normal monkeys and those that have been deprived of vision in one eye. **1.** This histogram is based on 1256 cells recorded from area 17 in the left hemisphere of normal adult and juvenile monkeys. The cells in layer 4 that received only monocular input were excluded. Most cells responded to input from both eyes. **2.** This histogram was obtained from the left hemisphere of a monkey in which the contralateral (right) eye was closed from age two weeks to 18 months and then reopened. Most of the cells responded only to stimulation of the ipsilateral eye. The hatched area represents cells with abnormal responses.

cells in the lateral geniculate nucleus that receive the projections from that eye indicate that these cells respond well to visual stimuli projected onto the deprived eye and have essentially normal receptive fields. In the visual cortex, however, most cells no longer respond to the deprived eye. The few cortical cells that can still be activated by the deprived eye are not sufficient for visual perception (Figure 60–2C,2). These effects of early deprivation are irrevers-

ible. In contrast to the severe effects of deprivation during this critical period of susceptibility, the first six months of life, comparable visual deprivation in an adult has no effect either on visual perception or on the visual responses of cortical cells to stimulation of one or the other eye. Yet during the peak of the critical period, the first six months of life, as little as one week of deprivation will lead to a nearly complete loss of vision and cortical responsiveness.

The Development of Ocular Dominance Columns Is an Important Example for Understanding the Development of Behavior

How do these permanent changes in the response properties of cortical cells come about? Are they accompanied by structural changes in the ocular dominance columns? Recall that each eye sends inputs to a distinct population of cells in the lateral geniculate nucleus. In turn, each population of cells in the lateral geniculate nucleus projects its axons to separate and alternating bands of cells in area 17 of the visual cortex, principally within layer 4c (see Figure 29–4). This segregation of endings is the anatomical basis for cortical ocular dominance columns of equal size for each eye. The cells in layer 4c then project to cells that lie in higher and lower layers of the same as well as adjacent columns. These projections from layer 4c are essential for the processing of convergent input from the two eyes by the cortical layers above and below.

To examine whether visual deprivation alters the architecture of the ocular dominance columns in the cerebral cortex, Hubel, Wiesel, and Simon LeVay deprived newborn monkeys of input from one eye. They then injected labeled amino acids into one or the other eye and, using autoradiography, observed the transport of the label to the cortex. After closure of one eye, they found that the columns receiving input from the normal eye were greatly

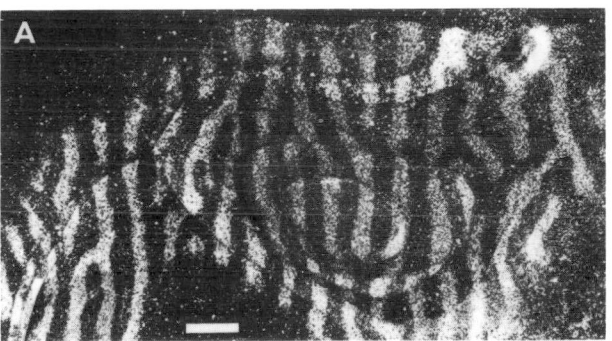

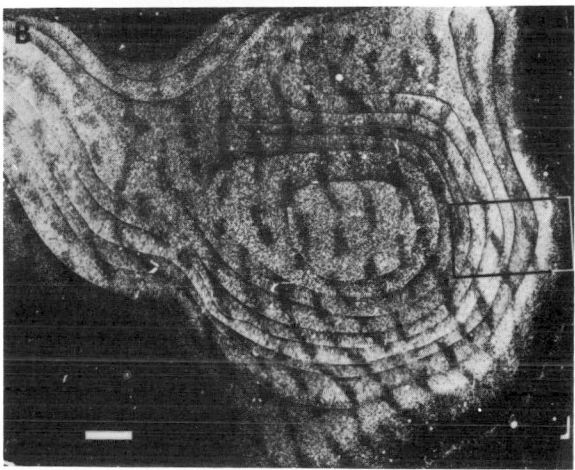

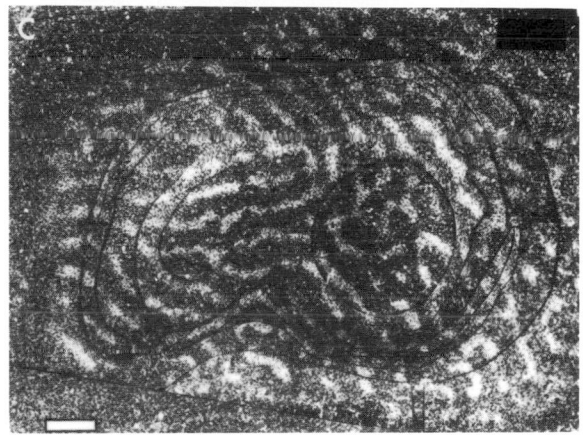

FIGURE 60–3

Visual deprivation of one eye reduces the size of the ocular dominance columns for that eye in the visual cortex of the monkey. (Adapted from Hubel, Wiesel, and LeVay, 1977.)

A. The right eye of a normal adult was injected with the radiolabeled amino acid *proline* (which is incorporated into protein) mixed with the labeled sugar *fucose* (which is incorporated into glycoprotein). This autoradiograph 10 days later is of a tangential section through the dome-shaped area 17 of the right hemisphere and was made with the technique of dark-field microscopy. Here the radioactivity can be seen forming white stripes, which correspond to the terminals in layer 4 of afferents from the lateral geniculate nucleus that carry input from the injected eye. The alternating dark stripes correspond to geniculate afferents from the uninjected eye. The section goes through layer 5, which is seen as the dark oval central area. Scale bars in micrographs of this part and parts B and C are 1 mm.

B. A comparable section through the visual cortex of an 18-month-old monkey whose right eye had been surgically closed at two weeks of age. The label was injected into the left eye. The plane of section cuts across layer 6, which is seen as the central oval shape. The white stripes of label correspond to afferent terminals from the open (**left**) eye, the narrower dark stripes to the closed (**right**) eye.

C. A section comparable to that in part B from an 18-month-old animal whose right eye had been shut at two weeks. In this case, however, the label was injected into the eye that had been closed, giving rise to narrow white stripes in the cortex and expanded dark ones.

D. Complete reconstruction of ocular dominance columns in area 17 of the right hemisphere showing the intricate organization of the complete map. (From S. LeVay, 1981.)

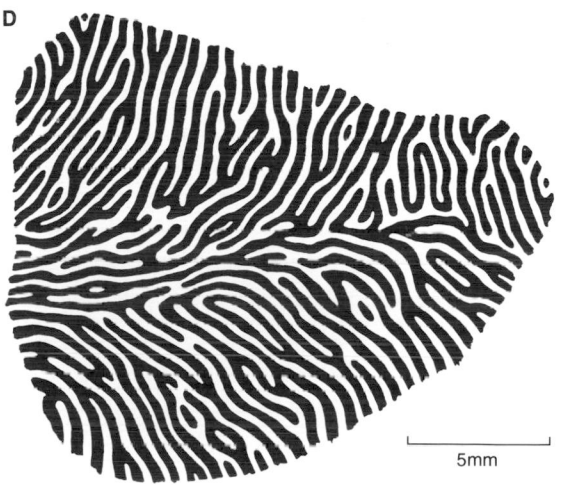

5mm

widened at the expense of those receiving input from the deprived eye (Figure 60–3B and C).

Here, then, is direct evidence that sensory deprivation early in life can alter the structure of the cerebral cortex! In 1965, when Hubel and Wiesel first discovered the existence of a critical period for binocular interaction, they had only a physiological indication of the effect of sensory deprivation. With the anatomical techniques then available, they were unable to find any morphological change in the visual cortex. Only after the development of autoradiographic labeling techniques involving axonal transport for mapping neuronal connections (see Box 4–1 and Chapter 18), were they able, in 1972, to demonstrate the structural features of the disturbance. In fact, we are just

beginning to develop the necessary techniques to explore the detailed structural organization of the brain and its possible alterations by experience and by disease. It is possible that social deprivation of the sort studied by the Harlows and their co-workers leads to a deterioration or distortion of connections in other areas of the brain.

Cooperation and Competition Are Important for Segregating Afferent Inputs into the Ocular Dominance Columns

How does monocular deprivation change the dimensions of ocular dominance columns in layer 4c of the visual cortex? When the afferent fibers from the lateral genicu-

FIGURE 60–4
Ocular dominance columns develop postnatally in the cat. These horizontal section dark-field autoradiographs (midline at the top, anterior to the left) illustrate four stages in the development of the visual cortex ipsilateral to an eye that was injected with [³H]proline. The geniculocortical afferents serving the injected eye are labeled by transneuronal transport. At about two weeks (15 days) postnatal, the afferents have spread uniformly along

layer 4, completely intermingled with the (unlabeled) afferents serving the contralateral eye. At 3 weeks and 5.5 weeks the emerging columns are visible but only as modest fluctuations in labeling density. At 13 weeks the borders of the labeled bands are more sharply defined as the afferents segregate—the anatomical basis for the physiologically described ocular dominance columns. (Adapted from LeVay, Stryker, and Shatz, 1978.)

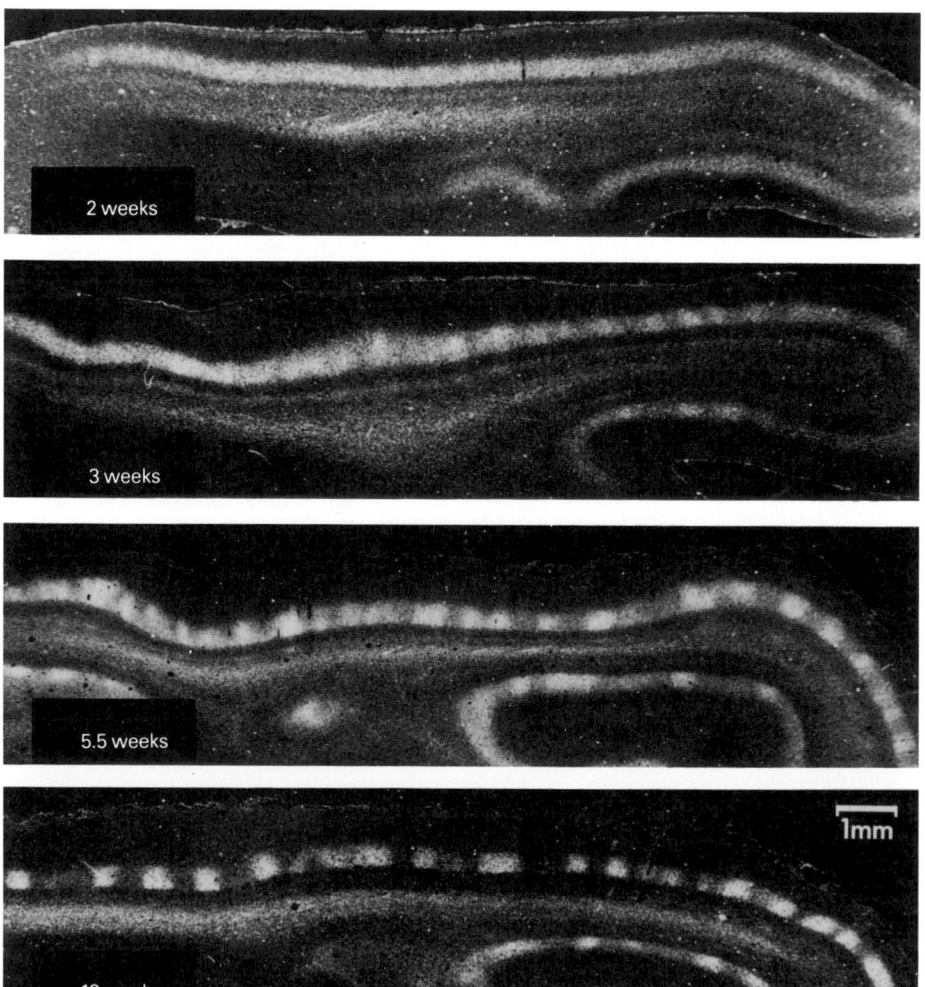

late nucleus reach layer 4c of the cortex, they at first overlap extensively. With further development, the inputs from each eye retract into ocular dominance columns. Monocular deprivation could interfere with this normal pattern of development. If the columns are not fully developed at birth, closing and thereby reducing the activity from one eye might put the axon terminals of the deprived eye at a selective disadvantage, and more of the terminals from the deprived eye would retract than under normal circumstances. Alternatively, if the columns are fully formed at birth, closing one eye might cause the geniculate axons from the normal eye to sprout and expand into the columns of the deprived eye and perhaps cause existing connections from the deprived eye to retract. To distinguish between these two types of mechanisms, it is important to know the developmental history of cortical columns.

Studies in the monkey and in the cat by Pasko Rakic and by Hubel and Wiesel and their associates have shown that ocular dominance columns are present at birth but only in a rudimentary form. In the monkey the columns do not form fully until six weeks after birth. It is only then that the afferent fibers from the lateral geniculate nucleus become completely segregated. In the cat segregation occurs even later (Figure 60–4).

The development of ocular dominance columns can be followed at the level of individual neurons by applying Golgi or other cellular stains to the afferent terminals of neurons of the lateral geniculate nucleus or by injecting a marker into their axons at different developmental stages and then following anatomically the segregation of the ocular dominance columns during development. These anatomical techniques show that a single afferent fiber from the lateral geniculate nucleus at first makes extensive branches in areas covering several future ocular dominance columns for each eye (Figure 60–5A). As the geniculate neuron matures, its afferent fiber loses some of its branches in a patterned way and expands and strengthens other branches so that ultimately the neuron connects powerfully only to the cells of the discrete ocular dominance columns for one eye (Figure 60–5B).

These features of normal development can be accounted for by the schema illustrated in Figure 60–6. At birth the terminals representing each eye have arrived in layer 4c but have not separated completely into the distinct bands characteristic of fully segregated columns. Initially the projections from each eye spread out within the full cortical space of layer 4c and try to form their own topographical map of the retina. During the first few weeks after birth a competitive interaction between the terminals from the two eyes sets in. This competition causes the two initially intermingled sets of incoming axons to arrange themselves in a regular pattern, presumably by the selective elimination of one or the other set of terminals. This is similar to the process of synapse retraction (or pruning) that we considered in Chapter 59.

In an animal deprived of the use of one eye during the *early* stages of this critical period of segregation, the axons of the lateral geniculate cells from the closed eye are at a competitive disadvantage and therefore retract to an ab-

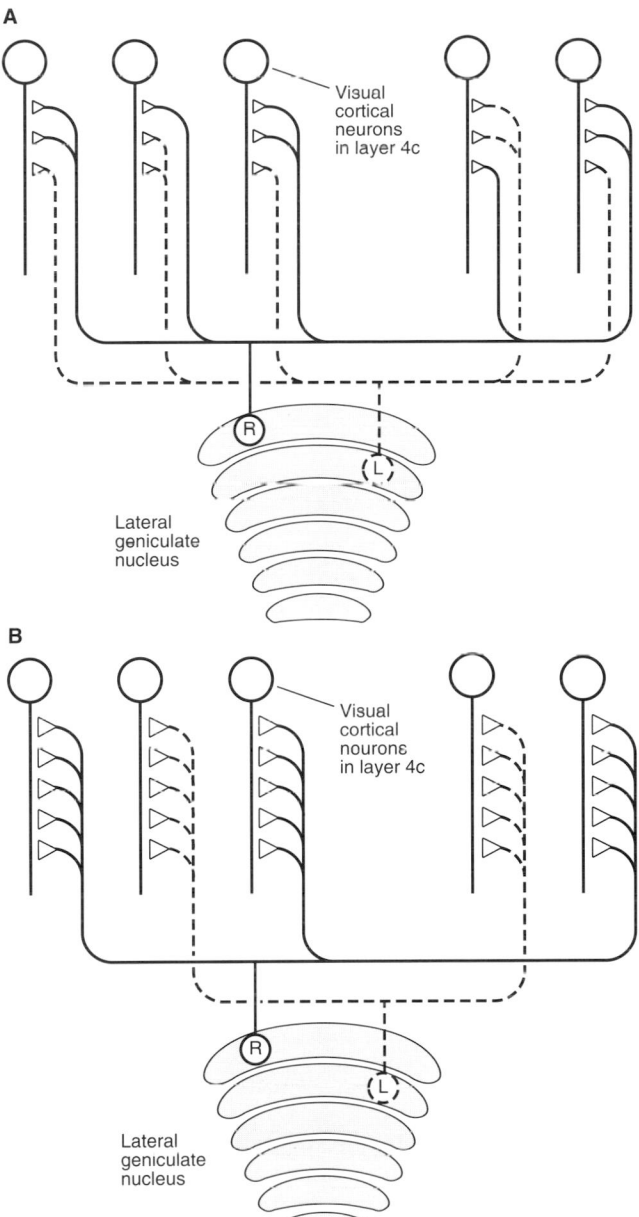

FIGURE 60–5

Segregation of ocular dominance columns in the monkey cortex based on injection of a tracer into single cells. (Based on unpublished experiments of Gilbert, Wiesel, and Katz.)

A. Early in development the afferent axons from the cells in the lateral geniculate nucleus receiving inputs from both eyes converge on common cortical neurons in layer 4c of the visual cortex. Because of genetic or possibly random developmental processes, this convergence is slightly biased so that alternating clusters of cells in layer 4c (illustrated here as single cells) receive slightly more connections from geniculate cells serving one rather than the other eye—indicated here as two synaptic endings rather than one.

B. As a result of the intrinsic bias illustrated in part A, axons from geniculate cells that have slightly more connections edge out competing axons carrying inputs from the other eye. The resulting dominance of inputs from one or the other eye gives rise to the characteristic stripes apparent in the autoradiographs of Figures 60–3 and 60–4.

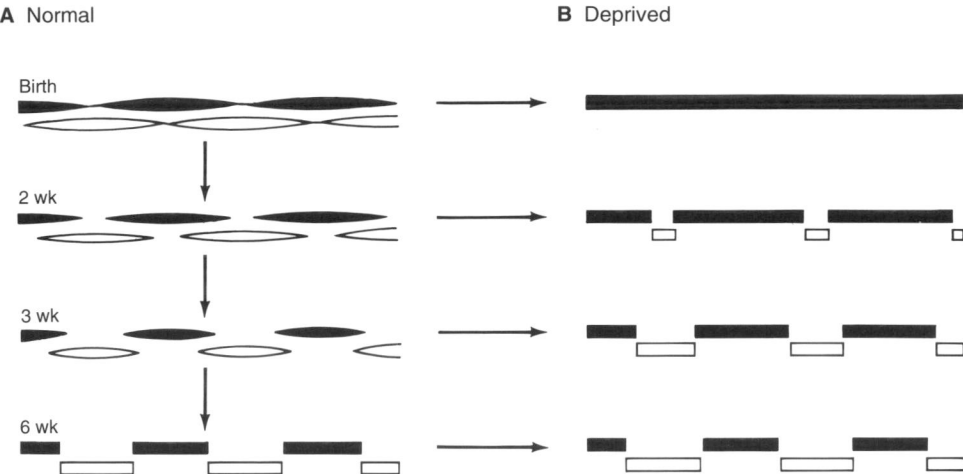

FIGURE 60–6

A comparison of normal development and of the effects of eye closure on columns in layer 4c, based on the assumption that the segregation of the eyes is not complete until some weeks after birth. The **black shapes** represent the terminations of geniculate afferents in layer 4c from one eye; the **unfilled shapes** represent the terminations from the other eye. The lengths of the shapes represent the density of the terminals at each point along layer 4c. The two sets of columns are shown here as one above the other for clarity. (Adapted from Hubel, Wiesel, and LeVay, 1977.)

A. According to this model, some periodic and regular variation in density of the afferent fibers is already present at birth. Because of the normal competition between inputs from the two eyes, the weaker input at any given point declines and the stronger is strengthened. As a result, the set of terminals that are weaker or fewer retract and die out. This works as follows. By a *spreading process* the afferent fibers from *each* eye form a complete topo-

graphical map within the same cortical space. This spreading mechanism is completed long before birth. A *grouping process* begins 3–6 weeks before birth. Cooperation among the fibers from each eye, thought to result from their tendency to fire together, leads to grouping of fibers from one eye and of their segregation from fibers from the other eye. By six weeks after birth this grouping process has led to a compromise: Layer 4c is divided into alternating groups of fibers from each eye.

B. The consequences of depriving one eye (**unfilled shapes**) depend on when that deprivation occurs. Deprivation at birth leads to complete dominance by the open eye (**black shapes**) because little segregation has occurred at this point. Deprivation at 2, 3, and 6 weeks has a progressively weaker effect on the ocular dominance columns since they become more segregated with time.

normal extent; by contrast, the terminals from the normal eye continue to occupy areas they normally would have relinquished. Closure of one eye during a *later* stage of this critical period, when the ocular dominance columns are almost fully segregated, brings a second mechanism into play. The remaining axons serving the open eye develop collateral branches that extend into areas they had earlier vacated (Figure 60–7).

Why do some terminals retract while others survive and grow stronger? The reason may be that at birth there are small, perhaps random, differences in the density of innervation from the afferent terminals from each eye onto common target cells (as indicated in Figures 60–6A and 60–4). As we shall learn below, neighboring axons from the same eye tend to fire synchronously and thereby cooperate with one another to depolarize and excite the target cell. Thus, when afferents from one eye are initially more numerous in one region, they are likely to have a competitive advantage. The cooperation between clustered fibers from the same eye allows them to grow and even to spread to adjacent cells. In contrast, competition between the afferent fibers from the two eyes acts to segregate fibers. Together, cooperation and competition pro-

vide a set of mechanisms that allows two populations of afferent fibers to share a common space without overlapping.

When one eye is closed, competition is reduced and cooperation among different fibers from the open eye dominates, so that the fibers from the open eye can spread to form a complete topographical map within the single neural space. This is indeed what happens in early stages of development, when the incoming fibers overlap extensively.

If the development of ocular dominance columns depends on competition between two sets of afferent fibers for representation on common cortical neurons, then it might be possible to induce the formation of columns where columns normally are not present by establishing competition between two sets of axons. Margaret Law and Martha Constantine-Paton examined this possibility in developing frogs. In the frog the retinal ganglion cells in one eye send their axons to the opposite side of the brain, where they terminate in the optic tectum in an orderly way that forms a map of the visual world. Here there is no competition from a second retina and indeed this map has no columnar organization. To establish a potential source

A Normal

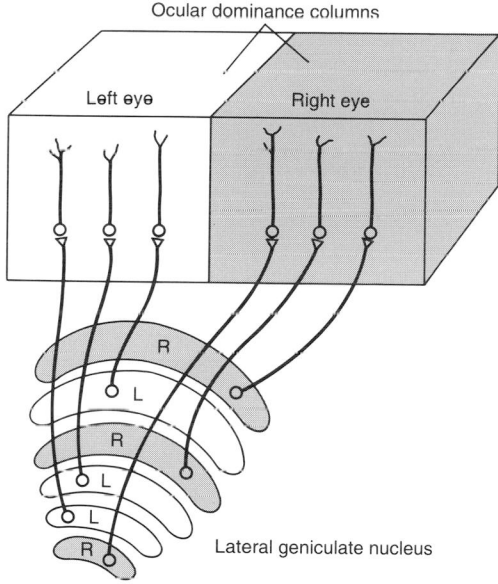

B Right eye closed

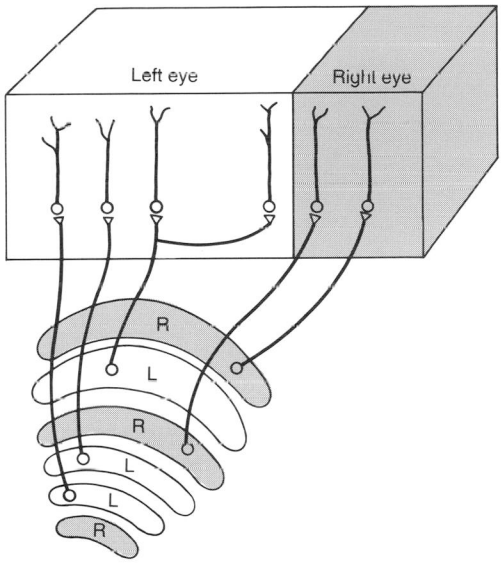

FIGURE 60–7

This drawing illustrates how lack of vision in one eye might affect development of the ocular dominance columns.

A. Ocular dominance columns are normally equal in size for each eye.

B. Without vision in the right eye, the columns devoted to the right eye become narrow compared to those of the left eye.

According to the hypothesis illustrated here, deprivation of one eye changes the normal balance between eyes so that the geniculate cells receiving input from the nonfunctional (right) eye regress and lose some of their connections with cortical cells, whereas the geniculate cells receiving input from the left eye sprout and connect to cortical cells previously occupied by geniculate neurons from the right eye.

of competition, Law and Constantine-Paton transplanted a third eye into a region of the head near one of the normal eyes. The retinal ganglion cells of the transplanted eye sent out axons that terminated in the contralateral optic tectum. This projection was mapped by injecting a radioactive tracer into the transplanted eye. The axons from the transplanted and normal eyes terminated in a regular pattern of alternating columns (Figure 60–8).

Thus, in the optic tectum, as in the cerebral cortex, columnar organization results when two sets of afferent fibers are forced to compete for the same population of postsynaptic cells. Because of this competition, those fibers that form the highest density of cooperating synapses and thus make the most effective contacts will retain their connections, whereas those fibers that make less extensive contact (perhaps because they arrive later) retract. The end result is that each set of fibers retracts from some cells and not others, thereby establishing alternating zones of dominance.

We earlier considered the cell adhesion and recognition signals that axons follow as they grow out from specific regions of the retina to the lateral geniculate nucleus and from that nucleus to the visual cortex (Chapters 58 and 59). On reaching their targets, the axons set up a *coarse* topographic map based on molecular recognition cues. Then a second set of mechanisms, based on cooperation and competition, takes over. This second set of mecha-

nisms matches each axon to its specific target neuron so as to create a *fine* topographic map.

Cooperation Requires Synchronous Activity

What factors lead to cooperation between adjacent fibers from the same eye and competition between afferent fibers from the two eyes? Experiments by Michael Stryker and others indicate that the critical factor regulating both competition and cooperation is neural activity. First, Stryker and William Harris found that ocular dominance columns do not form in kittens between the ages of two and eight weeks when all impulse activity in the retinal ganglion cells and optic nerves is blocked by injecting tetrodotoxin (which selectively blocks the voltage-sensitive Na^+ channel) into each eye. With activity blocked, Stryker next stimulated both optic nerves using implanted electrodes. When the two nerves were stimulated *synchronously*, formation of the ocular dominance columns was prevented. In contrast, when the optic nerves were stimulated *asynchronously*, ocular dominance columns formed. Thus, the formation and maintenance of normal binocular vision requires synchronous electrical activity among the optic nerve fibers *within* each eye and slightly asynchronous activity *between* the two eyes.

A similar mechanism appears to be present in the lateral geniculate nucleus. As we have seen in Chapter 29,

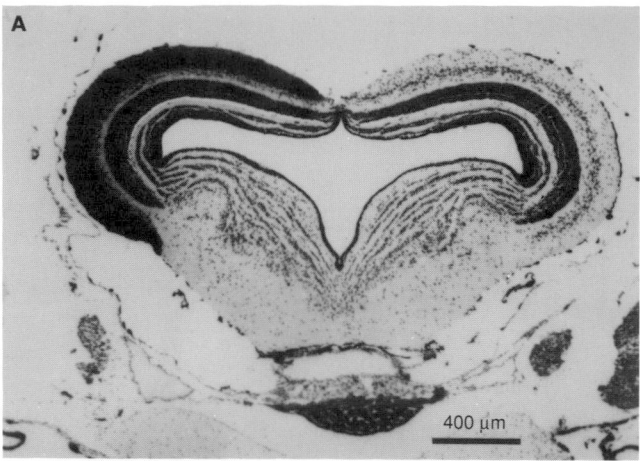

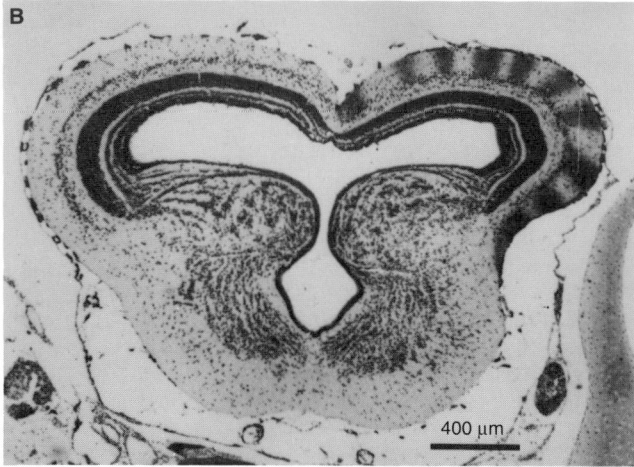

FIGURE 60–8

Ocular dominance columns can be induced by transplanting a third eye in frogs. Autoradiographs of a coronal section through the midbrain of frogs. (Adapted from Constantine-Paton, 1981.)

A. Normal frog. The left eye was injected with [³H]proline three days before the animal was sacrificed. The entire superficial neuropil of the right optic lobe (left side of the picture) is filled with silver grains, indicating the region occupied by synaptic terminals from the labeled (contralateral) eye.

B. Three-eyed frog. The normal right eye was injected with [³H]proline. The left optic lobe of this animal (right side of the picture) receives inputs from both the labeled eye and the supernumerary eye. The normally continuous retinotectal synaptic zone of the contralateral eye is divided into alternating bands of terminal endings from each eye.

inputs from each eye in the lateral geniculate nucleus are segregated in alternating layers, much as they are in the ocular dominance columns. Unlike the ocular dominance columns, however, this segregation is completed before birth, during prenatal development. Carla Shatz and Stryker found that the projections from each eye failed to segregate anatomically if they applied tetrodotoxin to the optic chiasm of a fetus and suppressed the generation of action potentials during the time axons still overlap extensively in the lateral geniculate nucleus.

There is, however, an important difference in the way

activity segregates afferents in the visual cortex and in the lateral geniculate nucleus. In the cortex the segregation occurs *after* birth, and the activity required for the formation of these connections is driven by visual experience. In the lateral geniculate nucleus segregation occurs *before* birth, while the infant is still *in utero*, so that the activity essential for segregating optic nerve fibers cannot be driven by visual experience. What then drives the retinal afferents? Lucia Galli and Lamberto Maffei and Shatz and her colleagues found that the retinal fibers of the optic nerve are spontaneously active *in utero*, independent of any visual information. Moreover, neighboring cells in the fetal retina tend to be active together, firing in synchronous bursts that are a few seconds in duration separated by silent periods lasting one to two minutes. Thus, spontaneous activity *in utero* may have an important instructive function in development, not only in the visual system but also generally. The spontaneous firing of a group of fibers and the resulting synchronous excitation of its target seem to strengthen those synapses whose presynaptic fibers are active together (cooperation) and to weaken those synapses whose presynaptic fibers are inactive or out of synchrony (competition).

These results in the lateral geniculate nucleus and cerebral cortex are consistent with an important idea first developed by the psychologist Donald Hebb: Coincident activity in the pre- and postsynaptic elements of a synapse leads to its strengthening. Hebb's idea has been incorporated into many neuronal models of competition, and we shall encounter them again in Chapter 65 in connection with cellular mechanisms of learning and memory. Indeed, based on the assumptions of a Hebbian coincidence mechanism, Kenneth Miller and Stryker have developed a mathematical model of activity-dependent competition between the two eyes that simulates quite accurately the segregation of ocular dominance columns during development (Figure 60–9).

A clue as to how this sort of cooperation might work has come from studies of the three-eyed frog (see above). As in the mammalian visual system, the formation of ocular dominance columns in the three-eyed frog also appears to require synchronous activity among neighboring neurons. Columns do not form in frogs when activity in the retinal ganglion cells of one eye is blocked by tetrodotoxin. The work of Constantine-Paton suggests that the critical feature in retinal activity is that neighboring fibers fire together. Temporal summation of synaptic excitation would assure a level of synaptic depolarization in the common target cell sufficient to remove the Mg^{2+} block from the *N*-methyl-D-aspartate (NMDA)-type glutamate receptors (Chapter 11). Removing the Mg^{2+} block allows Ca^{2+} to flow into the postsynaptic cell to activate Ca^{2+}-dependent second-messenger systems. These second-messenger systems might be essential for stabilizing the active synapses, thereby preserving neighbor relations of afferent fibers in the target during formation of the retinotopic map.

Consistent with this idea, Hollis Cline and Constantine-Paton found that segregation of columns is blocked by exposing the tectum to aminophosphonovaleric acid (APV), a selective antagonist of the NMDA receptor

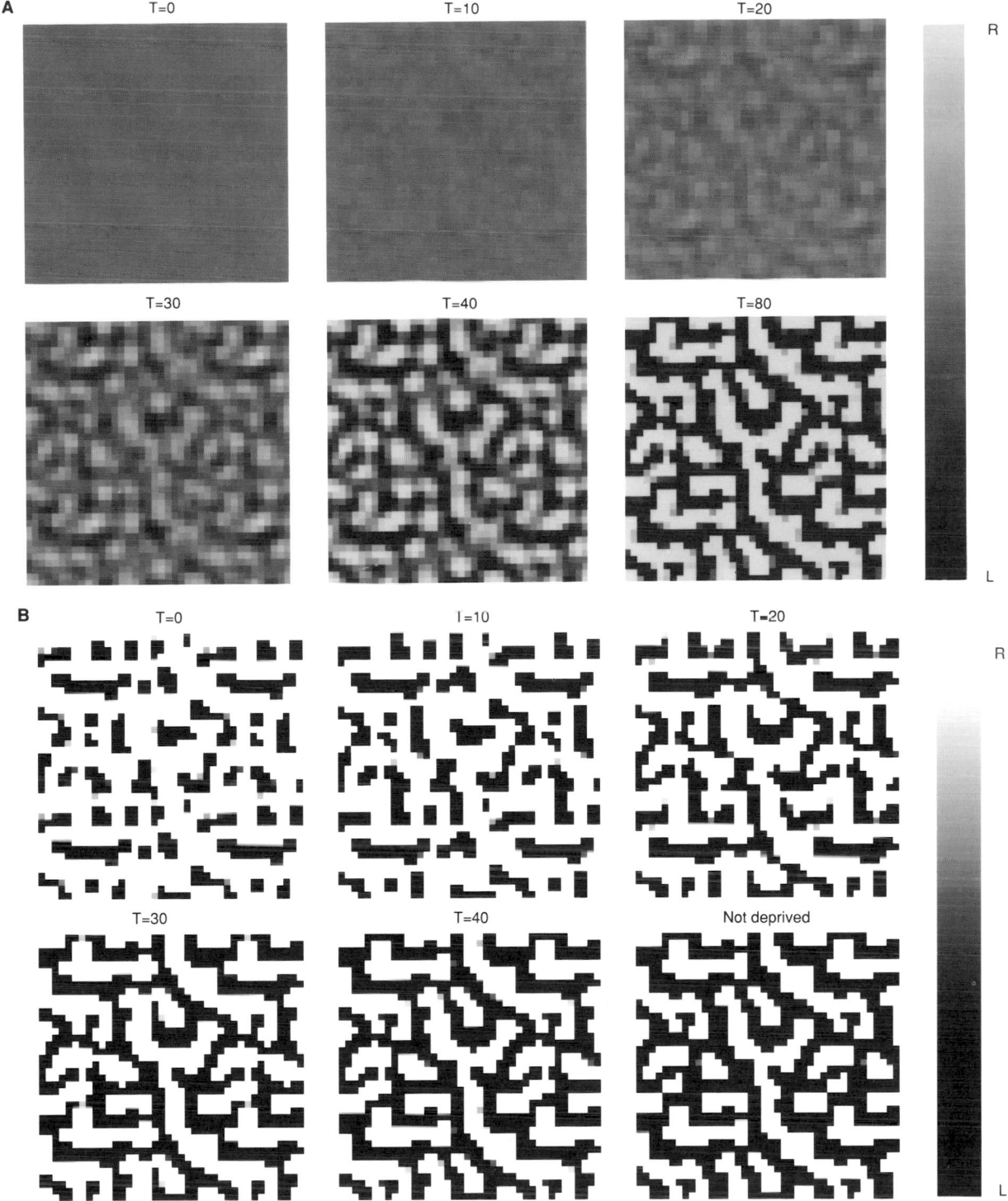

FIGURE 60-9

A computer generated simulation of the development of ocular dominance columns. (From Miller et al., 1989.)

A. These examples illustrate different stages in the normal development of ocular dominance columns. Each square represents a single cortical cell. **White** and **black** signify complete dominance of inputs from one or the other eye. Shades of **gray** indicate the degree of convergent input from both eyes. With time **(T)** in arbitrary units roughly comparable to days, this model generates a progressive segregation of inputs from each eye until at T = 80 there is almost no overlap. The resulting pattern is similar to that observed experimentally in Figure 60–3A.

B. Similar image showing the consequences for segregation of eye inputs when monocular deprivation has been carried out at various starting times **(T)** (ranging from 0 to 40). When segregation is started early (T = 0), the input of the remaining eye expands significantly during the initial period. As the onset of monocular deprivation is delayed (T = 10, 20, 30, 40), the expansion of the input of the intact eye decreases. In this example the critical period lasts from T = 0 to T = 20. After T = 30, monocular deprivation has little effect. This can be seen by comparison to the not deprived case in A.

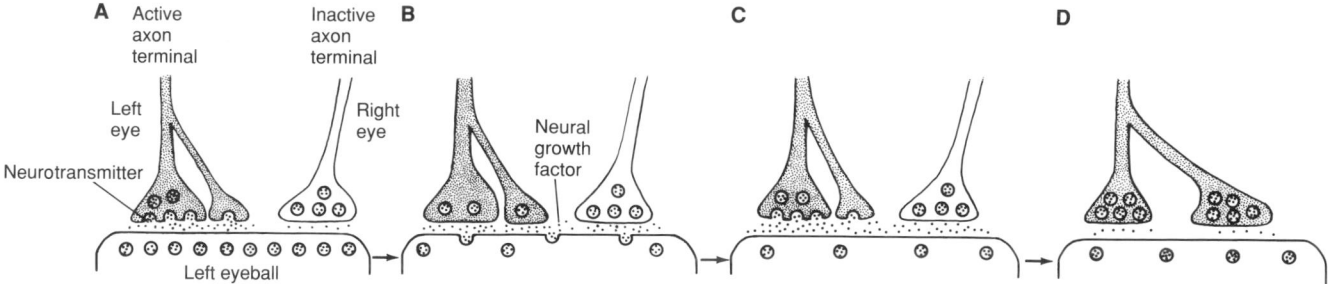

FIGURE 60–10

A possible mechanism for cooperation and competition. According to this model stabilization of a synapse depends on factors released from the postsynaptic cell (in this case a cell responding to the left eye) that act on and stimulate the growth of active presynaptic inputs. Synchronous release of the growth factor is triggered by action potentials in the postsynaptic cells. These are only produced when there is synchronous activity in the presynpatic input. In the visual system cells carrying information from neighboring regions in the retina tend to fire in synchrony.

In the absence of activity, there is only a low level of spontaneous release. The presynaptic terminal can take up the postsynaptic factor only when it is active, and it does so when it has just released neurotransmitter by exocytosis and is in the process of endocytic retrieval of the vesicle membrane (Chapter

13). Active axon terminals that take up the factor enlarge and grow additional terminals that thereby reinforce the strength of the synapse. The more frequently the postsynaptic cell is stimulated, the more its internal store of the factor is depleted and the lower is the rate of spontaneous release. Thus, inactive axon terminals competing with active ones will fail to obtain adequate amounts of growth factor and consequently will shrink and eventually withdraw (**B, C,** and **D**). When two axon terminals are active at diffcrent times they will compete with one another for the limited amount of growth factor that the postsynaptic cell contains. A large terminal will take up more growth factor, which in turn will make it larger still. The outcome of such competition may thus depend on slight differences in initial size of the synaptic terminal (**A**). (Modified from Alberts et al., 1989.)

(Chapter 11). In contrast, exposure of the tectum to NMDA, the agonist of this receptor, leads to a sharpening of the columnar organization. Experiments by Wolfgang Singer and his colleagues suggest that a similar mechanism might operate in the mammalian brain.

These considerations raise one final question: What are the molecular steps whereby synchronous activity strengthens the cooperating synapses and weakens that of neighboring inactive fibers? How do the Ca^{2+}-dependent second-messenger systems stabilize the cooperating synapses? We do not as yet know the answer to this question. But it is conceivable that the postsynaptic target cells in layer 4c release a growth or trophic factor, a protein with actions similar to nerve growth factor. This factor may be in short supply and the intermingled afferent fibers may spread over the entire target structure as they compete for the factor. Fibers that originate from neighboring neurons could, by acting in synergy to depolarize the target cell, increase the secretion of the growth factor from it. Axons from different eyes, or even axons from the same eye that originate from cells that are not neighbors, would not be able to enhance release because they are not activated in synchrony.

The growth factor might be released only when synchronous cooperating axons depolarize the postsynaptic cell sufficiently to activate the NMDA receptor-channel that allows Ca^{2+} inflow. Activation of Ca^{2+}-dependent second-messenger systems might then regulate the release of the growth factor. Moreover, only those presynaptic terminals that are active synchronously and participate cooperatively in the depolarization of the postsynaptic cell can take up the growth factor (Figure 60–10). Afferent

fibers from one eye that do not fire action potentials in phase with the neighboring afferents from the other eye might not be able to take up the trophic factor. They would be at a competitive disadvantage for survival and therefore would be eliminated (Figure 60–10).

Different Regions of the Brain Have Different Critical Periods of Development

It is becoming clear that, as with other aspects of behavior, the development of form perception and the binocular vision necessary for depth perception proceed in stages after birth. Each stage culminates in one or more developmental decisions, many of which are irreversible. In each stage appropriate sensory experiences are necessary to validate, shape, and update normal developmental processes. Consequently, the effects of sensory deprivation are most severe during a restricted and well-defined period early in postnatal life when these developmental decisions are still being made.

In the past it has been difficult to relate the development of behavior to the development of the nervous system. However, research on ocular dominance columns is providing an important bridge between the two. For example, developmental studies by Jack Pettigrew have shown that neurons in the visual cortex mature and become sensitive to ocular disparity toward the end of the fourth postnatal month. Psychophysical studies by Richard Held and his colleagues have shown that stereopsis develops at the same time. Thus, stereoscopic vision seems to parallel the maturation of the ocular dominance columns.

Critical periods of development generally do not have *sharp* time boundaries. Different layers within one region of the brain may have different critical periods of development, so that even after the critical period for one layer has passed, rearrangement of the layer may still be possible because the entire region has not yet fully developed. For example, 8 weeks after birth layer 4c in the visual cortex of the monkey is no longer affected by monocular deprivation, whereas the upper and lower layers continue to be susceptible for almost the entire first year. If each cortical area and each layer within each area has its own timetable for segregation of connections and its own critical period, this might account for the complex developmental consequences of disturbances in early experience. Experiences that interfere with the development of a primary sensory region of the brain, such as visual deprivation, might produce their behavioral consequences early in postnatal development, whereas other experiences, such as social deprivation, might act on association cortices and perhaps exert their actions later.

The existence of discrete stages in the formation of the ocular dominance columns is likely to represent a general feature of development of the nervous system. Different stages might explain two well-known features of intellectual and behavioral development: (1) certain capabilities—such as those for language, music, or mathematics—usually must be developed well before puberty if they are to develop at all; and (2) traumatic insults at certain stages of postnatal life affect one aspect of perceptual or character development while insults at other periods in development affect other aspects of behavior.

Studies of Development Are Important Clinically

Studies of maternal deprivation provide a striking example of how genetic factors, development, and experience interact inextricably in early life and how environmental deprivation can dramatically alter developmental processes. In addition to providing insights into the mechanisms governing development, these studies have obvious clinical relevance. For example, studies of strabismus and its effects on the development of visual perception have changed the clinical treatment of strabismus. Children with strabismus initially have good vision in each eye. However, because they cannot fuse the images in the two eyes, these children often tend to favor one eye.

Ophthalmologists used to delay correcting strabismus in children until they had reached the age of 8–9 years, long after the critical period. As a result, these children often lost useful vision in the neglected eye. Because of the work of Hubel and Wiesel, ophthalmologists now surgically correct the strabismus very early, when normal binocular vision can still be restored.

Overall View

The precise neural connections within the sensory areas of the brain are achieved by two very different sorts of mechanisms. First, as we have seen in Chapters 58 and 59,

various molecular guidance cues lead axons from specific regions of the periphery to particular, yet broadly defined target regions. Once this initial alignment is accomplished a second set of processes takes over based on cooperation and competition of the outgrowing axons.

This second set of processes matches each axon to a specific target neuron and thereby introduces a point-to-point order in the map of the target region. In the primary visual cortex, cooperation between the afferent fibers from the same eye and competition between afferents from the two eyes set up the alternating ocular dominance columns. In this precise matching, cooperation among afferent fibers from local regions of the retina enhances the ability of these afferents to group together on common target cells, thereby helping to segregate the axons from each of the two eyes. At the same time, competition between fibers from the two eyes also separates the axons because the weaker of the input from the two retinas onto a common target will decline until it withdraws, eliminating the overlap and leading to the almost complete segregation of the terminals. These two processes interact to establish a precise topographical map.

During a critical period in postnatal development this cooperation and competition are regulated by activity in the incoming fibers. As a result, the segregation of afferent fibers and the establishment of ocular dominance columns can be dramatically affected by experimentally changing the balance of input activity from the two eyes during this critical period. After the critical period, existing connections become stable and much less susceptible to modification. Studies of the development of the ocular dominance columns allow us to understand how other, more complex sensory experiences early in development may change the circuitry and structure of the growing brain. These studies also suggest that the use of drugs such as narcotics and alcohol during pregnancy can have profound effects on the wiring of the brain during infancy by interfering with activity-dependent development of neural connections.

Selected Readings

Constantine-Paton, M., Cline, H. T., and Debski, E. 1990. Patterned activity, synaptic convergence, and the NMDA receptor in developing visual pathways. Annu. Rev. Neurosci. 13: 129–154.

Harlow, H. F. 1958. The nature of love. Am. Psychol. 13:673–685.

Hebb, D. O. 1949. The Organization of Behavior: A Neuropsychological Theory. New York: Wiley.

Held, R. 1989. Perception and its neuronal mechanisms. Cognition 33:139–154.

Hubel, D. H. 1982. Exploration of the primary visual cortex, 1955–78. Nature 299:515–524.

Hubel, D. H. 1988. Eye, Brain, and Vision. New York: Scientific American Library.

Hubel, D. H., and Wiesel, T. N. 1977. Ferrier Lecture: Functional architecture of macaque monkey visual cortex. Proc. R. Soc. Lond. [Biol.] 198:1–59.

Knudsen, E. I. 1984. The role of auditory experience in the development and maintenance of sound localization. Trends Neurosci. 7:326–330.

Leiderman, P. H. 1981. Human mother-infant social bonding: Is there a sensitive phase? In K. Immelmann, G. W. Barlow, L. Petrinovich, and M. Main (eds.), Behavioral Development: The Bielepeld Interdisciplinary Project. Cambridge, England: Cambridge University Press, pp. 454–468.

Meister, M., Wong, R. O. L., Baylor, D. A., and Shatz, C. J. 1991. Synchronous bursts of action potentials in ganglion cells of the developing mammalian retina. Science 252:939–943.

Miller, K. D., Keller, J. B., and Stryker, M. P. 1989. Ocular dominance column development: Analysis and simulation. Science 245:605–615.

Rakic, P. 1981. Development of visual centers in the primate brain depends on binocular competition before birth. Science 214:928–931.

Riesen, A. H. 1958. Plasticity of behavior: Psychological aspects. In H. F. Harlow and C. N. Woolsey (eds.), Biological and Biochemical Bases of Behavior. Madison: University of Wisconsin Press, pp. 425–450.

Shatz, C. J. 1990. Impulse activity and the patterning of connections during CNS development. Neuron. 5:745–756.

Shatz, C. J., and Stryker, M. P. 1988. Prenatal tetrodotoxin infusion blocks segregation of retinogeniculate afferents. Science 242:87–89.

References

Bear, M. F., Kleinschmidt, A., Gu, Q., and Singer, W. 1990. Disruption of experience-dependent synaptic modifications in striate cortex by infusion of an NMDA receptor antagonist. J. Neurosci. 10:909–925.

Cline, H. T., and Constantine-Paton, M. 1990. NMDA receptor agonist and antagonists alter retinal ganglion cell arbor structure in the developing frog retinotectal projection. J. Neurosci. 10:1197–1216.

Constantine-Paton, M. 1981. Induced ocular-dominance zones in tectal cortex. In F. O. Schmitt, F. G. Worden, G. Adelman, S. G. Dennis (eds.), The Organization of the Cerebral Cortex: Proceedings of a Neurosciences Research Program Colloquium. Cambridge, Mass.: MIT Press, pp. 47–67.

Galli, L., and Maffei, L. 1988. Spontaneous impulse activity of rat retinal ganglion cells in prenatal life. Science 242:90–91.

Gilbert, C. D., and Wiesel, T. N. 1983. Clustered intrinsic connections in cat visual cortex. J. Neurosci. 3:1116–1133.

Harlow, H. F., Dodsworth, R. O., and Harlow, M. K. 1965. Total social isolation in monkeys. Proc. Natl. Acad. Sci. U.S.A. 54: 90–97.

Hubel, D. H., Wiesel, T. N., and LeVay, S. 1977. Plasticity of ocular dominance columns in monkey striate cortex. Philos. Trans. R. Soc. Lond [Biol.] 278:377–409.

Lane, H. 1976. The Wild Boy of Aveyron. Cambridge, Mass.: Harvard University Press.

LeVay, S., and Stryker, M. P. 1979. The development of ocular dominance columns in the cat. In J. A. Ferrendelli (ed.), Aspects of Developmental Neurobiology, Society for Neuro-

science Symposia, Vol. 4. Bethesda, Md.: Society for Neuroscience, pp. 83–98.

LeVay, S., Stryker, M. P., and Shatz, C. J. 1978. Ocular dominance columns and their development in layer IV of the cat's visual cortex: A quantitative study. J. Comp. Neurol. 179:223–244.

LeVay, S., Wiesel, T. N., and Hubel, D. H. 1980. The development of ocular dominance columns in normal and visually deprived monkeys. J. Comp. Neurol. 191:1–51.

LeVay, S., Wiesel, T. N., and Hubel, D. H. 1981. The postnatal development and plasticity of ocular-dominance columns in the monkey. In F. O. Schmitt, F. G. Worden, G. Adelman, and S. G. Dennis (eds.), The Organization of the Cerebral Cortex: Proceedings of a Neurosciences Research Program Colloquium. Cambridge, Mass.: MIT Press, pp. 29–45.

Lorenz, K. 1965. Evolution and Modification of Behavior. Chicago: University of Chicago Press.

Poggio, G. F., and Fischer, B. 1977. Binocular interaction and depth sensitivity in striate and prestriate cortex of behaving rhesus monkey. J. Neurophysiol. 40:1392–1405.

Rakic, P. 1976. Prenatal genesis of connections subserving ocular dominance in the rhesus monkey. Nature 261:467–471.

Rakic, P. 1977. Prenatal development of the visual system in rhesus monkey. Philos. Trans. R. Soc. Lond. [Biol.] 278:245–260.

Spitz, R. A. 1945. Hospitalism: An inquiry into the genesis of psychiatric conditions in early childhood. Psychoanal. Study Child 1:53–74.

Spitz, R. A. 1946. Hospitalism: A follow-up report on investigation described in Volume 1, 1945. Psychoanal. Study Child 2:113–117.

Spitz, R. A., and Wolf, K. M. 1946. Anaclitic depression: An inquiry into the genesis of psychiatric conditions in early childhood, II. Psychoanal. Study Child 2:313–342.

Stryker, M. P. 1991. Activity-dependent reorganization of afferents in the developing mammalian visual system. In D. M.-K. Lam and C. J. Shatz (eds.), Development of the Visual System. Cambridge, Mass.: MIT Press, pp. 267–287.

Stryker, M. P., and Harris, W. A. 1986. Binocular impulse blockade prevents the formation of ocular dominance columns in cat visual cortex. J. Neurosci. 6:2117–2133.

Stryker, M. P., and Strickland, S. L. 1984. Physiological segregation of ocular dominance columns depends on the pattern of afferent electrical activity. Invest. Ophthalmol. Visual Sci. (Suppl.) 25:278 (ARVO abstracts).

Suomi, S. J., and Harlow, H. F. 1975. The role and reason of peer relationships in rhesus monkeys. In M. Lewis and L. A. Rosenblum (eds.), Friendship and Peer Relations. New York: Wiley, pp. 153–185.

von Senden, M. 1932. Space and Sight. P. Heath (trans.) Glencoe, Ill.: Free Press, 1960.

Wiesel, T. N., and Hubel, D. H. 1963. Single-cell responses in striate cortex of kittens deprived of vision in one eye. J. Neurophysiol. 26:1003–1017.

61

Dennis D. Kelly

Sexual Differentiation of the Nervous System

The Gene for the Testes Determining Factor Is Located on the Y Chromosome

The Developing Gonads Are Embryologically Bipotential, Becoming Testes If the TDF Gene Is Present and Ovaries If It Is Not

Sexual Differentiation Is Regulated by Gonadal Hormones from Both Mother and Male Fetus

Gonadal Hormones Exert Both Organizational and Regulatory Effects upon Nervous Tissue Depending upon the Stage of the Life Cycle

Perinatal Hormones Impose a Permanent Sex-Specific Blueprint upon the Developing Nervous System

Fetal Exposure to Male Hormones Causes Pseudohermaphroditism in Genetic Females

Steroid Hormones Influence Perinatal Development Only During Critical Periods

The Brain Can Be Masculinized Not Only by Male Hormones But Also by Many Other Compounds

Alpha-Fetoprotein Binds Estrogen in the Rat and Thus Protects Female Fetuses from Masculinization

Receptors in the Cell Nucleus Mediate the Effects of Gonadal Steroid Hormones

Sexually Differentiated Brains Have Different Physiological Properties and Behavioral Tendencies

Perinatal Hormones Also Determine the Degree to Which Sex-Linked Behaviors Are Expressed by Normal Males and Females

Sexual Differentiation Is Reflected in the Structure of Certain Neurons

The Cellular Mechanisms Involved in the Development of Sex Differences in the Brain Can Be Studied *in Vitro*

A Wide Range of Behaviors Is Influenced by Sex Differences in the Organization of the Brain

Sexual Dimorphism Is Evident in Cognitive Development in Monkeys

Human Cerebral Asymmetry Is Sexually Dimorphic

An Overall View

Like cognitive behavior, reproductive behavior reflects the developmental plasticity of the brain. Here, too, the range of potential behaviors is genetically determined but the actual behaviors expressed are shaped by interactions with the environment. Like other forms of developmental plasticity, sexual differentiation of the neural network for reproductive behavior is characterized by *critical periods* during which specific interactions between developing cells and their environment determine future behavioral capacities. Critical periods are a part of the sequential nature of growth; at each stage of development a choice is made between a limited set of alterations. Once a time-dependent choice is made, it is nearly impossible to reverse the result.

Although males and females differ in many ways, the underlying developmental program, as we shall see, is the same for all aspects of sexual differentiation. A single gene determines the type of gonad. The gonad in turn influences the hormonal environment of the developing fetus or infant. Specific tissues develop along sexually dimorphic lines in response to the combination of sex hormones to which they are exposed. Developing target tissues are responsive to hormones only during certain critical phases of differentiation.

To understand this basic template of sexual differentiation we shall examine the following questions in sequence. Which gene determines gonad type? What and when do the developing gonads secrete? Which are the target tissues for sexual differentiation? When are the critical periods for these events? Finally, we shall examine the biological and behavioral consequences of sexually differentiated neuronal populations. As we shall see, these extend well beyond the domain of reproductive behavior.

The Gene for the Testes Determining Factor Is Located on the Y Chromosome

The chromosomal sex of an individual is established at conception when the sperm of the male contributes either an X or a Y chromosome. The genetic sex determines whether the bipotential embryonic gonad differentiates into an ovary or testis. Subsequent steps in sexual differentiation result from the action of hormones. If a Y chromosome is present, testes develop and their hormonal secretions result in the development of a phenotypic male. If only X chromosomes are present, ovaries develop and the female phenotype results. If only one sex chromosome is present (invariably an X), or if a gonad is absent, the individual also develops as a female. Thus, the pathway for developing the ovary is the normal (default) pathway. The function of the Y chromosome is to switch the developmental program of the precursor cells in undifferentiated gonads from the pathway for follicle cell development characteristic of the ovary to the pathway for Sertoli cells characteristic of the testis.

The existence of X and Y *sex chromosomes*, distinct from autosomes, was first demonstrated in humans in 1923, yet for nearly 40 years thereafter it was assumed that sex in mammals was decided by the number of X chromosomes, as it is in fruit flies (*Drosophila*). By 1959

the study of abnormal sex chromosome combinations, occurring in such syndromes as Klinefelter's (XXY) and Turner's (XO), revealed that mammalian embryos carrying a Y chromosome develop as males regardless of the number of X chromosomes. In 1966 the critical sex-determining region was narrowed down to the short arm of the Y chromosome. All sexually dimorphic characteristics, including the development of the brain, depend on the presence or absence of one or more genes on the short arm of chromosome Y. Thus, this segment of the mammalian Y chromosome constitutes a binary switch for sexual dimorphism. (The term *dimorphism* refers to the existence of two distinct forms within a species; *sexual dimorphism* refers to any characteristics that differ in males and females.)

In reality, sexual differentiation requires many genes that act in conjunction with the Y chromosome. Some of these genes are undoubtedly autosomal. Nevertheless, there must exist one or more genes on the Y chromosome whose products, directly or indirectly, determine gonadal form. This gene or set of genes is known to encode for the *testes determining factor*, or TDF.

Between 1986 and 1990 the search for the gene encoding TDF had focused on a progressively smaller region in the middle of the short arm of the Y chromosome. Detailed exploration of this critical 35 kilobase region by Peter Goodfellow, Robin Lovell-Badge, Andrew Sinclair, John Gubbay and their colleagues led to the discovery of a candidate gene for TDF. This gene is present on the Y chromosome of all mammals so far examined and encodes a transcript that is specifically expressed in the testes. The gene called *sex-determining region of Y* (SRY) encodes a protein that has a DNA-binding domain, suggesting that the protein serves as a transcription activator. In addition, the gene is deleted in female mice that are XY, of which we shall learn more later. The SRY gene is homologous to a gene in yeast that encodes for a transcriptional activator important in determining mating type, further supporting its function as a transcriptional activator. The mouse homolog of the SRY gene has been introduced into transgenic mice. Some XX mice transgenic for the SRY gene are phenotypically male even though they lack all the other genes on the Y chromosome. Thus the SRY gene alone can induce maleness.

Although males typically are XY, one male in 20,000 has two X chromosomes and no Y and yet is male. One female in 20,000 is XY. How does this come about? As outlined in Figure 61–1, genetic mapping and screening with Y-specific probes of the chromosomes of these XX males show that during meiosis of the paternal gamete there has been crossing over and transfer to the X chromosome of that portion of the Y chromosome that carries the TDF gene(s). It is the transfer of this part of the Y chromosome that confers maleness upon the individual. Conversely, XY females lack this segment of the Y chromosome. The region in the middle of the short arm of the Y chromosome that carries the TDG gene is homologous to the X chromosome, and therefore crossing over can occur during meiosis. The region of DNA on the normal Y chromosome essential for spermatogenesis, however, is

Preparation of radioactive probe
from cloned DNA from XY male genotype

Southern blot transfer of XX and XY DNA

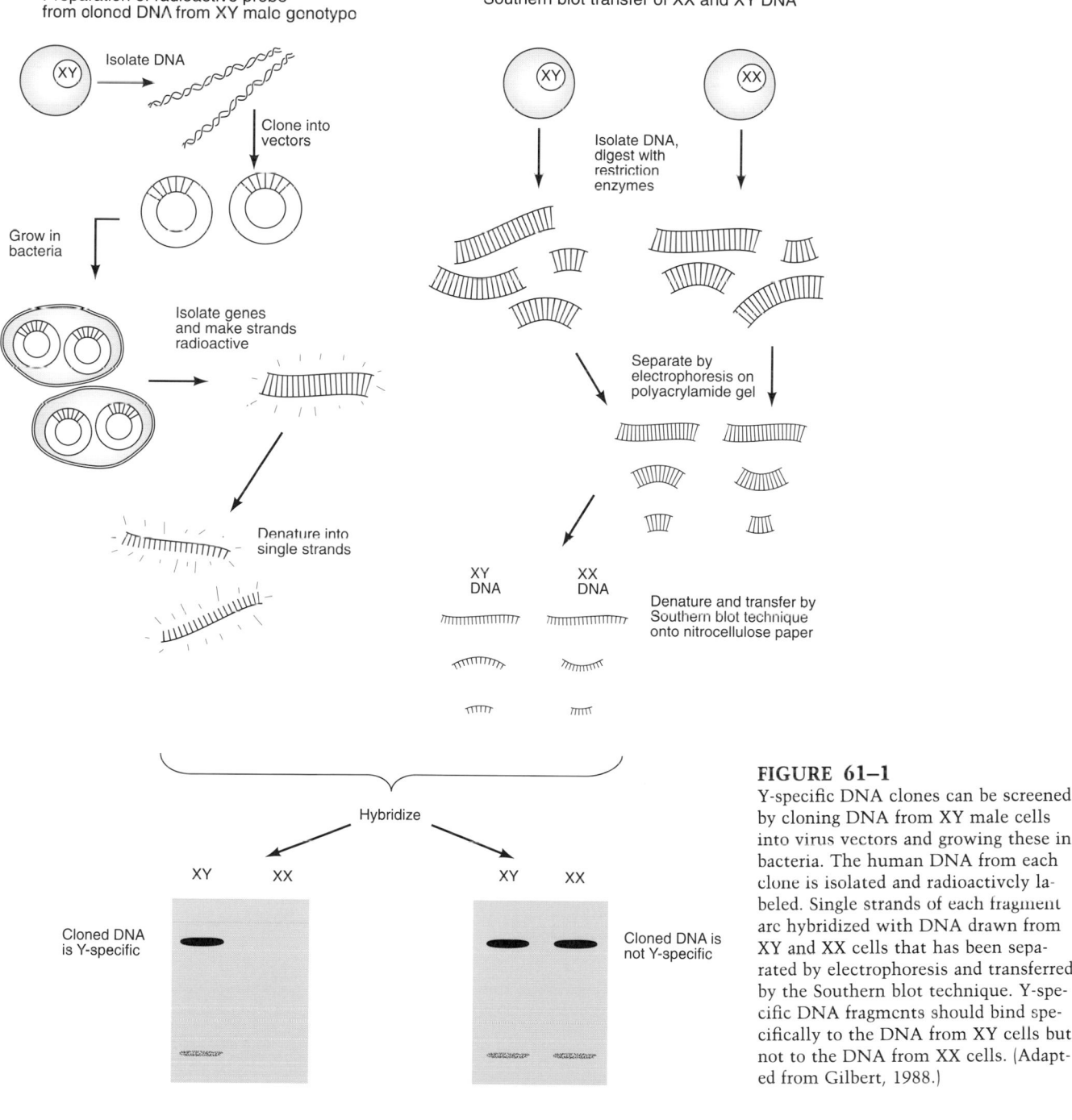

FIGURE 61-1

Y-specific DNA clones can be screened by cloning DNA from XY male cells into virus vectors and growing these in bacteria. The human DNA from each clone is isolated and radioactively labeled. Single strands of each fragment are hybridized with DNA drawn from XY and XX cells that has been separated by electrophoresis and transferred by the Southern blot technique. Y-specific DNA fragments should bind specifically to the DNA from XY cells but not to the DNA from XX cells. (Adapted from Gilbert, 1988.)

not transferred with the TDF gene; hence, XX males are not fertile.

The Developing Gonads Are Embryologically Bipotential, Becoming Testes If the TDF Gene Is Present and Ovaries If It Is Not

The TDF gene controls the option of whether the undifferentiated gonad becomes an ovary or testis. The secretions of the fetal testis in turn determine subsequent events

in the sexual differentiation of the male. However, the same is not true for the development of the ovary and the differentiation of the female. In 1953 Alfred Jost removed the gonadal tissue from early fetal rabbits, all of which later developed as females (with oviducts, uterus, cervix, and vagina), regardless of whether they were XX or XY. Thus, the female phenotype can develop in the absence of any gonadal tissue.

The fetal testes secrete two major hormones: (1) testosterone, a steroid secreted by Leydig cells, which masculinizes the sex organs, mammary gland rudiments, and nervous system, and (2) Müllerian duct-inhibiting substance (MIS), a glycoprotein secreted by Sertoli cells, which causes the resorption of the tissue that would otherwise become the oviducts, uterus, cervix, and vagina. The absence of these two hormones, or of receptors for them, results in female development.

Sexual Differentiation Is Regulated by Gonadal Hormones from Both Mother and Male Fetus

Although TDF genes determine whether the undifferentiated gonad will become a testis, later stages in the development of sexual phenotype result from the actions of the hormones of the fetal testes acting in concert with hormones from the mother. This principle was first appreciated and extended to the nervous system by the analysis of two syndromes that arise from spontaneously occurring hormonal deficiencies during early development.

The first is a congenital anhormonal condition in which only one X (and no Y) chromosome is present. In this disorder, known as *Turner's syndrome*, functional gonadal tissue does not form. Fetal ovaries bud, then atrophy. Wolffian ducts decay; Müllerian ducts develop. In the estrogen-dominated environment furnished by the mother and the placenta, a female genital tract forms. Patients with Turner's syndrome are usually regarded by their families as feminine before adolescence. Some are diagnosed at birth by such accompanying signs as webbing of the neck and impairment of hearing. Many cases are discovered only much later, when these children fail to show the signs of female puberty. If treated with ovarian hormones during adolescence, they respond as normal females. Moreover, the gender identity and sexual behavior of these patients do not differ significantly from normal females.

The second genetic anomaly involves individuals incapable of responding to androgens. This condition, called *androgen insensitivity syndrome*, occurs in XY individuals who possess the TDF gene. They develop testes, which secrete both testosterone and Müllerian duct inhibiting substance during fetal development. Because these genetic males cannot respond to the androgens they produce, they are indistinguishable from phenotypic females in their external appearance (Figure 61–2). However, they do respond to MIS, and so their Müllerian ducts degenerate. Although they develop as women, they lack both uterus and oviducts. Studies on mutant mice and rats with the same condition demonstrate that the deficiency is characterized by the often total absence of androgen receptors, whereas estrogen receptors are unaffected. As a result, even with normal production of androgens by the testes, the target cells of male sexual differentiation are unable to respond to the hormonal signal. Thus, despite the XY karyotype, the presence of testes and the absence of ovaries, these patients develop female secondary sex characteristics during adolescence in response to estrogens produced by both their adrenals and testes.

The implications of these clinical states is that the female form and gender identity can develop in the absence of

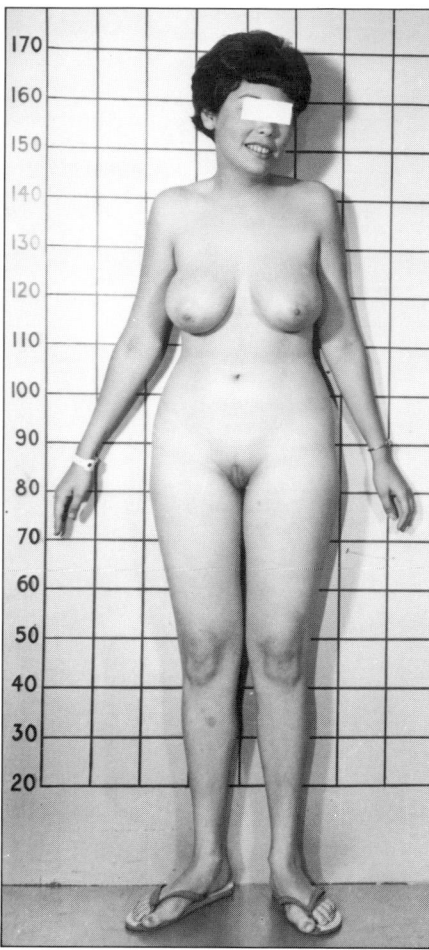

FIGURE 61–2
This adult patient with androgen insensitivity syndrome is a genetic XY male. Female pubertal development occurred under the influence of estrogens normally secreted by the testes, with no exogenous hormonal treatment. (From Money and Ehrhardt, 1972.)

hormonal influences from the fetal gonads. Moreover, under special circumstances individuals who are genetically male can develop feminine body characteristics. To integrate these clinical phenomena with experimental observations on the sexual differentiation of the nervous system *in utero*, we must first consider the differential actions of gonadal hormones upon the developing and mature nervous system.

Gonadal Hormones Exert Both Organizational and Regulatory Effects upon Nervous Tissue Depending upon the Stage of the Life Cycle

Vertebrate reproductive behavior, especially courtship behavior between prospective mates, is richly varied and often species distinctive. Whatever the behavioral ritual,

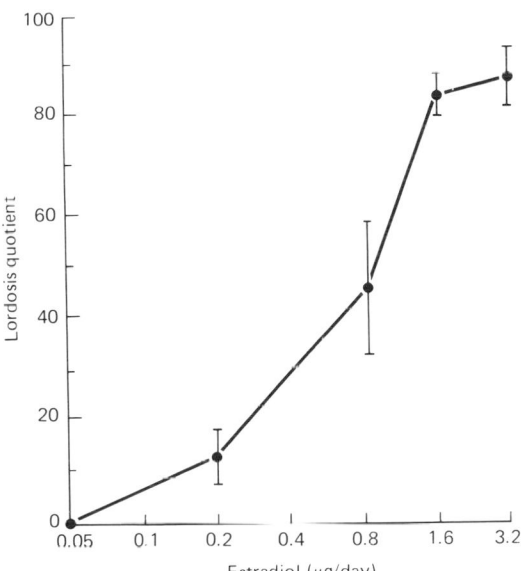

FIGURE 61–3

Estrogen induces sexual receptivity in ovariectomized female rats in a dose-dependent manner. After eight daily subcutaneous injections of estradiol benzoate, receptivity was measured by the lordosis quotient (the number of lordotic responses of the subject, divided by the number of mounts, multiplied by 100). (Data from Bermant and Davidson, 1974.)

it is virtually always sexually dimorphic. As examples, lordosis and mounting are two sexually dimorphic behavioral markers of neural differentiation frequently studied in rodents. The female elevates her rump and assumes a concave posture of the back; this is lordosis. The male mounts from the rear clasping her flanks with his forelimbs.

The secretions of the mature gonads (the ratio of steroids) are also sexually dimorphic. Testes secrete principally androgens, ovaries estrogens. Is it possible that the unique blend of testicular hormones produces male behavior and ovarian hormones female behavior equally well in adult males and females? If so, sex-related patterns of behavior could be explained by the type of hormones that are present in the adult. This line of reasoning was an accepted theory for many years. However, we now know that sexually dimorphic behavior patterns in many vertebrate species, including our own, depend upon the qualitatively different actions of gonadal hormones at two different stages in the life cycle.

In the adult, circulating steroid sex hormones primarily activate sexual responses. Thus, administration of estrogen increases sexual receptivity in female rats in a dose-dependent manner (Figure 61–3). In ovariectomized animals, however, the behavioral stimulation is short-lived. Receptivity declines as the hormone is metabolized. Thus, the actions of gonadal hormones upon the mature nervous system are *activational* and *transitory*.

In the developing nervous system, steroid hormones create a gender-specific blueprint, which in adulthood

leads to the expression of appropriate sexual behaviors in response to hormonal stimulation. As the clinical and genetic evidence suggests, the nervous system of a developing fetus is essentially undifferentiated and bipotential. Both male and female genotypes are compatible with either brain phenotype. To a remarkable degree, the sexual phenotype of the brain is determined by exposure to specific steroid hormones during an early critical period. Thus, the actions of gonadal hormones upon the developing nervous system are *organizational* and *permanent*. To understand the cellular mechanisms by which developing neural tissue is sexually differentiated by sex steroids, we must first consider the hormonal environment in which fetuses of both sexes develop.

Perinatal Hormones Impose a Permanent Sex-Specific Blueprint upon the Developing Nervous System

Although the mature gonads of both sexes are capable of synthesizing both androgens and estrogens, the steroid products of the testis and ovary differ in their ratio, timing, and some synthetic pathways. In considering the development of gender identity, it is helpful to distinguish experimentally between homotypical and heterotypical steroid sex hormones. *Homotypical hormones* are the prevalent hormones of a given sex administered to an individual of the same sex—for example, estrogens to a female. *Heterotypical hormones* are the dominant gonadal hormones of one sex given to the other. The same terms are also often applied to sex-specific behaviors: *homotypical behavior patterns* are those appropriate to the reference gender and *heterotypical behavior patterns* are those appropriate to the opposite sex.

This behavioral dimorphism is not all-or-none. In the limited repertoires of some species, apparently gender-specific reproductive behaviors often serve other purposes. Either sex may exhibit both male and female copulatory patterns in environmental circumstances that have little to do with reproduction. For instance, monkeys of both sexes use the female sexual posture as a submissive gesture during intraspecies encounters for dominance. But just as the ratio of androgens to estrogens differs between ovary and testis, certain behaviors are more likely to occur in one or the other sex, without falling within the exclusive domain of either.

Fetal Exposure to Male Hormones Causes Pseudohermaphroditism in Genetic Females

During pregnancy the fetuses of both sexes are exposed to the high levels of circulating estrogens in the maternal blood. Since estrogen is homotypical for female fetuses and heterotypical for male fetuses, the following simple question prompted a now classic experiment: What would happen if this normal relationship were reversed, bringing female fetuses under heterotypical hormone influences? Charles Phoenix and his co-workers found that injecting high doses of testosterone into guinea pig mothers had two consequences for genetically female offspring. First, they were born as pseudohermaphrodites: Their external genitalia were indistinguishable from those of normal males, but because they were not also exposed to MIS, a substance unknown at the time, the Müllerian duct derivatives were also present internally.

The second and more intriguing effect was that the adult sexual behavior of hermaphroditic females was also altered. When subsequently treated with estrogen and progesterone as adults, these XX guinea pigs showed some elements of homotypical sexual behaviors—lordosis, for example—but their capacity for this behavior was greatly reduced compared with that of control females. On the other hand, they displayed much more mounting behavior than normal females. When treated with testosterone as adults, these hermaphroditic females displayed a degree of heterotypical mounting comparable to that of normal males, and the female pattern of lordosis was suppressed. These observations led Phoenix to distinguish the effects of hormones present early in development from the effects of the same hormones circulating in the adult. The former were confined to a short critical period and might not become evident until adulthood.

Steroid Hormones Influence Perinatal Development Only During Critical Periods

As we have seen, the developing nervous system of either sex is bipotential. A female pattern of anatomical and behavioral organization can emerge in either an anhormonal or estrogen-dominated prenatal environment. The emergence of the male pattern, however, requires the influence of androgens. If androgens are needed for the development of normal male fetuses, where in the uterine environment do androgens come from? Most experiments on this question have been carried out in the rat, which has a 21-day gestation period. These studies show that the male testes begin to synthesize androgens as early as the 13th day of fetal development and androgen secretion continues in newborn rats until the 10th day after birth.

The possibility that the androgens produced by the immature gonads of the developing male rat are responsible for further masculinization can be checked simply by removing the testes. Even though castration on the day of birth deprives the male rat of testicular androgens for little more than one-half of the period that these hormones are normally present, it has profound effects on the sexual development of genotypic male rats: Rats castrated between one and five days of age develop behavioral characteristics of genetic females. If they are injected with estrogen and progesterone as adults, they display lordotic behavior when mounted by normal males. In contrast, males castrated later in development, after 10 or more days of age, show little or no tendency to display lordosis under comparable conditions.

Another source of steroids that might influence the developing fetuses of both sexes is the placenta, which acts

TABLE 61–1. Adult Gonadotropin Secretion Patterns in Rats Subjected to Neonatal Endocrine Manipulation

Genetic sex	Treatment	Age when treated	Adult luteinizing hormone secretion pattern
Female	None	—	Cyclical
	Testosterone*	4 days	Noncyclical
	Testosterone*	16 days	Cyclical
Male	None	—	Noncyclical
	Castration	1 day	Cyclical
	Castration	7 days	Noncyclical

*Single injection of 1.25 mg of testosterone propionate.
(From Raisman, 1974.)

as an endocrine gland thought to be essential for the maintenance of pregnancy. The role of placental secretions in sexual differentiation is not well understood. Maternal cholesterol is metabolized by the placenta into progesterone. To form other steroid hormones, placentally derived progesterone is transported to the fetal adrenal and liver and then returned to the placenta for transformation into estrogens and a group of androgens, including testosterone.

There is additional evidence that perinatal exposure to male hormones affects later sexual behavior by influencing the developing central nervous system rather than the peripheral sexual apparatus. Both males and females secrete two gonadotropins (or gonad-stimulating hormones) from the anterior pituitary: *luteinizing hormone* (LH) and *follicle-stimulating hormone* (FSH). In males these hormones are secreted at a steady level. In females, surges of the hormones underlie the cyclical activities of the reproductive tract.

In 1962 Charles Barraclough and Roger Gorski demonstrated that cyclical secretion of gonadotropin by the pituitary does not depend directly on the genetic sex of the animal, but rather on the absence of androgen during the perinatal period. Under normal circumstances androgen prevents cyclical secretion from developing in the male. An experiment by Geoffrey Raisman illustrates this point. Treatment of the normal genetic female rat with a single dose of androgen on the fourth day of postnatal life permanently abolishes the ability to ovulate. Conversely, a male castrated within one day of birth can exhibit cyclic ovulation and behavioral estrus if he receives transplanted ovaries as an adult (Table 61–1). The same manipulations carried out after the critical period do not affect the normal development and expression of homotypical behavior.

The Brain Can Be Masculinized Not Only by Male Hormones But Also by Many Other Compounds

The critical developmental period for sexual differentiation corresponds to a period in which the brain is sensitive to a broad spectrum of steroids, many of which are not normally present in the body. Experimental masculinization of the brain can be induced by exposure to such functionally diverse hormones as testosterone, androstenedione, estradiol, and diethylstilbestrol (DES), and even drugs, such as barbiturates, and pesticides, such as dichlorodiphenyltrichloroethane (DDT).

The principal active hormone that determines the normal male brain pattern in newborn rats is estradiol, one of the female sex hormones. Even though the hormone that reaches the brain is testosterone, much of it is converted there to estradiol by enzymes in the nerve cells that are the targets of sexual differentiation. When administered in experiments *in vitro*, estradiol has been found to be eight times more effective than testosterone in androgenization. This raises the question of why the high levels of maternal estrogen do not suffice to masculinize normal female fetuses *in utero*.

Alpha-Fetoprotein Binds Estrogen in the Rat and Thus Protects Female Fetuses from Masculinization

To understand the process by which the brain is sexually organized during the critical period, it is essential to understand what happens to testosterone when it reaches developing (as well as mature) neurons. As shown in Figure 61–4, there are two tissue-specific metabolic pathways: Testosterone can be reduced to 5α-dihydrotestosterone and can be aromatized to the female sex hormone, 17β-estradiol. The androgen-type reduction occurs preferentially in the cells of the pituitary gland and the brain stem, whereas aromatization occurs mostly in the neurons of the hypothalamus and limbic system. Aromatization into estradiol is also the major metabolic route by which behaviorally relevant neural circuits are permanently modified during the critical period. Inhibitors of steroidal aromatization inhibit the sexual differentiation of males and block the facilitation of normal adult sexual behavior induced by estradiol. Masculinization therefore involves estrogen receptors as well as androgen receptors.

For normal development to proceed in females the same estrogen receptors in the same target neurons as in the male must remain *unoccupied* during the critical period. Yet maternal blood is rich in estrogens from the gonads and placenta. What protects normal female fetuses from masculinization *in utero* by circulating estrogens? Normal rat fetuses of both sexes are protected from maternal estrogen by an estrogen-binding protein called α-fetoprotein. This protein is synthesized by the fetal liver and is present in blood and cerebrospinal fluid. Unlike estrogen, testosterone is not bound by α-fetoprotein, and thus in males it has free access to steroid-sensitive neurons during the critical period. Once taken up by a neuron, testosterone is aromatized to estradiol.

Receptors in the Cell Nucleus Mediate the Effects of Gonadal Steroid Hormones

Unlike receptors for neurotransmitters (see Chapters 11 and 12), some gonadal steroid receptors are not situated in the neuronal plasma membrane. Instead, they are located in the cell nucleus (Figure 61–5) where they act as transcriptional regulators. Steroids penetrate the cell membrane and can bind to the nuclear receptor. On binding with the hormone the receptor undergoes a conformational change, which enables it to bind to specific DNA recognition elements on the upstream regions of genes capable of being activated (or repressed) by steroid hormones. Hormone-receptor complexes bind with high affinity only to specific regions of the DNA, called *hormone-*

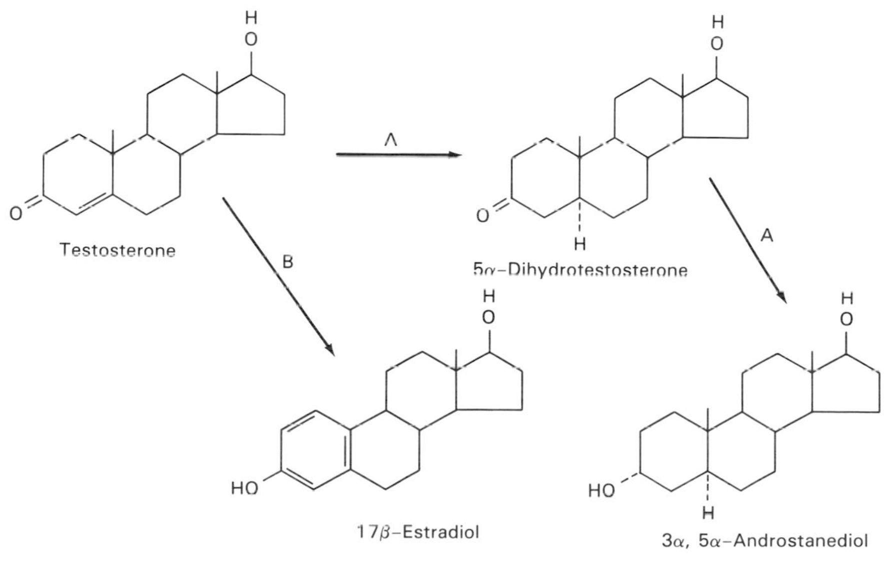

FIGURE 61–4
There are two metabolic pathways in neurons for testosterone: (A) an androgen-type reduction pathway, which requires the enzyme 5α-reductase, and (B) the aromatization route, by which testosterone is converted into the female sex hormone 17β-estradiol.

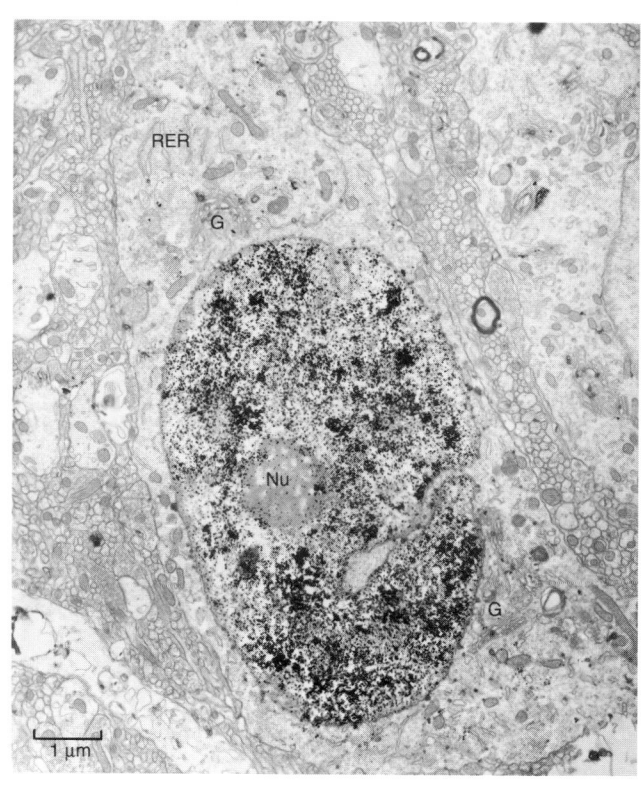

FIGURE 61–5
Gonadal steroid receptors are concentrated in the nucleus of the cell. The electron micrograph shows immunoreactivity to monoclonal antibodies to estrogen receptors in a cell from the hypothalamic ventrolateral nucleus of the guinea pig. This structure is equivalent to the ventrolateral portion of the rat hypothalamic ventromedial nucleus, a region essential for the expression of female reproductive behavior. The antibody in this electron micrograph is detected by a silver-intensified, horseradish peroxidase reaction. The prominent nucleolus (**Nu**), large Golgi apparatus (**G**), and extensive rough endoplasmic reticulum (**RER**) are characteristic of peptide-synthesizing cells. (Courtesy of Ann-Judith Silverman, Lydia DonCarlos, and Joan I. Morrell.)

responsive elements. In this manner, gonadal hormones can activate or inhibit transcription of certain genes, resulting in functional changes in the target cells.

In both sexes the same neuronal populations contain receptors for androgens, estrogens, and progesterone (Figure 61–6). Cells that express steroid receptors are found in the preoptic area, hypothalamus, amygdala, midbrain, and spinal cord (where their distribution differs most markedly between the sexes). They are also found in the frontal, prefrontal, and cingulate areas of the primate cerebral cortex. As we shall see later, these cortical receptors may be

important for the differentiation of nonreproductive but sexually dimorphic behavioral capacities. Depending upon receptor type and experimental method, estimates of the number of steroid receptor molecules present per cell range from 4,000 to 22,000.

Some cells contain receptors for more than one steroid hormone. As an important example, all progesterone-receptive cells also express estrogen receptors (although the opposite is not true). In these cells the binding of estrogen strongly enhances the expression of the progesterone receptor, which explains the interaction between the

FIGURE 61–6
The regional distribution of estradiol-sensitive neurons in the brain of an albino rat is shown in a sagittal section just adjacent to the midline. Within the diencephalon the greatest concentration of receptor sites (**dots**) is in the preoptic–suprachiasmatic area and the arcuate–ventromedial area. These are the areas responsible for controlling the release of luteinizing hormone by the pituitary. In more lateral sections (not shown) the amygdala and orbitofrontal cortex also appear as targets. (Adapted from McEwen, 1976.)

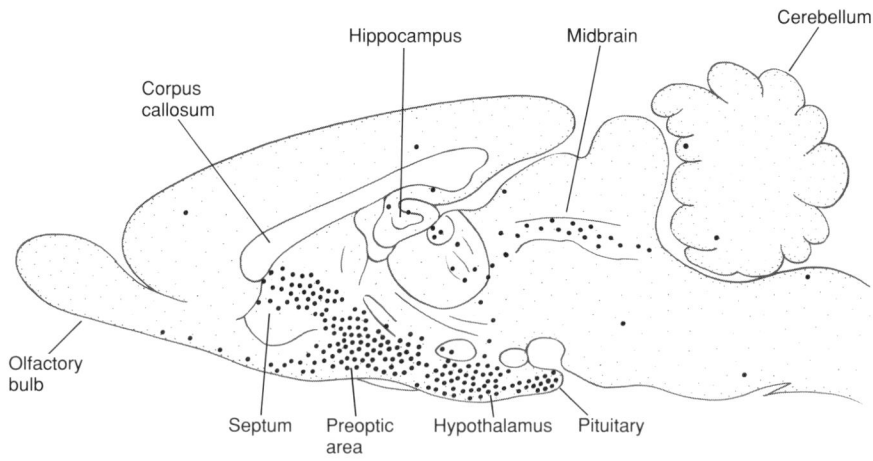

two hormones in controlling reproductive behaviors. For example, the induction of lordotic behavior by progesterone is greatly enhanced in rats primed with estrogen.

Sexually Differentiated Brains Have Different Physiological Properties and Behavioral Tendencies

How does a brain that mediates male behaviors differ from one that mediates female behaviors? As first illustrated by the experiment of Raisman (Table 60–1), a brain exposed to androgens during the critical period engenders an even pattern of LH secretion by the pituitary. In contrast, the secretory pattern generated by the female brain cycles over days. One explanation for this difference involves neurons in the preoptic area of the hypothalamus that project to the neurosecretory cells that produce LH-releasing hormone (LHRH). LHRH is a decapeptide that regulates the release of both LH and FSH from the anterior pituitary. Thus, LHRH is also known as gonadotropin-releasing hormone (GnRH). LHRH-producing cells do not express any steroid receptors; however, the preoptic cells from which LHRH cells receive synaptic input do contain estrogen receptors. In normal females the estrogen secreted by growing ovarian follicles activates the preoptic estrogen-sensitive cells, which in turn prompts a surge in the production of LHRH in the postsynaptic neurosecretory cells. In the androgenized brain, these preoptic cells are refractory to hormonal activation, and even direct electrical stimulation fails to alter release of LH from the pituitary.

Second, there is a significant sex difference in the effect of estrogen on the regulation of progesterone receptor levels in neurons of the hypothalamic ventromedial (HVM) nucleus. Bruce McEwen, Neil MacLusky, and their colleagues found significantly increased progestin binding in the HVM of female rats in response to injections of estradiol. In contrast, the same treatment had no effect on progestin binding in the male HVM. The HVM is the principal site for hormonal activation of lordosis (Figure 61–3).

Third, the mature animal with an androgenized brain exhibits male mounting behavior when androgens are administered systemically or implanted directly into the anterior hypothalamus. The same behavior cannot be activated by hormones in males that were castrated during the critical period. However, behavioral demasculinization can be prevented by administering replacement androgens within the critical period. A dramatic example of remasculinization in rats is shown in Figure 61–7 (broken line).

A fourth and separate property of mature androgenized brains is that they show little behavioral response to estrogens. In normal males there is an active suppression of the lordotic response, which in adult feminine brains may be elicited by estrogen. The display of adult lordosis following priming with estrogen is not genetic; it is either established or inhibited by the perinatal hormonal environment. This has been demonstrated in male rats in the castration-replacement paradigm shown in Figure 61–7

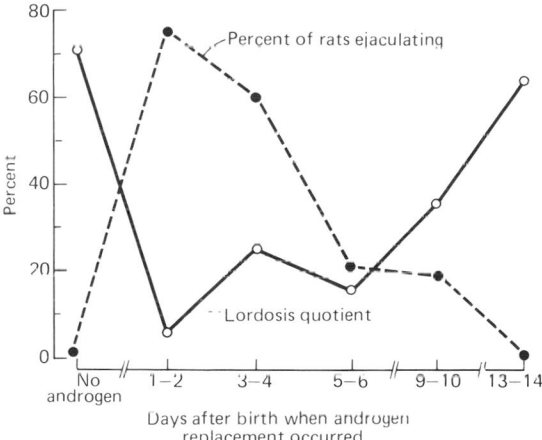

FIGURE 61–7

The adult sexual behavior of neonatally castrated male rats depends on the age at which testosterone replacement therapy is given. Therapy was administered to six groups at different ages. When the androgens were replaced within 2 days of birth, the castrated males exhibited as adults homotypical ejaculatory responses in the presence of testosterone (**broken line**). However, as the interval between castration and replacement increased, the remasculinizing effect of early androgen replacement therapy declines and heterotypical behavior increases. Heterotypical behavior was measured in terms of a lordosis quotient: the percentage of mounts by a stud male that elicited lordosis in the castrated males (**solid line**). (Adapted from Beach, Noble, and Orndoff, 1969.)

(solid line): Early androgen replacement during the critical period effectively suppresses adult heterotypical behavior in response to estrogen.

Although the critical periods for activating ejaculatory behavior and suppressing lordotic behavior appear to be roughly comparable in Figure 61–7, Richard Whalen and David Edwards provided strong evidence that the suppression in masculinized brains of female behavior patterns (*defeminization*) is a separate process from the active organization of male behavior patterns (masculinization). They castrated neonatal male rats and administered during the critical period replacement therapy consisting *only* of injections of androstenedione, an androgen produced primarily by the adrenal gland and also by the gonads of both sexes. Androstenedione is also normally produced in neurons as the final step in the enzymatic reduction of testosterone (Figure 61–4). As adults these animals displayed both male and female behavior. In addition to having different sensitivities to hormones, masculinization and defeminization occur at slightly different times during development.

Finally, events during the critical period result in strong sex differences in the nonreproductive behavioral repertoires of prepubertal juveniles. Because prepuberty is relatively anhormonal, these sex-specific behavior patterns do not depend on the contemporaneous presence of steroid hormones. Genetic female rhesus monkeys exposed to androgen during the critical period show more rough-and-tumble play, more aggressive encounters with normal males, and less maternal imitative behaviors than normal females. Also, animals exposed to androgen during the critical period spend more time playing with others who were similarly exposed, regardless of their genetic sex.

Perinatal Hormones Also Determine the Degree to Which Sex-Linked Behaviors Are Expressed by Normal Males and Females

Events during the critical period for sexual differentiation of the nervous system do not result in complete masculinization or feminization. Intermediate degrees are both possible and normal. Moreover, the same set of perinatal events that differentiates the brains and behaviors of males and females might also be responsible for determining the natural range of these behaviors in normal male and female populations.

In humans there is considerable variability in the amounts of testosterone and estrogen to which a developing normal fetus is exposed. Do these perinatal variations affect the degree to which sex-linked behaviors are expressed later in adulthood? Evidence for this possibility has come primarily from studies on rodents, which produce large litters. Positioning in the uterus is sexually random. Frederick vom Saal showed that female mice that develop between two male fetuses have a higher concentration of testosterone in both blood and amniotic fluid than do females that develop between one male and one female or between two other females. The three types of females—defined by intrauterine position as next to two males, one male, or zero males (2M, 1M, 0M)—differ in many characteristics after they are born, including activity, aggressiveness, and acceptability as mating partners to males. Although 2M females reproduce normally, they display erratic estrus cycles, begin to mate later, and cease to bear young earlier than females that develop between two females. Thus, normal variations in the reproductive

life spans of female mice appear to be related directly to position in the uterus and hence to variation in exposure to sex hormones.

Intrauterine position also has an important effect on certain male characteristics. The size and weight of the testes of males that develop between two other males are greater than those of males not surrounded by male siblings. The seminal vesicles of males surrounded by two male siblings are more sensitive to testosterone. The dosage of testosterone required to induce aggression in adult neonatally castrated males that developed between two male siblings is lower than that required for similarly castrated adults that developed between two females.

All of the behavioral variations displayed by 2M, 1M, and 0M offspring fall within the accepted, normal range of masculine or feminine behaviors. Indeed, together these subgroups define the normal range of behavioral expression in the whole population. The ways in which the 2M, 1M, and 0M offspring differ from each other are the same as those by which the two sexes differ from each other. The degree to which a normal male or female displays a sexually differentiated behavior may be determined by perinatal hormonal mechanisms similar to those that differentiate the two sexes from one another. Individual differences in any behavior with sexually dimorphic components might be due, at least in part, to hormonal exposure during the critical period.

Sexual Differentiation Is Reflected in the Structure of Certain Neurons

Is there a morphological basis for the androgen-dependent process in the developing central nervous system that underlies the sex-specific patterns of behavioral organization? In cells in the preoptic area and ventromedial hypothalamus, the size of the cell nucleus differs in males and females, as does the size of neuronal processes and synaptic terminals in the arcuate nucleus and the density of dendritic fields in the preoptic area. In 1971 Raisman and

FIGURE 61–8
The sexually dimorphic nucleus of the preoptic area (**SDN-POA**) in the rat brain is considerably smaller in females. **A.** Sagittal plane. **B.** Coronal plane. (Adapted from Gorski et al., 1978.)

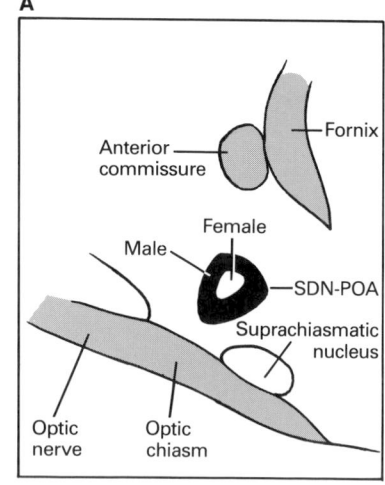
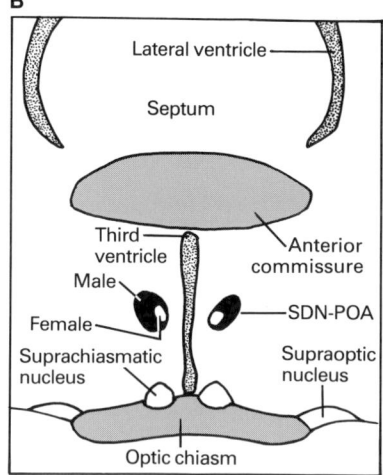

Pauline Field studied the ultrastructure of a sexually distinct synaptic organization of afferents to the preoptic area of the hypothalamus. They suggested that the number of synapses on dendritic spines as compared to the number on shafts might represent different patterns of connections in the two sexes. Until that time most scientists believed that perinatal exposure to steroids primarily altered the responsiveness of the brain, not its pattern of connections.

A salient morphological sex difference in mammals was described in rats by Gorski and his associates. Both the size and the number of neurons in a small part of the medial preoptic nucleus in the hypothalamic forebrain region are greater in males than in females. This region is now called the *sexually dimorphic nucleus of the preoptic area* (Figure 61–8). Irreversible sexual differentiation occurs during the perinatal period; in adults it is not dependent on the continued presence of gonadal hormones. Carol Jacobson and Gorski found that the size and number of neurons in the sexually dimorphic nucleus increase in the male rat around the time of birth and this continues during the first 10 days after birth. Although the function of this nucleus is not known, transplantation of the entire preoptic area from newborn males to female littermates enhances both homotypical and heterotypical adult sexual behaviors.

Sexually dimorphic areas have also been identified in the preoptic areas of gerbils, ferrets, guinea pigs, hamsters, mice, hyenas, and humans. The volume and number of cells occupied by the sexually dimorphic nucleus declines with age in both males and females (Figure 61–9).

The functions of the morphological sex differences in the superior cervical ganglion, the amygdala, the dorsal hippocampus, and the orbital frontal cortex are unknown, but one example of a sex difference in the spinal cord can be correlated directly with a sexually dimorphic behavior. Testicular androgen released during the critical period produces penile reflexes in the male rat. These behavioral reflexes are dependent on androgen. A discrete cluster of androgen-concentrating motor neurons in the sacral portion of the spinal cord of male rats innervates two striated muscles (the levator ani and bulbocavernosus) that move the penis. In female rats the same muscles are absent or vestigial, as is the corresponding spinal motor nucleus. However, as described by Marc Breedlove and Arthur Arnold, a single properly timed neonatal injection of testosterone can masculinize the spinal cord of female rats by preventing the death of neurons whose survival depends on the presence of androgens.

The Cellular Mechanisms Involved in the Development of Sex Differences in the Brain Can Be Studied in Vitro

The work of Dominique Toran-Allerand suggests that morphological sex differences reflect the growth-promoting effects of gonadal steroids on specific populations of neurons. Toran-Allerand maintained hypothalamic slices from newborn mouse brains for long periods in culture. In

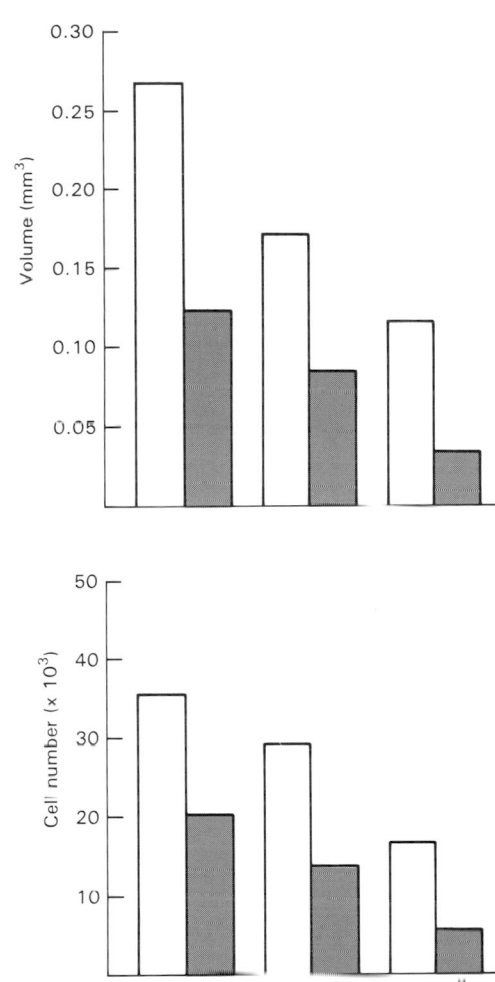

FIGURE 61–9

In humans there is a steady decline in both the number of cells and the volume of tissue occupied by the sexually dimorphic nucleus, but at each stage of life the structure is larger in men than in women. (Adapted from Swaab and Fliers, 1985.)

her initial experiments she exposed one-half of each slice to the masculinizing steroids, testosterone or estradiol, the other half serving as control. When she removed the meninges of the explant, she found a marked increase in the outgrowth of neurites (new axons and dendrites) as well as extensive new branching of existing processes in a small proportion of cells in the slices that were exposed to the androgenizing agent (Figure 61–10). The stimulation of neuritic growth by androgen is dose-dependent. Not all neurons are sensitive to steroids, however. Gonadal steroids were especially effective on cells located in the anterior preoptic region and in the infundibular-premammillary region.

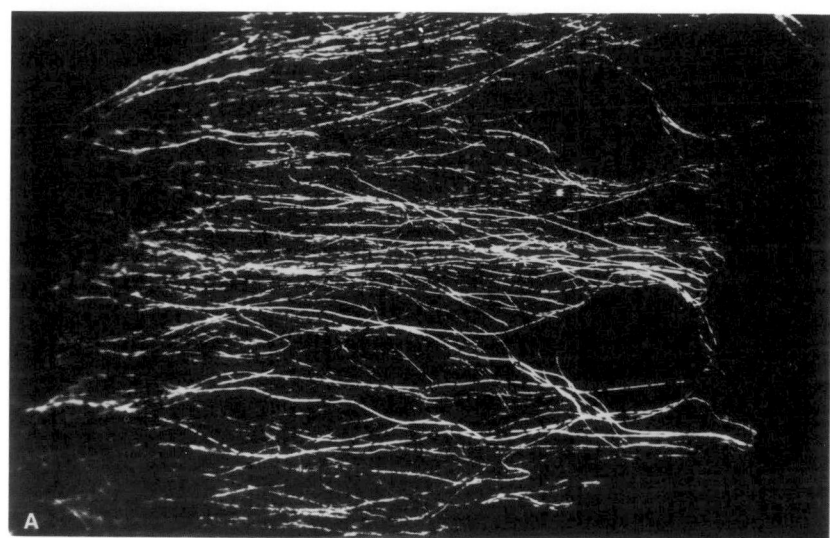

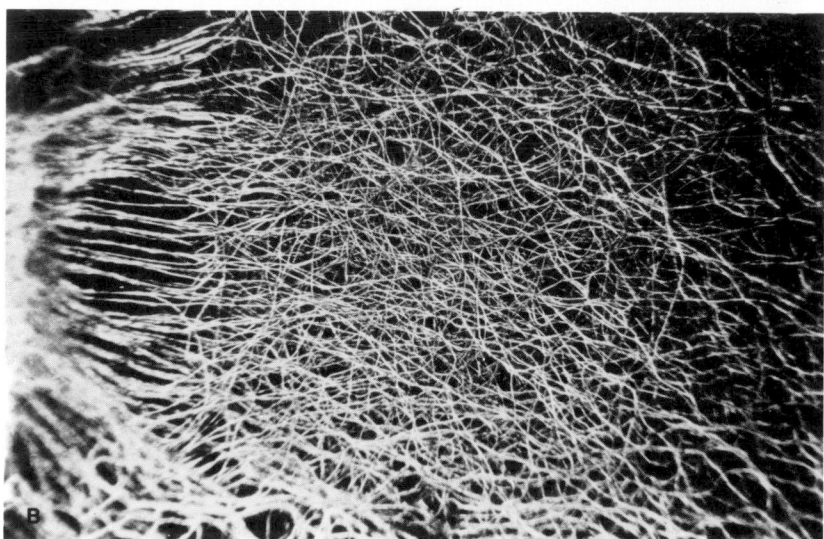

FIGURE 61–10

Gonadal steroids stimulate the growth of neuronal processes in hypothalamic explants from a newborn mouse. (From Toran-Allerand, 1978.)

A. The control culture shows silver-impregnated neurites coursing outward in hairlike wisps from the margin of the explant.

B. The neuritic growth of the other slice exhibits an extraordinarily dense plexus formation, which extends well beyond that of the control. This growth was stimulated by the addition of estradiol (100 ng/ml) to the fluid bathing the culture.

The principal implication of these developmental studies in tissue culture is that the different neuronal organization imposed on the brains of males and females by sex steroids may result from alterations in the growth rate of axons and dendrites of select steroid-sensitive cells. During the critical period, steroid sex hormones might bias the rate of axonal differentiation in different regional populations and thereby affect neural circuitry. Since postsynaptic space is limited, sexual differentiation of neural connections could occur as a result of competition for postsynaptic sites between axonal populations of different origins.

A Wide Range of Behaviors Is Influenced by Sex Differences in the Organization of the Brain

We have so far focused on the dimorphic reproductive behaviors of males and females as the primary behavioral markers of the sexual identity of the brain. Several recent lines of evidence suggest, however, that the repertoire of behaviors that are influenced by the perinatal hormonal environment may extend beyond reproductive behaviors. What other types of behavior might be influenced by sex differences in the cellular organization of the brain?

Sexual Dimorphism Is Evident in Cognitive Development in Monkeys

Patricia Goldman-Rakic has shown in rhesus monkeys that sexual dimorphism exists in the developmental processes that underlie certain cognitive functions of the frontal lobes. In both infant and adult male monkeys lesions of the orbital prefrontal cortex result in impaired performance in tests involving spatial discrimination and delayed responses. In contrast, identical lesions in infant females do not induce similar deficits until the animal has reached an age of 15–18 months. Thus, the effects of orbital prefrontal lesions are age dependent, and the age at which this part of the cortex becomes involved in spatial learning differs between the sexes. The earlier participation of the masculine frontal cortex in object-reversal learning may also be related to the later superiority of mature male monkeys in these learning tasks. Prenatal exposure of developing female monkey fetuses to androgens eliminates this sex difference in adults.

The frontal cortex of the monkey is sexually dimorphic in its rate of development. This may be related to the observation of steroid-sensitive neurons in the frontal cortex of infant rats, which, as McEwen has found, decline in number by puberty. If differences exist in the rate of cortical maturation in nonhuman primates, it is plausible that similar sex differences might occur in the brains of humans.

Human Cerebral Asymmetry Is Sexually Dimorphic

The specialization of cognitive functions in the left and right cerebral hemispheres of the mature human brain is described in Chapter 53. In brief, in most right-handed individuals the left hemisphere is specialized for language and related serial processing of information, and the right hemisphere is specialized for nonverbal processes, including three-dimensional visualization, mental rotation, face recognition, and understanding the meaning of facial expressions. Several lines of evidence suggest that the brains of the two sexes may differ in their patterns of cerebral asymmetry. As with the development of prefrontal cortical functions in the monkey, there is evidence that the two sexes differ in the rate of maturation of cognitive functions in the two hemispheres.

Sandra Witelson used a behavioral test that involved tactile perception to assess the relative participation of the two hemispheres in spatial processing. Children were given 10 seconds to manipulate out of view two objects differing in shape, each using only the index and middle fingers of one hand. The children then tried to identify these objects from pictures. Since tactile shape discrimination by adults depends mainly on the right hemisphere, to make the test as dependent as possible on the right hemisphere Witelson used objects with meaningless shapes, not readily labeled. As early as the age of six boys performed in a manner consistent with right-hemisphere specialization (left hand superiority). Girls showed no evidence of bilateral representation (no clear hand superiority) until the age of 13, suggesting that boys develop a greater hemispheric specialization at an earlier age. Therefore, during an extended period of development a sex difference may exist in the hemispheric allocation of cognitive functions.

Witelson also pointed out that the sexual dimorphism in neural organization underlying cognition may have educational implications. For instance, reading is considered to involve both visual and auditory processing. Males and females may be differentially organized for these cognitive processes at the time when they are learning to read. Different approaches in teaching reading, such as the whole-word and phonetic methods, which stress different cognitive strategies and by inference depend on different neural structures, may not be equally effective in girls and boys.

If the right hemisphere in girls is not specialized for a particular cognitive function, then it may retain greater plasticity for a longer period than in boys. Clinical impressions are consistent with this idea. Language functions appear to transfer more readily to the right hemisphere in females than in males after damage to the left hemisphere in childhood. The extended plasticity of the young female brain also suggests that females may have a lower incidence of developmental disorders associated with left-hemisphere dysfunction. Developmental dyslexia, developmental aphasia, and infantile autism are more frequent in males, and language deficits are prominent symptoms in all of these syndromes.

In addition, the degree of cerebral cognitive asymmetry differs in adult males and females. James Inglis and James Stuart Lawson discovered that in male neurological patients there is a strong association between the side of the brain that has been injured and the type of cognitive deficits observed: Verbal functions are disordered by left-hemisphere lesions, and nonverbal functions by right-hemisphere lesions. In female neurological patients, this association is much weaker, suggesting that the adult female brain is functionally less asymmetrical than the male brain.

These sex differences in the susceptibility of the developing human brain to early damage and in the cerebral asymmetry of the mature brain have not yet been related to perinatal hormonal events. Nor have sex differences been observed in cognitive abilities. Males often score higher in tests of mathematical reasoning and in understanding spatial relationships. Females score higher in tests of verbal fluency and in the meaning of facial expression.

Although understanding of sex differences in human neural organization is still limited, the range of sex-linked behavioral biases that may hinge upon perinatal events is clearly extensive and not limited to reproductive processes.

An Overall View

It is often tempting to view any intrinsic biological process, such as the perinatal differentiation of the nervous system, as a fixed and permanent constraint on behavior. Nevertheless, although strongly biased by neural organization, most behaviors remain flexible and open to modification. As we have seen, there are relatively few fixed-action patterns in the human repertoire. As an example, even though we inherit a finely tuned regulatory system for food consumption and body weight, certain experiences can override the homeostat for body weight and produce obesity in otherwise normal people—a person may develop a passionate interest in fine food and wines or get a job as a restaurant critic. Likewise, although the brain regulates aggressive behavior, individuals can, without apparent neuropathology, become pacifists or terrorists for ideological reasons.

Similarly, there is ample social evidence that the neural organization of reproductive behaviors, while *biased* by hormonal events during a critical prenatal period, does not exert an immutable influence over adult sexual behavior or even over an individual's sexual orientation. Within the life of the individual, religious, social, or economic motives can prompt biologically similar persons to diverge widely in their sexual habits.

Selected Readings

Arnold, A. P., Bottjer, S. W., Nordeen, E. J., Nordeen, K. W., and Sengelaub, D. R. 1987. Hormones and critical periods in behavioral and neural development. In J. P. Rauschecker and P. Marler (eds.), Imprinting and Cortical Plasticity: Comparative Aspects of Sensitive Periods. New York: Wiley, pp. 55–97.

Beato, M. 1989. Gene regulation by steroid hormones. Cell 56: 335–344.

Blaustein, J. D., and Olster, D. H. 1989. Gonadal steroid hormone receptors and social behaviors. In J. Balthazart (ed.), Advances in Comparative and Environmental Physiology, Vol. 3. Molecular and Cellular Basis of Social Behavior in Vertebrates. Berlin: Springer, pp. 31–104.

Breedlove, S. M. 1986. Cellular analyses of hormone influence on motoneuronal development and function. J. Neurobiol. 17: 157–176.

Eicher, E. M., and Washburn, L. L. 1986. Genetic control of primary sex determination in mice. Annu. Rev. Genet. 20:327–360.

Evans, R. M. 1988. The steroid and thyroid hormone receptor superfamily. Science 240:889–895.

Gilbert, S. F. 1988. Developmental Biology, 2nd Ed. Sunderland, Mass.: Sinauer, chap. 21, "Sex Determination."

Gorski, R. A. 1988. Sexual differentiation of the brain: Mechanisms and implications for neuroscience. In S. S. Easter, Jr., K. F. Barald, and B. M. Carlson (eds.), From Message to Mind: Directions in Developmental Neurobiology. Sunderland, Mass.: Sinauer, pp. 256–271.

Hines, M. 1982. Prenatal gonadal hormones and sex differences in human behavior. Psychol. Bull. 92:56–80.

Kelley, D. B. 1988. Sexually dimorphic behaviors. Annu. Rev. Neurosci. 11:225–251.

Knobil, E., and Neill, J. D. (eds.) 1988. The Physiology of Reproduction. New York: Raven Press, 2 vols.

McEwen, B. S., Luine, V. N., and Fischette, C. T. 1988. Developmental actions of hormones: From receptors to function. In S. S. Easter, Jr., K. F. Barald, and B. M. Carlson (eds.), From Message to Mind: Directions in Developmental Neurobiology. Sunderland, Mass.: Sinauer, pp. 272–287.

McLaren, A. 1990. What makes a man a man? Nature 346:216–217.

Pfaff, D. W., and McEwen, B. S. 1983. Actions of estrogens and progestins on nerve cells. Science 219:808–814.

Toran-Allerand, C. D. 1984. On the genesis of sexual differentiation of the central nervous system: Morphogenetic consequences of steroidal exposure and possible role of α-fetoprotein. In G. J. De Vries, J. P. C. De Bruin, H. B. M. Uylings, and M. A. Corner (eds.), Sex Differences in the Brain. The Relation Between Structure and Function. Prog. Brain Res. 61:63–98.

References

Andersson, M., Page, D. C., and de la Chapelle, A. 1986. Chromosome Y-specific DNA is transferred to the short arm of X chromosome in human XX males. Science 233:786–788.

Ayoub, D. M., Greenough, W. T., and Juraska, J. M. 1983. Sex differences in dendritic structure in the preoptic area of the juvenile macaque monkey brain. Science 219:197–198.

Barraclough, C. A., and Gorski, R. A. 1962. Studies on mating behaviour in the androgen-sterilized female rat in relation to the hypothalamic regulation of sexual behaviour. J. Endocrinol. 25:175–182.

Beach, F. A., Noble, R. G., and Orndoff, R. K. 1969. Effects of perinatal androgen treatment on responses of male rats to gonadal hormones in adulthood. J. Comp. Physiol. Psychol. 68: 490–497.

Bermant, G., and Davidson, J. M. 1974. Biological Bases of Sexual Behavior. New York: Harper & Row.

Breedlove, S. M., and Arnold, A. P. 1980. Hormone accumulation in a sexually dimorphic motor nucleus of the rat spinal cord. Science 210:564–566.

Breedlove, S. M., Jacobson, C. D., Gorski, R. A., and Arnold, A. P. 1982. Masculinization of the female rat spinal cord following a single neonatal injection of testosterone proprionate but not estradiol benzoate. Brain Res. 237:173–181.

Brown, T. J., Clark, A. S., and MacLusky, N. J. 1987. Regional sex differences in progestin receptor induction in the rat hypothalamus: Effects of various doses of estradiol benzoate. J. Neurosci. 7:2529–2536.

Brown, T. J., Hochberg, R. B., Zielinski, J. E., and MacLusky, N. J. 1988. Regional sex differences in cell nuclear estrogen-binding capacity in the rat hypothalamus and preoptic area. Endocrinology 123:1761–1770.

Goldman, P. S., Crawford, H. T., Stokes L. P., Galkin, T. W., and Rosvold, H. E. 1974. Sex-dependent behavioral effects of cerebral cortical lesions in the developing rhesus monkey. Science 186:540–542.

Gorski, R. A., Gordon, J. H., Shryne, J .E., and Southam, A. M. 1978. Evidence for a morphological sex difference within the medial preoptic area of the rat brain. Brain Res. 148:333–346.

Gould, E., Westlind-Danielsson, A., Frankfurt, M., and McEwen, B. S. 1990. Sex differences and thyroid hormone sensitivity of hippocampal pyramidal cells. J. Neurosci. 10:996–1003.

Gubbay, J., Collignon, J., Koopman, P., Capel, B., Economou, A., Münsterberg, A., Vivian, N., Goodfellow, P., and Lovell-Badge, R. 1990. A gene mapping to the sex-determining region of the mouse Y chromosome is a member of a novel family of embryonically expressed genes. Nature 346:245–250.

Inglis, J., and Lawson, J. S. 1981. Sex differences in the effects of unilateral brain damage on intelligence. Science 212:693–695.

Jacobson, C. D., and Gorski, R. A. 1981. Neurogenesis of the sexually dimorphic nucleus of the preoptic area in the rat. J. Comp. Neurol. 196:519–529.

Jost, A. 1953. Problems of fetal endocrinology: The gonadal and hypophyseal hormones. Recent Prog. Hormon. Res. 8:379–418.

Koopman, P., Gubbay, J., Vivian, N., Goodfellow, P., and Lovell-Badge, R. 1991. Male development of chromosomally female mice transgenic for Sry. Nature 351:117–121.

McEwen, B. S. 1976. Interactions between hormones and nerve tissue. Sci. Am. 235(1):48–58.

Money, J., and Ehrhardt, A. A. 1972. Man & Woman, Boy & Girl. Baltimore: Johns Hopkins University Press.

Morrell, J. I., Krieger, M. S., and Pfaff, D. W. 1986. Quantitative autoradiographic analysis of estradiol retention by cells in the preoptic area, hypothalamus and amygdala. Exp. Brain Res. 62:343–354.

Palmer, M. S., Sinclair, A. H., Berta, P., Ellis, N. A., Goodfellow, P. N., Abbas, N. E., and Fellous, M. 1989. Genetic evidence that ZFY is not the testis-determining factor. Nature 342:937–939.

Phoenix, C. H., Goy, R. W., Gerall, A. A., and Young, W. C. 1959. Organizing action of prenatally administered testosterone proprionate on the tissues mediating mating behavior in the female guinea pig. Endocrinology 65:369–382.

Rainbow, T. C., Parsons, B., and McEwen, B. S. 1982. Sex differences in rat brain oestrogen and progestin receptors. Nature 300:648–649.

Raisman, G., and Field, P. M. 1971. Sexual dimorphism in the preoptic area of the rat. Science 173:731–733.

Sinclair, A. H., Berta, P., Palmer, M. S., Hawkins, J. R., Griffiths, B. L., Smith, M. J., Foster, J. W., Frischauf, A.-M., Lovell-Badge, R., and Goodfellow, P. N. 1990. A gene from the human sex-determining region encodes a protein with homology to a conserved DNA-binding motif. Nature 346:240–244.

Swaab, D. F., and Fliers, E. 1985. A sexually dimorphic nucleus in the human brain. Science 228:1112–1115.

Toran-Allerand, C. D. 1978. Gonadal hormones and brain development: Cellular aspects of sexual differentiation. Am. Zool. 18:553–565.

vom Saal, F. S., and Bronson, F. H. 1980. Sexual characteristics of adult female mice are correlated with their blood testosterone levels during prenatal development. Science 208:597–599.

Weisz, J., and Ward, I. L. 1980. Plasma testosterone and progesterone titers of pregnant rats, their male and female fetuses and neonatal offspring. Endocrinology 106:306–316.

Whalen, R. E., and Edwards, D. A. 1967. Hormonal determinants of the development of masculine and feminine behavior in male and female rats. Anat. Rec. 157:173–180.

Witelson, S. F. 1976. Sex and the single hemisphere: Specialization of the right hemisphere for spatial processing. Science 193:425–427.

James Goldman
Lucien Côté

62

Aging of the Brain: Dementia of the Alzheimer's Type

Several Hypotheses Have Been Proposed for the Molecular Mechanisms of Aging

Normal Aging Produces Characteristic Changes in the Brain and Behavior

Progressive Decline in Mental Function Is Not An Inevitable Consequence of Aging

Alzheimer's Disease Is the Most Common Form of Dementia

There is a Genetic Component to Certain Forms of Alzheimer's Disease

Extracellular Plaques Containing Amyloid Deposition Are a Prominent Feature of Alzheimer's Disease

Neurofibrillary Tangles Are an Intracellular Characteristic of Alzheimer's Disease

There Are Neurotransmitter Deficits in Alzheimer's Disease

Other Degenerative Diseases Also Produce Dementia

An Overall View

A lthough the maximum number of years that human beings can live has not increased significantly in recorded history, the average life expectancy has increased, especially since the turn of this century (Figure 62–1). In 1900 the average life expectancy in the United States was about 50 years. Now the average life expectancy is approximately 73 years for men and 78 for women. This increase is largely due to medical advances, such as the reduction in infant mortality, the development of vaccines and antibiotics, and advances in the treatment and prevention of heart disease and stroke. But, as we shall see, this increase in life expectancy has unmasked a new epidemic: *dementia*, deterioration of mental function. Dementia accompanies aging in certain susceptible individuals. Even though these people now constitute a minority, they are becoming a larger proportion of the aging population.

Most people agree that lengthening life has little merit if its quality is not preserved. The ultimate goal of research on aging (senescence) therefore is not only to lengthen human life, but also to maintain and enhance its quality.

In this chapter we shall examine what is known about how aging affects the brain, and focus on some illnesses characteristic of age that produce severe memory loss and intellectual deterioration.

Several Hypotheses Have Been Proposed for the Molecular Mechanisms of Aging

Several lines of evidence suggest that senescence occurs as the result of changes in informational macromolecules. At

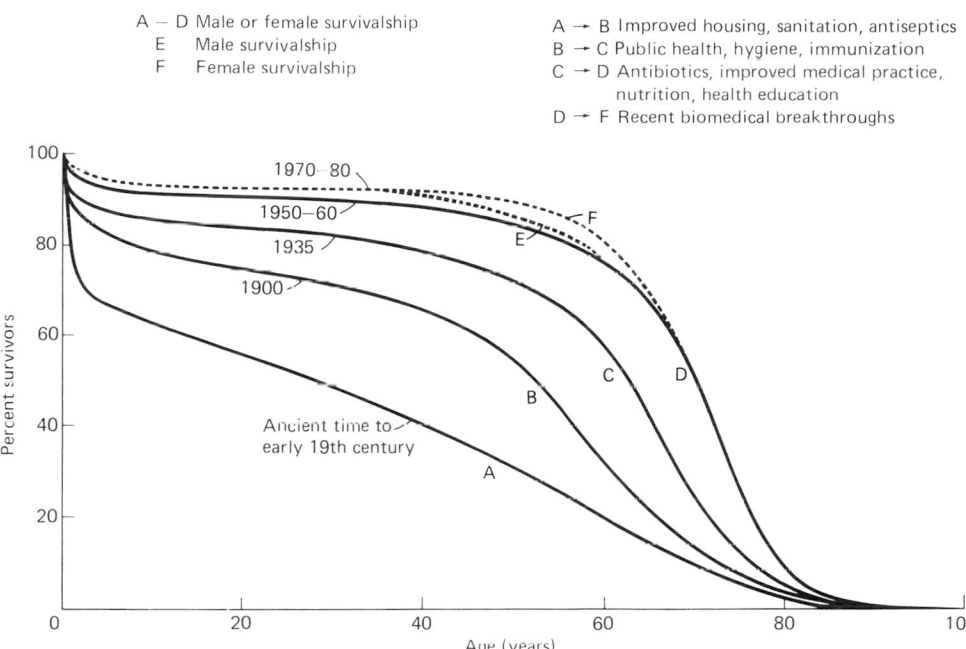

A – D Male or female survivalship
E   Male survivalship
F   Female survivalship

A → B Improved housing, sanitation, antiseptics
B → C Public health, hygiene, immunization
C → D Antibiotics, improved medical practice,
        nutrition, health education
D → F Recent biomedical breakthroughs

FIGURE 62–1

Trends in human longevity from ancient times to the present. These idealized curves illustrate the rapid approach to the limiting rectangular curve that has occurred during the past 150 years. The major factors responsible for these transitions are listed above the graph. Note that in men 50 years or older, the life expectancy has changed only slightly since 1950. However, female longevity has improved significantly during this period, in part because of better treatment of reproductive system malignancies. (Adapted from Strehler, 1975.)

least three hypotheses have been advanced that relate aging to changes in DNA and RNA. According to a theory proposed by Zhores Medvedev, mutations and chromosome anomalies accumulate with age. As these errors accumulate in functioning genes, reserve (redundant) DNA sequences, containing the same information take over until the redundancy is exhausted. Senescence then follows. An alternative hypothesis, supported by many researchers on aging, maintains that the genetic apparatus does not contain a specific program for senescence, but that errors in duplication of DNA increase with age because of random damage and insults that occur with time (wear and tear, radiation effects, and so on). When a significant number of errors accumulate, abnormal mRNA and protein molecules are formed that do not function normally. Senescence results from the accumulation of these errors. A third hypothesis, proposed by Bernard Strehler and his colleagues, is that aging is part of a larger developmental sequence. Just as some genes control embryonic development, other genes program aging processes in the organism. Thus, the changes of old age result from the normal expression of a genetic program that begins at conception and ends in death.

A particularly intriguing variant of these ideas, based on the work of Leonard Hayflick, is that cells possess a biological clock that dictates their life span. Hayflick found that normal human fibroblasts grown in culture divide regularly until they cover the entire surface of the culture flask. If the cells are transferred in equal numbers to two flasks containing fresh medium, they divide until they again become confluent and cover the surface of the flask. Normal cultured human fibroblasts can double only a limited number of times (about 50 times) over a period of 7–9 months. Starting at around the 35th passage, their ability to divide decreases; eventually they stop dividing and die. Fibroblasts from older human donors double significantly fewer times than those obtained from human embryos. The number of cell doublings is roughly related to the age of the donor whose cells are used.

The longevity of the species from which fibroblasts are obtained also is a factor in dictating the number of possible passages. Fibroblasts from mouse embryos (whose expected life span is three years) divide about 15 times before they die; fibroblasts from humans (with a life span of 70–80 years) divide about 50 times; and those from Galapagos tortoises (with a life span of 175 years) divide about 90 times. Thus, the number of passages is also roughly related to the longevity of the species.

If a nucleus from a young fibroblast is interchanged with that of an old fibroblast (a transfer technique made possible by using cytochalasin B and centrifugation), the newly formed hybrid cell divides according to the age of the nucleus, not that of the cytoplasm. Thus, the biological clock seems to be located in the nucleus of the fibroblast. These and other studies indicate that at least some aspects of aging are intrinsic or genetic.

Normal Aging Produces Characteristic Changes in the Brain and Behavior

Many behavioral changes occur with age, but they generally do not seriously compromise the quality of life. There are, for example, alterations in motor coordination, sleep, and mental functions. The gait of an elderly person is slower, with a shorter stride, and posture less erect than that of a young adult. Postural reflexes are often sluggish, making the individual more susceptible to losing his balance and falling. These motor changes involve both central nervous system mechanisms and peripheral alterations, such as reduced position sense, muscle weakness, and skeletal changes.

The sleep pattern changes with age. Older individuals awaken more frequently after falling asleep and have less sleep time. Stage 1 of slow-wave sleep is increased in the elderly while stages 3 and 4 are reduced, as well as rapid eye movement (REM) sleep. These changes can be troublesome and produce a chronic sleep deprivation state.

Age-related mental changes occur but they vary widely among individuals. There is a decline in the ability to retain a large new body of information over a long period of time. Semantic abilities, such as rapidly naming objects or naming as many words as possible that start with a specific letter of the alphabet, decreases with age. However, performance on the vocabulary subtest of the Wechsler Adult Intelligence Scale (WAIS) is well maintained into the eighties. Visuospatial ability, such as arranging blocks into a design or drawing a three-dimensional figure, is impaired in many older people. General intelligence declines somewhat in the sixties and continues with advancing age. Thus, several aspects of cognition change with age; however, they do not necessarily impair the quality of life significantly.

Several age-related changes occur in the brain. First, there often are gross changes, such as decreased brain weight and decreases in the level of proteins. Second, the human brain actually seems to lose neurons with age. For example, there is an age-related loss of neurons in several subcortical nuclei. In addition, cell counts in the cerebral cortex show a decrease in numbers of neurons in older people, although it is not clear whether the apparent loss of large neurons represents actual loss or shrinkage of neurons. Third, there are reductions in the enzymes that synthesize dopamine and norepinephrine and less severe changes in cholinergic function. This is at least in part due to loss of subcortical neurons that synthesize these transmitters. For example, there is a decrease with age in the number of neurons in the substantia nigra, a major dopaminergic center in the midbrain, and in the locus ceruleus, a noradrenergic nucleus in the pons. There are also reductions in the receptors for dopamine, norepinephrine, and acetylcholine. Age-related alterations in the synthesis and degradation of neurotransmitters and their receptors could explain some of the characteristics of senescence:

alterations in sleep pattern, mood, appetite, neuroendocrine functions, motor activity, and memory.

These chemical changes appear to be normal. At the same time, certain diseases that are selective for one or more neurotransmitters, such as Parkinson's disease, Huntington's disease, and Alzheimer's disease, occur more commonly with age. We have already seen that dopamine function is impaired in Parkinson's disease (Chapter 42). In Huntington's disease the levels of glutamic acid decarboxylase activity, γ-aminobutyric acid (GABA), and choline acetyltransferase are sharply reduced in the degenerating striatum.

Microscopic changes in the aging brain include senile plaques and neurofibrillary tangles (see below). The numbers of these lesions that accumulate in normal aging are less than those seen in Alzheimer's disease.

Progressive Decline in Mental Function Is Not An Inevitable Consequence of Aging

The word *dementia* denotes a progressive decline in mental function, in memory, and in acquired intellectual skills. Dementia can result from many causes, and therefore is not, by itself, diagnostic of a specific disease. Dementia is not an inevitable consequence of aging. Most people age without substantial loss of intellectual power. Nevertheless, dementia is age-related. It practically never occurs prior to age 45 and is rare between ages 45 and 65. About 11% of people in the United States over 65 years of age show mild to severe mental impairment. From age 75 on the incidence of dementia is 2% higher with each year of life. Currently over one million people in the United States suffer serious dementia and an estimated 120,000 of these will die each year of causes related to severe dementia. Thus, the value of any further increase in average life expectancy resulting from more effective modes of treatment for cancer and heart disease in the future may be diminished by the increased incidence of dementia with age.

Alzheimer's Disease Is the Most Common Form of Dementia

About 70% of all cases of dementia are due to Alzheimer's disease. About 15% are caused by strokes (sometimes many small infarcts). Thus, contrary to the popular notion of the past, hardening of the arteries of the brain (cerebral arteriosclerosis) is not the main cause of dementia. In some patients Alzheimer's disease occurs with vascular disease, and both contribute to the clinical picture. The remaining 15% of dementias are either associated with other neurodegenerative diseases, such as Huntington's disease or Parkinson's disease, or with conditions that can be corrected with treatment. This latter group includes patients with infections of the brain and the meninges, vitamin deficiencies, endocrine and metabolic diseases, intracranial mass lesions (such as tumors), chronically increased intracranial pressure, and normal pressure hydrocephalus.

A definitive diagnosis of Alzheimer's disease requires pathological examination of the brain, where the characteristic morphological features that we shall consider occur. Nevertheless, diagnosis on clinical grounds alone is correct in a majority of cases, especially if other causes have been ruled out. Computerized tomographic and magnetic resonance imaging of the brain of Alzheimer's patients show thin cortical gyri and enlarged ventricles. These findings are not specific, however, since other conditions produce atrophy of the brain. Furthermore, there is some degree of atrophy in normal aging. Imaging studies that measure cerebral blood flow, regional glucose utilization, or location of various receptors may improve diagnostic specificity and reveal functional abnormalities in the early stages of the disease. For example, low blood flow to the parietotemporal areas has been shown to occur early in the disease.

Alzheimer's disease is usually insidious in onset and it often becomes obvious to family members or co-workers only after the patient has experienced an episode of minor stress. Early manifestations include forgetfulness, untidiness, transient confusion, periods of restlessness and lethargy, and errors in judgment. The storage of new memory becomes impaired, but memory previously stored is less severely affected or for a time not affected at all. Patients eventually lose interest in their surroundings and become confined to wheelchair or bed. The course of the illness is highly variable. The final stages of the disease, marked by mental emptiness and loss of control of all body functions, may not occur until 5–10 years after onset.

There Is a Genetic Component to Certain Forms of Alzheimer's Disease

The risk of developing Alzheimer's disease is increased several-fold if a first-degree relative has the disease, even among individuals who do not have a clear-cut pattern of inheritance in their families. Since it is an age-related disease, the familial incidence of Alzheimer's disease has probably been underestimated. There presumably are many individuals who would in the past have developed Alzheimer's disease had they lived longer. The evidence for a genetic component is particularly strong in a form of Alzheimer's disease that has an early onset and strikes its victims when they are still in their 40's and 50's. In some of these families the disease is inherited in an autosomal dominant pattern. In a few families linkage analysis has demonstrated an association between this form of Alzheimer's disease and DNA markers on the long arm of chromosome 21. This location is of further interest because Alzheimer's disease is present in almost all people with Down's syndrome who live past the age of 35. (The syndrome is caused by an extra copy of chromosome 21.)

However, many patients with early onset Alzheimer's disease do not show linkage of the disease to chromosome 21, suggesting that even the familial form of the disease is genetically heterogeneous. Alterations in one of several genes or in more than one gene can likely cause this form

of the disease. Moreover, in the vast majority of late-onset cases of Alzheimer's disease, it is difficult to discern a pattern of inheritance for the disease.

Extracellular Plaques Containing Amyloid Deposition Are a Prominent Feature of Alzheimer's Disease

Several microscopic changes take place in the brains of Alzheimer patients. All of these can be found to some extent in the brains of elderly individuals who do not have impaired mental function, but the pathology in Alzheimer patients is far more severe. Moreover, these changes are found in much greater numbers in Alzheimer patients than in the brains of unimpaired people of similar ages.

One of the pathological hallmarks of Alzheimer's disease is *senile plaques*, that accumulate extra-cellularly in the brain. The major components of plaques are a form of *amyloid* and an irregular, loosely arranged aggregate of neuronal and glial processes (Figure 62–2). Amyloid is a general term for a variety of different proteins that accumulate as extracellular fibrils of 7–10 nm and have common structural features, including a β-pleated sheet conformation and the ability to bind such dyes as Congo red and thioflavine (see Figure 62–2). Different amyloids accumulate in different diseases and in a variety of tissues. The amyloid that accumulates in the brains of Alzheimer patients has properties similar to other amyloids seen in other systemic disorders, such as amyloid disease of the kidney or systemic vasculature, but is a different protein. The amyloid plaques in the brain are irregular, roughly spherical, and range in size from small, about 10 μm, to very large, or several hundred micrometers. They are found most characteristically in the gray matter of the neocortex and hippocampus, but also occur in the basal ganglia, thalamus, and cerebellum. A few are found in hemispheric white matter.

The amyloid peptide that accumulates in these plaques is a small, self-aggregating peptide (of 4,000 molecular weight) that forms filamentous arrays in the neuropil and in the walls of cerebral blood vessels. This peptide is part of a much larger, alternatively spliced, protein called the Amyloid β-Protein Precursor (APP). The amyloid β-protein precursor is a transmembrane protein with a large extracellular region and a small cytoplasmic tail. Different extracellular domains of the protein are thought to have different effects under normal and pathological conditions.

The amyloid gene that encodes the precursor is located on the long arm of chromosome 21. This location obviously is intriguing because, as we have seen, the genes for Down's syndrome and for a hereditary form of Alzheimer's disease also are located on chromosome 21. Two additional findings make this location of further interest. First, Blas Frangione and Efrat Levy have found that a single amino acid change in amyloid β-protein precursor leads to a rare human hereditary disorder—the Dutch type of human cerebral hemorrhage with amyloidosis. In this disease amyloid is deposited in the walls of cerebral blood vessels leading to strokes that are almost invariably fatal.

A

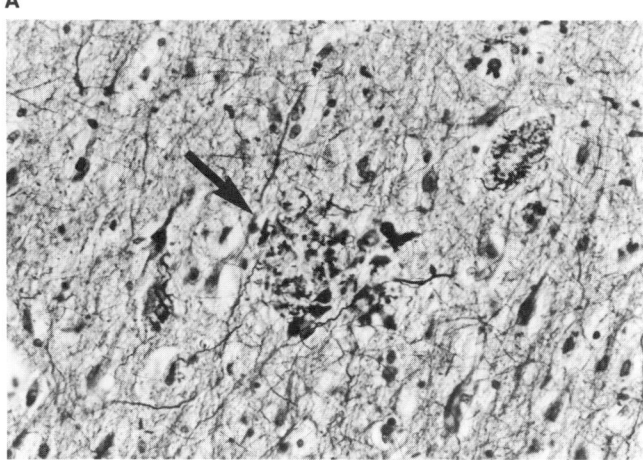

B

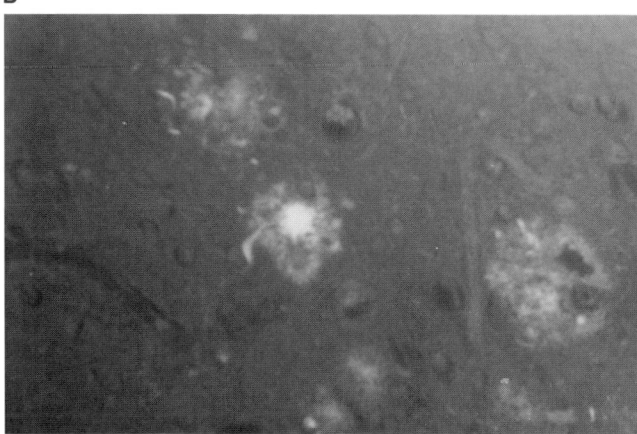

FIGURE 62–2
Cellular changes in Alzheimer's disease.

A. Abnormal, irregular cell processes in this cortical plaque are delineated by a silver stain (**arrow**).

B. The plaque in the center contains a dense core of amyloid and a more diffuse halo of amyloid deposits and neuronal processes. Other plaques in the figure do not show cores. The fluorescent dye, thioflavine S, binds to amyloid and to the abnormal neuronal processes.

Second, John Hardy and his colleagues have sequenced the APP genes in certain families in which the disease was known to be genetic and to be linked to chromosome 21. In affected individuals of two such families, they found a single base pair change—a valine to isoleucine substitution—in the amyloid β-protein precursor gene.

This point mutation is, however, extremely rare. Over 100 other families with the hereditary form of Alzheimer's disease do not have this mutation. Moreover, the valine to isoleucine substitution is conservative and may not alter the protein significantly. Nevertheless, the presence of this defect suggests that perhaps this mutation leads to an inappropriate processing of the precursor,

thereby producing an amyloid peptide that might be toxic to nerve cells. A similarly abnormally processed peptide might result from other mutations or perhaps nongenetically from environmentally-induced or age-related abnormalities such as covalent modifications due to abnormal patterns of phosphorylation.

The precursor proteins are synthesized by many types of cells in many organs, and in the central nervous system by both neurons and glia. Why a protein made in many different organs should form such striking deposits in the brains of patients with Alzheimer's disease is still a mystery. The answer must lie in the regulation of its synthesis, or perhaps even more likely in the mechanism by which the amyloid precursor is processed to form the small peptides that aggregate and accumulate. Large fragments of amyloid β-protein precursor normally are secreted by neurons in culture and may become associated with extracellular matrix. These normally secreted fragments are, however, different from the small amyloid generating peptides found in the plaques of patients with Alzheimer's disease. Therefore, it seems likely that with Alzheimer's disease, the protein is cleaved at an abnormal site to give rise to a small amyloid-producing peptide that accumulates to form fibrils, which then become resistant to further degradation and manifest neurotoxic properties.

Thus, the amyloid peptide presumably is generated by abnormal proteolytic cleavage of the precursor protein. In fact, the two largest amyloid precursors encode a protease inhibitor, and the amyloid plaques themselves contain another protease inhibitor (α-1-antichymotrypsin). These two inhibitors may contribute to the formation of amyloid deposits by inhibiting the proteolytic degradation of amyloid.

Despite the presence of large amounts of amyloid in Alzheimer's disease, it is not clear how amyloid deposition might contribute to degeneration of neurons or even if amyloid is the major causative agent in neuronal degeneration. It is possible that amyloid deposition in Alzheimer's disease is only an inert by-product of neuronal death.

Besides amyloid and ACT, the extra-cellularly located plaques contain axons and dendrites with twisted, kinked, irregular profiles. Many of these processes contain paired helical filaments (see below). The neuronal processes in plaques do not come from a specific class of neuron. A variety of neurotransmitters and neurotransmitter enzymes have been found in the neurites of plaques by immunocytochemistry, including acetylcholinesterase, choline acetyltransferase, tyrosine hydroxylase, somatostatin, vasoactive intestinal peptide, and substance P. Processes of astrocytes and microglia also take part in plaque formation.

Some patients with Alzheimer's disease have plaques with a large amount of amyloid but only a small number of or no cellular processes. Furthermore, large deposits of the amyloid peptide without abnormal processes have been detected in the cerebral cortex of individuals who are not suffering from dementia. Whether these individuals

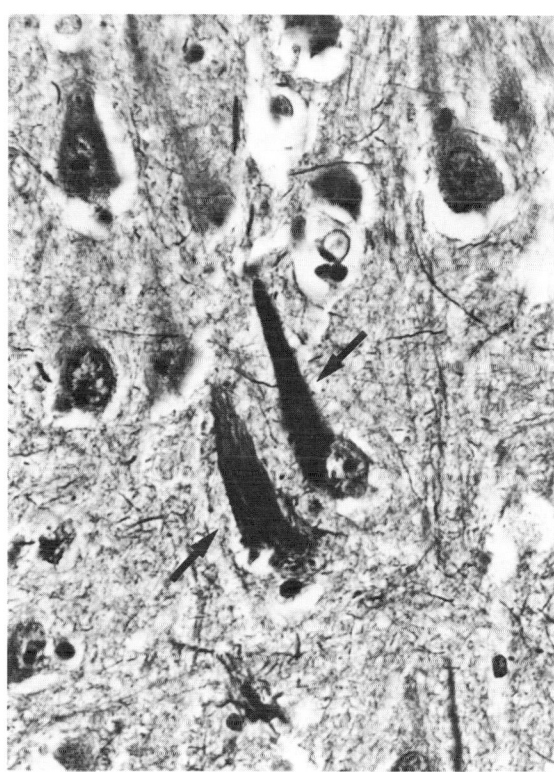

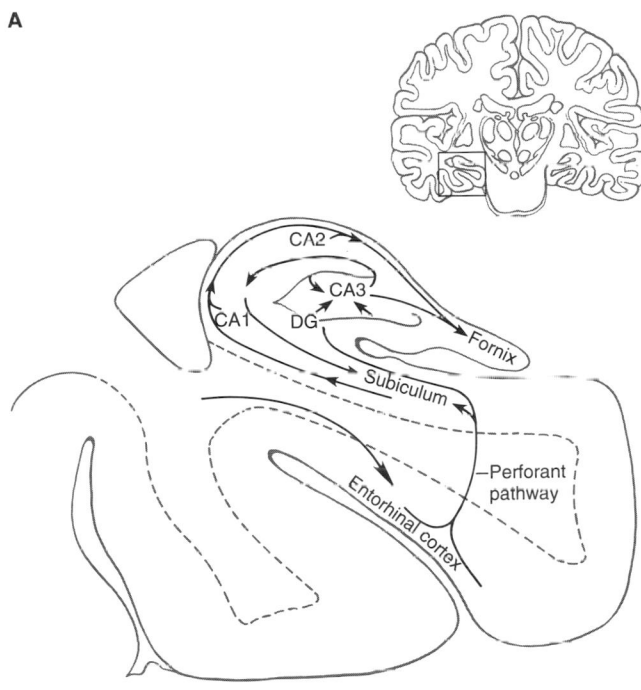

FIGURE 62–3
Neurofibrillary tangles in pyramidal neurons of the hippocampus (**arrows**). Bundles of paired helical filaments having an affinity for silver stains give these cytoskeletal abnormalities black profiles.

would have subsequently developed Alzheimer's disease is not known. If the generation of the amyloid peptide is in fact an initial and important event in the genesis of plaques, then the changes in axons and glial cells could be a later event, or even a delayed response to earlier pathological changes.

Neurofibrillary Tangles Are an Intracellular Characteristic of Alzheimer's Disease

Neurofibrillary tangles are bundles of abnormal filaments within neurons (Figure 62–3). Each filament consists of two thin filaments arranged in a helix (paired helical filament), measuring about 25 nm in diameter at its widest, with periodic constrictions every 80 nm. These structures do not resemble normal cytoskeletal proteins of neurons (see Chapter 4), but they appear to be derived from normal structures. For example, paired helical filaments contain *tau* proteins, microtubule-associated proteins that are a normal component of neurons. Paired helical filaments accumulate in a tangled mass in neuronal cell bodies, but these filaments are also found in many small neuronal processes and in axonal processes that are associated with plaques.

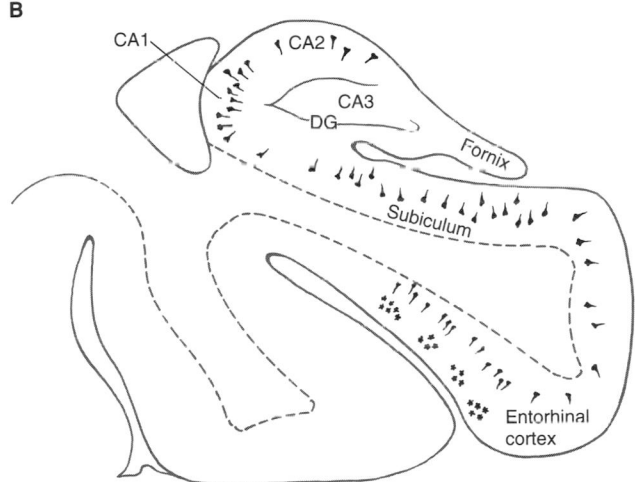

FIGURE 62–4
Alzheimer's pathology in the hippocampus.

A. The major divisions of the hippocampus and parahippocampal gyrus include the dentate gyrus (**DG**), the CA1, CA2, and CA3 divisions of Ammon's horn, the subiculum, and the entorhinal cortex. **Arrows** indicate the major synaptic pathways within the hippocampus. Major afferents to the entorhinal cortex come from the basal forebrain, neocortex, and amygdala. Major efferents from pyramidal neurons project to other limbic system areas via the fornix.

B. The major sites of neurofibrillary tangle formation in Alzheimer hippocampus. The most severe pathology is in the CA1 sector, subiculum, and entorhinal cortex. Large neurons in the entorhinal cortex, arranged in clusters in layer II, are especially affected.

Generally, tangles are formed by the large neurons of the brain—the pyramidal cells of the hippocampus and neocortex, the large neurons in the olfactory cortex, amygdala, basal forebrain nuclei, and several brain stem nuclei, including the locus ceruleus and the raphe nucleus. Tangles are not specific to Alzheimer's disease, since they are also found in the brains of patients with Down's syndrome, post-encephalitic parkinsonism, dementia pugilistica, and in a variety of degenerative, metabolic, and viral disorders. With the exception of Down's syndrome, amyloid plaques are not characteristic of these other tangle-bearing disorders. A small number of tangles is found in the brains of normal elderly people.

The Alzheimer brain also is characterized by neuronal cell loss and changes in neuronal morphology. This is reflected by a decreased brain weight and by atrophy of the cortex. Although the patterns and degrees of atrophy vary considerably from individual to individual, it is most prominent in frontal, anterior temporal, and parietal lobes. Neuronal loss is most notable in the hippocampus (see below), frontal, parietal, and anterior temporal cortices, amygdala, and the olfactory system. Profound loss also occurs in the nucleus basalis, a large cholinergic system at the base of the forebrain. This cell loss accounts for the severe cholinergic deficiency in the cortex of Alzheimer patients (see below). Cell loss occurs also in the locus ceruleus and is likely to account for reduction in brain level of norepinephrine noted in some Alzheimer patients. As might be expected, neuronal loss is generally seen in areas that show plaque or tangle pathology.

Which specific classes of neurons degenerate in Alzheimer's disease? Several patterns of degeneration are common to all Alzheimer patients. In the hippocampus the most prominently affected zones are the CA1 region, the subiculum, and the entorhinal cortex (Figure 62–4). The entorhinal cortex receives major innervation from the neocortex, basal forebrain, and amygdala. The large neurons of the entorhinal cortex (layer II), which project to the subiculum and dentate gyrus by means of the perforant pathway, are prominent sites of tangle formation in Alzheimer's disease. The major hippocampal output—to mammillary bodies, hypothalamus, and dorsomedial thalamus—arises from axons of the pyramidal cells which exit the hippocampus via the fornix. Thus, severe pathology occurs in those neuronal populations that receive input to the hippocampus or provide hippocampal efferents. This isolation probably accounts for a significant amount of the impairment of recent memory in Alzheimer's disease, since damage to both hippocampi or to their efferents by other processes (strokes, for example) produces memory deficits, particularly in the retention of recently acquired information.

Other areas of the limbic system are also affected. These include the olfactory bulbs, olfactory cortices, amygdala, cingulate gyrus, and hypothalamus. Limbic pathology may underlie some of the abnormal behavioral characteristics of some Alzheimer patients, such as uncontrollable violence and appetite. The profound olfactory pathology (tangle and neuronal loss) have led some investigators to speculate that the olfactory–limbic system con-

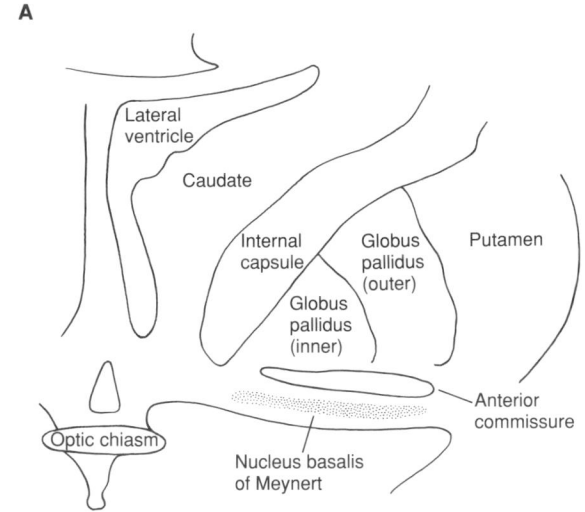

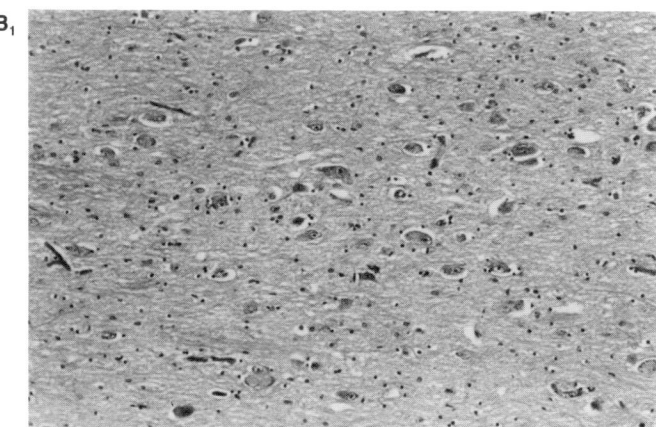

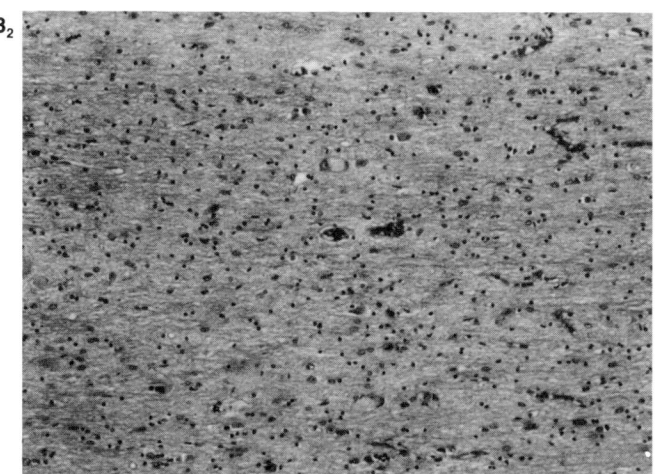

FIGURE 62–5

The nucleus basalis of Meynert in Alzheimer's disease.

A. The location of the nucleus within the basal forebrain system can be seen in this coronal section. Its main extent lies just under the anterior commissure (**AC**) and basal ganglia (globus pallidus, **GP**; and putamen, **P**).

B. Photomicrographs of the nucleus basalis of Meynert in a normal brain (**1**) and in an Alzheimer brain (**2**), in which marked neuronal loss has occurred.

nections may provide a pathway through which toxic substances or infectious agents could enter the central nervous system, either causing Alzheimer's or contributing to its features.

There Are Neurotransmitter Deficits in Alzheimer's Disease

Alzheimer's disease is associated with deficits in several neurotransmitter systems, both those that project to the neocortex and those that reside within the cortex. In the mid 1970s investigators discovered a 60–90% loss of choline acetyltransferase in the cerebral cortex and hippocampus of Alzheimer patients. This enzyme catalyzes the synthesis of acetylcholine (ACh) and is a specific marker for cholinergic neurons (Chapter 14). Most of the cholinergic activity in cortex and the hippocampus is contained in efferents from neurons of the *nucleus basalis of Meynert*, located beneath the globus pallidus in the substantia innominata of the basal forebrain (Figure 62–5).

The nucleus basalis is larger in humans than in other species and is a major component of the substantia innominata. Lesions of the basal forebrain in rats reduce the cortical choline acetyltransferase activity 60–70%. Cholinergic neurons in the nucleus basalis project widely, to neocortex and the hippocampus and to the amygdala, olfactory bulbs, thalamus, and brain stem. They receive afferents from many sources, including the hypothalamus, amygdala, peripeduncular nucleus, and midbrain. The nucleus basalis is therefore believed to play an important role in integrating subcortical function.

The nucleus basalis in patients with Alzheimer's disease was examined by Donald Price, Joseph Coyle, and Mahlon DeLong, who observed a profound (75%) loss of neurons, compared with age-matched controls. Consistent with the importance of cholinergic systems in cognition is the finding that anticholinergic drugs like scopolamine can produce memory disorders and confusion in normal individuals. The cholinergic deficit in Alzheimer's disease has led to attempts to improve the mental status of patients by administering a precursor to ACh, such as choline or lecithin. Although studies in animals indicate that the amount of ACh in the brain can be increased by administration of these precursors, these drug trials for Alzheimer's patients have not been successful. Cholinergic deficits are not the only transmitter deficit in Alzheimer's disease. There are cortical losses of norepinephrine and serotonin that can be traced to cell loss in the locus ceruleus and raphe nuclei.

In addition to deficits in systems that project to the cortex, there are abnormalities in pathways that are intrinsic to the cortex. A large number of peptide transmitters are found in cortical interneurons. Of these, losses of somatostatin, neuropeptide Y, corticotropin-releasing factor, and substance P have been described in Alzheimer cortex. These neurons are localized mainly to layer 2, upper layer 3, and layer 4. They do not send projections out of the cortex. There is some specificity in peptide loss, since other peptides appear normal (metencephalin and vasoactive intestinal peptide, for example.) Presumably,

the deficits in these various transmitter systems in Alzheimer's disease are all reflections of the degeneration and death of neuronal populations. Similarly, the cytoskeletal protein abnormalities are also manifestations of degenerative changes. Another indication of neuronal degeneration in Alzheimer's disease is the loss of synapses and presynaptic marker proteins in the neocortex and hippocampus. This loss is likely a result of both deafferentation of cortical and hippocampal neurons and of atrophy of the neurons themselves. Synaptic loss thus provides another neuroanatomic marker for the development and severity of dementia and may even be a better correlate of cognitive impairment than plaques or tangles.

The central question of why neurons die in Alzheimer's disease has yet to be answered. One of many speculations on the etiology of Alzheimer's disease is that neurons degenerate because specific growth factors diminish or neurons become less responsive to growth factors. One of the best studied of these, nerve growth factor, can bind to cholinergic neurons of the basal forebrain and help prevent their degeneration under certain experimental conditions. These ideas have led to the suggestion that some of the neuronal degeneration in Alzheimer's disease might be prevented or slowed if appropriate trophic factors could be applied.

Other Degenerative Diseases Also Produce Dementia

Although Alzheimer's disease is by far the most common form of dementia, several other disorders can produce dementia. Many are age-related, occurring in far greater incidence in older people than in younger ones. Several of these are degenerative diseases characterized by the death of neurons in various parts of the central nervous system, especially the cerebral cortex. However, some forms of dementia are associated with degeneration of the thalamus or the white matter underlying the cerebral cortex. Here the cognitive dysfunction results from the isolation of cortical areas by the degeneration of efferents and afferents.

Pick's disease is a severe neuronal degeneration in the neocortex of the frontal and anterior temporal lobes, sometimes accompanied by death of neurons in the striatum. Neurons contain a characteristic inclusion, the Pick body, a loose aggregate of abnormal, straight filaments. While these appear different from the neurofibrillary tangles of Alzheimer's disease, the filaments of Pick bodies are related to the paired helical filaments of tangles, since both kinds of abnormalities react with the same kinds of antibodies to neuronal cytoskeletal proteins. Thus, as in Alzheimer's disease, there is evidence for marked disorganization of the neuronal cytoskeleton.

Huntington's disease involves degeneration of the caudate nucleus and putamen (see Chapter 42) and produces cognitive deficits that often progress to frank dementia. The dementia probably results from degeneration of neurons in the neocortex.

Parkinson's disease also primarily affects subcortical structures, especially the substantia nigra and locus ceruleus (see Chapter 42). A significant number of Parkinson patients have cognitive deficits. Some have concomitant Alzheimer's disease. Others develop abnormal, filamentous inclusions in neurons of the hippocampus and neocortex, especially cortical areas such as the cingulate gyrus, linked closely to limbic systems.

An Overall View

Aging is of great interest scientifically and important clinically, but the neurobiological process responsible for aging is poorly understood. There now is evidence for a decrease in the number of neurons and of certain neurotransmitters during aging. However, our understanding of the aging of the central nervous system will only become clearer once we are able to study the process at the cellular level.

As the average age of the population increases, Alzheimer dementia and other age-related neurodegenerative diseases are becoming more common. Alzheimer's disease is characterized by memory loss associated with neuronal degeneration in the hippocampus, generation of amyloid plaques in many areas of gray matter, death of neurons with formation of abnormal cytoskeletal structures, and a profound cholinergic deficiency. Our knowledge of other neurodegenerative diseases that produce dementia is more rudimentary.

Selected Readings

Beal, M. F., and Martin, J. B. 1986. Neuropeptides in neurological disease. Ann. Neurol. 20:547–565.

Davies, P. 1986. The genetics of Alzheimer's disease: A review and a discussion of the implications. Neurobiol. Aging 7:459–466.

Hayflick, L. 1980. The cell biology of human aging. Sci. Am. 242(1):58–65.

Hooper, C. 1991. An exciting "if" in Alzheimer's. J. NIH Res. 3(4):65–70.

Katzman, R. 1986. Alzheimer's disease. N. Engl. J. Med. 314:964–973.

Selkoe, D. J. 1991. The molecular pathology of Alzheimer's disease. Neuron 6:487–498.

Tomlinson, B. E., and Henderson, G. 1976. Some quantitative cerebral findings in normal and demented old people. In R. D. Terry and S. Gershon (eds.), Aging, Vol. 3: Neurobiology of Aging. New York: Raven Press, pp. 183–204.

References

Abraham, C. R., Selkoe, D. J., and Potter, H. 1988. Immunochemical identification of the serine protease inhibitor α_1-antichymotrypsin in the brain amyloid deposits of Alzheimer's disease. Cell 52:487–501.

Côté, L. J., and Kremzner, L. T. 1983. Biochemical changes in normal aging in human brain. In R. Mayeux and W. G. Rosen (eds.), The Dementias. Advances in Neurology, Vol. 38. New York: Raven Press, pp. 19–30.

Crystal, H., Dickson, D., Fuld, P., Masur, D., Scott, R., Mehler, M., Masdeu, J., Kawas, C., Aronson, M., and Wolfson, L. 1988. Clinico-pathologic studies in dementia: Nondemented subjects with pathologically confirmed Alzheimer's disease. Neurology 38:1682–1687.

Dastur, D. K., Lane, M. H., Hansen, D. B., Kety, S. S., Butler, R. N., Perlin, S., and Sokoloff, L. 1963. Effects of aging on cerebral circulation and metabolism in man. In J. E. Birren, R. N. Butler, S. W. Greenhouse, L. Sokoloff, and M. R. Yarrow (eds.), Human Aging: A Biological and Behavioral Study. Public Health Service Publ. No. 986. Washington, D.C.: U.S. Government Printing Office, pp. 57–76.

Davies, P., and Maloney, A. J. F. 1976. Selective loss of central cholinergic neurons in Alzheimer's disease. Lancet 2:1403.

DeKosky, S. T., and Scheff, S. W. 1990. Synapse loss in frontal cortex biopsies in Alzheimer's disease: Correlation with cognitive severity. Ann. Neurol. 27:457–464.

Goate, A., Chartier-Harlin, M. C., Mullan, M., Brown, J., Crawford, F., Fidani, L., Giuffra, L., Haynes, A., Irving, N., James, L., Mant, R., Newton, P., Rooke, K., Roques, P., Talbot, C., Williamson, R., Rossor, M., Owen, M., and Hardy, J. 1991. Segregation of a missense mutation in the amyloid precursor protein gene with familial Alzheimer's disease. Nature 349: 704–706.

Glenner, G. G., and Wong, C. W. 1984. Alzheimer's disease: Initial report of the purification and characterization of a novel cerebrovascular amyloid protein. Biochem. Biophys. Res. Commun. 120:885–890.

Goldman, J. E., and Yen, S.-H. 1986. Cytoskeletal protein abnormalities in neurodegenerative diseases. Ann. Neurol. 19:209–223.

Hamos, J. E., DeGennaro, L. J., and Drachman, D. A. 1989. Synaptic loss in Alzheimer's disease and other dementias. Neurology 39:355–361.

Hansen, L. A., DeTeresa, R., Davies, P., and Terry, R. D. 1988. Neocortical morphometry, lesion counts, and choline acetyltransferase levels in the age spectrum of Alzheimer's disease. Neurology 38:48–54.

Hyman, B. T., Van Hoesen, G. W., Damasio, A. R., and Barnes, C. L. 1984. Alzheimer's disease: Cell-specific pathology isolates the hippocampal formation. Science 225:1168–1170.

Levy, E., Carman, M. D., Fernandez-Madrid, I. J., Power, M. D., Lieberburg, I., van Duinen, S. G., Bots, G. Th. A. M., Luyendijk, W., and Frangione, B. 1990. Mutation of the Alzheimer's disease amyloid gene in hereditary cerebral hemorrhage, Dutch type. Science 248:1124–1126.

Marsden, C. D., and Harrison, M. J. G. 1972. Outcome of investigation of patients with presenile dementia. Br. Med. J. 2:249–252.

Masliah, E., Terry, R. D., DeTeresa, R. M., and Hansen, L. A. 1989. Immunohistochemical quantification of the synapse-related protein synaptophysin in Alzheimer disease. Neurosci. Lett. 103:234–239.

Medvedev, Zh. A. 1972. Repetition of molecular–genetic information as a possible factor in evolutionary changes of life span. Exp. Gerontol. 7:227–238.

Olshansky, S. J., Carnes, B. A., and Cassel, C. 1990. In search of Methuselah: Estimating the upper limits to human longevity. Science 250:634–640.

Pearson, R. C. A., Esiri, M. M., Hiorns, R. W., Wilcock, G. K., and Powell, T. P. S. 1985. Anatomical correlates of the distribution of the pathological changes in the neocortex in Alzheimer disease. Proc. Natl. Acad. Sci. U.S.A. 82:4531–4534.

Perry, E. K., Perry, R. H., Blessed, G., and Tomlinson, B. E. 1977. Necropsy evidence of central cholinergic deficits in senile dementia. Lancet 1:189.

Price, D. L., Whitehouse, P. J., Struble, R. G., Clark, A. W., Coyle, J. T., DeLong, M. R., and Hedreen, J. C. 1982. Basal forebrain cholinergic systems in Alzheimer's disease and related dementia. Neurosci. Comment. 1(2):84–92.

Strehler, B., Hirsch, G., Gusseck, D., Johnson, R., and Bick, M. 1971. Codon-restriction theory of aging and development. J. Theor. Biol. 33:429–474.

Tanzi, R. E., Gusella, J. F., Watkins, P. C., Bruns, G. A. P., St George-Hyslop, P., Van Keuren, M. L., Patterson, D., Pagan, S., Kurnit, D. M., and Neve, R. L. 1987. Amyloid β protein gene: cDNA, mRNA distribution, and genetic linkage near the Alzheimer locus. Science 235:880–884.

Walford, R. L. 1974. Immunologic theory of aging: Current status. Fed. Proc. 33:2020–2027.

Weidemann, A., König, G., Bunke, D., Fischer, P., Salbaum, J. M., Masters, C. L., and Beyreuther, K. 1989. Identification, biogen-esis, and localization of precursors of Alzheimer's disease A4 amyloid protein. Cell 57:115–126.

White, P., Hiley, C. R., Goodhardt, M. J., Carrasco, L. H., Keet, J. P., Williams, I. E. I., and Bowen, D. M. 1977. Neocortical cholinergic neurons in elderly people. Lancet 1:668–671.

Yankner, B. A., Dawes, L. R., Fisher, S., Villa-Komaroff, L., Oster-Granite, M. L., and Neve, R. L. 1989. Neurotoxicity of a frag-ment of the amyloid precursor associated with Alzheimer's disease. Science 245:417–420.

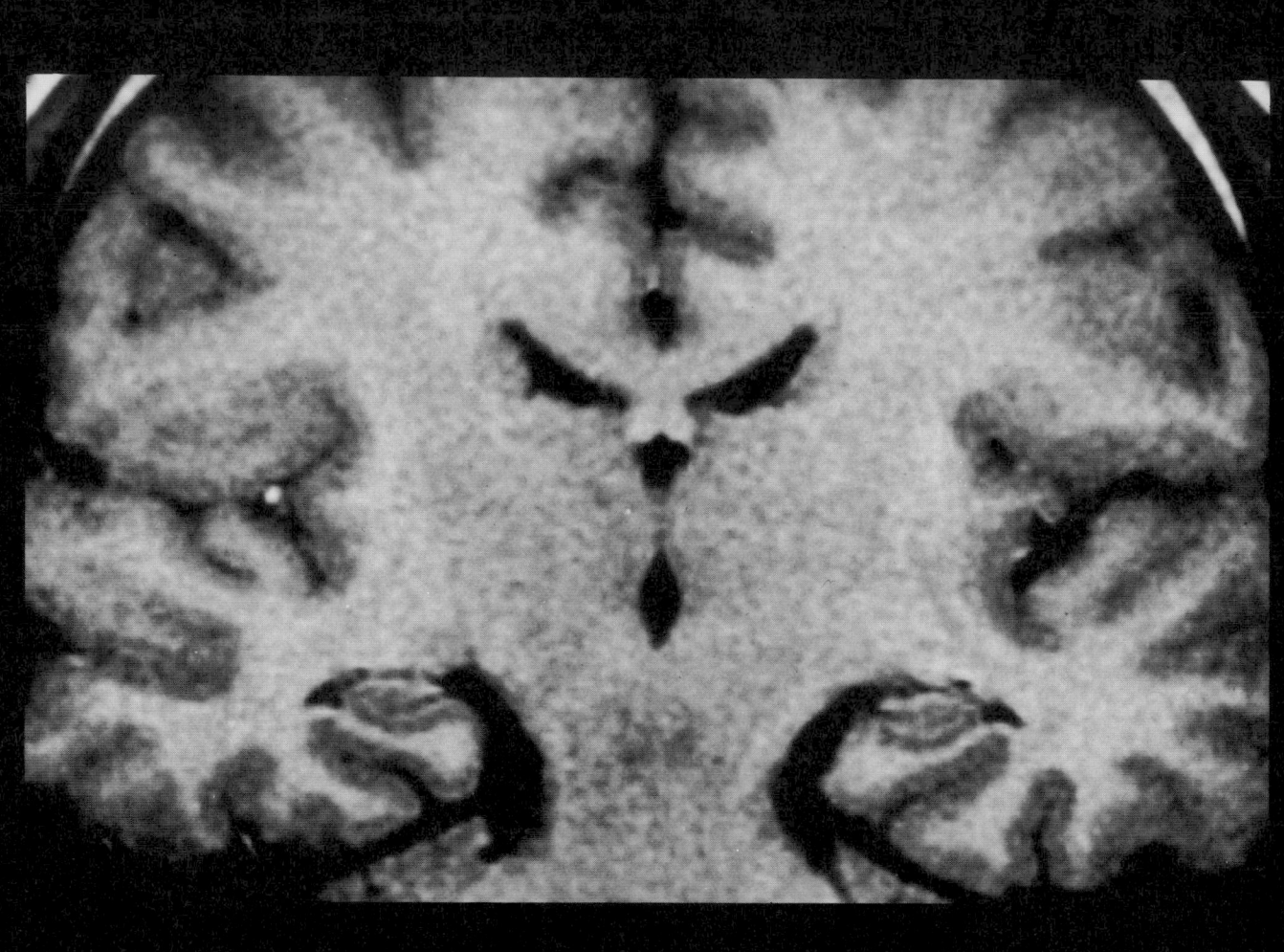

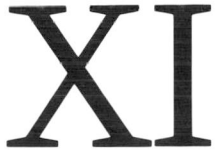

Genes, Environmental Experience, and the Mechanisms of Behavior

Behavior emerges gradually as the brain develops. At first the development of the brain is largely under the control of genetic and developmental programs. Influences from the environment begin to exert their effect *in utero*, and become of prime importance after birth. Knowledge of both innate (genetic and developmental) and environmental determinants is needed to understand behavior fully. This information is also essential for developing rational therapeutic strategies for treating psychiatric disorders.

In considering innate factors that control behavior, we need first to focus on aspects of behavior that are heritable. Clearly, no behavior is inherited: What is inherited is DNA. Genes encode proteins that are important for the development, maintenance, and regulation of the neural circuits that produce behavior. Therefore, we need to examine the interaction of genetic and environmental factors to understand behavior.

In considering behavior, careful and quantitative analysis of stimuli and responses is important because responses are *observable* indices of behavior. Stimuli and responses can be manipulated experimentally and measured objectively. By emphasizing observable actions, behaviorists focus on the questions of what an organism does and how it does it. The extreme behaviorist view is that observable indices of behavior are equivalent to mental life. This view narrowly defines all mental activity in terms of the scientific techniques available for studying it. The behaviorist view also denies the existence of consciousness as well as unconscious mentation, feelings, and motivation. However, as has been emphasized by cognitive psychologists and psychoanalysts, humans and other higher animals also possess knowledge of the surrounding world and past events. Thus, we need to ask the following question: What does the organism know and how does it come to know it? How is that knowledge

Few mental processes are as intriguing as memory. Neurobiological studies reveal that memory is not a single process, but can be divided into at least two types: reflexive and declarative. Reflexive memory is concerned with motor skills and strategies. Declarative memory is concerned with persons, places, or objects. Storage of declarative memories requires the hippocampus. A surprising feature of the human hippocampus, revealed by this magnetic resonance image, is how small it is: not much bigger than one's little finger. Despite its small size, when damaged by trauma or Alzheimer's disease, we suffer from forgetfulness. This photomicrograph illustrates high resolution imaging of a 5-mm slice through a human hippocampal formation. (From Press et al., 1989.)

represented in the brain? Is the representation of conscious mental activity or knowledge different from that of unconscious activity?

Neural science is only beginning to contribute to analyzing the richness of the internal representations that cognitive psychologists recognize as intervening between stimulus and response, and the dynamic mental processes experienced by all of us, processes that traditionally have been discussed within the framework of psychoanalysis or cognitive psychology. At the same time, neural science has so far not directly addressed the subjective sense of individuality, will, and purpose that is a common human experience. Yet are the issues most important to us as scientists, as physicians, and as people. In the past, ascribing a particular behavioral feature to an unobservable mental process essentially excluded the problem from direct study because the complexity of the brain posed a barrier to any kind of biological analysis. However, as the nervous system becomes more accessible to behavior experiments, internal representations of experience can be explored in a controlled manner, as illustrated in this section. Progress in this area encourages us to believe that cognition can now be explored directly and need no longer be merely inferred.

Modern neural science represents a merger of neurophysiology, anatomy, embryology, cell biology, and psychology. Along with astute clinical observation, neural science is providing renewed support for the idea first proposed by Hippocrates over two millennia ago that the proper study of mental processes begins with study of the brain. Cognitive psychology and psychoanalytic theory have emphasized the diversity and complexity of human mental experience. Both disciplines value the importance of genetic as well as learned factors in determining how the world is represented mentally, and they postulate that behavior is based on that representation. By emphasizing mental structure and internal representation, psychoanalysis served as a source of modern cognitive psychology, a psychology that has stressed the logic of mental operations and of internal representations. Experimental cognitive psychology and clinical psychotherapy can now be strengthened by insights into the cellular neurobiology of behavior. The task for the years ahead is to produce a psychology that—though still concerned with problems of internal representation, dynamics, and subjective states of mind—is firmly grounded in empirical neural science.

PART XI

Chapter 63:	**Genetic Determinants of Behavior**
Chapter 64:	**Learning and Memory**
Chapter 65:	**Cellular Mechanisms of Learning and the Biological Basis of Individuality**

Irving Kupfermann

Genetic Determinants of Behavior

Are Aspects of Behavior Genetically Determined?
  Ethologists Define Instincts as Inborn
  Motor Patterns
  Can a Behavior Be Inherited?

Some Species-Specific Behaviors Are Elicited by Sign Stimuli

Each Species Has a Repertory of Fixed-Action Patterns Generated by Central Programs

The Role of Genes in the Expression of Behavior Can Be Studied Directly

Higher Mammals and Humans Seem to Have Certain Innate Behavioral Patterns
  Certain Human Behavioral Traits Have a
  Hereditary Component
  Many Human Behaviors Are Universal
  Stereotyped Sequences of Movements Resemble
  Fixed-Action Patterns
  Certain Complex Patterns Require Little or
  No Learning

The Brain Sets Limits on the Structure of Language

An Overall View

Behavior in all organisms is shaped by the interaction of genes and environment. The relative importance of the two factors varies, but even the most stereotyped behavior can be modified by the environment, and the most plastic behavior, such as language, is influenced by innate factors. Because genetic factors are the substrate on which the environment acts, we shall consider the innate determinants of behavior first. In the next chapter we examine how behavior is modified by environmental factors through learning.

We begin by reviewing historical and current ideas about the innate determinants of behavior and then consider possible neural mechanisms underlying certain types of innate behaviors in animals. We shall address four questions: Are some aspects of behavior inherited? How do genes exert control over behavior? How do genetic processes interact with the environment? And finally, which aspects of human behavior are predominantly innate?

Are Aspects of Behavior Genetically Determined?

Traditionally, behavior has been divided into two categories, instinctive and learned. Instinctive behavior is that component of behavior most directly related to genetic endowment. A consideration of instinct is therefore a good starting point for examining the genetic determinants of behavior.

The study of instinctive behavior has a long and controversial history. Antecedents to the notion of instinctive behavior can be traced to the beginning of written history. The ancient Greek philosophers, and later Renaissance philosophers, sought to set humans apart from lower animals by arguing that much human behavior is guided by reason, whereas the behavior of animals, however complex, was thought to be entirely the result of natural instincts.

These early explanations of human and animal behavior were not based on experimental observations. Modern scientific thinking about instinctive behavior dates to the latter part of the nineteenth century and the influential writings of Charles Darwin. Darwin's work on the evolution of species indicated that there are no sharp discontinuities between the evolution of humans and simpler animals. Darwin therefore suggested that the behavior of animals must be guided not only by instinct but also by primitive forms of the same reasoning processes that guide human behavior. More important, if humans evolved from simpler animals, Darwin argued, human behavior also must be guided by instincts.

These notions were soon amplified by psychologists, who saw in the concept of instinct a way to explain much of human behavior on the basis of a few underlying principles. For example, Sigmund Freud suggested that all normal and abnormal human behavior is powerfully shaped by two fundamental, genetically determined strivings: a life (or sexual) instinct and a death (or aggressive) instinct. Freud maintained that these instincts provide an innate mental force that energizes all behavior. In *An Introduction to Social Psychology*, an influential book published in 1908, William McDougall postulated that humans have up to a dozen instincts: flight, repulsion, curiosity, pugnacity, self-abasement, self-assertion, parenting, reproduction, desire for food, gregariousness, acquisition, and construction.

These theories about human instincts were challenged by John Watson and other proponents of *behaviorism*. Watson rejected the idea of instinctive behavior for two reasons. First, Watson and his students had difficulty with the idea that behavior can be completely programmed and unlearned. Although some behaviorists admitted that stereotyped, unlearned motor patterns might exist in lower animals, they thought that one could never be sure a given behavior actually is free of learning. Even in a carefully controlled environment, unsuspected sources of environmental stimuli might still be responsible for an organism learning some aspects of behaviors. The more radical behaviorists felt that all behavior was built up from simple reflexes that were modified and shaped by experience.

Second, Freud, McDougall, and other psychologists argued that instincts were unlearned inner strivings that guide behavior. Viewed in this way, instincts were unobservable mechanisms—intervening variables—designed to explain behavior. The behaviorists argued that only the observable aspects of behavior can ever be studied experimentally, not its inner mechanisms. The behaviorists therefore rejected an analysis of behavior that relied on inner forces or mental processes to explain the manifestation of behavior.

Behaviorists argued that a true science of behavior must deal only with observable responses. According to the behaviorists, psychologists who attempted to explain behavior by relying on the concept of instincts were merely renaming phenomena and explaining nothing.

Under the pervasive influence of behavioristic philosophy, most experimental psychologists in the United States abandoned the consideration of innate determinants of behavior and focused almost exclusively on the study of learning. In many instances processes that were formerly called instincts were renamed *drives* (for example, hunger, sex, thirst, and curiosity) and were studied without consideration of whether they originated from innate factors or learning.

Ethologists Define Instincts as Inborn Motor Patterns

During the period from 1920 to 1950, while psychologists in the United States rejected the theory of instinctive behavior, European zoologists such as Konrad Lorenz and Nikolaas Tinbergen laid the groundwork for a comparative study of behavior under natural conditions, with particular emphasis on its mechanisms, ontogenesis, and evolution. This approach, known as ethology, advanced the study of instincts in two ways. First, whereas previously scientists had only speculated about the role of instinct in behavior, ethologists systematically observed and experimented on inborn behavior. Second, they limited their biological studies of instinct to stereotyped sequences of observable motor movements that are inborn. Ethological studies of a wide variety of species led to a partial reconciliation of the older mentalistic concepts of instinct with the behaviorist's insistence on explaining behavior only in terms of observed action.

While acknowledging some of the criticisms of the concept of instinct as unlearned behavior, ethologists emphasized that it is difficult to explain some behaviors of lower animals on the basis of learning alone. For example, a female bird that has been isolated from other birds since hatching is still able to build a perfect nest as an adult and can clean and care for its young. Although such behavior could not have been acquired while the animal was maturing, ethologists emphasized that it is also not completely unaffected by the environment, as all behavior is the result of the interaction between the genetic endowment of the animal and the internal and external environments. According to ethologists, if instinctive behavior is primarily genetically programmed, asking whether a behavior is instinctive is equivalent to asking whether the behavior is inherited. Thus the ethologists succeeded in reducing studies of instinct to the question: Is it possible to inherit a behavior?

Can a Behavior Be Inherited?

Psychologists have traditionally considered behavior to be a product of the mind. At one time the mind was thought to be nonphysical, and it was difficult to envisage how it could be inherited. Most neural scientists now believe that what we call the mind represents a set of strictly biological processes or functions. According to this view, the mind is not an entity of any kind, but rather a set of functions carried out by the brain. Mind is what the brain does, just as walking is one of the things that legs do. If mind and behavior are functions of the brain, then like the function of every other organ of the body it can be affected by genetic factors.

Nevertheless, there has been great resistance to the notion that behavior, particularly human behavior, can be inherited. Part of the reason for this resistance has been a mistaken notion of what inheritance of behavior really means. Take, for example, the question: Is mental illness inherited? The question is misleading if the aim is to demonstrate that a complex behavioral disorder is controlled entirely by a set of genes that are inherited. This is the case only rarely. The expression of inherited factors nearly always depends on an interaction of genetic and environmental factors. You can inherit genes that program you to grow tall, but if you are not raised with the appropriate diet you will be short.

Although learning may or may not be important for the expression of a genetic factor, one or more environmental factors (appropriate nutrition, light, etc.) will be important. Innate or inborn behaviors are responses that are not highly dependent on specific learning experiences. However, there is no sharp distinction between learned and innate behaviors. There is instead a continuous gradation, from stereotyped responses that are almost independent of the animal's history, to responses that are highly sensitive to environmental factors. What the ethologists call instinctive behaviors are a special class of innate behaviors that consist of relatively complex sequences of responses. Instinctive behaviors are now often called *species-specific behaviors* because they are inherited as characteristics of a species, much like morphological or physiological features. In the following sections we shall consider several examples of the influence of environment on the behavioral expression of genetic information.

Some Species-Specific Behaviors Are Elicited by Sign Stimuli

In the course of investigating examples of relatively stereotyped behavioral patterns that seem to require minimal experience for their expression, Lorenz, Tinbergen, and other ethologists developed a theoretical orientation based in part on two useful concepts: the sign stimulus and the fixed-action pattern.

Complex inborn behavioral patterns in lower animals typically are activated by specific stimuli. Behavioral analysis has shown that when animals are presented with a complex set of stimuli, they often respond to specific stimuli rather than to the situation as a whole. The effective stimulus is called a *sign stimulus* or releaser. The role of sign stimuli can be illustrated by a classic series of studies by Tinbergen on the sexual behavior of the stickleback fish. During the mating season the male stickleback develops a bright red abdomen. The red abdomen provokes fighting responses from other males but also elicits approach responses from females. The critical aspects of the stimulus can be characterized by the use of wax models. A model resembling a stickleback in every detail except the red belly does not elicit a response (Figure 63–1). On the other hand, a model that has a red un-

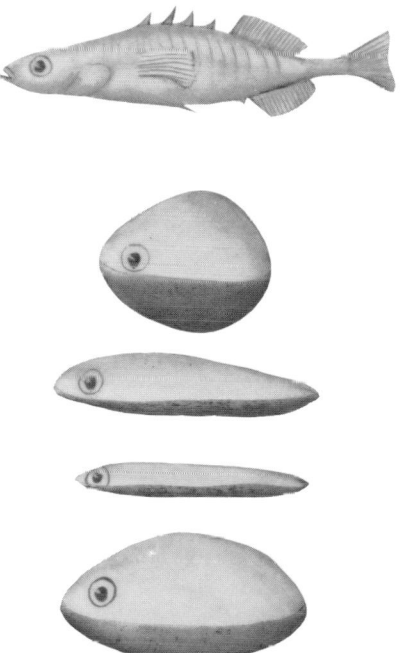

FIGURE 63–1
These models of the stickleback fish were used to identify the sign stimulus of mating and attack responses in this species. The model shown at the top is an accurate imitation of the male but lacks a red belly. The next four models, which have a red underside, are more frequently attacked by other males than the model at top. (Adapted from Tinbergen, 1951.)

derside but otherwise does not resemble a stickleback will effectively stimulate fighting behavior in males and mating behavior in females. For the color to be effective it must also occupy a specific relative location; if the model is turned upside down, for example, it will not elicit fighting responses. A similar analysis has revealed that the swollen abdomen of the female serves as a sign stimulus for the male and triggers mating behavior. Because the sign stimuli that elicit mating or attack are effective even in animals that have been raised in total isolation, mating and attack in stickleback fish are considered to be innately determined.

Each Species Has a Repertory of Fixed-Action Patterns Generated by Central Programs

Species-specific behavioral sequences typically begin with a phase of orienting or *appetitive behavior*, which consists of a variety of responses that aid the animal in finding environmental stimuli or goal objects (for example, a mate, food, water, or nesting material). Appetitive behavior is followed by a phase of *consummatory behavior*, which consists of chains of relatively stereotyped movements called *fixed-action patterns*. Each fixed-action pattern is triggered by a sign stimulus.

A fixed-action pattern resembles a reflex in that it is a behavioral response elicited by a specific stimulus and its

FIGURE 63–2

The intensity and duration of a stimulus strongly affects typical reflexes but have less influence on fixed-action patterns. Three hypothetical responses to three types of stimuli are shown: (**1**) a weak and brief stimulus; (**2**) a strong and brief stimulus, and (**3**) an even stronger and prolonged stimulus.

A. A simple reflex, for example pupillary constriction elicited by a light, reflects the nature of the stimulus.

B. A fixed-action pattern, such as courtship behaviors in fish or birds, is triggered by the stimulus but the nature of the response does not closely reflect the properties of the stimulus.

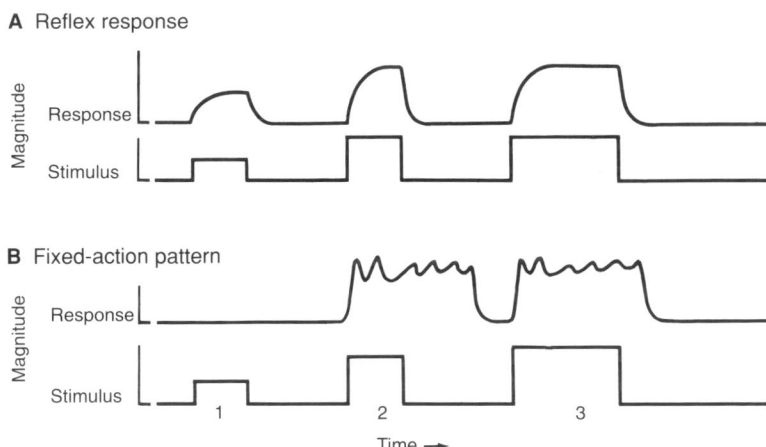

expression does not require previous learning. It differs from a simple reflex in that it is more complex and is preceded by orienting (appetitive) behavior. In addition, the sensory inputs for fixed-action patterns are transformed by the nervous system in complex ways. Whereas the strength and duration of reflexes often closely reflect the features of the evoking stimulus, the duration, latency, and intensity of fixed-action patterns generally are not precisely related to the stimulus parameters (Figure 63–2). Also, unlike reflexes, a fixed-action pattern sometimes can occur in the absence of any eliciting stimuli. This kind of behavior is referred to as *vacuum activity*. Finally, apparently inappropriate fixed-action patterns can occur when an animal is in a situation that elicits conflicting responses. For example, faced with a choice to fight or flee, a cat might momentarily groom itself instead. Such responses are referred to as *displacement activities*.

What is the neural basis of fixed-action patterns? Does the central nervous system determine the entire pattern and do stimuli only serve to release the pattern? Or are fixed-action patterns merely a complex series of reflexes, where each reflex in the series produces proprioceptive or other sensory feedback that elicits the next reflex response?

To approach this issue experimentally, it is necessary to eliminate all sources of external sensory input that could provide cues for the series of reflexes. Such experiments have been done in several invertebrate preparations in which the nervous system can be completely isolated. The nervous system thus receives no sensory feedback, but it remains alive, and its neurons are easily studied by intracellular recording electrodes. As we shall see below, the nervous systems of certain invertebrates contain command neurons that elicit complex behavioral sequences when stimulated. Experiments of this type have been done on flying, walking, swimming, and feeding behavior in insects, crustaceans, and molluscs. In all of these animals the isolated nervous system generates a motor output that is similar to that of the intact animal. Although sensory input typically modifies the strength or frequency of the central program, with rare exceptions the essential pattern does not require timing cues from sensory feedback.

Evidence that fixed-action patterns are controlled by central motor programs has also been obtained in vertebrates. For example, there is a central program for locomotion in cats (see Chapter 38). Many other responses in vertebrates, some quite complex, appear to involve built-in motor programs. These include swallowing, biting, grooming, orgasm, coughing, yawning, vomiting, and the startle reflex. Swallowing is a well-studied example. This response, triggered by stimulating the pharynx, involves sequential activation of at least 10 different muscles (Figure 63–3). Robert Doty and James Bosma studied the swallowing response of dogs by electrically stimulating the pharyngeal nerves. They examined the pattern of muscle contraction before and after anesthetizing the pharynx, or inactivating the various muscles either surgically or by application of a local anesthetic. The motor sequence was not significantly changed by altering or eliminating sources of peripheral feedback from the muscles or pharynx. However, the strength and duration of the motor output did vary with different levels of arousal or different degrees of pharyngeal stimulation. Thus, like locomotion, the details of the pattern of swallowing can be modified by external sensory feedback even though the basic pattern is regulated internally.

Certain complex behaviors of vertebrates, as well as invertebrates, consist of combinations of different fixed-action patterns in sequence. For example, John Fentress found that the grooming behavior of mice involves four types of movement, directed toward the face, belly, back, and tail. Grooming of the face is associated with six stereotyped motor patterns, including licking, single or parallel strokes with the forepaws, and shuddering of the body. The various patterns do not occur in random sequences, but in a predictable order, although the order is not absolutely fixed.

What are the neural mechanisms responsible for triggering fixed-action patterns? In 1938 C. A. G. Wiersma reported the important discovery that a complete complex motor output in crayfish can be triggered by stimulating individual *command neurons*. For example, the firing of a single command neuron elicits a complex defensive response involving dozens of different muscles. Command

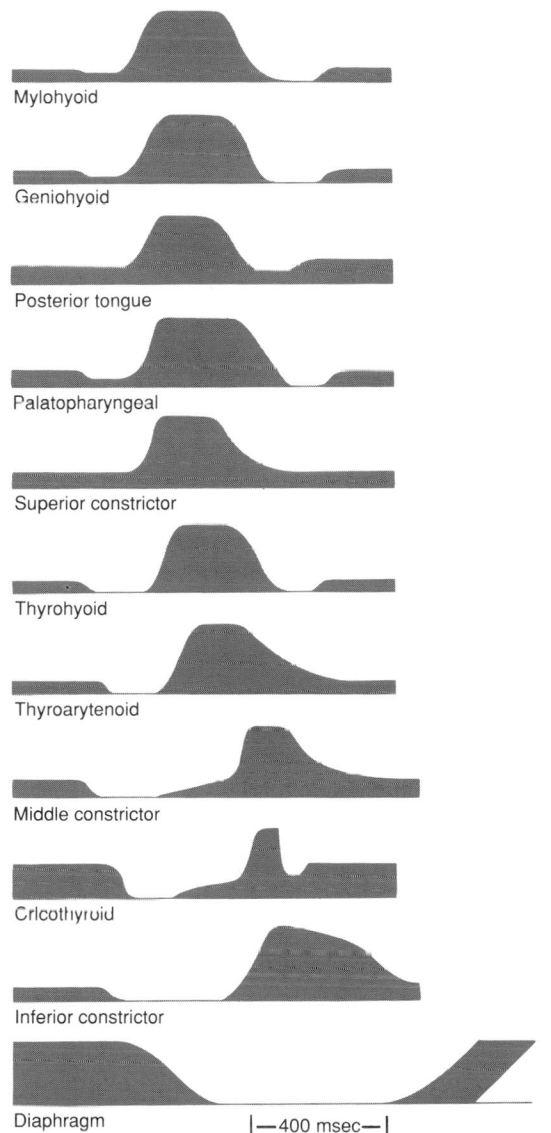

FIGURE 63-3

The sequential activation of several muscles during the swallowing reflex in the dog is typical of a fixed-action pattern. In this idealized summary of electromyographic activity the height of the trace for each muscle indicates the intensity of the action observed. (Adapted from Doty and Bosma, 1956.)

neurons have divergent synaptic outputs that excite some and inhibit other members in a population of follower neurons. These follower cells in turn are interconnected to generate specific patterns of motor output.

Individual neurons in invertebrates can elicit behavioral responses as well as modulate responsiveness in a manner similar to the effects of complex motivational states, such as hunger and arousal. For example, when the sea slug *Aplysia* is deprived of food and is then exposed to food stimuli, it exhibits a food-arousal state characterized by a constellation of behaviors—such as increased heart rate and head lifting—as well as modulation of responsive-

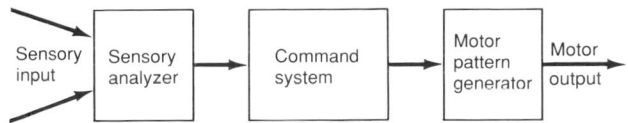

FIGURE 63-4

A simplified model of the neural organization that may underlie fixed-action patterns.

ness—such as suppression of withdrawal responses and potentiation of biting. Firing of a single neuron in the brain of the animal evokes activity in over a thousand neurons that are part of different systems, each of which could account for one or another aspect of the food-arousal state of the animal.

There is no evidence for command neurons in mammals. Nevertheless, there are in mammals specific groups of cells that trigger preprogrammed motor acts, and it is tempting to regard these cell groups as command systems that function like command neurons in invertebrates. In fact, even in invertebrates many complex motor acts may not be triggered by single command neurons; instead, different cells may trigger the component actions of a complete act. Just as perception in invertebrates depends on several feature detectors operating in parallel, the generation of a complex motor act may involve the operation of several command neurons, each of which is responsible for some limited aspect of the movement.

Certain command systems appear to be driven by neural mechanisms that are tuned to specific features of sensory input, for example, the red underside of the stickleback fish. Ethologists refer to this type of mechanism as the *innate releasing mechanism*. Although the neural structure of innate releasing mechanisms is largely unknown, it may include elements like the individual neurons in the sensory systems of vertebrates that respond to highly specific features of sensory input (see Chapter 30). A possible neural basis of fixed-action patterns is shown in the simplified model in Figure 63-4. Feature detection neurons, as part of a sensory system or innate releasing mechanism, are excited by specific sensory input and in turn excite command neurons or command systems. The command system in turn triggers a central motor program that generates a stereotyped behavioral sequence. Studies in invertebrates have shown that a given neuronal network can generate very different modes of stereotyped outputs, depending on which modulatory biogenic amine or peptide plays on the circuit. The modulators alter the circuit by changing both the membrane properties and the synaptic connectivity of the neurons.

The Role of Genes in the Expression of Behavior Can Be Studied Directly

Given that certain aspects of behavior are innate, how do genes code for behavior? The current revolution in molecular genetics has made it possible not only to delineate more precisely the central issues in this chapter, but also to look at simple instances in which the relationship between genes and behavior is unambiguous.

Clearly, genes do not code for behavior in a direct way; a single gene cannot code for a single behavior. Behavior is generated by neural circuits involving many nerve cells. Genes code for specific proteins, and many different proteins, both structural and enzymatic, are required for the development and functioning of a neural circuit. The fact that many genes are required does not mean, however, that individual genes are not critical for the expression of a behavior. The importance of particular genes for behavior can best be demonstrated in simple animals, such as the fruit fly *Drosophila*, in which mutations of single genes can be more easily studied. Such studies show that mutations of single genes can produce abnormalities of learned behavior (see Chapter 65) as well as instinctive behaviors such as courtship or locomotion.

An interesting and well-studied behavioral mutant of *Drosophila* is *shaker*. *Shaker* mutants exhibit spontaneous nonfunctional movements. The abnormal movements are due to prolonged action potentials in nerve and muscle cells. These abnormal action potentials result from a single gene mutation that deprives *shaker* of a particular K$^+$ channel (an early K$^+$ channel that we discussed in Chapter 8). In *Drosophila* this K$^+$ channel contributes importantly to the rapid repolarization of the action potential.

The sexual behavior of the fruit fly is a particularly instructive example of how genes can affect behavior. This behavior involves several acts that are under the control of different stimuli: visual, auditory, and olfactory. A large number of mutations that affect sexual behavior have been found. In some the behavior is disrupted in a rather simple fashion by mutations that interfere with motor responses or with sensory analysis. For example, the male normally excites the female by making a characteristic sound produced by fluttering of the wings. Thus, mutations that affect female hearing and mutations of the wing of the male can interfere with mating. The effects of other mutations do not have so simple an explanation. For example, it may seem surprising at first that a number of mutations that affect the learning abilities of the animals also affect their sexual behavior. *Drosophila* males normally attempt to mate with juvenile males and with already fertilized females; with experience, the adult male learns to avoid juvenile males and fertilized females. Animals with the learning mutations, however, fail to learn and persist in their inappropriate responses. Another mutation that affects sexual behavior involves the *per* gene, which modulates the circadian rhythms of the animals. Mutations of this gene, however, also alter the frequency modulation of the male wing song, resulting in a song that is less stimulating to the female.

Genes are essential not only for producing the appropriate neural circuitry of a behavior, but also for regulating the expression of the behavior in the adult, because genes code for the structural proteins necessary to maintain the neuronal circuitry as well as for enzymes—including the transmitter-synthesizing enzymes that are essential for normal synaptic transmission. Moreover, genes directly code for peptide hormones and modulators that trigger or inhibit the expression of behavior. For example, a fixed-action pattern can be triggered by a peptide hormone acting on the appropriate command elements in the neural circuitry.

An illustration of how genes can switch on a behavioral sequence comes from the study of egg-laying in *Aplysia* and the pond snail *Lymnaea*. Egg-laying is a fixed-action pattern with appetitive and consummatory phases. The appetitive phase includes cessation of walking, inhibition of feeding, and head waving, followed by an all-or-none consummatory phase in which the egg string is deposited. The consummatory phase and several aspects of the appetitive repertory are triggered by a peptide hormone, called egg-laying hormone, that is released by a cluster of identified neurons. The egg-laying hormone (see Chapter 14) acts directly on the smooth muscle of follicles in the ovotestes by a mechanism analogous to the action of oxytocin on the uterine musculature of mammals. In addition, the hormone excites and inhibits specific neurons throughout the nervous system of the animal.

Although the egg-laying hormone of *Aplysia* consists of only 36 amino acids, it is derived from a precursor polyprotein consisting of 271 amino acid residues. Thus, the synthesis of egg-laying hormone is similar to that of several well-studied neuropeptides in vertebrates, such as the proopiomelanocortin family of peptides that were considered in Chapter 14. Since the egg-laying hormone is synthesized as part of a larger precursor molecule, before it can be released it must be cleaved from the larger molecule at pairs of basic amino acid residues that flank its own sequence. Indeed, the precursor contains eight pairs of basic residues that serve as cleavage sites flanking other neuroactive peptides.

What are the functions of these peptides? A number of peptides have now been isolated from the precursor, and each appears to be released in a coordinated manner with the egg-laying hormone. Several of these peptides function as neurotransmitters that alter the activity of specific neurons involved in one or another aspect of egg-laying. Some of the peptides act on the neurons that secrete them, producing autoexcitation of the cell. This helps insure that once the neurons fire they will produce a prolonged discharge and release a substantial amount of hormone.

The study of egg laying allows us to pursue in a behavioral context the more general question that was examined in Chapter 14: Why are polyproteins used as precursors for peptide hormones and transmitters? One reason is that polyproteins provide a mechanism for coordinated expression and release of diverse peptides that may activate in a coherent manner the individual neuronal circuits responsible for the different components of a stereotyped behavior. Thus, in certain experimentally advantageous behaviors it is possible to relate specific genes to particular proteins in specific neural circuits and even to the controlling elements that act on those neural circuits to regulate the expression of a behavior.

Higher Mammals and Humans Seem to Have Certain Innate Behavioral Patterns

Most research on innate behavior has been done on non-mammalian species, but considerable evidence indicates that mammals, including primates, also exhibit innate behaviors. A particularly elegant example is the work done by Gene Sackett, who tried to determine whether the behavioral responses of monkeys to a specific visual stimulus are innate. He raised individual monkeys in complete isolation from their mothers and other monkeys. When these animals were given an opportunity to look at various types of photographs, they greatly preferred images of other infant monkeys over nonmonkey images. Until they were 10 weeks old, they preferred pictures of monkeys over other pictures even if the monkey in the picture showed threatening gestures. As they matured, however, their preference for monkeys with threatening gestures diminished abruptly and they began to be disturbed by them. Sackett's experiments clearly demonstrate that primates have innate releasing mechanisms.

What is the role of innate factors in determining human behavior? Because there are ethical limitations on the study of humans, one does not really know whether the primary determinants of complex human activities such as warfare, marriage, and religion are not definitely established but are thought to result largely from learning and culture. Certainly learning plays an enormous role in human behavior, and no clear-cut examples of complex inborn behaviors like those seen in lower animals have been demonstrated in humans. Nevertheless, the studies on the hormonal determinants of gender identity discussed in Chapter 61 indicate that some human behaviors are affected by innate factors. Four types of additional data support this conclusion: (1) the evidence for genetic factors influencing human behavior, (2) the universality of certain human behavioral patterns, (3) the existence of motor patterns that resemble fixed-action patterns, and (4) the existence of relatively complex motor patterns in the absence of any obvious specific learning experiences. We shall review each of these ideas in the following sections.

Certain Human Behavioral Traits Have a Hereditary Component

The issue of the role of genetic factors in human behavior can easily become clouded because of its profound social, ethical, and political implications. It is beyond the scope or purpose of this textbook to review these aspects of the problem. The point we wish to illustrate here is that all behavior, including human behavior, is mediated by components whose formation and organization are controlled by genes, and that therefore behavior must to *some* extent be under genetic control.

As we have seen in Chapter 55, there is substantial evidence for hereditary factors in human behaviors, particularly in severe mental illnesses such as schizophrenia. For many years neurobiologists were uneasy with the idea that schizophrenia, with its extreme disorder of thought and perception, is entirely due to the influence of a faulty environment. Studies of identical twins and adopted individuals have demonstrated conclusively that there is an important genetic component to this behavioral disorder.

There is also evidence for genetic factors in intelligence. Although exactly what is measured by intelligence tests is not clear, there is wide agreement (but not complete unanimity) that the measurements are a function of both inherited factors and learning. Several forms of severe mental retardation are linked to genetic factors. For example, as discussed in Chapter 62, Down's syndrome is known to be caused by the presence of an extra autosome, chromosome 21. *Phenylketonuria*, a metabolic disorder that also leads to mental retardation, is due to an autosomal recessive gene that codes for a type of phenylalanine hydroxylase that has reduced enzymatic activity, resulting in abnormally high levels of phenylalanine in the body fluids.

Many Human Behaviors Are Universal

All humans share many behaviors regardless of differences in their environmental or cultural backgrounds. These behaviors include the deep tendon reflexes, the eye blink response, and startle reflexes. In addition, we have common basic drives and needs, such as hunger, thirst, and sex. Equally important and widespread are human needs not related to simple tissue deficits. For example, to varying degrees, people of all cultures need social contact and variety of sensory experience.

One of the best examples of a complex set of human behaviors that is universal is emotional expression, first studied systematically by Darwin. The same facial expressions of anger, fear, disgust, and joy are universally recognized, even by people from different cultures that have had no contact. Thus, the recognition of certain emotional expressions probably has a strong innate component. Furthermore, the facial motor patterns themselves tend to be similar in diverse cultures.

Some human behavioral patterns appear to be analogous to the vacuum or displacement activities of animals. For example, during conflict situations or periods of stress, people, like animals, often exhibit grooming behavior, such as stroking their hair or scratching.

Stereotyped Sequences of Movements Resemble Fixed Action Patterns

Many emotional expressions, such as the startle response and smiling, involve a stereotyped sequence of movements. Smiling in human infants appears to be controlled by a specific sign stimulus. The eliciting stimulus has been studied by the use of models, similar to the colored wax models that have been used to study mating behavior in fish. Infant responses to inanimate models indicate that smiling is not a response to the face as a whole but rather

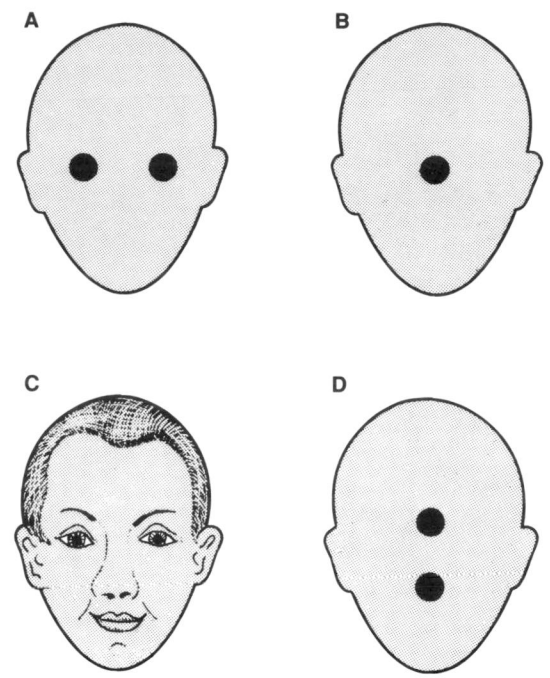

FIGURE 63–5
Patterns such as these are used to study the sign stimuli that elicit smiling in young babies. In babies of about six weeks of age, patterns A and D are more effective than B and C. Thus, the critical features appear to be multiple spots of high contrast. As the babies mature, the dot patterns become progressively less effective in eliciting a smile, while the face image (C) becomes more effective. (Adapted from Ahrens, 1954.)

to specific features. Contrasting elements (eyes, in the case of a real face) appear to be particularly important (Figure 63–5). As the child matures, however, other elements of the face have greater significance. Even in adults the eyes appear to function in some ways as a sign stimulus. A striking example is the brow flash response, studied in several cultures by Irenaus Eibl-Eibesfeldt. This stereotyped response, of which we are usually unaware, consists of rapidly raising and dropping the eyebrows. In widely different cultures it occurs as part of a greeting between individuals who know each other.

Certain Complex Patterns Require
Little or No Learning

Although there are numerous examples of behavioral patterns in humans that are unlikely to be entirely learned, the precise role of learning is difficult to assess in each and every instance. The role of learning can be studied in animals by raising them in restricted environments. In humans these types of experiments are not possible, but we can gain insights from natural experiments. For example, babies who are blind at birth have a limited opportu-

nity to learn facial expressions, yet their own facial responses can appear normal. Blind babies who smile in response to a sound may even turn their eyes toward the source of the sound, as sighted babies do. Other examples of abilities and disabilities in humans with limited environmental experiences are discussed in Chapter 60.

The Brain Sets Limits on the Structure of Language

The ability to speak sets humans apart from other animals. Since languages differ greatly from culture to culture, it might seem that language is not affected by innate determinants. This is clearly not so, however. Language is limited and shaped by our sensory–motor apparatus. For example, languages do not use frequencies of sound that we cannot hear or produce. More important, as we saw in Chapter 54, Noam Chomsky and many other linguists have proposed that, because widely different languages share common principles of grammar, the structure of languages is determined by conceptual constraints imposed by the structure of the brain.

It is difficult to distinguish experimentally the interaction of environmental factors and biological constraints in the development of human language. However, several informative models of communication have emerged from animal studies. Nonhuman primates can be taught a form of limited communication using sign language. Birds have a natural song, which is clearly not language in the human sense but which nevertheless is a highly complex auditory output that serves a primitive communicative function (Figure 63–6A). Studies of bird song provide fascinating and instructive examples of the interaction of innate factors with the environment. Early studies of whether songs were learned from other birds or inborn provided no simple answer. There are great differences between birds. Chickens can produce normal sounds even when they are raised in isolation and never hear another bird. On the other hand, songbirds, such as the chaffinch or white-crowned sparrow, produce distorted songs when raised in isolation.

In 1985 Masakazu Konishi discovered that the adult song of certain songbirds was more distorted if the birds were deafened at birth than if they were raised in isolation (Figure 63–6B, 5). This suggests that these birds must hear themselves sing to perfect their song. They must therefore have a built-in auditory template against which the song they produce is compared. This template is present even if the bird never hears another bird, because even the song of deafened birds is not random, but resembles, although imperfectly, the normal song. Variations in the song that a young bird hears result in similar variations in its own adult song but only within certain narrow limits. Most songbirds do not learn to imitate songs that deviate too far from their normal song commonly encountered in the wild (Figure 63–6B, 3).

These observations show that so-called biological con-

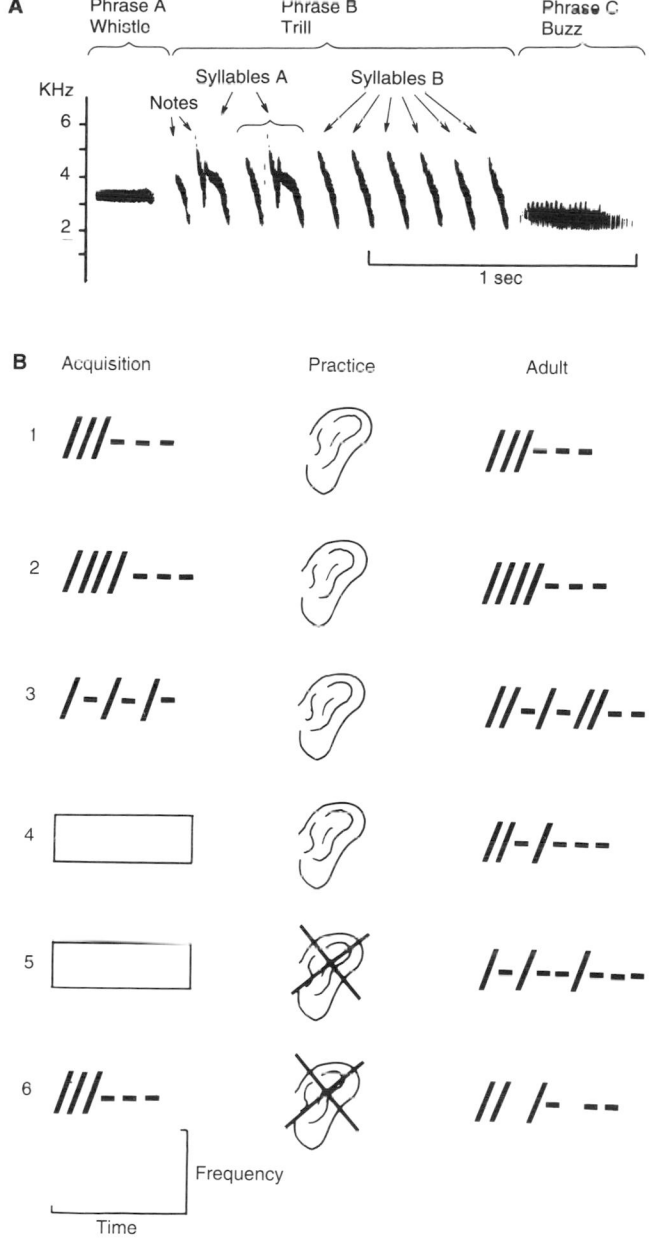

A

Phrase A — Whistle
Phrase B — Trill
Phrase C — Buzz

KHz
Notes
Syllables A
Syllables B

6
4
2

1 sec

B   Acquisition   Practice   Adult

1

2

3

4

5

6

Frequency

Time

FIGURE 63–6

Bird songs consist of a highly complex series of sounds and are highly dependent on the early experience of the animal.

A. The song of the white-crowned sparrow consists of a group of sounds separated by intervals of silence. A sound spectrogram shows the components of the sound, represented by the frequency of the tones over time. The spectrogram shows that the song consists of elementary notes, which are grouped into syllables, which in turn are grouped into phrases. (Data from Konishi, 1985.)

B. The normal adult songbird sings a song that is similar to the one heard during a time early in the life of the bird (acquisition phase). **1.** The first column illustrates a schematic sound spectrogram of a typical song that a particular species hears in the wild; the last column illustrates that the adult song is very similar to the typical song that the younger bird heard during the acquisition phase. **2.** If the bird hears a variant of the typical song during the acquisition phase, the adult song reflects that variation. **3.** If the bird is exposed to a very unusual song during the acquisition phase, the adult song does not closely resemble the one heard earlier. **4.** Birds that do not hear any song during the acquisition phase nevertheless develop a song that is somewhat similar to the normal pattern (the one shown in 1 and 2). **5.** If the birds also cannot hear themselves during the practice period, however, the song is highly abnormal. **6.** If birds hear a normal pattern during acquisition but cannot hear themselves during practice, their song is close to normal. Experiments 4 and 5 suggest that, even if not exposed to an appropriate song during acquisition, the birds can in effect teach themselves the appropriate song through auditory feedback. Thus, the birds have a built-in template of the song. As illustrated by experiments 1, 2, 3, and 6, the built-in template can be modified, within limits, by experience.

straints not only set limits on the effects that the environment can have, but also enormously facilitate the learning of certain things. In recent years there has been a growing appreciation that in each species, including humans, a unique set of biological constraints controls learning.

An Overall View

All behavior is shaped by an interaction of genetic and environmental factors, and there is no sharp distinction between learned and innate behaviors. Ethologists define species-specific behaviors as stereotyped responses that are characteristic of the species and relatively independent of specific learning experiences. Species-specific behaviors are made up of relatively stereotyped behavioral responses called fixed-action patterns. Fixed-action patterns are elicited by specific stimuli called sign stimuli. Sign stimuli trigger the activity of neural circuits that produce specific sequences of outputs of motor neurons, even in the absence of feedback stimuli. Species-specific behaviors are seen most clearly in invertebrates, but vertebrates including humans exhibit features of behavior that suggest the influence of innate factors. In lower animals the influence of specific genes on behavior can be shown, and there is also evidence for genetic factors in certain behaviors of higher animals.

Selected Readings

Boakes, R. 1984. From Darwin to Behaviourism: Psychology and the Minds of Animals. Cambridge, England: Cambridge University Press.

Camhi, J. M. 1984. Neuroethology: Nerve Cells and the Natural Behavior of Animals. Sunderland, Mass.: Sinauer.

Capron, C., and Duyme, M. 1989. Assessment of effects of socioeconomic status on IQ in a full cross-fostering study. Nature 340:552–554.

Delcomyn, F. 1980. Neural basis of rhythmic behavior in animals. Science 210:492–498.

Eibl-Eibesfeldt, I. 1970. Ethology: The Biology of Behavior. E. Klinghammer (trans.) New York: Holt, Rinehart and Winston.

Fieve, R. R., Rosenthal, D., and Brill, H. (eds.) 1975. Genetic Research in Psychiatry. Baltimore, Md.: Johns Hopkins University Press.

Gould, J. L. 1982. Ethology: The Mechanisms and Evolution of Behavior. New York: Norton.

Hirsch, J. (ed.) 1967. Behavior-Genetic Analysis. New York: McGraw-Hill.

Kupfermann, I., and Weiss, K. R. 1978. The command neuron concept. Behav. Brain Sci. 1:3–39.

Lewontin, R. 1982. Human Diversity. New York: Scientific American Books.

Manning, A. 1972. An Introduction to Animal Behavior, 2nd ed. Reading, Mass.: Addison-Wesley.

Plomin, R. 1990. The role of inheritance in behavior. Science 248:183–188.

Salkoff, L., and Wyman, R. 1983. Ion channels in Drosophila muscle. Trends Neurosci. 6:128–133.

Scheller, R. H., Jackson, J. F., McAllister, L. B., Schwartz, J. H., Kandel, E. R., and Axel, R. 1982. A family of genes that codes for ELH, a neuropeptide eliciting a stereotyped pattern of behavior in Aplysia. Cell 28:707–719.

Siegel, R. W., Hall, J. C., Gailey, D. A., and Kyriacou, C. P. 1984. Genetic elements of courtship in Drosophila: Mosaics and learning mutants. Behav. Genet. 14:383–410.

Teyke, T., Weiss, K. R., and Kupfermann, I. 1990. An identified neuron (CPR) evokes neuronal responses reflecting food arousal in Aplysia. Science 247:85–87.

References

Ahrens, R. 1954. Beitrag zur Entwicklung des Physiognomie-und Mimikerkennens. Z. Exp. Angew. Psychol. 2:412–454 and 599–633.

Chomsky, N. 1957. Syntactic Structures. The Hague: Mouton.

Darwin, C. 1872. The Expression of the Emotions in Man and Animals. London: Murray.

Doty, R. W., and Bosma, J. F. 1956. An electromyographic analysis of reflex deglutition. J. Neurophysiol. 19:44–60.

Fentress, J. C. 1972. Development and patterning of movement sequences in inbred mice. In J. A. Kiger, Jr. (ed.), The Biology of Behavior. Corvallis: Oregon State University Press, pp. 83–131.

Freud, S. 1940. An Outline of Psychoanalysis. J. Strachey (trans.) New York: Norton, 1949.

Kety, S. S., Rosenthal, D., Wender, P. H., and Schulsinger, F. 1968. The types and prevalence of mental illness in the biological and adoptive families of adopted schizophrenics. In D. Rosenthal and S. S. Kety (eds.), The Transmission of Schizophrenia. Oxford: Pergamon Press, pp. 345–362.

Konishi, M. 1985. Birdsong: From behavior to neuron. Annu. Rev. Neurosci. 8:125–170.

Lorenz, K. Z. 1950. The comparative method in studying innate behaviour patterns. Symp. Soc. Exp. Biol. 4:221–268.

Marler, P., and Hamilton, W. J., III. 1966. Mechanisms of Animal Behavior. New York: Wiley.

McDougall, W. 1908. An Introduction to Social Psychology. London: Methuen, 1960. New York: Barnes & Noble, 1960.

Sackett, G. P. 1966. Monkeys reared in isolation with pictures as visual input: Evidence for an innate releasing mechanism. Science 154:1468–1473.

Sherrington, C. 1947. The Integrative Action of the Nervous System, 2nd ed. New Haven: Yale University Press.

Thorpe, W. H. 1956. Learning and Instinct in Animals. Cambridge, Mass.: Harvard University Press.

Tinbergen, N. 1951. The Study of Instinct. Oxford: Clarendon Press.

Watson, J. B. 1930. Behaviorism, rev. ed. New York: Norton.

Wiersma, C. A. G. 1938. Function of the giant fibers of the central nervous system of the crayfish. Proc. Soc. Exp. Biol. Med. 38:661–662.

64

Irving Kupfermann

Learning and Memory

Certain Elementary Forms of Learning Are Nonassociative

Classical Conditioning Involves Associating a Conditioned and an Unconditioned Stimulus

Conditioning Involves the Learning of Predictive Relationships

Operant Conditioning Involves Associating an Animal's Own Behavior with a Subsequent Reinforcing Environmental Event

Food-Aversion Conditioning Illustrates How Biological Constraints Influence the Efficacy of Reinforcers

Conditioning Is Used as a Therapeutic Technique

Learning and Memory Can Be Classified as Reflexive or Declarative on the Basis of How Information Is Stored and Recalled

The Neural Basis of Memory Can Be Summarized in Four Generalizations

Memory Has Stages

Long-Term Memory May Be Represented by Plastic Changes in the Brain

The Plastic Changes Encoding Memory Are Often Localized in Different Places Throughout the Nervous System

Reflexive and Declarative Memories May Involve Different Neuronal Circuits

An Overall View

In Chapter 63 we considered how inborn and environmental factors interact to produce behavior. The most important means by which the environment alters behavior in humans is learning. Learning is the process of acquiring knowledge about the world. Memory is the retention or storage of that knowledge. The study of learning has taught us about the logical capabilities of the brain (for acquiring and storing information) and has proven a powerful approach to evaluating mental processing. In the study of learning we can ask several related questions: What types of environmental relationships are learned most easily? What conditions optimize learning? How many different forms of learning are there? What are the stages of memory formation?

Learning can occur in the absence of overt behavior but its occurrence can only be inferred from changes in behavior. Behavioral changes, as well as other changes that cannot be detected simply by observation of the organism's behavior, all reflect alterations in the brain produced by learning. Thus, although purely behavioral studies have defined many important principles of learning, many of the fundamental questions about learning require direct examination of the brain.

The study of learning is central to understanding both normal and abnormal behavior. Learning is thought to contribute to the genesis of certain mental and somatic diseases, and the principles governing learning that have emerged from laboratory studies are used in the treatment of patients with these diseases. Moreover, behavioral techniques based on learning are now used widely in neurobiological and clinical research to assess the effects of brain lesions and drugs.

Learning can be assessed by providing the subject with repeated learning experiences and observing progressive changes in performance. This provides an acquisition curve, an assessment of how performance improves as a function of learning trials and time. However, it is difficult to dissect the variables affecting the learning process using this method. Therefore, an alternative method for assessing learning has been developed. One group of subjects is provided with a learning experience while a second, control group is provided with a similar experience that lacks the ingredients needed for learning. The two groups are tested under identical conditions. The index of learning is the difference in performance of the two groups. For example, one group of rats is placed in a cage containing food in one corner; the control rats are placed in a cage that does not contain food. The next day both groups are placed in a new cage without food; the time spent in the corner where the food had been is then measured. This procedure controls for unspecified changes not due to learning, such as developmental changes. It also controls for *performance variables*, such as level of arousal, since the conditions for learning are separated from the conditions used to assess the learning.

Certain Elementary Forms of Learning Are Nonassociative

Psychologists study learning by exposing animals to information about the world, usually specific types of controlled sensory experience. Two major procedures (or paradigms) have emerged from such studies, and these procedures give rise to two major classes of learning: nonassociative and associative. Nonassociative learning results when the animal is exposed once or repeatedly to a single type of stimulus. This procedure provides an opportunity for the animal to learn about the properties of the stimulus. In associative learning the organism learns about the relationship of one stimulus to another (classical conditioning) or about the relationship of a stimulus to the organism's behavior (operant conditioning).

Two forms of nonassociative learning are very common in everyday life: habituation and sensitization. *Habituation* is a decrease in a behavioral response to a repeated, nonnoxious stimulus. An example of habituation is the failure of a person to show a startle response to a loud noise that has been repeatedly presented. *Sensitization* (or pseudoconditioning) is an increased response to a wide variety of stimuli following an intense or noxious stimulus. For example, a sensitized animal responds more vigorously to a mild tactile stimulus after it has received a painful pinch. Moreover, a sensitizing stimulus can override the effects of habituation. For example, after the startle response to a noise has become habituated, it can be restored by delivering a strong pinch. This process is called *dishabituation*. Sensitization and dishabituation occur independently of the timing of the intense stimulus relative to the weaker stimulus; no close association between the two stimuli is needed.

Not all examples of nonassociative learning are simple. Many types of more complex learning have no obvious associational element (although hidden forms of association may be present). These types of learning include sensory learning, in which a continuous record of sensory experience is formed, and imitative learning, which includes aspects of the acquisition of language.

One useful way to classify the many types of associative learning is on the basis of the experimental procedures used to establish the learning. Two experimental paradigms have been studied extensively and used clinically: classical and operant (or instrumental) conditioning. (Despite the widespread use of these models in research, not all associative learning readily fits into either operant or classical conditioning formats.)

Classical Conditioning Involves Associating a Conditioned and an Unconditioned Stimulus

Classical conditioning was introduced into behavioral science by Ivan Pavlov at the turn of the century, when he recognized that learning frequently consists of the acquisition of responsiveness to a stimulus that originally was ineffective. Aristotle had earlier suggested that learning involves the association of ideas, a proposal developed further by John Locke and the British empiricist philosophers, important forerunners of modern psychology. Pavlov's brilliant insight was to combine the philosophers' concept that learning involves the association of ideas with Sherrington's concept of the reflex act. With this framework Pavlov was able to deal with unobserved mental phenomena—ideas—and to study them objectively by examining behavioral acts, which are observable. Pavlov's work marked a permanent shift in the study of learning from introspective inferences about unobservable ideas to the objective analysis of stimulus and response. According to Pavlov, what animals and humans learn is not the association of ideas but the association of stimuli.

The essence of classical conditioning is the association or pairing of two stimuli, an unconditioned stimulus (US), and a conditioned stimulus (CS). The *conditioned stimulus*, such as a light or tone, is chosen because it produces either no overt responses or weak responses unrelated to the response that eventually will be learned. On the other hand, the *unconditioned stimulus* (sometimes termed reinforcement), such as food or a shock to the leg, is chosen because it always produces an overt response, the unconditioned response (UCR), such as salivation or leg withdrawal. Indeed, the reason the response is called unconditioned is because it is innate; it is produced by the eliciting (unconditioned) stimulus without learning. After the conditioned stimulus has been repeatedly followed by the unconditioned stimulus, the conditioned stimulus will begin to elicit responses called *conditioned responses* (CRs). Sometimes the conditioned response resembles the unconditioned response, but the two can also differ. Classical conditioning can be subdivided into appetitive conditioning and defensive conditioning. If the unconditioned stimulus is rewarding (e.g., food, water), the conditioning is termed *appetitive*; if the unconditioned stimulus is noxious (e.g., an electrical shock), the conditioning is termed *defensive*.

Upon repeated pairing of the conditioned and unconditioned stimulus, the conditioned stimulus appears to become an anticipatory signal for the occurrence of the unconditioned stimulus, and the animal responds to the conditioned stimulus as if it were preparing for the unconditioned stimulus. Thus, classical conditioning is a means by which animals learn to predict relationships between events in the environment. For example, if a light is followed repeatedly by the presentation of meat, after several learning trials the animal will respond to the light as if it predicts the taste of meat; the light itself will produce salivation.

As previously mentioned, Pavlov regarded classical conditioning not only as a way to study learning but also as a way to approach the mind—the inner workings of the brain. He was aware that if he could train animals to respond selectively to stimuli, he could discover which aspects of a stimulus an animal is capable of recognizing and processing. In fact, psychologists have used conditioning to explore whether an animal can recognize and distinguish colors, by determining whether lights of different colors can serve as discriminative stimuli for classical conditioning. During discriminative training, one stimulus (CS^+) is presented in association with reinforcement on some trials. On other trials, another stimulus (CS^-) is presented but is never followed close in time by reinforcement. If the CS^+ and CS^- are similar in certain respects, the animal will initially exhibit generalization; it will show conditioned responses to both the reinforced and nonreinforced stimuli. If the animal can discriminate between the stimuli, then after continued training it will show conditioned responses primarily or exclusively to the CS^+ and not to the CS^-. By appropriately manipulating the hue and intensity of visual stimuli, psychologists can determine whether the animal is responding to color rather than to differences in brightness. By this means they can use conditioning to determine the perceptual capacities of any animal capable of being conditioned.

An important principle of conditioning is that an established conditioned response decreases in intensity or probability of occurrence if the conditioned stimulus is repeatedly presented without the unconditioned stimulus. This process is known as *extinction*. Thus, a light that has been paired with an unconditioned stimulus of food will gradually cease to evoke salivation if the light is repeatedly presented in the absence of food. Extinction is just as important an adaptive mechanism as conditioning, because a continued response to cues that are no longer significant is maladaptive. The available evidence indicates that extinction does not simply involve the fading of previous learning. Rather, during the extinction process the animal learns something new—it learns that the conditioned stimulus no longer predicts that the unconditioned stimulus will occur; instead, the conditioned stimulus comes to predict that the unconditioned stimulus will not occur.

Conditioning Involves the Learning of Predictive Relationships

For many years most animal psychologists thought that classical conditioning depended only on temporal contiguity. According to this view, each time a conditioned stimulus is followed by a reinforcing or unconditioned stimulus, an internal connection between the stimulus and the response or between one stimulus and the others is strengthened, until eventually the bond becomes strong enough to produce conditioning. The only relevant variable determining the strength of conditioning was thought to be the number of contiguous CS–US pairing events. This theory proved inadequate for two reasons. First, it is maladaptive to depend solely on temporal contiguity. If animals learned to derive predictive information simply from the occurrence of any two events in close temporal contiguity, they might obtain erroneous information about the true causal relationship between signals in the environment. Second, a substantial body of empirical evidence indicates that learning cannot be adequately explained by such simple contiguity.

A striking example of the inadequacy of simple contiguity to produce conditioning is the so-called blocking phenomenon, described by Leon Kamin in 1968 in a three-part experiment. First, he conditioned a stimulus, a light, by pairing it repeatedly with an aversive unconditioned stimulus, a strong electric shock. He then assessed conditioning by determining to what degree the light suppressed ongoing behavior (a reflection of its ability to evoke a strong conditioned fear response in the animal similar to that initially evoked by the electrical shock). In the second part of the experiment, Kamin presented the conditioned stimulus simultaneously with a new stimulus, a tone, and the light–tone compound stimulus was then repeatedly paired with the shock. When, in the third part of the experiment, Kamin presented the tone alone, he found that little or no conditioning had occurred to the tone. Despite repeated pairings of the light–tone compound stimulus with shock, the tone presented alone failed to suppress behavior and did not evoke a fear response.

These findings were elaborated by Robert Rescorla and Alan Wagner in a theory of classical conditioning, according to which the amount of conditioning resulting from a trial is dependent on the degree to which the unconditioned stimulus is unexpected or surprising. If the unconditioned stimulus is completely novel and unexpected because it has not been previously paired with a conditioned stimulus, the rate of learning is maximal. But as the unconditioned stimulus gradually becomes expected because it is predicted by the conditioned stimulus, the rate of learning decreases until the unconditioned stimulus is fully expected, and the rate of learning becomes zero, so no further learning occurs. Thus, in the case of blocking, the tone component of the light–tone stimulus is an ineffective conditioning stimulus because the other element of the compound conditioned stimulus (the light) successfully and fully signals the occurrence of the unconditioned stimulus. This notion has been formalized in simple mathematical terms by Rescorla and Wagner, and predicts several properties of classical conditioning. Classical conditioning develops best when, in addition to contiguity of stimuli, there is also a *contingency* between the conditioned and the unconditioned stimulus—a truly predictive relationship. If an animal is presented with a long sequence of conditioned and unconditioned stimuli, each occurring randomly and completely independently, some contiguous CS–US sequences will occur just by chance. Nevertheless, a conditioned response to the CS does not develop. Clearly, the animal is not just counting the number of CS–US pairings, but rather determines the overall correlation or predictive relationship between the CS and US.

In fact, a stimulus that is repeatedly presented so that it specifically does not occur in association with a US will come to predict the absence of the US. When that stimulus is later paired with a US, conditioning occurs only very slowly, presumably because the animal must first unlearn the previous predictive property of the stimulus. In some instances stimuli that have been associated with the absence of the US actually acquire inhibitory properties. The inhibitory nature of a stimulus is inferred by observing what its presence does to the effectiveness of another stimulus that has been made excitatory by having been paired with a US. An inhibitory stimulus will suppress the response that the excitatory stimulus would have evoked in the absence of the concurrent inhibitory stimulus. Thus, in addition to being paired in time, the CS and reinforcer (the US) need to be positively correlated; the CS must indicate an increased probability that the US will occur.

These considerations suggest why animals and humans acquire classical conditioning so readily. It appears likely that classical conditioning, and perhaps all forms of associative learning, have evolved to enable animals to distinguish events that reliably and predictably occur together from those that are unrelated. In other words, the brain seems to have evolved to detect causal relationships in the environment.

All animals that exhibit associative conditioning, from snails to humans, seem to learn by detecting environmental contingencies rather than detecting the simple contiguity of a CS and US. Why is the recognition of contingent relationships similar in humans and in simpler animals? One good reason is that all animals face common problems of adaptation and survival, problems for which learning and flexible decision-making are useful. A successful biological solution to an environmental challenge, once evolved in a common primitive ancestor, continues to be inherited as long as it remains useful.

What environmental conditions might have shaped or maintained a common learning mechanism in a wide variety of species? To function effectively, all animals need to recognize key relationships between external events. They must be able to recognize prey and avoid predators; they must search out food that is nutritious and avoid food that is poisonous. There are two ways in which an animal arrives at such knowledge. The correct information can be preprogrammed into the animal's nervous system (as discussed in Chapter 63), or the ability to choose correctly among alternatives can be acquired through learning. Genetic and developmental programming may suffice for all of the behavior of very simple organisms, such as nematodes or parasitic invertebrates, but more complex animals must be capable of extensive learning to cope efficiently with varied or novel situations. Complex animals need to recognize order in the world. An effective way to do this is to be able to detect causal or predictive relationships between stimulus events, or between behavior and subsequent stimuli.

Operant Conditioning Involves Associating an Animal's Own Behavior with a Subsequent Reinforcing Environmental Event

A second major form of associational learning, discovered by Edward Thorndike and systematically studied by B. F. Skinner and others, is operant conditioning (also called instrumental conditioning or trial-and-error learning). In a typical laboratory example of operant conditioning an investigator begins by placing a hungry rat in a test chamber that has a lever protruding from one wall. Because of previous learning as well as innate response tendencies and random activity, the rat will occasionally press the lever. If the rat promptly receives food when it presses the lever, its subsequent rate of lever pressing will increase above the spontaneous rate. The animal can be described as having learned that a certain response (lever pressing) among the many it has made (for example, grooming, rearing, and walking) is rewarded with food. With this information, whenever the rat is hungry and finds itself in the same chamber, it is likely to make the appropriate responses.

If we think of classical conditioning as the formation of a predictive relationship between two stimuli (the conditioned stimulus and the unconditioned stimulus), operant conditioning can be considered to consist of the formation of a predictive relationship between a stimulus and a response. Unlike classical conditioning, which is restricted to specific reflex responses that are evoked by specific stimuli, operant conditioning involves behaviors (called operants) that apparently occur spontaneously or with no recognizable eliciting stimuli. Thus, operant behaviors are said to be emitted rather than elicited, and when the behaviors produce favorable changes in the environment (that is, when they either are rewarded, or lead to the removal of noxious stimuli), the animal tends to repeat them. A general observation is that behaviors that are rewarded tend to be repeated at the expense of behaviors that are not, whereas behaviors followed by aversive, though not necessarily painful, consequences (punishment) are usually not repeated. Experimental psychologists agree that this simple idea, called the *law of effect*, governs much voluntary behavior.

Superficially, operant and classical conditioning seem

to be dissimilar, involving completely different stimulus and response relationships. However, the laws that govern operant and classical conditioning are quite similar, suggesting that the two forms of learning may be manifestations of a set of common underlying neural mechanisms. For example, in both forms of conditioning, timing is critical: Typically, the reinforcer must closely follow the operant response. In operant conditioning, if the reinforcer (reward) is delayed too long, only weak conditioning occurs. There is an optimal interval between response and reinforcement, which varies depending on the specific task and the species. Similarly, in classical conditioning, depending on the task, there is an optimal interval between the conditioned stimulus and the unconditioned stimulus, and learning is generally poor when this interval is too long, or if the unconditioned stimulus precedes the conditioned stimulus. Finally, predictive relationships are equally important in both types of learning. In classical conditioning the subject learns that a certain stimulus predicts a subsequent event; in operant conditioning the animal learns to predict the consequences of its own behavior.

Food-Aversion Conditioning Illustrates How Biological Constraints Influence the Efficacy of Reinforcers

For many years it was thought that classical conditioning could occur simply by arbitrarily associating any two stimuli or, in the case of operant conditioning, any response and any reinforcer. More recent studies have shown, however, that there are important biological (evolutionary) constraints on learning. As we have seen, animals generally learn to associate stimuli that are relevant to their survival; they will not learn to associate events that are biologically meaningless. These findings illustrate nicely a principle we have encountered in the study of the development of behavior: The brain is not a tabula rasa, but is inherently predisposed to detect and manipulate certain environmental contingencies. For example, not all reinforcers are equally effective with all stimuli. This principle is dramatically illustrated in studies of food aversion (also called bait shyness, as it seems to be the means by which animals in their natural environment learn to avoid bait foods that contain poisons). As we saw in Chapter 34, if a distinctive taste stimulus, such as vanilla, is followed by nausea produced by a poison, an animal will quickly develop a strong aversion to the taste of vanilla. Unlike most other forms of conditioning, food aversion develops even when the unconditioned response (poison-induced nausea) occurs with a long delay (up to hours) after the conditioned stimulus (specific taste). This makes biological sense, since the ill effects of naturally occurring toxins usually follow ingestion only after some delay.

The food-aversion paradigm has been applied in the treatment of chronic alcoholism. The patient is first allowed to smell and taste alcoholic beverages, and then given a powerful emetic, such as apomorphine. The pairing of alcohol and nausea rapidly results in aversion to the taste of alcohol. Food-aversion learning has several other important implications in medicine. First, it may be a means by which people unintentionally learn to regulate their diets to avoid the unpleasant consequences of inappropriate or nonnutritious food. Second, the malaise associated with certain forms of cancer may induce aversive conditioning to foods in the ordinary diet of the patient. This, in part, might account for depressed appetites in cancer patients. Furthermore, the nausea that follows chemotherapy for cancer can produce aversion to foods that were tasted shortly before the treatment.

For most species, including humans, food-aversion conditioning occurs only when taste stimuli are associated with subsequent illness. Food aversion develops poorly, or not at all, if the taste is followed by a painful stimulus. Conversely, an animal does not develop an aversion to a visual or auditory stimulus that has been paired with nausea. Thus, the choice of an appropriate reinforcer depends on the nature of the response to be learned. Evolutionary pressures have predisposed the brains of different species of animals to learn an association between certain stimuli, or between a certain stimulus and a response, much more readily than between others. Within a given species, genetic and experiential factors also can modify the effectiveness of a reinforcer. The results obtained with a particular class of reinforcer vary enormously among species and among individuals within a species, particularly in humans.

Conditioning Is Used as a Therapeutic Technique

Various psychotherapeutic procedures involve reeducation of the patient in the context of a trusting relationship with the therapist. Aspects of therapeutic change are likely to involve components of classical and operant conditioning, but the specific contribution that each of these procedures makes to therapy has been delineated in only a few relatively simple instances.

The process of extinction, characteristic of classical conditioning, may underlie the therapeutic changes resulting from a clinical technique known as systematic desensitization (although other interpretations of this method have been offered). Systematic desensitization was introduced into psychiatry by Joseph Wolpe, who used it to decrease neurotic anxiety or phobias evoked by certain definable environmental situations, such as heights, crowds, or public speaking. The patient is first taught a technique of muscular relaxation. Then, over a period of days, the patient is told to imagine a series of progressively more severe anxiety-provoking situations while using relaxation to inhibit any anxiety that might be elicited. At the end of the series, the strongest potentially anxiety-provoking situations can be brought to mind without anxiety. This desensitization, induced in the therapeutic situation, often generalizes to real-life situations that the patient encounters.

Principles of operant conditioning also have been applied to the management of psychiatric disorders. One important therapeutic application is in the management of severely disturbed institutionalized patients with behavioral problems, such as shouting obscenities, messiness, or poor hygienic habits. The goal of conditioning these patients is to increase the frequency of positive, constructive behaviors. These behaviors are first defined precisely, and an effective reinforcement is found (compliments, privileges, money, or food). Nurses and orderlies are then trained to provide reinforcements when the patients behave in the desired way.

Biofeedback, another form of operant conditioning that has proved useful clinically, is used to enhance (or suppress) responses of which the patient is unaware. The behavior of interest, such as very slight muscle contractions in a stroke patient, is recorded by an electronic device that provides the patient with an immediate auditory or visual cue signaling that the response has occurred. If the patient desires to increase the frequency or strength of the response, the feedback cue can act as a positive reinforcement.

Learning and Memory Can Be Classified as Reflexive or Declarative on the Basis of How Information Is Stored and Recalled

The classification of associative learning into either operant or classical conditioning is based on the experimental procedures used to establish the conditioning. Alternative classification schemes of learning are based not on what the experimenter does, but rather on the type of knowledge acquired by the subject. Such classifications cut across the operant–classical distinction and take into account that a single training procedure may produce different forms of learning depending on how the experimental subject codes and recalls the information that is learned.

Many investigators have found it useful to distinguish between two types of learning—for example, one related to specific personal experiences and explicit factual knowledge, and another related to knowledge of rules and procedures, as reflected in skillful behavior that reflect habits or dispositions. As pointed out by Endel Tulving, different psychologists have used different terms to reflect this or closely related dichotomies, and it is not possible to determine the exact correspondence of different schemes. For our purposes, we shall refer to the two categories as reflexive and declarative memory. Later in this chapter we shall consider evidence indicating that these two types of memory can be differentially affected by brain damage and that they may involve different neuronal systems of the brain.

Reflexive memory has an automatic or reflexive quality, and its formation or readout is not dependent on awareness, consciousness, or cognitive processes such as comparison and evaluation. Reflexive memory accumulates slowly through repetition over many trials. This type of memory is expressed primarily by improved performance on certain tasks and is difficult to express in declarative sentences. Examples of reflexive memory include perceptual and motor skills and the learning of procedures and rules, such as those of grammar. Reflexive memory, however, is not limited to learning of procedures and skills. Certain verbal learning tasks, if repeated often enough, assume the characteristics of reflexive learning. These tasks can then be performed automatically without the participation of consciousness and other complex cognitive processes.

Declarative memory depends on conscious reflection for its acquisition and recall, and it relies on cognitive processes such as evaluation, comparison, and inference. Declarative memory encodes information about specific autobiographical events as well as the temporal and personal associations for those events. It often is established in a single trial or experience, and it can be concisely expressed in declarative statements, such as "I saw a yellow canary yesterday." Declarative memory involves the processing of bits and pieces of information that the brain can then use to reconstruct past events or episodes. As we saw earlier, constant repetition can transform declarative memory into the reflexive type. For example, learning to drive an automobile at first involves conscious linguistic processes, but eventually driving becomes an automatic and nonconscious motor activity.

How do elementary forms of learning such as classical conditioning fit into this scheme of reflexive and declarative memory? Although classical conditioning often results in reflexive memory, even this ostensibly simple form of conditioning may, under some circumstances, lead to declarative memory and involve mediation by cognitive processes. Consider the following experiment. A subject lays his hand, palm down, on an electrified grill; a light (conditioned stimulus) is turned on and he is immediately shocked on a finger. His hand lifts (unconditioned response), and, after several light–shock conditioning trials, he lifts his hand when the light alone is presented. The subject has been conditioned; but what exactly has been conditioned?

It appears as though the light is triggering a specific pattern of muscle activity that results in lifting of the hand. However, what if the subject now places his hand on the grill upside down, and the light is presented? If a specific pattern of muscle activity has been conditioned, the light should produce a response that moves the hand into the grill. On the other hand, if the subject has acquired the information that the light means grill shock, he may make a different response appropriate to that information. In fact, the subject will move his hand away from the grill; that is, he will make an adaptive response, even though it involves motor movements antagonistic to the original ones. Therefore, the subject did not originally learn a fixed response to a fixed stimulus, but rather acquired information that the brain could use to solve specific problems. In fact, many learning experiences have elements of both reflexive and declarative learning.

In another study of the nature of declarative memory, researchers analyzed remembered versions of stories. The versions that the subjects recalled were shorter and more coherent than the stories as originally told, containing reconstructions and syntheses of the original. The subjects were unaware that they were substituting, and they often felt most certain about reconstructed parts. The subjects were not confabulating; they were merely recalling in a way that interpreted the original material so it made sense.

Observations such as these lead us to believe that the accumulation of knowledge about past events is an active, cognitive process. Initially, what goes into the memory store is a representation of information that has been changed as a result of processing by our perceptual apparatus. We do not perceive the world precisely as it is but rather as a modified version that is altered on the basis of experience as well as the principles and limits of our perceptual analysis system. As we saw in Chapter 30, optical illusions nicely illustrate the difference between perception and the world as it is. Moreover, once the information is stored, what is recalled from the declarative memory store is not a faithful reproduction of the internal store. Recall of declarative memory involves a process in which past experiences are used in the present as clues to help the brain reconstruct a significant past event. During this reconstruction, the brain uses a variety of cognitive processes—comparison, inferences, shrewd guesses, and suppositions—to generate a consistent and coherent picture.

The Neural Basis of Memory Can Be Summarized in Four Generalizations

Although the literature on the neurobiology of memory is extensive, much of what is known can be summarized in just four generalizations: (1) memory has stages and is continually changing, (2) long-term memory may be represented by physical (or plastic) changes in the brain, (3) the physical changes coding memory are localized in multiple regions throughout the nervous system, and (4) reflexive and declarative memories may involve different neuronal circuits. Here we shall consider information obtained by gross techniques, such as brain lesions, electrical stimulation, and drugs. Studies of the cellular mechanisms of learning are considered in Chapter 65.

Memory Has Stages

It has long been known that a person who has been knocked unconscious can have selective memory loss for events that occurred before the blow (*retrograde amnesia*), as well as for events that occur after regaining consciousness (*anterograde amnesia*). This phenomenon has been documented thoroughly in animal studies using such traumatic agents as electroconvulsive shock, physical trauma to the brain, and drugs that depress neuronal activity or inhibit protein synthesis in the brain. Clinical studies also indicate that brain trauma can produce amnesia that is particularly prominent for recent events, typically within a few days of the trauma. Thus, recently acquired memories are readily disrupted, whereas older memories remain quite undisturbed. Once something has

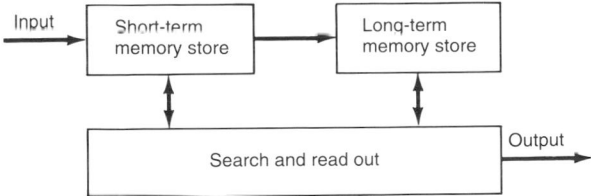

FIGURE 64–1
The rectangles represent a simplified model of processes that are thought to occur during a typical learning task, such as memorizing a list of nonsense syllables. The three processes indicated have been inferred primarily from the results of the time course of the decay of normal memory, and from the time course of the effects of brain trauma that results in the disruption of memory.

been learned, the extent of potential retrograde amnesia—the span of time during which memory is labile—varies from several seconds to several years, depending on the nature and strength of the learning, on the species of animal, and on the nature and severity of the disrupting event.

Studies of memory retention and of disruption of memory have contributed to a commonly used model of the memory storage system (Figure 64–1). Input to the brain is processed into a *short-term memory* store. This has very limited capacity (less than a dozen items) and, in the absence of rehearsal, persists only for minutes at most. The information is later transformed by some process into a more permanent *long-term store*. Sometimes the long-term memory is divided into an intermediate form that is relatively sensitive to disruption, and a truly long-term form, that is very insensitive to disruption. To complete the model, a system has been added that functions to search the memory store and to read out the information as demanded by specific tasks. According to this model, interference with the retention of experience can occur either by partial destruction of the contents of a memory store or by disruption of the search and read-out mechanism. In traumatic amnesia at least part of the interference must be due to a disturbance of the search and read-out mechanism. This conclusion stems from the observation that, after trauma, considerable memory for once-forgotten events gradually returns. If the stored memory had been completely destroyed, it obviously could not have been recovered.

Observations of patients undergoing a series of electroconvulsive treatments for depression have confirmed and extended the findings of experiments made on animals. Larry Squire and his associates used a memory test that could reliably quantify the degree of memory for relatively recent events (1–2 years old), old events (3–9 years old), and very old events (9–16 years old). Patients were asked to identify the names of various television programs that were broadcast during a single year between 1957 and 1972. The patients were initially tested and then tested again (with a different set of television programs) after the

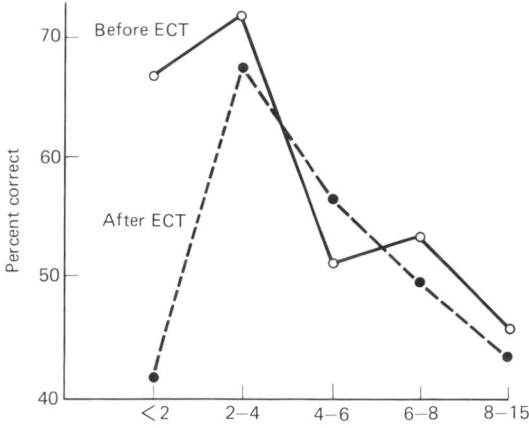

FIGURE 64–2

Recent memories are more susceptible than older memories to disruption by electroconvulsive shock therapy (**ECT**). The plot shows the percentage of correct responses of a group of patients who were tested on their ability to recognize the names of television programs that were on the air during a single year between 1957 and 1972. Testing was done before and after the patients received ECT for treatment of depression. After the ECT the patients showed a significant (but transitory) loss of memory for recent programs (1–2 years old) but not for older programs. (Adapted from Squire, Slater, and Chace, 1975.)

electroconvulsive therapy (ECT). The results of this experiment are shown in Figure 64–2. Both before and after ECT, correct memory for the programs steadily decreased with the time since the memory was first formed. This is a reflection of the all too familiar process of forgetting. After the ECT, however, the patients showed a significant but transitory memory loss for programs that had gone off the air one or two years previously, but their memory for the older programs was the same as it was before the ECT.

One interpretation of these observations is that the read-out of recent memories is easily disrupted until the memories have been converted into a long-term memory form. Once converted, they are relatively stable; but with time, even without external trauma, there is a gradual loss of the stored information or a diminished capacity to retrieve it. Thus, the memory process, at least as assessed by susceptibility to disruption, undergoes continual change with time.

Several experiments on the effects of drugs on learning support the idea that the memory process is time dependent and is subject to modification when the memory is first formed. James McGaugh and his colleagues have found that subconvulsant doses of excitant drugs, such as strychnine, can improve the retention of learning of animals even when the drug is administered after the training trials. If the drug is given to the animal soon after training, retention tested the next day is facilitated. If, however, the drug is given several hours after training, it has no effect.

Long-Term Memory May Be Represented by Plastic Changes in the Brain

How is information stored? There are probably several forms of short-term memory. One type of very brief short-term memory for visual events, called *iconic memory*, is probably due to brief retinal afterimages that follow exposure to visual stimuli. If a person is briefly allowed to view a matrix of many letters and numbers, he can accurately recall specific elements of the matrix; but, unlike most forms of learning, accuracy of recall diminishes extremely rapidly, typically in less than one second. The time before accuracy diminishes can be extended by increasing the brightness of the visual stimulus, and the time course for the decline of accuracy parallels the decay of the visual afterimages. Photochemical processes in the retina can account for visual afterimages. Thus, one very simple form of short-term memory appears to be encoded by a transient physical change in the sensory receptor.

Slightly longer lasting short-term memory that persists for minutes to hours could be mediated by a variety of short-term plastic change in synaptic transmissions that we considered in Chapter 13, such as posttetanic potentiation and presynaptic inhibition. Another possible mechanism for encoding short-term memory is the storage of information in the form of ongoing neural activity that is maintained by excitatory feedback connections between neurons (Figure 64–3). This type of activity could reverberate within the closed loop of neurons and might be sustained for some period of time. The idea of reverberatory circuits is interesting because it does not involve any enduring physical changes in nerve cells; the short-term memory for the event is maintained simply by ongoing neuronal activity.

But how is long-term memory stored? How are changes maintained for years? Two possibilities exist. First, but not likely, is the possibility that a dynamic change underlying short-term memory may persist and represent long-term memory as well. The second possibility is that long-term memory is related to some plastic rather than dynamic change—that is, to a persistent functional change in the brain. A simple experiment can distinguish between these alternatives. If all neuronal activity is tem-

FIGURE 64–3

A reverberating circuit might be used to encode short-term memory. Brief excitatory input can produce long-lasting neural activity through the circulation of activity among neurons that excite one another.

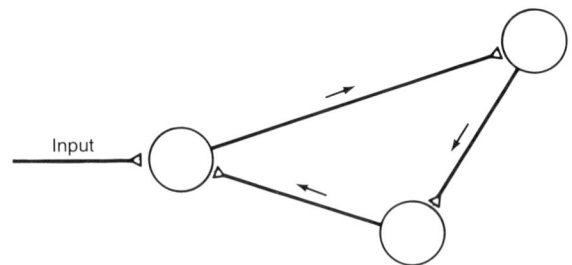

porarily stopped, memories represented by a dynamic mechanism, say reverberating circuits, should be permanently abolished. Neuronal activity can be silenced by the use of deep anesthesia, by anoxia, or by cooling the brain. When this is done, short-term or recent memories are disrupted, but older memories are not. Thus, it is safe to conclude that at least older memories are not mediated by dynamic change but, more likely, involve physical changes in the brain. Because of the enduring nature of memory, it seems reasonable to postulate that in some way the changes must be reflected in long-term alterations of the connections between neurons. We shall consider this question again in Chapter 65.

The Plastic Changes Encoding Memory Are Often Localized in Different Places Throughout the Nervous System

Whatever their nature, it seems clear that the memory traces for many different types of learning are not localized to any one brain structure. Pavlov believed that all learning processes are limited to the neocortex. The psychologist Karl Lashley did an extensive series of studies in which he made lesions in the cortex to define precisely where the representation of learning (called the *engram*) was located. He never succeeded. However, Lashley and others found that although cortical lesions can seriously disrupt learning, animals can relearn certain tasks even when they are completely decorticated. Classical conditioning of certain simple reflexes can be mediated by the spinal cord even after it has been isolated surgically from the brain, as was first shown by P. S. Shurrager and Elmer Culler in 1940. Thus, many, perhaps all, regions of the nervous system appear to contain neurons with the properties of plasticity needed for memory storage.

Even for a simple learning task, several parallel channels of information are used. There appear to be many ways for information to be stored in different regions of the brain. For example, David Cohen found that any one of three visual pathways sustained conditioned heart rate responses in pigeons. Although the neuronal code by which memories are stored is not known, neuronal models can be constructed in which a simple memory consists of patterns of changes of specific connections that are distributed throughout the network. As discussed in Chapter 53, these learning models perform in ways similar to learning exhibited by living animals. For example, the learning shows *generalization*, so that learning is exhibited even when tested with stimuli somewhat different from the original training stimulus. The information stored in distributed models also survives partial damage to the system.

Parallel processing may explain in part why a limited lesion does not eliminate specific learning, even for a simple task. Another important factor that may account for the resiliency of learning to small lesions may reside in the very nature of the learning process. As we have seen from behavioral studies, learning involves neither the simple formation of stimulus–response bonds nor a faithful reproduction of sensory experience. Although the plastic changes representing learning are likely to be localized to specific neurons, the complex nature of many learning tasks makes it likely that these neurons are widely distributed in the nervous system. Therefore, even after extensive lesions, some component of the plastic changes are likely to remain. Furthermore, the brain has the capacity to take even the limited information remaining, work it over, and reconstruct a relatively good reproduction of the original.

Reflexive and Declarative Memories May Involve Different Neuronal Circuits

Although many forms of memory seem to be widely distributed, some learning tasks are profoundly affected by circumscribed lesions of the brain. The most striking evidence of this comes from studies of the cerebellum and temporal lobes. These studies suggest the intriguing hypothesis that the brain may possess two classes of neural circuits, one primarily concerned with reflexive memory, the other with declarative memory.

Reflexive Memory. Lesions to several regions of the brain have been found to affect simple classically conditioned responses, and these regions probably represent loci for reflexive types of learning. For example, lesions of the amygdala interfere with conditioned heart rate responses, apparently by interrupting pathways close to the motor end of the reflex arc. Another example of a specific lesion affecting a classically conditioned response comes from the research of Richard Thompson and his associates. They studied the eye blink (or nictitating membrane) protective reflex in rabbits. By pairing an auditory stimulus with a puff of air to the eye, a conditioned eye blink reflex can be established to the auditory stimulus. The conditioned response is abolished by a lesion limited to the medial dentate and lateral interpositus nuclei of the cerebellum. After this region is lesioned, the previously effective conditioned auditory stimulus no longer produces an eyeblink, although an unconditioned eyeblink response can still be evoked by the unconditioned stimulus (air puff). Furthermore, the dentate-interpositus nuclei of the cerebellum also show learning-dependent increases in neuronal activity that closely parallel the development of the conditioned behavioral response.

The results of these experiments indicate that the cerebellum plays an important role in mediating conditioned eyeblink and perhaps other simple forms of classical conditioning. It has not yet been determined, however, whether the memory is actually stored in the cerebellum or in the brain stem or elsewhere, with the cerebellum needed for the adequate performance of the task.

Declarative Memory. Lesions of the temporal lobe or of the diencephalon dramatically affect declarative memory. These lesions interfere primarily with the retention of new memories; they have relatively weak effects on prior memories. Thus, these structures are not themselves registers or banks for memory storage, but are somehow involved in the process by which memories are placed into storage or are retrieved and read out from storage.

A significant clue that the temporal lobes are important for memory came from the observations by the neurosurgeon Wilder Penfield. Before carrying out temporal lobe surgery for the control of epilepsy, Penfield electrically stimulated the exposed temporal lobes in fully conscious patients. The patients reported vivid experiences of past events. For example, stimulation of one point on the temporal lobe caused a patient to hear a melody that she believed she had heard in the past. Later stimulation of the same point evoked experiences of hearing the same melody. Reginald Bickford and his colleagues found that in certain patients stimulation of the mid-temporal gyrus resulted in a brief anterograde and retrograde amnesia. Depending on the duration of stimulation, the retrograde amnesia extended back from several hours to several days, and recovered within 5 minutes to several hours.

Additional evidence of a role for the temporal lobes in memory has come from the study of a few epileptic patients who underwent bilateral removal of the hippocampus and associated structures in the temporal lobes. Brenda Milner found that these patients exhibited a profound and irreversible deficit of recent memory. New long-term memories could not be formed but previously acquired long-term (remote) memories remained relatively intact; for example, the patients remembered their own names and how to talk. Short-term memory was also unaffected in these patients; but the transition from short-term to long-term memory was virtually absent for most types of learning. For example, if the patient was told to remember the number 7, he could repeat the number immediately. However, if the patient was distracted, even briefly, he had no recollection of the number. The extent of the deficit is indicated by the observation that patients sometimes fail to recognize individuals whom they had known closely for years since the time of the surgery. In addition to anterograde amnesia, these patients often show some retrograde amnesia.

Often, memories that have been lost because of lesions or trauma gradually return, particularly those most distant in time from the insult. Bilateral damage largely limited to the hippocampus can also occur following anoxia, and this has also been reported to result in an amnesic syndrome in humans. Furthermore, Stuart Zola-Morgan and Larry Squire found that in monkeys experimental global ischemia produces damage to nerve cells, particularly in the hippocampus and can result in an enduring impairment on amnesia-sensitive tasks. Parts of the hippocampus were spared, indicating that even incomplete damage can result in memory impairments. As in humans with hippocampal damage, skill learning was unimpaired in these animals. Lesions of cortical tissue adjacent to the hippocampus result in similar memory impairments in monkeys.

Patients with Korsakoff's psychosis suffer from amnesia that is similar to that seen in patients who have had damage to temporal lobe structures. Korsakoff's psychosis, which results from chronic alcoholism and associated nutritional deficiency, is often characterized by signs of fron-

tal lobe dysfunction in addition to severe memory deficits. Patients exhibit pathological changes in diencephalic structures that are part of the limbic system. Typically, they have damage to the mammillary bodies of the hypothalamus as well as to the medial dorsal nucleus of the thalamus. Animal studies indicate that a large lesion of the medial thalamus is sufficient to produce learning deficits analogous to those exhibited by amnesic patients. Careful study of the memory deficit in patients with Korsakoff's psychosis supports the idea that the deficit is due, at least in part, to defective encoding at the time of original learning rather than exclusively to a defect in the retrieval mechanism.

Elizabeth Warrington and Lawrence Weiskrantz found that when patients with Korsakoff's psychosis are given a list of words to remember, they do poorly on a simple recall task, but their performance is greatly improved when retention is tested by the use of prompts or partial cues. For example, their performance is normal if, following the original learning, they are tested for retention by a completion task rather than being asked simply to recall the words. In the completion task the patients are given a list of letter sequences, each of which has the first few letters of a word in the original list. Then, on the basis of their memory for the words in the original list, the patients must complete the words. Some memories that are retrieved on the basis of prompts and partial cues may be a special type that has been termed *priming*. Priming has features of reflexive memory, and it appears to be largely intact in amnesic patients.

Peter Graf, George Mandler, and Patricia Haden found that this disjunction between performance on simple recall and completion tests can be demonstrated in normal subjects with no memory defects if the subjects are required to learn a list of words in a task that minimizes the opportunity to understand the meaning of the words. In this experiment a list of 20 words was presented with the instruction to detect certain vowels in the words. The subjects were not asked to memorize the words or to understand their meaning. After the vowel detection task they were unable to recall the words in the list. However, like the patients with Korsakoff's psychosis, the subjects were able to recall many of the words if they were given their initial letters and asked to complete them. Subjects in a second group were presented with a list of words and were instructed to determine if they liked each word, a task that requires an understanding of semantic content. When tested, these subjects remembered the words just as well on simple recall as on a completion task. These findings support the suggestion that patients with Korsakoff's psychosis fail to encode properly the semantic component of material on initial learning, although this deficit does not explain all of the features of memory loss of Korsakoff's psychosis or other amnesic syndromes.

Reflexive Versus Declarative Memory in Amnesic Patients. Amnesic patients with hippocampal lesions given a highly complex mechanical puzzle to solve may learn it as quickly as a normal person but later do not remember seeing the puzzle or having worked on it. Severely amnesic patients, either with temporal lobe or diencephalic damage can learn certain tasks perfectly well. Although these patients cannot master tasks involving declarative memory, they perform well on tasks involving reflexive memory. When a learning task involves both types of learning, amnesic patients remember some aspects of the problem but not others. Thus, amnesic patients can learn a complex skill and yet be unable to recall the specific events that allowed them to learn the rules and procedures that make up the skill. Furthermore, when they remember some experience of the past, the memory lacks the sense of familiarity that accompanies recall in normal individuals.

Warrington and Weiskrantz suggested that the fundamental deficit of amnesic patients is due to some type of disconnection between memory storage systems and a cognitive mediational system in the brain that aids in the retrieval and storage of memory. It is possible that in amnesic patients the cognitive system functions normally, but lacks access to the learning system that encodes declarative memory in the hippocampus, other areas in the temporal lobe, and diencephalon. Therefore, amnesic patients often show totally unimpaired intelligence and yet are virtually incapable of new declarative learning. This idea helps explain why amnesic patients, when they perform a particular task, are often not aware that they actually had learned it a few days or weeks earlier.

An Overall View

An understanding of the neurobiology of learning and memory requires an appreciation that there are different types. One important distinction has been drawn between declarative and reflexive memory. Declarative memory includes the learning of facts and experiences that can be reported verbally. Reflexive memory includes forms of perceptual and motor learning that are exhibited by alterations in the performance of tasks, but which cannot be expressed verbally.

Although there is an extensive literature on the neurobiology of memory it is possible to summarize much of what is known in just four generalizations: (1) memory has stages and its representation is continually changing, (2) long-term memory may be represented by plastic changes in the brain, (3) the plastic changes that encode memories are localized in multiple regions throughout the nervous system, and (4) reflexive and declarative memories may involve different neuronal circuits.

A major task confronting the neurobiology of learning is to determine how alterations in the brain are related to behavioral changes. A second task is to determine the mechanisms underlying the plastic changes. To this end, a number of simplified vertebrate and invertebrate animal preparations are being investigated, and some of these studies are reviewed in Chapter 65.

Selected Readings

Bellack, A. S., Hersen, M., and Kazdin, A. E. (eds.) 1990. International Handbook of Behavior Modification and Therapy, 2nd ed. New York: Plenum Press.

Dickinson, A. 1980. Contemporary Animal Learning Theory. Cambridge, England: Cambridge University Press.

Domjan, M., and Burkhard, B. 1982. The Principles of Learning and Behavior. Monterey, Calif.: Brooks/Cole.

Hilgard, E. R., and Bower, G. H. 1975. Theories of Learning, 4th ed. Englewood Cliffs, N.J.: Prentice-Hall.

Kanfer, F. H., and Phillips, J. S. 1970. Learning Foundations of Behavior Therapy. New York: Wiley.

Klatzky, R. L. 1980. Human Memory: Structures and Processes, 2nd ed. San Francisco: Freeman.

Lashley, K. S. 1950. In search of the engram. Symp. Soc. Exp. Biol. 4:454–482.

Mackintosh, N. J. 1983. Conditioning and Associative Learning. Oxford: Clarendon Press.

Rescorla, R. A. 1988. Behavioral studies of Pavlovian conditioning. Annu. Rev. Neurosci. 11:329–352.

Squire, L. R. 1987. Memory and Brain. New York: Oxford University Press.

Squire, L. R., Cohen, N. J., and Nadel, L. 1984. The medial temporal region and memory consolidation: A new hypothesis. In H. Weingartner and E. S. Parker (eds.), Memory Consolidation: Psychobiology of Cognition. Hillsdale, N. J.: Erlbaum, pp. 185–210.

Thompson, R. F. 1988. The neural basis of basic associative learning of discrete behavioral responses. Trends Neurosci. 11:152–155.

Tulving, E., and Schacter, D. L. 1990. Priming and human memory systems. Science 247:301–306.

References

Bickford, R. G., Mulder, D. W., Dodge, H. W., Jr., Svien, H. J., and Rome, H. P. 1958. Changes in memory function produced by electrical stimulation of the temporal lobe in man. Res. Publ. Assoc. Res. Nerv. Ment. Dis. 36:227–243.

Cohen, D. H. 1982. Central processing time for a conditioned response in a vertebrate model system. In C. D. Woody (ed.), Conditioning: Representation of Involved Neural Functions. New York: Plenum Press, pp. 517–534.

Graf, P., Mandler, G., and Haden, P. E. 1982. Simulating amnesic symptoms in normal subjects. Science 218:1243–1244.

Kamin, L. J. 1969. Predictability, surprise, attention, and conditioning. In B. A. Campbell and R. M. Church (eds.), Punishment and Aversive Behavior. New York: Appleton-Century-Crofts, pp. 279–296.

McGaugh, J. L. 1989. Involvement of hormonal and neuromodulatory systems in the regulation of memory storage. Annu. Rev. Neurosci. 12:255–287.

Milner, B. 1966. Amnesia following operation on the temporal lobes. In C. W. M. Whitty and O. L. Zangwill (eds.), Amnesia. London: Butterworths, pp. 109–133.

Pavlov, I. P. 1927. Conditioned Reflexes: An Investigation of the Physiological Activity of the Cerebral Cortex. G. V. Anrep (trans.) London: Oxford University Press.

Penfield, W. 1958. Functional localization in temporal and deep Sylvian areas. Res. Publ. Assoc. Res. Nerv. Ment. Dis. 36:210–226.

Rescorla, R. A., and Wagner, A. R. 1972. A theory of Pavlovian conditioning: Variations in the effectiveness of reinforcement and nonreinforcement. In A. H. Black and W. F. Prokasy (eds.),

Classical Conditioning II: Current Research and Theory. New York: Appleton-Century-Crofts, pp. 64–99.

Shurrager, P. S., and Culler, E. 1940. Conditioning in the spinal dog. J. Exp. Psychol. 26:133–159.

Skinner, B. F. 1938. The Behavior of Organisms: An Experimental Analysis. New York: Appleton-Century-Crofts.

Squire, L. R., Slater, P. C., and Chace, P. M. 1975. Retrograde amnesia: Temporal gradient in very long term memory following electroconvulsive therapy. Science 187:77–79.

Thompson, R. F., McCormick, D. A., Lavond, D. G., Clark, G. A., Kettner, R. E., and Mauk, M. D. 1983. The engram found? Initial localization of the memory trace for a basic form of associative learning. Prog. Psychobiol. Physiol. Psychol. 10: 167–196.

Thorndike, E. L. 1911. Animal Intelligence: Experimental Studies. New York: Macmillan.

Tulving, E. 1987. Multiple memory systems and consciousness. Human Neurobiol. 6:67–80.

Wagner, A. R., and Brandon, S. E. 1989. Evolution of a structured connectionist model of Pavlovian conditioning (AESOP). In S. B. Klein and R. R. Mowrer (eds.), Contemporary Learning Theories: Pavlovian Conditioning and the Status of Traditional Learning Theory. Hillsdale, N. J.: Erlbaum, pp. 149–189.

Warrington, E. K., and Weiskrantz, L. 1982. Amnesia: A disconnection syndrome? Neuropsychologia 20:233–248.

Wolpe, J. 1958. Psychotherapy by Reciprocal Inhibition. Stanford, Calif.: Stanford University Press.

Zola-Morgan, S., and Squire, L. R. 1990. Identification of the memory system damaged in medial temporal lobe amnesia. In L. R. Squire and E. Lindenlaub (eds.), The Biology of Memory. Stuttgart: Schattauer, pp. 509–522.

Zola-Morgan, S., Squire, L. R., and Amaral, D. G. 1986. Human amnesia and the medial temporal region: Enduring memory impairment following a bilateral lesion limited to field CA1 of the hippocampus. J. Neurosci. 6:2950–2967.

65

Eric R. Kandel

Cellular Mechanisms of Learning and the Biological Basis of Individuality

Simple Forms of Reflexive Learning Lead to Changes in the Effectiveness of Synaptic Transmission

Habituation Involves Depression of Synaptic Transmission

Sensitization Involves Enhancement of Synaptic Transmission

Long-Term Memory Requires Synthesis of New Proteins and the Growth of New Synaptic Connections

Classical Conditioning Involves an Associative Enhancement of Presynaptic Facilitation That Is Dependent on Activity

Long-Term Potentiation in the Hippocampus Is an Example for Both Associative and Nonassociative Learning in the Mammalian Brain

Long-Term Potentiation in the CA1 Region Is Associative

Associative Long-Term Potentiation Is Thought to Be Important for Spatial Memory

Long-Term Potentiation in the CA3 Region Is Nonassociative

Is There a Molecular Grammar for Learning?

The Somatotopic Map in the Brain Is Modifiable by Experience

Changes in the Somatotopic Map Produced by Learning May Contribute to the Biological Expression of Individuality

Changes in the Somatotopic Map May Reflect Common Cellular Mechanisms for Associative Plasticity

Studies of Neuronal Changes with Learning Provide Insights into Psychiatric Disorders

An Overall View

Throughout this book we have emphasized that all behavior is determined by the functioning of the brain and that malfunctions of the brain are expressed in characteristic disturbances of behavior. All functions of the brain, in turn, are the product of interactions between genetic and developmental processes on the one hand, and environmental factors, such as learning, on the other. Here we shall again examine the role of learning and memory in the generation of behavior, but now focusing on the mechanisms whereby learning alters the structure and function of nerve cells and their connections.

Many aspects of behavior result from the ability to learn from experience. Indeed, we are who we are largely because of what we learn and what we remember. Through learning we acquire languages that enable us to record experience and thereby create cultures that are maintained over generations. Learning also produces dysfunctional behaviors and these can, in the extreme, constitute psychological disorders. Fortunately, what is learned can sometimes be unlearned. Thus, insofar as psychotherapy is successful in treating behavioral disorders, it presumably does so because treatment provides a learning experience that allows the patient to change and to acquire new patterns of behavior.

The interface between biology and the study of mental processes presents some of the most challenging problems in neural science. In recent years neurobiology and cognitive psychology have begun to find a common ground. As a result, we are beginning to benefit from the increase in explanatory power that occurs when two initially disparate disciplines converge. The rewards of this merger are particularly evident in the study of memory and learning. Animal studies of learning and memory are yielding insights into mental processes—from the behavioral to the molecular level—that are providing the foundation for a science of mentation that promises to deepen our understanding of behavior and its abnormalities.

In this concluding chapter we first examine the cellular and molecular mechanisms that underlie simple forms of learning in both invertebrates and vertebrates. We shall then consider how these mechanisms may contribute to aspects of individuality through differences in life experience.

Simple Forms of Reflexive Learning Lead to Changes in the Effectiveness of Synaptic Transmission

Most of the progress in the cellular study of learning and memory has come from examining elementary forms of reflexive learning: habituation, sensitization, and classical conditioning. These elementary behavioral modifications have been analyzed both in the nervous system of invertebrates and in simple vertebrate preparations, such as the isolated spinal cord or brain slices of hippocampus. Most of these modifications involve *plastic change*, changes in the effectiveness of specific synaptic connections (Chapters 13 and 64).

Habituation Involves Depression of Synaptic Transmission

As we saw in Chapter 64, *habituation* is the simplest form of learning. It is a nonassociative form in which an animal learns about the properties of a novel, innocuous stimulus when that stimulus is repeated. An animal first responds to a new stimulus with a series of orienting reflexes. When the stimulus is repeated, the animal learns to recognize it and, if the stimulus is neither rewarding nor noxious, the animal learns to suppress its responses. The learned suppression of the response to a repeated stimulus is called *habituation*.

Habituation was first investigated in animals by Ivan Pavlov and Charles Sherrington. While studying posture and locomotion, Sherrington observed that certain reflex forms of behavior, such as the withdrawal of the limb in response to a tactile stimulus (a flexion reflex), habituated with repeated stimulation and only reoccurred after many seconds of rest. Sherrington suggested that the habituation was due to a functional decrease in the synaptic effectiveness of the pathways to the motor neurons that had been repeatedly activated.

This problem was later investigated at the cellular level by Alden Spencer and Richard Thompson. They first carried out a series of behavioral experiments and found close parallels between habituation of the spinal flexion reflex in the cat and habituation of more complex behavioral responses in humans. They thus felt confident that habituation of spinal reflexes is a good model for studying habituation. Next, by recording intracellularly from motor neurons in the spinal cord of cats, they found that habituation leads to a decrease in the synaptic activity between interneurons and motor neurons. The activity of the monosynaptic pathway underlying the stretch did not change, however. As described in Chapter 38, the organization of the interneurons in the spinal cord is quite complex, making it difficult to examine in detail the cellular

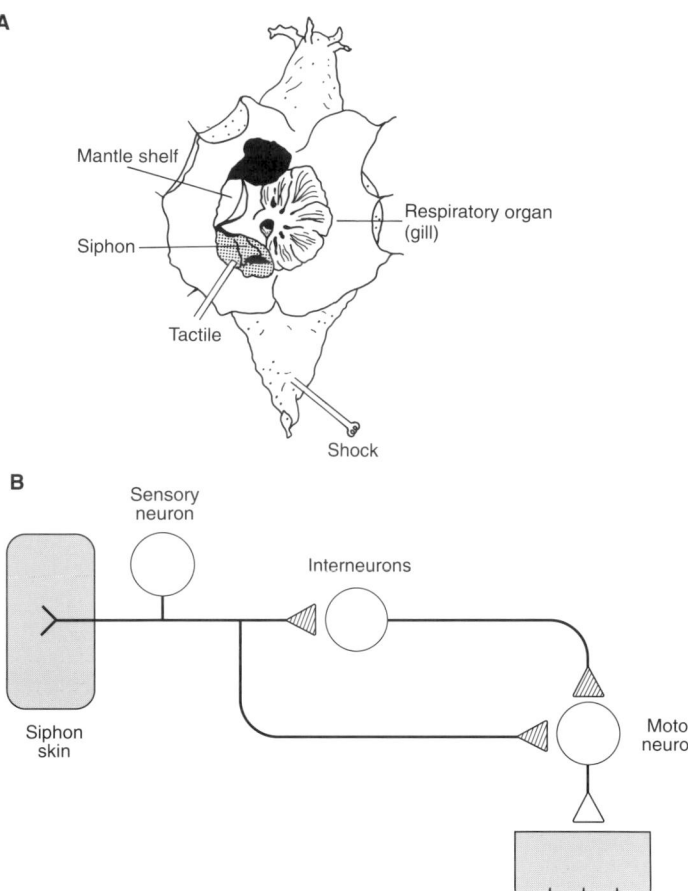

FIGURE 65–1

Habituation of the gill withdrawal reflex in the marine snail *Aplysia* is the result of reduced effectiveness of the synapse between sensory neurons and their central target cells in the neural circuit for the reflex.

A. This dorsal view of an *Aplysia* illustrates the respiratory organ, the gill, and the mantle shelf, which ends in a fleshy spout called the siphon.

B. This simplified circuit shows key elements involved in the gill-withdrawal reflex as well as sites involved in habituation. In this circuit, about 24 mechanoreceptor sensory neurons located in the abdominal ganglion innervate the siphon skin, only one of which is illustrated here for simplicity. These sensory cells terminate on a cluster of six motor neurons that innervate the gill and on several groups of excitatory and inhibitory interneurons (only one of which is illustrated here) that synapse on the motor neurons. Repeated stimulation of the siphon leads to a depression of synaptic transmission between the sensory and motor neurons as well as between certain interneurons and the motor cells.

mechanisms of habituation in the flexion reflex. As a result, further investigation of habituation has required still simpler systems in which the behavioral response can be examined in a series of monosynaptic connections.

This sort of analysis has been carried out in the marine snail *Aplysia californica*, which has a simple nervous system containing only about 20,000 central nerve cells. *Aplysia* has a set of defensive reflexes for withdrawing its tail, gill, and siphon, a small fleshy spout above the gill used to expel seawater and waste (Figure 65–1). These reflexes are similar to the leg-flexion reflex studied by Spencer and Thompson. For example, a mild tactile stimulus delivered to the siphon elicits withdrawal of both the siphon and gill; a tactile stimulus to the tail elicits tail withdrawal. With repeated stimulation these reflex withdrawals habituate. As we shall see later, these responses can also be sensitized and classically conditioned.

Gill withdrawal has been studied in detail. In response to a novel stimulus to the siphon, sensory neurons innervating the siphon generate excitatory synaptic potentials in the interneurons and motor cells (Figure 65–1). These synaptic potentials summate both temporally and spatially and cause the motor cells to discharge strongly, leading to a brisk reflex withdrawal of the gill. If the stimulus is repeatedly presented, the synaptic potentials produced by the sensory neurons in the interneurons and motor cells become progressively smaller. The synaptic potentials produced by some of the excitatory interneurons in the motor neurons also become weaker, with the net result that the strength of the reflex response is reduced.

The decrease in synaptic transmission in the sensory neurons results from a decrease in the amount of chemical transmitter released by each action potential from the presynaptic terminal. How this occurs is not fully understood. Part of the decrease is thought to be due to a reduction (inactivation) of an N-type Ca^{2+} channel in the presynaptic terminal. As a result, less Ca^{2+} flows into the terminals with each action potential, and therefore less transmitter is released (Chapter 12). In addition, and probably more important, habituation also decreases ability of transmitter vesicles to be mobilized into the active zone so as to be available for release.

This reduction in the effectiveness of the synaptic connections between the sensory neurons and their target cells (the interneurons and motor neurons) can last for many minutes. Similarly, enduring changes occur in the synaptic connections between several interneurons and motor neurons in this circuit. These *persistent* changes in the strength of a set of connections represent the components of the storage process for the short-term memory for habituation. Synaptic depression seems to be a general mechanism of habituation since a similar process accounts for short-term habituation of escape responses in crayfish and cockroaches and in the startle reflexes in vertebrates.

Synaptic changes similar to those that occur at the connections between sensory neurons and motor neurons also occur in interneurons and in a certain class of motor neurons. As we have seen in Chapter 64, the storage of even a simple reflexive memory is not restricted to one site but involves distributed sites. However, in all of these cases memory storage does not depend on *dynamic changes* in a closed chain of neurons (Chapter 64), but on *plastic changes* in the strength of preexisting connections. Reflexive learning also does not depend on specialized memory neurons whose only function is to store information, but instead memory storage results from changes in neurons that are integral components of a normal reflex

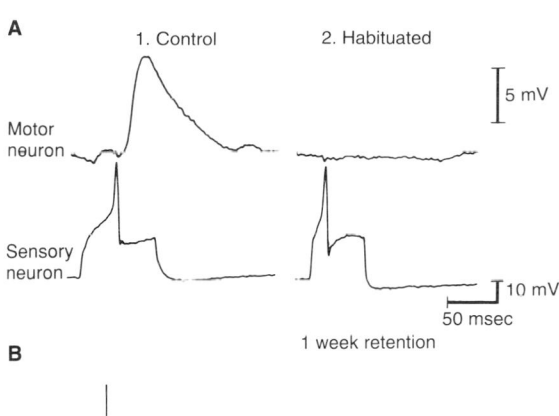

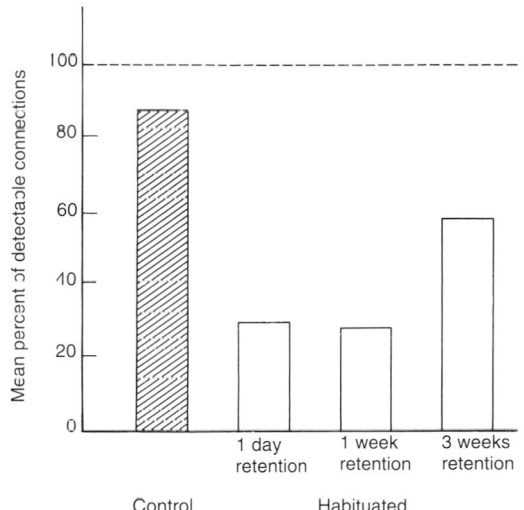

FIGURE 65–2

Long-term habituation of the gill-withdrawal reflex in *Aplysia* is reflected physiologically in a dramatic depression of synaptic effectiveness between the sensory and motor neurons. (Adapted from Castellucci, Carew, and Kandel, 1978.)

A. Comparison of a synaptic connection between a sensory neuron and a motor neuron in a control (untrained) animal and in an animal that had been subjected to long-term habituation. The synaptic potential in the motor neuron is still undetectable in the habituated animal one week after training.

B. The mean percentage of detectable connections in habituated animals at several points in time after long-term habituation training.

pathway. It is therefore likely that different types of experiences may be stored in different cells that have a variety of functions other than storing information.

What are the limits of this plasticity in neuronal function? How much can the effectiveness of a given synapse change and how long can the change last? Can changes in synaptic effectiveness also give rise to long-term memory lasting days, weeks, or years? A single training session of 10 stimuli in *Aplysia* leads to a short-term habituation lasting minutes, but four training sessions lead to a long-term change lasting up to 3 weeks (Figure 65–2). Whereas in control animals 90% of the sensory neurons make detectable connections onto a given motor neuron, in habituated animals the incidence of detectable connections between sensory neurons and the motor cell is reduced to

30%. This low incidence persists for one week and does not completely recover for three weeks after habituation training. As we shall see later, this long-term inactivation of synaptic transmission is accompanied by structural changes in the sensory cells.

Plastic change is not a feature of all synapses—some synaptic connections in the nervous system of *Aplysia* do not change their strength at all with repeated activation. However, at synapses involved in learning, such as the connections between the sensory neurons and the motor neurons as well as some of the interneuronal connections in the withdrawal reflex, a relatively small amount of training can produce large and enduring changes in synaptic strength.

Sensitization Involves Enhancement of Synaptic Transmission

In sensitization an animal learns about the properties of a noxious stimulus and as a result it remembers to respond more effectively to a variety of other stimuli, even innocuous ones. For example, following an aversive stimulus an animal learns to strengthen its defensive reflexes in preparation for withdrawal and escape. Sensitization is a more complex form of nonassociative learning than habituation but, like habituation, it has both a short-term form lasting minutes and a long-term form lasting days and weeks, depending on the number of stimuli presented to the animal.

Short-term sensitization in *Aplysia* has been examined at the cellular level. Following a single noxious stimulus to the head or tail, several synapses within the neural circuit of the gill-withdrawal reflex become modified, including the synapses made by the sensory neurons on the motor neurons and interneurons. Thus, a single set of synapses can participate in at least two different forms of learning. They can be depressed by habituation or enhanced by sensitization. Whereas habituation leads to a *homosynaptic depression*, a decrease in synaptic strength resulting from activity in the stimulated pathway, sensitization involves *heterosynaptic facilitation* (Figure 65–3A). The sensitizing stimulus activates a group of facilitating interneurons that synapse on the sensory neurons, including their terminals. The facilitating neurons make axo-axonal synapses of the sort we considered in Chapter 13. These facilitating neurons, some of which are serotonergic, enhance transmitter release from the sensory neurons by increasing the amount of the second messenger cAMP in the sensory neurons.

The likely sequence of biochemical steps in sensitization of this monosynaptic pathway of the gill-withdrawal reflex in *Aplysia* has been pieced together on the basis of pharmacological and biochemical studies (Figure 65–3B). Serotonin (and the other neurotransmitters released by facilitating neurons) activate receptors that engage a GTP-binding protein (G_s), which activates adenylyl cyclase and increases the concentration of cAMP in the sensory neurons. Cyclic AMP activates the cAMP-dependent protein kinase, which phosphorylates a number of substrate proteins. As discussed in Chapter 12, phosphorylation can

lead to an increase or decrease in the activity of a protein by changing its conformation. In sensitization, activation of cAMP-dependent protein kinase has at least three short-term consequences.

First, the protein kinase phosphorylates a K^+ channel protein, the serotonin-sensitive K^+ channel, or proteins associated with the channel. Phosphorylation of this channel reduces a component of the K^+ current that normally repolarizes the action potential. Reduction of this K^+ current thus prolongs the action potential and thereby allows the N-type Ca^{2+} channels to be activated for longer periods. More Ca^{2+} is able to enter the terminals, thereby enhancing transmitter release (Figure 65–3B). Second, serotonin and cAMP act to enhance transmitter mobilization through a Ca^{2+}-independent mechanism. Third, serotonin and cAMP alter an L-type Ca^{2+} channel. The Ca^{2+} influx through this channel does not directly affect release but also increases the availability of transmitter vesicles. In these two effects on mobilization, cAMP is thought to act in parallel with protein kinase C, which is also activated by serotonin (Figure 65–3B).

▷

FIGURE 65–3

Presynaptic facilitation is a factor in sensitization of the gill-withdrawal reflex in *Aplysia*.

A. Sensitization is produced by applying a noxious stimulus to another part of the body, such as the tail (Figure 65–1). Stimuli to the tail activate sensory neurons that excite facilitating interneurons. The facilitating cells, some of which use serotonin (5-hydroxytryptamine, or 5-HT) as their transmitter (indicated by dense core vesicles in the terminal of the facilitating neuron) in turn end on the synaptic terminals of the sensory neurons from the siphon skin, where they enhance transmitter release by means of presynaptic facilitation.

B. Postulated biochemical steps of presynaptic facilitation in the sensory neuron. The action of serotonin and other facilitating transmitters leads to enhanced transmitter release by modulating a number of steps in the release process; one of these is the closure of a special class of K^+ channels, which causes a consequent increase in Ca^{2+} influx through a (N-type) Ca^{2+} channel. Serotonin produces these actions by binding to a receptor that engages a G-protein, which increases the activity of adenylyl cyclase. The adenylyl cyclase converts ATP to cyclic AMP, thereby increasing the level of cyclic AMP in the terminal of the sensory neuron. The cAMP activates the cAMP-dependent protein kinase by attaching to its regulatory subunit, which releases its active catalytic subunit. The catalytic subunit then phosphorylates the K^+ channel (either directly or by acting on a regulatory protein associated with it), thereby changing the conformation of the channel and decreasing the K^+ current (**pathway 1**). This prolongs the action potential, increases the influx of Ca^{2+}, and thus augments transmitter release.

In addition to broadening the action potential (pathway 1), serotonin also leads to an increase in the availability of transmitter by mobilizing vesicles from a transmitter pool to the releasable pool at the active zone (**pathway 2**). This second pathway concerned with mobilization of transmitter vesicles reflects the joint action of the cAMP-dependent protein kinase and protein kinase C, a second kinase activated by 5-HT (**dotted line and pathway 2a**). Protein kinase C (PKC) is activated by 5-HT acting through another G-protein that activates a phospholipase that in turn stimulates diacylglycerol in the membrane. Diacylglycerol activates protein kinase C.

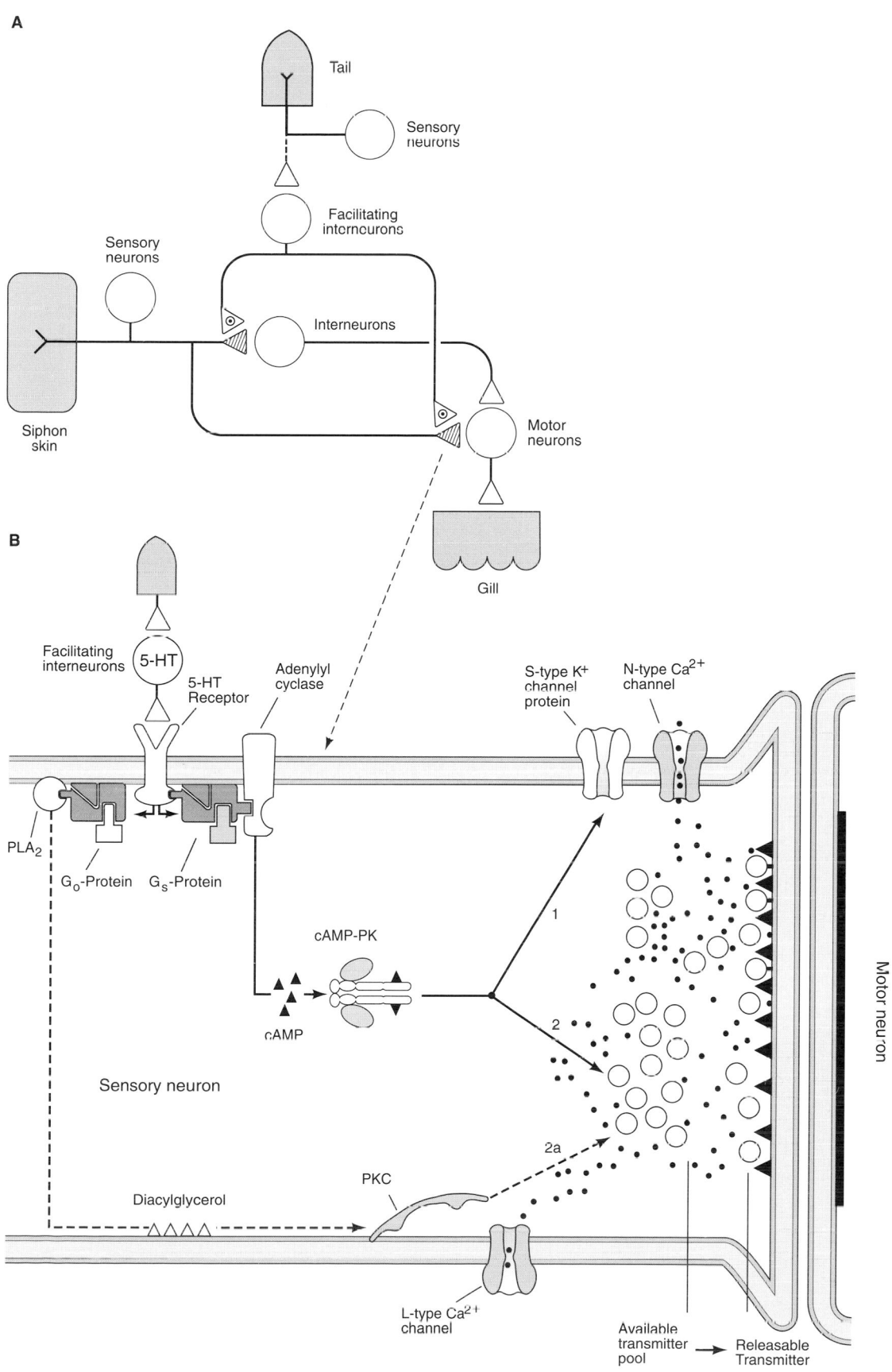

Long-Term Memory Requires Synthesis of New Proteins and the Growth of New Synaptic Connections

As with habituation and most other forms of reflexive learning, practice prolongs the memory for sensitization in a *graded* way. Whereas a single training trial (or a single application of serotonin) gives rise to short-term sensitization lasting minutes, four training trials produce long-term sensitization lasting one day, and further repetition produces sensitization that lasts one or more weeks. These behavioral studies in *Aplysia* and similar ones in vertebrates suggest that short- and long-term memory may be a single graded process. However, as we have seen in Chapter 64, certain clinical conditions such as seizure or head trauma can selectively affect either the short- or long-term memory process in human beings. An even clearer behavioral separation can be obtained in experimental animals. Here inhibitors of protein or mRNA synthesis selectively block long-term without affecting short-term memory.

These experiments raise the question: Is memory actually only a single graded process whose duration is related directly to the number of training trials, or does repetition during learning activate a different type of memory storage process? Cellular studies indicate that the long-term storage process appears to be a graded extension of the short-term process. First, long-term memory for sensitization is accompanied by changes in the strength of synaptic connections at the *same* locus involved in the short-term process: the connections between the sensory and motor neurons of the gill withdrawal reflex (Figure 65–4). Second, in the long-term as in the short-term process, this increase in synaptic strength again is due to the enhanced transmitter release. There is no change in the sensitivity of the postsynaptic receptor. Third, serotonin, a modulatory transmitter that produces the short-term facilitation following a single exposure, produces long-term facilitation following four or five repeated exposures. Finally, cAMP, the intracellular second messenger involved in the short-term facilitation, also turns on the long-term change.

However, despite these similarities on the cellular level there are important differences between the short- and long-term process that emerge on the molecular level. Specifically, whereas short-term facilitation of the synapse between the sensory and motor neurons involves covalent modification of pre-existing proteins and is not affected by inhibitors of protein or RNA synthesis, long-term facilitation requires the synthesis of new protein and mRNA. These findings suggest that genes and proteins not directly involved in short-term facilitation are required for long-term facilitation.

What is the function of these genes and proteins? Molecular studies indicate that with repeated training (or repeated application of serotonin), the cAMP dependent protein kinase acts on the nucleus of the sensory neurons to phosphorylate one or more cAMP-dependent transcriptional regulator proteins. These transcriptional regulators activate genes whose protein products have two long-term consequences.

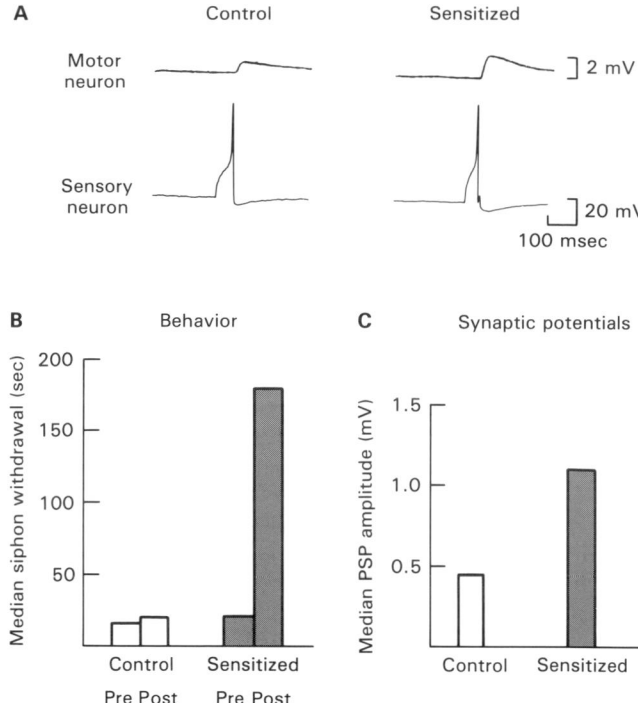

FIGURE 65–4

Long-term sensitization is associated with a facilitation of the connections between sensory and motor neurons. (Adapted from Frost et al., 1985.)

A. Representative synaptic potential from a siphon sensory neuron (**S.N.**) to a gill motor neuron (**M.N.**) in a control animal and an animal that had received long-term sensitization training. The record for the sensitized animal is one day after the end of training.

B. Group data from behavioral studies of animals receiving long-term sensitization training, illustrating median time to siphon withdrawal for the control and the experimental groups. (**Pre** = score before training; **post** = score after training.) The experimental group was tested one day after the end of training.

C. Median values of the synaptic potential from siphon sensory neuron to gill motor neuron for the control group and for sensitized animals one day after the end of training.

One consequence of gene activation is a persistent activation of the cAMP-dependent protein kinase. As we have seen in Chapter 12, the cAMP-dependent protein kinase is a heterodimer consisting of two regulatory subunits that inhibit the two catalytic subunits. With long-term training the amount of regulatory subunit in the sensory cells decreases relative to that of the catalytic subunit. This decrease in the regulatory subunit does not occur at the level of transcription but at the level of protein turnover. Thus, one of the proteins induced in long-term memory may perhaps be a protease that selectively enhances the degradation of the regulatory subunits (Figure 65–5). Moreover decrease in the regulatory subunit maintains the kinase constitutively active even at basal levels of cAMP. As a result, the same substrate proteins that are phosphorylated in the short-term can be maintained in a phosphorylated state in the long-term. This persistent

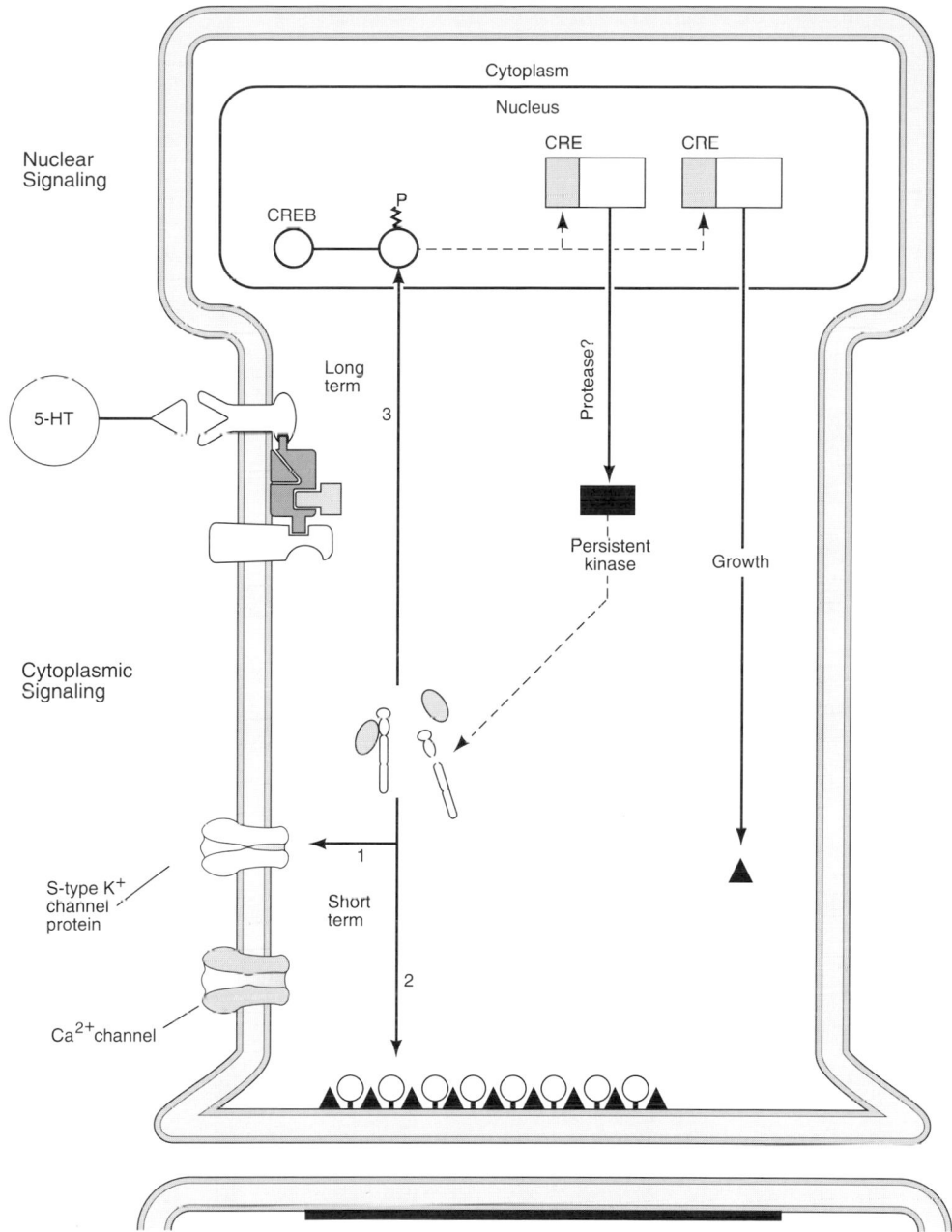

FIGURE 65–5

Schematic outline of the two major sets of changes in the sensory neurons of the gill-withdrawal reflex that accompany long-term memory for sensitization in *Aplysia:* persistent phosphorylation and structural changes. Serotonin (5-HT), a transmitter released by facilitatory neurons, acts on a sensory neuron to initiate both the short-term and the long-term facilitation that contribute to the memory processes.

Short-term facilitation (lasting minutes to hours), involves covalent modification of preexisting proteins (pathways 1 and 2). Serotonin acts on a transmembrane serotonin receptor to activate a GTP-binding protein that stimulates the amplifier, the enzyme adenylyl cyclase, to convert ATP to the second messenger cAMP. In turn, cAMP activates protein kinase A, which phosphorylates and covalently modifies a number of target proteins. These include closing a K^+ channel (pathway 1) as well as steps involved in transmitter availability and release (pathway 2). The duration of these modifications represents the retention or storage of a component of the short-term memory.

Long-term facilitation (lasting one or more days) involves the synthesis of new proteins. The switch for this inductive mechanism is initiated by the protein kinase A, which is thought to translocate to the nucleus where it is thought to phosphorylate one or more transcriptional activators that bind to cyclic AMP regulatory elements (CRE) located in the upstream region of cAMP-inducible genes. The transcriptional activators, thought to belong to the protein family of cyclic AMP response element binding (CREB) proteins, activate two classes of effector genes that encode two classes of proteins. (■ and ▲). Inhibiting protein synthesis during learning blocks the expression of these sets of induced proteins. These two sets of proteins have distinct functions. One set of proteins (■), one of which perhaps is a specific protease, leads to a down-regulation of the regulatory subunit. This results in persistent activity of kinase A, leading to persistent phosphorylation of the substrate proteins of pathways 1 and 2. The second set of proteins (▲) is important for the growth of new synaptic connections.

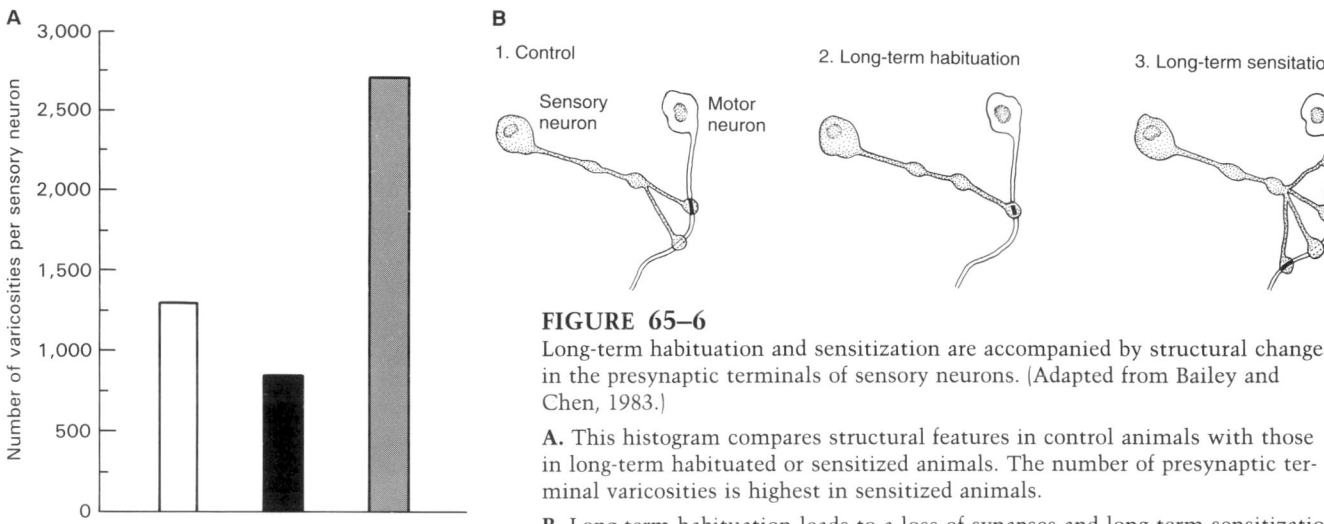

FIGURE 65–6

Long-term habituation and sensitization are accompanied by structural changes in the presynaptic terminals of sensory neurons. (Adapted from Bailey and Chen, 1983.)

A. This histogram compares structural features in control animals with those in long-term habituated or sensitized animals. The number of presynaptic terminal varicosities is highest in sensitized animals.

B. Long-term habituation leads to a loss of synapses and long-term sensitization to an increase.

phosphorylation may explain why long-term facilitation so resembles the short-term process as to seem a graded extension of it.

A second consequence of gene activation is the growth of synaptic connections. The growth change was first delineated by Craig Bailey and Mary Chen who injected the sensory and motor cells involved in the gill-withdrawal reflex in *Aplysia* with the electron-dense marker horseradish peroxidase and then examined the synaptic terminals with the electron microscope. They found that in trained animals the sensory neurons had twice as many postsynaptic terminals than in untrained animals. Moreover, in untrained animals only 40% of the synaptic terminals have active zones and seem capable of releasing transmitter. Long-term sensitization also increases the proportion of active zones to 65%. Finally, in the sensitized animals the dendrites of the motor neurons grow to accommodate the additional synaptic input.

Morphological changes seem to be a signature of the long-term process. These changes do not occur with short-term memory (Figure 65–6). Moreover, the structural changes that occur with the long-term process are not restricted to the growth. Long-term habituation leads to the opposite change—a regression and pruning of synaptic connections. With long-term habituation, where the functional connections between the sensory neurons and motor neurons are inactivated (Figure 65–2), the number of terminals per neuron is correspondingly reduced by one-third (Figure 65–6) and the proportion of terminals with active zones is reduced from 40% to 10%.

Classical Conditioning Involves an Associative Enhancement of Presynaptic Facilitation That Is Dependent on Activity

Classical conditioning is a more complex form of learning than sensitization. Rather than being concerned with learning about the properties of one stimulus (the sensitizing stimulus), the subject must learn the relationship between two stimuli and associate one type of stimulus with another (see Chapter 64). In classical conditioning an initially weak or ineffective stimulus becomes highly effective in producing a response after it has been paired or associated with a strong unconditioned stimulus. For reflexes that can be modified by both sensitization and classical conditioning, classical conditioning is more effective in enhancing the responsiveness of the reflex and lasts longer than sensitization. In fact, as we shall see in at least certain cases the mechanism of classical conditioning is an elaboration of the cellular strategy for sensitization.

The gill- and siphon-withdrawal reflexes of *Aplysia* are examples of behaviors that can be enhanced by both classical conditioning and sensitization. The withdrawal reflexes can be elicited by stimulating either the siphon or a nearby structure called the mantle shelf. Each of these areas is innervated by its own population of sensory neurons. Each pathway can be conditioned independently by pairing a stimulus to either the siphon or the mantle shelf with an unconditioned stimulus (a strong shock to the tail). The other pathway can then be stimulated as a control that is not paired with the tail shock. After such training the response to stimulation of the conditioned structure is significantly greater than that of the unconditioned structure.

Unlike nonassociative learning, time is critical to associative learning. For classical conditioning to work, the conditioned stimulus must *precede* the unconditioned stimulus and often, as with aversive unconditioned stimuli, it must do so within a critical interval of about 0.5 seconds. What cellular mechanisms are responsible for the temporal pairing of stimuli? In classical conditioning of the gill withdrawal reflex of *Aplysia* the temporal specificity in timing results from a convergence of the conditioned and unconditioned stimuli in individual sensory neurons. The facilitating interneurons that are activated by the unconditioned stimulus produce greater presynaptic facilitation of the sensory neurons only when they activate the sensory neurons immediately after the

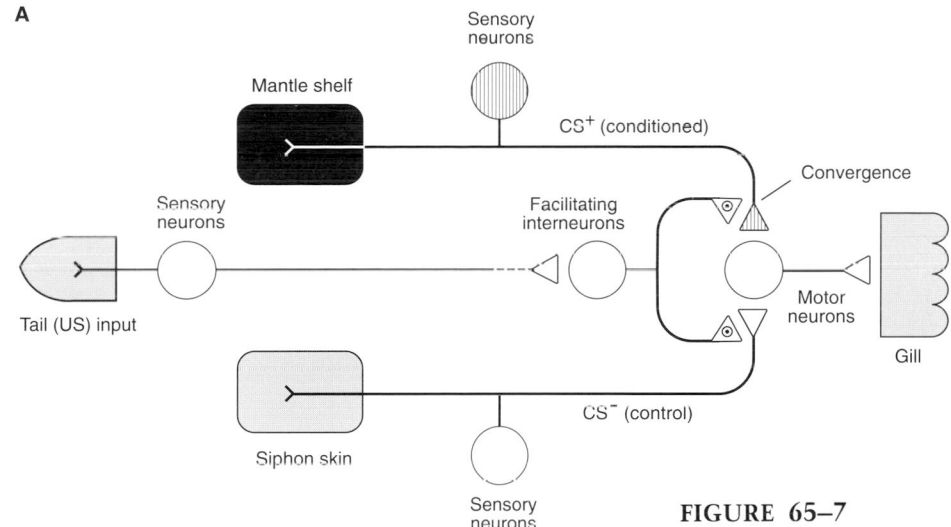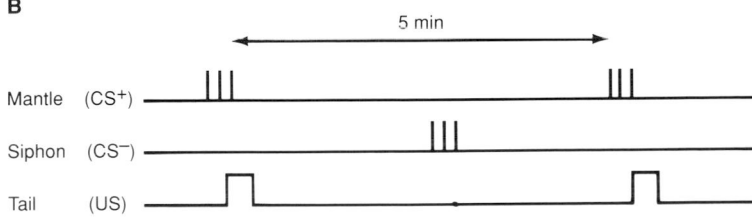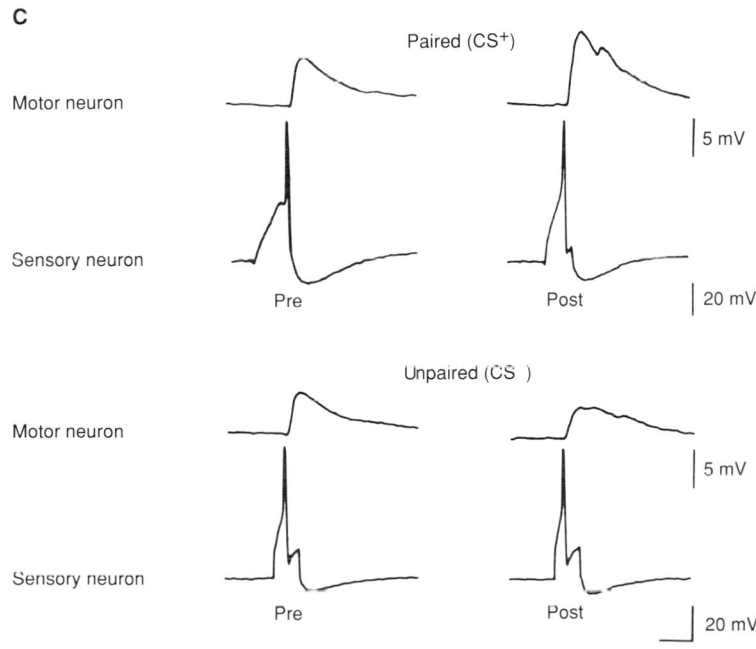

A

B

C

FIGURE 65–7

The cellular mechanism of classical conditioning. The sequence of pairing the conditioned stimulus and unconditioned stimulus establishes synaptic facilitation in the conditioned stimulus pathway.

A. This simplified diagram shows the pathways involved in classical conditioning of the gill withdrawal reflex in *Aplysia*. In this diagram a conditioned stimulus (**CS**) applied to the mantle is paired with an unconditioned stimulus (**US**) to the tail; as a control, a CS applied to the siphon is not paired with the US. A shock to the tail (US) excites facilitatory interneurons that synapse on the presynaptic terminals of sensory neurons in pathways from the mantle shelf and siphon. This is the mechanism of sensitization. However, when the mantle pathway is activated by a CS just prior to the US, the mantle sensory neurons are primed to respond in an amplified manner to subsequent stimulation from the facilitatory interneurons in the US pathway. This is the mechanism of classical conditioning; it both amplifies the response of the CS pathway and restricts the amplification to that pathway.

B. The experimental protocol for classical conditioning compares the responses of two conditioned stimuli (CSs) mediated by two sensory neurons, one (CS⁺) innervating the mantle and the other (CS⁻) innervating the siphon. Action potentials in the mantle sensory neurons (CS⁺) are paired with the US (tail stimulus). Action potentials in a siphon sensory neuron (CS⁻) are presented unpaired with the same US.

C. Examples of the excitatory postsynaptic potentials produced in an identified motor neuron by two sensory neurons mediating stimuli that were paired (mantle) or unpaired (siphon) with the tail shock, based on the protocol illustrated in part B. Electrical recordings were made before training (**Pre**) and one hour after training (**Post**). After training, facilitation of the excitatory postsynaptic potential from the paired sensory neuron is considerably greater than that from the unpaired neuron.

conditioned stimulus has caused the sensory neurons to fire action potentials (Figure 65–7). Thus, the facilitation is amplified if the conditioned stimulus produces action potentials in the sensory neurons just before the unconditioned stimulus arrives. This novel property of presynaptic facilitation is called *activity dependence*. In contrast, activity in the sensory neurons that *follows* the unconditioned stimulus has no facilitatory effect. Thus, the cellular mechanism of classical conditioning of the withdrawal reflex in *Aplysia* is an elaboration of presynaptic facilitation, the mechanism of sensitization of the reflex.

Edgar Walters and John Byrne found a similar enhancement for sensory neurons in the tail of *Aplysia*. Studies of classical conditioning in the mollusc *Hermissenda* by Daniel Alkon and in the cortex of the cat by Charles Woody suggest that modulation of K^+ channels may be critical for learning in many animals.

How is activity-dependent enhancement of presynaptic facilitation achieved? Tom Abrams and his colleagues found that action potentials allow Ca^{2+} to move into the sensory neuron. This influx of Ca^{2+} acting through calmodulin is thought to amplify the activation of the ade-

nylyl cyclase by serotonin and other modulatory transmitters (Figure 65–8). Much of the adenylyl cyclase in the brain is sensitive to Ca^{2+}/calmodulin, and generates more cAMP when it is bound to Ca^{2+}/calmodulin than when it is not. Thus, in *Aplysia* (and, as we shall see, in *Drosophila*) the stimulation of adenylyl cyclase by Ca^{2+}/calmodulin seems to be important for classical conditioning.

Genetic analyses of learning have also implicated the cAMP system. Seymour Benzer and his colleagues have explored how genes control behavior in *Drosophila*. They found that the fruit fly can be operantly or classically conditioned. Subsequently, William Quinn, Yadin Dudai, Duncan Byers, and Margaret Livingstone isolated single-gene mutants that were deficient in learning. Two of these mutants, called *dunce* and *rutabaga*, have been studied in detail. These mutants show two interesting features. First, neither mutant can be classically conditioned or sensitized. Second, both mutants have a defect in the cAMP cascade. The *dunce* mutant lacks a phosphodiesterase, an enzyme that degrades cAMP. As a result, this fly has abnormally high levels of cAMP that are thought to be out of the range of normal modulation. The *rutabaga* mutant has

FIGURE 65–8

A molecular model of the synaptic action underlying classical conditioning. The model is based on the hypothesis that activity in the sensory neurons of the conditioned stimulus (CS) pathway prior to the presentation of the unconditional stimulus (US) permits an influx of Ca^{2+} that enhances the activity of Ca^{2+}-dependent adenylyl cyclase.

A. In the unpaired pathway (CS) the sensory neuron is *not active* prior to presentation of the CS, so its Ca^{2+} channels are closed at the time the US input arrives.

B. In the paired pathway (CS$^+$) the sensory neuron *is active* prior to the CS and thus its Ca^{2+} channels are open when the US input arrives. Increased intracellular Ca^{2+} binds to calmodulin, which in turn binds to adenylyl cyclase, which undergoes a conformational change as a result. This change enhances the ability of the adenylyl cyclase to synthesize cAMP in response to serotonin released by the US. The greater amount of cAMP activates more cAMP-dependent protein kinase, and leads to a substantially greater amount of transmitter release than would occur normally (without paired activity).

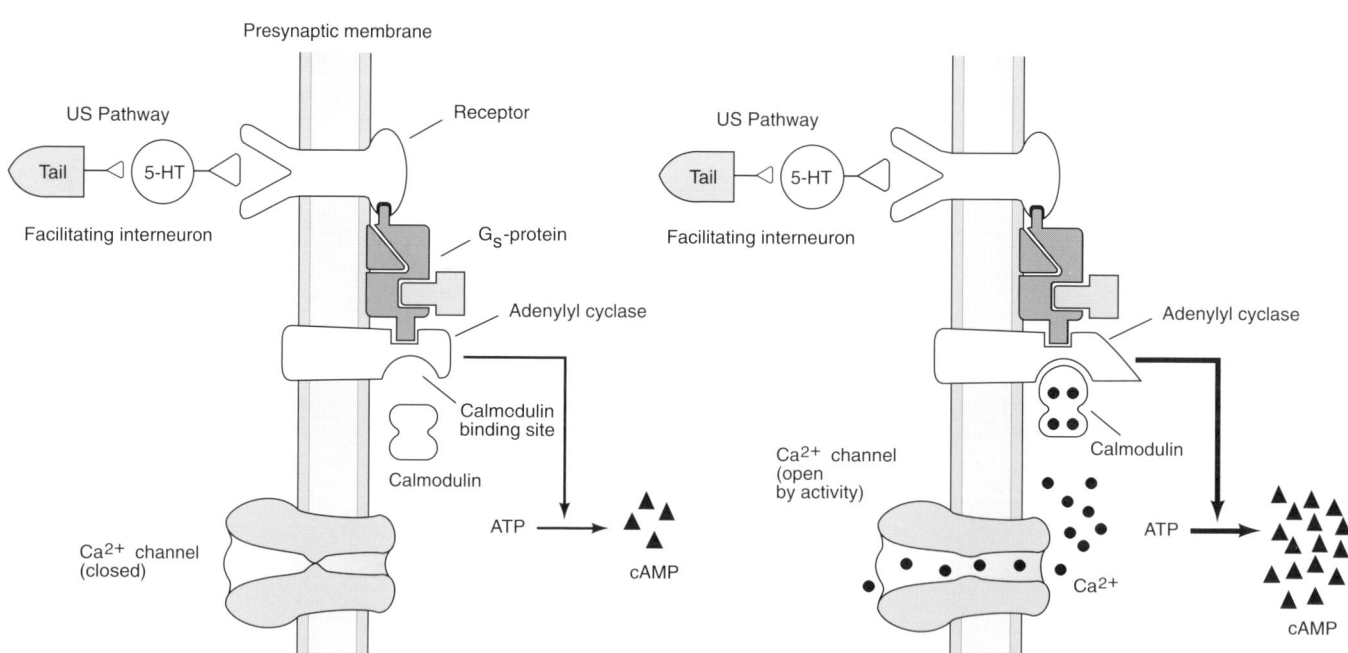

A   CS$^-$ Pathway (no preceding activity)

B   CS$^+$ Pathway (preceding activity)

a defect in the Ca^{2+}/calmodulin-dependent adenylyl cyclase and a low basal level of cAMP. Thus, both cellular studies of *Aplysia* and genetic studies of *Drosophila* indicate that the cAMP cascade is important for certain elementary forms of learning and memory storage. The cAMP cascade is not the only second-messenger system important for synaptic plasticity, however. As we shall see later in connection with long-term potentiation, other second messengers are important in other forms of plasticity.

That the cellular mechanisms of classical conditioning in *Aplysia* may be an elaboration of those involved in sensitization suggests that more complex forms of learning are built up from the molecular components of simpler forms. A variety of distinct forms of behavioral modifications could be achieved by combining a small set of molecular mechanisms.

Long-Term Potentiation in the Hippocampus Is an Example for Both Associative and Nonassociative Learning in the Mammalian Brain

As outlined in Chapter 64, the hippocampus is important for storage of declarative memory and there is evidence that neurons in the hippocampus show plastic capability of the sort that would be required for associative learning.

As first shown by Per Andersen, the hippocampus has three major excitatory pathways running from the subiculum to the CA1 region. The *perforant pathway* runs from the subiculum to the granule cells in the hilus of the dentate gyrus. The axons of the granule cells form a bundle, the *mossy fiber pathway*, that runs to the pyramidal cells lying in the CA3 region of the hippocampus. Finally, the pyramidal cells in the CA3 region send excitatory collaterals, the *Schaeffer collaterals*, to the pyramidal cells in CA1.

In 1973 Timothy Bliss and Terje Lømo demonstrated that a brief high-frequency train of stimuli to any one of the three afferent pathways to the hippocampus produces an increase in the excitatory synaptic potential in the postsynaptic hippocampal neurons, which can last for hours, and in the intact animal for days and even weeks. They called this facilitation *long-term potentiation* (LTP). Later studies showed that LTP at these different synapses is not identical. In the CA1 regions of the hippocampus, LTP has three interesting properties: (1) cooperativity (more than one fiber must be activated to obtain LTP), (2) associativity (the contributing fibers and the postsynaptic cell need to be active together, in an associative way), and (3) specificity (LTP is specific to the active pathway). In the CA3 region the LTP has different properties and is not associative (Figure 65–9).

Long-Term Potentiation in the CA1 Region Is Associative

In the CA1 region LTP cannot be produced by activating only one fiber; a minimum number of afferent fibers must

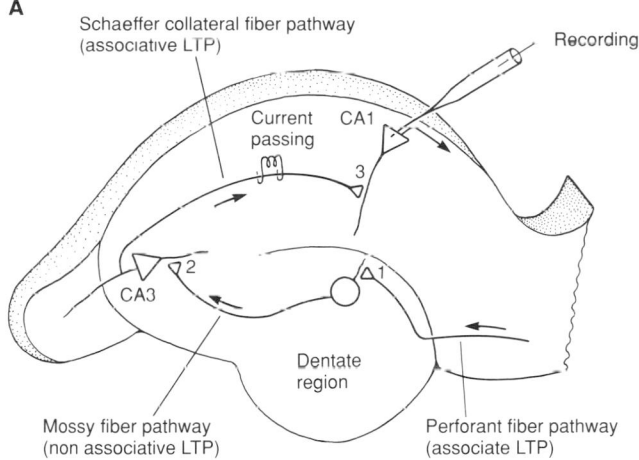

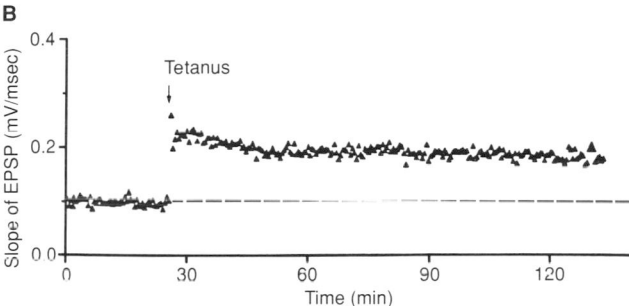

FIGURE 65–9

The major excitatory pathways in the hippocampus are capable of long-term potentiation.

A. The three major excitatory synaptic pathways in the hippocampus. The *perforant pathway* (1) from the subiculum forms excitatory connections with the granule cells of the dentate gyrus. The granule cells give rise to axons that form the *mossy fiber pathway* (2). This pathway connects with the pyramidal cells in area CA3 of the hippocampus. The CA3 cells project to the pyramidal cells in CA1 by means of the Schaeffer collaterals (3). (**Arrows** denote the direction of impulse flow.)

B. Long-term potentiation in the CA1 region of the hippocampus. The graph shows the slope of an excitatory synaptic potential (recorded extracellularly), an index of synaptic efficacy. The test stimulus was given every 10 seconds. To elicit long-term potentiation two trains of stimuli given for 1 second at 100 Hz tetani separated by 20 seconds were delivered to the Schaeffer collaterals. (Adapted from Nicoll et al., 1988.)

be activated together. This cooperative activity has *associative* features similar to those of classical conditioning. When separate weak and strong excitatory inputs arrive at the same region of the dendrite of a pyramidal cell, the weak input will become potentiated if it is activated in association with the strong one. Thus, LTP differs from conventional *posttetanic* potentiation (see Chapter 13) because, in addition to requiring high-frequency stimulation, it depends on cooperative and associative action. Finally, LTP is *specific* to those synapses that are activated by the stimulus. LTP produced by one input, for example

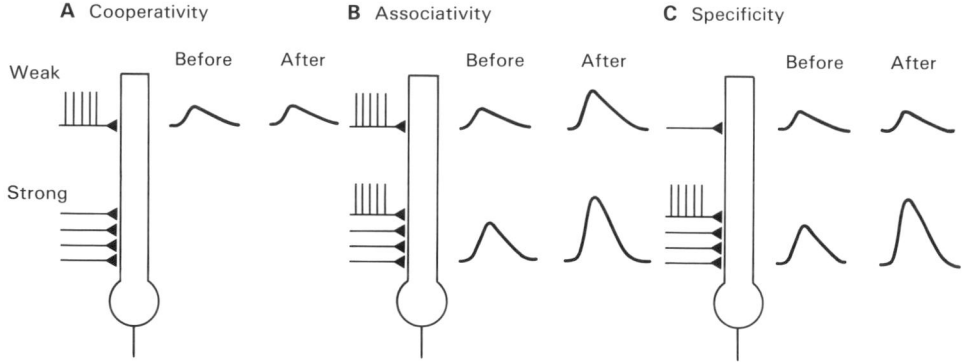

A Cooperativity   **B** Associativity   **C** Specificity

FIGURE 65–10

Long-term potentiation in area CA1 of the hippocampus shows cooperativity, associativity, and specificity. A single pyramidal cell is shown receiving weak and strong synaptic inputs by stimulating two different fascicles of the Schaffer collateral pathway. (Adapted from Nicoll et al., 1988.)

A. Tetanic stimulation of the weak input alone does not cause long-term potentiation in the pathway (compare the potential

before and after tetanus). A minimum number of axons must be activated.

B. Tetanic stimulation of the strong and weak pathways together causes long-term potentiation in both pathways.

C. Tetanic stimulation of the strong input alone causes long-term potentiation in the strong pathway but not in the weak.

---

an input to the apical dendrites, will not affect an independent input onto the basilar dendrites (Figure 65–10).

What accounts for these three features? Bengt Gustafsson and Holger Wigström found that the induction of LTP in the CA1 region of the hippocampus is postsynaptic. For example, LTP is greatly facilitated when postsynaptic inhibition is blocked by picrotoxin. Conversely, LTP can be reduced and even prevented by properly timed inhibitory inputs. Even more surprising, if the postsynaptic cell is hyperpolarized during the tetanus, LTP is prevented. Finally, LTP can be induced when a weak stimulus train, not sufficient to produce LTP, is paired repeatedly with a depolarizing current pulse injected in a single postsynaptic cell.

Thus, LTP requires depolarization of the postsynaptic cells coincident with activity in the presynaptic neuron. This finding provides the first direct evidence for *Hebb's rule*, proposed in 1949 by the Canadian psychologist Donald Hebb: "When an axon of cell A . . . excite[s] cell B and repeatedly or persistently takes part in firing it, some growth process or metabolic change takes place in one or both cells so that A's efficiency as one of the cells firing B is increased." As we have seen in Chapter 60, a similar principle seems to be involved in the fine tuning of synaptic connections during the late stages of development.

Why is the simultaneous firing of the pre- and postsynaptic cells important for LTP? The axons from the CA3 region of the hippocampus that terminate on the pyramidal cells of the CA1 region (by means of the Schaeffer collaterals) use glutamate as their transmitter. Glutamate acts on its target cells in the CA1 region by binding to both *N*-methyl-D-aspartate (NMDA) and non-NMDA receptors. The non-NMDA receptors dominate in normal synaptic transmission. However, the NMDA receptor-channel, which normally is blocked by Mg^{2+}, becomes unblocked and activated when the postsynaptic cell is adequately depolarized by a strong (cooperative) input from many pre-

synaptic neurons (see Chapter 11). Unblocking the channel allows the influx of Na^+ and Ca^{2+} into the cell.

Thus, the NMDA receptor is unique in being a *doubly gated channel*. It is gated by both transmitter and voltage. The Mg^{2+} blockade of the channel is removed only when both glutamate binds to the receptor *and* the membrane is depolarized. This critical membrane depolarization is normally achieved through the activation of many non-NMDA receptors by the firing of many presynaptic neurons (Figure 65–11). Artificially it can be obtained by simply depolarizing the postsynaptic cell.

The Ca^{2+} influx through the unblocked NMDA receptor-channel is critical for LTP. Blocking Ca^{2+} influx by injecting a Ca^{2+} chelator (such as EGTA or BABTA) prevents induction of LTP. Conversely, injecting Ca^{2+} into the postsynaptic cell initiates the early phase of LTP. In principle, Ca^{2+} could pass through either a voltage-gated Ca^{2+} channel or the NMDA-gated channel. There is now good evidence that the Ca^{2+} influx critical for LTP does not enter the cell through voltage-gated Ca^{2+} channels; rather, it comes only through the NMDA receptor-channel. Blocking this receptor-channel with the selective inhibitor aminophosphonovalerate (APV) also blocks LTP.

NMDA receptors seem to cluster on the heads of the spines of dendrites, not on their shafts (spines, as we have seen in Chapter 11, are lateral protrusions on the shafts of dendrites that are specialized to receive excitatory synaptic input). Activation of non-NMDA receptor-channels depolarizes the spines to the point where the Mg^{2+} blockade of the NMDA receptor-channels is removed, allowing Ca^{2+} to enter the spines. The spines then act as compartment that restrict the diffusion of Ca^{2+} to the spines, so that the synaptic action is restricted to the synapses that are active.

How does Ca^{2+} influx produce LTP? The work of Roger Nicoll and Richard Tsien and their colleagues indicates that Ca^{2+} initiates the persistent enhancement of synaptic

A   Normal synaptic transmission   **B**   During initiation

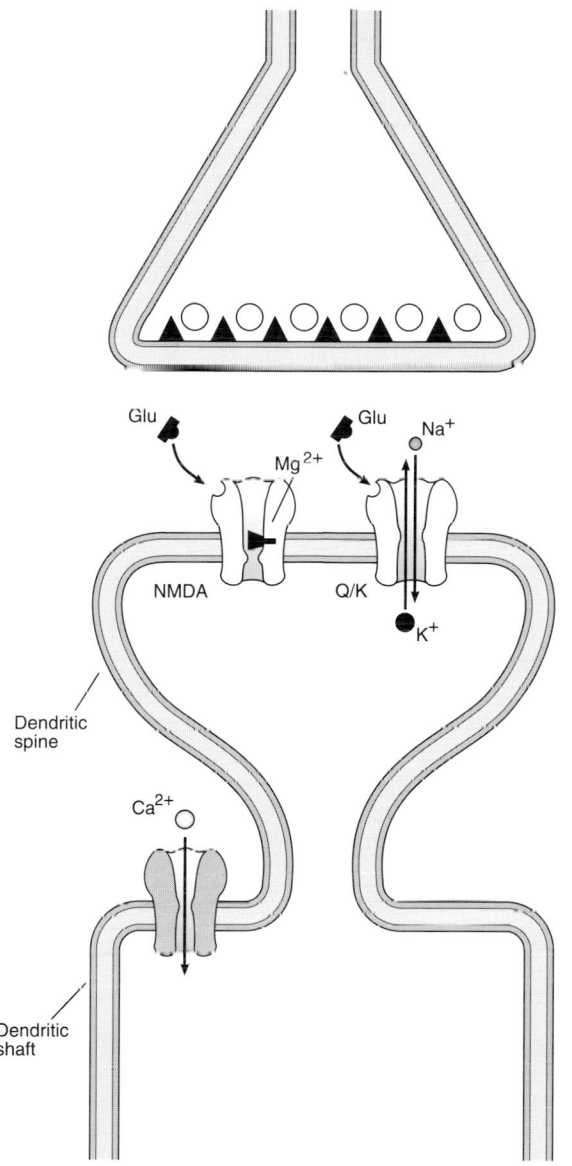
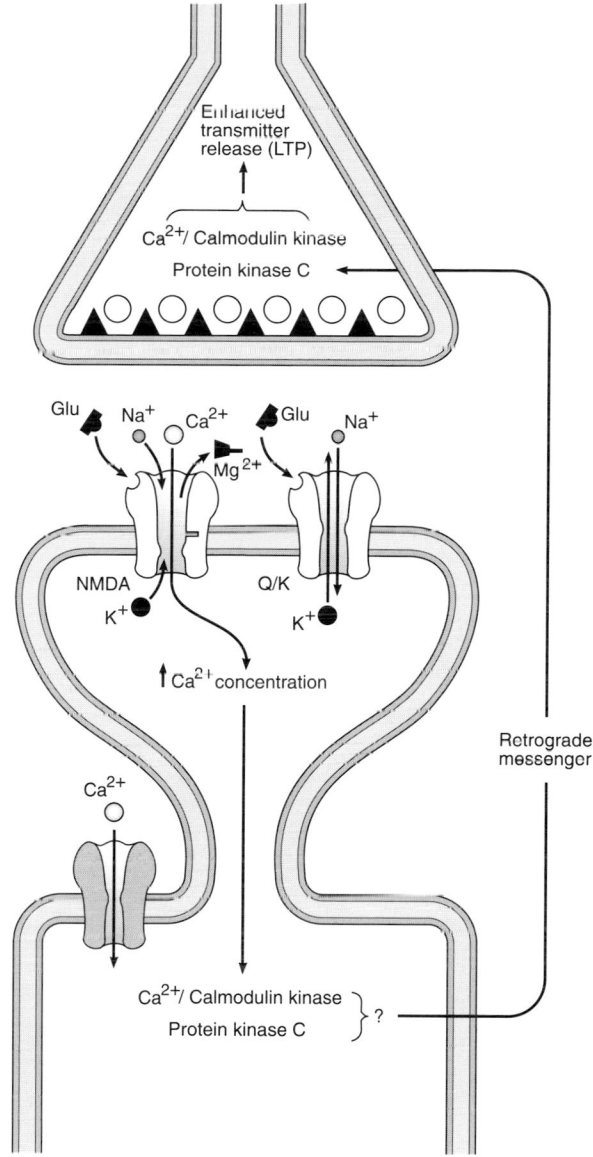

FIGURE 65–11

A model for the induction of LTP. According to this model NMDA and non-NMDA (quisqualate/kainate) receptor-channels (Q/K) are located near each other in dendritic spines. (Adapted from Gustafsson and Wigström, 1988.)

A. During normal low-frequency synaptic transmission, glutamate is released from the presynaptic terminal and acts on both the NMDA and non-NMDA (Q/K) receptors. Sodium and K^+ flow through the non-NMDA receptor-channels but not through the NMDA receptor-channels, due to Mg^{2+} blockade of this channel at the resting level of membrane potential.

B. When the postsynaptic membrane is depolarized by the actions of the non-NMDA receptor channels, as occurs during a high-frequency tetanus that induces LTP, the depolarization

relieves the Mg^{2+} blockade of the NMDA channel. This allows Na^+, K^+, and Ca^{2+} to flow through the NMDA channel. The resulting rise of Ca^{2+} in the dendritic spine triggers Ca^{2+}-dependent kinases (Ca^{2+}/calmodulin kinase and kinase C) that lead to induction of LTP. Once induced, the postsynaptic cell releases (in ways that are still not understood) a membrane permeable retrograde messenger that is thought to act on kinases in the presynaptic terminal (perhaps protein kinase C) to produce the sustained enhancement of transmitter release that underlies the persistence of LTP. Depolarization opens voltage-dependent Ca^{2+} channels in the dendritic shafts but not those in the spine; however, Ca^{2+} inflow through these voltage-dependent channels in the shaft does not seem to affect LTP which requires Ca^{2+} influx into the spine.

transmission by activating two Ca^{2+}-dependent protein kinases: the Ca^{2+}/calmodulin kinase and protein kinase C. These kinases then are thought to become persistently active.

Whereas the *induction* of LTP in the CA1 region appears to depend on postsynaptic depolarization, Ca^{2+} influx, and Ca^{2+} second-messenger activation, the *maintenance* of synaptic efficacy in LTP requires, in addition, an increase in *presynaptic* transmitter release. This idea is based on three lines of evidence. First, Bliss and his colleagues have found that LTP is accompanied by an enhancement of glutamate release. Second, quantal analyses of transmitter release by John Bekkers and Charles Stevens in cell culture and by them and by Roberto Malinow and Tsien in hippocampal tissue slices indicate that LTP involves an increased probability of transmitter release without a change in the sensitivity of the postsynaptic receptor. Third, imaging studies with voltage-sensitive dyes in hippocampal monolayer cultures by Tobias Bonhoeffer and his colleagues suggest that the induction of LTP by postsynaptic depolarization of a *single cell* produces LTP in a whole population of neurons. The LTP may not be restricted to the cell that was depolarized as might be expected from a strictly postsynaptic mechanism. Thus, not all postsynaptic cells of a population undergoing LTP need participate in the induction.

If the induction of LTP requires a postsynaptic event (activation of NMDA receptors) and maintenance of LTP involves a presynaptic event (increase in transmitter release), then some message must be sent from the postsynaptic to the presynaptic neurons. The Ca^{2+}-activated second messenger, or perhaps Ca^{2+} acting directly, is thought to cause release of *retrograde plasticity factor* from the dendritic spines of the active postsynaptic cell. This retrograde factor then diffuses to the presynaptic terminals to activate within them one or more second messengers that act to enhance transmitter release and thereby maintain LTP (Figure 65–12B). The actions of a membrane permeable retrograde message could be restricted to recently active presynaptic cells. Indeed, to account for the pathway specificity of LTP, the effects of this retrograde message must be restricted.

According to this view, LTP in CA1 may use two associative mechanisms in series: a Hebbian mechanism and activity-dependent presynaptic facilitation. However, LTP differs from the activity-dependent presynaptic facilitation found in *Aplysia* in that the facilitatory substance is released from the postsynaptic target cell by activation of NMDA receptors. Rather than activating diffusely projecting facilitator interneurons, as in *Aplysia*, the postsynaptic target cells in LTP act as facilitating neurons.

What might be the advantage of combining in the hippocampus two associative cellular mechanisms in series (the postsynaptic NMDA receptor and activity-dependent presynaptic facilitation)? One possible advantage is spatial amplification of the signal. The retrograde factor can recruit other, parallel presynaptic fibers in addition to those that synapse on the active postsynaptic cell.

Associative Long-Term Potentiation Is Thought to Be Important for Spatial Memory

The finding that LTP is involved in many areas of the brain including the hippocampus, a region known to be important for memory storage, raises the question: Is LTP involved in memory storage? Evidence for this has been provided by Richard Morris and his colleagues. They developed a spatial memory task in which a rat has to swim

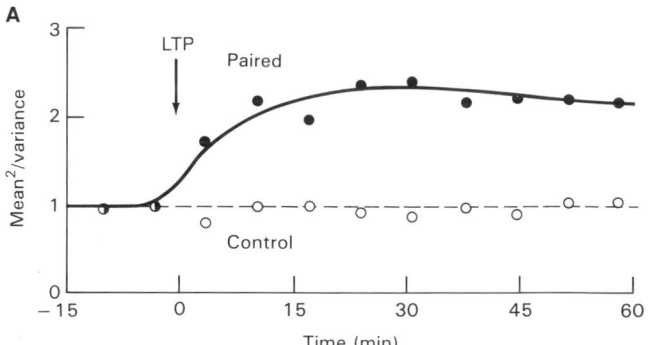

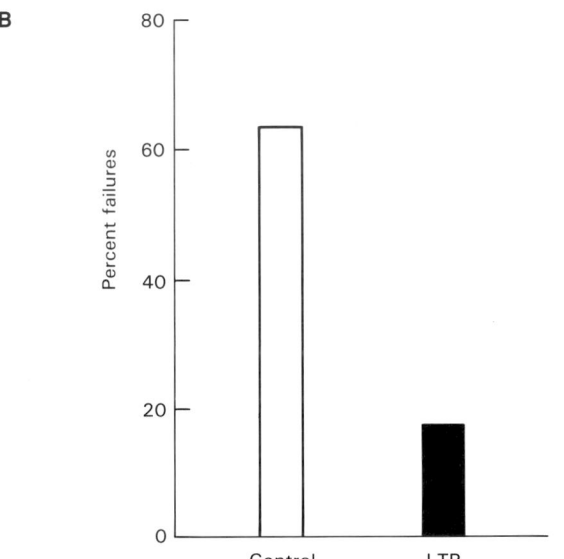

FIGURE 65–12

Evidence that the maintenance phase of LTP of the Schaffer precollateral synapses onto pyramidal cells in the CA1 region is presynaptic. Quantal analysis of long-term potentiation in area CA1 of the hippocampus is based on a coefficient of variation of evoked responses. This analysis assumes that the number of quanta of transmitter released by presynaptic impulse follows a binomial distribution, where the coefficient of variation (mean²/ variance) provides an index of transmitter release from the presynaptic terminal that is independent of quantal size. (From Malinow and Tsien, 1990.)

A. With long-term potentiation there is an increase in the ratio of the mean²/variance—indicating an increase in transmitter release. This increase only occurs in the pathway that is paired with depolarization of the postsynaptic cell (●). It does not occur in a control pathway that is not paired (○).

B. At normal rates of stimulation there is a significant number of failures in transmission (Chapter 13). Here in 60% of cases stimulation of the presynaptic axons leads to no release. Following LTP the percentage of failures decreases to 20%, another indication that LTP is presynaptic.

a water maze in a pool filled with an opaque fluid to find a platform hidden under the fluid. The animal is released at random locations around the pool and is required to navigate to the platform using spatial cues such as those that it can infer from the walls of the room in which the pool is located. In a visual (nonspatial) version of this task the platform is raised above the water surface so that it is visible. Here the rat can swim to the location where it sees the visible platform. When NMDA receptors in the hippocampus are blocked by injection into the ventricle of APV, animals can navigate the nonspatial version of the task using visual cues but they fail in the spatial version of the task. These experiments suggest that an NMDA receptor mechanism in the hippocampus, perhaps LTP, is involved in spatial learning.

Long-Term Potentiation in the CA3 Region Is Nonassociative

The capability for long-term potentiation has now been found in many regions of the cerebral cortex. Not all mechanisms for the induction of LTP are the same, however. Some do not work through the NMDA receptor and do not depend on either Ca^{2+} influx or the activation of Ca^{2+}-dependent kinases in the postsynaptic cell. For example, neurons in the CA3 region of the hippocampus receive excitatory synaptic connections from the mossy fibers of the granule cells in the dentate nucleus. Like the presynaptic cells that terminate in the CA1 region, these fibers release glutamate as their transmitter, but they do not end on NMDA receptors. In fact, LTP at the mossy fiber synapses is not blocked by the NMDA receptor antagonist APV. Moreover, this potentiation is not associative: It does not require cooperativity or associativity. The input need not be paired with another input or with the postsynaptic cells.

Robert Zalutsky and Nicoll have found that LTP in the CA3 region does not require Ca^{2+} influx into the postsynaptic cell; blocking Ca^{2+} influx into the postsynaptic cell does not affect LTP. Indeed, LTP can be obtained after dialyzing the postsynaptic cell with fluoride, which disrupts various intracellular second-messenger pathways. This form of LTP also involves an enhancement of transmitter release. The molecular mechanisms contributing to this form of LTP have not yet been delineated. But an interesting feature of the mossy fiber synapse, described by Daniel Johnston and his colleagues, is that both synaptic transmission and LTP are modulated by norepinephrine working through the cAMP cascade (Figure 65–13).

Is There a Molecular Grammar for Learning?

The learning-related changes in synaptic efficacy we have considered raise two surprisingly reductionist possibilities. First, the fact that in their most elementary forms synaptic changes can be associative without requiring complex neural networks may mean that the associative activity that contributes to associative conditioning represents a basic cellular process. This process may be mediated by proteins that are capable of responding to signals from the conditioned stimulus (CS) and unconditioned stimulus (US), such as the adenylyl cyclase or NMDA receptor. Second, the finding that the associative forms of synaptic plasticity in the hippocampus are related in certain instances to nonassociative forms suggests that there

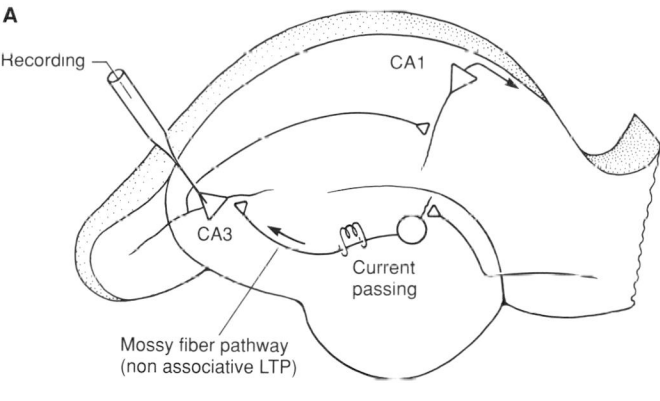

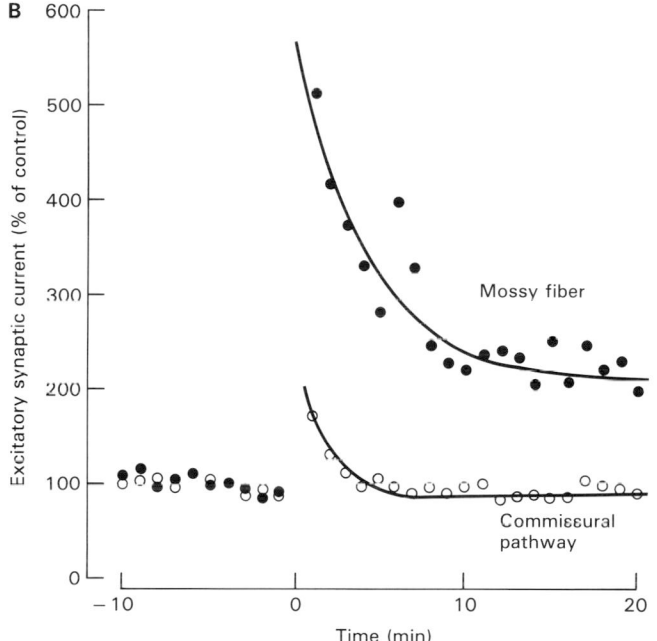

FIGURE 65–13

Evidence that long-term potentiation of the mossy fiber synapses on the pyramidal cells of the CA3 region in the hippocampus is presynaptic. (Adapted from Zalutsky and Nicoll, 1990.)

A. A diagram of the hippocampus showing the arrangement for studying LTP in the CA3 region.

B. Whole-cell voltage-clamp recording was carried out. This allowed injection into the cell body of the CA3 neuron of both fluoride and the Ca^{2+} chelator BAPTA (1,2-bis[o-amino-phenoxy] ethane-N,N,N', N'-tetraacetic acid). Together these two drugs are thought to block *all* second-messenger pathways in the postsynaptic cell. Despite this drastic biochemical blockade of the postsynaptic cell, the injections do not affect the expression of LTP in the mossy fiber pathway, which is therefore thought to be presynaptic. In contrast, these injections do block LTP in the association commissural pathway. This pathway ends on the NMDA receptor, and here induction of LTP is known to be postsynaptic.

may be a cellular grammar for synaptic plasticity, by which some elements are unique and others are shared and more complex forms of plasticity represent combinations of simpler forms. Of course, these mechanisms do not act in isolation. They are embedded in neural networks with considerable computational power, which can add substantial complexity to these elementary mechanisms.

The Somatotopic Map in the Brain Is Modifiable by Experience

Learning can lead to structural alterations in the brain. How important are these changes in determining the functional architecture of the brain?

We learned in Chapter 59 that the structure of the ocular dominance columns in area 17 of the cerebral cortex can be altered by experience during an early critical period. If one eye is closed during a critical period, the columns devoted to that eye shrink while those devoted to the open eye expand. This modifiability of the ocular dom-

inance columns is restricted to a relatively short period just after birth, but it raises an intriguing question: To what degree can altered sensory experience in later life produce changes in the architecture of the brain—in the size of cortical columns, or even in the precise details of the various sensory and motor maps?

The work we have just reviewed in simple animals indicates that learning produces structural and functional changes in specific nerve cells. In mammals, and especially in humans, in whom each functional component is represented by hundreds of thousands of nerve cells, learning is likely to lead to alterations in many nerve cells and is therefore likely to be reflected in changes in the pattern of interconnections of the various sensory and motor systems involved in a particular learning task. This is indeed

FIGURE 65–14

The innervation of the body surface is represented in more than one sensory map in the primary somatic sensory cortex. The illustration shows the hand areas represented in areas 3b and 1 of the owl monkey somatic sensory cortex. (Adapted from Merzenich and Kaas, 1982.)

A. The location of these two hand areas is shown in this dorsolateral view of the monkey brain.

B. 1. The ulnar and median nerves innervate different territories on the ventral surface of the hand. **2.** The areas innervated by the

two nerves are represented in adjacent area of cortex, areas 3b and 1. Cortex devoted to the representation of the ventral surface of the digits is indicated in **white**; that devoted to the dorsal surface is indicated by **shading**. In these cortical maps the five digits (D_1–D_5) and the four palmar pads (P_1–P_4) are arranged in an orderly sequence and their representations have been numbered in order. The insular (**I**) pads, the hypothenar (**H**) pads, and the thenar (**T**) pads are also indicated. **3.** The remarkable topographic organization of the cortical map can be appreciated by comparing the map in B_2 with this figurative representation of the hands.

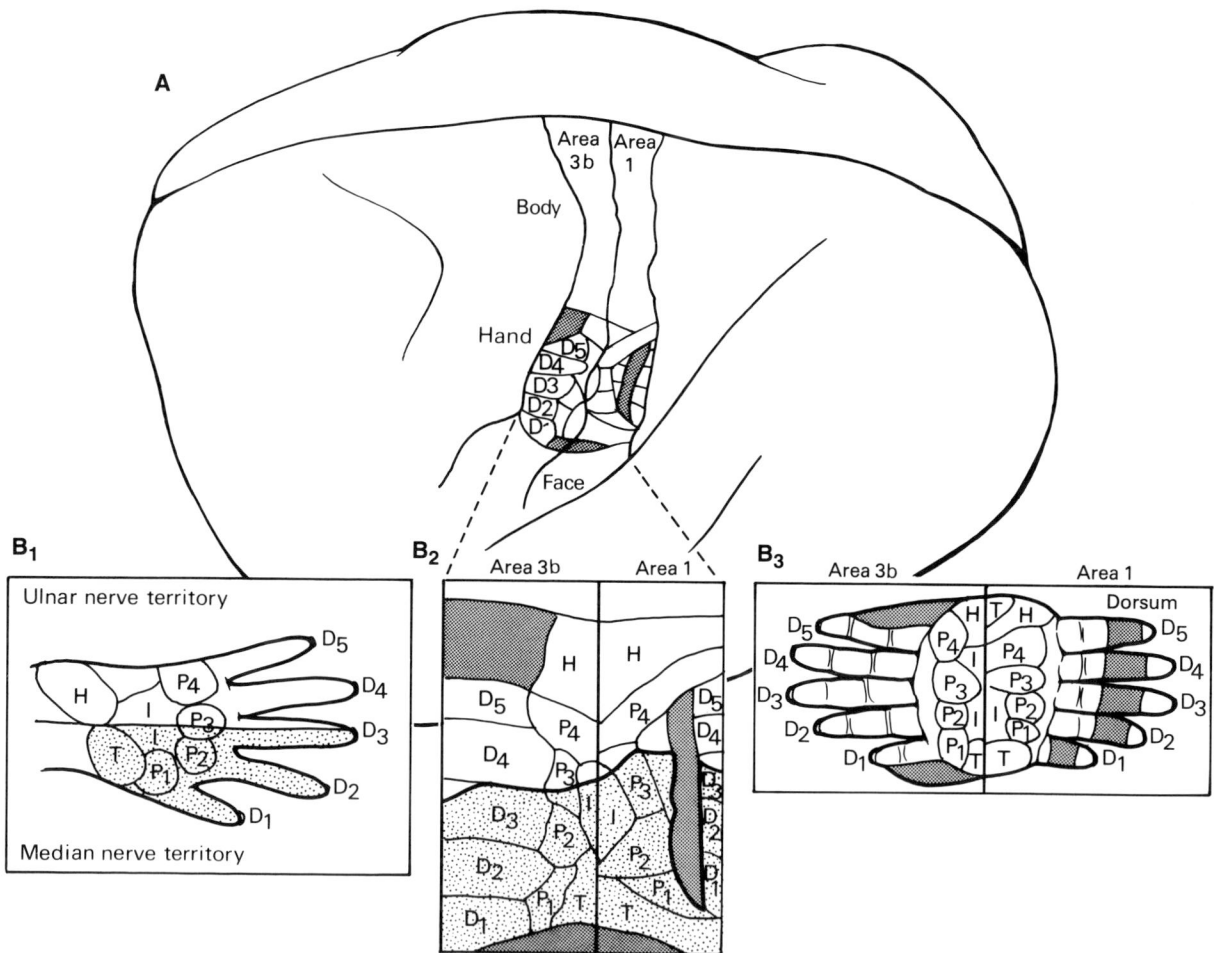

what appears to happen. The most detailed evidence has come from studies on the somatic sensory system.

The primary somatic sensory cortex consists of four Brodmann's areas (1, 2, 3a, and 3b) in the postcentral gyrus. Each of these areas represents a separate map of the body surface (see Chapter 27). Michael Merzenich and Jon Kaas and their colleagues have found that the cortical maps differ systematically among individuals in a manner that reflects their use. Merzenich and Kaas first encountered this phenomenon when examining the recovery of function after nerve injury in monkeys. They severed the median nerve in the hand, which innervates the cutaneous receptors on most of the ventral surface of the hand, palm, and glabrous portions of digits 1, 2, and 3 (Figure 65–14). One would expect that after cutting the nerve the cortical areas committed to the denervated parts of the hand would be unresponsive and silent. However, when the cortex was mapped before and after denervation, only a portion of the territory devoted to the median nerve was unresponsive.

Thus, a significant part of the cortical area of the median nerve could be activated following denervation by stimulating the neighboring parts of the hand outside the territory of the median nerve. Single nerve cells responding to stimuli on the hand in areas outside the territory of the median nerve had restricted, specific, and well-organized receptive fields. The dorsal surface of finger 2, which normally has a small representation in the cortical area of the median nerve, had a much larger representation after the median nerve had been cut. Similarly, areas on insular pads that normally were only modestly represented had substantially expanded representation after sectioning of the nerve (Figure 65–15). This additional representation was present immediately after denervation and expanded further in the weeks after sectioning of the nerve.

These findings indicate that maps derived from experiments record only the *dominant* functional organization in a particular region of the brain. The organization apparent in the maps of the somatic system (and perhaps all sensory and motor systems) reflects only part of the total pattern of anatomical connections. Other connections are revealed only when the dominant pathways are inactivated. Consistent with these findings, Peter Snow and his colleagues have demonstrated that thalamocortical neurons in the cat normally have projections to somatosensory cortex that are not organized in a strictly somatotopic way. Such projections may represent the necessary anatomical variations required for changing the somatotopic organization when functional reorganization is necessary.

Higher-order cortices may have an even greater capacity for reorganization than the primary sensory cortex. Mortimer Mishkin and his colleagues found that removal of the entire postcentral hand representation initially leaves the S-II representation of the hand unresponsive to somatic stimulation. Two months later, most of the region is responsive and is occupied by an expanded foot representation. This extensive somatotopic reorganization of S-II exceeds that observed in the postcentral gyrus after peripheral nerve damage and involves more than half the areal extent of S-II!

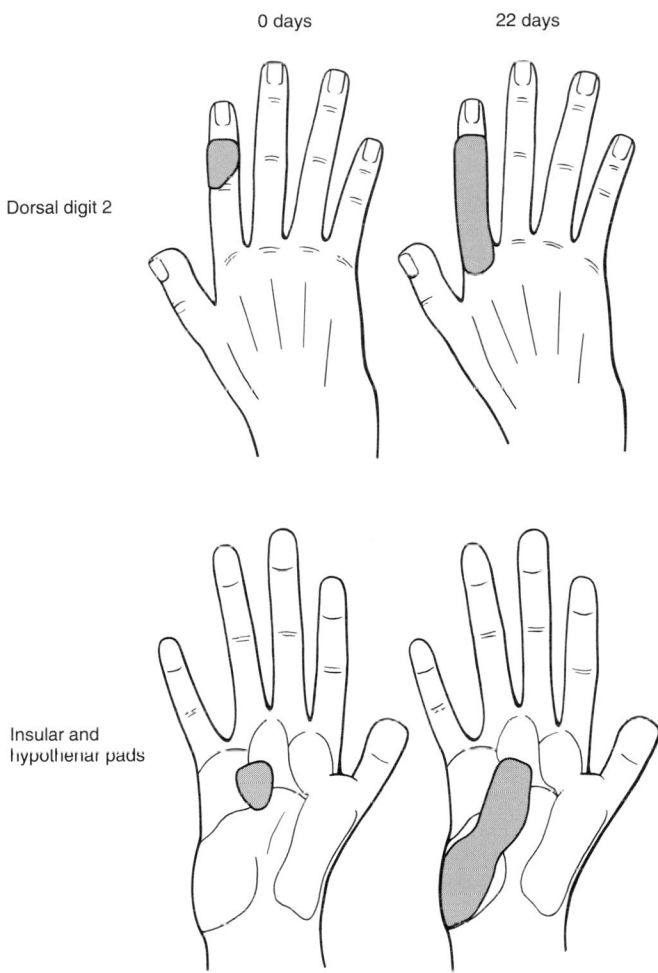

0 days   22 days

Dorsal digit 2

Insular and hypothenar pads

FIGURE 65–15

After the median nerve of a monkey is sectioned and prevented from regenerating, the cortical representation of the area of skin previously not innervated by the median nerve expands over time. The shaded regions represent the total region of the dorsum of digit 2 represented in area 3b (**upper** figure) and the region of the insular and hypothenar pads represented in areas 1 and 3b (**lower** figure) immediately after nerve section (**left**) and 22 days later (**right**). Regions of representation were determined from extracellular recordings of single units and evoked response. (Adapted from Merzenich et al., 1983.)

Changes in the Somatotopic Map Produced by Learning May Contribute to the Biological Expression of Individuality

The studies by Merzenich, Kaas, Mishkin, and their colleagues demonstrate that cortical somatic sensory maps are dynamic, not static. Functional connections can expand into nonfunctional sectors to represent, in greater detail, the skin regions bordering on a denervated area. Thus, even in adult monkeys there appears to be a use-dependent competition for cortical territory. Once a particular input becomes inactive, its former postsynaptic targets can be put to use by fibers from adjacent, normally innervated skin.

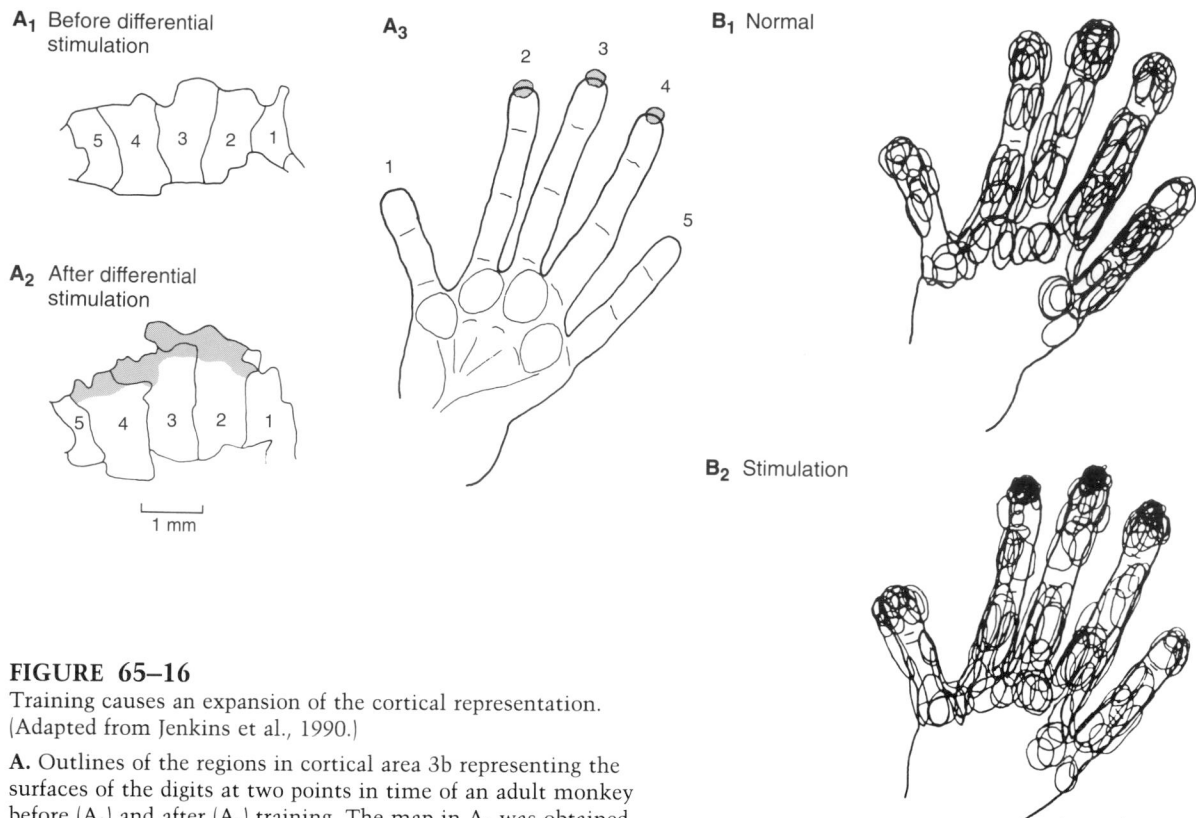

FIGURE 65–16

Training causes an expansion of the cortical representation. (Adapted from Jenkins et al., 1990.)

A. Outlines of the regions in cortical area 3b representing the surfaces of the digits at two points in time of an adult monkey before (A_1) and after (A_2) training. The map in A_1 was obtained three months prior to the onset of training. During the period of training the monkey performed a task that required repeated use, for one hour per day, of the tips of the distal phalanges of digits 2, 3, and occasionally 4 (**shaded** area at tip of digit in A_3). After a period of differential stimulation there is a substantial enlargement of the territory of representation (**shaded**) of the stimulated fingers (A_2).

B. A map of all glabrous receptive fields identified for recording sites within area 3b before differential stimulation (B_1) and after stimulation (B_2). Following the training behavior, a larger number of receptive fields is identified in the distal phalanges of the stimulated digits (2, 3, and 4).

The cortical maps of an adult are subject to constant modification on the basis of use or activity of the peripheral sensory pathways. Since all of us are brought up in somewhat different environments, are exposed to different combinations of stimuli, and are likely to exercise our motor skills in different ways, the architecture of each brain will be modified in special ways. This distinctive modification of brain architecture, along with a distinctive genetic make up, constitutes the biological basis for the expression of individuality.

Two further studies by Merzenich have provided evidence consistent with this view. First, he studied normal animals and found that the topographical maps vary considerably from one individual to another. This study, of course, did not separate the effects of different experiences from the consequences of different genetic endowment. Therefore, Merzenich, William Jenkins, and their colleagues next investigated the factors that underlie this variability. They encouraged monkeys to use their middle three fingers at the expense of other fingers by having them obtain food by contacting a rotating disc with only the middle fingers. After several thousand disc rotations, the area in the cortex devoted to the middle finger was greatly expanded. Practice, therefore, may act on preexisting patterns of connections and strengthen their effectiveness (Figure 65–16).

Reorganization is also evident at lower levels in the brain. As first illustrated by Patrick Wall and David Egger, reorganization occurs at least in part at the level of the dorsal column nuclei, which contain the first synapses of the somatic sensory system. Organizational changes are therefore probably a general property of the somatosensory system and occur throughout the somatic afferent pathway. The fact that anatomical changes occur so early in sensory processing suggests that higher centers are also capable of being influenced by experience.

Changes in the Somatotopic Map May Reflect Common Cellular Mechanisms for Associative Plasticity

What mechanisms underlie the changes in receptive fields? Recent evidence indicates that the input connections to cortical neurons in the somatic sensory system are formed on the basis of correlated activity, much as

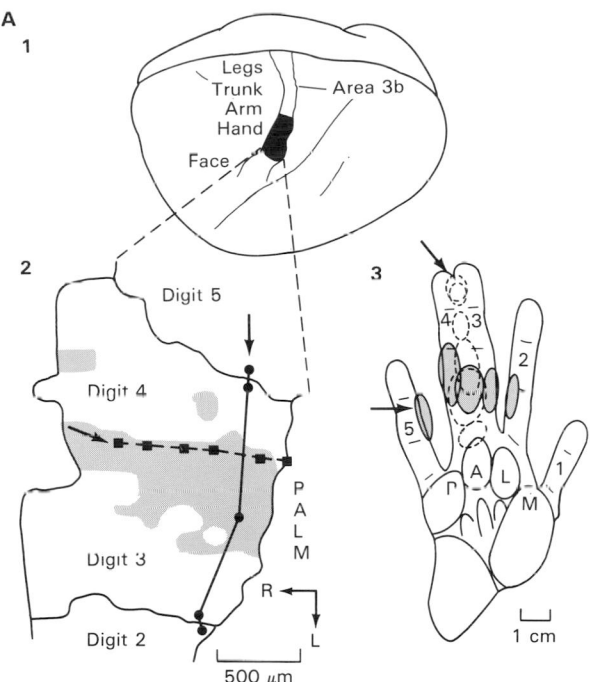

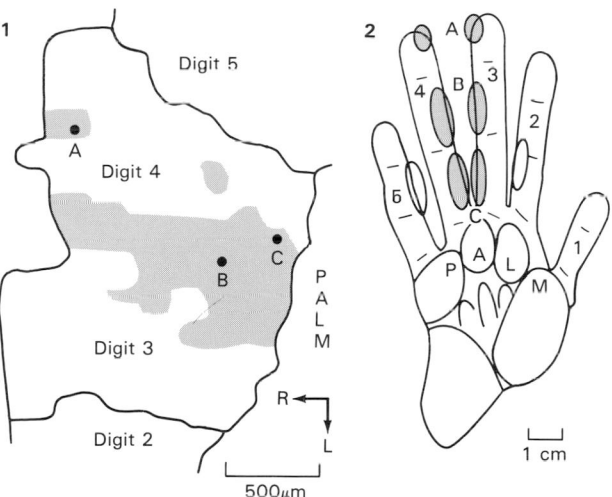

FIGURE 65–17

Cutaneous fusion of digits 3 and 4 in the adult owl monkey leads to loss of the normal discontinuities in the cortical representation of these digits. (Adapted from Clark et al., 1988.)

A. 1. Dorsolateral view of the neocortex of an owl monkey showing the representation of the contralateral skin surface, including that of the hand (shaded), in area 3b of the primary somatosensory cortex. **2.** Reconstruction of the cortical zones of representation of digits 3 and 4 and surrounding skin surfaces five and a half months after surgical fusion of these digits. The shaded area marks the representation following digit fusion. Instead of the discontinuities normally present between digits (as evident in Figures 65–14A and 65–16A), there is now a large common area, which represents the parts of the digits

that are jointly fused. Threshold stimulation of the surfaces of either one of the two fused digits evoked a cortical neuronal response within this zone. This zone ranged from 340 μm to 1000 μm in width. In contrast, the representation of the borders of the fused digits (3 and 4) with the adjacent free digits (2 and 5) remains sharp. **3.** The receptive fields for the neurons at the recording sites shown in A2.

B. Even after the fused digits are separated (**2**) the fused representations remain (**1**). Thus, the fusion of the representation of the common borders of digits 3 and 4 is achieved centrally, and does not result from peripheral regeneration that spares the site of contact.

cooperative activity shapes the development of ocular dominance columns in the visual system (Chapter 60). In each case the associative mechanisms involved seem similar to that of long-term potentiation and activity-dependent enhancement of presynaptic facilitation.

Merzenich and his colleagues tested this idea by surgically connecting the skin surfaces of the fingers of two adjacent digits on the hand of a monkey. This procedure assures that the connected fingers are always used together and therefore increases the correlation of inputs from the skin surfaces of the adjacent fingers. Increasing the correlation of activity from adjacent fingers in this way abolished the sharp discontinuity normally evident between the zones in area 3b in the somatosensory cortex that receive inputs from these digits. Thus, the *normal discontinuity* in the representation of adjacent fingers in the cortical map appears to be established not only by a genetically programmed demarcation in the pattern of connections, but also through learning, by temporal correlations in patterns of input. The normal discontinuity is

produced by synchronous activity much as are the ocular dominance columns (Figure 65–17).

Studies of Neuronal Changes with Learning Provide Insights into Psychiatric Disorders

The demonstration that learning is accompanied by changes in the effectiveness of neural connections suggests a new view of the relationship between social and biological processes in the generation of behavior. There is a tendency in medicine and psychiatry to think that biological and social determinants of behavior act on separate levels of the mind. For example, it is still customary to classify psychiatric illnesses into two major categories: organic and functional. *Organic* mental illnesses include the dementias and the toxic psychoses; *functional* mental illnesses include the various depressive syndromes, the schizophrenias, and the neurotic illnesses. This distinction dates to the nineteenth century, when neuropathologists examined the brains of patients coming to autopsy and found gross and readily demonstrable disturbances in the architecture of the brain in some psychiatric diseases but not in others. Diseases that produced anatomical evidence of brain lesions were called organic; those lacking these features were called functional.

The experiments reviewed in this chapter show that this distinction is unwarranted. Everyday events—sensory stimulation, deprivation, and learning—can cause an effective disruption of synaptic connections under some circumstances and a reactivation of connections under others. It is therefore incorrect to imply that certain diseases (organic diseases) affect mentation by producing biological changes in the brain, whereas other diseases (functional diseases) do not. The basis of contemporary neural science is that all mental processes are biological and any alteration in those processes is organic.

Rather than making the distinction along biological and nonbiological lines, it is more appropriate to ask the following questions for each type of mental illness: To what degree is this biological process determined by genetic and developmental factors, to what degree is it determined by a toxic or infectious agent, and to what degree is it environmentally or socially determined? Even those mental disturbances that are considered most socially determined must have a biological aspect, since it is the activity of the brain that is being modified. Insofar as social intervention works, whether through psychotherapy, counseling, or the support of family or friends, it must work by acting on the brain, and quite likely on the strength of connections between nerve cells. Moreover, the absence of demonstrable structural changes does not rule out the possibility that important biological changes are nevertheless occurring. They may simply be undetectable with the techniques available to us.

The work of David Hubel and Torsten Wiesel that we reviewed in Chapter 60 and the studies by Craig Bailey, William Greenough, and their colleagues make clear that demonstrating the biological nature of mental functioning will require more sophisticated anatomical methods than the light-microscopic histology of nineteenth-century pathologists. To clarify these issues it will be necessary to develop a neuropathology of mental illness that is based on anatomical function as well as on anatomical structure. Various new imaging techniques, such as positron emission tomography and magnetic resonance imaging described in Chapter 22, have opened the door to the noninvasive exploration of the human brain on a cell-biological level, the level of resolution that is required to understand the physical mechanisms of mentation and of mental disorders. As we have seen, this approach is now being pursued in the study of schizophrenia (Chapter 55).

Since structural changes in mental functions are likely to reflect alterations in gene expression, we should look for altered gene expression in all persistent mental states, normal as well as disturbed. There is now substantial evidence that the susceptibility to major psychotic illnesses—schizophrenia and manic-depressive disorders—are heritable. These illnesses reflect heritable alterations in the nucleotide sequence of DNA, leading to abnormal messenger RNA and abnormal protein. Whereas the genetic data on schizophrenia and depression indicate that these diseases involve alteration in the *structure* of genes, the cell-biological data on learning and long-term memory reviewed here suggest that neurotic illnesses, acquired by learning, are likely to involve alterations in the *regulation* of gene expression (Figure 65–18).

Development, hormones, stress, and learning are all factors that alter gene expression by modifying the binding of transcriptional activator proteins to each other and to the regulatory regions of genes. It is likely that at least some neurotic illnesses (or components of them) result from reversible defects in gene regulation, which are produced by learning and which may be due to altered binding of specific proteins to certain regulatory regions that control the expression of certain genes.

According to this view, schizophrenia and depression result primarily from heritable genetic changes in neuronal and synaptic function in a human population carrying one or more, likely several, abnormal alleles. In contrast, neurotic illnesses might result from alterations in neuronal and synaptic function produced by environmentally induced alterations in gene expression. It is intriguing to think, then, that insofar as psychotherapy is successful in bringing about substantive changes in behavior, it does so by producing alterations in gene expression.

A corollary to these arguments is that a neurotic illness should involve alterations in neuronal structure and function just as certain psychotic illnesses involve structural (anatomical) changes in the brain. Treatment of neurosis or character disorders by psychotherapeutic intervention should, if successful, also produce structural changes. Thus, we face the intriguing possibility that as brain imaging techniques improve, these techniques might ultimately be useful not only for diagnosis of various neurotic illnesses but also for evaluating the outcome of psychotherapy.

An Overall View

The cellular studies on synapse modulation reviewed here, and those on synapse formations discussed in Chapters 59 and 60, are consistent with three overlapping developmental stages of synaptic modification. The first stage, synapse formation, occurs primarily in the early stages of development and is under the control of genetic and developmental processes, commonly cell-cell interactions. The second stage, the fine tuning of newly developed synapses, occurs during critical early periods of development and requires an appropriately patterned activity in neurons usually provided by environmental stimulation. The third stage, the regulation of both the transient and long-term effectiveness of synapses, occurs daily throughout later life and also is determined by experience. An intriguing possibility is that the activity-dependent cellular mechanisms involved in associative learning may be similar to the activity-dependent mechanisms utilized during critical periods of development.

One of the implications of this view is that the potentialities for all behavior in an individual are created by genetic and developmental mechanisms acting on the

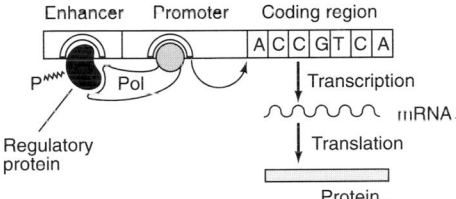

A Alteration in gene structure
in inherited psychiatric disease

1 Normal gene

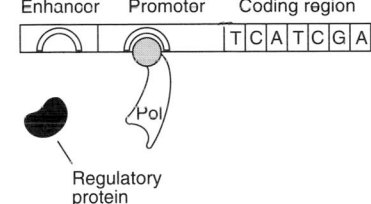

B Alteration in gene regulation
by acquired psychiatric disease

1 Gene is not expressed

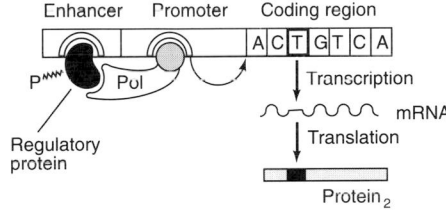

2 Mutation

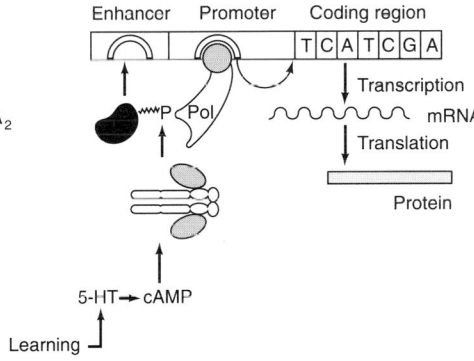

2 Gene is expressed

FIGURE 65–18

Comparison of mutation of a DNA sequence accompanying a genetic disease, leading to the expression of an altered gene, and the modulation of gene expression by environmental stimuli, leading to the activation of transcription of a previously inactive gene. For simplicity, a specific example is illustrated. The gene is illustrated as having two regions: a *coding region* that is transcribed by a mRNA and in turn is translated into a specific protein, and a *regulatory region* consisting of an *enhancer region* and a *promoter region* (see Chapter 12, Box 12–1). The enhancer and promoter are (commonly) located upstream from the coding region and regulate the initiation of the transcription of the structural gene. In this example the RNA polymerase can transcribe the gene only when families of regulatory proteins bind to the enhancer regions. For binding to occur, the regulatory protein that acts on the enhancer must first be phosphorylated.

A. 1. The phosphorylated regulatory protein binds to the enhancer segment, thereby activating the transcription of the structural gene, leading to the production of protein$_1$. **2.** A mutant form of the coding region of the structural gene is illustrated in which a single base change has occurred—a thymidine (**T**) has been substituted for cytosine (**C**). As a result, an altered mRNA is transcribed and an abnormal protein (protein$_2$) is produced, giving rise to the disease state. This alteration in gene structure is present in the germ line and is inherited.

B. 1. A specific example of alteration in expression of a normal structural gene that is not heritable. The regulatory protein is indicated in its dephosphorylated state; it therefore cannot bind to the promoter site and gene translation cannot be initiated. **2.** A learning or psychotherapeutic experience, acting in this case through serotonin and cAMP, activates the enzyme cAMP-dependent protein kinase. The catalytic unit phosphorylates the regulatory protein, which can now bind to the enhancer-segment and consequently initiates gene transcription.

brain. Environmental factors and learning bring out specific capabilities by altering the effectiveness (and anatomical connections) of preexisting pathways. It follows from this argument that everything that occurs in the brain—from the most private thoughts to commands for motor acts—are biological processes. We do not yet have the tools to examine complex ideas and feelings on the cellular level or even on the level of circuitry. But the pace of neurobiological research is quickening and in the not too distant future we may begin to have a cellular neuropsychology of human mentation, and with it a new and therapeutically more efficacious approach to mental illness.

The convergence of neurobiology and neuropsychology that we have emphasized throughout this book is filled with promise. Modern psychology has shown that the brain stores an internal representation of experience, while neurobiology has shown that this representation can be understood in terms of individual nerve cells and their interconnections. From this convergence we have gained a new perspective on perception, learning, and memory. We have also seen that the concept of mentation does not suffer by framing issues in terms of molecular biology.

Although early behaviorist psychology led the way in

exploring observable aspects of behavior, advances in modern cognitive psychology indicate that investigations that fail to consider internal representations of mental events are inadequate to account for behavior. The recognition of the importance of internal representations might have been discouraging as recently as 10 years ago, when internal mental processes were essentially inaccessible to experimental analysis. However, more recent developments in cell and molecular biology have made biological experiments on elementary aspects of internal mental processes feasible. Contrary to some expectations, biological analysis is unlikely to diminish our fascination with mentation or to make mentation trivial by reduction. Rather, cell and molecular biology have expanded our vision, allowing us to perceive previously unanticipated interrelationships between biological and psychological phenomena.

The boundary between behavioral studies and biology is arbitrary and changing. It has been imposed not by the natural contours of the disciplines, but by lack of knowledge. As our knowledge expands, the biological and behavioral disciplines will merge at certain points, and it is at these points that our understanding of mentation will rest on secure ground. As we have tried to illustrate in this book, the merger of biology and cognitive psychology is more than a sharing of methods and concepts. The joining of these two disciplines represents the emerging conviction that scientific descriptions of mentation at several different levels will all eventually contribute to a unified biological understanding of behavior.

Selected Readings

Bekkers, J. M., and Stevens, C. F. 1990. Presynaptic mechanism for long-term potentiation in the hippocampus. Nature 346: 724–728.

Bonhoeffer, T., Staiger, V., and Aertsen, A. 1989. Synaptic plasticity in rat hippocampal slice cultures: Local "Hebbian" conjunction of pre- and postsynaptic stimulation leads to distributed synaptic enhancement. Proc. Natl. Acad. Sci. U.S.A. 86:8113–8117.

Dudai, Y. 1989. The Neurobiology of Memory: Concepts, Findings, Trends. Oxford: Oxford University Press.

Kandel, E. R. 1989. Genes, nerve cells, and the remembrance of things past. J. Neuropsychiatry 1:103–125.

Kandel, E. R., and Schwartz, J. H. 1982. Molecular biology of learning: Modulation of transmitter release. Science 218:433–443.

Malinow, R. 1991. Transmission between pairs of hippocampal slice neurons: Quantal levels, oscillations and LTP. Science 252:722–724.

Merzenich, M. M., Recanzone, E. G., Jenkins, W. M., Allard, T. T., and Nudo, R. J. 1988. Cortical representational plasticity. In P. Rakic and W. Singer (eds.), Neurobiology of Neocortex. New York: Wiley, pp. 41–67.

Nicoll, R. A., Kauer, J. A., and Malenka, R. C. 1988. The current excitement in long-term potentiation. Neuron 1:97–103.

Pavlov, I. P. 1927. Conditioned Reflexes: An Investigation of the Physiological Activity of the Cerebral Cortex. G. V. Anrep (trans.) London: Oxford University Press.

Tsien, R. W., and Malinow, R. 1990. Long-term potentiation: Presynaptic enhancement following postsynaptic activation of Ca-dependent protein kinases. Cold Spring Harbor Symp. Quant. Biol. 55:147–159.

Zalutsky, R. A., and Nicoll, R. A. 1990. Comparison of two forms of long-term potentiation in single hippocampal neurons. Science 248:1619–1624.

References

Abrams, T. W., and Kandel, E. R. 1988. Is contiguity detection in classical conditioning a system or a cellular property? Learning in Aplysia suggests a possible molecular site. Trends Neurosci. 11:128–135.

Alkon, D. L. 1983. Learning in a marine snail. Sci. Am. 249(1): 70–84.

Andersen, P., Sundberg, S. H., Sveen, O., and Wigström, H. 1977. Specific long-lasting potentiation of synaptic transmission in hippocampal slices. Nature 266:736–737.

Bailey, C. H., and Chen, M. 1983. Morphological basis of long-term habituation and sensitization in Aplysia. Science 220: 91–93.

Benzer, S. 1973. Genetic dissection of behavior. Sci. Am. 229(6): 24–37.

Bergold, P. J., Sweatt, J. D., Winicov, I., Weiss, K. R., Kandel, E. R., and Schwartz, J. H. 1990. Protein synthesis during acquisition of long-term facilitation is needed for the persistent loss of regulatory subunits of the Aplysia cAMP-dependent protein kinase. Proc. Natl. Acad. Sci. U.S.A. 87:3788–3791.

Bliss, T. V. P., and Lømo, T. 1973. Long-lasting potentiation of synaptic transmission in the dentate area of the anaesthetized rabbit following stimulation of the perforant path. J. Physiol. (Lond.) 232:331–356.

Braha, O., Dale, N., Hochner, B., Klein, M., Abrams, T.W., and Kandel, E. R. 1990. Second messengers involved in the two processes of presynaptic facilitation that contribute to sensitization and dishabituation in Aplysia sensory neurons. Proc. Natl. Acad. Sci. U.S.A. 87:2040–2044.

Brons, J. F., and Woody, C. D. 1980. Long-term changes in excitability of cortical neurons after Pavlovian conditioning and extinction. J. Neurophysiol. 44:605–615.

Byrne, J. 1987. Cellular analysis of associative learning. Physiol. Rev. 67:329–439.

Carew, T. J., Hawkins, R. D., and Kandel, E. R. 1983. Differential classical conditioning of a defensive withdrawal reflex in Aplysia californica. Science 219:397–400.

Castellucci, V. F., Carew, T. J., and Kandel, E. R. 1978. Cellular analysis of long-term habituation of the gill-withdrawal reflex of Aplysia californica. Science 202:1306–1308.

Clark, S. A., Allard, T., Jenkins, W. M., and Merzenich, M. M. 1988. Receptive fields in the body-surface map in adult cortex defined by temporally correlated inputs. Nature 332:444–445.

Dash, P. K., Hochner, B., and Kandel, E. R. 1990. Injection of the cAMP responsive element into the nucleus of Aplysia sensory neurons blocks long-term facilitation. Nature 345:718–721.

Dudai, Y., Jan, Y.-N., Byers, D., Quinn, W. G., and Benzer, S. 1976. dunce, a mutant of Drosophila deficient in learning. Proc. Natl. Acad. Sci. U.S.A. 73:1684–1688.

Frost, W. N., Castellucci, V. F., Hawkins, R. D., and Kandel, E. R. 1985. Monosynaptic connections from the sensory neurons participate in the storage of long-term memory for sensitization of the gill- and siphon-withdrawal reflex in Aplysia. Proc. Natl. Acad. Sci. U.S.A. 82:8266–8269.

Greenberg, S. M., Castellucci, V. F., Bayley, H., and Schwartz, J. H. 1987. A molecular mechanism for long-term sensitization in Aplysia. Nature 329:62–65.

Greenough, W. T., and Bailey, C. H. 1988. The anatomy of a memory: Convergence of results across a diversity of tests. Trends Neurosci. 11:142–147.

Gustafsson, B., and Wigström, H. 1988. Physiological mechanisms underlying long-term potentiation. Trends Neurosci. 11:156–162.

Hawkins, R. D., Abrams, T. W., Carew, T. J., and Kandel, E. R. 1983. A cellular mechanism of classical conditioning in *Aplysia*: Activity-dependent amplification of presynaptic facilitation. Science 219:400–405.

Hebb, D. O. 1949. The Organization of Behavior: A Neuropsychological Theory. New York: Wiley.

Hoyle, G. 1979. Mechanisms of simple motor learning. Trends Neurosci. 2:153–159.

Jenkins, W. M., Merzenich, M. M., Ochs, M. T., Allard, T., and Guíc-Robles, E. 1990. Functional reorganization of primary somatosensory cortex in adult owl monkeys after behaviorally controlled tactile stimulation. J. Neurophysiol. 63:82–104.

Kaas, J. H., Nelson, R. J., Sur, M., Lin, C. S., and Merzenich, M. M. 1979. Multiple representations of the body within the primary somatosensory cortex of primates. Science 204:521–523.

Kandel, E. R., Abrams, T., Bernier, L., Carew, T. J., Hawkins, R. D., and Schwartz, J. H. 1983. Classical conditioning and sensitization share aspects of the same molecular cascade in *Aplysia*. Cold Spring Harbor Symp. Quant. Biol. 48:821–830.

Livingstone, M. S., Sziber, P. P., and Quinn, W. G. 1984. Loss of calcium/calmodulin responsiveness in adenylate cyclase of *rutabaga*, a Drosophila learning mutant. Cell 37:205–215.

Malinow, R., and Tsien, R. W. 1990. Presynaptic enhancement shown by whole-cell recordings of long-term potentiation in hippocampal slices. Nature 346:177–180.

Malinow, R., Madison, D. V., and Tsien, R. W. 1988. Persistent protein kinase activity underlying long-term potentiation. Nature 335:820–824.

Merzenich, M. M. 1984. Functional "maps" of skin sensations. In C. C. Brown (ed.), The Many Facets of Touch. The summary publication of Johnson & Johnson Pediatric Roundtable #10—Touch. Skillman, N. J.: Johnson & Johnson Baby Products Company, pp. 15–22.

Merzenich, M. M. 1985. Sources of intraspecies and interspecies cortical map variability in mammals: Conclusions and hypotheses. In M. J. Cohen and F. Strumwasser (eds.), Comparative Neurobiology: Modes of Communication in the Nervous System. New York: Wiley, pp. 105–116.

Merzenich, M. M., Kaas, J. H., Wall, J., Nelson, R. J., Sur, M., and Felleman, D. 1983. Topographic reorganization of somatosensory cortical areas 3B and 1 in adult monkeys following restricted deafferentation. Neuroscience 8:33–55.

Merzenich, M. M., Kaas, J. H., Wall, J. T., Sur, M., Nelson, R. J., and Felleman, D. J. 1983. Progression of change following median nerve section in the cortical representation of the hand in areas 3b and 1 in adult owl and squirrel monkeys. Neuroscience 10:639–665.

Merzenich, M. M., Nelson, R. J., Stryker, M. P., Cynander, M. S.,

Schoppmann, A., and Zook, J. M. 1984. Somatosensory cortical map changes following digit amputation in adult monkeys. J. Comp. Neurol. 224:591–605.

Montarolo, P. G., Goelet, P., Castellucci, V. F., Morgan, J., Kandel, E. R., and Schacher, S. 1986. A critical period for macromolecular synthesis in long-term heterosynaptic facilitation in *Aplysia*. Science 234:1249–1254.

Morris, R. G. M., Anderson, E., Lynch, G. S., and Baudry, M. 1986. Selective impairment of learning and blockade of long-term potentiation by an N-methyl-D-aspartate receptor antagonist, AP5. Nature 319:774–776.

Pons, T. P., Garraghty, P. E., and Mishkin, M. 1988. Lesion-induced plasticity in the second somatosensory cortex of adult macaques. Proc. Natl. Acad. Sci. U.S.A. 85:5279–5281.

Quinn, W. G. 1984. Work in invertebrates on the mechanisms underlying learning. In P. Marler and H. Terrace (eds.), The Biology of Learning. Dahlem Konferenzen. Berlin: Springer, pp. 197–246.

Sacktor, T. C., and Schwartz, J. H. 1990. Sensitizing stimuli cause translocation of protein kinase C in *Aplysia* sensory neurons. Proc. Natl. Acad. Sci. U.S.A. 87:2036–2039.

Sherrington, C. 1947. The Integrative Action of the Nervous System, 2nd ed. New Haven: Yale University Press.

Shuster, M. J., Camardo, J. S., Siegelbaum, S. A., and Kandel, E. R. 1985. Cyclic AMP-dependent protein kinase closes the serotonin-sensitive K^+ channels of *Aplysia* sensory neurones in cell-free membrane patches. Nature 313:392–395.

Siegelbaum, S. A., Camardo, J. S., and Kandel, E. R. 1982. Serotonin and cyclic AMP close single K^+ channels in *Aplysia* sensory neurones. Nature 299:413–417.

Snow, P. J., Nudo, R. J., Rivers, W., Jenkins, W. M., and Merzenich, M. M. 1988. Somatotopically inappropriate projections from thalamocortical neurons to the SI cortex of the cat demonstrated by the use of intracortical microstimulation. Somatosens. Res. 5:349–372.

Spencer, W. A., Thompson, R. F., and Neilson, D. R., Jr. 1966. Response decrement of the flexion reflex in the acute spinal cat and transient restoration by strong stimuli. J. Neurophysiol. 29:221–239.

Sweatt, J. D., and Kandel, E. R. 1989. Persistent and transcriptionally-dependent increase in protein phosphorylation in long-term facilitation of *Aplysia* sensory neurons. Nature 339:51–54.

Wall, P. D., and Egger, M. D. 1971. Formation of new connexions in adult rat brains after partial deafferentation. Nature 232:542–545.

Walters, E. T., and Byrne, J. H. 1983. Associative conditioning of single sensory neurons suggests a cellular mechanism for learning. Science 219:405–408.

Woody, C. D., Swartz, B. E., and Gruen, E. 1978. Effects of acetylcholine and cyclic GMP on input resistance of cortical neurons in awake cats. Brain Res. 158:373–395.

John Koester

Current Flow in Neurons

Definition of Electrical Parameters
  Potential Difference (V or E)
  Current (I)
  Conductance (g)
  Capacitance (C)

Rules for Circuit Analysis
  Conductance
  Current
  Capacitance
  Potential Difference

Current Flow in Circuits with Capacitance
  Circuit with Capacitor
  Circuit with Resistor and Capacitor in Series
  Circuit with Resistor and Capacitor in Parallel

This section reviews the basic principles of electrical circuit theory. Familiarity with this material is important for understanding the equivalent circuit model of the neuron developed in Chapters 5 through 9. The section is divided into three parts:

1. The definition of basic electrical parameters.
2. A set of rules for elementary circuit analysis.
3. A description of current flow in circuits with capacitance.

Definition of Electrical Parameters

Potential Difference (V or E)

Electrical charges exert an electrostatic force on other charges: Like charges repel, opposite charges attract. As the distance between two charges increases, the force that is exerted decreases. *Work* is done when two charges that initially are separated are brought together: *Negative work* is done if their polarities are opposite, and *positive work* if they are the same. The greater the values of the charges and the greater their initial separation, the greater the work that is done (work $- \int_r^0 f(t)\, dt$, where f is electrostatic force and r is the initial distance between the two charges). Potential difference is a measure of this work. The potential difference between two points is the work that must be done to move a unit of positive charge (1 coulomb), from one point to the other, i.e., it is the potential energy of the charge. One volt (V) is the energy required to move 1 coulomb a distance of 1 meter against a force of 1 newton.

Current (I)

A potential difference exists within a system whenever positive and negative charges are separated. Charge separation may be generated by a chemical reaction (as in a battery) or by diffusion between two electrolyte solutions with different ion concentrations across a permeability-selective barrier, such as a cell membrane. If a region of charge separation exists within a conducting medium, then charges move between the areas of potential difference: positive charges are attracted to the region with a more negative potential, and negative charges go to the regions of positive potential. The resulting movement of charges is *current flow*, which is defined as the net movement of positive charge per unit time. In metallic conductors current is carried by electrons, which move in the opposite direction of current flow. In nerve and muscle cells, current is carried by positive and negative ions in solution. One ampere (A) of current represents the movement of 1 coulomb (of charge) per second.

Conductance (g)

Any object through which electrical charges can flow is called a conductor. The unit of electrical conductance is the siemen (S). According to Ohm's law, the current that flows through a conductor is directly proportional to the potential difference imposed across it.[1]

$$I = V \times g$$

Current (A) = Potential difference (V) × Conductance (S).

As charge carriers move through a conductor, some of their potential energy is lost; it is converted into thermal energy due to the frictional interactions of the charge carriers with the conducting medium.

Each type of material has an intrinsic property called conductivity (σ), which is determined by its molecular structure. Metallic conductors have very high conductivities; they conduct electricity extremely well. Aqueous solutions with high ionized salt concentrations have somewhat lower values of σ, and lipids have very low conductivities—they are poor conductors of electricity and are therefore good insulators. The conductance of an object is proportional to σ times its cross-sectional area, divided by its length:

$$g = (\sigma) \times \frac{\text{Area}}{\text{Length}}$$

The length dimension is defined as the direction along

---

[1]Note the analogy of this formula for current flow to the other formulas for describing flow; e.g., bulk flow of a liquid due to a hydrostatic pressure; flow of a solute in response to a concentration gradient; flow of heat in response to a temperature gradient, etc. In each case flow is proportional to the product of a driving force times a conductance factor.

which one measures conductance (between *a* and *b*):

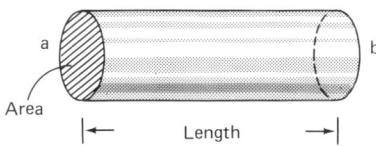

For example, the conductance measured across a piece of cell membrane is less if its length (thickness) is increased, e.g., by myelination. The conductance of a large area of membrane is greater than that of a small area of membrane.

Electrical resistance (R) is the reciprocal of conductance, and is a measure of the resistance provided by an object to current flow. Resistance is measured in ohms (Ω):

$$1 \text{ ohm} = (1 \text{ siemen})^{-1}.$$

Capacitance (C)

A capacitor consists of two conducting plates separated by an insulating layer. The fundamental property of a capacitor is its ability to store charges of opposite sign: positive charge on one plate, negative on the other.

A capacitor made up of two parallel plates with its two conducting surfaces separated by an insulator (an air gap) is shown in Figure A–1A, part 1. There is a net excess of positive charges on plate *x*, and an equal number of excess negative charges on plate *y*, resulting in a potential difference between the two plates. One can measure this potential difference by determining how much work is required to move a positive test charge from the surface of *y* to that of *x*. Initially, when the test charge is at *y*, it is attracted by the negative charges on *y*, and repelled less strongly by the more distant positive charges on *x*. The result of these electrostatic interactions is a force *f* that opposes the movement of the test charge from *y* to *x*. As the test charge is moved to the left across the gap, the attraction by the negative charges on *y* diminishes, but the repulsion by the positive charges on *x* increases, with the result that the net electrostatic force exerted on the test charge is constant everywhere between *x* and *y* (Figure A–1A, part 2). Work (*W*) is force times the distance (*D*) over which the force is exerted:

$$W = f \times D.$$

Therefore, it is simple to calculate the work done in moving the test charge from one side of the capacitor to the other. It is the shaded area under the curve in Figure A–1A, part 2. This work is equal to the difference in electrical potential energy, or potential difference, between *x* and *y*.

Capacitance is measured in farads (F). The greater the density of charges on the capacitor plates, the greater the force acting on the test charge, and the greater the resulting potential difference across the capacitor (Figure A–1B). Thus, for a given capacitor, there is a linear relationship

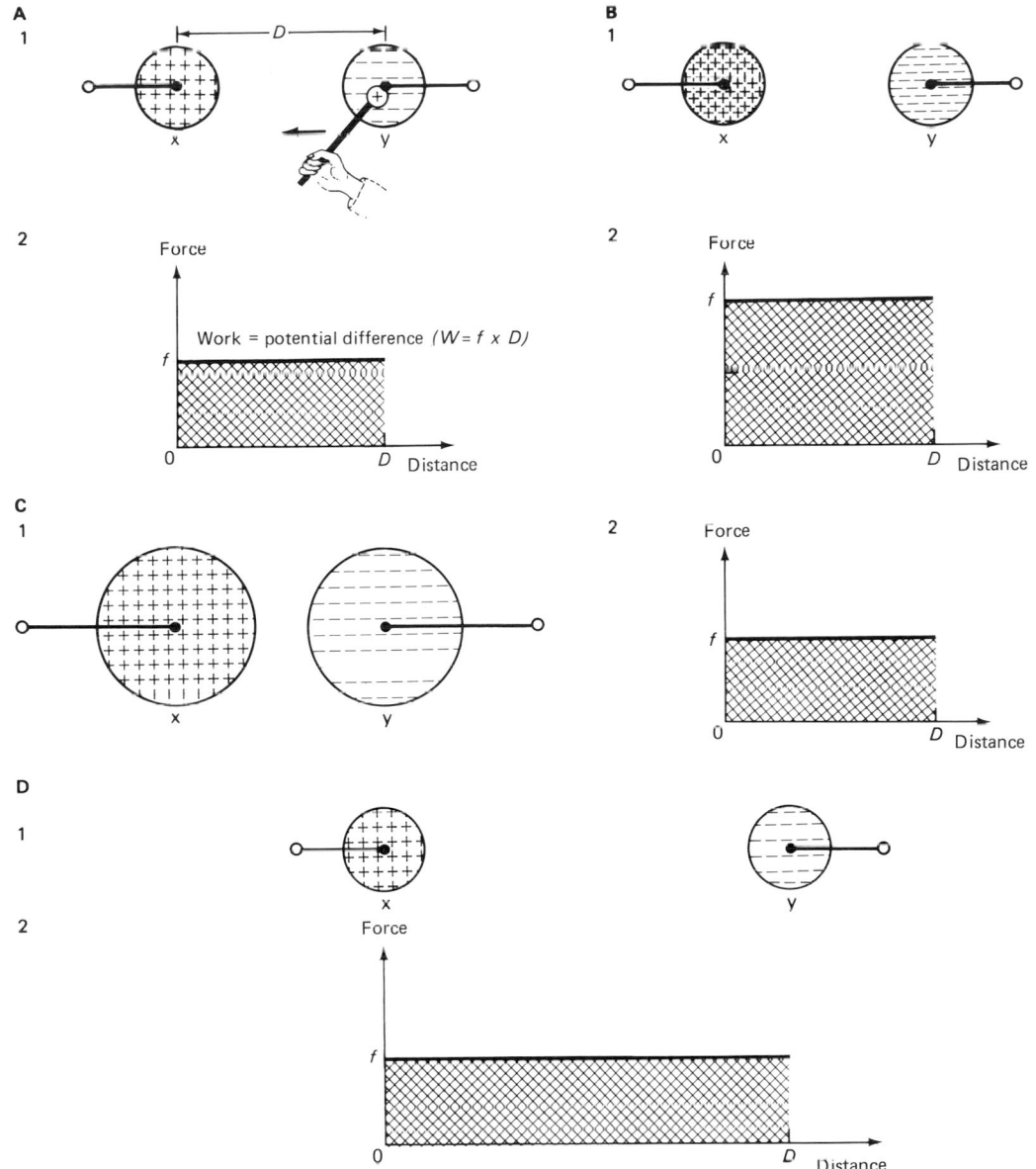

FIGURE A–1

The factors that affect the potential difference between two plates of a capacitor.

A. As a test charge is moved between two charged plates (**1**), it must overcome a force (**2**). The work done against this force is the potential difference between the two plates.

B. Increasing the charge density (**1**) increases the potential difference (**2**).

C. Increasing the area of the plates (**1**) increases the number of charges required to produce a given potential difference (**2**).

D. Increasing the distance between the two plates (**1**) increases the potential difference between them (**2**).

between the amount of charge (Q) stored on its plates and the potential difference across it:

$$Q \text{ (coulombs)} = C \text{ (farads)} \times V \text{ (volts)} \qquad (A\text{–}1)$$

where the capacitance, C, is a constant.

The capacitance of a parallel-plate capacitor is determined by two features of its geometry: the area (A) of the two plates, and the distance (D) between them. Increasing the area of the plates increases capacitance, because a greater amount of charge must be deposited on each side to produce the same charge density, which is what determines the force f acting on the test charge (Figure A 1A and C). Increasing the distance D between the plates does not change the force acting on the test charge, but it does increase the work that must be done to move it from one side of the capacitor to the other (Figures A–1A and D).

Therefore, for a given charge separation between the two plates, the potential difference between them is proportional to the distance. Put another way, the greater the distance the smaller the amount of charge that must be deposited on the plates to produce a given potential difference, and therefore the smaller the capacitance (Equation A–1). These geometrical determinants of capacitance can be summarized by the equation:

$$C \propto \frac{A}{D}.$$

As shown in Equation A–1, the separation of positive and negative charges on the two plates of a capacitor results in a potential difference between them. The converse of this statement is also true: The potential difference across a capacitor is determined by the excess of positive and negative charges on its plates. In order for the potential across a capacitor to change, the amount of electrical charges stored on the two conducting plates must change first.

Rules for Circuit Analysis

A few basic relationships that are used for circuit analysis are listed below. Familiarity with these rules will help in understanding the electric circuit examples that follow.

Conductance

This is the symbol for a conductor:

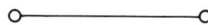

A variable conductor is represented this way:

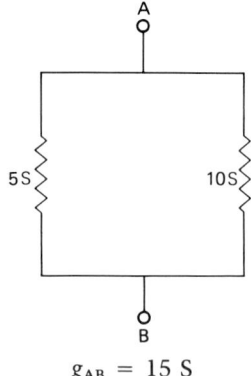

A pathway with infinite conductance (zero resistance) is called a short circuit, and is represented by a line:

Conductances in parallel add:

$g_{AB} = 15 \text{ S}$

Conductances in series add reciprocally:

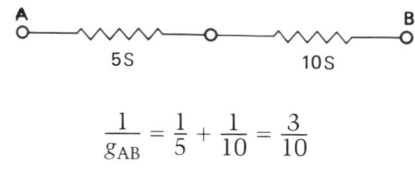

$$\frac{1}{g_{AB}} = \frac{1}{5} + \frac{1}{10} = \frac{3}{10}$$

$$g_{AB} = 3.3\text{S}.$$

Resistances in series add, while resistances in parallel add reciprocally.

Current

An *arrow* denotes the direction of current flow (net movement of positive charge).

Ohm's law is

$$I = V_g = \frac{V}{R}.$$

When current flows through a conductor, the end that the current enters is positive with respect to the end that it leaves:

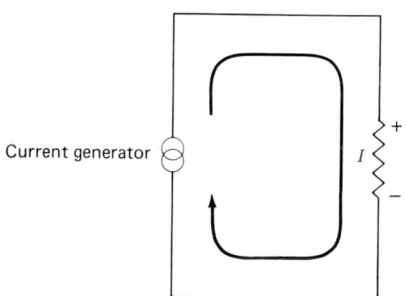

The algebraic sum of all currents entering or leaving a junction is zero (we arbitrarily define current approaching a junction as positive, and current leaving a junction as negative). In this circuit

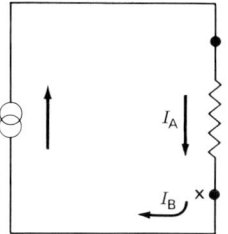

for junction x,

$$I_A = +5 \text{ A}$$

$$I_B = -5 \text{ A}$$

$$I_A + I_B = 0.$$

In this circuit

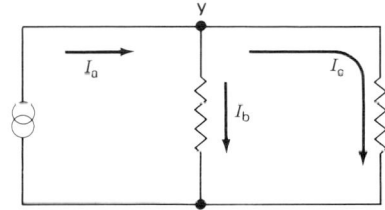

for junction y

$$I_a = +3 \text{ A}$$
$$I_b = -2 \text{ A}$$
$$I_c = -1 \text{ A}$$
$$I_a + I_b + I_c = 0.$$

Current follows the path of greatest conductance (least resistance). For conductance pathways in parallel, the current through each path is proportional to its conductance value divided by the total conductance of the parallel combination:

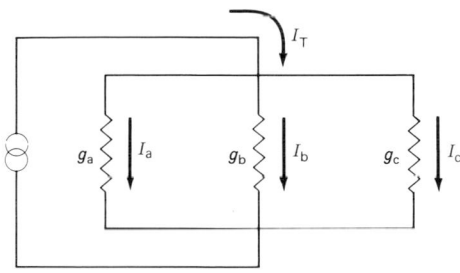

$$I_T = 10 \text{ A}$$
$$g_a = 3 \text{ S}$$
$$g_b = 2 \text{ S}$$
$$g_c = 5 \text{ S}$$

$$I_a = I_T \frac{g_a}{g_a + g_b + g_c} = 3 \text{ A}$$

$$I_b = I_T \frac{g_b}{g_a + g_b + g_c} = 2 \text{ A}$$

$$I_c = I_T \frac{g_c}{g_a + g_b + g_c} = 5 \text{ A}.$$

Capacitance

This is the symbol for a capacitor:

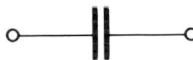

The potential difference across a capacitor is proportional to the charge stored on its plates:

$$V_C = \frac{Q}{C}.$$

Potential Difference

This is the symbol for a battery, or electromotive force. It is often abbreviated by the symbol E.

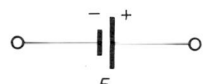

The positive pole is always represented by the longer bar.

Batteries in series add algebraically, but attention must be paid to their polarities. If their polarities are the same, their absolute values add:

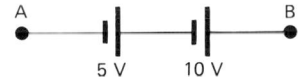

$$V_{AB} = -15 \text{ V}.$$

If their polarities are opposite, they subtract:

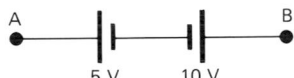

$$V_{AB} = -5 \text{ V}.$$

[The convention used here for potential difference is that $V_{AB} = (V_A - V_B)$.]

A battery drives a current around the circuit from its positive to its negative terminal:

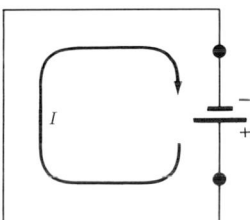

For purposes of calculating the total resistance of a circuit the internal resistance of a battery is set at zero.

The potential differences across parallel branches of a circuit are equal:

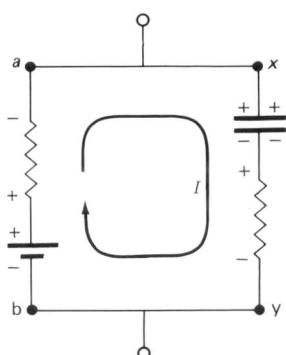

$$V_{ab} = V_{xy}.$$

As one goes around a closed loop in a circuit, the algebraic sum of all the potential differences is zero:

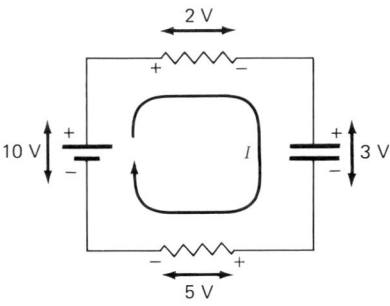

$$2\,V + 3\,V + 5\,V - 10\,V = 0.$$

Current Flow in Circuits with Capacitance

Circuits that have capacitive elements are much more complex than those that have only batteries and conductors. This complexity arises because current flow varies with time in capacitive circuits. The time dependence of the changes in current and voltage in capacitive circuits is illustrated qualitatively in the following three examples.

Circuit with Capacitor

Current does not actually flow across the insulating gap in a capacitor; rather it results in a build-up of positive and negative charges on the capacitor plates. However, we can measure a current flowing into and out of the terminals of a capacitor. Consider the circuit shown in Figure A–2A. When switch S is closed (Figure A–2B), a net positive charge is moved by the battery E onto plate a, and an equal amount of net positive charge is withdrawn from plate b. The result is current flowing counterclockwise in the circuit. Since the charges that carry this current flow into or out of the terminals of a capacitor, building up an excess of plus and minus charges on its plates, it is called a *capacitive current* (I_c). Because there is no resistance in this circuit, the battery E can generate a very large amplitude of current, which will charge the capacitance to a value $Q = E \times C$ in an infinitesimally short period of time (Figure A–2D).

Circuit with Resistor and Capacitor in Series

Now consider what happens if a resistor is added in series with the capacitor in the circuit shown in Figure A–3A. The maximum current that can be generated when switch

FIGURE A–2
Time course of charging a capacitor.
A. Circuit before the switch (S) is closed.
B. Immediately after the switch is closed.

C. After the capacitor has become fully charged.
D. Time course of changes in I_c and V_c in response to closing of the switch.

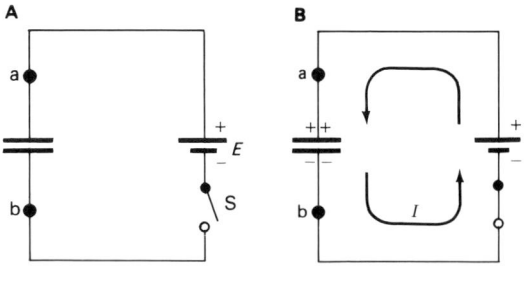
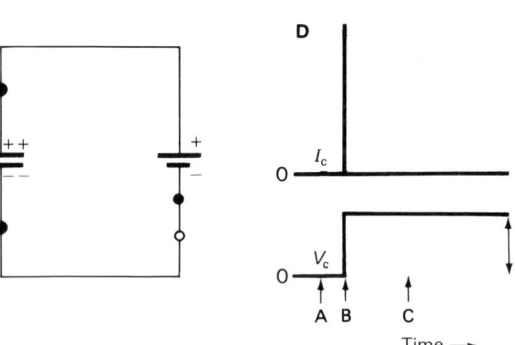

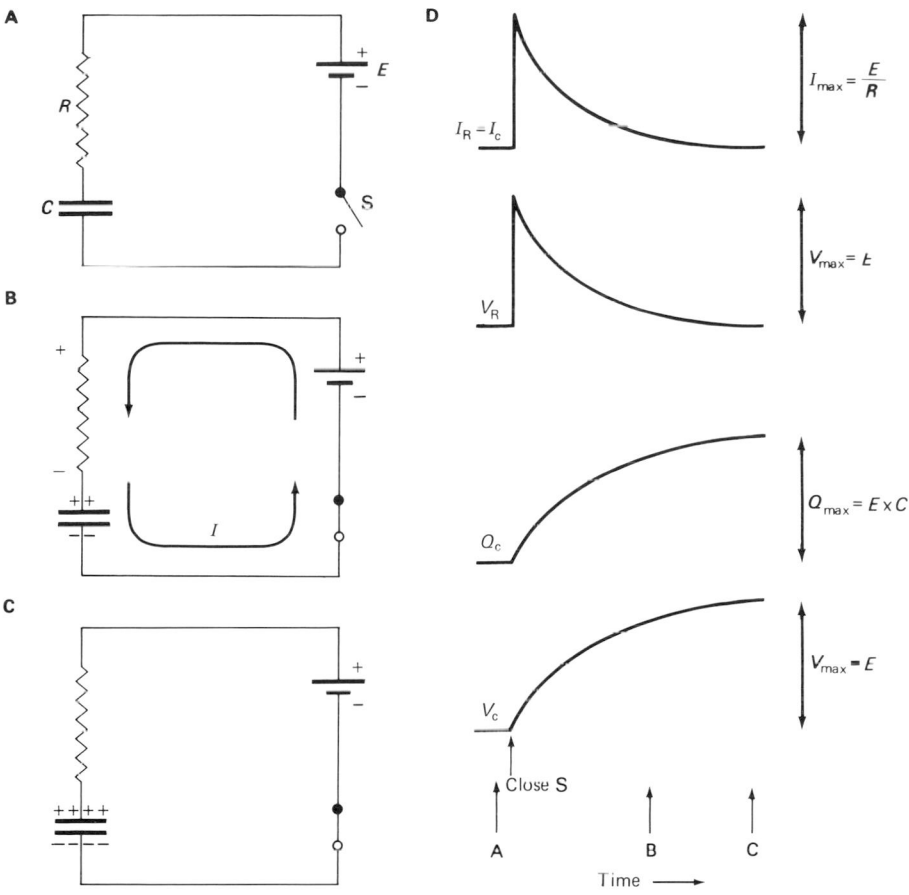

FIGURE A–3

Time course of charging a capacitor in series with a resistor, from a constant voltage source (**E**).

A. Circuit before the switch (**S**) is closed.

B. Shortly after the switch is closed.

C. After the capacitor has settled at its new potential.

D. Time course of current flow, of the increase in charge deposited on the capacitor, and of the increased potential differences across the resistor and the capacitor.

S is closed (Figure A–3B) is now limited by Ohm's law ($I = V/R$). Therefore, the capacitor charges more slowly. When the potential across the capacitor has finally reached the value $V_c = Q/C = E$ (Figure A–3C), there is no longer a difference in potential around the loop; i.e., the battery voltage (E) is equal and opposite to the voltage across the capacitor, V_c. The two thus cancel out, and there is no source of potential difference left to drive a current around the loop. Immediately after the switch is closed the potential difference is greatest, so current flow is at a maximum. As the capacitor begins to charge, however, the net potential difference ($V_c + E$) available to drive a current becomes smaller, so that current flow is reduced. The result is that an exponential change in voltage and in current flow occurs across the resistor and the capacitor.

Note that in this circuit resistive current must equal capacitative current at all times (see Rules for Circuit Analysis, above).

Circuit with Resistor and Capacitor in Parallel

Consider now what happens if we place a parallel resistor and capacitor combination in series with a constant current generator that generates a current I_T (Figure A–4). When switch S is closed (Figure A–4B), current starts to flow around the loop. Initially, in the first instant of time after the current flow begins, all of the current flows into the capacitor, i.e., $I_T = I_c$. However, as charge builds up on the plates of the capacitor, a potential difference V_c is gen-

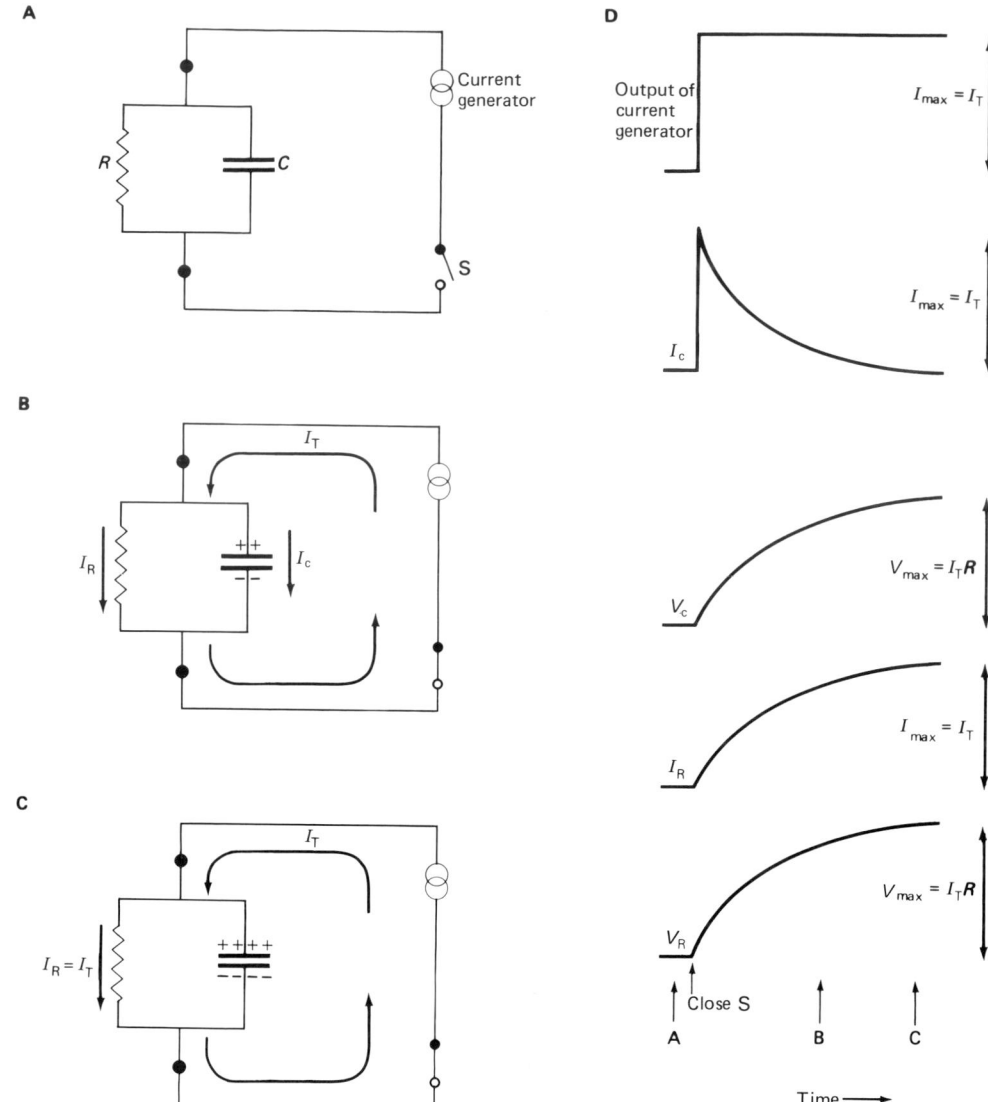

FIGURE A–4

Time course of charging a capacitor in parallel with a resistor, from a constant current source.

A. Circuit before the switch (**S**) is closed.

B. Shortly after the switch is closed.

C. After the charge deposited on the capacitor has reached its final value.

D. Time course of changes in I_c, V_c, I_R, and V_R in response to closing of the switch.

erated across it. Since the resistor and capacitor are in parallel, the potential across them must be equal; thus, part of the total current begins to flow through the resistor, such that $I_R R = V_R = V_c$. As less and less current flows into the capacitor, its rate of charging will become slower; this accounts for the exponential shape of the curve of voltage versus time. Eventually, a plateau is reached at which the voltage no longer changes. When this occurs, all of the current flows through the resistor, and $V_c = V_R = I_T R$.

John C. M. Brust

Cerebral Circulation: Stroke

The Blood Supply of the Brain Can Be Divided into Arterial Territories

The Cerebral Vessels Have Unique Physiological Responses

A Stroke Is the Result of Disease Involving Blood Vessels

Clinical Vascular Syndromes May Follow Vessel Occlusion, Hypoperfusion, or Hemorrhage

Infarction Can Occur in the Middle Cerebral Artery Territory

Infarction Can Occur in the Anterior Cerebral Artery Territory

Infarction Can Occur in the Posterior Cerebral Artery Territory

The Anterior Choroidal and Penetrating Arteries Can Become Occluded

The Carotid and Basilar Arteries Can Become Occluded

Diffuse Hypoperfusion Can Cause Ischemia or Infarction

The Rupture of Microaneurysms Causes Intraparenchymal Stroke

The Rupture of Saccular Aneurysms Causes Subarachnoid Hemorrhage

Stroke Alters the Vascular Physiology of the Brain

The brain is highly vulnerable to disturbance of the blood supply; anoxia and ischemia lasting only seconds can cause neurological symptoms and within minutes can cause irreversible neuronal damage.

Blood flow to the central nervous system must efficiently deliver oxygen, glucose, and other nutrients and remove carbon dioxide, lactic acid, and other metabolic products. The cerebral vasculature has unique anatomical and physiological features that serve to protect the brain from circulatory compromise. When these protective mechanisms fail the result is a stroke. Broadly defined, the term *stroke*, or *cerebrovascular accident*, refers to the neurological symptoms and signs, usually focal and acute, that result from diseases involving blood vessels.

The Blood Supply of the Brain Can Be Divided into Arterial Territories

Figure B–1 is a schematic illustration of the brain's blood vessels. Each cerebral hemisphere is supplied by an *internal carotid artery*, which arises from a common carotid artery beneath the angle of the jaw, enters the cranium through the carotid foramen, traverses the cavernous sinus (giving off the *ophthalmic* artery), penetrates the dura, and divides into the anterior and middle cerebral arteries. The large surface branches of the *anterior cerebral artery* supply the cortex and white matter of the inferior frontal lobe, the medial surface of the frontal and parietal lobes, and the anterior corpus callosum. Smaller penetrating branches supply the deeper cerebrum and diencephalon, including limbic structures, the head of the caudate, and the anterior limb of the internal capsule. The large surface branches of the *middle cerebral artery* supply most of the

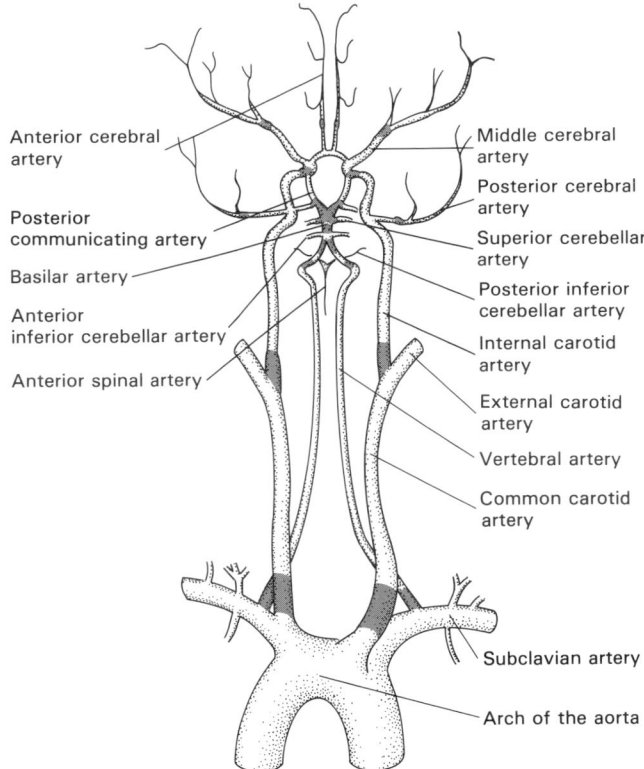

FIGURE B–1

The blood vessels of the brain. The circle of Willis is made up of the proximal posterior cerebral arteries, the posterior communicating arteries, the internal carotid arteries just before their bifurcations, the proximal anterior cerebral arteries, and the anterior communicating artery. **Dark areas:** common sites of atherosclerosis and occlusion. (Adapted from Barnett, 1988.)

cortex and white matter of the hemisphere's convexity, including the frontal, parietal, temporal, and occipital lobes, and the insula. Smaller penetrating branches (the lenticulostriate arteries) supply the deep white matter and diencephalic structures such as the posterior limb of the internal capsule, the putamen, the outer globus pallidus, and the body of the caudate. After the internal carotid emerges from the cavernous sinus, it also gives off the *anterior choroidal artery*, which supplies the anterior hippocampus and, at a caudal level, the posterior limb of the internal capsule.

Each vertebral artery arises from a subclavian artery, enters the cranium through the foramen magnum, and gives off an *anterior spinal artery* and a *posterior inferior cerebellar artery*. The vertebral arteries join at the junction of the pons and the medulla to form the *basilar artery*, which at the level of the pons gives off the *anterior inferior cerebellar artery* and the *internal auditory artery* and at the midbrain the *superior cerebellar artery*. The basilar artery then divides into the two *posterior cerebral arteries*, which supply the inferior temporal and medial occipital lobes and the posterior corpus callosum; the smaller penetrating branches of these vessels (the thalamoperforant and thalamogeniculate arteries) supply diencephalic structures, including the thalamus and the subthalamic nuclei, as well as parts of the midbrain.

These arterial territories are shown schematically in Figure B–2. Figures B–3, B–4, and B–5 are computerized tomography (CT) scans demonstrating infarctions in the territories of the anterior, middle, and posterior cerebral arteries, respectively.

Interconnections between blood vessels (anastomoses) protect the brain when part of its vascular supply is

FIGURE B–2

Cerebral arterial areas.

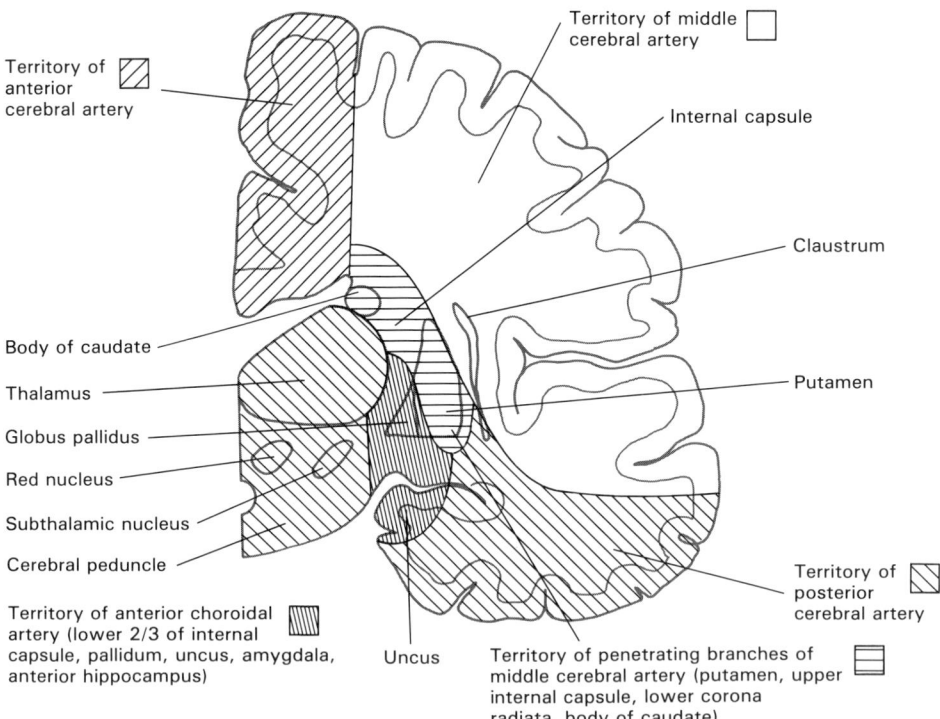

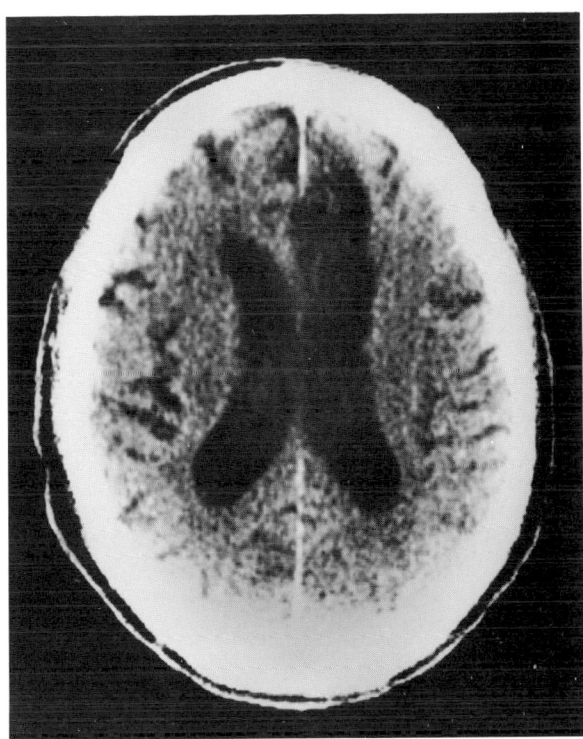

FIGURE B–3
CT scan showing infarction **(dark area)** in the territory of the anterior cerebral artery. (Courtesy Dr. Allan J. Schwartz.)

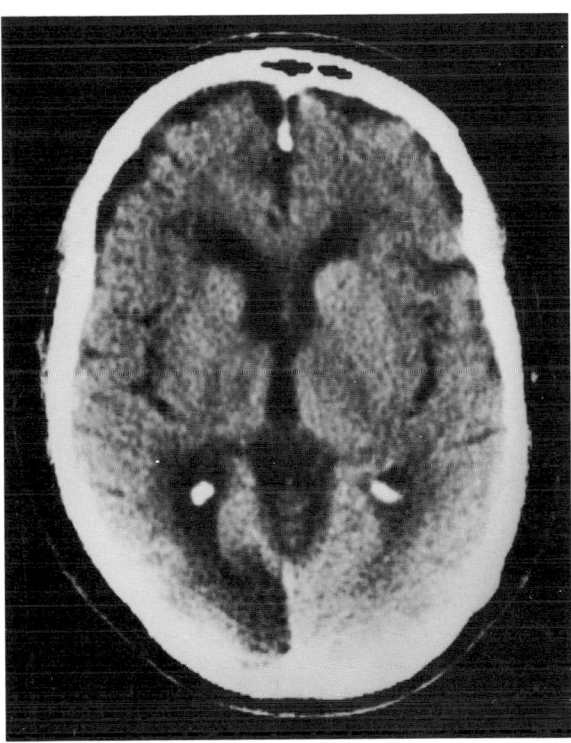

FIGURE B–5
CT scan showing infarction **(dark area)** in the territory of the posterior cerebral artery. (Courtesy Dr. Allan J. Schwartz.)

FIGURE B–4
CT scan showing infarction **(dark area)** in the territory of the middle cerebral artery. (Courtesy Dr. Allan J. Schwartz.)

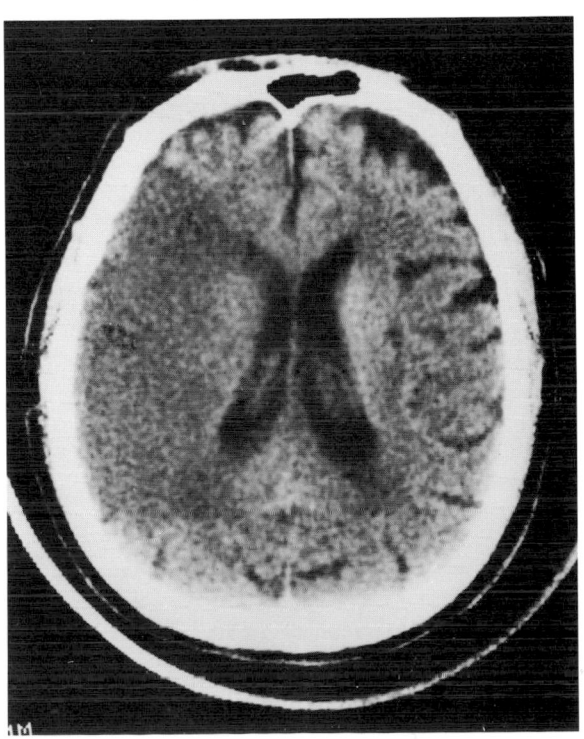

blocked. At the *circle of Willis* the two anterior cerebral arteries are connected by the anterior communicating artery, and the posterior cerebral arteries are connected to the internal carotid arteries by the posterior communicating arteries. The circle of Willis provides an overlapping blood supply. A congenitally incomplete circle, which is common in the general population, is much more frequent in patients who have had strokes. Other important anastomoses include connections between the ophthalmic artery and branches of the external carotid artery through the orbit, and connections at the brain surface between branches of the middle, anterior, and posterior cerebral arteries (sharing border-zones or watersheds). The angiograms in Figure B–6 show occlusion of the middle cerebral artery with retrograde filling through anastomoses. The small penetrating vessels arising from the circle of Willis and proximal major arteries tend to lack anastomoses. The deep brain regions they supply are therefore called endzones.

The Cerebral Vessels Have Unique Physiological Responses

Although the human brain constitutes only 2% of the total weight of the body, it receives about 15% of the cardiac output and its oxygen consumption is approxi-

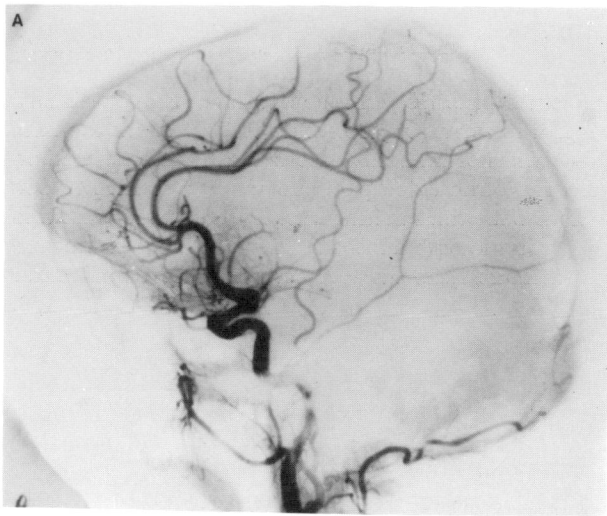

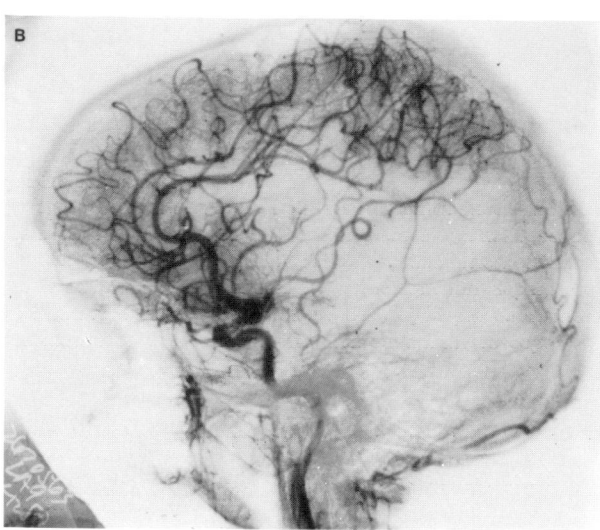

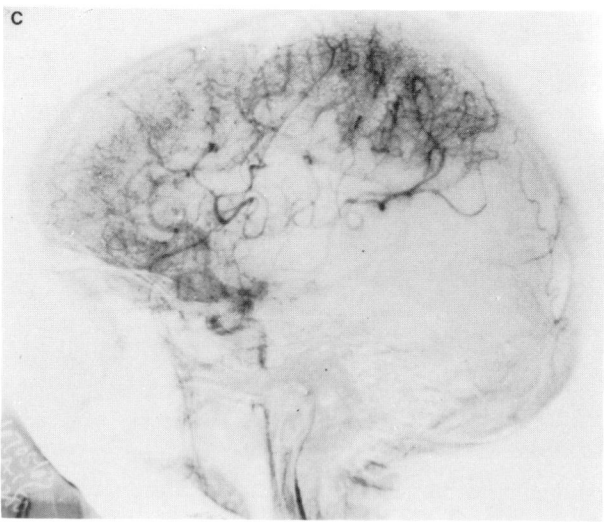

mately 20% of that for the total body. These values reflect the high metabolic rate and oxygen requirements of the brain. The total blood flow to the brain is about 750–1000 ml/min; about 350 ml of this amount flows through each carotid artery and about 100–200 ml flows through the vertebrobasilar system. Flow per unit mass of gray matter is approximately four times that of white matter.

Cerebral vessels are capable of altering their own diameter and can respond in a unique fashion to altered physiological conditions. Two main types of autoregulation exist. Brain arterioles constrict when the systemic blood pressure is raised and dilate when it is lowered. Both of these adjustments help to maintain optimal cerebral blood flow. The result is that normal individuals have a constant cerebral blood flow between mean arterial pressures of approximately 60–150 mm Hg. Above or below these pressures cerebral blood flow rises or falls linearly.

The second type of autoregulation involves blood or tissue gases and pH. When arterial P_{CO_2} is raised, brain arterioles dilate and cerebral blood flow increases; with hypocarbia there is vasoconstriction and cerebral blood flow decreases. The response is very sensitive: Inhalation of 5% CO_2 increases cerebral blood flow by 50% and 7% doubles it. Changing arterial P_{O_2} causes an opposite and less pronounced response: Breathing 100% O_2 lowers cerebral blood flow by about 13%; 10% O_2 raises it by 35%. The mechanism of these responses is uncertain. The influence of P_{CO_2} is probably mediated by alterations in extracellular pH. Local concentrations of K^+ and adenosine, both of which cause vasodilation in animals, may play a role. Whatever the mechanism, these responses not only protect the brain by increasing the delivery of oxygen and removal of acid metabolites in the presence of hypoxia, ischemia, or tissue damage; they also allow nearly instantaneous adjustments of regional cerebral blood flow to meet the demands of rapidly changing oxygen and glucose metabolism that accompany normal brain activities. For example, viewing a complex scene will increase oxygen and glucose consumption in the visual cortex of the occipital lobes (see Figure 22–6). The resulting increased carbon dioxide concentration and lowered pH in the area cause an immediate local increase in blood flow.

FIGURE B–6

These angiograms demonstrate the importance of anastomoses in that they allow retrograde filling after occlusion of the middle cerebral artery.

A. Occlusion of the middle cerebral artery results in no filling in the middle cerebral distribution.

B. Retrograde filling of the middle cerebral artery has begun via distal anastomotic branches of the anterior cerebral artery.

C. Retrograde filling of the middle cerebral artery continues at a time when little contrast material is seen in the anterior cerebral artery. (Courtesy Dr. Margaret Whelan and Dr. Sadek Hilal.)

A Stroke Is the Result of Disease Involving Blood Vessels

Diseases of the blood vessels are among the most frequent serious neurological disorders, ranking third as a cause of death in the adult population in the United States and probably first as a cause of chronic functional incapacity. Approximately 2,000,000 people living in the United States today are impaired by the neurological consequences of cerebrovascular disease. Many of them are between the ages of 25 and 64 years.

Strokes are either *occlusive* (due to closure of a blood vessel) or *hemorrhagic* (due to bleeding from a vessel). Insufficiency of blood supply is termed *ischemia*; if it is temporary, symptoms and signs may clear with little or no pathological evidence of tissue damage. *Ischemia* is not synonymous with *anoxia*, for a reduced blood supply deprives tissue not only of oxygen, but of glucose as well, and also prevents the removal of potentially toxic metabolites such as lactic acid. When ischemia is sufficiently severe and prolonged, neurons and other cellular elements die; this condition is called *infarction*.

Hemorrhage may occur at the brain surface (*extraparenchymal*), for example, from rupture of congenital aneurysms at the circle of Willis, causing *subarachnoid hemorrhage*. Alternatively, hemorrhage may be *intraparenchymal*—from rupture of vessels damaged by longstanding hypertension—and may cause a blood clot or *hematoma* within the cerebral hemispheres, in the brain stem, or in the cerebellum. Hemorrhage may result in ischemia or infarction. The mass effect of an intracerebral hematoma may limit the blood supply of adjacent brain tissue. By mechanisms that are not understood, subarachnoid hemorrhage may cause reactive vasospasm of cerebral surface vessels, leading to further ischemic brain damage.

Although most occlusive strokes are due to atherosclerosis and thrombosis and most hemorrhagic strokes are associated with hypertension or aneurysms, strokes of either type may occur at any age from many causes that include cardiac disease, trauma, infection, neoplasm, blood dyscrasia, vascular malformation, immunological disorder, and exogenous toxins. Diagnostic strategies and treatment should vary accordingly. We shall examine, however, the anatomical and physiological principles relevant to *any* occlusive or hemorrhagic stroke.

Clinical Vascular Syndromes May Follow Vessel Occlusion, Hypoperfusion, or Hemorrhage

Infarction Can Occur in the Middle Cerebral Artery Territory

Infarction in the territory of the middle cerebral artery (cortex and white matter) causes the most frequently encountered stroke syndrome, with contralateral weakness, sensory loss, and homonymous hemianopsia, and, depending on the hemisphere involved, either language distur-

bance or impaired spatial perception. Weakness and sensory loss affect the face and arm more than the leg because of the somatotopy of the motor and sensory cortex (pre- and postcentral gyri): The face and arm lie on the convexity, whereas the leg resides on the medial surface of the hemisphere. Motor and sensory loss are greatest in the hand, for the more proximal limbs and the trunk tend to have greater representation in both hemispheres. Paraspinal muscles, for example, are hardly ever weak in unilateral cerebral lesions. Similarly, the facial muscles of the forehead and the muscles of the pharynx and jaw are represented in both hemispheres and therefore are usually spared. Tongue weakness is variable. If weakness is severe (plegia), muscle tone is usually decreased at first but gradually increases over days or weeks to spasticity with hyperactive tendon reflexes. A Babinski sign, reflecting upper motor neuron disturbance (Chapter 35), is usually present from the outset. When weakness is mild, or during recovery, there may be clumsiness or slowness of movement out of proportion to loss of strength; such motor disability may resemble parkinsonian bradykinesia or even cerebellar ataxia.

Acutely, there is often weakness of contralateral conjugate gaze as a result of damage to the convexity of the cortex anterior to the motor cortex (the frontal eye field). The reason this gaze paralysis persists for only 1 or 2 days, even when other signs remain severe, is not clear.

Sensory loss tends to involve discriminative and proprioceptive modalities more than affective modalities. Pain and temperature sensation may be impaired or seem altered but are usually not lost. Joint position sense, however, may be severely disturbed, causing limb ataxia, and there may be loss of two-point discrimination, astereognosis (inability to recognize a held object by tactile sensation), or failure to appreciate a touch stimulus if another is simultaneously delivered to the normal side of the body (extinction).

Visual field impairment (homonymous hemianopsia) is the result of damage to the optic radiations, the deep fiber tracts connecting the thalamic lateral geniculate body to the visual (calcarine) cortex. If the parietal radiation is primarily involved, the visual field loss may be an inferior quadrantanopsia, whereas in temporal lobe lesions quadrantanopsia may be superior.

As we have seen in Chapter 53, in more than 95% of right-handed persons and in the majority of left-handed individuals, the left hemisphere is dominant for language. Destruction of left opercular (perisylvian) cortex in such patients causes aphasia, which may take several forms depending on the degree and distribution of the damage. Frontal opercular lesions tend to produce particular difficulty with speech output and writing with relative preservation of language comprehension (Broca's aphasia), whereas infarction of the posterior superior temporal gyrus tends to cause severe difficulty in speech comprehension and reading (Wernicke's aphasia). When opercular damage is widespread, there is severe disturbance of mixed type (global aphasia).

Left-hemisphere convexity damage, especially parietal, may also cause motor apraxia, a disturbance of learned motor acts not explained by weakness or incoordination, with the ability to perform the act when the setting is altered (Chapters 53 and 54). For example, a patient unable to imitate lighting a match might be able to perform the act normally if given an actual match to strike.

Right-hemisphere convexity infarction, especially parietal, tends to cause disturbances of spacial perception. There may be difficulty in copying simple pictures or diagrams (constructional apraxia), in interpreting maps or finding one's way about (topographagnosia), or in putting on one's clothes properly (dressing apraxia). Awareness of space and the patient's own body contralateral to the lesion may be particularly affected (hemi-inattention or hemineglect). Patients may fail to recognize their hemiplegia (anosognosia), left arm (asomatognosia), or any external object to the left of their own midline. Such phenomena may occur independently of visual field defects and in patients otherwise mentally quite intact.

Particular types of language or spatial dysfunction tend to follow occlusion, not of the proximal stem of the middle cerebral artery, but of one of its several main pial branches. In such circumstances, other signs (e.g., weakness or visual field loss) may not be present. Similarly, occlusion of the Rolandic branch of the middle cerebral artery may cause motor and sensory loss affecting the face and arm without disturbance of vision, language, or spatial perception.

Infarction Can Occur in the Anterior Cerebral Artery Territory

Infarction in the territory of the anterior cerebral artery causes weakness and sensory loss qualitatively similar to that of convexity lesions but affects mainly the distal contralateral leg. There may be urinary incontinence, but it is uncertain whether this is due to a lesion of the paracentral lobule (medial hemispheric motor and sensory cortices) or of a more anterior region concerned with the inhibition of bladder emptying. Damage to the supplementary motor cortex may cause speech disturbance, considered aphasic by some and a type of motor inertia by others. Involvement of the anterior corpus callosum may cause apraxia of the left arm (sympathetic apraxia), which is attributed to disconnection of the left (language-dominant) hemisphere from the right motor cortex.

Bilateral anterior cerebral artery territory infarction (occurring, for example, when both arteries arise anomalously from a single trunk) may cause a severe behavioral disturbance, with profound apathy, motor inertia, and muteness, attributed variably to destruction of the inferior frontal lobes (orbitofrontal cortex), deeper limbic structures, supplementary motor cortices, or cingulate gyri.

Infarction Can Occur in the Posterior Cerebral Artery Territory

Infarction in the territory of the posterior cerebral artery causes contralateral homonymous hemianopsia by destroying the calcarine cortex. Macular (central) vision tends to be spared because the occipital pole, where macular vision is represented, receives blood supply from the middle cerebral artery. If the lesion is on the left and the posterior corpus callosum is affected, there may be alexia (without aphasia or agraphia), attributed to disconnection of the seeing right occipital cortex from the language-dominant left hemisphere. If infarction is bilateral (e.g., following thrombosis at the point where both posterior cerebral arteries arise from the basilar artery), there may be cortical blindness with failure of the patient to recognize that he cannot see (Anton's syndrome), or, as a result of bilateral damage to the inferomedial temporal lobes, memory disturbance.

If posterior cerebral artery occlusion is proximal, the lesion may include, or especially affect, the following structures: the thalamus, causing contralateral hemisensory loss and sometimes spontaneous pain and dysesthesia (thalamic pain syndrome); the subthalamic nucleus, causing contralateral severe proximal chorea (hemiballismus); or even the midbrain, with ipsilateral oculomotor palsy and contralateral hemiparesis or ataxia from involvement of the corticospinal tract or the crossed superior cerebellar peduncle (dentatothalamic tract).

The Anterior Choroidal and Penetrating Arteries Can Become Occluded

Anterior choroidal artery occlusion can cause contralateral hemiplegia and sensory loss from involvement of the posterior limb of the internal capsule and homonymous hemianopsia from involvement of the thalamic lateral geniculate nucleus.

As mentioned above, the deeper cerebral white matter and diencephalon are supplied by small penetrating arteries, variably called the lenticulostriates, the thalamogeniculates, or the thalamoperforates, which arise from the circle of Willis or the proximal portions of the middle, anterior, and posterior cerebral arteries. These end-arteries lack anastomotic interconnections, and occlusion of individual vessels, usually in association with hypertensive damage to the vessel wall, causes small (less than 1.5 cm in diameter) infarcts (lacunes), which, if critically located, are followed by characteristic syndromes. For example, lacunes in the pyramidal tract area of the internal capsule cause pure hemiparesis, with arm and leg weakness of equal severity, but little or no sensory loss, visual field disturbance, aphasia, or spatial disruption. Lacunes in the ventral posterior nucleus of the thalamus produce pure hemisensory loss, with discriminative and affective modalities both involved and little motor, visual, language, or spatial disturbance. Most lacunes occur in redundant areas, e.g., nonpyramidal corona radiata, and so are asymptomatic. If bilateral and numerous, however, they may cause a characteristic syndrome (état lacunaire) of progressive dementia, shuffling gait, and pseudobulbar palsy (spastic dysarthria and dysphagia, with lingual and pharyngeal paralysis and hyperactive palate and gag reflexes, plus lability of emotional response, with abrupt crying or laughing out of proportion to mood).

The Carotid and Basilar Arteries Can Become Occluded

Atherothrombotic vessel occlusion often occurs in the internal carotid artery rather than the intracranial vessels. Particularly in a patient with an incomplete circle of Willis, infarction may then include the territories of both the middle and anterior cerebral arteries, with arm and leg weakness and sensory loss equally severe. Alternatively, infarction may be limited to the distal shared territory of these vessels (border zones), producing, by destruction of the motor cortex at the upper cerebral convexity, weakness limited to the arm or the leg. Another cause of leg weakness and sensory loss in association with a convexity syndrome is occlusion of the middle cerebral artery at its proximal stem; capsular (and other diencephalic) structures supplied by the middle cerebral artery's lenticulostriate branches are then affected in addition to the cortex of the cerebral convexity.

The medial and lateral syndromes of brain stem infarction have been discussed in Chapter 46. To recapitulate briefly, lateral syndromes—for example, following lateral medullary infarction, with vertigo, nystagmus, ipsilateral limb ataxia, loss of pain and temperature sensation on the ipsilateral face and contralateral arm and leg, and ipsilateral ptosis, miosis, and facial anhidrosis (Horner's syndrome)—result from the occlusion of large branches of the vertebral or basilar arteries supplying the lateral brain stem and cerebellum. Medial syndromes—for example, following medial pontine infarction with ipsilateral abducens, gaze or facial palsy and contralateral hemiparesis—result from occlusion of small paramedian penetrating vertebral or basilar artery branches.

In fact, most brain stem infarcts follow occlusion of the vertebral or basilar arteries, and the resulting symptoms and signs are less stereotyped than classical descriptions imply. Involvement of the posterior fossa structures in an infarct is suggested by (1) bilateral long tract (motor or sensory) signs, (2) crossed (e.g., left face and right limb) motor or sensory signs, (3) cerebellar signs, (4) stupor or coma (from involvement of the ascending reticular activating system), (5) disconjugate eye movements or nystagmus, including the syndrome of internuclear ophthalmoplegia (medial longitudinal fasciculus syndrome), and (6) involvement of cranial nerves not usually affected by single hemispheric infarcts (e.g., unilateral deafness or pharyngeal weakness).

Diffuse Hypoperfusion Can Cause Ischemia or Infarction

Brain ischemia or infarction may accompany diffuse hypoperfusion (shock), and in such circumstances the most vulnerable regions are often the border zones between large arterial territories and the end zones of deep penetrating vessels. Whatever the cause of reduced cerebral perfusion, signs tend to be bilateral. There may be paralysis and sensory loss in both arms (from bilateral infarction of the cortex at the junction of the middle and anterior arterial supply, affecting the arm area of the motor and sensory cortex). These may be disturbed vision or memory (from infarction of occipital or temporal lobes at the junction of middle and posterior cerebral arterial supply). There may also be ataxia (from cerebellar border zone infarction) or abnormal movements such as chorea or myoclonus (presumably from involvement of basal ganglia). Such signs may exist alone or in combination and may be accompanied by a variety of aphasic or other cognitive disturbances.

The Rupture of Microaneurysms Causes Intraparenchymal Stroke

The two most common causes of hemorrhagic stroke, hypertensive intra-axial hemorrhage and rupture of saccular aneurysm, tend to occur at particular sites and to cause recognizable syndromes. Hypertensive intercerebral hemorrhage is the result of damage to the same small penetrating vessels which, when occluded, cause lacunes; in this instance, however, the damaged vessels develop weakened walls (Charcot–Bouchard microaneurysms) that eventually rupture. The most common sites are the putamen, thalamus, pons, internal capsule and corona radiata, and cerebellum. Large diencephalic hemorrhages tend to cause stupor and hemiplegia and have a high mortality rate.

With lesions of the putamen, the eyes are usually deviated ipsilaterally (due to disruption of capsular pathways descending from the frontal eye field), whereas with thalamic hemorrhage the eyes tend to be deviated downward and the pupils may not react to light (due to involvement of midbrain pretectal structures essential for upward gaze and pupillary light reactivity—Parinaud syndrome). Small hemorrhages may not impair alertness; with thalamic hemorrhage, sensory loss may then be found to exceed weakness. Moreover, CT has shown that small thalamic hemorrhages may cause aphasia when on the left and hemi-inattention when on the right. Figures B–7 and B–8 are CT scans showing a putaminal and a thalamic hemorrhage, respectively.

Pontine hemorrhage, unless quite small, usually causes coma (by disrupting the reticular activating system) and quadriparesis (by transecting the corticospinal tracts). Eye movements, spontaneous or reflex (e.g., to ice water in either external auditory canal), are absent, and pupils are pinpoint in size, perhaps in part from transection of descending sympathetic pathways and in part from destruction of reticular inhibitory mechanisms on the Edinger–Westphal nucleus of the midbrain. Pupillary light reactivity, however, is usually preserved, for the pathway subserving this reflex, from retina to midbrain, is intact. Respirations may be irregular, presumably from reticular formation involvement. These strokes are nearly always fatal.

Cerebellar hemorrhage, which tends to occur in the region of the dentate nucleus, typically causes a sudden inability to stand or walk (atasia–abasia), with ipsilateral limb ataxia. There may be ipsilateral abducens or gaze palsy, or facial weakness, presumably from pontine compression. Long tract motor and sensory signs, however, are

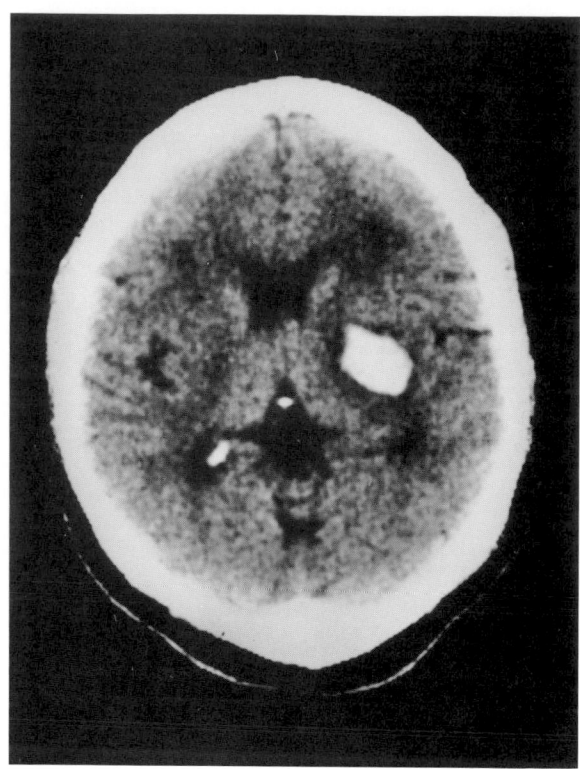

FIGURE B-7
CT scan showing hemorrhage (**white area**) in the putamen.
(Courtesy Dr. Allan J. Schwartz.)

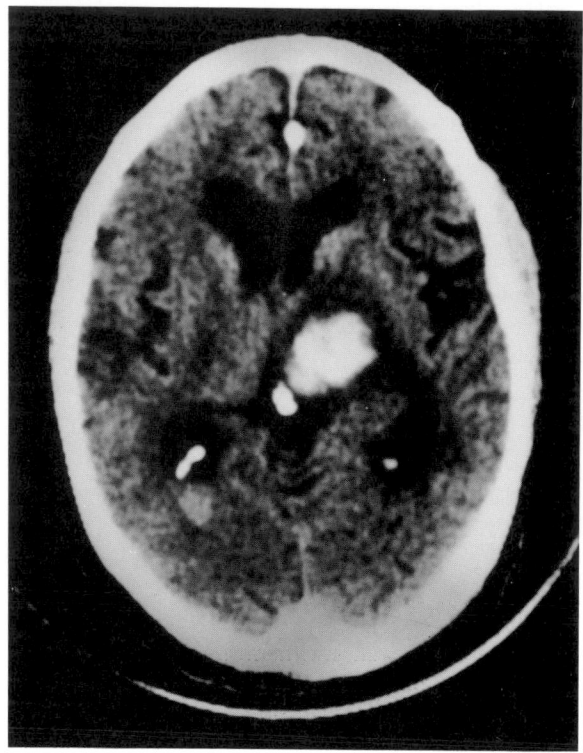

FIGURE B-8
CT scan showing thalamic hemorrhage. Hematoma is the
white area and is surrounded by a **darker zone** of edema or infarction. (Courtesy Dr. Allan J. Schwartz.)

usually absent. As swelling increases, further brain stem damage may cause coma, ophthalmoplegia, miosis, and irregular respiration, with fatal outcome.

The Rupture of Saccular Aneurysms Causes Subarachnoid Hemorrhage

Congenital saccular aneurysms (not to be confused with hypertensive Charcot–Bouchard aneurysms) are most often found at the junction of the anterior communicating artery with an anterior cerebral artery, at the junction of a posterior communicating artery with an internal carotid artery, and at the first bifurcation of a middle cerebral artery in the Sylvian fissure. Each, upon rupture, tends to cause not only sudden severe headache, but a characteristic syndrome. By producing a hematoma directly over the oculomotor nerve as it traverses the base of the brain, a ruptured posterior communicating artery aneurysm often causes ipsilateral pupillary dilation with loss of light reactivity. A middle cerebral artery aneurysm may, by either hematoma or secondary infarction, cause a clinical picture resembling that of middle cerebral artery occlusion. After rupture of an anterior communicating artery aneurysm, there may be no focal signs, but only decreased alertness or behavioral changes. Posterior fossa aneurysms most often occur at the rostral bifurcation of the basilar artery or

at the origin of the posterior inferior cerebellar artery. They cause a wide variety of cranial nerve and brain stem signs. Rupture of an aneurysm at any site may cause abrupt coma; the reason is uncertain but may be related to sudden increased intracranial pressure and functional disruption of vital pontomedullary structures.

Stroke Alters the Vascular Physiology of the Brain

After a stroke, cerebral blood flow and the responses to blood pressure or arterial gases are altered. The term *luxury perfusion* refers to the frequent appearance of hyperemia relative to demand after brain infarction. Red venous blood may be seen draining infarcts (reflecting decreased oxygen extraction), and regional cerebral blood flow may or may not be absolutely increased. In addition, there may be vasomotor paralysis with loss of autoregulation to blood pressure changes, and then blunted responses to alterations in P_{O_2} or P_{CO_2}. This kind of physiological abnormality occurs both within and around ischemic lesions. In such patients, carbon dioxide (or other cerebral vasodilators) may produce a paradoxical response, increasing cerebral blood flow in brain regions distant from the infarct without affecting the vessels around the lesion. Blood may therefore be shunted from ischemic to normal brain (intracerebral steal). On the other hand, cerebral vasoconstrictors, by decreasing cerebral blood flow in normal brain without affecting the vessels of ischemic brain, may shunt blood into the area of ischemia or infarction (inverse intracerebral steal).

There is controversy about the frequency of these phenomena. Hyperperfusion is not invariable in infarcted brain, and it may coexist with adjacent hypoperfusion with increased oxygen extraction. Similarly, intracerebral steal, while probably most frequent with very large infarcts, is quite unpredictable (particularly in duration) in any single patient. It is also not clear whether increasing cerebral blood flow to infarcted or ischemic areas improves matters by increasing oxygen delivery and the removal of tissue-damaging metabolites or makes matters worse by increasing edema, mass effect, and anastomotic compromise.

Selected Readings

Barnett, H. J. M. 1988. Cerebrovascular diseases. In J. B. Wyngaarden and L. H. Smith, (eds.), Cecil Textbook of Medicine, 18th ed. Philadelphia: Saunders, pp. 2159–2180.

Brust, J. C. M. 1989. Cerebral infarction. In L. P. Rowland (ed.), Merritt's Textbook of Neurology, 8th ed. Philadelphia: Lea & Febiger, pp. 206–214.

Lewis P. Rowland
Matthew E. Fink
Lee Rubin

APPENDIX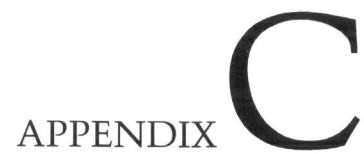

Cerebrospinal Fluid: Blood–Brain Barrier, Brain Edema, and Hydrocephalus

Cerebrospinal Fluid Is Secreted by the Choroid Plexus

Cerebrospinal Fluid Has Several Functions

Specific Permeability Barriers Exist Between Blood and Cerebrospinal Fluid and Between Blood and Brain

The Properties of the Brain Capillary Endothelial Cells Account for the Blood–Brain Barrier

The Blood–Brain Barrier Develops Early

Some Areas of the Brain Do Not Have a Blood–Brain Barrier

Why Is a Blood–Brain Barrier Necessary?

Disorders of the Blood–Brain Barrier

Drug Delivery to the Brain

The Composition of Cerebrospinal Fluid May Be Altered in Disease

Increased Intracranial Pressure May Harm the Brain

Brain Edema Is a State of Increased Brain Volume Due to Increased Water Content

    Vasogenic Edema Is a State of Increased Extracellular Fluid Volume

    Cytotoxic Edema Is the Swelling of Cellular Elements

    Interstitial Edema Is Attributed to Increased Sodium in Periventricular White Matter

Hydrocephalus Is an Increase in the Volume of the Cerebral Ventricles

I t is always surprising to realize that the brain is 80% water, and 20% of that water is extracellular. In addition to water, the cranial cavity contains blood and cerebrospinal fluid. Consideration of brain fluids and the cerebrospinal fluid (CSF) is therefore essential for understanding both the normal functions of the brain and the clinically important alterations in brain functions that arise from derangements in these fluid systems.

Cerebrospinal Fluid Is Secreted by the Choroid Plexus

The CSF is an important determinant of the extracellular fluid that bathes neurons and glia in the central nervous system. Most of the CSF is found within the four ventricles. It is secreted mainly by the *choroid plexus* in the lateral ventricles (Figure C–1A). This structure consists of capillary networks surrounded by cuboidal or columnar epithelium. CSF flows from the lateral ventricles through the interventricular foramina (of Monro) into the third ventricle. From here it flows into the fourth ventricle through the cerebral aqueduct (of Sylvius) and then through the foramina of Magendie and Luschka into the *subarachnoid space*. The subarachnoid space lies between the arachnoid and the pia mater, which together with the dura mater form the three meningeal layers that cover the brain (Figure C–1). Within the subarachnoid space, fluid flows down the spinal canal and also upward over the convexity of the brain (Figure C–1). The CSF flowing over the brain extends into the sulci and the depths of the cerebral cortex in extensions of the subarachnoid space along blood vessels called the *Virchow–Robin spaces*. Small solutes diffuse freely between the extracellular fluid and the CSF in these perivascular spaces and across the ependymal lining of the ventricular system, facilitating

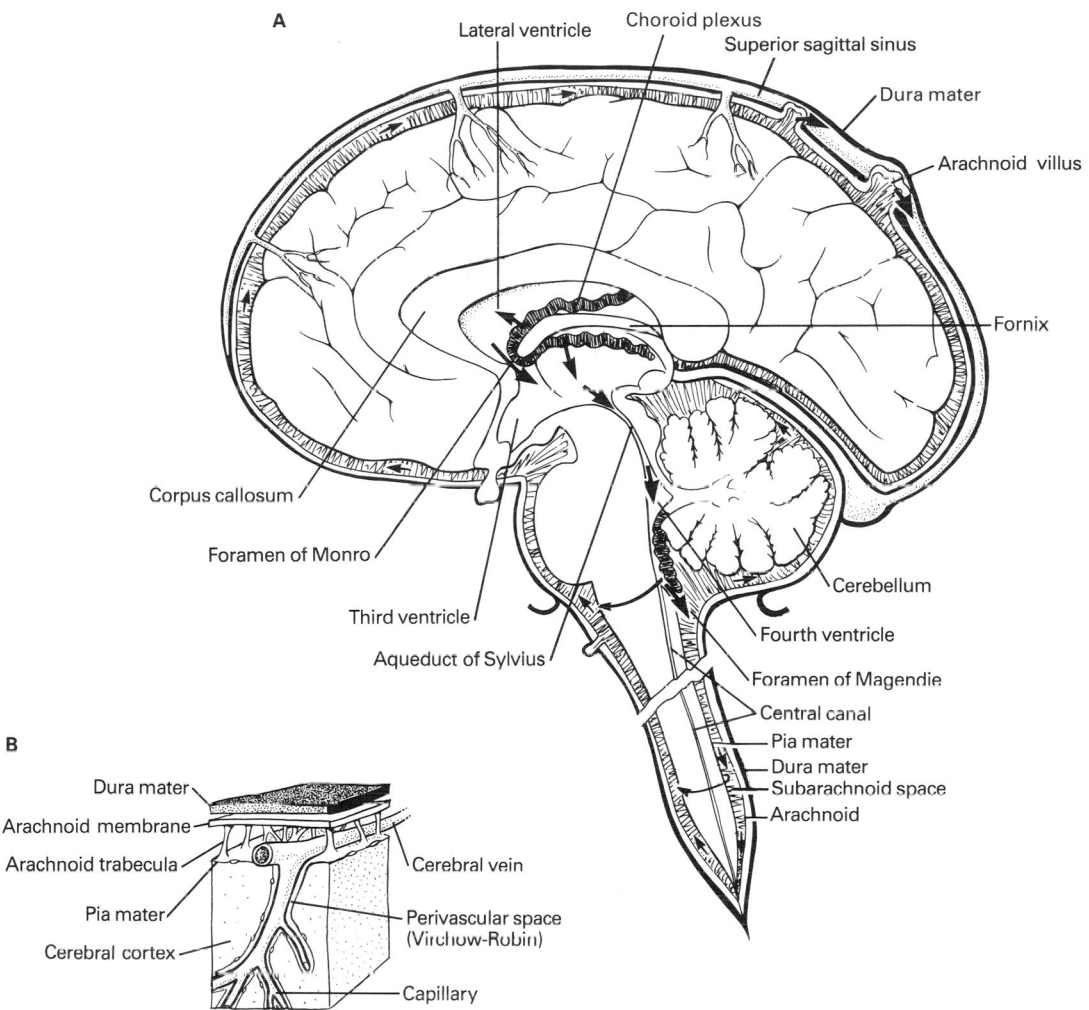

FIGURE C–1

Distribution of CSF. (Adapted from Kuffler and Nicholls, 1976; and Fishman, 1980.)

A. Sites of formation, circulation, and absorption of CSF. All spaces containing CSF communicate with each other. There are choroidal and extrachoroidal sources of the fluid within the ventricular system. The CSF circulates to the subarachnoid space and is absorbed into the venous system via the arachnoid villi. The presence of arachnoid villi adjacent to the spinal roots supplements the absorption into the intracranial venous sinuses.

B. The subarachnoid space is bounded internally by the pia mater and extends along the blood vessels that penetrate the surface of the brain. CSF flows from the lateral ventricles through the interventricular foramina (of Monro) into the third ventricle. From there it flows into the fourth ventricle through

the cerebral aqueduct (of Sylvius) and then through the foramina of Magendie and Luschka into the *subarachnoid space.* The subarachnoid space lies between the arachnoid membrane and the pia mater, which together with the dura mater form the three meninges that cover the brain (Figure C–1B). Within the subarachnoid space, fluid flows down the spinal canal and also upward through the tentorial notch around the midbrain, over the convexity of the brain (Figure C–1A). The CSF flowing over the brain extends into the sulci and the depths of the cerebral cortex in extensions of the subarachnoid space along blood vessels called the *Virchow–Robin spaces.* Small solutes diffuse freely across the pia mater between the extracellular fluid and the CSF in these perivascular spaces and across the ependymal lining of the ventricular system, facilitating the movement of metabolites from deep within the hemispheres to cortical subarachnoid spaces and the ventricular system.

the movement of metabolites from deep within the hemispheres to cortical subarachnoid spaces and the ventricular system.

The choroid plexus is structurally similar to the distal and collecting tubules of the kidney, and functions in a similar manner to maintain the chemical stability of the

CSF. However, the secretory capacities of the choroid plexus are bidirectional, accounting for both continuous production of CSF and active transport of metabolites out of the central nervous system and into the blood. The rest of the CSF not secreted by the choroid plexus is secreted by capillaries in the brain into the neuropil and enters the

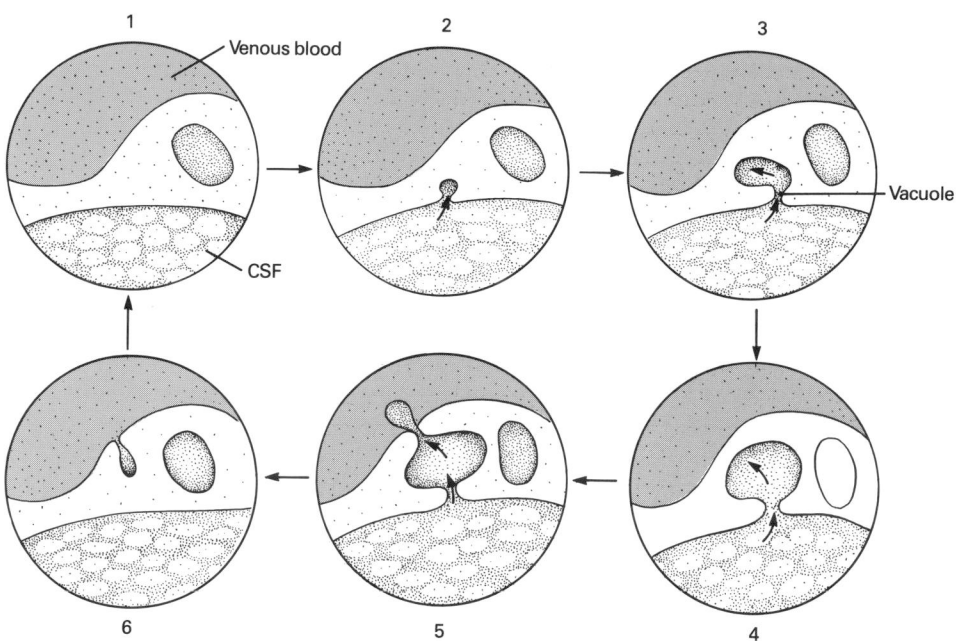

FIGURE C–2

It is postulated that giant vacuoles transport CSF within the arachnoid villus. This mechanism could account for the one-way bulk flow of CSF from the subarachnoid space to the venous system. The arachnoid cells have tight intercellular junctions. Some vesicles are large enough to encompass red blood cells. (Adapted from Fishman, 1980.)

ventricular system through a single layer of ependymal cells that line the walls of the ventricles.

The CSF is absorbed through the *pacchionian granulations*, or *arachnoid villi*. These structures are typically found in clusters that are visible herniations of the arachnoid membrane through the dura and into the lumen of the superior sagittal sinus and other venous structures (Figure C–1A). The villi themselves are visible microscop-

ically, but it is not clear whether they form a membrane that separates CSF and venous blood (a closed system), or whether a series of tubules within the villus communicates directly with venous blood (an open system). A third possibility is that vacuoles form within cells of the villus membrane to transport fluid from one side of the cell to the other, a form of vesicular transport that combines the characteristics of both a closed and an open system (Figure

FIGURE C–3

The structural and functional relationship involved in the blood–brain and blood–CSF barriers. Tissue elements that may participate in forming the barriers are indicated in parentheses. Substances entering the neurons and glial cells (i.e., intracellular compartment) must pass through the cell membrane. **Arrows:** direction of fluid flow under normal conditions. (Adapted from Carpenter, 1978.)

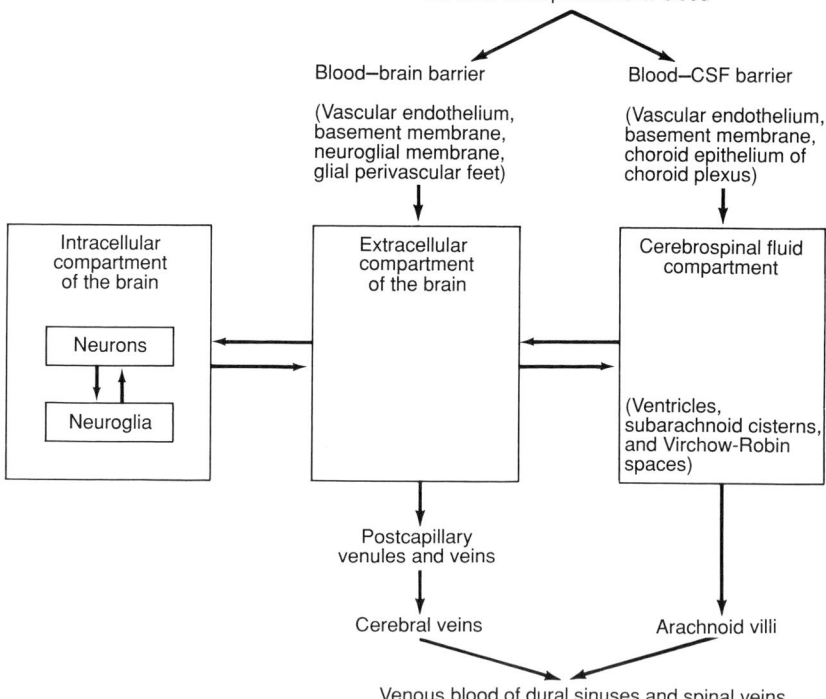

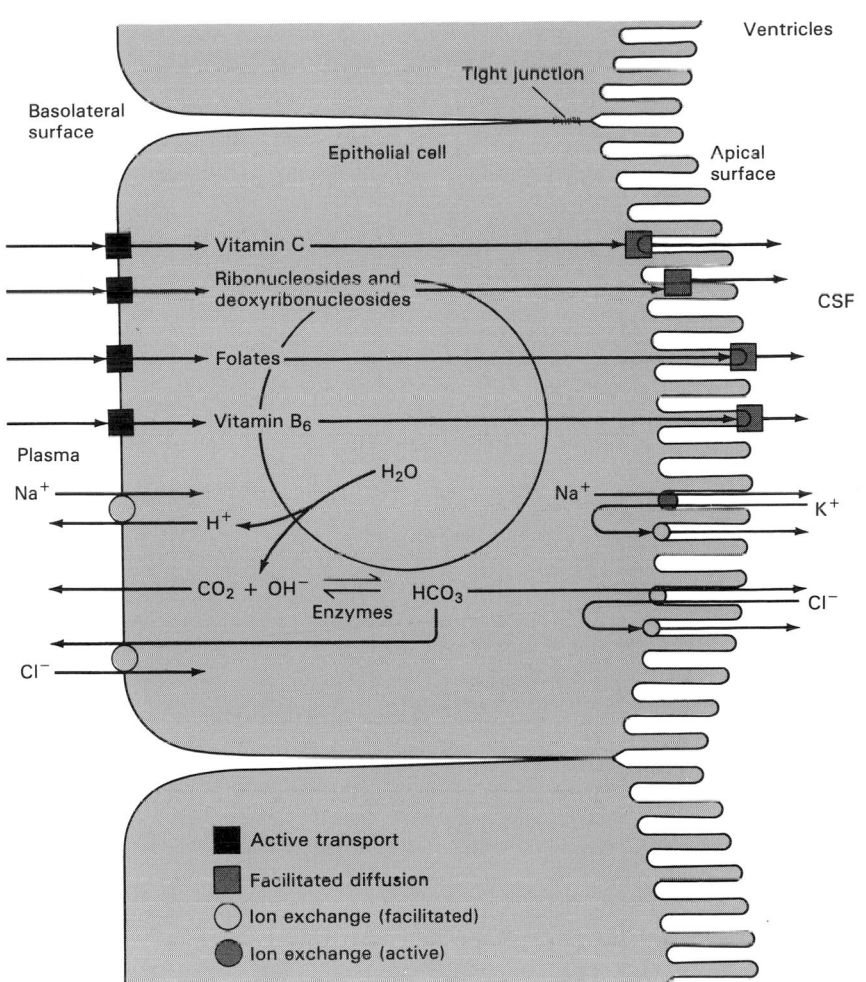

FIGURE C–4
Flow of molecules across the blood–CSF barrier is regulated by several mechanisms in the choroid plexus. Some micronutrients such as vitamin C are pulled into the epithelial cells at the basolateral surface by an energy-consuming process known as active transport; the micronutrients are released into the CSF at the apical surface by another regulated process, facilitated diffusion, which requires no energy. Essential ions are also controllably exchanged between the CSF and blood plasma. Transport of an ion in one direction is linked to the transport of a different ion in the opposite direction, as in the exchange of sodium (Na^+) ions for potassium (K^+) ions. (From Spector and Johanson, 1989.)

C–2). In any case, the granulations appear to function as valves that allow one-way flow of CSF from the subarachnoid spaces into venous blood. This one-way flow of CSF is sometimes called *bulk flow* because all constituents of CSF leave with the fluid, including small molecules, proteins, microorganisms, and red blood cells. The rate of formation of CSF in adults is about 0.35 ml/min or about 500 ml/day, so that the entire volume of CSF is turned over three to four times a day (Figure C–3).

The choroid plexus has both filtration and secretory functions that act together to maintain constant concentrations of CSF components. Much like capillary endothelial cells, the epithelial cells of the choroid plexus possess a specific set of transporters. The particular transporters are different in the two types of cells. For instance, a transport system for vitamin C is much more active in choroid plexus epithelial cells than in brain capillary endothelial cells (Figure C–4).

Cerebrospinal Fluid Has Several Functions

The composition of CSF is in a steady state with brain extracellular fluid and is therefore important in maintaining a constant external environment for neurons and glia. The primarily one-way flow of CSF from the ventricular system, around the spinal cord into the subarachnoid space around the brain, and into the venous sinuses is a major way potentially harmful brain metabolites are removed. The CSF also provides a mechanical cushion to protect the brain from impact with the bony calvarium when the head moves. By its buoyant action, the CSF allows the brain to float, thereby reducing its effective weight *in situ* to less than 50 g. The CSF may also serve as a lymphatic system for the brain and as a conduit for peptide hormones secreted by hypothalamic neurons, which act at remote sites in the brain. The pH of CSF affects both pulmonary ventilation and cerebral blood flow—another example of the homeostatic role of CSF.

Specific Permeability Barriers Exist Between Blood and Cerebrospinal Fluid and Between Blood and Brain

CSF and extracellular fluids of the brain are in a steady-state. For example, the concentrations of K^+, Ca^{2+}, bicarbonate, and glucose in the CSF are lower than in blood

TABLE C–1. Comparison of Serum and
Cerebrospinal Fluid

Component	CSF[a]	Serum[a]
Water content (%)	99	93
Protein (mg/dl)	35	7000
Glucose (mg/dl)	60	90
Osmolarity (mOsm/liter)	295	295
Na^+ (meq/liter)	138	138
K^+ (meq/liter)	2.8	4.5
Ca^{2+} (meq/liter)	2.1	4.8
Mg^{2+} (meq/liter)	0.3	1.7
Cl^- (meq/liter)	119	102
pH	7.33	7.41

[a]Average or representative values.
(From Fishman, 1980.)

plasma. The pH also is more acidic (Table C–1). These differences are due to regulation of the constituents of CSF by active transport. The formation of CSF in the choroid plexus involves both capillary filtration and active epithelial secretion. The capillaries that traverse the choroid plexus are freely permeable to plasma solutes. A barrier exists, however, at the level of the epithelial cells that make up the choroid plexus. This barrier is responsible for carrier-mediated active transport. Thus, normally, blood plasma and CSF are in osmotic balance, because water follows the osmotic gradient that is created by active transport of solutes.

The concept of a *blood–brain barrier* was developed by Paul Ehrlich, who found that intravenous injection of dyes stained tissues in most organs but not in the brain. The tracers used currently, such as trypan blue or Evans blue, are cationic vital dyes that bind to serum albumin. When administered intravenously, these dyes rapidly diffuse from capillaries and permeate most tissues, turning them blue. In contrast, most of the brain remains uncolored.

The Properties of the Brain Capillary Endothelial Cells Account for the Blood–Brain Barrier

What is the anatomical basis of the blood–brain barrier? Using electron microscopy and electron-dense tracers such as horseradish peroxidase (HRP) and lanthanum, Morris Karnovsky and Thomas Reese demonstrated that the blood–brain barrier of vertebrates is located in the specialized endothelial cells of the capillaries in the brain (Figures C–5 and C–6). These capillaries of the brain consist of overlapping endothelial cells that make frequent contact on their abluminal (brain) side with projections from *astrocytes*, referred to as glial end-feet (see Figure 2–3).

The endothelial cells of the capillaries in the brain differ from those in other organs in two important ways. These differences account for the ability of the blood–brain barrier to exclude certain molecules. First, peripheral endothelial cells are either fenestrated or have tight junctions of low resistance (5/10 ohm-cm^2) between the cells. In contrast, brain endothelial cells are joined by tight junctions of high electrical resistance (1000 ohm/cm^2 or more). These high resistance junctions present an effective barrier even to ions. Thus, in brain there is little movement of compounds between endothelial cells (Figure C–7).

Second, in peripheral endothelial cells there is good transcellular movement of compounds. In contrast, there is no such transport through brain endothelial cells. In peripheral endothelial cells molecules move across the cells by two means: (1) *fluid-phase endocytosis*, a relatively nonspecific process in which endothelial cells (and most other cells) first engulf molecules encountered in the extracellular environment and then internalize the molecules by means of vesicular endocytosis; (2) *receptor-mediated endocytosis*, a specific process in which a ligand first binds to a membrane receptor on one side of the cell. After binding the complex is internalized into a vesicle and transported across the cell, and the ligand may be

FIGURE C–5
Astrocytes are glial cells whose long processes (extensions) make contact with several other types of cells, as is shown schematically in this drawing (see also Chapter 2). The astrocyte processes touch neurons and the ependymal cells that line the ventricle, which are spaces at the center of the brain. In addition, each brain capillary is typically in contact with several astrocytes. Although the function of astrocytes is not yet fully understood, they are thought to influence capillary permeability.

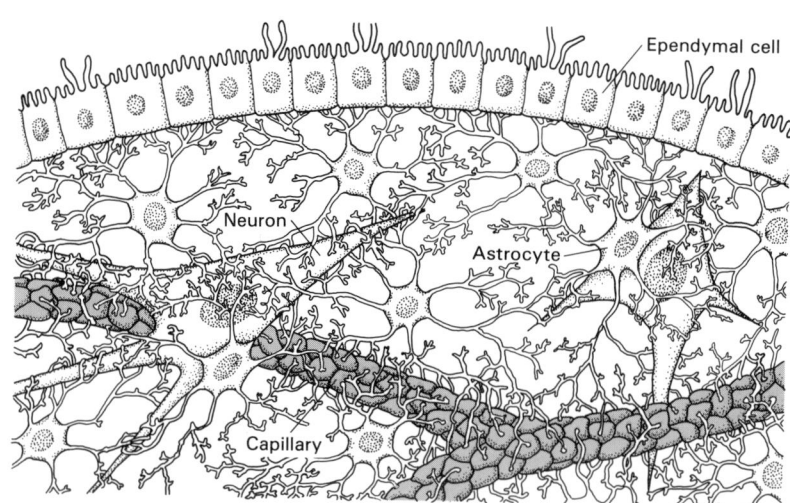

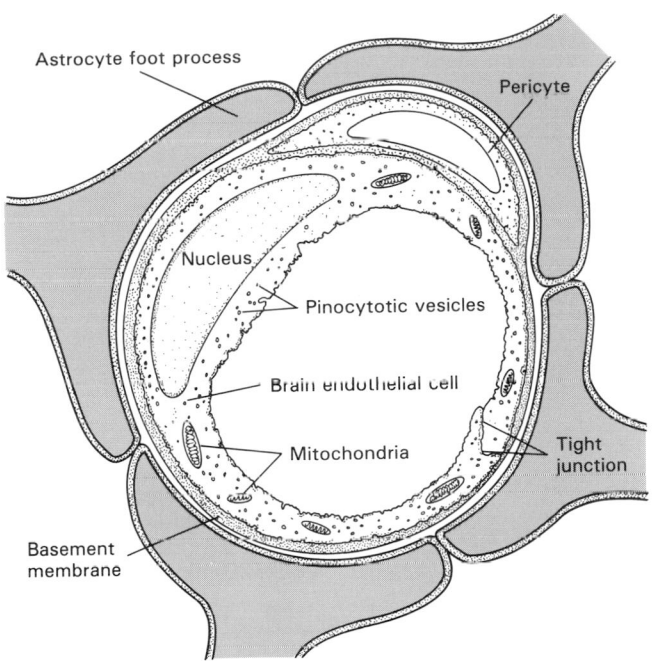

FIGURE C–6
The ultrastructural features of the capillary endothelial cells of the brain differ from those of general (systemic) capillaries. Note the relative absence of pinocytotic vesicles, the greatly increased number of mitochondria, and the presence of tight junctions in brain capillaries, whereas general capillaries have clefts, fenestrae, and prominent pinocytotic vesicles. (Adapted from Fishman, 1980.)

released. Endothelial cells of the brain lack both of these mechanisms.

The Blood–Brain Barrier Develops Early

The blood–brain barrier becomes established early in development when the endothelial cells in the brain first acquire these two differentiated properties. This was first shown by transplantation experiments using quail-chick chimeras. When avascular gut tissue was transplanted to the brain, the gut became vascularized by endothelial cells that migrated in from the brain. The capillaries that formed in the gut were leaky.

Conversely, when avascular brain was transplanted into gut it became vascularized from endothelial cells that originated in gut capillaries. The capillaries that formed in the transplanted brain tissue were impermeable to dye injection, thereby constituting a blood–brain barrier.

These experiments suggest that factors within the brain itself cause endothelial cells to adopt properties of the blood–brain barrier. The nature of these factors is still unknown. One of the most likely differences between brain and peripheral tissues that may influence endothelial cell differentiation is the astrocyte, which forms frequent contacts on endothelial cells. In the absence of other brain cell types, astrocytes cause endothelial cells to express some of the features characteristic of the blood–brain barrier.

Some Areas of the Brain Do Not Have a Blood–Brain Barrier

Not all cerebral blood vessels are entirely impermeant. Leaky areas include the posterior pituitary and circumventricular organs (CVOs), such as the area postrema and subfornical organ. In these regions, most of the capillaries are fenestrated, much like those in the periphery. In those capillaries that are not fenestrated there are many vesicles in the cytoplasm and these structures are thought to transport their contents across the cell. These structural features account for the enhanced transport across these cells.

Why are these regions not protected by the blood–brain barrier? In the pituitary, the blood–brain barrier seems to be absent because the neurosecretory products have to pass into the circulation. In the subfornical organ, a chemoreceptive area, the transcellular transport is required for water balance and other homeostatic functions.

These leaky regions are isolated from the rest of the brain (see also below) by specialized ependymal cells (called *tanycytes*) that line the structures located along the ventricular surface close to the midline. These *circumventricular* structures include: the vascular organ

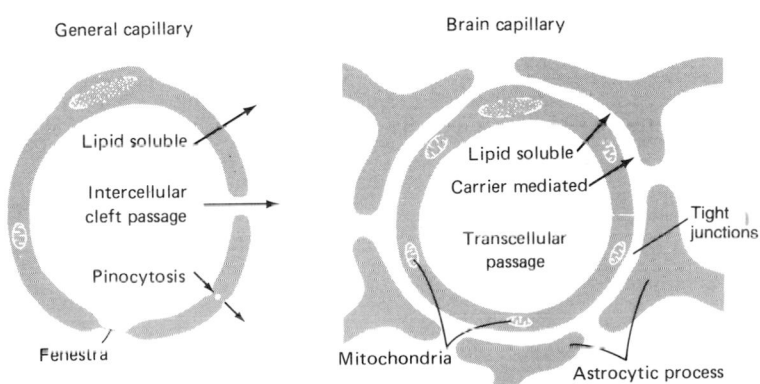

FIGURE C–7
Astrocyte foot processes almost completely surround the brain capillary. Because of this relationship it was once thought that the astrocytes form the blood–brain barrier. It is now known that the endothelial cells constitute the barrier. Endothelial cells selectively transport nutrients into the brain, and their many mitochondria probably provide energy for transport. The endothelial cells of the brain have few pinocytotic vesicles. In other organs such vesicles may provide relatively unselective transport across the capillary wall.

of the laminar terminalis, the subfornical organ, subcommissural organ, area postrema, median eminence, neurohypophysis, and the choroid plexus. The tanycytes are coupled by tight junctions and prevent free exchange between the circumventricular organs and the CSF.

Why Is a Blood–Brain Barrier Necessary?

Proper brain function depends on at least three environmental influences: extracellular ion concentrations, neurotransmitters, and growth factors that maintain neuronal and non-neuronal cells. Neurons must be protected as far as possible from extraneous changes in levels of any of these substances. For example, neurally active compounds such as epinephrine are released from the adrenal medulla and are normally found in circulating blood. Some neuronal and glial growth-promoting or growth-inhibiting factors are also found in the blood.

Moreover, ion levels in the serum may change abruptly. The blood–brain barrier protects the brain against surging fluctuations in ion concentrations. In addition, ionic regulation is influenced by local conditions. For instance, the abluminal membrane of brain endothelial cells has a relatively high concentration of Na-K-ATPase and astrocytic end-feet on the endothelial cells have an especially high concentration of K^+ channels. These channels may be used to remove the extracellular K^+ that might otherwise accumulate after intense neuronal activity (Chapter 2).

What molecules normally enter the brain? With the exception of molecules for which there are specific transport systems, only small lipophilic molecules enter the brain. For these small molecules the rate of entry parallels their lipophilicity (or hydrophobicity), as measured by their oil-water partition coefficients (Figure C–8). For instance, morphine is relatively hydrophilic and does not penetrate well into the brain. Heroin, a morphine derivative produced by acetylation of two polar hydroxyl groups, is more hydrophobic and enters the brain much more effectively. A hydrophobic compound presumably passes through the endothelial cell's luminal (blood side) lipid plasma membrane, crosses the cell, enters into the abluminal plasma membrane, and appears into the extracellular fluid of the brain. A concentration gradient between blood and brain creates a net movement into the brain.

The entry of some small hydrophilic molecules is higher than expected from the oil-water partition coefficients. For most of them, there are specific membrane transporters. These systems operate in one direction to transport compounds from blood into the endothelial cells and in the opposite direction to transport them out of the endothelial cells into the brain. For example, D-glucose is transported into the brain at high rates by a stereospecific glucose transporter. There are also three separate transport systems for amino acids—one for neutral amino acids, such as phenylalanine; one for basic amino acids, such as arginine; one for acidic amino acids, such as glutamate.

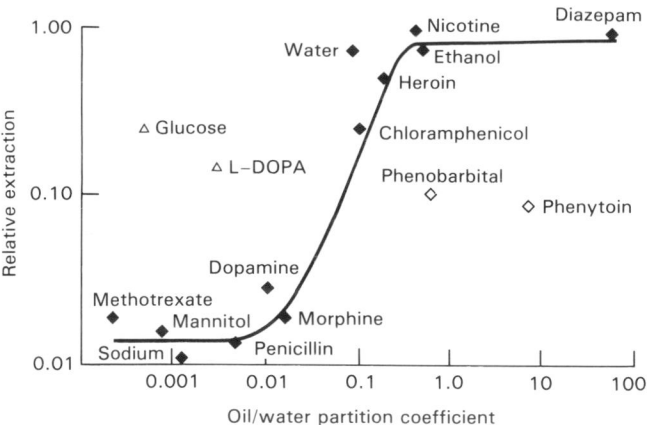

FIGURE C–8
The oil–water partition coefficient indicates the relationship between lipid solubility and brain uptake of selected compounds. The distribution into olive oil relative to water for each test substance serves as a measure of its lipid solubility. The brain uptake is determined by comparing the extraction of each test substance relative to a highly permeable tracer during a single passage through the cerebral circulation. In general, compounds with higher oil to water partition coefficients show increased entry into brain. Uptake of the two anticonvulsants, phenobarbital and phenytoin, is lower than predicted from their lipid solubility partly because of their binding to plasma proteins. This explains the slower onset of anticonvulsant activity of these agents compared with diazepam. Uptake of glucose and L-DOPA is greater than predicted by their lipid solubility because specific carriers facilitate their transport across the brain capillary. (Data from Oldendorf, 1977, 1983, except for diazepam and chloramphenicol, which are estimated.)

The clinical importance of these transport systems is seen with DOPA, the synthetic precursor of the neurotransmitter dopamine. In Parkinson's disease dopaminergic neurons are lost and the brain's content of dopamine is much reduced (see Chapter 42). Symptoms of the disease can be reduced by administration of L-DOPA, which is transported by the neutral amino acid transporter into the brain, where it is converted to dopamine. Dopamine itself, however, is therapeutically ineffective because it is not transported.

Disorders of the Blood–Brain Barrier

There are a variety of pathological situations that involve the blood–brain barrier. Brain tumors have a leaky vasculature, either because they lack normal astrocyte-capillary projections or because the tumor cells secrete factors that make the endothelial cells leaky. Presumably the absence of the normal barrier permits relatively rapid nutrient exchange between the blood and the tumor, facilitating the growth of the tumor.

Another interesting condition in which the blood–brain barrier is reduced is bacterial meningitis. Normally, the blood–brain barrier is impermeable to antibiotics such as penicillin. Bacterial meningitis causes a partial breakdown of the blood–brain barrier by unknown mechanisms, and this leads to enhanced antibiotic entry into the brain. The antibiotic can then act to suppress infection.

There are also situations in which leukocyte movement across the blood–brain barrier results in neurological disorders. Enhanced lymphocyte trafficking into the brain is associated with multiple sclerosis. Human immunodeficiency virus (HIV) enters the brain within infected macrophages and can produce HIV-dementia. Following stroke, neutrophils and monocytes can enter the brain and may be a source of neurotoxic agents.

Finally, the situation in which the blood–brain barrier is most obviously compromised is brain edema, a state of increased water content in the brain. In *cytotoxic brain edema*, which follows cerebral ischemia, for example, the edema follows damage to endothelial cells, neurons and glia. Cell damage causes membrane pumps, such as the ATP-dependent Na^+-K^+ pump to fail, and this leads to Na^+ and water accumulation inside the cells. Vasogenic brain edema, which often occurs in regions bordering those damaged during ischemia, results from increased influx across the blood–brain barrier of ions and proteins, again producing increased water content in the brain.

Drug Delivery to the Brain

A delivery system devised by Stanley Rapoport and his colleagues alters the tight junctions of the endothelial cells. A hypersomotic solution of mannitol (approximately 1.5 M) is first perfused through the carotid artery to shrink capillary endothelial cells in the brain, opening the tight junctions for several hours. Chemotherapeutic agents (which normally do not penetrate well into the brain) are then administered. Since the blood–brain barrier is already somewhat leaky in the region of the tumor itself, the goal of the procedure is to increase the total amount of drug loaded into the brain outside the tumor, providing a local drug reservoir. Unfortunately, the procedure is not always therapeutically effective and the procedures may have adverse effects.

The Composition of Cerebrospinal Fluid May Be Altered in Disease

The gross appearance of CSF has clinical significance. The fluid is normally clear and colorless. It may appear cloudy when it contains many leukocytes or has a high protein content. It may also appear grossly bloody or yellow (xanthochromia) when blood pigments are left behind after a hemorrhage or when CSF protein content is greater than 150 mg/dl, indicating that bilirubin (bound to albumin) has been brought from the plasma to the CSF.

Normally the CSF does not contain *red* or *white blood cells*. White blood cell counts greater than 3 per cubic milliliter are pathological. In acute bacterial meningitis, the count may be a thousand-fold greater. Cells may be increased moderately in viral infections or in response to cerebral infarction, brain tumor, or other cerebral tissue damage. Tumor cells in CSF can be collected on filters and identified by their characteristic morphology.

Protein content may be increased by many pathological processes of the brain or spinal cord, presumably because of changes in vascular permeability. Protein content greater than 500 mg/dl is usually a manifestation of a block in the spinal subarachnoid space by a tumor or other compressive lesion. The *gamma globulin content* is disproportionately increased to more than 13% of total protein in multiple sclerosis and a few other diseases. Because this may occur without a corresponding increase in blood gamma globulin content, the increased CSF is attributed to production of the immunoglobulins within the brain. In multiple sclerosis, the abnormal immunoglobulins can also be identified as *oligoclonal bands* by electrophoresis.

The concentration of *glucose* is decreased in acute bacterial infections and only exceptionally in viral infections. In chronic diseases, a CSF glucose content less than 40 mg/dl implies a tumor in the meninges—fungal, yeast, or tuberculous infection—or sarcoidosis. The basis for the reduced CSF glucose content is not clear. It may be due to impaired transport into CSF; to excessive utilization by organisms, blood cells, tumor cells, or the brain itself; or to combinations of these mechanisms. An inherited defect of the glucose transporter has also been identified as a cause of persistently low CSF glucose content.

Increased Intracranial Pressure May Harm the Brain

CSF pressure is ordinarily measured by lumbar puncture, a procedure in which a needle is inserted through the skin, between the fourth and fifth lumbar vertebrae, and into the lumbar subarachnoid space, with the patient lying sideways (lateral decubitus position). Because the spinal cord extends only to the first lumbar vertebra, there is no risk of injuring the cord. When the CSF flows freely through the needle, the hub of the needle is attached to a manometer and the fluid is allowed to rise. The normal pressure is 65–195 mm CSF (or water), or 5–15 mm Hg.

In measuring the lumbar CSF pressure as a guide to intracranial pressure, it is assumed that pressures are equal throughout the neuraxis. Normally, this is a reasonable assumption. In some pathological states (such as brain tumor or obstruction of CSF pathways), however, this may not be true. For this reason, and also because the lumbar needle cannot be left in place for prolonged periods, catheters are sometimes inserted into the lateral ventricles to measure pressure there (Figure C–9). Equally effective are pressure-sensitive transducers that can be inserted under the skull in the epidural or subarachnoid space for continuous monitoring of intracranial pressure.

In considering the factors that regulate intracranial pressure, the cranium and spinal canal may be regarded as a closed system. According to the *Monro–Kellie doctrine*,

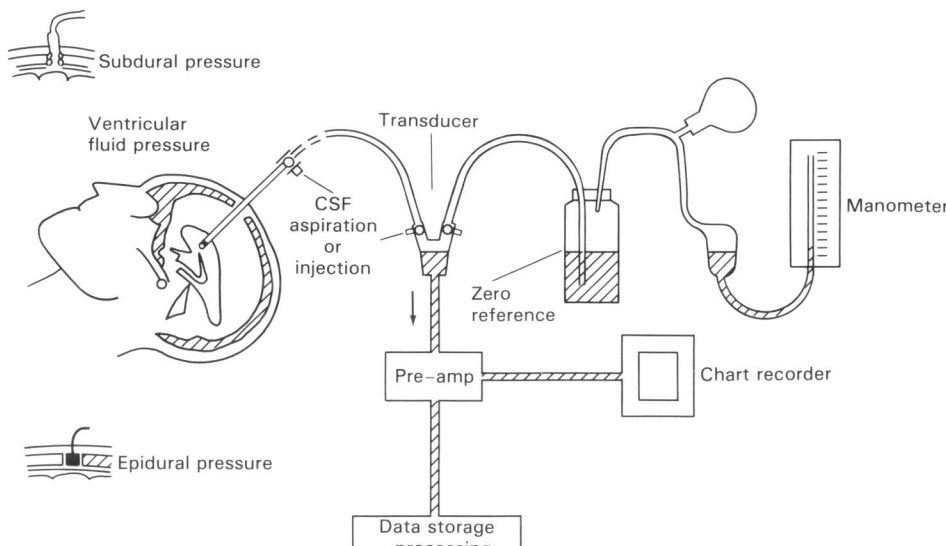

FIGURE C–9
Techniques for continuous measurement of intracranial pressure. (From Jennett and Teasdale, 1981.)

an increase in the volume of any one of the contents of the calvarium—brain tissue, blood, CSF, or brain fluids—must be accompanied by a decrease of another component or there will be a marked increase in intracranial pressure because the bony calvarium rigidly fixes the total cranial volume. If there is a sudden increase in intracranial blood volume—for example, during a voluntary Valsalva maneuver or a sneeze—CSF may surge into the cervical subarachnoid space momentarily, because the dura there is elastic. Increased CSF volume may partially compress cerebral blood vessels. Chronic changes may be compensated for by increased absorption or decreased formation of CSF. When these compensatory mechanisms fail, intracranial pressure rises, and cerebral blood flow falls. The relationship between intracranial pressure and cerebral blood flow can be described by the following equation: Cerebral Perfusion Pressure = Mean Arterial Blood Pressure − Intracranial Pressure. Several types of abnormalities lead to increased intracranial pressure, as described in the following sections.

Brain Edema Is a State of Increased Brain Volume Due to Increased Water Content

Brain edema may be local (surrounding contusion, infarct, or tumor) or generalized. Local brain edema may cause herniation of brain tissue (cingulate gyrus beneath falx, temporal lobe uncus across tentorium, cerebellar tonsils through foramen magnum, or cerebral cortex outward through calvarial defects after surgery or injury).

Vasogenic Edema Is a State of Increased Extracellular Fluid Volume

Vasogenic edema is the most common form of brain edema. It is attributed to increased permeability of brain capillary endothelial cells, which increases the volume of the extracellular fluid. White matter is affected more than gray matter. Vasogenic edema is demonstrated by intravenous contrast enhancement of computerized tomography and magnetic resonance imaging of brain tumor, abscess, infarct, or hemorrhage. Generalized forms of vasogenic edema occur in head injury, lead encephalopathy, and meningitis. Functional manifestations include focal neurological abnormalities, electroencephalographic slowing, intracranial hypertension, and impaired consciousness.

Cytotoxic Edema Is the Swelling of Cellular Elements

Cytotoxic edema implies intracellular swelling of neurons, glia, and endothelial cells, with a concomitant reduction of brain extracellular space. Cytotoxic edema occurs in hypoxia from asphyxia or global cerebral ischemia after cardiac arrest because failure of the ATP-dependent Na^+–K^+ pump allows Na^+, and therefore water, to accumulate within cells. Another cause of cytotoxic edema is water intoxication, a consequence of the acute systemic hypo-osmolarity that is caused by excessive ingestion of water or administration of hypotonic intravenous fluids. Acute hyponatremia, induced for example by inappropriate secretion of antidiuretic hormone or renal salt-wasting from secretion of atrial natriuretic hormone, can cause cellular swelling and brain edema. Under these circumstances water moves from extracellular to intracellular sites. Cytotoxic edema may also accompany other forms of edema in meningitis and encephalitis.

Interstitial Edema Is Attributed to Increased Sodium in Periventricular White Matter

In interstitial edema, best exemplified by obstructive hydrocephalus, water and Na^+ content increase in the periventricular white matter due to transependymal reab-

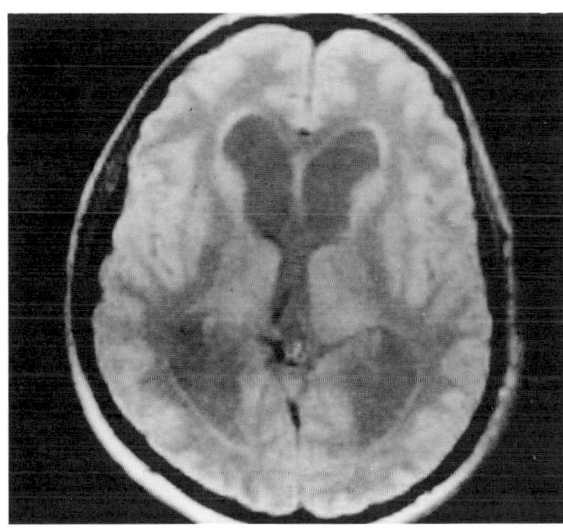

FIGURE C–10
Axial magnetic resonance image showing chronic hydrocephalus with transependymal CSF absorption (white rim around the frontal and occipital horns).

sorption of CSF. This is best observed by magnetic resonance imaging, which highlights areas of the brain that have increased water content (Figure C–10). The most effective treatment of interstitial edema from hydrocephalus is surgical shunting of CSF to relieve the obstruction.

Pseudotumor cerebri or *benign intracranial hypertension* is thought by some researchers to be a form of interstitial edema, but this has not been proved. In this condition, increased CSF pressure is usually attended by headaches and papilledema. Mental function, however, is not depressed, as often happens in generalized cerebral edema. Moreover, hydrocephalus does not occur in this condition (implying that CSF absorption is not impaired). Imaging studies have demonstrated both increased water content in the brain interstitium and an increased rate of CSF production by the choroid plexus. This combination of factors may account for the increased intracranial pressure, which may persist for months or years, but the condition often seems to be self-limited.

Hydrocephalus Is an Increase in the Volume of the Cerebral Ventricles

Hydrocephalus results from one of three possible causes: oversecretion of CSF, impaired absorption of CSF, or obstruction of CSF pathways.

Oversecretion of CSF is rare but is thought to occur in some functioning tumors of the choroid plexus (papillomas) because removal of the tumor may relieve the hydrocephalus. However, subarachnoid hemorrhage and high CSF protein content also characterize these tumors and could impair the absorption of CSF.

Impaired absorption of CSF could conceivably result from any condition that raises the venous pressure, such

as thrombosis and occlusion of cerebral venous sinuses, severe congestive heart failure, or removal of the jugular vein during radical neck dissections for tumors. However, well-documented cases of this type are rare. Impaired absorption is suspected as the cause of the more common *communicating hydrocephalus*, in which there is no obstruction of CSF flow from the lateral ventricles through the foramina of Luschka and Magendie and all four ventricles are enlarged. In this condition, CSF pressure may be high or normal.

In infants, CSF pressure may not rise because the cranial sutures have not yet fused and the cranium can expand. In adults, communicating hydrocephalus may occur in some patients who survive subarachnoid hemorrhage or meningitis. This type of hydrocephalus is attributed to impaired absorption of CSF because of mechanical obstruction or otherwise impaired function of the pacchionian granulations caused by protein and detritus. A similar mechanism is thought to explain the high CSF pressure in some patients with CSF protein content greater than 500 mg/dl due to acute peripheral neuropathy (Guillain–Barre syndrome) or spinal cord tumor.

Impaired absorption is also held responsible for the syndrome of *normal-pressure hydrocephalus*. This syndrome is of interest because it is a treatable cause of dementia. Dementia is a major, almost epidemic, public health problem. The dementia of this disorder is unusual in that it can be relieved by shunting of CSF; however, it is difficult to identify patients who will respond. In addition to dementia, the clinical syndrome comprises unsteady gait and urinary incontinence. In computerized tomography or magnetic resonance imaging, the ventricles are uniformly enlarged and there is no evidence of cortical atrophy or enlargement of the subarachnoid spaces over the convexity of the brain. In another test, the circulation of the CSF is assessed. In normal individuals, if ^{125}I-labeled albumin is injected into the lumbar subarachnoid space, the isotope can be traced by a gamma camera up to the arachnoid granulations, but it does not normally enter the ventricles. In patients with normal-pressure hydrocephalus the isotopic label does not follow the normal course to the convexities, may reflux into the ventricles, and takes longer to appear in the blood. In another test, there is an excessive rise of CSF pressure when saline is infused into the lumbar subarachnoid space at a rate of 0.3 ml/min.

Obstruction of CSF pathways may result from tumors, congenital malformations, or scarring. A particularly vulnerable site for all three mechanisms is the narrow aqueduct of Sylvius. *Aqueductal stenosis* may result from congenital malformations or gliosis due to intrauterine infection or hemorrhage. Later in life, the aqueduct may be occluded by tumor. In another condition, obstruction of the outlets of the fourth ventricle by congenital atresia of the foramina of Luschka and Magendie may lead to enlargement of all four ventricles (*Dandy–Walker syndrome*). In early life the cranial vault enlarges with the ventricles, but after the sutures fuse cranial volume is fixed and hydrocephalus develops at the expense of brain volume.

The ideal treatment of hydrocephalus would be to remove the causative factor. However, this can be done for only very few of the cases caused by tumors. In other cases, CSF can be diverted past the block or to a new site for absorption. Numerous ingenious variations have been attempted, but the most popular are ventriculoatrial, ventriculoperitoneal, and lumbar-peritoneal shunts. Complications include infection (meningitis or septicemia), obstruction of either end of the shunt, or subdural hematoma. Drug therapy directed toward decreasing CSF production or enhancing CSF absorption has not been successful in treating hydrocephalus, and ethical questions are raised in the treatment of infants with hydrocephalus and severe cortical atrophy.

Selected Readings

Bradbury, M. 1979. The Concept of a Blood–Brain Barrier. New York: Wiley.

Carpenter, M. B. 1985. Core Text of Neuroanatomy, 3rd ed. Baltimore: Williams & Wilkins.

Cervos-Navarro, J., and Ferszt, R. (eds.). 1980. Brain Edema: Pathology, Diagnosis, and Therapy. Advances in Neurology, Vol. 28. New York: Raven Press.

Cutler, R. W. P., and Spertel, R. B. 1982. Cerebrospinal fluid: A selective review. Ann. Neurol. 11:1–10.

Dauch, W. A., and Zimmermann, R. 1990. Der Normaldruck—Hydrocephalus: Eine Bilanz 25 Jahre nach der Erstbeschreibung. Fortschr. Neurol. Psychiatr. 58:178–190.

Fishman, R. A. 1975. Brain edema. N. Engl. J. Med. 293:706–711.

Fishman, R. A. 1980. Cerebrospinal Fluid in Diseases of the Nervous System. Philadelphia: Saunders.

Flitter, M. A. 1981. Techniques of intracranial pressure monitoring. Clin. Neurosurg. 28:547–563.

Friedland, R. P. 1989. Normal-pressure hydrocephalus and the saga of the treatable dementias. JAMA 262:2577–2581.

Goldstein, G. W., and Betz, A. L. 1986. The blood–brain barrier. Sci. Am. 255(3):74–83.

Graff-Radford, N. R., Godersky, J. C., and Jones, M. P. 1989. Variables predicting surgical outcome in symptomatic hydrocephalus in the elderly. Neurology 39:1601–1604.

Greer, M. 1988. Carrier Drugs: Presidential Address, American Academy of Neurology, 1987. Neurology 38:628–632.

Katzman, R., and Pappius, H. M. 1973. Brain Electrolytes and Fluid Metabolism. Baltimore: Williams & Wilkins.

Keck, P. J., Hauser, S. D., Krivi, G., Sanzo, K., Warren, T., Feder, J., and Connolly, D. T. 1989. Vascular permeability factor, an endothelial cell mitogen related to PDGF. Science 246:1309–1312.

Lyons, M. K., and Meyer, F. B. 1990. Cerebrospinal fluid physiology and the management of increased intracranial pressure. Mayo Clin. Proc. 65:684–707.

Miller, J. D. 1979. Barbiturates and raised intracranial pressure. Ann. Neurol. 6:189–193.

Mooradian, A. D. 1988. Effect of aging on the blood–brain barrier. Neurobiol. Aging 9:31–39.

Neuwelt, E. A. (ed.) 1989. Implications of the Blood–Brain Barrier and Its Manipulation, Vol. 1. Basic Science Aspects, Vol. 2. Clinical Aspects. New York: Plenum Press.

Rapoport, S. I. 1976. Blood–Brain Barrier in Physiology and Medicine. New York: Raven Press.

Springer, T. A. 1990. Adhesion receptors of the immune system. Nature 346:425–434.

Turner, D. A., and McGeachie, R. E. 1988. Normal pressure hydrocephalus and dementia—evaluation and treatment. Clin. Geriatr. Med. 4:815–830.

Wikkelsö, C., Andersson, H., Blomstrand, C., Matousek, M., and Svendsen, P. 1989. Computed tomography of the brain in the diagnosis of and prognosis in normal pressure hydrocephalus. Neuroradiology 31:160–165.

References

Betz, A. L., and Goldstein, G. W. 1986. Specialized properties and solute transport in brain capillaries. Annu. Rev. Physiol. 48: 241–250.

Borgesen, S. E., and Gjerris, F. 1982. The predictive value of conductance to outflow of CSF in normal pressure hydrocephalus. Brain 105:65–86.

Borgesen, S. E., and Gjerris, F. 1987. Relationships between intracranial pressure, ventricular size, and resistance to CSF outflow. J. Neurosurg. 67:535–539.

DeVivo, D. C., Trifiletti, R., Jacobson, R. I., and Harik, S. I. 1990. Glucose transporter deficiency causing persistent hypoglycorrhacia: A unique cause of infantile seizures and acquired microcephaly. Ann. Neurol. 29:414–415.

Ehrlich, P. 1885. Das Sauerstoff-Bedurfnis des Organismus. Eine Farbenanalytische Studie. Berlin: Hirschwold, cited by Friedemann, 1942.

Friedemann, U. 1942. Blood–brain barrier. Physiol. Rev. 22:125–145.

Janzer, R. C., and Raff, M. C. 1987. Astrocytes induce blood–brain barrier properties in endothelial cells. Nature 325:253–257.

Jennett, B., and Teasdale, G. 1981. Management of Head Injuries. Philadelphia: F.A. Davis.

Kudo, H., Tamaki, N., Kim, S., Shirataki, K., and Matsumoto, S. 1987. Intraspinal tumors associated with hydrocephalus. Neurosurgery 21:726–731.

Kuffler, S. M. W., and Nicholls, J. G., and Martin, A. R. 1984. From Neuron to Brain: A Cellular Approach to the Function of the Nervous System, 2nd ed. Sunderland, Mass.: Sinauer.

Resnick, L., Berger, J. R., Shapshak, P., and Tourtellotte, W. W. 1988. Early penetration of the blood–brain-barrier by HIV. Neurology 38:9–14.

Spector, R., and Johanson, C. E. 1989. The mammalian choroid plexus. Sci. Am. 261(5):68–74.

Stewart, P. A., and Wiley, M. J. 1981. Developing nervous tissue induces formation of blood–brain barrier characteristics in invading endothelial cells: A study using quail-chick transplantation chimeras. Dev. Biol. 84:183–192.

Wahl, M., Unterberg, A., Baethmann, A., and Schilling, L. 1988. Mediators of blood–brain barrier dysfunction and formation of vasogenic brain edema. J. Cereb. Blood Flow Metab. 8:621–634.

Index

Following page numbers:
d = definition, f – figure, t – table

A

A-delta fibers, release of glutamate and substance P, 390
A-type potassium channel, 111
    gene for, 117
Abducens nerve, 510f
    functions, 684t, 685f
    lesion, 667
    right, effect of lesion on eye movement, 722f
Abducens nuclei, in somatic motor column, 687–688
Abducens nucleus, 509f, 665
    interneurons drive medial rectus motor neurons, 668
Abduction, eye, vertical muscle action in, 666t
Absence seizure, 785
Absolute refractory period, 110d
Acceleration
    angular, semicircular ducts' response to, 506
    linear, utricle responds to, 506–508
Accessory oculomotor nucleus. See Edinger–Westphal nucleus
Accommodation
    threshold affected by modulatory transmitters, 185
    visual, 664d
Acetylcholine (ACh)
    amount stored in synaptic vesicle, 226
    biosynthetic pathway, 215
    channel activated by, pore diameter compared with
        voltage-gated Na⁺ and K⁺ channels, 141, 141f
    control of receptor synthesis, 939
    corelease
        with CGRP, 221–222
        with vasoactive intestinal peptide, 221
    effect
        of Ca²⁺ on the amount released, 199–201
        of on heart rate, 772
        of on L-type Ca²⁺ current, 772
        of on pacemaker current, 772
        on nociceptors, 387
    evokes fast EPSP in autonomic ganglia, 768
    and excitatory synaptic action, 183f
    first isolation of chemical transmitter, 773
    impaired release of in botulism, 242
    key biosynthetic enzyme, 215t
    as low-molecular-weight neurotransmitter, 215
    mediates IPSP in sympathetic and parasympathetic ganglia,
        769
    neurons that use, 215
    nicotinic receptors. See also Acetylcholine receptor, nicotinic
        change in functional properties after muscle innervation,
            939–940
        presynaptic neurons regulate development of, 941
    production of EPSP in sympathetic ganglia, 184f
    receptors, in autonomic ganglia, 768. See also Acetylcholine
        receptor release
        after stimulation of sympathetic or parasympathetic
            postganglionic axons, 769–770
        by leakage, 232
        of by motor neuron before making muscle contact, 936
    role
        of cells secreting in REM sleep, 803
        in fasciculations, 250
    and synaptic activation of skeletal muscle by motor neurons,
        138–139
    in synaptic vesicles, 136
Acetylcholine receptor
    agrin induces clustering of on muscle membrane, 938f
    bungarotoxin-binding site, 239
    change in channel properties due to change in subunit
        composition, 940
    effect of alpha-bungarotoxin on, 237
    identification of antibodies to, 237–238
    immunogenic peptide of, role in autoimmune reaction, 241
    inducing activity, produces increase in acetylcholine
        receptors on muscle surface, 938
    loss of from postjunctional folds characteristic of myasthenia
        gravis, 237
    mechanisms of autoimmune reaction directed against, 241f
    muscarinic and nicotinic, 183
    nicotinic
        antibodies against and myasthenia gravis, 235–243
        distribution of after innervation of skeletal muscle,
            937–939
        as membrane protein, 146–148
        mRNA sequence of alpha-subunit, 34f, 35
        structure, 146–148
    rate of destruction increased in myasthenia gravis, 240f

Acetylcholine receptor [*cont.*]
  tubocurarine binds to and blocks neuromuscular
      transmission, 138
Acetylcholine receptor–channel
  complex, EM image, 137f
  five subunits of, 165f
  and miniature end-plate potential, 199
  nicotinic, model of, 148
  subunits, 147f
  three-dimensional image, 147–148
Acetylcholinesterase
  loss of and myasthenia gravis, 242
  removal of ACh from synaptic cleft, 232
Achromatopsia, 449d, 849d
Acid hydrolase activity, and lysosomes, 56
Acoustic neuroma, extra-axial brain stem lesion, 720–721, 721f
Acquired immunodeficiency syndrome, and spinal cord
      degeneration, 719. *See also* Human immunodeficiency
      virus
Across-fiber pattern coding, taste perception, 527
ACT. *See* Alpha-1-antichymotrypsin
Actin, 549f
  association with plasma membrane, 62
  domains in growth cone, 913f
  interaction with myosin in muscle fiber contraction, 550
  neural, in microfilaments, 62
  polymerization of as regulating growth cone motility, 913
  role in
    cell motility, 59
    controlling activity of growth cone, 914f
    slow axonal transport, 58
Action potential, 19d, 26d, 28f, 82d. *See also* Excitability
  all-or-none behavior, 110
    propagated by conductile component, 29
  amplitude and duration affected by modulatory transmitters,
      185
  as series of independent binomial trials, 210
  basic mechanism of generation same in all neurons, 110–111
  chemical synaptic transmission, delay between action
      potentials in pre- and postsynaptic cells, 132f
  compound, 351
    amplitude decreased in myasthenia gravis, 236
  conducted, stimulus information transmitted to central
      nervous system by, 338–339
  conduction velocity and axonal diameter, 348–351
  decision to fire or not to fire, 166
  in demyelinating diseases, 102
  dendritic, types, 787
  effect of nodes of Ranvier on propagation, 101
  factors limiting duration, 110
  features, 29t
  followed by
    period of refractoriness, 110
    transient hyperpolarization, 110
  generation, 88
    by ion flow through voltage-gated Na⁺ and K⁺ channels,
        105
    of in spinal motor cells, 155–160
    and voltage-gated channels, 104–108
  Hodgkin–Huxley model of, 109–110
  increased and decreased ability to generate, 27
  information transmitted from ganglion cells as, 408
  initiation
    at end-plate, 142f
    of at axon hillock, 167f
  integrative component, 28–29
  ion channels and signal properties, 166f
  membrane potential driven to threshold of by temporal
      summation, 98f
  methods to increase propagation, 101–102
  only two types of ion channels needed to generate, 111–112
  pattern of as neural code, sensory receptors, 336

postsynaptic, time course, 199f
propagation
  affected by passive membrane properties and axon
      diameter, 100–102
  increased by myelination, 101–102
  and passive conduction of depolarization, 100f
  quantification with Goldman equation, 88–89
  rate and number evoked and stimulus intensity, 336
  reconstruction from known properties of neuron, 109–110
  recording, 83
    to determine motor nerve conduction velocity, 252f
  role
    of axonal trigger zone, 29
    of electrotonic conduction in propagation of, 100
  saltatory conduction, 101–102
  sequential steps, 194
  series of to present stimulus information in neural encoding,
      334
  shape of calculated from changes in K⁺ and Na⁺
      conductances, 110f
  threshold
    for generating elevated in electrically coupled neurons, 129
    for generation, 110
    for initiation, 167f
  to fire or not to fire, neuronal integration, 166
  triggered by recruitment by EPP of neighboring voltage-gated
      channels, 142
  and twitch in muscle fiber, 550
  variation in conduction with demyelination, 251–252
  velocity of related to density of voltage-gated Na⁺ ion
      channels, 112–113
  and vesicle release of neurotransmitter, 132f
Action tremor, 644d
Activator domain, 189d
Active sleep. *See* Rapid eye movement sleep
Active touch, spinal mechanism, 586
Active zone, 29d, 136d, 201, 201f
  electron microscopy view, 204f
  increased in long-term sensitization, 1016
  level of Ca²⁺ influx at, 206
  presynaptic terminal, 131
Activin, as mesoderm inducing factor, 895
Activity dependence, in presynaptic facilitation, 1018
Acute intermittent porphyria, as chronic neuropathy, 250
Adaptation
  long-term, vestibulo-ocular reflex, 671
  of sensory receptors, 337
  vestibulo-ocular and optokinetic reflexes, 663
Adaptive control, 535d
Adduction, eye, vertical muscle action in, 666t
Adenosine triphosphate
  activity as chemical messenger and purinergic transmission,
      223–224
  contained within synaptic vesicles, 226
  corelease with neuroactive peptides, 222–224
  effect on nociceptors, 387
  and Na⁺-K⁺ pump, 87–88
  requirement of in muscle contraction, 550
Adenylyl cyclase
  Ca²⁺ calmodulin, stimulation of in classical conditioning,
      1018
  coupling of serotonin receptors to, 875
  cycle, 176f
  odorants enhance activity of in olfactory epithelium, 515
  system, and synaptic second messengers, 174f
Adequate stimulus, 331d
Adhesion
  Ca²⁺ dependent, mechanism of axonal growth, 918f
  Ca²⁺ independent, mechanism of axonal growth, 918f
  cell substrate, proteins that mediate, 920f
  interaction between growth cone and environment, 917
  molecules, and axon extension, 917–921

neural cell
    classes of glycoprotein involved, 918–921
    role of fibronectin, 920–921
    role of integrins, 920
    role of laminin, 920–921
    substrate, mechanism of axonal growth, 918t
Adhesive gradient, along dorsoventral axis of retinotectal
        system, 922
Adipose tissue, cholinergic and noradrenergic responses, 771t
Adrenal cortex, hypersecretion of cortisol from in severe
        depression, 879
Adrenal insufficiency, hyposmia in conjunction with, 518
Adrenal medulla
    cholinergic and noradrenergic responses, 771t
    innervation, 764
Adrenergic, 214d
Adrenergic neurons, two populations of synaptic vesicles in,
        226
Adrenergic sweating, 771d
Adrenocorticotropic hormone, as neuroactive peptide, 218t
Affect, 869d
Affective disorders. See also Panic attack
    abnormality in biogenic amine transmission may contribute
        to, 875–879
    genetic predisposition, 871–872
    nongenetic factors, 872
    unipolar and bipolar, 870–871
Affective functions, localization, 823–838
Affective responses, examples, 869
Affective traits
    localization in temporal lobe, 13–15
    localization of in brain, 12–15
Afferent (sensory) dorsal root ganglion cell, role in knee jerk
        stretch reflex, 40f
Afferent input, modifies locomotor pattern, 593–594
Afferent nerve fibers
    activation by projection neurons in processing sensory
        information, 369
    conduction velocity and axonal diameter, 348–351
    distribution of different types in muscle and cutaneous
        tissue, 351f
    enter spinal cord through dorsal roots, 353–354
    gathered in peripheral nerves, 354f
    groups, fiber diameter and conduction velocity, 351t
    intensity function, 336–337
    muscle, mediate limb proprioception, 347–349
    neural activity regulates competition and cooperation,
        953–956
Afferent neurons, 22d. See also Primary sensory neurons
    characteristic signal produced by four components, 28f
    conductile component, 29
    input component, 27
    integrative component, 28–29
    output component, 29
Afferent pathways, 360fd
Afterpotential, follows action potential, 110
Age
    change in sleep pattern with, 795–796, 796f
    and sleep problems, 808
Aggregate field view. See also Mass action theory
    and theory of language, 10
    as dominant during first half of 20th century, 11
    early experimental support, 6
    versus cytoarchitectonic view, 20th century, 11
Aging
    brain, 974–983
    characteristic changes in brain and behavior, 976
    molecular mechanisms, 974–975
    progressive decline in mental function not inevitable, 976
Agnosia, 448d, 831d
    visual, 449t
Agranular cortex, 611d

primary motor cortex, 612f
Agraphias, disorders of writing, characteristics, 849–850
Agrin
    induces clustering of acetylcholine receptors on muscle
        membrane, 938, 938f
    localization in motor neurons and synaptic cleft, 939f
Akinesia, 653d
Alar plate
    cells develop into dorsal horn, 300
    embryonic development, 300f
Alcohol, suppresses REM sleep, 795
Alchoholism
    and cerebellar cortical degeneration, 644
    chronic, treatment using food-aversion paradigm, 1001
    as chronic neuropathy, 250
Alexias, 849d
    disorders of reading, characteristics, 849–850
All-or-none action potential, 28f
Allocortex, 292d
Allosteric proteins, 75d
Alpha activity, recording, 778f
Alpha coma, 816
Alpha motor axons, large-diameter, 566f
Alpha motor neurons
    connections with corticospinal neurons, 612
    innervate extrafusal fibers, 567
Alpha waves, 779
Alpha-1-antichymotrypsin, in amyloid plaques, 978
Alpha-adrenergic receptors, action of neurally released
        norepinephrine on, 772
Alpha-amidation, in prohormone processing, 221
Alpha-amino-3-hydroxy-5-methyl-4 isoxazole proprionic acid
    as glutamate agonist, 158
    receptor–channels, flip and flop modules, 163
Alpha-bungarotoxin
    as competitive inhibitor, 77–78
    binds nicotinic receptors and blocks ACh action, 142
    binds to alpha-subunit of ACh receptor–channel, 147
    binds to nicotinic ACh receptors, 137f
    effect on ACh receptors, 237
Alpha-fetoprotein, binds estrogen to protect female fetuses from
        masculinization, 965
Alpha–gamma coactivation, 572d
Alpha-helices
    membrane-spanning, ACh receptor-channel subunit, 147f
    S4 region of Na^+ voltage-gated ion channel, 116
Alpha-latroxin, and production of Ca^{2+}-independent exocytosis,
        231
Alpha-mating factor, precursor structure, 220f
Alpha-melanocyte-stimulating hormone, 218t
Alpha-methyltyrosine, site of action in noradrenergic
        transmission, 879f
Alpha-propyidopacetamide, site of action in serotonergic
        transmission, 878t
Alpha-subunit, of Na^+ voltage-gated ion channel, 115
Alternative splicing, in neuroactive peptides, 219
Alumina cream, induction of focal epilepsy with, 786
Alzheimer's disease
    causes, 976
    cellular changes, 978f
    dementia, 974–983
    diagnosis, 977
    disruptions in circadian rhythm, 808
    and extracellular plaques containing amyloid, 977–979
    genetic component, 977
    and levels of tropic factors in the brain, 263–264
    loss of neurons in nucleus basalis of Meynert in, 980f, 981
    neurofibrillary tangles, characteristics of, 979–981
    neurotransmitter deficits in, 981
    pathology of in hippocampus, 979f
    symptoms, 977
    ventricular enlargement in, 858

Amacrine cells, 408, 409f
  and responses of ganglion cells, 414
  role in shaping receptor field properties of specific classes of
      ganglion cells, 414
  similar function to horizontal cells, 414
Amacrine interneurons, 415f
Aminergic neurons, populations of synaptic vesicles in, 226
Aminergic pathway, 541
Aminergic receptor, electroconvulsive therapy and possible
      changes in sensitivity, 872
Amino acid neurotransmitters, 217
  in nociceptive primary afferent fibers, 389–390
  in retina, 401
Amino peptidases, role in processing polyproteins into
      neuroactive peptides, 221
2-Amino-5-phosphonovalerate, selectively blocks NMDA
      receptor, 159
Amitriptyline
  structure, 873f
  site of action in serotonergic transmission, 878f
Amnesia
  anterograde, 1003d
  fundamental deficit, 1007
  reflexive versus declarative memory in patients with, 1006
  retrograde, 1003d
Amnesic syndrome, following anoxia causing damage to
      hippocampus, 1006
AMPA. See Alpha-amino-3-hydroxy-5-methyl-4 isoxazole
      proprionic acid
Ampere, 1034d
Amphetamine
  increases dopamine levels and causes psychosis resembling
      schizophrenia, 861
  site of action in noradrenergic transmission, 879f
Amphipathic helical proteins, 189d
Amplification, property of chemical transmission, 131
Amplitude, miniature end-plate potential, 200f
Ampulla, semicircular duct, 501
Ampullary crest, semicircular duct, 501
Amygdala, 276, 277, 306, 738f
  connections to hypothalamus and limbic system, 737
  connects olfactory cortex with hypothalamus and midbrain,
      518
  cortical nucleus of, projections in olfactory tract to, 517
  damage, 747
  derived from telencephalon, 298
  direct connection with orbitofrontal cortex, 826
  expression of D2 dopamine receptors in, 860
  GABA/benzodiazepam receptors concentrated in, 882
  lesions, 739
    interfere with conditioned responses, 1005
  morphological sex differences, 969
  neurofibrillary tangles in, 979
  projections, 737
  role in emotion, 747
  steroid receptors in, 966
  stimulation of to produce focal epilepsy, 786
Amygdaloid nucleus, function, 9t
Amyloid, 977d
Amyloid beta-protein precursor, 977
  and Alzheimer's disease, 977–978
Amyloid peptide, generation of, 978
Amyloid plaques
  characteristic of Alzheimer's disease, 977–979
  contain alpha-1-antichymotrypsin, 978
  neurotransmitters in, 978
Amyloidosis, as chronic neuropathy, 250
Amyotrophic lateral sclerosis, 248–249
  as spinal cord disorder, 718
  involves upper and lower motor neurons, 246
  motor neuron disease, 249t
Anaclitic depression, 946

Analgesia
  effect of morphine on central nervous system, 394
  induction of by behavioral stress, 397–398
  and pain, 385–399
  produced by direct electrical stimulation of brain, 393
Anastomoses, 1042–1043
  cerebral arteries, 1044
Anatomical personology, based on anatomy of the brain, 6d
Anatomy, discipline contributing to study of brain, 6
Androgen
  insensitivity syndrome, symptoms, 962
  required for emergence of male pattern, 964
  secreted by testes, 963
  stimulation of neuritic growth, 969
Androstenedione
  masculinization of the brain, 965
  replacement therapy in castrated rats, behavior in, 967
Anemia
  macrocytic, and spinal cord degeneration, 719
  pernicious. See Anemia, macrocytic
Anencephaly, defect of neural tube formation, 297
Aneurysms, saccular, rupture of and subarachnoid hemorrhage,
      1048
Angel dust. See Phencyclidine
Angiography, 309, 310f
Angiotensin, function as hormone and neurotransmitter, 757
Angiotensin I, role in water regulation, 757
Angiotensin II
  as neuroactive peptide, 218t
  in hypothalamus, 743
Angular gyrus, 623
  left cerebral hemisphere, concerned with auditory
      representation of words, 850
  lesion, 849, 850
Anhedonia, 870d
Annexins, 227d, 228t
Anomic aphasia, characteristics, 847t, 848
Anosmia, specific and general, 513, 518
Anoxia, 1045d
Anterior cerebral artery, 1041
  infarction, 1043f, 1046
Anterior choroidal artery, 1042, 1046
Anterior choroidal and penetrating arteries, occlusion, 1046
Anterior commissure
  connects olfactory bulbs, 514f
  effect of cutting, 833
Anterior inferior cerebellar artery, 1042
Anterior nuclei, thalamic, 291f, 292
Anterior olfactory nucleus, 517f
Anterior spinal artery, 1042
Anterolateral system
  anatomy, 359
  comparison with dorsal column–medial lemniscal system,
      362, 364t
  conveys somatic sensory information to cerebral cortex,
      358–363
  mediates
    pain and tactile sensations, 333f
    pain and temperature sense, 362–363
  organization, 359f, 363f
  pathways, 362–363
Antibiotics, enhanced entry into brain with brain tumors, 1056
Antibodies, used to test ion channel structure, 73
Anticipatory mechanisms
  postural adjustment, 596
  and regulation of motivated behaviors, 758–759
Antidepressant drugs
  act on serotonergic and noradrenergic pathways, 875
  produce down-regulation in presynaptic beta-adrenergic
      autoreceptors, 877
  treatment
    for depression, 872

of panic attacks with, 881
sites of action
in noradrenergic transmission, 878f
in serotonergic transmission, 878f
Antipsychotic drugs
action of serotonin receptors, 866
block dopamine receptors, 860–861
dopaminergic system as primary site of action, 698
long-term treatment with and development of tardive
dyskinesia, 657
relationship between clinical potencies and ability to block
dopamine D2 receptors, 861
sites of action at dopaminergic synapse, 862f
structures, 859f
treatment of schizophrenia, 858–866
Anxiety
anticipatory, neuroanatomical correlates, 14f
and disturbed sleep, 807
treatment with systematic desensitization, 1001
Anxiety disorders, 880–882
acute. See Panic attack
generalized
symptoms, 881–882
treatment, 881–882
Aperture problem
and representation of motion in brain, 451, 451f
study of, 453f
Apes, and knowledge of causality, 841
Aphasias, 831d, 839–851
application of mass action theory to, 12
conduction, and destruction of arcuate fasciculus, 11
cortical, characteristics, 847t
and defects in affective components of language, 13–14
head trauma and stroke as most common causes, 843
impairment of comprehension, 10
in middle cerebral artery infarction, 1045
paraphasia, 11d
study of and localization of language function in brain, 10–11
types related to different anatomical systems, 846–848
Apical dendrites, 19f
Aplysia californica. See also Gill-withdrawal reflex;
Habituation; Inking; Sensitization
FMRFamide produces hyperpolarization and synaptic
inhibition in sensory neurons, 186
APP. See Amyloid beta-protein precursor
Apparent motion, 449–450
Appetitive behavior, 989
Appetitive conditioning, 998d
Apraxia, 619
types in middle cerebral artery infarction, 1046
Aprosodias, 14d, 848d
APV. See 2-Amino-5-phosphonovalerate;
Aminophosphonovaleric acid
Aqueduct of Sylvius, 1050, 1051f
development, 303
occlusion, 719
Aqueductal stenosis, and hydrocephalus, 1059
Arachidonic acid
cascade, release of arachidonic acid is through
receptor-mediated activation of a phospholipase, 181,
182f
release by diffusion, 232
Arachnoid mater, 304d
Arachnoid membrane, 1051f
Arachnoid trabecula, 1051f
Arachnoid villi, transport of cerebrospinal fluid, 1052f
Arcuate concavity, lesions of, 829
Arcuate fasciculus
destruction of and conduction aphasia, 11
lesion, 844, 848
Arcuate nucleus, 738f
origination of tuberoinfundibular dopaminergic system, 863

Arcuate sulcus, location, 827f
Arcuate–ventromedial area, concentration of estradiol-sensitive
neurons in, 966f
Area postrema, blood–brain barrier leaky, 1055
ARIA. See Acetylcholine receptor inducing activity
Arm, flexion, 560–561
Arm projection neurons, 623
Arousal
disorders, 805–819
levels of regulated by brain stem, 9t
maintenance, sensory information used for, 330
mediated by reticular formation in brain stem, 275
role
of hypothalamus and cerebral cortex, 733
of thalamic diffuse-projection nuclei in maintaining,
289–290
Arrestin, 187d, 406
Arterial areas, brain, 1042f
Arteries, major cerebral, 724, 724f
Arterioles, cholinergic and noradrenergic responses, 771t
Artificial intelligence, 32d
Ascending medial longitudinal fasciculus, 509f
Ascending pathways, convey nociceptive information to brain,
390–392
Ascending projection neurons, in dorsal horn of spinal cord, 354
Aspartate
as amino acid neurotransmitter, 217
neurotransmitter
in pyramidal cells of somatic sensory cortex, 365
in pyramidal and spinal stellate cells of primary visual
cortex, 427
Association areas, 824
cerebral cortex, 277
Association connections, in somatic sensory cortex, 364–365
Association cortex, 824t
integration of components of language, 11
Association cortices, 821
and localization of higher cognitive and affective functions,
823–838
locations, 825f
organizational principles, 826
Astereognosia, 831d
Asterixis, symptom of metabolic coma, 817
Astrocyte, 23f
fibrous, 22
functions, 23–24
as glial cell, 22
possible role in capillary permeability, 1054
protoplasmic, 22
type 1, control fate of O-2A progenitor cells, 898
type 2, differentiation promoted by ciliary neurotrophic
factor, 899
types, 22
types 1 and 2, macroglial cell class, 898
Astrotactin, granule cell-surface protein possibly involved in
adhesive interactions between radial glia and granule
cells, 911
Asymmetry, of structure and function of cerebral hemispheres,
8
Asynergia, 644d
Atasia–abasia, in cerebellar hemorrhage, 1047–1048
Ataxia, 644d
in acoustic neuroma, 721
limb, 726t
Athetosis, 653d
Atonia, during REM sleep, 794
eliminated by lesions in pons, 797
REM sleep without causes violent episodes, 811
Atrial natriuretic peptide, as neuroactive peptide, 218t
Atrophy, 245d
group, 248d
muscle, 546d

Attention
   and formation of associations between processing in different
      cortical areas, 459
   role of locus ceruleus, 681
   selective, cellular basis, 460–462
   spatial aspects of sensation, role of parietal cortex in, 831
Attentive process
   in visual perception, 460
   winner-take-all strategy, 460
Attenuation coefficients. *See* Computerized tomography
Auditory artery
   brain stem, 725f
   echolocating bat, 497f
Auditory cortex, phasic bursts of electrical activity in during
      REM sleep, 794
Auditory evoked potential, deflections, 780, 780f
Auditory nerve
   fibers making up, 489
   fibers terminate in cochlear nucleus, 491
   hair cell vibrations transformed into electrical signals in,
      489–491
   phase locking of fibers, 491
   place principle, 491
   response patterns to tone bursts, 490f, 490–491
   tuning of fibers, 489, 489f
   volley principle, 491
Auditory neurons, central, specialized to preserve time and
      frequency information, 491–492
Auditory pathways
   bilateral, and cues to localize sound, 493
   central, anatomy, 495f
   parallel processing of auditory information, 496
Auditory stimulation, brain regions activated by, 315–316f
Auditory system, feedback connections, 496
Auerbach's plexus. *See* Myenteric plexus
Autocoid, 217d
Autoimmune diseases. *See also* Myasthenia gravis;
      Guillain–Barré syndrome
Autoimmune neurological disorders, ion channels as targets in,
      79
Autoimmune reaction
   mechanisms of against ACh receptor, 241f
   molecular basis of, 241
Autonomic division, peripheral nervous system, 274
Autonomic function
   integration of in brain stem and spinal cord nuclei, role of
      lateral tegmental noradrenergic system, 696
   localized to medulla oblongata, 9t
   regulated by hypothalamus, 9t
Autonomic ganglia, functions, 768
Autonomic motor neurons. *See* Motor neurons, autonomic
Autonomic motor system, preganglionic sympathetic neurons
      of in spinal cord, 284
Autonomic nervous system, 761–776
   cellular level, 768–775
   central regulation of output, 767f
   control of target function is coordinately regulated, 770–775
   divisions, 761, 763–766
   enteric division, 766
   influenced by motivational system, 279
   output controlled by hypothalamus and nucleus of the
      solitary tract, 766–768
   parasympathetic division, 765f, 766
   preganglionic neurons, ACh is neurotransmitter used, 215
   regulation of by hypothalamus, 746–747
   response of target to nerve impulses and circulating
      catecholamines, 771t
   role of brain stem in coordinating functions, 767
   sympathetic division, 764, 764f, 766
   targets of regulated by cholinergic and noradrenergic inputs,
      769–770
   as visceral and involuntary motor system, 762–763

Autonomic reactions, role of thalamus, 288
Autonomic responses, coordinated with endocrine responses
      and emotional states by amygdaloid nucleus, 9t
Autonomic system. *See also* Amygdala
Autophosphorylation, cAMP cascade, 178
Autoradiography
   electron microscope, use in localizing transmitter substances
      in the nerve cell, 222
   functonal mapping of neurons, 694
Autoreceptors, 207d, 217d
   beta-adrenergic, presynaptic, electroconvulsive therapy and
      antidepressants produce delayed down-regulation of, 877
Awareness
   controlling levels of, role of reticular formation, 692
   dorsal root ganglion connection with reticular formation
      neurons mediates, 286
   levels regulated by brain stem, 9t
Axial resistance, 98d
Axo-axonic synapses
   depression or enhancement of transmitter release, 207
   distinguished from axosomatic, 207–208
   presynaptic facilitation, 208f
   presynaptic inhibition, 208f
Axo-axonic synaptic contact, 168
Axodendritic synapse, input from, 169f
Axodendritic synaptic contact, 168
Axolemma, 39f
   and retrograde transport system, 62f
   sensory neuron, 38d
Axon, 19. *See also* Growth cone
   adjacent membrane segments represented as electrical
      equivalent circuit, 101f
   as conducting portion of neuron, Cajao model, 171
   central nervous system
      damage is irreversible, 264–265
      peripheral nerve grafts to promote growth after injury,
         265–266, 266f
   competition for particular targets, 923
   conduction rate and diameter of, 349–351
   decision region, 915
   diameter affects current threshold, 100
   distal segment, 259
   effects of sectioning of in postganglionic sympathetic
      neurons, 263f
   error-correcting in growth toward target, 922–923
   extension
      molecules involved in promote adhesion, 917–921
      promoted by laminin, 264
   fasciculation, glycoproteins involved in are members of
      immunoglobulin superfamily, 921
   glial scars prevent regeneration, 265
   growth
      molecular mechanisms, 918f
      promoted by glycoproteins in extracellular matrix in
         central and peripheral nervous systems, 265
      rate not constant, 921
   guided to target by growth cone, 911–914
   increased diameter of core increases conduction velocity, 101
   injury
      degeneration of distal segment, 260
      effect on nerve cell body, 260
      synaptic transmission lost rapidly, 259–260
      Wallerian degeneration, 259f
   integrative component, 29
   in motor neuron, 40–41
   myelin sheath, 38
   nodes of Ranvier, 38
   pathfinding
      directed to specific targets, 914–915, 915f
      guided by chemotactic molecules, 916–917
      guidepost cells, 915–916, 916f
      influenced by cues in environment, 915

inhibitory guidance cues, 916
  precision of in invertebrates, 915–916
  specific cellular cues for in invertebrates, 915–916
peripheral, role of Schwann cells in regeneration of, 264
proximal segment, 259
pruning during development, 923, 924f
regeneration after injury, 258
as region of nerve cell, 19
retinal, discrimination of anterior and posterior tectal
    membranes, 923f
selectivity of connection with target, 924–926
severing
  causes degenerative changes in neuron, 259–261
  degenerative changes, 259f
target-finding, role of molecular gradients, 921–922
trigger zone, 29
unit lengths represented as electric equivalent circuit, 98f
Axon diameter, and velocity of action potential propagation,
    100–102
Axon extension, involvement of adhesion molecules, 917–921
Axon guidance, 908–928
Axon hillock, 19d, 40d
  initiation of action potential at, 167f
  site of neuronal integration process, 166
  threshold of, 166
  as region of nerve cell body, 19f
Axon reflex, 386d
Axon terminal
  as transmitting pole of neuron, Cajal model, 171
  synapses on are modulatory, 170
Axonal arcades, in cerebral cortex, 782f
Axonal conduction, nerve cell signaling mechanism, 123
Axonal transport
  distribution of membrane and secretory proteins in nerve
      cell, 57–60
  fast
    anterograde, 57–59
    neuroanatomical tracing based on, 61
Axons. See also Growth cones
  accuracy of pathways, 914–917
  corticospinal, terminate on motor neurons in spinal cord that
      innervate specific limb muscles on and motor
      neuron-associated interneurons, 294
  extension inhibited by oligodendrocytes, 916
  high specificity in formation of synaptic connections, 915
  in white matter of spinal cord, 284, 286
  motor and sensory neurons, insulated by myelin sheath, 44f
  myelinated, in spinal cord white matter, 356
  nonpyramidal cells of cerebral cortex, 292
  projection to targets, 922–923
  pyramidal cells of cerebral cortex, 292
  retinal
    precision of initial projection, 921
    projection to precise positions on tectum, 922f
    regeneration of after cutting optic nerve, 921–922
  sensory and motor neurons, ensheathed in myelin, 43–45
Axoplasmic resistance, effect on signal conduction efficiency,
    97–100
Axosomatic synapse
  distinguished from axo-axonic, 207–208
  input from, 169f
Axosomatic synaptic contact, 168
Axotomy. See also Axon, injury
  degeneration of peripheral neurons prevented by trophic
      factors, 262–264

B

Babinski sign
  lesion of corticospinal tract, 545f
  in middle cerebral artery infarction, 1045
  presence of in gaze disorders, 723f
  sign of damage to corticospinal tract, 717

Back propagation, 837d
Background, influence on perceived color of object, retinex
    method, 476
Bacterial meningitis, and reduced blood–brain barrier, 1056
Bacterial toxins, response of G-protein alpha-subunit, 178
Bacteriorhodopsin, membrane protein, 71
Bag cell peptides, as neuroactive peptide, 218t
Bag fibers, primary sensory nerves, 38f
Bait shyness, 1001d
Balance, 500–511
  control of by vestibular nuclei input to vestibulocerebellum,
      634
  and equilibrium, 500–511
  feedback information to maintain, 500
  inability to maintain in spinal cat, 593
  organs of located in inner ear, 501–503
  reflex control of by vestibulospinal tract, 541
Balint's syndrome, 831
  effect on saccadic movement, 675
Ballism, 653d
  as disorder of basal ganglia, 654t
Barbiturates
  increase GABA-induced Cl⁻ current, 162
  masculinization of the brain, 965
  suppress REM sleep, 795
  treatment of insomnia, 808–809
Baroreceptors, and autonomic control of blood pressure, 770
Barrel arrangement of S-I cortical cells, 707–708
Basal dendrites, 19f
Basal forebrain nuclei, neurofibrillary tangles in, 979
Basal ganglia, 276, 277, 647–659, 848. See also Caudate
    nucleus; Putamen; Globus pallidus
  anatomical connections, 649f
  appearance of amyloid plaques in, 977
  as component of subcortical feedback loops of motor system,
      650f
  components, 295
  control of cortical and brain stem motor systems, 539–540
  derived from telencephalon, 298
  different circuits use different neurotransmitters, 652–653
  diseases of, 540
    produce disorders in neurotransmitter metabolism, 653
  disorders, 654t
  function, 9t
  inhibit superior colliculus, 675
  inputs and output pathways, 648–651
  lesions, 652
  links to cortex, 652
  location, 648f
  motor circuit is subcortical feedback loop, 651f
  nuclei of, 648
  output, decreased in Huntington's disease and increased in
      Parkinson's disease, 656
  pathological changes in produce characteristic motor
      disturbances, 647
  pathways through, 652
    interactions of neurotransmitters, 653f
  projections to thalamus, 650–651
  requirement of for goal-directed locomotion, 593
  role in higher-order cognitive aspects of motor control, 651
  somatotopic organization of motor portion, 651
  topographic organization of internuclear connections, 650
Basal lamina. See also Basement membrane
  function in synapse formation, 941
  and organization of presynaptic nerve terminal, 942
Basal pedunculi, 288f
Basal plate
  cells develop into ventral horn, 300
  embryonic development, 300f
Basal synapses, 415f
  and calcium-independent nonvesicular release, 416
  retinal, 416

Basement membrane, 136d, 136f, 201f
Basilar artery, 724, 1042
    brain stem, 725f
    occlusion, 722, 1047
Basilar membrane, vibration of bends hair cell stereocilia, 486f
Basis pedunculi, 294f, 363f
Basket cells
    in cerebral cortex, 779, 782f
    inhibitory interneurons, 632
Basket neurons, in cerebellar cortex, 630
Batrachotoxin, 112
Battery, ion channel as, 89–90
BDNF. *See* Brain-derived neurotrophic factor
Becker muscular dystrophy
    dystrophin abnormal in, 256
    gene for, 256
Bed-wetting. *See* Nocturnal enuresis
Behavior
    adult sexual, effects of castration–replacement experiment,
        967f
    appetitive, 989
    as built up from reflexes shaped by experience, 988
    behaviorist view, 985
    and brain, overview, 5–17
    central effects of hormones on involve humoral and neural
        output, 745
    certain complex patterns require little or no learning, 994
    certain human traits have hereditary component, 993
    cognitive view, 985
    consummatory, 989
    cyclic, 733
    and development of the brain, 985
    development of ocular dominance columns as model for,
        949–956
    emotional and motivational aspects, and limbic area, 825
    feeding, regulatory mechanisms, 753–757
    feeding. *See* Feeding behavior
    fixed-action pattern, 989–991
    genetic determinants, 987–996
    genetic factors, 985
    homotypical versus heterotypical patterns, 963
    innate, in higher mammals and humans, 993–994
    instinctive
        development of, 946
        genetically programmed, 988
        study of, 987–988
    interaction between somatic sensory and motor systems to
        carry out, 280f
    involves sensory, motor, and motivational systems, 279
    localization of function in brain, history, 10–12
    motivated, factors that regulate, 758–759
    motivational system influences by acting on somatic and
        autonomic motor systems, 279
    and nerve cells, 18–32
    nerve cells as signaling units of, 24–25
    purposeful, 531
    question of inheritability, 988–989
    relationship to brain, alternative views of, 6–7
    relationship to development of nervous system, 885
    reproduction, sexual dimorphism of, 963
    role of genes in expression of, 991–992
    sex differences in brain influence wide range of, 970–971
    sex-linked, perinatal hormones determine degree of
        expression, 968
    sexual, affected by genes in *Drosophila*, 992
    species-specific, elicited by sign stimuli, 989
Behavioral act, participation of sensory, motor, and
        motivational systems, 281f
Behavioral arousal
    dorsal root ganglion connection with reticular formation
        neurons mediates, 286
    role of reticular formation, 692

Behavioral set, ability to change, role of lateral orbitofrontal
        circuit, 652
Behaviorism, 3
Behaviorist psychology, 330
Behaviors, human, many are universal, 993
Benign intracranial hypertension, 1059
Benzodiazepams, enhance activity of GABA receptors, 881–882
Benzodiazepines
    increase GABA-induced Cl⁻ current, 162
    lower core body temperature, 810
    and modulation of Cl⁻ flux through GABA receptor, 882
    receptor, and mechanism of flurazepam's sleep-inducing
        properties, 810
    reduce stage 4 slow-wave sleep, 795
    treatment
        anxiety disorders, 881–882
        insomnia, 809–810
Berger rhythm, 779
Beta activity, recording, 778f
Beta waves, 779
Beta-adrenergic autoreceptors, presynaptic, electroconvulsive
        therapy and antidepressants produce delayed
        down-regulation of, 877
Beta-adrenergic receptor
    and action of neurally released catecholamines on heart
        muscle cells, 771
    and desensitization by protein phosphorylation, 186
Beta-endorphin
    in hypothalamus, 743
    as neuroactive peptide, 218t
Between brain. *See* Diecephalon
Betz cells, in layer 5 of motor cortex, 611
Bicuculline, use of to generate spontaneous interictal spikes in
        hippocampus in vitro, 789
Binaural cells, primary auditory cortex, columnar groups, 494
Binocular disparity, 455d
    required for three-dimensional vision, 454–458
    responses of cells to, 457f
Binocular zone, 421d,f
Biofeedback, as form of operant conditioning used clinically,
        1002
Biogenic amines
    availability increased by monoamine oxidase inhibitors, 877
    contained within vesicles, 225
    degradation by catechol-O-methyltransferase, 232
    degradation by monoamine oxidases, 225
    as neurotransmitters, 215–217
    transmission, abnormality in may contribute to affective
        disorders, 875–879
    uptake blockers, structure, 873f
Biological clock
    and life span, 975
    suprachiasmatic nucleus for sleep–wake cycle, 800–801
Bipolar neurons, 21f, 408, 409f
    antagonism between center and surround areas, 414
    center–surround receptive fields, 412–414
    description, 20–21
    different populations contacted by rods and cones, 415f
    on-center and off-center, excitatory connections with
        ganglion cells, 414
    opposite actions of glutamate on two classes of, 413
    relay signals from photoreceptors to ganglion cells, 412
    respond to light with graded change in membrane potential,
        412
Bitemporal hemianopsia, 437d
Biting, central program for, 990
Bitterness, taste quality, 521
Bizarre delusions, in schizophrenia, 855
Bladder
    autonomic control, 773–774, 774f
    innervation, 764
    somatic motor control, 774, 774f

Blind sight, and perception of visual stimuli, 335
Blind spot, 402d, 422, 422f
Blindness, comparison with blind spot, 422
Blob regions
  primary visual cortex, 428
  striate cortex, 446
Blob zones
  double-opponent cells concentrated in, 475
  process color information in cortex, 473–476
Blobs, 434d
  primary visual cortex, 432, 432f
Blocking phenomenon, 999d
Blood
  and brain, specific permeability barrier, 1053–1054
  and cerebrospinal fluid, specific permeability barrier,
    1053–1054
Blood pressure
  autonomic control of, 770
  and carotid sinus reflex, 771f
Blood vessels
  innervation, 764
  magnetic resonance angiography, 321f
Blood–brain barrier
  and brain capillary endothelial cells, 1054
  development, 1055
  disorders, 1056–1057
  does not exist in some areas of brain, 1055
  function, 1056
  role of glial cells, 22
Blood–cerebrospinal fluid barrier
  mechanisms of molecular flow across, 1053f
  structural and functional relationship, 1052f
Bodian staining, based on degenerative changes in neurons, 262
Body, cortical representation, 370–374. See also Somatotopic
    map
Body image, function localized to parietal lobe of cerebral
    cortex, 7
Body plan, genetic control of during development, 897
Body regions, somatic sensibilities of different species, 373f
Body senses, 341
Body surface
  innervation of represented in more than one sensory map in
    primary somatic sensory cortex, 1024f
  map, in superior colliculus, 424. See also Somatotopic map
  and map of evoked potentials from surface of left postcentral
    gyrus of cerebral cortex, 370f
  neural maps of, 373–374
  representation of in brain, 370–374
Body sway, muscles contracting during, 598, 598f
Body temperature
  core, lowered by benzodiazepines, 810
  inability to regulate during REM sleep, 794
  in insomnia, 806–807, 807f
Body weight
  negative feedback system for regulation of fat stores, 754
  set point, 753–754
Bombesin
  as neuroactive peptide, 218t
  peptide in sympathetic neurons, 770t
Bone conduction, sound, 483
Bony labyrinth, 501
boss gene, Drosophila, and R8 photoreceptor, 902
Botulism, and impaired release of ACh, 242
Brachial plexus avulsions, 387d
Bradykinin
  and activation and sensitization of nociceptors, 387f
  effect on nociceptors, 387, 387t
  as neuroactive peptide, 218t
Braille, 326f
Brain
  adult, generation of new neurons, 268
  aging, 974–983

anatomical changes in some schizophrenia patients, 857–858
androgenized
  little behavioral response to estrogens, 967
  preoptic cells refractory to hormonal activation, 967
androgens exposed, even pattern of LH secretion, 967
antipyretic area in, 753
application of cell theory to, 20
association areas of cerebral cortex, 823–834
asymmetry revealed in conventional radiographs, 310–311
and behavior, overview, 5–17
biochemical processes imaged with positron emission
    tomography, 312–314
blood supply divided into arterial territories, 1041–1043
blood vessels, 1042f
cellular mechanisms of sex differences, 969–970
characteristics of in Alzheimer's disease, 980
chemical synaptic transmission in, 135
circulation, 1041–1049
connectionist approach, and principles of dynamic
    polarization and connectional specificity, 20
convergent versus divergent pathways, 271
critical periods of development for different regions, 956–957
death. See Death, cerebral
  criteria for, 818t
decision-making capacity, 166
decreased level of proteins with age, 976
decreased weight with age, 976
developing, mechanisms of segmentation, 302–303
development as guide to regional anatomy of, 296–308
disorders of function, 5
direct electrical stimulation produces analgesia, 393
divergence and convergence of neuronal connections, 25f
dopaminergic tracts in, 864f
drug delivery to, 1057
edema, 1057
enlarged lateral ventricles in some schizophrenia patients,
    857–858
enlarged third ventricles in some schizophrenia patients,
    857–858
female
  cyclical LH secretion pattern, 967
  LHRH secretion in, 967
function
  cellular connectionism view of, 7
  cytoarchitectonic view, 11–12
  distributed processing, 11
  evidence for localization of, 12
  mass action theory, 12
  parallel processing principle, 7
  phrenologic map of, 7f
functions of main parts, 9t
functional change in and long-term memory, 1004–1005
functional classification of nerve cells in, 22
glutamate as neurotransmitter in, 158–160
hemispheres, asymmetry and difference in capabilities, 832
hemorrhage, 1045
holistic view, 823
imaging, 309–324
  with computerized tomography, 311–312
immature neurons migrate on radial glial cells, 909–911
and increased intracranial pressure, 1057–1058
individual units of, 5
information processing in, 31
interconnections of language regions, 845
lateral view of cerebral cortex, 10f
and limits on structure of language, 994–995
localization
  of function, 823
  of mental processes, 12, 15–16
long-term memory and plastic changes in, 1004–1005
magnetic resonance image, 9f
major disciplines contributing to understanding of, 6–7

Brain [cont.]
  masculinization, 964–965
  mass not neuronal architecture important to function, 12
  mature, ventricular system, 306f
  metabolic rate and oxygen requirements, 1044
  midsagittal section, 9f
  noradrenergic pathways, 876f
  normal male pattern determined by estradiol, 965
  number of neurons in, 18
  number of synapses in, 121
  parts of, 8f
  pathways for processing word recognition, PET imaging, 13f
  PET scan of areas active during language task, 2f, 3
  primary language areas, 844f
  reduced cortical tissue in some schizophrenia patients,
      857–858
  and relationship to behavior, alternative views of, 6–7
  regions specialized for different function, 7
  representation of body surface in, 370–374
  and sense of self, 15–16
  sensory information processed in series of relay regions, 369
  sensory systems, 330–529
  separate perfusion of medulla, caudal pons, and posterior
      cerebellum in cat, 817
  serotonergic pathways, 874f
  sex differences in influence wide range of behaviors, 970–971
  sexually differentiated, physiological and behavioral
      tendencies, 967
  slice
    advantages in recording from neurons in, 788
    preparation, 788
  somatotopic map in is modifiable by experience, 1024–1027
  storage of knowledge as distinct categories, 15
  stimulation, as reinforcement of behavior, 759
  subcortical regions, projections to from retina, 423–426
  tissue localization of neuroactive peptides, 218t
  tissue slice preparation, 788
  tumors, and enhanced antibiotic entry into brain, 1056
  uptake of selected compounds and lipid solubility, 1055f
  vascular physiology altered by stroke, 1048–1049
  vasculature, 724, 724f
    imaging with angiography, 311
  ventricles, imaging with pneumoencephalogram, 311
  ventricular system and regional anatomy of diencephalon and
      cerebral hemispheres, 304–307
  vesicles
    cavities of become ventricular system of brain, 303–304
    formation from embryonic neural tube, 298, 298f
Brain-derived neurotrophic factor, 262
  receptor, trk B protein as, 933
  supports survival of sensory neurons not sensitive to nerve
      growth factor, 933
Brain stem. See also Cranial nuclei; Monoaminergic systems;
      Medulla; Pons; Midbrain
  activation of neurons responsible for descending inhibition of
      spinal motor neurons during REM sleep and narcolepsy,
      813
  active sleep-inducing neurons in, 799–800
  as rostral continuation of spinal cord, 681
  aspects of motor control by, 539
  caudal
    and active induction of sleep, 816
    developmental plan, 301
  classes of motor neurons in, 686–687
  clinical syndromes, 711–730
  cranial nerves in, 683–684
  cross sections at different levels, 288f
  damage to, 681
  depression of or damage to and impaired consciousness, 815
  descending pathways modulate motor neurons and
      interneurons in spinal cord, 541–543
  descending systems, level of motor control, 537–540

  developing, alar and basal plates, 686, 686f
  developmental plan similar to spinal cord, 300–302
  differentiation
    of alar plate cells, 302
    of vasal plate cells, 302
  divisions, 275
  dopaminergic cell groups in, 697f
  embryonic development, 300f
  evoked potentials, 780
  function, 9t, 275, 681, 719
  horizontal and longitudinal planes, 719–720
  lateral tegmental neurons provide primary noradrenergic
      input to, 696
  lateral view, emergence of cranial nerves, 685f
  lesions, 719–729
  lesions in and eye movement deficits, 673
  location of cranial nerves, 720f
  medial and lateral descending systems controlled by efferent
      spinocerebellar projections, 636–637
  medial and lateral syndromes of infarction, 1047
  mediate vestibular and neck reflexes, 600
  midsagittal section, MRI, 318f
  monoaminergic systems in, 693–697
  motor nuclei associated with individual cranial nerve, 691
  network coordinates horizontal vestibulo-ocular reflex,
      668–669
  noradrenergic neurons, 696
  nuclei, neurofibrillary tangles in, 979
    oculomotor nuclei, 667f
  organization, 683–700
    principles, 691–692
  pathways. See also Corticospinal tract; Corticobulbar tract
    descending, 542f
    of horizontal vestibulo-ocular reflex in, 670f
  phasic bursts of electrical activity in during REM sleep, 794
  preganglionic neurons of parasympathetic division located in,
      766
  reflexes, 565d
  role
    in coordinating autonomic functions, 767
    of regions of in triggering REM sleep, 801, 803
  saccade generator in controlled in cerebral cortex, 674–676
  sensory neurons, 687
  sensory nuclei, receive input from several cranial nerves, 691
  serotonergic cell groups in, 698f
  serotonin is neurotransmitter in cells at midline raphe
      nuclei, 217
  stimulation of inhibits nociceptive neurons in dorsal horn,
      394
  and stimulation of locomotion, 593
  structures at different levels, 288f
  syndromes produced by vascular lesions, 726t, 727f
  tonic descending signals activate spinal circuits for
      locomotion, 591–593
  transection
    above red nucleus, 604
    above vestibular nuclei causes decerebrate rigidity, 604
  transverse sections, cranial nerve nuclei, 689f
  traversed by all descending cortical and all somatic afferent
      projections, 691
  vascular lesions of, 723–729
  ventral view, origins of cranial nerves, 685f
  vertebral artery supply, 725f
  vestibulo-ocular reflex coordinated in, 667–671
Branchiomeric muscles, innervated by special visceral motor
      column, 687
Breathing
  function localized to medulla oblongata, 9t
  role of reticular formation in control of, 693
Brightness, color, total effect of object on all three cones, 477
Broca's aphasia
  characteristics, 847, 847t

in middle cerebral artery infarction, 1045
Broca's area
  and language perception, 11
  in lateral view of cerebral cortex, 10f
  lesion, 844
  localization of language function in brain, 10
  localization of word recognition during speaking, 13f
  perception of speech sounds, 495
Brodmann's areas of cerebral cortex, 11f
Brodmann's area 1
  evoked response mapping of body surface in, 371
  input from rapidly adapting cutaneous receptors dominant, 378
  lesions in produce defect in assessment of texture, 370
  somatosensory map, 373f
  spatial pattern of neuronal activity, cutaneous receptors, 379
Brodmann's area 2
  input from deep pressure receptors dominant, 377–378
  lesions in produce defect in ability to differentiate size and shape of objects, 370
Brodmann's areas 1 and 2
  complex response properties of neurons of to somatic stimulation, 380
  edge-orientation neurons and convergent projections from areas 3a and 3b, 380
  feature-detection neurons in, 380
Brodmann's areas 1, 2, and 3, postcentral gyrus, 11f
Brodmann's areas 1, 2, 3a, 3b, association connections in, 365.
    See also Primary somatic sensory cortex
  primary somatic sensory cortex, 368f
  removal of produces deficits in position sense and ability to discriminate size, texture, and shape, 370
Brodmann's area 3, somatosensory map, 373f
Brodmann's area 3a, input from muscle stretch receptors dominant, 377
Brodmann's area 3b
  gustatory region of postcentral gyrus, 525
  input from cutaneous receptors dominant, 377
  lesions in produce deficits in discrimination of texture, size, and shape, 370
  spatial pattern of neuronal activity, cutaneous receptors, 379
Brodmann's area 4
  facial area of motor cortex, 845f
  primary motor cortex, 844f
Brodmann's areas 4 and 6, corticospinal tracts originate in, 544f
Brodmann's area 5, retinotopic map in, 446
Brodmann's areas 5 and 7
  association connections in, 365
  posterior parietal cortex, 368f
Brodmann's area 6, stimulation of produces motor effects, 611
Brodmann's area 7, posterior parietal cortex, 675
Brodmann's area 8, frontal eye field, 675
Brodmann's areas 8, 9, and 10, prefrontal association cortex, 11f
Brodmann's area 17. See also Striate cortex
  primary visual cortex, 11f, 427–431, 825, 844, 845f
  projections from retina to, 423f
  response of cells in to ocular disparity, 458f
  retinotopic map in, 446
Brodmann's area 18, 849
  higher-order visual center, 825, 844, 845f
  projection of pyramidal cells of V1 to, 434
  retinotopic map in, 446
Brodmann's area 19, retinotopic map in, 446
Brodmann's areas 19, 21, 22, 37, 39, and 40, parietal–temporal–occipital association cortex, 11f
Brodmann's area 22, Wernicke's area, 844f, 845f
Brodmann's area 39, angular gyrus, 844, 845f
Brodmann's area 39, supramarginal gyrus, 623
Brodmann's area 40, angular gyrus, 623
Brodmann's area 41, primary auditory cortex, 844f
Brodmann's areas 41 and 42, primary auditory cortex, 11f
Brodmann's area 42, higher-order auditory cortex, 844

Brodmann's area 44, frontal gyrus, 847
Brodmann's area 45
  Broca's region, 844f
  frontal gyrus, 847
Brodmann's areas 18, 20, 21, 37, lesions of and visual agnosias, 449t
Brodmann's areas 41 and 42, primary auditory cortex, 494
Brodmann's layers, cytoarchitectonic areas of cerebral cortex, 293, 293f
Brow flash response, sign stimulus, 994
Brown–Séquard syndrome, 718
Buccalins, as neuroactive peptide, 218t
Burning pain, and activity of efferent fibers of sympathetic nervous system after peripheral nerve injury, 387
Burns, and production of primary and secondary hyperalgesia, 386f
Burst cells, role in horizontal saccades, 671
Burst-tonic cells, role in horizontal saccades, 671, 672
Bushy cells, cochlear nucleus, 492f
Butyrophenones
  long-term treatment with and development of tardive dyskinesia, 657
  structure, 859t, 859f
  treatment, schizophrenia, 858

C
C fibers, release of glutamate and substance P, 390
c-fos, as activity marker for neurons in vivo, 802
C-terminal recognition sequence, 55d
Ca²⁺/calmodulin-dependent protein kinase
  activation, 180f, 181
  domains, 179f
Cacosmia, 518d
Cadherins
  binding function dependent on Ca²⁺, 920
  involved in neural cell adhesion, 918
  role in neural cell adhesion, 919–920
Caenorhabditis elegans
  anatomy, 889f
  cell lineage and cell fate, 888
  cell–cell interaction, role in cell fate, 888, 889f, 890–891
  genetic analysis of differentiation of HSN neurons in, 890f
  genetically programmed death of neurons, 929–930
  lineage tree, 889f
  program of neural cell development in, 888
Calcarine cortex, 436f
Calcarine cortex, destroyed in posterior cerebral artery infarction, 1046
Calcarine fissure, 319f, 426f
Calcarine sulcus, effect of lesion, 437f
Calcineurin, and inactivation of Ca²⁺ channels, 111
Calcitonin, as neuroactive peptide, 218t
Calcitonin gene-related peptide
  contained within vesicles, 226
  corelease with ACh, 221–222
  increases acetylcholine receptor number on muscle surface, 938
  as neuroactive peptide, 218t
Calcium
  binding function of cadherins dependent on, 920
  binds to troponin, 550
  concentration
    and probability of quantum release, 200
    regulated by hyperpolarization and depolarization, 206–207
  enhanced influx as mechanism of presynaptic facilitation, 208
  entry into axon after injury, 259
  excess, and cell death, 657–658
  free, concentration of and plasticity of chemical synapse, 209
  free intracellular, regulated by synaptic connections on presynaptic terminals, 207
  functions, 197

Calcium [cont.]
  importance of in regulating neuronal function, 209
  increase in intracellular and muscle fiber contraction, 550
  influx
    affects exocytosis and mobilization of synaptic vesicles,
      205f
    and control of synaptic vesicle docking, fusion, and
      exocytosis, 203–206
    greatest at active zone region, 206
    and quantal release of neurotransmitter, 199–201
    required for neurotransmitter release, 197–198
    through NMDA receptor–channel critical for long-term
      potentiation, 1020
  inhibitory effect on guanylate cyclase, 408
  internal, and ion channel inactivation, 76f
  ions, intracellular, modulating effect on ion channels, 111
  intracellular
    and ion channel inactivation, 76f
    changes in and light adaptation in photoreceptors, 408
    effect of change in concentration on growth cone motility,
      913
  level of influx and modulation of number of synaptic vesicles
    released, 206–209
  and mobilization of synaptic vesicles from cytoskeleton,
    206
  NMDA receptor permeability to, 593
  release of triggered by bitter stimuli, 521
  residual, and potentiation, 207
  role
    in initiating persistent enhancement of synaptic
      transmission in LTP, 1021
    in mobilization of synaptic vesicles, 227
    in protein kinase C activity, 181
    in release of growth factor in synapse stabilization, 956
Calcium current
  L-type, effect of acetylcholine on, 772
  long-lasting, enhancement of by beta-adrenergic agonists
    mediated by cAMP, 771
  participation in electrical resonance of hair cells, 488, 488f
Calcium gluconate, promotes release of ACh, 242
Calcium influx, during depolarization and neurotransmitter
  release, experimental demonstration, 198f
Calcium ion channel. See Ion channel, calcium
Calcium-activated K⁺ channel, 111. See Ion channel,
  calcium-activated K⁺
Calcium-activated K⁺ current, participation in electrical
  resonance of hair cells, 488
Calcium-binding proteins
  examples, 228t
  role in synaptic vesicle mobilization, 227–228
Calcium-independent nonvesicular release, at basal synapses,
  416
Calculation with Ohm's law, through active ACh-gated
  channels and nongated membrane channels, 151
Caldesmin, and mobilization of synaptic vesicles, 227
Caldesmon, 228t
Calelectrin, 228t
Callosal connections, in somatic sensory cortex, 364–365
Calmodulin, 228t
  bound by GAP-43, 913
  role in axonal transport, 59
Calpactin I, 228t
Calpactin II, 228t
cAMP-dependent protein kinase, domains, 179f
Capacitance, 1034d. See also Membrane capacitance
  current flow in circuits with, 1038–1040
  and increase of plasma membrane surface area during fusion
    of synaptic vesicles, 203
  membrane, effect on time course of signal conductance,
    95–97
  as passive electrical property of nerve cell, 91
  symbol, 1037

Capacitive circuits, time dependence of changes in current and
  voltage, 1038
Capacitive current
  effect on amount of charge stored in cell membrane, 97
  study with voltage-clamp technique, 105
Capacitive membrane current, 96d
Capacitor
  factors affecting potential difference between two plates of,
    1035f
  properties, 91
  time course of charging, 1038
    in parallel with resistor, 1040f
    in series with resistor, 1039f
Capillary endothelial cells, brain
  and blood–brain barrier, 1054
  ultrastructural features, 1055f
Capsulotomy, internal capsule, 829
Carbachol, elicits REM sleep, 803
Carbamezapine, treatment of REM behavior disorder, 811
Carbon dioxide
  effects in brain after stroke, 1048
  and induction of panic attack, 881
Carboxypeptidase B, role in processing polyproteins into
  neuroactive peptides, 221
Carcinomas, examples of as chronic neuropathy, 250
Cardiac function, role of reticular formation, 693
Cardiac ganglion, innervation, 766
Cardiac peptides, small, as neuroactive peptide, 218t
Cardiovascular function
  autonomic control of, 770
  parasympathetic regulation, 772
  sympathetic regulation, 771–772
Carnosine, histamine as precursor, 217
Carotid artery
  brain stem, 725f
  occlusion, 1047
Carotid sinus reflex, and blood pressure control, 771, 771f
Castration, effect on sexual development of genotypic male
  rats, 964
Castration–replacement experiment, and adult sexual behavior,
  967f
Catalase, 64d
Cataplexy, narcoleptic symptom, 813d
Cataracts, effect on development of vision in newborn, 947
Catechol-O-methyltransferase, degrades biogenic amines, 232,
  879f
Catecholamine hypothesis, for depression, 875, 877
Catecholamines
  circulation, responses of autonomic target to, 771t
  as neurotransmitters, 216
  release of by sympathetic nervous system, 770
Catenins, interaction with cytoskeleton, 920
Cation channels, closing of in phototransduction, 404f
Cauda equina, 285f, 301
Caudal, in central nervous system, 274f
Caudate nucleus, 277, 290f
  C-shaped like lateral ventricles, 306–307
  cell death in Huntington's chorea, 306–307
  degeneration in Huntington's disease, 981
  development, 305f
  increased number of D2 dopamine receptors in schizophrenic
    patients, 861
  inputs to, 649f
  left, important for language, 845
  of basal ganglia, 648
  and regulating speed of movements, 295
  role in control of eye movements, 649
  selective loss of neurons in Huntington's disease, 656
  shape of parallels lateral ventricle, 307f
Caudate system, expression of D2 dopamine receptors in, 860
Causal relationships, detection of in classical conditioning,
  1000

Causalgia, 387d
Causalgic pain, relief, 388
Cell body, region of nerve cell, 19
Cell death
    genetically programmed, 657
    glutamate-induced, and Huntington's disease, 657–658
Cell differentiation
    fate depends of lineage in some cells, 888
    and gene activation, 887–888
Cell identity, control of in nervous system, 887–907
Cell membrane
    as capacitor in parallel with resistor, 96
    as leaky capacitor at rest, 92
    channels in allow ions to cross, 67–69
    charge within redistributed when voltage-gated Na$^+$ channels
        open, 113, 115
    electrical charge separation and alteration of polarization, 82
    equivalent circuit model for, 90–92
    lipid bilayer, as insulator separating two conductors, 92
    passive flux of ions across, 73–74
    passive properties, 95–103
    proteins, 52–55. See also Membrane-spanning proteins
    relationship between insulation and conducting properties, 99
    separation of charge across and membrane potential, 82
Cell motility, role of actin and dynein in, 59
Cell position, and identity of photoreceptors in *Drosophila* eye,
    899–902
Cell theory, application to the brain, 20
Cell–cell interactions, role in determining cell fate, 888, 889f,
    890–898
Cell-surface molecules, guide neurons by repelling growth
    cones, 916
Cells, two classes in nervous system, 19–25
Cellular connectionism, view of brain function, 7d
Central auditory neurons, specialized to preserve time and
    frequency information, 491–492
Central gyrus, 8
Central herniation, 817d
Central nerve cells, complex feature-detecting properties of in
    later stages of cortical processing, 380–381
Central nervous system. *See also* Brain; Brain stem; Retina;
        Spinal cord
    axes of organization, 274–275
    axonal damage is irreversible, 264–265
    basic plan established by migratory pattern of neurons,
        908–911
    bilateral auditory input, 494
    chemical synaptic transmission in, 153–172
    control of muscle spindle sensitivity through gamma motor
        neurons, 571–574
    decussation of neural pathways, 281–282
    degeneration of synapses after axonal injury, 260
    derived from endoderm, 296
    describing directions in, 274f
    developing, some neurons in dependent on nerve growth
        factor, 933
    dopaminergic cell groups in, 698
    elimination of synapses in, 943
    embryogenesis, 274f
    embryonic
        floor and roof plate in, 300
        long-axis view of flexure formation, 299f
        regional specialization, 297–299
        subdivisions and adult forms, 299t
    excitatory and inhibitory chemical synaptic transmission in,
        153–172
    expression of inhibitory glycoproteins, 265
    functional anatomy, 273–324
    functional mapping of neurons on basis of neurotransmitters,
        694
    functions of main parts, 9t
    high concentrations of GABA, 217

    mature, midsagittal view, 299f
    midsagittal section, 275f
    myelination, 43
    principles governing organization of, 279–282
    receptive field of sensory neurons in, 334, 335f
    recovery of function after damage, 261, 265–268
    regions, 275–279
    specificity of synaptic connections, 926
    spinal stretch reflex and synaptic transmission, 154–155
    stimulus information transmitted to by conducted action
        potentials, 338–339
    structure and functional state revealed by MRI, 314–321
    synapses, quantal analysis, 201
    transplantation of embryonic neurons to promote recovery of
        function after damage, 266–268
    trophic influence of NGF on cholinergic neurons of, 263
    vascular damage and chronic pain, 388
Central neurons, somatic sensory system, specific receptive
        fields, 374–377
Central pain syndromes, 388
Central pattern generator
    half-center model, 584
    elements include flexor reflex afferent pathways producing
        flexion and extension, 589
    interneuron networks, 582, 584
    spinal circuits as, 591
Central program
    generates fixed-action patterns, 989–991
    responses having, 990
Central sulcus, 278f
Central visual pathways, 420–439
Cephalic flexure, 298
Cerebellar artery, brain stem, 725f
Cerebellar cortex, 627d
    anterior lobe, stimulation of reduces decerebrate rigidity, 604
    inputs from raphe nuclei and locus ceruleus, 632
    mossy and climbing fibers as excitatory inputs, 631–632
    Purkinje cells provide output of, 631–632
Cerebellar flocculus, role in neural integration of
        vestibulo-ocular reflex, 671
Cerebellar hemisphere, intermediate, cortical projections, 637
Cerebellar hemorrhage, 1047
Cerebellar peduncles, 288f, 627d
Cerebellar tonsils, 628d
Cerebellar vermis, electrical stimulation of reduces decerebrate
        rigidity, 509
Cerebellopontine angle, tumors of, 720–721
Cerebellum, 8f, 626–646
    anatomy, dorsal, ventral, and midsagittal views, 628f, 629f
    appearance of amyloid plaques in, 977
    basket cells, release of GABA by, 217
    cellular organization, 630–632
    circuits modified during learning, 643f
    as component of subcortical feedback loops of motor system,
        650f
    control of cortical and brain stem motor systems, 539–540
    cortical layers, 630f
    deficits in diseases of, 643f
    derived from hindbrain, 298
    diseases of localized by clinical features, 644
    function, 9t, 276
    functional divisions, 632–634, 634f
    inputs, 627
        from cerebral cortex, 637
        to motor area of cerebral cortex, 611
    intermediate part of hemisphere, major input and output
        pathways, 636t
    involved in initiation and timing of movements, 295
    lateral part of hemisphere, major input and output pathways,
        636t
    lesions, 604–606, 671, 815
    lobes, 627–628

Cerebellum [cont.]
  longitudinal furrows, 628, 629
  major input and output pathways, 636t
  modulates
    decerebrate rigidity, 605f
    vestibulo-ocular reflex, 671
  mossy fiber pathways carry somatic sensory information to, 636
  neural mechanisms for role in learning of motor skills, 642
  output to motor and premotor cortices, 637
  part of brain stem, 275
  projections, 627
  Purkinje cells, release of GABA by, 217
  requirement of for goal-directed locomotion, 593
  somatotopic maps in, 634f, 635f
  structure of glomerulus in granular layer, 630f
Cerebral aqueduct, 288f
  development, 303
Cerebral arteries, 724, 724f
  border-zones, watersheds, and end-zones, 1043
  brain stem, 725f
Cerebral blood flow
  absence of as sign of brain death, 818
  decreased and transient loss of consciousness, 815
  increases in during behavior, 621f
  relationship to intracranial pressure, 1058
Cerebral circulation, 1041–1049
Cerebral cortex, 8f, 276. See also Visual cortex
  abnormal synchrony of neuronal discharge and epilepsy, 785
  anatomical features of lobes, 8
  areas of motor control, 539
  areas with steroid receptors, 966
  association areas, 823–838, 824t
  asymmetry of structure and function of hemispheres, 8
  bat, representation of constant frequency and frequency-modulated components of sounds, 496
  Brodmann's areas, 11f
  capability for long-term potentiation in, 1023
  collective electrical behavior of neurons and epilepsy, 777–791
  and contralateral control, 610
  contralateral control by hemispheres, 8
  controls saccade generator in brain stem, 674–676
  definition of cortical fields, 12
  derived from telencephalon, 298
  features of organization, 8
  function, 9t
  functional areas according to cytoarchitectonics, 11
  EEG generated by flow of synaptic currents through extracellular space, 780–783
  excitatory connections synchronize discharges in epileptic focus, 787, 789
  expression
    of D1 and D5 dopamine receptors, 860
    of D2 dopamine receptors in, 860
    of D3 and D4 dopamine receptors in, 860–861
  functional areas related to perception of speech sounds, 495
  inhibitory effects of serotonin on, 698
  input from integrated by reticulospinal tracts, 541
  intracortical connections, 826f
  language and other cognitive functions localized to, 7–12
  lateral view, 10f
  layering of neurons associated with neuronal birthdays, 909
  layers, 292f
  links from lateral geniculate nucleus to retinotopic maps in, 446
  lobes, 7–8, 276–279
  localization of function, 821
  location of highest level of information processing, 292–293
  major divisions, 278f
  medial and lateral descending systems controlled by efferent spinocerebellar projections, 636–637

  motor areas
    level of motor control, 537–540
    somatotopic organization, 610–613
  neurotransmitters in cells of, 782f
  phonetic symbols and ideographs localized to different regions, 849–850
  primary motor cortex, somatotopic organization, 293
  primary somatic sensory, somatotopy in, 361
  principal neuron types and their interconnections, 781f
  projections from retina to, 423f
  receives axons of thalamic relay nuclei, 289–290
  recording of alpha and beta activity, 778f
  reduction of tissue in some schizophrenia patients, 858
  regional specialization, 12
  representation
    of body, 370–374
    of taste in, 524–527
  sensory evoked potentials measure activity in specific sensory pathways, 780
  sensory information
    processed in thalamus, 280
    transmitted to by thalamus, 335
  sensory regions play critical role in perception, 335
  shared features of organization, 777
  sites of somatosensory processing, 364f
  somatic sensations localized to specific regions, 370–374
  somatic sensory information conveyed to by two ascending systems, 358–363
  somatotopic organization, 531
  striate and extrastriate regions, 445f
  thalamus as principal synaptic relay for information reaching, 287–292
  theory of cortical localization, 11
  training causes expansion of representation, 1026f
  types of cells in, 779, 782f
Cerebral death, determination of, 817–818
Cerebral disorders, metabolic and diffuse, and diagnosis of coma, 816t
Cerebral hemisphere
  left
    angular gyrus of is concerned with auditory representation of words, 850
    and cognitive capability for language, 843
    language and serial processing of information in right-handed individual, 971
    lesions, 843
  right
    anterior and posterior, lesion, 849
    damage to affects affective components of language, 848
    nonverbal processes in right-handed individual, 971
    plasticity of in females, 971
Cerebral hemispheres, 8f, 278f. See also Cerebral cortex; Basal ganglia; Hippocampus; Amygdaloid nucleus
  asymmetry of is sexually dimorphic, 971
  comparative for mammals, 824f
  coronal section, MRI, 320f
  deep-lying areas, 277
  derived from telencephalon, 298
  divisions, 276
  dominance of one over the other, 835
  evolution of in vertebrates, 277
  function, 9t, 276
  functional depression of and impaired consciousness, 815
  horizontal section, MRI, 319f
  lateralization of function, 835–836
  and localization of sense of self, 15–16
  midsagittal section, MRI, 318f
  performance after commissures are severed, 833–835
  regional anatomy of related to ventricular system, 304–307
  sex differences in dominance, 836
  signing localized to left, 843
Cerebral hemorrhage, Dutch-type, with amyloidosis, 977–978

Cerebral infarction
    cause of cortical lesions, 545
    revealed by sodium and phosphorus scans, 323
Cerebral peduncle, lesions, 728–729
Cerebral ventricles, hydrocephalus as increase in volume of,
        1059–1060
Cerebral vessels
    autoregulation, 1044
    unique physiological responses, 1043–1044
Cerebrocerebellum
    and coordination of planning of limb movements, 637–642
    functional region of cerebellum, 633
    input and output pathways, 640f
    lesions, 637, 640
        produce cognitive deficit, 640
    major input and output pathways, 636t
    role in preparation of movement, 642
Cerebrospinal fluid, 1050–1054, 1057, 1059
    drawn from lumbar cistern, 302
    and hydrocephalus, 304
    production by choroid plexus, 303
    secretion by choroid plexus, 1050–1051
    transport within arachnoid villus, 1052f
Ceruleospinal system, noradrenergic, 541
Cervical cord, 285f
Cervical flexure, 298
Cervical segments, spinal cord, 284
Cervicocollic reflexes, effect on neck and limb muscles,
        600–601
Cervicospinal reflexes, effect on neck and limb muscles,
        600–601
cGMP-dependent protein kinase, domains, 179f
CGRP. See Calcitonin gene-related peptide
Chain fibers, primary sensory nerves, 38f
Chandelier cells, in cerebral cortex, 782f
Channels. See Gap junctions; Ion channels
Chaperonins, 55d
Character traits, localization of in brain, 12–15
Charcot–Bouchard microaneurysms, 1047
Charcot–Marie–Tooth disease, as chronic neuropathy, 250
Charge
    amount stored in cell membrane, effect of capacitive current
        on, 97
    immobilization, Na+ ion channel, 115
    separation, 1034
        local, changes in change membrane potential, 91
Chemical mediators, and sensitization of nociceptors, 387f
Chemical messengers, as neurotransmitters, 213–224
Chemical stimuli, activate nociceptors, 386
Chemical structures, receptors that recognize, 513
Chemical synapse. See Synapse, chemical
    and quantal transmission, 200–201
    plasticity of due to regulation of free Ca2+ concentration in
        presynaptic terminal, 209
Chemical synaptic transmission, 123
    in autonomic ganglia, 768
    pharmacology as basis for study of, 6
Chemical transmitter, criteria for, 214–215
Chemiosmotic mechanism, and movement of
        neurotransmitters into synaptic vesicles, 226–227
Chemoaffinity hypothesis, 915
Chemoreceptor
    specialized sensory receptor, 338
    transduction by, 336, 336f
Chemotactic molecules
    guide growth cones, 916–917, 917f
    role of second-messenger pathways, 917
Chemotherapy, cancer, and food-aversion, 1001
Chemotropism, 917d
Cheyne–Stokes breathing, in coma due to supratentorial
        lesions, 817
Chimpanzees, and experiments in language, 840–841

Chlordiazepoxide, treatment, anxiety disorders, 881–882
Chloride ion channels. See Ion channels, chloride
Chloride ion
    concentrated outside the cell, 82
    distribution across cell membrane, 84
    electrical equivalent circuit of as passively distributed across
        membrane, 93f
    equation to determine contribution to resting membrane
        potential, 93–104
    flux across cell membrane, 87f
    increased conductance to as mechanism of presynaptic
        mechanism, 208
    nerve cells as rest permeable to, 85
    passive distribution, 88
Chloride pump, 88
Chloride receptor–channels, mediate inhibitory synaptic action,
        160
Chlorpromazine
    comparison of molecular structure with that of dopamine,
        860
    structure, 859f
    treatment, schizophrenia, 858
Chlorprothixene, structure, 859f
Cholecystokinin
    humoral signal for feeding behavior, 757
    in hypothalamus, 743
    as neuroactive peptide, 218t
    peptide in sympathetic neurons, 770t
Choline acetylcholine, loss of in cerebral cortex and
        hippocampus of Alzheimer's disease patients, 981
Choline acetyltransferase, decreased in striatum of patients
        with Huntington's disease, 656
Cholinergic, 214d. See also Acetylcholine
Cholinergic neurons, loss of in striatum in Huntington's
        disease, 656
Chopper response, stellate cells of cochlear nucleus, 492
Chorda tympani fibers, response profiles, 526f
Chorea, 653d
Choroid plexus
    cGMP-dependent protein phosphorylation in, 191
    filtration and secretory functions, 1053
    produces cerebrospinal fluid, 303
    secretion of cerebrospinal fluid, 1050–1051
    structural similarity to distal and collecting tubules of
        kidney, 1051
    tumors of and oversecretion of cerebrospinal fluid, 1059
Chromaffin cells, fibroblast growth factor promotes
        differentiation of into neurons, 904
Chromatic aberration, 469
Chromatolysis, indicator of axotomy, 259f, 260
Chromogranins, 226d
    and neurotransmitter release, 227
Chromosome 4, location of gene for Huntington's disease, 657
Chromosome 5, possible chromosomal location for
        schizophrenia, 857
Chromosome 21
    amyloid gene that encodes APP, 977
    marker for Alzheimer's disease, 977
Chromosome X, linked to biopolar depression in Ashkenazi
        Jews, 872
Chromosome Y, gene for testes determining factor located on,
        960
Chronic peripheral neuropathy, peripheral nerve disease, 249t
Chronic sensorimotor polyneuropathy, muscle histochemistry
        in, 248f
Chronic temporal lobe epilepsy, ictal phenomena during, 14
Ciliary ganglion, innervation, 424
Ciliary ganglion neurons, parasympathetic nervous system, and
        ciliary neuronotrophic factor, 933
Ciliary neuronotrophic factor
    promotes cholinergic differentiation of sympathetic neurons,
        905

Ciliary neuronotrophic factor [*cont.*]
  rescues brain stem motor neurons deprived of muscle targets,
    934
  supports survival of ciliary ganglion neurons in
    parasympathetic nervous system, 933
Ciliary neurotrophic factor, promotes astrocyte type 2
    differentiation, 899
Cingulate, and parahippocampal gyri, C-shaped, 307
Cingulate gyrus, 307f
  affected by Parkinson's disease, 981–982
  axons in, effect of severence, 829
  part of limbic lobe, 737
  role in emotional behavior, 829–830
  subarea of limbic association cortex, 829
Cingulate regions, in limbic association cortex, 826
Cingulum
  effect of severence, 829
  small lesion in, instead of frontal lobotomy, 830
Circadian clock, and light as zeitgeber, 800–801
Circadian light–dark cycles, metabolic activity of
    suprachiasmatic nucleus entrained to, 801f, 802f
Circadian rhythm, 758d
  altered, and temporary insomnia, 807–808
  biphasic pattern of sleepiness, 808f
  deliberate manipulation, 807–808
  disruptions in Alzheimer-type dementia, 808
  role of suprachiasmatic nucleus, 758f
  and *fos* oncoprotein expression in neurons of suprachiasmatic
    nucleus, 732f, 733
Circle of Willis, 1043
  incomplete, infarction, 1047
Circuit
  with capacitor, 1038
  with resistor and capacitor in parallel, 1039–1040
  with resistor and capacitor in series, 1038–1039
Circuit analysis, rules, 1036–1038
Circulation, brain, 1041–1049
Circumvallate papillate, 518
Circumventricular organs, blood–brain barrier leaky, 1055
cis-regulatory region, DNA, 188d
11-*cis*-retinal, light-absorbing, 404
Clarke's nucleus, 357f
  function, 286
  spinal cord, 286
    gray matter, 356
Clasp knife phenomenon, 606d
Classical conditioning. *See* Conditioning, classical
Clathrin
  role in recycling of synaptic vesicles, 228–231
  role in slow axonal transport, 59
Claustrum, 434
  possible role in mediating visual attention, 460
Climbing fibers
  as excitatory input to cerebellar cortex, 631–632
  during learning, 642
  effect of input on Purkinje cells, 642–644
  effect of on mossy fiber activity, 642
  role in motor learning, 640, 642
Clonazepam, treatment of REM behavior disorder, 811
Clonus, 578d, 606d, 717d
  sign of damage to corticospinal tract, 717, 718
Clozapine
  blocks several types of receptors, 866
  structure, 859f, 859t
  treatment, schizophrenia, 866
CNTF. *See* Ciliary neuronotrophic factor; Ciliary neurotrophic
    factor
Co-contraction, muscle, 561, 561f
Cocaine, increases dopamine levels and causes psychosis
    resembling schizophrenia, 861
Cochlea, 482d
  fluid waves in vibrate hair cells, 483–489

  organization, 486
    of compartments, 484f
  selective response to different sound frequencies, 486–487
  sound initiates traveling wave along length of, 487
  vibrations of conductive apparatus generate fluid waves in,
    482–483
Cochlear duct, 502f
  net potential difference between endolymph and perilymph,
    501
Cochlear nerve, 669f
Cochlear nucleus
  auditory fibers terminate in, 491
  axon pathways, 494
  cell types, 492f
  divisions of, 492
  location, 491f
  in special somatic afferent column, 690
  tonotopic organization, 492
Coeliac ganglion, autonomic nervous system, 764
Cognition, 886
Cognitive behavior, and association areas of frontal region, 826
Cognitive deficits, produced by cerebrocerebellar lesions, 640
Cognitive function
  localization, 823–838
  functions, sex difference in hemispheric allocation, 971
  simulation with parallel distributed processing networks,
    836–837
Cognitive psychology, combined with positron emission
    tomography, 3
Colchicine, abolishes retrograde transport, 263
Cold
  mediated by thermal receptors, 343–344
  paradoxical, 344
  receptor, 344f
Cold-sensitive neurons, hypothalamic, 753
Collicular syndrome, midbrain, symptoms, 729
Color
  detection of by comparison, 476
  detection of by parvocellular-interblob system, 447
  discrimination requires at least two types of photoreceptors,
    468–469
  information processed in cortex by double-opponent cells and
    blob zones, 473–476
  information transmitted by color-opponent cells, 472
  opponent process theory, 471
  processing by ganglion cells, 412
  role of parvocellular-blob system, 447
  subjective perception of, 476–477
  those not perceived in combination, perceptual cancellation,
    470–471
Color agnosia, 849d
Color blindness
  arrangement of red and green pigment genes on X
    chromosome in, 477f
  inherited or acquired, 477–479
  resulting from monochromatopsia, 469
Color constancy, 467
  key feature of color vision, 470–476
  role of double-opponent cells, 476
  examples, 471f
Color contrast, role of double-opponent cells, 476
Color opponency
  examples, 471f
  key feature of color vision, 470–476
  role of double-opponent cells, 476
Color perception, enhances contrast, 467
Color vision, 467–480
  as abstraction of physical parameters of light reflected from
    object's surface, 467
  defects, 477t
  mediated by cones, 402
  requirement of divariance, 469

role of primary visual cortex, 434
trivariancy, 468
Columnar organization
cranial nerve nuclei, 687–690
middle temporal region, 452
primary auditory cortex, 494
results in optic tectum from competition of two sets of
afferent fibers, 953
Columns
elementary functional module of cortex, 377
organization of primary visual cortex, 431–434
primary visual cortex
axis of orientation, 431–434
2-deoxyglucose visualization, 432f
hypercolumn, 432
ocular dominance columns, 432
Coma
alpha, 816
causes, 815–817
and cerebellar lesions, 815–817
decreased oxygen uptake in, 815
diagnosis, 816t
in pontine hemorrhage, 1047
irreversible, as sign of brain death, 818
metabolic, 817
versus deep sleep, 815
versus locked-in syndrome, 729
Command neurons, stimulation of complex motor output, role
in fixed-action pattern, 990
Command systems, in mammals, 991
Commissural nucleus, projections, 768
Commissures
in central nervous system, 281
hemispheric, functional role, 833
Communicating artery, brain stem, 725f
Comparator, 535d
Compensatory responses, postural adjustment, 596
Complete homonymous hemianopsia, 437d
Complex cells, in primary visual cortex, 430
Component direction-selective neurons, response to motion,
452
Compound action potential, 351
amplitude decreased in myasthenia gravis, 236
Compound sensations, 341
Computerized tomography
distinguishes gray and white matter, 312
mechanism, 311
COMT. See Catechol-O-methyltransferase
Concentration gradient, 84
Concentric broad-band cells, in retina and lateral geniculate
nucleus, 471
Concentric single-opponent cells
receptive fields concentrically organized with on-center and
off-surround, 473f
response to white or yellow light, 472
Concordance, 856d
Conditioned responses, lesions in amygdala interfere with, 1005
Conditioned stimulus, proteins capable of responding to signals
from and learning, 1023
Conditioning
associative, may not require complex neural networks, 1023
classical
associating a conditioned and unconditioned stimulus,
998–1001
and associative enhancement of presynaptic facilitation,
1016, 1017–1019
cellular mechanism of, 1017f
and detection of causal relationships, 1000
and enhancement of gill- and siphon-withdrawal reflex in
Aplysia, 1016
predictive relationship between two stimuli, 1000
requirement for contiguity of stimuli and contingency

between conditioned and unconditioned stimulus,
999–1000
food-aversion, 1001
and learning of predictive relationships, 999–1000
operant
associating behavior with subsequent reinforcing
environmental event, 1000–1001
predictive relationship between stimulus and response,
1000
treatment of psychiatric disorders, 1002
operant and classical, common underlying neural
mechanisms, 1001
use of as therapeutic technique, 1001–1002
Conductance, 1034
calculation of with Ohm's law, 108
change of in acetylcholine receptor-channels after skeletal
muscle innervation, 939
effect of Cl⁻ channel opening on, 160
effect of IPSP on, 162
end-plate, equivalent circuit for, 150
factors modulating at gap junction channels, 129
of fusion pore, 204
at gap junction channels, 129
increased to Cl⁻ as mechanism of presynaptic mechanism,
208
ion channel, influences current flow, 144–146
leakage, 107
measured as function of membrane potential by
voltage-clamp technique, 106
potassium, calculated from K⁺ current, 108–109
reciprocal relationship to resistance, 96–97
relative, use in determining reversal potential of EPSP, 140
sodium
calculated from Na⁺ current, 108–109
compared with potassium by voltage-clamp experiments,
109f
sodium and potassium, effect of depolarization on, 109f
total synaptic of ACh-activated channels, summed
conductance of all open channels, 144
two states of in voltage-gated ion channels, 113
versus permeability, 90
Conductances, Na⁺ and K⁺, calculation of shape of action
potential from, 110f
Conductile component, afferent neuron, propagates all-or-none
action potential, 28–29
Conducting signal, 26d
Conduction
demyelination slows velocity, 251–252
rate of and axonal diameter, 349–351
velocity increased by
increased diameter of axon core, 101
myelination, 101–102
Conduction aphasia, characteristics, 11d, 847–848, 847t
Conduction block, in demyelinating neuropathies, 251
Conduction velocity
axonal nomenclature based on, 349–351
and diagnosis of disease, 351
importance of, 351
Conductor, ion channel as, 89–90
Cones, 409f
absorption of light by visual pigments in, 403
compared with rods, 402t
comparison of amino acid sequences of visual pigments, 478f
desensitization and light adaptation, 408
disinhibition and depolarization, 414
genes, evolution, 478
mediate color vision, 402
opponent cells, code color in retina and lateral geniculate
nucleus, 471–473
photoreceptor, 402–403
pigments in, 468
response to visible light spectrum, 468

Cones [cont.]
in receptive field center of bipolar cell, 412
respond preferentially to different wavelengths of light, 469
signals transferred by direct or lateral pathways to ganglion cells, 412
spatial and temporal resolution, 402
spectral sensitivity, 469f
structure, 403f
univariance, 469
Connectional specificity, 20
Connectionist model, parallel distributed systems of neural function, 32
Connectionist view
brain, and principles of dynamic polarizaton and connectional specificity, 20
and theory of language, 10–11
Connectivity, nervous system, 271
Connexin, 129d
functions, 129
gene family, 131
Connexon, 129d
model of, 130f
Conscious awareness, analysis of visual attention as step in understanding, 462–464
Consciousness
disorders, 805–819
loss of, deep sleep versus coma, 815
role of thalamus in maintaining, 288
role of upper brain stem and diencephalic regions, 816
and split-brain experiments, 833–835
transient loss from decreased cerebral blood flow, 815
Consensual response, pupillary constriction, 424
Constructional apraxia, 831
Consummatory behavior, 989
Context, role in visual perception, 443–444
Contextual effect, 434d
Contraction
muscle. See Muscle, contraction
twitch, measurement of time of, 557
Contralateral control, feature of cerebral hemispheres organization, 8
Contralateral motor cortex, and limb movement, 10
Contrast, weak, detection of by ganglion cells, 411
Control systems, homeostatic processes analyzed in terms of, 751f
Controlled variable, 751d
Controlling elements, 751d
Convergence
group Ib inhibitory interneurons, 586
neural integration mechanism, 582d
neuronal, 25f
Convergence, and motor neurons, 25f
Convergent pathways, 271
Convulsant drugs, induction of focal epilepsy with, 786
Cordotomy, 713–714
Corollary discharge, 627d
Corpus callosum, 307d, 307f, 365
blood supply, 1041
commissure in brain, 281
effect of cutting, 833
effect of severing on sense of self, 15–16
in midsagittal brain section, 9f
midsagittal section, MRI, 318f
Corpus striatum, 277
role in regulating speed of movements, 295
structure, 307f
Cortex
blood supply, 1041
circuits connecting basal ganglia with, 652
color information relayed by parvocellular layers, 473
concentric double-opponent red-green contrast cells, sensitive to simultaneous color contrast, 475f

higher centers communicate with hypothalamus via limbic system, 737–739
inputs to basal ganglia, 648–651
left, effect of lesions of on eye movement, 722f
motor areas. See Motor cortex
representation of rodent whiskers in, 707–708
trigeminal sensory information mapped somatotopically in, 707
Cortical association areas, inputs to motor cortex, 611–612
Cortical connections, feature detection as property, 380
Cortical gyri, thin in Alzheimer's disease, 977
Cortical limbic areas, development, 305f
Cortical localization, theory of, 11
Cortical processing
dynamic properties of central neurons and receptors similar in early stages, 378–380
later stages, complex feature-detecting properties of central nerve cells, 380–381
Wernicke–Geschwind model of, 45f
Cortico-reticulospinal pathway, components, 541
Cortico-tectospinal pathways, 541
Corticobulbar fibers, 294
control cranial motor nerve nuclei, 543
Corticobulbar tract, 510f
Corticopontine fibers, 294
Corticopontine projections, pruning of axon branches during development, 924f
Corticopontine tract, 510f
Corticoreticular pathways, 603f
Corticospinal axons
act directly on motor neurons, interneurons, propriospinal neurons, and projection neurons, 543
connections with segmental motor neurons, 612–613
divergence, 613
Corticospinal fibers, control motor neurons innervating spinal fibers, 543
Corticospinal neurons
connections with alpha and gamma motor neurons, 612
direct influence on motor neurons, 612
Corticospinal projections, pruning of axon branches during development, 924f
Corticospinal tract neurons, role in movement, discharge frequency encodes amount of force, 614
Corticospinal tract, 510f, 712f
descends through basis pedunculi, 294f
as direct pathway for voluntary movement, 293
function, 294
lesions, 712
motor axons in, 611
origination in motor cortex, 294f
pattern of terminations, 545f
projections, 543
signs of lesion in, 718
and scarring in amyotrophic lateral sclerosis, 248
sources of axons in, 611
Corticostriate projection, input from cerebral cortex to basal ganglia, 649
Corticotropin-releasing factor
in hypothalamus, 743
loss of in Alzheimer's disease, 981
as neuroactive peptide, 218t
released by parvocellular neurons, 742
structure, 742f
Cortisol, hypersecretion of from adrenal cortex in severe depression, 879
Cotranslational transfer, 54d
Cotransmission, 222d
Coughing, central program for, 990
Coulomb, 1033d
Course topographic map, 953
Cranial bumps, use in describing character, 6
Cranial motor nerve nuclei, controlled by corticobulbar fibers, 543

Cranial muscles, affected by myasthenia gravis, 236f
Cranial nerve I. *See* Olfactory nerve
Cranial nerve II. *See* Optic nerve
Cranial nerve III. *See* Oculomotor nerve
Cranial nerve IV. *See* Trochlear nerve
Cranial nerve V. *See* Trigeminal nerve
Cranial nerve VI. *See* Abducens nerve
Cranial nerve VII. *See* Facial and intermediate nerves
Cranial nerve VIII. *See* Vestibulocochlear nerve
Cranial nerve IX. *See* Glossopharyngeal nerve
Cranial nerve X. *See* Vagus nerve
Cranial nerve XI. *See* Spinal accessory nerve
Cranial nerve XII. *See* Hypoglossal nerve
Cranial nerve, individual, brain stem motor nuclei associated
    with, 691
Cranial nerve nuclei, 683–700
    organization into columns, 687–690
    function, 9t
Cranial nerves, 681
    affected by acoustic neuroma, 720
    carry sensory input and motor output of brain stem, 275
    emergence from brain stem, lateral view, 685f
    fiber types intermingle in periphery of brain, 691
    functional classes, 687t
    functional organization, 686
    functions, 683, 684t
    in brain stem, 683–684, 685f
    lesions, 684
    location of in brain stem, 720f
    locations of nuclei in transverse sections of brain stem, 689f
    motor nuclei, 687–690
        somatic, special visceral, and general visceral motor
            columns, 687–690
        visceral, and somatic afferent fibers in, 684, 687
    nuclei, 683–700
        functional organization into columns, 688f
    origins, ventral view of brain stem, 685f
    sensory and motor nuclei, 686f
    sensory nuclei, 690
        in brain stem receive input from several, 691
        general and special visceral, special somatic, and general
            somatic afferent columns, 690
Cranial sensory ganglia, 286
Craniosacral division, autonomic nervous system. *See*
    Parasympathetic
Crayfish
    antidromic transmission at synapse, 127f
    electrical transmission at giant synapse, 126f
    giant motor synapse and evidence for electrical synaptic
        transmission, 125
    transmission at synapse, 127f
CRE-binding protein, transcriptional activator, 190–191
Creatine kinase, and diagnosis of myopathies, 246
Crib death. *See* Sudden infant death syndrome
Critical period
    sexual differentiation of nervous system, 959
    and steroid hormone influence on perinatal development, 964
Crossed extension reflex, 587d
CT. *See* Computerized tomography
Cuneate fascicle, 360d
Cuneate nucleus, 360d
    nociceptive and large-diameter myelinated primary afferent
        fiber axons terminate in, 390
Cupula, 502f
    and distortion of and displacement of sensory hairs, 503
Curare, and isolation of synaptic potential in intracellular
    voltage recordings, 138
Current, 1034d. *See also* Membrane current
    calculation of through each class of active conductance
        channel with Ohm's law, 108
    EPP, factors, 145
    excitatory, activated by glutamate, 163f

flow
    controlled by ion channels, 81
    during EPSP, equivalent circuit, 151
    in neurons, 1033–1040
    inhibitory, activated by GABA, 163f
    injected, illustration of differences in electrical and chemical
        synapses, 125f
    measurement
        as function of membrane potential with voltage-clamp
            technique, 109
        during EPSP, 155–158
        during IPSP, 160–162
    membrane, separation into ionic and capacitive components
        with voltage-clamp technique, 105–109
    recording flow from single ion channels with the patch-
        clamp technique, 71
    single channel, different reversal potentials of GABA- and
        glutamate-activated, 163f
    symbol, 1036
    synaptic, determination of reversal potential, 156f
Current clamp, 156d
    measuring current flow during IPSP, 160–162
Current flow
    in circuits with capacitance, 1038–1040
    distribution determined by three-dimensional geometry of
        nerve cell, 97–100
Cutaneous mechanoreceptors, 348, 349f
Cutaneous sensation, loss of on face, 726t
Cutaneous stimuli
    and complex reflexes serving protective and postural
        functions, 586–590
    modulate excitability of motor neuron pools, 586–587, 587f
Cyclic adenosine monophosphate pathway, 177–178, 177f
    importance of in classical conditioning, 1018–1019
    mediates enhancement of long-lasting calcium current by
        beta-adrenergic agonists, 771
    olfactory-specific Na$^+$ channel gated by, 515
    second-messenger pathway, 191
Cyclic guanosine monophosphatase, role in phototransduction
    cascade, 403, 406
Cyclopean perception, 454d
Cystic fibrosis, 79, 518
Cytoarchitectonics
    Brodmann's areas of cerebral cortex, 11f
    and functional areas of cerebral cortex, 11
Cytochalasins, effect on axonal growth cones, 913
Cytochrome oxidase, distribution in superficial layers of
    primary visual cortex, 432f
Cytochrome oxidase, stripes in occipital lobe, 446
Cytokeratins, 62d
Cytoskeleton, 50d, 60–64, 63f
    and mobilization of synaptic vesicles, 227
    synaptic vesicle anchored to, 206
Cytosol, 50d
Cytosol, and slow axonal transport, 58–59
Cytosolic proteins, 51–52

D

d-Amphetamine, treatment, narcolepsy, 814
d-Tubocurarine, effect of on miniature end-plate potentials, 198
Dale's law, mature nerve cell uses same transmitter at all of its
    synapses, 214
Dandy–Walker syndrome, and hydrocephalus, 1059
Dark adaptation, 408d
Dark current, 406–407, 407f
Dark-adapted eye, moderately and extremely, rod signals
    conveyed to ganglion cells by different pathways, 414
Darkness, prolonged exposure and sensitivity of ganglion cells,
    414
Day vision, cones, 402
Deafferentation, and injury to peripheral nerves, 387

Deafness, types, 483
Death
  cerebral
    determination of, 817–818
    isoelectric EEG as indication of, 818
    mimicked by reversible drug intoxication or other lesions, 818
  neuron
    genetically programmed, 929–930
    increasing target size reduces extent of, 934f
    preventing neuromuscular transmission reduces extent of, 934f
Decerebrate animals, 574, 575, 592f
Decerebrate preparation, 574d
Decerebrate rigidity, 604, 605f
  as symptom of coma, 816
  causes, 509
Decibel, 482d
Declarative memory, characteristics, 1002
Decorticate rigidity, 606d
Decortication, 746, 1005
Decreased-conductance postsynaptic potential, ion channels and signal properties, 166f
Deep tendon reflexes, universal human behavior, 993
Defensive conditioning, 999d
Degenerative changes, in injured nerve cells, 259–262
Deiter's cells, 485f
Deiter's nucleus. See Lateral vestibular nucleus
Delayed rectifier channel, 111
  gene for, 118
Delayed response tasks, role of principal sulcus of prefrontal association cortex, 828
Delta gene, neurogenic Drosophila gene, 896
Delta receptor, opiate, 395
Delta sleep, 806–807
  inducing peptide, 798, 799
  waves, 779
Delusions, 855d
Dematomyositis, acquired myopathy, 253
Dementia, 976d
  Alzheimer's disease, 974–983
  caused by normal pressure hydrocephalus, 1059
  produced by degenerative diseases, 981
Dementia praecox, 855
Demyelinating neuropathies, 250–251
  assessment of using EEG-derived sensory evoked potentials, 780
  evaluation of with measurement of evoked potentials, 716
Demyelination
  diseases causing, 102
  and slowing of conduction velocity, 251–252
Dendrites, 19f, 19d
  action potentials in, 787
  excitatory synaptic potential originating in, and threshold for initiation of action potential, 167f
  in motor neurons, 39–42
  NMDA receptors clustered on heads of spines, 1020
  protein synthesis in, 39
  structure of in spinal motor neuron, 41f
  trigger zones, 787
  unit lengths represented as electrical equivalent circuit, 98f
Dendrodentritic synaptic contact, 168
Dense bodies, 203
Dentate gyrus, 736f, 737
Dentate nuclei, 627d
  conveys output of cerebellum to motor and premotor cortices, 637
  effect of cooling on activity of, 640, 640f
Depolarization, 27d, 82d
  calcium influx during and neurotransmitter release, experimental demonstration, 198f
  effect

in neuron from nucleus tractus solitarius, 112f
  of noxious stimulus on nociceptor, 386
  on sodium and potassium conductances, 109f
  on steady-state Ca^{2+} conductance, 206
  local, and local-circuit flow, 100
  by motion of stereocilia of hair cells, 486, 488, 504
  of muscle fiber and contraction, 550
  and neurotransmitter release as function of Ca^{2+} influx, 197f
  of postsynaptic cells coincident with activity in presynaptic neuron as requirement of LTP, 1020
  passive conduction, 100–102, 100f
  permeability changes caused by, 105
  by receptor potential, 336
  recording, 83
  speed of at electrical synapse, 125, 126
  voltage-gated Ca^{2+} channels responding to, 111
Depolarization shift, underlies focal seizures, 787
Depression, 870–880
  anaclitic, 946
  atypical, 871
  bipolar, 871–879
  catecholamine hypothesis, 875, 877
  and disturbed sleep, 807
  endogenous, symptoms, 870
  genetic predisposition, 871–872
  homosynaptic, in habituation, 1012
  incidence of suicide among biological and adoptive relatives, 872f
  major. See Depression, unipolar
  nongenetic factors, 872
  reactive, symptoms, 870
  unipolar, 870–871
Deprivation, 946
  early sensory
    alters development of neural circuits, 947–948
    effect on perceptual development, 947
  visual, reduces size of ocular dominance columns in visual cortex, 949–956, 949f
Depth perception, 440–466
Dermatomes, 354d
  and determination of nerve root or segmental sensory loss, 715, 716f
  mapping, 355
  segmental arrangement, 716f
Dermatomyositis, myopathic disease, 249t
Descending brain stem neurons, release serotonin and suppress activity of spinothalamic tract neurons, 396
Descending systems, activity during locomotion, 593. See also Reticulospinal, Rubrospinal, and Corticospinal pathways
Desensitization, 77d, 186–187, 187f
Desipramine, site of action in noradrenergic transmission, 879f
Desynchronized sleep. See Rapid eye movement sleep
Deutanopia, 479d
Development
  and alteration of gene expression, 1028
  behavioral, stages, 957
  cognitive, sexual dimorphism in, 970–971
  critical periods of for different regions, 956–957
  intellectual, stages of, 957
  nerve–muscle synapse, 929–944
  nervous system, role of sensory experience and social interaction, 946–948
  perinatal, and steroid hormone influence during critical periods, 964
  role of homeobox genes, 884f, 885
Dexamethasone, suppression abnormal in depression, 880
Diabetes, as chronic neuropathy, 250
Diabetes, reduction of peak of compound action potential in, 351
Diacylglycerol, activates protein kinase C, 181
Diacylglycerol, as effector molecule, 173
Diagnostic and Statistical Manual of the American Psychiatric

Association, 855
Diazepam, 812, 881–882, 881f
Dichlorodiphenyltrichloroethane, masculinization of the brain, 965
Dichotic auditory task, performance according to handedness, 833
Dichromatopsia, 468
Diencephalic structures, pathological changes in Korsakoff's psychosis, 1006
Diencephalon, 8f, 288f. See also Hypothalamus; Thalamus
    formation, 298
    lesions of affect declarative memory, 1005
    regional anatomy of related to ventricular system, 304–307
    as thalamus and hypothalamus, 276
Diethylstilbestrol, masculinization of the brain, 965
Differentiation
    and cytological diversity in nervous system, 38
    glial cell, controlled by diffusible factors, 898
    in nervous system, 887–907
    neural crest cells, 902–904
    photoreceptor cells in Drosophila eye, 901f
    sexual, 959–973
    signals, membrane proteins as receptors for, 888
Diffuse-projection nuclei
    all functional divisions of cortex receive, 290
    thalamic, 289–290
Diffusion
    method of neurotransmitter release, 232
    removal of neurotransmitter from synaptic cleft, 232
Digestion, function localized to medulla oblongata, 9t
Dihydropyridine-binding channel, 117
Dimerization, of transcriptional regulatory proteins, 189
Dimorphism, sexual, 960
Diplopia, 667d
Direction-sensitive neurons, Brodmann's areas 1 and 2, 380
Discrimination, two-point, and location on body surface, 346f
Discs, in rods and cones, 403
Dishabituation, 998d
Disparity-selective neurons, in magnocellular pathway, 457–458
Displacement activity, 990d
Distal inhibition, in sensory relay nuclei, 369
Distal-to-proximal sequence, muscle contraction occurring during postural response, 597
Divergence, 582d, 583f
DNA-binding proteins, 894
Docking protein, 53d
Dopamine neurons, organization into four major subsystems in brain, 863–864
Dopamine
    age-related decrease in enzymes that synthesize, 976
    as catecholamine transmitter, 216
    basal ganglia, 648, 652
    beta-hydroxylase, contained within adrenergic vesicles, 226
    cell groups, 697–698
    comparison of molecular structure with that of chlorpromazine, 860
    dopaminergic receptors hypersensitive to after long-term treatment with antipsychotic drugs, 657
    innervation, in prefrontal cortex, 829
    neurons containing in brain stem, 693
    pathways, and reinforcing brain stimulation, 759
    receptors. See also Receptors
        areas of brain expressed in, 860–861
        blocked by antipsychotic drugs, 860–861
        brain, imaged by PET, 314f
    reduction of in brain in Parkinson's disease, 655
    sites of action of antipsychotic drugs, 862f
    synapse, 862f, 863–865
    synthesis and degradation, 862f
    system, 695f, 697–698
    tracts, in brain, 864f

uptake mechanism for, 233
Doppler shift, sound frequency, 496
Dorsal column, spinal cord, 284, 356, 360
    fibers, myelinated, stimulation of to suppress pain transmission, 393
    medial lemniscal system, 359–361, 712, 712f
    nociceptive neurons project axons in, 390
    nuclei, 287, 288f, 359, 360d, 369, 370
    organization, 359f
    principal pathway for somatosensory perception, 287
Dorsal horn
    localization of peptides to, 390f
    and nociceptive information, 388f, 389f, 390–392, 394, 396–397
    possible interactions between primary afferents, local interneurons, and descending neurons in, 396f
    spinal cord, enkephalin- and dynorphin-containing neuronal cell bodies and nerve terminals in, 395
    spinal cord gray matter, 283–284
    superficial, high levels of mu receptors, 395
Dorsal longitudinal fasciculus, 739
Dorsal raphe nucleus, activity or serotonergic neurons during REM sleep, 801
Dorsal root, 353–355
    fibers, branch in white matter, terminate in gray matter, 356–357
    ganglia, 286–287
    neuron, 342, 349–351
        central axons arranged somatotopically in dorsal column, 287
        and neurotrophin, 3
        primary sensory neurons, sensitive to trophic actions of NGF, 262
        types of connections determine how the sensory signal is used, 286
Dorsal vagal nucleus, parasympathetic preganglionic nucleus, 766
Dorsolateral prefrontal circuit, 652
Dorsolateral prefrontal cortex, role in saccades, 676
Dorsomedial hypothalamic nucleus, 738f
Double bouquet cells, in cerebral cortex, 782f
Double-opponent cells
    classes of, 476
    and color opponency, contrast, and constancy, 476
    concentrated in blob zones of cortex, 475–476
    process color information in cortex, 473–476
Double-vision. See Diplopia
Down's syndrome, and Alzheimer's disease, 977
Dreaming, 792–804
    during REM sleep, 795, 797, 812
    freudian interpretation, 792
    mental content linked to sleep physiology, 797–798
Drinking, regulation of, 757
Drives, 750d, 988d
Drug intoxication, mimics cerebral death, 818
Drugs
    delivery to brain, 1057
    and ion channel refractory state, 77–78
    mechanisms of action and sensory threshold, 332
Duchenne muscular dystrophy, 252, 257
    muscle histochemistry in, 248f
dunce mutant, Drosophila, defect in cAMP cascade in, 1018–1019
Dura mater, 304d, 1051f
    innervation by trigeminal nerve branch, 701–702
Duration, stimulus attribute expressed in sensation, 331
Dynamic instability, 63d
Dynamic nuclear bag, 566f
Dynamic polarization, and model neuron, 26
Dynein, 59
Dynorphin
    endogenous opioid peptides in brain, 394–396

Dynorphin [cont.]
  peptide in sympathetic neurons, 770t
  precursor structure, 220f
Dysarthria, 249d, 644d, 840d, 843d
Dyscalculia, 831
Dysdiadochokinesia, 643, 643f
Dysgraphia, 831
Dyslexia, 850
Dysmetria, 643f
Dysphagia, 249t
Dysphonia, 843d
Dystonia, 653d
Dystrophin, 256–257

E

E face, of lipid bilayer, 202f
Ear
  anatomy, 483f
  middle
    components of, 482
    phasic activity of muscles during REM sleep, 794
  as performing spectral analysis, 481
Echolalia, 848d
Echolocation, bats
  auditory cortex, 497f
  sound cues for, 495–496
Ecological constraints, and regulation of motivated behaviors, 758
ECT. See Electroconvulsive therapy
Ectoderm, 895–898
  embryonic cell layer, 296
Edema, brain, 1057–1059
Edge orientation, neurons in Brodmann's areas 1 and 2 and convergent projections from areas 3a and 3b, 380
Edges, orientation, detection by parvocellular-interblob system, 447
Edinger–Westphal nuclei
  in general visceral motor column, 690
  parasympathetic preganglionic nuclei, 766
  pretectal area cells project to, 424
EEG. See Electroencephalogram
Egg-laying hormone, 992
  precursor structure, 220f
Egg-laying, Aplysia, fixed-action pattern, 992
Eicosanoid metabolites, in arachidonic acid pathway, 181–182
Eicosanoids. See also Prostaglandins; Thromboxanes
  release by diffusion, 232
Eighth cranial nerve, axons of vestibular ganglion with, 508
Eighth nerve, vestibular portion, relays information from semicircular ducts and otolith organs, 501
Electrical charge separation, and alteration of membrane polarization, 82
Electrical circuit theory, basic principles, 1033–1040
Electrical current, behavior, 82
Electrical postsynaptic potential, ion channels and signal properties, 166f
Electrical potentials, features of different types, 166t
Electrical resonance, hair cells, 488
Electrical stimulation, induction of focal epilepsy with, 786
Electrical synapse. See Synapse, electrical
Electrical synaptic transmission, 123
Electrical transmission, mediated by gap junctions, 129
Electrochemical driving force, and ion flux across cell membranes, 73
Electroconvulsive shock therapy
  effect on memory, 1003–1004, 1004f
  produces downregulation in presynaptic beta-adrenergic autoreceptors, 877
  treatment for depression, 872
Electrocorticogram, 778d
  based on theory of volume conduction, 781

Electroencephalogram, 778d. See also Sensory evoked potential
Electrogenic pump, effect of, 94
Electromotive force, 90d
  symbol, 1037
Electromyography, 246–250
Electrotonic conduction, 99d
  effect on spatial summation, 99–100
  role in propagation of action potential, 100
Electrotonic potentials, 82d
Electrotonic transmission, 125d
Emboliform nuclei, 627d
Embryology. See also Development
  nervous system, 891–895
Embryonic axis, induction of in amphibian embryos, 893f
Emotion. See also Affective traits
  affects motor planning, and limbic association cortex, 826
  altered by stimulation or ablation of temporal portion of limbic association cortex, 831
  regulation of by hypothalamus, 746–747
Emotional behavior
  and limbic association cortex, 829–831
  role of orbitofrontal cortex and cingulate gyrus, 829–830
Emotional states, coordinated with autonomic and endocrine responses by amygdaloid nucleus, 9t
Empty speech, 847d
End-feet, 22d
End-plate channels, mean open time, 144
End-plate current
  calculation from equivalent circuit, 149–152
  total, summation, 144f
End-plate potential
  current for dependent on various factors, 145
  EPSP produced by ACh bound to receptors in muscle membrane, 136
  membrane potential during, 151
  produced by simultaneous Na^+ and K^+ flow, 139f
  recruits neighboring voltage-gated channels to trigger action potential, 142
  time course, 139f
    determined by active synaptic conductance and passive membrane properties, 150f
End-plate, 136d
  receptors in, 137f
  clustering of ACh receptor-channels at, 137f
  initiation of action potential, 142f
  synaptic channel at equally permeable to Na^+ and K^+, 140
Endocrine function, regulated by hypothalamus, 9t
Endocrine myopathies, myopathic disease, 249t
Endocrine responses, coordinated with autonomic responses and emotional state by amygdaloid nucleus, 9t
Endocrine system. See also Amygdala
  action of hypothalamus on, 767
  regulation of secretion by, 733
Endoderm, embryonic cell layer, 296
Endolymph, 502f
Endonexins, 228t
Endopeptidases, role in processing polyproteins into neuroactive peptides, 221
Endoplasmic reticulum, 49–56
Endosomes
  part of major membrane system of nerve cell, 49
  role in recycling of synaptic vesicle membranes, 229
engrailed homeobox protein, expression in *Drosophila* embryo, 884f, 885
Engram, 1005d
Enhancer region, DNA regulatory region, 189d
Enkephalins
  endogenous opioid peptides in brain, 394–396
  in hypothalamus, 743
  localized in interneurons in superficial dorsal horn, 390f
  mediate indirect pathway of basal ganglia, 652
  peptide in sympathetic neurons, 770t

precursor structure, 220f
Enteric division
    autonomic nervous system, 766
    innervation by parasympathetic and sympathetic systems, 766
    of autonomic nervous system, 761
    role in homeostasis, 766
Enteric system, peripheral nervous system (autonomic), 274
Entorhinal cortex, links neocortex and limbic system, 737
Enzymatic degradation, removal of neurotransmitter from synaptic cleft, 232
Ephaptic transmission, 251d
Epidermal cells, role of cell–cell interactions in determining fate, 891–898
Epidermal growth factor receptor, vertebrate, sequence similarity to membrane-spanning proteins encoded by *Drosophila* notch and delta genes, 896
Epigenetic influences, and neural cell differentiation, 885
Epilepsy, 777–791
    chronic temporal lobe, ictal phenomena during, 14
    excitatory connections in cerebral cortex synchronize discharges in focus, 787, 789
    focal, 785, 786, 789
    generalized, 785, 789, 790
    as interruption of normal brain function, 785–790
    types, 785–786
    temporal lobe, characteristic personality profile, 14
Epileptic lesions, discharging, and gaze disorders, 723f
Epinephrine
    as catecholamine transmitter, 216
    neurons in brain stem, 693
    reinforces effects of neurally released norepinephrine on cardiac function, 771
EPP. *See* End-plate potential
EPSP. *See* Excitatory postsynaptic potential
Equilibrium
    and balance, 500–511
    disturbance of by lesions of vestibulocerebellum, 635
Equilibrium point, for muscle, 551
Equilibrium potential, 84d. *See also* Nernst equation
    use in determining reversal potential of EPSP, 140
Equiluminance, perception of motion disappears at, 448
Equiluminant stimuli, to reduce contribution of magnocellular system, 448
Equivalent circuit
    calculation of end-plate current from, 149–152
    electrical, as model of current flow in neuron, 91f
    electrical
        model of nerve cell, 89–92
        of nerve cell under voltage-clamp conditions, 108f
Error detector, 751d
Error signal, 751d
Esophagus, innervation, 766
Estradiol, 965–966, 966f
Estrogen
    bound by alpha-fetoprotein to protect female fetuses from masculinization, 965
    induction of sexual receptivity in ovariectomized female, 963f
    litter behavioral response to in androgenized brain, 967
    secreted by ovaries, 963
Etat lacunaire, 1046d
Ethology, study of behavior, 988
Event-related potential, 779d
Evoked potentials, 371d
    auditory, 780, 781, 783
    brain stem, 780
        EEG recording, 780
    electrical activity of pyramidal cells as source of, 779
    polarity of, 783
    sensory, 779, 780
        use of to assess demyelinating diseases, 780
    visual, computer averaging of, 780
Evoked response method, mapping cortical response to tactile stimulation, 370–374
Excitability, 110–112
Excitation, interaction with inhibition on single nerve cell, 169f
Excitation–contraction coupling, 550d
Excitatory postsynaptic potential. *See also* End-plate potential; Postsynaptic potential, excitatory
    amplitude, 162
    and EEG recording, 780
    contribution of NMDA receptor-channel in hippocampus, 159f
    current flowing during, equivalent circuit, 140, 151
    dependence on activation of kainate and quisqualate receptors, 159
    determination of reversal potential, 155, 156f
    effect of conductance on amplitude, 160
    enhancement of generates depolarization shift, 787
    factors that affect size, 155
    fast, generated in autonomic ganglia, 768
    measurement of current flow during, 155–158, 159
    produced by ACh and LHRH in sympathetic ganglia, 184f
    produced by closing of channel (second-messenger modulated), characteristics, 185t
    produced by opening of channel (directly gated), characteristics, 185t
    relationship to resting membrane potential in nerve cell, 157
    reversal potential of, 140
    role in triggering dendritic action potentials, 787
    slow, in sympathetic and parasympathetic ganglia, 769
    temporal and spatial summation of, 168f
Excitatory synapse, distinctive ultrastructure, 170–171
Excitatory synaptic potential, in injured nerve cell, 261
Exocrine glands, controlled by autonomic nervous system, 762
Exocytosis, 29d, 56d, 203–206
    recycling of vesicle membranes, 57
    and release of chemical messengers, 225
    stages of, 230f
    versus glandular release, 227
Exogastrula, 893d
Extensor plantar reflex, sign of corticospinal damage, 545
Extensor thrust, 587d
Extensor tone, in decerebrate animals, 604
External auditory meatus, 482d
External feedback, 627d
External medullary lamina, 292
Extinction, 999d
Extracellular matrix molecules. *See* Fibronectin; Laminin
Extracellular potentials, 781, 783, 784f
Extrafusal fibers, 565f
    skeletal muscle fibers, 566
Extraocular motor neuron
    discharge frequency, 666
    lesions, 667
Extraocular muscles
    innervation, 665–667
    origins and insertions, 665f
Extrapyramidal tract syndrome, 647d
Extrastriate cortex, representations of retina in, 445
Eye. *See also* Retina
    ability to move during sleep paralysis and cataplexy, 813–814
    accommodation, 664
    anatomy, 401f
    autonomic control of, 772–773
    axes of rotation, 665
    cholinergic and noradrenergic responses, 771t
    complementary action of muscles, 666
    conjugate and disconjugate movements, 664
    directions of action of superior vertical muscles, 666f
    driven in direction of full-field motion by optokinetic system, 662

Eye. *See also* Retina [*cont.*]
  Drosophila, 899–902
  movements during REM sleep phasically activated by same
    neuronal spiking mechanism that generates dream
    imagery, 797
  muscles, 664–666
  position and velocity, signaled by extraocular motor neurons,
    665–667
  rapid movements during sleep, 794
  retinal disparity, 664
  stabilized by vestibular and neck reflexes, 600–602
  velocity, signal sent to brain stem by semicircular canals, 667
  vergence movement system aligns to look at targets with
    different depths, 664
Eye blink
  lesions that affect, 1005
  response, universal human behavior, 993
Eye closure, effect on development of ocular dominance
    columns, 951–952, 952f, 953f
Eye lens, projects inverted images on retina, 422f
Eye movement. *See also* Saccades; Smooth pursuit
  abnormalities of in brain stem lesions, 721, 722f
  control of by vestibular nuclei input to vestibulocerebellum,
    634
  cortical areas active in, 673f
  deficits in with brain stem lesions, 673
  functional classification, 661t
  role of association cortices, 828
  retinal input to superior colliculus, 423, 424–425
  saccadic, controlled by superior colliculus, 424–425
Eye position
  integrated signal carried by paramedian pontine reticular
    formation, 672
  maintained by neural integrator, 669–670
  reset by vestibular nystagmus during sustained rotation, 662

F

F11, structure, 919f
Face
  innervation by trigeminal nerve branch, 701–702
  recognition of occurs in inferior temporal cortex, 458–459
  tactile sensation from mediated by principal sensory nucleus
    of trigeminal nerve, 702
Facial and intermediate nerves, functions, 684t, 685f
Facial muscles, controlled by corticobulbar fibers, 543
Facial nerve, 510f, 669f
  affected by acoustic neuroma, 720–721
  lesion, 692
  peripheral course of, 691–692, 691f
Facial nucleus, 510f, 698
Facilitation
  heterosynaptic, in sensitization, 1012–1015
  presynaptic
    and activity dependence, 1018
    associative enhancement of in classical conditioning, 1016
    at axo-axonic synapses, 207–208, 208f
    biochemical steps in sensory neuron, 1012f
  short-term, biochemical steps in, 1015f
Facioscapulohumeral dystrophy, 252
  myopathic disease, 249t
Fainting, 815
False transmitters, 232d
Familiar size, monocular depth cue, 454f
Familiarity, monocular depth cue, 454
Far-field potentials, 780d
  EEG recording, 780
Farads, measurement of capacitance, 1034
Fasciculation
  axon, glycoproteins involved in are members of
    immunoglobulin superfamily, 921
  characteristic of neurogenic disease, 245
  mechanism of axonal growth, 918f

  in motor neuron diseases, 250
  muscle, 546d
Fasciculins, 919f
Fasciculus proprius, spinal cord white matter, 356
Fast anterograde transport, 57–59
Fast prepotentials
  dendritic action potentials, 787
  in pyramidal cells of hippocampus, 787
Fast retrograde transport
  use in study of axon distribution of neuron in CNS, 61f
Fast, transient K⁺ channel, 111
Fast, transient potassium channel, gene for, 117
Fastigial nuclei, 627d
  lesions of, 637
  projections, 636
Fate maps, neural crest cells, 902–903
Fatigue, caused by repeated muscle activation, 555
Feature abstraction, by progressive convergence in primary
    visual cortex, 431
Feature extraction, 338d
Feature maps, 460
Feature-detection neurons, as part of innate releasing
    mechanism, 991
Feed-forward control, 535d
  anticipatory
    coordinating posture with voluntary movement, 600
    and maintenance of postural stability during standing and
      walking, 597
  circuit, 536f
Feed-forward inhibition, in sensory relay nuclei, 369
Feed-forward inhibition, 30d
  in reflex systems, 31f
Feed-forward mechanisms
  for accuracy for rapid movements, 537
  to correct movement errors, 535–537
  deficits in with impaired proprioception, 537
  postural adjustment, 596
Feeding behavior
  altered by chemical stimulation of hypothalamus, 756–757
Female
  genetic, pseudohermaphroditism caused by fetal exposure to
    male hormones, 963–964
  phenotypic, development, 960, 961
  sex chromosomes, 960
Fetal cells, dopamine, transplantation into striatum to treat
    Parkinson's disease, 656
Fetal nerve cells, transplantation to central nervous system
    promotes recovery of function after damage, 266–268
Fetal neurons, form synaptic connections after transplantation
    into adult brain, 267f
FGF. *See* Fibroblast growth factor
Fiber-type grouping, 248d
Fibrillar elements, comprised of cytosolic proteins, 51
Fibrillary structures, 63f
Fibrillation
  characteristic of neurogenic disease, 245
  in motor neuron diseases, 250
Fibroblast growth factor
  induces sympatho-adrenal lineage cells to differentiate into
    sympathetic neurons, 904f
  as mesoderm inducing factor, 894
Fibroblasts, longevity of species and number of possible
    passages, 975
Fibronectin, 920f
  promotes axon growth in peripheral nervous system, 265
  role in migration of neural crest cells, 911
  role in neural cell adhesion, 920–921
Fictive reflexes, 590d
Fight and flight reaction, 761
Figure–ground alternation, 442, 442f, 443f
Filopodia, 911d
Finger agnosia, 831

Fink–Heimer staining, based on degenerative changes in neurons, 262
Fissures, 8d
  cerebellar, 276
Fixation plane, 455d
Fixation point, 455d
Fixed-action pattern, 989–992
FLA 63, site of action in noradrenergic transmission, 879f
Flexion reflexes
  modulation, 587
  and reciprocal innervation, 587
Flexion withdrawal, 587d
  reflex, pathways, 588f
  spinal circuits reponsible, 588
Flexor muscles, sequence of events in stretch reflex, 575–576
Flexor reflex afferent pathways, mutually inhibitory, 588
Flexor reflex afferents, 588d
Flexor-extension rule, spinal motor nuclei organization, 539
Flocculonodular lobe, 627. See also Vestibulocerebellum
  eighth nerve projects to, 501
  major input and output pathways, 636t
Flocculus, projects to oculomotor area, brain stem, 450
Floor plate, neural tube, 895d
Fluorescence, formaldehyde-induced, functional mapping of neurons, 694
Fluoxetine, antidepressant, 872
Flurazepam, treatment of insomnia, 809
FMRFamide. See also Phe-Met-Arg-Phe-NH$_2$
  as neuroactive peptide, 218t
  precursor structure, 220f
Focal attention, 460f
Focal epilepsy, studies of challenge aggregate field view of brain, 7
Focal motor seizures. See Epilepsy, focal
Fodrin, as anchoring protein, 62
Foldases, 55d
Folia, 627d
Foliate papillae, 518
Follicle-stimulating hormone, secreted by anterior pituitary, 964
Follower neurons, role in fixed-action patterns, 991
Food-aversion, 1001
Food intake
  adjustment of to maintain normal body weight, 754f
  controlling elements, 754–756
Foramen of Magendie, 304d
Foramina of Luschka, 304d
Foramina of Magendie and Luschka, 1050, 1051f
Foramina of Monro, 1050, 1051f
Force, produced by sarcomere contraction, 548–555
Forebrain, 8f
  formation, 298
  neurons, cholinergic, response to nerve growth factor in rats and are similar to cholinergic neurons in humans with Alzheimer's disease, 933
Form
  detection of by parvocellular-interblob system, 447
  perception of, 440–466
  processing by ganglion cells, 412
Fornix, 307f, 738f, 739
  relationship to subiculum and hypothalamus, 737
Fovea, 402d
  color vision in is divariant, 469
  neural mass devoted to representation of, 426f
  neuronal control systems, 661–664
  pointed toward object of interest by saccadic system, 664
  size of receptive field, 409
  smooth pursuit system keeps on target, 663
Foveola, 402d
Freeze-fracture electron micrographs, exocytosis, 204f
Freeze-fracture technique
  and structural details of synaptic membranes, 202

study of neurotransmitter release from synaptic vesicles, 203
Frequency code, stimulus strength and number and frequency of action potentials, 337
Frequency, hair cell, interaction of electrical and mechanical resonances, 488
Friedrich's ataxia, and spinal cord lesions, 719
From visual field, 451
Frontal association cortex
  proportion of brain taken up by, 827f
  subdivisions, 827f
Frontal cortex
  lesions, 829
  sexual dimorphism, 970
Frontal eye fields, 425d
  lesions, 676
  projections, 676
  role in generating saccades, 675
  sends movement signal superior colliculus, 675–676
Frontal granular cortex, 826d
Frontal lobe, 8f, 276, 278f
  association area, and cognitive behavior and motor planning, 826–829
  blood supply, 1041
  damage, and gaze disorders, 723f
  motor regions, thalamus transmits information to from cerebellum and basal ganglia, 288
  premotor area, associative functions, 825
  reduced blood flow in schizophrenics during intellectual tasks, 863
  size and blood flow in normal versus schizophrenic, 829
Frontal-limbic association connections, effect of severence, 829
FSH. See Follicle-stimulating hormone
Functional mental illness, 1027fd
Fungiform papillae, 518
Fusiform activity, level is according to type of behavior, 574f
Fusimotor set, 573d
Fusimotor system, 567d
  maintains muscle spindle sensitivity during muscle contraction, 571–573
  output adjusted independently of skeletomotor output, 573–574
Fusion pore, 204d
  structure, 205
Fusion proteins. See Synaptotagmin; Synaptophysin

                            G
G-proteins. See also GTP-binding protein
  alpha-subunit, response to bacterial toxins, 178
  bipolar cell glutamate receptor that activates, 413
  direct action on ion channels, 185–186
  direct gating of K$^+$ channels in heart, 772
  dopamine receptors coupled to, 860
  family, transducin as member of, 406
  hyperpolarization caused by in heart, 185
  p21^{ras}, role in guiding synaptic vesicles to release site, 206
  subunit structure, 177–178
  transducing, 175
G-protein coupled receptors, 174f
  olfactory receptors may belong to family of, 515
  structure, 175, 175f, 177
g. See Conductance
GABA. See Gamma-aminobutyric acid
GABA/benzodiazepine receptors, concentrated in limbic system, specifically the amygdala, 882
GABA-ergic neurons, loss of in striatum in Huntington's disease, 656
Gadolinium, and MRI of brain structures, 322
Gain, of feedback system, 577
Gait disorder, in spinal cord degeneration, 719
Galanin, as neuroactive peptide, 218t
Gall bladder
  cholinergic and noradrenergic responses, 771t

Gall bladder [*cont.*]
  innervation, 766
Gamma globulin, in cerebrospinal fluid, 1057
Gamma motor neurons. *See* Motor neurons, gamma
Gamma–aminobutyrate receptor, 162–164
Gamma–aminobutyric acid
  action on Cl^- ion channels, 162f
  biosynthesis, 217
  decrease in cortical inhibition by and focal seizures, 789
  and inhibition in cerebral cortex, 782
  inhibitory current activated by, 163f
  key biosynthetic enzyme, 215t
  mediate direct pathway from striatum, 652
  mediates indirect pathway of basal ganglia, 652
  neurotransmitter
    for Golgi neurons, 632
    in nonpyramidal cells in somatic sensory cortex, 365
    in nonpyramidal cells of cerebral cortex, 782f
    in smooth stellate cells of primary visual cortex, 427
  receptor
    benzodiazepines enhance activity of, 881–882
  reduction in inhibition mediated by and establishment of
    seizure, 790
  release by reversal of transporter carrier proteins, 232
  transporter protein for, 233
  uptake mechanism for, 233
Ganglion cell layer, retina, 412
Ganglion cells, 408–412, 409f
Gap junctions, 129d, 129–131
  in retina, rods, and cones, 414–415
GAP-42, growth-associated protein in peripheral nervous
    system, 265
GAP-43, expression in active growth cones, 913
Gasserian ganglia. *See* Trigeminal ganglia
Gastric intrinsic factor, loss of and spinal cord degeneration,
    719
Gastrin, as neuroactive peptide, 218t, 219t
Gastrin-releasing hormone, peptide in sympathetic neurons,
    770t
Gastrocnemius
  contraction, 553
  and postural responses, 597f
  types of motor units in, 557f
Gastrointestinal organs, innervation, 764
Gastrointestinal tract, innervation, 766
Gate control hypothesis, and modulation of pain, 392
Gated channels, 66d
Gating
  channel, from changes in charge distribution in Na^+ channel,
    114f
  charge, 113d
  current, 113d
  interneurons, 582d, 583f
  ion channel, 74–78, 74f
    molecular mechanism of, by chemical receptors, 132–133
  movement of S4 region during, 117f
  Na^+ channel, properties, 115
  presynaptic inhibition, 583f
  stimuli controlling, 75f
  voltage-sensitive ion channels, influenced by changes in
    intracellular ion concentrations, 111
Gaze
  centers, lesions, 721
    affecting, 673
    symptoms, 722f, 723f
  paralysis, 726t
    in middle cerebral artery infarction, 1045
  role of vestibulo-ocular reflex, 667
  stabilization of, role of hair cells in semicircular canals,
    661–662
Gender identity, development of, 963
General and special visceral afferent column, 690

General somatic afferent column, 690
General visceral motor column, 690
Generative grammar, 843d
Genes
  and behavior, 985, 987–996
  coding for Na^+ and K^+ voltage-gated ion channels, 115–118
  coding and regulatory regions, 188
  coding region, 1029f
  duplication, and K^+ channel diversity, 118
  enhancer region, 1029f
  expression
    alteration of in synaptic transmission by phosphorylation
      of transcriptional activator proteins, 187–191
    and transcriptional control, 188–189
  promoter region, 1029f
  regulatory region, 1029f
Genetic engineering, use to test ion channel structure, 73
Genetic factors, in schizophrenia, 856–857, 856t
Genetic linkage analysis, 254f. *See also* Restriction fragment
    length polymorphisms
Genetic markers, for Huntington's disease, 656–657
Genetic polymorphisms, methods for detecton, 254
Genetic predisposition, panic attacks, 881
Geniculate ganglion, 525f
Gerstmann's syndrome, 831
Gestalt psychology, 330, 441
Gigantocellular neuron, axonal plexus, 693f
Gigantocellular reticular neuron, 692
Gigantocellular tegmental field, firing of cholinoreceptive cells
    of, during REM sleep, 803
Gill-withdrawal reflex, *Aplysia*
  enhanced by classical conditioning and sensitization, 1016,
    1017
  habituation of, 1010–1012
Glandular release, and synaptic transmission, 227
Glial cells. *See also* Oligodendrocyte; Schwann cell
  brain, immature neurons migrate on, 909–911
  central nervous system, derived from neural plate of
    endoderm, 296
  class of cells in nervous cells, 22–24
  classes of, 22, 898–899
  differentiation controlled by diffusible factors, 898
  functions, 22
  location between synaptic terminals of injured neuron and
    postsynaptic element, 261f
  nongated channels in selective for K^+, 84
  permeability of to K^+, 23–24
  role in creation of blood–brain barrier, 22
  role in restoring damaged neurons, 260–261
  types in rat optic nerve, 23f
Glial scars, prevent axonal regeneration, 265
Global aphasia
  characteristics, 847t, 848
  in middle cerebral artery infarction, 1045
Globose nuclei, 627d
Globus pallidus, 277, 290f, 295
  of basal ganglia, 648
  basal ganglia, input to motor area of cerebral cortex, 611
Glomeruli, 516f
Glomeruli, specialized cells in olfactory bulb, 516–517
Glossopharyngeal nerve, functions, 684t, 685f
Glove-and-stocking pattern
  impaired perception of pain and temperature, 715
  paraesthesias, 250
Glucagon, as neuroactive peptide, 218t
Glucocorticoid response element, 189d
Glucocorticoids
  and differentiation of adrenal progenitor cells into chromaffin
    cells, 903–904, 904f
  variety of effects of in hippocampus, 746
Glucoreceptors, in hypothalamus, 757
Glucose

in cerebrospinal fluid, 1057
metabolism, mapping with PET, 312, 314
utilization by brain, PET scan, 315–316f
Glutamate
    agonists, 158
    as amino acid neurotransmitter, 217
    binds to NMDA receptors, 158
    cell death caused by, 657–658
    contribution to disease in nervous system, 160
    enhanced in long-term potentiation, 1022
    evokes fast synaptic potentials in superficial dorsal horn
        neurons, 390
    excitatory current activated by, 163f
    as excitatory neurotransmitter in brain, 158–160
    and excitatory synaptic action, 183f
    excitotoxicity, 58
    key biosynthetic enzyme, 215t
    mediates output nuclei of basal ganglia, 652
    neurotransmitter
        in A-delta and C fibers in superficial dorsal horn neurons,
            390
        in area CA1 hippocampal cells, 1020
        in pyramidal and spiny stellate cells of primary visual
            cortex, 427
        in pyramidal cells of cerebral cortex, 782f
        in pyramidal cells of somatic sensory cortex, 365
        in retina, 401
    receptors. See also Quisqualate B receptors
        as multisubunit transmembrane protein, 162–164
        NMDA, PCP binds to, 866
    regulation of excitatory synaptic actions in CNS neurons,
        157f
    release
        by cones in surround onto horizontal cells, 413f
        by cones, opposite effects on two classes of bipolar cells,
            413
        by reversal of transporter carrier proteins, 232
    toxicity, 160d
    transmitter versus metabolic, 217
    uptake mechanism for, 233
Glutamic acid decarboxylase
    decreased in striatum of patients with Huntington's disease,
        656
    decarboxylase, in terminals of cortical basket cells, 779
    in nonpyramidal cells of cerebral cortex, 782
Glycine
    action on Cl⁻ ion channels, 162f
    as amino acid neurotransmitter, 217
    as inhibitory neurotransmitter, 162
    key biosynthetic enzyme, 215t
    needed for efficient function of NMDA-activated channel,
        159
    receptor
        forms anion-selective channels, 164
        as multisubunit transmembrane protein, 162–164
        primary structure, 163
    uptake mechanism for, 233
Glycogen storage diseases, cause of muscular weakness in, 253
Glycoproteins
    classes involved in neural cell adhesion, 918–921
    and recognition of basal lamina by ingrowing nerve terminal,
        941
Glycosylation
    of membrane and secretory proteins, 55
    modification of NCAM, 919
Goldman equation, quantification of resting membrane
        potential and action potential, 88–89
Golgi apparatus
    part of major membrane system of nerve cell, 49
    role in protein distribution in nerve cell, 56
Golgi cells, inhibitory interneurons, 632
Golgi neurons, in cerebellar cortex, 630

Golgi staining, and identification of classes of neurons, 271
Golgi tendon organs, 565f
    arrangement within muscle and function, 568–569
    and group Ib inhibitory interneurons, 586
    innervation, 567–568
    as muscle receptor, 565
    response to muscle stretch and contraction, 567–568, 568f
Golgi's silver impregnation method, and neuronal structure,
        20
Gonadotropin
    cyclical secretion depends on absence of androgen during
        perinatal period, 964
    secretion patterns, adult, in rats subjected to neonatal
        endocrine manipulation, 964t
Gonadotropin-releasing hormone. See also Luteinizing
        hormone-releasing hormone
    as neuroactive peptide, 218t
Gonads
    developing, bipotentiality, 961–962
Gracile fascicle, 360d
Gracile nucleus, 360d
    nociceptive and large-diameter myelinated primary afferent
        fiber axons terminate in, 390
Gramicidin A, use of to study ion channel function, 69
Gramicidin ion channels, current through, 70f
Grand mal seizures, 785–786
Granular layer, cerebellar cortex, 630f
Granule cells, 516f
    in cerebellar cortex, 630
    function of affected in weaver mutant, 910
    migration in cerebellum of weaver mutant mice, 912f
Gray matter
    contain cell bodies of preganglionic neurons of sympathetic
        division, 764
    imaged with computerized tomography, 312, 312f
    midbrain periaqueductal, activity of serotonergic neurons
        during REM sleep, 801
    spinal cord, 283d
        contains nerve cell bodies, 354, 356
        termination of medial and lateral pathways in, 541
Gray type synapses, 171, 170f
Grooming, central program for, 990
Group atrophy, 248d
Group Ia afferent axon, 567
Group Ia afferent fiber
    innervate muscle spindles, 565
    innervation of intrafusal fiber, 566f
    monosynaptic connections to motor neurons, 575–576
    role in stretch reflex, 575
Group Ia inhibitory interneurons, coordinate opposing muscles
        in stretch reflex, 585
Group Ib afferent fiber
    innervates Golgi tendon organs, 565
    polysynaptic connections to motor neurons, 576–577
Group Ib inhibitory interneurons, convergent input from
        receptors, 586
Group II afferent axon, 567
Group II afferent fiber, polysynaptic connections to motor
        neurons, 576–577
Growth cone
    actin and microtubule domains, 913f
    activation of second-messenger pathways in, 913
    classes of interaction with, 914
    effect of change in intracellular Ca²⁺ concentration on
        motility, 913
    guided by chemotactic molecules, 916–917
    guides axon to target, 911–914
    morphology, 912f
    repelled by cells-surface molecules, 916
    stabilization and assembly of specialized structures, 935
    storing and release of neurotransmitter before contacting
        muscle, 936

Growth factors
  control differentiation of glial cells, 899f
  release of from postsynaptic cell and synaptic stabilization,
    956
  role
    in glial cell differentiation, 898
    in mesodermal and neural induction, 894, 896, 898
  as neuroactive peptide, 218t
Growth hormone-releasing hormone
  as neuroactive peptide, 218t
  released by parvocellular neurons, 742
  structure, 742f
GTP-binding protein, activates second messenger cascade to
    modulate ion channel activity, 133f
Guanidine, promotes release of ACh, 242
Guanylate cyclase, in cyclic GMP pathway, 191
Guidepost cells, 915d, 916f
Guillain-Barré syndrome
  as acute neuropathy, 250
  demyelinating disease, 102
  peripheral nerve disease, 249t
Gustatory nucleus, taste bud afferents project to, 524–525
Gustatory pathway, 519–521, 525f
Gustatory receptor cells, transduce information about taste,
    518–524
Gustatory sensation, stimulus qualities, 521–524
Gyri, 8d, 276f, 278f

H
Habituation
  and depression of synaptic transmission, 1010–1012
    and regression and pruning of synaptic connections, 1016
  of semicircular canals, 662
  type of nonassociative learning, 998
Hair cells, 484f
  arrangement in semicircular ducts, 504, 506
  inner ear, fluid waves in cochlea vibrate, 483–489
  innervation, 489
  neurotransmitter release with depolarization, 486
  semicircular canals, damage to and effect on stabilization of
    gaze, 661–662
  stimulation direction, 669f
  transduction processes of, 501
  tuned to different frequencies of sound, 487–489
  utricular, 507f, 508f
  variation in length, 488
  vestibular, 503–508
  vibrations transformed into electrical signals in auditory
    nerve, 489–491
Hair follicles
  innervation, 764
  receptor, 345
Hair receptors, 343f
Haldol. See Haloperidol
Half-center model, rhythmic alternating activity, 583f
Hallucinations, 855d
  in olfaction abnormalities, 518
  by stimulation of superior temporal gyrus, 830
  in schizophrenia, 855
Hallucinogens, act on serotonin receptors, 866
Haloperidol
  structure, 859f
  treatment, schizophrenia, 858
Hand manipulation neurons, 623
Handedness
  and cerebral asymmetry, 971
  deficits in left-handed populations, 835–836
  and dyslexia, 850
  and nature of hemispheric lateralization, 835
  and performance on dichotic auditory task, 833
  and performance on visuospatial test, 833
  relationship to lateralization of speech functions, 832

Head
  changes in movement or position of, vestibular hair cells
    respond to, 503–508
  and eye movements, coordinated by tectospinal tract, 541
  motor control of muscles, by brain stem, 9t
  stabilized by vestibular and neck reflexes, 600–602
  vestibular hair cells respond to changes in movement or
    position, 503–508
Head ganglion, hypothalamus as for autonomic nervous system,
    746
Head movement
  role of horizontal ducts to provide bilateral indication of,
    506f
  vestibulo-ocular and optokinetic reflexes compensate for,
    661–663
Hearing, 481–499. See also Ear
Heart
  cholinergic and noradrenergic responses, 771t
  muscle, controlled by autonomic nervous system, 762
  rate
    effect of acetylcholine, 772
    function for control localized to medulla oblongata, 9t
  sympathetic and parasympathetic innervation, 770
Heart pain, mediated by nociceptors, 344
Hebb's rule, 1020d
Hedonic factors, and regulation of motivated behaviors, 759
Heel-shin test, 644d
Helicotrema, 482d
Helix-turn-helix protein, 189d
Hematoma, 1045d
Hemianopsia
  contralateral homonymous, in posterior cerebral artery
    infarction, 1046
  types, 437d
Hemiballismus
  effect on direct and indirect pathways of basal ganglia, 653
  and pathological changes in basal ganglia, 647
Hemi-channel, model of, 130f
Hemichorea, 729
Hemiparesis, 726t
Hemiplegia, contralateral, in occlusion of anterior choroidal
    and penetrating arteries, 1046
Hemispheres, cerebral. See Cerebral hemispheres
Hemorrhage, 1045, 1048, 1048f
Hemorrhagic stroke, 1045
Hensen's cells, 485f
Hereditary achromatopsia, optokinetic reflex in, 671
Heredity
  and affective disorders, 871–872
  and alteration in gene structure in inherited psychiatric
    disease, 1029f
  and Alzheimer's disease, 977
  and certain human behavioral traits, 993
Herniation, uncal and central, 817d
Heroin, and blood–brain barrier, 1056
Herpes simplex virus, fast retrograde transport, 60
Hertz, 482d
Heterodimers, transcriptional, 189d
Hindbrain, 8f
  formation, 298
  segmental organization, 303, 303f
Hippocampal pyramidal cell, as multipolar cell, 21f
Hippocampus, 277, 307f, 736f
  activation of cAMP by norepinephrine in, 183–184, 184f
  Alzheimer's pathology in, 979f
  appearance of amyloid plaques in, 977
  area CA1, associative mechanisms used in series in long-term
    potentiation, 1022
  area CA3
    long-term potentiation is nonassociative, 1023
    long-term potentiation of mossy fiber synapses, 1023f
  basket cells, release of GABA by, 217

bilateral removal, and deficit of recent memory, 1006

contribution of NMDA receptor-channel to EPSP in, 159f

developing, synthesizes nerve growth factor and its receptor, 933

dorsal, morphological sex differences, 969

expression of D1 and D5 dopamine receptors, 860

expression of D2 dopamine receptors in, 860

fast prepotentials in pyramidal cells of, 787

and fornix, C-shaped, 307

function, 9t

generation of theta rhythm during REM sleep, 794

inhibitory effects of serotonin on, 698

long-term potentiation in
  area CA1, 1020f
  example of associative and nonassociative learning, 1019–1024

magnetic resonance image of, 984f

major excitatory pathways and long-term potentiation, 1019f

neurofibrillary tangles in pyramidal neurons of, 979, 979f

norepinephrine increases excitability of neurons of, 696

projections in olfactory tract to, 517

quantal analysis, of long-term potentiation in CA1 area of, 1022f

variety of glucocorticoid effects in, 746

Histamine
  as biogenic amine, 216–217
  effect on nociceptors, 387, 387t

Hodgkin–Huxley model, applicability of, 110–112

Hoffmann sign, sign of corticospinal tract lesion, 718

Homeobox domain, 894d
  Drosophila, 897

Homeobox genes
  clusters, sequence comparison of in Drosophila and mouse, 897
  role in development, 884f, 885
  role in establishing regional differences in early nervous system, 894

Homeostasis, 735d
  role of enteric nervous system, 766
  role of hypothalamus, 733

Homeostatic processes
  analyzed in terms of control systems, 751f
  correspondence to motivational states, 751–752

Homocarnosine, histamine as precursor, 217

Homodimers, transcriptional, 189d

Homunculus
  motor, 372f
  sensory, 372f

Horizontal cells, 408, 409f, 415f
  depolarized, release inhibitory transmitter, 413f
  and lateral pathways in retina, 412
  respond to light with graded change in membrane potential, 412

Horizontal ducts, orientation within head, 507f

Hormone secretion, chemical synaptic transmission as modified form, 131

Hormone-responsive elements, 966

Hormones. See also specific names
  and alteration of gene expression, 1028
  central effects on behavior involve humoral and neural output, 745
  effect of on feeding behavior, 756
  and gating of ion channels, 75
  gonadal
    actions on developing and mature nervous system, 963
    organizational and regulatory effects on nervous tissue during development, 962
    regulation of sexual differential in fetus, 962
    steroid, effective on anterior preoptic region and infundibular-premammillary region, 969
    steroid, receptors for, located in cell nucleus, 965–967, 966f

male, fetal exposure to causes pseudohermaphroditism in genetic females, 963–964

perinatal, and degree to which sex-linked behavior is expressed, 968

production of involves feedback loops, 744–745

sex, homotypical versus heterotypical, 963

steroid
  influence perinatal development only during critical periods, 964
  manufacture by fetus, 964

structures of precursors, 220f

Horner syndrome, 718, 726t, 1047

Horseradish peroxidase
  retrograde accumulation in frog triceps motor neuron pools, 530f
  and study of axon distribution of neuron in CNS, 61f
  use in neuroanatomical tracing based on fast axonal transport, 61

Hospitalism, abandoned children, 946

HPETE. See Hydroperoxyeicosatrienoic acid

Hue, color, determined by proportion in which cones are activated by object and background, 476

Human immunodeficiency virus, enters brain with infected macrophages, 1057. See also Acquired immunodeficiency syndrome

Human lymphotropic virus type I, and spinal cord degeneration, 719

Huntington's chorea. See Huntington's disease

Huntington's disease
  and cell death in caudate nucleus, 306–307
  characteristics, 981
  as disorder of basal ganglia, 654t
  genetic markers for, 656–657
  and glutamate toxicity, 160
  and glutamate-induced neuronal cell death, 657–658
  and loss of striatal neurons, 656
  and pathological changes in basal ganglia, 647
  pre- and postsynaptic mechanisms of NMDA receptor-mediated toxicity in, 658
  symptoms, 656

HVM. See Hypothalamic ventromedial nucleus

Hybrid figures, in experiments with commissurotomized patients, 835

Hybridization, use in detecting chemical messengers within the nerve cell, 222

Hydra head activator, as neuroactive peptide, 218t

Hydrocephalus
  in acoustic neuroma, 721
  cause, 304
    obstruction of cerebrospinal fluid pathways, 1059
  as increase in volume of cerebral ventricles, 1059–1060

Hydroperoxyeicosatrienoic acid, in arachidonic acid cascade, 182

Hydrophobicity plot, for study of membrane-spanning regions of ion channel, 72, 72f

5-Hydroxytryptamine, and presynaptic facilitation, 208

Hyperalgesia, 386d

Hypercolumns, regions of visual field in primary visual cortex, 432, 433f

Hyperlexia, disorder of reading, 850

Hypermetamorphosis, and bilateral temporal lobe removal, 747

Hyperpolarization, 27d, 82d
  Cl^- influx into cell, 161f
  effect on steady-state Ca^{2+} conductance, 206
  hair cells, 488
  and limitation of focal seizure, 789
  by motion of stereocilia of hair cells, 486
  photoreceptor membrane, caused by closing of cGMP-gated ion channels, 407f
  recording, 83
  vestibular hair cells, 504

Hyperreflexia, 249d

Hypersomnia, 816d
Hypersomnolent apnea syndrome, 812
Hyperthermia, chronic, after lesions of anterior hypothalamus, 752
Hypertonus, 578d
Hypnagogic hallucinations, narcoleptic symptom, 813d
Hypoglossal nerve, functions, 684t, 685f
Hypoglossal nuclei, in somatic motor column, 687–688
Hypoglossal nucleus, 288f
Hypoglycemia, and coma, 817
Hypoperfusion, diffuse, as cause of ischemia or infarction, 1047
Hyposmia, 518d
Hypothalamic hormones, release of regulated by limbic system, 279
Hypothalamic sulcus, 290f
Hypothalamic ventromedial nucleus
    principal site for hormonal activation of lordosis, 967
    sex difference in effect of estrogen on progesterone receptor levels in, 967
Hypothalamohypophyseal tract, 739
Hypothalamus, 290f. See also Suprachiasmatic nucleus
    action of steroid and thyroid hormones in, 745
    acts on endocrine, autonomic nervous, and limbic systems, 735, 767
    anatomy, 736–740
    beta-endorphin in, 395
    classes of peptidergic neuroendocrine cells in, 740–744
    cold-sensitive neurons, 753
    derived from diencephalon, 298
    disturbance of in depression, 879–880
    and emotions, 746–747
    fiber systems of, 739–740
    function, 9t, 276, 733, 739–740, 752, 756, 766–768
    gluco-receptors in, 757
    higher cortical centers communicate with via limbic system, 737–739
    histamine as transmitter in cells of, 217
    lesions, 746, 752, 755, 756
    and limbic system, 735–749
    location and structure, 738f
    as main control center for autonomic nervous system, 279
    nuclei, 738f, 739
    paraventricular nucleus, 739f
    plasticity of neurons in, 746
    preoptic area, sexual differentiation, 969
    projections, 766–767
    regions concerned with heat conservation and dissipation, 752
    regulation
        of autonomic nervous system, 746–747
        of behavioral aspects of drinking, 757
        temperature, 752–753
        of vital functions, 736
    relationship to pituitary, 738f
    role
        in homeostasis, 733, 735
        in motivation, 750–760
    steroid receptors in, 966
Hypotonia, 637d, 644d

I

I. See Current
Ia afferent neurons, quantal analysis, 201
Iconic memory, 1004
Ictal phenomena, 14d
I$_g$. See Gating current
Illumination, monocular depth cue, 455
Imaging
    localization of language in cerebral cortex with PET, 12
    magnetic resonance image of brain, 9f
    PET, and brain pathways for word recognition, 13f
    techniques, and study of higher brain function, 272

Imipramine
    antidepressant, 872
    site of action in serotonergic transmission, 878f
    structure, 873f
Immediate-early genes, induced by growth factors and neurotransmitters, 802. See also c-fos
Immune system, interaction with sleep factors, 798–799
Immunocytochemistry
    functional mapping of neurons, 694
    use in localizing transmitter substances in the nerve cell, 222–223
Immunoglobulin superfamily
    members include glycoproteins involved in axon fasciculation, 921
    neural cell glycoproteins, 918
Immunogold technique, use in localizing transmitter substances in the nerve cell, 222
Impaired proprioception, deficits in feedback and feedforward mechanisms, 537
Imprinting, 946d
In situ hybridization, use in detecting chemical messengers within the nerve cell, 222
Inactivation, and ion channel refractory state, 77d
Increased-conductance postsynaptic potential, ion channels and signal properties, 166f
Incus, 482d
Indirect immunofluorescence, use in localizing transmitter substances in the nerve cell, 222
Infarction, 1043f, 1045–1047, 1045d
Inferior cerebellar peduncle, location of cochlear nucleus on, 491f
Inferior colliculus, 494, 509f
    feedback connection in auditory system, 496
Inferior frontal cortex, localization of word recognition during thinking, 13f
Inferior prefrontal convexity
    lesions in interfere with motor responses, 829
    location, 827f
    subdivision of prefrontal cortex, 826
Inferior temporal cortex
    cellular basis of visual attention in, 462
    parvocellular-blob and parvocellular-interblob systems terminate, 447
    recognition of faces, 458–459
Inferior temporal lobe, lesions, 447
Inferior temporal region, lesions, 830
Inferior vestibular nucleus, integrates input from vestibular labyrinth and cerebellum, 510
Inferotemporal cortex
    large receptive fields, 358–359
    not organized retinotopically, 458–459
Information processing
    highest level occurs in cerebral cortex, 292–293
    in retina, 400–417
Information
    neural, transformation of in signaling, 30–31
    unique, patterns of interconnection allow nerve cells to convey, 31–32
Infratentorial lesions, and coma, 815–816
Infundibular-premammillary region, effect of gonadal steroid hormones on, 969
Infundibulum, 739d
Inheritance, pattern of in schizophrenia, 856–857
Inhibition
    cells responsible for in cerebral cortex, 782f
    and contrast between stimuli, 376–377
    interaction with excitation on single nerve cell, 169f
    postsynaptic, decrease in may synchronize neuronal ensembles in focal epilepsy, 789
    presynaptic, at axo-axonic synapses, 207–208, 208f
    short-circuiting or shunting action, 162
    shunting action of, 169f

in stretch reflex, 30
synaptic
    and limit of seizure spread, 789
    sculpturing role of, 155, 155f
Inhibitory channels, not influenced by membrane voltage, 162
Inhibitory inputs, synapses on nerve cell body, 168
Inhibitory interneurons, feedforward and feedback connections, 31f
Inhibitory postsynaptic potential. See Postsynaptic potential, inhibitory
Inhibitory synapse, distinction ultrastructure, 170–171
Inhibitory synaptic action
    integrated with excitatory synaptic actions at common trigger zone, 165–167
    mediated by receptor-channels selective for Cl⁻, 160–162
Initial segment, 40d
Injury, reaction of nerve cells, 258–269
Inking, Aplysia, 128–129
Inner ear, 501–503, 502f
Inner nuclear layer, retina, contains bipolar, horizontal, and amacrine cells, 412
Inner pillar cells, 485f
Inner plexiform layer, retina, 412
Innervation ratio, 555d
Inositol phosphates, metabolism, 181
Inositol polyphosphate, as effector molecule, 173
Inositol-lipid pathway, activation, 180f
Input component, afferent neuron, produces graded local signal, 28
Input signal, 26d
Insomnia, 806–810
Instinctive behavior, study of, 987–988
Instincts
    development of, 946
    human, 988
Insular cortex, 276, 304d
Insulin
    as neuroactive peptide, 218t, 219t
    precursor structure, 220f
Integrative component, 29d
    afferent neuron, decision to generate action potential, 28–29
Integrative zone, 103d
Integrator, 751d
Integrins, 62d
    involved in neural cell adhesion, 918
    mediate adhesion of neural cells to glycoproteins in extracellular matrix, 920
    structure, 920f
Intelligence, hereditary component, 993
Intensity, stimulus attribute expressed in sensation, 331
Intensity function, afferent fiber, 336–337
Intention tremor, 644d
    in acoustic neuroma, 721
Interaural time difference, and sound localization, 493
    in medial superior olive, 494
Interblob regions, striate cortex, 446
Interferon-alpha-2, sleep-promoting, 798
Interhemispheric fissure, 276, 278f
Interictal phenomena, 14d
Interictal spikes, 787d
    first abnormal electrical event in focal seizures, 787
    spontaneous, with application of bicuculline to hippocampus in vitro, 789
Interleukin 1
    evokes synthesis of NGF in Schwann cells, 264
    sleep-promoting, 798
Intermediate acoustic stria, 494
Intermediate filaments, relationship of neurofilaments to, 62
Intermediate hemisphere, input and output pathways, 638f
Intermediate zone
    input and output pathways, 638f
    spinal cord, 284

Intermediolateral cell column, spinal cord, 284, 286
Intermediolateral nucleus, 357f
    spinal cord gray matter, 356
Internal arcuate fibers, 360d
Internal auditory artery, 1042
Internal capsule, 288f, 290f, 359, 361
    carries axons from and to cerebral hemisphere, 288–289
    stimulating electrodes reduce pain, 393
Internal carotid artery, 1041
Internal granular layer, 611d, 612f
Internal medullary lamina, separates thalamic nuclei, 290
Interneuron, 540d
    in cerebral cortex, 782f
    input signal is the synaptic potential, 27
Interneurons, 22d. See Bipolar cells; Renshaw cells
    activation by projection neurons in processing sensory information, 369
    between photoreceptors and ganglion cells, 408
    component of reflex pathway, 582
    as component of spinal reflexes, 582–584
    convergence of descending signals, 582
    cortical, 779
    gating, 582d
    group Ia inhibitory, coordinate opposing muscles in stretch reflex, 585
    group Ib inhibitory, convergent input from receptors, 586
    inhibitory, 42
        coordinate muscle action around a joint, 584–586
        role in reflex pathways, 584
    local
        inhibit Purkinje cells, 632
        projections for axial muscle control, 540
    modulated by descending brain stem pathways, 541–543
    multisensory convergence onto, 588
    network, tonic input and excitability, 584
    networks of as central pattern generators, 582, 584
    reverberating circuits, 582
    spinal, mediation of reflexes, 539
    synaptic changes in habituation, 1011
    types, 279
Internuclear ophthalmoplegia, 721
    in multiple sclerosis, 674
Interposed nuclei, 627d
    lesions of, 637
Interposition, monocular depth cue, 454, 454f
Intersegmental reflexes, 357
Interventricular foramen, 303d
Intestine, cholinergic and noradrenergic responses, 771t
Intracellular potentials
    recording configuration, 783
    versus extracellular potentials, 781, 783
Intracortical connections, in somatic sensory cortex, 364–365
Intracranial pressure, relationship to cerebral blood flow, 1058
Intrafusal creep, 570d, 571f
Intrafusal fibers, 38d, 566f
    effect of muscle stretch, 571f
    innervation by spindle afferents and efferents, 570–571
    of muscle spindle, 566
    nonuniform characteristics, 570
Intralaminar nuclei, thalamic, 291f, 292
Intraparietal sulcus, third-part connections, 828f
Intrasegmental reflexes, 357
Intrauterine position, and effect on male characteristics, 968
Invaginating synapses, 415f
Ion, physical chemistry of in solution, 67
Ion channels, 35, 66–70. See also Gap junctions; Membrane-spanning proteins; Receptors
    ACh activated, 141–143, 141f, 143f, 146f
    active, calculation of conductance for with Ohm's law, 108
    allosteric modulators and gating transition, 78
    allosteric proteins, 74
    arrayed according to neuronal function, 112

Ion channels [*cont.*]
  A-type K$^+$ channel, 111
  behaves as
    rectifier, 73
    simple resistor, 69
  binding of exogenous ligands, 77f
  blocked, 74f
  calcium, 111, 117, 185
    voltage-gated, 111, 116f, 117
  change in functional properties over course of development, 78
  chloride
    action of GABA on, 162f
    action of glycine on, 162f
    GABA/benzodiazepine, subunit types, 882f
    opening of by chemical inhibitory synaptic action hyperpolarizes postsynaptic cell, 161f
    transmitter-gated, mediate inhibitory synaptic action, 160
  cGMP-gated
    closing of hyperpolarizes photoreceptor membrane, 406–408, 407f
    opening of in phototransduction cascade, 404
  common characteristics, 73–78
  as conductor and battery, 89–90
  control current flow, 81
  cross cell membrane, 67–69
  current flow and changes in membrane voltage, 96
  conformational changes to open and close, 75–78
  delayed rectifier, voltage-gated K$^+$ channel, 111
  direct action
    of G-proteins, 185–186
    of second messengers, 185–186
  direct gating mediated by transmitter receptor, 133f
  directly gated
    characteristics, 185t
    involved in synaptic excitation of skeletal muscle by motor neurons, 138–139
  distribution of types in photoreceptors, 407
  end-plate
    mean open time, 144
    permeable to Na$^+$ and K$^+$, 139–140
  fast, transient K$^+$ channel, 111
  formation of at site of fusion of secretory vesicle to plasma membrane, 203
  functional states, 76
  gap junction
    comparison with transmitter- and voltage-gated channels, 164
    molecular structure, 165f
  gated, 66d, 81
  gating, 74–78
    stimuli controlling, 75f
  gene superfamilies for, 164
  genes encoding are grouped into families, 78
  genes for, 70–71
  gramicidin, current through, 70f
  indirect gating mediated by second messenger, 133f
  inhibitory, not influenced by membrane voltage, 162
  ion selectivity related to number of subunits and pore diameter, 164
  ionophoric receptors gate directly, 132–133
  kinetics of ion flow, 73
  ligand-gated, 75f
  L-type Ca^{2+}, role in sensitization, 1012, 1013f
  M channel, 769
  mechanically activated, and change in conformation, 77
  molecular biology study approaches, 697
  molecular mechanisms of gating by chemical receptors, 132–133
  M-type K$^+$ channel, 111, 183
  N-type Ca^{2+}
    inactivation of in habituation, 1011

    role in sensitization, 1012, 1013f
  nongated, 81
    in glial cells, selective for K$^+$, 84
    passive fluxes of Na$^+$ and K$^+$ balanced by active pumping, 86–88
    selective for several ion species in nerve cells, 84–86
  number open influences current flow, 144–146
  and passive flux of ions across cell membrane, 73–74
  pharmacological blockade, 107
  photoreceptor plasma membrane, gated by cGMP, 406
  physical models for gating, 74f
  potassium
    abnormal in *Drosophila shaker* mutant, 992
    Ca^{2+}-dependent, and limitation of focal seizure, 789
    direct gating of by G-protein in heart, 772
    modulating effect of G-protein, 185
    modulation of as important in learning, 1018
    P region, 117
    PCP binds to, 866
    pore-forming region, 117
    -selective nongated, role in driving photoreceptor membrane potential, 406
    serotonin sensitive, role in sensitization, 1012
    voltage-gated, hydrophobicity analysis of subunit, 116f
    voltage-sensitive, and limitation of focal seizure, 789
  produce electrical signals resulting from movement of ions down their electrochemical gradients, 164
  properties, 66
  protein, phosphorylation of by second messengers, 182–185
  protein structure, 70
  as proteins, 67
  and rate of ion transfer across membranes, 68
  receptors, directly gated, 174f
  refractory state and competitive inhibitors, 77–78
  in refractory states, 76f
  relation between single-channel current and ionic concentration saturates, 74
  relative proportions of determine membrane selectivity, 84
  second-messenger modulated, characteristics, 185t
  second-messenger-regulated, and olfactory transduction, 515
  secondary structure, 71–72
  selectivity, 66, 67–69, 73
    filter, 68
    for Na$^+$, K$^+$, Cl$^-$, as battery in series with conductor, 91f
    permeable to K$^+$, as battery in series with conductor, 89f
  signaling potentials, 166t
  similarity of molecular structure, 165f
  simultaneous closure of Ca^{2+} and opening of voltage-gated K$^+$ as mechanism of presynaptic mechanism, 208
  single, recording current flow from with patch-clamp technique, 71
  sodium
    and generation of action potential, 28–29
    schematic diagram, 69f
    -selective, voltage-independent, and transduction of sweet taste, 522
    selectivity filter, 69f
    voltage-gated, hydrophobicity analysis of subunit, 116f
    voltage-gated, postulated tertiary structure, 116f
  speed of directly gated versus G-protein coupled, 175
  stimuli that open and close, 164
  study methods, 68–73
    single-channel recording, 69
  structure, 72–73
  S-type K$^+$ channel, 183
  subunit basis of structure, 72f
  as target in autoimmune neurological disorders, 79
  transitions between open and closed state, 77
  transmitter-gated
    ACh receptor, molecular structure, 165f
    binding of ACh, 142f
    and change in conformation, 77

different from voltage-gated channels, 140–142
individual channels conduct unitary current, 144
permeable to Na⁺ and K⁺ ions, 141f
and permeable to Na⁺ and K⁺, mediate EPSP, 155–160
study of single channel, 142–146
versus voltage-gated, 162
and voltage-gated are structurally similar, 164
and voltage-gated, pharmacological differences, 142
type of gated by transmitter in postsynaptic cell determines sign of synaptic potential, 170
voltage-dependent
and closed by second messengers, 184–185
leaking K⁺, and transduction of sweet taste, 522
and transduction of sour taste, 522
voltage-dependent Ca²⁺, opening in response to
voltage gated
applicability of Hodgkin–Huxley model of excitability, 110–112
and change in conformation, 76
different from transmitter-gated channels, 140–142
existence of two types demonstrated by voltage-clamp experiment, 107f
functions in presynaptic cell at electrical synapse, 124–125
and generation of action potential, 88, 104–118
generation of action potential by ion flow through Na⁺ and K⁺, 105
K⁺ and Na⁺ belong to gene family, 115–118
molecular properties, 112–118
Na⁺ flux through is regenerative, 142
open in all-or-none fashion, 113, 113f
recruited by EPP to trigger action potential, 142
selectivity for cations, 141f
study with voltage-clamp technique, 105–109
variety of in nervous system, 111
voltage-gated Ca²⁺
antibodies to and Lambert–Eaton syndrome, 242
and neurotransmitter release, 136
voltage-gated Na⁺
convert end plate potential into action potential, 136
molecular structure, 165f
tetrodotoxin blocks, 142
voltage-gated Na⁺ and K⁺, pore diameter compared with ACh-activated channel, 141, 141f
voltage-gated Na⁺, K⁺, and Ca²⁺, in taste cells, 520–521
voltage-independent
and release of Ca²⁺ in muscle fiber contraction process, 550
and transduction of saltiness, 523
voltage-sensitive, gating influenced by changes in intracellular ion concentrations, 111
voltage-sensitive Ca²⁺, classes of, 198
Ion flow
electrodiffusion model, 74
kinetics of through ion channel, 73
saturation, 74
Ion flux, and electrochemical driving force, 73
Ionic conductance, neurotransmitter modulation of through second messenger, 771
Ionic current, study of with voltage-clamp technique, 105
Ionic gradients, dissipation of with Na⁺-K⁺ pump, 87–88
Ionic membrane current, 96d
Ionophoric receptors, 132d
Iproniazid
antidepressant, 877
site of action in serotonergic transmission, 878f
Iron
distribution of altered by movement disorders, 322
paramagnetic effects of allow imaging of specific neural systems, 321–323
Ischemia, 1045d
diffuse hypoperfusion as cause of, 1047
Isocarboxazid, structure, 873f
Isolation syndrome, 946–947

J

Jacksonian motor seizures, 785d
characteristics, 610
progression of and arrangement of sensory projections in brain, 372
Jaw muscles
activity controlled by trigeminal motor nucleus, 706–707
mesencephalic nucleus mediates proprioceptive responses from, 705–706
Jaw reflex, 706
Jet lag, and temporary insomnia, 807, 808f
Jitter, 239d
Joint
afferents, and limb proprioception, 348
angle
and muscle spindle receptors, 348
strategies that produce, 560–561
sensitivity of knee joint afferents to, 348
co-contraction and reciprocal innervation, 585d
muscle action around coordinated by inhibitory interneurons, 584–586
proprioceptors in, 535
receptors, 349f
Junctional fold, 136d, 136f
Just noticeable difference, 332d
Juxtaglomerular cells, cholinergic and noradrenergic responses, 771t

K

Kainate receptor
channel regulation by, 157f
glutamate binding to, 158
Kana, phonetic Japanese writing system, localization to region of cerebral cortex, 849–850
Kanjii, ideographic Japanese writing system, localization to region of cerebral cortex, 849–850
Kappa receptor, opiate, 395
Kindling, 786d
Kinesin
association with microtubules, 59f
role in fast anterograde transport, 58
Kinesthesia, 347
Kinocilium
arrangement on surface of vestibular hair cell and polarization, 504f
characteristics, 503
Kleiber's rule, 754d
Klinefelter's syndrome, abnormal sex chromosomes in, 960
Klüver–Bucy syndrome, 747
Knee-jerk reflex
as involuntary stretch reflex, 24–25
role of sensory and motor neurons in, 38–43
Knee-jerk stretch reflex, nerve cells that participate in, 40f
Knowledge, storage of in brain as distinct categories, 14
Korsakoff's psychosis, memory deficits, 1006

L

L-3,4-Hydroxyphenylalanine, and amelioration of Parkinson's disease symptoms, 655
L1, structure, 919f
Labeled line code
encodes stimulus modality, 338
paradoxical cold as example, 344
Labeled line system, in taste pathway, 525
Labeling techniques, and organization of neural circuits, 271–272
Labyrinth, inner ear, parts, 501
Lacrimal glands
cholinergic and noradrenergic responses, 771t
innervation, 764
Lactate dehydrogenase, and diagnosis of myopathies, 246
Lacunes, 1046d

Lambert–Eaton syndrome
  and facilitating neuromuscular block, 242
  ion channels as targets in, 79
Lamellipodia, 911d
Lamina terminalis, 303d
Laminae, of spinal cord gray matter, 354, 356
Laminar nucleus, contains neurons that detect interaural
      timing differences, 493
Laminectomy, 714
Laminin
  and axon extension, 264
  promotes axon growth in peripheral nervous system, 265
  role in migration of neural crest cells, 911
  structure, 920f
Language
  affective components, 13–14, 848
  anatomical organization, 12
  aprosodias localized to right hemisphere, 14
  auditory comprehension center in Wernicke's area, 844f
  cognitive capability for in left cerebral hemisphere, 843
  cognitive studies, 845
  comprehension of emotional content localized to Wernicke's
      area in left hemisphere, 14
  cytoarchitectonic areas of brain, 844
  deficit, 831, 835, 971
  disorders of, 839–851
  as distinctive from other forms of communication, 840–843
  experiments, 12, 840–841
  expression of emotional aspects localized to right frontal area
  gestural theories, 841
  importance of left caudate nucleus, 845
  as innate skill or as learned, 842
  integration with sensory function by
      parietal–temporal–occipital area, 825
  interconnections of regions of brain involved with, 845
  as involving separate motor and sensory brain regions, 11
  localization of, 7–12
  models of, 840–841
  motor–speech area, Broca's area, 844f
  movements of articulation, facial expression, and phonation
      in precentral gyrus, 844f
  neural pathways involved in production and comprehension,
      845f
  origin of, 841
  pathways, 844, 845
  PET scan of areas of brain active during different tasks, 2f, 3
  processing is both serial and parallel, 12
  role of association areas of parietal lobes in, 831
  stages in acquisition of, 842t
  and structure of brain, 842–843, 994–995
  universals that characterize, 843
  vocal theories, 841
  Wernicke–Geschwind model, 11, 843–844
Large-fiber sensory neuropathy
  examples, 538f
  and impaired proprioception, 537
Lateral brain stem pathways
  role in motor function, 541
  termination, 541
Lateral columns
  white matter of spinal cord, 284, 356
Lateral geniculate neurons, classification according to cone
      inputs, 472f
Lateral geniculate nucleus
  afferent fibers from terminate in primary visual cortex, 428f
  broad-band cells in, 471
  cone opponent cells code color in, 471–473
  input, 431, 954
  layers, 426
  link between parvo- and magnocellular layers and retinotopic
      maps in cortex, 446
  neurons have circular receptive fields, 426

processes visual information, 423, 425–426
  projections, 423f, 425f, 433f, 949
  receptive fields of neurons in compared with primary visual
      cortex, 428f
  role in optokinetic reflex, 671
  thalamic, 290, 291f
Lateral horn, spinal cord, 286
Lateral lemniscus, 494d
Lateral medullary syndrome, manifestations, 728
Lateral nuclear group, thalamus, receives nociceptive input, 391
Lateral nucleus, thalamic, 290, 291f
Lateral orbitofrontal circuit, 652
Lateral premotor area, 539
  firing of neurons in before voluntary finger movement, 619f
  inputs to, 620
  lesions, 619
  projections, 620
  role in controlling proximal movements, 620–622
Lateral reticulospinal tract, 603
Lateral sclerosis, 248d
Lateral sulcus, 278f
Lateral superior olive, and interaural differences in sound
      intensity, 494
Lateral syndrome of lower pons, manifestations, 728
Lateral tegmental neurons
  projections, 695f, 696
  provide primary noradrenergic input to brain stem and spinal
      cord, 697
Lateral tegmental nucleus, noradrenergic neurons in, 696
Lateral tegmentum, noradrenergic cell groups, 695f
Lateral tuberal nucleus, 738f
Lateral ventricle, development, 305f
Lateral vestibular nucleus
  role in control of posture, 508–509
  selective reponse of neurons to tilting of head, 508
Lateral vestibulospinal tract, 508, 509f
Lateralization, of functions in brain, 832
Law of effect, 1000d
Layered network, 836d
LDH. See Lactate dehydrogenase
L-Dihydroxyphenylalanine
  effect on flexor reflex afferent pathways, 589
  effect of in spinal cats, 591
  increases dopamine levels and causes psychosis resembling
      schizophrenia, 861
L-DOPA. See also L-3,4-Hydroxyphenylalanine
  and blood–brain barrier, 1056
Lead intoxication, chronic neuropathy, 250
Leakage
  conductance, 107d
  method of neurotransmitter release, 232
Learning, 997–1008. See also Habituation; Sensitization
  and alteration
    of gene expression, 1028
    in nerve cells and patterns of interconnections of sensory
        and motor systems, 1024–1025
  associational. See also Conditioning, operant
  associative, 998d
    importance of timing, 1016, 1018
    long-term potentiation in CA1 region of hippocampus,
        1019–1022
  associative and nonassociative, long-term potentiation in
      hippocampus as example of, 1019–1024
  cellular mechanisms, 1009–1031
  changes in somatotopic map produced by may contribute to
      biological expression of individuality, 1025–1026
  and changes in synaptic strength, 1012
  conditioning and predictive relationships, 999–1000
  declarative, amnesia patients not capable of, 1006
  and decortication, 1005
  function localized to temporal lobe of cerebral cortex, 7
  importance of cAMP cascade in, 1019

index of, 998d
and modification of cerebellar circuits, 642, 643f
modulation of K⁺ channel may be critical for, 1018
molecular grammar for, 1023
motor skills, role of cerebellum, 642
neuronal changes and understanding of psychiatric disorders, 1027–1028
nonassociative, 998d
  elementary forms, 998
  types, 998
and parallel channels of information, 1005
reflexive, changes in effectiveness of synaptic transmission, 1010–1013
as reflexive or declarative, 1002–1003
resiliency of, 1005
role of amygdala in, 739
spatial, involvement of NMDA receptor mechanism, 1023
trial-and-error, 1000
Left abducens neurons, action, 668
Left hemifield, 421d,f
Left homonymous hemianopsia, 437d
Left medial longitudinal fasciculus, effect of lesion on eye movement, 722f
Left-right confusion, 831
Lenticulostriates, 1046d
Leucine-enkephalin, 218t
Leucine zippers, 189d
Leukemia inhibitory factor, comparison with CNTF, 905
Leukotrienes, effect on nociceptors, 387t
LH. See Luteinizing hormone
LHRH. See Luteinizing hormone-releasing hormone
Librium. See Chlordiazepoxide
Light. See also Phototransduction
  absorption
    by cones triggers isomerization of retinal from 11-cis to all-trans form, 469
    by visual pigments in rods and cones, 403
  adaptation
    and cone desensitization, 408
    role of Ca²⁺ in mediating, 408
  and alteration of circadian rhythm, 808
  and change in photoreceptor membrane potential, 406
  and closure of cGMP-gated ion channels and hyperpolarization, 407–408
  different cones respond preferentially to different wavelengths, 469
  intensity of and effect on inward current and membrane potential of photoreceptor, 407f
  response of ganglion cells to, 408–412
  as zeitgeber for circadian clock, 800–801
Limb movement
  coordinated by flexion reflex pathways, 587
  coordination by flexion withdrawal reflexes, 588
Limb position
  classes of receptors, 349f
  illusion of and muscle vibration, 350f
  psychophysical studies, 348
Limb proprioception
  mediated by muscle afferent fibers, 347–349
Limb-girdle dystrophy, 249t, 253
Limbic association cortex, 277, 824, 825f
  role in memory and emotional behavior, 829–831
  stimulation or ablation of temporal portion alters emotions, 831
Limbic lobe, 276, 736f, 737
Limbic system, 276. See also Motivational system
  ablation of and sham rage phenomena, 747
  affected by Alzheimer's disease, 980
  anatomy, 736–740
  components, 736f
    develop C shape, 307
  dopaminergic system, 697–698

dopamine receptors in, 860–861
higher cortical centers communicate with hypothalamus via, 737–739
and hypothalamus, 735–749
role in motivation, 750–760
Limbs
  effect of vestibulospinal reflexes, 600
  individual pattern generators for, 591
  sensory and motor innervation of by spinal cord, 283–287
  sensory neurons that innervate originate in dorsal root ganglia, 286–287
Lin-12 gene
  C. elegans, sequence similarity to membrane-spanning proteins encoded by Drosophila notch and delta genes, 896
Lineage, and differentiated fate of cells, 888
Linear motion, otolith reflexes compensate for, 663
Linear perspective, monocular depth cue, 454f
Linguistic information, processed by left posterior parietal cortex, 623
Lipid bilayer, and separation of charge across membrane, 82
Lipopolysaccharides, sleep-promoting, 798
Lipoxygenases, in arachidonic acid cascade, 182
Lithium, mechanism of action, 880f
Lithium salts, treatment for depression, 872
Lobotomy, 829
  frontal, early results, 829–830
Local interneurons, 22d, 279
Local sign, 586d
Local-circuit current flow, and local depolarization, 100
Location, stimulus attribute expressed in sensation, 331
Locked-in syndrome, versus coma, 729
Locomotion
  automaticity of, 591
  goal-directed, requirement of intact supraspinal systems, 593
  migrating neurons, 911, 913
  reticular neurons produce extension during stance phase, 604
  rhythmic pattern generated by spinal circuits, 591–594
Locomotor pattern
  NMDA receptors role in generating, 593
  rhythmic, modified by afferent information, 593–594
Locus ceruleus
  activity of monoaminergic cells in during REM sleep, 803
  affected by Parkinson's disease, 981–982
  aminergic pathways from modulate excitability of spinal neurons, 541
  input, 696
  loss
    of nerve cells and depigmentation of in Parkinson's disease, 655
    noradrenergic neurons in Parkinson's disease, 655
  neurofibrillary tangles in, 979
  noradrenergic cell groups, 694f, 696
  as noradrenergic nucleus, 876f
  noradrenergic pathways originate in, 216, 875
  and possible role in panic attacks, 881
  projections, 694f, 696
    to cerebellar cortex, 632
  provide principal aminergic input to neocortex, 696
  visualized by immunofluorescence histochemical localization of tyrosine hydroxylase, 680f
Logorrhea, 846d
Long-term potentiation, model for induction, 1021f
Lordosis
  active suppression of in male brain, 967
  female sexually dimorphic behavior, 963
  HVM principal site for hormonal activation of, 967
Lou Gehrig's disease. See Amyotrophic lateral sclerosis
LSD. See Lysergic acid diethylamide
LTP. See Potentiation, long-term
Lumbar cistern, 301, 302
Lumbar puncture, cerebrospinal fluid, 1057

Lung, cholinergic and noradrenergic responses, 771t
Lung cancer, small-cell, and occurrence of Lambert–Eaton
    syndrome, 242
Luteinizing hormone
    as neuroactive peptide, 218t
    secreted by anterior pituitary, 964
Luteinizing hormone-releasing hormone
    -like peptide, colocalization with acetylcholine in
        sympathetic chain ganglia, 769
    production of EPSP in sympathetic ganglia, 184f
    regulates release of LH and FSH, 967
    released by parvocellular neurons, 742
    structure, 742f
Lymphocytes, enhanced trafficking into brain with multiple
    sclerosis, 1056–1057
Lysergic acid diethylamide
    acts on serotonin receptors, 866
    site of action in serotonergic transmission, 878f
Lysosomes
    part of major membrane system of nerve cell, 49
    protein distribution to, 56
    and synaptic vesicle recycling, 230

M

M cells
    lateral geniculate nucleus, projection to primary visual
        cortex, 428f
    retinal ganglion cells, 412
        input to magnocellular layers of lateral geniculate nucleus,
        426
M pathway, lateral geniculate nucleus, initial analysis of
        movement of visual image, 427
M-type potassium channel, 111
M2 region
    in GABA- and glycine-activated channels, 164
    membrane-spanning region of ACh receptor-channel subunit,
        147, 148
    in transmitter-gated ion channels, 164
Macroelectrodes, for study of collective behavior of neurons,
        778–779
Macroglia, 22d
    principal types, 23f
    role in restoring nerve cells after injury, 260–261
Macrophages, role in restoring damaged neurons, 260–261
Macula, on floor of utricle, 503
MAG. See Myelin-associated glycoprotein
Magnesium
    blockade and NMDA channel, 593
    blocks Ca²⁺ channels, 197
Magnetic resonance angiography, imaging of blood vessels, 321
Magnetic resonance imaging
    of brain, 9f
    can distinguish body tissues, 314
    mechanism, 317
    pons lesion, 728f
    sagittal section of brain, 318f
    used to reveal structure and functional state of central
        nervous system, 314–321
Magnocellular layers
    lateral geniculate nucleus, 426
Magnocellular neuroendocrine neurons, release oxytocin and
        vasopressin, 741
Magnocellular neurons, hypothalamic, contain multiple
        peptides, 743–744
Magnocellular pathway, disparity–selective neurons in,
        457–458
Magnocellular system, pathway, 446–447
Magnocellular–interblob system, role in visual perception, sees
        whole image and movements at low resolution, 448
Major histocompatibility complex, class II antigen, narcolepsy
        associated with inheritance of, 814
Major histocompatibility complex, class II molecules, role in

    autoimmune reaction, 241
Male
    pattern, androgen required for, 964
    sex chromosomes, 960
    sex organs, cholinergic and noradrenergic responses, 771t
Malleus, 482d
Mammillary body, 738f, 739
Mammillotegmental tract, 739
Mammillothalamic tract, 738f
Mandibular nerve, branch of trigeminal nerve, 701
Manic–depressive disorders, 855. See also Depression, bipolar
MAP–IC, microtubule–associated ATPase. See Dynein
MAP. See Microtubule–associated proteins
Marijuana, increases pain threshold, 332
Masculinization, 967d
    alpha–fetoprotein binds estrogen to protect female fetuses
        from, 965
Mass action theory, of brain function, 12
Mauthner neuron, electrical synapses permit rapid
        depolarization, 126
Maxillary nerve, branch of trigeminal nerve, 701
Mechanical nociceptors, 343, 386
    different responses to different types of stimulus, 343f
Mechanical resonance, hair cells, 488
Mechanical stimuli, activate nociceptors, 386
Mechanoreceptors. See also Receptors, somatic
    as A-beta and A-alpha fibers, 350
    cutaneous and subcutaneous, types, 342t
    differing abilities to resolve spatial and temporal features of
        stimuli, 346
    muscle and skeletal, 342t
    pathways, anatomically distinct, 378–380
    peripheral receptor, 347–348
    single-point stimulus, sequence of events, 375–376
    in skin, mediate touch, 344
    two-point discrimination, 376–377
    types for glabrous versus hairy skin, 345–346
Medial brain stem pathways
    components, 541
    role in motor function, 541
Medial forebrain bundle, 739, 759
Medial geniculate body, 494
Medial geniculate nucleus
    feedback connection in auditory system, 496
    thalamic, 290, 291f
Medial lemniscus, 287, 359, 363f, 510f
    anatomy, 360
    fibers of synapse on neurons in thalamus, 360
    path from medulla to thalamus, 289f
    somatotopic organization, 360
Medial longitudinal fasciculus, 509
    lesion of, 674
    location in relation to medial vestibular nucleus, 510f
Medial nuclear group, thalamus, receives nociceptive input, 391
Medial nuclei, thalamic, 291f, 292
Medial reticular formation, 542f
Medial reticulospinal tract, 603
Medial superior olive, 494
Medial superior temporal area, 673
    motion represented in, 450–452
    retinotopic map in, 446
    role in optokinetic reflex, 671
Medial thalamus, lesion, 1006
Medial vestibular nucleus
    location in relation to medial longitudinal fasciculus, 510f
    role in neural integration of vestibulo-ocular reflex, 671
Medial vestibulospinal tract, 509f
Median eminence, 738f
Median nerve, effect of severing on cortical organization, 1025
Mediodorsal nuclei, thalamic, 650
Medulla, 8f, 288f
    blood supply, 727f

derived from myelencephalon, 298
features of syndromes common to, 726t
lateral syndromes, 726–729
medial lesions, 724, 726
path of medial lemniscus from to thalamus, 289f
Medulla oblongata, function, 9t
Medullary pyramid, 543d
Medullary reticular nuclei, produce facilitation and inhibition, 602–604
Medullary reticulospinal tract, 693
Meissner's corpuscle, 343f, 368
rapidly adapting receptor in fingertip skin, 345
sensitive to low-frequency mechanical stimuli, 347f
Meissner's plexus, enteric nervous system, 766
Melanin, 401d
Membrane
continuity of in nerve cell, 50f
model for anchoring protein to, 56f
pathways for recapture in epithelial cell, 229f
synaptic vesicle
pathways for recycling at neuromuscular junction, 229f
proteins associated, 227–228
recycling of, 228–231
Membrane capacitance
electrical equivalent circuit, 96f
and rate of change in membrane potential, 96f
and time course of signal conduction, 95–97
value for, 91
Membrane current
capacitive, 96d
ionic, 96d
resistive, 96d
separation into ionic and capacitive components with voltage–clamp technique, 105–109
Membrane potential, 81–94. See also Reversal potential
calculation
from equivalent circuit model of neuron, 92–93
with equivalent circuit model, 90
change in ion channel refractory state, 76f
changed by changes in local charge separation, 91
changes of in presynaptic terminal affect intracellular concentration of Ca^{2+}, 207f
conductance measured as function of by voltage–clamp technique, 106
decrease in as depolarization, 27
effect on ACh-activated single-channel currents, total synaptic current, and EPP, 145f
exponential decay with distance along neuronal process, 99f
increase in as hyperpolarization, 27
influences current flow, 144–146
photoreceptor, change in during illumination, 406
positive feedback cycle driving to action potential, 105
rate of change
in relation to amount of charge stored on membrane, 97
in relation to time, 97
relationship with external K^+ concentration, 85f
rods and cones respond to light with graded changes in, 402
as separation charge across cell membrane, 82
time course of change in, 97, 97f
variations in membrane Na^+ and K^+ conductances as function of, 109
Membrane properties, passive, affect velocity of action potential propagation, 100–102
Membrane proteins. See also Membrane–spanning proteins;
Receptors as receptors for differentiation signals, 888
distribution by axonal transport, 57–60
modification of after translation, 55
Na^+-K^+ pump, 87–88
sorting, modification, and distribution of in nerve cell, 55–56
Membrane resistance, 98d
effect on signal conduction efficiency, 97–100
Membrane systems, in nerve cell, 49–56

Membrane time constant (tau), 97f
effect on integration of synaptic input, 97
Membrane voltage
changes in and ion channel gating, 75f
does not influence inhibitory channels, 162
Membrane–spanning proteins. See also G-protein coupled receptor; See also Ion channels
alpha–helices of ion channels, 116f
formation of in association with endoplasmic reticulum, 54f
structure, 72
neurotransmitter transporters, 233
receptors for chemical transmitters as, 132
rhodopsin, 405
secondary structure, 72
visual pigments, 478
Membrane–spanning regions, rod and cone opsins, 406
Membranous labyrinth, 501
Memory, 997–1008
declarative, 1005–1006
effect of electroconvulsive treatments on, 1003–1004, 1004f
function localized to temporal lobe of cerebral cortex, 7
and limbic area, 825
and limbic association cortex, 829–831
localization of plastic changes encoding throughout nervous system, 1005
long-term
and functional change in brain, 1004–1005
impairment with removal of left and right temporal lobes, 830
and plastic changes in the brain, 1004–1005
synthesis of new proteins and growth of new synaptic connections, 1014–1016
neural basis, 1003–1007
and orientation in space, role of dorsolateral prefrontal circuit, 652
reflexive
and declarative, 985
and declarative involve different neuronal circuits, 1005–1007
spatial, importance of associative long-term potentiation, 1022–1023
storage. See also Hippocampus
importance of cAMP cascade in, 1019
involvement of hippocampus, 9t
role of long-term potentiation, 1022–1023
system, 1003
time-dependent nature of, 1004
Meniere's syndrome, disturbance of auditory and vestibular function, 501
Meninges, 304d
Meningovascular syphilis, and vascular brain lesions that affect corticospinal tract, 545
Mental activity, intense, beta waves associated with, 779
Mental function
localization in brain, 12
progressive decline in aging not inevitable, 976
nonlocalization of, aggregate field view of brain, 6
Mental illness, clinical criteria for classifying, 854
Mental processes, localization of in brain, 15–16
Mental retardation, hereditary component, 993
Merkel's cells, 368
encodes spatial characteristics of stimuli, 346
receptive field, 345
slowly adapting receptor in fingertip skin, 345
Merkel's receptors, 343f
as slowly adapting receptor, 337
Mesaxon, 43d
Mesencephalic locomotor region, 591
in midbrain, 593
Mesencephalic nucleus, trigeminal nerve, 702
mediates proprioceptive responses from jaw muscles, 705–706

Mesencephalic periaqueductal gray region, axons of spinomesencephalic tract end in, 362

Mesencephalic reticular formation, vertical saccades generated in, 672

Mesencephalic trigeminal nucleus, 703f, 704f

Mesencephalon, formation, 298. *See also* Midbrain

Mesenteric ganglia, autonomic nervous system, 764

Mesocortical dopaminergic pathway
  decrease in transmission in Parkinson's disease, 863
  function and role in schizophrenia, 863
  role in response to stress, 865

Mesoderm
  control of differentiation within neural plate, 895
    as source of signals required for neural induction, 894f
  embryonic cell layer, 296
  -inducing factors, peptides, 894
  role in inducing the embryonic nervous system, 891–895

Mesolimbic dopaminergic system, function and role in schizophrenia, 863

Mesolimbic dopaminergic tract, 864f

Mesolimbic system, projections, 698

Mesopharyngeal glands, cholinergic and noradrenergic responses, 771t

Mesostriatal system
  destruction of degeneration of dopaminergic cells in Parkinson's disease, 698
  projections, 698

Messenger RNA, three classes of proteins encoded by, 49–56

Metabolic coma, 817

Metabolic mapping, use of nuclear proteins for, 802

Metabolism, brain, revealed by sodium and phosphorus scans, 323

Metarhodopsin II, active form of rhodopsin, 404

Metencephalon, formation, 298

Methionine–enkephalin, 218t

Methylphenidate, treatment, narcolepsy, 814

Meyer's loop, 436d, 436f

Microaneurysms, rupture of as cause of intraparenchymal stroke, 1047–1048

Microfilaments
  component of cytoskeleton, 62
  structure, 63f

Microglia, 22d
  role in restoring nerve cells after injury, 260–261

Microtubule-associated ATPase. *See* Dynein

Microtubule-associated proteins, and polymerization and assembly of microtubules, 61–62

Microtubules
  association with kinesin, 59f
  component of cytoskeleton, 61
  domains in growth cone, 913f
  role in fast anterograde transport, 58
  structure, 63f
    as cytoskeletal fiber, 61

Mid-temporal gyrus, stimulation of results in brief anterograde and retrograde amnesia, 1006

Midbrain, 8f, 288f
  axons of anterolateral system terminate in, 359
  derived from mesencephalon, 298
  dopaminergic system originates in, 697–698
  formation, 298
  function, 9t, 276
  lesions, 797
  organizes vergence, 673–674
  pretectal region, controls pupillary reflexes, 424
  projections from retina to, 423f
  steroid receptors in, 966
  syndromes of, 728–729
  tectum, axons of spinomesencephalic tract end in, 362
  vascular lesions of, 723–729

Midbrain cat, 604

Midbrain nuclei, spinocervical tract terminates in, 390

Midbrain periaqueductal gray matter, activity of serotonergic neurons during REM sleep, 801

Middle cerebellar peduncle, 510f

Middle cerebral artery, 1041
  infarction in, 1043f, 1045–1046

Middle temporal area
  lesions, 673
  motion represented in, 450–452
  retinotopic map in, 446

Middle temporal region
  columnar organization, 452
  effect of lesions, 452
  and perceptual judgment of motion direction, 452, 454
  role in detecting motion, 452
  role in optokinetic reflex, 671

Midline nuclei, thalamic, 291f, 292

Migration, neuronal, 908–928

MII. *See* Secondary motor cortex

Milk ejection, regulation by oxytocin release, 744

Mind
  and preknowledge, 330
  as range of functions carried out by brain, 5

Miniature end-plate potential, 198d
  amplitude reduced in myasthenia gravis, 238f
  characteristics, 198
  and opening of ACh receptor-channels, 199
  reduction in amplitude characteristic of myasthenia gravis, 237
  requirement of summation of elementary conductance, 199
  spontaneous, 199, 200f

Miosis, 718d

MIS. *See* Mullerian duct-inhibiting substance

Mitochondria
  membrane system of nerve cell, 49
  nerve cell, and generation of energy, 47

Mitochondrial proteins, 52

Mitral cells, 516, 517f
  projection of, 517

Mitral valve prolapse, association with panic disorders, 881

Mixed aphasia, 847t

Mobilization, and neurotransmitter release, 227

Modality, stimulus attribute expressed in sensation, 331

Modality coding, in somatic sensory system, 341–352

Model neuron, 26

Modiolus, 482d

Molecular layer, cerebellar cortex, 630f

Monoamine oxidase inhibitors
  antidepressant, 872
  block degradation of amine transmitters, 232
  can extinguish REM sleep, 795
  effective as antidepressants, 877
  increase availability of serotonin and biogenic amines, 877
  structure, 873f
  treatment, panic attacks, 881

Monoamine oxidases, and degradation of biogenic amines, 225

Monoaminergic systems, 683–700
  in brain stem, 693–697

Monochromatopsia, 468

Monocular zone, 421d,f

Monosynaptic reflex, 25d

Monosynaptic reflex system, knee-jerk reflex as, 24f

Monro–Kellie doctrine, 1057d

Mood, 869d
  disorders of, 869–883

Morphine
  activates descending pathways that control nociceptive inputs, 396
  agonist at mu receptor, 395
  analgesic effect on spinal cord, 396
  elevation of pain threshold, 332
  regions of brain sensitive to, 394

Morphogenetic furrow, *Drosophila* eye, 900f
Mossy fiber pathway
  carry somatic sensory information to cerebellum, 636
  hippocampus, excitatory synaptic pathway, 1019f
Mossy fiber synapse
  long-term potentiation, CA3 region in hippocampus, 1023f
  norepinephrine and cAMP cascade modulate synaptic
    transmission and LTP, 1023
Mossy fibers
  during learning, 642
  effect of climbing fiber input on effectiveness, 642–644
  as excitatory input to cerebellar cortex, 631–632
Motilin, as neuroactive peptide, 218t
Motion
  actual versus apparent, perception of, 451f
  apparent, 449–450
  detection of in visual field, 449–454
  extraction of information
  methods of detecting in visual field, 450
  parallax, monocular depth cue, 455
  pathway, 450
  perception of, 440–466
  perceptual judgment of direction, middle temporal region,
    452, 454
  representation in brain, 451–452
  represented in middle temporal area and medial superior
    temporal area, 450–452
  role of magnocellular pathway, 446–447
Motion–sensitive neurons, Brodmann's areas 1 and 2, 380
Motivation
  as hypothetical state, 750–751
  role of hypothalamus and limbic system, 750–760
Motivational states, correspondence to homeostatic processes,
    751–752
Motivational system
  distinct pathways in, 280
  influences autonomic nervous system, 279
  influences voluntary movement, 279
  receives direct input from thalamic nuclei, 290
Motor actions, complex, and prefrontal cortex, 825
Motor apraxia, in middle cerebral artery infarction, 1046
Motor areas, cerebral cortex, 276
Motor axons, carried by ventral roots, 275
Motor circuit, basal ganglia, 651f, 652
Motor component, language, 11
Motor control
  role of putamen, 649
  role of thalamus in, 287–292
Motor coordination, spinal mechanisms, 581–595
Motor cortex, 278f, 825f
  cytoarchitecture, 611
  electrical stimulation of leads to activation of alpha and
    gamma motor neurons, 572
  functions in parallel with spinal stretch reflex, 617
  homotopic nature of connections with somatic sensory
    cortices, 612
  indirect control over spinal motor neurons, 613
  inputs to, 611–612
  primary and higher-order, 824t
  requirement of for goal-directed locomotion, 593
  seizures of, 785
  subcortical and corticocortical input, 613f
  unexpected load and activity of neurons in, 618
Motor decussation, 294f
Motor disturbances, produced by pathological changes in basal
    ganglia, 647
Motor equivalence, 609d
Motor function
  biochemical level, 531
  motor unit as basic unit, 244
  nervous system structure subserving, 531
  roles of medial and lateral brain stem pathways, 541

precentral gyrus, 8
Motor learning
  role of cerebellum, 642–644
  vestibulo-ocular reflex and modification of cerebellar circuits,
    641
Motor level, focal weakness as indicator as site of spinal cord
    lesion, 715
Motor loss, in middle cerebral artery infarction, 1045
Motor map, 281
  in superior colliculus, 424
Motor molecules. *See* Dynein; Actin; Myosin; Kinesin
Motor nerve
  influence on acetylcholine receptor distribution on muscle
    membrane, 938–939
  recording of action potential to determine conduction
    velocity, 252f
Motor neurons, 22d
  alpha
    innervate intrafusal fibers, provide equivalent of
      alpha-gamma coactivation, 573
    role in stretch reflex, 575
    and gamma, connections with corticospinal neurons,
      612
  autonomic. *See also* Postganglionic neurons
    located peripherally within autonomic ganglia outside the
      central nervous system, 762
    receive inhibitory inputs, 763
  axial and limb, vestibulospinal projections to, 603f
  axon innervates muscle membrane end-plate, 136
  axon that runs in peripheral nerve as part of motor unit, 244
  axons ensheathed in myelin, 43–45
  cell body as part of motor unit, 244
  collateral branches of, 42–43
  component of reflex pathway, 582
  connection with sensory neurons, 41f
  diseases, 244–257
    acute and chronic, 248–250
    fasciculation and fibrillation are characteristics, 250
    mechanism, 247f
  dendrites in, 39–42
  distinction between lower and upper, 245
  excitability, effect of group Ib inhibitory interneuron on, 586
  excitatory action of glutamate on, 158–160
  extraocular, eye position and velocity, 665–667
  flexor and extensor, half-center model of rhythmic
    alternating activity, 583f
  gamma
    activity reduced after lesion of interposed and fastigial
      nuclei, 637
    central nervous system controls sensitivity of muscle
      spindles through, 571–574
    co-activation, 573
    connections with corticospinal neurons, 612
    independent fusimotor system, 573
    innervate intrafusal fibers, 567
    selective stimulation, 570f
    types of alter responsiveness of muscle spindles, 570
  innervating fast muscle fibers, progressive drop in firing rate,
    557
  input signal is the synaptic potential, 27
  limb, input to mediated by lateral vestibular nucleus, 602
  localization of agrin, 939f
  location of synaptic inputs, 42
  lower, disorders of, 245
  monsynaptic connections of group Ia afferents to, 575–576
  with muscle fibers it innervates constitutes motor unit,
    555–556
  neck, input to mediated by medial and inferior vestibular
    nuclei, 602
  one innervates many muscle fibers, 557f
  parallel control and recovery of function following lesions,
    546

Motor neurons [cont.]
  polysynaptic connections of group II and group Ia afferents, 576–577
  pontine reticular nuclei facilitate, 602–604
  pools, 539d
    excitability modulated by cutaneous stimuli, 586–587, 587f
  postsynaptic muscle cell regulates differentiation of terminal, 941–942
  presynaptic terminal triggers changes in postsynaptic membrane, 937–941
  release of acetylcholine before muscle contact, 936
  removal of developing limb results in decrease in number, 933f
  Renshaw cells as part of negative feedback loop, 585–586
  role in knee-jerk reflex, 38–43
  spinal
    as multipolar cell, 21f
    recording of inhibitory postsynaptic potential, 782f
    trophic factors support survival, 934
  spinal cord, complex input, 153
  synapse with skeletal muscle, and study of gated transmission, 135–138
  synaptic excitation of skeletal muscle involving directly gated ion channels, 138–139
  somatic
    excitatory, 763
    located in central nervous system, 762
    spinal cord, 686
  specific connection with developing muscle spindle afferents, 925f
  spinal
    disturbances can cause muscle weakness, 546
    excitability modulated by aminergic pathways from locus ceruleus and raphe nuclei, 541–543
    levels of control, 537–540
    modulated by descending brain stem pathways, 541–543
    motor cortical areas influence via corticospinal and corticobulbar tracts, 543–544
    organization, 540f
    subject to afferent input and descending control, 539–540
    survival regulated by activity of target muscle, 933–934
    topographic organization, 539
  spinal cord, ACh is neurotransmitter used, 215
  synaptic changes in habituation, 1011
  topographic organization, 543
  types of interneuronal circuits acting on, 583f
  upper, disorders of, 245
  ventral horn, and recurrent inhibition, 585
  visceral (autonomic), spinal cord, 686
Motor nuclei, 357f, 539d
  cranial nerves, 687–690
  lateral, interconnected by short propriospinal neurons, 541f
  medial, interconnected by long propriospinal neurons, 541f
  proximal-distal rule and flexor-extensor rule, 539
  trigeminal nerve, 704f
  in ventral horn of spinal cord, 284
Motor performance, regulated by basal ganglia, 9t
Motor planning, and association areas of frontal region, 826
Motor plant, 534
Motor responses, effect of lesions in inferior prefrontal convexity, 829
Motor skills, learning of and cerebellum, 9t
Motor system
  basal ganglia and cerebellum as components of two subcortical feedback loops of, 650f
  classes of movements, 534
  cortical and brain stem, control by cerebellum and basal ganglia, 539–540
  distinct pathways in, 280
  involuntary, 762
  muscles as effectors of, 548–563
  ocular, 660–678
  organizational features, 534
  somatic versus autonomic, 762–763, 762f
  somatotopic maps, 539
  synaptic relays in, 279
  transform neural information into physical energy, 534
  voluntary, 762
  voluntary movements depend on integration with sensory system, 294–295
Motor tasks, effect of lesions of principal sulcus on, 827–829
Motor unit, 246f
  as basic unit of motor function, 244
  assessment of force, 557
  characteristics of diseases of, 245
  diseases of, 244–257
  distribution of muscle fibers in, 247–248
  functional components, 244–245
  gastrocnemius, types, 557f
  increased firing rate and increased force output, 559–560
  motor neuron and muscle fibers it innervates, 555–556
  size principle, 556
  types distinguished by muscle fiber properties, 555–556
  variability of twitch tetanic force and fatigability, 556f
Mounting
  and androgen effects on anterior hypothalamus, 967
  male sexually dimorphic behavior, 963
Movement disorders, disturb iron distribution in brain, 322
Movement fields, in neurons of paramedian pontine reticular formation, 675
Movement
  amount and rate of change of force encoded by neurons in primary motor cortex, 614
  arm and hand, three-dimensional reconstruction, 620
  axons of pontine nuclei participate in cerebellar control of, 287
  bilateral, role of supplementary motor area in coordinating, 619–620
  cerebellum as comparator, 627
  control of, 533–547
  coordinated with posture by reticulospinal system, 604
  cortical control achieved late in phylogeny, 543–544
  direction encoded by specific motor cortical neurons, 614–616
  execution of, controlled by spinocerebellum, 637
  eye
    and body equilibrium during stance and gait, role of vestibulocerebellum, 633
    cortical areas active in, 673f
    role of caudate nucleus, 649
  force and range modulated by cerebellum, 9t
  fractionation of, 546
  higher-order aspects, role of basal ganglia, 651–652
  initiation
    delays produced by cerebrocerebellar lesions, 637, 640
    and premotor area, 825
    role of cerebellum, 642f
    and timing of involves cerebellum, 295
  involuntary
    can be caused by imbalance in dopamine, acetylcholine, or GABA systems, 656
    in diseases of basal ganglia, 653
  limb
    delays in coordination produced by cerebrocerebellar lesions, 637, 640
    neurons in putamen selective for direction of, 652
    role of cerebrocerebellum in coordination of planning, 637–642
  muscle properties determine strategies of control, 650–563
  neural basis of, 296–308
  ongoing
    reflex action during modulated by medial and lateral reticulospinal fibers, 603–604
    role of spinocerebellum in adjusting, 634–637

planning and initiation, role of cerebrocerebellum, 633

pons conveys information about from cerebral hemisphere to cerebellum, 9t

produced by sarcomere contraction, 548–555

proximal, role of lateral premotor area in controlling, 620–622

rapid, accuracy achieved by feedforward mechanisms, 527

role
  of basal ganglia in controlling, 295
  of individual corticospinal tract neurons, 614
  of premotor cortex in preparing motor systems for, 619–622
  of primary motor cortex in initiation or triggering of, 614

sensory input to primary motor cortex informs consequences of, 616–619

slow, regulation by feedback mechanisms, 536

stereotypes sequences resemble fixed-action patterns, 993–994

targeted, role of posterior lobe in providing spatial information for, 622–624

voluntary, 609–625
  and firing of neurons in lateral premotor area, 619f
  corticospinal tract as direct pathway for, 293
  dependence of postural reflexes on, 622f
  difference from reflex movements, 609
  isometric contraction, distinctive patterns of neuron firing during, 615f
  recruits actions of entire motor system, 294–295
  role of mesostriatal system, 698
  wrist, recordings of pyramidal tract neurons during, 615f

MPTP. See 1-Methyl-4-phenyl-1,2,3,6-tetrahydropyridine

MRA. See Magnetic resonance angiography

MRI. See Magnetic resonance imaging

MST. See Medial superior temporal area contraction

MT. See Middle temporal area

Mu receptor, opiate, 395

Muller–Lyer illusion, 443, 443f

Mullerian duct-inhibiting substance, secreted by fetal testes, 961

Multiple sclerosis
  as cause of internuclear ophthalmoplegia, 721
  demyelinating disease, 102
  and enhanced lymphocyte trafficking into brain, 1056–1057
  experimental allergic encephalomyelitis as model for, 44

Multipolar cells, 21f

Multipolar neurons, description, 21–22

Muramyl peptides, sleep-promoting, 798, 799

Muscarinic receptors
  ACh, 183
  activation, 769

Muscle. See also End-plate; Neuromuscular junction; Nerve–muscle synapse
  action around a joint coordinated by inhibitory interneurons, 584–586
  agonist versus antagonist, 562, 562f
  agonists and antagonists, 534
  axial, coordination during postural adjustment, 541
  contractile element and rack and pinion analogy, 552
  contractile properties changed by innervation, 941
  contraction
    amount of active tension depends on degree of overlap of thick and thin filaments, 551
    and activation of gamma motor neurons, 572f
    and shortening of sarcomere, 550f
    force of and relative rates of movements of thick and thin filaments, 552–553
    force of graded in two ways by nervous system, 556–560
    mechanics, 552
    rapid stretch causes length–tension relationship to break

down, 553f
    sequence of events, 550
    size and strength reflect stimulus intensity, 587
    sliding filament theory, 549
    spindle sensitivity during maintained by fusimotor system, 571–573
    tension during depends on muscle length, 553f
  contraction and relaxation, 534
  disease of, 249t
  distal limb, control by propriospinal systems, 540–541
  distal, of fingers, control of by corticospinal tract, 612–613
  damaged, reinnervation of, 940f
  disease of, 244–257
  distribution of nicotinic acetylcholine receptors after innervation, 937–939
  effectors of motor systems, 548–563
  extraocular
    innervation, 665–667
    origins and insertions, 665f
  eye, 664–666
  fiber biopsy, 247–248
  flexion, 560–561, 561f
  generation of restoring force, 551
  heart, controlled by autonomic nervous system, 762
  immature, ion channel functional properties, 78f
  innervation
    of fast versus slow, 941
    of slow and fast by tonic and phase neurons, 942f
  jaw, activity controlled by trigeminal motor nucleus, 706–707
  limb
    effect of neck reflex on, 601f
    opposing actions of vestibular and neck reflexes, 601f
  length
    and activation of static gamma motor neurons, 570
    controlled variable in negative feedback loop of stretch reflex, 577f
  mature, ion channel functional properties, 78f
  nocturnal myoclonus, 806d
  postsynaptic, presynaptic motor nerve triggers changes in, 937–941
  postsynaptic cell, regulates differentiation of motor neuron terminal, 941–942
  properties determine movement control strategies, 560–563
  proprioceptors in, 535
  proximal and distal innervated by medial and lateral groups of spinal motor neurons, 539
  receptors and stretch reflexes, 564–580
  repeated activation causes fatigue, 555
  skeletal
    components, 565f
    composition, 548–549
    fiber properties, 555
    and filtering of information in neural spikes trains, 561–563, 562f
    as low-pass filters of neural input, 561–562
    steps in synaptic connection, 936
    striations, 549f
  slow, 941
  smooth
    controlled by autonomic nervous system, 762
    innervation, 764
  smooth response to stretch and release, 578
  spring analogy, 552
  stimulation increases death of motor neurons, 934
  stretch
    and activation of dynamic gamma motor neurons, 570
    and different firing properties of primary and secondary endings of afferents in, 569, 569f
    muscle spindles sensitive to aspects of, 569–571
  synaptic excitation of by motor neurons involving directly gated ion channels, 138–139

Muscle [*cont.*]
  synergist and antagonist, innervation by muscle spindle
      afferents, 584
  tension
    changes represent transformation of neural impulses, 562
    increases in proportion to amount of stretch, 578
    regulated by Ib afferent fibers from Golgi tendon organs,
        negative feedback system, 586f
  tone, contribution of stretch reflexes, 577–578
  twitch, 941
  vibration of and illusion of limb position, 350f
  weakness results from disturbances in descending motor
      pathways or spinal motor neurons, 546
Muscle afferent fibers, mediate limb proprioception, 347–349
Muscle diseases, mechanisms, 247f. *See also* specific names
Muscle fibers, 548d
  amount of force produced, 554
Muscle length, changes signaled by muscle spindles, 565
Muscle proprioceptors, trigger postural responses, 597–598
Muscle spindles, 25d, 38d, 565f
  afferents
    direct connections to motor neurons and interneurons,
        activation of synergist and antagonist muscles, 584
    specific connection with motor neurons, 925f
  arranged in parallel with extrafusal fibers, 568
  arrangement within muscle and function, 568–569
  biochemical distinction, 247–248
  central nervous system control through gamma motor
      neurons, 571–574
  components, 565–566, 566f
  different firing properties of primary and secondary endings of
      afferents in, 569, 569f
  discharge of afferents produces stretch reflex, 574–577
  excitation of and stretch reflex, 576f
  fast-twitch (type I), 247
  fine-tuning of, 574
  and joint angle, 348
  respond to stretch of muscle fibers, 565–567
  sensitive to aspects of muscle stretch, 569–571
  sensitivity during muscle contraction maintained by
      fusimotor system, 571–573
  sliding of filamentous proteins in results in contraction,
      548–550
  transducer characteristics, 578
Muscle stretch receptors, types, 568f
Muscle tension
  changes signaled by Golgi tendon organs, 565
  tension, Golgi tendon organs sensitive to changes in,
      567–568
Muscle tone
  controlled by spinocerebellum, 637
  modulation by reticular formation, 692–693
  role of stretch reflexes in maintaining, 604
Muscular dystrophy, types, 252–253
Music, as higher cognitive function, 821
Myalgia, 245d
Myasthenia gravis
  association with rheumatoid arthritis, 237
  basis of antibody binding in, 239–240
  and density of ACh receptors in muscle fibers, 237f
  as disease of chemical transmission at nerve–muscle synapse,
      235–243
  experimental model of, 237–238
  as heterogeneous syndrome, 241–242
  ion channels as targets in, 79
  morphological changes in neuromuscular junction reduce
      likelihood of synaptic transmission, 239f
  rate of destruction of ACh receptors increased in, 240f
  therapy for, 242
  types, congenital versus autoimmune, 241–242
Mydriasis, 667d
Myelencephalon, formation, 298

Myelin, 20d. *See also* Nodes of Ranvier; Saltatory conduction
  central, proteolipid in, 43
  diseases affecting, 102
  effect on regenerative mechanism for action potential
      propagation, 101
  ensheathes axons of sensory and motor neurons, 43–45
  on motor and sensory neurons, 44f
Myelin-associated glycoprotein, characteristics, 43
Myelin basic protein, 44
  and experimental allergic encephalomyelitis, 44
Myelin sheath, 19f
MAG, structure, 919f
Myelinated axons, in spinal cord white matter, 356
Myelination
  central versus peripheral nervous system, 43
  cerebral, and ontogenetic pattern of REM sleep, 796
  increases conduction velocity, 101
  role of Schwann cells, 43
  in shiverer mice, 45, 45f
Myelogram, thoracic schwannoma, 717f
Myelography, diagnosis of spinal cord lesions, 715
Myelopathic diseases, mechanisms, 247f
Myenteric plexus, enteric nervous system, 766
Myocardial infarction, referred pain in, 389
Myoclonus
  palatal, 726t
Myofibrils, 548d, 549
Myogenic diseases, laboratory criteria, 246–248
Myoglobinuria, 245d, 249t
Myomodulins, as neuroactive peptide, 218t
Myopathic diseases,
  clinical and laboratory criteria for, 245–248
  differential diagnosis from neurogenic diseases, 249t
  symptoms, 245
Myopathies, causes of weakness in, 253
Myosin, 549f
  heads
    as ATPases, 549
    attachment to actin, 550f
  interaction with actin in muscle fiber contraction, 550
  neural, role in slow axonal transport, 59
  thick filament component, 549
Myotatic reflex, in decerebrate animal, 575
Myotatic unit, 584d
Myotonia, 245d, 252d
Myotonic dystrophy, 249t
Myotonic muscular dystrophy, 252
Mystacial vibrissae, 702d

N

N-acetylation, cotranslational modification of polypeptide,
    52
N-cadherin
  expressed in neural ectoderm after induction, 894
  expression in nervous system, 920
  involved in neural cell adhesion, 918
N-Methyl-D-aspartate
  receptor, 158
    channel regulation by, 157f
    receptor-channel, properties, 159–160, 159f
    receptor mechanism, involvement in spatial learning, 1023
    receptor-mediated toxicity, pre- and postsynaptic
        mechanisms of in Huntington's disease, 658
    receptors, role in generating locomotor pattern, 593
Na-K pump. *See* Sodium-potassium pump in photoreceptors,
    407
Naloxone
  blocks morphine-induced analgesia, 394
  as opiate antagonist, 396
Narcolepsy
  associated with inheritance of class II antigen of major
      histocompatibility complex, 814

and drugs that enhance transmission at central catecholaminergic synapses, 814

enter REM sleep directly from waking state, 814f

sleep attacks accompanied by REM-related symptoms, 813–815

Nauta staining, based on degenerative changes in neurons, 262

NCAM. *See* Neural cell adhesion molecule

Neck, effect of vestibulocollic reflexes, 600

Neck reflexes

effect on limb muscles, 601f

in newborns, 602f

stabilize head and eyes, 600–602

Negative feedback, stretch reflex regulation of muscle tone, 577–578

Neglect syndrome, 831d

Neocortex, 292d

affected by Pick's disease, 981

appearance of amyloid plaques in, 977

dopaminergic system projects to, 697–698

layers, 292–293

neurofibrillary tangles in, 979

principal aminergic input is from locus ceruleus, 696

role in emotion, 747

Neologisms, 846d

Neoplastic changes, revealed by sodium and phosphorus scans, 323

Neospinothalamic tract, 392

Neostigmine

effects of treatment, mouse, 237f

reverses symptoms of myasthenia gravis, 236

Neostriatum

anatomic and functional organization, 651

basal ganglia, 648d

inhibitory effects of serotonin on, 698

inputs mediated by glutamatergic neurons, 652

Nernst equation, and determination of equilibrium potential, 84

Nernst potential, 84d

Nerulation, 297

Nerve cells

afferent, 22d

afferent, characteristic signal produced by four components, 28f

as electrical equivalent circuit, 89–92

brain, functional classification, 22

Cajal model of, 171

classified according to shape, 20–22

components of cytoskeletal structure, 61–62

continuity of major membrane system, 50f

current in modeled by electrical equivalent circuit, 91f

cytology, 37–48

cytosolic proteins, 51–52

degenerative changes in those having synaptic connections with injured cell, 261–262

each primarily sensitive to one type of stimulus, 331

electrically coupled

elevated threshold for action potential in, 129

tendency to fire synchronously, 129

electrical equivalent circuit of under voltage-clamp conditions, 108

excitability modulated by slow synaptic actions produced by second messengers, 185

features of different electrical potentials in, 166t

flow of information conveyed by electrical and chemical signals, 81

fibrillar proteins of cytoskeleton responsible for shape, 60–62

functional components, 26

integrative zone, 103

interaction of excitation and inhibition on, 169t

interneuronal, 22d

ion channels, 66–79

mature, uses same transmitter at all of its synapses, 214

membrane systems in, 49–56

morphological regions, 19–20

motor, 22d

myelinated, saltatory conduction, 102f

neurogenesis in adult brain, 268

nongated channels in selective for several ion species, 84–86

nucleus, 46–47

one of two classes of cells in nervous system, 19–22

passive membrane properties, 95–103

and temporal and spatial summation, 167

permeability of membrane and action potential, 26–27

reaction to injury, 258–269

reconstruction of action potential from known properties of, 109–110

recovery of function after damage, 266–268

regeneration of axons in peripheral nervous system, 262–264

relationship of resting membrane potential to EPSP, 157

resting membrane potential of, 26, 157

role of glial cells and macrophage in restoring after injury, 260–261

sarcoma tissue evokes extensive growth of sensory fibers into tumor, 930–931

severing of axon causes degenerative changes in, 259–261

sites of synaptic contact, 168–171

three-dimensional geometry and distribution of current flow, 97–100

variation

in excitability properties, 111–112

in repetitive firing properties, 112f

vertebrate, main features, 19f

Nerve growth factor

binding to its receptor triggers second-messenger pathways, 932

fast retrograde transport of, 60

increases synthesis of enzymes involved in neurotransmitter synthesis, 933

induces sympatho-adrenal cells to differentiate into sympathetic neurons, 904f

influence on neurite growth in vitro, 932f

localization in whisker target field of mouse embryo, 932f

and neuronal survival, 930–933

and neurotrophic activity, 931

neurotrophic factor, 262

produced by target tissues of sensory and sympathetic neurons, 932

retrograde transport, 263

role in survival of sensory and sympathetic neurons, 931–933

secretion by Schwann cells, 264

subunits, 931

trk encodes receptor, 933

Nerve roots, lesions, 715

Nerve terminal, presynaptic, organization by basal lamina, 942

Nerve–muscle synapse

directly gated transmission at, 135–152

mechanisms of transmission, pharmacological versus physiological, 124

myasthenia gravis as disease of chemical transmission at, 235–243

presynaptic thickening at, 201

synaptic potential generated by inward current confined to end-plate region, 138

Nervous system

actions of gonadal hormones on, 963

anatomical organization, 273–282

classes of cells in, 19–24

control of cell identity, 887–907

embryonic development, 296–308

epigenetic influences on development, 885

glial cells, 22–24

histology of, history, 6

integrative action, 531

parallel processing as organizational principle, 7

Nervous system [cont.]
  relationship of development of and behavior, 885
  sexual differentiation, 959–973
  two types of chemical substances for signaling, 215
Nervous tissue
  anatomical complexity, early views, 6
  developing, organizational and regulatory effects of gonadal
    hormones on, 962
  as glandular in function, early view, 6
Networks
  interneuronal, coordinate timing of reflex components, 582,
    584
  parallel distributed processing, 836–837
  recurrent, 837
  self-correcting, 837
Neural adhesion molecules, structures, 919f
Neural cell adhesion molecule, 918
  binding function of, 919
  expressed in neural ectoderm after its induction, 894
  major forms, 918
  structure, 919f
Neural cell fate, role of local cell interactions, 896
Neural cells
  fate not determined by cell lineage in most species, 891
  methods for tracing lineage, 891
  program of development in C. elegans, 888
  role of cell–cell interactions in determining fate, 891–898
Neural code
  pattern of action potentials in sensory receptor transduction,
    336
  stimulus energy translated into by sensory receptors, 336–338
Neural crest
  classes of committed progenitor cells derived from, 903f
  development, 297f
  form sensory and autonomic neurons in peripheral ganglia
    and other tissues, 297
  pathways of cell migration, 902f
Neural crest cells
  differentiation into neurons, 904
  fate controlled by signals from neighboring cells, 902–904
  fate influenced by signals from neighboring cells, 902–903
  migration, role of laminin and fibronectin, 911
  multipotentiality, 903
  sympatho-adrenal lineage, developmental potential, 904, 904f
Neural ectoderm
  depends on proximity of axial mesoderm and overlying
    ectoderm, 893
  genes expressed in after its induction, 894
Neural encoding, 334d
Neural function
  parallel distributed systems of as connectionist models, 32
  plasticity, 1011–1012
Neural groove, formation, 297f
Neural growth factor, release of from postsynaptic cell and
    synapse stabilization, 956f
Neural induction, 297
  quantitative assay to measure in Xenopus, 895
  role of signaling molecules, 894
  sources of signals required, 894f
  steps, 894–895
Neural integration, convergence and divergence as mechanisms,
    582–584
Neural integrator, maintains eye position, 669–670
Neural maps, body surface, 373–374
Neural networks, and learning, 1023
Neural plate, 891d
  activation by neural induction, 297f
  development of neural tube from, 296–297
  differentiation within controlled by mesoderm, 895
  induction from ectoderm is dependent on interactions with
    mesoderm, 891–895
Neural spectrin, as anchoring protein, 62

Neural tube, 891d
  as embryonic precursor of brain regions, 296–299
  development of from neural plate, 297
  formation in embryo, 297f
Neuroactive peptides, 215, 217–221
  contained within vesicles, 226
  corelease
    of ATP, 222–224
    with small-molecule neurotransmitters, 221–224
  derived from processing of secretory proteins in endoplasmic
    reticulum, 218
  histochemical detection, 222–223
  mechanisms for diversification, 219
  processing, 219
  rate of removal after release, 232
  receptor recognition, 219
  role in modulating sensibility and emotions, 218
  structural analysis, 219
  structures of precursors, 220f
  synthesized in nerve cell body, 221
Neuroanatomical tracing
  based on fast axonal transport, 61
  techniques based on degenerative changes in neurons, 262
Neuroanatomy, 271
Neuroendocrine function, disturbances of in depression,
    879–880
Neuroepithelium, gives rise to all neurons and glial cells of
    central nervous system, 297–299
Neurofibrillary tangles, 979f
  in aging brain, 967
  intracellular characteristics of Alzheimer's disease, 979–981
Neurofilaments
  cytoskeletal component, 62
  structure, 63f
Neurogenic diseases, 245d
  clinical and laboratory criteria for, 245–248
  denervated muscle spontaneously active at rest, 246
  differential diagnosis from myopathic diseases, 249t
  distal limb weakness characteristic, 245
  mechanisms, 247f
Neurogenic genes, identification of in Drosophila, 896
Neurogenic region, grasshopper, differentiation controlled by
    local cell interactions, 898f
Neurogliaform cells, in cerebral cortex, 782f
Neurohormones, synthesis of in hypothalamic cells, 740f
Neurohypophyseal peptides, neuroactive, 219t
Neurokinin. See Substance K
Neurological disease, 121
Neuromuscular block, presynaptic (facilitating)
  and Lambert–Eaton syndrome, 242
  and small-cell lung cancers, 242
Neuromuscular junction, 43d
  and study of gated transmission, 135–138
  failure of transmission at in myasthenia gravis, 238f
  morphological changes in reduce likelihood of synaptic
    transmission in myasthenia gravis, 239f
  regeneration of, 940f
  topography of transmitter release site at, 201f
Neuromuscular synapse, organization, 935f
Neuromuscular transmission
  blockage increases number of surviving motor neurons, 934
  blocked by tubocurarine binding to ACh receptor, 138
  diseases of, 242
  disorders, myasthenia gravis, 236
Neuron doctrine, 20d
  doctrine, statement of, 6d
Neuron. See also Nerve cell
  birthday establishes eventual position and properties, 909
  c-fos as activity marker for in vivo, 802
  central nervous system, derived from neural plate of
    endoderm, 296
  current flow, 1033–1040

death enhanced when neuronal target is removed, 930
developing, effect of testosterone, 965
ensemble activity, 777–791
estradiol–sensitive, regional distribution in brain, 966f
genetically programmed death, 929–930
model, 26
number of synaptic connections formed by, 121
presynaptic, regulate development of nicotinic acetylcholine
    receptors, 941
recording from in brain slices, 788
retroviruses used to trace migratory paths, 910f
sexual differentiation reflected in structure of, 968–969
study of collective behavior of, 778–779
survival
    and nerve growth factor, 930–933
    regulated by interaction with target, 929–930
    and synapse formation, 929–944
Neuronal assemblies, model for coding for coherent features,
    463f
Neuronal connections, establishment of, 887–907
Neuronal death, gene products involved in, 264
Neuronal divergence, 25d
Neuronal integration, 166d
    effects of temporal and spatial summation on, 168f
    and summation of synaptic potentials, 167
Neuronal proteins, synthesis and trafficking, 49–65
Neuropathies, 245. See also Peripheral nerves, diseases
    as demyelinating or axonal, 250–251
    positive or negative symptoms, 251
Neuropeptide Y
    loss of in Alzheimer's disease, 981
    as neuroactive peptide, 218t
    in sympathetic neurons, 770t
Neurophysin, release of, 741
Neurophysiology, history, 6
Neurosecretion, 740
Neurotensin
    in hypothalamus, 743
    as neuroactive peptide, 218t
    peptide in sympathetic neurons, 770t
Neurotic illnesses, and alterations in regulation of gene
    expression, 1028
Neurotoxin, snake venom. See Alpha–Bungarotoxin
Neurotransmission
    diseases, myasthenia gravis, 235–243
    evidence for, 121
Neurotransmitters, 121
Neurotransmitters, acetylcholine, 215
Neurotransmitters, age-related alterations in synthesis and
    degradation, 976
Neurotransmitters, amino acid, 217
Neurotransmitters, 217
    active uptake by synaptic vesicle, 226–227
    amount released as reflection of properties of presynaptic
        cell, 211
    in basal ganglial circuits, 652–653
    biogenic amine, 215–217
    bound by autoreceptors, 207
    calculating probability of release, 210–211
    in cell types of cerebral cortex, 782f
    chemical
        criteria for, 214–215
        synaptic action produced by, 190f
        in synaptic vesicles, 131
    chemical messengers as, 213–224
    complex with ATP and chromogranin in synaptic vesicles to
        decrease osmotic pressure, 226
    deficits in Alzheimer's disease, 981
    discharge from synaptic vesicles by exocytosis, 203
    disorders in metabolism of in diseases of basal ganglia,
        653–657
    each quantum stored in synaptic vesicle, 201, 203

excitatory. See Glutamate; Quisqualate; Kainate; NMDA
    Kainate;
functional mapping of neurons on basis of, 694
GABA
    and glycine as inhibitory, 162
    in Purkinje neurons, 630
    used by Golgi neurons, 632
and gating of ion channels, 75
interference with can produce psychotic behavior, 866
modulation of ionic conductance through second messenger,
    771
in nociceptive primary afferent fibers, 389–390
quantal release
    and Ca²⁺ influx, 199–201
    and fixed-amplitude response, 200f
presence of in amyloid plaques, 978
and receptors, 132
    major functions, 173
release, 194–212
    and calcium influx during depolarization, experimental
        demonstration, 198f
    by carrier mechanisms, 232
    as function of Ca²⁺ influx, 197f
    depression or enhancement of at axo–axonic synapses, 207
removal from synaptic cleft terminates synaptic
    transmission, 232–233
role of synaptic vesicle in release of, 227
secretory process coupled to electrical events in presynaptic
    terminals, 194–212
small-molecule, 215–217
    biosynthetic enzymes, 215t
    corelease with neuroactive peptides, 221–224
    histochemical detection, 222–223
    rate of removal after release, 232
    synthesized at nerve terminals, 221
storage in synaptic vesicles, 225–227
storing and release of by growth cone before contacting
    muscle, 936
synthesis of enzymes involved in increased by nerve growth
    factor, 933
transporter proteins, 233
Neurotrophic factors, prevent degeneration of peripheral
    neurons after axotomy, 262–264
Neurotrophin 3, 262
    receptor, trk B and C proteins as, 933
    supports survival of dorsal root ganglion neurons, 933
    supports survival of proprioceptive neurons of trigeminal
        mesencephalic nucleus, 933
Neurotropic diseases, 250d. See also Motor neuron diseases
    laboratory criteria, 246–248
Neurotropic viruses, fast retrograde transport, 60
Neurulation, 891d
Newborn infants, rhythmic pattern generation in, 594
NGF. See Nerve growth factor
Nicotinic receptor, ACh, 183
Night blindness, 402
    and nutritional deficiency in vitamin A, 404
Night terrors, during REM or slow-wave sleep, 811–812
Night vision, rods, 402
Nightmares
    during REM or slow-wave sleep, 811–812
Nigrostriatal dopaminergic system, function and role in
        schizophrenia, 863
Nigrostriatal dopaminergic tract, 864f
Nissl substance, 52d, 260d
Nitric oxide, role in cGMP synthesis, 191
NMDA. See N-Methyl-D-aspartate
Nociception, distinguished from pain, 385
Nociceptive afferent fibers, form connections with three types
    of neurons in dorsal horn, 389
Nociceptive afferent input, modulated by local dorsal horn
    circuits, 396–397

Nociceptive control pathways, descend to spinal cord, 393–394
Nociceptive fibers, pathway, dorsal horn, 389
Nociceptive information, major ascending pathways, 391f
Nociceptive input, relayed to brain by ascending pathways, 390–392
Nociceptive primary afferent fibers, low-theshold myelinated, activation of reduces activity of projection neuron, 392
Nociceptive receptors, activated by noxious insults, 386–388
Nociceptive transmission
    coordinately modulated by supraspinal and spinal networks, 396
    modulated by opiate alkaloids and endogenous opioid peptides, 397
Nociceptors
    as A-delta and C fibers, 350
    afferent fibers terminate on projection neurons in dorsal horn of spinal cord, 388f
    change in sensitivity and hyperalgesia, 386
    damage to and local pain, 387
    sensitization of by chemical mediators, 387f
    sensitized by tissue damage, 386–388
    signals from in viscera felt as pain elsewhere in body, 388f
Nocturnal enuresis, 810
Nocturnal myoclonus, 806d
Nodes of Ranvier, 19f, 20d. See also Saltatory conduction
    effect on action potential propagation, 101
    on sensory neuron, 38
Nodose ganglion, 525f
Nonpyramidal cells
    cerebral cortex, 292, 782f
    neurons in somatic sensory cortex, 364–365
    primary visual cortex, 427
Nonspiny neurons, in cerebral cortex, 782
Noradrenergic neurons, in brain stem, 696
Noradrenergic pathways, 876f
    antidepressant drugs act on, 875
    originate in locus ceruleus, 875
Noradrenergic receptors, linked to second-messenger systems, 877t
Noradrenergic transmission, sites of antidepressant drug action, 879f
Norepinephrine
    action on cardiac muscle, 771
    activation of cAMP in hippocampal neurons, 183–184, 184f
    age-related decrease in enzymes that synthesize, 976
    biosynthesis, 216
    cortical loss of in Alzheimer's disease, 981
    increases excitability of hippocampal neurons, 696
    measurement of in depressed patients, 877
    neurally released
        action on alpha-adrenergic receptors, 772
        action on beta-adrenergic receptors, 771
    neurons containing in brain stem, 693
    regulation of in cholinergic presynaptic neuron, 187, 190
    release after stimulation of sympathetic or parasympathetic postganglionic axons, 769–770
    slow EPSP, Ca^{2+}-activated K^+ channel, 183–184
    synthesis and release stimulated by L-DOPA, 591
    transmitter
        in descending pathway from pons, 396
        in locus ceruleus, 216
    uptake mechanism for, 233
Notch gene, neurogenic Drosophila gene, 896
Notochord, and induction of floor plate cells in neural tube, 895
Noxious stimuli
    neurons in ventrobasal complex in lateral thalamus respond to, 391
    transduction mechanisms for each type are distinct, 386
NT3. See Neurotrophin 3
Nuclear bag fibers

dynamic, and dynamic sensitivity of primary afferent fibers, 570
    innervation, 570
    mechanical properties and dynamic sensitivity of primary endings, 571
Nuclear chain fibers, 566f
Nuclear envelope, 46–47d
Nuclear membrane, part of major membrane system of nerve cell, 49
Nuclear proteins, 52
    appearance of after physiological stimulation as metabolic mapping technique, 802
    control of gene activation, 887–888
    Drosophila, transcriptional activators, 897
Nuclei of lateral lemniscus, 494
Nuclei, 283d
    of basal ganglia, 648
    cranial nerve, 683–700, 688f, 687–690
    dentate, 627d, 637
    emboliform, 627d
    fastigial, 627d
        projections of, 636
    globose, 627d
    hypothalamus, 738f, 739
    interposed, 627d
    oculomotor, 666, 667f
    pontine, 637
    serotonergic, in brain stem, 698f
    thalamic, 650
Nucleolus, 46d
Nucleus, solitary tract, and sleep induction, 800
Nucleus, suprachiasmatic, as biological clock for sleep–wake cycle, 800–801
Nucleus accumbens
    effect of addictive drugs, 759
    electrical stimulation, 759
    expression of D2 dopamine receptors in, 860
    increased number of D2 dopamine receptors in schizophrenic patients, 861
    projections of mesolimbic system to and importance in schizophrenia, 863
Nucleus ambiguus, 690
    parasympathetic preganglionic nucleus, 766
Nucleus basalis of Meynert
    profound loss of neurons in Alzheimer's disease, 981
Nucleus basalis
    cell bodies synthesize ACh, 215
    cholinergic neurons, sensitive to trophic actions of NGF, 262
Nucleus caudalis, 703, 703f
    nociceptive neurons in, 705
    somatotopic organization, 705
Nucleus hypoglossi prepositus, projection to locus ceruleus, 696
Nucleus interpolaris, 703f, 704
    trigeminal nerve, role in mediating sensation from teeth, 705
Nucleus interpositus neurons, modulation of, 637
Nucleus of the solitary tract, modulates autonomic function, 767
Nucleus oralis, 703f, 704
Nucleus paragigantocellularis, projection to locus ceruleus, 696
Nucleus prepositus hypoglossi
    lesions in, 671
    role in neural integration of vestibulo-ocular reflex, 671
Nucleus proprius, 357f
    spinal cord gray matter, 356
Nucleus reticularis pontis oralis, 603d
Nucleus X, input to motor cortex, 611
Nystagmus, 662d, 726t
    abducting, 722
    in acoustic neuroma, 721
    and brain stem lesions, 721
    caused by disease of vestibular system, 668–669

gaze-evoked, 726t
result of lesions of vestibulocerebellum, 635
vestibular, resets eye position during sustained rotation, 662

O

O-2A progenitor, 22d
  fate controlled by type 1 astrocytes, 898
  precursor cell for oligodendrocytes and type 2 astrocytes, 898
  role of PDGF in proliferation, 898
Oblique muscles, eye, 665, 665f
Occipital lobe, 8f, 276, 278f
  cerebral cortex, function, 7
  retinotopic maps in, 446
Occipital cortex, left, damage to and alexia, 849
Occlusion
  anterior choroidal and penetrating arteries, 1046
  basilar arteries, 1047
  carotid arteries, 1047
Occlusive stroke, 1045
Octopamine, neurotransmitter in invertebrate nervous systems, 216
Ocular disparity, response of cells in area 17 to, 458f
Ocular dominance columns, 434d
  activity-dependent competition between two eyes stimulates segregation of, 954
  area 17 of cerebral cortex, altered by experience, 1024
  development of as model for development of behavior, 949–956
  effect of eye closure on development of, 951–952, 952f, 953f
  induction of by transplanting third eye in frogs, 954
  maturation of parallel stereoscopic vision, 956–957
  neural activity regulates formation of, 953–956
  postnatal development, 950–953, 950f
  primary visual cortex, 432, 433f
  projections from lateral geniculate nucleus, 433f
  and segregation of afferent inputs into, 950–953, 951f
  segregation blocked by exposure of tectum to aminophosphonovaleric acid, 956
  visual deprivation reduces size of in visual cortex, 949–956, 949f
Ocular motor system, 660–678
Oculomotor circuit, 652
Oculomotor nerve, 294f
  functions, 684t, 685f
  left, effect of lesion on eye movement, 722f
Oculomotor neurons, compared with spinal motor neurons, 667
Oculomotor nucleus, 288f, 509f, 665
  in brain stem, 667f
  dense serotonergic projections in, 698
  in somatic motor column, 687–688
Oculomotor system, and superior colliculus, 674
Odorants
  changes induced by in second messengers, 515
  enhance activity of adenyl cyclase in olfactory epithelium, 515
  individual olfactory neurons respond to variety of, 516
  presentation to receptor may involve olfactory binding protein, 514–515
Odors, affective component of mediated by limbic pathway, 518
Ohm's law, 1036
  calculation of current flowing
    through active ACh-gated channels, 151
    through each class of active conductance channel, 108
    through nongated membrane channels, 151
  calculation of voltage difference between potentials recorded intra- and extracellularly, 783
  current responsible for EPSP, 140
Ohm's, measurement of resistance, 1034d
Olfaction, abnormalities, 518
Olfactory binding protein
  analogy to retinol-binding proteins, 514–515
  and presentation of odorants to receptor, 514–515

Olfactory bulb
  anatomy, 514f
  different odors eliciting different degrees of activity in different regions of glomerular layer, 518f
  organization, 516f
  processing of olfactory information, 517
Olfactory cortex, 517f
  divisions, 517
  neurofibrillary tangles in, 979
Olfactory epithelium
  neurons in transduce sensation of smell, 513–516
  structure, 514f
Olfactory knob, 513
Olfactory nerve, functions, 684t, 685f
Olfactory neurons, 514–517
Olfactory pathways, to limbic system, 518
Olfactory receptors, location, 513f
Olfactory system, transmits sensory information directly to primitive cortex of medial temporal lobe, bypassing the thalamus, 335
Olfactory tract, neural connections, 517f
Olfactory transduction, and second-messenger-regulated ion channels, 515
Olfactory tubercle, 517f
  increased number of D2 dopamine receptors in schizophrenic patients, 861
Oligodendrocyte, 23f, 43d
  as glial cell, 22
  inhibits axon extension, 916
Olivocochlear bundle, 497
Operant conditioning. See Conditioning, operant
Ophthalmic artery, 1041
Ophthalmic nerve, branch of trigeminal nerve, 701
Ophthalmoplegia, internuclear, 726t
Opiates. See also Morphine
  analgesic effects by direct action on central nervous system, 394
  antagonists, 396
  electrophysiological analysis of action on sensory and dorsal horn neurons, 397f
  intrathecal administration, 396
  receptors, classes, 395–396
  regulate nociceptive transmission by inhibiting release of glutamate, substance P, and other transmitters from sensory neurons, 397
Opioid peptides
  endogenous
    amino acid sequences of, 395t
    anatomical distribution, 395
  neuroactive, 219t
Opioid receptors, endogenous, in brain, 394–396
Opponent process theory, color, 471
Opsin, 405f
  cone, 404
  protein portion of rhodopsin, 404
  rod and cone, membrane-spanning regions, 406
Opsin kinase, 406
Optic ataxia, 831
Optic chiasm, 123d
  commissure in visual system, 281
  effect of lesion, 437f
Optic cup, 298
Optic disc, 402d, 423d
  no photoreceptors, 422
Optic nerve, 294f, 423d
  axons of retinal ganglion cells, 408
  effect of lesion, 437f
  functions, 684t, 685f
  number of fibers, 420
  projection, 408
  retinal fibers spontaneously active in utero, 954
  types of glial cells in, 23f

Optic radiation, course of fibers, 436, 436f
Optic radiation fibers, effect of lesion, 437f
Optic tectum, columnar organization in results from
    competition of two sets of afferent fibers, 953
Optic tract, 423d
    role in optokinetic reflex, 671
Optical imaging, for study of collective behavior of neurons,
    779
Optokinetic movement, 661t
Optokinetic reflex, 662f
    compensates for head movement, 661–663
    in hereditary achromatopsia, 671
    role of subcortical and cortical structures, 671
    under adaptive control, 662–663
Optokinetic system, use of visual information to complement
    vestibulo-ocular reflex, 662
Oral cavity, innervation by trigeminal nerve branch, 701–702
Orbital frontal cortex, morphological sex differences, 969
Orbital prefrontal cortex, lesions, 970
Orbitofrontal cortex
    and conscious perception of smell, 518
    as part of limbic association cortex, 826
    effect of electrical stimulation, 829
    in limbic association cortex, 826
    in prefrontal association area, 826
    location, 827f
    role in emotional behavior, 829–830
    seizures involving limbic structures in, 785
Organ of Corti, 483, 484f
    electron microscopy of, 485f
    frequency selectivity determined by hair cells, 487
    hair cells in, 483
    vibration of bends hair cell stereocilia, 486f
Organelles, recycling, 57f
Organic anions
    concentrated inside the cell, 82
    distribution across cell membrane, 84
Organic mental illness, 1027d
Organizer region, 892
    as source of signals required for neural induction, 894f
Orgasm, central program for, 990
Orientation columns, 434d
    in primary visual cortex, 431–434
Orientation-sensitive neurons, Brodmann's areas 1 and 2, 380
Oscillators, primary, functions controlled by, 758–759
Osmotic activity, decreased by ATP and chromogranin
    complexes with neurotransmitter in synaptic vesicles,
    226
Ossicles, 482d
Otoacoustic emissions, 489
Otolith organs
    detect linear acceleration, 501
    input to vestibulocerebellum, 634
    role in vestibulo-ocular reflex, 667
Otolith reflex, compensates for linear motion, 663
Otoliths, deformation of gelatinous mass and displacement of
    hairs of receptor cells, 503
Otosclerosis, 483
Outer plexiform layer, retina, 412
Oxytocin
    as neuroactive peptide, 218t
    recordings from cells releasing during suckling, 745f
    released by magnocellular neuroendocrine neurons, 741
    role in milk ejection and uterine contraction, 744
    structure and function, 741

P

P cells
    lateral geniculate nucleus, projection to primary visual
        cortex, 428f
    retinal, input to parvocellular layers of lateral genicular
        nucleus, 426

retinal ganglion cells, 412
P face, of lipid bilayer, 202f
P pathway, lateral geniculate nucleus, analysis of fine structure
    and color vision, 427
P region, 164
    ion channel subunit, 116f
    K^+ ion channel, 117
P-alpha cells. *See* M cells
P-beta cells. *See* P cells
p-Chlorophenylalanine, site of action in serotonergic
    transmission, 878f
p29, 228t
p65, 228t
Pacchionian granulations. *See* Arachnoid villi
Pacemaker current, effect of acetylcholine on, 772
Pacinian corpuscle, 343f, 368
    as rapidly adapting receptor, 337
    sensitive to high-frequency mechanical stimuli, 346
    structure, 338
Pain
    and analgesia, 385–399
    burning, 387–388
    chronic
        diagnosis and treatment using somatotopic organization of
            spinothalamic tract, 713–714
        intractable, reduced by lesions that include the limbic
            association cortex, 829
        from spontaneous lesions to central sites in nociceptive
            pathways, 388
    control of by central mechanisms, 393–397
    deep referred, mechanism of, 388
    descending pathway modulating, 394
    due to injury of peripheral nerves, 387
    gate control hypothesis for explanation of modulation, 392
    and hyperactivity of dorsal horn neurons in deafferented
        region, 387
    induction of analgesia by behavioral stress, 397–398
    information about carried by ventral columns of spinal cord,
        284
    mechanical thresholds for before and after burns, 386f
    mediated by
        anterolateral system, 333f, 362–363
        by nociceptors, 343
    mediation by different classes of nociceptive afferent fibers,
        386
    modulating by activity balance between nociceptive and
        other afferent inputs, 392
    processing in somatosensory cortex, 392
    referred, 389
    role of neuroactive peptides in perception of, 218
    sensation, mediated by spinal nucleus of trigeminal nerve,
        702–703, 705
    sense of modulated by reticulospinal pathways, 693
    as somatic modality, 341
    subjective nature of, 385
    syndromes
        interpretation, 389
        resulting from surgery to alleviate pain, 388
    threshold and mechanisms of drug action, 332
Painful stimuli, transmission modulated by raphe–spinal
    system, 543
Paleospinothalamic tract, 392
Pancreas
    cholinergic and noradrenergic responses, 771t
    innervation, 766
Panic attack
    and abnormality in right parahippocampal gyrus, 14
    abnormality of temporal poles in, 881
    genetic predisposition, 881
    induction of with sodium lactate or carbon dioxide, 882
    localized to temporal lobe, 14
    symptoms, 881

treatment with antidepressants, 881
Parachlorophenylalanine, inhibits sleep, 799
Paradoxical cold, 344
Paradoxical sleep. *See* Rapid eye movement sleep
Parahippocampal area, in limbic association cortex, 826
Parahippocampal gyrus, 307f
  part of limbic lobe, 737
  right, abnormality in patients with panic attacks, 14
Parallel control, motor neurons, and recovery of function
      following lesions, 546
Parallel distributed processing networks, simulation of
      cognitive functions with, 836–837
Parallel organization, motor system, 539
Parallel pathways
  mediation of vision by, 445–449
  processing of visual information by ganglion cells, 409–411
  in spinal cord, 359–360
  synchrony as possible mechanism for binding, 462
  visual, psychological evidence supporting, 448
  visual system, 447f
Parallel processing
  auditory information, 496
  and conveyance of information in the nervous system, 31
  lateral geniculate nucleus, 427
  as organizational principle of nervous system, 7
  perception, 328
  and resiliency of learning, 1005
  sensory and motor information, 784
  visual information, clinical evidence, 448–449
Parallelism, motor cortex and spinal stretch reflex, 617
Paralysis
  gaze, 726t
  ipsilateral facial, 726t
  ipsilateral lateral rectus, 726t
Paralysis agitans. *See* Parkinson's disease
Paramagnetic substances, and MRI of brain structures, 322
Paraphasia, 846d
Paraphrasia, 11d
Parasomnias, 810–812
Parasthesias, positive symptoms of peripheral neuropathies, 251
Parasympathetic division, autonomic nervous system,
    projections of pre- and postganglionic neurons, 765f
    regulation of cardiovascular function, 772
Parasympathetic division
  of autonomic nervous system, 761
  embryonic development of neurons, 300
  preganglionic neurons are located in brain stem and spinal
      cord, 766
Parasympathetic ganglia
  cholinergic synaptic transmission in, 768–769
  slow postsynaptic potentials in, 769
Parasympathetic nervous system, 763f
Parasympathetic postganglionic neurons, ACh is
      neurotransmitter used, 215
Parasympathetic system, peripheral nervous system
    (autonomic), 274
Paraventricular nucleus, 738f
  hypothalamic, oxytocin release by regulates milk ejection
      and uterine contraction, 744
  peptidergic projections, 743
  role in feeding behavior, 756
  vasopressin release by regulates urine flow, 744
Paravertebral chain ganglia, 764
Paresthesias, 250d
Pargyline, site of action in noradrenergic transmission, 879f
Parietal association area, projections, 828f
Parietal cortex
  controls visual attention, 675
  left, damage to inferior regions causes Gerstmann's
      syndrome, 831
  postcentral gyrus, somatic sensory and motor connections
      from body arranged in somatotopic order, 372, 372f

role in attention to spatial aspects of sensation, 831
Parietal lobe, 8f, 276, 278f
  association area, role in higher sensory functions and
      language, 831–832
  blood supply, 1041
  cerebral cortex, function, 7
  effect of damage to, 831
  nondominant, effect of lesions, 831
Parietal-temporal-occipital association cortex, 277, 278f, 824,
      825f
  associative function, 825
  pulvinar projects to, 290
Parietal–temporal–occipital cortex, 821
Parietal–temporal–occipital junction, 848
Parieto-occipital regions, and Balint's syndrome, 831
Parinaud syndrome, 1047
  midbrain, symptoms, 729
Parkinson's disease
  characteristics, 981–982
  effect on direct and indirect pathways of basal ganglia, 653
  experimental, 653
  hyposmia in conjunction with, 518
  loss of dopaminergic cells, 654–655
  and pathological changes in basal ganglia, 647
  possible role of environmental toxin, 655
  rigidity, 606
  symptoms, 654
    reflect decrease in transmission in mesocortical
        dopaminergic pathways, 863
  treatment, transplantation of fetal dopamine cells, 656
Parkinson's syndrome, produced by MPTP, 655–656
Parkinsonism, 531
Pars compacta, 648d
Pars reticulata, 648d
Parvocellular layers
  lateral geniculate nucleus, 426
  lesions, 448
  relay color information to cortex, 473
Parvocellular neuroendocrine neurons, peptide secreting, 741
Parvocellular neurons, hypothalamic, contain multiple
      peptides, 743–744
Parvocellular-blob system
  processes color information, 474f
  role in visual perception, concern with fine detail and color,
      448
  specialized for color, 447
Parvocellular-interblob system
  detection of form and color, 447
  pathway, 447
  projection of, 447
  shape recognition represented in and conveyed to inferior
      temporal cortex, 458
Patch-clamp technique
  demonstration of all-or-none opening of voltage-gated ion
      channels, 113
  for determination of functional properties of single ion
      channels, method, 71
  as refinement of voltage-clamp technique, 106. *See also*
      Patch-clamp technique
  study of elementary current through single ACh activated
      channel, 144
Pattern
  code, different patterns of firing by uncommitted sensory
      receptor, 338
  coding, across-fiber, in taste perception, 527
  direction-selective neurons, response to motion, 452
  discrimination, clues of similarity and proximity, 442
  generators, for each limb, 591
Pause cells, role in horizontal saccades, 671, 672
Pavor nocturnus. *See* Night terror
PCP. *See* Phencyclidine
PDGF. *See* Platelet-derived growth factor

PDP. *See* Parallel distributed processing
Peduncles, 9t
Pendular reflexes, 644d
Penicillin
    high dose, and experimental petit mal epilepsy, 789
    induction of focal epilepsy with, 786
    induction of generalized epilepsy, 787
Peptide A, precursor structure, 220f
Peptidergic neuroendocrine cells, classes of in hypothalamus,
        740–744
Peptides
    and alteration of neuronal excitability in autonomic ganglia,
        769
    coreleased with acetylcholine in preganglionic fibers of
        autonomic nervous system, 769
    elicits slow excitatory postsynaptic potential, nociceptive
        afferents, 390
    functioning as neurotransmitters in egg-laying, 992
    neurotransmitters in nociceptive primary afferent fibers,
        389–390
    regions of in paraventricular nucleus, 739f
    release of by peptides, 387
    in sympathetic neurons, 770t
Perception, 330d
    dorsal root ganglion connection with neurons whose output
        connects with thalamus mediates, 286
    neural basis of, 296–308
    parallel processing, 328
    roles of dorsal column–medial lemniscal system and parts of
        anterolateral system, 360
    sensory information for integrated by pulvinar, 290
    sensory regions of cerebral cortex play critical role in, 335
    somatosensory, principal pathway for is dorsal
        column–medial lemniscal system, 287
    versus physical properties of stimuli, 330
    voluntary movement, 347
Perceptions, produced by preattentive scanning, 460f
Perceptual cancellation, color, 470–471
Perceptual development, effect of early sensory deprivation on,
        947
Perforant pathway, hippocampus, excitatory synaptic pathway,
        1019f
Performance variables, 998d
Perfusion, separate, of medulla, caudal pons, and posterior
        cerebellum in cat, 817f
Periaqueductal gray matter, 288f
    enkephalin- and dynorphin-containing neuronal cell bodies
        and nerve terminals in, 395
    high levels of mu receptors in, 395
    sensitive to morphine, 394
Periglomerular cells, 516f
Perilymph, 484f, 502f
    in space surrounding membranous labyrinth, 501
Peripheral cutaneous nerve, effect of damage to, 354
Peripheral motor axons, conduction velocities in neuropathies
        and myelopathies, 246
Peripheral nerves
    afferent fibers bundled together in convey sensory
        information to spinal cord, 353
    consist of afferent and efferent nerve fibers for same general
        body part, 353
    detection of damage with Tinel sign, 251
    diseases of, 244–257, 249t
        chronic and acute diseases of, 250
    injury
        and activity of efferent fibers of sympathetic nervous
            system triggers burning pain, 387
    lesions, 715
    redistribution among dorsal roots, 354f
Peripheral nervous system
    autonomic ganglia, elimination of synapses during
        development, 942–943

    derived from endoderm, 296
    divisions, 273–274
    grafts from promote growth in central nervous system after
        injury, 265–266, 266f
    growth-promoting proteins in, 265
    myelination, 43
    rearrangement of synaptic connections, 943f
    recovery after injury, 261
    regeneration of axons in nerve cells of, 262–264
Peripheral neurons, neurotransmitter choice is controlled by
        signals from neighboring cells, 904
Peripheral neuropathy
    motor disorder of, 250
    symptoms, 250
Peripheral receptors
    perception of limb position and movement, 347
    types, 347–348
Perisylvian region, lesion, 848
Periventricular gray region, brain, stimulating electrodes reduce
        pain, 393
Permeability
    of leakage channels, 107
    membrane, changes in caused by depolarization, 105
    versus conductance, 90
Permeation, inhibition of through ion channel, 75
Peroxisomal proteins, 52
Peroxisomes, part of membrane system of nerve cell, 49
Personality, characteristic profile for temporal lobe epilepsy, 14
Perspectives, linear and size, monocular depth cue, 454
PET. *See* Positron emission tomography
Petit mal seizures, 785
Petrosal ganglion, 525f
PGO spikes. *See* Pontine–geniculate–occipital spikes
pH gradient, and movement of neurotransmitters into synaptic
        vesicles, 226
Phantom pain, 387d
Pharmacology, as basis for study of chemical synaptic
        transmission, 6
Phase locking, auditory nerve fiber, 491
Phe-Met-Arg-Phe-NH2, and hyperpolarization and synaptic
        inhibition in sensory neurons, 186
Phencyclidine
    inhibits NMDA receptor, 159
    molecular targets in the brain, 866
    produces psychosis similar to schizophrenia, 866
Phenelzine, antidepressant, 872, 873f
Phenothiazines
    long-term treatment with and development of tardive
        dyskinesia, 657
    response of schizophrenic symptoms to, 858t
    structure, 859f
    treatment, schizophrenia, 858
Phenoxybenzamine, site of action in noradrenergic
        transmission, 879f
Phentolamine, site of action in noradrenergic transmission,
        879f
Phenylethylamines, mechanism of action, 232
Phenylketonuria, genetic basis for, 993
Phenylthiorea, tasters and nontasters, 513
Phobias, treatment with systematic desensitization, 1001
Phorbol ester response element, 189d
Phosphene, 331d
Phosphoinositol linkage, and anchoring proteins to membranes,
        56
Phospholipase A2
    activation by G-proteins, 178–179
    system, and synaptic second messengers, 174f
    receptors that activate cause release of arachidonic acid, 181
Phospholipase C
    activation
        by G-proteins, 178–179
        produces diacylglycerol-IP3 system, 181

activity stimulated by quisqualate-B receptor, 157f
system, and synaptic second messengers, 174f
Phospholipids
hydrolysis of and generation of second messengers, 178–181
structure, 180–181
Phosphorus scans, reveal cerebral infarcts, neoplastic changes,
and metabolism in brain, 323
Phosphorylation
in adenylyl cyclase cycle, 176f, 177
cAMP cascade, 178
cGMP-dependent, in brain, 191
domain, 189d
effect on protein conformation, 177
and ion channel gating, 75f
of MAPs, 61–62
protein, 52
and desensitization, 186–187
regulatory consequences, 182
second messenger systems and effect on other receptors,
187f
sequence, 178d
of substrate proteins in long-term training, 1014, 1016
Phosphatidylinosodtide turnover, coupling of serotonin
receptors to, 875
Photon absorbency, brain structures with large differences
imaged with X-rays, 309–312
Photoreceptors, 401d
cGMP gates ion channels in plasma membrane of, 406
closing of cGMP-gated channels causes hyperpolarization,
407f
connected by gap junctions, 415
Drosophila,
classification according to opsin pigment expression and
axon projection, 900
differentiation, 901f
hyperpolarized by closing of cGMP-gated ion channel,
406–408
light adaptation in and changes in intracellular Ca^{2+}, 408
role of cell position in controlling identity of in Drosophila,
899–902
signals relayed to ganglion cells by bipolar cells, 412
specialized sensory receptor, 338
spectral responses of trivariant, divariant, and monovariant
systems, 470f
transduction by, 336, 336f
types, 402–403
Phototransduction
cascade of biochemical events in photoreceptors, 403–408
closing of cation channels in, 404f
in retina, 400–417
Phrenologists, and localization of mental functions in brain, 15
Phrenology, 823
early study of the brain, 6
map of skull and brain function, 7f
Physostigmine, reverses symptoms of myasthenia gravis, 236
Pia mater, 1051f, 304d
Pick body, 981
Pick's disease, characteristics, 981
Pigment epithelium, 401d
Pigment molecules, photoreceptor
activated by light, 404–406
and control of cGMP phosphodiesterase, 406
structural similarity with family of hormone and transmitter
receptors that activate effector enzymes via G-proteins,
406
Pineal gland
cholinergic and noradrenergic responses, 771t
imaging with conventional radiography, 311
Pituitary
anterior
gonadotropins secreted, 964
hypothalamic substances that release or inhibit hormones

of, 743t
regulation of release of, 742
control of by hypothalamus, 739–740, 741f
posterior, blood–brain barrier leaky, 1055
relationship to hypothalamus, 738f
Pituitary–hypophyseal–portal system, vascular link between
hypothalamus and pituitary, 740
Place principle, auditory nerve, 491
Placenta, as source of steroid hormones influencing developing
fetus, 964
Plantar reflex, 587d
Planum temporale
anatomical asymmetry, 832, 832f
cytoarchitectonic abnormalities in dyslexia, 850
Plasma cell disease, as chronic neuropathy, 250
Plasma membrane
incorporation of synaptic vesicle membranes into during
recycling, 230, 231f
part of major membrane system of nerve cell, 49
renovation of by vesicles, 56
Plasmapheresis, 238d
Plasticity
associative, changes in somatotopic map may reflect
common cellular mechanisms for, 1026–1027
brain, and long-term memory, 1004–1005
encoding memory, localization throughout nervous system,
1005
of neurons in hypothalamus, 746
right cerebral hemisphere in females, 971
synaptic
cellular grammar for, 1023
importance of cAMP cascade in, 1018–1019
synaptic connections, and learning, 1010
synaptic transmissions and short-term memory, 1004
Platelet-derived growth factor, role in O-2A progenitor cell
proliferation, 898
Pleasure, and regulation of motivated behaviors, 759
Pneumoencephalography, 309, 310f
P_o, protein in mature peripheral myelin, 43
Polarization, dynamic, 20
Polio virus, fast retrograde transport, 60
Poliomyelitis, affects motor neurons, 250
Polymerization
of cytoskeletal proteins, 62–64
directional, 63
states of, 64f
Polymodal nociceptors, 343, 386
Polymyositis syndrome, myopathic disease, 249t
Polyneuropathy, 715d
Polypeptides, cytosolic, cotranslational and posttranslational
modifications, 51–52
Polyprotein, 55d
Polyribosomes, and protein manufacture in nerve cells, 51, 53.
See also Polysomes
Polysomnograms, 806d
POMC. See Proopiomelanocortin
Pons, 8f, 288f
and location of medial longitudinal fasciculus in relation to
medial vestibular nucleus, 510f
contains pontine nuclei, axons participate in cerebellar
control of movement and posture, 287
derived from hindbrain, 298
features of syndromes common to, 726t
function, 9t, 276
lateral syndromes, 726–729
lesions in eliminate atonia during REM sleep, 797
medial lesions, 724, 726
part of brain stem, 275
role in smooth pursuit, 672
stimulation of nuclei in facilitates spinal reflexes, 602
Pontine flexure, 298
Pontine hemorrhage, 1047

Pontine nuclei, 288f, 510f
  axons participate in cerebellar control of movement and
      posture, 287
  brain stem, MT and MST neurons project to, 450
  conveys input of cerebral cortex to cerebellum, 637
Pontine reticular formation, 603d
  formation, saccade-related neurons, spike discharge patterns,
      672f
  generates horizontal saccades, 671–672
Pontine reticular nuclei, facilitates motor neurons, 602–604
Pontine reticulospinal tract, 693
Pontine–geniculate–occipital spikes, generation of during REM
      sleep, 795
Population code, activity of population of responding sensory
      receptors, 337
Population vector, and directional tuning of motor cortical
      neurons, 616
Position sense
  deficits of in tabes dorsalis, 370
  loss of, 726t
Positional invariance, 431d
Positivism, 329d, 330
Positron emission tomography
  brain regions activated
      by auditory stimulation, 315–316f
      by visual stimuli, 315–316f
  combined with cognitive psychology, 3
  demonstration of increased D2 dopamine receptors in
      schizophrenia patients, 861
  images biochemical processes of brain, 312–314
  local utilization of glucose by brain, 315–316f
  localization of language in cerebral cortex, 12, 13f
  mechanism, 313
  resolution, 313
Postcentral gyrus, 8, 278f
  projection of somatosensory information from arms, trunk,
      and legs, 707
  somatotopic organization, 707f
Posterior cerebral arteries, 1042
Posterior cerebral artery territory, infarction, 1043f, 1046
Posterior fossa structures, in infarct, 1047
Posterior hypothalamic area, 738f
Posterior inferior cerebellar artery, 1042
Posterior nucleus, hypothalamic, 739
Posterior parietal cortex, 276–277, 368f, 825f
  cellular basis of visual attention in, 460–462
  damage causes complex abnormalities in attending sensations
      from contralateral half of body, 370
  inputs to, 623
  lesions, 619, 623, 675
  receives somatic inputs, 364
  role in generating saccades, 675
  role in providing spatial information for targeted movements,
      622–624
Postganglionic axons, sympathetic or parasympathetic, release
      of acetylcholine or norepinephrine at target sites after
      stimulation, 769
Postganglionic neurons, 763
  autonomic nervous system
      dual expression of slow inhibitory and excitatory
          mechanisms, 769
      pathways, 764, 764f, 765f
Postganglionic sympathetic neurons, effects of axonal
      sectioning, 263f
Postjunctional folds, smoothing of characteristic of myasthenia
      gravis, 237
Postsaccadic drift, 673f
Postsynaptic inhibition, 208d
Postsynaptic membranes, three-dimensional view, 202f
Postsynaptic neuron
  competing inputs integrated by neuronal integration, 166
  inhibitory effect of Cl⁻ channel opening on, 160, 161f, 162

passive membrane properties and neuronal summation, 167
Postsynaptic potential
  excitatory, directions of deflection in EEG recordings, 785t
  increase in amplitude after high rate of stimulation of
      presynaptic neuron, 207f
  increased and decreased potential, ion channels and signal
      properties, 166f
  inhibitory
      counteracts EPSP, 161f
      current flow during, 150–161
      directions of deflection in EEG recordings, 785t
      recording from hippocampal pyramidal cells compared with
          one from spinal motor neuron, 782f
      reverses at equilibrium potential for chloride, 161f
      slow, in sympathetic and parasympathetic ganglia, 769
Postsynaptic response, to neurotransmitter release, time course,
      199f
Posttetanic potentiation, 207d, 207f
Posttranslational importation, 52d
Postural control, role of experience, 598–599
Postural responses
  arm and leg muscles, 599f
  dependence on voluntary movement, 622f
  latency, 598
  postural set, 599d
      descending influences generated by, 600
  rapid, topography dependent on context, 598–599
  triggered
      centrally before voluntary movements, 599–600
      by sensory input, 597–598
Posture, 596–607, 596d
  axons of pontine nuclei participate in cerebellar control of, 287
  cerebellar lesions modify vestibular and reticular influences
      on, 604–606
  coordinated with movement by reticulospinal system, 604
  decerebrate, mechanism, 604
  feedback information to maintain, 500
  maintenance by feedback mechanisms, 536
  maintenance during standing and walking, 597–600
  maintenance of by reticulospinal tracts, 541
  mechanisms of adjustment, 596
  motor axons that control carried by ventral columns of spinal
      cord, 284
  and movable platform experiments, 597f
  problems in maintaining in decerebrate animal, 604
  reflex control of by vestibulospinal tract, 541
  role of brain stem and spinal mechanisms, 602–606
  role
      of lateral vestibular nucleus in control of, 508–509
      of muscle tone, 577
      of supplementary motor area in coordinating with
          voluntary movement, 620
Potassium conductance. See also Conductance
  calculated from K⁺ current, 109–110
  compared with sodium in voltage-clamp experiments, 109f
  effect of acetylcholine on in heart, 772
  effect of depolarization on, 109f
  similarities with Na⁺ conductance, 108
Potassium current
  as battery, 89f
  delayed-rectifier-type, and activation of beta-adrenergic
      receptors, 771
  effect of ACh on in sympathetic ganglion cells, 183
  voltage-sensitive delayed, participation in electrical resonance
      of hair cells, 488
Potassium channels. See also Ion channel, potassium
  during afterpolarization, 110
  as battery in series with conductor, 90f
  and falling phase of action potential, 105
  molecular structure, 117
  during refractoriness following action potential, 110
  and resting potential, 86

transmitter-gated, mediates EPSP, 155–160
voltage-gated
 belongs to same gene family as Na$^+$ channel, 115–119
 display, types of, 111
 and generation of action potential, 105
 kinetics, 105, 107
 secondary structure in cell membrane, 116f
Potassium ion
 calculation of passive flux and Na$^+$-K$^+$ pump, 94
 channel selectivity for, 68f
 concentrated inside the cell, 82
 diffusion of, 85–86
 distribution across cell membrane, 84t
 effect on nociceptors, 387t
 efflux not necessary for neurotransmitter release, 196–197
 flux across cell membrane, 87f
 generation of resting potential in cell permeable to, 85f
 glial cells permeable to at rest, 85
 ion channel at end-plate permeable to, 139–140
 nerve cells at rest permeable to, 85
 nongated in glial cells selective for, 84
 passive flux through nongated channels balanced by active
  pumping, 86–88
 permeability of glial cells to, 23–24
 relationship with membrane potential, 85f
 resting conductance, increased by serotonin in pyramidal
  cells, 698
 synaptic channel at end-plate permeable to, 140
 voltage-gated channel selective for, 141
 voltage-gated channels selective for and generation of action
  potential, 88
Potential difference, 1033
 symbol, 1037
Potentiation, 207d, 207f
 associative long-term, importance for spatial memory,
  1022–1023
 long-term, 207d
  in area CA1 of hippocampus, 1020f
  in CA1 region of hippocampus is associative, 1019–1022
  calcium influx through NMDA receptor-channel critical
   form, 1020
  capability for in cerebral cortex, 1023
  and enhanced glutamate release, 1022
  enhancement, 1020
  in hippocampus, example of associative and nonassociative
   learning, 1019–1024
  as increase in excitatory synaptic potential in postsynaptic
   hippocampal neurons, 1019
  induction, 1020
  maintenance of synaptic efficiency in requires increase in
   presynaptic transmitter release, 1021–1022
  maintenance phase, 1022f
  maintenance phase of Schaffer collateral synapses, 1022f
  model for induction, 1021f
  nonassociative in area CA3 of hippocampus, 1023
  requirement of depolarization of postsynaptic cells
   coincident with activity in presynaptic neuron, 1020
Preattentive scanning, 460f
 process in visual perception, 460
Precentral gyrus, 8, 278f
 and eliciting motor effects, 610
Perceptions, produced by focal attention, 460f
Prefrontal association cortex, 277, 278f, 824, 825f
 projections, 828f
 subregions, 826
Prefrontal cortex, 821
 dopaminergic innervation, 829
 dorsolateral, modulatory pathway form mesocortical
  dopaminergic system essential for normal function,
  863
 possible role in mediating visual attention, 460
 schizophrenia as disorder in activation of, 864–865

subdivisions, 826
Prefrontal sulcus, electrical stimulation interferes with delayed
  spatial response tasks, 828
Preganglionic neurons
 activate autonomic motor neurons, 763
 autonomic nervous system
  corelease of acetylcholine and peptides, 769
 pathways, 764, 764f, 765f
Preknowledge, 330
Premotor cortex
 monkey, 611f
 role in preparing motor systems for movement, 619–622
Premotor neurons, upper motor neurons, 245
Preoptic area, steroid receptors in, 966
 anterior, effect of gonadal steroid hormones on, 969, 970f
Preoptic nuclei, hypothalamic, 739
Press of speech, 846d
Pressure
 and ion channel gating, 75f
 intracranial, increased in brain, 1057–1058
 transmission of in ear, 483
Presynaptic facilitation, 207
 mechanisms, 208
Presynaptic inhibition, 207, 208d
 mechanisms, 208
Presynaptic membranes, three-dimensional view, 202f
Presynaptic neurons, 20d
 electrical synapse and function of voltage-gated channels,
  124–125
 electrical synapse, significance of size of cell, 124–125
 focus on target cell by convergence, 25f
 properties of and amount of neurotransmitter released, 211
Presynaptic terminal, 19f, 20d
 active zone, 131
 boutons, 935f
 as region of nerve cell, 19
 synaptic connections on regulate intracellular free Ca^{2+},
  207–209
Pretectum, projections from retina to, 423f
Prevertebral ganglia, autonomic nervous system, 764
Primal sketch, 431d
Primary afferent neurons
 component of reflex pathway, 582
 electrophysiological analysis of action of opiates, 397f
 fibers, 357–358, 358f
  nociceptive, 389–390
 innervate taste receptors, 519–521
 transmits stimulus information from dorsal root ganglion
  neuron to central nervous system, 342
Primary afferent synapses, presynaptic and postsynaptic
  inhibitory actions exerted by enkephalin-containing
  interneurons, 396
Primary auditory cortex, 276, 278f, 494
 callosal connections, 494
 lesions, 494–495
 organization into columns, 494
 tonotopic maps of frequency spectrum in, 494–497
Primary motor cortex (areas), 276, 278f, 539, 824t, 825f
 agranular cortex, 612f
 areas projecting to, 539
 cerebral cortex, somatotopic organization, 293
 descending fiber tracts, 543, 544f
 detailed somatotopic map in, 613–614
 directional tuning of neurons in, 614–616, 616f
 and initiation or triggering of movement, 614
 internal granular layer, 612f
 layer 4, 612f
 layer 5, 612f
 monkey, 611f
 motor map of body, 610
 neurons encode direction of force exerted, 613–619
 receptive fields, 617

Primary motor cortex (areas) [*cont.*]
  recordings of pyramidal tract neurons during wrist movement, 615f
  sensory input to inform of consequences of movement, 616–619
  somatotopic organization, 610, 610f
Primary sensory areas, 276, 278f, 824t
Primary sensory nerve endings, soleus muscle, 38
Primary somatic sensory cortex, 276, 361d, 368f, 825f
  functional areas, 363–364
  GABA agonist disrupts finger coordination, 383f
  innervation of body surface represented in more than one sensory map, 1024f
  one somatic sensory modality dominates in each area, 377–378
  projections of neurons in different layers of, 365
  representation of body surface in each region of, 373f
  responses in to tactile stimulation, 371f
  responses of three types of cortical neurons to stimulation on hand, 381f
  termination of thalamic fibers in, 368, 368f
Primary visual cortex, 276, 825f, *See also* Striate cortex; VI
  classes of cells, 427
  contains map of visual field, 426f
  cross section, 436f
  damage to causes blindness, 335
  decomposition of outlines of visual image into short line segments, 430–431
  distribution of cytochrome oxidase in superficial layers, 432f
  each hemisphere receives information from contralateral field, 427
  feature abstraction accomplished by progressive convergence, 431
  functions, 434
  horizontal connections linking columns, 434, 435d
  layers, 427, 428f, 434
  localization of word recognition during reading, 13f
  neural mass devoted to representation of fovea, 426
  organization into vertical columns, 431–434
  receives input from magnocellular and parvocellular pathways of lateral geniculate nucleus, 431
  receptive field of simple cell in, 429f
  role in detecting motion, 452
  site where information from both eyes is combined, 457–458
  transforms concentric receptive fields into linear segments and boundaries, 427–431
  types of neurons, 428f
  visual field as hypercolumns in, 433f
Priming, and memory retrieval, 1006
Principal sensory trigeminal nucleus, 703f, 704f
  analogy to dorsal column–medial lemniscal system, 702
  nerve, mediates tactile sensation from face, 702
Principal sulcus
  lesions, 827–829
  location, 827f
  prefrontal association cortex, role in delay response tasks, 828
  subdivision of prefrontal cortex, 826
  third-party connections, 828f
Principle of connectional specificity, 20d
Principle of dynamic polarization, 20d
Probst's commissure, 494
Processes, neuronal, and classification of nerve cells, 21f
Prochlorperazine, structure, 859f
Proctolin, as neuroactive peptide, 218t
Prodynorphin, precursor molecules, 395
Proenkephalin, precursor molecules, 395
Progressive bulbar palsy, 249t
Progressive convergence, method of feature abstraction in primary visual cortex, 431
Projection connections, descending projections, 365
Projection interneurons (neurons), 22d, 279

Projection neurons
  in central nervous system, processing sensory information, 369
  conduct stimulus energy transduced by sensory receptors to central nervous system, 339
  process nociceptive information in dorsal horn, 389
Prolactin
  as neuroactive peptide, 218t
  precursor structure, 220f
Promoter region, DNA regulatory region, 188d
Proopiomelanocortin
  differential processing, 221
  endogenous opioid peptide in brain, 394–396
  precursor molecules, 395
  precursor structure, 220f
Proprioception
  arm, mediated by dorsal column–medial lemniscal system, 360–361
  impaired
    compensation for with vision, 537
    deficits in feedback and feedforward mechanisms, 537
  limb, mediated by muscle afferent fibers, 347–349
  pathways for arm and leg, 360
  processing of, 360
  sensitivity, dependent on combined actions of muscle, joint, and cutaneous receptors, 349, 350f
  as somatic modality, 341
Proprioceptors, muscles and joints, 535
Propriospinal neurons, 540d
  medial, pathway, 540
  projections, 540
  vestibular and neck afferents converge on, 602
Prosody, 13d, 848d
Prosopagnosia, 449d, 458
Prostaglandin E2, effect on nociceptors, 387
Prostaglandins
  and activation and sensitization of nociceptors, 387f
  effect on nociceptors, 387t
  sleep-promoting, 798
  synthesis, 181–182
Prostigmine, effect of on miniature end-plate potentials, 198
Protanopia, 479d
Protease, one of proteins induced in long-term memory, 1014
Protein II, 228t
Protein kinases
  A, role in short- and long-term facilitation, 1015f
  C
    activated by diacylglycerol
    activation, 180f
    domains, 179f
    GAP-43 as substrate for, 913
    isoforms, 181
    role in sensitization, 1012
  cAMP-dependent
    activation of in repeated training, 1014
    activation of in sensitization, 1012
    and phosphorylation of receptor, 187
    regulatory subunits, 178
  modulate ion channel activity by phosphorylation, 133
  mediation of second messenger activity in inactivation of ion channels, 76
  molecular relationships, 179f
  novel synaptic action of those activated by second messengers, 182
  reaction, in cAMP cascade, 178
Proteins
  allosteric, ion channels as, 74
  anchored, 50
  anchoring, 62
  associated with membranes of synaptic vesicles, 228t
  associated, 50
  cell membrane, 52–55

in cerebrospinal fluid, 1057
classes of made by nerve cell, 50–51
configurations, 54–55
cotranslational and posttranslational modifications, 51–52
covalent modification of in short-term facilitation, 1015f
cytoskeletal, polymerization of, 62–64
cytosolic, 51–52
distribution by axonal transport in nerve cell, 57–60
effect of phosphorylation on conformation, 177
formation in association with endoplasmic reticulum, 54f
fibrillar, responsible for shape of nerve cell, 60–62
glycosylation, 55
hydrophobicity plot, 72, 72f
ion channel structure, 70
ion channels, 67
membrane. *See also* Bacteriorhodopsin
membrane and secretory, distribution in nerve cell by axonal
    transport, 57–60
membrane-spanning, 50f
    structure, 72f
mitochondrial, 52
model for anchoring to membrane, 56f
in myelin, 43
N-myristoylated, 52
nerve cell, manufacture, 52–55
neuronal, synthesis and trafficking, 49–56
new synthesis in long-term facilitation, 1015f
nuclear, 52
nuclear uptake, 52
organelles that synthesize and process, 53f
peroxisomal, 52
phosphorylation, 52
proteolytic cleavage, 55
secondary structure, 55
secretory, 52–55
slow axonal transport, 61f
sodium-potassium pump as transport, 68
study of single molecules with single-channel recording, 68
synthesis and processing of in nerve cell, 51f
three classes encoded by nerve cell mRNA, 49–56
transcriptional activator, phosphorylation of in synaptic
    transmission, 187–191
transport, 57–60
Proteolipid, in central myelin, 43
Proteolytic cleavage, of membrane and secretory proteins, 55
Proton images, of brain lesions, 321
Proximal–distal rule
motor nuclei, 539
spinal motor nuclei organization, 539
Pseudo-affective reflexes, 747
Pseudo-athetosis, 537f
Pseudo-unipolar neurons, 38d
    description, 21, 21F
Pseudohermaphroditism, caused by fetal exposure of genetic
    females to male hormones, 963–964
Pseudoinsomnia, 806d
Pseudosubstrate, 178d
Pseudotumor cerebri, 1059
Psychiatric disease. *See also* Mental illness
acquired, and alteration in gene regulation, 1029f
inherited, alteration in gene structure, 1029f
altered gene expression in, 1028
categories, 1027–1028
correlation with demonstrable pathology, 854
and diagnosis of coma, 816t
diagnosis with imaging techniques, 1028
as disease processes, 854
and neuronal changes produced by learning, 1027–1028
organic versus functional, 1028
syndrome, defining, 853–854
treatment with operant conditioning, 1002
Psychoactive agents, effect on sleep stages, 795

Psychology
as discipline for understanding brain function, 6
emergence as distinct discipline, 329–330
Psychometric function, frequency of stimulus detection as
    function of stimulus intensity, 331, 331f
Psychomotor seizures, 785d
Psychopathology, and disturbed sleep, 807
Psychophysics, 327, 330
Psychotic behavior
episodes, 855d
produced by interfering with transmitter systems, 866
Psychotropic drugs, block uptake mechanism for
    neurotransmitters, 233
Ptosis, 236f, 667d, 718d
Pulvinar, 434
possible role in mediating visual attention, 460
thalamic nucleus, 290, 291f
Pumps, method of neurotransmitter release, 232. *See*
    Sodium-potassium pump
Pupil, constriction of with light, 424
autonomic control, 772–773
reflex pathway mediating, 424f
during REM sleep, 794
reflexes
    clinical importance, 424
    in pontine hemorrhage, 1047
    retinal input to pretectal area of midbrain, 423, 424
response
    to light in coma as result of supratentorial lesions, 817
    in metabolic coma, 817
Pupils, parasympathetic and sympathetic innervation, 772–773
Purinergic transmission, role of ATP, 223–224
Purines
role as autocoid in presynaptic receptors for adenosine, 223
role in synaptic transmission, 223–224
Purkinje cell layer, cerebellar cortex, 630f
inputs and projections, 630
Purkinje cells
in cerebellar cortex, 630
cerebellum, as multipolar cell, 21f
cGMP-dependent protein phosphorylation in, 191
complex spike evoked by climbing fiber activation, 631, 631f
effect of climbing fiber input, 642–644
excitation of on-beam and inhibition of off-beam, 632f
GABA as neurotransmitter in, 630
inhibition by local interneurons, 632
simple spike evoked by mossy fiber activation, 631, 631f
Purposeful action, information for integrated by association
    areas of cerebral cortex, 277
Pursuit eye movements, 450
Putamen, 277, 290f
activity of neurons in, versus those in cortex and
    supplementary motor area, 652
of basal ganglia, 648
CT scan of hemorrhage, 1048f
degeneration of in Huntington's disease, 981
development, 305f
inputs to, 649f
involved in regulating speed of movements, 295
lesions, 1047
neurons in selective for direction of limb movement, 652
role in motor control, 649
PVN. *See* Paraventricular nucleus
Pyramidal cells
cerebral cortex, 292, 779, 781f, 782f
    as projection interneurons, 292
dendritic organization, 779
hippocampus, recording of inhibitory postsynaptic potential,
    782f
neurons in somatic sensory cortex, 364–365
output cells of primary visual cortex, 434
primary visual cortex, 427

Pyramidal cells [*cont.*]
  projections, 779
  serotonin increases resting potassium conductance in, 698
  synaptic potentials in recorded by EEGs, 784–785
Pyramidal decussation, 543d
Pyramidal tract, 294
  as pathway in motor system, 280
  syndrome, 647d
Pyriform cortex, 517f
Pyrogens, 753d

Q

Quadratic field defect, 437d
Quadriceps muscle
  connections of neurons mediating stretch reflex, 154f
  production of EPSP and IPSP in motor neurons innervating, 155
Quadriparesis, in pontine hemorrhage, 1047
Quantum. *See also* Synaptic versicles
  each stored in synaptic vesicle, 201, 203
  neurotransmitter, 198d
    release of as binomial or Bernoulli trial, 210
Quick phase, 662d
Quisqualate receptor
  channel regulation by, 157f
  glutamate binding to, 158
Quisqualate B receptor, 158
  coupled to second-messenger pathway, 171

R

Ra. *See* Axial resistance
rab 3A, 228t
rab 3B, 228t
Rabies virus, fast retrograde transport, 60
Radial glial cells
  migration of immature neurons on, 909–911
  misaligned in weaver mutant, 910
  organization of dependent on interactions with granule cells, 910
Radiography, 309, 310f
  conventional
    high spatial resolution, 310–311
    reveals brain asymmetry, 310–311
Raphe nuclei
  activity of monoaminergic cells in during REM sleep, 803
  aminergic pathways from modulate excitability of spinal neurons, 541
  brain stem, serotonergic pathways originate in, 875
  loss of serotonergic neurons in Parkinson's disease, 655
  neurofibrillary tangles in, 979
  principal descending serotonergic projections to spinal cord, 698
  in reticular formation, 692
  rostral, serotonergic projections from, 874f
  serotonergic projection to cerebellar cortex, 632
  serotonergic system originates in, 698
  and sleep induction, 800
  spinal system, serotonergic, 541
Rapid changes, detection of by ganglion cells, 411
Rapid eye movement sleep, 794–795
  behavior disorder, 811
  fragmentation, in narcolepsy, 814
  rebound, 809
Rate modulation, 559d
Reaction time, to stimuli, simple versus choice, 619
Reading
  brain pathway to process word recognition, PET imaging, 13f
  disorders, localization, 849–850
Reafference, 627d
Receptive fields, 409d
  center–surround in bipolar cells, 412–414
    central neurons of somatic sensory system, 374–377
    cerebral cortex, mechanisms, 1026–1027
    circular in neurons of lateral geniculate nucleus, 426
    comparison of in retina, lateral geniculate nucleus, and primary visual cortex, 428f
    complex cells in primary visual cortex, 430
    concentric, transformation into linear segments and boundaries by primary visual cortex, 427–431
    concentric arrangement in concentric single-opponent cells, 473f
    gradient of excitatory activity, 374
    gradient of inhibitory activity, 374
    large in inferotemporal cortex, 358–359
    larger in neurons involved in later stages of cortical processing, 380
    P and M cells of retinal ganglion cells, 412
    retinal ganglion cells, 408–411
    of sensory receptor, 334d
    simple cell in primary visual cortex, 429f
Receptor activation, in chemical synaptic transmission, 131–132
Receptor-channels. *See* Ion channels, transmitter gated
Receptor neurons, and relay nuclei, 334
Receptor potential, 26d, 28f, 336d
  features, 29t
  input signal in sensory neurons, 27
  ion channels and signal properties, 166f
Receptor proteins
  synaptic, 27
  transducing, 27
Receptor theory, development of, 132
Receptors. *See also* Autoreceptors; Sensory receptors
  acetylcholine, 136
    and acetylcholine receptor inducing activity, 938
    agrin induces clustering of on muscle membrane, 938f
    in autonomic ganglia, 768
    change in channel properties due to change in subunit composition, 940
    control of synthesis, 939
    identification of antibodies to, 237–238
    loss of extrajunctional, 938
    muscarinic and nicotinic, 183
    nicotinic, antibodies against and myasthenia gravis, 235–243
    nicotinic, cAMP protein kinase phosphorylates subunits of, 187
    nicotinic, change in functional properties after muscle innervation, 939–940
    nicotinic, distribution of after innervation of skeletal muscle, 937–939
    nicotinic, mRNA sequence of alpha-subunit, 34f, 35
    nicotinic, presynaptic neurons regulate development of, 941
    nicotinic, structure, 146–148
    number increased on muscle surface by calcitonin gene-related peptide, 938
  activated by norepinephrine in hippocampus, 696
  activation
    by movements, 588
    for smell and taste, 513
  alpha-adrenergic, action of neurally released norepinephrine on, 772
  aminergic, electroconvulsive therapy and possible changes in sensitivity, 872
  AMPA, mediate EPSP produced in motor neurons by Ia afferent fibers, 158
  androgen, absence of in androgen insensitivity syndrome, 962
  benzodiazepine, and mechanism of flurazepam's sleep-inducing properties, 810
  beta-adrenergic
    and action of neurally released catecholamines on heart muscle cells, 771

and desensitization by protein phosphorylation, 186
chemical transmitters
   biochemical features, 132
   molecular mechanisms of gating ion channels, 132–133
cutaneous
   dynamic properties of are matched by those of central
      neurons to which they are connected, 379
   and spatial pattern of neuronal activity in peripheral fibers
      and Brodmann's areas 3b and 1, 379f
directly gated ion channel, 174f
dopamine
   blocked by antipsychotic drugs, 860–861
   in brain, imaged by PET, 314f
   types, 861f
dopaminergic, effects of long-term treatment with
      antipsychotic drugs on, 657
effect of phosphorylation, 187f
endogenous opioid, in brain, 394–396
GABA
   as multisubunit transmembrane protein, 162–164
   benzodiazepines enhance activity of, 881–882
   primary structure, 162–163
G-protein-coupled family, 174f, 175f. *See also*
      Alpha-adrenergic receptor; Beta-adrenergic receptor;
      Serotonin receptor; Dopamine receptor; Muscarinic ACh
      receptor; Neuropeptide receptor; Rhodopsin receptor
   and olfactory receptors, 515
glucocorticoid, concentration of in hippocampus, 746
glutamate
   binding to, 158
   as multisubunit transmembrane protein, 162–164
   NMDA, PCP binds to, 866
   regulation of excitatory synaptic actions in CNS neurons,
      157f
   types, 158
glycine
   as multisubunit transmembrane protein, 162–164
   primary structure, 163
gonadal steroid, location in cell nucleus, 965–967, 966f
gustatory, 518–524
   types, 521–524
hair follicle, 345
inner ear, hair cells, 483–489
ionophoric, 132
kainate, channel regulation by, 157f
membrane proteins for differentiation signal, 888
muscle, and stretch reflexes, 564–580
nerve growth factor, transmembrane protein, 931
neurotransmitter
   determines action of transmitter, 132
   major functions, 173
NMDA
   blocked by APV, 159
   channel regulation by, 157f
   as doubly gated channel, 1020
   excessive activation, 658
   glutamate binds to, 158
   inhibited by PCP, 159
   role in generating locomotor pattern, 593
nociceptive, activated by noxious insults, 386–388
noradrenergic, linked to second-messenger system, 877t
olfactory
   activate second-messenger pathways, 515
   as bipolar neurons, 513
   location, 513f
   may belong to family of G-protein-coupled receptors, 515
   presentation of odorants may involve olfactory binding
      protein, 514–515
   project to olfactory bulbs, 514f
   responses to isoamylacetate and camphor, 515f
opiate, classes, 395–396

quisqualate, channel regulation by, 157f
quisqualate B, coupled to second-messenger pathway,
   171
postsynaptic dopamine, types, 862t
sensory
   and recruitment of postural mechanisms, 597
   sensitivity to physical energy, 333–334
serotonin
   action of antipsychotic drugs on, 866
   classification, 875t
   hallucinogens acts on, 866
   and second-messenger system, 875
sevenless gene of *Drosophila* as for signal transmitted from
      neighboring photoreceptor cells, 901
skin, 367–368
   of face, 702
somatic, density of, 374. *See also* Mechanoreceptors
specificity, 327
steroid, cells expressing in nervous system, 966
taste
   in taste buds, 520
   innervation by primary afferent neurons, 519–521
that gate ion channels directly, 173. *See also* Glutamate
      receptors; ACh; GABA; NMDA; Glycine;
      Kainate-Quisqualate
that gate ion channels indirectly, 173. *See also*
      G-protein-coupled receptors
transmitter, and desensitization, 186–187
trk encodes for NGF, 933
trk B protein, for BDNF and NT3, 933
unique stimulus activating is adequate stimulus, 331
vestibular hair cells, 503
warmth, 344f
Reciprocal innervation, 585d
   muscle, 561, 561f
Reciprocal interpretation, method to study neural activity
      distribution across population of neurons, 375
Rectifier
   behavior of electrical synapse as, 125
   ion channel behavior as, 73
Rectus muscles, eye, 665, 665f
Recurrent inhibition, 585d
Red nucleus, 288f, 542f
   lesion, 729
   origin of rubrospinal tract, 541
   projection of dentate nucleus to, 637
   transection of brain stem about, 604
Reeler mutant, use in defining properties and projections of
      cerebral cortex neurons, 909
Referred pain, mechanism, 388, 389
Reflexes, 565d
   automatic and stereotypes, mediated by spinal cord neuronal
      circuits, 539
   carotid sinus, and blood pressure control, 771f
   circuit
      as negative feedback loop, 577
      and nucleus of the solitary tract, 767
   closed loop or open loop control, 663
   components, timing coordinated by interneuronal networks,
      582, 584
   coordination of visual and auditory by midbrain, 9t
   dorsal root ganglion connection with interneurons and motor
      neurons of spinal cord mediate, 286
   hyperactive, sign of damage to corticospinal tract, 717
   jaw, 706
   pupillary light, autonomic control, 772–773
   responses, 534
   reversal, 594
   signals that produce, 30f
   spatial and temporal organization, 582, 584
   spinal

Reflexes [cont.]
  adaptability to body postures, 590
  after transection of spinal cord dependent on conditions of postural support, 590f, 600
  consisting of rhythmic movements, 589–590
  stimulation of nuclei in medulla inhibits, 602
  stimulation of nuclei in pons facilitates, 602
  the stretch reflex, 564–580
  stretch, 564–580
    sympathetic dystrophy syndrome, 387–388d
    systems, 31, 31f
Reflexive memory, characteristics, 1002
Refractoriness, following action potential, 110
Regeneration, peripheral axons, role of Schwann cells, 264
Reinnervation, of damaged muscle, 940f
Reissner's membrane, 483f, 484f
Relative refractory period, 110d
Relay interneurons, 22d
Relay nuclei, 334d
  in central nervous system, processing sensory information, 369
  process sensory information about touch, 367–370
  sensory
    complex inputs in dorsal column, 369f
    inhibitory pathways, 369
  thalamic, 289–290
  types, 279
Release phenomena, 545d
REM sleep. See Sleep, rapid eye movement
Renin, role in water regulation, 757
Renshaw cells, 42d
  divergent connections, 586
  inhibitory connections with Ia inhibitory interneurons acting on antagonist motor neurons, 585–586
  as part of negative feedback loop in motor neurons, 585–586
Reorganization
  capacity of cerebral cortex for, 1025
  at level of dorsal column nuclei, 1026
Reserpine
  precipitates depressive symptoms, 875
  site of action
    in noradrenergic transmission, 879f
    in serotonergic transmission, 878f
  treatment, schizophrenia, 858
Resistance, (resistor) 1034d
  axoplasmic, effect on signal conduction efficiency, 97–100
  behavior of electrical synapse as, 125
  ion channel behavior as, 69
  membrane, effect on efficiency of signal conduction, 97–100
  reciprocal relationship to conductance, 95–96
Resistive membrane current, 96d
Resonance hypothesis, 914d
Respiration, spontaneous, lack of as sign of brain death, 818
Response
  conditioned, 998d
  unconditioned, 998d
Response elements, enhancer elements, 189d
Rest and digest reaction, 761
Restiform body, 510f
Resting length, 552d
Resting membrane potential, 26d, 82d
  as baseline, 27
  and Cl^-, 88
  CNS neuron, 160
  determination of, 82–84
  and effect of electrogenic pump, 94
  equation to describe as function of Na^+, K^+, and Cl^- permeant ions, 93–94
  generation of in cell permeable only to K^+, 85f
  ion channels and signal properties, 166t
  and nongated Na^+ and K^+ channels, 86f
  quantification with Goldman equation, 88–89

as signaling mechanism, 26
  steady, requirements for, 86–87
Restless leg syndrome, 806d
Restoring force, 552d
Restriction enzymes, use in RFLP detection, 254
Restriction fragment length polymorphisms
  identification of genes responsible for disease, 253
  methods for detection, 254
Reticular formation, 288f, 363f, 681
  axons in spinoreticular tract end on neurons of, 362
  axons of anterolateral system terminate in, 359
  contains networks of nuclei, 692–693
  and control of posture, 602
  distribution, 692f
  lesions, 799
  mesencephalic, organizes vertical component of saccades and smooth pursuit, 671–674
  modulation of segmental stretch reflexes and muscle tone, 692–693
  part of brain stem, mediates aspects of arousal, 275
  pontine, organizes horizontal component of saccades and smooth pursuit, 671–674
  projections of spinal nucleus to, 704
  role in
    behavioral arousal and levels of awareness, 692
    control of breathing and cardiac function, 693
    sleep, 799
  spinoreticular tract terminates in, 390
Reticular neurons
  produce extension during stance phase of locomotion, 604
  projections, 602
Reticular nuclei, thalamic, 291f, 292
Reticulospinal pathways, 542f, 603f
  components of medial brain stem pathway, 541
  coordination of posture and movement, 604
  medial and lateral, modulate reflex action during ongoing movements, 603
  mediate decerebrate rigidity, 542f, 605f
  modulation of sense of pain, 693
Retina. See also Ganglion cells
  amacrine cells, release of GABA by, 217
  anatomy, 401f
  classes of neurons, 409f
  concentric broad-band cells in, 471
  cone opponent cells code color in, 471–473
  development, 401
  distinctive morphologies of chemical synapses, 415–416
  fovea, and fine spatial discrimination, 333
  ganglion cells are output neurons of, 408–412
  gradient of TOP antigen in, 923f
  image on is inversion of visual field, 420–423
  information processing in, 400–417
  lesion of and transneuronal degeneration, 262f
  maps of in striate and extrastriate cortices and occipital lobe, 446
  neurons organized into three nuclear layers, 412
  neurotransmitters in, 401
  phototransduction in, 400–417
  projections to
    subcortical regions of brain, 423–426
    visual areas of thalamus, midbrain, and cerebral cortex, 423f
  receptive fields of neurons in compared with primary visual cortex, 428f
  regenerating axons form functional connections with target neurons in brain, 267f
  regeneration of axons after cutting optic nerve, 921–922
  regions, 421
  vertebrate
    determination of developmental fate of cells in, 892f
    differentiation of cells depends on signals received from neighboring cell groups, 891

Retinal, 405f
  isomeric conformations, 404
  isomers, structure, 405f
  light-absorbing portion of rhodopsin, 404
Retinal bipolar cell, 21f
Retinal disparity, 664d
Retinal image, correspondence with visual field, 423
Retinal neurons, classification according to cone inputs, 472f
Retinex, method for predicting colors of objects from responses
  of cone mechanisms, 476
Retinol-binding proteins, analogy of olfactory binding protein
  to, 514–515
Retinotectal system, adhesive gradient along dorsoventral axis,
  922
Retinotopy, 336d
Retrograde plasticity factor, 1022d
Retrograde transport system, and axolemma, 62f
Retrovirus
  use in tracing neural cell lineage, 891
  use to trace migratory paths of neurons, 910f
Reuptake, removal of neurotransmitter from synaptic cleft,
  232–233
Reverberating circuits
  illustration, 583f
  interneurons, 582
  and short-term memory, 1004, 1004f
Reversal potential, 139d, 139f
  determination of for EPSP, 155, 156f
  determination of for synaptic current, 156f
  of EPSP, 140
  same for single-channel current and total end-plate current,
  144f
RFLP. See Restriction fragment length polymorphisms
Rheumatoid arthritis, association of myasthenia gravis
  with, 237
Rhodopsin
  amino acid sequence, 478f
  genes, evolution, 478
  location and structure, 405f
  photoactivation initiates biochemical cascade, 406
  visual pigment in rod cells, 404
Rhombomeres, and segmental organization of hindbrain, 303,
  303f
Rhythmic pattern generation, in newborn infants, 594
Ribbon synapses, 415f
  retinal, 416
Ribosomal RNA, in rough endoplasmic reticulum, 53
Ribosomes, 46d
Right hemifield, 421d,f
Rigidity, 606d
Rigor mortis, 550d
Rinne's test, to reveal origin of hearing abnormalities, 483
rm. See Membrane resistance
RNA polymerase, role in transcription, 188–189
RNA splicing, alternative, in neuroactive peptides, 219
Rod signals, conveyed to ganglion cells by different pathways
  for moderately and extremely dark-adapted eye, 414
Rods, 409f
  absorption of light by visual pigments in, 403
  as convergent system, 402
  compared with cones, 402t
  comparison of amino acid sequences of visual pigments, 478f
  function regions, 403
  photoreceptor, 402–403
  structure, 403f
Rolpram, as antidepressant, 878–879
Rostral, in central nervous system, 274f
Rostroventral medulla
  enkephalin- and dynorphin-containing neuronal cell bodies
    and nerve terminals in, 395
  excitatory connections in as part of descending pathway
    modulating pain, 394
  and inhibitory connections in the dorsal horn, 394
  sensitive to morphine, 394
Rough endoplasmic reticulum, 52d
Rubrospinal tract, 541, 542f
Ruffini's corpuscles, 343f, 368
  slowly adapting subcutaneous receptor, 345
Rupture, saccular aneurysms, and subarachnoid hemorrhage,
  1048
rutabaga mutant, Drosophila, defect in cAMP cascade in,
  1018–1019
Ryanodine, bound by non-voltage-gated Ca^{2+} channel, 117

S

S-I. See Primary somatic sensory cortex
S-II. See Secondary somatic sensory cortex
s-Laminin, role in formation and operation of neuromuscular
  synapses, 941
S4 region
  charge movement in and gating, site-directed mutagenesis
    studies of, 117
  movement of during gating, 117f
  of Na^+ voltage-gated ion channel, and control of activation
    gate, 116–117
  of voltage-gated Na^+ channel, conservation of, 115–116
Saccadic eye movements, 661d, 661t, 663f, 664d
  controlled by superior colliculus, 424–425
  fish, extraocular motor neurons mediated by electrical
    synapses, 129
  generator, brain stem, controlled by cerebral cortex, 674–676
  higher control of, 674f
  horizontal, generated in pontine reticular formation, 671–672
  hypermetric, 672
  neurons for in pontine reticular formation, spike discharge
    patterns, 672f
  organized in pontine and mesencephalic reticular centers,
    671–674
  points fovea toward object of interest, 664
  role of dorsolateral prefrontal cortex and supplementary eye
    field, 676
  role of cerebellum in modulation of, by experience, 672
  role of oculomotor circuit, 652
  role of posterior parietal cortex and frontal eye field in
    generating, 675
  vertical, generated in mesencephalic reticular formation, 672
Saccule, 501d, 502f
  receptors respond selectively to vertically directed linear
    force, 503
Sacculus endolymphalicus, 669f
Sacral segments, spinal cord, 284, 285f
Sacral sparing, 713d
Saliency map, 460
Salivary glands
  autonomic control, 773
  cholinergic and noradrenergic responses, 771t
  innervation, 764
  protein. See von Ebner's gland protein
Salivatory nuclei
  parasympathetic preganglionic nuclei, 766
  superior and inferior, in general visceral motor column, 690
Salt, innate hunger for, 527
Saltatory conduction, 101–102d
Saltiness, taste quality, 523
Sapid stimuli, 518d
  response of taste buds to, 518, 521f
Sarcoma tissue, evokes extensive growth of sensory fibers into
  tumor, 930–931
Sarcomere
  contraction of produces movement and force, 548–555
  cross section, 549f
  fibrillar proteins composing, 549
  shortening and muscle contraction, 550f
  structure, 549

Sarcoplasmic reticulum, 549d
Saturation, color, determined by degree to which all three cones are stimulated to the same degree by object and background, 476
Saxitoxin, 112
Scala media, 482d
Scala tympani, 482d
  perilymph in, 484f
Scala vestibuli, 482d
  perilymph in, 484f
Scalae, 482d
Scalp recording. See Electroencephalogram
Scanning-speech, 644d
Scarpa's ganglia, 669f. See also Vestibular ganglion
Schaffer collateral synapses
  hippocampus, 1019
  maintenance phase, long-term potentiation of, 1022f
Schizophrenia, 853–868, 855d
  and alteration of structure of genes, 1028
  anatomical changes in brain in some patients, 857–858
  as disorder in prefrontal cortical activation, 864–865
  catatonic, 855
  diagnosis, 855–856
  different disturbances in dopaminergic transmission, 863
  differentiation from drug-induced psychoses, manic depressive illness, paranoid states, 855
  excess dopaminergic transmission may contribute to development of, 861–863
  future research, 867
  genetic predisposition, 856–857, 856t
  hereditary component, 993
  linkage studies of families with, 857
  neuroanatomical model, 865f
  other factors, 865–866
  paranoid, 855
  possible chromosomal location for, 857
  prodromal signs, psychotic epidsodes, and residual symptoms, 855–856
  reduced blood flow in frontal lobe during intellectual tasks, 863
  size and blood flow abnormalities in frontal lobe, 829
  symptoms associated with anatomical components of dopaminergic synapse, 863–865
  treatment, with antipsychotic drugs, 858–866
Schizotypal personality disorder, 854d, 857
Schwann cell, 23f, 39f, 43d, 935f
  as glial cell, 22
  origination of acoustic neuroma from, 720
  and regeneration of peripheral axons, 264
  secretion of laminin, 264
  synthesis of NGF, 264f
Scorpion toxin, 112, 115
Scratch reflex, 589d
  fictive, 590
Sculpturing, role of synaptic inhibition, 155, 155f
Secobarbital, treatment of insomnia, 808–809
Second messengers
  activated by G-protein to modulate ion channel activity, 133f
  activation by Ca^{2+} in NMDA-activated channel, 160
  activated by olfactory receptors, 515
  activation of in growth cones, 913
  Ca^{2+}-dependent, and release of growth factor in synapse stabilization, 956
  cAMP, increased in sensory neurons in sensitization, 1012
  common molecular logic, 175–182
  and desensitization, 186–187
  diffusible, water-soluble in cAMP pathway, 177–178
  direct action on ion channels, 185–186
  generated through hydrolysis of phospholipids, 178–181
  involvement in
    olfactory and gustatory receptor transduction, 336
    photoelectric transduction, 336, 336f
  and ion channel gating, 75
  interaction, 182
  ion channels regulated by, and olfactory transduction, 515
  linked to noradrenergic receptors, 877t
  mediate synaptic transmission, 173–193
  modulatory actions, 185
  neurotransmitter modulation of ionic conductance through, 771
  phosphoinositide, affect of lithium on, 880f
  and phosphorylation of ion channel protein, 182–185
  protein phosphorylation versus directly gated synaptic actions, comparison, 185
  quisqualate channel stimulates formation of, 157f, 158
  and regulation of gene expression, 187–191
  and regulation of transcription factor activity, 888
  role in chemotactic factor response, 917
  role of cGMP in phototransduction, 406
  and serotonin receptors, 875
  and stabilization of synapses, 954
  and taste transduction, 524f
  triggered by nerve growth factor binding to its receptor, 932
  synaptic, 174f, 175
Secondary motor cortex, 611d
Secondary somatic sensory cortex, 364, 368f
  removal causes impairment in discrimination of shape and texture, 370
Secretin, as neuroactive peptide, 218t, 219t
Secretory granules, part of major membrane system of nerve cell, 49
Secretory potential, Ca^{2+} current responsible for transmitter secretion into synaptic cleft, 197
Secretory proteins, 52–55
  distribution by axonal transport, 57–60
  formation of in association with endoplasmic reticulum, 54, 60
  modification of, after translation, 55
Seizures. See also Epilepsy
  absence, 785
  epileptic, large populations of neurons activated syncronously during, 786
  focal
    depolarization shift underlying, 787
    epileptic, scalp recording, 786f
  generalized, 786f, 787
  grand mal, 785–786
  induction of with electroconvulsant therapy for treatment of depression, 872
  Jacksonian motor, 785d
  petit mal, 785
  psychomotor, 785d
  temporal lobe, ictal phenomena during, 14
Selective attention, early study, 462, 464
Selective perception, sensory stimuli, 369
Self, sense of, neuroanatomic correlates of in brain, 15–16
Self-assembly, polymerization method, 62–63
Self-awareness, and split-brain experiments, 833–835
Semantic abilities, and aging, 976
Semicircular canals, 501
  effects on eye muscles, 669t
  habituation, 662
  in head movement, 661
  input to vestibulocerebellum, 634
  send eye velocity signal to brain stem, 667
Semicircular ducts, 502f
  arrangement of hair cells, 504, 506
  detect angular acceleration, 501
  organization of ampulla, 502f
  orientation within head, 507f
  response to angular acceleration, 506
Semilunar ganglia. See Trigeminal ganglia
Senile plaques, 977d
  in aging brain, 976

Sensory inputs, integration of in later stages of cortical
    processing, 380–381
Sensation
    duration, 333
    intensity, 331
    location, 331
    modality, 331
    relationship between intensity experienced and intensity of
        stimulus, 332
    role of thalamus in, 287–292
    sensory information used for, 330
Senses, steps common to all, 330
Sensibility, role of neuroactive peptides in modulating, 218
Sensilla, and detection of odorants and pheromones in insects,
    515
Sensitization
    biochemical sequence of steps, 1012
    and classical conditioning, 1016
    enhancement of synaptic transmission, 1012–1013
    long-term
        and facilitation of connections between sensory and motor
            neurons, 1014
        memory for, 1014
    molecular basis of in nociceptors, 387
    role of presynaptic facilitation in gill-withdrawal reflex in
        Aplysia, 1012f
    type of nonassociative learning, 998
Sensory aphasia, characteristics, 847t
Sensory association areas, inputs to motor cortex, 612
Sensory ataxia, spinal cord disorder, 719
Sensory axons, in dorsal root ganglia, innervate trunk and
    limbs, 286–287
Sensory component, language, 11
Sensory cortices, 276
    higher order, projections, 825
    inputs to motor cortex, 612
    primary and higher-order, 824t
Sensory evoked potential, 779d
Sensory experience
    as construction of the brain, 330
    not a direct encounter with physical properties of stimulus,
        330
    role in nervous system development, 946–948
    with no stimulus, 332
Sensory function
    integration with language by parietal–temporal–occipital
        area, 825
    postcentral gyrus, 8
    role of association areas of parietal lobes in, 831
Sensory fusion, 455d
Sensory information
    carried into spinal cord by dorsal roots, 275
    coding and processing, 329–340
    modalities. See Hearing; Smell; Taste; Touch; Vision
    necessary for control of movement, 535–537
    physiology, 330
    psychophysics, 331
    processed by projection neurons and interneurons, 369
    processed in series of relay regions in brain, 369
    processed by spinal cord, 9t
    processed by thalamus and transmitted to cerebral cortex,
        335
    threshold, 331, 332
    stimuli, selective perception, 369
    to correct movement errors through feedback and feedforward
        mechanisms, 534–537
    used for sensation, control of movement, and maintaining
        arousal, 330
Sensory input
    and triggering of postural responses, 597–598
    types of triggering postural responses, 597–598
Sensory level, pattern of sensory level as indicator of site of

spinal cord lesion, 715
Sensory loss
    in middle cerebral artery infarction, 1045
    in occlusion of anterior choroidal and penetrating arteries,
        1046
    in olfaction abnormalities, 518
Sensory nerve cell
    axons ensheathed in myelin, 43–45
    brain stem, 687
    central nervous system, receptive field, 334, 335f
    connection with motor neurons, 41f
    and divergence, 25f
    feature extraction by, 338
    frequency of discharge as function of stimulus intensity, 337f
    increase in stimulus intensity paralleled by increase in
        discharge rate of, 333
    innervating hamstring, stimulation of produces IPSP
        innervating quadriceps, 155
    input signal is the receptor potential, 27
    location of synaptic inputs, 42
    role in knee-jerk reflex, 38
    role of nerve growth factor in survival of, 931–933
    stimulation of produces EPSP in motor neuron innervating
        quadriceps muscle, 155
    synaptic changes in habituation, 1011
Sensory nuclei
    cranial nerves, 690
    in dorsal horn of spinal cord, 284
Sensory pathways, 327, 360d
Sensory perception, role of thalamus in generating, 289–290
Sensory receptors. See also Merkel receptor; Pacinian
        corpuscle; Nociceptors
    adaptation from constant stimulation, 337
    adequate stimulus, 338
    classes of specialized, 338
    committed versus noncommitted, 338
    dorsal root ganglion neuron, 342
    distinguishing anatomical features, 342
    mechanisms of neural coding, 334
    morphologies and organization, 333f
    population code, 337
    range of intensity of energy responded to, 338f
    receptive field, 334
    relationship between type and action potential conduction
        velocity, 349–351
    receptive fields and spatial discrimination, 345–346
    and recruitment of postural mechanisms, 597
    response to constant or sustained stimulation, 337f
    sensitivities, 334
        to physical energy, 333–334
    size of population stimulated, 337
    slowly versus rapidly adapting, 337
    specificity of, 338
    stimulus transduction, 334
    thermal, 343–344
    transformation of stimulus energy into electrochemical
        energy, 333
    translate stimulus energy into neural codes, 336–338
    tuning curve, 338
    types, 342t
        in hairy versus glabrous skin, 343f
Sensory relay nucleus. See Relay nuclei, sensory
Sensory systems, 327, 334t
    attributed mediated by, 331–333
    of brain, 330–529
    distinct pathways in, 280
    hierarchical and parallel organization, 333f, 335
    plan common to all, 333–336
    and quantification of stimulus intensity, 332–333
    somatic, modality coding, 341–352
    somatotopic maps, 328
    synaptic relays in, 279

Sensory systems [*cont.*]
  topographical organization, 280–281, 335–336
Septum pellucidum, 305d, 307f
Septum, cholinergic neurons, sensitive to trophic actions of
    NGF, 262
Serial processing, sensory and motor information, 784
Serine proteases, processing of neuroactive peptides, 219, 221
Serotonergic cell groups, in brain stem, 698f
Serotonergic pathways (system)
  antidepressant drugs act on, 875
  brain, 874f
  origin in raphe nuclei of brain stem, 698, 875
Serotonergic transmission, sites of antidepressant drug action,
    878f
Serotonin
  availability increased by monoamine oxidase inhibitors, 877
  biosynthesis, 216
  cortical loss of in Alzheimer's disease, 981
  effect on nociceptors, 387, 387t
  excitatory effects, 698
  and excitatory synaptic action, 183f
  and hypothesis for sleep, 800
  and induction of slow-wave sleep, 800
  inhibitory effects, 698
  key biosynthetic enzyme, 215t
  measurement of in depressed patients, 877
  mechanism of synaptic action produced by, 190f
  neurons containing in brain stem, 693
  neurotransmitter in cells at midline raphe nuclei of brain
      stem, 217
  production of short- and long-term facilitation, 1013, 1014
  and presynaptic facilitation, 208
  as neurotransmitter, 216
  receptors
    classification, 875t
    and second-messenger system, 875
  role in sensitization, 1012
  sleep-inducing, 798
  slow synaptic excitation, S-type K$^+$ channel, 183
  transmitter in rostroventral medullary neurons, 396
  uptake blockers
    antidepressant, 872
    structure, 873f
  uptake mechanism for, 233
Sertoli cells, and testes development, 960
Serum, comparison with cerebrospinal fluid, 1054t
Serum enzyme activity, to distinguish neurotropic from
    myotropic diseases, 246
Serum glutamic oxaloacetic transaminase, and diagnosis of
    myopathies, 246
Serum response element, 189d
Servomechanisms, analysis of homeostatic mechanisms in
    terms of, 751
Set point, 552d
  body weight, 753–754
    alteration by hypothalamic lesions, 755, 756f
  temperature, 753
Set-related neurons, 622d
sevenless gene, *Drosophila*
  cytoplasmic domain functions as tyrosine kinase, 901
  encodes membrane-spanning protein, 901
  receptor function, 901
  role in R7 photoreceptor cell development in *Drosophila*, 901
Sex chromosomes, 960. *See also* X chromosome; Y
    chromosome
Sex determining region of Y, gene induces maleness, 960
Sex hormones. *See* Hormones, sex
Sexual dimorphism
  asymmetry of cerebral hemispheres, 971
  in cognitive development, 970–971
  hemispheric allocation of cognitive functions, 971
  preoptic area of hypothalamus, 969

SGOT. *See* Serum glutamic oxaloacetic transaminase
Shadows
  monocular depth cue, 455
  perception of shape from, 444
shaker mutant, behavioral *Drosophila* mutant, 992
Sham rage, 747d
Shape
  perception of from shadows, 444
  represented in parvocellular–blob system and conveyed to
      inferior temporal cortex, 458
Shingles, use of to map areas of innervation of dorsal root
    fibers, 355
Shiverer mice, myelination in, 45, 45f
SI. *See* Primary somatic sensory cortex
Sialic acid, levels of in NCAM, 919
Sialylation, changes in levels of in NCAM, 919
Siemen, unit of electrical conductance, 1034d
SIF. *See* Small intensely fluorescent cells
Sign stimuli
  brow flash response, 994
  elicit species-specific behaviors, 989
  and smiling in babies, 994f
  in stickleback fish, 989f
Signal, transformation of signal carried by, 30–31
Signal conduction, 95–100
Signal detection theory, 332d
Signal peptidase, 53d
Signal receptor particle, 53d
Signal sequence, polypeptide, 53d
Signaling molecules, role in neural induction, 894
Signaling. *See also* Action potential
  local cell
    determinant of neural and epidermal cell fate, 898
    mediated by growth factors and their receptors, 898
  meaning carried by, 29
  neuronal
    cellular mechanisms, 121
    and ion channels, 66–79
  organization of in nerve cells, 26
Signals, as changes in electrical properties of nerve cells, 26–29
Signs, 854d
SII. *See* Secondary somatic sensory cortex
Silent areas, association cortices, 824
Simple cells, in primary visual cortex, 429–430
Simultaneous color contrast, key feature of color vision,
    470–476
Single-channel current
  has same reversal potential as total end-plate current, 144f
  recording, 68–69
Single-fiber electromyography, assessment of efficacy of
    neuromuscular transmission, 239
Sinoatrial node, action sympathetic and vagal transmitters on
    electrical activity of cardiocytes from, 772f
Siphon-withdrawal reflex, *Aplysia*, enhanced by classical
    conditioning and sensitization, 1016
Site-directed mutagenesis, use to test ion channel structure, 73
Size
  illusions of, 443–444, 444f
  perspective, monocular depth cue, 454f
Skeletal muscle. *See* Muscle, skeletal
Skeletal myotubes, clustering of acetylcholine receptors on
    induced by presynaptic neurons, 937f
Skeletofusimotor efferents, 567d
Skeletomotor system, 567d
  output, fusimotor output adjusted independently of, 573–574
Skew deviation, 667d
Skilled movements, involvement of primary motor cortex,
    somatic sensory cortex, 380–381
Skin
  cholinergic and noradrenergic responses, 771t
  glabrous, specific mechanoreceptors for, 345–346
  hairy, specific mechanoreceptors for, 345–346

mechanoreceptors in mediate touch, 344
receptors in, 367–368
receptors, innervation, 368
subcutaneous receptor types, 345
types of sensory receptors in hairy versus glabrous, 343f
Skin senses, 341
Sleep
active induction, and caudal brain stem, 816
as active process, 795
apnea, 812–813, 813f
attacks. *See* Narcolepsy
center, 800
characteristics of mental activity during, 798t
delta and theta waves associated with, 779
disorders, 805–819
disturbed, and psychopathology, 807
and dreaming, 792–804
factors that promote, 798–799
features of, 792
inducing neurons, in brain stem, 799–800
interaction with immune system, 798–799
mechanism for cyclical nature, 803
medications for, 808–810
misperception syndrome, 806d
normal range of, 806
onset REM, 813
paralysis, narcoleptic symptom, 813d
parasomnias associated with, 810–812
passive theory of, 793
pattern of, 795
and aging, 976
peptides, as neuroactive peptide, 218t
periodicity, 793
physiology linked to mental content of dreams, 797–798
problems magnified in elderly, 808
rapid eye movement, 794–795
behavior disorder, 811
biological importance, 795–797
decline for need during maturation, 795–796
deprivation and rebound, 795
entered directly from waking state by narcoleptic patient, 814f
fragmentation of in narcoleptics, 814
genetic programming of, 797
mental activity during, 798t
narcoleptic patients enter directly, 813
need for differs across species, 796–797
nightmares during, 812
pattern of, 795
penile erection during, 797
pontine–geniculate–occipital spikes during, 795
and recall of dreaming, 795
role of brain stem regions in triggering, 801, 803
role of cholinergic cells in, 803
shortened in endogenous depression, 870
suppressed by barbiturates, 809
suppression of sympathetic activity during, 794
threshold for arousal, 795
without atonia causes violent episodes, 811
serotonin hypothesis, 800
slow-wave, 793–794
incubus as parasomnia during, 812
mental activity during, 798, 798t
parasympathetic activity is predominant, 794
pattern of, 795
sleep terror nightmares during, 798
suppression of by benzodiazepines, 809
threshold for arousal, 794
stages of in which nocturnal enuresis occurs, 810
stages, 793–795
suprachiasmatic nucleus as biological clock for, 800–801
terror nightmares, during slow-wave sleep, 798

wake cycle, 793f, 798–801
Sleepwalking, 810–811
electrooculogram, electromyogram, and electroencephalogram during, 811f
Sliding filament theory, muscle contraction, 549
Slow axonal transport, 61f
components of, 58
and transport of cytosol in axon, 58–59
Slow-channel syndrome, and myasthenia gravis, 242
Slow-wave sleep, 793–794
sleepwalking triggered by arousal from, 810–811
Small intensely fluorescent cells, 903d
Small-cell lung cancer, and disorders of neuromuscular transmission, 242
Smell, 512–529
and activation of receptors, 513
conscious perception of involves orbitofrontal cortex, 518
conscious perception of involves thalamus-neocortex projection, 518
neural mechanisms associate it with nausea and stomach illness, 527
transduced by neurons in olfactory epithelium, 513–516
Smiling, as stereotyped sequence of movements, 993
Smooth endoplasmic reticulum, 53d
Smooth muscle, controlled by autonomic nervous system, 762
Smooth pursuit movement, 661t
organized in pontine and mesencephalic reticular centers, 671–674
role of cerebral cortex, cerebellum, and pons, 672
systems, 663f, 673f
Social behavior, effect of isolation on development of, 946–947
Social interaction, role in nervous system development, 946–948
Sodium amytal test
effect on mood, 832
to determine dominant hemisphere for speech function, 832
Sodium conductance (membrane conductance)
compared with potassium in voltage-clamp experiments, 109f
effect of depolarization on, 109f
similarities with K^+ conductance, 108
Sodium ion
calculation of passive flux and Na^+-K^+ pump, 94
channel at end-plate permeable to, 139–140
concentrated outside the cell, 82
conductance, calculated from Na^+ current, 108–109
diffusion of, 85–86
distribution across cell membrane, 84t
equilibrium potential for, 86
flux across cell membrane, 87f
flux through voltage-gated channel is regenerative, 142
and generation of action potential, 28–29
increase at site of cerebral infarct, shown in MRI scan, 323
increased in preventricular white matter causes interstitial edema, 1058–1059
local field strength, 68f
MRI scan showing distribution in brain, 322f
nerve cells at rest permeable to, 85
not required for neurotransmitter release, 195–196
passive flux through nongated channels balanced by active pumping, 86–88
synaptic channel at end-plate permeable to, 140
voltage-gated channel selective for, 141
and generation of action potential, 88
Sodium ion channel. *See also* Ion channels, sodium
activation and inactivation gates, 108–109
changes in charge distribution in give rise to gating current, 114f
charge immobilization, 115
nongated, and resting potential, 86f
opened by depolarization, 105
during refractoriness following action potential, 110

Sodium ion channel. *See also* Ion channels, sodium [*cont.*]
  relationship of density of with action potential velocity,
    112–113
  states of, 108–109
  time course of recovery from inactivation, 109f
  transmitter-gated, mediates EPSP, 155–160
  voltage-gated
    charges redistributed within membrane when open, 113, 115
    and generation of action potential, 105
    high density in node of Ranvier, 101
    belongs to same gene family as K$^+$ channel, 115–118
    kinetics, 105, 107
    mechanism for selection for sodium, 115–118
    methods for estimating number of, 112–113
    molecular features, 115–117
    role of S4 region in control of activation gate, 116–117
    secondary structure in cell membrane, 116f
    sparse distribution, 112–113
    subunits of, 115
Sodium lactate, and induction of panic attack, 881
Sodium scans, reveal cerebral infarcts, neoplastic changes, and
    metabolism in brain, 323
Sodium–potassium pump
  and calculation of counteraction of passive Na$^+$ and K$^+$
    fluxes, 94
  and dissipation ionic gradients, 87–88
  as electrogenic, 87
  and hydrolysis of ATP, 87
  in photoreceptors, 407
  and resting membrane potential, 26
  as transport protein, 68
Solitary tract and nucleus, 288f, 690
Solitary tract nucleus
  controls output of the autonomic nervous system, 766–768
  nucleus, modulates autonomic function, 767
  and sleep induction, 800
Somasomatic synaptic contact, 168
Somatic afferent neurons, spinal cord, 686
Somatic division, peripheral nervous system, 273–274
Somatic modalities, 341
  submodalities, 341
Somatic motor column, innervate somatic muscles of head, 687
Somatic motor neurons. *See also* Motor neurons, somatic
  brain stem, muscles innervated by, 686
  spinal cord, 686
Somatic muscles, head, innervated by somatic motor column,
    687
Somatic sensation
  afferent fibers that carry synapse on cells in dorsal column
    nuclei, 287
  Brodmann's areas concerned with, 370
  carried by dorsal columns of spinal cord, 284
  conveyed to cerebral cortex by two ascending systems,
    358–363
  function localized to parietal lobe of cerebral cortex, 7
  labeled line coding and pattern coding, 342
  localized to specific regions of cerebral cortex, 370–374
  pathways, ascending, 333f
  perception, principal pathway for is dorsal column-medial
    lemniscal system, 287
Somatic sensory cortex, 278f
  barrel arrangement, 708–709f
  Brodmann's areas 1 and 2, complex response properties of
    neurons, 380
  cell types, 364–365
  divisions of, 368f
  functional organization based on experience, 1025
  functional similarities with visual cortex, 436
  inputs
    by region, 378f
    organized into columns by submodality, 377–378
  neuronal connections in, 364–365

organization in columns, 378f
  primary. *See* Primary somatic sensory cortex
  processing of pain, 392
  recording potentials from noninvasively, 372
  secondary. *See* Secondary somatic sensory cortex
  spinal cord as first relay point, 354–358
Somatic sensory evoked potentials, measurement to diagnose
    spinal cord lesions, 716
Somatic sensory fibers, organization of in dorsal column of
    spinal cord, 360
Somatic sensory system
  anatomy, 353–366
  cellular level, 374
  cortical maps are dynamic, 1025–1026
  cortical representation, 370–374
  dorsal root ganglion neuron as sensory receptor, 342
  inhibitory interactions, 369–370
  integration of sensory inputs in later stages of cortical
    processing, 380–381
  modalities, 367
  modality coding by, 341–352
Somatic stimulus, detailed features communicated to brain,
    378–381
Somatosensory submodalities, conveyed by anatomically
    separate pathways, 378–380
Somatostatin
  as neuroactive peptide, 218t, 219t
  loss of in Alzheimer's disease, 981
  peptide in sympathetic neurons, 770t
  released by parvocellular neurons, 742
  structure, 742f
Somatotopic organization, 634–635
  cerebellar surface, 634f
  changes in may reflect common cellular mechanisms for
    associative plasticity, 1026–1027
  cortical, 707f
  maintained throughout ascending somatosensory pathway,
    287
  modification of by experience, 1024–1027
  motor areas of cerebral cortex, 610–613
  of motor portion of basal ganglia, 651
  motor system, 539
  nucleus caudalis, 705
  primary trigeminal fibers, 702–703
  spinothalamic tract, 713–714
  trigeminal sensory information in cortex, 707
  ventral posterior lateral and medial thalamus, 706f
Somites, 302d
Somnambulism. *See* Sleep-walking
Song, bird
  built-in auditory template for, 994
  dependence on early experience, 995f
Sound
  bone conduction, 483
  cues to localize provided by bilateral auditory pathways, 493
  frequency changes as result of motion of source or receiver,
    496
  frequency spectrum, tonotopic maps of in primary auditory
    cortex, 494–497
  individual hair cells tuned to different frequencies, 487–489
  localization
    neural model of excitatory and inhibitory interactions
      underlying, 494f
    role of medial and superior olive, 494
  pathway through ear, 482
  produced by vibration, 481–482
  range over which ear responds, 482
  resonance theory of encoding frequencies into neural signals,
    486
  selective response of cochlea to different frequencies,
    486–487
  in space map, in superior colliculus, 424

time and intensity as cues for localization, 493
wave
    amplitude correlated with loudness, 482
    frequency determines pitch, 482
    relationship to temperature and pressure, 482
Sourness, taste quality, 521
Southern blot hybridization, 254f
Spasms, sign of damage to corticospinal tract, 717
Spasticity, 546d, 578d, 606d
    and supraspinal lesions, 606
Spatial discrimination
    and receptive fields of sensory receptors, 345–346
    two-point, 374–375
        mechanism of in somatic sensory system, 376–377
        and separation of signals, 377f
Spatial event plots, 379d
Spatial information, processed by right posterior parietal cortex,
    623
Spatial integration, 103d
Spatial perception, disturbed in middle cerebral artery
    infarction, 1046
Spatial relationships, role of magnocellular pathway, 446–447
Spatial response tasks, electrical stimulation of prefrontal
    sulcus interferes with, 828
Spatial summation, 99d, 167d
    effect on neuronal integration, 168f
Speaking, brain pathway for processing word recognition, PET
    imaging, 13f
Special somatic afferent column, 690
Special visceral motor column, 688, 690
    innervate branchiomeric muscles, 687
Species-specific behaviors, 989
Specific hunger, 527
Specific pathway theory, taste perception, 526
Speech
    formants, 491
    perception of sounds, functional areas in cerebral cortex, 495
    relationship of lateralization of functions to handedness, 832
    sodium amytal test to determine dominant hemisphere for,
        832
    sounds, detection, 491
Spike generation, threshold affected by modulatory
    transmitters, 185
Spike-triggered averaging, 557d
Spike-wave pattern, characteristic of generalized epilepsy, 789
Spina bifida, defect of neural tube formation, 297
Spinal accessory nerve, functions, 684t, 685f
Spinal accessory nucleus, in special visceral motor column, 690
Spinal angiography, diagnosis of spinal cord lesions, 715
Spinal artery, brain stem, 725f
Spinal cat, and maintenance of balance, 593
Spinal circuits
    as central pattern generators, 591
    generation of rhythmic locomotor pattern, 591–594
    for locomotion, activated by tonic descending signals from
        brain stem, 591–593
    stretch reflex, 575
        adjust muscle tone according to behavioral task, 577
Spinal cord, 8f, 288f
    ascending pathways, 275
    clinical syndromes, 711–730
    clinically important ascending and descending tracts,
        712–713, 712f
    cross section, 284f
    descending pathways, 275
    developing
        alar and basal plates, 300
        mechanisms of segmentation, 302–303
        developmental plan similar to brain stem, 300–302
        direct analgesic effect of morphine on, 396
    disorders
        amyotrophic lateral sclerosis, 718

Friedrich's ataxia, 719
    multiple sclerosis, 718
    subacute combined degeneration, 719
    syringomyelia, 718
    as division of central nervous system, 275
    dorsal column
        anatomy, 360
        organization of somatic sensory fibers, 360
    dorsal horn, contains ascending projection neurons, 354
    effect of amyotrophic lateral sclerosis, 248
    effect of hemisection, 363
    embryonic development, 300f
        in neural tube, 297f
    female, masculinization by neonatal injection of testosterone,
        969
    as first relay point for somatic sensory information, 354–358
    formation from embryonic nerual tube, 298f
    function, 9t
    gray matter
        anatomy, 357f
        contains nerve cell bodies, 354, 356
        dorsal root fibers terminate in, 356
        layers of functionally distinct nuclei, 356f
        layers of, 354, 356
        structure, 283–284
    hemisection, 718
    intermediate zone, contain autonomic preganglionic neurons,
        354
    internal structure varies at different levels, 284, 286
    intra-axial versus extra-axial lesions, 715–716
    laminae, functions, 356
    lateral tegmental neurons provide primary noradrenergic
        input to, 696
    lesions
        diagnosis by measuring evoked potentials, 716
        produce characteristic syndromes, 716–719
        radiographic diagnosis, 715
    level of motor control, 537–540
    longitudinal disorders, 719
    mediate vestibular and neck reflexes, 600
    and mediation of some simple reflexes, 1005
    midsagittal section, MRI, 318f
    motor nuclei of, organization, 540f
    neuronal circuits mediate automatic and stereotyped reflexes,
        539
    nociceptive control pathways descend to, 393–394
    organization at different levels, 285f
    parasympathetic neurons of parasympathetic division located
        in, 766
    partial transection, 717
    raphe nuclei are principal descending serotonergic projections
        to, 698
    regions of, 284, 286
    sacral, parasympathetic preganglionic cell bodies in, 766
    segmental lesions, 719
    sensory and motor innervation of trunk and limbs, 283–287
    sensory and motor neuron classes, 686
    size in relation to vertebral column during development, 301,
        301f
    steroid receptors in, 966
    structure, 283–286
    transection, 717
    transverse lesion, 714–715
    ventral horn, contains interneurons and motor neurons
        controlling muscles of trunk and limbs, 354
    white matter
        afferent and efferent axons, 356f
        dorsal root fibers branch in, 356
        matter, myelinated axons in, 356
        structure, 284, 286
Spinal loop, as parallel mechanism, 617f
Spinal motor neuron. See also Motor neurons, spinal

Spinal motor neuron. *See also* Motor neurons, spinal [*cont.*]
  contact of axon with interneurons, 42f
  compared with oculomotor neurons, 667
  dendritic structure, 41f
  generation of action potential in, 155–160
  as multipolar cell, 21f
  role in knee jerk stretch reflex, 40f
  structure, 42f
  and synthesis of macromolecules, 46f
  transmitter-gated channels in, 155, 157
Spinal muscular atrophy, 249t
Spinal nerves, 275, 285f
  dorsal and ventral roots, 286
  as groups of peripheral nerves, 353
Spinal neurons. *See also* Interneuron; Propriospinal neurons
  divergence, 582
  functional organization, 705
Spinal nucleus, trigeminal nerve
  mediates pain and temperature sensation, 702–703, 705
  projections, 704
  subdivisions, 703, 704
Spinal reflexes, 565d
  for clinical diagnosis, 565
  habituation, 1010
  interneurons as component, 582–584
  and motor coordination, 581–595
  neural integration, convergence and divergence, 582–584
  role of inhibitory interneurons, 584
  stretch reflex, motor cortex functions in parallel with, 617
Spinal shock, 717d
Spinal tract, trigeminal nerve, 704f
Spines, dendritic, 39
Spinocerebellar tracts, 712f, 713
  affected by Friedrich's ataxia, 719
  cuneo and rostral, carry somatic sensory information to cerebellum, 636
  dorsal and ventral, carry somatic sensory information to cerebellum, 636
Spinocerebellum
  complete somatosensory maps of body in, 634–635
  functional region of cerebellum, 633
  input and output pathways, 638f
  major input and output pathways, 636t
  projection from primary motor and somatic sensory cortex, 635
  projections control medial and lateral descending systems in brain stem and cerebral cortex, 636–637
  role in movement execution and feedback adjustments, 642
  sensory input and role in adjusting ongoing movements, 634–637
  use of sensory feedback to control muscle tone and execution of movement, 637
Spinocervical tract, ascending nociceptive pathway in spinal cord, 390
Spinomesencephalic tract
  anterolateral system, 362
  ascending nociceptive pathway in spinal cord, 390
  ascending pathway transmitting nociceptive information, 391f
Spinoreticular tract
  anterolateral system, 362
  ascending nociceptive pathway in spinal cord, 390
  ascending pathway transmitting nociceptive information, 391f
Spinothalamic tract
  anterolateral system, 362
  ascending nociceptive pathway in spinal cord, 390
  ascending pathway transmitting nociceptive information, 391f
  evolution, 392
  lateral, 712f, 713
  neurons, descending inhibition of mediated partly by

activation of enkephalin interneurons in dorsal horn, 396
  signs of lesion, 718
  using somatotopic organization to diagnose chronic pain, 713–714
Spiny stellate cells, primary visual cortex, 427
Spiral ganglion cells, innervate hair cells, 489
Spiral sulcus cells, 485f
Spleen capsule, cholinergic and noradrenergic responses, 771t
Splenium, damage to and alexia, 849
Split-brain experiments, and consciousness and self-awareness, 833–835
SRY. *See* Sex-determining region of Y
SRY gene, induces maleness, 960
Stance phase
  of stepping pattern during locomotion, 591
  stimulation of reticular nuclei produces extension during, 604
Stapes, 482d
Startle reflex
  central program for, 990
  universal human behavior, 993
Startle response, as stereotypes sequence of movements, 993
Static bag fibers, innervation, 570
Static nuclear bag, 566f
Status epileptics, and glutamate toxicity, 160
Stelazine. *See* Triflupromazine
Stellate cells
  of cerebral cortex, 779, 781f
  chopper response, 492
  cochlear nucleus, 492f
  inhibitory interneurons, 632
  spiny, 779
Stellate neurons, in cerebellar cortex, 630
Stereocilia
  arrangement on surface of vestibular hair cell and polarization, 504f
  characteristics, 503
  organ of Corti, 485d, 485f
Stereognosis, 380d
Stereopsis
  demonstration of requirements for, 456f
  retinal disparity required for, 455–456
  role of magnocellular pathway, 446–447
  roles of magnocellular and parvocellular systems in, 448
Stereoscope, 455d
Stereoscopic cues, for depth perception, 455–457
Stereoscopic vision, 455
  parallels maturation of ocular dominance columns, 956–957
Stimulus
  adequate, as unique stimulus activating specific receptor, 331
  affects on reflexes, 990f
  attributes of, 331–333
  awareness of spatial aspects, 333
  conditioned, 998d
    as anticipatory signal for unconditioned signal, 999
  differing abilities of mechanoreceptors to resolve spatial and temporal features of, 346
  discriminative, 999
  duration, encoded in discharge patterns of receptors, 337–338
  information
    presented in series of action potentials by neural encoding, 334
    transmitted to central nervous system by conducted action potentials, 338–339
  intensity
    encoded by frequency and population codes, 336–337
    of and perceived intensity, 333
    coding increases in, 337
    sensory neuron frequency of discharge is function of, 337
  modality, encoded by labeled line code, 338
  physical properties of versus perception, 330
  quantification of intensity by sensory system, 332–333

relationship between intensity and intensity of sensation experienced, 332
transduction
  of energy into neural code by sensory receptor, 336–338
  into neural activity, 336f
  by sensory receptors, 334
unconditioned, 998d
Stomach, cholinerigc and noradrenergic responses, 771t
Stop transfer segment, polypeptide, 54d
Strabismus, correction early in life, 957
Streptomycin, toxicity to hair cells of semicircular canals, 661–662
Stress
  and alteration of gene expression, 1028
  behavioral, and induction of analgesia, 397–398
  and reactive depression, 870
  role of mesocortical dopaminergic pathway, 865
  role of neuroactive peptides in response to, 218
Stretch reflex, 574d
  amplitude and duration, 30–31
  contribution to muscle tone, 577–578, 604
  and discharge of muscle spindle afferents, 574–577
  flexor muscles, sequence of events, 575–576
  group Ia inhibitory interneurons coordinate opposing muscles in, 585
  hyperactive
    in extensor muscles in decerebrate posture, 604
    and spasticity, 606
  hypoactive and hyperactive, clinical diagnosis, 576
  input signal in, 27
  knee jerk, two-neuron circuit as, 24–25, 575–576
  modulation of gain in, 577
  as negative feedback loop, 577f
  neurons that mediate differ in morphology and transmitter substance, 38–43
  quadriceps muscle, neurons mediating, 154f
  segmental, modulation by reticular formation, 692–693
  spinal, and synaptic transmission between central neurons, 154–155
  spinal circuit, structure of, 575
  tonic and phasic components, 574–575
Stretch, and ion channel gating, 75f
Stria terminalis, 739
  descending projection of the amygdala, 737
Stria vascularis, 501
Striate cortex. See also Primary visual cortex; VI
  blob and interblob regions of, 446
  cellular basis of visual attention in, 460–461
  origin of stereopsis, 457
  retinotopic map in, 445
  role in optokinetic reflex, 671
Striatonigral pathway, 650
Striatopallidal pathway, 650
Striatum
  dopaminergic system projects to, 697–698
  loss of neurons in Huntington's disease, 656
Striola, 508d
Striosomes, modules of neostriatum, 651
Stripe of Gennari, primary visual cortex, 427
Stroke
  alters vascular physiology of brain, 1048–1049
  disease involving blood vessels, 1045
  effects of carbon dioxide in brain after, 1048
  intraparenchymal, rupture of microaneurysms as cause, 1047–1048
  neutrophils and monocytes enter brain after, 1057
  types, 1045
Stumble corrective reaction, 593
Stupor, 815d
Subarachnoid space, 304d, 1050d, 1051f
Subcallosal gyrus, part of limbic lobe, 737
Subcellular fractionation, for study of synaptic vesicles, 226

Subcortical aphasia, characteristics, 848
Subcutaneous receptors, types, 345
Subfornical organ
  action of angiotensin on, 757
  blood–brain barrier leaky, 1055
Subiculum
  part of hippocampal formation, 737
  receives input from hippocampus, 737
Submucous plexus, enteric nervous system, 766
Substance K
  as neuroactive peptide, 218t
  precursor structure, 220f
Substance P
  and activation of nociceptors, 387f
  concentration in primary afferent fibers in superficial dorsal horn, 390f
  contained with vesicles, 226
  in hypothalamus, 743
  loss of in Alzheimer's disease, 981
  mediate direct pathway from striatum, 652
  as neuroactive peptide, 218t
  peptide in sympathetic neurons, 770t
  precursor structure, 220f
  synthesis increased by nerve growth factor, 933
Substantia gelatinosa, 357f
  spinal cord gray matter, 356
Substantia nigra, 288f, 363f
  affected by Parkinson's disease, 981–982
  of basal ganglia, 648
  dense serotonergic projections in, 698
  inhibitory projection to colliculus, role in saccadic eye movements, 674
  loss of nerve cells and depigmentation of in Parkinson's disease, 655
  nigra, origination of nigrostriatal dopaminergic system, 863
Substantia nigra pars reticulata, projection to superior colliculus, 675
Subtentorial lesions, types, and diagnosis of coma, 816t
Subthalamic nucleus, 290f
  of basal ganglia, 648
  reduction of activity in Huntington's disease, 656
Subthalamus, derived from diencephalon, 298
Sudden infant death syndrome, and sleep apnea, 813
Sugar linkage, anchoring of protein to membrane, 55, 56f
Suicide, incidence among biological and adoptive relatives of depressed patients, 872
Sulci, 8d, 276d, 278f
  widened in some schizophrenia patients, 857–858
Sulcus limitans, 686, 690
Summation
  and convergent input to motor neurons and interneurons, 582
  excitatory and inhibitory synaptic currents, 169f
  extracellular currents, and alternation of neuronal excitability in focal seizures, 789
  of elementary conductance to produce miniature end-plate potential, 199
  of impulses in muscle contraction, 553, 554d
  in rods, 402
  in somatic sensory system, 376–377
  synaptic potentials in activated pyramidal cells of cerebral cortex, 778, 785
  synaptic potentials and neuronal integration, 167
  of temperature information in the hypothalamus, 753f
  temporal, 97d
  temporal and spatial, 167
  total end-plate current, 144f
  of visual input, 458
Summation columns, primary auditory cortex, 494
Superior cerebellar artery, 1042
Superior cervical ganglion
  accuracy of preganglionic innervation, 926
  morphological sex differences, 969

Superior colliculus, 288f, 509f
  axons distributed to descending tracts, 425
  controls saccadic eye movements, 424–425
  inhibited by basal ganglia, 675
  inputs and outputs, 674
  lesions, 674
  possible role in mediating visual attention, 460–461
  projections from retina to, 423f
  sensory maps within layers of, 424
  specific visual receptive fields in neurons of, 674
  transmits cortical oculomotor signals to brain stem, 674–675
  as visuomotor integration region, 674
Superior olivary nucleus, 510f
  trapezoid fibers terminate in, 494
Superior prefrontal convexity
  location, 827f
  subdivision of prefrontal cortex, 826
Superior temporal gyrus, stimulation of produces
    hallucinations, 830
Supplementary eye field, role in saccades, 676
Supplementary motor area, 539, 611d
  lesions, 619, 620
  role in programming motor sequences and coordinating
      bilateral movements, 619–620
  unilateral lesion, 621f
Suppression columns, primary auditory cortex, 494
Suprachiasmatic nuclei, hypothalamic, 739
Suprachiasmatic nucleus
  as biological clock for sleep–wake cycle, 800–801
  lesions, 758
  metabolic activity entrained to circadian light–dark cycle,
      801f, 802f
  role in regulating rhythm, 758–759
  sexually dimorphic, 968f
Supramarginal gyrus, 623
  lesion, 849
Supraoptic nucleus, 738f
  hypothalamic, oxytocin release by regulates milk ejection
      and uterine contraction, 744
  vasopressin release by regulates urine flow, 744
Supraspinal lesions, and spasticity, 606
Supraspinal system, requirement of for goal-directed
    locomotion, 593
Supratentorial lesions, and coma, 817
Supratentorial mass lesions, types, and diagnosis of coma, 816t
Surface texture, neural representation, 380
Surround inhibition, 779d
Swallowing, central program for, 990
Sweat glands, innervation, 764
Sweetness, taste quality, 521
Swing phase
  of reticular nuclei produces flexion during, 604
  of stepping pattern during locomotion, 591
Sylvian fissure, 278f
Sympathectomized animal, characteristics, 762
Sympathetic crisis, in panic attack, 881
Sympathetic division, autonomic nervous system, 764, 766
  activity of efferent fibers after peripheral nerve injury and
      burning pain, 387
  coordinate innervation of target organs with parasympathetic
      nervous system, 763f
  embryonic development of neurons, 300
  overactivity in panic attack, 881
  pre- and postganglionic neurons, 764, 764f
  projections of pre- and postganglion neurons, 764f
  regulation of cardiovascular function, 771–772
  release of catecholamines by, 770
Sympathetic ganglia
  cholinergic synaptic transmission in, 768–769
  functions, 768
  independent convergent excitatory connections, role of ACh
      and LHRH, 184f
  slow postsynaptic potentials in, 769
Sympathetic neurons
  CNTF promotes cholinergic differentiation, 905
  differentiation of from sympatho-adrenal lineage of neural
      crest cells, 904f
  growth conditions influence choice of neurotransmitter,
      904–905
  morphology of synaptic vesicles, 905f
  peptides in, 770t
  role of nerve growth factor in survival of, 931–933
  sensitive to trophic actions of NGF, 262
Symptoms, 854d
Synapse, 20d, 124d
  axo-axonic, depression or enhancement of transmitter release,
      207
  chemical
    current injection illustrated difference from electrical
        synapse, 125f
    plasticity of due to regulation of free Ca^{2+} concentration in
        presynaptic terminal, 209
    synaptic delay at, 131
  central nervous system
    directly gated transmission at, 153–172
    quantal analysis, 201
  chemical
    characteristics, 123
    distinctive morphologies of in retina, 415–416
    distinguishing properties, 124t
    pre- and postsynaptic elements separated by synaptic cleft,
        131–133
    synaptic delay at, 131
  common morphological types in CNS, 170–171, 170f
  developing, biochemical and morphological changes in,
      936–937
  distinctive ultrastructures of excitatory and inhibitory,
      170–171
  early experience and fine tuning, 945–958
  electrical. See also Gap junctions
    behavior as rectifier or resistor, 125
    bidirectional current flow in nonrectifying, 127f
    characteristics, 123
    current injection illustrates difference from chemical
        synapse, 125f
    distinguishing properties, 124t
    as either unidirectional or bidirectional, 124–125
    electrotonic transmission, 125
    features of behavior mediated by, 129
    gap junctions bridge pre- and postsynaptic elements,
        129–131
    rapid transmission across, 125, 127
  electrotonic, spread of inhibitory current from synapses along
      postsynaptic neuron, 169f
  as element of neuron doctrine, 6d
  excitatory on dendritic spines, 168, 170
  formation
    and neuronal survival, 929–933
    of is a gradual process, 935–937
  growth cone stabilization, 935
  inhibitory on cell body, 168
  modulatory on axon terminals, 170
  mechanism of cooperation and competition for stabilization
      of, 956f
  nociceptive, electron-dense translucent vesicles in, 389f
  number in brain, 121
  nerve–muscle
    components regulated by innervation of muscle, 940–941
    directly gated transmission at, 135–152
    elimination of during development, 942–943
    role of basal lamina, 941
    role of s-laminin in formation and operation of, 941
  role in transmitting developmental or regulatory signals
      between cells, 129

sites of on nerve cell, 168–171
stabilization by second-messenger systems, 954
types, 123
ultrastructure, 120f
Synapsin Ia,b, 228t
Synapsin IIa,b, 228t
Synapsins, inhibit synaptic vesicle mobilization, 227
Synaptic action
produced by chemical transmitter, 190f
mediating versus modulating, 185
second messenger-mediated, time course, 185
speed of influenced by transmitter receptor function, 133
Synaptic boutons, 42d, 136d, 136f
and transmitter release, 136
Synaptic cleft, 19d, 20d, 131f, 136f, 935f
localization of agrin, 939f
removal of neurotransmitter from terminates synaptic
transmission, 232–233
separates pre- and postsynaptic elements in chemical
synapse, 131–133
Synaptic connections
accurate formation of, 923–926
growth of new ones in long-term memory, 1014, 1016
high specificity of in formation, 915
selectivity of, 924–926
steps in, 936–937
Synaptic contact
sites of, 168f
types, 168
Synaptic inhibition, sculpturing role of, 155, 155f
Synaptic input
effect of membrane time constant on, 97
neuronal response to, 111
Synaptic membranes, structural details revealed by
freeze-fracture technique, 202
Synaptic plasticity, importance of cAMP cascade in, 1018–1019
Synaptic potentials, 26d
composition, 198
features, 29t
generated by inward current to end-plate region, 138
initiated by input onto dendrites, spatial decay of, 167f
input signal
in interneurons, 27
in motor neurons, 27
largest at site of origin at end-plate region, 138f
overlapping, 97
sign determined by type of ion channels gated by transmitter
in postsynaptic cell, 170
spatial summation, 99–100
time course of, 97
Synaptic relays, in sensory, motor, and motivational systems,
279
Synaptic terminal, degeneration of after axonal injury, 260f
Synaptic transmission, 123–134. See also Synapse
changes in effectiveness of in reflexive learning, 1010–1013
cholinergic in sympathetic and parasympathetic ganglia,
768–769
depression in habituation, 1010–1012
directly gated
at CNS synapses, 153–172
at nerve–muscle synapse, 135–152
enhanced in sensitization, 1012–1013
exocytosis versus glandular release, 227
facilitating effect of Ca²⁺ on, 197–198
four biochemical steps, 214f
mediated by second messengers, 173–193
and phosphorylation of transcriptional activator proteins
altering gene expression, 187–191
plastic changes in strength of connections, 1011
rapid loss of after injury to axon, 259–260
termination by removal of transmitter from synaptic cleft,
232–233

time course of events related to, 199f
types, 123
Synaptic vesicles, 199, 225–234
active uptake of neurotransmitter by, 226–227
ATP and chromogranin complexes with neurotransmitter to
decrease osmotic activity, 226
biochemical characterization, 226
calcium influx affects exocytosis and mobilization of, 205f
discharge of neurotransmitter from by exocytosis, 203
docking, controlled by influx of Ca²⁺, 203–206
electron microscopy view, 204f
filled with chemical neurotransmitter, 131
fusion, controlled by influx of Ca²⁺, 203–206
fusion proteins associated, 205–206
inhibition of mobilization by synapsins, 227
location, 201
membranes
differ according to neuron type, 231–232
proteins associated, 227–228, 228t
and membrane retrieval after exocytosis, 204–205, 204f
mobilization, 227
from cytoskeletal filaments by Ca²⁺, 206
number released modulated by level of calcium influx,
206–209
populations of, 225
quantum of neurotransmitter stored in, 201, 203
recycling of, 228–231, 57f
role
of Ca²⁺ in mobilization, 227
of p21ʳᵃˢ G proteins in guiding to release site, 206
in transmitter release, 227
stages of exocytosis and membrane retrieval, 230f
study by subcellular fractionation, 226
two populations in adrenergic neurons, 226
Synaptophysin, 228t
Ca²⁺-binding protein associated with synaptic vesicles, 228
role in synaptic vesicle recycling, 231
synaptic vesicle fusion protein, 206
Synaptosomes, 226d
Synaptotagmin, synaptic vesicle fusion protein, 206
Synchrony, possible mechanism for binding parallel pathways,
462
Syncope. See Fainting
Syndrome, validation of, 854
Synexin I, 228t
Syringomyelia
effects, 718f
symptoms, 718
Systematic desensitization, 1001
Systemic veins, cholinergic and noradrenergic responses,
771t

T
T-cell receptor, antigen-specific, role in autoimmune reaction,
241
T-tubule system, association with myofibrils, 549
Tabes dorsalis, deficits of touch and position sense in, 370
Tabula rasa, 329d
Tachykinins, as neuroactive peptides, 219t
Tactile information
information about conveyed to cerebral cortex, 359
mediated by dorsal column-medial lemniscal system and
anterolateral system, 333f
Tactile sensation, information about conveyed to cerebral
cortex by dorsal column–medial lemniscal system, 359,
360–361
Tactile stimulation, cortical responses in monkeys, 371f. See
also Cutaneous stimuli
TAG-1, structure, 919f
Tanycytes, 1055d
Tardive dyskinesia, 863d
as disorder of basal ganglia, 654t

Tardive dyskinesia [*cont.*]
  response to long-term treatment with antipsychotic drugs, 657
Target cells, influence of single cell on by divergence, 25f
Taste, 512–529
  and activation of receptors, 513
  inborn and learned preferences, 527
  information transduced by gustatory receptor cells, 518–524
  mechanism of coding as general principle of sensory perception, 527
  neural mechanisms associate it with nausea and stomach illness, 527
  representations in thalamus and cortex, 524–527
  transduction mechanisms, 524f
Taste buds
  afferents project to gustatory nucleus, 524–525
  location, 518
  response to sapid stimuli, 521f
Taste cells, electrically excitable, 520–521
Taste perception
  across-fiber pattern vs. specific pathway, coding, 526, 527
Taste pore, 519d
TATA box, DNA regulatory region, 188d
Tau, as membrane time constant, 97d
Tau proteins, in neurofibrillary tangles, 979
TDF. *See* Testes determining factor
TEA. *See* Tetraethylammonium
Tectopontine tract, descending, relays visual input to cerebellus, coordination of eye–head movements, 425
Tectorial membrane, 484f, 485d
Tectospinal tract, descending, reflex control of head and neck movements, 425
Tectospinal tracts, 542f
  component of medial brain stem pathway, 541
Tectum
  axon-repellent molecule in, 921
  precision of retinal axon projection onto, 921
Tegmental syndrome, midbrain, symptoms, 729
Telencephalon
  connection to hypothalamus, 747
  formation, 298
Temperature
  information about conveyed to cerebral cortex by anterolateral system, 359
  loss of sensation, 726t
  regulation requires integration of autonomic, endocrine, and skeletomotor responses, 752–753
  sensation, mediated by spinal nucleus of trigeminal nerve, 702–703, 705
  sense, mediated by anterolateral system, 362–363
  sensitivity, punctate nature of, 343
  set point mechanism, alteration of, 753
Temporal crescent, 421d,f
Temporal hemiretina, 421d,f
Temporal integration, 103d
Temporal lobe, 8f, 276, 278f
  bilateral destruction, 739
  bilateral removal and resulting behavioral syndrome, 747
  cerebral cortex, function, 7
  effect of electrical stimulation, 1006
  left
    deficits in patient with limited lesion, 15t
    lesion produces problems with memory of verbal material, 830
  lesions
    affect declarative memory, 1005
    in and aphasia, 10
  localization of affective traits, 13–15
  localization of word recognition during listening, 13f
  neuroanatomical correlation with normal anticipatory anxiety, 14f
  panic attack localized to, 14
  personality, 831
  posterior aspect of left inferior, lesion, 848
  removal of impairs long-term memory, 830
  right, lesion impairs memory of patterns of sensory input, 830
  role, in memory functions, 830, 1006
  seizures
    ictal phenomena during, 14
    involving limbic structures in, 785
  subarea of limbic association cortex, 829
Temporal resolution, 402d
Temporal summation, 97d, 167d
  drive membrane potential to threshold for action potential, 98
  effect on neuronal integration, 168f
Temporal–parietal cortex junction, localization of word recognition during listening, 13f
Tendon jerk, 576d
Terror. *See* Nightmares; Night terrors; Panic attacks
Testes, fetal
  hormones act in concert with maternal hormones, 962
  hormones secreted by, 961–962
Testes determining factor, gene for is on Y chromosome, 960
Testosterone
  effect on developing neurons, 965
  masculinization of the brain, 965
  metabolic pathways, 965f
  neonatal injection masculinizes female spinal cord, 969
  secreted by fetal testes, 961–962
Tetanic stimulation, 206d, 207f, 553, 554
Tetanus toxin, fast retrograde transport, 60
Tetrabenazine
  site of action in noradrenergic transmission, 879f
  site of action in serotonergic transmission, 878f
Tetraethylammonium
  blockade of voltage-gated K^+ channel, 107
  blocks voltage-gated K^+ channel, 194–195
  effect on pre- and postsynaptic action potentials, 196f
Tetrahydrobiopterin, required for tyrosine hydroxylase activity, 187, 190
Tetrodotoxin
  blockade of voltage-gated Na^+ channel, 107
  blocks voltage-gated Na^+ channel, 142
  blocks voltage-gated Na^+ channel, 194–195
  and determination of density of voltage-gated Na^+ channels, 112
  effect on pre- and postsynaptic action potentials, 196f
  effect on presynaptic voltage-gated Na^+ channels, 195f
TGF-beta. *See* Transforming growth factor-beta
Thalamic syndrome, 388
Thalamotomy, treatment, Parkinson's disease, 656
Thalamus, 288f
  appearance of amyloid plaques in, 977
  axons
    of anterolateral system terminate in, 359
    from terminate on pyramidal cells of primary somatic sensory cortex, 361, 362f
  circuits connecting basal ganglia with, 652
  in coronal section through diencephalon, 290f
  CT scan of hemorrhage, 1048f
  degeneration of postsynaptic cells in after retinal lesion, 261–262, 262f
  derived from diencephalon, 298
  fibers
    of anterolateral system synapse on neurons in, 362–363
    from solitary nucleus synapse in, 690
  function, 9t, 276
  input
    activates cortical neurons synchronously, 784
    to amygdala, 747
    to basal ganglia, 648–651
    to motor cortex, 611–612

lesions, 848
  and chronic pain, 388
major nuclei of, 291f
medial, as part of nonspecific arousal system, 392
medial dorsal nucleus, in olfactory tract, 517f
medial lemniscus
  fibers synapse on neurons in, 360
  terminates in, 287
mediates motor function by transmitting information to
    motor regions of frontal lobe, 288
nuclei of, 289–290, 291f, 291t, 292, 650
path of medial lemniscus to from the medulla, 289f
phasic bursts of electrical activity in during REM sleep, 794
as principal synaptic relay for information reaching the
    cerebral cortex, 287–292
processes sensory information and transmits to cerebral
    cortex, 335
projections
  of basal ganglia to, 650–651
  from retina to, 423f
as relay structure, 279–280
representation of taste in, 524–527
role
  in autonomic reactions, 288
  in maintenance of consciousness, 288
somatic sensory nuclei and projections to primary somatic
    sensory cortex, 362f
spinocervical tract terminates in, 390
spinoreticular tract terminates in, 390
spinothalamic tract terminates in, 390
as target of basal ganglial projections, 649f
ventral posterior lateral and medial, somatotopic
    organization, 706f
ventrobasal complex, stimulating electrodes reduce pain,
    393
Thalamus-neocortex projection, and conscious perception of
    smell, 518
Thermal sensation
  information about carried by ventral columns of spinal cord,
    284
  nociceptors, 343, 386
  as somatic modality, 341
  stimuli, activate nociceptors, 386
  receptors
    A-delta and C fibers, 350
    mediate warmth and cold, 343–344
    in skin of face, 702
    specialized sensory receptor, 338
Theta rhythm, hippocampal, during REM sleep, 794
Theta waves, 779
Thiamine deficiency, as chronic neuropathy, 250
Thick filament, fibrillar sarcomeric protein, 549
Thin filament, fibrillar sarcomeric protein, 549
Thinking, brain pathway for processing word recognition, PET
    imaging, 13f
Thiothixene, structure, 859f
Thioxanthenes, structure, 859t, 859f
  treatment, schizophrenia, 858
Third-messenger system, nuclear, 802
Thirst, regulation, 757–758
Thoracic segments, spinal cord, 284
Thoracolumbar division; autonomic nervous system. See
    Sympathetic division; Thorazine. See Chlorpromazine
Thought
  disorders of, 853–868
    versus disorders of mood, 869
  disordered in schizophrenia, 855
Threshold, 82d
  action potential, determination, 110
Thromboxanes, synthesis, 181–182
Thymectomy, as treatment for myasthenia gravis, 242
Thymic motor patterns, 534

Thymomas, and myasthenia gravis, 236–237
Thymus, benign tumors of and myasthenia gravis, 236–237
Thyrotropin, as neuroactive peptide, 218t
Thyrotropin-releasing hormone
  as neuroactive peptide, 218t
  released by parvocellular neurons, 742
  structure, 742f
Timing, importance of in associative learning, 1016, 1018
Tinel sign, and detection of peripheral nerve damage, 251
Tinnitus, 489
Tissue damage, sensitizes nociceptors, 386–388
Tissue osmolality, and control of drinking, 757
Titubation, 644d
Tongue
  gustatory receptors on, 518, 519f
  innervation of, 519f
  ipsilateral hemiparalysis, 726t
  loss of taste, 726t
Tonic cells, role in horizontal saccades, 671
Tonotopic neural map, 280
Tonotopy, 336d
Topographical maps, variation in from one individual to
    another, 1026
Touch, 367–384. See also Tactile information
  as somatic modality, 341
  deficits of in tabes dorsalis, 370
  mediated by mechanoreceptors in skin, 344
  sensory information processed by relay nuclei, 367–370
Toxins
  fast retrograde transport, 60
  and ion channel refractory state, 77–78
Tract of Lissauer
  and nociceptive fibers, 389
  spinal cord white matter, 356
Training
  causes expansion of cortical representation, 1026f
  long-term
    activation of cAMP-dependent protein kinase, 1014
    substrate proteins maintained in phosphorylated state,
      1014, 1016
Trans-regulatory region, DNA, 188d
Transcortical aphasias, characteristics, 848
Transcription, and regulation of gene expression, 188–189
  activator proteins, phosphorylation of in synaptic
    transmission, 187–191
  and altered gene expression in psychiatric disorders, 1028,
    1029f
  factors
    activity regulated by second-messenger pathways, 888
    control regions, 189
  regulated by
    gonadal steroid receptors, 965–967
    nuclear and cellular signaling proteins, 888
    in nucleus, 888
Transcytosis, and recycling pathway for synaptic vesicle
    membranes, 229
Transdermal microneurography, for study of relation between
    touch sensations and mechanoreceptor properties, 345
Transducin
  and amplification of cGMP by photoactivation, 406
  as member of G-protein family, 406
Transduction
  chemoelectric, 336f
  mechanoelectric, 336f
  olfactory, and second-messenger-regulated ion channels, 515
  photoelectric, 336f
Transformation, of neural information during stretch reflex,
    30–31
Transforming growth factor-beta, as mesoderm inducing factor,
    894
Transient gaze paralysis, 676
Transient hyperpolarization, follows action potential, 110

Transmembrane glycoprotein, neural cell adhesion molecule form, 918
Transmembrane proteins. *See also* Membrane-spanning proteins
  amyloid beta-protein precursor, 977–978
  nerve growth factor receptor, 931
  receptors for GABA, glycine, and glutamate as, 162–164
Transmission. *See* Synaptic transmission
Transmitter receptors, and desensitization, 186–187
Transmitter release, in chemical synaptic transmission, 131–132
Transmitter, 214d
Transmitter. *See* Neurotransmitter
Transneuronal degeneration, 261–262
Transport proteins, 57–60
Transporter carrier proteins, method of neurotransmitter release, 232
Transporter proteins, for GABA-1, 233
Transsynaptic degeneration, 261–262
Transverse myelitis, and spinal cord transection, 717
Tranylcypromine, structure, 873f
Trapezoid body, 494, 510f
Trazodone, antidepressant, 872
Treadmilling
  as directional polymerization, 63
  state of polymerization, 64f
Tremor, 653d
  cerebellar, 644
  symptom of metabolic coma, 817
Trial-and-error learning, 1000
Triazolam, treatment of insomnia, 809
Tricyclic antidepressants
  structure, 873f
  treatment, cataplexy, 814
Tricyclic compounds
  antidepressant, 872, 877
  block active reuptake of transmitter released by serotonergic and noradrenergic neurons, 877
  treatment, panic attacks, 881
Triflupromazine, structure, 859f
Trigeminal fibers, primary, somatotopic organization, 702–703
Trigeminal ganglion neurons, peripheral axons of, 702
Trigeminal mesencephalic nucleus, proprioceptive neurons of and neurotrophin, 3
Trigeminal motor nucleus and tract, 288f, 702, 707, 708f
  controls jaw muscle activity, 706–707
  in special visceral motor column, 688
Trigeminal nerve 288f, 294f, 360d
  branches, 701–702
  fibers, projections, 702–706
  functions, 684t, 685f
  innervaton of facial skin by, 702f
  mesencephalic nucleus, 702
  nuclei, locations, 704f
  nucleus, 510f
  sensory nucleus of, in general somatic afferent column, 690
Trigeminal neuralgia, 705d
Trigeminal sensory information, mapped somatotopically in cortex, 707
Trigeminal system, 701–710
  afferent and efferent components, 703f
  lesions, 705
Trigeminal tractotomy of Sjoqvist, 705
Trigger zone, 29d, 40d
  and control of membrane potential, 166
  within the dendritic tree, 166
Trimolecular complex, as molecular basis of autoimmune reaction, 241
Tritanopia, 479d
trk B protein, as receptor for BDNF and NT3, 933
Trochlear nerve
  functions, 684t, 685f

lesion, 667
Trochlear nuclei, in somatic motor column, 509f, 665, 687–688
Trophic, 929d
Trophic factors
  regulation of supply to motor neurons, 934
  role in regulating number of synapses, 943
  support survival of spinal motor neurons, 934
Tropic spastic paraparesis, and spinal cord degeneration, 719
Tropolone, site of action in noradrenergic transmission, 879f
Tropomyosin, thin filament protein, 549
Troponin
  calcium binds to, 550
  thin filament protein, 549
True equilibrium, state of polymerization, 64f
Trunk
  sensory and motor innervation of by spinal cord, 283–287
  sensory neurons that innervate originate in dorsal root ganglia, 286–287
TTX. *See* Tetrodotoxin
Tuberoinfundibular dopaminergic system, function and role in schizophrenia, 863, 864f
Tubocurarine, binds to ACh receptor and blocks neuromuscular transmission, 138
Tufted cells, 516f, 517f
  projection of, 517
Tumor necrosis factor, sleep-promoting, 798
Tuning curve, for sensory receptor, 338
Turner's syndrome
  abnormal sex chromosomes in, 960
  characteristics, 962
Twin studies, and genetic predisposition for schizophrenia, 856–857
Twitch, muscle, time required, 553, 554d
Twitch contraction time, measurement, 558
Two-point threshold, 333
Tympanic membrane, 482d
Tyramine, neurotransmitter in invertebrate nervous systems, 216
Tyrosine hydroxylase
  and immunofluorescence histochemical localization of, 680f
  and synthesis of norepinephrine, 187
  synthesis increased by nerve growth factor, 933
Tyrosine kinases
  cytoplasmic domain of *Drosophila sevenless* protein functions as, 901
  domains, 179f
  second-messenger pathway, 191

U

Ubiquitin, posttranslational modification, 52
unc-86, gene encoding DNA binding protein that regulates gene transcription in *C. elegans*, 891
Uncal herniation, 817d
Unconditioned stimulus, proteins capable of responding to signals from and learning, 1023
Unipolar neurons, description, 20, 21f
Unit synaptic potential, 198d
  effect of external Ca^{2+} concentration on, 200
Upper motor neuron syndrome, 546
Ureter, cholinergic and noradrenergic responses, 771t
Urinary bladder, cholinergic and noradrenergic responses, 771t
Urine flow, regulated by vasopressin release, 744
Uterine contraction, regulation by oxytocin release, 744
Uterus, cholinergic and noradrenergic responses, 771t
Utricle, 501d, 502f
  macula of, 507f
  reponds to linear acceleration, 506–508

V

V1. *See* Striate cortex; Primary visual cortex
V2, striped regions as relay points for visual pathways, 446. *See* Visual cortex

V5. *See* Middle temporal area
V5a. *See* Medial superior temporal area
Vacuolar myopathy, spinal cord degeneration in AIDS patients, 719
Vacuum activity, 990d
Vafusstoff, vagus substance. *See* Acetylcholine
Vagus nerve, functions, 684t, 685f
    dorsal motor nucleus of, in general visceral motor column, 690
    motor nucleus, activation of and decrease in heart rate and cardiac contractility, 772
Valium. *See* Diazepam
VAMP-1,2, 228t
Vascular lesions. *See* Lesions, vascular
Vascular syndromes, 1045–1048
Vascular volume, and control of drinking, 757
Vasculature, brain, 724f
Vasoactive intestinal peptide
    corelease with ACH, 221
    as neuroactive peptide, 218t
    sleep-inducing, 798
    in sympathetic neurons, 770t
Vasogenic brain edema, 1057
Vasopressin
    effect of on antipyretic area of brain, 753
    as neuroactive peptide, 218t
    release of regulates urine flow, 744
    released by magnocellular neuroendocrine neurons, 741
    strong release of associated with vomiting, 744
    structure and function, 741
Vasovagal syncope, 815
VAT-1, 228t
Ventral, in central nervous system, 274f
Ventral anterior nucleus, thalamic, 650
Ventral columns
    spinal cord white matter, 356
    white matter of spinal cord, 284
Ventral commissure
    development from floor plate, 300
    spinal cord, 284
Ventral horn, spinal cord gray matter, 283–284
Ventral lateral nucleus, thalamic, 650
    inputs to primary motor cortex, 611–612
Ventral posterior lateral nucleus, 360d
Ventral posterior medial nucleus, 360d
    projections, 707
Ventral posterior nucleus, 360d
Ventral posterolateral nucleus, inputs to primary motor cortex, 611–612
Ventral roots, of spinal nerves, 275
Ventral syndrome, midbrain, symptoms, 728–729
Ventral tegmental area, 738f
    lesions, 863
    origination of mesocortical dopaminergic system, 863
    origination of mesolimbic dopaminergic system, 863
Ventricles, brain, 306f
    arise from cavities of embryonic brain vesicles, 303–304
    imaging with pneumoencephalogram, 311
    enlarged in Alzheimer's disease, 858, 977
    lateral, enlarged in some schizophrenia patients, 857–858
    third, enlarged in some schizophrenia patients, 857–858
Ventromedial hypothalamic nucleus, 738f
    lesion, 755
    role in control of food intake, 754–755
Vergence system
    aligns eyes to look at targets with different depths, 661t, 664
    organized in midbrain, 673–674
Vermis, 628d
    input and output pathways, 638f
    major input and output pathways, 636t
Vertebral arteries, blood supply to brain stem, 725f
Vertebral column, size in relation to spinal cord during

development, 301, 301f
Vestibular apparatus, receptor system, 503
Vestibular end organs, 669f
Vestibular ganglion, anatomy, 508
Vestibular hair cells. *See* Hair cells, vestibular
Vestibular labyrinth
    central connections, 508–510
    in head movement, 661
Vestibular nerve, 510f, 669f
    cutting reduces decerebrate rigidity, 604
    firing of in relation to direction of hair cell bending, 506f
    left, effect of lesion on eye movement, 722f
    projections, 602
Vestibular nuclei, 288f, 603f
    central connections, 509f
    connections with central nervous system, 508
    eighth nerve projects to, 501
    input from
        ampullae of semicircular ducts, 509
        integrated by reticulospinal tracts, 541
    input to vestibulocerebellum, 634
    nuclei of, 508
    projections, 667
    transection of brain stem above level of causes decerebrate rigidity, 604
    vestibular and neck afferents converge on, 602
Vestibular nucleus
    interneurons drive lateral rectus motor neurons, 668
    role in optokinetic reflex, 671
    in special somatic afferent column, 690
Vestibular receptors, trigger postural responses, 597–598
Vestibular reflexes, stabilize head and eyes, 600–602
Vestibular system
    disease of causes nystagmus, 668–669
    role in maintaining balance and posture, 500
Vestibulocerebellum
    diseases of, 635
    functional region of cerebellum, 633
    input to and projection from, 634, 634f
    major input and output pathways, 636t
Vestibulocochlear nerve, 508
    functions, 684t, 685f
Vestibulocollic reflexes, maintain head vertical, 600
Vestibulo-ocular reflex, 661t, 662f, 669f
    changes head velocity signal into eye velocity signal, 670–671
    compensates for head movement, 661–663
    coordinated in brain stem, 667–671
    horizontal, brain stem network coordinates, 668–669
    horizontal, pathways of in brain stem, 670f
    input is head movement and output is eye movement, 663
    mediated by medial and superior vestibular nuclei, 509–510
    and modification of cerebellar circuits in motor learning, 641
    modulated by cerebellum, 671
    under adaptive control, 662–663
Vestibulo-ocular system, plasticity, 510
Vestibulospinal pathway, 542f, 603f
    to axial and limb motor neurons, 603f
    components of medial brain stem pathway, 541
    maintain head vertical, 600
    mediates decerebrate rigidity, 605f
Vibration
    loss of sense of, 726t
    produce sound, 481–482
Vibrissal nerve, structure and projections, 707
Virchow–Robin spaces, 1050d, 1051f
Virus, infection, and spinal cord degeneration, 719
Visceral (autonomic) afferent neurons, spinal cord, 686
Visceral (autonomic) motor neurons, spinal cord, 686
Visceral function, regulated by hypothalamus, 9t
Visceral motor neurons, brain stem, muscles innervated by, 686
Vision
    affected in Broca's aphasia, 847

Vision [cont.]
  color, role of P pathways in lateral geniculate nucleus, 427
  compensation for loss of proprioceptive sensation, 537
  cone-mediated, acuity, 402
  creation of three-dimensional perception of world versus
    two-dimensional images projected onto retina, 441
  effect of early sensory deprivation on development, 947–948
  effects of lesions in retino-geniculate cortical pathway,
    436–437
  function localized to occipital lobe of cerebral cortex, 7
  mediation by parallel pathways, 445–449
  perception
    actual versus apparent motion, 451f
    attributes of disappear at equiluminance, 448
    context, 443–444
    creative process, 441–445
    hypothetical model of stages in, 461f
    illusions of size, 443–444, 444f
    image built up by scanning, 450f
    Muller–Lyer illusion, 443–443f
    stages, 401
    two distinct processes in, 460
    visual information processed in lateral geniculate nucleus,
      423
    winner-take-all strategy, 442
  processing
    conversion of concentric receptive fields into linear
      segments and boundaries, 427–431
    path of parallel processing, 446
  rod-mediated, acuity, 402
  stereoscopic, 455–457
  three-dimensional, requirements, 454–458
Visual association cortex, localization of word recognition
  during reading, 13f
Visual attention
  cellular basis of selective attention, 460–462
  controlled by parietal cortex, 675
  focusing perception, the binding problem, 459
  mediated by subcortical structures, 460
  role of claustrum and pulvinar, 434
  step in understanding conscious awareness, 462–464
Visual cortex, 278f, 445f. See also Ocular dominance columns
  area 17, binocular interaction and plasticity in, 948f
  direction selectivity of neurons, 453f
  effect of lesion, 437f
  effects of early visual deprivation on cellular responses in
    area 17 of, 947–948
  functional similarities with somatic sensory cortex, 436
  left, damage to and alexia, 849
  phasic bursts of electrical activity in during REM sleep, 794
  postnatal development of ocular dominance columns, 950f
  projections of lateral geniculate nucleus to, 949
  and segregation of input from two eyes, 947f
  visual deprivation reduces size of ocular dominance columns
    in, 949–956, 949f
Visual field, 421d,f
  correspondence with retinal image, 423
  impairment, in middle cerebral artery infarction, 1045
  map of contained in primary visual cortex, 426f
  retinal image is inversion, 420–423
  right, image in stimulates left temporal retina and right nasal
    retina, 833f
  zones, 421f
Visual illusions, Gestalt illlustrations, 441, 442f
Visual image
  detection
    of rapid changes, 411
    of weak contrasts, 411
  outlines decomposed into short line segments by simple and
    complex cells of primary visual cortex, 430–431
Visual inputs, trigger postural responses, 597–598
Visual map, in superior colliculus, 424

Visual pathway
  hierarchy of relay points, 431
  lesions, 437f
Visual pigments, 403
  amino acid sequences, 478f
Visual stimulation, glucose metabolism during assessed by
  PET, 314
Visual stimuli, brain regions activated by, 315–316f
Visual system
  detection of color of objects by comparison, 476
  Gestalt view of, 441
  parallel pathways, 447f
  pathways in, 280
  retrograde degeneration in, 262
  transneuronal degeneration in, 261–262
Visuospatial ability, and aging, 976
Visuotopic neural map, 280
Vitamin A, nutritional deficiency in and night blindness, 404
Vitamin B12 deficiency
  as chronic neuropathy, 250
  and degeneration of spinal cord, 719
VLc. See Ventrolateral nucleus
Vm. See Membrane potential
Volley principle, auditory nerve, 491
Volt, 1033d
Voltage amplifier, use in voltage-clamp technique, 106
Voltage changes, passive spread along neuron as electrotonic
  conduction, 99
Voltage, as resting membrane potential, 82
Voltage-clamp technique, 105. See also Patch-clamp technique
  demonstration of existence of two types of voltage-gated
    channels, 107
  electrical equivalent circuit, 108f
  and measurement of current flow during EPSP, 155–158
  as negative feedback system, 106
  study of time course and properties of current generating
    EPP, 138–139
  for study of voltage-gated channels, 105–109
  use of to measure conductance as function of membrane
    potential, 106
Voltage-gated ion channels, and generation of action potential,
  104–118
Voltage-sensitive dyes, 779
Volume conduction, theory of, 781d
Voluntary movements, 534
  proprioceptive sensations as consequence of, 347
Vomiting
  associated with vasopressin release, 744
  central program for, 990
von Ebner's gland protein, may deliver molecules to gustatory
  receptors, 515
VPLo. See Ventral posterolateral nucleus
VR. See Resting membrane potential
VT. See Threshold

W

Wakefulness, relaxed, alpha waves associated with, 779
Wallenberg syndrome, manifestations, 728
Wallerian degeneration
  after axonal injury, 260
  axonal injury, 259f
Warm-sensitive neurons, hypothalamic, 753
Warmth, mediated by thermal receptors, 343–344, 344f
Water intoxication, 1058
Water regulation, feedback signals for, 757
Waters of hydration, 67d
Watershed area, cerebral arteries, 848
Weaver mutant
  affects function of granule cells, 910
  granule cell migration in cerebellum of, 912f
  misaligned radial glial cells in, 910
Weber syndrome, midbrain, symptoms, 728–729

Weber–Fechner law
  applied to hearing, 482
  quantitative relationship between stimulus intensity and
    discrimination, 332–333
Weigert staining, based on degenerative changes in neurons,
    262
Wernicke's aphasia, characteristics, 846–847, 847t
  in middle cerebral artery infarction, 1045
Wernicke's area
  and language perception, 11
  in lateral view of cerebral cortex, 10f
  lesion, 844
  perception of speech sounds, 495
Whiskers, rodents. *See also* Vibrissae
  field, plasticity of central representation of, 708
  representation in cortex, 707–708
  target field, mouse embryo, localization of nerve growth
    factor, 932f
White blood cell count, cerebrospinal fluid, 1057
White matter, 276
  cerebellar cortex, 630f
  imaged with computerized tomography, 312, 312f
  spinal cord, 283d
White rami communicantes, 764d
Wide dynamic range neurons, process nociceptive information
    in dorsal horn, 389
Wiping reflex, nature of, 590

Wisconsin Card Sort Test, results with lobotomized patients,
    830
Wisconsin General Testing Apparatus, 828f
Word blindness. *See* Alexias
Word recognition, brain pathways for processing, PET imaging,
    13f
Work, negative versus positive, electrical charges, 1033d
Working memory, 827d
Writing disorders, localization, 849–850

X

X-rays, imaging brain with, 309–312
Xhox-3 gene, expressed as posterior-anterior gradient in
    Xenopus axial mesoderm, 895

Y

Y chromosome, gene for testes determining factor located on,
    960
Y-specific DNA clones, screening, 961f
Yawning, central program for, 990

Z

Z disc, separate sarcomeres, 549
Zeitgeber, 800d
Zinc finger, 189d
  proteins, 897

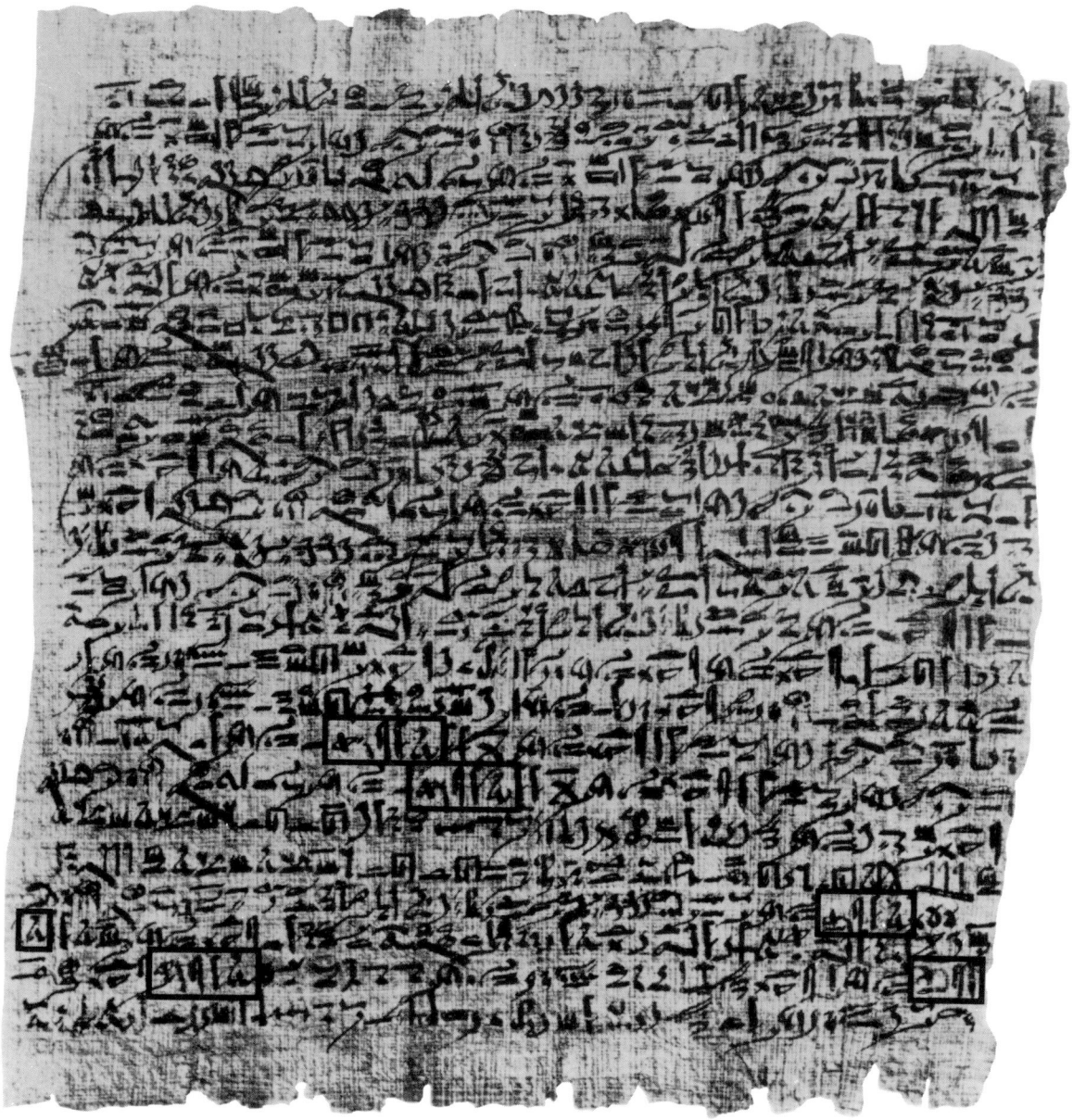

Columns II (left) and IV (right) of the Edwin Smith Surgical Papyrus

This papryus, written in the Seventeenth Century B.C., contains the earliest reference to the brain anywhere in human records. According to James Breasted, who translated and published the document in 1930, the word brain 𓄹𓏭𓏤 ('yś) occurs only 8 times in ancient Egyptian, 6 of them on these pages of the Smith Papyrus describing the symptoms, diagnosis and prognosis of two patients, wounded in the head, who had compound fractures of the skull. The entire treatise is now in the Rare Book Room of the New York Academy of Medicine.

Reference: Breasted, James Henry. The Edwin Smith Surgical Papyrus, 2 volumes. The University of Chicago Press, Chicago. 1930.

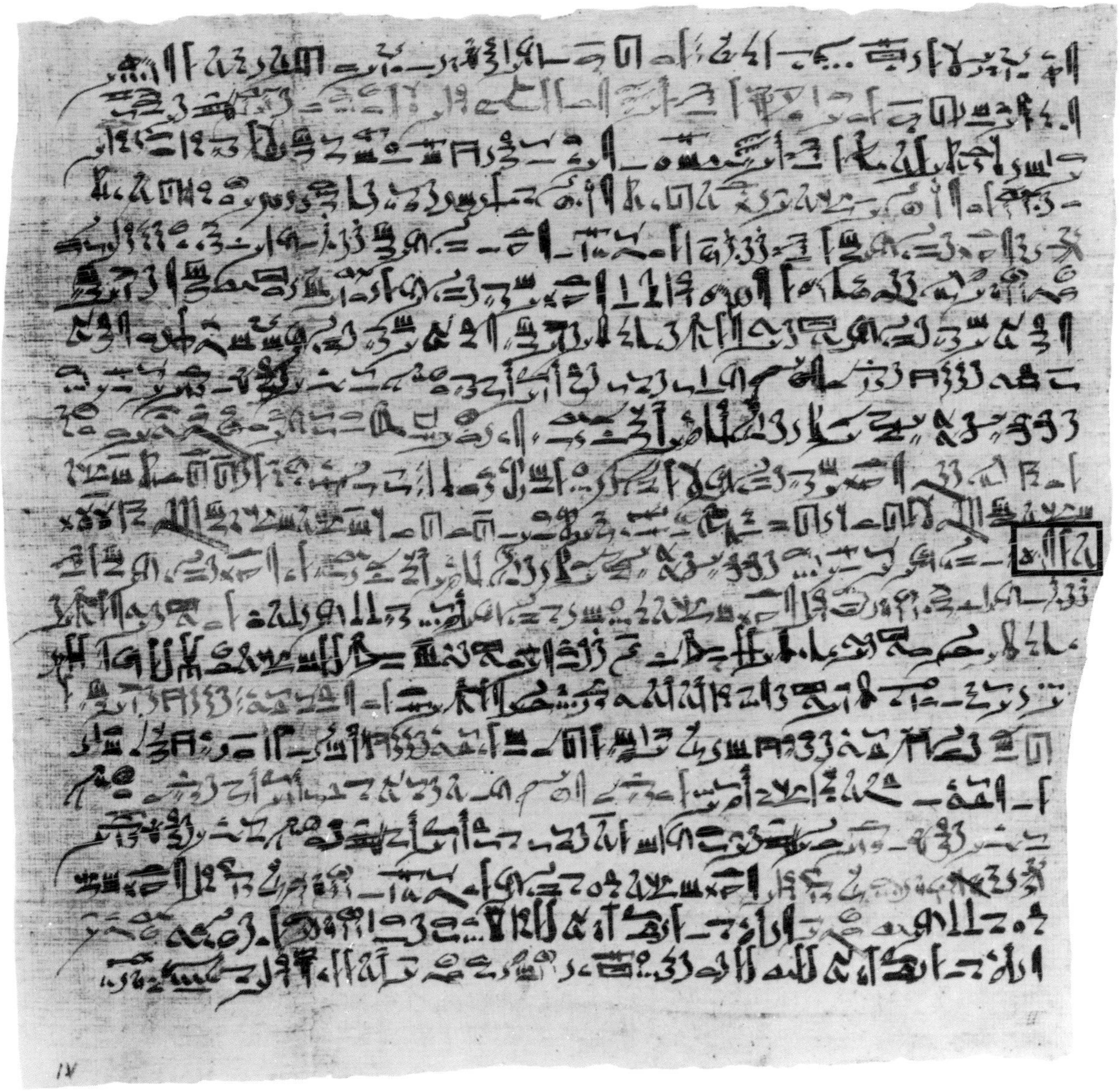

Part I: Concepts and Techniques for Crafting and Executing Strategy

Section A:
Introduction and Overview

Section B:
Concepts and Analytical Tools

Section C:
Crafting a Strategy

Section D:
Executing the Strategy

What Is Strategy and Why Does It Matter?

The Managerial Process of Crafting and Executing Strategies

Concepts and Analytical Tools for Evaluating a Company's Situation

Tailoring Strategy to Various Company Situations

Should Company Strategies Be Ethical and/or Socially Responsible?

Managerial Keys to Successfully Executing the Chosen Strategy

Chapter 1

Chapter 2

Chapters 3 and 4

Chapter 10

Chapters 11,12, and 13

Single-Business Companies

Chapters 5,6,7, and 8

Multi-business or Diversified Companies

Chapter 9

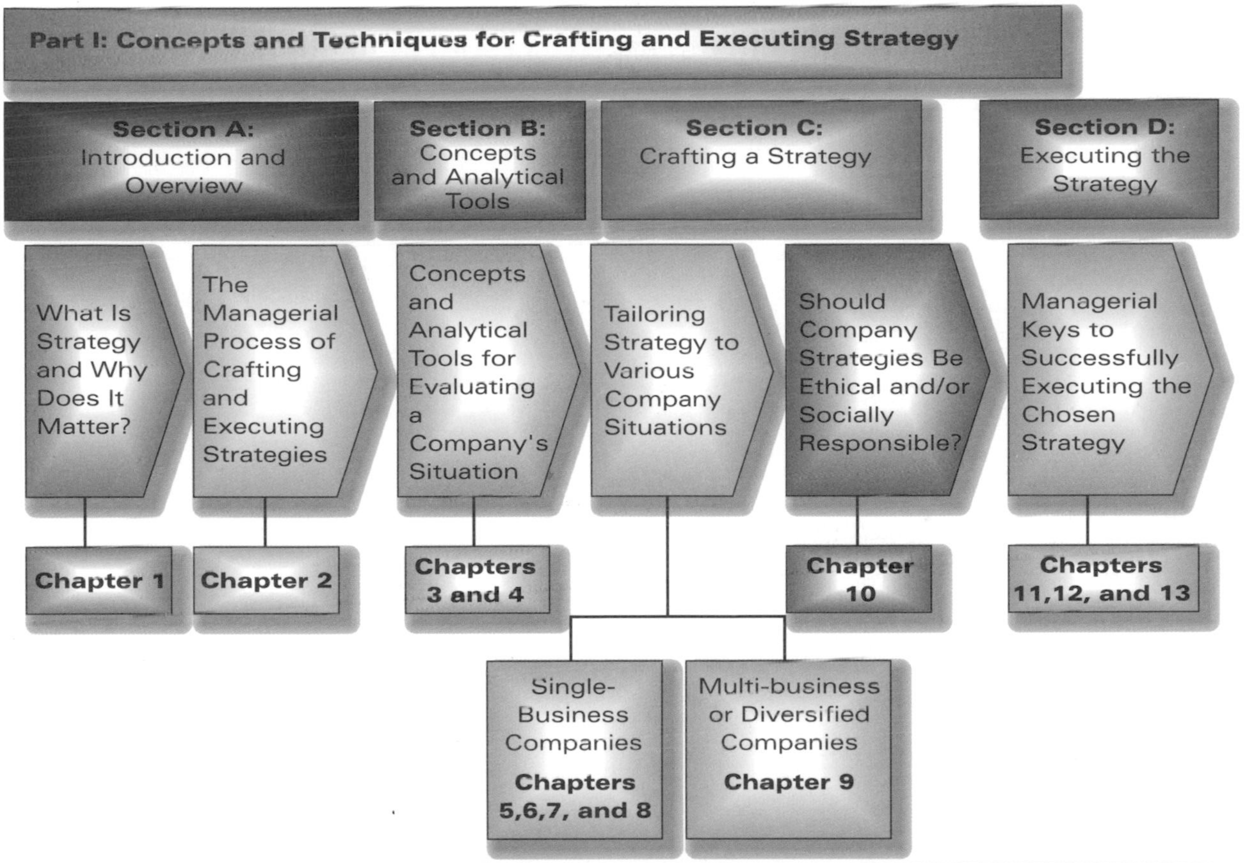

Part II: Cases in Crafting and Executing Strategy

Section A: Crafting Strategy in Single-Business Companies (20 cases)
Section B: Crafting Strategy in Diversified Companies (2 cases)
Section C: Implementing and Executing Strategy (8 cases)
Section D: Strategy, Ethics, and Social Responsibility (3 cases)

IMPORTANT

HERE IS YOUR REGISTRATION CODE TO ACCESS MCGRAW-HILL
PREMIUM CONTENT AND MCGRAW-HILL ONLINE RESOURCES

For key premium online resources you need THIS CODE to
gain access. Once the code is entered, you will be able to
use the web resources for the length of your course.

Access is provided only if you have purchased a new book.

If the registration code is missing from this book, the registration screen on our
website, and within your WebCT or Blackboard course will tell you how to obtain
your new code. Your registration code can be used only once to establish
access. It is not transferable

To gain access to these online resources

1. USE your web browser to go to: **http://www.mhhe.com/thompson**

2. CLICK on "First Time User"

3. ENTER the Registration Code printed on the tear-off bookmark on the right

4. After you have entered your registration code, click on "Register"

5. FOLLOW the instructions to setup your personal UserID and Password

6. WRITE your UserID and Password down for future reference. Keep it in a safe place.

If your course is using WebCT or Blackboard, you'll be able to use this code to
access the McGraw-Hill content within your instructor's online course.

To gain access to the McGraw-Hill content in your instructor's WebCT or
Blackboard course simply log into the course with the user ID and Password
provided by your instructor. Enter the registration code exactly as it appears to
the right when prompted by the system. You will only need to use this code the
first time you click on McGraw-Hill content.

These instructions are specifically for student access. Instructors are not required
to register via the above instructions.

The McGraw·Hill Companies

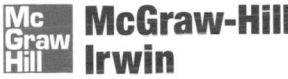

**McGraw-Hill
Irwin**

Thank you, and welcome to your
McGraw-Hill/Irwin Online Resources.

Thompson/Strickland/Gamble

Crafting & Executing Strategy: The Quest for Competitive Advantage: Concepts & Cases. 15/e
Crafting & Executing Strategy: Text and Readings. 15/e
ISBN 13: 978 0-07-326939-9; ISBN 10: 0-07-326939-5

3QW9-GKNP-HJNH-PHPG-JQNQ

REGISTRATION CODE
REGISTRATION CODE

The McGraw·Hill Companies

**McGraw-Hill
Irwin**

THE PREMIMUM CONTENT INCLUDES:

- **Case-TUTOR**—Downloadable software w/assignment questions for all 35 cases in the text, plus analytically-structured exercises for 11 of the cases

- **PowerWeb**—Articles, Weekly Update Archive, and News Feeds

- **Build Your Management Skills**—Interactive self-assessment and concept review exercises

Crafting and Executing Strategy

The Quest for Competitive Advantage

Concepts and Cases

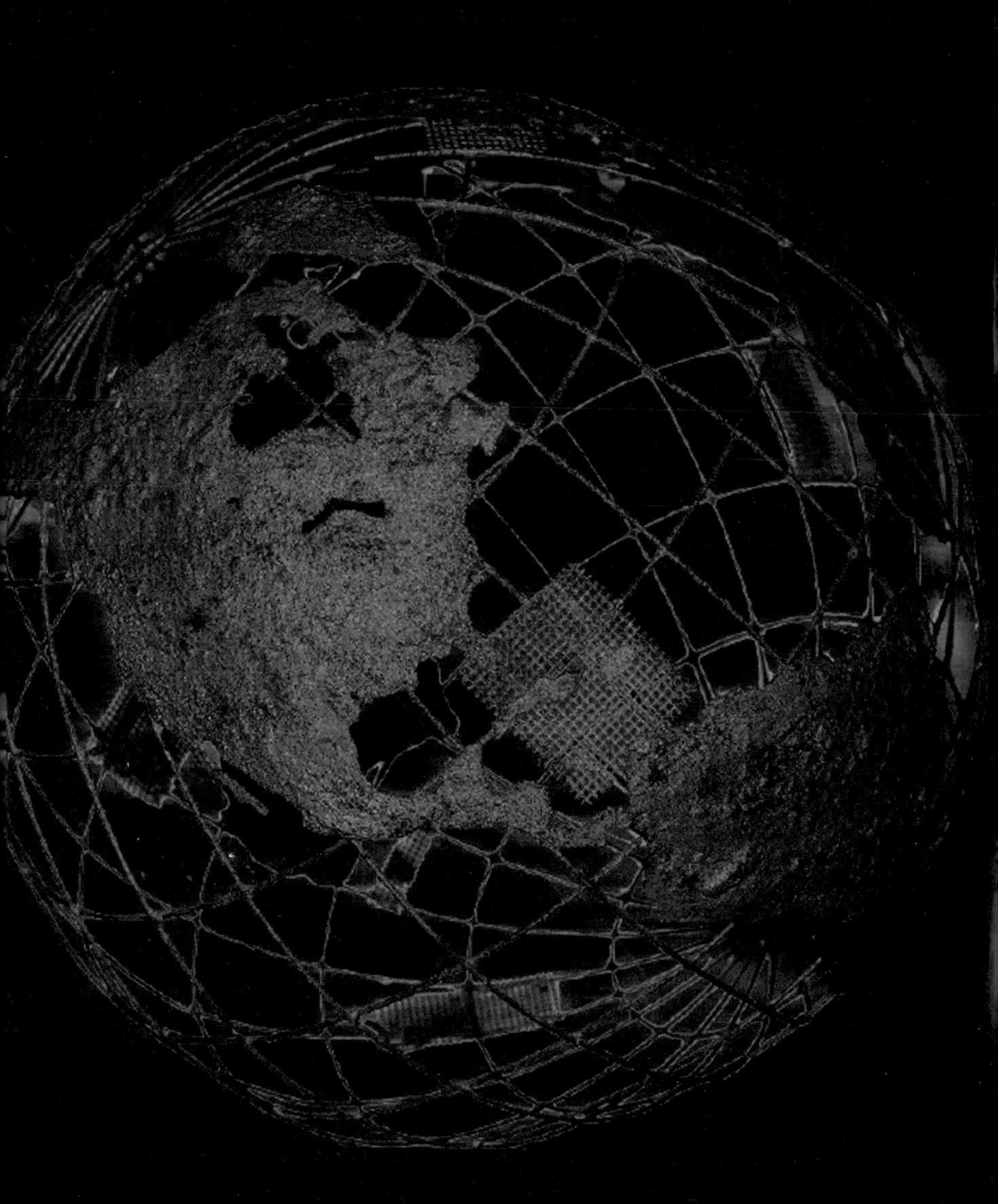

Crafting and Executing Strategy

The Quest for Competitive Advantage

Concepts and Cases

15th Edition

Arthur A. Thompson, Jr.
University of Alabama

A. J. Strickland III
University of Alabama

John E. Gamble
University of South Alabama

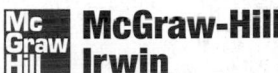

McGraw-Hill Irwin

Boston   Burr Ridge, IL   Dubuque, IA   Madison, WI   New York
San Francisco   St. Louis   Bangkok   Bogotá   Caracas   Kuala Lumpur
Lisbon   London   Madrid   Mexico City   Milan   Montreal   New Delhi
Santiago   Seoul   Singapore   Sydney   Taipei   Toronto

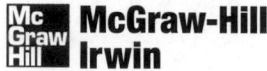
McGraw-Hill
Irwin

CRAFTING AND EXECUTING STRATEGY: THE QUEST FOR COMPETITIVE ADVANTAGE: CONCEPTS AND CASES

Published by McGraw-Hill/Irwin, a business unit of The McGraw-Hill Companies, Inc., 1221 Avenue of the Americas, New York, NY, 10020. Copyright © 2007 by The McGraw-Hill Companies, Inc. All rights reserved. No part of this publication may be reproduced or distributed in any form or by any means, or stored in a database or retrieval system, without the prior written consent of The McGraw-Hill Companies, Inc., including, but not limited to, in any network or other electronic storage or transmission, or broadcast for distance learning.

Some ancillaries, including electronic and print components, may not be available to customers outside the United States.

This book is printed on acid-free paper.

2 3 4 5 6 7 8 9 0 DOW/DOW 0 9 8 7 6

ISBN-13: 978-0-07-296943-6
ISBN-10: 0-07-296943-1

Editorial director: *John E. Biernat*
Executive editor: *John Weimeister*
Managing developmental editor: *Laura Hurst Spell*
Marketing director: *Ellen Cleary*
Media producer: *Benjamin Curless*
Project manager: *Harvey Yep*
Lead production supervisor: *Rose Hepburn*
Designer: *Cara David*
Photo research coordinator: *Lori Kramer*
Media project manager: *Joyce J. Chappetto*
Cover design: *Cara David*
Interior design: *Cara David*
Typeface: *10.5/12 Times New Roman*
Compositor: *Laserwords Private Limited*
Printer: *R. R. Donnelley*
Cover Image: *(c) Stockbyte*

Library of Congress Cataloging-in-Publication Data

Thompson, Arthur A., 1940-
    Crafting and executing strategy : the quest for competitive advantage : concepts and cases / Arthur A. Thompson, A. J. Strickland, John E. Gamble. -- 15th ed.
        p. cm.
    Includes bibliographical references and index.
    ISBN-13: 978-0-07-296943-6 (alk. paper)
    ISBN-10: 0-07-296943-1 (alk. paper)
    1. Strategic planning. 2. Strategic planning--Case studies. I. Strickland, A. J.
(Alonzo J.) II. Gamble, John (John E.) III. Title.
    HD30.28.T53 2007
    658.4' 012--dc22

                                                                    2006011853

www.mhhe.com

To our families and especially our wives:
Hasseline, Kitty, and Debra

About the Authors

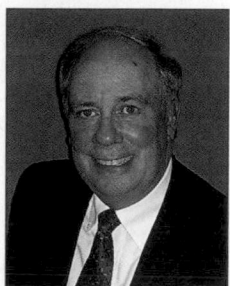

Arthur A. Thompson, Jr., earned his B.S. and Ph.D. degrees in economics from The University of Tennessee, spent three years on the economics faculty at Virginia Tech, and served on the faculty of The University of Alabama's College of Commerce and Business Administration for 24 years. In 1974 and again in 1982, Dr. Thompson spent semester-long sabbaticals as a visiting scholar at the Harvard Business School.

His areas of specialization are business strategy, competition and market analysis, and the economics of business enterprises. In addition to publishing over 30 articles in some 25 different professional and trade publications, he has authored or co-authored five textbooks and six computer-based simulation exercises that are used in colleges and universities worldwide.

Dr. Thompson spends much of his off-campus time giving presentations, putting on management development programs, working with companies, and helping operate a business simulation enterprise in which he is a major partner.

Dr. Thompson and his wife of 45 years have two daughters, two grandchildren, and two Yorkshire terriers.

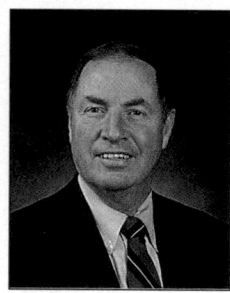

Dr. A. J. (Lonnie) Strickland, a native of North Georgia, attended the University of Georgia, where he received a bachelor of science degree in math and physics in 1965. Afterward he entered the Georgia Institute of Technology, where he received a master of science in industrial management. He earned a PhD in business administration from Georgia State University in 1969. He currently holds the title of Professor of Strategic Management in the Graduate School of Business at The University of Alabama.

Dr. Strickland's experience in consulting and executive development is in the strategic management area, with a concentration in industry and competitive analysis. He has developed strategic planning systems for such firms as the Southern Company, BellSouth, South Central Bell, American Telephone and Telegraph, Gulf States Paper, Carraway Methodist Medical Center, Delco Remy, Mark IV Industries, Amoco Oil Company, USA Group, General Motors, and Kimberly Clark Corporation (Medical Products). He is a very popular speaker on the subject of implementing strategic change and serves on several corporate boards.

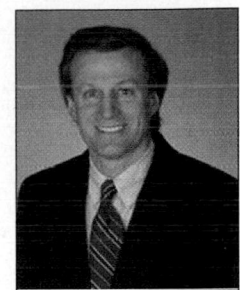

John E. Gamble is currently Associate Dean and Professor of Management in the Mitchell College of Business at the University of South Alabama. His teaching specialty at USA is strategic management and he also conducts a course in strategic management in Germany, which is sponsored by the University of Applied Sciences in Worms.

Dr. Gamble's research interests center on strategic issues in entrepreneurial, health care, and manufacturing settings. His work has been published in various scholarly journals and he is the author or co-author of more than 30 case studies published in an assortment of strategic management and strategic marketing texts. He has done consulting on industry and market analysis for clients in a diverse mix of industries.

Professor Gamble received his Ph.D. in management from The University of Alabama in 1995. Dr. Gamble also has a Bachelor of Science degree and a Master of Arts degree from The University of Alabama.

The Preface

The hallmark of this 15th edition is a fresh, refined presentation in every chapter and a powerhouse collection of cases. A bigger portion of each chapter has been revised and rewritten than in any previous edition. Coverage was trimmed in some areas, expanded in others. Every paragraph on every page of the 14th edition was revisited, producing a host of both major and minor changes in exposition. Pains were taken to improve and enliven the explanations of core concepts and analytical tools. The latest research findings from the literature and cutting-edge strategic practices of companies have been incorporated to keep step with both theory and practice. Scores of new examples have been added to complement the new and updated Illustration Capsules. More chapter-end exercises have been included. The result is a text treatment with more punch, greater clarity, and improved classroom effectiveness. But none of the changes have altered the fundamental character that has driven the text's success over the years. The chapter content continues to be solidly mainstream and balanced, mirroring *both* the best academic thinking and the pragmatism of real-world strategic management.

Complementing the text presentation is a truly appealing lineup of 33 diverse, timely, and thoughtfully crafted cases. Many involve high-profile companies, and all are framed around issues and circumstances tightly linked to the content of the 13 chapters, thus pushing students to apply the concepts and analytical tools they have read about. We are confident you will be impressed with how well these cases will teach and the amount of student interest they will spark. And there's a comprehensive package of support materials that are a breeze to use, highly effective, and flexible enough to fit most any course design.

A TEXT WITH ON-TARGET CONTENT

In our view, for a senior/MBA-level strategy text to qualify as having on-target content, it must:

- Explain core concepts in language that students can grasp and provide examples of their relevance and use by actual companies.
- Take care to thoroughly describe the tools of strategic analysis, how they are used, and where they fit into the managerial process of crafting and executing strategy.
- Be up-to-date and comprehensive, with solid coverage of the landmark changes in competitive markets and company strategies being driven by globalization and Internet technology.
- Focus squarely on what every student needs to know about crafting, implementing, and executing business strategies in today's market environments.
- Contain freshly researched, value-adding cases that feature interesting products and companies, illustrate the important kinds of strategic challenges managers face, link closely to the chapter content, contain valuable teaching points, and ignite lively class discussions.

We believe this 15th edition measures up on all five of these criteria. Chapter discussions cut straight to the chase about what students really need to know. Our explanations of core concepts and analytical tools are covered in enough depth to make them understandable and usable, the rationale being that a shallow explanation carries little punch and has almost no instructional value. All the chapters are flush with convincing examples that students can easily relate to. There's a straightforward, integrated flow from one chapter to the next. All the latest research findings pertinent to a first course in strategy have been woven into the chapters. We have deliberately adopted a pragmatic, down-to-earth writing style, not only to better communicate to an audience of students (who, for the most part, will soon be practicing managers) but also to convince readers that the subject matter deals directly with what managers and companies do in the real world.

And, thanks to the excellent case research and case writing being done by colleagues in strategic management, this edition contains a set of high-interest cases with an unusual ability to work magic in the classroom. Great cases make it far easier for you to drive home valuable lessons in the whys and hows of successfully crafting and executing strategy.

ORGANIZATION, CONTENT, AND FEATURES OF THE TEXT CHAPTERS

The 13 chapters in this edition are arranged in the same order as the 14th edition and cover essentially the same topics. But every chapter has been given a refreshing facelift that includes the latest thinking and evidence from the literature, more refined presentations, and a greater number of current examples. The latest developments in the theory and practice of strategic management have been ingrained in every chapter to keep the content solidly in the mainstream of contemporary strategic thinking. You'll find up-to-date coverage of the continuing march of industries and companies to wider globalization, the growing scope and strategic importance of collaborative alliances, the spread of high-velocity change to more industries and company environments, and how online technology is driving fundamental changes in both strategy and internal operations in companies across the world.

No other leading strategy text comes close to matching our coverage of the resource-based theory of the firm. The resource-based view of the firm is prominently and comprehensively integrated into our coverage of crafting both single-business and multibusiness strategies. Chapters 3 through 9 emphasize that a company's strategy must be matched *both* to its external market circumstances and to its internal resources and competitive capabilities. Moreover, Chapters 11, 12, and 13, on various aspects of executing strategy, have a strong resource-based perspective that makes it unequivocally clear how and why the tasks of assembling intellectual capital and building core competencies and competitive capabilities are absolutely critical to successful strategy execution and operating excellence.

No other leading strategy text comes close to matching our coverage of business ethics, values, and social responsibility. We have embellished the highly important Chapter 10, "Strategy, Ethics, and Social Responsibility," with new discussions and material so that it can better fulfill the important functions of (1) alerting students to the role and importance of incorporating business ethics and social responsibility into decision making and (2) addressing the accreditation requirements of the AACSB that business ethics be visibly and thoroughly embedded in the core curriculum. Moreover, there are discussions of the roles of values and ethics in Chapters 1, 2, 11, and 13, thus providing you with a meaty, comprehensive treatment of business ethics and socially responsible behavior as they apply to crafting and executing company strategies.

The following rundown summarizes the noteworthy chapter features and topical emphasis in this edition:

- Chapter 1 continues to focus on the central questions of "What is strategy?" and "Why is it important?" It defines what is meant by the term *strategy,* identifies the different elements of a company's strategy, and explains why management efforts to craft a company's strategy entail a quest for competitive advantage. Following Henry Mintzberg's pioneering research, we stress how and why a company's strategy is partly planned and partly reactive, and why a company's strategy tends to evolve over time. There's an enhanced discussion of what is meant by the term *business model* and how it relates to the concept of strategy. The thrust of this first chapter is to convince students that good strategy + good strategy execution = good management. The chapter is a perfect accompaniment for your opening-day lecture on what the course is all about and why it matters.

- Chapter 2 delves into the managerial process of actually crafting and executing a strategy—it makes a great assignment for the second day of class and is a perfect follow-on to your first day's lecture. The focal point of the chapter is the five-step managerial process of crafting and executing strategy: (1) forming a strategic vision of where the company is headed and why, (2) setting objectives and performance targets that measure the company's progress, (3) crafting a strategy to achieve these targets and move the company toward its market destination, (4) implementing and executing the strategy, and (5) monitoring progress and making corrective adjustments as needed. Students are introduced to such core concepts as strategic visions, mission statements, strategic versus financial objectives, and strategic intent. There's a section underscoring that *all managers are on a company's strategy-making, strategy-executing team* and that a company's strategic plan is a collection of strategies devised by different managers at different levels in the organizational hierarchy. The chapter winds up with a substantially expanded section on corporate governance.

- Chapter 3 sets forth the now-familiar analytical tools and concepts of industry and competitive analysis and demonstrates the importance of tailoring strategy to fit the circumstances of a company's industry and competitive environment. The standout feature of this chapter is a presentation of Michael E. Porter's "five-forces model of competition" that we think is the clearest, most straightforward discussion of any text in the field. Globalization and Internet technology are treated as potent driving forces capable of reshaping industry competition—their roles as change agents have become factors that most companies in most industries must reckon with in forging winning strategies.

- Chapter 4 establishes the equal importance of doing solid company situation analysis as a basis for matching strategy to organizational resources, competencies, and competitive capabilities. The roles of core competencies and organizational resources and capabilities in creating customer value and helping build competitive advantage are *center stage* in the discussions of company resource strengths and weaknesses. SWOT analysis is cast as a simple, easy-to-use way to assess a company's resources and overall situation. There is much-clearer coverage of value chain analysis, benchmarking, and competitive strength assessments—standard tools for appraising a company's relative cost position and market standing vis-à-vis rivals. *An important addition to this chapter is a table showing how key financial and operating ratios are calculated and how to interpret them;* students will find this table handy in doing the number-crunching needed to evaluate whether a company's strategy is delivering good financial performance.

- Chapter 5 deals with a company's quest for competitive advantage and is framed around the five generic competitive strategies—low-cost leadership, differentiation, best-cost provider, focused differentiation, and focused low-cost provider.

- Chapter 6 extends the coverage of the previous chapter and deals with what *other strategic actions* a company can take to complement its choice of a basic competitive strategy. The chapter features sections on what use to make of strategic alliances and collaborative partnerships; merger and acquisition strategies; vertical integration strategies; outsourcing strategies; offensive and defensive strategies; and the different types of Web site strategies that companies can employ to position themselves in the marketplace. The discussion of offensive strategies has been totally overhauled and features a new section on blue ocean strategy. The concluding section of this chapter provides a much enhanced treatment of first-mover advantages and disadvantages.

- Chapter 7 explores the full range of strategy options for competing in foreign markets: export strategies; licensing; franchising; multicountry strategies; global strategies; and collaborative strategies involving heavy reliance on strategic alliances and joint ventures. The spotlight is trained on two strategic issues unique to competing multinationally: (1) whether to customize the company's offerings in each different country market to match the tastes and preferences of local buyers or whether to offer a mostly standardized product worldwide, and (2) whether to employ essentially the same basic competitive strategy in the markets of all countries where it operates or whether to modify the company's competitive approach country by country as needed to fit the specific market conditions and competitive circumstances it encounters. There's also coverage of the concepts of profit sanctuaries and cross-market subsidization, the ways to achieve competitive advantage by operating multinationally, the special issues of competing in the markets of emerging countries; and the strategies that local companies in emerging countries can use to defend against global giants.

- The role of Chapter 8 is to hammer home the points made in Chapters 3 and 4 that winning strategies have to be matched both to industry and competitive conditions and to company resources and capabilities. The first portion of the chapter covers the broad strategy options for companies competing in six representative industry and competitive situations: (1) emerging industries; (2) rapid-growth industries; (3) mature, slow-growth industries; (4) stagnant or declining industries; (5) turbulent, high-velocity industries; and (6) fragmented industries. The second portion of the chapter looks at matching strategy to the resources and capabilities of four representative types of companies: (1) companies pursuing rapid growth, (2) companies in industry-leading positions, (3) companies in runner-up positions, and (4) companies in competitively weak positions or plagued by crisis conditions. The detail with which these 10 concrete examples are covered in Chapter 8 should enable you to convince students why it is management's job to craft a strategy that is tightly matched to a company's internal and external circumstances.

- Our rather meaty treatment of diversification strategies for multibusiness enterprises in Chapter 9 begins by laying out the various paths for becoming diversified, explains how a company can use diversification to create or compound competitive advantage for its business units, and examines the strategic options an already-diversified company has to improve its overall performance. In the middle part of the chapter, the analytical spotlight is on the techniques and procedures for assessing the strategic attractiveness of a diversified company's business portfolio—the relative attractiveness of the various businesses the company has diversified into, a multi-industry company's competitive strength in each of its lines of business, and the *strategic fits* and *resource fits* among a diversified company's different businesses. The chapter concludes with a brief survey of a company's four main postdiversification strategy alternatives: (1) broadening the diversification base, (2) divesting some businesses and retrenching to a narrower diversification base, (3) restructuring the makeup of the company's business lineup, and (4) multinational diversification.

- Chapter 10 reflects the very latest in the literature on (1) whether and why a company has a *duty* to operate according to ethical standards and (2) whether and why a company has a *duty* or *obligation* to contribute to the betterment of society independent of the needs and preferences of the customers it serves. Is there a credible business case for operating ethically and/or operating in a socially responsible manner? The opening section of the chapter addresses whether ethical standards are universal (as maintained by the school of ethical universalism) or dependent on local norms and situational circumstances (as maintained by the school of ethical relativism) or a combination of both (as maintained by integrative social contracts theory). Following this is a section on the three categories of managerial morality (moral, immoral, and amoral), a section on the drivers of unethical strategies and shady business behavior, a section on the approaches to managing a company's ethical conduct, a section on linking a company's strategy to its ethical principles and core values, a section on the concept of a "social responsibility strategy," and sections that explore the business case for ethical and socially responsible behavior. The chapter will give students some serious ideas to chew on and, hopefully, will make them far more ethically conscious. It has been written as a stand-alone chapter that can be assigned in the early, middle, or late part of the course.

- The three-chapter module on executing strategy (Chapters 11–13) is anchored around a pragmatic, compelling conceptual framework: (1) building the resource strengths and organizational capabilities needed to execute the strategy in competent fashion; (2) allocating ample resources to strategy-critical activities; (3) ensuring that policies and procedures facilitate rather than impede strategy execution; (4) instituting best practices and pushing for continuous improvement in how value chain activities are performed; (5) installing information and operating systems that enable company personnel to better carry out their strategic roles proficiently; (6) tying rewards and incentives directly to the achievement of performance targets and good strategy execution; (7) shaping the work environment and corporate culture to fit the strategy; and (8) exerting the internal leadership needed to drive execution forward.

  We have reworked and refreshed the content all three chapters. You will see thoroughly overhauled discussions of staffing the organization, building capabilities, instilling a corporate culture, leading the strategy-execution process, and adopting best practices and Six Sigma in facilitating the drive for operating excellence.

As with the 14th edition, the recurring theme of these Chapters 11–13 is that implementing and executing strategy entails figuring out the specific actions, behaviors, and conditions that are needed for a smooth strategy-supportive operation and then following through to get things done and deliver results—the goal here is to ensure that students understand the strategy-implementing/strategy-executing phase is a make-things-happen and make-them-happen-right kind of managerial exercise.

We have done our best to ensure that the 13 chapters hit the bull's-eye in covering the essentials of a senior/MBA course in strategy and convey the best thinking of academics and practitioners. The number of examples in each chapter has been dramatically expanded. There are new and updated "strategy in action" capsules in each chapter that tie core concepts to real-world management practice. We've provided a host of interesting chapter-end exercises that you can use as a basis for class discussion or written assignments or team presentations. We are confident you'll find this 13-chapter presentation superior to our prior editions as concerns coverage, readability, and convincing examples. The ultimate test of the text, of course, is the positive pedagogical impact it has in the classroom. If this edition sets a more effective stage for your lectures and does a better job of helping you persuade students that the discipline of strategy merits their rapt attention, then it will have fulfilled its purpose.

THE CASE COLLECTION

The 33 cases included in this edition are the very latest and best that we could find. The lineup is flush with interesting companies and valuable lessons for students in the art and science of crafting and executing strategy. And there's a good blend of cases from a length perspective—close to one-third are under 15 pages yet offer plenty for students to chew on; about one-third are medium-length cases; and one-third are longer, detail-rich cases, the 33 cases average just under 17 pages in length.

At least 26 of the 33 cases involve companies, products, or people that students will have heard of, know about from personal experience, or can easily identify with. There are four dot-com company cases, plus several others that will provide students with insight into the special demands of competing in industry environments where technological developments are an everyday event, product life cycles are short, and competitive maneuvering among rivals comes fast and furious. Over 20 of the cases involve situations where company resources and competitive capabilities play as large a role in the strategy-making, strategy-executing scheme of things as industry and competitive conditions do. Scattered throughout the lineup are 10 cases concerning non-U.S. companies, globally competitive industries, and/or cross-cultural situations; these cases, in conjunction with the globalized content of the text chapters, provide ample material for linking the study of strategic management tightly to the ongoing globalization of the world economy. You'll also find 7 cases dealing with the strategic problems of family-owned or relatively small entrepreneurial businesses and 23 cases involving public companies about which students can do further research on the Internet. Eleven of the cases (Starbucks, JetBlue Airways, Competition in the MP3 Player Industry, Netflix, Krispy Kreme Doughnuts, eBay, Google, Harley-Davidson, Wal-Mart, Monsanto, and Merck-Vioxx) have accompanying videotape segments.

We believe you will find the collection of 33 cases quite appealing, eminently teachable, and very suitable for drilling students in the use of the concepts and analytical treatments in Chapters 1 through 13. With this case lineup, you should have no difficulty whatsoever choosing a set of cases to assign that will capture the interest of students from start to finish.

TWO ACCOMPANYING ONLINE, FULLY-AUTOMATED SIMULATION EXERCISES—*THE BUSINESS STRATEGY GAME* AND *GLO-BUS*

The Business Strategy Game and *GLO-BUS: Developing Winning Competitive Strategies*—two competition-based strategy simulations that are delivered online and that feature automated processing of decisions and grading of performance—are being marketed by the publisher as companion supplements for use with this and other texts in the field. *The Business Strategy Game* is the world's leading strategy simulation, having been played by well over 400,000 students at universities across the world. *GLO-BUS,* a somewhat simpler online simulation introduced in 2004, has been played by over 15,000 students at more than 125 universities across the world.

We think there are compelling reasons for using a simulation as a cornerstone, if not a centerpiece, of strategy courses for seniors and MBA students:

- Assigning students to run a company that competes head-to-head against companies run by other class members *gives students immediate opportunity to experiment with various strategy options and to gain proficiency in applying the core concepts and analytical tools that they have been reading about in the chapters.* The whole teaching/learning enterprise is facilitated when what the chapters have to say about the managerial tasks of crafting and executing strategy matches up with the strategy-making challenges that students confront in the simulation.

- Most *students desperately need the experience of actively managing a close-to-real-life company where they can practice and hone their skills* in thinking strategically, evaluating changing industry and competitive conditions, assessing a company's financial and competitive condition, and crafting and executing a strategy that delivers good results and produces sustainable competitive advantage. Strategy simulations put students through a drill where they can improve (1) their business acumen, (2) their ability to make good bottom-line decisions in the face of uncertain market and competitive conditions, and (3) their proficiency in weaving functional area decisions into a cohesive strategy. *Such skills building is the essence of senior and MBA courses in business strategy.*

- Students are *more motivated* to buckle down and figure out what strategic moves will make their simulation company perform better than they are to wrestle with the strategic issues posed in an assigned case (which entails reading the case thoroughly, diagnosing the company's situation, and proposing well-reasoned action recommendations). In a strategy simulation, students have to take the analysis of market conditions, the strategies and actions of competitors, and the condition of their company *seriously*—they are held fully accountable for their decisions and their company's performance. It is to students' advantage to avoid faulty analysis and flawed strategies—*nothing gets students' attention quicker than the adverse grade consequences of a decline in their company's performance or the loss of an industry position.* And no other type of assignment does a better job of spurring students to fully exercise their strategic wits and analytical prowess—*company co-managers have a strong grade incentive to spend quality time debating and deciding how best to boost the performance of their company.*

In class discussions of cases, however, students take on the more passive and detached role of outside observers providing their thoughts about a company's situation. It is sometimes hard to get students to think long and hard about the company in the assigned case or what needs to be done to improve its future performance. They may well not see an immediate or alarming impact on their grade if their case preparation is skimpy or their analysis of the company's situation is deficient or their recommendations about what the company should do are suboptimal or even off-the-wall. Thus, while case analysis absolutely needs to be an essential part of senior/MBA courses in strategy, case assignments fall short of strategy simulations in their capacity to motivate students to do first-rate strategic analysis and come up with insightful action recommendations.

- *A competition-based strategy simulation adds an enormous amount of student interest and excitement*—a head to-head competitive battle for market share and industry leadership *stirs students' competitive juices and emotionally engages them in the subject matter.* Being an active manager in running a company in which they have a stake makes their task of learning about crafting and executing winning strategies more enjoyable. Their company becomes "real" and takes on a life of its own as the simulation unfolds—and it doesn't take long for students to establish a healthy rivalry with other class members who are running rival companies. Because the competition in the simulation typically gets very personal, most students become immersed in what's going on in their industry—as compared to the more impersonal engagement that occurs when they are assigned a case to analyze.

- A first-rate simulation produces a "Wow! Not only is this fun, but I am learning a lot" reaction from students. *The element of competition ingrained in strategy simulations stirs students' competitive juices and emotionally engages them in the subject matter.* Most students will thoroughly enjoy the *learn-by-doing* character of a simulation, recognize the practical value of having to make all kinds of decisions and run a whole company, and gain confidence from working with all the financial and operating statistics—all of which tends to (1) make the strategy course *a livelier, richer learning experience,* and (2) result in higher instructor evaluations at the end of the course.

- Strategy simulations like *The Business Strategy Game* or *GLO-BUS* that have exceptionally close ties between the industry and company circumstances in the simulation and the topics covered in the text chapters *provide instructors with a host of first-rate examples of how the material in the text applies both to the experience that students are having in running their companies and to real-world management.* Since *students can easily relate to these examples,* they are much more apt to say "Aha! Now I see how this applies and why I need to know about it and use it." The host of examples the simulation experience provides to create this "Aha!" effect thus adds real value. (There is information posted in the Instructor Centers for both *The Business Strategy Game* and *GLO-BUS* showing specific links between the pages of this text and the simulation.)

- Because a simulation involves making decisions relating to production operations, worker compensation and training, sales and marketing, distribution, customer service, and finance and requires analysis of company financial statements and market data, *the simulation helps students synthesize the knowledge gained in a variety of different business courses. The cross-functional, integrative nature of a strategy simulation helps make courses in strategy much more of a true capstone experience.*

In sum, *a three-pronged text–case–simulation course model has significantly more teaching/learning power than the traditional text–case combination.* Indeed, a very convincing argument can be made that a competition-based strategy simulation is *the single most powerful vehicle that instructors can use to effectively teach the discipline of business and competitive strategy and to build student proficiencies in crafting and executing a winning strategy.* Mounting instructor recognition of the teaching/learning effectiveness of a good strategy simulation accounts for why strategy simulations have earned a prominent place in so many of today's strategy courses.

And, happily, there's another positive side benefit to using a simulation—*it lightens the grading burden for instructors.* Since a simulation can entail 20 or more hours of student time over the course of a term (depending on the number of decisions and the extent of accompanying assignments), most adopters compensate by trimming the total number of assigned cases or substituting the simulation for one (or two) written cases and/or an hour exam. This results in less time spent grading, because both *The Business Strategy Game* and *GLO-BUS* have built-in grading features that require no instructor effort (beyond setting the grading weights).

A Bird's-Eye View of The Business Strategy Game

The setting for *The Business Strategy Game* (*BSG*) is the global athletic footwear industry (there can be little doubt in today's world that a globally competitive strategy simulation is *vastly superior* to a simulation with a domestic-only setting). Global market demand for footwear grows at the rate of 7–9 percent annually for the first five years and 5–7 percent annually for the second five years. However, market growth rates vary by geographic region—North America, Latin America, Europe-Africa, and Asia-Pacific.

Companies begin the simulation producing branded and private-label footwear in two plants, one in North America and one in Asia. They have the option to establish production facilities in Latin America and Europe-Africa, either by constructing new plants or buying previously constructed plants that have been sold by competing companies. Company co-managers exercise control over production costs based on the styling and quality they opt to manufacture, plant location (wages and incentive compensation vary from region to region), the use of best practices and Six Sigma programs to reduce the production of defective footwear and to boost worker productivity, and compensation practices.

All newly produced footwear is shipped in bulk containers to one of four geographic distribution centers. All sales in a geographic region are made from footwear inventories in that region's distribution center. Costs at the four regional distribution centers are a function of inventory storage costs, packing and shipping fees, import tariffs paid on incoming pairs shipped from foreign plants, and exchange rate impacts. At the start of the simulation, import tariffs average $4 per pair in Europe-Africa, $6 per pair in Latin America, and $8 in the Asia-Pacific region. However, the Free Trade Treaty of the Americas allows tariff-free movement of footwear between North America and Latin America. Instructors have the option to alter tariffs as the game progresses.

Companies market their brand of athletic footwear to footwear retailers worldwide and to individuals buying online at the company's Web site. Each company's sales and market share in the branded footwear segments hinge on its competitiveness on 11 factors: attractive pricing, footwear styling and quality, product-line breadth, advertising, the use of mail-in rebates, the appeal of celebrities endorsing a company's brand, success in convincing footwear retailers dealers to carry its brand, the number of weeks it takes to fill retailer orders, the effectiveness of a company's online sales effort at its Web site, and customer loyalty. Sales of private-label footwear hinge solely on being the low-price bidder.

All told, company co-managers make 47 types of decisions each period that cut across production operations (up to 10 decisions each plant, with a maximum of 4 plants), plant capacity additions/sales/upgrades (up to 6 decisions per plant), worker compensation and training (3 decisions per plant), shipping (up to 8 decisions each plant), pricing and marketing (up to 10 decisions in 4 geographic regions), bids to sign celebrities (2 decision entries per bid), and financing of company operations (up to 8 decisions).

Each time company co-managers make a decision entry, an assortment of on-screen calculations instantly shows the projected effects on unit sales, revenues, market shares, unit costs, profit, earnings per share, ROE, and other operating statistics. The on-screen calculations help team members evaluate the relative merits of one decision entry versus another and put together a promising strategy.

Companies can employ any of the five generic competitive strategy options in selling branded footwear—low-cost leadership, differentiation, best-cost provider, focused low-cost, and focused differentiation. They can pursue essentially the same strategy worldwide or craft slightly or very different strategies for the Europe-Africa, Asia-Pacific, Latin America, and North America markets. They can strive for competitive advantage based on more advertising or a wider selection of models or more appealing styling/quality, or bigger rebates, and so on.

Any well-conceived, well-executed competitive approach is capable of succeeding, provided it is not overpowered by the strategies of competitors or defeated by the presence of too many copycat strategies that dilute its effectiveness. The challenge for each company's management team is to craft and execute a competitive strategy that produces good performance on five measures: earnings per share, return on equity investment, stock price appreciation, credit rating, and brand image.

All activity for *The Business Strategy Game* takes place at www.bsg-online.com.

A Bird's-Eye View of GLO-BUS

The industry setting for *GLO-BUS* is the digital camera industry. Global market demand grows at the rate of 8–10 percent annually for the first five years and 4–6 percent annually for the second five years. Retail sales of digital cameras are seasonal, with about 20 percent of consumer demand coming in each of the first three quarters of each calendar year and 40 percent coming during the big fourth-quarter retailing season.

Companies produce entry-level and upscale, multifeatured cameras of varying designs and quality in a Taiwan assembly facility and ship assembled cameras directly to retailers in North America, Asia-Pacific, Europe-Africa, and Latin America. All cameras are assembled as retail orders come in and shipped immediately upon completion of the assembly process—companies maintain no finished-goods inventories, and all parts and components are delivered on a just-in-time basis (which eliminates the need to track inventories and simplifies the accounting for plant operations and costs). Company co-managers exercise control over production costs based on the designs and components they specify for their cameras, workforce compensation and training, the length of warranties offered (which affects warranty costs), the amount spent for technical support provided to buyers of the company's cameras, and their management of the assembly process.

Competition in each of the two product market segments (entry-level and multifeatured digital cameras) is based on 10 factors: price, camera performance and quality, number of quarterly sales promotions, length of promotions in weeks, the size of the promotional discounts offered, advertising, the number of camera models, size of retail dealer network, warranty period, and the amount/caliber of technical support provided to camera buyers. Low-cost leadership, differentiation strategies, best-cost provider strategies, and focus strategies are all viable competitive options. Rival companies can strive to be the clear market leader in either entry-level cameras, upscale multifeatured cameras, or both. They can focus on one or two geographic regions or strive for geographic balance. They can pursue essentially the same strategy worldwide or craft slightly or very different strategies for the Europe-Africa, Asia-Pacific, Latin America, and North America markets. Just as with *The Business Strategy Game,* most any well-conceived, well-executed competitive approach is capable of succeeding, *provided it is not overpowered by the strategies of competitors or defeated by the presence of too many copycat strategies that dilute its effectiveness.*

Company co-managers make 44 types of decisions each period, ranging from R&D, camera components, and camera performance (10 decisions) to production operations and worker compensation (15 decisions) to pricing and marketing (15 decisions) to the financing of company operations (4 decisions). Each time participants make a decision entry, an assortment of on-screen calculations instantly shows the projected effects on unit sales, revenues, market shares, unit costs, profit, earnings per share, ROE, and other operating statistics. These on-screen calculations help team members evaluate the relative merits of one decision entry versus another and stitch the separate decisions into a cohesive and promising strategy. Company performance is judged on five criteria: earnings per share, return on equity investment, stock price, credit rating and brand image.

All activity for *GLO-BUS* occurs at www.glo-bus.com.

Administration and Operating Features of the Two Simulations

The online delivery and user-friendly designs of both *BSG* and *GLO-BUS* make them incredibly easy to administer, even for first-time users. And the menus and controls are so similar that you can readily switch between the two simulations or use one in your undergraduate class and the other in a graduate class. If you have not yet used either of the two simulations, you may find the following of particular interest:

- Time requirements for instructors are minimal. Setting up the simulation for your course is done online and takes about 10–15 minutes. Once setup is completed, no other administrative actions are required beyond that of moving participants to a different team (should the need arise) and monitoring the progress of the simulation (to whatever extent desired).

- There's no software for students or administrators to download and no disks to fool with. All work must be done online and the speed for participants using dial-up modems is quite satisfactory. The servers dedicated to hosting the two simulations have appropriate back-up capability and are maintained by a prominent Web-hosting service that guarantees 99.99 percent reliability on a 24/7/365 basis—as long as students or instructors are connected to the Internet, the servers are virtually guaranteed to be operational.

- Participant's Guides are delivered at the Web site—students can read the Guide on their monitors or print out a copy, as they prefer.

- There are extensive built-in "Help" screens explaining (1) each decision entry, (2) the information on each page of the Industry Reports, and (3) the numbers presented in the Company Reports. *The Help screens allow company co-managers to figure things out for themselves, thereby curbing the need for students to always run to the instructor with questions about "how things work."*

- The results of each decision are processed automatically and are typically available to all participants *15 minutes* after the decision deadline specified by the instructor/game administrator.

- Participants and instructors are notified via e-mail when the results are ready.

- Decision schedules are instructor-determined. Decisions can be made once per week, twice per week, or even twice daily, depending on how instructors want to conduct the exercise. One popular decision schedule involves 1 or 2 practice decisions, 6–10 regular decisions, and weekly decisions across the whole term. A second popular schedule is 1 or 2 practice decisions, 6–8 regular decisions, and biweekly decisions, all made during the last 4 to 6 weeks of the course (when it can be assumed that students have pretty much digested the contents of Chapters 1–6, gotten somewhat comfortable with what is involved in crafting strategy for a single-business company situation, and have prepared several assigned cases). A third popular schedule is to use the simulation as a "final exam" for the course, with daily decisions (Monday through Friday) for the last two weeks of the term.

- Instructors have the flexibility to prescribe 0, 1, or 2 practice decisions and from 3 to 10 regular decisions.

- Company teams can be composed of 1 to 5 players each and the number of companies in a single industry can range from 4 to 12. If your class size is too large for a single industry, then it is a simple matter to create two or more industries for a single class section.

- Following each decision, participants are provided with a complete set of reports—a six-page Industry Report, a one-page Competitive Intelligence report for each geographic region that includes strategic group maps and bulleted lists of competitive strengths and weaknesses, and a set of Company Reports (income statement, balance sheet, cash flow statement, and assorted production, marketing, and cost statistics).

- Two "open-book" multiple-choice tests of 20 questions (optional, but strongly recommended) are included as part of each of the two simulations. The quizzes are taken online and automatically graded, with scores reported instantaneously to participants and automatically recorded in the instructor's electronic gradebook. Students are automatically provided with three sample questions for each test.

- Both simulations contain a three-year strategic plan option that you can assign. Scores on the plan are automatically recorded in the instructor's online gradebook.
- At the end of the simulation, you can have students complete online peer evaluations. (Again, the scores are automatically recorded in your online gradebook.)
- Both simulations have a Company Presentation feature that enables students to easily prepare PowerPoint slides for use in describing their strategy and summarizing their company's performance in a presentation either to the class, the instructor, or an "outside" board of directors.

For more details on either simulation, please consult the Instructor's Manual or visit the simulation Web sites (www.bsg-online.com and www.glo-bus.com). The Web sites provide a wealth of information, including a "Guided Tour" link that takes about five minutes. Once you register (there's no obligation), you'll be able to access the Instructor's Guide and a set of PowerPoint Presentation slides that you can skim to preview the two simulations in some depth. The simulation authors will be glad to provide you with a personal tour of either or both Web sites (while you are on your PC) and walk you through the many features that are built into the simulations. We think you'll be quite impressed with the capabilities that have been programmed into *The Business Strategy Game and GLO-BUS,* the simplicity with which both simulations can be administered, and their exceptionally tight connection to the text chapters, core concepts, and standard analytical tools.

Adopters of the text who also want to incorporate use of either of the two simulation supplements should instruct their bookstores to order the "book-simulation package"—the publisher has a special ISBN for new texts that contain a special card shrink-wrapped with each text; printed on the enclosed card is a prepaid access code that student can use to register for either simulation and gain full access to the student portion of the Web site.

STUDENT SUPPORT MATERIALS FOR THE 15TH EDITION

Key Points Summaries

At the end of each chapter is a synopsis of the core concepts, analytical tools, and other key points discussed in the chapter. These chapter-end synopses, along with the margin notes scattered throughout each chapter, help students focus on basic strategy principles, digest the messages of each chapter, and prepare for tests.

Chapter-End Exercises

Each chapter contains a much-embellished set of exercises that you can use as the basis for class discussion, oral presentation assignments, and/or short written reports. A few of the exercises (and many of the Illustration Capsules) qualify as "mini-cases"; these can be used to round out the rest of a 75-minute class period should your lecture on a chapter only last for 50 minutes.

A Value-Added Web Site

Students use the code that comes on the inside page of each new copy of the text to gain access to the publisher's Web site for the 15th edition; students having a used text can purchase access to the site for a very modest fee. The student section of www. mhhe.com/thompson contains a number of helpful aids:

- Self-scoring 20-question chapter tests that students can take to measure their grasp of the material presented in each of the 13 chapters.
- A "Guide to Case Analysis" containing sections on what a case is, why cases are a standard part of courses in strategy, preparing a case for class discussion, doing a written case analysis, doing an oral presentation, and using financial ratio analysis to assess a company's financial condition. We suggest having students read this Guide prior to the first class discussion of a case.
- A select number of PowerPoint slides for each chapter.

PowerWeb

With each new book, students gain access to the publisher's PowerWeb site offering current news, articles from 6,300 premium sources, a Web research guide, current readings from annual editions, and links to related sites.

Case-Tutor Software

One of the most important and useful student aids at the 15th edition's Web site is a set of downloadable files called Case-Tutor that consists of (1) files containing assignment questions for all 35 cases in the text and (2) files containing analytically structured exercises for 11 of the cases—these 11 "case preparation exercises" coach students in doing the strategic thinking needed to arrive at solid answers to the assignment questions for that case. Conscientious completion of the case preparation exercises helps students gain quicker command of the concepts and analytical techniques and points them toward doing good strategic analysis. The 11 cases with an accompanying case preparation exercise are indicated by the Case-Tutor logo in the case listing section of the Table of Contents. (The Case-Tutor logo also appears on the first page of cases for which there is an exercise.)

INSTRUCTOR SUPPORT MATERIALS FOR THE 15TH EDITION

Instructor's Manual

The accompanying Instructor's Manual contains a section on suggestions for organizing and structuring your course, sample syllabi and course outlines, a set of lecture notes on each chapter, a copy of the test bank, and comprehensive teaching notes for each of cases.

Test Bank

There is a test bank prepared by the co-authors containing over 1,200 multiple-choice questions and short-answer/essay questions.

EZ-Test

A computerized version of the test bank, EZ-Test allows you to generate tests quite conveniently and to add in your own questions.

PowerPoint Slides

To facilitate delivery preparation of your lectures and to serve as chapter outlines, you'll have access to approximately 500 colorful and professional-looking slides displaying core concepts, analytical procedures, key points, and all the figures in the text chapters. The slides, prepared in close collaboration with the text authors, are the creation of Professor Jana Kuzmicki of Troy State University.

Accompanying Case Videos

Eleven of the cases (Starbucks, JetBlue Airways, Netflix, Krispy Kreme Doughnuts, Competition in the MP3 Player Industry, eBay, Google, Harley-Davidson, Wal-Mart, Monsanto, and Merck-Vioxx) have accompanying videotape segments that can be shown in conjunction with the case discussions. Suggestions for using each video are contained in the teaching note for that case.

The Business Strategy Game *and* GLO-BUS
Online Simulations

Using one of the two companion simulations is a powerful and constructive way of emotionally connecting students to the subject matter of the course. We know of no more effective and interesting way to stimulate the competitive energy of students and prepare them for the rigors of real-world business decision making than to have them match strategic wits with classmates in running a company in head-to-head competition for global market leadership.

Instructor's Resource CD-ROM

The complete Instructor's Manual and the accompanying PowerPoint slides have been installed on an Instructor's Resource CD that the publisher provides to adopters.

We've done our level best in this 15th edition to provide you with a full-featured teaching/learning package that squarely targets what every business student needs to know about crafting and executing business strategies, that is diverse enough to keep the nature of student assignments varied and interesting, and that wins the applause of students. The intent has been to raise the bar for what a text package in the discipline of strategy ought to deliver and to equip you with all the resources and materials you'll need to design and deliver a course that is on the cutting-edge and pedagogically effective.

ACKNOWLEDGMENTS

We heartily acknowledge the contributions of the case researchers whose case-writing efforts appear herein and the companies whose cooperation made the cases possible. To each one goes a very special thank-you. We cannot overstate the importance of timely, carefully researched cases in contributing to a substantive study of strategic management issues and practices. From a research standpoint, strategy-related cases are invaluable in exposing the generic kinds of strategic issues that companies face, in forming hypotheses about strategic behavior, and in drawing experienced-based generalizations about the practice of strategic management. From an instructional standpoint, strategy cases give students essential practice in diagnosing and evaluating the strategic situations of companies and organizations, in applying the concepts and tools of strategic analysis, in weighing strategic options and crafting strategies, and in tackling the challenges of successful strategy execution. Without a continuing stream of fresh, well-researched, and well-conceived cases, the discipline of strategic management would lose its close ties to the very institutions whose strategic actions and behavior it is aimed at explaining. There's no question, therefore, that first-class case research constitutes a valuable scholarly contribution to the theory and practice of strategic management.

In addition, a great number of colleagues and students at various universities, business acquaintances, and people at McGraw-Hill provided inspiration, encouragement, and counsel during the course of this project. Like all text authors in the strategy field, we are intellectually indebted to the many academics whose research and writing have blazed new trails and advanced the discipline of strategic management. The following reviewers provided seasoned advice and splendid suggestions for improving the chapters in this 15th edition:

Lynne Patten, *Clark Atlanta University*

Nancy E. Landrum, *Morehead State University*

Jim Goes, *Walden University*

Jon Kalinowski, *Minnesota State University–Mankato*

Rodney M. Walter Jr., *Western Illinois University*

Judith D. Powell, *Virginia Union University*

We also express our thanks to Seyda Deligonul, David Flanagan, Esmerelda Garbi, Mohsin Habib, Kim Hester, Jeffrey E. McGee, Diana J. Wong, F. William Brown, Anthony F. Chelte, Gregory G. Dess, Alan B. Eisner, John George, Carle M. Hunt, Theresa Marron-Grodsky, Sarah Marsh, Joshua D. Martin, William L. Moore, Donald Neubaum, George M. Puia, Amit Shah, Lois M. Shelton, Mark Weber, Steve Barndt, J. Michael Geringer, Ming-Fang Li, Richard Stackman, Stephen Tallman, Gerardo R. Ungson, James Boulgarides, Betty Diener, Daniel F. Jennings, David Kuhn, Kathryn Martell, Wilbur Mouton, Bobby Vaught, Tuck Bounds, Lee Burk, Ralph Catalanello, William Crittenden, Vince Luchsinger, Stan Mendenhall, John Moore, Will Mulvaney, Sandra Richard, Ralph Roberts, Thomas Turk, Gordon VonStroh, Fred Zimmerman, S. A. Billion, Charles Byles, Gerald L. Geisler, Rose Knotts, Joseph Rosenstein, James B. Thurman, Ivan Able, W. Harvey Hegarty, Roger Evered, Charles B. Saunders, Rhae

M. Swisher, Claude I. Shell, R. Thomas Lenz, Michael C. White, Dennis Callahan, R. Duane Ireland, William E. Burr II, C. W. Millard, Richard Mann, Kurt Christensen, Neil W. Jacobs, Louis W. Fry, D. Robley Wood, George J. Gore, and William R. Soukup. These reviewers provided valuable guidance in steering our efforts to improve earlier editions.

As always, we value your recommendations and thoughts about the book. Your comments regarding coverage and contents will be taken to heart, and we always are grateful for the time you take to call our attention to printing errors, deficiencies, and other shortcomings. Please e-mail us at athompso@cba.ua.edu, astrickl@cba.ua.edu, or jgamble@usouthal.edu; fax us at (205) 348-6695; or write us at P.O. Box 870225, Department of Management and Marketing, The University of Alabama, Tuscaloosa, Alabama 35487-0225.

Arthur A. Thompson

A. J. Strickland

John E. Gamble

Guided Tour

Chapter Structure and Organization

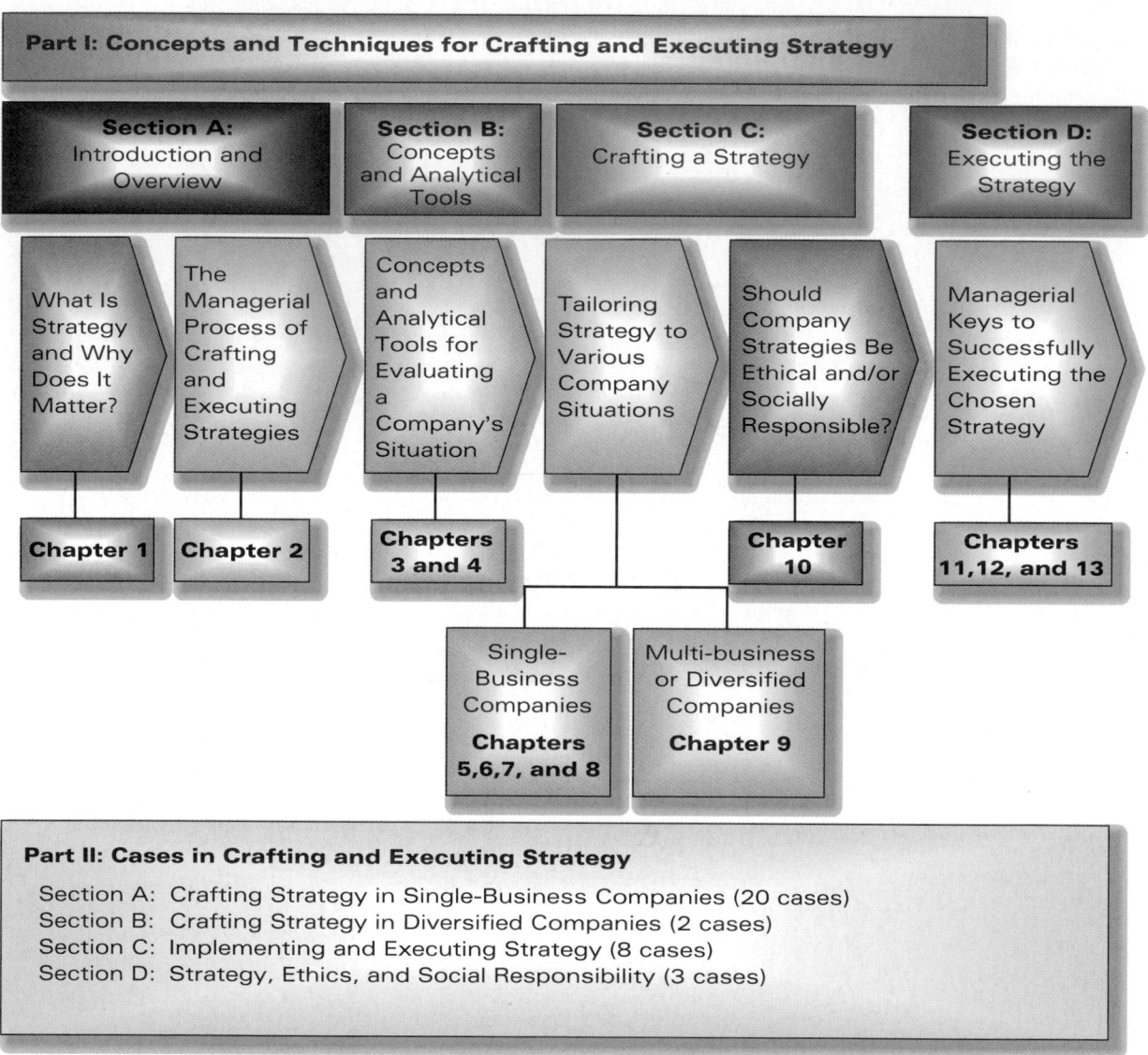

Part I: Concepts and Techniques for Crafting and Executing Strategy

Section A: Introduction and Overview

Section B: Concepts and Analytical Tools

Section C: Crafting a Strategy

Section D: Executing the Strategy

What Is Strategy and Why Does It Matter?

The Managerial Process of Crafting and Executing Strategies

Concepts and Analytical Tools for Evaluating a Company's Situation

Tailoring Strategy to Various Company Situations

Should Company Strategies Be Ethical and/or Socially Responsible?

Managerial Keys to Successfully Executing the Chosen Strategy

Chapter 1

Chapter 2

Chapters 3 and 4

Chapter 10

Chapters 11,12, and 13

Single-Business Companies

Chapters 5,6,7, and 8

Multi-business or Diversified Companies

Chapter 9

Part II: Cases in Crafting and Executing Strategy

Section A: Crafting Strategy in Single-Business Companies (20 cases)
Section B: Crafting Strategy in Diversified Companies (2 cases)
Section C: Implementing and Executing Strategy (8 cases)
Section D: Strategy, Ethics, and Social Responsibility (3 cases)

chapter one

What Is Strategy and Why Is It Important?

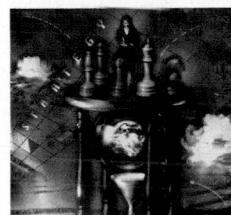

Strategy means making clear-cut choices about how to compete.
—**Jack Welch**
Former CEO, General Electric

A strategy is a commitment to undertake one set of actions rather than another.
—**Sharon Oster**
Professor, Yale University

The process of developing superior strategies is part planning, part trial and error, until you hit upon something that works.
—**Costas Markides**
Professor, London Business School

Without a strategy the organization is like a ship without a rudder.
—**Joel Ross and Michael Kami**
Authors and Consultants

M anagers face three central questions in evaluating their company's business prospects: What's the company's present situation? Where does the company need to go from here? How should it get there? Arriving at a probing answer to the question "What's the company's present situation?" prompts managers to evaluate industry conditions and competitive pressures, the company's current performance and market standing, its resource strengths and capabilities, and its competitive weaknesses. The question "Where does the company need to go from here?" pushes managers to make choices about the direction the company should be headed—what new or different customer groups and customer needs it should endeavor to satisfy, what market positions it should be staking out, what changes in its business makeup are needed. The question "How should it get there?" challenges managers to craft and execute a strategy capable of moving the company in the intended direction, growing its business, and improving its financial and market performance.

In this opening chapter, we define the concept of strategy and describe its many facets. We shall indicate the kinds of actions that determine what a company's strategy is, why strategies are partly proactive and partly reactive, and why company strategies tend to evolve over time. We will look at what sets a winning strategy apart from ho-hum or flawed strategies and why the caliber of a company's strategy determines whether it will enjoy a competitive advantage or be burdened by competitive disadvantage. By the end of this chapter, you will have a pretty clear idea of why the tasks of crafting and executing strategy are core management functions and why excellent execution of an excellent strategy is the most reliable recipe for turning a company into a standout performer.

WHAT DO WE MEAN BY *STRATEGY*?

A company's **strategy** is management's action plan for running the business and conducting operations. The crafting of a strategy represents a managerial *commitment to pursue a particular set of actions* in growing the business, attracting and pleasing customers, competing successfully, conducting operations, and improving the company's financial and market performance. Thus a company's strategy is all about *how*—how management intends to grow the business, *how* it will build a loyal clientele and outcompete rivals, *how* each functional piece of the business (research and development,

---

Each chapter begins with a series of pertinent **quotes** and an introductory preview of its contents.

Illustration Capsule 1.2

Microsoft and Red Hat: Two Contrasting Business Models

The strategies of rival companies are often predicated on strikingly different business models. Consider, for example, the business models for Microsoft and Red Hat in operating system software for personal computers (PCs).

Microsoft's business model for making money from its Windows operating system products is based on the following revenue-cost-profit economics:

- Employ a cadre of highly skilled programmers to develop proprietary code; keep the source code hidden so as to keep the inner workings of the software proprietary.

- Sell the resulting operating system and software package to PC makers and to PC users at relatively attractive prices (around $75 for PC makers and about $100 at retail to PC users); strive to maintain a 90 percent or more market share of the 150 million PCs sold annually worldwide.

- Strive for big-volume sales. Most of Microsoft's costs arise on the front end in developing the software and are thus fixed; the variable costs of producing and packaging the CDs provided to users are only a couple of dollars per copy—once the break-even volume is reached, Microsoft's revenues from additional sales are almost pure profit.

- Provide a modest level of technical support to users at no cost.

- Keep rejuvenating revenues by periodically introducing next-generation software versions with features that will induce PC users to upgrade the operating system on previously purchased PCs to the new version.

Red Hat, a company formed to market its own version of the Linux open-source operating system, employs a business model based on sharply different revenue-cost-profit economics:

- Rely on the collaborative efforts of volunteer programmers from all over the world who contribute bits and pieces of code to improve and polish the Linux system. The global community of thousands of programmers who work on Linux in their spare time do what they do because they love it, because they are fervent believers that all software should be free (as in free speech), and in some cases because they are anti-Microsoft and want to have a part in undoing what they see as a Microsoft monopoly.

- Collect and test enhancements and new applications submitted by the open-source community of volunteer programmers. Linux's originator, Linus Torvalds, and a team of 300-plus Red Hat engineers and software developers evaluate which incoming submissions merit inclusion in new releases of Linux—the evaluation and integration of new submissions are Red Hat's only upfront product development costs.

- Market the upgraded and tested family of Red Hat products to large enterprises and charge them a subscription fee that includes 24/7 support within one hour in seven languages. Provide subscribers with updated versions of Linux every 12–18 months to maintain the subscriber base.

- Make the source code open and available to all users, allowing them to create a customized version of Linux.

- Capitalize on the specialized expertise required to use Linux in multiserver, multiprocessor applications by providing fees-based training, consulting, software customization, and client-directed engineering to Linux users. Red Hat offers Linux certification training programs at all skill levels at more than 60 global locations—Red Hat certification in the use of Linux is considered the best in the world.

Microsoft's business model—sell proprietary code software and give service away free—is a proven moneymaker that generates billions in profits annually. In contrast, the jury is still out on Red Hat's business model of selling subscriptions to open-source software to large corporations and deriving substantial revenues from the sales of technical support (included in the subscription cost), training, consulting, software customization, and engineering to generate revenues sufficient to cover costs and yield a profit. Red Hat posted losses of $140 million on revenues of $79 million in fiscal year 2002 and losses of $6.6 million on revenues of $91 million in fiscal year 2003, but it earned $14 million on revenues of $126 million in fiscal 2004. The profits came from a shift in Red Hat's business model that involved putting considerably more emphasis on getting large corporations to purchase subscriptions to the latest Linux updates. In 2005, about 75 percent of Red Hat's revenues came from large enterprise subscriptions, compared to about 53 percent in 2003.

Source: Company documents and information posted on www.microsoft.com and www.redhat.com. (accessed August 10, 2005).

In-depth examples—**Illustration Capsules**—appear in boxes throughout each chapter to illustrate important chapter topics, connect the text presentation to real world companies, and convincingly demonstrate "strategy in action." Some can be used as "mini-cases" for purposes of class discussion.

Margin notes define core concepts and call attention to important ideas and principles.

Strategy and the Quest for Competitive Advantage

The heart and soul of any strategy are the actions and moves in the marketplace that managers are taking to improve the company's financial performance, strengthen its long-term competitive position, and gain a competitive edge over rivals. A creative, distinctive strategy that sets a company apart from rivals and yields a competitive advantage is a company's most reliable ticket for earning above-average profits. Competing in the marketplace with a competitive advantage tends to be more profitable than competing with no advantage. And a company is almost certain to earn significantly higher profits when it enjoys a competitive advantage as opposed to when it is hamstrung by competitive disadvantage. Furthermore, if a company's competitive edge holds promise for being durable and sustainable (as opposed to just temporary), then so much the better for both the strategy and the company's future profitability. It's nice when a company's strategy produces at least a temporary competitive edge, but a **sustainable competitive advantage** is plainly much better. What makes a competitive advantage sustainable as opposed to temporary are actions and elements in the strategy that cause an attractive number of buyers to have a *lasting preference* for a company's products or services as compared to the offerings of competitors. Competitive advantage is the key to above-average profitability and financial performance because strong buyer preferences for the company's product offering translate into higher sales volumes (Wal-Mart) and/or the ability to command a higher price (Häagen-Dazs), thus driving up earnings, return on investment, and other measures of financial performance.

> **Core Concept**
> A company achieves **sustainable competitive advantage** when an attractive number of buyers prefer its products or services over the offerings of competitors and when the basis for this preference is durable.

Four of the most frequently used and dependable strategic approaches to setting a company apart from rivals, building strong customer loyalty, and winning a sustainable competitive advantage are:

Figures scattered throughout the chapters provide conceptual and analytical frameworks.

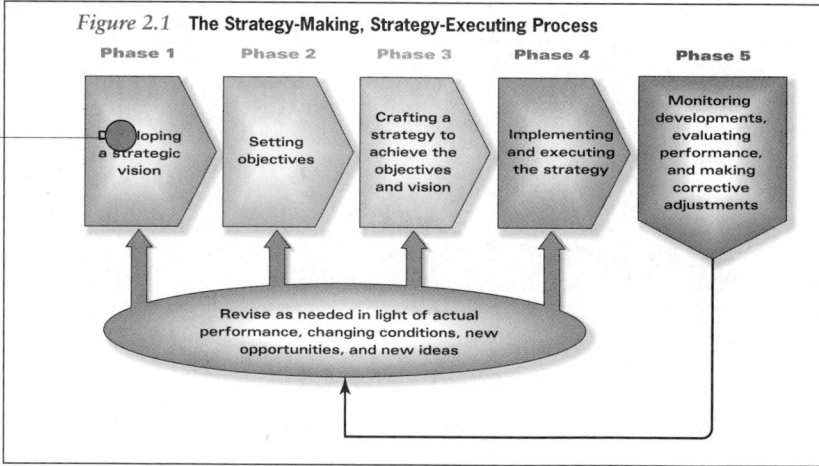

Figure 2.1   **The Strategy-Making, Strategy-Executing Process**

Phase 1 — Developing a strategic vision
Phase 2 — Setting objectives
Phase 3 — Crafting a strategy to achieve the objectives and vision
Phase 4 — Implementing and executing the strategy
Phase 5 — Monitoring developments, evaluating performance, and making corrective adjustments

Revise as needed in light of actual performance, changing conditions, new opportunities, and new ideas ist and poet Ralph Waldo Emerson: "Commerce is a game of skill which many people play, but which few play well." If the content of this book helps you become a more savvy player and equips you to succeed in business, then your journey through these pages will indeed be time well spent.

Key Points

The tasks of crafting and executing company strategies are the heart and soul of managing a business enterprise and winning in the marketplace. A company's strategy is the game plan management is using to stake out a market position, conduct its operations, attract and please customers, compete successfully, and achieve organizational objectives. The central thrust of a company's strategy is undertaking moves to build and strengthen the company's long-term competitive position and financial performance and, ideally, gain a competitive advantage over rivals that then becomes a company's ticket to above-average profitability. A company's strategy typically evolves and re-forms over time, emerging from a blend of (1) proactive and purposeful actions on the part of company managers and (2) as-needed reactions to unanticipated developments and fresh market conditions.

Key Points sections at the end of each chapter provide a handy summary of essential ideas and things to remember.

the company's product offerings and competitive approaches will generate a revenue stream and have an associated cost structure that produces attractive earnings and return on investment—in effect, a company's business model sets forth the economic logic for making money in a particular business, given the company's current strategy.

A winning strategy fits the circumstances of a company's external situation and its internal resource strengths and competitive capabilities, builds competitive advantage, and boosts company performance.

Crafting and executing strategy are core management functions. Whether a company wins or loses in the marketplace is directly attributable to the caliber of a company's strategy and the proficiency with which the strategy is executed.

Exercises

1. Go to Red Hat's Web site (www.redhat.com) and check whether the company's recent financial reports indicate that its business model is working. Is the company sufficiently profitable to validate its business model and strategy? Is its revenue stream from selling training, consulting, and engineering services growing or declining as a percentage of total revenues? Does your review of the company's recent financial performance suggest that its business model and strategy are changing? Read the company's latest statement about its business model and about why it is pursuing the subscription approach (as compared to Microsoft's approach of selling copies of its operating software directly to PC manufacturers

Value-added **exercises** at the end of each chapter provide a basis for class discussion, oral presentations, and written assignments. Several chapters have exercises that qualify as "mini-cases."

Case 6

Competition in the MP3 Player Industry in 2005

Louis D. Marino
The University of Alabama

Katy Beth Jackson
The University of Alabama

The earliest portable music players were transistor radios introduced by Regency in 1954. While these radios allowed their owners to listen to broadcasts on the go, they generally suffered from relatively weak signal reception, poor sound quality, and the ability to only receive AM stations. It was not until the mid-1970s that consumers had access to portable personal stereos; the smallest of these were slightly larger than a shoebox and allowed users not only to listen to both AM and FM radio but also to carry their personal music collections, recorded on cassette tapes, with them. However, it was not until 1979 that consumers could purchase the first truly portable personal music player, the Sony Walkman, which only played cassettes and did not offer radio reception. By 1984, the cassette tape was beginning to be supplanted by the compact disc (CD), and Sony led the way again with the development of the portable CD player, the CD Walkman or the Discman.

The portable CD player, and its more advanced cousin the minidisc player, were the mechanical precursors to the modern digital music players. These were referred to as mechanical players since they had moving parts that were involved in playing the music. The main drawbacks to these players were that they could hold only a relatively limited amount of music and were subject to skipping if the player was bumped or jostled. In an effort to overcome these weaknesses, and to capitalize on the growing popularity of digitally encoded music that individuals were storing on their computers in the form of MP3s, in 1997 SaeHan information systems developed the MPMan F10, the world's first nonmechanical digital audio player.[1]

The MPMan player was introduced to the U.S. market in the summer of 1998 as the Eiger Labs MPMan F10, a 32-megabyte digital audio player (DAP) that could only be expanded by returning it to the manufacturer. The second DAP (also known as an MP3 player) introduced in the U.S. market was the Rio PMP300, which was brought to market by Diamond Multimedia in September 1998. The Rio was so successful in the 1998 Christmas season that it led to significant investment in the MP3 player industry by other players and to a lawsuit by the Recording Industry Association of America for enabling the illegal copying of music. This suit was resolved in Diamond's favor; thus, digital music players were ruled legal. By the end of 1999, Remote Solutions had introduced the first hard-drive-based player, the Personal Jukebox, which had a 4.8-gigabyte (GB) internal hard drive and could hold about 1,200 songs consumers could choose from flash memory, hard drive, and in-dash digital audio players from a variety of manufacturers.[2]

Growth in the MP3 player market continued fairly slowly until Apple released its legendary iPod in the latter half of 2001. Apple's original hard-drive player virtually revolutionized the MP3 market single-handedly, spurring the development of many look-alike models from competing manufacturers. By 2004, sales of portable audio players had reached 27.8 million units. Just over the Christmas season of 2004 (a five-week period), MP3 player sales reached $270 million, up 147.5 percent from Christmas 2003, and most analysts predicted continued rapid growth in the industry for the foreseeable future. The research firm Gartner predicted that over 150 million units would be shipped in 2010 (see Exhibit 1).[3] With the percentage of the U.S. population owning

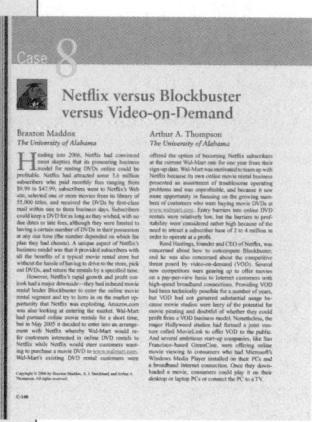

Case 8

Netflix versus Blockbuster versus Video-on-Demand

Braxton Maddox
The University of Alabama

Arthur A. Thompson
The University of Alabama

Case 11

Zoës Kitchen: Making Cents of the Fast-Casual Dining Industry

Braxton Maddox
The University of Alabama

Jennifer Traywick
The University of Alabama

As the globed lights illuminated the glass storefront of the newest Zoës Kitchen in Brentwood, Tennessee, curious passers-by could see a multitude of activities late that night. John Cassimus, president and CEO of Zoës Kitchen, knew every detail had to be perfect for opening day. Required were sweeping, mopping, cleaning, prepping food, and double-checking every inch of the store. The success of the entire Zoës Kitchen brand depended on how well the next few restaurants performed. As Cassimus carefully placed T-shirts, hats, and "Zoës Life" booklets, on the merchandising racks, his thoughts wandered from the cheerful, inviting store that was now almost complete to the challenges on the road ahead.

Zoës Kitchen was the natural extension of Zoë Cassimus's own kitchen—a place livened by her love of family and warm hospitality. Zoë had carefully created all the recipes from scratch, producing fresh food that also promoted good health. Her son John had carefully grown Zoës Kitchen from a single family restaurant into what could soon be one of the leading concepts in the fast-casual restaurant industry.

The fast-casual dining classification was the newest segment to emerge in the maturing restaurant industry. Year after year of double-digit sales growth was proving that fast-casual was not just a fad, and many of the major food companies had begun to take notice. With new, larger competitors

looking to enter the market, John Cassimus was convinced that now was the time for Zoës Kitchen to make its strategic move.

ZOËS STORY

Marcus and Zoë Cassimus opened the first Zoës Kitchen in Homewood, Alabama, in 1995, serving lunch five days a week. Zoës Kitchen quickly became a favorite spot for both mothers with children and primarily white-collar employees in the area. As of December 2005, Zoës Kitchen operated 16 locations in five states, and each store had helped build a brand synonymous with fresh ingredients, family recipes, and homemade food. Zoës menu included a healthy selection of chicken sandwiches, rollups, pitas, dinner plates, and an assortment of salads including chicken, potato, pasta, and egg (see Exhibit 1). Customers could also purchase many salads and sides by the pound to take home. Most menu items had a Greek influence, reflecting the heritage of the Cassimus family.

John Cassimus graduated from the University of Alabama in 1990 as a four-time football letterman. After graduation, he began work with Pittman Financial Partners in Birmingham, Alabama, and honed his marketing and sales skills. Cassimus was often described as a hard worker, optimist, excellent salesman, true entrepreneur, and visionary—attributes that contributed much to his success in the business arena. His first start-up, launched in

This case was prepared under the supervision of Professor A. J. Strickland, The University of Alabama. Copyright © 2006 by Braxton Maddox, Jennifer Traywick, and A. J. Strickland. All rights reserved.

C-182

33 cases detailing the strategic circumstances of actual companies and providing practice in applying the concepts and tools of strategic analysis.

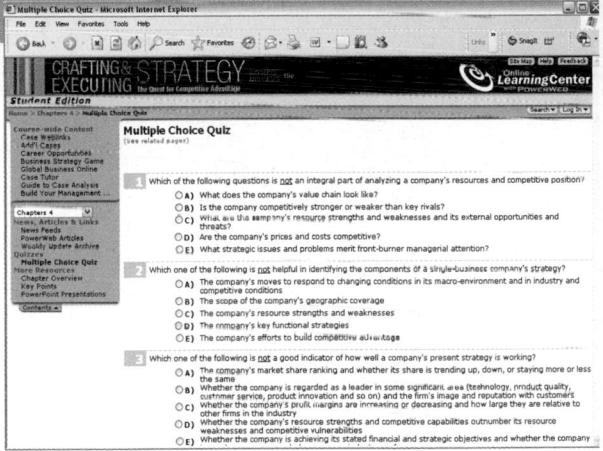

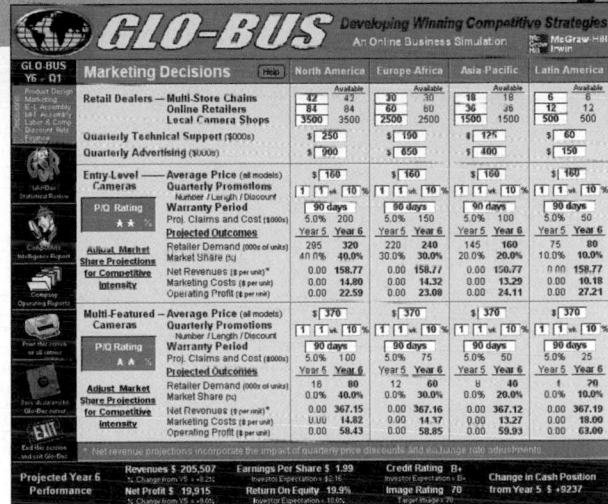

Web site: www.mhhe.com/thompson

The student portion of the Web site features a "Guide to Case Analysis," with special sections on what a case is, why cases are a standard part of courses in strategy, preparing a case for class discussion, doing a written case analysis, doing an oral presentation, and using financial ratio analysis to assess a company's financial condition. In addition, there are 20-question self-scoring chapter tests and a select number of PowerPoint slides for each chapter.

The Business Strategy Game or GLO-BUS Simulation Exercises Either one of these text supplements involves teams of students managing companies in a head-to-head contest for global market leadership. Company co-managers have to make decisions relating to product quality, production, work force compensation and training, pricing and marketing, and financing of company operations. The challenge is to craft and execute a strategy that is powerful enough to deliver good financial performance despite the competitive efforts of rival companies. Each company competes in North America, Latin America, Europe-Africa, and Asia-Pacific.

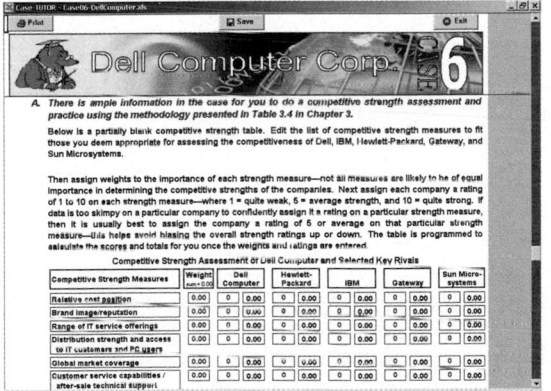

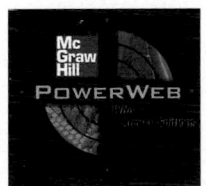

PowerWeb With each new book, students gain access to publisher's PowerWeb site offering current news, articles from 6,300 premium sources, a Web research guide, current readings from annual editions, and links to related sites.

Case-TUTOR: A set of downloadable files containing assignment questions for each of the 33 cases in the text, plus analytically-structured exercises for 11 of the cases that coach students in doing the strategic thinking needed to arrive at solid answers to the assignment questions for that case. Conscientious completion of the 11 case exercises aids quicker command of the concepts and analytical techniques and facilitates good strategic analysis and thorough preparation of assigned cases.

Brief Contents

Part One Concepts and Techniques for Crafting
and Executing Strategy

Section A: Introduction and Overview

1. What Is Strategy and Why Is It Important? 2
2. The Managerial Process of Crafting and Executing Strategy 18

Section B: Core Concepts and Analytical Tools

3. Evaluating a Company's External Environment 48
4. Evaluating a Company's Resources and Competitive Position 94

Section C: Crafting a Strategy

5. The Five Generic Competitive Strategies: Which One to Employ? 132
6. Supplementing the Chosen Competitive Strategy: *Other Important Strategy Choices* 160
7. Competing in Foreign Markets 194
8. Tailoring Strategy to Fit Specific Industry and Company Situations 230
9. Diversification: *Strategies for Managing a Group of Businesses* 266
10. Strategy, Ethics, and Social Responsibility 316

Section D: Executing the Strategy

11. Building an Organization Capable of Good Strategy Execution 358
12. Managing Internal Operations: Actions that Promote Good Strategy Execution 388
13. Corporate Culture and Leadership: Keys to Good Strategy Execution 414

Part Two Cases in Crafting and Executing Strategy

Section A: Crafting Strategy in Single Business Companies

1. Whole Foods Market in 2006: Mission, Core Values, and Strategy C-2
2. Oliver's Markets C-28
3. JetBlue Airways: Can It Survive in a Turbulent Industry? C-48
4. Competition in the Golf Equipment Industry in 2005 C-68
5. Dell Inc. in 2006: Can Rivals Beat Its Strategy? C-89
6. Competition in the MP3 Player Industry in 2005 C-116
7. Apple Computer in 2006 C-130
8. Netflix versus Blockbuster versus Video-on-Demand C-148

9. easyCar.com C-162

10. Smithfield Foods' Vertical Integration Strategy: Harmful to the Environment? C-171

11. Zoës Kitchen: Making Cents of the Fast-Casual Dining Industry C-182

12. Krispy Kreme Doughnuts in 2006: Is a Turnaround Possible? C-193

13. Kodak at a Crossroads: The Transition from Film-Based to Digital Photography C-219

14. Adam Aircraft C-235

15. KRCB Television and Radio: The Canary in the Coal Mine? C-251

16. Western States Insurance Agency C-273

17. eBay: Facing the Challenge of Global Growth C-286

18. Google Inc. in 2006: Can the Strategy Support the Lofty Stock Price? C-312

19. Copperfield's Books Inc. C-328

20. Harley-Davidson in 2004 C-356

Section B: Crafting Strategy in Diversified Companies

21. adidas: Will Restructuring Its Business Lineup Allow It to Catch Nike? C-376

22. Procter & Gamble's Acquisition of Gillette C-392

Section C: Executing Strategy and Strategic Leadership

23. Robin Hood C-405

24. Dilemma at Devil's Den C-407

25. Wal-Mart Stores Inc.: Combating Critics and Sustaining Growth C-410

26. Outback Steakhouse C-436

27. Moses at the Red Sea C-454

28. Implementing Strategic Change: Monica Ashley's Experience C-458

29. Starbucks' Global Quest in 2006: Is the Best Yet to Come? C-468

30. Leadership at TDC Sunrise: "Always a Smile" or "Communication Is Life"? C-496

Section D: Strategy, Ethics, and Social Responsibility

31. Merck and the Recall of Vioxx C-518

32. Kimpton Hotels: Balancing Strategy and Environmental Sustainability C-533

33. Monsanto and the Genetic Engineering on Agricultural Seeds C-547

Endnotes EN-1

Indexes

Organization I-1

Name I-10

Subject I-17

Table of Contents

Part One Concepts and Techniques for Crafting
and Executing Strategy 1

Section A: Introduction and Overview

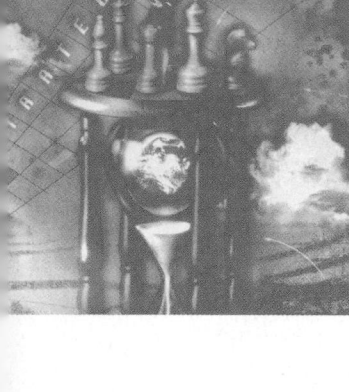

1. What Is Strategy and Why Is It Important? 2

What Do We Mean by *Strategy?* 3
   Strategy and the Quest for Competitive Advantage 6
   Identifying a Company's Strategy 7
   Why a Company's Strategy Evolves over Time 8
   A Company's Strategy Is Partly Proactive and Partly Reactive 9
Strategy and Ethics: Passing the Test of Moral Scrutiny 10
The Relationship between a Company's Strategy and Its Business Model 12
What Makes a Strategy a Winner? 13
Why Are Crafting and Executing Strategy Important? 15
   Good Strategy + Good Strategy Execution = Good Management 15

Illustration Capsules
1.1. Comcast's Strategy to Revolutionize the Cable Industry 5
1.2. Microsoft and Red Hat: Two Contrasting Business Models 14

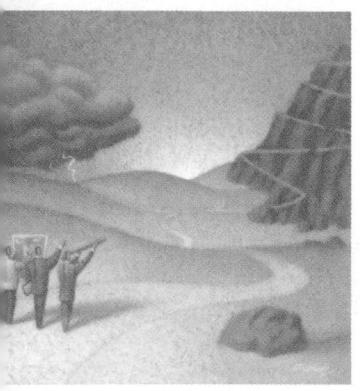

2. The Managerial Process of Crafting and Executing Strategy 18

What Does the Strategy-Making, Strategy-Executing Process Entail? 19
Developing a Strategic Vision: Phase 1 of the Strategy-Making, Strategy-Executing Process 20
   A Strategic Vision Covers Different Ground than the Typical Mission Statement 23
   Communicating the Strategic Vision 25
   Linking the Vision/Mission with Company Values 27
Setting Objectives: Phase 2 of the Strategy-Making, Strategy-Executing Process 29
   What Kinds of Objectives to Set: The Need for a Balanced Scorecard 31
Crafting a Strategy: Phase 3 of the Strategy-Making, Strategy-Executing Process 35
   Who Participates in Crafting a Company's Strategy? 35
   A Company's Strategy-Making Hierarchy 37
   Uniting the Strategy-Making Effort 40
   A Strategic Vision + Objectives + Strategy = A Strategic Plan 41

Implementing and Executing the Strategy: Phase 4 of the Strategy-Making, Strategy-Executing Process   42

Evaluating Performance and Initiating Corrective Adjustments: Phase 5 of the Strategy-Making, Strategy-Executing Process   43

Corporate Governance: The Role of the Board of Directors in the Strategy-Making, Strategy-Executing Process   44

Illustration Capsules

2.1. Examples of Strategic Visions—How Well Do They Measure Up?   23

2.2. Intel's Two Strategic Inflection Points   27

2.3. The Connection between Yahoo's Mission and Core Values   30

2.4. Examples of Company Objectives   33

Section B: Core Concepts and Analytical Tools

3. Evaluating a Company's External Environment   48

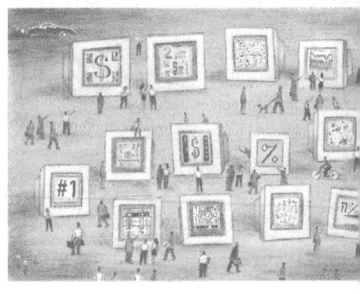

The Strategically Relevant Components of a Company's External Environment   49

Thinking Strategically about a Company's Industry and Competitive Environment   51

Question 1: What Are the Industry's Dominant Economic Features?   52

Question 2: What Kinds of Competitive Forces Are Industry Members Facing?   54

Competitive Pressures Associated with Jockeying among Rival Sellers   55

Competitive Pressures Associated with the Threat of New Entrants   60

Competitive Pressures from the Sellers of Substitute Products   64

Competitive Pressures Stemming from Supplier Bargaining Power and Supplier–Seller Collaboration   66

Competitive Pressures Stemming from Buyer Bargaining Power and Seller–Buyer Collaboration   69

Is the Collective Strength of the Five Competitive Forces Conducive to Good Profitability?   72

Question 3: What Factors Are Driving Industry Change and What Impacts Will They Have?   74

The Concept of Driving Forces   74

Identifying an Industry's Driving Forces   74

Assessing the Impact of the Driving Forces   80

Developing a Strategy That Takes the Impacts of the Driving Forces into Account   81

Question 4: What Market Positions Do Rivals Occupy—Who Is Strongly Positioned and Who Is Not?   81

Using Strategic Group Maps to Assess the Market Positions of Key Competitors   82

What Can Be Learned from Strategic Group Maps?   83

Question 5: What Strategic Moves Are Rivals Likely to Make Next?   85

Identifying Competitors' Strategies and Resource Strengths and Weaknesses   85

Predicting Competitors' Next Moves   86

Question 6: What Are the Key Factors for Future Competitive Success?   87

Question 7: Does the Outlook for the Industry Present the Company
with an Attractive Opportunity?   89

Illustration Capsules

3.1. Comparative Market Positions of Selected Retail Chains: A Strategic
Group Map Application   83

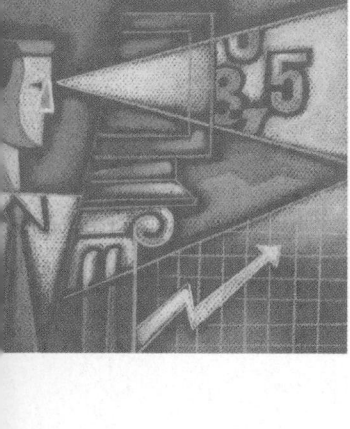

4. Evaluating a Company's Resources and Competitive Position   94

Question 1: How Well Is the Company's Present Strategy Working?   95

Question 2: What Are the Company's Resource Strengths and Weaknesses,
and Its External Opportunities and Threats?   97

Identifying Company Resource Strengths and Competitive Capabilities   97

Identifying Company Resource Weaknesses and Competitive Deficiencies   104

Identifying a Company's Market Opportunities   104

Identifying the External Threats to a Company's Future Profitability   106

What Do the SWOT Listings Reveal?   107

Question 3: Are the Company's Prices and Costs Competitive?   109

The Concept of a Company Value Chain   110

Why the Value Chains of Rival Companies Often Differ   112

The Value Chain System for an Entire Industry   113

*Activity-Based Costing: A Tool for Assessing a Company's Cost
Competitiveness   114*

*Benchmarking: A Tool for Assessing Whether a Company's
Value Chain Costs Are in Line   116*

Strategic Options for Remedying a Cost Disadvantage   117

*Translating Proficient Performance of Value Chain
Activities into Competitive Advantage   120*

Question 4: Is the Company Competitively Stronger or Weaker
Than Key Rivals?   122

Interpreting the Competitive Strength Assessments   124

Question 5: What Strategic Issues and Problems Merit Front-Burner
Managerial Attention?   125

Illustration Capsules

4.1. Estimated Value Chain Costs for Recording and Distributing Music CDs
through Traditional Music Retailers   115

4.2. Benchmarking and Ethical Conduct   118

Section C: Crafting a Strategy

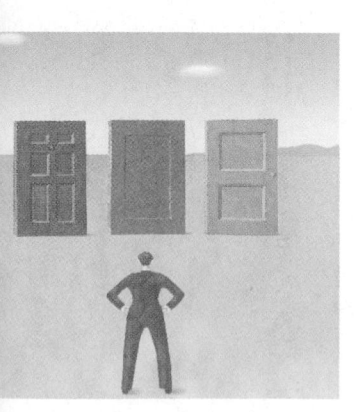

5. The Five Generic Competitive Strategies: Which One to Employ?   132

The Five Generic Competitive Strategies   134

Low-Cost Provider Strategies   135

The Two Major Avenues for Achieving a Cost Advantage   135

The Keys to Success in Achieving Low-Cost Leadership   142

When a Low-Cost Provider Strategy Works Best   143

The Pitfalls of a Low-Cost Provider Strategy   144

Broad Differentiation Strategies   144

Types of Differentiation Themes   145

Where along the Value Chain to Create the Differentiating Attributes   145

The Four Best Routes to Competitive Advantage via a Broad Differentiation Strategy   146

The Importance of Perceived Value and Signaling Value   147

When a Differentiation Strategy Works Best   148

The Pitfalls of a Differentiation Strategy   148

Best-Cost Provider Strategies   150

When a Best-Cost Provider Strategy Works Best   151

The Big Risk of a Best-Cost Provider Strategy   151

Focused (or Market Niche) Strategies   151

A Focused Low-Cost Strategy   153

A Focused Differentiation Strategy   153

When a Focused Low-Cost or Focused Differentiation Strategy Is Attractive   154

The Risks of a Focused Low-Cost or Focused Differentiation Strategy   156

The Contrasting Features of the Five Generic Competitive Strategies: A Summary   156

Illustration Capsules

5.1. Nucor Corporation's Low-Cost Provider Strategy   136

5.2. How Wal-Mart Managed Its Value Chain to Achieve a Huge Low-Cost Advantage over Rival Supermarket Chains   141

5.3. Toyota's Best-Cost Producer Strategy for Its Lexus Line   152

5.4. Motel 6's Focused Low-Cost Strategy   154

5.5. Progressive Insurance's Focused Differentiation Strategy in Auto Insurance   155

6. Supplementing the Chosen Competitive Strategy: *Other Important Strategy Choices*   160

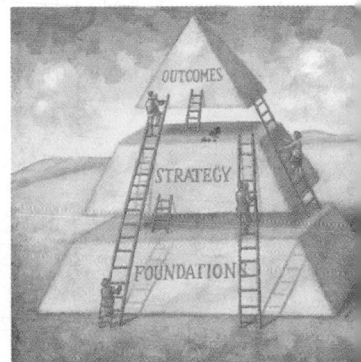

Collaborative Strategies: Alliances and Partnerships   163

Why and How Strategic Alliances Are Advantageous   164

Capturing the Benefits of Strategic Alliances   166

Why Many Alliances Are Unstable or Break Apart   167

The Strategic Dangers of Relying Heavily on Alliances and Collaborative Partnerships   167

Merger and Acquisition Strategies   168

Vertical Integration Strategies: Operating across More Stages of the Industry Value Chain   171

The Advantages of a Vertical Integration Strategy   172

The Disadvantages of a Vertical Integration Strategy   173

Outsourcing Strategies: Narrowing the Boundaries of the Business   175

When Outsourcing Strategies Are Advantageous   175

The Big Risk of an Outsourcing Strategy   177

Offensive Strategies: Improving Market Position and Building Competitive
Advantage   177
    Blue Ocean Strategy: A Special Kind of Offensive   180
    Choosing Which Rivals to Attack   181
    Choosing the Basis for Competitive Attack   181

Defensive Strategies: Protecting Market Position and Competitive
Advantage   182
    Blocking the Avenues Open to Challengers   182
    Signaling Challengers that Retaliation Is Likely   182

Web Site Strategies   183
    Product Information–Only Web Strategies: Avoiding Channel Conflict   183
    Web Site e-Stores as a Minor Distribution Channel   184
    Brick-and-Click Strategies   184
    Strategies for Online Enterprises   185

Choosing Appropriate Functional-Area Strategies   187

First-Mover Advantages and Disadvantages   188
    The Potential for Late-Mover Advantages or First-Mover Disadvantages   189
    To Be a First-Mover or Not   189

Illustration Capsules

6.1. Clear Channel Communications: Using Mergers and Acquisitions to
Become a Global Market Leader   170

6.2. Brick-and-Click Strategies in the Office Supplies Industry   186

6.3. The Battle in Consumer Broadband: First-Movers versus
Late-Movers   190

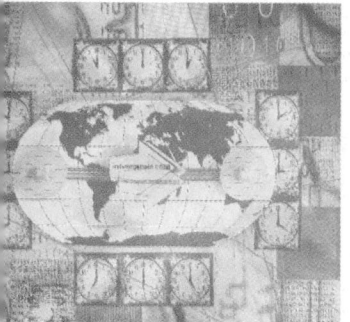

7. Competing in Foreign Markets   194

Why Companies Expand into Foreign Markets   196
    The Difference between Competing Internationally and Competing Globally   196

Cross-Country Differences in Cultural, Demographic, and Market
Conditions   197
    Gaining Competitive Advantage Based on Where Activities Are Located   198
    The Risks of Adverse Exchange Rate Shifts   199
    Host Governments' Policies   200

The Concepts of Multicountry Competition and Global Competition   201

Strategy Options for Entering and Competing in Foreign Markets   202
    Export Strategies   203
    Licensing Strategies   203
    Franchising Strategies   204
    Localized Multicountry Strategies or a Global Strategy?   204

The Quest for Competitive Advantage in Foreign Markets   209
    Using Location to Build Competitive Advantage   209
    *Using Cross-Border Transfers of Competencies and
Capabilities to Build Competitive Advantage   211*
    Using Cross-Border Coordination to Build Competitive Advantage   212

Profit Sanctuaries, Cross-Market Subsidization, and Global Strategic
Offensives   213

*Using Cross-Market Subsidization to Wage a Strategic
Offensive   214*

Offensive Strategies Suitable for Competing in Foreign Markets   215

Strategic Alliances and Joint Ventures with Foreign Partners   217

The Risks of Strategic Alliances with Foreign Partners   218

When a Cross-Border Alliance May Be Unnecessary   220

Strategies That Fit the Markets of Emerging Countries   220

Strategy Options   222

*Defending against Global Giants: Strategies for Local Companies
in Emerging Markets   224*

Illustration Capsules

7.1. Multicountry Strategies at Electronic Arts and Coca-Cola   209

7.2. Six Examples of Cross-Border Strategic Alliances   219

7.3. Coca-Cola's Strategy for Growing Its Sales in China and India   221

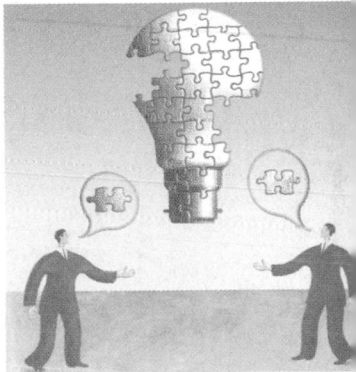

8. Tailoring Strategy to Fit Specific Industry and
   Company Situations   230

Strategies for Competing in Emerging Industries   231

The Unique Characteristics of an Emerging Industry   232

Strategy Options for Emerging Industries   233

Strategies for Competing in Rapidly Growing Markets   234

Strategies for Competing in Maturing Industries   236

How Slowing Growth Alters Market Conditions   236

Strategies that Fit Conditions in Maturing Industries   237

Strategic Pitfalls in Maturing Industries   238

Strategies for Competing in Stagnant or Declining Industries   239

End-Game Strategies for Declining Industries   241

Strategies for Competing in Turbulent, High-Velocity Markets   241

Ways to Cope with Rapid Change   242

Strategy Options for Fast-Changing Markets   242

Strategies for Competing in Fragmented Industries   245

Reasons for Supply-Side Fragmentation   245

Competitive Conditions in a Fragmented Industry   246

Strategy Options for Competing in a Fragmented Industry   247

Strategies for Sustaining Rapid Company Growth   249

The Risks of Pursuing Multiple Strategy Horizons   250

Strategies for Industry Leaders   251

Strategies for Runner-Up Firms   254

Obstacles for Firms with Small Market Shares   254

Offensive Strategies to Build Market Share   254

Other Strategic Approaches for Runner-Up Companies   255

Strategies for Weak and Crisis-Ridden Businesses 257
  Turnaround Strategies for Businesses in Crisis 257
  Harvest Strategies for Weak Businesses 260
  Liquidation: The Strategy of Last Resort 261
10 Commandments for Crafting Successful Business Strategies 261

Illustration Capsules

8.1. Exertris's Focus Strategy in the Fragmented Exercise Equipment
     Industry 248
8.2. ESPN's Strategy to Dominate Sports Entertainment 252
8.3. Sony's Turnaround Strategy—Will It Work? 259

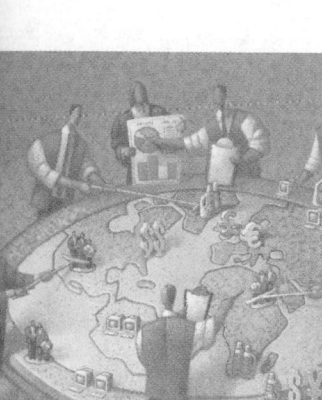

9. Diversification: *Strategies for Managing a Group
   of Businesses* 266

When to Diversify 269
Building Shareholder Value: The Ultimate Justification for Diversifying 269
Strategies for Entering New Businesses 270
  Acquisition of an Existing Business 271
  Internal Start-Up 271
  Joint Ventures 271
Choosing the Diversification Path: Related versus Unrelated Businesses 272
The Case for Diversifying into Related Businesses 272
  Identifying Cross-Business Strategic Fits along the Value Chain 274
  Strategic Fit, Economies of Scope, and Competitive Advantage 277
The Case for Diversifying into Unrelated Businesses 279
  The Merits of an Unrelated Diversification Strategy 280
  The Drawbacks of Unrelated Diversification 283
Combination Related–Unrelated Diversification Strategies 284
Evaluating the Strategy of a Diversified Company 285
  Step 1: Evaluating Industry Attractiveness 286
  Step 2: Evaluating Business-Unit Competitive Strength 289
  *Step 3: Checking the Competitive Advantage Potential of Cross-Business
  Strategic Fits 294*
  Step 4: Checking for Resource Fit 294
  *Step 5: Ranking the Performance Prospects of Business Units and Assigning
  a Priority for Resource Allocation 298*
  *Step 6: Crafting New Strategic Moves to Improve Overall Corporate
  Performance 299*
After a Company Diversifies: The Four Main Strategy Alternatives 300
  Strategies to Broaden a Diversified Company's Business Base 300
  *Divestiture Strategies Aimed at Retrenching to a
  Narrower Diversification Base 303*
  Strategies to Restructure a Company's Business Lineup 306
  Multinational Diversification Strategies 308

Illustration Capsules

9.1. Related Diversification at L'Oréal, Johnson & Johnson, PepsiCo, and Darden Restaurants   277

9.2. Unrelated Diversification at General Electric, United Technologies, American Standard, and Lancaster Colony   281

9.3. Managing Diversification at Johnson & Johnson: The Benefits of Cross-Business Strategic Fits   302

9.4. Lucent Technology's Retrenchment Strategy   304

9.5. The Global Scope of Four Prominent Diversified Multinational Corporations   309

10. Strategy, Ethics, and Social Responsibility   316

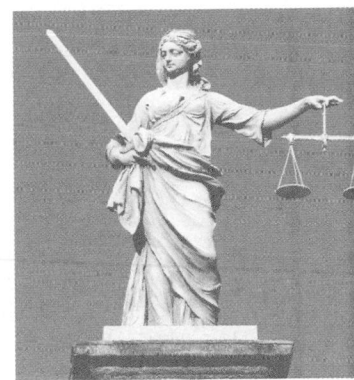

What Do We Mean by *Business Ethics?*   317

Where Do Ethical Standards Come From—Are They Universal or Dependent on Local Norms and Situational Circumstances?   318

The School of Ethical Universalism   318

The School of Ethical Relativism   319

Ethics and Integrative Social Contracts Theory   322

The Three Categories of Management Morality   323

Evidence of Managerial Immorality in the Global Business Community   325

Do Company Strategies Need to Be Ethical?   327

What Are the Drivers of Unethical Strategies and Business Behavior?   328

Approaches to Managing a Company's Ethical Conduct   333

Why Should Company Strategies Be Ethical?   338

The Moral Case for an Ethical Strategy   338

The Business Case for an Ethical Strategy   338

Linking a Company's Strategy to Its Ethical Principles and Core Values   341

Strategy and Social Responsibility   342

What Do We Mean by Social Responsibility?   342

Crafting a Social Responsibility Strategy: The Starting Point for Demonstrating a Social Conscience   345

The Moral Case for Corporate Social Responsibility   346

The Business Case for Socially Responsible Behavior   347

The Well-Intentioned Efforts of Do-Good Executives Can Be Controversial   349

How Much Attention to Social Responsibility Is Enough?   351

Linking Social Performance Targets to Executive Compensation   352

Illustration Capsules

10.1. Marsh & McLennan's Ethically Flawed Strategy   329

10.2. Philip Morris USA's Strategy for Marlboro Cigarettes: Ethical or Unethical?   334

10.3. A Test of Your Business Ethics   340

Section D: Executing the Strategy

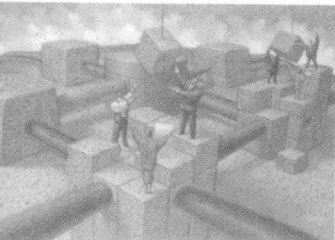

11. Building an Organization Capable of Good Strategy Execution   358

A Framework for Executing Strategy   361

The Principal Managerial Components of the Strategy Execution Process   361

Building an Organization Capable of Good Strategy Execution   363

Staffing the Organization   364

   Putting Together a Strong Management Team   364

   Recruiting and Retaining Capable Employees   365

Building Core Competencies and Competitive Capabilities   368

   The Three-Stage Process of Developing and Strengthening Competencies and Capabilities   368

   The Strategic Role of Employee Training   371

   From Competencies and Capabilities to Competitive Advantage   373

Execution-Related Aspects of Organizing the Work Effort   373

   Deciding Which Value Chain Activities to Perform Internally and Which to Outsource   373

   Making Strategy-Critical Activities the Main Building Blocks of the Organization Structure   376

   Determining the Degree of Authority and Independence to Give Each Unit and Each Employee   378

   Providing for Internal Cross-Unit Coordination   381

   Providing for Collaboration with Outside Suppliers and Strategic Allies   383

Current Organizational Trends   383

Illustration Capsules

11.1. How General Electric Develops a Talented and Deep Management Team   366

11.2. Toyota's Legendary Production System: A Capability That Translates into Competitive Advantage   372

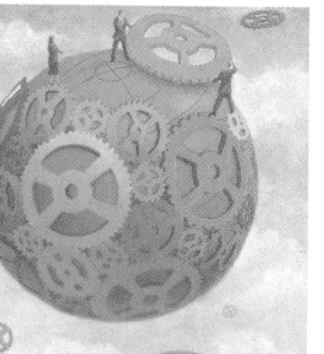

12. Managing Internal Operations: Actions That Promote Good Strategy Execution   388

Marshaling Resources behind the Drive for Good Strategy Execution   389

Instituting Policies and Procedures That Facilitate Good Strategy Execution   390

Adopting Best Practices and Striving for Continuous Improvement   393

   How the Process of Identifying and Incorporating Best Practices Works   393

   Business Process Reengineering, Six Sigma Quality Programs, and TQM: Tools for Promoting Operating Excellence   395

   Capturing the Benefits of Initiatives to Improve Operations   399

Installing Information and Operating Systems   401

    Instituting Adequate Information Systems,
    Performance Tracking, and Controls   402

    Exercising Adequate Controls over Empowered Employees   403

Tying Rewards and Incentives to Good Strategy Execution   404

    Strategy-Facilitating Motivational Practices   404

    Striking the Right Balance between Rewards and Punishment   406

    Linking the Reward System to Strategically Relevant Performance Outcomes   408

Illustration Capsules

12.1. Granite Construction's Short-Pay Policy: An Innovative Way to Drive
    Better Strategy Execution   392

12.2. Whirlpool's Use of Six Sigma to Promote Operating Excellence   398

12.3. What Companies Do to Motivate and Reward Employees   407

12.4. Nucor and Bank One: Two Companies That Tie Incentives
    Directly to Strategy Execution   409

13. Corporate Culture and Leadership: Keys to Good Strategy Execution   414

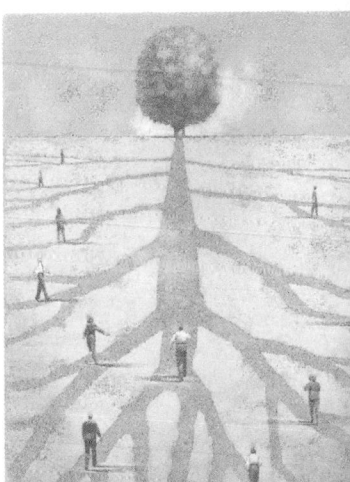

Instilling a Corporate Culture That Promotes Good Strategy Execution   415

    Identifying the Key Features of a Company's Corporate Culture   416

    Strong versus Weak Cultures   420

    Unhealthy Cultures   422

    High-Performance Cultures   424

    Adaptive Cultures   425

    Culture: Ally or Obstacle to Strategy Execution?   426

    Changing a Problem Culture   428

    Grounding the Culture in Core Values and Ethics   434

    Establishing a Strategy–Culture Fit in Multinational
    and Global Companies   437

Leading the Strategy Execution Process   439

    Staying on Top of How Well Things Are Going   439

    Putting Constructive Pressure on the Organization to Achieve Good Results
    and Operating Excellence   441

    Leading the Development of Better Competencies and Capabilities   442

    Displaying Ethical Integrity and Leading Social Responsibility Initiatives   443

    Leading the Process of Making Corrective Adjustments   445

Illustration Capsules

13.1. The Corporate Cultures at Google and Alberto-Culver   417

13.2. Changing the Culture in Alberto-Culver's North American Division   433

Part Two   Cases in Crafting and Executing Strategy   451

Section A: Crafting Strategy in Single Business Companies

1. Whole Foods Market in 2006: Mission, Core Values, and Strategy   C-2
   Arthur A. Thompson, The University of Alabama

2. Oliver's Markets   C-28
   Armand Gilinsky Jr., Sonoma State University
   John Moore, Sonoma State University
   Richard L. McCline, San Francisco State University

3. JetBlue Airways: Can It Survive in a Turbulent Industry?   C-48
   Janet Rovenpor, Manhattan College

4. Competition in the Golf Equipment Industry in 2005   C-68
   John E. Gamble, University of South Alabama

5. Dell Inc. in 2006: Can Rivals Beat Its Strategy?   C-89
   Arthur A. Thompson, The University of Alabama
   John E. Gamble, University of South Alabama

6. Competition in the MP3 Player Industry in 2005   C-116
   Lou Marino, The University of Alabama
   Kay Beth Jackson, The University of Alabama

7. Apple Computer in 2006   C-130
   Louis D. Marino, The University of Alabama
   John Hattaway, The University of Alabama
   Katy Beth Jackson, The University of Alabama

8. Netflix versus Blockbuster versus Video-on-Demand   C-148
   Braxton Maddox, The University of Alabama
   Arthur A. Thompson, The University of Alabama

9. easyCar.com   C-162
   John J. Lawrence, University of Idaho
   Luis Solis, Instituto de Empresa

10. Smithfield Foods' Vertical Integration Strategy:
    Harmful to the Environment?   C-171
    LaRue T. Hosmer, The University of Michigan

11. Zoës Kitchen: Making Cents of the Fast-Casual Dining Industry   C-182
    Braxton Maddox, The University of Alabama
    Jennifer Traywick, The University of Alabama

12. Krispy Kreme Doughnuts in 2006: Is a Turnaround Possible?   C-193
    Arthur A. Thompson, The University of Alabama
    Amit J. Shah, Frostburg State University

13. Kodak at a Crossroads: The Transition from Film-Based to Digital Photography   C-219

Boris Morozov, University of Nebraska at Omaha
Rebecca J. Morris, University of Nebraska at Omaha

14. Adam Aircraft   C-235

Carl Hedberg, Babson College
John Hamilton, Babson College
William Bygrave, Babson College

15. KRCB Television and Radio: The Canary in the Coal Mine?   C-251

Armand Gilinsky Jr., Sonoma State University
Teresa M. Shern, Sonoma State University
Robert H. Girling, Sonoma State University

16. Western States Insurance Agency   C-273

Jeffrey P. Shay, University of Montana
Tony Crawford, University of Montana
Keith Jakob, University of Montana
Sally Baack, San Francisco State University

 17. eBay: Facing the Challenge of Global Growth   C-286

Lou Marino, The University of Alabama
Patrick Kreiser, Ohio University

18. Google Inc. in 2006: Can the Strategy Support the Lofty Stock Price?   C-312

John E. Gamble, University of South Alabama

19. Copperfield's Books Inc.   C-328

Armand Gilinsky, Sonoma State University
Tom Scott, Sonoma State University

20. Harley-Davidson in 2004   C-356

John E. Gamble, University of South Alabama
Roger Schäfer, University of South Alabama

Section B: Crafting Strategy in Diversified Companies

 21. adidas: Will Restructuring Its Business Lineup Allow It to Catch Nike?   C-376

John E. Gamble, University of South Alabama

 22. Procter & Gamble's Acquisition of Gillette   C-392

John E. Gamble, University of South Alabama

Section C: Executing Strategy and Strategic Leadership

 23. Robin Hood   C-405

Joseph Lampel, New York University

24. Dilemma at Devil's Den   C-407

Allen Cohen, Babson College
Kim Johnson, Babson College

25. Wal-Mart Stores Inc.: Combating Critics and Sustaining Growth   C-410
   Arthur A. Thompson, The University of Alabama

26. Outback Steakhouse   C-436
   Sarah June Gauntlett, The University of Alabama

27. Moses at the Red Sea   C-454
   Mark Meckler, University of Portland
   Howard Feldman, University of Portland
   Michele Snead, University of Portland

28. Implementing Strategic Change: Monica Ashley's Experience   C-458
   Allen R. Cohen, Babson College
   David L. Bradford, Stanford University

29. Starbucks' Global Quest in 2006: Is the Best Yet to Come?   C-468
   Amit J. Shah, Frostburg State University
   Arthur A. Thompson, The University of Alabama
   Thomas F. Hawk, Frostburg State University

30. Leadership at TDC sunrise: "Always a Smile" or "Communication Is Life"?   C-496
   Preston Bottger, International Institute for Management Development
   George Rädler, International Institute for Management Development

Section D: Strategy, Ethics, and Social Responsibility

31. Merck and the Recall of Vioxx   C-518
   Arthur A. Thompson, The University of Alabama

32. Kimpton Hotels: Balancing Strategy and Environmental Sustainability   C-533
   Murray Silverman, San Francisco State University
   Tom Thomas, San Francisco State University

33. Monsanto and the Genetic Engineering on Agricultural Seeds   C-547
   Lisa Johnson, The University of Puget Sound

Endnotes   EN-1

Indexes

   Organization   I-1

   Name   I-10

   Subject   I-17

part one

1

Concepts and Techniques for Crafting and Executing Strategy

What Is Strategy and Why Is It Important?

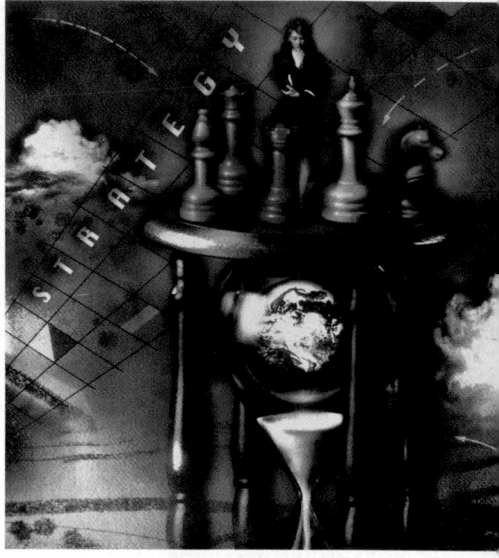

Strategy means making clear-cut choices about how to compete.

—Jack Welch

Former CEO, General Electric

A strategy is a commitment to undertake one set of actions rather than another.

—Sharon Oster

Professor, Yale University

The process of developing superior strategies is part planning, part trial and error, until you hit upon something that works.

—Costas Markides

Professor, London Business School

Without a strategy the organization is like a ship without a rudder.

—Joel Ross and Michael Kami

Authors and Consultants

Managers face three central questions in evaluating their company's business prospects: What's the company's present situation? Where does the company need to go from here? How should it get there? Arriving at a probing answer to the question "What's the company's present situation?" prompts managers to evaluate industry conditions and competitive pressures, the company's current performance and market standing, its resource strengths and capabilities, and its competitive weaknesses. The question "Where does the company need to go from here?" pushes managers to make choices about the direction the company should be headed —what new or different customer groups and customer needs it should endeavor to satisfy, what market positions it should be staking out, what changes in its business makeup are needed. The question "How should it get there?" challenges managers to craft and execute a strategy capable of moving the company in the intended direction, growing its business, and improving its financial and market performance.

In this opening chapter, we define the concept of strategy and describe its many facets. We shall indicate the kinds of actions that determine what a company's strategy is, why strategies are partly proactive and partly reactive, and why company strategies tend to evolve over time. We will look at what sets a winning strategy apart from ho-hum or flawed strategies and why the caliber of a company's strategy determines whether it will enjoy a competitive advantage or be burdened by competitive disadvantage. By the end of this chapter, you will have a pretty clear idea of why the tasks of crafting and executing strategy are core management functions and why excellent execution of an excellent strategy is the most reliable recipe for turning a company into a standout performer.

WHAT DO WE MEAN BY *STRATEGY?*

A company's **strategy** is management's action plan for running the business and conducting operations. The crafting of a strategy represents a managerial *commitment to pursue a particular set of actions* in growing the business, attracting and pleasing customers, competing successfully, conducting operations, and improving the company's financial and market performance. Thus a company's strategy is all about *how—how* management intends to grow the business, *how* it will build a loyal clientele and outcompete rivals, *how* each functional piece of the business (research and development, supply chain activities, production, sales and marketing, distribution, finance, and human resources) will be operated, *how* performance will be boosted. In choosing a strategy, management is in effect saying, "Among all the many different business approaches and ways of competing we could have chosen, we have decided to employ this particular combination of competitive and operating approaches in moving the company in the intended direction, strengthening its market position and competitiveness, and boosting performance." The strategic choices a company makes are seldom easy decisions, and some of them may turn out to be wrong—but that is not an excuse for not deciding on a concrete course of action.[1]

In most industries companies have considerable freedom in choosing the hows of strategy.[2] Thus, some rivals strive to improve their performance and market standing by achieving lower costs than rivals, while others pursue product superiority or personalized customer service or the development of competencies and capabilities that rivals cannot match. Some target the high end of the market, while others go after the middle or low end; some opt for wide product lines, while others concentrate their energies on a narrow product lineup. Some competitors position themselves in only one part of the industry's chain of production/distribution activities (preferring to be just in manufacturing or wholesale distribution or retailing), while others are partially or fully integrated, with operations ranging from components production to manufacturing and assembly to wholesale distribution or retailing. Some competitors deliberately confine their operations to local or regional markets; others opt to compete nationally, internationally (several countries), or globally (all or most of the major country markets worldwide). Some companies decide to operate in only one industry, while others diversify broadly or narrowly, into related or unrelated industries, via acquisitions, joint ventures, strategic alliances, or internal start-ups.

At companies intent on gaining sales and market share at the expense of competitors, managers typically opt for offensive strategies, frequently launching fresh initiatives of one kind or another to make the company's product offering more distinctive and appealing to buyers. Companies already in a strong industry position are more prone to strategies that emphasize gradual gains in the marketplace, fortifying the company's market position, and defending against the latest maneuvering of rivals and other developments that threaten the company's well-being. Risk-averse companies often prefer conservative strategies, preferring to follow the successful moves of pioneering companies whose managers are more entrepreneurial and willing to take the risks of being first to make a bold and perhaps pivotal move that reshapes the contest among market rivals.

There is no shortage of opportunity to fashion a strategy that both tightly fits a company's own particular situation and is discernibly different from the strategies of rivals. In fact, a company's managers normally attempt to make strategic choices about the key building blocks of its strategy that differ from the choices made by competitors—not 100 percent different but at least different in several important respects. A strategy stands a better chance of succeeding when it is predicated on actions, business approaches, and competitive moves aimed at (1) appealing to buyers in ways that set a company apart from rivals and (2) carving out its own market position. Simply copying what successful companies in the industry are doing and trying to mimic their market position rarely works. Rather, there needs to be some distinctive "aha" element to the strategy that draws in customers and produces a competitive edge. Carbon-copy strategies among companies in the same industry are the exception rather than the rule.

For a concrete example of the actions and approaches that comprise strategy, see Illustration Capsule 1.1, which describes Comcast's strategy to revolutionize the cable TV business.

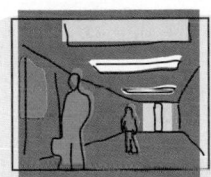

Illustration Capsule 1.1

Comcast's Strategy to Revolutionize the Cable Industry

In 2004–2005 cable TV giant Comcast put the finishing touches on a bold strategy to change the way people watched television and to grow its business by introducing Internet phone service. With revenues of $18 billion and almost 22 million of the 74 million U.S. cable subscribers, Comcast became the industry leader in the U.S. market in 2002 when it acquired AT&T Broadband, along with its 13 million cable subscribers, for about $50 billion. Comcast's strategy had the following elements:

- *Continue to roll out high-speed Internet or broadband service to customers via cable modems.* With more than 8 million customers that generated revenues approaching $5 billion annually, Comcast was already America's number one provider of broadband service. It had recently upgraded its broadband service to allow download speeds of up to six megabits per second— considerably faster than the DSL-type broadband service available over telephone lines.

- *Continue to promote a relatively new video-on-demand service that allowed digital subscribers to watch TV programs whenever they wanted to watch them.* The service allowed customers to use their remotes to choose from a menu of thousands of programs, stored on Comcast's servers as they were first broadcast, and included network shows, news, sports, and movies. Viewers with a Comcast DVR set-top box had the ability to pause, stop, restart, and save programs, without having to remember to record them when they were broadcast. Comcast had signed up more than 10 million of its cable customers for digital service, and it was introducing enhanced digital and high-definition television (HDTV) service in additional geographic markets at a brisk pace.

- *Promote a video-on-demand service whereby digital customers with a set-top box could order and watch pay-per-view movies using a menu on their remote.* Comcast's technology enabled viewers to call up the programs they wanted with a few clicks of the remote. In 2005, Comcast had almost 4000 program choices and customers were viewing about 120 million videos per month.

- *Partner with Sony, MGM, and others to expand Comcast's library of movie offerings.* In 2004, Comcast agreed to develop new cable channels using MGM and Sony libraries, which had a combined 7,500 movies and 42,000 TV shows—it took about 300 movies to feed a 24-hour channel for a month.

- *Use Voice over Internet Protocol (VoIP) technology to offer subscribers Internet-based phone service at a fraction of the cost charged by other providers.* VoIP is an appealing low-cost technology widely seen as the most significant new communication technology since the invention of the telephone. Comcast was on track to make its Comcast Digital Voice (CDV) service available to 41 million homes by year-end 2006. CDV had many snazzy features, including call forwarding, caller ID, and conferencing, thus putting Comcast in position to go after the customers of traditional telephone companies.

- *Use its video-on-demand and CDV offerings to combat mounting competition from direct-to-home satellite TV providers.* Satellite TV providers such as EchoStar and DIRECTV had been using the attraction of lower monthly fees to steal customers away from cable TV providers. Comcast believed that the appeal of video-on-demand and low-cost CDV service would overcome its higher price. And satellite TV providers lacked the technological capability to provide either two-way communications connection to homes (necessary to offer video-on-demand) or reliable high-speed Internet access.

- *Employ a sales force (currently numbering about 3,200 people) to sell advertising to businesses that were shifting some of their advertising dollars from sponsoring network programs to sponsoring cable programs.* Ad sales generated revenues of about $1.6 billion, and Comcast had cable operations in 21 of the 25 largest markets in the United States.

- *Significantly improve Comcast's customer service.* Most cable subscribers were dissatisfied with the caliber of customer service offered by their local cable companies. Comcast management believed that service would be a big issue given the need to support video-on-demand, cable modems, HDTV, phone service, and the array of customer inquiries and problems such services entailed. In 2004, Comcast employed about 12,500 people to answer an expected volume of 200 million phone calls. Newly hired customer service personnel were given five weeks of classroom training, followed by three weeks of taking calls while a supervisor listened in—it cost Comcast about $7 to handle each call. The company's goal was to answer 90 percent of calls within 30 seconds.

Sources: Information posted at www.comcast.com (accessed August 6, 2005); Marc Gunter, "Comcast Wants to Change the World, But Can It Learn to Answer the Phone?" *Fortune,* October 16, 2004, pp. 140–56; and Stephanie N. Mehta, "The Future Is on the Line," *Fortune,* July 26, 2004, pp. 121–30.

Strategy and the Quest for Competitive Advantage

The heart and soul of any strategy are the actions and moves in the marketplace that managers are taking to improve the company's financial performance, strengthen its long-term competitive position, and gain a competitive edge over rivals. A creative, distinctive strategy that sets a company apart from rivals and yields a competitive advantage is a company's most reliable ticket for earning above-average profits. Competing in the marketplace with a competitive advantage tends to be more profitable than competing with no advantage. And a company is almost certain to earn significantly higher profits when it enjoys a competitive advantage as opposed to when it is hamstrung by competitive disadvantage. Furthermore, if a company's competitive edge holds promise for being durable and sustainable (as opposed to just temporary), then so much the better for both the strategy and the company's future profitability. It's nice when a company's strategy produces at least a temporary competitive edge, but

Core Concept

A company achieves *sustainable competitive advantage* when an attractive number of buyers prefer its products or services over the offerings of competitors and when the basis for this preference is durable.

a **sustainable competitive advantage** is plainly much better. What makes a competitive advantage sustainable as opposed to temporary are actions and elements in the strategy that cause an attractive number of buyers to have a *lasting preference* for a company's products or services as compared to the offerings of competitors. Competitive advantage is the key to above-average profitability and financial performance because strong buyer preferences for the company's product offering translate into higher sales volumes (Wal-Mart) and/or the ability to command a higher price (Häagen-Dazs), thus driving up earnings, return on investment, and other measures of financial performance.

Four of the most frequently used and dependable strategic approaches to setting a company apart from rivals, building strong customer loyalty, and winning a sustainable competitive advantage are:

1. *Striving to be the industry's low-cost provider, thereby aiming for a cost-based competitive advantage over rivals.* Wal-Mart and Southwest Airlines have earned strong market positions because of the low-cost advantages they have achieved over their rivals and their consequent ability to underprice competitors. Achieving lower costs than rivals can produce a durable competitive edge when rivals find it hard to match the low-cost leader's approach to driving costs out of the business. Despite years of trying, discounters like Kmart and Target have struck out trying to match Wal-Mart's frugal operating practices, super-efficient distribution systems, and its finely honed supply chain approaches that allow it to obtain merchandise from manufacturers at super-low prices.

2. *Outcompeting rivals based on such differentiating features as higher quality, wider product selection, added performance, value-added services, more attractive styling, technological superiority, or unusually good value for the money.* Successful adopters of differentiation strategies include Johnson & Johnson in baby products (product reliability), Harley-Davidson (bad-boy image and king-of-the-road styling), Chanel and Rolex (top-of-the-line prestige), Mercedes-Benz and BMW (engineering design and performance), L. L. Bean (good value), and Amazon.com (wide selection and convenience). Differentiation strategies can be powerful so long as a company is sufficiently innovative to thwart clever rivals in finding ways to copy or closely imitate the features of a successful differentiator's product offering.

3. *Focusing on a narrow market niche and winning a competitive edge by doing a better job than rivals of serving the special needs and tastes of buyers comprising*

the niche. Prominent companies that enjoy competitive success in a specialized market niche include eBay in online auctions, Jiffy Lube International in quick oil changes, McAfee in virus protection software, Starbucks in premium coffees and coffee drinks, Whole Foods Market in natural and organic foods, CNBC and The Weather Channel in cable TV.

4. *Developing expertise and resource strengths that give the company competitive capabilities that rivals can't easily imitate or trump with capabilities of their own.* FedEx has superior capabilities in next-day delivery of small packages. Walt Disney has hard-to-beat capabilities in theme park management and family entertainment. Over the years, Toyota has developed a sophisticated production system that allows it to produce reliable, largely defect-free vehicles at low cost. IBM has wide-ranging expertise in helping corporate customers develop and install cutting-edge information systems. Ritz-Carlton and Four Seasons have uniquely strong capabilities in providing their hotel guests with an array of personalized services. Very often, winning a durable competitive edge over rivals hinges more on building competitively valuable expertise and capabilities than it does on having a distinctive product. Clever rivals can nearly always copy the attributes of a popular or innovative product, but for rivals to match experience, know-how, and specialized competitive capabilities that a company has developed and perfected over a long period of time is substantially harder to duplicate and takes much longer.

The tight connection between competitive advantage and profitability means that the quest for sustainable competitive advantage always ranks center stage in crafting a strategy. The key to successful strategy making is to come up with one or more differentiating strategy elements that act as a magnet to draw customers and yield a lasting competitive edge. Indeed, what separates a powerful strategy from a run-of-the-mill or ineffective one is management's ability to forge a series of moves, both in the marketplace and internally, that sets the company apart from its rivals, tilts the playing field in the company's favor by giving buyers reason to prefer its products or services, and produces a sustainable competitive advantage over rivals. The bigger and more sustainable the competitive advantage, the better the company's prospects for winning in the marketplace and earning superior long-term profits relative to its rivals. Without a strategy that leads to competitive advantage, a company risks being outcompeted by stronger rivals and/or locked in to mediocre financial performance. Hence, company managers deserve no gold stars for coming up with a ho-hum strategy that results in ho-hum financial performance and a ho-hum industry standing.

Identifying a Company's Strategy

The best indicators of a company's strategy are its actions in the marketplace and the statements of senior managers about the company's current business approaches, future plans, and efforts to strengthen its competitiveness and performance. Figure 1.1 shows what to look for in identifying the key elements of a company's strategy.

Once it is clear what to look for, the task of identifying a company's strategy is mainly one of researching information about the company's actions in the marketplace and business approaches. In the case of publicly owned enterprises, the strategy is often openly discussed by senior executives in the company's annual report and 10-K report, in press releases and company news (posted on the company's Web site), and in the information provided to investors at the company's Web site. To maintain the confidence of investors and Wall Street, most public companies have to be fairly open about their strategies. Company executives typically lay out key elements of their strategies in

Figure 1.1   **Identifying a Company's Strategy—What to Look for**

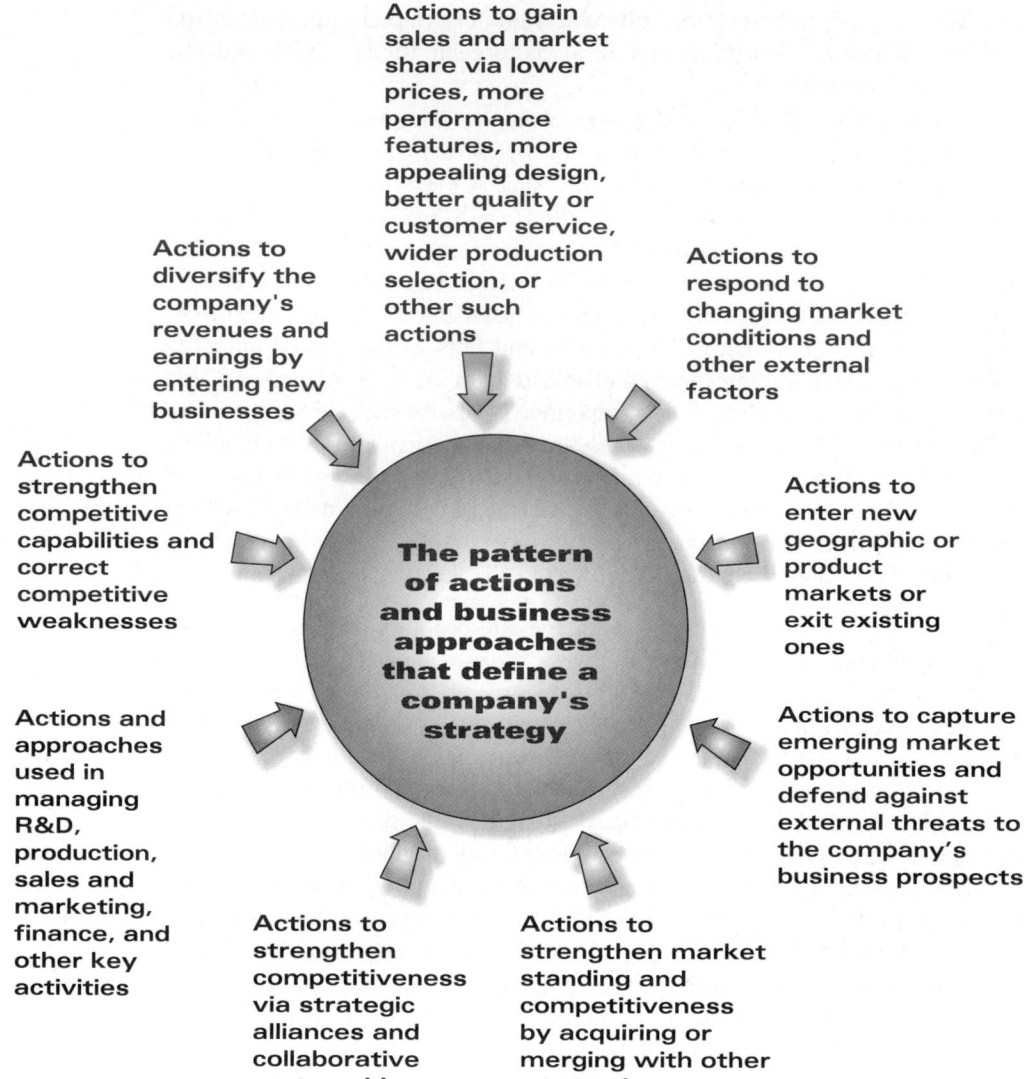

Actions to gain sales and market share via lower prices, more performance features, more appealing design, better quality or customer service, wider production selection, or other such actions

Actions to diversify the company's revenues and earnings by entering new businesses

Actions to respond to changing market conditions and other external factors

Actions to strengthen competitive capabilities and correct competitive weaknesses

Actions to enter new geographic or product markets or exit existing ones

The pattern of actions and business approaches that define a company's strategy

Actions and approaches used in managing R&D, production, sales and marketing, finance, and other key activities

Actions to capture emerging market opportunities and defend against external threats to the company's business prospects

Actions to strengthen competitiveness via strategic alliances and collaborative partnerships

Actions to strengthen market standing and competitiveness by acquiring or merging with other companies

presentations to securities analysts (the accompanying PowerPoint slides are sometimes posted in the investor relations section of the company's Web site), and stories in the business media about the company often include aspects of the company's strategy. Hence, except for some about-to-be-launched moves and changes that remain under wraps and in the planning stage, there's usually nothing secret or undiscoverable about a company's present strategy.

Why a Company's Strategy Evolves over Time

Irrespective of where the strategy comes from—be it the product of top executives or the collaborative product of numerous company personnel—it is unlikely that the strategy, as originally conceived, will prove entirely suitable over time. Every company must be willing and ready to modify its strategy in response to changing market conditions, advancing technology, the fresh moves of competitors, shifting buyer needs and preferences, emerging market opportunities, new ideas for improving the strategy, and mounting evidence that the strategy is not working well. Thus, *a company's strategy is always a work in progress.*

Most of the time a company's strategy evolves incrementally from management's ongoing efforts to fine-tune this or that piece of the strategy and to adjust certain strategy elements in response to unfolding events. But, on occasion, major strategy shifts are called for, such as when a strategy is clearly failing and the company faces a financial crisis, when market conditions or buyer preferences change significantly, or when important technological breakthroughs occur. In some industries, conditions change at a fairly slow pace, making it feasible for the major components of a good strategy to remain in place for long periods. But in industries where industry and competitive conditions change frequently and in sometimes dramatic ways, the life cycle of a given strategy is short. Industry environments characterized by *high-velocity change* require companies to rapidly adapt their strategies.[3] For example, companies in industries with rapid-fire advances in technology—like medical equipment, electronics, and wireless devices—often find it essential to adjust one or more key elements of their strategies several times a year, sometimes even finding necessary to reinvent their approach to providing value to their customers. Companies in online retailing and the travel and resort industries find it necessary to adapt their strategies to accommodate sudden bursts of new spending or sharp drop-offs in demand, often updating their market prospects and financial projections every few months.

But regardless of whether a company's strategy changes gradually or swiftly, the important point is that a company's present strategy is always temporary and on trial, pending new ideas for improvement from management, changing industry and competitive conditions, and any other new developments that management believes warrant strategy adjustments. Thus, a company's strategy at any given point is fluid, representing the temporary outcome of an ongoing process that, on the one hand, involves reasoned and creative management efforts to craft an effective strategy and, on the other hand, involves ongoing responses to market change and constant experimentation and tinkering. Adapting to new conditions and constantly learning what is working well enough to continue and what needs to be improved is consequently a normal part of the strategy-making process and results in an evolving strategy.

A Company's Strategy Is Partly Proactive and Partly Reactive

The evolving nature of a company's strategy means that the typical company strategy is a blend of (1) proactive actions to improve the company's financial performance and secure a competitive edge and (2) as-needed reactions to unanticipated developments and fresh market conditions (see Figure 1.2).[4] The biggest portion of a company's current strategy flows from previously initiated actions and business approaches that are working well enough to merit continuation and newly launched initiatives aimed at boosting financial performance and edging out rivals. Typically, managers proactively modify this or that aspect of their strategy as new learning emerges about which pieces of the strategy are working well and which aren't, and as they hit upon new ideas for strategy improvement. This part of management's action plan for running the company is deliberate and proactive, standing as the current product of management's latest and best strategy ideas.

> **Core Concept**
> Changing circumstances and ongoing management efforts to improve the strategy cause a company's strategy to evolve over time—a condition that makes the task of crafting a strategy a work in progress, not a one-time event.

> A company's strategy is shaped partly by management analysis and choice and partly by the necessity of adapting and learning by doing.

Figure 1.2   **A Company's Strategy Is a Blend of Proactive Initiatives and Reactive Adjustments**

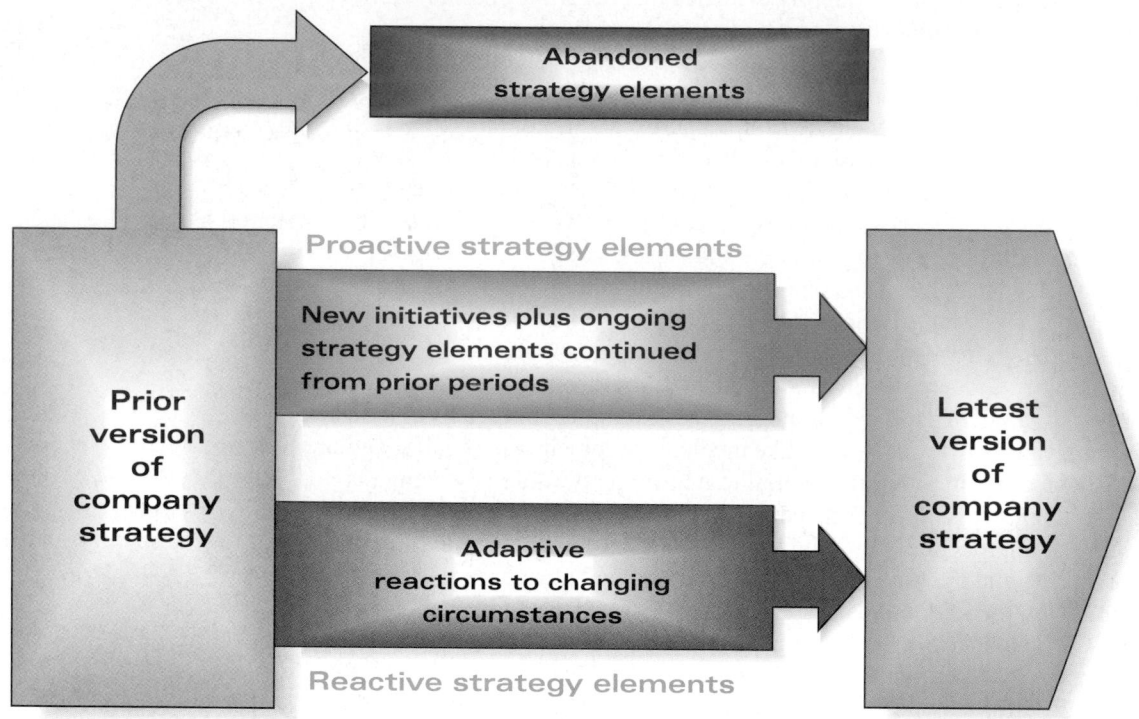

But managers must always be willing to supplement or modify all the proactive strategy elements with as-needed reactions to unanticipated developments. Inevitably, there will be occasions when market and competitive conditions take an unexpected turn that calls for some kind of strategic reaction or adjustment. Hence, a portion of a company's strategy is always developed on the fly, coming as a response to fresh strategic maneuvers on the part of rival firms, unexpected shifts in customer requirements and expectations, fast-changing technological developments, newly appearing market opportunities, a changing political or economic climate, or other unanticipated happenings in the surrounding environment. These adaptive strategy adjustments form the reactive strategy elements.

As shown in Figure 1.2, a company's strategy evolves from one version to the next as managers abandon obsolete or ineffective strategy elements, settle upon a set of *proactive/intended strategy elements*, and then adapt the strategy as new circumstances unfold, thus giving rise to *reactive/adaptive strategy elements*. A company's strategy thus tends to be a *combination* of proactive and reactive elements. In the process, some strategy elements end up being abandoned because they have become obsolete or ineffective.

STRATEGY AND ETHICS: PASSING THE TEST OF MORAL SCRUTINY

In choosing from among strategic alternatives, company managers are well advised to embrace actions that are aboveboard and can pass the test of moral scrutiny. Just keeping a company's strategic actions within the bounds of what is legal does not mean the strategy is ethical. Ethical and moral standards are not governed by what is legal. Rather, they involve issues of both right versus wrong and *duty*—what one *should* do. A strategy is ethical only if (1) it does not entail actions and behaviors that cross the line from "should do" to "should not do" (because such actions are unsavory, unconscionable, or injurious to other people or unnecessarily harmful to the environment) and (2) it allows management to fulfill its ethical duties to all stakeholders— owners/shareholders, employees, customers, suppliers, the communities in which it operates, and society at large.

> **Core Concept**
> A strategy cannot be considered ethical just because it involves actions that are legal. To meet the standard of being ethical, a strategy must entail actions that can pass moral scrutiny and that are aboveboard in the sense of not being shady, unconscionable, injurious to others, or unnecessarily harmful to the environment.

Admittedly, it is not always easy to categorize a given strategic behavior as definitely ethical or definitely unethical. Many strategic actions fall in a gray zone in between, and whether they are deemed ethical or unethical hinges on how clearly the boundaries are defined. For example, is it ethical for advertisers of alcoholic products to place ads in media having an audience of as much as 50 percent underage viewers? (In 2003, growing concerns about underage drinking prompted some beer and distilled spirits companies to agree to place ads in media with an audience at least 70 percent adult, up from a standard of 50 percent adult.) Is it ethical for an apparel retailer attempting to keep prices attractively low to source clothing from foreign manufacturers who pay substandard wages, use child labor, or subject workers to unsafe working conditions? Many people would say no, but some might argue that a company is not unethical simply because it does not police the business practices of its suppliers. Is it ethical for the makers of athletic uniforms, shoes, and other sports equipment to pay coaches large sums of money to induce them to use the manufacturer's products in their sport? (The compensation contracts of many college coaches include substantial payments from sportswear and sports equipment manufacturers, and the teams subsequently end up wearing the uniforms and using the products of those manufacturers.) Is it ethical for manufacturers of life-saving drugs to charge higher prices in some countries than they charge in others? (This is a fairly common practice that has recently come under scrutiny because it raises the costs of health care for consumers who are charged higher prices.) Is it ethical for a company to turn a blind eye to the damage its operations do to the environment even though its operations are in compliance with current environmental regulations—especially if it has the know-how and the means to alleviate some of the environmental impacts by making relatively inexpensive changes in its operating practices?

Senior executives with strong ethical convictions are generally proactive in linking strategic action and ethics: They forbid the pursuit of ethically questionable business opportunities and insist that all aspects of company strategy reflect high ethical standards.[5] They make it clear that all company personnel are expected to act with integrity, and they put organizational checks and balances into place to monitor behavior, enforce ethical codes of conduct, and provide guidance to employees regarding any gray areas. Their commitment to conducting the company's business in an ethical manner is genuine, not hypocritical.

Instances of corporate malfeasance, ethical lapses, and fraudulent accounting practices at Enron, WorldCom, Tyco, Adelphia, HealthSouth, and other companies leave no room to doubt the damage to a company's reputation and business that can result from ethical misconduct, corporate misdeeds, and even criminal behavior on the part of company personnel. Aside from just the embarrassment and black marks that accompany headline exposure of a company's unethical practices, the hard fact is that many customers and many suppliers are wary of doing business with a company that engages in sleazy practices or that turns a blind eye to illegal or unethical behavior on the part of employees. They are turned off by unethical strategies or behavior and, rather than become victims or get burned themselves, wary customers will quickly take their business elsewhere and wary suppliers will tread carefully. Moreover, employees with character and integrity do not want to work for a company whose strategies are shady or whose executives lack character and integrity. There's little lasting benefit to unethical strategies and behavior, and the downside risks can be substantial. Besides, such actions are plain wrong.

THE RELATIONSHIP BETWEEN A COMPANY'S STRATEGY AND ITS BUSINESS MODEL

Core Concept
A company's **business model** explains the rationale for why its business approach and strategy will be a moneymaker. Absent the ability to deliver good profitability, the strategy is not viable and the survival of the business is in doubt.

Closely related to the concept of strategy is the concept of a company's **business model.** While the word *model* conjures up images of ivory-tower ideas that may be loosely connected to the real world, such images do not apply here. A company's business model is management's story line for how the strategy will be a moneymaker. The story line sets forth the key components of the enterprise's business approach, indicates how revenues will be generated, and makes a case for why the strategy can deliver value to customers in a profitable manner.[6] A company's business model thus explains why its business approach and strategy will generate ample revenues to cover costs and capture a profit.

The nitty-gritty issue surrounding a company's business model is whether the chosen strategy makes good business sense. Why is there convincing reason to believe that the strategy is capable of producing a profit? How will the business generate its revenues? Will those revenues be sufficient to cover operating costs? Will customers see enough value in what the business does for them to pay a profitable price? The concept of a company's business model is, consequently, more narrowly focused than the concept of a company's business strategy. A company's strategy *relates broadly to its competitive initiatives and action plan for running the business* (but it may or may not lead to profitability). However, a company's business model zeros in on *how and why the business will generate revenues sufficient to cover costs and produce attractive profits and return on investment.* Absent the ability to deliver good profits, the strategy is not viable, the business model is flawed, and the business itself is in jeopardy of failing.

Companies that have been in business for a while and are making acceptable profits have a proven business model—because there is hard evidence that their strategies are capable of profitability. Companies that are in a start-up mode or that are losing money have questionable business models; their strategies have yet to produce good bottom-line results, putting their story line about how they intend to make money and their viability as business enterprises in doubt.

Magazines and newspapers employ a business model based on generating sufficient subscriptions and advertising to cover the costs of delivering their products to readers. Cable TV companies, cell-phone providers, record clubs, satellite radio companies, and Internet service providers also employ a subscription-based business model. The business model of network TV and radio broadcasters entails providing free programming to audiences but charging advertising fees based on audience size. McDonald's invented the business model for fast food—economical quick-service meals at clean, convenient locations. Wal-Mart has perfected the business model for big-box discount retailing—a model also used by Home Depot, Costco, and Target. Gillette's business model in razor blades involves selling a "master product"—the razor—at an attractively low price and then making money on repeat purchases— the razor blades. Printer manufacturers like Hewlett-Packard, Lexmark, and Epson pursue much the same business model as Gillette—selling printers at a low (virtually break-even) price and making large profit margins on the repeat purchases of printer supplies, especially ink cartridges. Companies like Dell and Avon employ a direct sales business model that helps keep prices low by cutting out the costs of reaching consumers through distributors and retail dealers. Illustration Capsule 1.2 discusses the contrasting business models of Microsoft and Red Hat.

WHAT MAKES A STRATEGY A WINNER?

Three questions can be used to test the merits of one strategy versus another and distinguish a winning strategy from a so-so or flawed strategy:

1. *How well does the strategy fit the company's situation?* To qualify as a winner, a strategy has to be well matched to industry and competitive conditions, a company's best market opportunities, and other aspects of the enterprise's external environment. At the same time, it has to be tailored to the company's resource strengths and weaknesses, competencies, and competitive capabilities. Unless a strategy exhibits tight fit with both the external and internal aspects of a company's overall situation, it is likely to produce less than the best possible business results.

> **Core Concept**
> A winning strategy must fit the enterprise's external and internal situation, build sustainable competitive advantage, and improve company performance.

2. *Is the strategy helping the company achieve a sustainable competitive advantage?* Winning strategies enable a company to achieve a competitive advantage that is durable. The bigger and more durable the competitive edge that a strategy helps build, the more powerful and appealing it is.

3. *Is the strategy resulting in better company performance?* A good strategy boosts company performance. Two kinds of performance improvements tell the most about the caliber of a company's strategy: (*a*) gains in profitability and financial strength, and (*b*) gains in the company's competitive strength and market standing.

Once a company commits to a particular strategy and enough time elapses to assess how well it fits the situation and whether it is actually delivering competitive advantage and better performance, then one can determine what grade to assign that strategy. Strategies that come up short on one or more of the above questions are plainly less appealing than strategies that pass all three test questions with flying colors.

Managers can also use the same questions to pick and choose among alternative strategic actions. A company evaluating which of several strategic options to employ can evaluate how well each option measures up against each of the three questions. The strategic option with the highest prospective passing scores on all three questions can be regarded as the best or most attractive strategic alternative.

Other criteria for judging the merits of a particular strategy include internal consistency and unity among all the pieces of strategy, the degree of risk the strategy poses as compared to alternative strategies, and the degree to which it is flexible and adaptable to changing circumstances. These criteria are relevant and merit consideration, but they seldom override the importance of the three test questions posed above.

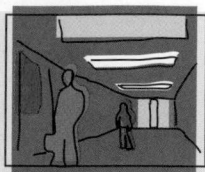

Illustration Capsule 1.2

Microsoft and Red Hat: Two Contrasting Business Models

The strategies of rival companies are often predicated on strikingly different business models. Consider, for example, the business models for Microsoft and Red Hat in operating system software for personal computers (PCs).

Microsoft's business model for making money from its Windows operating system products is based on the following revenue-cost-profit economics:

- Employ a cadre of highly skilled programmers to develop proprietary code; keep the source code hidden so as to keep the inner workings of the software proprietary.

- Sell the resulting operating system and software package to PC makers and to PC users at relatively attractive prices (around $75 to PC makers and about $100 at retail to PC users); strive to maintain a 90 percent or more market share of the 150 million PCs sold annually worldwide.

- Strive for big-volume sales. Most of Microsoft's costs arise on the front end in developing the software and are thus fixed; the variable costs of producing and packaging the CDs provided to users are only a couple of dollars per copy—once the break-even volume is reached, Microsoft's revenues from additional sales are almost pure profit.

- Provide a modest level of technical support to users at no cost.

- Keep rejuvenating revenues by periodically introducing next-generation software versions with features that will induce PC users to upgrade the operating system on previously purchased PCs to the new version.

Red Hat, a company formed to market its own version of the Linux open-source operating system, employs a business model based on sharply different revenue-cost-profit economics:

- Rely on the collaborative efforts of volunteer programmers from all over the world who contribute bits and pieces of code to improve and polish the Linux system. The global community of thousands of programmers who work on Linux in their spare time do what they do because they love it, because they are fervent believers that all software should be free (as in free speech), and in some cases because they are anti-Microsoft and want to have a part in undoing what they see as a Microsoft monopoly.

- Collect and test enhancements and new applications submitted by the open-source community of volunteer programmers. Linux's originator, Linus Torvalds, and a team of 300-plus Red Hat engineers and software developers evaluate which incoming submissions merit inclusion in new releases of Linux—the evaluation and integration of new submissions are Red Hat's only upfront product development costs.

- Market the upgraded and tested family of Red Hat products to large enterprises and charge them a subscription fee that includes 24/7 support within one hour in seven languages. Provide subscribers with updated versions of Linux every 12–18 months to maintain the subscriber base.

- Make the source code open and available to all users, allowing them to create a customized version of Linux.

- Capitalize on the specialized expertise required to use Linux in multiserver, multiprocessor applications by providing fees-based training, consulting, software customization, and client-directed engineering to Linux users. Red Hat offers Linux certification training programs at all skill levels at more than 60 global locations—Red Hat certification in the use of Linux is considered the best in the world.

Microsoft's business model—sell proprietary code software and give service away free—is a proven moneymaker that generates billions in profits annually. In contrast, the jury is still out on Red Hat's business model of selling subscriptions to open-source software to large corporations and deriving substantial revenues from the sales of technical support (included in the subscription cost), training, consulting, software customization, and engineering to generate revenues sufficient to cover costs and yield a profit. Red Hat posted losses of $140 million on revenues of $79 million in fiscal year 2002 and losses of $6.6 million on revenues of $91 million in fiscal year 2003, but it earned $14 million on revenues of $126 million in fiscal 2004. The profits came from a shift in Red Hat's business model that involved putting considerably more emphasis on getting large corporations to purchase subscriptions to the latest Linux updates. In 2005, about 75 percent of Red Hat's revenues came from large enterprise subscriptions, compared to about 53 percent in 2003.

Source: Company documents and information posted on www.microsoft.com and www.redhat.com. (accessed August 10, 2005).

WHY ARE CRAFTING AND EXECUTING STRATEGY IMPORTANT?

Crafting and executing strategy are top-priority managerial tasks for two very big reasons. First, there is a compelling need for managers to *proactively shape*, or *craft*, how the company's business will be conducted. A clear and reasoned strategy is management's prescription for doing business, its road map to competitive advantage, its game plan for pleasing customers and improving financial performance. Winning in the marketplace requires a well-conceived, opportunistic strategy, usually one characterized by strategic offensives to outinnovate and outmaneuver rivals and secure sustainable competitive advantage, then using this market edge to achieve superior financial performance. A powerful strategy that delivers a home run in the marketplace can propel a firm from a trailing position into a leading one, clearing the way for its products/services to become the industry standard. High-achieving enterprises are nearly always the product of astute, creative, proactive strategy making that sets a company apart from its rivals. Companies don't get to the top of the industry rankings or stay there with imitative strategies or with strategies built around timid actions to try to do better. And only a handful of companies can boast of strategies that hit home runs in the marketplace due to lucky breaks or the good fortune of having stumbled into the right market at the right time with the right product. There can be little argument that a company's strategy matters—and matters a lot.

Second, a *strategy-focused enterprise* is more likely to be a strong bottom-line performer than a company whose management views strategy as secondary and puts its priorities elsewhere. There's no escaping the fact that the quality of managerial strategy making and strategy execution has a highly positive impact on revenue growth, earnings, and return on investment. A company that lacks clear-cut direction, has vague or undemanding performance targets, has a muddled or flawed strategy, or can't seem to execute its strategy competently is a company whose financial performance is probably suffering, whose business is at long-term risk, and whose management is sorely lacking. In contrast, when crafting and executing a winning strategy drive management's whole approach to operating the enterprise, the odds are much greater that the initiatives and activities of different divisions, departments, managers, and work groups will be unified into a *coordinated, cohesive effort*. Mobilizing the full complement of company resources in a total team effort behind good execution of the chosen strategy and achievement of the targeted performance allows a company to operate at full power. The chief executive officer of one successful company put it well when he said:

> In the main, our competitors are acquainted with the same fundamental concepts and techniques and approaches that we follow, and they are as free to pursue them as we are. More often than not, the difference between their level of success and ours lies in the relative thoroughness and self-discipline with which we and they develop and execute our strategies for the future.

Good Strategy + Good Strategy Execution = Good Management

Crafting and executing strategy are core management functions. Among all the things managers do, nothing affects a company's ultimate success or failure more fundamentally than how well its management team charts the company's direction, develops

Core Concept

Excellent execution of an excellent strategy is the best test of managerial excellence—and the most reliable recipe for turning companies into standout performers.

competitively effective strategic moves and business approaches, and pursues what needs to be done internally to produce good day-in, day-out strategy execution and operating excellence. Indeed, *good strategy and good strategy execution are the most trustworthy signs of good management.* Managers don't deserve a gold star for designing a potentially brilliant strategy but failing to put the organizational means in place to carry it out in high-caliber fashion—weak implementation and execution undermine the strategy's potential and pave the way for shortfalls in customer satisfaction and company performance. Competent execution of a mediocre strategy scarcely merits enthusiastic applause for management's efforts either. The rationale for using the twin standards of good strategy making and good strategy execution to determine whether a company is well managed is therefore compelling: *The better conceived a company's strategy and the more competently it is executed, the more likely that the company will be a standout performer in the marketplace.*

Throughout the text chapters to come and the accompanying case collection, the spotlight is trained on the foremost question in running a business enterprise: What must managers do, and do well, to make a company a winner in the marketplace? The answer that emerges, and that becomes the message of this book, is that doing a good job of managing inherently requires good strategic thinking and good management of the strategy-making, strategy-executing process.

The mission of this book is to provide a solid overview of what every business student and aspiring manager needs to know about crafting and executing strategy. This requires exploring what good strategic thinking entails; presenting the core concepts and tools of strategic analysis; describing the ins and outs of crafting and executing strategy; and, through the cases, helping you build your skills both in diagnosing how well the strategy-making, strategy-executing task is being performed in actual companies and in prescribing actions for how the companies in question can improve their approaches to crafting and executing their strategies. At the very least, we hope to convince you that capabilities in crafting and executing strategy are basic to managing successfully and merit a place in a manager's tool kit.

As you tackle the following pages, ponder the following observation by the essayist and poet Ralph Waldo Emerson: "Commerce is a game of skill which many people play, but which few play well." If the content of this book helps you become a more savvy player and equips you to succeed in business, then your journey through these pages will indeed be time well spent.

Key Points

The tasks of crafting and executing company strategies are the heart and soul of managing a business enterprise and winning in the marketplace. A company's strategy is the game plan management is using to stake out a market position, conduct its operations, attract and please customers, compete successfully, and achieve organizational objectives. The central thrust of a company's strategy is undertaking moves to build and strengthen the company's long-term competitive position and financial performance and, ideally, gain a competitive advantage over rivals that then becomes a company's ticket to above-average profitability. A company's strategy typically evolves and reforms over time, emerging from a blend of (1) proactive and purposeful actions on the part of company managers and (2) as-needed reactions to unanticipated developments and fresh market conditions.

Closely related to the concept of strategy is the concept of a company's business model. A company's business model is management's story line for how and why the company's product offerings and competitive approaches will generate a revenue stream and have an associated cost structure that produces attractive earnings and return on investment —in effect, a company's business model sets forth the economic logic for making money in a particular business, given the company's current strategy.

A winning strategy fits the circumstances of a company's external situation and its internal resource strengths and competitive capabilities, builds competitive advantage, and boosts company performance.

Crafting and executing strategy are core management functions. Whether a company wins or loses in the marketplace is directly attributable to the caliber of a company's strategy and the proficiency with which the strategy is executed.

Exercises

1. Go to Red Hat's Web site (www.redhat.com) and check whether the company's recent financial reports indicate that its business model is working. Is the company sufficiently profitable to validate its business model and strategy? Is its revenue stream from selling training, consulting, and engineering services growing or declining as a percentage of total revenues? Does your review of the company's recent financial performance suggest that its business model and strategy are changing? Read the company's latest statement about its business model and about why it is pursuing the subscription approach (as compared to Microsoft's approach of selling copies of its operating software directly to PC manufacturers and individuals).

2. From your perspective as a cable or satellite service consumer, does Comcast's strategy as described in Illustration Capsule 1.1 seem to be well matched to industry and competitive conditions? Does the strategy seem to be keyed to maintaining a cost advantage, offering differentiating features, serving the unique needs of a niche, or developing resource strengths and competitive capabilities rivals can't imitate or trump (or a mixture of these)? Do you think Comcast's strategy has evolved in recent years? Why or why not? What is there about Comcast's strategy that can lead to sustainable competitive advantage?

3. In 2003, Levi Strauss & Company announced it would close its two remaining U.S. apparel plants to finalize its transition from a clothing manufacturer to a marketing, sales, and design company. Beginning in 2004, all Levi's apparel would be produced by contract manufacturers located in low-wage countries. As recently as 1990, Levi Strauss had produced 90 percent of its apparel in company-owned plants in the United States employing over 20,000 production workers. With every plant closing, Levi Strauss & Company provided severance and job retraining packages to affected workers and cash payments to small communities where its plants were located. However, the economies of many small communities had yet to recover and some employees had found it difficult to match their previous levels of compensation and benefits.

    Review Levi Strauss & Company's discussion of its Global Sourcing and Operating Guidelines at www.levistrauss.com/responsibility/conduct. Does the company's strategy fulfill the company's ethical duties to all stakeholders—owners/shareholders, employees, customers, suppliers, the communities in which it operates, and society at large? Does Levi Strauss's strategy to outsource all of its manufacturing operations to low-wage countries pass the moral scrutiny test given that 20,000 workers lost their jobs?

The Managerial Process of Crafting and Executing Strategy

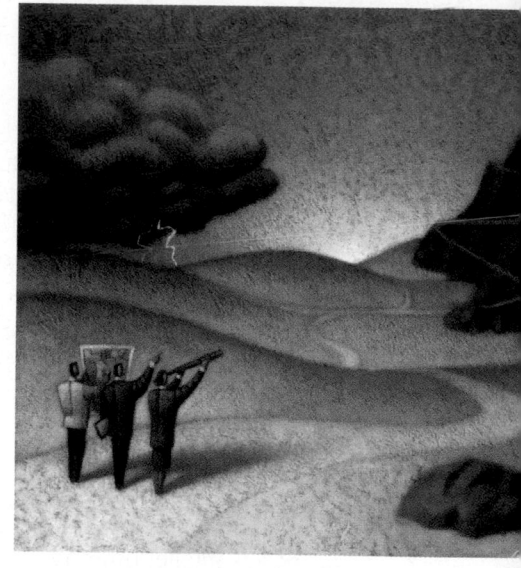

Unless we change our direction we are likely to end up where we are headed.

—Ancient Chinese proverb

If we can know where we are and something about how we got there, we might see where we are trending—and if the outcomes which lie naturally in our course are unacceptable, to make timely change.

—Abraham Lincoln

If you don't know where you are going, any road will take you there.

—The Koran

Management's job is not to see the company as it is . . . but as it can become.

—John W. Teets
Former CEO

Crafting and executing strategy are the heart and soul of managing a business enterprise. But exactly what is involved in developing a strategy and executing it proficiently? What are the various components of the strategy-making, strategy-executing process? And to what extent are company personnel—aside from top executives—involved in the process? In this chapter we present an overview of the managerial ins and outs of crafting and executing company strategies. Special attention will be given to management's direction-setting responsibilities—charting a strategic course, setting performance targets, and choosing a strategy capable of producing the desired outcomes. We will also examine which kinds of strategic decisions are made at which levels of management and the roles and responsibilities of the company's board of directors in the strategy-making, strategy-executing process.

WHAT DOES THE STRATEGY-MAKING, STRATEGY-EXECUTING PROCESS ENTAIL?

The managerial process of crafting and executing a company's strategy consists of five interrelated and integrated phases:

1. *Developing a strategic vision* of where the company needs to head and what its future product/market/customer technology focus should be.
2. *Setting objectives* and using them as yardsticks for measuring the company's performance and progress.
3. *Crafting a strategy to achieve the objectives* and move the company along the strategic course that management has charted.
4. *Implementing and executing the chosen strategy efficiently and effectively.*
5. *Evaluating performance and initiating corrective adjustments* in the company's long-term direction, objectives, strategy, or execution in light of actual experience, changing conditions, new ideas, and new opportunities.

Figure 2.1 displays this five-phase process. Let's examine each phase in enough detail to set the stage for the forthcoming chapters and give you a bird's-eye view of what this book is about.

Figure 2.1   **The Strategy-Making, Strategy-Executing Process**

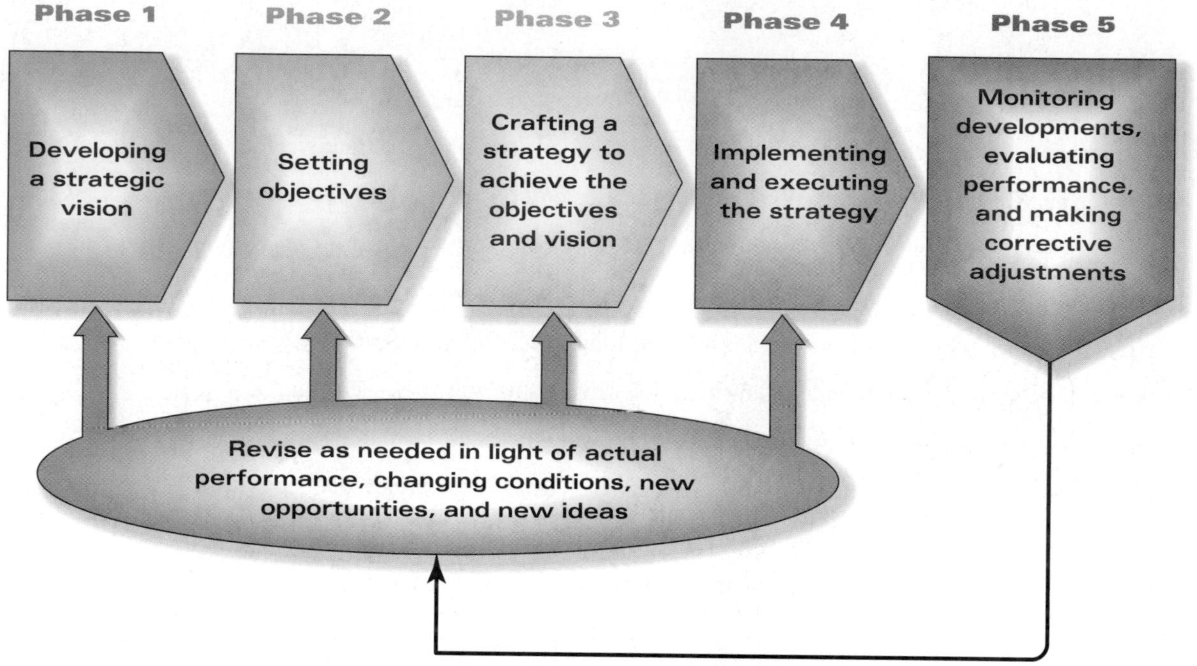

DEVELOPING A STRATEGIC VISION: PHASE 1 OF THE STRATEGY-MAKING, STRATEGY-EXECUTING PROCESS

Very early in the strategy-making process, a company's senior managers must wrestle with the issue of what path the company should take and what changes in the company's product/market/customer/technology focus would improve its market position and future prospects. Deciding to commit the company to one path versus another pushes managers to draw some carefully reasoned conclusions about how to modify the company's business makeup and what market position it should stake out. A number of direction-shaping factors need to be considered in deciding where to head and why such a direction makes good business sense—see Table 2.1.

Top management's views and conclusions about the company's direction and future product/market/customer/technology focus constitute a **strategic vision** for the company. A strategic vision delineates management's aspirations for the business, providing a panoramic view of "where we are going" and a convincing rationale for why this makes good business sense for the company. A strategic vision thus points an organization in a particular direction, charts a strategic path, and molds organizational identity. A clearly articulated strategic vision communicates management's aspirations to stakeholders and helps steer the energies of company personnel in a common direction. For instance, Henry Ford's vision of a car in every garage had power because it captured the imagination of others, aided internal efforts to mobilize the Ford Motor Company's resources, and served as a reference point for gauging the merits of the company's strategic actions.

Core Concept
A ***strategic vision*** describes the route a company intends to take in developing and strengthening its business. It lays out the company's strategic course in preparing for the future.

Table 2.1   **Factors to Consider in Deciding to Commit the Company to One Path versus Another**

External Considerations	Internal Considerations
• Is the outlook for the company promising if it simply maintains its product/market/customer/technology focus? Does sticking with the company's current strategic course present attractive growth opportunities? • Are changes under way in the market and competitive landscape acting to enhance or weaken the company's prospects? • What, if any, new customer groups and/or geographic markets should the company get in position to serve? • Which emerging market opportunities should the company pursue? Which ones should not be pursued? • Should the company plan to abandon any of the markets, market segments, or customer groups it is currently serving?	• What are the company's ambitions? What industry standing should the company have? • Will the company's present business generate sufficient growth and profitability in the years ahead to please shareholders? • What organizational strengths ought to be leveraged in terms of adding new products or services and getting into new businesses? • Is the company stretching its resources too thin by trying to compete in too many markets or segments, some of which are unprofitable? • Is the company's technological focus too broad or too narrow? Are any changes needed?

Well-conceived visions are *distinctive* and *specific* to a particular organization; they avoid generic feel-good statements like "We will become a global leader and the first choice of customers in every market we choose to serve"—which could apply to any of hundreds of organizations.[1] And they are not the product of a committee charged with coming up with an innocuous but well-meaning one-sentence vision that wins consensus approval from various stakeholders. Nicely worded vision statements with no specifics about the company's product/market/customer/technology focus fall well short of what it takes for a vision to measure up. A strategic vision proclaiming management's quest "to be the market leader" or "to be the first choice of customers" or "to be the most innovative" or "to be recognized as the best company in the industry" offers scant guidance about a company's direction and what changes and challenges lie on the road ahead.

For a strategic vision to function as a valuable managerial tool, it must (1) provide understanding of what management wants its business to look like and (2) provide managers with a reference point in making strategic decisions and preparing the company for the future. It must say something definitive about how the company's leaders intend to position the company beyond where it is today. A good vision always needs to be a bit beyond a company's reach, but progress toward the vision is what unifies the efforts of company personnel. Table 2.2 lists some characteristics of an effectively worded strategic vision.

A sampling of strategic visions currently in use shows a range from strong and clear to overly general and generic. A surprising number of the visions found on company Web sites and in annual reports are vague and unrevealing, saying very little about the company's future product/market/customer/technology focus. Some are nice-sounding but say little. Others read like something written by a committee to win the support of different stakeholders. And some are so short on specifics as to apply to most any company in any industry. Many read like a public relations statement—high-sounding words that someone came up with because it is fashionable for companies to have an official vision statement.[2] Table 2.3 provides a list of the most

Table 2.2   **Characteristics of an Effectively Worded Strategic Vision**

Graphic	Paints a picture of the kind of company that management is trying to create and the market position(s) the company is striving to stake out.
Directional	Is forward-looking; describes the strategic course that management has charted and the kinds of product/market/customer/technology changes that will help the company prepare for the future.
Focused	Is specific enough to provide managers with guidance in making decisions and allocating resources.
Flexible	Is not a once-and-for-all-time statement—the directional course that management has charted may have to be adjusted as product/market/customer/technology circumstances change.
Feasible	Is within the realm of what the company can reasonably expect to achieve in due time.
Desirable	Indicates why the chosen path makes good business sense and is in the long-term interests of stakeholders (especially shareowners, employees, and customers).
Easy to communicate	Is explainable in 5–10 minutes and, ideally, can be reduced to a simple, memorable slogan (like Henry Ford's famous vision of "a car in every garage").

Source: Based partly on John P. Kotter, *Leading Change* (Boston: Harvard Business School Press, 1996), p. 72.

common shortcomings in strategic vision statements. The one- or two-sentence vision statements most companies make available to the public, of course, provide only a glimpse of what company executives are really thinking and the strategic course they have charted—company personnel nearly always have a much better understanding of where the company is headed and why that is revealed in the official vision. But the real purpose of a strategic vision is to serve as a management tool for giving the organization a sense of direction. Like any tool, it can be used properly or improperly, either clearly conveying a company's strategic course or not.

Table 2.3   **Common Shortcomings in Company Vision Statements**

Vague or incomplete	Is short on specifics about where the company is headed or what the company is doing to prepare for the future.
Not forward-looking	Does not indicate whether or how management intends to alter the company's current product/market/customer/technology focus.
Too broad	Is so umbrella-like and all-inclusive that the company could head in most any direction, pursue most any opportunity, or enter most any business.
Bland or uninspiring	Lacks the power to motivate company personnel or inspire shareholder confidence about the company's direction or future prospects.
Not distinctive	Provides no unique company identity; could apply to companies in any of several industries (or at least several rivals operating in the same industry or market arena).
Too reliant on superlatives	Does not say anything specific about the company's strategic course beyond the pursuit of such lofty accolades as *best, most successful, recognized leader, global or worldwide leader,* or *first choice of customers.*

Sources: Based on information in Hugh Davidson, *The Committed Enterprise: How to Make Vision and Values Work* (Oxford: Butterworth Heinemann, 2002), Chapter 2, and Michel Robert, *Strategy Pure and Simple II* (New York: McGraw-Hill, 1992), Chapters 2, 3, and 6.

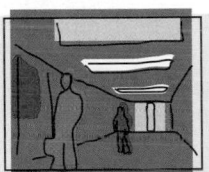

Illustration Capsule 2.1

Examples of Strategic Visions—How Well Do They Measure Up?

Using the information in Tables 2.2 and 2.3, critique the following strategic visions and rank them from 1 (best) to 7 (in need of substantial improvement).

RED HAT

To extend our position as the most trusted Linux and open source provider to the enterprise. We intend to grow the market for Linux through a complete range of enterprise Red Hat Linux software, a powerful Internet management platform, and associated support and services.

WELLS FARGO

We want to satisfy all of our customers' financial needs, help them succeed financially, be the premier provider of financial services in every one of our markets, and be known as one of America's great companies.

HILTON HOTELS CORPORATION

Our vision is to be the first choice of the world's travelers. Hilton intends to build on the rich heritage and strength of our brands by.

- Consistently delighting our customers
- Investing in our team members
- Delivering innovative products and services
- Continuously improving performance
- Increasing shareholder value

- Creating a culture of pride
- Strengthening the loyalty of our constituents

THE DENTAL PRODUCTS DIVISION OF 3M CORPORATION

Become THE supplier of choice to the global dental professional markets, providing world-class quality and innovative products.
[*Note:* All employees of the division wear badges bearing these words, and whenever a new product or business procedure is being considered, management asks "Is this representative of THE leading dental company?"]

CATERPILLAR

Be the global leader in customer value.

eBAY

Provide a global trading platform where practically anyone can trade practically anything.

H. J. HEINZ COMPANY

Be the world's premier food company, offering nutritious, superior tasting foods to people everywhere. Being the premier food company does not mean being the biggest but it does mean being the best in terms of consumer value, customer service, employee talent, and consistent and predictable growth.

Sources: Company documents and Web sites.

Illustration Capsule 2.1 provides examples of strategic visions of several prominent companies. See if you can tell which ones are mostly meaningless or nice-sounding and which ones are managerially useful in communicating "where we are headed and the kind of company we are trying to become".

A Strategic Vision Covers Different Ground than the Typical Mission Statement

The defining characteristic of a well-conceived *strategic vision* is what it says about the company's *future strategic course*—"the direction we are headed and what our future product/market/customer/technology focus will be."

In contrast, the *mission statements* that one finds in company annual reports or posted on company Web sites typically provide a brief overview of the company's *present* business purpose and raison d'être, and sometimes its geographic coverage or standing as a market leader. They may or may not single out the company's present products/services, the buyer needs it is seeking to satisfy, the customer groups it serves, or its technological and business capabilities. But rarely do company mission statements say anything about where the company is headed, the anticipated changes in its business, or its aspirations; hence, they lack the essential forward-looking quality of a strategic vision in specifying a company's direction and *future* product/market/customer/technology focus.

Consider, for example, the mission statement of Trader Joe's (a specialty grocery chain):

> The mission of Trader Joe's is to give our customers the best food and beverage values that they can find anywhere and to provide them with the information required for informed buying decisions. We provide these with a dedication to the highest quality of customer satisfaction delivered with a sense of warmth, friendliness, fun, individual pride, and company spirit.

Note that Trader Joe's mission statement does a good job of conveying "who we are, what we do, and why we are here," but provides no sense of "where we are headed." (Some companies use the term *business purpose* instead of *mission statement* in describing themselves; in practice, there seems to be no meaningful difference between the terms *mission statement* and *business purpose*—which one is used is a matter of preference.)

The distinction between a strategic vision and a mission statement is fairly clear-cut: A strategic vision portrays a company's *future* business scope ("where we are going"), whereas a company's mission typically describes its *present* business and purpose ("who we are, what we do, and why we are here").

There is value in distinguishing between the forward-looking concept of a strategic vision and the here-and-now theme of the typical mission statement. Thus, to mirror actual practice, we will use the term *mission statement* to refer to an enterprise's description of its *present* business and its purpose for existence. Ideally, a company mission statement is sufficiently descriptive to *identify the company's products/services and specify the buyer needs it seeks to satisfy, the customer groups or markets it is endeavoring to serve, and its approach to pleasing customers.* Not many company mission statements fully reveal *all* of these facets (and a few companies have worded their mission statements so obscurely as to mask what they are about), but most company mission statements do a decent job of indicating "who we are, what we do, and why we are here."

An example of a well-formed mission statement with ample specifics is that of the U.S. government's Occupational Safety and Health Administration (OSHA): "to assure the safety and health of America's workers by setting and enforcing standards; providing training, outreach, and education; establishing partnerships; and encouraging continual improvement in workplace safety and health." Google's mission statement, while short, still captures the essence of the company: "to organize the world's information and make it universally accessible and useful." Likewise, Blockbuster has a brief mission statement that cuts right to the chase: "To help people transform ordinary nights into BLOCKBUSTER nights by being their complete source for movies and games."

An example of a not-so-revealing mission statement is that of the present-day Ford Motor Company: "We are a global family with a proud heritage passionately committed to providing personal mobility for people around the world. We anticipate consumer need and deliver outstanding products and services that improve people's lives." A person who has never heard of Ford would not know from reading the company's mission statement that it is a global producer of motor vehicles. Similarly, Microsoft's mission statement—"to help people and businesses throughout the world realize their full potential"—says nothing about its products or business makeup and could apply to many companies in many different industries. Coca-Cola, which markets nearly 400 beverage brands in over 200 countries, also has an overly general mission statement: "to benefit and refresh everyone it touches." A mission statement that provides scant indication of "who we are and what we do" has no substantive value.

Occasionally, companies couch their mission statements in terms of making a profit. This is misguided. Profit is more correctly an *objective* and a *result* of what a company does. Moreover, earning a profit is the obvious intent of every commercial enterprise. Such companies as BMW, McDonald's, Shell Oil, Procter & Gamble, Nintendo, and Nokia are each striving to earn a profit for shareholders; but plainly the fundamentals of their businesses are substantially different when it comes to "who we are and what we do." It is management's answer to "Make a profit doing what and for whom?" that reveals a company's true substance and business purpose. *A well-conceived mission statement distinguishes a company's business makeup from that of other profit-seeking enterprises in language specific enough to give the company its own identity.*

Communicating the Strategic Vision

Effectively communicating the strategic vision down the line to lower-level managers and employees is as important as choosing a strategically sound long-term direction. Not only do people have a need to believe that senior management knows where it's trying to take the company and understand what changes lie ahead both externally and internally, but unless and until frontline employees understand why the strategic course that management has charted is reasonable and beneficial, they are unlikely to rally behind managerial efforts to get the organization moving in the intended direction.

Winning the support of organization members for the vision nearly always means putting "where we are going and why" in writing, distributing the written vision organizationwide, and having executives personally explain the vision and its rationale to as many people as feasible. Ideally, executives should present their vision for the company in a manner that reaches out and grabs people. An engaging and convincing strategic vision has enormous motivational value—for the same reason that a stonemason is more inspired by "building a great cathedral for the ages" than by "laying stones to create floors and walls." When managers articulate a vivid and compelling case for where the company is headed, organization members begin to say, "This is interesting and has a lot of merit. I want to be involved and do my part to helping make it happen." The more that a vision evokes positive support and excitement, the greater its impact in terms of arousing a committed organizational effort and getting company personnel to move in a common direction.[3] Thus executive ability to paint a convincing and inspiring picture of a company's journey and destination is an important element of effective strategic leadership.

> **Core Concept**
> An effectively communicated vision is a valuable management tool for enlisting the commitment of company personnel to actions that get the company moving in the intended direction.

Expressing the Essence of the Vision in a Slogan   The task of effectively conveying the vision to company personnel is assisted when management can capture the vision of where to head in a catchy or easily remembered slogan. A number of organizations have summed up their vision in a brief phrase:

- Levi Strauss & Company: "We will clothe the world by marketing the most appealing and widely worn casual clothing in the world."
- Nike: "To bring innovation and inspiration to every athlete in the world."

- Mayo Clinic: "The best care to every patient every day."
- Scotland Yard: "To make London the safest major city in the world."
- Greenpeace: "To halt environmental abuse and promote environmental solutions."
- Charles Schwab: "To provide customers with the most useful and ethical financial services in the world."

Strategic visions become real only when the vision statement is imprinted in the minds of organization members and then translated into hard objectives and strategies.

Creating a short slogan to illuminate an organization's direction and purpose and then using it repeatedly as a reminder of "where we are headed and why" helps rally organization members to hurdle whatever obstacles lie in the company's path and maintain their focus.

Breaking Down Resistance to a New Strategic Vision   It is particularly important for executives to provide a compelling rationale for a dramatically *new* strategic vision and company direction. When company personnel don't understand or accept the need for redirecting organizational efforts, they are prone to resist change. Hence, reiterating the basis for the new direction, addressing employee concerns head-on, calming fears, lifting spirits, and providing updates and progress reports as events unfold all become part of the task of mobilizing support for the vision and winning commitment to needed actions.

Just stating the case for a new direction once is not enough. Executives must repeat the reasons for the new direction often and convincingly at company gatherings and in company publications, and they must reinforce their pronouncements with updates about how the latest information confirms the choice of direction and the validity of the vision. Unless and until more and more people are persuaded of the merits of management's new vision and the vision gains wide acceptance, it will be a struggle to move the organization down the newly chosen path.

Recognizing Strategic Inflection Points   Sometimes there's an order-of-magnitude change in a company's environment that dramatically alters its prospects and mandates radical revision of its strategic course. Intel's former chairman Andrew Grove has called such occasions *strategic inflection points*—Illustration Capsule 2.2 relates Intel's two encounters with strategic inflection points and the resulting alterations in its strategic vision. As the Intel example forcefully demonstrates, when a company reaches a strategic inflection point, management has some tough decisions to make about the company's course. Often it is a question of what to do to sustain company success, not just how to avoid possible disaster. Responding quickly to unfolding changes in the marketplace lessens a company's chances of becoming trapped in a stagnant or declining business or letting attractive new growth opportunities slip away.

Understanding the Payoffs of a Clear Vision Statement   In sum, a well-conceived, forcefully communicated strategic vision pays off in several respects: (1) it crystallizes senior executives' own views about the firm's long-term direction; (2) it reduces the risk of rudderless decision making; (3) it is a tool for winning the support of organizational members for internal changes that will help make the vision a reality; (4) it provides a beacon for lower-level managers in forming departmental missions, setting departmental objectives, and crafting functional and departmental strategies that are in sync with the company's overall strategy; and (5) it helps an organization prepare for the future. When management is able to demonstrate significant progress in achieving these five benefits, the first step in organizational direction setting has been successfully completed.

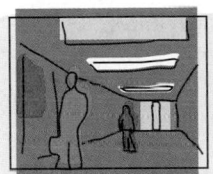

Illustration Capsule 2.2
Intel's Two Strategic Inflection Points

Intel Corporation has encountered two strategic inflection points within the past 20 years. The first came in the mid-1980s, when memory chips were Intel's principal business and Japanese manufacturers, intent on dominating the memory chip business, began cutting their prices 10 percent below the prices charged by Intel and other U.S. memory chip manufacturers. Each time U.S. companies matched the Japanese price cuts, the Japanese manufacturers responded with another 10 percent price cut. Intel's management explored a number of strategic options to cope with the aggressive pricing of its Japanese rivals—building a giant memory chip factory to overcome the cost advantage of Japanese producers, investing in research and development (R&D) to come up with a more advanced memory chip, and retreating to niche markets for memory chips that were not of interest to the Japanese.

At the time, Gordon Moore, Intel's chairman and cofounder, and Andrew Grove, Intel's chief executive officer (CEO), jointly concluded that none of these options offered much promise and that the best long-term solution was to abandon the memory chip business even though it accounted for 70 percent of Intel's revenue. Grove, with the concurrence of both Moore and the board of directors, then proceeded to commit Intel's full energies to the business of developing ever more powerful microprocessors for personal computers. Intel had invented microprocessors in the early 1970s but had recently been concentrating on memory chips because of strong competition and excess capacity in the market for microprocessors.

Grove's bold decision to withdraw from memory chips, absorb a $173 million write-off in 1986, and go all out in microprocessors produced a new strategic vision for Intel—becoming the preeminent supplier of microprocessors to the personal computing industry, making the personal computer (PC) the central appliance in the workplace and the home, and being the undisputed leader in driving PC technology forward. Grove's new vision for Intel and the strategic course he charted in 1985 produced spectacular results. Since 1996, over 80 percent of the world's PCs have been made with Intel microprocessors and Intel has become the world's most profitable chip maker.

Intel encountered a second inflection point in 1998, opting to refocus on becoming the preeminent building-block supplier to the Internet economy and spurring efforts to make the Internet more useful. Starting in early 1998 and responding to the mushrooming importance of the Internet, Intel's senior management launched major new initiatives to direct attention and resources to expanding the capabilities of both the PC platform and the Internet. It was this strategic inflection point that led to Intel's latest strategic vision of playing a major role in getting a billion computers connected to the Internet worldwide, installing millions of servers, and building an Internet infrastructure that would support trillions of dollars of e-commerce and serve as a worldwide communication medium.

Source: Andrew S. Grove, *Only the Paranoid Survive* (New York: Doubleday-Currency, 1996), company documents and press releases, and information posted at www.intel.com.

Linking the Vision/Mission with Company Values

Many companies have developed a statement of values to guide the company's pursuit of its vision/mission, strategy, and ways of operating. By **values** (or *core values,* as they are often called), we mean the beliefs, traits, and ways of doing things that management has determined should guide the pursuit of its vision and strategy, the conduct of company's operations, and the behavior of company personnel.

Values, good and bad, exist in every organization. They relate to such things as fair treatment, integrity, ethical behavior, innovation, teamwork, top-notch quality, superior customer service, social responsibility, and community citizenship. Most companies have built their statements of values around four to eight traits that company personnel are expected to display and that are supposed to be mirrored in how the company conducts its business.

> **Core Concept**
> A company's **values** are the beliefs, traits, and behavioral norms that company personnel are expected to display in conducting the company's business and pursuing its strategic vision and strategy.

At Kodak, the core values are respect for the dignity of the individual, uncompromising integrity, unquestioned trust, constant credibility, continual improvement and personal renewal, and open celebration of individual and team achievements. Home Depot embraces eight values (entrepreneurial spirit, excellent customer service, giving back to the community, respect for all people, doing the right thing, taking care of people, building strong relationships, and creating shareholder value) in its quest to be the world's leading home improvement retailer by operating warehouse stores filled with a wide assortment of products at the lowest prices with trained associates giving absolutely the best customer service in the industry. Toyota preaches respect for and development of its employees, teamwork, getting quality right the first time, learning, continuous improvement, and embracing change in its pursuit of low-cost, top-notch manufacturing excellence in motor vehicles.[4] DuPont stresses four values—safety, ethics, respect for people, and environmental stewardship; the first three have been in place since the company was founded 200 years ago by the DuPont family. Heinz uses the acronym PREMIER to identify seven values that "define to the world and to ourselves who we are and what we stand for":

- **P**assion . . . to be passionate about winning and about our brands, products and people, thereby delivering superior value to our shareholders.
- **R**isk Tolerance . . . to create a culture where entrepreneurship and prudent risk taking are encouraged and rewarded.
- **E**xcellence . . . to be the best in quality and in everything we do.
- **M**otivation . . . to celebrate success, recognizing and rewarding the achievements of individuals and teams.
- **I**nnovation . . . to innovate in everything, from products to processes.
- **E**mpowerment . . . to empower our talented people to take the initiative and to do what's right.
- **R**espect . . . to act with integrity and respect towards all.

Do companies practice what they preach when it comes to their professed values? Sometimes no, sometimes yes—at runs the gamut. At one extreme are companies with window-dressing values; the values statement is merely a collection of nice words and phrases that may be given lip service by top executives but have little discernible impact on either how company personnel behave or how the company operates. Such companies have values statements because such statements are in vogue and are seen as making the company look good. At the other extreme are companies whose executives take the stated values very seriously—the values are widely adopted by company personnel, are ingrained in the corporate culture, and are mirrored in how company personnel conduct themselves and the company's business on a daily basis. Top executives at companies on this end of the values-statement gamut genuinely believe in the importance of grounding company operations on sound values and ways of doing business. In their view, holding company personnel accountable for displaying the stated values is a way of infusing the company with the desired character, identity, and behavioral norms—the values become the company's equivalent of DNA.

At companies where the stated values are real rather than cosmetic, managers connect values to the pursuit of the strategic vision and mission in one of two ways. In companies with long-standing values that are deeply entrenched in the corporate culture, senior managers are careful to craft a vision, mission, and strategy that match established values, and they reiterate how the values-based behavioral norms contribute to the company's business success. If the company changes to a different vision or strategy, executives take care to explain how and why the core values continue to be relevant. Few companies with sincere commitment to established core values ever undertake strategic moves that conflict with ingrained values.

In new companies or companies with weak or incomplete sets of values, top management considers what values, behaviors, and business conduct should characterize the company and that will help drive the vision and strategy forward. Then values and behaviors that complement and support vision are drafted and circulated among managers and employees for discussion and possible modification. A final values statement that incorporates the desired behaviors and traits and that connects to the vision/mission is then officially adopted. Some companies combine their vision and values into a single statement or document, circulate it to all organization members, and in many instances post the vision/mission and values statement on the company's Web site. Illustration Capsule 2.3 describes the connection between Yahoo's mission and its core values.

Of course, a wide gap sometimes opens between a company's stated values and its actual business practices. Enron, for example, touted four corporate values—respect, integrity, communication, and excellence—but some top officials engaged in dishonest and fraudulent maneuvers that were concealed by "creative" accounting; the lack of integrity on the part of Enron executives and their deliberate failure to accurately communicate with shareholders and regulators in the company's financial filings led directly to the company's dramatic bankruptcy and implosion over a six-week period, along with criminal indictments, fines, or jail terms for over a dozen Enron executives. Once one of the world's most distinguished public accounting firms, Arthur Andersen was renowned for its commitment to the highest standards of audit integrity, but its high-profile audit failures and ethical lapses at Enron, WorldCom, and other companies led to Andersen's demise—in 2002, it was indicted for destroying Enron-related documents to thwart investigators.

SETTING OBJECTIVES: PHASE 2 OF THE STRATEGY-MAKING, STRATEGY-EXECUTING PROCESS

The managerial purpose of setting **objectives** is to convert the strategic vision into specific performance targets—results and outcomes the company's management wants to achieve. Objectives represent a managerial commitment to achieving particular results and outcomes. Well-stated objectives are *quantifiable,* or *measurable,* and contain a *deadline for achievement.* As Bill Hewlett, cofounder of Hewlett-Packard, shrewdly observed, "You cannot manage what you cannot measure. . . . And what gets measured gets done."[5] Concrete, measurable objectives are managerially valuable because they serve as yardsticks for tracking a company's performance and progress—a company that consistently meets or beats its performance targets is generally a better overall performer than a company that frequently falls short of achieving its objectives. Indeed, the experiences of countless companies and managers teach that precisely spelling out *how much* of *what kind* of performance *by when* and then pressing forward with actions and incentives calculated to help achieve the targeted outcomes greatly improve a company's actual performance. Such an approach definitely beats setting vague targets like "maximize profits," "reduce costs," "become more efficient," or "increase sales," which specify neither how much nor when. Similarly, exhorting

Core Concept
Objectives are an organization's performance targets—the results and outcomes management wants to achieve. They function as yardsticks for measuring how well the organization is doing.

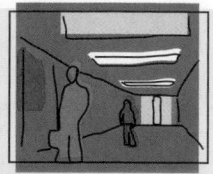

Illustration Capsule 2.3

The Connection between Yahoo's Mission and Core Values

Our mission is to be the most essential global Internet service for consumers and businesses. How we pursue that mission is influenced by a set of core values—the standards that guide interactions with fellow Yahoos, the principles that direct how we service our customers, the ideals that drive what we do and how we do it. Many of our values were put into practice by two guys in a trailer some time ago; others reflect ambitions as our company grows. All of them are what we strive to achieve every day.

EXCELLENCE

We are committed to winning with integrity. We know leadership is hard won and should never be taken for granted. We aspire to flawless execution and don't take shortcuts on quality. We seek the best talent and promote its development. We are flexible and learn from our mistakes.

INNOVATION

We thrive on creativity and ingenuity. We seek the innovations and ideas that can change the world. We anticipate market trends and move quickly to embrace them. We are not afraid to take informed, responsible risk.

CUSTOMER FIXATION

We respect our customers above all else and never forget that they come to us by choice. We share a personal responsibility to maintain our customers' loyalty and trust. We listen and respond to our customers and seek to exceed their expectations.

TEAMWORK

We treat one another with respect and communicate openly. We foster collaboration while maintaining individual accountability. We encourage the best ideas to surface from anywhere within the organization. We appreciate the value of multiple perspectives and diverse expertise.

COMMUNITY

We share an infectious sense of mission to make an impact on society and empower consumers in ways never before possible. We are committed to serving both the Internet community and our own communities.

FUN

We believe humor is essential to success. We applaud irreverence and don't take ourselves too seriously. We celebrate achievement. We yodel.

WHAT YAHOO DOESN'T VALUE

At the end of its values statement, Yahoo made a point of singling out 54 things that it did not value, including bureaucracy, losing, good enough, arrogance, the status quo, following, formality, quick fixes, passing the buck, micromanaging, Monday morning quarterbacks, 20/20 hindsight, missing the boat, playing catch-up, punching the clock, and "shoulda coulda woulda."

Source: http://docs.yahoo.com/info/values (accessed August 20, 2005).

company personnel to try hard or do the best they can, and then living with whatever results they deliver, is clearly inadequate.

The Imperative of Setting Stretch Objectives   Ideally, managers ought to use the objective-setting exercise as a tool for *stretching an organization to perform at its full potential and deliver the best possible results.* Challenging company personnel to go all out and deliver "stretch" gains in performance pushes an enterprise to be more inventive, to exhibit more urgency in improving both its financial performance and its business position, and to be more intentional and focused in its actions. Stretch objectives spur exceptional performance and help companies guard against contentment with modest gains in organizational performance. As Mitchell Leibovitz, former CEO of the auto parts and service retailer Pep Boys, once said, "If you want to have ho-hum results, have ho-hum objectives." *There's no better way to avoid ho-hum results than by setting stretch objectives and*

Setting stretch objectives is an effective tool for avoiding ho-hum results.

using compensation incentives to motivate organization members to achieve the stretch performance targets.

What Kinds of Objectives to Set: The Need for a Balanced Scorecard

Two very distinct types of performance yardsticks are required: those relating to *financial performance* and those relating to *strategic performance*—outcomes that indicate a company is strengthening its marketing standing, competitive vitality, and future business prospects. Examples of commonly used **financial objectives** and **strategic objectives** include the following:

> **Core Concept**
> ***Financial objectives*** relate to the financial performance targets management has established for the organization to achieve. ***Strategic objectives*** relate to target outcomes that indicate a company is strengthening its market standing, competitive vitality, and future business prospects.

Financial Objectives	Strategic Objectives
• An *x* percent increase in annual revenues	• Winning an *x* percent market share
• Annual increases in after-tax profits of *x* percent	• Achieving lower overall costs than rivals
• Annual increases in earnings per share of *x* percent	• Overtaking key competitors on product performance or quality or customer service
• Annual dividend increases	• Deriving *x* percent of revenues from the sale of new products introduced within the past five years
• Larger profit margins	
• An *x* percent return on capital employed (ROCE) or return on equity (ROE)	• Achieving technological leadership
	• Having better product selection than rivals
• Increased shareholder value—in the form of an upward trending stock price and annual dividend increases	• Strengthening the company's brand-name appeal
• Strong bond and credit ratings	• Having stronger national or global sales and distribution capabilities than rivals
• Sufficient internal cash flows to fund new capital investment	• Consistently getting new or improved products to market ahead of rivals
• Stable earnings during periods of recession	

Achieving acceptable financial results is a must. Without adequate profitability and financial strength, a company's pursuit of its strategic vision, as well as its long-term health and ultimate survival, is jeopardized. Furthermore, subpar earnings and a weak balance sheet not only alarm shareholders and creditors but also put the jobs of senior executives at risk. However, good financial performance, by itself, is not enough. Of equal or greater importance is a company's strategic performance—outcomes that indicate whether a company's market position and competitiveness are deteriorating, holding steady, or improving.

The Case for a Balanced Scorecard: Improved Strategic Performance Fosters Better Financial Performance   A company's financial performance measures are really *lagging indicators* that reflect the results of past decisions and organizational activities.[6] But a company's past or current financial performance is not a reliable indicator of its future prospects—poor financial performers often turn things around and do better, while good financial performers can fall on hard times. The best and most reliable *leading indicators* of a company's future financial performance and business prospects are strategic outcomes that indicate whether the

> **Core Concept**
> A company that pursues and achieves strategic outcomes that boost its competitiveness and strength in the marketplace is in much better position to improve its future financial performance.

company's competitiveness and market position are stronger or weaker. For instance, if a company has set aggressive strategic objectives and is achieving them—such that its competitive strength and market position are on the rise, then there's reason to expect that its *future* financial performance will be better than its current or past performance. If a company is losing ground to competitors and its market position is slipping—outcomes that reflect weak strategic performance (and, very likely, failure to achieve its strategic objectives), then its ability to maintain its present profitability is highly suspect. Hence, the degree to which a company's managers set, pursue, and achieve stretch strategic objectives tends to be a reliable leading indicator of whether its future financial performance will improve or stall.

Consequently, a *balanced scorecard* for measuring company performance—one that tracks the achievement of both financial objectives and strategic objectives—is optimal.[7] Just tracking a company's financial performance overlooks the fact that what ultimately enables a company to deliver better financial results from its operations is the achievement of strategic objectives that improve its competitiveness and market strength. Indeed, *the surest path to boosting company profitability quarter after quarter and year after year is to relentlessly pursue strategic outcomes that strengthen the company's market position and produce a growing competitive advantage over rivals.*

Roughly 36 percent of global companies and over 100 nonprofit and governmental organizations used the balanced scorecard approach in 2001.[8] A more recent survey of 708 companies on five continents found that 62 percent were using a balanced scorecard to track performance.[9] Organizations that have adopted the balanced scorecard approach to setting objectives and measuring performance include Exxon Mobil, CIGNA, United Parcel Service, Sears, Nova Scotia Power, BMW, AT&T Canada, Chemical Bank, DaimlerChrysler, DuPont, Motorola, Siemens, Wells Fargo, Wendy's, Saatchi & Saatchi, Duke Children's Hospital, U.S. Department of the Army, Tennessee Valley Authority, the United Kingdom's Ministry of Defense, the University of California at San Diego, and the City of Charlotte, North Carolina.[10]

Illustration Capsule 2.4 shows selected objectives of five prominent companies—all employ a combination of strategic and financial objectives.

Both Short-Term and Long-Term Objectives Are Needed   As a rule, a company's set of financial and strategic objectives ought to include both near-term and longer-term performance targets. Having quarterly and annual objectives focuses attention on delivering immediate performance improvements. Targets to be achieved within three to five years prompt considerations of what to do *now* to put the company in position to perform better later. A company that has an objective of doubling its sales within five years can't wait until the third or fourth year to begin growing its sales and customer base. By spelling out annual (or perhaps quarterly) performance targets, management indicates the *speed* at which longer range targets are to be approached. Long-term objectives take on particular importance because it is generally in the best interest of shareholders for companies to be managed for optimal long-term performance. When trade-offs have to be made between achieving long-run objectives and achieving short-run objectives, long-run objectives should take precedence (unless the achievement of one or more short-run performance targets have unique importance). Shareholders are seldom well-served by repeated management actions that sacrifice better long-term performance in order to make quarterly or annual targets.

Strategic Intent: Relentless Pursuit of an Ambitious Strategic Objective
Very ambitious companies often establish a long-term strategic objective that clearly

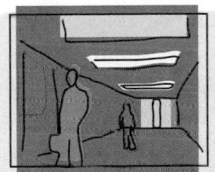

Illustration Capsule 2.4
Examples of Company Objectives

NISSAN

Increase sales to 4.2 million cars and trucks by 2008 (up from 3 million in 2003); cut purchasing costs 20% and halve the number of suppliers; have zero net debt; maintain a return on invested capital of 20%; maintain a 10% or better operating margin.

McDONALD'S

Place more emphasis on delivering an exceptional customer experience; add approximately 350 net new McDonald's restaurants; reduce general and administrative spending as a percent of total revenues; achieve systemwide sales and revenue growth of 3% to 5%, annual operating income growth of 6% to 7%, and annual returns on incremental invested capital in the high teens.

H. J. HEINZ COMPANY

Achieve 4–6% sales growth, 7–10% growth in operating income, EPS in the range of $2.35 to $2.45, and operating free cash flow of $900 million to $1 billion in fiscal 2006; pay dividends equal to 45–50 percent of earnings, increase the focus on the company's 15 power brands and give top resource priority to those brands with number one and two market positions; continue to introduce new and improved food products; add to the Heinz portfolio of brands by acquiring companies with brands that complement

existing brands; increase sales in Russia, Indonesia, China and India by 50 percent in fiscal year 2006 to roughly 6 percent of total sales; and by the end of fiscal 2008, derive approximately 50 percent of sales and profits from North America, 30 percent from Europe, and 20 percent from all other markets.

SEAGATE TECHNOLOGY

Solidify the company's No. 1 position in the overall market for hard-disk drives; get more Seagate drives into popular consumer electronics products; take share away from Western Digital in providing disk drives for Microsoft's Xbox; maintain leadership in core markets and achieve leadership in emerging markets; grow revenues by 10 percent per year; maintain gross margins of 24–26 percent; hold internal operating expenses to 13–13.5 percent of revenue.

3M CORPORATION

To achieve long term sales growth of 5–8% organic plus 2–4% from acquisitions; annual growth in earnings per share of 10% or better, on average; a return on stockholders' equity of 20%–25%; a return on capital employed of 27% or better; double the number of qualified new 3M product ideas and triple the value of products that win in the marketplace; and build the best sales and marketing organization in the world.

Sources: Information posted on company Web sites (accessed August 21, 2005); and "Nissan's Smryna Plant Produces 7 Millionth Vehicle," *Automotive Intelligence News,* August 2, 2005, p. 5.

---

signals **strategic intent** to be a winner in the marketplace, often against long odds.[11] A company's strategic intent can entail unseating the existing industry leader, becoming the dominant market share leader, delivering the best customer service of any company in the industry (or the world), or turning a new technology into products capable of changing the way people work and live. Nike's strategic intent during the 1960s was to overtake Adidas; this intent connected nicely with Nike's core purpose "to experience the emotion of competition, winning, and crushing competitors." Canon's strategic intent in copying equipment was to "beat Xerox." For some years, Toyota has been driving to overtake General Motors as the world's largest motor vehicle producer—and it surpassed Ford Motor Company in total vehicles sold in 2003, to move into second place. Toyota has expressed its strategic intent in the form of a global market share objective of 15 percent by 2010, up from 5 percent in 1980 and 10 percent in 2003. Starbucks' strategic intent is to make the Starbucks brand the world's most recognized and respected brand.

> **Core Concept**
> A company exhibits ***strategic intent*** when it relentlessly pursues an ambitious strategic objective, concentrating the full force of its resources and competitive actions on achieving that objective.

Ambitious companies that establish exceptionally bold strategic objectives and have an unshakable commitment to achieving them almost invariably begin with strategic intents that are out of proportion to their immediate capabilities and market grasp. But they pursue their strategic target relentlessly, sometimes even obsessively. They rally the organization around efforts to make the strategic intent a reality. They go all out to marshal the resources and capabilities to close in on their strategic target (which is often global market leadership) as rapidly as they can. They craft potent offensive strategies calculated to throw rivals off-balance, put them on the defensive, and force them into an ongoing game of catch-up. They deliberately try to alter the market contest and tilt the rules for competing in their favor. As a consequence, capably managed up-and-coming enterprises with strategic intents exceeding their present reach and resources are a force to be reckoned with, often proving to be more formidable competitors over time than larger, cash-rich rivals that have modest strategic objectives and market ambitions.

The Need for Objectives at All Organizational Levels

Objective setting should not stop with top management's establishing of companywide performance targets. Company objectives need to be broken down into performance targets for each of the organization's separate businesses, product lines, functional departments, and individual work units. Company performance can't reach full potential unless each organizational unit sets and pursues performance targets that contribute directly to the desired companywide outcomes and results. Objective setting is thus a top-down process that must extend to the lowest organizational levels. And it means that each organizational unit must take care to set performance targets that support—rather than conflict with or negate—the achievement of companywide strategic and financial objectives.

The ideal situation is a team effort in which each organizational unit strives to produce results in its area of responsibility that contribute to the achievement of the company's performance targets and strategic vision. Such consistency signals that organizational units know their strategic role and are on board in helping the company move down the chosen strategic path and produce the desired results.

Objective Setting Needs to Be Top-Down Rather than Bottom-Up

To appreciate why a company's objective-setting process needs to be more top-down than bottom-up, consider the following example. Suppose the senior executives of a diversified corporation establish a corporate profit objective of $500 million for next year. Suppose further that, after discussion between corporate management and the general managers of the firm's five different businesses, each business is given a stretch profit objective of $100 million by year-end (i.e., if the five business divisions contribute $100 million each in profit, the corporation can reach its $500 million profit objective). A concrete result has thus been agreed on and translated into measurable action commitments at two levels in the managerial hierarchy. Next, suppose the general manager of business unit A, after some analysis and discussion with functional area managers, concludes that reaching the $100 million profit objective will require selling 1 million units at an average price of $500 and producing them at an average cost of $400 (a $100 profit margin times 1 million units equals $100 million profit). Consequently, the general manager and the manufacturing manager settle on a production objective of 1 million units at a unit cost of $400; and the general manager and the marketing manager agree on a sales objective of 1 million units and a target selling price of $500. In turn, the marketing manager, after consultation with regional sales personnel, breaks the sales objective of 1 million units into unit sales targets for each sales territory, each item in the product line, and each salesperson. It is logical for organizationwide objectives and strategy to be established first so they can guide objective setting and strategy making at lower levels.

A top-down process of setting companywide performance targets first and then insisting that the financial and strategic performance targets established for business units, divisions, functional departments, and operating units be directly connected to the achievement of company objectives has two powerful advantages: One, it helps produce *cohesion* among the objectives and strategies of different parts of the organization. Two, it helps *unify internal efforts* to move the company along the chosen strategic path. If top management, desirous of involving many organization members, allows objective setting to start at the bottom levels of an organization without the benefit of companywide performance targets as a guide, then lower-level organizational units have no basis for connecting their performance targets to the company's. Bottom-up objective setting, with little or no guidance from above, nearly always signals an absence of strategic leadership on the part of senior executives.

CRAFTING A STRATEGY: PHASE 3 OF THE STRATEGY-MAKING, STRATEGY-EXECUTING PROCESS

The task of crafting a strategy entails answering a series of hows: *how* to grow the business, *how* to please customers, *how* to outcompete rivals, *how* to respond to changing market conditions, *how* to manage each functional piece of the business and develop needed competencies and capabilities, *how* to achieve strategic and financial objectives. It also means exercising astute entrepreneurship in choosing among the various strategic alternatives—proactively searching for opportunities to do new things or to do existing things in new or better ways.[12] The faster a company's business environment is changing, the more critical the need for its managers to be good entrepreneurs in diagnosing the direction and force of the changes under way and in responding with timely adjustments in strategy. Strategy makers have to pay attention to early warnings of future change and be willing to experiment with dare-to-be-different ways to alter their market position in preparing for new market conditions. When obstacles unexpectedly appear in a company's path, it is up to management to adapt rapidly and innovatively. *Masterful strategies come partly (maybe mostly) by doing things differently from competitors where it counts—outinnovating them, being more efficient, being more imaginative, adapting faster—rather than running with the herd.* Good strategy making is therefore inseparable from good business entrepreneurship. One cannot exist without the other.

Who Participates in Crafting a Company's Strategy?

A company's senior executives obviously have important strategy-making roles. The chief executive officer (CEO) wears the mantles of chief direction setter, chief objective setter, chief strategy maker, and chief strategy implementer for the total enterprise. Ultimate responsibility for *leading* the strategy-making, strategy-executing process rests with the CEO. In some enterprises the CEO functions as strategic visionary and chief architect of strategy, personally deciding what the key elements of the company's strategy will be, although others may well assist with data gathering and analysis, and the CEO may seek the advice of other senior managers and key employees in fashioning an overall strategy and deciding on important strategic moves. A CEO-centered approach to strategy development is characteristic of small owner-managed companies and sometimes large corporations that have been founded by the present CEO or that have CEOs with strong strategic leadership skills. Meg Whitman at eBay, Andrea Jung at Avon, Jeffrey Immelt at General Electric, and Howard Schultz at Starbucks are prominent examples of corporate CEOs who have wielded a heavy hand in shaping their company's strategy.

In most companies, however, strategy is the product of more than just the CEO's handiwork. Typically, other senior executives—business unit heads, the chief financial officer, and vice presidents for production, marketing, human resources, and other functional departments—have influential strategy-making roles and help fashion the chief strategy components. Normally, a company's chief financial officer (CFO) is in charge of devising and implementing an appropriate financial strategy; the production vice president takes the lead in developing the company's production strategy; the marketing vice president orchestrates sales and marketing strategy; a brand manager is in charge of the strategy for a particular brand in the company's product lineup; and so on.

But even here it is a mistake to view strategy making as a *top* management function, the exclusive province of owner-entrepreneurs, CEOs, and other senior executives. The more that a company's operations cut across different products, industries, and geographical areas, the more that headquarters executives have little option but to delegate considerable strategy-making authority to down-the-line managers in charge of particular subsidiaries, divisions, product lines, geographic sales offices, distribution centers, and plants. On-the-scene managers with authority over specific operating units are in the best position to evaluate the local situation in which the strategic choices must be made and can be expected to have detailed familiarity with local market and competitive conditions, customer requirements and expectations, and all the other aspects surrounding the strategic issues and choices in their arena of authority. This gives them an edge over headquarters executives in keeping the local aspects of the company's strategy responsive to local market and competitive conditions.

Take a company like Toshiba, a $43 billion corporation with 300 subsidiaries, thousands of products, and operations extending across the world. While top-level Toshiba executives may well be personally involved in shaping Toshiba's *overall* strategy and fashioning *important* strategic moves, it doesn't follow that a few senior executives at Toshiba headquarters have either the expertise or a sufficiently detailed understanding of all the relevant factors to wisely craft all the strategic initiatives taken for 300 subsidiaries and thousands of products. They simply cannot know enough about the situation in every Toshiba organizational unit to decide upon every strategy detail and direct every strategic move made in Toshiba's worldwide organization. Rather, it takes involvement on the part of Toshiba's whole management team—top executives, subsidiary heads, division heads, and key managers in such geographic units as sales offices, distribution centers, and plants—to craft the thousands of strategic initiatives that end up comprising the whole of Toshiba's strategy. The same can be said for a company like General Electric, which employs 300,000 people in businesses ranging from jet engines to plastics, power generation equipment to appliances, medical equipment to TV broadcasting, and locomotives to financial services (among many others) and that sells to customers in over 100 countries.

While managers farther down in the managerial hierarchy obviously have a narrower, more specific strategy-making role than managers closer to the top, the important understanding here is that in most of today's companies *every company manager typically has a strategy-making role—ranging from minor to major—for the area he or she heads.* Hence, any notion that an organization's strategists are at the top of the management hierarchy and that midlevel and frontline personnel merely carry out the strategic directives of senior managers needs to be cast aside. In companies with wide-ranging operations, it is far more accurate to view strategy making as a *collaborative or team effort* involving managers (and sometimes key employees) down through the whole organizational hierarchy.

> **Core Concept**
> In most companies, crafting and executing strategy is a team effort in which every manager has a role for the area he or she heads. It is flawed thinking to view crafting and executing strategy as something only high-level managers do.

In fact, the necessity of delegating some strategy-making authority to down-the-line managers has resulted in it being fairly common for key pieces of a company's strategy to originate in a company's middle and lower ranks.[13] Electronic Data Systems conducted a yearlong strategy review involving 2,500 of its 55,000 employees and coordinated by a core of 150 managers and staffers from all over the world.[14] J. M. Smucker, best-known for its jams and jellies, formed a team of 140 employees (7 percent of its 2,000-person workforce) who spent 25 percent of their time over a six-month period looking for ways to rejuvenate the company's growth. Involving teams of people to dissect complex situations and come up with strategic solutions is an often-used component of the strategy-making process because many strategic issues are complex or cut across multiple areas of expertise and operating units, thus calling for the contributions of many disciplinary experts and the collaboration of managers from different parts of the organization. A valuable strength of collaborative strategy-making is that the team of people charged with crafting the strategy can easily include the very people who will also be charged with implementing and executing it. Giving people an influential stake in crafting the strategy they must later help implement and execute not only builds motivation and commitment but also means those people can be held accountable for putting the strategy into place and making it work— the excuse of "It wasn't my idea to do this" won't fly.

The Strategy-Making Role of Corporate Intrapreneurs   In some companies, top management makes a regular practice of encouraging individuals and teams to develop and champion proposals for new product lines and new business ventures. The idea is to unleash the talents and energies of promising "corporate intrapreneurs," letting them try out untested business ideas and giving them the room to pursue new strategic initiatives. Executives judge which proposals merit support, give the chosen intrapreneurs the organizational and budgetary support they need, and let them proceed freely. Thus, important pieces of company strategy can originate with those intrapreneurial individuals and teams who succeed in championing a proposal through the approval stage and then end up being charged with the lead role in launching new products, overseeing the company's entry into new geographic markets, or heading up new business ventures. W. L. Gore and Associates, a privately owned company famous for its Gore-Tex waterproofing film, is an avid and highly successful practitioner of the corporate intrapreneur approach to strategy making. Gore expects all employees to initiate improvements and to display innovativeness. Each employee's intrapreneurial contributions are prime considerations in determining raises, stock option bonuses, and promotions. Gore's commitment to intrapreneurship has produced a stream of product innovations and new strategic initiatives that have kept the company vibrant and growing for nearly two decades.

A Company's Strategy-Making Hierarchy

It thus follows that *a company's overall strategy is a collection of strategic initiatives and actions* devised by managers and key employees up and down the whole organizational hierarchy. The larger and more diverse the operations of an enterprise, the more points of strategic initiative it has and the more managers and employees at more levels of management that have a relevant strategy-making role. Figure 2.2 shows who is generally responsible for devising what pieces of a company's overall strategy.

In diversified, multibusiness companies where the strategies of several different businesses have to be managed, the strategy-making task involves four distinct types or levels of strategy, each of which involves different facets of the company's overall strategy:

1. *Corporate strategy* consists of the kinds of initiatives the company uses to establish business positions in different industries, the approaches corporate executives pursue to boost the combined performance of the set of businesses the company has diversified into, and the means of capturing cross-business synergies and turning them into competitive advantage. Senior corporate executives normally have lead responsibility for devising corporate strategy and for choosing from among whatever recommended actions bubble up from the organization below. Key business-unit heads may also be influential, especially in strategic decisions affecting the businesses they head. Major strategic decisions are usually reviewed and approved by the company's board of directors. We will look deeper into the strategy-making process at diversified companies when we get to Chapter 9.

2. *Business strategy* concerns the actions and the approaches crafted to produce successful performance in one specific line of business. The key focus is crafting responses to changing market circumstances and initiating actions to strengthen market position, build competitive advantage, and develop strong competitive capabilities. Orchestrating the development of business-level strategy is the responsibility of the manager in charge of the business. The business head has at least two other strategy-related roles: (*a*) seeing that lower-level strategies are well conceived, consistent, and adequately matched to the overall business strategy, and (*b*) getting major business-level strategic moves approved by corporate-level officers (and sometimes the board of directors) and keeping them informed of emerging strategic issues. In diversified companies, business-unit heads may have the additional obligation of making sure business-level objectives and strategy conform to corporate-level objectives and strategy themes.

3. *Functional-area strategies* concern the actions, approaches, and practices to be employed in managing particular functions or business processes or key activities within a business. A company's marketing strategy, for example, represents the managerial game plan for running the sales and marketing part of the business. A company's product development strategy represents the managerial game plan for keeping the company's product lineup fresh and in tune with what buyers are looking for. Functional strategies add specifics to the hows of business-level strategy. Plus, they aim at establishing or strengthening a business unit's competencies and capabilities in performing strategy-critical activities so as to enhance the business's market position and standing with customers. The primary role of a functional strategy is to *support* the company's overall business strategy and competitive approach.

   Lead responsibility for functional strategies within a business is normally delegated to the heads of the respective functions, with the general manager of

Figure 2.2   **A Company's Strategy-Making Hierarchy**

Orchestrated by
the CEO and
other senior
executives.

**Corporate
Strategy**

The companywide
game plan for managing a
set of businesses

In the case of a
single-business
company, these
two levels of
the strategy-
making
hierarchy
merge into one
level—*business
strategy*—that
is orchestrated
by the
company's
CEO and other
top executives.

Two-Way Influence

Orchestrated by the
general managers
of each of the
company's different
lines of business,
often with advice
and input from the
heads of functional
area activities
within each
business and
other key people.

**Business Strategy
(one for each business the
company has diversified into)**

- How to strengthen market position
  and build competitive advantage
- Actions to build competitive
  capabilities

Two-Way Influence

Crafted by the
heads of major
functional
activities within
a particular
business—often in
collaboration with
other key people.

**Functional-area
strategies within
each business**

- Add relevant detail to the hows of
  overall business strategy
- Provide a game plan for managing
  a particular activity in ways that
  support the overall business
  strategy

Two-Way Influence

Crafted by brand
managers; the
operating
managers of
plants, distribution
centers, and
geographic units;
and the managers
of strategically
important activities
like advertising and
Web site
operations—often
key employees are
involved.

**Operating
strategies within
each business**

- Add detail and completeness to business
  and functional strategy
- Provide a game plan for managing specific
  lower-echelon activities with strategic
  significance

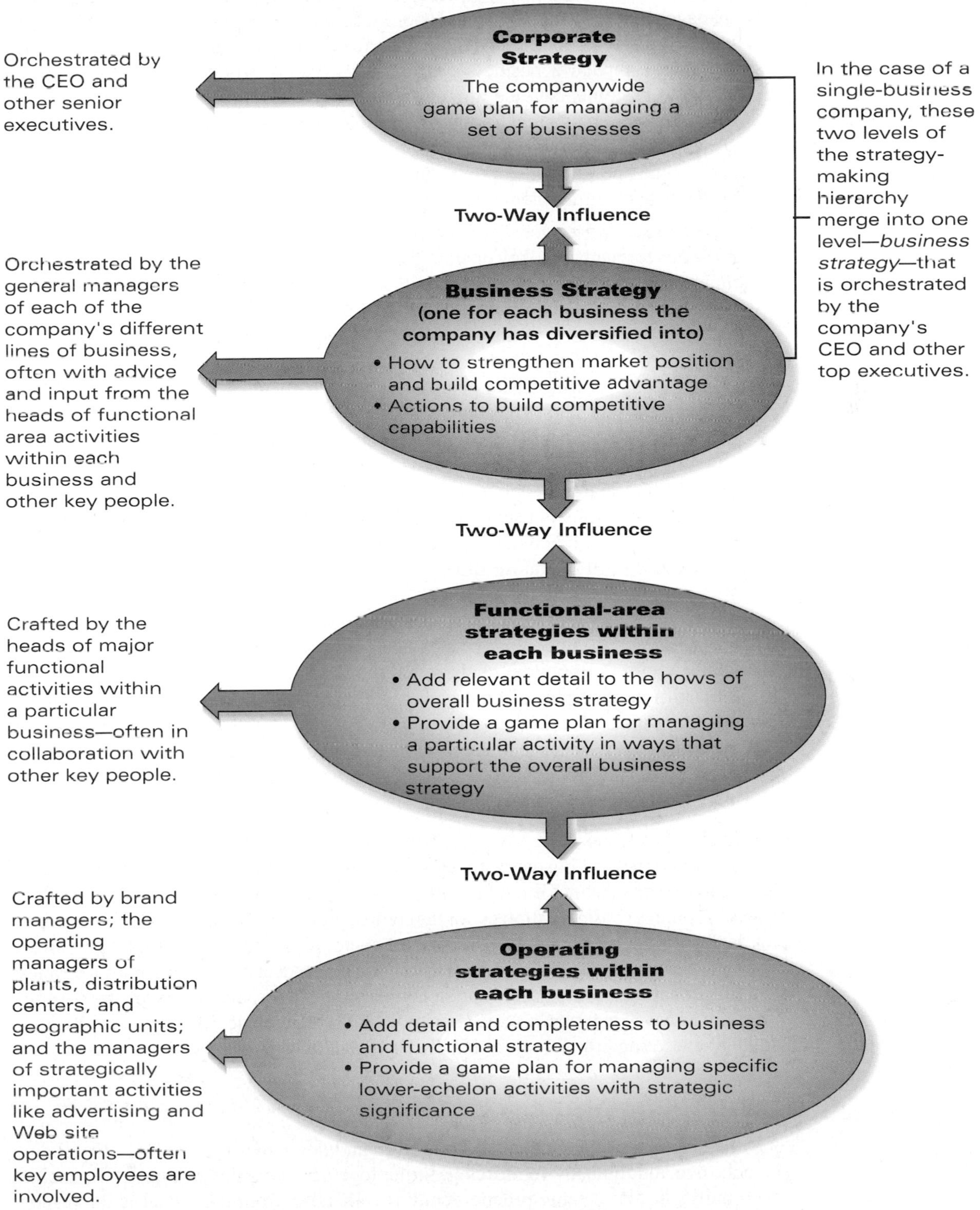

the business having final approval and perhaps even exerting a strong influence over the content of particular pieces of the strategies. To some extent, functional managers have to collaborate and coordinate their strategy-making efforts to avoid uncoordinated or conflicting strategies. For the overall business strategy to have maximum impact, a business's marketing strategy, production strategy, finance strategy, customer service strategy, product development strategy, and human resources strategy should be compatible and mutually reinforcing rather than each serving its own narrower purposes. If inconsistent functional-area strategies are sent up the line for final approval, the business head is responsible for spotting the conflicts and getting them resolved.

4. *Operating strategies* concern the relatively narrow strategic initiatives and approaches for managing key operating units (plants, distribution centers, geographic units) and specific operating activities with strategic significance (advertising campaigns, the management of specific brands, supply chain–related activities, and Web site sales and operations). A plant manager needs a strategy for accomplishing the plant's objectives, carrying out the plant's part of the company's overall manufacturing game plan, and dealing with any strategy-related problems that exist at the plant. A company's advertising manager needs a strategy for getting maximum audience exposure and sales impact from the ad budget. Operating strategies, while of limited scope, add further detail and completeness to functional strategies and to the overall business strategy. Lead responsibility for operating strategies is usually delegated to frontline managers, subject to review and approval by higher-ranking managers.

Even though operating strategy is at the bottom of the strategy-making hierarchy, its importance should not be downplayed. A major plant that fails in its strategy to achieve production volume, unit cost, and quality targets can undercut the achievement of company sales and profit objectives and wreak havoc with strategic efforts to build a quality image with customers. Frontline managers are thus an important part of an organization's strategy-making team because many operating units have strategy-critical performance targets and need to have strategic action plans in place to achieve them. One cannot reliably judge the strategic importance of a given action simply by the strategy level or location within the managerial hierarchy where it is initiated.

In single-business enterprises, the corporate and business levels of strategy making merge into one level—business strategy—because the strategy for the whole company involves only one distinct line of business. Thus, a single-business enterprise has three levels of strategy: business strategy for the company as a whole, functional-area strategies for each main area within the business, and operating strategies undertaken by lower-echelon managers to flesh out strategically significant aspects for the company's business and functional-area strategies. Proprietorships, partnerships, and owner-managed enterprises may have only one or two strategy-making levels since their strategy-making, strategy-executing process can be handled by just a few key people.

Uniting the Strategy-Making Effort

Ideally, the pieces of a company's strategy up and down the strategy hierarchy should be cohesive and mutually reinforcing, fitting together like a jigsaw puzzle. To achieve such unity, the strategizing process requires leadership from the top. It is the responsibility of top executives to provide strategy-making direction and clearly articulate key strategic themes that paint the white lines for lower-level strategy-making efforts. *Mid-level and frontline managers cannot craft unified strategic moves without first understanding the company's long-term direction and knowing the major components of the overall and business strategies that their strategy-making efforts are supposed to support and enhance.* Thus, as a general rule, strategy making must start at the top of the organization and then proceed downward through the hierarchy from the corporate level to the business level and then from the business level to the associated functional and operating levels. Strategy cohesion requires that business-level strategies complement and be compatible with the overall corporate strategy. Likewise, functional and operating strategies have to complement and support the overall business-level strategy of which they are a part. When the strategizing process is mostly top-down, with lower-level strategy-making efforts taking their cues from the higher-level strategy elements they are supposed to complement and support, there's less potential for strategy conflict between different levels. An absence of strong strategic leadership from the top sets the stage for some degree of strategic disunity. The strategic disarray that occurs in an organization when there is weak leadership and too few strategy guidelines coming from top executives is akin to what would happen to a football team's offensive performance if the quarterback decided not to call a play for the team but instead let each player do whatever he/thought would work best at his respective position. In business, as in sports, all the strategy makers in a company are on the same team and the many different pieces of the overall strategy crafted at various organizational levels need to be in sync. *Anything less than a unified collection of strategies weakens the overall strategy and is likely to impair company performance.*

> **Core Concept**
> A company's strategy is at full power only when its many pieces are united.

There are two things that top-level executives can do to drive consistent strategic action down through the organizational hierarchy. One is to effectively communicate the company's vision, objectives, and major strategy components to down-the-line managers and key personnel. The greater the numbers of company personnel who know, understand, and buy into the company's long-term direction and overall strategy, the smaller the risk that organization units will go off in conflicting strategic directions when strategy making is pushed down to frontline levels and many people are given a strategy-making role. The second is to exercise due diligence in reviewing lower-level strategies for consistency and support of higher level strategies. Any strategy conflicts must be addressed and resolved, either by modifying the lower-level strategies with conflicting elements or by adapting the higher-level strategy to accommodate what may be more appealing strategy ideas and initiatives bubbling from below. Thus, the process of synchronizing the strategy initiatives up and down the organizational hierarchy does not necessarily mean that lower-level strategies must be changed whenever conflicts and inconsistencies are spotted. When more attractive strategies ideas originate at lower organizational levels, it makes sense to adapt higher-level strategies to accommodate them.

A Strategic Vision + Objectives + Strategy = A Strategic Plan

Developing a strategic vision and mission, setting objectives, and crafting a strategy are basic direction-setting tasks. They map out where a company is headed, the targeted strategic and financial outcomes, and the competitive moves and internal action approaches to be used in achieving the desired business results. Together, they constitute a **strategic plan** for coping with industry and competitive conditions, the expected actions of the industry's key players, and the challenges and issues that stand as obstacles to the company's success.[15]

> **Core Concept**
> A **strategic plan** lays out the company's future direction, performance targets, and strategy.

In companies that do regular strategy reviews and develop explicit strategic plans, the strategic plan usually ends up as a written document that is circulated to most managers and perhaps selected employees. Near-term performance targets are the part of the strategic plan most often spelled out explicitly and communicated to managers and employees. A number of companies summarize key elements of their strategic plans in the company's annual report to shareholders, in postings on their Web site, or in statements provided to the business media. Other companies, perhaps for reasons of competitive sensitivity, make only vague, general statements about their strategic plans. In small, privately owned companies, it is rare for strategic plans to exist in written form. Small companies' strategic plans tend to reside in the thinking and directives of owners/executives, with aspects of the plan being revealed in meetings and conversations with company personnel, and the understandings and commitments among managers and key employees about where to head, what to accomplish, and how to proceed.

IMPLEMENTING AND EXECUTING THE STRATEGY: PHASE 4 OF THE STRATEGY-MAKING, STRATEGY-EXECUTING PROCESS

Managing the implementation and execution of strategy is an operations-oriented, make-things-happen activity aimed at performing core business activities in a strategy-supportive manner. It is easily the most demanding and time-consuming part of the strategy management process. Converting strategic plans into actions and results tests a manager's ability to direct organizational change, motivate people, build and strengthen company competencies and competitive capabilities, create and nurture a strategy-supportive work climate, and meet or beat performance targets. Initiatives to put the strategy in place and execute it proficiently have to be launched and managed on many organizational fronts.

Management's action agenda for implementing and executing the chosen strategy emerges from assessing what the company will have to do differently or better, given its particular operating practices and organizational circumstances, to execute the strategy competently and achieve the targeted financial and strategic performance. Each company manager has to think through the answer to "What has to be done in my area to execute my piece of the strategic plan, and what actions should I take to get the process under way?" How much internal change is needed depends on how much of the strategy is new, how far internal practices and competencies deviate from what the strategy requires, and how well the present work climate/culture supports good strategy execution. Depending on the amount of internal change involved, full implementation and proficient execution of company strategy (or important new pieces thereof) can take several months to several years.

In most situations, managing the strategy execution process includes the following principal aspects:

- Staffing the organization with the needed skills and expertise, consciously building and strengthening strategy-supportive competencies and competitive capabilities, and organizing the work effort.
- Allocating ample resources to those activities critical to strategic success.
- Ensuring that policies and procedures facilitate rather than impede effective execution.

- Using best practices to perform core business activities and pushing for continuous improvement. Organizational units have to periodically reassess how things are being done and diligently pursue useful changes and improvements.
- Installing information and operating systems that enable company personnel to better carry out their strategic roles day in and day out.
- Motivating people to pursue the target objectives energetically and, if need be, modifying their duties and job behavior to better fit the requirements of successful strategy execution.
- Tying rewards and incentives directly to the achievement of performance objectives and good strategy execution.
- Creating a company culture and work climate conducive to successful strategy execution.
- Exerting the internal leadership needed to drive implementation forward and keep improving on how the strategy is being executed. When stumbling blocks or weaknesses are encountered, management has to see that they are addressed and rectified in timely and effective fashion.

Good strategy execution requires diligent pursuit of operating excellence. It is a job for a company's whole management team. And success hinges on the skills and cooperation of operating managers who can push needed changes in their organization units and consistently deliver good results. Strategy implementation can be considered successful if things go smoothly enough that the company meets or beats its strategic and financial performance targets and shows good progress in achieving management's strategic vision.

EVALUATING PERFORMANCE AND INITIATING CORRECTIVE ADJUSTMENTS: PHASE 5 OF THE STRATEGY-MAKING, STRATEGY-EXECUTING PROCESS

The fifth phase of the strategy management process—monitoring new external developments, evaluating the company's progress, and making corrective adjustments—is the trigger point for deciding whether to continue or change the company's vision, objectives, strategy, or strategy execution methods. So long as the company's direction and strategy seem well matched to industry and competitive conditions, and performance targets are being met, company executives may well decide to stay the course. Simply fine-tuning the strategic plan and continuing with efforts to improve strategy execution are sufficient.

> **Core Concept**
> A company's vision, objectives, strategy, and approach to strategy execution are never final; managing strategy is an ongoing process, not an every-now-and-then task.

But whenever a company encounters disruptive changes in its environment, questions need to be raised about the appropriateness of its direction and strategy. If a company experiences a downturn in its market position or persistent shortfalls in performance, then company managers are obligated to ferret out the causes—do they relate to poor strategy, poor strategy execution, or both?—and take timely corrective action. A company's direction, objectives, and strategy have to be revisited anytime external or internal conditions warrant. It is to be expected that a company will modify its strategic vision, direction, objectives, and strategy over time.

Likewise, it is not unusual for a company to find that one or more aspects of its strategy implementation and execution are not going as well as intended. Proficient strategy execution is always the product of much organizational learning. It is achieved unevenly—coming quickly in some areas and proving nettlesome in others. It is both normal and desirable to periodically assess strategy execution to determine which aspects are working well and which need improving. Successful strategy execution entails vigilantly searching for ways to improve and then making corrective adjustments whenever and wherever it is useful to do so.

CORPORATE GOVERNANCE: THE ROLE OF THE BOARD OF DIRECTORS IN THE STRATEGY-MAKING, STRATEGY-EXECUTING PROCESS

Although senior managers have *lead responsibility* for crafting and executing a company's strategy, it is the duty of the board of directors to exercise *strong oversight* and see that the five tasks of strategic management are done in a manner that benefits shareholders (in the case of investor-owned enterprises) or stakeholders (in the case of not-for-profit organizations). In watching over management's strategy-making, strategy-executing actions and making sure that executive actions are not only proper but also aligned with the interests of stakeholders, a company's board of directors has four important obligations to fulfill:

1. *Be inquiring critics and oversee the company's direction, strategy, and business approaches.* Board members must ask probing questions and draw on their business acumen to make independent judgments about whether strategy proposals have been adequately analyzed and whether proposed strategic actions appear to have greater promise than alternatives. If executive management is bringing well-supported and reasoned strategy proposals to the board, there's little reason for board members to aggressively challenge or pick apart everything put before them. Asking incisive questions is usually sufficient to test whether the case for management's proposals is compelling. However, when the company's strategy is failing or is plagued with faulty execution, and certainly when there is a precipitous collapse in profitability, board members have a duty to express their concerns about the validity of the strategy and/or operating methods, initiate debate about the company's strategic path, hold one-on-one discussions with key executives and other board members, and perhaps directly intervene as a group to alter the company's executive leadership and, ultimately, its strategy and business approaches.

2. *Evaluate the caliber of senior executives' strategy-making and strategy-executing skills.* The board is always responsible for determining whether the current CEO is doing a good job of strategic leadership (as a basis for awarding salary increases and bonuses and deciding on retention or removal). Boards must also exercise due diligence in evaluating the strategic leadership skills of other senior executives in line to succeed the CEO. When the incumbent CEO steps down or leaves for a position elsewhere, the board must elect a successor, either going with an insider or deciding that a better-qualified outsider is needed to perhaps radically change the company's strategic course.

3. *Institute a compensation plan for top executives that rewards them for actions and results that serve stakeholder interests, and most especially those of shareholders.* A basic principle of corporate governance is that the owners of a corporation delegate operating authority and managerial control to top management in return for compensation. In their role as an *agent* of shareholders, top executives have a

clear and unequivocal duty to make decisions and operate the company in accord with shareholder interests (but this does not mean disregarding the interests of other stakeholders, particularly those of employees, with whom they also have an agency relationship). Most boards of directors have a compensation committee, composed entirely of outside directors, to develop a salary and incentive compensation plan that makes it in the self-interest of executives to operate the business in a manner that benefits the owners; the compensation committee's recommendations are presented to the full board for approval. But in addition to creating compensation plans intended to align executive actions with owner interests, the board of directors must put a halt to self-serving executive perks and privileges that simply line the financial pockets of executives. Numerous media reports have recounted instances in which boards of directors have gone along with opportunistic executive efforts to secure excessive, if not downright obscene, compensation of one kind or another (multimillion-dollar interest-free loans, personal use of corporate aircraft, lucrative severance and retirement packages, outsized stock incentive awards, and so on).

4. *Oversee the company's financial accounting and financial reporting practices.* While top managers, particularly the company's CEO and CFO, are primarily responsible for seeing that the company's financial statements fairly and accurately report the results of the company's operations, it is well established that board members have a fiduciary duty to protect shareholders by exercising oversight of the company's financial practices, ensuring that generally accepted accounting principles (GAAP) are properly used in preparing the company's financial statements, and determining whether proper financial controls are in place to prevent fraud and misuse of funds. Virtually all boards of directors monitor the financial reporting activities by appointing an audit committee, always composed entirely of outside directors. The members of the audit committee have lead responsibility for overseeing the company's financial officers and consulting with both internal and external auditors to ensure accurate financial reporting and adequate financial controls.

   The number of prominent companies penalized because of the actions of scurrilous or out-of-control CEOs and CFOs, the growing propensity of disgruntled stockholders to file lawsuits alleging director negligence, and the escalating costs of liability insurance for directors all underscore the responsibility that a board of directors has for overseeing a company's strategy-making, strategy-executing process and ensuring that management actions are proper and responsible. Moreover, holders of large blocks of shares (mutual funds and pension funds), regulatory authorities, and the financial press consistently urge that board members, especially outside directors, be active and diligent in their oversight of company strategy and maintain a tight rein on executive actions.

Every corporation should have a strong, independent board of directors that (1) is well informed about the company's performance, (2) guides and judges the CEO and other top executives, (3) has the courage to curb inappropriate or unduly risky management actions, (4) certifies to shareholders that the CEO is doing what the board expects, (5) provides insight and advice to management, and (6) is intensely involved in debating the pros and cons of key decisions and actions.[14] Boards of directors that lack the backbone to challenge a strong-willed or imperial CEO or that rubber-stamp most anything the CEO recommends without probing inquiry and debate (perhaps because the board is stacked with the CEO's cronies) abdicate their duty to represent and protect shareholder interests. The whole fabric of effective corporate governance is undermined when boards of directors shirk their responsibility to maintain ultimate control over the company's strategic direction, the major elements of its strategy, the business approaches management is using to implement and execute the strategy, executive compensation, and the financial reporting process. Thus, even though lead responsibility for crafting and executing strategy falls to top executives, boards of directors have a very important oversight role in the strategy-making, strategy-executing process.

Key Points

The managerial process of crafting and executing a company's strategy consists of five interrelated and integrated phases:

1. *Developing a strategic vision* of where the company needs to head and what its future product/market/customer/technology focus should be. This managerial step provides long-term direction, infuses the organization with a sense of purposeful action, and communicates management's aspirations to stakeholders.

2. *Setting objectives* to spell out for the company *how much* of *what kind* of performance is expected, and *by when.* The objectives need to require a significant amount of organizational stretch. A balanced scorecard approach for measuring company performance entails setting both *financial objectives* and *strategic objectives.*

3. *Crafting a strategy to achieve the objectives* and move the company along the strategic course that management has charted. Crafting strategy is concerned principally with forming responses to changes under way in the external environment, devising competitive moves and market approaches aimed at producing sustainable competitive advantage, building competitively valuable competencies and capabilities, and uniting the strategic actions initiated in various parts of the company. The more that a company's operations cut across different products, industries, and geographical areas, the more that strategy making becomes a *team effort* involving managers and company personnel at many organizational levels. The total strategy that emerges in such companies is really a collection of strategic actions and business approaches initiated partly by senior company executives, partly by the heads of major business divisions, partly by functional-area managers, and partly by frontline operating managers. The larger and more diverse the operations of an enterprise, the more points of strategic initiative it has and the more managers and employees at more levels of management that have a relevant strategy-making role. A single business enterprise has three levels of strategy—business strategy for the company as a whole, functional-area strategies for each main area within the business, and operating strategies undertaken by lower-echelon managers to flesh out strategically significant aspects for the company's business and functional-area strategies. In diversified, multibusiness companies, the strategy-making task involves four distinct types or levels of strategy: corporate strategy for the company as a whole, business strategy (one for each business the company has diversified into), functional-area strategies within each business, and operating strategies. Typically, the strategy-making task is more top-down than bottom-up, with higher-level strategies serving as the guide for developing lower-level strategies.

4. *Implementing and executing the chosen strategy efficiently and effectively.* Managing the implementation and execution of strategy is an operations-oriented, make-things-happen activity aimed at shaping the performance of core business activities in a strategy-supportive manner. Management's handling of the strategy implementation process can be considered successful if things go smoothly

enough that the company meets or beats its strategic and financial performance targets and shows good progress in achieving management's strategic vision.

5. *Evaluating performance and initiating corrective adjustments* in vision, long-term direction, objectives, strategy, or execution in light of actual experience, changing conditions, new ideas, and new opportunities. This phase of the strategy management process is the trigger point for deciding whether to continue or change the company's vision, objectives, strategy, and/or strategy execution methods.

A company's strategic vision, objectives, and strategy constitute a *strategic plan* for coping with industry and competitive conditions, outcompeting rivals, and addressing the challenges and issues that stand as obstacles to the company's success.

Boards of directors have a duty to shareholders to play a vigilant role in overseeing management's handling of a company's strategy-making, strategy-executing process. A company's board is obligated to (1) critically appraise and ultimately approve strategic action plans; (2) evaluate the strategic leadership skills of the CEO and others in line to succeed the incumbent CEO; (3) institute a compensation plan for top executives that rewards them for actions and results that serve stakeholder interests, most especially those of shareholders; and (4) ensure that the company issues accurate financial reports and has adequate financial controls.

Exercises

1. Go to the Investors section of Heinz's Web site (www.heinz.com) and read the letter to the shareholders in the company's fiscal 2003 annual report. Is the vision for Heinz articulated by Chairman and CEO William R. Johnson sufficiently clear and well defined? Why or why not? Are the company's objectives well stated and appropriate? What about the strategy that Johnson outlines for the company? If you were a shareholder, would you be satisfied with what Johnson has told you about the company's direction, performance targets, and strategy?

2. Consider the following mission statement of the American Association of Retired People (AARP):

AARP Mission Statement

- AARP is a nonprofit, nonpartisan membership organization for people age 50 and over.
- AARP is dedicated to enhancing quality of life for all as we age. We lead positive social change and deliver value to members through information, advocacy and service.
- AARP also provides a wide range of unique benefits, special products, and services for our members. These benefits include AARP Web site at www.aarp.org, "AARP The Magazine," the monthly "AARP Bulletin," and a Spanish-language newspaper, "Segunda Juventud."
- Active in every state, the District of Columbia, Puerto Rico, and the U.S. Virgin Islands, AARP celebrates the attitude that age is just a number and life is what you make it.

Is AARP's mission statement well-crafted? Does it do an adequate job of indicating "who we are, what we do, and why we are here"? Why or why not?

3. How would you rewrite/restate the strategic vision for Caterpillar in Illustration Capsule 2.1 so as to better exemplify the characteristics of effective vision statements presented in Tables 2.2 and 2.3? Visit www.caterpillar.com to get more information about Caterpillar and figure out how a more appropriate strategic vision might be worded.

Evaluating a Company's External Environment

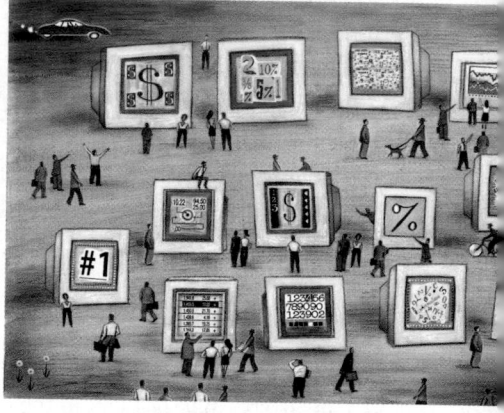

Analysis is the critical starting point of strategic thinking.

—Kenichi Ohmae
Consultant and Author

Things are always different—the art is figuring out which differences matter.

—Laszlo Birinyi
Investments Manager

Competitive battles should be seen not as one-shot skirmishes but as a dynamic multiround game of moves and countermoves.

—Anil K. Gupta
Professor

anagers are not prepared to act wisely in steering a company in a different direction or altering its strategy until they have a deep understanding of the pertinent factors surrounding the company's situation. As indicated in the opening paragraph of Chapter 1, one of the three central questions that managers must address in evaluating their company's business prospects is "What's the company's present situation?" Two facets of a company's situation are especially pertinent: (1) the industry and competitive environment in which the company operates and the forces acting to reshape this environment, and (2) the company's own market position and competitiveness—its resources and capabilities, its strengths and weaknesses vis-à-vis rivals, and its windows of opportunity.

Insightful diagnosis of a company's external and internal environment is a prerequisite for managers to succeed in crafting a strategy that is an excellent fit with the company's situation, is capable of building competitive advantage, and holds good prospect for boosting company performance—the three criteria of a winning strategy. As depicted in Figure 3.1, the task of crafting a strategy thus should always begin with an appraisal of the company's external and internal situation (as a basis for developing strategic vision of where the company needs to head), then move toward an evaluation of the most promising alternative strategies and business models, and culminate in choosing a specific strategy.

This chapter presents the concepts and analytical tools for zeroing in on those aspects of a single-business company's external environment that should be considered in making strategic choices. Attention centers on the competitive arena in which a company operates, the drivers of market change, and what rival companies are doing. In Chapter 4 we explore the methods of evaluating a company's internal circumstances and competitiveness.

THE STRATEGICALLY RELEVANT COMPONENTS OF A COMPANY'S EXTERNAL ENVIRONMENT

All companies operate in a "macroenvironment" shaped by influences emanating from the economy at large; population demographics; societal values and lifestyles; governmental legislation and regulation; technological factors; and, closer to home, the

Figure 3.1   **From Thinking Strategically about the Company's Situation to Choosing a Strategy**

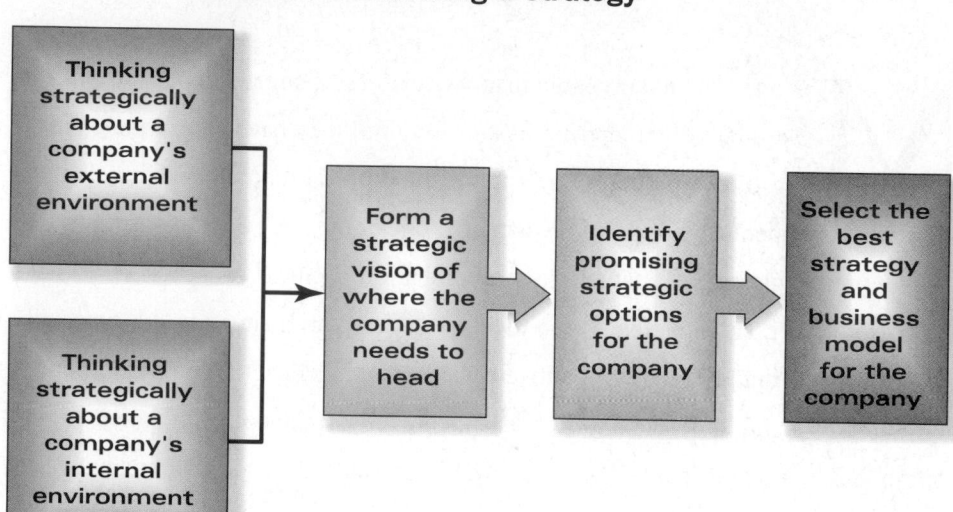

industry and competitive arena in which the company operates (see Figure 3.2). Strictly speaking, a company's macroenvironment includes *all relevant factors and influences* outside the company's boundaries; by relevant, we mean important enough to have a bearing on the decisions the company ultimately makes about its direction, objectives, strategy, and business model. Strategically relevant influences coming from the outer ring of the macroenvironment can sometimes have a high impact on a company's business situation and have a very significant impact on the company's direction and strategy. The strategic opportunities of cigarette producers to grow their business are greatly reduced by antismoking ordinances and the growing cultural stigma attached to smoking. Motor vehicle companies must adapt their strategies (especially as concerns the fuel mileage of their vehicles) to customer concerns about gasoline prices. The demographics of an aging population and longer life expectancies are having a dramatic impact on the business prospects and strategies of health care and prescription drug companies. Companies in most all industries have to craft strategies that are responsive to environmental regulations, growing use of the Internet and broadband technology, and energy prices. Companies in the food-processing, restaurant, sports, and fitness industries have to pay special attention to changes in lifestyles, eating habits, leisure-time preferences, and attitudes toward nutrition and exercise in fashioning their strategies.

Happenings in the outer ring of the macroenvironment may occur rapidly or slowly, with or without advance warning. The impact of outer-ring factors on a company's choice of strategy can range from big to small. But even if the factors in the outer ring of the macroenvironment change slowly or have such a comparatively low impact on a company's situation that only the edges of a company's direction and strategy are affected, there are enough strategically relevant outer-ring trends and events to justify a watchful eye. As company managers scan the external environment, they must be alert for potentially important outer-ring developments, assess their impact and influence, and adapt the company's direction and strategy as needed.

Figure 3.2   **The Components of a Company's Macroenvironment**

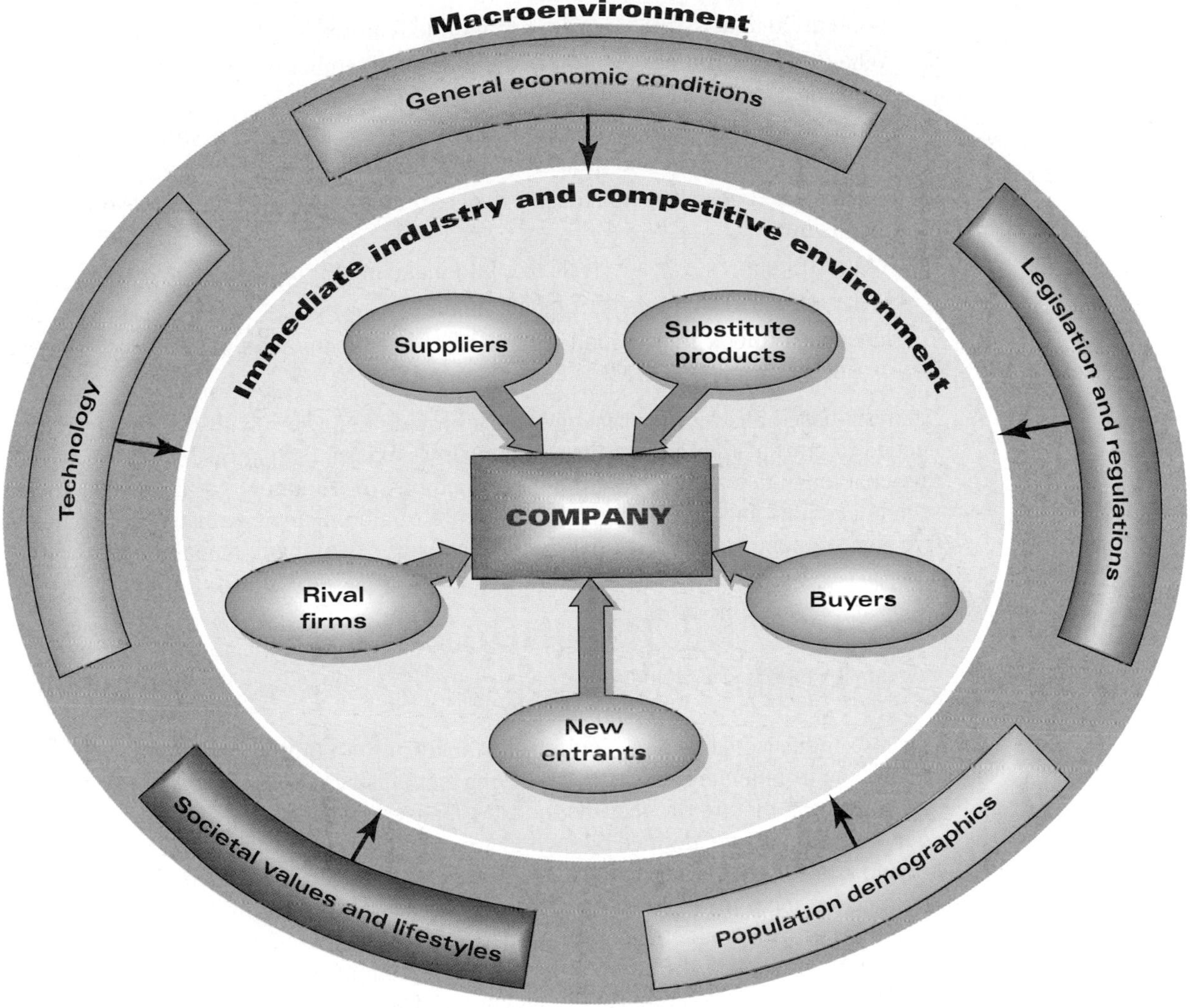

However, the factors and forces in a company's macroenvironment having the *biggest* strategy-shaping impact typically pertain to the company's immediate industry and competitive environment—competitive pressures, the actions of rivals firms, buyer behavior, supplier-related considerations, and so on. Consequently, it is on a company's industry and competitive environment that we concentrate our attention in this chapter.

THINKING STRATEGICALLY ABOUT A COMPANY'S INDUSTRY AND COMPETITIVE ENVIRONMENT

To gain a deep understanding of a company's industry and competitive environment, managers do not need to gather all the information they can find and spend lots of time digesting it. Rather, the task is much more focused. Thinking strategically about a company's industry and competitive environment entails using some well-defined concepts and analytical tools to get clear answers to seven questions:

1. What are the industry's dominant economic features?
2. What kinds of competitive forces are industry members facing and how strong is each force?
3. What forces are driving industry change and what impacts will they have on competitive intensity and industry profitability?
4. What market positions do industry rivals occupy—who is strongly positioned and who is not?
5. What strategic moves are rivals likely to make next?
6. What are the key factors for future competitive success?
7. Does the outlook for the industry present the company with sufficiently attractive prospects for profitability?

Analysis-based answers to these questions provide managers with the understanding needed to craft a strategy that fits the company's external situation. The remainder of this chapter is devoted to describing the methods of obtaining solid answers to the seven questions and explaining how the nature of a company's industry and competitive environment weighs upon the strategic choices of company managers.

QUESTION 1: WHAT ARE THE INDUSTRY'S DOMINANT ECONOMIC FEATURES?

Because industries differ so significantly, analyzing a company's industry and competitive environment begins with identifying an industry's dominant economic features and forming a picture of what the industry landscape is like. An industry's dominant economic features are defined by such factors as market size and growth rate, the number and sizes of buyers and sellers, the geographic boundaries of the market (which can extend from local to worldwide), the degree to which sellers' products are differentiated, the pace of product innovation, market supply/demand conditions, the pace of technological change, the extent of vertical integration, and the extent to which costs are affected by scale economies (i.e., situations in which large-volume operations result in lower unit costs) and learning/experience curve effects (i.e., situations in which costs decline as a company gains knowledge and experience). Table 3.1 provides a convenient summary of what economic features to look at and the corresponding questions to consider in profiling an industry's landscape.

Getting a handle on an industry's distinguishing economic features not only sets the stage for the analysis to come but also promotes understanding of the kinds of strategic moves that industry members are likely to employ. For example, in industries characterized by one product advance after another, companies must invest in research and development (R&D) and develop strong product innovation capabilities—a strategy of continuous product innovation becomes a condition of survival in such industries as video games, mobile phones, and pharmaceuticals. An industry that has recently passed through the rapid-growth stage and is looking at single-digit percentage increases in buyer demand is likely to be experiencing a competitive shake-out and much stronger strategic emphasis on cost reduction and improved customer service.

In industries like semiconductors, strong *learning/experience curve effects* in manufacturing cause unit costs to decline about 20 percent each time *cumulative* production

Table 3.1   **What to Consider in Identifying an Industry's Dominant Economic Features**

Economic Feature	Questions to Answer
Market size and growth rate	• How big is the industry and how fast is it growing? • What does the industry's position in the life cycle (early development, rapid growth and takeoff, early maturity and slowing growth, saturation and stagnation, decline) reveal about the industry's growth prospects?
Number of rivals	• Is the industry fragmented into many small companies or concentrated and dominated by a few large companies? • Is the industry going through a period of consolidation to a smaller number of competitors?
Scope of competitive rivalry	• Is the geographic area over which most companies compete local, regional, national, multinational, or global? • Is having a presence in the foreign country markets becoming more important to a company's long-term competitive success?
Number of buyers	• Is market demand fragmented among many buyers? • Do some buyers have bargaining power because they purchase in large volume?
Degree of product differentiation	• Are the products of rivals becoming more differentiated or less differentiated? • Are increasingly look-alike products of rivals causing heightened price competition?
Product innovation	• Is the industry characterized by rapid product innovation and short product life cycles? • How important is R&D and product innovation? • Are there opportunities to overtake key rivals by being first-to-market with next-generation products?
Supply/demand conditions	• Is a surplus of capacity pushing prices and profit margins down? • Is the industry overcrowded with too many competitors? • Are short supplies creating a sellers' market?
Pace of technological change	• What role does advancing technology play in this industry? • Are ongoing upgrades of facilities/equipment essential because of rapidly advancing production process technologies? • Do most industry members have or need strong technological capabilities?
Vertical integration	• Do most competitors operate in only one stage of the industry (parts and components production, manufacturing and assembly, distribution, retailing) or do some competitors operate in multiple stages? • Is there any cost or competitive advantage or disadvantage associated with being fully or partially integrated?
Economies of scale	• Is the industry characterized by economies of scale in purchasing, manufacturing, advertising, shipping, or other activities? • Do companies with large-scale operations have an important cost advantage over small-scale firms?
Learning/experience curve effects	• Are certain industry activities characterized by strong learning/experience curve effects ("learning by doing") such that unit costs decline as a company's experience in performing the activity builds? • Do any companies have significant cost advantages because of their learning/experience in performing particular activities?

volume doubles. With a 20 percent experience curve effect, if the first 1 million chips cost $100 each, the unit cost would be $80 (80 percent of $100) by a production volume of 2 million, the unit cost would be $64 (80 percent of $80) by a production volume of 4 million, and so on.[1] The bigger the learning/experience curve effect, the bigger the cost advantage of the company with the largest *cumulative* production volume.

Thus, when an industry is characterized by important learning/experience curve effects (or by economies of scale), industry members are strongly motivated to adopt volume-increasing strategies to capture the resulting cost-saving economies and maintain their competitiveness. Unless small-scale firms succeed in pursuing strategic options that allow them to grow sales sufficiently to remain cost-competitive with larger-volume rivals, they are unlikely to survive. The bigger the learning/experience curve effects and/or scale economies in an industry, the more imperative it becomes for competing sellers to pursue strategies to win additional sales and market share—the company with the biggest sales volume gains sustainable competitive advantage as the low-cost producer.

QUESTION 2: WHAT KINDS OF COMPETITIVE FORCES ARE INDUSTRY MEMBERS FACING?

The character, mix, and subtleties of the competitive forces operating in a company's industry are never the same from one industry to another. Far and away the most powerful and widely used tool for systematically diagnosing the principal competitive pressures in a market and assessing the strength and importance of each is the *five-forces model of competition.*[2] This model, depicted in Figure 3.3, holds that the state of competition in an industry is a composite of competitive pressures operating in five areas of the overall market:

1. Competitive pressures associated with the market maneuvering and jockeying for buyer patronage that goes on among *rival sellers* in the industry.
2. Competitive pressures associated with the threat of *new entrants* into the market.
3. Competitive pressures coming from the attempts of companies in other industries to win buyers over to their own *substitute products.*
4. Competitive pressures stemming from *supplier* bargaining power and supplier–seller collaboration.
5. Competitive pressures stemming from *buyer* bargaining power and seller–buyer collaboration.

The way one uses the five-forces model to determine the nature and strength of competitive pressures in a given industry is to build the picture of competition in three steps:

- *Step 1:* Identify the specific competitive pressures associated with each of the five forces.
- *Step 2:* Evaluate how strong the pressures comprising each of the five forces are (fierce, strong, moderate to normal, or weak).
- *Step 3:* Determine whether the collective strength of the five competitive forces is conducive to earning attractive profits.

Figure 3.3   **The Five-Forces Model of Competition: A Key Analytical Tool**

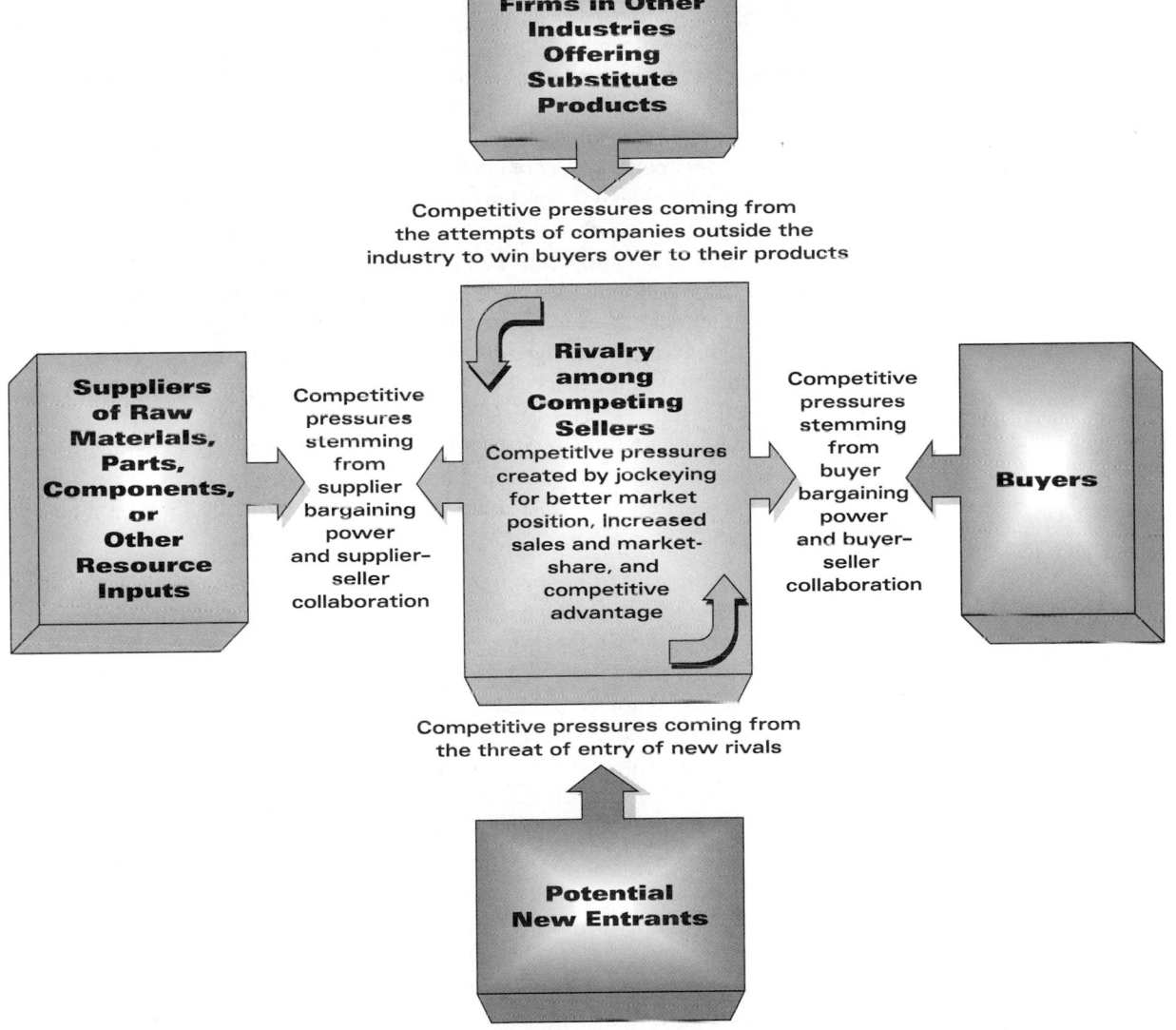

Source: Adapted from Michael E. Porter, "How Competitive Forces Shape Strategy," *Harvard Business Review* 57, no. 2 (March–April 1979), pp. 137–45.

Competitive Pressures Associated with the Jockeying among Rival Sellers

The strongest of the five competitive forces is nearly always the market maneuvering and jockeying for buyer patronage that goes on among rival sellers of a product or service. In effect, *a market is a competitive battlefield* where there's no end to the jockeying for buyer patronage. Rival sellers are prone to employ whatever weapons they have in their business arsenal to improve their market positions, strengthen their market position with buyers, and earn good profits. The challenge is to craft a competitive strategy that, at the very least, allows a company to hold its own against rivals and that, ideally, *produces a competitive edge over rivals.* But competitive contests are ongoing and dynamic. When one firm makes a strategic move that produces good results, its rivals typically respond with offensive or defensive countermoves, shifting their strategic emphasis from one combination of product attributes, marketing tactics, and capabilities to another. This pattern of action and reaction, move and countermove, adjust and readjust produces a continually evolving competitive landscape in which the market battle ebbs and flows, sometimes takes unpredictable twists and turns, and produces winners and losers. But the winners—the current market leaders—have no guarantees of continued leadership; their market success is no more durable than the power of their strategies to fend off the strategies of ambitious challengers. In every industry, the ongoing jockeying of rivals leads to one or another companies gaining or losing momentum in the marketplace according to whether their latest strategic maneuvers succeed or fail.

Figure 3.4 shows a sampling of competitive weapons that firms can deploy in battling rivals and indicates the factors that influence the intensity of their rivalry. A brief discussion of some of the factors that influence the tempo of rivalry among industry competitors is in order:[3]

- *Rivalry intensifies when competing sellers are active in launching fresh actions to boost their market standing and business performance.* One indicator of active rivalry is lively price competition, a condition that puts pressure on industry members to drive costs out of the business and threatens the survival of high-cost companies. Another indicator of active rivalry is rapid introduction of next-generation products—when one or more rivals frequently introduce new or improved products, competitors that lack good product innovation capabilities feel considerable competitive heat to get their own new and improved products into the marketplace quickly. Other indicators of active rivalry among industry members include:

  - Whether industry members are racing to differentiate their products from rivals by offering better performance features or higher quality or improved customer service or a wider product selection.

  - How frequently rivals resort to such marketing tactics as special sales promotions, heavy advertising, rebates, or low-interest-rate financing to drum up additional sales.

  - How actively industry members are pursuing efforts to build stronger dealer networks or establish positions in foreign markets or otherwise expand their distribution capabilities and market presence.

  - How hard companies are striving to gain a market edge over rivals by developing valuable expertise and capabilities that rivals are hard pressed to match.

  Normally, competitive jockeying among rival sellers is active and fairly intense because competing companies are highly motivated to launch whatever fresh actions and creative market maneuvers they can think of to try to strengthen their market positions and business performance.

- *Rivalry intensifies as the number of competitors increases and as competitors become more equal in size and capability.* Rivalry is not as vigorous in microprocessors for PCs, where Advanced Micro Devices (AMD) is one of the few

Figure 3.4 **Weapons for Competing and Factors Affecting the Strength of Rivalry**

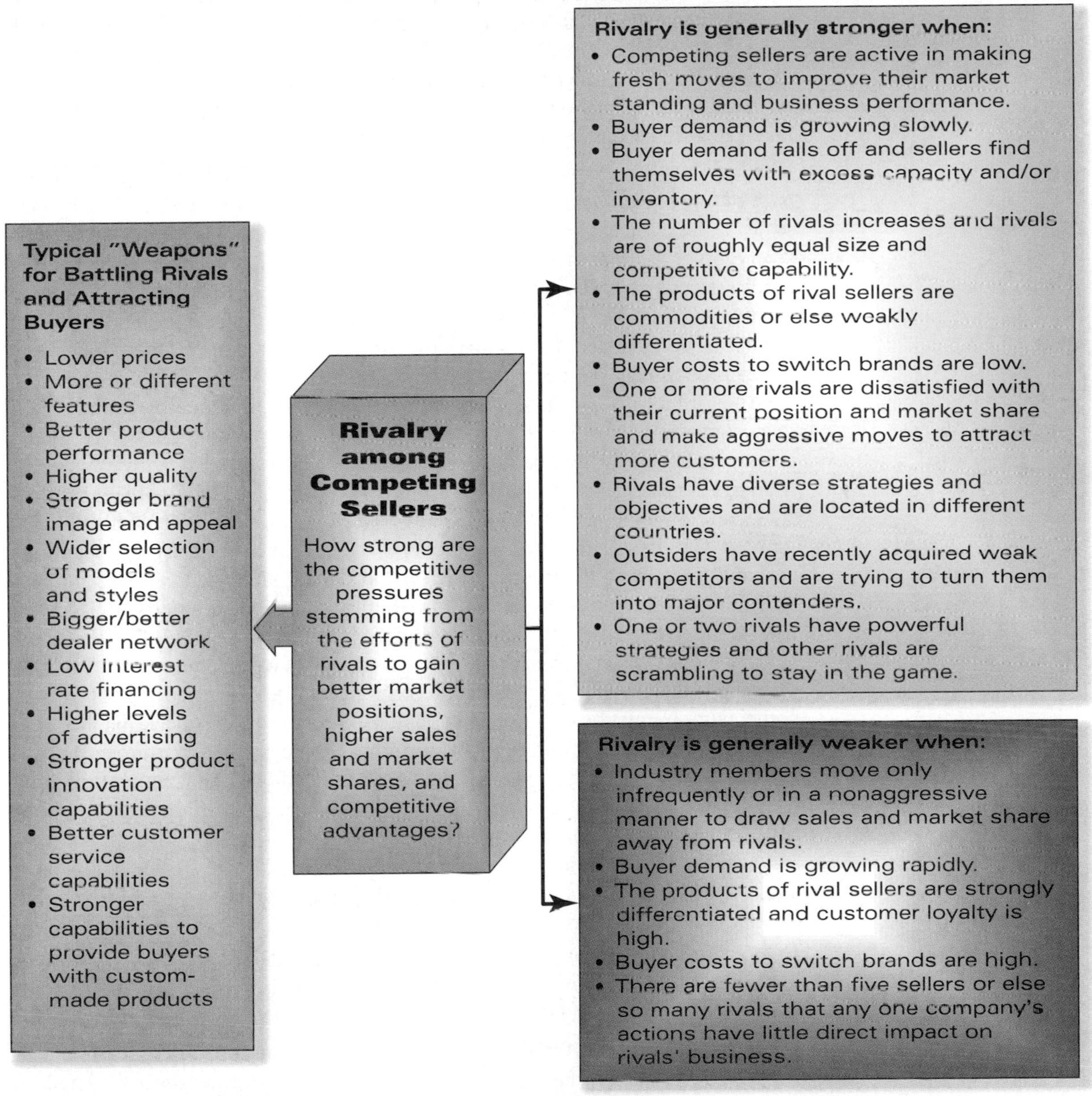

Typical "Weapons" for Battling Rivals and Attracting Buyers

- Lower prices
- More or different features
- Better product performance
- Higher quality
- Stronger brand image and appeal
- Wider selection of models and styles
- Bigger/better dealer network
- Low interest rate financing
- Higher levels of advertising
- Stronger product innovation capabilities
- Better customer service capabilities
- Stronger capabilities to provide buyers with custom-made products

Rivalry among Competing Sellers

How strong are the competitive pressures stemming from the efforts of rivals to gain better market positions, higher sales and market shares, and competitive advantages?

Rivalry is generally stronger when:

- Competing sellers are active in making fresh moves to improve their market standing and business performance.
- Buyer demand is growing slowly.
- Buyer demand falls off and sellers find themselves with excess capacity and/or inventory.
- The number of rivals increases and rivals are of roughly equal size and competitive capability.
- The products of rival sellers are commodities or else weakly differentiated.
- Buyer costs to switch brands are low.
- One or more rivals are dissatisfied with their current position and market share and make aggressive moves to attract more customers.
- Rivals have diverse strategies and objectives and are located in different countries.
- Outsiders have recently acquired weak competitors and are trying to turn them into major contenders.
- One or two rivals have powerful strategies and other rivals are scrambling to stay in the game.

Rivalry is generally weaker when:

- Industry members move only infrequently or in a nonaggressive manner to draw sales and market share away from rivals.
- Buyer demand is growing rapidly.
- The products of rival sellers are strongly differentiated and customer loyalty is high.
- Buyer costs to switch brands are high.
- There are fewer than five sellers or else so many rivals that any one company's actions have little direct impact on rivals' business.

challengers to Intel, as it is in fast-food restaurants, where numerous sellers are actively jockeying for buyer patronage. Up to a point, the greater the number of competitors, the greater the probability of fresh, creative strategic initiatives. In addition, when rivals are nearly equal in size and capability, they can usually compete on a fairly even footing, making it harder for one or two firms to win commanding market shares and confront weaker market challenges from rivals.

- *Rivalry is usually stronger in slow-growing markets and weaker in fast-growing markets.* Rapidly expanding buyer demand produces enough new business for all industry members to grow. Indeed, in a fast-growing market, a company may find itself stretched just to keep abreast of incoming orders, let alone devote resources to stealing customers away from rivals. But in markets where growth is sluggish or where buyer demand drops off unexpectedly, expansion-minded firms and firms with excess capacity often are quick to cut prices and initiate other sales-increasing tactics, thereby igniting a battle for market share that can result in a shake-out of weak, inefficient firms.

- *Rivalry is usually weaker in industries comprised of so many rivals that the impact of any one company's actions is spread thin across all industry members; likewise, it is often weak when there are fewer than five competitors.* A progressively larger number of competitors can actually begin to weaken head-to-head rivalry once an industry becomes populated with so many rivals that the impact of successful moves by any one company is spread thin across many industry members. To the extent that a company's strategic moves ripple out to have little discernible impact on the businesses of its many rivals, then industry members soon learn that it is not imperative to respond every time one or another rival does something to enhance its market position—an outcome that weakens the intensity of head-to-head battles for market share. Rivalry also *tends* to be weak if an industry consists of just two or three or four sellers. In a market with few rivals, each competitor soon learns that aggressive moves to grow its sales and market share can have immediate adverse impact on rivals' businesses, almost certainly provoking vigorous retaliation and risking an all-out battle for market share that is likely to lower the profits of all concerned. Companies that have a few strong rivals thus come to understand the merits of *restrained* efforts to wrest sales and market share from competitors as opposed to undertaking hard-hitting offensives that escalate into a profit-eroding arms-race or price war. However, some caution must be exercised in concluding that rivalry is weak just because there are only a few competitors. Thus, although occasional warfare can break out (the fierceness of the current battle between Red Hat and Microsoft and the decades-long war between Coca-Cola and Pepsi are prime examples), competition among the few normally produces a live-and-let-live approach to competing because rivals see the merits of restrained efforts to wrest sales and market share from competitors as opposed to undertaking hard-hitting offensives that escalate into a profit-eroding arms race or price war.

- *Rivalry increases when buyer demand falls off and sellers find themselves with excess capacity and/or inventory.* Excess supply conditions create a "buyers' market," putting added competitive pressure on industry rivals to scramble for profitable sales levels (often by price discounting).

- *Rivalry increases as it becomes less costly for buyers to switch brands.* The less expensive it is for buyers to switch their purchases from the seller of one brand to the s eller of another brand, the easier it is for sellers to steal customers away from rivals. But the higher the costs buyers incur to switch brands, the less prone they are to brand switching. Even if consumers view one or more rival brands as more attractive, they may not be inclined to switch because of the added time and inconvenience or the psychological costs of abandoning a familiar brand. Distributors and retailers may not switch to the brands of rival manufacturers because they are hesitant to sever long-standing supplier relationships, incur any technical support costs or retraining expenses in making the switchover, go to the trouble of testing the quality and reliability of the rival brand, or devote resources to marketing the new brand (especially if the brand is lesser known).

Apple Computer, for example, has been unable to convince PC users to switch from Windows-based PCs because of the time burdens and inconvenience associated with learning Apple's operating system and because so many Windows-based applications will not run on a MacIntosh due to operating system incompatibility. Consequently, unless buyers are dissatisfied with the brand they are presently purchasing, high switching costs can significantly weaken the rivalry among competing sellers.

- *Rivalry increases as the products of rival sellers become more standardized and diminishes as the products of industry rivals become more strongly differentiated.* When the offerings of rivals are identical or weakly differentiated, buyers have less reason to be brand-loyal—a condition that makes it easier for rivals to convince buyers to switch to their offering. And since the brands of different sellers have comparable attributes, buyers can shop the market for the best deal and switch brands at will. In contrast, strongly differentiated product offerings among rivals breed high brand loyalty on the part of buyers—because many buyers view the attributes of certain brands as better suited to their needs. Strong brand attachments make it tougher for sellers to draw customers away from rivals. Unless meaningful numbers of buyers are open to considering new or different product attributes being offered by rivals, the high degrees of brand loyalty that accompany strong product differentiation work against fierce rivalry among competing sellers. *The degree of product differentiation also affects switching costs.* When the offerings of rivals are identical or weakly differentiated, it is usually easy and inexpensive for buyers to switch their purchases from one seller to another. Strongly differentiated products raise the probability that buyers will find it costly to switch brands.

- *Rivalry is more intense when industry conditions tempt competitors to use price cuts or other competitive weapons to boost unit volume.* When a product is perishable, seasonal, or costly to hold in inventory, competitive pressures build quickly anytime one or more firms decide to cut prices and dump supplies on the market. Likewise, whenever fixed costs account for a large fraction of total cost, such that unit costs tend to be lowest at or near full capacity, then firms come under significant pressure to cut prices or otherwise try to boost sales whenever they are operating below full capacity. Unused capacity imposes a significant cost-increasing penalty because there are fewer units over which to spread fixed costs. The pressure of high fixed costs can push rival firms into price concessions, special discounts, rebates, low-interest-rate financing, and other volume-boosting tactics.

- *Rivalry increases when one or more competitors become dissatisfied with their market position and launch moves to bolster their standing at the expense of rivals.* Firms that are losing ground or in financial trouble often pursue aggressive (or perhaps desperate) turnaround strategies that can involve price discounts, more advertising, acquisition of or merger with other rivals, or new product introductions—such strategies can turn competitive pressures up a notch.

- *Rivalry becomes more volatile and unpredictable as the diversity of competitors increases in terms of visions, strategic intents, objectives, strategies, resources, and countries of origin.* A diverse group of sellers often contains one or more mavericks willing to try novel or high-risk or rule-breaking market approaches, thus generating a livelier and less predictable competitive environment. Globally competitive markets often contain rivals with different views about where the industry is headed and a willingness to employ perhaps radically different competitive approaches. Attempts by cross-border rivals to gain stronger footholds in each other's domestic markets usually boost the intensity of rivalry, especially when the aggressors have lower costs or products with more attractive features.

- *Rivalry increases when strong companies outside the industry acquire weak firms in the industry and launch aggressive, well-funded moves to transform their newly acquired competitors into major market contenders.* A concerted effort to turn a weak rival into a market leader nearly always entails launching well-financed strategic initiatives to dramatically improve the competitor's product offering, excite buyer interest, and win a much bigger market share—actions that, if successful, put added pressure on rivals to counter with fresh strategic moves of their own.

- *A powerful, successful competitive strategy employed by one company greatly intensifies the competitive pressures on its rivals to develop effective strategic responses or be relegated to also-ran status.*

Rivalry can be characterized as *cutthroat* or *brutal* when competitors engage in protracted price wars or habitually employ other aggressive tactics that are mutually destructive to profitability. Rivalry can be considered *fierce* to *strong* when the battle for market share is so vigorous that the profit margins of most industry members are squeezed to bare-bones levels. Rivalry can be characterized as *moderate* or *normal* when the maneuvering among industry members, while lively and healthy, still allows most industry members to earn acceptable profits. Rivalry is *weak* when most companies in the industry are relatively well satisfied with their sales growth and market shares, rarely undertake offensives to steal customers away from one another, and have comparatively attractive earnings and returns on investment.

Competitive Pressures Associated with the Threat of New Entrants

Several factors determine whether the threat of new companies entering the marketplace poses significant competitive pressure (see Figure 3.5). One factor relates to the size of the pool of likely entry candidates and the resources at their command. As a rule, the bigger the pool of entry candidates, the stronger the threat of potential entry. This is especially true when some of the likely entry candidates have ample resources and the potential to become formidable contenders for market leadership. Frequently, the strongest competitive pressures associated with potential entry come not from outsiders, but from current industry participants looking for growth opportunities. *Existing industry members are often strong candidates for entering market segments or geographic areas where they currently do not have a market presence.* Companies already well established in certain product categories or geographic areas often possess the resources, competencies, and competitive capabilities to hurdle the barriers of entering a different market segment or new geographic area.

A second factor concerns whether the likely entry candidates face high or low entry barriers. High barriers reduce the competitive threat of potential entry, while low barriers make entry more likely, especially if the industry is growing and offers attractive profit opportunities. The most widely encountered barriers that entry candidates must hurdle include:[4]

- *The presence of sizable economies of scale in production or other areas of operation*—When incumbent companies enjoy cost advantages associated with

Figure 3.5   **Factors Affecting the Threat of Entry**

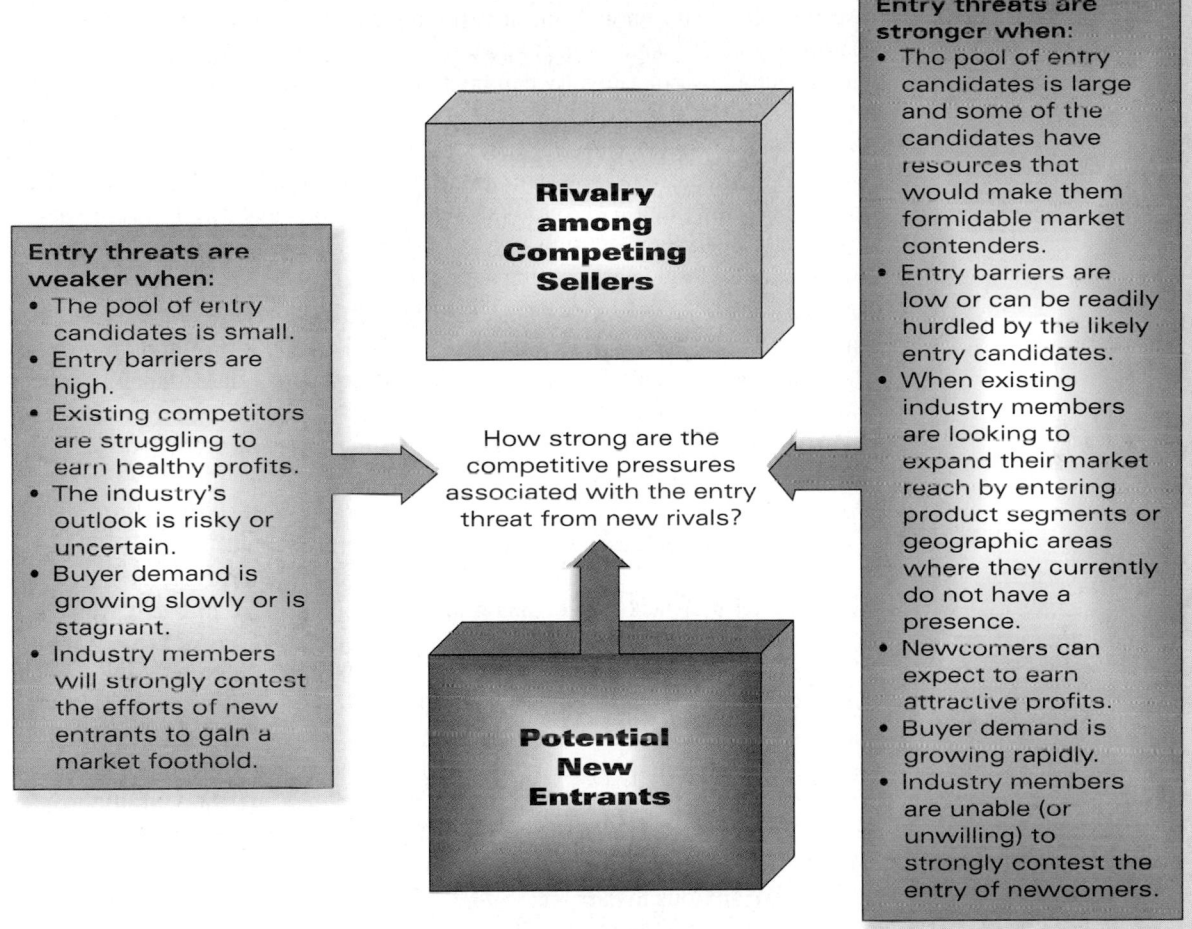

Entry threats are weaker when:
- The pool of entry candidates is small.
- Entry barriers are high.
- Existing competitors are struggling to earn healthy profits.
- The industry's outlook is risky or uncertain.
- Buyer demand is growing slowly or is stagnant.
- Industry members will strongly contest the efforts of new entrants to gain a market foothold.

Rivalry among Competing Sellers

How strong are the competitive pressures associated with the entry threat from new rivals?

Potential New Entrants

Entry threats are stronger when:
- The pool of entry candidates is large and some of the candidates have resources that would make them formidable market contenders.
- Entry barriers are low or can be readily hurdled by the likely entry candidates.
- When existing industry members are looking to expand their market reach by entering product segments or geographic areas where they currently do not have a presence.
- Newcomers can expect to earn attractive profits.
- Buyer demand is growing rapidly.
- Industry members are unable (or unwilling) to strongly contest the entry of newcomers.

large-scale operation, outsiders must either enter on a large scale (a costly and perhaps risky move) or accept a cost disadvantage and consequently lower profitability. Trying to overcome the disadvantages of small size by entering on a large scale at the outset can result in long-term overcapacity problems for the new entrant (until sales volume builds up), and it can so threaten the market shares of existing firms that they launch strong defensive maneuvers (price cuts, increased advertising and sales promotion, and similar blocking actions) to maintain their positions and make things hard on a newcomer.

- *Cost and resource disadvantages not related to scale of operation*—Aside from enjoying economies of scale, there are other reasons why existing firms may have low unit costs that are hard to replicate by newcomers. Industry incumbents can have cost advantages that stem from learning/experience curve effects, the possession of key patents or proprietary technology, partnerships with the best and cheapest suppliers of raw materials and components, favorable locations, and low fixed costs (because they have older facilities that have been mostly depreciated).

- *Strong brand preferences and high degrees of customer loyalty*—The stronger the attachment of buyers to established brands, the harder it is for a newcomer to break into the marketplace. In such cases, a new entrant must have the financial resources to spend enough on advertising and sales promotion to overcome customer loyalties and build its own clientele. Establishing brand recognition and building customer loyalty can be a slow and costly process. In addition, if it is difficult or costly for a customer to switch to a new brand, a new entrant must persuade buyers that its brand is worth the switching costs. To overcome switching-cost barriers, new entrants may have to offer buyers a discounted price or an extra margin of quality or service. All this can mean lower expected profit margins for new entrants, which increases the risk to start-up companies dependent on sizable early profits to support their new investments.

- *High capital requirements*—The larger the total dollar investment needed to enter the market successfully, the more limited the pool of potential entrants. The most obvious capital requirements for new entrants relate to manufacturing facilities and equipment, introductory advertising and sales promotion campaigns, working capital to finance inventories and customer credit, and sufficient cash to cover start-up costs.

- *The difficulties of building a network of distributors or retailers and securing adequate space on retailers' shelves*—A potential entrant can face numerous distribution channel challenges. Wholesale distributors may be reluctant to take on a product that lacks buyer recognition. Retailers have to be recruited and convinced to give a new brand ample display space and an adequate trial period. When existing sellers have strong, well-functioning distributor or retailer networks, a newcomer has an uphill struggle in squeezing its way in. Potential entrants sometimes have to "buy" their way into wholesale or retail channels by cutting their prices to provide dealers and distributors with higher markups and profit margins or by giving them big advertising and promotional allowances. As a consequence, a potential entrant's own profits may be squeezed unless and until its product gains enough consumer acceptance that distributors and retailers are anxious to carry it.

- *Restrictive regulatory policies*—Government agencies can limit or even bar entry by requiring licenses and permits. Regulated industries like cable TV, telecommunications, electric and gas utilities, radio and television broadcasting, liquor retailing, and railroads entail government-controlled entry. In international markets, host governments commonly limit foreign entry and must approve all foreign investment applications. Stringent government-mandated safety regulations and environmental pollution standards are entry barriers because they raise entry costs.

- *Tariffs and international trade restrictions*—National governments commonly use tariffs and trade restrictions (antidumping rules, local content requirements, quotas, etc.) to raise entry barriers for foreign firms and protect domestic producers from outside competition.

- *The ability and inclination of industry incumbents to launch vigorous initiatives to block a newcomer's successful entry*—Even if a potential entrant has or can acquire the needed competencies and resources to attempt entry, it must still worry about the reaction of existing firms.[5] Sometimes, there's little that incumbents can do to throw obstacles in an entrant's path—for instance, existing restaurants have little in their arsenal to discourage a new restaurant from opening or to dissuade people from trying the new restaurant. But there are times when incumbents do all they can to make it difficult for a new entrant, using price cuts, increased advertising, product improvements, and whatever else they can think of to prevent the entrant from building a clientele. Cable TV companies vigorously fight the entry of satellite TV companies; Sony and Nintendo have mounted strong defenses to thwart Microsoft's entry in videogames with its Xbox; existing hotels try to combat the opening of new hotels with loyalty programs, renovations of their own, the addition of new services, and so on. A potential entrant can have second thoughts when financially strong incumbent firms send clear signals that they will give newcomers a hard time.

Whether an industry's entry barriers ought to be considered high or low depends on the resources and competencies possessed by the pool of potential entrants. Companies with sizable financial resources, proven competitive capabilities, and a respected brand name may be able to hurdle an industry's entry barriers rather easily. Small start-up enterprises may find the same entry barriers insurmountable. Thus, how hard it will be for potential entrants to compete on a level playing field is always relative to the financial resources and competitive capabilities of likely entrants. For example, when Honda opted to enter the U.S. lawn-mower market in competition against Toro, Snapper, Craftsman, John Deere, and others, it was easily able to hurdle entry barriers that would have been formidable to other newcomers because it had long-standing expertise in gasoline engines and because its well-known reputation for quality and durability gave it instant credibility with shoppers looking to buy a new lawn mower. Honda had to spend relatively little on advertising to attract buyers and gain a market foothold, distributors and dealers were quite willing to handle the Honda lawn-mower line, and Honda had ample capital to build a U.S. assembly plant.

In evaluating whether the threat of additional entry is strong or weak, company managers must look at (1) how formidable the entry barriers are for each type of potential entrant—start-up enterprises, specific candidate companies in other industries, and current industry participants looking to expand their market reach—and (2) how attractive the growth and profit prospects are for new entrants. Rapidly growing market demand and high potential profits act as magnets, motivating potential entrants to commit the resources needed to hurdle entry barriers.[6] When profits are sufficiently attractive, entry barriers are unlikely to be an effective entry deterrent. At most, they limit the pool of candidate entrants to enterprises with the requisite competencies and resources and with the creativity to fashion a strategy for competing with incumbent firms.

Hence, *the best test of whether potential entry is a strong or weak competitive force in the marketplace is to ask if the industry's growth and profit prospects are strongly attractive to potential entry candidates.* When the answer is no, potential entry is a weak competitive force. When the answer is yes and there are entry candidates with sufficient expertise and resources, then potential entry adds significantly to competitive pressures in the marketplace. The stronger the threat of entry, the more that incumbent firms are driven to seek ways to fortify their positions against newcomers, pursuing strategic moves not only to protect their market shares but also to make entry more costly or difficult.

One additional point: *The threat of entry changes as the industry's prospects grow brighter or dimmer and as entry barriers rise or fall.* For example, in the pharmaceutical industry the expiration of a key patent on a widely prescribed drug virtually guarantees that one or more drug makers will enter with generic offerings of their own. Growing use of the Internet for shopping is making it much easier for Web-based retailers to enter into competition

> High entry barriers and weak entry threats today do not always translate into high entry barriers and weak entry threats tomorrow.

against such well-known retail chains as Sears, Circuit City, and Barnes and Noble. In international markets, entry barriers for foreign-based firms fall as tariffs are lowered, as host governments open up their domestic markets to outsiders, as domestic whole-salers and dealers seek out lower-cost foreign-made goods, and as domestic buyers become more willing to purchase foreign brands.

Competitive Pressures from the Sellers of Substitute Products

Companies in one industry come under competitive pressure from the actions of companies in a closely adjoining industry whenever buyers view the products of the two industries as good substitutes. For instance, the producers of sugar experience competitive pressures from the sales and marketing efforts of the makers of artificial sweeteners. Similarly, the producers of eyeglasses and contact lenses are currently facing mounting competitive pressures from growing consumer interest in corrective laser surgery. Newspapers are feeling the competitive force of the general public turning to cable news channels for late-breaking news and using Internet sources to get information about sports results, stock quotes, and job opportunities. The makers of videotapes and VCRs have watched demand evaporate as more and more consumers have been attracted to substitute use of DVDs and DVD recorders/players. Traditional providers of telephone service like BellSouth, AT&T, Verizon, and Qwest are feeling enormous competitive pressure from cell phone providers, as more and more consumers find cell phones preferable to landline phones.

Just how strong the competitive pressures are from the sellers of substitute products depends on three factors:

1. *Whether substitutes are readily available and attractively priced.* The presence of readily available and attractively priced substitutes creates competitive pressure by placing a ceiling on the prices industry members can charge without giving customers an incentive to switch to substitutes and risking sales erosion.[7] This price ceiling, at the same time, puts a lid on the profits that industry members can earn unless they find ways to cut costs. When substitutes are cheaper than an industry's product, industry members come under heavy competitive pressure to reduce their prices and find ways to absorb the price cuts with cost reductions.

2. *Whether buyers view the substitutes as being comparable or better in terms of quality, performance, and other relevant attributes.* The availability of substitutes inevitably invites customers to compare performance, features, ease of use, and other attributes as well as price. For example, ski boat manufacturers are experiencing strong competition from personal water-ski craft because water sports enthusiasts see personal water skis as fun to ride and less expensive. The users of paper cartons constantly weigh the performance trade-offs with plastic containers and metal cans. Camera users consider the convenience and performance trade-offs when deciding whether to substitute a digital camera for a film-based camera. Competition from good-performing substitutes unleashes competitive pressures on industry participants to incorporate new performance features and attributes that makes their product offerings more competitive.

3. *Whether the costs that buyers incur in switching to the substitutes are high or low.* High switching costs deter switching to substitutes, while low switching costs make it easier for the sellers of attractive substitutes to lure buyers to their offering.[8] Typical switching costs include the time and inconvenience that may be involved, the costs of additional equipment, the time and cost in testing the quality

Figure 3.6   **Factors Affecting Competition from Substitute Products**

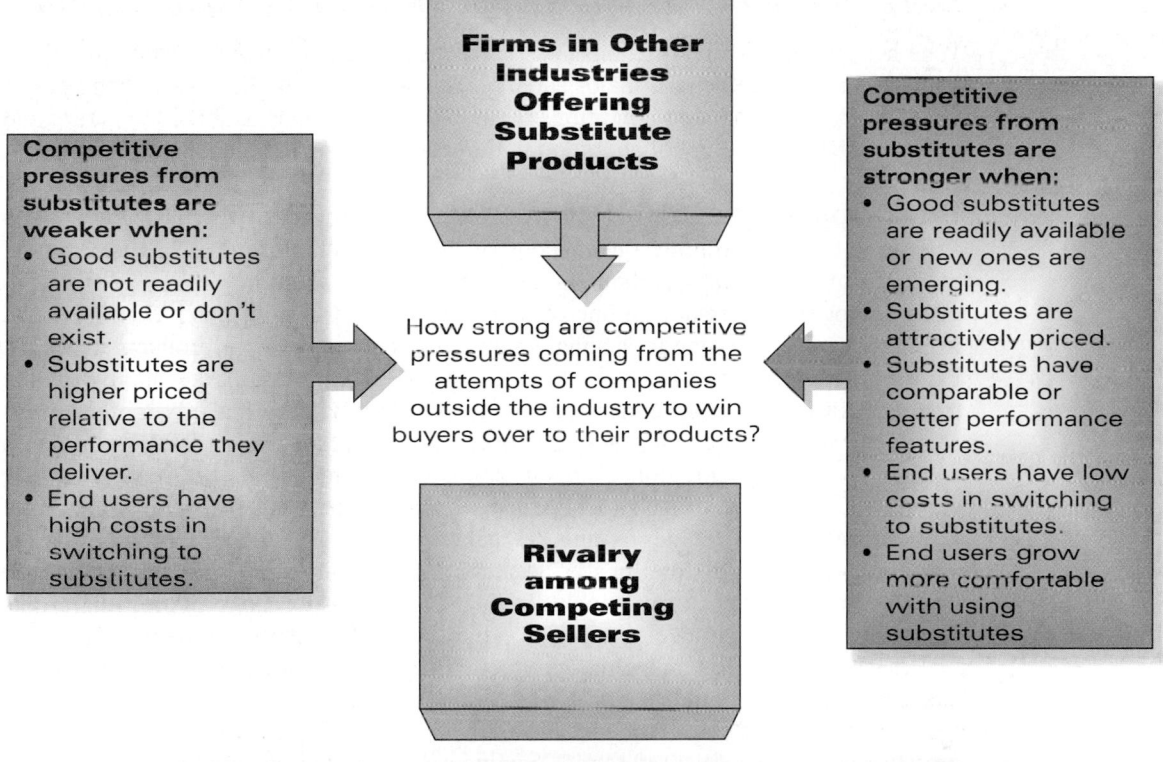

Signs That Competition from Substitutes Is Strong
- Sales of substitutes are growing faster than sales of the industry being analyzed (an indication that the sellers of substitutes are drawing customers away from the industry in question).
- Producers of substitutes are moving to add new capacity.
- Profits of the producers of substitutes are on the rise.

and reliability of the substitute, the psychological costs of severing old supplier relationships and establishing new ones, payments for technical help in making the changeover, and employee retraining costs. High switching costs can materially weaken the competitive pressures that industry members experience from substitutes unless the sellers of substitutes are successful in offsetting the high switching costs with enticing price discounts or additional performance enhancements.

Figure 3.6 summarizes the conditions that determine whether the competitive pressures from substitute products are strong, moderate, or weak.

As a rule, the lower the price of substitutes, the higher their quality and performance, and the lower the user's switching costs, the more intense the competitive pressures posed by substitute products. Other market indicators of the competitive strength of substitute products include (1) whether the sales of substitutes are growing faster than the sales of the industry being analyzed (a sign that the sellers of substitutes may be drawing customers away from the industry in question), (2) whether the producers of substitutes are moving to add new capacity, and (3) whether the profits of the producers of substitutes are on the rise.

Competitive Pressures Stemming from Supplier Bargaining Power and Supplier–Seller Collaboration

Whether supplier–seller relationships represent a weak or strong competitive force depends on (1) whether the major suppliers can exercise sufficient bargaining power to influence the terms and conditions of supply in their favor, and (2) the nature and extent of supplier–seller collaboration in the industry.

How Supplier Bargaining Power Can Create Competitive Pressures

Whenever the major suppliers to an industry have considerable leverage in determining the terms and conditions of the item they are supplying, then they are in a position to exert competitive pressure on one or more rival sellers. For instance, Microsoft and Intel, both of which supply personal computer (PC) makers with products that most PC users consider essential, are known for using their dominant market status not only to charge PC makers premium prices but also to leverage PC makers in other ways. Microsoft pressures PC makers to load only Microsoft products on the PCs they ship and to position the icons for Microsoft software prominently on the screens of new computers that come with factory-loaded software. Intel pushes greater use of Intel microprocessors in PCs by granting PC makers sizable advertising allowances on PC models equipped with "Intel Inside" stickers; it also tends to give PC makers that use the biggest percentages of Intel chips in their PC models top priority in filling orders for newly introduced Intel chips. Being on Intel's list of preferred customers helps a PC maker get an allocation of the first production runs of Intel's latest and greatest chips and thus get new PC models equipped with these chips to market ahead of rivals who are heavier users of chips made by Intel's rivals. The ability of Microsoft and Intel to pressure PC makers for preferential treatment of one kind or another in turn affects competition among rival PC makers.

Several other instances of supplier bargaining power are worth citing. Small-scale retailers must often contend with the power of manufacturers whose products enjoy prestigious and well-respected brand names; when a manufacturer knows that a retailer needs to stock the manufacturer's product because consumers expect to find the product on the shelves of retail stores where they shop, the manufacturer usually has some degree of pricing power and can also push hard for favorable shelf displays. Motor vehicle manufacturers typically exert considerable power over the terms and conditions with which they supply new vehicles to their independent automobile dealerships. The operators of franchised units of such chains as McDonald's, Dunkin' Donuts, Pizza Hut, Sylvan Learning Centers, and Hampton Inns must frequently agree not only to source some of their supplies from the franchisor at prices and terms favorable to that franchisor but also to operate their facilities in a manner largely dictated by the franchisor.

Strong supplier bargaining power is a competitive factor in industries where unions have been able to organize the workforces of some industry members but not others; those industry members that must negotiate wages, fringe benefits, and working conditions with powerful unions (which control the supply of labor) often find themselves with higher labor costs than their competitors with nonunion labor forces. The bigger the gap between union and nonunion labor costs in an industry, the more that unionized industry members must scramble to find ways to relieve the competitive pressure associated with their disadvantage on labor costs. High labor costs are proving a huge competitive liability to unionized supermarket chains like Kroger and Safeway in trying to combat the market share gains being made by Wal-Mart in supermarket retailing—Wal-Mart has a nonunion workforce, and the prices for supermarket items at its Supercenters tend to run 5 to 20 percent lower than those at unionized supermarket chains.

The factors that determine whether any of the suppliers to an industry are in a position to exert substantial bargaining power or leverage are fairly clear-cut:[9]

- *Whether the item being supplied is a commodity that is readily available from many suppliers at the going market price.* Suppliers have little or no bargaining power or leverage whenever industry members have the ability to source their requirements at competitive prices from any of several alternative and eager suppliers, perhaps dividing their purchases among two or more suppliers to promote lively competition for orders. The suppliers of commodity items have market power only when supplies become quite tight and industry members are so eager to secure what they need that they agree to terms more favorable to suppliers.

- *Whether a few large suppliers are the primary sources of a particular item.* The leading suppliers may well have pricing leverage unless they are plagued with excess capacity and are scrambling to secure additional orders for their products. Major suppliers with good reputations and strong demand for the items they supply are harder to wring concessions from than struggling suppliers striving to broaden their customer base or more fully utilize their production capacity.

- *Whether it is difficult or costly for industry members to switch their purchases from one supplier to another or to switch to attractive substitute inputs.* High switching costs signal strong bargaining power on the part of suppliers, whereas low switching costs and ready availability of good substitute inputs signal weak bargaining power. Soft-drink bottlers, for example, can counter the bargaining power of aluminum can suppliers by shifting or threatening to shift to greater use of plastic containers and introducing more attractive plastic container designs.

- *Whether certain needed inputs are in short supply.* Suppliers of items in short supply have some degree of pricing power, whereas a surge in the availability of particular items greatly weakens supplier pricing power and bargaining leverage.

- *Whether certain suppliers provide a differentiated input that enhances the performance or quality of the industry's product.* The more valuable that a particular input is in terms of enhancing the performance or quality of the products of industry members or of improving the efficiency of their production processes, the more bargaining leverage its suppliers are likely to possess.

- *Whether certain suppliers provide equipment or services that deliver valuable cost-saving efficiencies to industry members in operating their production processes.* Suppliers who provide cost-saving equipment or other valuable or necessary production-related services are likely to possess bargaining leverage. Industry members that do not source from such suppliers may find themselves at a cost disadvantage and thus under competitive pressure to do so (on terms that are favorable to the suppliers).

- *Whether suppliers provide an item that accounts for a sizable fraction of the costs of the industry's product.* The bigger the cost of a particular part or component, the more opportunity for the pattern of competition in the marketplace to be affected by the actions of suppliers to raise or lower their prices.

- *Whether industry members are major customers of suppliers.* As a rule, suppliers have less bargaining leverage when their sales to members of this one industry constitute a big percentage of their total sales. In such cases, the well-being of suppliers is closely tied to the well-being of their major customers.

Suppliers then have a big incentive to protect and enhance their customers' competitiveness via reasonable prices, exceptional quality, and ongoing advances in the technology of the items supplied.

- *Whether it makes good economic sense for industry members to integrate backward and self-manufacture items they have been buying from suppliers.* The make-or-buy issue generally boils down to whether suppliers who specialize in the production of a particular part or component and make them in volume for many different customers have the expertise and scale economies to supply as good or better component at a lower cost than industry members could achieve via self-manufacture. Frequently, it is difficult for industry members to self-manufacture parts and components more economically than they can obtain them from suppliers who specialize in making such items. For instance, most producers of outdoor power equipment (lawn mowers, rotary tillers, leaf blowers, etc.) find it cheaper to source the small engines they need from outside manufacturers who specialize in small-engine manufacture rather than make their own engines because the quantity of engines they need is too small to justify the investment in manufacturing facilities, master the production process, and capture scale economies. Specialists in small-engine manufacture, by supplying many kinds of engines to the whole power equipment industry, can obtain a big enough sales volume to fully realize scale economies, become proficient in all the manufacturing techniques, and keep costs low. As a rule, suppliers are safe from the threat of self-manufacture by their customers *until* the volume of parts a customer needs becomes large enough for the customer to justify backward integration into self-manufacture of the component. Suppliers also gain bargaining power when they have the resources and profit incentive to integrate forward into the business of the customers they are supplying and thus become a strong rival.

Figure 3.7 summarizes the conditions that tend to make supplier bargaining power strong or weak.

How Seller–Supplier Partnerships Can Create Competitive Pressures   In more and more industries, sellers are forging strategic partnerships with select suppliers in efforts to (1) reduce inventory and logistics costs (e.g., through just-in-time deliveries), (2) speed the availability of next-generation components, (3) enhance the quality of the parts and components being supplied and reduce defect rates, and (4) squeeze out important cost savings for both themselves and their suppliers. Numerous Internet technology applications are now available that permit real-time data sharing, eliminate paperwork, and produce cost savings all along the supply chain. The many benefits of effective seller–supplier collaboration can translate into competitive advantage for industry members that do the best job of managing supply chain relationships.

Dell Computer has used strategic partnering with key suppliers as a major element in its strategy to be the world's lowest-cost supplier of branded PCs, servers, and workstations. Because Dell has managed its supply chain relationships in ways that contribute to a low-cost, high-quality competitive edge in components supply, it has put enormous pressure on its PC rivals to try to imitate its supply chain management practices. Effective partnerships with suppliers on the part of one or more industry members can thus become a major source of competitive pressure for rival firms.

The more opportunities that exist for win–win efforts between a company and its suppliers, the less their relationship is characterized by who has the upper hand in

Figure 3.7   **Factors Affecting the Bargaining Power of Suppliers**

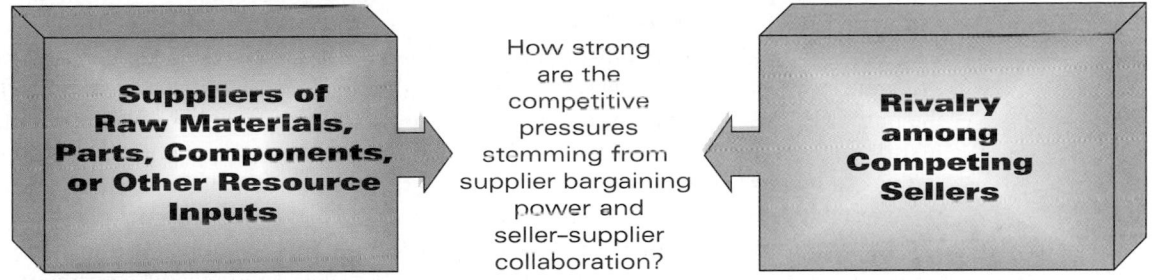

Supplier bargaining power is stronger when:
- Industry members incurs high costs in switching their purchases to alternative suppliers.
- Needed inputs are in short supply (which gives suppliers more leverage in setting prices).
- A supplier has a differentiated input that enhances the quality or performance of sellers' products or is a valuable or critical part of sellers' production process.
- There are only a few suppliers of a particular input.
- Some suppliers threaten to integrate forward into the business of industry members and perhaps become a powerful rival.

Supplier bargaining power is weaker when:
- The item being supplied is a commodity that is readily available from many suppliers at the going market price.
- Seller switching costs to alternative suppliers are low.
- Good substitute inputs exist or new ones emerge.
- There is a surge in the availability of supplies (thus greatly weakening supplier pricing power).
- Industry members account for a big fraction of suppliers' total sales and continued high volume purchases are important to the well-being of suppliers.
- Industry members are a threat to integrate backward into the business of suppliers and to self-manufacture their own requirements.
- Seller collaboration or partnering with selected suppliers provides attractive win–win opportunities.

bargaining with the other. Collaborative partnerships between a company and a supplier tend to last so long as the relationship is producing valuable benefits for both parties. Only if a supply partner is falling behind alternative suppliers is a company likely to switch suppliers and incur the costs and trouble of building close working ties with a different supplier.

Competitive Pressures Stemming from Buyer Bargaining Power and Seller–Buyer Collaboration

Whether seller–buyer relationships represent a weak or strong competitive force depends on (1) whether some or many buyers have sufficient bargaining leverage to obtain price concessions and other favorable terms and conditions of sale, and (2) the extent and competitive importance of seller–buyer strategic partnerships in the industry.

How Buyer Bargaining Power Can Create Competitive Pressures   As with suppliers, the leverage that certain types of buyers have in negotiating favorable terms can range from weak to strong. Individual consumers, for example, rarely have much bargaining power in negotiating price concessions or other favorable terms with sellers; the primary exceptions involve situations in which price haggling is customary, such as the purchase of new and used motor vehicles, homes, and certain big-ticket items like luxury watches, jewelry, and pleasure boats. For most consumer goods and services, individual buyers have no bargaining leverage—their option is to pay the seller's posted price or take their business elsewhere.

In contrast, large retail chains like Wal-Mart, Best Buy, Staples, and Home Depot typically have considerable negotiating leverage in purchasing products from manufacturers because of manufacturers' need for broad retail exposure and the most appealing shelf locations. Retailers may stock two or three competing brands of a product but rarely all competing brands, so competition among rival manufacturers for visibility on the shelves of popular multistore retailers gives such retailers significant bargaining strength. Major supermarket chains like Kroger, Safeway, and Royal Ahold, which provide access to millions of grocery shoppers, have sufficient bargaining power to demand promotional allowances and lump-sum payments (called slotting fees) from food products manufacturers in return for stocking certain brands or putting them in the best shelf locations. Motor vehicle manufacturers have strong bargaining power in negotiating to buy original equipment tires from Goodyear, Michelin, Bridgestone/Firestone, Continental, and Pirelli not only because they buy in large quantities but also because tire makers believe they gain an advantage in supplying replacement tires to vehicle owners if their tire brand is original equipment on the vehicle. "Prestige" buyers have a degree of clout in negotiating with sellers because a seller's reputation is enhanced by having prestige buyers on its customer list.

Even if buyers do not purchase in large quantities or offer a seller important market exposure or prestige, they gain a degree of bargaining leverage in the following circumstances:[10]

- *If buyers' costs of switching to competing brands or substitutes are relatively low*—Buyers who can readily switch brands or source from several sellers have more negotiating leverage than buyers who have high switching costs. When the products of rival sellers are virtually identical, it is relatively easy for buyers to switch from seller to seller at little or no cost and anxious sellers may be willing to make concessions to win or retain a buyer's business.

- *If the number of buyers is small or if a customer is particularly important to a seller*—The smaller the number of buyers, the less easy it is for sellers to find alternative buyers when a customer is lost to a competitor. The prospect of losing a customer not easily replaced often makes a seller more willing to grant concessions of one kind or another.

- *If buyer demand is weak and sellers are scrambling to secure additional sales of their products*—Weak or declining demand creates a "buyers' market"; conversely, strong or rapidly growing demand creates a "sellers' market" and shifts bargaining power to sellers.

- *If buyers are well informed about sellers' products, prices, and costs*—The more information buyers have, the better bargaining position they are in. The mushrooming availability of product information on the Internet is giving added bargaining power to individuals. Buyers can easily use the Internet to compare prices and features of vacation packages, shop for the best interest rates on mortgages and loans, and find the best prices on big-ticket items such as digital cameras. Bargain-hunting individuals can shop around for the best deal on the Internet and use that information to negotiate a better deal from local retailers; this method is becoming commonplace in buying new and used motor vehicles. Further, the Internet has created opportunities for manufacturers, wholesalers, retailers, and sometimes individuals to join online buying groups to pool their purchasing power and approach vendors for better terms than could be gotten individually. A multinational manufacturer's geographically scattered purchasing groups can use Internet technology to pool their orders with parts and components suppliers and bargain for volume discounts. Purchasing agents at some companies are banding together at third-party Web sites to pool corporate purchases to get better deals or special treatment.

- *If buyers pose a credible threat of integrating backward into the business of sellers*—Companies like Anheuser-Busch, Coors, and Heinz have integrated backward into metal can manufacturing to gain bargaining power in obtaining the balance of their can requirements from otherwise powerful metal can manufacturers. Retailers gain bargaining power by stocking and promoting their own private-label brands alongside manufacturers' name brands. Wal-Mart, for example, has elected to compete against Procter & Gamble (P&G), its biggest supplier, with its own brand of laundry detergent, called Sam's American Choice, which is priced 25 to 30 percent lower than P&G's Tide.

- *If buyers have discretion in whether and when they purchase the product*—Many consumers, if they are unhappy with the present deals offered on major appliances or hot tubs or home entertainment centers, may be in a position to delay purchase until prices and financing terms improve. If business customers are not happy with the prices or security features of bill-payment software systems, they can either delay purchase until next-generation products become available or attempt to develop their own software in-house. If college students believe that the prices of new textbooks are too high, they can purchase used copies.

Figure 3.8 highlights the factors causing buyer bargaining power to be strong or weak.

A final point to keep in mind is that *not all buyers of an industry's product have equal degrees of bargaining power with sellers*, and some may be less sensitive than others to price, quality, or service differences. For example, independent tire retailers have less bargaining power in purchasing tires than do Honda, Ford, and DaimlerChrysler (which buy in much larger quantities), and they are also less sensitive to quality. Motor vehicle manufacturers are very particular about tire quality and tire performance because of the effects on vehicle performance, and they drive a hard bargain with tire manufacturers on both price and quality. Apparel manufacturers confront significant bargaining power when selling to big retailers like JCPenney, Macy's, or L. L. Bean but they can command much better prices selling to small owner-managed apparel boutiques.

How Seller–Buyer Partnerships Can Create Competitive Pressures Partnerships between sellers and buyers are an increasingly important element of the competitive picture in *business-to-business relationships* (as opposed to business-to-consumer relationships). Many sellers that provide items to business customers have found it in their mutual interest to collaborate closely on such matters as just-in-time deliveries, order processing, electronic invoice payments, and data sharing. Wal-Mart, for example, provides the manufacturers with which it does business (like Procter & Gamble) with daily sales at each of its stores so that the manufacturers can maintain sufficient inventories at Wal-Mart's distribution centers to keep the shelves at each Wal-Mart store amply stocked. Dell has partnered with its largest PC customers to create

Figure 3.8 **Factors Affecting the Bargaining Power of Buyers**

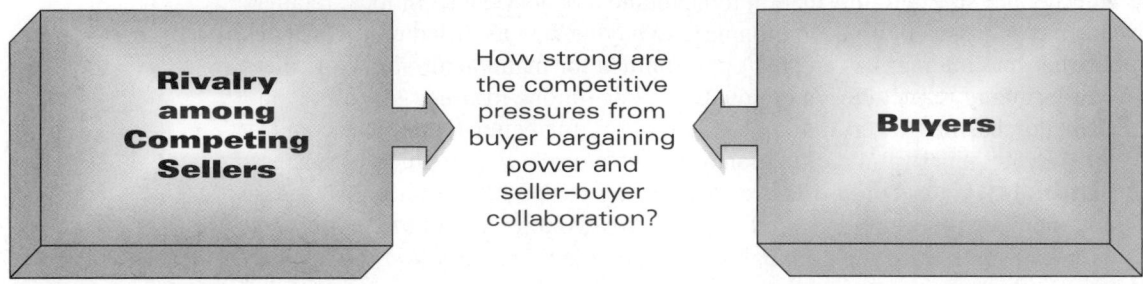

Buyer bargaining power is stronger when:
- Buyer switching costs to competing brands or substitute products are low.
- Buyers are large and can demand concessions when purchasing large quantities.
- Large-volume purchases by buyers are important to sellers.
- Buyer demand is weak or declining.
- There are only a few buyers—so that each one's business is important to sellers.
- Identity of buyer adds prestige to the seller's list of customers.
- Quantity and quality of information available to buyers improves.
- Buyers have the ability to postpone purchases until later if they do not like the present deals being offered by sellers.
- Some buyers are a threat to integrate backward into the business of sellers and become an important competitor.

Buyer bargaining power is weaker when:
- Buyers purchase the item infrequently or in small quantities.
- Buyer switching costs to competing brands are high.
- There is a surge in buyer demand that creates a "sellers' market."
- A seller's brand reputation is important to a buyer.
- A particular seller's product delivers quality or performance that is very important to buyer and that is not matched in other brands.
- Buyer collaboration or partnering with selected sellers provides attractive win–win opportunities.

online systems for over 50,000 corporate customers, providing their employees with information on approved product configurations, global pricing, paperless purchase orders, real-time order tracking, invoicing, purchasing history, and other efficiency tools. Dell loads a customer's software at the factory and installs asset tags so that customer setup time is minimal; it also helps customers upgrade their PC systems to next-generation hardware and software. Dell's partnerships with its corporate customers have put significant competitive pressure on other PC makers.

Is the Collective Strength of the Five Competitive Forces Conducive to Good Profitability?

Scrutinizing each of the five competitive forces one by one provides a powerful diagnosis of what competition is like in a given market. Once the strategist has gained an understanding of the specific competitive pressures comprising each force and determined whether these pressures constitute a strong, moderate, or weak competitive force, the next step is to evaluate the collective strength of the five forces and determine whether the state of competition is conducive to good profitability. Is the collective impact of the five competitive forces stronger than "normal"? Are some of the competitive forces sufficiently strong to undermine industry profitability? Can companies in this industry reasonably expect to earn decent profits in light of the prevailing competitive forces?

Is the Industry Competitively Attractive or Unattractive?   *As a rule, the stronger the collective impact of the five competitive forces, the lower the combined profitability of industry participants.* The most extreme case of a competitively unattractive industry is when all five forces are producing strong competitive pressures: Rivalry among sellers is vigorous, low entry barriers allow new rivals to gain a market foothold, competition from substitutes is intense, and both suppliers and customers are able to exercise considerable bargaining leverage. Fierce to strong competitive pressures coming from all five directions nearly always drive industry profitability to unacceptably low levels, frequently producing losses for many industry members and forcing some out of business. But an industry can be competitively unattractive even when not all five competitive forces are strong. Intense competitive pressures from just two or three of the five forces may suffice to destroy the conditions for good profitability and prompt some companies to exit the business. The manufacture of disk drives, for example, is brutally competitive; IBM recently announced the sale of its disk drive business to Hitachi, taking a loss of over $2 billion on its exit from the business. Especially intense competitive conditions seem to be the norm in tire manufacturing and apparel, two industries where profit margins have historically been thin.

> The stronger the forces of competition, the harder it becomes for industry members to earn attractive profits.

In contrast, when the collective impact of the five competitive forces is moderate to weak, an industry is competitively attractive in the sense that industry members can reasonably expect to earn good profits and a nice return on investment. The ideal competitive environment for earning superior profits is one in which both suppliers and customers are in weak bargaining positions, there are no good substitutes, high barriers block further entry, and rivalry among present sellers generates only moderate competitive pressures. Weak competition is the best of all possible worlds for also-ran companies because even they can usually eke out a decent profit—if a company can't make a decent profit when competition is weak, then its business outlook is indeed grim.

In most industries, the collective strength of the five competitive forces is somewhere near the middle of the two extremes of very intense and very weak, typically ranging from slightly stronger than normal to slightly weaker than normal and typically allowing well-managed companies with sound strategies to earn attractive profits.

Matching Company Strategy to Competitive Conditions   Working through the five-forces model step by step not only aids strategy makers in assessing whether the intensity of competition allows good profitability but also promotes sound strategic thinking about how to better match company strategy to the specific competitive character of the marketplace. Effectively matching a company's strategy to prevailing competitive conditions has two aspects:

> A company's strategy is increasingly effective the more it provides some insulation from competitive pressures and shifts the competitive battle in the company's favor.

1. Pursuing avenues that shield the firm from as many of the different competitive pressures as possible.
2. Initiating actions calculated to produce sustainable competitive advantage, thereby shifting competition in the company's favor, putting added competitive pressure on rivals, and perhaps even defining the business model for the industry.

But making headway on these two fronts first requires identifying competitive pressures, gauging the relative strength of each of the five competitive forces, and gaining a deep enough understanding of the state of competition in the industry to know which strategy buttons to push.

QUESTION 3: WHAT FACTORS ARE DRIVING INDUSTRY CHANGE AND WHAT IMPACTS WILL THEY HAVE?

An industry's present conditions don't necessarily reveal much about the strategically relevant ways in which the industry environment is changing. All industries are characterized by trends and new developments that gradually or speedily produce changes important enough to require a strategic response from participating firms. A popular hypothesis states that industries go through a life cycle of takeoff, rapid growth, early maturity and slowing growth, market saturation, and stagnation or decline. This hypothesis helps explain industry change—but it is far from complete.[11] There are more causes of industry change than an industry's normal progression through the life cycle—these need to be identified and their impacts understood.

The Concept of Driving Forces

Core Concept
Industry conditions change because important forces are *driving* industry participants (competitors, customers, or suppliers) to alter their actions; the **driving forces** in an industry are the *major underlying causes* of changing industry and competitive conditions—they have the biggest influence on how the industry landscape will be altered. Some driving forces originate in the outer ring of macroenvironment and some originate from the inner ring.

While it is important to track where an industry is in the life cycle, there's more analytical value in identifying the other factors that may be even stronger drivers of industry and competitive change. The point to be made here is that industry and competitive conditions change because forces are enticing or pressuring certain industry participants (competitors, customers, suppliers) to alter their actions in important ways.[12] The most powerful of the change agents are called **driving forces** because they have the biggest influences in reshaping the industry landscape and altering competitive conditions. Some driving forces originate in the outer ring of the company's macroenvironment (see Figure 3.2), but most originate in the company's more immediate industry and competitive environment.

Driving-forces analysis has three steps: (1) identifying what the driving forces are; (2) assessing whether the drivers of change are, on the whole, acting to make the industry more or less attractive; and (3) determining what strategy changes are needed to prepare for the impacts of the driving forces. All three steps merit further discussion.

Identifying an Industry's Driving Forces

Many developments can affect an industry powerfully enough to qualify as driving forces. Some drivers of change are unique and specific to a particular industry situation, but most drivers of industry and competitive change fall into one of the following categories:[13]

- *Emerging new Internet capabilities and applications*—Since the late 1990s, the Internet has woven its way into everyday business operations and the social fabric of life all across the world. Mushrooming Internet use, growing acceptance of Internet shopping, the emergence of high-speed Internet service and Voice over Internet Protocol (VoIP) technology, and an ever-growing series of Internet applications and capabilities have been major drivers of change in industry after industry. Companies are increasingly using online technology (1) to collaborate closely with suppliers and streamline their supply chains and (2) to revamp internal operations and squeeze out cost savings. Manufacturers can use their Web sites to access customers directly rather than distribute exclusively through traditional wholesale and retail channels. Businesses of all types can use Web stores to extend their geographic reach and vie for sales in areas where they formerly did not have a presence. The ability of companies to reach consumers via the Internet increases the number of rivals a company faces and often escalates rivalry by pitting pure online sellers against combination brick-and-click sellers against pure brick-and-mortar sellers. The Internet gives buyers unprecedented ability to research the product offerings of competitors and shop the market for the best value. Mounting ability of consumers to download music from the Internet via either file sharing or online music retailers has profoundly and reshaped the music industry and the business of traditional brick-and-mortar music retailers. Widespread use of e-mail has forever eroded the business of providing fax services and the first-class mail delivery revenues of government postal services worldwide. Videoconferencing via the Internet can erode the demand for business travel. Online course offerings at universities have the potential to revolutionize higher education. The Internet of the future will feature faster speeds, dazzling applications, and over a billion connected gadgets performing an array of functions, thus driving further industry and competitive changes. But Internet-related impacts vary from industry to industry. The challenges here are to assess precisely how emerging Internet developments are altering a particular industry's landscape and to factor these impacts into the strategy-making equation.

- *Increasing globalization*—Competition begins to shift from primarily a regional or national focus to an international or global focus when industry members begin seeking out customers in foreign markets or when production activities begin to migrate to countries where costs are lowest. Globalization of competition really starts to take hold when one or more ambitious companies precipitate a race for worldwide market leadership by launching initiatives to expand into more and more country markets. Globalization can also be precipitated by the blossoming of consumer demand in more and more countries and by the actions of government officials in many countries to reduce trade barriers or open up once-closed markets to foreign competitors, as is occurring in many parts of Europe, Latin America, and Asia. Significant differences in labor costs among countries give manufacturers a strong incentive to locate plants for labor-intensive products in low-wage countries and use these plants to supply market demand across the world. Wages in China, India, Singapore, Mexico, and Brazil, for example, are about one-fourth those in the United States, Germany, and Japan. The forces of globalization are sometimes such a strong driver that companies find it highly advantageous, if not necessary, to spread their operating reach into more and more country markets. Globalization is very much a driver of industry change in such industries as credit cards, cell phones, digital cameras, golf and ski equipment, motor vehicles, steel, petroleum, personal computers, video games, public accounting, and textbook publishing.

- *Changes in an industry's long-term growth rate*—Shifts in industry growth up or down are a driving force for industry change, affecting the balance between industry supply and buyer demand, entry and exit, and the character and strength of competition. An upsurge in buyer demand triggers a race among established firms and newcomers to capture the new sales opportunities; ambitious companies with trailing market shares may see the upturn in demand as a golden opportunity to launch offensive strategies to broaden their customer base and move up several notches in the industry standings. A slowdown in the rate at which demand is growing nearly always portends mounting rivalry and increased efforts by some firms to maintain their high rates of growth by taking sales and market share away from rivals. If industry sales suddenly turn flat or begin to shrink after years of rising at double-digit levels, competition is certain to intensify as industry members scramble for the available business and as mergers and acquisitions result in industry consolidation to a smaller number of competitively stronger participants. Stagnating sales usually prompt both competitively weak and growth-oriented companies to sell their business operations to those industry members who elect to stick it out; as demand for the industry's product continues to shrink, the remaining industry members may be forced to close inefficient plants and retrench to a smaller production base—all of which results in a much-changed competitive landscape.

- *Changes in who buys the product and how they use it*—Shifts in buyer demographics and new ways of using the product can alter the state of competition by opening the way to market an industry's product through a different mix of dealers and retail outlets; prompting producers to broaden or narrow their product lines; bringing different sales and promotion approaches into play; and forcing adjustments in customer service offerings (credit, technical assistance, maintenance, and repair). The mushrooming popularity of downloading music from the Internet, storing music files on PC hard drives, and burning custom discs has forced recording companies to reexamine their distribution strategies and raised questions about the future of traditional retail music stores; at the same time, it has stimulated sales of disc burners and blank discs. Longer life expectancies and growing percentages of relatively well-to-do retirees are driving changes in such industries as health care, prescription drugs, recreational living, and vacation travel. The growing percentage of households with PCs and Internet access is opening opportunities for banks to expand their electronic bill-payment services and for retailers to move more of their customer services online.

- *Product innovation*—Competition in an industry is always affected by rivals racing to be first to introduce one new product or product enhancement after another. An ongoing stream of product innovations tends to alter the pattern of competition in an industry by attracting more first-time buyers, rejuvenating industry growth, and/or creating wider or narrower product differentiation among rival sellers. Successful new product introductions strengthen the market positions of the innovating companies, usually at the expense of companies that stick with their old products or are slow to follow with their own versions of the new product. Product innovation has been a key driving force in such industries as digital cameras, golf clubs, video games, toys, and prescription drugs.

- *Technological change and manufacturing process innovation*—Advances in technology can dramatically alter an industry's landscape, making it possible to produce new and better products at lower cost and opening up whole new industry frontiers. For instance, Voice over Internet Protocol (VoIP) technology has spawned low-cost, Internet-based phone networks that are stealing large numbers of customers away from traditional telephone companies worldwide (whose higher cost technology depends on hardwired connections via overhead and underground telephone lines). Flat-screen technology for PC monitors is killing the demand for conventional cathode ray tube (CRT) monitors. Liquid crystal display (LCD), plasma screen technology, and high-definition technology are precipitating a revolution in the television industry and driving use of cathode ray technology (CRT) into the background. MP3 technology is transforming how people listen to music. Digital technology is driving huge changes in the camera and film industries. Satellite radio technology is allowing satellite radio companies with their largely commercial-free programming to draw millions of listeners away from traditional radio stations whose revenue streams from commercials are dependent on audience size. Technological developments can also produce competitively significant changes in capital requirements, minimum efficient plant sizes, distribution channels and logistics, and learning/experience curve effects. In the steel industry, ongoing advances in electric arc minimill technology (which involve recycling scrap steel to make new products) have allowed steelmakers with state-of-the-art minimills to gradually expand into the production of more and more steel products, steadily taking sales and market share from higher-cost integrated producers (which make steel from scratch using iron ore, coke, and traditional blast furnace technology). Nucor Corporation, the leader of the minimill technology revolution in the United States, began operations in 1970 and has ridden the wave of technological advances in minimill technology to become the biggest U.S. steel producer (as of 2004) and rank among the lowest-cost producers in the world. In a space of 30 years, advances in minimill technology have changed the face of the steel industry worldwide.

- *Marketing innovation*—When firms are successful in introducing new ways to *market* their products, they can spark a burst of buyer interest, widen industry demand, increase product differentiation, and lower unit costs—any or all of which can alter the competitive positions of rival firms and force strategy revisions. Online marketing is shaking up competition in electronics (where there are dozens of online electronics retailers, often with deep-discount prices) and office supplies (where Office Depot, Staples, and Office Max are using their Web sites to market office supplies to corporations, small businesses, schools and universities, and government agencies). Increasing numbers of music artists are marketing their recordings at their own Web sites rather than entering into contracts with recording studios that distribute through online and brick-and-mortar music retailers.

- *Entry or exit of major firms*—The entry of one or more foreign companies into a geographic market once dominated by domestic firms nearly always shakes up competitive conditions. Likewise, when an established domestic firm from another industry attempts entry either by acquisition or by launching its own start-up venture, it usually applies its skills and resources in some innovative fashion that pushes competition in new directions. Entry by a major firm thus often produces a new ball game, not only with new key players but also with new rules for competing. Similarly, exit of a major firm changes the competitive structure by reducing the number of market leaders (perhaps increasing the dominance of the leaders who remain) and causing a rush to capture the exiting firm's customers.

- *Diffusion of technical know-how across more companies and more countries*—As knowledge about how to perform a particular activity or execute a particular manufacturing technology spreads, the competitive advantage held by firms originally possessing this know-how erodes. Knowledge diffusion can occur through scientific journals, trade publications, on-site plant tours, word of mouth among suppliers and customers, employee migration, and Internet sources. It can also occur when those possessing technological knowledge license others to use that knowledge for a royalty fee or team up with a company interested in turning the technology into a new business venture. Quite often, technological know-how can be acquired by simply buying a company that has the wanted skills, patents, or manufacturing capabilities. In recent years, *rapid technology transfer across national boundaries has been a prime factor in causing industries to become more globally competitive.* As companies worldwide gain access to valuable technical know-how, they upgrade their manufacturing capabilities in a long-term effort to compete head-on with established companies. Cross-border technology transfer has made the once domestic industries of automobiles, tires, consumer electronics, telecommunications, computers, and others increasingly global.

- *Changes in cost and efficiency*—Widening or shrinking differences in the costs among key competitors tend to dramatically alter the state of competition. The low cost of fax and e-mail transmission has put mounting competitive pressure on the relatively inefficient and high-cost operations of the U.S. Postal Service—sending a one-page fax is cheaper and far quicker than sending a first-class letter; sending e-mail is faster and cheaper still. In the steel industry, the lower costs of companies using electric-arc furnaces to recycle scrap steel into new steel products has forced traditional manufacturers that produce steel from iron ore using blast furnace technology to overhaul their plants and to withdraw totally from making those steel products where they could no longer be cost competitive. Shrinking cost differences in producing multifeatured mobile phones is turning the mobile phone market into a commodity business and causing more buyers to base their purchase decisions on price.

- *Growing buyer preferences for differentiated products instead of a commodity product (or for a more standardized product instead of strongly differentiated products)*—When buyer tastes and preferences start to diverge, sellers can win a loyal following with product offerings that stand apart from those of rival sellers. In recent years, beer drinkers have grown less loyal to a single brand and have begun to drink a variety of domestic and foreign beers; as a consequence, beer manufacturers have introduced a host of new brands and malt beverages with different tastes and flavors. Buyer preferences for motor vehicles are becoming increasingly diverse, with few models generating sales of more than 250,000 units annually. When a shift from standardized to differentiated products occurs, the driver of change is the contest among rivals to cleverly outdifferentiate one another.

    However, buyers sometimes decide that a standardized, budget-priced product suits their requirements as well as or better than a premium-priced product with lots of snappy features and personalized services. Online brokers, for example, have used the lure of cheap commissions to attract many investors willing to place their own buy–sell orders via the Internet; growing acceptance of online trading has put significant competitive pressures on full-service brokers whose business model has always revolved around convincing clients of the value of asking for personalized advice from professional brokers and paying their high commission fees to make trades. Pronounced shifts toward greater product standardization usually spawn lively price competition and force rival sellers to drive down their costs to maintain profitability. The lesson here is that competition is driven partly by whether the market forces in motion are acting to increase or decrease product differentiation.

- *Reductions in uncertainty and business risk*—An emerging industry is typically characterized by much uncertainty over potential market size, how much time and money will be needed to surmount technological problems, and what distribution channels and buyer segments to emphasize. Emerging industries tend to attract only risk-taking entrepreneurial companies. Over time, however, if the business model of industry pioneers proves profitable and market demand for the product appears durable, more conservative firms are usually enticed to enter the market. Often, these later entrants are large, financially strong firms looking to invest in attractive growth industries.

  Lower business risks and less industry uncertainty also affect competition in international markets. In the early stages of a company's entry into foreign markets, conservatism prevails and firms limit their downside exposure by using less risky strategies like exporting, licensing, joint marketing agreements, or joint ventures with local companies to accomplish entry. Then, as experience accumulates and perceived risk levels decline, companies move more boldly and more independently, making acquisitions, constructing their own plants, putting in their own sales and marketing capabilities to build strong competitive positions in each country market, and beginning to link the strategies in each country to create a more globalized strategy.

- *Regulatory influences and government policy changes*—Government regulatory actions can often force significant changes in industry practices and strategic approaches. Deregulation has proved to be a potent pro-competitive force in the airline, banking, natural gas, telecommunications, and electric utility industries. Government efforts to reform Medicare and health insurance have become potent driving forces in the health care industry. In international markets, host governments can drive competitive changes by opening their domestic markets to foreign participation or closing them to protect domestic companies. Note that this driving force is spawned by forces in a company's macroenvironment.

- *Changing societal concerns, attitudes, and lifestyles*—Emerging social issues and changing attitudes and lifestyles can be powerful instigators of industry change. Growing antismoking sentiment has emerged as a major driver of change in the tobacco industry; concerns about terrorism are having a big impact on the travel industry. Consumer concerns about salt, sugar, chemical additives, saturated fat, cholesterol, carbohydrates, and nutritional value have forced food producers to revamp food-processing techniques, redirect R&D efforts into the use of healthier ingredients, and compete in developing nutritious, good-tasting products. Safety concerns have driven product design changes in the automobile, toy, and outdoor power equipment industries, to mention a few. Increased interest in physical fitness has spawned new industries in exercise equipment, biking, outdoor apparel, sports gyms and recreation centers, vitamin and nutrition supplements, and medically supervised diet programs. Social concerns about air and water pollution have forced industries to incorporate expenditures for controlling pollution into their cost structures. Shifting societal concerns, attitudes, and lifestyles alter the pattern of competition, usually favoring those

Table 3.2   **The Most Common Driving Forces**

1. Emerging new Internet capabilities and applications
2. Increasing globalization
3. Changes in an industry's long-term growth rate
4. Changes in who buys the product and how they use it
5. Product innovation
6. Technological change and manufacturing process innovation
7. Marketing innovation
8. Entry or exit of major firms
9. Diffusion of technical know-how across more companies and more countries
10. Changes in cost and efficiency
11. Growing buyer preferences for differentiated products instead of a commodity product (or for a more standardized product instead of strongly differentiated products)
12. Reductions in uncertainty and business risk
13. Regulatory Influences and government policy changes
14. Changing societal concerns, attitudes, and lifestyles

players that respond quickly and creatively with products targeted to the new trends and conditions. As with the preceding driving force, this driving force springs from factors at work in a company's macroenvironment.

Table 3.2 lists these 14 most common driving forces.

That there are so many different potential driving forces explains why it is too simplistic to view industry change only in terms of moving through the different stages in an industry's life cycle and why a full understanding of all types of change drivers is a fundamental part of industry analysis. However, while many forces of change may be at work in a given industry, no more than three or four are likely to be true driving forces powerful enough to qualify as the *major determinants* of why and how the industry is changing. Thus company strategists must resist the temptation to label every change they see as a driving force; the analytical task is to evaluate the forces of industry and competitive change carefully enough to separate major factors from minor ones.

Assessing the Impact of the Driving Forces

An important part of driving-forces analysis is to determine whether the collective impact of the driving forces will be to increase or decrease market demand, make competition more or less intense, and lead to higher or lower industry profitability.

Just identifying the driving forces is not sufficient, however. The second, and more important, step in driving-forces analysis is to determine whether the prevailing driving forces are, on the whole, acting to make the industry environment more or less attractive. Answers to three questions are needed here:

1. Are the driving forces collectively acting to cause demand for the industry's product to increase or decrease?
2. Are the driving forces acting to make competition more or less intense?
3. Will the combined impacts of the driving forces lead to higher or lower industry profitability?

Getting a handle on the collective impact of the driving forces usually requires looking at the likely effects of each force separately, since the driving forces may not all be pushing change in the same direction. For example, two driving forces may be acting to spur demand for the industry's product while one driving force may be working to curtail demand. Whether the net effect on industry demand is up or down hinges on which driving forces are the more powerful. The analyst's objective here is to get a good grip on what external factors are shaping industry change and what difference these factors will make.

Developing a Strategy That Takes the Impacts of the Driving Forces into Account

The third step of driving-forces analysis—where the real payoff for strategy making comes—is for managers to draw some conclusions about what strategy adjustments will be needed to deal with the impacts of the driving forces. The real value of doing driving-forces analysis is to gain better understanding of what strategy adjustments will be needed to cope with the drivers of industry change and the impacts they are likely to have on market demand, competitive intensity, and industry profitability. In short, the strategy-making challenge that flows from driving-forces analysis is what to do to prepare for the industry and competitive changes being wrought by the driving forces. Indeed, without understanding the forces driving industry change and the impacts these forces will have on the character of the industry environment and on the company's business over the next one to three years, managers are ill-prepared to craft a strategy tightly matched to emerging conditions. Similarly, if managers are uncertain about the implications of one or more driving forces, or if their views are incomplete or off base, it's difficult for them to craft a strategy that is responsive to the driving forces and their consequences for the industry. So driving-forces analysis is not something to take lightly; it has practical value and is basic to the task of thinking strategically about where the industry is headed and how to prepare for the changes ahead.

> Driving-forces analysis, when done properly, pushes company managers to think about what's around the corner and what the company needs to be doing to get ready for it.

> The real payoff of driving-forces analysis is to help managers understand what strategy changes are needed to prepare for the impacts of the driving forces.

QUESTION 4: WHAT MARKET POSITIONS DO RIVALS OCCUPY—WHO IS STRONGLY POSITIONED AND WHO IS NOT?

Since competing companies commonly sell in different price/quality ranges, emphasize different distribution channels, incorporate product features that appeal to different types of buyers, have different geographic coverage, and so on, it stands to reason that some companies enjoy stronger or more attractive market positions than other companies. Understanding which companies are strongly positioned and which are weakly positioned is an integral part of analyzing an industry's competitive structure. The best technique for revealing the market positions of industry competitors is **strategic group mapping**.[14] This analytical tool is useful for comparing the market positions of each firm separately or for grouping them into like positions when an industry has so many competitors that it is not practical to examine each one in depth.

> **Core Concept**
> *Strategic group mapping* is a technique for displaying the different market or competitive positions that rival firms occupy in the industry.

Using Strategic Group Maps to Assess the Market Positions of Key Competitors

A **strategic group** consists of those industry members with similar competitive approaches and positions in the market.[15] Companies in the same strategic group can resemble one another in any of several ways: They may have comparable product-line breadth, sell in the same price/quality range, emphasize the same distribution channels, use essentially the same product attributes to appeal to similar types of buyers, depend on identical technological approaches, or offer buyers similar services and technical assistance.[16] An industry contains only one strategic group when all sellers pursue essentially identical strategies and have comparable market positions. At the other extreme, an industry may contain as many strategic groups as there are competitors when each rival pursues a distinctively different competitive approach and occupies a substantially different market position.

> **Core Concept**
> A **strategic group** is a cluster of industry rivals that have similar competitive approaches and market positions.

The procedure for constructing a *strategic group map* is straightforward:

- Identify the competitive characteristics that differentiate firms in the industry. Typical variables are price/quality range (high, medium, low); geographic coverage (local, regional, national, global); degree of vertical integration (none, partial, full); product-line breadth (wide, narrow); use of distribution channels (one, some, all); and degree of service offered (no-frills, limited, full).
- Plot the firms on a two-variable map using pairs of these differentiating characteristics.
- Assign firms that fall in about the same strategy space to the same strategic group.
- Draw circles around each strategic group, making the circles proportional to the size of the group's share of total industry sales revenues.

This produces a two-dimensional diagram like the one for the retailing industry in Illustration Capsule 3.1.

Several guidelines need to be observed in mapping the positions of strategic groups in the industry's overall strategy space.[17] First, the two variables selected as axes for the map should *not* be highly correlated; if they are, the circles on the map will fall along a diagonal and strategy makers will learn nothing more about the relative positions of competitors than they would by considering just one of the variables. For instance, if companies with broad product lines use multiple distribution channels while companies with narrow lines use a single distribution channel, then looking at broad versus narrow product lines reveals just as much about who is positioned where as looking at single versus multiple distribution channels; that is, one of the variables is redundant. Second, the variables chosen as axes for the map should expose big differences in how rivals position themselves to compete in the marketplace. This, of course, means analysts must identify the characteristics that differentiate rival firms and use these differences as variables for the axes and as the basis for deciding which firm belongs in which strategic group. Third, the variables used as axes don't have to be either quantitative or continuous; rather, they can be discrete variables or defined in terms of distinct classes and combinations. Fourth, drawing the sizes of the circles on the map proportional to the combined sales of the firms in each strategic group allows the map to reflect the relative sizes of each strategic group. Fifth, if more than two good competitive variables can be used as axes for the map, several maps can be drawn to give different exposures to the competitive positioning relationships present

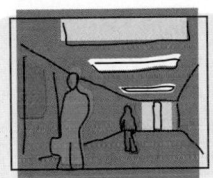

Illustration Capsule 3.1

Comparative Market Positions of Selected Retail Chains: A Strategic Group Map Application

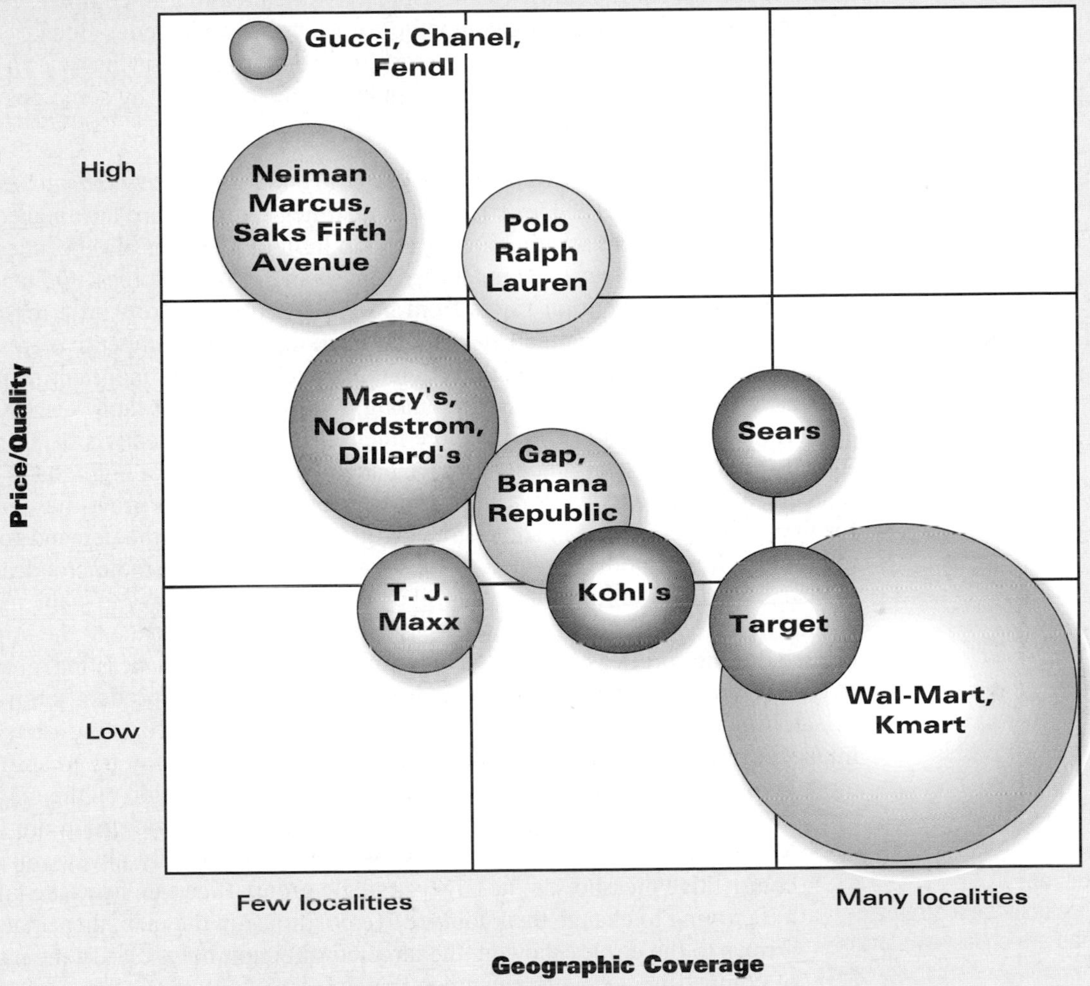

High

Low

Price/Quality

Gucci, Chanel, Fendl

Neiman Marcus, Saks Fifth Avenue

Polo Ralph Lauren

Macy's, Nordstrom, Dillard's

Gap, Banana Republic

Sears

T. J. Maxx

Kohl's

Target

Wal-Mart, Kmart

Few localities

Many localities

Geographic Coverage

Note: Circles are drawn roughly proportional to the sizes of the chains, based on revenues.

in the industry's structure. Because there is not necessarily one best map for portraying how competing firms are positioned in the market, it is advisable to experiment with different pairs of competitive variables.

What Can Be Learned from Strategic Group Maps?

Strategic group maps are revealing in several respects. The most important has to do with which rivals are similarly positioned and are thus close rivals and which are distant rivals. Generally speaking, *the closer strategic groups are to each other on the map, the stronger the cross-group competitive rivalry tends to be.* Although firms in the same strategic group are the closest rivals, the next closest rivals are in the immediately adjacent groups.[18] Often, firms in strategic groups that are far apart on the map hardly compete at all. For instance, Wal-Mart's clientele, merchandise selection, and pricing points are much too different to justify calling them close competitors of Neiman Marcus or Saks Fifth Avenue in retailing. For the same reason, Timex is not a meaningful competitive rival of Rolex, and Subaru is not a close competitor of Lincoln or Mercedes-Benz.

The second thing to be gleaned from strategic group mapping is that *not all positions on the map are equally attractive.* Two reasons account for why some positions can be more attractive than others:

1. *Prevailing competitive pressures and industry driving forces favor some strategic groups and hurt others.*[19] Discerning which strategic groups are advantaged and disadvantaged requires scrutinizing the map in light of what has also been learned from the prior analysis of competitive forces and driving forces. Quite often the strength of competition varies from group to group—there's little reason to believe that all firms in an industry feel the same degrees of competitive pressure, since their strategies and market positions may well differ in important respects. For instance, the competitive battle among Wal-Mart, Target, and Sears/Kmart (Kmart acquired Sears in 2005) is more intense (with consequently smaller profit margins) than the rivalry among Gucci, Chanel, Fendi, and other high-end fashion retailers. Likewise, industry driving forces may be acting to grow the demand for the products of firms in some strategic groups and shrink the demand for the products of firms in other strategic groups—as is the case in the radio broadcasting industry where satellite radio firms like XM and Sirius stand to gain market ground at the expense of commercial-based radio broadcasters due to the impacts of such driving forces as technological advances in satellite broadcasting, growing buyer preferences for more diverse radio programming, and product innovation in satellite radio devices. Firms in strategic groups that are being adversely impacted by intense competitive pressures or driving forces may try to shift to a more favorably situated group. But shifting to a different position on the map can prove difficult when entry barriers for the target strategic group are high. Moreover, attempts to enter a new strategic group nearly always increase competitive pressures in the target strategic group. If certain firms are known to be trying to change their competitive positions on the map, then attaching arrows to the circles showing the targeted direction helps clarify the picture of competitive maneuvering among rivals.

2. *The profit potential of different strategic groups varies due to the strengths and weaknesses in each group's market position.* The profit prospects of firms in different strategic groups can vary from good to ho-hum to poor because of differing growth rates for the principal buyer segments served by each group, differing degrees of competitive rivalry within strategic groups, differing degrees of exposure to competition from substitute products outside the industry, and differing degrees of supplier or customer bargaining power from group to group.

Thus, part of strategic group map analysis always entails drawing conclusions about where on the map is the "best" place to be and why. Which companies/strategic groups are destined to prosper because of their positions? Which companies/strategic groups seem destined to struggle because of their positions? What accounts for why some parts of the map are better than others?

QUESTION 5: WHAT STRATEGIC MOVES ARE RIVALS LIKELY TO MAKE NEXT?

Unless a company pays attention to what competitors are doing and knows their strengths and weaknesses, it ends up flying blind into competitive battle. As in sports, scouting the opposition is essential. *Competitive intelligence* about rivals' strategies, their latest actions and announcements, their resource strengths and weaknesses, the efforts being made to improve their situation, and the thinking and leadership styles of their executives is valuable for predicting or anticipating the strategic moves competitors are likely to make next in the marketplace. Having good information to predict the strategic

> Good scouting reports on rivals provide a valuable assist in anticipating what moves rivals are likely to make next and outmaneuvering them in the marketplace.

direction and likely moves of key competitors allows a company to prepare defensive countermoves, to craft its own strategic moves with some confidence about what market maneuvers to expect from rivals, and to exploit any openings that arise from competitors' missteps or strategy flaws.

Identifying Competitors' Strategies and Resource Strengths and Weaknesses

Keeping close tabs on a com.petitor's strategy entails monitoring what the rival is doing in the marketplace, what its management is saying in company press releases, information posted on the company's Web site (especially press releases and the presentations management has recently made to securities analysts), and such public documents as annual reports and 10-K filings, articles in the business media, and the reports of securities analysts. (Figure 1.1 in Chapter 1 indicates what to look for in identifying a company's strategy.) Company personnel may be able to pick up useful information from a rival's exhibits at trade shows and from conversations with a rival's customers, suppliers, and former employees.[20] Many companies have a competitive intelligence unit that sifts through the available information to construct up-to-date strategic profiles of rivals—their current strategies, resource strengths and competitive capabilities, competitive shortcomings, press releases, and recent executive pronouncements. Such profiles are typically updated regularly and made available to managers and other key personnel.

Those who gather competitive intelligence on rivals, however, can sometimes cross the fine line between honest inquiry and unethical or even illegal behavior. For example, calling rivals to get information about prices, the dates of new product introductions, or wage and salary levels is legal, but misrepresenting one's company affiliation during such calls is unethical. Pumping rivals' representatives at trade shows is ethical only if one wears a name tag with accurate company affiliation indicated. Avon Products at one point secured information about its biggest rival, Mary Kay Cosmetics (MKC), by having its personnel search through the garbage bins outside MKC's headquarters.[21] When MKC officials learned of the action and sued, Avon claimed it did nothing illegal, since a 1988 Supreme Court case had ruled that trash left on public property (in this case, a sidewalk) was anyone's for the taking. Avon even produced a videotape of its removal of the trash at the MKC site. Avon won the lawsuit—but Avon's action, while legal, scarcely qualifies as ethical.

In sizing up competitors, it makes sense for company strategists to make three assessments:

1. Which competitor has the best strategy? Which competitors appear to have flawed or weak strategies?

2. Which competitors are poised to gain market share, and which ones seem destined to lose ground?

3. Which competitors are likely to rank among the industry leaders five years from now? Do one or more up-and-coming competitors have powerful strategies and sufficient resource capabilities to overtake the current industry leader?

The industry's *current* major players are generally easy to identify, but some of the leaders may be plagued with weaknesses that are causing them to lose ground; other notable rivals may lack the resources and capabilities to remain strong contenders given the superior strategies and capabilities of up-and-coming companies. In evaluating which competitors are favorably or unfavorably positioned to gain market ground, company strategists need to focus on why there is potential for some rivals to do better or worse than other rivals. Usually, a competitor's prospects are a function of whether it is in a strategic group that is being favored or hurt by competitive pressures and driving forces, whether its strategy has resulted in competitive advantage or disadvantage, and whether its resources and capabilities are well suited for competing on the road ahead.

> Today's market leaders don't automatically become tomorrow's.

Predicting Competitors' Next Moves

Predicting the next strategic moves of competitors is the hardest yet most useful part of competitor analysis. Good clues about what actions a specific company is likely to undertake can often be gleaned from how well it is faring in the marketplace, the problems or weaknesses it needs to address, and how much pressure it is under to improve its financial performance. Content rivals are likely to continue their present strategy with only minor fine-tuning. Ailing rivals can be performing so poorly that fresh strategic moves are virtually certain. Ambitious rivals looking to move up in the industry ranks are strong candidates for launching new strategic offensives to pursue emerging market opportunities and exploit the vulnerabilities of weaker rivals.

Since the moves a competitor is likely to make are generally predicated on the views their executives have about the industry's future and their beliefs about their firm's situation, it makes sense to closely scrutinize the public pronouncements of rival company executives about where the industry is headed and what it will take to be successful, what they are saying about their firm's situation, information from the grapevine about what they are doing, and their past actions and leadership styles. Other considerations in trying to predict what strategic moves rivals are likely to make next include the following:

- Which rivals badly need to increase their unit sales and market share? What strategic options are they most likely to pursue: lowering prices, adding new models and styles, expanding their dealer networks, entering additional geographic markets, boosting advertising to build better brand-name awareness, acquiring a weaker competitor, or placing more emphasis on direct sales via their Web site?

- Which rivals have a strong incentive, along with the resources, to make major strategic changes, perhaps moving to a different position on the strategic group map? Which rivals are probably locked in to pursuing the same basic strategy with only minor adjustments?

- Which rivals are good candidates to be acquired? Which rivals may be looking to make an acquisition and are financially able to do so?

- Which rivals are likely to enter new geographic markets?
- Which rivals are strong candidates to expand their product offerings and enter new product segments where they do not currently have a presence?

To succeed in predicting a competitor's next moves, company strategists need to have a good feel for each rival's situation, how its managers think, and what the rival's best strategic options are. Doing the necessary detective work can be tedious and time-consuming, but scouting competitors well enough to anticipate their next moves allows managers to prepare effective countermoves (perhaps even beat a rival to the punch) and to take rivals' probable actions into account in crafting their own best course of action.

> Managers who fail to study competitors closely risk being caught napping when rivals make fresh and perhaps bold strategic moves.

QUESTION 6: WHAT ARE THE KEY FACTORS FOR FUTURE COMPETITIVE SUCCESS?

An industry's **key success factors (KSFs)** are those competitive factors that most affect industry members' ability to prosper in the marketplace—the particular strategy elements, product attributes, resources, competencies, competitive capabilities, and market achievements that spell the difference between being a strong competitor and a weak competitor—and sometimes between profit and loss. KSFs by their very nature are so important to future competitive success that *all firms* in the industry must pay close attention to them or risk becoming an industry also-ran. To indicate the significance of KSFs another way, how well a company's product offering, resources, and capabilities measure up against an industry's KSFs determines just how financially and competitively successful that company will be. Identifying KSFs, in light of the prevailing and anticipated industry and competitive conditions, is therefore always a top-priority analytical and strategy-making consideration. Company strategists need to understand the industry landscape well enough to separate the factors most important to competitive success from those that are less important.

> **Core Concept**
> **Key success factors** are the product attributes, competencies, competitive capabilities, and market achievements with the greatest impact on future competitive success in the marketplace.

In the beer industry, the KSFs are full utilization of brewing capacity (to keep manufacturing costs low), a strong network of wholesale distributors (to get the company's brand stocked and favorably displayed in retail outlets where beer is sold), and clever advertising (to induce beer drinkers to buy the company's brand and thereby pull beer sales through the established wholesale/retail channels). In apparel manufacturing, the KSFs are appealing designs and color combinations (to create buyer interest) and low-cost manufacturing efficiency (to permit attractive retail pricing and ample profit margins). In tin and aluminum cans, because the cost of shipping empty cans is substantial, one of the keys is having can-manufacturing facilities located close to end-use customers. Key success factors thus vary from industry to industry, and even from time to time within the same industry, as driving forces and competitive conditions change. Table 3.3 lists the most common types of industry key success factors.

An industry's key success factors can usually be deduced from what was learned from the previously described analysis of the industry and competitive environment. Which factors are most important to future competitive success flow directly from the industry's dominant characteristics, what competition is like, the impacts of the driving forces, the comparative market positions of industry members, and the likely

Table 3.3   **Common Types of Industry Key Success Factors**

Technology-related KSFs	• Expertise in a particular technology or in scientific research (important in pharmaceuticals, Internet applications, mobile communications, and most high-tech industries) • Proven ability to improve production processes (important in industries where advancing technology opens the way for higher manufacturing efficiency and lower production costs)
Manufacturing-related KSFs	• Ability to achieve scale economies and/or capture learning/experience curve effects (important to achieving low production costs) • Quality control know-how (important in industries where customers insist on product reliability) • High utilization of fixed assets (important in capital-intensive, high-fixed-cost industries) • Access to attractive supplies of skilled labor • High labor productivity (important for items with high labor content) • Low-cost product design and engineering (reduces manufacturing costs) • Ability to manufacture or assemble products that are customized to buyer specifications
Distribution-related KSFs	• A strong network of wholesale distributors/dealers • Strong direct sales capabilities via the Internet and/or having company-owned retail outlets • Ability to secure favorable display space on retailer shelves
Marketing-related KSFs	• Breadth of product line and product selection • A well-known and well-respected brand name • Fast, accurate technical assistance • Courteous, personalized customer service • Accurate filling of buyer orders (few back orders or mistakes) • Customer guarantees and warranties (important in mail-order and online retailing, big-ticket purchases, new product introductions) • Clever advertising
Skills and capability-related KSFs	• A talented workforce (important in professional services like accounting and investment banking) • National or global distribution capabilities • Product innovation capabilities (important in industries where rivals are racing to be first-to-market with new product attributes or performance features) • Design expertise (important in fashion and apparel industries) • Short delivery time capability • Supply chain management capabilities • Strong e-commerce capabilities—a user-friendly Web site and/or skills in using Internet technology applications to streamline internal operations
Other types of KSFs	• Overall low costs (not just in manufacturing) so as to be able to meet customer expectations of low price • Convenient locations (important in many retailing businesses) • Ability to provide fast, convenient after-the-sale repairs and service • A strong balance sheet and access to financial capital (important in newly emerging industries with high degrees of business risk and in capital-intensive industries) • Patent protection

next moves of key rivals. In addition, the answers to three questions help identify an industry's key success factors:

1. On what basis do buyers of the industry's product choose between the competing brands of sellers? That is, what product attributes are crucial?

2. Given the nature of competitive rivalry and the competitive forces prevailing in the marketplace, what resources and competitive capabilities does a company need to have to be competitively successful?

3. What shortcomings are almost certain to put a company at a significant competitive disadvantage?

Only rarely are there more than five or six key factors for future competitive success. And even among these, two or three usually outrank the others in importance. Managers should therefore bear in mind the purpose of identifying key success factors— to determine which factors are most important to future competitive success— and resist the temptation to label a factor that has only minor importance a KSF. To compile a list of every factor that matters even a little bit defeats the purpose of concentrating management attention on the factors truly critical to long-term competitive success.

Correctly diagnosing an industry's KSFs raises a company's chances of crafting a sound strategy. The goal of company strategists should be to design a strategy aimed at stacking up well on all of the industry's future KSFs and trying to be *distinctively better* than rivals on one (or possibly two) of the KSFs. Indeed, companies that stand out or excel on a particular KSF are likely to enjoy a stronger market position—*being distinctively better than rivals on one or two key success factors tends to translate into competitive advantage.* Hence, using the industry's KSFs as *cornerstones* for the company's strategy and trying to gain sustainable competitive advantage by excelling at one particular KSF is a fruitful competitive strategy approach.[22]

> **Core Concept**
> A sound strategy incorporates the intent to stack up well on all of the industry's key success factors and to excel on one or two KSFs.

QUESTION 7: DOES THE OUTLOOK FOR THE INDUSTRY PRESENT THE COMPANY WITH AN ATTRACTIVE OPPORTUNITY?

The final step in evaluating the industry and competitive environment is to use the preceding analysis to decide whether the outlook for the industry presents the company with a sufficiently attractive business opportunity. The important factors on which to base such a conclusion include:

- The industry's growth potential.
- Whether powerful competitive forces are squeezing industry profitability to subpar levels and whether competition appears destined to grow stronger or weaker.
- Whether industry profitability will be favorably or unfavorably affected by the prevailing driving forces.
- The degrees of risk and uncertainty in the industry's future.
- Whether the industry as a whole confronts severe problems—regulatory or environmental issues, stagnating buyer demand, industry overcapacity, mounting competition, and so on.

- The company's competitive position in the industry vis-à-vis rivals. (Being a well-entrenched leader or strongly positioned contender in a lackluster industry may present adequate opportunity for good profitability; however, having to fight a steep uphill battle against much stronger rivals may hold little promise of eventual market success or good return on shareholder investment, even though the industry environment is attractive.)

- The company's potential to capitalize on the vulnerabilities of weaker rivals, perhaps converting a relatively unattractive *industry* situation into a potentially rewarding *company* opportunity.

- Whether the company has sufficient competitive strength to defend against or counteract the factors that make the industry unattractive.

- Whether continued participation in this industry adds importantly to the firm's ability to be successful in other industries in which it may have business interests.

Core Concept
The degree to which an industry is attractive or unattractive is not the same for all industry participants and all potential entrants; the attractiveness of the opportunities an industry presents depends heavily on whether a company has the resource strengths and competitive capabilities to capture them.

As a general proposition, *if an industry's overall profit prospects are above average, the industry environment is basically attractive; if industry profit prospects are below average, conditions are unattractive.* However, it is a mistake to think of a particular industry as being equally attractive or unattractive to all industry participants and all potential entrants. Attractiveness is relative, not absolute, and conclusions one way or the other have to be drawn from the perspective of a particular company. Industries attractive to insiders may be unattractive to outsiders. Companies on the outside may look at an industry's environment and conclude that it is an unattractive business for them to get into, given the prevailing entry barriers, the difficulty of challenging current market leaders with their particular resources and competencies, and the opportunities they have elsewhere. Industry environments unattractive to weak competitors may be attractive to strong competitors. A favorably positioned company may survey a business environment and see a host of opportunities that weak competitors cannot capture.

When a company decides an industry is fundamentally attractive and presents good opportunities, a strong case can be made that it should invest aggressively to capture the opportunities it sees and to improve its long-term competitive position in the business. When a strong competitor concludes an industry is relatively unattractive and lacking in opportunity, it may elect to simply protect its present position, investing cautiously if at all and looking for opportunities in other industries. A competitively weak company in an unattractive industry may see its best option as finding a buyer, perhaps a rival, to acquire its business.

Key Points

Thinking strategically about a company's external situation involves probing for answers to the following seven questions:

1. *What are the industry's dominant economic features?* Industries differ significantly on such factors as market size and growth rate, the number and relative sizes of both buyers and sellers, the geographic scope of competitive rivalry, the degree of product differentiation, the speed of product innovation, demand–supply conditions, the extent of vertical integration, and the extent of scale economies and learning-curve effects. In addition to setting the stage for the analysis to come,

identifying an industry's economic features also promotes understanding of the kinds of strategic moves that industry members are likely to employ.

2. *What kinds of competitive forces are industry members facing, and how strong is each force?* The strength of competition is a composite of five forces: (1) competitive pressures stemming from the competitive jockeying and market maneuvering among industry rivals, (2) competitive pressures associated with the market inroads being made by the sellers of substitutes, (3) competitive pressures associated with the threat of new entrants into the market, (4) competitive pressures stemming from supplier bargaining power and supplier–seller collaboration, and (5) competitive pressures stemming from buyer bargaining power and seller–buyer collaboration. The nature and strength of the competitive pressures associated with these five forces have to be examined force by force to identify the specific competitive pressures they each comprise and to decide whether these pressures constitute a strong or weak competitive force. The next step in competition analysis is to evaluate the collective strength of the five forces and determine whether the state of competition is conducive to good profitability. Working through the five-forces model step by step not only aids strategy makers in assessing whether the intensity of competition allows good profitability but also promotes sound strategic thinking about how to better match company strategy to the specific competitive character of the marketplace. Effectively matching a company's strategy to the particular competitive pressures and competitive conditions that exist has two aspects: (1) pursuing avenues that shield the firm from as many of the prevailing competitive pressures as possible, and (2) initiating actions calculated to produce sustainable competitive advantage, thereby shifting competition in the company's favor, putting added competitive pressure on rivals, and perhaps even defining the business model for the industry.

3. *What factors are driving industry change and what impact will they have on competitive intensity and industry profitability?* Industry and competitive conditions change because forces are in motion that create incentives or pressures for change. The first phase is to identify the forces that are driving change in the industry; the most common driving forces include the Internet and Internet technology applications, globalization of competition in the industry, changes in the long-term industry growth rate, changes in buyer composition, product innovation, entry or exit of major firms, changes in cost and efficiency, changing buyer preferences for standardized versus differentiated products or services, regulatory influences and government policy changes, changing societal and lifestyle factors, and reductions in uncertainty and business risk. The second phase of driving-forces analysis is to determine whether the driving forces, taken together, are acting to make the industry environment more or less attractive. Are the driving forces causing demand for the industry's product to increase or decrease? Are the driving forces acting to make competition more or less intense? Will the driving forces lead to higher or lower industry profitability?

4. *What market positions do industry rivals occupy—who is strongly positioned and who is not?* Strategic group mapping is a valuable tool for understanding the similarities, differences, strengths, and weaknesses inherent in the market positions of rival companies. Rivals in the same or nearby strategic groups are close competitors, whereas companies in distant strategic groups usually pose little or no immediate threat. The lesson of strategic group mapping is that some positions on the map are more favorable than others. The profit potential of different strategic groups varies due to strengths and weaknesses in each group's market

position. Often, industry driving forces and competitive pressures favor some strategic groups and hurt others.

5. *What strategic moves are rivals likely to make next?* This analytical step involves identifying competitors' strategies, deciding which rivals are likely to be strong contenders and which are likely to be weak, evaluating rivals' competitive options, and predicting their next moves. Scouting competitors well enough to anticipate their actions can help a company prepare effective countermoves (perhaps even beating a rival to the punch) and allows managers to take rivals' probable actions into account in designing their own company's best course of action. Managers who fail to study competitors risk being caught unprepared by the strategic moves of rivals.

6. *What are the key factors for future competitive success?* An industry's key success factors (KSFs) are the particular strategy elements, product attributes, competitive capabilities, and business outcomes that spell the difference between being a strong competitor and a weak competitor—and sometimes between profit and loss. KSFs by their very nature are so important to competitive success that *all firms* in the industry must pay close attention to them or risk becoming an industry also-ran. Correctly diagnosing an industry's KSFs raises a company's chances of crafting a sound strategy. The goal of company strategists should be to design a strategy aimed at stacking up well on all of the industry KSFs and trying to be *distinctively better* than rivals on one (or possibly two) of the KSFs. Indeed, using the industry's KSFs as *cornerstones* for the company's strategy and trying to gain sustainable competitive advantage by excelling at one particular KSF is a fruitful competitive strategy approach.

7. *Does the outlook for the industry present the company with sufficiently attractive prospects for profitability?* If an industry's overall profit prospects are above average, the industry environment is basically attractive; if industry profit prospects are below average, conditions are unattractive. Conclusions regarding industry attractive are a major driver of company strategy. When a company decides an industry is fundamentally attractive and presents good opportunities, a strong case can be made that it should invest aggressively to capture the opportunities it sees and to improve its long-term competitive position in the business. When a strong competitor concludes an industry is relatively unattractive and lacking in opportunity, it may elect to simply protect its present position, investing cautiously if at all and looking for opportunities in other industries. A competitively weak company in an unattractive industry may see its best option as finding a buyer, perhaps a rival, to acquire its business. On occasion, an industry that is unattractive overall is still very attractive to a favorably situated company with the skills and resources to take business away from weaker rivals.

A competently conducted industry and competitive analysis generally tells a clear, easily understood story about the company's external environment. Different analysts can have varying judgments about competitive intensity, the impacts of driving forces, how industry conditions will evolve, how good the outlook is for industry profitability, and the degree to which the industry environment offers the company an attractive business opportunity. However, while no method can guarantee that all analysts will come to identical conclusions about the state of industry and competitive conditions and an industry's future outlook, this doesn't justify shortcutting hardnosed strategic analysis and relying instead on opinion and casual observation. Managers become better strategists when they know what questions to pose and what tools to use. This is why this chapter has concentrated on suggesting the right questions to ask, explaining concepts and analytical approaches, and indicating the kinds of things to look for. There's no substitute for doing cutting edge strategic thinking about a company's external situation—anything less weakens managers' ability to craft strategies that are well matched to industry and competitive conditions.

Exercises

1. As the owner of a fast-food enterprise seeking a loan from a bank to finance the construction and operation of three new store locations, you have been asked to provide the loan officer with a brief analysis of the competitive environment in fast food. Draw a five-forces diagram for the fast-food industry, and briefly discuss the nature and strength of each of the five competitive forces in fast food. Do whatever Internet research is required to expand your understanding of competition in the fast-food industry and do a competent five-forces analysis.

2. Based on the strategic group map in Illustration Capsule 3.1: Who are Polo Ralph Lauren's closest competitors? Between which two strategic groups is competition the strongest? Why do you think no retailers are positioned in the upper right-hand corner of the map? Which company/strategic group faces the weakest competition from the members of other strategic groups?

3. With regard to the ice cream industry, which of the following factors might qualify as possible driving forces capable of causing fundamental change in the industry's structure and competitive environment?

    a. Increasing sales of frozen yogurt and frozen sorbets.

    b. The potential for additional makers of ice cream to enter the market.

    c. Growing consumer interest in low-calorie/low-fat/low-carb/sugar-free dessert alternatives.

    d. A slowdown in consumer purchases of ice cream products.

    e. Rising prices for milk, sugar, and other ice cream ingredients.

    f. A decision by Häagen-Dazs to increase its prices by 10 percent.

    g. A decision by Ben & Jerry's to add five new flavors to its product line.

chapter four

Evaluating a Company's Resources and Competitive Position

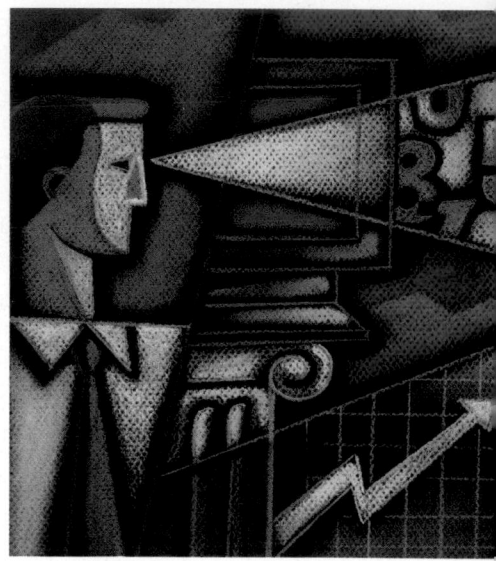

Before executives can chart a new strategy, they must reach common understanding of the company's current position.
—**W. Chan Kim and Rene Mauborgne**

The real question isn't how well you're doing today against your own history, but how you're doing against your competitors.
—**Donald Kress**

Organizations succeed in a competitive marketplace over the long run because they can do certain things their customers value better than can their competitors.
—**Robert Hayes, Gary Pisano, and David Upton**

Only firms who are able to continually build new strategic assets faster and cheaper than their competitors will earn superior returns over the long term.
—**C. C. Markides and P. J. Williamson**

In Chapter 3 we described how to use the tools of industry and competitive analysis to assess a company's external environment and lay the groundwork for matching a company's strategy to its external situation. In this chapter we discuss the techniques of evaluating a company's resource capabilities, relative cost position, and competitive strength vis-á-vis its rivals. The analytical spotlight will be trained on five questions:

1. How well is the company's present strategy working?

2. What are the company's resource strengths and weaknesses, and its external opportunities and threats?

3. Are the company's prices and costs competitive?

4. Is the company competitively stronger or weaker than key rivals?

5. What strategic issues and problems merit front-burner managerial attention?

We will describe four analytical tools that should be used to probe for answers to these questions—SWOT analysis, value chain analysis, benchmarking, and competitive strength assessment. All four are valuable techniques for revealing a company's competitiveness and for helping company managers match their strategy to the company's own particular circumstances.

QUESTION 1: HOW WELL IS THE COMPANY'S PRESENT STRATEGY WORKING?

In evaluating how well a company's present strategy is working, a manager has to start with what the strategy is. Figure 4.1 shows the key components of a single-business company's strategy. The first thing to pin down is the company's competitive approach. Is the company striving to be a low-cost leader *or* stressing ways to differentiate its product offering from rivals? Is it concentrating its efforts on serving a broad spectrum of customers *or* a narrow market niche? Another strategy-defining consideration is the firm's competitive scope within the industry—what its geographic market coverage is and whether it operates in just a single stage of the industry's production/distribution chain or is vertically integrated across several stages. Another good indication of the company's strategy is whether the company has made moves recently to improve its competitive position and performance—for instance, by cutting prices, improving design, stepping up advertising, entering a new geographic market (domestic or foreign),

Figure 4.1   **Identifying the Components of a Single-Business Company's Strategy**

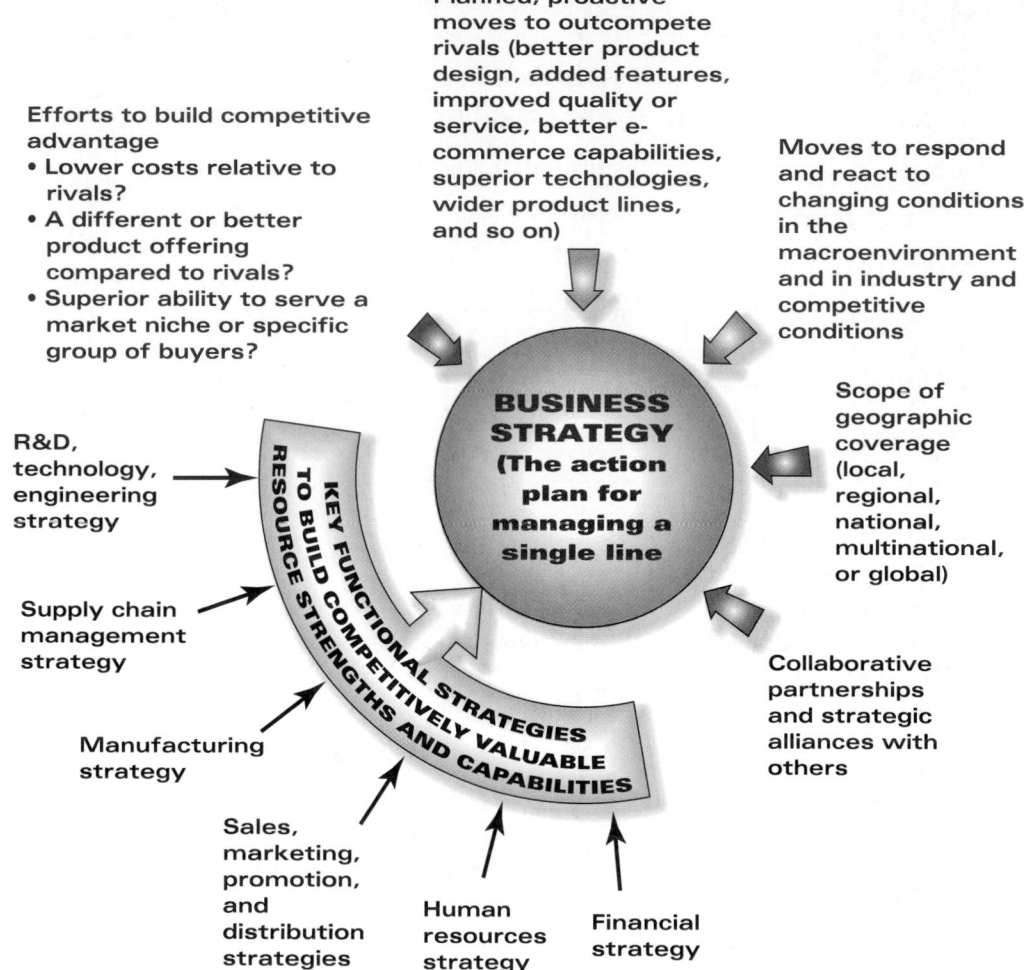

or merging with a competitor. The company's functional strategies in R&D, production, marketing, finance, human resources, information technology, and so on further characterize company strategy.

While there's merit in evaluating the strategy from a *qualitative* standpoint (its completeness, internal consistency, rationale, and relevance), the best *quantitative* evidence of how well a company's strategy is working comes from its results. The two best empirical indicators are (1) whether the company is achieving its stated financial and strategic objectives, and (2) whether the company is an above-average industry performer. Persistent shortfalls in meeting company performance targets and weak performance relative to rivals are reliable warning signs that the company suffers from poor strategy making, less-than-competent strategy execution, or both. Other indicators of how well a company's strategy is working include:

- Whether the firm's sales are growing faster, slower, or about the same pace as the market as a whole, thus resulting in a rising, eroding, or stable market share.

- Whether the company is acquiring new customers at an attractive rate as well as retaining existing customers.
- Whether the firm's profit margins are increasing or decreasing and how well its margins compare to rival firms' margins.
- Trends in the firm's net profits and return on investment and how these compare to the same trends for other companies in the industry.
- Whether the company's overall financial strength and credit rating are improving or on the decline.
- Whether the company can demonstrate continuous improvement in such internal performance measures as days of inventory, employee productivity, unit cost, defect rate, scrap rate, misfilled orders, delivery times, warranty costs, and so on.
- How shareholders view the company based on trends in the company's stock price and shareholder value (relative to the stock price trends at other companies in the industry).
- The firm's image and reputation with its customers.
- How well the company stacks up against rivals on technology, product innovation, customer service, product quality, delivery time, price, getting newly developed products to market quickly, and other relevant factors on which buyers base their choice of brands.

The stronger a company's current overall performance, the less likely the need for radical changes in strategy. The weaker a company's financial performance and market standing, the more its current strategy must be questioned. Weak performance is almost always a sign of weak strategy, weak execution, or both.

Table 4.1 provides a compilation of the financial ratios most commonly used to evaluate a company's financial performance and balance sheet strength.

> The stronger a company's financial performance and market position, the more likely it has a well-conceived, well-executed strategy.

QUESTION 2: WHAT ARE THE COMPANY'S RESOURCE STRENGTHS AND WEAKNESSES AND ITS EXTERNAL OPPORTUNITIES AND THREATS?

Appraising a company's resource strengths and weaknesses and its external opportunities and threats, commonly known as **SWOT analysis,** provides a good overview of whether the company's overall situation is fundamentally healthy or unhealthy. Just as important, a first-rate SWOT analysis provides the basis for crafting a strategy that capitalizes on the company's resources, aims squarely at capturing the company's best opportunities, and defends against the threats to its well-being.

> **Core Concept**
> **SWOT analysis** is a simple but powerful tool for sizing up a company's resource capabilities and deficiencies, its market opportunities, and the external threats to its future well-being.

Identifying Company Resource Strengths and Competitive Capabilities

A *resource strength* is something a company is good at doing or an attribute that enhances its competitiveness in the marketplace. Resource strengths can take any of several forms:

Table 4.1   **Key Financial Ratios: How to Calculate Them and What They Mean**

Ratio	How Calculated	What It Shows
Profitability ratios		
1. Gross profit margin	$\dfrac{\text{Sales} - \text{cost of goods sold}}{\text{Sales}}$	Shows the percentage of revenues available to cover operating expenses and yield a profit. Higher is better, and the trend should be upward.
2. Operating profit margin (or return on sales)	$\dfrac{\text{Sales} - \text{Operating expenses}}{\text{Sales}}$ or $\dfrac{\text{Operating income}}{\text{Sales}}$	Shows the profitability of current operations without regard to interest charges and income taxes. Higher is better, and the trend should be upward.
3. Net profit margin (or net return on sales)	$\dfrac{\text{Profits after taxes}}{\text{Sales}}$	Shows after-tax profits per dollar of sales. Higher is better, and the trend should be upward.
4. Return on total assets	$\dfrac{\text{Profits after taxes} + \text{Interest}}{\text{Total assets}}$	A measure of the return on total investment in the enterprise. Interest is added to after-tax profits to form the numerator since total assets are financed by creditors as well as by stockholders. Higher is better, and the trend should be upward.
5. Return on stockholders' equity	$\dfrac{\text{Profits after taxes}}{\text{Total stockholders' equity}}$	Shows the return stockholders are earning on their investment in the enterprise. A return in the 12–15 percent range is average, and the trend should be upward.
6. Earnings per share	$\dfrac{\text{Profits after taxes}}{\text{Number of shares of common stock outstanding}}$	Shows the earnings for each share of common stock outstanding. The trend should be upward, and the bigger the annual percentage gains, the better.
Liquidity ratios		
1. Current ratio	$\dfrac{\text{Current assets}}{\text{Current liabilities}}$	Shows a firm's ability to pay current liabilities using assets that can be converted to cash in the near term. Ratio should definitely be higher than 1.0; ratios of 2 or higher are better still.
2. Quick ratio (or acid-test ratio)	$\dfrac{\text{Current assets} - \text{Inventory}}{\text{Current liabilities}}$	Shows a firm's ability to pay current liabilities without relying on the sale of its inventories.
3. Working capital	Current assets − Current liabilities	Bigger amounts are better because the company has more internal funds available to (1) pay its current liabilities on a timely basis and (2) finance inventory expansion, additional accounts receivable, and a larger base of operations without resorting to borrowing or raising more equity capital.
Leverage ratios		
1. Debt-to-assets ratio	$\dfrac{\text{Total debt}}{\text{Total assets}}$	Measures the extent to which borrowed funds have been used to finance the firm's operations. Low fractions or ratios are better—high fractions indicate overuse of debt and greater risk of bankruptcy.

(Continued)

Table 4.1   **Continued**

Ratio	How Calculated	What It Shows
2. Debt-to-equity ratio	$\dfrac{\text{Total debt}}{\text{Total stockholders' equity}}$	Should usually be less than 1.0. High ratios (especially above 1.0) signal excessive debt, lower creditworthiness, and weaker balance sheet strength.
3. Long-term debt-to-equity ratio	$\dfrac{\text{Long-term debt}}{\text{Total stockholders' equity}}$	Shows the balance between debt and equity in the firm's *long-term* capital structure. Low ratios indicate greater capacity to borrow additional funds if needed.
4. Times-interest-earned (or coverage) ratio	$\dfrac{\text{Operating income}}{\text{Interest expenses}}$	Measures the ability to pay annual interest charges. Lenders usually insist on a minimum ratio of 2.0, but ratios above 3.0 signal better creditworthiness.
Activity ratios		
1. Days of inventory	$\dfrac{\text{Sales} \div 365}{\text{Inventory}}$	Measures inventory management efficiency. Fewer days of inventory are usually better.
2. Inventory turnover	$\dfrac{\text{Sales}}{\text{Inventory}}$	Measures the number of inventory turns per year. Higher is better.
3. Average collection period	$\dfrac{\text{Accounts receivable}}{\text{Total sales} \div 365}$ or $\dfrac{\text{Accounts receivable}}{\text{Average daily sales}}$	Indicates the average length of time the firm must wait after making a sale to receive cash payment. A shorter collection time is better.
Other important measures of financial performance		
1. Dividend yield on common stock	$\dfrac{\text{Annual dividends per share}}{\text{Current market price per share}}$	A measure of the return that shareholders receive in the form of dividends. A "typical" dividend yield in 2–3%. The dividend yield for fast-growth companies in often below 1% (may be even 0); the dividend yield for slow-growth companies can run 4–5%.
2. Price/earnings ratio	$\dfrac{\text{Current market price per share}}{\text{Earnings per share}}$	P/E ratios above 20 indicate strong investor confidence in a firm's outlook and earnings growth; firms whose future earnings are at risk or likely to grow slowly typically have ratios below 12.
3. Dividend payout ratio	$\dfrac{\text{Annual dividends per share}}{\text{Earnings per share}}$	Indicates the percentage of after-tax profits paid out as dividends.
4. Internal cash flow	After tax profits + Depreciation	A quick and rough estimate of the cash a company's business is generating after payment of operating expenses, interest, and taxes. Such amounts can be used for dividend payments or funding capital expenditures.

- *A skill, specialized expertise, or competitively important capability*—skills in low-cost operations, technological expertise, expertise in defect-free manufacture, proven capabilities in developing and introducing innovative products, cutting-edge supply chain management capabilities, expertise in getting new products to market quickly, strong e-commerce expertise, expertise in providing consistently good customer service, excellent mass merchandising skills, or unique advertising and promotional talents.

- *Valuable physical assets*—state-of-the-art plants and equipment, attractive real estate locations, worldwide distribution facilities, or ownership of valuable natural resource deposits.

- *Valuable human assets and intellectual capital*—an experienced and capable workforce, talented employees in key areas, cutting-edge knowledge in technology or other important areas of the business, collective learning embedded in the organization and built up over time, or proven managerial know-how.[1]

- *Valuable organizational assets*—proven quality control systems, proprietary technology, key patents, state-of-the-art systems for doing business via the Internet, ownership of important natural resources, a cadre of highly trained customer service representatives, a strong network of distributors or retail dealers, sizable amounts of cash and marketable securities, a strong balance sheet and credit rating (thus giving the company access to additional financial capital), or a comprehensive list of customers' e-mail addresses.

- *Valuable intangible assets*—a powerful or well-known brand name, a reputation for technological leadership, or strong buyer loyalty and goodwill.

- *An achievement or attribute that puts the company in a position of market advantage*—low overall costs relative to competitors, market share leadership, a superior product, a wider product line than rivals, wide geographic coverage, or award-winning customer service.

- *Competitively valuable alliances or cooperative ventures*—fruitful partnerships with suppliers that reduce costs and/or enhance product quality and performance; alliances or joint ventures that provide access to valuable technologies, specialized know-how, or geographic markets.

Core Concept
A company's resource strengths represent *competitive assets* and are big determinants of its competitiveness and ability to succeed in the marketplace.

A company's resource strengths represent its endowment of *competitive assets*. The caliber of a firm's resource strengths is a big determinant of its competitiveness—whether it has the wherewithal to be a strong competitor in the marketplace or whether its capabilities and competitive strengths are modest, thus relegating it to a trailing position in the industry.[2] Plainly, a company's resource strengths may or may not enable it to improve its competitive position and financial performance.

Assessing a Company's Competencies and Capabilities—What Activities Does It Perform Well?   One of the most important aspects of appraising a company's resource strengths has to do with its competence level in performing key pieces of its business—such as supply chain management, research and development (R&D), production, distribution, sales and marketing, and customer service. Which activities does it perform especially well? And are there any activities it performs better than rivals? A company's proficiency in conducting different facets of its operations can range from merely a competence in performing an activity to a core competence to a distinctive competence:

1. A **competence** is something an organization is good at doing. It is nearly always the product of experience, representing an accumulation of learning and the buildup

of proficiency in performing an internal activity. Usually a company competence originates with deliberate efforts to develop the organizational ability to do something, however imperfectly or inefficiently. Such efforts involve selecting people with the requisite knowledge and skills, upgrading or expanding individual abilities as needed, and then molding the efforts and work products of individuals into a cooperative group effort to create organizational ability. Then, as experience builds, such that the company gains proficiency in performing the activity consistently well and at an acceptable cost, the ability evolves into a true competence and company capability. Some competencies relate to fairly specific skills and expertise (like just-in-time inventory control or low-cost manufacturing efficiency or picking locations for new stores or designing an unusually appealing and user-friendly Web site); they spring from proficiency in a single discipline or function and may be performed in a single department or organizational unit. Other competencies, however, are inherently multidisciplinary and cross-functional—they are the result of effective collaboration among people with different expertise working in different organizational units. A competence in continuous product innovation, for example, comes from teaming the efforts of people and groups with expertise in market research, new product R&D, design and engineering, cost-effective manufacturing, and market testing.

> **Core Concept**
> A ***competence*** is an activity that a company has learned to perform well.

2. A **core competence** is a proficiently performed internal activity that is *central* to a company's strategy and competitiveness. A core competence is a more valuable resource strength than a competence because of the well-performed activity's core role in the company's strategy and the contribution it makes to the company's success in the marketplace. A core competence can relate to any of several aspects of a company's business: expertise in integrating multiple technologies to create families of new products, know-how in creating and operating systems for cost-efficient supply chain management, the capability to speed new or next-generation products to market, good after-sale service capabilities, skills in manufacturing a high-quality product at a low cost, or the capability to fill customer orders accurately and swiftly. A company may have more than one core competence in its resource portfolio, but rare is the company that can legitimately claim more than two or three core competencies. Most often, *a core competence is knowledge-based, residing in people and in a company's intellectual capital and not in its assets on the balance sheet.* Moreover, a core competence is more likely to be grounded in cross-department combinations of knowledge and expertise rather than being the product of a single department or work group. 3M Corporation has a core competence in product innovation—its record of introducing new products goes back several decades and new product introduction is central to 3M's strategy of growing its business. Ben & Jerry's Homemade, a subsidiary of Unilever, has a core competence in creating unusual flavors of ice cream and marketing them with catchy names like Chunky Monkey, Wavy Gravy, Chubby Hubby, The Gobfather, Dublin Mudslide, and Marsha Marsha Marshmallow.

> **Core Concept**
> A ***core competence*** is a *competitively important* activity that a company performs better than other internal activities.

3. A **distinctive competence** is a competitively valuable activity that a company *performs better than its rivals.* A distinctive competence thus signifies even greater proficiency than a core competence. But what is especially important about a distinctive competence is that the company enjoys *competitive superiority*

Core Concept
A **distinctive competence** is a competitively important activity that a company performs better than its rivals—it thus represents *a competitively superior resource strength.*

in performing that activity—a distinctive competence represents a level of proficiency that rivals do not have. Because a distinctive competence represents uniquely strong capability relative to rival companies, it qualifies as a *competitively superior resource strength* with competitive advantage potential. This is particularly true when the distinctive competence enables a company to deliver standout value to customers (in the form of lower costs and prices or better product performance or superior service). Toyota has worked diligently over several decades to establish a distinctive competence in low-cost, high-quality manufacturing of motor vehicles; its "lean production" system is far superior to that of any other automaker's, and the company is pushing the boundaries of its production advantage with a new type of assembly line—called the Global Body line—that costs 50 percent less to install and can be changed to accommodate a new model for 70 percent less than its previous production system.[3] Starbucks' distinctive competence in innovative coffee drinks and store ambience has propelled it to the forefront among coffee retailers.

The conceptual differences between a competence, a core competence, and a distinctive competence draw attention to the fact that a company's resource strengths and competitive capabilities are not all equal.[4] Some competencies and competitive capabilities merely enable market survival because most rivals have them—indeed, not having a competence or capability that rivals have can result in competitive disadvantage. If an apparel company does not have the competence to produce its apparel items cost-efficiently, it is unlikely to survive given the intensely price-competitive nature of the apparel industry. Every Web retailer requires a basic competence in designing an appealing and user-friendly Web site.

Core competencies are *competitively* more important resource strengths than competencies because they add power to the company's strategy and have a bigger positive impact on its market position and profitability. Distinctive competencies are even more competitively important. A distinctive competence is a competitively potent resource strength for three reasons: (1) it gives a company competitively valuable capability that is unmatched by rivals, (2) it has potential for being the cornerstone of the company's strategy, and (3) it can produce a competitive edge in the marketplace since it represents a level of proficiency that is superior to rivals. It is always easier for a company to build competitive advantage when it has a distinctive competence in performing an activity important to market success, when rival companies do not have offsetting competencies, and when it is costly and time-consuming for rivals to imitate the competence. A distinctive competence is thus potentially the mainspring of a company's success—unless it is trumped by more powerful resources possessed by rivals.

Core Concept
A distinctive competence is a competitively potent resource strength for three reasons: (1) it gives a company competitively valuable capability that is unmatched by rivals, (2) it can underpin and add real punch to a company's strategy, and (3) it is a basis for sustainable competitive advantage.

What Is the Competitive Power of a Resource Strength?

It is not enough to simply compile a list of a company's resource strengths and competitive capabilities. What is most telling about a company's resource strengths, individually and collectively, is how powerful they are in the marketplace. The competitive power of a resource strength is measured by how many of the following four tests it can pass:[5]

1. *Is the resource strength hard to copy?* The more difficult and more expensive it is to imitate a company's resource strength, the greater its potential competitive

value. Resources tend to be difficult to copy when they are unique (a fantastic real estate location, patent protection), when they must be built over time in ways that are difficult to imitate (a brand name, mastery of a technology), and when they carry big capital requirements (a cost-effective plant to manufacture cutting-edge microprocessors). Wal-Mart's competitors have failed miserably in their attempts over the past two decades to match Wal-Mart's super-efficient state-of-the-art distribution capabilities. Hard-to-copy strengths and capabilities are valuable competitive assets, adding to a company's market strength and contributing to sustained profitability.

2. *Is the resource strength durable—does it have staying power?* The longer the competitive value of a resource lasts, the greater its value. Some resources lose their clout in the marketplace quickly because of the rapid speeds at which technologies or industry conditions are moving. The value of Eastman Kodak's resources in film and film processing is rapidly being undercut by the growing popularity of digital cameras. The investments that commercial banks have made in branch offices is a rapidly depreciating asset because of growing use of direct deposits, debit cards, automated teller machines, and telephone and Internet banking options.

3. *Is the resource really competitively superior?* Companies have to guard against pridefully believing that their core competencies are distinctive competencies or that their brand name is more powerful than the brand names of rivals. Who can really say whether Coca-Cola's consumer marketing prowess is better than Pepsi-Cola's or whether the Mercedes-Benz brand name is more powerful than that of BMW or Lexus? Although many retailers claim to be quite proficient in product selection and in-store merchandising, a number run into trouble in the marketplace because they encounter rivals whose competencies in product selection and in-store merchandising are better than theirs. Apple's operating system for its MacIntosh PCs is by most accounts a world beater (compared to Windows XP), but Apple has failed miserably in converting its resource strength in operating system design into competitive success in the global PC market—it is an also-ran with a paltry 2–3 percent market share worldwide.

4. *Can the resource strength be trumped by the different resource strengths and competitive capabilities of rivals?* Many commercial airlines have invested heavily in developing the resources and capabilities to offer passengers safe, reliable flights at convenient times, along with an array of in-flight amenities. However, Southwest Airlines and JetBlue in the United States and Ryanair and easyJet in Europe have been quite successful deploying their resources in ways that enable them to provide commercial air services at radically lower fares. Amazon.com's strengths in online retailing of books have put a big dent in the business prospects of brick-and-mortar bookstores. Whole Foods Market has a resource lineup that enables it to merchandise a dazzling array of natural and organic food products in a supermarket setting, thus putting strong competitive pressure on Kroger, Safeway, Albertson's, and other prominent supermarket chains. The prestigious brand names of Cadillac and Lincoln have faded because Mercedes, BMW, Audi, and Lexus have used their resources to design, produce, and market more appealing luxury vehicles.

The vast majority of companies are not well endowed with standout resource strengths, much less with one or more competitively superior resources (or distinctive competencies) capable of passing all four tests with high marks. Most firms have a mixed bag of resources—one or two quite valuable, some good, many satisfactory to mediocre.

Companies in the top tier of their industry may have as many as two core competencies in their resource strength lineup. But only a few companies, usually the strongest industry leaders or up-and-coming challengers, have a resource strength that truly qualifies as a distinctive competence. Even so, a company can still marshal the resource strengths to be competitively successful without having a competitively superior resource or distinctive competence. A company can achieve considerable competitive vitality, maybe even competitive advantage, from a collection of good-to-adequate resource strengths that collectively give it competitive power in the marketplace. A number of fast-food chains—for example, Wendy's, Taco Bell, and Subway—have achieved a respectable market position competing against McDonald's with satisfactory sets of resource strengths and no apparent distinctive competence. The same can be said for Lowe's, which competes against industry leader Home Depot, and such regional banks as Compass, State Street, Keybank, PNC, BB&T, and AmSouth, which increasingly find themselves in competition with the top five U.S. banks—JPMorgan Chase, Bank of America, Citibank, Wachovia, and Wells Fargo.

> **Core Concept**
> A company's ability to succeed in the marketplace hinges to a considerable extent on the competitive power of its resources—the set of competencies, capabilities, and competitive assets at its command.

Identifying Company Resource Weaknesses and Competitive Deficiencies

A *resource weakness,* or *competitive deficiency,* is something a company lacks or does poorly (in comparison to others) or a condition that puts it at a disadvantage in the marketplace. A company's resource weaknesses can relate to (1) inferior or unproven skills, expertise, or intellectual capital in competitively important areas of the business; (2) deficiencies in competitively important physical, organizational, or intangible assets; or (3) missing or competitively inferior capabilities in key areas. *Internal weaknesses are thus shortcomings in a company's complement of resources and represent competitive liabilities.* Nearly all companies have competitive liabilities of one kind or another. Whether a company's resource weaknesses make it competitively vulnerable depends on how much they matter in the marketplace and whether they are offset by the company's resource strengths.

> **Core Concept**
> A company's resource strengths represent competitive assets; its resource weaknesses represent competitive liabilities.

Table 4.2 lists the kinds of factors to consider in compiling a company's resource strengths and weaknesses. Sizing up a company's complement of resource capabilities and deficiencies is akin to constructing a *strategic balance sheet,* where resource strengths represent *competitive assets* and resource weaknesses represent *competitive liabilities.* Obviously, the ideal condition is for the company's competitive assets to outweigh its competitive liabilities by an ample margin—a 50–50 balance is definitely not the desired condition!

Identifying a Company's Market Opportunities

Market opportunity is a big factor in shaping a company's strategy. Indeed, managers can't properly tailor strategy to the company's situation without first identifying its market opportunities and appraising the growth and profit potential each one holds. Depending on the prevailing circumstances, a company's opportunities can be plentiful or scarce, fleeting or lasting, and can range from wildly attractive (an absolute "must" to pursue) to marginally interesting (because the growth and profit potential are questionable) to unsuitable (because there's not a good match with the company's

Table 4.2   **What to Look for in Identifying a Company's Strengths, Weaknesses, Opportunities, and Threats**

Potential Resource Strengths and Competitive Capabilities	Potential Resource Weaknesses and Competitive Deficiencies
<ul><li>A powerful strategy</li><li>Core competencies in _____</li><li>A distinctive competence in _____</li><li>A product that is strongly differentiated from those of rivals</li><li>Competencies and capabilities that are well matched to industry key success factors</li><li>A strong financial condition; ample financial resources to grow the business</li><li>Strong brand-name image/company reputation</li><li>An attractive customer base</li><li>Economy of scale and/or learning/experience curve advantages over rivals</li><li>Proprietary technology/superior technological skills/important patents</li><li>Superior intellectual capital relative to key rivals</li><li>Cost advantages over rivals</li><li>Strong advertising and promotion</li><li>Product innovation capabilities</li><li>Proven capabilities in improving production processes</li><li>Good supply chain management capabilities</li><li>Good customer service capabilities</li><li>Better product quality relative to rivals</li><li>Wide geographic coverage and/or strong global distribution capability</li><li>Alliances/joint ventures with other firms that provide access to valuable technology, competencies, and/or attractive geographic markets</li></ul>	<ul><li>No clear strategic direction</li><li>Resources that are not well matched to industry key success factors</li><li>No well-developed or proven core competencies</li><li>A weak balance sheet; burdened with too much debt</li><li>Higher overall unit costs relative to key competitors</li><li>Weak or unproven product innovation capabilities</li><li>A product/service with ho-hum attributes or features inferior to those of rivals</li><li>Too narrow a product line relative to rivals</li><li>Weak brand image or reputation</li><li>Weaker dealer network than key rivals and/or lack of adequate global distribution capability</li><li>Behind on product quality, R&D, and/or technological know-how</li><li>In the wrong strategic group</li><li>Losing market share because . . .</li><li>Lack of management depth</li><li>Inferior intellectual capital relative to leading rivals</li><li>Subpar profitability because . . .</li><li>Plagued with internal operating problems or obsolete facilities</li><li>Behind rivals in e-commerce capabilities</li><li>Short on financial resources to grow the business and pursue promising initiatives</li><li>Too much underutilized plant capacity</li></ul>

Potential Market Opportunities	Potential External Threats to a Company's Future Prospects
<ul><li>Openings to win market share from rivals</li><li>Sharply rising buyer demand for the industry's product</li><li>Serving additional customer groups or market segments</li><li>Expanding into new geographic markets</li><li>Expanding the company's product line to meet a broader range of customer needs</li><li>Using existing company skills or technological know-how to enter new product lines or new businesses</li><li>Online sales</li><li>Integrating forward or backward</li><li>Falling trade barriers in attractive foreign markets</li><li>Acquiring rival firms or companies with attractive technological expertise or capabilities</li><li>Entering into alliances or joint ventures to expand the firm's market coverage or boost its competitive capability</li><li>Openings to exploit emerging new technologies</li></ul>	<ul><li>Increasing intensity of competition among industry rivals—may squeeze profit margins</li><li>Slowdowns in market growth</li><li>Likely entry of potent new competitors</li><li>Loss of sales to substitute products</li><li>Growing bargaining power of customers or suppliers</li><li>A shift in buyer needs and tastes away from the industry's product</li><li>Adverse demographic changes that threaten to curtail demand for the industry's product</li><li>Vulnerability to unfavorable industry driving forces</li><li>Restrictive trade policies on the part of foreign governments</li><li>Costly new regulatory requirements</li></ul>

resource strengths and capabilities). A checklist of potential market opportunities is included in Table 4.2.

While stunningly big or "golden" opportunities appear fairly frequently in volatile, fast-changing markets (typically due to important technological developments or rapidly shifting consumer preferences), they are nonetheless hard to see before most all companies in the industry identify them. The more volatile and thus unpredictable market conditions are, the more limited a company's ability to do market reconnaissance and spot important opportunities much ahead of rivals—there are simply too many variables in play for managers to peer into the fog of the future, identify one or more upcoming opportunities, and get a jump on rivals in pursuing it.[6] In mature markets, unusually attractive market opportunities emerge sporadically, often after long periods of relative calm—but future market conditions may be less foggy, thus facilitating good market reconnaissance and making emerging opportunities easier for industry members to detect. But in both volatile and stable markets, the rise of a golden opportunity is almost never under the control of a single company or manufactured by company executives—rather, it springs from the simultaneous alignment of several external factors. For instance, in China the recent upsurge in demand for motor vehicles was spawned by a convergence of many factors—increased disposable income, rising middle-class aspirations, a major road-building program by the government, the demise of employer-provided housing, and easy credit.[7] But golden opportunities are nearly always seized rapidly—and the companies that seize them are usually those that have been actively waiting, staying alert with diligent market reconnaissance, and preparing themselves to capitalize on shifting market conditions by patiently assembling an arsenal of competitively valuable resources—talented personnel, technical know-how, strategic partnerships, and a war chest of cash to finance aggressive action when the time comes.[8]

> A company is well advised to pass on a particular market opportunity unless it has or can acquire the resources to capture it.

In evaluating a company's market opportunities and ranking their attractiveness, managers have to guard against viewing every *industry* opportunity as a *company* opportunity. Not every company is equipped with the resources to successfully pursue each opportunity that exists in its industry. Some companies are more capable of going after particular opportunities than others, and a few companies may be hopelessly outclassed. *The market opportunities most relevant to a company are those that match up well with the company's financial and organizational resource capabilities, offer the best growth and profitability, and present the most potential for competitive advantage.*

Identifying the External Threats to a Company's Future Profitability

Often, certain factors in a company's external environment pose *threats* to its profitability and competitive well-being. Threats can stem from the emergence of cheaper or better technologies, rivals' introduction of new or improved products, the entry of lower-cost foreign competitors into a company's market stronghold, new regulations that are more burdensome to a company than to its competitors, vulnerability to a rise in interest rates, the potential of a hostile takeover, unfavorable demographic shifts, adverse changes in foreign exchange rates, political upheaval in a foreign country where the company has facilities, and the like. A list of potential threats to a company's future profitability and market position is shown in Table 4.2.

External threats may pose no more than a moderate degree of adversity (all companies confront some threatening elements in the course of doing business), or they may be so imposing as to make a company's situation and outlook quite tenuous. On rare occasions, market shocks can give birth to a *sudden-death* threat that throws a company into an immediate crisis and battle to survive. Many of the world's major airlines have been plunged into unprecedented financial crisis by the perfect storm of the September 11, 2001, terrorist attacks, rising prices for jet fuel, mounting competition from low-fare carriers, shifting traveler preferences for low fares as opposed to lots of in-flight amenities, and out-of-control labor costs. It is management's job to identify the threats to the company's future prospects and to evaluate what strategic actions can be taken to neutralize or lessen their impact.

What Do the SWOT Listings Reveal?

SWOT analysis involves more than making four lists. The two most important parts of SWOT analysis are *drawing conclusions* from the SWOT listings about the company's overall situation, and *translating these conclusions into strategic actions* to better match the company's strategy to its resource strengths and market opportunities, to correct the important weaknesses, and to defend against external threats. Figure 4.2 shows the three steps of SWOT analysis.

> Simply making lists of a company's strengths, weaknesses, opportunities, and threats is not enough; the payoff from SWOT analysis comes from the conclusions about a company's situation and the implications for strategy improvement that flow from the four lists.

Just what story the SWOT listings tell about the company's overall situation is often revealed in the answers to the following sets of questions:

- Does the company have an attractive set of resource strengths? Does it have any strong core competencies or a distinctive competence? Are the company's strengths and capabilities well matched to the industry key success factors? Do they add adequate power to the company's strategy, or are more or different strengths needed? Will the company's current strengths and capabilities matter in the future?

- How serious are the company's weaknesses and competitive deficiencies? Are they mostly inconsequential and readily correctable, or could one or more prove fatal if not remedied soon? Are some of the company's weaknesses in areas that relate to the industry's key success factors? Are there any weaknesses that if uncorrected, would keep the company from pursuing an otherwise attractive opportunity? Does the company have important resource gaps that need to be filled for it to move up in the industry rankings and/or boost its profitability?

- Do the company's resource strengths and competitive capabilities (its competitive assets) outweigh its resource weaknesses and competitive deficiencies (its competitive liabilities) by an attractive margin?

- Does the company have attractive market opportunities that are well suited to its resource strengths and competitive capabilities? Does the company lack the resources and capabilities to pursue any of the most attractive opportunities?

- Are the threats alarming, or are they something the company appears able to deal with and defend against?

Figure 4.2   **The Three Steps of SWOT Analysis: Identify, Draw Conclusions, Translate into Strategic Action**

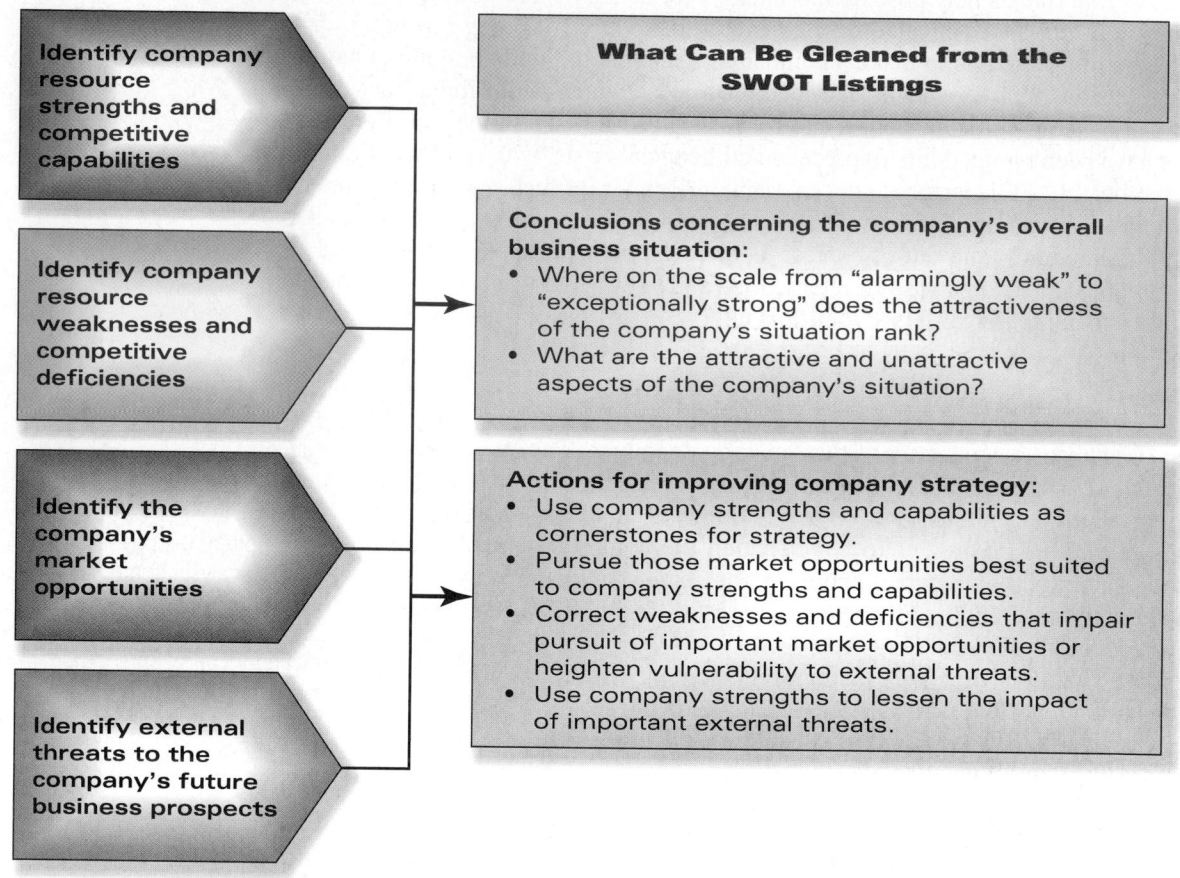

All things considered, how strong is the company's overall situation? Where on a scale of 1 to 10 (1 being alarmingly weak and 10 exceptionally strong) should the firm's position and overall situation be ranked? What aspects of the company's situation are particularly attractive? What aspects are of the most concern?

The final piece of SWOT analysis is to translate the diagnosis of the company's situation into actions for improving the company's strategy and business prospects. The following questions point to implications the SWOT listings have for strategic action:

- Which competitive capabilities need to be strengthened immediately, so as to add greater power to the company's strategy and boost sales and profitability? Do new types of competitive capabilities need to be put in place to help the company better respond to emerging industry and competitive conditions? Which resources and capabilities need to be given greater emphasis, and which merit less emphasis? Should the company emphasize leveraging its existing resource strengths and capabilities, or does it need to create new resource strengths and capabilities?

- What actions should be taken to reduce the company's competitive liabilities? Which weaknesses or competitive deficiencies are in urgent need of correction?

- Which market opportunities should be top priority in future strategic initiatives (because they are good fits with the company's resource strengths and competitive capabilities, present attractive growth and profit prospects, and/or offer the best potential for securing competitive advantage)? Which opportunities should be ignored, at least for the time being (because they offer less growth potential or are not suited to the company's resources and capabilities)?
- What should the company be doing to guard against the threats to its well-being?

A company's resource strengths should generally form the cornerstones of strategy because they represent the company's best chance for market success.[9] As a rule, strategies that place heavy demands on areas where the company is weakest or has unproven ability are suspect and should be avoided. If a company doesn't have the resources and competitive capabilities around which to craft an attractive strategy, managers need to take decisive remedial action either to upgrade existing organizational resources and capabilities and add others as needed or to acquire them through partnerships or strategic alliances with firms possessing the needed expertise. Plainly, managers have to look toward correcting competitive weaknesses that make the company vulnerable, hold down profitability, or disqualify it from pursuing an attractive opportunity.

At the same time, sound strategy making requires sifting through the available market opportunities and aiming strategy at capturing those that are most attractive and suited to the company's circumstances. Rarely does a company have the resource depth to pursue all available market opportunities simultaneously without spreading itself too thin. How much attention to devote to defending against external threats to the company's market position and future performance hinges on how vulnerable the company is, whether there are attractive defensive moves that can be taken to lessen their impact, and whether the costs of undertaking such moves represent the best use of company resources.

QUESTION 3: ARE THE COMPANY'S PRICES AND COSTS COMPETITIVE?

Company managers are often stunned when a competitor cuts its price to "unbelievably low" levels or when a new market entrant comes on strong with a very low price. The competitor may not, however, be "dumping" (an economic term for selling at prices that are below cost), buying its way into the market with a super-low price, or waging a desperate move to gain sales—it may simply have substantially lower costs. One of the most telling signs of whether a company's business position is strong or precarious is whether its prices and costs are competitive with industry rivals. For a company to compete successfully, its costs must be *in line* with those of close rivals.

> The higher a company's costs are above those of close rivals, the more competitively vulnerable it becomes.

Price–cost comparisons are especially critical in a commodity-product industry where the value provided to buyers is the same from seller to seller, price competition is typically the ruling market force, and low-cost companies have the upper hand. But even in industries where products are differentiated and competition centers on the different attributes of competing brands as much as on price, rival companies have to keep their costs in line and make sure that any added costs they incur, and any price premiums they charge, create ample value that buyers are willing to pay extra for.

While some cost disparity is justified so long as the products or services of closely competing companies are sufficiently differentiated, a high-cost firm's market position becomes increasingly vulnerable the more its costs exceed those of close rivals.

Two analytical tools are particularly useful in determining whether a company's prices and costs are competitive: value chain analysis and benchmarking.

The Concept of a Company Value Chain

Core Concept

A company's **value chain** identifies the primary activities that create customer value and the related support activities.

Every company's business consists of a collection of activities undertaken in the course of designing, producing, marketing, delivering, and supporting its product or service. All of the various activities that a company performs internally combine to form a **value chain**—so called because the underlying intent of a company's activities is to do things that ultimately *create value for buyers*. A company's value chain also includes an allowance for profit because a markup over the cost of performing the firm's value-creating activities is customarily part of the price (or total cost) borne by buyers—unless an enterprise succeeds in creating and delivering sufficient value to buyers to produce an attractive profit, it can't survive for long.

As shown in Figure 4.3, a company's value chain consists of two broad categories of activities: the *primary activities* that are foremost in creating value for customers and the requisite *support activities* that facilitate and enhance the performance of the primary activities.[10] For example, the primary value-creating activities for a maker of bakery goods include supply chain management, recipe development and testing, mixing and baking, packaging, sales and marketing, and distribution; related support activities include quality control, human resource management, and administration. A wholesaler's primary activities and costs deal with merchandise selection and purchasing, inbound shipping and warehousing from suppliers, and outbound distribution to retail customers. The primary activities for a department store retailer include merchandise selection and buying, store layout and product display, advertising, and customer service; its support activities include site selection, hiring and training, and store maintenance, plus the usual assortment of administrative activities. A hotel chain's primary activities and costs are in site selection and construction, reservations, operation of its hotel properties (check-in and check-out, maintenance and housekeeping, dining and room service, and conventions and meetings), and managing its lineup of hotel locations; principal support activities include accounting, hiring and training hotel staff, advertising, building a brand and reputation, and general administration. Supply chain management is a crucial activity for Nissan and Amazon.com but is not a value chain component at Google or a TV and radio broadcasting company. Sales and marketing are dominant activities at Procter & Gamble and Sony but have minor roles at oil drilling companies and natural gas pipeline companies. Delivery to buyers is a crucial activity at Domino's Pizza but comparatively insignificant at Starbucks. Thus, what constitutes a primary or secondary activity varies according to the specific nature of a company's business, meaning that you should view the listing of the primary and support activities in Figure 4.3 as illustrative rather than definitive.

A Company's Primary and Support Activities Identify the Major Components of Its Cost Structure   Segregating a company's operations into different types of primary and support activities is the first step in understanding its cost structure. Each activity in the value chain gives rise to costs and ties up assets.

Figure 4.3   **A Representative Company Value Chain**

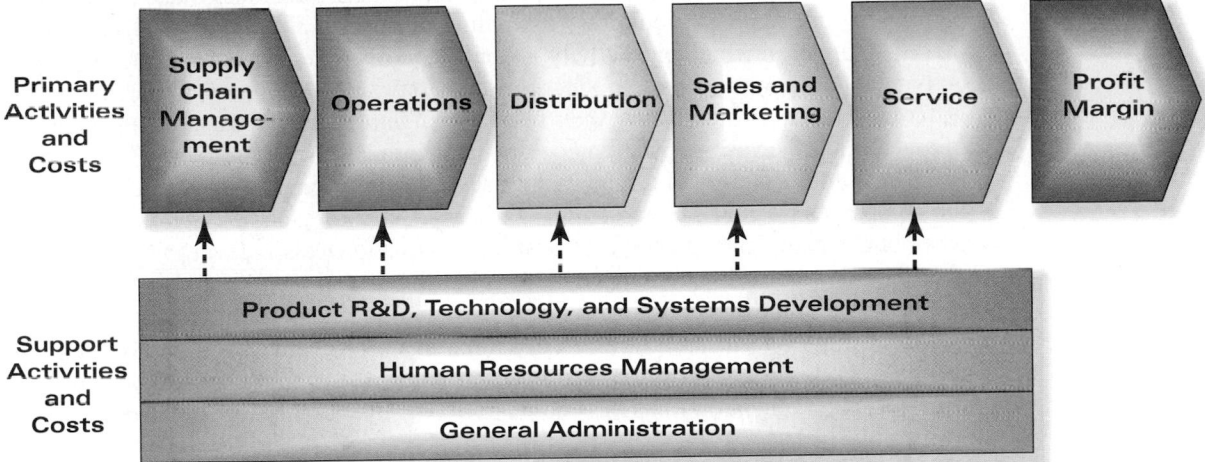

PRIMARY ACTIVITIES
- **Supply chain management**—activities, costs, and assets associated with purchasing fuel, energy, raw materials, parts and components, merchandise, and consumable items from vendors; receiving, storing, and disseminating inputs from suppliers; inspection; and inventory management.

- **Operations**—activities, costs, and assets associated with converting inputs into final product from (production, assembly, packaging, equipment maintenance, facilities, operations, quality assurance, environmental protection).

- **Distribution**—activities, costs, and assets dealing with physically distributing the product to buyers (finished goods warehousing, order processing, order picking and packing, shipping, delivery vehicle operations, establishing and maintaining a network of dealers and distributors).

- **Sales and marketing**—activities, costs, and assets related to sales force efforts, advertising and promotion, market research and planning, and dealer/distributor support.

- **Service**—activities, costs, and assets associated with providing assistance to buyers, such as installation, spare parts delivery, maintenance and repair, technical assistance, buyer inquiries, and complaints.

SUPPORT ACTIVITIES
- **Product R&D, technology, and systems development**—activities, costs, and assets relating to product R&D, process R&D, process design improvement, equipment design, computer software development, telecommunications systems, computer-assisted design and engineering, database capabilities, and development of computerized support systems.

- **Human resources management**—activities, costs, and assets associated with the recruitment, hiring, training, development, and compensation of all types of personnel; labor relations activities; and development of knowledge-based skills and core competencies.

- **General administration**—activities, costs, and assets relating to general management, accounting and finance, legal and regulatory affairs, safety and security, management information systems, forming strategic alliances and collaborating with strategic partners, and other overhead functions.

Source: Based on the discussion in Michael E. Porter, *Competitive Advantage* (New York: Free Press, 1985), pp. 37–43.

Assigning the company's operating costs and assets to each individual activity in the chain provides cost estimates and capital requirements—a process that accountants call activity-based cost accounting. Quite often, there are links between activities such that the manner in which one activity is done can affect the costs of performing other activities. For instance, how a product is designed has a huge impact on the number of different parts and components, their respective manufacturing costs, and the expense of assembling the various parts and components into a finished product.

The combined costs of all the various activities in a company's value chain define the company's internal cost structure. Further, the cost of each activity contributes to whether the company's overall cost position relative to rivals is favorable or unfavorable. The tasks of value chain analysis and benchmarking are to develop the data for comparing a company's costs activity-by-activity against the costs of key rivals and to learn which internal activities are a source of cost advantage or disadvantage. A company's relative cost position is a function of how the overall costs of the activities it performs in conducting business compare to the overall costs of the activities performed by rivals.

Why the Value Chains of Rival Companies Often Differ

A company's value chain and the manner in which it performs each activity reflect the evolution of its own particular business and internal operations, its strategy, the approaches it is using to execute its strategy, and the underlying economics of the activities themselves.[11] Because these factors differ from company to company, the value chains of rival companies sometimes differ substantially—a condition that complicates the task of assessing rivals' relative cost positions. For instance, music retailers like Blockbuster and Musicland, which purchase CDs from recording studios and wholesale distributors and sell them in their own retail store locations, have value chains and cost structures different from those of rival online music stores like Apple's iTunes and Musicmatch, which sell downloadable music files directly to music shoppers. Competing companies may differ in their degrees of vertical integration. The operations component of the value chain for a manufacturer that *makes* all of its own parts and assembles them into a finished product differs from the operations component of a rival producer that *buys* the needed parts from outside suppliers and performs assembly operations only. Likewise, there is legitimate reason to expect value chain and cost differences between a company that is pursuing a low-cost/low-price strategy and a rival that is positioned on the high end of the market. The costs of certain activities along the low-cost company's value chain should indeed be relatively low, whereas the high-end firm may understandably be spending relatively more to perform those activities that create the added quality and extra features of its products.

Moreover, cost and price differences among rival companies can have their origins in activities performed by suppliers or by distribution channel allies involved in getting the product to end users. Suppliers or wholesale/retail dealers may have excessively high cost structures or profit margins that jeopardize a company's cost-competitiveness even though its costs for internally performed activities are competitive. For example, when determining Michelin's cost-competitiveness vis-à-vis Goodyear and Bridgestone in supplying replacement tires to vehicle owners, we have to look at more than whether Michelin's tire manufacturing costs are above or below Goodyear's and Bridgestone's. Let's say that a motor vehicle owner looking for a new set of tires has to pay $400 for a set of Michelin tires and only $350 for a set of Goodyear or Bridgestone tires. Michelin's $50 price disadvantage can stem not only from higher manufacturing costs (reflecting, perhaps, the added costs of Michelin's strategic efforts to build a better-quality tire with more performance features) but also from (1) differences in what the three tire makers pay their suppliers for materials and tire-making components, and (2) differences in the operating efficiencies, costs, and markups of Michelin's wholesale–retail dealer outlets versus those of Goodyear and Bridgestone.

The Value Chain System for an Entire Industry

As the tire industry example makes clear, a company's value chain is embedded in a larger system of activities that includes the value chains of its suppliers and the value chains of whatever distribution channel allies it uses in getting its product or service to end users.[12] Suppliers' value chains are relevant because suppliers perform activities and incur costs in creating and delivering the purchased inputs used in a company's own value-creating activities. The costs, performance features, and quality of these inputs influence a company's own costs and product differentiation capabilities. Anything a company can do to help its suppliers' drive down the costs of their value chain activities or improve the quality and performance of the items being supplied can enhance its own competitiveness—a powerful reason for working collaboratively with suppliers in managing supply chain activities.[13]

The value chains of forward channel partners and/or the customers to whom a company sells are relevant because (1) the costs and margins of a company's distributors and retail dealers are part of the price the ultimate consumer pays, and (2) the activities that distribution allies perform affect customer satisfaction. For these reasons, companies normally work closely with their forward channel allies (who are their direct customers) to perform value chain activities in mutually beneficial ways. For instance, motor vehicle manufacturers work closely with their local automobile dealers to keep the retail prices of their vehicles competitive with rivals' models and to ensure that owners are satisfied with dealers' repair and maintenance services. Some aluminum can producers have constructed plants next to beer breweries and deliver cans on overhead conveyors directly to the breweries' can-filling lines; this has resulted in significant savings in production scheduling, shipping, and inventory costs for both container producers and breweries.[14] Many automotive parts suppliers have built plants near the auto assembly plants they supply to facilitate just-in-time deliveries, reduce warehousing and shipping costs, and promote close collaboration on parts design and production scheduling. Irrigation equipment companies, suppliers of grape-harvesting and winemaking equipment, and firms making barrels, wine bottles, caps, corks, and labels all have facilities in the California wine country to be close to the nearly 700 winemakers they supply.[15] The lesson here is that a company's value chain activities are often closely linked to the value chains of their suppliers and the forward allies or customers to whom they sell.

> A company's cost-competitiveness depends not only on the costs of internally performed activities (its own value chain) but also on costs in the value chains of its suppliers and forward channel allies.

As a consequence, *accurately assessing a company's competitiveness from the perspective of the consumers who ultimately use its products or services thus requires that company managers understand an industry's entire value chain system for delivering a product or service to customers, not just the company's own value chain.* A typical industry value chain that incorporates the value chains of suppliers and forward channel allies (if any) is shown in Figure 4.4. However, industry value chains

Figure 4.4   **Representative Value Chain for an Entire Industry**

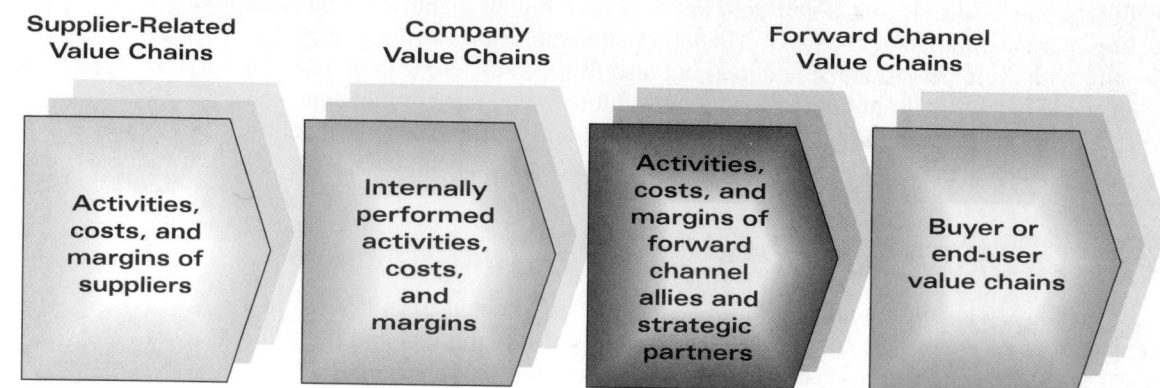

Source: Based in part on the single-industry value chain displayed in Michael E. Porter, *Competitive Advantage* (New York: Free Press, 1985), p. 35.

vary significantly by industry. The primary value chain activities in the pulp and paper industry (timber farming, logging, pulp mills, and papermaking) differ from the primary value chain activities in the home appliance industry (parts and components manufacture, assembly, wholesale distribution, retail sales). The value chain for the soft-drink industry (processing of basic ingredients and syrup manufacture, bottling and can filling, wholesale distribution, advertising, and retail merchandising) differs from that for the computer software industry (programming, disk loading, marketing, distribution). Producers of bathroom and kitchen faucets depend heavily on the activities of wholesale distributors and building supply retailers in winning sales to homebuilders and do-it-yourselfers, but producers of papermaking machines internalize their distribution activities by selling directly to the operators of paper plants. Illustration Capsule 4.1 shows representative costs for various activities performed by the producers and marketers of music CDs.

Activity-Based Costing: A Tool for Assessing a Company's Cost Competitiveness

Once the company has identified its major value chain activities, the next step in evaluating its cost competitiveness involves determining the costs of performing specific value chain activities, using what accountants call activity-based costing.[16] Traditional accounting identifies costs according to broad categories of expenses—wages and salaries, employee benefits, supplies, maintenance, utilities, travel, depreciation, R&D, interest, general administration, and so on. But activity-based cost accounting involves establishing expense categories for specific value chain activities and assigning costs to the activity responsible for creating the cost. An illustrative example is shown in Table 4.3. Perhaps 25 percent of the companies that have explored the feasibility of activity-based costing have adopted this accounting approach.

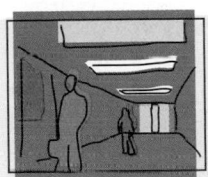

Illustration Capsule 4.1

Estimated Value Chain Costs for Recording and Distributing Music CDs through Traditional Music Retailers

The following table presents the representative costs and markups associated with producing and distributing a music CD retailing for $15 in music stores (as opposed to Internet sources).

Value Chain Activities and Costs in Producing and Distributing a CD		
1. Record company direct production costs:		$2.40
Artists and repertoire	$0.75	
Pressing of CD and packaging	1.65	
2. Royalties		0.99
3. Record company marketing expenses		1.50
4. Record company overhead		1.50
5. Total record company costs		6.39
6. Record company's operating profit		1.86
7. Record company's selling price to distributor/wholesaler		8.25
8. Average wholesale distributor markup to cover distribution activities and profit margins		1.50
9. Average wholesale price charged to retailer		9.75
10. Average retail markup over wholesale cost		5.25
11. Average price to consumer at retail		$15.00

Source: Developed from information in "Fight the Power," a case study prepared by Adrian Aleyne, Babson College, 1999.

The degree to which a company's costs should be disaggregated into specific activities depends on how valuable it is to develop cross-company cost comparisons for narrowly defined activities as opposed to broadly defined activities. Generally speaking, cost estimates are needed at least for each broad category of primary and secondary activities, but finer classifications may be needed if a company discovers that it has a cost disadvantage vis-à-vis rivals and wants to pin down the exact source or activity causing the cost disadvantage. It can also be necessary to develop cost estimates for activities performed in the competitively relevant portions of suppliers' and customers' value chains—which requires going to outside sources for reliable cost information.

Once a company has developed good cost estimates for each of the major activities in its value chain, and perhaps has cost estimates for subactivities within each primary/ secondary value chain activity, then it is ready to see how its costs for these activities compare with the costs of rival firms. This is where benchmarking comes in.

Table 4.3   **The Difference between Traditional Cost Accounting and Activity-Based Cost Accounting: A Supply Chain Activity Example**

Traditional Cost Accounting Categories for Supply Chain Activities		Cost of Performing Specific Supply Chain Activities Using Activity-Based Cost Accounting	
Wages and salaries	$450,000	Evaluate supplier capabilities	$150,000
Employee benefits	95,000	Process purchase orders	92,000
Supplies	21,500	Collaborate with suppliers on just-in-time deliveries	180,000
Travel	12,250		
Depreciation	19,000	Share data with suppliers	69,000
Other fixed charges (office space, utilities)	112,000	Check quality of items purchased	94,000
Miscellaneous operating expenses	40,250	Check incoming deliveries against purchase orders	50,000
	$750,000	Resolve disputes	15,000
		Conduct internal administration	100,000
			$750,000

Source: Developed from information in Terence P. Par, "A New Tool for Managing Costs," *Fortune,* June 14, 1993, pp. 124–29.

Benchmarking: A Tool for Assessing Whether a Company's Value Chain Costs Are in Line

Core Concept
Benchmarking is a potent tool for learning which companies are best at performing particular activities and then using their techniques (or "best practices") to improve the cost and effectiveness of a company's own internal activities.

Many companies today are **benchmarking** their costs of performing a given activity against competitors' costs (and/or against the costs of a noncompetitor that efficiently and effectively performs much the same activity in another industry). *Benchmarking is a tool that allows a company to determine whether its performance of a particular function or activity represents the "best practice" when both cost and effectiveness are taken into account.*

Benchmarking entails comparing how different companies perform various value chain activities—how materials are purchased, how suppliers are paid, how inventories are managed, how products are assembled, how fast the company can get new products to market, how the quality control function is performed, how customer orders are filled and shipped, how employees are trained, how payrolls are processed, and how maintenance is performed—and then making cross-company comparisons of the costs of these activities.[17] The objectives of benchmarking are to identify the best practices in performing an activity, to learn how other companies have actually achieved lower costs or better results in performing benchmarked activities, and to take action to improve a company's competitiveness whenever benchmarking reveals that its costs and results of performing an activity are not on a par with what other companies (either competitors or noncompetitors) have achieved.

Xerox became one of the first companies to use benchmarking when, in 1979, Japanese manufacturers began selling midsize copiers in the United States for $9,600 each—less than Xerox's production costs.[18] Xerox management suspected its Japanese competitors were dumping, but it sent a team of line managers to Japan, including the head of manufacturing, to study competitors' business processes and costs. With the aid of Xerox's joint venture partner in Japan, Fuji-Xerox, which knew the competitors well, the team found that Xerox's costs were excessive due to gross inefficiencies in the company's manufacturing processes and business practices. The findings triggered a major internal effort at Xerox to become cost-competitive and prompted Xerox to begin benchmarking 67 of its key work processes against companies identified as employing the best practices. Xerox quickly decided not to restrict its benchmarking efforts to its office equipment rivals but to extend them to any company regarded as world class in performing *any activity* relevant to Xerox's business. Other companies quickly picked up on Xerox's approach. Toyota managers got their idea for just-in-time inventory deliveries by studying how U.S. supermarkets replenished their shelves. Southwest Airlines reduced the turnaround time of its aircraft at each scheduled stop by studying pit crews on the auto racing circuit. Over 80 percent of Fortune 500 companies reportedly use benchmarking for comparing themselves against rivals on cost and other competitively important measures.

The tough part of benchmarking is not whether to do it, but rather how to gain access to information about other companies' practices and costs. Sometimes benchmarking can be accomplished by collecting information from published reports, trade groups, and industry research firms and by talking to knowledgeable industry analysts, customers, and suppliers. Sometimes field trips to the facilities of competing or noncompeting companies can be arranged to observe how things are done, ask questions, compare practices and processes, and perhaps exchange data on productivity, staffing levels, time requirements, and other cost components—but the problem here is that such companies, even if they agree to host facilities tours and answer questions, are unlikely to share competitively sensitive cost information. Furthermore, comparing one company's costs to another's costs may not involve comparing apples to apples if the two companies employ different cost accounting principles to calculate the costs of particular activities.

> Benchmarking the costs of company activities against rivals provides hard evidence of whether a company is cost-competitive.

However, a third and fairly reliable source of benchmarking information has emerged. The explosive interest of companies in benchmarking costs and identifying best practices has prompted consulting organizations (e.g., Accenture, A. T. Kearney, Benchnet—The Benchmarking Exchange, Towers Perrin, and Best Practices) and several councils and associations (e.g., the American Productivity and Quality Center, the Qualserve Benchmarking Clearinghouse, and the Strategic Planning Institute's Council on Benchmarking) to gather benchmarking data, distribute information about best practices, and provide comparative cost data without identifying the names of particular companies. Having an independent group gather the information and report it in a manner that disguises the names of individual companies avoid having the disclosure of competitively sensitive data and lessens the potential for unethical behavior on the part of company personnel in gathering their own data about competitors.Illustration Capsule 4.2 presents a widely recommended code of conduct for engaging in benchmarking that is intended to help companies avoid any improprieties in gathering and using benchmarking data.

Strategic Options for Remedying a Cost Disadvantage

Value chain analysis and benchmarking can reveal a great deal about a firm's cost competitiveness. Examining the costs of a company's own value chain activities and comparing them to rivals' indicates who has how much of a cost advantage or

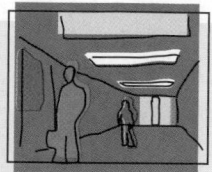

Illustration Capsule 4.2
Benchmarking and Ethical Conduct

Because discussions between benchmarking partners can involve competitively sensitive data, conceivably raising questions about possible restraint of trade or improper business conduct, many benchmarking organizations urge all individuals and organizations involved in benchmarking to abide by a code of conduct grounded in ethical business behavior. Among the most widely used codes of conduct is the one developed by the American Productivity and Quality Center and advocated by the Qualserve Benchmarking Clearinghouse; it is based on the following principles and guidelines:

- Avoid discussions or actions that could lead to or imply an interest in restraint of trade, market and/or customer allocation schemes, price fixing, dealing arrangements, bid rigging, or bribery. Don't discuss costs with competitors if costs are an element of pricing.

- Refrain from the acquisition of trade secrets from another by any means that could be interpreted as improper including the breach or inducement of a breach of any duty to maintain secrecy. Do not disclose or use any trade secret that may have been obtained through improper means or that was disclosed by another in violation of duty to maintain its secrecy or limit its use.

- Be willing to provide the same type and level of information that you request from your benchmarking partner to your benchmarking partner.

- Communicate fully and early in the relationship to clarify expectations, avoid misunderstanding, and establish mutual interest in the benchmarking exchange.

- Be honest and complete.

- Treat benchmarking interchange as confidential to the individuals and companies involved. Information must not be communicated outside the partnering organizations without the prior consent of the benchmarking partner who shared the information.

- Use information obtained through benchmarking only for purposes stated to the benchmarking partner.

- The use or communication of a benchmarking partner's name with the data obtained or practices observed requires the prior permission of that partner.

- Respect the corporate culture of partner companies and work within mutually agreed-on procedures.

- Use benchmarking contacts designated by the partner company, if that is the company's preferred procedure.

- Obtain mutual agreement with the designated benchmarking contact on any hand-off of communication or responsibility to other parties.

- Make the most of your benchmarking partner's time by being fully prepared for each exchange.

- Help your benchmarking partners prepare by providing them with a questionnaire and agenda prior to benchmarking visits.

- Follow through with each commitment made to your benchmarking partner in a timely manner.

- Understand how your benchmarking partner would like to have the information he or she provides handled and used, and handle and use it in that manner.

Note: Identification of firms, organizations, and contacts visited is prohibited without advance approval from the organization.

Sources: The American Productivity and Quality Center, www.apqc.org, and the Qualserve Benchmarking Clearinghouse, www.awwa.org (accessed September 14, 2005).

disadvantage and which cost components are responsible. Such information is vital in strategic actions to eliminate a cost disadvantage or create a cost advantage. One of the fundamental insights of value chain analysis and benchmarking is that *a company's competitiveness on cost depends on how efficiently it manages its value chain activities relative to how well competitors manage theirs.*[19] There are three main areas in a company's overall value chain where important differences in the costs of competing firms can occur: a company's own activity segments, suppliers' part of the industry value chain, and the forward channel portion of the industry chain.

Remedying an Internal Cost Disadvantage   When a company's cost disadvantage stems from performing internal value chain activities at a higher cost than key rivals, then managers can pursue any of several strategic approaches to restore cost parity:[20]

1.   Implement the use of best practices throughout the company, particularly for high-cost activities.

2.   Try to eliminate some cost-producing activities altogether by revamping the value chain. Examples include cutting out low-value-added activities or bypassing the value chains and associated costs of distribution allies and marketing directly to end users. Dell has used this approach in PCs, and airlines have begun bypassing travel agents by getting passengers to purchase their tickets directly at airline Web sites.

3.   Relocate high-cost activities (such as manufacturing) to geographic areas—such as China, Latin America, or Eastern Europe—where they can be performed more cheaply.

4.   See if certain internally performed activities can be outsourced from vendors or performed by contractors more cheaply than they can be done in-house.

5.   Invest in productivity-enhancing, cost-saving technological improvements (robotics, flexible manufacturing techniques, state-of-the-art electronic networking).

6.   Find ways to detour around the activities or items where costs are high—computer chip makers regularly design around the patents held by others to avoid paying royalties; automakers have substituted lower-cost plastic and rubber for metal at many exterior body locations.

7.   Redesign the product and/or some of its components to facilitate speedier and more economical manufacture or assembly.

8.   Try to make up the internal cost disadvantage by reducing costs in the supplier or forward channel portions of the industry value chain—usually a last resort.

Remedying a Supplier-Related Cost Disadvantage   Supplier-related cost disadvantages can be attacked by pressuring suppliers for lower prices, switching to lower-priced substitute inputs, and collaborating closely with suppliers to identify mutual cost-saving opportunities.[21] For example, just-in-time deliveries from suppliers can lower a company's inventory and internal logistics costs and may also allow its suppliers to economize on their warehousing, shipping, and production scheduling costs—a win–win outcome for both. In a few instances, companies may find that it is cheaper to integrate backward into the business of high-cost suppliers and make the item in-house instead of buying it from outsiders. If a company strikes out in wringing savings out of its high-cost supply chain activities, then it must resort to finding cost savings either in-house or in the forward channel portion of the industry value chain to offset its supplier-related cost disadvantage.

Remedying a Cost Disadvantage Associated with Activities Performed by Forward Channel Allies   There are three main ways to combat a cost disadvantage in the forward portion of the industry value chain:

1.   Pressure dealer-distributors and other forward channel allies to reduce their costs and markups so as to make the final price to buyers more competitive with the prices of rivals.

2. Work closely with forward channel allies to identify win–win opportunities to reduce costs. For example, a chocolate manufacturer learned that by shipping its bulk chocolate in liquid form in tank cars instead of 10-pound molded bars, it could not only save its candy bar manufacturing customers the costs associated with unpacking and melting but also eliminate its own costs of molding bars and packing them.

3. Change to a more economical distribution strategy, including switching to cheaper distribution channels (perhaps direct sales via the Internet) or perhaps integrating forward into company-owned retail outlets.

If these efforts fail, the company can either try to live with the cost disadvantage or pursue cost-cutting earlier in the value chain system.

Translating Proficient Performance of Value Chain Activities into Competitive Advantage

Performing value chain activities in ways that give a company the capabilities to either outmatch the competencies and capabilities of rivals or else beat them on costs are two good ways to secure competitive advantage.

A company that does a *first-rate job* of managing its value chain activities *relative to competitors* stands a good chance of achieving sustainable competitive advantage. As shown in Figure 4.5, outmanaging rivals in performing value chain activities can be accomplished in either or both of two ways: (1) by astutely developing core competencies and maybe a distinctive competence that rivals don't have or can't quite match and that are instrumental in helping it deliver attractive value to customers, and/or (2) by simply doing an overall better job than rivals of lowering its combined costs of performing all the various value chain activities, such that it ends up with a low-cost advantage over rivals.

The first of these two approaches begins with management efforts to build more organizational expertise in performing certain competitively important value chain activities, deliberately striving to develop competencies and capabilities that add power to its strategy and competitiveness. If management begins to make selected competencies and capabilities cornerstones of its strategy and continues to invest resources in building greater and greater proficiency in performing them, then over time one (or maybe several) of the targeted competencies/capabilities may rise to the level of a core competence. Later, following additional organizational learning and investments in gaining still greater proficiency, a core competence could evolve into a distinctive competence, giving the company superiority over rivals in performing an important value chain activity. Such superiority, if it gives the company significant competitive clout in the marketplace, can produce an attractive competitive edge over rivals and, more important, prove difficult for rivals to match or offset with competencies and capabilities of their own making. As a general rule, it is substantially harder for rivals to achieve best-in-industry proficiency in performing a key value chain activity than it is for them to clone the features and attributes of a hot-selling product or service.[22] This is especially true when a company with a distinctive competence avoids becoming complacent and works diligently to maintain its industry-leading expertise and capability. GlaxoSmithKline, one of the world's most competitively capable pharmaceutical companies, has built its business position around expert performance of a few competitively crucial activities: extensive R&D to achieve first discovery of new drugs, a carefully constructed approach to patenting, skill in gaining rapid and thorough clinical clearance through regulatory bodies, and unusually strong distribution and sales-force

Figure 4.5   **Translating Company Performance of Value Chain Activities into Competitive Advantage**

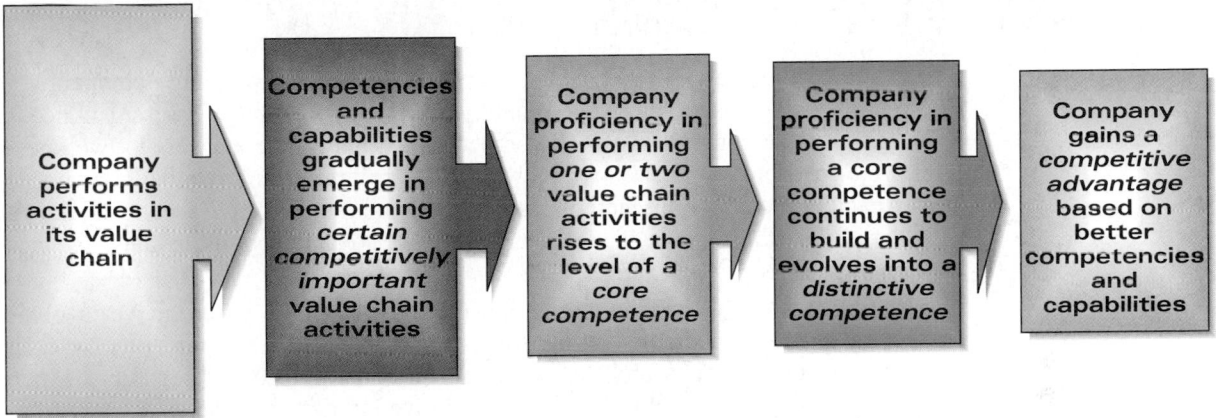

Option 1: Beat rivals in performing value chain activities more proficiently

Company performs activities in its value chain → Competencies and capabilities gradually emerge in performing *certain competitively important* value chain activities → Company proficiency in performing *one or two* value chain activities rises to the level of a *core competence* → Company proficiency in performing a core competence continues to build and evolves into a *distinctive competence* → Company gains a *competitive advantage* based on better competencies and capabilities

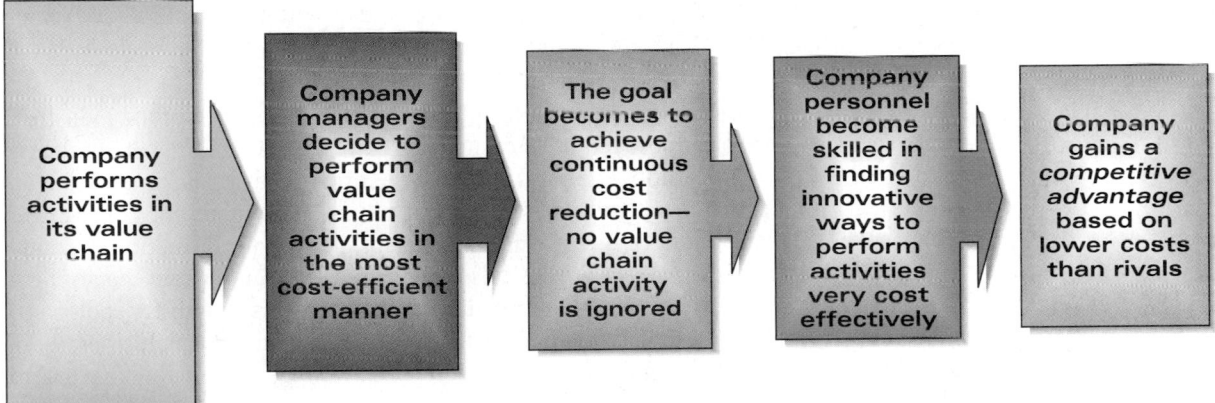

Option 2: Beat rivals in performing value chain activities more cheaply

Company performs activities in its value chain → Company managers decide to perform value chain activities in the most cost-efficient manner → The goal becomes to achieve continuous cost reduction—no value chain activity is ignored → Company personnel become skilled in finding innovative ways to perform activities very cost effectively → Company gains a *competitive advantage* based on lower costs than rivals

capabilities.[23] FedEx's astute management of its value chain has produced unmatched competencies and capabilities in overnight package delivery.

The second approach to building competitive advantage entails determined management efforts to be cost-efficient in performing value chain activities. Such efforts have to be ongoing and persistent, and they have to involve each and every value chain activity. The goal must be continuous cost reduction, not a one-time or on-again/off-again effort. Companies whose managers are truly committed to low-cost performance of value chain activities and succeed in engaging company personnel to discover innovative ways to drive costs out of the business have a real chance of gaining a durable low-cost edge over rivals. It is not as easy as it seems to imitate a company's low-cost practices. Companies like Wal-Mart, Dell, Nucor Steel, Southwest Airlines,

Toyota, and French discount retailer Carrefour have been highly successful in managing their values chains in a low-cost manner.

QUESTION 4: IS THE COMPANY COMPETITIVELY STRONGER OR WEAKER THAN KEY RIVALS?

Using value chain analysis and benchmarking to determine a company's competitiveness on price is necessary but not sufficient. A more comprehensive assessment needs to be made of the company's overall competitive strength. The answers to two questions are of particular interest: First, how does the company rank relative to competitors on each of the important factors that determine market success? Second, all things considered, does the company have a net competitive advantage or disadvantage versus major competitors?

An easy-to-use method for answering the two questions posed above involves developing quantitative strength ratings for the company and its key competitors on each industry key success factor and each competitively pivotal resource capability. Much of the information needed for doing a competitive strength assessment comes from previous analyses. Industry and competitive analysis reveals the key success factors and competitive capabilities that separate industry winners from losers. Benchmarking data and scouting key competitors provide a basis for judging the competitive strength of rivals on such factors as cost, key product attributes, customer service, image and reputation, financial strength, technological skills, distribution capability, and other competitively important resources and capabilities. SWOT analysis reveals how the company in question stacks up on these same strength measures.

Step 1 in doing a competitive strength assessment is to make a list of the industry's key success factors and most telling measures of competitive strength or weakness (6 to 10 measures usually suffice). Step 2 is to rate the firm and its rivals on each factor. Numerical rating scales (e.g., from 1 to 10) are best to use, although ratings of stronger (+), weaker (−), and about equal (=) may be appropriate when information is scanty and assigning numerical scores conveys false precision. Step 3 is to sum the strength ratings on each factor to get an overall measure of competitive strength for each company being rated. Step 4 is to use the overall strength ratings to draw conclusions about the size and extent of the company's net competitive advantage or disadvantage and to take specific note of areas of strength and weakness.

Table 4.5 provides two examples of competitive strength assessment, using the hypothetical ABC Company against four rivals. The first example employs an *unweighted rating system.* With unweighted ratings, each key success factor/competitive strength measure is assumed to be equally important (a rather dubious assumption). Whichever company has the highest strength rating on a given measure has an implied competitive edge on that factor; the size of its edge is mirrored in the margin of difference between its rating and the ratings assigned to rivals—a rating of 9 for one company versus ratings of 5, 4, and 3, respectively, for three other companies indicates a bigger advantage than a rating of 9 versus ratings of 8, 7, and 6. Summing a company's ratings on all the measures produces an overall strength rating. The higher a company's overall strength rating, the stronger its overall competitiveness versus rivals. The bigger the difference between a company's overall rating and the scores of *lower-rated* rivals, the greater its implied *net competitive advantage.* Conversely, the bigger the difference between a company's overall rating and the scores of *higher-rated* rivals, the greater its implied

Table 4.5 **Illustrations of Unweighted and Weighted Competitive Strength Assessments**

A. An Unweighted Competitive Strength Assessment

Key Success Factor/Strength Measure	ABC Co.	Strength Rating (Scale: 1 = Very weak; 10 = Very strong)			
		Rival 1	Rival 2	Rival 3	Rival 4
Quality/product performance	8	5	10	1	6
Reputation/image	8	7	10	1	6
Manufacturing capability	2	10	4	5	1
Technological skills	10	1	7	3	8
Dealer network/distribution capability	9	4	10	5	1
New product innovation capability	9	4	10	5	1
Financial resources	5	10	7	3	1
Relative cost position	5	10	3	1	4
Customer service capabilities	5	7	10	1	4
Unweighted overall strength rating	61	58	71	25	32

B. A Weighted Competitive Strength Assessment
(Rating Scale: 1 = Very weak; 10 = Very strong)

Key Success Factor/Strength Measure	Importance Weight	ABC Co.		Rival 1		Rival 2		Rival 3		Rival 4	
		Strength Rating	Score	Strength Rating	Score	Strength Rating	Score	Strength Rating	Score	Strength Rating	Score
Quality/product performance	0.10	8	0.80	5	0.50	10	1.00	1	0.10	6	0.60
Reputation/image	0.10	8	0.80	7	0.70	10	1.00	1	0.10	6	0.60
Manufacturing capability	0.10	2	0.20	10	1.00	4	0.40	5	0.50	1	0.10
Technological skills	0.05	10	0.50	1	0.05	7	0.35	3	0.15	8	0.40
Dealer network/distribution capability	0.05	9	0.45	4	0.20	10	0.50	5	0.25	1	0.05
New product innovation capability	0.05	9	0.45	4	0.20	10	0.50	5	0.25	1	0.05
Financial resources	0.10	5	0.50	10	1.00	7	0.70	3	0.30	1	0.10
Relative cost position	0.30	5	1.50	10	3.00	3	0.95	1	0.30	4	1.20
Customer service capabilities	0.15	5	0.75	7	1.05	10	1.50	1	0.15	4	0.60
Sum of importance weights	1.00										
Weighted overall strength rating		61	**5.95**	58	**7.70**	71	**6.85**	25	**2.10**	32	**3.70**

net competitive disadvantage. Thus, ABC's total score of 61 (see the top half of Table 4.5) signals a much greater net competitive advantage over Rival 4 (with a score of 32) than over Rival 1 (with a score of 58) but indicates a moderate net competitive disadvantage against Rival 2 (with an overall score of 71).

However, a better method is a *weighted rating system* (shown in the bottom half of Table 4.5) because the different measures of competitive strength are unlikely to be equally important. In an industry where the products/services of rivals are virtually identical, for instance, having low unit costs relative to rivals is nearly always the most important determinant of competitive strength. In an industry with strong product differentiation, the most significant measures of competitive strength

> A weighted competitive strength analysis is conceptually stronger than an unweighted analysis because of the inherent weakness in assuming that all the strength measures are equally important.

may be brand awareness, amount of advertising, product attractiveness, and distribution capability. In a weighted rating system each measure of competitive strength is assigned a weight based on its perceived importance in shaping competitive success. A weight could be as high as 0.75 (maybe even higher) in situations where one particular competitive variable is overwhelmingly decisive, or a weight could be as low as 0.20 when two or three strength measures are more important than the rest. Lesser competitive strength indicators can carry weights of 0.05 or 0.10. No matter whether the differences between the importance weights are big or little, *the sum of the weights must equal 1.0.*

Weighted strength ratings are calculated by rating each competitor on each strength measure (using the 1 to 10 rating scale) and multiplying the assigned rating by the assigned weight (a rating of 4 times a weight of 0.20 gives a weighted rating, or score, of 0.80). Again, the company with the highest rating on a given measure has an implied competitive edge on that measure, with the size of its edge reflected in the difference between its rating and rivals' ratings. The weight attached to the measure indicates how important the edge is. Summing a company's weighted strength ratings for all the measures yields an overall strength rating. Comparisons of the weighted overall strength scores indicate which competitors are in the strongest and weakest competitive positions and who has how big a net competitive advantage over whom.

Note in Table 4.5 that the unweighted and weighted rating schemes produce different orderings of the companies. In the weighted system, ABC Company drops from second to third in strength, and Rival 1 jumps from third to first because of its high strength ratings on the two most important factors. Weighting the importance of the strength measures can thus make a significant difference in the outcome of the assessment.

Interpreting the Competitive Strength Assessments

> High competitive strength ratings signal a strong competitive position and possession of competitive advantage; low ratings signal a weak position and competitive disadvantage.

Competitive strength assessments provide useful conclusions about a company's competitive situation. The ratings show how a company compares against rivals, factor by factor or capability by capability, thus revealing where it is strongest and weakest, and against whom. Moreover, the overall competitive strength scores indicate how all the different factors add up—whether the company is at a net competitive advantage or disadvantage against each rival. The firm with the largest overall competitive strength rating enjoys the strongest competitive position, with the size of its net competitive advantage reflected by how much its score exceeds the scores of rivals.

In addition, the strength ratings provide guidelines for designing wise offensive and defensive strategies. For example, consider the ratings and weighted scores in the bottom half of Table 4.5. If ABC Company wants to go on the offensive to win additional sales and market share, such an offensive probably needs to be aimed directly at winning customers away from Rivals 3 and 4 (which have lower overall strength scores) rather than Rivals 1 and 2 (which have higher overall strength scores). Moreover, while ABC has high ratings for quality/product performance (an 8 rating), reputation/image (an 8 rating), technological skills (a 10 rating), dealer network/distribution capability (a 9 rating), and new product innovation capability (a 9 rating), these strength measures have low importance weights—meaning that ABC has strengths in areas that don't translate into much competitive clout in the marketplace. Even so, it outclasses Rival 3 in all five areas, plus it enjoys lower costs than Rival 3: On relative cost position ABC has a 5 rating versus a 1 rating for Rival 3—and relative cost position carries the highest importance weight of all the strength measures. ABC also has greater competitive strength than Rival 3 as concerns customer service capabilities (which carries the second-highest importance weight). Hence, because ABC's strengths are in the very areas where Rival 3 is weak, ABC is in good position to attack Rival 3—it may well be able to persuade a number of Rival 3's customers to switch their purchases over to ABC's product.

But in mounting an offensive to win customers away from Rival 3, ABC should note that Rival 1 has an excellent relative cost position—its rating of 10, combined with the importance weight of 0.30 for relative cost, means that Rival 1 has meaningfully lower costs in an industry where low costs are competitively important. Rival 1 is thus strongly positioned to retaliate against ABC with lower prices if ABC's strategy offensive ends up drawing customers away from Rival 1. Moreover, Rival 1's very strong relative cost position vis-à-vis all the other companies arms it with the ability to use its lower-cost advantage to underprice all of its rivals and gain sales and market share at their expense. If ABC wants to defend against its vulnerability to potential price cutting by Rival 1, then it needs to aim a portion of its strategy at lowering its costs.

The point here is that a competitively astute company should use the strength assessment in deciding what strategic moves to make—which strengths to exploit in winning business away from rivals and which competitive weaknesses to try to correct. When a company has important competitive strengths in areas where one or more rivals are weak, it makes sense to consider offensive moves to exploit rivals' competitive weaknesses. When a company has important competitive weaknesses in areas where one or more rivals are strong, it makes sense to consider defensive moves to curtail its vulnerability.

> A company's competitive strength scores pinpoint its strengths and weaknesses against rivals and point directly to the kinds of offensive/defensive actions it can use to exploit its competitive strengths and reduce its competitive vulnerabilities.

QUESTION 5: WHAT STRATEGIC ISSUES AND PROBLEMS MERIT FRONT-BURNER MANAGERIAL ATTENTION?

The final and most important analytical step is to zero in on exactly what strategic issues that company managers need to address—and resolve—for the company to be more financially and competitively successful in the years ahead. This step involves drawing on the results of both industry and competitive analysis and the evaluations of the company's own competitiveness. The task here is to get a clear fix on exactly what strategic and competitive challenges confront the company, which of the company's competitive shortcomings need fixing, what obstacles stand in the way of improving the company's competitive position in the marketplace, and what specific problems

Zeroing in on the strategic issues a company faces and compiling a "worry list" of problems and roadblocks creates a strategic agenda of problems that merit prompt managerial attention.

Actually deciding upon a strategy and what specific actions to take is what comes *after* developing the list of strategic issues and problems that merit front-burner management attention.

A good strategy must contain ways to deal with all the strategic issues and obstacles that stand in the way of the company's financial and competitive success in the years ahead.

merit front-burner attention by company managers. *Pinpointing the precise things that management needs to worry about sets the agenda for deciding what actions to take next to improve the company's performance and business outlook.*

The "worry list" of issues and problems that have to be wrestled with can include such things as *how* to stave off market challenges from new foreign competitors, *how* to combat the price discounting of rivals, *how* to reduce the company's high costs and pave the way for price reductions, *how* to sustain the company's present rate of growth in light of slowing buyer demand, *whether* to expand the company's product line, *whether* to correct the company's competitive deficiencies by acquiring a rival company with the missing strengths, *whether* to expand into foreign markets rapidly or cautiously, *whether* to reposition the company and move to a different strategic group, *what to do* about growing buyer interest in substitute products, and *what to do* to combat the aging demographics of the company's customer base. The worry list thus always centers on such concerns as "how to . . .," "what to do about . . .," and "whether to . . ."—the purpose of the worry list is to identify the specific issues/problems that management needs to address, not to figure out what specific actions to take. Deciding what to do—which strategic actions to take and which strategic moves to make—comes later (when it is time to craft the strategy and choose from among the various strategic alternatives).

If the items on the worry list are relatively minor—which suggests the company's strategy is mostly on track and reasonably well matched to the company's overall situation—then company managers seldom need to go much beyond fine-tuning of the present strategy. If, however, the issues and problems confronting the company are serious and indicate the present strategy is not well suited for the road ahead, the task of crafting a better strategy has got to go to the top of management's action agenda.

Key Points

There are five key questions to consider in analyzing a company's own particular competitive circumstances and its competitive position vis-à-vis key rivals:

1. *How well is the present strategy working?* This involves evaluating the strategy from a qualitative standpoint (completeness, internal consistency, rationale, and suitability to the situation) and also from a quantitative standpoint (the strategic and financial results the strategy is producing). The stronger a company's current overall performance, the less likely the need for radical strategy changes. The weaker a company's performance and/or the faster the changes in its external situation (which can be gleaned from industry and competitive analysis), the more its current strategy must be questioned.

2. *What are the company's resource strengths and weaknesses, and its external opportunities and threats?* A SWOT analysis provides an overview of a firm's situation and is an essential component of crafting a strategy tightly matched to the company's situation. The two most important parts of SWOT analysis are (*a*) drawing conclusions about what story the compilation of strengths, weaknesses, opportunities, and threats tells about the company's overall situation, and

(b) acting on those conclusions to better match the company's strategy, to its resource strengths and market opportunities, to correct the important weaknesses, and to defend against external threats. A company's resource strengths, competencies, and competitive capabilities are strategically relevant because they are the most logical and appealing building blocks for strategy; resource weaknesses are important because they may represent vulnerabilities that need correction. External opportunities and threats come into play because a good strategy necessarily aims at capturing a company's most attractive opportunities and at defending against threats to its well-being.

3. *Are the company's prices and costs competitive?* One telling sign of whether a company's situation is strong or precarious is whether its prices and costs are competitive with those of industry rivals. Value chain analysis and benchmarking are essential tools in determining whether the company is performing particular functions and activities cost-effectively, learning whether its costs are in line with competitors, and deciding which internal activities and business processes need to be scrutinized for improvement. Value chain analysis teaches that how competently a company manages its value chain activities relative to rivals is a key to building a competitive advantage based on either better competencies and competitive capabilities or lower costs than rivals.

4. *Is the company competitively stronger or weaker than key rivals?* The key appraisals here involve how the company matches up against key rivals on industry key success factors and other chief determinants of competitive success and whether and why the company has a competitive advantage or disadvantage. Quantitative competitive strength assessments, using the method presented in Table 4.5, indicate where a company is competitively strong and weak, and provide insight into the company's ability to defend or enhance its market position. As a rule a company's competitive strategy should be built around its competitive strengths and should aim at shoring up areas where it is competitively vulnerable. When a company has important competitive strengths in areas where one or more rivals are weak, it makes sense to consider offensive moves to exploit rivals' competitive weaknesses. When a company has important competitive weaknesses in areas where one or more rivals are strong, it makes sense to consider defensive moves to curtail its vulnerability.

5. *What strategic issues and problems merit front-burner managerial attention?* This analytical step zeros in on the strategic issues and problems that stand in the way of the company's success. It involves using the results of both industry and competitive analysis and company situation analysis to identify a "worry list" of issues to be resolved for the company to be financially and competitively successful in the years ahead. The worry list always centers on such concerns as "how to . . .," "what to do about . . .," and "whether to . . ."—the purpose of the worry list is to identify the specific issues/problems that management needs to address. Actually deciding upon a strategy and what specific actions to take is what comes after the list of strategic issues and problems that merit front-burner management attention is developed.

Good company situation analysis, like good industry and competitive analysis, is a valuable precondition for good strategy making. A competently done evaluation of a company's resource capabilities and competitive strengths exposes strong and weak points in the present strategy and how attractive or unattractive the company's competitive position is and why. Managers need such understanding to craft a strategy that is well suited to the company's competitive circumstances.

Exercises

1. Review the information in Illustration Capsule 4.1 concerning the costs of the different value chain activities associated with recording and distributing music CDs through traditional brick-and-mortar retail outlets. Then answer the following questions:

   a. Does the growing popularity of downloading music from the Internet give rise to a new music industry value chain that differs considerably from the traditional value chain? Explain why or why not.

   b. What costs are cut out of the traditional value chain or bypassed when *online music retailers* (Apple, Sony, Microsoft, Musicmatch, Napster, Cdigix, and others) sell songs directly to online buyers? (Note: In 2005, online music stores were selling download-only titles for $0.79 to $0.99 per song and $9.99 for most albums.)

   c. What costs would be cut out of the traditional value chain or bypassed in the event that *recording studios* sell downloadable files of artists' recordings directly to online buyers?

   d. What happens to the traditional value chain if more and more music lovers use peer-to-peer file-sharing software to download music from the Internet to play music on their PCs or MP3 players or make their own CDs? (Note: It was estimated that, in 2004, about 1 billion songs were available for online trading and file sharing via such programs as Kazaa, Grokster, Shareaza, BitTorrent, and eDonkey, despite the fact that some 4,000 people had been sued by the Recording Industry Association of America for pirating copyrighted music via peer-to-peer file sharing.)

2. Using the information in Table 4.1 and the following financial statement information for Avon Products, calculate the following ratios for Avon for both 2003 and 2004:

   a. Gross profit margin.

   b. Operating profit margin.

   c. Net profit margin.

   d. Return on total assets.

   e. Return on stockholders' equity.

   f. Debt-to-equity ratio.

   g. Times-interest-earned.

   h. Days of inventory.

   i. Inventory turnover ratio.

   j. Average collection period.

   Based on these ratios, did Avon's financial performance improve, weaken, or remain about the same from 2003 to 2004?

Avon Products Inc., Consolidated Statements of Income
(in millions, except per share data)

	Years Ended December 31	
	2004	2003
Net sales	$7,656.2	$6,773.7
Other revenue	91.6	71.4
Total revenue	7,747.8	6,845.1
Costs, expenses and other:		
Cost of sales	2,911.7	2,611.8
Marketing, distribution and administrative expenses	3,610.3	3,194.4
Special charges, net	(3.2)	(3.9)
Operating profit	1,229.0	1,042.8
Interest expense	33.8	33.3
Interest Income	(20.6)	(12.6)
Other expense (income), net	28.3	28.6
Total other expenses	41.5	49.3
Income before taxes and minority interest	1,187.5	993.5
Income taxes	330.6	318.9
Income before minority interest	856.9	674.6
Minority interest	(10.8)	(9.8)
Net income	$ 846.1	$ 664.8
Earnings per share:		
Basic	$ 1.79	$ 1.41
Diluted	$ 1.77	$ 1.39
Weighted-average shares outstanding (in millions):		
Basic	472.35	471.08
Diluted	477.96	483.13

Avon Products Inc. Consolidated Balance Sheets (in millions)

| | December 31 | |
	2004	2003
Current assets		
Cash, including cash equivalents of $401.2 and $373.8	$ 769.6	$ 694.0
Accounts receivable (less allowances of $101.0 and $81.1)	599.1	553.2
Inventories	740.5	653.4
Prepaid expenses and other	397.2	325.5
Total current assets	$2,506.4	$2,226.1
Property, plant and equipment, at cost:		
Land	$ 61.7	$ 58.6
Buildings and improvements	886.8	765.9
Equipment	1,006.7	904.4
	1,955.2	1,728.9
Less accumulated depreciation	(940.4)	(873.3)
	1,014.8	855.6
Other assets	626.9	499.9
Total assets	$4,148.1	$3,581.6
Liabilities and shareholders' equity		
Current liabilities		
Debt maturing within one year	$ 51.7	$ 244.1
Accounts payable	490.1	400.1
Accrued compensation	164.5	149.5
Other accrued liabilities	360.1	332.6
Sales and taxes other than income	154.4	139.5
Income taxes	304.7	341.2
Total current liabilities	$1,525.5	$1,607.0
Long-term debt	$ 866.3	$ 877.7
Employee benefit plans	620.6	502.1
Deferred income taxes	12.1	50.6
Other liabilities (including minority interest of $42.5 and $46.0)	173.4	172.9
Total liabilities	$3,197.9	$3,210.3

(*Continued*)

	December 31	
	2004	2003
Shareholders' equity		
Common stock, par value $.25—authorized 1,500 shares; issued 728.61 and 722.25 shares	182.2	90.3
Additional paid-in capital	1,356.8	1,188.4
Retained earnings	2,693.5	2,202.4
Accumulated other comprehensive loss	(679.5)	(729.4)
Treasury stock, at cost—257.08 and 251.66 shares	(2,602.8)	(2,380.4)
Total shareholders' equity	950.2	371.3
Total liabilities and shareholders' equity	$4,148.1	$3,581.6

Source: Avon Products Inc., 2004 10-K

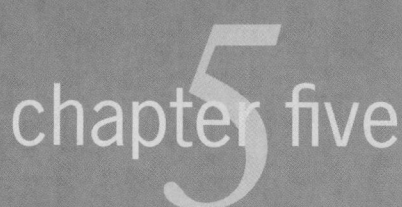
The Five Generic Competitive Strategies

Which One to Employ?

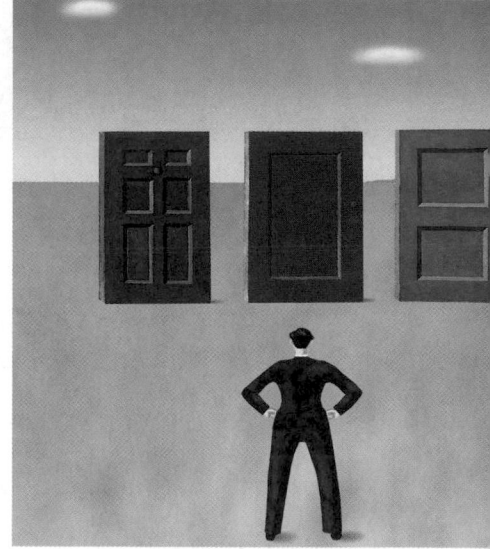

Competitive strategy is about being different. It means deliberately choosing to perform activities differently or to perform different activities than rivals to deliver a unique mix of value.

—**Michael E. Porter**

Strategy . . . is about first analyzing and then experimenting, trying, learning, and experimenting some more.

—**Ian C. McMillan and Rita Gunther McGrath**

Winners in business play rough and don't apologize for it. The nicest part of playing hardball is watching your competitors squirm.

—**George Stalk Jr. and Rob Lachenauer**

The essence of strategy lies in creating tomorrow's competitive advantages faster than competitors mimic the ones you possess today.

—**Gary Hamel and C. K. Prahalad**

This chapter describes the *five basic competitive strategy options*—which of the five to employ is a company's first and foremost choice in crafting an overall strategy and beginning its quest for competitive advantage. A company's **competitive strategy** deals exclusively with the specifics of management's game plan for competing successfully—its specific efforts to please customers, its offensive and defensive moves to counter the maneuvers of rivals, its responses to whatever market conditions prevail at the moment, its initiatives to strengthen its market position, and its approach to securing a competitive advantage vis-à-vis rivals. Companies the world over are imaginative in conceiving competitive strategies to win customer favor. At most companies the aim, quite simply, is to do a significantly better job than rivals of providing what buyers are looking for and thereby secure an upper hand in the marketplace.

> **Core Concept**
> A **competitive strategy** concerns the specifics of management's game plan for competing successfully and securing a competitive advantage over rivals.

A company achieves competitive advantage whenever it has some type of edge over rivals in attracting buyers and coping with competitive forces. There are many routes to competitive advantage, but they all involve giving buyers what they perceive as superior value compared to the offerings of rival sellers. Superior value can mean a good product at a lower price; a superior product that is worth paying more for; or a best-value offering that represents an attractive combination of price, features, quality, service, and other appealing attributes. Delivering superior value—whatever form it takes—nearly always requires performing value chain activities differently than rivals and building competencies and resource capabilities that are not readily matched.

> **Core Concept**
> The objective of competitive strategy is to knock the socks off rival companies by doing a better job of satisfying buyer needs and preferences.

THE FIVE GENERIC COMPETITIVE STRATEGIES

There are countless variations in the competitive strategies that companies employ, mainly because each company's strategic approach entails custom-designed actions to fit its own circumstances and industry environment. The custom-tailored nature of each company's strategy makes the chances remote that any two companies—even companies in the same industry—will employ strategies that are exactly alike in every detail. Managers at different companies always have a slightly different spin on future market conditions and how to best align their company's strategy with these conditions; moreover, they have different notions of how they intend to outmaneuver rivals and what strategic options make the most sense for their particular company. However, when one strips away the details to get at the real substance, the biggest and most important differences among competitive strategies boil down to (1) whether a company's market target is broad or narrow, and (2) whether the company is pursuing a competitive advantage linked to low costs or product differentiation. Five distinct competitive strategy approaches stand out:[1]

1. A *low-cost provider strategy*—striving to achieve lower overall costs than rivals and appealing to a broad spectrum of customers, usually by underpricing rivals.

2. A *broad differentiation strategy*—seeking to differentiate the company's product offering from rivals' in ways that will appeal to a broad spectrum of buyers.

3. A *best-cost provider strategy*—giving customers more value for their money by incorporating good-to-excellent product attributes at a lower cost than rivals; the target is to have the lowest (best) costs and prices compared to rivals offering products with comparable attributes.

Figure 5.1   **The Five Generic Competitive Strategies: Each Stakes Out a Different Market Position**

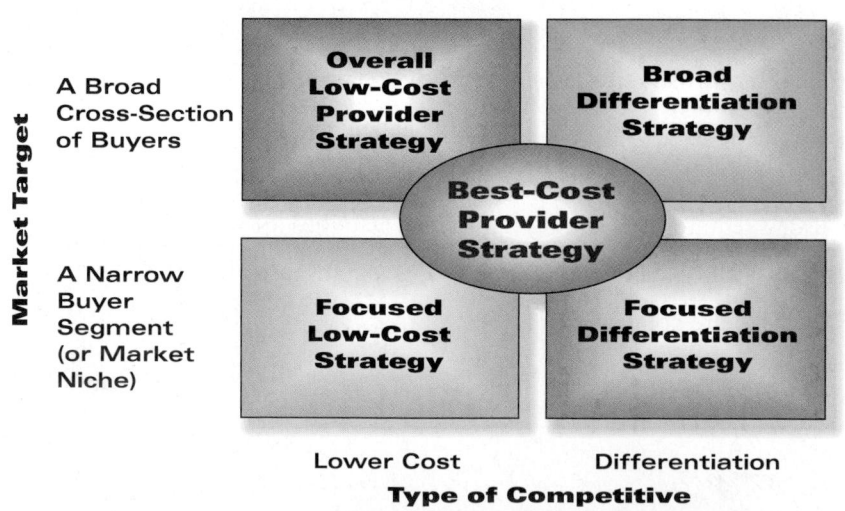

Source: This is an author-expanded version of a three-strategy classification discussed in Michael E. Porter, *Competitive Strategy: Techniques for Analyzing Industries and Competitors* (New York: Free Press, 1980), pp. 35–40.

4. *A focused (or market niche) strategy based on low costs*—concentrating on a narrow buyer segment and outcompeting rivals by having lower costs than rivals and thus being able to serve niche members at a lower price.

5. *A focused (or market niche) strategy based on differentiation*—concentrating on a narrow buyer segment and outcompeting rivals by offering niche members customized attributes that meet their tastes and requirements better than rivals' products.

Each of these five generic competitive approaches stakes out a different market position, as shown in Figure 5.1. Each involves distinctively different approaches to competing and operating the business. The remainder of this chapter explores the ins and outs of the five generic competitive strategies and how they differ.

LOW-COST PROVIDER STRATEGIES

Striving to be the industry's overall low-cost provider is a powerful competitive approach in markets with many price-sensitive buyers. A company achieves low-cost leadership when it becomes the industry's lowest-cost provider rather than just being one of perhaps several competitors with comparatively low costs. A low-cost provider's strategic target is meaningfully lower costs than rivals—but not necessarily the absolutely lowest possible cost. In striving for a cost advantage over rivals, managers must take care to include features and services that buyers consider essential—*a product offering that is too frills-free sabotages the attractiveness of the company's product and can turn buyers off even if it is priced lower than competing products.* For maximum effectiveness, companies employing a low-cost provider strategy need to achieve their cost advantage in ways difficult for rivals to copy or match. If rivals find it relatively easy or inexpensive to imitate the leader's low-cost methods, then the leader's advantage will be too short-lived to yield a valuable edge in the marketplace.

> **Core Concept**
> A low-cost leader's basis for competitive advantage is lower overall costs than competitors. Successful low-cost leaders are exceptionally good at finding ways to drive costs out of their businesses.

A company has two options for translating a low-cost advantage over rivals into attractive profit performance. Option 1 is to use the lower-cost edge to underprice competitors and attract price-sensitive buyers in great enough numbers to increase total profits. The trick to profitably underpricing rivals is either to keep the size of the price cut smaller than the size of the firm's cost advantage (thus reaping the benefits of both a bigger profit margin per unit sold and the added profits on incremental sales) or to generate enough added volume to increase total profits despite thinner profit margins (larger volume can make up for smaller margins provided the underpricing of rivals brings in enough extra sales). Option 2 is to maintain the present price, be content with the present market share, and use the lower-cost edge to earn a higher profit margin on each unit sold, thereby raising the firm's total profits and overall return on investment.

Illustration Capsule 5.1 describes Nucor Corporation's strategy for gaining low-cost leadership in manufacturing a variety of steel products.

The Two Major Avenues for Achieving a Cost Advantage

To achieve a low-cost edge over rivals, a firm's cumulative costs across its overall value chain must be lower than competitors' cumulative costs—and the means of achieving

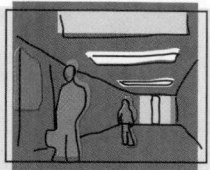

Illustration Capsule 5.1

Nucor Corporation's Low-Cost Provider Strategy

Nucor Corporation is the world's leading minimill producer of such steel products as carbon and alloy steel bars, beams, sheet, and plate; steel joists and joist girders; steel deck; cold finished steel; steel fasteners; metal building systems; and light gauge steel framing. In 2004, it had close to $10 billion in sales, 9,000 employees, and annual production capacity of nearly 22 million tons, making it the largest steel producer in the United States and one of the 10 largest in the world. The company has pursued a strategy that has made it among the world's lowest-cost producers of steel and has allowed the company to consistently outperform its rivals in terms of financial and market performance.

Nucor's low-cost strategy aims to give it a cost and pricing advantage in the commodity-like steel industry and leaves no part of the company's value chain neglected. The key elements of the strategy include the following:

- Using electric arc furnaces where scrap steel and directly reduced iron ore are melted and then sent to a continuous caster and rolling mill to be shaped into steel products, thereby eliminating an assortment of production processes from the value chain used by traditional integrated steel mills. Nucor's minimill value chain makes the use of coal, coke, and iron ore unnecessary; cuts investment in facilities and equipment (eliminating coke ovens, blast furnaces, basic oxygen furnaces, and ingot casters); and requires fewer employees than integrated mills.

- Striving hard for continuous improvement in the efficiency of its plants and frequently investing in state-of-the-art equipment to reduce unit costs. Nucor is known for its technological leadership and its aggressive pursuit of production process innovation.

- Carefully selecting plant sites to minimize inbound and outbound shipping costs and to take advantage of low rates for electricity (electric arc furnaces are heavy users of electricity). Nucor tends to avoid locating new plants in geographic areas where labor unions are a strong influence.

- Hiring a nonunion workforce that uses team-based incentive compensation systems (often opposed by unions). Operating and maintenance employees and supervisors are paid weekly bonuses based on the productivity of their work group. The size of the bonus is based on the capabilities of the equipment employed and ranges from 80 percent to 150 percent of an employee's base pay; no bonus is paid if the equipment is not operating. Nucor's compensation program has boosted the company's labor productivity to levels nearly double the industry average while rewarding productive employees with annual compensation packages that exceed what their union counterparts earn by as much as 20 percent. Nucor has been able to attract and retain highly talented, productive, and dedicated employees. In addition, the company's healthy culture and results-oriented self-managed work teams allow the company to employ fewer supervisors than what would be needed with an hourly union workforce.

- Heavily emphasizing consistent product quality and has rigorous quality systems.

- Minimizing general and administrative expenses by maintaining a lean staff at corporate headquarters (fewer than 125 employees) and allowing only four levels of management between the CEO and production workers. Headquarters offices are modestly furnished and located in an inexpensive building. The company minimizes reports, paperwork, and meetings to keep managers focused on value-adding activities. Nucor is noted not only for its streamlined organizational structure but also for its frugality in travel and entertainment expenses—the company's top managers set the example by flying coach class, avoiding pricey hotels, and refraining from taking customers out for expensive dinners.

In 2001–2003, when many U.S. producers of steel products were in dire economic straits because of weak demand for steel and deep price discounting by foreign rivals, Nucor began acquiring state-of-the-art steelmaking facilities from bankrupt or nearly bankrupt rivals at bargain-basement prices, often at 20 to 25 percent of what it cost to construct the facilities. This has given Nucor much lower depreciation costs than rivals having comparable plants.

Nucor management's outstanding execution of its low-cost strategy and its commitment to drive down costs throughout its value chain has allowed it to compete aggressively on price, earn higher profit margins than rivals, and grow its business at a considerably faster rate than its integrated steel mill rivals.

Source: Company annual reports, news releases, and Web site.

the cost advantage must be durable. There are two ways to accomplish this:[2]

1. Do a better job than rivals of performing value chain activities more cost-effectively.
2. Revamp the firm's overall value chain to eliminate or bypass some cost-producing activities.

Let's look at each of the two approaches to securing a cost advantage.

Cost-Efficient Management of Value Chain Activities   For a company to do a more cost-efficient job of managing its value chain than rivals, managers must launch a concerted, ongoing effort to ferret out cost-saving opportunities in every part of the value chain. No activity can escape cost-saving scrutiny, and all company personnel must be expected to use their talents and ingenuity to come up with innovative and effective ways to keep costs down. All avenues for performing value chain activities at a lower cost than rivals have to be explored. Attempts to outmanage rivals on cost commonly involve such actions as:

1. *Striving to capture all available economies of scale.* Economies of scale stem from an ability to lower unit costs by increasing the scale of operation—there are many occasions when a large plant is more economical to operate than a small or medium-size plant or when a large distribution warehouse is more cost efficient than a small warehouse. Often, manufacturing economics can be achieved by using common parts and components in different models and/or by cutting back on the number of models offered (especially slow-selling ones) and then scheduling longer production runs for fewer models. In global industries, making separate products for each country market instead of selling a mostly standard product worldwide tends to boost unit costs because of lost time in model changeover, shorter production runs, and inability to reach the most economic scale of production for each country model.
2. *Taking full advantage of learning/experience curve effects.* The cost of performing an activity can decline over time as the learning and experience of company personnel builds. Learning/experience curve economies can stem from debugging and mastering newly introduced technologies, using the experiences and suggestions of workers to install more efficient plant layouts and assembly procedures, and the added speed and effectiveness that accrues from repeatedly picking sites for and building new plants, retail outlets, or distribution centers. Aggressively managed low-cost providers pay diligent attention to capturing the benefits of learning and experience and to keeping these benefits proprietary to whatever extent possible.
3. *Trying to operate facilities at full capacity.* Whether a company is able to operate at or near full capacity has a big impact on units costs when its value chain contains activities associated with substantial fixed costs. Higher rates of capacity utilization allow depreciation and other fixed costs to be spread over a larger unit volume, thereby lowering fixed costs per unit. The more capital-intensive the business, or the higher the percentage of fixed costs as a percentage of total costs, the more important that full-capacity operation becomes because there's such a stiff unit-cost penalty for underutilizing existing capacity. In such cases, finding ways to operate close to full capacity year-round can be an important source of cost advantage.
4. *Pursuing efforts to boost sales volumes and thus spread such costs as R&D, advertising, and selling and administrative costs out over more units.* The more units

a company sells, the more it lowers its unit costs for R&D, sales and marketing, and administrative overhead.

5. *Improving supply chain efficiency.* Many companies pursue cost reduction by partnering with suppliers to streamline the ordering and purchasing process via online systems, reduce inventory carrying costs via just-in-time inventory practices, economize on shipping and materials handling, and ferret out other cost-saving opportunities. A company with a core competence (or better still a distinctive competence) in cost-efficient supply chain management can sometimes achieve a sizable cost advantage over less adept rivals.

6. *Substituting the use of low-cost for high-cost raw materials or component parts.* If the costs of raw materials and parts are too high, a company can either substitute the use of lower-cost items or maybe even design the high-cost components out of the product altogether.

7. *Using online systems and sophisticated software to achieve operating efficiencies.* Data sharing, starting with customer orders and going all the way back to components production, coupled with the use of enterprise resource planning (ERP) and manufacturing execution system (MES) software, can make custom manufacturing just as cheap as mass production—and sometimes cheaper. Online systems and software can also greatly reduce production times and labor costs. Lexmark used ERP and MES software to cut its production time for inkjet printers from four hours to 24 minutes. Southwest Airlines uses proprietary software to schedule flights and assign flight crews cost-effectively.

8. *Adopting labor-saving operating methods.* Examples of ways for a company to economize on labor costs include the following: installing labor-saving technology, shifting production from geographic areas where labor costs are high to geographic areas where labor costs are low, avoiding the use of union labor where possible (because of work rules that can stifle productivity and because of union demands for above-market pay scales and costly fringe benefits), and using incentive compensation systems that promote high labor productivity.

9. *Using the company's bargaining power vis-à-vis suppliers to gain concessions.* Many large enterprises (e.g., Wal-Mart, Home Depot, the world's major motor vehicle producers) have used their bargaining clout in purchasing large volumes to wrangle good prices on their purchases from suppliers. Having greater buying power than rivals can be an important source of cost advantage.

10. *Being alert to the cost advantages of outsourcing and vertical integration.* Outsourcing the performance of certain value chain activities can be more economical than performing them in-house if outside specialists, by virtue of their expertise and volume, can perform the activities at lower cost. Indeed, outsourcing has in recent years become a widely used cost-reduction approach. However, there can be times when integrating the activities of either suppliers or distribution channel allies can allow an enterprise to detour suppliers or buyers who have an adverse impact on costs because of their considerable bargaining power.

In addition to the above means of achieving lower costs than rivals, managers can also achieve important cost savings by deliberately opting for an inherently economical strategy keyed to a frills-free product offering. For instance, a company can bolster its attempts to open up a durable cost advantage over rivals by:

- Having lower specifications for purchased materials, parts, and components than rivals do. Thus, a maker of personal computers (PCs) can use the cheapest hard drives, microprocessors, monitors, DVD drives, and other components it can find so as to end up with lower production costs than rival PC makers.

- Distributing the company's product only through low-cost distribution channels and avoiding high-cost distribution channels.
- Choosing to use the most economical method for delivering customer orders (even if it results in longer delivery times).

These strategy-related means of keeping costs low don't really involve "outmanaging" rivals, but they can nonetheless contribute materially to becoming the industry's low-cost leader.

Revamping the Value Chain to Curb or Eliminate Unnecessary Activities

Dramatic cost advantages can emerge from finding innovative ways to cut back on or entirely bypass certain cost-producing value chain activities. There are six primary ways companies can achieve a cost advantage by reconfiguring their value chains:

1. *Cutting out distributors and dealers by selling directly to customers.* Selling directly and bypassing the activities and costs of distributors or dealers can involve (1) having the company's own direct sales force (which adds the costs of maintaining and supporting a sales force but may well be cheaper than accessing customers through distributors or dealers) and/or (2) conducting sales operations at the company's Web site (Web site operations may be substantially cheaper than distributor or dealer channels). Costs in the wholesale/retail portions of the value chain frequently represent 35–50 percent of the price final consumers pay. There are several prominent examples in which companies have instituted a sell-direct approach to cutting costs out of the value chain. Software developers allow customers to download new programs directly from the Internet, eliminating the costs of producing and packaging CDs and cutting out the host of activities, costs, and markups associated with shipping and distributing software through wholesale and retail channels. By cutting all these costs and activities out of the value chain, software developers have the pricing room to boost their profit margins and still sell their products below levels that retailers would have to charge. The major airlines now sell most of their tickets directly to passengers via their Web sites, ticket counter agents, and telephone reservation systems, allowing them to save hundreds of millions of dollars in commissions once paid to travel agents.

2. *Replacing certain value chain activities with faster and cheaper online technology.* In recent years the Internet and Internet technology applications have become powerful and pervasive tools for conducting business and reengineering company and industry value chains. For instance, Internet technology has revolutionized supply chain management, turning many time-consuming and labor-intensive activities into paperless transactions performed instantaneously. Company procurement personnel can—with only a few mouse clicks—check materials inventories against incoming customer orders, check suppliers' stocks, check the latest prices for parts and components at auction and e-sourcing Web sites, and check FedEx delivery schedules. Various e-procurement software packages streamline the purchasing process by eliminating paper documents such as requests for quotations, purchase orders, order acceptances, and shipping notices. There's software that permits the relevant details of incoming customer orders to be instantly shared with the suppliers of needed parts and components. All this facilitates

just-in-time deliveries of parts and components and matching the production of parts and components to assembly plant requirements and production schedules, cutting out unnecessary activities and producing savings for both suppliers and manufacturers. Retailers can install online systems that relay data from cash register sales at the check-out counter back to manufacturers and their suppliers. Manufacturers can use online systems to collaborate closely with parts and components suppliers in designing new products and shortening the time it takes to get them into production. Online systems allow warranty claims and product performance problems involving supplier components to be instantly relayed to the relevant suppliers so that corrections can be expedited. Online systems have the further effect of breaking down corporate bureaucracies and reducing overhead costs. The whole back-office data management process (order processing, invoicing, customer accounting, and other kinds of transaction costs) can be handled fast, accurately, and with less paperwork and fewer personnel.

3. *Streamlining operations by eliminating low-value-added or unnecessary work steps and activities.* Examples include using computer-assisted design techniques, standardizing parts and components across models and styles, having suppliers collaborate to combine parts and components into modules so that products can be assembled in fewer steps, and shifting to an easy-to-manufacture product design. At Wal-Mart, some items supplied by manufacturers are delivered directly to retail stores rather than being routed through Wal-Mart's distribution centers and delivered by Wal-Mart trucks; in other instances, Wal-Mart unloads incoming shipments from manufacturers' trucks arriving at its distribution centers directly onto outgoing Wal-Mart trucks headed to particular stores without ever moving the goods into the distribution center. Many supermarket chains have greatly reduced in-store meat butchering and cutting activities by shifting to meats that are cut and packaged at the meat-packing plant and then delivered to their stores in ready-to-sell form.

4. *Relocating facilities so as to curb the need for shipping and handling activities.* Having suppliers locate facilities adjacent to the company's plant or locating the company's plants or warehouses near customers can help curb or eliminate shipping and handling costs.

5. *Offering a frills-free product.* Deliberately restricting a company's product offering to the essentials can help the company cut costs associated with snazzy attributes and a full lineup of options and extras. Activities and costs can also be eliminated by incorporating fewer performance and quality features into the product and by offering buyers fewer services. Stripping extras like first-class sections, meals, and reserved seating is a favorite technique of budget airlines like Southwest, Ryanair (Europe), easyJet (Europe), and Gol (Brazil).

6. *Offering a limited product line as opposed to a full product line.* Pruning slow-selling items from the product lineup and being content to meet the needs of most buyers rather than all buyers can eliminate activities and costs associated with numerous product versions and wide selection.

Illustration Capsule 5.2 describes how Wal-Mart has managed its value chain in the retail grocery portion of its business to achieve a dramatic cost advantage over rival supermarket chains and become the world's biggest grocery retailer.

Examples of Companies That Revamped Their Value Chains to Reduce Costs   Iowa Beef Packers (IBP), now a subsidiary of Tyson Foods, pioneered the

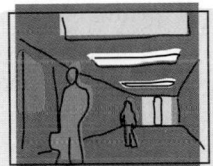

Illustration Capsule 5.2

How Wal-Mart Managed Its Value Chain to Achieve a Huge Low-Cost Advantage over Rival Supermarket Chains

Wal-Mart has achieved a very substantial cost and pricing advantage over rival supermarket chains both by revamping portions of the grocery retailing value chain and by out-managing its rivals in efficiently performing various value chain activities. Its cost advantage stems from a series of initiatives and practices:

- Instituting extensive information sharing with vendors via online systems that relay sales at its check-out counters directly to suppliers of the items, thereby providing suppliers with real-time information on customer demand and preferences (creating an estimated 6 percent cost advantage). It is standard practice at Wal-Mart to collaborate extensively with vendors on all aspects of the purchasing and store delivery process to squeeze out mutually beneficial cost savings. Procter & Gamble, Wal-Mart's biggest supplier, went so far as to integrate its enterprise resource planning (ERP) system with Wal-Mart's.

- Pursuing global procurement of some items and centralizing most purchasing activities so as to leverage the company's buying power (creating an estimated 2.5 percent cost advantage).

- Investing in state-of-the-art automation at its distribution centers, efficiently operating a truck fleet that makes daily deliveries to Wal-Mart's stores, and putting assorted other cost-saving practices into place at its headquarters, distribution centers, and stores (resulting in an estimated 4 percent cost advantage).

- Striving to optimize the product mix and achieve greater sales turnover (resulting in about a 2 percent cost advantage).

- Installing security systems and store operating procedures that lower shrinkage rates (producing a cost advantage of about 0.5 percent).

- Negotiating preferred real estate rental and leasing rates with real estate developers and owners of its store sites (yielding a cost advantage of 2 percent).

- Managing and compensating its workforce in a manner that produces lower labor costs (yielding an estimated 5 percent cost advantage)

Altogether, these value chain initiatives give Wal-Mart an approximately 22 percent cost advantage over Kroger, Safeway, and other leading supermarket chains. With such a sizable cost advantage, Wal-Mart has been able to underprice its rivals and become the world's leading supermarket retailer in little more than a decade.

Source: Developed by the authors from information at www.wal-mart.com (accessed September 15, 2004) and in Marco Iansiti and Roy Levien, "Strategy as Ecology," *Harvard Business Review* 82, no. 3 (March 2004), p. 70.

development of a cheaper value chain system in the beef-packing industry.[3] The traditional cost chain involved raising cattle on scattered farms and ranches; shipping them live to labor-intensive, unionized slaughtering plants; and then transporting whole sides of beef to grocery retailers whose butcher departments cut them into smaller pieces and packaged them for sale to grocery shoppers. IBP revamped the traditional chain with a radically different strategy: It built large automated plants employing nonunion workers near cattle supplies. Near the plants it arranged to set up large feed lots (or holding pens) where cattle were fed grain for a short time to fatten them up prior to slaughter. The meat was butchered at the processing plant into small, high-yield cuts. Some of the trimmed and boned cuts were vacuum-sealed in plastic casings for further butchering in supermarket meat departments, but others were trimmed and/or boned, put in plastic-sealed ready-to-sell trays, boxed, and shipped to retailers. IBP's strategy was to increase the volume of prepackaged, "case-ready" cuts that retail grocers could unpack from boxes and place directly into the meat case. In addition, IBP provided meat retailers with individually wrapped quick-frozen steaks, as well as precooked roasts, beef tip, and meatloaf selections that could be prepared in a matter of minutes. Iowa Beef's inbound cattle transportation expenses, traditionally a major cost item, were cut significantly by avoiding the weight losses that occurred when live animals were shipped long distances just prior to slaughter. Sizable major outbound shipping cost savings were achieved by not having to ship whole sides of beef, which had a high waste factor. Meat retailers had to do far less butchering to stock their meat cases. IBP value chain revamping was so successful that the company became the largest U.S. meatpacker.

Southwest Airlines has reconfigured the traditional value chain of commercial airlines to lower costs and thereby offer dramatically lower fares to passengers. Its mastery of fast turnarounds at the gates (about 25 minutes versus 45 minutes for rivals) allows its planes to fly more hours per day. This translates into being able to schedule more flights per day with fewer aircraft, allowing Southwest to generate more revenue per plane on average than rivals. Southwest does not offer in-flight meals, assigned seating, baggage transfer to connecting airlines, or first-class seating and service, thereby eliminating all the cost-producing activities associated with these features. The company's fast, user-friendly online reservation system facilitates e-ticketing and reduces staffing requirements at telephone reservation centers and airport counters. Its use of automated check-in equipment reduces staffing requirements for terminal check-in.

Dell has created the best, most cost-efficient value chain in the global personal computer industry. Whereas Dell's major rivals (Hewlett-Packard, Lenovo, Sony, and Toshiba) produce their models in volume and sell them through independent resellers and retailers, Dell has elected to market directly to PC users, building its PCs to customer specifications as orders come in and shipping them to customers within a few days of receiving the order. Dell's value chain approach has proved cost-effective in coping with the PC industry's blink-of-an-eye product life cycle. The build-to-order strategy enables the company to avoid misjudging buyer demand for its various models and being saddled with quickly obsolete excess components and finished-goods inventories—all parts and components are obtained on a just-in-time basis from vendors, many of which deliver their items to Dell assembly plants several times a day in volumes matched to the Dell's daily assembly schedule. Also, Dell's sell-direct strategy slices reseller/retailer costs and margins out of the value chain (although some of these savings are offset by the cost of Dell's direct marketing and customer support activities—functions that would otherwise be performed by resellers and retailers). Partnerships with suppliers that facilitate just-in-time deliveries of components and minimize Dell's inventory costs, coupled with Dell's extensive use of e-commerce technologies further reduce Dell's costs. Dell's value chain approach is widely considered to have made it the global low-cost leader in the PC industry.

The Keys to Success in Achieving Low-Cost Leadership

To succeed with a low-cost-provider strategy, company managers have to scrutinize each cost-creating activity and determine what factors cause costs to be high or low. Then they have to use this knowledge to keep the unit costs of each activity low, exhaustively pursuing cost efficiencies throughout the value chain. They have to be proactive in restructuring the value chain to eliminate nonessential work steps and low-value activities. Normally, low-cost producers work diligently to create cost-conscious corporate cultures that feature broad employee participation in continuous cost improvement efforts and limited perks and frills for executives. They strive to operate with exceptionally small corporate staffs to keep administrative costs to a minimum.

Many successful low-cost leaders also use benchmarking to keep close tabs on how their costs compare with rivals and firms performing comparable activities in other industries.

> Success in achieving a low-cost edge over rivals comes from outmanaging rivals in figuring out how to perform value chain activities most cost effectively and eliminating or curbing non essential value chain activities

But while low-cost providers are champions of frugality, they are usually aggressive in investing in resources and capabilities that promise to drive costs out of the business. Wal-Mart, one of the foremost practitioners of low-cost leadership, employs state-of-the-art technology throughout its operations—its distribution facilities are an automated showcase, it uses online systems to order goods from suppliers and manage inventories, it equips its stores with cutting-edge sales-tracking and check-out systems, and it sends daily point-of-sale data to 4,000 vendors. Wal-Mart's information and communications systems and capabilities are more sophisticated than those of virtually any other retail chain in the world.

Other companies noted for their successful use of low-cost provider strategies include Lincoln Electric in arc welding equipment, Briggs & Stratton in small gasoline engines, Bic in ballpoint pens, Black & Decker in power tools, Stride Rite in footwear, Beaird-Poulan in chain saws, and General Electric and Whirlpool in major home appliances.

When a Low-Cost Provider Strategy Works Best

A competitive strategy predicated on low-cost leadership is particularly powerful when:

1. *Price competition among rival sellers is especially vigorous*—Low-cost providers are in the best position to compete offensively on the basis of price, to use the appeal of lower price to grab sales (and market share) from rivals, to win the business of price-sensitive buyers, to remain profitable in the face of strong price competition, and to survive price wars.

2. *The products of rival sellers are essentially identical and supplies are readily available from any of several eager sellers*—Commodity-like products and/or ample supplies set the stage for lively price competition; in such markets, it is less efficient, higher-cost companies whose profits get squeezed the most.

3. *There are few ways to achieve product differentiation that have value to buyers*—When the differences between brands do not matter much to buyers, buyers are nearly always very sensitive to price differences and shop the market for the best price.

4. *Most buyers use the product in the same ways*—With common user requirements, a standardized product can satisfy the needs of buyers, in which case low selling price, not features or quality, becomes the dominant factor in causing buyers to choose one seller's product over another's.

5. *Buyers incur low costs in switching their purchases from one seller to another*—Low switching costs give buyers the flexibility to shift purchases to lower-priced sellers having equally good products or to attractively priced substitute products. A low-cost leader is well positioned to use low price to induce its customers not to switch to rival brands or substitutes.

6. *Buyers are large and have significant power to bargain down prices*—Low-cost providers have partial profit-margin protection in bargaining with high-volume buyers, since powerful buyers are rarely able to bargain price down past the survival level of the next most cost-efficient seller.

7. *Industry newcomers use introductory low prices to attract buyers and build a customer base*—The low-cost leader can use price cuts of its own to make it harder

A low-cost provider is in the best position to win the business of price-sensitive buyers, set the floor on market price, and still earn a profit.

for a new rival to win customers; the pricing power of the low-cost provider acts as a barrier for new entrants.

As a rule, the more price-sensitive buyers are, the more appealing a low-cost strategy becomes. A low-cost company's ability to set the industry's price floor and still earn a profit erects protective barriers around its market position.

The Pitfalls of a Low-Cost Provider Strategy

Perhaps the biggest pitfall of a low-cost provider strategy is getting carried away with overly aggressive price cutting and ending up with lower, rather than higher, profitability. A low-cost/low-price advantage results in superior profitability only if (1) prices are cut by less than the size of the cost advantage or (2) the added gains in unit sales are large enough to bring in a bigger total profit despite lower margins per unit sold. A company with a 5 percent cost advantage cannot cut prices 20 percent, end up with a volume gain of only 10 percent, and still expect to earn higher profits!

A second big pitfall is not emphasizing avenues of cost advantage that can be kept proprietary or that relegate rivals to playing catch-up. The value of a cost advantage depends on its sustainability. Sustainability, in turn, hinges on whether the company achieves its cost advantage in ways difficult for rivals to copy or match.

A low-cost provider's product offering must always contain enough attributes to be attractive to prospective buyers—low price, by itself, is not always appealing to buyers.

A third pitfall is becoming too fixated on cost reduction. Low cost cannot be pursued so zealously that a firm's offering ends up being too features-poor to generate buyer appeal. Furthermore, a company driving hard to push its costs down has to guard against misreading or ignoring increased buyer interest in added features or service, declining buyer sensitivity to price, or new developments that start to alter how buyers use the product. A low-cost zealot risks losing market ground if buyers start opting for more upscale or features-rich products.

Even if these mistakes are avoided, a low-cost competitive approach still carries risk. Cost-saving technological breakthroughs or the emergence of still-lower-cost value chain models can nullify a low-cost leader's hard-won position. The current leader may have difficulty in shifting quickly to the new technologies or value chain approaches because heavy investments lock it in (at least temporarily) to its present value chain approach.

BROAD DIFFERENTIATION STRATEGIES

Core Concept
The essence of a broad differentiation strategy is to be unique in ways that are valuable to a wide range of customers.

Differentiation strategies are attractive whenever buyers' needs and preferences are too diverse to be fully satisfied by a standardized product or by sellers with identical capabilities. A company attempting to succeed through differentiation must study buyers' needs and behavior carefully to learn what buyers consider important, what they think has value, and what they are willing to pay for. Then the company has to incorporate buyer-desired attributes into its product or service offering that will clearly set it apart from rivals. Competitive advantage results once a sufficient number of buyers become strongly attached to the differentiated attributes.

Successful differentiation allows a firm to:

- Command a premium price for its product, and/or
- Increase unit sales (because additional buyers are won over by the differentiating features), and/or

- Gain buyer loyalty to its brand (because some buyers are strongly attracted to the differentiating features and bond with the company and its products).

Differentiation enhances profitability whenever the extra price the product commands outweighs the added costs of achieving the differentiation. Company differentiation strategies fail when buyers don't value the brand's uniqueness and when a company's approach to differentiation is easily copied or matched by its rivals.

Types of Differentiation Themes

Companies can pursue differentiation from many angles: a unique taste (Dr Pepper, Listerine); multiple features (Microsoft Windows, Microsoft Office); wide selection and one-stop shopping (Home Depot, Amazon.com); superior service (FedEx); spare parts availability (Caterpillar); engineering design and performance (Mercedes, BMW); prestige and distinctiveness (Rolex); product reliability (Johnson & Johnson in baby products); quality manufacture (Karastan in carpets, Michelin in tires, Toyota and Honda in automobiles); technological leadership (3M Corporation in bonding and coating products); a full range of services (Charles Schwab in stock brokerage); a complete line of products (Campbell's soups); and top-of-the-line image and reputation (Ralph Lauren and Starbucks).

The most appealing approaches to differentiation are those that are hard or expensive for rivals to duplicate. Indeed, resourceful competitors can, in time, clone almost any product or feature or attribute. If Coca-Cola introduces a vanilla-flavored soft drink, so can Pepsi; if Ford offers a 50,000-mile bumper-to-bumper warranty on its new vehicles, so can Volkswagen and Nissan. If Nokia introduces cell phones with cameras and Internet capability, so can Motorola and Samsung. As a rule, differentiation yields a longer-lasting and more profitable competitive edge when it is based on product innovation, technical superiority, product quality and reliability, comprehensive customer service, and unique competitive capabilities. Such differentiating attributes tend to be tough for rivals to copy or offset profitably, and buyers widely perceive them as having value.

> Easy-to-copy differentiating features cannot produce sustainable competitive advantage; differentiation based on competencies and capabilities tend to be more sustainable.

Where along the Value Chain to Create the Differentiating Attributes

Differentiation is not something hatched in marketing and advertising departments, nor is it limited to the catchalls of quality and service. Differentiation opportunities can exist in activities all along an industry's value chain; possibilities include the following:

- *Supply chain activities* that ultimately spill over to affect the performance or quality of the company's end product. Starbucks gets high ratings on its coffees partly because it has very strict specifications on the coffee beans purchased from suppliers.
- *Product R&D activities* that aim at improved product designs and performance features, expanded end uses and applications, more frequent first-on-the-market victories, wider product variety and selection, added user safety, greater recycling capability, or enhanced environmental protection.
- *Production R&D and technology-related activities* that permit custom-order manufacture at an efficient cost; make production methods safer for the

environment; or improve product quality, reliability, and appearance. Many manufacturers have developed flexible manufacturing systems that allow different models and product versions to be made on the same assembly line. Being able to provide buyers with made-to-order products can be a potent differentiating capability.

- *Manufacturing activities* that reduce product defects, prevent premature product failure, extend product life, allow better warranty coverages, improve economy of use, result in more end-user convenience, or enhance product appearance. The quality edge enjoyed by Japanese automakers stems partly from their distinctive competence in performing assembly-line activities.

- *Distribution and shipping activities* that allow for fewer warehouse and on-the-shelf stockouts, quicker delivery to customers, more accurate order filling, and/or lower shipping costs.

- *Marketing, sales, and customer service activities* that result in superior technical assistance to buyers, faster maintenance and repair services, more and better product information provided to customers, more and better training materials for end users, better credit terms, quicker order processing, or greater customer convenience.

Managers need keen understanding of the sources of differentiation and the activities that drive uniqueness to evaluate various differentiation approaches and design durable ways to set their product offering apart from those of rival brands.

The Four Best Routes to Competitive Advantage via a Broad Differentiation Strategy

While it is easy enough to grasp that a successful differentiation strategy must entail creating buyer value in ways unmatched by rivals, the big issue in crafting a differentiation strategy is which of four basic routes to take in delivering unique buyer value via a broad differentiation strategy. Usually, building a sustainable competitive advantage via differentiation involves pursuing one of four basic routes to delivering superior value to buyers.

One route is to *incorporate product attributes and user features that lower the buyer's overall costs of using the company's product.* Making a company's product more economical for a buyer to use can be done by reducing the buyer's raw materials waste (providing cut-to-size components), reducing a buyer's inventory requirements (providing just-in-time deliveries), increasing maintenance intervals and product reliability so as to lower a buyer's repair and maintenance costs, using online systems to reduce a buyer's procurement and order processing costs, and providing free technical support. Rising costs for gasoline have dramatically spurred the efforts of motor vehicle manufacturers worldwide to introduce models with better fuel economy and reduce operating costs for motor vehicle owners.

A second route is to *incorporate features that raise product performance.*[4] This can be accomplished with attributes that provide buyers greater reliability, ease of use, convenience, or durability. Other performance-enhancing options include making the company's product or service cleaner, safer, quieter, or more maintenance-free than rival brands. Cell phone manufacturrs are in a race to introduce next-generation phones with trendsetting features and options.

A third route to a differentiation-based competitive advantage is to *incorporate features that enhance buyer satisfaction in noneconomic or intangible ways.* Goodyear's Aquatread tire design appeals to safety-conscious motorists wary of slick roads. Rolls Royce, Ralph Lauren, Gucci, Tiffany, Cartier, and Rolex have differentiation-based competitive advantages linked to buyer desires for status, image, prestige, upscale fashion, superior craftsmanship, and the finer things in life. L. L. Bean makes its mail-order customers feel secure in their purchases by providing an unconditional guarantee with no time limit: "All of our products are guaranteed to give 100 percent satisfaction in every way. Return anything purchased from us at any time if it proves otherwise. We will replace it, refund your purchase price, or credit your credit card, as you wish."

> **Core Concept**
> A differentiator's basis for competitive advantage is either a product/service offering whose attributes differ significantly from the offerings of rivals or a set of capabilities for delivering customer value that rivals don't have.

The fourth route is to *deliver value to customers by differentiating on the basis of competencies and competitive capabilities that rivals don't have or can't afford to match.*[5] The importance of cultivating competencies and capabilities that add power to a company's resource strengths and competitiveness comes into play here. Core and/or distinctive competencies not only enhance a company's ability to compete successfully in the marketplace but can also be unique in delivering value to buyers. There are numerous examples of companies that have differentiated themselves on the basis of capabilities. Because Fox News and CNN have the capability to devote more air time to breaking news stories and get reporters on the scene very quickly compared to the major networks, many viewers turn to the cable networks when a major news event occurs. Microsoft has stronger capabilities to design, create, distribute, and advertise an array of software products for PC applications than any of its rivals. Avon and Mary Kay Cosmetics have differentiated themselves from other cosmetics and personal care companies by assembling a sales force numbering in the hundreds of thousands that gives them direct sales capability—their sales associates can demonstrate products to interested buyers, take their orders on the spot, and deliver the items to buyers' homes. Japanese automakers have the capability to satisfy changing consumer preferences for one vehicle style versus another because they can bring new models to market faster than American and European automakers.

The Importance of Perceived Value and Signaling Value

Buyers seldom pay for value they don't perceive, no matter how real the unique extras may be.[6] Thus, the price premium commanded by a differentiation strategy reflects *the value actually delivered* to the buyer and *the value perceived* by the buyer (even if not actually delivered). Actual and perceived value can differ whenever buyers have trouble assessing what their experience with the product will be. Incomplete knowledge on the part of buyers often causes them to judge value based on such signals as price (where price connotes quality), attractive packaging, extensive ad campaigns (i.e., how well-known the product is), ad content and image, the quality of brochures and sales presentations, the seller's facilities, the seller's list of customers, the firm's market share, the length of time the firm has been in business, and the professionalism, appearance, and personality of the seller's employees. Such signals of value may be as important as actual value (1) when the nature of differentiation is subjective or hard to quantify, (2) when buyers are making a first-time purchase, (3) when repurchase is infrequent, and (4) when buyers are unsophisticated.

When a Differentiation Strategy Works Best

Differentiation strategies tend to work best in market circumstances where:

- *Buyer needs and uses of the product are diverse*—Diverse buyer preferences present competitors with a bigger window of opportunity to do things differently and set themselves apart with product attributes that appeal to particular buyers. For instance, the diversity of consumer preferences for menu selection, ambience, pricing, and customer service gives restaurants exceptionally wide latitude in creating a differentiated product offering. Other companies having many ways to strongly differentiate themselves from rivals include the publishers of magazines, the makers of motor vehicles, and the manufacturers of cabinetry and countertops.

- *There are many ways to differentiate the product or service and many buyers perceive these differences as having value*—There is plenty of room for retail apparel competitors to stock different styles and quality of apparel merchandise but very little room for the makers of paper clips, copier paper, or sugar to set their products apart. Likewise, the sellers of different brands of gasoline or orange juice have little differentiation opportunity compared to the sellers of high-definition TVs, patio furniture, or breakfast cereal. Unless different buyers have distinguishably different preferences for certain features and product attributes, profitable differentiation opportunities are very restricted.

- *Few rival firms are following a similar differentiation approach*—The best differentiation approaches involve trying to appeal to buyers on the basis of attributes that rivals are not emphasizing. A differentiator encounters less head-to-head rivalry when it goes its own separate way in creating uniqueness and does not try to outdifferentiate rivals on the very same attributes—when many rivals are all claiming "Ours tastes better than theirs" or "Ours gets your clothes cleaner than theirs," the most likely result is weak brand differentiation and "strategy overcrowding"—a situation in which competitors end up chasing the same buyers with very similar product offerings.

- *Technological change is fast-paced and competition revolves around rapidly evolving product features*—Rapid product innovation and frequent introductions of next-version products not only provide space for companies to pursue separate differentiating paths but also heighten buyer interest. In video game hardware and video games, golf equipment, PCs, cell phones, and MP3 players, competitors are locked into an ongoing battle to set themselves apart by introducing the best next-generation products—companies that fail to come up with new and improved products and distinctive performance features quickly lose out in the marketplace. In network TV broadcasting in the United States, NBC, ABC, CBS, Fox, and several others are always scrambling to develop a lineup of TV shows that will win higher audience ratings and pave the way for charging higher advertising rates and boosting ad revenues.

The Pitfalls of a Differentiation Strategy

Differentiation strategies can fail for any of several reasons. *A differentiation strategy is always doomed when competitors are able to quickly copy most or all of the appealing product attributes a company comes up with.* Rapid imitation means that no rival achieves differentiation, since whenever one firm introduces some aspect of uniqueness that strikes the fancy of buyers, fast-following copycats quickly reestablish similarity. This is why a firm must search out sources of uniqueness that are time-consuming or burdensome for rivals to match if it hopes to use differentiation to win a competitive edge over rivals.

*A second pitfall is that the company's differentiation strategy produces a ho-hum market reception because buyers see little value in the unique attributes of a company's produc*t. Thus, even if a company sets the attributes of its brand apart from the brands of rivals, its strategy can fail because of trying to differentiate on the basis of something that does not deliver adequate value to buyers (such as lowering a buyer's cost to use the product or enhancing a buyer's well-being). Anytime many potential buyers look at a company's differentiated product offering and conclude "So what?" the company's differentiation strategy is in deep trouble—buyers will likely decide the product is not worth the extra price, and sales will be disappointingly low.

The third big pitfall of a differentiation strategy is overspending on efforts to differentiate the company's product offering, thus eroding profitability. Company efforts to achieve differentiation nearly always raise costs. The trick to profitable differentiation is either to keep the costs of achieving differentiation below the price premium the differentiating attributes can command in the marketplace (thus increasing the profit margin per unit sold) or to offset thinner profit margins per unit by selling enough additional units to increase total profits. If a company goes overboard in pursuing costly differentiation efforts and then unexpectedly discovers that buyers are unwilling to pay a sufficient price premium to cover the added costs of differentiation, it ends up saddled with unacceptably thin profit margins or even losses. The need to contain differentiation costs is why many companies add little touches of differentiation that add to buyer satisfaction but are inexpensive to institute. Upscale restaurants often provide valet parking. Ski resorts provide skiers with complimentary coffee or hot apple cider at the base of the lifts in the morning and late afternoon. FedEx, UPS, and many catalog and online retailers have installed software capabilities that allow customers to track packages in transit. Some hotels and motels provide free continental breakfasts, exercise facilities, and in-room coffeemaking amenities. Publishers are using their Web sites to deliver supplementary educational materials to the buyers of their textbooks. Laundry detergent and soap manufacturers add pleasing scents to their products.

Other common pitfalls and mistakes in crafting a differentiation strategy include:[7]

- *Overdifferentiating so that product quality or service levels exceed buyers' needs.* Even if buyers like the differentiating extras, they may not find them sufficiently valuable for their purposes to pay extra to get them. Many shoppers shy away from buying top-of-the-line items because they have no particular interest in all the bells and whistles; for them, a less deluxe model or style makes better economic sense.

- *Trying to charge too high a price premium.* Even if buyers view certain extras or deluxe features as nice to have, they may still conclude that the added cost is excessive relative to the value they deliver. A differentiator must guard against turning off would-be buyers with what is perceived as price gouging. Normally, the bigger the price premium for the differentiating extras, the harder it is to keep buyers from switching to the lower-priced offerings of competitors.

- *Being timid and not striving to open up meaningful gaps in quality or service or performance features vis-à-vis the products of rivals.* Tiny differences between rivals' product offerings may not be visible or important to buyers. If a company wants to generate the fiercely loyal customer following needed to earn superior profits and open up a differentiation-based competitive advantage over rivals, then its strategy must result in strong rather than weak product differentiation. In markets where differentiators do no better than achieve weak product differentiation (because the attributes of rival brands are fairly similar in the minds of many buyers), customer loyalty to any one brand is weak, the costs of buyers to switch to rival brands are fairly low, and no one company has enough of a market edge that it can get by with charging a price premium over rival brands.

A low-cost provider strategy can defeat a differentiation strategy when buyers are satisfied with a basic product and don't think extra attributes are worth a higher price.

BEST-COST PROVIDER STRATEGIES

Core Concept
The competitive advantage of a best-cost provider is lower costs than rivals in incorporating upscale attributes, putting the company in a position to underprice rivals whose products have similar upscale attributes.

Best-cost provider strategies aim at giving customers *more value for the money.* The objective is to deliver superior value to buyers by satisfying their expectations on key quality/features/performance/service attributes and beating their expectations on price (given what rivals are charging for much the same attributes). *A company achieves best-cost status from an ability to incorporate attractive or upscale attributes at a lower cost than rivals.* The attractive attributes can take the form of appealing features, good-to-excellent product performance or quality, or attractive customer service. When a company has the resource strengths and competitive capabilities to incorporate these upscale attributes into its product offering *at a lower cost than rivals,* it enjoys best-cost status—it is the low-cost provider *of an upscale product.*

Being a best-cost provider is different from being a low-cost provider because the additional upscale features entail additional costs (that a low-cost provider can avoid by offering buyers a basic product with few frills). As Figure 5.1 indicates, best-cost provider strategies stake out a middle ground between pursuing a low-cost advantage and a differentiation advantage and between appealing to the broad market as a whole and a narrow market niche. From a competitive positioning standpoint, best-cost strategies are thus a *hybrid,* balancing a strategic emphasis on low cost against a strategic emphasis on differentiation (upscale features delivered at a price that constitutes superior value).

The competitive advantage of a best-cost provider is its capability to include upscale attributes at a lower cost than rivals whose products have comparable attributes. A best-cost provider can use its low-cost advantage to underprice rivals whose products have similar upscale attributes—it is usually not difficult to entice customers away from rivals charging a higher price for an item with highly comparable features, quality, performance, and/or customer service attributes. To achieve competitive advantage with a best-cost provider strategy, it is critical that a company have the resources and capabilities to incorporate upscale attributes at a lower cost than rivals. In other words, it must be able to (1) incorporate attractive features at a lower cost than rivals whose products have similar features, (2) manufacture a good-to-excellent quality product at a lower cost than rivals with good-to-excellent product quality, (3) develop a product that delivers good-to-excellent performance at a lower cost than rivals whose products also entail good-to-excellent performance, or (4) provide attractive customer service at a lower cost than rivals who provide comparably attractive customer service.

What makes a best-cost provider strategy so appealing is being able to incorporate upscale attributes at a lower cost than rivals and then using the company's low-cost advantage to underprice rivals whose products have similar upscale attributes.

The target market for a best-cost provider is value-conscious buyers—buyers that are looking for appealing extras at an appealingly low price. Value-hunting buyers (as distinct from buyers looking only for bargain-basement prices) often constitute a very sizable part of the overall market. Normally, value-conscious buyers are willing to pay a fair price for extra features, but they shy away from paying top dollar for items havingall the bells and whistles. It is the desire to cater to *value-conscious buyers* as opposed to *budget-conscious buyers* that sets a best-cost provider apart from a low-cost provider—the two strategies aim at distinguishably different market targets.

When a Best-Cost Provider Strategy Works Best

A best-cost provider strategy works best in markets where buyer diversity makes product differentiation the norm and where many buyers are also sensitive to price and value. This is because a best-cost provider can position itself near the middle of the market with either a medium-quality product at a below-average price or a high-quality product at an average or slightly higher price. Often, substantial numbers of buyers prefer midrange products rather than the cheap, basic products of low-cost producers or the expensive products of top-of-the-line differentiators. But unless a company has the resources, know-how, and capabilities to incorporate upscale product or service attributes at a lower cost than rivals, adopting a best-cost strategy is ill advised—a winning strategy must always be matched to a company's resource strengths and capabilities.

Illustration Capsule 5.3 describes how Toyota has applied the principles of a best-cost provider strategy in producing and marketing its Lexus brand.

The Big Risk of a Best-Cost Provider Strategy

A company's biggest vulnerability in employing a best-cost provider strategy is getting squeezed between the strategies of firms using low-cost and high-end differentiation strategies. Low-cost providers may be able to siphon customers away with the appeal of a lower price (despite their less appealing product attributes). High-end differentiators may be able to steal customers away with the appeal of better product attributes (even though their products carry a higher price tag). Thus, to be successful, a best-cost provider must offer buyers *significantly* better product attributes in order to justify a price above what low-cost leaders are charging. Likewise, it has to achieve *significantly* lower costs in providing upscale features so that it can outcompete high-end differentiators on the basis of a *significantly* lower price.

FOCUSED (OR MARKET NICHE) STRATEGIES

What sets focused strategies apart from low-cost leadership or broad differentiation strategies is concentrated attention on a narrow piece of the total market. The target segment, or niche, can be defined by geographic uniqueness, by specialized requirements in using the product, or by special product attributes that appeal only to niche members. Community Coffee, the largest family-owned specialty coffee retailer in the United States, is a company that focused on a geographic market niche; despite having a national market share of only 1.1 percent, Community has won a 50 percent share of the coffee business in supermarkets in southern Louisiana in competition

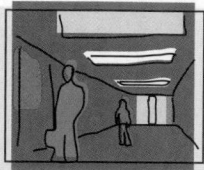

Illustration Capsule 5.3

Toyota's Best-Cost Producer Strategy for Its Lexus Line

Toyota Motor Company is widely regarded as a low-cost producer among the world's motor vehicle manufacturers. Despite its emphasis on product quality, Toyota has achieved low-cost leadership because it has developed considerable skills in efficient supply chain management and low-cost assembly capabilities, and because its models are positioned in the low-to-medium end of the price spectrum, where high production volumes are conducive to low unit costs. But when Toyota decided to introduce its new Lexus models to compete in the luxury-car market, it employed a classic best-cost provider strategy. Toyota took the following four steps in crafting and implementing its Lexus strategy:

- Designing an array of high-performance characteristics and upscale features into the Lexus models so as to make them comparable in performance and luxury to other high-end models and attractive to Mercedes, BMW, Audi, Jaguar, Cadillac, and Lincoln buyers.

- Transferring its capabilities in making high-quality Toyota models at low cost to making premium-quality Lexus models at costs below other luxury-car makers. Toyota's supply chain capabilities and low-cost assembly know-how allowed it to incorporate high-tech performance features and upscale quality into Lexus models at substantially less cost than comparable Mercedes and BMW models.

- Using its relatively lower manufacturing costs to underprice comparable Mercedes and BMW models. Toyota believed that with its cost advantage it could price attractively equipped Lexus cars low enough to draw price-conscious buyers away from Mercedes and BMW and perhaps induce dissatisfied Lincoln and Cadillac owners to switch to a Lexus. Lexus's pricing advantage over Mercedes and BMW was sometimes quite significant. For example, in 2006 the Lexus RX 330, a midsized SUV, carried a sticker price in the $36,000–$45,000 range (depending on how it was equipped), whereas variously equipped Mercedes M-class SUVs had price tags in the $50,000–$65,000 range and a BMW X5 SUV could range anywhere from $42,000 to $70,000, depending on the optional equipment chosen.

- Establishing a new network of Lexus dealers, separate from Toyota dealers, dedicated to providing a level of personalized, attentive customer service unmatched in the industry.

Lexus models have consistently ranked first in the widely watched J. D. Power & Associates quality survey, and the prices of Lexus models are typically several thousand dollars below those of comparable Mercedes and BMW models—clear signals that Toyota has succeeded in becoming a best-cost producer with its Lexus brand.

---

against Starbucks, Folger's, Maxwell House, and asserted specialty coffee retailers. Community Coffee's geographic version of a focus strategy has allowed it to capture sales in excess of $100 million annually by catering to the tastes of coffee drinkers across an 11-state region. Examples of firms that concentrate on a well-defined market niche keyed to a particular product or buyer segment include Animal Planet and the History Channel (in cable TV); Google (in Internet search engines); Porsche (in sports cars); Cannondale (in top-of-the-line mountain bikes); Domino's Pizza (in pizza delivery); Enterprise Rent-a-Car (a specialist in providing rental cars to repair garage customers); Bandag (a specialist in truck tire recapping that promotes its recaps aggressively at over 1,000 truck stops), CGA Inc. (a specialist in providing insurance to cover the cost of lucrative hole-in-one prizes at golf tournaments); Match.com (the world's largest online dating service); and Avid Technology (the world leader in digital technology products to create 3D animation and to edit films, videos, TV broadcasts, video games, and audio recordings). Microbreweries, local bakeries, bed-and-breakfast inns, and local owner-managed retail boutiques are all good examples of enterprises that have scaled their operations to serve narrow or local customer segments.

A Focused Low-Cost Strategy

A focused strategy based on low cost aims at securing a competitive advantage by serving buyers in the target market niche at a lower cost and lower price than rival competitors. This strategy has considerable attraction when a firm can lower costs significantly by limiting its customer base to a well-defined buyer segment. The avenues to achieving a cost advantage over rivals also serving the target market niche are the same as for low-cost leadership—outmanage rivals in keeping the costs of value chain activities contained to a bare minimum and search for innovative ways to reconfigure the firm's value chain and bypass or reduce certain value chain activities. The only real difference between a low-cost provider strategy and a focused low-cost strategy is the size of the buyer group that a company is trying to appeal to—the former involves a product offering that appeals broadly to most all buyer groups and market segments whereas the latter at just meeting the needs of buyers in a narrow market segment.

Focused low-cost strategies are fairly common. Producers of private-label goods are able to achieve low costs in product development, marketing, distribution, and advertising by concentrating on making generic items imitative of name-brand merchandise and selling directly to retail chains wanting a basic house brand to sell to price-sensitive shoppers. Several small printer-supply manufacturers have begun making low-cost clones of the premium-priced replacement ink and toner cartridges sold by Hewlett-Packard, Lexmark, Canon, and Epson; the clone manufacturers dissect the cartridges of the name-brand companies and then reengineer a similar version that won't violate patents. The components for remanufactured replacement cartridges are aquired from various outside sources, and the clones are then marketed at prices as much as 50 percent below the name-brand cartridges. Cartridge remanufacturers have been lured to focus on this market because replacement cartridges constitute a multibillion-dollar business with considerable profit potential given their low costs and the premium pricing of the name-brand companies. Illustration Capsule 5.4 describes how Motel 6 has kept its costs low in catering to budget-conscious travelers.

A Focused Differentiation Strategy

A focused strategy keyed to differentiation aims at securing a competitive advantage with a product offering carefully designed to appeal to the unique preferences and needs of a narrow, well-defined group of buyers (as opposed to a broad differentiation strategy aimed at many buyer groups and market segments). Successful use of a focused differentiation strategy depends on the existence of a buyer segment that is looking for special product attributes or seller capabilities and on a firm's ability to stand apart from rivals competing in the same target market niche.

Companies like Godiva Chocolates, Chanel, Gucci, Rolls-Royce, Häagen-Dazs, and W. L. Gore (the maker of Gore-Tex) employ successful differentiation-based focused strategies targeted at upscale buyers wanting products and services with world-class attributes. Indeed, most markets contain a buyer segment willing to pay a big price premium for the very finest items available, thus opening the strategic window for some competitors to pursue differentiation-based focused strategies aimed at the very top of the market pyramid. Another successful focused differentiator is Trader Joe's, a 150-store East and West Coast "fashion food retailer" that is a combination gourmet deli and grocery warehouse.[8] Customers shop Trader Joe's as much for entertainment as for conventional grocery items—the store stocks out-of-the-ordinary culinary treats like raspberry salsa, salmon burgers, and jasmine fried rice,

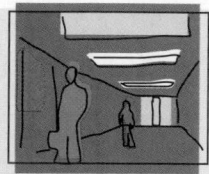

Illustration Capsule 5.4
Motel 6's Focused Low-Cost Strategy

Motel 6 caters to price-conscious travelers who want a clean, no-frills place to spend the night. To be a low-cost provider of overnight lodging, Motel 6 (1) selects relatively inexpensive sites on which to construct its units (usually near interstate exits and high-traffic locations but far enough away to avoid paying prime site prices); (2) builds only basic facilities (no restaurant or bar and only rarely a swimming pool); (3) relies on standard architectural designs that incorporate inexpensive materials and low-cost construction techniques; and (4) provides simple room furnishings and decorations. These approaches lower both investment costs and operating costs. Without restaurants,

bars, and all kinds of guest services, a Motel 6 unit can be operated with just front-desk personnel, room cleanup crews, and skeleton building-and-grounds maintenance.

To promote the Motel 6 concept with travelers who have simple overnight requirements, the chain uses unique, recognizable radio ads done by nationally syndicated radio personality Tom Bodett; the ads describe Motel 6's clean rooms, no-frills facilities, friendly atmosphere, and dependably low rates (usually under $40 a night).

Motel 6's basis for competitive advantage is lower costs than competitors in providing basic, economical overnight accommodations to price-constrained travelers.

as well as the standard goods normally found in supermarkets. What sets Trader Joe's apart is not just its unique combination of food novelties and competitively priced grocery items but also its capability to turn an otherwise mundane grocery excursion into a whimsical treasure hunt that is just plain fun.

Illustration Capsule 5.5 describes Progressive Insurance's focused differentiation strategy.

When a Focused Low-Cost or Focused Differentiation Strategy Is Attractive

A focused strategy aimed at securing a competitive edge based on either low cost or differentiation becomes increasingly attractive as more of the following conditions are met:

- The target market niche is big enough to be profitable and offers good growth potential.
- Industry leaders do not see that having a presence in the niche is crucial to their own success—in which case focusers can often escape battling head-to-head against some of the industry's biggest and strongest competitors.
- It is costly or difficult for multisegment competitors to put capabilities in place to meet the specialized needs of buyers comprising the target market niche and at the same time satisfy the expectations of their mainstream customers.
- The industry has many different niches and segments, thereby allowing a focuser to pick a competitively attractive niche suited to its resource strengths and capabilities. Also, with more niches, there is more room for focusers to avoid each other in competing for the same customers.

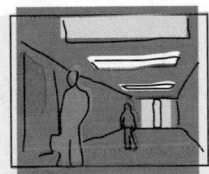

Illustration Capsule 5.5
Progressive Insurance's Focused Differentiation Strategy in Auto Insurance

Progressive Insurance has fashioned a strategy in auto insurance focused on people with a record of traffic violations who drive high-performance cars, drivers with accident histories, motorcyclists, teenagers, and other so-called high-risk categories of drivers that most auto insurance companies steer away from. Progressive discovered that some of these high-risk drivers are affluent and pressed for time, making them less sensitive to paying premium rates for their car insurance. Management learned that it could charge such drivers high enough premiums to cover the added risks, plus it differentiated Progressive from other insurers by expediting the process of obtaining insurance and decreasing the annoyance that such drivers faced in obtaining insurance coverage. Progressive pioneered the low-cost direct sales model of allowing customers to purchase insurance online and over the phone.

Progressive also studied the market segments for insurance carefully enough to discover that some motorcycle owners were not especially risky (middle-aged suburbanites who sometimes commuted to work or used their motorcycles mainly for recreational trips with their friends). Progressive's strategy allowed it to become a leader in the market for luxury-car insurance for customers who appreciated Progressive's streamlined approach to doing business.

In further differentiating and promoting Progressive policies, management created teams of roving claims adjusters who would arrive at accident scenes to assess claims and issue checks for repairs on the spot. Progressive introduced 24-hour claims reporting, now an industry standard. In addition, it developed a sophisticated pricing system so that it could quickly and accurately assess each customer's risk and weed out unprofitable customers.

By being creative and excelling at the nuts and bolts of its business, Progressive has won a 7 percent share of the $150 billion market for auto insurance and has the highest underwriting margins in the auto-insurance industry.

Sources: www.progressiveinsurance.com; Ian C. McMillan, Alexander van Putten, and Rita Gunther McGrath, "Global Gamesmanship," *Harvard Business Review* 81, no. 5 (May 2003), p. 68; and *Fortune,* May 16, 2005, p. 34.

- Few, if any, other rivals are attempting to specialize in the same target segment—a condition that reduces the risk of segment overcrowding.
- The focuser has a reservoir of customer goodwill and loyalty (accumulated from having catered to the specialized needs and preferences of niche members over many years) that it can draw on to help stave off ambitious challengers looking to horn in on its business.

The advantages of focusing a company's entire competitive effort on a single market niche are considerable, especially for smaller and medium-sized companies that may lack the breadth and depth of resources to tackle going after a broad customer base with a "something for everyone" lineup of models, styles, and product selection. eBay has made a huge name for itself and very attractive profits for shareholders by focusing its attention on online auctions—at one time a very small niche in the overall auction business that eBay's focus strategy turned into the dominant piece of the global auction industry. Google has capitalized on its specialized expertise in Internet search engines to become one of the most spectacular growth companies of the past 10 years. Two hippie entrepreneurs, Ben Cohen and Jerry Greenfield, built Ben & Jerry's Homemade into an impressive business by focusing their energies and resources solely on the superpremium segment of the ice cream market.

The Risks of a Focused Low-Cost or Focused Differentiation Strategy

Focusing carries several risks. One is the chance that competitors will find effective ways to match the focused firm's capabilities in serving the target niche—perhaps by coming up with products or brands specifically designed to appeal to buyers in the target niche or by developing expertise and capabilities that offset the focuser's strengths. In the lodging business, large chains like Marriott and Hilton have launched multibrand strategies that allow them to compete effectively in several lodging segments simultaneously. Marriott has flagship hotels with a full complement of services and amenities that allow it to attract travelers and vacationers going to major resorts, it has J. W. Marriot hotels usually located in downtown metropolitan areas that cater to business travelers; the Courtyard by Marriott brand is for business travelers looking for moderately priced lodging; Marriott Residence Inns are designed as a home away from home for travelers staying five or more nights; and the 530 Fairfield Inn locations cater to travelers looking for quality lodging at an affordable price. Similarly, Hilton has a lineup of brands (Conrad Hotels, Doubletree Hotels, Embassy Suite Hotels, Hampton Inns, Hilton Hotels, Hilton Garden Inns, and Homewood Suites) that enable it to operate in multiple segments and compete head-to-head against lodging chains that operate only in a single segment. Multibrand strategies are attractive to large companies like Marriott and Hilton precisely because they enable a company to enter a market niche and siphon business away from companies that employ a focus strategy.

A second risk of employing a focus strategy is the potential for the preferences and needs of niche members to shift over time toward the product attributes desired by the majority of buyers. An erosion of the differences across buyer segments lowers entry barriers into a focuser's market niche and provides an open invitation for rivals in adjacent segments to begin competing for the focuser's customers. A third risk is that the segment may become so attractive it is soon inundated with competitors, intensifying rivalry and splintering segment profits.

THE CONTRASTING FEATURES OF THE FIVE GENERIC COMPETITIVE STRATEGIES: A SUMMARY

Deciding which generic competitive strategy should serve as the framework for hanging the rest of the company's strategy is not a trivial matter. Each of the five generic competitive strategies positions the company differently in its market and competitive environment. Each establishes a central theme for how the company will endeavor to outcompete rivals. Each creates some boundaries or guidelines for maneuvering as market circumstances unfold and as ideas for improving the strategy are debated. Each points to different ways of experimenting and tinkering with the basic strategy—for example, employing a low-cost leadership strategy means experimenting with ways that costs can be cut and value chain activities can be streamlined, whereas a broad differentiation strategy means exploring ways to add new differentiating features or to perform value chain activities differently if the result is to add value for customers in ways they are willing to pay for. Each entails differences in terms of product line, production emphasis, marketing emphasis, and means of sustaining the strategy—as shown in Table 5.1.

Table 5.1 **Distinguishing Features of the Five Generic Competitive Strategies**

	Low-Cost Provider	Broad Differentiation	Best-Cost Provider	Focused Low-Cost Provider	Focused Differentiation
Strategic target	• A broad cross-section of the market	• A broad cross-section of the market	• Value-conscious buyers	• A narrow market niche where buyer needs and preferences are distinctively different	• A narrow market niche where buyer needs and preferences are distinctively different
Basis of competitive advantage	• Lower overall costs than competitors	• Ability to offer buyers something attractively different from competitors	• Ability to give customers more value for the money	• Lower overall cost than rivals in serving niche members	• Attributes that appeal specifically to niche members
Product line	• A good basic product with few frills (acceptable quality and limited selection)	• Many product variations, wide selection; emphasis on differentiating features	• Items with appealing attributes; assorted upscale features	• Features and attributes tailored to the tastes and requirements of niche members	• Features and attributes tailored to the tastes and requirements of niche members
Production emphasis	• A continuous search for cost reduction without sacrificing acceptable quality and essential features	• Build in whatever differentiating features buyers are willing to pay for; strive for product superiority	• Build in upscale features and appealing attributes at lower cost than rivals	• A continuous search for cost reduction while incorporating features and attributes matched to niche member preferences	• Custom-made products that match the tastes and requirements of niche members
Marketing emphasis	• Try to make a virtue out of product features that lead to low cost	• Tout differentiating features • Charge a premium price to cover the extra costs of differentiating features	• Tout delivery of best value • Either deliver comparable features at a lower price than rivals or else match rivals on prices and provide better features	• Communicate attractive features of a budget-priced product offering that fits niche buyers' expectations	• Communicate how product offering does the best job of meeting niche buyers' expectations
Keys to sustaining the strategy	• Economical prices/good value • Strive to manage costs down, year after year, in every area of the business	• Stress constant innovation to stay ahead of imitative competitors • Concentrate on a few key differentiating features	• Unique expertise in simultaneously managing costs down while incorporating upscale features and attributes	• Stay committed to serving the niche at lowest overall cost; don't blur the firm's image by entering other market segments or adding other products to widen market appeal	• Stay committed to serving the niche better than rivals; don't blur the firm's image by entering other market segments or adding other products to widen market appeal

Thus, a choice of which generic strategy to employ spills over to affect several aspects of how the business will be operated and the manner in which value chain activities must be managed. Deciding which generic strategy to employ is perhaps the most important strategic commitment a company makes—it tends to drive the rest of the strategic actions a company decides to undertake.

One of the big dangers in crafting a competitive strategy is that managers, torn between the pros and cons of the various generic strategies, will opt for *stuck-in-the-middle strategies* that represent compromises between lower costs and greater differentiation and between broad and narrow market appeal. Compromise or middle-ground strategies rarely produce sustainable competitive advantage or a distinctive competitive position—a well-executed best-cost producer strategy is the only compromise between low cost and differentiation that succeeds. Usually, companies with compromise strategies end up with a middle-of-the-pack industry ranking—they have average costs, some but not a lot of product differentiation relative to rivals, an average image and reputation, and little prospect of industry leadership. Having a competitive edge over rivals is the single most dependable contributor to above-average company profitability. Hence, only if a company makes a strong and unwavering commitmentto one of the five generic competitive strategies does it stand much chance of achieving sustainable competitive advantage that such strategies can deliver if properly executed.

Key Points

Early in the process of crafting a strategy company managers have to decide which of the five basic competitive strategies to employ—overall low-cost, broad differentiation, best-cost, focused low-cost, or focused differentiation.

In employing a low-cost provider strategy and trying to achieve a low-cost advantage over rivals, a company must do a better job than rivals of cost-effectively managing value chain activities and/or find innovative ways to eliminate or bypass cost-producing activities. Low-cost provider strategies work particularly well when the products of rival sellers are virtually identical or very weakly differentiated and supplies are readily available from eager sellers, when there are not many ways to differentiate that have value to buyers, when many buyers are price sensitive and shop the market for the lowest price, and when buyer switching costs are low.

Broad differentiation strategies seek to produce a competitive edge by incorporating attributes and features that set a company's product/service offering apart from rivals in ways that buyers consider valuable and worth paying for. Successful differentiation allows a firm to (1) command a premium price for its product, (2) increase unit sales (because additional buyers are won over by the differentiating features), and/or (3) gain buyer loyalty to its brand (because some buyers are strongly attracted to the differentiating features and bond with the company and its products). Differentiation strategies work best in markets with diverse buyer preferences where there are big windows of opportunity to strongly differentiate a company's product offering from those of rival brands, in situations where few other rivals are pursuing a similar differentiation approach, and in circumstances where companies are racing to bring out the most appealing next-generation product. A differentiation strategy is doomed when competitors are able to quickly copy most or all of the appealing product attributes a company comes up with, when a company's differentiation efforts meet with a ho-hum or so what market reception, or when a company erodes profitability by overspending on efforts to differentiate its product offering.

Best-cost provider strategies combine a strategic emphasis on low cost with a strategic emphasis on more than minimal quality, service, features, or performance. The aim is to create competitive advantage by giving buyers more value for the money—an approach that entails matching close rivals on key quality/service/features/performance attributes and beating them on the costs of incorporating such attributes into the product or service. A best-cost provider strategy works best in markets where buyer diversity makes product differentiation the norm and where many buyers are also sensitive to price and value.

A focus strategy delivers competitive advantage either by achieving lower costs than rivals in serving buyers comprising the target market niche or by developing specialized ability to offer niche buyers an appealingly differentiated offering than meets their needs better than rival brands. A focused strategy based on either low cost or differentiation becomes increasingly attractive when the target market niche is big enough to be profitable and offers good growth potential, when it is costly or difficult for multi-segment competitors to put capabilities in place to meet the specialized needs of the target market niche and at the same time satisfy the expectations of their mainstream customers, when there are one or more niches that present a good match with a focuser's resource strengths and capabilities, and when few other rivals are attempting to specialize in the same target segment.

Deciding which generic strategy to employ is perhaps the most important strategic commitment a company makes—it tends to drive the rest of the strategic actions a company decides to undertake and it sets the whole tone for the pursuit of a competitive advantage over rivals.

Exercises

1. Go to www.google.com and do a search for "low-cost producer." See if you can identify five companies that are pursuing a low-cost strategy in their respective industries.

2. Using the advanced search function at www.google.com, enter "best-cost producer" in the exact-phrase box and see if you can locate three companies that indicate they are employing a best-cost producer strategy.

3. Go to BMW's Web site (www.bmw.com) click on the link for BMW Group. The site you find provides an overview of the company's key functional areas, including R&D and production activities. Explore each of the links on the Research & Development page—People & Networks, Innovation & Technology, and Mobility & Traffic—to better understand the company's approach. Also review the statements under Production focusing on vehicle production and sustainable production. How do these activities contribute to BMW's differentiation strategy and the unique position in the auto industry that BMW has achieved?

4. Which of the five generic competitive strategies do you think the following companies are employing (do whatever research at the various company Web sites might be needed to arrive at and support your answer):
   a. The Saturn division of General Motors
   b. Abercrombie & Fitch
   c. Amazon.com
   d. Home Depot
   e. Mary Kay Cosmetics
   f. *USA Today*

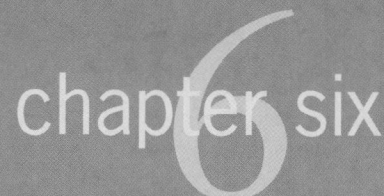

chapter six

Supplementing the Chosen Competitive Strategy

Other Important Strategy Choices

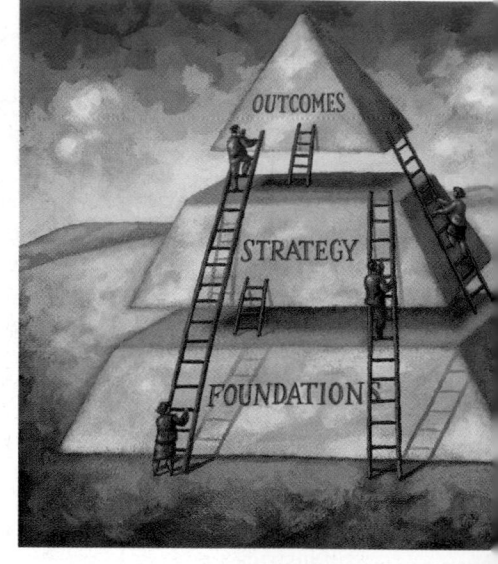

Don't form an alliance to correct a weakness and don't ally with a partner that is trying to correct a weakness of its own. The only result from a marriage of weaknesses is the creation of even more weaknesses.

—Michel Robert

Strategies for taking the hill won't necessarily hold it.

—Amar Bhide

The sure path to oblivion is to stay where you are.

—Bernard Fauber

Successful business strategy is about actively shaping the game you play, not just playing the game you find.

—Adam M. Brandenburger and Barry J. Nalebuff

O nce a company has settled on which of the five generic strategies to employ, attention turns to what other *strategic actions* it can take to complement its choice of a basic competitive strategy. Several decisions have to be made:

- What use to make of strategic alliances and collaborative partnerships.
- Whether to bolster the company's market position via merger or acquisitions.
- Whether to integrate backward or forward into more stages of the industry value chain.
- Whether to outsource certain value chain activities or perform them in-house.
- Whether and when to employ offensive and defensive moves.
- Which of several ways to use the Internet as a distribution channel in positioning the company in the marketplace.

This chapter contains sections discussing the pros and cons of each of the above complementary strategic options. The next-to-last section in the chapter discusses the need for strategic choices in each functional area of a company's business (R&D, production, sales and marketing, finance, and so on) to support its basic competitive approach and complementary strategic moves. The chapter concludes with a brief look at the competitive importance of timing strategic moves—when it is advantageous to be a first-mover and when it is better to be a fast-follower or late-mover.

Figure 6.1 shows the menu of strategic options a company has in crafting a strategy and the order in which the choices should generally be made. The portion of Figure 6.1 below the five generic competitive strategy options illustrates the structure of this chapter and the topics that will be covered.

Figure 6.1   **A Company's Menu of Strategy Options**

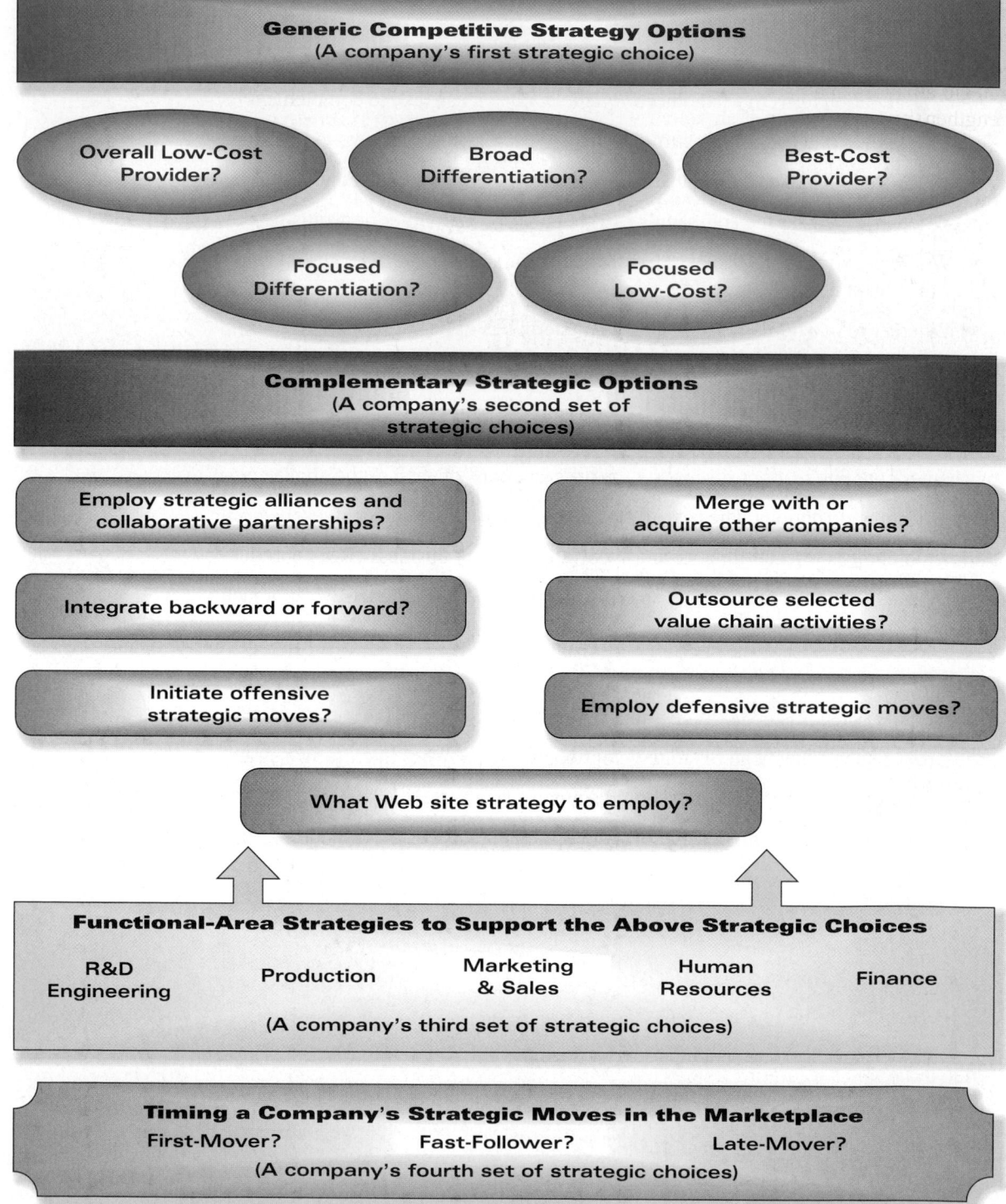

COLLABORATIVE STRATEGIES: ALLIANCES AND PARTNERSHIPS

Companies in all types of industries and in all parts of the world have elected to form strategic alliances and partnerships to complement their own strategic initiatives and strengthen their competitiveness in domestic and international markets. This is an about-face from times past, when the vast majority of companies were content to go it alone, confident that they already had or could independently develop whatever resources and know-how were needed to be successful in their markets. But globalization of the world economy; revolutionary advances in technology across a broad front; and untapped opportunities in Asia, Latin America, and Europe—whose national markets are opening up, deregulating, and/or undergoing privatization—have made strategic partnerships of one kind or another integral to competing on a broad geographic scale.

Many companies now find themselves thrust into two very demanding competitive races: (1) *the global race to build a market presence in many different national markets* and join the ranks of companies recognized as global market leaders, and (2) *the race to seize opportunities on the frontiers of advancing technology* and build the resource strengths and business capabilities to compete successfully in the industries and product markets of the future.[1] Even the largest and most financially sound companies have concluded that simultaneously running the races for global market leadership and for a stake in the industries of the future requires more diverse and expansive skills, resources, technological expertise, and competitive capabilities than they can assemble and manage alone. Such companies, along with others that are missing the resources and competitive capabilities needed to pursue promising opportunities, have determined that the fastest way to fill the gap is often to form alliances with enterprises having the desired strengths. Consequently, these companies form strategic alliances or collaborative partnerships in which two or more companies jointly work to achieve mutually beneficial strategic outcomes. Thus, a **strategic alliance** is a formal agreement between two or more separate companies in which there is strategically relevant collaboration of some sort, joint contribution of resources, shared risk, shared control, and mutual dependence. Often, alliances involve joint marketing, joint sales or distribution, joint production, design collaboration, joint research, or projects to jointly develop new technologies or products. The relationship between the partners may be contractual or merely collaborative; the arrangement commonly stops short of formal ownership ties between the partners (although there are a few strategic alliances where one or more allies have minority ownership in certain of the other alliance members). Five factors make an alliance strategic, as opposed to just a convenient business arrangement:[2]

> **Core Concept**
> **Strategic alliances** are collaborative arrangements where two or more companies join forces to achieve mutually beneficial strategic outcomes.

1. It is critical to the company's achievement of an important objective.
2. It helps build, sustain, or enhance a core competence or competitive advantage.
3. It helps block a competitive threat.
4. It helps open up important new market opportunities.
5. It mitigates a significant risk to a company's business.

Strategic cooperation is a much-favored, indeed necessary, approach in industries where new technological developments are occurring at a furious pace along many different paths and where advances in one technology spill over to affect others (often blurring industry boundaries). Whenever industries are experiencing high-velocity technological advances in many areas simultaneously, firms find it virtually essential to have cooperative relationships with other enterprises to stay on the leading edge of technology and product performance even in their own area of specialization.

Companies in many different industries all across the world have made strategic alliances a core part of their overall strategy; U.S. companies alone announced nearly 68,000 alliances from 1996 through 2003.[3] In the personal computer (PC) industry, alliances are pervasive because the different components of PCs and the software to run them are supplied by so many different companies—one set of companies provides the microprocessors, another group makes the motherboards, another the monitors, another the disk drives, another the memory chips, and so on. Moreover, their facilities are scattered across the United States, Japan, Taiwan, Singapore, Malaysia, and parts of Europe. Strategic alliances among companies in the various parts of the PC industry facilitate the close cross-company collaboration required on next-generation product development, logistics, production, and the timing of new product releases.

> Company use of alliances is quite widespread.

Toyota has forged long-term strategic partnerships with many of its suppliers of automotive parts and components, both to achieve lower costs and to improve the quality and reliability of its vehicles. Microsoft collaborates very closely with independent software developers to ensure that their programs will run on the next-generation versions of Windows. Genentech, a leader in biotechnology and human genetics, has a partnering strategy to increase its access to novel biotherapeutics products and technologies and has formed alliances with over 30 companies to strengthen its research and development (R&D) pipeline. During the 1998–2004 period, Samsung Electronics, a South Korean corporation with $54 billion in sales, entered into over 50 major strategic alliances involving such companies as Sony, Yahoo, Hewlett-Packard, Nokia, Motorola, Intel, Microsoft, Dell, Mitsubishi, Disney, IBM, Maytag, and Rockwell Automation; the alliances involved joint investments, technology transfer arrangements, joint R&D projects, and agreements to supply parts and components—all of which facilitated Samsung's strategic efforts to transform itself into a global enterprise and establish itself as a leader in the worldwide electronics industry.

Studies indicate that large corporations are commonly involved in 30 to 50 alliances and that some have hundreds of alliances. One recent study estimated that about 35 percent of corporate revenues in 2003 came from activities involving strategic alliances, up from 15 percent in 1995.[4] Another study reported that the typical large corporation relied on alliances for 15 to 20 percent of its revenues, assets, or income.[5] Companies that have formed a host of alliances have a need to manage their alliances like a portfolio—terminating those that no longer serve a useful purpose or that have produced meager results, forming promising new alliances, and restructuring certain existing alliances to correct performance problems and/or redirect the collaborative effort.[6]

Why and How Strategic Alliances Are Advantageous

The most common reasons why companies enter into strategic alliances are to expedite the development of promising new technologies or products, to overcome deficits in their own technical and manufacturing expertise, to bring together the personnel and expertise needed to create desirable new skill sets and capabilities, to improve supply chain efficiency, to gain economies of scale in production and/or marketing, and to acquire or improve market access through joint marketing agreements.[7] In bringing together firms with different skills and knowledge bases, alliances open up learning opportunities that help partner firms better leverage their own resource strengths.[8] In industries where technology is advancing rapidly, alliances are all about fast cycles of learning, staying abreast of the latest developments, and gaining quick access to the latest round of technological know-how and capability.

> The best alliances are highly selective, focusing on particular value chain activities and on obtaining a particular competitive benefit. They tend to enable a firm to build on its strengths and to learn.

There are several other instances in which companies find strategic alliances particularly valuable. A company that is racing for *global market leadership* needs alliances to:

- Get into critical country markets quickly and accelerate the process of building a potent global market presence.

- *Gain inside knowledge about unfamiliar markets and cultures* through alliances with local partners. For example, U.S., European, and Japanese companies wanting to build market footholds in the fast-growing Chinese market have pursued partnership arrangements with Chinese companies to help in getting products through the tedious and typically corrupt customs process, to help guide them through the maze of government regulations, to supply knowledge of local markets, to provide guidance on adapting their products to better match the buying preferences of Chinese consumers, to set up local manufacturing capabilities, and to assist in distribution, marketing, and promotional activities. The Chinese government has long required foreign companies operating in China to have a state-owned Chinese company as a minority or maybe even 50 percent partner—only recently has it backed off this requirement for foreign companies operating in selected parts of the Chinese economy.

- *Access valuable skills and competencies* that are concentrated in particular geographic locations (such as software design competencies in the United States, fashion design skills in Italy, and efficient manufacturing skills in Japan and China).

A company that is racing to *stake out a strong position in an industry of the future* needs alliances to:

- *Establish a stronger beachhead* for participating in the target industry.

- *Master new technologies and build new expertise and competencies* faster than would be possible through internal efforts.

- *Open up broader opportunities* in the target industry by melding the firm's own capabilities with the expertise and resources of partners.

Allies can learn much from one another in performing joint research, sharing technological know-how, and collaborating on complementary new technologies and products—sometimes enough to enable them to pursue other new opportunities on their own.[9] Manufacturers frequently pursue alliances with parts and components suppliers to gain the efficiencies of better supply chain management and to speed new products to market. By joining forces in components production and/or final assembly, companies may be able to realize cost savings not achievable with their own small volumes—German automakers Volkswagen, Audi, and Porsche formed a strategic alliance to spur mutual development of a gasoline-electric hybrid engine and transmission system that they could each then incorporate into their motor vehicle models; BMW, General

> The competitive attraction of alliances is in allowing companies to bundle competencies and resources that are more valuable in a joint effort than when kept separate.

Motors, and DaimlerChrysler formed a similar partnership. Both alliances were aimed at closing the gap on Toyota, generally said to be the world leader in fuel-efficient hybrid engines. Information systems consultant Accenture has developed strategic alliances with such leading technology providers as SAP, Oracle, Siebel, Microsoft, BEA, and Hewlett-Packard to give it greater capabilities in designing and integrating information systems for its corporate clients. Johnson & Johnson and Merck entered into an alliance to market Pepcid AC; Merck developed the stomach distress remedy, and Johnson & Johnson functioned as marketer—the alliance made Pepcid products the best-selling remedies for acid indigestion and heartburn. United Airlines, American Airlines, Continental, Delta, and Northwest created an alliance to form Orbitz, an Internet travel site to compete head-to-head against Expedia and Travelocity, thereby strengthening their access to travelers and vacationers shopping online for airfares, rental cars, lodging, cruises, and vacation packages.

Capturing the Benefits of Strategic Alliances

The extent to which companies benefit from entering into alliances and collaborative partnerships seems to be a function of six factors:[10]

1. *Picking a good partner*—A good partner not only has the desired expertise and capabilities but also shares the company's vision about the purpose of the alliance. Experience indicates that it is generally wise to avoid a partnership in which there is strong potential of direct competition because of overlapping product lines or other conflicting interests—agreements to jointly market each other's products hold much potential for conflict unless the products are complements rather than substitutes and unless there is good chemistry among key personnel. Experience also indicates that alliances between strong and weak companies rarely work because the alliance is unlikely to provide the strong partner with useful resources or skills and because there's a greater chance of the alliance producing mediocre results.

2. *Being sensitive to cultural differences*—Unless the outsider exhibits respect for the local culture and local business practices, productive working relationships are unlikely to emerge.

3. *Recognizing that the alliance must benefit both sides*—Information must be shared as well as gained, and the relationship must remain forthright and trustful. Many alliances fail because one or both partners grow unhappy with what they are learning. Also, if either partner plays games with information or tries to take advantage of the other, the resulting friction can quickly erode the value of further collaboration.

4. *Ensuring that both parties live up to their commitments*—Both parties have to deliver on their commitments for the alliance to produce the intended benefits. The division of work has to be perceived as fairly apportioned, and the caliber of the benefits received on both sides has to be perceived as adequate.

5. *Structuring the decision-making process so that actions can be taken swiftly when needed*—In many instances, the fast pace of technological and competitive changes dictates an equally fast decision-making process. If the parties get bogged down in discussion or in gaining internal approval from higher-ups, the alliance can turn into an anchor of delay and inaction.

6. *Managing the learning process and then adjusting the alliance agreement over time to fit new circumstances*—One of the keys to long-lasting success is adapting the nature and structure of the alliance to be responsive to shifting market conditions, emerging technologies, and changing customer requirements. Wise allies are quick

to recognize the merit of an evolving collaborative arrangement, where adjustments are made to accommodate changing market conditions and to overcome whatever problems arise in establishing an effective working relationship. Most alliances encounter troubles of some kind within a couple of years—those that are flexible enough to evolve are better able to recover.

Most alliances that aim at technology sharing or providing market access turn out to be temporary, fulfilling their purpose after a few years because the benefits of mutual learning have occurred and because the businesses of both partners have developed to the point where they are ready to go their own ways. In such cases, it is important for each partner to learn thoroughly and rapidly about the other partner's technology, business practices, and organizational capabilities and then promptly transfer valuable ideas and practices into its own operations. Although long-term alliances sometimes prove mutually beneficial, most partners don't hesitate to terminate the alliance and go it alone when the payoffs run out.

Alliances are more likely to be long-lasting when (1) they involve collaboration with suppliers or distribution allies and each party's contribution involves activities in different portions of the industry value chain, or (2) both parties conclude that continued collaboration is in their mutual interest, perhaps because new opportunities for learning are emerging or perhaps because further collaboration will allow each partner to extend its market reach beyond what it could accomplish on its own.

Why Many Alliances Are Unstable or Break Apart

The stability of an alliance depends on how well the partners work together, their success in responding and adapting to changing internal and external conditions, and their willingness to renegotiate the bargain if circumstances so warrant. A successful alliance requires real in-the-trenches collaboration, not merely an arm's-length exchange of ideas. Unless partners place a high value on the skills, resources, and contributions each brings to the alliance and the cooperative arrangement results in valuable win–win outcomes, it is doomed. A surprisingly large number of alliances never live up to expectations. A 1999 study by Accenture, a global business consulting organization, revealed that 61 percent of alliances were either outright failures or "limping along." In 2004, McKinsey & Company estimated that the overall success rate of alliances was around 50 percent, based on whether the alliance achieved the stated objectives.[11] Many alliances are dissolved after a few years. The high "divorce rate" among strategic allies has several causes—diverging objectives and priorities, an inability to work well together (an alliance between Disney and Pixar came apart because of clashes between high-level executives —in 2005, after one of the feuding executives retired, Disney acquired Pixar), changing conditions that render the purpose of the alliance obsolete, the emergence of more attractive technological paths, and marketplace rivalry between one or more allies.[12] Experience indicates that *alliances stand a reasonable chance of helping a company reduce competitive disadvantage, but very rarely have they proved a strategic option for gaining a durable competitive edge over rivals.*

The Strategic Dangers of Relying Heavily on Alliances and Collaborative Partnerships

The Achilles heel of alliances and collaborative partnerships is dependence on another company for *essential* expertise and capabilities. To be a market leader (and perhaps even a serious market contender), a company must ultimately develop its own capabilities in areas where internal strategic control is pivotal to protecting its competitiveness and building competitive advantage. Moreover, some alliances hold only limited potential because the partner guards its most valuable skills and expertise; in such instances, acquiring or merging with a company possessing the desired know-how and resources is a better solution.

MERGER AND ACQUISITION STRATEGIES

Mergers and acquisitions are much-used strategic options—for example, U.S. companies alone made 90,000 acquisitions from 1996 through 2003.[13] Mergers and acquisitions are especially suited for situations in which alliances and partnerships do not go far enough in providing a company with access to needed resources and capabilities.[14] Ownership ties are more permanent than partnership ties, allowing the operations of the merger/acquisition participants to be tightly integrated and creating more in-house control and autonomy. A *merger* is a pooling of equals, with the newly created company often taking on a new name. An *acquisition* is a combination in which one company, the acquirer, purchases and absorbs the operations of another, the acquired. The difference between a merger and an acquisition relates more to the details of ownership, management control, and financial arrangements than to strategy and competitive advantage. The resources, competencies, and competitive capabilities of the newly created enterprise end up much the same whether the combination is the result of acquisition or merger.

> Combining the operations of two companies, via merger or acquisition, is an attractive strategic option for achieving operating economies, strengthening the resulting company's competences and competitiveness, and opening up avenues of new market opportunity.

Many mergers and acquisitions are driven by strategies to achieve any of five strategic objectives:[15]

1. *To create a more cost-efficient operation out of the combined companies*—When a company acquires another company in the same industry, there's usually enough overlap in operations that certain inefficient plants can be closed or distribution activities partly combined and downsized (when nearby centers serve some of the same geographic areas), or sales-force and marketing activities combined and downsized (when each company has salespeople calling on the same customer). The combined companies may also be able to reduce supply chain costs because of buying in greater volume from common suppliers and from closer collaboration with supply chain partners. Likewise, it is usually feasible to squeeze out cost savings in administrative activities, again by combining and downsizing such administrative activities as finance and accounting, information technology, and human resources. The merger that formed DaimlerChrysler was motivated in large part by the fact that the motor vehicle industry had far more production capacity worldwide than was needed; top executives at both Daimler-Benz and Chrysler believed that the efficiency of the two companies could be significantly improved by shutting some plants and laying off workers; realigning which models were produced at which plants; and squeezing out efficiencies by combining supply chain activities, product design, and administration. Quite a number of acquisitions are undertaken with the objective of transforming two or more otherwise high-cost companies into one lean competitor with average or below-average costs.

2. *To expand a company's geographic coverage*—One of the best and quickest ways to expand a company's geographic coverage is to acquire rivals with operations in the desired locations. And if there is some geographic overlap, then a side benefit is being able to reduce costs by eliminating duplicate facilities in those geographic areas where undesirable overlap exists. Banks like Wells Fargo, Bank

of America, Wachovia, and Suntrust have pursued geographic expansion by making a series of acquisitions over the years, enabling them to establish a market presence in an ever-growing number of states and localities. Many companies use acquisitions to expand internationally; for example, food products companies like Nestlé, Kraft, Unilever, and Procter & Gamble—all racing for global market leadership—have made acquisitions an integral part of their strategies to widen their geographic reach.

3. *To extend the company's business into new product categories*—Many times a company has gaps in its product line that need to be filled. Acquisition can be a quicker and more potent way to broaden a company's product line than going through the exercise of introducing a company's own new product to fill the gap. PepsiCo acquired Quaker Oats chiefly to bring Gatorade into the Pepsi family of beverages. While Coca-Cola has expanded its beverage lineup by introducing its own new products (like Powerade and Dasani), it has also expanded its lineup by acquiring Fanta (carbonated fruit beverages), Minute Maid (juices and juice drinks), Odwalla (juices), and Hi-C (ready-to-drink fruit beverages).

4. *To gain quick access to new technologies or other resources and competitive capabilities*—Making acquisitions to bolster a company's technological know-how or to fill resource holes is a favorite of companies racing to establish a position in an industry or product category about to be born. Making acquisitions aimed at filling meaningful gaps in technological expertise allows a company to bypass a time-consuming and perhaps expensive R&D effort (which might not succeed). Cisco Systems purchased over 75 technology companies to give it more technological reach and product breadth, thereby buttressing its standing as the world's biggest supplier of systems for building the infrastructure of the Internet. Intel has made over 300 acquisitions in the past five or so years to broaden its technological base, obtain the resource capabilities to produce and market a variety of Internet-related and electronics-related products, and make it less dependent on supplying microprocessors for PCs.

5. *To try to invent a new industry and lead the convergence of industries whose boundaries are being blurred by changing technologies and new market opportunities*—Such acquisitions are the result of a company's management betting that two or more distinct industries are converging into one and deciding to establish a strong position in the consolidating markets by bringing together the resources and products of several different companies. Examples include the merger of AOL and media giant Time Warner—a move predicated on the belief that entertainment content would ultimately converge into a single industry (much of which would be distributed over the Internet) —and News Corporation's purchase of satellite TV companies to complement its media holdings in TV broadcasting (the Fox network and TV stations in various countries); cable TV (Fox News, Fox Sports, and FX); filmed entertainment (Twentieth Century Fox and Fox Studios); and newspaper, magazine, and book publishing.

Numerous companies have employed an acquisition strategy to catapult themselves from the ranks of the unknown into positions of market leadership. During the 1990s, North Carolina National Bank (NCNB) pursued a series of acquisitions to transform itself into a major regional bank in the Southeast. But NCNB's strategic vision was to become a bank with offices across most of the United States, so the company changed its name to NationsBank. In 1998, NationsBank acquired Bank of America for $66 billion and adopted its name. In 2004, Bank of America acquired Fleet Boston Financial for $48 billion. Then in mid-2005, Bank of America spent $35 billion to acquire MBNA,

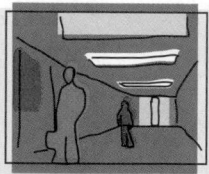

Illustration Capsule 6.1

Clear Channel Communications: Using Mergers and Acquisitions to Become a Global Market Leader

Going into 2006, Clear Channel Communications was the world's fourth largest media company, behind Disney, Time Warner, and Viacom/CBS. The company, founded in 1972 by Lowry Mays and Billy Joe McCombs, got its start by acquiring an unprofitable country-music radio station in San Antonio, Texas. Over the next 10 years, Mays learned the radio business and slowly bought other radio stations in a variety of states. Going public in 1984 helped the company raise the equity capital needed to continue acquiring radio stations in additional geographic markets.

In the late 1980s, when the Federal Communications Commission loosened the rules regarding the ability of one company to own both radio and TV stations, Clear Channel broadened its strategy and began acquiring small, struggling TV stations. By 1998, Clear Channel had used acquisitions to build a leading position in radio and television stations. Domestically, it owned, programmed, or sold airtime for 69 AM radio stations, 135 FM stations, and 18 TV stations in 48 local markets in 24 states. Clear Channel's big move was to begin expanding internationally, chiefly by acquiring interests in radio station properties in a variety of countries.

In 1997, Clear Channel used acquisitions to establish a major position in outdoor advertising. Its first acquisition was Phoenix-based Eller Media Company, an outdoor advertising company with over 100,000 billboard facings. This was quickly followed by additional acquisitions of outdoor advertising companies, the most important of which were ABC Outdoor in Milwaukee, Wisconsin; Paxton Communications (with operations in Tampa and Orlando, Florida); Universal Outdoor; the More Group, with outdoor operations and 90,000 displays in 24 countries; and the Ackerley Group.

Then in October 1999, Clear Channel made a major move by acquiring AM-FM Inc. and changed its name to

Clear Channel Communications; the AM-FM acquisition gave Clear Channel operations in 32 countries, including 830 radio stations, 19 TV stations, and more than 425,000 outdoor displays.

Additional acquisitions were completed during the 2000–2003 period. The emphasis was on buying radio, TV, and outdoor advertising properties with operations in many of the same local markets, which made it feasible to (1) cut costs by sharing facilities and staffs, (2) improve programming, and (3) sell advertising to customers in packages for all three media simultaneously. Packaging ads for two or three media not only helped Clear Channel's advertising clients distribute their messages more effectively but also allowed the company to combine its sales activities and have a common sales force for all three media, achieving significant cost savings and boosting profit margins. But in 2000 Clear Channel broadened its media strategy by acquiring SFX Entertainment, one of the world's largest promoters, producers, and presenters of live entertainment events.

At year-end 2005, Clear Channel owned radio and television stations, outdoor displays, and entertainment venues in 66 countries around the world. It operated approximately 1,200 radio and 40 television stations in the United States and had equity interests in over 240 radio stations internationally. It also operated a U.S. radio network of syndicated talk shows with about 180 million weekly listeners. In addition, the company owned or operated over 820,000 outdoor advertising displays, including billboards, street furniture, and transit panels around the world. In late 2005, the company spun off its Clear Channel Entertainment division (which was a leading promoter, producer, and marketer of about 32,000 live entertainment events annually and also owned leading athlete management and sports marketing companies) as a separate entity via an initial public offering of stock.

Sources: Information posted at www.clearchannel.com (accessed September 2005), and *BusinessWeek,* October 19, 1999, p. 56.

a leading credit card company. Going into 2006, Bank of America had a network of 5,900 branch banks in 29 states and the District of Columbia, and was managing $140 billion in credit card balances. It was the largest U.S. bank in terms of deposits, the second largest in terms of assets, and the fifth most profitable company in the world (with 2005 profits of about $17 billion).

Illustration Capsule 6.1 describes how Clear Channel Worldwide has used acquisitions to build a leading global position in outdoor advertising and radio and TV broadcasting.

All too frequently, mergers and acquisitions do not produce the hoped-for outcomes.[16] Cost savings may prove smaller than expected. Gains in competitive capabilities may take substantially longer to realize or, worse, may never materialize at all. Efforts to mesh the corporate cultures can stall due to formidable resistance from organization members. Managers and employees at the acquired company may argue forcefully for continuing to do certain things the way they were done prior to the acquisition. Key employees at the acquired company can quickly become disenchanted and leave; morale can drop to disturbingly low levels because personnel who remain disagree with newly instituted changes. Differences in management styles and operating procedures can prove hard to resolve. The managers appointed to oversee the integration of a newly acquired company can make mistakes in deciding what activities to leave alone and what activities to meld into their own operations and systems.

A number of previously applauded mergers/acquisitions have yet to live up to expectations—the merger of America Online (AOL) and Time Warner, the merger of Daimler-Benz and Chrysler, Hewlett-Packard's acquisition of Compaq Computer, Ford's acquisition of Jaguar, and Kmart's acquisition of Sears are prime examples. The AOL-Time Warner merger has proved to be mostly a disaster, partly because AOL's once-rapid growth has evaporated, partly because of a huge clash of corporate cultures, and partly because most of the expected benefits from industry convergence have yet to materialize. Ford paid a handsome price to acquire Jaguar but has yet to make the Jaguar brand a major factor in the luxury-car segment in competition against Mercedes, BMW, and Lexus. Novell acquired WordPerfect for $1.7 billion in stock in 1994, but the combination never generated enough punch to compete against Microsoft Word and Microsoft Office—Novell sold WordPerfect to Corel for $124 million in cash and stock less than two years later. In 2001 electronics retailer Best Buy paid $685 million to acquire Musicland, a struggling 1,300-store music retailer that included stores operating under the names Musicland, Sam Goody, Suncoast, Media Play, and On Cue. But Musicland's sales, already declining, dropped even further. In June 2003, Best Buy "sold" Musicland to a Florida investment firm—no cash changed hands and the "buyer" received shares of stock in Best Buy in return for assuming Musicland's liabilities.

VERTICAL INTEGRATION STRATEGIES: OPERATING ACROSS MORE STAGES OF THE INDUSTRY VALUE CHAIN

Vertical integration extends a firm's competitive and operating scope within the same industry. It involves expanding the firm's range of activities backward into sources of supply and/or forward toward end users. Thus, if a manufacturer invests in facilities to produce certain component parts that it formerly purchased from outside suppliers, it remains in essentially the same industry as before. The only change is that it has operations in two stages of the industry value chain. Similarly, if a paint manufacturer, Sherwin-Williams for example, elects to integrate forward by opening 100 retail stores to market its paint products directly to consumers, it remains in the paint business even though its competitive scope extends from manufacturing to retailing.

Vertical integration strategies can aim at *full integration* (participating in all stages of the industry value chain) or *partial integration* (building positions in selected stages of the industry's total value chain). A firm can pursue vertical integration by starting its own operations in other stages in the industry's activity chain or by acquiring a company already performing the activities it wants to bring in-house.

The Advantages of a Vertical Integration Strategy

The two best reasons for investing company resources in vertical integration are to strengthen the firm's competitive position and/or boost its profitability.[17] Vertical integration has no real payoff profitwise or strategywise unless it produces sufficient cost savings or profit increases to justify the extra investment, adds materially to a company's technological and competitive strengths, or helps differentiate the company's product offering.

Integrating Backward to Achieve Greater Competitiveness   It is harder than one might think to generate cost savings or boost profitability by integrating backward into activities such as manufacturing parts and components (which could otherwise be purchased from suppliers with specialized expertise in making these parts and components). For backward integration to be a viable and profitable strategy, a company must be able to (1) achieve the same scale economies as outside suppliers and (2) match or beat suppliers' production efficiency with no drop-off in quality. Neither outcome is a slam-dunk. To begin with, a company's in-house requirements are often too small to reach the optimum size for low-cost operation—for instance, if it takes a minimum production volume of 1 million units to achieve mass-production economies and a company's in-house requirements are just 250,000 units, then the company falls way short of being able to capture the scale economies of outside suppliers (which may readily find buyers for 1 million or more units). Furthermore, matching the production efficiency of suppliers is fraught with problems when suppliers have considerable production experience of their own, when the technology they employ has elements that are hard to master, or when substantial R&D expertise is required to develop next-version parts and components or keep pace with advancing technology in parts/components production.

But that being said, there are still occasions when a company can improve its cost position and competitiveness by performing a broad range of value chain activities in-house. The best potential for being able to reduce costs via a backward integration strategy exists in situations where suppliers have outsized profit margins, where the item being supplied is a major cost component, and where the requisite technological skills are easily mastered or can be gained by acquiring a supplier with the desired technological know-how. Furthermore, when a company has proprietary know-how that it is beneficial to keep away from rivals, then in-house performance of value chain activities related to this know-how is beneficial even if such activities could be performed by outsiders. For example, Krispy Kreme Doughnuts has successfully employed a backward vertical integration strategy that involves internally producing both the doughnut-making equipment and ready-mixed doughnut ingredients that company-owned and franchised retail stores used in making Krispy Kreme doughnuts—the company earned substantial profits from producing these items internally rather than having them supplied by outsiders. Furthermore, Krispy Kreme's vertical integration strategy made good competitive sense because both its doughnut-making equipment and its doughnut recipe were proprietary; keeping its equipment manufacturing know-how and its secret recipe out of the hands of outside suppliers helped Krispy Kreme protect its doughnut offering from would-be imitators.

Backward vertical integration can produce a differentiation-based competitive advantage when a company, by performing activities internally rather than using outside suppliers, ends up with a better-quality product/service offering, improves the caliber of its customer service, or in other ways enhances the performance of its final product. On occasion, integrating into more stages along the industry value chain can add to a company's differentiation capabilities by allowing the company to build or strengthen its core competencies, better master key skills or strategy-critical technologies, or add features that deliver greater customer value. Other potential advantages of backward integration include sparing a company the uncertainty of being dependent on suppliers for crucial components or support services and lessening a company's vulnerability to powerful suppliers inclined to raise prices at every opportunity.

Integrating Forward to Enhance Competitiveness   The strategic impetus for forward integration is to gain better access to end users and better market visibility. In many industries, independent sales agents, wholesalers, and retailers handle competing brands of the same product; having no allegiance to any one company's brand, they tend to push whatever sells and earns them the biggest profits. An independent insurance agency, for example, represents a number of different insurance companies—in trying to find the best match between a customer's insurance requirements and the policies of alternative insurance companies, there's plenty of opportunity for independent agents to end up promoting certain insurance companies' policies ahead of others'. An insurance company may therefore conclude that it is better off setting up its own local sales offices with its own local agents to exclusively promote its policies. Likewise, a manufacturer can be frustrated in its attempts to win higher sales and market share or get rid of unwanted inventory or maintain steady, near-capacity production if it must distribute its products through distributors and/or retailers who are only halfheartedly committed to promoting and marketing its brand as opposed to those of rivals. In such cases, it can be advantageous for a manufacturer to integrate forward into wholesaling or retailing via company-owned distributorships or a chain of retail stores. For instance, both Goodyear and Bridgestone opted to integrate forward into tire retailing rather than to use independent distributors and retailers that stocked multiple brands because the independent distributors/retailers stressed selling the tire brands on which they earned the highest profit margins. A number of housewares and apparel manufacturers have integrated forward into retailing so as to move seconds, overstocked items, and slow-selling merchandise through their own branded retail outlet stores located in discount malls. Some producers have opted to integrate forward into retailing by selling directly to customers at the company's Web site. Bypassing regular wholesale/retail channels in favor of direct sales and Internet retailing can have appeal if it lowers distribution costs, produces a relative cost advantage over certain rivals, and results in lower selling prices to end users.

The Disadvantages of a Vertical Integration Strategy

Vertical integration has some substantial drawbacks, however.[18] As it boosts a firm's capital investment in the industry, it increases business risk (what if industry growth and profitability go sour?) and increases the company's vested interests in sticking with its vertically integrated value chain (what if some aspects of its technology and production facilities become obsolete before they are worn out or fully depreciated?). Vertically integrated companies that have invested heavily in a particular technology or in parts/components manufacture are often slow to embrace technological advances or more efficient production methods compared to partially integrated or nonintegrated firms. This is because less integrated firms can pressure suppliers to provide only the latest and best parts and components (even going so far as to shift their purchases from one supplier to another if need be), whereas a vertically integrated firm that is saddled with older technology or facilities that make items it no longer needs is looking at the high costs of premature abandonment. Second, integrating forward or backward locks a firm into relying on its own in-house activities and sources of supply (which later may prove more costly than outsourcing) and potentially results in less flexibility in accommodating shifting buyer preferences or a product design that doesn't include parts and components that it makes in-house. *In today's world of close working relationships with suppliers and efficient supply chain management systems, very few businesses can make a case for integrating backward into the business of suppliers to ensure a reliable supply of materials and components or to reduce production costs.* The best materials and components suppliers stay abreast of advancing technology and are adept in boosting their efficiency and keeping their costs and prices as low as possible. A company that pursues a vertical integration strategy and tries to produce many parts and components in-house is likely to find itself hard-pressed to keep up with technological advances and cutting-edge production practices for each part and component used in making its product.

Third, vertical integration poses all kinds of capacity-matching problems. In motor vehicle manufacturing, for example, the most efficient scale of operation for making axles is different from the most economic volume for radiators, and different yet again for both engines and transmissions. Building the capacity to produce just the right number of axles, radiators, engines, and transmissions in-house—and doing so at the lowest unit cost for each—is much easier said than done. If internal capacity for making transmissions is deficient, the difference has to be bought externally. Where internal capacity for radiators proves excessive, customers need to be found for the surplus. And if by-products are generated—as occurs in the processing of many chemical products—they require arrangements for disposal. Consequently, integrating across several production stages in ways that achieve the lowest feasible costs is not as easy as it might seem.

Fourth, integration forward or backward often calls for radical changes in skills and business capabilities. Parts and components manufacturing, assembly operations, wholesale distribution and retailing, and direct sales via the Internet are different businesses with different key success factors. Managers of a manufacturing company should consider carefully whether it makes good business sense to invest time and money in developing the expertise and merchandising skills to integrate forward into wholesaling and retailing. Many manufacturers learn the hard way that company-owned wholesale/retail networks present many headaches, fit poorly with what they do best, and don't always add the kind of value to their core business they thought they would. Selling to customers via the Internet poses still another set of problems—it is usually easier to use the Internet to sell to business customers than to consumers.

Finally, integrating backward into parts and components manufacture can impair a company's operating flexibility when it comes to changing out the use of certain parts and components. It is one thing to design out a component made by a supplier and another to design out a component being made in-house (which can mean laying off employees and writing off the associated investment in equipment and facilities). Companies that alter designs and models frequently in response to shifting buyer preferences often find that outsourcing the needed parts and components is cheaper and less complicated than producing them in-house. Most of the world's automakers, despite their expertise in automotive technology and manufacturing, have concluded that purchasing many of their key parts and components from manufacturing specialists results in higher quality, lower costs, and greater design flexibility than does the vertical integration option.

Weighing the Pros and Cons of Vertical Integration   All in all, therefore, a strategy of vertical integration can have both important strengths and weaknesses. The tip of the scales depends on (1) whether vertical integration can enhance the performance of strategy-critical activities in ways that lower cost, build expertise, protect proprietary know-how, or increase differentiation; (2) the impact of vertical integration on investment costs, flexibility and response times, and the administrative costs of coordinating operations across more value chain activities; and (3) whether vertical integration substantially enhances a company's competitiveness and profitability. *Vertical integration strategies have merit according to which capabilities and value-chain activities truly need to be performed in-house and which can be performed better or cheaper by outsiders.* Absent solid benefits, integrating forward or backward is not likely to be an attractive strategy option.

OUTSOURCING STRATEGIES: NARROWING THE BOUNDARIES OF THE BUSINESS

Outsourcing involves a conscious decision to abandon or forgo attempts to perform certain value chain activities internally and instead to farm them out to outside specialists and strategic allies. The two big drivers for outsourcing are that (1) outsiders can often perform certain activities better or cheaper and (2) outsourcing allows a firm to focus its entire energies on those activities at the center of its expertise (its core competencies) and that are the most critical to its competitive and financial success.

> **Core Concept**
> *Outsourcing* involves farming out certain value chain activities to outside vendors.

The current interest of many companies in making outsourcing a key component of their overall strategy and their approach to supply chain management represents a big departure from the way that companies used to deal with their suppliers and vendors. In years past, it was common for companies to maintain arm's-length relationships with suppliers and outside vendors, insisting on items being made to precise specifications and negotiating long and hard over price.[19] Although a company might place orders with the same supplier repeatedly, there was no expectation that this would be the case; price usually determined which supplier was awarded an order, and companies used the threat of switching suppliers to get the lowest possible prices. To enhance their bargaining power and, to make the threat of switching credible, it was standard practice for companies to source key parts and components from several suppliers as opposed to dealing with only a single supplier. But today most companies are abandoning such approaches in favor of forging alliances and strategic partnerships with a small number of highly capable suppliers. Collaborative relationships are replacing contractual, purely price-oriented relationships because companies have discovered that many of the advantages of performing value chain activities in-house can be captured and many of the disadvantages avoided by forging close, long-term cooperative partnerships with able suppliers and vendors and tapping into the expertise and capabilities that they have painstakingly developed.

When Outsourcing Strategies Are Advantageous

Outsourcing pieces of the value chain to narrow the boundaries of a firm's business makes strategic sense whenever:

- *An activity can be performed better or more cheaply by outside specialists.* Many PC makers, for example, have shifted from assembling units in-house to using contract assemblers because of the sizable scale economies associated with purchasing PC components in large volumes and assembling PCs. German shoemaker Birkenstock, by outsourcing the distribution of shoes made in its two plants in Germany to UPS, cut the time for delivering orders to U.S. footwear retailers from seven weeks to three weeks.[20]

- *The activity is not crucial to the firm's ability to achieve sustainable competitive advantage and won't hollow out its core competencies, capabilities, or technical know-how.* Outsourcing of maintenance services, data processing and data storage, fringe benefit management, Web site operations, and similar administrative support activities to specialists has become commonplace. American Express, for instance, recently entered into a seven-year, $4 billion deal whereby IBM's Services division would host American Express's Web site, network servers, data storage, and help desk; American Express indicated that it would save several hundred million dollars by paying only for the services it needed when it needed them (as opposed to funding its own full-time staff). A number of companies have begun outsourcing their call center operations to foreign-based contractors who have access to lower-cost labor supplies and can employ lower-paid call center personnel to respond to customer inquiries or requests for technical support.

  - *It reduces the company's risk exposure to changing technology and/ or changing buyer preferences.* When a company outsources certain parts, components, and services, its suppliers must bear the burden of incorporating state-of-the-art technologies and/or undertaking redesigns and upgrades to accommodate a company's plans to introduce next-generation products. If what a supplier provides falls out of favor with buyers or is designed out of next-generation products, it is the supplier's business that suffers rather than a company's own internal operations.

- *It improves a company's ability to innovate.* Collaborative partnerships with world-class suppliers who have cutting-edge intellectual capital and are early adopters of the latest technology give a company access to ever better parts and components—such supplier-driven innovations, when incorporated into a company's own product offering, fuel a company's ability to introduce its own new and improved products.

- *It streamlines company operations in ways that improve organizational flexibility and cuts the time it takes to get new products into the marketplace.* Outsourcing gives a company the flexibility to switch suppliers in the event that its present supplier falls behind competing suppliers. To the extent that its suppliers can speedily get next-generation parts and components into production, then a company can get its own next-generation product offerings into the marketplace quicker. Moreover, seeking out new suppliers with the needed capabilities already in place is frequently quicker, easier, less risky, and cheaper than hurriedly retooling internal operations to replace obsolete capabilities or try to install and master new technologies.

- *It allows a company to assemble diverse kinds of expertise speedily and efficiently.* A company can nearly always gain quicker access to first-rate capabilities and expertise by partnering with suppliers who already have them in place than it can by trying to build them from scratch with its own company personnel.

- *It allows a company to concentrate on its core business, leverage its key resources, and do even better what it already does best.* A company is better able to build and develop its own competitively valuable competencies and capabilities when it concentrates its full resources and energies on performing those activities internally that it can perform better than outsiders and/or that it needs to have under its direct control. Cisco Systems, for example, devotes its energy to designing new generations of switches, routers, and other Internet-related equipment, opting to outsource the more mundane activities of producing and assembling its routers and switching equipment to contract manufacturers that together operate 37 factories, all closely monitored and overseen by Cisco personnel via online systems. Cisco's contract suppliers work so closely with Cisco that they can ship Cisco products to Cisco customers without a Cisco employee ever touching the gear. This system of alliances saves $500 million to $800 million annually.[21]

Dell Computer's partnerships with the suppliers of PC components have allowed it to operate with only three days of inventory (just a couple of hours of inventory in the case of some components), to realize substantial savings in inventory costs, and to get PCs equipped with next-generation components into the marketplace in less than a week after the newly upgraded components start shipping. Hewlett-Packard, IBM, Silicon Graphics (now SGI), and others have sold plants to suppliers and then contracted to purchase the output. Starbucks has found purchasing coffee beans from independent growers far more advantageous than trying to integrate backward into the coffee-growing business.

The Big Risk of an Outsourcing Strategy

The biggest danger of outsourcing is that a company will farm out too many or the wrong types of activities and thereby hollow out its own capabilities.[22] In such cases, a company loses touch with the very activities and expertise that over the long run determine its success. But most companies are alert to this danger and take actions to protect against being held hostage by outside suppliers. Cisco Systems guards against loss of control and protects its manufacturing expertise by designing the production methods that its contract manufacturers must use. Cisco keeps the source code for its designs proprietary, thereby controlling the initiation of all improvements and safeguarding its innovations from imitation. Further, Cisco uses the Internet to monitor the factory operations of contract manufacturers around the clock and can therefore know immediately when problems arise and whether to get involved.

OFFENSIVE STRATEGIES: IMPROVING MARKET POSITION AND BUILDING COMPETITIVE ADVANTAGE

Most every company must at times go on the offensive to improve its market position and try to build a competitive advantage or widen an existing one. Companies like Dell, Wal-Mart, and Toyota play hardball, aggressively pursuing competitive advantage and trying to reap the benefits a competitive edge offers—a leading market share, excellent profit margins and rapid growth (as compared to rivals), and all the intangibles of being known as a company on the move and one that plays to win.[23] The best offensives tend to incorporate several behaviors and principles: (1) focusing relentlessly on building competitive advantage and then striving to convert competitive advantage into decisive advantage, (2) employing the element of surprise as opposed to doing what rivals expect and are prepared for, (3) applying resources where rivals are least able to defend themselves, and (4) being impatient with the status quo and displaying a strong bias for swift, decisive actions to boost a company's competitive position vis-à-vis rivals.[24]

Offensive strategies are also important when a company has no choice but to try to whittle away at a strong rival's competitive advantage and when it is possible to gain profitable market share at the expense of rivals despite whatever resource strengths and capabilities they have. How long it takes for an offensive to yield good results varies with the competitive circumstances.[25] It can be short if buyers respond immediately (as can occur with a dramatic price cut, an imaginative ad campaign, or an especially appealing new product). Securing a competitive edge can take much longer if winning consumer acceptance of an innovative product will take some time or if the firm may need several years to debug a new technology or put new production capacity in place or develop and perfect new competitive capabilities. Ideally, an offensive move will improve a company's market standing or result in a competitive edge fairly quickly; the longer it takes, the more likely it is that rivals will spot the move, see its potential, and begin a counterresponse.

The principal offensive strategy options include the following:

1. *Offering an equally good or better product at a lower price.* This is the classic offensive for improving a company's market position vis-à-vis rivals. Advanced Micro Devices (AMD), wanting to grow its sales of microprocessors for PCs, has on several occasions elected to attack Intel head-on, offering a faster alternative to Intel's Pentium chips at a lower price. Believing that the company's survival depends on eliminating the performance gap between AMD chips and Intel chips, AMD management has been willing to risk that a head-on offensive might prompt Intel to counter with lower prices of its own and accelerated development of next-generation chips. Lower prices can produce market share gains if competitors don't respond with price cuts of their own and if the challenger convinces buyers that its product is just as good or better. However, such a strategy increases total profits only if the gains in additional unit sales are enough to offset the impact of lower prices and thinner margins per unit sold. Price-cutting offensives generally work best when a company *first achieves a cost advantage and then hits competitors with a lower price.*[26]

2. *Leapfrogging competitors by being the first adopter of next-generation technologies or being first to market with next-generation products.* In 2004–2005, Microsoft waged an offensive to get its next-generation Xbox to market four to six months ahead of Sony's PlayStation 3, anticipating that such a lead time would allow help it convince video gamers to switch to the Xbox rather than wait for the new PlayStation to hit the market in 2006.

3. *Pursuing continuous product innovation to draw sales and market share away from less innovative rivals.* Aggressive and sustained efforts to trump the products of rivals by introducing new or improved products with features calculated to win customers away from rivals can put rivals under tremendous competitive pressure, especially when their new product development capabilities are weak or suspect. But such offensives work only if a company has potent product innovation skills of its own and can keep its pipeline full of ideas that are consistently well received in the marketplace.

4. *Adopting and improving on the good ideas of other companies (rivals or otherwise).*[27] The idea of warehouse-type hardware and home improvement centers did not

originate with Home Depot founders Arthur Blank and Bernie Marcus; they got the big-box concept from their former employer Handy Dan Home Improvement. But they were quick to improve on Handy Dan's business model and strategy and take Home Depot to the next plateau in terms of product line breadth and customer service. Casket maker Hillenbrand greatly improved its market position by adapting Toyota's production methods to casket making. Ryanair has succeeded as a low-cost airline in Europe by imitating many of Southwest Airlines' operating practices and applying them in a different geographic market. Companies that like to play hardball are willing to take any good idea (not nailed down by a patent or other legal protection), make it their own, and then aggressively apply it to create competitive advantage for themselves.[28]

5. *Deliberately attacking those market segments where a key rival makes big profits.*[29] Dell Computer's recent entry into printers and printer cartridges—the market arena where number-two PC maker Hewlett-Packard (HP) enjoys hefty profit margins and makes the majority of its profits—while mainly motivated by Dell's desire to broaden its product line and save its customers money (because of Dell's lower prices), nonetheless represented a hardball offensive calculated to weaken HP's market position in printers. To the extent that Dell might be able to use lower prices to woo away some of HP's printer customers, the move would erode HP's "profit sanctuary," distract HP's attention away from PCs, and reduce the financial resources HP has available for battling Dell in the global market for PCs.

6. *Attacking the competitive weaknesses of rivals.* Offensives aimed at rivals' weaknesses present many options. One is to go after the customers of those rivals whose products lag on quality, features, or product performance. If a company has especially good customer service capabilities, it can make special sales pitches to the customers of those rivals who provide subpar customer service. Aggressors with a recognized brand name and strong marketing skills can launch efforts to win customers away from rivals with weak brand recognition. There is considerable appeal in emphasizing sales to buyers in geographic regions where a rival has a weak market share or is exerting less competitive effort. Likewise, it may be attractive to pay special attention to buyer segments that a rival is neglecting or is weakly equipped to serve.

7. *Maneuvering around competitors and concentrating on capturing unoccupied or less contested market territory.* Examples include launching initiatives to build strong positions in geographic areas where close rivals have little or no market presence and trying to create new market segments by introducing products with different attributes and performance features to better meet the needs of selected buyers.

8. *Using hit-and-run or guerrilla warfare tactics to grab sales and market share from complacent or distracted rivals.* Options for "guerrilla offensives" include occasional lowballing on price (to win a big order or steal a key account from a rival); surprising key rivals with sporadic but intense bursts of promotional activity (offering a 20 percent discount for one week to draw customers away from rival brands); or undertaking special campaigns to attract buyers away from rivals plagued with a strike or problems in meeting buyer demand.[30] Guerrilla offensives are particularly well suited to small challengers who have neither the resources nor the market visibility to mount a full-fledged attack on industry leaders.

9. *Launching a preemptive strike to secure an advantageous position that rivals are prevented or discouraged from duplicating.*[31] What makes a move preemptive

is its one-of-a-kind nature—whoever strikes first stands to acquire competitive assets that rivals can't readily match. Examples of preemptive moves include (1) securing the best distributors in a particular geographic region or country; (2) moving to obtain the most favorable site along a heavily traveled thoroughfare, at a new interchange or intersection, in a new shopping mall, in a natural beauty spot, close to cheap transportation or raw material supplies or market outlets, and so on; (3) tying up the most reliable, high-quality suppliers via exclusive partnership, long-term contracts, or even acquisition; and (4) moving swiftly to acquire the assets of distressed rivals at bargain prices. To be successful, a preemptive move doesn't have to totally block rivals from following or copying; it merely needs to give a firm a prime position that is not easily circumvented.

Blue Ocean Strategy: A Special Kind of Offensive

A "blue ocean strategy" seeks to gain a dramatic and durable competitive advantage *by abandoning efforts to beat out competitors in existing markets and, instead, inventing a new industry or distinctive market segment (a wide-open blue ocean of possibility) that renders existing competitors largely irrelevant and allows a company to create and capture altogether new demand.*[32] This strategy views the business universe as consisting of two distinct types of market space. One is where industry boundaries are defined and accepted, the competitive rules of the game are well understood by all industry members, and companies try to outperform rivals by capturing a bigger share of existing demand; in such markets, lively competition constrains a company's prospects for rapid growth and superior profitability since rivals move quickly to either imitate or counter the successes of competitors. In the second type of market space, the industry does not really exist yet, is untainted by competition, and offers wide-open opportunity for profitable and rapid growth if a company can come up with a product offering and strategy that allows it to create new demand rather than fight over existing demand. A terrific example of such a blue ocean market space is the online auction industry that eBay created and now dominates.

Another company that has employed a blue ocean strategy is Cirque du Soleil, which increased its revenues by 22 times during the 1993–2003 period in the circus business, an industry that had been in long-term decline for 20 years. How did Cirque du Soleil pull this off against legendary industry leader Ringling Bros. and Barnum & Bailey? By reinventing the circus, creating a distinctively different market space for its performances (Las Vegas nightclubs and theater-type settings), and pulling in a whole new group of customers—adults and corporate clients—who were noncustomers of traditional circuses and were willing to pay several times more than the price of a conventional circus ticket to have an "entertainment experience" featuring sophisticated clowns and star-quality acrobatic acts in a comfortable big-tent atmosphere. Cirque studiously avoided the use of animals because of costs and because of concerns over their treatment by traditional circus organizations. Cirque's market research led management to conclude that the lasting allure of the traditional circus came down to just three factors: the clowns, classic acrobatic acts, and a tentlike stage. As of 2005, Cirque du Soleil was presenting nine different shows, each with its own theme and story line; was performing before audiences of about 7 million people annually; and had performed 250 engagements in 100 cities before 50 million spectators since its formation in 1984.

Other examples of companies that have achieved competitive advantages by creating blue ocean market spaces include AMC via its pioneering of megaplex movie theaters, The Weather Channel in cable TV, Home Depot in big-box retailing of hardware and building supplies, and FedEx in overnight package delivery. Companies that create blue ocean market spaces can usually sustain their initially won competitive advantage without encountering major competitive challenge for 10 to 15 years because of high barriers to imitation and the strong brand-name awareness that a blue ocean strategy can produce.

Choosing Which Rivals to Attack

Offense-minded firms need to analyze which of their rivals to challenge as well as how to mount that challenge. The following are the best targets for offensive attacks:[33]

- *Market leaders that are vulnerable*—Offensive attacks make good sense when a company that leads in terms of size and market share is not a true leader in terms of serving the market well. Signs of leader vulnerability include unhappy buyers, an inferior product line, a weak competitive strategy with regard to low-cost leadership or differentiation, strong emotional commitment to an aging technology the leader has pioneered, outdated plants and equipment, a preoccupation with diversification into other industries, and mediocre or declining profitability. Offensives to erode the positions of market leaders have real promise when the challenger is able to revamp its value chain or innovate to gain a fresh cost-based or differentiation-based competitive advantage.[34] To be judged successful, attacks on leaders don't have to result in making the aggressor the new leader; a challenger may "win" by simply becoming a stronger runner-up. Caution is well advised in challenging strong market leaders— there's a significant risk of squandering valuable resources in a futile effort or precipitating a fierce and profitless industrywide battle for market share.

- *Runner-up firms with weaknesses in areas where the challenger is strong*— Runner-up firms are an especially attractive target when a challenger's resource strengths and competitive capabilities are well suited to exploiting their weaknesses.

- *Struggling enterprises that are on the verge of going under*—Challenging a hard-pressed rival in ways that further sap its financial strength and competitive position can weaken its resolve and hasten its exit from the market.

- *Small local and regional firms with limited capabilities*—Because small firms typically have limited expertise and resources, a challenger with broader capabilities is well positioned to raid their biggest and best customers—particularly those who are growing rapidly, have increasingly sophisticated requirements, and may already be thinking about switching to a supplier with more full-service capability.

Choosing the Basis for Competitive Attack

As a rule, challenging rivals on competitive grounds where they are strong is an uphill struggle.[35] Offensive initiatives that exploit competitor weaknesses stand a better chance of succeeding than do those that challenge competitor strengths, especially if the weaknesses represent important vulnerabilities and weak rivals can be caught by surprise with no ready defense.[36]

Strategic offensives should, as a general rule, be grounded in a company's competitive assets and strong points—its core competencies, competitive capabilities, and such resource strengths as a better-known brand name, a cost advantage in manufacturing or distribution, greater technological capability,

> **Core Concept**
> The best offensives use a company's resource strengths to attack rivals in those competitive areas where they are weak.

or a superior product. If the attacker's resource strengths give it a competitive advantage over the targeted rivals, so much the better. Ignoring the need to tie a strategic offensive to a company's competitive strengths is like going to war with a popgun—the prospects for success are dim. For instance, it is foolish for a company with relatively high costs to employ a price-cutting offensive—price-cutting offensives are best left to financially strong companies whose costs are relatively low in comparison to those of the companies being attacked. Likewise, it is ill advised to pursue a product innovation offensive without having proven expertise in R&D, new product development, and speeding new or improved products to market.

DEFENSIVE STRATEGIES: PROTECTING MARKET POSITION AND COMPETITIVE ADVANTAGE

It is just as important to discern when to fortify a company's present market position with defensive actions as it is to seize the initiative and launch strategic offensives.

In a competitive market, all firms are subject to offensive challenges from rivals. The purposes of defensive strategies are to lower the risk of being attacked, weaken the impact of any attack that occurs, and influence challengers to aim their efforts at other rivals. While defensive strategies usually don't enhance a firm's competitive advantage, they can definitely help fortify its competitive position, protect its most valuable resources and capabilities from imitation, and defend whatever competitive advantage it might have. Defensive strategies can take either of two forms: actions to block challengers and signaling the likelihood of strong retaliation.

Blocking the Avenues Open to Challengers

There are many ways to throw obstacles in the path of would-be challengers.

The most frequently employed approach to defending a company's present position involves actions that restrict a challenger's options for initiating competitive attack. There are any number of obstacles that can be put in the path of would-be challengers.[37] A defender can participate in alternative technologies as a hedge against rivals attacking with a new or better technology. A defender can introduce new features, add new models, or broaden its product line to close off gaps and vacant niches to opportunity-seeking challengers. It can thwart the efforts of rivals to attack with a lower price by maintaining economy-priced options of its own. It can try to discourage buyers from trying competitors' brands by lengthening warranties, offering free training and support services, developing the capability to deliver spare parts to users faster than rivals can, providing coupons and sample giveaways to buyers most prone to experiment, and making early announcements about impending new products or price changes to induce potential buyers to postpone switching. It can challenge the quality or safety of rivals' products. Finally, a defender can grant volume discounts or better financing terms to dealers and distributors to discourage them from experimenting with other suppliers, or it can convince them to handle its product line *exclusively* and force competitors to use other distribution outlets.

Signaling Challengers that Retaliation Is Likely

The goal of signaling challengers that strong retaliation is likely in the event of an attack is either to dissuade challengers from attacking at all or to divert them to less threatening options. Either goal can be achieved by letting challengers know the battle will cost more than it is worth. Would-be challengers can be signaled by:[38]

- Publicly announcing management's commitment to maintain the firm's present market share.
- Publicly committing the company to a policy of matching competitors' terms or prices.
- Maintaining a war chest of cash and marketable securities.
- Making an occasional strong counterresponse to the moves of weak competitors to enhance the firm's image as a tough defender.

WEB SITE STRATEGIES

One of the biggest strategic issues facing company executives across the world is just what role the company's Web site should play in a company's competitive strategy. In particular, to what degree should a company use the Internet as a distribution channel for accessing buyers? Should a company use its Web site *only as a means of disseminating product information* (with traditional distribution channel partners making all sales to end users), as a *secondary or minor channel* for selling directly to buyers of its product, as *one of several important distribution channels* for accessing customers, as *the primary distribution channel* for accessing customers, or as *the exclusive channel* for transacting sales with customers?[39] Let's look at each of these strategic options in turn.

> Companies today must wrestle with the strategic issue of how to use their Web sites in positioning themselves in the marketplace—whether to use their Web sites just to disseminate product information or whether to operate an e-store to sell direct to online shoppers.

Product Information–Only Web Strategies: Avoiding Channel Conflict

Operating a Web site that contains extensive product information but that relies on click-throughs to the Web sites of distribution channel partners for sales transactions (or that informs site users where nearby retail stores are located) is an attractive market positioning option for manufacturers and/or wholesalers that have invested heavily in building and cultivating retail dealer networks and that face nettlesome channel conflict issues if they try to sell online in direct competition with their dealers. A manufacturer or wholesaler that aggressively pursues online sales to end users is signaling both a weak strategic commitment to its dealers and a willingness to cannibalize dealers' sales and growth potential.

To the extent that strong partnerships with wholesale and/or retail dealers are critical to accessing end users, selling directly to end users via the company's Web site is a very tricky road to negotiate. A manufacturer's efforts to use its Web site to sell around its dealers is certain to anger its wholesale distributors and retail dealers, which may respond by putting more effort into marketing the brands of rival manufacturers that don't sell online. In sum, the manufacturer may stand to lose more sales by offending its dealers than it gains from its own online sales effort. Moreover, dealers may be in better position to employ a brick-and-click strategy than a manufacturer is because dealers have a local presence to complement their online sales approach (which consumers may find appealing). Consequently, in industries where the strong support and goodwill of dealer networks is essential, manufacturers may conclude that their Web site should be designed to partner with dealers rather than compete with them—just as the auto manufacturers are doing with their franchised dealers.

Web Site e-Stores as a Minor Distribution Channel

A second strategic option is to use online sales as a relatively minor distribution channel for achieving incremental sales, gaining online sales experience, and doing marketing research. If channel conflict poses a big obstacle to online sales, or if only a small fraction of buyers can be attracted to make online purchases, then companies are well advised to pursue online sales with the strategic intent of gaining experience, learning more about buyer tastes and preferences, testing reaction to new products, creating added market buzz about their products, and boosting overall sales volume a few percentage points. Sony and Nike, for example, sell most all of their products at their Web sites without provoking resistance from their retail dealers since most buyers of their products prefer to do their buying at retail stores rather than online. They use their Web site not so much to make sales as to glean valuable marketing research data from tracking the browsing patterns of Web site visitors. The behavior and actions of Web surfers are a veritable gold mine of information for companies seeking to keep their finger on the market pulse and respond more precisely to buyer preferences and interests.

Despite the channel conflict that exists when a manufacturer sells directly to end users at its Web site in head-to-head competition with its distribution channel allies, manufacturers might still opt to pursue online sales at their Web sites and try to establish online sales as an important distribution channel because (1) their profit margins from online sales are bigger than they earned from selling to their wholesale/retail customers; (2) encouraging buyers to visit the company's Web site helps educate them to the ease and convenience of purchasing online and, over time, prompts more and more buyers to purchase online (where company profit margins are greater)—which makes incurring channel conflict in the short term and competing against traditional distribution allies potentially worthwhile—and (3) selling directly to end users allows a manufacturer to make greater use of build-to-order manufacturing and assembly, which, if met with growing buyer acceptance of and satisfaction, would increase the rate at which sales migrate from distribution allies to the company's Web site—such migration could lead to streamlining the company's value chain and boosting its profit margins.

Brick-and-Click Strategies

Brick-and-click strategies have two big strategic appeals for wholesale and retail enterprises: They are an economic means of expanding a company's geographic reach, and they give both existing and potential customers another choice of how to communicate with the company, shop for product information, make purchases, or resolve customer service problems. Software developers, for example, have come to rely on the Internet as a highly effective distribution channel to complement sales through brick-and-mortar wholesalers and retailers. Selling online directly to end users has the advantage of eliminating the costs of producing and packaging CDs, as well as cutting out the costs and margins of software wholesalers and retailers (often 35 to 50 percent of the retail price). However, software developers are still strongly motivated to continue to distribute their products through wholesalers and retailers (to maintain broad access to existing and potential users who, for whatever reason, may be reluctant to buy online). Chain retailers like Wal-Mart and Circuit City operate online stores for their products primarily as a convenience to customers who want to buy online rather than making a shopping trip to nearby stores.

Many brick-and-mortar companies can enter online retailing at relatively low cost—all they need is a Web store and systems for filling and delivering individual customer orders. Brick-and-mortar distributors and retailers (as well as manufacturers with company-owned retail stores) can employ brick-and-click strategies by using their current distribution centers and/or retail stores for picking orders from on-hand inventories and making deliveries. Blockbuster, the world's largest chain of video and DVD rental stores, uses the inventories at its stores to fill orders for its online subscribers, who pay a monthly fee for unlimited DVDs delivered by mail carrier; using local stores to fill orders typically allows delivery in 24 hours versus 48 hours for shipments made from a regional shipping center. Walgreen's, a leading drugstore chain, allows customers to order a prescription online and then pick it up at the drive-through window or inside counter of a local store. In banking, a brick-and-click strategy allows customers to use local branches and ATMs for depositing checks and getting cash while using online systems to pay bills, check account balances, and transfer funds. Many industrial distributors are finding it efficient for customers to place their orders over the Web rather than phoning them in or waiting for salespeople to call in person. Illustration Capsule 6.2 describes how office supply chains like Office Depot, Staples, and OfficeMax have successfully migrated from a traditional brick-and-mortar distribution strategy to a combination brick-and-click distribution strategy.

Strategies for Online Enterprises

A company that elects to use the Internet as its exclusive channel for accessing buyers is essentially an online enterprise from the perspective of the customer. The Internet becomes the vehicle for transacting sales and delivering customer services; except for advertising, the Internet is the sole point of all buyer–seller contact. Many so-called pure dot-com enterprises have chosen this strategic approach—prominent examples include eBay, Yahoo, Amazon.com, Buy.com, Overstock.com, and Priceline.com. For a company to succeed in using the Internet as its exclusive distribution channel, its product or service must be one for which buying online holds strong appeal.

A company that decides to use online sales as its exclusive method for sales transactions must address several strategic issues:

- *How it will deliver unique value to buyers*—Online businesses must usually attract buyers on the basis of low price, convenience, superior product information, build-to-order options, or attentive online service.

- *Whether it will pursue competitive advantage based on lower costs, differentiation, or better value for the money*—For an online-only sales strategy to succeed in head-to-head competition with brick-and-mortar and brick-and-click rivals, an online seller's value chain approach must hold potential for a low-cost advantage, competitively valuable differentiating attributes, or a best-cost provider advantage. If an online firm's strategy is to attract customers by selling at cut-rate prices, then it must possess cost advantages in those activities it performs, and it must outsource the remaining activities to low-cost specialists. If an online seller is going to differentiate itself on the basis of a superior buying experience and top-notch customer service, then it needs to concentrate on having an easy-to-navigate Web site, an array of functions and conveniences for customers, Web reps who can answer questions online, and logistical capabilities to deliver products quickly and accommodate returned merchandise. If it is going to deliver more value for the money, then it must manage value chain activities so as to deliver upscale products and services at lower costs than rivals.

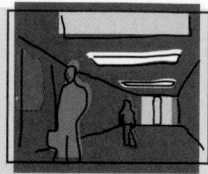

Illustration Capsule 6.2

Brick-and-Click Strategies in the Office Supplies Industry

Office Depot was in the first wave of retailers to adopt a combination brick-and-click strategy. Management quickly saw the merits of allowing business customers to use the Internet to place orders instead of having to make a call, generate a purchase order, and pay an invoice—while still getting same-day or next-day delivery from one of Office Depot's local stores.

Office Depot already had an existing network of retail stores, delivery centers and warehouses, delivery trucks, account managers, sales offices, and regional call centers that handled large business customers. In addition, it had a solid brand name and enough purchasing power with its suppliers to counter discount-minded online rivals trying to attract buyers of office supplies on the basis of super-low prices. Office Depot's incremental investment to enter the e-commerce arena was minimal since all it needed to add was a Web site where customers could see pictures and descriptions of the 14,000 items it carried, their prices, and in-stock availability. Marketing costs to make customers aware of its Web store option ran less than $10 million.

Office Depot's online prices were the same as its store prices, the strategy being to promote Web sales on the basis of service, convenience, and lower customer costs for order processing and inventories. Customers reported that doing business with Office Depot online cut their transaction costs by up to 80 percent; plus, Office Depot's same-day or next-day delivery capability allowed them to reduce office supply inventories.

The company set up customized Web pages for 37,000 corporate and educational customers that allowed the customer's employees varying degrees of freedom to buy supplies. A clerk might be able to order only copying paper, toner cartridges, computer disks, and paper clips up to a preset dollar limit per order, while a vice president might have carte blanche to order any item Office Depot sold.

Web site sales cost Office Depot less than $1 per $100 of goods ordered, compared with about $2 for phone and fax orders. And since Web sales eliminate the need to key in transactions, order-entry errors were virtually eliminated and product returns cut by 50 percent. Billing is handled electronically.

In 2005, over 50 percent of Office Depot's major customers were ordering most of their supplies online. Online sales accounted for almost $3 billion in 2004 (about 24 percent of Office Depot's total revenues), up from $982 million in 2000 and making Office Depot the third-largest online retailer. Its online operations were profitable from the start.

Office Depot's successful brick-and-click strategy prompted its two biggest rivals—Staples and OfficeMax—to adopt brick-and-click strategies too. In 2005, all three companies were enjoying increasing success with selling online to business customers and using local stores to fill orders and make deliveries.

Sources: Information posted at www.officedepot.com (accessed September 28, 2005); "Office Depot's e-Diva," *BusinessWeek Online* (www.businessweek.com), August 6, 2001; Laura Lorek, "Office Depot Site Picks Up Speed," *Interactive Week* (www.zdnet.com/intweek), June 25, 2001; "Why Office Depot Loves the Net," *BusinessWeek,* September 27, 1999, pp. EB 66, EB 68; and *Fortune,* November 8, 1999, p. 17.

- *Whether it will have a broad or a narrow product offering*—A one-stop shopping strategy like that employed by Amazon.com (which offers over 30 million items for sale at its Web sites in the United States, Britain, France, Germany, Denmark, and Japan) has the appealing economics of helping spread fixed operating costs over a wide number of items and a large customer base. Other e-tailers, such as E-Loan and Hotel.com, have adopted classic focus strategies and cater to a sharply defined target audience shopping for a particular product or product category.

- *Whether to perform order fulfillment activities internally or to outsource them*—Building central warehouses, stocking them with adequate inventories, and developing systems to pick, pack, and ship individual orders all require substantial start-up capital but may result in lower overall unit costs than would paying the fees of order fulfillment specialists who make a business of providing warehouse space, stocking inventories, and shipping orders for e-tailers. However, outsourcing order fulfillment activities is likely to be more economical unless an e-tailer has high unit volume and the capital to invest in its own order fulfillment capabilities. Buy.com, an online superstore consisting of some 30,000 items, obtains products from name-brand manufacturers and uses outsiders to stock and ship those products; thus, its focus is not on manufacturing or order fulfillment but rather on selling.

- *How it will draw traffic to its Web site and then convert page views into revenues*—Web sites have to be cleverly marketed. Unless Web surfers hear about the site, like what they see on their first visit, and are intrigued enough to return again and again, the site is unlikely to generate adequate revenues. Marketing campaigns that result only in heavy site traffic and lots of page views are seldom sufficient; the best test of effective marketing and the appeal of an online company's product offering is the ratio at which page views are converted into revenues (the "look-to-buy" ratio). For example, in 2001 Yahoo's site traffic averaged 1.2 *billion* page views daily but generated only about $2 million in daily revenues; in contrast, the traffic at brokerage firm Charles Schwab's Web site averaged only 40 *million* page views per day but resulted in an average of $5 million daily in online commission revenues.

CHOOSING APPROPRIATE FUNCTIONAL-AREA STRATEGIES

A company's strategy is not complete until company managers have made strategic choices about how the various functional parts of the business—R&D, production, human resources, sales and marketing, finance, and so on—will be managed in support of its basic competitive strategy approach and the other important competitive moves being taken. Normally, functional-area strategy choices rank third on the menu of choosing among the various strategy options, as shown in Figure 6.1 (see p. 162). But whether commitments to particular functional strategies are made before or after the choices of complementary strategic options shown in Figure 6.1 is beside the point—what's really important is what the functional strategies are and how they mesh to enhance the success of the company's higher-level strategic thrusts.

In many respects, the nature of functional strategies is dictated by the choice of competitive strategy. For example, a manufacturer employing a low-cost provider strategy needs an R&D and product design strategy that emphasizes cheap-to-incorporate features and facilitates economical assembly and a production strategy that stresses capture of scale economies and actions to achieve low-cost manufacture (such as high labor productivity, efficient supply chain management, and automated production processes), and a low-budget marketing strategy. A business pursuing a high-end differentiation strategy needs a production strategy geared to top-notch quality and a marketing strategy aimed at touting differentiating features and using advertising and a trusted brand name to "pull" sales through the chosen distribution channels. A company using a focused differentiation strategy needs a marketing strategy that stresses growing the niche. For example, the Missouri-based franchise Panera Bread has been growing its business by getting more people hooked on fresh-baked specialty breads and patronizing its bakery-cafés, keeping buyer interest in Panera's all-natural specialty breads at a high level, and protecting its specialty bread niche against invasion by outsiders.

Beyond very general prescriptions, it is difficult to say just what the content of the different functional-area strategies should be without first knowing what higher-level strategic choices a company has made, the industry environment in which it operates, the resource strengths that can be leveraged, and so on. Suffice it to say here that company personnel—both managers and employees charged with strategy-making responsibility down through the organizational hierarchy—must be clear about which higher-level strategies top management has chosen and then must tailor the company's functional-area strategies accordingly.

FIRST-MOVER ADVANTAGES AND DISADVANTAGES

Core Concept
Because of first-mover advantages and disadvantages, competitive advantage can spring from *when* a move is made as well as from *what* move is made.

When to make a strategic move is often as crucial as *what* move to make. Timing is especially important when *first-mover advantages* or *disadvantages* exist.[40] Being first to initiate a strategic move can have a high payoff when (1) pioneering helps build a firm's image and reputation with buyers; (2) early commitments to new technologies, new-style components, new or emerging distribution channels, and so on can produce an absolute cost advantage over rivals; (3) first-time customers remain strongly loyal to pioneering firms in making repeat purchases; and (4) moving first constitutes a preemptive strike, making imitation extra hard or unlikely. The bigger the first-mover advantages, the more attractive making the first move becomes.[41] In e-commerce, companies like America Online, Amazon.com, Yahoo, eBay, and Priceline.com that were first with a new technology, network solution, or business model enjoyed lasting first-mover advantages in gaining the visibility and reputation needed to remain market leaders. However, other first-movers such as Xerox in fax machines, eToys (an online toy retailer), Webvan and Peapod (in online groceries), and scores of other dot-com companies never converted their first-mover status into any sort of competitive advantage. Sometimes markets are slow to accept the innovative product offering of a first-mover; sometimes, a fast-follower with greater resources and marketing muscle can easily overtake the first-mover (as Microsoft was able to do when it introduced Internet Explorer against Netscape, the pioneer of Internet browsers with the lion's share of the market); and sometimes furious technological change or product innovation makes a first-mover vulnerable to quickly appearing next-generation technology or products. Hence, just being a first-mover by itself is seldom enough to win a sustainable competitive advantage.[42]

To sustain any advantage that may initially accrue to a pioneer, a first-mover needs to be a fast learner and continue to move aggressively to capitalize on any initial pioneering advantage. It helps immensely if the first-mover has deep financial pockets, important competencies and competitive capabilities, and astute managers. If a first-mover's skills, know-how, and actions are easily copied or even surpassed, then fast-followers and even late-movers can catch or overtake the first-mover in a relatively short period. What makes being a first-mover strategically important is not being the first company to do something but rather being the first competitor to put together the precise combination of features, customer value, and sound revenue/cost/profit economics that gives it an edge over rivals in the battle for market leadership.[43] If the marketplace quickly takes to a first-mover's innovative product offering, a first-mover must have large-scale production, marketing, and distribution capabilities if it is to stave off fast-followers who possess these resources capabilities. If technology is advancing at torrid pace, a first-mover cannot hope to sustain its lead without having strong capabilities in R&D, design, and new product development, along with the financial strength to fund these activities.

The Potential for Late-Mover Advantages or First-Mover Disadvantages

There are instances when there are actually *advantages* to being an adept follower rather than a first-mover. Late-mover advantages (or *first-mover disadvantages*) arise in four instances:

- When pioneering leadership is more costly than imitating followership and only negligible learning/experience curve benefits accrue to the leader—a condition that allows a follower to end up with lower costs than the first-mover.
- When the products of an innovator are somewhat primitive and do not live up to buyer expectations, thus allowing a clever follower to win disenchanted buyers away from the leader with better-performing products.
- When the demand side of the marketplace is skeptical about the benefits of a new technology or product being pioneered by a first-mover.
- When rapid market evolution (due to fast-paced changes in either technology or buyer needs and expectations) gives fast-followers and maybe even cautious late-movers the opening to leapfrog a first-mover's products with more attractive next-version products.

To Be a First-Mover or Not

In weighing the pros and cons of being a first-mover versus a fast-follower versus a slow-mover, it matters whether the race to market leadership in a particular industry is a marathon or a sprint. In marathons, a slow-mover is not unduly penalized—first-mover advantages can be fleeting, and there is ample time for fast-followers and sometimes even late-movers to play catch-up.[44] Thus, the speed at which the pioneering innovation is likely to catch on matters considerably as companies struggle with whether to pursue a particular emerging market opportunity aggressively (as a first-mover or fast-follower) or cautiously (as a late-mover). For instance, it took 18 months for 10 million users to sign up for Hotmail, 5.5 years for worldwide mobile phone use to grow from 10 million to 100 million worldwide, 7 years for videocassette recorders to find their way into 1 million U.S. homes, and close to 10 years for the number of at-home broadband subscribers to grow to 100 million worldwide. The lesson here is that there is a market-penetration curve for every emerging opportunity; typically, the curve has an inflection point at which all the pieces of the business model fall into place, buyer demand explodes, and the market takes off. The inflection point can come early on a fast-rising curve (like use of e-mail) or further up on a slow-rising curve (like the use of broadband). Any company that seeks competitive advantage by being a first-mover thus needs to ask some hard questions:

- Does market takeoff depend on the development of complementary products or services that currently are not available?
- Is new infrastructure required before buyer demand can surge?
- Will buyers need to learn new skills or adopt new behaviors? Will buyers encounter high switching costs?
- Are there influential competitors in a position to delay or derail the efforts of a first-mover?

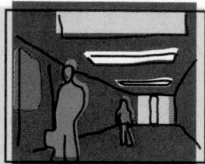

Illustration Capsule 6.3

The Battle in Consumer Broadband: First-Movers versus Late-Movers

In 1988 an engineer at the Bell companies' research labs figured out how to rush signals along ordinary copper wire at high speed using digital technology, thus creating the digital subscriber line (DSL). But the regional Bells, which dominated the local telephone market in the United States, showed little interest over the next 10 years, believing it was more lucrative to rent T-1 lines to businesses that needed fast data transmission capability and rent second phone lines to households wanting an Internet connection that didn't disrupt their regular telephone service. Furthermore, telephone executives were skeptical about DSL technology— there were a host of technical snarls to overcome, and early users encountered annoying glitches. Many executives doubted that it made good sense to invest billions of dollars in the infrastructure needed to roll out DSL to residential and small business customers, given the success they were having with T-1 and second-line rentals. As a consequence, the Bells didn't seriously begin to market DSL until the late 1990s, two years after the cable TV companies began their push to market cable broadband.

Cable companies were more than happy to be the first-movers in marketing broadband service via their copper cable wires, chiefly because their business was threatened by satellite TV technology and they saw broadband as an innovative service they could provide that the satellite companies could not. (Delivering broadband service via satellite has yet to become a factor in the marketplace, winning only a 1 percent share in 2003.) Cable companies were able to deploy broadband on their copper wire economically because during the 1980s and early 1990s most cable operators had spent about $60 billion to upgrade their systems with fiber-optic technology in order to handle two-way traffic rather than just one-way TV signals and thereby make good on their promises to local governments to develop "interactive" cable systems if they were awarded franchises. Although the early interactive services were duds, technicians discovered in the mid-1990s that the two-way systems enabled high-speed Internet hookups.

With Internet excitement surging in the late 1990s, cable executives saw high-speed Internet service as a no-brainer and began rolling it out to customers in 1998, securing about 362,000 customers by year-end versus only about 41,000 for DSL. Part of the early success of cable broadband was due to a cost advantage in modems—cable executives, seeing the potential of cable broadband several years earlier, had asked CableLabs to standardize the technology for cable modems, a move that lowered costs and made cable modems marketable in consumer electronics stores. DSL modems were substantially more complicated, and it took longer to drive the costs down from several hundred dollars each to under $100—in 2004, both cable and phone companies paid about $50 for modems, but cable modems got there much sooner.

As cable broadband began to attract more and more attention in the 1998–2002 period, the regional Bells continued to move slowly on DSL. The technical problems lingered, and early users were disgruntled by a host of annoying and sometimes horrendous installation difficulties and service glitches. Not only did providing users with convenient and reliable service prove to be a formidable challenge, but some regulatory issues stood in the way as well. Even in 2003 phone company executives found it hard to justify multibillion-dollar investments to install the necessary equipment and support systems to offer, market, manage, and maintain DSL service on the vast scale of a regional Bell company. SBC Communications figured it would cost at least $6 billion to roll out DSL to its customers. Verizon estimated that it would take 3.5 to 4 million customers to make DSL economics work, a number it would probably not reach until the end of 2005.

In 2003–2004, high-speed consumer access to the Internet was a surging business with a bright outlook—the number of U.S. Internet users upgrading to high-speed service increased by close to 500,000 monthly. In 2005, cable broadband was the preferred choice—70 percent of U.S. broadband users had opted for cable modems supplied by cable TV companies, with cable modem subscribers outnumbering DSL subscribers 30 million to 10.6 million. Its late start made it questionable whether DSL would be able to catch cable broadband in the U.S. marketplace, although DSL providers added 1.4 million subscribers in the first three months of 2005 compared to 1.2 million new subscribers for cable. In the rest of the world, however, DSL was the broadband connection of choice—there were an estimated 200 million broadband subscribers worldwide at the end of 2005.

Source: Developed from information in Shawn Young and Peter Grant, "How Phone Firms Lost to Cable in Consumer Broadband Market," *The Wall Street Journal,* March 13, 2003, pp. A1, A6, and Cnet's www.news.com site (accessed September 22, 2005).

When the answers to any of these questions are yes, then a company must be careful not to pour too many resources into getting ahead of the market opportunity—the race is likely going to be more of a 10-year marathon than a 2-year sprint. Being first out of the starting block is competitively important only when pioneering early introduction of a technology or product delivers clear and substantial benefits to early adopters and buyers, thus winning their immediate support, perhaps giving the pioneer a reputational head-start advantage, and forcing competitors to quickly follow the pioneer's lead. In the remaining instances where the race is more of a marathon, the companies that end up capturing and dominating new-to-the-world markets are almost never the pioneers that gave birth to those markets—there is time for a company to marshal the needed resources and to ponder its best time and method of entry.[45] Furthermore, being a late-mover into industries of the future has the advantages of being less risky and skirting the costs of pioneering.

But while a company is right to be cautious about quickly entering virgin territory, where all kinds of risks abound, rarely does a company have much to gain from consistently being a late-mover whose main concern is avoiding the mistakes of first-movers. Companies that are habitual late-movers regardless of the circumstances, while often able to survive, can find themselves and scrambling to keep pace with more progressive and innovative rivals and fighting to retain their customers. For a habitual late-mover to catch up, it must count on first-movers to be slow learners and complacent in letting their lead dwindle. It also has to hope that buyers will be slow to gravitate to the products of first-movers, again giving it time to catch up. And it has to have competencies and capabilities that are sufficiently strong to allow it to close the gap fairly quickly once it makes its move. Counting on all first-movers to stumble or otherwise be easily overtaken is usually a bad bet that puts a late-mover's competitive position at risk.

Illustration Capsule 6.3 describes the challenges that late-moving telephone companies have in winning the battle to supply at-home high-speed Internet access and overcoming the first-mover advantages of cable companies.

Key Points

Once a company has selected which of the five basic competitive strategies to employ in its quest for competitive advantage, then it must decide whether to supplement its choice of a basic competitive strategy approach, as shown in Figure 6.1 (p. 162).

Many companies are using strategic alliances and collaborative partnerships to help them in the race to build a global market presence or be a leader in the industries of the future. Strategic alliances are an attractive, flexible, and often cost-effective means by which companies can gain access to missing technology, expertise, and business capabilities.

Mergers and acquisitions are another attractive strategic option for strengthening a firm's competitiveness. When the operations of two companies are combined via merger or acquisition, the new company's competitiveness can be enhanced in any of several ways—lower costs; stronger technological skills; more or better competitive capabilities; a more attractive lineup of products and services; wider geographic coverage; and/or greater financial resources with which to invest in R&D, add capacity, or expand into new areas.

Vertically integrating forward or backward makes strategic sense only if it strengthens a company's position via either cost reduction or creation of a differentiation-based advantage. Otherwise, the drawbacks of vertical integration (increased investment, greater business risk, increased vulnerability to technological changes, and less flexibility in making product changes) are likely to outweigh any advantages.

Outsourcing pieces of the value chain formerly performed in-house can enhance a company's competitiveness whenever an activity (1) can be performed better or more cheaply by outside specialists; (2) is not crucial to the firm's ability to achieve sustainable competitive advantage and won't hollow out its core competencies, capabilities, or technical know-how; (3) reduces the company's risk exposure to changing technology or changing buyer preferences; (4) streamlines company operations in ways that improve organizational flexibility, cut cycle time, speed decision making, and reduce coordination costs; or (5) allows a company to concentrate on its core business and do what it does best.

One of the most pertinent strategic issues that companies face is how to use the Internet in positioning the company in the marketplace—whether to use the Internet as *only a means of disseminating product information* (with traditional distribution channel partners making all sales to end users), as *a secondary or minor channel*, as *one of several important distribution channels*, as *the company's primary distribution channel,* or as *the company's exclusive channel for accessing customers.*

Companies have a number of offensive strategy options for improving their market positions and trying to secure a competitive advantage: offering an equal or better product at a lower price, leapfrogging competitors by being first to adopt next-generation technologies or the first to introduce next-generation products, pursuing sustained product innovation, attacking competitors weaknesses, going after less contested or unoccupied market territory, using hit-and-run tactics to steal sales away from unsuspecting rivals, and launching preemptive strikes. A blue ocean strategy seeks to gain a dramatic and durable competitive advantage by abandoning efforts to beat out competitors in existing markets and, instead, inventing a new industry or distinctive market segment that renders existing competitors largely irrelevant and allows a company to create and capture altogether new demand.

Defensive strategies to protect a company's position usually take the form of making moves that put obstacles in the path of would-be challengers and fortify the company's present position while undertaking actions to dissuade rivals from even trying to attack (by signaling that the resulting battle will be more costly to the challenger than it is worth).

Once all the higher-level strategic choices have been made, company managers can turn to the task of crafting functional and operating-level strategies to flesh out the details of the company's overall business and competitive strategy.

The timing of strategic moves also has relevance in the quest for competitive advantage. Company managers are obligated to carefully consider the advantages or disadvantages that attach to being a first-mover versus a fast-follower versus a late-mover.

Exercises

1. Go to Google or another Internet search engine and do a search on "strategic alliances." Identify at least two companies in different industries that are making a significant use of strategic alliances as a core part of their strategies. In addition, identify who their alliances are with and describe the purpose of the alliances.

2. Go to Google or another Internet search engine and do a search on "acquisition strategy." Identify at least two companies in different industries that are using

acquisitions to strengthen their market positions. Identify some of the companies that have been acquired, and research the purpose behind the acquisitions.

3. Go to www.goodyear.com/investor and read Goodyear's most recent annual report. To what extent is the company vertically integrated? What segments of the industry value chain has the company chosen to perform? Based on the company's discussion of business unit performance, does it appear the company is becoming more vertically integrated or choosing to narrow its range of internally performed activities?

4. Illustration Capsule 6.3 describes how cable companies used fiber-optic networks to gain a first-mover advantage over telephone companies in providing high-speed Internet access to home subscribers. Telephone companies are attempting to catch up with cable companies in the broadband access market with the widespread rollout of DSL to telephone customers. In addition, phone companies are pursuing fiber-to-the-premises (FTTP) and outdoor wireless networks (outdoor WLAN) technologies to supplement or replace DSL. Conduct Web searches on FTTP and outdoor WLAN, and discuss how use of these technologies by telephone companies might offset the first-mover advantage currently held by cable companies in the high-speed Internet market.

5. Go to the Web sites of various companies (such as those appearing on the Fortune 500) and identify two companies using each of the following Web site strategies and explain why the approach is well matched to the company's business model:

   a. Product information only.

   b. E-store as a minor distribution strategy.

   c. Brick-and-click.

   d. Online enterprise.

Competing in Foreign Markets

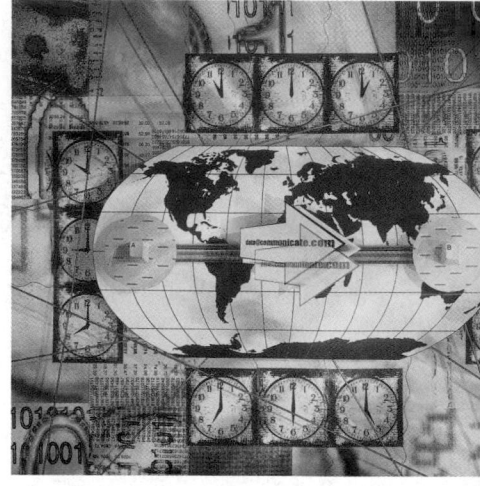

You have no choice but to operate in a world shaped by globalization and the information revolution. There are two options: Adapt or die.

—Andrew S. Grove

Former Chairman, Intel Corporation

You do not choose to become global. The market chooses for you; it forces your hand.

—Alain Gomez

CEO, Thomson SA

[I]ndustries actually vary a great deal in the pressures they put on a company to sell internationally.

—Niraj Dawar and Tony Frost

Professors, Richard Ivey School of Business

Any company that aspires to industry leadership in the 21st century must think in terms of global, not domestic, market leadership. The world economy is globalizing at an accelerating pace as countries previously closed to foreign companies open up their markets, as the Internet shrinks the importance of geographic distance, and as ambitious growth-minded companies race to build stronger competitive positions in the markets of more and more countries. Companies in industries that are already globally competitive or in the process of becoming so are under the gun to come up with a strategy for competing successfully in foreign markets.

This chapter focuses on strategy options for expanding beyond domestic boundaries and competing in the markets of either a few or a great many countries. The spotlight will be on four strategic issues unique to competing multinationally:

1. Whether to customize the company's offerings in each different country market to match the tastes and preferences of local buyers or to offer a mostly standardized product worldwide.

2. Whether to employ essentially the same basic competitive strategy in all countries or modify the strategy country by country.

3. Where to locate the company's production facilities, distribution centers, and customer service operations so as to realize the greatest location advantages.

4. How to efficiently transfer the company's resource strengths and capabilities from one country to another in an effort to secure competitive advantage.

In the process of exploring these issues, we will introduce a number of core concepts—multicountry competition, global competition, profit sanctuaries, and cross-market subsidization. The chapter includes sections on cross-country differences in cultural, demographic, and market conditions; strategy options for entering and competing in foreign markets; the growing role of alliances with foreign partners; the importance of locating operations in the most advantageous countries; and the special circumstances of competing in such emerging markets as China, India, Brazil, Russia, and Eastern Europe.

WHY COMPANIES EXPAND INTO FOREIGN MARKETS

A company may opt to expand outside its domestic market for any of four major reasons:

1. *To gain access to new customers*—Expanding into foreign markets offers potential for increased revenues, profits, and long-term growth and becomes an especially attractive option when a company's home markets are mature. Firms like Cisco Systems, Dell, Sony, Nokia, Avon, and Toyota, which are racing for global leadership in their respective industries, are moving rapidly and aggressively to extend their market reach into all corners of the world.

2. *To achieve lower costs and enhance the firm's competitiveness*—Many companies are driven to sell in more than one country because domestic sales volume is not large enough to fully capture manufacturing economies of scale or learning/experience curve effects and thereby substantially improve the firm's cost-competitiveness. The relatively small size of country markets in Europe explains why companies like Michelin, BMW, and Nestlé long ago began selling their products all across Europe and then moved into markets in North America and Latin America.

3. *To capitalize on its core competencies*—A company may be able to leverage its competencies and capabilities into a position of competitive advantage in foreign markets as well as just domestic markets. Nokia's competencies and capabilities in mobile phones have propelled it to global market leadership in the wireless telecommunications business. Wal-Mart is capitalizing on its considerable expertise in discount retailing to expand into China, Latin America, and parts of Europe— Wal-Mart executives believe the company has tremendous growth opportunities in China.

4. *To spread its business risk across a wider market base*—A company spreads business risk by operating in a number of different foreign countries rather than depending entirely on operations in its domestic market. Thus, if the economies of certain Asian countries turn down for a period of time, a company with operations across much of the world may be sustained by buoyant sales in Latin America or Europe.

In a few cases, companies in industries based on natural resources (e.g., oil and gas, minerals, rubber, and lumber) often find it necessary to operate in the international arena because attractive raw material supplies are located in foreign countries.

The Difference Between Competing Internationally and Competing Globally

Typically, a company will start to compete internationally by entering just one or maybe a select few foreign markets. Competing on a truly global scale comes later, after the company has established operations on several continents and is racing against rivals for global market leadership. Thus, there is a meaningful distinction between the competitive scope of a company that operates in a few foreign countries (with perhaps modest ambitions to enter several more country markets) and a company that markets its products in 50 to 100 countries and is expanding its operations into additional country markets annually. The former is most accurately termed an *international competitor,* whereas the latter qualifies as a *global competitor.* In the discussion that follows, we'll continue to make a distinction between strategies for competing internationally and strategies for competing globally.

CROSS-COUNTRY DIFFERENCES IN CULTURAL, DEMOGRAPHIC, AND MARKET CONDITIONS

Regardless of a company's motivation for expanding outside its domestic markets, the strategies it uses to compete in foreign markets must be situation-driven. Cultural, demographic, and market conditions vary significantly among the countries of the world.[1] Cultures and lifestyles are the most obvious areas in which countries differ; market demographics and income levels are close behind. Consumers in Spain do not have the same tastes, preferences, and buying habits as consumers in Norway; buyers differ yet again in Greece, Chile, New Zealand, and Taiwan. Less than 20 percent of the populations of Brazil, India, and China have annual purchasing power equivalent to $25,000. Middle-class consumers represent a much smaller portion of the population in these and other emerging countries than in North America, Japan, and much of Western Europe—China's middle class numbers about 125 million out of a population of 1.3 billion.[2]

Sometimes product designs suitable in one country are inappropriate in another—for example, in the United States electrical devices run on 110-volt systems, but in some European countries the standard is a 240-volt system, necessitating the use of different electrical designs and components. In France consumers prefer top-loading washing machines, while in most other European countries consumers prefer front-loading machines. Northern Europeans want large refrigerators because they tend to shop once a week in supermarkets; southern Europeans can get by on small refrigerators because they shop daily. In parts of Asia refrigerators are a status symbol and may be placed in the living room, leading to preferences for stylish designs and colors—in India bright blue and red are popular colors. In other Asian countries household space is constrained and many refrigerators are only four feet high so that the top can be used for storage. In Hong Kong the preference is for compact European-style appliances, but in Taiwan large American-style appliances are more popular. In Italy, most people use automatic washing machines but prefer to hang the clothes out to dry on a clothesline—there is a strongly entrenched tradition and cultural belief that sun-dried clothes are fresher, which virtually shuts down any opportunities for appliance makers to market clothes dryers in Italy. In China, many parents are reluctant to purchase personal computers (PCs) even when they can afford them because of concerns that their children will be distracted from their schoolwork by surfing the Web, playing PC-based video games, and downloading and listening to pop music.

Similarly, market growth varies from country to country. In emerging markets like India, China, Brazil, and Malaysia, market growth potential is far higher than in the more mature economies of Britain, Denmark, Canada, and Japan. In automobiles, for example, the potential for market growth is explosive in China, where 2005 sales of new vehicles amounted to less than 5 million in a country with 1.3 billion people. In India there are efficient, well-developed national channels for distributing trucks, scooters, farm equipment, groceries, personal care items, and other packaged products to the country's 3 million retailers, whereas in China distribution is primarily local and there is no national network for distributing most products. The marketplace is intensely competitive in some countries and only moderately contested in others. Industry driving forces may be one thing in Spain, quite another in Canada, and different yet again in Turkey or Argentina or South Korea.

One of the biggest concerns of companies competing in foreign markets is whether to customize their offerings in each different country market to match the tastes and preferences of local buyers or whether to offer a mostly standardized product worldwide. While making products that are closely matched to local tastes makes them more appealing to local buyers, customizing a company's products country by country may have the effect of raising production and distribution costs due to the greater variety of designs and components, shorter production runs, and the complications of added inventory handling and distribution logistics. Greater standardization of a global company's product offering, however, can lead to scale economies and experience/learning curve effects, thus contributing to the achievement of a low-cost advantage. *The tension between the market pressures to localize a company's product offerings country by country and the competitive pressures to lower costs is one of the big strategic issues that participants in foreign markets have to resolve.*

Aside from the basic cultural and market differences among countries, a company also has to pay special attention to location advantages that stem from country-to-country variations in manufacturing and distribution costs, the risks of adverse shifts in exchange rates, and the economic and political demands of host governments.

Gaining Competitive Advantage Based on Where Activities Are Located

Differences in wage rates, worker productivity, inflation rates, energy costs, tax rates, government regulations, and the like create sizable variations in manufacturing costs from country to country. Plants in some countries have major manufacturing cost advantages because of lower input costs (especially labor), relaxed government regulations, the proximity of suppliers, or unique natural resources. In such cases, the low-cost countries become principal production sites, with most of the output being exported to markets in other parts of the world. Companies that build production facilities in low-cost countries (or that source their products from contract manufacturers in these countries) have a competitive advantage over rivals with plants in countries where costs are higher. The competitive role of low manufacturing costs is most evident in low-wage countries like China, India, Pakistan, Cambodia, Vietnam, Mexico, Brazil, Guatemala, the Philippines, and several countries in Africa that have become production havens for manufactured goods with high labor content (especially textiles and apparel). Labor costs in China averaged about $0.70 an hour in 2004–2005 versus about $1.50 in Russia, $4.60 in Hungary, $4.90 in Portugal, $16.50 in Canada, $21.00 in the United States, $23.00 in Norway, and $25.00 in Germany.[3] China is fast becoming the manufacturing capital of the world—virtually all of the world's major manufacturing companies now have facilities in China, and China attracted more foreign direct investment in 2002 and 2003 than any other country in the world. Likewise, concerns about short delivery times and low shipping costs make some countries better locations than others for establishing distribution centers.

The quality of a country's business environment also offers locational advantages—the governments of some countries are anxious to attract foreign investments and go all out to create a business climate that outsiders will view as favorable. A good example is Ireland, which has one of the world's most pro-business environments. Ireland offers companies very low corporate tax rates, has a government that is responsive to the needs of industry, and aggressively recruits high-tech manufacturing facilities and multinational companies. Such policies were a significant force in making Ireland the most dynamic, fastest-growing nation in Europe during the 1990s. Ireland's policies were a major factor in Intel's decision to choose Leixlip, County Kildare, as the site for a $2.5 billion chip manufacturing plant that employs over 4,000 people. Another locational advantage is the clustering of suppliers of components and capital equipment; infrastructure suppliers (universities, vocational training providers, research enterprises); trade associations; and makers of complementary products in a geographic area—such clustering can be an important source of cost savings in addition to facilitating close collaboration with key suppliers.

The Risks of Adverse Exchange Rate Shifts

The volatility of exchange rates greatly complicates the issue of geographic cost advantages. Currency exchange rates often move up or down 20 to 40 percent annually. Changes of this magnitude can either totally wipe out a country's low-cost advantage or transform a former high-cost location into a competitive-cost location. For instance, in the mid-1980s, when the dollar was strong relative to the Japanese yen (meaning that $1 would purchase, say, 125 yen as opposed to only 100 yen), Japanese heavy-equipment maker Komatsu was able to undercut U.S.-based Caterpillar's prices by as much as 25 percent, causing Caterpillar to lose sales and market share. But starting in 1985, when exchange rates began to shift and the dollar grew steadily weaker against the yen (meaning that $1 was worth fewer and fewer yen, and that a Komatsu product made in Japan at a cost of 20 million yen translated into costs of many more dollars than before), Komatsu had to raise its prices to U.S. buyers six times over two years. With its competitiveness against Komatsu restored because of the weaker dollar and Komatsu's higher prices, Caterpillar regained sales and market share. *The lesson of fluctuating exchange rates is that companies that export goods to foreign countries always gain in competitiveness when the currency of the country in which the goods are manufactured is weak. Exporters are disadvantaged when the currency of the country where goods are being manufactured grows stronger.* Sizable long-term shifts in exchange rates thus shuffle the global cards of which rivals have the upper hand in the marketplace and which countries represent the low-cost manufacturing location.

> **Core Concept**
> Companies with manufacturing facilities in a particular country are more cost-competitive in exporting goods to world markets when the local currency is weak (or declines in value relative to other currencies); their competitiveness erodes when the local currency grows stronger relative to the currencies of the countries to which the locally made goods are being exported.

As a further illustration of the risks associated with fluctuating exchange rates, consider the case of a U.S. company that has located manufacturing facilities in Brazil (where the currency is reals—pronounced *ray-alls*) and that exports most of the Brazilian-made goods to markets in the European Union (where the currency is euros). To keep the numbers simple, assume that the exchange rate is 4 Brazilian reals for 1 euro and that the product being made in Brazil has a manufacturing cost of 4 Brazilian reals (or 1 euro). Now suppose that for some reason the exchange rate shifts from 4 reals per euro to 5 reals per euro (meaning that the real has declined in value and that the euro is stronger). Making the product in Brazil is now more cost-competitive because a Brazilian good costing 4 reals to produce has fallen to only 0.8 euros at the new exchange rate. If, in contrast, the value of the Brazilian real grows stronger in relation to the euro—resulting in an exchange rate of 3 reals to 1 euro—the same good costing 4 reals to produce now has a cost of 1.33 euros. Clearly, the attraction of manufacturing a good in Brazil and selling it in Europe is far greater when the euro is strong (an exchange rate of 1 euro for 5 Brazilian reals) than when the euro is weak and exchanges for only 3 Brazilian reals.

Insofar as U.S.-based manufacturers are concerned, declines in the value of the U.S. dollar against foreign currencies act to reduce or eliminate whatever cost advantage foreign manufacturers might have over U.S. manufacturers and can even prompt foreign companies to establish production plants in the United States. Likewise, a weak euro enhances the cost competitiveness of companies manufacturing goods in Europe for export to foreign markets; a strong euro versus other currencies weakens the cost competitiveness of European plants that manufacture goods for export.

In 2002, when the Brazilian real declined in value by about 25 percent against the dollar, the euro, and several other currencies, the ability of companies with manufacturing plants in Brazil to compete in world markets was greatly enhanced—of course, in the future years this windfall gain in cost advantage might well be eroded by sustained rises in the value of the Brazilian real against these same currencies. Herein lies the risk: *Currency exchange rates are rather unpredictable, swinging first one way and then another way, so the competitiveness of any company's facilities in any country is partly dependent on whether exchange rate changes over time have a favorable or unfavorable cost impact.* Companies producing goods in one country for export abroad always improve their cost competitiveness when the country's currency grows weaker relative to currencies of the countries where the goods are being exported to, and they find their cost competitiveness eroded when the local currency grows stronger. In contrast, domestic companies that are under pressure from lower-cost imported goods become more cost competitive when their currency grows weaker in relation to the currencies of the countries where the imported goods are made—in other words, a U.S. manufacturer views a weaker U.S. dollar as a *favorable exchange rate shift* because such shifts help make its costs more competitive versus those of foreign rivals.

Core Concept

Fluctuating exchange rates pose significant risks to a company's competitiveness in foreign markets. Exporters win when the currency of the country where goods are being manufactured grows weaker, and they lose when the currency grows stronger. Domestic companies under pressure from lower-cost imports are benefited when their government's currency grows weaker in relation to the countries where the imported goods are being made.

Host Governments' Policies

National governments enact all kinds of measures affecting business conditions and the operation of foreign companies in their markets. Host governments may set local content requirements on goods made inside their borders by foreign-based companies, have rules and policies that protect local companies from foreign competition, put restrictions on exports to ensure adequate local supplies, regulate the prices of imported and locally produced goods, enact deliberately burdensome procedures and requirements for imported goods to pass customs inspection, and impose tariffs or quotas on the imports of certain goods—until 2002, when it joined the World Trade Organization, China imposed a 100 percent tariff on motor vehicle imports. The European Union imposes quotas on textile and apparel imports from China, as a measure to protect European producers in southern Europe. India imposed excise taxes on newly purchased motor vehicles in 2005 ranging from 24 to 40 percent—a policy that has significantly dampened the demand for new vehicles in India (though down from as much as 50 percent in prior years). Governments may or may not have burdensome tax structures, stringent environmental regulations, or strictly enforced worker safety standards. Sometimes outsiders face a web of regulations regarding technical standards, product certification, prior approval of capital spending projects, withdrawal of funds from the country, and required minority (sometimes majority) ownership of foreign company operations by local companies or investors. A few governments may be hostile to or suspicious of foreign companies operating within their borders. Some governments provide subsidies and low-interest loans to domestic companies to help them compete against foreign-based companies. Other governments, anxious to obtain new plants and jobs, offer foreign companies a helping hand in the form of subsidies, privileged market access, and technical assistance. All of these possibilities explain why the managers of companies opting to compete in foreign markets have to take a close look at a country's politics and policies toward business in general, and foreign companies in particular, in deciding which country markets to participate in and which ones to avoid.

THE CONCEPTS OF MULTICOUNTRY COMPETITION AND GLOBAL COMPETITION

There are important differences in the patterns of international competition from industry to industry.[4] At one extreme is **multicountry competition,** in which there's so much cross-country variation in market conditions and in the companies contending for leadership that the market contest among rivals in one country is not closely connected to the market contests in other countries. The standout features of multicountry competition are that (1) buyers in different countries are attracted to different product attributes, (2) sellers vary from country to country, and (3) industry conditions and competitive forces in each national market differ in important respects. Take the banking industry in Italy, Brazil, and Japan as an example—the requirements and expectations of banking customers vary among the three countries, the lead banking competitors in Italy differ from those in Brazil or in Japan, and the competitive battle going on among the leading banks in Italy is unrelated to the rivalry taking place in Brazil or Japan. Thus, with multicountry competition, rival firms battle for national championships, and winning in one country does not necessarily signal the ability to fare well in other countries. In multicountry competition, the power of a company's strategy and resource capabilities in one country may not enhance its competitiveness to the same degree in other countries where it operates. Moreover, any competitive advantage a company secures in one country is largely confined to that country; the spillover effects to other countries are minimal to nonexistent. Industries characterized by multicountry competition include radio and TV broadcasting, consumer banking, life insurance, apparel, metals fabrication, many types of food products (coffee, cereals, breads, canned goods, frozen foods), and retailing.

> **Core Concept**
> **Multicountry competition** exists when competition in one national market is not closely connected to competition in another national market—there is no global or world market, just a collection of self-contained country markets.

At the other extreme is **global competition,** in which prices and competitive conditions across country markets are strongly linked and the term *global market* has true meaning. In a globally competitive industry, much the same group of rival companies competes in many different countries, but especially so in countries where sales volumes are large and where having a competitive presence is strategically important to building a strong global position in the industry. Thus, a company's competitive position in one country both affects and is affected by its position in other countries. In global competition, a firm's overall competitive advantage grows out of its entire worldwide operations; the competitive advantage it creates at its home base is supplemented by advantages growing out of its operations in other countries (having plants in low-wage countries, being able to transfer expertise from country to country, having the capability to serve customers who also have multinational operations, and brand-name recognition in many parts of the world). Rival firms in globally competitive industries vie for worldwide leadership. Global competition exists in motor vehicles, television sets, tires, mobile phones, personal computers, copiers, watches, digital cameras, bicycles, and commercial aircraft.

> **Core Concept**
> **Global competition** exists when competitive conditions across national markets are linked strongly enough to form a true international market and when leading competitors compete head to head in many different countries.

An industry can have segments that are globally competitive and segments in which competition is country by country.[5] In the hotel/motel industry, for example, the low- and medium-priced segments are characterized by multicountry competition—competitors serve travelers mainly within the same country. In the business and luxury segments, however, competition is more globalized. Companies like Nikki, Marriott, Sheraton, and Hilton have hotels at many international locations, use worldwide reservation systems, and establish common quality and service standards to gain marketing advantages in serving businesspeople and other travelers who make frequent international trips. In lubricants, the marine engine segment is globally competitive—ships move from port to port and require the same oil everywhere they stop. Brand reputations in marine lubricants have a global scope, and successful marine engine lubricant producers (Exxon Mobil, BP Amoco, and Shell) operate globally. In automotive motor oil, however, multicountry competition dominates—countries have different weather conditions and driving patterns, production of motor oil is subject to limited scale economies, shipping costs are high, and retail distribution channels differ markedly from country to country. Thus, domestic firms—like Quaker State and Pennzoil in the United States and Castrol in Great Britain—can be leaders in their home markets without competing globally.

It is also important to recognize that an industry can be in transition from multicountry competition to global competition. In a number of today's industries—beer and major home appliances are prime examples—leading domestic competitors have begun expanding into more and more foreign markets, often acquiring local companies or brands and integrating them into their operations. As some industry members start to build global brands and a global presence, other industry members find themselves pressured to follow the same strategic path—especially if establishing multinational operations results in important scale economies and a powerhouse brand name. As the industry consolidates to fewer players, such that many of the same companies find themselves in head-to-head competition in more and more country markets, global competition begins to replace multicountry competition.

At the same time, consumer tastes in a number of important product categories are converging across the world. Less diversity of tastes and preferences opens the way for companies to create global brands and sell essentially the same products in most all countries of the world. Even in industries where consumer tastes remain fairly diverse, companies are learning to use "custom mass production" to economically create different versions of a product and thereby satisfy the tastes of people in different countries.

In addition to taking the obvious cultural and political differences between countries into account, a company has to shape its strategic approach to competing in foreign markets according to whether its industry is characterized by multicountry competition, global competition, or a transition from one to the other.

STRATEGY OPTIONS FOR ENTERING AND COMPETING IN FOREIGN MARKETS

There are a host of generic strategic options for a company that decides to expand outside its domestic market and compete internationally or globally:

1. *Maintain a national (one-country) production base and export goods to foreign markets*, using either company-owned or foreign-controlled forward distribution channels.

2. *License foreign firms to use the company's technology or to produce and distribute the company's products.*

3. *Employ a franchising strategy.*

4. *Follow a multicountry strategy,* varying the company's strategic approach (perhaps a little, perhaps a lot) from country to country in accordance with local conditions and differing buyer tastes and preferences.

5. *Follow a global strategy,* using essentially the same competitive strategy approach in all country markets where the company has a presence.

6. *Use strategic alliances or joint ventures with foreign companies as the primary vehicle for entering foreign markets* and perhaps also using them as an ongoing strategic arrangement aimed at maintaining or strengthening its competitiveness.

The following sections discuss the first five options in more detail; the sixth option is discussed in a separate section later in the chapter.

Export Strategies

Using domestic plants as a production base for exporting goods to foreign markets is an excellent initial strategy for pursuing international sales. It is a conservative way to test the international waters. The amount of capital needed to begin exporting is often quite minimal; existing production capacity may well be sufficient to make goods for export. With an export strategy, a manufacturer can limit its involvement in foreign markets by contracting with foreign wholesalers experienced in importing to handle the entire distribution and marketing function in their countries or regions of the world. If it is more advantageous to maintain control over these functions, however, a manufacturer can establish its own distribution and sales organizations in some or all of the target foreign markets. Either way, a home-based production and export strategy helps the firm minimize its direct investments in foreign countries. Such strategies are commonly favored by Chinese, Korean, and Italian companies—products are designed and manufactured at home and then distributed through local channels in the importing countries; the primary functions performed abroad relate chiefly to establishing a network of distributors and perhaps conducting sales promotion and brand awareness activities.

Whether an export strategy can be pursued successfully over the long run hinges on the relative cost competitiveness of the home-country production base. In some industries, firms gain additional scale economies and experience/learning curve benefits from centralizing production in one or several giant plants whose output capability exceeds demand in any one country market; obviously, a company must export to capture such economies. However, an export strategy is vulnerable when (1) manufacturing costs in the home country are substantially higher than in foreign countries where rivals have plants, (2) the costs of shipping the product to distant foreign markets are relatively high, or (3) adverse shifts occur in currency exchange rates. Unless an exporter can both keep its production and shipping costs competitive with rivals and successfully hedge against unfavorable changes in currency exchange rates, its success will be limited.

Licensing Strategies

Licensing makes sense when a firm with valuable technical know-how or a unique patented product has neither the internal organizational capability nor the resources to enter foreign markets. Licensing also has the advantage of avoiding the risks of committing resources to country markets that are unfamiliar, politically volatile, economically unstable, or otherwise risky. By licensing the technology or the production rights to foreign-based firms, the firm does not have to bear the costs and risks of entering foreign markets on its own, yet it is able to generate income from royalties. The big disadvantage of licensing is the risk of providing valuable technological know-how to foreign companies and thereby losing some degree of control over its use; monitoring licensees and safeguarding the company's proprietary know-how can prove quite difficult in some circumstances. But if the royalty potential is considerable and the companies to whom the licenses are being granted are both trustworthy and reputable, then licensing can be a very attractive option. Many software and pharmaceutical companies use licensing strategies.

Franchising Strategies

While licensing works well for manufacturers and owners of proprietary technology, franchising is often better suited to the global expansion efforts of service and retailing enterprises. McDonald's, Yum! Brands (the parent of Pizza Hut, KFC, and Taco Bell), The UPS Store, Jani-King International (the world's largest commercial cleaning franchisor), Roto-Rooter, 7-Eleven, and Hilton Hotels have all used franchising to build a presence in foreign markets. Franchising has much the same advantages as licensing. The franchisee bears most of the costs and risks of establishing foreign locations; a franchisor has to expend only the resources to recruit, train, support, and monitor franchisees. The big problem a franchisor faces is maintaining quality control; foreign franchisees do not always exhibit strong commitment to consistency and standardization, especially when the local culture does not stress the same kinds of quality concerns. Another problem that can arise is whether to allow foreign franchisees to make modifications in the franchisor's product offering so as to better satisfy the tastes and expectations of local buyers. Should McDonald's allow its franchised units in Japan to modify Big Macs slightly to suit Japanese tastes? Should the franchised KFC units in China be permitted to substitute spices that appeal to Chinese consumers? Or should the same menu offerings be rigorously and unvaryingly required of all franchisees worldwide?

Localized Multicountry Strategies or a Global Strategy?

The issue of whether to vary the company's competitive approach to fit specific market conditions and buyer preferences in each host country or whether to employ essentially the same strategy in all countries is perhaps the foremost strategic issue that companies must address when they operate in two or more foreign markets. Figure 7.1 shows a company's options for resolving this issue.

Core Concept

A *localized* or *multicountry strategy* is one where a company varies its product offering and competitive approach from country to country in an effort to be responsive to differing buyer preferences and market conditions.

Think-Local, Act-Local Approaches to Strategy Making The bigger the differences in buyer tastes, cultural traditions, and market conditions in different countries, the stronger the case for a think-local, act-local approach to strategy-making, in which a company tailors its product offerings and perhaps its basic competitive strategy to fit buyer tastes and market conditions in each country where it opts to compete. The strength of employing a set of *localized* or *multicountry strategies* is that the company's actions and business approaches are deliberately crafted to accommodate the

Figure 7.1   **A Company's Strategic Options for Dealing with Cross-Country Variations in Buyer Preferences and Market Conditions**

Strategic Posturing Options	**Ways to Deal with Cross-Country Variations in Buyer Preferences and Market Conditions**
Think Local, Act Local	**Employ localized strategies—one for each country market:** ■ Tailor the company's competitive approach and product offering to fit specific market conditions and buyer preferences in each host country. ■ Delegate strategy making to local managers with firsthand knowledge of local conditions.
Think Global, Act Global	**Employ same strategy worldwide:** ■ Pursue *the same basic competitive strategy theme* (low-cost, differentiation, best-cost, or focused) *in all country markets*—a global strategy. ■ Offer the same products worldwide, with only very minor deviations from one country to another when local market conditions so dictate. ■ Utilize the same capabilities, distribution channels, and marketing approaches worldwide. ■ Coordinate strategic actions from central headquarters
Think Global, Act Local	**Employ a combination global-local strategy:** ■ Employ essentially *the same basic competitive strategy theme* (low-cost, differentiation, best-cost, or focused) in *all country markets*. ■ Develop the capability to customize product offerings and sell different product versions in different countries (perhaps even under different brand names). ■ Give local managers the latitude to adapt the global approach as needed to accommodate local buyer preferences and be responsive to local market and competitive conditions.

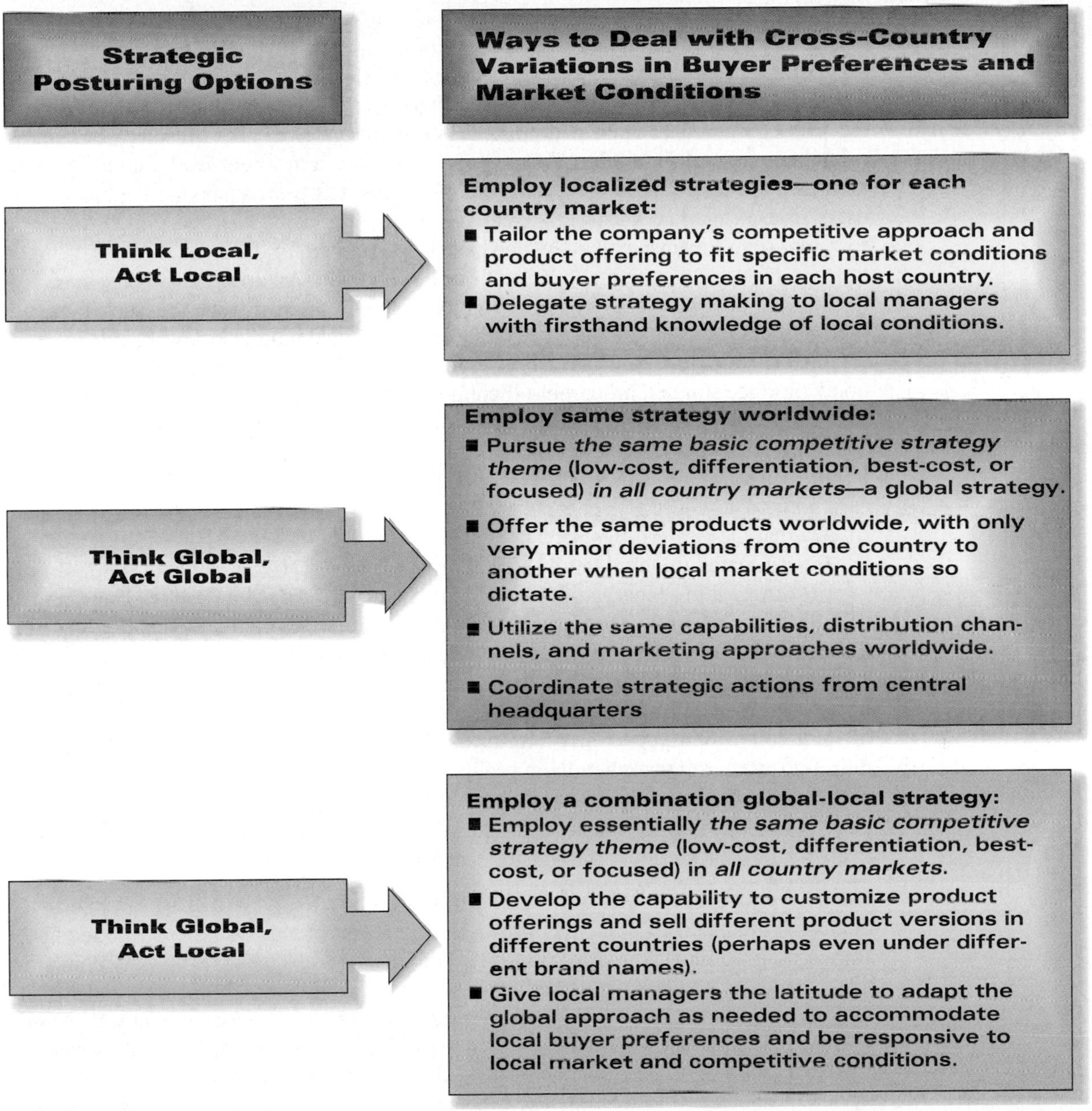

differing tastes and expectations of buyers in each country and to stake out the most attractive market positions vis-à-vis local competitors. A think-local, act-local approach means giving local managers considerable strategy-making latitude. It means having plants produce different product versions for different local markets, and adapting marketing and distribution to fit local customs and cultures. The bigger the country-to-country variations, the more that a company's overall strategy is a collection of its localized country strategies rather than a common or global strategy.

A think-local, act-local approach to strategy making is essential when there are significant country-to-country differences in customer preferences and buying habits, when there are significant cross-country differences in distribution channels and marketing methods, when host governments enact regulations requiring that products sold locally meet strict manufacturing specifications or performance standards, and when the trade restrictions of host governments are so diverse and complicated that they preclude a uniform, coordinated worldwide market approach. With localized strategies, a company often has different product versions for different countries and sometimes sells them under different brand names. Sony markets a different Walkman in Norway than in Sweden to better meet the somewhat different preferences and habits of the users in each market. Castrol, a specialist in oil lubricants, has over 3,000 different formulas of lubricants, many of which have been tailored for different climates, vehicle types and uses, and equipment applications that characterize different country markets. In the food products industry, it is common for companies to vary the ingredients in their products and sell the localized versions under local brand names in order to cater to country-specific tastes and eating preferences. Motor vehicle manufacturers routinely produce smaller, more fuel-efficient vehicles for markets in Europe where roads are often narrower and gasoline prices two or three times higher than they produce for the North American market; the models they manufacture for the Asian market are different yet again. DaimlerChrysler, for example, equips all of the Jeep Grand Cherokees and many of its Mercedes cars sold in Europe with fuel-efficient diesel engines. The Buicks that General Motors sells in China are small compacts, whereas those sold in the United States are large family sedans and SUVs.

However, think-local, act-local strategies have two big drawbacks: They hinder transfer of a company's competencies and resources across country boundaries (since the strategies in different host countries can be grounded in varying competencies and capabilities), and they do not promote building a single, unified competitive advantage—especially one based on low cost. Companies employing highly localized or multicountry strategies face big hurdles in achieving low-cost leadership *unless* they find ways to customize their products and *still* be in position to capture scale economies and experience/learning curve effects. Companies like Dell Computer and Toyota, because they have mass customization production capabilities, can cost effectively adapt their product offerings to local buyer tastes.

Think-Global, Act-Global Approaches to Strategy Making

While multicountry or localized strategies are best suited for industries where multicountry competition dominates and a fairly high degree of local responsiveness is competitively imperative, global strategies are best suited for globally competitive industries. A *global strategy* is one in which the company's approach is predominantly the same in all countries—it sells the same products under the same brand names everywhere, uses much the same distribution channels in all countries, and competes on the basis of the same capabilities and marketing approaches worldwide. Although the company's strategy or product offering may be adapted in very minor ways to accommodate specific situations in a few host countries, the company's fundamental competitive approach (low-cost, differentiation, best-cost, or focused) remains very much intact worldwide, and local managers stick close to the global strategy. A think-global, act-global strategic theme prompts company managers to integrate and coordinate the company's strategic moves worldwide and to expand into most if not all nations where there is significant buyer demand. It puts considerable strategic

Core Concept

A *global strategy* is one where a company employs the same basic competitive approach in all countries where it operates, sells much the same products everywhere, strives to build global brands, and coordinates its actions worldwide.

emphasis on building a *global* brand name and aggressively pursuing opportunities to transfer ideas, new products, and capabilities from one country to another.[6] Indeed, with a think global, act global approach to strategy making, a company's operations in each country can be viewed as experiments that result in learning and in capabilities that may merit transfer to other country markets.

Whenever country-to-country differences are small enough to be accommodated within the framework of a global strategy, a global strategy is preferable to localized strategies because a company can more readily unify its operations and focus on establishing a brand image and reputation that is uniform from country to country. Moreover, with a global strategy a company is better able to focus its full resources on building the resource strengths and capabilities to secure a sustainable low-cost or differentiation-based competitive advantage over both domestic rivals and global rivals racing for world market leadership. Figure 7.2 summarizes the basic differences between a localized or multicountry strategy and a global strategy.

Think-Global, Act-Local Approaches to Strategy Making   Often, a company can accommodate cross-country variations in buyer tastes, local customs, and market conditions with a think-global, act-local approach to developing strategy. This middle-ground approach entails using the same basic competitive theme (low-cost, differentiation, best-cost, or focused) in each country but allowing local mangers the latitude to (1) incorporate whatever country-specific variations in product attributes are needed to best satisfy local buyers and (2) make whatever adjustments in production, distribution, and marketing are needed to be responsive to local market conditions and compete successfully against local rivals. Slightly different product versions sold under the same brand name may suffice to satisfy local tastes, and it may be feasible to accommodate these versions rather economically in the course of designing and manufacturing the company's product offerings. The build-to-order component of Dell's strategy in PCs for example, makes it simple for Dell to be responsive to how buyers in different parts of the world want their PCs equipped. However, Dell has not wavered in its strategy to sell directly to customers rather than through local retailers, even though the majority of buyers in countries such as China are concerned about ordering online and prefer to personally inspect PCs at stores before making a purchase.

As a rule, most companies that operate multinationally endeavor to employ as global a strategy as customer needs and market conditions permit. Philips Electronics, the Netherlands-based electronics and consumer products company, operated successfully with localized strategies for many years but has recently begun moving more toward a unified strategy within the European Union and within North America.[7] Whirlpool has been globalizing its low-cost leadership strategy in home appliances for over 15 years, striving to standardize parts and components and move toward worldwide designs for as many of its appliance products as possible. But it has found it necessary to continue producing significantly different versions of refrigerators, washing machines, and cooking appliances for consumers in different regions of the world because the needs and tastes of local buyers for appliances of different sizes and designs have not converged sufficiently to permit standardization of Whirlpool's product offerings worldwide. General Motors began an initiative in 2004 to insist that its worldwide units share basic parts and work together to design vehicles that can be sold, with modest variations, anywhere around the world; by reducing the types of radios used in its cars and trucks from 270 to 50, it expected to save 40 percent in radio costs.

Illustration Capsule 7.1 on page 209 describes how two companies localize their strategies for competing in country markets across the world.

Figure 7.2   **How a Localized or Multicountry Strategy Differs from a Global Strategy**

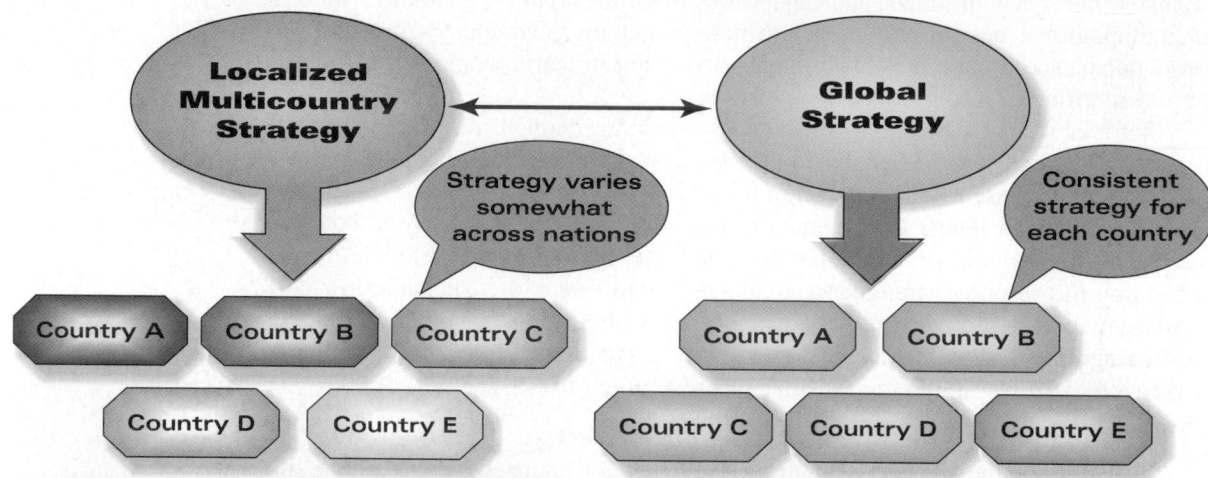

- Customize the company's competitive approach as needed to fit market and business circumstances in each host country—strong responsiveness to local conditions.
- Sell different product versions in different countries under different brand names—adapt product attributes to fit buyer tastes and preferences country by country.
- Scatter plants across many host countries, each producing product versions for local markets.
- Preferably use local suppliers (some local sources may be required by host government).
- Adapt marketing and distribution to local customs and culture of each country.
- Transfer competencies and capabilities from country to country where feasible.
- Give country managers fairly wide strategy-making latitude and autonomy over local operations.

- Pursue same basic competitive strategy worldwide (low-cost, differentiation, best-cost, focused low-cost, focused differentiation), with minimal responsiveness to local conditions.
- Sell same products under same brand name worldwide; focus efforts on building global brands as opposed to strengthening local/regional brands sold in local/regional markets.
- Locate plants on basis of maximum locational advantage, usually in countries where production costs are lowest but plants may be scattered if shipping costs are high or other locational advantages dominate.
- Use best suppliers from anywhere in world.
- Coordinate marketing and distribution worldwide; make minor adaptation to local countries where needed.
- Compete on basis of same technologies, competencies, and capabilities worldwide; stress rapid transfer of new ideas, products, and capabilities to other countries.
- Coordinate major strategic decisions worldwide; expect local managers to stick close to global strategy.

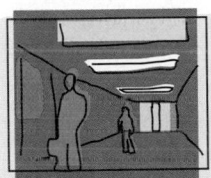

Illustration Capsule 7.1

Multicountry Strategies at Electronic Arts and Coca-Cola

ELECTRONIC ARTS' MULTICOUNTRY STRATEGY IN VIDEO GAMES

Electronic Arts (EA), the world's largest independent developer and marketer of video games, designs games that are suited to the differing tastes of game players in different countries and also designs games in multiple languages. EA has two major design studios—one in Vancouver, British Columbia, and one in Los Angeles—and smaller design studios in San Francisco, Orlando, London, and Tokyo. This dispersion of design studios helps EA to design games that are specific to different cultures—for example, the London studio took the lead in designing the popular FIFA Soccer game to suit European tastes and to replicate the stadiums, signage, and team rosters; the U.S. studio took the lead in designing games involving NFL football, NBA basketball, and NASCAR racing. No other game software company had EA's ability to localize games or to launch games on multiple platforms in multiple countries in multiple languages. EA's game Harry Potter and the Chamber of Secrets was released simultaneously in 75 countries, in 31 languages, and on seven platforms.

COCA-COLA'S MULTICOUNTRY STRATEGY IN BEVERAGES

Coca-Cola strives to meet the demands of local tastes and cultures, offering 300 brands in some 200 countries. Its network of bottlers and distributors is distinctly local, and the company's products and brands are formulated to cater to local tastes. The ways in which Coca-Cola's local operating units bring products to market, the packaging that is used, and the company's advertising messages are all intended to match the local culture and fit in with local business practices. Many of the ingredients and supplies for Coca-Cola's products are sourced locally.

Sources: Information posted at www.ea.com and www.cocacola.com (accessed September 2004).

THE QUEST FOR COMPETITIVE ADVANTAGE IN FOREIGN MARKETS

There are three important ways in which a firm can gain competitive advantage (or offset domestic disadvantages) by expanding outside its domestic market:[8] One, it can use location to lower costs or achieve greater product differentiation. Two, it can transfer competitively valuable competencies and capabilities from its domestic markets to foreign markets. And three, it can use cross-border coordination in ways that a domestic-only competitor cannot.

Using Location to Build Competitive Advantage

To use location to build competitive advantage, a company must consider two issues: (1) whether to concentrate each activity it performs in a few select countries or to disperse performance of the activity to many nations, and (2) in which countries to locate particular activities.[9]

> Companies that compete multinationally can pursue competitive advantage in world markets by locating their value chain activities in whatever nations prove most advantageous.

When to Concentrate Activities in a Few Locations   Companies tend to concentrate their activities in a limited number of locations in the following circumstances:

- *When the costs of manufacturing or other activities are significantly lower in some geographic locations than in others*—For example, much of the world's athletic footwear is manufactured in Asia (China and Korea) because of low labor costs; much of the production of motherboards for PCs is located in Taiwan because of both low costs and the high-caliber technical skills of the Taiwanese labor force.

- *When there are significant scale economies*—The presence of significant economies of scale in components production or final assembly means that a company can gain major cost savings from operating a few superefficient plants as opposed to a host of small plants scattered across the world. Important marketing and distribution economies associated with multinational operations can also yield low-cost leadership. In situations where some competitors are intent on global dominance, being the worldwide low-cost provider is a powerful competitive advantage. Achieving low-cost provider status often requires a company to have the largest worldwide manufacturing share, with production centralized in one or a few world-scale plants in low-cost locations. Some companies even use such plants to manufacture units sold under the brand names of rivals. Manufacturing share (as distinct from brand share or market share) is significant because it provides more certain access to production-related scale economies. Japanese makers of VCRs, microwave ovens, TVs, and DVD players have used their large manufacturing share to establish a low-cost advantage.[10]

- *When there is a steep learning curve associated with performing an activity in a single location*—In some industries experience/learning curve effects in parts manufacture or assembly are so great that a company establishes one or two large plants from which it serves the world market. The key to riding down the learning curve is to concentrate production in a few locations to increase the accumulated volume at a plant (and thus the experience of the plant's workforce) as rapidly as possible.

- *When certain locations have superior resources, allow better coordination of related activities, or offer other valuable advantages*—A research unit or a sophisticated production facility may be situated in a particular nation because of its pool of technically trained personnel. Samsung became a leader in memory chip technology by establishing a major R&D facility in Silicon Valley and transferring the know-how it gained back to headquarters and its plants in South Korea. Where just-in-time inventory practices yield big cost savings and/or where an assembly firm has long-term partnering arrangements with its key suppliers, parts manufacturing plants may be clustered around final assembly plants. An assembly plant may be located in a country in return for the host government's allowing freer import of components from large-scale, centralized parts plants located elsewhere. A customer service center or sales office may be opened in a particular country to help cultivate strong relationships with pivotal customers located nearby.

When to Disperse Activities Across Many Locations   There are several instances when dispersing activities is more advantageous than concentrating them. Buyer-related activities—such as distribution to dealers, sales and advertising, and after-sale service—usually must take place close to buyers. This means physically locating the capability to perform such activities in every country market where a global firm has major customers (unless buyers in several adjoining countries can be served quickly from a nearby central location). For example, firms that make mining and oil-drilling equipment maintain operations in many international locations to support customers' needs for speedy equipment repair and technical assistance. The four biggest public accounting firms have numerous international offices to service the foreign operations of their multinational corporate clients. A global competitor that effectively disperses its buyer-related activities can gain a service-based competitive edge in world markets over rivals whose buyer-related activities are more concentrated—this is one reason the Big Four public accounting firms (PricewaterhouseCoopers, KPMG, Deloitte & Touche, and Ernst & Young) have been so successful relative to regional and national firms. Dispersing activities to many locations is also competitively advantageous when high transportation costs, diseconomies of large size, and trade barriers make it too expensive to operate from a central location. Many companies distribute their products from multiple locations to shorten delivery times to customers. In addition, it is strategically advantageous to disperse activities to hedge against the risks of fluctuating exchange rates; supply interruptions (due to strikes, mechanical failures, and transportation delays); and adverse political developments. Such risks are greater when activities are concentrated in a single location.

The classic reason for locating an activity in a particular country is low cost.[11] Even though multinational and global firms have strong reason to disperse buyer-related activities to many international locations, such activities as materials procurement, parts manufacture, finished goods assembly, technology research, and new product development can frequently be decoupled from buyer locations and performed wherever advantage lies. Components can be made in Mexico; technology research done in Frankfurt; new products developed and tested in Phoenix; and assembly plants located in Spain, Brazil, Taiwan, or South Carolina. Capital can be raised in whatever country it is available on the best terms.

Using Cross-Border Transfers of Competencies and Capabilities to Build Competitive Advantage

One of the best ways for a company with valuable competencies and resource strengths to secure competitive advantage is to use its considerable resource strengths to enter additional country markets. A company whose resource strengths prove particularly potent in competing successfully in newly entered country markets not only grows sales and profits but also may find that its competitiveness is sufficiently enhanced to produce competitive advantage over one or more rivals and contend for global market leadership. Transferring competencies, capabilities, and resource strengths from country to country contributes to the development of broader or deeper competencies and capabilities—ideally helping a company achieve dominating depth in some competitively valuable area. Dominating depth in a competitively valuable capability, resource, or value chain activity is a strong basis for sustainable competitive advantage over other multinational or global competitors, and especially so over domestic-only competitors. A one-country customer base is often too small to support the resource buildup needed to achieve such depth; this is particularly true when the market is just emerging and sophisticated resources have not been required.

Whirlpool, the leading global manufacturer of home appliances, with plants in 14 countries and sales in 170 countries, has used the Internet to create a global information technology platform that allows the company to transfer key product innovations and production processes across regions and brands quickly and effectively. Wal-Mart is slowly but forcefully expanding its operations with a strategy that involves transferring its considerable domestic expertise in distribution and discount retailing to store operations recently established in China, Japan, Latin America, and Europe. Its status as the largest, most resource-deep, and most sophisticated user of distribution/retailing know-how has served it well in building its foreign sales and profitability. But Wal-Mart is not racing madly to position itself in many foreign markets; rather, it is establishing a strong presence in select country markets and learning how to be successful in these before tackling entry into other countries well-suited to its business model.

However, cross-border resource transfers are not a guaranteed recipe for success. Philips Electronics sells more color TVs and DVD recorders in Europe than any other company does; its biggest technological breakthrough was the compact disc, which it invented in 1982. Philips has worldwide sales of about 38 billion euros, but as of 2005 Philips had lost money for 17 consecutive years in its U.S. consumer electronics business. In the United States, the company's color TVs and DVD recorders (sold under the Magnavox and Philips brands) are slow sellers. Philips notoriously lags in introducing new products into the U.S. market and has been struggling to develop an able sales force that can make inroads with U.S. electronics retailers and change its image as a low-end brand.

Using Cross-Border Coordination to Build Competitive Advantage

Coordinating company activities across different countries contributes to sustainable competitive advantage in several different ways.[12] Multinational and global competitors can choose where and how to challenge rivals. They may decide to retaliate against an aggressive rival in the country market where the rival has its biggest sales volume or its best profit margins in order to reduce the rival's financial resources for competing in other country markets. They may also decide to wage a price-cutting offensive against weak rivals in their home markets, capturing greater market share and subsidizing any short-term losses with profits earned in other country markets.

If a firm learns how to assemble its product more efficiently at, say, its Brazilian plant, the accumulated expertise can be quickly communicated via the Internet to assembly plants in other world locations. Knowledge gained in marketing a company's product in Great Britain can readily be exchanged with company personnel in New Zealand or Australia. A global or multinational manufacturer can shift production from a plant in one country to a plant in another to take advantage of exchange rate fluctuations, to enhance its leverage with host-country governments, and to respond to changing wage rates, components shortages, energy costs, or changes in tariffs and quotas. Production schedules can be coordinated worldwide; shipments can be diverted from one distribution center to another if sales rise unexpectedly in one place and fall in another.

Using online systems, companies can readily gather ideas for new and improved products from customers and company personnel all over the world, permitting informed decisions about what can be standardized and what should be customized. Likewise, online systems enable multinational companies to involve their best design and engineering personnel (wherever they are located) in collectively coming up with next-generation products—it is easy for company personnel in one location to use the Internet to collaborate closely with personnel in other locations in performing all sorts of strategically relevant activities. Efficiencies can also be achieved by shifting workloads from where they are unusually heavy to locations where personnel are underutilized. Whirlpool's efforts to link its product R&D and manufacturing operations in North America, Latin America, Europe, and Asia allowed it to accelerate the discovery of innovative appliance features, coordinate the introduction of these features in the appliance products marketed in different countries, and create a cost-efficient worldwide supply chain. Whirlpool's conscious efforts to integrate and coordinate its various operations around the world have helped it become a low-cost producer and also speed product innovations to market, thereby giving Whirlpool an edge over rivals in designing and rapidly introducing innovative and attractively priced appliances worldwide.

Furthermore, a multinational company that consistently incorporates the same differentiating attributes in its products worldwide has enhanced potential to build a global brand name with significant power in the marketplace. The reputation for quality that Honda established worldwide first in motorcycles and then in automobiles gave it competitive advantage in positioning Honda lawn mowers at the upper end of the U.S. outdoor power equipment market—the Honda name gave the company immediate credibility with U.S. buyers of power equipment and enabled it to become an instant market contender without all the fanfare and cost of a multimillion-dollar ad campaign to build brand awareness.

PROFIT SANCTUARIES, CROSS-MARKET SUBSIDIZATION, AND GLOBAL STRATEGIC OFFENSIVES

Profit sanctuaries are country markets (or geographic regions) in which a company derives substantial profits because of its strong or protected market position. McDonald's serves about 50 million customers daily at nearly 32,000 locations in 119 countries on five continents; not surprisingly, its biggest profit sanctuary is the United States, which generated 61.2 percent of 2004 profits, despite accounting for just 34.2 percent of 2004 revenues. Nike, which markets its products in 160 countries, has two big profit sanctuaries: the United States (where it earned 41.5 percent of its operating profits in 2005) and Europe, the Middle East, and Africa (where it earned 34.8 percent of 2005 operating profits). Discount retailer Carrefour, which has stores across much of Europe plus stores in Asia and the Americas, also has two principal profit sanctuaries; its biggest is in France (which in 2004 accounted for 49.2 percent of revenues and 60.8 percent of earnings before interest and taxes), and its second biggest is Europe outside of France (which in 2004 accounted for 37.3 percent of revenues and 33.1 percent of earnings before interest and taxes). Japan is the chief profit sanctuary for most Japanese companies because trade barriers erected by the Japanese government effectively block foreign companies from competing for a large share of Japanese sales. Protected from the threat of foreign competition in their home market, Japanese companies can safely charge somewhat higher prices to their Japanese customers and thus earn attractively large profits on sales made in Japan. In most cases, a company's biggest and most strategically crucial profit sanctuary is its home market, but international and global companies may also enjoy profit sanctuary status in other nations where they have a strong competitive position, big sales volume, and attractive profit margins. Companies that compete globally are likely to have more profit sanctuaries than companies that compete in just a few country markets; a domestic-only competitor, of course, can have only one profit sanctuary (see Figure 7.3).

> **Core Concept**
> Companies with large, protected **profit sanctuaries** have competitive advantage over companies that don't have a protected sanctuary. Companies with multiple profit sanctuaries have a competitive advantage over companies with a single sanctuary.

Figure 7.3   **Profit Sanctuary Potential of Domestic-Only, International, and Global Competitors**

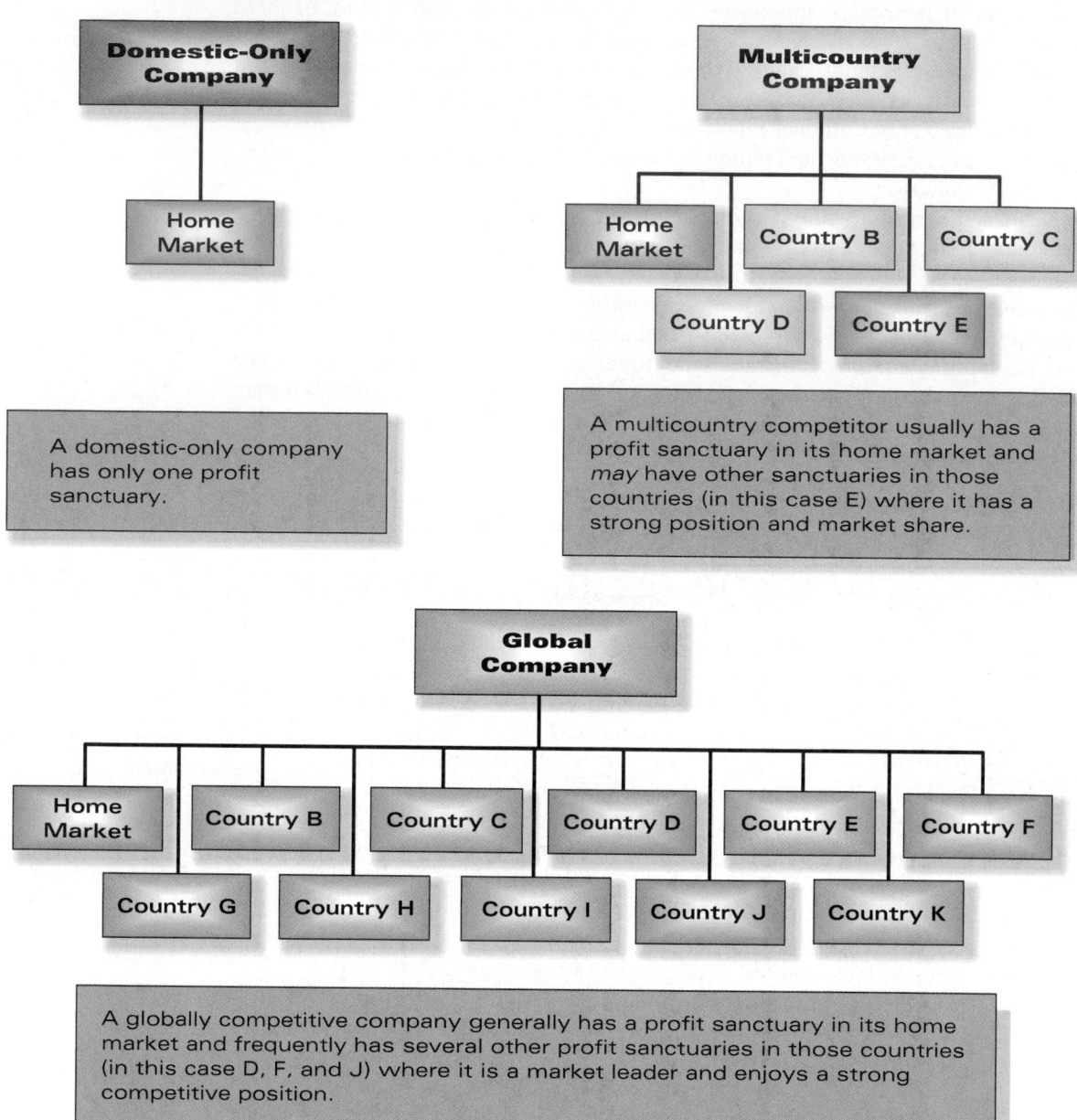

Using Cross-Market Subsidization to Wage a Strategic Offensive

Profit sanctuaries are valuable competitive assets, providing the financial strength to support strategic offensives in selected country markets and fuel a company's race for global market leadership. The added financial capability afforded by multiple profit sanctuaries gives a global or multicountry competitor the financial strength to wage a market offensive against a domestic competitor whose only profit sanctuary is its home market. Consider the case of a purely domestic company in competition with a company that has multiple profit sanctuaries and that is racing for global market leadership. The global company has the flexibility of lowballing its prices in the domestic company's home market and grabbing market share at the domestic company's expense, subsidizing razor-thin margins or even losses with the healthy profits earned in its profit sanctuaries—a practice called **cross-market subsidization.** The global company can adjust the depth of its price cutting to move in and capture market share quickly, or it can shave prices slightly to make gradual market inroads (perhaps over a decade or more) so as not to threaten domestic firms precipitously or trigger protectionist government actions. If the domestic company retaliates with matching price cuts, it exposes its entire revenue and profit base to erosion; its profits can be squeezed substantially and its competitive strength sapped, even if it is the domestic market leader.

> **Core Concept**
> ***Cross-market subsidization—***
> supporting competitive offensives in one market with resources and profits diverted from operations in other markets—is a powerful competitive weapon.

Offensive Strategies Suitable for Competing in Foreign Markets

Companies that compete in multiple foreign markets can, of course, fashion an offensive strategy based on any of the approaches discussed in Chapter 6 (pages 160–193)—these types of offensive strategies are universally applicable and are just as suitable for competing in foreign markets as for domestic markets. But there are three additional types of offensive strategies that are suited to companies competing in foreign markets:[13]

- *Attack a foreign rival's profit sanctuaries.* Launching an offensive in a country market where a rival earns its biggest profits can put the rival on the defensive, forcing it to perhaps spend more on marketing/advertising, trim its prices, boost product innovation efforts, or otherwise undertake actions that raise its costs and erode its profits. If a company's offensive succeeds in eroding a rival's profits in its chief profit sanctuary, the rival's financial resources may be sufficiently weakened to enable the attacker to gain the upper hand and build market momentum. While attacking a rival's profit sanctuary violates the principle of attacking competitor weaknesses instead of competitor strengths, it can nonetheless prove valuable when there is special merit in pursuing actions that cut into a foreign rival's profit margins and force it to defend a market that is important to its competitive well-being. This is especially true when the attacker has important resource strengths and profit sanctuaries of its own that it can draw on to support its offensive.

- *Employ cross-market subsidization to win customers and sales away from select rivals in select country markets.* This can be a particularly attractive offensive strategy for companies that compete in multiple country markets with multiple products (several brands of cigarettes or different brands of food products). Competing in multiple country markets gives a company the luxury of drawing upon the resources, profits, and cash flows derived from particular country markets (especially its profit sanctuaries) to support offensives aimed at winning customers away from select rivals in those country markets that it wants either to enter or to boost its sales and market share. Alternatively, a company whose product lineup consists of different items can shift resources from a product category where it is competitively strong and resource deep (say soft drinks) to add firepower to an offensive in those countries with bright growth prospects in another product category (say bottled water or fruit juices).

- *Dump goods at cut-rate prices in the markets of foreign rivals.* A company is said to be dumping when it sells its goods in foreign markets at prices that are (1) well below the prices at which it normally sells in its home market or (2) well below its full costs per unit. Companies that engage in dumping usually keep their selling prices high enough to cover variable costs per unit, thereby limiting their losses on each unit to some percentage of fixed costs per unit. Dumping can be an appealing offensive strategy in either of two instances. One is when dumping drives down the price so far in the targeted country that domestic firms are quickly put in dire financial straits and end up declaring bankruptcy or being driven out of business—for dumping to pay off in this instance, however, the dumping company needs to have deep enough financial pockets to cover any losses from selling at below-market prices, and the targeted domestic companies need to be financially weak. The second instance in which dumping becomes an attractive strategy is when a company with unused production capacity

Core Concept
Three strategy offensives that are particularly suitable for competing in foreign markets involve (1) attacking a foreign rival's profit sanctuaries, (2) employing cross-market subsidization, and (3) dumping.

discovers that it is cheaper to keep producing (as long as the selling prices cover average variable costs per unit) than it is to incur the costs associated with idle plant capacity. By keeping its plants operating at or near capacity, a dumping company not only may be able to cover variable costs and earn a contribution to fixed costs but also may be able to use its below-market prices to draw price-sensitive customers away from foreign rivals, then attentively court these new customers and retain their business when prices later begin a gradual rise back to normal market levels. Thus, dumping may prove useful as a way of entering the market of a particular foreign country and establishing a customer base.

However, dumping strategies run a high risk of host government retaliation on behalf of the adversely affected domestic companies. Indeed, as the trade among nations has mushroomed over the past 10 years, most governments have joined the World Trade Organization (WTO), which promotes fair trade practices among nations and actively polices dumping. The WTO allows member governments to take actions against dumping wherever there is material injury to domestic competitors. In 2002, for example, the U.S. government imposed tariffs of up to 30 percent on selected steel products that Asian and European steel manufacturers were said to be selling at ultra-low prices in the U.S. market. Canada recently investigated charges that companies in Austria, Belgium, France, Germany, Poland and China were dumping supplies of laminate flooring in Canada to the detriment of Canadian producers and concluded that companies in France and China were indeed selling such flooring in Canada at unreasonably low prices.[14] Most all governments can be expected to retaliate against dumping by imposing special tariffs on goods being imported from the countries of the guilty companies. Companies deemed guilty of dumping frequently come under pressure from their government to cease and desist, especially if the tariffs adversely affect innocent companies based in the same country or if the advent of special tariffs raises the specter of a trade war.

A company desirous of employing some type of offensive strategy in foreign markets is well advised to observe the principles for employing offensive strategies in general. For instance, it usually wise to attack foreign rivals on grounds that pit the challenger's competitive strengths against the defender's weaknesses and vulnerabilities. As a rule, trying to steal customers away from foreign rivals with strategies aimed at besting rivals where they are strongest stand a lower chance of succeeding than strategies that attack their competitive weaknesses, especially when the challenger has resource strengths that enable it to exploit rivals' weaknesses and when its attack involves an element of surprise.[15] It nearly always makes good strategic sense to use the challenger's core competencies and best competitive capabilities to spearhead the offensive. Furthermore, strategic offensives in foreign markets should, as a general rule, be predicated on exploiting the challenger's core competencies and best competitive capabilities. The ideal condition for a strategic offensive is when the attacker's resource strengths give it a competitive advantage over the targeted foreign rivals. The only two exceptions to these offensive strategy principles come when a competitively strong company with deep financial pockets sees considerable benefit in attacking a foreign rival's profit sanctuary and/or has the ability to employ cross-market subsidization—both of these offensive strategies can involve attacking a foreign rival's strengths (but they also are grounded in important strengths of the challenger and don't fall into the trap of challenging a competitively strong rival with a strategic offensive based on unproven expertise or inferior technology or a relatively unknown brand name or other resource weaknesses).

STRATEGIC ALLIANCES AND JOINT VENTURES WITH FOREIGN PARTNERS

Strategic alliances, joint ventures, and other cooperative agreements with foreign companies are a favorite and potentially fruitful means for entering a foreign market or strengthening a firm's competitiveness in world markets.[16] Historically, export-minded firms in industrialized nations sought alliances with firms in less-developed countries to import and market their products locally—such arrangements were often necessary to win approval for entry from the host country's government. Both Japanese and American companies are actively forming alliances with European companies to strengthen their ability to compete in the 25-nation European Union (and the five countries that are seeking to become EU members) and to capitalize on the opening up of Eastern European markets. Many U.S. and European companies are allying with Asian companies in their efforts to enter markets in China, India, Malaysia, Thailand, and other Asian countries. Companies in Europe, Latin America, and Asia are using alliances and joint ventures as a means of strengthening their mutual ability to compete across a wider geographical area—for instance, all the countries in the European Union or whole continents or most all country markets where there is sizable demand for the industry's product. Many foreign companies, of course, are particularly interested in strategic partnerships that will strengthen their ability to gain a foothold in the U.S. market.

> Cross-border alliances have proved to be popular and viable vehicles for companies to edge their way into the markets of foreign countries.

However, cooperative arrangements between domestic and foreign companies have strategic appeal for reasons besides gaining better access to attractive country markets.[17] A second big appeal of cross-border alliances is to capture economies of scale in production and/or marketing—cost reduction can be the difference that allows a company to be cost-competitive. By joining forces in producing components, assembling models, and marketing their products, companies can realize cost savings not achievable with their own small volumes. A third motivation for entering into a cross-border alliance is to fill gaps in technical expertise and/or knowledge of local markets (buying habits and product preferences of consumers, local customs, and so on). Allies learn much from one another in performing joint research, sharing technological know-how, studying one another's manufacturing methods, and understanding how to tailor sales and marketing approaches to fit local cultures and traditions. Indeed, one of the win–win benefits of an alliance is to learn from the skills, technological know-how, and capabilities of alliance partners and implant the knowledge and know-how of these partners in personnel throughout the company.

A fourth motivation for cross-border alliances is to share distribution facilities and dealer networks, thus mutually strengthening their access to buyers. A fifth benefit is that cross-border allies can direct their competitive energies more toward mutual rivals and less toward one another; teaming up may help them close the gap on leading companies. A sixth driver of cross-border alliances comes into play when companies desirous of entering a new foreign market conclude that alliances with local companies are an effective way to tap into a partner's local market knowledge and help it establish working relationships with key officials in the host-country government.[18] And, finally, alliances can be a particularly useful way for companies across the world to gain agreement on important technical standards—they have been used to arrive at standards for DVD players, assorted PC devices, Internet-related technologies, high-definition televisions, and mobile phones.

> Cross-border alliances enable a growth-minded company to widen its geographic coverage and strengthen its competitiveness in foreign markets while, at the same time, offering flexibility and allowing a company to retain some degree of autonomy and operating control.

What makes cross-border alliances an attractive strategic means of gaining the above types of benefits (as compared to acquiring or merging with foreign-based companies to gain much the same benefits) is that entering into alliances and strategic partnerships to gain market access and/ or expertise of one kind or another allows a company to preserve its independence (which is not the case with a merger), retain veto power over how the alliance operates, and avoid using perhaps scarce financial resources to fund acquisitions. Furthermore, an alliance offers the flexibility to readily disengage once its purpose has been served or if the benefits prove elusive, whereas an acquisition is more permanent sort of arrangement (although the acquired company can, of course, be divested).[19]

Illustration Capsule 7.2 provides six examples of cross-border strategic alliances.

The Risks of Strategic Alliances with Foreign Partners

Alliances and joint ventures with foreign partners have their pitfalls, however. Cross-border allies typically have to overcome language and cultural barriers and figure out how to deal with diverse (or perhaps conflicting) operating practices. The communication, trust-building, and coordination costs are high in terms of management time.[20] It is not unusual for there to be little personal chemistry among some of the key people on whom success or failure of the alliance depends—the rapport such personnel need to work well together may never emerge. And even if allies are able to develop productive personal relationships, they can still have trouble reaching mutually agreeable ways to deal with key issues or resolve differences. There is a natural tendency for allies to struggle to collaborate effectively in competitively sensitive areas, thus spawning suspicions on both sides about forthright exchanges of information and expertise. Occasionally, the egos of corporate executives can clash—an alliance between Northwest Airlines and KLM Royal Dutch Airlines resulted in a bitter feud among both companies' top officials (who, according to some reports, refused to speak to each other).[21] In addition, there is the thorny problem of getting alliance partners to sort through issues and reach decisions fast enough to stay abreast of rapid advances in technology or fast-changing market conditions.

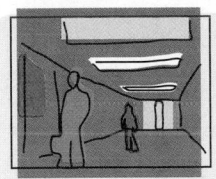

Illustration Capsule 7.2

Six Examples of Cross-Border Strategic Alliances

1. Two auto firms, Renault of France and Nissan of Japan, formed a broad-ranging global partnership in 1999 and then strengthened and expanded the alliance in 2002. The initial objective was to gain sales for new Nissan vehicles introduced in the European market, but the alliance now extends to full cooperation in all major areas, including the use of common platforms, joint development and use of engines and transmissions, fuel cell research, purchasing and use of common suppliers, and exchange of best practices. When the alliance was formed in 1999, Renault acquired a 36.8 percent ownership stake in Nissan; this was extended to 44.4 percent in 2002 when the alliance was expanded. Also, in 2002, the partners formed a jointly and equally owned strategic management company, named Renault-Nissan, to coordinate cooperative efforts.

2. Intel, the world's largest chip maker, has formed strategic alliances with leading software application providers and computer hardware providers to bring more innovativeness and expertise to the architecture underlying Intel's family of microprocessors and semiconductors. Intel's partners in the effort to enhance Intel's next-generation products include SAP, Oracle, SAS, BEA, IBM, Hewlett-Packard, Dell, Microsoft, Cisco Systems, and Alcatel. One of the alliances between Intel and Cisco involves a collaborative effort in Hong Kong to build next-generation infrastructure for Electronic Product Code/Radio Frequency Identification (EPC/RFID) solutions used to link manufacturers and logistics companies in the Hong Kong region with retailers worldwide. Intel and France-based Alcatel (a leading provider of fixed and mobile broadband access products, marketed in 130 countries) formed an alliance in 2004 to advance the definition, standardization, development, integration, and marketing of WiMAX broadband services solutions. WiMAX was seen as a cost-effective wireless or mobile broadband solution for deployment in both emerging markets and developed countries when, for either economic or technical reasons, it was not feasible to provide urban or rural customers with hardwired DSL broadband access.

3. Verio, a subsidiary of Japan-based NTT Communications and one of the leading global providers of Web hosting services and IP data transport, operates with the philosophy that in today's highly competitive and challenging technology market, companies must gain and share skills, information, and technology with technology leaders across the world. Believing that no company can be all things to all customers in the Web hosting industry, Verio executives have developed an alliance-oriented business model that combines the company's core competencies with the skills and products of best-of-breed, technology partners. Verio's strategic partners include Accenture, Cisco Systems, Microsoft, Sun Microsystems, Oracle, Arsenal Digital Solutions (a provider of worry-free tape backup, data restore, and data storage services), Internet Security Systems (a provider of firewall and intrusion detection systems), and Mercantec (a developer of storefront and shopping cart software). Verio management believes that its portfolio of strategic alliances allows it to use innovative, best-of-class technologies in providing its customers with fast, efficient, accurate data transport and a complete set of Web hosting services. An independent panel of 12 judges recently selected Verio as the winner of the Best Technology Foresight Award for its efforts in pioneering new technologies.

4. Toyota and First Automotive Works, China's biggest automaker, entered into an alliance in 2002 to make luxury sedans, sport-utility vehicles (SUVs), and minivehicles for the Chinese market. The intent was to make as many as 400,000 vehicles annually by 2010, an amount equal to the number that Volkswagen, the company with the largest share of the Chinese market, was making as of 2002. The alliance envisioned a joint investment of about $1.2 billion. At the time of the announced alliance, Toyota was lagging behind Honda, General Motors, and Volkswagen in setting up production facilities in China. Capturing a bigger share of the Chinese market was seen as crucial to Toyota's success in achieving its strategic objective of having a 15 percent share of the world's automotive market by 2010.

5. Airbus Industrie was formed by an alliance of aerospace companies from Britain, Spain, Germany, and France that included British Aerospace, Daimler-Benz Aerospace, and Aerospatiale. The objective of the alliance was to create a European aircraft company capable of competing with U.S.-based Boeing Corporation. The alliance has proved highly successful, infusing Airbus with the know-how and resources to compete head-to-head with Boeing for world leadership in large commercial aircraft (over 100 passengers).

6. General Motors, DaimlerChrysler, and BMW have entered into an alliance to develop a hybrid gasoline-electric engine that is simpler and less expensive to produce than the hybrid engine technology being pioneered by Toyota. Toyota, the acknowledged world leader in hybrid engines, is endeavoring to establish its design as the industry standard by signing up other automakers to use it. But the technology favored by the General Motors/DaimlerChrysler/BMW alliance is said to be less costly to produce and easier to configure for large trucks and SUVs than Toyota's (although it is also less fuel efficient). Europe's largest automaker, Volkswagen, has allied with Porsche to pursue the development of hybrid engines. Ford Motor and Honda, so far, have elected to go it alone in developing hybrid engine technology.

Sources: Company Web sites and press releases; Yves L. Doz and Gary Hamel, *Alliance Advantage: The Art of Creating Value through Partnering* (Boston, MA: Harvard Business School Press, 1998); and Norihiko Shirouzu and Jathon Sapsford, "As Hybrid Cars Gain Traction, Industry Battles over Designs," *The Wall Street Journal,* October 19, 2005, pp. A1, A9B.

It requires many meetings of many people working in good faith over time to iron out what is to be shared, what is to remain proprietary, and how the cooperative arrangements will work. Often, once the bloom is off the rose, partners discover they have conflicting objectives and strategies, deep differences of opinion about how to proceed, or important differences in corporate values and ethical standards. Tensions build up, working relationships cool, and the hoped-for benefits never materialize.[22]

Even if the alliance becomes a win–win proposition for both parties, there is the danger of becoming overly dependent on foreign partners for essential expertise and competitive capabilities. If a company is aiming for global market leadership and needs to develop capabilities of its own, then at some juncture cross-border merger or acquisition may have to be substituted for cross-border alliances and joint ventures.

> Strategic alliances are more effective in helping establish a beachhead of new opportunity in world markets than in achieving and sustaining global leadership.

One of the lessons about cross-border alliances is that they are more effective in helping a company establish a beachhead of new opportunity in world markets than they are in enabling a company to achieve and sustain global market leadership. Global market leaders, while benefiting from alliances, usually must guard against becoming overly dependent on the assistance they get from alliance partners—otherwise, they are not masters of their own destiny.

When a Cross-Border Alliance May Be Unnecessary

Experienced multinational companies that market in 50 to 100 or more countries across the world find less need for entering into cross-border alliances than do companies in the early stages of globalizing their operations.[23] Multinational companies make it a point to develop senior managers who understand how "the system" works in different countries; these companies can also avail themselves of local managerial talent and know-how by simply hiring experienced local managers and thereby detouring the hazards of collaborative alliances with local companies. If a multinational enterprise with considerable experience in entering the markets of different countries wants to detour the hazards and hassles of allying with local businesses, it can simply assemble a capable management team consisting of both senior managers with considerable international experience and local managers. The responsibilities of its own in-house managers with international business savvy are (1) to transfer technology, business practices, and the corporate culture into the company's operations in the new country market, and (2) to serve as conduits for the flow of information between the corporate office and local operations. The responsibilities of local managers are (1) to contribute needed understanding of the local market conditions, local buying habits, and local ways of doing business, and (2) in many cases, to head up local operations.

Hence, one cannot automatically presume that a company needs the wisdom and resources of a local partner to guide it through the process of successfully entering the markets of foreign countries. Indeed, experienced multinationals often discover that local partners do not always have adequate local market knowledge—much of the so-called experience of local partners can predate the emergence of current market trends and conditions, and sometimes their operating practices can be archaic.[24]

STRATEGIES THAT FIT THE MARKETS OF EMERGING COUNTRIES

Companies racing for global leadership have to consider competing in emerging markets like China, India, Brazil, Indonesia, and Mexico—countries where the business risks are considerable but where the opportunities for growth are huge, especially as their

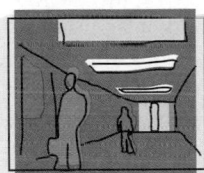

Illustration Capsule 7.3

Coca-Cola's Strategy for Growing Its Sales in China and India

In 2004, Coca-Cola developed a strategy to dramatically boost its market penetration in such emerging countries as China and India, where annual growth had recently dropped from about 30 percent in 1994–1998 to 10–12 percent in 2001–2003. Prior to 2003, Coca-Cola had focused its marketing efforts in China and India on making its drinks attractive to status-seeking young people in urbanized areas (cities with populations of 500,000 or more), but as annual sales growth steadily declined in these areas during the 1998–2003 period, Coca-Cola's management decided that the company needed a new, bolder strategy aimed at more rural areas of these countries. It began promoting the sales of 6.5-ounce returnable glass bottles of Coke in smaller cities and outlying towns with populations in the 50,000 to 250,000 range. Returnable bottles (which could be reused about 20 times) were much cheaper than plastic bottles or aluminum cans, and the savings in packaging costs were enough to slash the price of single-serve bottles to one yuan in China and about five rupees in India,

the equivalent in both cases of about 12 cents. Initial results were promising. Despite the fact that annual disposable incomes in these rural areas were often less than $1,000, the one-yuan and five-rupee prices proved attractive. Sales of the small bottles of Coke for one local Coca-Cola distributor in Anning, China, soon accounted for two-thirds of the distributor's total sales; a local distributor in India boosted sales from 9,000 cases in 2002 to 27,000 cases in 2003 and was expecting sales of 45,000 cases in 2004. Coca-Cola management expected that greater emphasis on rural sales would boost its growth rate in Asia to close to 20 percent and help boost worldwide volume growth to the 3–5 percent range as opposed to the paltry 1 percent rate experienced in 2003.

However, Pepsi, which had a market share of about 27 percent in China versus Coca-Cola's 55 percent, was skeptical of Coca-Cola's rural strategy and continued with its all-urban strategy of marketing to consumers in China's 165 cities with populations greater than 1 million people.

Sources. Based on information in Gabriel Kahn and Eric Bellman, "Coke's Big Gamble in Asia: Digging Deeper in China, India," *The Wall Street Journal,* August 11, 2004, pp. A1, A4, plus information at www.cocacola.com (accessed September 20, 2004 and October 6, 2005).

economies develop and living standards climb toward levels in the industrialized world.[25] With the world now comprising more than 6 billion people—fully one-third of whom are in India and China, and hundreds of millions more in other less-developed countries of Asia and in Latin America—a company that aspires to world market leadership (or to sustained rapid growth) cannot ignore the market opportunities or the base of technical and managerial talent such countries offer. For example, in 2003 China's population of 1.3 billion people consumed nearly 33 percent of the world's annual cotton production, 51 percent of the world's pork, 35 percent of all the cigarettes, 31 percent of worldwide coal production, 27 percent of the world's steel production, 19 percent of the aluminum, 23 percent of the TVs, 20 percent of the cell phones, and 18 percent of the washing machines.[26] China is the world's largest consumer of copper, aluminum, and cement and the second largest importer of oil; it is the world's biggest market for mobile phones and the second biggest for PCs, and it is on track to become the second largest market for motor vehicles by 2010.

Illustration Capsule 7.3 describes Coca-Cola's strategy to boost its sales and market share in China.

Tailoring products to fit conditions in an emerging-country market, however, often involves more than making minor product changes and becoming more familiar with local cultures.[27] Ford's attempt to sell a Ford Escort in India at a price of $21,000—a luxury-car price, given that India's best-selling Maruti-Suzuki model sold at the time for $10,000 or less, and that fewer than 10 percent of Indian households have annual purchasing power greater than $20,000—met with a less-than-enthusiastic market response. McDonald's has had to offer vegetable burgers in parts of Asia and to rethink its prices, which are often high by local standards and affordable only by the well-to-do. Kellogg has struggled to introduce its cereals successfully because consumers in many less-developed countries do not eat cereal for breakfast—changing habits is difficult and expensive. In several emerging countries, Coca-Cola has found that advertising its world image does not strike a chord with the local populace in a number of emerging-country markets. Single-serving packages of detergents, shampoos, pickles, cough syrup, and cooking oils are very popular in India because they allow buyers to conserve cash by purchasing only what they need immediately. Thus, many companies find that trying to employ a strategy akin to that used in the markets of developed countries is hazardous.[28] Experimenting with some, perhaps many, local twists is usually necessary to find a strategy combination that works.

Strategy Options

Several strategy options for tailoring a company's strategy to fit the sometimes unusual or challenging circumstances presented in emerging-country markets:

- *Prepare to compete on the basis of low price.* Consumers in emerging markets are often highly focused on price, which can give low-cost local competitors the edge unless a company can find ways to attract buyers with bargain prices as well as better products.[29] For example, when Unilever entered the market for laundry detergents in India, it realized that 80 percent of the population could not afford the brands it was selling to affluent consumers there (or the brands it was selling in wealthier countries). To compete against a low-priced detergent made by a local company, Unilever came up with a low-cost formula that was not harsh to the skin, constructed new low-cost production facilities, packaged the detergent (named Wheel) in single-use amounts so that it could be sold very cheaply, distributed the product to local merchants by handcarts, and crafted an economical marketing campaign that included painted signs on buildings and demonstrations near stores—the new brand quickly captured $100 million in sales and was the number one detergent brand in India in 2004 based on dollar sales. Unilever later replicated the strategy with low-priced packets of shampoos and deodorants in India and in South America with a detergent brand named Ala.

- *Be prepared to modify aspects of the company's business model to accommodate local circumstances (but not so much that the company loses the advantage of global scale and global branding).*[30] For instance when Dell entered China, it discovered that individuals and businesses were not accustomed to placing orders through the Internet (in North America, over 50 percent of Dell's sales in 2002–2005 were online). To adapt, Dell modified its direct sales model to rely more heavily on phone and fax orders and decided to be patient in getting Chinese customers to place Internet orders. Further, because numerous Chinese government departments and state-owned enterprises insisted that hardware vendors make their bids through distributors and systems integrators (as opposed to dealing directly with Dell salespeople as did large enterprises in other countries), Dell opted to use third parties in marketing its products to this buyer segment (although it did sell through its own sales force where it could). But Dell was careful not to abandon those parts of its business model that gave it a competitive edge over rivals. When McDonald's moved into Russia in the 1990s, it was forced to alter its practice of obtaining needed supplies from outside vendors because capable local suppliers were not available; to supply its Russian outlets and stay true to its core principle of serving consistent quality fast food, McDonald's set up its own vertically integrated supply chain (cattle were imported from Holland, russet potatoes were imported from the United States), worked with a select number of Russian bakers for its bread; brought in agricultural specialists from Canada and Europe to improve the management practices of Russian farmers; built its own 100,000-square-foot McComplex to produce hamburgers, French fries, ketchup, mustard, and Big Mac sauce; and set up a trucking fleet to move supplies to restaurants.

- *Try to change the local market to better match the way the company does business elsewhere.*[31] A multinational company often has enough market clout to drive major changes in the way a local country market operates. When Hong Kong–based STAR launched its first satellite TV channel in 1991, it profoundly impacted the TV marketplace in India: The Indian government lost its monopoly on TV broadcasts, several other satellite TV channels aimed at Indian audiences quickly emerged, and the excitement of additional channels triggered a boom in TV manufacturing in India. When Japan's Suzuki entered India in 1981, it triggered a quality revolution among Indian auto parts manufacturers. Local parts and components suppliers teamed up with Suzuki's vendors in Japan and worked with Japanese experts to produce higher-quality products. Over the next two decades, Indian companies became very proficient in making top-notch parts and components for vehicles, won more prizes for quality than companies in any country other than Japan, and broke into the global market as suppliers to many automakers in Asia and other parts of the world.

- *Stay away from those emerging markets where it is impractical or uneconomic to modify the company's business model to accommodate local circumstances.*[32] Home Depot has avoided entry into most Latin American countries because its value proposition of good quality, low prices, and attentive customer service relies on (1) good highways and logistical systems to minimize store inventory costs, (2) employee stock ownership to help motivate store personnel to provide good customer service, and (3) high labor costs for housing construction and home repairs to encourage homeowners to engage in do-it-yourself projects. Relying on these factors in the U.S. market has worked spectacularly for Home Depot, but the company has found that it cannot count on these factors in much of Latin America. Thus, to enter the market in Mexico, Home Depot switched to an acquisition strategy; it has acquired two building supply retailers in Mexico with a total of 40-plus stores. But it has not tried to operate them in the style of its U.S. big-box stores, and it doesn't have retail operations in any other developing nations (although it is exploring entry into China).

Company experiences in entering developing markets like China, India, Russia, and Brazil indicate that profitability seldom comes quickly or easily. Building a market for the company's products can often turn into a long-term process that involves reeducation of consumers, sizable investments in advertising and promotion to alter tastes and buying habits, and upgrades of the local infrastructure (the supplier base, transportation systems, distribution channels, labor markets, and capital markets). In such cases, a company must be patient, work within the system to improve the infrastructure, and lay the foundation for generating sizable revenues and profits once conditions are ripe for market takeoff.

> Profitability in emerging markets rarely comes quickly or easily—new entrants have to adapt their business models and strategies to local conditions and be patient in earning a profit.

Figure 7.4   **Strategy Options for Local Companies in Competing Against Global Companies**

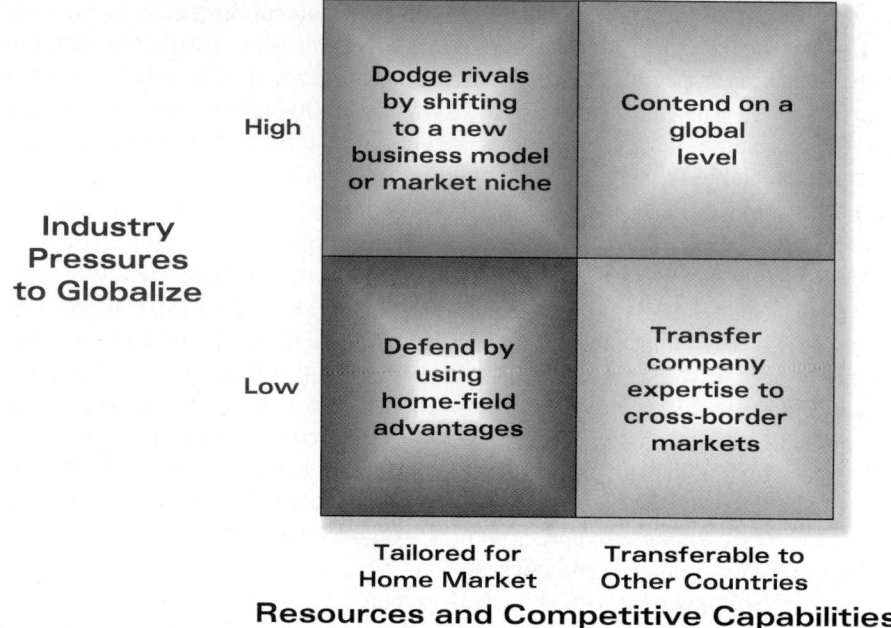

Source: Adapted from Niroj Dawar and Tony Frost, "Competing with Giants: Survival Strategies for Local Companies in Emerging Markets," *Harvard Business Review* 77, no. 1 (January–February 1999), p. 122.

Defending Against Global Giants: Strategies for Local Companies in Emerging Markets

If opportunity-seeking, resource-rich multinational companies are looking to enter emerging markets, what strategy options can local companies use to survive? As it turns out, the prospects for local companies facing global giants are by no means grim. They can employ any of four generic strategic approaches depending on (1) whether their competitive assets are suitable only for the home market or can be transferred abroad, and (2) whether industry pressures to move toward global competition are strong or weak, as shown in Figure 7.4.

Using Home-Field Advantages   When the pressures for competing globally are low and a local firm has competitive strengths well suited to the local market, a good strategy option is to concentrate on the advantages enjoyed in the home market, cater to customers who prefer a local touch, and accept the loss of customers attracted to global brands.[33] A local company may be able to astutely exploit its local orientation— its familiarity with local preferences, its expertise in traditional products, its long-standing customer relationships. In many cases, a local company enjoys a significant cost advantage over global rivals (perhaps because of simpler product design or lower operating and overhead costs), allowing it to compete on the basis of price. Its global competitors often aim their products at upper- and middle-income urban buyers, who tend to be more fashion-conscious, more willing to experiment with new products, and more attracted to global brands.

Another competitive approach is to cater to the local market in ways that pose difficulties for global rivals. A small Middle Eastern cell phone manufacturer competes
successfully against industry giants Nokia, Samsung, and Motorola by selling a model
designed especially for Muslims—it is loaded with the Koran, alerts people at prayer
times, and is equipped with a compass that points them toward Mecca. Several Chinese
PC makers have been able to retain customers in competition against global leader Dell
because Chinese PC buyers strongly prefer to personally inspect PCs before making a
purchase; local PC makers with their extensive retailer networks that allow prospective
buyers to check out their offerings in nearby stores have a competitive edge in winning
the business of first-time PC buyers vis-à-vis Dell with its build-to-order, sell-direct
business strategy (where customers are encouraged to place their orders online or via
phone or fax). Bajaj Auto, India's largest producer of scooters, has defended its turf
against Honda (which entered the Indian market with local joint venture partner Hero
Group to sell scooters, motorcycles, and other vehicles on the basis of its superior technology, quality, and the appeal) by focusing on buyers who wanted low-cost, durable
scooters and easy access to maintenance in the countryside. Bajaj designed a rugged,
cheap-to-build scooter for India's rough roads, increased its investments in R&D to
improve reliability and quality, and created an extensive network of distributors and
roadside-mechanic stalls, a strategic approach that allowed it to remain the market
leader with a 70–75 percent market share through 2004 despite growing unit sales of
Hero Honda motorcycles and scooters.

Transferring the Company's Expertise to Cross-Border Markets   When
a company has resource strengths and capabilities suitable for competing in other
country markets, launching initiatives to transfer its expertise to cross-border markets
becomes a viable strategic option.[34] Televisa, Mexico's largest media company, used
its expertise in Spanish culture and linguistics to become the world's most prolific
producer of Spanish-language soap operas. Jollibee Foods, a family-owned company
with 56 percent of the fast-food business in the Philippines, combated McDonald's
entry first by upgrading service and delivery standards and then by using its expertise
in seasoning hamburgers with garlic and soy sauce and making noodle and rice meals
with fish to open outlets catering to Asian residents in Hong Kong, the Middle East,
and California.

Shifting to a New Business Model or Market Niche   When industry pressures to globalize are high, any of the following three options makes the most sense:
(1) shift the business to a piece of the industry value chain where the firm's expertise
and resources provide competitive advantage, (2) enter into a joint venture with a globally competitive partner, or (3) sell out to (be acquired by) a global entrant into the home
market who concludes the company would be a good entry vehicle.[35] When Microsoft
entered China, local software developers shifted from cloning Windows products to
developing Windows application software customized to the Chinese market. When the
Russian PC market opened to IBM, Compaq, and Hewlett-Packard, local Russian PC
maker Vist focused on assembling low-cost models, marketing them through exclusive
distribution agreements with selected local retailers, and opening company-owned full-
service centers in dozens of Russian cities. Vist focused on providing low-cost PCs,
giving lengthy warranties, and catering to buyers who felt the need for local service and
support. Vist's strategy allowed it to remain the market leader, with a 20 percent share.

An India-based electronics company has been able to carve out a market niche for itself by developing an all-in-one business machine designed especially for India's 1.2 million small shopkeepers that tolerates heat, dust, and power outages and that sells for a modest $180 for the smallest of its three models.[36]

Contending on a Global Level   If a local company in an emerging market has transferable resources and capabilities, it can sometimes launch successful initiatives to meet the pressures for globalization head-on and start to compete on a global level itself.[37] Lenovo, China's biggest PC maker, recently purchased IBM's PC business, moved its headquarters to New York City, put the Lenovo brand on IBM's PCs, and launched initiative to become a global PC maker alongside leaders Dell and Hewlett-Packard. When General Motors (GM) decided to outsource the production of radiator caps for all of its North American vehicles, Sundaram Fasteners of India pursued the opportunity; it purchased one of GM's radiator cap production lines, moved it to India, and became GM's sole supplier of radiator caps in North America—at 5 million units a year. As a participant in GM's supplier network, Sundaram learned about emerging technical standards, built its capabilities, and became one of the first Indian companies to achieve QS 9000 certification, a quality standard that GM now requires for all suppliers. Sundaram's acquired expertise in quality standards enabled it then to pursue opportunities to supply automotive parts in Japan and Europe. Chinese communications equipment maker Huawei has captured a 16 percent share in the global market for Internet routers because its prices are up to 50 percent lower than those of industry leaders like Cisco Systems; Huawei's success in low-priced Internet networking gear has allowed it to expand aggressively outside China, into such country markets as Russia and Brazil, and achieve the number two worldwide market share in broadband networking gear.[38] In 2005 Chinese automakers were laying plans to begin exporting fuel-efficient small cars to the United States and begin the long-term process of competing internationally against the world's leading automakers.

Key Points

Most issues in competitive strategy that apply to domestic companies apply also to companies that compete internationally. But there are four strategic issues unique to competing across national boundaries:

1. Whether to customize the company's offerings in each different country market to match the tastes and preferences of local buyers or offer a mostly standardized product worldwide.

2. Whether to employ essentially the same basic competitive strategy in all countries or modify the strategy country by country to fit the specific market conditions and competitive circumstances it encounters.

3. Where to locate the company's production facilities, distribution centers, and customer service operations so as to realize the greatest locational advantages.

4. Whether and how to efficiently transfer the company's resource strengths and capabilities from one country to another in an effort to secure competitive advantage.

Multicountry competition refers to situations where competition in one national market is largely independent of competition in another national market—there is no "international market," just a collection of self-contained country (or maybe regional) markets. Global competition exists when competitive conditions across national markets are linked strongly enough to form a true world market and when leading competitors compete head-to-head in many different countries.

In posturing to compete in foreign markets, a company has three basic options: (1) a think-local, act-local approach to crafting a strategy, (2) a think-global, act-global approach to crafting a strategy, and (3) a combination think-global, act-local approach. A think-local, act-local, or multicountry, strategy is appropriate for industries where multicountry competition dominates; a localized approach to strategy making calls for a company to vary its product offering and competitive approach from country to country in order to accommodate differing buyer preferences and market conditions. A think-global, act-global approach (or global strategy) works best in markets that are globally competitive or beginning to globalize; global strategies involve employing the same basic competitive approach (low-cost, differentiation, best-cost, focused) in all country markets and marketing essentially the same products under the same brand names in all countries where the company operates. A think-global, act-local approach can be used when it is feasible for a company to employ essentially the same basic competitive strategy in all markets but still customize its product offering and some aspect of its operations to fit local market circumstances.

Other strategy options for competing in world markets include maintaining a national (one-country) production base and exporting goods to foreign markets, licensing foreign firms to use the company's technology or produce and distribute the company's products, employing a franchising strategy, and using strategic alliances or other collaborative partnerships to enter a foreign market or strengthen a firm's competitiveness in world markets.

Strategic alliances with foreign partners have appeal from several angles: gaining wider access to attractive country markets, allowing capture of economies of scale in production and/or marketing, filling gaps in technical expertise and/or knowledge of local markets, saving on costs by sharing distribution facilities and dealer networks, helping gain agreement on important technical standards, and helping combat the impact of alliances that rivals have formed. Cross-border strategic alliances are fast reshaping competition in world markets, pitting one group of allied global companies against other groups of allied global companies.

There are three ways in which a firm can gain competitive advantage (or offset domestic disadvantages) in global markets. One way involves locating various value chain activities among nations in a manner that lowers costs or achieves greater product differentiation. A second way involves efficient and effective transfer of competitively valuable competencies and capabilities from its domestic markets to foreign markets. A third way draws on a multinational or global competitor's ability to deepen or broaden its resource strengths and capabilities and to coordinate its dispersed activities in ways that a domestic-only competitor cannot.

Profit sanctuaries are country markets in which a company derives substantial profits because of its strong or protected market position. They are valuable competitive assets. A company with multiple profit sanctuaries has the financial strength to support competitive offensives in one market with resources and profits diverted from its operations in other markets—a practice called *cross-market subsidization*. The ability of companies with multiple profit sanctuaries to employ cross-subsidization gives them a powerful offensive weapon and a competitive advantage over companies with a single sanctuary.

Companies racing for global leadership have to consider competing in emerging markets like China, India, Brazil, Indonesia, and Mexico—countries where the business risks are considerable but the opportunities for growth are huge. To succeed in these markets, companies often have to (1) compete on the basis of low price, (2) be prepared to modify aspects of the company's business model to accommodate local circumstances (but not so much that the company loses the advantage of global scale and global branding), and/or (3) try to change the local market to better match the way the company does business elsewhere. Profitability is unlikely to come quickly or easily in emerging markets, typically because of the investments needed to alter buying habits and tastes and/or the need for infrastructure upgrades. And there may be times when a company should simply stay away from certain emerging markets until conditions for entry are better suited to its business model and strategy.

Local companies in emerging country markets can seek to compete against multinational companies by (1) defending on the basis of home-field advantages, (2) transferring their expertise to cross-border markets, (3) dodging large rivals by shifting to a new business model or market niche, or (4) launching initiatives to compete on a global level themselves.

Exercises

1.   Go to Caterpillar's Web site (www.caterpillar.com) and search for information about the company's strategy in foreign markets. Is Caterpillar pursuing a global strategy or a localized multicountry strategy? Support your answer.

2.   Assume you are in charge of developing the strategy for a multinational company selling products in some 50 different countries around the world. One of the issues you face is whether to employ a multicountry strategy or a global strategy.

   a.   If your company's product is personal computers, do you think it would make better strategic sense to employ a multicountry strategy or a global strategy? Why?

   b.   If your company's product is dry soup mixes and canned soups, would a multicountry strategy seem to be more advisable than a global strategy? Why?

   c.   If your company's product is washing machines, would it seem to make more sense to pursue a multicountry strategy or a global strategy? Why?

   d.   If your company's product is basic work tools (hammers, screwdrivers, pliers, wrenches, saws), would a multicountry strategy or a global strategy seem to have more appeal? Why?

3.   The Hero Group is among the 10 largest corporations in India, with 19 business segments and annual revenues of $2.75 billion in fiscal 2004–2005. Many of the corporation's business units have used strategic alliances with foreign partners to compete in new product and geographic markets. Review the company's statements concerning its alliances and international business operations at www.herogroup.com and prepare a two-page report that outlines Hero's successful use of international strategic alliances.

4. Using this chapter's discussion of strategies for local companies competing against global rivals and Figure 7.4, develop a strategic approach for a manufacturer or service company in your community that might be forced to compete with a global firm. How might the local company exploit a home-field advantage? Would it make sense for the local company to attempt to transfer its capabilities or expertise to cross-border markets? Or change its business model or market niche? Or join the fight on a global level? Explain.

Tailoring Strategy to Fit Specific Industry and Company Situations

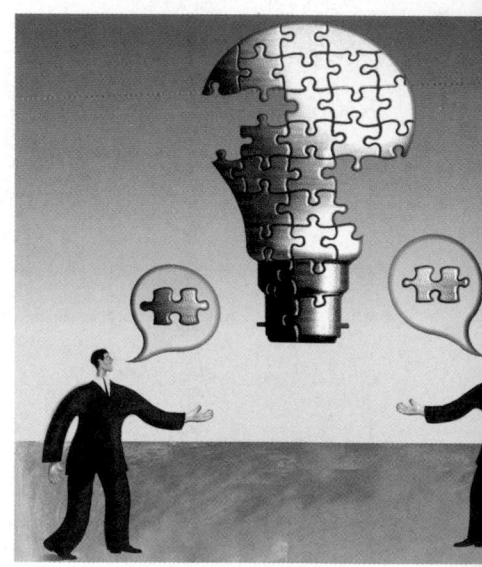

Strategy is all about combining choices of what to do and what not to do into a system that creates the requisite fit between what the environment needs and what the company does.
—Costas Markides

Competing in the marketplace is like war. You have injuries and casualties, and the best strategy wins.
—John Collins

It is much better to make your own products obsolete than allow a competitor to do it.
—Michael A. Cusamano and Richard W. Selby

In a turbulent age, the only dependable advantage is reinventing your business model before circumstances force you to.
—Gary Hamel and Liisa Välikangas

P rior chapters have emphasized the analysis and options that go into matching a company's choice of strategy to (1) industry and competitive conditions and (2) its own resource strengths and weaknesses, competitive capabilities, opportunities and threats, and market position. But there's more to be revealed about the hows of matching the choices of strategy to a company's circumstances. This chapter looks at the strategy-making task in 10 commonly encountered situations:

1. Companies competing in emerging industries.

2. Companies competing in rapidly growing markets.

3. Companies competing in maturing industries.

4. Companies competing in stagnant or declining industries.

5. Companies competing in turbulent, high-velocity markets.

6. Companies competing in fragmented industries.

7. Companies striving to sustain rapid growth.

8. Companies in industry leadership positions.

9. Companies in runner-up positions.

10. Companies in competitively weak positions or plagued by crisis conditions.

We selected these situations to shed still more light on the factors that managers need to consider in tailoring a company's strategy. When you finish this chapter, you will have a stronger grasp of the factors that managers have to weigh in choosing a strategy and what the pros and cons are for some of the heretofore unexplored strategic options that are open to a company.

STRATEGIES FOR COMPETING IN EMERGING INDUSTRIES

An emerging industry is one in the formative stage. Examples include Voice over Internet Protocol (VoIP) telephone communications, high-definition TV, assisted living for the elderly, online education, organic food products, e-book publishing, and electronic banking. Many companies striving to establish a strong foothold in an emerging industry are start-up enterprises busily engaged in perfecting technology, gearing up operations, and trying to broaden distribution and gain buyer acceptance. Important product design issues or technological problems may still have to be worked out. The business models and strategies of companies in an emerging industry are unproved—they may look promising but may or may not ever result in attractive profitability.

The Unique Characteristics of an Emerging Industry

Competing in emerging industries presents managers with some unique strategy-making challenges:[1]

- Because the market is in its infancy, there's usually much speculation about how it will function, how fast it will grow, and how big it will get. The little historical information available is virtually useless in making sales and profit projections. There's lots of guesswork about how rapidly buyers will be attracted and how much they will be willing to pay. For example, there is much uncertainty about how many users of traditional telephone service will be inclined to switch over to VoIP telephone technology and how rapidly any such switchovers will occur.

- In many cases, much of the technological know-how underlying the products of emerging industries is proprietary and closely guarded, having been developed in-house by pioneering firms. In such cases, patents and unique technical expertise are key factors in securing competitive advantage. In other cases, numerous companies have access to the requisite technology and may be racing to perfect it, often in collaboration with others. In still other instances, there can be competing technological approaches, with much uncertainty over whether multiple technologies will end up competing alongside one another or whether one approach will ultimately win out because of lower costs or better performance—such a battle is currently under way in the emerging market for gasoline-electric hybrid engines (where demand is mushrooming because of greater fuel efficiency without a loss of power and acceleration). Toyota has pioneered one design; an alliance among General Motors, DaimlerChrysler, and BMW is pursuing another design; a Volkswagen-Porsche alliance is looking at a third technological approach; and Ford and Honda have their own slightly different hybrid engine designs.

- Just as there may be uncertainties surrounding an emerging industry's technology, there may also be no consensus regarding which product attributes will prove decisive in winning buyer favor. Rivalry therefore centers on each firm's efforts to get the market to ratify its own strategic approach to technology, product design, marketing, and distribution. Such rivalry can result in wide differences in product quality and performance from brand to brand.

- Since in an emerging industry all buyers are first-time users, the marketing task is to induce initial purchase and to overcome customer concerns about product features, performance reliability, and conflicting claims of rival firms.

- Many potential buyers expect first-generation products to be rapidly improved, so they delay purchase until technology and product design mature and second- or third-generation products appear on the market.

- Entry barriers tend to be relatively low, even for entrepreneurial start-up companies. Large, well-known, opportunity-seeking companies with ample resources and competitive capabilities are likely to enter if the industry has promise for explosive growth or if its emergence threatens their present business. For instance, many traditional local telephone companies, seeing the potent threat of wireless communications technology and VoIP, have opted to enter the mobile communications business and begin offering landline customers a VoIP option.

- Strong experience/learning curve effects may be present, allowing significant price reductions as volume builds and costs fall.

- Sometimes firms have trouble securing ample supplies of raw materials and components (until suppliers gear up to meet the industry's needs).

- Undercapitalized companies, finding themselves short of funds to support needed R&D and get through several lean years until the product catches on, end up merging with competitors or being acquired by financially strong outsiders looking to invest in a growth market.

Strategy Options for Emerging Industries

The lack of established rules of the game in an emerging industry gives industry participants considerable freedom to experiment with a variety of different strategic approaches. Competitive strategies keyed either to low cost or differentiation are usually viable. Focusing makes good sense when resources and capabilities are limited and the industry has too many technological frontiers or too many buyer segments to pursue at once. Broad or focused differentiation strategies keyed to technological or product superiority typically offer the best chance for early competitive advantage.

Core Concept
Companies in an emerging industry have wide latitude in experimenting with different strategic approaches.

In addition to choosing a competitive strategy, companies in an emerging industry usually have to fashion a strategy containing one or more of the following actions:[2]

1. Push to perfect the technology, improve product quality, and develop additional attractive performance features. Out-innovating the competition is often one of the best avenues to industry leadership.

2. Consider merging with or acquiring another firm to gain added expertise and pool resource strengths.

3. As technological uncertainty clears and a dominant technology emerges, try to capture any first-mover advantages by adopting it quickly. However, while there's merit in trying to be the industry standard-bearer on technology and to pioneer the dominant product design, firms have to beware of betting too heavily on their own preferred technological approach or product design—especially when there are many competing technologies, R&D is costly, and technological developments can quickly move in surprising new directions.

4. Acquire or form alliances with companies that have related or complementary technological expertise as a means of helping outcompete rivals on the basis of technological superiority.

5. Pursue new customer groups, new user applications, and entry into new geographical areas (perhaps using strategic partnerships or joint ventures if financial resources are constrained).

6. Make it easy and cheap for first-time buyers to try the industry's first-generation product.

7. As the product becomes familiar to a wide portion of the market, shift the advertising emphasis from creating product awareness to increasing frequency of use and building brand loyalty.

8. Use price cuts to attract the next layer of price-sensitive buyers into the market.

9. Form strategic alliances with key suppliers whenever effective supply chain management provides important access to specialized skills, technological capabilities, and critical materials or components.

Young companies in emerging industries face four strategic hurdles: (1) raising the capital to finance initial operations until sales and revenues take off, profits appear, and cash flows turn positive; (2) developing a strategy to ride the wave of industry growth(what market segments and competitive advantages to go after?); (3) managing the rapid expansion of facilities and sales in a manner that positions them to contend for industry leadership; and (4) defending against competitors trying to horn in on their success.[3] Up-and-coming companies can help their cause by selecting knowledgeable members for their boards of directors and by hiring entrepreneurial managers with experience in guiding young businesses through the start-up and takeoff stages. *A firm that develops solid resource capabilities, an appealing business model, and a good strategy has a golden opportunity to shape the rules and establish itself as the recognized industry front-runner.*

But strategic efforts to win the early race for growth and market share leadership in an emerging industry have to be balanced against the longer-range need to build a durable competitive edge and a defendable market position.[4] The initial front-runners in a fast-growing emerging industry that shows signs of good profitability will almost certainly have to defend their positions against ambitious challengers striving to overtake the current market leaders. Well-financed outsiders can be counted on to enter with aggressive offensive strategies once industry sales take off, the perceived risk of investing in the industry lessens, and the success of current industry members becomes apparent. Sometimes a rush of new entrants, attracted by the growth and profit potential, overcrowds the market and forces industry consolidation to a smaller number of players. Resource-rich latecomers, aspiring to industry leadership, may become major players by acquiring and merging the operations of weaker competitors and then using their own perhaps considerable brand name recognition to draw customers and build market share. Hence, the strategies of the early leaders must be aimed at competing for the long haul and making a point of developing the resources, capabilities, and market recognition needed to sustain early successes and stave off competition from capable, ambitious newcomers.

STRATEGIES FOR COMPETING IN RAPIDLY GROWING MARKETS

Companies that have the good fortune to be in an industry growing at double-digit rates have a golden opportunity to achieve double-digit revenues and profit growth.

In a fast-growing market, a company needs a strategy predicated on growing faster than the market average, so that it can boost its market share and improve its competitive standing vis-à-vis rivals.

If market demand is expanding 20 percent annually, a company can grow 20 percent annually simply by doing little more than contentedly riding the tide of market growth—it has to simply be aggressive enough to secure enough new customers to realize a 20 percent gain in sales, not a particularly impressive strategic feat. What is more interesting, however, is to craft a strategy that enables sales to grow at 25 or 30 percent when the overall market is growing by 20 percent, such that the company's market share and competitive position improve relative to rivals, on average. Should a company's strategy only deliver sales growth of 12 percent in a market growing at

20 percent, then it is actually losing ground in the marketplace—a condition that signals a weak strategy and an unappealing product offering. The point here is that, in a rapidly growing market, a company must aim its strategy at producing gains in revenue that exceed the market average; otherwise, the best it can hope for is to maintain its market standing (if it is able to boost sales at a rate equal to the market average) and its market standing may indeed erode if its sales rise by less than the market average.

To be able to grow at a pace exceeding the market average, a company generally must have a strategy that incorporates one or more of the following elements:

- *Driving down costs per unit so as to enable price reductions that attract droves of new customers.* Charging a lower price always has strong appeal in markets where customers are price-sensitive, and lower prices can help push up buyers demand by drawing new customers into the marketplace. But since rivals can lower their prices also, a company must really be able to drive its unit costs down *faster than rivals*, such that it can use its low-cost advantage to underprice rivals. The makers of liquid crystal display (LCD) and high-definition TVs are aggressively pursuing cost reduction to bring the prices of their TV sets down under $1,000 and thus make their products more affordable to more consumers.

- *Pursuing rapid product innovation, both to set a company's product offering apart from rivals and to incorporate attributes that appeal to growing numbers of customers.* Differentiation strategies, when keyed to product attributes that draw in large numbers of new customers, help bolster a company's reputation for product superiority and lay the foundation for sales gains in excess of the overall rate of market growth. If the market is one where technology is advancing rapidly and product life cycles are short, then it becomes especially important to be first-to-market with next-generation products. But product innovation strategies require competencies in R&D and new product development and design, plus organizational agility in getting new and improved products to market quickly. At the same time they are pursuing cost reductions, the makers of LCD and high-definition TVs are pursuing all sorts of product improvements to enhance product quality and performance and boost screen sizes, so as to match or beat the picture quality and reliability of conventional TVs (with old-fashioned cathode-ray tubes) and drive up sales at an even faster clip.

- *Gaining access to additional distribution channels and sales outlets.* Pursuing wider distribution access so as to reach more potential buyers is a particularly good strategic approach for realizing above-average sales gains. But usually this requires a company to be a first-mover in positioning itself in new distribution channels and forcing rivals into playing catch-up.

- *Expanding the company's geographic coverage.* Expanding into areas, either domestic or foreign, where the company does not have a market presence can also be an effective way to reach more potential buyers and pave the way for gains in sales that outpace the overall market average.

- *Expanding the product line to add models/styles that appeal to a wider range of buyers.* Offering buyers a wider selection can be an effective way to draw new customers in numbers sufficient to realize above-average sales gains. Makers of MP3 players and cell phones are adding new models to stimulate buyer demand; Starbucks is adding new drinks and other menu selections to build store traffic; and marketers of VoIP technology are rapidly introducing a wider variety of plans to broaden their appeal to customers with different calling habits and needs.

STRATEGIES FOR COMPETING IN MATURING INDUSTRIES

A *maturing industry* is one that is moving from rapid growth to significantly slower growth. An industry is said to be *mature* when nearly all potential buyers are already users of the industry's products and growth in market demand closely parallels that of the population and the economy as a whole. In a mature market, demand consists mainly of replacement sales to existing users, with growth hinging on the industry's abilities to attract the few remaining new buyers and to convince existing buyers to up their usage. Consumer goods industries that are mature typically have a growth rate under 5 percent—roughly equal to the growth of the customer base or economy as a whole.

How Slowing Growth Alters Market Conditions

An industry's transition to maturity does not begin on an easily predicted schedule. Industry maturity can be forestalled by the emergence of new technological advances, product innovations, or other driving forces that keep rejuvenating market demand. Nonetheless, when growth rates do slacken, the onset of market maturity usually produces fundamental changes in the industry's competitive environment:[5]

1. *Slowing growth in buyer demand generates more head-to-head competition for market share.* Firms that want to continue on a rapid-growth track start looking for ways to take customers away from competitors. Outbreaks of price cutting, increased advertising, and other aggressive tactics to gain market share are common.

2. *Buyers become more sophisticated, often driving a harder bargain on repeat purchases.* Since buyers have experience with the product and are familiar with competing brands, they are better able to evaluate different brands and can use their knowledge to negotiate a better deal with sellers.

3. *Competition often produces a greater emphasis on cost and service.* As sellers all begin to offer the product attributes buyers prefer, buyer choices increasingly depend on which seller offers the best combination of price and service.

4. *Firms have a "topping-out" problem in adding new facilities.* Reduced rates of industry growth mean slowdowns in capacity expansion for manufacturers—adding too much plant capacity at a time when growth is slowing can create oversupply conditions that adversely affect manufacturers' profits well into the future. Likewise, retail chains that specialize in the industry's product have to cut back on the number of new stores being opened to keep from saturating localities with too many stores.

5. *Product innovation and new end-use applications are harder to come by.* Producers find it increasingly difficult to create new product features, find further uses for the product, and sustain buyer excitement.

6. *International competition increases.* Growth-minded domestic firms start to seek out sales opportunities in foreign markets. Some companies, looking for ways to cut costs, relocate plants to countries with lower wage rates. Greater product standardization and diffusion of technological know-how reduce entry barriers and make it possible for enterprising foreign companies to become serious market contenders in more countries. Industry leadership passes to companies that succeed in building strong competitive positions in most of the world's major geographic markets and in winning the biggest global market shares.

7. *Industry profitability falls temporarily or permanently.* Slower growth, increased competition, more sophisticated buyers, and occasional periods of overcapacity put pressure on industry profit margins. Weaker, less-efficient firms are usually the hardest hit.

8. *Stiffening competition induces a number of mergers and acquisitions among former competitors, driving industry consolidation to a smaller number of larger players.* Inefficient firms and firms with weak competitive strategies can achieve respectable results in a fast-growing industry with booming sales. But the intensifying competition that accompanies industry maturity exposes competitive weakness and throws second- and third-tier competitors into a survival-of-the-fittest contest.

Strategies that Fit Conditions in Maturing Industries

As the new competitive character of industry maturity begins to hit full force, any of several strategic moves can strengthen a firm's competitive position: pruning the product line, improving value chain efficiency, trimming costs, increasing sales to present customers, acquiring rival firms, expanding internationally, and strengthening capabilities.[6]

Pruning Marginal Products and Models A wide selection of models, features, and product options sometimes has competitive value during the growth stage, when buyers' needs are still evolving. But such variety can become too costly as price competition stiffens and profit margins are squeezed. Maintaining many product versions works against achieving design, parts inventory, and production economies at the manufacturing levels and can increase inventory stocking costs for distributors and retailers. In addition, the prices of slow-selling versions may not cover their true costs. Pruning marginal products from the line opens the door for cost savings and permits more concentration on items whose margins are highest and/or where a firm has a competitive advantage. General Motors has been cutting slow-selling models and brands from its lineup of offerings—it has eliminated the entire Oldsmobile division and is said to be looking at whether it can eliminate its Saab lineup. Textbook publishers are discontinuing publication of those books that sell only a few thousand copies annually (where profits are marginal at best) and instead focusing their resources on texts that generate sales of at least 5,000 copies per edition.

Improving Value Chain Efficiency Efforts to reinvent the industry value chain can have a fourfold payoff: lower costs, better product or service quality, greater capability to turn out multiple or customized product versions, and shorter design-to-market cycles. Manufacturers can mechanize high-cost activities, redesign production lines to improve labor efficiency, build flexibility into the assembly process so that customized product versions can be easily produced, and increase use of advanced technology (robotics, computerized controls, and automated assembly). Suppliers of parts and components, manufacturers, and distributors can collaboratively deploy online systems and product coding techniques to streamline activities and achieve cost savings all along the value chain—from supplier-related activities all the way through distribution, retailing, and customer service.

Trimming Costs   Stiffening price competition gives firms extra incentive to drive down unit costs. Company cost-reduction initiatives can cover a broad front. Some of the most frequently pursued options are pushing suppliers for better prices, implementing tighter supply chain management practices, cutting low-value activities out of the value chain, developing more economical product designs, reengineering internal processes using e-commerce technology, and shifting to more economical distribution arrangements.

Increasing Sales to Present Customers   In a mature market, growing by taking customers away from rivals may not be as appealing as expanding sales to existing customers. Strategies to increase purchases by existing customers can involve adding more sales promotions, providing complementary items and ancillary services, and finding more ways for customers to use the product. Convenience stores, for example, have boosted average sales per customer by adding video rentals, automated teller machines, gasoline pumps, and deli counters.

Acquiring Rival Firms at Bargain Prices   Sometimes a firm can acquire the facilities and assets of struggling rivals quite cheaply. Bargain-priced acquisitions can help create a low-cost position if they also present opportunities for greater operating efficiency. In addition, an acquired firm's customer base can provide expanded market coverage and opportunities for greater scale economies. The most desirable acquisitions are those that will significantly enhance the acquiring firm's competitive strength.

Expanding Internationally   As its domestic market matures, a firm may seek to enter foreign markets where attractive growth potential still exists and competitive pressures are not so strong. Many multinational companies are expanding into such emerging markets as China, India, Brazil, Argentina, and the Philippines, where the long-term growth prospects are quite attractive. Strategies to expand internationally also make sense when a domestic firm's skills, reputation, and product are readily transferable to foreign markets. For example, even though the U.S. market for soft drinks is mature, Coca-Cola has remained a growth company by upping its efforts to penetrate emerging markets where soft-drink sales are expanding rapidly.

Building New or More Flexible Capabilities   The stiffening pressures of competition in a maturing or already mature market can often be combated by strengthening the company's resource base and competitive capabilities. This can mean adding new competencies or capabilities, deepening existing competencies to make them harder to imitate, or striving to make core competencies more adaptable to changing customer requirements and expectations. Microsoft has responded to challenges by such competitors as Google and Linux by expanding its competencies in search engine software and revamping its entire approach to programming next-generation operating systems. Chevron has developed a best-practices discovery team and a best-practices resource map to enhance the speed and effectiveness with which it is able to transfer efficiency improvements from one oil refinery to another.

Strategic Pitfalls in Maturing Industries

Perhaps the biggest strategic mistake a company can make as an industry matures is steering a middle course between low cost, differentiation, and focusing—blending efforts to achieve low cost with efforts to incorporate differentiating features and efforts to focus on a limited target market. Such strategic compromises typically leave the firm *stuck in the middle* with a fuzzy strategy, too little commitment to winning a competitive advantage, an average image with buyers, and little chance of springing into the ranks of the industry leaders.

Other strategic pitfalls include being slow to mount a defense against stiffening competitive pressures, concentrating more on protecting short-term profitability than on building or maintaining long-term competitive position, waiting too long to respond to price cutting by rivals, overexpanding in the face of slowing growth, overspending on advertising and sales promotion efforts in a losing effort to combat the growth slow-down, and failing to pursue cost reduction soon enough or aggressively enough.

STRATEGIES FOR COMPETING IN STAGNANT OR DECLINING INDUSTRIES

Many firms operate in industries where demand is growing more slowly than the economy-wide average or is even declining. The demand for an industry's product can decline for any of several reasons: (1) advancing technology gives rise to better-performing substitute products (slim LCD monitors displace bulky CRT monitors; DVD players replace VCRs; wrinkle-free fabrics replace the need for laundry/dry-cleaning services) or lower costs (cheaper synthetics replace expensive leather); (2) the customer group shrinks (baby foods are in less demand when birthrates fall); (3) changing lifestyles and buyer tastes (cigarette smoking and wearing dress hats go out of vogue); (4) the rising costs of complementary products (higher gasoline prices drive down purchases of gas-guzzling vehicles).[7] The most attractive declining industries are those in which sales are eroding only slowly, there are pockets of stable or even growing demand, and some market niches present good profit opportunities. But in some stagnant or declining industries, decaying buyer demand precipitates a desperate competitive battle among industry members for the available business, replete with price discounting, costly sales promotions, growing amounts of idle plant capacity, and fast-eroding profit margins. It matters greatly whether buyer demand falls gradually or sharply and whether competition proves to be fierce or moderate.

Businesses competing in stagnant or declining industries have to make a fundamental strategic choice—whether to remain committed to the industry for the long term despite the industry's dim prospects or whether to pursue an end-game strategy to withdraw gradually or quickly from the market. Deciding to stick with the industry despite eroding market demand can have considerable merit. Stagnant demand by itself is not enough to make an

> It is erroneous to assume that companies in a declining industry are doomed to having declining revenues and profits.

industry unattractive. Market demand may be decaying slowly. Some segments of the market may still present good profit opportunities. Cash flows from operations may still remain strongly positive. Strong competitors may well be able to grow and boost profits by taking market share from weaker competitors.[8] Furthermore, the acquisition or exit of weaker firms creates opportunities for the remaining companies to capture greater market share. On the one hand, striving to become the market leader and be one of the few remaining companies in a declining industry can lead to above-average profitability even though overall market demand is stagnant or eroding. On the other hand, if the market environment of a declining industry is characterized by bitter warfare for customers and lots of overcapacity, such that companies are plagued with heavy operating losses, then an early exit makes much more strategic sense.

If a company decides to stick with a declining industry—because top management is encouraged by the remaining opportunities or sees merit in striving for market share leadership (or even just being one of the few remaining companies in the industry), then its three best strategic alternatives are usually the following:[9]

1. *Pursue a focused strategy aimed at the fastest-growing or slowest-decaying market segments within the industry.* Stagnant or declining markets, like other markets, are composed of numerous segments or niches. Frequently, one or more of these segments is growing rapidly (or at least decaying much more slowly), despite stagnation in the industry as a whole. An astute competitor who zeros in on fast-growing segments and does a first-rate job of meeting the needs of buyers comprising these segments can often escape stagnating sales and profits and even gain decided competitive advantage. For instance, both Ben & Jerry's and Häagen-Dazs have achieved success by focusing on the growing luxury or superpremium segment of the otherwise stagnant market for ice cream; revenue growth and profit margins are substantially higher for high-end ice creams sold in supermarkets and in scoop shops than is the case in other segments of the ice cream market. Companies that focus on the one or two most attractive market segments in a declining business may well decide to ignore the other segments altogether—withdrawing from them entirely or at least gradually or rapidly disinvesting in them. But the key is to *move aggressively* to establish a strong position in the most attractive parts of the stagnant or declining industry.

2. *Stress differentiation based on quality improvement and product innovation.* Either enhanced quality or innovation can rejuvenate demand by creating important new growth segments or inducing buyers to trade up. Successful product innovation opens up an avenue for competing that bypasses meeting or beating rivals' prices. Differentiation based on successful innovation has the additional advantage of being difficult and expensive for rival firms to imitate. New Covent Garden Soup has met with success by introducing packaged fresh soups for sale in major supermarkets, where the typical soup offerings are canned or dry mixes. Procter & Gamble has rejuvenated sales of its toothbrushes with its new line of Crest battery-powered spin toothbrushes, and it has revitalized interest in tooth care products with a series of product innovations related to teeth whitening. Bread makers are fighting declining sales of white breads that use bleached flour by introducing all kinds of whole-grain breads (which have far more nutritional value).

3. *Strive to drive costs down and become the industry's low-cost leader.* Companies in stagnant industries can improve profit margins and return on investment by pursuing innovative cost reduction year after year. Potential cost-saving actions include (*a*) cutting marginally beneficial activities out of the value chain; (*b*) outsourcing functions and activities that can be performed more cheaply by outsiders; (*c*) redesigning internal business processes to exploit cost-reducing e-commerce technologies; (*d*) consolidating underutilized production facilities; (*e*) adding more distribution channels to ensure the unit volume needed for low-cost production; (*f*) closing low-volume, high-cost retail outlets; and (*g*) pruning marginal products from the firm's offerings. Japan-based Asahi Glass (a low-cost producer of flat glass), PotashCorp and IMC Global (two low-cost leaders in potash production), Alcan Aluminum, Nucor Steel, and Safety Components International (a low-cost producer of air bags for motor vehicles) have all been successful in driving costs down in competitively tough and largely stagnant industry environments.

These three strategic themes are not mutually exclusive.[10] Introducing innovative versions of a product can create a fast-growing market segment. Similarly, relentless pursuit of greater operating efficiencies permits price reductions that create price-conscious growth segments. Note that all three themes are spinoffs of the five generic competitive strategies, adjusted to fit the circumstances of a tough industry environment.

End-Game Strategies for Declining Industries

An *end-game strategy* can take either of two paths: (1) a *slow-exit strategy* that involves a gradual phasing down of operations coupled with an objective of getting the most cash flow from the business even if it means sacrificing market position or profitability and (2) a *fast-exit* or *sell-out-quickly strategy* to disengage from the industry during the early stages of the decline and recover as much of the company's investment as possible for deployment elsewhere.[11]

A Slow-Exit Strategy With a slow-exit strategy, *the key objective is to generate the greatest possible harvest of cash from the business for as long as possible.* Management either eliminates or severely curtails new investment in the business. Capital expenditures for new equipment are put on hold or given low financial priority (unless replacement needs are unusually urgent); instead, efforts are made to stretch the life of existing equipment and make do with present facilities as long as possible. Old plants with high costs may be retired from service. The operating budget is chopped to a rock-bottom level. Promotional expenses may be cut gradually, quality reduced in not-so-visible ways, nonessential customer services curtailed, and maintenance of facilities held to a bare minimum. The resulting increases in cash flow (and perhaps even bottom-line profitability and return on investment) compensate for whatever declines in sales might be experienced. Withering buyer demand is tolerable if sizable amounts of cash can be reaped in the interim. If and when cash flows dwindle to meager levels as sales volumes decay, the business can be sold or, if no buyer can be found, closed down.

A Fast-Exit Strategy The challenge of a sell-out-quickly strategy is to find a buyer willing to pay an agreeable price for the company's business assets. Buyers may be scarce since there's a tendency for investors to shy away from purchasing a stagnant or dying business. And even if willing buyers appear, they will be in a strong bargaining position once it's clear that the industry's prospects are permanently waning. How much prospective buyers will pay is usually a function of how rapidly they expect the industry to decline, whether they see opportunities to rejuvenate demand (at least temporarily), whether they believe that costs can be cut enough to still produce attractive profit margins or cash flows, whether there are pockets of stable demand where buyers are not especially price sensitive, and whether they believe that fading market demand will weaken competition (which could enhance profitability) or trigger strong competition for the remaining business (which could put pressure on profit margins). Thus, the expectations of prospective buyers will tend to drive the price they are willing to pay for the business assets of a company wanting to sell out quickly.

STRATEGIES FOR COMPETING IN TURBULENT, HIGH-VELOCITY MARKETS

Many companies operate in industries characterized by rapid technological change, short product life cycles, the entry of important new rivals, lots of competitive maneuvering by rivals, and fast-evolving customer requirements and expectations—all occurring in a manner that creates swirling market conditions. Since news of this or that important competitive development arrives daily, it is an imposing task just to monitor and assess developing events. High-velocity change is plainly the prevailing condition in computer/server hardware and software, video games, networking, wireless tele-communications, medical equipment, biotechnology, prescription drugs, and online retailing.

Ways to Cope with Rapid Change

The central strategy-making challenge in a turbulent market environment is managing change.[12] As illustrated in Figure 8.1, a company can assume any of three strategic postures in dealing with high-velocity change:[13]

- *It can react to change.* The company can respond to a rival's new product with a better product. It can counter an unexpected shift in buyer tastes and buyer demand by redesigning or repackaging its product, or shifting its advertising emphasis to different product attributes. Reacting is a defensive strategy and is therefore unlikely to create fresh opportunity, but it is nonetheless a necessary component in a company's arsenal of options.

- *It can anticipate change.* The company can make plans for dealing with the expected changes and follow its plans as changes occur (fine-tuning them as may be needed). Anticipation entails looking ahead to analyze what is likely to occur and then preparing and positioning for that future. It entails studying buyer behavior, buyer needs, and buyer expectations to get insight into how the market will evolve, then lining up the necessary production and distribution capabilities ahead of time. Like reacting to change, anticipating change is still fundamentally defensive in that forces outside the enterprise are in the driver's seat. Anticipation, however, can open up new opportunities and thus is a better way to manage change than just pure reaction.

- *It can lead change.* Leading change entails initiating the market and competitive forces that others must respond to—it is an offensive strategy aimed at putting a company in the driver's seat. Leading change means being first to market with an important new product or service. It means being the technological leader, rushing next-generation products to market ahead of rivals, and having products whose features and attributes shape customer preferences and expectations. It means proactively seeking to shape the rules of the game.

A sound way to deal with turbulent market conditions is to try to lead change with proactive strategic moves while at the same time trying to anticipate and prepare for upcoming changes and being quick to react to unexpected developments.

As a practical matter, a company's approach to managing change should, ideally, incorporate all three postures (though not in the same proportion). The best-performing companies in high-velocity markets consistently seek to lead change with proactive strategies that often entail the flexibility to pursue any of several strategic options, depending on how the market actually evolves. Even so, an environment of relentless change makes it incumbent on any company to anticipate and prepare for the future and to react quickly to unpredictable or uncontrollable new developments.

Strategy Options for Fast-Changing Markets

Competitive success in fast-changing markets tends to hinge on a company's ability to improvise, experiment, adapt, reinvent, and regenerate as market and competitive conditions shift rapidly and sometimes unpredictably.[14] It has to constantly reshape its

Figure 8.1   **Meeting the Challenge of High-Velocity Change**

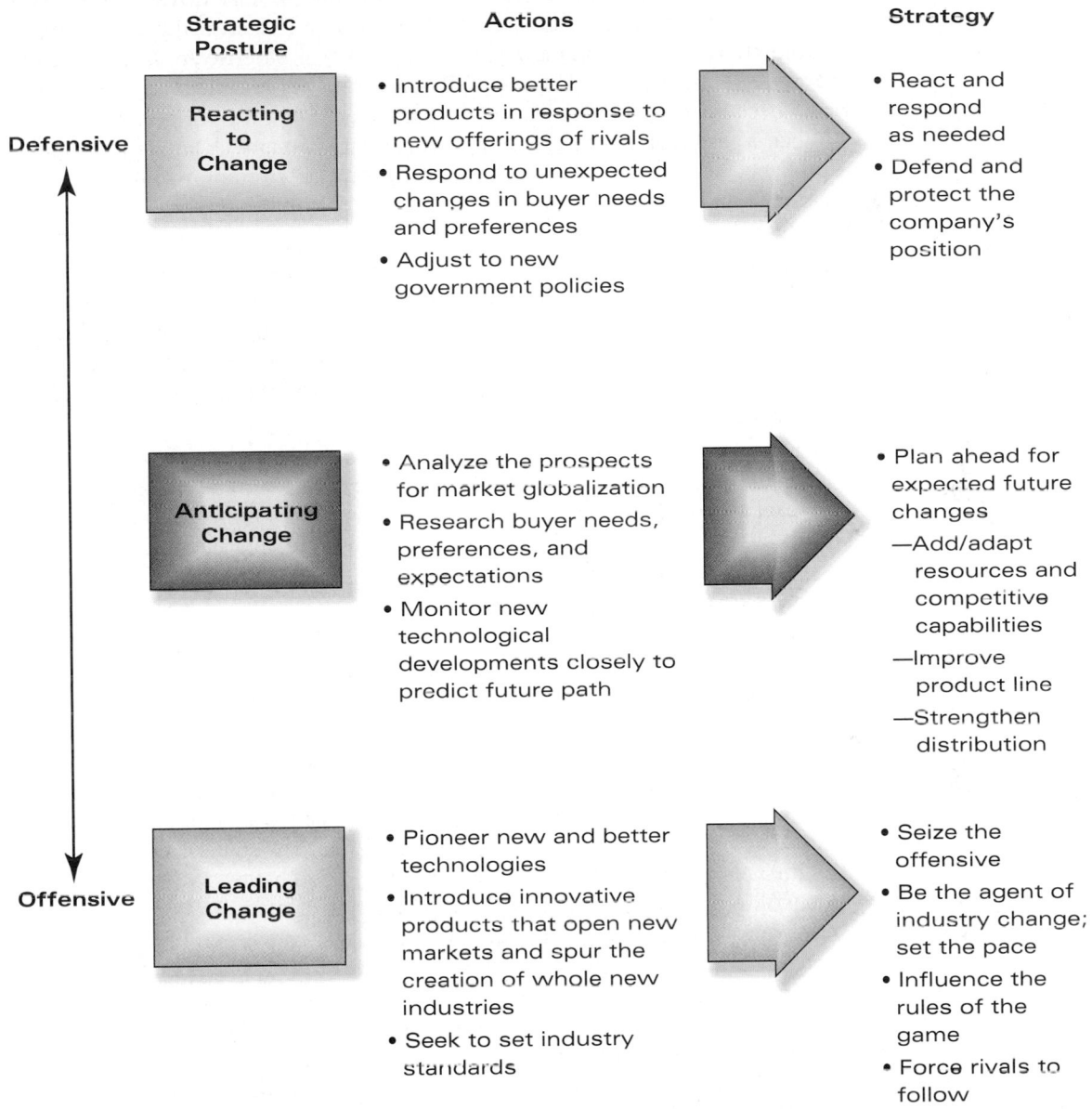

	Strategic Posture	Actions	Strategy

Defensive

Reacting to Change

- Introduce better products in response to new offerings of rivals
- Respond to unexpected changes in buyer needs and preferences
- Adjust to new government policies

- React and respond as needed
- Defend and protect the company's position

Anticipating Change

- Analyze the prospects for market globalization
- Research buyer needs, preferences, and expectations
- Monitor new technological developments closely to predict future path

- Plan ahead for expected future changes
  —Add/adapt resources and competitive capabilities
  —Improve product line
  —Strengthen distribution

Offensive

Leading Change

- Pioneer new and better technologies
- Introduce innovative products that open new markets and spur the creation of whole new industries
- Seek to set industry standards

- Seize the offensive
- Be the agent of industry change; set the pace
- Influence the rules of the game
- Force rivals to follow

Source: Adapted from Shona L. Brown and Kathleen M. Eisenhardt, *Competing on the Edge: Strategy as Structured Chaos* (Boston, MA: Harvard Business School Press, 1998) p. 5.

strategy and its basis for competitive advantage. While the process of altering offensive and defensive moves every few months or weeks to keep the overall strategy closely matched to changing conditions is inefficient, the alternative—a fast-obsolescing strategy—is worse. The following five strategic moves seem to offer the best payoffs:

1. *Invest aggressively in R&D to stay on the leading edge of technological know-how.* Translating technological advances into innovative new products (and remaining close on the heels of whatever advances and features are pioneered by rivals) is a necessity in industries where technology is the primary driver of change. But it is often desirable to focus the R&D effort on a few critical areas, not only to avoid stretching the company's resources too thin but also to deepen the firm's expertise, master the technology, fully capture experience/learning curve effects, and become the dominant leader in a particular technology or product category.[15] When a fast-evolving market environment entails many technological areas and product categories, competitors have little choice but to employ some type of focus strategy and concentrate on being the leader in a particular product/technology category.

2. *Keep the company's products and services fresh and exciting enough to stand out in the midst of all the change that is taking place.* One of the risks of rapid change is that products and even companies can get lost in the shuffle. The marketing challenge here is to keep the firm's products and services in the limelight and, further, to keep them innovative and well matched to the changes that are occurring in the marketplace.

3. *Develop quick-response capability.* Because no company can predict all of the changes that will occur, it is crucial to have the organizational capability to be able to react quickly, improvising if necessary. This means shifting resources internally, adapting existing competencies and capabilities, creating new competencies and capabilities, and not falling far behind rivals. Companies that are habitual late-movers are destined to be industry also-rans.

4. *Rely on strategic partnerships with outside suppliers and with companies making tie-in products.* In many high-velocity industries, technology is branching off to create so many new technological paths and product categories that no company has the resources and competencies to pursue them all. Specialization (to promote the necessary technical depth) and focus (to preserve organizational agility and leverage the firm's expertise) are desirable strategies. Companies build their competitive position not just by strengthening their own internal resource base but also by partnering with those suppliers making state-of-the-art parts and components and by collaborating closely with both the developers of related technologies and the makers of tie-in products. For example, personal computer companies like Gateway, Dell, Compaq, and Acer rely heavily on the developers and manufacturers of chips, monitors, hard drives, DVD players, and software for innovative advances in PCs. None of the PC makers have done much in the way of integrating backward into parts and components because they have learned that the most effective way to provide PC users with a state-of-the-art product is to outsource the latest, most advanced components from technologically sophisticated suppliers who make it their business to stay on the cutting edge of their specialization and who can achieve economies of scale by mass-producing components for many PC assemblers. An outsourcing strategy also allows a company the flexibility to replace suppliers that fall behind on technology or product features or that cease to be competitive on price. The managerial challenge here is to strike a good balance between building a rich internal resource base that, on the one hand, keeps the firm from being at the mercy of its suppliers and allies and, on the other hand, maintains organizational agility by relying on the resources and expertise of capable (and perhaps best-in-world) outsiders.

5. *Initiate fresh actions every few months, not just when a competitive response is needed.* In some sense, change is partly triggered by the passage of time rather

than solely by the occurrence of events. A company can be proactive by making time-paced moves—introducing a new or improved product every four months, rather than when the market tapers off or a rival introduces a next-generation model.[16] Similarly, a company can expand into a new geographic market every six months rather than waiting for a new market opportunity to present itself; it can also refresh existing brands every two years rather than waiting until their popularity wanes. The keys to successfully using time pacing as a strategic weapon are choosing intervals that make sense internally and externally, establishing an internal organizational rhythm for change, and choreographing the transitions. 3M Corporation has long pursued an objective of having 25 percent of its revenues come from products less than four years old, a force that established the rhythm of change and created a relentless push for new products. Recently, the firm's CEO upped the tempo of change at 3M by increasing the goal from 25 to 30 percent.

Cutting-edge know-how and first-to-market capabilities are very valuable competitive assets in fast-evolving markets. Moreover, action-packed competition demands that a company have quick reaction times and flexible, adaptable resources—organizational agility is a huge competitive asset. Even so, companies will make mistakes and take some actions that do not work out well. When a company's strategy doesn't seem to be working well, it has to quickly regroup—probing, experimenting, improvising, and trying again and again until it finds something that strikes the right chord with buyers and that puts it in sync with market and competitive realities.

STRATEGIES FOR COMPETING IN FRAGMENTED INDUSTRIES

A number of industries are populated by hundreds, even thousands, of small and medium-sized companies, many privately held and none with a substantial share of total industry sales.[17] The standout competitive feature of a fragmented industry is the absence of market leaders with king-sized market shares or widespread buyer recognition. Examples of fragmented industries include book publishing, landscaping and plant nurseries, real estate development, convenience stores, banking, health and medical care, mail order catalog sales, computer software development, custom printing, kitchen cabinets, trucking, auto repair, restaurants and fast food, public accounting, apparel manufacture and apparel retailing, paperboard boxes, hotels and motels, and furniture.

Reasons for Supply-Side Fragmentation

Any of several reasons can account for why the supply side of an industry comprises hundreds or even thousands of companies:

- *The product or service is delivered at neighborhood locations so as to be conveniently accessible to local residents.* Retail and service businesses, for example, are inherently local—gas stations and car washes, pharmacies, dry-cleaning services, nursing homes, auto repair firms, furniture stores, flower shops, and lawn care enterprises. Whenever it takes thousands of locations to adequately serve the market, the way is opened for many enterprises to be engaged in providing products/services to local residents and businesses (and such enterprises can operate at just one location or at multiple locations).

- *Buyer preferences and requirements are so diverse that very large numbers of firms can easily coexist trying to accommodate differing buyer tastes, expectations, and pocketbooks.* This is true in the market for apparel, where there are thousands of apparel manufacturers making garments of various styles and price ranges. There's a host of different hotels and restaurants in places like New York City, London, Buenos Aires, Mexico City, and Tokyo. The software development industry is highly fragmented because there are so many types of software applications and because the needs and expectations of software users are so highly diverse—hence, there's ample market space for a software company to concentrate its attention on serving a particular market niche.

- *Low entry barriers allow small firms to enter quickly and cheaply.* Such tends to be the case in many areas of retailing, residential real estate, insurance sales, beauty shops, and the restaurant business.

- *An absence of scale economies permits small companies to compete on an equal cost footing with larger firms.* The markets for business forms, interior design, kitchen cabinets, and picture framing are fragmented because buyers require relatively small quantities of customized products; since demand for any particular product version is small, sales volumes are not adequate to support producing, distributing, or marketing on a scale that yields cost advantages to a large-scale firm. A locally owned pharmacy can be cost competitive with the pharmacy operations of large drugstore chains like Walgreen's or Rite Aid or CVS. Small trucking companies can be cost-competitive with companies that have huge truck fleets. A local pizzeria is not cost-disadvantaged in competing against such chains as Pizza Hut, Domino's, and Papa John's.

- *The scope of the geographic market for the industry's product or service is transitioning from national to global.* A broadening of geographic scope puts companies in more and more countries in the same competitive market arena (as in the apparel industry, where increasing numbers of garment makers across the world are shifting their production operations to low-wage countries and then shipping their goods to retailers in several countries).

- *The technologies embodied in the industry's value chain are exploding into so many new areas and along so many different paths that specialization is essential just to keep abreast in any one area of expertise.* Technology branching accounts for why the manufacture of electronic parts and components is fragmented and why there's fragmentation in prescription drug research.

- *The industry is young and crowded with aspiring contenders.* In most young industries, no firm has yet developed the resource base, competitive capabilities, and market recognition to command a significant market share (as in online e-tailing).

Competitive Conditions in a Fragmented Industry

Competitive rivalry in fragmented industries can vary from moderately strong to fierce. Low barriers tend to make entry of new competitors an ongoing threat. Competition from substitutes may or may not be a major factor. The relatively small size of companies in fragmented industries puts them in a relatively weak position to bargain with powerful suppliers and buyers, although sometimes they can become members of a cooperative formed for the purpose of using their combined leverage to negotiate better sales and purchase terms. In such an environment, the best a firm can expect is to cultivate a loyal customer base and grow a bit faster than the industry average.

Some fragmented industries consolidate over time as growth slows and the market matures. The stiffer competition that accompanies slower growth produces a shake-out of weak, inefficient firms and a greater concentration of larger, more visible sellers. Others remain atomistic because it is inherent in their businesses. And still others remain stuck in a fragmented state because existing firms lack the resources or ingenuity to employ a strategy powerful enough to drive industry consolidation.

Strategy Options for Competing in a Fragmented Industry

In fragmented industries, firms generally have the strategic freedom to pursue broad or narrow market targets and low-cost or differentiation-based competitive advantages. Many different strategic approaches can exist side by side (unless the industry's product is highly standardized or a commodity—like concrete blocks, sand and gravel, or paperboard boxes). Fragmented industry environments are usually ideal for focusing on a well-defined market niche—a particular geographic area or buyer group or product type. In an industry that is fragmented due to highly diverse buyer tastes or requirements, focusing usually offers more competitive advantage potential than trying to come up with a product offering that has broad market appeal.

Some of the most suitable strategy options for competing in a fragmented industry include:

- *Constructing and operating "formula" facilities*—This strategic approach is frequently employed in restaurant and retailing businesses operating at multiple locations. It involves constructing standardized outlets in favorable locations at minimum cost and then operating them cost-effectively. This is a favorite approach for locally owned fast-food enterprises and convenience stores that have multiple locations serving a geographically limited market area. Major fast-food chains like Yum! Brands—the parent of Pizza Hut, Taco Bell, KFC, Long John Silver's, and A&W restaurants—and big convenience store retailers like 7-Eleven have, of course, perfected the formula facilities strategy.

- *Becoming a low-cost operator*—When price competition is intense and profit margins are under constant pressure, companies can stress no-frills operations featuring low overhead, high-productivity/low-cost labor, lean capital budgets, and dedicated pursuit of total operating efficiency. Successful low-cost producers in a fragmented industry can play the price-discounting game and still earn profits above the industry average. Many e-tailers compete on the basis of bargain prices; so do budget motel chains like Econo Lodge, Super 8, and Days Inn.

- *Specializing by product type*—When a fragmented industry's products include a range of styles or services, a strategy to focus on one product or service category can be effective. Some firms in the furniture industry specialize in only one furniture type such as brass beds, rattan and wicker, lawn and garden, or Early American. In auto repair, companies specialize in transmission repair, body work, or speedy oil changes.

- *Specializing by customer type*—A firm can stake out a market niche in a fragmented industry by catering to those customers who are interested in low prices,

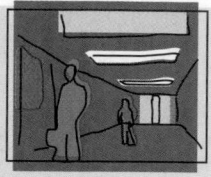

Illustration Capsule 8.1

Exertris's Focus Strategy in the Fragmented Exercise Equipment Industry

The exercise equipment industry is largely fragmented from a global perspective—there are hundreds of companies across the world making exercise and fitness products of one kind or another. The window of opportunity for employing a focus strategy is big. In 2001, three fitness enthusiasts in Great Britain came up with a novel way to make exercise more interesting. Their idea was to create an exercise bike equipped with a video game console, a flat-screen display, and an on-board PC that allowed users to play a video game while doing their workout.

After creating a prototype and forming a company called Exertris, the three fitness entrepreneurs approached a product design company for help in turning the prototype into a marketable product. The design company quickly determined that the task was not trivial and required significant additional product development. But the company was enthusiastic about the product and put up the capital to fund the venture as a minority partner. The partners set a goal of having six prototypes ready in time for a major leisure products trade show scheduled to be held in the United Kingdom in several months. The design company assumed responsibility for engineering the product, finding a contract manufacturer, and managing the supply chain; certain other specialty tasks were outsourced. The three cofounders concentrated on developing gaming software where the exerciser's pedaling performance had direct consequences for particular elements of the game; for example, the exerciser had to pedal harder to power a spaceship's weapon systems or move cards around in a game of Solitaire.

The Exertris bike won the "best new product" award at the trade show. It featured four games (Gems, Orbit, Solitaire, and Space Tripper), and new games and features could be added as they were released. Exercisers could play solo or competitively against other people, with the option of handicapping for multiplayer games. The recommended workout included an automatic warm-up and cool-down period. The bike had an armrest, a monitor, and a seat that optimized posture. The LCD display used the latest 3D graphics, and the on-board PC (positioned under the mounting step) used Microsoft Windows XP Embedded and was compatible with Polar heart rate monitors. Earphones were optional, and the game pad and menu control were sweat-proof and easy to clean.

Production by contract manufacturers started soon after the show. In the ensuing months, the Exertris bike was well received by gyms and fitness enthusiasts (for whom the addictive nature of video games broke the monotony and made exercise time fly by). The first interactive fitness arcade featuring 25 linked Exertris Interactive Bikes opened in Great Britain in April 2003. In 2005, the Exertris exercise bike was being marketed online in Great Britain at Amazon's Web site (www.amazon-leisure.co.uk) at a price of £675 (or about $1,150); it could also be purchased at Broadcast Vision Entertainment's online store. Exertris's strategy of focusing on this one niche product in exercise equipment was, however, producing unexpectedly weak results—sales were much slower than initially expected.

Sources: Information posted at www.betterproductdesign.com (accessed October 14, 2005), www.embedded-resources.com (accessed October 14, 2005), and www.broadcastvision.com (accessed December 31, 2005).

unique product attributes, customized features, carefree service, or other extras. A number of restaurants cater to take-out customers; others specialize in fine dining, and still others cater to the sports bar crowd. Bed-and-breakfast inns cater to a particular type of traveler/vacationer (and also focus on a very limited geographic area).

- *Focusing on a limited geographic area*—Even though a firm in a fragmented industry can't win a big share of total industrywide sales, it can still try to dominate a local or regional geographic area. Concentrating company efforts on a limited territory can produce greater operating efficiency, speed delivery and customer services, promote strong brand awareness, and permit saturation advertising, while avoiding the diseconomies of stretching operations out over a much wider area. Several locally owned banks, drugstores, and sporting goods retailers successfully operate multiple locations within a limited geographic area. Numerous local restaurant operators have pursued operating economies by opening anywhere from 4 to 10 restaurants (each with each its own distinctive theme and menu) scattered across a single metropolitan area like Atlanta or Denver or Houston.

Illustration Capsule 8.1 describes how a new start-up company in Great Britain has employed a product niche type of focus strategy in the fragmented exercise equipment industry.

STRATEGIES FOR SUSTAINING RAPID COMPANY GROWTH

Companies that strive to grow their revenues and earnings at double-digit rates year after year (or at rates exceeding the overall market average so that they are growing faster than rivals and gaining market share) generally have to craft *a portfolio of strategic initiatives* covering three horizons:[18]

- *Horizon 1: "Short-jump" strategic initiatives to fortify and extend the company's position in existing businesses*—Short-jump initiatives typically include adding new items to the company's present product line, expanding into new geographic areas where the company does not yet have a market presence, and launching offensives to take market share away from rivals. The objective is to capitalize fully on whatever growth potential exists in the company's present business arenas.

- *Horizon 2: "Medium-jump" strategic initiatives to leverage existing resources and capabilities by entering new businesses with promising growth potential*— Growth companies have to be alert for opportunities to jump into new businesses where there is promise of rapid growth and where their experience, intellectual capital, and technological know-how will prove valuable in gaining rapid market penetration. While Horizon 2 initiatives may take a back seat to Horizon 1 initiatives as long as there is plenty of untapped growth in the company's present businesses, they move to the front as the onset of market maturity dims the company's growth prospects in its present business(es).

- *Horizon 3: "Long-jump" strategic initiatives to plant the seeds for ventures in businesses that do not yet exist*—Long-jump initiatives can entail pumping funds into long-range R&D projects, setting up an internal venture capital fund to invest in promising start-up companies attempting to create the industries of the future, or acquiring a number of small start-up companies experimenting with technologies and product ideas that complement the company's present businesses. Intel, for example, set up a multibillion-dollar venture fund to invest in over 100 different projects and start-up companies, the intent being to plant seeds for Intel's future, broadening its base as a global leader in supplying building blocks for PCs and the worldwide Internet economy. Royal Dutch/ Shell, with over $140 billion in revenues and over 100,000 employees, spent over $20 million on rule-breaking, game-changing ideas put forth by free-thinking employees; the objective was to inject a new spirit of entrepreneurship into the company and sow the seeds of faster growth.[19]

Figure 8.2   **The Three Strategy Horizons for Sustaining Rapid Growth**

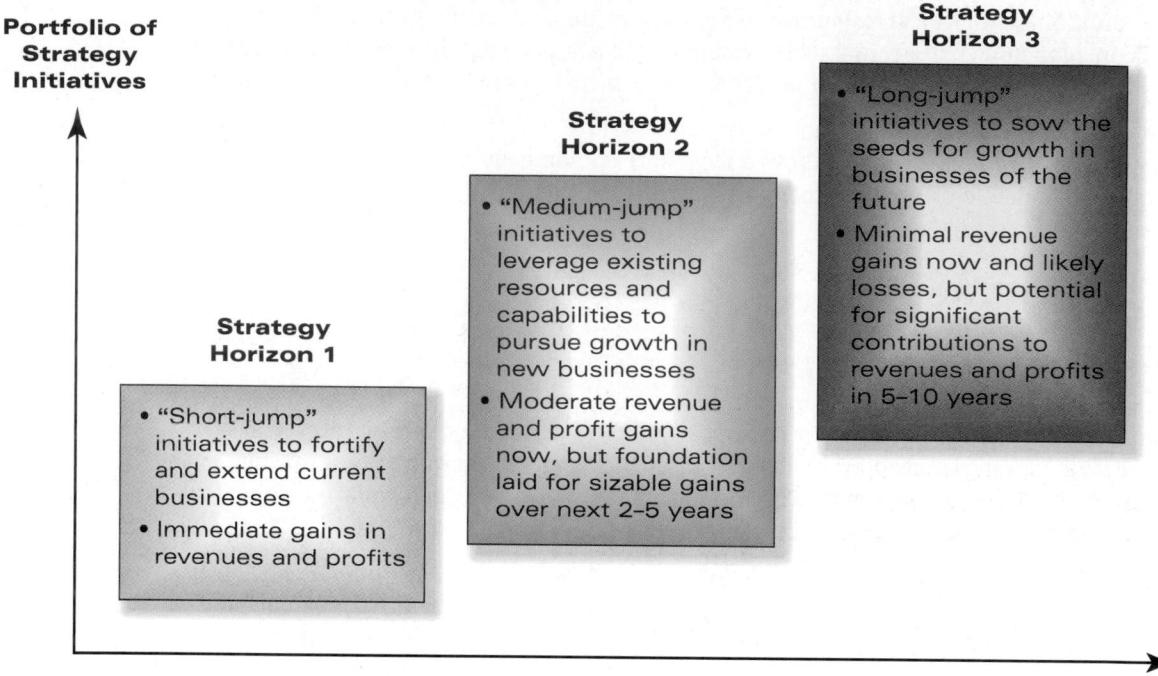

Source: Adapted from Eric D. Beinhocker, "Robust Adaptive Strategies," *Sloan Management Review* 40. No. 3 (Spring 1999), p. 101.

The three strategy horizons are illustrated in Figure 8.2. Managing such a portfolio of strategic initiatives to sustain rapid growth is not easy, however. The tendency of most companies is to focus on Horizon 1 strategies and devote only sporadic and uneven attention to Horizon 2 and 3 strategies. But a recent McKinsey & Company study of 30 of the world's leading growth companies revealed a relatively balanced portfolio of strategic initiatives covering all three horizons. The lesson of successful growth companies is that keeping a company's record of rapid growth intact over the long term entails crafting a diverse population of strategies, ranging from short-jump incremental strategies to grow present businesses to long-jump initiatives with a 5- to 10-year growth payoff horizon.[20] Having a mixture of short-jump, medium-jump, and long-jump initiatives not only increases the odds of hitting a few home runs but also provides some protection against unexpected adversity in present or newly entered businesses.

The Risks of Pursuing Multiple Strategy Horizons

There are, of course, risks to pursuing a diverse strategy portfolio aimed at sustained growth. A company cannot, of course, place bets on every opportunity that appears on its radar screen, lest it stretch its resources too thin. And medium-jump and long-jump initiatives can cause a company to stray far from its core competencies and end up trying to compete in businesses for which it is ill-suited. Moreover, it can be difficult to achieve competitive advantage in medium- and long-jump product families and businesses that prove not to mesh well with a company's present businesses and resource strengths. The payoffs of long-jump initiatives often prove elusive; not all of the seeds a company sows will bear fruit, and only a few may evolve into truly significant contributors to the company's revenue and profit growth. The losses from those long-jump ventures that do not take root may significantly erode the gains from those that do, resulting in disappointingly modest gains in overall profits.

STRATEGIES FOR INDUSTRY LEADERS

The competitive positions of industry leaders normally range from "stronger than average" to "powerful." Leaders typically are well known, and strongly entrenched leaders have proven strategies (keyed either to low-cost leadership or to differentiation). Some of the best-known industry leaders are Anheuser-Busch (beer), Starbucks (coffee drinks), Microsoft (computer software), Callaway (golf clubs), McDonald's (fast food), Procter & Gamble (laundry detergents and soaps), Campbell's (canned soups), Gerber (baby food), Hewlett-Packard (printers), Sony (video game consoles), Black & Decker (power tools), Intel (semiconductors and chip sets), Wal-Mart and Carrefour (discount retailing), Amazon.com (online shopping), eBay (online auctions), Apple (MP3 players), and Ocean Spray (cranberries).

The main strategic concern for a leader revolves around how to defend and strengthen its leadership position, perhaps becoming the dominant leader as opposed to just a leader. However, the pursuit of industry leadership and large market share is primarily important because of the competitive advantage and profitability that accrue to being the industry's biggest company. Three contrasting strategic postures are open to industry leaders:[21]

1. *Stay-on-the-offensive strategy*—The central goal of a stay-on-the-offensive strategy is to be a first-mover and a proactive market leader.[22] It rests on the principle that playing hardball, moving early and frequently, and forcing rivals into a catch-up mode is the surest path to industry prominence and potential market dominance—as the saying goes, the best defense is a good offense. Furthermore, *an offensive-minded industry leader relentlessly concentrates on achieving a competitive advantage over rivals and then widening this advantage over time to achieve extreme competitive advantage.*[23] Being the industry standard setter thus requires being impatient with the status quo, seizing the initiative, and pioneering continuous improvement and innovation—this can mean being first-to-market with technological improvements, new or better products, more attractive performance features, quality enhancements, or customer service improvements. It can mean aggressively seeking out ways to cut operating costs, ways to establish competitive capabilities that rivals cannot match, or ways to make it easier and less costly for potential customers to switch their purchases from runner-up firms to the leader's own products. It can mean aggressively attacking the profit sanctuaries of important rivals, perhaps with bursts of advertising or price-cutting or approaching its customers with special deals.[24]

> The governing principle underlying an industry leader's use of a stay-on-the-offensive strategy is to be an action-oriented first-mover, impatient with the status quo.

A low-cost leader must set the pace for cost reduction, and a differentiator must constantly initiate new ways to keep its product set apart from the brands of imitative rivals in order to be the standard against which rivals' products are judged. The array of options for a potent stay-on-the-offensive strategy can also include initiatives to expand overall industry demand—spurring the creation of new families of products, making the product more suitable for consumers in emerging-country markets, discovering new uses for the product, attracting new users of the product, and promoting more frequent use.

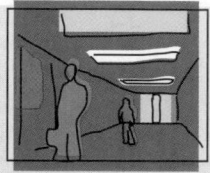

Illustration Capsule 8.2
ESPN's Strategy to Dominate Sports Entertainment

Via a series of offensive initiatives over the past 10 years, ESPN has parlayed its cable TV sports programming franchise into a dominating and pervasive general store of sports entertainment. The thrust of ESPN's strategy has been to stay on the offensive by (1) continually enhancing its program offerings and (2) extending the ESPN brand into a host of cutting-edge sports businesses. Examples of ESPN's enhanced product offering include the ESPY Awards for top achievements in sports, the X Games (an annual extreme sports competition for both winter and summer sports), the addition of *Monday Night Football* (starting in 2006), making new movies to show on ESPN, and producing its own shows (such as *ESPN Hollywood, Cold Pizza,* and *Bound for Glory*). The appeal of ESPN's programming was so powerful that ESPN was able to charge cable operators an estimated $2.80 per subscriber per month—nearly twice as much as the next most popular cable channel (CNN, for instance, was only able to command a monthly fee of roughly $0.40 per subscriber).

But the most important element of ESPN's strategic offensive had been to start up a series of new ESPN-branded businesses—all of which were brainstormed by ESPN's entrepreneurially talented management team. The company's brand extension offensive has produced nine TV channels (the most prominent of which are ESPN, ESPN2, ESPN Classic, ESPNews, and ESPN Desportes); the ESPN radio network, with 700 affiliate stations; ESPN.com (which in 2005 attracted some 16 million unique visitors monthly to view its bazaar of wide-ranging sports stories and information); *ESPN: The Magazine* (with a fast-growing base of 1.8 million subscribers that could in time overtake the barely growing 3.3 million subscriber

base of longtime leader *Sports Illustrated*); ESPN Motion (an online video service); ESPN360 (which offers sports information and video-clip programming tailored for broadband providers—it had 5 million subscribers in 2005 and was available from 14 broadband providers); Mobile ESPN (an ESPN-branded cell phone service provided in partnership with Sprint Nextel); ESPN Zones (nine sports-themed restaurants in various cities); ESPN branded video games (video game developer Electronic Arts has 15-year licensing rights to use the ESPN name for a series of sports-related games), and a business unit that distributes ESPN sports programming in 11 languages in over 180 countries.

In 2005, the empire of ESPN consisted of some 50 different businesses that generated annual revenues in excess of $5 billion and hefty annual operating profits of about $2 billion—about 40 percent of its revenues came from advertising and 60 percent from subscriptions and distribution fees. ESPN, a division of Disney, was one of Disney's most profitable and fastest-growing operations (Disney was also the parent of ABC Broadcasting).

So far, ESPN's stay-a-step-ahead strategy had left lesser rivals in the dust. But Comcast, the largest U.S. cable operator, with 22 million subscribers, was maneuvering to create its own cable TV sports channel; Comcast already owned the Philadelphia 76ers, the Philadelphia Flyers, and a collection of regional sports networks in cities from Philadelphia to Chicago to Los Angeles. And Rupert Murdoch's expansion-minded News Corporation, a worldwide media conglomerate whose many businesses included Fox Broadcasting and DIRECTV, was said to be looking at melding its 15 regional U.S. sports channels into a national sports channel.

Source: Developed from information in Tom Lowry, "ESPN the Zone," *BusinessWeek,* October 17, 2005, pp. 66–78.

A stay-on-the-offensive strategy cannot be considered successful unless it results in growing sales and revenues faster than the industry as a whole and wresting market share from rivals—a leader whose sales growth is only 5 percent in a market growing at 8 percent is losing ground to some of its competitors. Only if an industry's leader's market share is already so dominant that it presents a threat of antitrust action (a market share under 60 percent is usually safe) should an industry leader deliberately back away from aggressively pursuing market share gains.

Illustration Capsule 8.2 describes ESPN's stay-on-the-offensive strategy to dominate the sports entertainment business.

   2.   *Fortify-and-defend strategy*—The essence of "fortify and defend" is to make it harder for challengers to gain ground and for new firms to enter. The goals of a strong defense are to hold on to the present market share, strengthen current market position, and protect whatever competitive advantage the firm has. Specific defensive actions can include:

- Attempting to raise the competitive ante for challengers and new entrants via increased spending for advertising, higher levels of customer service, and bigger R&D outlays.
- Introducing more product versions or brands to match the product attributes that challenger brands have or to fill vacant niches that competitors could slip into.
- Adding personalized services and other extras that boost customer loyalty and make it harder or more costly for customers to switch to rival products.
- Keeping prices reasonable and quality attractive.
- Building new capacity ahead of market demand to discourage smaller competitors from adding capacity of their own.
- Investing enough to remain cost-competitive and technologically progressive.
- Patenting the feasible alternative technologies.
- Signing exclusive contracts with the best suppliers and dealer/distributors.

A fortify-and-defend strategy best suits firms that have already achieved industry dominance and don't wish to risk antitrust action. It is also well suited to situations where a firm wishes to milk its present position for profits and cash flow because the industry's prospects for growth are low or because further gains in market share do not appear profitable enough to go after. But a fortify-and-defend strategy always entails trying to grow as fast as the market as a whole (to stave off market-share slippage) and requires reinvesting enough capital in the business to protect the leader's ability to compete.

3. *Muscle-flexing strategy*—Here a dominant leader plays competitive hardball (presumably in an ethical and competitively legal manner) when smaller rivals rock the boat with price cuts or mount new market offensives that directly threaten its position. Specific responses can include quickly matching and perhaps exceeding challengers' price cuts, using large promotional campaigns to counter challengers' moves to gain market share, and offering better deals to their major customers. Dominant leaders may also court distributors assiduously to dissuade them from carrying rivals' products, provide salespersons with documented information about the weaknesses of competing products, or try to fill any vacant positions in their own firms by making attractive offers to the better executives of rivals that get out of line.

The leader may also use various arm-twisting tactics to pressure present customers not to use the products of rivals. This can range from simply forcefully communicating its displeasure should customers opt to use the products of rivals to pushing them to agree to exclusive arrangements in return for better prices to charging them a higher price if they use any competitors' products. As a final resort, a leader may grant certain customers special discounts or preferred treatment if they do not use any products of rivals.

The obvious risks of a muscle-flexing strategy are running afoul of laws prohibiting monopoly practices and unfair competition and using bullying tactics that arouse adverse public opinion. Microsoft paid Real Networks $460 million in 2005 to resolve all of Real Network's antitrust complaints and settle a long-standing feud over Microsoft's repeated bullying of PC makers to include Windows Media Player instead of Real's media player as standard installed software on their PCs. In 2005 AMD filed an antitrust suit against Intel, claiming that Intel unfairly and monopolistically coerced 38 named companies on three continents in efforts to get them to use Intel chips instead of AMD chips in the computer products they manufactured or marketed. Consequently, a company that throws its weight around to protect and enhance its market dominance has got to be judicious, lest it cross the line from allowable muscle-flexing to unethical or illegal competitive bullying.

STRATEGIES FOR RUNNER-UP FIRMS

Runner-up, or second-tier, firms have smaller market shares than first-tier industry leaders. Some runner-up firms are often advancing market challengers, employing offensive strategies to gain market share and build a stronger market position. Other runner-up competitors are focusers, seeking to improve their lot by concentrating their attention on serving a limited portion of the market. There are, of course, always a number of firms in any industry that are destined to be perennial runners-up, either because they are content to follow the trendsetting moves of the market leaders or because they lack the resources and competitive strengths to do much better in the marketplace than they are already doing. But it is erroneous to view runner-up firms as inherently less profitable or unable to hold their own against the biggest firms. Many small and medium-sized firms earn healthy profits and enjoy good reputations with customers.

Obstacles for Firms with Small Market Shares

There are times when runner-up companies face significant hurdles in contending for market leadership. In industries where big size is definitely a key success factor, firms with small market shares have four obstacles to overcome: (1) less access to economies of scale in manufacturing, distribution, or marketing and sales promotion; (2) difficulty in gaining customer recognition (since the products and brands of the market leaders are much better known); (3) less money to spend on mass-media advertising; and (4) limited funds for capital expansion or making acquisitions.[25] Some runner-up companies may be able to surmount these obstacles. Others may not. When significant scale economies give large-volume competitors a dominating cost advantage, small-share firms have only two viable strategic options: initiate offensive moves aimed at building sufficient sales volume to approach the scale economies and lower unit costs enjoyed by larger rivals or withdraw from the business (gradually or quickly) because of the inability to achieve low enough costs to compete effectively against the market leaders.

Offensive Strategies to Build Market Share

A runner-up company desirous of closing in on the market leaders has to make some waves in the marketplace if it wants to make big market share gains—this means coming up with distinctive strategy elements that set it apart from rivals and draw buyer attention. If a challenger has a 5 percent market share and needs a 15 to 20 percent share to contend for leadership and earn attractive profits, it requires a more creative approach to competing than just "Try harder" or "Follow in the footsteps of current industry leaders." Rarely can a runner-up significantly improve its competitive position by imitating the strategies of leading firms. A cardinal rule in offensive strategy is to avoid attacking a leader head-on with an imitative strategy, regardless of the resources and staying power an underdog may have.[26] What an aspiring challenger really needs is a strategy aimed at building a competitive advantage of its own (and certainly a strategy capable of quickly eliminating any important competitive disadvantages).

The best "mover-and-shaker" offensives for a second-tier challenger aiming to join the first-tier ranks usually involve one of the following five approaches:

1. Making a series of acquisitions of smaller rivals to greatly expand the company's market reach and market presence. *Growth via acquisition* is perhaps the most frequently used strategy employed by ambitious runner-up companies to form an enterprise that has greater competitive strength and a larger share of the overall market. For an enterprise to succeed with this strategic approach, senior management must be skilled in quickly assimilating the operations of the acquired companies, eliminating duplication and overlap, generating efficiencies and cost savings, and structuring the combined resources in ways that create substantially stronger competitive capabilities. Many banks and public accounting firms owe their growth during the past decade to acquisition of smaller regional and local banks. Likewise, a number of book publishers have grown by acquiring small publishers, and public accounting firms have grown by acquiring lesser-sized accounting firms with attractive client lists.

2. Finding innovative ways to dramatically drive down costs and then using the attraction of lower prices to win customers from higher-cost, higher-priced rivals. This is a necessary offensive move when a runner-up company has higher costs than larger-scale enterprises (either because the latter possess scale economies or have benefited from experience/learning curve effects). A challenger firm can pursue aggressive cost reduction by eliminating marginal activities from its value chain, streamlining supply chain relationships, improving internal operating efficiency, using various e-commerce techniques, and merging with or acquiring rival firms to achieve the size needed to capture greater scale economies.

3. Crafting an attractive differentiation strategy based on premium quality, technological superiority, outstanding customer service, rapid product innovation, or convenient online shopping options.

4. Pioneering a leapfrog technological breakthrough—an attractive option if an important technological breakthrough is within a challenger's reach and rivals are not close behind.

5. Being first-to-market with new or better products and building a reputation for product leadership. A strategy of product innovation has appeal if the runner-up company possesses the necessary resources—cutting-edge R&D capability and organizational agility in speeding new products to market.

Other possible, but likely less effective, offensive strategy options include (1) outmaneuvering slow-to-change market leaders in adapting to evolving market conditions and customer expectations and (2) forging productive strategic alliances with key distributors, dealers, or marketers of complementary products.

Without a potent offensive strategy to capture added market share, runner-up companies have to patiently nibble away at the lead of market leaders and build sales at a moderate pace over time.

Other Strategic Approaches for Runner-Up Companies

There are five other strategies that runner-up companies can employ.[27] While none of the five is likely to move a company from second-tier to first-tier status, all are capable of producing attractive profits and returns for shareholders.

Vacant-Niche Strategy   A version of a focused strategy, the vacant-niche strategy involves concentrating on specific customer groups or end-use applications that market leaders have bypassed or neglected. An ideal vacant niche is of sufficient size and scope to be profitable, has some growth potential, is well suited to a firm's own capabilities, and for one reason or another is hard for leading firms to serve. Two examples where vacant-niche strategies have worked successfully are (1) regional commuter airlines serving cities with too few passengers to fill the large jets flown by major airlines and (2) health-food producers (like Health Valley, Hain, and Tree of Life) that cater to local health-food stores—a market segment that until recently has been given little attention by such leading companies as Kraft, Nestlé, and Unilever.

Specialist Strategy   A specialist firm trains its competitive effort on one technology, product or product family, end use, or market segment (often one in which buyers have special needs). The aim is to train the company's resource strengths and capabilities on building competitive advantage through leadership in a specific area. Smaller companies that successfully use this focused strategy include Formby's (a specialist in stains and finishes for wood furniture, especially refinishing); Blue Diamond (a California-based grower and marketer of almonds); Cuddledown (a specialty producer and retailer of down and synthetic comforters, featherbeds, and other bedding products); and American Tobacco (a leader in chewing tobacco and snuff). Many companies in high-tech industries concentrate their energies on being the clear leader in a particular technological niche; their competitive advantage is superior technological depth, technical expertise that is highly valued by customers, and the capability to consistently beat out rivals in pioneering technological advances.

Superior Product Strategy   The approach here is to use a differentiation-based focused strategy keyed to superior product quality or unique attributes. Sales and marketing efforts are aimed directly at quality-conscious and performance-oriented buyers. Fine craftsmanship, prestige quality, frequent product innovations, and/or close contact with customers to solicit their input in developing a better product usually undergird the superior product approach. Some examples include Samuel Adams in beer, Tiffany in diamonds and jewelry, Chicago Cutlery in premium-quality kitchen knives, Baccarat in fine crystal, Cannondale in mountain bikes, Bally in shoes, and Patagonia in apparel for outdoor recreation enthusiasts.

Distinctive-Image Strategy   Some runner-up companies build their strategies around ways to make themselves stand out from competitors. A variety of distinctive-image strategies can be used: building a reputation for charging the lowest prices (Dollar General), providing high-end quality at a good price (Orvis, Lands' End, and L. L. Bean), going all out to give superior customer service (Four Seasons hotels), incorporating unique product attributes (Omega-3 enriched eggs), making a product with disctinctive styling (General Motors' Hummer), or devising unusually creative advertising (AFLAC's duck ads on TV). Other examples include Dr Pepper's strategy in calling attention to its distinctive taste, Apple Computer's making it easier and more interesting for people to use its Macintosh PCs, and Mary Kay Cosmetics' distinctive use of the color pink.

Content Follower Strategy   Content followers deliberately refrain from initiating trendsetting strategic moves and from aggressive attempts to steal customers away from the leaders. Followers prefer approaches that will not provoke competitive retaliation, often opting for focus and differentiation strategies that keep them out of the leaders' paths. They react and respond rather than initiate and challenge. They prefer defense to offense. And they rarely get out of line with the leaders on price. They are content to simply maintain their market position, albeit sometimes struggling to do so. Followers have no urgent strategic questions to confront beyond "What strategic changes are the leaders initiating and what do we need to do to follow along and maintain our present position?" The marketers of private-label products tend to be followers, imitating many of the newly introduced features of name brand products and content to sell to price-conscious buyers at prices modestly below those of well-known brands.

STRATEGIES FOR WEAK AND CRISIS-RIDDEN BUSINESSES

A firm in an also-ran or declining competitive position has four basic strategic options. If it can come up with the financial resources, it can launch a turnaround strategy keyed either to "low-cost" or "new" differentiation themes, pouring enough money and talent into the effort to move up a notch or two in the industry rankings and become a respectable market contender within five years or so. It can employ a fortify-and-defend strategy, using variations of its present strategy and fighting hard to keep sales, market share, profitability, and competitive position at current levels. It can opt for a fast-exit strategy and get out of the business, either by selling out to another firm or by closing down operations if a buyer cannot be found. Or it can employ an end-game or slow-exit strategy, keeping reinvestment to a bare-bones minimum and taking actions to maximize short-term cash flows in preparation for orderly market withdrawal.

Turnaround Strategies for Businesses in Crisis

Turnaround strategies are needed when a business worth rescuing goes into crisis. The objective is to arrest and reverse the sources of competitive and financial weakness as quickly as possible. Management's first task in formulating a suitable turnaround strategy is to diagnose what lies at the root of poor performance. Is it an unexpected downturn in sales brought on by a weak economy? An ill-chosen competitive strategy? Poor execution of an otherwise viable strategy? High operating costs? Important resource deficiencies? An overload of debt? The next task is to decide whether the business can be saved or whether the situation is hopeless. Understanding what is wrong with the business and how serious its strategic problems are is essential because different diagnoses lead to different turnaround strategies.

Some of the most common causes of business trouble are taking on too much debt, overestimating the potential for sales growth, ignoring the profit-depressing effects of an overly aggressive effort to "buy" market share with deep price cuts, being burdened with heavy fixed costs because weak sales don't permit near-full capacity utilization, betting on R&D efforts but failing to come up with effective innovations, betting on technological long shots, being too optimistic about the ability to penetrate new markets, making frequent changes in strategy (because the previous strategy didn't work out), and being overpowered by more successful rivals. Curing these kinds of problems and achieving a successful business turnaround can involve any of the following actions:

- Selling off assets to raise cash to save the remaining part of the business.
- Revising the existing strategy.
- Launching efforts to boost revenues.

- Pursuing cost reduction.
- Using a combination of these efforts.

Selling Off Assets   Asset-reduction strategies are essential when cash flow is a critical consideration and when the most practical ways to generate cash are (1) through sale of some of the firm's assets (plant and equipment, land, patents, inventories, or profitable subsidiaries) and (2) through retrenchment (pruning of marginal products from the product line, closing or selling older plants, reducing the workforce, withdrawing from outlying markets, cutting back customer service). Sometimes crisis-ridden companies sell off assets not so much to unload losing operations as to raise funds to save and strengthen the remaining business activities. In such cases, the choice is usually to dispose of noncore business assets to support strategy renewal in the firm's core businesses.

Strategy Revision   When weak performance is caused by bad strategy, the task of strategy overhaul can proceed along any of several paths: (1) shifting to a new competitive approach to rebuild the firm's market position; (2) overhauling internal operations and functional-area strategies to better support the same overall business strategy; (3) merging with another firm in the industry and forging a new strategy keyed to the newly merged firm's strengths; and (4) retrenching into a reduced core of products and customers more closely matched to the firm's strengths. The most appealing path depends on prevailing industry conditions, the firm's particular strengths and weaknesses, its competitive capabilities vis-à-vis rival firms, and the severity of the crisis. A situation analysis of the industry, the major competitors, and the firm's own competitive position is a prerequisite for action. As a rule, successful strategy revision must be tied to the ailing firm's strengths and near-term competitive capabilities and directed at its best market opportunities.

Boosting Revenues   Revenue-increasing turnaround efforts aim at generating increased sales volume. The chief revenue-building options include price cuts, increased advertising, a bigger sales force, added customer services, and quickly achieved product improvements. Attempts to increase revenues and sales volumes are necessary (1) when there is little or no room in the operating budget to cut expenses and still break even, and (2) when the key to restoring profitability is increased use of existing capacity. If buyers are not especially price-sensitive (because many are strongly attached to various differentiating features in the company's product offering), the quickest way to boost short-term revenues may be to raise prices rather than opt for volume-building price cuts. A price increase in the 2–4 percent range may well be feasible if the company's prices are already below those of key rivals.

Cutting Costs   Cost-reducing turnaround strategies work best when an ailing firm's value chain and cost structure are flexible enough to permit radical surgery, when operating inefficiencies are identifiable and readily correctable, when the firm's costs are obviously bloated, and when the firm is relatively close to its break-even point. Accompanying a general belt-tightening can be an increased emphasis on paring administrative overheads, elimination of nonessential and low-value-added activities in the firm's value chain, modernization of existing plant and equipment to gain greater productivity, delay of nonessential capital expenditures, and debt restructuring to reduce interest costs and stretch out repayments.

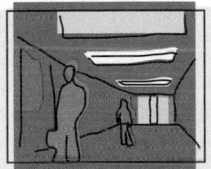

Illustration Capsule 8.3
Sony's Turnaround Strategy—Will It Work?

Electronics was once Sony's star business, but Sony's electronics business was a huge money-loser in 2003–2004, pushing the company's stock price down about 65 percent. Once the clear leader in top-quality TVs, in 2005 Sony lagged miserably behind Samsung, Panasonic, and Sharp in popular flat-panel LCD and plasma TVs, where sales were growing fastest. Apple Computer's iPod players had stolen the limelight in the handheld music market, where Sony's Walkman had long ruled.

In the fall of 2005, Sony management announced a turnaround strategy. Howard Stringer, a dual American and British citizen who was named Sony's CEO in early 2005 and was the first foreigner ever to head Sony, unveiled a plan centered on cutting 10,000 jobs (about 6 percent of Sony's workforce), closing 11 of Sony's 65 manufacturing plants, and shrinking or eliminating 15 unprofitable

electronics operations by March 2008 (the unprofitable operations were not identified). These initiatives were projected to reduce costs by $1.8 billion. In addition to the cost cuts, Sony said it would focus on growing its sales of "champion products" like the next-generation Sony PlayStation 3 video game console, a newly introduced line of Bravia LCD TVs, and Walkman MP3 music players.

Analysts were not impressed by the turnaround plan. Standard & Poor's cut its credit rating for Sony, citing doubts about the company's turnaround strategy and forecasting "substantially" lower profitability and cash flow in fiscal 2005. Moody's put Sony on its watch list for a credit rating downgrade. Other analysts said Stringer's strategy lacked vision and creativity because it was in the same mold as most corporate streamlining efforts.

Sources: Company press releases; Yuri Kageyama, "Sony Announcing Turnaround Strategy," www.yahoo.com (accessed October 20, 2005); *Mainichi Daily News*, October 14, 2005 (accessed on Google News, October 20, 2005); and "Sony to Cut 10,000 Jobs," www.cnn.com (accessed October 20, 2005).

Combination Efforts   Combination turnaround strategies are usually essential in grim situations that require fast action on a broad front. Likewise, combination actions frequently come into play when new managers are brought in and given a free hand to make whatever changes they see fit. The tougher the problems, the more likely it is that the solutions will involve multiple strategic initiatives—see the story of turnaround efforts at Sony in Illustration Capsule 8.3.

The Chances of a Successful Turnaround Are Not High   Turnaround efforts tend to be high-risk undertakings; some return a company to good profitability, but most don't. A landmark study of 64 companies found no successful turnarounds among the most troubled companies in eight basic industries.[28] Many of the troubled businesses waited too long to begin a turnaround. Others found themselves short of both the cash and entrepreneurial talent needed to compete in a slow-growth industry characterized by a fierce battle for market share. Better-positioned rivals simply proved too strong to defeat in a long, head-to-head contest. Even when successful, turnaround may involve numerous attempts and management changes before long-term competitive viability and profitability are finally restored. A recent study found that troubled companies that did nothing and elected to wait out hard times had only a 10 percent chance of recovery.[29] This same study also found that, of the companies studied, the chances of recovery were boosted 190 percent if the turnaround strategy involved buying assets that strengthened the company's business in its core markets; companies that both bought assets or companies in their core markets while selling off noncore assets increased their chances of recovery by 250 percent.

Harvest Strategies for Weak Businesses

When a struggling company's chances of pulling off a successful turnaround are poor, the wisest option may be to forget about trying to restore the company's competitiveness and profitability and, instead employ a *harvesting strategy* that aims at generating the largest possible cash flows from the company's operations for as long as possible. A losing effort to transform a competitively weak company into a viable market contender has little appeal when there are opportunities to generate potentially sizable amounts of cash by running the business in a manner calculated to either maintain the status quo or even let the business slowly deteriorate over a long period.

As is the case with a slow-exit strategy, a harvesting strategy entails trimming operating expenses to the bone and spending the minimum amount on capital projects to keep the business going. Internal cash flow becomes the key measure of how well the company is performing, and top priority is given to cash-generating actions. Thus,

> The overriding objective of a harvesting strategy is to maximize short-term cash flows from operations.

advertising and promotional costs are kept at minimal levels; personnel who leave for jobs elsewhere or retire may not be replaced; and maintenance is performed with an eye toward stretching the life of existing facilities and equipment. Even though a harvesting strategy is likely to lead to a gradual decline in the company's business over time, the ability to harvest sizable amounts of cash in the interim makes such an outcome tolerable.

The Conditions That Make a Harvesting Strategy Attractive   A strategy of harvesting the cash flows from a weak business is a reasonable option in the following circumstances:[30]

1. *When industry demand is stagnant or declining and there's little hope that either market conditions will improve*—The growing popularity of digital cameras has forever doomed market demand for camera film.

2. *When rejuvenating the business would be too costly or at best marginally profitable*—A struggling provider of dial-up Internet access is likely to realize more benefit from harvesting than from a losing effort to grow its business in the face of the unstoppable shift to high-speed broadband service.

3. *When trying to maintain or grow the company's present sales is becoming increasingly costly*—A money-losing producer of pipe tobacco and cigars is unlikely to make market headway in gaining sales and market share against the top-tier producers (which have more resources to compete for the business that is still available).

4. *When reduced levels of competitive effort will not trigger an immediate or rapid falloff in sales*—the makers of corded telephones will not likely experience much of a decline in sales if they spend all of their R&D and marketing budgets on wireless phone systems.

5. *When the enterprise can redeploy the freed resources in higher-opportunity areas*—The makers of food products with "bad-for-you" ingredients (saturated fats, high transfats, and sugar) are better off devoting their resources to the development, production, and sale of "good-for-you" products (those with no transfats, more fiber, and good types of carbohydrates).

6. *When the business is not a crucial or core component of a diversified company's overall lineup of businesses*—Harvesting a sideline business and perhaps hastening

its decay is strategically preferable to harvesting a mainline or core business (where even a gradual decline may not be a very attractive outcome).

The more of these six conditions that are present, the more ideal the business is for harvesting.

Liquidation: The Strategy of Last Resort

Sometimes a business in crisis is too far gone to be salvaged and presents insufficient harvesting potential to be interesting. Closing down a crisis-ridden business and liquidating its assets is sometimes the best and wisest strategy. But it is also the most unpleasant and painful strategic alternative due to the hardships of job eliminations and the economic effects of business closings on local communities. Nonetheless, in hopeless situations, an early liquidation effort usually serves owner-stockholder interests better than an inevitable bankruptcy. Prolonging the pursuit of a lost cause further erodes an organization's resources and leaves less to salvage, not to mention the added stress and potential career impairment for all the people involved. The problem, of course, is differentiating between when a turnaround is achievable and when it isn't. It is easy for owners or managers to let their emotions and pride overcome sound judgment when a business gets in such deep trouble that a successful turnaround is remote.

10 COMMANDMENTS FOR CRAFTING SUCCESSFUL BUSINESS STRATEGIES

Company experiences over the years prove again and again that disastrous strategies can be avoided by adhering to good strategy-making principles. We've distilled the lessons learned from the strategic mistakes companies most often make into 10 commandments that serve as useful guides for developing sound strategies:

1. *Place top priority on crafting and executing strategic moves that enhance the company's competitive position for the long term.* The glory of meeting one quarter's or one year's financial performance targets quickly fades, but an ever-stronger competitive position pays off year after year. Shareholders are never well served by managers who let short-term financial performance considerations rule out strategic initiatives that will meaningfully bolster the company's longer-term competitive position and competitive strength. The best way to ensure a company's long-term profitability is with a strategy that strengthens the company's long-term competitiveness and market position.

2. *Be prompt in adapting to changing market conditions, unmet customer needs, buyer wishes for something better, emerging technological alternatives, and new initiatives of competitors.* Responding late or with too little often puts a company in the precarious position of having to play catch-up. While pursuit of a consistent strategy has its virtues, adapting strategy to changing circumstances is normal and necessary. Moreover, long-term strategic commitments to achieve top quality or lowest cost should be interpreted relative to competitors' products as well as customers' needs and expectations; the company should avoid singlemindedly striving to make the absolute highest-quality or lowest-cost product no matter what.

3. *Invest in creating a sustainable competitive advantage.* Having a competitive edge over rivals is the single most dependable contributor to above-average profitability.

As a general rule, a company must play aggressive offense to build competitive advantage and aggressive defense to protect it.

4. *Avoid strategies capable of succeeding only in the most optimistic circumstances.* Expect competitors to employ countermeasures and expect times of unfavorable market conditions. A good strategy works reasonably well and produces tolerable results even in the worst of times.

5. *Consider that attacking competitive weakness is usually more profitable and less risky than attacking competitive strength.* Attacking capable, resourceful rivals is likely to fail unless the attacker has deep financial pockets and a solid basis for competitive advantage despite the strengths of the competitor being attacked.

6. *Strive to open up very meaningful gaps in quality or service or performance features when pursuing a differentiation strategy.* Tiny differences between rivals' product offerings may not be visible or important to buyers.

7. *Be wary of cutting prices without an established cost advantage.* Price cuts run the risk that rivals will retaliate with matching or deeper price cuts of their own. The best chance for remaining profitable if the price-cutting contest turns into a price war is to have lower costs than rivals.

8. *Don't underestimate the reactions and the commitment of rival firms.* Rivals are most dangerous when they are pushed into a corner and their well-being is threatened.

9. *Avoid stuck-in-the-middle strategies that represent compromises between lower costs and greater differentiation and between broad and narrow market appeal.* Compromise strategies rarely produce sustainable competitive advantage or a distinctive competitive position—a well-executed best-cost producer strategy is the only exception in which a compromise between low cost and differentiation succeeds. Companies with compromise strategies most usually end up with average costs, an average product, an average reputation, and *no distinctive image in the marketplace.* Lacking any strategy element that causes them to stand out in the minds of buyers, companies with compromise strategies are destined for a middle-of-the-pack industry ranking, with little prospect of ever becoming an industry leader.

10. *Be judicious in employing aggressive moves to wrest market share away from rivals often provoke retaliation in the form of escalating marketing and sales promotion, a furious race to be first-to-market with next-version products or a price war—to the detriment of everyone's profits.* Aggressive moves to capture a bigger market share invite cutthroat competition, especially when many industry members, plagued with high inventories and excess production capacity, are also scrambling for additional sales.

Key Points

The lessons of this chapter are that (1) some strategic options are better suited to certain specific industry and competitive environments than others and (2) some strategic options are better suited to certain specific company situations than others. Crafting a strategy tightly matched to a company's situation thus involves being alert to which strategy alternatives are likely to work well and which alternatives are unlikely to work well. Specifically:

1. What basic type of industry environment (emerging, rapid-growth, mature/slow-growth, stagnant/declining, high-velocity/turbulent, fragmented) does the company operate in? What strategic options and strategic postures are usually best suited to this generic type of environment?

2. What position does the firm have in the industry (leader, runner-up, or weak/distressed)? Given this position, which strategic options merit strong consideration and which options should definitely be ruled out?

In addition, creating a tight strategy-situation fit entails considering all the external and internal situational factors discussed in Chapters 3 and 4 and then revising the list of strategy options accordingly to take account of competitive conditions, industry driving forces, the expected moves of rivals, and the company's own competitive strengths and weaknesses. Listing the pros and cons of the candidate strategies is nearly always a helpful step. In weeding out the least attractive strategic alternatives and weighing the pros and cons of the most attractive ones, the answers to four questions often help point to the best course of action:

1. What kind of competitive edge can the company realistically achieve, given its resource strengths, competencies, and competitive capabilities? Is the company in a position to lead industry change and set the rules by which rivals must compete?

2. Which strategy alternative best addresses all the issues and problems the firm confronts.

3. Are any rivals particularly vulnerable and, if so, what sort of an offensive will it take to capitalize on these vulnerabilities? Will rivals counterattack? What can be done to blunt their efforts?

4. Are any defensive actions needed to protect against rivals' likely moves or other external threats to the company's future profitability?

In picking and choosing among the menu of strategic options, there are four pitfalls to avoid:

1. Designing an overly ambitious strategic plan—one that overtaxes the company's resources and capabilities.

2. Selecting a strategy that represents a radical departure from or abandonment of the cornerstones of the company's prior success—a radical strategy change need not be rejected automatically, but it should be pursued only after careful risk assessment.

3. Choosing a strategy that goes against the grain of the organization's culture.

4. Being unwilling to commit wholeheartedly to one of the five competitive strategies—picking and choosing features of the different strategies usually produces so many compromises between low cost, best cost, differentiation, and focusing that the company fails to achieve any kind of advantage and ends up stuck in the middle.

Table 8.1 provides a generic format for outlining a strategic action plan for a single-business enterprise. It contains all of the pieces of a comprehensive strategic action plan that we discussed at various places in these first eight chapters.

Table 8.1   **Sample Format for a Strategic Action Plan**

1. Strategic Vision and Mission	**5.** Supporting Functional Strategies • Production
2. Strategic Objectives • Short-term	 • Marketing/sales
  • Long-term	 • Finance
3. Financial Objectives • Short-term	 • Personnel/human resources
  • Long-term	 • Other
4. Overall Business Strategy	**6.** Recommended Actions to Improve Company Performance • Immediate
	  • Longer-range

Exercises

1. Listed below are 10 industries. Classify each one as (*a*) emerging, (*b*) rapid-growth, (*c*) mature/slow-growth, (*d*) stagnant/declining, (*e*) high-velocity/turbulent, and (*f*) fragmented. Do research on the Internet, if needed, to locate information on industry conditions and reach a conclusion on what classification to assign each of the following:

   a. Exercise and fitness industry.

   b. Dry-cleaning industry.

   c. Poultry industry.

   d. Camera film and film-developing industry.

   e. Wine, beer, and liquor retailing.

   f. Watch industry.

   g. Cell-phone industry.

   h. Recorded music industry (DVDs, CDs, tapes).

   i. Computer software industry.

   j. Newspaper industry.

2. Toyota overtook Ford Motor Company in 2003 to become the world's second-largest maker of motor vehicles, behind General Motors. Toyota is widely regarded as having aspirations to overtake General Motors as the global leader in motor vehicles within the next 10 years. Do research on the Internet or in the library to determine what strategy General Motors is pursuing to maintain its status as the industry leader. Then research Toyota's strategy to overtake General Motors.

3. Review the discussion in Illustration Capsule 8.1 concerning the focused differentiation strategy that Exertris has employed in the exercise equipment industry. Then answer the following:

   a. What reasons can you give for why sales of the Exertris exercise bike have not taken off?

   b. What strategic actions would you recommend to the cofounders of Exertris to spark substantially greater sales of its innovative exercise bike and overcome the apparent market apathy for its video-game-equipped exercise bike? Should the company consider making any changes in its product offering? What distribution channels should it emphasize? What advertising and promotional approaches should be considered? How can it get gym owners to purchase or at least try its bikes?

   c. Should the company just give up on its product innovation (because the bike is not ever likely to get good reception in the marketplace)? Or should the cofounders try to sell their fledgling business to another exercise equipment company with a more extensive product line and wider geographic coverage?

4. Review the information in Illustration Capsule 8.3 concerning the turnaround strategy Sony launched in the fall of 2005. Go to the company's Web site and check out other Internet sources to see how Sony's strategy to revitalize its electronics business is coming along. Does your research indicate that Sony's turnaround strategy is a success or a failure, or is it still too early to tell? Explain.

5. Yahoo competes in an industry characterized by high-velocity change. Read the company's press releases at http://yhoo.client.shareholder.com/releases.cfm and answer the following questions:

   a. Does it appear that the company has dealt with change in the industry by reacting to change, anticipating change, or leading change? Explain.

   b. What are its key strategies for competing in fast-changing markets? Describe them.

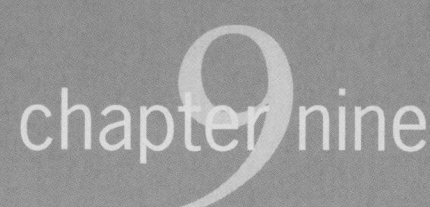

chapter nine

Diversification

Strategies for Managing a Group of Businesses

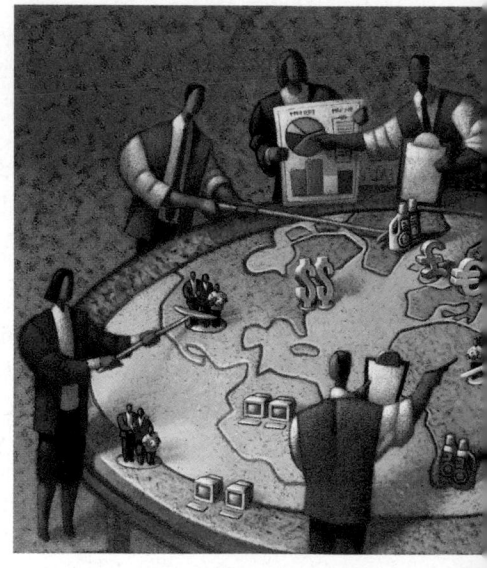

To acquire or not to acquire: that is the question.

—Robert J. Terry

Fit between a parent and its businesses is a two-edged sword: a good fit can create value; a bad one can destroy it.

—Andrew Campbell, Michael Goold, and Marcus Alexander

Achieving superior performance through diversification is largely based on relatedness.

—Philippe Very

Make winners out of every business in your company. Don't carry losers.

—Jack Welch
Former CEO, General Electric

We measure each of our businesses against strict criteria: growth, margin, and return-on-capital hurdle rate, and does it have the ability to become number one or two in its industry? We are quite pragmatic. If a business does not contribute to our overall vision, it has to go.

—Richard Wambold
CEO, Pactiv

In this chapter, we move up one level in the strategy-making hierarchy, from strategy making in a single-business enterprise to strategy making in a diversified enterprise. Because a diversified company is a collection of individual businesses, the strategy-making task is more complicated. In a one-business company, managers have to come up with a plan for competing successfully in only a single industry environment—the result is what we labeled in Chapter 2 as *business strategy* (or *business-level strategy*). But in a diversified company, the strategy-making challenge involves assessing multiple industry environments and developing a *set* of business strategies, one for each industry arena in which the diversified company operates. And top executives at a diversified company must still go one step further and devise a company-wide or *corporate strategy* for improving the attractiveness and performance of the company's overall business lineup and for making a rational whole out of its diversified collection of individual businesses.

In most diversified companies, corporate-level executives delegate considerable strategy-making authority to the heads of each business, usually giving them the latitude to craft a business strategy suited to their particular industry and competitive circumstances and holding them accountable for producing good results. But the task of crafting a diversified company's overall or corporate strategy falls squarely in the lap of top-level executives and involves four distinct facets:

1. *Picking new industries to enter and deciding on the means of entry*—The first concerns in diversifying are what new industries to get into and whether to enter by starting a new business from the ground up, acquiring a company already in the target industry, or forming a joint venture or strategic alliance with another company. A company can diversify narrowly into a few industries or broadly into many industries. The choice of whether to enter an industry via a start-up operation; a joint venture; or the acquisition of an established leader, an up-and-coming company, or a troubled company with turnaround potential shapes what position the company will initially stake out for itself.

2. *Initiating actions to boost the combined performance of the businesses the firm has entered*—As positions are created in the chosen industries, corporate strategists typically zero in on ways to strengthen the long-term competitive positions and profits of the businesses the firm has invested in. Corporate parents can help their business subsidiaries by providing financial resources, by supplying missing skills or technological know-how or managerial expertise to better perform key value chain activities, and by providing new avenues for cost reduction. They can also acquire another company in the same industry and merge the two operations into a stronger business, or acquire new businesses that strongly complement existing businesses. Typically, a company will pursue rapid-growth strategies in its most promising businesses, initiate turnaround efforts in weak-performing businesses with potential, and divest businesses that are no longer attractive or that don't fit into management's long-range plans.

3. *Pursuing opportunities to leverage cross-business value chain relationships and strategic fits into competitive advantage*—A company that diversifies into businesses with competitively important value chain matchups (pertaining to technology, supply chain logistics, production, overlapping distribution channels, or common customers) gains competitive advantage potential not open to a company that diversifies into businesses whose value chains are totally unrelated. Capturing this competitive advantage potential requires that corporate strategists spend considerable time trying to capitalize on such cross-business opportunities as transferring skills or technology from one business to another, reducing costs via sharing use of common facilities and resources, and using the company's well-known brand names and distribution muscle to grow the sales of newly acquired products.

4. *Establishing investment priorities and steering corporate resources into the most attractive business units*—A diversified company's different businesses are usually not equally attractive from the standpoint of investing additional funds. It is incumbent on corporate management to (*a*) decide on the priorities for investing capital in the company's different businesses, (*b*) channel resources into areas where earnings potentials are higher and away from areas where they are lower, and (*c*) divest business units that are chronically poor performers or are in an increasingly unattractive industry. Divesting poor performers and businesses in unattractive industries frees up unproductive investments either for redeployment to promising business units or for financing attractive new acquisitions.

The demanding and time-consuming nature of these four tasks explains why corporate executives generally refrain from becoming immersed in the details of crafting and implementing business-level strategies, preferring instead to delegate lead responsibility for business strategy to the heads of each business unit.

In the first portion of this chapter we describe the various means a company can use to become diversified and explore the pros and cons of related versus unrelated diversification strategies. The second part of the chapter looks at how to evaluate the attractiveness of a diversified company's business lineup, decide whether it has a good diversification strategy, and identify ways to improve its future performance. In the chapter's concluding section, we survey the strategic options open to already-diversified companies.

WHEN TO DIVERSIFY

So long as a company has its hands full trying to capitalize on profitable growth opportunities in its present industry, there is no urgency to pursue diversification. The big risk of a single-business company, of course, is having all of the firm's eggs in one industry basket. If demand for the industry's product is eroded by the appearance of alternative technologies, substitute products, or fast-shifting buyer preferences, or if the industry becomes competitively unattractive and unprofitable, then a company's prospects can quickly dim. Consider, for example, what digital cameras have done to erode the revenues of companies dependent on making camera film and doing film processing, what CD and DVD technology have done to business outlook for producers of cassette tapes and 3.5-inch disks, and what cell-phone companies with their no-long-distance-charge plans and marketers of Voice over Internet Protocol (VoIP) are doing to the revenues of such once-dominant long-distance providers as AT&T, British Telecommunications, and NTT in Japan.

Thus, diversifying into new industries always merits strong consideration whenever a single-business company encounters diminishing market opportunities and stagnating sales in its principal business—most landline-based telecommunications companies across the world are quickly diversifying their product offerings to include wireless and VoIP services. But there are four other instances in which a company becomes a prime candidate for diversifying:[1]

1. When it spots opportunities for expanding into industries whose technologies and products complement its present business.
2. When it can leverage existing competencies and capabilities by expanding into businesses where these same resource strengths are key success factors and valuable competitive assets.
3. When diversifying into closely related businesses opens new avenues for reducing costs.
4. When it has a powerful and well-known brand name that can be transferred to the products of other businesses and thereby used as a lever for driving up the sales and profits of such businesses.

The decision to diversify presents wide-open possibilities. A company can diversify into closely related businesses or into totally unrelated businesses. It can diversify its present revenue and earning base to a small extent (such that new businesses account for less than 15 percent of companywide revenues and profits) or to a major extent (such that new businesses produce 30 or more percent of revenues and profits). It can move into one or two large new businesses or a greater number of small ones. It can achieve multibusiness/multi-industry status by acquiring an existing company already in a business/industry it wants to enter, starting up a new business subsidiary from scratch, or forming a joint venture with one or more companies to enter new businesses.

BUILDING SHAREHOLDER VALUE: THE ULTIMATE JUSTIFICATION FOR DIVERSIFYING

Diversification must do more for a company than simply spread its business risk across various industries. In principle, diversification cannot be considered a success unless it results in *added shareholder value*—value that shareholders cannot capture on their own by purchasing stock in companies in different industries or investing in mutual funds so as to spread their investments across several industries.

For there to be reasonable expectations that a company's diversification efforts can produce added value, a move to diversify into a new business must pass three tests:[2]

1. *The industry attractiveness test*—The industry to be entered must be attractive enough to yield consistently good returns on investment. Whether an industry is attractive depends chiefly on the presence of industry and competitive conditions that are conducive to earning as good or better profits and return on investment than the company is earning in its present business(es). It is hard to justify diversifying into an industry where profit expectations are *lower* than in the company's present businesses.

2. *The cost-of-entry test*—The cost to enter the target industry must not be so high as to erode the potential for good profitability. A catch-22 can prevail here, however. The more attractive an industry's prospects are for growth and good long-term profitability, the more expensive it can be to get into. Entry barriers for start-up companies are likely to be high in attractive industries; were barriers low, a rush of new entrants would soon erode the potential for high profitability. And buying a well-positioned company in an appealing industry often entails a high acquisition cost that makes passing the cost-of-entry test less likely. For instance, suppose that the price to purchase a company is $3 million and that the company is earning after-tax profits of $200,000 on an equity investment of $1 million (a 20 percent annual return). Simple arithmetic requires that the profits be tripled if the purchaser (paying $3 million) is to earn the same 20 percent return. Building the acquired firm's earnings from $200,000 to $600,000 annually could take several years—and require additional investment on which the purchaser would also have to earn a 20 percent return. Since the owners of a successful and growing company usually demand a price that reflects their business's profit prospects, it's easy for such an acquisition to fail the cost-of-entry test.

3. *The better-off test*—Diversifying into a new business must offer potential for the company's existing businesses and the new business to perform better together under a single corporate umbrella than they would perform operating as independent, stand-alone businesses. For example, let's say that company A diversifies by purchasing company B in another industry. If A and B's consolidated profits in the years to come prove no greater than what each could have earned on its own, then A's diversification won't provide its shareholders with added value. Company A's shareholders could have achieved the same $1 + 1 = 2$ result by merely purchasing stock in company B. Shareholder value is not created by diversification unless it produces a $1 + 1 = 3$ effect where sister businesses *perform better together* as part of the same firm than they could have performed as independent companies.

Core Concept
Creating added value for shareholders via diversification requires building a multibusiness company where the whole is greater than the sum of its parts.

Diversification moves that satisfy all three tests have the greatest potential to grow shareholder value over the long term. Diversification moves that can pass only one or two tests are suspect.

STRATEGIES FOR ENTERING NEW BUSINESSES

The means of entering new businesses can take any of three forms: acquisition, internal start-up, or joint ventures with other companies.

Acquisition of an Existing Business

Acquisition is the most popular means of diversifying into another industry. Not only is it quicker than trying to launch a brand-new operation, but it also offers an effective way to hurdle such entry barriers as acquiring technological know-how, establishing supplier relationships, becoming big enough to match rivals' efficiency and unit costs, having to spend large sums on introductory advertising and promotions, and securing adequate distribution. Buying an ongoing operation allows the acquirer to move directly to the task of building a strong market position in the target industry, rather than getting bogged down in going the internal start-up route and trying to develop the knowledge, resources, scale of operation, and market reputation necessary to become an effective competitor within a few years.

The big dilemma an acquisition-minded firm faces is whether to pay a premium price for a successful company or to buy a struggling company at a bargain price.[3] If the buying firm has little knowledge of the industry but ample capital, it is often better off purchasing a capable, strongly positioned firm—unless the price of such an acquisition flunks the cost-of-entry test. However, when the acquirer sees promising ways to transform a weak firm into a strong one and has the resources, the know-how, and the patience to do it, a struggling company can be the better long-term investment.

Internal Start-Up

Achieving diversification through *internal start-up* involves building a new business subsidiary from scratch. This entry option takes longer than the acquisition option and poses some hurdles. A newly formed business unit not only has to overcome entry barriers but also has to invest in new production capacity, develop sources of supply, hire and train employees, build channels of distribution, grow a customer base, and so on. Generally, forming a start-up subsidiary to enter a new business has appeal only when (1) the parent company already has in-house most or all of the skills and resources it needs to piece together a new business and compete effectively; (2) there is ample time to launch the business; (3) internal entry has lower costs than entry via acquisition; (4) the targeted industry is populated with many relatively small firms such that the new start-up does not have to compete head-to-head against larger, more powerful rivals; (5) adding new production capacity will not adversely impact the supply–demand balance in the industry; and (6) incumbent firms are likely to be slow or ineffective in responding to a new entrant's efforts to crack the market.[4]

> The biggest drawbacks to entering an industry by forming an internal start-up are the costs of overcoming entry barriers and the extra time it takes to build a strong and profitable competitive position.

Joint Ventures

Joint ventures entail forming a new corporate entity owned by two or more companies, where the purpose of the joint venture is to pursue a mutually attractive opportunity. The terms and conditions of a joint venture concern joint operation of a mutually owned business, which tends to make the arrangement more definitive and perhaps more durable than a strategic alliance—in a strategic alliance, the arrangement between the partners is one of limited collaboration for a limited purpose and a partner can choose to simply walk away or reduce its commitment at any time.

A joint venture to enter a new business can be useful in at least three types of situations.[5] First, a joint venture is a good vehicle for pursuing an opportunity that is too complex, uneconomical, or risky for one company to pursue alone. Second, joint ventures make sense when the opportunities in a new industry require a broader range of competencies and know-how than a company can marshal. Many of the opportunities in satellite-based telecommunications, biotechnology, and network-based systems that blend hardware, software, and services call for the coordinated development of complementary innovations and tackling an intricate web of financial, technical, political, and regulatory factors simultaneously. In such cases, pooling the resources and competencies of two or more companies is a wiser and less risky way to proceed.

Third, companies sometimes use joint ventures to diversify into a new industry when the diversification move entails having operations in a foreign country—several governments require foreign companies operating within their borders to have a local partner that has minority, if not majority, ownership in the local operations. Aside from fulfilling host government ownership requirements, companies usually seek out a local partner with expertise and other resources that will aid the success of the newly established local operation.

However, as discussed in Chapters 6 and 7, partnering with another company—in either a joint venture or a collaborative alliance—has significant drawbacks due to the potential for conflicting objectives, disagreements over how to best operate the venture, culture clashes, and so on. Joint ventures are generally the least durable of the entry options, usually lasting only until the partners decide to go their own ways.

CHOOSING THE DIVERSIFICATION PATH: RELATED VERSUS UNRELATED BUSINESSES

Core Concept
Related businesses possess competitively valuable cross-business value chain matchups; **unrelated businesses** have dissimilar value chains, containing no competitively useful cross-business relationships.

Once a company decides to diversify, its first big strategy decision is whether to diversify into related businesses, unrelated businesses, or some mix of both (see Figure 9.1). *Businesses are said to be related when their value chains possess competitively valuable cross-business relationships that present opportunities for the businesses to perform better under the same corporate umbrella than they could by operating as stand-alone entities.* The big appeal of related diversification is to build shareholder value by leveraging these cross-business relationships into competitive advantage, thus allowing the company as a whole to perform better than just the sum of its individual businesses. *Businesses are said to be unrelated when the activities comprising their respective value chains are so dissimilar that no competitively valuable cross-business relationships are present.*

The next two sections of this chapter explore the ins and outs of related and unrelated diversification.

THE CASE FOR DIVERSIFYING INTO RELATED BUSINESSES

A related diversification strategy involves building the company around businesses whose value chains possess competitively valuable strategic fits, as shown in Figure 9.2. **Strategic fit** exists whenever one or more activities comprising the value chains of different businesses are sufficiently similar as to present opportunities for:[6]

- Transferring competitively valuable expertise, technological know-how, or other capabilities from one business to another.

Figure 9.1   **Strategy Alternatives for a Company Looking to Diversify**

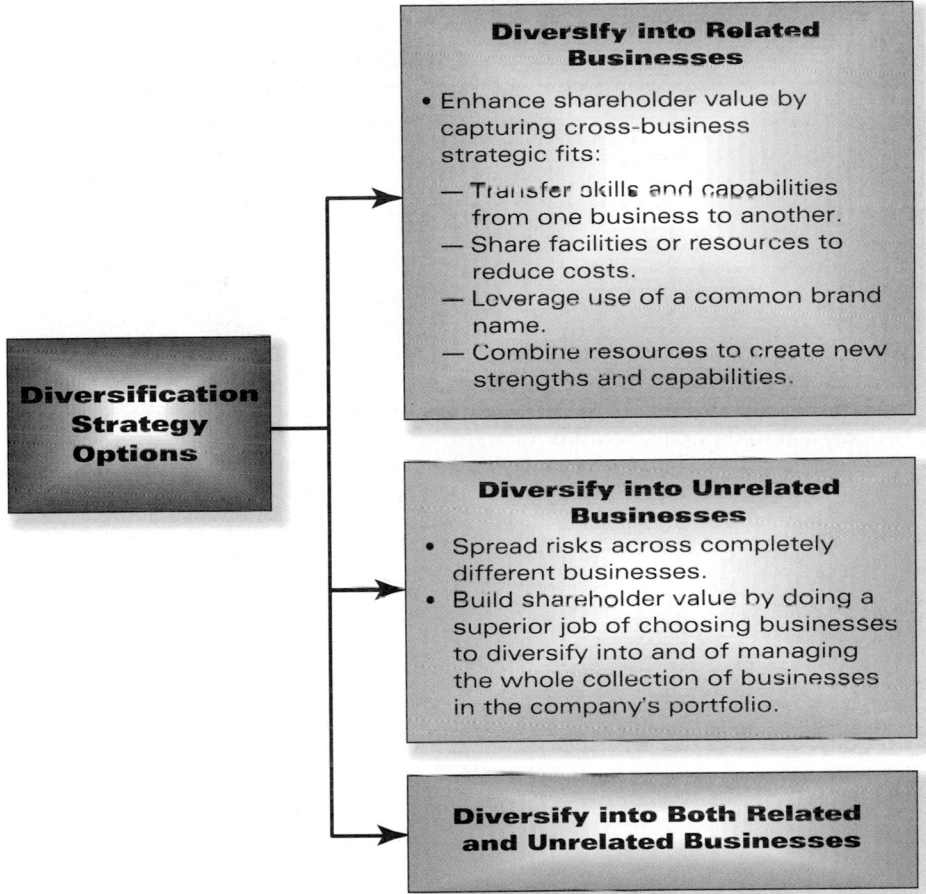

- Combining the related value chain activities of separate businesses into a single operation to achieve lower costs. For instance, it is often feasible to manufacture the products of different businesses in a single plant or use the same warehouses for shipping and distribution or have a single sales force for the products of different businesses (because they are marketed to the same types of customers).
- Exploiting common use of a well-known and potent brand name. For example, Honda's name in motorcycles and automobiles gave it instant credibility and recognition in entering the lawn-mower business, allowing it to achieve a significant market share without spending large sums on advertising to establish a brand identity for its lawn mowers. Canon's reputation in photographic equipment was a competitive asset that facilitated the company's diversification into copying equipment. Sony's name in consumer electronics made it easier and cheaper for Sony to enter the market for video games with its PlayStation console and lineup of PlayStation video games.
- Cross-business collaboration to create competitively valuable resource strengths and capabilities.

> **Core Concept**
> **Strategic fit** exists when the value chains of different businesses present opportunities for cross business resource transfer, lower costs through combining the performance of related value chain activities, cross-business use of a potent brand name, and cross-business collaboration to build new or stronger competitive capabilities.

Figure 9.2   **Related Businesses Possess Related Value Chain Activities and Competitively Valuable Strategic Fits**

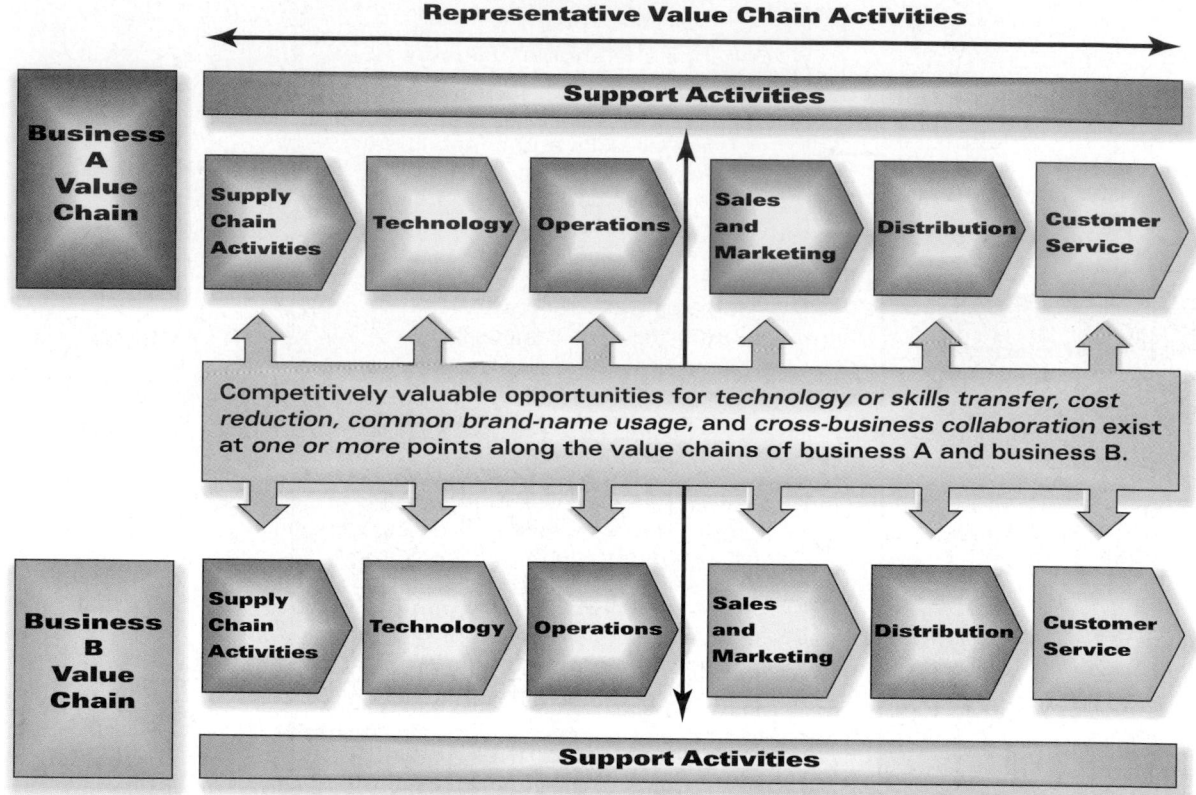

Related diversification thus has strategic appeal from several angles. It allows a firm to reap the competitive advantage benefits of skills transfer, lower costs, a powerful brand name, and/or stronger competitive capabilities and still spread investor risks over a broad business base. Furthermore, the relatedness among the different businesses provides sharper focus for managing diversification and a useful degree of strategic unity across the company's various business activities.

Identifying Cross-Business Strategic Fits along the Value Chain

Cross-business strategic fits can exist anywhere along the value chain—in R&D and technology activities, in supply chain activities and relationships with suppliers, in manufacturing, in sales and marketing, in distribution activities, or in administrative support activities.[7]

Strategic Fits in R&D and Technology Activities   Diversifying into businesses where there is potential for sharing common technology, exploiting the full range of business opportunities associated with a particular technology and its derivatives, or transferring technological know-how from one business to another has considerable appeal. Businesses with technology-sharing benefits can perform better together than apart because of potential cost savings in R&D and potentially shorter times in getting new products to market; also, technological advances in one business can lead to increased sales for both. Technological innovations have been the driver behind the efforts of cable TV companies to diversify into high-speed Internet access (via the use of cable modems) and, further, to explore providing local and long-distance telephone service to residential and commercial customers in either a single wire or using VoIP technology.

Strategic Fits in Supply Chain Activities   Businesses that have supply chain strategic fits can perform better together because of the potential for skills transfer in procuring materials, greater bargaining power in negotiating with common suppliers, the benefits of added collaboration with common supply chain partners, and/or added leverage with shippers in securing volume discounts on incoming parts and components. Dell Computer's strategic partnerships with leading suppliers of microprocessors, motherboards, disk drives, memory chips, flat-panel displays, wireless capabilities, long-life batteries, and other PC-related components have been an important element of the company's strategy to diversify into servers, data storage devices, MP3 players, and LCD TVs—products that include many components common to PCs and that can be sourced from the same strategic partners that provide Dell with PC components.

Manufacturing-Related Strategic Fits   Cross-business strategic fits in manufacturing-related activities can represent an important source of competitive advantage in situations where a diversifier's expertise in quality manufacture and cost-efficient production methods can be transferred to another business. When Emerson Electric diversified into the chain-saw business, it transferred its expertise in low-cost manufacture to its newly acquired Beaird-Poulan business division; the transfer drove Beaird-Poulan's new strategy—to be the low-cost provider of chain-saw products—and fundamentally changed the way Beaird-Poulan chain saws were designed and manufactured. Another benefit of production-related value chain matchups is the ability to consolidate production into a smaller number of plants and significantly reduce overall production costs. When snowmobile maker Bombardier diversified into motorcycles, it was able to set up motorcycle assembly lines in the same manufacturing facility where it was assembling snowmobiles. When Smuckers acquired Procter & Gamble's Jif peanut butter business, it was able to combine the manufacture of its own Smucker's peanut butter products with those of Jif; in addition, it gained greater leverage with vendors in purchasing its peanut supplies.

Distribution-Related Strategic Fits   Businesses with closely related distribution activities can perform better together than apart because of potential cost savings in sharing the same distribution facilities or using many of the same wholesale distributors and retail dealers to access customers. When Sunbeam acquired Mr. Coffee, it was able to consolidate its own distribution centers for small household appliances with those of Mr. Coffee, thereby generating considerable cost savings. Likewise, since Sunbeam products were sold to many of the same retailers as Mr. Coffee products (Wal-Mart, Kmart, Target, department stores, home centers, hardware chains, supermarket chains, and drugstore chains), Sunbeam was able to convince many of the retailers carrying Sunbeam appliances to also take on the Mr. Coffee line and vice versa.

Strategic Fits in Sales and Marketing Activities Various cost-saving opportunities spring from diversifying into businesses with closely related sales and marketing activities. The same distribution centers can be used for warehousing and shipping the products of different businesses. When the products are sold directly to the same customers, sales costs can often be reduced by using a single sales force and avoiding having two different salespeople call on the same customer. The products of related businesses can be promoted at the same Web site, and included in the same media ads and sales brochures. After-sale service and repair organizations for the products of closely related businesses can often be consolidated into a single operation. There may be opportunities to reduce costs by consolidating order processing and billing and using common promotional tie-ins (cents-off couponing, free samples and trial offers, seasonal specials, and the like). When global power-tool maker Black & Decker acquired General Electric's domestic small household appliance business, it was able to use its own global sales force and distribution facilities to sell and distribute the newly acquired GE line of toasters, irons, mixers, and coffeemakers because the types of customers that carried its power tools (discounters like Wal-Mart and Target, home centers, and hardware stores) also stocked small appliances. The economies Black & Decker achieved for both product lines were substantial.

A second category of benefits arises when different businesses use similar sales and marketing approaches; in such cases, there may be competitively valuable opportunities to transfer selling, merchandising, advertising, and product differentiation skills from one business to another. Procter & Gamble's product lineup includes Folgers coffee, Tide laundry detergent, Crest toothpaste, Ivory soap, Charmin toilet tissue, Gillette razors and blades, Duracell batteries, Oral-B toothbrushes, and Head & Shoulders shampoo. All of these have different competitors and different supply chain and production requirements, but they all move through the same wholesale distribution systems, are sold in common retail settings to the same shoppers, are advertised and promoted in much the same ways, and require the same marketing and merchandising skills.

Strategic Fits in Managerial and Administrative Support Activities Often, different businesses require comparable types managerial know-how, thereby allowing know-how in one line of business to be transferred to another. At General Electric (GE), managers who were involved in GE's expansion into Russia were able to expedite entry because of information gained from GE managers involved in expansions into other emerging markets. The lessons GE managers learned in China were passed along to GE managers in Russia, allowing them to anticipate that the Russian government would demand that GE build production capacity in the country rather than enter the market through exporting or licensing. In addition, GE's managers in Russia were better able to develop realistic performance expectations and make tough upfront decisions since experience in China and elsewhere warned them (1) that there would likely be increased short-term costs during the early years of start-up and (2) that if GE committed to the Russian market for the long term and aided the country's economic development it could eventually expect to be given the freedom to pursue profitable penetration of the Russian market.[8]

Likewise, different businesses can often use the same administrative and customer service infrastructure. For instance, an electric utility that diversifies into natural gas, water, appliance sales and repair services, and home security services can use the same customer data network, the same customer call centers and local offices, the same

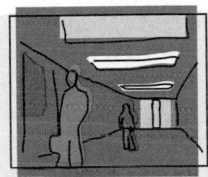

Illustration Capsule 9.1

Related Diversification at L'Oréal, Johnson & Johnson, PepsiCo, and Darden Restaurants

See if you can identify the value chain relationships that make the businesses of the following companies related in competitively relevant ways. In particular, you should consider whether there are cross-business opportunities for (1) transferring skills/technology, (2) combining related value chain activities to achieve lower costs, (3) leveraging use of a well-respected brand name, and/or (4) establishing cross-business collaboration to create new resource strengths and capabilities.

L'ORÉAL

- Maybelline, Lancôme, Helena Rubenstein, Kiehl's, Garner, and Shu Uemura cosmetics.
- L'Oréal and Soft Sheen/Carson hair care products.
- Redken, Matrix, L'Oréal Professional, and Kerastase Paris professional hair care and skin care products.
- Ralph Lauren and Giorgio Armani fragrances.
- Biotherm skin care products.
- La Roche–Posay and Vichy Laboratories dermocosmetics.

JOHNSON & JOHNSON

- Baby products (powder, shampoo, oil, lotion).
- Band-Aids and other first-aid products.
- Women's health and personal care products (Stayfree, Carefree, Sure & Natural).
- Neutrogena and Aveeno skin care products.

- Nonprescription drugs (Tylenol, Motrin, Pepcid AC, Mylanta, Monistat).
- Prescription drugs.
- Prosthetic and other medical devices.
- Surgical and hospital products.
- Accuvue contact lenses.

PEPSICO

- Soft drinks (Pepsi, Diet Pepsi, Pepsi One, Mountain Dew, Mug, Slice).
- Fruit juices (Tropicana and Dole).
- Sports drinks (Gatorade).
- Other beverages (Aquafina bottled water, SoBe, Lipton ready-to-drink tea, Frappucino—in partnership with Starbucks, international sales of 7UP).
- Snack foods (Fritos, Lay's, Ruffles, Doritos, Tostitos, Santitas, Smart Food, Rold Gold pretzels, Chee-tos, Grandma's cookies, Sun Chips, Cracker Jack, Frito-Lay dips and salsas).
- Cereals, rice, and breakfast products (Quaker oatmeal, Cap'n Crunch, Life, Rice-A-Roni, Quaker rice cakes, Aunt Jemima mixes and syrups, Quaker grits).

DARDEN RESTAURANTS

- Olive Garden restaurant chain (Italian-themed).
- Red Lobster restaurant chain (seafood-themed).
- Bahama Breeze restaurant chain (Caribbean-themed).

Source: Company Web sites, annual reports, and 10-K reports.

billing and customer accounting systems, and the same customer service infrastructure to support all of its products and services.

Illustration Capsule 9.1 lists the businesses of five companies that have pursued a strategy of related diversification.

Strategic Fit, Economies of Scope, and Competitive Advantage

What makes related diversification an attractive strategy is the opportunity to convert cross-business strategic fits into a competitive advantage over business rivals whose operations do not offer comparable strategic-fit benefits. The greater the relatedness among a diversified company's sister businesses, the bigger a company's window for converting strategic fits into competitive advantage via (1) skills transfer, (2) combining related value chain activities to achieve lower costs, (3) leveraging use of a well-respected brand name, and/or (4) cross-business collaboration to create new resource strengths and capabilities.

Economies of Scope: A Path to Competitive Advantage

One of the most important competitive advantages that a related diversification strategy can produce is lower costs than competitors. Related businesses often present opportunities to eliminate or reduce the costs of performing certain value chain activities; such cost savings are termed **economies of scope**—a concept distinct from *economies of scale*. Economies of *scale* are cost savings that accrue directly from a larger-sized operation; for example, unit costs may be lower in a large plant than in a small plant, lower in a large distribution center than in a small one, and lower for large-volume purchases of components than for small-volume purchases. Economies of *scope,* however, stem directly from cost-saving strategic fits along the value chains of related businesses. Such economies are open only to a multibusiness enterprise and are the result of a related diversification strategy that allows sister businesses to share technology, perform R&D together, use common manufacturing or distribution facilities, share a common sales force or distributor/dealer network, use the same established brand name, and/or share the same administrative infrastructure. *The greater the cross-business economies associated with cost-saving strategic fits, the greater the potential for a related diversification strategy to yield a competitive advantage based on lower costs than rivals.*

> **Core Concept**
> *Economies of scope* are cost reductions that flow from operating in multiple businesses; such economies stem directly from strategic fit efficiencies along the value chains of related businesses.

From Competitive Advantage to Added Profitability and Gains in Shareholder Value

The competitive advantage potential that flows from economies of scope and the capture of other strategic-fit benefits is what enables a company pursuing related diversification to achieve $1 + 1 = 3$ financial performance and the hoped-for gains in shareholder value. The strategic and business logic is compelling: Capturing strategic fits along the value chains of its related businesses gives a diversified company a clear path to achieving competitive advantage over undiversified competitors and competitors whose own diversification efforts don't offer equivalent strategic-fit benefits.[9] Such competitive advantage potential provides a company with a dependable basis for earning profits and a return on investment that exceed what the company's businesses could earn as stand-alone enterprises. Converting the competitive advantage potential into greater profitability is what fuels $1 + 1 = 3$ gains in shareholder value—the necessary outcome for satisfying the better-off test and proving the business merit of a company's diversification effort.

> **Core Concept**
> Diversifying into related businesses where competitively valuable strategic fit benefits can be captured puts sister businesses in position to perform better financially as part of the same company than they could have performed as independent enterprises, thus providing a clear avenue for boosting shareholder value.

There are three things to bear in mind here. One, capturing cross-business strategic fits via a strategy of related diversification builds shareholder value in ways that shareholders cannot undertake by simply owning a portfolio of stocks of companies in different industries. Two, the capture of cross-business strategic-fit benefits is possible only via a strategy of related diversification. Three, the benefits of cross-business strategic fits are not automatically realized when a company diversifies into related businesses; *the benefits materialize only after management has successfully pursued internal actions to capture them.*

Figure 9.3   **Unrelated Businesses Have Unrelated Value Chains and No Strategic Fits**

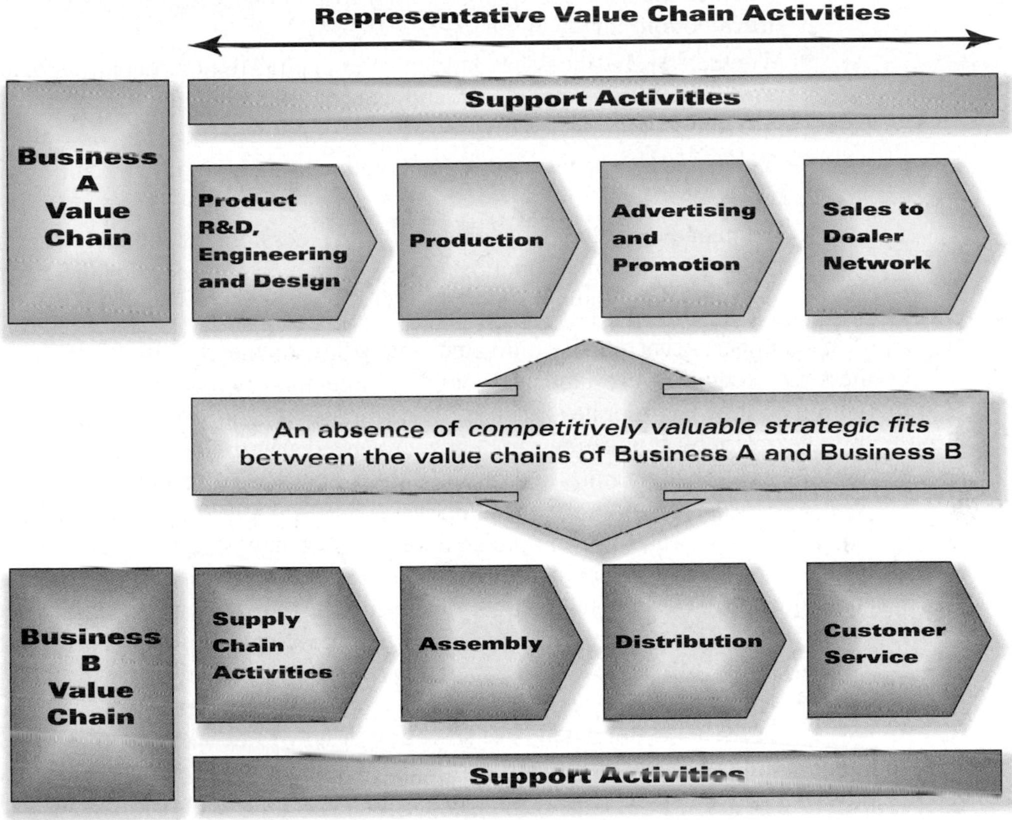

Representative Value Chain Activities

Business A Value Chain

Support Activities

Product R&D, Engineering and Design → Production → Advertising and Promotion → Sales to Dealer Network

An absence of competitively valuable strategic fits *between the value chains of Business A and Business B*

Business B Value Chain

Supply Chain Activities → Assembly → Distribution → Customer Service

Support Activities

THE CASE FOR DIVERSIFYING INTO UNRELATED BUSINESSES

An unrelated diversification strategy discounts the merits of pursuing cross-business strategic fits and, instead, focuses squarely on entering and operating businesses in industries that allow the company as a whole to grow its revenues and earnings. Companies that pursue a strategy of unrelated diversification generally exhibit a willingness to diversify into *any industry* where senior managers see *opportunity* to realize consistently good financial results— *the basic premise of unrelated diversification is that any company or business that can be acquired on good financial terms and that has satisfactory growth and earnings potential represents a good acquisition and a good business opportunity.* With a strategy of unrelated diversification, the emphasis is on satisfying the attractiveness and cost-of-entry tests and each business's prospects for good financial performance. As indicated in Figure 9.3, there's no deliberate effort to satisfy the better-off test in the sense of diversifying only into businesses having strategic fits with the firm's other businesses.

Thus, with an unrelated diversification strategy, company managers spend much time and effort screening acquisition candidates and evaluating the pros and cons of keeping or divesting existing businesses, using such criteria as:

- Whether the business can meet corporate targets for profitability and return on investment.

- Whether the business is in an industry with attractive growth potential.
- Whether the business is big enough to contribute *significantly* to the parent firm's bottom line.
- Whether the business has burdensome capital requirements (associated with replacing out-of-date plants and equipment, growing the business, and/or providing working capital).
- Whether the business is plagued with chronic union difficulties and labor problems.
- Whether there is industry vulnerability to recession, inflation, high interest rates, tough government regulations concerning product safety or the environment, and other potentially negative factors.

Companies that pursue unrelated diversification nearly always enter new businesses by acquiring an established company rather than by forming a start-up subsidiary within their own corporate structures. The premise of acquisition-minded corporations is that growth by acquisition can deliver enhanced shareholder value through upward-trending corporate revenues and earnings and a stock price that *on average* rises enough year after year to amply reward and please shareholders. Three types of acquisition candidates are usually of particular interest: (1) businesses that have bright growth prospects but are short on investment capital—cash-poor, opportunity-rich businesses are highly coveted acquisition targets for cash-rich companies scouting for good market opportunities; (2) undervalued companies that can be acquired at a bargain price; and (3) struggling companies whose operations can be turned around with the aid of the parent company's financial resources and managerial know-how.

A key issue in unrelated diversification is how wide a net to cast in building a portfolio of unrelated businesses. In other words, should a company pursuing unrelated diversification seek to have few or many unrelated businesses? How much business diversity can corporate executives successfully manage? A reasonable way to resolve the issue of how much diversification comes from answering two questions: "What is the least diversification it will take to achieve acceptable growth and profitability?" and "What is the most diversification that can be managed, given the complexity it adds?"[10] The optimal amount of diversification usually lies between these two extremes.

Illustration Capsule 9.2 lists the businesses of three companies that have pursued unrelated diversification. Such companies are frequently labeled *conglomerates* because their business interests range broadly across diverse industries.

The Merits of an Unrelated Diversification Strategy

A strategy of unrelated diversification has appeal from several angles:

1. Business risk is scattered over a set of truly *diverse* industries. In comparison to related diversification, unrelated diversification more closely approximates *pure* diversification of financial and business risk because the company's investments are spread over businesses whose technologies and value chain activities bear no close relationship and whose markets are largely disconnected.[11]

2. The company's financial resources can be employed to maximum advantage by (*a*) investing in *whatever industries* offer the best profit prospects (as opposed to considering only opportunities in industries with related value chain activities) and (*b*) diverting cash flows from company businesses with lower growth and profit prospects to acquiring and expanding businesses with higher growth and profit potentials.

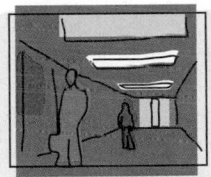

Illustration Capsule 9.2

Unrelated Diversification at General Electric, United Technologies, American Standard, and Lancaster Colony

The defining characteristic of unrelated diversification is few competitively valuable cross-business relationships. Peruse the business group listings for General Electric, United Technologies, American Standard, and Lancaster Colony and see if you can confirm why these four companies have unrelated diversification strategies.

GENERAL ELECTRIC

- Advanced materials (engineering thermoplastics, silicon-based products and technology platforms, and fused quartz and ceramics)—revenues of $8.3 billion in 2004.
- Commercial and consumer finance (loans, operating leases, financing programs and financial services provided to corporations, retailers, and consumers in 38 countries)—revenues of $39.2 billion in 2004.
- Major appliances, lighting, and integrated industrial equipment, systems and services—revenues of $13.8 billion in 2004.
- Commercial insurance and reinsurance products and services for insurance companies, Fortune 1000 companies, self-insurers, health care providers and other groups—revenues of $23.1 billion in 2004.
- Jet engines for military and civil aircraft, freight and passenger locomotives, motorized systems for mining trucks and drills, and gas turbines for marine and industrial applications—revenues of $15.6 billion in 2004.
- Electric power generation equipment, power transformers, high-voltage breakers, distribution transformers and breakers, capacitors, relays, regulators, substation equipment, metering products—revenues of $17.3 billion in 2004.
- Medical imaging and information technologies, medical diagnostics, patient monitoring systems, disease research, drug discovery and biopharmaceuticals—revenues of $13.5 billion in 2004.
- NBC Universal—owns and operates the NBC television network, a Spanish-language network (Telemundo), several news and entertainment networks (CNBC, MSNBC, Bravo, Sci-Fi Channel, USA Network), Universal Studios, various television production operations, a group of television stations, and theme parks—revenues of $12.9 billion in 2004.
- Chemical treatment programs for water and industrial process systems; precision sensors; security and safety systems for intrusion and fire detection, access and building control, video surveillance, explosives and drug detection; and real estate services—revenues of $3.4 billion in 2004.
- Equipment services, including Penske truck leasing; operating leases, loans, sales, and asset management services for owners of computer networks, trucks, trailers, railcars, construction equipment, and shipping containers—revenues of $8.5 billion in 2004.

UNITED TECHNOLOGIES

- Pratt & Whitney aircraft engines—2005 revenues of $9.3 billion.
- Carrier heating and air-conditioning equipment—2005 revenues of $12.5 billion.
- Otis elevators and escalators—2005 revenues of $9.6 billion.
- Sikorsky helicopters and Hamilton Sunstrand aerospace systems—2005 revenues of $7.2 billion.
- Chubb fire detection and security systems—2005 revenues of $4.3 billion.

AMERICAN STANDARD

- Trane and American Standard furnaces, heat pumps, and air conditioners—2005 revenues of $6.0 billion.
- American Standard, Ideal Standard, Standard, and Porcher lavatories, toilets, bath tubs, faucets, whirlpool baths, and shower basins—2005 revenues of $2.4 billion.
- Commercial and utility vehicle braking and control systems—2005 revenues of $1.8 billion.

LANCASTER COLONY

- Specialty food products: Cardini, Marzetti, Girard's, and Pheiffer salad dressings; Chatham Village croutons; New York Brand, Sister Schubert, and Mamma Bella frozen breads and rolls; Reames and Aunt Vi's frozen noodles and pastas; Inn Maid and Amish dry egg noodles; and Romanoff caviar—fiscal 2005 revenues of $674 million.
- Candles and glassware: Candle-lite candles; Indiana Glass and Fostoria drinkware and tabletop items; Colony giftware; and Brody floral containers—fiscal 2005 revenues of $234 million.
- Automotive products: Rubber Queen automotive floor mats; Dee Zee aluminum accessories and running boards for light trucks; Protecta truck bed mats; and assorted other truck accessories—fiscal 2005 revenues of $224 million.

Source: Company Web sites, annual reports, and 10-K reports.

3. To the extent that corporate managers are exceptionally astute at spotting bargain-priced companies with big upside profit potential, shareholder wealth can be enhanced by buying distressed businesses at a low price, turning their operations around fairly quickly with infusions of cash and managerial know-how supplied by the parent company, and then riding the crest of the profit increases generated by the newly acquired businesses.

4. Company profitability may prove somewhat more stable over the course of economic upswings and downswings because market conditions in all industries don't move upward or downward simultaneously—in a broadly diversified company, there's a chance that market downtrends in some of the company's businesses will be partially offset by cyclical upswings in its other businesses, thus producing somewhat less earnings volatility. (In actual practice, however, there's no convincing evidence that the consolidated profits of firms with unrelated diversification strategies are more stable or less subject to reversal in periods of recession and economic stress than the profits of firms with related diversification strategies.)

Unrelated diversification certainly merits consideration when a firm is trapped in or overly dependent on an endangered or unattractive industry, especially when it has no competitively valuable resources or capabilities it can transfer to an adjacent industry. A case can also be made for unrelated diversification when a company has a strong preference for spreading business risks widely and not restricting itself to investing in a family of closely related businesses.

Building Shareholder Value via Unrelated Diversification   Given the absence of cross-business strategic fits with which to capture added competitive advantage, the task of building shareholder value via unrelated diversification ultimately hinges on the business acumen of corporate executives. To succeed in using a strategy of unrelated diversification to produce companywide financial results above and beyond what the businesses could generate operating as stand-alone entities, corporate executives must:

- Do a superior job of diversifying into new businesses that can produce consistently good earnings and returns on investment (thereby satisfying the attractiveness test).

- Do an excellent job of negotiating favorable acquisition prices (thereby satisfying the cost-of-entry test).

- Do such a good job overseeing the firm's business subsidiaries and contributing to how they are managed—by providing expert problem-solving skills, creative strategy suggestions, and high caliber decision-making guidance to the heads of the various business subsidiaries—that the subsidiaries perform at a higher level than they would otherwise be able to do through the efforts of the business-unit heads alone (a possible way to satisfy the better-off test).

- Be shrewd in identifying when to shift resources out of businesses with dim profit prospects and into businesses with above-average prospects for growth and profitability.

- Be good at discerning when a business needs to be sold (because it is on the verge of confronting adverse industry and competitive conditions and probable declines in long-term profitability) and also finding buyers who will pay a price higher than the company's net investment in the business (so that the sale of divested businesses will result in capital gains for shareholders rather than capital losses).

To the extent that corporate executives are able to craft and execute a strategy of unrelated diversification that produces enough of the above outcomes to result in a stream of dividends and capital gains for stockholders greater than a $1 + 1 = 2$ outcome, a case can be made that shareholder value has truly been enhanced.

The Drawbacks of Unrelated Diversification

Unrelated diversification strategies have two important negatives that undercut the pluses: demanding managerial requirements and limited competitive advantage potential.

Demanding Managerial Requirements Successfully managing a set of fundamentally different businesses operating in fundamentally different industry and competitive environments is an exceptionally challenging proposition for corporate-level managers. It is difficult because key executives at the corporate level, while perhaps having personally worked in one or two of the company's businesses, rarely have the time and expertise to be sufficiently familiar with all the circumstances surrounding each of the company's businesses to be in a position to give high-caliber guidance to business-level managers. Indeed, the greater the number of businesses a company is in and the more diverse they are, the harder it is for corporate managers to (1) stay abreast of what's happening in each industry and each subsidiary and thus judge whether a particular business has bright prospects or is headed for trouble, (2) know enough about the issues and problems facing each subsidiary to pick business-unit heads having the requisite combination of managerial skills and know-how, (3) be able to tell the difference between those strategic proposals of business-unit managers that are prudent and those that are risky or unlikely to succeed, and (4) know what to do if a business unit stumbles and its results suddenly head downhill.[12]

> **Core Concept**
> The two biggest drawbacks to unrelated diversification are the difficulties of competently managing many different businesses and being without the added source of competitive advantage that cross-business strategic fit provides.

In a company like General Electric (see Illustration Capsule 9.2) or Tyco International (which acquired over 1,000 companies during the 1990–2001 period), corporate executives are constantly scrambling to stay on top of fresh industry developments and the strategic progress and plans of each subsidiary, often depending on briefings by business-level managers for many of the details. As a rule, the more unrelated businesses that a company has diversified into, the more corporate executives are dependent on briefings from business unit heads and "managing by the numbers"—that is, keeping a close track on the financial and operating results of each subsidiary and assuming that the heads of the various subsidiaries have most everything under control so long as the latest key financial and operating measures look good. Managing by the numbers works if the heads of the various business units are quite capable and consistently meet their numbers. But the problem comes when things start to go awry in a business despite the best effort of business-unit managers and corporate management has to get deeply involved in turning around a business it does not know all that much about—as the former chairman of a Fortune 500 company advised, "Never acquire a business you don't know how to run." Because every business tends to encounter rough sledding, a good way to gauge the merits of acquiring a company in an unrelated industry is to ask, "If the business got into trouble, is corporate management likely to know how to bail it out?" When the answer is no (or even a qualified yes or maybe), growth via acquisition into unrelated businesses is a chancy strategy.[13] Just one or two unforeseen declines or big strategic mistakes (misjudging the importance of certain competitive forces or the impact of driving forces or key success factors, encountering unexpected problems in a newly acquired business, or being too optimistic about turning around a struggling subsidiary) can cause a precipitous drop in corporate earnings and crash the parent company's stock price.

> Relying solely on the expertise of corporate executives to wisely manage a set of unrelated businesses is *a much weaker foundation for enhancing shareholder value* than is a strategy of related diversification where corporate performance can be boosted by competitively valuable cross-business strategic fits.

Hence, competently overseeing a set of widely diverse businesses can turn out to be much harder than it sounds. In practice, comparatively few companies have proved up to the task. There are far more companies whose corporate executives have failed at delivering consistently good financial results with an unrelated diversification strategy than there are companies with corporate executives who have been successful.[14] It is simply very difficult for corporate executives to achieve $1 + 1 = 3$ gains in shareholder value based on their expertise in (*a*) picking which industries to diversify into and which companies in these industries to acquire, (*b*) shifting resources from low-performing businesses into high-performing businesses, and (*c*) giving high-caliber decision-making guidance to the general managers of their business subsidiaries. The odds are that the result of unrelated diversification will be $1 + 1 = 2$ or less.

Limited Competitive Advantage Potential   The second big negative is that *unrelated diversification offers no potential for competitive advantage beyond what each individual business can generate on its own.* Unlike a related diversification strategy, there are no cross-business strategic fits to draw on for reducing costs, beneficially transferring skills and technology, leveraging use of a powerful brand name, or collaborating to build mutually beneficial competitive capabilities and thereby *adding to any competitive advantage possessed by individual businesses.* Yes, a cash-rich corporate parent pursuing unrelated diversification can provide its subsidiaries with much-needed capital and maybe even the managerial know-how to help resolve problems in particular business units, but otherwise it has little to offer in the way of enhancing the competitive strength of its individual business units. *Without the competitive advantage potential of strategic fits, consolidated performance of an unrelated group of businesses stands to be little or no better than the sum of what the individual business units could achieve if they were independent.*

COMBINATION RELATED–UNRELATED DIVERSIFICATION STRATEGIES

There's nothing to preclude a company from diversifying into both related and unrelated businesses. Indeed, in actual practice the business makeup of diversified companies varies considerably. Some diversified companies are really *dominant-business enterprises*—one major "core" business accounts for 50 to 80 percent of total revenues and a collection of small related or unrelated businesses accounts for the remainder. Some diversified companies are *narrowly diversified* around a few (two to five) related or unrelated businesses. Others are *broadly diversified* around a wide-ranging collection of related businesses, unrelated businesses, or a mixture of both. And a number of multibusiness enterprises have diversified into unrelated areas but have a collection of related businesses within each area—thus giving them a business portfolio consisting of *several unrelated groups of related businesses*. There's ample room for companies to customize their diversification strategies to incorporate elements of both related and unrelated diversification, as may suit their own risk preferences and strategic vision.

Figure 9.4   **Identifying a Diversified Company's Strategy**

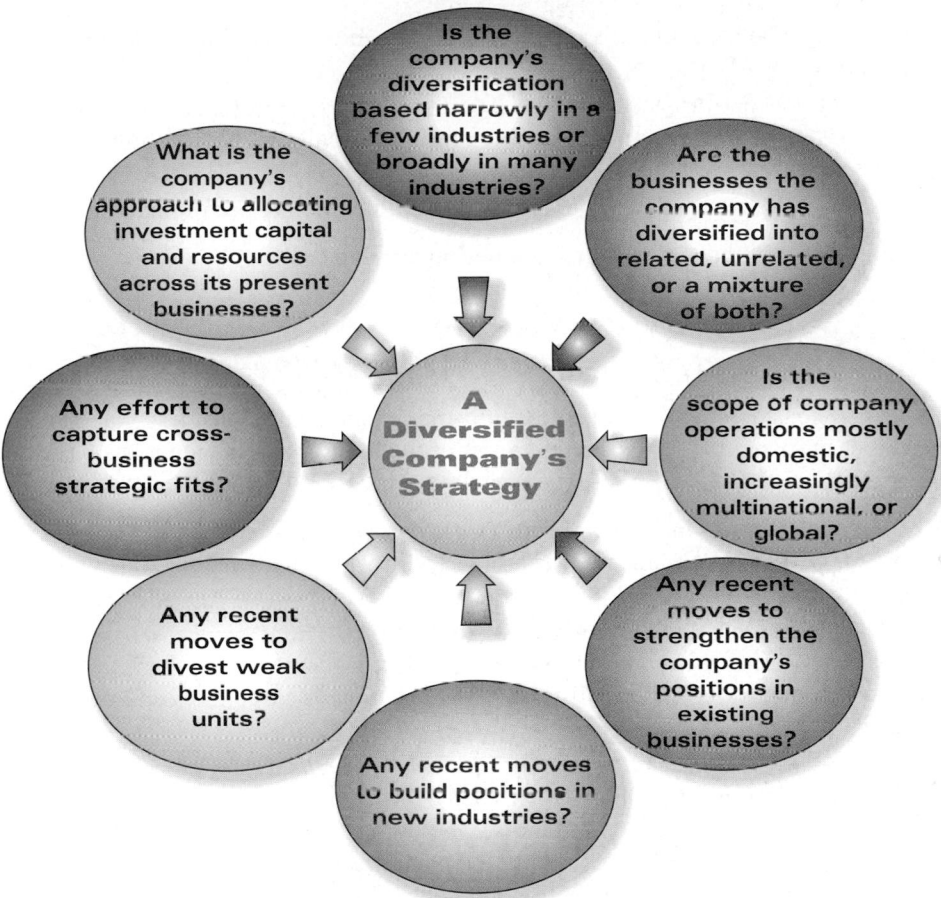

Figure 9.4 indicates what to look for in identifying the main elements of a company's diversification strategy. Having a clear fix on the company's current corporate strategy sets the stage for evaluating how good the strategy is and proposing strategic moves to boost the company's performance.

EVALUATING THE STRATEGY OF A DIVERSIFIED COMPANY

Strategic analysis of diversified companies builds on the concepts and methods used for single-business companies. But there are some additional aspects to consider and a couple of new analytical tools to master. The procedure for evaluating the pluses and minuses of a diversified company's strategy and deciding what actions to take to improve the company's performance involves six steps:

1. Assessing the attractiveness of the industries the company has diversified into, both individually and as a group.
2. Assessing the competitive strength of the company's business units and determining how many are strong contenders in their respective industries.

3. Checking the competitive advantage potential of cross-business strategic fits among the company's various business units.

4. Checking whether the firm's resources fit the requirements of its present business lineup.

5. Ranking the performance prospects of the businesses from best to worst and determining what the corporate parent's priority should be in allocating resources to its various businesses.

6. Crafting new strategic moves to improve overall corporate performance.

The core concepts and analytical techniques underlying each of these steps merit further discussion.

Step 1: Evaluating Industry Attractiveness

A principal consideration in evaluating a diversified company's business makeup and the caliber of its strategy is the attractiveness of the industries in which it has business operations. Answers to several questions are required:

1. *Does each industry the company has diversified into represent a good business for the company to be in?* Ideally, each industry in which the firm operates will pass the attractiveness test.

2. *Which of the company's industries are most attractive and which are least attractive?* Comparing the attractiveness of the industries and ranking them from most to least attractive is a prerequisite to wise allocation of corporate resources across the various businesses.

3. *How appealing is the whole group of industries in which the company has invested?* The answer to this question points to whether the group of industries holds promise for attractive growth and profitability. A company whose revenues and profits come chiefly from businesses in relatively unattractive industries probably needs to look at divesting businesses in unattractive industries and entering industries that qualify as highly attractive.

The more attractive the industries (both individually and as a group) a diversified company is in, the better its prospects for good long-term performance.

Calculating Industry Attractiveness Scores for Each Industry into Which the Company Has Diversified   A simple and reliable analytical tool involves calculating quantitative industry attractiveness scores, which can then be used to gauge each industry's attractiveness, rank the industries from most to least attractive, and make judgments about the attractiveness of all the industries as a group.

The following measures are typically used to gauge an industry's attractiveness:

- *Market size and projected growth rate*—Big industries are more attractive than small industries, and fast-growing industries tend to be more attractive than slow-growing industries, other things being equal.

- *The intensity of competition*—Industries where competitive pressures are relatively weak are more attractive than industries where competitive pressures are strong.

- *Emerging opportunities and threats*—Industries with promising opportunities and minimal threats on the near horizon are more attractive than industries with modest opportunities and imposing threats.

- *The presence of cross-industry strategic fits*—The more the industry's value chain and resource requirements match up well with the value chain activities of other industries in which the company has operations, the more attractive the industry is to a firm pursuing related diversification. However, cross-industry strategic fits may be of no consequence to a company committed to a strategy of unrelated diversification.

- *Resource requirements*—Industries having resource requirements within the company's reach are more attractive than industries where capital and other resource requirements could strain corporate financial resources and organizational capabilities.

- *Seasonal and cyclical factors*—Industries where buyer demand is relatively steady year-round and not unduly vulnerable to economic ups and downs tend to be more attractive than industries where there are wide swings in buyer demand within or across years. However, seasonality may be a plus for a company that is in several seasonal industries, if the seasonal highs in one industry correspond to the lows in another industry, thus helping even out monthly sales levels. Likewise, cyclical market demand in one industry can be attractive if its up-cycle runs counter to the market down-cycles in another industry where the company operates, thus helping reduce revenue and earnings volatility.

- *Social, political, regulatory, and environmental factors*—Industries with significant problems in such areas as consumer health, safety, or environmental pollution or that are subject to intense regulation are less attractive than industries where such problems are not burning issues.

- *Industry profitability*—Industries with healthy profit margins and high rates of return on investment are generally more attractive than industries where profits have historically been low or unstable.

- *Industry uncertainty and business risk*—Industries with less uncertainty on the horizon and lower overall business risk are more attractive than industries whose prospects for one reason or another are quite uncertain, especially when the industry has formidable resource requirements.

After settling on a set of attractiveness measures that suit a diversified company's circumstances, each attractiveness measure is assigned a weight reflecting its relative importance in determining an industry's attractiveness—it is weak methodology to assume that the various attractiveness measures are equally important. The intensity of competition in an industry should nearly always carry a high weight (say, 0.20 to 0.30). Strategic-fit considerations should be assigned a high weight in the case of companies with related diversification strategies; but, for companies with an unrelated diversification strategy, strategic fits with other industries may be given a low weight or even dropped from the list of attractiveness measures altogether. Seasonal and cyclical factors generally are assigned a low weight (or maybe even eliminated from the analysis) unless a company has diversified into industries strongly characterized by seasonal demand and/or heavy vulnerability to cyclical upswings and downswings. The importance weights must add up to 1.0.

Next, each industry is rated on each of the chosen industry attractiveness measures, using a rating scale of 1 to 10 (where a *high* rating signifies *high* attractiveness and a *low* rating signifies *low* attractiveness). *Keep in mind here that the more intensely competitive an industry is, the lower the attractiveness rating for that industry.* Likewise, the higher the capital and resource requirements associated with being in a particular industry, the lower the attractiveness rating. And an industry that is subject

Table 9.1   **Calculating Weighted Industry Attractiveness Scores**

Industry Attractiveness Measure	Importance Weight	Industry A Rating/ Score	Industry B Rating/ Score	Industry C Rating/ Score	Industry D Rating/ Score
Market size and projected growth rate	0.10	8/0.80	5/0.50	7/0.70	3/0.30
Intensity of competition	0.25	8/2.00	7/1.75	3/0.75	2/0.50
Emerging opportunities and threats	0.10	2/0.20	9/0.90	4/0.40	5/0.50
Cross-industry strategic fits	0.20	8/1.60	4/0.80	8/1.60	2/0.40
Resource requirements	0.10	9/0.90	7/0.70	10/1.00	5/0.50
Seasonal and cyclical influences	0.05	9/0.45	8/0.40	10/0.50	5/0.25
Societal, political, regulatory, and environmental factors	0.05	10/1.00	7/0.70	7/0.70	3/0.30
Industry profitability	0.10	5/0.50	10/1.00	3/0.30	3/0.30
Industry uncertainty and business risk	0.05	5/0.25	7/0.35	10/0.50	1/0.05
Sum of the assigned weights	1.00				
Overall industry attractiveness scores		**7.70**	**7.10**	**5.45**	**3.10**

Rating scale: 1 = Very unattractive to company; 10 = Very attractive to company.

to stringent pollution control regulations or that causes societal problems (like cigarettes or alcoholic beverages) should usually be given a low attractiveness rating. Weighted attractiveness scores are then calculated by multiplying the industry's rating on each measure by the corresponding weight. For example, a rating of 8 times a weight of 0.25 gives a weighted attractiveness score of 2.00. The sum of the weighted scores for all the attractiveness measures provides an overall industry attractiveness score. This procedure is illustrated in Table 9.1.

Interpreting the Industry Attractiveness Scores   Industries with a score much below 5.0 probably do not pass the attractiveness test. If a company's industry attractiveness scores are all above 5.0, it is probably fair to conclude that the group of industries the company operates in is attractive as a whole. But the group of industries takes on a decidedly lower degree of attractiveness as the number of industries with scores below 5.0 increases, especially if industries with low scores account for a sizable fraction of the company's revenues.

For a diversified company to be a strong performer, a substantial portion of its revenues and profits must come from business units with relatively high attractiveness scores. It is particularly important that a diversified company's principal businesses be in industries with a good outlook for growth and above-average profitability. Having a big fraction of the company's revenues and profits come from industries with slow growth, low profitability, or intense competition tends to drag overall company performance down. Business units in the least attractive industries are potential candidates for divestiture, unless they are positioned strongly enough to overcome the unattractive aspects of their industry environments or they are a strategically important component of the company's business makeup.

The Difficulties of Calculating Industry Attractiveness Scores   There are two hurdles to calculating industry attractiveness scores. One is deciding on appropriate weights for the industry attractiveness measures. Not only may different analysts have diffcrent views about which weights are appropriate for the different attractiveness measures but also different weightings may be appropriate for diffcrent companies—based on their strategies, performance targets, and financial circumstances. For instance, placing a low weight on industry resource requirements may be justifiable for a cash-rich company, whereas a high weight may be more appropriate for a financially strapped company. The second hurdle is gaining sufficient command of the industry to assign accurate and objective ratings. Generally, a company can come up with the statistical data needed to compare its industries on such factors as market size, growth rate, seasonal and cyclical influences, and industry profitability. Cross-industry fits and resource requirements are also fairly easy to judge. But the attractiveness measure where judgment weighs most heavily is that of intensity of competition. It is not always easy to conclude whether competition in one industry is stronger or weaker than in another industry because of the different types of competitive influences that prevail and the differences in their relative importance. In the event that the available information is too skimpy to confidently assign a rating value to an industry on a particular attractiveness measure, then it is usually best to use a score of 5, which avoids biasing the overall attractiveness score either up or down.

But despite the hurdlcs, calculating industry attractiveness scores is a systcmatic and reasonably reliable method for ranking a diversified company's industries from most to least attractive—numbers like those shown for the four industries in Table 9.1 help pin down the basis for judging which industries are more attractive and to what degree.

Step 2: Evaluating Business-Unit Competitive Strength

The second stcp in evaluating a diversified company is to appraise how strongly positioned each of its business units are in their respective industry. Doing an appraisal of each business unit's strength and competitive position in its industry not only reveals its chances for industry success but also provides a basis for ranking the units from competitively strongest to competitively weakest and sizing up the competitive strength of all the business units as a group.

Calculating Competitive Strength Scores for Each Business Unit   Quantitative measures of each business unit's competitive strength can be calculated using a procedure similar to that for measuring industry attractiveness. The following factors are using in quantifying the compctitive strengths of a diversified company's business subsidiaries:

- *Relative market share*—A business unit's *relative market share* is defined as the ratio of its market share to the market share held by the largest rival firm in the industry, with market share measured in unit volume, not dollars. For instance, if business A has a market-leading share of 40 percent and its largest rival has 30 percent, A's relative market share is 1.33. (Note that only business units that are market share leaders in their respective industries can have relative market shares greater then 1.0.) If business B has a 15 percent market share and B's largest rival has 30 percent, B's relative market share is 0.5. *The further below 1.0 a business unit's relative market share is, the weaker its competitive strength and market position vis-à-vis rivals.* A 10 percent market share, for example, does not signal much competitive strength if the leader's share is 50 percent

Using relative market share to measure competitive strength is analytically superior to using straight-percentage market share.

(a 0.20 relative market share), but a 10 percent share is actually quite strong if the leader's share is only 12 percent (a 0.83 relative market share)—this is why a company's relative market share is a better measure of competitive strength than a company's market share based on either dollars or unit volume.

- *Costs relative to competitors' costs*—Business units that have low costs relative to key competitors' costs tend to be more strongly positioned in their industries than business units struggling to maintain cost parity with major rivals. Assuming that the prices charged by industry rivals are about the same, there's reason to expect that business units with higher relative market shares have lower unit costs than competitors with lower relative market shares because their greater unit sales volumes offer the possibility of economies from larger-scale operations and the benefits of any experience/learning curve effects. Another indicator of low cost can be a business unit's supply chain management capabilities. The only time when a business unit's competitive strength may not be undermined by having higher costs than rivals is when it has incurred the higher costs to strongly differentiate its product offering and its customers are willing to pay premium prices for the differentiating features.

- *Ability to match or beat rivals on key product attributes*—A company's competitiveness depends in part on being able to satisfy buyer expectations with regard to features, product performance, reliability, service, and other important attributes.

- *Ability to benefit from strategic fits with sister businesses*—Strategic fits with other businesses within the company enhance a business unit's competitive strength and may provide a competitive edge.

- *Ability to exercise bargaining leverage with key suppliers or customers*—Having bargaining leverage signals competitive strength and can be a source of competitive advantage.

- *Caliber of alliances and collaborative partnerships with suppliers and/or buyers*—Well-functioning alliances and partnerships may signal a potential competitive advantage vis-à-vis rivals and thus add to a business's competitive strength. Alliances with key suppliers are often the basis for competitive strength in supply chain management.

- *Brand image and reputation*—A strong brand name is a valuable competitive asset in most industries.

- *Competitively valuable capabilities*—Business units recognized for their technological leadership, product innovation, or marketing prowess are usually strong competitors in their industry. Skills in supply chain management can generate valuable cost or product differentiation advantages. So can unique production capabilities. Sometimes a company's business units gain competitive strength because of their knowledge of customers and markets and/or their proven managerial capabilities. *An important thing to look for here is how well a business unit's competitive assets match industry key success factors.* The more a business unit's resource strengths and competitive capabilities match the industry's key success factors, the stronger its competitive position tends to be.

- *Profitability relative to competitors*—Business units that consistently earn above-average returns on investment and have bigger profit margins than their rivals usually have stronger competitive positions. Moreover, above-average profitability signals competitive advantage, while below-average profitability usually denotes competitive disadvantage.

Table 9.2   **Calculating Weighted Competitive Strength Scores for a Diversified Company's Business Units**

Competitive Strength Measure	Importance Weight	Business A in Industry A Rating/ Score	Business B in Industry B Rating/ Score	Business C in Industry C Rating/ Score	Business D in Industry D Rating/ Score
Relative market share	0.15	10/1.50	1/0.15	6/0.90	2/0.30
Costs relative to competitors' costs	0.20	7/1.40	2/0.40	5/1.00	3/0.00
Ability to match or beat rivals on key product attributes	0.05	9/0.45	4/0.20	8/0.40	4/0.20
Ability to benefit from strategic fits with sister businesses	0.20	8/1.60	4/0.80	8/0.80	2/0.60
Bargaining leverage with suppliers/ buyers; caliber of alliances	0.05	9/0.90	3/0.30	6/0.30	2/0.10
Brand image and reputation	0.10	9/0.90	2/0.20	7/0.70	5/0.50
Competitively valuable capabilities	0.15	7/1.05	2/0.20	5/0.75	3/0.45
Profitability relative to competitors	0.10	5/0.50	1/0.10	4/0.40	4/0.40
Sum of the assigned weights	1.00				
Overall industry attractiveness scores		**8.30**	**2.35**	**5.25**	**3.15**

Rating scale: 1 = Very weak; 10 = Very strong.

After settling on a set of competitive strength measures that are well matched to the circumstances of the various business units, weights indicating each measure's importance need to be assigned. A case can be made for using different weights for different business units whenever the importance of the strength measures differs significantly from business to business, but otherwise it is simpler just to go with a single set of weights and avoid the added complication of multiple weights. As before, the importance weights must add up to 1.0. Each business unit is then rated on each of the chosen strength measures, using a rating scale of 1 to 10 (where a *high* rating signifies competitive *strength* and a *low* rating signifies competitive *weakness*). In the event that the available information is too skimpy to confidently assign a rating value to a business unit on a particular strength measure, then it is usually best to use a score of 5, which avoids biasing the overall score either up or down. Weighted strength ratings are calculated by multiplying the business unit's rating on each strength measure by the assigned weight. For example, a strength score of 6 times a weight of 0.15 gives a weighted strength rating of 0.90. The sum of weighted ratings across all the strength measures provides a quantitative measure of a business unit's overall market strength and competitive standing. Table 9.2 provides sample calculations of competitive strength ratings for four businesses.

Interpreting the Competitive Strength Scores   Business units with competitive strength ratings above 6.7 (on a scale of 1 to 10) are strong market contenders in their industries. Businesses with ratings in the 3.3 to 6.7 range have moderate competitive strength vis-à-vis rivals. Businesses with ratings below 3.3 are in competitively weak market positions. If a diversified company's business units all have competitive strength scores above 5.0, it is fair to conclude that its business units are all fairly strong market contenders in their respective industries. But as the number of business units with scores below 5.0 increases, there's reason to question whether the company can perform well with so many businesses in relatively weak competitive positions. This concern takes on even more importance when business units with low scores account for a sizable fraction of the company's revenues.

Using a Nine-Cell Matrix to Simultaneously Portray Industry Attractiveness and Competitive Strength   The industry attractiveness and competitive strength scores can be used to portray the strategic positions of each business in a diversified company. Industry attractiveness is plotted on the vertical axis, and competitive strength on the horizontal axis. A nine-cell grid emerges from dividing the vertical axis into three regions (high, medium, and low attractiveness) and the horizontal axis into three regions (strong, average, and weak competitive strength). As shown in Figure 9.5, high attractiveness is associated with scores of 6.7 or greater on a rating scale of 1 to 10, medium attractiveness to scores of 3.3 to 6.7, and low attractiveness to scores below 3.3. Likewise, high competitive strength is defined as a score greater than 6.7, average strength as scores of 3.3 to 6.7, and low strength as scores below 3.3. *Each business unit is plotted on the nine-cell matrix according to its overall attractiveness score and strength score, and then shown as a bubble.* The size of each bubble is scaled to what percentage of revenues the business generates relative to total corporate revenues. The bubbles in Figure 9.5 were located on the grid using the four industry attractiveness scores from Table 9.1 and the strength scores for the four business units in Table 9.2.

The locations of the business units on the attractiveness–strength matrix provide valuable guidance in deploying corporate resources to the various business units. In general, *a diversified company's prospects for good overall performance are enhanced by concentrating corporate resources and strategic attention on those business units having the greatest competitive strength and positioned in highly attractive industries*—specifically, businesses in the three cells in the upper left portion of the attractiveness–strength matrix, where industry attractiveness and competitive strength/market position are both favorable. The general strategic prescription for businesses falling in these three cells (for instance, business A in Figure 9.5) is "grow and build," with businesses in the high–strong cell standing first in line for resource allocations by the corporate parent.

Next in priority come businesses positioned in the three diagonal cells stretching from the lower left to the upper right (businesses B and C in Figure 9.5). Such businesses usually merit medium or intermediate priority in the parent's resource allocation ranking. However, some businesses in the medium-priority diagonal cells may have brighter or dimmer prospects than others. For example, a small business in the upper right cell of the matrix (like business B), despite being in a highly attractive industry, may occupy too weak a competitive position in its industry to justify the investment and resources needed to turn it into a strong market contender and shift its position leftward in the matrix over time. If, however, a business in the upper right cell has attractive opportunities for rapid growth and a good potential for winning a much stronger market position over time, it may merit a high claim on the corporate parent's resource allocation ranking and be given the capital it needs to pursue a grow-and-build strategy–the strategic objective here would be to move the business leftward in the attractiveness–strength matrix over time.

Businesses in the three cells in the lower right corner of the matrix (like business D in Figure 9.5) typically are weak performers and have the lowest claim on corporate resources. Most such businesses are good candidates for being divested (sold to other companies) or else managed in a manner calculated to squeeze out the maximum cash flows from operations—the cash flows from low-performing/low-potential businesses

Figure 9.5   A Nine-Cell Industry Attractiveness–Competitive Strength Matrix

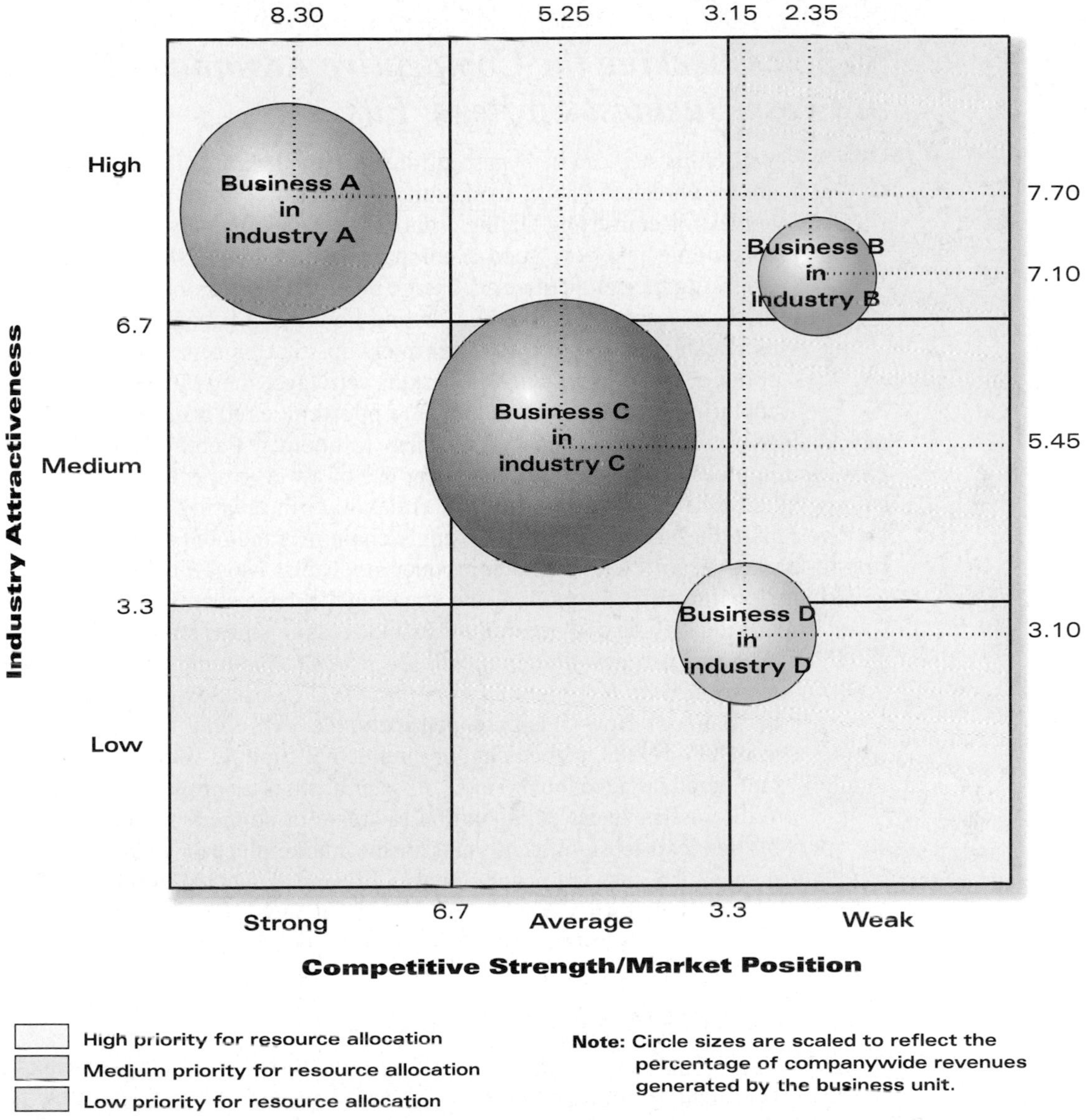

can then be diverted to financing expansion of business units with greater market opportunities. In exceptional cases where a business located in the three lower right cells is nonetheless fairly profitable (which it might be if it is in the low–average cell) or has the potential for good earnings and return on investment, the business merits retention and the allocation of sufficient resources to achieve better performance.

The nine-cell attractiveness–strength matrix provides clear, strong logic for why a diversified company needs to consider both industry attractiveness and business strength in allocating resources and investment capital to its different businesses. A good case can be made for concentrating resources in those businesses that enjoy higher degrees of attractiveness and competitive strength, being very selective in making investments in businesses with intermediate positions on the grid, and withdrawing resources from businesses that are lower in attractiveness and strength unless they offer exceptional profit or cash flow potential.

Step 3: Checking the Competitive Advantage Potential of Cross-Business Strategic Fits

> **Core Concept**
> A company's related diversification strategy derives its power in large part from the presence of competitively valuable strategic fits among its businesses.

While this step can be bypassed for diversified companies whose businesses are all unrelated (since, by design, no strategic fits are present), a high potential for converting strategic fits into competitive advantage is central to concluding just how good a company's related diversification strategy is. Checking the competitive advantage potential of cross-business strategic fits involves searching for and evaluating how much benefit a diversified company can gain from value chain matchups that present (1) opportunities to combine the performance of certain activities, thereby reducing costs and capturing economies of scope; (2) opportunities to transfer skills, technology, or intellectual capital from one business to another, thereby leveraging use of existing resources; (3) opportunities to share use of a well-respected brand name; and (4) opportunities for sister businesses to collaborate in creating valuable new competitive capabilities (such as enhanced supply chain management capabilities, quicker first-to-market capabilities, or greater product innovation capabilities).

Figure 9.6 illustrates the process of comparing the value chains of sister businesses and identifying competitively valuable cross-business strategic fits. *But more than just strategic fit identification is needed. The real test is what competitive value can be generated from these fits.* To what extent can cost savings be realized? How much competitive value will come from cross-business transfer of skills, technology, or intellectual capital? Will transferring a potent brand name to the products of sister businesses grow sales significantly? Will cross-business collaboration to create or strengthen competitive capabilities lead to significant gains in the marketplace or in financial performance? Absent significant strategic fits and dedicated company efforts to capture the benefits, one has to be skeptical about the potential for a diversified company's businesses to perform better together than apart.

> **Core Concept**
> The greater the value of cross-business strategic fits in enhancing a company's performance in the marketplace or on the bottom line, the more competitively powerful is its strategy of related diversification.

Step 4: Checking for Resource Fit

> **Core Concept**
> Sister businesses possess *resource fit* when they add to a company's overall resource strengths and when a company has adequate resources to support their requirements.

The businesses in a diversified company's lineup need to exhibit good **resource fit.** Resource fit exists when (1) businesses add to a company's overall resource strengths and (2) a company has adequate resources to support its entire group of businesses without spreading itself too thin. One important dimension of resource fit concerns whether a diversified company can generate the internal cash flows sufficient to fund the capital requirements of its businesses, pay its dividends, meet its debt obligations, and otherwise remain financially healthy.

Financial Resource Fits: Cash Cows versus Cash Hogs   Different businesses have different cash flow and investment characteristics. For example, business units in rapidly growing industries are often **cash hogs**—so labeled because the cash flows they are able to generate from internal operations aren't big enough to fund their expansion. To keep pace with rising buyer demand, rapid-growth businesses frequently need sizable annual capital investments—for new facilities and equipment, for

Figure 9.6   **Identifying the Competitive Advantage Potential of Cross-Business Strategic Fits**

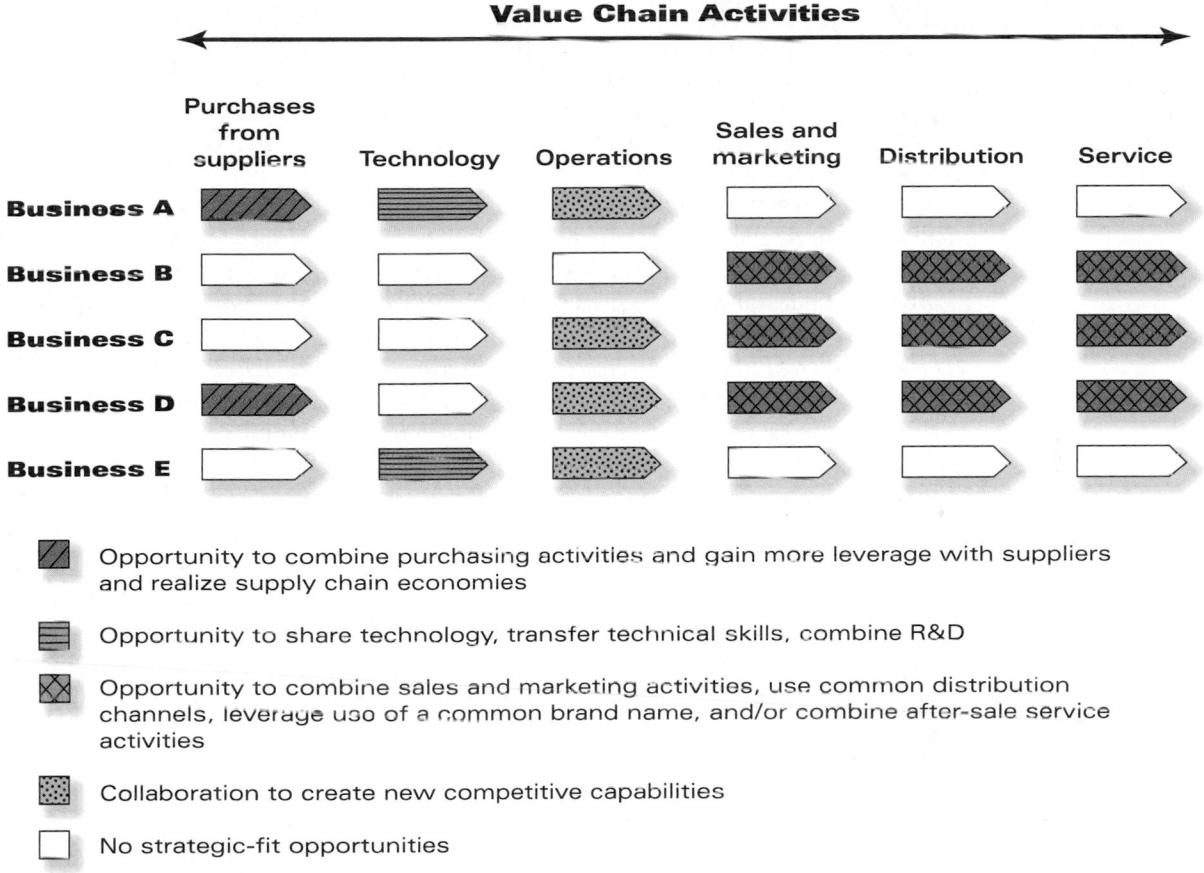

Opportunity to combine purchasing activities and gain more leverage with suppliers and realize supply chain economies

Opportunity to share technology, transfer technical skills, combine R&D

Opportunity to combine sales and marketing activities, use common distribution channels, leverage use of a common brand name, and/or combine after-sale service activities

Collaboration to create new competitive capabilities

No strategic-fit opportunities

new product development or technology improvements, and for additional working capital to support inventory expansion and a larger base of operations. A business in a fast-growing industry becomes an even bigger cash hog when it has a relatively low market share and is pursuing a strategy to become an industry leader. Because a cash hog's financial resources must be provided by the corporate parent, corporate managers have to decide whether it makes good financial and strategic sense to keep pouring new money into a business that continually needs cash infusions.

In contrast, business units with leading market positions in mature industries may, however, be **cash cows**—businesses that generate substantial cash surpluses over what is needed to adequately fund their operations. Market leaders in slow-growth industries often generate sizable positive cash flows *over and above what is needed for growth and reinvestment* because their industry-leading positions tend to give them the sales volumes and reputation to earn attractive profits and because the slow-growth nature of their industry often entails relatively modest annual investment requirements. Cash cows, though not always attractive from a growth standpoint, are valuable businesses from a financial resource perspective. The surplus cash flows they generate can be used to pay corporate dividends, finance acquisitions, and provide

> **Core Concept**
> A **cash hog** generates cash flows that are too small to fully fund its operations and growth; a cash hog requires cash infusions to provide additional working capital and finance new capital investment.

funds for investing in the company's promising cash hogs. It makes good financial and strategic sense for diversified companies to keep cash cows in healthy condition, fortifying and defending their market position so as to preserve their cash-generating capability over the long term and thereby have an ongoing source of financial resources to deploy elsewhere. The cigarette business is one of the world's biggest cash cows. General Electric, whose business lineup is shown in Illustration Capsule 9.2, considers that its advanced materials, equipment services, and appliance and lighting businesses are cash cows.

Viewing a diversified group of businesses as a collection of cash flows and cash requirements (present and future) is a major step forward in understanding what the financial ramifications of diversification are and why having businesses with good financial resource fit is so important. For instance, *a diversified company's businesses exhibit good financial resource fit when the excess cash generated by its cash cows is sufficient to fund the investment requirements of promising cash hogs*. Ideally, investing in promising cash hog businesses over time results in growing the hogs into self-supporting *star businesses* that have strong or market-leading competitive positions in attractive, high-growth markets and high levels of profitability. Star businesses are often the cash cows of the future—when the markets of star businesses begin to mature and their growth slows, their competitive strength should produce self-generated cash flows more than sufficient to cover their investment needs. The "success sequence" is thus cash hog to young star (but perhaps still a cash hog) to self-supporting star to cash cow.

If, however, a cash hog has questionable promise (either because of low industry attractiveness or a weak competitive position), then it becomes a logical candidate for divestiture. Pursuing an aggressive invest-and-expand strategy for a cash hog with an uncertain future seldom makes sense because it requires the corporate parent to keep pumping more capital into the business with only a dim hope of eventually turning the cash hog into a future star and realizing a good return on its investments. Such financially draining businesses fail the resource fit test because they strain the corporate parent's ability to adequately fund its other businesses. Divesting a cash hog is usually the best alternative unless (1) it has valuable strategic fits with other business units or (2) the capital infusions needed from the corporate parent are modest relative to the funds available and there's a decent chance of growing the business into a solid bottom-line contributor yielding a good return on invested capital.

Other Tests of Resource Fit   Aside from cash flow considerations, there are four other factors to consider in determining whether the businesses comprising a diversified company's portfolio exhibit good resource fit:

- *Does the business adequately contribute to achieving companywide performance targets?* A business has good financial fit when it contributes to the achievement of corporate performance objectives (growth in earnings per share, above-average return on investment, recognition as an industry leader, etc.) and when it materially enhances shareholder value via helping drive increases in the company's stock price. A business exhibits poor financial fit if it soaks up a disproportionate share of the company's financial resources, makes subpar or inconsistent bottom-line contributions, is unduly risky and failure would jeopardize the entire enterprise, or remains too small to make a material earnings contribution even though it performs well.

- *Does the company have adequate financial strength to fund its different businesses and maintain a healthy credit rating?* A diversified company's strategy fails the resource fit test when its financial resources are stretched across so many businesses that its credit rating is impaired. Severe financial strain sometimes occurs when a company borrows so heavily to finance new acquisitions that it has to trim way back on capital expenditures for existing businesses and use the big majority of its financial resources to meet interest obligations and to pay down debt. Time Warner, Royal Ahold, and AT&T, for example, have found themselves so financially overextended that they have had to sell off some of their business units to raise the money to pay down burdensome debt obligations and continue to fund essential capital expenditures for the remaining businesses.

- *Does the company have or can it develop the specific resource strengths and competitive capabilities needed to be successful in each of its businesses?*[15] Sometimes the resource strengths a company has accumulated in its core or mainstay business prove to be a poor match with the key success factors and competitive capabilities needed to succeed in one or more businesses it has diversified into. For instance, BTR, a multibusiness company in Great Britain, discovered that the company's resources and managerial skills were quite well suited for parenting industrial manufacturing businesses but not for parenting its distribution businesses (National Tyre Services and Texas-based Summers Group); as a consequence, BTR decided to divest its distribution businesses and focus exclusively on diversifying around small industrial manufacturing.[16] One company with businesses in restaurants and retailing decided that its resource capabilities in site selection, controlling operating costs, management selection and training, and supply chain logistics would enable it to succeed in the hotel business and in property management; but what management missed was that these businesses had some significantly different key success factors—namely, skills in controlling property development costs, maintaining low overheads, product branding (hotels), and ability to recruit a sufficient volume of business to maintain high levels of facility use.[17] Thus, a mismatch between the company's resource strengths and the key success factors in a particular business can be serious enough to warrant divesting an existing business or not acquiring a new business. In contrast, when a company's resources and capabilities are a good match with the key success factors of industries it is not presently in, it makes sense to take a hard look at acquiring companies in these industries and expanding the company's business lineup.

- *Are recently acquired businesses acting to strengthen a company's resource base and competitive capabilities or are they causing its competitive and managerial resources to be stretched too thin?* A diversified company has to guard against overtaxing its resource strengths, a condition that can arise when (1) it goes on an acquisition spree and management is called on to assimilate and oversee many new businesses very quickly or (2) when it lacks sufficient resource depth to do a creditable job of transferring skills and competences from one of its businesses to another (especially, a large acquisition or several lesser ones). The broader the diversification, the greater the concern about whether the company has sufficient managerial depth to cope with the diverse range of operating problems its wide business lineup presents. And the more a company's diversification strategy is tied to transferring its existing know-how or technologies to new businesses, the more it has to develop a big enough and deep enough resource pool to supply these businesses with sufficient capability to create competitive advantage.[18] Otherwise its strengths end up being thinly spread across many businesses and the opportunity for competitive advantage slips through the cracks.

A Cautionary Note About Transferring Resources from One Business to Another   Just because a company has hit a home run in one business doesn't mean it can easily enter a new business with similar resource requirements and hit a second home run.[19] Noted British retailer Marks & Spencer, despite possessing a range of impressive resource capabilities (ability to choose excellent store locations, having a supply chain that gives it both low costs and high merchandise quality, loyal employees, an excellent reputation with consumers, and strong management expertise) that have made it one of Britain's premier retailers for 100 years, has failed repeatedly in its efforts to diversify into department store retailing in the United States. Even though Philip Morris (now named Altria) had built powerful consumer marketing capabilities in its cigarette and beer businesses, it floundered in soft drinks and ended up divesting its acquisition of 7UP after several frustrating years of competing against strongly entrenched and resource-capable rivals like Coca-Cola and PepsiCo. Then in 2002 it decided to divest its Miller Brewing business—despite its long-standing marketing successes in cigarettes and in its Kraft Foods subsidiary—because it was unable to grow Miller's market share in head-to-head competition against the considerable marketing prowess of Anheuser-Busch.

Step 5: Ranking the Performance Prospects of Business Units and Assigning a Priority for Resource Allocation

Once a diversified company's strategy has been evaluated from the perspective of industry attractiveness, competitive strength, strategic fit, and resource fit, the next step is to rank the performance prospects of the businesses from best to worst and determine which businesses merit top priority for resource support and new capital investments by the corporate parent.

The most important considerations in judging business-unit performance are sales growth, profit growth, contribution to company earnings, and return on capital invested in the business. Sometimes cash flow is a big consideration. Information on each business's past performance can be gleaned from a company's financial records. While past performance is not necessarily a good predictor of future performance, it does signal whether a business already has good-to-excellent performance or has problems to overcome.

Furthermore, the industry attractiveness/business strength evaluations provide a solid basis for judging a business's prospects. Normally, strong business units in attractive industries have significantly better prospects than weak businesses in unattractive industries. And, normally, the revenue and earnings outlook for businesses in fast-growing industries is better than for businesses in slow-growing industries—one important exception is when a business in a slow-growing industry has the competitive strength to draw sales and market share away from its rivals and thus achieve much faster growth than the industry as whole. As a rule, the prior analyses, taken together, signal which business units are likely to be strong performers on the road ahead and which are likely to be laggards. And it is a short step from ranking the prospects of business units to drawing conclusions about whether the company as a whole is capable of strong, mediocre, or weak performance in upcoming years.

Figure 9.7   The Chief Strategic and Financial Options for Allocating a Diversified Company's Financial Resources

Strategic Options for Allocating Company Financial Resources	Financial Options for Allocating Company Financial Resources
Invest in ways to strengthen or grow existing businesses	Pay off existing long-term or short-term debt
Make acquisitions to establish positions in new industries or to complement existing businesses	Increase dividend payments to shareholders
Fund long-range R&D ventures aimed at opening market opportunities in new or existing businesses	Repurchase shares of the company's common stock
	Build cash reserves; invest in short-term securities

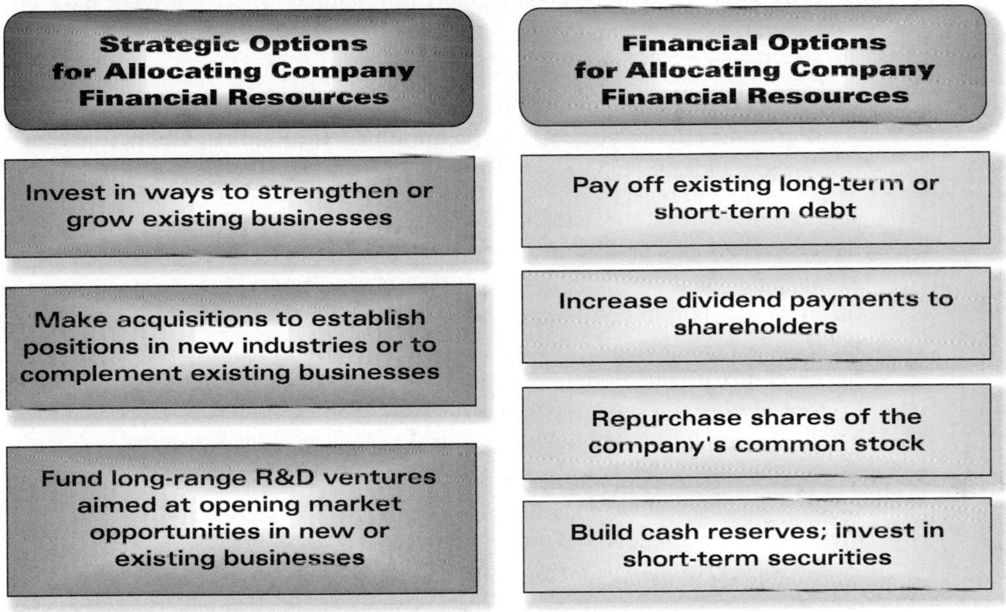

The rankings of future performance generally determine what priority the corporate parent should give to each business in terms of resource allocation. The task here is to decide which business units should have top priority for corporate resource support and new capital investment and which should carry the lowest priority. *Business subsidiaries with the brightest profit and growth prospects and solid strategic and resource fits generally should head the list for corporate resource support.* More specifically, corporate executives need to consider whether and how corporate resources can be used to enhance the competitiveness of particular business units. And they must be diligent in steering resources out of low-opportunity areas and into high-opportunity areas. Divesting marginal businesses is one of the best ways of freeing unproductive assets for redeployment. Surplus funds from cash cows also add to the corporate treasury.

Figure 9.7 shows the chief strategic and financial options for allocating a diversified company's financial resources. Ideally, a company will have enough funds to do what is needed, both strategically and financially. If not, strategic uses of corporate resources should usually take precedence unless there is a compelling reason to strengthen the firm's balance sheet or divert financial resources to pacify shareholders.

Step 6: Crafting New Strategic Moves to Improve Overall Corporate Performance

The diagnosis and conclusions flowing from the five preceding analytical steps set the agenda for crafting strategic moves to improve a diversified company's overall performance. The strategic options boil down to five broad categories of actions:

1. Sticking closely with the existing business lineup and pursuing the opportunities these businesses present.

2. Broadening the company's business scope by making new acquisitions in new industries.

3. Divesting certain businesses and retrenching to a narrower base of business operations.

4. Restructuring the company's business lineup and putting a whole new face on the company's business makeup.

5. Pursuing multinational diversification and striving to globalize the operations of several of the company's business units.

The option of sticking with the current business lineup makes sense when the company's present businesses offer attractive growth opportunities and can be counted on to generate good earnings and cash flows. As long as the company's set of existing businesses puts it in good position for the future and these businesses have good strategic and/or resource fits, then rocking the boat with major changes in the company's business mix is usually unnecessary. Corporate executives can concentrate their attention on getting the best performance from each of its businesses, steering corporate resources into those areas of greatest potential and profitability. The specifics of "what to do" to wring better performance from the present business lineup have to be dictated by each business's circumstances and the preceding analysis of the corporate parent's diversification strategy.

However, in the event that corporate executives are not entirely satisfied with the opportunities they see in the company's present set of businesses and conclude that changes in the company's direction and business makeup are in order, they can opt for any of the four other strategic alternatives listed above. These options are discussed in the following section.

AFTER A COMPANY DIVERSIFIES: THE FOUR MAIN STRATEGY ALTERNATIVES

Diversifying is by no means the final chapter in the evolution of a company's strategy. Once a company has diversified into a collection of related or unrelated businesses and concludes that some overhaul is needed in the company's present lineup and diversification strategy, there are four main strategic paths it can pursue (see Figure 9.8). To more fully understand the strategic issues corporate managers face in the ongoing process of managing a diversified group of businesses, we need to take a brief look at the central thrust of each of the four postdiversification strategy alternatives.

Strategies to Broaden a Diversified Company's Business Base

Diversified companies sometimes find it desirable to build positions in new industries, whether related or unrelated. There are several motivating factors. One is sluggish growth that makes the potential revenue and profit boost of a newly acquired business look attractive. A second is vulnerability to seasonal or recessionary influences or to threats from emerging new technologies. A third is the potential for transferring resources and capabilities to other related or complementary businesses. A fourth is rapidly changing conditions in one or more of a company's core businesses brought on by technological, legislative, or new product innovations that alter buyer requirements and preferences. For instance, the passage of legislation in the United States allowing

Figure 9.8 **A Company's Four Main Strategic Alternatives After It Diversifies**

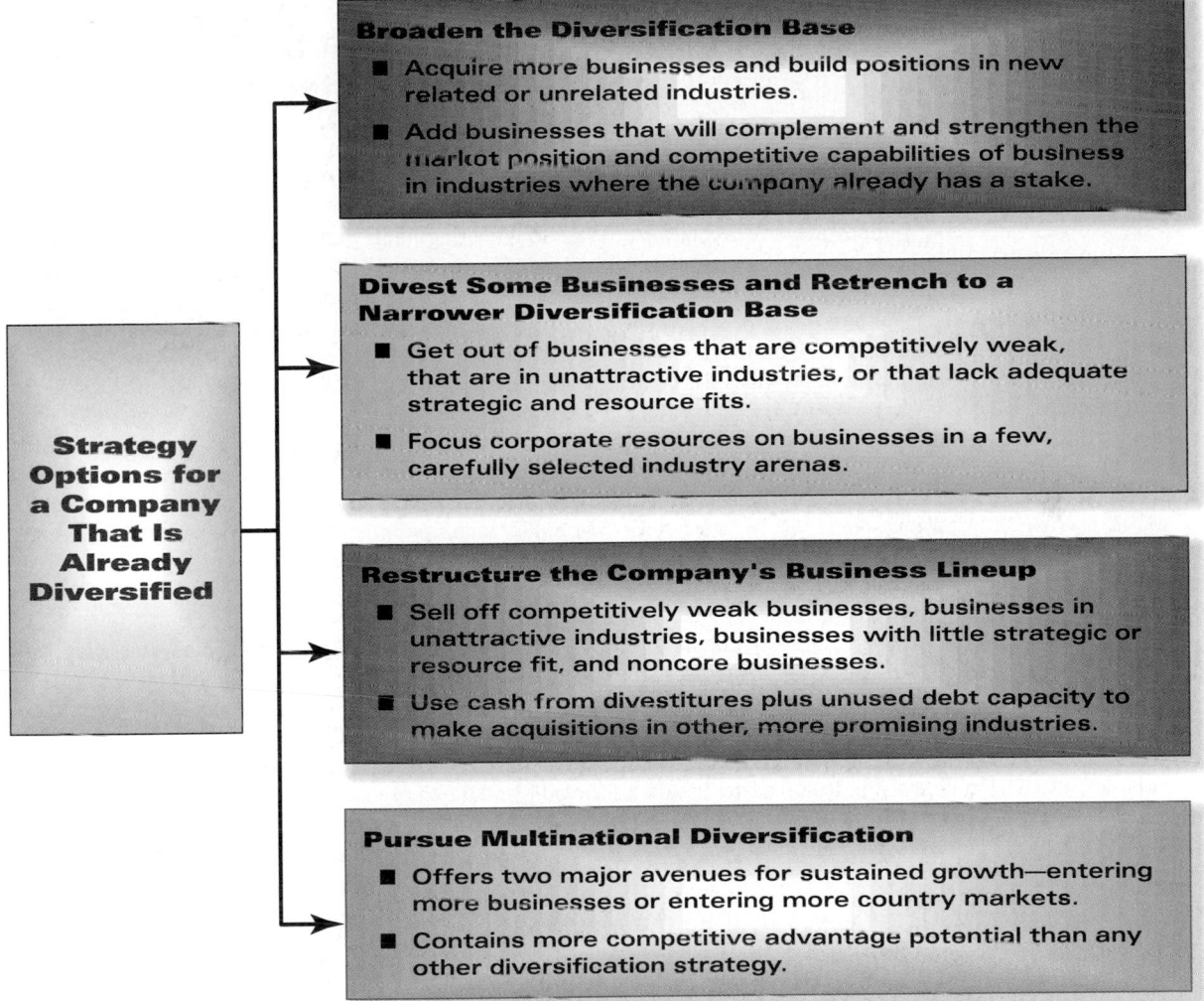

Strategy Options for a Company That Is Already Diversified

Broaden the Diversification Base
■ Acquire more businesses and build positions in new related or unrelated industries.
■ Add businesses that will complement and strengthen the market position and competitive capabilities of business in industries where the company already has a stake.

Divest Some Businesses and Retrench to a Narrower Diversification Base
■ Get out of businesses that are competitively weak, that are in unattractive industries, or that lack adequate strategic and resource fits.
■ Focus corporate resources on businesses in a few, carefully selected industry arenas.

Restructure the Company's Business Lineup
■ Sell off competitively weak businesses, businesses in unattractive industries, businesses with little strategic or resource fit, and noncore businesses.
■ Use cash from divestitures plus unused debt capacity to make acquisitions in other, more promising industries.

Pursue Multinational Diversification
■ Offers two major avenues for sustained growth—entering more businesses or entering more country markets.
■ Contains more competitive advantage potential than any other diversification strategy.

banks, insurance companies, and stock brokerages to enter each other's businesses spurred a raft of acquisitions and mergers to create full-service financial enterprises capable of meeting the multiple financial needs of customers. Citigroup, already the largest U.S. bank, with a global banking franchise, acquired Salomon Smith Barney to position itself in the investment banking and brokerage business and acquired insurance giant Travelers Group to enable it to offer customers insurance products.

A fifth, and often very important, motivating factor for adding new businesses is to complement and strengthen the market position and competitive capabilities of one or more of its present businesses. Procter & Gamble's recent acquisition of Gillette strengthened and extended P&G's reach into personal care and household products— Gillette's businesses included Oral-B toothbrushes, Gillette razors and razor blades, Duracell batteries, Braun shavers and small appliances (coffeemakers, mixers, hair dryers, and electric toothbrushes), and toiletries (Right Guard, Foamy, Soft & Dry, White Rain, and Dry Idea). Unilever, a leading maker of food and personal care products, expanded its business lineup by acquiring SlimFast, Ben & Jerry's Homemade,

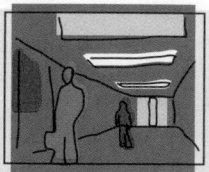

Illustration Capsule 9.3

Managing Diversification at Johnson & Johnson: The Benefits of Cross-Business Strategic Fits

Johnson & Johnson (J&J), once a consumer products company known for its Band-Aid line and its baby care products, has evolved into a $42 billion diversified enterprise consisting of some 200-plus operating companies organized into three divisions: drugs, medical devices and diagnostics, and consumer products. Over the past decade J&J has acquired 56 businesses at a cost of about $30 billion; about 10 to 15 percent of J&J's annual growth in revenues has come from acquisitions. Much of the company's recent growth has been in the pharmaceutical division, which in 2004 accounted for 47 percent of J&J's revenues and 57 percent of its operating profits.

While each of J&J's business units sets its own strategies and operates with its own finance and human resource departments, corporate management strongly encourages cross-business cooperation and collaboration, believing that many of the advances in 21st century medicine will come from applying advances in one discipline to another. J&J had 9,300 scientists working in 40 research labs in 2003, and the frequency of cross-disciplinary collaboration was increasing. One of J&J's new drug-coated stents grew out of a discussion between a drug researcher and a researcher in the company's stent business. (When stents are inserted to prop open arteries following angioplasty, the drug coating helps prevent infection.) A gene technology database compiled by the company's gene research lab was shared with personnel from the diagnostics division, who developed a test that the drug R&D people could use to predict which patients would most benefit from an experimental cancer therapy. J&J experts in various diseases have been meeting quarterly for the past five years to share information, and top management is setting up cross-disciplinary groups to focus on new treatments for particular diseases. J&J's new liquid Band-Aid product (a liquid coating applied to hard-to-cover places like fingers and knuckles) is based on a material used in a wound-closing product sold by the company's hospital products company.

J&J's corporate management maintains that close collaboration among people in its diagnostics, medical devices, and pharmaceuticals businesses—where numerous cross-business strategic fits exist—gives J&J an edge on competitors, most of whom cannot match the company's breadth and depth of expertise.

Sources: Amy Barrett, "Staying on Top," *BusinessWeek,* May 5, 2003, pp. 60–68, and www.jnj.com (accessed October 19, 2005).

and Bestfoods (whose brands included Knorr's soups, Hellman's mayonnaise, Skippy peanut butter, and Mazola cooking oils). Unilever saw these businesses as giving it more clout in competing against such other diversified food and household products companies as Nestlé, Kraft, Procter & Gamble, Campbell Soup, and General Mills.

Usually, expansion into new businesses is undertaken by acquiring companies already in the target industry. Some companies depend on new acquisitions to drive a major portion of their growth in revenues and earnings, and thus are always on the acquisition trail. Cisco Systems built itself into a worldwide leader in networking systems for the Internet by making 95 technology-based acquisitions during 1993–2005 to extend its market reach from routing and switching into Internet Protocol (IP) telephony, home networking, wireless local-area networking (LAN), storage networking, network security, broadband, and optical and broadband systems. Tyco International, now recovering from charges of looting on the part of several top executives, transformed itself from an obscure company in the early 1990s into a $40 billion global manufacturing enterprise with operations in over 100 countries as of 2005 by making over 1,000 acquisitions; the company's far-flung diversification includes businesses in electronics, electrical components, fire and security systems, health care products, valves, undersea telecommunications systems, plastics, and adhesives. Tyco made over 700 acquisitions of small companies in the 1999–2001 period alone. As a group, Tyco's businesses were cash cows, generating a combined free cash flow in 2005 of around $4.4 billion.

Illustration Capsule 9.3 describes how Johnson & Johnson has used acquisitions to diversify far beyond its well-known Band-Aid and baby care businesses and become a major player in pharmaceuticals, medical devices, and medical diagnostics.

Divestiture Strategies Aimed at Retrenching to a Narrower Diversification Base

A number of diversified firms have had difficulty managing a diverse group of businesses and have elected to get out of some of them. Retrenching to a narrower diversification base is usually undertaken when top management concludes that its diversification strategy has ranged too far afield and that the company can improve long-term performance by concentrating on build-ing stronger positions in a smaller number of core businesses and industries. Hewlett-Packard spun off its testing and measurement businesses into a stand-alone company called Agilent Technologies so that it could better concen-trate on its PC, workstation, server, printer and peripherals, and electronics businesses. PepsiCo divested its cash-hog group of restaurant businesses, consisting of KFC, Pizza Hut, Taco Bell, and California Pizza Kitchens, to provide more resources for strength-ening its soft-drink business (which was losing market share to Coca-Cola) and growing its more profitable Frito-Lay snack foods business. Kmart divested OfficeMax, Sports Authority, and Borders Bookstores in order to refocus management attention and all of the company's resources on restoring luster to its distressed discount retailing business, which was (and still is) being totally outclassed in the marketplace by Wal-Mart and Target. In 2003–2004, Tyco International began a program to divest itself of some 50 businesses, including its entire undersea fiber-optics telecommunications network and an assortment of businesses in its fire and security division; the initiative also involved consolidating 219 manufacturing, sales, distribution, and other facilities and reducing its workforce of some 260,000 people by 7,200. Lucent Technology's retrenchment strategy is described in Illustration Capsule 9.4.

> Focusing corporate resources on a few core and mostly related businesses avoids the mistake of diversifying so broadly that resources and management attention are stretched too thin.

But there are other important reasons for divesting one or more of a company's present businesses. Sometimes divesting a business has to be considered because mar-ket conditions in a once-attractive industry have badly deteriorated. A business can become a prime candidate for divestiture because it lacks adequate strategic or re-source fit, because it is a cash hog with questionable long-term potential, or because it is weakly positioned in its industry with little prospect the corporate parent can realize a decent return on its investment in the business. Sometimes a company acquires busi-nesses that, down the road, just do not work out as expected even though management has tried all it can think of to make them profitable—mistakes cannot be completely avoided because it is hard to foresee how getting into a new line of business will actu-ally work out. Subpar performance by some business units is bound to occur, thereby raising questions of whether to divest them or keep them and attempt a turnaround. Other business units, despite adequate financial performance, may not mesh as well with the rest of the firm as was originally thought.

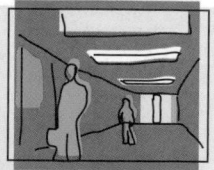

Illustration Capsule 9.4
Lucent Technology's Retrenchment Strategy

At the height of the telecommunications boom in 1999–2000, Lucent Technology was a company with $38.3 billion in revenues and 157,000 employees; it was the biggest maker of telecommunications equipment in the United States and a recognized leader worldwide. The company's strategy was to build positions in a number of blossoming technologies and industry arenas and achieve 20 percent annual revenue growth in each of 11 different business groups. But when customers' orders for new equipment began to evaporate in 2000–2001, Lucent's profits vanished and the once-growing company found itself battling to overcome bloated costs, deep price discounting, and customer defaults on the $7.5 billion in loans Lucent had made to finance their purchases. As it became clear that equipment sales and prices would never return to former levels, Lucent executives concluded that the company had overextended itself trying to do too many things and needed to pare its lineup of businesses.

Alongside efforts to curtail lavish spending at the company's fabled Bell Labs research unit, make deep workforce cutbacks, streamline order-taking and billing systems, shore up the balance sheet, and conserve cash by ending dividend payments, management launched a series of retrenchment initiatives:

- Of the 40 businesses Lucent acquired since 1996, 27 were sold, closed, or spun off.

- Lucent ceased all manufacturing operations, opting to outsource everything.

- It stopped making gear for wireless phone networks based on global system for mobile communication (GSM) technology (the dominant technology used in Europe and much of the world) in order to focus more fully on wireless gear using code division multiple

access (CDMA) technology (a technology prevalent in the United States and some developing nations). As of 2004 Lucent had an estimated 45 percent share in the CDMA market and the CDMA gear division was the company's chief revenue and profit producer.

- The wireline and wireless business units were combined to form a single, unified organization called Network Solutions.

- All the remaining businesses were grouped into a unit called Lucent Worldwide Services that was engaged in designing, implementing, integrating, and managing sophisticated voice and data networks for service providers in 45 countries.

- The role of Bell Labs was narrowed to supporting the efforts of both the Network Solutions group and the Worldwide Services group.

Lucent's strategic moves to retrench stemmed a string of 13 straight money-losing quarters. In fiscal 2004 Lucent reported profits of $2 billion from continuing operations (equal to EPS of $0.47 but still far below the levels of $0.93 in 2000 and $1.12 in 1999). In May 2004, Lucent announced its first acquisition in four years, buying a maker of Internet transmission technology for $300 million to help it become a leader in Internet telephony technology. Going into 2006, Lucent was a company with sales of about $9 billion (versus $38 billion in 1999) and a workforce of about 30,000 (versus 157,000 in 1999). The company's stock price, which reached a high of $62 in 1999 before crashing to below $1 in 2002, languished in the $3–$4 range for most of 2004–2005, indicating continuing investor skepticism about Lucent's prospects despite its having retreated to businesses where it was strongest.

Sources: Shawn Young, "Less May Be More," *The Wall Street Journal,* October 23, 2004, p. R10, and www.lucent.com (accessed October 19, 2005).

On occasion, a diversification move that seems sensible from a strategic-fit stand point turns out to be a poor *cultural fit.*[20] Several pharmaceutical companies had just this experience. When they diversified into cosmetics and perfume, they discovered their personnel had little respect for the "frivolous" nature of such products compared to the far nobler task of developing miracle drugs to cure the ill. The absence of shared values and cultural compatibility between the medical research and chemical-compounding expertise of the pharmaceutical companies and the fashion/marketing orientation of the cosmetics business was the undoing of what otherwise was diversification into businesses with technology-sharing potential, product-development fit, and some overlap in distribution channels.

There's evidence indicating that pruning businesses and narrowing a firm's diversification base improves corporate performance.[21] Corporate parents often end up selling off businesses too late and at too low a price, sacrificing shareholder value.[22] A useful guide to determine whether or when to divest a business subsidiary is to ask, "If we were not in this business today, would we want to get into it now?"[23] When the answer is no or probably not, divestiture should be considered. Another signal that a business should become a divestiture candidate is whether it is worth more to another company than to the present parent; in such cases, shareholders would be well served if the company sells the business and collects a premium price from the buyer for whom the business is a valuable fit.[24]

> Diversified companies need to divest low-performing businesses or businesses that don't fit in order to concentrate on expanding existing businesses and entering new ones where opportunities are more promising.

The Two Options for Divesting a Business: Selling It or Spinning It Off as an Independent Company   Selling a business outright to another company is far and away the most frequently used option for divesting a business. But sometimes a business selected for divestiture has ample resource strengths to compete successfully on its own. In such cases, a corporate parent may elect to spin the unwanted business off as a financially and managerially independent company, either by selling shares to the investing public via an initial public offering or by distributing shares in the new company to existing shareholders of the corporate parent. When a corporate parent decides to spin off one of its businesses as a separate company, it must decide whether or not to retain partial ownership. Retaining partial ownership makes sense when the business to be divested has a hot product or technological capabilities that give it good profit prospects. When 3Com elected to divest its PalmPilot business, which investors then saw as having very promising profit potential, it elected to retain a substantial ownership interest so as to provide 3Com shareholders a way of participating in whatever future market success that PalmPilot (now Palm Inc.) might have on its own. In 2001, when Philip Morris (now Altria) became concerned that its popular Kraft Foods subsidiary was suffering because of its affiliation with Philip Morris's cigarette business (antismoking groups were leading a national boycott of Kraft macaroni and cheese, and a Harris poll revealed that about 16 percent of people familiar with Philip Morris had boycotted its products), Philip Morris executives opted to spin Kraft Foods off as an independent public company but retained a controlling ownership interest. R. J. Reynolds Tobacco was also spun off from Nabisco Foods in 1999 in an effort to distance the tobacco operations part of the company from the food operations part. (Nabisco was then acquired by Philip Morris in 2000 and integrated into Kraft Foods.) In 2005, Cendant announced it would split its diversified businesses into four separate publicly traded companies—one for vehicle rental services (which consisted of Avis and Budget car rental companies); one for real estate and mortgage services (which included Century 21, Coldwell Banker, ERA, Sotheby's International Realty, and NRT—a residential real estate brokerage company); one for hospitality and lodging (consisting of such hotels and motel chains as Wyndam, Ramada, Days Inn, Howard Johnson, Travelodge, AmeriHost Inn, and Knights Inn, plus an assortment of time-share resort properties); and one for travel (consisting of various travel agencies, online ticket and vacation travel sites like Orbitz and Cheap Tickets, and vacation rental operations handling some 55,000 villas and condos). Cendant said the reason for the split-up was that shareholders would realize more value from operating the businesses independently—a clear sign that Cendant's diversification strategy had failed to deliver added shareholder value and that the parts were worth more than the whole.

Selling a business outright requires finding a buyer. This can prove hard or easy, depending on the business. As a rule, a company selling a troubled business should not ask, "How can we pawn this business off on someone, and what is the most we can get for it?"[25] Instead, it is wiser to ask, "For what sort of company would this business be a good fit, and under what conditions would it be viewed as a good deal?" Enterprises for which the business is a good fit are likely to pay the highest price. Of course, if a buyer willing to pay an acceptable price cannot be found, then a company must decide whether to keep the business until a buyer appears; spin it off as a separate company; or, in the case of a crisis-ridden business that is losing substantial sums, simply close it down and liquidate the remaining assets. Liquidation is obviously a last resort.

Strategies to Restructure a Company's Business Lineup

Core Concept
Restructuring involves divesting some businesses and acquiring others so as to put a whole new face on the company's business lineup.

Restructuring strategies involve divesting some businesses and acquiring others so as to put a whole new face on the company's business lineup. Performing radical surgery on a company's group of businesses is an appealing strategy alternative when its financial performance is being squeezed or eroded by:

- Too many businesses in slow-growth, declining, low-margin, or otherwise unattractive industries (a condition indicated by the number and size of businesses with industry attractiveness ratings below 5 and located on the bottom half of the attractiveness–strength matrix—see Figure 9.5).
- Too many competitively weak businesses (a condition indicated by the number and size of businesses with competitive strength ratings below 5 and located on the right half of the attractiveness–strength matrix).
- Ongoing declines in the market shares of one or more major business units that are falling prey to more market-savvy competitors.
- An excessive debt burden with interest costs that eat deeply into profitability.
- Ill-chosen acquisitions that haven't lived up to expectations.

Restructuring can also be mandated by the emergence of new technologies that threaten the survival of one or more of a diversified company's important businesses or by the appointment of a new CEO who decides to redirect the company. On occasion, restructuring can be prompted by special circumstances—as when a firm has a unique opportunity to make an acquisition so big and important that it has to sell several existing business units to finance the new acquisition, or when a company needs to sell off some businesses in order to raise the cash for entering a potentially big industry with wave-of-the-future technologies or products.

Candidates for divestiture in a corporate restructuring effort typically include not only weak or up-and-down performers or those in unattractive industries but also business units that lack strategic fit with the businesses to be retained, businesses that are cash hogs or that lack other types of resource fit, and businesses incompatible with the company's revised diversification strategy (even though they may be profitable or in an attractive industry). As businesses are divested, corporate restructuring generally involves aligning the remaining business units into groups with the best strategic fits and then redeploying the cash flows from the divested business to either pay down debt or make new acquisitions to strengthen the parent company's business position in the industries it has chosen to emphasize.[26]

Over the past decade, corporate restructuring has become a popular strategy at many diversified companies, especially those that had diversified broadly into many different industries and lines of business. For instance, one struggling diversified company over a two-year period divested four business units, closed down the operations of four others, and added 25 new lines of business to its portfolio (16 through acquisition and 9 through internal start-up). PerkinElmer used a series of divestitures and new acquisitions to transform itself from a supplier of low-margin services sold to the government agencies into an innovative high-tech company with operations in over 125 countries and businesses in four industry groups—life sciences (drug research and clinical screening), optoelectronics, medical instruments, and fluid control and containment services (for customers in aerospace, power generation, and semiconductors). In 2005, PerkinElmer took a second restructuring step by divesting its entire fluid control and containment business group so that it could concentrate on its higher-growth health sciences and optoelectronics businesses; the company's CEO said, "While fluid services is an excellent business, it does not fit with our long-term strategy."[27] Before beginning a restructuring effort in 1995, British-based Hanson PLC owned companies with more than $20 billion in revenues in industries as diverse as beer, exercise equipment, tools, construction cranes, tobacco, cement, chemicals, coal mining, electricity, hot tubs and whirlpools, cookware, rock and gravel, bricks, and asphalt. By early 1997, Hanson had restructured itself into a $3.8 billion enterprise focused more narrowly on gravel, crushed rock, cement, asphalt, bricks, and construction cranes; the remaining businesses were divided into four groups and divested.

During Jack Welch's first four years as CEO of General Electric (GE), the company divested 117 business units, accounting for about 20 percent of GE's assets; these divestitures, coupled with several important acquisitions, provided GE with 14 major business divisions and led to Welch's challenge to the managers of GE's divisions to become number one or number two in their industry. Ten years after Welch became CEO, GE was a different company, having divested operations worth $9 billion, made new acquisitions totaling $24 billion, and cut its workforce by 100,000 people. Then, during the 1990–2001 period, GE continued to reshuffle its business lineup, acquiring over 600 new companies, including 108 in 1998 and 64 during a 90-day period in 1999. Most of the new acquisitions were in Europe, Asia, and Latin America and were aimed at transforming GE into a truly global enterprise. In 2003, GE's new CEO, Jeffrey Immelt, began a further restructuring of GE's business lineup with three initiatives: (1) spending $10 billion to acquire British-based Amersham and extend GE's Medical Systems business into diagnostic pharmaceuticals and biosciences, thereby creating a $15 billion business designated as GE Healthcare; (2) acquiring the entertainment assets of debt-ridden French media conglomerate Vivendi Universal Entertainment (Universal Studios, five Universal theme parks, USA Network, Sci-Fi Channel, the Trio cable channel, and Spanish-language broadcaster Telemundo) and integrate its operations into GE's NBC division (the owner of NBC, 29 television stations, and cable networks CNBC, MSNBC, and Bravo), thereby creating a broad-based $13 billion media business positioned to compete against Walt Disney, Time Warner, Fox, and Viacom; and (3) beginning a withdrawal from the insurance business by divesting several companies in its insurance division and preparing to spin off its remaining life and mortgage insurance businesses through an initial public offering of stock for a new company called Genworth Financial.

In a study of the performance of the 200 largest U.S. corporations from 1990 to 2000, McKinsey & Company found that those companies that actively managed their business portfolios through acquisitions and divestitures created substantially more shareholder value than those that kept a fixed lineup of businesses.[28]

Multinational Diversification Strategies

The distinguishing characteristics of a multinational diversification strategy are a *diversity of businesses* and a *diversity of national markets.*[29] Such diversity makes multinational diversification a particularly challenging and complex strategy to conceive and execute. Managers have to develop business strategies for each industry (with as many multinational variations as conditions in each country market dictate). Then they have to pursue and manage opportunities for cross-business and cross-country collaboration and strategic coordination in ways calculated to result in competitive advantage and enhanced profitability.

Moreover, the geographic operating scope of individual businesses within a diversified multinational corporation (DMNC) can range from one country only to several countries to many countries to global. Thus, each business unit within a DMNC often competes in a somewhat different combination of geographic markets than the other businesses do—adding another element of strategic complexity, and perhaps an element of opportunity.

Illustration Capsule 9.5 shows the scope of four prominent DMNCs.

The Appeal of Multinational Diversification: More Opportunities for Sustained Growth and Maximum Competitive Advantage Potential

Despite their complexity, multinational diversification strategies have great appeal. They contain *two major avenues* for growing revenues and profits: One is to grow by entering additional businesses, and the other is to grow by extending the operations of existing businesses into additional country markets. Moreover, a strategy of multinational diversification also contains six attractive paths to competitive advantage, *all of which can be pursued simultaneously:*

1. *Full capture of economies of scale and experience/learning curve effects.* In some businesses, the volume of sales needed to realize full economies of scale and/or benefit fully from experience/learning curve effects is rather sizable, often exceeding the volume that can be achieved operating within the boundaries of a single country market, especially a small one. *The ability to drive down unit costs by expanding sales to additional country markets is one reason why a diversified multinational may seek to acquire a business and then rapidly expand its operations into more and more foreign markets.*

2. *Opportunities to capitalize on cross-business economies of scope.* Diversifying into related businesses offering economies of scope can drive the development of a low-cost advantage over less diversified rivals. For example, a DMNC that uses mostly the same distributors and retail dealers worldwide can diversify into new businesses using these same worldwide distribution channels at relatively little incremental expense. The cost savings of piggybacking distribution activities can be substantial. Moreover, with more business selling more products in more countries, a DMNC acquires more bargaining leverage in its purchases from suppliers and more bargaining leverage with retailers in securing attractive display space for its products. Consider, for example, the competitive power that Sony derived

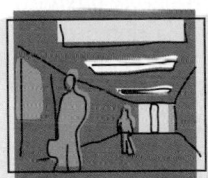

Illustration Capsule 9.5

The Global Scope of Four Prominent Diversified Multinational Corporations

Company	Global Scope	Businesses into Which the Company Has Diversified
Sony	Operations in more than 100 countries and sales offices in more than 200 countries	• Televisions, VCRs, DVD players, Walkman MP3 players, radios, digital cameras and video equipment, Vaio PCs, and Trinitron computer monitors; PlayStation game consoles and video game software; Columbia, Epic, and Sony Classical pre-recorded music; Columbia TriStar motion pictures; syndicated television programs; entertainment complexes, and insurance
Nestlé	Operations in 70 countries and sales offices in more than 200 countries	• Beverages (Nescafé and Taster's Choice coffees, Nestea, Perrier, Arrowhead, & Calistoga mineral and bottled waters); milk products (Carnation, Gloria, Neslac, Coffee Mate, Nestlé ice cream and yogurt); pet foods (Friskies, Alpo, Fancy Feast, Mighty Dog); Contadina, Libby's, and Stouffer's food products and prepared dishes; chocolate and confectionery products (Nestlé Crunch, Smarties, Baby Ruth, Butterfinger, KitKat); and pharmaceuticals (Alcon opthalmic products, Galderma dermatological products)
Siemens	Operations in 160 countries and sales offices in more than 190 countries	• Electrical power generation, transmission, and distribution equipment and products; manufacturing automation systems; industrial motors, machinery, and tools; plant construction and maintenance; corporate communication networks; telephones; PCs, mainframes, computer network products, consulting services; mass transit and light rail systems, rail cars, locomotives, lighting products (bulbs, lamps, theater and television lighting systems); semiconductors; home appliances; vacuum cleaners; and financial, procurement, and logistics services
Samsung	Operations in more than 60 countries and sales in more than 200 countries	• Notebook computers, hard disk drives, CD/DVD-ROM drives, monitors, printers, and fax machines; televisions (big-screen TVs, plasma-screen TVs, and LCD-screen TVs); DVD and MP3 players; Cell phones and various other telecommunications products; compressors; home appliances; DRAM chips, flash memory chips, and graphics memory chips; and optical fibers, fiber-optic cables, and fiber-optic connectors

Source: Company annual reports and Web sites.

from these very sorts of economies of scope when it decided to diversify into the video game business with its PlayStation product line. Sony had in place capability to go after video game sales in all country markets where it presently did business in other electronics product categories (TVs, computers, DVD players, VCRs, radios, CD players, and camcorders). And it had the marketing clout and brand-name credibility to persuade retailers to give Sony's PlayStation products prime shelf space and visibility. These strategic-fit benefits helped Sony quickly overtake long-time industry leaders Nintendo and Sega and defend its market leadership against Microsoft's new Xbox.

3. *Opportunities to transfer competitively valuable resources both from one business to another and from one country to another.* A company pursuing related diversification can gain a competitive edge over less diversified rivals by transferring competitively valuable resources from one business to another; a multinational company can gain competitive advantage over rivals with narrower geographic coverage by transferring competitively valuable resources from one country to another. But a strategy of multinational diversification enables simultaneous pursuit of both sources of competitive advantage.

4. *Ability to leverage use of a well-known and competitively powerful brand name.* Diversified multinational companies whose businesses have brand names that are well known and respected across the world possess a valuable strategic asset with competitive advantage potential. For example, Sony's well-established global brand-name recognition gives it an important marketing and advertising advantage over rivals with lesser-known brands. When Sony goes into a new marketplace with the stamp of the Sony brand on its product families, it can command prominent display space with retailers. It can expect to win sales and market share simply on the confidence that buyers place in products carrying the Sony name. While Sony may spend money to make consumers aware of the availability of its new products, it does not have to spend nearly as much on achieving brand recognition and market acceptance as would a lesser-known competitor looking at the marketing and advertising costs of entering the same new product/business/country markets and trying to go head-to-head against Sony. Further, if Sony moves into a new country market for the first time and does well selling Sony PlayStations and video games, it is easier to sell consumers in that country Sony TVs, digital cameras, PCs, MP3 players, and so on—plus, the related advertising costs are likely to be less than they would be without having already established the Sony brand strongly in the minds of buyers.

5. *Ability to capitalize on opportunities for cross-business and cross-country collaboration and strategic coordination.*[30] A multinational diversification strategy allows competitively valuable cross-business and cross-country coordination of certain value chain activities. For instance, by channeling corporate resources directly into a combined R&D/technology effort for all related businesses, as opposed to letting each business unit fund and direct its own R&D effort however it sees fit, a DMNC can merge its expertise and efforts *worldwide* to advance core technologies, expedite cross-business and cross-country product improvements, speed the development of new products that complement existing products, and pursue promising technological avenues to create altogether new businesses—all significant contributors to competitive advantage and better corporate performance.[31] Honda has been very successful in building R&D expertise in gasoline engines and transferring the resulting technological advances to its businesses in automobiles, motorcycles, outboard engines, snow blowers, lawn mowers, garden tillers, and portable power generators. Further, a DMNC can reduce costs through cross-business and cross-country coordination of purchasing and procurement from suppliers, from collaborative introduction and shared use of e-commerce technologies and online sales efforts, and from coordinated product introductions and promotional campaigns. Firms that are less diversified and less global in scope have less such cross-business and cross-country collaborative opportunities.

6. *Opportunities to use cross-business or cross-country subsidization to outcompete rivals.* A financially successful DMNC has potentially valuable organizational resources and multiple profit sanctuaries in both certain country markets and certain businesses that it can draw on to wage a market offensive. In comparison, a one-business domestic company has only one profit sanctuary—its home market. A diversified one-country competitor may have profit sanctuaries in several businesses, but all are in the same country market. A one-business multinational company may have profit sanctuaries in several country markets, but all are in the same business. All three are vulnerable to an offensive in their more limited profit sanctuaries by an aggressive DMNC willing to lowball its prices or spend extravagantly on advertising to win market share at their expense. A DMNC's ability to keep hammering away at competitors with low prices year after year may reflect either a cost advantage growing out of its related diversification strategy or a willingness to accept low profits or even losses in the market being attacked because it has ample earnings from its other profit sanctuaries. For example, Sony's global-scale diversification strategy gives it unique competitive strengths in outcompeting Nintendo and Sega, neither of which are diversified. If need be, Sony can maintain low prices on its PlayStations or fund high-profile promotions for its latest video game products, using earnings from its other business lines to fund its offensive to wrest market share away from Nintendo and Sega in video games. At the same time, Sony can draw on its considerable resources in R&D, its ability to transfer electronics technology from one electronics product family to another, and its expertise in product innovation to introduce better and better video game players, perhaps players that are multifunctional and do more than just play video games. Such competitive actions not only enhance Sony's own brand image but also make it very tough for Nintendo and Sega to match Sony's prices, advertising, and product development efforts and still earn acceptable profits.

The Combined Effects of These Advantages Is Potent
A strategy of diversifying into *related* industries and then competing *globally* in each of these industries thus has great potential for being a winner in the marketplace because of the long-term growth opportunities it offers and the multiple corporate-level competitive advantage opportunities it contains. Indeed, *a strategy of multinational diversification contains more competitive advantage potential* (above and beyond what is achievable through a particular business's own competitive strategy) *than any other diversification strategy.*
The strategic key to maximum competitive advantage is for a DMNC to concentrate its diversification efforts in those industries where there are resource-sharing and resource-transfer opportunities and where there are important economies of scope and brand-name benefits. The more a company's diversification strategy yields these kinds of strategic-fit benefits, the more powerful a competitor it becomes and the better its profit and growth performance is likely to be.

Core Concept
A strategy of multinational diversification has more built-in potential for competitive advantage than any other diversification strategy.

However, it is important to recognize that while, in theory, a DMNC's cross-subsidization capabilities are a potent competitive weapon, cross-subsidization can, in actual practice, be used only sparingly. It is one thing to *occasionally* divert a portion of the profits and cash flows from existing businesses to help fund entry into a new business or country market or wage a competitive offensive against select rivals. It is quite another thing to *regularly* use cross-subsidization tactics and thereby weaken overall company performance. A DMNC is under the same pressures as any other company to demonstrate consistently acceptable profitability across its whole operation.[32] At some juncture, every business and every country market needs to make a profit contribution or become a candidate for abandonment. As a general rule, *cross-subsidization tactics are justified only when there is a good prospect that the short-term impairment to corporate profitability will be offset by stronger competitiveness and better overall profitability over the long term.*

Key Points

The purpose of diversification is to build shareholder value. Diversification builds shareholder value when a diversified group of businesses can perform better under the auspices of a single corporate parent than they would as independent, stand-alone businesses—the goal is not to achieve just a $1 + 1 = 2$ result, but rather to realize important $1 + 1 = 3$ performance benefits. Whether getting into a new business has potential to enhance shareholder value hinges on whether a company's entry into that business can pass the attractiveness test, the cost-of-entry test, and the better-off test.

Entry into new businesses can take any of three forms: acquisition, internal start-up, or joint venture/strategic partnership. Each has its pros and cons, but acquisition is the most frequently used; internal start-up takes the longest to produce home-run results, and joint venture/strategic partnership, though used second most frequently, is the least durable.

There are two fundamental approaches to diversification—into related businesses and into unrelated businesses. The rationale for *related* diversification is *strategic*: Diversify into businesses with strategic fits along their respective value chains, capitalize on strategic-fit relationships to gain competitive advantage, and then use competitive advantage to achieve the desired $1 + 1 = 3$ impact on shareholder value.

The basic premise of unrelated diversification is that any business that has good profit prospects and can be acquired on good financial terms is a good business to diversify into. Unrelated diversification strategies surrender the competitive advantage potential of strategic fit in return for such advantages as (1) spreading business risk over a variety of industries and (2) providing opportunities for financial gain (if candidate acquisitions have undervalued assets, are bargain priced and have good upside potential given the right management, or need the backing of a financially strong parent to capitalize on attractive opportunities). However, the greater the number of businesses a company has diversified into and the more diverse these businesses are, the harder it is for corporate executives to select capable managers to run each business, know when the major strategic proposals of business units are sound, or decide on a wise course of recovery when a business unit stumbles.

Analyzing how good a company's diversification strategy is a six-step process:

1. *Evaluate the long-term attractiveness of the industries into which the firm has diversified.* Industry attractiveness needs to be evaluated from three angles: the attractiveness of each industry on its own, the attractiveness of each industry relative to the others, and the attractiveness of all the industries as a group.

2. *Evaluate the relative competitive strength of each of the company's business units.* Again, quantitative ratings of competitive strength are preferable to subjective

judgments. The purpose of rating the competitive strength of each business is to gain clear understanding of which businesses are strong contenders in their industries, which are weak contenders, and the underlying reasons for their strength or weakness. The conclusions about industry attractiveness can be joined with the conclusions about competitive strength by drawing an industry attractiveness–competitive strength matrix that helps identify the prospects of each business and what priority each business should be given in allocating corporate resources and investment capital.

3. *Check for cross-business strategic fits.* A business is more attractive strategically when it has value chain relationships with sister business units that offer potential to (*a*) realize economies of scope or cost-saving efficiencies; (*b*) transfer technology, skills, know-how, or other resource capabilities from one business to another; (*c*) leverage use of a well-known and trusted brand name; and (*d*) to build new or stronger resource strengths and competitive capabilities via cross-business collaboration. Cross-business strategic fits represent a significant avenue for producing competitive advantage beyond what any one business can achieve on its own.

4. *Check whether the firm's resource strengths fit the resource requirements of its present business lineup.* Resource fit exists when (*a*) businesses add to a company's resource strengths, either financially or strategically; (*b*) a company has the resources to adequately support the resource requirements of its businesses as a group without spreading itself too thin; and (*c*) there are close matches between a company's resources and industry key success factors. One important test of financial resource fit involves determining whether a company has ample cash cows and not too many cash hogs.

5. *Rank the performance prospects of the businesses from best to worst and determine what the corporate parent's priority should be in allocating resources to its various businesses.* The most important considerations in judging business-unit performance are sales growth, profit growth, contribution to company earnings, and the return on capital invested in the business. Sometimes, cash flow generation is a big consideration. Normally, strong business units in attractive industries have significantly better performance prospects than weak businesses or businesses in unattractive industries. Business subsidiaries with the brightest profit and growth prospects and solid strategic and resource fits generally should head the list for corporate resource support.

6. *Crafting new strategic moves to improve overall corporate performance.* This step entails using the results of the preceding analysis as the basis for devising actions to strengthen existing businesses, make new acquisitions, divest weak-performing and unattractive businesses, restructure the company's business lineup, expand the scope of the company's geographic reach multinationally or globally, and otherwise steer corporate resources into the areas of greatest opportunity.

Once a company has diversified, corporate management's task is to manage the collection of businesses for maximum long-term performance. There are four different strategic paths for improving a diversified company's performance: (1) broadening the firm's business base by diversifying into additional businesses, (2) retrenching to a narrower diversification base by divesting some of its present businesses, (3) restructuring the company, and (4) diversifying multinationally.

Exercises

1. Consider the business lineup of General Electric (GE) shown in Illustration Capsule 9.2. What problems do you think the top executives at GE encounter in trying to stay on top of all the businesses the company is in? How might they decide the merits of adding new businesses or divesting poorly performing businesses? What types of advice might they be in a position to give to the general managers of each of GE's business units?

2. The Walt Disney Company is in the following businesses:
    *   Theme parks.
    *   Disney Cruise Line.
    *   Resort properties.
    *   Movie, video, and theatrical productions (for both children and adults).
    *   Television broadcasting (ABC, Disney Channel, Toon Disney, Classic Sports Network, ESPN and ESPN2, E!, Lifetime, and A&E networks).
    *   Radio broadcasting (Disney Radio).
    *   Musical recordings and sales of animation art.
    *   Anaheim Mighty Ducks NHL franchise.
    *   Anaheim Angels major league baseball franchise (25 percent ownership).
    *   Books and magazine publishing.
    *   Interactive software and Internet sites.
    *   The Disney Store retail shops.

    Given the above listing, would you say that Walt Disney's business lineup reflects a strategy of related or unrelated diversification? Explain your answer in terms of the extent to which the value chains of Disney's different businesses seem to have competitively valuable cross-business relationships.

3. Newell Rubbermaid is in the following businesses:
    *   Cleaning and organizations businesses: Rubbermaid storage, organization, and cleaning products; Blue Ice ice substitute; Roughneck storage itemmms; Stain Shield and TakeAlongs food storage containers; and Brute commercial-grade storage and cleaning products (25 percent of annual revenues).
    *   Home and family businesses: Calphalon cookware and bakeware, Cookware Europe, Graco strollers, Little Tikes children's toys and furniture, and Goody hair accessories (20 percent of annual sales).
    *   Home fashions: Levolor and Kirsch window blinds, shades, and hardware in the United States; Swish, Gardinia and Harrison Drape home furnishings in Europe (15 percent of annual revenues).
    *   Office products businesses: Sharpie markers, Sanford highlighters, Eberhard Faber and Berol ballpoint pens, Paper Mate pens and pencils, Waterman and Parker fine writing instruments, and Liquid Paper (25 percent of annual revenues).

    Would you say that Newell Rubbermaid's strategy is one of related diversification, unrelated diversification or a mixture of both? Explain.

4. Explore the Web sites of the following companies and determine whether the company is pursuing a strategy of related diversification, unrelated diversification, or a mixture of both:

- Berkshire Hathaway
- News Corporation
- Dow Jones & Company
- Kimberly Clark

10

Strategy, Ethics, and Social Responsibility

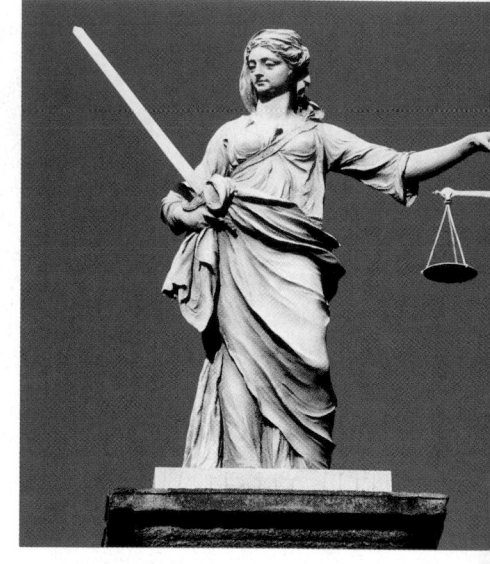

When morality comes up against profit, it is seldom profit that loses.

—Shirley Chisholm
Former Congresswoman

But I'd shut my eyes in the sentry box so I didn't see nothing wrong.

—Rudyard Kipling
Author

Values can't just be words on a page. To be effective, they must shape action.

—Jeffrey R. Immelt
CEO, General Electric

Leaders must be more than individuals of high character. They must "lead" others to behave ethically.

**—Linda K. Treviño
and Michael E. Brown**
Professors

Integrity violations are no-brainers. In such cases, you don't need to hesitate for a moment before firing someone or fret about it either. Just do it, and make sure the organization knows why, so that the consequences of breaking the rules are not lost on anyone.

—Jack Welch
Former CEO, General Electric

There is one and only one social responsibility of business—to use its resources and engage in activities designed to increase its profits so long as it stays within the rules of the game, which is to say engages in free and open competition, without deception or fraud.

—Milton Friedman
Nobel Prize–winning economist

Corporations are economic entities, to be sure, but they are also social institutions that must justify their existence by their overall contribution to society.

—Henry Mintzberg, Robert Simons, and Kunal Basu
Professors

lready, a company has a responsibility to make a profit and grow the business—in capitalistic, or market, economies, management's fiduciary duty to create value for shareholders is not a matter for serious debate. Just as clearly, a company and its personnel also have a duty to obey the law and play by the rules of fair competition. But does a company have a duty to operate according to the ethical norms of the societies in which it operates—should it be held to some standard of ethical conduct? And does it have a duty or obligation to contribute to the betterment of society independent of the needs and preferences of the customers it serves? Should a company display a social conscience and devote a portion of its resources to bettering society?

The focus of this chapter is to examine what link, if any, there should be between a company's efforts to craft and execute a winning strategy and its duties to (1) conduct its activities ethically and (2) demonstrate socially responsible behavior by being a committed corporate citizen and directing corporate resources to the betterment of employees, the communities in which it operates, and society as a whole.

WHAT DO WE MEAN BY *BUSINESS ETHICS?*

Business ethics is the application of ethical principles and standards to business behavior.[1] Business ethics does not really involve a special set of ethical standards applicable only to business situations. Ethical principles in business are not materially different from ethical principles in general. Why? Because business actions have to be judged in the context of society's standards of right and wrong, not by a special set of rules that businesspeople decide to apply to their own conduct. If dishonesty is considered to be unethical and immoral, then dishonest behavior in business—whether it relates to customers, suppliers, employees or shareholders—qualifies as equally unethical and immoral. If being ethical entails not deliberately harming others, then recalling a defective or unsafe product is ethically necessary and failing to undertake such a recall or correct the problem in future shipments of the product is likewise unethical. If society deems bribery to be unethical, then it is unethical for company personnel to make payoffs to government officials to facilitate business transactions or bestow gifts and other favors on prospective customers to win or retain their business.

Core Concept
Business ethics concerns the application of general ethical principles and standards to the actions and decisions of companies and the conduct of company personnel.

WHERE DO ETHICAL STANDARDS COME FROM—ARE THEY UNIVERSAL OR DEPENDENT ON LOCAL NORMS AND SITUATIONAL CIRCUMSTANCES?

Notions of right and wrong, fair and unfair, moral and immoral, ethical and unethical are present in all societies, organizations, and individuals. But there are three schools of thought about the extent to which the ethical standards travel across cultures and whether multinational companies can apply the same set of ethical standards in any and all of the locations where they operate.

The School of Ethical Universalism

According to the school of **ethical universalism,** some concepts of what is right and what is wrong are *universal*; that is, they transcend all cultures, societies, and religions.[2] For instance, being truthful (or not lying, or not being deliberately deceitful) is considered right by the peoples of all nations. Likewise, demonstrating integrity of character, not cheating, and treating people with dignity and respect are concepts that resonate with people of most cultures and religions. In most societies, people believe that companies should not pillage or degrade the environment in the course of conducting their operations. In most societies, people would concur that it is unethical to knowingly expose workers to toxic chemicals and hazardous materials or to sell products known to be unsafe or harmful to the users. *To the extent that there is common moral agreement about right and wrong actions and behaviors across multiple cultures and countries, there exists a set of universal ethical standards to which all societies, all companies, and all individuals can be held accountable.* These universal ethical principles or norms put limits on what actions and behaviors fall inside the boundaries of what is right and which ones fall outside. They set forth the traits and behaviors that are considered virtuous and that a good person is supposed to believe in and to display.

> **Core Concept**
> According to the school of ***ethical universalism,*** the same standards of what's ethical and what's unethical resonate with peoples of most societies regardless of local traditions and cultural norms; hence, common ethical standards can be used to judge the conduct of personnel at companies operating in a variety of country markets and cultural circumstances.

Many ethicists believe that the most important moral standards travel well across countries and cultures and thus are *universal*—universal norms include honesty or trustworthiness, respecting the rights of others, practicing the Golden Rule, avoiding unnecessary harm to workers or to the users of the company's product or service, and respect for the environment.[3] In all such instances where there is cross-cultural agreement as to what actions and behaviors are inside and outside ethical and moral boundaries, adherents of the school of ethical universalism maintain that the conduct of personnel at companies operating in a variety of country markets and cultural circumstances can be judged against the resulting set of common ethical standards.

The strength of ethical universalism is that it draws on the collective views of multiple societies and cultures to put some clear boundaries on what constitutes ethical business behavior and what constitutes unethical business behavior no matter what country market or culture a company or its personnel are operating in. This means that whenever basic moral standards really do not vary significantly according to local cultural beliefs, traditions, religious convictions, or time and circumstance, a multinational company can apply a code of ethics more or less evenly across its worldwide operations.[4] It can avoid the slippery slope that comes from having different ethical standards for different company personnel depending on where in the world they are working.

The School of Ethical Relativism

Apart from select universal basics—honesty, trustworthiness, fairness, a regard for worker safety, and respect for the environment—there are meaningful variations in what societies generally agree to be right and wrong in the conduct of business activities. Divergent religious beliefs, historic traditions, social customs, and prevailing political and economic doctrines (whether a country leans more toward a capitalistic market economy or one heavily dominated by socialistic or communistic principles) frequently produce ethical norms that vary from one country to another. The school of **ethical relativism** holds that when there are cross-country or cross-cultural differences in what is deemed fair or unfair, what constitutes proper regard for human rights, and what is considered ethical or unethical in business situations, it is appropriate for local moral standards to take precedence over what the ethical standards may be elsewhere—for instance, in a company's home market. The thesis is that whatever a culture thinks is right or wrong really is right or wrong for that culture.[5] Hence, the school of ethical relativism contends that there are important occasions when cultural norms and the circumstances of the situation determine whether certain actions or behaviors are right or wrong. Consider the following examples.

> **Core Concept**
> According to the school of *ethical relativism* different societal cultures and customs have divergent values and standards of right and wrong— thus what is ethical or unethical must be judged in the light of local customs and social mores and can vary from culture or nation to another.

The Use of Underage Labor   In industrialized nations, the use of underage workers is considered taboo; social activists are adamant that child labor is unethical and that companies should neither employ children under the age of 18 as full-time employees nor source any products from foreign suppliers that employ underage workers. Many countries have passed legislation forbidding the use of underage labor or, at a minimum, regulating the employment of people under the age of 18. However, in India, Bangladesh, Botswana, Sri Lanka, Ghana, Somalia, Turkey, and 100-plus other countries, it is customary to view children as potential, even necessary, workers.[6] Many poverty-stricken families cannot subsist without the income earned by young family members, and sending their children to school instead of having them participate in the workforce is not a realistic option. In 2000, the International Labor Organization estimated that 211 million children ages 5 to 14 were working around the world.[7] If such children are not permitted to work—due to pressures imposed by activist groups in industrialized nations—they may be forced to seek work in lower-wage jobs in "hidden" parts of the economy of their countries, beg on the street, or even traffic in drugs or engage in prostitution.[8] So if all businesses succumb to the protests of activist groups and government organizations that, based on their values and beliefs, loudly proclaim that underage labor is unethical, then have either businesses or the protesting groups really done something good on behalf of society in general?

The Payment of Bribes and Kickbacks   A particularly thorny area facing multinational companies is the degree of cross-country variability in paying bribes.[9] In many countries in Eastern Europe, Africa, Latin America, and Asia, it is customary to pay bribes to government officials in order to win a government contract, obtain a license or permit, or facilitate an administrative ruling.[10] Senior managers in China often use their power to obtain kickbacks and offer bribes when they purchase materials or other products for their companies.[11] In some developing nations, it is difficult for any company, foreign or domestic, to move goods through customs without paying off low-level officials.[12] Likewise, in many countries it is normal to make payments to prospective customers in order to win or retain their business. A *Wall Street Journal* article reported that 30 to 60 percent of all business transactions in Eastern Europe involved paying bribes, and the costs of bribe payments averaged 2 to 8 percent of revenues.[13] Three recent annual issues of the *Global Corruption Report*, sponsored by Berlin-based Transparency International, provide credible evidence that corruption among public officials and in business transactions is widespread across the world.[14] Some people stretch to justify the payment of bribes and kickbacks on grounds that bribing government officials to get goods through customs or giving kickbacks to customers to retail their business or win an order is simply a payment for services rendered, in the same way that people tip for service at restaurants.[15] But this argument rests on moral quicksand, even though it is a clever and pragmatic way to rationalize why such facilitating payments should be viewed as a normal and maybe unavoidable cost of doing business in some countries.

Companies that forbid the payment of bribes and kickbacks in their codes of ethical conduct and that are serious about enforcing this prohibition face a particularly vexing problem in those countries where bribery and kickback payments have been entrenched as a local custom for decades and are not considered unethical by the local population.[16] Refusing to pay bribes or kickbacks (so as to comply with the company's code of ethical conduct) is very often tantamount to losing business. Frequently, the sales and profits are lost to more unscrupulous companies, with the result that both ethical companies and ethical individuals are penalized. However, winking at the code of ethical conduct and going along with the payment of bribes or kickbacks not only undercuts enforcement of and adherence to the company's code of ethics but can also risk breaking the law. U.S. companies are prohibited by the Foreign Corrupt Practices Act (FCPA) from paying bribes to government officials, political parties, political candidates, or others in all countries where they do business; the FCPA requires U.S. companies with foreign operations to adopt accounting practices that ensure full disclosure of a company's transactions so that illegal payments can be detected. The 35 member countries of the Organization for Economic Cooperation and Development (OECD) in 1997 adopted a convention to combat bribery in international business transactions; the Anti-Bribery Convention obligated the countries to criminalize the bribery of foreign public officials, including payments made to political parties and party officials. So far, however, there has been only token enforcement of the OECD convention and the payment of bribes in global business transactions remains a common practice in many countries.

Ethical Relativism Equates to Multiple Sets of Ethical Standards   The existence of varying ethical norms such as those cited above explains why the adherents of ethical relativism maintain that there are few absolutes when it comes to business ethics and thus few ethical absolutes for consistently judging a company's conduct in various countries and markets. Indeed, the thesis of ethical relativists is that while there are sometimes general moral prescriptions that apply in most every society and business circumstance there are plenty of situations where ethical norms must be contoured to fit the local customs, traditions, and the notions of fairness shared by the parties involved. They argue that a one-size-fits-all template for judging the ethical appropriateness of business actions and the behaviors of company personnel simply does not exist—in other words, ethical problems in business cannot be fully resolved without appealing to the shared convictions of the parties in question.[17] European and American managers may want to impose standards of business conduct that give heavy weight to such core human rights as personal freedom, individual security, political participation, the ownership of property, and the right to subsistence as well as the obligation to respect the dignity of each human person, adequate health and safety standards for all employees, and respect for the environment; managers in China have a much weaker commitment to these kinds of human rights. Japanese managers may prefer ethical standards that show respect for the collective good of society. Muslim managers may wish to apply ethical standards compatible with the teachings of Mohammed. Individual companies may want to give explicit recognition to the importance of company personnel living up to the company's own espoused values and business principles. Clearly, there is merit in the school of ethical relativism's view that what is deemed right or wrong, fair or unfair, moral or immoral, ethical or unethical in business situations depends partly on the context of each country's local customs, religious traditions, and societal norms. Hence, there is a kernel of truth in the argument that businesses need some room to tailor their ethical standards to fit local situations. A company has to be very cautious about exporting its home-country values and ethics to foreign countries where it operates—"photocopying" ethics is disrespectful of other cultures and neglects the important role of moral free space.

> Under ethical relativism, there can be no one-size-fits-all set of authentic ethical norms against which to gauge the conduct of company personnel.

Pushed to Extreme, Ethical Relativism Breaks Down   While the relativistic rule of "When in Rome, do as the Romans do" appears reasonable, it nonetheless presents a big problem—when the envelope starts to be pushed, as will inevitably be the case, *it is tantamount to rudderless ethical standards.* Consider, for instance, the following example: In 1992, the owners of the SS *United States,* an aging luxury ocean liner constructed with asbestos in the 1940s, had the liner towed to Turkey, where a contractor had agreed to remove the asbestos for $2 million (versus a far higher cost in the United States, where asbestos removal safety standards were much more stringent).[18] When Turkish officials blocked the asbestos removal because of the dangers to workers of contracting cancer, the owners had the liner towed to the Black Sea port of Sevastopol, in the Crimean Republic, where the asbestos removal standards were quite lax and where a contractor had agreed to remove more than 500,000 square feet of carcinogenic asbestos for less than $2 million. There are no moral grounds for arguing that exposing workers to carcinogenic asbestos is ethically correct, irrespective of what a country's law allows or the value the country places on worker safety.

A company that adopts the principle of ethical relativism and holds company personnel to local ethical standards necessarily assumes that what prevails as local morality is an adequate guide to ethical behavior. This can be ethically dangerous—it leads to the conclusion that if a country's culture is accepting of bribery or environmental degradation or exposing workers to dangerous conditions (toxic chemicals or bodily harm), then so much the worse for honest people and protection of the environment and safe working conditions. Such a position is morally unacceptable. Even though bribery of government officials in China is a common practice, when Lucent Technologies found that managers in its Chinese operations had bribed government officials, it fired the entire senior management team.[19]

> Managers in multinational enterprises have to figure out how to navigate the gray zone that arises when operating in two cultures with two sets of ethics.

Moreover, from a global markets perspective, ethical relativism results in a maze of conflicting ethical standards for multinational companies wanting to address the very real issue of what ethical standards to enforce companywide. On the one hand, multinational companies need to educate and motivate their employees worldwide to respect the customs and traditions of other nations, and, on the other hand, they must enforce compliance with the company's own particular code of ethical behavior. It is a slippery slope indeed to resolve such ethical diversity without any kind of higher-order moral compass. Imagine, for example, that a multinational company in the name of ethical relativism takes the position that it is okay for company personnel to pay bribes and kickbacks in countries where such payments are customary but forbids company personnel from making such payments in those countries where bribes and kickbacks are considered unethical or illegal. Or that the company says it is ethically fine to use underage labor in its plants in those countries where underage labor is acceptable and ethically inappropriate to employ underage labor at the remainder of its plants. Having thus adopted conflicting ethical standards for operating in different countries, company managers have little moral basis for enforcing ethical standards companywide—rather, the clear message to employees would be that the company has no ethical standards or principles of its own, preferring to let its practices be governed by the countries in which it operates. This is scarcely strong moral ground to stand on.

Ethics and Integrative Social Contracts Theory

Core Concept
According to *integrated social contracts theory,* universal ethical principles or norms based on the collective views of multiple cultures and societies combine to form a "social contract" that all individuals in all situations have a duty to observe. Within the boundaries of this social contract, local cultures or groups can specify other impermissible actions; however, universal ethical norms always take precedence over local ethical norms.

Social contract theory provides a middle position between the opposing views of universalism (that the same set of ethical standards should apply everywhere) and relativism (that ethical standards vary according to local custom).[20] According to **integrative social contracts theory,** the ethical standards a company should try to uphold are governed both by (1) a limited number of universal ethical principles that are widely recognized as putting legitimate ethical boundaries on actions and behavior in *all* situations and (2) the circumstances of local cultures, traditions, and shared values that further prescribe what constitutes ethically permissible behavior and what does not. However, *universal ethical norms take precedence over local ethical norms.* In other words, universal ethical principles apply in those situations where most all societies—endowed with rationality and moral knowledge—have common moral agreement on what is wrong and thereby put limits on what actions and behaviors fall inside the boundaries of what is right and which ones fall outside. *These mostly uniform agreements about what is morally right and wrong form a "social contract" or contract with society that is binding on all individuals, groups, organizations, and businesses in terms of establishing right and wrong and in drawing the line between ethical and unethical behaviors.* But these universal ethical principles or norms nonetheless still leave some moral free space for the people in a particular country (or local culture or even a company) to make specific interpretations of what other actions may or may not be permissible within the bounds defined by universal ethical principles. Hence, while firms, industries, professional associations, and other business-relevant groups are contractually obligated to society to observe universal ethical norms, they have the discretion to go beyond these universal norms and specify other behaviors that are out of bounds and place further limitations on what is considered ethical. Both the legal and medical professions have standards regarding what kinds of advertising are ethically permissible and what kinds are not. Food products companies are beginning to establish ethical guidelines for judging what is and is not appropriate advertising for food products that are inherently unhealthy and may cause dietary or obesity problems for people who eat them regularly or consume them in large quantities.

The strength of integrated social contracts theory is that it accommodates the best parts of ethical universalism and ethical relativism. It is indisputable that cultural differences impact how business is conducted in various parts of the world and that these cultural differences sometimes give rise to different ethical norms. But it is just as indisputable that some ethical norms are more authentic or universally applicable than others, meaning that, in many instances of cross-country differences, one side may be more "ethically correct" or "more right" than another. In such instances, resolving cross-cultural differences entails applying universal, or first-order, ethical norms and overriding the local, or second-order, ethical norms. A good example is the payment of bribes and kickbacks. Yes, bribes and kickbacks seem to be common in some countries, but does this justify paying them? Just because bribery flourishes in a country does not mean that it is an authentic or legitimate ethical norm. Virtually all of the world's major religions (Buddhism, Christianity, Confucianism, Hinduism, Islam, Judaism, Sikhism, and Taoism) and all moral schools of thought condemn bribery and corruption.[21] Bribery is commonplace in India but interviews with Indian CEOs whose companies constantly engaged in payoffs indicated disgust for the practice and they expressed no illusions about its impropriety.[22] Therefore, a multinational company might reasonably conclude that the right ethical standard is one of refusing to condone bribery and kickbacks on the part of company personnel no matter what the local custom is and no matter what the sales consequences are.

Granting an automatic preference to local country ethical norms presents vexing problems to multinational company managers when the ethical standards followed in a foreign country are lower than those in its home country or are in conflict with the company's code of ethics. Sometimes there can be no compromise on what is ethically permissible and what is not. *This is precisely what integrated social contracts theory maintains—universal or first-order ethical norms should always take precedence over local or second-order norms.* Integrated social contracts theory offers managers in multinational companies clear guidance in resolving cross-country ethical differences: Those parts of the company's code of ethics that involve universal ethical norms must be enforced worldwide, but within these boundaries there is room for ethical diversity and opportunity for host country cultures to exert *some* influence in setting their own moral and ethical standards. Such an approach detours the somewhat scary case of a self-righteous multinational company trying to operate as the standard-bearer of moral truth and imposing its interpretation of its code of ethics worldwide no matter what. And it avoids the equally scary case for a company's ethical conduct to be no higher than local ethical norms in situations where local ethical norms permit practices that are generally considered immoral or when local norms clearly conflict with a company's code of ethical conduct. But even with the guidance provided by integrated social contracts theory, there are many instances where cross-country differences in ethical norms create gray areas in which it is tough to draw a line in the sand between right and wrong decisions, actions, and business practices.

THE THREE CATEGORIES OF MANAGEMENT MORALITY

Three categories of managers stand out with regard to ethical and moral principles in business affairs:[23]

- *The moral manager*—Moral managers are dedicated to high standards of ethical behavior, both in their own actions and in their expectations of how the company's business is to be conducted. They see themselves as stewards of ethical behavior and believe it is important to exercise ethical leadership. Moral managers may well be ambitious and have a powerful urge to succeed, but they pursue success in business within the confines of both the letter and the spirit of what is ethical and legal—they typically regard the law as an ethical minimum and have a habit of operating well above what the law requires.

- *The immoral manager*—Immoral managers have no regard for so-called ethical standards in business and pay no attention to ethical principles in making decisions and conducting the company's business. Their philosophy is that good businesspeople cannot spend time watching out for the interests of others and agonizing over "the right thing to do." In the minds of immoral managers, nice guys come in second and the competitive nature of business requires that you either trample on others or get trampled yourself. They believe what really matters is single-minded pursuit of their own best interests—they are living examples of capitalistic greed, caring only about their own or their organization's gains and successes. Immoral managers may even be willing to short-circuit legal and regulatory requirements if they think they can escape detection. And they are always on the lookout for legal loopholes and creative ways to get around rules and regulations that block or constrain actions they deem in their own or their company's self-interest. Immoral managers are thus the bad guys—they have few scruples, little or no integrity, and are willing to do most anything they believe they can get away with. It doesn't bother them much to be seen by others as wearing the black hats.

- *The amoral manager*—Amoral managers appear in two forms: the intentionally amoral manager and the unintentionally amoral manager. Intentionally amoral managers are of the strong opinion that business and ethics are not to be mixed. They are not troubled by failing to factor ethical considerations into their decisions and actions because it is perfectly legitimate for businesses to do anything they wish so long as they stay within legal and regulatory bounds—in other words, if particular actions and behaviors are legal and comply with existing regulations, then they qualify as permissible and should not be seen as unethical. Intentionally amoral managers view the observance of high ethical standards (doing more than what is required by law) as too Sunday-schoolish for the tough competitive world of business, even though observing some higher ethical considerations may be appropriate in life outside of business. Their concept of right and wrong tends to be lawyer-driven—how much can we get by with and can we go ahead even if it is borderline? Thus intentionally amoral managers hold firmly to the view that anything goes, so long as actions and behaviors are not clearly ruled out by prevailing legal and regulatory requirements.

Core Concept

Amoral managers believe that businesses ought to be able to do whatever current laws and regulations allow them to do without being shackled by ethical considerations—they think that what is permissible and what is not is governed entirely by prevailing laws and regulations, not by societal concepts of right and wrong.

Unintentionally amoral managers do not pay much attention to the concept of business ethics either, but for different reasons. They are simply casual about, careless about, or inattentive to the fact that certain kinds of business decisions or company activities are unsavory or may have deleterious effects on others—in short, they go about their jobs as best they can without giving serious thought to the ethical dimension of decisions and business actions. They are ethically unconscious when it comes to business matters, partly or mainly because they have just never stopped to consider whether and to what extent business decisions or company actions sometimes spill over to create adverse impacts on others. Unintentionally amoral managers may even see themselves as people of integrity and as personally ethical. But, like intentionally amoral managers, they are of the firm view that businesses ought to be able to do whatever the current legal and regulatory framework allows them to do without being shackled by ethical considerations.

By some accounts, the population of managers is said to be distributed among all three types in a bell-shaped curve, with immoral managers and moral managers occupying the two tails of the curve, and the amoral managers (especially the intentionally amoral managers) occupying the broad middle ground.[24] Furthermore, within the population of managers, there is experiential evidence to support that while the average manager may be amoral most of the time, he or she may slip into a moral or immoral mode on occasion, based on a variety of impinging factors and circumstances.

Evidence of Managerial Immorality in the Global Business Community

There is considerable evidence that a sizable majority of managers are either amoral or immoral. The *2005 Global Corruption Report,* sponsored by Transparency International, found that corruption among public officials and in business transactions is widespread across the world. Table 10.1 shows some of the countries where corruption is believed to be lowest and highest—even in the countries where business practices are deemed to be least corrupt, there is considerable room for improvement in the extent to which managers observe ethical business practices. Table 10.2 presents data showing the perceived likelihood that companies in the 21 largest exporting countries are paying bribes to win business in the markets of 15 emerging-country markets—Argentina, Brazil, Colombia, Hungary, India, Indonesia, Mexico, Morocco, Nigeria, the Philippines, Poland, Russia, South Africa, South Korea, and Thailand.

Table 10.1   Corruption Perceptions Index, Selected Countries, 2004

Country	2004 CPI Score*	High–Low Range	Number of Surveys Used	Country	2004 CPI Score*	High–Low Range	Number of Surveys Used
Finland	9.7	9.2–10.0	9	Taiwan	5.6	4.7–6.0	15
New Zealand	9.6	9.2–9.7	9	Italy	4.8	3.4–5.6	10
Denmark	9.5	8.7–9.8	10	South Africa	4.6	3.4–5.8	11
Sweden	9.2	8.7–9.5	11	South Korea	4.5	2.2–5.8	14
Switzerland	9.1	8.6–9.4	10	Brazil	3.9	3.5–4.8	11
Norway	8.9	8.0–9.5	9	Mexico	3.6	2.6–4.5	11
Australia	8.8	6.7–9.5	15	Thailand	3.6	2.5–4.5	14
Netherlands	8.7	8.3–9.4	10	China	3.4	2.1–5.6	16
United Kingdom	8.6	7.8–9.2	12	Saudi Arabia	3.4	2.0–4.5	5
Canada	8.5	6.5–9.4	12	Turkey	3.2	1.9–5.4	13
Germany	8.2	7.5–9.2	11	India	2.8	2.2–3.7	15
Hong Kong	8.0	3.5–9.4	13	Russia	2.8	2.0–5.0	15
United States	7.5	5.0–8.7	14	Philippines	2.6	1.4–3.7	14
Chile	7.4	6.3–8.7	11	Vietnam	2.6	1.6–3.7	11
France	7.1	5.0–9.0	12	Argentina	2.5	1.7–3.7	11
Spain	7.1	5.6–8.0	11	Venezuela	2.3	2.0–3.0	11
Japan	6.9	3.5–9.0	15	Pakistan	2.1	1.2–3.3	7
Israel	6.4	3.5–8.1	10	Nigeria	1.6	0.9–2.1	9
Uruguay	6.2	5.6–7.3	6	Bangladesh	1.5	0.3–2.4	5

* The CPI scores range between 10 (highly clean) and 0 (highly corrupt); the data were collected between 2002 and 2004 and reflects a composite of 18 data sources from 12 institutions, as indicated in the number of surveys used. The CPI score represents the perceptions of the degree of corruption as seen by businesspeople, academics, and risk analysts. CPI scores were reported for 146 countries.

Source: Transparency International, *2005 Global Corruption Report,* www.globalcorruptionreport.org (accessed October 31, 2005), pp. 235–38.

Table 10.2   **The Degree to Which Companies in Major Exporting Countries Are Perceived to Be Paying Bribes in Doing Business Abroad**

Rank/Country	Bribe-Payer Index (10 = Low; 0 = High)	Rank/Country	Bribe-Payer Index (10 = Low; 0 = High)
1. Australia	8.5	12. France	5.5
2. Sweden	8.4	13. United States	5.3
3. Switzerland	8.4	14. Japan	5.3
4. Austria	8.2	15. Malaysia	4.3
5. Canada	8.1	16. Hong Kong	4.3
6. Netherlands	7.8	17. Italy	4.1
7. Belgium	7.8	18. South Korea	3.9
8. Britain	6.9	19. Taiwan	3.8
9. Singapore	6.3	20. China (excluding Hong Kong)	3.5
10. Germany	6.3	21. Russia	3.2
11. Spain	5.8		

Note: The bribe-payer index is based on a questionnaire developed by Transparency International and a survey of some 835 private-sector leaders in 15 emerging countries accounting for 60 percent of all imports into non-Organization for Economic Cooperation and Development countries—actual polling was conducted by Gallup International.

Source: Transparency International, *2003 Global Corruption Report*, www.globalcorruptionreport.org (accessed November 1, 2005), p. 267.

The *2003 Global Corruption Report* cited data indicating that bribery occurred most often in (1) public works contracts and construction, (2) the arms and defense industry, and (3) the oil and gas industry. On a scale of 1 to 10, where 10 indicates negligible bribery, even the "cleanest" industry sectors—agriculture, light manufacturing, and fisheries—only had "passable" scores of 5.9, indicating that bribes are quite likely a common occurrence in these sectors as well (see Table 10.3).

The corruption, of course, extends beyond just bribes and kickbacks. For example, in 2005, four global chip makers (Samsung and Hynix Semiconductor in South Korea, Infineon Technologies in Germany, and Micron Technology in the United States) pleaded guilty to conspiring to fix the prices of dynamic random access memory (DRAM) chips sold to such companies as Dell, Apple Computer, and Hewlett-Packard—DRAM chips generate annual worldwide sales of around $26 billion and are used in computers, electronics products, and motor vehicles.[25] So far, the probe has resulted in fines of $730 million, jail terms for nine executives, and pending criminal charges for three more employees for their role in the global cartel; the guilty companies face hundreds of millions of dollars more in damage claims from customers and from consumer class-action lawsuits.

A global business community that is apparently so populated with unethical business practices and managerial immorality does not bode well for concluding that many companies ground their strategies on exemplary ethical principles or for the vigor with which company managers try to ingrain ethical behavior into company personnel. And, as many business school professors have noted, there are considerable numbers of amoral business students in our classrooms. So efforts to root out shady and corrupt business practices and implant high ethical principles into the managerial process of crafting and executing strategy is unlikely to produce an ethically strong global business climate anytime in the near future, barring major effort to address and correct the ethical laxness of company managers.

Table 10.3   **Bribery in Different Industries**

Business Sector	Bribery Score (10 = Low; 0 = High)
Agriculture	5.9
Light manufacturing	5.9
Fisheries	5.9
Information technology	5.1
Forestry	5.1
Civilian aerospace	4.9
Banking and finance	4.7
Heavy manufacturing	4.5
Pharmaceuticals/medical care	4.3
Transportation/storage	4.3
Mining	4.0
Power generation/transmission	3.7
Telecommunications	3.7
Real estate/property	3.5
Oil and gas	2.7
Arms and defense	1.9
Public works/construction	1.3

Note: The bribery scores for each industry are based on a questionnaire developed by Transparency International and a survey of some 835 private sector leaders in 15 emerging countries accounting for 60 percent of all imports into non-Organization for Economic Cooperation and Development countries—actual polling was conducted by Gallup International.

Source: Transparency International, *2003 Global Corruption Report*, www.globalcorruption report.org (accessed November 1, 2005), p. 268.

DO COMPANY STRATEGIES NEED TO BE ETHICAL?

Company managers may formulate strategies that are ethical in all respects, or they may decide to employ strategies that, for one reason or another, have unethical or at least gray-area components. While most company managers are usually careful to ensure that a company's strategy is within the bounds of what is legal, the available evidence indicates they are not always so careful to ensure that all elements of their strategies are within the bounds of what is generally deemed ethical. Senior executives with strong ethical convictions are normally proactive in insisting that all aspects of company strategy fall within ethical boundaries. In contrast, senior executives who are either immoral or amoral may use shady strategies and unethical or borderline business practices, especially if they are clever at devising schemes to keep ethically questionable actions hidden from view.

During the past five years, there has been an ongoing series of revelations about managers who have ignored ethical standards, deliberately stepped out of bounds, and been called to account by the media, regulators, and the legal system. Ethical misconduct has occurred at Enron, Tyco International, HealthSouth, Rite Aid, Citicorp, Bristol-Myers, Squibb, Adelphia, Royal Dutch/Shell, Parmalat (an Italy-based food products company), Mexican oil giant Pemex, Marsh & McLennan and other insurance brokers, several leading brokerage houses and investment banking firms, and a host of mutual fund companies. The consequences of crafting strategies that cannot pass the test of moral scrutiny are manifested in the sharp drops in the stock prices of the guilty companies that have cost shareholders billions of dollars; the frequently devastating public relations hits that the accused companies have taken, the sizes of the fines that have been levied (often amounting to several hundred million dollars); the growing legion of criminal indictments and convictions of company executives; and the numbers of executives who have either been dismissed from their jobs, shoved into early retirement, and/or suffered immense public embarrassment. The fallout from all these scandals has resulted in heightened management attention to legal and ethical considerations in crafting strategy. Illustration Capsule 10.1 details the ethically flawed strategy at the world's leading insurance broker, and the consequences to those concerned.

What Are the Drivers of Unethical Strategies and Business Behavior?

The apparent pervasiveness of immoral and amoral businesspeople is one obvious reason why ethical principles are an ineffective moral compass in business dealings and why companies may resort to unethical strategic behavior. But apart from thinking that maintains "The business of business is business, not ethics," three other main drivers of unethical business behavior also stand out:[26]

- Faulty oversight such that overzealous or obsessive pursuit of personal gain, wealth, and other selfish interests is overlooked by or escapes the attention of higher-ups (most usually the board of directors).
- Heavy pressures on company managers to meet or beat performance targets.
- A company culture that puts the profitability and good business performance ahead of ethical behavior.

Overzealous Pursuit of Personal Gain, Wealth, and Selfish Interests
People who are obsessed with wealth accumulation, greed, power, status, and other selfish interests often push ethical principles aside in their quest for self-gain. Driven by their ambitions, they exhibit few qualms in skirting the rules or doing whatever is necessary to achieve their goals. The first and only priority of such corporate bad apples is to look out for their own best interests and if climbing the ladder of success means having few scruples and ignoring the welfare of others, so be it. A general disregard for business ethics can prompt all kinds of unethical strategic maneuvers and behaviors at companies. Top executives, directors, and majority shareholders at cable-TV company Adelphia Communications ripped off the company for amounts totaling well over $1 billion, diverting hundreds of millions of dollars to fund their Buffalo Sabres hockey team, build a private golf course, and buy timber rights—among other things—and driving the company into bankruptcy. Their actions, which represent one of the biggest instances of corporate looting and self-dealing in American business, took place despite the company's public pontifications about the principles it would observe in trying to care for customers, employees, stockholders, and the local communities where it operated. Andrew Fastow, Enron's chief financial officer (CFO), set himself up as the manager of one of Enron's off-the-books partnerships and as the part-owner of another, allegedly earning extra compensation of $30 million for his owner-manager roles in the two partnerships; Enron's board of directors agreed to suspend the company's conflict-of-interest rules designed to protect the company from this very kind of executive self-dealing (but directors and perhaps Fastow's superiors were kept in the dark about how much Fastow was earning on the side).

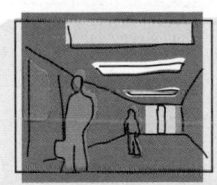

Illustration Capsule 10.1

Marsh & McLennan's Ethically Flawed Strategy

In October 2004, *Wall Street Journal* headlines trumpeted that a cartel among insurance brokers had been busted. Among the ringleaders was worldwide industry leader Marsh & McLennan Companies Inc., with 2003 revenues of $11.5 billion and a U.S. market share of close to 20 percent. The gist of the brokers' plan was to cheat corporate clients by rigging the bids brokers solicited for insurance policies and thereby collecting big fees (called contingent commissions) from major insurance companies for steering business their way. Two family members of Marsh & McLennan CEO Jeffery Greenberg were CEOs of major insurance companies to which Marsh sometimes steered business. Greenberg's father was CEO of insurance giant AIG (which had total revenues of $81 billion and insurance premium revenues of $28 billion in 2003), and Greenberg's younger brother was CEO of ACE Ltd., the 24th biggest property-casualty insurer in the United States, with 2003 revenues of $10.7 billion and insurance premium revenues of more than $5 billion worldwide. Prior to joining ACE, Greenberg's younger brother had been president and chief operating officer of AIG, headed by his father.

Several months prior to the cartel bust, a Marsh subsidiary, Putnam Investments, had paid a $110 million fine for securities fraud and another Marsh subsidiary, Mercer Consulting, was placed under Securities and Exchange Commission (SEC) investigation for engaging in pay-to-play practices that forced investment managers to pay fees in order to secure Mercer's endorsement of their services when making recommendations to Mercer's pension fund clients.

The cartel scheme arose from the practice of large corporations to hire the services of such brokers as Marsh & McLennan, Aon Corporation, A. J. Gallaher & Company, Wells Fargo, or BB&T Insurance Services to manage their risks and take out appropriate property and casualty insurance on their behalf. The broker's job was to solicit bids from several insurers and obtain the best policies at the lowest prices for the client.

Marsh's insurance brokerage strategy was to solicit artificially high bids from some insurance companies so that it could guarantee that the bid of a preferred insurer on a given deal would win the bid. Marsh brokers called underwriters at various insurers, often including AIG and ACE, and asked for "B" quotes—bids that were deliberately high. Insurers asked for B quotes knew that Marsh wanted another insurer to win the business, but they were willing to participate because on other policy solicitations Marsh could end up steering the business to them via Marsh's same strategy. Sometimes Marsh even asked underwriters that were providing B quotes to attend a meeting with Marsh's client and make a presentation regarding their policy to help bolster the credibility of their inflated bid.

Since it was widespread practice among insurers to pay brokers contingent commissions based on the volume or profitability of the business the broker directed to them, Marsh's B-quote solicitation strategy allowed it to steer business to those insurers paying the largest contingent commissions—these contingent commissions were in addition to the fees the broker earned from the corporate client for services rendered in conducting the bidding process for the client. A substantial fraction of the policies that Marsh unlawfully steered were to two Bermuda-based insurance companies that it helped start up and in which it also had ownership interests (some Marsh executives also indirectly owned shares of stock in one of the companies); indeed, these two insurance companies received 30–40 percent of their total business from policies steered to them by Marsh.

At Marsh, steering business to insurers paying the highest contingent commission was a key component of the company's overall strategy. Marsh's contingent commissions generated revenues of close to $1.5 billion over the 2001–2003 period, including $845 million in 2003. Without these commission revenues, Marsh's $1.5 billion in net profits would have been close to 40 percent lower in 2003.

Within days of headlines about the cartel bust, Marsh's stock price had fallen by 48 percent (costing shareholders about $11.5 billion in market value) and the company was looking down the barrel of a criminal indictment. To stave off the criminal indictment (something no insurance company had ever survived), board members forced Jeffrey Greenberg to resign as CEO. Another top executive was suspended. Criminal charges against several Marsh executives for their roles in the bid-rigging scheme were filed several weeks thereafter.

In an attempt to lead industry reform, Greenberg's successor quickly announced a new business model for Marsh that included not accepting any contingent commissions from insurers. Marsh's new strategy and business model involved charging fees only to its corporate clients for soliciting bids, placing their insurance, and otherwise managing clients' risks and crises. This eliminated Marsh's conflict of interest in earning fees from both sides of the transactions it made on behalf of its corporate clients. Marsh also committed to provide up-front disclosure to clients of the fees it would earn on their business (in the past such fees had been murky and incomplete). Even so, there were indications that close to 10 lawsuits, some involving class action, would soon be filed against the company.

Meanwhile, all major commercial property-casualty insurers were scrambling to determine whether their payment of contingent commissions was ethical, since such arrangements clearly gave insurance brokers a financial incentive to place insurance with companies paying the biggest contingent commissions, not those with the best prices or terms. Prosecutors of the cartel had referred to the contingent commissions as kickbacks.

Sources: Monica Langley and Theo Francis, "Insurers Reel from Bust of a 'Cartel,' " *The Wall Street Journal,* October 18, 2004, pp. A1, A14; Monica Langley and Ian McDonald, "Marsh Averts Criminal Case with New CEO," *The Wall Street Journal,* October 26, 2004, pp. A1, A10; Christopher Oster and Theo Francis, "Marsh and Aon Have Holdings in Two Insurers," *The Wall Street Journal,* November 1, 2004, p. C1; and Marcia Vickers, "The Secret World of Marsh Mac," *BusinessWeek,* November 1, 2004, pp. 78–89.

According to a civil complaint filed by the Securities and Exchange Commission, the CEO of Tyco International, a well-known $35.6 billion manufacturing and services company, conspired with the company's CFO to steal more than $170 million, including a company-paid $2 million birthday party for the CEO's wife held on Sardinia, an island off the coast of Italy; a $7 million Park Avenue apartment for his wife; and secret low-interest and interest-free loans to fund private businesses and investments and purchase lavish artwork, yachts, estate jewelry, and vacation homes in New Hampshire, Connecticut, Massachusetts, and Utah. The CEO allegedly lived rent-free in a $31 million Fifth Avenue apartment that Tyco purchased in his name, directed millions of dollars of charitable contributions in his own name using Tyco funds, diverted company funds to finance his personal businesses and investments, and sold millions of dollars of Tyco stock back to Tyco itself through Tyco subsidiaries located in offshore bank-secrecy jurisdictions. Tyco's CEO and CFO were further charged with conspiring to reap more than $430 million from sales of stock, using questionable accounting to hide their actions, and engaging in deceptive accounting practices to distort the company's financial condition from 1995 to 2002. At the trial on the charges filed by the SEC, the prosecutor told the jury in his opening statement, "This case is about lying, cheating and stealing. These people didn't win the jackpot—they stole it." Defense lawyers countered that "every single transaction . . . was set down in detail in Tyco's books and records" and that the authorized and disclosed multimillion-dollar compensation packages were merited by the company's financial performance and stock price gains. The two Tyco executives were convicted and sentenced to jail.

Prudential Securities paid a total of about $2 billion in the 1990s to settle misconduct charges relating to practices that misled investors on the risks and rewards of limited-partnership investments. Providian Financial Corporation, despite an otherwise glowing record of social responsibility and corporate citizenship, paid $150 million in 2001 to settle claims that its strategy included systematic attempts to cheat credit card holders. Ten prominent Wall Street securities firms in 2003 paid $1.4 billion to settle charges that they knowingly issued misleading stock research to investors in an effort to prop up the stock prices of client corporations. A host of mutual-fund firms made under-the-table arrangements to regularly buy and sell stock for their accounts at special after-hours trading prices that disadvantaged long-term investors and had to pay nearly $2.0 billion in fines and restitution when their unethical practices were discovered by authorities during 2002–2003. Salomon Smith Barney, Goldman Sachs, Credit Suisse First Boston, and several other financial firms were assessed close to $2 billion in fines and restitution for the unethical manner in which they contributed to the scandals at Enron and WorldCom and for the shady practice of allocating shares of hot initial public offering stocks to a select list of corporate executives who either steered or were in a position to steer investment banking business their way.

Heavy Pressures on Company Managers to Meet or Beat Earnings Targets   When companies find themselves scrambling to achieve ambitious earnings growth and meet the quarterly and annual performance expectations of Wall Street analysts and investors, managers often feel enormous pressure to do whatever it takes to sustain the company's reputation for delivering good financial performance. Executives at high-performing companies know that investors will see the slightest sign of a slowdown in earnings growth as a red flag and drive down the company's stock price. The company's credit rating could be downgraded if it has used lots of debt to finance its growth. The pressure to watch the scoreboard and never miss a quarter—so as not to upset the expectations of Wall Street analysts and fickle stock market investors—prompts managers to cut costs wherever savings show up immediately, squeeze extra sales out of early deliveries, and engage in other short-term maneuvers to make the numbers. As the pressure builds to keep performance numbers looking good, company personnel start stretching the rules further and further, until the limits of ethical conduct are overlooked.[27] Once ethical boundaries are crossed in efforts to "meet or beat the numbers," the threshold for making more extreme ethical compromises becomes lower.

Several top executives at WorldCom (the remains of which is now part of Verizon Communications), a company built with scores of acquisitions in exchange for WorldCom stock, allegedly concocted a fraudulent $11 billion accounting scheme to hide costs and inflate revenues and profit over several years; the scheme was said to have helped the company keep its stock price propped up high enough to make additional acquisitions, support its nearly $30 billion debt load, and allow executives to cash in on their lucrative stock options. At Qwest Communications, a company created by the merger of a go-go telecom start-up and U.S. West (one of the regional Bell companies), management was charged with scheming to improperly book $2.4 billion in revenues from a variety of sources and deals, thereby inflating the company's profits and making it appear that the company's strategy to create a telecommunications company of the future was on track when, in fact, it was faltering badly behind the scenes. Top-level Qwest executives were dismissed, and in 2004 new management agreed to $250 million in fines for all the misdeeds.

At Bristol-Myers Squibb, the world's fifth-largest drug maker, management apparently engaged in a series of numbers-game maneuvers to meet earnings targets, including such actions as:

- Offering special end-of-quarter discounts to induce distributors and local pharmacies to stock up on certain prescription drugs—a practice known as channel stuffing.
- Issuing last-minute price increase alerts to spur purchases and beef up operating profits.
- Setting up excessive reserves for restructuring charges and then reversing some of the charges as needed to bolster operating profits.
- Making repeated asset sales small enough that the gains could be reported as additions to operating profit rather than being flagged as one-time gains. (Some accountants have long used a rule of thumb that says a transaction that alters quarterly profits by less than 5 percent is "immaterial" and need not be disclosed in the company's financial reports.)

Such numbers games were said to be a common "earnings management" practice at Bristol-Myers and, according to one former executive, "sent a huge message across the organization that you make your numbers at all costs."[28]

Company executives often feel pressured to hit financial performance targets because their compensation depends heavily on the company's performance. During the late 1990s, it became fashionable for boards of directors to grant lavish bonuses, stock option awards, and other compensation benefits to executives for meeting specified performance targets. So outlandishly large were these rewards that executives had strong personal incentives to bend the rules and engage in behaviors the allowed the targets to be met. Much of the accounting hocus-pocus at the root of recent corporate scandals has entailed situations in which executives benefited enormously from misleading accounting or other shady activities that allowed them to hit the numbers and receive incentive awards ranging from $10 million to $100 million. At Bristol-Myers Squibb, for example, the pay-for-performance link spawned strong rules-bending incentives. About 94 percent of one top executive's $18.5 million in total compensation in 2001 came from stock-option grants, a bonus, and long-term incentive payments linked to corporate performance; about 92 percent of a second executive's $12.9 million of compensation was incentive-based.[29]

The fundamental problem with a "make the numbers and move on" syndrome is that a company doesn't really serve its customers or its shareholders by going overboard in pursuing bottom-line profitability. In the final analysis, shareholder interests are best served by doing a really good job of serving customers (observing the rule that customers are king) and by improving the company's competitiveness in the marketplace—these outcomes are the most reliable drivers of higher profits and added shareholder value. Cutting ethical corners or stooping to downright illegal actions in the name of profits first carries exceptionally high risk for shareholders—the steep stock-price decline and tarnished brand image that accompany the discovery of scurrilous behavior leaves shareholders with a company worth much less than before—and the rebuilding task can be arduous, taking both considerable time and resources.

Company Cultures That Put the Bottom Line Ahead of Ethical Behavior

When a company's culture spawns an ethically corrupt or amoral work climate, people have a company-approved license to ignore what's right and engage in most any behavior or employ most any strategy they think they can get away with. Such cultural norms as "No one expects strict adherence to ethical standards," "Everyone else does it," and "It is politic to bend the rules to get the job done" permeate the work environment.[30] At such companies, ethically immoral or amoral people play down observance of ethical strategic actions and business conduct. Moreover, the pressures to conform to cultural norms can prompt otherwise honorable people to make ethical mistakes and succumb to the many opportunities around them to engage in unethical practices.

A perfect example of a company culture gone awry on ethics is Enron.[31] Enron's leaders encouraged company personnel to focus on the current bottom line and to be innovative and aggressive in figuring out what could be done to grow current revenues and earnings. Employees were expected to pursue opportunities to the utmost. Enron executives viewed the company as a laboratory for innovation; the company hired the best and brightest people and pushed them to be creative, look at problems and opportunities in new ways, and exhibit a sense of urgency in making things happen. Employees were encouraged to make a difference and do their part in creating an entrepreneurial environment in which creativity flourished, people could achieve their full potential, and everyone had a stake in the outcome. Enron employees got the message—pushing the limits and meeting one's numbers were viewed as survival skills. Enron's annual "rank and yank" formal evaluation process, in which the 15 to 20 percent lowest-ranking employees were let go or encouraged to seek other employment, made it abundantly clear that hitting earnings targets and being *the* mover and shaker -in the marketplace were what counted. The name of the game at Enron became devising clever ways to boost revenues and earnings, even if it sometimes meant operating outside established policies and without the knowledge of superiors. In fact, outside-the-lines behavior was celebrated if it generated profitable new business. Enron's energy contracts and its trading and hedging activities grew increasingly more complex and diverse as employees pursued first this avenue and then another to help keep Enron's financial performance looking good.

As a consequence of Enron's well-publicized successes in creating new products and businesses and leveraging the company's trading and hedging expertise into new market arenas, Enron came to be regarded as exceptionally innovative. It was ranked by its corporate peers as the most innovative U.S. company for three consecutive years in *Fortune* magazine's annual surveys of the most-admired companies. A high-performance/high-rewards climate came to pervade the Enron culture, as the best workers (determined by who produced the best bottom-line results) received impressively large incentives and bonuses (amounting to as much as $1 million for traders and even more for senior executives). On Car Day at Enron, an array of luxury sports cars arrived for presentation to the most successful employees. Understandably, employees wanted to be seen as part of Enron's star team and partake in the benefits that being one of Enron's best and smartest employees entailed. The high monetary rewards, the ambitious and hard-driving people that the company hired and promoted, and the competitive, results-oriented culture combined to give Enron a reputation not only for trampling competitors at every opportunity but also for practicing internal ruthlessness. The company's super-aggressiveness and win-at-all-costs mind-set nurtured a culture that gradually and then more rapidly fostered the erosion of ethical standards, eventually making a mockery of the company's stated values of integrity and respect. When it became evident in the fall of 2001 that Enron was a house of cards propped up by deceitful accounting and a myriad of unsavory practices, the company imploded in a matter of weeks—the biggest bankruptcy of all time cost investors $64 billion in losses (between August 2000, when the stock price was at its five-year high, and November 2001), and Enron employees lost their retirement assets, which were almost totally invested in Enron stock.

More recently, a team investigating an ethical scandal at oil giant Royal Dutch/ Shell Group that resulted in the payment of $150 million in fines found that an ethically flawed culture was a major contributor to why managers made rosy forecasts that they couldn't meet and why top executives engaged in maneuvers to mislead investors by overstating Shell's oil and gas reserves by 25 percent (equal to 4.5 billion barrels of oil). The investigation revealed that top Shell executives knew that a variety of internal practices, together with unrealistic and unsupportable estimates submitted by overzealous, bonus-conscious managers in Shell's exploration and production group, were being used to overstate reserves. An e-mail written by Shell's top executive for exploration and production (who was caught up in the ethical misdeeds and later forced to resign) said, "I am becoming sick and tired about lying about the extent of our reserves issues and the downward revisions that need to be done because of our far too aggressive/optimistic bookings."[32]

Illustration Capsule 10.2 describes Philip Morris USA's new strategy for growing the sales of its leading Marlboro cigarette brand—judge for yourself whether the strategy is ethical or shady in light of the undisputed medical links between smoking and lung cancer.

Approaches to Managing a Company's Ethical Conduct

The stance a company takes in dealing with or managing ethical conduct at any given point can take any of four basic forms:[33]

- The unconcerned, or nonissue, approach.
- The damage control approach.
- The compliance approach.
- The ethical culture approach.

The differences in these four approaches are discussed briefly below and summarized in Table 10.4 on page 335.

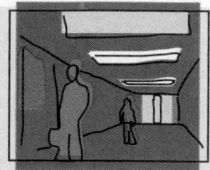

Illustration Capsule 10.2

Philip Morris USA's Strategy for Marlboro Cigarettes: Ethical or Unethical?

In late 2005, Philip Morris USA and its corporate parent, Altria Group Inc., wrapped up a year of promotions and parties to celebrate the 50th year of selling Marlboro cigarettes. Marlboro commanded a 40 percent share of the U.S. market for cigarettes and was also one of the world's top cigarette brands. Despite sharp advertising restrictions agreed to by cigarette marketers in 1998 and a big jump in state excise taxes on cigarettes since 2002, Marlboro's sales and market share were climbing, thanks to a new trailblazing marketing strategy.

Marlboro had become a major brand in the 1960s and 1970s via a classic mass-marketing strategy anchored by annual ad budgets in the millions of dollars. The company's TV, magazine, and billboard ads for Marlboros always featured a rugged cowboy wearing a Stetson, riding a horse in a mountainous area, and smoking a Marlboro—closely connecting the brand with the American West gave Marlboro a distinctive and instantly recognized brand image. The Marlboro ad campaign was a gigantic success, making Marlboro one of the world's best-known and valuable brands.

But following the ad restrictions in 1998, Philip Morris had to shift to a different marketing strategy to grow Marlboro's sales. It opted for an approach aimed at generating all kinds of marketing buzz for the Marlboro brand and creating a larger cadre of loyal Marlboro smokers (who often felt persecuted by social pressures and antismoking ordinances). Philip Morris directed company field reps to set up promotions at local bars where smokers could sign up for promotional offers like price discounts on Marlboro purchases, a Marlboro Miles program that awarded points for each pack purchased, and sweepstakes prizes that included cash, trips, and Marlboro apparel; some prizes could be purchased with Marlboro Miles points. It also began to sponsor live concerts and other events to generate additional sign-ups among attendees. A Web site was created to spur Internet chatter among the Marlboro faithful and to encourage still more sign-ups

for special deals and contests (some with prizes up to a $1 million)—an online community quickly sprang up around the brand. Via all the sign-ups and calls to an 800 number, Philip Morris created a database of Marlboro smokers that by 2005 had grown to 26 million names. Using direct mail and e-mail, the company sent the members of its database a steady stream of messages and offers, ranging from birthday coupons for free breakfasts to price discounts to chances to attend local concerts, enjoy a day at nearby horse tracks, or win a trip to the company's ranch in Montana (where winners got gifts, five-course meals, massages, and free drinks and could go snowmobiling, fly fishing, or horseback riding).

Meanwhile, Philip Morris also became considerably more aggressive in retail stores, launching an offensive initiative to give discounts and incentives to retailers who utilized special aisle displays and signage for its cigarette brands. One 22-store retail chain reported that, by agreeing to a deal to give Philip Morris brands about 66 percent of its cigarette shelf space, it ended up paying about $5.50 per carton less for its Marlboro purchases than it paid for cartons of Camels supplied by rival R. J. Reynolds. Some Wal-Mart stores were said to have awarded Philip Morris as much as 80 percent of its cigarette shelf space.

Thus, despite being besieged by the costs of defending lawsuits and paying out billions to governments as compensation for the increased health care costs associated with smoking, Philip Morris and other cigarette makers were making very healthy profits: operating margins of nearly 28 percent in 2005 (up from 26 percent in 2004) and net income of about $11.4 billion on sales of $66.3 billion in the United States and abroad.

However, health care officials were highly critical of Philip Morris's marketing tactics for Marlboro, and the U.S. Department of Justice had filed a lawsuit claiming, among other things, that the company knowingly marketed Marlboros to underage people in its database, a charge denied by the company.

Source: Based largely on information in Nanette Byrnes, "Leader of the Packs," *BusinessWeek,* October 31, 2005, pp. 56, 58.

The Unconcerned, or Nonissue, Approach   The unconcerned approach is prevalent at companies whose executives are immoral and unintentionally amoral. Senior executives at companies using this approach ascribe to the view that notions of right and wrong in matters of business are defined entirely by government via the prevailing laws and regulations. They maintain that trying to enforce ethical standards above and beyond what is legally required is a nonissue because businesses are entitled to conduct their affairs in whatever

Table 10.4   **Four Approaches to Managing Business Ethics**

	Unconcerned, or Nonissue Approach	Damage Control Approach	Compliance Approach	Ethical Culture Approach
Underlying beliefs	• The business of business is business, not ethics. • All that matters is whether an action is legal. • Ethics has no place in the conduct of business. • Companies should not be morally accountable for their actions.	• The company needs to make a token gesture in the direction of ethical standards (a code of ethics)	• The company must be committed to ethical standards and monitoring ethics performance. • Unethical behavior must be prevented and punished if discovered. • It is important to have a reputation for high ethical standards.	• Ethics is basic to the culture. • Behaving ethically must be a deeply held corporate value and become a way of life. • Everyone is expected to walk the talk.
Ethics management approaches	• There's no need to make decisions concerning business ethics—if its legal, it is okay. • No intervention regarding the ethical component of decisions is needed.	• The company must act to protect against the dangers of unethical strategies and behavior. • Ignore unethical behavior or allow it to go unpunished unless the situation is extreme and requires action.	• The company must establish a clear, comprehensive code of ethics. • The company must provide ethics training for all personnel. • Have formal ethics compliance procedures, an ethics compliance office, and a chief ethics officer.	• Ethical behavior is ingrained and reinforced as part of the culture. • Much reliance on co-worker peer pressure—"That's not how we do things here." • Everyone is an ethics watchdog—whistle-blowing is required. • Ethics heroes are celebrated; ethics stories are told.
Challenges	• Financial consequences can become unaffordable. • Some stakeholders are alienated.	• Credibility problems with stakeholders can arise. • The company is susceptible to ethical scandal. • The company has a subpar ethical reputation—executives and company personnel don't walk the talk.	• Organizational members come to rely on the existing rules for moral guidance—fosters a mentality of what is not forbidden is allowed. • Rules and guidelines proliferate. • The locus of moral control resides in the code and in the ethics compliance system rather than in an individual's own moral responsibility for ethical behavior.	• New employees must go through strong ethics induction program. • Formal ethics management systems can be underutilized. • Relying on peer pressures and cultural norms to enforce ethical standards can result in eliminating some or many of the compliance trappings and, over time, induce moral laxness.

Source: Adapted from Gedeon J. Rossouw and Leon J. van Vuuren, "Modes of Managing Morality: A Descriptive Model of Strategies for Managing Ethics," *Journal of Business Ethics* 46, no. 4 (September 2003), pp. 392–93.

manner they wish so long as they comply with the letter of what is legally required. Hence, there is no need to spend valuable management time trying to prescribe and enforce standards of conduct that go above and beyond legal and regulatory requirements. In companies where senior managers are immoral, the prevailing view may well be that under-the-table dealing can be good business if it can be kept hidden or if it can be justified on grounds that others are doing it too. Companies in this mode usually engage in most any business practices they believe they can get away with, and the strategies they employ may well embrace elements that are either borderline from a legal perspective or ethically shady and unsavory.

The Damage Control Approach   Damage control is favored at companies whose managers are intentionally amoral but who are wary of scandal and adverse public relations fallout that could cost them their jobs of tarnish their careers. Companies using this approach, not wanting to risk tarnishing the reputations of key personnel or the company, usually make some concession to window-dressing ethics, going so far as to adopt a code of ethics—so that their executives can point to it as evidence of good-faith efforts to prevent unethical strategy making or unethical conduct on the part of company personnel. But the code of ethics exists mainly as nice words on paper, and company personnel do not operate within a strong ethical context—there's a notable gap between talking ethics and walking ethics. Employees quickly get the message that rule bending is tolerated and may even be rewarded if the company benefits from their actions.

> The main objective of the damage control approach is to protect against adverse publicity and any damaging consequences brought on by headlines in the media, outside investigation, threats of litigation, punitive government action, or angry or vocal stakeholders.

Company executives that practice the damage control approach are prone to look the other way when shady or borderline behavior occurs—adopting a kind of "See no evil, hear no evil, speak no evil" stance (except when exposure of the company's actions put executives under great pressure to redress any wrongs that have been done). They may even condone questionable actions that help the company reach earnings targets or bolster its market standing—such as pressuring customers to stock up on the company's product (channel stuffing), making under-the-table payments to win new business, stonewalling the recall of products claimed to be unsafe, bad-mouthing the products of rivals, or trying to keep prices low by sourcing goods from disreputable suppliers in low-wage countries that run sweatshop operations or use child labor. But they are usually careful to do such things in a manner that lessens the risks of exposure or damaging consequences. This generally includes making token gestures to police compliance with codes of ethics and relying heavily on spin to help extricate the company or themselves from claims that the company's strategy has unethical components or that company personnel have engaged in unethical practices.

The Compliance Approach   Anywhere from light to forceful compliance is favored at companies whose managers (1) lean toward being somewhat amoral but are highly concerned about having ethically upstanding reputations or (2) are moral and see strong compliance methods as the best way to impose and enforce ethical rules and high ethical standards. Companies that adopt a compliance mode usually do some or all of the following to display their commitment to ethical conduct: make the code of ethics a visible and regular part of communications with employees, implement ethics training programs, appoint a chief ethics officer or ethics ombudsperson, have ethics committees to give guidance on ethics matters, institute formal procedures for investigating alleged ethics violations, conduct ethics audits to measure and document compliance, give ethics awards to employees for outstanding efforts to create an ethical climate and improve ethical performance, and/or try to deter violations by setting up ethics hotlines for anonymous callers to use in reporting possible violations.

Emphasis here is usually on securing broad compliance and measuring the degree to which ethical standards are upheld and observed. However, violators are disciplined and sometimes subjected to public reprimand and punishment (including dismissal), thereby sending a clear signal to company personnel that complying with ethical standards needs to be taken seriously. The driving force behind the company's commitment to eradicate unethical behavior normally stems from a desire to avoid the cost and damage associated with unethical conduct or else a quest to gain favor from stakeholders (especially ethically conscious customers, employees, and investors) for having a highly regarded reputation for ethical behavior. One of the weaknesses of the compliance approach is that moral control resides in the company's code of ethics and in the ethics compliance system rather than in (1) the strong peer pressures for ethical behavior that come from ingraining a highly ethical corporate culture and (2) an individual's own moral responsibility for ethical behavior.[34]

The Ethical Culture Approach   At some companies, top executives believe that high ethical principles must be deeply ingrained in the corporate culture and function as guides for "how we do things around here." A company using the ethical culture approach seeks to gain employee buy-in to the company's ethical standards, business principles, and corporate values. The ethical principles embraced in the company's code of ethics and/or in its statement of corporate values are seen as integral to the company's identity and ways of operating—they are at the core of the company's soul and are promoted as part of business as usual. The integrity of the ethical culture approach depends heavily on the ethical integrity of the executives who create and nurture the culture—it is incumbent on them to determine how high the bar is to be set and to exemplify ethical standards in their own decisions and behavior. Further, it is essential that the strategy be ethical in all respects and that ethical behavior be ingrained in the means that company personnel employ to execute the strategy. Such insistence on observing ethical standards is what creates an ethical work climate and a workplace where displaying integrity is the norm.

Many of the trappings used in the compliance approach are also manifest in the ethical culture mode, but one other is added—strong peer pressure from coworkers to observe ethical norms. Thus, responsibility for ethics compliance is widely dispersed throughout all levels of management and the rank-and-file. Stories of former and current moral heroes are kept in circulation, and the deeds of company personnel who display ethical values and are dedicated to walking the talk are celebrated at internal company events. The message that ethics matters—and matters a lot—resounds loudly and clearly throughout the organization and in its strategy and decisions. However, one of the challenges to overcome in the ethical culture approach is relying too heavily on peer pressures and cultural norms to enforce ethics compliance rather than on an individual's own moral responsibility for ethical behavior—absent unrelenting peer pressure or strong internal compliance systems, there is a danger that over time company personnel may become lax about its ethical standards. Compliance procedures need to be an integral part of the ethical culture approach to help send the message that management takes the observance of ethical norms seriously and that behavior that falls outside ethical boundaries will have negative consequences.

Why a Company Can Change Its Ethics Management Approach
Regardless of the approach they have used to managing ethical conduct, a company's executives may sense that they have exhausted a particular mode's potential for managing ethics and that they need to become more forceful in their approach to ethics management. Such changes typically occur when the company's ethical failures have made the headlines and created an embarrassing situation for company officials or when the business climate changes. For example, the recent raft of corporate scandals, coupled with aggressive enforcement of anticorruption legislation such as the Sarbanes-Oxley Act of 2002 (which addresses corporate governance and accounting practices), has prompted numerous executives and boards of directors to clean up their acts in accounting and financial reporting, review their ethical standards, and tighten up ethics compliance procedures. Intentionally amoral managers using the unconcerned approach to ethics management may see less risk in shifting to the damage control approach (or, for appearance's sake, maybe a "light" compliance mode). Senior managers who have employed the damage control mode may be motivated by bad experiences to mend their ways and shift to a compliance mode. In the wake of so many corporate scandals, companies in the compliance mode may move closer to the ethical culture approach.

WHY SHOULD COMPANY STRATEGIES BE ETHICAL?

There are two reasons why a company's strategy should be ethical: (1) because a strategy that is unethical in whole or in part is morally wrong and reflects badly on the character of the company personnel involved and (2) because an ethical strategy is good business and in the self-interest of shareholders.

The Moral Case for an Ethical Strategy

Managers do not dispassionately assess what strategic course to steer. Ethical strategy making generally begins with managers who themselves have strong character (i.e., who are honest, have integrity, are ethical, and truly care about how they conduct the company's business). Managers with high ethical principles and standards are usually advocates of a corporate code of ethics and strong ethics compliance, and they are typically genuinely committed to certain corporate values and business principles. They walk the talk in displaying the company's stated values and living up to its business principles and ethical standards. They understand that there is a big difference between adopting values statements and codes of ethics that serve merely as window dressing and those that truly paint the white lines for a company's actual strategy and business conduct. As a consequence, ethically strong managers consciously opt for strategic actions that can pass moral scrutiny—they display no tolerance for strategies with ethically controversial components.

The Business Case for an Ethical Strategy

There are solid business reasons to adopt ethical strategies even if most company managers are not of strong moral character and personally committed to high ethical standards. Pursuing unethical strategies not only damages a company's reputation but can also have costly, wide-ranging consequences. Some of the costs are readily visible; others are hidden and difficult to track down—as shown in Figure 10.1. The costs of

Figure 10.1 **The Business Costs of Ethical Failures**

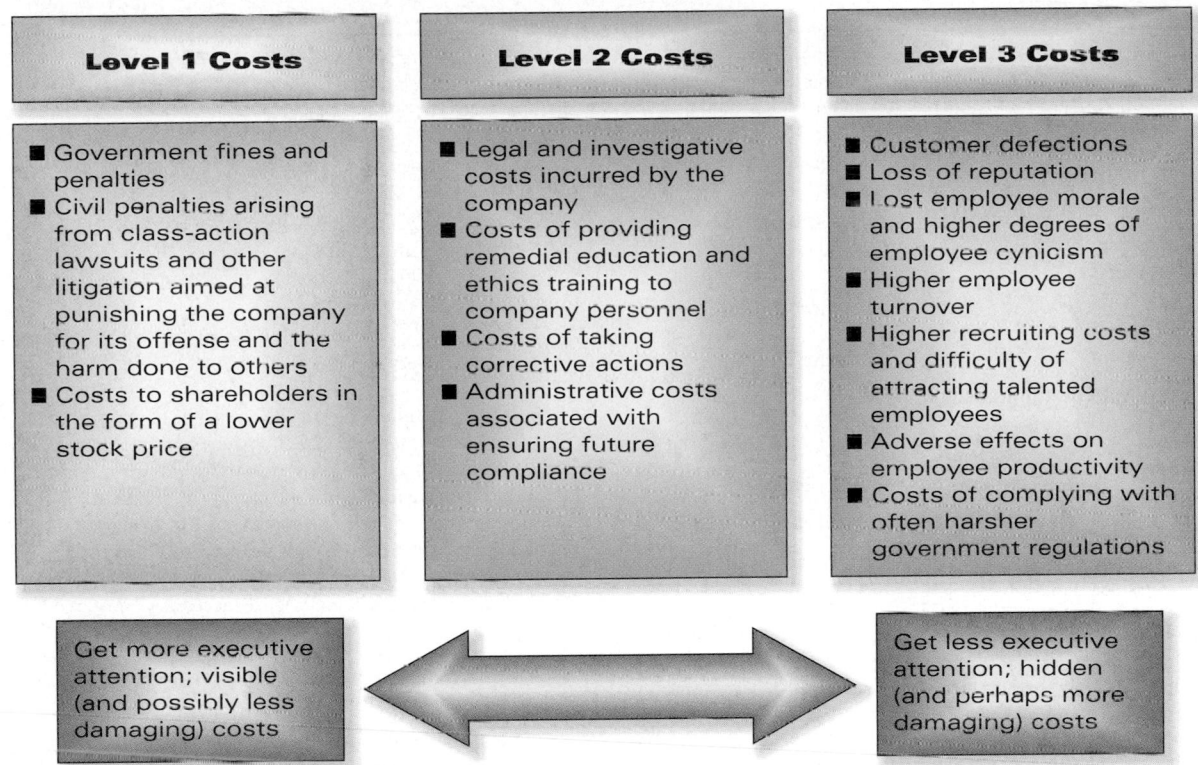

Level 1 Costs	**Level 2 Costs**	**Level 3 Costs**
■ Government fines and penalties ■ Civil penalties arising from class-action lawsuits and other litigation aimed at punishing the company for its offense and the harm done to others ■ Costs to shareholders in the form of a lower stock price	■ Legal and investigative costs incurred by the company ■ Costs of providing remedial education and ethics training to company personnel ■ Costs of taking corrective actions ■ Administrative costs associated with ensuring future compliance	■ Customer defections ■ Loss of reputation ■ Lost employee morale and higher degrees of employee cynicism ■ Higher employee turnover ■ Higher recruiting costs and difficulty of attracting talented employees ■ Adverse effects on employee productivity ■ Costs of complying with often harsher government regulations

Get more executive attention; visible (and possibly less damaging) costs ⟷ Get less executive attention; hidden (and perhaps more damaging) costs

Source: Adapted from Terry Thomas, John R. Schermerhorn, and John W. Dienhart, "Strategic Leadership of Ethical Behavior," *Academy of Management Executive* 18, no. 2 (May 2004), p. 58.

fines and penalties and any declines in the stock price are easy enough to calculate. The administrative cleanup (or Level 2) costs are usually buried in the general costs of doing business and can be difficult to ascribe to any one ethical misdeed. Level 3 costs can be quite difficult to quantify but can sometimes be the most devastating— the aftermath of the Enron debacle left Arthur Andersen's reputation in shreds and led to the once-revered accounting firm's almost immediate demise, and it remains to be seen whether Marsh & McLennan can overcome the problems described in Illustration Capsule 10.1. Merck, once one of the world's most respected pharmaceutical firms, has been struggling against the revelation that senior management deliberately concealed that its Vioxx painkiller, which the company pulled off the market in September 2004, was tied to much greater risk of heart attack and strokes—some 20 million people in the United States had taken Vioxx over the years, and Merck executives had reason to suspect as early as 2000 (and perhaps earlier) that Vioxx had dangerous side effects.[35]

Rehabilitating a company's shattered reputation is time-consuming and costly. Customers shun companies known for their shady behavior. Companies with reputations for unethical conduct have considerable difficulty in recruiting and retaining talented employees. Most hardworking, ethically upstanding people are repulsed by a work environment where unethical behavior is condoned; they don't want to get entrapped in a compromising

Conducting business in an ethical fashion is in a company's enlightened self-interest.

As a gauge of your own ethical and moral standards, take the following quiz and see how you stack up against other members of your class. For the test to be valid, you need to answer the questions candidly, not on the basis of what you think the ethically correct answer is.

1. Do you think that it would be unethical for you to give two Super Bowl tickets to an important customer? Would your answer be different if the customer is likely to place a large order that would qualify you for a large year-end sales bonus?

_____Yes   _____No   _____Unsure (it depends)

_____Need more information

2. Would it be wrong to accept a case of fine wine from an important customer? Would your answer be different if you have just convinced your superiors to authorize a special price discount on a big order that the customer has just placed?

_____Yes   _____No   _____Unsure (it depends)

_____Need more information

3. Is it unethical for a high school or college coach to accept a "talent fee" or similar type of payment from a maker of sports apparel or sports equipment when the coach has authority to determine which brand of apparel or equipment to use for his or her team and subsequently chooses the brand of the company making the payment? Is it unethical for the maker of the sports apparel or equipment to make such payments in expectation that the coach will reciprocate by selecting the company's brand? (Would you answer be different if everybody else is doing it?)

_____Yes   _____No   _____Unsure (it depends)

_____Need more information

4. Is it unethical to accept an invitation from a supplier to spend a holiday weekend skiing at the supplier company's resort home in Colorado? (Would your answer be different if you were presently considering a proposal from that supplier to purchase $1 million worth of components?)

_____Yes   _____No   _____Unsure (it depends)

_____Need more information

5. Is it unethical for a food products company to incorporate ingredients that have trans fats in its products, given that trans fats are known to be very unhealthy for consumers and that alternative ingredients (which might be somewhat more expensive) can be used in producing the product?

_____Yes   _____No   _____Unsure (it depends)

_____Need more information

6. Would it be wrong to keep quiet if you, as a junior financial analyst, had just calculated that the projected return on a possible project was 18 percent and your boss (a) informed you that no project could be approved without the prospect of a 25 percent return and (b) told you to go back and redo the numbers and "get them right"?

_____Yes   _____No   _____Unsure (it depends)

_____Need more information

7. Would it be unethical to allow your supervisor to believe that you were chiefly responsible for the success of a new company initiative if it actually resulted from a team effort or major contributions by a co-worker?

_____Yes   _____No   _____Unsure (it depends)

_____Need more information

8. Would it be unethical for you, as the chief company official in India to (a) authorize a $25,000 payment to a local government official to facilitate governmental approval to construct a $200 million petrochemical plant and (b) disguise this payment by instructing accounting personnel to classify the payment as part of the cost of obtaining a building permit? (As you can see from Table 10.1, corruption is the norm in India, and bribes and kickbacks are often a "necessary" cost of doing business there.)

_____Yes   _____No   _____Unsure (it depends)

_____Need more information

9. Is it unethical for a motor vehicle manufacturer to resist recalling some of its vehicles when governmental authorities present it with credible evidence that the vehicles have safety defects?

_____Yes   _____No   _____Unsure (it depends)

_____Need more information

10. Is it unethical for a credit card company to aggressively try to sign up new accounts when, after an introductory period of interest-free or low-interest charges on unpaid monthly balances, the interest rate on unpaid balances jumps to 1.5 percent or more monthly (even though such high rates of 18 percent or more annually are disclosed in fine print)?

_____Yes   _____No   _____Unsure (it depends)

_____Need more information

11. Is it unethical to bolster your résumé with exaggerated claims of your credentials and prior job accomplishments in hopes of improving your chances of gaining employment at another company?

_____Yes   _____No   _____Unsure (it depends)

_____Need more information

12. Is it unethical for a company to spend as little as possible on pollution control when, with some extra effort and expenditures, it could substantially reduce the amount of pollution caused by its operations?

_____Yes   _____No   _____Unsure (it depends)

_____Need more information

Answers: The answers to questions 1, 2, and 4 probably shift from no/unsure to a definite yes when the second part of the circumstance comes into play. We think a strong case can be made that the answers to the remaining 9 questions are yes, although it can be argued that more information about the circumstances might be needed in responding to questions 5, 7, 9, and 12.

situation, nor do they want their personal reputations tarnished by the actions of an unsavory employer. A 1997 survey revealed that 42 percent of the respondents took into account a company's ethics when deciding whether to accept a job.[36] Creditors are usually unnerved by the unethical actions of a borrower because of the potential business fallout and subsequent risk of default on any loans. To some significant degree, therefore, companies recognize that ethical strategies and ethical conduct are good business. Most companies have strategies that pass the test of being ethical, and most companies are aware that both their reputations and their long-term well-being are tied to conducting their business in a manner that wins the approval of suppliers, employees, investors, and society at large.

As a test your own business ethics and where you stand on the importance of companies having an ethical strategy, take the test on page 340.

LINKING A COMPANY'S STRATEGY TO ITS ETHICAL PRINCIPLES AND CORE VALUES

Many companies have officially adopted a code of ethical conduct and a statement of company values—in the United States, the Sarbannes-Oxley Act, passed in 2002, requires that companies whose stock is publicly traded have a code of ethics or else explain in writing to the Securities and Exchange Commission why they do not. But there's a big difference between having a code of ethics and a values statement that serve merely as a public window dressing and having ethical standards and corporate values that truly paint the white lines for a company's actual strategy and business conduct. If ethical standards and statements of core values are to have more than a cosmetic role, boards of directors and top executives must work diligently to see that they are scrupulously observed in crafting the company's strategy and conducting every facet of the company's business. In other words, living up to the ethical principles and displaying the core values in actions and decisions must become a way of life at the company.

Indeed, the litmus test of whether a company's code of ethics and statement of core values are cosmetic is the extent to which they are embraced in crafting strategy and in operating the business day to day. It is up to senior executives to walk the talk and make a point of considering two sets of questions whenever a new strategic initiative is under review:

- Is what we are proposing to do fully compliant with our code of ethical conduct? Is there anything here that could be considered ethically objectionable?
- Is it apparent that this proposed action is in harmony with our core values? Are any conflicts or concerns evident?

Unless questions of this nature are posed—either in open discussion or by force of habit in the minds of strategy makers, then there's room for strategic initiatives to become disconnected from the company's code of ethics and stated core values. If a company's executives are ethically principled and believe strongly in living up to the company's stated core values, there's a good chance they will pose these types of questions and reject strategic initiatives that don't measure up. There's also a good chance that strategic actions will be scrutinized for their compatibility with ethical standards and core values when the latter are so deeply ingrained in a company's culture and in the

> **Core Concept**
> More attention is paid to linking strategy with ethical principles and core values in companies headed by moral executives and in companies where ethical principles and core values are a way of life.

everyday conduct of company personnel that they are automatically taken into account in all that the company does. However, in companies with window-dressing ethics and core values or in companies headed by immoral or amoral managers, any strategy-ethics-values link stems mainly from a desire to avoid the risk of embarrassment, scandal, and possible disciplinary action should strategy makers get called on the carpet and held accountable for approving an unethical strategic initiative.

STRATEGY AND SOCIAL RESPONSIBILITY

The idea that businesses have an obligation to foster social betterment, a much-debated topic in the past 40 years, took root in the 19th century when progressive companies in the aftermath of the industrial revolution began to provide workers with housing and other amenities. The notion that corporate executives should balance the interests of all stakeholders –shareholders, employees, customers, suppliers, the communities in which they operated, and society at large—began to blossom in the 1960s. A group of chief executives of America's 200 largest corporations, calling themselves the Business Roundtable, promoted the concept of corporate social responsibility. In 1981, the Roundtable's "Statement on Corporate Responsibility" said:[37]

> Balancing the shareholder's expectations of maximum return against other priorities is one of the fundamental problems confronting corporate management. The shareholder must receive a good return but the legitimate concerns of other constituencies (customers, employees, communities, suppliers and society at large) also must have the appropriate attention . . . [Leading managers] believe that by giving enlightened consideration to balancing the legitimate claims of all its constituents, a corporation will best serve the interest of its shareholders.

Today, corporate social responsibility is a concept that resonates in Western Europe, the United States, Canada, and such developing nations as Brazil and India.

What Do We Mean by Social Responsibility?

Core Concept

The notion of *social responsibility* as it applies to businesses concerns a company's *duty* to operate in an honorable manner, provide good working conditions for employees, be a good steward of the environment, and actively work to better the quality of life in the local communities where it operates and in society at large.

The essence of socially responsible business behavior is that a company should balance strategic actions to benefit shareholders against the *duty* to be a good corporate citizen. The thesis is that company managers are obligated to display a *social conscience* in operating the business and specifically take into account how management decisions and company actions affect the well-being of employees, local communities, the environment, and society at large. Acting in a socially responsible manner thus encompasses more than just participating in community service projects and donating money to charities and other worthy social causes. Demonstrating social responsibility also entails undertaking actions that earn trust and respect from all stakeholders—operating in an honorable and ethical manner, striving to make the company a great place to work, demonstrating genuine respect for the environment, and trying to make a difference in bettering society. As depicted in Figure 10.2, the menu for demonstrating a social conscience and choosing specific ways to exercise social responsibility includes:

- *Efforts to employ an ethical strategy and observe ethical principles in operating the business*—A sincere commitment to observing ethical principles is

Figure 10.2   **Demonstrating a Social Conscience: The Five Components of Socially Responsible Business Behavior**

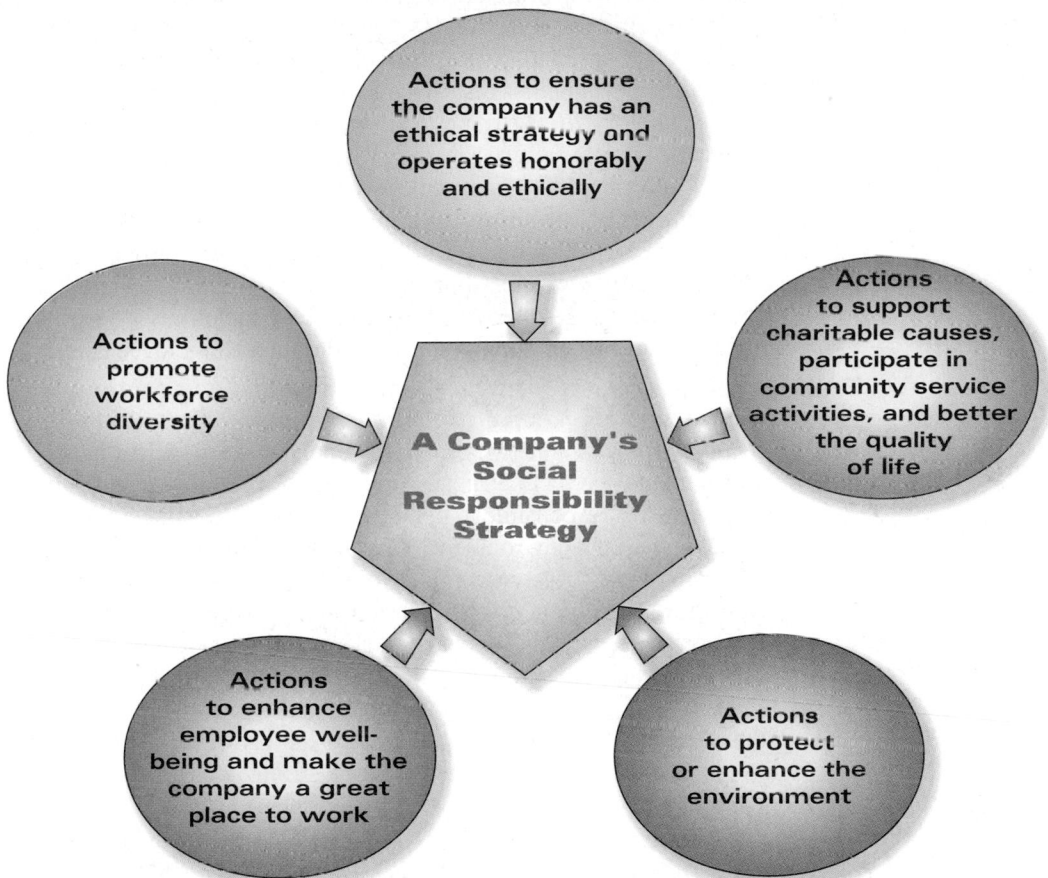

Source: Adapted from material in Ronald Paul Hill, Debra Stephens, and Iain Smith, "Corporate Social Responsibility: An Examination of Individual Firm Behavior," *Business and Society Review* 108, no. 3 (September 2003), p. 348.

necessary here simply because unethical strategies and conduct are incompatible with the concept of good corporate citizenship and socially responsible business behavior.

• *Making charitable contributions, donating money and the time of company personnel to community service endeavors, supporting various worthy organizational causes, and reaching out to make a difference in the lives of the disadvantaged*—Some companies fulfill their corporate citizenship and community outreach obligations by spreading their efforts over a multitude of charitable and community activities; for instance, Microsoft and Johnson & Johnson support a broad variety of community art, social welfare, and environmental programs. Others prefer to focus their energies more narrowly. McDonald's, for example, concentrates on sponsoring the Ronald McDonald House program (which provides a home away from home for the families of seriously ill children receiving treatment at nearby hospitals), preventing child abuse and neglect, and participating in local community service activities; in 2004, there were 240 Ronald McDonald Houses in 25 countries and more than 6,000 bedrooms available nightly. British Telecom gives 1 percent of its profits directly to communities, largely for education—teacher training, in-school workshops, and digital technology. Leading prescription drug maker GlaxoSmithKline and other pharmaceutical companies either donate or heavily discount medicines for distribution in the least-developed nations. Numerous health-related businesses take a leading role in community activities that promote effective health care. Many companies work closely with community officials to minimize the impact of hiring large numbers of new employees (which could put a strain on local schools and utility services) and to provide outplacement services for laid-off workers. Companies frequently reinforce their philanthropic efforts by encouraging employees to support charitable causes and participate in community affairs, often through programs to match employee contributions.

- *Actions to protect or enhance the environment and, in particular, to minimize or eliminate any adverse impact on the environment stemming from the company's own business activities*—Social responsibility as it applies to environmental protection means doing more than what is legally required. From a social responsibility perspective, companies have an obligation to be stewards of the environment. This means using the best available science and technology to achieve higher-than-required environmental standards. Even more ideally, it means putting time and money into improving the environment in ways that extend past a company's own industry boundaries— such as participating in recycling projects, adopting energy conservation practices, and supporting efforts to clean up local water supplies. Retailers such as Home Depot in the United States and B&Q in the United Kingdom have pressured their suppliers to adopt stronger environmental protection practices.[38]

> Business leaders who want their companies to be regarded as exemplary corporate citizens must not only see that their companies operate ethically but they must personally display a social conscience in making decisions that affect employees, the environment, the communities in which they operate, and society at large.

- *Actions to create a work environment that enhances the quality of life for employees and makes the company a great place to work*—Numerous companies go beyond providing the ordinary kinds of compensation and exert extra efforts to enhance the quality of life for their employees, both at work and at home. This can include varied and engaging job assignments, career development programs and mentoring, rapid career advancement, appealing compensation incentives, ongoing training to ensure future employability, added decision-making authority, onsite day care, flexible work schedules for single parents, workplace exercise facilities, special leaves to care for sick family members, work-at-home opportunities, gender pay equity, showcase plants and offices, special safety programs, and the like.

- *Actions to build a workforce that is diverse with respect to gender, race, national origin, and perhaps other aspects that different people bring to the workplace*— Most large companies in the United States have established workforce diversity programs, and some go the extra mile to ensure that their workplaces are attractive to ethnic minorities and inclusive of all groups and perspectives. The pursuit of workforce diversity can be good business—Johnson & Johnson, Pfizer, and Coca-Cola believe that a reputation for workforce diversity makes recruiting employees easier (talented employees from diverse backgrounds often seek out such companies). And at Coca-Cola, where strategic success depends on getting people all over the world to become loyal consumers of the company's beverages, efforts to build a public persona of inclusiveness for people of all races, religions, nationalities, interests, and talents has considerable strategic value. Multinational companies are particularly inclined to make workforce diversity a visible strategic component; they recognize that respecting individual differences and promoting inclusiveness resonate well with people all around the world. At a few companies the diversity initiative extends to suppliers—sourcing items from small businesses owned by women or ethnic minorities.

Crafting a Social Responsibility Strategy: The Starting Point for Demonstrating a Social Conscience

While striving to be socially responsible entails choosing from the menu outlined in the preceding section, there's plenty of room for every company to make its own statement about what charitable contributions to make, what kinds of community service projects to emphasize, what environmental actions to support, how to make the company a good place to work, where and how workforce diversity fits into the picture, and what else it will do to support worthy causes and projects that benefit society. The particular combination of socially responsible endeavors a company elects to pursue defines its **social responsibility strategy.** However, unless a company's social responsibility initiatives become part of the way it operates its business every day, the initiatives are unlikely to catch fire and be fully effective. As an executive at Royal Dutch/Shell put it, corporate social responsibility "is not a cosmetic; it must be rooted in our values. It must make a difference to the way we do business."[39] Thus some companies are integrating social responsibility objectives into their missions and overall performance targets—they see social performance and environmental metrics as an essential component of judging the company's overall future performance. Some 2,500 companies around the world are not only articulating their social responsibility strategies and commitments but they are also issuing annual social responsibility reports (much like an annual report) that set forth their commitments and the progress they are making for all the world to see and evaluate.[40]

> **Core Concept**
> A company's *social responsibility strategy* is defined by the specific combination of socially beneficial activities it opts to support with its contributions of time, money, and other resources.

At Starbucks, the commitment to social responsibility is linked to the company's strategy and operating practices via the tag line "Giving back to our communities is the way we do business"; top management makes the theme come alive via the company's extensive community-building activities, efforts to protect the welfare of coffee growers and their families (in particular, making sure they receive a fair price), a variety of recycling and environmental conservation practices, and the financial support it provides to charities and the disadvantaged through the Starbucks Foundation. At Green Mountain Coffee Roasters, social responsibility includes fair dealing with suppliers and trying to do something about the poverty of small coffee growers; in its dealings with suppliers at small farmer cooperatives in Peru, Mexico, and Sumatra, Green Mountain pays "fair trade" prices for coffee beans (in 2002, the fair trade prices were a minimum of $1.26 per pound for conventional coffee and $1.41 for organically grown versus market prices of 24 to 50 cents per pound). Green Mountain also purchases about 25 percent of its coffee direct from farmers so as to cut out intermediaries and see that farmers realize a higher price for their efforts—coffee is the world's second most heavily traded commodity after oil, requiring the labor of some 20 million people, most of whom live at the poverty level.[41] At Whole Foods Market, a $5 billion supermarket chain specializing in organic and natural foods, the social responsibility emphasis is on supporting organic farming and

> Many companies tailor their strategic efforts to operate in a socially responsible manner to fit their core values and business mission, thereby making their own statement about "how we do business and how we intend to fulfill our duties to all stakeholders and society at large."

sustainable agriculture, recycling, sustainable seafood practices, giving employees paid time off to participate in worthy community service endeavors, and donating 5 percent of after-tax profits in cash or products to charitable causes. At General Mills the social responsibility focus is on service to the community and bettering the employment opportunities for minorities and women. Stonyfield Farm, a producer of yogurt and ice cream products, employs a social responsibility strategy focused on wellness, good nutrition, and earth-friendly actions (10 percent of profits are donated to help protect and restore the earth, and yogurt lids are used as miniature billboards to help educate people about environmental issues); in addition, it is stressing the development of an environmentally friendly supply chain, sourcing from farmers that grow organic products and refrain from using artificial hormones in milk production. Chick-Fil-A, an Atlanta-based fast-food chain with over 1,200 outlets in 38 states, has a charitable foundation; supports 14 foster homes and a summer camp (for some 1,600 campers from 22 states and several foreign countries); funds two scholarship programs (including one for employees that has awarded more than $20 million in scholarships); and maintains a closed-on-Sunday policy to ensure that every Chick-Fil-A employee and restaurant operator has an opportunity to worship, spend time with family and friends, or just plain rest from the workweek.[42] Toys "R" Us supports initiatives addressing the issues of child labor and fair labor practices around the world. Community Pride Food Stores is assisting in revitalizing the inner city of Richmond, Virginia, where the company is based.

It is common for companies engaged in natural resource extraction, electric power production, forestry and paper products, motor vehicles, and chemicals production to place more emphasis on addressing environmental concerns than, say, software and electronics firms or apparel manufacturers. Companies whose business success is heavily dependent on high employee morale or attracting and retaining the best and brightest employees are somewhat more prone to stress the well-being of their employees and foster a positive, high-energy workplace environment that elicits the dedication and enthusiastic commitment of employees, thus putting real meaning behind the claim "Our people are our greatest asset." Ernst & Young, one of the four largest global accounting firms, stresses its "People First" workforce diversity strategy, which focuses on respecting differences, fostering individuality, and promoting inclusiveness so that its 105,000 employees in 140 countries can feel valued, engaged, and empowered in developing creative ways to serve the firm's clients.

Thus, while the strategies and actions of all socially responsible companies have a sameness in the sense of drawing on the five categories of socially responsible behavior shown in Figure 10.2, each company's version of being socially responsible is unique.

The Moral Case for Corporate Social Responsibility

Every action a company takes can be interpreted as a statement of what it stands for.

The moral case for why businesses should actively promote the betterment of society and act in a manner that benefits all of the company's stakeholders—not just the interests of shareholders—boils down to the fact that it's the right thing to do. Ordinary decency, civic-mindedness, and contributing to the well-being of society should be expected of any business. In today's social and political climate, most business leaders can be expected to acknowledge that socially responsible actions are important and that businesses have a duty to be good corporate citizens. But there is a complementary school of thought that business operates on the basis of an implied social contract with the members of society. According to this contract, society grants a business the right to conduct its business affairs and agrees not to unreasonably restrain its pursuit of a fair profit for the goods or services it sells; in return for this "license to operate," a business is obligated to act as a responsible citizen and do its fair share to promote the general welfare. Such a view clearly puts a moral burden on a company to take corporate citizenship into consideration and to do what's best for shareholders within the confines of discharging its duties to operate honorably, provide good working conditions to employees, be a good environmental steward, and display good corporate citizenship.

The Business Case for Socially Responsible Behavior

Whatever the merits of the moral case for socially responsible business behavior, it has long been recognized that it is in the enlightened self-interest of companies to be good citizens and devote some of their energies and resources to the betterment of employees, the communities in which they operate, and society in general. In short, there are several reasons why the exercise of social responsibility is good business:

- *It generates internal benefits (particularly as concerns employee recruiting, workforce retention, and training costs)*—Companies with deservedly good reputations for contributing time and money to the betterment of society are better able to attract and retain employees compared to companies with tarnished reputations. Some employees just feel better about working for a company committed to improving society.[43] This can contribute to lower turnover and better worker productivity. Other direct and indirect economic benefits include lower costs for staff recruitment and training. For example, Starbucks is said to enjoy much lower rates of employee turnover because of its full benefits package for both full-time and part-time employees, management efforts to make Starbucks a great place to work, and the company's socially responsible practices. When a U.S. manufacturer of recycled paper, taking eco-efficiency to heart, discovered how to increase its fiber recovery rate, it saved the equivalent of 20,000 tons of waste paper—a factor that helped the company become the industry's lowest-cost producer.[44] Various benchmarking and measurement mechanisms have shown that workforce diversity initiatives promote the success of companies that stay behind them. Making a company a great place to work pays dividends in recruiting talented workers, more creativity and energy on the part of workers, higher worker productivity, and greater employee commitment to the company's business mission/vision and success in the marketplace.

- *It reduces the risk of reputation-damaging incidents and can lead to increased buyer patronage*—Firms may well be penalized by employees, consumers, and shareholders for actions that are not considered socially responsible. When a major oil company suffered damage to its reputation on environmental and social grounds, the CEO repeatedly said that the most negative impact the company suffered—and the one that made him fear for the future of the company—was that bright young graduates were no longer attracted to work for the company.[45] Consumer, environmental, and human rights activist groups are quick to criticize businesses whose behavior they consider to be out of line, and they are adept at getting their message into the media and onto the Internet. Pressure groups can generate widespread adverse publicity, promote boycotts, and influence like-minded or sympathetic buyers to avoid an offender's products.

> The higher the public profile of a company or brand, the greater the scrutiny of its activities and the higher the potential for it to become a target for pressure-group action.

Research has shown that product boycott announcements are associated with a decline in a company's stock price.[46] Outspoken criticism of Royal Dutch/Shell by environmental and human rights groups and associated boycotts were said to be major factors in the company's decision to tune in to its social responsibilities. For many years, Nike received stinging criticism for not policing sweatshop conditions in the Asian factories of its contractors, causing Nike CEO Phil Knight to observe that "Nike has become synonymous with slave wages, forced overtime, and arbitrary abuse."[47] In 1997, Nike began an extensive effort to monitor conditions in the 800 overseas factories from which it outsourced its shoes; Knight said, "Good shoes come from good factories, and good factories have good labor relations." Nonetheless, Nike has continually been plagued by complaints from human rights activists that its monitoring procedures are flawed and that it is not doing enough to correct the plight of factory workers. In contrast, to the extent that a company's socially responsible behavior wins applause from consumers and fortifies its reputation, the company may win additional patronage; Ben & Jerry's, Whole Foods Market, Stonyfield Farm, and the Body Shop have definitely expanded their customer bases because of their visible and well-publicized activities as socially conscious companies. More and more companies are recognizing the strategic value of social responsibility strategies that reach out to people of all cultures and demographics—in the United States, women are said to having buying power of $3.7 trillion, retired and disabled people close to $4.1 trillion, Hispanics nearly $600 billion, African Americans some $500 billion, and Asian Americans about $255 billion.[48] So reaching out in ways that appeal to such groups can pay off at the cash register. Some observers and executives are convinced that a strong, visible social responsibility strategy gives a company an edge in differentiating itself from rivals and in appealing to those consumers who prefer to do business with companies that are solid corporate citizens. Yet there is only limited evidence that consumers go out of their way to patronize socially responsible companies if it means paying a higher price or purchasing an inferior product.[49]

- *It is in the best interest of shareholders*—Well-conceived social responsibility strategies work to the advantage of shareholders in several ways. Socially responsible business behavior helps avoid or preempt legal and regulatory actions that could prove costly and otherwise burdensome. Increasing numbers of mutual funds and pension benefit managers are restricting their stock purchases to companies that meet social responsibility criteria. According to one survey, one out of every eight dollars under professional management in the United States involved socially responsible investing.[50] Moreover, the growth in socially responsible investing and identifying socially responsible companies has led to a substantial increase in the number of companies that publish formal reports on their social and environmental activities.[51] The stock prices of companies that rate high on social and environmental performance criteria have been found to perform 35 to 45 percent better than the average of the 2,500 companies comprising the Dow Jones Global Index.[52] A two-year study of leading companies found that improving environmental compliance and developing environmentally friendly products can enhance earnings per share, profitability, and the likelihood of winning contracts.[53] Nearly 100 studies have examined the relationship between corporate citizenship and corporate financial performance over the past 30 years; the majority point to a positive relationship. Of the 80 studies that examined whether a company's social performance is a good predictor of its financial performance, 42 concluded yes, 4 concluded

There's little hard evidence indicating shareholders are disadvantaged in any meaningful way by a company's actions to be socially responsible.

no, and the remainder reported mixed or inconclusive findings.[54] To the extent that socially responsible behavior is good business, then, a social responsibility strategy that packs some punch and is more than rhetorical flourish turns out to be in the best interest of shareholders.

In sum, companies that take social responsibility seriously can improve their business reputations and operational efficiency while also reducing their risk exposure and encouraging loyalty and innovation. Overall, companies that take special pains to protect the environment (beyond what is required by law), are active in community affairs, and are generous supporters of charitable causes and projects that benefit society are more likely to be seen as good investments and as good companies to work for or do business with. Shareholders are likely to view the business case for social responsibility as a strong one, even though they certainly have a right to be concerned whether the time and money their company spends to carry out its social responsibility strategy outweighs the benefits and reduces the bottom line by an unjustified amount.

Companies are, of course, sometimes rewarded for bad behavior—a company that is able to shift environmental and other social costs associated with its activities onto society as a whole can reap large short-term profits. The major cigarette producers for many years were able to earn greatly inflated profits by shifting the health-related costs of smoking onto others and escaping any responsibility for the harm their products caused to consumers and the general public. Most companies will, of course, try to evade paying for the social harms of their operations for as long as they can. Calling a halt to such actions usually hinges upon (1) the effectiveness of activist social groups in publicizing the adverse consequences of a company's social irresponsibility and marshaling public opinion for something to be done, (2) the enactment of legislation or regulations to correct the inequity, and (3) widespread actions on the part of socially conscious buyers to take their business elsewhere.

The Well-Intentioned Efforts of Do-Good Executives Can Be Controversial

While there is substantial agreement that businesses have obligations to non-owner stakeholders and to society at large, and that these must be factored into a company's overall strategy and into the conduct of its business operations, there is much less agreement about the extent to which "do-good" executives should pursue their personal vision of a better world using company funds. One view holds that any money executives authorize for so-called social responsibility initiatives is effectively theft from a company's shareholders who can, after all, decide for themselves what and how much to give to charity and other causes they deem worthy. A related school of thought says that companies should be wary of taking on an assortment of societal obligations because doing so diverts valuable resources and weakens a company's competitiveness. Many academics and businesspeople believe that businesses best satisfy their social responsibilities through conventional business activities, primarily producing needed goods and services at prices that people can afford. They further argue that spending shareholders' or customers' money for social causes not only muddies decision making by diluting the focus on the company's business mission but also thrusts business executives into the role of social engineers—a role more appropriately performed by charitable and nonprofit organizations and duly elected government officials. Do we really want corporate executives deciding how to best balance the different interests of stakeholders and functioning as social engineers? Are they competent to make such judgments?

Take the case of Coca-Cola and Pepsi bottlers. Local bottlers of both brands have signed contracts with public school districts that provide millions of dollars of support for local schools in exchange for vending-machine distribution rights in the schools.[55] While such contracts would seem to be a win–win proposition, protests from parents concerned about children's sugar-laden diets and commercialism in the schools make such contracts questionable. Opponents of these contracts claim that it is the role of government to provide adequate school funding and that the learning environment in local schools should be free of commercialism and the self-serving efforts of businesses to hide behind providing support for education.

In September 1997, the Business Roundtable changed its stance from one of support for social responsibility and balanced consideration of stakeholder interests to one of skepticism with regard to such actions:

> The notion that the board must somehow balance the interests of stockholders against the interests of other stakeholders fundamentally misconstrues the role of directors. It is, moreover, an unworkable notion because it would leave the board with no criteria for resolving conflicts between the interest of stockholders and of other stakeholders or among different groups of stakeholders.[56]

The new Business Roundtable view implied that the paramount duty of management and of boards of directors is to the corporation's stockholders. Customers may be "king," and employees may be the corporation's "greatest asset" (at least in the rhetoric), but the interests of shareholders rule.[57]

However, there are real problems with disconnecting business behavior from the well-being of non-owner stakeholders and the well-being of society at large.[58] Isolating business from the rest of society when the two are inextricably intertwined is unrealistic. Many business decisions spill over to impact non-owner stakeholders and society. Furthermore, the notion that businesses must be managed solely to serve the interests of shareholders is something of a stretch. Clearly, a business's first priority must be to deliver value to customers. Unless a company does a creditable job of satisfying buyer needs and expectations of reliable and attractively priced goods and services, it cannot survive. While shareholders provide capital and are certainly entitled to a return on their investment, fewer and fewer shareholders are truly committed to the companies whose stock they own. Shareholders can dispose of their holdings in a moment's whim or at the first sign of a downturn in the stock price. Mutual funds buy and sell shares daily, adding and dropping companies whenever they see fit. Day traders buy and sell within hours. Such buying and selling of shares is nothing more than a financial transaction and results in no capital being provided to the company to fund operations except when it entails the purchase of newly issued shares of stock. So why should shareholders—a group distant from the company's operations and adding little to its operations except when new shares of stock are purchased—lay such a large claim on how a company should be managed? Are most shareholders really interested in or knowledgeable about the companies they own? Or do they just own a stock for whatever financial returns it is expected to provide?

While there is legitimate concern about the use of company resources for do-good purposes and the motives and competencies of business executives in functioning as social engineers, it is tough to argue that businesses have no obligations to nonowner stakeholders or to society at large. If one looks at the category of activities that fall under the umbrella of socially responsible behavior (Figure 10.2), there's really very little for shareholders or others concerned about the do-good attempts of executives to object to in principle. Certainly, it is legitimate for companies to minimize or eliminate any adverse impacts of their operations on the environment. It is hard to argue against efforts to make the company a great place to work or to promote workforce diversity. And with regard to charitable contributions, community service projects, and the like, it would be hard to find a company where spending on such activities is so out of control that shareholders might rightfully complain or that the company's competitiveness is being eroded. What is likely to prove most objectionable in the social responsibility arena are the specific activities a company elects to engage in and/or the manner in which a company carries out its attempts to behave in a socially responsible manner.

How Much Attention to Social Responsibility Is Enough?

What is an appropriate balance between the imperative to create value for shareholders and the obligation to proactively contribute to the larger social good? What fraction of a company's resources ought to be aimed at addressing social concerns and bettering the well-being of society and the environment? A few companies have a policy of setting aside a specified percentage of their profits (typically 5 percent or maybe 10 percent) to fund their social responsibility strategy; they view such percentages as a fair amount to return to the community as a kind of thank-you or a tithe to the betterment of society. Other companies shy away from a specified percentage of profits or revenues because it entails upping the commitment in good times and cutting back on social responsibility initiatives in hard times (even cutting out social responsibility initiatives entirely if profits temporarily turn into losses). If social responsibility is an ongoing commitment rooted in the corporate culture and enlists broad participation on the part of company personnel, then a sizable portion of the funding for the company's social responsibility strategy has to be viewed as simply a regular and ongoing cost of doing business.

But judging how far a particular company should go in pursuing particular social causes is a tough issue. Consider, for example, Nike's commitment to monitoring the workplace conditions of its contract suppliers.[59] The scale of this monitoring task is significant: in 2005, Nike had over 800 contract suppliers employing over 600,000 people in 50 countries. How frequently should sites be monitored? How should it respond to the use of underage labor? If only children above a set age are to be employed by suppliers, should suppliers still be required to provide schooling opportunities? At last count, Nike had some 80 people engaged in site monitoring. Should Nike's monitoring budget be $2 million, $5 million, $10 million, or whatever it takes?

Consider another example: If pharmaceutical manufacturers donate or discount their drugs for distribution to low-income people in less-developed nations, what safeguards should they put in place to see that the drugs reach the intended recipients and are not diverted by corrupt local officials for reexport to markets in other countries? Should drug manufacturers also assist in drug distribution and administration in these less-developed countries? How much should a drug company invest in R&D to develop medicines for tropical diseases commonly occurring in less-developed countries when it is unlikely to recover its costs in the foreseeable future?

And how much should a company allocate to charitable contributions? Is it falling short of its responsibilities if its donations are less than 1 percent of profits? Is a company going too far if it allocates 5 percent or even 10 percent of its profits to worthy causes of one kind or another? The point here is that there is no simple or widely accepted standard for judging when a company has or has not gone far enough in fulfilling its citizenship responsibilities.

Linking Social Performance Targets to Executive Compensation

Perhaps the most surefire way to enlist a genuine commitment to corporate social responsibility initiatives is to link the achievement of social performance targets to executive compensation. If a company's board of directors is serious about corporate citizenship, then it will incorporate measures of the company's social and environmental performance into its evaluation of top executives, especially the CEO. And if the CEO uses compensation incentives to further enlist the support of down-the-line company personnel in effectively crafting and executing a social responsibility strategy, the company will over time build a culture rooted in social responsible and ethical behavior. According to one survey, 80 percent of surveyed CEOs believe that environmental and social performance metrics are a valid part of measuring a company's overall performance. At Verizon Communications, 10 percent of the annual bonus of the company's top 2,500 managers is tied directly to the achievement of social responsibility targets; for the rest of the staff, there are corporate recognition awards in the form of cash for employees who have made big contributions towards social causes. The corporate social responsibility reports being issued annually by 2,500 companies across the world that detail social responsibility initiatives and the results achieved are a good basis for compensating executives and judging the effectiveness of their commitment to social responsibility.

Key Points

Ethics involves concepts of right and wrong, fair and unfair, moral and immoral. Beliefs about what is ethical serve as a moral compass in guiding the actions and behaviors of individuals and organizations. Ethical principles in business are not materially different from ethical principles in general.

There are three schools of thought about ethical standards:

1. According to the *school of ethical universalism*, the same standards of what's ethical and what's unethical resonate with peoples of most societies regardless of local traditions and cultural norms; hence, common ethical standards can be used to judge the conduct of personnel at companies operating in a variety of country markets and cultural circumstances.

2. According to the *school of ethical relativism* different societal cultures and customs have divergent values and standards of right and wrong—thus, what is ethical or unethical must be judged in the light of local customs and social mores and can vary from culture or nation to another.

3. According to *integrated social contracts theory*, universal ethical principles or norms based on the collective views of multiple cultures and societies combine to form a "social contract" that all individuals in all situations have a duty to observe. Within the boundaries of this social contract, local cultures can specify other impermissible actions; however, universal ethical norms always take precedence over local ethical norms.

Three categories of managers stand out as concerns their prevailing beliefs in and commitments to ethical and moral principles in business affairs: the moral manager; the immoral manager, and the amoral manager. By some accounts, the population of managers is said to be distributed among all three types in a bell-shaped curve, with immoral managers and moral managers occupying the two tails of the curve, and the amoral managers, especially the intentionally amoral managers, occupying the broad middle ground.

The apparently large numbers of immoral and amoral businesspeople are one obvious reason why some companies resort to unethical strategic behavior. Three other main drivers of unethical business behavior also stand out:

1. Overzealous or obsessive pursuit of personal gain, wealth, and other selfish interests.
2. Heavy pressures on company managers to meet or beat earnings targets.
3. A company culture that puts the profitability and good business performance ahead of ethical behavior.

The stance a company takes in dealing with or managing ethical conduct at any given time can take any of four basic forms:

1. The unconcerned, or nonissue, approach.
2. The damage control approach.
3. The compliance approach.
4. The ethical culture approach.

There are two reasons why a company's strategy should be ethical: (1) because a strategy that is unethical in whole or in part is morally wrong and reflects badly on the character of the company personnel involved, and (2) because an ethical strategy is good business and in the self-interest of shareholders.

The term *corporate social responsibility* concerns a company's *duty* to operate in an honorable manner, provide good working conditions for employees, be a good steward of the environment, and actively work to better the quality of life in the local communities where it operates and in society at large. The menu of actions and behavior for demonstrating social responsibility includes:

1. Employing an ethical strategy and observing ethical principles in operating the business.
2. Making charitable contributions, donating money and the time of company personnel to community service endeavors, supporting various worthy organizational causes, and making a difference in the lives of the disadvantaged. Corporate commitments are further reinforced by encouraging employees to support charitable and community activities.
3. Protecting or enhancing the environment and, in particular, striving to minimize or eliminate any adverse impact on the environment stemming from the company's own business activities.
4. Creating a work environment that makes the company a great place to work.
5. Employing a workforce that is diverse with respect to gender, race, national origin, and perhaps other aspects that different people bring to the workplace.

There is ample room for every company to tailor its social responsibility strategy to fit its core values and business mission, thereby making their own statement about "how we do business and how we intend to fulfill our duties to all stakeholders and society at large."

The moral case for social responsibility boils down to a simple concept: It's the right thing to do. The business case for social responsibility holds that it is in the enlightened self-interest of companies to be good citizens and devote some of their energies and resources to the betterment of such stakeholders as employees, the communities in which it operates, and society in general.

Exercises

1. Given the description of Marsh & McLennan's strategy presented in Illustration Capsule 10.1, would it be fair to characterize the payment of contingent commissions by property-casualty insurers as nothing more than thinly disguised kickbacks? Why or why not? If you were the manager of a company that hired Marsh & McLennan to provide risk management services, would you see that Marsh had a conflict of interest in steering your company's insurance policies to insurers in which it has an ownership interest? Given Marsh's unethical and illegal foray into rigging the bids on insurance policies for its corporate clients, what sort of fines and penalties would you impose on the company for its misdeeds (assuming you were asked to recommend appropriate penalties by the prosecuting authorities). In arriving at a figure, bear in mind that Prudential Securities paid a total of about $2 billion in the 1990s to settle civil regulatory charges and private lawsuits alleging that it misled investors on the risks and rewards of limited-partnership investments. Ten Wall Street securities firms in 2003 paid $1.4 billion to settle civil charges for issuing misleading stock research to investors. Prominent mutual-fund firms were assessed nearly $2 billion in fines and restitution for engaging in after-hours stock trading at prearranged prices that were contrary to the interests of long-term shareholders. And several well-known financial institutions, including Citigroup, Merrill Lynch, Goldmans Sachs, and Credit Suisse First Boston agreed to pay several billion dollars in fines and restitution for their role in scandals at Enron and WorldCom and for improperly allocating initial public offerings of stock. Using Internet research tools, determine what Marsh & McLennan ended up paying in fines and restitution for its unethical and illegal strategic behavior and assess the extent to which the conduct of company personnel damaged shareholders.

2. Consider the following portrayal of strategies employed by major recording studios:[60]

> Some recording artists and the Recording Artists' Coalition claim that the world's five major music recording studios—Universal, Sony, Time Warner, EMI/Virgin, and Bertelsmann—deliberately employ strategies calculated to take advantage of musicians who record for them. One practice to which they strenuously object is that the major-label record companies frequently require artists to sign contracts committing them to do six to eight albums, an obligation that some artists say can entail an indefinite term of indentured servitude. Further, it is claimed that audits routinely detect unpaid royalties to musicians under contract; according to one music industry attorney, record companies misreport and underpay artist royalties by 10 to 40 percent and are "intentionally fraudulent." One music writer was recently quoted as saying the process was "an entrenched system whose prowess and conniving makes Enron look like amateur hour." Royalty calculations are based on complex formulas that are paid only after artists pay for recording costs and other expenses and after any advances are covered by royalty earnings.
>
> A *Baffler* magazine article outlined a hypothetical but typical record deal in which a promising young band is given a $250,000 royalty advance on a new album. The album subsequently sells 250,000 copies, earning $710,000 for the

record company; but the band, after repaying the record company for $264,000 in expenses ranging from recording fees and video budgets to catering, wardrobe, and bus tour costs for promotional events related to the album, ends up $14,000 in the hole, owes the record company money, and is thus paid no royalties on any of the $710,000 in revenues the recording company receives from the sale of the band's music. It is also standard practice in the music industry for recording studios to sidestep payola laws by hiring independent promoters to lobby and compensate radio stations for playing certain records. Record companies are often entitled to damages for undelivered albums if an artist leaves a recording studio for another label after seven years. Record companies also retain the copyrights in perpetuity on all music recorded under contract, a practice that artists claim is unfair. The Dixie Chicks, after a year-long feud with Sony over contract terms, ended up refusing to do another album; Sony sued for breach of contract, prompting a countersuit by the Dixie Chicks charging "systematic thievery" to cheat them out of royalties. The suits were settled out of court. One artist said, "The record companies are like cartels."

Recording studios defend their strategic practices by pointing out that fewer than 5 percent of the signed artists ever deliver a hit and that they lose money on albums that sell poorly. According to one study, only 1 of 244 contracts signed during 1994–1996 was negotiated without the artists being represented by legal counsel, and virtually all contracts renegotiated after a hit album added terms more favorable to the artist.

a.   If you were a recording artist, would you be happy with some of the strategic practices of the recording studios? Would you feel comfortable signing a recording contract with studios engaging in any of the practices?

b.   Which, if any, of the practices of the recording studios do you view as unethical?

3.   Recently, it came to light that three of the world's four biggest public accounting firms may have overbilled clients for travel-related expenses. Pricewaterhouse Coopers, KPMG, and Ernst & Young were sued for systematically charging their clients full price for airline tickets, hotel rooms and car-rental expenses, even though they received volume discounts and rebates of up to 40 percent under their contracts with various travel companies. Large accounting firms, law firms, and medical practices have in recent years used their size and purchasing volumes to negotiate sizable discounts and rebates on up-front travel costs; some of these contracts apparently required that the discounts not be disclosed to other parties, which seemingly included clients.

However, it has long been the custom for accounting and law firms to bill their clients for actual out-of-pocket expenses. The three accounting firms, so the lawsuit alleges, billed clients for the so-called full prices of the airline tickets, hotel rooms, and car-rental expenses rather than for the out-of-pocket discounted amounts. They pocketed the differences to the tune of several million dollars annually in additional profits. Several clients, upon learning of the full-price billing practices, claimed fraud and sued.

Do you consider the accounting firms' billing practice to be unethical? Why or why not?

4.   Suppose you found yourself in the following situation: In preparing a bid for a multimillion-dollar contract in a foreign country, you are introduced to a "consultant" who offers to help you in submitting the bid and negotiating with the customer company. You learn in conversing with the consultant that she is well connected in local government and business circles and knows key personnel in the customer company extremely well. The consultant quotes you a six-figure fee.

Later, your local co-workers tell you that the use of such consultants is normal in this country—and that a large fraction of the fee will go directly to people working for the customer company. They further inform you that bidders who reject the help of such consultants have lost contracts to competitors who employed them. What would you do, assuming your company's code of ethics expressly forbids the payments of bribes or kickbacks in any form?

5. Assume that you are the sales manager at a European company that makes sleepwear products for children. Company personnel discover that the chemicals used to flameproof the company's line of children's pajamas might cause cancer if absorbed through the skin. Following this discovery, the pajamas are then banned from sale in the European Union and the United States, but senior executives of your company learn that the children's pajamas in inventory and the remaining flameproof material can be sold to sleepwear distributors in certain East European countries where there are no restrictions against the material's use. Your superiors instruct you to make the necessary arrangements to sell the inventories of banned pajamas and flameproof materials to East European distributors. Would you comply if you felt that your job would be in jeopardy if you didn't?

6. At Salomon Smith Barney (a subsidiary of Citigroup), Credit Suisse First Boston (CSFB), and Goldman Sachs (three of the world's most prominent investment banking companies), part of the strategy for securing the investment banking business of large corporate clients (to handle the sale of new stock issues or new bond issues or advise on mergers and acquisitions) involved (*a*) hyping the stocks of companies that were actual or prospective customers of their investment banking services, and (*b*) allocating hard-to-get shares of hot new initial public offerings (IPOs) to select executives and directors of existing and potential client companies, who then made millions of dollars in profits when the stocks went up once public trading began.[61] Former WorldCom CEO Bernard Ebbers reportedly made more than $11 million in trading profits over a four-year period on shares of IPOs received from Salomon Smith Barney; Salomon served as WorldCom's investment banker on a variety of deals during this period. Jack Grubman, Salomon's top-paid research analyst at the time, enthusiastically touted WorldCom stock and was regarded as the company's biggest cheerleader on Wall Street.

To help draw in business from new or existing corporate clients, CSFB established brokerage accounts for corporate executives who steered their company's investment banking business to CSFB. Apparently, CSFB's strategy for acquiring more business involved promising the CEO and/or CFO of companies about to go public for the first time or needing to issue new long-term bonds that if CSFB was chosen to handle their company's IPO of common stock or a new bond issue, then CSFB would ensure they would be allocated shares at the initial offering price of all subsequent IPOs in which CSFB was a participant. During 1999–2000, it was common for the stock of a hot new IPO to rise 100 to 500 percent above the initial offering price in the first few days or weeks of public trading; the shares allocated to these executives were then sold for a tidy profit over the initial offering price. According to investigative sources, CSFB increased the number of companies whose executives were allowed to participate in its IPO offerings from 26 companies in January 1999 to 160 companies in early 2000; executives received anywhere from 200 to 1,000 shares each of every IPO in which CSFB was a participant in 2000. CSFB's accounts for these executives reportedly generated profits of about $80 million for the participants. Apparently, it was CSFB's practice to curtail access to IPOs for some executives if their companies didn't come through with additional securities business for CSFB or if CSFB concluded that other securities offerings by these companies would be unlikely.

Goldman Sachs also used an IPO-allocation scheme to attract investment banking business, giving shares to executives at 21 companies—among the participants were the CEOs of eBay, Yahoo, and Ford Motor Company. eBay's CEO was a participant in over 100 IPOs managed by Goldman during the 1996–2000 period and was on Goldman's board of directors part of this time; eBay paid Goldman Sachs $8 million in fees for services during the 1996–2001 period.

a. If you were a top executive at Salomon Smith Barney, CSFB, or Goldman Sachs, would you be proud to defend your company's actions?

b. Would you want to step forward and take credit for having been a part of the group who designed or approved of the strategy for gaining new business at any of these three firms?

c. Is it accurate to characterize the allocations of IPO shares to "favored" corporate executives as bribes or kickbacks?

Building an Organization Capable of Good Strategy Execution

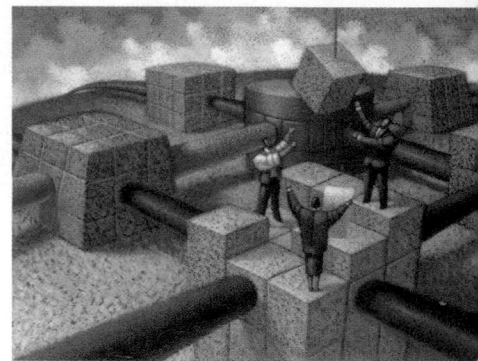

The best game plan in the world never blocked or tackled anybody.

—Vince Lombardi
Hall of Fame football coach

Strategies most often fail because they aren't executed well.

—Larry Bossidy and Ram Charan
CEO Honeywell International; author and consultant

A second-rate strategy perfectly executed will beat a first-rate strategy poorly executed every time.

—Richard M. Kovacevich
Chairman and CEO, Wells Fargo

Any strategy, however brilliant, needs to be implemented properly if it is to deliver the desired results.

—Costas Markides
Professor

People are *not* your most important asset. The right people are.

—Jim Collins
Professor and author

Organizing is what you do before you do something, so that when you do it, it is not all mixed up.

—A. A. Milne
Author

O nce managers have decided on a strategy, the emphasis turns to converting it into actions and good results. Putting the strategy into place and
getting the organization to execute it well call for different sets of managerial skills. Whereas crafting strategy is largely a market-driven activity, implementing and executing strategy is primarily an operations-driven activity revolving around
the management of people and business processes. Whereas successful strategy making
depends on business vision, solid industry and competitive analysis, and shrewd market positioning, successful strategy execution depends on doing a good job of working
with and through others, building and strengthening competitive capabilities, motivating and rewarding people in a strategy-supportive manner, and instilling a discipline
of getting things done. Executing strategy is an action-oriented, make-things-happen
task that tests a manager's ability to direct organizational change, achieve continuous improvement in operations and business processes, create and nurture a strategy-
supportive culture, and consistently meet or beat performance targets.

Experienced managers are emphatic in declaring that it is a whole lot easier to
develop a sound strategic plan than it is to execute the plan and achieve the desired
outcomes. According to one executive, "It's been rather easy for us to decide where
we wanted to go. The hard part is to get the organization to act on the new priorities."[1]
*Just because senior managers announce a new strategy doesn't mean that organiza-
tional members will agree with it or enthusiastically move forward in implementing
it.* Senior executives cannot simply direct immediate subordinates to abandon old
ways and take up new ways, and they certainly cannot expect the needed actions
and changes to occur in rapid-fire fashion and lead to the desired outcomes. Some
managers and employees may be skeptical about the merits of the strategy, seeing
it as contrary to the organization's best interests, unlikely to succeed, or threatening to their departments or careers. Moreover, different employees may interpret
the new strategy differently or have different ideas about what internal changes are
needed to execute it. Long-standing attitudes, vested interests, inertia, and ingrained
organizational practices don't melt away when managers decide on a new strategy
and begin efforts to implement it—especially when only comparatively few people have been involved in crafting the strategy and when the rationale for strategic
change has to be sold to enough organizational members to root out the status quo.

It takes adept managerial leadership to convincingly communicate the new strategy and the reasons for it, overcome pockets of doubt and disagreement, secure the commitment and enthusiasm of concerned parties, identify and build consensus on all the hows of implementation and execution, and move forward to get all the pieces into place. Company personnel have to understand—in their heads and in their hearts—why a new strategic direction is necessary and where the new strategy is taking them.[2] Instituting change is, of course, easier when the problems with the old strategy have become obvious and/or the company has spiraled into a financial crisis.

But the challenge of successfully implementing new strategic initiatives goes well beyond managerial adeptness in overcoming resistance to change. What really makes executing strategy a tougher, more time-consuming management challenge than crafting strategy are the wide array of managerial activities that have to be attended to, the many ways that managers can proceed, and the number of bedeviling issues that must be worked out. It takes first-rate "managerial smarts" to zero in on what exactly needs to be done to put new strategic initiatives in place and, further, how best to get these things done in a timely fashion and in a manner that yields good results. Demanding people-management skills are required. Plus, it takes follow-through and perseverance to get a variety of initiatives launched and moving and to integrate the efforts of many different work groups into a smoothly functioning whole. Depending on how much consensus building and organizational change is involved, the process of implementing strategy changes can take several months to several years. And it takes still longer to achieve *real proficiency* in executing the strategy.

Like crafting strategy, *executing strategy is a job for the whole management team, not just a few senior managers.* While an organization's chief executive officer and the heads of major units (business divisions, functional departments, and key operating units) are ultimately responsible for seeing that strategy is executed successfully, the process typically affects every part of the firm, from the biggest operating unit to the smallest frontline work group. Top-level managers have to rely on the active support and cooperation of middle and lower managers to push strategy changes into functional areas and operating units and to see that the organization actually operates in accordance with the strategy on a daily basis. Middle and lower-level managers not only are responsible for initiating and supervising the execution process in their areas of authority but also are instrumental in getting subordinates to continuously improve on how strategy-critical value chain activities are being performed and in producing the operating results that allow company performance targets to be met—their role on the company's strategy execution team is by no means minimal.

Core Concept

Good strategy execution requires a *team effort*. All managers have strategy-executing responsibility in their areas of authority, and all employees are participants in the strategy execution process.

Strategy execution thus requires every manager to think through the answer to "What does my area have to do to implement its part of the strategic plan, and what should I do to get these things accomplished effectively and efficiently?" The bigger the organization or the more geographically scattered its operating units, the more that successful strategy execution depends on the cooperation and implementing skills of operating managers who can push the needed changes at the lowest organizational levels and, in the process, deliver good results. Only in small organizations can top-level managers get around the need for a team effort on the part of management and personally orchestrate the actions steps required for good strategy execution and operating excellence.

A FRAMEWORK FOR EXECUTING STRATEGY

Implementing and executing strategy entails figuring out all the hows—the specific techniques, actions, and behaviors that are needed for a smooth strategy-supportive operation—and then following through to get things done and deliver results. The idea is to make things happen and make them happen right. The first step in implementing strategic changes is for management to communicate the case for organizational change so clearly and persuasively to organizational members that a determined commitment takes hold throughout the ranks to find ways to put the strategy into place, make it work, and meet performance targets. The ideal condition is for managers to arouse enough enthusiasm for the strategy to turn the implementation process into a companywide crusade. *Management's handling of the strategy implementation process can be considered successful if and when the company achieves the targeted strategic and financial performance and shows good progress in making its strategic vision a reality.*

The specific hows of executing a strategy—the exact items that need to be placed on management's action agenda—always have to be customized to fit the particulars of a company's situation. Making minor changes in an existing strategy differs from implementing radical strategy changes. The hot buttons for successfully executing a low-cost provider strategy are different from those in executing a high-end differentiation strategy. Implementing and executing a new strategy for a struggling company in the midst of a financial crisis is a different job from that of improving strategy execution in a company where the execution is already pretty good. Moreover, some managers are more adept than others at using this or that approach to achieving the desired kinds of organizational changes. Hence, there's no definitive managerial recipe for successful strategy execution that cuts across all company situations and all types of strategies or that works for all types of managers. Rather, the specific hows of implementing and executing a strategy—the to-do list that constitutes management's agenda for action—must always be custom-tailored to fit an individual company's own circumstances and represents management's judgment about how best to proceed.

THE PRINCIPAL MANAGERIAL COMPONENTS OF THE STRATEGY EXECUTION PROCESS

Despite the need to tailor a company's strategy-executing approaches to the particulars of its situation, certain managerial bases have to be covered no matter what the circumstances. Eight managerial tasks crop up repeatedly in company efforts to execute strategy (see Figure 11.1):

1. Building an organization with the competencies, capabilities, and resource strengths to execute strategy successfully.
2. Marshaling sufficient money and people behind the drive for strategy execution.
3. Instituting policies and procedures that facilitate rather than impede strategy execution.
4. Adopting best practices and pushing for continuous improvement in how value chain activities are performed.
5. Installing information and operating systems that enable company personnel to carry out their strategic roles proficiently.

Figure 11.1   **The Eight Components of the Strategy Execution Process**

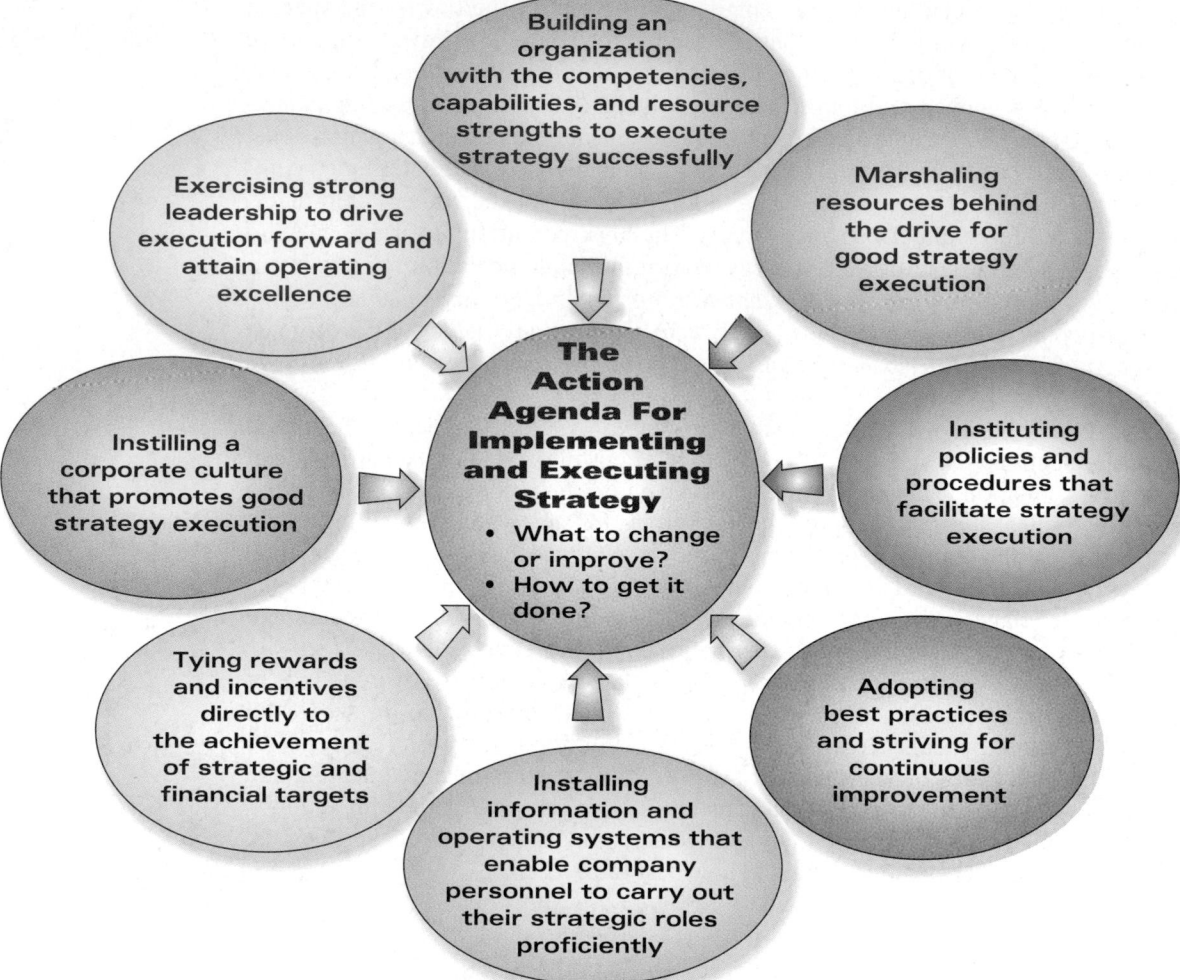

6. Tying rewards directly to the achievement of strategic and financial targets and to good strategy execution.

7. Instilling a corporate culture that promotes good strategy execution.

8. Exercising strong leadership to drive execution forward, keep improving on the details of execution, and achieve operating excellence as rapidly as feasible.

How well managers perform these eight tasks has a decisive impact on whether the outcome is a spectacular success, a colossal failure, or something in between.

In devising an action agenda for implementing and executing strategy, the place for managers to start is with *a probing assessment of what the organization must do differently and better to carry out the strategy successfully*. They should then consider *precisely how to make the necessary internal changes* as rapidly as possible. Successful strategy implementers have a knack for diagnosing what their organizations need to do to execute the chosen strategy well and figuring out how to get things done—they are

When strategies fail, it is often because of poor execution—things that were supposed to get done slip through the cracks.

masters in promoting results-oriented behaviors on the part of company personnel and following through on making the right things happen in a timely fashion.[3]

In big organizations with geographically scattered operating units, the action agenda of senior executives mostly involves communicating the case for change to others, building consensus for how to proceed, installing strong allies in positions where they can push implementation along in key organizational units, urging and empowering subordinates to keep the process moving, establishing measures of progress and deadlines, recognizing and rewarding those who achieve implementation milestones, directing resources to the right places, and personally leading the strategic change process. Thus, the bigger the organization, the more successful strategy execution depends on the cooperation and implementing skills of operating managers who can push needed changes at the lowest organizational levels and deliver results. In small organizations, top managers can deal directly with frontline managers and employees, personally orchestrating the action steps and implementation sequence, observing firsthand how implementation is progressing, and deciding how hard and how fast to push the process along. Regardless of the organization's size and whether implementation involves sweeping or minor changes, the most important leadership traits are a strong, confident sense of what to do and how to do it. Having a strong grip on these two things comes from understanding the circumstances of the organization and the requirements for effective strategy execution. Then it remains for those managers and company personnel in strategy-critical areas to step up to the plate and produce the desired results.

What's Covered in Chapters 11, 12, and 13   In the remainder of this chapter and the next two chapters, we will discuss what is involved in performing the eight key managerial tasks (shown in Figure 11.1) that shape the process of implementing and executing strategy. This chapter explores building an organization with the competencies, capabilities, and resource strengths to execute the strategy successfully. Chapter 12 looks at marshaling resources, instituting strategy-facilitating policies and procedures, adopting best practices, installing operating systems, and tying rewards to the achievement of good results. Chapter 13 deals with creating a strategy-supportive corporate culture and exercising the leadership needed to drive the execution process forward.

BUILDING AN ORGANIZATION CAPABLE OF GOOD STRATEGY EXECUTION

Proficient strategy execution depends heavily on competent personnel, better-than-adequate competitive capabilities, and effective internal organization. Building a capable organization is thus always a top priority in strategy execution. As shown in Figure 11.2, three types of organization-building actions are paramount:

1. *Staffing the organization*—putting together a strong management team, and recruiting and retaining employees with the needed experience, technical skills, and intellectual capital.

2. *Building core competencies and competitive capabilities*—developing proficiencies in performing strategy-critical value chain activities and updating them to match changing market conditions and customer expectations.

3. *Structuring the organization and work effort*—organizing value chain activities and business processes and deciding how much decision-making authority to push down to lower-level managers and frontline employees.

Figure 11.2   **The Three Components of Building an Organization Capable of Proficient Strategy Execution**

Staffing the Organization

- Putting together a strong management team
- Recruiting and retaining talented employees

Building Core Competencies and Competitive Capabilities

- Developing a set of competencies and capabilities suited to the current strategy
- Updating and revising this set as external conditions and strategy change
- Training and retraining employees as needed to maintain skills-based competencies

Matching the Organization Structure to Strategy

- Instituting organizational arrangements that facilitate good strategy execution
- Deciding how much decision-making authority to push down to lower-level managers and front line employees

A Company with the Competencies and Capabilities Needed for Proficient Strategy Execution

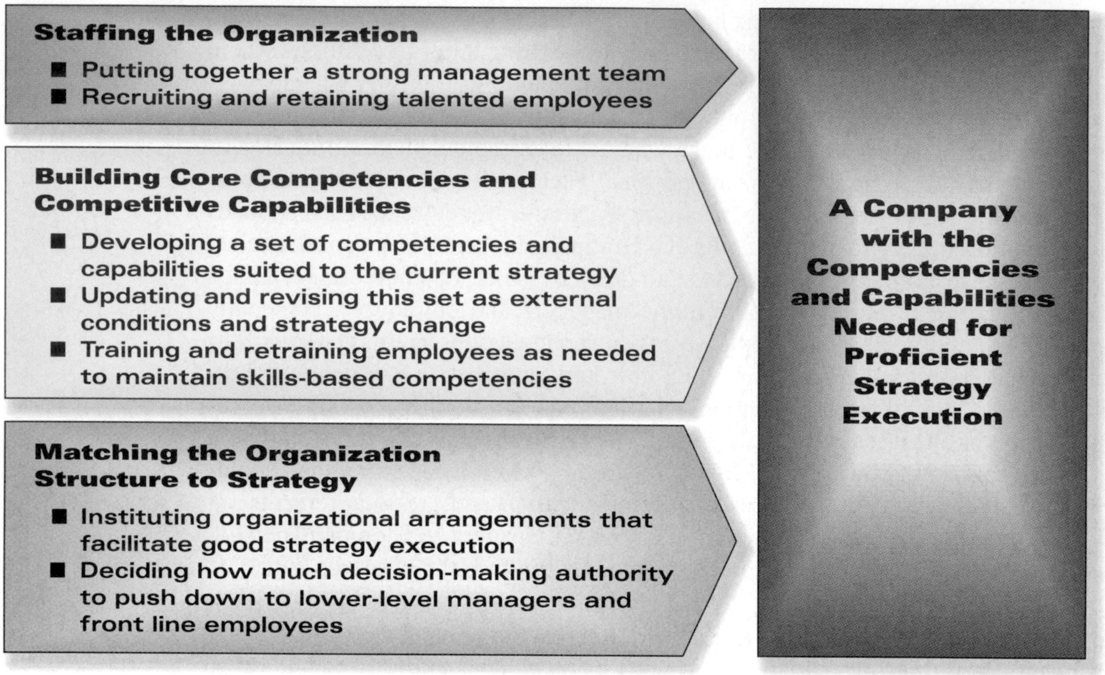

STAFFING THE ORGANIZATION

No company can hope to perform the activities required for successful strategy execution without attracting and retaining talented managers and employees with suitable skills and *intellectual capital.*

Putting Together a Strong Management Team

Assembling a capable management team is a cornerstone of the organization-building task.[4] While different strategies and company circumstances sometimes call for different mixes of backgrounds, experiences, values, beliefs, management styles, and know-how, *the most important consideration is to fill key managerial slots with smart people who are clear thinkers, good at figuring out what needs to be done, and skilled in "making it happen" and delivering good results.*[5] The task of implementing and executing challenging strategic initiatives must be assigned to executives who have the skills and talents to handle them and who can be counted on to turn their decisions and actions into results that meet or beat the established performance targets. It helps enormously when a company's top management team has several people who are particularly good change agents—true believers who champion change, know how to make it happen, and love every second of the process.[6] Without a smart, capable, results-oriented management team, the implementation-execution process ends up being hampered by missed deadlines, misdirected or wasteful efforts, and/or managerial ineptness.[7] Weak executives are serious impediments to getting

Core Concept
Putting together a talented management team with the right mix of experiences, skills, and abilities to get things done is one of the first strategy-implementing steps.

optimal results because they are unable to differentiate between ideas and approaches that have merit and those that are misguided—the caliber of work done under their supervision suffers.[8] In contrast, managers with strong strategy-implementing capabilities have a talent for asking tough, incisive questions. They know enough about the details of the business to be able to challenge and ensure the soundness of the approaches and decisions of the people around them, and they can discern whether the resources people are asking for to put the strategy in place make sense. They are good at getting things done through others, typically by making sure they have the right people under them and that these people are put in the right jobs.[9] They consistently follow through on issues, monitor progress carefully, make adjustments when needed, and not let important details slip through the cracks. In short, they understand how to drive organizational change, and they have the managerial discipline requisite for first-rate strategy execution.

Sometimes a company's existing management team is suitable; at other times it may need to be strengthened or expanded by promoting qualified people from within or by bringing in outsiders whose experiences, talents, and leadership styles better suit the situation. In turnaround and rapid-growth situations, and in instances when a company doesn't have insiders with the requisite know-how, filling key management slots from the outside is a fairly standard organization-building approach. In addition, it is important to ferret out and replace managers who, for whatever reasons, prefer the status quo and who either do not buy into the case for making organizational changes or do not see ways to make things better.[10] For a top management team to be truly effective, it has got to consist of "true believers" who recognize that organizational changes are needed and are ready to get on with the process. Weak executives and diehard resisters have to be replaced or sidelined (by shifting them to positions of lesser influence where they cannot hamper or derail new strategy execution initiatives).

The overriding aim in building a management team should be to assemble a *critical mass* of talented managers who can function as agents of change and further the cause of first-rate strategy execution—every manager's success is enhanced (or limited) by the quality of their managerial colleagues and the degree to which they freely exchange ideas, debate how to improve approaches that have merit, and join forces to tackle issues and solve problems.[11] When a first-rate manager enjoys the help and support of other first-rate managers, it's possible to create a managerial whole that is greater than the sum of individual efforts—talented managers who work well together as a team can produce organizational results that are dramatically better than what one or two star managers acting individually can achieve. The chief lesson here is that *a company needs to get the right executives on the bus—and the wrong executives off the bus—before trying to drive the bus in the desired direction.*[12]

Illustration Capsule 11.1 describes General Electric's widely acclaimed approach to developing a top-caliber management team.

Recruiting and Retaining Capable Employees

Assembling a capable management team is not enough. Staffing the organization with the right kinds of people must go much deeper than managerial jobs in order for value chain activities to be performed competently. *The quality of an organization's people is always an essential ingredient of successful strategy execution—knowledgeable, engaged employees are a company's best source of creative ideas for the nuts-and-bolts operating improvements that lead to operating excellence.* Companies

Core Concept
In many industries, adding to a company's talent base and building intellectual capital is more important to good strategy execution than additional investments in plants, equipment, and capital projects.

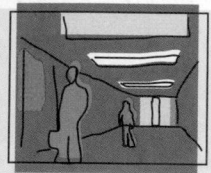

Illustration Capsule 11.1

How General Electric Develops a Talented and Deep Management Team

General Electric (GE) is widely considered to be one of the best-managed companies in the world, partly because of its concerted effort to develop outstanding managers. For starters, GE strives to hire talented people with high potential for executive leadership; it then goes to great lengths to expand the leadership, business, and decision-making capabilities of all its managers. Four key elements undergird GE's efforts to build a talent-rich stable of managers:

- GE makes a practice of transferring managers across divisional, business, or functional lines for sustained periods of time. Such transfers allow managers to develop relationships with colleagues in other parts of the company, help break down insular thinking in business "silos," and promote the sharing of cross-business ideas and best practices. There is an enormous emphasis at GE on transferring ideas and best practices from business to business and making GE a "boundaryless" company.

- In selecting executives for key positions, GE is strongly disposed to candidates who exhibit what are called the four E's—enormous personal *energy,* the ability to motivate and *energize* others, *edge* (a GE code word for instinctive competitiveness and the ability to make tough decisions in a timely fashion, saying yes or no, and not maybe), and *execution* (the ability to carry things through to fruition). Considerable attention is also paid to problem-solving ability, experience in multiple functions or businesses, and experience in driving business growth (as indicated by good market instincts, in-depth knowledge of particular markets, customer touch, and technical understanding).

- All managers are expected to be proficient at what GE calls *workout*—a process in which managers and employees come together to confront issues as soon as they come up, pinpoint the root cause of the issues, and bring about quick resolutions so the business can move forward. Workout is GE's way of training its managers to diagnose what to do and how to do it.

- Each year GE sends about 10,000 newly hired and long-time managers to its Leadership Development Center (generally regarded as one of the best corporate training centers in the world), for a three-week course on the company's Six Sigma quality initiative. Close to 10,000 "master black belt" and "black belt" Six Sigma experts have graduated from the program to drive forward thousands of quality initiatives throughout GE. Six Sigma training is an ironclad requirement for promotion to any professional and managerial position and any stock option award. GE's Leadership Development Center also offers advanced courses for senior managers that may focus on a single management topic for a month. All classes involve managers from different GE businesses and different parts of the world. Some of the most valuable learning comes in between formal class sessions when GE managers from different businesses trade ideas about how to improve processes and better serve the customer. This knowledge sharing not only spreads best practices throughout the organization but also improves each GE manager's knowledge.

All of GE's 85,000 managers and professionals are graded in an annual process that divides them into five tiers: the top 10 percent, the next 15 percent, the middle 50 percent, the next 15 percent, and the bottom 10 percent. Everyone in the top tier gets stock awards, nobody in the fourth tier gets shares of stock, and most of those in the fifth tier become candidates for being weeded out. Business heads are pressured to wean out "C" players. GE's CEO personally reviews the performance of the top 3,000 managers. Senior executive compensation is heavily weighted toward Six Sigma commitment and successful business results.

According to Jack Welch, GE's CEO from 1980 to 2001, "The reality is, we simply cannot afford to field anything but teams of 'A' players."

Sources: General Electric's 1998 and 2003 annual reports; www.ge.com; John A. Byrne, "How Jack Welch Runs GE," *BusinessWeek,* June 8, 1998, p. 90; Miriam Leuchter, "Management Farm Teams," *Journal of Business Strategy,* May 1998, pp. 29–32; and "The House That Jack Built, *The Economist,* September 18, 1999.

like Microsoft, McKinsey & Company, Southwest Airlines, Cisco Systems, Amazon.com, Procter & Gamble, PepsiCo, Nike, Electronic Data Systems, Google, and Intel make a concerted effort to recruit the best and brightest people they can find and then retain them with excellent compensation packages, opportunities for rapid advancement and professional growth, and challenging and interesting assignments. Having a pool of "A players" with strong skill sets and lots of brainpower is essential to their business. Microsoft makes a point of hiring the very brightest and most talented programmers it can find and motivating them with both good monetary incentives and the challenge of working on cutting-edge software design projects. McKinsey & Company, one of the world's premier management consulting companies, recruits only cream-of-the-crop MBAs at the nation's top 10 business schools; such talent is essential to McKinsey's strategy of performing high-level consulting for the world's top corporations. The leading global accounting firms screen candidates not only on the basis of their accounting expertise but also on whether they possess the people skills needed to relate well with clients and colleagues. Southwest Airlines goes to considerable lengths to hire people who can have fun and be fun on the job; it uses special interviewing and screening methods to gauge whether applicants for customer-contact jobs have outgoing personality traits that match its strategy of creating a high-spirited, fun-loving, in-flight atmosphere for passengers; it is so selective that only about 3 percent of the people who apply are offered jobs.

In high-tech companies, the challenge is to staff work groups with gifted, imaginative, and energetic people who can bring life to new ideas quickly and inject into the organization what one Dell Inc. executive calls "hum."[13] The saying "People are our most important asset" may seem hollow, but it fits high-technology companies dead-on. Besides checking closely for functional and technical skills, Dell tests applicants for their tolerance of ambiguity and change, their capacity to work in teams, and their ability to learn on the fly. Companies like Amazon.com, Google, Yahoo, and Cisco Systems have broken new ground in recruiting, hiring, cultivating, developing, and retaining talented employees—most of whom are in their 20s and 30s. Cisco goes after the top 10 percent, raiding other companies and endeavoring to retain key people at the companies it acquires so as to maintain a cadre of star engineers, programmers, managers, salespeople, and support personnel in executing its strategy to remain the world's leading provider of Internet infrastructure products and technology.

In instances where intellectual capital greatly aids good strategy execution, companies have instituted a number of practices aimed at staffing jobs with the best people they can find:

1. Spending considerable effort in screening and evaluating job applicants, selecting only those with suitable skill sets, energy, initiative, judgment, and aptitudes for learning and adaptability to the company's work environment and culture.

2. Putting employees through training programs that continue throughout their careers.

3. Providing promising employees with challenging, interesting, and skill-stretching assignments.

4. Rotating people through jobs that not only have great content but also span functional and geographic boundaries. Providing people with opportunities to gain experience in a variety of international settings is increasingly considered an essential part of career development in multinational or global companies.

5. Encouraging employees to challenge existing ways of doing things, to be creative and innovative in proposing better ways of operating, and to push their ideas for new products or businesses. Progressive companies work hard at creating an environment in which ideas and suggestions bubble up from below and employees are made to feel that their views and suggestions count.

6. Making the work environment stimulating and engaging such that employees will consider the company a great place to work.

7. Striving to retain talented, high-performing employees via promotions, salary increases, performance bonuses, stock options and equity ownership, fringe benefit packages, and other perks.

> The best companies make a point of recruiting and retaining talented employees—the objective is to make the company's entire workforce (managers and rank-and-file employees) a genuine resource strength

8. Coaching average performers to improve their skills and capabilities, while weeding out underperformers and benchwarmers.

It is very difficult for a company to competently execute its strategy and achieve operating excellence without a large band of capable employees who are actively engaged in the process of making ongoing operating improvements.

BUILDING CORE COMPETENCIES AND COMPETITIVE CAPABILITIES

High among the organization-building priorities in the strategy implementing/executing process is the need to build and strengthen competitively valuable core competencies and organizational capabilities. Whereas managers identify the desired competencies and capabilities in the course of crafting strategy, good strategy execution requires putting the desired competencies and capabilities in place, upgrading them as needed, and then modifying them as market conditions evolve. Sometimes a company already has some semblance of the needed competencies and capabilities, in which case managers can concentrate on strengthening and nurturing them to promote better strategy execution. More usually, however, company managers have to significantly broaden or deepen certain capabilities or even add entirely new competencies in order to put strategic initiatives in place and execute them proficiently.

A number of prominent companies have succeeded in establishing core competencies and capabilities that have been instrumental in making them winners in the marketplace. Intel's core competence is in the design and mass production of complex chips for personal computers, servers, and other electronic products. Procter & Gamble's core competencies reside in its superb marketing/distribution skills and its R&D capabilities in five core technologies—fats, oils, skin chemistry, surfactants, and emulsifiers. Ciba Specialty Chemicals has technology-based competencies that allow it to quickly manufacture products for customers wanting customized products relating to coloration, brightening and whitening, water treatment and paper processing, freshness, and cleaning. General Electric has a core competence in developing professional managers with broad problem-solving skills and proven ability to grow global businesses. Disney has core competencies in theme park operation and family entertainment. Dell Inc. has the capabilities to deliver state-of-the-art products to its customers within days of next-generation components coming available—and to do so at attractively low costs (it has leveraged its collection of competencies and capabilities into being the global low-cost leader in PCs). Toyota's success in motor vehicles is due, in large part, to its legendary "production system," which it has honed and perfected and which gives it the capability to produce high-quality vehicles at relatively low costs.

The Three-Stage Process of Developing and Strengthening Competencies and Capabilities

Building core competencies and competitive capabilities is a time-consuming, managerially challenging exercise. While some organization-building assist can be gotten from discovering how best-in-industry or best-in-world companies perform a particular activity, trying to replicate and then improve on the competencies and capabilities of others is, however, much easier said than done—for the same reasons that one is unlikely to ever become a good golfer just by studying what Tiger Woods does. Putting a new capability in place is more complicated than just forming a new team or department and charging it with becoming highly competent in performing the desired activity, using whatever it can learn from other companies having similar competencies or capabilities. Rather, it takes a series of deliberate and well orchestrated organizational steps to achieve mounting proficiency in performing an activity. The capability-building process has three stages:

> **Core Concept**
> Building competencies and capabilities is a multistage process that occurs over a period of months and years, not something that is accomplished overnight.

Stage 1—First, the organization must develop the *ability* to do something, however imperfectly or inefficiently. This entails selecting people with the requisite skills and experience, upgrading or expanding individual abilities as needed, and then molding the efforts and work products of individuals into a collaborative effort to create organizational ability.

Stage 2—As experience grows and company personnel learn how to perform the activity *consistently well and at an acceptable cost,* the ability evolves into a tried-and-true *competence* or *capability.*

Stage 3—Should company personnel continue to polish and refine their know-how and otherwise sharpen their performance of an activity such that the company eventually becomes *better than rivals* at performing the activity, the core competence rises to the rank of a *distinctive competence* (or the capability becomes a competitively superior capability), thus providing a path to competitive advantage.

Many companies are able to get through stages 1 and 2 in performing a strategy-critical activity, but comparatively few achieve sufficient proficiency in performing strategy-critical activities to qualify for the third stage.

Managing the Process   Four traits concerning core competencies and competitive capabilities are important in successfully managing the organization-building process:[14]

1. *Core competencies and competitive capabilities are bundles of skills and know-how that most often grow out of the combined efforts of cross-functional work groups and departments performing complementary activities at different locations in the firm's value chain.* Rarely does a core competence or capability consist of narrow skills attached to the work efforts of a single department. For instance, a core competence in speeding new products to market involves the collaborative efforts of personnel in research and development (R&D), engineering and design, purchasing, production, marketing, and distribution. Similarly, the capability to provide superior customer service is a team effort among people in customer call centers (where orders are taken and inquiries are answered), shipping and delivery, billing and accounts receivable, and after-sale support. Complex activities (like designing and manufacturing a sports-utility vehicle or creating the capability for secure credit card transactions over the Internet) usually involve a number of component skills, technological disciplines, competencies, and capabilities—some performed in-house and some provided by suppliers/allies. An important part of the organization-building function is to think about which activities of which groups need to be linked and made mutually reinforcing and then to forge the necessary collaboration both internally and with outside resource providers.

2. *Normally, a core competence or capability emerges incrementally out of company efforts either to bolster skills that contributed to earlier successes or to respond to customer problems, new technological and market opportunities, and the*

competitive maneuverings of rivals. Migrating from the one-time ability to do something up the ladder to a core competence or competitively valuable capability is usually an organization-building process that takes months and often years to accomplish—it is definitely not an overnight event.

3. *The key to leveraging a core competence into a distinctive competence (or a capability into a competitively superior capability) is concentrating more effort and more talent than rivals on deepening and strengthening the competence or capability, so as to achieve the dominance needed for competitive advantage.* This does not necessarily mean spending more money on such activities than competitors, but it does mean consciously focusing more talent on them and striving for best-in-industry, if not best-in-world, status. To achieve dominance on lean financial resources, companies like Cray in large computers and Honda in gasoline engines have leveraged the expertise of their talent pool by frequently re-forming high-intensity teams and reusing key people on special projects. The experiences of these and other companies indicate that the usual keys to successfully building core competencies and valuable capabilities are superior employee selection, thorough training and retraining, powerful cultural influences, effective cross-functional collaboration, empowerment, motivating incentives, short deadlines, and good databases—not big operating budgets.

4. *Evolving changes in customers' needs and competitive conditions often require tweaking and adjusting a company's portfolio of competencies and intellectual capital to keep its capabilities freshly honed and on the cutting edge.* This is particularly important in high-tech industries and fast-paced markets where important developments occur weekly. As a consequence, wise company managers work at anticipating changes in customer-market requirements and staying ahead of the curve in proactively building a package of competencies and capabilities that can win out over rivals.

Managerial actions to develop core competencies and competitive capabilities generally take one of two forms: either strengthening the company's base of skills, knowledge, and intellect, or coordinating and networking the efforts of the various work groups and departments. Actions of the first sort can be undertaken at all managerial levels, but actions of the second sort are best orchestrated by senior managers who not only appreciate the strategy-executing significance of strong competencies/capabilities but also have the clout to enforce the necessary networking and cooperation among individuals, groups, departments, and external allies.

One organization-building question is whether to develop the desired competencies and capabilities internally or to outsource them by partnering with key suppliers or forming strategic alliances. The answer depends on what can be safely delegated to outside suppliers or allies versus what internal capabilities are key to the company's long-term success. Either way, though, calls for action. Outsourcing means launching initiatives to identify the most attractive providers and to establish collaborative relationships. Developing the capabilities in-house means marshaling personnel with relevant skills and experience, collaboratively networking the individual skills and related cross-functional activities to form organizational capability, and building the desired levels of proficiency through repetition (practice makes perfect).[15]

Sometimes the tediousness of internal organization building can be shortcut by buying a company that has the requisite capability and integrating its competencies into the firm's value chain. Indeed, a pressing need to acquire certain capabilities quickly is one reason to acquire another company—an acquisition aimed at building greater capability can be every bit as competitively valuable as an acquisition aimed at adding new products or services to the company's business lineup. Capabilities-motivated acquisitions are essential (1) when a market opportunity can slip by faster than a needed capability can be created internally, and (2) when industry conditions, technology, or competitors are moving at such a rapid clip that time is of the essence. But usually there's no good substitute for ongoing internal efforts to build and strengthen the company's competencies and capabilities in performing strategy-critical value chain activities.

Updating and Remodeling Competencies and Capabilities as External Conditions and Company Strategy Change Even after core competencies and competitive capabilities are in place and functioning, company managers can't relax. Competencies and capabilities that grow stale can impair competitiveness unless they are refreshed, modified, or even phased out and replaced in response to ongoing market changes and shifts in company strategy. Indeed, the buildup of knowledge and experience over time, coupled with the imperatives of keeping capabilities in step with ongoing strategy and market changes, makes it appropriate to view a company as *a bundle of evolving competencies and capabilities*. Management's organization-building challenge is one of deciding when and how to recalibrate existing com petencies and capabilities, and when and how to develop new ones. Although the task is formidable, ideally it produces a dynamic organization with "hum" and momentum as well as a distinctive competence. Toyota, aspiring to overtake General Motors as the global leader in motor vehicles, has been aggressively upgrading its capabilities in fuel-efficient hybrid engine technology and is constantly fine-tuning its famed Toyota Production System to enhance its already proficient capabilities in manufacturing top-quality vehicles at relatively low costs—see Illustration Capsule 11.2. Likewise, Honda, which has long had a core competence in gasoline engine technology and small engine design, has accelerated its efforts to broaden its expertise and capabilities in hybrid engines so as to stay close behind Toyota. TV broadcasters are upgrading their capabilities in digital broadcasting technology in readiness for the upcoming switchover from analog to digital signal transmission. Microsoft has totally retooled the manner in which its programmers attack the task of writing code for its new operating systems for PCs and servers (the first wave of which was due out in 2006).

The Strategic Role of Employee Training

Training and retraining are important when a company shifts to a strategy requiring different skills, competitive capabilities, managerial approaches, and operating methods. Training is also strategically important in organizational efforts to build skills-based competencies. And it is a key activity in businesses where technical know-how is changing so rapidly that a company loses its ability to compete unless its skilled people have cutting-edge knowledge and expertise. Successful strategy implementers see to it that the training function is both adequately funded and effective. If the chosen strategy calls for new skills, deeper technological capability, or building and using new capabilities, training should be placed near the top of the action agenda.

The strategic importance of training has not gone unnoticed. Over 600 companies have established internal "universities" to lead the training effort, facilitate continuous organizational learning, and help upgrade company competencies and capabilities. Many companies conduct orientation sessions for new employees, fund an assortment

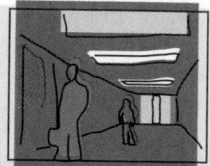

Illustration Capsule 11.2

Toyota's Legendary Production System: A Capability That Translates into Competitive Advantage

The heart of Toyota's strategy in motor vehicles is to outcompete rivals by manufacturing world-class, quality vehicles at lower costs and selling them at competitive price levels. Executing this strategy requires top-notch manufacturing capability and super-efficient management of people, equipment, and materials. Toyota began conscious efforts to improve its manufacturing competence more than 50 years ago. Through tireless trial and error, the company gradually took what started as a loose collection of techniques and practices and integrated them into a full-fledged process that has come to be known as the Toyota Production System (TPS). The TPS drives all plant operations and the company's supply chain management practices. TPS is grounded in the following principles, practices, and techniques:

- *Deliver parts and components just-in-time to the point of vehicle assembly.* The idea here is to cut out all the bits and pieces of transferring materials from place to place and to discontinue all activities on the part of workers that don't add value (particularly activities where nothing ends up being made or assembled).

- *Develop people who can come up with unique ideas for production improvements.*

- *Emphasize continuous improvement.* Workers are expected to use their heads and develop better ways of doing things, rather than mechanically follow instructions. Toyota managers tell workers that the *T* in TPS also stands for "Thinking." The thesis is that a work environment where people have to think generates the wisdom to spot opportunities for making tasks simpler and easier to perform, increasing the speed and efficiency with which activities are performed, and constantly improving product quality.

- *Empower workers to stop the assembly line when there's a problem or a defect is spotted.* Toyota views worker efforts to purge defects and sort out the problem immediately as critical to the whole concept of building quality

into the production process. According to TPS, "If the line doesn't stop, useless defective items will move on to the next stage. If you don't know where the problem occurred, you can't do anything to fix it." The tool for halting the assembly line is the *andon* electric light board, which is visible to everyone on the production floor.

- *Deal with defects only when they occur.* TPS philosophy holds that when things are running smoothly, they should not be subject to control; if attention is directed to fixing problems that are found, quality control along the assembly line can be handled with fewer personnel.

- *Ask yourself "Why?" five times.* While errors need to be fixed whenever they occur, the value of asking "Why?" five times enables identifying the root cause of the error and correcting it so that the error won't recur.

- *Organize all jobs around human motion to create a production/assembly system with no wasted effort.* Work organized in this fashion is called standardized work, and people are trained to observe standardized work procedures (which include supplying parts to each process on the assembly line at the proper time, sequencing the work in an optimal manner, and allowing workers to do their jobs continuously in a set sequence of subprocesses).

- *Find where a part is made cheaply and use that price as a benchmark.*

The TPS uses unique terms (such as *kanban, takt time, jikoda, kaizen, heijunka, monozukuri, poka yoke,* and *muda*) that facilitate precise discussion of specific TPS elements. In 2003, Toyota established a Global Production Center to efficiently train large numbers of shop-floor experts in the latest TPS methods and better operate an increasing number of production sites worldwide. There's widespread agreement that Toyota's ongoing effort to refine and improve on its renowned TPS gives it important manufacturing capabilities that are the envy of other motor vehicle manufacturers.

Sources: Information posted at www.toyotageorgetown.com, and Taiichi Ohno, *Toyota Production System: Beyond Large-Scale Production* (New York: Sheridan, 1988).

of competence-building training programs, and reimburse employees for tuition and other expenses associated with obtaining additional college education, attending professional development courses, and earning professional certification of one kind or another. A number of companies offer online, just-in-time training courses to employees around the clock. Increasingly, employees at all levels are expected to take an active role in their own professional development, assuming responsibility for keeping their skills and expertise up-to-date and in sync with the company's needs.

From Competencies and Capabilities to Competitive Advantage

While strong core competencies and competitive capabilities are a major assist in executing strategy, they are an equally important avenue for securing a competitive edge over rivals in situations where it is relatively easy for rivals to copy smart strategies. Any time rivals can readily duplicate successful strategy features, making it difficult or impossible to outstrategize rivals and beat them in the marketplace with a superior strategy, the chief way to achieve lasting competitive advantage is to outexecute them (beat them by performing certain value chain activities in a superior fashion). *Building core competencies and competitive capabilities that are very difficult or costly for rivals to emulate and that push a company closer to true operating excellence promotes very proficient strategy execution.* Moreover, because cutting-edge core competencies and competitive capabilities represent resource strengths that are often time-consuming and expensive for rivals to match or trump, any competitive edge they produce tends to be sustainable and pave the way for above-average company performance.

> **Core Concept**
> Building competencies and capabilities that are very difficult or costly for rivals to emulate has a huge payoff—improved strategy execution and a potential for competitive advantage.

It is easy to cite instances where companies have gained a competitive edge based on superior competencies and capabilities. Toyota's production capabilities (see Illustration Capsule 11.2) have given it a decided market edge over such rivals as General Motors, Ford, DaimlerChrysler, and Volkswagen. Dell's competitors have spent years and millions of dollars in what so far is a futile effort to match Dell's cost-efficient supply chain management capabilities. FedEx has unmatched capabilities in reliable overnight delivery of documents and small parcels. Various business news media have been unable to match the competence of Dow-Jones in gathering and reporting business news via *The Wall Street Journal.*

EXECUTION-RELATED ASPECTS OF ORGANIZING THE WORK EFFORT

There are few hard-and-fast rules for organizing the work effort to support good strategy execution. Every firm's organization chart is partly a product of its particular situation, reflecting prior organizational patterns, varying internal circumstances, executive judgments about reporting relationships, and the politics of who gets which assignments. Moreover, every strategy is grounded in its own set of key success factors and value chain activities. But some organizational considerations are common to all companies. These are summarized in Figure 11.3 and discussed in turn in the following sections.

Deciding Which Value Chain Activities to Perform Internally and Which to Outsource

The advantages of a company having an outsourcing component in its strategy were discussed in Chapter 6 (pp. 160–193), but there is also a need to consider the role of outsourcing in executing the strategy. Aside from the fact than an outsider, because of

Figure 11.3   **Structuring the Work Effort to Promote Successful Strategy Execution**

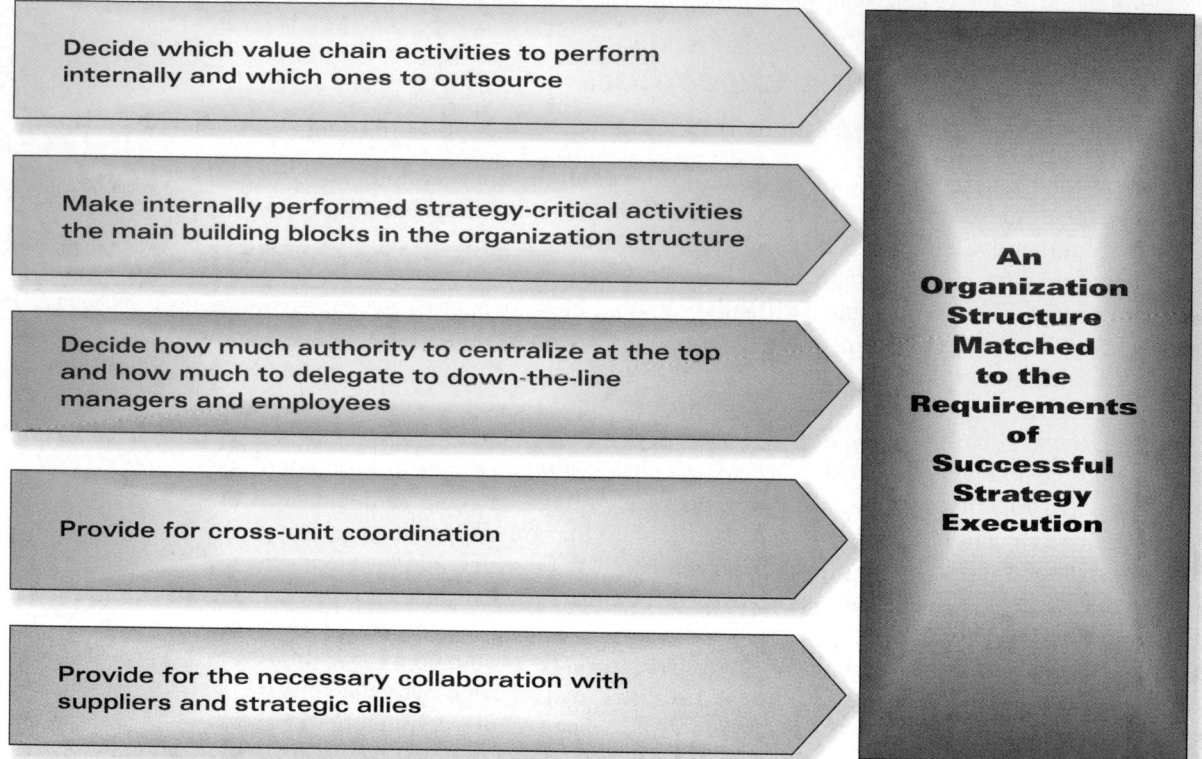

its expertise and specialized know-how, may be able to perform certain value chain activities better or cheaper than a company can perform them internally, outsourcing can also have several organization-related benefits. Managers too often spend inordinate amounts of time, mental energy, and resources haggling with functional support groups and other internal bureaucracies over needed services, leaving less time for them to devote to performing strategy-critical activities in the most proficient manner. One way to reduce such distractions is to outsource the performance of assorted administrative support functions and perhaps even selected core or primary value chain activities to outside vendors, thereby enabling the company to *heighten its strategic focus and concentrate its full energies and resources on even more competently performing those value chain activities that are at the core of its strategy and for which it can create unique value.* For example, E. & J. Gallo Winery outsources 95 percent of its grape production, letting farmers take on the weather and other grape-growing risks while it concentrates its full energies on wine production and sales.[16] A number of personal computer (PC) makers outsource the mundane and highly specialized task of PC assembly, concentrating their energies instead on product design, sales and marketing, and distribution.

When a company uses outsourcing to zero in on ever better performance of those truly strategy-critical activities where its expertise is most needed, then it may be able to realize three very positive benefits:

1. *The company improves its chances for outclassing rivals in the performance of strategy-critical activities and turning a core competence into a distinctive competence.* At the very least, the heightened focus on performing a select few value chain activities should meaningfully strengthen the company's existing core competences and promote more innovative performance of those activities—either of which could lower costs or materially improve competitive capabilities. Eastman Kodak, Ford, Exxon Mobil, Merrill Lynch, and Chevron have outsourced their data processing activities to computer service firms, believing that outside specialists can perform the needed services at lower costs and equal or better quality. A relatively large number of companies outsource the operation of their Web sites to Web design and hosting enterprises. Many business that get a lot of inquiries from customers or that have to provide 24/7 technical support to users of their products across the world have found that it is considerably less expensive to outsource these functions to specialists (often located in foreign countries where skilled personnel are readily available and worker compensation costs are much lower) than to operate their own call centers.

2. *The streamlining of internal operations that flows from outsourcing often acts to decrease internal bureaucracies, flatten the organization structure, speed internal decision making, and shorten the time it takes to respond to changing market conditions.*[17] In consumer electronics, where advancing technology drives new product innovation, organizing the work effort in a manner that expedites getting next-generation products to market ahead of rivals is a critical competitive capability. Motor vehicle manufacturers have found that they can shorten the cycle time for new models, improve the quality and performance of those models, and lower overall production costs by outsourcing the big majority of their parts and components from independent suppliers and then working closely with their vendors to advance the design and functioning of the items being supplied, to swiftly incorporate new technology, and to better integrate individual parts and components to form engine cooling systems, transmission systems, and electrical systems.

3. *Outsourcing the performance of certain value chain activities to able suppliers can add to a company's arsenal of capabilities and contribute to better strategy execution.* By building, continually improving, and then leveraging its partnerships with able suppliers, a company enhances its overall organizational capabilities and builds resource strengths—strengths that deliver value to customers and consequently pave the way for competitive success. Soft-drink and beer manufacturers all cultivate their relationships with their bottlers and distributors to strengthen access to local markets and build the loyalty, support, and commitment for corporate marketing programs, without which their own sales and growth are weakened. Similarly, fast-food enterprises like McDonald's and Taco Bell find it essential to work hand-in-hand with franchisees on outlet cleanliness, consistency of product quality, in-store ambience, courtesy and friendliness of store personnel, and other aspects of store operations. Unless franchisees continuously deliver sufficient customer satisfaction to attract repeat business, a fast-food chain's sales and competitive standing will suffer quickly. Companies like Boeing, Aerospatiale, Verizon Communications, and Dell have learned that their central R&D groups cannot begin to match the innovative capabilities of a well-managed network of supply chain partners having the ability to advance the technology, lead the development of next-generation parts and components, and supply them at a relatively low price.[18]

As a general rule, companies refrain from outsourcing those value chain activities over which they need direct strategic and operating control in order to build core competencies, achieve competitive advantage, and effectively manage key customer–supplier–distributor relationships. It is the strategically less important activities—like handling customer inquiries and providing technical support, doing the payroll,

Core Concept
Wisely choosing which activities to perform internally and which to outsource can lead to several strategy-executing advantages—lower costs, heightened strategic focus, less internal bureaucracy, speedier decision making, and a better arsenal of competencies and capabilities.

administering employee benefit programs, providing corporate security, managing stockholder relations, maintaining fleet vehicles, operating the company's Web site, conducting employee training, and managing an assortment of information and data processing functions—where outsourcing is most used.

Even so, a number of companies have found ways to successfully rely on outside vendors to perform strategically significant value chain activities.[19] Broadcom, a global leader in chips for broadband communications systems, outsources the manufacture of its chips to Taiwan Semiconductor, thus freeing company personnel to focus their full energies on R&D, new chip design, and marketing. For years Polaroid Corporation bought its film from Eastman Kodak, its electronics from Texas Instruments, and its cameras from Timex and others, while it concentrated on producing its unique self-developing film packets and designing its next-generation cameras and films. Nike concentrates on design, marketing, and distribution to retailers, while outsourcing virtually all production of its shoes and sporting apparel. Cisco Systems outsources virtually all manufacturing of its routers, switches, and other Internet gear, yet it protects its market position by retaining tight internal control over product design and closely monitors the daily operations of its manufacturing vendors. Large numbers of electronics companies outsource the design, engineering, manufacturing, and shipping of their products to such companies as Flextronics and Solectron, both of which have built huge businesses as providers of such services to companies worldwide. So while performing *core* value chain activities in-house normally makes good sense, there can be times when outsourcing some of them works to good advantage.

The Dangers of Excessive Outsourcing Critics contend that a company can go overboard on outsourcing and so hollow out its knowledge base and capabilities as to leave itself at the mercy of outside suppliers and short of the resource strengths to be a master of its own destiny.[20] The point is well taken, but most companies appear alert to the danger of taking outsourcing to an extreme or failing to maintain control of the work performed by specialist vendors or offshore suppliers. Many companies refuse to source key components from a single supplier, opting to use two or three suppliers as a way of avoiding single supplier dependence or giving one supplier too much bargaining power. Moreover, they regularly evaluate their suppliers, looking not only at the supplier's overall performance but also at whether they should switch to another supplier or even bring the activity back in-house. To avoid loss of control, companies typically work closely with key suppliers, meeting often and setting up online systems to share data and information, collaborate on work in progress, monitor performance, and otherwise document that suppliers' activities are closely integrated with their own requirements and expectations. Indeed, sophisticated online systems permit companies to work in "real time" with suppliers 10,000 miles away, making rapid response possible whenever concerns or problems arise. Hence *the real debate surrounding outsourcing is not about whether too much outsourcing risks loss of control, but about how to use outsourcing in a manner that produces greater competitiveness.*

Making Strategy-Critical Activities the Main Building Blocks of the Organization Structure

In any business, some activities in the value chain are always more critical to strategic success and competitive advantage than others. For instance, hotel/motel enterprises have to be good at fast check-in/check-out, housekeeping and facilities maintenance, food service, and the creation of a pleasant ambience. For a manufacturer of chocolate bars, buying quality cocoa beans at low prices is vital and reducing production costs by a fraction of a cent per bar can mean a seven-figure improvement in the bottom line. In discount stock brokerage, the strategy-critical activities are fast access to information, accurate order execution, efficient record keeping and transactions processing, and good customer service. In specialty chemicals, the critical activities are R&D, product innovation, getting new products onto the market quickly, effective marketing, and expertise in assisting customers. Where such is the case, it is important for management to build its organization structure around proficient performance of these activities, making them the centerpieces or main building blocks on the organization chart.

The rationale for making strategy-critical activities the main building blocks in structuring a business is compelling: If activities crucial to strategic success are to have the resources, decision-making influence, and organizational impact they need, they have to be centerpieces in the organizational scheme. Plainly, implementing a new or changed strategy is likely to entail new or different key activities, competencies, or capabilities and therefore to require new or different organizational arrangements. If workable organizational adjustments are not forthcoming, the resulting mismatch between strategy and structure can open the door to execution and performance problems.[21] Hence, attempting to carry out a new strategy with an old organization structure is usually unwise.

What Types of Organization Structures Fit Which Strategies?   It is generally agreed that some type of functional structure is the best organizational arrangement when a company is in just one particular business (irrespective of which of the five competitive strategies it opts to pursue). The primary organizational building blocks within a business are usually *traditional functional departments* (R&D, engineering and design, production and operations, sales and marketing, information technology, finance and accounting, and human resources) and *process departments* (where people in a single work unit have responsibility for all the aspects of a certain process like supply chain management, new product development, customer service, quality control, or selling direct to customers via the company's Web site). For instance, a technical instruments manufacturer may be organized around research and development, engineering, supply chain management, assembly, quality control, marketing, technical services, and corporate administration. A hotel may have a functional organization based on front-desk operations, housekeeping, building maintenance, food service, convention services and special events, guest services, personnel and training, and accounting. A discount retailer may organize around such functional units as purchasing, warehousing and distribution, store operations, advertising, merchandising and promotion, customer service, and corporate administrative services.

In enterprises with operations in various countries around the world (or with geographically scattered organizational units within a country), the basic building blocks may also include *geographic organizational units,* each of which has profit/loss responsibility for its assigned geographic area. In vertically integrated firms, the major building blocks are *divisional units performing one or more of the major processing steps along the value chain* (raw materials production, components manufacture, assembly, wholesale distribution, retail store operations); each division in the value chain may operate as a profit center for performance measurement purposes. The typical building blocks of a diversified company are its *individual businesses,* with each business unit usually operating as an independent profit center and with corporate headquarters performing assorted support functions for all of its business units. But a divisional business-unit structure can present problems to a company pursuing related diversification.

Determining the Degree of Authority and Independence to Give Each Unit and Each Employee

In executing the strategy and conducting daily operations, companies must decide how much authority to delegate to the managers of each organization unit—especially the heads of business subsidiaries; functional and process departments; and plants, sales offices, distribution centers, and other operating units—and how much decision-making latitude to give individual employees in performing their jobs. The two extremes are to *centralize decision making* at the top (the CEO and a few close lieutenants) or to *decentralize decision making* by giving managers and employees considerable decision-making latitude in their areas of responsibility. As shown in Table 11.1, the two approaches are based on sharply different underlying principles and beliefs, with each having its pros and cons.

Centralized Decision Making: Pros and Cons *In a highly centralized organization structure, top executives retain authority for most strategic and operating decisions and keep a tight rein on business-unit heads, department heads, and the*

Table 11.1 **Advantages and Disadvantages of Centralized versus Decentralized Decision Making**

Centralized Organizational Structures	Decentralized Organizational Structures
Basic tenets • Decisions on most matters of importance should be pushed to managers up the line who have the experience, expertise, and judgment to decide what is the wisest or best course of action. • Frontline supervisors and rank-and-file employees can't be relied on to make the right decisions—because they seldom know what is best for the organization and because they do not have the time or the inclination to properly manage the tasks they are performing (letting them decide "what to do" is thus risky).	**Basic tenets** • Decision-making authority should be put in the hands of the people closest to and most familiar with the situation and these people should be trained to exercise good judgment. • A company that draws on the combined intellectual capital of all its employees can outperform a command-and-control company.
Chief advantage • Fixes accountability.	**Chief advantages** • Encourages lower level managers and rank-and-file employees to exercise initiative and act responsibly. • Promotes greater motivation and involvement in the business on the part of more company personnel. • Spurs new ideas and creative thinking. • Allows fast response times. • Entails fewer layers of management.
Primary disadvantages • Lengthens response times because management bureaucracy must decide on a course of action. • Does not encourage responsibility among lower level managers and rank-and-file employees. • Discourages lower level managers and rank-and-file employees from exercising any initiative—they are expected to wait to be told what to do.	**Primary disadvantages** • Puts the organization at risk if many bad decisions are made at lower levels—top management lacks full control. • Impedes cross-business coordination and capture of strategic fits in diversified companies.

managers of key operating units; comparatively little discretionary authority is granted to frontline supervisors and rank-and-file employees. The command-and-control paradigm of centralized structures is based on the underlying assumption that frontline personnel have neither the time nor the inclination to direct and properly control the work they are performing, and that they lack the knowledge and judgment to make wise decisions about how best to do it—hence the need for managerially prescribed policies and procedures, close supervision, and tight control. The thesis underlying authoritarian structures is that strict enforcement of detailed procedures backed by rigorous managerial oversight is the most reliable way to keep the daily execution of strategy on track.

The big advantage of an authoritarian structure is tight control by the manager in charge—it is easy to know who is accountable when things do not go well. But there are some serious disadvantages. Hierarchical command-and-control structures make an organization sluggish in responding to changing conditions because of the time it takes for the review/approval process to run up all the layers of the management bureaucracy. Furthermore, to work well, centralized decision making requires top-level managers to gather and process whatever information is relevant to the decision. When the relevant knowledge resides at lower organizational levels (or is technical, detailed, or hard to express in words), it is difficult and time-consuming to get all of the facts and nuances in front of a high-level executive located far from the scene of the action—full understanding of the situation cannot be readily copied from one mind to another. Hence, centralized decision making is often impractical—the larger the company and the more scattered its operations, the more that decision-making authority has to be delegated to managers closer to the scene of the action.

> There are disadvantages to having a small number of top-level managers micromanage the business either by personally making decisions or by requiring lower-level subordinates to gain approval before taking action.

Decentralized Decision Making: Pros and Cons   *In a highly decentralized organization, decision-making authority is pushed down to the lowest organizational level capable of making timely, informed, competent decisions.* The objective is to put adequate decision-making authority in the hands of the people closest to and most familiar with the situation and train them to weigh all the factors and exercise good judgment. Decentralized decision making means that the managers of each organizational unit are delegated lead responsibility for deciding how best to execute strategy (as well as some role in shaping the strategy for the units they head). Decentralization thus requires selecting strong managers to head each organizational unit and holding them accountable for crafting and executing appropriate strategies for their units. Managers who consistently produce unsatisfactory results have to be weeded out.

The case for empowering down-the-line managers and employees to make decisions related to daily operations and executing the strategy is based on the belief that a company that draws on the combined intellectual capital of all its employees can outperform a command-and-control company.[22] Decentralized decision making means, for example, that in a diversified company the various business-unit heads have broad authority to execute the agreed-on business strategy with comparatively little interference from corporate headquarters; moreover, the business-unit heads delegate considerable decision-making latitude to functional and process department heads and the heads of the various operating units (plants, distribution centers, sales offices) in implementing and executing their pieces of the strategy. In turn, work teams may be empowered to manage and improve their assigned value chain activity, and employees with customer contact may be empowered to do what it takes to please customers.

The ultimate goal of decentralized decision making is to put decision-making authority in the hands of those persons or teams closest to and most knowledgeable about the situation.

At Starbucks, for example, employees are encouraged to exercise initiative in promoting customer satisfaction—there's the story of a store employee who, when the computerized cash register system went offline, enthusiastically offered free coffee to waiting customers.[23] *With decentralized decision making, top management maintains control by limiting empowered managers' and employees' discretionary authority and holding people accountable for the decisions they make.*

Decentralized organization structures have much to recommend them. Delegating greater authority to subordinate managers and employees creates a more horizontal organization structure with fewer management layers. Whereas in a centralized vertical structure managers and workers have to go up the ladder of authority for an answer, in a decentralized horizontal structure they develop their own answers and action plans—making decisions in their areas of responsibility and being accountable for results is an integral part of their job. Pushing decision-making authority down to middle and lower-level managers and then further on to work teams and individual employees shortens organizational response times and spurs new ideas, creative thinking, innovation, and greater involvement on the part of subordinate managers and employees. In worker-empowered structures, jobs can be defined more broadly, several tasks can be integrated into a single job, and people can direct their own work. Fewer managers are needed because deciding how to do things becomes part of each person's or team's job. Further, today's online communication systems make it easy and relatively inexpensive for people at all organizational levels to have direct access to data, other employees, managers, suppliers, and customers. They can access information quickly (via the Internet or company intranet), readily check with superiors or coworkers as needed, and take responsible action. Typically, there are genuine gains in morale and productivity when people are provided with the tools and information they need to operate in a self-directed way. Decentralized decision making not only can shorten organizational response times but also can spur new ideas, creative thinking, innovation, and greater involvement on the part of subordinate managers and employees.

The past decade has seen a growing shift from authoritarian, multilayered hierarchical structures to flatter, more decentralized structures that stress employee empowerment. There's strong and growing consensus that authoritarian, hierarchical organization structures are not well suited to implementing and executing strategies in an era when extensive information and instant communication are the norm and when a big fraction of the organization's most valuable assets consists of intellectual capital and resides in the knowledge and capabilities of its employees. Many companies have therefore begun empowering lower-level managers and employees throughout their organizations, giving them greater discretionary authority to make strategic adjustments in their areas of responsibility and to decide what needs to be done to put new strategic initiatives into place and execute them proficiently.

Maintaining Control in a Decentralized Organization Structure

Pushing decision-making authority deep down into the organization structure and empowering employees presents its own organizing challenge: *how to exercise adequate control over the actions of empowered employees so that the business is not put at risk at the same time that the benefits of empowerment are realized.*[24] Maintaining adequate organizational control over empowered employees is generally accomplished by placing limits on the authority that empowered personnel can exercise, holding people accountable for their decisions, instituting compensation incentives that reward people for doing their jobs in a manner that contributes to good company performance, and creating a corporate culture where there's strong peer pressure on individuals to act responsibly.

Capturing Strategic Fits in a Decentralized Structure   Diversified companies striving to capture cross-business strategic fits have to beware of giving business heads full rein to operate independently when cross-business collaboration is essential in order to gain strategic fit benefits. Cross-business strategic fits typically have to be captured either by enforcing close cross-business collaboration or by centralizing performance of functions having strategic fits at the corporate level.[25] For example, if businesses with overlapping process and product technologies have their own independent R&D departments—each pursuing their own priorities, projects, and strategic agendas—it's hard for the corporate parent to prevent duplication of effort, capture either economies of scale or economies of scope, or broaden the company's R&D efforts to embrace new technological paths, product families, end-use applications, and customer groups. Where cross-business R&D fits exist, the best solution is usually to centralize the R&D function and have a coordinated corporate R&D effort that serves both the interests of individual businesses and the company as a whole. Likewise, centralizing the related activities of separate businesses makes sense when there are opportunities to share a common sales force, use common distribution channels, rely on a common field service organization to handle customer requests or provide maintenance and repair services, use common e-commerce systems and approaches, and so on.

The point here is that efforts to decentralize decision making and give organizational units leeway in conducting operations have to be tempered with the need to maintain adequate control and cross-unit coordination—decentralization doesn't mean delegating authority in ways that allow organization units and individuals to do their own thing. There are numerous instances when decision-making authority must be retained at high levels in the organization and ample cross-unit coordination strictly enforced.

Providing for Internal Cross-Unit Coordination

The classic way to coordinate the activities of organizational units is to position them in the hierarchy so that the most closely related ones report to a single person (a functional department head, a process manager, a geographic area head, a senior executive). Managers higher up in the ranks generally have the clout to coordinate, integrate, and arrange for the cooperation of units under their supervision. In such structures, the chief executive officer, chief operating officer, and business-level managers end up as central points of coordination because of their positions of authority over the whole unit. When a firm is pursuing a related diversification strategy, coordinating the related activities of independent business units often requires the centralizing authority of a single corporate-level officer. Also, diversified companies commonly centralize such staff support functions as public relations, finance and accounting, employee benefits, and information technology at the corporate level both to contain the costs of support activities and to facilitate uniform and coordinated performance of such functions within each business unit.

However, close cross-unit collaboration is usually needed to build core competencies and competitive capabilities in strategically important activities—such as speeding new products to market and providing superior customer service—that involve employees scattered across several internal organization units (and perhaps the employees of outside strategic partners or specialty vendors). A big weakness of traditional functionally organized structures is that pieces of strategically relevant activities and capabilities often end up scattered across many departments, with the result that no one group or manager is accountable. Consider, for example, how the following strategy-critical activities cut across different functions:

- *Filling customer orders accurately and promptly*—a process that involves personnel from sales (which wins the order); finance (which may have to check credit terms or approve special financing); production (which must produce the goods and replenish warehouse inventories as needed); warehousing (which has to verify whether the items are in stock, pick the order from the warehouse, and package it for shipping); and shipping (which has to choose a carrier to deliver the goods and release the goods to the carrier).[26]

- *Fast, ongoing introduction of new products*—a cross-functional process involving personnel in R&D, design and engineering, purchasing, manufacturing, and sales and marketing.

- *Improving product quality*—a process that entails the collaboration of personnel in R&D, design and engineering, purchasing, in-house components production, manufacturing, and assembly.

- *Supply chain management*—a collaborative process that cuts across such functional areas as purchasing, inventory management, manufacturing and assembly, and warehousing and shipping.

- *Building the capability to conduct business via the Internet*—a process that involves personnel in information technology, supply chain management, production, sales and marketing, warehousing and shipping, customer service, finance, and accounting.

- *Obtaining feedback from customers and making product modifications to meet their needs*—a process that involves personnel in customer service and after-sale support, R&D, design and engineering, purchasing, manufacturing and assembly, and marketing research.

Handoffs from one department to another lengthen completion time and frequently drive up administrative costs, since coordinating the fragmented pieces can soak up hours of effort on the parts of many people.[27] This is not a fatal flaw of functional organization—organizing around specific functions normally works to good advantage in support activities like finance and accounting, human resource management, and engineering, and in such primary activities as R&D, manufacturing, and marketing. But the tendency for pieces of a strategy-critical activity to be scattered across several functional departments is an important weakness of functional organization and accounts for why a company's competencies and capabilities are typically cross-functional.

Many companies have found that rather than continuing to scatter related pieces of a strategy-critical business process across several functional departments and scrambling to integrate their efforts, it is better to reengineer the work effort and pull the people who performed the pieces in functional departments into a group that works together to perform the whole process, thus creating *process departments* (like customer service or new product development or supply chain management). And sometimes the coordinating mechanisms involve the use of cross-functional task forces, dual reporting relationships, informal organizational networking, voluntary cooperation, incentive compensation tied to measures of group performance, and strong executive-level insistence on teamwork and cross-department cooperation (including removal of recalcitrant managers who stonewall collaborative efforts). At one European-based company, a top executive promptly replaced the managers of several plants who were not fully committed to collaborating closely on eliminating duplication in product development and production efforts among plants in several different countries. Earlier, the executive, noting that negotiations among the managers had stalled on which labs and plants to close, had met with all the managers, asked them to cooperate to find a solution, discussed with them which options were unacceptable, and given them a deadline to find a solution. When the asked-for teamwork wasn't forthcoming, several managers were replaced.

Providing for Collaboration with Outside Suppliers and Strategic Allies

Someone or some group must be authorized to collaborate as needed with each major outside constituency involved in strategy execution. Forming alliances and cooperative relationships presents immediate opportunities and opens the door to future possibilities, but nothing valuable is realized until the relationship grows, develops, and blossoms. Unless top management sees that constructive organizational bridge building with strategic partners occurs and that productive working relationships emerge, the value of alliances is lost and the company's power to execute its strategy is weakened. If close working relationships with suppliers are crucial, then supply chain management must be given formal status on the company's organization chart and a significant position in the pecking order. If distributor/dealer/franchisee relationships are important, someone must be assigned the task of nurturing the relationships with forward channel allies. If working in parallel with providers of complementary products and services contributes to enhanced organizational capability, then cooperative organizational arrangements have to be put in place and managed to good effect.

Building organizational bridges with external allies can be accomplished by appointing "relationship managers" with responsibility for making particular strategic partnerships or alliances generate the intended benefits. Relationship managers have many roles and functions: getting the right people together, promoting good rapport, seeing that plans for specific activities are developed and carried out, helping adjust internal organizational procedures and communication systems, ironing out operating dissimilarities, and nurturing interpersonal cooperation. Multiple cross-organization ties have to be established and kept open to ensure proper communication and coordination.[28] There has to be enough information sharing to make the relationship work and periodic frank discussions of conflicts, trouble spots, and changing situations.[29]

CURRENT ORGANIZATIONAL TRENDS

Many of today's companies are winding up the task of remodeling their traditional hierarchical structures once built around functional specialization and centralized authority. Much of the corporate downsizing movement in the late 1980s and early 1990s was aimed at recasting authoritarian, pyramidal organizational structures into flatter, decentralized structures. The change was driven by growing realization that command-and-control hierarchies were proving a liability in businesses where customer preferences were shifting from standardized products to custom orders and special features, product life cycles were growing shorter, custom mass-production methods were replacing standardized mass-production techniques, customers wanted to be treated as individuals, technological change was ongoing, and market conditions were fluid. Layered management hierarchies with lots of checks and controls that required people to look upward in the organizational structure for answers and approval were failing to deliver responsive customer service and timely adaptations to changing conditions.

The organizational adjustments and downsizing of companies in 2001–2005 brought further refinements and changes to streamline organizational activities and shake out inefficiencies. The goals have been to make companies leaner, flatter, and more responsive to change. Many companies are drawing on five tools of organizational design: (1) managers and workers empowered to act on their own judgments, (2) work process redesign (to achieve greater streamlining and tighter cohesion), (3) self-directed work teams, (4) rapid incorporation of Internet technology applications, and (5) networking with outsiders to improve existing organization capabilities and create new ones. Considerable management attention is being devoted to building a company capable of outcompeting rivals on the basis of superior resource strengths and competitive capabilities—capabilities that are increasingly based on intellectual capital and cross-unit collaboration.

Several other organizational characteristics are emerging:

- Extensive use of Internet technology and e-commerce business practices—real-time data and information systems; greater reliance on online systems for transacting business with suppliers and customers; and Internet-based communication and collaboration with suppliers, customers, and strategic partners.
- Fewer barriers between different vertical ranks, between functions and disciplines, between units in different geographic locations, and between the company and its suppliers, distributors/dealers, strategic allies, and customers—an outcome partly due to pervasive use of online systems.
- Rapid dissemination of information, rapid learning, and rapid response times—also an outcome partly due to pervasive use of online systems.
- Collaborative efforts among people in different functional specialties and geographic locations—essential to create organization competencies and capabilities.

Key Points

Implementing and executing strategy is an operation-driven activity revolving around the management of people and business processes. The managerial emphasis is on converting strategic plans into actions and good results. *Management's handling of the process of implementing and executing the chosen strategy can be considered successful if and when the company achieves the targeted strategic and financial performance and shows good progress in making its strategic vision a reality.* Shortfalls in performance signal weak strategy, weak execution, or both.

The place for managers to start in implementing and executing a new or different strategy is with *a probing assessment of what the organization must do differently and better to carry out the strategy successfully.* They should then consider *precisely how to make the necessary internal changes* as rapidly as possible.

Like crafting strategy, executing strategy is a job for a company's whole management team, not just a few senior managers. Top-level managers have to rely on the active support and cooperation of middle and lower managers to push strategy changes into functional areas and operating units and to see that the organization actually operates in accordance with the strategy on a daily basis.

Eight managerial tasks crop up repeatedly in company efforts to execute strategy:

1. Building an organization with the competencies, capabilities, and resource strengths to execute strategy successfully.

2. Marshaling sufficient money and people behind the drive for strategy execution.

3. Instituting policies and procedures that facilitate rather than impede strategy execution.

4. Adopting best practices and pushing for continuous improvement in how value chain activities are performed.

5. Installing information and operating systems that enable company personnel to carry out their strategic roles proficiently.

6. Tying rewards directly to the achievement of strategic and financial targets and to good strategy execution.

7. Shaping the work environment and corporate culture to fit the strategy.

8. Exercising strong leadership to drive execution forward, keep improving on the details of execution, and achieve operating excellence as rapidly as feasible.

Building an organization capable of good strategy execution entails three types of organization-building actions: (1) *staffing the organization*—assembling a talented, can-do management team, and recruiting and retaining employees with the needed experience, technical skills, and intellectual capital; (2) *building core competencies and competitive capabilities* that will enable good strategy execution and updating them as strategy and external conditions change; and (3) *structuring the organization and work effort*—organizing value chain activities and business processes and deciding how much decision-making authority to push down to lower-level managers and frontline employees.

Building core competencies and competitive capabilities is a time-consuming, managerially challenging exercise that involves three stages: (1) developing the *ability to do something, however imperfectly or inefficiently*, by selecting people with the requisite skills and experience, upgrading or expanding individual abilities as needed, and then molding the efforts and work products of individuals into a collaborative group effort; (2) coordinating group efforts to learn how to perform the activity *consistently well and at an acceptable cost,* thereby transforming the ability into a tried-and-true *competence or capability;* and (3) continuing to polish and refine the organization's know-how and otherwise sharpen performance such that it becomes *better than rivals* at performing the activity, thus raising the core competence (or capability) to the rank of a *distinctive competence* (or competitively superior capability) and opening an avenue to competitive advantage. Many companies manage to get through stages 1 and 2 in performing a strategy-critical activity but comparatively few achieve sufficient proficiency in performing strategy-critical activities to qualify for the third stage.

Strong core competencies and competitive capabilities are an important avenue for securing a competitive edge over rivals in situations where it is relatively easy for rivals to copy smart strategies. Any time rivals can readily duplicate successful strategy features, making it difficult or impossible to *outstrategize* rivals and beat them in the marketplace with a superior strategy, the chief way to achieve lasting competitive advantage is to *outexecute* them (beat them by performing certain value chain activities in superior fashion). *Building core competencies and competitive capabilities that are very difficult or costly for rivals to emulate and that push a company closer to true operating excellence is one of the best and most reliable ways to achieve a durable competitive edge.*

Structuring the organization and organizing the work effort in a strategy-supportive fashion has five aspects: (1) deciding which value chain activities to perform internally and which ones to outsource; (2) making internally performed strategy-critical activities the main building blocks in the organization structure; (3) deciding how much authority to centralize at the top and how much to delegate to down-the-line managers and employees; (4) providing for internal cross-unit coordination and collaboration to build and strengthen internal competencies/capabilities; and (5) providing for the necessary collaboration and coordination with suppliers and strategic allies.

Exercises

1. As the new owner of a local ice cream store located in a strip mall adjacent to a university campus, you are contemplating how to organize your business—whether to make your ice cream in-house or outsource its production to a nearby ice cream manufacturer whose brand is most of the local supermarkets, and how much authority to delegate to the two assistant store managers and to employees working the counter and the cash register. You plan to sell 20 flavors of ice cream.

    a. What are the pros and cons of contracting with the local company to custom-produce your product line?

    b. Since you do not plan to be in the store during all of the hours it is open, what specific decision-making authority would you delegate to the two assistant store managers?

    c. To what extent, if any, should store employees—many of whom will be university students working part-time—be empowered to make decisions relating to store operations (opening and closing, keeping the premises clean and attractive, keeping the work area behind the counter stocked with adequate supplies of cups, cones, napkins, and so on)?

    d. Should you create a policies and procedures manual for the assistant managers and employees, or should you just give oral instructions and have them learn their duties and responsibilities on the job?

    e. How can you maintain control during the times you are not in the store?

2. Go to Home Depot's corporate home page (www.homedepot.com/corporate) and review the information under the headings About The Home Depot, Investor Relations, and Careers. How does Home Depot go about building core competencies and competitive capabilities? Would any of Home Depot's competencies qualify as a distinctive competence? Please use the chapter's discussion of building core competencies and competitive capabilities as a guide for preparing your answer.

3. Using Google Scholar or your access to EBSCO, InfoTrac, or other online database of journal articles and research in your university's library, do a search for recent writings on self-directed or empowered work teams. According to the articles you found in the various management journals, what are the conditions for the effective use of such teams? Also, how should such teams be organized or structured to better ensure their success?

Managing Internal Operations

Actions That Promote Good Strategy Execution

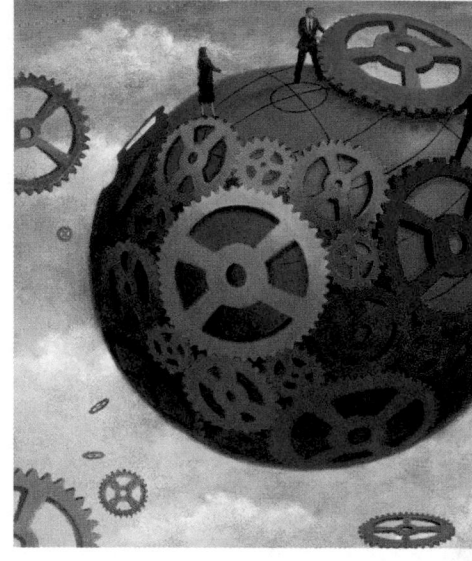

Winning companies know how to do their work better.

—Michael Hammer and James Champy

Companies that make best practices a priority are thriving, thirsty, learning organizations. They believe that everyone should always be searching for a better way. Those kinds of companies are filled with energy and curiosity and a spirit of can-do.

—Jack Welch
Former CEO, General Electric

If you want people motivated to do a good job, give them a good job to do.

—Frederick Herzberg

You ought to pay big bonuses for premier performance . . . Be a top payer, not in the middle or low end of the pack.

—Lawrence Bossidy
CEO, Honeywell International

In Chapter 11 we emphasized the importance of building organization capabilities and structuring the work effort so as to perform strategy-critical activities in a coordinated and highly competent manner. In this chapter we discuss five additional managerial actions that promote the success of a company's strategy execution efforts:

1. Marshaling resources behind the drive for good strategy execution.

2. Instituting policies and procedures that facilitate strategy execution.

3. Adopting best practices and striving for continuous improvement in how value chain activities are performed.

4. Installing information and operating systems that enable company personnel to carry out their strategic roles proficiently.

5. Tying rewards and incentives directly to the achievement of strategic and financial targets and to good strategy execution.

MARSHALING RESOURCES BEHIND THE DRIVE FOR GOOD STRATEGY EXECUTION

Early in the process of implementing and executing a new or different strategy, managers need to determine what resources will be needed and then consider whether the current budgets of organizational units are suitable. Plainly, organizational units must have the budgets and resources for executing their parts of the strategic plan effectively and efficiently. Developing a strategy-driven budget requires top management to determine what funding is needed to execute new strategic initiatives and to strengthen or modify the company's competencies and capabilities. This includes careful screening of requests for more people and more or better facilities and equipment, approving those that hold promise for making a cost-justified contribution to strategy execution, and turning down those that don't. Should internal cash flows prove insufficient to fund the planned strategic initiatives, then management must raise additional funds through borrowing or selling additional shares of stock to willing investors.

A company's ability to marshal the resources needed to support new strategic initiatives and steer them to the appropriate organizational units has a major impact on the strategy execution process. Too little funding (stemming either from constrained financial resources or from sluggish management action to adequately increase the budgets of strategy-critical organizational units) slows progress and impedes the efforts of organizational units to execute their pieces of the strategic plan proficiently. Too much funding wastes organizational resources and reduces financial performance. Both outcomes argue for managers to be deeply involved in reviewing budget proposals and directing the proper kinds and amounts of resources to strategy-critical organization units.

A change in strategy nearly always calls for budget reallocations and resource shifting. Units important in the prior strategy but having a lesser role in the new strategy may need downsizing. Units that now have a bigger and more critical strategic role may need more people, new equipment, additional facilities, and above-average increases in their operating budgets. More resources may have to be devoted to quality control or to adding new product features or to building a better brand image or to cutting costs or to employee retraining. Strategy implementers need to be active and forceful in shifting resources, downsizing some functions and upsizing others, not only to amply fund activities with a critical role in the new strategy but also to avoid inefficiency and achieve profit projections. They have to exercise their power to put enough resources behind new strategic initiatives to make things happen, and they have to make the tough decisions to kill projects and activities that are no longer justified.

Visible actions to reallocate operating funds and move people into new organizational units signal a determined commitment to strategic change and frequently are needed to catalyze the implementation process and give it credibility. Microsoft has made a practice of regularly shifting hundreds of programmers to new high-priority programming initiatives within a matter of weeks or even days. At Harris Corporation, where the strategy was to diffuse research ideas into areas that were commercially viable, top management regularly shifted groups of engineers out of government projects and into new commercial venture divisions. Fast-moving developments in many markets are prompting companies to abandon traditional annual or semiannual budgeting and resource allocation cycles in favor of cycles that match the strategy changes a company makes in response to newly developing events.

The bigger the change in strategy (or the more obstacles that lie in the path of good strategy execution), the bigger the resource shifts that will likely be required. Merely fine-tuning the execution of a company's existing strategy seldom requires big movements of people and money from one area to another. The desired improvements can usually be accomplished through above-average budget increases to organizational units launching new initiatives and below-average increases (or even small cuts) for the remaining organizational units. The chief exception occurs where all the strategy changes or new execution initiatives need to be made without adding to total expenses. Then managers have to work their way through the existing budget line-by-line and activity-by-activity, looking for ways to trim costs in some areas and shift the resources to higher priority activities where new execution initiatives are needed.

INSTITUTING POLICIES AND PROCEDURES THAT FACILITATE GOOD STRATEGY EXECUTION

A company's policies and procedures can either assist the cause of good strategy execution or be a barrier. Anytime a company moves to put new strategy elements in place or improve its strategy execution capabilities, managers are well advised to undertake a careful review of existing policies and procedures, proactively revising or discarding those that are out of sync. A change in strategy or a push for better strategy execution generally requires some changes in work practices and the behavior of company personnel. One way of promoting such changes is by instituting a select set of new policies and procedures deliberately aimed at steering the actions and behavior of company personnel in a direction more conducive to good strategy execution and operating excellence.

Figure 12.1   **How Prescribed Policies and Procedures Facilitate Strategy Execution**

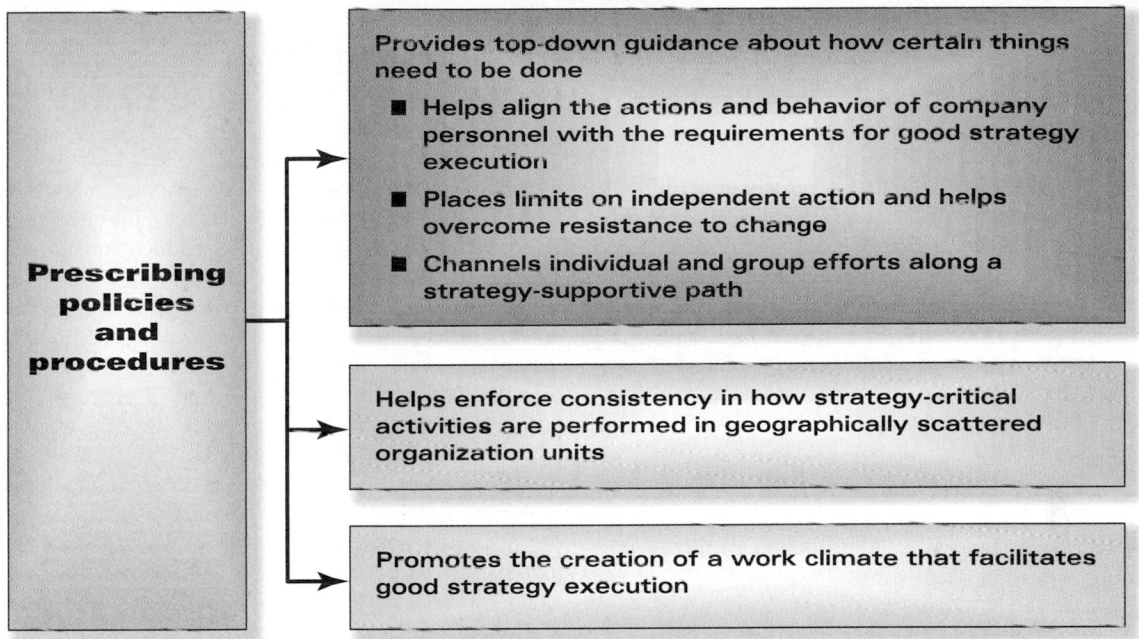

As shown in Figure 12.1, prescribing new policies and operating procedures acts to facilitate strategy execution in three ways:

1. *Instituting new policies and procedures provides top-down guidance regarding how certain things now need to be done.* Asking people to alter established habits and procedures, of course, always upsets the internal order of things. It is normal for pockets of resistance to develop and for people to exhibit some degree of stress and anxiety about how the changes will affect them, especially when the changes may eliminate jobs. But when existing ways of doing things pose a barrier to improving strategy execution, actions and behaviors have to be changed. The managerial role of establishing and enforcing new policies and operating practices is to paint a different set of white lines, place limits on independent behavior, and channel individual and group efforts along a path more conducive to executing the strategy. Policies are a particularly useful way to counteract tendencies for some people to resist change—most people refrain from violating company policy or going against recommended practices and procedures without first gaining clearance or having strong justification.

2. *Policies and procedures help enforce needed consistency in how particular strategy-critical activities are performed in geographically scattered operating units.* Standardization and strict conformity are sometimes desirable components of good strategy execution. Eliminating significant differences in the operating practices of different plants, sales regions, customer service centers, or the individual outlets in a chain operation helps a company deliver consistent product quality and service to customers. Good strategy execution nearly always entails an ability to replicate product quality and the caliber of customer service at every location where the company does business—anything less blurs the company's image and fails to meet customer expectations.

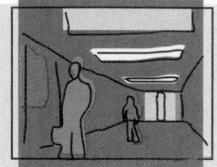

Illustration Capsule 12.1

Granite Construction's Short-Pay Policy: An Innovative Way to Drive Better Strategy Execution

In 1987, the owners of Granite Construction, a 100-plus-year-old supplier of crushed gravel, sand, concrete, and asphalt in Watsonville, California, decided to pursue two strategic targets: total customer satisfaction and a reputation for superior service. To drive the internal efforts to achieve these two objectives and signal both employees and customers that it was deadly serious about these two strategic commitments, top management instituted a short-pay policy that appeared on the bottom of every Granite Construction invoice:

> If you are not satisfied for any reason, don't pay us for it. Simply scratch out the line item, write a brief note about the problem, and return a copy of this invoice along with your check for the balance.

Customers did not have to call and complain and were not expected to return the product. They were given complete discretionary power to decide whether and how much to pay based on their satisfaction level. Management believed that empowering customers not to pay for items or service they found lacking would provide unmistakable feedback and spur company personnel to correct any problems quickly in order to avoid repeated short payments.

The short-pay policy had the desired impact, focusing the attention of company personnel on avoiding short payments by customers and boosting customer satisfaction significantly. Granite has enjoyed compound annual sales gains of 12.2 percent since 2000, while charging a 6 percent price premium for its commodity products in competition against larger rivals.

In addition to its short-pay policy, Granite employs two other policies to help induce company personnel to do their very best to satisfy the company's customers. It has a no-lay-off policy (no employees have been laid off in over 80 years), and it sends positive customer comments about employees home for families to read. To make sure its workforce force is properly trained, company employees go through training programs averaging 43 hours per employee annually. And compensation is attractive: Entry-level employees, called job owners, start at $16 an hour and progress to such positions as "accomplished job owner" and "improvement champion" (base pay of $26 an hour); all employees are entitled to 12 company-paid massages annually.

Granite won the prestigious Malcolm Baldrige National Quality Award in 1992, about five years after instituting the short-pay policy. *Fortune* rated Granite as one of the 100 best companies to work for in America in eight of the nine years from 1998 to 2006 (its highest ranking was 16th in 2002, and its lowest was 90th in 2004). The company was on *Fortune*'s "Most Admired Companies" list in 2005 and 2006.

Source: Based on information in Jim Collins, "Turning Goals into Results: The Power of Catalytic Mechanisms," *Harvard Business Review* 77, no. 4 (July–August 1999), pp. 72–73; Robert Levering and Milton Moskowitz, "The 100 Best Companies to Work For," *Fortune,* February 4, 2004, p. 73; Robert Levering and Milton Moskowitz, "The 100 Best Companies to Work For," *Fortune,* January 12, 2005, p. 78; and www.fortune.com (accessed November 11, 2005).

3. *Well-conceived policies and procedures promote the creation of a work climate that facilitates good strategy execution.* Because discarding old policies and procedures in favor of new ones invariably alters the internal work climate, managers can use the policy-changing process as a powerful lever for changing the corporate culture in ways that produce a stronger fit with the new strategy. The trick here, obviously, is to hit upon a new policy that will catch the immediate attention of the whole organization, quickly shift their actions and behavior, and then become embedded in how things are done—as with Granite Construction's short-pay policy discussed in Illustration Capsule 12.1.

In an attempt to steer "crew members" into stronger quality and service behavior patterns, McDonald's policy manual spells out detailed procedures that personnel in each McDonald's unit are expected to observe; for example, "Cooks must turn, never flip, hamburgers," "If they haven't been purchased, Big Macs must be discarded in 10 minutes after being cooked and French fries in 7 minutes," and "Cashiers must make eye contact with and smile at every customer."

Nordstrom's strategic objective is to make sure that each customer has a pleasing shopping experience in its department stores and returns time and again; to get store personnel to dedicate themselves to outstanding customer service, Nordstrom has a policy of promoting only those people whose personnel records contain evidence of "heroic acts" to please customers—especially customers who may have made "unreasonable requests" that require special efforts. To keep its R&D activities responsive to customer needs and expectations, Hewlett-Packard (HP) requires R&D people to make regular visits to customers to learn about their problems and learn their reactions to HP's latest new products.

One of the big policymaking issues concerns what activities need to be rigidly prescribed and what activities ought to allow room for independent action on the part of empowered personnel. Few companies need thick policy manuals to direct the strategy execution process or prescribe exactly how daily operations are to be conducted. Too much policy can erect as many obstacles as wrong policy or be as confusing as no policy. There is wisdom in a middle approach: *Prescribe enough policies to give organization members clear direction in implementing strategy and to place desirable boundaries on their actions; then empower them to act within these boundaries however they think makes sense.* Allowing company personnel to act anywhere between the "white lines" is especially appropriate when individual creativity and initiative are more essential to good strategy execution than standardization and strict conformity. Instituting strategy-facilitating policies can therefore mean more policies, fewer policies, or different policies. It can mean policies that require things to be done a certain way or policies that give employees leeway to do activities the way they think best.

ADOPTING BEST PRACTICES AND STRIVING FOR CONTINUOUS IMPROVEMENT

Company managers can significantly advance the cause of competent strategy execution by pushing organization units and company personnel to identify and adopt the best practices for performing value chain activities and, further, insisting on continuous improvement in how internal operations are conducted. One of the most widely used and effective tools for gauging how well a company is executing pieces of its strategy entails benchmarking the company's performance of particular activities and business processes against best-in-industry and best-in-world performers.[1] It can also be useful to look at best-in-company performers of an activity if a company has a number of different organizational units performing much the same function at different locations. Identifying, analyzing, and understanding how top companies or individuals perform particular value chain activities and business processes provides useful yardsticks for judging the effectiveness and efficiency of internal operations and setting performance standards for organization units to meet or beat.

Core Concept
Managerial efforts to identify and adopt best practices are a powerful tool for promoting operating excellence and better strategy execution.

How the Process of Identifying and Incorporating Best Practices Works

A **best practice** is a technique for performing an activity or business process that at least one company has demonstrated works particularly well. To qualify as a legitimate best practice, the technique must have a proven record in significantly lowering costs, improving quality or performance, shortening time requirements, enhancing safety, or delivering some other highly positive operating outcome. Best practices thus identify a path to operating excellence. For a best practice to be valuable and transferable, it must demonstrate success over time, deliver quantifiable and highly positive results, and be repeatable.

Benchmarking is the backbone of the process of identifying, studying, and implementing outstanding practices. A company's benchmarking effort looks outward to find best practices and then proceeds to develop the data for measuring how well a company's own performance of an activity stacks up against the best-practice standard. Informally, benchmarking involves being humble enough to admit that others have come up with world-class ways to perform particular activities yet wise enough to try to learn how to match, and even surpass, them. But, as shown in Figure 12.2, the payoff of benchmarking comes from adapting the top-notch approaches pioneered by other companies in the company's own operation and thereby boosting, perhaps dramatically, the proficiency with which value chain tasks are performed.

However, benchmarking is more complicated than simply identifying which companies are the best performers of an activity and then trying to imitate their approaches—especially if these companies are in other industries. Normally, the outstanding practices of other organizations have to be *adapted* to fit the specific circumstances of a company's own business and operating requirements. Since most companies believe their work is unique, the telling part of any best-practice initiative is how well the company puts its own version of the best practice into place and makes it work.

Indeed, a best practice remains little more than another company's interesting success story unless company personnel buy into the task of translating what can be learned from other companies into real action and results. The agents of change must be frontline employees who are convinced of the need to abandon the old ways of doing things and switch to a best-practice mind-set. *The more that organizational units use best practices in performing their work, the closer a company moves toward performing its value chain activities as effectively and efficiently as possible.* This is what operational excellence is all about.

Legions of companies across the world now engage in benchmarking to improve their strategy execution efforts and, ideally, gain a strategic, operational, and financial advantage over rivals. Scores of trade associations and special interest organizations have undertaken efforts to collect best-practice data relevant to a particular industry or business function and make their databases available online to members—good

Figure 12.2 **From Benchmarking and Best-Practice Implementation to Operating Excellence**

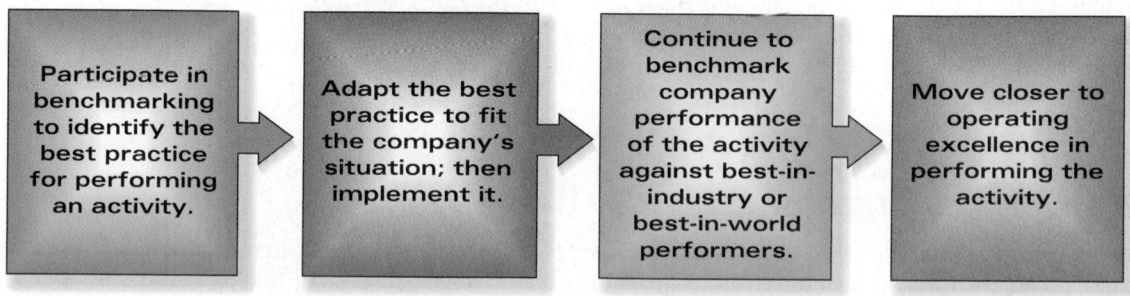

examples include The Benchmarking Exchange's BenchNet (www.benchnet.com), Best Practices LLC (www.best-in-class.com), and the American Productivity and Quality Center (www.apqc.org). Benchmarking and best-practice implementation have clearly emerged as legitimate and valuable managerial tools for promoting operational excellence.

Business Process Reengineering, Six Sigma Quality Programs, and TQM: Tools for Promoting Operating Excellence

In striving for operating excellence, many companies have also come to rely on three other potent management tools: business process reengineering, Six Sigma quality control techniques, and total quality management (TQM) programs. Indeed, these three tools have become globally pervasive techniques for implementing strategies keyed to cost reduction, defect-free manufacture, superior product quality, superior customer service, and total customer satisfaction. The following sections describe how business process reengineering, Six Sigma, and TQM can contribute to operating excellence and better strategy execution.

Business Process Reengineering   Companies scouring for ways to improve their operations have sometimes discovered that the execution of strategy-critical activities is hindered by an organizational arrangement where pieces of the activity are performed in several different functional departments, with no one manager or group being accountable for optimum performance of the entire activity. This can easily occur in such inherently cross-functional activities as customer service (which can involve personnel in order filling, warehousing and shipping, invoicing, accounts receivable, after-sale repair, and technical support), new product development (which can typically involve personnel in R&D, design and engineering, purchasing, manufacturing, and sales and marketing), and supply chain management (which cuts across such areas as purchasing, inventory management, manufacturing and assembly, warehousing, and shipping). Even if personnel in all the different departments and functional areas are inclined to collaborate closely, the activity may not end up being performed optimally or cost-efficiently, such that performance is adversely affected.

To address such shortcomings in strategy execution, many companies during the past decade have opted to *reengineer the work effort* by pulling the pieces of strategy-critical activities out of different departments and unifying their performance in a single department or cross-functional work group. Reorganizing the people who performed the pieces in functional departments into a close-knit group that has charge over the whole process and that can be held accountable for performing the activity in a cheaper, better, and/or more strategy-supportive fashion is called *business process reengineering.*[2] When done properly, business process reengineering can produce dramatic operating benefits. In the order-processing section of General Electric's circuit breaker division, elapsed time from order receipt to delivery was cut from three weeks to three days by consolidating six production units into one, reducing a variety of former inventory and handling steps, automating the design system to replace a human custom-design process, and cutting the organizational layers between managers and workers from three to one. Productivity rose 20 percent in one year, and unit manufacturing costs dropped 30 percent. Northwest Water, a British utility, used business process reengineering to eliminate 45 work depots that served as home bases to crews who installed and repaired water and sewage lines and equipment. Now crews work directly from their vehicles, receiving assignments and reporting work completion from computer terminals in their trucks. Crew members are no longer employees but rather contractors to Northwest Water. These reengineering efforts not only eliminated the need for the work depots but also allowed Northwest Water to eliminate a big percentage of the bureaucratic personnel and supervisory organization that managed the crews.[3]

Since the early 1990s, reengineering of value chain activities has been undertaken at many companies in many industries all over the world, with excellent results being achieved at some companies.[4] While reengineering has produced only modest results in some instances, usually because of ineptness or lack of wholehearted commitment, reengineering has nonetheless proved itself as a useful tool for streamlining a company's work effort and moving closer to operational excellence.

Total Quality Management Programs   Total quality management (TQM) is a philosophy of managing a set of business practices that emphasizes continuous improvement in all phases of operations, 100 percent accuracy in performing tasks, involvement and empowerment of employees at all levels, team-based work design, benchmarking, and total customer satisfaction.[5] While TQM concentrates on the production of quality goods and fully satisfying customer expectations, it achieves its biggest successes when it is also extended to employee efforts in *all departments*—human resources, billing, R&D, engineering, accounting and records, and information systems—that may lack pressing, customer-driven incentives to improve. It involves reforming the corporate culture and shifting to a total quality/continuous improvement business philosophy that permeates every facet of the organization.[6] TQM aims at instilling enthusiasm and commitment to doing things right from the top to the bottom of the organization. Management's job is to kindle an companywide search for ways to improve, a search that involves all company personnel exercising initiative and using their ingenuity. TQM doctrine preaches that there's no such thing as "good enough" and that everyone has a responsibility to participate in continuous improvement. TQM is thus a race without a finish. Success comes from making little steps forward each day, a process that the Japanese call *kaizen*.

Core Concept
TQM entails creating a total quality culture bent on continuously improving the performance of every task and value chain activity.

TQM takes a fairly long time to show significant results—very little benefit emerges within the first six months. The long-term payoff of TQM, if it comes, depends heavily on management's success in implanting a culture within which TQM philosophies and practices can thrive. TQM is a managerial tool that has attracted numerous users and advocates over several decades, and it can deliver good results when used properly.

Six Sigma Quality Control   Six Sigma quality control consists of a disciplined, statistics-based system aimed at producing not more than 3.4 defects per million iterations for any business process—from manufacturing to customer transactions.[7] The Six Sigma process of define, measure, analyze, improve, and control (DMAIC) is an improvement system for existing processes falling below specification and needing incremental improvement. The Six Sigma process of define, measure, analyze, design, and verify (DMADV) is used to develop *new* processes or products at Six Sigma quality levels. Both Six Sigma processes are executed by personnel who have earned Six Sigma "green belts" and Six Sigma "black belts," and are overseen by personnel who have completed Six Sigma "master black belt" training. According to the Six Sigma Academy, personnel with black belts can save companies approximately $230,000 per project and can complete four to six projects a year.[8]

The statistical thinking underlying Six Sigma is based on the following three principles: All work is a process, all processes have variability, and all processes create data that explains variability.[9] To illustrate how these three principles drive the metrics of DMAIC, consider the case of a janitorial company that wants to improve the caliber of work done by its cleaning crews and thereby boost customer satisfaction. The janitorial company's Six Sigma team can pursue quality enhancement and continuous improvement via the DMAIC process as follows:

- *Define.* Because Six Sigma is aimed at reducing defects, the first step is to define what constitutes a defect. Six Sigma team members might decide that leaving streaks on windows is a defect because it is a source of customer dissatisfaction.

- *Measure.* The next step is to collect data to find out why, how, and how often this defect occurs. This might include a process flow map of the specific ways that cleaning crews go about the task of cleaning a commercial customer's windows. Other metrics may include recording what tools and cleaning products the crews use to clean windows.

- *Analyze.* After the data are gathered and the statistics analyzed, the company's Six Sigma team discovers that the tools and window-cleaning techniques of certain employees are better than those of other employees because their tools and procedures leave no streaked windows—a "best practice" for avoiding window streaking is thus identified and documented.

- *Improve.* The Six Sigma team implements the documented best practice as a standard way of cleaning windows.

- *Control.* The company teaches new and existing employees the best practice technique for window cleaning. Over time, there's significant improvement in customer satisfaction and increased business.

Six Sigma's DMAIC process is a particularly good vehicle for improving performance when there are *wide variations* in how well an activity is performed.[10] For instance, airlines striving to improve the on-time performance of their flights have more to gain from actions to curtail the number of flights that are late by more then 30 minutes than from actions to reduce the number of flights that are late by less than 5 minutes. Likewise, an overnight delivery service might have a 16-hour average delivery time, but if the actual delivery time varies around the 16-hour average from a low of 12 hours to a high of 26 hours such that 10 percent of its packages are delivered more than 6 hours late, then the company has a huge *reliability* problem.

Since the mid-1990s, thousands of companies and nonprofit organizations around the world have begun using Six Sigma programs to promote operating excellence. Such manufacturers as Motorola, Allied Signal, Caterpillar, DuPont, Xerox, Alcan Aluminum, BMW, Volkswagen, Nokia, Owens Corning, and Emerson Electric have employed Six Sigma techniques to good advantage in improving production quality. General Electric (GE), one of the most successful companies implementing Six Sigma training and pursuing Six Sigma perfection, estimated benefits on the order of $10 billion during the first five years of implementation. GE first began Six Sigma in 1995 after Motorola and Allied Signal blazed the Six Sigma trail. One of GE's successes was in its Lighting division, where Six Sigma was used to cut invoice defects and disputes by 98 percent, a particular benefit to Wal-Mart, the division's largest customer. GE Capital Mortgage improved the chances of a caller reaching a "live" GE person from 76 to 99 percent.[11] Illustration Capsule 12.2 describes Whirlpool's use of Six Sigma in its appliance business.

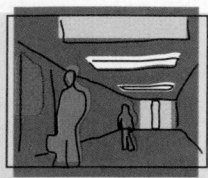

Illustration Capsule 12.2

Whirlpool's Use of Six Sigma to Promote Operating Excellence

Top management at Whirlpool Corporation, the leading global manufacturer and marketer of home appliances in 2005 with 50 manufacturing and technology centers aound the globe and sales in some 170 countries, has a vision of Whirlpool appliances in "Every Home, Everywhere." One of management's chief objectives in pursuing this vision is to build unmatched customer loyalty to the Whirlpool brand. Whirlpool's strategy to win the hearts and minds of appliance buyers the world over has been to produce and market appliances with top-notch quality and innovative features that users will find appealing. In addition, Whirlpool's strategy has been to offer a wide selection of models (recognizing that buyer tastes and needs differ) and to strive for low-cost production efficiency, thereby enabling Whirlpool to price its products competitively. Executing this strategy at Whirlpool's operations in North America (where it is the market leader), Latin America (where it is also the market leader), Europe (where it is ranks third), and Asia (where it is number one in India and has a foothold with huge growth opportunities elsewhere) has involved a strong focus on continuous improvement, lean manufacturing capabilities, and a drive for operating excellence. To marshal the efforts of Whirlpool's 68,000 employees in executing the strategy successfully, management developed a comprehensive Operational Excellence program with Six Sigma as one of the centerpieces.

The Operational Excellence initiative, which began in the 1990s, incorporated Six Sigma techniques to improve the quality of Whirlpool products, while at the same time lowering costs and trimming the time it took to get product innovations into the marketplace. The Six Sigma program helped Whirlpool save $175 million in manufacturing costs in its first three years.

To sustain the productivity gains and cost savings, Whirlpool embedded Six Sigma practices within each of its manufacturing facilities worldwide and instilled a culture based on Six Sigma and lean manufacturing skills and capabilities. Beginning in 2002, each of Whirlpool's operating units began taking the Six Sigma initiative to a higher level by first placing the needs of the customer at the center of every function—R&D, technology, manufacturing, marketing, and administrative support—and then striving to consistently improve quality levels while eliminating all unnecessary costs. The company systematically went through every aspect of its business with the view that company personnel should perform every activity at every level in a manner that delivers value to the customer and that leads to continuous improvement on how things are done.

Whirlpool management believes that the company's Operational Excellence process has been a major contributor in sustaining the company's global leadership in appliances.

Source: Information posted at www.whirlpool.com (accessed September 25, 2003, and November 15, 2005).

Six Sigma is, however, not just a quality-enhancing tool for manufacturers. At one company, product sales personnel typically wined and dined customers to close their deals.[12] But the costs of such entertaining were viewed as excessively high in many instances. A Six Sigma project that examined sales data found that although face time with customers was important, wining, dining, and other types of entertainment were not. The data showed that regular face time helped close sales, but that time could be spent over a cup of coffee instead of golfing at a resort or taking clients to expensive restaurants. In addition, analysis showed that too much face time with customers was counterproductive. A regularly scheduled customer picnic was found to be detrimental to closing sales because it was held at a busy time of year, when customers preferred not to be away from their offices. Changing the manner in which prospective customers were wooed resulted in a 10 percent increase in sales.

A Milwaukee hospital used Six Sigma to map the process as prescriptions originated with a doctor's writeup, were filled by the hospital pharmacy, and then administered by nurses. DMAIC analysis revealed that most mistakes came from misreading the doctor's handwriting.[13] The hospital implemented a program requiring doctors to type the prescription into a computer, which slashed the number of errors dramatically.

A problem tailor-made for Six Sigma occurs in the insurance industry, where it is common for top agents to outsell poor agents by a factor of 10 to 1 or more. If insurance executives offer a trip to Hawaii in a monthly contest to motivate low-performing agents, the typical result is to motivate top agents to be even more productive and make the performance gap even wider. A DMAIC Six Sigma project to reduce the variation in the performance of agents and correct the problem of so many low-performing agents would begin by measuring the performance of all agents, perhaps discovering that the top 20 percent sell 7 times more policies than the bottom 40 percent. Six Sigma analysis would then consider such steps as mapping how top agents spend their day, investigating the factors that distinguish top performers from low performers, learning what techniques training specialists have employed in converting low-performing agents into high performers, and examining how the hiring process could be improved to avoid hiring underperformers in the first place. The next step would be to *test* proposed solutions—better training methods or psychological profiling to identify and weed out candidates likely to be poor performers--to identify and measure which alternative solutions really work, which don't, and why. Only those actions that prove statistically beneficial are then introduced on a wide scale. The DMAIC method thus entails empirical analysis to diagnose the problem (*design, measure, analyze*), test alternative solutions (*improve*) and then *control* the variability in how well the activity is performed by implementing actions shown to truly fix the problem.

A company that systematically applies Six Sigma methods to its value chain, activity by activity, can make major strides in improving the proficiency with which its strategy is executed. As is the case with TQM, obtaining managerial commitment, establishing a quality culture, and fully involving employees are the three most intractable challenges encountered in the implementation of Six Sigma quality programs.[14]

The Difference between Business Process Reengineering and Continuous Improvement Programs Like Six Sigma and TQM Business process reengineering and continuous improvement efforts like TQM and Six Sigma both aim at improved efficiency and reduced costs, better product quality, and greater customer satisfaction. The essential difference between business process reengineering and continuous improvement programs is that reengineering aims at *quantum gains* on the order of 30 to 50 percent or more whereas total quality programs stress *incremental progress,* striving for inch-by-inch gains again and again in a never-ending stream. The two approaches to improved performance of value chain activities and operating excellence are not mutually exclusive; it makes sense to use them in tandem. Reengineering can be used first to produce a good basic design that yields quick, dramatic improvements in performing a business process. Total quality programs can then be used as a follow-on to reengineering and/or best-practice implementation, delivering gradual improvements. Such a two-pronged approach to implementing operational excellence is like a marathon race in which you run the first four miles as fast as you can, then gradually pick up speed the remainder of the way.

> Business process reengineering aims at one-time quantum improvement; continuous improvement programs like TQM and Six Sigma aim at ongoing incremental improvements.

Capturing the Benefits of Initiatives to Improve Operations

Usually, the biggest beneficiaries of benchmarking and best-practice initiatives, reengineering, TQM, and Six Sigma are companies that view such programs not as ends in themselves but as tools for implementing and executing company strategy more effectively. The skimpiest payoffs occur when company managers seize them as something worth trying—novel ideas that could improve things. In most such instances, they result in strategy-blind efforts to simply manage better. There's an important lesson here. Best practices, TQM, Six Sigma quality, and reengineering all need to be seen and used as part of a bigger-picture effort to execute strategy proficiently. Only strategy can point to which value chain activities matter and what performance targets make the most sense. Absent a strategic framework, managers lack the context in which to fix things that really matter to business-unit performance and competitive success.

Core Concept
The purpose of using benchmarking, best practices, business process reengineering, TQM, Six Sigma, or other operational improvement programs is to improve the performance of strategy-critical activities and enhance strategy execution.

To get the most from initiative to better execute strategy, managers must have a clear idea of what specific outcomes really matter. Is it a Six Sigma or lower defect rate, high on-time delivery percentages, low overall costs relative to rivals, high percentages of pleased customers and few customer complaints, shorter cycle times, a higher percentage of revenues coming from recently introduced products, or what? Benchmarking best-in-industry and best-in-world performance of most or all value chain activities provides a realistic basis for setting internal performance milestones and longer-range targets.

Then comes the managerial task of building a total quality culture genuinely committed to achieving the performance outcomes that strategic success requires.[15] Managers can take the following action steps to realize full value from TQM or Six Sigma initiatives:[16]

1. Visible, unequivocal, and unyielding commitment to total quality and continuous improvement, including a quality vision and specific, measurable objectives for boosting quality and making continuous improvement.

2. Nudging people toward quality-supportive behaviors by:
   a. Screening job applicants rigorously and hiring only those with attitudes and aptitudes right for quality-based performance.
   b. Providing quality training for most employees.
   c. Using teams and team-building exercises to reinforce and nurture individual effort (the creation of a quality culture is facilitated when teams become more cross-functional, multitask-oriented, and increasingly self-managed).
   d. Recognizing and rewarding individual and team efforts regularly and systematically.
   e. Stressing prevention (doing it right the first time), not inspection (instituting ways to correct mistakes).

3. Empowering employees so that authority for delivering great service or improving products is in the hands of the doers rather than the overseers—*improving quality has to be seen as part of everyone's job.*

4. Using online systems to provide all relevant parties with the latest best practices and actual experiences with them, thereby speeding the diffusion and adoption of best practices throughout the organization and also allowing them to exchange data and opinions about how to upgrade the prevailing best practices.

5. Preaching that performance can, and must, be improved because competitors are not resting on their laurels and customers are always looking for something better.

If the targeted performance measures are appropriate to the strategy and if all organizational members (top executives, middle managers, professional staff, and line employees) buy into a culture of operating excellence, then a company's work climate becomes decidedly more conducive to proficient strategy execution. Benchmarking, best-practice implementation, reengineering, TQM, and Six Sigma initiatives can greatly enhance a company's product design, cycle time, production costs, product quality, service, customer satisfaction, and other operating capabilities—and they can even deliver competitive advantage.[17] Not only do improvements from such initiatives add up over time and strengthen organizational capabilities, but the benefits they produce have hard-to-imitate aspects. While it is relatively easy for rivals to undertake benchmarking, process improvement, and quality training, it is much more difficult and time-consuming for them to instill a deeply ingrained culture of operating excellence (as occurs when such techniques are religiously employed) and top management exhibits lasting commitment to operational excellence throughout the organization.

INSTALLING INFORMATION AND OPERATING SYSTEMS

Company strategies can't be executed well without a number of internal systems for business operations. Southwest, American, Northwest, Delta, and other major airlines cannot hope to provide passenger-pleasing service without a user-friendly online reservation system, an accurate and speedy baggage handling system, and a strict aircraft maintenance program that minimizes equipment failures requiring at-the-gate service and delaying plane departures. FedEx has internal communication systems that allow it to coordinate its over 70,000 vehicles in handling an average of 5.5 million packages a day. Its leading edge flight operations systems allow a single controller to direct as many as 200 of FedEx's 650 aircraft simultaneously, overriding their flight plans should weather or other special emergencies arise. In addition, FedEx has created a series of e-business tools for customers that allow them to ship and track packages online (either at FedEx's Web site or on their own company intranets or Web sites), create address books, review shipping history, generate custom reports, simplify customer billing, reduce internal warehousing and inventory management costs, purchase goods and services from suppliers, and respond quickly to changing customer demands. All of FedEx's systems support the company's strategy of providing businesses and individuals with a broad array of package delivery services (from premium next-day to economical five-day deliveries) and boosting its competitiveness against United Parcel Service, Airborne Express, and the U.S. Postal Service.

Otis Elevator, the world's largest manufacturer of elevators, has 24-hour communications service centers for customers called OtisLine to coordinate its maintenance efforts for some 1.5 million elevators and escalators it has installed worldwide.[18] Electronic monitors installed on each user's site can detect when an elevator or escalator has any of 325 problems and will automatically place a service call to the nearest service center location. Trained operators take all trouble calls, input critical information on a computer screen, and can dispatch trained mechanics from 325 locations across the world to the local trouble spot when needed. All customers have online access to performance data on each of their Otis elevators. More than 80 percent of mechanics in North America carry Web-enabled phones connected to e*Service that transport needed information quickly and allow mechanics to update data in Otis computers for future reference. The OtisLine system helps keep outage times to less than two and a half hours. All the trouble-call data is relayed to design and manufacturing personnel, allowing them to quickly alter design specifications or manufacturing procedures when needed to correct recurring problems.

Amazon.com ships customer orders from fully computerized, 1,300-by-600-foot warehouses containing about 3 million books, CDs, toys, and houseware items.[19] The warehouses are so technologically sophisticated that they require about as many lines of code to run as Amazon's Web site does. Using complex picking algorithms, computers initiate the order-picking process by sending signals to workers' wireless receivers, telling them which items to pick off the shelves in which order. Computers also generate data on misboxed items, chute backup times, line speed, worker productivity, and shipping weights on orders. Systems are upgraded regularly, and productivity improvements are aggressively pursued. In 2003 Amazon's six warehouses were able to handle three times the volume handled in 1999 at costs averaging 10 percent of revenues (versus 20 percent in 1999); in addition, they turned their inventory over 20 times annually in an industry whose average was 15 turns. Amazon's warehouse efficiency and cost per order filled was so low that one of the fastest-growing and most profitable parts of Amazon's business was using its warehouses to run the e-commerce operations of Toys "R" Us and Target.

Most telephone companies, electric utilities, and TV broadcasting systems have online monitoring systems to spot transmission problems within seconds and increase the reliability of their services. At eBay, there are systems for real-time monitoring of new listings, bidding activity, Web site traffic, and page views. Kaiser Permanente spent $3 billion to digitize the medical records of its 8.2 million members so that it could manage patient care more efficiently.[20] IBM has created a database of 36,000 employee profiles that enable it to better assign the most qualified IBM consultant to the projects it is doing for clients. In businesses such as public accounting and management consulting, where large numbers of professional staff need cutting-edge technical know-how, companies have developed systems that identify when it is time for certain employees to attend training programs to update their skills and know-how. Many companies have cataloged best-practice information on their intranets to promote faster transfer and implementation throughout the organization.[21]

Well-conceived state-of-the-art operating systems not only enable better strategy execution but also strengthen organizational capabilities—perhaps enough to provide a competitive edge over rivals. For example, a company with a differentiation strategy based on superior quality has added capability if it has systems for training personnel in quality techniques, tracking product quality at each production step, and ensuring that all goods shipped meet quality standards. A company striving to be a low-cost provider is competitively stronger if it has a benchmarking system that identifies opportunities to implement best practices and drive costs out of the business. Fast-growing companies get an important assist from having capabilities in place to recruit and train new employees in large numbers and from investing in infrastructure that gives them the capability to handle rapid growth as it occurs. It is nearly always better to put infrastructure and support systems in place before they are actually needed than to have to scramble to catch up to customer demand.

> **Core Concept**
> State-of-the-art support systems can be a basis for competitive advantage if they give a firm capabilities that rivals can't match.

Instituting Adequate Information Systems, Performance Tracking, and Controls

Accurate and timely information about daily operations is essential if managers are to gauge how well the strategy execution process is proceeding. Information systems need to cover five broad areas: (1) customer data, (2) operations data, (3) employee data, (4) supplier/partner/collaborative ally data, and (5) financial performance data. All key strategic performance indicators have to be tracked and reported as often as practical. Monthly profit-and-loss statements and monthly statistical summaries, long the norm, are fast being replaced by daily statistical updates and even up-to-the-minute performance monitoring that online technology makes possible. Many retail companies have automated online systems that generate daily sales reports for each store and maintain up-to-the-minute inventory and sales records on each item. Manufacturing plants typically generate daily production reports and track labor productivity on every shift. Many retailers and manufacturers have online data systems connecting them with their suppliers that monitor the status of inventories, track shipments and deliveries, and measure defect rates.

Real-time information systems permit company managers to stay on top of implementation initiatives and daily operations, and to intervene if things seem to be drifting off course. Tracking key performance indicators, gathering information from operating personnel, quickly identifying and diagnosing problems, and taking corrective actions are all integral pieces of the process of managing strategy implementation and execution and exercising adequate organization control. A number of companies have recently begun creating "electronic scorecards" for senior managers that gather daily or weekly statistics from different databases about inventory, sales, costs, and sales trends; such information enables these managers to easily stay abreast of what's happening and make better decisions on a real-time basis.[22] Telephone companies have elaborate information systems to measure signal quality, connection times, interrupts, wrong connections, billing errors, and other measures of reliability that affect customer service and satisfaction. To track and manage the quality of passenger service, airlines have information systems to monitor gate delays, on-time departures and arrivals, baggage handling times, lost baggage complaints, stockouts on meals and drinks, overbookings, and maintenance delays and failures. Continental Airlines has an online system that alerts the company when planes arrive late and assesses whether connecting flights needs to be delayed slightly for late-arriving passengers and carts sent to the gate to shorten the time it will take for passengers to reach their connecting flight. British Petroleum (BP) has outfitted rail cars carrying hazardous materials with sensors and global positioning system (GPS) devices so that it can track the status, location, and other information about these shipments via satellite and relay the data to its corporate intranet. Companies that rely on empowered customer-contact personnel to act promptly and creatively in pleasing customers have installed online information systems that put essential customer data on their computer monitors with a few keystrokes so that they can respond effectively to customer inquiries and deliver personalized customer service.

Statistical information gives managers a feel for the numbers, briefings and meetings provide a feel for the latest developments and emerging issues, and personal contacts add a feel for the people dimension. All are good barometers. Managers have to identify problem areas and deviations from plan before they can take actions to get the organization back on course, by either improving the approaches to strategy execution or fine-tuning the strategy. Jeff Bezos, Amazon's CEO, is an ardent proponent of managing by the numbers—as he puts it, "Math-based decisions always trump opinion and judgment. The trouble with most corporations is that they make judgment-based decisions when data-based decisions could be made."[23]

> **Core Concept**
> Having good information systems and operating data are integral to competent strategy execution and operating excellence.

Exercising Adequate Controls over Empowered Employees

Another important aspect of effectively managing and controlling the strategy execution process is monitoring the performance of empowered workers to see that they are acting within the specified limits.[24] Leaving empowered employees to their own devices in meeting performance standards without appropriate checks and balances can expose an organization to excessive risk.[25] Instances abound of employees' decisions or behavior having gone awry, sometimes costing a company huge sums or producing lawsuits aside from just generating embarrassing publicity.

Managers shouldn't have to devote big chunks of their time to making sure that the decisions and behavior of empowered employees stay between the white lines—this would defeat the major purpose of empowerment and, in effect, lead to the reinstatement of a managerial bureaucracy engaged in constant over-the-shoulder supervision. Yet managers have a clear responsibility to exercise sufficient control over empowered employees to protect the company against out-of-bounds behavior and unwelcome surprises. Scrutinizing daily and weekly operating statistics is one of the important ways in which managers can monitor the results that flow from the actions of empowered subordinates—if the operating results flowing from the actions of empowered employees look good, then it is reasonable to assume that empowerment is working.

But close monitoring of real-time or daily operating performance is only one of the control tools at management's disposal. Another valuable lever of control in companies that rely on empowered employees, especially in those that use self-managed work groups or other such teams, is peer-based control. Most team members feel responsible for the success of the whole team and tend to be relatively intolerant of any team member's behavior that weakens team performance or puts team accomplishments at risk (especially when team performance has a big impact on each team member's compensation). Because peer evaluation is such a powerful control device, companies organized into teams can remove some layers of the management hierarchy and rely on strong peer pressure to keep team members operating between the white lines. This is especially true when a company has the information systems capability to monitor team performance daily or in real time.

TYING REWARDS AND INCENTIVES TO GOOD STRATEGY EXECUTION

It is important for both organization units and individuals to be enthusiastically committed to executing strategy and achieving performance targets. Managers typically use an assortment of motivational techniques and rewards to enlist companywide commitment to executing the strategic plan. A manager has to do more than just talk to everyone about how important new strategic practices and performance targets are to the organization's well-being. No matter how inspiring, talk seldom commands people's best efforts for long. *To get employees' sustained, energetic commitment, management has to be resourceful in designing and using motivational incentives—both monetary and nonmonetary.* The more a manager understands what motivates subordinates and the more he or she relies on motivational incentives as a tool for achieving the targeted strategic and financial results, the greater will be employees' commitment to good day-in, day-out strategy execution and achievement of performance targets.[26]

> **Core Concept**
> A properly designed reward structure is management's most powerful tool for mobilizing organizational commitment to successful strategy execution.

Strategy-Facilitating Motivational Practices

Financial incentives generally head the list of motivating tools for trying to gain wholehearted employee commitment to good strategy execution and operating excellence. Monetary rewards generally include some combination of base pay increases, performance bonuses, profit-sharing plans, stock awards, company contributions to employee

401(k) or retirement plans, and piecework incentives (in the case of production workers). But successful companies and managers normally make extensive use of such nonmonetary carrot-and-stick incentives as frequent words of praise (or constructive criticism), special recognition at company gatherings or in the company newsletter, more (or less) job security, stimulating assignments, opportunities to transfer to attractive locations, increased (or decreased) autonomy, and rapid promotion (or the risk of being sidelined in a routine or dead-end job). In addition, companies use a host of other motivational approaches to make their workplaces more appealing and spur stronger employee commitment to the strategy execution process; the following are some of the most important:[27]

> **Core Concept**
> One of management's biggest strategy-executing challenges is to employ motivational techniques that build wholehearted commitment to operating excellence and winning attitudes among employees.

- *Providing attractive perks and fringe benefits*—The various options here include full coverage of health insurance premiums; full tuition reimbursement for work on college degrees; paid vacation time of three or four weeks; on-site child care at major facilities; on-site gym facilities and massage therapists; getaway opportunities at company-owned recreational facilities (beach houses, ranches, resort condos); personal concierge services; subsidized cafeterias and free lunches; casual dress every day; personal travel services; paid sabbaticals; maternity leaves; paid leaves to care for ill family members; telecommuting; compressed workweeks (four 10-hour days instead of five 8-hour days); reduced summer hours; college scholarships for children; on-the-spot bonuses for exceptional performance; and relocation services.

- *Relying on promotion from within whenever possible*—This practice helps bind workers to their employer and employers to their workers; plus, it is an incentive for good performance. Promotion from within also helps ensure that people in positions of responsibility actually know something about the business, technology, and operations they are managing.

- *Making sure that the ideas and suggestions of employees are valued and that those with merit are promptly acted on*—Many companies find that their best ideas for nuts-and-bolts operating improvements come from the suggestions of employees. Moreover, research indicates that the moves of many companies to push decision making down the line and empower employees increases employee motivation and satisfaction, as well as boosting their productivity. The use of self-managed teams has much the same effect.

- *Creating a work atmosphere in which there is genuine sincerity, caring, and mutual respect among workers and between management and employees*—A "family" work environment in which people are on a first-name basis and there is strong camaraderie promotes teamwork and cross-unit collaboration.

- *Stating the strategic vision in inspirational terms that make employees feel they are a part of doing something very worthwhile in a larger social sense*—There's strong motivating power associated with giving people a chance to be part of something exciting and personally satisfying. Jobs with noble purpose tend to turn employees on. At Pfizer, Merck, and most other pharmaceutical companies, it is the notion of helping sick people get well and restoring patients to full life. At Whole Foods Market (a natural foods grocery chain), it is helping customers discover good eating habits and thus improving human health and nutrition.

- *Sharing information with employees about financial performance, strategy, operational measures, market conditions, and competitors' actions*—Broad disclosure and prompt communication send the message that managers trust their workers. Keeping employees in the dark denies them information useful to performing their job, prevents them from being "students of the business," and usually turns them off.

- *Having knockout facilities*—A workplace with appealing features and amenities usually has decidedly positive effects on employee morale and productivity.

- *Being flexible in how the company approaches people management (motivation, compensation, recognition, recruitment) in multinational, multicultural environments*—There is usually some merit in giving local managers in foreign operations to adapt their motivation, compensation, recognition, and recruitment practices to fit local customs, habits, values, and business practices rather than insisting on consistent people-management practices worldwide. But the one area where consistency is essential is conveying the message that the organization values people of all races and cultural backgrounds and that discrimination of any sort will not be tolerated.

For specific examples of the motivational tactics employed by several prominent companies (many of which appear on *Fortune*'s list of "The 100 Best Companies to Work for in America"), see Illustration Capsule 12.3.

Striking the Right Balance between Rewards and Punishment

While most approaches to motivation, compensation, and people management accentuate the positive, companies also embellish positive rewards with the risk of punishment. At General Electric, McKinsey & Company, several global public accounting firms, and other companies that look for and expect top-notch individual performance, there's an "up-or-out" policy—managers and professionals whose performance is not good enough to warrant promotion are first denied bonuses and stock awards and eventually weeded out. A number of companies deliberately give employees heavy workloads and tight deadlines—personnel are pushed hard to achieve "stretch" objectives and expected to put in long hours (nights and weekends if need be). At most companies, senior executives and key personnel in underperforming units are pressured to boost performance to acceptable levels and keep it there or risk being replaced.

As a general rule, it is unwise to take off the pressure for good individual and group performance or play down the stress, anxiety, and adverse consequences of shortfalls in performance. There is no evidence that a no-pressure/no-adverse-consequences work environment leads to superior strategy execution or operating excellence. As the CEO of a major bank put it, "There's a deliberate policy here to create a level of anxiety. Winners usually play like they're one touchdown behind."[28] *High-performing organizations nearly always have a cadre of ambitious people who relish the opportunity to climb the ladder of success, love a challenge, thrive in a performance-oriented environment, and find some competition and pressure useful to satisfy their own drives for personal recognition, accomplishment, and self-satisfaction.*

However, if an organization's motivational approaches and reward structure induce too much stress, internal competitiveness, job insecurity, and unpleasant consequences, the impact on workforce morale and strategy execution can be counterproductive. Evidence shows that managerial initiatives to improve strategy execution should incorporate more positive than negative motivational elements because when cooperation is

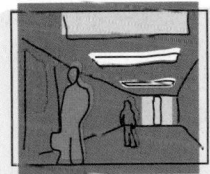

Illustration Capsule 12.3
What Companies Do to Motivate and Reward Employees

Companies have come up with an impressive variety of motivational and reward practices to help create a work environment that energizes employees and promotes better strategy execution. Here's a sampling of what companies are doing:

- Google has a sprawling four-building complex known as the Googleplex where the company's roughly 1,000 employees are provided with free food, unlimited ice cream, pool and Ping-Pong tables, and complimentary massages—management built the Googleplex to be "a dream environment." Moreover, the company gives its employees the ability to spend 20 percent of their work time on any outside activity.

- Lincoln Electric, widely known for its piecework pay scheme and incentive bonus plan, rewards individual productivity by paying workers for each nondefective piece produced. Workers have to correct quality problems on their own time—defects in products used by customers can be traced back to the worker who caused them. Lincoln's piecework plan motivates workers to pay attention to both quality and volume produced. In addition, the company sets aside a substantial portion of its profits above a specified base for worker bonuses. To determine bonus size, Lincoln Electric rates each worker on four equally important performance measures: dependability, quality, output, and ideas and cooperation. The higher a worker's merit rating, the higher the incentive bonus earned; the most highly rated workers in good profit years receive bonuses of as much as 110 percent of their piecework compensation.

- At JM Family Enterprises, a Toyota distributor in Florida, employees get a great lease on new Toyotas and are flown to the Bahamas for cruises on the 172-foot company yacht. The company's office facility has such amenities as a heated lap pool, a fitness center, and a free nail salon. Employees get free prescriptions delivered by a "pharmacy concierge" and professionally made take-home dinners.

- Amazon.com hands out Just Do It awards to employees who do something they think will help Amazon *without* getting their boss's permission. The action has to be well thought through but doesn't have to succeed.

- Nordstrom, widely regarded for its superior in-house customer service experience, typically pays its retail salespeople an hourly wage higher than the prevailing rates paid by other department store chains plus a commission on each sale. Spurred by a culture that encourages salespeople to go all out to satisfy customers and to seek out and promote new fashion ideas, Nordstrom salespeople often earn twice the average incomes of sales employees at competing stores. Nordstrom's rules for employees are simple: "Rule #1: Use your good judgment in all situations. There will be no additional rules."

- At W. L. Gore (the maker of Gore-Tex), employees get to choose what project/team they work on and each team member's compensation is based on other team members' rankings of his or her contribution to the enterprise.

- At Ukrop's Super Markets, a family-owned chain, stores stay closed on Sunday; the company pays out 20 percent of pretax profits to employees in the form of quarterly bonuses; and the company picks up the membership tab for employees if they visit their health club 30 times a quarter.

- At biotech leader Amgen, employees get 16 paid holidays, generous vacation time, tuition reimbursements up to $10,000, on-site massages, a discounted car wash, and the convenience of shopping at on-site farmers' markets.

- At Synovus, a financial services and credit card company, the company adds as much as 20 percent annually to each employee's compensation via a "wealth-building" program that includes a 401(k) and profit sharing; plus, it holds an annual bass fishing tournament.

- At specialty chipmaker Xilinx, new hires receive stock option grants; the CEO responds promptly to employee e-mails, and during hard times management takes a 20 percent pay cut instead of laying off employees.

Sources: Fortune's lists of the 100 best companies to work for in America, 2002, 2004, and 2005 (accessed November 14, 2005); Jefferson Graham, "The Search Engine that Could," *USA Today,* August 26, 2003, p. B3; and Fred Vogelstein, "Winning the Amazon Way," *Fortune* (May 26, 2003), p. 73.

positively enlisted and rewarded, rather than strong-armed by orders and threats (implicit or explicit), people tend to respond with more enthusiasm, dedication, creativity, and initiative. Something of a middle ground is generally optimal—not only handing out decidedly positive rewards for meeting or beating performance targets but also imposing sufficiently negative consequences (if only withholding rewards) when actual performance falls short of the target. But the negative consequences of underachievement should never be so severe or demoralizing as to impede a renewed and determined effort to overcome existing obstacles and hit the targets in upcoming periods.

Linking the Reward System to Strategically Relevant Performance Outcomes

The most dependable way to keep people focused on strategy execution and the achievement of performance targets is to *generously* reward and recognize individuals and groups who meet or beat performance targets and deny rewards and recognition to those who don't. *The use of incentives and rewards is the single most powerful tool management has to win strong employee commitment to diligent, competent strategy execution and operating excellence.* Decisions on salary increases, incentive compensation, promotions, key assignments, and the ways and means of awarding praise and recognition are potent attention-getting, commitment-generating devices.

Core Concept

A properly designed reward system aligns the well-being of organization members with their contributions to competent strategy execution and the achievement of performance targets.

Such decisions seldom escape the closest employee scrutiny, saying more about what is expected and who is considered to be doing a good job than about any other factor. Hence, when meeting or beating strategic and financial targets become *the dominating basis* for designing incentives, evaluating individual and group efforts, and handing out rewards, company personnel quickly grasp that it is in their own self-interest to do their best in executing the strategy competently and achieving key performance targets.[29] Indeed, it is usually through the company's system of incentives and rewards that workforce members emotionally ratify their commitment to the company's strategy execution effort.

Ideally, performance targets should be set for every organization unit, every manager, every team or work group, and perhaps every employee—targets that measure whether strategy execution is progressing satisfactorily. If the company's strategy is to be a low-cost provider, the incentive system must reward actions and achievements that result in lower costs. If the company has a differentiation strategy predicated on superior quality and service, the incentive system must reward such outcomes as Six Sigma defect rates, infrequent need for product repair, low numbers of customer complaints, speedy order processing and delivery, and high levels of customer satisfaction. If a company's growth is predicated on a strategy of new product innovation, incentives should be tied to factors such as the percentages of revenues and profits coming from newly introduced products.

Illustration Capsule 12.4 provides two vivid examples of how companies have designed incentives linked directly to outcomes reflecting good strategy execution.

The Importance of Basing Incentives on Achieving Results, Not on Performing Assigned Duties   To create a strategy-supportive system of rewards and incentives, a company must emphasize rewarding people for accomplishing results, not for just dutifully performing assigned tasks. Focusing jobholders' attention and energy on what to *achieve* as opposed to what to *do* makes the work

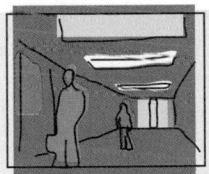

Illustration Capsule 12.4

Nucor and Bank One: Two Companies that Tie Incentives Directly to Strategy Execution

The strategy at Nucor Corporation, now the biggest steel producer in the United States, is to be *the* low-cost producer of steel products. Because labor costs are a significant fraction of total cost in the steel business, successful implementation of Nucor's low-cost leadership strategy entails achieving lower labor costs per ton of steel than competitors' costs. Nucor management uses an incentive system to promote high worker productivity and drive labor costs per ton below rivals'. Each plant's workforce is organized into production teams (each assigned to perform particular functions), and weekly production targets are established for each team. Base pay scales are set at levels comparable to wages for similar manufacturing jobs in the local areas where Nucor has plants, but workers can earn a 1 percent bonus for each 1 percent that their output exceeds target levels. If a production team exceeds its weekly production target by 10 percent, team members receive a 10 percent bonus in their next paycheck; if a team exceeds its quota by 20 percent, team members earn a 20 percent bonus. Bonuses, paid every two weeks, are based on the prior two weeks' actual production levels measured against the targets.

Nucor's piece-rate incentive plan has produced impressive results. The production teams put forth exceptional effort; it is not uncommon for most teams to beat their weekly production targets anywhere from 20 to 50 percent. When added to their base pay, the bonuses earned by Nucor workers make Nucor's workforce among the highest-paid in the U.S. steel industry. From a management perspective, the incentive system has resulted in Nucor having labor productivity levels 10 to 20 percent above the average of the unionized workforces at several of its largest rivals, which in turn has given Nucor a significant labor cost advantage over most rivals.

At Bank One (recently acquired by JP Morgan Chase), management believed it was strategically important to boost its customer satisfaction ratings in order to enhance its competitiveness vis-à-vis rivals. Targets were set for customer satisfaction and monitoring systems for measuring customer satisfaction at each branch office were put in place. Then, to motivate branch office personnel to be more attentive in trying to please customers and also to signal that top management was truly committed to achieving higher levels of overall customer satisfaction, top management opted to tie pay scales in each branch office to that branch's customer satisfaction rating—the higher the branch's ratings, the higher that branch's pay scales. Management believed its shift from a theme of equal pay for equal work to one of equal pay for equal performance contributed significantly to its customer satisfaction priority.

environment results-oriented. It is flawed management to tie incentives and rewards to satisfactory performance of duties and activities in hopes that the by-products will be the desired business outcomes and company achievements.[30] In any job, performing assigned tasks is not equivalent to achieving intended outcomes. Diligently showing up for work and attending to one's job assignment does not, by itself, guarantee results. As any student knows, the fact that an instructor teaches and students go to class doesn't necessarily mean that the students are learning. The enterprise of education would no doubt take on a different character if teachers were rewarded for the result of student learning rather than for the activity of teaching.

> It is folly to reward one outcome in hopes of getting another outcome.

Incentive compensation for top executives is typically tied to such financial measures as revenue and earnings growth, stock price performance, return on investment, and creditworthiness and perhaps such strategic measures as market share, product quality, or customer satisfaction. However, incentives for department heads, teams, and individual workers may be tied to performance outcomes more closely related to their strategic area of responsibility. In manufacturing, incentive compensation may be tied to unit manufacturing costs, on-time production and shipping, defect rates,

Core Concept
The role of the reward system is to align the well-being of organization members with realizing the company's vision, so that organization members benefit by helping the company execute its strategy competently and fully satisfy customers.

the number and extent of work stoppages due to labor disagreements and equipment breakdowns, and so on. In sales and marketing, there may be incentives for achieving dollar sales or unit volume targets, market share, sales penetration of each target customer group, the fate of newly introduced products, the frequency of customer complaints, the number of new accounts acquired, and customer satisfaction. Which performance measures to base incentive compensation on depends on the situation—the priority placed on various financial and strategic objectives, the requirements for strategic and competitive success, and what specific results are needed in different facets of the business to keep strategy execution on track.

Guidelines for Designing Incentive Compensation Systems   The concepts and company experiences discussed above yield the following prescriptive guidelines for creating an incentive compensation system to help drive successful strategy execution:

1. *Make the performance payoff a major, not minor, piece of the total compensation package.* Payoffs must be at least 10 to 12 percent of base salary to have much impact. Incentives that amount to 20 percent or more of total compensation are big attention-getters, likely to really drive individual or team effort; incentives amounting to less than 5 percent of total compensation have comparatively weak motivational impact. Moreover, the payoff for high-performing individuals and teams must be meaningfully greater than the payoff for average performers, and the payoff for average performers meaningfully bigger than for below-average performers.

2. *Have incentives that extend to all managers and all workers, not just top management.* It is a gross miscalculation to expect that lower-level managers and employees will work their hardest to hit performance targets just so a few senior executives can get lucrative rewards.

3. *Administer the reward system with scrupulous objectivity and fairness.* If performance standards are set unrealistically high or if individual/group performance evaluations are not accurate and well documented, dissatisfaction with the system will overcome any positive benefits.

4. *Tie incentives to performance outcomes directly linked to good strategy execution and financial performance.* Incentives should never be paid just because people are thought to be "doing a good job" or because they "work hard." Performance evaluation based on factors not tightly related to good strategy execution signal that either the strategic plan is incomplete (because important performance targets were left out) or management's real agenda is something other than the stated strategic and financial objectives.

5. *Make sure that the performance targets each individual or team is expected to achieve involve outcomes that the individual or team can personally affect.* The role of incentives is to enhance individual commitment and channel behavior in beneficial directions. This role is not well served when the performance measures by which company personnel are judged are outside their arena of influence.

6. *Keep the time between achieving the target performance outcome and the payment of the reward as short as possible.* Companies like Nucor and Continental Airlines have discovered that weekly or monthly payments for good performance work much better than annual payments. Nucor pays weekly bonuses based on

prior-week production levels; Continental awards employees a monthly bonus for each month that on-time flight performance meets or beats a specified percentage companywide. Annual bonus payouts work best for higher-level managers and for situations where target outcome relates to overall company profitability or stock price performance.

7. *Make liberal use of nonmonetary rewards; don't rely solely on monetary rewards.* When used properly, money is a great motivator, but there are also potent advantages to be gained from praise, special recognition, handing out plum assignments, and so on.

8. *Absolutely avoid skirting the system to find ways to reward effort rather than results.* Whenever actual performance falls short of targeted performance, there's merit in determining whether the causes are attributable to subpar individual/group performance or to circumstances beyond the control of those responsible. An argument can be made that exceptions should be made in giving rewards to people who've tried hard, gone the extra mile, yet still come up short because of circumstances beyond their control. The problem with making exceptions for unknowable, uncontrollable, or unforeseeable circumstances is that once good excuses start to creep into justifying rewards for subpar results, the door is open for all kinds of reasons why actual performance failed to match targeted performance. A "no excuses" standard is more evenhanded and certainly easier to administer.

Once the incentives are designed, they have to be communicated and explained. Everybody needs to understand how their incentive compensation is calculated and how individual/group performance targets contribute to organizational performance targets. The pressure to achieve the targeted strategic and financial performance and continuously improve on strategy execution should be unrelenting, with few (if any) loopholes for rewarding shortfalls in performance. People at all levels have to be held accountable for carrying out their assigned parts of the strategic plan, and they have to understand their rewards are based on the caliber of results that are achieved. But with the pressure to perform should come meaningful rewards. Without an ample payoff, the system breaks down, and managers are left with the less workable options of barking orders, trying to enforce compliance, and depending on the goodwill of employees.

> **Core Concept**
> The unwavering standard for judging whether individuals, teams, and organizational units have done a good job must be whether they meet or beat performance targets that reflect good strategy execution.

Performance-Based Incentives and Rewards in Multinational Enterprises

In some foreign countries, incentive pay runs counter to local customs and cultural norms. Professor Steven Kerr cites the time he lectured an executive education class on the need for more performance-based pay and a Japanese manager protested, "You shouldn't bribe your children to do their homework, you shouldn't bribe your wife to prepare dinner, and you shouldn't bribe your employees to work for the company."[31] Singling out individuals and commending them for unusually good effort can also be a problem; Japanese culture considers public praise of an individual an affront to the harmony of the group. In some countries, employees have a preference for nonmonetary rewards—more leisure time, important titles, access to vacation villages, and nontaxable perks. Thus, multinational companies have to build some degree of flexibility into the design of incentives and rewards in order to accommodate cross-cultural traditions and preferences.

Key Points

Managers implementing and executing a new or different strategy must identify the resource requirements of each new strategic initiative and then consider whether the current pattern of resource allocation and the budgets of the various subunits are suitable.

Anytime a company alters its strategy, managers should review existing policies and operating procedures, proactively revise or discard those that are out of sync, and formulate new ones to facilitate execution of new strategic initiatives. Prescribing new or freshly revised policies and operating procedures aids the task of strategy execution (1) by providing top-down guidance to operating managers, supervisory personnel, and employees regarding how certain things need to be done and what the boundaries are on independent actions and decisions; (2) by enforcing consistency in how particular strategy-critical activities are performed in geographically scattered operating units; and (3) by promoting the creation of a work climate and corporate culture that promotes good strategy execution.

Competent strategy execution entails visible, unyielding managerial commitment to best practices and continuous improvement. Benchmarking, the discovery and adoption of best practices, reengineering core business processes, and continuous improvement initiatives like total quality management (TQM) or Six Sigma programs, all aim at improved efficiency, lower costs, better product quality, and greater customer satisfaction. *These initiatives are important tools for learning how to execute a strategy more proficiently.*

Company strategies can't be implemented or executed well without a number of support systems to carry on business operations. Well-conceived state-of-the-art support systems not only facilitate better strategy execution but also strengthen organizational capabilities enough to provide a competitive edge over rivals. Real-time information and control systems further aid the cause of good strategy execution.

Strategy-supportive motivational practices and reward systems are powerful management tools for gaining employee commitment. The key to creating a reward system that promotes good strategy execution is to make strategically relevant measures of performance *the dominating basis* for designing incentives, evaluating individual and group efforts, and handing out rewards. Positive motivational practices generally work better than negative ones, but there is a place for both. There's also a place for both monetary and nonmonetary incentives.

For an incentive compensation system to work well (1) the monetary payoff should be a major percentage of the compensation package, (2) the use of incentives should extend to all managers and workers, (3) the system should be administered with care and fairness, (4) the incentives should be linked to performance targets spelled out in the strategic plan, (5) each individual's performance targets should involve outcomes the person can personally affect, (6) rewards should promptly follow the determination of good performance, (7) monetary rewards should be supplemented with liberal use of nonmonetary rewards, and (8) skirting the system to reward nonperformers or subpar results should be scrupulously avoided. Companies with operations in multiple countries often have to build some degree of flexibility into the design of incentives and rewards in order to accommodate cross-cultural traditions and preferences.

Exercises

1. Go to Google or another Internet search engine and, using the advanced search feature, enter "best practices." Browse through the search results to identify at least five organizations that have gathered a set of best practices and are making the best-practice library they have assembled available to members. Explore at least one of the sites to get an idea of the kind of best-practice information that is available.

2. Do an Internet search on "Six Sigma" quality programs. Browse through the search results and (*a*) identify at least three companies that offer Six Sigma training and (*b*) find lists of companies that have implemented Six Sigma programs in their pursuit of operational excellence—you should be able to cite at least 25 companies that are Six Sigma users. Prepare a one-page report to your instructor detailing the experiences and benefits that one company has realized from employing Six Sigma methods in its operations. To learn more about how Six Sigma works, go to www.isixsigma.com and explore the Q&A menu option.

3. Do an Internet search on "total quality management." Browse through the search results and (*a*) identify 10 companies that offer TQM training, (*b*) identify 5 books on TQM programs, and (*c*) find lists of companies that have implemented TQM programs in their pursuit of operational excellence—you should be able to name at least 20 companies that are TQM users.

4. Consult the latest issue of *Fortune* containing the annual "100 Best Companies to Work For" (usually a late-January or early-February issue, or else use a search engine to locate the list online) and identify at least five compensation incentives and work practices that these companies use to enhance employee motivation and reward them for good strategic and financial performance. Choose compensation methods and work practices that are different from those cited in Illustration Capsule 12.3.

5. Review the profiles and applications of the latest Malcolm Baldrige National Quality Award recipients at www.quality.nist.gov. What are the standout features of the companies' approaches to managing operations? What do you find impressive about the companies' policies and procedures, use of best practices, emphasis on continuous improvement, and use of rewards and incentives?

6. Using Google Scholar or your access to online business periodicals in your university's library, search for the term "incentive compensation" and prepare a report of one to two pages to your instructor discussing the successful (or unsuccessful) use of incentive compensation plans by various companies. According to your research, what factors seem to determine whether incentive compensation plans succeed or fail?

chapter thirteen

13

Corporate Culture and Leadership

Keys to Good Strategy Execution

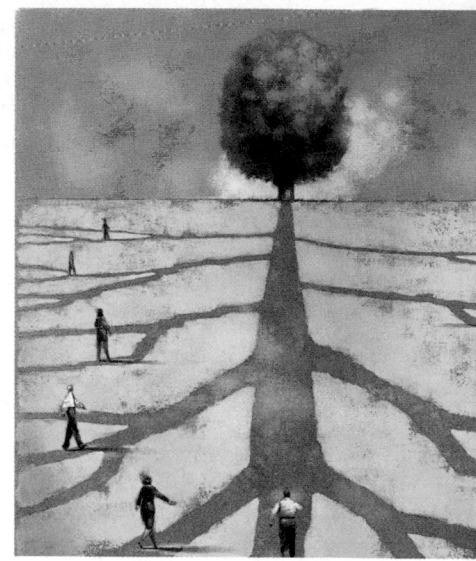

The biggest levers you've got to change a company are strategy, structure, and culture. If I could pick two, I'd pick strategy and culture.

—Wayne Leonard
CEO, Entergy

An organization's capacity to execute its strategy depends on its "hard" infrastructure—its organizational structure and systems—and on its "soft" infrastructure—its culture and norms.

—Amar Bhide

Weak leadership can wreck the soundest strategy; forceful execution of even a poor plan can often bring victory.

—Sun Zi

Leadership is accomplishing something through other people that wouldn't have happened if you weren't there . . . Leadership is being able to mobilize ideas and values that energize other people . . . Leaders develop a story line that engages other people.

—Noel Tichy

Seeing people in person is a big part of how you drive any change process. You have to show people a positive view of the future and say "we can do it."

—Jeffrey R. Immelt
CEO, General Electric

In the previous two chapters we examined six of the managerial tasks important to good strategy execution and operating excellence—building a capable organization, marshaling the needed resources and steering them to strategy-critical operating units, establishing policies and procedures that facilitate good strategy execution, adopting best practices and pushing for continuous improvement in how value chain activities are performed, creating internal operating systems that enable better execution, and employing motivational practices and compensation incentives that gain wholehearted employee commitment to the strategy execution process. In this chapter we explore the two remaining managerial tasks that shape the outcome of efforts to execute a company's strategy: creating a strategy-supportive corporate culture and exerting the internal leadership needed to drive the implementation of strategic initiatives forward and achieve higher plateaus of operating excellence.

INSTILLING A CORPORATE CULTURE THAT PROMOTES GOOD STRATEGY EXECUTION

Every company has its own unique culture. The character of a company's culture or work climate is a product of the core values and business principles that executives espouse, the standards of what is ethically acceptable and what is not, the work practices and behaviors that define "how we do things around here," the approach to people management and style of operating, the "chemistry" and the "personality" that permeates the work environment, and the stories that get told over and over to illustrate and reinforce the company's values, business practices, and traditions. The meshing together of stated beliefs, business principles, styles of operating, ingrained behaviors and attitudes, and work climate define a company's **corporate culture.** A company's culture is important because it influences the organization's actions and approaches to conducting business—in a very real sense, the culture is the company's "operating system" or organizational DNA.[1]

> **Core Concept**
> **Corporate culture** refers to the character of a company's internal work climate and personality—as shaped by its core values, beliefs, business principles, traditions, ingrained behaviors, work practices, and styles of operating.

The psyche of corporate cultures varies widely. For instance, the bedrock of Wal-Mart's culture is dedication to customer satisfaction, zealous pursuit of low costs and frugal operating practices, a strong work ethic, ritualistic Saturday-morning headquarters meetings to exchange ideas and review problems, and company executives' commitment to visiting stores, listening to customers, and soliciting suggestions from employees. General Electric's culture is founded on a hard-driving, results-oriented atmosphere (where all of the company's business divisions are held to a standard of being number one or two in their industries as well as achieving good business results); extensive cross-business sharing of ideas, best practices, and learning; the reliance on "workout sessions" to identify, debate, and resolve burning issues; a commitment to Six Sigma quality; and globalization of the company. At Occidental Petroleum, the culture is grounded in entrepreneurship on the part of employees; the company's empowered employees are encouraged to be innovative, excel in their fields of specialization, respond quickly to strategic opportunities, and creatively apply state-of-the-art technology in a manner that promotes operating excellence and sets Occidental apart from its competitors. At Nordstrom, the corporate culture is centered on delivering exceptional service to customers; the company's motto is "Respond to unreasonable customer requests"—each out-of-the-ordinary request is seen as an opportunity for a "heroic" act by an employee that can further the company's reputation for a customer-pleasing shopping environment. Nordstrom makes a point of promoting employees noted for their heroic acts and dedication to outstanding service; the company motivates its salespeople with a commission-based compensation system that enables Nordstrom's best salespeople to earn more than double what other department stores pay.

Illustration Capsule 13.1 relates how Google and Alberto-Culver describe their corporate cultures.

Identifying the Key Features of a Company's Corporate Culture

A company's corporate culture is mirrored in the character or "personality" of its work environment—the factors that underlie how the company tries to conduct its business and the behaviors that are held in high esteem. The chief things to look for include the following:

- *The values, business principles, and ethical standards that management preaches and practices.* Actions speak much louder than words here.
- *The company's approach to people management* and the official policies, procedures, and operating practices that paint the white lines for the behavior of company personnel.
- *The spirit and character that pervade the work climate.* Is the workplace vibrant and fun, methodical and all-business, tense and harried, or highly competitive and politicized? Are people excited about their work and emotionally connected to the company's business or are they just there to draw a paycheck? Is there an emphasis on empowered worker creativity or do people have little discretion in how jobs are done?
- *How managers and employees interact and relate to each other.* How much reliance is there on teamwork and open communication? To what extent is there good camaraderie? Are people called by their first names? Do coworkers spend little or lots of time together outside the workplace? What are the dress codes (the accepted styles of attire and whether there are casual days)?
- *The strength of peer pressure to do things in particular ways and conform to expected norms.* What actions and behaviors are approved (and rewarded by management in the form of compensation and promotion) and which ones are frowned on?

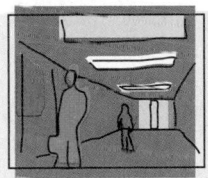

Illustration Capsule 13.1

The Corporate Cultures at Google and Alberto-Culver

GOOGLE

Founded in 1998 by Larry Page and Sergey Brin, two Ph.D. students in computer science at Stanford University, Google has beome world-renowned for its search engine technology. Google.com is one of the five most popular sites on the Internet, attracting over 380 million unique visitors monthly from around the world. Google has some unique ways of operating, and its culture is rather quirky. The company describes its culture as follows:

> Though growing rapidly, Google still maintains a small company feel. At the Googleplex headquarters almost everyone eats in the Google café (known as "Charlie's Place"), sitting at whatever table has an opening and enjoying conversations with Googlers from all different departments. Topics range from the trivial to the technical, and whether the discussion is about computer games or encryption or ad serving software, it's not surprising to hear someone say, "That's a product I helped develop before I came to Google."
>
> Google's emphasis on innovation and commitment to cost containment means each employee is a hands-on contributor. There's little in the way of corporate hierarchy and everyone wears several hats. The international webmaster who creates Google's holiday logos spent a week translating the entire site into Korean. The chief operations engineer is also a licensed neurosurgeon. Because everyone realizes they are an equally important part of Google's success, no one hesitates to skate over a corporate officer during roller hockey.
>
> Google's hiring policy is aggressively non-discriminatory and favors ability over experience. The result is a staff that reflects the global audience the search engine serves. Google has offices around the globe and Google engineering centers are recruiting local talent in locations from Zurich to Bangalore. Dozens of languages are spoken by Google staffers, from Turkish to Telugu. When not at work, Googlers pursue interests from cross-country cycling to wine tasting, from flying to Frisbee. As Google expands its development team, it continues to look for those who share an obsessive commitment to creating search perfection and having a great time doing it.

ALBERTO-CULVER

The Alberto-Culver Company, with fiscal 2005 revenues of about $3.5 billion, is the producer and marketer of Alberto VO5, TRESemmé, Consort, and Just for Me hair care products; St. Ives skin care, hair care, and facial care products; and such brands as Molly McButter, Mrs. Dash, Sugar Twin, and Static Guard. Alberto-Culver brands are sold in 120 countries. Its Sally Beauty Company, with over 3,250 stores and 1,250 professional sales consultants, is the largest marketer of professional beauty care products in the world.

At the careers section of its Web site, the company described its culture in the following words:

> Building careers is as important to us as building brands. We believe that passionate people create powerful growth. We believe in a workplace built on values and believe our best people display those same values in their families and their communities. We believe in recognizing and rewarding accomplishment and celebrating our victories.
>
> We believe the best ideas work their way—quickly—up an organization, not down. We believe that we should take advantage of every ounce of your talent on teams and cross-functional activities, not just assign you to a box.
>
> We believe in open communication. We believe that you can improve what you measure, so we survey and spot check all the time. For that same reason, every one has specific goals so that their expectations are in line with their managers' and the company's.
>
> We believe that victory is a team accomplishment. We believe in personal development. We believe if you talk with us you will catch our enthusiasm and want to be a part of the Alberto-Culver team.

Sources: Information posted at www.google.com and www.alberto.com (accessed November 16, 2005).

- *The company's revered traditions and oft-repeated stories.* Do people talk a lot about "heroic acts" and "how we do things around here"?
- *The manner in which the company deals with external stakeholders (particularly vendors and local communities where it has operations).* Does it treat suppliers as business partners or does it prefer

hardnosed, arm's-length business arrangements? How strong and genuine is its commitment to corporate citizenship?

Some of these sociological forces are readily apparent, and others operate quite subtly.

The values, beliefs, and practices that undergird a company's culture can come from anywhere in the organization hierarchy, most often representing the business philosophy and managerial style of influential executives but also resulting from exemplary actions on the part of company personnel and consensus agreement about "how we ought to do things around here."[2] Typically, key elements of the culture originate with a founder or certain strong leaders who articulated them as a set of business principles, company policies, operating approaches, and ways of dealing with employees, customers, vendors, shareholders, and local communities where the company has operations. Over time, these cultural underpinnings take root, become embedded in how the company conducts its business, come to be accepted by company managers and employees alike, and then persist as new employees are encouraged to adopt and follow the professed values, behaviors, and work practices.

The Role of Stories   Frequently, a significant part of a company's culture is captured in the stories that get told over and over again to illustrate to newcomers the importance of certain values and the depth of commitment that various company personnel have displayed. One of the folktales at FedEx, world renowned for the reliability of its next-day package delivery guarantee, is about a deliveryman who had been given the wrong key to a FedEx drop box. Rather than leave the packages in the drop box until the next day when the right key was available, the deliveryman unbolted the drop box from its base, loaded it into the truck, and took it back to the station. There, the box was pried open and the contents removed and sped on their way to their destination the next day. Nordstrom keeps a scrapbook commemorating the heroic acts of its employees and uses it as a regular reminder of the beyond-the-call-of-duty behaviors that employees are encouraged to display. At Frito-Lay, there are dozens of stories about truck drivers who went to extraordinary lengths in overcoming adverse weather conditions in order to make scheduled deliveries to retail customers and keep store shelves stocked with Frito-Lay products. At Microsoft, there are stories of the long hours programmers put in, the emotional peaks and valleys in encountering and overcoming coding problems, the exhilaration of completing a complex program on schedule, the satisfaction of working on cutting-edge projects, the rewards of being part of a team responsible for a popular new software program, and the tradition of competing aggressively. Such stories serve the valuable purpose of illustrating the kinds of behavior the company encourages and reveres. Moreover, each retelling of a legendary story puts a bit more peer pressure on company personnel to display core values and do their part in keeping the company's traditions alive.

Perpetuating the Culture   Once established, company cultures are perpetuated in six important ways: (1) by screening and selecting new employees that will mesh well with the culture, (2) by systematic indoctrination of new members in the culture's fundamentals, (3) by the efforts of senior group members to reiterate core values in daily conversations and pronouncements, (4) by the telling and retelling of company legends, (5) by regular ceremonies honoring members who display desired cultural behaviors, and (6) by visibly rewarding those who display cultural norms and penalizing those who don't.[3] *The more new employees a company is hiring, the more important it becomes to screen job applicants every bit as much for how well their values, beliefs, and personalities match up with the culture as for their technical skills and experience.*

For example, a company that stresses operating with integrity and fairness has to hire people who themselves have integrity and place a high value on fair play. A company whose culture revolves around creativity, product innovation, and leading change has to screen new hires for their ability to think outside the box, generate new ideas, and thrive in a climate of rapid change and ambiguity. Southwest Airlines—whose two core values, "LUV" and fun, permeate the work environment and whose objective is to ensure that passengers have a positive and enjoyable flying experience— goes to considerable lengths to hire flight attendants and gate personnel who are witty, cheery, and outgoing and who display whistle-while-you-work attitudes. Fast-growing companies risk creating a culture by chance rather than by design if they rush to hire employees mainly for their talents and credentials and neglect to screen out candidates whose values, philosophies, and personalities aren't a good fit with the organizational character, vision, and strategy being articulated by the company's senior executives.

As a rule, companies are attentive to the task of hiring people who will fit in and who will embrace the prevailing culture. And, usually, job seekers lean toward accepting jobs at companies where they feel comfortable with the atmosphere and the people they will be working with. Employees who don't hit it off at a company tend to leave quickly, while employees who thrive and are pleased with the work environment stay on, eventually moving up the ranks to positions of greater responsibility. The longer people stay at an organization, the more they come to embrace and mirror the corporate culture—their values and beliefs tend to be molded by mentors, fellow workers, company training programs, and the reward structure. Normally, employees who have worked at a company for a long time play a major role in indoctrinating new employees into the culture.

Forces That Cause a Company's Culture to Evolve   However, even stable cultures aren't static; just like strategy and organization structure, they evolve. New challenges in the marketplace, revolutionary technologies, and shifting internal conditions—especially eroding business prospects, an internal crisis, or top executive turnover—tend to breed new ways of doing things and, in turn, cultural evolution. An incoming CEO who decides to shake up the existing business and take it in new directions often triggers a cultural shift, perhaps one of major proportions. Likewise, diversification into new businesses, expansion into foreign countries, rapid growth, an influx of new employees, and merger with or acquisition of another company can all precipitate cultural changes of one kind or another.

Company Subcultures: The Problems Posed by New Acquisitions and Multinational Operations   Although it is common to speak about corporate culture in the singular, it is not uncommon for companies to have multiple cultures (or subcultures).[4] Values, beliefs, and practices within a company sometimes vary significantly by department, geographic location, division, or business unit. A company's subcultures can clash, or at least not mesh well, if they embrace conflicting business philosophies or operating approaches, if key executives employ different approaches to people management, or if important differences between a company's culture and those of recently acquired companies have not yet been ironed out. *Global and multinational companies tend to be at least partly multicultural* because cross-country organization units have different operating histories and work climates, as well as members who have grown up under different social customs and traditions and who have different sets of values and beliefs. The human resources manager of a global pharmaceutical company who took on an assignment in the Far East discovered, to his surprise, that one of his biggest challenges was to persuade his company's managers in China,

Korea, Malaysia, and Taiwan to accept promotions—their cultural values were such that they did not believe in competing with their peers for career rewards or personal gain, nor did they relish breaking ties to their local communities to assume cross-national responsibilities.[5] Many companies that have merged with or acquired foreign companies have to deal with language- and custom-based cultural differences.

Nonetheless, the existence of subcultures does not preclude important areas of commonality and compatibility. For example, General Electric's cultural traits of boundarylessness, workout, and Six Sigma quality can be implanted and practiced successfully in different countries. AES, a global power company with operations in over 25 countries, has found that the four core values of integrity, fairness, fun, and social responsibility underlying its culture are readily embraced by people in most countries. Moreover, AES tries to define and practice its cultural values the same way in all of its locations while still being sensitive to differences that exist among various people groups across the world; top managers at AES express the views that people across the world are more similar than different and that the company's culture is as meaningful in Buenos Aires or Kazakhstan as in Virginia.

In today's globalizing world, multinational companies are learning how to make strategy-critical cultural traits travel across country boundaries and create a workably uniform culture worldwide. Likewise, company managements are quite alert to the importance of cultural compatibility in making acquisitions and the need to address how to merge and integrate the cultures of newly acquired companies—cultural due diligence is often as important as financial due diligence in deciding whether to go forward on an acquisition or merger. On a number of occasions, companies have decided to pass on acquiring particular companies because of culture conflicts that they believed would be hard to resolve.

Strong versus Weak Cultures

Company cultures vary widely in strength and influence. Some are strongly embedded and have a big impact on a company's practices and behavioral norms. Others are weak and have comparatively little influence on company operations.

Strong-Culture Companies   The hallmark of a strong-culture company is the dominating presence of certain deeply rooted values and operating approaches that "regulate" the conduct of a company's business and the climate of its workplace.[6] Strong cultures emerge over a period of years (sometimes decades) and are never an overnight phenomenon. In strong culture companies, senior managers make a point of reiterating these principles and values to organization members and explaining how they relate to its business environment. But, more important, they make a conscious effort to display these principles in their own actions and behavior—they walk the talk, and they *insist that company values and business principles be reflected in the decisions and actions taken by all company personnel.* An unequivocal expectation that company personnel will act and behave in accordance with the adopted values and ways of doing business leads to two important outcomes: (1) Over time, the values come to be widely shared by rank-and-file employees—people who dislike the culture tend to leave—and (2) individuals encounter strong peer pressure from coworkers to observe the culturally approved norms and behaviors. Hence, a strongly implanted corporate culture ends up having a powerful influence on "how we

Core Concept
In a strong-culture company, culturally-approved behaviors and ways of doing things are nurtured while culturally-disapproved behaviors and work practices get squashed.

do things around here" because so many company personnel are accepting of cultural traditions and because this acceptance is reinforced both by management expectations and coworker peer pressure to conform to cultural norms. Since cultural traditions and norms have such a dominating influence in strong-culture companies, the character of the culture becomes the the company's soul or psyche.

Three factors contribute to the development of strong cultures: (1) a founder or strong leader who establishes values, principles, and practices that are consistent and sensible in light of customer needs, competitive conditions, and strategic requirements; (2) a sincere, long-standing company commitment to operating the business according to these established traditions, thereby creating an internal environment that supports decision making and strategies based on cultural norms; and (3) a genuine concern for the well-being of the organization's three biggest constituencies—customers, employees, and shareholders. Continuity of leadership, small group size, stable group membership, geographic concentration, and considerable organizational success all contribute to the emergence and sustainability of a strong culture.[7]

During the time a strong culture is being implanted, there's nearly always a good strategy–culture fit (which partially accounts for the organization's success). Mismatches between strategy and culture in a strong-culture company tend to occur when a company's business environment undergoes significant change, prompting a drastic strategy revision that clashes with the entrenched culture. A strategy–culture clash can also occur in a strong-culture company whose business has gradually eroded; when a new leader is brought in to revitalize the company's operations, he or she may push the company in a strategic direction that requires substantially different cultural and behavioral norms. In such cases, a major culture-changing effort has to be launched.

In strong-culture companies, values and behavioral norms are so ingrained that they can endure leadership changes at the top—although their strength can erode over time if new CEOs cease to nurture them or move aggressively to institute cultural adjustments. And the cultural norms in a strong-culture company may not change much as strategy evolves and the organization acts to make strategy adjustments, either because the new strategies are compatible with the present culture or because the dominant traits of the culture are somewhat strategy-neutral and compatible with evolving versions of the company's strategy.

> In a strong-culture company, values and behavioral norms are like crabgrass: deeply rooted and hard to weed out.

Weak-Culture Companies   In direct contrast to strong-culture companies, weak-culture companies lack values and principles that are consistently preached or widely shared (usually because the company has had a series of CEOs with differing values and differing views about how the company's business ought to be conducted). As a consequence, the company has few widely revered traditions and few culture-induced norms are evident in operating practices. Because top executives at a weak-culture company don't repeatedly espouse any particular business philosophy, exhibit long-standing commitment to particular values, or extol particular operating practices and behavioral norms, individuals encounter little coworker peer pressure to do things in particular ways. Moreover, a weak company culture breeds no strong employee allegiance to what the company stands for or to operating the business in well-defined ways. While individual employees may well have some bonds of identification with and loyalty toward their department, their colleagues, their union, or their boss, there is neither passion about the company nor emotional commitment to what it is trying to accomplish—a condition that often results in many employees viewing their company as just a place to work and their job as just a way to make a living. Very often, cultural weakness stems from moderately entrenched subcultures that block the emergence of a well-defined companywide work climate.

As a consequence, *weak cultures provide little or no assistance in executing strategy* because there are no traditions, beliefs, values, common bonds, or behavioral norms that management can use as levers to mobilize commitment to executing the chosen strategy. The only plus of a weak culture is that it does not usually pose a strong barrier to strategy execution, but the negative of not providing any support means that culture-building has to be high on management's action agenda. Absent a work climate that channels organizational energy in the direction of good strategy execution, managers are left with the options of either using compensation incentives and other motivational devices to mobilize employee commitment or trying to establish cultural roots that will in time start to nurture the strategy execution process.

Unhealthy Cultures

The distinctive characteristic of an unhealthy corporate culture is the presence of counterproductive cultural traits that adversely impact the work climate and company performance.[8] The following four traits are particularly unhealthy:

1. A highly politicized internal environment in which many issues get resolved and decisions made on the basis of which individuals or groups have the most political clout to carry the day.
2. Hostility to change and a general wariness of people who champion new ways of doing things.
3. An insular "not-invented-here" mind-set that makes company personnel averse to looking outside the company for best practices, new managerial approaches, and innovative ideas.
4. A disregard for high ethical standards and overzealous pursuit of wealth and status on the part of key executives.

Politicized Cultures   What makes a politicized internal environment so unhealthy is that political infighting consumes a great deal of organizational energy, often with the result that what's best for the company takes a backseat to political maneuvering. In companies where internal politics pervades the work climate, empire-building managers jealously guard their decision-making prerogatives. They have their own agendas and operate the work units under their supervision as autonomous "fiefdoms," and the positions they take on issues is usually aimed at protecting or expanding their turf. Collaboration with other organizational units is viewed with suspicion (What are "they" up to? How can "we" protect "our" flanks?), and cross-unit cooperation occurs grudgingly. When an important proposal moves to the front burner, advocates try to ram it through and opponents try to alter it in significant ways or else kill it altogether. The support or opposition of politically influential executives and/or coalitions among departments with vested interests in a particular outcome typically weigh heavily in deciding what actions the company takes. All this maneuvering takes away from efforts to execute strategy with real proficiency and frustrates company personnel who are less political and more inclined to do what is in the company's best interests.

Change-Resistant Cultures   In less-adaptive cultures where skepticism about the importance of new developments and resistance to change are the norm, managers prefer waiting until the fog of uncertainty clears before steering a new course, making fundamental adjustments to their product line, or embracing a major new technology. They believe in moving cautiously and conservatively, preferring to follow others rather than taking decisive action to be in the forefront of change. Change-resistant cultures place a premium on not making mistakes, prompting managers to lean toward safe, don't-rock-the-boat options that will have only a ripple effect on the status quo, protect or advance their own careers, and guard the interests of their immediate work groups.

Change-resistant cultures encourage a number of undesirable or unhealthy behaviors—avoiding risks, not making bold proposals to pursue emerging opportunities, a lax approach to both product innovation and continuous improvement in performing value chain activities, and following rather than leading market change. In change-resistant cultures, word quickly gets around that proposals to do things differently face an uphill battle and that people who champion them may be seen as either something of a nuisance or a troublemaker. Executives who don't value managers or employees with initiative and new ideas put a damper on product innovation, experimentation, and efforts to improve. At the same time, change-resistant companies have little appetite for being first-movers or fast-followers, believing that being in the forefront of change is too risky and that acting too quickly increases vulnerability to costly mistakes. They are more inclined to adopt a wait-and-see posture, carefully analyze several alternative responses, learn from the missteps of early movers, and then move forward cautiously and conservatively with initiatives that are deemed safe. Hostility to change is most often found in companies with multilayered management bureaucracies that have enjoyed considerable market success in years past and that are wedded to the "We have done it this way for years" syndrome.

When such companies encounter business environments with accelerating change, going slow on altering traditional ways of doing things can be become a liability rather than an asset. General Motors, IBM, Sears, and Eastman Kodak are classic examples of companies whose change-resistant bureaucracies were slow to respond to fundamental changes in their markets; clinging to the cultures and traditions that made them successful, they were reluctant to alter operating practices and modify their business approaches. As strategies of gradual change won out over bold innovation and being an early mover, all four lost market share to rivals that quickly moved to institute changes more in tune with evolving market conditions and buyer preferences. These companies are now struggling to recoup lost ground with cultures and behaviors more suited to market success—the kinds of fit that caused them to succeed in the first place.

Insular, Inwardly Focused Cultures   Sometimes a company reigns as an industry leader or enjoys great market success for so long that its personnel start to believe they have all the answers or can develop them on their own. There is a strong tendency to neglect what customers are saying and how their needs and expectations are changing. Such confidence in the correctness of how it does things and in the company's skills and capabilities breeds arrogance—company personnel discount the merits of what outsiders are doing and what can be learned by studying best-in-class performers. Benchmarking and a search for the best practices of outsiders are seen as offering little payoff. Any market share gains on the part of up-and-coming rivals are regarded as temporary setbacks, soon to be reversed by the company's own forthcoming initiatives (which, it is confidently predicted, will be an instant market hit with customers).

Insular thinking, internally driven solutions, and a must-be-invented-here mindset come to permeate the corporate culture. An inwardly focused corporate culture gives rise to managerial inbreeding and a failure to recruit people who can offer fresh thinking and outside perspectives. The big risk of insular cultural thinking is that the company can underestimate the competencies and accomplishments of rival companies and overestimate its own progress—with a resulting loss of competitive advantage over time.

Unethical and Greed-Driven Cultures   Companies that have little regard for ethical standards or that are run by executives driven by greed and ego gratification are scandals waiting to happen. Enron's collapse in 2001 was largely the product of an ethically dysfunctional corporate culture—while the culture embraced the positives of product innovation, aggressive risk taking, and a driving ambition to lead global change in the energy business, its executives exuded the negatives of arrogance, ego, greed, and an ends-justify-the-means mentality in pursuing stretched revenue and profitability targets.[9] A number of Enron's senior managers were all too willing to wink at unethical behavior, to cross over the line to unethical (and sometimes criminal) behavior themselves, and to deliberately stretch generally accepted accounting principles to make Enron's financial performance look far better than it really was. In the end, Enron came unglued because a few top executives chose unethical and illegal paths to pursue corporate revenue and profitability targets—in a company that publicly preached integrity and other notable corporate values but was lax in making sure that key executives walked the talk. Unethical cultures and executive greed have also produced scandals at WorldCom, Qwest, HealthSouth, Adelphia, Tyco, McWane, Parmalat, Rite Aid, Hollinger International, Refco, and Marsh & McLennan, with executives being indicted and/or convicted of criminal behavior. The U.S. Attorney's office elected not to prosecute the accounting firm KPMG with "systematic" criminal acts to market illegal tax shelters to wealthy clients (which KPMG tried mightily to cover up) because a criminal indictment would have resulted in the immediate collapse of KPMG and cut the number of global public accounting firms from four to just three; instead, criminal charges were filed against the company officials deemed most responsible. In 2005, U.S. prosecutors elected not to press criminal charges against Royal Dutch Petroleum (Shell Oil) for repeatedly and knowingly reporting inflated oil reserves to the U.S. Securities and Exchange Commission and not to indict Tommy Hilfiger USA for multiple tax law violations—but both companies agreed to sign nonprosecution agreements, the terms of which were not made public but which almost certainly involved fines and a long-term company commitment to cease and desist.

High-Performance Cultures

Some companies have high-performance cultures, in which the standout cultural traits are a can-do spirit, pride in doing things right, no-excuses accountability, and a pervasive results-oriented work climate in which people go the extra mile to meet or beat stretch objectives. In high-performance cultures, there is a strong sense of involvement on the part of company personnel and emphasis on individual initiative and creativity. Performance expectations are clearly delineated for the company as a whole, for each organizational unit, and for each individual. Issues and problems are promptly addressed—a strong bias exists for being proactive instead of reactive. There is a razor-sharp focus on what needs to be done. The clear and unyielding expectation is that all company personnel, from senior executives to frontline employees will display high-performance behaviors and a passion for making the company successful. There is respect for the contributions of individuals and groups.

A high-performance culture is a valuable contributor to good strategy execution and operating excellence. High performance, results-oriented cultures are permeated with a spirit of achievement and have a good track record in meeting or beating performance targets.

The challenge in creating a high-performance culture is to inspire high loyalty and dedication on the part of employees, such that they are both energized and preoccupied with putting forth their very best efforts to do things right and be unusually productive. Managers have to reinforce constructive behavior, reward top performers, and purge habits and behaviors that stand in the way of high productivity and good results. They must work at knowing the strengths and weaknesses of their subordinates, so as to better match talent with task and enable people to make meaningful contributions by doing what they do best.[10] They have to stress correcting and learning from mistakes, and they must put an unrelenting emphasis on moving forward and making good progress—in effect, there has to be a disciplined, performance-focused approach to managing the organization.

Adaptive Cultures

The hallmark of adaptive corporate cultures is willingness on the part of organizational members to accept change and take on the challenge of introducing and executing new strategies.[11] Company personnel share a feeling of confidence that the organization can deal with whatever threats and opportunities come down the pike; they are receptive to risk taking, experimentation, and innovation. In direct contrast to change-resistant cultures, adaptive cultures are very supportive of managers and employees at all ranks who propose or help initiate useful change. Internal entrepreneurship on the part of individuals and groups is encouraged and rewarded. Senior executives seek out, support, and promote individuals who exercise initiative, spot opportunities for improvement, and display the skills to implement them. Managers openly evaluate ideas and suggestions, fund initiatives to develop new or better products, and take prudent risks to pursue emerging market opportunities. As in high-performance cultures, the adaptive company exhibits a proactive approach to identifying issues, evaluating the implications and options, and quickly moving ahead with workable solutions. Strategies and traditional operating practices are modified as needed to adjust to or take advantage of changes in the business environment.

> **Core Concept**
> In adaptive cultures, there is a spirit of doing what's necessary to ensure long-term organizational success provided the new behaviors and operating practices that management is calling for are seen as legitimate and consistent with the core values and business principles underpinning the culture.

But why is change so willingly embraced in an adaptive culture? Why are organization members not fearful of how change will affect them? Why does an adaptive culture not become unglued with ongoing changes in strategy, operating practices, and behavioral norms? The answers lie in two distinctive and dominant traits of an adaptive culture: (1) Any changes in operating practices and behaviors must *not* compromise core values and long-standing business principles, and (2) the changes that are instituted must satisfy the legitimate interests of stakeholders—customers, employees, shareowners, suppliers, and the communities in which the company operates.[12] In other words, what sustains an adaptive culture is that organization members perceive the changes that management is trying to institute as legitimate and in keeping with the core values and business principles that form the heart and soul of the culture.

Thus, for an adaptive culture to remain intact over time, top management must orchestrate organizational changes in a manner that (1) demonstrates genuine care for the well-being of all key constituencies and (2) tries to satisfy all their legitimate interests simultaneously. Unless fairness to all constituencies is a decision-making principle and a commitment to doing the right thing is evident to organization members, the changes are not likely to be seen as legitimate and thus be readily accepted and implemented wholeheartedly.[13] Making changes that will please customers and that protect, if not enhance, the company's long-term well-being are generally seen as legitimate and are often seen as the best way of looking out for the interests of employees, stockholders, suppliers, and communities where the company operates. At companies with adaptive cultures, management concern for the well-being of employees is nearly always a big factor in gaining employee support for change—company personnel are usually receptive to change as long as employees understand that changes in their job assignments are part of the process of adapting to new conditions and that their employment security will not be threatened unless the company's business unexpectedly reverses direction. In cases where workforce downsizing becomes necessary, management concern for employees dictates that separation be handled humanely, making employee departure as painless as possible. Management efforts to make the process of adapting to change fair and equitable for customers, employees, stockholders, suppliers, and communities where the company operates, keeping adverse impacts to a minimum insofar as possible, breeds acceptance of and support for change among all organization stakeholders.

> Adaptive cultures are exceptionally well suited to companies with fast-changing strategies and market environments.

Technology companies, software companies, and today's dot-com companies are good illustrations of organizations with adaptive cultures. Such companies thrive on change—driving it, leading it, and capitalizing on it (but sometimes also succumbing to change when they make the wrong move or are swamped by better technologies or the superior business models of rivals). Companies like Google, Intel, Cisco Systems, eBay, Nokia, Amazon.com, and Dell cultivate the capability to act and react rapidly. They are avid practitioners of entrepreneurship and innovation, with a demonstrated willingness to take bold risks to create altogether new products, new businesses, and new industries. To create and nurture a culture that can adapt rapidly to changing to shifting business conditions, they make a point of staffing their organizations with people who are proactive, who rise to the challenge of change, and who have an aptitude for adapting.

In fast-changing business environments, a corporate culture that is receptive to altering organizational practices and behaviors is a virtual necessity. However, adaptive cultures work to the advantage of all companies, not just those in rapid-change environments. Every company operates in a market and business climate that is changing to one degree or another and that, in turn, requires internal operating responses and new behaviors on the part of organization members. *As a company's strategy evolves, an adaptive culture is a definite ally in the strategy-implementing, strategy-executing process as compared to cultures that have to be coaxed and cajoled to change.*

Culture: Ally or Obstacle to Strategy Execution?

A company's present culture and work climate may or may not be compatible with what is needed for effective implementation and execution of the chosen strategy. *When a company's present work climate promotes attitudes and behaviors that are well suited to first-rate strategy execution, its culture functions as a valuable ally in the strategy execution process.* When the culture is in conflict with some aspect of the company's direction, performance targets, or strategy, the culture becomes a stumbling block.[14]

How a Company's Culture Can Promote Better Strategy Execution   A culture grounded in strategy-supportive values, practices, and behavioral norms adds significantly to the power and effectiveness of a company's strategy execution effort.

For example, a culture where frugality and thrift are values widely shared by organizational members nurtures employee actions to identify cost-saving opportunities—the very behavior needed for successful execution of a low-cost leadership strategy. A culture built around such business principles as pleasing customers, fair treatment, operating excellence, and employee empowerment promotes employee behaviors and an esprit de corps that facilitate execution of strategies keyed to high product quality and superior customer service. A culture in which taking initiative, challenging the status quo, exhibiting creativity, embracing change, and collaborating with team members pervade the work climate promotes a company's drive to lead market change—outcomes that are conducive to successful execution of product innovation and technological leadership strategies.[15] Good alignment between ingrained cultural norms and the behaviors needed for good strategy execution makes the culture a valuable ally in the strategy-execution process. In a company where strategy and culture are misaligned, some of the very behaviors needed to execute strategy successfully run contrary to the behaviors and values imbedded in the prevailing culture. Such a clash nearly always produces a roadblock from employees whose actions and behaviors are strongly linked to the present culture. Culture-bred resistance to the actions and behaviors needed for good execution, if strong and widespread, poses a formidable hurdle that has to be cleared for strategy execution to get very far.

> **Core Concept**
> The tighter the culture–strategy fit, the more that the culture steers company personnel into displaying behaviors and adopting operating practices that promote good strategy execution.

A tight culture–strategy matchup furthers a company's strategy execution effort in three ways:[16]

1. *A culture that encourages actions, behaviors, and work practices supportive of good strategy execution not only provides company personnel with clear guidance regarding "how we do things around here" but also produces significant peer pressure from coworkers to conform to culturally acceptable norms.* The stronger the admonishments from top executives about "how we need to do things around here" and the stronger the peer pressure from coworkers, the more the culture influences people to display behaviors and observe operating practices that support good strategy execution.

2. *A deeply embedded culture tightly matched to the strategy aids the cause of competent strategy execution by steering company personnel to culturally approved behaviors and work practices and thus makes it far simpler to root out any operating practice that is a misfit.* This is why it is very much in management's best interests to build and nurture a deeply rooted culture where ingrained behaviors and operating practices marshal organizational energy behind the drive for good strategy execution.

3. *A culture imbedded with values and behaviors that facilitate strategy execution promotes strong employee identification with and commitment to the company's vision, performance targets, and strategy.* When a company's culture is grounded in many of the needed strategy-executing behaviors, employees feel genuinely better about their jobs, the company they work for, and the merits of what the company is trying to accomplish. As a consequence, greater numbers of company personnel exhibit some passion about their work and exert their best efforts to execute the strategy and achieve performance targets. All this helps move the company closer to realizing its strategic vision and, from employees' standpoint, makes the company a more engaging place to work.

These aspects of culture–strategy alignment say something important about the task of managing the strategy executing process: *Closely aligning corporate culture with the requirements for proficient strategy execution merits the full attention of senior executives.* The culture-building objective is to create a work climate and style of operating that mobilize the energy and behavior of company personnel squarely behind efforts to execute strategy competently. The more deeply that management can embed strategy-supportive ways of doing things, the more that management can rely on the culture to automatically steer company personnel toward behaviors and work practices that aid good strategy execution and away from ways of doing things that impede it.

Furthermore, culturally astute managers understand that nourishing the right cultural environment not only adds power to their push for proficient strategy execution but also promotes strong employee identification with and commitment to the company's vision, performance targets, and strategy. A culture–strategy fit prompts employees with emotional allegiance to the culture to feel genuinely better about their jobs, the company they work for, and the merits of what the company is trying to accomplish. As a consequence, their morale is higher and their productivity is higher. In addition, greater numbers of company personnel exhibit passion for their work and exert their best efforts to make the strategy succeed and achieve performance targets. All this helps move the company closer to realizing its strategic vision and, from the employees' standpoint, makes the company a more engaging place to work.

The Perils of Strategy–Culture Conflict   Conflicts between behaviors approved by the culture and behaviors needed for good strategy execution pose a real dilemma for company personnel. Should they be loyal to the culture and company traditions (to which they are likely to be emotionally attached) and thus resist or be indifferent to actions and behaviors that will promote better strategy execution—a choice that will certainly weaken the drive for good strategy execution? Or should they go along with the strategy execution effort and engage in actions and behaviors that run counter to the culture—a choice that will likely impair morale and lead to less-than-wholehearted commitment to management's strategy execution efforts? Neither choice leads to desirable outcomes, and the solution is obvious: eliminate the conflict.

When a company's culture is out of sync with the actions and behaviors needed to execute the strategy successfully, the culture has to be changed as rapidly as can be managed—this, of course, presumes that it is one or more aspects of the culture that are out of whack rather than the strategy executions approaches management wishes to institute. While correcting a strategy–culture conflict can occasionally mean revamping a company's approach to executing the strategy to produce good cultural fit, more usually it means altering aspects of the mismatched culture to ingrain new behaviors and work practices that will enable first-rate strategy execution. The more entrenched the mismatched aspects of the culture, the greater the difficulty of implementing and executing new or different strategies until better strategy–culture alignment emerges. A sizable and prolonged strategy–culture conflict weakens and may even defeat managerial efforts to make the strategy work.

Changing a Problem Culture

Changing a company culture that impedes proficient strategy execution is among the toughest management tasks because of the heavy anchor of ingrained behaviors and ways of doing things. It is natural for company personnel to cling to familiar practices and to be wary, if not hostile, to new approaches of how things are to be done. Consequently, it takes concerted management action over a period of time to root out certain unwanted behaviors and replace an out-of-sync culture with different behaviors and ways of doing things deemed more conducive to executing the strategy. *The single most visible factor that distinguishes successful culture-change efforts from failed attempts is competent leadership at the top.* Great power is needed to force major cultural change and overcome the springback resistance of entrenched cultures—and great power is possessed only by the most senior executives, especially the CEO. However, while top management must be out front leading the effort, marshaling support for a new culture and, more important, instilling new cultural behaviors are tasks for the whole management team. Middle managers and frontline supervisors play a key role in implementing the new work practices and operating approaches, helping win rank-and-file acceptance of and support for the changes, and instilling the desired behavioral norms.

As shown in Figure 13.1, the first step in fixing a problem culture is for top management to identify those facets of the present culture that are dysfunctional and pose obstacles to executing new strategic initiatives and meeting or beating company performance targets. Second, managers have to clearly define the desired new behaviors and features of the culture they want to create. Third, managers have to convince company personnel why the present culture poses problems and why and how new behaviors and operating approaches will improve company performance—the case for cultural change and the benefits of a reformed culture have to be persuasive. Finally, and most important, all the talk about remodeling the present culture has to be followed swiftly by visible, forceful actions to promote the desired new behaviors and work practices—actions that company personnel will interpret as a determined top management commitment to alter the culture and instill a different work climate and different ways of operating.

Making a Compelling Case for Culture Change   The place for management to begin a major remodeling of the corporate culture is by selling company personnel on

Figure 13.1   **Changing a Problem Culture**

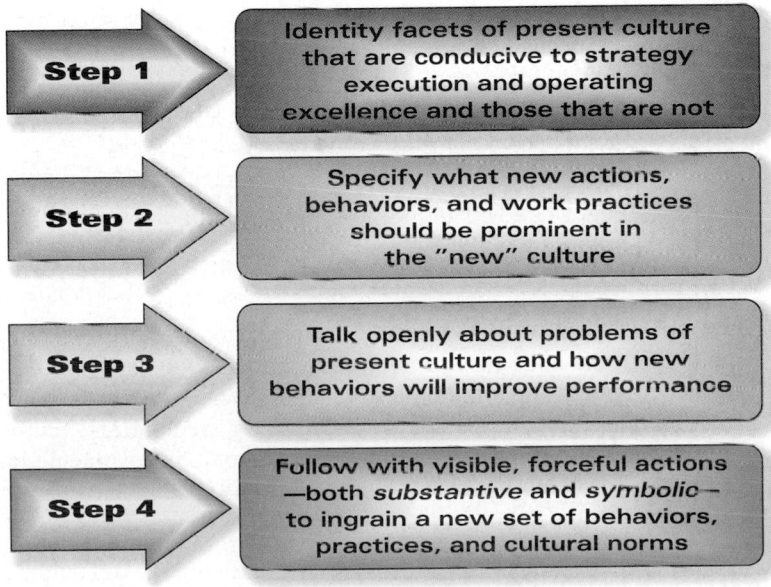

the need for new-style behaviors and work practices. This means making a compelling case for why the company's new strategic direction and culture-remodeling efforts are in the organization's best interests and why company personnel should wholeheartedly join the effort to doing things somewhat differently. Skeptics and opinion leaders have to be convinced that all is not well with the status quo. This can be done by:

- Citing reasons why the current strategy has to be modified and why new strategic initiatives that are being undertaken will bolster the company's competitiveness and performance. The case for altering the old strategy usually needs to be predicated on its shortcomings—why sales are growing slowly, why rivals are doing so much better, why too many customers are opting to go with the products of rivals, why costs are too high, why the company's price has to be lowered, and so on. There may be merit in holding events where managers and other key personnel are forced to listen to dissatisfied customers, the complaints of strategic allies, alienated employees, or disenchanted stockholders
- Citing why and how certain behavioral norms and work practices in the current culture pose obstacles to good execution of new strategic initiatives.
- Explaining how certain new behaviors and work practices that are to be introduced and have important roles in the new culture will be more advantageous and produce better results.

It is essential for the CEO and other top executives to personally talk to company personnel all across the company about the reasons for modifying work practices and culture-related behaviors. Senior officers and department heads have to play the lead role in explaining the behaviors, practices, and operating approaches that are to be introduced and why they are beneficial—and the explanations will likely have to be repeated many times. For the culture-change effort to be successful, frontline supervisors and employee opinion leaders must be won over to the cause, which means convincing them of the merits of *practicing* and *enforcing* cultural norms at the lowest levels in the organization. Until a big majority of employees accept the need for a new culture and agree that different work practices and behaviors are called for, there's more work to be done in selling company personnel on the whys and wherefores of culture change. Building widespread organizational support requires taking every opportunity to repeat the messages of why the new work practices, operating approaches, and behaviors are good for company stakeholders (particularly customers, employees, and shareholders). Effective culture-change leaders are good at telling stories to describe the new values and desired behaviors and connect them to everyday practices.

Management's efforts to make a persuasive case for changing what is deemed to be a problem culture must be *quickly followed* by forceful, high-profile actions across several fronts. The actions to implant the new culture must be both substantive and symbolic.

Substantive Culture-Changing Actions   No culture change effort can get very far with just talk about the need for different actions, behaviors, and work practices. Company executives have to give the culture-change effort some teeth by initiating *a series of actions* that company personnel will see as credible and unmistakably indicative of the seriousness of management's commitment to new strategic initiatives and the associated cultural changes. The strongest signs that management is truly committed to instilling a new culture include:

1. Replacing key executives who are strongly associated with the old culture and are stonewalling needed organizational and cultural changes.

2. Promoting individuals who are known to possess the desired cultural traits, who have stepped forward to advocate the shift to a different culture, and who can serve as role models for the desired cultural behavior.

3. Appointing outsiders with the desired cultural attributes to high-profile positions—bringing in new-breed managers to serve as role models and help drive the culture-change movement sends an unmistakable message that a new era is dawning and acts to reinforce company personnel who have already gotten on board the culture-change effort.

4. Screening all candidates for new positions carefully, hiring only those who appear to fit in with the new culture—this helps build a critical mass of people to help turn the tide in favor of the new culture.

5. Mandating that all company personnel attend culture-training programs to learn more about the new work practices and operating approaches and to better understand the cultured-related actions and behaviors that are expected.

6. Pushing hard to implement new-style work practices and operating procedures.

7. Designing compensation incentives that boost the pay of teams and individuals who display the desired cultural behaviors and hit change resisters in the pocketbook—company personnel are much more inclined to exhibit the desired kinds of actions and behaviors when it is in their financial best interest to do so.

8. Granting generous pay raises to individuals who step out front, lead the adoption of the desired work practices, display the new-style behaviors, and achieve pace-setting results.

9. Revising policies and procedures in ways that will help drive cultural change.

Executives must take care to launch enough companywide culture change actions at the outset to leave no room for doubt that management is dead serious about changing the present culture and that a cultural transformation is inevitable. To convince doubters and skeptics that they cannot just wait in hopes the culture-change initiative will soon die out, the series of actions initiated by top management must create lots of hallway talk across the whole company, get the change process off to a fast start, and be followed by unrelenting efforts to firmly establish the new work practices and style of operating as standard.

Symbolic Culture-Changing Actions Symbolic managerial actions are necessary to alter a problem culture and tighten the strategy–culture fit. The most important symbolic actions are those that top executives take to *lead by example*. For instance, if the organization's strategy involves a drive to become the industry's low-cost producer, senior managers must display frugality in their own actions and decisions: inexpensive decorations in the executive suite, conservative expense accounts and entertainment allowances, a lean staff in the corporate office, scrutiny of budget requests, few executive perks, and so on. At Wal-Mart, all the executive offices are simply decorated; executives are habitually frugal in their own actions, and they are zealous in their own efforts to control costs and promote greater efficiency. At Nucor, one of the world's low-cost producers of steel products, executives fly coach class and use taxis at airports rather than limousines. If the culture change imperative is to be more responsive to customers' needs and to pleasing customers, the CEO can instill greater customer awareness by requiring all officers and executives to spend a significant portion of each week talking with customers about their needs. Top executives must be alert to the fact that company personnel will be watching their actions and decisions to see if they are walking the talk. Hence, they need to make sure that their current decisions will be construed as consistent with new-culture values and behaviors.[17]

Another category of symbolic actions includes holding ceremonial events to single out and honor people whose actions and performance exemplify what is called for in the new culture. A point is made of holding events to celebrate each culture-change success (and any other outcome that management would like to see happen again). Executives sensitive to their role in promoting strategy–culture fits make a habit of appearing at ceremonial functions to praise individuals and groups that get with the program. They show up at employee training programs to stress strategic priorities, values, ethical principles, and cultural norms. Every group gathering is seen as an opportunity to repeat and ingrain values, praise good deeds, expound on the merits of the new culture, and cite instances of how the new work practices and operating approaches have worked to good advantage.

The use of symbols in culture building is widespread. Many universities give outstanding teacher awards each year to symbolize their commitment to good teaching and their esteem for instructors who display exceptional classroom talents. Numerous businesses have employee-of-the-month awards. The military has a long-standing custom of awarding ribbons and medals for exemplary actions. Mary Kay Cosmetics awards an array of prizes—from ribbons to pink automobiles—to its beauty consultants for reaching various sales plateaus.

How Long Does It Take to Change a Problem Culture?   Planting and growing the seeds of a new culture require a determined effort by the chief executive and other senior managers. Neither charisma nor personal magnetism is essential. But a sustained and persistent effort to reinforce the culture at every opportunity through both word and deed is very definitely required. Changing a problem culture is never a short-term exercise. It takes time for a new culture to emerge and prevail. Overnight transformations simply don't occur. And it takes even longer for a new culture to become deeply embedded The bigger the organization and the greater the cultural shift needed to produce a strategy–culture fit, the longer it takes. In large companies, fixing a problem culture and instilling a new set of attitudes and behaviors can take two to five years. In fact, it is usually tougher to reform an entrenched problematic culture than it is to instill a strategy-supportive culture from scratch in a brand-new organization. Sometimes executives succeed in changing the values and behaviors of small groups of managers and even whole departments or divisions, only to find the changes eroded over time by the actions of the rest of the organization—what is communicated, praised, supported, and penalized by an entrenched majority undermines the new emergent culture and halts its progress. Executives, despite a series of well-intended actions to reform a problem culture, are likely to fail at weeding out embedded cultural traits when widespread employee skepticism about the company's new directions and culture-change effort spawns covert resistance to the cultural behaviors and operating practices advocated by top management. This is why management must take every opportunity to convince employees of the need for culture change and communicate to them how new attitudes, behaviors, and operating practices will benefit the interests of organizational stakeholders.

A company that succeeded in fixing a problem culture is Alberto-Culver—see Illustration Capsule 13.2.

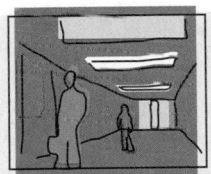

Illustration Capsule 13.2
Changing the Culture in Alberto-Culver's North American Division

In 1993, Carol Bernick—vice chairperson of Alberto-Culver, president of its North American division, and daughter of the company's founders— concluded that her division's existing culture had four problems: Employees dutifully waited for marching orders from their bosses, workers put pleasing their bosses ahead of pleasing customers, some company policies were not family-friendly, and there was too much bureaucracy and paperwork. What was needed, in Bernick's opinion, was a culture in which company employees had a sense of ownership and an urgency to get things done, welcomed innovation, and were willing to taking risks.

Alberto-Culver's management undertook a series of actions to introduce and ingrain the desired cultural attributes:

- In 1993, a new position, called growth development leader (GDL), was created to help orchestrate the task of fixing the culture deep in the ranks (there were 70 GDLs in Alberto-Culver's North American division). GDLs came from all ranks of the company's managerial ladder and were handpicked for such qualities as empathy, communication skills, positive attitude, and ability to let their hair down and have fun. GDLs performed their regular jobs in addition to taking on the GDL roles; it was considered an honor to be chosen. Each GDL mentored about 12 people from both a career and a family standpoint. GDLs met with senior executives weekly, bringing forward people's questions and issues and then, afterward, sharing with their groups the topics and solutions that were discussed. GDLs brought a group member as a guest to each meeting. One meeting each year is devoted to identifying "macros and irritations"— attendees are divided into four subgroups and given 15 minutes to identify the company's four biggest challenges (the macros) and the four most annoying aspects of life at the company (the irritations); the whole group votes on which four deserve the company's attention. Those selected are then addressed, and assignments made for follow-up and results.

- Changing the culture was made an issue across the company, starting in 1995 with a two-hour State of the Company presentation to employees covering where the company was and where it wanted to be. The State of the Company address then became an annual event.

- Management created ways to measure the gains in changing the culture. One involved an annual all-employee survey to assess progress against cultural goals and to get 360-degree feedback—the 2000 survey had 180 questions, including 33 relating to the performance of each respondent's GDL. A bonfire celebration was held in the company parking lot to announce that paperwork would be cut by 30 percent.

- A list of 10 cultural imperatives was formalized in 1998—honesty, ownership, trust, customer orientation, commitment, fun, innovation, risk taking, speed and urgency, and teamwork. These imperatives came to be known internally as HOT CC FIRST.

- Numerous celebrations and awards programs were instituted. Most celebrations are scheduled, but some are spontaneous (an impromptu thank-you party for a good fiscal year). Business Builder Awards (initiated in 1997) are given to individuals and teams that make a significant impact on the company's growth and profitability. The best-scoring GDLs on the annual employee surveys are awarded shares of company stock. The company notes all work anniversaries and personal milestones with "Alberto-appropriate" gifts; appreciative company employees sometimes give thank-you gifts to their GDLs. According to Carol Bernick, "If you want something to grow, pour champagne on it. We've made a huge effort—maybe even an over-the-top effort—to celebrate our successes and, indeed, just about everything we'd like to see happen again."

The culture change effort at Alberto-Culver North America was viewed as a major contributor to improved performance. From 1993 (when the effort first began) to 2001, the division's sales increased from just under $350 million to over $600 million and pretax profits rose from $20 million to almost $50 million. Carol Bernick was elevated to chairman of Alberto-Culver's board of directors in 2004.

Source: Based on information in Carol Lavin Bernick, "When Your Culture Needs a Makeover," Harvard Business Review 79, no. 6 (June 2001), p. 61 and information posted at the company's Web site, www.alberto.com (accessed November 10, 2005).

Grounding the Culture in Core Values and Ethics

The foundation of a company's corporate culture nearly always resides in its dedication to certain core values and the bar it sets for ethical behavior. The culture-shaping significance of core values and ethical behaviors accounts for why so many companies have developed a formal values statement and a code of ethics—see Table 13.1 for representative core values and the ground usually covered in codes of ethics. Many companies today convey their values and codes of ethics to stakeholders and interested parties in their annual reports and on their Web sites. The trend of making stakeholders aware of a company's commitment to core values and ethical business conduct is attributable to three factors: (1) greater management understanding of the role these statements play in culture building, (2) a renewed focus on ethical standards stemming from the numerous corporate scandals that hit the headlines during 2001–2005, and (3) the sizable fraction of consumers and suppliers who prefer doing business with ethical companies.

> **Core Concept**
> A company's culture is grounded in and shaped by its core values and the bar it sets for ethical behavior.

At Darden Restaurants—the world's largest casual dining company, which employs more than 150,000 people and serves 300 million meals annually at 1,400 Red Lobster, Olive Garden, Bahama Breeze, Smokey Bones Barbeque & Grill, and Seasons 52 restaurants in North America—the core values are operating with integrity and fairness, caring and respect, being of service, teamwork, excellence, always learning and teaching, and welcoming and celebrating workforce diversity. Top executives at

Table 13.1   **Representative Content of Company Values Statements and Codes of Ethics**

Typical Core Values	Areas Covered by Codes of Ethics
• Satisfying and delighting customers	• Expecting all company personnel to display honesty and integrity in their actions and avoid conflicts of interest
• Dedication to superior customer service, top-notch quality, product innovation, and/or technological leadership	• Mandating full compliance with all laws and regulations, specifically:
• A commitment to excellence and results	—Antitrust laws prohibiting anticompetitive practices, conspiracies to fix prices, or attempts to monopolize
• Exhibiting such qualities as integrity, fairness, trustworthiness, pride of workmanship, Golden Rule behavior, respect for coworkers, and ethical behavior	—Foreign Corrupt Practices Act
• Creativity, exercising initiative, and accepting responsibility	—Securities laws and prohibitions against insider trading
• Teamwork and cooperative attitudes	—Environmental and workplace safety regulations
• Fair treatment of suppliers	—Discrimination and sexual harassment regulations
• Making the company a great place to work	—Political contributions and lobbying activities
• A commitment to having fun and creating a fun work environment	• Prohibiting giving or accepting bribes, kickbacks, or gifts
• Being stewards of shareholders' investments and remaining committed to profits and growth	• Engaging in fair selling and marketing practices
• Exercising social responsibility and being a good community citizen	• Not dealing with suppliers that employ child labor or engage in other unsavory practices
• Caring about protecting the environment	• Being above-board in acquiring and using competitively sensitive information about rivals and others
• Having a diverse workforce	• Avoiding use of company assets, resources, and property for personal or other inappropriate purposes
	• Responsibility to protect proprietary information and not divulge trade secrets

Darden believe the company's practice of these values has been instrumental in creating a culture characterized by trust, exciting jobs and career opportunities for employees, and a passion to provide "a terrific dining experience to every guest, every time, in every one of our restaurants."[18]

Of course, sometimes a company's stated core values and codes of ethics are cosmetic, existing mainly to impress outsiders and help create a positive company image. But more usually they have been developed to shape the culture. Many executives want the work climate at their companies to mirror certain values and ethical standards, partly because they are personally committed to these values and ethical standards but mainly because they are convinced that adherence to such values and ethical principles will make the company a much better performer *and* improve its image. As discussed earlier, values-related cultural norms promote better strategy execution and mobilize company personnel behind the drive to achieve stretch objectives and the company's strategic vision. Hence, a corporate culture grounded in well-chosen core values and high ethical standards contributes mightily to a company's long-term strategic success.[19] And, not incidentally, strongly ingrained values and ethical standards reduce the likelihood of lapses in ethical and socially-approved behavior that mar a company's reputation and put its financial performance and market standing at risk.

> A company's values statement and code of ethics communicate expectations of how employees should conduct themselves in the workplace.

The Culture-Building Role of Values and Codes of Ethics   At companies where executives believe in the merits of practicing the values and ethical standards that have been espoused, *the stated core values and ethical principles are the cornerstones of the corporate culture.* As depicted in Figure 13.2, a company's stated core values and ethical principles have two roles in the culture-building process. One, a company that works hard at putting its stated core values and ethical principles into practice fosters a work climate where company personnel share common and strongly held convictions about how the company's business is to be conducted. Second, the stated values and ethical principles provide company personnel with guidance about the manner in which

Figure 13.2   **The Two Culture-Building Roles of a Company's Core Values and Ethical Standards**

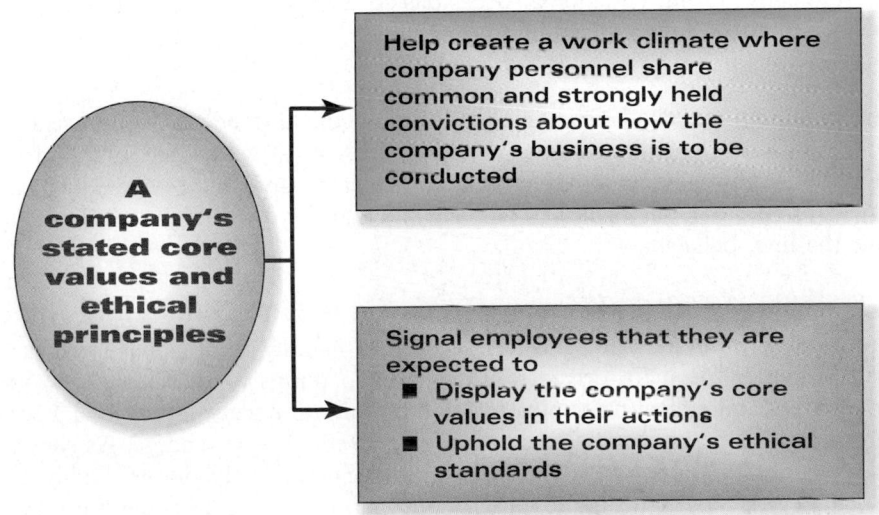

they are to do their jobs—which behaviors and ways of doing things are approved (and expected) and which are out-of-bounds.

Transforming Core Values and Ethical Standards into Cultural Norms

Once values and ethical standards have been formally adopted, they must be institutionalized in the company's policies and practices and embedded in the conduct of company personnel. This can be done in a number of different ways.[20] Tradition-steeped companies with a rich folklore rely heavily on word-of-mouth indoctrination and the power of tradition to instill values and enforce ethical conduct. But most companies employ a variety of techniques to hammer in core values and ethical standards, using some or all of the following:

1. Giving explicit attention to values and ethics in recruiting and hiring to screen out applicants who do not exhibit compatible character traits.

2. Incorporating the statement of values and the code of ethics into orientation programs for new employees and training courses for managers and employees.

3. Having senior executives frequently reiterate the importance and role of company values and ethical principles at company events and internal communications to employees.

4. Using values statements and codes of ethical conduct as benchmarks for judging the appropriateness of company policies and operating practices.

5. Making the display of core values and ethical principles a big factor in evaluating each person's job performance—there's no better way to win the attention and commitment of company personnel than by using the degree to which individuals observe core values and ethical standards as a basis for compensation increases and promotion.

6. Making sure that managers, from the CEO down to frontline supervisors, are diligent in stressing the importance of ethical conduct and observance of core values. Line managers at all levels must give serious and continuous attention to the task of explaining how the values and ethical code apply in their areas.

7. Encouraging everyone to use their influence in helping enforce observance of core values and ethical standards—strong peer pressures to exhibit core values and ethical standards are a deterrent to outside-the-lines behavior.

8. Periodically having ceremonial occasions to recognize individuals and groups who display the values and ethical principles.

9. Instituting ethics enforcement procedures.

To deeply ingrain the stated core values and to high ethical standards, companies must turn them into *strictly enforced cultural norms*. They must put a stake in the ground, making it unequivocally clear that living up to the company's values and ethical standards has to be a way of life at the company and that there will be little toleration of outside-the-lines behavior.

The Benefits of Cultural Norms Grounded in Core Values and Ethical Principles

The more that managers succeed in making the espoused values and ethical principles the main drivers of "how we do things around here," the more that the values and ethical principles function as cultural norms. Over time, a strong culture grounded in the display of core values and ethics may emerge. As shown in Figure 13.3, *cultural norms* rooted in core values and ethical behavior are highly beneficial in three respects.[21] One, the advocated core values and ethical standards accurately

Figure 13.3   **The Benefits of Cultural Norms Strongly Grounded in Core Values and Ethical Principles**

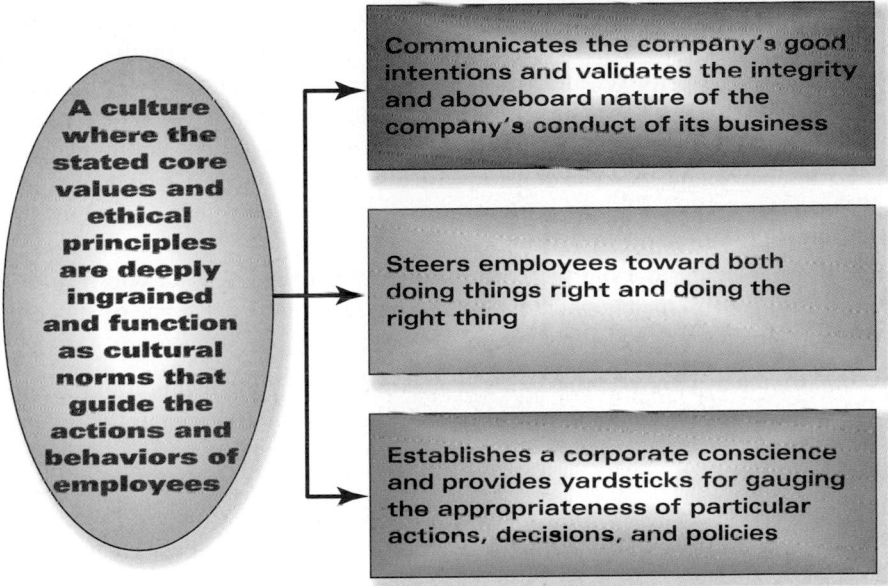

communicate the company's good intentions and validate the integrity and above-board character of its business principles and operating methods. There's nothing cosmetic or fake about the company's values statement and code of ethics— company personnel actually strive to practice what is being preached. Second, the values-based and ethics-based cultural norms steer company personnel toward both doing things right and doing the right thing. Third, they establish a "corporate conscience" and provide yardsticks for gauging the appropriateness of particular actions, decisions, and policies.

Establishing a Strategy–Culture Fit in Multinational and Global Companies

In multinational and global companies, establishing a tight strategy–culture fit is complicated by the diverse societal circumstances surrounding the company's operations in different countries. The nature of the local economies, living conditions, per capita incomes, and lifestyles can give rise to considerable cross-border diversity in a company's workforce and to subcultures within the corporate culture. Leading cross-border culture-change initiatives requires sensitivity to prevailing differences in local circumstances; company managers must discern when local subcultures have to be accommodated and when cross-border differences in the company's corporate culture can be and should be narrowed.[22] Cross-border diversity in a multinational enterprise's corporate culture is more tolerable if the company is pursuing a multicountry strategy and if the company's culture in each country is well aligned with its strategy in that country. But significant cross-country differences in a company's culture are likely to impede execution of a global strategy and have to be addressed.

As discussed earlier in this chapter, *the trick to establishing a workable strategy– culture fit in multinational companies is to ground the culture in strategy-supportive values and operating practices that travel well across country borders* and strike a

Core Concept
A multinational company needs to build its corporate culture around values and operating practices that travel well across borders.

chord with managers and workers in many different areas of the world, despite varying local customs and traditions. A multinational enterprise with a misfit between its strategy and culture in certain countries where it operates can attack the problem by rewording its values statement so as to express core values in ways that have universal appeal. The alternative is to allow *some leeway* for certain core values to be reinterpreted or de-emphasized or applied somewhat differently from country to country whenever local customs and traditions in a few countries really need to be accommodated. But such accommodation needs to be done in ways that do not impede good strategy execution. Sometimes certain offending operating styles can be modified to good advantage in all locations where the company operates.

Aside from trying to build the corporate culture around a set of core values that have universal appeal, management can seek to minimize the existence of subcultures and promote greater cross-country cultural uniformity by:

- *Instituting culture training in each country.* The goals of this training should be to (1) communicate the meaning of core values in language that resonates with company personnel in that country and (2) explain the case for common operating approaches and work practices. The use of uniform work practices becomes particularly important when the company's work practices are efficient and aid good strategy execution—in such instances, local managers have to find ways to skirt local preferences and win support for "how we do things around here."

- *Creating a cultural climate where the norm is to adopt best practices, use common work procedures, and pursue operating excellence.* Companies may find that a values-based corporate culture is less crucial to good strategy execution that an operations-based, results-oriented culture in which the dominant cultural norm is an all-out effort to do things in the best possible manner, achieve continuous improvement, and meet or beat performance targets. A results-oriented culture keyed to operating excellence and meeting stretch objectives sidesteps many of the problems with trying to get people from different societies and traditions to embrace common values.

- *Giving local managers the flexibility to modify people management approaches or operating styles.* In some situations, adherence to companywide cultural traditions simply doesn't work well. However, local modifications have to be infrequent and done in a manner that doesn't undermine the establishment of a mostly uniform corporate culture.

- *Giving local managers discretionary authority to use somewhat different motivational and compensation incentives to induce local personnel to adopt and practice the desired cultural behaviors.* Personnel in different countries may respond better to some compensation structures and reward systems than to others.

Generally, a high degree of cross-country homogeneity in a multinational company's corporate culture is desirable and has to be pursued, particularly when it comes to ingraining universal core values and companywide enforcement of such ethical standards as the payment of bribes and kickbacks, the use of underage labor, and environmental stewardship. Having too much variation in the culture from country to country not only makes it difficult to use the culture in helping drive the strategy execution process but also works against the establishment of a one-company mind-set and a consistent corporate identity.

LEADING THE STRATEGY EXECUTION PROCESS

The litany of managing the strategy process is simple enough: Craft a sound strategic plan, implement it, execute it to the fullest, adjust it as needed, and win! But the leadership challenges are significant and diverse. Exerting take-charge leadership, being a "spark plug," ramrodding things through, and achieving results thrusts a manager into a variety of leadership roles in managing the strategy execution process: resource acquirer and allocator, capabilities builder, motivator, policymaker, policy enforcer, head cheerleader, crisis solver, decision maker, and taskmaster, to mention a few. There are times when leading the strategy execution process entails being hard-nosed and authoritarian, times when it is best to be a perceptive listener and a compromising decision maker, times when matters are best delegated to people closest to the scene of the action, and times when mentoring or coaching is appropriate. Many occasions call for the manager in charge to assume a highly visible role and put in long hours guiding the process, while others entail only a brief ceremonial performance with the details delegated to subordinates.

For the most part, leading the strategy execution process is a top-down responsibility driven by mandates to get things on the right track and show good results. It must start with a perceptive diagnosis of the requirements for good strategy execution, given the company's circumstances. Then comes diagnosis of the organization's capabilities and preparedness to execute the necessary strategic initiatives and decisions as to which of several ways to proceed to get things done and achieve the targeted results.[23] In general, leading the drive for good strategy execution and operating excellence calls for five actions on the part of the manager-in-charge:

1. Staying on top of what is happening, closely monitoring progress, ferreting out issues, and learning what obstacles lie in the path of good execution.
2. Putting constructive pressure on the organization to achieve good results and operating excellence.
3. Leading the development of stronger core competencies and competitive capabilities.
4. Displaying ethical integrity and leading social responsibility initiatives.
5. Pushing corrective actions to improve strategy execution and achieve the targeted results.

Staying on Top of How Well Things Are Going

To stay on top of how well the strategy execution process is going, a manager needs to develop a broad network of contacts and sources of information, both formal and informal. The regular channels include talking with key subordinates, attending meetings and quizzing the presenters, reading reviews of the latest operating results, talking to customers, watching the competitive reactions of rival firms, exchanging e-mail and holding telephone conversations with people in outlying locations, making on-site visits, and listening to rank-and-file employees. However, some information is more trustworthy than the rest, and the views and perspectives offered by different people can vary widely. Presentations and briefings by subordinates may be colored by wishful thinking or shoddy analysis rather than representing the unvarnished truth. Bad news is sometimes filtered, minimized, or distorted by people pursuing their own agendas, and in some cases not reported at all as subordinates delay conveying failures and problems in hopes that they can turn things around in time. Hence, managers have to decide which information is trustworthy and get an accurate feel for the existing situation. They have to confirm whether things on track, identify problems, learn what obstacles lie in the path of good strategy execution, ruthlessly assess whether the organization has the talent and attitude needed to drive the required changes, and develop a basis for determining what, if anything, they can personally do to move the process along.[24]

One of the best ways for executives to stay on top of the strategy execution process is by making regular visits to the field and talking with many different people at many different levels—a technique often labeled **managing by walking around (MBWA).** Wal-Mart executives have had a long-standing practice of spending two to three days every week visiting Wal-Mart's stores and talking with store managers and employees. Sam Walton, Wal-Mart's founder, insisted, "The key is to get out into the store and listen to what the associates have to say." Jack Welch, the highly effective CEO of General Electric (GE) from 1980 to 2001, not only spent several days each month personally visiting GE operations and talking with major customers but also arranged his schedule so that he could spend time exchanging information and ideas with GE managers from all over the world who were attending classes at the company's leadership development center near GE's headquarters.

> **Core Concept**
> *Management by walking around (MBWA)* is one of the techniques that effective leaders use to stay informed about how well the strategy execution process is progressing.

Often, customers and suppliers can provide valuable perspectives on how well a company's strategy execution process is going. Joe Tucci, chief operating officer at data-storage leader EMC, when confronted with an unexpected dropoff in EMC's sales in 2001 and not sure whether the downturn represented a temporary slump or a structural market change went straight to the source for hard information: the chief executive officers and chief financial officers to whom chief information officers at customer companies reported and to the consultants who advised them. The information he got was eye-opening—fundamental market shifts were occurring, and the rules of market engagement now called for major strategy changes at EMC followed by quick implementation.

To keep their fingers on the company's pulse, managers at some companies host weekly get-togethers (often on Friday afternoons) to create a regular opportunity for tidbits of information to flow freely between down-the-line employees and executives. Many manufacturing executives make a point of strolling the factory floor to talk with workers and meeting regularly with union officials. Some managers operate out of open cubicles in big spaces so that they can interact easily and frequently with coworkers. Jeff Bezos, Amazon.com's CEO, is noted for his practice of MBWA, firing off a battery of questions when he tours facilities and insisting that Amazon managers spend time in the trenches with their people to avoid abstract thinking and getting disconnected from the reality of what's happening.[25]

Most managers practice MBWA, attaching great importance to spending time with people at various company facilities and gathering information and opinions firsthand from diverse sources about how well various aspects of the strategy execution process are going. They believe facilities visits and face-to-face contacts give them a good feel for what progress is being made, what problems are being encountered, and whether additional resources or different approaches may be needed. Just as important, MBWA provides opportunities to talk informally to many different people at different organizational levels, give encouragement, lift spirits, shift attention from the old to the new priorities, and create some excitement—all of which generate positive energy and help mobilize organizational efforts behind strategy execution.

Putting Constructive Pressure on the Organization to Achieve Good Results and Operating Excellence

Managers have to be out front in mobilizing organizational energy behind the drive for good strategy execution and operating excellence. Part of the leadership requirement here entails nurturing a results-oriented work climate, where performance standards are high and a spirit of achievement is pervasive. The intended outcome is an organization with a good track record in meeting or beating stretch performance targets. A high-performance culture in which there is constructive pressure to achieve good results is a valuable contributor to good strategy execution and operating excellence. If management wants to drive the strategy execution effort by instilling a results-oriented work climate, then senior executives have to take the lead in promoting certain enabling cultural drivers: a strong sense of involvement on the part of company personnel, emphasis on individual initiative and creativity, respect for the contribution of individuals and groups, and pride in doing things right.

Organizational leaders who succeed in creating a results-oriented work climate typically are intensely people-oriented, and they are skilled users of people-management practices that win the emotional commitment of company personnel and inspire them to do their best.[26] They understand that treating employees well generally leads to increased teamwork, higher morale, greater loyalty, and increased employee commitment to making a contribution. All of these foster an esprit de corps that energizes organizational members to contribute to the drive for operating excellence and proficient strategy execution.

Successfully leading the effort to instill a spirit of high achievement into the culture generally entails such leadership actions and managerial practices as:

- *Treating employees with dignity and respect.* This often includes a strong company commitment to training each employee thoroughly, providing attractive career opportunities, emphasizing promotion from within, and providing a high degree of job security. Some companies symbolize the value of individual employees and the importance of their contributions by referring to them as cast members (Disney), crew members (McDonald's), coworkers (Kinko's and CDW Computer Centers), job owners (Granite Construction), partners (Starbucks), or associates (Wal-Mart, Lenscrafters, W. L. Gore, Edward Jones, Publix Supermarkets, and Marriott International). At a number of companies, managers at every level are held responsible for developing the people who report to them.

- *Making champions out of the people who turn in winning performances.* This must be done in ways that promote teamwork and cross-unit collaboration as opposed to spurring an unhealthy footrace among employees to best one another. Would-be champions who advocate radical or different ideas must not be looked on as disruptive or troublesome. The best champions and change agents are persistent, competitive, tenacious, committed, and fanatic about seeing their idea through to success. It is particularly important that people who champion an unsuccessful idea not be punished or sidelined but rather encouraged to try again—encouraging lots of "tries" is important since many ideas won't pan out.

- *Encouraging employees to use initiative and creativity in performing their work.* Operating excellence requires that everybody be expected to contribute ideas, exercise initiative, and pursue continuous improvement. The leadership trick is to keep a sense of urgency alive in the business so that people see change and innovation as necessities. Moreover, people with maverick ideas or out-of-the-ordinary proposals have to be tolerated and given room to operate; anything less tends to squelch creativity and initiative.

- *Setting stretch objectives.* Managers must clearly communicate an expectation that company personnel are to give their best in achieving performance targets.

- *Using the tools of benchmarking, best practices, business process reengineering, TQM, and Six Sigma quality to focus attention on operating excellence.* These are proven approaches to getting better operating results and facilitating better strategy execution.

- *Using the full range of motivational techniques and compensation incentives to inspire company personnel, nurture a results-oriented work climate, and enforce high-performance standards.* Managers cannot mandate innovative improvements by simply exhorting people to "be creative," nor can they make continuous progress toward operating excellence with directives to "try harder." Rather, they have to foster a culture where innovative ideas and experimentation with new ways of doing things can blossom and thrive. Individuals and groups need to be strongly encouraged to brainstorm, let their imaginations fly in all directions, and come up with proposals for improving how things are done. This means giving company personnel enough autonomy to stand out, excel, and contribute. And it means that the rewards for successful champions of new ideas and operating improvements should be large and visible.

- *Celebrating individual, group, and company successes.* Top management should miss no opportunity to express respect for individual employees and their appreciation of extraordinary individual and group effort.[27] Companies like Mary Kay Cosmetics, Tupperware, and McDonald's actively seek out reasons and opportunities to give pins, buttons, badges, and medals for good showings by average performers—the idea being to express appreciation and give a motivational boost to people who stand out in doing ordinary jobs. General Electric and 3M Corporation make a point of ceremoniously honoring individuals who believe so strongly in their ideas that they take it on themselves to hurdle the bureaucracy, maneuver their projects through the system, and turn them into improved services, new products, or even new businesses.

While leadership efforts to instill a results-oriented, high performance culture usually accentuate the positive, there are negative reinforcers too. Managers whose units consistently perform poorly have to be replaced. Low-performing workers and people who reject the results-oriented cultural emphasis have to be weeded out or at least moved to out-of-the-way positions. Average performers have to be candidly counseled that they have limited career potential unless they show more progress in the form of additional effort, better skills, and improved ability to deliver good results.

Leading the Development of Better Competencies and Capabilities

A third avenue to better strategy execution and operating excellence is proactively strengthening core competencies and competitive capabilities to better perform value chain activities and pave the way for better bottom-line results. This often requires top management intervention for two reasons. One, senior managers are more likely to recognize and appreciate the strategy-executing significance of stronger capabilities; this is especially true in multinational companies where it is top executives are in the best position to spot opportunities to leverage existing competencies and competitive capabilities across geographical borders. Two, senior managers usually have to *lead* the strengthening effort because core competencies and competitive capabilities typically reside in the combined efforts of different work groups, departments, and strategic allies and only senior managers have the organizational clout to enforce the necessary networking and collaboration.

Aside from leading efforts to strengthen *existing* competencies and capabilities, effective strategy leaders try to anticipate changes in customer-market requirements and proactively build *new* competencies and capabilities that offer a competitive edge over rivals. Again, senior managers are in the best position to see the need and potential of new capabilities and then to play a lead role in the capability-building, resource-enhancing process. Proactively building new competencies and capabilities ahead of rivals to gain a competitive edge is strategic leadership of the best kind, but strengthening the company's resource base in reaction to newly developed capabilities of pioneering rivals occurs more frequently.

Displaying Ethical Integrity and Leading Social Responsibility Initiatives

For an organization to avoid the pitfalls of scandal and disgrace and consistently display the intent to conduct its business in a principled manner, the CEO and those around the CEO must be openly and unswervingly committed to ethical conduct and socially redeeming business principles and core values. Leading the effort to operate the company's business in an ethically principled fashion has three pieces. First and foremost, the CEO and other senior executives must set an excellent example in their own ethical behavior, demonstrating character and personal integrity in their actions and decisions. The behavior of senior executives sends a clear message to company personnel regarding what the "real" standards of personal conduct are. Moreover, the company's strategy and operating decisions have to be seen as ethical—actions always speak far louder than the words in a company's code of ethics. Second, top management must declare unequivocal support of the company's ethical code and take an uncompromising stand on expecting all company personnel to conduct themselves in an ethical fashion at all times. This means iterating and reiterating to employees that it is their duty to observe the company's ethical codes. Third, top management must be prepared to act as the final arbiter on hard calls; this means removing people from key positions or terminating them when they are guilty of a violation. It also means reprimanding those who have been lax in monitoring and enforcing ethical compliance. Failure to act swiftly and decisively in punishing ethical misconduct is interpreted as a lack of real commitment.

Establishing an Effective Ethics Compliance and Enforcement Process

If a company's executives truly aspire for company personnel to behave ethically, they must personally see to it that strong and effective procedures for enforcing ethical standards and handling potential violations are put in place. Even in an ethically strong company, there can be bad apples—and some of the bad apples may be executives. So it is rarely enough to rely on either the exhortations of senior executives or an ethically principled culture to produce ethics compliance.

Executive action to institute formal ethics compliance and enforcement mechanisms can entail forming an ethics committee to give guidance on ethics matters, appointing an ethics officers to head the compliance effort, establishing an ethics hotline or Web site that employees can use to either anonymously report a possible violation or get confidential advice on a troubling ethics-related situation, and having an annual ethics audit to measure the extent of ethical behavior and identify problem areas. If senior executives are really serious about enforcing ethical behavior, they probably need to do five things:[28]

1. Have mandatory ethics training programs for employees. Company personnel have to be educated about what is ethical and what is not and given guidance about the gray areas. Special training programs probably are needed for personnel in such ethically vulnerable areas as procurement, sales, and lobbying. Company personnel assigned to subsidiaries in foreign countries can find themselves trapped in ethical dilemmas if bribery and corruption of public officials are common practices or if suppliers or customers are accustomed to kickbacks of one kind or another.

2. Openly encourage company personnel to report possible infractions via anonymous calls to a hotline or e-mails sent to a designated address. Ideally, the company's culture will be sufficiently ethically principled that most company personnel will feel it is their obligation and duty to report possible ethical violations (not so much to get someone in trouble but to prevent further damage and help the company avoid the dire consequences of a debilitating scandal. Furthermore, everyone must be encouraged to raise issues about ethically gray areas and to get confidential advice from the company's ethics specialists.

3. Conduct an annual audit of each manager's efforts to uphold ethical standards and require formal reports on the actions taken by managers to remedy deficient conduct.

4. Require all employees to sign a statement annually certifying that they have complied with the company's code of ethics.

5. Make sure that ethical violations carry appropriate punishment, including dismissal if the violation is sufficiently egregious.

While these actions may seem extreme, they leave little room to doubt the seriousness of executive commitment to ethics compliance. Openly encouraging people to report possible ethical violations heightens awareness of operating within ethical bounds. And while violators have to be disciplined, *the main purpose of the various means of enforcement is to encourage compliance rather than administer punishment.* Most company personnel will think twice about knowingly engaging in unethical conduct when their actions could be reported by watchful coworkers. The same is true when they know their actions will be audited and/or when they have to sign statements certifying compliance with the company's code of ethics.

Top executives in multinational companies face big challenges in enforcing strict ethical standards companywide because what is considered ethical often varies substantially or subtly from country to country. There are shades and variations in what societies generally agree to be right and wrong based on the prevailing circumstances, local customs, and predominant religious convictions. And certainly there are cross-country variations in the *degree* to which certain behaviors are considered unethical.[29] Thus, transnational companies have to make a fundamental decision regarding whether to try to enforce common ethical standards across their operations in all countries or whether to allow some rules to be bent in some cases.

Leading Social Responsibility Initiatives   The exercise of social responsibility, just as with observance of ethical principles, requires top executive leadership. *What separates companies that make a sincere effort to carry their weight in being good corporate citizens from companies that are content to do only what is legally required of them are company leaders who believe strongly that just making a profit is not good enough. Such leaders are committed to a higher standard of performance that includes social and environmental metrics as well as financial and strategic metrics.* Thus, it is up to the CEO and other senior executives to insist that the company go past the rhetoric and cosmetics of corporate citizenship and implement social responsibility initiatives.

> CEOs who are committed to a core value of corporate social responsibility move beyond the rhetorical flourishes and enlist the full support of company personnel behind the execution of social responsibility initiatives.

Among the leadership responsibilities of the CEO and other senior managers, therefore, are to *step out front,* to wave the flag of socially responsible behavior for all to see, to marshal the support of company personnel, and to make social responsibility initiatives an everyday part of how the company conducts its business affairs. Top executives have to use social and environmental metrics in evaluating performance and, ideally, the company's board of directors will elect to tie the company's social and environmental performance to executive compensation—a surefire way to make sure that social responsibility efforts are more than window dressing. To help ensure that it has commitment from senior managers, Verizon Communications ties 10 percent of the annual bonus of the company's top 2,500 managers directly to the achievement of social responsibility targets. One survey found over 60 percent of senior managers believed that a portion of executive compensation should be linked to a company's performance on social and environmental measures. The strength of the commitment from the top—typically a company's CEO and board of directors—ultimately determines whether a company will implement and execute a full-fledged strategy of social responsibility that embraces some customized combination of actions to protect the environment (beyond what is required by law), actively participate in community affairs, be a generous supporter of charitable causes and projects that benefit society, and have a positive impact on workforce diversity and the overall well-being of employees. One of the most reliable signs that company executives are leading an authentic effort to carry out fruitful social responsibility initiatives is whether the company issues an annual report on its social responsibility efforts that cites quantitative and qualitative evidence of the company accomplishments.

Leading the Process of Making Corrective Adjustments

The leadership challenge of making corrective adjustments is twofold: deciding when adjustments are needed and deciding what adjustments to make. Both decisions are a normal and necessary part of managing the strategy execution process, since no scheme for implementing and executing strategy can foresee all the events and problems that will arise. There comes a time at every company when managers have to fine-tune or overhaul the approaches to strategy execution and push for better results. Clearly, when a company's strategy execution effort is not delivering good results and making measurable progress toward operating excellence, it is the leader's responsibility to step forward and push corrective actions.

The *process* of making corrective adjustments varies according to the situation. In a crisis, it is typical for leaders to have key subordinates gather information, identify and evaluate options (crunching whatever numbers may be appropriate), and perhaps prepare a preliminary set of recommended actions for consideration. The organizational leader then usually meets with key subordinates and personally presides over extended discussions of the proposed responses, trying to build a quick consensus among members of the executive inner circle. If no consensus emerges and action is required immediately, the burden falls on the manager in charge to choose the response and urge its support.

When the situation allows managers to proceed more deliberately in deciding when to make changes and what changes to make, most managers seem to prefer a process of incrementally solidifying commitment to a particular course of action.[30] The process that managers go through in deciding on corrective adjustments is essentially the same for both proactive and reactive changes: They sense needs, gather information, broaden and deepen their understanding of the situation, develop options and explore their pros and cons, put forth action proposals, generate partial (comfort-level) solutions, strive for a consensus, and finally formally adopt an agreed-on course of action.[31] Deciding what corrective changes to initiate can take a few hours, a few days, a few weeks, or even a few months if the situation is particularly complicated.

Success in initiating corrective actions usually hinges on thorough analysis of the situation, the exercise of good business judgment in deciding what actions to take, and good implementation of the corrective actions that are initiated. Successful managers are skilled in getting an organization back on track rather quickly; they (and their staffs) are good at discerning what actions to take and in ramrodding them through to a successful conclusion. Managers that struggle to show measurable progress in generating good results and improving the performance of strategy-critical value chain activities are candidates for being replaced.

The challenges of leading a successful strategy execution effort are, without question, substantial.[32] But the job is definitely doable. Because each instance of executing strategy occurs under different organizational circumstances, the managerial agenda for executing strategy always needs to be situation-specific—there's no neat generic procedure to follow. And, as we said at the beginning of Chapter 11, executing strategy is an action-oriented, make-the-right-things-happen task that challenges a manager's ability to lead and direct organizational change, create or reinvent business processes, manage and motivate people, and achieve performance targets. If you now better understand what the challenges are, what approaches are available, which issues need to be considered, and why the action agenda for implementing and executing strategy sweeps across so many aspects of administrative and managerial work, then we will look on our discussion in Chapters 11, 12, and 13 as a success.

A Final Word on Managing the Process of Crafting and Executing Strategy   In practice, it is hard to separate the leadership requirements of executing strategy from the other pieces of the strategy process. As we emphasized in Chapter 1, the job of crafting, implementing, and executing strategy is a five-phase process with much looping and recycling to fine-tune and adjust strategic visions, objectives, strategies, capabilities, implementation approaches, and cultures to fit one another and to fit changing circumstances. The process is continuous, and the conceptually separate acts of crafting and executing strategy blur together in real-world situations. The best tests of good strategic leadership are whether the company has a good strategy and whether the strategy execution effort is delivering the hoped-for results. If these two conditions exist, the chances are excellent that the company has good strategic leadership.

Key Points

The character of a company's culture is a product of the core values and business principles that executives espouse, the standards of what is ethically acceptable and what is not, the work practices and behaviors that define "how we do things around here," its approach to people management and style of operating, the "chemistry" and the "personality" that permeates its work environment, and the stories that get told over and over to illustrate and reinforce the company's values, business practices, and traditions. A company's culture is important because it influences the organization's actions and approaches to conducting business—in a very real sense, the culture is the company's "operating system" or organizational DNA.

The psyche of corporate cultures varies widely. Moreover, company cultures vary widely in strength and influence. Some are strongly embedded and have a big impact on a company's practices and behavioral norms. Others are weak and have comparatively little influence on company operations. There are four types of unhealthy cultures: (1) those that are highly political and characterized by empire building, (2) those that are change resistant, (3) those that are insular and inwardly focused, and (4) those that are ethically unprincipled and are driven by greed. High-performance cultures and adaptive cultures both have positive features that are conducive to good strategy execution.

A culture grounded in values, practices, and behavioral norms that match what is needed for good strategy execution helps energize people throughout the company to do their jobs in a strategy-supportive manner, adding significantly to the power of a company's strategy execution effort and the chances of achieving the targeted results. But when the culture is in conflict with some aspect of the company's direction, performance targets, or strategy, the culture becomes a stumbling block. Thus, an important part of the managing the strategy execution process is establishing and nurturing a good fit between culture and strategy.

A company's present culture and work climate may or may not be compatible with what is needed for effective implementation and execution of the chosen strategy. *When a company's present work climate promotes attitudes and behaviors that are well suited to first-rate strategy execution, its culture functions as a valuable ally in the strategy execution process.* When the culture is in conflict with some aspect of the company's direction, performance targets, or strategy, the culture becomes a stumbling block.

Changing a company's culture, especially a strong one with traits that don't fit a new strategy's requirements, is a tough and often time-consuming challenge. Changing a culture requires competent leadership at the top. It requires symbolic actions and substantive actions that unmistakably indicate serious commitment on the part of top management. The more that culture-driven actions and behaviors fit what's needed for good strategy execution, the less managers have to depend on policies, rules, procedures, and supervision to enforce what people should and should not do.

The taproot of a company's corporate culture nearly always is its dedication to certain core values and the bar it sets for ethical behavior. Of course, sometimes a company's stated core values and codes of ethics are cosmetic, existing mainly to impress outsiders and help create a positive company image. But more usually they have been developed to shape the culture. If management practices what it preaches, a company's core values and ethical standards nurture the corporate culture in three highly positive ways: (1) They communicate the company's good intentions and validate the integrity and above-board character of its business principles and operating methods; (2) they steer company personnel toward both doing the right thing and doing things right; and (3) they establish a corporate conscience that gauges the appropriateness of particular actions, decisions, and policies. Companies that really care about how they conduct their business put a stake in the ground, making it unequivocally clear that company personnel are expected to live up to the company's values and ethical standards—how well individuals display core values and adhere to ethical standards is often part of the job performance evaluations. Peer pressures to conform to cultural norms are quite strong, acting as an important deterrent to outside-the-lines behavior.

Leading the drive for good strategy execution and operating excellence calls for five actions on the part of the manager-in-charge:

1. Staying on top of what is happening, closely monitoring progress, ferreting out issues, and learning what obstacles lie in the path of good execution.

2. Putting constructive pressure on the organization to achieve good results and operating excellence.

3. Leading the development of stronger core competencies and competitive capabilities.

4. Displaying ethical integrity and leading social responsibility initiatives.

5. Pushing corrective actions to improve strategy execution and achieve the targeted results.

Exercises

1. Go to Herman Miller's Web site (www.hermanmiller.com) and read what the company has to say about its corporate culture in its careers sections. Do you think this statement is just public relations, or, based on what else you can learn about the Herman Miller Company from browsing this Web site, is there reason to believe that management has truly built a culture that makes the stated values and principles come alive?

2. Go to the careers section at Qualcomm's Web site (www.qualcomm.com) and see what this company, one of the most prominent companies in mobile communications technology, has to say about life at Qualcomm. Is what's on this Web site just recruiting propaganda, or does it convey the type of work climate that management is actually trying to create? If you were a senior executive at Qualcomm, would you see merit in building and nurturing a culture like what is described in the section "Life at Qualcomm"? Would such a culture represent a tight fit with Qualcomm's high-tech business and strategy? (You can get an overview of the Qualcomm's strategy by exploring the section for investors and some of the recent press releases.) Is your answer consistent with what is presented in the "Awards and Honors" menu selection in the "About Qualcomm" portion of the Web site?

3. Go to the Web site of Johnson & Johnson (www.jnj.com) and read the "J&J Credo," which sets forth the company's responsibilities to customers, employees, the community, and shareholders. Then read the "Our Company" section. Why do you think the credo has resulted in numerous awards and accolades that recognize the company as a good corporate citizen?

4. Do an Internet search or use the resources of your university's library to identify at least five companies that have experienced a failure of strategic leadership on the part of the CEO since 2000. Three candidate companies you might want to research are Adelphia Communications, AIG, and HealthSouth. Then determine which, if any, of the five factors discussed in this chapter's section titled "Leading the Strategy Execution Process" came into play in the CEOs' failure.

5. Dell Inc. has been listed as one of *Fortune*'s most admired companies for several years. Click on the "About Dell" link at www.dell.com. What is your assessment of the company's extensive discussion of accountability, concern for the environment, and community involvement? Does it appear these programs have the support of upper-level management? Is there evidence that this is more than a public relations initiative?

6. Review the material in Illustration Capsule 13.1 on Google's corporate culture; then go to the company's Web site, click on the "About Google" link, then on the "Corporate Info" link and read the "Ten things Google has found to be true" in the "Our Philosophy" section. What relationships do you see between these 10 things and Google's description of its culture? Are the two closely connected? Why or why not? Explain.

part two

2

Cases in Crafting and Executing Strategy

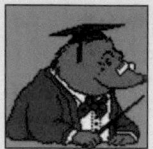

Whole Foods Market in 2006: Mission, Core Values, and Strategy

Arthur A. Thompson
The University of Alabama

Founded in 1980 as a local supermarket for natural and health foods in Austin, Texas, Whole Foods Market had by 2006 evolved into the world's largest retail chain of natural and organic foods supermarkets. The company had 180 stores in the United States, Canada, and Great Britain and 2005 sales of $4.7 billion; revenues had grown at a compound annual rate of 20 percent since 1998. John Mackey, the company's cofounder and CEO, believed that Whole Foods' rapid growth and market success had much to do with having "remained a uniquely mission-driven company—highly selective about what we sell, dedicated to our core values and stringent quality standards and committed to sustainable agriculture." The company's stated mission was to promote vitality and well-being for all individuals by offering the highest quality, least processed, most flavorful natural and naturally preserved foods available. But as the company's motto—"Whole Foods, Whole People, Whole Planet"—implied, its core mission extended well beyond food retailing (see Exhibit 1).

John Mackey's vision was for Whole Foods to become a national brand synonymous not just with natural and organic foods but also with being the best food retailer in every community it served. In pursuit of this vision, the company's strategic plan aimed at expanding its retail operations to offer the highest quality and most nutritious foods to more and more customers and promoting organically grown foods, food safety concern, and sustainability of the entire

ecosystem. During its 25-year history, Whole Foods Market had been a leader in the natural and organic foods movement across the United States, helping the industry gain acceptance among growing numbers of consumers. The company's long-term objectives were to have 400 stores and sales of $12 billion by 2010.

THE NATURAL AND ORGANIC FOODS INDUSTRY

The combined sales of natural and organic foods—about $43 billion in 2003—represented 5.5 percent of the roughly $775 billion in total U.S. grocery store sales. *Natural foods* are defined as foods that are minimally processed; largely or completely free of artificial ingredients, preservatives, and other non–naturally occurring chemicals; and as near to their whole, natural state as possible. The U.S. Department of Agriculture's Food and Safety Inspection Service defines *natural food* as "a product containing no artificial ingredient or added color and that is minimally processed." While sales of natural foods products had increased at double-digit rates in the 1990s, growth had slowed to the 7–9 percent range in 2001–2005.

Organic foods were a special subset of the natural foods category and had to be grown and processed without the use of pesticides, antibiotics, hormones,

Exhibit 1   **Whole Foods Market's Motto: Whole Foods, Whole People, Whole Planet**

Whole Foods

We obtain our products locally and from all over the world, often from small, uniquely dedicated food artisans. We strive to offer the highest quality, least processed, most flavorful and naturally preserved foods. Why? Because food in its purest state—unadulterated by artificial additives, sweeteners, colorings and preservatives—is the best tasting and most nutritious food available.

Whole People

We recruit the best people we can to become part of our team. We empower them to make their own decisions, creating a respectful workplace where people are treated fairly and are highly motivated to succeed. We look for people who are passionate about food. Our team members are also well-rounded human beings. They play a critical role in helping build the store into a profitable and beneficial part of its community.

Whole Planet

We believe companies, like individuals, must assume their share of responsibility as tenants of Planet Earth. On a global basis we actively support organic farming—the best method for promoting sustainable agriculture and protecting the environment and the farm workers. On a local basis, we are actively involved in our communities by supporting food banks, sponsoring neighborhood events, compensating our team members for community service work, and contributing at least five percent of total net profits to not-for-profit organizations.

Source: Information posted at www.wholefoodsmarket.com (accessed November 28, 2005).

synthetic chemicals, artificial fertilizers, preservatives, dyes or additives, or genetic engineering. Organic foods included fresh fruits and vegetables, meats, and processed foods that had been produced using:

1. Agricultural management practices that promoted a healthy and renewable ecosystem that used no genetically engineered seeds or crops, sewage sludge, long-lasting pesticides, herbicides, or fungicides.

2. Livestock management practices that involved organically grown feed, fresh air and outdoor access for the animals, and no use of antibiotics or growth hormones.

3. Food processing practices that protected the integrity of the organic product and did not involve the use of radiation, genetically modified organisms, or synthetic preservatives.

In 1990, passage of the Organic Food Production Act started the process of establishing national standards for organically grown products in the United States, a movement that included farmers, food activists, conventional food producers, and consumer groups. In October 2002, the U.S. Department of Agriculture (USDA) officially established labeling standards for organic products, overriding both the patchwork of inconsistent state regulations for what could be labeled as organic and the different rules of some

43 agencies for certifying organic products. The new USDA regulations established four categories of food with organic ingredients and varying levels of organic purity:

1. *100 percent organic products:* Such products were usually whole foods, such as fresh fruits and vegetables, grown by organic methods— which meant that the product had been grown without the use of synthetic pesticides or sewage-based fertilizers, had not been subjected to irradiation, and had not been genetically modified or injected with bioengineered organisms, growth hormones, or antibiotics. Products that were 100 percent organic could carry the green USDA organic certification seal, provided the merchant could document that the food product had been organically grown (usually by a certified organic producer).

2. *Organic products:* Such products, often processed, had to have at least 95 percent organically certified ingredients. These could also carry the green USDA organic certification seal.

3. *Made with organic ingredients:* Such products had to have at least 70 percent organic ingredients; they could be labeled "made with organic ingredients" but could not display the USDA seal.

4. *All other products with organic ingredients:* Products with less than 70 percent organic ingredients could not use the word *organic* on the front of a package, but organic ingredients could be listed among other ingredients in a less prominent part of the package.

An official with the National Organic Program, commenting on the appropriateness and need for the new USDA regulations, said, "For the first time, when consumers see the word *organic* on a package, it will have consistent meaning."[1] The new labeling program was not intended as a health or safety program (organic products have not been shown to be more nutritious than conventionally grown products, according to the American Dietetic Association), but rather as a marketing solution. An organic label has long been a selling point for shoppers wanting to avoid pesticides or to support environmentally friendly agricultural practices. However, the new regulations required additional documentation on the part of growers, processors, exporters, importers, shippers, and merchants to verify that they were certified to grow, process, or handle organic products carrying the USDA's organic seal. In 2003, Whole Foods was designated as the first national "Certified Organic" grocer by Quality Assurance International, a federally recognized independent third-party certification organization. In 2005, major food processors were lobbying to make the definition of organic foods less restrictive and permit the use of synthetics in so-called 100 percent organic products.

Organic farmland in the United States was estimated at close to 3 million acres, with an estimated 14,000 mostly small-scale farmers growing organic products in 2004. The amount of certified organic cropland had doubled between 1997 and 2001, and livestock pastures increased at an even faster rate. However, less than 1 percent of U.S. farmland was certified organic in 2004. The Rodale Institute, a Pennsylvania-based advocate of organic farming, had set a goal of 100,000 certified organic U.S. farmers by 2013, a number equal to 5 percent of the 2 million U.S. farmers.[2]

A 2004 survey conducted by the Organic Trade Association found that U.S. manufacturers' sales of organic food products hit $10.4 billion in 2003, up from $1 billion in 1990; sales were expected to reach $30 billion in 2007.[3] In 2005, organic products were sold in about 14,500 natural foods stores in the United States and over 75 percent of the nation's conventional grocery stores and supermarkets. Organic foods and beverages were available in nearly every food category in 2005.

RETAILING OF NATURAL AND ORGANIC FOODS

According to the USDA, 2000 was the first year in which more organic food was sold in conventional U.S. supermarkets than in the nation's 14,500 natural foods stores. Since 2002, most mainstream supermarkets had been expanding their selections of natural and organic products, which ranged from potato chips to fresh produce to wines, cereals, pastas, cheeses, yogurt, vinegars, beef, chicken, and canned and frozen fruits and vegetables. Fresh produce was the most popular organic product— lettuce, broccoli, cauliflower, celery, carrots, and apples were the biggest sellers. Meat, dairy, bread, and snack foods were among the fastest-growing organic product categories. Most supermarket chains stocked a selection of natural and organic food items, and the number and variety of items they carried was growing. Leading supermarket chains like Wal-Mart, Kroger, Publix, Safeway, Albertson's, and Supervalu/Save-a-Lot had created special organic and health food sections for nonperishable foods in most of their stores. Kroger, Publix, and several other chains also had special sections for fresh organic fruits and vegetables in their produce cases in many of their stores in 2005. Kroger had reopened several of its supermarkets as Fresh Fare stores, offering shoppers items such as sushi, gourmet takeout food, organic produce, and an extensive selection of fine wines and cheeses; in 2004–2005, there were 20 Fresh Fare stores in California operating under the Ralph's Fresh Fare name and the Fresh Fare concept was being tested in five Michigan locations. A Kroger official indicated that Fresh Fare was not aimed at the customer who shopped exclusively at upscale, natural foods chains like Whole Foods, but rather at the customer who already shopped Kroger but might travel to Whole Foods for things like vegetables, meats, and prepared foods. Two chains— upscale Harris Teeter in the southeastern United States and Whole Foods Market—had launched their own private-label brands of organics. Exhibit 2 shows 2004–2005 data for the leading supermarket retailers in North America.

Exhibit 2   **Leading North American Supermarket Chains, 2004–2005 (ranked by sales revenues)**

Rank/Company	Number of Stores	2004–2005 Sales Revenues (in billions)	Share of Total U.S. Grocery Sales ($775 billion)
1. Wal-Mart Supercenters	1,713	$70.8	9.1%
2. Kroger	2,530	56.2	7.3
3. Albertson's	1,810	39.7	5.1
4. Safeway	1,817	35.8	4.6
5. Costco	434	29.3	3.8
6. Ahold USA*	1,489	27.4	3.5
7. Sam's Clubs	551	22.3	2.9
8. Loblaw	1,050	21.7	n.a.‡
9. Supervalu/Save-a-Lot	1,544	19.5	2.5
10. Publix Super Markets	847	18.6	2.4
11. Delhaize†	1,494	15.8	2.0
27. Whole Foods Market	171	4.7	0.6

Note: Sales revenue numbers represent estimated sales of supermarket items only in the case of Wal-Mart, Sam's Club, and Costco. Sales data for Kroger's (whose supermarket brands also include City Market, King Sooper, Ralph's, and 11 smaller chains) and Albertson's include revenues from company-owned retail outlets (fuel centers, drugstores, apparel, and jewelry) that are not supermarket related.

*Ahold USA , the U.S. division of Netherlands-based Ahold, includes 339 Stop & Shops, 197 Giant Foods (Landover, Maryland), 180 Bruno's units, 292 Bi-Los, 116 Giant Foods (Carlisle, Pennsylvania), and 365 Tops Friendly Markets.

†Delhaize includes 1,214 Food Lion stores, 123 Hannaford Bros. stores, 103 Kash 'n Karry stores, and 54 Harvey's stores.

‡**n.a.** = Not applicable. Loblaw is a Canadian chain, and market shares are based on U.S. supermarket sales.

Sources: Top 75, www.supermarketnews.com (accessed November 28, 2005); www.walmartstores.com (accessed November 28, 2005); and Whole Foods Market press release, November 9, 2005.

Most industry observers expected that conventional supermarkets would continue to expand their offerings and selection as demand for natural and organic foods expanded. Supermarkets were attracted to merchandising natural and organic foods for two reasons: Consumer demand for natural and organic foods was growing at 7–9 percent annually and was expected to accelerate; meanwhile, retail sales of general food products were growing slowly because of intense price pressures and because more and more consumers were eating out rather than cooking at home.

Leading food processors were showing greater interest in organics as well. Heinz had introduced an organic ketchup and owned a 19 percent stake in Hain Celestial Group, one of the largest organic and natural foods producers. Campbell Soup had introduced organic tomato juice. Starbucks, Green Mountain Coffee, and several other premium coffee marketers were marketing organically grown coffees; Coca-Cola's Odwalla juices were organic; and Tyson Foods and several other chicken producers had introduced organic chicken products. Producers of organically grown beef were selling all they could produce, and sales were expected to grow 30 percent annually through 2008. Safeway, Publix, and Kroger were stocking organic beef and chicken in a number of their stores. Whole Foods was struggling to find organic beef and chicken suppliers big enough to supply all its stores. Lite House organic salad dressings had recently been added to the shelves of several mainstream supermarkets. Major food-processing companies like Kraft, General Mills, Groupe Danone (the parent of Dannon Yogurt), Dean Foods, and Kellogg had all purchased organic food producers in an effort to capitalize on sales-growth opportunities for healthy foods that taste good. In the fall of 2005, McDonald's began marketing organic coffee in

650 units in New England. Most observers saw the trend toward organics as in its infancy, believing that organic products had staying power in the marketplace and were not a fad marching by in the night.

Several factors had combined to transform natural and organic foods retailing, once a niche market, into the fastest-growing segment of U.S. food sales:

- Healthier eating patterns on the part of a populace that was becoming better educated about foods, nutrition, and good eating habits. Among those most interested in organic products were aging affluent people concerned about health and better-for-you foods.

- Increasing consumer concerns over the purity and safety of food due to the presence of pesticide residues, growth hormones, artificial ingredients and other chemicals, and genetically engineered ingredients.

- Environmental concerns due to the degradation of water and soil quality.

- A wellness, or health-consciousness, trend among people of many ages and ethnic groups.

An August 2004 report by Mintel indicated that 10 percent of consumers purchased organic products frequently enough to be "organically obsessed" and another 34 percent purchased them "at least occasionally." All age groups were at least as likely to buy organics in 2004 as they were in 2002, but the largest increases were among young adults, ages 18 to 24 (49 percent versus 34 percent in 2002), and 55- to 64-year-olds (45 percent, up from 25 percent in 2002).[4]

A 2005 survey commissioned by Whole Foods found that 65 percent of U.S. consumers had tried organic foods and beverages, up from 54 percent in both 2003 and 2004; 27 percent of respondents indicated they consumed more organic foods and beverages than they did one year ago.[5] Ten percent consumed organic foods several times per week, up from just 7 percent in 2004. The top three reasons why consumers were buying organic foods and beverages were avoidance of pesticides (70.3 percent), freshness (68.3 percent), and health and nutrition (67.1 percent); 55 percent reported buying organic to avoid genetically modified foods. Also, many respondents agreed that organic foods and beverages were "better for my health" (52.8 percent) and better for the environment (52.4 percent). The categories of organic foods and beverages that were purchased most frequently by those participating in the Whole Foods survey were fresh fruits and vegetables (73 percent), nondairy beverages (32 percent), bread or baked goods (32 percent), dairy items (24.6 percent), packaged goods such as soup or pasta (22.2 percent), meat (22.2 percent), snack foods (22.1 percent), frozen foods (16.6 percent), prepared and ready-to-eat meals (12.2 percent), and baby food (3.2 percent).

The higher prices of organic products were the primary barrier for most consumers in trying or using organic products—75 percent of those participating in the 2005 Whole Foods survey believed organics were too expensive. Other reasons for not consuming more organics were availability (46.1 percent) and loyalty to non-organic brands (36.7 percent).

WHOLE FOODS MARKET

Whole Foods Market was founded in Austin, Texas, when John Mackey, the current CEO, and two other local natural foods grocers in Austin decided the natural foods industry was ready for a supermarket format. The original Whole Foods Market opened in 1980 with a staff of only 19. It was an immediate success. At the time, there were less than half a dozen natural foods supermarkets in the United States. By 1991, the company had 10 stores, revenues of $92.5 million, and net income of $1.6 million. Whole Foods became a public company in 1992, with its stock trading on the Nasdaq; Whole Foods stock was added to the Standard & Poor's (S&P) Mid-Cap 400 Index in May 2002 and to the Nasdaq-100 Index in December 2002. The company had 32,000 employees in 2005 and expected sales of around $5.6 billion in 2006; Mackey believed the company's cash flow from operations in upcoming years would prove more than sufficient to cover the capital costs of the company's aggressive store expansion plan. In November 2005, the company announced a 20 percent increase in its quarterly dividend to $0.30, a special dividend of $4.00 per share, a 2-for-1 stock split, and a $200 million four-year stock buyback program.

Core Values

In 1997, when Whole Foods developed the "Whole Foods, Whole People, Whole Planet" slogan, John

Mackey, known as a go-getter with a "cowboy way of doing things," said:

> This slogan taps into perhaps the deepest purpose of Whole Foods Market. It's a purpose we seldom talk about because it seems pretentious, but a purpose nevertheless felt by many of our Team Members and by many of our customers (and hopefully many of our shareholders too). Our deepest purpose as an organization is helping support the health, well-being, and healing of both people (customers and Team Members) and of the planet (sustainable agriculture, organic production and environmental sensitivity). When I peel away the onion of my personal consciousness down to its core in trying to understand what has driven me to create and grow this company, I come to my desire to promote the general well-being of everyone on earth as well as the earth itself. This is my personal greater purpose with the company and the slogan perfectly reflects it.

Complementing the slogan were five core values shared by both top management and company personnel (see Exhibit 3 on page C-8). In the company's 2003 annual report, John Mackey said:

> Our core values reflect the sense of collective fate among our stakeholders and are the soul of our company. Our Team Members, shareholders, vendors, community and environment must flourish together through their affiliation with us or we are not succeeding as a business. It is leadership's role to balance the needs and desires of all our stakeholders and increase the productivity of Whole Foods Market. By growing the collective pie, we create larger slices for all of our shareholders.

Growth Strategy

Prior to 2002, Whole Foods' growth strategy had been to expand via a combination of opening its own new stores and acquiring small, owner-managed chains. About 35 percent of the company's store base had come from acquisitions; since 1991, the company had acquired 14 chains with 67 stores (see Exhibit 4 on page C-9). Since the natural foods industry was highly fragmented, consisting of close to 20,000 mostly one-store operations and small and regional chains, Whole Foods' management had continued to explore acquisitions that provided access to desirable locations and markets and that had capable personnel that would fit in with Whole Foods. However, since 2002 the company's growth strategy had shifted markedly to opening its own large stores

(50,000 square feet and larger) rather than be acquiring small chains having stores in the range of 5,000 to 20,000 square feet—very few natural foods competitors had stores bigger than 20,000 square feet.

Store Sizes and Locations

Whole Foods' 180 stores (as of January 2006) had an open format and generated average annual sales of about $26 million. Stores opened in fiscal 2004–2005 were averaging sales of over $30 million annually. Stores more than eight years old averaged about 30,000 square feet, stores less than eight years old averaged about 36,000 square feet, and the company's newest stores ranged between 25,000 and 80,000 square feet. The three Harry's Farmers Market stores in Atlanta that Whole Foods acquired in 2001 each measured 75,000–80,000 square feet. Whole Foods' newly opened 58,000-square-foot store on Columbus Circle in New York City was the largest grocery in Manhattan and the company's biggest revenue producer in 2005; Whole Foods opened a three-story 48,500-square-foot store in the Union Square area of Manhattan in March 2005. Whole Foods had a new 74,500-square-foot store in Columbus, Ohio; a flagship 78,000-square-foot store in Austin, Texas; a 62,500-square-foot store in Princeton, New Jersey; a 62,200-square-foot store in Plano, Texas; a 61,000-square-foot store in Omaha, Nebraska; a 56,000-square-foot store in Bellevue, Washington; and a 53,000-square-foot store in Torrance, California. The company was on the verge of opening a 75,000-square-foot store in London, England; a 60,000-square-foot store in Chandler (outside Phoenix); and a 65,000-square-foot store in Plymouth Meeting (a suburb of Philadelphia). In early 2006, 113 of the company's 180 stores were 30,000 square feet or larger. It was the company's practice each year to relocate some of its smaller stores to larger sites with improved visibility and parking. Exhibit 5 on page C-10 provides store-related statistics.

Whole Foods sought to locate its new stores in the upscale areas of urban metropolitan centers—86 percent of the U.S. stores were in the top 50 statistical metropolitan areas. In 2005, Whole Foods had stores in 31 states and 38 of the top 50 U.S. metropolitan areas. In 2002, the company entered Toronto, Canada, and expanded into London and Bristol, England, in 2004. In November 2005, the company had 64 stores averaging 55,000 square feet

Exhibit 3 **Whole Foods Market's Core Values**

Our Core Values

The following list of core values reflects what is truly important to us as an organization. These are not values that change from time to time, situation to situation or person to person, but rather they are the underpinning of our company culture. Many people feel Whole Foods is an exciting company of which to be a part and a very special place to work. These core values are the primary reasons for this feeling, and they transcend our size and our growth rate. By maintaining these core values, regardless of how large a company Whole Foods becomes, we can preserve what has always been special about our company. These core values are the soul of our company.

Selling the Highest Quality Natural and Organic Products Available

- **Passion for Food**—We appreciate and celebrate the difference natural and organic products can make in the quality of one's life.
- **Quality Standards**—We have high standards and our goal is to sell the highest quality products we possibly can. We define quality by evaluating the ingredients, freshness, safety, taste, nutritive value and appearance of all of the products we carry. We are buying agents for our customers and not the selling agents for the manufacturers.

Satisfying and Delighting Our Customers

- **Our Customers**—They are our most important stakeholders in our business and the lifeblood of our business. Only by satisfying our customers first do we have the opportunity to satisfy the needs of our other stakeholders.
- **Extraordinary Customer Service**—We go to extraordinary lengths to satisfy and delight our customers. We want to meet or exceed their expectations on every shopping trip. We know that by doing so we turn customers into advocates for our business. Advocates do more than shop with us, they talk about Whole Foods to their friends and others. We want to serve our customers competently, efficiently, knowledgeably and with flair.
- **Education**—We can generate greater appreciation and loyalty from all of our stakeholders by educating them about natural and organic foods, health, nutrition and the environment.
- **Meaningful Value**—We offer value to our customers by providing them with high quality products, extraordinary service and a competitive price. We are constantly challenged to improve the value proposition to our customers.
- **Retail Innovation**—We value retail experiments. Friendly competition within the company helps us to continually improve our stores. We constantly innovate and raise our retail standards and are not afraid to try new ideas and concepts.
- **Inviting Store Environments**—We create store environments that are inviting and fun, and reflect the communities they serve. We want our stores to become community meeting places where our customers meet their friends and make new ones.

Team Member Happiness and Excellence

- **Empowering Work Environments**—Our success is dependent upon the collective energy and intelligence of all of our Team Members. We strive to create a work environment where motivated Team Members can flourish and succeed to their highest potential. We appreciate effort and reward results.
- **Self-Responsibility**—We take responsibility for our own success and failures. We celebrate success and see failures as opportunities for growth. We recognize that we are responsible for our own happiness and success.
- **Self-Directed Teams**—The fundamental work unit of the company is the self-directed Team. Teams meet regularly to discuss issues, solve problems and appreciate each others' contributions. Every Team Member belongs to a Team.
- **Open & Timely Information**—We believe knowledge is power and we support our Team Members' right to access information that impacts their jobs. Our books are open to our Team Members, including our annual individual compensation report. We also recognize everyone's right to be listened to and heard regardless of their point of view.
- **Incremental Progress**—Our company continually improves through unleashing the collective creativity and intelligence of all of our Team Members. We recognize that everyone has a contribution to make. We keep getting better at what we do.
- **Shared Fate**—We recognize there is a community of interest among all of our stakeholders. There are no entitlements; we share together in our collective fate. To that end we have a salary cap that limits the compensation (wages plus profit incentive bonuses) of any Team Member to fourteen times the average total compensation of all full-time Team Members in the company.

(Continued)

Exhibit 3   **Continued**

Creating Wealth Through Profits & Growth

- **Stewardship**—We are stewards of our shareholders' investments and we take that responsibility very seriously. We are committed to increasing long term shareholder value.
- **Profits**—We earn our profits everyday through voluntary exchange with our customers. We recognize that profits are essential to creating capital for growth, prosperity, opportunity, job satisfaction and job security.

Caring About Our Communities & Our Environment

- **Sustainable Agriculture**—We support organic farmers, growers and the environment through our commitment to sustainable agriculture and by expanding the market for organic products.
- **Wise Environmental Practices**—We respect our environment and recycle, reuse, and reduce our waste wherever and whenever we can.
- **Community Citizenship**—We recognize our responsibility to be active participants in our local communities. We give a minimum of 5% of our profits every year to a wide variety of community and non-profit organizations. In addition, we pay our Team Members to give of their time to community and service organizations.
- **Integrity in All Business Dealings**—Our trade partners are our allies in serving our stakeholders. We treat them with respect, fairness and integrity at all times and expect the same in return.

Source: Information posted at www.wholefoodsmarket.com (accessed November 29, 2005).

in varying stages of development (the new stores of supermarket chains like Safeway and Kroger averaged around 55,000 square feet).

Most stores were in high-traffic shopping locations, some were freestanding, and some were in strip centers. Whole Foods had its own internally developed model to analyze potential markets according to education levels, population density, and income. After picking a target metropolitan area, the company's site consultant did a comprehensive site study and developed sales projections; potential sites had to pass certain financial hurdles. New stores opened 12 to 24 months after a lease was signed.

The cash investment needed to ready a new Whole Foods Market for opening varied with the metropolitan area, site characteristics, store size, and amount of work performed by the landlord; totals ranged from as little as $2 million to as much as $16 million—the average for the past five years was $8.6 million. In addition to the cost of readying a

Exhibit 4   **Major Acquisitions by Whole Foods Market**

Year	Company Acquired	Location	Number of Stores	Acquisition Costs
1992	Bread & Circus	Northeast United States	6	$20 million plus $6.2 million in common stock
1993	Mrs. Gooch's	Southern California	7	2,970,596 shares of common stock
1996	Fresh Fields Markets	East Coast and Chicago area	22	4.8 million shares of stock plus options for 549,000 additional shares
1997	Merchant of Vino	Detroit area	6	Approximately 1 million shares of common stock
1997	Bread of Life	South Florida	2	200,000 shares of common stock
1999	Nature's Heartland	Boston area	4	$24.5 million in cash
2000	Food 4 Thought (Natural Abilities Inc.)	Sonoma County, California	3	$25.7 million in cash, plus assumption of certain liabilities
2001	Harry's Farmer's Market	Atlanta	3	Approximately $35 million in cash
2004	Fresh & Wild	Great Britain	7	$20 million in cash plus 239,000 shares of common stock

Source: Investor relations section of www.wholefoodsmarket.com (accessed November 18, 2004).

t 5 Number of Stores in the Whole Foods Markets Chain, 1991–2005, and Selected Store Operating Statistics, 2000–2005

Year	Number of Stores at End of Fiscal Year
1991	10
1992	25
1993	42
1994	49
1995	61
1996	68
1997	75
1998	87
1999	100
2000	117
2001	126
2002	135
2003	145
2004	163
2005	178

Store Counts	1998	1999	2000	2001	2002	2003	2004	2005
Beginning of fiscal year	75	87	100	117	126	135	145	163
New stores opened	9	9	17	12	11	12	12	15
Stores acquired	6	5	3	0	3	0	7	0
Relocations and closures	(2)	(3)	(1)	(3)	(3)	(5)	(2)	(1)
End of fiscal year	87	100	117	126	135	145	163	178

	Fiscal Year					
	2000	2001	2002	2003	2004	2005
Store sales (000s)	$1,838,630	$2,272,231	$2,690,475	$3,148,593	$3,864,950	$4,701,289
Average weekly sales	$324,710	$353,024	$392,837	$424,095	$482,061	$536,986
Comparable store sales growth	8.6%	9.2%	10.0%	8.6%	14.9%	12.8%
Total square footage of all stores, end of year	3,180,207	3,598,469	4,098,492	4,545,433	5,145,261	5,819,843
Average store size, end of year, in square feet	27,181	28,559	30,359	31,348	31,566	33,200
Gross margin, all-store average	34.5%	34.7%	34.6%	34.2%	34.2%	35.1%
Store contribution, all-store average*	9.4%	9.5%	9.6%	9.2%	9.3%	9.6%

*Defined as gross profit minus direct store expenses, where gross profit equals store revenues less cost of goods sold.

Source: Information posted at www.wholefoodsmarket.com (accessed November 18, 2004, and November 29, 2005).

store for operation, it took approximately $750,000 to stock the store with inventory, a portion of which was financed by vendors. Preopening expenses had averaged approximately $600,000 per store over the past five years.

Product Line

While product and brand selections varied from store to store (because of differing store sizes and clientele), Whole Foods' product line included some 30,000 natural, organic, and gourmet food and non-food items:

- Fresh produce—fruits and vegetables; displays of fresh-cut fruits; and a selection of seasonal, exotic, and specialty products like cactus pears and cippolini onions.

- Meat and poultry—natural and organic meats, house-made sausages, and poultry products from animals raised on wholesome grains, pastureland, and well water (and not grown with the use of by-products, hormones, or steroids).

- Fresh seafood—a selection of fresh fish; shrimp; oysters; clams; mussels; homemade marinades; and exotic items like octopus, sushi, and black-tip shark. A portion of the fresh fish selections at the seafood station came from the company's Pigeon Cove and Select Fish seafood processing subsidiaries. Seafood items coming from distant supply sources were flown in to stores to ensure maximum freshness.

- A selection of daily baked goods—breads, cakes, pies, cookies, bagels, muffins, and scones.

- Prepared foods—soups, canned and packaged goods, oven-ready meals, rotisserie meats, hearth-fired pizza, pastas, patés, salad bars, a sandwich station, and a selection of entrées and side foods prepared daily.

- Fine-quality cheeses, olives (up to 40 varieties in some stores), and chocolates and confections.

- Frozen foods, juices, yogurt and dairy products, smoothies, and bottled waters.

- A wide selection of bulk items in bins.

- Beer and wines—the selection of domestic and imported wines varied from store to store; organic wines were among those available.

- A body care and nutrition department containing a wide selection of natural and organic body care and cosmetics products, along with assorted vitamin supplements, homeopathic remedies, yoga supplies, and aromatherapy products. All items entailed the use of non-animal testing methods and contained no artificial ingredients.

- Natural and organic pet foods (including the company's own private-label line), treats, toys, and pest control remedies.

- Grocery and household products—canned and packaged goods, pastas, soaps, cleaning products, and other conventional household items. Whole Foods' larger stores stocked conventional household products in order to make Whole Foods a one-stop grocery-shopping destination.

- A floral department with sophisticated flower bouquets.

- A 365 Every Day Value line of private-label products that included over 440 items at very competitive price points, a 365 Organic line consisting of 200 items, a 29-item Whole X line of best-of-class premium and superpremium organic products, and a 50-item organic food product line developed for children under the Whole Kids label. Most recently, the company had begun using four other private brands—Whole Catch (for frozen seafood selections), Whole Ranch (for frozen meats), Whole Treats (for candies, cookies, and frozen desserts), and Whole Kitchen (a wide selection of frozen entrées and appetizers).

- Educational products (information on alternative health care) and books relating to healing, cookery, diet, and lifestyle. In some stores, there were cooking classes and nutrition sessions.

Whole Foods was the world's biggest seller of organic produce. Perishables accounted for about 65 percent of Whole Foods' sales, considerably higher than the 40–50 percent that perishables represented at conventional supermarkets. The acquisition of the three 75,000-plus-square-foot Harry's Market superstores in Atlanta, where 75 percent of sales were perishables, had provided the company with personnel having valuable intellectual capital in creatively merchandising all major perishables categories. Management believed that the company's emphasis on fresh fruits and vegetables, bakery goods, meats, seafood, and other perishables differentiated Whole Foods stores from other supermarkets and attracted a broader customer base. According to John Mackey:

First-time visitors to Whole Foods Market are often awed by our perishables. We devote more space to fresh fruits and vegetables, including an extensive selection of organics, than most of our competitors. Our meat and poultry products are natural—no artificial ingredients, minimal processing, and raised without the use of artificial growth hormones, antibiotics or animal by-products in their feed. Our seafood is either wild-caught or sourced from aquaculture farms where environmental concerns are a priority. Also, our seafood is never treated with chlorine or other chemicals, as is common practice in the food retailing industry. With each new store or renovation, we challenge ourselves to create more entertaining, theatrical, and scintillatingly appetizing prepared foods areas. We bake daily, using whole grains and unbleached, unbromated flour and feature European-style loaves, pastries, cookies and cakes as well as gluten-free baked goods for those allergic to wheat. We also offer many vegetarian and vegan products for our customers seeking to avoid all animal products. Our cheeses are free of artificial flavors, colors, and synthetic preservatives, and we offer an outstanding variety of both organic cheeses and cheeses made using traditional methods.[6]

Whole Foods' three-story showcase Union Square store in Manhattan carried locally made New York offerings, seasonal items from the nearby Greenmarket farmers' market, and numerous exotic and gourmet items. A 28-foot international section featured such items as Lebanese fig jam, preserved lemons from Morocco, Indian curries, Thai rice, stuffed grape leaves from Greece, and goulash from Hungary. The prepared foods section had a Grilling Station where shoppers could get grilled-to-order dishes such as swordfish in red pepper Romesco sauce and steak with a mushroom demi-glace.

One of Whole Foods Market's foremost commitments to its customers was to sell foods that met strict standards and that were of high quality in terms of nutrition, freshness, appearance, and taste. (Exhibit 6 shows the company's quality standards.) Whole Foods guaranteed 100 percent satisfaction on all items purchased and went to great lengths to live up to its core value of satisfying and delighting customers. Buyers personally visited the facilities of many of the company's suppliers and were very picky about the items they chose and the ingredients they contained. For the benefit of prospective food suppliers, the company maintained a list of ingredients it considered unacceptable in food products (see Exhibit 6).

Pricing

Because the costs of growing and marketing organic foods ran 25 to 75 percent more than those of conventionally grown items, prices at Whole Foods were higher than at conventional supermarkets. For the most part, Whole Foods sold premium products at premium prices. Because the prices for price-sensitive consumers and some media critics had dubbed Whole Foods as "Whole Paycheck," chiefly because some of its exotic items had eye-popping price tags—for example, Graffitti eggplants grown in Holland were $4 per pound, lobster mushrooms from Oregon were $25 per pound, and a three-ounce can of organic pearl jasmine tea was $14.[7] Its earth-friendly detergents, toilet papers, and other household items frequently were priced higher than the name brands of comparable products found in traditional supermarkets. However, as one analyst noted, "If people believe that the food is healthier and they are doing something good for themselves, they are willing to invest a bit more, particularly as they get older. It's not a fad."[8] Another grocery industry analyst noted that while Whole Foods served a growing niche, it had managed to attract a new kind of customer, one who was willing to pay a premium to dabble in health food without being totally committed to vegetarianism or an organic lifestyle.[9]

Store Description and Merchandising

Whole Foods Market did not have a standard store design. Instead, each store's layout was customized to fit the particular site and building configuration and to best show off the particular product mix for the store's target clientele. For instance, the new 78,000-square-foot Austin store opened in March 2005 was already a top Central Texas tourist destination and downtown Austin landmark; it had an intimate village-style layout; six mini-restaurants within the store; a raw food and juice bar; more than 600 varieties of cheese and 40 varieties of olives; a selection of 1,800 wines; a Candy Island with handmade lollipops and popcorn balls; a hot nut bar with an in-house nut roaster; a World Foods section; a walk-in beer cooler with 800 selections; 14 pastry chefs making a variety of items; a Natural Home

Exhibit 6 **Whole Foods Market's Product Quality Standards and Customer Commitments**

Our business is to sell the highest quality foods we can find at the most competitive prices possible. We evaluate quality in terms of nutrition, freshness, appearance, and taste. Our search for quality is a never-ending process involving the careful judgment of buyers throughout the company.

- We carefully evaluate each and every product we sell.
- We feature foods that are free from artificial preservatives, colors, flavors and sweeteners.
- We are passionate about great tasting food and the pleasure of sharing it with each other.
- We are committed to foods that are fresh, wholesome and safe to eat.
- We seek out and promote organically grown foods.
- We provide food and nutritional products that support health and well-being.

Whole Foods Market's Quality Standards team maintains an extensive list of unacceptable ingredients (see below). However, creating a product with no unacceptable ingredients does not guarantee that Whole Foods Market will sell it. Our buyers are passionate about seeking out the freshest, most healthful, minimally processed products available.

As of December 2005, the following 83 chemicals were on Whole Foods' list of unacceptable ingredients:

- acesulfame-K (acesulfame potassium)
- acetylated esters of mono- and diglycerides
- ammonium chloride
- artificial colors
- artificial flavors
- aspartame
- azodicarbonamide
- benzoates in food
- benzoyl peroxide
- BHA (butylated hydroxyanisole)
- BHT (butylated hydroxytoluene)
- bleached flour
- bromated flour
- brominated vegetable oil (BVO)
- calcium bromate
- calcium disodium EDTA
- calcium peroxide
- calcium propionate
- calcium saccharin
- calcium sorbate
- calcium stearoyl-2-lactylate
- caprocaprylobehenin
- carmine (see cochineal)
- certified colors
- cochineal (carmine)
- cyclamates
- cysteine (l-cysteine), as an additive for bread products
- DATEM (diacetyl tartaric and fatty acid esters of mono and diglycerides)
- dimethylpolysiloxane

- dioctyl sodium sulfosuccinate (DSS)
- disodium calcium EDTA
- disodium dihydrogen EDTA
- disodium guanylate
- disodium inosinate
- EDTA
- ethyl vanillin
- ethylene oxide
- ethyoxyquin
- FD & C colors
- fois gras
- GMP (disodium guanylate)
- hexa-, hepta- and octa- esters of sucrose
- hydrogenated oil
- IMP (disodium inosinate)
- irradiated foods
- lactylated esters of mono- and diglycerides
- lead soldered cans
- methyl silicon
- methylparaben
- microparticularized whey protein derived fat substitute
- monosodium glutamate (MSG)
- natamycin
- nitrates/nitrites
- partially hydrogenated oil
- polydextrose
- potassium benzoate

- potassium bisulfite
- potassium bromate
- potassium metabisulfite
- potassium sorbate
- propionates
- propyl gallate
- propylparaben
- saccharin
- sodium aluminum phosphate
- sodium aluminum sulfate
- sodium benzoate
- sodium bisulfite
- sodium diacetate
- sodium glutamate
- sodium metabisulfite
- sodium nitrate/nitrite
- sodium propionate
- sodium stearoyl-2-lactylate
- sodium sulfite
- solvent extracted oils, as standalone single-ingredient oils (except grapeseed oil)
- sorbic acid
- sucralose
- sucroglycerides
- sucrose polyester
- sulfites (sulfur dioxide)
- TBHQ (tertiary butylhydroquinone)
- tetrasodium EDTA
- vanillin

Whole Foods reserved the right to alter its list of unacceptable ingredients at any time.

Source: Information posted at www.wholefoodsmarket.com (accessed November 29, 2005).

section with organic cotton apparel and household linens; an extensive meat department with an in-house smoker and 50 oven-ready items prepared by in-house chefs; and a theater-like seafood department with more than 150 fresh seafood items and on-the-spot shucking, cooking, smoking, slicing, and frying to order. The Columbus Circle store in Manhattan had a 248-seat café where shoppers could enjoy restaurant-quality prepared foods while relaxing in a comfortable community setting; a Jamba Juice smoothie station that served freshly blended-to-order fruit smoothies and juices; a full-service sushi bar by Genji Express where customers sat on bar stools wrapped in nori enjoying fresh-cut sushi wrapped in organic seaweed; a walk-in greenhouse showcasing fresh-cut and exotic flowers; a wine shop with more than 700 varieties of wine from both large and small vineyards and family estates; and a chocolate enrobing station in the bakery where customers could request just about anything covered in chocolate.

The driving concept of Whole Foods' merchandising strategy was to create an inviting and interactive store atmosphere that turned shopping for food into a fun, pleasurable experience. Management at Whole Foods wanted customers to view company stores as a "third place" (besides home and office) where people could gather, learn, and interact while at the same time enjoying an intriguing food-shopping and eating experience. Stores had a colorful décor, and products were attractively merchandised (see Exhibit 7). According to one industry analyst, Whole Foods had "put together the ideal model for the foodie who's a premium gourmet and the natural foods buyer. When you walk into a Whole Foods store, you're overwhelmed by a desire to look at everything you see."[10]

Most stores featured hand-stacked produce, in-store chefs and open kitchens, scratch bakeries, prepared foods stations, European-style charcuterie departments, Whole Body departments with a wide selection of natural cosmetics (as well as a makeup station) and personal care items, salad bars, sit-down dining areas, gourmet food sections with items from around the world, and ever-changing selections and merchandise displays. Many stores had recipe cards at the end of key aisles. A few stores offered valet parking, home delivery, and massages. Management believed that the extensive and attractive displays of fresh produce, seafood, meats and house-made sausages (up to 40 varieties), baked goods, and prepared

foods in its larger stores appealed to a broader customer base and were responsible for the stores bigger than 30,000 square feet showing higher performance than the smaller stores.

Whole Foods got very high marks from merchandising experts and customers for its presentation—from the bright colors of the produce displays, to the quality of the foods and customer service, to the wide aisles and cleanliness. Management was continually experimenting with new merchandising concepts to keep stores fresh and exciting for customers. According to a Whole Foods regional manager, "We take the best ideas from each of our stores and try to incorporate them in all our other stores. We're constantly making our stores better."[11] Whole Foods' merchandising skills were said to be a prime factor in its success in luring shoppers back time and again—Whole Foods stores had annual sales averaging more than $800 per square foot of space about double the sales per square foot of Kroger and Safeway.

To further a sense of community and interaction with customers, stores typically included customer comment boards and Take Action centers for customers who wanted information on such topics as sustainable agriculture, organics, the sustainability of seafood supplies and overfishing problems, and the environment in general. The Toronto store had biographies of farmers suspended from the ceiling on placards and a board calling attention to Whole Foods' Sustainable Seafood Policy hung above the seafood station.

Marketing and Customer Service

Whole Foods spent about 0.5 percent of its revenues on advertising, a much smaller percentage than conventional supermarkets spent, preferring instead to rely primarily on word-of-mouth recommendations from customers. The corporate marketing budget was allocated to regionwide programs, marketing efforts for individual stores, a national brand awareness initiative, and consumer research. Stores spent most of their marketing budgets on in-store signage and store events such as taste fairs, classes, and product samplings. Store personnel were encouraged to extend company efforts to encourage the adoption of a natural and organic lifestyle by going out into the community and conducting a proactive public relations campaign. Each store also had a separate

Exhibit 7 **Scenes from Whole Foods Stores**

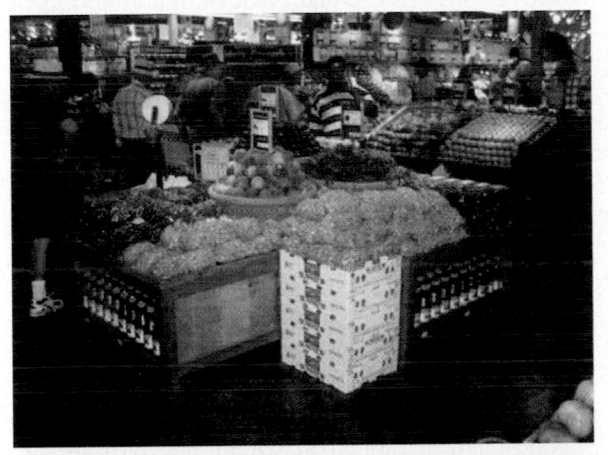
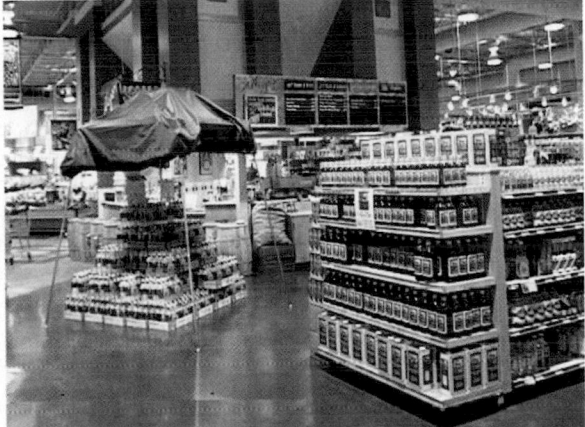
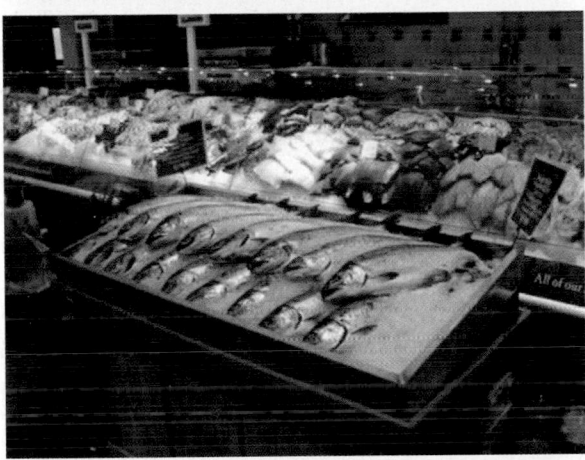
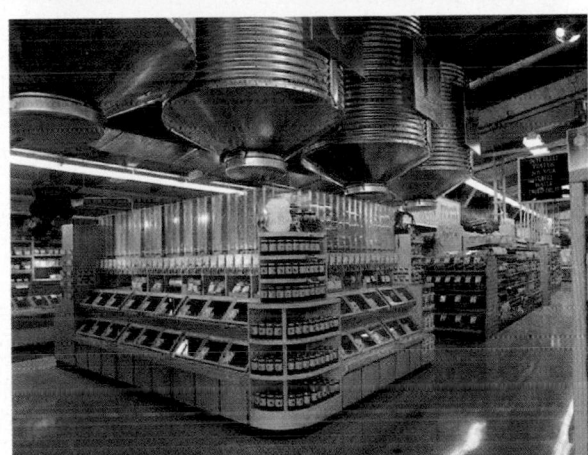
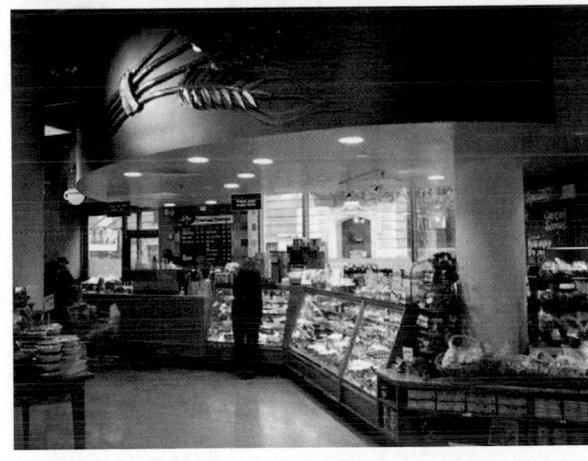
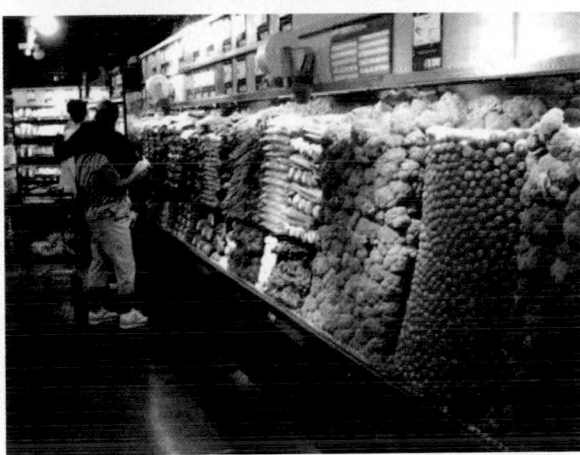

budget for making contributions to philanthropic activities and community outreach programs.

Since one of its core values was to satisfy and delight customers (see Exhibit 3), Whole Foods Market strove to meet or exceed customer expectations on every shopping trip. Competent, knowledgeable, and friendly service was a hallmark of shopping at a Whole Foods Market. The aim was to turn highly satisfied customers into advocates for Whole Foods who talked to close friends and acquaintances about their positive experiences with the company. Store personnel were personable and chatty with shoppers. Customers could get personal attention in every department of the store. When customers asked where an item was located, team members often took them to the spot, making conversation along the way and offering to answer any questions. Team members were quite knowledgeable and enthusiastic about the products in their particular department and tried to take advantage of opportunities to inform and educate customers about natural foods, organics, healthy eating, and food-related environmental issues. They took pride in helping customers navigate the extensive variety to make the best choices. Meat department personnel provided customers with custom cuts, cooking instructions, and personal recommendations.

Store Operations

Depending on store size and traffic volume, Whole Foods stores employed between 80 and 500 team members, who were organized into up to 11 teams, each led by a team leader. Each team within a store was responsible for a different product category or aspect of store operations such as customer service and customer check-out stations. Team leaders screened candidates for job openings on their team, but a two-thirds majority of the team had to approve a new hire—approval came only after a 30-day trial for the candidate.

Whole Foods practiced a decentralized team approach to store operations, with many personnel, merchandising, and operating decisions made by teams at the individual store level. Management believed that the decentralized structure made it critical to have an effective store team leader. The store team leader worked with one or more associate store team leaders, as well as with all the department team leaders, to operate the store as efficiently and profitably as possible. Store team leaders were paid a salary plus a bonus based on the store's economic value added

(EVA) contribution; they were also eligible to receive stock options.[12] Store team leaders reported directly to one of the 10 regional presidents.

Management believed its team members were inspired by the company's mission because it complemented their own views about the benefits of a natural and organic foods diet. In management's view, many Whole Foods team members felt good about their jobs because they saw themselves as contributing to the welfare of society and to the company's customers by selling clean and nutritious foods, by helping advance the cause of long-term sustainable agriculture methods, and by promoting a healthy, pesticide-free environment.

In December 2005, the company had some 32,000 team members, of which approximately 86 percent were full-time. None were represented by unions, although there had been a couple of unionization attempts. John Mackey was viewed as fiercely anti-union and had once said: "The union is like having herpes. It doesn't kill you, but it's unpleasant and inconvenient and it stops a lot of people from becoming your lover."[13] Union leaders were critical of the company's anti-union stance and a Web site (www.wholeworkersunite.org) was devoted to criticizing Mackey, explaining why unionization was good for Whole Foods employees, and compiling instances of the company's anti-union actions. A second Web site (www.michaelbluejay.com) touted so-called scandals at Whole Foods; the material consisted of two articles from publications that criticized Whole Foods' wage rates and Mackey's anti-union stance.

Whole Foods had been ranked by *Fortune* magazine for eight consecutive years (1998–2006) as one of the top 100 companies to work for in America—Whole Foods was one of only 22 companies to make the list every year since its inception. Whole Foods was the only national supermarket chain to ever make the list, although the regional supermarket chain Wegman's was the top-ranked company on the 2005 list. (In scoring companies, *Fortune* places a two-thirds weight on responses to a random survey of employees and a one-third weight on its evaluation of a company's benefits and practices.) A team member at Whole Foods' store in Austin, Texas, said, "I really feel like we're a part of making the world a better place. When I joined the company 17 years ago, we only had four stores. I have always loved—as a customer and now as a Team Member—the camaraderie, support for others, and progressive atmosphere at Whole Foods Market."[14] According to the company's vice president of human resources, "Team members who love to take initiative, while enjoying working as part of a team and being rewarded through shared fate, thrive here."

During 2002, team members across the company actively contributed ideas about the benefits they would like the company to offer; the suggestions were compiled and, through three subsequent votes, put into package form. The benefits plan that was adopted for three years was approved by 83 percent of the 79 percent of the team members participating in the benefits vote. Under the adopted plan, each team member could select his or her own benefits package. The resulting health insurance plan that the company put in place in January 2003 involved the company paying 100 percent of the premium for full-time employees and the establishment of company-funded "personal wellness accounts" that team members could use to pay the higher deductibles; any unused balances in a team member's account could roll over and accumulate for future expenses. Whole Foods expected to repeat its benefits vote every three years.

Every year, management gave team members an opportunity to complete a morale survey covering job satisfaction, opportunity and empowerment, pay, training, and benefits. In 2004, the overall participation rate was 63 percent (versus 71 percent in 2003). Of the team members responding in 2004, 86 percent said they almost always or frequently enjoyed their job (the same percentage as in 2003), and 82 percent said they almost always or frequently felt empowered to do their best work at Whole Foods Market (up slightly from 81 percent in 2003). In response to the question "What is the best thing about working at Whole Foods Market?" common responses included coworkers, customers, flexibility, work environment, growth and learning opportunities, the products Whole Foods sold, benefits, the team concept, and the culture of empowerment.

Compensation and Incentives

Whole Foods' management strove to create a "shared-fate consciousness" on the part of team members by uniting the self-interests of team members with those of shareholders. One way management reinforced this concept was through a gain-sharing program that rewarded a store's team members according to their store's contribution to operating profit (store sales less cost of goods sold less store operating expenses)—gain-sharing distributions added 5–7 percent to team member wages. The company also encouraged stock ownership on the part of team members through three other programs:

1. *A team member stock option plan*—Team members were eligible for stock options based on seniority, promotion, or the discretion of regional or national executives. Roughly 85 percent of the company's stock options in 2004 were held by non-executives.

2. *A team member stock purchase plan*—Team members could purchase a restricted number of shares at a discount from the market price through payroll deductions.

3. *A team member 401(k) plan*—Whole Foods Market stock was one of the investment options in the 401(k) plan.

All the teams at each store were continuously evaluated on measures relating to sales, operations, and morale; the results were made available to team members and to headquarters personnel.[15] Teams competed not only against the goals they had set for themselves but also against other teams at their stores or in their region—competition among teams was encouraged. In addition, stores went through two review processes—a store tour and a "customer snapshot." Each store was toured periodically and subjected to a rigorous evaluation by a group of 40 personnel from another region; the group included region heads, store team leaders, associate team leaders, and leaders from two operating teams. Customer snapshots involved a surprise inspection by a headquarters official or regional president who rated the store on 300 items; each store had 10 surprise inspections annually, with the results distributed to every store and included in the reward system. Rewards were team-based and tied to performance metrics—all compensation was publicly disclosed.

Whole Foods had a salary cap that limited the compensation (wages plus profit incentive bonuses) of any team member to 14 times the average total compensation of all full-time team members in the company—a policy mandated in the company's core values (see Exhibit 3). The salary cap was raised from 10 to 14 times the average total compensation in 2005—it had been 8 times in 2003; the increases stemmed from the need to attract and retain key executives. For example, if the average total compensation was $50,000, then a cap of

10 times the average meant that an executive could not be paid more than $500,000. Such an amount was below top-level salaries at companies of comparable size and growing as rapidly as Whole Foods. In 2005, the average annual compensation was $73,061 for salaried workers and $25,451 for hourly workers. Any employee could look up anyone else's pay.

Promotions were primarily from within, with people often moving up to assume positions at stores soon to be opened or at stores in other regions.

The Use of Economic Value Added   In 1999, Whole Foods adopted an economic value added (EVA) management and incentive system. EVA is defined as net operating profits after taxes minus a charge for the cost of capital necessary to generate that profit. EVA at the store level was based on store contribution (store revenues minus cost of goods sold minus store operating expenses) relative to store investment over and above the cost of capital—see Exhibit 5 for average store contribution percentages. Senior executives managed the company with the goal of *improving* EVA at the store level and companywide; they believed that an EVA-based bonus system was the best financial framework for team members to use in helping make decisions that created sustainable shareholder value. The teams in all stores were challenged to find ways to boost store contribution and EVA—the team member bonuses paid on EVA improvement averaged 6 percent in 2003.

In 2005, over 500 senior executives, regional managers, and the store leaders were on EVA-based incentive compensation plans. The primary measure for payout was EVA improvement. In fiscal year 2001, the company's overall EVA was a negative $30.4 million, but companywide EVA was $2.6 million in fiscal 2003, $15.6 million in fiscal 2004, and a record $25.8 million in 2005.

In addition, management used EVA calculations to determine whether the sales and profit projections for new stores would yield a positive and large enough EVA to justify the investment; EVA was also used to guide decisions on store closings and to evaluate new acquisitions.

Purchasing and Distribution

Whole Foods' buyers purchased most of the items retailed in the company's stores from local, regional, and national wholesale suppliers and vendors. In recent years, the company had shifted much of the buying responsibility from the store level to the regional and national levels in order to put the company in a better position to negotiate volume discounts with major vendors and distributors. Whole Foods Market was the largest account for many suppliers of natural and organic foods. United Natural Foods was the company's biggest supplier, accounting for about 20 percent of Whole Foods' purchases.

Whole Foods owned two produce procurement centers and procured and distributed the majority of its produce itself. However, where feasible, local store personnel sourced produce items from local organic farmers as part of the company's commitment to promote and support organic farming methods. Two subsidiaries, the Pigeon Cove seafood processing facility in Massachusetts and Select Fish, a West Coast seafood processing facility, supplied a portion of the company's seafood requirements. A regional seafood distribution facility had recently been established in Atlanta.

The company operated eight regional distribution centers to supply its stores. The largest distribution center in Austin supplied a full range of natural products to the company's stores in Texas, Louisiana, Colorado, Kansas, and New Mexico; the other seven regional centers distributed mainly produce and private-label goods to area stores. Twelve regional bake houses and five regional commissary kitchens supplied area stores with various prepared foods. A central coffee-roasting operation supplied stores with the company's Allegro brand of coffees.

Community Citizenship and Social Activism

Whole Foods demonstrated its social conscience and community citizenship in two ways: (1) by donating at least 5 percent of its after-tax profits in cash or products to nonprofit or educational organizations and (2) by giving each team member 20 hours of paid community service hours to use for volunteer work for every 2,000 hours worked. Team members at every store were heavily involved in such community citizenship activities as sponsoring blood donation drives, preparing meals for seniors and the homeless, holding fund-raisers to help the disadvantaged, growing vegetables for a domestic violence shelter, participating in housing renovation projects, and working as deliverypeople for Meals on Wheels.

Further, John Mackey indicated the company was sincere in living up to its core values as they related to healthy eating habits and protection of environmental ecosystems. In an effort to "walk the talk," Mackey had initiated the gathering of information about key issues that could affect people's health and well-being—the genetic engineering of food supplies, food irradiation practices, and the organic standards process; Whole Foods disseminated this information via in-store brochures, presentations to groups, and postings on its Web site. Mackey had also charged company personnel with developing position statements on sustainable seafood practices (see Exhibit 8), the merits of organic farming, and wise environmental practices. Whole Foods regularly publicized its position statements in its stores and on its Web site, along with the company's commitment to selling only those meats that had been raised without the use of growth hormones, antibiotics, and animal by-products. Company personnel were conscientious in identifying and implementing "green" actions on Whole Foods' part that enhanced the health of the planet's ecosystems. The company's Web site had a legislative action center that alerted people to pending legislation on these types of issues and made it easy for them to send their comments and opinions to legislators and government officials.

In 2004, *Business Ethics* named Whole Foods Market to its list "100 Best Corporate Citizens."

Whole Foods Market's Financial Performance

From 1991 to 2005, Whole Foods Market's net income rose at a compound average rate of 37.4 percent. The company had been profitable every year except one since 1991, when it became a public company. The one money-losing year in 2000, which involved a net loss of $8.5 million, stemmed from a decision to divest a nutritional supplement business and losses in two affiliated dot-com enterprises (Gaiam.com and WholePeople.com) in which Whole Foods owned a minority interest. The company's stock price had jumped from $30 in December 2000 to $152.50 as of December 1, 2005, and was set for a 2-for-1 stock split in January 2006.

Whole Foods paid its first quarterly dividend of $0.15 per share in January 2004; the quarterly dividend was increased to $0.19 per share in January 2005, to $0.25 per share in April 2005, and to $0.30 per share starting in January 2006 (before the scheduled stock split). The company's business was generating strong, positive cash flows. In fiscal 2004, for instance, cash flow from operations was $330 million, allowing Whole Foods to self-fund $265 million in capital expenditures (of which $155 million was for new stores) and cover cash outlays of $28 million for dividends. In fiscal 2005, Whole Foods realized $411 million in cash flow from operations, which more than covered $324 million

---

Exhibit 8   **Whole Foods' Position on Seafood Sustainability**

The simple fact is our oceans are soon to be in trouble. Our world's fish stocks are disappearing from our seas because they have been overfished or harvested using damaging fishing practices. To keep our favorite seafood plentiful for us to enjoy and to keep it around for future generations, we must act now.

As a shopper, you have the power to turn the tide. When you purchase seafood from fisheries using ocean-friendly methods, you reward their actions and encourage other fisheries to operate responsibly.

At Whole Foods Market, we demonstrate our long-term commitment to seafood preservation by:

- Supporting fishing practices that ensure the ecological health of the ocean and the abundance of marine life.
- Partnering with groups who encourage responsible practices and provide the public with accurate information about the issue.
- Operating our own well-managed seafood facility and processing plant, Pigeon Cove Seafood, located in Gloucester, Massachusetts.
- Helping educate our customers on the importance of practices that can make a difference now and well into the future.
- Promoting and selling the products of well-managed fisheries.

Source: Information posted at www.wholefoodsmarket.com (accessed November 26, 2004).

it 9   Whole Foods Market, Statement of Operations, Fiscal Years 2002–2005 (in thousands)

	Fiscal Year 2005	Fiscal Year 2004	Fiscal Year 2003	Fiscal Year 2002
Sales	$4,701,289	$3,864,950	$3,148,593	$2,690,475
Cost of goods sold and occupancy costs	3,048,870	2,523,816	2,070,334	1,758,281
Gross profit	1,652,419	1,341,134	1,078,259	932,194
Direct store expenses	1,199,870	986,040	794,422	677,704
Store contribution	452,549	355,094	283,837	254,490
General and administrative expenses	149,364	119,800	100,693	95,871
Share-based compensation*	19,896			
Pre-opening and relocation costs	37,035	18,648	15,765	17,934
Natural disaster costs†	16,521	—	—	—
Operating income	229,733	216,646	167,379	140,985
Interest expense, net	2,223	7,249	8,114	10,384
Investment and other income (loss)	9,623	6,456	5,593	2,056
Income before income taxes	237,133	215,853	164,858	132,657
Provision for income taxes	100,782	86,341	65,943	53,063
Net income	$ 136,351	$ 129,512	$ 98,915	$ 79,594
Basic earnings per share	$2.10	$2.11	$1.68	$1.41
Weighted average shares outstanding	65,045	61,324	59,035	56,385
Diluted earnings per share	$1.98	$1.98	$1.58	$1.32
Weighted average shares outstanding, diluted basis	69,975	67,727	65,330	63,340

*The company began expensing the costs of stock option compensation in 2005.

†Costs associated with damage to two stores in New Orleans resulting from Hurricane Katrina.

Sources: Company press release, November 9, 2005, and 2004 10K/A report.

in capital expenditures (of which $208 million was related to opening new stores) and dividend payments of $55 million. During fiscal 2005, Whole Foods also reduced its long-term debt from $164.7 million to $12.9 million. Exhibits 9 and 10 present the company's recent statements of operations and consolidated balance sheets.

COMPETITORS

The food retailing business was intensely competitive. The degree of competition Whole Foods faced varied from locality to locality, and to some extent from store location to store location within a given locale. Competitors included local, regional, and national supermarkets, along with specialty grocery stores and health and natural foods stores. Most supermarkets had offered at least a limited selection of natural and organic foods and some had chosen to expand their offerings aggressively. Whole Foods' executives had said it was to the company's benefit for conventional supermarkets to offer natural and organic foods for two reasons: First, it helped fulfill the company's mission of improving the health and well-being of people and the planet, and, second, it helped create new customers for Whole Foods by providing a gateway experience. They contended that as more

Exhibit 10   **Whole Foods Market, Consolidated Balance Sheet, Fiscal Years 2004–2005 (in thousands)**

	September 25, 2005	September 26, 2004
Assets		
Current assets:		
Cash and cash equivalents	$ 308,524	$ 194,747
Restricted cash	36,922	26,790
Trade accounts receivable	66,682	64,972
Merchandise inventories	174,848	152,912
Deferred income taxes	39,588	29,974
Prepaid expenses and other current assets	45,965	16,702
Total current assets	$ 672,529	$ 486,097
Property and equipment, net of accumulated depreciation and amortization	1,054,605	873,397
Goodwill	112,476	112,186
Intangible assets, net of accumulated amortization	21,990	24,831
Deferred income taxes	22,452	4,193
Other assets	5,244	20,302
Total assets	$1,889,296	$1,521,006
Liabilities and shareholders' equity		
Current liabilities:		
Current installments of long-term debt and capital lease obligations	$ 5,932	$ 5,973
Trade accounts payable	103,348	90,751
Accrued payroll, bonus and other benefits due team members	126,981	100,536
Dividends payable	17,208	9,361
Other current liabilities	164,914	128,329
Total current liabilities	$ 418,383	$ 334,950
Long-term debt and capital lease obligations, less current installments	12,932	164,770
Deferred rent liability	91,775	70,067
Other long-term liabilities	530	1,581
Total liabilities	$ 523,620	$ 571,368
Shareholders' equity:		
Common stock, no par value, 300,000 and 150,000 shares authorized; 68,009 and 62,771 shares issued; 67,954 and 62,407 shares outstanding in 2005 and 2004, respectively	874,972	535,107
Accumulated other comprehensive income	4,405	2,053
Retained earnings	486,299	412,478
Total shareholders' equity	$1,365,676	$ 949,638
Commitments and contingencies		
Total liabilities and shareholders' equity	$1,889,296	$1,521,006

Source: Company press release, November 9, 2005.

people were exposed to natural and organic products, they were more likely to become a Whole Foods customer because Whole Foods was the category leader for natural and organic products, offered the largest selection at competitive prices, and provided the most well-informed customer service.

Whole Foods Market's two biggest competitors in the natural foods and organics segment of the food retailing industry were Wild Oats Markets and Fresh Market. Another competitor with some overlap in products and shopping ambience was Trader Joe's. Supervalu/Save-a-Lot, the ninth largest supermarket chain in North America (see Exhibit 2), had begun an initiative to launch a chain of small natural and organic foods stores called Sunflower Markets.

Wild Oats Markets

Wild Oats Markets—a 113-store natural foods chain based in Boulder, Colorado—ranked second behind Whole Foods in the natural foods and organics segment. The company's stores were in 24 states and British Columbia, Canada; stores were operated under four names: Wild Oats Natural Marketplace, Henry's Marketplace, Sun Harvest, and Capers Community Markets. Founded in 1987, Wild Oats had sales of $1.05 billion in 2004, up from $969 million in 2003. In 1993 and 1994, Wild Oats was named one of the "500 Fastest-Growing Private Companies in America" by *Inc.* magazine. Interest quickly spread to Wall Street, and in 1996 Wild Oats became a public company traded on the Nasdaq under the symbol OATS. Grocery analysts believed that Wild Oats had close to a 3 percent market share of the natural and organic foods market in 2000, compared to about 14 percent for Whole Foods.

Wild Oats' CEO, Perry Odak, formerly the CEO of Ben & Jerry's Homemade until it was acquired by Unilever in 2000, joined the company in 2001 and had launched a turnaround strategy, which was still in progress in 2005. The company's prior CEO and founder, Mike Gilliland, had gone on an aggressive acquisition streak during the late 1990s to expand Wild Oats' geographic coverage; store growth peaked in 1999 with the acquisition of 47 stores. But Gilliland's acquisition binge piled up extensive debt and dropped the company into a money-losing position with too many stores, a dozen different store names, and a dozen different ways of operating. Product selection

and customer service were inconsistent from one location to another.

When Odak arrived in March 2001, he streamlined operations, closed 28 unprofitable stores, cut prices, trimmed store staffing by 100 employees, and launched a new, smaller prototype store with a heavier emphasis on fresh food. Merchandising and marketing were revamped. The strategy was to draw in more "crossover" shoppers with lower-priced produce, meat, and seafood, along with a Fresh Look program stressing freshness and affordability to increase store traffic and raise the average purchase above the current $19 level. While the lower prices cut into the company's gross profit margin, management had tried to restore margins by concentrating purchases with fewer vendors and getting better discounts. An agreement was reached in September 2002 for Wild Oats to obtain a substantial part of its store inventories from Tree of Life, one of the leading natural foods distributors. Another of Odak's strategic thrusts was to drive a customer service mindset throughout the organization via training programs and enhanced employee communication. Odak wanted to position Wild Oats as a resource for value-added services and education about health and well-being. In 2002 Wild Oats sold close to 4.45 million shares at $11.50 to raise capital for opening 58 stores in the next three years (13 in 2003, 20 in 2004, and 25 in 2005) and remodeling a number of existing stores. While both Whole Foods and Wild Oats had stores in some of the same urban areas and were targeting some of the same areas for expansion, Wild Oats was targeting city and metropolitan neighborhoods for its new stores where there were no Whole Foods stores.

Wild Oats' new prototype stores were 22,000 to 24,000 square feet and featured a grocery-store layout where produce, dairy, meat, seafood, and baked goods were around the perimeters of the store), an expanded produce section at the front of the store, a deli, a sushi bar, a juice and java bar, a reduced selection of canned and packaged items, and store-within-a-store sections for supplements and specialty personal care products. Wild Oats had completed the remodeling of six stores (as part of its overall store remodeling initiative begun in 2003); it opened 12 new stores in 2004 and closed, sold, or relocated 7 others; it was planning to open 12 stores and remodel 10 others in 2005—both new store numbers were below the original target set when new shareholder capital had been raised in 2002. Wild Oats ended 2004 with 2.45 million square feet of floor space in its 113 stores (versus 5.8 million for Whole Foods); its expansion plans called for a total of 2.6 million square feet of floor space by year-end 2006. Also, in 2004, Wild Oats (1) completed a transition to using United Natural Foods as its primary distributor; (2) consolidated its smaller produce warehouse facilities into a single, 240,000-square-foot, state-of-the-art perishables distribution center in Riverside, California; and (3) completed the centralization and reorganization of its operations to improve efficiency. Like Whole Foods, Wild Oats was expanding its private-label offerings—400 Wild Oats and Henry's products were scheduled for introduction in 2005.

As was the case at Whole Foods, Perry Odak believed that while conventional supermarkets would continue to expand their offerings of natural and organic products, the competitive threat posed by conventional supermarkets was only moderate because their selection was more limited than what Wild Oats stores offered and because they lacked the knowledge and high level of service provided by a natural foods supermarket. In his view, "They are introducing conventional shoppers to natural brands, which will benefit us in the long run."

Wild Oats' sales in 2004 were adversely affected by conventional grocers' overly aggressive promotional activity in Southern California and by intense competition in Texas. This competition resulted in negative comparable store sales throughout the third quarter in approximately one-third of the company's store base. As a result, comparable store customer traffic in the third quarter of 2004 was a negative 4.1 percent. Wild Oats management took "aggressive action" in the form of lower prices and additional promotions to rebuild its customer traffic and sales in regions affected by intense competitive activity. But despite all of the moves that had been made under Perry Odak's leadership, the company was still struggling. After reporting losses of $15.0 million in 2000 before Odak became CEO, Wild Oats recorded losses of $43.9 million in 2001, net income of $5.1 million in 2002, net income of $1.6 million in 2003, and a loss of $40.0 million in 2004. It was expecting a small profit for 2005—through the first nine months of fiscal 2005, Wild Oats reported a small net loss of $148,000 on sales of $841.2 million

(compared to sales of $766.2 million in the first nine months of 2004). Gross margins (sales minus cost of goods sold) at Wild Oats averaged about 28.5 percent in 2002–2005, compared to 34.5 percent at Whole Foods (see Exhibit 5). Wild Oats stores averaged sales per square foot of about $440 annually versus just over $800 for Whole Foods.

Odak's latest initiatives to improve Wild Oats Markets' performance were to offer Wild Oats branded products in other retail environments. The company had reached agreement to test two alternative retail concepts. The first—a test in the Chicago market with Peapod, the country's leading Internet grocer—began in October 2004 and involved offering more than 200 private-label products on the Peapod site to consumers in the greater Chicago metropolitan area. The second, which began in June 2005, was a three-to-five store test of a Wild Oats branded store-within-a-store concept with Stop & Shop, the largest food retailer in the northeastern United States.

In a June 2004 financial move, Wild Oats sold $100 million in 3.25 percent convertible debentures to private investors; the debentures were convertible into Wild Oats common stock, at the option of the holders, at an initial price of $17.70 per share and could be redeemed starting in May 2011. Management intended to use proceeds of the offering to accelerate its growth plans, fund the repurchase of $25 million in common stock, and finance other "general corporate purposes." Wild Oats stock had traded in the $6–$16 range since 2002 and in December 2005 was trading in the $11–$13 range.

Fresh Market

Fresh Market, headquartered in Greensboro, North Carolina, was a 50-store chain operating in 12 southeastern and midwestern states (Alabama, Florida, Georgia, North Carolina, South Carolina, Tennessee, Virginia, Louisiana, Indiana, Illinois, Ohio, and Kentucky).[16] The company was founded by Ray Berry, a former vice president with Southland Corporation who had responsibility over some 3,600 7-Eleven stores. The first Fresh Market store opened in 1982 in Greensboro. Berry borrowed ideas from stores he had seen all over the United States and, as the chain expanded, used his convenience-store experience to replicate the store format and shape the product lines. During the 1982–2000 period, Fresh Market's sales revenues grew at a 25.2 percent compound rate, reaching $193 million in 2000; revenues were an estimated $280 million in 2004. Fresh Market's goal was to be the food destination store for people who enjoy cooking and good eating. The company was founded on the premise of getting customers to return again and again by offering quality products at reasonable prices and providing top-notch customer service.

Fresh Market's product line included meats, seafood, fresh produce, fresh-baked goods, prepared foods, 40 varieties of coffees, a selection of grocery and dairy items, bulk products, cheeses and deli meats, wine and beer, and floral and gift items. Fresh Market stores averaged 18,000 square feet and were located in neighborhoods near educated, high-income residents. Fresh Market differentiated itself with "upscale grocery boutique" items such as free-range chicken; pick-and-pack spices; gourmet coffees; chocolates; hard-to-get H&H bagels from New York City; Ferrara's New York cheesecake; fresh Orsini parmesan cheese; Acqua della Madonna bottled water; and an extended selection of olive oils, mustards, bulk products (granolas, nuts, beans, dried fruits, spices, and snack mixes), wine, and beer. Stores also stocked a small assortment of floral items and gifts (cookbooks, gift cards, cutting boards, and gift baskets) and a bare lineup of general grocery products. None of the meats and seafood and few of the deli products were prepackaged, and each department had at least one employee in the area constantly to help shoppers—the idea was to force interaction between store employees and shoppers. Fresh Market's warm lights, classical background music and terra-cotta-colored tiles made it a cozier place to shop than a typical grocery store. From time to time, stores had cooking classes, wine tastings, and food-sampling events. Fresh Market sponsored an annual fund-raiser for the Juvenile Diabetes Research Foundation called the Root Beer Float. The average store had 75 employees, resulting in labor costs about double those of typical supermarkets.

Merchandisers at Fresh Market's headquarters selected the stores' products, but store managers placed orders directly from third-party distributors. According to Berry, Fresh Market didn't have the concentration of stores that would make running its own warehouses profitable; Berry believed some grocers' distribution operations had grown so big that they drove the retail business, rather than the other way around.

Since 2000, the company had opened 3 to 5 new stores each year, but going forward the company planned to open 8 to 10 new stores annually. Expansion was funded by internal cash flows and bank debt. Financial data was not available because the company was privately owned, but Fresh Market's profitability was believed to be above the industry average. Several public companies had shown interest in buying the chain. In 2001 Ray Berry, then age 60, had said, "If I can get what I think the company's worth three years from now, I'll sell it. But I won't sell it for what it's worth today because I'm having too much fun."

Trader Joe's

Based in Pasadena, California, Trader Joe's was a specialty supermarket chain with over 200 stores in Arizona, California, Connecticut, Delaware, Illinois, Indiana, Maryland, Massachusetts, Michigan, Missouri, Nevada, New Jersey, New Mexico, New York, Ohio, Oregon, Pennsylvania, Virginia, and Washington. Management described the company's mission and business as follows:

> At Trader Joe's, our mission is to bring our customers the best food and beverage values and the information to make informed buying decisions. There are more than 2000 unique grocery items in our label, all at honest everyday low prices. We work hard at buying things right: Our buyers travel the world searching for new items and we work with a variety of suppliers who make interesting products for us, many of them exclusive to Trader Joe's. All our private label products have their own "angle," i.e., vegetarian, Kosher, organic or just plain decadent, and all have minimally processed ingredients.
>
> Customers tell us, "I never knew food shopping could be so much fun!" Some even call us "The home of cheap thrills!" We like to be part of our neighborhoods and get to know our customers. And where else do you shop that even the CEO, Dan Bane, wears a loud Hawaiian shirt.
>
> Our tasting panel tastes every product before we buy it. If we don't like it, we don't buy it. If customers don't like it, they can bring it back for a no-hassle refund.
>
> We stick to the business we know: good food at the best prices! Whenever possible we buy direct from our suppliers, in large volume. We bargain hard and manage our costs carefully. We pay in cash, and on time, so our suppliers like to do business with us.
>
> Trader Joe's Crew Members are friendly, knowledgeable and happy to see their customers. They

taste our items too, so they can discuss them with their customers. All our stores regularly cook up new and interesting products for our customers to sample.[17]

Plans called for ongoing development and introduction of new, one-of-a-kind food items at value prices, and continued expansion of store locations across the country.

Prices and product offerings varied somewhat by region and state. Customers could choose from a variety of baked goods, organic foods, fresh fruits and vegetables, imported and domestic cheeses, gourmet chocolates and candies, coffees, fresh salads, meatless entrées and other vegan products, low-fat and low-carbohydrate foods, frozen fish and seafood, heat-and-serve entrées, packaged meats, juices, wine and beer, snack foods, energy bars, vitamins, nuts and trail mixes, and whatever other exotic items the company's buyers had come upon. About 10–15 new, seasonal, or one-time-buy items were introduced each week. Products that weren't selling well were dropped. Trader Joe's had recently worked with its vendors to remove genetically modified ingredients from all of its private-label products. It had also discontinued sale of duck meat because of the cruel conditions under which ducks were grown.

Stores were open, with wide aisles, appealing displays, cedar plank walls, a nautical decor, and crew members wearing colorful Hawaiian shirts. Because of its combination of low prices, emporium-like atmosphere, intriguing selections, and friendly service, customers viewed shopping at Trader Joe's as an enjoyable experience. The company was able to keep the prices of its unique products attractively low (relative to those at Whole Foods, Fresh Market, and Wild Oats) partly because its buyers were always on the lookout for exotic items they could buy at a discount (all products had to pass a taste test and a cost test) and partly because most items were sold under the Trader Joe's label.

Sunflower Markets

Sunflower Markets, out to establish a discount niche in organic and natural foods, entered the market in 2003 with four stores—two in Phoenix, one in Albuquerque, and one in Denver.[18] As of November 2004 the company had opened three additional stores in Arizona and one in Colorado. Based in Longmont, Colorado, Sunflower's strategy borrowed from concepts employed by Trader Joe's and

small farmers' market–type stores. The company's mission statement described its four-pronged strategic approach:

- We Will Always Offer the Best Quality Food at the Lowest Prices in Town. "Better-than-supermarket quality at better-than-supermarket prices" is our motto.

- We Keep Our Overhead Low. No fancy fixtures or high rent. No corporate headquarters . . . just regular people, like you, looking for the best deals we can find.

- We Buy Big. We source directly, we pay our vendors quickly and we buy almost everything by the pallet or truckload. That buying power means big savings for you!

- We Keep It Simple. We don't charge our vendors "slotting allowances" or shelf space fees. Just honest-to-goodness negotiating for the lowest possible price and we pass the savings on to you.

The company's tag line was "Serious Food . . . Silly Prices." According to founding partner Mark Gilliland, "The last thing we want to be is another wanna-be Whole Foods." Gilliland was formerly the founder and president of Wild Oats but was forced out when his aggressive expansion strategy put Wild Oats in a financial bind.

Each Sunflower Market was about 40,000 square feet and had a warehouse-like atmosphere, with no customer service except for check-out personnel. Stores featured many one-of-a-kind items purchased in large lots from brokers. Pallets of goods were placed wherever floor space was available.

In late 2005, Sunflower had begun downsizing some of its stores to the 30,000-square-foot range and reducing the number of sections within each category—for instance, it was decreasing its selections of capers from 19 to 2 varieties.

Supervalu/Save-a-Lot

In early 2006, Minneapolis-based Supervalu, a Fortune 500 company with 2005 sales of $19.5 billion that operated 649 corporate stores (under eight brands) and 841 licensed Save-A-Lot stores in 40 states, was on the front end of launching a new 12,000- to 15,000-square-foot grocery format called Sunflower Market. The first Sunflower Market opened in January 2006 in Indianapolis as a value-priced organic and natural food store. The stores were modeled after Supervalu's Save-A-Lot small-box, limited-assortment format but had a focus on natural and organic products. Sunflower's offerings consisted of 8,000 to 12,000 stock-keeping units (SKUs) of grocery, frozen and dairy items, produce, deli and cheese, bakery, café, hormone- and antibiotic-free meat and seafood, beer and wine, and wellness products. All Sunflower Market stores were to be operated by Supervalu. Supervalu's venture had no connection to Mike Gilliland's Sunflower Market chain; Supervalu had trademarked the Sunflower name some years earlier and had licensed it to Gilliland for use in the Southwest. It was expected that the first wave of Supervalu's Sunflower Market stores would be opened in the Midwest, where Wild Oats and Whole Foods had comparatively few stores.

Jeff Noddle, Supervalu's chairman and CEO, said, "Across the nation, we are seeing a growing demand for affordable organic foods with exceptional taste and nutritional quality. Sunflower Market draws on our expertise in small-box formats, and leverages our supply chain expertise, which enables us to deliver outstanding natural and organic products at a price point consistent with consumer expectations."[19] Supervalu decided to enter the natural and organics market because the 17 to 21 percent annual growth in sales of natural and organic products was eight times higher than the growth of the conventional food market and because of the success of Whole Foods and Wild Oats. Supervalu's research indicated that 96 percent of consumers purchased organic products occasionally and 27 percent of grocery shoppers bought organics weekly. Another Supervalu executive noted, "Organics is not a fad. It is fast becoming a constant in consumers' lives. By offering these items in a convenient neighborhood market at a value price point, we create a compelling proposition for the middle-market consumer." Supervalu management believed that the company's ownership of specialty produce company W. Newell & Co. would enable Sunflower's prices to run 10 to 15 percent below that of conventional and natural food stores. Supervalu was also launching a new 100-plus-item line of private-label organic and natural products under the Nature's Best brand at Sunflower Market and planned to also make the brand available to Supervalu's 2,200 distribution customers.

Independent Natural and Health Food Grocers

In 2005 there were approximately 14,000 small, independent retailers of natural and organic foods, vitamins/supplements, and beauty and personal care products. Most were single-store, owner-managed enterprises. Combined sales of the 14,000 independents were in the $15 billion range in 2004. Two other vitamin/supplement chains, General Nutrition and Vitamin World, dominated the vitamin/supplement segment with about 7,500 store locations. Most of the independent stores had less than 2,500 square feet of retail sales space and generated revenues of less than $1 million annually, but there were roughly 850 natural foods and organic retailers with store sizes exceeding 6,000 square feet and sales of between $1 million and $5 million annually.

Product lines and range of selection at the stores of independent natural and health foods retailers varied from narrow to moderately broad, depending on a store's market focus and the shopper traffic it was able to generate. Inventories at stores under 1,000 square feet could run as little as $10,000, while those at stores of 6,000 square feet or more often ranged from $400,000 to $1.2 million. Many of the independents had some sort of deli or beverage bar, and some even had a small dine-in area with a limited health food menu. Revenues and customer traffic at most independent stores were trending upward, reflecting growing buyer interest in natural and organic products. Most independent retailers had average annual sales per square foot of store space of $200 (for stores under 2,000 square feet) to as much as $470 (for stores greater than 6,000 square feet)—Whole Foods' average was over $800 per square foot in 2005.[20]

Endnotes

[1]As quoted in Elizabeth Lee, "National Standards Now Define Organic Food," *Atlanta Journal and Constitution,* October 21, 2002.

[2]Press release, May 22, 2003, www.newfarm.org (accessed November 24, 2004).

[3]Organic Trade Association, "2004 Manufacturer Survey," www.ota.com (accessed November 28, 2005).

[4]Cited in the Trendspotting section of *Natural Foods Buyer,* Fall 2004, www.newhope.com (accessed November 26, 2004).

[5]Company press release, November 18, 2005.

[6]Letter to shareholders, 2003 annual report.

[7]Prices cited in "Eating Too Fast at Whole Foods," *BusinessWeek,* October 24, 2005, p. 84.

[8]Hollie Shaw, "Retail-Savvy Whole Foods Opens in Canada," *National Post,* May 1, 2002, p. FP9.

[9]See Karin Schill Rives, "Texas-Based Whole Foods Market Makes Changes to Cary, N.C., Grocery Store," *News and Observer,* March 7, 2002.

[10]As quoted in Marilyn Much, "Whole Foods Markets: Austin, Texas Green Grocer Relishes Atypical Sales," *Investors Business Daily,* September 10, 2002.

[11]As quoted in "Whole Foods Market to Open in Albuquerque, N.M.," *Santa Fe New Mexican,* September 10, 2002.

[12]EVA at the store level was based on store contribution (store revenues minus cost of goods sold minus store operating expenses) relative to store investment over and above the cost of capital.

[13]As quoted in John K. Wilson, "Going Whole Hog with Whole Foods," Bankrate.com, December 23, 1999. Mackey made the statement in 1991 when efforts were being made to unionize the company's store in Berkeley, California.

[14]Company press release, January 21, 2003.

[15]Information contained in John R. Wells and Travis Haglock, "Whole Foods Market, Inc." Harvard Business School case study 9-705-476.

[16]Much of the information in this section is based on M. E. Lloyd, "Specialty-Grocer Fresh Market Cultivates Upscale Consumers, Reaps Big Returns," *The Wall Street Journal,* February 20, 2001, p. B11, and information posted at www.freshmarket.com (accessed December 1, 2005).

[17]Information posted at www.traderjoes.com (accessed December 1, 2005).

[18]This section is based on information posted at www.sunflowermarkets.com and in Joe Lewandowski, "Naturals Stores Freshen Their Strategies," *Natural Foods Merchandiser,* January 1, 2004 (accessed November 19, 2004, at www.naturalfoodsmerchandiser.com).

[19] Company press release, October 19, 2005.

[20]*Natural Foods Merchandiser,* June 2004, p. 27.

Oliver's Markets

Armand Gilinsky Jr.
Sonoma State University

Richard L. McCline
San Francisco State University

John Moore
Sonoma State University

In September 2005, Oliver's Markets was nearing completion of an estimated $500,000 remodel of its original Cotati, California, store when its top management team, consisting of Steve Maass (owner) and Tom Scott (general manager), quickly had to decide whether or not to bid on an expansion opportunity. Oliver's Markets consisted of two supermarkets in Sonoma County, one in Cotati and the other in nearby Santa Rosa, which together generated about $40 million in sales per year. Sonoma County was situated at the northern fringe of the San Francisco Bay Area, about an hour's driving time from the Golden Gate Bridge. Oliver's had just been informed by its grocery wholesaler that Kroger's, a national chain, was selling 20 supermarkets in the San Francisco Bay Area. Within a week of receiving the list of Kroger's locations for sale, Steve and Tom narrowed the choice to two stores—Ralph's Supermarket in Santa Rosa and Bell's Market in Novato. Novato was in Marin County, about 30 minutes south of Santa Rosa. Oliver's had one week to tender a bid on one or both of the Kroger stores, either of which could cost an estimated $2 million to retrofit, in addition to the ongoing lease and operating costs.

In deciding whether or not to purchase and retrofit the new site(s), Steve and Tom were primarily guided by logistics, that is, proximity to existing stores, and by expected leasehold costs. Of greater concern, perhaps, was how to continue to differentiate Oliver's Markets from other supermarket chains. Prominent among these rivals, Trader Joe's,

Costco, and Whole Foods had recently entered Oliver's Markets' sales territory with brand-new stores; Wal-Mart and Target had also announced plans to develop regional supercenters, that is, large-format discount supermarkets, in California. See Exhibit 1 for an explanation of supermarket terms.

OLIVER'S HISTORY

In 1988, Steve Oliver Maass purchased the then bankrupt Cotati Farmer's Market. He recalled:

> We came in here and it was just the worst store I'd ever seen. I looked at it and I said I know I can do a better job than this store has been doing. There's just no way I'd do this bad a job. But I had absolutely no grocery experience, none. I worked in the produce department of a grocery store, which isn't the same. We went to bankruptcy court and bought it for $200,000, I mortgaged my house. There wasn't a lot of money so we painted, and cleaned, and cleaned. What Farmer's had done is they had eliminated things that didn't work, instead of trying to figure out how to make them work. They wouldn't carry lamb because they wouldn't sell it. They had very little to offer. The first question I asked was, "Why would anyone want to shop here?"

Steve named his new store Oliver's Market, using his middle name because he thought that would sound more upscale than Steve's Market. His wife, Ruth, worked in the store for about the first four years, much of the time as a self-trained bookkeeper. Oliver's was organized as a Subchapter S corporation. Steve Maass was president, and Ruth Maass was vice president and secretary. They were co-owners.

Exhibit 1   **Glossary of Supermarket Terms**

Grocery store—Any retail store selling a line of dry grocery, canned goods, or nonfood items as well as some perishable items.

Supermarket—Any full-line self-service grocery store generating a sales volume of $2 million or more annually.

Convenience store—Any full-line, self-service grocery store that is open long hours, is easy to access, and offers limited line of high-convenience items. The majority sell gasoline with an annual sales of $2 million or more.

Independent—An operator of fewer than 11 retail stores.

Chain—An operator of 11 or more retail stores.

Wholesale club—A membership retail/wholesale hybrid with a varied selection and limited variety of products presented in a warehouse-type environment. These 120,000-square-foot stores have 60 percent to 70 percent general merchandise/health and beauty care and a grocery line dedicated to large sizes and bulk sales. Memberships include both business accounts and consumer groups. Examples are Sam's Club, Costco, and BJ's.

Supercenter—A large food/drug combination store and mass merchandiser under a single roof. The supercenters offer a wide variety of food, as well as nonfood merchandise. These stores average more than 170,000 square feet and typically devote as much as 40 percent of the space to grocery items. Examples are Wal-Mart, Kmart, Super Target, Meijer, and Fred Meyer.

Sources: Progressive Grocer's 2003 Marketing Guidebook and Bishop Consulting, 2003.

Oliver's added a deli in 1990, and an aisle of health foods in 1991. In 1994, the city of Cotati offered Steve and Ruth Maass a low-interest redevelopment loan of $500,000. They used the money to expand by taking over the adjacent space and adding an additional 11,000 square feet, for a total of 36,000 square feet with about 28,000 square feet of selling space. Steve recalled:

> At that time I decided that, in every aisle, we would have the same things that Whole Foods did. We would give people a choice in all their health foods and we would integrate it throughout the store. There isn't a section you can go to where you won't have a good selection of organic or health foods and conventional. We didn't mirror Whole Foods so much as Whole Foods did a wonderful job on health foods, and people were going in there and buying it. But we couldn't sell health foods. The only reason we couldn't sell it was because we weren't doing it well enough. So, we learned how to do it well enough, and we did it everywhere.

Oliver's opened a second store in Santa Rosa on April 4, 2000, and thenceforth changed its name to Oliver's Markets. Steve recalled:

> The landlord came to us. I wasn't really that interested in expanding at the time. It was a good deal, as we didn't have to pay anything for the store. We considered hiring a nationally known retail architect, but decided that was too costly, so we just sort of designed it ourselves. We picked the colors out and figured out what we wanted for a deli. I think the deli was to a large degree fashioned after Woodlands Market, the best little market I've seen.[1]

In 2005, Oliver's began a remodel of its Cotati store. Steve had hoped to invest $2 million in the remodel, but uncertainty over the future of the lease forced him to scale back his plans. He recounted, "Our landlords wouldn't talk to us. I couldn't even get a meeting going with them. I wanted to get another ten years on the lease so we could put a couple million dollars in here and do a really good job. Even with nine years left on this lease we're putting in $500,000, because otherwise we'll get down to the sixth or seventh year and be in trouble."

Steve himself was now 59 years old and had been in the business since 1988. Ruth was ill with cancer. Steve and Ruth's only child, Eva, 40, had worked full-time for Oliver's for about four years, primarily as the scan coordinator at the Cotati store. She had worked part-time as needed, doing an assortment of jobs—such as bookkeeper and gift buyer. Steve reflected that Eva was extremely smart and quite capable, but as a musician and painter she was more interested in Oliver's design and decor than in the business side. She had, for example, designed and purchased new fixtures for a remodeled gift department. Steve and Tom were both working to involve her more in various aspects of the operation.

Exhibit 2 presents milestones in Oliver's Markets' history. Oliver's recent track record is shown

Exhibit 2   **Oliver's Markets' Milestones**

1988	Oliver's in Cotati opened
1990	Service deli added
1991	Health foods added
1994	Cotati store enlarged with an additional 11,000 square feet; natural and organic products added in every category throughout store
2000	Oliver's in Santa Rosa opened
2004	5,000-square-foot warehouse opened adjacent to the Santa Rosa store
2005	Cotati store remodeling started in May
2005	Oliver's named one of six Outstanding Retailers of 2005 by the National Association for the Specialty Food Trade.

Source: Oliver's Markets Inc.

in Exhibits 3 and 4, containing 2000–2004 income statements for the two Oliver's Markets. The financial condition of Oliver's as a consolidated entity is shown in Exhibit 5, presenting 2003 and 2004 consolidated balance sheets. Exhibit 6 provides a comparison of Oliver's performance to selected industry standards. Exhibit 7 provides comparisons of Oliver's performance to industrywide statistics on cost items, including labor and rent.

FOOD RETAILING IN THE UNITED STATES

Supermarkets had become the dominant form of food retailer in the United States throughout the second half of the 20th century, but by the early 2000s, that dominance was being challenged by five major trends: (1) the increasing dominance of warehouse club stores and discount supercenters such as Costco and Wal-Mart's Sam's Clubs, (2) increased purchases of prepared foods away from home in restaurants and fast-food outlets, (3) chronic overcapacity in the supermarket industry, (4) changing shopping patterns due to the emergence of "lifestyle" food operators and Internet delivery services, and (5) higher labor costs, particularly for chains that had a unionized labor force.

Discount Supermarkets

Owing to a growing number of price-sensitive and time-pressed customers, traditional supermarkets struggled to protect their market share against discount supercenters or "hypermarkets," warehouse club stores, dollar stores, and drugstores. Such non-traditional retail outlets increased their share of consumers' food-at-home expenditures from 17.7 percent in 1998 to 30.8 percent in 2003. According to the U.S. Department of Agriculture (USDA), traditional retailers' market share declined from 82.3 percent to 69.2 percent over the same period.[2] Wal-Mart was both a driver and a beneficiary of this change in shopping patterns: its share of U.S. supermarket sales reached 15.2 percent by 2003.[3] In 2004, Wal-Mart opened its first California supercenter, marking the format's entry into the country's most populous state. By 2007, the number of Wal-Mart supercenters nationwide was forecast by *Progressive Grocer* to approach 2,000, translating into a 35 percent share of food store industry sales.[4] Union Bank of Switzerland (UBS) predicted that traditional supermarkets' share of food sales would drop to 63 percent by 2006, as shown in Exhibit 8.[5]

Food Prepared Away from Home

Food-service operators—including restaurants and fast-food outlets—were increasing their share of consumers' total food dollars. Long-term trends showed that increases in household incomes, due in part to the growth of dual-income households, had raised the share of food spending devoted to prepared foods and meals. By 2002, food-service outlets accounted for 46.1 percent of all food spending, up from 45.4 percent in 1990 and 39 percent in 1980.[6] According to *American Demographics,* from 1996 to 2001, married couples with children reduced the fraction of their food budget spent on food to

(*Continued on page C-35*)

Exhibit 3 Oliver's Markets' Five-Year Income Statements, 2000–2004—Cotati Store (in thousands)

	2000	2001	2002	2003	2004
Sales					
Grocery	$ 5,929.2	$ 6,192.4	$ 6,154.9	$ 5,835.4	$ 5,658.2
Floral	211.8	236.2	249.4	223.3	196.8
Liquor	2,016.0	2,038.2	2,090.8	1,902.7	1,823.3
Meat	1,696.6	1,761.4	1,795.1	1,745.1	1,678.9
Natural foods	3,051.8	3,296.7	3,692.1	3,743.3	3,788.6
Produce	1,886.5	2,059.9	2,235.9	2,205.3	2,254.0
Deli	1,806.1	2,041.1	2,537.8	2,725.6	2,619.4
Bakery	1,007.4	1,086.8	1,158.8	1,149.2	1,046.8
Sushi bar	274.8	260.4	270.4	270.5	232.6
Billbacks	108.0	78.1	45.5	51.8	56.4
Total sales	$ 17,988.3	$ 19,051.4	$ 20,230.8	$ 19,852.2	$ 19,355.3
Cost of sales					
Grocery	$ 4,150.9	4,294.4	4,249.1	4,008.1	3,961.1
Floral	153.3	172.5	174.9	143.4	135.4
Liquor	1,415.1	1,440.8	1,480.0	1,379.6	1,374.0
Meat	1,177.3	1,142.5	1,202.6	1,209.4	1,141.4
Natural foods	1,942.0	2,099.9	2,394.3	2,465.6	2,487.5
Produce	1,159.7	1,244.6	1,325.0	1,317.8	1,364.5
Deli	877.7	1,006.4	1,198.5	1,348.9	1,295.5
Bakery	579.9	643.5	656.0	628.8	595.5
Sushi bar	208.6	195.4	202.8	202.9	174.7
Total cost of sales	$ 11,664.5	$ 12,240.0	$ 12,883.2	$ 12,704.5	$ 12,529.6
Gross profit	$ 6,323.8	$ 6,811.3	$ 7,347.6	$ 7,147.7	$ 6,825.7
Operating expenses					
Wages	$ 2,640.4	$ 2,925.3	$ 3,137.1	$ 3,298.7	$ 214.8
Benefits	593.5	684.7	1,014.7	1,163.7	1,256.3
Supplies	324.1	304.7	295.2	314.1	300.1
Rent	320.8	334.0	364.1	350.1	378.3
Telephone	10.9	12.7	7.4	6.6	6.9
Utilities	172.8	291.9	264.1	259.3	256.7
Garbage	32.3	34.5	42.1	46.2	49.0
Repair	179.1	144.5	165.2	149.9	167.4
Customer refunds	0.4	0.4	0.2	0.4	0.2
Depreciation	111.8	60.0	93.0	162.0	165.0
Taxes and licenses	27.9	19.1	32.9	23.5	23.4
Administrative	456.4	476.1	467.7	496.3	503.7
Other costs	108.0	131.9	179.2	209.1	224.6
Total operating expense	$ 4,978.5	$ 5,419.8	$ 6,062.9	$ 6,479.9	$ 6,546.3
Income from operations	$ 1,345.3	$ 1,391.5	$ 1,284.8	$ 667.8	$ 279.4
Other income and expense					
Interest expense	12.2	11.6	11.3	11.1	10.8
Other income	—	(11.0)	(15.9)	(14.9)	(12.7)
Total other income (expense)	12.2	0.6	(4.6)	(3.9)	(1.9)
Pretax income (loss)	$ 1,357.4	$ 1,392.1	$ 1,280.2	$ 664.0	$ 277.5

Note: Fiscal year is same as calendar year.

Source: Oliver's Markets Inc.

Exhibit 4 **Oliver's Markets' Five-Year Income Statements, 2000–2004 —Santa Rosa Store (in thousands)**

	2000	2001	2002	2003	2004
Sales					
Grocery	$ 2,988.9	$ 4,287.1	$ 4,569.0	$ 4,935.7	$ 5,090.3
Floral	58.9	200.5	223.8	251.9	248.6
Liquor	962.1	1,389.1	1,548.5	1,576.7	1,647.2
Meat	1,206.6	1,766.9	1,933.9	2,226.5	2,318.2
Natural foods	1,278.6	2,112.5	2,503.5	2,930.0	3,252.8
Produce	1,056.7	1,651.7	2,037.0	2,400.5	2,544.1
Deli	1,310.4	2,177.3	2,640.7	3,200.7	3,546.4
Bakery	493.9	786.5	924.5	990.1	981.0
Sushi bar	146.5	200.8	226.6	235.3	229.9
Billbacks	24.8	55.7	29.5	28.1	43.7
Total sales	$ 9,527.4	$ 14,628.0	$ 16,636.9	$ 18,775.4	$ 19,902.1
Cost of sales					
Grocery	$ 2,193.5	$ 2,984.1	$ 3,162.7	$ 3,365.5	$ 3,470.5
Floral	50.2	171.5	171.9	162.6	161.3
Liquor	732.5	1,003.6	1,080.5	1,154.3	1,252.9
Meat	856.7	1,167.6	1,211.5	1,498.1	1,558.8
Natural foods	802.6	1,383.6	1,605.5	1,958.6	2,142.1
Produce	722.9	1,055.4	1,252.4	1,472.3	1,517.8
Deli	714.7	1,096.8	1,187.0	1,505.1	1,656.6
Bakery	304.0	473.3	542.1	583.0	570.7
Sushi bar	107.4	152.3	168.1	176.5	172.3
Total cost of sales	$ 6,484.7	$ 9,488.3	$ 10,381.6	$ 11,876.0	$ 12,503.0
Gross profit	$ 3,042.7	$ 5,139.7	$ 6,255.2	$ 6,899.3	$ 7,399.1
Operating expenses					
Wages	$ 1,890.4	$ 2,527.0	$ 2,764.5	$ 3,128.3	$ 3,320.1
Benefits	321.7	574.8	898.7	1,118.5	1,309.3
Supplies	245.2	242.0	246.4	286.6	292.8
Rent	196.5	288.5	337.0	377.4	410.0
Telephone	5.9	5.8	6.9	5.9	6.2
Utilities	119.1	185.1	181.0	213.0	200.2
Garbage	21.9	35.0	28.1	33.1	44.2
Repair	74.7	106.4	103.0	113.6	127.4
Customer refunds	0.3	0.2	0.3	0.6	0.2
Depreciation	266.0	144.0	197.0	250.0	279.0
Taxes and licenses	17.8	28.7	22.3	25.8	28.3
Administrative	287.2	356.9	386.0	468.7	517.6
Other costs	64.1	91.9	108.7	165.3	207.7
Total operating expense	$ 3,510.8	$ 4,586.5	$ 5,279.8	$ 6,186.9	$ 6,742.8
Income from operations	$ (468.1)	$ 553.3	$ 975.5	$ 712.4	$ 656.3
Other income and expense					
Interest expense	$ 126.0	$ 157.5	$ 144.2	$ 103.1	$ 85.8
Other income	3.2	—	(7.6)	(7.9)	(7.9)
Total other income (expense)	$ 129.2	$ 157.5	$ 136.5	$ 95.2	$ 77.9
Pretax income (loss)	$ (338.9)	$ 710.7	$ 1,112.0	$ 807.6	$ 734.2

Source: Oliver's Markets Inc.

Exhibit 5 Oliver's Markets, Consolidated Balance Sheets, 2003–2004

	Fiscal Year Ending 12/31	
	2003	2004
Assets		
Current assets		
Cash and marketable securities	$2,411,598	$2,310,120
Inventory	2,276,374	2,461,271
Note receivable		100,000
Prepaid expenses	534,718	345,883
Other current assets	742	5,673
Total current assets	$5,223,433	$5,222,948
Fixed assets		
Equipment	$3,218,389	$3,568,810
Less accumulated amortization	(2,482,489)	(2,861,360)
Total fixed assets	$ 735,900	$ 707,450
Other assets		
Goodwill and intangible assets	$ 71,441	$ 71,441
Less accumulated amortization	(11,730)	(11,730)
Total other assets	59,711	59,711
Total assets	$6,019,043	$5,990,109
Liabilities and stockholders' equity		
Current liabilities		
Accounts payable	$1,135,870	$1,144,713
Accrued payroll	211,522	124,076
Other accrued liabilities	620,746	597,420
Total current liabilities	$1,968,138	$1,866,209
Long-term debt		
Note payable	$1,000,331	$ 809,585
Stockholder loans	121,841	118,669
Total long-term debt	$1,122,172	$ 928,254
Stockholders' equity		
Common stock	$ 200,000	$ 200,000
Retained earnings	2,424,774	2,728,733
Accumulated adjustments	(703,976)	(624,929)
Current-year income	1,007,935	891,842
Total equity	$2,928,733	$3,195,646
Total liabiities and stockholders' equity	$6,019,043	$5,990,109

Source: Oliver's Markets Inc.

Exhibit 6   **Oliver's Markets Versus National Average Supermarket Performance, 2004**

	National Average	Oliver's Cotati	Oliver's Santa Rosa
Average supermarket:			
Selling area in square feet	31,245	28,000	17,500
Volume in millions	$ 13.35	$ 19.36	$ 19.90
Number of check-outs	9	8	6
Number of full-time equivalent employees	69	110	115
Weekly sales per:			
Store	$256,730	$372,217	$382,733
Check-out line	$ 28,414	$ 46,527	$ 63,789
Full-time equivalent employee	$ 3,730	$ 3,384	$ 3,328
Employee hour	$ 93.25	$ 84.59	$ 83.21
Square foot	$ 8.22	$ 13.29	$ 21.87

Source: Progressive Grocer, April 2004, p. 32. Oliver's Markets figures: supplied by Oliver's, for fiscal year 2004.

Exhibit 7   **Oliver's Markets Versus National Average Supermarket Operating Costs, 2003**

	National Average % of Sales	Oliver's Markets, Consolidated 2003
Gross margin	27.6%	36.4%
Expenses		
Payroll	11.4	16.6
Employee benefits	3.5	5.9
Utilities	1.3	1.2
Property rentals	1.8	1.9
Taxes and licenses	0.4	0.1
Insurance	0.3	0.2
Depreciation and amortization	1.3	1.1
Maintenance and repairs	0.7	0.7
Supplies	1.1	1.6
Other operating costs	3.8	3.5
Total expenses	25.7	36.4
Operating profit	1.6	3.6
Other income (expense)	0.1	0.1
Income before taxes	2.0	3.8

Sources: FMI Speaks 2004 Key Industry Facts—Prepared by FMI Information Service, July 2004, p. 16.

Exhibit 8   **Traditional Supermarket Share of U.S. Retail Food Dollars 1995–2006 (estimated)**

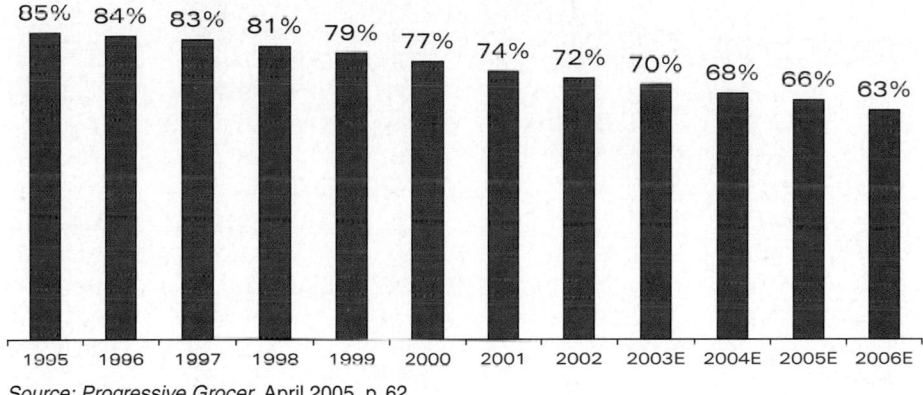

Source: Progressive Grocer, April 2005, p. 62.

be prepared at home from 62 percent to 59 percent, translating into a reduction of over $7 billion a year in food spending at retail outlets.[7]

Industry Overcapacity

Declining market share combined with growing store counts contributed to poor year-on-year comparable store sales growth results for the major supermarket chains. Many food retailers struggled with comparable store sales that had, at best, increased by 1 to 2 percent and, in some cases, decreased. Exhibit 9 presents 2000–2004 financial results for several national chains. With a net increase of 411 supermarkets in 2004, many industry analysts considered the industry to be at overcapacity.[8]

Changing Shopping Patterns

Nearly one-third (31 percent) of households shopped in 29 or more retailers or retail channels per year.[9] Due to increased competition from nontraditional food retailers, supermarkets suffered from a decline in shopping trips. In 1999, the average household made 83 trips to supermarkets; by 2004, that statistic had fallen to 69 trips, as shown in Exhibit 10.

Early in 2005, household penetration of supermarkets was below 100 percent for the first time in recent memory. One percent of shoppers, over a period of a year, had found that they could live without visiting a supermarket. That is, a tiny minority of consumers acquired all their food for home preparation without visiting a traditional supermarket. They did this by shopping at warehouse club stores, supercenters, dollar stores, and niche operators such as Trader Joe's. Some also shopped over the Internet, but the demise of Webvan and the sale of Peapod had largely left this market to traditional retailers, with perhaps the sole exception of FreshDirect, a rapidly growing Internet-based delivery service in New York City. Although many chains offered Internet shopping, Albertson's advertisements proclaimed that it was the largest Internet grocery provider in terms of geographic reach.

Labor Costs

Many traditional supermarkets faced another obstacle—higher labor costs—in their attempts to compete with Wal-Mart, Costco, and other nontraditional food retailers. The higher labor costs were due to the fact that traditional retailers were predominantly union shops. Three major Southern California supermarket chains, Safeway, Albertson's, and Kroger's settled a prolonged costly dispute with unionized workers in March 2004.[10]

The food retailing industry in Sonoma County and throughout northern California prior to 2005

Exhibit 9 Food Retail Chain Store Financial Statistics, 2000–2004

(\$ figures are in millions and include international operations)

	2000	2001	2002	2003	2004
Safeway[1]					
Comp store sales growth (%)	2.8%	2.3%	−0.7%	−2.4%	0.9%
Revenue	\$ 32,103	\$ 34,434	\$ 34,917	\$ 35,727	\$ 35,823
Gross profit	\$ 9,666	\$ 10,776	\$ 10,996	\$ 10,724	\$ 10,595
Gross margin %	30.11%	31.30%	31.49%	30.02%	29.58%
EBIT	\$ 2,282	\$ 2,589	\$ 948	\$ 574	\$ 1,173
Net income	\$ 1,092	\$ 1,254	\$ (828)	\$ (170)	\$ 560
Kroger[2]					
Comp store sales growth (%)	1.9%	1.5%	0.8%	0.3%	1.7%
Revenue	\$ 49,000	\$ 50,098	\$ 51,760	\$ 53,791	\$ 56,434
Gross profit	\$ 13,196	\$ 13,700	\$ 13,950	\$ 14,154	\$ 14,294
Gross margin %	26.93%	27.35%	26.95%	26.31%	25.33%
EBIT	\$ 2,183	\$ 2,359	\$ 2,569	\$ 1,370	\$ 847
Net Income	\$ 874	\$ 1,040	\$ 1,202	\$ 312	−\$ 100
Albertson's[3]					
Comp store sales growth (%)	0.6%	1.3%	−0.4%	−2.4%	0.2%
Revenue	\$ 35,221	\$ 36,294	\$ 35,316	\$ 35,107	\$ 39,897
Gross profit	\$ 9,989	\$ 10,337	\$ 10,298	\$ 10,048	\$ 11,187
Gross margin %	28.36%	28.48%	29.16%	28.62%	28.04%
EBIT	\$ 1,588	\$ 1,248	\$ 1,801	\$ 1,316	\$ 1,229
Net Income	\$ 765	\$ 501	\$ 485	\$ 556	\$ 444
Costco[4]					
Comp store sales growth (%)	11.0%	4.0%	6.0%	5.0%	10.0%
Revenue	\$ 32,169	\$ 34,797	\$ 38,762	\$ 42,456	\$ 48,107
Gross profit	\$ 3,847	\$ 4,199	\$ 4,779	\$ 5,221	\$ 6,015
Gross margin %	11.96%	12.07%	12.33%	12.30%	12.50%
EBIT	\$ 1,037	\$ 992	\$ 1,132	\$ 1,157	\$ 1,385
Net Income	\$ 631	\$ 602	\$ 700	\$ 721	\$ 882
Whole Foods[5]					
Comp store sales growth (%)	8.6%	9.2%	10.0%	8.6%	14.9%
Revenue	\$ 1,839	\$ 2,272	\$ 2,698	\$ 3,149	\$ 3,865
Gross profit	\$ 633	\$ 789	\$ 932	\$ 1,078	\$ 1,341
Gross margin %	34.42%	34.73%	34.54%	34.23%	34.70%
EBIT	\$ 94	\$ 104	\$ 141	\$ 167	\$ 216
Net Income	−\$ 5	\$ 65	\$ 82	\$ 100	\$ 132
Wal-Mart[6]					
Comp store sales growth (%)	5.0%	6.0%	5.0%	4.0%	3.0%
Revenue	\$180,787	\$204,011	\$229,616	\$256,320	\$285,222
Gross profit	\$ 40,067	\$ 44,914	\$ 51,317	\$ 57,573	\$ 65,249
Gross margin %	22.16%	22.02%	22.35%	22.46%	22.88%
EBIT	\$ 9,245	\$ 9,767	\$ 11,334	\$ 12,664	\$ 14,144
Net Income	\$ 6,235	\$ 6,592	\$ 7,955	\$ 9,054	\$ 10,267

[1] Safeway opened 34 "Lifestyle" stores in 2003 and remodeled 108 stores to the format by the end of that year.

[2] Kroger Co. includes advertising expense in cost of goods sold.

[3] Comp store sales for 2003 were down 0.1% for stores not affected by southern CA strike.

[4] Costco includes membership sales in total revenue; data also includes all products, not just supermarket items.

[5] Whole Foods includes occupancy expense in cost of goods sold.

[6] Comp store sales figures are for U.S. stores only; other figures include all products, not just supermarket items.

Sources: Annual reports as found on company Web sites and the U.S. Securities and Exchange Commission's Web site.

Exhibit 10   **Shopping Trip and Basket Size Statistics**

	1999	2000	2001	2002	2003	2004	Five-Year Change (%)
Percent of Households That Shop at Selected Retail Outlets							
Supermarkets	100%	100%	100%	100%	100%	99%	−1%
Mass merchants	95	94	95	93	91	89	−6
Drugstores	87	86	86	86	85	84	−3
Supercenters*	52	51	51	54	54	54	2
Dollar stores	52	55	59	62	66	67	15
Warehouse	50	49	50	52	51	51	1
Convenience/gas	50	48	45	46	45	44	−6
Annual Trips Made per Household							
Supermarkets	83	78	75	73	72	69	−14%
Mass merchants	26	25	24	23	21	20	−6
Drugstores	15	15	15	15	15	15	0
Supercenters*	15	17	20	22	25	27	12
Dollar stores	10	10	11	12	13	13	3
Warehouse	9	10	10	11	11	11	2
Convenience/gas	13	14	15	14	15	15	2
Total	171	169	170	169	172	170	−1%
Basket $ Size							
Supermarkets	$31	$32	$32	$33	$33	$34	3%
Mass merchants	36	38	39	41	41	42	6
Drugstores	18	19	19	20	20	20	2
Supercenters*	45	49	51	53	55	56	11
Dollar stores	10	11	11	11	11	11	1
Warehouse	82	83	82	83	83	83	1
Convenience/gas	9	10	10	10	11	12	3

* Includes Kmart, Target, and Wal-Mart supercenters.

Source: Progressive Grocer, April 2005, p. 60.

appeared to mirror the national scene with one major exception—the absence of Wal-Mart supercenters. Exhibit 11 shows store counts and estimated sales for selected retailers. In 2003, Safeway was the number one food retailer in Sonoma County; Oliver's ranked ninth in sales (Exhibit 12).

OLIVER'S STORE OPERATIONS

Oliver's flagship operation in Cotati was one part traditional supermarket, one part natural foods store, and one part gourmet foods store. The main entrance led directly into the health and beauty aids (HABA)

area of the store, which featured vitamins, homeo-pathic treatments, essential oils, and other natural HABA products. The department hired an in-store therapist four evenings a week to do massages. The placement and size of the department gave the store its predominant feel as a natural foods retailer. In virtually every area of the store, shoppers could find natural products, including organic baby food, or-ganic spices, and organic pet food.

Gourmet foods were also in abundance. In June 2005, Oliver's was one of just six retailers to be honored with an Outstanding Retailer Award by the National Association for the Specialty Food Trade. Oliver's had 108 stock-keeping units of olive oil, ranging from a 17-ounce bottle of Star Extra Virgin for $3.79, to a 101-ounce tin of Spectrum Naturals

Exhibit 11   **Store Counts and Estimated Grocery Sales, Northern California Food Retailers, 2004**

	Number of Stores	Estimated Grocery Sales ($ millions)
Safeway	251	$4,688
Albertson's	158	3,230
Raley's	113	2,320
Costco	35	2,250
Trader Joe's	44	340
Whole Foods	18	320
Ralph's (Kroger's)	17	363

Sources: Sales estimated using figures from *Progressive Grocer*'s annual list of the 50 largest food retailers (May 2005) and from information found on company Web sites.

Organic Spanish that retailed for $35.89. The store's cheese department featured cheeses imported from England, Italy, France, and Spain that sold for as much as $26.99 per pound. Steve stated, "Nobody has good cheese in this area and we're doing a phenomenal business in good cheese. I mean $21, $22 a pound, and we can hire someone for $50 an hour that's going to double our cheese business, because she's unique enough and *we're* unique enough." The cheese department in Cotati did $15,000–$20,000

Exhibit 12   **Sonoma County Retail Food Sales, 2003**

Rank*		Number of Stores	Total Sales ($ millions)	Estimated Grocery Sales ($ millions)
1	Safeway	12	$ 240	$ 240
2	Costco†	2	340	211
3	Albertson's	7	108	108
4	FoodMaxx	2	78	78
5	Raley's	3	73	73
6	Whole Foods	3	65	65
7	Ralph's (Kroger)	3	61	61
8	G&G	2	50	50
9	Oliver's	2	40	40
10	Wal-Mart‡	2	121	36
11	Fiesta	2	20	20
12	Petaluma	1	13	13
13	Andy's Produce	1	11	11
14	Molsberry	1	10	10
15	Big John's	1	8	8
16	Berry's	6	8	8

† Estimated grocery sales for Costco were determined using *Supermarket News*' estimate that 62% of Costco's sales are derived from traditional grocery categories.

‡ Estimated grocery sales for Wal-Mart were derived using *Supermarket News*' estimate that 30% of Wal-Mart's discount store sales are derived from traditional grocery categories.

Source: Figures derived from the *Santa Rosa Press Democrat's Outlook 2004* survey of Sonoma County businesses, www.pressdemo.com. The businesses listed above all made the paper's list of the 350 largest companies in Sonoma County.

in sales per week. The store also featured a 3,000-square-foot wine department staffed with two full-time employees every day and a biweekly wine tasting. Wine buyer Renay Santero said,

> On a good day, we'll do $16,000 in wine. The wine tasting is most beneficial to the customer. Because I have an on-site license, I get every restaurant wine. What makes me a little different is that I get wines that other places cannot get.

The deli included a taqueria, a salad bar, and an inside seating area. Tom said, "When Safeway took out their salad bar, we put one in." The deli benefited from a front-end cold case used to sell Oliver's branded take-and-heat entrées, such as beef stroganoff and vegetarian lasagna, which were produced in the kitchen of the deli in the Santa Rosa store.

Deli manager Roxanne "Rocky" Abruzzo said, "It's the closest to homemade you're going to get without takeout . . . We do an easy $1,000 a day." The sushi bar located next to the deli was contracted to an outside vendor, AFC, and Oliver's received 25 percent of the gross sales as profit. The bakery featured gourmet store-baked desserts and a coffee bar that served mochas and lattes in addition to brewed organic coffees. Produce included a large organics section, and the department tried to source as much local produce as possible. The full-service meat department carried lamb, veal, and buffalo in addition to three grades of beef. Tom stated, "We feel that we need to have a better quality of meat . . . It's the same in produce. They're told to buy the best and charge what they have to get for it . . . So, having a steak that's twice the price of our competition is kind of a way of doing business in the summer here. This is a secondary shop for a lot of people in this neighborhood. They'll do their pantry loading at Costco or FoodMaxx and come here and buy their perishables." As evidence of this, Oliver's experienced a significant increase in sales during the 2004 holidays, jumping from an average of about $369,000 per week to $525,000 the week before Christmas.

Oliver's Santa Rosa

While the layout of the Cotati store provided an "organic, health foods store" feel, the size and design of the Santa Rosa store provided more of an upscale, gourmet market ambience. The most significant difference between the two stores was size, as the Santa Rosa store occupied only 22,000 square feet with 17,500 in selling space. In 2004, Oliver's opened a 5,000-square-foot warehouse to alleviate space constraints in Santa Rosa. The other significant difference was the focus on food service, bakery, deli, and taqueria, which ran almost the entire length of the left-hand wall. Tom stated, "The customers at the Santa Rosa store have the disposable income to just basically ask us to cook for them."

Marketing Strategy

Pricing   In 2002, Oliver's changed its pricing strategy to a program that involved setting its merchandise at prices relative to Safeway's, chosen because it was the dominant supermarket retailer in Sonoma County. Safeway was a traditional "hi-lo" retailer, meaning that low ad prices were used to offset high regular prices. For example, in early May 2005, Safeway advertised Clorox bleach for $1.00 when the regular retail was $2.59. Safeway was able to do this by negotiating special deals with its suppliers for ad periods. Oliver's set its everyday prices on traditional grocery items approximately 8 to 10 percent below Safeway's prices, having determined that being below Safeway by that amount provided acceptable margins while providing value to customers. Similarly, pricing in the natural foods department was maintained at just below the prices found at Whole Foods. Oliver's management considered the Whole Foods store in Santa Rosa to be its primary competitor in that market. Point-of-sale (POS) coordinator Laurie Tuxhorn reflected, "[Our pricing strategy] has proven to be really good to us. When I first took over this department and started doing printouts, we were so out of line. It was incredible how much lower we were." Department managers were responsible for setting prices in perishables departments such as deli, bakery, meat and produce. They were given a gross margin goal as part of the budget process and priced products to attain that goal. In line with Oliver's overall strategy, they tended to focus more on uniqueness and quality than on price.

Wine department manager Renay Santero said, "We've considered adjusting our margins to be more competitive. What makes sense to me is to turn people on to something that maybe nobody else can get a hold of."

Tom stated that Oliver's price strategy was "to try to communicate value amidst the perception of quality. We don't have a problem selling the idea that our product is better. We try to do that in a way that allows customers to feel that they're getting value." Tom admitted that his pricing strategy was not communicated well to customers and that Oliver's was perceived to have higher prices than Safeway. He opined that typical consumers could not believe that an apparently upscale two-store independent could have lower prices than a major chain store given the chain store's clear advantages in economies of scale.

Promotion   Oliver's also offered a weekly ad, an in-store flyer featuring items at no more than 10 percent above cost and temporary price reductions provided by vendors. Tom stated, "We pass through virtually everything we get . . . The one big price impact program is the 'Direct to You' program that's geared at . . . the kind of thing you'd buy at Trader Joes's." Oliver's offered a 10 percent discount to seniors on Wednesdays before 4:00 p.m. The Santa Rosa store was quite successful with this program due to its proximity to an affluent senior community, Oakmont. In 2004, Oliver's began experimenting with an everyday-low-price program on key items. Laurie, the POS coordinator, recalled,

> We have a program that Tom started a while back called the "staples program" where he compares our prices to Safeway for everyday items such as Tide, Nabisco crackers, things like that. We just want to show the customer that even with the Safeway Club card going on, we're still cheaper than them on everyday items.

Steve expressed his concerns about the mixed messages Oliver's might be sending to customers: "We have all these pricing programs like 'Direct to You' and 'staples,' which we stopped temporarily while we try and figure out whether we are price or quality focused."

Oliver's Private Label   Oliver's had a small private-label program that included vitamins, spices, and juices. The take-and-heat entrées from the deli also carried the Oliver's label. The private-label program was generally used as a way to provide value to their customers rather than as a way to build the Oliver's brand; there were no plans to significantly expand the private-label line.

Customer Service   Oliver's prided itself on its willingness to try to get any product a customer requested. According to Steve:

Most stores look at how many turns they get on an item to determine if the product is worth carrying. We almost do the opposite. If somebody wants it, we're going to have it . . . so we become the place that people call and say, "Somebody said if anybody would have it, you would." It's not the item we look at, it's the overall picture . . . It's not whether that one item sells well, it's what it adds to the rest of the store.

Stores had a special-request kiosk against the front wall near the check-out counters. Tom noted:

> We were the first store around here to carry Glaceau Vitamin Water. We're always looking for something new to add to the mix. If a customer wants us to carry something, we'll at least slot one case and see how it goes, and it only falls off the shelf due to competition from other items.

Mission and Culture

Oliver's mission statement, written by Tom, was printed on the back of the stores' item locator maps; thus, it was readily available to employees and customers. It read:

> Our mission is to provide the communities we serve with the finest grocery store in the marketplace. To this end we seek out our customer's specific needs and tailor our products and services to meet those needs. We carry the largest possible selection of natural, conventional and gourmet products. We carry only the highest quality meat, produce and deli products, buying locally whenever possible. We also strive to provide merchandise at the lowest possible cost so that we can offer value to our customers and maintain fair price. We treat each customer like a guest in our own home and we strive to exceed our customer's expectations every time they shop with us.
>
> We believe that our employees work to live, not live to work. We believe that each employee's talents and creativity contribute to making Oliver's successful. We also support employees in their life goals by offering competitive wage and benefit packages and special scheduling whenever possible.
>
> Oliver's is committed to playing an active role in the communities we serve. We support local schools and civic groups. Whenever possible, we fill staffing needs from the local neighborhood.

Oliver's offered a casual, relaxed shopping environment. Most employees, including management, wore blue jeans and company-supplied T-shirts or baseball caps with the Oliver's logo. Male employees were allowed to wear earrings and facial hair.

Employees played classic rock-and-roll on the in-store compact disc system.

Human Resources

Department managers ran their departments as if they were independent businesses. Tom stated that the performance of the individual departments, and of the company as a whole, was driven very much by the managers' individual personalities. Each was given the autonomy to decide what products to carry and how to price them. Each was expected to look for innovative ways to grow his or her department and to enhance the store's position in the market. Renay, formerly a Lucky's manager, said, "There's a lot of autonomy. They allow us to do what we think is best for the store. We negotiate price. We set our own prices. We have our own business plans. It's not like working in a chain where I was told what to do."

Rocky, a veteran of 22 years as a deli manager with Safeway, agreed: "There, I was just the most experienced clerk in the department. Here, it's like the Safeway corporate job and the deli manager job all tied into one. It enables me to use my brain, and still get behind the counter and help customers."

Oliver's maintained department-level fiscal accountability by requiring department managers to turn in financial statements every week. The department managers reported figures on cost of sales, labor, gross margin, and supplies to their store managers. The accounting department generated monthly statements, which were compared to the departments' weekly statements. All departments that sold perishable products were inventoried twice per year, as opposed to the industry standard of monthly inventories. Early in 2005, Tom put the cheese department in Cotati on a monthly inventory schedule and reiterated his preference that all departments selling perishable items conduct inventory as often.

Tom, 46, in addition to being general manager, was the manager of the Cotati Oliver's. Eric Meuse, 32, had started with Oliver's as a courtesy clerk in 1989. He had worked his way up through grocery management; Steve had promoted him to store manager when Oliver's expanded into Santa Rosa. Tom and Eric functioned as business coaches for the department managers. This was a role that had evolved over time, and it had been facilitated by the development of the employment contracts for department managers. Tom and Eric were able to

approach issues as mentors, sharing their observations in terms that related to the manager's contract and potential bonus. They helped them to reach goals, rather than ordering them to do specific things. The coaching role was considered successful, first of all, to the extent that financial goals were achieved. The second measure was the professional growth of the department managers in terms of their business acumen and their leadership of their own crews. Renay commented, "It's like family. They're dedicated to helping me with my career."

Rocky amplified this view, stating with a grin, "I always tell Tom, my worst day here is better than my best day at Safeway."

Eric noted, "The fun part about Oliver's is that we all set the standards. Everyone works as a team in creating the vision for Oliver's. Together, we decide which road we're going to take. Everybody has a little bit of say in it."

Tom agreed: "Ultimately, I think, we find good places in that tension, in that sort of give and take between all of us here."

As store managers, Tom and Eric had responsibility for tracking financial performance and for maintaining Oliver's standards in such areas as merchandising, customer service and cleanliness. In conjunction with their department heads, the two store managers oversaw all human resource functions. They were responsible for recruiting, training, and evaluating all employees. Whenever possible, Oliver's promoted from within. According to Tom, "There's a certain cultural learning curve in coming to work for us. Guys who come from the chain stores have a real problem with the entrepreneurial nature." Tom stated that all department managers in Santa Rosa had been promoted from within, and he estimated that this was also true of over 70 percent of the managers in Cotati.

The key component of Oliver's human resource program was its use of an employment contract with all department managers. Oliver's had been using these contracts since about 1998. Tom said, "It's one thing to say, 'If you hit this number, I'll give you this much money,' but the ritual of signing the contract has power to it." The contracts spelled out required hours, personal time off, holidays, and bonuses. Company management structured the bonuses so as to address the needs of the individual departments as they fit in with overall strategy. The primary factor in the bonus calculation was net profit percentage, defined as sales minus cost of goods and minus all operating expenses, including labor. Other factors, such as inventory control, were also included in the bonus calculations for particular managers.

Of her contract, Renay said, "You're on contract to make *this*. If you don't, you don't bonus, and potentially, you don't have a job."

Being a non-union operator gave Oliver's flexibility in pay structure. In a typical unionized Northern California supermarket, deli clerks reached top scale at about $13.50 per hour while journeyman grocery clerks, including checkers, made over $19.00. Union stores were also required to provide benefits to all courtesy clerks who worked over 16 hours per week and to all other clerks who worked more than 24 hours. At Oliver's top level, deli clerks made about the same amount as cashiers, $14 to $15 per hour. Oliver's benefited from additional cost savings as only employees who worked over 32 hours per week were eligible for benefits.

Eric felt that he needed more help with human resource issues: "I think if we had a dedicated professional, just one for the two stores, they could take care of a lot of issues we have, such as hiring people we shouldn't have." Tom agreed with Eric that more help was needed and that poor hiring practices and ignorance about the details of worker's compensation laws had cost Oliver's dearly. It had suffered a number of injuries in the year the Santa Rosa store opened and the change in their accident rate contributed to an increase in their premiums from $200,000 to $1.2 million in one year's time. The rates had since come down, but they were still at a 30 percent premium over industry standards. Tom also cited the need to improve Oliver's training program, especially in the meat department, where Oliver's needed to develop its own apprentice program if it was to remain non-union throughout the store. Most butchers were trained either in family shops or through the apprentice program at the local union meat hall. However, Steve did not feel that there was enough work for a 40-hour professional and instead outsourced training to a consulting firm.

The General Manager's Role

Tom's role as general manager required him to do tasks beyond that of store manager. With input from Eric and the department managers, Tom was responsible for writing all department budgets and for negotiating them with Steve. Tom also wrote the ad budget and ran Oliver's advertising program, coordinating newsprint and radio ads with respective agencies on a weekly basis. He was responsible for the quarterly "Direct to You" mailer. He actively pursued co-op money from vendors to support additional radio advertising during the holidays, and spent an additional $25,000–$30,000 during that period. Tom was also responsible for maintaining all training materials. He spoke about his background:

> I began working at Alpha Beta (the ancestor of the current Albertson's Chain) in 1975 as a bagger in high school. I worked my way through my undergraduate studies at Cal-State San Bernardino (BA in political science 1982) at Alpha Beta. In 1985, while working as an assistant store manager, I enrolled at Sonoma State University and took a sufficient number of accounting courses to sit for and pass the CPA exam. I then went to work for Eckhoff Accountancy Corp. in San Rafael in 1988. I never received certification due to lack of audit experience. In 1989, I became a minority owner and controller for Montecito Markets. We opened a store in Rincon Valley and shortly thereafter one in Lakeport. In 1991, I sold my shares and went to work for Steve as the general manager in Cotati. When we opened the Santa Rosa store, I moved up there and ran it for the first five years. I was brought down to Cotati in October of 2004, to shore up some management problems and coordinate the limited remodeling we've been doing. Eric was promoted to store manager in Cotati and transferred to Santa Rosa when I came down here.

A recent graduate with an MBA degree from a local state university, Tom had been directly involved in all aspects of opening the Santa Rosa store, in the Cotati store remodel, and performing the financial analysis for the potential new store acquisitions.

Tom assumed that if a second Oliver's in Santa Rosa were opened, he would be replaced as Cotati store manager and be freed up to function solely as general manager. Due to the time-consuming nature of his duties as store manager, Tom had had little opportunity to coach Eric and the other managers in the Santa Rosa store. He felt that he was successful in his role as store manager but that his general manager duties suffered from the demands put on a store manager. Additionally, Tom's entire salary was charged to the Cotati store and his bonus was based solely on that store.

Nevertheless, Tom expressed some frustration stemming from his uncertainty about what direction Steve wanted to take Oliver's for the long term. If Steve wanted to own Oliver's for 20 more years, then Tom thought he was doing the right things. If he wanted to sell in five years, they needed to make some changes. At the same time, Tom was comfortable with the level of supervision he received, noting that "Steve is very generous . . . He knows when to be involved and when not to."

THE EXPANSION DECISION

In weighing the decision to bid on one or both Kroger-owned supermarkets, Steve and Tom compiled demographic data and financial data for each location. Tom explained Oliver's site-selection criteria:

> We are looking for existing buildings with older leases that are renting below current market value. We look for an area that is growing in population with at least 10,000 households making over $75,000 per year, with at least 25 percent of the population having had college educations, all within a three-mile radius. An important criterion is the absence of Whole Foods within the trade area as they appeal directly to the same demographic. We do not currently cater to Hispanic shoppers, which could be an issue for the proposed Stony Point Road (Santa Rosa) location.

Tom estimated that they would need to invest approximately $2 million in each store to make it an Oliver's Market. Exhibit 13 presents selected demographic data for the Oliver's Markets in Cotati and Santa Rosa, Exhibit 14 presents comparative demographic data for the Santa Rosa Ralph's supermarket and Novato Bell Market, and Exhibit 15 summarizes information about existing and potential competitors in each location.

Kroger's Santa Rosa supermarket, Ralph's, was a traditional market, with deli, bakery, dry and frozen grocery, produce, meat, and liquor sections. Tom thought that he could run the store in its current condition, incorporating natural and organic items, and be profitable. He estimated that the market rate rent for this site would be about $360,000 per year. Ralph's was located in a center that was fully occupied and that had more than 20 other businesses, including a Longs' Drugs, Radio Shack, Carl's Jr., KFC, Subway

and Domino's Pizza. There was also a Chinese restaurant, a Mexican restaurant, a hair salon, a mail center, and a bank.

Kroger's had decided to put two Bell Markets in Novato up for sale. Oliver's management was interested in the South Novato Boulevard site because it had a very favorable lease and because it was the southernmost store in central Novato, meaning that approximately half the population would have to go past that store to get to its competitors. Estimated market rate rent for this location was about $460,000 per year. This Bell Market was located in a center considered tiny by comparison to the Vintage Oaks Mall that housed Costco across the freeway; still, the site housed the only post office in Novato. It also featured an Ace hardware, a bicycle shop, and a couple of small restaurants.

Oliver's Future

Steve and Tom had previously considered expanding to three stores, even making an offer on one, but nothing had come of these bids. Steve stated unequivocally that he would not open a third store on his own. He was interested in the possibility, however, because it would provide the opportunity to explore some sort of ownership position for Tom. Tom's future was a concern to Steve. He was comfortable with Tom's leadership style and with his decision making. He felt that he and Tom were very much alike and that Tom ran Oliver's Markets the way he, Steve, would run it. That allowed Steve to be as involved as he wanted to be, with no particular day-to-day responsibility.

Steve felt that his days of working 60 to 80 hours per week were past and admitted that he was uncertain what he would do if Tom left to pursue something else. He stated that perhaps then it would be time to sell. If Oliver's expanded, however, Tom could buy into the company and become a minority partner; Tom would also relinquish his position as store manager and function solely as general manager. Steve was nervous about the decision to bid on either (or both) supermarkets, and debated whether or not Oliver's should expand at all. Also, as his wife was ill and his daughter was not actively involved in running the family business, Steve wondered if perhaps a new expansion initiative might provide the impetus for him to begin to step aside and thereby allow his trusted general manager, Tom, to buy into and eventually take over the business. Steve said,

(Continued on page C-47)

Exhibit 13   **Selected Demographic Data for Oliver's Markets, Cotati and Santa Rosa**

	Cotati	Santa Rosa
Population	50,458	34,966
Number of households	15,867	14,777
Average household size	3.18	2.37
Under 14	20.8%	16.6%
15 to 24 years	18.7	9.7
25 to 44 years	32.3	21.5
45 to 64 years	20.2	28.1
Over 65	8.0	24.1
	100.0%	100.0%
Race		
White	80.9%	90.1%
Black	2.0	0.9
Asian	5.2	2.5
Other	11.9	6.5
Hispanic or Latino of any race	13.3	6.4
Educational Attainment for Population 25 Years and Over		
Less than high school grad	12.3%	7.3%
High school grad	23.3	17.9
Some college	30.0	26.9
Associate degree	9.8	8.8
Bachelor's degree	17.8	23.8
Graduate or professional degree	6.7	15.2
Percent high school graduate or higher	87.7	92.7
Percent bachelor's degree or higher	24.5	39.0
Household Income		
Less than $10,000	6.0%	3.3%
$10,000 to $14,999	4.2	3.5
$15,000 to $24,999	8.9	7.7
$25,000 to $34,999	11.3	10.8
$35,000 to $49,999	16.5	15.0
$50,000 to $74,999	25.1	20.1
$75,000 to $99,999	14.3	13.1
$100,000 to $149,999	10.1	15.2
$150,000 to $199,999	1.9	5.3
$200,000 or more	1.7	6.0
	100.0%	100.0%
Median household income (dollars)	$52,010	$62,067

Source: American Fact Finder on www.census.gov.

Exhibit 14 **Demographic Data: Ralph's Santa Rosa and Bell Markets, Novato**

	Ralph's Market, 461 Stony Point Rd., Santa Rosa, CA (0–3 mile radius)	Bell Market, 1535 S. Novato Blvd. Novato, CA (0–3 mile radius)
Population		
2010 projection	122,986	47,700
2005 estimate	114,839	46,905
2000 census	106,307	46,114
Growth 2005–2010	7.09%	1.69%
Growth 2000–2005	8.03%	1.72%
2005 Estimated Population by Race Classification		
White alone	75,395	38,393
Black or African American alone	3,042	852
American Indian and Alaska Native alone	2,269	229
Asian alone	5,489	2,553
Hispanic or Latino	38,236	6,676
2005 Estimated Population by Age		
Age 0–14 (%)	21.46%	17.87%
Age 15–24 (%)	14.28	11.49
Age 25–44 (%)	31.95	24.54
Age 45–64 (%)	22.93	32.09
Age 65 and over (%)	9.38	14.01
2005 estimated median age	33.72	42.39
2005 estimated average age	35.17	40.63
2005 Estimated Population Age 25 by Educational Attainment		
Less than high school graduate	16,886	3,093
High school graduate (or GED)	16,705	5,953
Some college, no degree	19,490	9,092
Associate degree	6,487	2,688
Bachelor's degree	10,159	8,150
Master's degree	2,476	2,611
Professional school degree or doctorate	1,584	1,545
Households		
2010 projection	41,870	18,686
2005 estimate	39,745	18,238
2000 census	37,534	17,824
Growth, 2005–2010	5.35%	2.46%
Growth, 2000–2005	5.89%	2.32%
2005 Estimated Households by Household Income	39,745	18,238
Income less than $15,000	4,154	1,043
Income, $15,000–$24,999	3,917	1,039
Income, $25,000–$34,999	3,971	1,119
Income, $35,000–$49,999	6,367	2,133
Income, $50,000–$74,999	8,880	3,446

(Continued)

Exhibit 14   **Continued**

	Ralph's Market, 461 Stony Point Rd., Santa Rosa, CA (0–3 mile radius)	Bell Market, 1535 S. Novato Blvd. Novato, CA (0–3 mile radius)
Income, $75,000–$99,999	5,598	2,763
Income, $100,000–$149,999	5,050	3,500
Income, $150,000 and more	1,809	3,193
2005 estimated average household income	$64,736	$102,150
2005 estimated median household income	$54,123	$78,062
2005 estimated per capita income	$22,942	$40,153
2005 estimated average household size	2.80	2.52

Source: Claritas online demographics database, www.claritas.com, supplied by Oliver's Markets.

Exhibit 15   **Competitor Stores Near Proposed Locations for Oliver's Markets**

Store	Estimated Square Feet of Selling Space	Estimated Weekly Sales (in thousands)	Estimated Distance in Miles	Notes
Santa Rosa Location				
Ralph's/proposed Oliver's	20,848	n/a	—	Could run as is and remodel while open. Estimated $1–$2 million to remodel.
FoodMaxx	50,000	$840	0.5	Former Food 4 Less
G&G	53,000	750	1.0	Plus 25,000 square feet of warehouse
Lola's	6,000	220	1.2	Hispanic market, originally a carniceria
Safeway	35,000	500	1.4	Marketplace format
Raley's	38,000	500	2.3	Includes pharmacy
Novato Location				
Bell Market/proposed Oliver's	16,917	n/a	—	Some cases need to be replaced. Could remodel while open.
Whole Foods	39,000	n/a	0.6	Anticipated opening— early 2007
Trader Joe's	10,000	n/a	1.0	Scheduled to open November 2005
Safeway				
900 Diablo Ave	60,000	900	0.1	One block north
470 Ignacio Blvd	25,000	500	3.5	South off Highway 101
Albertson's	45,000	300	1.2	North on same major road
Bell Market	20,000	131		Also for sale
Apple Market	26,000	230	3.2	Out-of-state ownership
Costco	137,000	2,028	1.5	South off U.S. 101 on opposite side of freeway

n/a = Not available.

Source: Oliver's Markets.

"We have grown every year except the last two years. I attribute it to us not doing as good a job as we could do. I can't do anything about Costco, but I can do something about the job we're doing here. I don't think the age of smaller stores like ours is gone."

Bibliography

American Factfinder. Available at www.census.gov (accessed May to July 2005).

"Consumers Continue to Shift Shopping Away from Grocery Stores." Available at http://retailindustry. about.com/library/bl/03q1/bl_acn030403a.htm (accessed April 10, 2005).

Currie, Neil. "UBS Q-Series Report: Do Supermarkets Have a Future?" *Progressive Grocer* 84, no. 6 (2005), pp. 62–79.

D'Aveni, Richard A. *Hypercompetition: Managing the Dynamics of Strategic Maneuvering.* New York: The Free Press, 1994.

Economic Research Service of the U.S. Department of Agriculture. "Food Market Structures: Food Retailing." Available at www.ers.usda.gov/briefing.htm (accessed June 15, 2005).

FMI Speaks 2004 Key Industry Facts. Prepared by FMI Information Service, July 2004, p. 16. Available at www.fmi.org (accessed June 2005).

Food Marketing Institute. "Facts and Figures." Available at www.fmi.org (accessed June and July 2005).

Francese, Peter. "Trend Ticker: Trouble in Store." *American Demographics* 25, no. 10 (December 2003–January 2004), p. 36.

Goll, David. "Grocers, Union Reach Tentative Agreement." *East Bay Business Times,* February 27, 2004.

Available at www.bizjournals.com/eastbay/ stories/2004/02/23/daily36.html (accessed October 20, 2005).

Heller, Walter, and Jenny McTaggart. "The Search for Growth: 71st Annual Report of the Grocery Industry." *Progressive Grocer* 83, no. 6 (2004), pp. 31–41.

Lasher, William. *Process to Profits: Strategic Planning for a Growing Business.* Mason, OH: Texere, 2005.

McTaggart, Jenny, and Walter Heller. "Forces of Change: 72nd Annual Report of the Grocery Industry." *Progressive Grocer* 84, no. 6 (2005), pp. 48–60.

Naumes, William, and Margaret J. Naumes. *The Art & Craft of Case Writing.* Thousand Oaks, California: Sage, 1999.

"Outlook 2004." *Santa Rosa Press Democrat.* Available at www1.pressdemocrat.com/apps/pbcs. dll/section?Category = BUSINESS06 (accessed May 2005).

Porter, Michael E. *Competitive Strategy: Techniques for Analyzing Industries and Competitors.* New York: Free Press, 1980.

"SN's Top 75." *Supermarket News.* Available at www.supermarketnews.com/sntop752004.htm (accessed March 21, 2005).

"Store Definitions." *Progressive Grocer's 2003 Marketing Guidebook and Bishop Consulting, 2003.* Available at www.fmi.org/facts_figs/superfact.htm (accessed June 2005).

"The Super 50: Views from the Top." *Progressive Grocer* 84, no. 7 (2005), pp. 74–84.

Tarnowski, Joseph, and Walter Heller. "The Super 50." *Progressive Grocer* 83, no. 7 (2004), pp. 59–66.

Turock, Art. "Alternative Formats: Teflon Retailing." *Progressive Grocer* 84, no. 7 (2005), pp. 22–24.

Endnotes

[1] Woodlands Market was located in Kentfield, a town with upscale demographics in affluent Marin County, approximately 40 miles south of Santa Rosa.

[2] Economic Research Service of the U.S. Department of Agriculture, www.ers.usda.gov/briefing.

[3] *Progressive Grocer* 83, no. 7 (May 1, 2004), p. 59.

[4] *Progressive Grocer* 83, no. 6 (April 15, 2004), pp. 31–32.

[5] Neil Currie, analyst for UBS, advised against opening stores solely for the pursuit of market share. In a report published in *Progressive Grocer,* he wrote, "There's too much capacity in the marketplace, leading to poor sales densities. While short-term sacrifices may have to be made to take out weaker competition, stores will be much more efficient if there are less around." *Progressive Grocer* 84, no. 6 (April 15, 2005), p. 70.

[6] www.ers.usda.gov.

[7] *American Demographics* 25, no. 10 (December 2003–January 2004), p. 36.

[8] *Progressive Grocer,* 84(6), April 15, 2005, p. 70.

[9] Report found on www.retailindustryabout.com on April 10, 2005.

[10] The bitter dispute, which affected 852 stores from San Diego in the south to Mammoth Lakes in the north, had begun on October 11, 2003, when 21,000 union workers walked off their jobs at Safeway's 329 Vons and Pavilions supermarkets. Later the same day, it expanded to include a total of 70,000 grocery employees throughout the region when Albertson's and Kroger, which owned the Ralph's chain, locked out their union workers. The standoff centered on reductions in employee health care benefits proposed by the grocers, as well as a two-tiered compensation package that would result in lower pay and benefits for newly hired workers. Union leaders characterized the health care cuts as excessive. Safeway CEO Steve Burd told industry analysts that major cuts in expenses were necessary for his and other traditional grocery companies to compete with nonunion rivals such as Wal-Mart Stores Inc. Losses suffered by the grocers as a result of the strike were estimated at $2.5 billion. D. Goll, "Grocers, Union Reach Tentative Settlement," *East Bay Business Times,* February 27, 2004, www.bizjournals.com/eastbay/stories/2004/02/23/daily36.html (accessed October 20, 2005).

JetBlue Airways: Can It Survive in a Turbulent Industry?

Janet Rovenpor
Manhattan College

It was the night of February 17, 2005. Snowfall in the Boston area had already reached 55 inches for the season, with several more major storms on the way. People started to line up at the Prudential Center's Terrace Food Court on Boylston Street. One woman was dressed in a Winnie-the-Pooh costume. A man a few steps behind her wore a straw hat and a colorful lei. Still others carried donations of canned food intended for the Greater Boston Food Bank. What brought these Bostonians out on such a cold winter night? Dressed to represent a JetBlue Airways travel destination, they arrived early for a chance to win the free airline tickets that had been promised to the first 250 people. In all, 1,000 people showed up for the event. JetBlue rose to the occasion and rewarded them with double the number of tickets originally planned. JetBlue tickets were especially coveted at this time of year, providing travelers with an opportunity to fly to such sunny destinations as Tampa and West Palm Beach.

The JetBlue giveaway program in Boston was meant to demonstrate the airline's commitment to expanding its operations at Logan Airport. More significantly, it was part of the company's fifth anniversary celebration. JetBlue had a lot to celebrate. Annual revenues in 2004 surpassed $1 billion. The company thus met the U.S. Transportation Department's definition of a major airline carrier

and became the youngest airline ever to achieve such status. JetBlue organized other celebratory promotions, including one in which passengers could win a variety of prizes by logging on to the company's Web site. Prizes included 12 XM satellite radio systems (to feature the airline's new XM digital radio in-flight service) and five La-Z-Boy recliners (in honor of the airline's leather seats and extra leg room). Here was one of the company's strategies for success—a dedicated effort to make air travel fun and comfortable.

COMPANY BACKGROUND

David Neeleman, a Salt Lake City entrepreneur, founded JetBlue Airways when he was 39 years old. His vision was to "bring humanity back to air travel."[1] He had raised $130 million in capital—a record high for an airline industry start-up—to do just that. In its first full year in business, JetBlue operated 64 flights a day and served 12 destinations in four states. It had 11 Airbus A320 aircraft and employed 1,028 employees. By late 2005, JetBlue was operating 318 flights a day and serving 33 destinations in 14 states, Puerto Rico, the Dominican Republic, and the Bahamas. It had a fleet of 82 Airbus A320 aircraft and employed approximately 8,600 employees. It won several awards, including "Best U.S. Airline" by *Conde Nast Traveler* readers and "Best Overall Airline" for onboard service.

David Neeleman's Entrepreneurial Spirit

Using his wristwatch calculator, David Neeleman (pronounced Neel-uh-man), the CEO of JetBlue, could punch in some numbers and predict to his colleagues that a competitor was not going to break even because it operated too many flights in and out of small markets.[2] He might have been found once a week on a JetBlue flight serving biscotti, animal crackers, or Terra-Blue potato chips to passengers. Passengers were surprised when they learned that the crew member nicknamed "Snack Boy" was actually the CEO.[3] Neeleman would ask passengers if they were comfortable and jot down their suggestions for improvement on a cocktail napkin. He also loved giving interviews and explaining how JetBlue got its start.

Contrary to popular notions, JetBlue did not enter the airline industry as an overnight sensation that simply benefited from the good fortune of having the right strategy at the right time. The company's success took years of planning and preparation on the part of its founder. Some of Neeleman's insights came from careful study of the airline industry; others came in a roundabout way as he tried to find a suitable occupation that would hold his interest. Over the course of his career, Neeleman would develop skills in accounting, salesmanship, and technology. He would use his own air travel experiences as lessons regarding how to provide superior customer service. He would learn that he suffered from attention deficit disorder (ADD), a situation that had its advantages and disadvantages. Neeleman attributed his creativity and high levels of energy to ADD, yet he also recognized that he had difficulty writing memos and keeping track of his belongings. He knew he needed to work with other individuals who could handle details.

Neeleman was born in São Paulo, Brazil, in 1959. His father worked there as a foreign correspondent for United Press International. The family moved to Sandy, Utah, when Neeleman was five years old. One of Neeleman's first jobs was in his grandfather's grocery store in downtown Salt Lake City.[4] As a teenager he would order items, cut the meat, and stack the beer. He learned from his grandfather never to disappoint customers. Satisfied customers would return. Neeleman even pushed elderly customers' shopping carts home for them. Later, when Neeleman became CEO of JetBlue, he performed similar good deeds. He once drove an elderly couple from New York's JFK Airport to their home in Connecticut (to where he had relocated) to save them $200 for a taxi. His customer service message was communicated throughout the company. It was common, for example, for a pilot to buy dozens of McDonald's Happy Meals for children whose flight was delayed.[5]

As a young man, Neeleman studied accounting at the University of Utah. He did not complete four consecutive years of study. After his freshman year, he spent time in Brazil as a Mormon missionary. There, he learned to be frugal, saving $1,300 out of the $3,000 his parents had given him.[6] Neeleman dropped out of college for good in his junior year and opened up his own travel agency near Salt Lake City. He sold vacation packages to Hawaii that included airfare and a stay in a time-share. His company grew to 20 employees and brought in $8 million in business.[7] Unfortunately, the air charter company with which he had an agreement to transport his customers, Pineapple Express, went bankrupt. Neeleman was forced to close his business in 1983, but he took away with him two lessons: (1) Never rely on someone who could put you out of business, and (2) use funds wisely so that they will be available during tough times.[8]

In 1984, Neeleman joined Morris Air, a small local carrier based in Salt Lake City. Working there for about eight years, he held the titles of executive vice president and later president. The carrier's most popular routes provided service from Salt Lake City to Los Angeles, from Salt Lake City to Hawaii, and from Salt Lake City to Cancun, Mexico. Neeleman solicited business from shoppers in malls and sold honeymoon packages to couples during weddings he attended. He convinced venture capitalists to invest $15 million and expanded Morris Air's operations to 300 flights a day with a fleet of 22 Boeing 737 airplanes. He introduced electronic ticketing and allowed reservation agents to work from home.

Neeleman's early ideas at Morris Air were later implemented at JetBlue Airways. Take, for example, the unconventional way in which he sold airline tickets at shopping malls and weddings. When JetBlue started service out of Long Beach, California, in 2001, paid college interns rode local streets in nine Volkswagen Beatles painted in the airline's logo and colors. For a month, they handed out bumper stickers, buttons, and tote bags to potential passengers in hotels, movie studios, and restaurants. It was especially important to talk to bartenders and hotel concierges—people whom vacationers sought out for all kinds of advice.[9] Off-beat guerrilla advertising was always part of the company's approach to marketing.

Like Morris Air, JetBlue also issued electronic tickets. Travelers printed boarding passes at check-in kiosks at the airport. This was convenient for people like Neeleman who often forgot their paper tickets at home. Reservation agents worked from home, serving six-hour shifts with two 15-minute breaks. By February 2005, 900 agents worked from their homes in the Salt Lake City area. The company thus saved money on paper tickets, on postage needed to mail out paper tickets, and on rent for office space. Neeleman raised capital for JetBlue from some of the same investors in Morris Air.

In 1993, Southwest Airlines purchased Morris Air for $129 million. The deal made Neeleman $20 million wealthier. Investors got back two and a half times their investment. Southwest hired Neeleman, but his tenure as a member of the executive planning committee was very brief. Unable to get used to the company's policies and procedures, he was fired. At Southwest Airlines, though, Neeleman learned that it was important to treat employees with respect and that it was better to purchase new airplanes instead of leasing them.[10]

Because he had signed a five-year noncompete agreement with Southwest Airlines, Neeleman had to wait before he could start up another airline company. He kept himself busy in the meantime. With a college student, he developed a computerized system called "Open Skies" that could handle electronic ticketing, Internet bookings, and revenue management. He sold the system to Hewlett-Packard in 1999 for $22 million. Neeleman also served as a consultant to a low-fare Canadian carrier, WestJet.

By 1998, Neeleman was ready to move on and start JetBlue. He contributed $5 million of his own money and raised $130 million from investors, including George Soros, Weston Presidio, and Chase Manhattan Bank's venture capital group. When he began JetBlue, Neeleman and his wife moved to New Canaan, Connecticut, with their nine children. His salary in 2004 was $200,000, with a bonus of $90,000. He owned 7.3 million JetBlue shares, worth about $150 million as of December 2005.[11]

THE JETBLUE CONCEPT

Neeleman envisioned that JetBlue would combine the low fares of a discount airline carrier with the comforts of a cozy den in people's homes. Passengers would be able to save money while they sat in leather seats, munched on gourmet snacks, and watched television. Individual monitors were installed in all seats so that passengers had access to 24-channel live television via satellite—for free. Neeleman wanted leather seats because they were more durable and easier to clean (he had once had the unfortunate personal experience of having been assigned a fabric seat soaked with urine). Having been on a flight forced to land because of engine failure, and not receiving any information or compensation afterward, Neeleman also made sure that inconvenienced JetBlue travelers would get discount coupons for future flights as well as food and accommodations.

Neeleman's customer service philosophy fit in well with the sociocultural and political environment of the times. In 1999, the House Transportation Committee held hearings in which passengers told horror stories of being kept on a Northwest Airlines plane during a blizzard in Detroit for hours as toilets overflowed, hungry infants cried, and chronically ill travelers went without medication. One woman complained that her six-year-old son, who was traveling as a unaccompanied minor, was put in a hotel room with a sexually abusive teenager.[12] As a result of such complaints, the Clinton administration tried to enact a passenger "bill of rights" that would have doubled the minimum payment for lost baggage to $2,500, doubled the maximum compensation for being bumped from an overbooked flight to $800, required airlines to tell customers whether they must change planes during a trip, and required airlines to hire an ombudsman.

Airline companies were opposed to the bill but voluntarily agreed to make improvements to customer service on their own. Their 12-point plan included a pledge to quote the lowest available fare on their telephone reservation systems; to notify passengers of delays, cancellations, and diversions; and to make an effort to provide food, water, restrooms, and medical attention to on-board passengers held on the tarmac for extended periods.[13] Following the terrorist attacks of September 11, 2001, however, the nation's attention shifted from issues related to customer satisfaction to issues related to airline security.

BUILDING A STRONG TOP MANAGEMENT TEAM

Neeleman took the staffing of his senior management team very seriously. He did not hesitate to recruit top talent from other airline companies. As Ann Roades, executive vice president of human resources, said, "He realized that if you hire A-players, you don't have to sit on them and tell them what to do."[14] David Barger was hired as president and chief operating officer. With 10 years' experience in the airline industry, Barger had been the vice president at Continental Airlines and was responsible for running its Newark, New Jersey, hub. Barger helped Neeleman make the decision to purchase all new aircraft of a single body type and to eventually operate point-to-point service instead of the more costly hub and spoke system.[15]

John Owen was hired as executive vice president and chief financial officer. His career began as a financial analyst at American Airlines. He later worked at Southwest Airlines as vice president of operations/planning and analysis, and then as treasurer. Every morning, Owen received the previous day's financial and operating statistics. He evaluated such information as the number of seats sold, revenues generated from every passenger mile flown, take-off and landing times, and the length of time it took to unload baggage. He traveled to Europe in an attempt to raise capital to finance the purchase of new jets. He was opposed to installing live television in airplanes, viewing it as an expense that would never be recovered. He realized, however, that sometimes financial officers needed to see the big picture. He learned that service was an essential part of the JetBlue experience and that it contributed to "loyalty and passenger buzz that will result in higher demand."[16]

Neeleman's longtime business partner Thomas Kelly became JetBlue's executive vice president and general counsel. Kelly had left private law practice to join Morris Air in 1990. Ann Rhoades was hired as executive vice president to handle human resources. She had been the head of the people department at Southwest Airlines and was the one who had fired Neeleman from the carrier back in 1993. She implemented many of the company's highly successful human resource strategies to hire, retain, and motivate high quality employees. Out of all five original members of the top management team, she was the only one to leave JetBlue, doing so in 2005 to devote time to her own consulting company, People Ink, in Arizona. She remained, however, a member of JetBlue's board of directors.

JETBLUE'S NEW YORK CITY ROOTS

On February 11, 2000, JetBlue launched its first ceremonial flight between Buffalo and New York City, making John F. Kennedy International Airport (JFK) its hub. The one-way fare for the first month was set at $25, which would then go up to $98 round-trip. Fares available from other carriers at that time were as high as $600 round-trip.[17] Although the flight was delayed for three hours because of heavy fog, David Neeleman was exuberant. His vision was about to become a reality. Senator Charles Schumer, who had been instrumental in helping the airline obtain its 75 take-off and landing slots at JFK, and Mayor Rudolph Guiliani were among the celebrity passengers. Schumer wanted to make good on a campaign promise that he would help stimulate the stagnant economy in upper New York State. Given low-fare accessibility to such cities as Buffalo and Syracuse, outside employers might be encouraged to open up new businesses.

Later that day, JetBlue introduced its first commercial flight from JFK to Fort Lauderdale, Florida, with 152 passengers aboard. The fare was $159 one-way, which was 70 percent less than the fares of other carriers. JetBlue would soon fly to Tampa, Orlando, West Palm Beach, and Fort Myers, Florida. David Barger viewed Florida as "the sixth borough of New York."[18] It became JetBlue's most popular destination.

The decision to start up service at JFK was a risky one. The airport was called the "black sheep of New York airports" because of its crowded skies, high costs, and inevitable hassles.[19] Even Southwest Airlines had entered the region by choosing to fly in and out of a secondary airport, MacArthur Airport in Islip, Long Island, instead of JFK. Yet Neeleman saw an opportunity at JFK that no one else saw. While airlines faced heavy delays during the 3:00–8:00 p.m. time period (when most international flights arrived and departed), the morning hours were relatively free. Neeleman noted that only 15 flights left JFK between the hours of 8:00 and 9:00 a.m.[20] JFK had an average gate utilization of 2.7 flights a day, much lower than La Guardia's 5.5 flights a day.[21]

In addition, the demographics were great. Neeleman originally thought that JetBlue's target market consisted of the 8 million people in a five-mile radius around JFK. He later found that his service also appealed to young, affluent professionals with Manhattan zip codes. "You have this large population that makes a lot of money per capita, and everyone in New York would like to get out. At the same time, everyone outside New York would like to get in. It's truly the nirvana of all markets," said Neeleman.[22] New York City travelers had not had access to a low-fare carrier since People Express folded in 1986.

JETBLUE'S RAPID EXPANSION

From the beginning, JetBlue introduced a simple fare structure. All passengers flew coach and purchased one-way, nonrefundable tickets. The average one-way fare in 2000 was $88.84; in 2004, it was $103.61. No Saturday stay was required. A $25 fee was charged to passengers who wanted to change their departure times.

Exhibit 1 shows JetBlue's rapid growth. By the end of 2000, JetBlue was flying to 12 cities and had boarded its millionth passenger. It had 1,174 employees and a fleet of 10 Airbus A320 airplanes. In addition to its Florida destinations, JetBlue provided service from JFK to Buffalo and Rochester, New York; to Burlington, Vermont; to Salt Lake City, Utah; and to Oakland and Ontario, California. One of its goals was to balance out short-haul routes with transcontinental routes.

In April 2001, JetBlue boarded its 2 millionth passenger. It had more than doubled the number of its aircraft from the previous year. It also added service from JFK to Syracuse, New York; to Seattle, Washington; to Denver, Colorado; to Long Beach, California; and to New Orleans, Louisiana. More important, it started direct service between Washington, D.C. (Dulles International Airport), and Fort Lauderdale, Florida—on the first flight, 133 out of 162 seats were full. Fares ranged from $79 to $199 one-way. This marked the beginning of the company's plans to operate as a point-to-point carrier. JetBlue wanted be the preferred carrier for Washington-area businesses. Executives mailed letters, along with free round-trip tickets, to corporate travel managers and chief financial officers of the top 100 local companies.[23]

On March 7, 2002, JetBlue flew its 5 millionth passenger. On April 12, JetBlue raised $182 million from its first public offering of stock, selling 5.87 million shares at a starting price of $27 a share. In September, JetBlue acquired LiveTV LLC, its provider of in-flight satellite entertainment systems. JetBlue added service from Washington, D.C., to Oakland and Long Beach, California. It significantly expanded its operations out of Long Beach by offering nine flights to Oakland, California; five daily flights to Las Vegas, Nevada; and one daily flight to Salt Lake City, Utah. This brought JetBlue into close competition with Southwest Airlines, which had dominated the California market for many years. JetBlue opportunistically launched its service between JFK and Las Vegas two months ahead of schedule, filling a void left by National Airlines, a Las Vegas–based discount carrier, which had halted all flights as part of its liquidation efforts.

On January 1, 2003, JetBlue flew its 10 millionth passenger. It also launched service that year between JFK and San Diego, Long Beach, Fort Lauderdale,

Exhibit 1   **JetBlue Airways' Expansion from 2000 to 2004**

	2000	2001	2002	2003	2004
Number of cities served	12	18	20	21	30
Number of departures	10,265	26,334	44,144	66,920	90,532
Number of aircraft (owned and leased)	10	21	37	53	69
Number of full-time and part-time employees	1,174	2,361	4,011	5,433	7,211
Percentage of sales through JetBlue.com	28.7%	44.1%	63%	73%	75.4%

Source: 2005 10-K report, JetBlue Web site.

and it ordered a new type of plane, the Embraer 190, and started construction on a new hangar complex at JFK. It pulled out of Atlanta, Georgia, because of competition from Delta and AirTran on its transcontinental routes to Oakland and Long Beach.

In 2004, JetBlue added satellite radio and movie channels to its in-flight entertainment systems. It had 7,211 employees and 69 airplanes. It was a big year for route expansion. JetBlue started service out of Boston (with flights to Long Beach, Denver, Fort Lauderdale, Orlando, and Tampa) and out of New York's LaGuardia Airport (with flights to Fort Lauderdale). It launched service out of JFK to seven new cities, including Aguadillo, Puerto Rico; Santiago, Dominican Republic; and Nassau, the Bahamas.

In 2005, JetBlue added flights from Boston to San Jose, California; Las Vegas, Nevada; and Seattle, Washington. It started a new service between Washington's Dulles Airport and San Diego, California. In the New York area, it added flights out of JFK to Burbank, California; to Portland, Oregon; and to Ponce, Puerto Rico; and out of La Guardia to West Palm Beach, Florida, and to San Juan, Puerto Rico. In September, people were glued to their television sets as they watched the pilot of JetBlue flight 292 successfully make an emergency landing at Los Angeles International airport (with the wheel of the aircraft's front landing gear skewed sideways). In a first in aviation history, passengers on the airplane watched their own predicament on live television. In November, JetBlue started service between New York's JFK Airport and Boston's Logan Airport with its Embraer 190 airplanes. To celebrate the introduction of a new type of airplane into its fleet, JetBlue employees randomly distributed free tickets to pedestrians walking in Manhattan who were wearing the color blue. On the first day of service, most of the Embraer flights were delayed due to minor maintenance issues.

JETBLUE'S COMMITMENT TO LOW COSTS AND SERVICE QUALITY

Over the years, JetBlue had developed an excellent reputation for on-time performance, few reports from passengers about mishandled baggage, and a low number of passenger complaints (see Exhibit 2). For the 12 months ending in January 2004, 84 percent of JetBlue's flights arrived within 15 minutes of their scheduled times (earning JetBlue third place for this measure among major U.S. airlines). For the 12 months ending in January 2005, 80.3 percent of JetBlue's flights arrived within 15 minutes of their scheduled times (fourth place). In 2003, JetBlue received 3.21 reports of mishandled baggage (baggage that was lost or damaged) per 1,000 passengers, putting it in fourth place among 18 other carriers. In 2004, that number went down to 2.99 (third place). In 2003, JetBlue had 0.31 complaints per 100,000 passengers (for such things as cancelled flights, poor customer service, discrimination); in 2004 it had 0.27, which moved it from fourth place to third place among the major airlines.

JetBlue modeled itself after the pioneering discount carrier Southwest Airlines. Managers at Southwest had figured out how to operate an airline company successfully by keeping its costs down. Both carriers offered passengers low fares and operated point-to-point systems. Flight attendants wore casual uniforms and created a relaxed atmosphere for passengers. The carriers became highly efficient by using one type of aircraft, serving only snacks and maintaining quick turnaround times. Exhibit 3 displays comparative operating cost statistics for 10 major airline carriers.

Southwest Airlines flew only Boeing 737s; JetBlue flew only Airbus A320s. The Airbus model had 30 additional seats and was more fuel efficient and less costly to operate than a Boeing 737.[24] Costs were kept down since pilots and maintenance technicians were trained for only one aircraft. The same spare parts could be stored in inventory. Delta, in comparison, operated 16 different kinds of aircraft. It needed larger and more expensive planes to fly on its international routes. Eight weeks of extra training were required to transfer a pilot from one type of aircraft to another. In addition, Delta had to pay another pilot to cover the pilot-in-training's existing route.[25] This got expensive since pilots earned more than $100 an hour.

Most large airlines required an hour on the ground to service their aircraft and board passengers before taking off again. JetBlue's turnaround time ranged from 20 to 30 minutes. Because no meals were served, JetBlue did not have to wait for catering services to replenish the aircraft. To save time, flight attendants themselves stowed carry-on bags

Exhibit 2 On-Time Flights, Mishandled Baggage, and Passenger Complaints of Major U.S. Airlines, 2003–2005

Percentage of Flights Arriving within 15 Minutes of the Scheduled Time, and Carrier Rank

| Airline | 12 Months Ending January 2005 | | 12 Months Ending January 2004 | |
	%	Rank	%	Rank
AirTran	77.4	(10)	77.4	(15)
Alaska	76.7	(12)	79.9	(10)
America West	75.4	(17)	81.9	(6)
American	76.9	(11)	80.3	(9)
American Eagle	73.1	(19)	77.4	(14)
ATA	80.4	(3)	79.3	(13)
Atlantic Southeast	75.2	(18)	75.7	(16)
Comair	76.7	(13)		
Continental	78.7	(8)	81.6	(8)
Delta	75.9	(15)	81.6	(7)
Express Jet	76.5	(14)	79.3	(12)
Hawaiian	94.3	(1)		
Independence Air	75.6	(16)	74.4	(17)
JetBlue	**80.3**	**(4)**	**84.0**	**(3)**
Northwest	79.0	(7)	82.0	(4)
Skywest	82.5	(2)	86.6	(1)
Southwest	79.4	(6)	86.0	(2)
United	79.6	(5)	81.9	(5)
US Airways	78.2	(9)	79.5	(1)
Average	77.8		81.2	

Mishandled Baggage Reports Filed by Passengers

| Airline | January–December 2004 | | January–December 2003 | |
	Reports per 1,000 Passengers	Rank	Reports per 1,000 Passengers	Rank
AirTran	2.82	(1)	2.84	(2)
Alaska	3.51	(5)	2.56	(1)
America West	3.98	(9)	3.30	(5)
American	4.73	(11)	4.45	(12)
American Eagle	8.95	(15)	8.42	(14)
ATA	3.82	(7)	4.06	(11)
Atlantic Southeast	14.49	(19)	15.41	(17)
Comair	10.66	(17)		
Continental	3.58	(6)	3.11	(3)
Delta	5.17	(12)	3.84	(9)
Express Jet	5.70	(14)	4.51	(13)
Hawaiian	2.85	(2)		
Independence Air	10.68	(18)	9.23	(16)
JetBlue	**2.99**	**(3)**	**3.21**	**(4)**
Northwest	4.22	(10)	3.42	(7)
Skywest	10.00	(16)	8.62	(15)
Southwest	3.35	(4)	3.35	(6)
United	3.93	(8)	3.93	(10)
US Airways	5.33	(13)	3.55	(8)
Average	4.91		4.19	

(Continued)

Exhibit 2   Continued

Passenger Complaints				
	January–December 2004		January–December 2003	
Airline	Complaints per 100,000 Passengers Boarded	Rank	Complaints per 100,000 Passengers Boarded	Rank
AirTran	0.89	(13)	0.83	(12)
Alaska	3.51	(5)	0.52	(6)
America West	3.98	(9)	0.84	(13)
American	0.88	(12)	0.88	(14)
American Eagle	0.54	(6)	0.51	(5)
ATA	0.79	(10)	0.66	(8)
Atlantic Southeast	0.40	(4)	0.59	(7)
Comair	1.10	(18)		
Continental	0.82	(11)	0.95	(3)
Delta	0.79	(9)	0.78	(17)
Express Jet	0.16	(1)	0.21	(2)
Hawaiian	0.46	(5)		
Independence Air	0.95	(17)	0.76	(9)
JetBlue	**0.27**	**(3)**	**0.31**	**(4)**
Northwest	0.89	(15)	3.42	(7)
Skywest	0.56	(7)	0.30	(3)
Southwest	0.18	(2)	0.14	(1)
United	0.88	(12)	0.83	(11)
US Airways	1.21	(19)	3.55	(8)
Average	0.74		0.71	

Source: U.S. Department of Transportation, Air Travel Consumer Report, www.airconsumer.ost.dot.gov/reports, February 2005.

and coats in the overhead bins. Everyone—pilots, flight attendants, and passengers—helped throw away the trash after each flight. JetBlue's aircraft were the most productive of all U.S. fleets and operated almost 14 hours per day.[26]

There were some differences between JetBlue and Southwest. JetBlue exhibited a stronger commitment to service quality than Southwest. JetBlue offered assigned seats to make boarding a more orderly process. It equipped its planes with leather seats at an additional cost of $15,000 per airplane before Southwest did. The live television was another unique benefit. Southwest did not even offer in-flight movies. JetBlue wanted to ensure that its flights arrived at their destinations on time. It spent extra funds for emergency equipment—life rafts and beacons—so that it could fly over water and avoid traffic along its East Coast routes. It flew at 10,000 feet instead of 18,000 feet to avoid congestion in upstate New York. This added $400 to the cost of operating the flight.[27]

JetBlue paid attention to the little details customers found special. It added amenities while other airlines were cutting back. Delta Air Lines stopped providing hot meals to passengers in 2003. It announced that it would not even sell food on board starting in 2005, nor would it continue to provide pillows. American Airlines also eliminated pillows on its domestic and Caribbean flights to save over $300,000 a year.[28] It reversed its "More Room Throughout Coach" program by adding 12,000 seats back into its fleet of jets in 2005. JetBlue, in contrast, kept its promise to give passengers more legroom. In 2003, it removed a row of seats from its planes, increasing legroom by two inches.[29] Exhibit 4 shows that JetBlue's aircraft "seat pitch" (a measure of the distance from one point on a seat to the same point on the seat in front) was favorable compared to that of other carriers. JetBlue worked with a unit of Bally Total Fitness to offer in-flight yoga cards in seat pockets. Passengers received instruction on how they could hold four yoga poses without removing

(Continued on page C-58)

Exhibit 3 **Comparative Operating Cost Statistics, JetBlue versus Major U.S. Airlines, 1995, 2000–2004 (in cents per available seat mile)***

Carrier	Year	Food	Salaries & Benefits	Aircraft Fuel & Oil	Commissions	Landing Fees	Advertising	Other Operating & Maintenance Expenses	Total Operating Expenses	Rent & Leasing Fees
JetBlue	2003	0.06¢	2.12¢	1.08¢	0.00¢	0.22¢	0.18¢	1.90¢	6.06¢	0.72¢
	2004	0.05	1.95	1.35	0.00	0.22	0.13	2.38	6.08	0.63
American	1995	0.41¢	3.70¢	1.01¢	0.80¢	0.15¢	0.15¢	3.23¢	9.45¢	0.73¢
	2000	0.44	4.18	1.48	0.60	0.17	0.13	3.49	10.49	0.74
	2001	0.44	4.55	1.57	0.47	0.19	0.13	4.53	11.89	0.78
	2002	0.40	4.97	1.33	0.35	0.22	0.11	3.75	11.12	0.87
	2003	0.37	4.31	1.57	0.25	0.23	0.09	4.24	11.41	0.83
	2004	0.32	3.72	2.10	0.25	0.23	0.08	4.23	10.94	0.72
Alaska	1995	0.31¢	2.60¢	1.07¢	0.55¢	0.15¢	0.12¢	3.10¢	7.89¢	1.17¢
	2000	0.29	3.53	1.76	0.38	0.18	0.38	3.72	10.25	1.08
	2001	0.31	3.81	1.45	0.35	0.25	0.21	3.78	10.17	1.07
	2002	0.32	3.83	1.21	0.30	0.21	0.10	3.98	9.95	1.02
	2003	0.28	3.94	1.42	0.24	0.25	0.10	3.10	9.79	0.96
	2004	0.21	3.65	1.94	0.12	0.19	0.19	3.30	9.61	0.89
Continental	1995	0.22¢	2.45¢	1.11¢	0.74¢	0.18¢	0.16¢	3.82¢	8.67¢	1.20¢
	2000	0.28	3.30	1.62	0.54	0.18	0.07	4.21	10.20	1.23
	2001	0.27	3.44	1.39	0.37	0.21	0.02	4.52	10.23	1.32
	2002	0.26	3.52	1.10	0.28	0.25	0.00	5.18	10.57	1.42
	2003	0.24	3.63	1.46	0.16	0.23	0.00	3.04	9.60	1.29
	2004	0.23	3.34	1.83	0.14	0.27	0.00	4.50	10.15	1.18
Delta	1995	0.26¢	3.25¢	1.11¢	0.85¢	0.20¢	0.13¢	3.06¢	8.86¢	0.81¢
	2000	0.27	3.73	1.27	0.42	0.16	0.08	3.51	9.43	0.72
	2001	0.28	4.10	1.20	0.36	0.16	0.11	3.81	10.02	0.76
	2002	0.25	4.37	1.10	0.28	0.18	0.10	4.03	10.30	0.81
	2003	0.23	4.79	1.44	0.17	0.19	0.11	5.28	12.75	0.90
	2004	0.23	4.38	1.98	0.16	0.18	0.11	5.87	12.91	0.82

America West	1995	0.19¢	2.08¢	0.96¢	0.64¢	0.16¢	0.19¢	3.07¢	7.29¢	1.30¢
	2000	0.12	2.21	1.54	0.32	0.13	0.09	4.17	3.57	1.58
	2001	0.10	2.42	1.35	0.28	0.15	0.06	4.50	8.86	1.72
	2002	0.06	2.36	1.09	0.19	0.16	0.08	4.67	8.61	1.56
	2003	0.05	2.47	1.44	0.08	0.16	0.03	2.44	7.89	1.46
	2004	0.04	2.30	1.94	0.06	0.17	0.03	3.37	8.31	1.40
Northwest	1995	0.28¢	3.47¢	1.24¢	0.93¢	0.27¢	0.16¢	2.80¢	9.15¢	0.70¢
	2000	0.29	3.65	1.80	0.61	0.24	0.13	3.24	9.96	0.67
	2001	0.27	4.15	1.73	0.45	0.27	0.11	3.55	10.52	0.70
	2002	0.24	4.18	1.40	0.36	0.27	0.10	3.60	10.15	0.77
	2003	0.24	4.45	1.68	0.27	0.31	0.08	3.38	10.62	0.80
	2004	0.24	4.27	2.37	0.30	0.32	0.18	5.11	12.79	0.82
Southwest	1995	0.02¢	2.56¢	1.01¢	0.39¢	0.23¢	0.27¢	2.61¢	7.09¢	0.71¢
	2000	0.03	2.99	1.38	0.30	0.22	0.26	2.55	7.72	0.55
	2001	0.03	3.01	1.29	0.18	0.22	0.24	2.51	7.48	0.54
	2002	0.03	3.02	1.17	0.10	0.24	0.22	2.58	7.36	0.55
	2003	0.02	3.25	1.28	0.08	0.23	0.23	2.28	7.59	0.54
	2004	0.02	3.34	1.44	0.02	0.24	0.21	2.50	7.76	0.52
United	1995	0.37¢	3.34¢	1.06¢	0.93¢	0.21¢	0.13¢	2.84¢	8.89¢	0.94¢
	2000	0.38	4.16	1.43	0.59	0.20	0.20	3.64	10.60	0.88
	2001	0.37	4.73	1.50	0.43	0.22	0.13	4.54	12.02	0.90
	2002	0.35	4.87	1.21	0.32	0.22	0.11	4.27	11.35	1.07
	2003	0.30	4.07	1.52	0.22	0.26	0.12	4.06	10.95	0.87
	2004	0.30	3.60	2.03	0.23	0.26	0.15	5.04	11.61	0.77
US Airways	1995	0.25¢	4.93¢	1.04¢	0.90¢	0.19¢	0.11¢	4.18¢	11.61¢	1.16¢
	2000	0.28	5.35	1.72	0.51	0.20	0.08	5.73	13.88	1.11
	2001	0.28	5.62	1.56	0.39	0.20	0.08	6.00	14.13	1.31
	2002	0.21	5.93	1.20	0.25	0.23	0.06	6.57	14.45	1.30
	2003	0.17	4.76	1.50	0.23	0.24	0.03	6.18	13.94	1.31
	2004	0.15	4.17	1.87	0.18	0.23	0.04	7.11	13.75	1.27

*The airline industry statistic "available seat miles" is calculated by multiplying the number of seats on each aircraft by the number of miles flown by each aircraft.

Source: U.S. Department of Transportation, Bureau of Transportation Statistics, Office of Airline Information, Form 41B, Form 41P, Form T100.

Exhibit 4   **Airline Seat Pitch as of April 2005**

Airline Company	Type of Aircraft	Seat Pitch
AirTran	Boeing 717	31"
Alaska	Boeing 737-400	31
America West	Airbus A320	31
American	McDonald Douglas MD80	31
Continental	Boeing 737-800	31
Delta	Boeing 757-200	31
Delta Song	Boeing 757	33
Frontier	Airbus A319	33
JetBlue—rear rows	**Airbus A320**	**34**
JetBlue—front rows		**32**
Midwest	Boeing 717	33
Northwest	DC9-30	30
Southwest	Boeing 737-700	32
United—regular coach	Airbus A320, Boeing 757	31
United—economy plus*		36
US Airways	Boeing 737-300	31

*Offers roomier coach seats with limited availability.

Source: Scott McCartney, "The Middle Seat: Discounters Win the Legroom Wars," *The Wall Street Journal*, April 5, 2005, p. D1.

their seatbelts. JetBlue wanted to avoid the "cattle-car image of discount flying."[30]

Even JetBlue's terminals had several unique features. The company used a simple queue program at its check-in counters so that the next person in line knew which agent was available. Average check-in times were under a minute.[31] In 2005, JetBlue partnered with Oasis Day Spa to offer private massages, manicures, and hair styling to travelers at JetBlue's JFK Terminal 6. It was "just another way we look to take the stress and hassle out of traveling," said JetBlue's spokesperson, Gareth Edmondson-Jones.[32] A children's play area and a big-screen television could be found near its gates. Free wireless Internet access was also available.

JETBLUE'S INNOVATIVE USE OF TECHNOLOGY

JetBlue's operating costs per seat mile were historically low. In the first quarter of 2005, for example, it spent only 6.74 cents to fly one seat one mile. This compared to 7.70 cents for Southwest, 9.80 cents for American, 10.12 cents for United, 10.56 cents for Continental, 10.89 cents for U S Airways, and 11.62 cents for Delta.[33] Jet Blue used technology to help improve efficiency and minimize costs.

JetBlue operated "Open Skies" software to handle electronic ticketing, Internet bookings, and revenue management. It cost 25 cents to process an e-ticket compared to $25 for a paper ticket.[34] JetBlue's Web site was responsible for 75 percent of ticket sales. Since it did not sell its tickets through such online reservation systems as Expedia, it saved money on booking fees.

JetBlue hired reservation agents to sell tickets over the telephone. They worked at home with company-supplied computers and second telephone lines. The home offices had certain advantages. During a blizzard one winter, for example., the agents of a competing carrier found it difficult to reach their call centers in the Northeast; such events did not affect JetBlue's agents. JetBlue needed to operate only a small office in Salt Lake City for training. Average pay for the agents was $8.25 per hour.[35] Southwest Airlines, in contrast, operated 10 call centers across the country, but three were closed in 2004 because of the growing popularity of Internet reservations. Call centers cost about $10 more per employee hour to operate than a network of home-based operators. Agents who worked at home were more satisfied and had much lower rates of turnover than call center agents. Turnover was as low as 4 percent at JetBlue.[36]

JetBlue pilots did not have to carry heavy flight manuals with them into the cockpit. All instruction books were computerized and loaded onto laptop computers. Before a flight, pilots used their laptops in an airport lounge to log on to the Internet wirelessly or via a high-speed connection. They could also download the latest manual updates and technical notices. Pilots at other carriers had flight manuals in three- or five-ring binders; they inserted paper updates and removed the old pages manually. The electronic system saved JetBlue $600,000 a year in printing and distribution costs.[37]

Once in the cockpit, JetBlue pilots read from a printout from the airline's dispatch department and entered basic information, including the outside temperature, destination, weight of the aircraft, fuel load, and number of passengers. The takeoff-calculation software program determined how much engine thrust the pilot should apply and which runways could be used. Pilots did not have to rely on dispatchers at headquarters for the calculations, saving 4,800 worker-hours a year.[38] If an air traffic controller changed a runway at the last minute, the pilot could redo the calculations in 15 seconds, often jumping ahead of other planes still waiting for their numbers. The program detected human errors; if a grossly wrong number was entered, a warning flashed on the screen. The program also helped save on fuel and engine wear. With a paper system, pilots used rules of thumb and thus had to add extra thrust and speed to widen the safety margin.[39]

JETBLUE'S CORPORATE CULTURE

JetBlue had a delicate balancing act to perform. The most significant cost for airlines was labor, which accounted for 36 to 40 percent of total operating expenses.[40] Historically, relations between unions and management were contentious. Unions could shut down an airline if they told their members to go out on strike. JetBlue had to find ways to keep costs down and make employees happy. It wanted to prevent unionization of its employees by offering attractive working conditions. By keeping employees happy, JetBlue managers could then motivate them

to take the next crucial step, which was to provide extraordinary service to passengers. The following are some excerpts from David Neeleman's letter to shareholders in JetBlue's 2003 annual report:

> JetBlue has turned the airline industry upside-down. We set out with the revolutionary idea to create an airline that would treat customers with humanity and provide everyone with high-quality service at affordable fares. We also aspired to build a company with a positive environment where crewmembers would feel respected and excited to come to work every day . . .
>
> At JetBlue, we live by our belief in the 3 P's: great **people** drive solid **performance** which generates **prosperity** for all . . .
>
> At the heart of our company is a conviction that the airline business is fundamentally one of customer service. As such, our crewmembers work hard to exceed expectations on every flight. Our job is to "get it right" every step of the way, from the initial reservation booking with our friendly home-based Reservation team or via www.jetblue.com, to the efficient delivery of the last bag at the customer's destination by our Customer Service team. Our Inflight Crew, Pilots, Technicians and everyone else working to support our front-line crewmembers are central to delivering "the JetBlue experience."

David Neeleman served as a role model to JetBlue employees in a myriad of ways. He constantly strove to make flying a safe, memorable, and satisfying experience for passengers. His goal was for JetBlue to be the best "customer service" company, not necessarily the best "airline" company. He felt that it was too easy to outperform major industry competitors because most of them, including Southwest Airlines, were run in a mediocre fashion. During a speech at an executive breakfast at the Graduate Center of the City University of New York in May 2005, Neeleman said that the foundations for excellent customer service were rooted in (1) crew members who were ambassadors of a brand; (2) flawless execution in which reservation agents who worked from home got what they wanted (e.g., a uniform consisting of JetBlue logo slippers) and in which passengers were told the truth and were compensated for air-travel hassles; and (3) a leader who made sure that his or her company mattered (that customers cared about it and would be distraught if it one day disappeared).

Neeleman tried to create an egalitarian culture at JetBlue. When he went on business trips, he rented a standard midsized automobile, not a limousine. There was no reserved parking, and there were no special perquisites for managers at JetBlue's corporate offices. Passengers were also on an equal footing with one another. There was only one class of airplanes, and the same types of gourmet snacks were offered to all passengers. Neeleman attributed his personal value system, and its subsequent impact on Jet-Blue's culture, to the time he spent in his youth in the slums of Brazil. He was keenly aware of the differences between the "haves" and the "have-nots"; he did not feel that wealthy people were entitled to consider themselves better than those who were poor. As Neeleman liked to tell his pilots, "There are people who make more money at this company than others, but that doesn't mean you should flaunt it."[41]

Neeleman flew on a JetBlue flight once a week so that he could talk to passengers about what they liked and did not like about the airline. He proudly reported that it once took him as long as three and a half hours to walk through the entire cabin. He never had time to watch the live television broadcasts on board. Neeleman also remembered how he felt on September 11, 2001, after the attacks on the World Trade Center and the Pentagon. Since he himself no longer wanted to fly on an airplane, how could he expect his passengers to want to fly? He acted quickly and made sure that six weeks after the attacks, Kevlar® bulletproof cockpit doors (with titanium bolts that could be opened only from the inside) were installed in all JetBlue airplanes. Camera surveillance devices were connected to the onboard DIRECTV system so that the captain and co-pilot could monitor the activities of passengers in the cabin.

Teamwork was important too. It was JetBlue's vice president for marketing, Amy Curtis-McIntyre, who came up with the company name. Her help was important because a series of proposals from outside agencies had been rejected and discussions among senior executives were stalled. While the name Blue was popular because it suggested something airy, futuristic, and vague; and it was in the public domain and could not be protected by a trademark. Curtis-McIntyre thought of the name JetBlue during a conversation with Neeleman.

Often, Neeleman was overruled by his managers. After the September 11 attacks, JetBlue managers faced the difficult task of developing an appropriate marketing message for its customers, many of whom were based in New York City. Neeleman drafted a personal letter that would appear as a full-page advertisement, but his team criticized it for being too "self-conscious." Instead, the carrier ran an ad that suggested understanding and patience: "We know you need time to heal. JetBlue will be here when you're ready to fly again."[42]

Ann Rhoades, JetBlue's first executive vice president of human resources, helped Neelman put in place a strong organizational culture. She believed that "people can accomplish the extraordinary when they are give the authority and responsibility to succeed."[43] She helped the company achieve extraordinary results from its employees by implementing five steps.

The first step for the company was to determine its values. At JetBlue, these values were safety, caring, integrity, fun, and passion. Safety was the company's number one priority, with the other four values being approximately equal in importance.[44] The values guided employees in the decision-making process.

- The carrier's concern over safety was exhibited early on when it signed an agreement with Medaire Inc. that enabled crew members to immediately consult with land-based emergency physicians anytime a passenger fell ill during a flight. JetBlue's Web site featured a link called "inflight health," which offered tips on such topics as what to do if flying caused ear pain and how to prevent deep-vein thrombosis, a rare condition that occurred when blood clots formed in the leg and pelvic veins.

- Caring, according to Rhoades, was exhibited after the September 11 terrorist attacks when the company did not lay off anyone and continued paying salaries and benefits.[45] Both the CEO and the president/chief operating officer donated part of their salaries to a "crisis fund." It might pay the medical bills of an employee's wife who was sick with cancer or replace the personal belongings of an employee whose home was destroyed by a fire.[46] Neeleman once helped a widowed employee make a down payment on a house.[47]

- CEO Neeleman responded with integrity when JetBlue's security department violated company policy and released passenger data to a U.S. Defense Department contractor. Neeleman took personal responsibility for the incident. He either e-mailed, called, or wrote letters to passengers whose information had been released, and he sent out free airline tickets. He hired Deloitte & Touche to analyze and further develop the carrier's privacy policies.

- Fun was apparent at JetBlue's JFK terminal. Employees used George Foreman grills for barbecues. Passengers could hit yellow punching bags to relieve stress. The bags were tagged with such humorous sayings as "Forget where you parked?" and "Left the iron on?"

- The company demonstrated a passion for many things. Employees were passionate about providing excellent service to customers. Once, a passenger who had landed at JFK could not board a connecting flight to Italy because she had left her passport at home in Buffalo. A JetBlue customer service agent telephoned a colleague in Buffalo who went to the woman's home, collected her passport, and put it on a flight to JFK. The passenger was able to depart for Italy.[48] Managers were passionate about showing that they cared about employees. When employees in Burlington, Vermont, complained that there were not enough health care providers in their area, the company added a second health insurance plan. The company was passionate about the larger community; it distributed information about the American Red Cross to its customers during the month of March 2003.

The second step was for managers to hire employees who mirrored company values. An example of an outstanding flight attendant who embodied the values of safety and caring was a 63-year-old former firefighter who had rescued people during the 1993 World Trade Center bombing. An example of someone who was not hired was a pilot who promoted himself by saying that he had 15,000 hours of experience in the cockpit and could fly a plane anywhere, anytime. Yet when asked by the recruiter what else he had done, he could not provide an answer. JetBlue wanted to hear that a candidate had done something special for someone else.

Rhoades encouraged managers to be creative during the hiring process. Instead of asking, "How should we do a better job of screening flight attendants?" one might ask, "Why don't people want to be flight attendants?" College graduates did not want to commit themselves to a long-term contract, so Rhoades agreed to hire them for a year. That way, they could meet people and visit places. Parents with children did not want to be away from home for long periods of time. She created the Friends Crew Program, which allowed two people to train and share a job. This was perfect for a mother and daughter.

When the daughter worked, the mother cared for her grandchild. Rhoades developed three different paths: one for traditional flight attendants, one for college students, and one for friends.

The third and fourth steps were for the company to continually exceed employee expectations and to listen to its customers. JetBlue pilots received immediate benefits and profit-sharing opportunities in their first year of service. Passengers told JetBlue that they wanted television shows free of charge and low-carb snacks such as almonds. They indicated that there was no need for separate restrooms for men and women. The fifth step was for the company to create a "disciplined culture of excellence." It had to continually improve its services and differentiate itself from its competitors.

JETBLUE'S HUMAN RESOURCE MANAGEMENT PRACTICES

Rhoades laid the foundations for JetBlue's focus on people. Employees were called "crew members"; passengers were referred to as "customers"; vendors were addressed as "business partners." Vincent Stabile, who replaced Rhoades as executive vice president of human resources, made sure the company values became an integral part of JetBlue's human resource management practices. His first day at JetBlue was September 11, 2001. He witnessed firsthand how JetBlue employees put their values into action. Soon after the attacks on the World Trade Center, crew members realized that the airports would be closing. At the company's expense, they booked blocks of hotel rooms and reserved buses to transport passengers to their accommodations. They extended the same courtesy to stranded passengers who were booked on the flights of their competitors.[49]

Hiring

According to Stabile, JetBlue received over 100,000 applications and hired between 2,400 and 2,500 employees a year. To screen applicants, JetBlue used a guide created by Development Dimensions International. Every candidate was interviewed by a recruiter, a line manager, and a person from the unit (e.g., customer service) in which he or she might work. The interviewers kept notes, scored the interview, and then met as a group to decide whether the candidate should be hired.

The company looked for employees who were energetic, had a positive attitude, and showed a breadth of skills. For some jobs, candidates did not need experience in the airline industry. If an employee were to have direct contact with customers, he or she needed to have a minimum of two years in a similar service environment. Candidates could have worked at a Ritz-Carlton Hotel or a Nordstrom's department store.[50] In a flight attendant class, one could find a woman in her 50s with a law degree or with a background in the financing of exotic cars. There might be a man in his early 20s who had worked part-time as an emergency medical technician or a man in his 40s who had been an elementary school physical education teacher.[51]

Pilots were encouraged to do more than just fly a plane skillfully. One created diagrams to help orient colleagues to an airport's physical layout, another performed financial analyses, and yet another developed an inventory of pilot skills to screen job applicants.[52] Every executive was assigned to one of the JetBlue's destinations and was expected to tour the airport, visit with JetBlue's staff, and thoroughly check out how well things were going. This was a way for managers at headquarters to learn the names of their subordinates, show that they cared, and develop good working relationships with employees in the field.

Training

JetBlue's director of training was Mike Barger (whose brother David was the president). Initially, Mike Barger ran his program as most airline companies did: Training was tailored to each specific discipline. Worried that the system was fragmented, he proposed bringing all of JetBlue's resources together so that a common philosophy could be developed and standardized. This led to the creation of JetBlue University, which was responsible for the orientation and training of new hires, annual refresher sessions, and leadership courses. The company spent $30 million a year (or 3 percent of its operating budget) on training.[53]

During the new-hire orientation, Mike Barger discussed JetBlue's brand, Neeleman indicated how airline companies made money, and Stabile focused on the company's culture and its values. New hires also learned about the company's informal and formal communication processes. The need for leadership courses arose in 2002 after the company conducted its annual "Speak-Up" survey of all its crew members. One-third of the respondents said they were unhappy with their supervisors, who were abrasive and showed favoritism. The company realized it had promoted people without proper training. It developed a five-day program called "Principles of Leadership," taught by its senior executives. The program emphasized that effective managers were expected to inspire greatness in others.

In 2004, JetBlue formed an educational partnership with New York University (NYU) to teach its trainers at JetBlue University. NYU faculty developed a customized curriculum for JetBlue. It taught trainers how to write a lesson plan, how to conduct assessments, how to design systems, and how to develop facilitation skills. It offered opportunities for trainers to apply their newly acquired knowledge to practical situations. The curriculum was also designed to include specialized training.

In 2005, JetBlue completed construction on a 107,000-square-foot building at Orlando International Airport that became the new home for the airline's training center. It had the capacity for eight flight simulators, two cabin simulators, classrooms, a training pool, a firefighting training station, and a cafeteria. Pilots and in-flight crew would receive all their training there. JetBlue planned to phase out its training with Airbus in Miami in two years. The new facility was situated 2,000 feet away from a LiveTV hangar completed earlier in the year. The firm planned to add a lodge to the location with 300 rooms to house crew members during their training. Total costs for the related projects were estimated at $160 million.

Compensation

JetBlue paid employees lower base salaries than its competitors. Flight attendants started at $25 an hour, mechanics at $26 an hour, and pilots at $108 an hour. US Airways, after implementing cuts, paid its flight attendants $39.95 an hour, its mechanics $28 an hour, and its pilots $134 an hour.[54] JetBlue also had a health coverage plan for employees, as well as profit-sharing and 401(k) retirement plans. Employees who participated in profit sharing received payouts equivalent to seven weeks of pay in 2000 and

2001, eight weeks of pay in 2002, and nine weeks of pay in 2003; 84 percent of the company's employees were JetBlue shareholders. The company had a no-layoff policy.[55]

JETBLUE'S FINANCIAL AND OPERATING PERFORMANCE

Was it too good to be true? The JetBlue story was amazing. It had a CEO who admitted he had ADD but who worked hard to run a company with a caring attitude toward employees and customers. It had a great set of values, including integrity and passion. Passengers liked its hip image and expressed enthusiasm for its service. Nonetheless, JetBlue needed to demonstrate that it was profitable too. It needed to assure shareholders that its long-term prospects were good, not an easy thing to do in an industry where Chapter 11 bankruptcy filings had become common and industrywide losses had totaled over $20 billion during 2001–2005.

Among the major airlines, only Southwest had established that it could remain profitable in tough and turbulent times. JetBlue's performance was encouraging, but scarcely comforting (see Exhibit 5). Sharply rising fuel prices were a particular concern to all the airlines. Eclat Consulting estimated that an increase of one cent per gallon of fuel meant an increase of approximately $2.6 million a year in operating expenses for JetBlue.[56] The summer hurricanes in the Gulf Coast—Katrina and Rita—had further disrupted the jet fuel market. Crude oil prices surged to $70 a barrel, while jet fuel prices rose to $109 a barrel (from $48.82 a barrel in January 2005). The increased fuel costs prompted Neeleman to issue a "grave warning" in October 2005 that the company would report a fourth-quarter loss and a loss for the entire year. Standard & Poor's Rating Services placed JetBlue Airways on a credit watch. In November, the company issued 7 million new shares of its common stock to raise equity.

In 2000, airlines sold tickets for 73.2 percent of the available seats on all flights. Due to flight cutbacks, grounding of some planes, assorted bankruptcy filings, and growing passenger traffic, the number of empty seats on flights in 2004 was down substantially, thus producing a load factor of 83.2 percent.

JetBlue did a good job filling its planes to near capacity, thus helping to lower its operating costs per available seat mile from 9.17 cents to 6.10 cents (refer back to Exhibit 3).

JetBlue's load factors and operating costs (if fuel costs were excluded) were good for most of 2005. JetBlue did, however, encounter a significant problem with delays. Its on-time performance during the months starting from December 2004 and ending in July 2005 put it into 14th place among 19 U.S. carriers. In July 2005, for example, only 61.5 percent of its flights arrived on time. The delays were attributed to bad weather, runway construction at both JFK and Boston's Logan airports; and the firm's preference to proceed with a delayed flight instead of canceling it.[57]

JETBLUE'S POSITION IN THE AIRLINE INDUSTRY

For two consecutive years, a seat at the Phoenix Sky Harbor International Airport Aviation Symposium was left empty.[58] In 2004, the seat was intended for David Siegel, the CEO of US Airways, who resigned under pressure two days before the conference began. US Airways was undergoing Chapter 11 restructuring, and Siegel was unpopular with labor because he had pushed for further employee wage and benefit concessions. In 2005, the seat was vacant because Doug Parker, CEO of America West, was negotiating a merger with US Airways. His attorneys advised him not to attend. The unfilled seats were symbolic of the significant challenges facing the U.S. airline industry, which was said to be at a tipping point.[59]

Several of the so-called legacy carriers (United, Delta, and US Airways) had sustained financial losses over a period of four years and were struggling to survive. In addition to US Airways, UAL Corporation, the parent company of United Airlines, was in bankruptcy. Delta Air Lines and Northwest Airlines filed for bankruptcy protection in September 2005. Restructuring efforts entailed salary cuts, benefits trimming, layoffs, and heavier workloads for remaining employees. The human toll was evident. Employees experienced job-related stresses and frustrations. In 2004, a large flight attendant's union considered an industrywide strike. The FBI investigated employees at US Airways for possibly sabotaging airplanes by punching small

Exhibit 5 **Summary of JetBlue Airways' Financial and Operating Performance, 2000–2004 (in thousands, except per share data)**

	2004	2003	2002	2001	2000
Operating revenues	$1,265,972	$998,351	$635,191	$320,414	$104,618
Operating expenses	1,153,029	829,518	530,204	293,607	125,806
Operating income (loss)	112,943	168,833	104,987	26,807	(21,188)
Government compensation	—	22,761	407	18,706	—
Other income (expense)	(36,121)	(16,155)	(10,370)	(3,598)	(381)
Income (loss) before income taxes	76,822	175,439	95,024	41,915	(21,569)
Income tax expense (benefit)	29,355	71,541	40,116	3,378	(239)
Net income	47,467	103,898	54,908	38,537	(21,330)
Earnings (loss) per share, basic	0.46	1.07	0.73	4.39	(11.85)
Earnings (loss) per share, diluted	0.43	0.96	0.56	0.51	(11.85)
Cash, cash equivalents and investment securities	449,162	607,305	257,853	117,522	34,403
Total assets	2,798,644	2,185,757	1,378,923	673,773	344,128
Total debt	1,544,812	1,108,595	711,931	374,431	177,048
Common stockholders' equity (deficit)	$ 756,200	$671,136	$414,673	$ (32,167)	$ (54,153)
Revenue passengers	11,782,625	9,011,552	5,752,105	3,116,817	1,144,421
Revenue passenger miles (000)	15,730,302	11,526,945	6,835,828	3,281,835	1,004,496
Available seat miles (ASMs) (000)	18,911,051	13,639,488	8,239,938	4,208,267	1,371,836
Load factor	83.2%	84.5%	83.0%	78.0%	73.2%
Aircraft utilization (hours per day)	13.4	13.0	12.9	12.6	12.0
Average fare	$ 103.61	$ 107.09	$ 106.95	$ 99.62	$ 88.84
Passenger revenue per ASM	6.46¢	7.08¢	7.47¢	7.38¢	7.41¢
Operating revenue per ASM	6.69¢	7.32¢	7.71¢	7.61¢	7.63¢
Operating expense per ASM	6.10¢	6.08¢	6.43¢	6.98¢	9.17¢
Fuel gallons consumed (000)	241,087	173,157	105,515	55,095	18,340

Source: 2005 10-K report.

holes into three jets. ComPysch, an employee assistance provider, received 20 percent more calls for help from baggage handlers, flight attendants, and pilots in 2004 compared to 2003. Demoralized employees tended to be less pleasant to passengers. Not surprisingly, customer satisfaction with service provided by the major carriers, went down.[60]

Small carriers were in trouble too. Hawaiian Airlines, a unit of Hawaiian Holdings, had been in bankruptcy since March 2003. As part of its restructuring under Chapter 11, ATA Airlines sold the leasing rights to 6 of its 14 gates at Midway Airport to Southwest Airlines; it also announced plans to sell its Chicago Express regional airline. In June 2004, Flyi Incorporated, the parent of Independence Air, tried to transform itself from a regional feeder for larger airlines into a low-cost carrier. It lost millions of dollars every quarter, its stock price on the Nasdaq fell to $0.07, and it finally filed for bankruptcy protection in November 2005.

Meanwhile, three of the better-positioned low-cost carriers—Southwest Airlines, JetBlue Airways, and AirTran Holdings—were able to increase their

market shares and seemed strong enough to expand their operations into new cities. The future seemed promising—until crude oil prices surged to an all-time high of $70 a barrel in September 2005. In October and November, as the refineries shut down by the Gulf hurricanes went back into service and as the East Coast experienced warmer-than-expected temperatures, crude oil prices fell into a more reasonable price range of between $56 to $60 per barrel. Nonetheless, airlines were expected to pay a total of $30 billion on fuel in 2005 (up from $21 billion in 2004 and $15 billion in 2003).[61]

Southwest Airlines employed the best hedging strategy to lock in lower jet fuel prices (see Exhibit 6). During 2005, it paid $26 a barrel for 85 percent of its fuel and it would pay $32 a barrel for 65 percent of its fuel in 2006. JetBlue, in contrast, had contracts to purchase only 22 percent of its fuel at $30 a barrel for 2005. It did not have any hedges in place for subsequent years. It did the next best thing. It purchased "caps" to ensure that it would not pay more than $65 a barrel for 20 percent of its fuel needs in August and $66 a barrel for 15 percent of its fuel

Exhibit 6   **Fuel Hedge Positions of Major U.S. Air Carriers (crude-equivalent prices)**

	2005		2006		2007		2008		2009	
	% Hedged	Price/ Barrel	% Hedged	Price/ Barrel	% Hedged	Price/ Barrel	% Hedged	Price/ Barrel	% Hedged	Price/ Barrel
AirTran Airways	74%	$50	23%	$55	16%	$31	0%		0%	
Alaska Airways	50	30	43	40	20	45	7	$49	0	
American Airlines	6	40	0		0		0		0	
America West	57	55	12	60	0		0		0	
Continental Airlines	0		0		0		0		0	
Delta Air Lines	0		0		0		0		0	
Frontier Airlines	17	51	0		0		0		0	
JetBlue Airways	22	30	0		0		0		0	
Northwest Airlines	6	42	0		0		0		0	
Southwest Airlines	85	26	65	32	45	31	30	33	25	$35
United Airlines	0		0		0		0		0	

Source: Bear Stearns as Reported to Subcommittee on Aviation, Hearing on Current Situation and Future Outlook of US Commercial Airline Industry (www.house.gov/transportation/aviation/09-28-05/09-28-05memo.html).

needs in September.[62] Some carriers—Continental, Delta, and United—had no hedges. It was not just a lack of foresight. Even if carriers could have gone back in time to purchase hedging contracts with reasonable prices for crude oil, most of them would not have had the funds to afford them.

Energy conservation became crucial. To save fuel, airlines used one engine instead of two to taxi on runways, installed wing fins to minimize drag, flew at slower speeds to reduce the burn rate, and carried less fuel on long flights to decrease weight. Other strategies included flying at higher altitudes, where the air was thinner (and there was less resistance so planes used less fuel), and "tankering" (filling up with more fuel than needed at locations where fuel was less expensive). Many carriers imposed fuel surcharges—between $10 to $50—on one-way fares. Others resorted to canceling flights. American Airlines eliminated 15 daily flights from its hubs in Chicago and Dallas. JetBlue eliminated one round-trip flight from New York to seven Florida destinations on Tuesdays and Thursdays during the month of December. In September 2005, airline industry executives asked Congress to suspend a federal fuel tax for just one year. Suspension of the tax—4.3 cents per gallon—would help the industry save $600 million.

Besides the volatility of jet fuel prices, airline companies faced the prospects of increased competition from new entrants. The British entrepreneur Richard Branson prepared to launch a low-fare carrier, Virgin America, with a hub in San Francisco and administrative offices in New York City. Since foreign ownership of a U.S. airline was limited by law to 25 percent, Branson was in the process of raising funds and finding American investors. David Spurlock, a former executive at British Airways, filed a Department of Transportation application to offer low-fare international service from JFK to Europe on Atlantic Express. Mark Morris, former head of DHL Air Group, formed a plan to start Primaris Airlines, which would offer first-class service in and out of Las Vegas.

Would JetBlue be able to compete? In 2005, JetBlue was still considered a relatively small airline company. Domestically, it ranked 10th in terms of the number of passengers transported per mile and 10th in terms of its 2003 operating revenues. Worldwide, it held the 62nd place for its 2003 revenues.[63] JetBlue faced significant challenges. What would it do if jet fuel prices rose sharply again in 2006? Would it be able to integrate its fleet of smaller Embraer jetliners smoothly into its existing operations? Could it continue to afford investments in the construction of new facilities at the airports in Orlando and New York (JFK)? JetBlue's managers spoke confidently of the future and outlined an aggressive growth strategy. Efforts were under way to recruit 3,500 new employees in 2006. Route expansion was announced for 2006 that would start service between such destinations as New York and Cancun, Mexico; New York and Richmond, Virginia; and New York and Austin, Texas. Airline consultant, Julius Maldutis, however, issued the following warning to airline executives: "You'd better have a very unique business plan that will give you sufficient financial leverage to survive the Armageddon that is already underway in the airline business."[64]

Endnotes

[1]R. Newman, "Loyal Clients Key, JetBlue CEO Says," *Knight Ridder Tribune Business News*, November, 2003, p. 1. Retrieved May 5, 2005, from ABI/INFORM (Proquest) database.

[2]R. Newman, "Preaching JetBlue," *Chief Executive* 202 (October 2004), pp. 26–29. Retrieved March 5, 2005, from ABI/INFORM (Proquest) database.

[3]S. Prasso, "Piloting JetBlue and eBay," *BusinessWeek*, March 17, 2003, p. 16. Retrieved March 24, 2003, from ABI/INFORM (Proquest) database.

[4]D. Neeleman, "From Milk Crates to High Altitudes," *New York Times*, November 5, 2000, p. 3. Retrieved March 12, 2005, from ABI/INFORM (Proquest) database.

[5]C. Salter, "And Now the Hard Part," *Fast Company* 82 (May 2004), p. 67. Retrieved March 12, 2005, from ABI/INFORM (Proquest) database.

[6]S. B. Donnelly, "Blue Skies," *Time*, July 30, 2001, pp. 24–26. Retrieved March 13, 2005, from ABI/INFORM (Proquest) database.

[7]"On the Record: David Neeleman," *San Francisco Chronicle*, September 12, 2004, p. J1. Retrieved March 6, 2005, from ABI/INFORM (Proquest) database.

[8]Newman, "Preaching Jet Blue."

[9]C. Woodyard, "JetBlue Turns to Beetles, Beaches, Bars," *USA Today*, August 22, 2001, p. B3. Retrieved March 6, 2005, from ABI/INFORM (Proquest) database.

[10]Newman, "Preaching JetBlue."

[11]W. Zellner, "Is JetBlue's Flight Plan Flawed?" *BusinessWeek*, February 16, 2004, p. 72. Retrieved March 5, 2005, from ABI/INFORM (Proquest) database.

[12]R. Alonso-Zaldivar, "Frustrated Air Travelers May Get 'Bill of Rights,'" *Los Angeles Times*, March 11, 1999, p. 10. Retrieved March 1, 2005, from ABI/INFORM (Proquest) database.

[13]P. Mann, "Passenger Bill of Rights Loses Luster in Congress," *Aviation Week & Space Technology*, September 27, 1999, p. 41. Retrieved March 1, 2005, from ABI/INFORM (Proquest) database.

[14]Salter, "And Now the Hard Part."

[15]S. Overby, "JetBlue Skies Ahead," *CIO*, July 1, 2002, pp. 72–78. Retrieved January 22, 2003, from ABI/INFORM (Proquest) database.

[16]R. Harris, "The Long Haul," *CIO*, February 1, 2005, p. 1. Retrieved May 5, 2005, from ABI/INFORM (Proquest) database.

[17]R. Smothers, "New Airline to Emphasize More Flights for Upstate," *New York Times*, February 11, 2000, p. B8. Retrieved March 2, 2005, from ABI/INFORM (Proquest) database.

[18]J. M. Feldman, "JetBlue Loves New York," *Air Transport World* 38 (June 2001), pp. 78–80. Retrieved March 3, 2005, from ABI/INFORM (Proquest) database.

[19]E. Brown, "A Smokeless Herb," *Fortune*, May 28, 2001, pp. 78–79. Retrieved May 5, 2005, from ABI/INFORM (Proquest) database.

[20]A. Williams, "SuperFly," *New York Magazine On the Web*, January 31, 2000. Retrieved March 2, 2005, from www.newyorkmetro.com/nymetro/news/bizfinance/biz/features/1879.

[21]R. Dwyer, "Blue Skies," *AirFinance Journal*, 227 (April 2000), p. 26. Retrieved March 15, 2005, from ADI/INFORM (Proquest) database.

[22]Williams, "SuperFly."

[23]K. L. Alexander, "It's Advantage JetBlue in Race for California," *Washington Post*, November 6, 2002, p. F1. Retrieved April 1, 2003, from ABI/INFORM (Proquest) database.

[24]D. Armstrong, "David Neeleman, Founder and CEO of JetBlue Airways, Has a Successful Flight Plan," *San Francisco Chronicle*, December 28, 2002, p. B1. Retrieved January 20, 2003, from ABI/INFORM (Proquest) database.

[25] K. L. Alexander, "The Math Flies," *Washington Post*, February 29, 2004, p. F1. Retrieved March 17, 2005, from ABI/INFORM (Proquest) database.

[26]S. Lott and A. Taylor, "Arrivals: As Planes Go Up, Costs Come Down," *Aviation Daily*, November 16, 2005, p. 5. Retrieved November 25, 2005, from ABI/INFORM (Proquest) database.

[27]Donnelly, "Blue Skies."

[28]K. L. Alexander, "In-Flight Perks Are Steadily Disappearing," *Washington Post*, March 1, 2005, p. E01. Retrieved March 18, 2005, from ABI/INFORM (Proquest) database.

[29]E. Wong, "JetBlue Gives More Passengers 2 Inches More Legroom," *New York Times*, November 14, 2003, p. C3. Retrieved February 28, 2005, from ADI/INFORM (Proquest) database.

[30]R. Smothers, "New Airline to Emphasize More Flights for Upstate," *New York Times*, February 11, 2000, p. B8. Retrieved March 2, 2005, from ABI/INFORM (Proquest) database.

[31]Overby, "JetBlue Skies Ahead."

[32]W. Woodberry, "JFK's Spa Has Riders on Cloud 9," *New York Daily News*, February 8, 2005. Retrieved March 5, 2005, from www.nydailynews.com.

[33]S. Carey, "UAL Hopes Latest Cost Cuts Will Yield Needed Efficiencies," *The Wall Street Journal*, May 12, 2005, p. A10. Retrieved May 26, 2005, from ABI/INFORM (Proquest) database.

[34]M. Walker, "The Thrill Is Gone," *Los Angeles Times*, December 14, 2003, p. I22. Retrieved March 20, 2005, from ABI/INFORM (Proquest) database.

[35]Alexander, "The Math Flies."

[36]D. Whelan, "The Slipper Solution," *Forbes*, May 24, 2004, p. 64. Retrieved March 17, 2005, from ABI/INFORM (Proquest) database.

[37]C. J. Dickinson, "JetBlue CIO Shares Secrets at Technology 2003," *Business Journal—Central New York*, May 9, 2003, p. A2. Retrieved March 17, 2005, from ABI/INFORM (Proquest) database.

[38]Overby, "JetBlue Skies Ahead."

[39]S. Carey and D. Michaels, "At Some Airlines, Laptops Replace Pilots' 'Brain Bags,'" *The Wall Street Journal*, March 26, 2002, p. B1. Retrieved March 20, 2005, from ABI/INFORM (Proquest) database.

[40]*Standard & Poor's Industry Surveys: Airlines*, November 25, 2004.

[41]D. Wademan, "Lessons from the Slums of Brazil," *Harvard Business Review* 83 (March 2005), p. 24.

[42]P. Judge, "How Will Your Company Adapt?" *Fast Company*, December 2001, pp. 128–138. Retrieved March 17, 2005, from ABI/INFORM (Proquest) database.

[43]J. Ginovsky, "Corporate Excellence," *ABA Bankers News* 12 (March 16, 2004), pp 1–2. Retrieved March 17, 2005, from ABI/INFORM (Proquest) database.

[44]"Corporate Culture," *Air Safety Week*, November 12, 2001, p. 1. Retrieved March 17, 2005, from ABI/INFORM (Proquest) database.

[45]"Find a Way to Yes! SLA Keynoter's Tips," *Information Outlook* 8 (March 2004). Retrieved March 17, 2005, from ABI/INFORM (Proquest) database.

[46]B. Finn and D. Neeleman, "How to Turn Managers into Leaders," *Business 2.0* 5 (September 2004), p. 70. Retrieved March 17, 2005, from ABI/INFORM (Proquest) database.

[47]M. Wells, "Lord of the Skies," *Forbes*, October 14, 2002, pp. 130–136. Retrieved April 1, 2003, from ABI/INFORM (Proquest) database.

[48]E. Sanger, "JetBlue Flying High with Service," *New York Newsday*, June 14, 2004. Retrieved March 18, 2005, from www.nynewsday.com.

[49]E. Tahmincioglu, "True Blue," *Workforce Management* 84 (February 2005), pp. 47–50. Retrieved March 17, 2005, from ABI/INFORM (Proquest) database.

[50]P. Flint, "It's a Blue World After All," *Air Transport World* 40 (June 2003), p. 36. Retrieved March 15, 2005, from ABI/INFORM (Proquest) database.

[51]R. Kennedy, "The Skies Are Blue and the Chips Are, Too," *New York Times*, March 18, 2001, p. 9.1. Retrieved March 17, 2005, from ABI/INFORM (Proquest) database.

[52]Salter, "And Now the Hard Part."

[53]Sanger, "JetBlue Flying High."

[54]M. Maynard, "Coffee, Tea or Job?" *New York Times*, September 3, 2004, p. C1.

[55]F. Campailla, "JetBlue Founder Believes Happy Employees Make Successful Companies," *QU Daily*, November 17, 2004. Retrieved March 19, 2005, from www.quinnipiac.edu/x13967.xml.

[56]J. W. Peters, "Rougher Times Amid Higher Costs at JetBlue," *New York Times*, November 11, 2004, p. C1. Retrieved March 5, 2005, from ABI/INFORM (Proquest) database.

[57]S. Lott, "JetBlue Plans Operational Changes to Recover from Chronic Delays," *Aviation Daily*, August 25, 2005, p. 1. Retrieved November 3, 2005, from ABI/INFORM (Proquest) database.

[58]C. Daniel, "Aviation Needs More Than Mergers to Rise Again," *Financial Times*, May 3, 2005, p. 27. Retrieved May 21, 2005, from LexisNexis Academic.

[59]*Standard & Poor's Industry Surveys*, p. 1.

[60]B. De Lollis, "Job Stress Beginning to Take Toll on Some Airline Workers," *USA Today*, November 30, 2004, p. B1. Retrieved November 3, 2005, from ABI/INFORM (Proquest) database.

[61]J. Mouawad and M. Maynard, "On Wall and Main, Worries about Oil," *New York Times*, October 6, 2005, p. C1. Retrieved November 25, 2005, from ABI/INFORM (Proquest) database.

[62]D. McDonald, "A Hard Landing," *New York Magazine*, October 17, 2005, p. 38. Retrieved November 3, 2005, from ABI/INFORM (Proquest) database.

[63]C. Baker, "Challenges Ahead," *Airline Business* 20 (August 2004), pp. 50–58.

[64]D. Reed, "Start-ups Risk It All to Be the Next Southwest," *USA Today*, March 1, 2005, p. B1. Retrieved March 5, 2005, from ABI/INFORM (Proquest) database.

Case 4

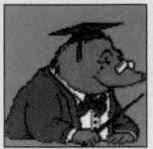

Competition in the Golf Equipment Industry in 2005

John E. Gamble
University of South Alabama

It is not known with certainty when the game of golf originatcd, but historians believe it evolved from ball-and-stick games played throughout Europe in the Middle Ages. The first known reference to golf in historical documents was a 1452 decree by King James II of Scotland banning the game. The ban was instituted because King James believed his archers were spending too much time playing golf and not enough time practicing archery. King James III and King James IV reaffirmed the ban in 1471 and 1491, respectively, but King James IV ultimately repealed the ban in 1502 after he himself became hooked on the game. The game became very popular with royalty and commoners alike, with the Archbishop of Saint Andrews decreeing in 1553 that the local citizenry had the right to play on the links of Saint Andrews and King James VI declaring in 1603 that his subjects had the right to play golf on Sundays.

The first known international golf tournament was played in Leith, Scotland, in 1682 when Scotsmen George Patterson and James VII prevailed over two Englishmen. By the 1700s golf had become an established sport in the British Isles, complete with golfing societies, published official rules, regularly held tournaments, full-time equipment manufacturers, and equipment exports from Scotland to the American colonies. The course at Saint Andrews became a private golf society in 1754 and was bestowed the title of Royal & Ancient Golf Club of Saint Andrews by King William IV in 1834. The first golf society in the United States was founded in Charleston, South Carolina, in 1786.

By 2000, the U.S. golf economy accounted for approximately $62 billion worth of goods and services. The golf economy involved core industries such as golf equipment manufacturers, course designers, turf maintenance services, and club management services. The golf economy also included such enabled industries as residential golf communities and hospitality and tourism. In 2000, the size of golf-enabled industries was estimated at approximately $23 billion. The overall size of core golf industries was estimated at nearly $39 billion, with retail sales of golfing supplies totaling nearly $6 billion. The largest segment of the golfing supply industry was golf equipment, at approximately $4 billion in retail sales, followed by golf apparel, at $989 million; golf magazines, at $737 million; and golf books, at $160 million in retail sales.

Even though golf had grown to have a greater total effect on the U.S. economy than, for example, the motion picture industry or the mining industry, at $57.8 billion and $51.6 billion, respectively, the golf equipment industry was faced with serious troubles in 2005. The retail value of the golf equipment industry had declined from approximately $4 billion in 2000 to $3.2 billion projected for 2005. In addition, the number of golfers in the United States playing eight or more times per year had declined by 3 percent between 2000 and 2004. Industry sales were keyed to the number of core golfers playing eight or more times per year since these frequent golfers accounted for the majority of equipment sales. In addition, equipment manufacturers were finding it more difficult to develop technological innovations that would encourage occasional and core golfers to purchase new equipment. Golf's governing body in North America, the United States Golf Association (USGA), had ruled in 1998 that some clubs planned for introduction at that time were too technologically advanced and posed a threat to the game. The primary concern of the USGA was that technologically advanced driving clubs might produce a spring-like effect to help launch the ball as it was struck by a golfer. As a result of its concern, the USGA established a coefficient of restitution (COR) club face performance limitation that created a technology ceiling; all major manufacturers had reached this ceiling by 2005. Once the USGA felt comfortable that it was able to hold golf club innovation in check, it turned its attention to golf balls. In June 2005, the USGA asked all golf ball manufacturers to develop prototypes of golf balls that would fly 25 yards shorter than current models. USGA officials asked that these prototypes be submitted for evaluation by golf's governing body.

The combined effect of technological limitations imposed by the USGA, slowing growth in the number of new golfers, a decline in the number of core golfers, and blurred differentiation between golf equipment brands had set off some notable price competition in the industry and had led to significant declines in industry profitability and market value. Industry leader Callaway Golf Company, which had earned a record $132 million when it enjoyed a large technology-based competitive advantage over rivals in 1997, experienced a $10.1 million loss in 2004. The company's share price declined from a peak of $35 in 1997 to approximately $15 in late 2005. The company's shares had traded as low as $10 before the company was rumored to be an acquisition target during mid-2005. TaylorMade Golf, which was an adidas-Salomon business unit and another technological leader in the industry, suffered a 1 percent decline in sales and an 11 percent decline in operating profits between 2003 and 2004. Industry rivals with less-developed technological capabilities had actually benefited from the USGA COR limitation, since it provided those companies with an opportunity to catch up to TaylorMade and Callaway Golf from a technology standpoint. Revenues for Adams Golf, which had been a niche seller with limited technological capabilities, increased from $41.7 million in 2000 to $56.8 million in 2004 after its products eventually matched the COR of those offered by such industry leaders as Callaway Golf and TaylorMade. The sizable increase in revenues allowed Adams Golf to swing from a $37 million loss in 2000 to a $3.1 million profit in 2004.

Even though the equalization of technological capabilities and market shares had resulted in increased profits for some golf equipment manufacturers, the overall slim operating profit margins in the industry and emergence of price competition were troubling signs for investors seeking growth and preservation of principal. Golf equipment retail sales, units sold, and average selling price by product category for 1997–2004 are presented in Exhibit 1.

INDUSTRY CONDITIONS IN 2005

In 2005, approximately 27.5 million Americans played golf at least once per year. About one-third of golfers were considered core golfers—those playing at least eight times per year and averaging 37 rounds per year. In 2004, there were 10.2 million adult male core golfers and 2.5 million adult female core golfers in the United States. One million of the 2.9 million junior golfers in the United States played eight or more rounds per year. Minority participation was relatively low in the United States, with only 1.3 million African American golfers, 1.1 million Asian American golfers, and 1.0 million Hispanic American golfers participating in 2003. Ninety-one percent of rounds played per year were accounted for by core golfers. Core golfers also accounted for 87 percent of the industry equipment sales, membership fees, and greens fees.

A large percentage of the sales of gloves, shoes, and bags were replacement purchases by existing golfers since those products tended to wear out over time. Similarly, golf balls needed to be replaced regularly because they were frequently lost. However, the sales of new golf clubs were usually dependent on whether existing golfers believed new clubs would improve their games. Many golfers new to the game tended either to purchase used clubs or to borrow a set, but it was not uncommon for core golfers to spend considerable amounts of money on new equipment in anticipation of lower scores. Even though core golfers might play once a week or more, only a small fraction of golfers might be confused for Professional Golfers' Association (PGA) touring professionals while on the course. The average score for adult male golfers on an 18-hole course was 95, with only 8 percent of adult male golfers regularly

(*Continued on page C-72*)

Exhibit 1 Retail Value, Units Sold, and Average Selling Price of Golf Equipment in the United States, 1997–2004 (dollar amounts and units in millions)

Drivers and Woods

Year	Retail Value	Drivers/Woods Sold	Average Selling Price
1997	$676.8	2.93 million	$231
1998	601.1	2.81	214
1999	583.8	2.91	201
2000	599.1	2.94	204
2001	626.6	2.99	210
2002	608.7	3.09	197
2003	660.4	3.28	201
2004	654.1	3.56	184
2004 vs. 2003	−1.0%	8.5%	−8.7%

Irons

Year	Retail Value	Irons Sold	Average Selling Price
1997	$533.4	7.12 million	$74.90
1998	485.4	6.87	70.71
1999	447.9	6.97	64.28
2000	475.3	7.14	66.57
2001	459.3	7.17	64.06
2002	456.4	7.42	61.50
2003	461.4	7.66	60.23
2004	482.6	8.06	59.88
2004 vs. 2003	4.6%	4.6%	−0.6%

Putters

Year	Retail Value	Putters Sold	Average Selling Price
1997	$142.1	1.70 million	$83.49
1998	150.3	1.68	89.20
1999	160.1	1.68	95.13
2000	161.5	1.67	96.52
2001	167.2	1.65	101.44
2002	184.3	1.65	111.38
2003	195.2	1.60	121.92
2004	188.6	1.58	119.67
2004 vs. 2003	−3.4%	−1.6%	−1.8%

Wedges

Year	Retail Value	Wedges Sold	Average Selling Price
1997	$67.6	0.78 million	$86.17
1998	64.3	0.79	81.79
1999	65.0	0.81	80.45
2000	68.3	0.82	82.88
2001	69.4	0.82	84.78
2002	71.2	0.83	85.24
2003	77.0	0.88	86.99
2004	79.3	0.93	85.58
2004 vs. 2003	3.1%	4.8%	−1.6%

(Continued)

Exhibit 1 **Continued**

Golf Balls

Year	Retail Value	Golf Balls Sold	Average Selling Price per Dozen
1997	$458.7	19.97 million	$22.97
1998	487.4	20.06	24.30
1999	518.1	20.46	25.32
2000	530.8	20.80	25.52
2001	555.6	21.32	26.06
2002	529.9	20.81	25.46
2003	496.4	19.85	25.01
2004	506.3	19.98	25.34
2004 vs. 2003	2.0%	0.7%	1.3%

Footwear

Year	Retail Value	Pairs Sold	Average Selling Price
1997	$214.3	2.48 million	$86.49
1998	204.3	2.43	84.13
1999	206.9	2.47	83.77
2000	220.8	2.52	87.68
2001	217.8	2.57	84.62
2002	211.7	2.68	78.95
2003	217.1	2.82	76.97
2004	234.4	3.00	78.22
2004 vs. 2003	8.0%	6.2%	1.6%

Gloves

Year	Retail Value	Gloves Sold	Average Selling Price
1997	$156.7	12.81 million	$12.23
1998	160.6	12.79	12.56
1999	161.6	12.98	12.46
2000	165.4	13.20	12.53
2001	169.2	13.42	12.61
2002	163.7	13.36	12.26
2003	157.1	12.92	12.16
2004	159.3	13.15	12.11
2004 vs. 2003	1.4%	1.8%	−0.4%

Golf Bags

Year	Retail Value	Golf Bags Sold	Average Selling Price
1997	$171.8	1.37 million	$125.82
1998	165.6	1.32	125.13
1999	165.4	1.32	125.22
2000	165.1	1.31	125.56
2001	163.2	1.32	124.02
2002	153.4	1.32	116.27
2003	145.5	1.32	110.58
2004	146.8	1.34	109.55
2004 vs. 2003	0.9%	1.8%	−0.9%

Source: Golf Datatech

breaking a score of 80. The average score for adult female golfers was 106. Throughout the 1990s, it was very common for core golfers to purchase a new driver at $400–$500 at least every other year as clubs with new technological advances were introduced. Most core golfers seemed to believe it was worth the cost of new drivers, putters, and irons if technology could help offset their modest skill levels.

Key Competitive Capabilities in the Golf Equipment Industry

Competitive rivalry in the industry centered on technological innovation in clubhead and shaft design, product performance, company image, and tour exposure. The pace of technological innovation had increased rapidly during the late 1990s as industry leaders Callaway Golf, Ping Golf, TaylorMade Golf, and Titlelist each attempted to beat the other to market with clubs touting unique performance characteristics. The breakneck pace of technological change caused product life cycles to decline from about three to four years during the early 1990s to about 12–18 months by 2000. Similarly, the manufacturers of golf balls introduced new products at intervals of 12–18 months to keep the interest of golfers who were looking for products that included innovations and improved performance.

The innovations in clubhead design focused on the use of lightweight metal or carbon composite materials to increase clubhead size without adding weight, to improve weight distribution within the clubhead, and to create a larger club face. After Callaway Golf Company's 1991 launch of the oversized Big Bertha driver, golf equipment manufacturers began to search for materials that would allow the clubhead to increase further in size and have a thinner face. The larger clubhead size and thinness of the club face created a larger "sweet spot," which reduced the negative effects of mis-hit shots. Beginning in the early 2000s, clubhead designers began to reposition weight in the clubhead to produce higher launch angles and to create a draw bias. Higher launch angles tended to help golfers achieve greater distance, while a draw bias helped many golfers hit straighter shots.

A golf club manufacturer's image was based in large part on its reputation for innovation and on endorsements from touring professionals. Most recreational golfers who watched televised golf tournaments or read golf magazines were very aware of what brands of clubs and golf balls their favorite touring professionals used. Also, it was not unusual for recreational golfers to base purchase decisions on the equipment choices of successful golfers on the PGA Tour. All leading golf equipment companies had long-term endorsement agreements with well-known touring professionals and also went to great lengths to make sure their products were used by lesser-known golfers as well.

The Darrell Survey counted and recorded the brand and model of each club in every golfer's bag during every professional tournament. Many golf equipment companies would pay tournament entrants a "tee-up fee" of $1,000 to $2,000 to put a club in their bag during the day of the Darrell Survey count. The tee-up fees allowed some golf club manufacturers to make factual, although misleading, claims in upcoming ads in golf magazines that their products were "number one on the PGA Tour." Endorsements paid to professional golfers totaled nearly $255 million in 2000. The best players in the game commanded multimillion-dollar contracts. Ernie Els's contract with Titleist was worth $3 million per year, while Callaway Golf paid Phil Mickelson a reported $8 million per year to use its clubs in PGA tournaments. Tiger Woods's $125 million five-year contract inked with Nike in 2003 far exceeded that provided to any other PGA touring professional in 2005. Woods's total endorsements were estimated to be worth more than $50 million per year.

Golf equipment companies also relied on personalized service in addition to lucrative endorsement fees to retain endorsements from key touring professionals. All golf equipment companies supported their touring staff members with equipment trailers during tournaments that could make adjustments to clubs prior to and during a tournament or make club substitutions at the pro's request. Some professionals' requests during the tournament might be as simple as asking the manufacturer's support staff to substitute a long iron for an additional fairway wood, while others, who might have struggled during the day, might ask that the shafts be replaced in all of their clubs before the next day's round. Touring staff members also frequented the manufacturer's headquarters to give designers feedback during the development process and to have their equipment customized to their preference. For example, when Tiger Woods became a Nike Golf staff player in 1999, his Nike irons were so highly customized they did not even resemble Nike irons offered to consumers.

Suppliers to the Industry

Most club makers' manufacturing activities were restricted to club assembly since clubhead production was contracted out to investment casting houses located in Asia and shafts and grips were usually purchased from third-party suppliers. Casting houses, such as Advanced International Multitech Company in Taiwan, produced clubheads to manufacturers' specifications and shipped the clubheads to the United States for assembly. Manufacturers were quite selective in establishing contracts with offshore casting houses since the quality of clubhead greatly affected consumers' perception of overall golf club quality and performance. Poor casting could result in clubheads that could easily break or fail to perform to the developers' expectations. Ping Golf was the only golf club producer vertically integrated into clubhead casting.

Differentiation based on shaft performance became more important to golf club manufacturers as technological differences between brands of golf clubs decreased after the USGA enacted its limitation on clubhead size and performance. Most golf club manufacturers developed modestly sized lines of proprietary shafts, which were also produced by outside suppliers. The relatively narrow line of shafts bearing the club manufacturer's name was supplemented with branded shafts produced and marketed by companies such as UST, Fujikura, or Graffaloy. Even though third-party branded shafts were equally available to all manufacturers, they were important in attracting sales to highly discriminating consumers, since these golfers might have as strong a preference for a particular shaft as for a clubhead design. For example, the purchase decision made by a low-handicap golfer considering two drivers might come down to which club could be ordered with a specific shaft.

The USGA limitation on clubhead size and club face performance had helped shaft manufacturers record higher revenues and profits. Like many shaft manufacturers, Aldila had struggled during years when consumers' greatest interest was on clubhead innovations, but a shifting consumer focus on shafts had allowed the company to swing from a $1.7 million loss in 2003 to a $9.3 million profit in 2004. At the end of the company's second quarter 2005, its net profit margins had soared to nearly 19 percent, its current ratio was nearly 4.0, and its stock price had improved to $25 per share from $1 per share in late 2002. Grips had yet to prove to be a point of differentiation, and few golfers showed a strong preference for one brand of grip over another.

Golf Equipment Retailers and the Distribution and Sale of Golf Equipment

Leading golf equipment manufacturers distributed their products through on-course pro shops, off-course pro shops such as Edwin Watts and Nevada Bob's, and online golf retailers such as Golfsmith.com and TGW.com. Most on-course pro shops sold only to members and carried few clubs since their members purchased golf clubs infrequently. Off-course pro shops accounted for the largest portion of retail golf club sales because they carried a wider variety of brands and marketed more aggressively than on-course shops. Off-course pro shops held an advantage over online retailers as well, since golf equipment consumers could inspect clubs and try out demo models before committing to a purchase. Also, both on-course and off-course pro shops were able to offer consumers custom fitting and advice from a PGA member or other individual with the training necessary to properly match equipment to the customer. Most consumers making online purchases had already decided on a brand and model, choosing to buy online to get a lower price or to avoid sales taxes. However, most of the top brands required online retailers to sell their equipment at the same prices as those offered by traditional retailers.

Custom fitting was offered by most manufacturers and large off-course pro shops with the use of specialized computer equipment. Common swing variables recorded and evaluated in determining the proper clubs for golfers included clubhead speed and path, club face angle at impact, ball position, the golfer's weight distribution, ball flight pattern, and ball flight distance. Custom fitting had become very important as golf equipment companies expanded shaft flex options during the early 2000s. In 2005, most iron sets could be equipped with shafts in senior, regular, stiff, or extra-stiff flex. Manufacturers offered drivers with dozens of different shaft configurations. For example, the Callaway Golf Big Bertha Fusion FT-3 Driver could be ordered with Aldila, Fujikura, Graffaloy, UST, or Graphite Design shafts. There were 20 different Aldila shafts available for the Fusion FT-3, each with a unique flex, weight, torque, and kick point. A wide variety of shafts from UST, Graphite Design, Fujikura, and Graffaloy were also available on the Fusion FT-3 driver.

Pro shops generally chose to stock only equipment produced by leading manufacturers and did not carry less expensive, less technologically advanced equipment. Low-end manufacturers sold their products mainly through discounters, mass merchandisers, and large sporting goods stores. These retailers had no custom fitting capabilities and rarely had sales personnel knowledgeable about the performance features of the different brands and models of golf equipment carried in the store. Such retail outlets offered the appeal of low price; they mainly attracted beginning golfers and occasional golfers who were unwilling to invest in more expensive equipment.

RECENT TRENDS IN THE GOLF EQUIPMENT INDUSTRY

Limited Opportunities for Innovation in Clubface Design

Not long after Callaway Golf Company's introduction of the Great Big Bertha titanium driver in 1995, the United States Golf Association (USGA) began to show concern that technologically advanced golf equipment might change the game of golf. The driving distance of John Daly, Tiger Woods, and other PGA members had overwhelmed some golf courses designed in the age of persimmon woods, and it was not unusual for the average driving distance of professional tournament golfers to exceed 300 yards. Many golfers playing on the Champions Tour claimed that new, technologically advanced drivers had helped them hit the longest drives of their careers even though they might be age 60 or over. The USGA believed that the added distance was a product of ultra-thin driver clubfaces that produced a springlike or trampoline effect that could help propel the ball forward.

Beginning in 1998, the USGA limited the coefficient of restitution (COR) for drivers to 0.83 to prevent manufacturers from developing clubs with a so-called springlike effect. The COR—the ratio of incoming to outgoing velocity—was calculated by firing a golf ball at a driver out of a cannonlike machine at 109 miles per hour. The speed that the ball returned to the cannon could not exceed 83 percent of its initial speed (90.47 miles per hour). Drivers that did not conform to the USGA 0.83 COR threshold were barred from use by recreational or professional golfers in the United States, Canada, and Mexico who intended to play by the USGA's Rules of Golf. The USGA refused to calculate handicaps for golfers who had used nonconforming equipment, but it did not attempt to restrict the club's usage among players who did not choose to establish or maintain handicaps.

A discrepancy existed between the USGA's limitation on driver performance and the Rules of Golf as published by the Royal and Ancient (R&A) Golf Club of Saint Andrews, Scotland, which governed play in most countries outside of North America. The R&A did not measure the COR for driving clubs at the time of the USGA's ruling and did not have a COR limitation for clubhead performance. The two organizations agreed to develop a common worldwide standard for clubhead performance in May 2002, but the USGA unexpectedly withdrew its support from the compromise standard in August 2002. In December 2003, the R&A announced its policy regarding driver performance that would become effective in January 2004. The R&A developed a less complex test for a springlike or trampoline effect that used a pendulum to drop a weight onto the clubface of the driver. The R&A pendulum test required that the clubface and the weight remain in contact for 239 microseconds, with a tolerance of 18 microseconds. The pendulum test was applied only to drivers used in elite professional tournaments. The R&A ruled that recreational golfers and those competing in lesser tournaments were not subject to its Driving Club Condition of Competition. The USGA developed a similar pendulum test to replace its test for COR after the R&A made its December 2003 announcement. However, the USGA's use of a pendulum test did not change its specifications for drivers or make nonconforming drivers available to recreational golfers wishing to maintain a handicap.

Golf club manufacturers disagreed that a springlike effect could be produced by a metal golf club and believed that the USGA's ruling, which affected recreational as well as professional tournament golfers, would discourage new golfers from taking up the game. During the 2000 Masters Tournament in Augusta, Georgia, Callaway Golf's chief engineer, Richard Helmstetter, challenged the suggestion that clubs with a high COR could produce a springlike effect:

> We do a great deal of research at Callaway Golf and I think we are the most technologically advanced golf company in the world. We have been unable to find any evidence at all that a club face, no matter how thin, plays a role like a trampoline in striking the ball. We do think that certain kinds of construction and materials will reduce the loss of energy in the golf ball at impact and give the golfer longer drives, but this is quite different from a trampoline. The club face vibrates during impact at a speed so high that it cannot be timed, we believe, to the compression and release of a golf ball. Consequently, we think that trampoline effect is a misnomer, if not a myth entirely.[1]

Callaway Golf challenged the USGA's COR limitation in 2000 when it introduced for sale in the United States the ERC II driver with a COR of 0.86. The company's management believed that the 6–10 additional yards of carry achieved by recreational golfers using the ERC II posed no threat to the game of golf. Callaway Golf executives did concede that equipment limitations might be set for professional golfers, but saw no need to limit the performance of equipment used by recreational golfers who might gain more pleasure from hitting longer drives. Callaway Golf founder Ely Callaway suggested there were "two games of golf—tournament golf and recreational golf, and the two games differ in many respects . . . We believe that recreational golfers should not be denied the benefits of modern technology that can bring them added enjoyment that comes from occasionally hitting the ball a little bit further."[2]

Upon the announcement that Callaway Golf would make the club available to golfers in the United States, Arnold Palmer supported the company's decision by saying, "I think what Callaway is doing is just right. I have given a lot of thought to conforming and nonconforming clubs. If my daughter, who is a 100s shooter can shoot 90 with a nonconforming driver, I can't imagine that there would be anything wrong with that."[3]

The ERC II was a failure in the United States since the USGA did not agree with Callaway Golf's arguments and recreational golfers were hesitant to purchase a nonconforming club. The club did sell in large numbers in markets where the R&A Rules of Golf governed play. In 2005, all major golf club producers produced two versions of their drivers—high-COR drivers for markets outside North America and a version with a COR of 0.83 for the United States, Mexico, and Canada.

Slowing Growth in the Number of New Golfers and Rounds Played

Golf was the 12th most popular form of recreation in the United States, with approximately 27.5 million participants. In 2003, there were approximately 6.3 million golfers in Europe and 16.7 million golfers in Asia. The industry had seemingly reached maturity as a sport, with the number of new participants each year barely exceeding the number who were giving up the sport. Asia's 2–3 percent annual growth in the number of new golfers made it the only geographic region to experience growth between 1999 and 2003. Poor economic conditions in the United States during 2000 caused many frequent golfers to scale back their participation levels that year, but the number of core and avid core golfers rebounded in 2001 through 2004. However, the overall number of rounds played by golfers declined until 2004, when the number of rounds played increased by nearly 7 percent. Exhibits 2 and 3 present trends in frequency of play and rounds played for the U.S. golf market for various years between 1991 and 2004.

A survey of golfers conducted in June 2003 by the National Golf Foundation found that golfers of all types were finding it more difficult to play golf often. Golfers who were married with children were most likely to comment that job responsibilities, lack of free time, and family responsibilities prohibited them from playing golf on a more regular basis. Job responsibilities and lack of free time were also barriers to playing golf more frequently for married or single golfers who had no children. Older golfers who were either retired or who were working less than 40 hours per week had fewer job and family responsibilities and had ample free time, but were frequently troubled with heath concerns or injuries. About 30 percent of golfers said that high golf fees prevented them from playing golf more often. In fact, a different study on golf participation conducted by the National Golf Foundation in 2003 found that income was the primary predictor of golf participation.

The 2003 National Golf Foundation study on minority golf participation in the United States found there were differences in participation rates

Exhibit 2 **Number of U.S. Golfers by Frequency of Play, 1991, 1994, 1997, 2000–2003 (in thousands)**

Year	Occasional Golfers (1–7 rounds/year)	Core Golfers (8–24 rounds/year)	Avid Core Golfers (25+ rounds per year)	Total Golfers
1991	11,480	6,133	5,348	22,961
1994	11,463	6,058	5,113	22,634
1997	10,619	7,897	5,602	24,118
2000	10,961	7,399	6,276	24,636
2001	14,190	5,676	5,934	25,800
2002	13,624	6,812	5,764	26,200
2003	14,184	7,083	6,133	27,400

Source: National Golf Foundation

among races, but income tended to reduce those differences. For golfers with household incomes lower than $100,000, white non-Hispanics and Asians were nearly twice as likely to play golf as African Americans or Hispanic Americans. Nearly 15 percent of white non-Hispanic Americans and 12.4 percent of Asian Americans with household incomes of less than $100,000 per year played golf, whereas only 8.4 percent of African Americans and 8.0 percent of Hispanic Americans with incomes under $100,000 played golf. However, the percentage of individuals with household incomes less than $100,000 interested in playing golf did not vary to a great degree among U.S. citizens of different races. White non-Hispanic Americans were most interested in golf (29.6 percent), but 23.8 percent of African Americans, 24.2 percent of Asian Americans, and 20.2 percent of Hispanic Americans were also interested in playing golf. About 28 percent of adults with household incomes exceeding $100,000 played golf, regardless of race. At household incomes exceeding $150,000, the National Golf Foundation

study found that Hispanic Americans had the highest golf participation rate, at 32 percent.

Foretelling the findings of the National Golf Foundation's studies on golf participation, former Callaway Golf CEO Ron Drapeau said in a 2002 interview with *Smart Money*, "The cost of golf is a concern: We need to see more affordable municipal-type golf courses, including alternative facilities; 9-hole courses, pitch-and-putt, and par 3 courses. The time it takes to play is also an issue."[4]

The Rise of Counterfeiting in the Golf Equipment Industry

Knockoffs of branded golf equipment had been produced by Chinese manufacturers and sold in the United States since the early 1990s, but they weren't a serious threat to the industry because knockoffs only appeared similar to legitimate products. For example, knockoffs like the Canterbury Big Bursar looked similar to the Callaway Big Bertha driver but

Exhibit 3 **Total Rounds of Golf Played in the United States, 2001–2004 (in millions)**

Year	Rounds Played (in millions)	Percent Change
2001	518.1	—
2002	502.4	−3.0%
2003	494.9	−1.5
2004	528.6	6.8

Source: National Golf Foundation

would never pass for a Big Bertha upon close inspection. Beginning golfers were most likely to purchase knockoffs since they looked similar to brand-name clubs but sold for as much as 75 percent less than clubs made by Callaway Golf, Cobra, TaylorMade, Ping, or Titleist. Serious golfers tended not to purchase knockoff clubs since they were made from poor-quality alloy metals, did not perform as well as branded clubs, and were prone to breaking.

Counterfeit clubs were a much greater threat to the industry since good counterfeits were nearly exact copies of legitimate products and could only be identified as counterfeits by very knowledgeable golfers, trained personnel of golf equipment retailers, or golf equipment producers. Like knockoffs, counterfeits were made from inferior materials, were not produced to the standards of legitimate equipment manufacturers, and were not very durable. However, the extraordinarily low prices that counterfeit clubs were offered at were too great a temptation for many bargain-hunter golfers. In 2005, it was not unusual to see complete sets of new Callaway Golf, TaylorMade, Ping, Titleist, Nike, or Cobra clubs that would retail for more than $2,000 sell on eBay or similar auction Web sites for $150 to $400. Sellers who dealt in counterfeit merchandise could purchase counterfeit sets complete with eight irons, a driver, two or three fairway woods, a putter, a golf bag, and a travel bag for as little as $100 in China. Callaway Golf Company alerted visitors to its Web site to counterfeit clubs sold on eBay or other Internet sites with the following warning: "A full set of authentic Callaway Golf clubs, depending on the models, will retail for $2,500–$3,000 or more. If the deal looks too good to be true, it probably is."[5]

The rise in counterfeiting was attributable to the improved manufacturing capabilities of companies in China and the decision by golf equipment companies to source components from Chinese manufacturers. In 2005, about 60 percent of all golf equipment was produced in China and more than 90 percent of counterfeits came from China. Counterfeiters were able to make very accurate copies of branded golf clubs through reverse engineering or by enticing employees of contract manufacturers to steal clubhead molds that could be used to produce counterfeit clubheads. Similarly, counterfeit shafts and grips could be fabricated to produce complete sets of counterfeit golf clubs. Counterfeiters even copied the details of the packaging golf clubs were shipped in to better disguise the fakes. It was estimated that counterfeiters in China could produce golf clubs for less than $3 per club.

The golf equipment industry's six leading manufacturers created an alliance in December 2003 to identify and pursue counterfeiters and sellers of counterfeit clubs. TaylorMade Golf, Fortune Brands (parent of Titleist and Cobra Golf), Callaway Golf, Ping Golf, Cleveland Golf, and Nike Golf had successfully shut down many Internet auction sellers in the United States and Canada that listed counterfeit clubs and had gained cooperation from the Chinese government to confiscate counterfeit goods produced in that country. The Chinese government conducted two raids in 2004 that netted approximately $3 million worth of counterfeit golf equipment and the Chinese seized more than $1 million worth of counterfeit clubs in 2005. However, the efforts to shut down Internet sellers of counterfeits and manufacturers of counterfeits had achieved limited success. A Nike executive explained, "Often these aren't legitimate businesses, so you can't take the case to a court of law, you have to hunt them down. Many times it isn't even worth the effort. They simply create a new company and move. It's really frustrating."[6]

PROFILES OF THE LEADING MANUFACTURERS AND MARKETERS OF GOLF EQUIPMENT

Callaway Golf Company

Callaway Golf Company began to take form in 1983 when Ely Reeves Callaway Jr. purchased a 50 percent interest in a Temecula, California, manufacturer and marketer of hickory-shafted wedges and putters for $400,000. Upon acquiring an interest in Hickory Stick USA, Callaway became the company's president and CEO and soon began to transform the little-known maker of reproductions of antique clubs into the world's largest producer of golf clubs. Callaway knew from the outset that the company's prospects for outstanding profits were limited as long as its product line was restricted to hickory-shafted clubs. Callaway noticed that most golf equipment had changed very little since the 1920s and believed that, due to the difficulty of the game of golf (there was so much room for variation in *each* swing of the club and for off-center contact with the ball), recreational golfers would be willing to invest in high-tech, premium-priced equipment if such clubs could improve their game by being more forgiving of a less-than-optimum swing. Ely Callaway's vision was at odds with that of the company's founders and eventually resulted in Callaway's outright purchase of the company. In 1985 Ely Callaway hired Richard C. Helmstetter as the company's chief club designer, who was aided by a team of five aerospace and metallurgical engineers, to develop what Callaway termed a "demonstrably superior and pleasingly different" line of clubs that was set apart from competing brands by its technological innovation. Helmstetter and his team introduced the company's S2H2 (short, straight, hollow hosel) line of irons in 1988 and an S2H2 line of metal woods in 1989. The 1988 S2H2 launch was accompanied by a name change from Callaway Hickory Stick USA to Callaway Golf Company. The S2H2 line of clubs was well received by professional and recreational golfers alike and became the number one driver on the Senior PGA Tour by year-end 1989.

The company's engineers followed up the successful S2H2 line with the Big Bertha—named by Callaway after the World War I German long-distance cannon—which was launched in 1991. The Big Bertha was revolutionary in that it was much larger than conventional woods and lacked a hosel so that the weight could be better distributed throughout the clubhead. This innovative design gave the clubhead a larger sweet spot, which allowed a player to mis-hit or strike the golf ball off-center and not suffer much loss of distance or accuracy. By 1992 Big Bertha drivers were number one on the Senior PGA, LPGA, and Hogan Tours. Callaway Golf Company became a public company on February 28, 1992. By year-end 1992 its annual revenues had doubled to $132 million, and by 1996 Callaway Golf had become the world's largest manufacturer and marketer of golf clubs, with annual sales of more than $683 million.

The company's technological leadership and financial performance eroded during a brief retirement by Ely Callaway between 1996 and 1998, but rebounded soon after Ely Callaway returned as CEO in October 1998. The founder's first efforts upon his return to active management at Callaway Golf were to "direct [the company's] resources—talent,

energy, and money—in an ever-increasing degree toward the creation, design, production, sale and service of new and better products."[7] As part of his turnaround strategy Ely Callaway also initiated a $54.2 million restructuring program that involved a number of cost-reduction actions and operational improvements. Ely's strategies allowed the company to regain its technological leadership with the introduction of Callaway Golf Company's low center-of-gravity Steelhead line of metal woods in 1998, the ERC Forged Titanium Driver in 1999, and variable face thickness X-14 irons and the ERC II Forged Titanium Driver in 2000. Also, the company acquired Odyssey, a leading brand of putters, in 1996 and began manufacturing and marketing golf balls in 2000. Ely Callaway believed that golf balls were a natural product-line extension for the company, pointing out, "We have 7 million people out there playing our products, and 80% of them think they're the best clubs in the world—we have almost a guaranteed 'try' on our new products."[8]

In February 2000 a survey of golf equipment company executives voted Callaway's Big Bertha driver the best golf product of the century by a 2-to-1 margin. The same group of executives called Ely Callaway the most influential golf trade person of the 1990s. Ely Callaway stepped down as president and CEO of the company on May 15, 2001, after being diagnosed with pancreatic cancer. He was replaced by the company's senior executive vice president of manufacturing, Ron Drapeau, and passed away at his home in Rancho Santa Fe, California, on July 5, 2001. Drapeau began his employment with Callaway Golf in late 1996 and had headed the company's Odyssey Golf unit for 18 months before becoming responsible for all of the company's manufacturing operations as vice president of manufacturing in February 1999.

As it had during Ely Callaway's 1996 retirement, the company's performance declined soon after his death in 2001. Callaway's share of drivers began to decline after the USGA instituted its 0.83 COR limitation in 1998, but the company's share of the driver market fell at a faster rate under Drapeau. The 0.83 limitation left Callaway with fewer innovation options since the company had already met the 0.83 threshold at the time the rule went into effect. The key innovation of Callaway's highly successful Great Big Bertha driver launched in 1995 was its titanium construction. Titanium was a much lighter metal than stainless steel, which allowed Callaway

Golf's engineers to create a larger clubhead featuring an expanded sweet spot. After competitors had matched Callaway Golf Company's titanium construction, the company's research and development efforts steered toward identifying materials lighter than titanium. In 2002, Callaway Golf introduced the C4 driver— a 360-cubic-centimeter (cc) driver made from a carbon composite material. The carbon composite material performed exceptionally well and was 75 percent lighter than titanium, which allowed golfers to generate more clubhead speed than with heavier titanium clubs.

Even though the C4 performed up to the R&D staff's expectations, the driver was a failure in the marketplace. The driver met the 0.83 COR limit, as did competing drivers, but golfers were much more impressed with the drivers offered by Titleist, Ping, Cobra, and TaylorMade. The C4 had two shortcomings in the minds of many golfers. First, most of Callaway's rivals chose to push the size of their drivers toward the USGA size limit of 460 cc rather than experiment with lighter materials. The larger clubhead tended to give some golfers more confidence at the tee and produced a higher launch angle, which equated to greater distance. Also, golfers were dissatisfied with the sound of the carbon composite driver, which was rather muffled when it struck a ball. The extra-large, hollow titanium drivers produced by Callaway Golf's rivals tended to produce an exceptionally loud noise when they made contact with the ball. Golf retailers found that many customers that tried C4 and competing demo drivers returned the C4 to their stores stating that "even though they hit the club very well, it didn't sound like they hit it well."

The company also misjudged the importance of a new type of club introduced by rivals that was a substitute for low-lofted, long irons. Hybrid clubs had a clubhead smaller than, but similar to, a fairway wood with a shaft the length of that used in a midlength iron. Golfers of all abilities (even touring professionals) found the hybrid clubs much easier to hit than long irons. TaylorMade's Rescue was the first hybrid to gain a widespread appeal, but almost all manufacturers raced to quickly get hybrid clubs to the market. Callaway Golf's inability to get its hybrid club to market before 2005 caused it to lose significant sales as many golfers purchased TaylorMade, Nike Golf, Adams Golf, and Cobra hybrid clubs to replace 2-, 3-, and 4-irons from their bags. Some golfers replaced fairway woods with hybrids as well.

As Callaway Golf struggled with its golf club business, its golf ball operations also failed to perform to management's expectations. When Ely Callaway announced that the company would enter the golf ball business, the company expected to gain a 10 percent market share within two years and eventually become one of the two top brands of golf balls. The company missed its projections, with its sales growing to just $66 million and its share reaching only 5.7 percent in 2002. In addition, Callaway Golf's golf ball business had lost $90 million between 2000 and 2002 and showed little hope of providing a return on its $170 million investment in golf ball development and plant and equipment. In 2003, the company acquired Top-Flite Golf for $125 million to give it the volume necessary to achieve economies of scale in golf ball production. At the time of its acquisition by Callaway Golf, the maker of Top-Flite golf balls, Strata golf balls, and Ben Hogan golf clubs had sales of $250 million and was in bankruptcy. About $175 million of the company's 2002 revenues were generated from the sale of golf balls.

Even though the Top-Flite acquisition made Callaway Golf the number two golf ball producer behind Titleist, the acquisition led to further financial problems for the company. Integrating Top-Flite's operations into Callaway's golf ball business was more troublesome than expected. Callaway Golf's golf balls were the most technologically advanced in the industry in 2003 and were produced at its state-of-the-art production facility in Carlsbad, California. Top-Flite primarily produced lower-end golf balls for mass merchandisers using an older golf ball production facility with few technological capabilities. Callaway was unable to use Top-Flite's production facility to produce Callaway Golf golf balls until 2005 because Callaway's high-tech golf balls were too complex to be produced in the older Top-Flite plant. In addition, the integration of Top-Flite and Callaway personnel was a challenge because the two companies had dramatically different cultures. Ely Callaway had developed a professional, technology-based culture that encouraged employees to exhibit the highest levels of gentlemanly behavior, while some retailers had likened Top-Flite's freewheeling sales force to carnival barkers.

With Callaway's growing problems in its golf club operations and golf ball business, pressure began to mount on Ron Drapeau to produce results acceptable to investors. Under Drapeau, the company did introduce the highly successful Odyssey 2-Ball putter, which allowed the company to increase its share of the putter market from 30.7 percent in 1999 to 40.2 percent in 2002. In fact, the sales of 2-Ball putters alone were greater than the total revenues for any golf company except Titleist/Cobra, TaylorMade, and Ping in 2003. Callaway Golf had also achieved acceptable results in the irons category of the golf equipment industry, where its share grew from 14.4 percent in 1999 to 16.1 percent in 2002, but its inventory of fairway woods and drivers grew to unacceptable levels as its share of those products declined from 30.9 percent in 1999 to 21.6 percent in 2002. In 2003 and 2004, Drapeau dropped retail prices on its drivers by as much as $100 and even gave some products away to retailers. The price cut on current models was a first in the company's history. Typically, the company did not discount products until a new generation was launched and available in retail stores.

Ron Drapeau stepped down as Callaway Golf CEO in August 2004 to be replaced on an interim basis by longtime board member 71-year-old William Baker. The company did not name a permanent replacement until August 2005, when it hired former Revlon CEO George Fellows to lead the company. While at Revlon as CEO between 1997 and 1999, Fellows had been credited for producing a turnaround year in 1997 after years of losses. However, the company returned to a loss in 1998 and recorded its worst-ever loss in 1999. Some analysts suggested that Fellows did "not [have] a strong résumé" for the job, and others claimed that while Fellows was at Revlon, he "was handed a deck that didn't have 52 cards."[9]

During William Baker's tenure as interim CEO, Callaway Golf continued to struggle with excessive inventory and integration of Top-Flite and Ben Hogan Golf operations. However, the company was able to develop some of its most innovative products prior to George Fellows's arrival. The company's titanium-faced Big Bertha Fusion irons were unlike any made by other golf equipment manufacturers at the time and were said by some retailers to be the best product Callaway Golf had ever developed. The company had also launched new X-18 and X-Tour irons, which contributed to a 28 percent increase in the sales of its irons between the second quarter of 2004 and the second quarter of 2005. The two-piece X-Tour iron was Callaway Golf's first forged iron, which was the preference of touring professionals and some low-handicap golfers. The company also

developed new versions of its 2-Ball putter that produced a 16 percent increase in putter sales between the second quarter of 2004 and the second quarter of 2005 and had created a 460-cc replacement to its ERC Fusion driver. The Fusion FT-3, like the original Big Bertha Fusion featured a titanium clubface and carbon composite shell, but also featured prepositioned weights to produce a draw, fade, or neutral ball path. The success of the FT-3 in the marketplace was critical to Callaway's turnaround since its Big Bertha 454 had met with limited success—leading to a 32 percent decline in net sales of woods for the six months ending June 30, 2005, when compared to the months ending June 30, 2004.

Callaway Golf also added the state-of-the-art HX Tour 56 golf ball to its lineup of Top-Flite and Callaway golf balls in June 2005. The HX Tour 56 was Callaway Golf's most technologically advanced golf ball and accounted for nine victories across all six professional tours since it was released to touring professionals in early 2005. The Tour 56 also was used in three of Phil Mickelson's lowest career 18-hole scores. In addition to the HX Tour 56's nine pro tour wins in 2005, the company's HX Tour golf ball had accounted for 46 global tour wins between 2003 and 2005. Callaway Golf expected the HX Tour 56 to help the golf ball division reverse an 11 percent decline in sales during the first six months of 2005. However, in mid-2005 the company was unable to get large quantities of its HX Tour 56 golf ball to retailers because of production problems in its Top-Flite plant. The company was also unable to ship sufficient quantities of its Fusion FT-3 drivers to retailers due to production problems at supplier foundries. As of late 2005, it was unknown how successful the FT-3 would be in allowing Callaway to recapture lost market share in the driver segment of the golf equipment industry since Callaway had not made the driver available to many retailers.

Even though Callaway Golf had significant hurdles to clear to return to its late-1990s glory, the company's stock price rose by nearly 50 percent in mid-2005 amid talks of a possible takeover. At least two separate groups of investors were pursuing the company with offers as high as $1.2 billion, or $16.25 per share. Prior to the hiring of George Fellows as Callaway Golf's CEO, its board had hired an investment bank to evaluate strategic alternatives for the company. However, upon his acceptance of the job, Fellows commented that the company was worth substantially more than the amounts of the two buyout bids and that he had been hired to turn around the company, not to prepare it for sale. At the end of the company's third quarter in 2005, Fellows announced a broad restructuring plan that would reduce expenses by $70 million by year-end 2006 by consolidating all golf ball operations; integrating sales functions of Callaway, Odyssey, Top-Flite, and Ben Hogan brands; and eliminating an unspecified number of jobs. The restructuring program would result in charges against 2005 and 2006 earnings of $12 million. A financial summary for Callaway Golf Company is presented in Exhibit 4. Exhibit 5 provides the company's revenues by product group for the period 1999 to 2004.

TaylorMade-adidas Golf

TaylorMade was founded in 1979 when Gary Adams mortgaged his home and began production of his "metalwoods" in an abandoned car dealership building in McHenry, Illinois. Both touring pros and golf retailers alike were skeptical of the new club design until they found that the metal woods actually hit the ball higher and farther than persimmon woods. By 1984, TaylorMade metalwoods were the number one wood on the PGA Tour and the company had grown to be the third-largest golf equipment company in the United States. The company was acquired by France-based Salomon SA in 1984, which provided the capital necessary for the company to continue to develop innovative new lines of metal woods. The company also produced irons and putters, but most of TaylorMade's sales were derived from high-margin drivers and fairway woods.

TaylorMade's metalwood drivers were the most technologically advanced in the industry until Callaway Golf's 1991 introduction of the oversized Big Bertha metalwood. During the entire decade of the 1990s, TaylorMade was unable to leapfrog Callaway Golf's innovations and remained a runner-up in the driver segment. Even though TaylorMade was unable to beat Callaway to the market with latest technology, the company was always able to launch drivers nearing the performance of Callaway products within months of a Callaway product introduction. Taylor-Made and its parent were acquired by athletic footwear and apparel company adidas in 1997.

TaylorMade's introduction of a 400-cc driver in 2003 gave it the innovation it had long sought to become the largest seller of drivers and fairway woods. The company's R580 driver was 40 cc larger than Callaway's competing Great Big Bertha II driver and matched consumers' preference for the largest possible driver. TaylorMade expanded its lead over Callaway Golf in drivers with its 2004 introduction of its r5 series and r7 Quad drivers. The r5 was a 450 cc driver that came in three varieties and used prepositioned weights to produce a draw, slight fade, or straight shots. The r5 was one of the best-selling drivers in the marketplace but was less technologically advanced (and lower-priced) than TaylorMade's r7 Quad driver. The r7's movable weight technology allowed users to use a special tool move four tungsten weights with a total weight of 48 grams to ports in various positions in the clubhead to produce whatever bias the golfer found necessary on a given day. For example, a golfer who was struggling with a low fade could move the heaviest of the four weights to the toe of the clubhead favor a high draw. The golfer could later move the weights to a different position if he or she experienced a different ball flight on a different day. The movable weight system allowed golfers to have a single driver that could produce six ball flight paths.

TaylorMade was also the leading seller of hybrid clubs. TaylorMade introduced its Rescue line of hybrid clubs in 1999, but the clubs did not become a huge success in the marketplace until 2002. In 2005, TaylorMade extended its Rescue line by adding models that featured its movable weight technology. Retailers were uncertain that movable weights would be a strong selling point in hybrids, since hybrids were already marketed as clubs that were easier to hit with than woods or long irons.

TaylorMade had traded positions with Titleist and Ping as the second-largest brand of irons, but it had never challenged Callaway Golf for market share leadership in the category. In late 2005, the company introduced its r7 irons in hopes of repeating the success of the r7 driver. The r7 irons were designed much like Callaway Golf's Fusion irons, with a titanium face mounted to a stainless-steel perimeter-weighted frame. The r7 irons also featured prepositioned tungsten cartridges imbedded into the stainless-steel clubhead to improve launch angles.

TaylorMade was a relatively weak competitor in the putter segment. Its Maxfli golf ball business produced successful models such as the Noodle—which sold more than 2 million dozen per year—but the division had yet to post a profit since its acquisition by adidas-Salomon in 2002. In 2005, the Maxfli brand accounted for less than 5 percent golf ball sales worldwide.

Exhibit 4 **Callaway Golf Company, Financial Summary, 1992–2004 (in thousands, except per share amounts)**

	2004	2003	2002	2001	2000	1999	1998	1997	1996	1995	1994	1993	1992
Net sales	$934,564	$514,032	$792,064	$816,163	$837,627	$719,038	$703,060	$848,941	$683,536	$557,048	$451,779	$256,376	$132,956
Pretax income	(23,713)	67,883	111,671	98,192	128,365	85,497	(38,899)	213,765	195,595	158,401	129,405	69,600	33,175
Pretax income as a percent of sales	−3%	13%	14%	12%	15%	12%	−6%	25%	29%	29%	29%	27%	25%
Net income	$ 10,103	$ 45,523	$ 69,446	$ 58,375	$ 80,999	$ 55,322	($25,564)	$13 2,704	$122,337	$ 97,736	$ 78,022	$ 42,862	$ 19,280
Net income as a percent of sales	1%	9%	9%	7%	10%	8%	−4%	16%	18%	18%	17%	17%*	15%
Fully diluted earnings per share	($0.15)	$0.68	$1.03	$0.82	$1.13	$0.78	($0.38)	$1.85	$1.73	$1.40	$1.07	$0.62	$0.32
Shareholders' equity	$586,317	$589,383	$543,387	$514,349	$511,744	$499,934	$453,096	$481,425	$362,267	$224,934	$186,414	$116,577	$ 49,750

Source: Callaway Golf Company annual reports.

Exhibit 5   **Callaway Golf Company's Net Sales by Product Group, 1999–2004 (in thousands)**

Product Group	2004	2003	2002	2001	2000	1999
Woods	$238.6	$252.4	$310.00	$392.90	$403.00	$429.00
Irons	259.1	280.7	243.5	248.9	299.9	221.3
Balls	231.3	78.4	66.0	54.9	34.0	—
Putters, accessories and other	205.6	202.5	172.6	119.5	100.8	68.7
Net sales	$934.6	$814.0	$792.10	$816.20	$837.60	$719.00

Source: Callaway Golf Company annual reports.

TaylorMade's net sales on a currency-neutral basis grew by 5 percent between 2003 and 2004, but declined by 1 percent after the effects of exchange rates were taken into account. The company's growth in sales was attributable to the popularity of its r7 Quad driver, which recorded wins in the U.S. Open and the PGA Championship. Growth in adidas golf footwear and apparel also contributed to the 5 percent revenue increase. In 2004, the company's Asian sourcing allowed its gross margins to improve to 47.0 percent, from 45.5 percent in 2003, but its operating margins declined from 10.5 percent in 2003 to 9.5 percent in 2004 because of increased marketing expenses. Exhibit 6 presents net sales and operating profit between 2001 and 2004 for TaylorMade-adidas Golf. The table also presents the adidas-Salomon golf division's sales by product category in 2004. Market shares for the leading sellers of drivers and fairway woods, irons, and golf shoes between January 2002 and July 2004 are presented in Exhibit 7.

Titleist/Cobra

The Acushnet Company was a rubber deresinating company founded in 1910 in Acushnet, Massachusetts. The company opened a golf ball division in 1932 when founder Phil Young believed that a bad putt during a round of golf he was playing was a result of a faulty ball rather than his poor putting. Young took the ball to a dentist's office to have it X-rayed and found that the core of the ball was indeed off-center. Believing that Acushnet could develop and manufacture high-quality golf balls, Young teamed with a fellow Massachusetts Institute of Technology graduate, Fred Bommer, to create the Titleist line of balls. Young and Bommer introduced their first Titleist golf ball in 1935, and by 1949 Titleist had become the most played ball on the PGA Tour.

Acushnet's acquisition of John Reuter Jr. Inc. in 1958 and Golfcraft Inc. in 1969 put Titleist into the golf club business. Titleist's Reuter Bulls Eye

Exhibit 6   **Selected Data for Taylor Made-adidas Golf**

	2004	2003	2002	2001
Net sales (in millions)	€633	€637	€707	€545
Operating profit (in millions)	60	67	74	63
Sales by Product				
Metalwoods	48%			
Irons	19			
Apparel	11			
Footwear	7			
Golf balls	6			
Accessories	6			
Putters	3			

Source: adidas-Salomon annual reports.

Exhibit 7   **Market Shares of Leading Sellers of Golf Equipment for Drivers and Fairway Woods, Irons, and Footwear, January 2002–July 2004**

Drivers and fairway woods

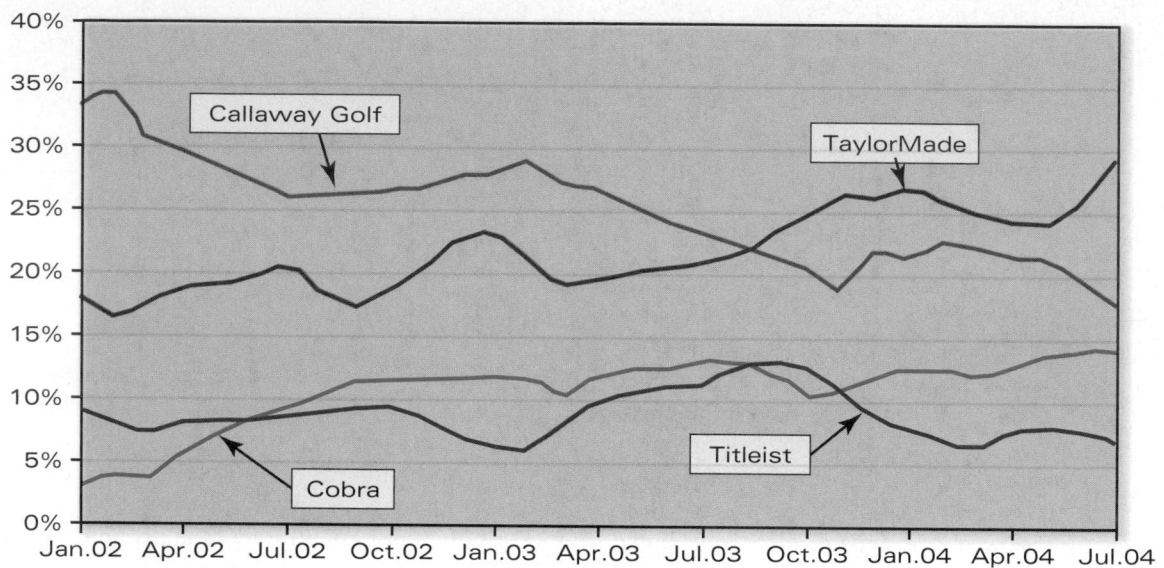

Irons

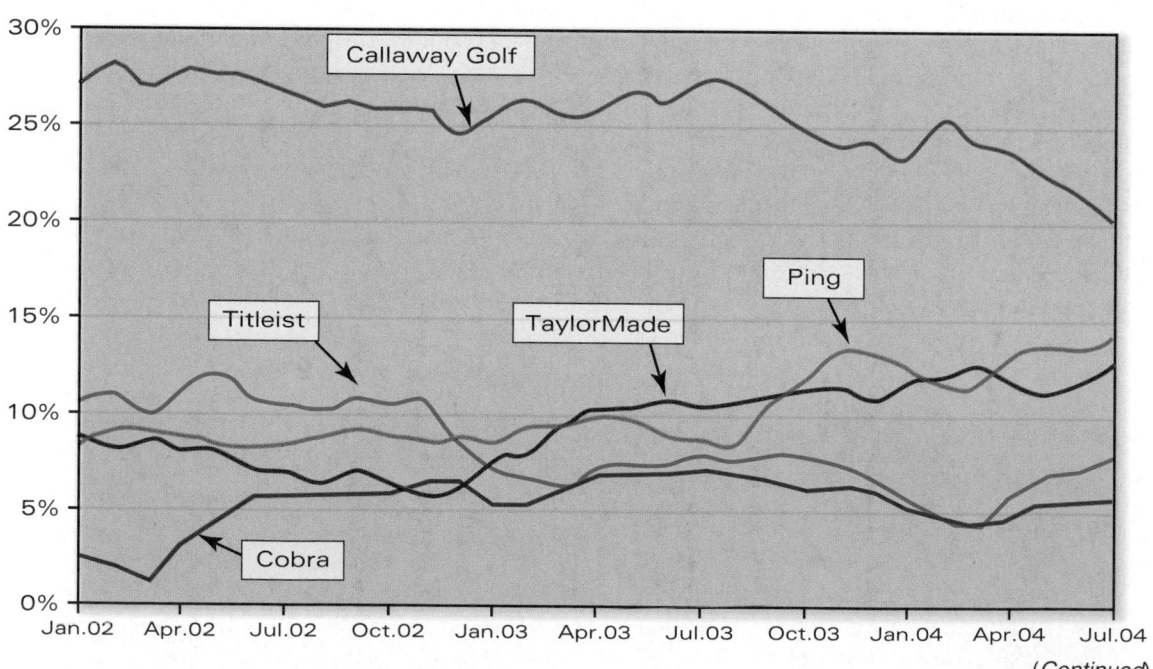

(*Continued*)

Exhibit 7   Continued

Footwear

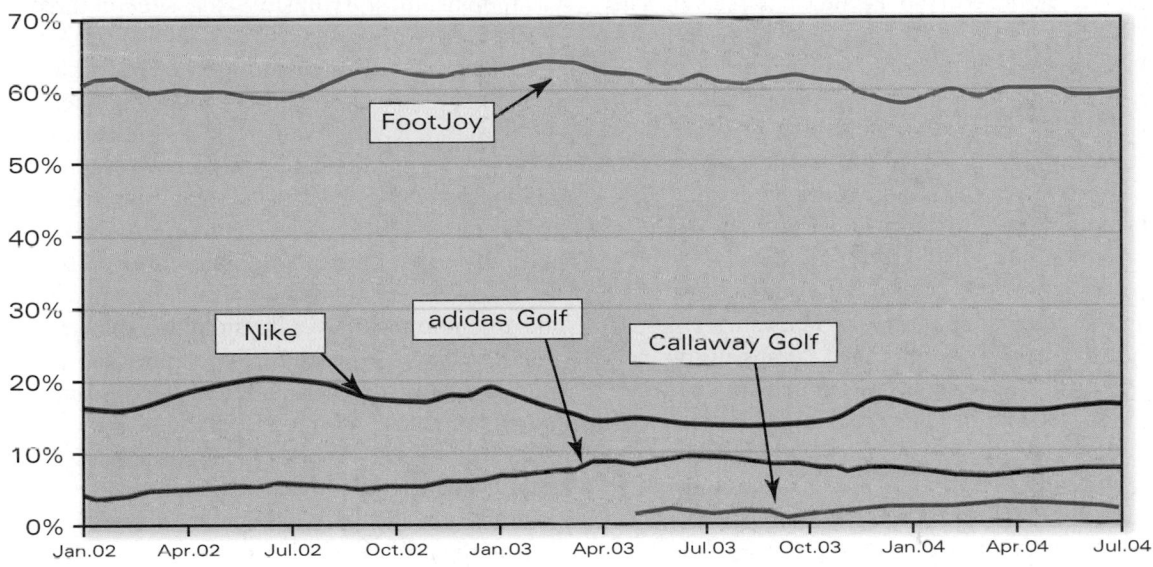

Source: Adidas-Salomon AG Investor Day 2004 Presentation, October 5, 2004.

putter became a favorite on the PGA Tour during the 1960s, and its AC-108 heel-toe weighted irons were among the most popular brands of irons during the early 1970s. The company's Pinnacle line of golf balls was developed in 1980 as a lower-priced alternative to Titleist-branded golf balls. In 1996, The Acushnet Company was acquired by tobacco and spirits producer and marketer American Brands. American Brands increased its presence in the golf equipment industry in 1985 when it acquired Foot-Joy, the number one seller of golf gloves and shoes. In 1996 American Brands acquired Cobra Golf for $715 million. The company changed its name to Fortune Brands in 1997 when it completed the divestiture of tobacco businesses begun in 1994. Fortune Brands' golf and leisure products division had an operating profit of $154 million on sales of $1.2 billion in 2004.

At year-end 2004, Titleist and Cobra were ranked third and fourth, respectively, in total equipment sales, with the sales of each brand totaling nearly $200 million. The sales of Titlist and Pinnacle golf balls amounted to approximately $485 million and accounted for more than 70 percent of industry sales. In addition, FootJoy led the industry in the sale of golf shoes, golf gloves, and golf outerwear, with revenues of $363 million.

Most golfers considered Titleist golf balls to be technologically superior to other brands, although industry analysts and golf retailers considered Callaway Golf's HX technology equally impressive. Titleist's Pro V1 golf ball was the company's most advanced and expensive golf ball and was able to offer maximum distance along with spin rates that allowed low-handicap golfers to stop approach shots near the pin. Lower-grade golf balls were able to offer golfers distance off the tee but were likely to roll across the green on approach shots to the hole. Titleist's line of golf clubs was targeted toward low-handicap golfers. Titleist produced only forged irons, which were difficult for all but the best recreational golfers to hit with since they had a small sweet spot and were very unforgiving of mis-hits. Titleist offered one driver model—the 905, which was a 400-cc driver and a popular choice with professionals and better recreational golfers.

Titleist offered only one hybrid club, which was more ironlike in its design than hybrids offered by Callaway or TaylorMade. Titleist's Vokey forged wedges were frequently used on the PGA Tour and were favorites of many low-handicap golfers. The Titleist Scotty Cameron putter line sold at the highest price points in the industry. Scotty Cameron putter models sold between $270 and $300 and were status symbols at country clubs and golf resorts throughout North America and Asia.

Fortune Brands' Cobra line of golf clubs was targeted to golfers of an average skill level. The brand's drivers pushed the regulatory limits in terms of clubhead size. In 2005, Cobra offered a 460-cc driver with the largest clubface among all major brands, a 454-cc driver, and 414-cc driver. All of the company's King Cobra drivers featured carbon composite top plates and milled titanium clubfaces. Cobra emphasized distance and forgiveness in its advertisements and fielded a long-drive team, which competed in various long-drive competitions held throughout the United States. King Cobra irons sold at slight lower price points than competing brands and were mostly perimeter-weighted models. The Cobra Baffler hybrid club was similar in design to the TaylorMade Rescue and Callaway Golf Heavenwood and sold at a slightly lower price point than models offered by key rivals. The company's wedges and putters were not widely used on the PGA Tour or among recreational golfers.

Titleist management's biggest concern in late 2005 centered on the USGA's interest in lesser-performing golf balls. In a special equipment issue of *Inside the USGA* published in October 2005, the editors worried openly that technology might endanger some of golf's most historic courses. The editors recalled how the wound, rubber-cored Haskell ball developed in 1898 and popularized during the early 1900s eventually "removed for consideration the Myopia Hunt Club, which hosted four U.S. Opens between 1898 and 1908."[10] The USGA editorial staff continued to speculate that the "confluence of golf science and commercial investment . . . accelerated by the injection of large amounts of capital" might possibly have the same effect on such championship courses as Merion or Oakland Hills.[11] The USGA believed it had a responsibility to the protect the game of golf and pointed out in its special issue that the average driving distance of touring professionals had increased by 26 yards between 1990 and 2005. In addition, the USGA commented that improvements in golf clubs and golf balls had contributed to a 1.5 stroke improvement in average handicaps between 1994 and 2005. Titleist management responded to such concerns by pointing out that the average score per round during PGA tournaments had improved by only one stroke between 1980 and 1997. In addition, Titleist management also disagreed with the contention that historic courses were likely to become obsolete because of technology. Titleist noted on its Web site that the average score during the 2005 PGA Championship at Baltusrol—the site of three U.S Opens dating back to 1967—was .345 higher than the average score posted during when the Springfield, New Jersey, course hosted the 1993 U.S. Open.

Titleist's CEO, Wally Uihlein, attributed the overall scoring improvement among recreational and tournament golfers to "six contributing factors: 1) the introduction of low-spinning high performance golf balls, 2) the introduction of oversize, thin-faced drivers, 3) improved golf course conditioning and agronomy; 4) player physiology—they're bigger and stronger; 5) improved techniques and instruction; and 6) launch monitors and the customization of equipment."[12] In a tit-for-tat reply, the USGA quoted famous golf course designer Pete Dye, who commented, "It's not the strength of the players. My good friend John Daly hits the ball 30 yards farther in 2005 than he did in 1991. Now John will be the first one to tell you he hasn't done too many push-ups in the last 15 years."[13]

Ping Golf

Perimeter weighting came about due to the poor putting of Karsten Solheim, a General Electric mechanical engineer, who took up golf at the age of 47 in 1954. Solheim designed a putter for himself that he found provided more "feel" when he struck the ball. Solheim moved much of the clubhead weight to the heel and toe, leaving a cavity at the rear and center of the club. Perimeter-weighted, or cavity-back, clubs had a larger sweet spot because of a higher moment of inertia or resistance to twisting. The resistance to twisting reduced the gear effect of the clubhead and resulted in straighter, longer shots with irons. In addition to perimeter weighting, Solheim also developed the investment-casting manufacturing process. This process allowed clubheads to be formed from molds rather than forged from steel—the traditional manufacturing process.

Solheim made his putters by hand from 1959 until 1967, when he left GE and founded Karsten Manufacturing. By the 1970s, Karsten manufactured a full line of perimeter-weighted putters and irons that carried the Ping brand. Solheim named the brand Ping because of the sound the perimeter-weighted clubhead made when it struck the ball. Karsten Manufacturing's Ping putters and irons were thought to be among the most technologically advanced throughout the 1980s and reigned as the market leaders. Karsten Manufacturing was renamed Ping Inc. in 1999.

Karsten Solheim was also the pioneer of custom fitting, with his fitting activities predating the official founding of the company. During the 1960s, touring professionals would meet with Solheim to have him custom-fit putters to their body measurements, and by the 1970s Solheim had developed a fitting system for irons. His system used the golfer's physical measurements, stance and swing, and ball flight to select irons with the optimal lie. The company's irons were sold in 10 color-coded lie configurations to best match recreational golfers' unique fit conditions. In a 2005 golf consumer survey, Ping was rated as the industry leader in custom fitting by a 3-to-1 margin. In addition to producing 10 configurations of iron models, Ping invited retailers to three-day training programs in its plant in Phoenix to become better skilled at custom fitting. By 2005, Ping had trained thousands of retailers.

Ping remained an industry leader in the iron segment in 2005, with a number two position in irons behind Callaway Golf. The company offered three lines of irons —the traditional blade S59 irons, which featured minimal perimeter weighting; the i5 line, with a medium degree of perimeter weighting; and the G5 line, which had expanded perimeter weighting. The S59 line was suitable for professionals and low-handicap recreational golfers, while the i5 was designed for average players looking for a lower ball flight. The G5 produced a higher ball flight than other models and was intended for average golfers who were able to produce only modest amounts of clubhead speed. The company produced a broad line of putters and regularly traded positions with Odyssey as the number one brand of putters.

Even though Ping had been known at one time for only its irons and putters, in late 2005 the privately owned company had become the maker of the most sought-after driver in the industry. The company's 460-cc G5 titanium driver had become the best-selling driver in late 2005 as golfers began to question the merit of the r7's movable weight system and found it difficult to locate Callaway Golf's FT-3 Fusion on retailer shelves. The company had failed to develop a hybrid until late 2005, but retailers expected Ping's G5 hybrid to become one of the best-selling hybrid clubs during equipment upgrades in the spring of 2006. The company's wedges were not big sellers in the market.

Nike Golf

Nike management believed that Tiger Woods could not only generate interest in golf but also help generate substantial revenues for a golf equipment company. Nike seized on the instant popularity of Tiger Woods in 1996 by signing the young star to a five-year, $40 million contract to endorse Nike shoes and apparel. In 1999 Woods extended the contract for an additional five years for $90 million to endorse Nike's new golf ball and forthcoming golf clubs. As with its athletic and apparel and footwear, Nike outsourced the production of its golf balls (in this instance to Bridgestone), while it hired a custom-club designer to design and lead its new golf club business. Nike's new driver, irons, and wedges were introduced during the 2002 PGA Merchandise Show. The company's 2002 line of golf clubs achieved only modest success and an improved line, including a 400-cc forged titanium driver, was introduced during the 2003 PGA Merchandise Show. Tiger Woods began endorsing the company's golf ball in 2000 and began using its driver and irons in 2002. Woods again extended his contract to endorse Nike's golf equipment, golf balls, apparel, and footwear in 2003 for $25 million per year for five years.

Nike management's 1996 assessment of Tiger Woods's enduring worldwide popularity was on the mark with PGA tournament viewership doubling when Woods was in contention for a Sunday win. However, Woods's appeal with television viewers did not translate into equipment sales. Nike's entry into the golf equipment industry had proved successful in terms of apparel and footwear sales, where it was the second leading seller of golf shoes behind FootJoy, but Nike Golf held only a 2.6 percent share of the golf club market in 2004. Nike Golf had achieved nearly a 10 percent market share in golf balls in 2004 and might likely benefit from Tiger Woods's miracle chip shot on the 16th hole of the 2005 Masters that put him in a playoff with Chris DiMarco and led to an eventual win. While an estimated television audience of 15 million watched, Woods's Nike Platinum One golf ball slowly rolled across the 16th green, where it clung to the edge of the hole for what seemed like eternity. As the ball perched at the edge of the cup, the Nike logo could not have been aligned with the camera more perfectly if it had been placed there by the company's advertising agency. After being tracked by CBS's cameras for 17 seconds, the ball fell into the cup.

Nike also boasted after the 2005 Masters Tournament that its brand of irons was the most widely used during the tournament. However, with the exception of those used by Woods, all Nike irons were used by former champions who were not expected to be in contention for a win at the Masters, including Billy Casper, who withdrew from the tournament after shooting a first-round score of 106. Casper's withdrawal from the tournament prevented his score from being recorded as an official statistic. It was reported that Nike paid $20,000 tee-up fees during the Masters practice rounds to those willing to use the company's irons during the day. As of late 2005, Nike's 460-cc SasQuatch and Ignite drivers; Slingshot, NDS, Forged, and Combo irons; and CPR hybrids remained poor sellers. Demand for the company's putters and wedges was also low. Nike had more recently signed 13 additional professional golfers to endorsement contracts, including 15-year-old Michelle Wie. Nike's October 2005 agreement with Wie would pay the teenager, who had yet to win a tournament competing against professionals in her 30 attempts, $20 million over four years. Nike did not disclose in its financial statements what percentage of its 2004 revenues of $12.3 billion was made up of golf equipment and apparel sales.

End notes

[1] As quoted in *The Callaway Connection*, Spring 2000, p. 7.

[2] As quoted in "Callaway Golf Introduced ERC II Forged Titanium Driver—Its Hottest and Most Forgiving Driver Ever," *PR Newswire*, October 24, 2000.

[3] Ibid.

[4] As quoted in *Smart Money*, August 2002, p. 34.

[5] Posted at www.callawaygolf.com/EN/customerservice.aspx?pid=9ways.

[6] As quoted in "Teed Off: Counterfeiters Are Cashing In on Big-Name Clubs by Hawking Bogus Merchandise on the Internet," *St. Louis Post-Dispatch*, May 18, 2005, p. C1.

[7] Callaway Golf Company 1998 annual report.

[8] "Callaway Enters the Ball Game," *Show News*, February 5, 2000.

[9] As quoted in "Looking for the Sweet Spot: Prospects Are Rosier for Carlsbad's Callaway Golf, but Some Wonder If New CEO Can Complete the Turnaround," *San Diego Union-Tribune*, August 28, 2005, p. H-1.

[10] As quoted in "Keeping Our Eye on the Ball," *Inside the USGA, Special Issue: Equipment*, October 2005, p. 1.

[11] Ibid, p. 9.

[12] As quoted in a reprint of "Mr. Titleist Talks," *Travel & Leisure Golf*, posted at www.titleist.com, 2005.

[13] As quoted in "Keeping Our Eye on the Ball," p. 16.

Case 5

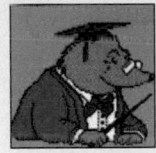

Dell Inc. in 2006: Can Rivals Beat Its Strategy?

Arthur A. Thompson
The University of Alabama

John E. Gamble
University of South Alabama

In 1984, at the age of 19, Michael Dell invested $1,000 of his own money and founded Dell Computer with a simple vision and business concept—that personal computers (PCs) could be built to order and sold directly to customers. Michael Dell believed his approach to the PC business had two advantages: (1) bypassing distributors and retail dealers eliminated the markups of resellers, and (2) building to order greatly reduced the costs and risks associated with carrying large stocks of parts, components, and finished goods. Between 1986 and 1993 the company worked to refine its strategy, build an adequate infrastructure, and establish market credibility against better-known rivals. In the mid- and late 1990s, Dell's strategy started to click into full gear. By 2003, Dell's sell-direct and build-to-order business model and strategy had provided the company with the most efficient procurement, manufacturing, and distribution capabilities in the global PC industry and given Dell a substantial cost and profit margin advantage over rival PC vendors. During 2004–2005, the company solidified its position as the global market leader in PCs.

Dell had a commanding 33.9 percent share of PC sales in the United States in the first nine months of 2005, comfortably ahead of Hewlett-Packard (19.1 percent), Gateway (6.0 percent), and IBM/Lenovo (4.3 percent)—and its lead over rivals was increasing. Dell had moved ahead of IBM into second place during 1998 and then overtaken Compaq Computer as the U.S. sales leader in the third quarter of 1999. Its market share leadership in the United States had widened every year since 2000. Dell had

eclipsed Compaq as the global market leader in 2001. But when Hewlett-Packard (HP), the third-ranking PC seller in the world, acquired Compaq, the second-ranking PC vendor in 2002, Dell found itself in a tight battle with HP for the top spot globally. Dell was the world leader in unit sales in the first and third quarters of 2002, and HP was the sales leader in the second and fourth quarters. However, Dell opened a clear market share gap over HP in 2003–2005. Nonetheless, Dell trailed HP in PC sales outside the United States; HP's non-U.S. share had been in the 12.5 to 14.1 percent range since late 2001, with Dell's overall share of sales outside the United States climbing from about 7.5 percent in late 2001 to 11.6 percent in 2005. Exhibit 1 shows the shifting domestic and global sales and market share rankings in PCs during 1998–2005.

Since the late 1990s, Dell had also been driving for industry leadership in servers. In 2004 Dell was the number one domestic seller of servers, with close to a 33 percent market share (up from about 3–4 percent in the mid-1990s). It was number two in the world in server shipments, with a 24.5 percent share in the third quarter of 2004, within striking distance of global market leadership. Dell was the leader in servers (based on unit volume) in the three largest server markets—the United States, Japan, and China. In the mid- to late-1990s, a big fraction of the servers sold were proprietary machines running on customized Unix operating systems and carrying price tags ranging from $30,000 to $1 million or more. But a seismic shift in server technology, coupled with growing cost-consciousness on the part of server users, produced a radical shift away from more costly, proprietary, Unix-based servers during

Exhibit 1 **U.S. and Global Market Shares of Leading PC Vendors, 1998–2005**

A. U.S. Market Shares of the Leading PC Vendors, 1998–2005

2003 Rank	Vendor	First Nine Months of 2005		2004		2003		2002		2001		2000		1998	
		Shipments (in 000s)	Market Share	Shipments (in 000s)	Market Share	Shipments (in 000s)	Market Share	Shipments (in 000s)	Market Share	Shipments (in 000s)	Market Share	Shipments (in 000s)	Market Share	Shipments (in 000s)	Market Share
1	Dell	15,725	33.1%	19,296	33.1%	16,319	30.9%	13,324	27.9%	10,817	23.5%	9,645	19.7%	4,799	13.2%
	Compaq*	—	—	—	—	—	—	—	—	5,341	11.6	7,761	15.9	6,052	16.7
2	Hewlett-Packard*	8,869	19.1	11,600	19.9	10,851	20.6	8,052	16.8	4,374	9.5	5,630	11.5	2,832	7.8
3	Gateway	2,802	6.0	2,945	5.1	1,987	3.8	2,725	5.7	3,219	7.0	4,237	8.7	3,039	8.4
4	IBM/Lenovo	1,995	4.3	2,932	5.0	2,748	5.2	2,531	5.3	2,461	5.3	2,668	5.5	2,983	8.2
5	Apple	n.a.	n.a.	1,935	3.3	1,675	3.2	1,693	3.5	1,665	3.6	n.a	n.a.	n.a.	n.a.
	Others	n.a.	n.a.	19,548	33.6	19,158	36.3	19,514	40.8	23,509	51.0	18,959	38.8	16,549	45.6
	All vendors	46,337	100.0%	58,256	100.0%	52,739	100.0%	47,839	100.0%	46,051	100.0%	48,900	100.0%	36,254	100.0%

B. Worldwide Market Shares of the Leading PC Vendors, 1998–2005

2003 Rank	Vendor	First Nine Months of 2005		2004		2003		2002		2001		2000		1998	
		Shipments (in 000s)	Market Share	Shipments (in 000s)	Market Share	Shipments (in 000s)	Market Share	Shipments (in 000s)	Market Share	Shipments (in 000s)	Market Share	Shipments (in 000s)	Market Share	Shipments (in 000s)	Market Share
1	Dell	27,192	18.7%	31,771	17.9%	25,833	16.9%	20,672	15.2%	17,231	12.9%	14,801	10.6%	7,770	8.5%
	Compaq*	—	—	—	—	—	—	—	—	14,673	11	17,399	12.5	13,266	14.5
2	Hewlett-Packard*	22,825	15.7	28,063	15.8	25,009	16.4	18,432	13.6	9,309	7	10,327	7.4	5,743	6.3
3	IBM/Lenovo	9,942	6.8	10,492	5.9	9,000	5.9	7,996	5.9	8,292	6.2	9,308	6.7	7,946	8.7
4	Fujitsu Siemens	—	—	7,182	4.0	6,375	4.2	5,822	4.3	6,022	4.5	6,582	4.7	n.a.	n.a.
5	Acer	—	—	6,461	3.6	n.a.	n.a.	n.a	n.a	n.a	n.a	n.a.	n.a	n.a	n.a
	Others	—	—	93,511	52.7	81,271	53.3	78,567	57.8	73,237	54.9	80,640	58	50,741	55.5
	All vendors	145,542	100.0%	177,480	100.0%	152,568	100.0%	136,022	100.0%	133,466	100.0%	139,057	100.0%	91,442	100.0%

n.a. = Not available.

*Compaq was acquired by Hewlett-Packard in May 2002. The 2002 data for Hewlett-Packard includes both Compaq-branded and Hewlett-Packard-branded PCs for the last three quarters of 2002 plus only Hewlett-Packard-branded PCs for Q1 2002.

1999–2004. In 2003–2004, about 8 out of 10 servers sold carried price tags below $10,000, were based on standardized components and technology, and ran on either Windows or Linux operating systems. The overall share of Unix-based servers shipped in 2003–2004 was under 10 percent, down from about 18 percent in 1997. Dell's rise to prominence in servers came from its focus on low- and midrange servers that used standard technology.

In addition, Dell was making market inroads in other product categories. Its sales of data storage devices had grown to over $2 billion annually, aided by a strategic alliance with EMC, a leader in data storage. In 2001–2002, Dell began selling low-cost, data-routing switches—a product category in which Cisco Systems was the dominant global leader. In late 2002, Dell introduced a new line of handheld PCs— the Axim X5—to compete against the higher-priced products of Palm, HP, and others; the Axim offered a solid but not trendsetting design, was packed with features, and was priced roughly 50 percent below the best-selling models of rivals. Starting in 2003, Dell began marketing Dell-branded printers and printer cartridges, product categories that provided global leader HP with the lion's share of its profits—the company was on track to sell over 5 million printers and generate more than $1 billion in imaging and printing revenues in 2004. Also in 2003, Dell began selling flat-screen LCD TVs and retail-store systems, including electronic cash registers, specialized software, services, and peripherals required to link retail-store check-out lanes to corporate information systems. Dell's MP3 player, the Dell DJ, was number two behind the Apple iPod. Dell added plasma-screen TVs to its TV product line in 2004. Since the late 1990s, Dell had been marketing CD and DVD drives, printers, scanners, modems, monitors, digital cameras, memory cards, data storage devices, and speakers made by a variety of manufacturers.

So far, Dell's foray into new products and businesses had proved profitable. According to Michael Dell, "We believe that all our businesses should make money. If a business doesn't make money, if you can't figure out how to make money in that business, you shouldn't be in that business."[1] In 2003 and 2004, Dell earned a profit in each of its product categories, customer segments, and geographic markets. Dell products were sold in more than 170 countries, but sales in 60 countries accounted for about 95 percent of total revenues.

COMPANY BACKGROUND

At age 12, Michael Dell was running a mail order stamp-trading business, complete with a national catalog, and grossing $2,000 a month. At 16 he was selling subscriptions to the *Houston Post*, and at 17 he bought his first BMW with money he had earned. He enrolled at the University of Texas in 1983 as a premed student (his parents wanted him to become a doctor), but he soon became immersed in computers and started selling PC components out of his college dormitory room. He bought random-access memory (RAM) chips and disk drives for IBM PCs at cost from IBM dealers, who at the time often had excess supplies on hand because they were required to order large monthly quotas from IBM. Dell resold the components through newspaper ads (and later through ads in national computer magazines) at 10–15 percent below the regular retail price.

By April 1984 sales were running about $80,000 per month. Michael decided to drop out of college and form a company, PCs Ltd., to sell both PC components and PCs under the brand name PCs Limited. He obtained his PCs by buying retailers' surplus stocks at cost, then powering them up with graphics cards, hard disks, and memory before reselling them. His strategy was to sell directly to end users; by eliminating the retail markup, Dell's new company was able to sell IBM clones (machines that copied the functioning of IBM PCs using the same or similar components) about 40 percent below the price of IBM's best-selling PCs. The discounting strategy was successful, attracting price-conscious buyers and generating rapid revenue growth. By 1985, the company was assembling its own PC designs with a few people working on six-foot tables. The company had 40 employees, and Michael Dell worked 18-hour days, often sleeping on a cot in his office. By the end of fiscal 1986, sales had reached $33 million.

During the next several years, however, PCs Limited was hampered by growing pains—specifically, a lack of money, people, and resources. Michael Dell sought to refine the company's business model; add needed production capacity; and build a bigger, deeper management staff and corporate infrastructure while at the same time keeping costs low. The company was renamed Dell Computer in 1987, and the first international offices were opened that same year. In 1988 Dell added a sales force to serve large customers, began selling to government agencies, and became a public company—raising $34.2 million in its first offering of common stock. Sales to large customers quickly became the dominant part of Dell's business. By 1990 Dell Computer had sales of $388 million, a market share of 2–3 percent, and a research and development (R&D) staff of over 150 people. Michael Dell's vision was for Dell Computer to become one of the top three PC companies.

Thinking its direct sales business would not grow fast enough, in 1990–93 the company began distributing its computer products through Soft Warehouse Superstores (now CompUSA), Staples (a leading office products chain), Wal-Mart, Sam's Club, and Price Club (now Price/Costco). Dell also sold PCs through Best Buy stores in 16 states and through Xerox in 19 Latin American countries. But when the company learned how thin its margins were in selling through such distribution channels, it realized it had made a mistake and withdrew from selling to retailers and other intermediaries in 1994 to refocus on direct sales. At the time, sales through retailers accounted for only about 2 percent of Dell's revenues.

In 1993, further problems emerged: Dell reportedly lost $38 million in a risky foreign-currency hedging, quality difficulties arose with certain PC lines made by the company's contract manufacturers, profit margins declined, and buyers were turned off by the company's laptop PC models. To get laptop sales back on track, the company took a charge of $40 million to write off its laptop line and suspended sales of laptops until it could get redesigned models into the marketplace.

Because of higher costs and unacceptably low profit margins in selling to individuals and households, Dell did not pursue the consumer market aggressively until sales to individuals at the company's Internet site took off in 1996 and 1997. It became clear that PC-savvy individuals, who were buying their second and third computers, wanted powerful computers with multiple features; did not need much technical support; and liked the convenience of buying direct from Dell, ordering exactly what they wanted, and having it delivered to their door within a matter of days. In early 1997, Dell created an internal sales and marketing group dedicated to serving the individual consumer segment and introduced a product line designed especially for individual users. In 2005, sales to consumers accounted for 15 percent of Dell's worldwide PC business, with sales to business, government, and educational institutions accounting for 85 percent.

By late 1997, Dell had become a low-cost leader among PC vendors by wringing greater and greater efficiency out of its direct sales and build-to-order business model. Since then, the company had continued driving hard to reduce its costs and, in 2003–2005, was considered the lowest-cost producer among all the leading vendors of PCs and servers. The company was a pioneer and an acknowledged world leader in incorporating e-commerce technology and use of the Internet into its everyday business practices. Michael Dell's goal was to stitch Dell's business together with its supply partners and customers in real time such that all three appeared to be part of the same organizational team.[3]

In its 2005 fiscal year, Dell posted revenues of $49.2 billion and profits of $3.0 billion. Since fiscal 1995, revenues had grown at a compound average growth rate of 30.6 percent and profits had grown at 36.0 percent compound rate. Dell reported close to $56 billion in sales in its fiscal year ending January 2006. A $100 investment in Dell's stock at its initial public offering in June 1988 would have been worth close to $40,000 in December 2005. Based on 2004 data, Dell ranked number 28 on the Fortune 500, number 84 on the Fortune Global 500, and number 3 on the Fortune Global "most admired" list. In February 2006, Dell Computer had 65,200 employees worldwide, up from 16,000 at year-end 1997; over 60 percent of Dell's employees were located in countries outside the United States, and this percentage was growing. The company's headquarters and main office complex was in Round Rock, Texas (an Austin suburb). The company changed its name from Dell Computer to Dell Inc. in 2003 to reflect the company's growing business base outside of PCs. Exhibits 2 and 3 provide information about Dell's financial performance and geographic operations.

Michael Dell

In the company's early days Michael Dell hung around mostly with the company's engineers. He was so shy that some employees thought he was stuck up because he never talked to them. But people who worked with him closely described him as a likable young man who was slow to warm up to strangers.[4] He was a terrible public speaker and wasn't good at running meetings. But Lee Walker, a 51-year-old venture capitalist brought in by Michael Dell to provide much-needed managerial and financial experience during the

Exhibit 2   **Selected Financial Statement Data for Dell Inc., Fiscal Years 1998–2006 (in millions, except per share data)**

	Fiscal Year Ended						
	February 3, 2006	January 28, 2005	January 30, 2004	January 31, 2003	February 1, 2002	January 28, 2000	February 1, 1998
Results of operations:							
Net revenue	$55,908	$49,205	$41,444	$35,404	$31,168	$25,265	$12,327
Cost of revenue	45,958	40,190	33,892	29,055	25,661	20,047	9,605
Gross margin	9,950	9,015	7,552	6,349	5,507	5,218	2,722
Operating expenses:							
Selling, general and administrative	5,140	4,298	3,544	3,050	2,784	2,387	1,202
Research, development and engineering	463	463	464	455	452	374	204
Special charges	—	—	—	—	482	194	—
Total operating expenses	5,603	4,761	4,008	3,505	3,718	2,955	1,406
Operating income	4,347	4,254	3,544	2,844	1,789	2,263	1,316
Investment and other income (loss), net	227	191	180	183	(58)	188	52
Income before income taxes, extraordinary loss, and cumulative effect of change in accounting principle	4,574	4,445	3,724	3,027	1,731	2,451	1,368
Provision for Income taxes	1,002	1,402	1,079	905	485	785	424
Net income	$ 3,572	$ 3,043	$ 2,645	$ 2,122	$ 1,246	$ 1,666	$ 944
Earnings per common share:							
Basic	$1,49	$1.21	$1.03	$0.82	$0.48	$0.66	$0.36
Diluted	$1,46	$1.18	$1.01	$0.80	$0.46	$0.61	$0.32
Weighted average shares outstanding:							
Basic	2,403	2,509	2,565	2,584	2,602	2,536	2,631
Diluted	2,449	2,568	2,619	2,644	2,726	2,728	2,952
Cash flow and balance sheet data							
Net cash provided by operating activities	$ 4,839	$ 5,310	$ 3,670	$ 3,538	$ 3,797	$ 3,926	$ 1,592
Cash, cash equivalents, and investments	11,749	14,101	11,922	9.905	8,287	6,853	1,844
Total assets	23,109	23,215	19,311	15,470	13,535	11,560	4,268
Long-term debt	504	505	505	506	520	508	17
Total stockholders' equity	$ 4,129	$ 6,485	$ 6,280	$ 4,873	$ 4,694	$ 5,308	$ 1,293

*Includes effect of $59 million adjustment due to the cumulative effect of a change in accounting principle.

Source: Dell Inc. 2005 10-K report, 1999 annual report, and press release on February 16, 2006.

Exhibit 3 **Dell's Geographic Area Performance, Fiscal Years 2000–2006 (in millions of dollars)**

	February 3, 2006	January 28, 2005	January 30, 2004	January 31, 2003	February 1, 2002	January 28, 2000
Net revenues						
Americas						
Business	$28,481	$25,339	$21,888	$19,394	$17,275	$15,160
U.S. consumer	7,930	7,601	6,715	5,653	4,485	2,719
Total Americas	36,411	32,940	28,603	25,047	21,760	17,879
Europe*	12,873	10,787	8,495	6,912	6,429	5,590
Asia Pacific-Japan	6,624	5,478	4,436	3,445	2,979	1,796
Total net revenues	$55,908	$49,205	$41,444	$35,404	$31,168	$25,265
Operating income						
Americas						
Business	$ 3,015	$ 2,579	$ 2,124	$ 1,945	$ 1,482	$ 1,800
U.S. consumer	414	399	400	308	260	204
Total Americas	3,429	2,978	2,594	2,253	1,742	2,004
Europe*	857	818	637	388	377	359
Asia Pacific-Japan	503	458	313	203	152	94
Special charges	—	—	—	—	(482)	(194)
Total operating income	$ 4,789	$ 4,254	$ 3,544	$ 2,844	$ 1,789	$ 2,263

*Includes Africa and the Middle East.

Source: Dell Inc. 10-K reports 2006, 2005, and 2002.

company's organization-building years, became Michael Dell's mentor, built up his confidence, and was instrumental in turning him into a polished executive.[5] Walker served as the company's president and chief operating officer during the 1986–1990 period; he had a fatherly image, knew everyone by name, and played a key role in implementing Michael Dell's marketing ideas. Under Walker's tutelage, Michael Dell became intimately familiar with all parts of the business, overcame his shyness, learned to control his ego, and turned into a charismatic leader with an instinct for motivating people and winning their loyalty and respect.

When Walker had to leave the company in 1990 for health reasons, Dell turned to Morton Meyerson, former CEO and president of Electronic Data Systems, for advice and guidance on how to transform Dell Computer from a fast-growing medium-sized company into a billion-dollar enterprise. Though sometimes given to displays of impatience, Michael Dell usually spoke in a quiet, reflective manner and came across as a person with maturity and seasoned

judgment far beyond his age. His prowess was based more on an astute combination of technical knowledge and marketing know-how than on being a technological wizard. In 1992, at the age of 27, Michael Dell became the youngest CEO ever to head a Fortune 500 company; he was a billionaire at the age of 31.

By the late 1990s, Michael Dell had become one of the most respected executives in the PC industry. Media journalists had described him as "the quintessential American entrepreneur" and "the most innovative guy for marketing computers." He was a much-sought-after speaker at industry and company conferences. His views and opinions about the future of PCs, the Internet, and e-commerce practices carried considerable weight both in the PC industry and among executives worldwide. In early 2005, the once pudgy and bespectacled 40-year-old Michael Dell was physically fit, considered good-looking, wore contact lenses, ate only health foods, and lived in a three-story 33,000-square-foot home on a 60-acre estate in Austin, Texas, with his wife and four children. In 2005, he owned about 9 percent of Dell's common stock, worth about $8.7 billion.

Michael Dell was considered a very accessible CEO and a role model for young executives because he had done what many of them were trying to do. He delegated authority to subordinates, believing that the best results came from turning loose "talented people who can be relied upon to do what they're supposed to do." Business associates viewed Michael Dell as an aggressive personality, an extremely competitive risk taker who had always played close to the edge. He spent about 30 percent of his time traveling to company operations and meeting with customers. In a typical year, he would make two or three trips to Europe and two trips to Asia.

In mid-2004, Michael Dell, the company's first and only CEO, transferred his title of CEO to Kevin Rollins, the company's president and chief operating officer. Dell remained as chairman of the board. Dell and Rollins had run the company for the past seven years under a shared leadership structure. The changes were primarily ones of title, not of roles or responsibilities.

DELL'S STRATEGY AND BUSINESS MODEL

In orchestrating Dell's rise to global prominence, company executives had come to believe strongly that five tenets were the key to delivering superior customer value:[6]

1. A direct relationship is the most efficient path to the customer because it eliminates wholesale and retail dealers that impede Dell's understanding of customer needs and expectations and that add unnecessary time and cost.
2. Allowing customers to purchase custom-built products and custom-tailored services is the most effective way to meet customer needs.
3. Nonproprietary, standardized technologies deliver the best value to customers.
4. A highly efficient supply chain and manufacturing organization, grounded in the use of standardized technologies and selling direct, paves the way for a low-cost structure where cost-savings can be passed along to customers in the form of lower prices.

5. Dell should endeavor to deliver added value to customers by (a) researching all the technological options, (b) trying to determine which ones are "optimal" in the sense of delivering the best combination of performance and efficiency, and (c) being accountable to customers for helping them obtain the highest return on their investment in information technology (IT) products and services.

In accordance with these tenets, Dell's strategy during the 2002–2005 period had seven core elements: a cost-efficient approach to build-to-order manufacturing, partnerships with suppliers aimed at squeezing cost savings out of the supply chain, direct sales to customers, award-winning customer service and technical support, customer-driven R&D, emphasis on using standardized technologies, and product-line expansion aimed at capturing a bigger share of the dollars its customers spent for IT products and services.

The business model on which the strategy was predicated was powerful: Use the company's strong capabilities in supply chain management, low-cost manufacturing, and direct sales capabilities to expand into product categories where Dell could provide added value to its customers in the form of lower prices. The standard pattern of attack was to identify an IT product with good margins; figure out how to build it (or else have it built by others) cheaply enough to be able to significantly underprice competitive products; and then market the new product to Dell's steadily growing customer base and watch the market share points, incremental revenues, and incremental profits pile up.

Cost-Efficient Build-to-Order Manufacturing

Dell built its computers, workstations, and servers to order; none were produced for inventory. Dell customers could order custom-equipped servers and workstations according to the needs of their applications. Desktop and laptop customers ordered whatever configuration of microprocessor speed, random-access memory, hard disk capacity, CD or DVD drives, fax/modem/wireless capabilities, graphics cards, monitor size, speakers, and other accessories they preferred. The orders were directed to the nearest factory. In 2005 Dell had assembly plants in Austin, Texas; Nashville, Tennessee; Limerick,

Ireland; Xiamen, China; Penang, Malaysia; and El Dorado do Sul, Brazil. A seventh manufacturing plant with capacity to make 15,000 to 20,000 desktops per day opened outside Winston-Salem, North Carolina, in late 2005—it was Dell's largest plant to date and could turn out a new PC every five seconds. Dell opened a second plant in Xiamen in January 2006, and an additional plant in Europe was in the planning stages. At all locations, the company had the capability to assemble PCs, workstations, and servers; Dell assembled its data storage products at its Austin, Limerick, and Penang plants. All plants used the same production systems and procedures. In 2002–2005, typical orders were built and delivered in three to five days; however, the new North Carolina plant was expected to be able to deliver orders to customers on the eastern coast of the United States in one to three days. Dell believed in building its plants close to customers because the labor costs to assemble a PC were about $10, whereas the logistics costs to move parts and ship a finished PC were about $40 per unit.[7]

Until 1997, Dell operated its assembly lines in traditional fashion, with workers performing a single operation. An order form accompanied each metal chassis across the production floor; drives, chips, and ancillary items were installed to match customer specifications. As a partly assembled PC arrived at a new workstation, the operator, standing beside a tall steel rack with drawers full of components, was instructed what to do by little red and green lights flashing beside the drawers. When the operator was finished, the drawers containing the used components were automatically replenished from the other side, and the PC chassis glided down the line to the next workstation. However, Dell had reorganized its plants in 1997, shifting to "cell manufacturing" techniques whereby a team of workers operating at a group workstation (or cell) assembled an entire PC according to customer specifications. The shift to cell manufacturing reduced Dell's assembly times by 75 percent and doubled productivity per square foot of assembly space. Assembled computers were first tested and then loaded with the desired software, shipped, and typically delivered five to six business days after the order was placed.

At Dell's newest plant in Austin, the cell manufacturing approach had been abandoned in favor of an even more efficient assembly-line approach. Workers at the new plant in 2004 could turn out close to 800 desktop PCs per hour on three assembly lines that took half the floor space of the older cell manufacturing process, where production had run about 120 units per hour. Although the new Austin plant was originally designed for production of 400 units per hour (1 PC every 9 seconds), management expected to boost hourly production to 1,000 units per hour. The gains in productivity were being achieved partly by redesigning the PCs to permit easier and faster assembly, partly by innovations in the assembly process, and partly by reducing the number of times a computer was touched by workers during assembly and shipping by 50 percent. In 2005 it took about 66 minutes to assemble and test a PC. Moreover, just-in-time inventory practices that left pallets of parts sitting around everywhere had been tweaked to just-in-the-nick-of-time delivery by suppliers of the exact parts needed every couple of hours; double-decker conveyor belts moved parts and components to designated assembly points. Newly assembled PCs were routed on conveyors to shipping, where they were boxed and shipped to customers the same day.

Dell's new 750,000-square-foot plant in North Carolina featured a production layout that allowed computers to be tested as its components and software were installed. This "instantaneous build and test" operation permitted team members to identify and correct any problems on the spot, rather than waiting until the PC was fully assembled. The assembly innovations pioneered in the Austin and North Carolina plants were in the process of being instituted in Dell's other plants. Workers at all Dell plants competed with each other to come up with more efficient assembly methods. New cost-saving ideas at one plant were quickly implemented worldwide.

Dell was regarded as a world-class manufacturing innovator and a pioneer in how to mass-produce a customized product—its methods were routinely studied in business schools worldwide. Most of Dell's PC rivals—notably, IBM and HP/Compaq—had given up on trying to produce their own PCs as cheaply as Dell and shifted to outsourcing their PCs from contract manufacturers. Dell management believed that its in-house manufacturing delivered about a 6 percent cost advantage versus outsourcing. Dell's build-to-order strategy meant that the company had no in-house stock of finished goods inventories and that, unlike competitors using the traditional value chain model, it did not have to wait for resellers to clear out their own inventories before it could push new models into the marketplace—resellers typically operated with 30 to 60 days inventory of prebuilt models (see Exhibit 4). Equally important was the fact that customers who bought from Dell got the satisfaction

Exhibit 4   **Comparative Value Chain Models of PC Vendors**

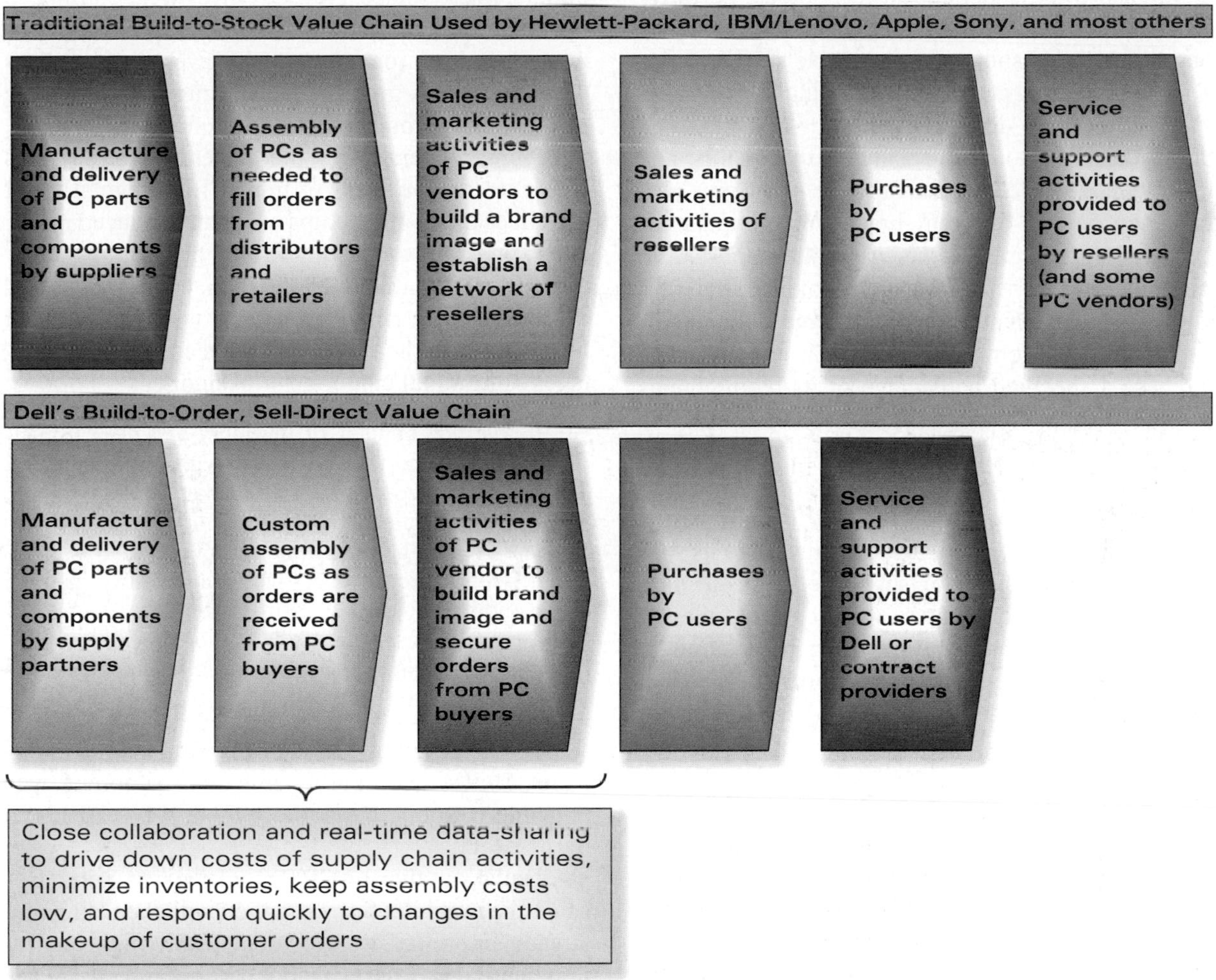

Traditional Build-to-Stock Value Chain Used by Hewlett-Packard, IBM/Lenovo, Apple, Sony, and most others

| Manufacture and delivery of PC parts and components by suppliers | Assembly of PCs as needed to fill orders from distributors and retailers | Sales and marketing activities of PC vendors to build a brand image and establish a network of resellers | Sales and marketing activities of resellers | Purchases by PC users | Service and support activities provided to PC users by resellers (and some PC vendors) |

Dell's Build-to-Order, Sell-Direct Value Chain

| Manufacture and delivery of PC parts and components by supply partners | Custom assembly of PCs as orders are received from PC buyers | Sales and marketing activities of PC vendor to build brand image and secure orders from PC buyers | Purchases by PC users | Service and support activities provided to PC users by Dell or contract providers |

Close collaboration and real-time data-sharing to drive down costs of supply chain activities, minimize inventories, keep assembly costs low, and respond quickly to changes in the makeup of customer orders

of having their computers customized to their particular liking and pocketbook.

Quality Control

All assembly plants had the capability to run testing and quality control processes on components, parts, and subassemblies obtained from suppliers, as well as on the finished products Dell assembled. Suppliers were urged to participate in a quality certification program that committed them to achieving defined quality specifications. Quality control activities were undertaken at various stages in the assembly process. In addition, Dell's quality control program included testing of completed units after assembly, ongoing production reliability audits, failure tracking for early identification of problems associated with new models shipped to customers,

and information obtained from customers through its service and technical support programs. All of the company's plants had been certified as meeting ISO 9002 quality standards.

Partnerships with Suppliers

Michael Dell believed that it made much better sense for the company to partner with reputable suppliers of PC parts and components than to integrate backward and get into parts and components manufacturing on its own. He explained why:

> If you've got a race with 20 players all vying to make the fastest graphics chip in the world, do you want to be the twenty-first horse, or do you want to evaluate the field of 20 and pick the best one?[8]

Dell management evaluated the various makers of each component; picked the best one or two as suppliers; and then stuck with them as long as they maintained their leadership in technology, performance, quality, and cost. Management believed that long-term partnerships with reputable suppliers had at least five advantages. First, using name-brand processors, disk drives, modems, speakers, and multimedia components enhanced the quality and performance of Dell's PCs. Because of varying performance among different brands of components, the brand of the components was quite important to customers concerned about performance and reliability. Second, because Dell partnered with suppliers for the long term and because it committed to purchase a specified percentage of its requirements from each supplier, Dell was assured of getting the volume of components it needed on a timely basis even when overall market demand for a particular component temporarily exceeded the overall market supply. Third, Dell's long-run commitment to its suppliers made it feasible for suppliers to locate their plants or distribution centers within a few miles of Dell assembly plants, putting them in position to make deliveries daily or every few hours, as needed. Dell supplied data on inventories and replenishment needs to its suppliers at least once a day—hourly in the case of components being delivered several times daily from nearby sources.

Fourth, long-term supply partnerships facilitated having some of the supplier's engineers assigned to Dell's product design teams and being treated as part of Dell. When new products were launched, suppliers' engineers were stationed in Dell's plants; if early buyers called with a problem related to design, further assembly and shipments were halted while the supplier's engineers and Dell personnel corrected the flaw on the spot.[9] Fifth, long-term partnerships enlisted greater cooperation on the part of suppliers to seek new ways to drive costs out of the supply chain. Dell openly shared its daily production schedules, sales forecasts, and new model introduction plans with vendors. Dell also did a three-year plan with each of its key suppliers and worked with suppliers to minimize the number of different stock-keeping units of parts and components in its products and to identify ways to drive costs down.

Commitment to Just-in-Time Inventory Practices

Dell's just-in-time inventory emphasis yielded major cost advantages and shortened the time it took for Dell to get new generations of its computer models into the marketplace. New advances were coming so fast in certain computer parts and components (particularly microprocessors, disk drives, and wireless devices) that any given item in inventory was obsolete in a matter of months, sometimes quicker. Moreover, rapid-fire reductions in the prices of components were not unusual—for example, Intel regularly cut the prices on its older chips when it introduced newer chips, and it introduced new chip generations about every three months. In 2003–2004, component costs declined an average of 0.5 percent weekly.[10] Michael Dell explained the competitive and economic advantages of minimal component inventories:

> If I've got 11 days of inventory and my competitor has 80 and Intel comes out with a new chip, that means I'm going to get to market 69 days sooner. In the computer industry, inventory can be a pretty massive risk because if the cost of materials is going down 50 percent a year and you have two or three months of inventory versus eleven days, you've got a big cost disadvantage. And you're vulnerable to product transitions, when you can get stuck with obsolete inventory.[11]

For a growing number of parts and components, Dell's close partnership with suppliers was allowing it to operate with no more than two hours of inventory.

Dell's supplier of CRT monitors was Sony. Because the monitors Sony supplied with the Dell name already imprinted were of dependably high quality (a defect rate of fewer than 1,000 per million), Dell didn't even open up the monitor boxes to test them at its Reno, Nevada, monitor distribution center.[12] Using sophisticated data exchange systems, Dell arranged for its shippers (Airborne Express and United Parcel Service) to pick up computers at U.S. assembly plants, then pick up the accompanying monitors at its Reno distribution center and deliver both to the customer simultaneously. The savings in time and cost were significant. Dell had been working hard for the past several years to refine and improve its relationships with suppliers and its procedures for operating with smaller inventories.

In fiscal year 1995, Dell averaged an inventory turn cycle of 32 days. By the end of fiscal 1997 (January 1997), the average was down to 13 days. In fiscal 1998 Dell's inventory averaged 7 days, which compared very favorably with Gateway's 14-day average, Compaq's 23-day average, and the estimated industrywide average of over 50 days. In fiscal years

1999 and 2000, Dell operated with an average of six days' supply in inventory; the average dropped to 5 days' supply in fiscal year 2001, 4 days' supply in 2002, and 3 to 4 days' supply in 2003–2006.

Dell's Direct Sales Strategy and Marketing Efforts

With thousands of phone, fax, and Internet orders daily and ongoing field sales force contact with customers, the company kept its finger on the market pulse, quickly detecting shifts in sales trends, design problems, and quality glitches. If the company got more than a few of the same complaints, the information was relayed immediately to design engineers who checked out the problem. When design flaws or components defects were found, the factory was notified and the problem corrected within a few days. Management believed Dell's ability to respond quickly gave it a significant advantage over PC makers that operated on the basis of large production runs of variously configured and equipped PCs and sold them through retail channels. Dell saw its direct sales approach as a totally customer-driven system, with the flexibility to transition quickly to new generations of components and PC models.

Dell's Customer-Based Sales and Marketing Focus

Whereas many technology companies organized their sales and marketing efforts around product lines, Dell was organized around customer groups. Dell had placed managers in charge of developing sales and service programs appropriate to the needs and expectations of each customer group. Up until the early 1990s, Dell operated with sales and service programs aimed at just two market segments—high-volume corporate and governmental buyers and low-volume business and individual buyers. But as sales took off in 1995–97, these segments were subdivided into finer, more homogeneous categories that by 2000 included global enterprise accounts, large and midsize companies (over 400 employees), small companies (under 400 employees), health care businesses (over 400 employees), federal government agencies, state and local government agencies, educational institutions, and individual consumers. Many of these customer segments were further subdivided—for instance, in education, there were separate sales and marketing programs for K–12 schools; higher education institutions; and personal-use purchases by faculty, staff, and students.

Dell had a field sales force that called on large business and institutional customers throughout the world. Dell's largest global enterprise accounts were assigned their own dedicated sales force—for example, Dell had a sales force of 150 people dedicated to meeting the needs of General Electric's facilities and personnel scattered across the world. Individuals and small businesses could place orders by telephone or at Dell's Web site. Dell had call centers in the United States, Canada, Europe, and Asia with toll-free lines; customers could talk with a sales representative about specific models, get information faxed or mailed to them, place an order, and pay by credit card. The Asian and European call centers were equipped with technology that routed calls from a particular country to a particular call center. Thus, for example, a customer calling from Lisbon, Portugal, was automatically directed to a Portuguese-speaking sales rep at the call center in Montpelier, France.

Dell in Japan   Dell's share in Japan had climbed steadily from 1.0 percent in 1995 to 7.7 percent in 2002 to close to 12 percent in 2005, making it the number three provider of computer systems in Japan (behind NEC and Toshiba). Other competitors in Japan included Sony, Fujitsu, Hitachi, IBM/Lenovo, Sharp, and Matshusita. Based on units sold, however, Dell was number one in business desktop computers and number two in entry-level and midrange servers. Dell's 2004 sales in Japan were up about 30 percent, in a market where overall sales were flat, and its sales in 2005 were up around 20 percent. Dell's technical and customer support for PCs, servers, and network storage devices was ranked the best in Japan in 2002 and 2003. Dell had 1,100 personnel in Japan and was tracking Japanese buying habits and preferences with its proprietary software. The head of Dell's consumer PC sales group in Japan had installed 34 kiosks in leading electronics stores around Japan, allowing shoppers to test Dell computers, ask questions of staff, and place orders—close to half the sales were to people who did not know about Dell prior to visiting the kiosk. The kiosks proved quite popular and were boosting Dell's share of PC sales to consumers in Japan. Dell believed that it was more profitable than any other PC-server vendor selling in the Japanese market. Dell's profit margins in Japan were higher than those in the U.S. market.

Dell in China   Dell Computer entered China in 1998 and achieved faster growth there than in any other foreign market it had entered. The market for PCs in China was the third largest in the world, behind the United States and Japan, and was on the verge of being the second largest. PC sales in China were growing 20–30 percent annually and, with a population of 1.4 billion people (of which some 400 million lived in metropolitan areas where computer use was growing rapidly), the Chinese market for PCs was expected to become the largest in the world by 2010. Dell's shipments in China rose 60 percent in fiscal 2004 (four times the rest of the industry) and its revenues were up 40 percent, making China Dell's fourth largest market. Sales growth in 2005 was almost as strong—unit sales rose 46 percent in the third quarter of 2005 and revenues were up 29 percent, with the strongest gains coming in the home and small business segment.

The market leader in China was Lenovo with a 25.0 percent share in 2005; Lenovo was a company on the move, having acquired the PC business of IBM in 2004 to become the third largest PC maker in the world. Other major local PC producers were Founder (with about a 10 percent share) and Great Wall (with about a 9.0 percent share). Dell had close to a 10 percent share in 2005. Other competitors in China included Hewlett-Packard, Toshiba, Acer, and NEC Japan. All of the major contenders except Dell relied on resellers to handle sales and service; in 2005, Lenovo had more than 4,800 retail outlets carrying its PCs in China. Dell sold directly to customers in China just as it did elsewhere.

Dell's primary target market in China consisted of large corporate accounts. Management believed that many Chinese companies would find the savings from direct sales appealing, that they would like the idea of having Dell build PCs and servers to their requirements and specifications, and that—once they became a Dell customer—they would like the convenience of Internet purchases and the company's growing array of products and services. In 2005, Dell had 5,000 employees in China. It operated a call center in Xiamen, a city of over 1 million people on China's southeast coast, where sales representatives took most of Dell's orders via telephone. In nine other cities in China, Dell had sales representatives who called on large business and government customers, relaying orders back to their colleagues in Xiamen. Dell had contracted with service providers in 40 cities in China to provide onsite service in no more than four hours.

Dell recognized that its direct sales approach put it at a short-term disadvantage in appealing to small business customers and individual consumers, since most of these customers were reluctant to place orders by phone or over the Internet. According to an executive from rival Lenovo, "It takes two years of a person's savings to buy a PC in China. And when two years of savings is at stake, the whole family wants to come out to a store to touch and try the machine."[13] But Dell believed that over time, as Chinese consumers became more familiar with PCs and more comfortable with making online purchases, growing numbers of small business customers and consumers would become comfortable with placing Internet and telephone orders. In 2005, more than 100 million Chinese consumers had access to the Internet at home or at work and the numbers were growing rapidly. In 2005, about 6 percent of Dell's sales in China were over the Internet. Dell believed its business in China was two to three times more profitable than Lenovo's business in China.

Dell in Latin America   In 2002, PC sales in Latin America exceeded 5 million units. Latin America had a population of 450 million people. Dell management believed that in the next few years PC use in Latin America would reach 1 for every 30 people (one-tenth the penetration in the United States), pushing annual sales up to 15 million units. The company's plant in Brazil, the largest market in Latin America, was opened to produce, sell, and provide service and technical support for customers in Brazil, Argentina, Chile, Uruguay, and Paraguay.

Using Dell Direct Store Kiosks to Access Individual Consumers   Inspired by the success of kiosks in Japan, Dell began installing Dell Direct Store kiosks in a variety of U.S. retail settings as a hands-on complement to Internet and phone sales in 2002. The stores showcased Dell's newest notebook and desktop computers, plasma and LCD TVs, printers, and music players. The kiosks did not carry inventory, but customers could talk face-to-face with a knowledgeable Dell sales representative, inspect Dell's products, and place an order via the Internet while at the kiosk. The kiosks were considered a success in getting consumers to try Dell products, and more kiosks had been added. In December 2005, Dell had 145 Dell Direct Store kiosks in 20 states, within reach of more than 50 percent of the U.S. population.

Customer Service and Technical Support

Service became a feature of Dell's strategy in 1986 when the company began providing a year's free onsite service with most of its PCs after users complained about having to ship their PCs back to Austin for repairs. Dell contracted with local service providers to handle customer requests for repairs; onsite service was provided on a four-hour basis to large customers and on a next-day basis to small customers. In 2005, Dell had five Enterprise Command Centers (ECCs) coordinating around-the-clock service globally for large customers; 350 hubs in cities around the world with four-hour service capability; 52,000 people worldwide who were trained to service Dell products; and 81 million active contracts to service PCs, servers, and other equipment it had sold to customers. Dell used the ECCs to monitor and manage the repair service and support effectiveness of Dell's field engineers and contract service personnel. If business or institutional customers preferred to work with their own service provider, Dell supplied the provider of choice with training and spare parts needed to service customers' equipment. When individuals or small businesses purchased their PCs, they could obtain a service contract for At Home service (usually the next day). Dell also offered Complete-Care accidental damage service, had a help desk for all software and peripherals support, and Gold Technical Support for advanced technical service. Dell's online training programs featured over 1,200 courses for consumer, business, and IT professionals.

Customers needing technical support could contact Dell via a toll-free phone number or e-mail. Dell received 6 to 8 million phone calls and 500,000 to 600,000 e-mail messages annually requesting service and support. Dell was aggressively pursuing initiatives to enhance its online technical support tools and reduce the number and cost of telephone support calls. The company was adding Web-based customer service and support tools to make customers' online experiences pleasant and satisfying. In 2003–2005, over 50 percent of Dell's technical support activities were conducted via the Internet. Dell had instituted a First Call Resolution initiative to strengthen its capabilities to resolve customer inquiries or difficulties on the first call; First Call Resolution percentages were made an important measure in evaluating the company's technical support performance. Dell had recently opened new customer contact and distribution facilities in Oklahoma and Ohio.

Value-Added Services   Dell kept close track of the purchases of its large global customers, country by country and department by department—and customers themselves found this purchase information valuable. Dell's sales and support personnel used their knowledge about a particular customer's needs to help that customer plan PC purchases, to configure the customer's PC networks, and to provide value-added services. For example, for its large customers Dell loaded software and placed ID tags on newly ordered PCs at the factory, thereby eliminating the need for the customer's IT personnel to unpack the PC, deliver it to an employee's desk, hook it up, place asset tags on the PC, and load the needed software from an assortment of CD-ROMs and diskettes—a process that could take several hours and cost $200–$300.[14] While Dell charged an extra $15 or $20 for the software-loading and asset-tagging services, the savings to customers were still considerable—one large customer reported savings of $500,000 annually from this service.[15]

Premier Pages   Dell had developed customized, password-protected Web sites called Premier Pages for over 50,000 corporate, governmental, and institutional customers worldwide. These Premier Pages gave customers' personnel online access to information about all Dell products and configurations the company had purchased or that were currently authorized for purchase. Employees could use Premier Pages to (1) obtain customer-specific pricing for whatever machines and options the employee wanted to consider, (2) place an order online that would be electronically routed to higher-level managers for approval and then on to Dell for assembly and delivery, and (3) seek advanced help desk support. Customers could also search and sort all invoices and obtain purchase histories. These features eliminated paper invoices, cut ordering time, and reduced the internal labor customers needed to staff corporate purchasing and accounting functions. Customer use of Premier Pages had boosted the productivity of Dell salespeople assigned to these accounts by 50 percent. Dell was providing Premier Page service to thousands of additional customers annually and adding more features to further improve functionality.

www.dell.com   Dell operated one of the world's highest-volume Internet commerce sites, with nearly 8 billion page requests annually at 81 country sites in 28 languages/dialects and 26 currencies. Dell began Internet sales at its Web site (www.dell.com) in 1995, achieving sales of $1 million a day almost overnight. By early 2003, over 50 percent of Dell's sales were Web-enabled—and the percentage was increasing, especially for sales to small businesses and consumers. Dell's Web site sales exceeded $60 million a day in 2004, up from $35 million daily in early 2000 and $5 million daily in early 1998. The revenues generated at Dell.com were greater than those of Yahoo, Google, eBay, and Amazon.com combined.[16] Its Web site was averaging 300 million visits by some 100 million unique visitors per quarter in 2005.

At the company's Web site, prospective buyers could review Dell's entire product line in detail, configure and price customized PCs, place orders, and track orders from manufacturing through shipping. The closing rate on sales at Dell's Web site was 20 percent higher than that on sales inquiries received via telephone. Management believed that enhancing Dell.com to shrink transaction and order fulfillment times, increase accuracy, and provide more personalized content resulted in a higher degree of "e-loyalty" than traditional attributes like price and product selection.

On-Site Services   Corporate customers paid Dell fees to provide technical support, on-site service, and help with migrating to new IT technologies. Services were one of the fastest-growing part of Dell, with revenues climbing from $1.7 billion in 2002 to about $5 billion in 2005. Dell's service business was split about 50–50 between what Michael Dell called close-to-the-box services and management and professional services—but the latter were growing faster, at close to 25 percent annually. Dell estimated that close-to-the-box support services for Dell products represented about a $50 billion market, whereas the market for management and professional services (IT life-cycle services, deployment of new technology, and solutions for greater IT productivity) was about $90 billion. IT consulting services were becoming more standardized, driven primarily by growing hardware and software standardization, reduction in on-site service requirements (partly because of online diagnostic and support tools, growing ease of repair and maintenance, increased customer knowledge, and increased remote management

capabilities), and declines in the skills and know-how that were required to perform service tasks on standardized equipment and install new, more standardized systems.

Dell's strategy in services, like its strategy in hardware products, was to bring down the cost of IT consulting services for its large enterprise customers. The providers of on-site service, technical support, and other types of IT consulting typically charged premium prices and realized hefty profits for their efforts. According to Michael Dell, customers who bought the services being provided by Dell saved 40 to 50 percent over what they would have paid other providers of IT services.

Top management expected services to play an expanding role in the company's growth. Kevin Rollins, Dell's president and CEO, indicated the company's business model "isn't just about making cheap boxes, it's also about freeing customers from overpriced relationships" with such vendors as IBM, Sun Microsystems, and Hewlett- Packard.[17] While a number of Dell's corporate accounts were large enough to justify dedicated on-site teams of Dell support personnel, Dell generally contracted with third-party providers to make the necessary on-site service calls. Customers notified Dell when they had problems; such notices triggered two electronic dispatches—one to ship replacement parts from Dell's factory to the customer sites, and one to notify the contract service provider to prepare to make the needed repairs as soon as the parts arrived.[18] Bad parts were returned so that Dell could determine what went wrong and how to prevent such problems from happening again. Problems relating to faulty components or flawed components design were promptly passed along to the relevant supplier for correction.

Customer Forums   In addition to using its sales and support mechanisms to stay close to customers, Dell periodically held regional forums for its best customers. The company formed Platinum and Gold Councils composed of its largest customers in the United States, Europe, Japan, and the Asia-Pacific region; regional meetings were held every six to nine months.[19] Some regions had two meetings—one for chief information officers and one for technical personnel. At the meetings, which frequently included a presentation by Michael Dell, Dell's senior technologists shared their views on the direction of the latest technological developments, what the flow of technology really meant for customers, and Dell's plans for introducing new and upgraded products over the next two years. There were also breakout sessions on topics of current interest. Dell found that the information gleaned from customers at these meetings assisted the company in forecasting demand for its products.

In a 2005 survey of IT executives by *CIO Magazine,* Dell was rated number one among leading vendors for providing "impeccable customer service."

Customer-Driven Research and Development and Standardized Technology

Dell's R&D focus was to track and test new developments in components and software, ascertain which ones would prove most useful and cost-effective for customers, and then design them into Dell products. Management's philosophy was that it was Dell's job on behalf of its customers to sort out all the new technology coming into the marketplace and help steer customers to options and solutions most relevant to their needs. The company talked to its customers frequently about "relevant technology," listening carefully to customers' needs and problems and endeavoring to identify the most cost-effective solutions.

Dell was a strong advocate of incorporating standardized components in its products so as not to tie either it or its customers to one company's proprietary technology and components, which almost always carried a price premium and increased costs for its customers. Dell actively promoted the use of industrywide standards and regularly pressed its suppliers of a particular part or component to agree on common standards. Dell executives saw standardized technology as beginning to take over the largest part of the $800 billion spent annually on IT—standardization was particularly evident in servers, storage, networking, and high-performance computing. One example of the impact of standardized technology was at the University of Buffalo, where Dell had installed a 5.6 teraflop cluster of about 2,000 Dell servers containing 4,000 microprocessors that was being used to decode the human genome. The cluster of servers, which were the same as those Dell sold to its business customers, had been installed in about 60 days at a cost of a few million dollars and represented the third most powerful supercomputer in the world. High-performance clusters of PCs and servers were replacing mainframe computers

and custom-designed supercomputers because of their much lower cost. Amerada Hess, attracted by Dell's use of standardized and upgradable parts and components, installed a cluster of several hundred Dell workstations and allocated about $300,000 a year to upgrade and maintain it; the cluster had replaced an IBM supercomputer that cost $1.5 million a year to lease and operate. Studies conducted by Dell indicated that, over time, products incorporating standardized technology delivered about twice the performance per dollar of cost as products based on proprietary technology.

Dell's R&D group included about 4,000 engineers, and its annual R&D budget had been in the $450 to $465 million range for the past four years (see Exhibit 2). The company's R&D unit also studied and implemented ways to control quality and to streamline the assembly process. In 2005, Dell had a portfolio of 1,128 U.S. patents and another 719 patent applications were pending—at least 10 percent of Dell's U.S. patents were ranked "elite."

Expansion into New Products

Dell's recent expansion into data storage hardware, switches, handheld PCs, printers, and printer cartridges represented an effort to diversify the company's product base and to use its competitive capabilities in PCs and servers to pursue revenue growth opportunities. Michael Dell explained why Dell had decided to expand into products and services that complemented its sales of PCs and servers:

> We tend to look at what is the next big opportunity all the time. We can't take on too many of these at once, because it kind of overloads the system. But we believe fundamentally that if you think about the whole market, it's about an $800 billion market, all areas of technology over time go through a process of standardization or commoditization. And we try to look at those, anticipate what's happening, and develop strategies that will allow us to get into those markets. In the server market in 1995 we had a 2 percent market share, today we have over a 30 percent share, we're number 1 in the U.S. How did that happen? Well, first of all it happened because we started to have a high market share for desktops and notebooks. Then customers said, oh yes, we know Dell, those are the guys who have really good desktops and notebooks. So they have servers, yes, we'll test those, we'll test them around the periphery, maybe not in the most critical applications at first, but we'll test them here.

[Then they discover] these are really good and Dell provides great support . . . and I think to some extent we've benefited from the fact that our competitors have underestimated the importance of value, and the power of the relationship and the service that we can create with the customer.

And, also, as a product tends to standardize there's not an elimination of the requirement for custom services, there's a reduction of it. So by offering some services, but not the services of the traditional proprietary computer company, we've been able to increase our share. And, in fact, what tends to happen is customers embrace the standards, because they know that's going to save them costs. Let me give you an example . . . about a year ago we entered into the data networking market. So we have Ethernet switches, layer 2 switches. So if you have PCs and servers, you need switches; every PC attaches to a switch, every server attaches to a switch. It's a pretty easy sale, switches go along with computer systems. We looked at this market and were able to come up with products that are priced about 2½ times less than the market leader today, Cisco, and as a result the business has grown very, very quickly. We shipped 1.8 million switch ports in a period of about a year, when most people would have said that's not going to work and come up with all kinds of reasons why we can't succeed.[20]

As Dell's sales of data-routing switches accelerated in 2001–2002 and Dell management mulled whether to expand into other networking products and Internet gear, Cisco elected to discontinue supplying its switches to Dell for resale as of October 2002. Dell's family of PowerConnect switches—simple commodity-like products generally referred to as layer 2 switches in the industry—carried a price of $20 per port, versus $70–$100 for comparable Cisco switches and $38 for comparable 3Com switches.

Michael Dell and Kevin Rollins saw external storage devices as a growth opportunity because the company's corporate and institutional customers were making increasing use of high-speed data storage and retrieval devices. Dell's PowerVault line of storage products had data protection and recovery features that made it easy for customers to add and manage storage and simplify consolidation. The PowerVault products used standardized technology and components (which were considerably cheaper than customized ones), allowing Dell to underprice rivals and drive down storage costs for its customers

by about 50 percent. Dell's competitors in storage devices included Hewlett-Packard and IBM.

Some observers saw Dell's 2003 entry into the printer market as a calculated effort to go after Hewlett-Packard's biggest and most profitable business segment and believed the Dell offensive was deliberately timed to throw a wrench into HP's efforts to resolve the many challenges of successfully merging its operations with those of Compaq. One of the reasons that Dell had entered the market for servers back in 1995 was that Compaq Computer, then its biggest rival in PCs, had been using its lucrative profits on server sales to subsidize charging lower prices on Compaq computers and thus be more price competitive against Dell's PCs—at the time Compaq was losing money on its desktop and notebook PC business. According to Michael Dell:

> Compaq had this enormous profit pool that they were using to fight against us in the desktop and notebook business. That was not an acceptable situation. Our product teams knew that the servers weren't that complicated or expensive to produce, and customers were being charged unfair prices.[21]

Dell management believed that HP was doing much the same thing in printers and printer products, where it had a dominant market share worldwide and generated about 75 percent of its operating profits. Dell believed HP was using its big margins on printer products to subsidize selling its PCs at prices comparable to Dell's, even though Dell had costs that were about 8 percent lower than HP. HP's PC operations were either in the red or barely in the black during most of 2003–2004, while Dell consistently had profit margins of 8 percent or more on PCs. Dell management believed the company's entry into the printer market would add value for its customers. Michael Dell explained:

> We think we can drive down the entire cost of owning and using printing products. If you look at any other market Dell has gone into, we have been able to significantly save money for customers. We know we can do that in printers; we have looked at the supply chain all the way through its various cycles and we know there are inefficiencies there. I think the price of the total offering when we include the printer and the supplies . . . can come down quite considerably.[22]

Dell's entry and market success in printer products had put pricing pressure on HP in the printer market and had helped erode HP's share of the printer market worldwide from just under 50 percent to around 46 percent. Kevin Rollins believed that Dell's decision to enter the printer market as as a head-to-head rival of HP served two purposes: "Any strategist is going to try to develop a strategy that is going to help them and hurt competitors. Our whole vision here was to do both: improve the revenues and profits of our own business, and at the same time put our competitors at a disadvantage."[23] As of the fall of 2005, Dell had sold over 10 million printers and had an estimated 20 percent of the market for color network lasers and color inkjet printers in the United States.[24]

When Dell announced it had contracted with Lexmark to make printers and printer and toner cartridges for sale under the Dell label beginning in 2003, HP immediately discontinued supplying HP printers to Dell for resale at Dell's Web site. Dell had been selling Lexmark printers for two years and since 2000 had resold about 4 million printers made by such vendors as HP, Lexmark, and other vendors to its customers. Lexmark designed and made critical parts for its printers but used offshore contract manufacturers for assembly. Gross profit margins on printers (sales minus cost of goods sold) were said to be in single digits in 2002–2004, but the gross margins on printer supplies were in the 50–60 percent range—brand-name ink cartridges for printers typically ran $25 to $35.

To further keep the pricing pressure on HP in 2003, Dell had priced its new Axim line of handheld PCs at about 50 percent less than HP's popular iPaq line of handhelds, and Dell's storage and networking products also carried lower prices than comparable HP products.

Exhibit 5 shows a breakdown of Dell's sales by product type. Exhibit 6 shows trends in Dell's market shares in various categories.

Other Elements of Dell's Business Strategy

Dell's strategy had three other elements that assisted the company's drive for industry leadership: the use of the Internet and e-commerce technologies, entry into the white-box segment of the PC industry, and advertising.

Pioneering Leadership in Use of the Internet and E-Commerce Technology   Dell was a leader in using the Internet and e-commerce technologies to squeeze greater efficiency out of its supply chain activities, to streamline the order-to-delivery process, to encourage greater customer use of its Web site, and to gather and use all types of information. In a 1999 speech to 1,200 customers, Michael Dell said:

Exhibit 5   **Dell's Revenues by Product Category, First Nine Months, Fiscal 2006 versus Fiscal 2005**

| | Nine Months Ended | | | |
| | October 28, 2005 | | October 29, 2004 | |
Product Category	Revenues (in billions)	% of Total Revenues	Revenues (in billions)	% of Total Revenues
Desktop PCs	$15.5	38%	$15.2	43%
Mobility products (notebook PCs, Dell DJ, Axim)	10.3	25	8.7	24
Printers, monitors, TVs, projectors, ink and toner cartridges	6.1	15	4.7	13
Servers and networking hardware	4.0	10	3.6	10
Professional consulting and support services	3.5	9	2.6	7
Storage products	1.3	3	0.9	3
Totals	$40.7	100%	$35.7	100%

Source: Dell's 10-Q report, third quarter, fiscal 2006.

Exhibit 6   **Trends in Dell's Market Shares in PCs, 1994–2005**

Market Segment	Dell's Market Share						
	2005*	2004	2002	2000	1998	1996	1994
Worldwide share	18.7%	17.7%	14.9%	10.5%	8.0%	4.1%	2.7%
United States	33.1	33.1	28.0	18.4	12.0	6.4	4.2
Europe/Middle East/Africa	13.0	11.5	9.6	7.8	7.0	3.8	2.4
Asia-Pacific	8.0	7.0	4.8	3.4	2.4	1.3	0.3
Japan	12.1	11.3	7.7	4.0	3.0	1.6	1.1
Desktop PCs	18.5%	18.0%	14.8%	10.1%	7.8%	4.3%	3.0%
Notebook PCs	17.6	16.2	14.4	11.3	8.5	3.4	1.1
x86 Servers	26.8	24.8	21.7	15.4	9.7	3.4	3.1
U.S segment share	33.1%	33.1%	28.0%	18.4%	12.0%	6.4%	4.2%
Education	45.2	44.3	34.9	26.2	11.0	3.9	1.1
Government	34.8	32.9	33.7	22.9	14.6	6.5	7.1
Home	28.8	29.7	22.7	6.5	3.5	2.1	1.2
Large business	44.9	44.2	39.9	31.3	21.6	11.2	6.9
Small/medium business	29.1	28.5	24.2	22.6	14.3	7.9	5.4

*First nine months.

Source: Information posted at www.dell.com (accessed December 12, 2005).

The world will be changed forever by the Internet . . . The Internet will be your business. If your business isn't enabled by providing customers and suppliers with more information, you're probably already in trouble. The Internet provides a dramatic reduction in the cost of transactions and the cost of interaction among people and businesses, and it creates dramatic new opportunities and destroys old competitive advantages. The Internet is like a weapon sitting on a table ready to be picked up by either you or your competitors.[25]

Dell's use of its Web site and various Internet technology applications had proved instrumental in helping the company become the industry's low-cost provider and drive costs out of its business. Internet technology applications were a cornerstone of Dell's collaborative efforts with suppliers. The company provided order-status information quickly and conveniently over the Internet, thereby eliminating tens of thousands of order-status inquiries coming in by phone. It used its Web site as a powerful sales and technical support tool. Few companies could match Dell's competencies and capabilities in the use of Internet technology to improve operating efficiency and gain new sales in a cost-efficient manner.

Dell's Entry into the White-Box PC Segment   In 2002 Dell announced it would begin making so-called white-box (i.e., unbranded) PCs for resale under the private labels of retailers. PC dealers that supplied white-box PCs to small businesses and price-conscious individuals under the dealer's own brand name accounted for about one-third of total PC sales and about 50 percent of sales to small businesses. According to one industry analyst, "Increasingly, Dell's biggest competitor these days isn't big brand-name companies like IBM or HP, it's white-box vendors." Dell's thinking in entering the white-box PC segment was that it was cheaper to reach many small businesses through the white-box dealers that already served them than by using its own sales force and support groups to sell and service businesses with fewer than 100 employees. Dell believed its low-cost supply chain and assembly capabilities would allow it to build generic machines cheaper than white-box resellers could buy components and assemble a customized machine. Management forecasted that Dell would achieve $380 million in sales of white-box PCs in 2003 and would generate profit margins equal to those on Dell-branded PCs. Some industry analysts were skeptical of Dell's move into white-box PCs because they expected white-box dealers to be reluctant to buy their PCs from a company that had a history of taking their clients. Others believed this was a test effort by Dell to develop the capabilities to take on white-box dealers in Asia and especially in China, where the sellers of generic PCs were particularly strong.

Advertising   Michael Dell was a strong believer in the power of advertising and frequently espoused its importance in the company's strategy. He insisted that the company's ads be communicative and forceful, not soft and fuzzy. The company regularly had prominent ads describing its products and prices in such leading computer publications as *PC Magazine* and *PC World,* as well as in *USA Today, The Wall Street Journal,* and other business publications. From time to time, the company ran ads on TV to promote its products to consumers and small businesses. Catalogs of about 25–30 pages describing Dell's latest desktop and laptop PCs, along with its printers, TVs, MP3 players, handheld PCs, and other related products were periodically mailed to consumers who had bought Dell products. Other direct marketing initiatives included sending their newsletters and promotional pieces to customers via the Internet.

DELL'S PERFORMANCE IN 2005

Dell shipped about 27 million units during the first nine months of 2005, and it had a record shipment of 9.2 million units in the third quarter of fiscal 2006. Despite steadily eroding average selling prices— $1,540 in fiscal 2004, down from $1,640 in 2003, $1,700 in 2002, $2,050 in 2001, $2,250 in 2000, and $2,600 in 1998—Dell's revenues were climbing as the company gained volume and market share in virtually all product categories and geographic areas where it competed.

Worldwide revenues, which reached $40.7 billion in the first nine months of fiscal 2006, were expected to run 10–12 percent higher than fiscal 2005 levels and total about $55 billion for the full year. Dell's sales increases were strongest in outside the United States (non-U.S. sales were up 20 percent), in servers (where shipments were up 21 percent), storage products (where sales were up 35 percent, three times the industrywide rate). Unit

sales of "mobility" products (laptop PC and work-stations, Dell DJ MP3 players, and Axim handheld computers) were up 41 percent and produced revenues gains of 18 percent (the lower growth rate for revenues was due to falling prices industrywide for virtually all types of mobile devices). Dell's shipments of printers were up 8 percent and sales of replacement ink and toner cartridges doubled.

Dell ended fiscal 2006 with $11.7 billion in cash and investments. The company had invested about $500 million in property, plant, and equipment in fiscal 2005 and expected that total capital expenditures for all of fiscal 2006 would approximate $700 million.

MARKET CONDITIONS IN THE INFORMATION TECHNOLOGY INDUSTRY IN LATE 2005

Analysts expected the $800 billion worldwide IT industry to grow roughly 6–9 percent in 2005, following nearly a 10 percent increase in 2004, a single-digit increase in 2003, a 2.3 percent decline in 2002, and close to a 1 percent decline in 2001— corporate spending for IT products accounted for about 45 percent of all capital expenditures of U.S. businesses. From 1980 to 2000, IT spending had grown at an average annual rate of 12 percent and then flattened. The slowdown in IT spending reflected a combination of factors: sluggish economic growth worldwide that was prompting businesses to delay IT upgrades and hold on to aging equipment longer, overinvestment in IT in the 1995–99 period, declining unit prices for many IT products (especially PCs and servers), and a growing preference for lower-priced, standard-component hardware that was good enough to perform a variety of functions using off-the-shelf Windows or Linux operating systems (as opposed to relying on proprietary hardware and customized Unix software). The selling points that appealed most to IT customers were standardization, flexibility, modularity, simplicity, economy of use, and value.

Exhibit 7 shows actual and projected PC sales for 1980–2009 as compiled by industry researcher International Data Corporation (IDC). According to Gartner Research, the billionth PC was shipped sometime in July 2002; of the billion, an estimated

Exhibit 7 **Worldwide Shipments of PCs, Actual and Forecasted, 1980–2009**

Year	PCs Shipped (millions)	Year	PCs Shipped (millions)
1980	1	2001	133
1985	11	2002	136
1990	24	2003	153
1995	58	2004	177
1996	69	2005*	205
1997	80	2006*	223
1998	91	2007*	243
1999	113	2008*	265
2000	139	2009*	286

*Forecasted.

Source: International Data Corporation.

550 million were still in use. Nearly 82 percent of the 1 billion PCs that had been shipped were desktops, and 75 percent were sold to businesses. With a world population of 6 billion, most industry participants believed there was ample opportunity for further growth in the PC market. Computer usage in Europe was half of that in the United States, even though the combined economies of the European countries were a bit larger than the U.S. economy. Growth potential for PCs was particularly strong in China, India, several other Asian countries, and portions of Latin America. Forrester Research estimated that the numbers of PCs in use worldwide would approach 1.3 billion by 2010, up from 575 million in 2004, with the growth being driven by the emerging markets in China, India, and Russia. IDC had predicted that notebook PC sales would grow from 26.9 percent of PC shipments in 2003 to 37.3 percent in 2007.

Currently, there was growing interest in notebook computers equipped wireless capability; many businesses were turning to notebooks equipped with wireless data communications devices to improve worker productivity and keep workers connected to important information. The emergence of Wireless Fidelity (Wi-Fi) networking technology, along with the installation of wireless home and office networks, was fueling the trend. Wi-Fi systems were being used in businesses, on college campuses, in airports, and other locations to link users to the Internet and to private networks. Three other devices—flat-panel LCD monitors, DVD recorders, and portable music players like Apple's iPod—were also stimulating sales of new PCs.

At the same time, forecasters expected full global build-out of the Internet to continue, which would require the installation of millions of servers. But since 2000 IT customers had been switching from the use of expensive high-end servers running customized Unix operating systems to the use of low-cost servers running on standardized Intel/Windows/Linux technologies; the switch to stands-based servers had caused a slowdown in dollar revenues from server sales despite rapidly increasing unit volume. A number of industry observers believed that the days of using expensive, proprietary Unix-based servers were numbered. The Unix share of the server operating system market (based on unit shipments) was said to have decreased by nearly 50 percent over the past five years, whereas Windows and Linux servers had tripled in use.

HOW DELL'S STRATEGY PUTS RIVALS IN A COMPETITIVE BIND

When the personal computer industry first began to take shape in the early 1980s, the founding companies manufactured many of the components themselves—disk drives, memory chips, graphics chips, microprocessors, motherboards, and software. Subscribing to a philosophy that mandated in-house development of key components, they built expertise in a variety of PC-related technologies and created organizational units to produce components as well as handle final assembly. While certain noncritical items were typically outsourced, if a computer maker was not at least partially vertically integrated and produced some components for its PCs, then it was not taken seriously as a manufacturer. But as the industry grew, technology advanced quickly in so many directions on so many parts and components that the early personal computer manufacturers could not keep pace as experts on all fronts. There were too many technologies and manufacturing intricacies to master for a vertically integrated manufacturer to keep its products on the cutting edge.

As a consequence, companies emerged that specialized in making particular components. Specialists could marshal enough R&D capability and resources to either lead the technological developments in their area of specialization or else quickly match the advances made by their competitors.

Moreover, specialist firms could mass-produce the component and supply it to several computer manufacturers far cheaper than any one manufacturer could fund the needed component R&D and then make only whatever smaller volume of components it needed for assembling its own brand of PCs. Thus, in the early 1990s, such computer makers as Compaq Computer, IBM, Hewlett-Packard, Sony, Toshiba, and Fujitsu-Siemens began to abandon vertical integration in favor of a strategy of outsourcing most components from specialists and concentrating on efficient assembly and marketing their brand of computers. They adopted the build-to-stock value chain model (shown in the top section of Exhibit 4). It featured arm's-length transactions between specialist suppliers, manufacturer/assemblers, distributors and retailers, and end users. However, a few others, most notably Dell and Gateway, employed a shorter value chain model, selling directly to customers and eliminating the time and costs associated with distributing through independent resellers. Building to order avoided (1) having to keep many differently equipped models on retailers' shelves to fill buyer requests for one or another configuration of options and components, and (2) having to clear out slow-selling models at a discount before introducing new generations of PCs (for instance, Hewlett-Packard's retail dealers had an average of 43 days of HP products in stock as of October 2004). Direct sales eliminated retailer costs and markups (retail dealer margins were typically in the range of 4 to 10 percent).

Because of Dell's success in using its business model and strategy to become the low-cost leader, most other PC makers in 2002–2005 were endeavoring to emulate various aspects of Dell's strategy, but with only limited success. Nearly all vendors were trying to cut days of inventory out of their supply chains and reduce their costs of goods sold and operating expenses to levels that would make them more cost competitive with Dell. In an effort to cut their assembly costs, Hewlett-Packard, IBM, and several others had begun outsourcing assembly to contract manufacturers and refocused their internal efforts on product design and marketing. Virtually all vendors were trying to minimize the amount of finished goods in dealer/distributor inventories and shorten the time it took to replenish dealer stocks. Collaboration with contract manufacturers was increasing to develop the capabilities to build and deliver PCs equipped to customer specifications within 7 to 14 days, but these efforts were hampered by the use of Asia-based contract manufacturers—delivering built-to-order PCs to North American and European customers within a two-week time frame required the use of costly air freight from Asia-based assembly plants.

While most PC vendors would have liked to adopt Dell's sell direct strategy for at least some of their sales, they confronted big channel conflict problems: if they started to push direct sales hard, they would almost certainly alienate the independent dealers on whom they depended for the bulk of their sales and service to customers. Dealers saw sell-direct efforts on the part of a manufacturer whose brand they represented as a move to cannibalize their business and to compete against them. However, Dell's success in gaining large enterprise customers with its direct sales force had forced growing numbers of PC vendors to supplement the efforts of their independent dealers with direct sales and service efforts of their own. During 2003–2005 several of Dell's rivals were selling 15 to 25 percent of their products direct.

PROFILES OF SELECTED COMPETITORS IN THE PC INDUSTRY

This section presents brief profiles of three of Dell's principal competitors. Exhibit 8 summarizes Dell's principal competitors in the various product categories where it competed and the sizes of these product markets.

Hewlett-Packard

In one of the most contentious and controversial acquisitions in U.S. history, Hewlett-Packard shareholders voted by a narrow margin in early 2002 to approve the company's acquisition of Compaq Computer, the world's second largest full-service global computing company (behind IBM) and a company with 2001 revenues of $33.6 billion and a net loss of $785 million. Compaq had passed IBM to become the world leader in PCs in 1995 and remained in first place until it was overtaken by Dell in late 1999. Compaq had acquired Tandem Computer in 1997 and Digital Equipment Corporation in 1998 to give it capabilities, products, and service offerings that allowed it to compete in every sector of the computer industry—PCs, servers, workstations, mainframes, peripherals, and such services as business and e-commerce solutions, hardware and software support, systems integration, and technology consulting.[26] In 2000, Compaq spent $370 million to acquire certain assets of Inacom Corporation that management believed would help Compaq reduce inventories, speed cycle time, and enhance its capabilities to do business with customers via the Internet. Nonetheless, at the time of its acquisition by HP, Compaq was struggling to compete successfully in all of its many product and service arenas where it operated.

Carly Fiorina, who became HP's CEO in 1999, explained why the acquisition of Compaq was strategically sound:

> With Compaq, we become No. 1 in Windows, No. 1 in Linux and No. 1 in Unix . . . With Compaq, we become the No. 1 player in storage, and the leader in the fastest growing segment of the storage market—storage area networks. With Compaq, we double our service and support capacity in the area of mission-critical infrastructure design, outsourcing and support . . . Let's talk about PCs . . . Compaq has been

able to improve their turns in that business from 23 turns of inventory per year to 62—100 percent improvement year over year—and they are coming close to doing as well as Dell does. They've reduced operating expenses by $130 million, improved gross margins by three points, reduced channel inventory by more than $800 million. They ship about 70 percent of their commercial volume through their direct channel, comparable to Dell. We will combine our successful retail PC business model with their commercial business model and achieve much more together than we could alone. With Compaq, we will double the size of our sales force to 15,000 strong. We will build our R&D budget to more than $4 billion a year, and add important capabilities to HP Labs. We will become the No. 1 player in a whole host of countries around the world—HP operates in more than 160 countries, with well over 60 percent of our revenues coming from outside the U.S. The new HP will be the No. 1 player in the consumer and small- and medium-business segments . . . We have estimated cost synergies of $2.5 billion by 2004 . . . It is a rare opportunity when a technology company can advance its market position substantially and reduce its cost structure substantially at the same time. And this is possible because Compaq and HP are in the same

Exhibit 8   **Dell's Principal Competitors and Dell's Estimated Market Shares by Product Category, 2004–2005**

Product Category	Dell's Principal Competitors	Estimated Size of Worldwide Market, 2003–2004 (in billions)	Dell's Estimated Worldwide Share, 2004–2005
PCs	Hewlett-Packard (maker of both Compaq and HP brands); IBM/Lenovo, Gateway, Apple, Acer, Sony, Fujitsu-Siemens (in Europe and Japan)	$175	18.5%
Servers	Hewlett-Packard, IBM, Sun Microsystems, Fujitsu	$50	≈11%
Data storage devices	Hewlett-Packard, IBM, EMC, Hitachi	$40	≈5%
Networking switches and related equipment	Cisco Systems, Enterasys, Nortel, 3Com	$58	2–3%
Handheld PCs	Palm, Sony, Hewlett-Packard, Toshiba, Casio	$4	≈2–3%
Printers and printer cartridges	Hewlett-Packard, Lexmark, Canon, Epson	≈$50	≈6%
Cash register systems	IBM, NCR, Wincor Nixdorf, Hewlett-Packard, Sun Microsystems	$4 (in North America)	≈1–2%
Services	Accenture, IBM, Hewlett-Packard, many others	$350	≈2%

Source: Compiled by the case authors from a variety of sources, including International Data Corporation and www.dell.com.

businesses, pursuing the same strategies, in the same markets, with complementary capabilities.

However, going into 2005 the jury was still out on whether HP's acquisition of Compaq was the success that Carly Fiorina had claimed it would be. The company's only real bright spot was its $24 billion crown jewel printer business, which still reigned as the unchallenged world leader (largely because of a highly productive $1 billion investment in printer R&D). But the rest of HP's businesses were underachievers. Its PC and server businesses were struggling, losing money in most quarters and barely breaking even in others—and HP was definitely losing ground to Dell in PCs and low-priced servers. In servers, HP was being squeezed on the low end by Dell's low prices and on the high end by strong competition from IBM. Most observers saw IBM as overshadowing HP in corporate computing—high-end servers and IT services. In data storage and technical support services, HP had been able to grow revenues but profit margins and total operating profits were declining. While HP had successfully cut annual operating costs by $3.5 billion—beating the $2.5 billion target set at the time of the Compaq acquisition—the company had missed its earnings forecasts in 7 of the past 20 quarters.

With the company's stock price stuck in the $18–$23 price range, impatient investors in 2004 began clamoring for the company to break itself up and create two separate companies, one for its printer business and one for all the rest of the businesses (PCs, servers, storage devices, digital cameras, calculators, and IT services). While HP's board of directors had looked at breaking up the company into smaller pieces, Carly Fiorina had been opposed, arguing that HP's broad product/business lineup paid off in the form of added sales and lower costs.

HP reported total revenues of $79.9 billion and net profits of $3.5 billion for fiscal 2004, versus total revenues of $73.1 billion and earnings of $2.5 billion in 2003. However, a substantial portion of the increase in net earnings in 2004 was due to cutbacks in R&D spending and a lower effective tax rate. Moreover, the company's EPS of $1.16 in 2004 was substantially below the EPS of $1.80 reported in 2000. In February 2005, with HP's financial performance continuing to lag and mounting differences with HP's board of directors, Carly Fiorina resigned her post as HP's CEO.

Mark Hurd, president and CEO of NCR (formerly National Cash Resister Systems), was brought in to replace Fiorina, effective April 1, 2005; Hurd had been at NCR for 25 years in a variety of management positions and was regarded as a no-nonsense executive who underpromised and overdelivered on results.[27] Hurd immediately sought to bolster HP's competitiveness and financial performance by bringing in new managers and attacking bloated costs. In his first seven months as CEO, the results were somewhat encouraging. HP posted revenues of $86.7 billion and net profits of $2.4 billion for the fiscal year ending October 31, 2005. HP had the number one ranking worldwide for server shipments (a position it had held for 14 consecutive quarters) and disk storage systems; plus, it was the world leader in server revenues for Unix, Windows, and Linux systems. Since Hurd had taken over, the company's stock price had risen about 25 percent.

Exhibit 9 shows the performance of HP's four major business groups for the 2001–2005 period.

IBM/Lenovo

IBM was seen as a "computer solutions" company and had the broadest and deepest capabilities in customer service, technical support, and systems integration of any company in the world. IBM's Global Services business group was the world's largest information technology services provider, with sales of $46.2 billion in 2004. In addition to its IT services business, IBM had 2004 hardware sales of $31.3 billion and software sales of $15.1 billion. IBM conducted business in 170 countries and had total sales of $96.3 billion and earnings of $8.4 billion in 2004. Once the world's undisputed king of computing and information processing, IBM was struggling to remain a potent contender in PCs, servers, storage products, and other hardware-related products. In 2003–2005, IBM's only remaining strength in IT hardware was in high-end servers.

IBM's Troubles in PCs Formerly the dominant global and U.S. market leader, with a market share exceeding 50 percent in the late 1980s and early 1990s, IBM had become an also-ran in PCs, with a global market share of only 5.9 percent in 2004 (see Exhibit 1). IBM had lost about $750 million in PCs in the last three years. Its last stronghold in PCs was in laptop computers, where its ThinkPad line was a

Exhibit 9   **Performance of Hewlett-Packard's Four Major Business Groups, Fiscal Years 2001–2005 (in billions of dollars)**

	Printing and Imaging	Personal Computing Systems*	Enterprise Systems*	HP Services
2005 (fiscal year ending October 31)				
Net revenue	$25,155	$26,741	$17,778	$15,536
Operating income (loss)	3,413	657	751	1,151
2004 (fiscal year ending October 31)				
Net revenue	$24,199	$24,622	$16,074	$13,778
Operating income (loss)	3,847	210	28	1,263
2003 (fiscal year ending October 31)				
Net revenue	$22,569	$21,210	$15,367	$12,357
Operating income (loss)	3,596	22	(48)	1,362
2002 (fiscal year ending October 31)*				
Net revenue	$20,358	$21,895	$11,105	$12,326
Operating income (loss)	3,365	(372)	(656)	1,369
2001 (fiscal year ending October 31)*				
Net revenue	$19,602	$26,710	$20,205	$12,802
Operating income (loss)	2,103	(728)	(579)	1,617

*Results for 2001 and 2002 represent the combined results of both HP and Compaq Computer.

Source: 2004 10-K report, 2003 10-K report, and company press release, November 17, 2005.

consistent award winner on performance, features, and reliability—but it was losing money on ThinkPad sales as well. The vast majority of IBM's laptop and desktop sales were to long-standing IBM customers that had IBM mainframe computers. IBM's PC group had higher costs than rivals, making it virtually impossible to match rivals on price and make a profit. IBM distributed its PCs, workstations, and servers through reseller partners, but used its own sales force to market to large enterprises. IBM competed against rival hardware vendors by emphasizing confidence in the IBM brand and the company's long-standing strengths in software applications, IT services and support, and systems integration capabilities. IBM had responded to the direct sales inroads Dell had made in the corporate market by allowing some of its resellers to economize on costs by custom-assembling IBM PCs to buyer specifications.

The Sale of IBM's PC Business to Lenovo in Late 2004

In December 2004, IBM agreed to sell its money-losing PC business to Lenovo Group Ltd., the number one computer maker in China, in a $1.75 billion business deal that made Lenovo the world's third-biggest PC maker, with a global market share of close to 7 percent. As part of the deal, IBM had an 18.9 percent ownership interest in Lenovo. The head of IBM's PC operations became CEO of Lenovo, with Lenovo's current CEO (who did not speak English) assuming the role of chairman. Shortly after the transaction was finalized, Lenovo moved its corporate headquarters from Beijing to New York City.

The new company had about $10 billion in annual sales and 20,000 employees, including about 10,000 IBM employees that would be a part of the new company—about 2,500 of the IBM employees that became part of Lenovo were in North Carolina, about half were in China, and the rest were scattered around the world. The new company had the rights to use the IBM name on its PCs for a maximum of five years, but in the months following the acquisition

Lenovo began co-branding efforts. The new company planned to continue to sell its PCs through the efforts of an internal sales force for large accounts and its network of distributors and retail outlets.

Prior to the acquisition of IBM's PC business, Lenovo had little reputation for innovation, and it usually followed the technology lead of Intel and Microsoft, the PC industry's standard setters. It was regarded as a made-in-China-for-China producer of PCs. It had previously tried to enter the PC market outside China without success and was under competitive pressure in its home market, particularly from Dell (which was said to have lower costs). However, the company's original parent, the government's Chinese Academy of Sciences, was still a major shareholder, which gave Lenovo access to loans from state banks.

Some observers believed that one of management's major challenges would be integrating the cultures of the operations. Twice daily at Lenovo's headquarters, the sound system broadcast "Number Six Broadcast Exercises," a set of stretches and knee bends—participation was voluntary but highly encouraged.[28] The company song was played every morning at 8:00 a.m. and sung by workers at the start of widely attended meetings. Lenovo employees who were late to meetings had to stand behind their chairs for a minute (as an attempt to humiliate them into being punctual). Employees' activities were strictly monitored; time spent outside the work area during work hours had to be accounted for, and deductions were made from employees' paychecks if the explanations were unsatisfactory. Most employees were young and had worked at Lenovo since graduating from college; few spoke English and most had never met a foreigner.

Lenovo's new management team had its sights set on using the acquisition of IBM's PC business as the platform for becoming a global competitor in PCs and for making Lenovo a recognized international brand. The company was pursuing initiatives to cut its costs closer to Dell's level. It was experimenting with selling directly to a few of its largest customers in China. It had opened a telephone sales center in China to handle orders from small customers and was trying to match Dell's speedy four-hour service capability. Lenovo had implemented new processes and systems that cut its inventory levels from about 30 days in 2000–2002 to about 16–19 days in 2004–2005. Although Lenovo reported earnings of $47 million for the 2005 fourth quarter

on revenue of about $4 billion, in 2006 the company announced it was cutting 1,000 jobs, taking a $100 million restructuring charge to pay for restructuring, moving its headquarters from New York City to North Carolina to reduce expenses. A new president took over in late 2005.

Gateway

Founded in 1985, Gateway had grown from a two-person start-up into a Fortune 500 company with $3.6 billion in revenues in 2004. It was battling with IBM/Lenovo for third place in the U.S. market and was one of the top 10 sellers of PCs worldwide. However, as shown in Exhibit 1, its unit sales and market share had been sliding since 2000. Gateway's all-time peak revenues were $9.6 billion in 2000, and its peak-year profits were $428 million; the company reported a loss every year during the 2001–2004 period.

After a series of failed turnaround efforts during 2001–2003, Gateway acquired eMachines, one of the world's fastest-growing and most efficient PC makers, in early 2004, for 50 million shares of Gateway stock and $30 million in cash. eMachines was a $1.1 billion producer of low-end computers and had distribution capabilities in Japan, Great Britain, and parts of Western Europe. The two companies had combined sales of $4.5 billion in 2003. Gateway management believed the eMachines acquisition would allow it to better compete in the low end of the PC market and also give it the resources and competitive strength to reenter markets outside the United States. As part of the deal, the founder and CEO of eMachines, Wayne Inouye, became the CEO of Gateway, with Ted Waitt, Gateway's founder and former CEO, functioning as chairman. The company moved its headquarters from South Dakota to Irvine, California, in September 2004.

Inouye immediately refocused the company's efforts on its core PC business and products like Media Center PCs, MP3 players, and digital displays. As of 2005, the company's value-based eMachines PC brand was sold exclusively by leading retailers worldwide, while the premium Gateway line was available at major retailers, over the phone and Web, and through the company's direct sales force. In 2004–2005, Gateway made several moves to restore the company to profitability:

- All 188 company-owned Gateway stores were closed, and distribution of Gateway PCs was shifted to selling through some 3,000 retailers, including Best Buy, Circuit City, Comp USA, Costco, Micro Center, and Office Depot in the United States as well as Best Buy and Future Shop in Canada. In total, Gateway and eMachines products were sold in more than 6,300 retail locations in North America alone in 2005.

- A new, more efficient manufacturing model was instituted.
- The company began expanding internationally, reentering the Japanese market with the Gateway brand and introducing eMachines in the Mexican retail market.
- The workforce was cut to about 1,900 (compared with 7,400 at the start of 2004).
- The company's supply base and service and support relationships were consolidated to further drive business efficiencies, ensure quality, and optimize the overall customer experience.
- Product development and sales operations were consolidated in centers in North Sioux City, South Dakota, and Kansas City, Missouri.
- Selling, general, and administrative (SG&A) costs were reduced significantly—fourth-quarter 2004 SG&A costs were 57 percent lower than the 2003 quarterly average. SG&A expenses for the first nine months of 2005 were $252.5 million versus $803.3 million in the comparable period for 2004.

The results of Inouye's turnaround strategy were encouraging. In the fourth quarter of 2004, unit sales were 128 percent higher than during the fourth quarter of 2003. During the first nine months of 2005, the company sold about 3.2 million units and had become profitable—Gateway reported sales of $2.7 billion and net income of $27.1 million (compared to sales of $2.6 billion and a loss of $576 million for the first nine months of 2004). Gateway expected that full-year revenues for 2005 would approach $4 billion and that net earnings would be about $45 million.

DELL'S FUTURE PROSPECTS

In a February 2003 article in *Business 2.0,* Michael Dell said, "The best way to describe us now is as a broad computer systems and services company. We have a pretty simple system. The most important thing is to satisfy our customers. The second most important thing is to be profitable. If we don't do the first one well, the second one won't happen."[29] For the most part, Michael Dell was not particularly concerned about the efforts of competitors to copy many aspects of Dell's build-to-order, sell-direct strategy. He explained why:

> The competition started copying us seven years ago. That's when we were a $1 billion business . . . And they haven't made much progress to be honest with you. The learning curve for them is difficult. It's like going from baseball to soccer.[30]
>
> I think a lot of people have analyzed our business model, a lot of people have written about it and tried to understand it. This is an 18½ year process . . . It comes from many, many cycles of learning . . . It's very, very different than designing products to be built to stock . . . Our whole company is oriented around a very different way of operating . . . I don't, for any second, believe that they are not trying to catch up. But it is also safe to assume that Dell is not staying in the same place. You know, this past year we've driven a billion dollars of cost out of our supply chain, and certainly next year we plan to drive quite a bit of cost out as well.[31]

On other occasions, Michael Dell spoke about the size of the company's future opportunities:

> When technologies begin to standardize or commoditize, the game starts to change. Markets open up to be volume markets and this is very much where Dell has made its mark—first in the PC market in desktops and notebooks and then in the server market and the storage market and services and data networking. We continue to expand the array of products that we sell, the array of services and, of course, expand on a geographic basis. The way we think about it is that there are all of these various technologies out there . . . What we have been able to do is build a business system that takes those technological ingredients, translates them into products and services and gets them to the customer more efficiently than any company around.[32]
>
> We have only seven percent market share in an $800 billion market. There are enormous opportunities for us to grow across multiple dimensions in terms of products, with servers, storage, printing and services, representing a huge realm of expansion for us. There's geographic expansion and market share expansion back in the core business. The primary focus for us is picking those opportunities, seizing on them, and making sure we have the talent and the

leadership growing inside the company to support all that growth. And there's also a network effect here. As we grow our product lines and enter new markets, we see a faster ability to gain share in new markets versus ones we've previously entered.[33]

A great portion of our growth will come from key markets outside the U.S. We have about 10 percent market share outside the United States, so there's definitely room to grow. We'll grow in the enterprise with servers, storage, and services. Our growth will come from new areas like printing. And, quite frankly, those are really enough. There are other things that I could mention, other things we do, but those opportunities I mentioned can drive us to $80 billion and beyond.[34]

Endnotes

[1]As quoted in "Dell Puts Happy Customers First," *Nikkei Weekly,* December 16, 2002.

[3]Joan Magretta, "The Power of Virtual Integration: An Interview with Dell Computer's Michael Dell, *Harvard Business Review,* March–April 1998, p. 75.

[4]"Michael Dell: On Managing Growth," *MIS Week,* September 5, 1988, p. 1.

[5]"The Education of Michael Dell," *BusinessWeek,* March 22, 1993, p. 86.

[6]Dell's 2005 10-K report, pp. 1–2.

[7]Remarks by Kevin Rollins in a speech at Peking University, November 2, 2005, and posted at www.dell.com.

[8]As quoted in Magretta, "The Power of Virtual Integration," p. 74.

[9]Magretta, "The Power of Virtual Integration," p. 75.

[10]Speech by Michael Dell at University of Toronto, September 21, 2004, posted at www.dell.com (accessed December 15, 2004).

[11]Ibid., p. 76.

[12]Ibid.

[13]Quoted in Neel Chowdhury, "Dell Cracks China," *Fortune,* June 21, 1999, p. 121.

[14]Magretta, "The Power of Virtual Integration," p. 79.

[15]"Michael Dell Rocks," *Fortune,* May 11, 1998, p. 61.

[16]Remarks by Michael Dell, Gartner Symposium, Orlando, Florida, October 20, 2005, and posted at www.dell.com.

[17]Quoted in Kathryn Jones, "The Dell Way," *Business 2.0,* February 2003.

[18]Kevin Rollins, "Using Information to Speed Execution," *Harvard Business Review,* March–April, 1998, p. 81.v

[19]Magretta, "The Power of Virtual Integration," p. 80.

[20]Remarks by Michael Dell, Gartner Fall Symposium, Orlando, Florida, October 9, 2002; posted at www.dell.com.

[21]Remarks by Michael Dell at the University of Toronto, September 21, 2004; posted at www.dell.com.

[22]Quoted in the *Financial Times* Global News Wire, October 10, 2002

[23]Quoted in Adam Lashinsky, "Where Dell Is Going Next," *Fortune,* October 18, 2004, p. 116.

[24]Remarks by Michael Dell, Gartner Symposium, Orlando, Florida, October 20, 2005; posted at www.dell.com.

[25]Keynote speech given on August 25, 1999, in Austin, Texas, at Dell's DirectConnect Conference and posted at www.dell.com.

[26]"Can Compaq Catch Up?" *BusinessWeek,* May 3, 1999, p. 163.

[27]Louise Lee and Peter Burrows, "What's Dogging Dell's Stock," *BusinessWeek,* September 5, 2005, p. 90.

[28]Julie Chao, "Chinese Computer Maker Lenovo Shoots for Leadership in the World," *Atlanta Journal-Constitution,* December 14, 2004, pp. F1, F8.

[29]*Business 2.0,* February 2003; posted at www.business2.com.

[30]Comments made to students at the University of North Carolina and reported in the *Raleigh News & Observer,* November 16, 1999.

[31]Remarks by Michael Dell, Gartner Fall Symposium, Orlando, Florida, October 9, 2002; posted at www.dell.com.

[32]Remarks by Michael Dell, MIT Sloan School of Management, September 26, 2002; posted at www.dell.com.

[33]Remarks by Michael Dell, University of Toronto, September 21, 2004; posted at www.dell.com.

[34]Remarks by Michael Dell, Gartner Symposium, Orlando, Florida, October 20, 2005; posted at www.dell.com.

Case 6

Competition in the MP3 Player Industry in 2005

Louis D. Marino
The University of Alabama

Katy Beth Jackson
The University of Alabama

The earliest portable music players were transistor radios introduced by Regency in 1954. While these radios allowed their owners to listen to broadcasts on the go, they generally suffered from relatively weak signal reception, poor sound quality, and the ability to only receive AM stations. It was not until the mid-1970s that consumers had access to portable personal stereos; the smallest of these were slightly larger than a shoebox and allowed users not only to listen to both AM and FM radio but also to carry their personal music collections, recorded on cassette tapes, with them. However, it was not until 1979 that consumers could purchase the first truly portable personal music player, the Sony Walkman, which only played cassettes and did not offer radio reception. By 1984, the cassette tape was beginning to be supplanted by the compact disc (CD), and Sony led the way again with the development of the portable CD player, the CD Walkman or the Discman.

The portable CD player, and its more advanced cousin the minidisc player, were the mechanical precursors to the modern digital music players. These were referred to as mechanical players since they had moving parts that were involved in playing the music. The main drawbacks to these players were that they could hold only a relatively limited amount of music and were subject to skipping if the player was bumped or jostled. In an effort to overcome these weaknesses, and to capitalize on the growing popularity of digitally encoded music that individuals were storing on their computers in the form of MP3s, in 1997 SaeHan information systems developed the MPMan F10, the world's first nonmechanical digital audio player.[1]

The MPMan player was introduced to the U.S. market in the summer of 1998 as the Eiger Labs MPMan F10, a 32-megabyte digital audio player (DAP) that could only be expanded by returning it to the manufacturer. The second DAP (also known as an MP3 player) introduced in the U.S. market was the Rio PMP300, which was brought to market by Diamond Multimedia in September 1998. The Rio was so successful in the 1998 Christmas season that it led to significant investment in the MP3 player industry by other players and to a lawsuit by the Recording Industry Association of America for enabling the illegal copying of music. This suit was resolved in Diamond's favor; thus, digital music players were ruled legal. By the end of 1999, Remote Solutions had introduced the first hard-drive-based player, the Personal Jukebox, which had a 4.8-gigabyte (GB) internal hard drive and could hold about 1,200 songs consumers could choose from flash memory, hard drive, and in-dash digital audio players from a variety of manufacturers.[2]

Growth in the MP3 player market continued fairly slowly until Apple released its legendary iPod in the latter half of 2001. Apple's original hard-drive player virtually revolutionized the MP3 market single-handedly, spurring the development of many look-alike models from competing manufacturers. By 2004, sales of portable audio players had reached 27.8 million units. Just over the Christmas season of 2004 (a five-week period), MP3 player sales reached $270 million, up 147.5 percent from Christmas 2003, and most analysts predicted continued rapid growth in the industry for the foreseeable future. The research firm Gartner predicted that over 150 million units would be shipped in 2010 (see Exhibit 1).[3] With only 11 percent of the U.S. population owning

Exhibit 1   **MP3 Player Forecast (millions of units shipped)**

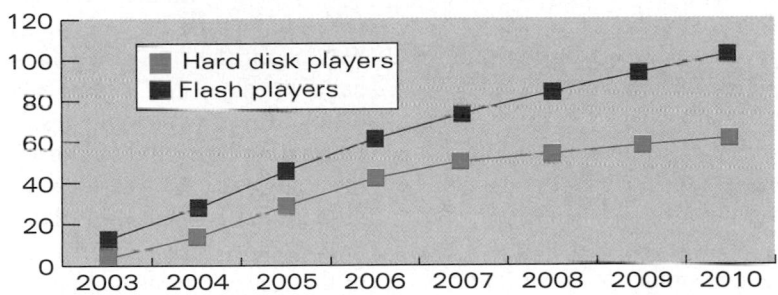

Gartner expects sales of MP3 players to remain strong for several years before slowing by the end of the decade.

Source: Gartner.

an MP3 player in 2004, and much lower penetration rates worldwide, normally conservative analysts were using descriptors such as *boom* and *explosive* to describe growth in MP3 player industry. While sales were expected to grow in each of the main categories of players (flash-based and hard-drive players), the clear winners, in terms of millions of units shipped, were expected to be flash memory players such as the iPod Nano and the iRiver U10.

TRENDS IN THE MP3 PLAYER INDUSTRY

One important factor that had remained fairly constant in the MP3 industry since its beginnings was the pace of technological innovation. MP3 player manufacturers were continuously working to develop players that were physically smaller, with larger storage capacity, a longer battery life, and a simpler user interface. In developing their offerings, MP3 player manufacturers typically purchased component pieces from various computer hardware vendors and assembled them into the end product. There was not a significant differentiation between the types of batteries used, and many firms developed their user interfaces in-house. However, the key element of a player that influenced the unit's size and weight was the memory used in the player. Firms such as Toshiba, Samsung, and Hitachi that supplied the hard drives and flash memory to the MP3 player manufacturers were constantly trying to cut down the size of their

hardware component so that MP3 player manufacturers could ultimately make their product as small and lightweight as possible. Likewise, memory card manufacturers were continuously investigating ways to make their flash cards smaller while maintaining a fairly high level of capacity. While there were numerous manufacturers of hard drives and flash memory, the leading MP3 player manufacturers preferred to partner with the leading memory manufacturers so that they could use the newest and most innovative memory in their players.

Another important trend in the industry was increasing convergence between consumer electronics devices. In response to consumers' changing lifestyles and increasing frustration at having to carry multiple devices, manufacturers of electronic devices, including MP3 players, had recently begun to combine as many features as possible into a single, portable unit. Combinations of cameras, MP3s, Personal digital assistants (PDAs), and even cell phones were becoming abundantly popular. Consumers were leading increasingly busy lives, and with more people constantly on the go—spending more time in the car, exercising, or waiting in line to accomplish some other task—there was an increasing demand for products that would let people carry their music with them so they could essentially "listen while they live." By 2005, MP3 players had evolved into another piece of technology that many busy consumers could hardly live without; that box the size of a deck of cards could hold their entire record collection and allow them to listen to it anytime, anywhere. With the boom of the cell phone industry, many MP3 companies were scrambling to partner with the successful phone brands to incorporate MP3 players into new cell phones that were already able to act as cameras and camcorders as well.

In response to consumers' increasing demands for convergence, MP3 player manufacturers were seeking ways to increase their players' multifunctional usage capabilities. Many of the competing models available in 2005 could be used not only for managing and listening to music but also as calendar/appointment books, data storage devices, and alarm clocks, as well as other functions similar to those found on PDAs. For example, hard-drive-based iPods could be used as an external hard drive when attached to a computer and also had photo storage capabilities; the ability to be used as an alarm clock, a calendar, an appointment book, and a gaming device; and voice-recording abilities (with the purchase of an accessory). Other attributes that MP3 player manufacturers were adding included a built-in radio tuner and sound-manipulating hardware. Some of the MP3 players also had the ability to store and display videos.

The growing size of, access to, and comfort of consumers with the Internet was also fueling the MP3 player boom. Not every electronics company had access to retail outlets, and the Internet allowed consumers to shop for just about any MP3 player on the market at the lowest price, no matter where the unit was physically located. After purchasing the player itself online, users could then go online to shop for brand-new songs to load onto the unit. Hordes of legitimate subscription and pay-as-you-go online music stores had begun appearing on the Internet. Between January and July 2005, over 184 million tracks were sold online, more than twice the sales in January–July 2004. Growth of the online digital music market not only facilitated but also was facilitated by the increasing popularity of MP3 players. Some MP3 manufacturers operated their own online music stores. This was especially important for Apple, which used a proprietary audio format in programming its MP3 players so that only music purchased from its online store would work on an Apple player. A host of other online music stores were owned by various industry players, including RealNetworks and Wal-Mart.

As MP3 players increasingly became a part of everyday life, they were also changing from being mere music players to becoming fashion statements and status symbols. MP3 players were being seen as the new toy for the young and old alike to sport in their daily lives, and generally, the smaller, lighter, and "prettier" models were the most popular. Apple's product design and color schemes were nearly famous for their elegance and simplicity; the original iPod (about the size of a box of cigarettes) had distinctive white headphones that were easily distinguished, and the Mini's colorful pastel models (about the size of a credit card) were equally unique and popular. Said one article, "iPod has become so popular it is now a fashion statement."[4] The popularity of those players was due partly to Apple's excellent marketing scheme and partly to the many very famous celebrities who had been photographed or seen with an Apple player or happened to mention their iPod during interviews.[5] Additionally, other players were literally being incorporated as fashion. For example, Oakley, a sunglasses maker, had introduced a line of sunglasses called Oakley Thump, which had tiny MP3 players built into them and were priced between $395 and $495.[6] As another example of these tiny wearable players, Virgin had one so small that it could be worn as a necklace. There were a few reasons why MP3 players were becoming more fashion-oriented, including the fact that they were actually worn on the body, which made their appearance important, and that MP3 players were extremely popular with younger consumers, a group that often demanded that the products they bought look just as good as they function.

Finally, with the increasing competition in the MP3 player industry, some major producers were deciding to exit the market. Specifically, Rio, the company that brought the second MP3 player to the U.S. market, closed its doors in September 2005. Rio was owned by Digital Networks North America (a subsidiary of D&M Holdings U.S.). In the fiscal year ended in March 2005, D&M reported an increase in revenues of almost 5 percent over the previous year and an increase in net income of 123 percent over the same year (it reported a large net loss in 2004). However, in July 2005, D&M sold the technology underlying its Rio MP3 players in an effort to recoup some of the losses the Rio subsidiary had generated but the parent corporation had not yet decided whether to completely terminate the Rio division.[7] At that point, the company was still manufacturing its current-generation players and shipping them out while making final decisions about Rio's future in the MP3 industry. Early in September 2005,

D&M decided to discontinue all Rio products by the end of the month. The company's reason for exiting the MP3 industry was that management felt any investment would be eroded by the high level of competition facing the market.[8]

COMPETITION IN THE MP3 PLAYER INDUSTRY

Although well over 100 companies manufactured MP3 players by the end of 2005, only about 7 could legitimately claim real importance in this market: Apple, Archos, Creative, Dell, iRiver, SanDisk, and Sony. However, the market was clearly dominated by Apple, with estimates of the company's market share ranging from 65 to 80 percent and each of the other manufacturers having less than 6 percent of the market. All MP3 manufacturers, however, realized that their continued success depended, in large part, on how well they could satisfy their current customers as well as their ability to attract new ones. Research showed that most buyers shopped for players on the basis of song capacity (some users required significantly more capacity than the average user), availability of and compatibility with online music stores, unit battery life, physical size and weight specifications, and ease of use. While price was factor in some consumer purchases, Apple's success had proved that many consumers were willing to pay a premium for some perceived benefit, whether it was higher quality, more technological sophistication, or greater ease of use. However, industry experts predicted that as competition and rivalry became tougher, price would be likely to play a more central role in the buyer's decision. Exhibit 2 provides information on the MP3 players offered by the major players in the industry and consumer satisfaction with the players.

Apple

In fiscal year 2005 (ended in September 2005), Apple reported net revenues of $13.9 billion, a 68 percent increase over 2004. Net income over the same period increased from $276 million to $1.34 billion, a whopping 384 percent increase over the span of a year. For much of the company's history, Apple had been very good at being the first company to introduce a concept or a new product but had then struggled to maintain control of its market share for that product line. Although Apple didn't introduce the first portable MP3 player, it did introduce the first one that gained widespread attention and widespread popularity—the iPod, which came on the market in October 2001. At first, many critics did not give the iPod much of a chance for success, as its launch came about one month after the September 11 terrorist attacks and carried a fairly hefty price tag of $399. However, the success of the iPod had reached phenomenal proportions, such that "it is now a fashion statement, and any other digital music player is considered 'Brand X' for many consumers."[9] What Sony did for portable cassette devices with the Walkman in the 1980s, Apple was doing for the digital music industry with the iPod line.

The iPod accounted for over $4.5 billion, or 32.3 percent, of Apple's total sales in 2005. Unit sales of the iPods had increased by 410 percent since 2004, to almost 22.5 million units in 2005 alone (total unit sales since the product's introduction were 28 million units). Apple's strategy with regard to its iPods centered largely on quick product innovation and marketing. By July 2004, the regular iPod was in its fourth-generation model. The Mini had been introduced in January of that year; by mid-2005, it no longer existed, but the iPod Nano and iPod Shuffle did. Each successive product or model improved on previous ones, in terms of both features and price. Apple had used unique and creative television and magazine ads as well as several brand alliances—with BMW, Hewlett-Packard, Motorola, and U2—in an effort to make the iPod *the* choice for buyers in this industry. After the company's success skyrocketed, the MP3 player industry exploded and competition became widespread and intense. Both computer industry regulars and newcomers solely devoted to the MP3 player product moved into the market, quickly making competition intense. As the technology continued to evolve, even traditional cellular phone manufacturers had become potential rivals in this fast-paced market.

Some analysts felt that Apple was merely "making a careful gamble" with regard to the company's tentative entry into the MP3 player/cell phone market by teaming with Motorola to offer a phone that could hold 100 songs.[10] That judgment was based on the fact that other cell phone companies like Nokia and Samsung had introduced phones that could

Exhibit 2   **Customer Satisfaction with MP3 Players**

	Customer Satisfaction (out of 10)	Quality of Sound (out of 10)	Ease of Use (out of 10)	Reliability (out of 10)	Percent Needing Repair
All MP3 Players					
Apple	8.6	8.8	8.8	8.5	9%
Archos	7.5	8.0	7.1	7.5	3
Creative	7.6	8.2	7.5	7.9	5
Dell	7.7	8.1	7.9	7.9	7
iRiver	7.9	8.6	7.2	8.3	3
RCA	6.8	7.4	7.0	7.3	1
Rio	7.1	7.8	7.5	7.5	6
SanDisk	7.1	7,7	6.9	7.7	4
Sony	7.3	8.0	7.4	7.7	1
Average	7.6	8.1	7.5	7.9	5%
MP3 Players with Flash Drives (1 GB or Less)					
Apple	8.2	8.6	8.4	8.4	3%
Creative	7.3	7.8	7.4	7.8	2
iRiver	7.7	8.3	7.2	8.2	2
Rio	6.8	7.5	7.3	7.3	4
SanDisk	7.0	7.6	6.8	7.6	3
Sony	7.1	7.9	7.2	7.6	1
Average	7.3	7.9	7.3	7.8	3%
MP3 Players with Micro Drives (More than 1 GB but Less Than 10 GB)					
Apple	8.5	8.7	8.6	8.4	9%
Creative	8.0	8.6	7.7	8.0	9
Rio	7.9	8.4	8.2	8.1	8
Sony	7.6	8.0	7.6	7.9	2
Average	8.0	8.4	8.0	8.1	7%
MP3 Players with 10 GB or Larger Hard Drives					
Apple	8.8	9.0	9.0	8.6	11
Archos	7.7	8.2	7.2	7.7	2
Creative	7.8	8.6	7.4	7.9	7
Dell	8.1	8.5	8.3	8.3	9
iRiver	8.3	9.2	7.2	8.6	5
Average	8.2	8.7	7.8	8.2	7%

Source: Developed by the case authors from infromation in a *PC Magazine* customer survey, *PC Magazine*, November 8, 2005, available at www.pcmag.com.

hold up to 3,000 songs and were meant to replace the user's regular MP3 player. The last thing Apple wanted was Motorola users, or any others for that matter, to use their cell phones as a replacement for the iPod. However, the possibilities offered by the huge and booming cell phone market were too big to be ignored by any MP3 company. Only time would tell whether users would prefer to carry an all-in-one unit or would opt to keep their phones and music players separate. However, other analysts felt these new cell phone company additions to the industry and the copycat products would soon break Apple's stride with the iPod and cut deeply into the product's astounding success.[11]

Archos

For the six months ended in June 2004, Archos, headquartered in France, reported net revenues of 17.9 million euros (€), a 14.7 percent decrease over the same period in 2003. Net income for that time period was a net loss of € 3.5 million, a 4.3 percent decrease over the same six months during 2003. The company's U.S. and German subsidiaries also reported net losses for the year, while the UK subsidiary posted a modest net income. Also during 2004, the company had laid off 25 percent of its employees in its U.S. subsidiary and began work on restructuring management and sales and marketing.

Archos had paired with a broadband video service that would allow users of its portable players to access the movies and other video files they would want to store on the player. In addition, with the Gmini XS 100 player, the company had offered support for a subscription-based online music store as part of what users get in the box when they bought that particular player. For that last initiative, Archos teamed with Microsoft's subscription-based download service called Janus to allow users to transfer any available video and audio files to their portable players as long as they continued to pay the subscription fee. The company's wide product line and reputation for offering players with many features made the company stand apart from others. Most players offered by Archos had audio, video, radio, and numerous recording abilities built in to the unit. One drawback was that many of the company's products were priced at a premium. However, Archos was very quick to get a foot into emerging technologies and incorporate as many of those as possible into single units to appeal to consumers who demanded the convenience offered by multifunction media products.

Creative

Creative Technology, founded in 1981 in Singapore, reported fiscal year 2005 (ending June 2005) revenues of $1.2 billion (up 50 percent from fiscal 2004) and net income of $588 million (down 99 percent from 2004). Creative first gained success and fame with its Sound Blaster audio cards for computers and was the first Singapore company listed on the Nasdaq. Since that time, the company had expanded its product lines to include audio as well as graphics, video, and music products. Several of the company's MP3 players had won industry awards—including the Zen Portable Media Center, the Zen Micro, and the Zen Micro Photo—and Creative introduced the world's first MP3 player with a hard drive.

Creative had announced early that it would play tough in the MP3 market, specifically referencing competition with Apple. During Christmas 2004, the company sold 2 million units, during the first quarter of 2005, it sold another 2 million (the iPod sold about 4.5 million and 5.3 million over the same periods, respectively). Creative had announced plans for aggressive advertising campaigns and had focused on offering an extremely extensive product line in the MP3 player market. Many of its portable players had been designed to appeal to consumers' demand for a fashionable and easy-to-use music player. Many analysts felt that Creative's biggest problems were not its wide product line, but its brand appeal, brand image, and other marketing issues. One said, "The biggest lesson learnt is that no matter how good your product is, if it's not branded properly, it's going to fail. Especially with the style-conscious audience it's targeted at."[12]

Dell

Headquartered in Round Rock, Texas, Dell had become famous for its successful direct business model in the personal computer industry. In fiscal year 2006 (ending February 3, 2006), Dell reported net revenues of $55.9 billion (a 14 percent increase from 2004) and net income of $3.6 billion (up 17 percent from the year before). A longtime supplier of customized PCs, Dell was a relatively new entry to the personal electronics market. In October 2003, Dell entered the digital music market in direct competition with a host of rivals by offering its Dell Digital Jukebox (Dell DJ), a personal, portable MP3 player. With the DJ, users could either download music from the Internet to the device or "rip" tracks from the CD collection they already owned.

Although later than some to enter the MP3 player market, Dell had long recognized consumers' interest in and demand for electronics that catered to digital music fans. As early as 1999, it began offering PC customization features such as a CD-recordable disk drive, specialized software for managing a digital music library, and, of course, the jukebox software necessary to play all the digital music on the PC. So with Dell's recent forays into computer peripherals and other electronics, the Dell DJ was a natural extension of the company's product line, and one that placed Dell in a market with a perhaps more constant and steady stream of income than personal computers, which most consumers only purchased once every few years.

In a recent press release, an executive at Dell mentioned that the company had not yet established plans to enter the market for portable entertainment units that included MP3 players as well as video capabilities.[13] However, Dell had established other advantages in the MP3 market that stemmed primarily from the company's pared-down players that afforded consumers a price advantage on the rather expensive hard-drive players by cutting out a lot of the extra features offered in other players. With few or no exceptions, Dell offered a fairly significant price savings in their 30 GB model. Most players with that much capacity cost at least $50 to $100 more than Dell's price. That, of course, stemmed from Dell's direct-sales strategy, which cut out retail intermediaries entirely.

When Dell did decide to enter the already very competitive MP3 market in late 2003, it realized that style was a very important selling point for these players, but rather than focusing on just making an aesthetically pleasing product, it examined the way customers used a variety of preexisting MP3 players and noted the good points and problem areas encountered with each player.[14] During this research, Dell discovered that a prominent button for volume control was lacking in many competitors' players, so it made that a more dominant feature of the DJ. Dell also found customers to be easily annoyed by fingerprints on their MP3 player, so it chose to use aluminum for the body of the DJ in hopes that that material would resist smudges easier than other players did. This approach to entering the market reinforced Dell's history of commitment to customer service and to discovering what product features its customers valued and which were considered unnecessary.

Overall, Dell's product stacked up well against other competitors, especially given the size and strength of the company and its success in other electronics areas. Although some critics would argue that the Dell DJ just was not as aesthetically pleasing or quite as easy to use as others, it was generally considered a solid contender in the MP3 player market.

iRiver

The manufacturer iRiver Inc. was owned by Reigncom Ltd. (based in South Korea), which reported in 2003 sales growth of over 182 percent from 2002. The company had been involved in many portable device products and had at one time released the world's thinnest MP3-compatible portable CD player. More recently, its large product line had offered flash-based and hard-drive MP3 players as well as multifunction players with video and audio capabilities. iRiver had partnered with many important players in the computer and electronics industries, including Microsoft, Samsung, Philips, Hitachi, and Texas Instruments.

In a survey of Asian consumers, iRiver won in Korea, with over 46 percent of respondents preferring the brand above all others.[15] The company also saw the increasing necessity of competing head-to-head with Apple as executives specifically named that company in announcements about future plans for competing in the MP3 player industry. To achieve that, at the beginning of 2005, the company initiated greater spending on marketing—one ad even featured a person listening to music on an iRiver player while eating an Apple, perhaps a deliberate stab at Apple. The company had also underestimated prices for component parts at the beginning of 2005 and had some issues with lower-than-expected profitability at that time. The underestimates of budget were partly the failure of company executives to correctly assess the popularity of the iPod Shuffle and the ensuing increase in demand for flash-based component parts, demand that would not allow component prices to fall as low as iRiver had expected.[16]

Recently, the company had teamed up with Soundbuzz, an online music provider based in Singapore. Following the alliance, iRiver purchasers would also receive the software that would allow them to load Soundbuzz's music database onto their computers and search for songs to download for a fee. The company's catalog of songs ranged above 300,000 and had selections from American, Mandarin, and Canto pop music. In addition, Reigncom had planned to license Soundbuzz the rights to any Korean music that it already owned.[17]

SanDisk

SanDisk was founded in 1988 and had become one of the world's leading suppliers of flash memory data storage products such as USB storage drives, flash storage cards, and memory sticks for use in digital cameras and digital music players. SanDisk designed, developed, and manufactured its products and sold them to consumers and to manufacturers of electronic products. SanDisk also licensed its technology to other memory manufacturers. On January 6, 2005, SanDisk announced that it would leverage its experience in manufacturing flash-based memory and memory products to vertically integrate into the flash memory segment of the MP3 player market. SanDisk designed its MP3 players to be small and light, and to be expandable through Secure Digital (SD) cards, a form of flash-based memory manufactured by SanDisk and other flash memory manufacturers. To provide software for its products, SanDisk partnered with Rhapsody, AudioFeast, and Audible. Rhasody provided SanDisk MP3 player users with a digital jukebox that allowed them to manage their music on their MP3 players and purchase music from Rhapsody's library of over 850,000 songs. AudioFeat was a commercial-free digital radio service that allowed users to update music, news, sports, and entertainment programs and news on their MP3 players and to listen to the content on the go. Finally, Audible was a provider of digital audiobooks, radio programs, and newspapers that users could download to their MP3 players for listening on the go. Analysts applauded SanDisk's expansion into the MP3 player market as a natural extension for the company. The first SanDisk MP3 players were shipped in May 2005, and by June 2005 the company had captured 8.9 percent of the flash memory digital music player market.

Sony

In fiscal year 2005 (ending in March), Sony Corporation brought in $66.9 billion in revenue (down 4.5 percent from fiscal 2004) and $1.5 billion in net income (up 85 percent from 2004). The company's net revenues specifically from the electronics segment had fallen every year since fiscal year 2002; from 2004 to 2005, sales in the electronics segment fell by a little less than 0.5 percent. In the 1980s, Sony revolutionized mobile music technology when it introduced the Walkman, a portable cassette tape player that spawned dozens of imitations and look-alikes. Unfortunately, Sony was relatively late to enter the new digital music/MP3 player revolution and was forced to be one of the look-alikes in that market. The Sony Network Walkman was released in August 2004— nearly three years after the iPod, and the iPod was not even the first MP3 player out on the market.

According to some critics, the Network Walkman's user interface was confusing and difficult to use and the accompanying computer software for unloading and managing the music was weaker than the competition. One other point that could potentially work against Sony was that the Network Walkman could not play MP3 files or any other standard music format files like WMA. The Walkman would only play a special format unique to Sony called ATRAC3. Therefore, when the user transferred MP3 or any other type of files to the device, the software had to painstakingly convert each file into the ATRAC format so that it could play on the Network Walkman. Sony claimed to use this unusual format because it improved sound quality and helped extend battery life.

In March 2005, the chairman, the CEO, and the chief operating officer resigned from the company. At the same time, other officers were shuffled, with some demoted. The head of the company was replaced with Sir Howard Stringer, the first non-Japanese person ever placed in the position (he does not speak Japanese). Sony had opted for these drastic measures because it faced intense competition in many of its market segments, including MP3 players, video game equipment, DVD players, and because other electronics companies had gained market share. Sony walkman devices had dominated the portable music player market for more than a decade. However, while the company was not looking, MP3 technology took over the portable music industry and Sony had been late to join in. Now the huge conglomerate was forced to compete with significantly smaller companies just to regain some amount of market share in this fast-growing market. One analyst stated, "Sony's failure to recognize the digital music revolution is classic big-company myopia. As the leading manufacturer of portable CD players and boom boxes, it's easy to see how it could reflexively dismiss MP3 players as a passing fad."[18] In most of Sony's product lines, other Asian electronics manufacturers had forced the company to cut prices since the other companies were making the same electronics for much cheaper. The only product line where Sony was still able to charge a premium price was in the video game segment, with its PlayStation products.

Types of MP3 Payers

Most of the major players in the industry offered products in both of the industry's major segments: hard-drive players and flash memory players. While some analysts included other types of MP3 players in the market—CD players; hard-drive players, which could be separated into microdrive or minidrive players (those with less than 10 GB of storage); and larger players sometimes referred to as digital jukeboxes—flash memory players comprised over 99 percent of the MP3 player market.

Hard-Drive Players

MP3 players with very large levels of capacity typically contained internal hard drives that could be as small as 1.5 GB or as large as 100 GB. These players behaved similarly to real computers in the way they stored and retrieved files from their hard drives. In fact, some players (such as the iPod) would actually function as an external computer hard drive when connected to a computer. Literally thousands of songs as well as other types of files could be stored in players no larger than a deck of cards—for the average user, that meant an entire record collection could be carried in a pocket or purse. Most MP3 manufacturers' product lines included at least one hard-drive player, and many of them had at least one option at the microdrive level and one at a higher-capacity level. This segment of the market also included portable video players (PVPs), which worked much like MP3 players but could store and display video and photo files in addition to audio files. At the end of 2004, Apple controlled 83.7 percent of the hard-drive MP3 player market, followed by Hewlett-Packard (HP), whose iPod device had 3.6 percent of the market. Rio controlled 2.8 percent of the hard-drive MP3 player market at this time, with Creative controlling 2.6 percent and iRiver with 1.5 percent of the market.

Apple　Since the legendary Apple iPod's October 2001 introduction, Apple had altered the product several times, always adding some new feature while consistently lowering the price to keep up with heavy competition. In early 2006, the iPod was available in black or white and in two hard-drive capacities: 30 GB (7,500 songs) and 60 GB (15,000 songs). The smaller model could last for up to 14 hours of playback time, while the larger model boasted up to 20 hours of playback time. The iPods supported several audio formats, including MP3, Apple Lossless, WAV, and Apple's own AAC. All iPods other than the Shuffle included Apple's unique "click wheel" for navigation through the simple interface. With a single finger, the user could adjust volume and move along the intuitive menus, tapping at the center of the wheel to select an option. The color screen displayed a picture of the album cover of whatever song was currently playing. In the newest-generation iPod, Apple had built in up to 150 hours of video capability. That allowed the user to purchase music videos at the online iTunes store for $1.99 each and watch them on the go. Users could also buy ad-free ABC and Disney television shows to watch at any time, and the store also offered a selection of audio books for users to purchase and listen to on the iPod. Whenever they finished listening for the day, they could set a "book marker" at that location and pick up there later. Another feature on the iPod was the Podcast—radio talk shows to which buyers could subscribe from the iPod interface. The iPod could also hold up to 25,000 photos, which could be viewed in thumbnail or full-screen size or in a slide show, on the iPod itself or on any television. Extra features offered by Apple included a calendar, a contact list, a world clock (which included a sleep timer and an alarm clock), a stopwatch, password protection, four games, and the ability to create custom playlists from the unit itself (users did not have to wait until they could connect to a computer). The 30 GB and 60 GB iPods retailed for $299 and $399, respectively. Users could purchase music for the iPod, iPod Nano, and iPod shuffle only at iTunes, Apple's online music store.

Archos　The Gmini XS 202 was a 20 GB hard-drive MP3 player that could store about 10,000 songs. The unit could play back WMA, MP3, and WAV audio files for up to 17 hours. The XS 202 had an internal battery that could be charged though an included AC adapter. When connected with a computer, the product could automatically sync with Windows Media Player to allow the user to transfer songs or playlists from the PC to the player. This player used a double browser to help the user organize music files without a computer—a sort of split screen appeared that had files and folders on one side and playlists and songs on the other. That feature facilitated the user in moving, copying, deleting, renaming, and creating new files and folders. Any online music stores that sold songs in the previously mentioned formats could be used to buy new songs for the XS 202. In addition, Archos had the Gmini 400, a combination video, photo, game, and music player. Its 20 GB hard drive could hold 80 hours of video, 200,000 photos, or 10,000 songs. The 400 supported the same audio formats as the XS 202 and could play up to 10 hours of music or 4 hours of video. In addition, users could record audio directly into the device at stereo quality. For photo viewing, users could download their pictures directly to the player from a compact flash reader. An optional adapter could be purchased to allow the unit the ability to read all types of flash memory cards. The company boasted near-DVD-quality video storage and viewing capability. The XS 202 retailed for about $249, while the Gmini 400 sold for $329.

In the microdrive segment of the market, Archos offered the XS 100 model. This 3 GB hard-drive player could hold up to 1,500 songs and was the lightest and smallest model offered by Archos. The product was available in pink, blue, gray, and black and offered features similar to the larger hard-drive models. The XS 100 automatically synced with Windows Media Player, used the split-screen feature, and allowed the user to connect the player to his or her home stereo for playback purposes. This smaller player retailed for $169.

Creative   Creative Labs offered a vast product selection in both the hard-drive and microdrive segments. The Zen Vision had a 30 GB hard drive with the ability to store and view thousands of photos, 120 hours of video, or 15,000 songs. Its wide array of features included photo slide-show abilities, direct transfer of photos through the compact flash reader (optional adapter for other types of flash cards), an FM tuner and live radio recording ability, a voice recorder, and a personal organizer. The battery supported 13 hours of music listening and 4.5 hours of video playback. The Vision was available in black or white and sold for $399. Another player was the Zen Sleek, a 20 GB hard-drive player that held up to 10,000 WMA-formatted songs or 5,000 MP3 songs. With an 18-hour battery and a built-in FM tuner and recording ability, the Sleek was similar to other Creative products. The player also offered a

vertical touchpad that allowed users to select options with their fingertips. Creative's Zen Sleek sold for $269. Next, Creative's Zen Touch took the idea of the touchpad and made an entirely new product line out of it. The Touch is a model that reduced the size of the regular Play, Stop, Rewind, and Fast Forward buttons and made the touchpad a more predominant feature on the front of the player. The streamlined Touch was offered in a 20 GB model (10,000 WMA songs/5,000 MP3 songs) or a 40 GB model (16,000 WMA songs/10,000 MP3 songs). The battery could last for up to 32 hours of play time. Playlists could be created on the go, without a computer, and the unique search function allowed users to locate a specific artist, song, or album. The 20 GB and 40 GB Zen Touch models sold for $229 and $299, respectively.

Creative's primary microdrive players were the Zen Micro and Zen Micro Photo. The Micro was offered in a 4, 5, or 6 GB model (holding 1,000, 1,250, and 1,500 MP3 songs, respectively). This model had a contoured shape, designed with portability and pocketability in mind. Available in 10 fashionable colors, the Micro could appeal to many consumers. Like Creative's many other models, the Micro had an FM tuner, a voice and radio recorder, a vertical touchpad, a personal organizer, a sleep timer, an alarm clock, a customizable menu, and various song shuffling features. In order of size, this model's variations sold for $179, $199, and $229. The only significant changes made to the Zen Micro Photo were the size upgrade (to 8 GB) and, of course, the ability to view still images or slide shows. The increased capacity allowed 4,000 songs to be stored, and the model was still offered in 10 colors and sold for $249.

Dell   The Dell Digital Jukebox (DJ) was offered in a 30 GB size (15,000 songs). The DJ was in its second generation and lasted for about 12 hours of listening. Very few additional features were offered; the model had a backlit blue screen just under two inches wide and navigational buttons on the front. The model sold for $239.

The Dell Pocket DJ offered a microdrive alternative with 5 GB of capacity, or 2,500 songs. With battery life of 10 hours and a small, sleek design, the Pocket DJ was a slightly shrunken version of the Dell DJ and sold for $169. Both the DJ and Pocket DJ could be customized with accessories such as jackets, premium headphones, armbands or other carrying cases, and various auto accessories.

iRiver   The 20 GB iRiver H10 model played up to 600 hours of music and had a color screen display. In a feature similar to Apple's Click Wheel, the H10 had a touch strip that allowed the user's finger to move up and down to navigate the menu options. Young Se Kim, the designer of the H10, got the idea for the vertical touch strip by watching people use the iPod in a coffee shop. He noticed that most people only used about one-fourth of the circular wheel on the front of the iPod, so he though a short vertical strip made more sense.[19] Battery life claimed to be 16 hours (it was rechargeable) and the player could also display digital photos on the screen. Supported files included WMA, MP3, TXT, and JPEG files. Two extra, unique features were an FM radio tuner and a built-in voice recorder. The iRiver II10 sold for about $299. In addition, iRiver offered the PMC-120, a 20 GB multimedia portable unit that could play video, music, and photos. This model had a 3.5-inch color widescreen and played up to 600 hours of music or 80 hours of video, but it did not offer the FM tuner or voice-recording ability of the H10. The removable, rechargeable battery could last for 14 hours of audio use or 5 hours of video use. It retailed for $499.

Among its H10 products, iRiver also offered two microdrive models, either a 5 GB or a 6 GB option. The former played up to 150 hours of music; the latter, up to 180 hours. Both supported WMA, MP3, and ASF audio files as well as JPEG and TXT data files and had built-in FM radio tuners and voice recorders. The smaller model sold for around $249, while the larger was priced at $279.

Rio   The Rio Karma was a 20 GB player that could hold about 10,000 songs (5,000 if in WMA format). Special features included Cross-Fader, which blended the end of one song seamlessly with the beginning of the next, an Ogg Vorbis audio format (different from either MP3 or WMA), and a large display screen that had animated menus and visualizations. The auto-synchronization function meant that whenever the unit was connected to the user's computer, it would automatically update its playlist with any missing songs. The Karma also had a DJ capability that let it find the user's 10 most-played songs, rarely played songs, or songs downloaded to the unit in a certain time period. Rio's Karma sold for about $199.

Rio's microdrive offerings included the ce2100, a small 2.5 GB player. In addition, the Rio Carbon was sold in a 5 GB or 6 GB capacity. This model's tapered design had won awards; the unit was about the size of a business card. Extra features included voice recording through a built-in microphone. All Rio players included software called Rio Music Manager, which could play MP3 files and manage playlists. In order of size, Rio's three microdrive players retailed for approximately $125, $149, and $179.

Sony   Sony's hard-drive player, the Network Walkman, was offered in a single capacity: 20 GB, or 13,000 songs, according to Sony. The unit could store audio and data files and supported MP3, WMA, WAV, and ATRAC3 (Sony's own format) audio formats. The Network Walkman could last for up to 40 hours of playback time, and the removable battery could charge through a USB cable or an AC adapter, both provided with the unit. The newest model offered the user a choice for the viewing screen—it could be switched between horizontal or vertical viewing. Another unique feature of the Network Walkman was G-Sensor Shock Protection, a system that could react quickly to changes in gravity and velocity to protect the hard drive's surface. The product also had built-in technology to help prevent music skipping caused by forceful impact. Songs for the unit could only be purchased through Sony's online Connect music store. The Network Walkman was available in black, silver, or red and retailed for $279.

Flash-Based Players

Flash-based MP3 players used either an internal or external source of memory to store and retrieve audio files. The most common type of storage media used was a memory card, available in a wide variety of sizes and capacities, usually ranging from 128 MB to 1 GB for portable music players. However, some manufacturers had players with as much as 4 GB of flash memory. The players could be as large as some of the smaller hard-drive players or as small as a pack of gum. Although flash players stored fewer songs than hard-drive players, their primary advantage over the larger-capacity players was that they had no moving parts, which made them ideal for physical activity. Even with jostling and shaking, they were less likely to skip during songs. All of the manufacturers previously discussed in this case had at least one flash-based player in their product lines. According to the market research firm NPD Group, the top manufacturers of flash memory players in June 2005, were Apple, which had captured 46.3 percent of the market; SanDisk, which controlled 8.9 percent of the market; Rio, with 2.9 percent of the market; and Creative Labs, with 2.4 percent of the total market.

Apple   Apple had recently stopped making the iPod Mini, a micro drive player, and replaced it with the 62 percent smaller iPod Nano, which used a built-in USB flash drive and was available in sizes of 2 GB (500 songs in AAC format) and 4 GB (1,000 songs). The Nano was also able to store and display up to 25,000 photos on its color screen. Apple incorporated its click wheel into the design of the Nano, which made navigation simple and easy. The player could play songs in shuffle mode, or the user could browse for a specific song by title, artist, composer, genre, album, or playlist. In addition, for whatever song was currently playing, the cover art of song's album was displayed on the Nano's screen. Like the larger iPods, the Nano also had the capability to allow the user to subscribe to Podcasts. Other features included the ability to purchase and listen to audio books from the iTunes store, to display photos individually, as thumbnails, or in a slideshow, and to maintain a calendar with appointments and an address book. The Nano also had games, a world clock, a stopwatch, and password protection, and it allowed the user to create custom playlists without a computer. The 2 GB model retailed for $199, while the 4 GB model sold for $249.

Apple also offered one other flash player, the tiny Shuffle, about the size of a pack of chewing gum. The Shuffle came in 512 MB (120 songs) or 1 GB (240 songs) capacities. With this player, Apple eliminated the screen altogether and offered users two options: play the songs in order or shuffle the songs to play randomly. The songs stored on the player could be changed as often as the user liked, and the user could choose a specific playlist to load for the day from his or her purchased collection at the iTunes store. Any Podcasts the user had purchased could also be loaded onto the player. The only thing on the front of the Shuffle was a small circular control pad that had buttons for play/pause, fast forward, rewind, and volume up and down. The back side of the player contained a simple switch that moved vertically to turn the power off, to choose in-order playing mode, or to choose shuffle mode. The 512 MB model sold for $99, while the 1 GB Shuffle sold for $129.

Creative   Creative also offered an extremely extensive product line; the MuVo players were Creative's flash-based MP3 players. The MuVo Vidz was offered in 512 MB or 1 GB models but was not yet available in North America. Small enough to wear around the neck, the Vidz could hold music, photos, or video and had a 1.8-inch widescreen color display. The player could hold up to 500 songs (WMA or MP3 format), eight hours of video, or 999 photos in its largest capacity. With a 10-hour battery life, the Vidz offered extra features such as an FM radio and recorder, a voice recorder, and the ability to store any other type of computer file (Word documents, spreadsheets, etc.).

The MuVo Chameleon was also unavailable in North America but came in a 1 GB model that could hold 500 songs. The Chameleon's special feature was that it came with 10 interchangeable color pieces that snapped onto the front of the player and allowed the user to coordinate "every outfit, every occasion, and every mood," according to Creative's Web site. The Chameleon, like the Vidz, had an FM tuner and recorder, a voice recorder, and the ability to function as a flash memory drive for storage of all types of computer files. With an 18-hour battery life, this player also offered some other unique features, such as random playback mode and a reversible LCD screen that could adapt to a left- or right-handed user.

For the sports enthusiast, the MuVo Sport C100 was a small flash-based player that could stand physical jostling and moderate exposure to moisture. The player came in 128 MB or 256 MB ($99) models and included three sport timers: a lap timer, a split timer, and a countdown timer. The player also had an FM radio tuner and an expansion slot for an optional memory card that could hold up to an additional 1 GB of memory. The player came with a carrying case and an armband and ran on a AAA battery.

Dell   Dell offered one flash-based player, the DJ Ditty, the size of a pack of gum and available in a 512 MB capacity (220 songs in WMA format) for $99. With a small LCD screen, the Ditty had an FM tuner and a built-in rechargeable battery that lasted up to 14 hours. Like all of Dell's players, the Ditty was compatible with several online music stores and operated in regular or random playback mode. One end of the Ditty was a USB port that facilitated the player's connection to a computer, and Dell had recently started selling colorful caps for the port (the player came with a black cap). Like other manufacturers' tiny flash players, the Ditty was ideal for physical activity because of its size, light weight, and lack of moving parts.

iRiver   The extensive iRiver collection of flash-based MP3 players included the U10 player, which came in 512 MB ($199) or 1 GB ($249) sizes and featured a two-inch color screen. The U10 could play music, video, or photo files for up to 28 hours of battery life (according to iRiver). This player supported WMA and MP3 formatted files, among others. Extra features the iRiver incorporated into the U10 included an FM tuner, a voice recorder, and an alarm clock.

Another flash-based player offered by iRiver was the T10, also in 512 MB ($149) and 1 GB ($199) sizes. The company claimed a whopping 45 hours of battery life, and music could be purchased for any of iRiver's players from almost any online music store including subscription-based and pay-as-you-go stores (excluding the iTunes and Connect stores). The T10 also had an FM tuner, an FM recorder, and a color screen. Made for physical activity, the U10 had a sport clip that allowed the user to attach the player to his or her clothing and also featured skip-free song play. Finally, iRiver also included a voice recorder with the U10 players.

The company's N10 flash-based series came in three sizes: 512 MB ($239), 256 MB ($169), and 128 MB ($139). A tiny player about the size of a pack of gum, the N10 was meant to be worn either around the neck or on the arm or wrist. With up to 11 hours of battery life, the N10 series had a small display screen that provided song titles and the artist's name. Finally, iRiver was able to incorporate its voice recorder into this player as well. Although iRiver's product line included several other flash-based players, those mentioned were representative of the types of capacities, prices, and features the company offered in its players.

Rio   Rio had two flash-based players. The first was the Rio Forge Sport, available in 128, 256 (about $150), or 512 MB (about $189) capacities. With a unique circular design, the Forge Sport had a rubber grip around its perimeter to allow the user to get a better hold on it. Features included an FM radio, 20 hours of battery life, and a stopwatch and lap timer. The player also had a slot for memory card expansion, which meant the user could buy up to 1 GB of

additional song capacity for this player. The player came boxed with sport clip earphones, a carrying case, and an armband. Like Rio's hard-drive players, the Forge also came with Rio Music Manager software for managing a music library.

Rio's other flash player was the se510 sport player, which had a similar design to the Forge. This player was only available in the 512 MB capacity and sold for $129. Like the Forge, the se510 lasted up to 20 hours and included a sports armband and stopwatch and lap timer. The primary difference between Rio's flash-based players was that the se510 did not offer an expandable memory card slot.

SanDisk   In May 2005 SanDisk shipped its first flash MP3 players, the 512 MB Sansa e130 (up to 240 songs in WMA format) and the 1GB Sansa e140 (up to 480 songs in WMA format). Each of these players had an SD slot for additional storage; supported MP3, WMA, and audible files; had a digital FM radio receiver; and could purportedly last up to 17 hours on a single AAA battery. The front of each unit offered a multiline backlit LCD that provided the title, artists, and album of the song currently being played. In September 2005, SanDisk began offering a car transmitter that would allow the user to play MP3 music through a car radio, and a portable speaker dock for Sansa MP3 players.

Sony   Sony offered two flash-based MP3 players. The first was the Network Walkman NW-E407, available in 512 MB (345 songs in ATRAC3 format) and 1 GB (695 songs) capacities. About the size of a pack of chewing gum, the player had built-in flash memory and could serve as an MP3 player or as an FM tuner. The front of the unit had a small, three-line display screen that revealed information like the song title. Sony claimed that the internal battery on the flash Network Walkman could last up to 50 hours and could be charged for just three minutes to provide 3 hours of playback time (under certain playing conditions, such as when the unit was in super-power-saving mode). The 512 MB Network Walkman sold for $119; the 1 GB model sold for $179.

Sony's other flash player was the Walkman Bean, also available in a 512 MB or 1 GB model (song capacities were the same as for the flash Network Walkman). Similar in overall size to Sony's other flash player, the Walkman Bean had a curved shape, like a kidney bean. The Bean also had an FM tuner with preset station capability and a one-line display screen. The battery power and charging ability of the Bean was the same as for the flash Network Walkman. While the smaller Bean player sold for $119, the larger sold for $149. Music for all of Sony's MP3 players (including the hard-drive players) could only be purchased through Sony's online music store, Sony Connect.

Endnotes

[1] http://en.wikipedia.org/wiki/MP3_player (accessed December 23, 2005).

[2] Ibid.

[3] Russ Arensman, "MP3 Leaders Face Off," *Electronic Business,* June 1, 2005, www.reed-electronics.com/eb-mag/article/CA603499.html?industryid-43314 (accessed December 16, 2005).

[4] Steve Smith, "iPod's Lessons," *Twice,* July 26, 2004, p. 12.

[5] Steven Levy, "iPod Nation." *Newsweek,* July 26, 2004, pp. 42–50.

[6] Paul Hansell, "Battle of Form (and Function) in MP3 Players," *New York Times,* October 4, 2004.

[7] Joseph Palenchar, "Rio Foresees Delay for Next Generation Devices," *Twice,* August 8, 2005, p. 6.

[8] Antony Bruno, "No More Rio," *Billboard,* September 10, 2005, p. 6.

[9] Smith, "iPod's Lessons."

[10] Peter Burrows and Roger O. Crockett, "Apple's Phones Isn't Ringing Any Chimes," *BusinessWeek,* September 19, 2005, p. 58.

[11] Steve Maich, "Nowhere to Go but Down," *Maclean's,* May 9, 2005, p. 32.

[12] Arun Sudhaman, "Bid to Beat Apple Has Creative Striking Out," *Media Asia,* June 17, 2005, p. 18.

[13] Mark Hachman, "Dell Brings Dling to Gaming Notebook," *ExtremeTech.com,* February 24, 2005, p. 1.

[14] Jennifer Vilaga, "Fast Talk," *Fast Company,* June 2005, p. 43.

[15] Aki Tsukioka, "Info Plant Announces Results of Survey of Youth in East Asia on MP3 Players," *JCN Newswire,* October 3, 2005, p. 1.

[16] Evan Ramstad, "An iPod Casually: The Rio Digital Music Player," *The Wall Street Journal,* September 1, 2005, p. B3.

[17] "Soundbuzz Seals iRiver Music Deal," *Media,* August 12, 2005, p. 8.

[18] "Executive Shake-Up at Sony," *Knight Ridder Tribune Business News,* March 8, 2005, p. 1.

[19] Jennifer Vilaga, "Fast Talk," *Fast Company,* June 2005, p. 43.

Apple Computer in 2006

Lou Marino
The University of Alabama

John Hattaway
The University of Alabama

Katy Beth Jackson
The University of Alabama

When Steve Jobs unveiled the fifth-generation iPod on October 12, 2005, he called it the "evolution of a revolution." In this statement, Jobs perfectly described the progress of Apple's flagship iPod line, and the progress of Apple itself. Adding video playback to its popular music player was a natural step in Apple's transformation from an innovative computer manufacturer to a state-of-the-art consumer electronics company. Entering the video sector signaled that Apple would not be content to stop with music and that the company intended to further its penetration into the vast consumer electronics market. With this step, analysts and Apple enthusiasts agreed that the company had come a long way from its personal computing history.

HISTORY OF APPLE

Steven Wozniak and Steven Jobs founded Apple Computer in 1976 by introducing the initial version of what was to become the first highly successful mass-produced personal computer, the Apple I. Alth-ough the original Apple I needed some refinement (it lacked a monitor, a keyboard, or even a case), it eventually influenced the computer industry immeasurably. Wozniak and Jobs had attended high school together and maintained contact after graduation despite taking jobs with different companies in Silicon Valley (at Hewlett-Packard and Atari, respectively). Wozniak was the true designer of the Apple I, but Jobs recognized its commercial potential and insisted that they sell the computer. Although the original model was certainly no rousing success, Wozniak was already designing the Apple II, which was introduced at a local trade show in 1977 and launched in April 1978. This second machine was instantly much more popular than its predecessor and included a plastic case and color graphics. Apple's president, Michael Scott, and chairman of the board, Mike Markkula, were happy with the computer's sales; by the end of 1980, Apple had sold more than 10,000 Apple IIs.

While the Apple II was relatively successful, the next revision of the product line, which was code-named Macintosh (or Mac), was already in the works by 1979 under the direction of Jeff Raskin, a former professor the University of California at San Diego and a researcher at Xerox's Palo Alto Research Center (PARC) who had proposed the project to Mike Markkula. Raskin's ambitious goal was to design a user-friendly computer that would feature a graphical user interface (GUI) and would cost less than $500. At Raskin's urging, in the same year, Jobs visited PARC, where he saw researchers using a GUI to simplify their computing. Jobs immediately recognized the importance of the interface and decided to use it in the project he was spearheading with project manager Ken Rothmuller, the Apple Lisa, named after Jobs's daughter. However, Jobs's constant drive for innovation and demands for refinements of, and additional features for, the Lisa drove up costs for the system, delayed the shipping date, and resulted in Jobs's frustration with the process. Apple's president, Michael Scott, eventually removed Jobs from the project when Jobs tried to take it over. Due to excessive cost, the Lisa never performed up to Apple's expectations and was retired from the market soon after it was introduced.

Undeterred, Jobs took his passion for the GUI to Raskin's Macintosh project. Jobs's 11 percent share of Apple's equity helped convince Scott to allow him to take over the Macintosh project, and personality conflicts between Jobs and Raskin eventually forced Raskin to leave Apple in 1981. In the same year, Scott resigned as president of Apple and became the vice chairman of the board. Scott was replaced by Mike Markkula, who became president and CEO, while Jobs became the chairman of the board. Under Jobs, the Macintosh team was challenged to make something "insanely great," and by many accounts they succeeded. The Macintosh, introduced in 1984, was hailed as a breakthrough in user-friendly computing. It was also the first computer to use a 3.5-inch disk drive. Unfortunately, the Macintosh did not have the speed, power, or software availability to compete with the personal computer (PC) that had been introduced by IBM in 1981. One of the reasons the Macintosh lacked the necessary software was that Apple put strict restrictions on the Apple Certified Developer Program, which made it difficult for software developers to obtain Macs at a discount and receive informational materials about the operating system that they could use to develop software for the Macintosh.

Back in 1981, Jobs had begun actively working to replace Mike Markkula with John Sculley, then president of Pepsi-Cola, as president and CEO of Apple. In April 1983, Sculley assumed the head position at Apple Computer and Markkula became the associate chairman. In 1984, when Apple introduced the Macintosh and it was not as well received as initially expected, Jobs (a volatile individual) and Sculley began to have personal disputes. Finally, in 1985, Jobs staged an unsuccessful "boardroom coup" to replace Sculley as Sculley was planning a trip to China. Sculley found out about the coup and canceled his trip. After Apple's board voted unanimously to keep Sculley in his position, Jobs, who was retained as chairman of the company but stripped of all decision-making authority, resigned. During the remainder of 1985, Apple continued to encounter problems and laid off one-fifth of its employees while posting its first-ever quarterly loss. In addition, Sculley entered a legal battle with Microsoft's Bill Gates over the introduction of Windows 1.0, which used technology similar to the Mac's GUI. Gates eventually signed a document that in effect ensured that Microsoft would not use Mac technology in Windows 1.0, but he made no such promises for any later versions of Windows. Essentially, Apple had lost the exclusive right to use its own GUI.

Despite these setbacks, Apple kept bringing innovative products to the market, realizing that innovation would have to be its strategy against big companies like IBM and Microsoft, especially since Microsoft had made its technology available to any PC company that wanted to incorporate that software into its own hardware components. However, Apple had always been famous for closely guarding the secrets behind its technology. In 1987, Apple released the second version of the unsuccessful Macintosh computer, but this machine, like the Apple II, was a phenomenal success. The Mac II was easy to use, making it a favorite at schools and in homes. In addition, it had excellent graphics capabilities. However, by 1990, PCs with Microsoft software had flooded the marketplace and Windows technology was far more prevalent than Mac because Microsoft had licensed its software for use on computers built by many different companies.

In 1991, Apple released the first generation of its notebook computers, the PowerBook, which was successful. In the meantime, Sculley began to push for the completion of a project that was under way to develop a new type of computer system called the personal digital assistant (PDA). Apple's version of the PDA was called the Newton, and under Sculley's persistence the product was completed and released to the market in August 1993. However, the machines did not sell well, partly because they failed to successfully recognize handwriting. Also in 1993, Sculley began to lose interest in Apple's daily operations; in June, the board of directors opted to remove Sculley from the position of CEO. The board chose to place the chief operating officer, Michael Spindler, in the vacated spot. Sculley was allowed to keep his position as chairman, but he chose to resign from the company altogether a few months later.

Although Spindler was not a personable, accessible leader, he did oversee the development of several important Apple products. First, in 1994, Apple released the PowerMac family of PCs, the first Macs to incorporate the PowerPC chip, a very fast processor co-developed with Motorola and IBM. For the first time since Intel technology had become prevalent, Apple could compete with, and sometimes even surpass, the speed of Intel's processors in its computers. Spindler also made a somewhat half-hearted attempt to license the Mac operating system (OS) to other companies. However, few companies ever chose to license the Mac OS because many felt the licensing agreements were far too restrictive. By 1995, Apple had bigger problems than selling computers: It had $1 billion in back orders and insufficient parts to build those machines. And worse, in the late summer of 1995, Microsoft released its Windows 95 OS, which was well suited to compete with the strengths of the Mac OS. During the winter between 1995 and 1996, Apple made some misguided judgments concerning its product line and as a result posted a loss for that quarter. In January 1996, Apple asked Spindler to resign and chose Gil Amelio, former president of National Semiconductor, to take his place.

During his first 100 days in office, Amelio announced many sweeping changes for the company. He split Apple into seven distinct divisions, each responsible for its own profit or loss, and he tried to better inform software developers and consumers of Apple's products and projects. Although Apple announced a staggering first-quarter loss of $740 million in 1996, it brought that down to a $33 million loss for the second quarter, an achievement the financial experts had not imagined the company could accomplish. And in the third quarter, Apple again beat the best estimates, reporting a $30 million profit for that period. At the end of 1996, the company astonished the industry when it announced that it planned to acquire Steve Jobs's new venture, NeXT Software Inc., and rehire Jobs. The acquisition was chosen in order to control NeXTstep, a software design Apple planned to use for its next-generation operating system, Rhapsody. During the summer of 1997, after announcing another multimillion-dollar quarterly loss, Apple determined that Gil Amelio had made many significant improvements in Apple's operations but that he had done all he could. No permanent replacement was announced, but Fred Anderson, chief financial officer, was placed in charge of daily operations; Jobs was also given an expanded role in the company.

Jobs's "expanded role" soon became more clear in terms of his responsibilities—Apple had no CEO, stock prices were at a five-year low, and important decisions needed to be made. Jobs soon began to be referred to as interim CEO, and 1997 proved to be a landmark year for his company. A conference called MacWorld Boston was held in August of that year, and Jobs was the keynote speaker. He used that event to make several significant announcements that would turn Apple around. An almost entirely new board of directors was announced, an aggressive advertising campaign was planned, and an alliance with Microsoft was revealed. Microsoft received $150 million in Apple stock, Apple received a five-year patent cross-license, and the long legal battle between the two companies started to taper off. As part of the legal dispute resolution, Microsoft paid an undisclosed amount to Apple to quiet the allegations that it had stolen Apple's intellectual property (the Mac GUI). By year's end, Microsoft's Windows 1998 was available for Mac users. Jobs also effectively ended Apple's licensing agreements with other companies, buying out all but one, with the understanding that company would only serve the low-end market for computers (under $1,000). At a late 1997 press conference, Jobs announced that Apple would begin selling direct to consumers over the Web and by phone. Within a week, the Apple e-store was the third-largest e-commerce site on the Web.

Jobs continued to make several changes during 1998, a year in which Apple reported four quarters of profitable earnings, a full year of profitability. Apple's stock price was on the rise, and Apple had released the iMac, an all-new design for the Macintosh that was meant to serve the lower-end consumer market. The iMac had more processing capabilities than most consumers would ever need and was priced affordably. In the fall of that year, the iMac was the best-selling computer in the country. Apple followed up that success by introducing the iBook in 1999, the portable counterpart to the iMac, a laptop meant to be stylish, affordable, and powerful. Throughout 1999, Apple's stock continued to soar, and in the fall was as high as the upper $70s.

In early 2000, Jobs announced that he was now permanent CEO of Apple. The remainder of that year was a slow one for Apple and for the rest of the computer industry. As a result, Apple reported its first quarterly loss in three years. In late 2000 the company cut prices across the board, and in early 2001 it released a new set of PowerMacs with optical drives that let consumers choose whether to burn or listen to CDs or read or write DVDs as well. In May 2001, Jobs announced that Apple would open several retail stores that would sell Apple products as well as third-party products, including MP3 players, digital cameras, and digital video cameras. In October

2001, Apple released its first noncomputer product in years, the iPod. This small machine was a portable MP3 player that stored songs on a hard drive and could be taken anywhere. Apple took quite a risk in pricing the small machine at a premium, but it felt that consumers would be willing to pay more for the unique style, design, and technology.

Over the next few years, Apple made adjustments and additions to its product line, both on the software side and on the hardware side. Although the latter half of 2002 was a poor time for the entire economy as a whole, Apple did well, with net earnings of $65 million. The company's other products sold well and also enjoyed success, but it was the iPod that would revolutionize the company and the industry. In 2003, when the company released iTunes, the online retail store where consumers could purchase individual songs legally, the success of the venture skyrocketed. The iTunes technology was available only for Macs at first, but has since become available for PC users as well. By July 2004, 100 million songs had been sold and iTunes had a 70 percent market share among all legal online music download services.

APPLE'S CURRENT SITUATION

By 2005, Jobs's leadership had placed Apple at the forefront of the MP3 player industry and had established the company as a player once again in the computer industry. Jobs had idea after idea for how to improve the company and turn its performance around. He not only consistently pushed for innovative ideas and products but also enforced several structural changes, including ridding the company of unprofitable segments and divisions. His leadership style, which epitomized the spirit and standards upon which Apple was founded, blended with the business discipline that was lacking in the younger Jobs. Jobs also credited Apple's success to its skill management team, which included Peter Oppenheimer and Timothy Cook.

Peter Oppenheimer started with Apple in 1996 as controller for the Americas and was senior vice president and chief financial officer for the company. He was promoted to these positions after less than two years with the company, due to his extensive experience in business and financial

areas. Oppenheimer, who reported to the CEO, was responsible for the supervision of the controller, trea-sury, investor relations, tax, information systems, internal audit, corporate development, and human resources departments, and he helped return a healthy fiscal discipline to the company. Timothy D. Cook, Apple's executive vice president of worldwide sales and operations, also reported to the CEO. Cook was responsible for managing Apple's supply chain, sales activities, and service and support in all markets and countries. His position was accountable for maintaining Apple's flexibility in serving more-demanding consumers. Cook had extensive experience in technological industries and had worked previously for IBM and then for Compaq. The skill management team, along with the other members of the executive staff and the board of directors, was responsible for ensuring that all operations of Apple ran efficiently and smoothly, while Jobs provided the vision for the organization. Together they worked to ensure that Apple could continue to be a vital, innovative company in a competitive environment.

In February 2005, Apple's stock prices reached record highs (prices were in the $80s, though just a year before a record low of $21.89 had been hit) and the company announced a 2-for-1 stock split. Investor confidence in the company was rewarded as, during Apple's fiscal fourth quarter of 2005, which ended September 24, 2005, Apple reported the highest revenue and earnings in the company's history, with revenues of $3.68 billion and a net quarterly profit of $430 million, up from revenues of $2.35 billion and a net profit of $106 million, or $.13 per diluted share, in the same quarter of the previous year. In the fourth quarter of 2005, Apple shipped 1,236,000 Macintosh units (up 48 percent from the same quarter the previous year) and 6,451,000 iPods (up 48 percent from the same quarter the previous year). As of October 2005, the price of a share of Apple stock was above $55. Apple's financial performance is shown in Exhibit 1.

Jobs reported that these figures represented the company's highest-ever quarterly revenue and income. With 10 million iPod units already sold by 2005, and with Apple's plans to continue to grow and design innovative products in the iPod line, the enormous success of the iPod line really could not be overstated. As a result of the introduction of the iPod, Apple's sales and financial information had consistently surpassed expectations since 2001.

Exhibit 1   **Apple Computer's Financial Performance, Fiscal Years 2001–2005 (in millions, except share amounts)**

Results of Operations	2005	2004	2003	2002	2001
Net sales					
Domestic	$ 8,334	$4,893	$3,626	$3,272	$2,936
International	5,597	3,386	2,581	2,470	2,427
Total net sales	13,931	8,279	6,207	5,742	5,363
Costs and expenses					
Cost of sales	9,888	6,020	4,499	4,139	4,128
Research and development (R&D)	534	489	471	446	430
Selling, general and administrative (SG&A)	1,859	1,421	1,212	1,111	1,138
Operating expenses before special charges	2,393	1,910	1,683	1,557	1,568
Special charges					
Executive bonus	—	—	—	−2	—
In-process research and development	—	—	—	1	11
Restructuring costs and other	—	23	26	30	—
Total operating expenses	2,393	1,933	1,709	1,586	1,579
Operating income (loss)	1,650	326	−1	17	−344
Interest and other income (expense) net	165	57	93	70	292
Income (loss) before provision (benefit) for income taxes	1,815	383	92	87	−52
Provision (benefit) for income taxes	480	107	24	22	−15
Cumulative income of accounting change, net of income taxes of	5	0	0	1	12
Net earnings (loss)	$ 1,335	$ 276	$ 69	$ 65	$ (25)
Diluted earnings (loss) per common and common equivalent share	$1.56	$0.36	$0.09	$0.09	$(0.04)
Diluted common and common equivalent shares used in the calculations of earnings (loss) per share (in thousands)	856,780	774,622	726,932	723,570	691,226
Financial position					
Cash, cash equivalents and short-term investments	$8,261	$5,464	$4,566	$4,337	$4,336
Accounts receivable, net	895	774	766	565	466
Inventories	165	101	56	45	11
Net property, plant and equipment	817	707	669	621	564
Total assets	11,551	8,050	6,815	6,298	6,021
Current liabilities	3,484	2,680	2,357	1,658	1,518
Long-term debt	—	—	—	316	317
Deferred tax liabilities and other noncurrent liabilities	601	294	235	229	266
Shareholders' equity	$7,466	$5,076	$4,223	$4,095	$3,920

Source: Company 2005 10-K report.

Further, some analysts believed that sales of iPods would create permanent consumer converts to the entire line of Apple products, including PCs. While a few analysts believed that interest in a portable MP3 player could not possibly generate a significant amount of interest in Apple's computers, at least one source reported that as many as 11 percent of iPod users intended to purchase an Apple Mac, and "in a November [2004] survey, money managers Piper Jaffray & Co., found that 6 percent of iPod users had switched from a standard personal computer running Microsoft Corp.'s Windows operating software to an Apple Mac, and another 7 percent planned to switch in the coming year."[1]

Most of the actions Apple had taken over its history were consistent with its underlying philosophy that innovation and improvement of existing products was essential for the growth and development of the company and its continued success. Since 2002, Apple had determined that the digital electronics market was converging with the computer market and that consumers would begin to demand more synchronization and harmony between the two. That belief had led Apple to release the iPod and iTunes, as well as to improve the software and available options on its computers to incorporate more closely the two areas of demand.

In Apple's fiscal-year 2005, the company had $13.93 billion in sales, with about $6 billion of that from sales of all Macintosh computers and approximately $4.5 billion from iPod sales (see Exhibit 2). Apple's unit sales for the same fiscal year, broken down by product, revealed that approximately 4.5 million Mac units were sold in 2005, while approximately 22.5 million iPods, including all types of iPods, were sold over the same time period.

One other impressive feature of Apple's financial statements was that although the company had some minimal long-term debt in recent years, in February 2004, the company retired $300 million of outstanding debt and reduced long-term liabilities to $0. In retiring this debt, Apple did not deprive key operating areas of the necessary levels of funding and additional funds were allocated to research and development (see Exhibit 2). Spending more on R&D was consistent with the company's philosophy that its continued achievement would depend heavily on its ability to improve existing products, introduce new products, offer the items at competitive prices to achieve widespread popularity, and perhaps even more importantly, to convince investors and consumers that Apple products were better than those of competitors in the two main industries in which it competed, personal computers and MP3 players.

PERSONAL COMPUTER INDUSTRY

In the third quarter of 2005, the worldwide PC market experienced its 10th consecutive quarter of double-digit growth. The PC industry was relatively consolidated. The U.S. market was dominated by five main players (see Exhibit 3), who controlled 64.2 percent of the market. Internationally, the top five controlled over 40 percent of the market, and Apple only accounted for 2 percent of international volume. While the market had experienced substantial growth, experts predicted that the market in the United States, as well as the market throughout the world with the exception of Asia, would experience a slowdown to 8 percent unit sales growth from 2006 to 2009, with flat revenue growth. In the face of these flat margins, it was predicted that the marginal players were likely to be forced out of the market.

Apple's Computer Operations

Even though Apple's revenues were increasingly coming from noncomputer products, primarily the iPod, Apple still remained a company with computers at its core. Apple's approach of handling every facet of the computer in-house differentiated it from its primary competitors in the PC market but left out many of the synergies that Windows/Intel (Wintel) PC makers benefited from. Many analysts still projected that Apple's greatest opportunity for growth would come from the projected halo effect of iPods (i.e., consumers switching to Apple computers after being exposed to the iPod/iTunes combination), rather than from just iPod sales.

Apple's computer product line consisted of several models in various configurations. Its desktop lines included the Power Mac (aimed at professional users), the iMac (home and educational use), and the eMac (made specifically for educational use). Apple had two notebook product lines as well: PowerBook (for professional and business users) and iBook (for

Exhibit 2   **Apple's Net Sales by Operating Segment, Fiscal Years 2003–2005**

	September 24, 2005	Percent Change	September 25, 2004	Percent Change	September 27, 2003
Net sales by operating segment:					
Americas	$ 6,950	64%	$4,019	26%	$3,181
Europe	3,073	71	1,799	37	1,309
Japan	920	36	677	−3	698
Retail	2,350	98	1,185	91	621
Other segments[a]	998	67	599	51	398
Total net sales	$13,931	68%	$8,279	33%	$6,207
Net sales by product:					
Desktops[b]	$ 3,436	45%	$2,373	−4%	$2,475
Portables[c]	2,839	11	2,550	26	2,016
Total Macintosh sales	$ 6,275	27%	$4,923	10%	$4,491
iPod	4,540	248	1,306	279	345
Other music-related products and services[d]	899	223	278	672	36
Peripherals and other hardware[e]	1,126	18	951	38	691
Software, service, and other products[f]	1,091	33	821	27	644
Total	$13,931	68%	$8,279	33%	$6,207
Unit sales by product:					
Desktops[b]	$ 2,520	55%	$1,625	−8%	$1,761
Portables[c]	2,014	21	1,665	33	1,251
Total Macintosh unit sales	$ 4,534	38%	$3,290	9%	$3,012
Net sales per Macintosh unit sold[g]	$1,384	−7%	$1,496	0%	$1,491
iPod unit sales(in 000s)	22,497	409%	4,416	370%	939
Net revenue per iPod unit sold[h]	$202	−32%	$296	−19%	$367

Notes:

[a]Other Segments include Asia Pacific and FileMaker.

[b]Includes iMac, eMac, Mac mini, Power Mac and Xserve product lines.

[c]Includes iBook and PowerBook product lines.

[d]Consists of iTunes Music Store sales, iPod services, and Apple-branded and third-party iPod accessories.

[e]Includes sales of Apple-branded and third-party displays, wireless connectivity and networking solutions, and other hardware accessories.

[f]Includes sales of Apple-branded operating system, application software, third-party software, AppleCare, and Internet services.

[g]Derived by dividing total Macintosh net sales by total Macintosh unit sales.

[h]Derived by dividing total iPod net sales by total iPod unit sales.

Source: 2005 10-K report.

consumers and students). In both cases, the Power products were higher-end and offered more computing power at a premium price. The other models were lower on the price scale but still high relative to Wintel sellers, but had less power and fewer features.

To help drive customers toward its products, Apple released its first truly low-end computer in January 2005, the Mac Mini. This small computer, about the size of five CD cases, started at $499, but came without a keyboard or monitor. Sales of the Mini took off and lifted Apple's share of the U.S. PC market almost overnight. However, even with the large increase in sales, Apple remained a small player in the PC market as a whole (see Exhibit 3).

Exhibit 3   **U.S. Market Shares of Leading Personal Computer Manufacturers, Third-Quarter 2005 versus Third-Quarter 2004**

Company	Q3 2005	Q3 2004
Dell Inc.	30.7%	30.3%
Hewlett-Packard	19.1	19.1
Gateway	6.0	4.9
Lenovo/IBM	4.2	4.4
Apple Computer	4.2	3.2

Source: www.gartner.com (accessed October 25, 2005).

COMPETITORS IN THE PC MARKET

Dell

Dell, the industry leader in PC sales, recorded net revenues of almost $50 billion for the fiscal year ending in January 2005. Dell's revenues had been consistently growing, and this trend would continue into 2005. Of this revenue, about 40 percent came from sales of desktop PCs (see Exhibit 4). These PCs ranged from low-end bargain desktops to high-end gaming setups with the latest hardware and software. However, competition in the desktop market was lowering the profitability of desktop sales. Dell, a company that attempted to be a low-cost provider through supply chain and distribution logistics, was beginning to see a shift in consumer demand toward mobility products: laptops, MP3 players, and PDAs. Dell's notebook computers, like its desktops, ranged from low-end and low-priced to state-of-the-art and high-priced. The notebook segment showed promising revenue growth for Dell. The company also offered peripherals such as LCD televisions as it attempted to move into a role as a consumer electronics provider along with its role as a PC manufacturer.

Hewlett-Packard

Hewlett-Packard's Personal Systems Group, which included sales of PCs, accounted for about one-third

Exhibit 4   **Dell's Revenues by Product Category, First Nine Months, Fiscal 2006 versus Fiscal 2005**

Product Category	Percentage of Total Revenues for Nine Months Ended	
	October 28, 2005	October 29, 2004
Desktop PCs	38%	43%
Mobility products (notebook PCs, Dell DJ, Axim)	25	24
Printers, monitors, TVs, projectors, ink and toner cartridges	15	13
Servers and networking hardware	10	10
Professional consulting and support services	9	7
Storage products	3	3
Total	100%	100%

Source: Dell's 10-Q report for the third quarter of 2005.

of the company's revenues in fiscal year 2004. HP's biggest revenue producers were printers, printer supplies, other imaging products, servers, and information systems consulting services. The Personal Systems Group provided half of the company's net revenue growth from 2003 to 2004, however. Earnings from the division were only 0.9 percent of net revenues, though ($210 million in earnings on $24.6 billion in net revenues). Overall revenue growth in the Personal Systems Group broke down as shown in Exhibit 5.

The desktop and notebook lines were the key growth areas for HP. At one point, HP offered a branded version of Apple's iPod, but that relationship ended because the partnership wasn't helping HP as much as had been hoped. HP then moved to Microsoft-compatible devices but did not develop its own product for this market. Like Dell, HP offered desktops and notebooks in various configurations, with prices determined by the features offered and hardware contained in the systems. HP also offered peripherals such as televisions and related media devices.

Gateway

Gateway initially set itself apart from Dell, HP, and other PC brands by selling its wares through proprietary stores designed to give consumers a chance to test the systems they were considering purchasing. While this tactic worked for a time, by 2004 the stores were losing money for the company. Because of this, the company closed its stores and began focusing on selling through third-party retailers and online. Gateway also purchased eMachines in early 2004, acquiring a company that had a cost structure comparable to Dell's. This was important to Gateway, as the

company was not profitable, with a net loss of $568 million during fiscal 2004. Much of the increase in desktop sales during 2004 (see Exhibit 6) was due to the acquisition of eMachines. However, unlike many of its competitors, Gateway was not showing strong growth in the mobile (laptop) market.

Like its competitors, Gateway included high- and low-priced desktops and notebooks in its product line. Gateway also made a strong effort to sell its computers as media centers, using Microsoft's Media Center version of Windows XP. Gateway was one of the first computer manufacturers to venture into the consumer electronics side of the business, selling TVs and related peripherals to tie in to the media-center hub. Gateway, like HP, sold MP3 players from companies like Creative rather than developing its own product for the category.

MP3 PLAYER INDUSTRY

The personal electronics industry existed long before the iPod was popular. However, much of the history of the industry was related to the iPod's ancestors: portable music devices. Sony, with its Walkman product line, was one of the early giants in this sector of the personal electronics industry. The first Walkman appeared in 1979 in Japan. This device was a tape player that, notably, did not have a record function and was an innovative gamble by Sony's management. After a slow start, sales skyrocketed and music history was made. By 1995, over 150 million Walkman products had been sold worldwide. The Walkman line eventually included CD-playing devices.

The history of personal digital assistants (PDAs) reaches back almost as far as the history of portable

Exhibit 5 **Weighted Average Revenue Growth, Hewlett-Packard's Personal Systems Group, 2003–2004**

Product	Weighted Average Growth	
	2004	2003
Desktop PCs	7.9%	21.9%
Notebook PCs	7.1	19.6
Handhelds	0.7	2.0
Workstations	0.4	1.1
Other	—	(0.1)
Total Personal Systems Group growth	16.1%	44.5%

Source: Company records.

Exhibit 6   **Gateway's Sales of Personal Computer Products, 2002–2004 (in millions of $)**

Product Line	2004		2003		2002	
	Sales Revenues	% of Revenues	Sales Revenues	% of Revenues	Sales Revenues	% of Revenues
Desktop PCs	$1,982	54.3%	$1,649	48.4%	$2,600	62.3%
Mobile PCs	790	21.7	755	22.2	731	17.5
Servers	54	1.5	53	1.6	52	1.3
Non-PC products	823	22.5	946	27.0	788	18.9
Total	$3,650	100.0%	$3,402	100.0%	$4,171	100.0%

Source: Company financial reports.

music players. While Apple is often credited with making and distributing the first true PDA, there were many forerunners to Apple's Newton. Sharp, Toshiba, and Casio, among others, had products that mimicked the functions of PDAs. However, Apple's Newton was the first product to successfully bring the functionality into a package for mass marketing.[2]

As PDAs have become more and more functional in recent years, the line between them and portable computers has blurred. Microsoft's specialized edition of Windows for PDAs has further blurred this line. PDAs can sync with PC software and hold calendar events, task lists, and even documents. However, despite this increase in functionality, pure PDA sales declined leading up to 2005 and were expected to continue to fall. This decline was due not to a lack of demand for portable devices, but to a convergence between PDAs and other devices—particularly the cell phone.

The other major consumer electronics product of the past 25 years sector was the cellular telephone. The first public testing of cell phones was in Chicago in 1977, although a successful demonstration of cell phone technology had occurred as early as 1973. In 1982, the U.S. Federal Communications Commission (FCC) authorized commercial cellular service in the United States. By 1987, demand was so high (over 1 million users) that the original allocations for bandwidth were no longer sufficient. Changes and improvements were made to the technology, and the FCC allowed broader innovation in the industry. By 2000, there were over 100 million cell phone users in the United States.[3] The market for cell phones was expected to near 800 million units worldwide in 2005.[4]

The last 30 years of consumer electronics history were filled with companies expanding functionality and portability in products. At the same time, personal computers were getting smaller and creeping toward the market that these consumer electronics products historically filled. Apple's foray into the consumer electronics market with its iPod was a perfect example of this movement. The iPod had the functionality of a Walkman and many of the features found in PDAs: calendar, calculator, address book, and more. Microsoft's partnership with PDA market leader Palm, which put Windows in Palm's products, was another example of this convergence. Apple even moved toward the cell phone market through a partnership with Cingular and Motorola. The Motorola ROKR, though not the first phone to play music, was the first to have a portable version of Apple's iTunes built in.

While a number of the major computer manufacturers had entered the MP3 player industry, there were over 100 manufacturers offering MP3 players in the United States in 2006. Apple was the undisputed leader of the young market. In fact, it was the introduction of the user-friendly iPod in 2001 that spurred growth in the MP3 industry. By 2004, sales of portable audio players had reached 27.8 million units and Gartner, a U.S.-based research firm, predicted that over 150 million units would be shipped in 2010.

It was estimated that by the end of 2004, Apple had captured 83.7 percent of the hard-drive MP3 player market. HP, selling its own version of the iPod, followed with 3.6 percent of the market. Rio had 2.8 percent of the hard-drive MP3 player market, while Creative and iRiver had 2.6 percent and 1.5 percent of the market, respectively. In the flash-based segment, the top manufacturers of flash memory players were Apple (which controlled 46.3 percent of the market), SanDisk (which had captured 8.9 percent of the market), Rio (with 2.9 percent of the market), and Creative Labs (with 2.4 percent of the market).

The substantial growth in the market was fueled by (1) the increasing availability of digital music, both paid and pirated; (2) consumers' increasing familiarity with MP3 technology; and (3) the fact that in 2004 only 11 percent of the U.S. population owned an MP3 player. While the phenomenal growth in the MP3 player industry was expected to favor both of the main categories of players (flash-based and hard-drive players), flash-based players such as the iPod Nano were expected to disproportionately benefit from the growth.

IPOD AND ITUNES

Aside from the iPod's ease of use, one of the primary factors that contributed to the popularity of the iPod was Apple's iPod/iTunes combination. In fact, some analysts believed that, despite the acclaim that had been heaped on the iPod, the device would not achieved its dominant position without iTunes.

Apple first released the iTunes digital music management software for Macintosh computers in 2001. It was innovative, but not alone. Originally, the software was intended to allow users to store music from their compact discs (CDs) to their computer hard drives and make the content easily accessible. As features such as the ability to burn custom CDs were added to the software, iTunes became more and more useful to consumers.

When the iPod was released in 2001, iTunes was quickly adjusted to allow for syncing between the music management software and the new music player. This interface made it easy for consumers to move content from their computer to their iPod, an essential part of the product value of the iPod. While the iTunes software was a key component in Apple's strategy, it did not have a significant impact on iPod sales until the iTune's fourth edition was released in April 2003.

With the release of iTunes' fourth edition, Steve Jobs announced that he had reached a deal with the music industry's five major recording labels to sell their content in a copy-protected form via the iTunes online music store—and the world took notice. This announcement marked the first time that such a large library of popular music was available in one place via a simple method. Jobs was able to negotiate the agreement with the music companies for two main

reasons: First, the recording labels were eager to offer a legitimate online source for their music that would reduce the flow of pirated music. Second, the music Apple provided at iTunes was compressed using Apple's proprietary Advanced Audio Coding (ACC) and was protected with Apple's Fairplay Digital Rights Management system, one of the strongest in the country.

In October 2003, a version of the iTunes software, including the iTunes music store, was released for Windows users. This immediately opened up Apple's music store to millions of users who had previously been shut out. By October 2005, Apple had introduced a new version of iTunes that sold not only music but video as well. This version of iTunes was released in conjunction with Apple's video iPods. As with the original launch of iTunes, Apple formed partnerships with major networks such as ABC, NBC, ESPN, and Disney to make content such as television shows, sports programming, newscasts, and children's shows available in a secure, encoded format. In the first 20 days of offering video, Apple reported that it sold over 1 million videos. Most important, Apple's innovative iTunes was again the first company to really enter the digital music market, and the digital video industry, in a big way. When Apple's iTunes became a major hit in 2003, it ushered in the digital music era for mainstream computer users and encouraged new competitors to enter the market. There was little doubt that competition for the digital video segment would be significant as well.

Apple: The iPod and the iPod Mini

In fiscal year 2003, Apple Computer Inc. reported net revenues of $6.2 billion (up 8.1 percent from 2002) and net income of $69 million. For much of the company's history, Apple had excelled at being the first company to introduce a concept or a new product but had then struggled to maintain its market share in that product line. Although Apple didn't introduce the first portable MP3 player (EigerLabs did in 1998), its iPod, introduced in October 2001, was the first such device to gain widespread attention and popularity.

Many critics did not give the iPod much of a chance for success, because its launch came about one month after the September 11 terrorist attacks and because it carried a fairly hefty price tag of

$399. However, the success of the iPod reached phenomenal proportions, leading one analyst to say that "it is now a fashion statement, and any other MP3 player is considered 'Brand X' for many consumers."[5] Industry experts agreed that the iPod's success revolutionized the portable music industry as the Sony Walkman had in 1980.

By June 2005, Apple's iPod models accounted for well over 70 percent of the hard-drive MP3 player market and more than 40 percent of the flash-based player market. In December 2005, the iPod was available in many models:

- The iPod Shuffle, a flash memory player with no screen that was about the size of a pack of chewing gum, was offered in either a 512 megabyte (MB) model with the capacity for about 120 songs ($99), and in a 1 gigabyte (GB) model that could hold 240 songs ($149).

- The iPod Nano, a flash-based player that was about the size of a credit card, but thicker, was offered in a 2GB model that held 500 songs ($199) and a 4GB model that held 100 songs ($249). The Nano also had games, a calendar with an appointment scheduler, a contact manager, a world clock, a stopwatch, and password protection. It allowed the user to create custom playlists without a computer and could hold up to 25,000 photos.

- The iPod, a hard-drive player, was offered in a 30GB version that could hold 7,500 songs, 25,000 photos, or 75 hours of video ($299) and in a 60GB version that could hold 15,000 songs, 25,000 photos, or over 150 hours of video. Like the Nano, the iPod had games, a calendar with an appointment scheduler, a contact manager, a world clock, a stopwatch, and password protection, and it allowed the user to create custom playlists without a computer. However, the iPod also allowed users to play video.

All of Apple's iPods featured a thumb wheel, a concept that Apple first introduced in MP3 players, which served as the tool for scrolling through playlists and other menus on the iPod interfaces. When comparing the iPod with other competing products, most critics agreed that Apple's simple and elegant interface was superior to most competitors' and made the product especially attractive to consumers who were new to the MP3 player industry and were willing to pay a premium for the simplicity. Another fairly unique feature was that the iPod included a calendar, a contact list, and a to-do list. These features allowed the iPods to meet both the music and PDA needs of their owners, who thus did not have to carry two separate units to accomplish both tasks. The iPod also featured some unique antipiracy software: If the iPod was connected to a foreign computer (one that it did not recognize) and the user tried to transfer music files either to or from the computer, the software would give the user a choice—either stop the transfer or proceed with it and the newly transferred music would delete every file that was on the iPod, essentially overwriting it and replacing it.

While each new version of the iPod offered innovative technology, the introductions were not without their challenges. The original iPods were criticized for poor battery life, and eventually users brought a class-action lawsuit against Apple claiming that Apple had misrepresented the life of the rechargeable battery used in the iPod. Although Apple denied this claim, it offered a battery replacement service for $99 and offered to settle the suit in June 2005, offering purchasers of first-, second-, and third-generation iPods an extended warranty and a $50 voucher. Apple also experienced problems with the launch of the Nano in 2005, with customer complaints related to the tendency of the device to freeze and to the ease with the device, especially the screen, scratched or stopped functioning. Apple offered a repair and replacement service for these devices, but it expected to face a class-action suit similar to the one filed over battery-life problem.

Regardless of these challenges, a 2005 customer survey by *PC Magazine* showed that Apple iPods ranked significantly higher than other brands of MP3 players in terms of overall quality, sound quality, ease of use, and overall reliability (see Exhibit 7). By the end of 2005, many iPod fans were eagerly awaiting the next version of the iPod, and the competition was working diligently to take a bite out of Apple's market share.

COMPETITION IN THE MP3 PLAYER INDUSTRY

Creative Labs

Creative Labs first became famous for its Sound Blaster sound cards, which set the standard in PC audio in 1989. Since that time, Creative had been an

Exhibit 7   **Customer Satisfaction with MP3 Players, Based on a Reader Survey by *PC Magazine*, 2005 (Scale: 10 = High; 1 = Low)**

Brand of MP3 Players	Sound Quality	Ease of Use	Reliability	Overall Satisfaction
Apple	8.8	8.8	8.5	8.6
Creative	8.2	7.5	7.9	7.6
Dell	8.1	7.9	7.9	7.7
iRiver	8.6	7.2	8.3	7.9
RCA	7.4	7.0	7.3	6.8
Rio	7.8	7.5	7.5	7.1
SanDisk	7.7	6.9	7.7	7.1
Sony	8.0	7.4	7.7	7.3
Average	8.1	7.5	7.9	7.6

Source: Compiled by the case authors from information in *PC Magazine* November 8, 2005, www.pcmag.com (accessed January 8, 2006).

industry leader in PC audio technology and had built a large user base and strong brand name in this area. Leveraging this position, Creative offered the broadest and most diverse product line of MP3 players. Additionally, Creative had won the prestigious Best of CES (Consumer Electronics Show) Award three years in a row with its Zen Portable Media Center in 2004, the Zen Microphoto in 2005, and the Zen Vision:M in 2006. The 30GB Zen Vision:M ($299), which also was named the best overall product at CES in 2006, was about the same size as an iPod 30GB, although twice as thick, and could play back music, video, and photos; it also included a personal organizer that would sync with Microsoft Outlook to transfer the user's calendar, contacts, and task list. This player was viewed as the first real competition to the iPod video, as it would hold about as much content as the iPod but had a superior screen, a battery that lasted twice as long as the iPod's, an FM tuner, and a voice recorder.

Creative's product line also included:

- The 30GB Zen Vision ($399) multimedia player, which used Windows Media Center Edition software and allowed users to listen to, record, and play back WMAs and MP3s (up to 16,000 songs) and movies and television shows (up to 120 hours of video), to view photos (over 20,000), and to listen to and record FM radio.

- The 20GB Zen Sleek ($230) photo player, which held up to 10,000 songs or thousands of photos and featured a 19-hour rechargeable battery, a voice recorder, an FM radio tuner, and an organizer that would sync with Microsoft Outlook.

- The 8GB Zen Microphoto ($249), which featured a 15-hour rechargeable battery, a color screen, 10 different colors, an FM radio and recorder, a personal organizer that synced with Microsoft Outlook, a sleep timer, and a capacity of 4,000 songs

- The 5GB Zen Neeon ($199), which was offered in six colors and had an LED that had seven color options. This player held 2,500 songs, included a 16-hour rechargeable battery, an FM tuner and recorder, a voice recorder, and a line-in port that allowed users to recorder directly from a CD player, a record player, or a mixing turntable.

- The flash-based 512MB ($109) or 1GB ($139.99) Zen Nano Plus, which was about the size of the iPod shuffle, was offered in 10 colors, used a single AAA battery (for up to 18 hours of playback), and held up to 500 songs. The Zen Nano offered a monochrome LED, an FM tuner, a voice recorder, and a line-in recorder.

Like the other hard-drive models, the Nomad Zen Xtra players doubled as external hard drives and could carry any type of files, not just music or MP3 files. Creative's players also allowed users to slow down a song while it was playing without ruining the pitch or to speed up an audio file (such as a book) without making it sound nonsensical.[6] Downsides to the Creative products were that the car adapter kit had to be purchased separately and that the user had to purchase online music from other sources.

Creative also offered nine MP3 players under the MuVo brand, ranging from the Creative MuVo Micro, which was offered in eight colors, claimed a

15-hour battery life from a single AAA battery, and included an FM tuner and the ability to record from the tuner, to the MuVo Sport ($99), which was a splash-proof 256MB player that offered memory expansion through SD or MMC cards and included a stopwatch, an armband, and a case as well as an FM tuner.

In Creative's fiscal year ending June 30, 2005, the company experienced an operating loss of $68.5 million on a net sales of $1.2 billion, as compared to an operating income of $44.2 million on net sales of $814 million in 2004. However, the company had strongly reinforced its dedication to the MP3 player market in 2006 and beyond, and had declared its intention to be a leader in this dynamic market.

Dell

Dell was best known for its direct business model in the personal computer industry and had the leading market share in the United States and worldwide in 2005. In fiscal year 2006, Dell reported a net income of approximately $3.6 billion on net revenues of $55.9 billion (a 14 percent increase in net revenue from 2005). A longtime supplier of customized PCs, Dell was a relatively new entry to the personal electronics market, introducing the Dell Digital Jukebox (Dell DJ), a personal MP3 player that was a direct competitor to Apple's hard-drive players, in October 2003.

As with most other MP3 players, Dell DJ users could either download music from the Internet to the device or "rip" tracks from their CD collection and load them onto the device. The Dell DJ was both physically and technically similar to the iPod and, in early 2005, was available in three hard-drive models. The 5GB Pocket DJ (similar to the iPod Mini) held 2,500 songs ($179); the 20GB DJ held about 9,900 songs (128-bit rate) and sold for $179; and the 30GB model held up to 15,000 songs compressed at the same bit rate and sold regularly for $299 (but was occasionally sold by Dell for as low as $254). The Dell DJ also claimed 12 hours of battery life with continuous play, although some consumers found that the device could last for up to 23 hours of play.[7] Additionally, the Dell DJ, like any other voice recorder, allowed the user to record sound, while the iPod users had to purchase a kit that allowed external sound recording.

Although a relatively late entrant to the MP3 player market, Dell had long recognized consumers' interest in, and demand for, electronics that catered to digital music fans. As early as 1999, Dell had begun offering PC customization features such as a CD-recordable disk drive, specialized software for managing a digital music library, and of course the jukebox software necessary to play all the digital music on a PC. Dell saw its recent forays into computer peripherals and other electronics such as the Digital Jukebox as a natural extension of its product line. Dell was committed to building a relatively diversified product line to afford the company a more constant and steady stream of income than it realized on personal computers alone. Overall, Dell's product rated well against Apple and other competitors, especially given the size and strength of the company and its success in other electronics areas. Although some critics argued that it was not as aesthetically pleasing or quite as easy to use as the iPod, the Dell DJ was considered a very solid contender in the MP3 player market. With Dell's price advantage and much more flexibility concerning where users could shop for their digital music, it was suggested that many consumers might decide the iPod was not worth the extra cash and lack of options.

In September 2005, Dell introduced the DJ Ditty, a 512MB flash player that was about the size of an iPod shuffle but included a screen and an integrated FM tuner. The Ditty weighed only 1.29 ounces, held 220 songs, and would play for up to 14 hours. In October 2005, Dell announced that in 2006 it would offer a third-generation Dell DJ and Pocket DJ that would be capable of receiving XM radio, with the appropriate docking equipment, and would be able to play recorded XM radio streams. It was expected that the third-generation DJs would offer a color screen, as opposed to the second-generation's monochrome blue display. However, in January 2006, the only Dell-branded MP3 player offered at the company's Web site was the Ditty, but customers could purchase a variety of 5GB, 8GB, 20GB, and 30GB Creative Labs MP3 players from Dell's site. While Dell had announced a 2006 launch of its third generation of players in October 2005, the lack of any Dell micro-drive or hard-drive players on the company's site left its future in the MP3 player industry unclear.

iRiver

In 2005, iRiver produced multimedia players, hard-drive-based players, flash-based players, and CD players. The company's 20GB multimedia player, the PMC-120 ($499.99), offered a widescreen color display (3.5 inches) and used Microsoft's Media Center interface to connect with Windows Media Player. The PMC-120 held 80 hours of video or

600 hours of music and offered a rechargeable battery that provided 5 hours of video playback or up to 14 hours of audio playback. The iRiver H10 audio jukebox players included two 20GB ($299) models, as well as a 6GB ($279) and a 5GB ($229) player. The H10 MP3 players were the first to be fully compatible with Microsoft's PlaysForSure platform and allowed users to play music or view photos; they also included an integrated FM tuner and recorder, an integrated voice recorder, and a rechargeable battery that lasted approximately 16 hours. Furthermore, the user interface of the iRiver models was versatile, allowing users to customize the buttons and the method of scrolling through the music. Like RCA, Rio, and Creative, iRiver users could shop for music at almost any online store other than Sony's or Apple's. Additionally, the screens of iRiver's players included a significant amount of information about the song currently playing, as well as the status of the machine, such as volume and battery levels.

In its Ultra Portable Players category, iRiver also offered seven flash players, ranging from the u10 multimedia player, offered in 1GB and 512MB models, to the 100 series, offered in 256MB and 128MB models. All of the players in this category played WMA and MP3 music and offered an integrated FM tuner and recorder, and a voice recorder. The 1GB u10 ($249) played music (up to 34 hours of WMA or MP3) and video, displayed photos, and included some limited games, an ultrabright 2.2-inch screen, and a rechargeable battery that would last up to 28 hours. The T30 series, offered in 1GB ($149.99) and 512MB ($99.99) models, offered up to 24 hours of battery life on a single AAA battery and could record music from any source, with no PC required. The T10 series, offered in 1GB ($199.99) and 512MB models ($149.99), had a color display and played for up to 45 hours on a single AA battery. The 700 series ranged in size from 1GB ($179.99) to 128MB ($79.99), but also offered a waterproof case ($99.99) that allowed users to take their iRiver player swimming or surfing. At the low end, iRiver offered its 100 series in 256MB ($99.99) and 128MB ($79.99) models. Even these low-end players offered a screen, an FM tuner, an integrated voice and FM recorder, and long battery life from a single AA battery.

At the end of 2005, iRiver had a dominant position in Korea's MP3 player market. The Korea-based ReignCom, iRiver's parent company, estimated that the company controlled 50 percent of the Korean market. In the U.S. market, ReignCom acknowledged that it was having a more difficult time, but it intended for iRiver to capture 15 percent of the North American and global hard-drive MP3 player market. Additionally, ReignCom intended future iRiver portable media players to be Wi-Fi enabled and to include more portable Internet and gaming applications.

RCA

RCA was owned and manufactured by Thomson Worldwide, which earned a net income of 373 million euros in 2004, up from 26 million euros in 2003. Thompson's RCA division released its first portable MP3 player, called the Lyra, in 1999. In 2005, RCA offered a relatively broad range of players, including the Lyra.2780 portable multimedia player, flash players (ranging from 128MB to 1G, some with secure digital expansion slots), hard-drive players (with 5GB or less of capacity except the Lyra 2780, with 20GB capacity), and the Lyra CD player with MP3 playback. RCA's Lyra players supported either MP3 or WMA music files, which allow users to shop for music from any online music store or subscription service.

Similar to other MP3 players with internal hard drives, the Lyra players could be used for file or data storage, similar to a computer hard drive. The Lyra 2780 ($399.99) featured a 20B hard drive that could store up to 80 hours of video and a compact flash slot to allow users to easily transfer audio or video to the player, or to view pictures from a digital camera. Lyra's other three models of hard-drive players were similar to other industry offerings and included the 5GB RD2763 ($179.99), which featured a built-in FM transmitter for playing music in a car; the 4GB RD2762 ($199.99), which featured a color screen; and the 5GB RD2765 ($229.99), which offered a color screen with icons, a JPG viewer for album art, and upgraded earphones.

RCA's line of flash-based players offered more variety than its hard-drive players. The flash-based Lyras included:

- The M100 ($119.99) series, which was a 1GB player that had a screen and plugged directly into a computer like a thumb drive.
- The RD 22 series, which ranged in size from 256MB ($99.99) to 1GB ($169.99) and featured an LCD screen, a 50-hour battery life, a digital FM tuner with FM record, a stopwatch, a calorie counter, and a pulse rate monitor.
- The RD10 series, which ranged in size from 128MB ($89.99) to 256MB ($149.99) and in-

cluded a digital FM turner and an expansion card slot for external SD/MMC memory.

- The RD 23 series, which featured a dual orientation backlit LCD screen that allowed users to view the LCD from multiple angles, and ranged in size from 256MB ($99.99) to 1GB ($169.99). These players also included a digital FM tuner with FM record and allowed for voice recording and line-in recording form multiple sources.

RCA's Lyras shipped with MusicMatch Jukebox software, which users could install on their computer to allow music to be loaded and unloaded from their MP3 player. The MusicMatch software also played the music on the PC itself and allowed users to convert and transfer music from their own CDs to their MP3 players.

Rio

Rio was the second company to introduce an MP3 player in the United States when it launched the Rio in 1998, but by 2005 the company was fighting to survive in the dynamic industry. Recognizing Rio's position, its parent company D&M Holdings Inc. decided to exit the business and sold Rio's assets to SigmaTel Inc., a leading supplier of integrated circuits for the portable digital audio player market. With this acquisition, one of the founders of the MP3 player industry was out of the game. SigmaTel believed that it could leverage its production efficiencies and Rio's brand name to revive the struggling MP3 player manufacturer, and by January 2006 the company listed four models of MP3 players on its site. However, these models were not available from major online retailers such as Amazon.com. The models listed on Rio's site, all MP3 and WMA compatible, included:

- The 5GB Rio Carbon ($130), a 5GB player (competitive with the iPod Mini) that held about 1,250 songs compressed at 128 Kbps. The unit could be charged through an electrical outlet or through a computer's USB port, and the rechargeable battery's life was claimed to be 20 hours. The Carbon also allowed voice recordings, like the Dell, and was supported on either PC or Mac operating systems. The carbon was available in a pearl-colored casing.
- The 2.5GB Rio ce2100, a hard-drive model that held about 625 songs. Its 20-hour rechargeable battery could be charged either from a computer or an electrical wall outlet.

- The Rio Forge, a flash-based player ranging from 128MB to 512MB and included a memory expansion slot, a stopwatch and lap timer, an FM tuner, and a battery life of up to 20 hours.
- Rio's se510, was basically the same as the Forge. While it did not offer an FM tuner, it did include an armband for wearing the unit while working out.

SanDisk

A new entrant in the flash-based MP3 player market, SanDisk, a leader in digital memory manufacturing, shipped its first players in May 2005. SanDisk's original offerings included the 512MB Sansa e130 (240 songs in WMA format) and the 1GB Sansa e140 (up to 480 songs in WMA format). SanDisk's players featured an SD slot for additional storage and a digital FM radio receiver, and they were claimed to be able to last up to 17 hours on a single AAA battery. SanDisk's players also offered a multiline backlit LCD that provided the title, artists, and album of the song currently being played. In September 2005, SanDisk began offering a car transmitter that would allow users to play MP3 music through a car radio, and a portable speaker dock for Sansa MP3 players. In 2006, SanDisk planned aggressively expand its product line to include:

- The SanDisk Sansa e200, which would be offered in 2GB (480 songs), 4GB (960 songs), and 6GB (1,440 songs) capacities. The e200 series would feature a metal case, a color screen, a removable rechargeable battery, a microSD memory expansion slot, and a digital FM tuner and recorder.
- The SanDisk Sansa c10, which SanDisk planned to offer in 1GB (240 songs) and 2B (480 songs) capacities. The c10 models featured a color screen, a digital FM tuner and recorder, and one AAA battery.
- The Sansa m200, which became available in January 2006 and was offered in 512MB ($79.99, 120 songs), 1GB ($119.99, 240 songs) and 2GB ($159.99, 480 songs) capacities. The m200 series featured 19 hours of play from a single AAA battery, an FM tuner and recorder, a voice recorder with a built-in microphone, and a backlit LCD display.
- The SanDisk Sansa e100 series, which was introduced in January 2006 and was offered in 512MB ($79.99, 120 songs) and 1GB ($119.99,

240 songs) capacities. The e10 players featured a backlit multiline LCD display, a digital FM tuner, and up to 17 hours of play from a single AAA battery.

- The SanDisk digital audio player, which was introduced in January 2006 in 256MB ($49.99, 60 songs), 512MB ($79.99, 120 songs), and 1GB ($119.99, 240 songs) capacities. The digital audio players featured 15 hours of play from a single AAA battery, a digital FM tuner, a voice recorder with a built-in microphone, and a backlit multiline display.

While SanDisk operated only in the flash-based seg-ment, there was little doubt that the company intended to leverage its expertise in flash-based manufacturing and distribution to compete vigorously in the MP3 player industry.

Sony

In fiscal-year 2005, Sony Corporation earned $1.5 billion in net income (up 85 percent from 2004) on revenues of $66.9 billion in revenue (down 4.5 percent from 2004). Sony became the original pioneer in the portable music industry when it introduced the Walkman portable cassette tape player in the 1980s. That product spawned dozens of imitations and look-alikes. Prior to 2004, Sony had been active in the digital music industry but had resisted selling portable players that were MP3-compatible, arguing that its proprietary compression technology, Acoustic TRansform Adaptive Coding (ATRAC3), was superior to MP3. However, in the face of declining sales, Sony relented in August 2004 and released its first hard-drive-based MP3-compatible player, the 20GB Sony Network Walkman, and released an MP3-compatible flash player by year's end. Additionally, Sony allowed users of some earlier hard-drive-based players to upgrade to MP3 compatibility for a fee of $20. However, by this time roles were reversed and Sony was viewed as one of the imitators in the digital music industry.

In 2004 and 2005, Sony expanded its line of MP3 players. New offerings included 40GB Vaio Pocket Digital Music Player ($399), which allowed users to download photos as well as music, and the Psyc Network Walkman, which was intended to be a direct competitor to Apple's Shuffle. The Psyc had the option to shuffle songs and was available in a

256MB model ($89), a 512MB model ($99), and a 1GB model ($149).

This move meant Sony was finally competing on a more level playing field with Apple in terms of the price of the models and their capacities. In terms of physical characteristics, the 20GB Walkman was about 10 percent smaller than the iPod in total volume, was about one-third lighter than the iPod, and had a much better battery life (up to 30 hours).[8] However, critics generally viewed the Network Walkman as somewhat inferior to other MP3 players. The user interface on the machine was found by some to be confusing and difficult to use, and the accompanying computer software for unloading and managing the music was thought to be weaker than the competition. Critics believed that these perceived weaknesses coupled with the company's late entry to the digital music market indicated that the company would encounter significant trouble in overcoming the competition.

In the face of competitive pressures, by January 2006, Sony no longer offered a hard-drive-based MP3 player, but did offer three models of flash-based players, a CD player, a minidisc player, and a boom box that were all MP3 and ATRAC compatible and that were compatible with Sony's Connect online music store. Sony's flash-based models included the Walkman Core, the Walkman Bean, and the Walkman Circ. The Walkman Core was available in 512MB ($129.95, 345 songs) and 1GB models ($149.95, 695 songs) and included a three-line display and a rechargeable battery that lasted up to 50 hours and could be quick-charged in 3 minutes for 3 hours of play. The Walkman Bean was a small, ergonomic player that was shaped like a bean and came in white, pink, black, and blue. This model was offered in 512MB ($109.95, 345 songs) and 1GB ($139.95, 695 songs) options and featured a one-line display, a built-in FM tuner and a rechargeable battery that lasted 50 hours and could be quick-charged in 3 minutes for 3 hours of play. The Walkman Circ was a round player that had a diameter about twice the size of a quarter. The Circ was powered by an AA battery that would last up to 70 hours and was offered in both 512MB ($89.95, 345 songs) and 1GB ($119.95, 695 songs) sizes, which both included a two-line display.

Sony's CD-based MP3 players included a portable CD player, a minidisc player, and a boom box. Sony's MP3 CD Walkman ($39.95) featured a compact full-circle design and MP3 playback of prerecorded tracks or user-recorded CD-R/RW media. The Hi-MD Walkman Digital Music Player ($299.95) offered a six-line display, a remote control, the ability to record from multiple sources using the line-in, mic-in capabilities, a digital amplifier, and a rechargeable battery that would last up to 33 hours. The Psyc ($79.95) MP3/ATRAC3 CD/Tuner Boom-box included a two-line display, a remote control with 10-key direct access, an AM/FM digital tuner, and AC/DC power; it could hold 490 songs (compressed with Sony's proprietary ATRAC3plus) on a single CD.

THE FUTURE

Heading into 2006, Apple had much to be excited about. During the 2005 holiday season, the company had sold 14 million digital media players, up from 4.5 million in the same period of 2004, and reported record revenues for the quarter of $5.7 billion compared to $3.5 billion in the same quarter of 2004. In the digital music segment, Apple had also expanded its agreements with automobile manufacturers to build iPod accessories, such as iPod docks, into new cars. Additionally, Apple introduced a new line of Apple computers that were based on Intel chips six months ahead of schedule. Apple also announced that, in February 2006, it would ship its new MacBook Pro, which was four times faster than the company's current PowerBooks and was designed in a manner consistent with the company's dedication to products that were powerful, easy to use, and aesthetically pleasing. These new Macs included a program named iLife '06, which included tools to enable users to edit movies, digital photographs, and homegrown music, as well as iWeb, which allowed users to easily create and upload Web sites, blogs, and podcasts. Additionally, the new MacBooks were expected to have a new piece of software named Front Row, which was targeted squarely at Microsoft's Media Center. This software served as a simple user interface for accessing digital media on the computer.

However, Apple also faced some significant challenges. Microsoft planned on releasing its new operating system, Vista, late in 2006. Vista was designed to enhance the ease of use of Windows-based computers and to make multimedia content development and editing easier. Additionally, in the rush to provide digital entertainment to the living room, competitors were becoming more diverse. Microsoft's new gaming console, the Xbox 360, integrated the gaming console and the PC and was set to become even more widely available. Sony's and Nintendo's counters to the new Xbox 360 were expected sometime early in 2006. In the digital music market, Microsoft partnered with MTV to announce a new online media service named Urge, which was targeted directly at Apple's iTunes. Microsoft planned, upon Urge's launch, to have 2 million songs available for purchase, and to offer video clips. Unlike iTunes, Urge was expected to offer a subscription service as well as allowing customers to purchase individual songs.

In assessing Apple's future, most analysts agreed that Apple would undoubtedly continue its well-established track record of introducing innovative, high-quality consumer electronics to the masses. However, many believed that it would be very difficult for Apple to maintain its substantial market share indefinitely, recognizing that it was much easier to control 60 percent of the digital music player market when only 11 percent of the U.S. population owned the devices than it would be when they were more common. Additionally, analysts acknowledged that Apple had once lost a big lead in the operating systems market because it refused to license to others and it appeared that Apple was making the same gamble in the MP3 player and digital music industries. The question was whether Apple had enough of a lead to maintain its status as the market leader. Would the company's refusal to license its technology to others eventually relegate it to the same niche position in the MP3 player industry that the company occupied in computers?

Endnotes

[1]Peter J. Howe, "Powered by iPod, Apple Splits Stock," *Knight Ridder Tribune Business News*, February 12, 2005, p. 1.
[2]www.snarc.net/pda/pda-treatise.htm.
[3]www.inventors.about.com.
[4]www.redherring.com.
[5]Steve Smith, "iPod's Lessons," *Twice New York* 19, no. 5 (July 26, 2004), p. 12.

[6]Bill Machrone, "New Music Players Gun for the iPod," *PC Magazine*, August 17, 2004, pp. 34–35.
[7]Peter Rojas, "Feeding Power-Hungry Gadgets," *Money* 33, no. 5 (May 2004), pp. 131–32.
[8]Walter S. Mossberg, "The Mossberg Solution: Sony's iPod Killer," *The Wall Street Journal (Eastern Ed.)*, July 28, 2004, p. D1.

Case 8

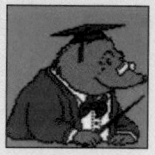

Netflix versus Blockbuster versus Video-on-Demand

Braxton Maddox
The University of Alabama

Arthur A. Thompson
The University of Alabama

Heading into 2006, Netflix had convinced most skeptics that its pioneering business model for renting DVDs online could be profitable. Netflix had attracted some 3.6 million subscribers who paid monthly fees ranging from $9.99 to $47.99; subscribers went to Netflix's Web site, selected one or more movies from its library of 55,000 titles, and received the DVDs by first-class mail within one to three business days. Subscribers could keep a DVD for as long as they wished, with no due dates or late fees, although they were limited to having a certain number of DVDs in their possession at any one time (the number depended on which fee plan they had chosen). A unique aspect of Netflix's business model was that it provided subscribers with all the benefits of a typical movie rental store but without the hassle of having to drive to the store, pick out DVDs, and return the rentals by a specified time.

However, Netflix's rapid growth and profit outlook had a major downside—they had induced movie rental leader Blockbuster to enter the online movie rental segment and try to horn in on the market opportunity that Netflix was exploiting. Amazon.com was also looking at entering the market. Wal-Mart had pursued online movie rentals for a short time, but in May 2005 it decided to enter into an arrangement with Netflix whereby Wal-Mart would refer customers interested in online DVD rentals to Netflix while Netflix would steer customers wanting to purchase a movie DVD to www.walmart.com. Wal-Mart's existing DVD rental customers were offered the option of becoming Netflix subscribers at the current Wal-Mart rate for one year from their sign-up date. Wal-Mart was motivated to team up with Netflix because its own online movie rental business presented an assortment of troublesome operating problems and was unprofitable, and because it saw more opportunity in focusing on the growing numbers of customers who were buying movie DVDs at www.walmart.com. Entry barriers into online DVD rentals were relatively low, but the barriers to profitability were considered rather high because of the need to attract a subscriber base of 2 to 4 million in order to operate at a profit.

Reed Hastings, founder and CEO of Netflix, was concerned about how to outcompete Blockbuster, and he was also concerned about the competitive threat posed by video-on-demand (VOD). Several new competitors were gearing up to offer movies on a pay-per-view basis to Internet customers with high-speed broadband connections. Providing VOD had been technically possible for a number of years, but VOD had not garnered substantial usage because movie studios were leery of the potential for movie pirating and doubtful of whether they could profit from a VOD business model. Nonetheless, the major Hollywood studios had formed a joint venture called MovieLink to offer VOD to the public. And several ambitious start-up companies, like San Francisco–based GreenCine, were offering online movie viewing to consumers who had Microsoft's Windows Media Player installed on their PCs and a broadband Internet connection. Once they downloaded a movie, consumers could play it on their desktop or laptop PCs or connect the PC to a TV.

Hastings's challenge was how to sustain Netflix's growth and put together a strategy that would protect Netflix's industry-leading position against mounting competition. In Hastings's view, "No one is going to out-hare Netflix. Our danger is in a tortoise attack."

COMPANY BACKGROUND AND STRATEGY

After successfully founding his first company, Pure Software, in 1991, Reed Hastings engineered several acquisitions and grew Pure Software into one of the 50 largest software companies in the world—the company's principal product was a debugging tool for engineers. When Pure Software was acquired by Rational Software in 1997 for $750 million, Hastings used the money from selling his shares of Pure Software to help fund his pursuit of another, entirely different business venture. Sensing the opportunity for online movie rentals in a climate where the popularity of the Interet was mushrooming, he founded Netflix in 1997, launched the online subscription service in 1999, and attracted a subscriber base of over 2 million in just four years (America Online took six years to acquire the same number of subscribers). Exhibit 1 shows trends in Netflix's subscriber growth.

By 2005, in what proved to be a rapidly evolving marketplace, Netflix had made a name for itself. It was the world's largest online DVD movie rental service, with 2005 revenues approaching $700 million and a selection of movie titles that far exceeded those available in local brick-and-mortar movie rental stores. Its strategy and market success were predicated on providing an expansive selection of DVDs, an easy way to choose movies, and fast, free delivery—the goal was to deliver customer value by eliminating the hassle involved in choosing, renting, and returning movies. Netflix's DVD lineup included everything from the latest big Hollywood releases to hard-to-locate documentaries to independent films to TV shows and how-to videos.

Exhibit 1   **Subscriber Data for Netflix, 2000–2005**

	1999	2000	2001	2002	2003	2004	First Nine Months, 2005
Total subscribers at beginning of period	0	107,000	292,000	456,000	857,000	1,487,000	2,610,000
Gross subscriber additions during period	127,000	515,000	566,000	1,140,000	1,571,000	2,716,000	2,573,000
Subscriber cancellations during the period	20,000	330,000	402,000	739,000	941,000	1,593,000	1,591,000
Total subscribers at end of period	107,000	292,000	456,000	857,000	1,487,000	2,610,000	3,592,000
Net subscriber additions during the period	107,000	185,000	164,000	401,000	630,000	1,123,000	982,000
Free trial subscribers*	n.a.	n.a.	56,000	61,000	71,000	124,000	169,000
Subscriber acquisition cost	$110.79	$49.96	$37.16	$31.39	$31.79	$36.09	$36.92

n.a. = Not available.

*First-time subscribers automatically were eligible for a free two-week trial; membership fees began after the two-week trial expired (unless the membership was canceled).

Members had the choice of eight subscription plans:

- $9.99, unlimited DVDs, one title out at a time.
- $11.99, four DVDs a month, two titles out at a time.
- $14.99, unlimited DVDs, two titles out at a time.
- $17.99, unlimited DVDs, three titles out at a time.
- $23.99, unlimited DVDs, four titles out at a time.
- $29.99, unlimited DVDs, five titles out at a time.
- $35.99, unlimited DVDs, six titles out at a time.
- $41.99, unlimited DVDs, seven titles out at a time.
- $47.99, unlimited DVDs, eight titles out at a time.

The most popular plan in 2005 was $17.99 a month. Subscribers could cancel anytime. Subscribers were drawn to Netflix's policies of no late fees and no due dates (which eliminated the hassle of getting DVDs back to local rental stores by the designated due date), and the convenience of being provided a postage-paid return envelope for mailing the DVDs back to Netflix. Netflix provided subscribers extensive information about DVD movies, including critic reviews, member reviews, online trailers, ratings, and personalized movie recommendations. Subscribers could create a "wish list" of all the movies they wanted to see, change the list at any time, and use the list to order their next round of movies.

Netflix's Cinematch Software Technology

Netflix had developed proprietary software technology, called Cinematch, which enabled it to provide subscribers with personalized movie recommendations every time they visited the Netflix Web site. These personalized recommendations were based on a subscriber's individual likes and dislikes (determined by their wish list, rental history, and movie ratings). Cinematch was an Oracle database that organized Netflix's library of movies into clusters of similar movies and analyzed how customers rated

them after they rented them. Those customers who rated similar movies in similar clusters were then matched as like-minded viewers. When a customer was online, Cinematch looked at the clusters the subscriber had rented from in the past, determined which movies the customer had yet to rent in that cluster, and recommended only those movies in the cluster that had been highly rated by viewers. The recommendations helped subscribers quickly identify films they might like to rent and allowed Netflix to promote lesser-known, high-quality films to subscribers who otherwise might have missed spotting them in the company's massive 55,000-film library (to which new titles were continuously being added).

In December 2005 Netflix had more than 1 billion movie ratings from customers in its database, and the average subscriber had rated more than 200 movies. On average, more than 85 percent of the movie titles in the Netflix library of offerings were rented each quarter, an indication of the effectiveness of the company's Cinematch software in steering subscribers to movies of interest. Netflix management believed that over 50 percent of its rentals came from the recommendations generated by Cinematch.

Shipping

Netflix had 37 regional shipping centers scattered across the United States, giving it one-business-day delivery capability for 90 percent of its subscribers. Additional shipping centers were on the drawing board.

Netflix had developed sophisticated software to track its inventory and minimize delivery times. Netflix's system allowed the distribution centers to communicate to determine the fastest way of getting DVDs to customers. When a customer placed an order for a specific DVD, the system first looked for that DVD at the shipping center closest to the customer. If that center didn't have the DVD in stock, the system then moved the next closest center and checked there. The search continued until the DVD was found, at which point the shipping center was provided with the information needed to initiate the order fulfillment and shipping process. If the DVD was unavailable anywhere in the system, it was waitlisted. The system then moved to the customer's next choice and the process started all over. And no matter where the DVD was sent from, the system knew to print the return label on the prepaid envelope to send the DVDs to the shipping center closest to the customer to reduce return mail times and permit more efficient use of the company's DVD inventory.

In 2005, Netflix was shipping more than 1 million DVDs a day. It had an inventory of around 20 million DVDs (which was growing as the subscriber base increased). In the first nine months of 2005, Netflix spent $84.2 million on the acquisition of new DVDs; it had an arrangement with movie studios to purchase new-release DVDs for an upfront fee plus a percentage of revenue earned from rentals for a defined period. The company's September 30, 2005, balance sheet indicated that its DVD holdings had a net value of $52.7 million (after depreciation). New-release DVDs were amortized over one year; the useful life of back-library titles (some of which qualified as classics) were amortized over periods of one to three years (since they continued to be rented from time to time because of the Cinematch recommendations). DVDs that the company expected to sell at the end of their useful lives carried a salvage value of $3 per DVD; DVDs that the company did not expect to sell were assigned a salvage value of zero.

Target Customers and Customer Satisfaction

The company's subscriber base consisted of three types of customers: those who liked the convenience of home delivery, bargain hunters who were enthused about being able to watch 10 or more movies a month at an economical price (on the $17.99 plan, 12 movies a month equated to a rental fee of $1.50 per movie), and movie buffs who wanted access to a wide selection of films.

In a survey by Netflix, customers said they rented twice as many movies per month as they did prior to joining Netflix. New Netflix customers also said they were immediately more satisfied with their home-entertainment experience than they were prior to joining Netflix. And 9 out of 10 customers said they were so satisfied with the service that they recommended the service to family and friends. Netflix was the top-rated Web site for customer satisfaction according to a spring 2005 survey by ForeSee Results and FGI Research. In the fall of 2005, *Fast Company* magazine named Netflix the winner of its annual Customers First Award.

Growth Strategy

Netflix's growth strategy had three primary components:

- Continue to innovate and enhance the consumer experience.
- Use Netflix's market-leading position to lead the transition to high-definition DVDs and eventually digital downloading.
- Focus on rapid subscriber growth in order to
  —Maintain market leadership.
  —Realize economies of scale.

Netflix's strategic intent was to be the world's largest and most influential movie supplier.

Netflix's Performance

The company's recent operating statistics and financial statement data are shown in Exhibits 2 and 3. Netflix's decline in profit in 2005 reflected the adverse effects of lower subscription prices that had been instituted in late 2004. Concerned about mounting competitive pressures—particularly from Blockbuster, which announced its entry into the online rental segment in August 2004—Netflix had halted expansion into Britain and Canada and dropped the monthly subscription price on its most popular plan from $21.99 to $17.99 starting November 1, 2004. At the lower $17.99 price, Netflix believed it could continue to grow its subscriber base but would only be able to break even (given the $48 per year revenue loss for many of its subscribers). Blockbuster responded in December 2004 with a price drop from $19.99 to $14.99 per month on its most popular plan, which allowed three DVDs out at a time.

Following Blockbuster's announced entry into online movie rentals and Netflix's November price cut, investors immediately grew nervous about Netflix's profitability and competitive staying power—the company's stock price dropped sharply from around $35 per share in late July 2004 to $10 to $12 per share in the November 2004–February 2005 period. Starting March 2005, the stock began a climb back to the $25 to $30 range, as investors took comfort in Netflix's continued growth in subscribers, the partnership arrangement with Wal-Mart (which had eliminated a prime competitive threat), the company's return to profitability in the second and third quarters of 2005, and upbeat management forecasts for 2006.

Exhibit 2   **Netflix's Statement of Operations, 2000–2005 (in thousands of $, except per share data)**

	Year Ended December 31,					First Nine Months, 2005
	2000	2001	2002	2003	2004	
Statement of Operations Data						
Revenues:						
Subscriptions	$ 35,894	$ 74,255	$150,818	$270,410	$500,611	$489,213
Sales	—	1,657	1,988	1,833	5,617	3,741
Total revenues	35,894	75,912	152,806	272,243	506,228	492,954
Cost of revenues:						
Subscriptions	24,861	49,088	77,044	147,736	273,401	291,821
Sales	—	819	1,092	624	3,057	2,542
Total cost of revenues	24,861	49,907	78,136	148,360	276,458	294,363
Gross profit	11,033	26,005	74,670	123,883	229,770	198,591
Operating expenses:						
Fulfillment	10,247	13,452	19,366	31,274	56,609	51,798
Technology and development	16,823	17,734	14,625	17,884	22,906	22,674
Marketing	25,727	21,031	35,783	49,949	98,027	95,008
General and administrative	6,990	4,658	6,737	9,585	16,287	17,925
Restructuring charges	—	671	—	—	—	—
Stock-based compensation	9,714	6,250	8,832	10,719	16,587	10,995
Total operating expenses	69,501	63,796	85,343	119,411	210,416	198,400
Operating income (loss)	(58,468)	(37,791)	(10,673)	4,472	19,354	191
Other income (expense):						
Interest and other income	1,645	461	1,697	2,457	2,592	3,788
Interest and other expense	(1,451)	(1,852)	(11,972)	(417)	(170)	(54)
Net income before income taxes	(58,274)	(39,182)	(20,948)	6,512	21,776	3,925
Provision for income taxes	—	—	—	—	181	109
Net income (loss)	$(58,274)	$(39,182)	$ (20,948)	$ 6,512	$ 21,595	$ 3,816
Net income (loss) per share:						
Basic	$ (20.61)	$ (10.73)	$ (0.74)	$ 0.14	$ 0.42	$ 0.07
Diluted	(20.61)	(10.73)	(0.74)	0.10	0.33	0.06
Weighted-average shares outstanding:						
Basic	2,828	3,652	28,204	47,786	51,988	53,237
Diluted	2,828	3,652	28,204	62,884	64,713	64,928

Source: Netflix's 2004 10-K Report and company press release, October 19, 2005.

Netflix expected to end 2005 with about 4 million subscribers, revenues of close to $685 million (versus $506 million in 2004), and net income of $5 to $10 million (versus $21.6 million in 2004); the lower profits in 2005 were a direct result of having lowered subscription fees in November 2004.

Netflix reported a loss of $8.8 million in the first quarter of 2005, a profit of $5.7 million in the second quarter, and a profit of $6.9 million in the third quarter. Management's latest forecast for 2006 called for 5.65 million subscribers at year-end, revenues of at least $940 million, and pretax income

Exhibit 3   **Selected Balance Sheet and Cash Flow Data for Netflix, 2000–2005 (in thousands of $)**

	2000	2001	2002	2003	2004	September 30, 2005
Selected Balance Sheet Data						
Cash and cash equivalents	$ 14,895	$ 16,131	$ 59,814	$ 89,894	$174,461	$181,886
Short-term investments	—		43,796	45,297	—	—
Current assets	n.a.	19,552	107,075	138,946	187,346	191,198
Net investment in DVD library	n.a.	3,633	9,972	22,238	42,158	52,735
Total assets	52,488	41,630	130,530	176,012	251,793	278,302
Current liabilities	n.a.	26,208	40,426	63,019	94,910	98,755
Working capital*	(1,655)	(6,656)	66,649	75,927	92,436	93,163
Notes payable, less current portion	1,843	—	—	—	—	—
Subordinated notes payable	—	2,799	—	—	—	—
Redeemable convertible preferred stock	101,830	101,830	—	—	—	—
Stockholders' equity	(73,267)	(90,504)	89,356	112,708	156,283	178,672
Cash flow data						
Net cash provided by operating activities	$(22,706)	$ 4,847	$ 40,114	$ 89,792	$147,571	$ 99,245
Net cash used in investing activities	(24,972)	(12,670)	(67,301)	(64,677)	(68,381)	(99,307)
Net cash provided by financing activities	48,375	9,059	70,870	4,965	5,599	7,487

*Defined as current assets minus current liabilities.

Sources: 2002 10-K report, 2004 10-K report, and company press release October 19, 2005.

of $50 to $60 million. One Wall Street analyst had recently forecast that Netflix could have 7 million subscribers by the end of 2007. Adams Media Research and Netflix had projected that there would be more than 20 million online subscribers for DVD movie rentals within the next five to seven years.

MARKET TRENDS IN MOVIE DVDs

The digital video disc (DVD) player was one of the most successful consumer electronic products of all time. As of December 2005, more than 160 million DVD players had been sold since launch and more than 80 million U.S. households had DVD players (many had more than one). DVD playback had

worked its way into a number of electronic devices, and DVD recording was expected to be an essential driver of the DVD market. DVD recorders were forecast to surpass sales of play-only DVD players by 2007, with an expected compound annual growth rate of 126 percent.

Consumers could obtain movie DVDs through a wide variety of channels:

- Retail outlets such as Wal-Mart, Target, Circuit City, Best Buy, Office Depot, and Staples.
- Rental outlets such as Blockbuster and Movie Gallery.
- Web sites of both brick-and-mortar retailers (Wal-Mart) and Internet-only retailers such as Amazon.com.
- Online rental services such as Netflix and GreenCine.

- PC downloads from Web sites such as Movielink or file-sharing programs such as Kazaa.

According to Kagan Research, consumer spending for in-home movie viewing increased from about $22.6 billion in 2003 to about $25.1 billion in 2004 and was projected to increase to about $33.8 billion by 2009.[1] These numbers represented rental fees and household purchases of videocassettes and DVDs. According to Adams Media Research, DVD sales and rentals amounted to a $23.4 billion market in the United States in 2005, up from $22.0 billion in 2004.[2]

But despite growing sales of DVD players, there were some other factors at work in the marketplace:[3]

- Growth in the sales of DVDs was slowing from double-digit growth to forecasts of single-digit growth in 2006. Online rentals of movie DVDs, computer downloads of music and movie files, video-on-demand (VOD) services, and growing popularity of high-definition TV programs were cited as factors.

- The flood of new and old TV shows on DVDs that had recently hit the marketplace had cut into the sales of movie DVDs—the multidisc sets of TVs shows were more expensive than many new releases of movie DVDs.

- A growing number of households were purchasing digital video recorders (DVRs), which made it simple to record a TV program or movie and then replay it at a convenient time. Many DVR owners were highly attracted to recording movies (and other programs) shown in high definition and then watching them at their convenience.

- Cable companies like Comcast were offering VOD options for many of their premium movie channels. The Starz Entertainment Group claimed that its research showed that Comcast customers who were using the Starz on Demand VOD service tended to reduce their purchases and rentals of movie DVDs due to the ease of using the VOD service.

- Cable and satellite TV companies were expected to expand their VOD services over the next several years and make many more movie titles available to their customers.

- Cable customers with DVRs could readily substitute use of VOD movie offerings from their cable TV provider for purchasing or renting movie DVDs.

- Online rentals and VOD services were not only cutting into sales of movie DVDs but also taking business away from video rental stores. Just as Netflix posed a competitive threat to Blockbuster and Movie Gallery in the United States, market research in Great Britain indicated that one out of every five DVDs rented was rented online.

- Hollywood movie producers were hoping that next-generation, high-definition optical-disc-format DVDs would rejuvenate sales of movie DVDs, but it remained to be seen whether such hopes were well founded, given the growing popularity of DVRs, VOD, and online rentals.

Another factor acting to spur watching movies at home was rapidly growing sales of wide-screen TVs with a 16:9 scale as opposed to the old-style 4:3 scale. Most TV manufacturers had introduced a variety of high-tech TV models with screen sizes up to 72 inches. Prices for wide-screen TVs were dropping rapidly, and picture quality was exceptionally good, if not stunning, on increasing numbers of models. Consumers with wide-screen TVs typically found watching movies at home much more appealing, as compared to those having TVs with 27-inch to 36-inch screens.

BLOCKBUSTER INC.

Blockbuster was the world leader in the videocassette, DVD, and video game rental market, with an estimated 40 percent share of the roughly $13 billion rental market. Founded in Dallas, Texas, in 1985, Blockbuster had grown to over 9,000 company-operated and franchised stores worldwide—in 2005, it had 4,660 company-operated stores in the United States, 2,585 company-operated stores outside the United States, and 1,831 franchised stores (400 of which were in the United States). The company's revenues were derived from rentals of videocassettes for VCRs (11.4 percent of 2004 revenues), DVDs (53.5 percent), video games (8.2 percent), and sales of videotapes, DVDs, and video games (25.3 percent). Revenue from rentals and sales of tapes for VCRs was falling sharply, mainly because more and more households were converting from VCRs to DVD players. Blockbuster's rental revenues from tapes for VCRs had fallen from $1.43 billion in 2003 to $692 million in 2004 to just $150 million in the first nine months of 2005. Its DVD rental revenues had risen from $2.6 billion in 2003 to $3.24 billion in 2004 and accounted for 61.8 percent of rental revenues in first nine months of 2005 (up from 54.9 percent for the comparable period in 2004).

Recent Strategic Moves at Blockbuster's Retail Stores

In September 2000, Blockbuster began marketing DIRECTV system equipment in its U.S. stores; in June 2001, the partnership with DIRECTV was extended to marketing a co-branded pay-per-view movie service that made Blockbuster one of the early entrants into the pay-per-view segment of the home entertainment industry.

In 2002, Blockbuster announced a strategic vision of becoming the complete source for movies and games—rental and retail. Already the leader in movie and game rental market, the company set its sights on increasing its share of the growing retail market by launching a variety promotional programs and expanding its in-store selection of movies and gaming equipment, including hardware, software and accessories. In 2003, it began offering an in-store movie rental subscription program, the Blockbuster Freedom Pass, in approximately 25 percent of its stores. For a flat monthly fee, the Freedom Pass allowed members to rent an unlimited supply of movies without due dates or extended viewing fees for as long as they subscribed to the pass. The Freedom Pass program was rolled out to all U.S. company-operated stores in 2004, and the name was changed to Blockbuster Movie Pass. For $24.99 per month, members could take up to two movies out at a time; for $29.99 per month, they could choose the three-movies-at-a-time option. Both plans entitled customers to watch all the movies they wanted, with no specified return dates and no extended viewing fees. Once customers purchased the pass, their credit card or check card was automatically charged the monthly fee; subscriptions could be cancelled at any time.

To expand its presence in the gaming marketplace, in 2002 Blockbuster purchased the U.K.-based video game retailer Gamestation and proceeded to grow the chain from 64 to more than 150 stores. In the United States, the company began offering a Game Freedom Pass rental subscription program in all of its U.S. company-operated stores. Customers could purchase a single-month pass for just $19.99 and get unlimited game rentals for 30 consecutive days with a maximum of one game rented at any given time, and no extended viewing fees during the 30 days; a gamer could keep one game for the entire 30 consecutive days or change out the game daily—or even multiple times a day.

Several other initiatives in video games were launched in 2004–2005. Blockbuster began carrying PlayStation portable handheld games for rent in all stores. And it had boosted its games offering by creating a special "Game Rush" section within certain high-traffic Blockbuster stores where customers could rent, sell, and buy new and used game software and hardware. During peak hours, Game Rush sections were staffed by trained game specialists. Blockbuster believed that about half its U.S. stores were suited to having a Game Rush section.

However, despite all these and other strategic initiatives, Blockbuster was a troubled company in 2005. Sales revenues were stagnant at around $6 billion annually (see Exhibit 4), and the company had lost money in five of the past six years. Blockbuster reported net losses of $1.62 billion in 2002, $979 million in 2003, $1.25 billion in 2004, and $606 million through the first nine months of 2005. It had split off from media conglomerate Viacom in October 2004; part of the split-off arrangement involved paying a special one-time $5 dividend (totaling $905 million) to all shareholders, including Viacom (which owned 81.5 percent of Blockbuster's shares prior to the divestiture deal).

Blockbuster's Online Rental Business

Blockbuster entered the online rental segment in August 2004, offering customers a choice of three monthly plans (all with unlimited rentals and no due dates or late fees): (1) a $19.99 plan with three DVDs out at a time, (2) a $29.99 plan with five DVDs out at a time, and (3) a $39.99 plan with eight DVDs out at a time. Customers could choose from 25,000 titles, ranging from classics to new releases. In addition, subscribers were e-mailed two "e-coupons" each month for two free in-store rentals; all Blockbuster Online members were eligible for exclusive deals and discounts at participating Blockbuster stores.

Exhibit 4   Selected Financial and Operating Statistics for Blockbuster Inc., 2002–2005 ($ in millions, except for per share data)

	First Nine Months, 2005	2004	2003	2002
Selected statement of operations data				
Revenues				
Rentals	$3,165.2	$ 4,428.6	$4,533.5	$4,460.4
Merchandise sales	1,114.0	1,532.6	1,281.6	1,019.7
Other	54.6	92.0	96.6	85.8
Total	4,333.8	6,053.2	5,911.7	5,565.9
Cost of rental revenues	1,046.8	1,250.7	1,362.1	1,513.8
Gross margin on rentals	66.9%	71.8%	70.0%	66.1%
Cost of merchandise sold	861.9	1,190.7	1,027.7	844.9
Gross margin on merchandise sales	22.6%	22.3%	19.8%	17.1%
Gross profit	2,425.1	3,611.8	3,521.9	3,207.2
Gross profit margin	56.0%	59.7%	59.6%	57.6%
Operating expenses				
General and administrative	2,147.4	2,835.2	2,605.9	2,369.5
Share-based compensation	—	18.3		
Advertising	227.1	257.4	179.4	249.2
Depreciation	173.0	247.4	266.0	239.1
Impairment of goodwill and other long-lived assets	356.8	1,504.4	1,304.9	—
Amortization of intangibles	1.8	2.3	2.4	1.7
Total	2,906.1	4,865.0	4,358.6	2,859.5
Operating income	(481.0)	(1,253.2)	(836.7)	347.7
Interest expense	(70.0)	(38.1)	(33.1)	(49.5)
Interest income	2.8	3.6	3.1	4.1
Income (loss) before income taxes	(551.0)	(1,286.1)	(867.1)	305.2
Net profit (loss)	$ (606.1)	$(1,248.8)	$ (978.7)	$ 195.9
Earnings per share (diluted)	$(3.30)	$(6.89)	$(5.41)	$1.08
Dividends per share	$0.04	$5.08	$0.08	$0.08
Selected balance sheet data				
Cash and cash equivalents	$ 190.2	$ 330.3	$ 233.4	$ 152.5
Merchandise inventories	352.2	516.6	415.1	452.1
Current assets	866.5	1,217.7	960.3	958.9
Total assets	3,030.4	3,863.4	4,822.0	6,243.8
Current liabilities	1,989.5	1,449.4	1,323.4	1,477.6
Long-term debt, less current portion	300.0	1,044.9	0.7	328.9
Stockholders' equity	465.9	1,062.9	3,188.4	4,100.9
Selected cash flow data				
Net cash flow provided by operations	$ 492.4	$ 1,215.4	$1,430.3	$ 1,462.3
Net cash flow (used for)/provided by investing activities	(741.2)	(1,112.3)	(1,024.6)	(1,314.6)
Net cash flow (used for)/provided by financing activities	112.8	(18.8)	(335.5)	(199.2)
Worldwide Store Data				
Same-store revenue increase (decrease)	(2.9)%	(3.2)%	(2.2)%	5.1%
Company-owned stores, end-of-year	7,245	7,265	7,105	6,907
Franchised stores, end-of-year	1,831	1,829	1,762	1,638
Total stores, end-of-year	9,076	9,094	8,867	8,545

Source: Blockbuster's 2003 10-K report, 2004 10-K report, and third-quarter 2005 10-Q report.

Rentals were shipped from 11 distribution centers to subscribers via first-class mail and usually arrived in one to three business days. Subscribers were provided with a postage-paid envelope for returning the DVDs. Subscribers could create and maintain a personal queue of movies they wished to rent at Blockbuster's Web site. When Blockbuster received return DVDs from subscribers, it automatically shipped the next available titles in the subscriber's rental queue. Management said the online rental service was the latest in a series of initiatives being implemented by Blockbuster to transform itself from a neighborhood movie rental store into an "anywhere, anytime" entertainment destination that eventually would enable customers to rent, buy, or trade movies and games, new or used, in-store and online. The initial response to Blockbuster Online was promising; John Antonico, Blockbuster's CEO, said, "After six weeks, we had more subscribers than Netflix had in a year and a half of existence."

On December 22, 2004, Blockbuster cut the price on its most popular subscription plan from $19.99 per month to $14.99 and announced it was expanding the copy-depth of new-release movies, boosting the number of titles available for online rental to 30,000, and expanding the selection of TV shows, anime, Hollywood classics, Asian cinema, music performance, documentaries, fitness, and how-to categories among others. It also announced that it was increasing the number of shipping centers to 23 and implementing new technology with the U.S. Postal Service that would shorten delivery times.

Developments at Blockbuster in 2005

In a move to revitalize stagnant store sales (see the worldwide store data section of Exhibit 4) and combat the attractiveness of the no-due-dates/no-late-fees policies of Netflix, Blockbuster in January 2005 discontinued its practice of charging late fees on DVD rental returns at its retail stores. However, it held on to the practice of specified due dates—one week for games and two days or one week for movies. If customers kept the rental beyond the due date, they were automatically granted an extra one-week goodwill period at no additional charge. If a customer chose to keep his or her rental past the end of the seventh day after the due date per the posted rental terms, Blockbuster converted the rental to

a sale and charged the customer for the movie or game, minus the original rental fee. If the customer later decided he or she did not want to own the movie or game and returned the product within 30 days, Blockbuster reversed the sale and charged a minimal restocking fee of $1.25 (some franchise stores charged a higher restocking fee).

Blockbuster ran extensive ads in December 2004 and January 2005 touting its new no-late-fee policy. To help compensate for the estimated $250 to $300 million that late fees were expected to contribute to Blockbuster's revenues in 2005, management planned to lower its ongoing marketing, operating, and promotional costs. Nonetheless, John Antioco, CEO of Blockbuster, was under fire from shareholders and some members of the company's board of directors for instituting the no-late-fee policy, given the big revenue erosion impact, Blockbuster's string of huge losses, and the need to increase store inventories of DVDs to compensate for the extra time that customers were keeping the DVDs. Investors and board members were also skeptical about Blockbuster's move in the online rental market segment because of the heavy costs (estimated at $100 to $200 million) and what some considered as dim prospects for profitability. About 160 Blockbuster franchisees decided to discontinue the no-late-fees policy in 2005, even though the program was popular with customers, because of the extra expenses involved in stocking additional copies of popular titles.

In May 2005, disgruntled Blockbuster shareholders ignored management's recommendations and elected an opposing slate of three new directors to the company's board, one of whom was running against CEO John Antioco. When Antioco indicated that he would leave his position as CEO as a consequence of being defeated in his reelection bid, the newly constituted board opted to expand from six to eight members, appointed Antioco to one of the two newly created seats, and made him chairman. It was understood, however, that Antioco would not continue on as CEO past 2005 if the board was not satisfied with the progress being made to restore Blockbuster to profitability.

During his contentious campaign against the opposing slate of directors, Antonico had defended his strategy for Blockbuster:

A key feature of our growth strategy is the recently introduced "End of Late Fees" program, which directly addresses the major problem customers had with their movie rental experience. The program also positions us better to compete with home entertainment options that do not have late fees, including retail DVD, pay-per-view and VOD. To date, the "End of Late Fees" program is producing the desired results. Since the first of January when we introduced the program, we have had positive growth in active membership for the first time in nearly two years.

Another critically important initiative—and the only significant investment we intend to make this year—is our online rental business. Blockbuster is uniquely positioned to compete in this fast growing business. Given the views of leading industry experts that within three years online rental could represent 20% to 30% of movie rental revenues, it is imperative that we pursue this opportunity, which we believe will mean hundreds of millions of dollars in future operating income for our company.

We are prioritizing new initiatives, investing wisely for the future and cutting costs aggressively. We have cut 2005 capital spending by over $100 million from last year and reduced corporate overhead by $70 million on an annualized basis. Additionally, to reduce costs further and better focus our resources, we have put our game initiative, as well as the marketing of our movie trading business, on hold until 2006.

Regarding our dividend policy, during 2004 Blockbuster paid a one-time dividend of $5 per share in addition to its normal quarterly dividends. As a result, our shareholders received a total of $920 million in dividends in 2004. We have consistently said that once we have successfully executed our business initiatives and delivered on our strategic plan, we would consider paying increased quarterly dividends or repurchasing stock.[4]

In characterizing the company's direction, Antonico said, "Our mission right now is to transform Blockbuster from a place you go to rent movies to a place you go to rent or buy movies or games new or used, pay by the day, pay by the month, online or in-store."

In August 2005, Blockbuster Online's pricing was raised. Customers could choose from among three plans:

- $9.99, unlimited DVDs, one title out at a time.
- $14.99, unlimited DVDs, two titles out at a time.
- $17.99, unlimited DVDs, three titles out at a time.

The $17.99 plan was the most popular; all plans included a free two-week trial. The company said it had 1 million online subscribers and during 2005 had added about as many net new subscribers as Netflix. As of mid-2005, online subscribers could choose from over 40,000 titles, with new titles added weekly. Blockbuster had 30 distribution centers, and more than 200 local Blockbuster stores were fulfilling online orders for nearby customers (to help shorten delivery times). More local stores were being added daily to fulfill online orders.

Also in 2005, Blockbuster integrated its in-store and online subscription programs—members paid the same fees and had the same privileges. To conserve cash and bolster Blockbuster's lackluster balance sheet, the company's board of directors elected not to pay the $0.02 per share dividend for the third quarter of 2005. Blockbuster management had plans to reduce costs by over $100 million in 2006 and an additional $50 million in 2007 through a combination of overhead reductions, lower marketing expenditures, and operational savings from divesting a subsidiary that acquired and distributed products for the theatrical, home entertainment, and television markets. Management further planned to cut capital expenditures from $140 million in 2005 to $90 million in 2006, principally because of fewer new store openings.

MOVIE GALLERY INC.

In 2005, Movie Gallery was the second-largest North American home video retailer, with more than 4,700 stores located in all 50 U.S. states, Mexico, and Canada. It specialized in the rental and sale of DVD and VHS movies and video games. Since the company's initial public offering in August 1994, Movie Gallery had grown from 97 stores in 1994 to nearly 2,500 stores at year-end 2004 via new store openings and a series of acquisitions. It had revenues of $791 million in 2004 and earnings of $49.5 million. In April 2005, Movie Gallery beat out Blockbuster in a bidding war to acquire Hollywood Entertainment, which had 2004 revenues of $1.78 billion and operated 2,000 Hollywood Video stores and 700 Game Crazy stores.

The company's stores operating under the Movie Gallery brand primarily targeted small towns and suburban areas. Movie Gallery's scale of operations and resource capabilities enabled it to compete effectively against the independently owned stores and small regional chains in these areas; it was regarded as the industry's lowest-cost operator. The strategy of the Movie Gallery stores was to take advantage of purchasing economics, effective labor strategies, and a strong, proven business model to generate cash flow and continued growth.

The stores operating under the Hollywood Video and Game Crazy brands primarily targeted urban centers and surrounding suburban neighborhoods—much the same places that Blockbuster targeted. The strategy of these stores was predicated on exceptional customer service, innovative marketing and merchandising programs, a strong brand image, and solid in-store execution.

Movie Gallery was formed in 1985 by Joe Malugen and Harrison Parrish in Dothan, Alabama. Through its wholly owned subsidiary M.G.A., the company's founders began operating video specialty stores in southern Alabama and the Florida panhandle, and franchising the Movie Gallery store concept. By June 1987 the company owned five stores and had a franchise operation of 45 stores. In 1988, Movie Gallery began to consolidate the franchisees into company-owned stores; by 1992, it had a total of 37 stores and annual revenues of $6 million.

In August 1994, Movie Gallery completed an initial public offering of its stock and used the proceeds to acquire small video chains, primarily in the Southeast. Additional shares were issued in 1995 to open new stores and continue making acquisitions. By mid-1996 Movie Gallery had made over 100 separate acquisitions and built a chain of over 850 stores. In 1999, Movie Gallery announced plans to build 100 new stores and completed an 88-store acquisition of Blowout Entertainment; it went into 2000 with more than 950 locations in 31 states.

In 2000, Movie Gallery again set its goal at opening 100 new stores and relocating 25. This goal was met and surpassed. In late 2001, Movie Gallery expanded its store base by 30 percent by acquiring Video Update, its largest single-chain acquisition to date. The Video Update acquisition, which included 100 retail locations in Canada, marked Movie Gallery's emergence as a leader in video rentals in North America. Movie Gallery continued to execute an aggressive growth strategy, reaching the 2,000-store mark in 2003.

Following the April 2005 acquisition of Hollywood Entertainment, Movie Gallery strengthened its presence in Western Canada by acquiring the

61-store VHQ Entertainment chain. VHQ also operated VHQ Online (www.VHQonline.ca), a flat-fee, direct-to-home movie delivery service.

Movie Gallery had not launched an online DVD rental service, but its large and diverse geographic spread and its ambitions to be "the dominant entertainment source for video and video game rental and sale in rural and secondary markets in the United States" made it a likely entry candidate.

In the first nine months of 2005, Movie Gallery reported revenues of $1.31 billion and a net loss of $6.3 million. Movie Gallery anticipated fourth-quarter 2005 revenues of $675 to $705 million and same-store revenues in the range of −5 to −9 percent, as compared to the fourth quarter of 2004. In June 2005, management revised the new store development plan for the Movie Gallery and Hollywood Entertainment, cutting the plans for 500 new stores in 2005 to 300 stores; in the fall of 2005 it was on track to meet the target of 300 new store openings. Movie Gallery intended to further reduce its annual capital expenditures for new store development and open approximately 150 new stores in 2006, primarily in rural and secondary markets. It was also exploring various strategic alternatives for its Game Crazy business, including a potential sale, strategic partnership, or joint venture.

VIDEO-ON-DEMAND

Some analysts saw video-on-demand as a huge threat to Netflix because it could kill the market for DVD rentals. Growing numbers of households had high-speed Internet access, thus allowing technologically-savvy consumers to download movies to their PCs and then use the capabilities of Windows Media Center (which was standard on many newly purchased PCs shipped in 2005) to show the downloaded movies on their TVs. Alternatively, they could simply use a credit card to pay a fee to online movie suppliers to watch the movie on their PCs via streaming video.

However, VOD was materializing more slowly than expected because of wrangles with getting movie studios to license more movies for digital downloads—most movie studios feared that any contribution on their part to wider digital downloading of movies would facilitate even greater movie pirating (via file-sharing software) and cause them to lose significant revenues from both declining movie attendance and movie DVD sales. The file-sharing software used to pirate music files over the Internet also allowed people to pirate movies—in 2004, an estimated 400,000 to 600,000 movies were being illegally downloaded each day, costing film companies hundreds of millions in lost sales. More than half of the college-educated adults 35 and under in the United States had broadband connections at home, making it easy to trade copyrighted music and movie files. To try to deter illegal movie downloading, the Motion Picture Association of America in 2004 launched a major ad campaign in daily newspapers and consumer magazines across the country, as well as in more than 100 college newspapers, explaining why movie piracy was illegal, how it impacted jobs and the economy, and what the consequences were for engaging in illegal trafficking. Additionally, antipiracy messages appeared in motion picture theaters across the country.

Movielink's VOD Service

In 2005, Movielink (www.movielink.com), headquartered in Santa Monica, California, was the leading broadband video-on-demand (VOD) service. It offered an extensive selection of new and classic hit movies, foreign films, and other hard-to-find content. The business was a joint venture of Metro-Goldwyn-Mayer Studios, Paramount Pictures, Sony Pictures Entertainment, Universal Studios, and Warner Bros. Studios. Movielink drew its content offerings from the vast libraries of those studios, as well as Walt Disney Pictures, Twentieth Century Fox, Miramax, Artisan, and others on a non-exclusive basis.

After browsing the selection of movies, customers registered and rented movies using a valid credit card. There were no late fees or return times, and Movielink did not require a subscription or membership. Instead, each movie was independently priced by the content provider and charged per rental—fees were as low as $1.99 per movie. "We're excited about the opportunity to work with Movielink and its growing customer base of broadband households," said Peter Levinsohn, Fox's president of worldwide pay television and digital media.

Movielink was available to U.S. Internet users with broadband connections. Consumers could browse Movielink's site and view trailers of available titles without charge. Once customers were ready to rent a title, they registered with Movielink and paid for their rental via credit card. Movielink's Movies in Minutes software let customers either begin watching titles within 2–10 minutes after beginning the download or store them on their hard drives for up to 30 days and experience unlimited viewing for any 24-hour period on a PC, a television connected to the PC, or a laptop computer. Customers could also use Movielink's MultiPlay software feature to re-rent titles for additional 24-hour viewing periods for up to 30 days after the initial rental. Thirty days after the download, movie files were automatically deleted from the customer's hard drive.

Movielink had partnered with Verizon to launch a co-branded movie downloading service for Verizon Online's consumer broadband subscribers. Verizon Online's consumer DSL and FiOS Internet Service customers could purchase and download movies to watch at home or rent movies through Verizon's special agreement with Movielink.

GreenCine's Combination Online Rental-VOD Movie Offering

GreenCine was an online DVD rental company that also offered its subscribers two other options for watching movies—VOD and DivX downloads, both priced at $4.99 per movie and both allowing customers to watch the movie as many times as they wished over a 10-day period (GreenCine's adult movies had a 30-day use period). GreenCine had 10,000 on-demand movie titles that included independent, international, documentary, classic, and adult movies covering 32 genres.

GreenCine's online rental customers could select from a library of 25,000 titles and choose from among seven plans:

- $9.95, unlimited DVDs, 1 title out at a time.
- $14.95, unlimited DVDs, 2 titles out at a time.
- $21.95, unlimited DVDs, 3 titles out at a time.
- $27.95, unlimited DVDs, 4 titles out at a time.
- $33.95, unlimited DVDs, 5 titles out at a time.
- $49.95, unlimited DVDs, 8 titles out at a time.
- $59.95, unlimited DVDs, 10 titles out at a time.

Like Netflix, GreenCine offered a free two-week trial period. It had one distribution center and delivery could run two to three days. GreenCine sent members an e-mail alert when a movie was mailed out and when it received a movie that the member had returned.

Headquartered in the San Francisco Bay area, GreenCine touted itself as a movie source for people who liked the arts and were fond of off-the-wall, offbeat, eclectic, and unusual movies. Its collection featured independent, foreign, anime, and art house movies, as well as HK action and classic titles. The company's Web site said, "If what you like to see is off-center, or dead center, in terms of taste, Green-Cine is for you."

NETFLIX'S OUTLOOK

Reed Hastings believed that Netflix's prospects were exceptionally bright. In a December 2005 interview with *Inc.* magazine, he said:

> Netflix has at least another decade of dominance ahead of it. But movies over the Internet are coming, and at some point it will become big business. We started investing 1% to 2% of revenue every year in downloading, and I think it's tremendously exciting because it will fundamentally lower our mailing costs. We want to be ready when video-on-demand happens. That's why the company is called Netflix, not DVD-by-Mail.[5]

But two new developments cast shadows on this prognosis. In January 2006, *The Wall Street Journal* reported that cable TV companies and major movie studios were considering strategies to release movies through VOD cable services the same day that the DVDs were available in retail stores and rental outlets.[6] The move was precipitated by deals that Walt Disney and NBC Universal had recently made to make television shows available on Apple Computer's video-capable iPod. With movie box-office attendance and revenues lagging, movie studios were anxious to pursue highly lucrative sales of movie DVDs and prevent that revenue stream from eroding. Historically, movie studios had released new movies first to theaters and then several weeks or months later made them available on DVD, cable video-on-demand services, and other platforms (each a few weeks apart)—a strategy that they believed maximized revenue.

Also in January 2006, Google announced that it would begin allowing consumers to buy videos from major content partners through the Google site.[7] Consumers would be able to pay to download and view videos, such as television shows, on their computers from Google content partners that included CBS Corporation, the National Basketball Association, and other partners soon to be named.

Endnotes

[1] As cited in Blockbuster's 2004 10-K report, p. 1.

[2] As cited in Sarah McBride, Peter Grant, and Merissa Marr, "Movies May Hit DVD Cable Simultaneously," *The Wall Street Journal,* January 4, 2006, p. B1.

[3] Based on information in Shane C. Buettner, "DVD Sales Peaking," posted at Ultimate AV, www.guidetohometheater.com (accessed December 29, 2005).

[4] Excerpt from company press release, April 18, 2005.

[5] Interview with *Inc.* magazine's Patrick J. Sauer, posted at www.inc.com (accessed December 29, 2005).

[6] McBride, Grant, and Marr, "Movies May Hit DVD Cable Simultaneously," p. B1.

[7] Kevin J. Delaney and Nick Wingfield, "Google to Offer Video, Software That Rivals Microsoft's," *The Wall Street Journal,* January 5, 2006, p. A9.

easyCar.com

John J. Lawrence
University of Idaho

Luis Solis
Instituto de Empresa

In 2003 easyCar.com had become the fastest-growing rental car company in Europe by offering a minimal selection of cars that could be booked at low daily rates via the company's Web site. Its mission was "to offer you outstanding value for money. To us value for money means a reliable service at a low price. We achieve this by simplifying the product we offer, and passing on the benefits to you in the form of lower prices."[1]

EasyCar was a member of the easyGroup family of companies, founded by the flamboyant Greek entrepreneur Stelios Haji-Ioannou, who was known simply as Stelios to most. Stelios founded low-cost air carrier easyJet.com in 1995 after convincing his father, a Greek shipping billionaire, to loan him the £5 million to start the business.[2] (Note: In January 2003, £1 = €1.52 = U.S.$1.61.) EasyJet was one of the early low-cost, no-frills air carriers in the European market and was built on a foundation of simple point-to-point flights, Internet-only flight reservations, and the aggressive use of yield management policies. The company proved highly successful, and as a result Stelios expanded the easyJet business model to industries with characteristics similar to the airline industry. One such business was easyCar, which was founded in 2000 with a £10 million initial investment.

EasyCar's business model was quite different than that of traditional rental car companies. EasyCar rented only a single vehicle type at each location it operated, while most of its competitors rented a wide variety of vehicle types. EasyCar did not work with agents—over 95 percent of its bookings were made through the company's Web site, with the remainder of bookings being made directly through the company's phone reservation system (at a cost to the customer of €0.95/minute for the call). Most rental car companies worked with a variety of intermediaries, with their own Web sites accounting for less than 10 percent of their total booking.[3] And like easyJet, easyCar managed rental rates in an attempt to have its fleet rented out 100 percent of the time and to generate the maximum revenue from its rentals. EasyCar's information system constantly evaluated projected demand and expected utilization at each site, and adjusted price accordingly. Because of its aggressive pricing, easyCar was able to achieve a fleet utilization rate in excess of 90 percent[4]—much higher than other major rental car companies. Industry leader Avis Europe, for example, had a fleet utilization rate of 68 percent.[5]

EasyCar's business model was showing signs of success by fiscal year-end 2002, when it broke even on revenues of £27 million[6] after losing £7.5 million on revenues of £18.5 million in 2001.[7] Pleased with the company's early performance, Stelios announced the company would open an average of two new sites a week through 2003 and 2004 to reach a total of 180 sites by the end of 2004.[8] Stelios expected new locations would allow easyCar to quadruple revenues to £100 million in revenue and earn profits of £10 million by year-end 2004 in preparation for a planned initial public offering (IPO) that same year. The company's management and financial advisers projected the IPO might yield as much as £250 million to fund future growth in the European rental car market.[9]

THE RENTAL CAR INDUSTRY IN WESTERN EUROPE

The western European rental car industry consisted of many different national markets that were only semi-integrated. While there were many companies that competed within this industry, a handful of companies held dominant positions, either across a number of national markets or within one or a few national markets. Industry experts saw the sector as ripe for consolidation.[10] Several international companies—notably Avis, Europcar, and Hertz—had strong positions across most major European markets. Within most countries, there was also a primarily national or regional company that had a strong position in its home market and perhaps moderate market share in neighboring markets. Sixt was the market leader in Germany, for example, while Atesa (in partnership with National) was the market leader in Spain. Generally these major players accounted for more than half of the market. In Germany, for example, Sixt, Europcar, Avis, and Hertz had a combined 60 percent of the €2.5 billion German rental car market.[11] In Spain, the top five firms accounted for 60 percent of the €920 million Spanish rental car market. Generally, these top firms targeted both business and vacation travelers and offered a wide range of vehicles for rent. Exhibit 1 provides basic information on these market-leading companies.

In addition to these major companies in each market, there were many smaller rental companies operating in each market. In Germany, for example, there were over 700 smaller companies,[12] while in Spain there were more than 1,600 smaller companies. Many of these smaller companies operated at only one or a few locations and were particularly prevalent in tourist locations. Also operating in the sector were a number of brokers, like Holiday Autos. Brokerage companies did not own their own fleet of cars but instead managed the excess inventory of other companies and matched customers with rental companies with excess fleet capacity.

Overall, the rental car market could be thought of as composed of two broad segments, a business segment and a tourist/leisure segment. Depending on the market, the leisure segment represented somewhere between 45 and 65 percent of the overall market, and a large part of this segment was very price-conscious. The business segment made up the remaining 35 to 55 percent of the market. It was less price-sensitive than the tourist segment and more

Exhibit 1   Information on easyCar's Major European Competitors, 2002

	easyCar	Avis Europe	Europcar	Hertz	Sixt
Number of rental outlets	46	3,100	2,650	7,000	1,250
2002 fleet size	7,000	120,000	220,000	700,000	(46,700)
Number of countries	5	107	118	150	50
Largest market	United Kingdom	France	France	United States	Germany
Who owns company	EasyGroup/ Stelios Haji-Ioannou	D'Ieteren (Belgium) is majority shareholder	Volkswagen AG	Ford Motor Company	Publicly traded
European revenues	€41 million	€1.25 billion	€1.12 billion	€910 million	€600 million
Company Web site	www.easycar.com	www.avis-europe.com	www.europcar.com	www.hertz.com	ag.sixt.com

Source: Information in this table came from each company's Web site and online annual reports. European revenues are for vehicle rental in Europe and are estimated on the basis of market share estimates for 2001 from Avis Europe's Web site.

concerned about service quality, convenience, and flexibility.

THE GROWTH OF EASYCAR

EasyCar opened its first location in London, in April 2000, under the name easyRentacar. In the same week, easyCar opened locations in Glasgow and Barcelona. All three locations were popular easyJet destinations. Vehicles initially could be rented for as low as €15 a day plus a one-time car preparation fee of €8. Each of these locations had a fleet consisting entirely of Mercedes A-class vehicles, which was the smallest car manufactured by the German automaker. It was the only vehicle that easyCar rented at the time. Exhibit 2 presents images of easyCar's Spanish home page, an A-class model, and its Mercedes MPV rental fleet.

Exhibit 2   **Images of easyCar's Spanish Home Page, A-Class Mercedes Rental Car, and Its Mercedes MPV Rental Fleet**

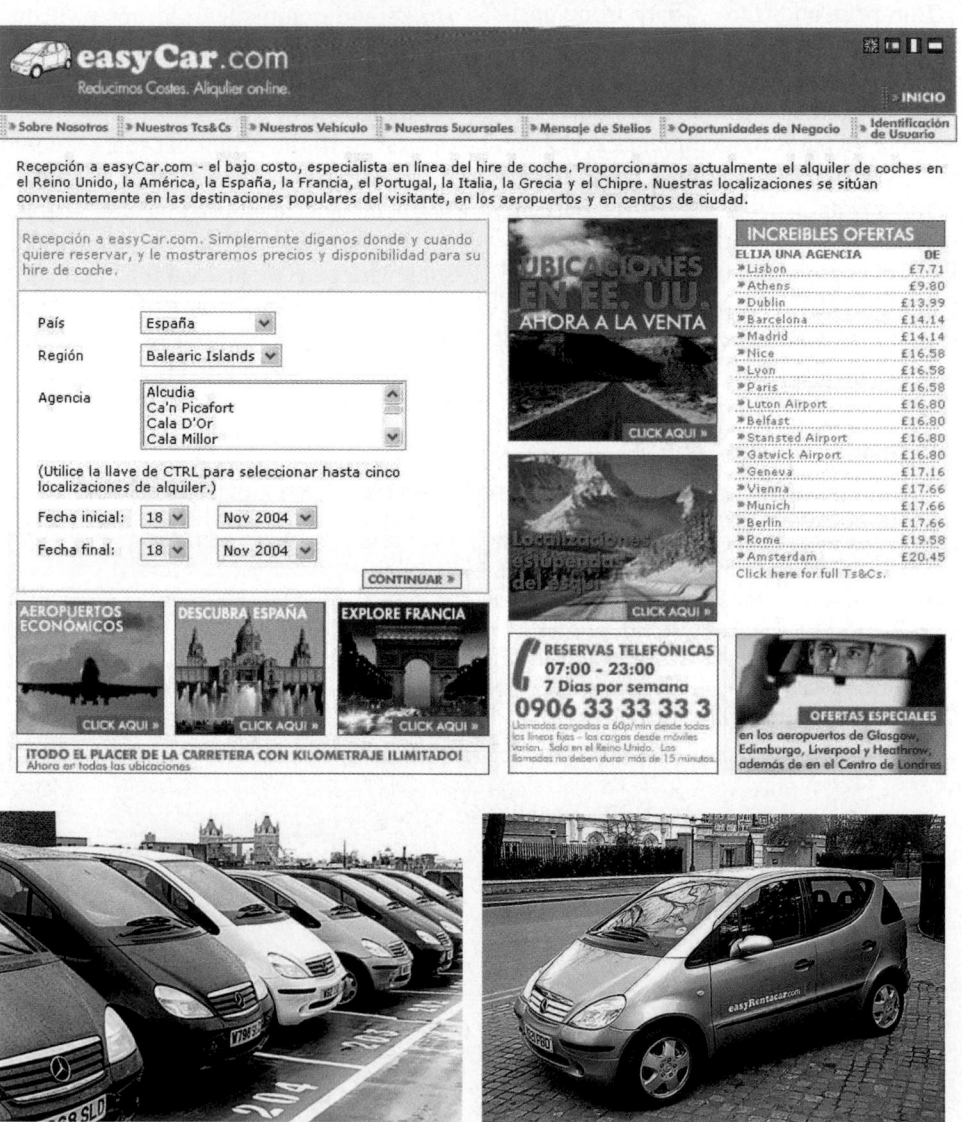

Source: easyCar.com's Web site (accessed October and November 2004).

EasyCar had signed a deal with Mercedes, amid much fanfare, at the Geneva Motor Show earlier in the year to purchase a total of 5,000 A-class vehicles. The vehicles, which came with guaranteed buy-back terms, cost easyCar's parent company a little over £6 million.[13] Many in the car rental industry were surprised by the choice, expecting easyCar to rely on less expensive compact models.[14] In describing the acquisition of the 5,000 Mercedes vehicles, Stelios had said:

> The choice of Mercedes reflects the easyGroup brand. EasyRentacar will use brand new Mercedes cars in the same way that easyJet uses brand new Boeing aircraft. We do not compromise on the hardware, we just use innovation to substantially reduce costs. The car hire industry is where the airline industry was five years ago, a cartel feeding off the corporate client. EasyRentacar will provide a choice for consumers who pay out of their own pockets and who will not be ripped off for traveling mid-week.[15]

EasyCar quickly expanded to other locations, focusing first on those locations popular with easy-Jet customers, including Amsterdam, Geneva, Nice, and Malagra. By July 2001, a little over a year after its initial launch, easyCar had fleets of Mercedes A-class vehicles in 14 locations in the United Kingdom, Spain, France, and the Netherlands. At this point, EasyCar secured £27 million from a consortium of Bank of Scotland Corporate Banking and NBGI Private Equity to further expand its operations. The package consisted of a combination of equity and loan stock.

While easyCar added a few sites in the second half of 2001 and early 2002, volatile demand in the wake of the September 11, 2001, terrorist attacks forced easyCar to roll out new rental locations somewhat slower than originally expected.[16] Growth accelerated, however, in the spring of 2002. Between May 2002 and January 2003, EasyCar opened 30 new locations, going from 18 to 48 sites. This acceleration in growth also coincided with a change in easyCar's policy regarding the makeup of its fleet. By May 2002, easyCar's fleet consisted of 6,000 Mercedes A-class vehicles across 18 sites. Beginning in May, however, easyCar began to stock its fleet with other types of vehicles. It still maintained its policy of offering only a single type of vehicle at each location, but now the vehicle the customer received depended on the location. The first new vehicle easyCar introduced was the Vauxhall Corsa. According to Stelios,

> Vauxhall Corsas cost easyCar £2 a day less than Mercedes A-Class so we can pass this saving on to customers. Customers themselves will decide if they want to pay a premium for a Mercedes. EasyGroup companies benefit from economies of scale where relevant but we also want to create contestable markets among our suppliers so that we can keep the cost to our customers as low as possible.[17]

By January 2003, EasyCar was also using Ford Focuses (4 locations), Renault Clios (3 locations), Toyota Yarises (3 locations), and Smart cars (2 locations) in addition to the Vauxhall Corsas (7 locations) and the Mercedes A-Class vehicles (28 locations). Plans called for a further expansion of the fleet, from the 7,000 vehicles that easyCar had in January to 24,000 vehicles across 180 rental sites by the end of 2004.[18]

In addition to making vehicles available at more locations, easyCar had also changed its policies for 2003 to allow rentals for as little as one hour, and with as little as one hour's notice of rental. By making this change, Stelios felt that easyCar could be a serious competitor to local taxis, buses, trains, and even car ownership. EasyCar expected that if it made car rental simple enough and cheap enough, that some people living in traffic-congested European cities who only used their car occasionally would give up the costs and hassles of car ownership and simply hire an easyCar when they needed a vehicle. Tapping into this broader transportation market would help the company reach its ambitious future sales goals.

FACILITIES

In January 2003 easyCar had facilities in a total of 17 cities in five European countries, as shown in Exhibit 3. It primarily located its facilities near bus and train stations in the major European cities, seeking out sites that offered lower lease costs. It generally avoided prime airport locations, as the cost for space at, and in some cases near, airports was significantly higher than most other locations. When easyCar did locate near an airport, it generally chose sites off the airport, in order to reduce the cost of the lease. Airport locations also tended to require longer hours to satisfy customers arriving on late flights or departing on very early flights. EasyCar kept its airport locations open 24 hours a day, whereas its other locations were generally only open from 7:00 a.m. to 11:00 p.m.

Exhibit 3   **easyCar Locations in January 2003**

Country	City	Number	Number Near an Airport
France	Nice	1	1
France	Paris	8	0
Netherlands	Amsterdam	3	1
Spain	Barcelona	2	0
Spain	Madrid	2	0
Spain	Majorca	1	1
Spain	Malagra	1	1
Switzerland	Geneva	1	1
United Kingdom	Birmingham	2	0
United Kingdom	Bromley	1	0
United Kingdom	Croydon	1	1
United Kingdom	Glasgow	2	1
United Kingdom	Kingston-upon-Thames	1	0
United Kingdom	Liverpool	2	1
United Kingdom	London	15	0
United Kingdom	Manchester	2	1
United Kingdom	Waterford	1	0
Total	5 Countries, 17 Cities	46	9

Source: www.easyCar.com, January 2003.

The physical facilities at all locations were kept to a minimum. In many locations, easyCar leased space in an existing parking garage. Employees worked out of a small, self-contained cubicle within the garage. The cubicle, depending on the location, might be no more than 15 square meters and included little more than a small counter and a couple of computers at which staff processed customers as they came to pick up or return their vehicles. EasyCar also leased a number of spaces within the garage for its fleet of cars. However, because easyCar's vehicles were rented 90 percent of the time, only 15 to 20 spaces were required at an average site, which had a fleet of about 150 cars.[19] To speed up the opening of new sites, easyCar had equipped a number of vans with all the needed computer and telephone equipment to run a site.[20] From an operational perspective, it could open a new location by simply leasing 20 or so spaces in a parking garage, hiring a small staff, driving a van to the location, and adding the location to the company's Web site. Depending on the fleet size at a location, easyCar typically had only one or two people working at a site at a time.

VEHICLE PICKUP AND RETURN PROCESSES

Customers arrived to a site to pick up a vehicle within a prearranged one-hour period. They selected this time slot when they booked the vehicles. EasyCar adjusted the first day's rental price according to the pickup time. Customers who picked their cars up earlier in the day or at popular times were charged more than were customers picking up their cars later in the day or at less busy times. Customers were required to bring a printed copy of their contract, along with the credit card they used to make the booking and identification. Given the low staffing levels, customers occasionally had to wait 30 minutes or more to be processed and receive their vehicles, particularly at peak times of the day. Processing a customer began with the employee accessing the customer's contract online. If the customer was new to the site, the basic policies and possible additional charges were briefly explained. The employee then made copies of the customer's identification and credit card and took a digital photo of the customer. The customer put down an €80 refundable deposit, signed the contract, and drove the car away.

All vehicles were rented with more or less empty fuel tanks, with the exact level dependent on how much gasoline was left in the vehicle when the previous renter returned it. Customers were provided with a small map of the immediate area around the rental site, showing the locations and hours of nearby gas stations. Customers could return vehicles with any amount of gas in them as long as the low-fuel indicator light in the vehicle was not on. Customers who returned vehicles with the low-fuel indicator light on were charged a fueling fee of €16.

Customers were also expected to return the vehicle within a prearranged one-hour period, which they also selected at the time of booking. While customers did not have to worry about refueling the car before returning it, they were expected to thoroughly clean the car. This clean car policy was implemented in May 2002 as a way to further reduce the price customers could pay for their vehicle. Prior to this change, all customers paid a fixed preparation fee of €11 each time they rented a vehicle (up from the €8 preparation fee when the company started operations in 2000). The new policy reduced this up-front preparation fee to €4 but required customers to either return the vehicle clean or pay an additional cleaning fee of €16. In order to avoid any misunderstanding, easyCar provided customers with an explicit description of what constituted a clean car, both for the interior and the exterior. It had to be apparent, for example, that the exterior of the car had been washed. The maps showing nearby gas stations also showed nearby car washes. While easyCar had received some bad press in relation to the policy,[21] 85 percent of customers returned their vehicles clean as a result of it.

When a customer returned the vehicle, an easyCar employee would check to make sure that the vehicle was clean and undamaged and that the low-fuel indicator light was not on. The employee would also check the kilometers driven. The customer would then be notified of any additional charges. These charges would be subtracted from the €80 deposit and the difference refunded to the customer's credit card (or, if additional charges exceeded the €80 deposit, the customer's credit card would be charged the difference).

PRICING

EasyCar's low pricing was a major point of distinction from rival car rental companies. EasyCar advertised prices as low as €5 a day plus a per rental preparation fee of €4. Prices, however, varied by the location and dates of the rental, by when the booking was made, and by what time the car was to be picked up and returned. EasyCar's systems constantly evaluated projected demand and expected use at each site, and adjusted price accordingly. Achieving the €5 a day rate usually required customers to book well in advance, and these rates were typically available only on weekdays. Weekend rates, when booked well in advance, typically started a few euros higher than the weekday rates. As a given rental date approached, however, the price typically went up significantly as easyCar approached 100 percent fleet use for that day. Rates could triple overnight if there was sufficient booking activity. Generally, however, easyCar's price was less than half that of its major competitors. EasyCar, unlike most other rental car companies, required customers to pay in full at the time of booking, and once a booking was made, it was nonrefundable.

EasyCar's base price covered only the core rental of the vehicle—the total price customers paid was in many cases much higher and depended on how the customer reserved, paid for, used, and returned the vehicle. EasyCar's price was based on customers booking through the company's Web site and paying for their rental with their easyMoney credit card. EasyMoney was the easyGroup's credit and financial services company. Customers who chose to book through the company's phone reservation system were charged an additional €0.95 a minute for the call, and those who used other credit cards were charged €5 extra. All vehicles had to be paid for by a credit or debit card—cash was not accepted. The base rental price allowed customers to drive vehicles 100 kilometers per day—additional kilometers were charged at a rate of €0.12 per kilometer. In addition, customers were expected to return their cars clean and on time. Customers who returned cars that did not meet easyCar's standards for clean were charged a €16 cleaning fee. Those who returned their cars late were immediately charged €120 and subsequently charged an additional €120 for each subsequent

24-hour period in which the car was not returned. EasyCar explained the high late fee as representing the cost that the company would likely incur in providing another vehicle to the next customer. Customers wishing to make any changes to their bookings were also charged a change fee of €16. Changes could be made either before the rental started or during the rental period, but were limited to changing the dates, times, and location of the rental, and were subject to the prices and vehicle availability at the time the change was made. If the change resulted in an overall lower price for the rental, however, no refund was provided for the difference.

Beginning in 2003, for an additional charge of €4 a day, all customers were also required to purchase loss/damage insurance that eliminated the customer's liability for loss or damage to the vehicle (excluding damage to the tires or windshield of the vehicle). Through 2002, customers were able to choose whether or not to purchase additional insurance from easyCar to eliminate any financial liability in the event that the rental vehicle was damaged. The cost of this optional insurance had been €6 a day, and approximately 60 percent of easyCar's customers had purchased it. Those not purchasing this insurance either had assumed the liability for the first €800 in damages personally or had had their own insurance through some other means (e.g., some credit card companies provide this insurance to their cardholders at no additional charge for short-term rentals paid for with the credit card).

EasyCar's Web site attempted to make all of these additional charges clear to customers at the time of the booking. EasyCar had received a fair amount of bad press when it first opened for business after many renters complained about having to pay undisclosed charges when they returned their cars.[22] In response, easyCar had revamped its Web site in an effort to make these charges more transparent to customers and to explain the logic behind many of them.

PROMOTION

EasyCar's promotional efforts through 2002 had focused primarily on posters and press advertising. Posters were particularly prevalent in metro systems and bus and train stations in cities where easyCar

had operations. All of this advertising focused on easyCar's low price. According to founder Stelios:

> You will never see an advert for an easy company offering an experience—it's about price. If you create expectations you can't live up to, then you will ultimately suffer as a result.[23]

The company allocated £1.43 million to advertising in 2002.[24]

EasyCar also promoted itself by displaying its name, phone number, and Web address prominently on the doors and rear window of its entire fleet of vehicles, and took advantage of free publicity when the opportunity presented itself. An example of seeking out such publicity occurred when Hertz complained that easyCar's comparative advertising campaign in the Netherlands that featured the line "The best reason to use easyCar.com can be found at hertz.nl" violated Dutch law that required comparative advertising to be exact, not general. In response, Stelios and a group of easyCar employees, dressed in orange boiler suits and with a fleet of easyCar vehicles, protested outside the Hertz Amsterdam office with signs asking "What is Hertz frightened of?"[25]

In an effort to help reach its goal of quadrupling sales in the next two years, easyCar had recently hired Jennifer Mowat into the new position of commercial director to take over responsibility for easyCar's European marketing. Mowat had previously been eBay's UK country manager and had recently completed an MBA in Switzerland. Previously, Stelios and easyCar's managing director, Andrew Fitzmaurice, had handled the marketing function themselves.[26] As part of this stepped-up marketing effort, easyCar also planned to double its advertising budget for 2003, to £3 million, and to begin to advertise on television. The television advertising campaign was to feature easyCar's founder, Stelios.[27]

LEGAL CHALLENGES

EasyCar faced several challenges to its approaches. The most significant dealt with a November 2002 ruling made by the Office of Fair Trading (OFT) that easyCar had to grant customers seven days from the time they made a booking to cancel their booking and receive a full refund. The OFT was a

UK governmental agency responsible for protecting UK consumers from unfair and/or anticompetitive business practices. The ruling against easyCar was based on the 2000 Consumer Protection Distance Selling Regulations. These regulations stipulated that companies that sell at a distance (e.g., by Internet or phone) must provide customers with a seven-day cooling-off period, during which time customers can cancel their contracts with the company and receive a full refund. The law exempted accommodation, transportation, catering, and leisure service companies from this requirement. The OFT's ruling concluded that easyCar did not qualify as a transportation service company because the consumer had to drive themselves, and therefore they were not receiving a transport service, just a car.[28]

EasyCar had appealed the OFT's decision to the UK High Court on the grounds that it was indeed a transportation service company and was entitled to an exemption from this requirement. EasyCar was hopeful that it would eventually win this legal challenge. EasyCar had argued that this ruling would destroy the company's book-early-pay-less philosophy and could lead to a tripling of prices.[29] Chairman Stelios was quoted as saying:

> It is very serious. My fear is that as soon as we put in the seven-day cooling off periods our utilization-rate will fall from 90% to 65%. That's the difference between a profitable company and an unprofitable one.[30]

EasyCar was also concerned that prolonged legal action on this point could interfere with its plans for a 2004 IPO.

The OFT, for its part, had also applied to the UK High Court for an injunction to make the company comply with the ruling. Other rental car companies were generally unconcerned about the ruling, because few offered big discounts for early bookings or nonrefundable bookings.[31]

EasyCar's new policy of posting the pictures of customers whose cars were 15 days or more overdue was also drawing legal criticism. EasyCar had recently received public warnings from lawyers that this new policy might violate data protection, libel, privacy, confidentiality, and human rights laws.[32] Of particular concern to some lawyers was the possibility that easyCar might post the wrong person's picture, given the large number of customers the company dealt with.[33] Such a mistake could open the company to costly libel suits. The policy of posting the pictures of overdue customers on the easyCar Web site, initiated in November 2002, was designed to reduce the losses associated with customers renting a vehicle and never returning it. The costs were significant, according to Stelios:

> These cars are expensive, £15,000 each, and we have 6,000 of them. At any given time we are looking for as many as several tens which are overdue. If we don't get one back, it's a write-off. We are writing off an entire car, and it's uninsurable.[34]

Stelios was also convinced of the legality of the new policy. In a letter to the editor responding to the legal concerns raised in the press, Stelios said:

> From a legal perspective, we have been entirely factual and objective and are merely reporting the details of the overdue car and the person who collected it. In addition, our policy is made very clear in our terms and conditions and the photo is taken both overtly and with the consent of the customer . . . I estimate the total cost of overdue cars to be 5 percent of total easyCar costs, or 50p on every car rental day for all customers. In 2004, when I intend to float easyCar, this cost will amount to £5 million unless we can reduce our quantity of overdue cars.[35]

In the past, easyCar had simply provided pictures to police when a rental was 15 or more days overdue. It was hoped that posting the picture would both discourage drivers from not returning vehicles and shame those drivers who currently had overdue cars into returning them. In fact, the first person whose photo was posted on the easyCar Web site did indeed return his car two days later. The vehicle was 29 days late.[36]

THE FUTURE

At the end of 2002, Stelios had stepped down as the CEO of easyJet so that he could devote more of his time to the other easyGroup companies, including easyCar. He had three priorities for the new year. One was to turn around the money-losing easyInternetCafe business, which Stelios had described as "the worst mistake of my career."[37] The 22-store chain had lost £80 million in the last two years. Stelios's second priority was to oversee the planned launch of another new easyGroup business, easy-Cinema, in the spring of 2003. And the third was to oversee the rapid expansion of the easyCar chain so that it would be ready for an initial public offering by year-end 2004.

Endnotes

[1] www.easyCar.com

[2] "The Big Picture—an Interview with Stelios," *Sunday Herald* (UK), March 16, 2003.

[3] "Click to Fly," *The Economist,* May 13, 2004.

[4] E. Simpkins, "Stelios Isn't Taking It Easy," *Sunday Telegraph* (UK), December 15, 2002.

[5] Avis Europe plc 2002 annual report, p. 10, http://ir.avis-europe.com/avis/reports, accessed August 16, 2004.

[6] "Marketing: Former eBay UK Chief Lands Top easyCar Position," *Financial Times* Information Limited, January 9, 2003.

[7] T. Burt, "EasyCar Agrees Deal with Vauxhall," *Financial Times,* April 30, 2002, p. 24.

[8] Simpkins, "Stelios Isn't Taking It Easy."

[9] N. Hodgson, "Stelios Plans easyCar Float," *Liverpool Echo,* September 24, 2002.

[10] "Marketing Week: Don't Write Off the Car Rental Industry," *Financial Times* Information Limited, September 26, 2002.

[11] "EasyCar Set to Shake Up German Car Rental Market," European Intelligence Wire, February 22, 2002.

[12] Ibid.

[13] Hodgson, "Stelios Plans easyCar Float."

[14] A. Felsted, "EasyCar Courts Clio for Rental Fleet," *Financial Times,* February 11, 2002, p. 26.

[15] EasyCar.com news release, March 1, 2000, www.easyCar.com.

[16] T. Burt, "EasyCar Agrees Deal with Vauxhall."

[17] EasyCar.com news release, May 2, 2002, www.easyCar.com.

[18] "Marketing Week: EasyCar Appoints Head of European Marketing," *Financial Times* Information Limited, January 9, 2003.

[19] Simpkins, "Stelios Isn't Taking It Easy."

[20] Ibid.

[21] J. Hyde, "Travel View: Clearing Up on the Extras," *The Observer* (UK), July 7, 2002.

[22] J. Stanton, "The Empire That's Easy Money," *Edinburgh Evening News,* November 26, 2002.

[23] "The Big Picture."

[24] "EasyCar Appoints Head of European Marketing."

[25] EasyCar.com news release, April 22, 2002, www.easyCar.com.

[26] "EasyCar Appoints Head of European Marketing."

[27] "Campaigning: EasyGroup Appoints Publicist for easyCar TV Advertising Brief," *Financial Times* Information Limited, January 31, 2003.

[28] J. Macintosh, "EasyCar Sues OFT amid Threat to Planned Flotation," *Financial Times,* November 22, 2002, p. 4.

[29] "EasyCar Appoints Head of European Marketing."

[30] Mackintosh, "EasyCar Sues OFT amid Threat.

[31] Ibid.

[32] B. Sherwood & A. Wendlandt, "EasyCar May Be in Difficulty over Naming Ploy," *Financial Times,* November 14, 2002, p. 2.

[33] Ibid.

[34] "E-Business: Internet Fraudsters Fail to Steal Potter Movie's Magic & Other News," *Financial Times* Information Limited, November 19, 2002.

[35] S. Haji-Ioannou, "Letters to the Editor: Costly Effect of Late Car Return," *Financial Times,* November 16, 2002, p. 10.

[36] M. Hookham, "How Stelios Nets Return of His Cars," *Daily Post* (Liverpool, UK), November 14, 2002.

[37] S. Bentley, "The Worst Mistake of My Career, by Stelios" *Financial Times,* December 24, 2002.

Smithfield Foods' Vertical Integration Strategy

LaRue T. Hosmer
The University of Michigan

In 2005 Smithfield Foods was the largest hog producer and pork processor in the world. The company raised 14 million hogs domestically (a 14 percent U.S. share) and processed 27 million hogs annually (a 27 percent U.S. share). Smithfield marketed chops, roasts, ribs, loins, ground pork, bacon, hams, sausages, and sliced deli meats under such brands as Smithfield, Smithfield Lean Generation, John Morrell, Gwaltney, Patrick Cudahy, Stefano's, Farmland, Quick-n-Easy, and Jean Caby (France), plus it had the two best-known meat brands in Poland—Krakus and Morliny. Smithfield specialized in producing exceptionally lean hogs; the company had exclusive U.S. franchise rights to a proprietary breed of SPG sows that accounted for about 55 percent of its herd and provided live hogs for its best-selling Smithfield Lean Generation Pork products. In 2005 Smithfield operated 52 pork processing plants and 7 beef processing plants. A new state-of-the-art ham processing plant opened in 2005.

Since 1981, the company had made some 32 acquisitions to expand geographically, diversify into new product segments, and vertically integrate its pork business. Smithfield's acquisitions of Moyer Packing Company and Packerland Holdings in 2002 made it the fifth largest beef producer in the United States. In 1998, Smithfield began expanding into foreign markets, making acquisitions in Canada, France, Romania, and Poland and establishing joint ventures in Mexico, Spain, and China. Two meat processors in Poland and Romania were acquired in 2004, along with a Romanian hog farming operation with 15,000 sows producing 200,000 market hogs

annually. Management believed its acquisitions and joint ventures gave the company strong market positions, high-quality manufacturing facilities, and excellent growth and exporting potential to serve regions that already had high pork consumption levels and that were emerging as major meat consumers. Executives were particularly excited about the company's opportunities in the European Union.

In pork, Smithfield had pursued a vertical integration strategy, establishing operations in hog farming, feed mills, meat packing plants, and distribution. Smithfield's hog processing group, the chief subsidiary of which was Murphy-Brown LLC, owned and operated hog farms with close to 900,000 sows in North Carolina, South Carolina, Virginia, Utah, Colorado, Texas, Oklahoma, South Dakota, Iowa, Missouri, Illinois, Mexico, Romania, and Poland.

Smithfield Foods was headquartered in Smithfield, Virginia, where it operated two large hog processing plants. But large parts of the company's operations were in North Carolina—Smithfield's biggest pork processing plant was in Bladen County, North Carolina, and the company's Murphy-Brown hog production subsidiary had a very sizable hog farming operation in eastern North Carolina. Smithfield opened a new state-of-the-art ham processing plant in Kinston, North Carolina, in 2005 that employed 206 workers; the Kinston plant was expected to be the most efficient premier-cooked-ham plant in the United States, employing the newest technologies available and meeting the highest food standards in the industry. Smithfield's large southern base provided low wages and relatively low operating costs across much of its integrated operations, factors that helped pave the

Exhibit 1   **Financial and Operating Summary, Smithfield Foods, 1995–2004 (in millions, except per share amounts)**

	2004	2003	2001	1999	1995
Operations					
Sales revenues	$9,267.0	$7,135.4	$5,123.7	$3,550.0	$1,526.5
Gross profit	938.9	602.2	762.3	448.6	126.9
Selling, general, and administrative expenses	570.8	497.9	416.2	280.4	62.4
Depreciation expense	167.5	151.5	114.5	59.3	19.7
Interest expenses	121.3	87.8	81.5	38.4	14.1
Income from continuing operations	162.7	11.9	214.3	89.6	31.9
Net income	$ 227.1	$ 26.3	$ 223.5	$ 94.9	$ 27.8
Earnings per share	$2.03	$0.24	$2.03	$1.16	$0.40
Financial position					
Working capital	$1,056.6	$ 833.0	$ 635.4	$ 215.9	$ 60.9
Total assets	4,813.7	4,410.6	3,250.9	1,771.6	550.2
Total debt	1,801.5	1,642.3	1,188.7	610.3	234.7
Shareholders' equity	1,617.2	1,299.2	1,053.1	542.2	184.0
Current ratio	2.09	2.02	2.01	1.46	1.35
Total debt to total capitalization	52.7%	55.8%	53.0%	53.0%	58.4%
Other statistics					
Capital expenditures	$151.4	$172.0	$113.3	$92.0	$90.6
Number of employees	46,400	44,100	34,000	33,000	9,000

Source: 2004 annual report.

way for Smithfield's competitive prices and strong growth.

The company's longtime chairman and CEO, Joseph W. Luter III, continually emphasized the need to drive down costs and push up sales. Top executives at Smithfield Foods wanted to continue the company's rapid and profitable expansion and were constantly on the lookout for opportunities to grow the company's business. Going into 2006, Smithfield had annualized sales of close to $11 billion, up from $1.5 billion in 1995; revenues had grown at a compound average rate of close to 24 percent during the past decade. Exhibit 1 provides historical financial data.

OPPOSITION TO SMITHFIELD'S EXPANSION

Over the last decade, Smithfield Foods had met with mounting opposition to expansion of its business,

particularly in hog farming. The chief pockets of opposition to Smithfield's hog farming activities came from rural residents in eastern North Carolina, where there were some 8,000 hog farms. Neighboring residents complained that commercial hog farming had essentially been imposed on them and that it entailed substantial adverse impacts in the form of low wages and environmental discharges.

Eastern North Carolina and Smithfield's Hog Farming Operations

Eastern North Carolina, essentially the area extending about 150 miles from Raleigh (the state capital) to the Atlantic coast, is a region of flat land, sandy soil, and ample rainfall. At one time it was a relatively prosperous region, with thousands of small family farms, each of which had a tobacco allotment. During the 1930s far more tobacco had been grown than was needed, and the price plummeted. One of the government initiatives of the Depression era was a restriction on the total amount of tobacco that could be grown, and this total amount was divided up among the existing growers by restricting each to a set percentage of the amount of their land that had been devoted to the crop during a given base year. These restrictions on growth first stabilized and later increased the price, and the possession of an allotment almost guaranteed the financial prosperity of the farm.

The typical family farm would have 150 to 200 acres. Perhaps 15 acres would be devoted to tobacco, and the balance would be sown in corn, wheat, rye, or soybeans, or left as pasture for cattle or—more frequently—hogs. The grains grown locally would be trucked to the nearest town within the region to be milled into feed and then returned to the farm for the livestock. The cattle and hogs produced locally would be trucked to the nearest town to be sold at auction, and then slaughtered and processed at a nearby packing plant. These towns were also relatively prosperous, as the farmers and their families purchased clothing and household goods at local stores and automobiles and farm machinery at local dealers.

This prosperity started downhill in the 1970s as the national campaigns against smoking led to continual reductions in the size, and consequently the profitability, of the tobacco allotments, which eventually came almost to an end. Local prosperity continued to decline in the 1980s as very large feed lots in Nebraska, Iowa, and Kansas developed a much less costly means of raising hogs prior to slaughter; the piglets spent only the first 12 to 15 months of their lives on the farms where they were bred before being brought to fenced open-air corrals where they were closely confined but fed continuously to gain weight. Farmers in eastern North Carolina had to compete against this new and far more efficient production process. Prices for the hogs raised in eastern North Carolina declined sharply, and many of the local packing plants went out of business.

Local prosperity stabilized to some extent in the 1990s, though with a greatly changed distribution of income, as Smithfield Foods introduced the concept of the factory farm. Large metal sheds with concrete floors were built, each designed to hold up to 1,000 hogs. Feeding was by means of a mechanized conveyor that carried food alongside both walls. Waste was removed by hosing it off the floors to a central

trough that carried it to a storage lagoon. Temperature was controlled by huge fans at each end of each shed. Every effort was made to reduce costs. Feed grains were no longer grown, purchased, and milled locally; instead most grains were grown, purchased, and milled in the Midwest and transported to eastern North Carolina by unit feed trains, which were strings of covered hopper cars that moved as a unit, without switching, from the feed mill in Nebraska or Iowa directly to one of the company's distribution centers in North Carolina. Some feed grains were grown and purchased even more cheaply abroad, primarily in Australia and Argentina, and then carried by ship to a company-leased milling facility and distribution center in Wilmington (a port in southeastern North Carolina, near the South Carolina border).

Limited farm machinery was needed for this new method of raising hogs, given that few feed grains were grown locally, but the little that was needed was purchased by the Smithfield headquarters office directly from the manufacturer. Many farm equipment dealers within the region were forced to close. Even diesel fuel, needed for the trucks that transported the feed grains to the farms and the mature hogs to the packing plants, was purchased from the refinery, transported by railway tank cars to large storage tanks at the distribution centers, and pumped directly into the trucks. Local fuel dealers got little or none of this business. All truck purchases were arranged by bid from national dealers located in Detroit (auto companies had refused to sell outside their dealer chains, but they allegedly gave favored prices to very large dealers near their corporate headquarters) at very low prices, and all subsequent truck repairs were done at company-owned repair shops located at the company-owned distribution centers. Some truck dealers in the region were forced to close.

Executives at Smithfield Foods did not apologize for the business model that they had created. Their attitude could be summed up as follows: "This is the way the world is going and this is what the market demands. All we have done is to create a competitive system that works. Moreover, we have saved farms and brought jobs to the eastern North Carolina region through this system, and we have provided better (leaner) pork products at lower prices to our customers." Smithfield's development of a "competitive system that works" had won Joseph Luter an award as Master Entrepreneur of the Year in 2002;

a Smithfield news release dated December 21, 2002, said:

> Joseph W. Luter III has been named the Ernst & Young 2002 Virginia Master Entrepreneur of the Year. The Ernst & Young program recognizes entrepreneurs who have demonstrated excellence and extraordinary success in such areas as innovation, financial performance and personal commitment to their businesses and communities . . .
>
> Since becoming chairman and chief executive officer of Smithfield Foods, Inc. in 1975, Mr. Luter transformed the company from a small, regional meat packer with sales of $125 million and net worth of $1 million to an international concern with annual sales of $8 billion and a net worth of $1.4 billion.

Smithfield Foods did not own the farms that raised the hogs. Instead, company representatives would select a reasonably large farm, one that had been successful in the past and therefore was financially solvent now, and negotiate a contract with the owning family to raise hogs at a set price per animal. The farm family would frequently use a loan provided through the Smithfield Corporation and a contractor licensed by the Smithfield Corporation to build metal barns with concrete floors, feed conveyors, ventilation fans, and waste systems; connect the waste systems to storage lagoons (five to eight acres in size); construct feed bins and loading ramps; and be ready for business. Smithfield Corporation would then deliver the hogs at piglet stage, provide a constant supply of feed grains mixed with antibiotics (to prevent disease in the crowded conditions of the metal barns), and offer free veterinarian service. The responsibility of the farm family was to raise those hogs to marketable weight as quickly and as efficiently as possible. This was termed *contract farming*; it was described in the following terms in a five-part investigative series that ran February 19–26, 1995, in the *Raleigh News and Observer*:

> Greg Stephens is the 1995 version of the North Carolina hog farmer. He owns no hogs. Stephens carries a mortgage on four new confinement barns that cost him $300,000 to build. The 4,000 hogs inside belong to a company called Prestage Farms, Inc. (one of the larger suppliers of Smithfield Foods). Prestage simply pays Stephens a fee to raise them . . .
>
> This arrangement is called contract farming, and it's hardly risk-free. But for anyone wanting to

break into the swine business these days, it's the only game in town. "Without a contract, there's no way I'd be raising hogs," says Stephens, "and even if I had somehow gotten in, my pockets aren't nearly deep enough to let me stay in."

> Welcome to corporate livestock production, the force behind the swine industry's explosive growth in North Carolina. The backbone of the new system is a network of hundreds of contractors like Stephens, the franchise owners in a system that more closely resembles a fast-food chain than traditional agriculture.
>
> Nowhere in the nation has this change been as dramatic, or as officially embraced, as in North Carolina. As a result, the hog population has more than doubled in four years, and nearly all of that growth has occurred on farms controlled by the big companies. Meanwhile, independent farmers have left the business by the thousands.

In 1998 Smithfield Foods reportedly had a two-year waiting list of farmers wishing to obtain hog farming contracts. Industry observers, however, worried about the practice of saddling hundreds of small farmers with thousands of dollars of debt. As one elected state representative said, "Why invest your capital when you can get a farmer to take the risk? Why own the farm when you can own the farmer?"[1]

The problem foreseen by industry observers was the possibility that a company could cancel its contract with only 30 days' notice, leaving the farmer with the debt and no income to repay it, or could threaten to cancel and then renew the contract only with a sharply lower price per animal. Both sudden cancellations and lower prices were said to have happened frequently in the poultry industry:

> The changes that are sweeping the swine industry today were pioneered by chicken and turkey growers in the 1960s and '70s. Total confinement housing, vertical integration, and contract farming are all standard practices in the feather world. As a result, you need only look at chickens to see where pork is headed.
>
> The poultry industry today is fully integrated—meaning a handful of companies control all phases of production—and the labor is performed by an army of contract growers, some of them decidedly unhappy. "It's sharecropping, that's what it is," said Larry Holder, a chicken farmer and president of the Contract Poultry Growers Association.

The *Raleigh News and Observer* interviewed a number of farmers with hog-growing contracts in

North Carolina. One farmer with 10 years of experience growing for Carroll Farms (another large supplier of Smithfield Foods), said, "They've been nothing but good to me."[2] Greg Stephens, the farmer quoted earlier, told the *News and Observer* that in his case the biggest selling point had been his freedom from market risk: "If hog prices go south, as they did two months ago, the contract farmer is barely affected. The company that owns the pigs takes on more risk than you do."[3]

The survival of over 1,000 family farms as contract hog growers is cited as one of the major benefits of the industrialization of agriculture in eastern North Carolina. Another is the creation of new agricultural jobs. Each of the contract farms averages 7,500 animals. The owning families cannot care for all those animals, even though the hogs are closely confined and automatically fed and watered. The typical farm will employ five people from the community at wages of $7 to $8 an hour; working conditions are hard and unpleasant. Most of the people filling such jobs are untrained and poorly educated area residents.

Smithfield's three newest slaughterhouses in North Carolina employed about 3,200 people. Many of the jobs at these plants were regarded as hard and unpleasant; some involved killing and disemboweling the hogs. The killing was said to be painless, and much of the early processing (scraping the carcass to remove the hair, and dealing with the internal organs) was automated. One of the more labor-intensive tasks involved preparing cuts of meat for packaged sale at grocery chains. Most grocery chains, to reduce their internal costs, had eliminated the position of store butchers, opting instead to buy their fresh meats cut, wrapped, packaged, and ready for sale. The cutting at meatpacking facilities was done on a high-speed assembly line, using very sharp laser-guided knives; workers were under continual pressure to perform and were exposed to dangers of injury. Workers who became skilled at this cutting and were able to endure the stress earned $10 to $12 an hour; turnover was relatively high because of the strenuous job demands. Many of the workers at the high-volume packing plants in eastern North Carolina were immigrants from Central or South America. The jobs were described in the following terms by an undercover reporter for the *New York Times* who worked at one of the Smithfield packing plants for three weeks on what was termed the picnic line:

One o'clock means it is getting near the end of the workday [for the first shift]. Quota has to be met, and the workload doubles. The conveyor belt always overflows with meat around 1 o'clock. So the workers redouble their pace, hacking pork from shoulder bones with a driven single-mindedness. They stare blankly, like mules in wooden blinders, as the butchered slabs pass by.

It is called the picnic line: 18 workers lined up on both sides of a belt, carving meat from bone. Up to 16 million shoulders a year come down that line here at Smithfield Packing Co., the largest pork production plant in the world. That works out to about 32,000 per shift, 63 a minute, one every 17 seconds for each worker for eight and a half hours a day. The first time you stare down at that belt you know your body is going to give in way before the machine ever will.[4]

Smithfield's vertical integration strategy, which had resulted in very limited purchasing of feed, machinery, and fuel from local sources; the debt-laden nature of the farm contracts, which fueled concerns about the possibility of future contract cancellations or price reductions; and the low-pay/low-quality nature of the jobs that had been created at both the farms and the packing plants had combined to create strong, often vocal, opposition on the part of many local residents to any planned expansion of Smithfield Foods within eastern North Carolina.

A much bigger and far more intense issue, however, was the alleged impact of a concentrated cluster of hog farms on the environment:

Imagine a city as big as New York suddenly grafted onto North Carolina's Coastal Plain. Double it. Now imagine that this city has no sewage treatment plants. All the wastes from 15 million inhabitants are simply flushed into open pits and sprayed onto fields.

Turn those humans into hogs, and you don't have to imagine at all. It's already here. A vast city of swine has risen practically overnight in the counties east of Interstate 95. It's a megalopolis of 7 million animals that live in metal confinement barns and produce two to four times as much waste, per hog, as the average human.

All that manure—about 9.5 million tons a year—is stored in thousands of earthen pits called lagoons, where it is decomposed and sprayed or spread on crop lands. The lagoon system is the source of most hog farm odor, but industry officials say it's a proven and effective way to keep harmful chemicals and bacteria out of water supplies. New evidence says otherwise:

- The *News and Observer* has obtained new scientific studies showing that contaminants from hog lagoons are getting into groundwater. One N.C. State University report estimates that as many as half of existing lagoons—perhaps hundreds—are leaking badly enough to contaminate ground water.

- The industry also is running out of places to spread or spray the waste from lagoons. On paper, the state's biggest swine counties already are producing more phosphorous-rich manure than available land can absorb, state Agriculture Department records show.

- Scientists are discovering that hog farms emit large amounts of ammonia gas, which returns to earth in rain. The ammonia is believed to be contributing to an explosion of algae growth that's choking many of the state's rivers and estuaries.[5]

Raising hogs is admitted even by farm families to be a messy and smelly business. Hogs eat more than other farm animals, and they excrete more. And those excretions smell far, far worse. Having 50 to 100 hogs running free in a fenced pasture is one thing. The odor is clearly noticeable, but that sharp and pungent smell is felt to be part of rural living. Having 5,000 to 10,000 hogs closely confined in metal barns, with large ventilation fans moving the air continually from each barn, and the wastes from those hogs collected in huge open-air lagoons is something else. People who live near one of the large hog farms say that, unless you've experienced it, you just can't know what it is like:

> At 11 o'clock sharp on a Sunday morning the choir marched into the sanctuary of New Brown's Chapel Baptist Church. And the stench of 4,800 hogs rolled right in with them.
>
> The odor hung oppressively in the vestibule, clinging to church robes, winter coats and fancy hats. It sent stragglers scurrying indoors from the parking lot, some holding their noses. Sherry Leveston, 4, pulled her fancy white sweater over her face as she ran. "It stinks," she cried.
>
> It was another Sunday morning in Brownsville, a Greene County North Carolina hamlet that's home to 200 people and one hog farm. Like many of its counterparts throughout the eastern portion of the state, the town hasn't been the same since the hogs moved in a couple of years ago.

> To some, each new gust from the south [the direction of the farm] is a reminder of serious wrongs committed for which there has been no redress. "We've basically given up," said the Rev. Charles White, pastor at New Brown's Chapel.
>
> In scores of rural neighborhoods down east [the eastern portion of North Carolina] the talk is the same. There's something new in the air, and people are furious about it.
>
> Hog odor is by far the most emotional issue facing the pork industry—and the most divisive. Growers assert their right to earn a living; neighbors say they have a right to odor-free air. Hog company officials, meanwhile, accuse activists of exaggerating the problem to stir up opposition . . .
>
> For other residents [of Brownsville, close to New Brown's Chapel] hog odor has simply become an inescapable part of their daily routine. It's usually heaviest about 5 a.m., when Lisa Hines leaves the house for her factory job. It seeps into her car and follows her on her commute to work. It clings to her hair and clothes during the day. And it awaits her when she returns home in the afternoon.
>
> "It makes me so mad," she said. "The owner lives miles away from here, and he can go home and smell apples and cinnamon if he wants to. But we have no choice."[6]

The 7 million hogs in eastern North Carolina currently generate about 9.5 million tons of manure each year. This waste was stored in large earthen pits called lagoons. These pits were open so that sunlight would decompose the wastes and kill the harmful bacteria; the manure was then spread on farm fields as organic fertilizer. This had been the accepted means for disposing of animal wastes on small family farms for centuries. It was a method fully protected by federal, state, and local laws; a hog farmer—whether a small family or large contract farm—could not be sued for any inconveniences brought about by the hogs, unless those inconveniences were the result of clear negligence in caring for the hogs.

The difference now, of course, comes from the huge expansion of scale. Again, the wastes of 50 to 100 animals were easily accommodated. There was a noticeable effect on air quality, but that was felt to be a natural consequence of living in the country, and the smell came from your own farm, or that of your neighbor, or that of a person who had been there for years. There was a probable effect on water quality, but farm wells were always located uphill and a substantial distance from manure piles, and it was thought that neighbors would be protected by natural filtration through the clay subsoils of the region. No one worried very much about possible public health effects of small numbers of farm animals.

The wastes from 5,000 to 10,000 animals could not be so easily accommodated, and people did worry about the possible public health effects of very large numbers of farm animals. Debilitating asthma had become a much more frequent condition among young children who lived near large hog farms, and there was concern that waste was leaking from the lagoons and contaminating the groundwater. The conventional wisdom about the lagoons was that the heavier sludge was supposed to settle on the bottom and form a seal that would prevent the escape of harmful bacteria or destructive chemicals:

> As recently as two years ago, the U.S. Division of Environmental Management told state lawmakers in a briefing that lagoons effectively self-seal within months with "little or no groundwater contamination." Wendell H. Murphy, a former state senator who was also [in partnership with Smithfield Corporation] the nation's largest producer of hogs, said in an interview this month that "lagoons will seal themselves" and that "there is not one shred, not one piece of evidence anywhere in this nation that any groundwater is being contaminated by any hog lagoon."
>
> What Murphy didn't know was that a series of brand-new studies, conducted among Eastern North Carolina hog farms, showed that large numbers of lagoons are leaking, some of them severely.[7]

The *Raleigh News and Observer* had reported that researchers at North Carolina State University had dug test wells near 11 lagoons that were at least seven years old. They found that more than half of the lagoons were leaking moderately to severely; even those lagoons that were described as leaking only moderately still produced groundwater nitrate levels up to three times the allowable limit. The researchers also found that lagoons were not the only source of groundwater contamination. They dug test wells and examined water quality in fields where hog waste had been sprayed as fertilizer, and found evidence of widespread bacterial and chemical contamination. It was felt that fully as much water contamination came from the practice of attempting to dispose of the decomposed waste through spraying on crops as from the earlier storage of decomposing waste in the lagoons. According to the *Raleigh*

News and Observer reporter, too much waste was being sprayed on too few fields, even though almost all farmers in the region now accepted this natural fertilizer in lieu of buying commercial products.

The researchers from North Carolina State University, however, did not urge rural residents to rush out to buy bottled water. In most of the cases they concluded that the contaminants appeared to be migrating laterally toward the nearest ditch or stream, and they found no evidence that a private well had been contaminated. But they did find evidence that numerous streams had been contaminated, partially from leakage but primarily from spills and overflows:

> Frequently major spills are cleaned up quickly so that the public never hears about them. That's what happened in May 1995 when a 10-acre lagoon ruptured on Murphy's Farms' 8,000-hog facility in Magnolia, North Carolina. A limestone layer beneath the lagoon collapsed, sending tons of waste cascading into nearby Millers Creek in an accident that was never reported to state water-quality officials.
>
> An employee of the town's water department discovered the problem when he saw corn kernels and hog waste floating by in the creek that runs through the center of town. He alerted the company, and within hours a task force had been assembled to plug the leak.
>
> It took four days to find the source and fix the problem. But neither Magnolia town officials nor Murphy Farms executives ever notified the state about the spill.
>
> "In retrospect, maybe we should have," Wendell Murphy said, "but I would also say that to my knowledge no harm has ever come of it."
>
> Former employees of hog companies, however, told *News and Observer* reporters that spills were a common occurrence. "Hardly a week goes by," said a former manager for one of the largest hog farms in the state, "that there isn't some sort of leak or overflow. Almost any heavy rain will bring an overflow. When that happens, workers do the best they can to clean it up. After that it's just pray no one notices and keep your mouth shut," he explained.[8]

The waste lagoons could not be covered with a roof to prevent overflows associated with heavy rains, or enclosed with a building to prevent the escape of odors; They were simply too large—five to eight acres—and it was necessary to have direct sunlight to create the natural conditions that would break down the toxic chemicals and kill the harmful bacteria in the wastes. Company officials seemed to believe that there was no possible solution to the problem of the extremely bad odors; essentially they said it would just be necessary for people to learn to live with the smell, which extends up to two miles from the open lagoons and the sprayed fields. According to the *Raleigh News and Observer,*

> Wendell Murphy, chairman of Murphy Family Farms [part of the Murphy Brown hog farming subsidiary of Smithfield Foods] said that while the hog industry is extremely sensitive to the odor problem, he thinks the industry's economic importance should be considered in the equation. "Should we expect the odor to never drift off the site to a neighbor's house? If so, then we're out of business. We all have to have some inconvenience once in a while for the benefits that come with it."[9]

As the *Raleigh News and Observer* reported, feelings ran high among eastern North Carolina residents in opposing further expansion of hog farming in the region:

> Three weeks ago, the tiny town of Faison held a referendum of sorts on whether its residents wanted a new industrial plant, with 1,500 new jobs, built in their community. The jobs lost.
>
> Because the industry in question was a hog-processing plant, people packed the local fire station an hour early to blast the idea. They jeered and hissed every time the county's industrial recruiter mentioned pigs or the plant. "I want to know two things," thundered one burly speaker thrusting a finger at that much smaller industrial recruiter, Woody Brinson. "How can we stop this thing, and how can we get you fired?"
>
> The town council's eventual 3–0 vote against the proposed IBP [a subsidiary of Smithfield Foods] hog slaughterhouse may have little effect on whether the plant is built. [Zoning within rural North Carolina is controlled by the county, not the municipality, and agriculturally related zoning has always been very loosely applied, to benefit local farmers.] What was striking about this meeting, and this vote, was that both occurred in the heart of Duplin County, an economic showcase for the hog industry.
>
> With a pigs-per-person ratio of 32-to-1, Duplin has seen big payoffs from eastern North Carolina's hog revolution in the past decade. The county's revenues from sales and property taxes have soared, and Duplin's per capita income has risen from the lowest 25 percent statewide to about the middle.

Pork production also has spawned jobs in support businesses in Duplin and neighboring counties. People in the hog business say farm odor—"the smell of money"—is a small price to pay for a big benefit. "These hog farms are putting money in people's pockets," says Woody Brinston [the county's director of industrial development]. "Duplin County is booming."

But even here, some bitterly resent the way the industry has transformed the way the countryside looks and smells. Some say that their property has gone down in value. Others note the contrasts in the economic picture. In Duplin County, just 70 miles east of the booming Research Triangle [an area located between Raleigh, Durham, and Chapel Hill with a large number of advanced electronic and biotechnology firms], the population hasn't grown in 10 years. Farm jobs are dwindling despite the rise in hog production.

Daryl Walker, a newly elected Duplin County commissioner, says he hears these arguments all the time. "If this is prosperity," he says, "many of my constituents would just as soon do without it. They are scared to death that there are just going to be more and more hogs, and more and more of the problems that come with those hogs.[10]

A subsequent letter to the editor of the *Raleigh News and Observer* said:

> Last Sunday, returning from a weekend at Wrightsville Beach, we stopped at an Interstate 40 rest area near Clinton. When we stepped from our car the stench brought tears to our eyes. So add to the ever-mounting environment damage the poor image our state now leaves with tourists heading towards our beautiful coast. We'll never know how many big tourism bucks are now and soon will be going elsewhere.[11]

SMITHFIELD'S EFFORTS TO ADDRESS CONCERNS ABOUT THE ENVIRONMENTAL IMPACT OF ITS VERTICAL INTEGRATION STRATEGY

Smithfield management was endeavoring to combat opposition to its operations in eastern North Carolina and elsewhere and to respond to the environmental challenges that its pork business presented.

Exhibit 2   **Examples of Smithfield Foods' Environmental Projects, 2000–2004**

- In 2000, Smithfield signed an agreement with the Office of the North Carolina Attorney General to contribute $2 million per year for 25 years to a fund used for such environmental enhancement projects as constructing and maintaining wetlands, preserving environmentally sensitive lands, and promoting similar projects. In 2003, the attorney general used Smithfield's contributions for grants to five recipients: the Cape Fear River Assembly, Save Our State, the Green Trust Alliance, the North Carolina Coastal Land Trust, and the North Carolina Foundation for Soil and Water Conservation Districts.

- Smithfield had funded a $15 million research project at North Carolina State University to investigate 18 different technologies to modify or replace current methods of swine waste removal at hog farms. A major goal of the project was to achieve cleaner air by finding ways to reduce methane and ammonia emissions of the swine waste lagoons. Smithfield had agreed to implement the recommended technologies, if they were commercially feasible, at all of its hog farms.

- In 2001, all of Murphy-Brown's company-owned swine production farms in North Carolina, South Carolina, and Virginia implemented "environmental management systems" (EMSs) to identify and manage parts of Smithfield's activities that have, or could have, an impact on the environment—the objective was to monitor environmental performance, pinpoint problem areas, and implement any needed preventive and corrective action. These farms then went an extra step and achieved ISO 14001 certification, making Murphy-Brown the first livestock operation in the world to do so—ISO 14001 certification was considered the gold standard for environmental excellence in implementing methods to monitor and measure the environmental impact of production operations and pinpoint problem areas. Since that time, Murphy-Brown has completed EMS implementation and achieved ISO 14001 certification for all company-owned farms in the United States.

- Smithfield was investing up to $20 million in a majority-owned subsidiary, BEST BioFuels, to build a waste collection system and a central treatment facility in southwestern Utah that used proprietary technology to convert livestock waste (which contained methane, a greenhouse gas) into biomethanol. Biomethanol could be processed with a variety of vegetable- or animal-based oils to create biodiesel, an environmentally friendly alternative to petroleum diesel. The waste-to-biomethanol treatment facility in Utah, which began operations in 2004, was connected by an underground sewage network to 23 area farms and received waste from approximately 257,000 hogs over the course of a year. The Utah plant shipped much of its 2.7 million gallons of biomethanol to a newly constructed BEST Biofuels plant in Texas, where it was processed with used cooking oil, rendered animal fat, or other oil foodstock to create biodiesel, an environmentally friendly alternative to petroleum diesel that emitted nearly 50 percent less carbon monoxide and hazardous particulate matter than regular petroleum diesel. Fuel distributors then blended biodiesel with conventional petroleum diesel in a 20/80 ratio to create a cleaner diesel fuel.

- Cooling towers were installed at four of Smithfield's company processing plants to recirculate water needed in operating the plants; these water conservation measures reduced use of groundwater and relieved stresses on local water tables.

- Smithfield had partnered with its primary corrugated packaging suppliers to pursue cardboard recycling in its operations. Since 2002, close to 50,000 tons of cardboard had been recycled rather than being sent to landfills.

- Several Smithfield plants had modified their facilities to allow biogas—a fuel source derived from plant wastewater—to be used as an energy source. Most all Smithfield plants were pursuing projects to conserve on the use of electric energy.

Source: Information contained in Smithfield's 2003 Stewardship Report and information posted at www.smithfieldfoods.com (accessed December 26, 2002, and November 23, 2004).

Exhibit 2 describes examples of Smithfield's environmental improvement projects during 2000–2004. Exhibit 3 presents Smithfield Foods' environmental policy statement. Exhibit 4 presents senior management's statement regarding the company's "Strategy for Responsible Growth." Exhibit 5 presents excerpts from the company's Code of Business Conduct.

During the spring of 2003, the highest seasonal rainfall in North Carolina's recorded history caused elevated lagoon levels at many eastern North Carolina hog farms. Farmers reported the levels to the state agency, as was the standard practice, but officials at North Carolina's Department of Environment and Natural Resources nonetheless sent out hundreds of notices of violations (NOVs), 55 of which were

Exhibit 3 **Smithfield Foods' Environmental Policy Statement, 2004**

It is the corporate policy of Smithfield Foods, Inc., and its subsidiaries to conduct business in a manner consistent with continual improvement in regard to protecting the environment.

- Smithfield Foods, Inc., is committed to protecting the environment through pollution prevention and continual improvement of our environmental practices.
- Smithfield Foods, Inc., seeks to demonstrate its responsible corporate citizenship by complying with relevant environmental legislation and regulations, and with other requirements to which we subscribe. We will create, implement, and periodically review appropriate environmental objectives and targets.
- Protection of the environment is the responsibility of all Smithfield Foods, Inc., employees.

Source: www.smithfieldfoods.com (accessed November 23, 2004).

to farms operated by Smithfield's Murphy-Brown subsidiary. While elevated lagoon levels did not compromise the structural integrity of the lagoons, they did decrease the reserve designated for storage

of rainfall accumulated over a 24-hour period from intense storms. Many farmers and legislative leaders protested the number of NOVs issued, prompting the Department of Environment and Natural Resources

Exhibit 4 **Statement of Smithfield Foods' Management Regarding the Company's Strategy for Responsible Growth**

Over the past few years, our company has set the foundations for continuous improvement in our stewardship responsibilities, which include our environmental, employee safety and animal welfare–related performance. We have firmly established the necessary policies, organizations, management systems, programs, funding, and expertise.

This foundation is now in place within the majority of our U.S. operations. We continue to move forward guided by the principles of accountability, transparency, and sustainability, and by our primary objectives:

- Achieve 100 percent regulatory compliance, 100 percent of the time.
- Move well beyond compliance in stewardship responsibilities.
- Reduce the frequency and severity of injuries to employees.
- Enhance communications and transparency with external stakeholders.
- Continue to expand community involvement.

We also have a more ambitious vision, and that is to be recognized as the industry leader for stewardship. To do this, we will continue to explore approaches to the issues that are unique to our industry. We will continue to find ways to participate productively in key industry and multi-stakeholder groups where we can help facilitate win–win solutions. We will share our experiences and best practices with our peers and other interested parties. We will also work toward policy changes that promote industry innovation and enable our company to better deliver financial, environmental, and social value.

In 2003, Smithfield embarked on a major project, committing to invest $20 million to implement technology beneficial to the environment and that will also play a key role in the solution for our global energy needs. We are using the untapped energy stored in livestock waste to create a fully renewable motor fuel—biodiesel. Our renewable fuel project at Circle Four Farms in Utah will produce in excess of 7,000 gallons of biomethanol per day. Blended with rendered fats, this biomethanol is converted to biodiesel that would meet the daily fuel requirements for about 300 over-the-road trucks, offsetting the need to import crude oil to produce that quantity of traditional diesel fuel. The project is highlighted in more detail in other sections of this report and is expected to be in full operation in late spring 2004.

We are very encouraged by the results we have seen over the past few years. Moving forward, Smithfield's strategy for responsible growth can be summed up as follows: more of the same. And by that we mean more management systems, more measurement and target setting, more innovative thinking and partnering, further support of environmentally superior waste management technologies, more communication, transparency and relationship building, more improvement—and more listening. This is what Smithfield will strive to accomplish.

Source: Smithfield Foods, *2003 Stewardship Report*, pp. 11–12.

Exhibit 5   **Excerpts from Smithfield Foods' Code of Business Conduct, 2004**

Smithfield is committed to compliance with the laws, rules, and regulations applicable to the conduct of our business wherever we operate. Our ultimate goal is 100% compliance, 100% of the time. Employees must avoid activities that could involve or lead to involvement of Smithfield or its personnel in any unlawful practice.

Employee awareness of Smithfield operating practices must include knowledge of the environmental laws and Smithfield policies governing their operations. Employees must immediately control and report all spills and releases as required by applicable regulations and facility rules.

The nature of Smithfield's business requires it to conduct various monitoring, inspecting, and testing to ensure compliance with applicable laws and regulations. Such monitoring, inspecting, and testing must be performed, and accurate records thereof made and retained, in compliance with all applicable legal requirements. Employees who have questions about legal requirements applicable to such areas should consult their supervisor or a member of the Smithfield Law Department.

Smithfield employees are expected to comply with all federal, state, local, and foreign environmental laws and all Smithfield policies related to environmental affairs. We expect 100% compliance 100% of the time. It is each employee's responsibility to know and understand the legal, policy, and operating practice requirements applicable to his or her job and to notify management when the employee believes that a violation of law or Smithfield policies has occurred. Any employee who has concerns regarding compliance in this area should immediately consult with the environmental contact for his or her facility or subsidiary, a senior environmental officer, or the Smithfield Law Department. The Smithfield Foods, Inc. Employee Hotline (1-877-237-5270) is available for reporting employee concerns anonymously.

Compliance with environmental laws and all Smithfield policies is the single highest priority for the company's environmental program. Our employees' job performance is important to us, and is evaluated not only on business results achieved, but also on whether our employees, and particularly our management team, operate within our expectations for environmental performance. We hold all of our employees to a high standard of conduct and accountability for environmental performance.

Compliance with the Smithfield Foods, Inc., Code of Business Conduct and Ethics is a condition of employment. Failure to comply may result in a range of disciplinary actions, including termination. Failure by any Smithfield employee to disclose violations of these standards and practices by other Smithfield employees or contract workers is also grounds for disciplinary action.

Source: Smithfield Foods' Code of Business Conduct, www.smithfieldfoods.com (accessed November 23, 2004).

to reconsider their having issued so many NOVs; a substantial number were subsequently reclassified as notices of deficiency (NODs). Following the severe weather, Smithfield moved swiftly to get its lagoon levels back to compliance levels and no further regulatory actions were taken. All told, Smithfield received 77 notices of violations or noncompliance in 2003, resulting in fines of $124,204. The biggest fine ($77,000) was for a wastewater incident at its Moyer beef processing plant in Pennsylvania, and a $17,875 fine was imposed for an ammonia release at a Georgia plant.

Endnotes

[1]Quoted in the five-part series by Joby Warrick and Pat Stith, "Boss Hog: North Carolina's Pork Revolution—Hog Waste Is Polluting the Ground Water," *Raleigh News and Observer,* February 19, 1995. This series, based on a seven-month investigation and run in the *News and Observer,* February 19–26, 1995, was awarded the Pulitzer Prize for Public Service Journalism in 1996.
[2]Ibid.
[3]Ibid.
[4]Charlie LeDuff, "At a Slaughterhouse, Some Things Never Die," *New York Times,* June 16, 2000, p. A1.

[5]*Raleigh News and Observer,* February 19, 1995.
[6]Joby Warrick and Pat Stith, "Boss Hog: North Carolina's Pork Revolution—Money Talks," *Raleigh News and Observer,* February 24, 1995, p. A9.
[7]Ibid.
[8]Ibid.
[9]Ibid.
[10]Joby Warrick and Pat Stith, "Boss Hog: North Carolina's Pork Revolution—Pork Barrels," *Raleigh News and Observer,* February 26, 1995.
[11]*Raleigh News and Observer,* March 4, 1995, p. A10.

Zoës Kitchen: Making Cents of the Fast-Casual Dining Industry

Braxton Maddox
The University of Alabama

Jennifer Traywick
The University of Alabama

As the globed lights illuminated the glass storefront of the newest Zoës Kitchen in Brentwood, Tennessee, curious passers-by could see a multitude of activities late that night. John Cassimus, president and CEO of Zoës Kitchen, knew every detail had to be perfect for opening day. Required were sweeping, mopping, cleaning, prepping food, and double-checking every inch of the store. The success of the entire Zoës Kitchen brand depended on how well the next few restaurants performed. As Cassimus carefully placed T-shirts, hats, and "Zoës Life" booklets, on the merchandising racks, his thoughts wandered from the cheerful, inviting store that was now almost complete to the challenges on the road ahead.

Zoës Kitchen was the natural extension of Zoë Cassimus's own kitchen—a place livened by her love of family and warm hospitality. Zoë had carefully created all the recipes from scratch, producing fresh food that also promoted good health. Her son John had carefully grown Zoës Kitchen from a single family restaurant into what could soon be one of the leading concepts in the fast-casual restaurant industry.

The fast-casual dining classification was the newest segment to emerge in the maturing restaurant industry. Year after year of double-digit sales growth was proving that fast-casual was not just a fad, and many of the major food companies had begun to take notice. With new, larger competitors looking to enter the market, John Cassimus was convinced that now was the time for Zoës Kitchen to make its strategic move.

ZOËS STORY

Marcus and Zoë Cassimus opened the first Zoës Kitchen in Homewood, Alabama, in 1995, serving lunch five days a week. Zoës Kitchen quickly became a favorite spot for both mothers with children and primarily white-collar employees in the area. As of December 2005, Zoës Kitchen operated 16 locations in five states, and each store had helped build a brand synonymous with fresh ingredients, family recipes, and homemade food. Zoës menu included a healthy selection of chicken sandwiches, rollups, pitas, dinner plates, and an assortment of salads including chicken, potato, pasta, and egg (see Exhibit 1). Customers could also purchase many salads and sides by the pound to take home. Most menu items had a Greek influence, reflecting the heritage of the Cassimus family.

John Cassimus graduated from the University of Alabama in 1990 as a four-time football letterman. After graduation, he began work with Pittman Financial Partners in Birmingham, Alabama, and honed his marketing and sales skills. Cassimus was often described as a hard worker, optimist, excellent salesman, true entrepreneur, and visionary—attributes that contributed much to his success in the business arena. His first start-up, launched in

Exhibit 1   **Zoës Kitchen Menu**

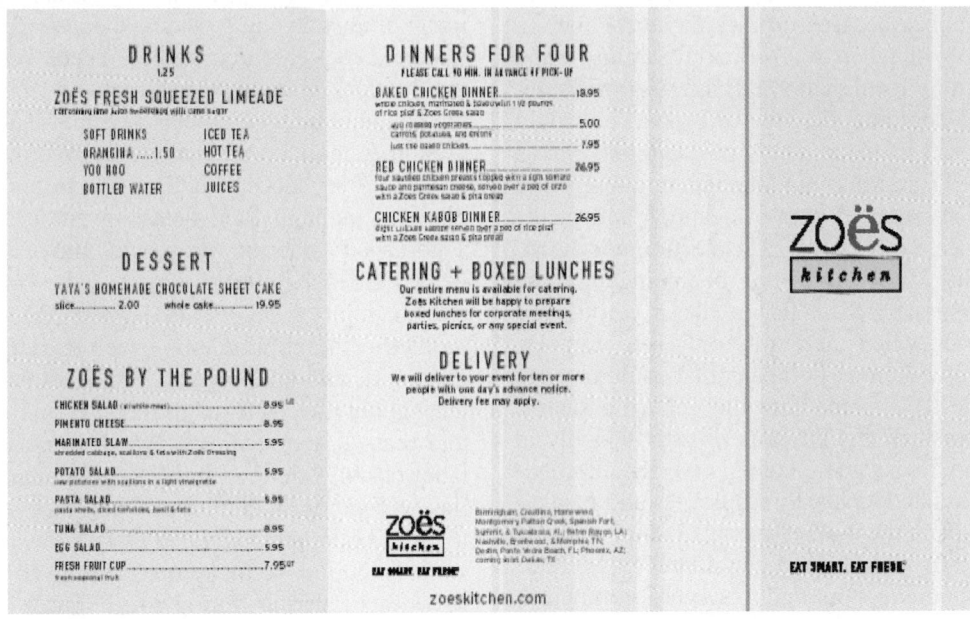

the fall of 1993, was an apparel company named J-Rag Inc. After J-Rag became the leader in imprinted sportswear to cycling manufacturers, Cassimus sold the company in 1996. He spent the next two years traveling extensively in his efforts to direct a new venture called Compensation Management Associates, and during that time he successfully

tripled the company's sales. Recognizing national trends and the success of the first Zoës Kitchen, Cassimus turned his attention to growing his family's restaurant business.

Under Cassimus's leadership, Zoës Kitchen quickly expanded from its original location, adding three more Zoës Kitchen locations in Birmingham;

one in Tuscaloosa; and two in Nashville, Tennessee. Franchises were also developed successfully in Memphis, Tennessee; Destin, Florida; and Phoenix, Arizona. Zoës Kitchen was quickly gaining brand awareness and a loyal customer base. Cassimus decided that to continue the pace of growth he would need his pilot's license. The Zoës Kitchen Sirrus plane allowed Cassimus and his team to quickly and easily visit stores in disparate locations and facilitated the process of making site-selection decisions.

Cassimus knew from the beginning that he wanted to operate Zoës Kitchen like a world-class company, even when there was only one unit. He also wanted to develop a company that could one day be sold, if he so desired. With the goal of a steady, predictable cash flow, Cassimus invested heavily in people, brand image, and systems. Zoës Kitchen generally compensated its hourly employees and managers at rates above the market average, which allowed the company to recruit good candidates and reduce turnover. A bonus system tied managers' compensation to their performance based on key metrics. Morale was high in stores, and many employees had been with the company for much of its existence.

In 2001, as Cassimus was speaking to a class at the University of Alabama, a student suggested redesigning the original logo to enhance the Zoës Kitchen brand image. Cassimus was initially opposed to the idea, primarily because the logo had been designed by his mother Zoë and because the cost to effect widespread image change would be high. However, after Cassimus's mentor from Chick-Fil-A made the same recommendation, he reconsidered.

A marketing survey the University of Alabama conducted for Zoës Kitchen indicated that customer loyalty to Zoës Kitchen was strong. Customers surveyed most often selected four words to describe Zoës Kitchen: fresh, healthy, tasty, and unique. Respondents also indicated that those who ate at Zoës Kitchen more than once a week told their friends and family about their experience. Of the 242 customers surveyed, nearly 50 percent of the respondents had discovered the restaurant through friends and family, 21 percent were enticed by seeing the store, 9 percent had been recommended by coworkers, and only 3 percent were influenced by advertising. Customers also placed the highest value on service and quality of menu offerings, so Zoës Kitchen did not compete primarily on price. After analyzing the survey results, Zoës Kitchen underwent an extensive brand redesign in 2002. Cassimus hired an architectural design company to create an identity for Zoës Kitchen. After many brainstorming sessions, the new Zoës Kitchen look and feel emerged. Simple decor, bright colors, vivid stripes, a trademarked logo, and Zoës Kitchen merchandise became crucial elements of all locations. Customers noticed, and sales improved immediately.

By 2006, Zoës Kitchen had strong systems in place to manage food costs, inventory, and labor. Tight food ordering processes and cash controls helped Zoës Kitchen mitigate risk. Zoës Kitchen used a point-of-sale (POS) system that featured a biometric thumbprint employees used to clock in, clock out, and take orders. Managers were assisted throughout the day by a "dashboard" in the POS system that allowed them to easily monitor sales and labor costs. A defined training program and job duties helped hourly employees succeed every day.

Zoës Kitchen remained close to what Zoë Cassimus pictured, with approximately 70 percent of its sales occurring during lunch. Most stores were open seven days a week from 10:00 a.m. to 8:00 p.m. While nearly half of the food purchased was consumed off premises, there were still significant growth opportunities available in developing the catering and dinner business.

THE RESTAURANT INDUSTRY IN THE UNITED STATES

In 2005, the United States restaurant industry included over 870,000 restaurants and employed 11.6 million workers. According to an article by Lori Dahm titled "Fast-Casual: Positioned for Growth" in *Stagnito's New Products Magazine,* fast-casual chains in the United States grew by 13 percent in 2004, while overall the restaurant industry grew by 4.5 percent. Fast-casual restaurants brought in $7.5 billion in sales in 2004, or 2.5 percent of the $300 billion restaurant industry (see Exhibit 2). Despite being dominated by giant fast-food chains, most restaurants in the industry were small operations. More than 70 percent were independent, single-unit businesses with fewer than 20 employees. One out of every three was owned by a sole proprietor or a partnership. While the restaurant industry had grown

Exhibit 2   **Share of Restaurant Meal Occasions by Segment**

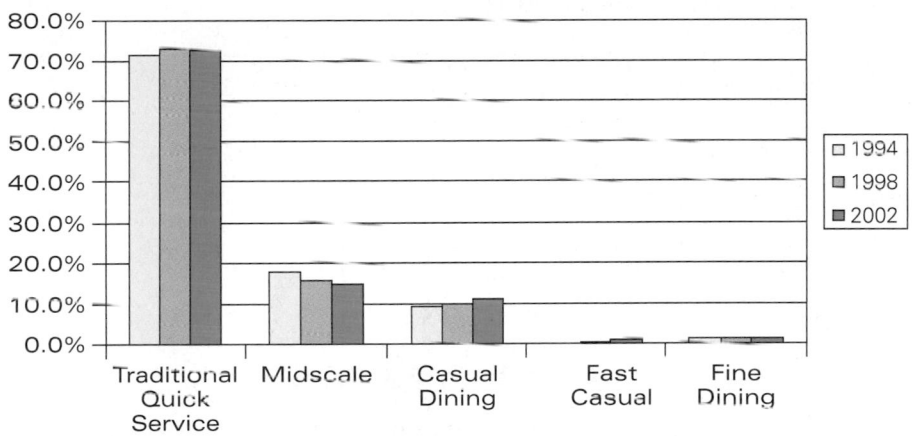

Source: Zoës Kitchen.

rapidly from 1970 to 2005 (see Exhibit 3), it was now regarded as mature, and unfortunately the outlook for overall restaurant industry growth had become rather bleak. A report in the *McKinsey Quarterly* projected annual growth of only 2 percent until 2010. Many large players were suffering because they could not profitably offer what consumers desired: fresh food served quickly in a distinctive, casual environment. The growth in the industry was expected to come from the middle ground—a segment with strong potential called fast-casual.

The fast-casual segment of the restaurant industry emerged in the mid-1990s, beginning with high-end bakeries and cafés including Panera Bread and Corner Bakery. There was no exact, agreed-on definition of fast-casual in the industry, typically because each chain is so distinctive. However, there were some

characteristics that most chains shared: high quality, fresh food, and a wide variety of menu items. Many innovative menu items could be rotated seasonally and tailored to customers' requests, which helped preserve the "fresh" connotation. Customers usually ordered at a counter, and a server brought food to their table. The restaurants often focused on dining-room ambiance, creating a warm environment for customers. Even though fast-casual was a small part of the overall restaurant industry, the fast-casual chains were able to grow by adapting their offerings to consumer demands. Most consumers had time-starved lifestyles, leaving little time to visit a sit-down restaurant (see Exhibit 4). However, consumers did want to eat healthy, high-quality foods. Fast-casual chains overcame this dilemma by offering quality food in a unique environment at a speed close to that of fast-food restaurants.

Exhibit 3   **Restaurant Industry Sales (billions of dollars)**

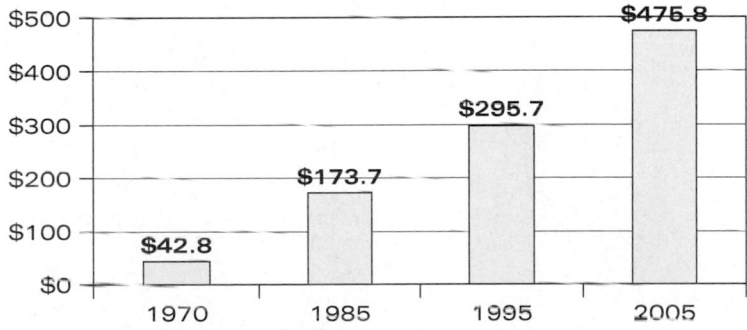

Source: National Restaurant Association.

Exhibit 4   **Distribution of Fast-Casual Visits (where consumers came from), 2004**

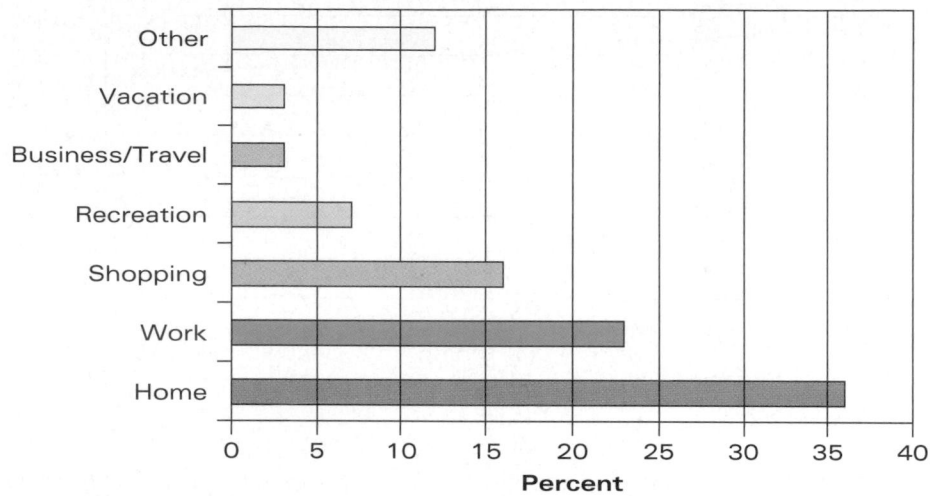

Source: "The Casual Dining Evolution and the Rise of Fast Casual," presentation prepared by Dan White, Coca-Cola Fountain Marketing.

Therefore, many consumers frequented fast-casual restaurants several times each week because they saw the experience as a valuable use of time and money (see Exhibit 5). The fast-casual segment was expected to be worth approximately $35 billion by the end of the decade and to account for more than half of all food-service growth.

Consumers welcomed fast-casual with open arms because it met their lifestyle demands by providing an alternative to traditional fast food and offering more choices. "They woke up the industry to what consumers want when they eat out," said Michele Schmal, vice president of product management for NPD Foodworld. Each fast-casual restaurant had a personality all its own and a menu to match. Before fast-casual, there were two ends of the dining-out spectrum: fast food and sit-down casual dining. Fast-casual brought the two together and essentially bridged the gap in quality, taste, ambiance, price, and convenience for quick service (see Exhibit 6).

According the NPD Group's latest "Fast-Casual Report", fast-casual restaurants were continuing to see increases in units (locations), traffic, and sales. Unit expansion increased by 17 percent in 2003, while the total number of restaurants nationally remained constant. The segment's expansion slowed to 13 percent

Exhibit 5   **Average Income of Fast-Casual Customers, 2004**

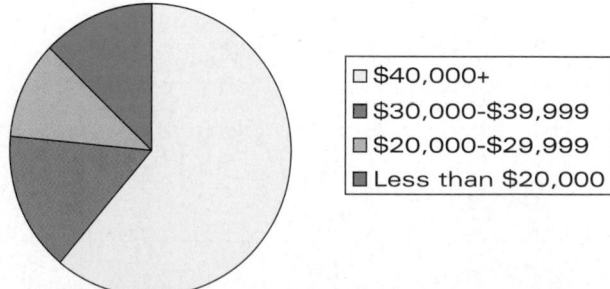

☐ $40,000+
■ $30,000-$39,999
■ $20,000-$29,999
■ Less than $20,000

Source: "The Casual Dining Evolution and the Rise of Fast-Casual," presentation prepared by Dan White, Coca-Cola Fountain Marketing.

Exhibit 6 **Fast-Casual Consumer Demographics Compared with Other Food-Service Providers, 2004**

	Quick-Service Restaurant	Fast-Casual	Casual Dining
Ages 35–64	40%	47%	47%
Professional/white collar	39	54	48
Female	52	54	52

Source: "The Casual Dining Evolution and the Rise of Fast Casual," presentation prepared by Dan White, Coca-Cola Fountain Marketing.

in 2004, but customer traffic rose 7 percent in 2004 versus 5 percent in 2003.

This change in the industry resulted from changing lifestyles and subsequent demands those lifestyles placed on consumers. The typical consumer was strapped for time, especially during meals, and valued control, personality, and healthy choices from food providers. Kasey Burleson, chief financial officer of Zoës Kitchen, said, "People are more educated than ever on health and global cuisine, and their acumen of quality, freshness, and value is becoming more precise. People demand extremely high levels of quality, service, and speed, and the fast-casual dining segment is poised to grow and change with consumers." A fast-paced society valued quick service and increasingly more health-conscious meals. Consumers were also increasingly unwilling or unable to cook, a factor that had the most profound effect on dinner (see Exhibit 7). In the last 10 years, consumers had increasingly shifted from home-prepared dinners to restaurant-prepared meals either served at the restaurant or consumed off-premises (see Exhibit 8).

These factors naturally left a gap with regard to both speed and quality of food, giving rise to fast-casual providers. Since most of the large quick-service food providers were struggling to reach this segment,

most of the unit supply was expected to come from small, specialized food establishments. Naturally, the biggest challenge for these small competitors was reaching a critical mass of customers that would enable fast-casual restaurants to enjoy the economies of scale of mass fast-food chains while maintaining the quality consumers wanted.

The atmosphere of fast-casual stores often attempted to reflect the brand. For instance, Corner Bakery Café aimed for a comfortable, old-fashioned bistro feel, while Panera Bread strategically positioned fireplaces in the middle of the restaurant to project coziness. The fluorescent lights and plastic utensils often seen in fast-food restaurants were considered taboo. Customers were often served on high-end plastic plates with metal silverware, even though they were expected to bus their own tables.

Offering fresh food instead of frozen, hiring talented labor, and constructing each restaurant with character could be very expensive. While fast-casual chains offered high-quality products at relatively low prices compared to sit-down restaurants, expenses could quickly erode profit margins. Even the best service would fail if it lacked the scale or operational efficiency. For example, Cosi, a New York–based bread and coffee chain, generated $70 million

Exhibit 7 **Total Meal Occasions for Meals Prepared Outside the Home (in percent)**

Meal Occasion	1987	1999	2005
Breakfast	14%	12%	11%
Lunch	41	39	38
Dinner	45	49	51
Total	100%	100%	100%

Source: Technomic; McKinsey analysis.

Exhibit 8 **Average Expenditures for Food Away from Home by Households with Two or More Persons, 2003**

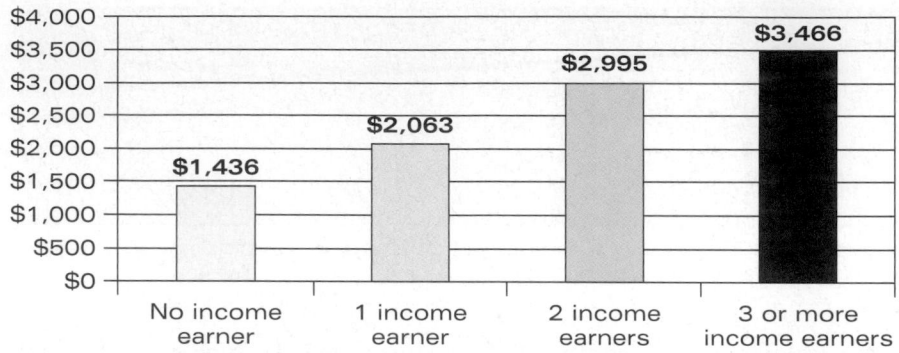

Source: National Restaurant Association.

in sales in 2001 from more than 60 restaurants but recorded a net loss of $35 million. Therefore, fast-casual restaurants sought growth in number of units to capitalize quickly on economies of scale.

Fast-food companies, also known as quick-service restaurants (QSRs), seemed likely to move into the fast-casual segment because their operations were streamlined and operationally efficient. They possessed strong distribution networks, and most carried heavy purchasing clout. However, they had scant experience beyond their current offerings, and their supplier network was not tuned for the shipment of fresh products. Moreover, their image and value proposition of fast food was seen as a liability as far as consumers were concerned. To compete, fast-food chains were likely to find it more beneficial to enter the market through a buyout or other form of a merger. Full-service restaurants offered similar products, but their service was slower than consumers desired.

COMPETITION

For Zoës Kitchen, trying to identify close competitors was somewhat challenging because of the number and variety of choices consumers had for dining out. Zoës Kitchen experienced the most direct competition with other restaurants in a five-minute radius of each location. On a national scale, Zoës Kitchen did not have any competitors that emulated its format and menu. However, several fast-food chains had added more healthful offerings to their menus—a move that might prove trendsetting for the entire fast-casual dining segment.

The recent success of the fast-casual segment had turned heads in the quick-service segment (see Exhibit 9). Various fast-casual brands had popped up around the nation, most with strong regional appeal (see Exhibit 10). The fast-food giants found it very difficult to break into this market with their existing operations. The features consumers wanted—including

Exhibit 9 **Top Fast-Casual Restaurants (ranked by 2004 sales)**

Rank	Chain	Sales (in $ millions)	% Change 2003 to 2004
1	Panera Bread	$1,241	+23%
2	Chipotle Mexican Grill	430	+34
3	Baja Fresh Mexican Grill	348	+11
4	Atlanta Bread	220	+22
5	Qdoba Mexican Grill	133	+53

Source: Technomic; figures for year-end 2004.

Exhibit 10   **Comparisons of Select Restaurant Industry Competitors**

Competitor	Menu Options	Decor/Target Customers	Growth and Growth Potential	Geographic Placement
Panera Bread	Baked breads, sandwiches, paninis, salads, soups, bagels	Mimicked Starbucks (bold colors, varied seating options, contemporary fixtures, young professionals)	478 current locations and 346 franchised in 30 states	Locations were in high-traffic areas with visibility
Qdoba Mexican Grill	Generous portions of Mexican food; all food prepared in front of customer	Slightly industrial decor (deep reds and dark woods and aluminum tabletops)/targeted the trend-seeking consumer	100 locations in 15 states; 301 locations in development (due to acquisition of Jack in the Box)	Tuscaloosa, Alabama, location had high visibility near university of Alabama campus
Baja Fresh	Fresh Mexican food	Contemporary decor with black-and-white theme lends itself to attracting the modern consumer	210 locations in18 states (acquired by Wendy's in 2002)	None in Alabama, on the West Coast, or in the Midwest
Moe's Southwestern Grill	Restaurant claimed to not even own a freezer, supporting its claim that all food was fresh and made to order; all food was prepared in front of customer	Muted tones covered the walls, icons from the 1960s and 70s were featured throughout	115 locations	Birmingham locations were in strip malls and usually surrounded by other restaurants

Source: Zoës Kitchen.

healthy, wide-ranging product offerings and an up-scale atmosphere—could not be replicated profitably by most of the larger quick-service companies. In response, companies such as Wendy's, McDonald's, and Jack in the Box acquired smaller companies in hopes of fueling growth in this illusive segment with their strong financial resources (see Exhibit 11).

Wendy's spent $9 million to purchase a 45 percent stake in Café Express, a fast-casual chain owned by the Schiller Del Grande Restaurant Group in Houston. Wendy's was planning to expand the current 13 Café Express locations in Houston, Dallas, and Phoenix to 50 units nationwide. In 2002, Wendy's acquired Baja Fresh, which still operated as a wholly owned subsidiary and remained loyal to the vision of becoming the leading name and defining standard in fresh Mexican food. Wendy's also changed its own menu in response to fast-casual by adding a choice

of sides including salad, fruit, baked potato, and yogurt, in addition to the traditional fries.

McDonald's was also trying to break into fast-casual. Looking for relief from its sliding sales and profit margins, it purchased a minority interest in Chipotle Mexican Grill, headquartered in Denver, in 1998. In 2004, McDonald's expanded its stake in Chipotle to a majority interest. Chipotle showed phenomenal success with its 150 units in more than 20 markets. Same-store sales growth had increased annually by 15 percent for the last three years, with an average unit volume estimated to be $1.05 million per unit. In the fourth quarter of 2005, McDonald's filed with the Securities Exchange Commission to spin off Chipotle into a separate, publicly held company.

Subway was the only company experimenting with completely refashioning itself as a fast-casual brand. Subway had recently opened its own

Exhibit 11   **The 10 Fastest-Growing Restaurant Chains (ranked by sales increase)**

Rank	Chain	Sales Increase 2002–2003 ($000)	% Sales Change	2003 U.S. Sales ($000)
1	McDonald's	$1,816,100	8.9%	$22,121,800
2	Starbucks	759,694	25.8	3,699,972
3	Wendy's	525,000	7.7	7,350,000
4	Subway	499,000	9.6	5,699,000
5	Applebee's	336,404	10.6	3,518,961
6	Dunkin' Donuts	300,000	11.1	3,000,000
7	Chili's Grill	246,553	11.4	2,402,517
8	Panera Bread	221,689	29.3	977,099
9	International House of Pancakes	212,459	14.5	1,676,026
10	Krispy Kreme	207,708	26.3	997,708
	Total top 10	$5,124,607	11.1%	$51,443,083

Source: Technomic.

Tuscan-themed restaurant, which was the first major brand overhaul in a decade. The new restaurant, located in Chicago, sported soft gold tones, instead of the company's trademark bright yellow, and earth-toned tiles instead of linoleum floors. Since making these changes, Subway had noticed a new wave of customer traffic, including more suits and ties for lunch.

Panera Bread

Panera Bread was founded as Au Bon Pain in 1981 by Louis Kane and Ron Shaich. The company prospered along the East Coast and internationally during the 1980s and 1990s and became the dominant operator in the bakery-café segment. In 1993, Au Bon Pain purchased Saint Louis Bread Company, then a chain of 20 bakery-cafés located in the Saint Louis area. The management conducted a restaging of Saint Louis Bread, and ultimately the name was changed to Panera Bread. In May 1999, Au Bon Pain was renamed Panera Bread, and it sold all its business units with the exception of its namesake. As of 2006 the company was publicly held, with numerous locations across the country, and had a market capitalization of $1.8 billion.

Panera Bread had seen strong growth, and it planned to expand into New York and California. Of its 741 bakery-cafés in 35 states, 226 were company-owned; the rest were franchised. There were 155 Panera bakery-cafés projected to open in 2005.

The primary basis of Panera's product offering was, simply, bread. The company claimed that it baked more bread from scratch each day than any other restaurant chain and operated with the goal of making quality bread broadly available to everyone in the United States. Panera was highly recognized nationwide for its specialty breads and had among the highest rankings in terms of customer loyalty and quality food.

Qdoba Mexican Grill

In 1995, Anthony Miller and Robert Hauser opened the first Qdoba Mexican Grill restaurant in Denver, Colorado. Since its beginning, Qdoba had won over both customers and critics with its big portions and big flavors. The *Denver Post* and *Westward* named Qdoba's the "best burrito," and *Gabby Gourmet* recognized Qdoba as one of the top 15 inexpensive restaurants in Colorado. In just a few years, Qdoba grew to over 100 locations in more than 30 states. In 2003, Qdoba was acquired by Jack in the Box Inc., the first major drive-through hamburger chain. Jack in the Box has more than 1,900 franchised restaurants.

Baja Fresh

Jim and Linda Magglos introduced the first all-fresh, fire-grilled, fast-casual concept as Baja Fresh in August 1990. The product offering included fresh flavors and generous portions that quickly drew a loyal following of customers. The idea was a restaurant that catered to the more mature tastes for healthy, vibrant, flavorful foods in a festive atmosphere. The restaurants were designed to involve many senses with bright, contemporary decor, artistic lighting, and clean, crisp design. The resulting customer following helped Baja Fresh expand rapidly from a regional to a national scope, with a high volume of requests for franchises resulting in over 288 locations. In an effort to take full advantage of this new concept, Greg Dollarhyde and Pete Siracusa, with over 60 collective years of restaurant experience, were hired to help manage the growth.

Moe's Southwestern Grill

Emphasizing simplicity, Moe's Southwestern Grill was the fastest-growing fast-casual concept in the country. The founder wanted to create a place that combined his favorite flavors from road trips through the Southwest with the music of days gone by. Moe's stressed freshness; it even claimed not to own a freezer. It made every menu item on the day that a customer ordered it. The atmosphere paid tribute to Moe's musical heroes with relics from the 1960s and 70s.

Moe's recently announced that it had signed a 20-store deal for the northern Virginia/greater Washington, D.C., territory. The company had over 800 franchise deals in development and was on pace to open 150 additional units in 2005. Moe's was part of Raving Brands, which also franchised Mama Fu's Asian House, Planet Smoothie, PJ's Coffee, Shane's Rib Shack, Doc Green's Gourmet Salads, and Bonehead's Seafood.

FRANCHISES

Offering franchises allowed many companies to rapidly expand after their start-up stage. Most of the fast-casual concepts had seen such strong growth due to franchising that they continued to increase the number of franchises planned to open each year. In a market when numbers of units counted, franchising had become a catalyst for growth.

Franchisees were able to run their own business, gaining instant brand recognition, training, and other support as needed to succeed. The franchisee typically paid a franchising fee, which could cost several thousand dollars. The franchisor provides the franchisee with the format to use in operating the business, the right to use the company's name for a limited amount of time, and other assistance that

varied greatly. Company systems for cash control, inventory management, labor, and technology were usually included as well. The franchisee could reduce investment risk by associating with an established company. Only 2 percent of franchises discontinued operations within three years of opening. However, franchising could have high intangible costs. A franchisor could require franchisees to relinquish significant control over operations and take on contractual obligations. Other payments often included continued royalties and advertising fees.

Zoës Kitchen had expanded primarily through company-owned stores and had not yet tapped too deeply into the franchising aspect of the business. With systems in place to control food costs, inventory costs, labor, and cash, Zoës was positioned well to take advantage of franchise opportunities in the future.

ZOËS GROWTH

This was an exciting time for fast-casual and even more so for Zoës Kitchen. With the industry still young and scale economies a core aspect of gaining fast-casual supremacy, strategic growth was Zoës main priority. "Zoës Kitchen is positioned in the fastest growing sector of the food service industry. Offering a fresh, tasty, healthy, and unique menu, more profitable business model, and differentiation from any of our peers allows us to replicate our menu for success in strategically planned markets," said John Cassimus.

Whether operating as company-owned stores or franchises, Zoës Kitchen had to have a sound, executable plan for entering new markets, focusing first on excellent site selection (see Exhibit 12). The desire to grow and achieve economies of scale had to be balanced with the desire to find outstanding locations, and growth had to be deferred if only sub-par sites were available. When looking for new sites, Zoës Kitchen primarily considered the following criteria:

- Well-located space in dense, affluent markets.
- Average household income above $75,000 in a three-mile radius.
- Premier end-cap or similar positions.
- Minimum of 25 feet of storefront footage.
- Parking ratio of 10 per 1,000 square feet.
- Excellent visibility and signage to primary traffic corridors.

Exhibit 12   **Zoës Kitchen Locations, as of December 2005, and Scheduled 2006 Openings**

Locations as of December 2005

Birmingham, AL—Crestline
Birmingham, AL—Downtown
Birmingham, AL—Summit
Homewood, AL
Montgomery, AL
Hoover, AL
Spanish Fort, AL
Tuscaloosa, AL
Phoenix, AZ—Central Avenue
Phoenix, AZ—West McDowell
Destin, FL
Ponte Vedra Beach, FL
Baton Rouge, LA
Brentwood, TN
Nashville, TN
Memphis, TN

2006 Scheduled Openings

Mobile, AL
Phoenix, AZ—Camelback
Dallas, TX

- Daytime population within two miles above 50,000.
- Co-tenancy that generated daily traffic (i.e., groceries, gyms, schools).
- Real estate projects that promoted the quality and uniqueness of the Zoës Kitchen brand.

In the restaurant industry, sales were often measured in average unit volumes (AUV), with company value often based on a multiple of its AUV. To increase the AUV of each restaurant, Zoës Kitchen had to increase its dinner sales by further developing its dinner dine-in and dinner take-out business. In 2005, Zoës Kitchen added three new menu items targeted at this segment: chicken kabobs, a red chicken sandwich, and a red chicken plate. Zoës Kitchen also developed "Dinners for Four," which allowed customers to take home a meal that could be served on family-style platters with no preparation time. While Zoës Kitchen offered its entire menu for catering, a menu specifically designed to increase catering sales was expected to be introduced in the first quarter of 2006. Zoës Catering was to feature more platters, trays, and new menu items aimed directly at the catering segment of the industry.

The year 2006 was expected to be a year for concept validation, and success would largely determine Zoës ability to continue to grow. Zoës Kitchen sought to position itself to best capitalize on market opportunities. Expansion in the fast-casual segment had remained strong, but growth had already seen a decline while the industry was still seemingly in its infancy. Even so, fast-casual had made such a dramatic impact on current and new quick-service providers that everyone wanted to be poised to take advantage of growth opportunities.

As John Cassimus flew over the Brentwood, Tennessee, location after a successful grand opening, he believed that the newest Zoës restaurant was positioned for success. His employees, brand image, and systems gave him confidence that everything would run smoothly. A true visionary at heart, Cassimus focused his attention on the future of Zoës Kitchen. When would he be ready and able to sell the company? How much growth needed to occur, and when? What was the best mechanism for growth, and how could the value of the company continue to increase?

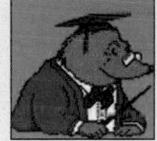

Krispy Kreme Doughnuts in 2006: Is a Turnaround Possible?

Arthur A. Thompson
The University of Alabama

Amit J. Shah
Frostburg State University

We think we're the Stradivarius of doughnuts.
—*Scott Livengood, former president, chairman, and CEO*

How can a company firing on all cylinders until 2003, with revenue and earnings growth running at 20–25 percent per year and the stock price more than tripling since its initial public offering, go so wrong so quickly? In 2004–2005 Krispy Kreme Doughnuts was besieged with declining doughnut sales, falling revenues, the prospect of store closings and failed franchises, problems with the U.S. Securities and Exchange Commission over false and misleading financial statements, and lawsuits from shareholders and franchisees. The stock price in late 2005 was trading at around $6 per share, down 88 percent from its all-time high of close to $50 per share.

Until May 2004, Krispy Kreme's prospects appeared bright. With 357 Krispy Kreme stores in 45 states, Canada, Great Britain, Australia, and Mexico, the company was riding the crest of customer enthusiasm for its light, warm, melt-in-your-mouth doughnuts. During the past four years, consumer purchases of Krispy Kreme's doughnut products had taken off, with sales reaching 7.5 million doughnuts a day. Considerable customer excitement—approaching a cult-like frenzy—often surrounded the opening of the first store in an area. When a new Krispy Kreme opened in Rochester, New York, in 2000, more than 100 people

lined up in a snowstorm before 5:00 a.m. to get some of the first hot doughnuts coming off the conveyor line; within an hour there were 75 cars in the drive-through lane. Three TV stations and a radio station broadcast live from the store site. The first Krispy Kreme store in Denver, Colorado, opened in 2001, grossed $1 million in revenues in its first 22 days of operation, commonly had lines running out the door with a one-hour wait for doughnuts, and, according to local newspaper reports, one night had 150 cars in line for the drive-through window at 1:30 a.m.— opening day was covered by local TV and radio stations, and off-duty sheriff's deputies were brought in to help with traffic jams for a week following the grand opening.

The first Minnesota store, just outside of Minneapolis, had opening-week sales of $480,693—the company record for fiscal 2002. In July 2003, the first store to open in the Massachusetts market—in Medford, outside Boston—had a record opening-day revenue of $73,813 and a record opening-week sales volume of $506,917; sales at the Medford store exceeded $2 million in the first seven weeks. At the June 2003 opening of the company's first store in Australia, in the outskirts of Sydney, customers camped overnight in anticipation of the opening and others waited in line for hours to experience their first Krispy Kreme hot doughnut—the store, about an hour from downtown Sydney, attracted more than 500,000 customers from Sydney in its first six months of operations. In South Bend, Indiana, one exuberant customer camped out in the parking lot for 17 days to be the first in line for the Krispy Kreme Store's grand opening.

To capitalize on all the buzz and customer excitement, Krispy Kreme had been adding new stores at a record pace throughout 2002–2003. The company's strategy and business model were aimed at opening a sufficient number of new stores and boosting sales at existing stores to achieve 20 percent annual revenue growth and 25 percent annual growth in earnings per share. In the just-completed 2004 fiscal year, total company revenues rose by 35.4 percent, to $665.6 million compared with $491.5 million in the fiscal 2003. Net income in fiscal 2004 increased by 70.4 percent, from $33.5 million to $57.1 million. Krispy Kreme's stock price had increased eightfold since it went public in April 2000, giving the company a high profile with investors and Wall Street analysts. In February 2004, Krispy Kreme stock was trading at 30 times the consensus earnings estimates for fiscal 2005, a price/earnings ratio that was "justified" only if the company continued to grow 20–25 percent annually.

A number of securities analysts doubted whether Krispy Kreme's strategy and growth potential would continue to push the company's stock price upward. According to one analyst, "The odds are against this stock for long-term success." Another commented, "I think the market is overly optimistic about the long-term opportunities of the growth of the doughnut business." A third said, "Single-product concepts only have so many years to run." Indeed, restaurants with quick-service products presently had the slowest revenue growth of any restaurant type. The Krispy Kreme bears were particularly concerned about reports from franchisees that, as the number of Krispy Kreme stores expanded in choice markets, average-store sales were slowing and newly opened stores were not performing as well as the first one or two stores. After the initial buying frenzy at high-profile store openings in a major market, the buzz tended to fade as the fourth, fifth, and sixth outlets opened; moreover, new stores started to cannibalize sales from existing stores, thus moderating the potential for new stores to boost overall sales. Several franchisees in California, Michigan, New York, Canada and a few other places were said to be in financial difficulty because of overexpansion and disappointing sales at newly opened stores.

COMPANY BACKGROUND

In 1933, Vernon Rudolph bought a doughnut shop in Paducah, Kentucky, from Joe LeBeau. His purchase included the company's assets, goodwill, the Krispy Kreme name, and rights to a secret yeast-raised doughnut recipe that LeBeau had created in New Orleans years earlier. Several years thereafter, Rudolph and his partner, looking for a larger market, moved their operations to Nashville, Tennessee; other members of the Rudolph family joined the enterprise, opening doughnut shops in Charleston, West Virginia, and Atlanta, Georgia. The business consisted of producing, marketing, and delivering fresh-made doughnuts to local grocery stores. Then, during the summer of 1937, Rudolph decided to quit the family business and left Nashville, taking with him a 1936 Pontiac, $200 in cash, doughnut-making equipment, and the secret recipe; after some disappointing efforts to find another location, he settled on opening the first Krispy Kreme Doughnuts shop in Winston-Salem, North Carolina. Rudolph was drawn to Winston-Salem because the city was developing into a tobacco and textiles hub in the Southeast, and he thought a doughnut shop would make a good addition to the thriving local economy. Rudolph and his two partners, who accompanied him from Nashville, used their last $25 to rent a building across from Salem College and Academy. With no money left to buy ingredients, Rudolph convinced a local grocer to lend them what they needed, promising payment once the first doughnuts were sold. To deliver the doughnuts, he took the backseat out of the 1936 Pontiac and installed a delivery rack. On July 13, 1937, the first Krispy Kreme doughnuts were made at Rudolph's new Winston-Salem shop and delivered to grocery retailers.

Soon afterward, people began stopping by the shop to ask if they could buy hot doughnuts. There were so many requests that Rudolph decided to cut a hole in the shop's wall so that he could sell doughnuts at retail to passersby. Krispy Kreme doughnuts proved highly popular in Winston-Salem, and Rudolph's shop prospered. By the late 1950s, Krispy Kreme had 29 shops in 12 states, with each shop having the capacity to produce 500 dozen doughnuts per hour.

In the early 1950s, Vernon Rudolph met Mike Harding, who was then selling powdered milk to bakeries. Rudolph was looking for someone to help grow the business, and Harding joined the company as a partner in 1954. Starting with six employees, the two began building an equipment department and a plant for blending doughnut mixes. They believed the key to Krispy Kreme's expansion was to have control over each step of the doughnut-making process and to be able to deliver hot doughnuts to customers as soon as they emerged from the frying and sugar-glazing process. In 1960, they decided to standardize all Krispy Kreme shops with a green roof, a red-glazed brick exterior, a viewing window inside, an overhead conveyor for doughnut production, and bar stools—creating a look that became Krispy Kreme's trademark during that era.

Harding focused on operations, while Rudolph concentrated on finding promising locations for new stores and getting bank financing to support expansion into other southeastern cities and towns. Harding became Krispy Kreme's president in 1958, and he became chief executive officer when Rudolph died in 1973. Under Rudolph and then Harding, Krispy Kreme's revenues grew from less than $1 million in 1954 to $58 million by the time Harding retired in 1974. Corporate headquarters remained in Winston-Salem.

In 1976, Beatrice Foods bought Krispy Kreme and proceeded to make a series of changes. The recipe was changed, and the company's script-lettered signs were altered to produce a more modern look. As customers reacted negatively to Beatrice's changes, business declined. A group of franchisees, led by Joseph McAleer, bought the company from Beatrice in 1982 in a $22 million leveraged buyout. The new owners quickly reinstated the original recipe and the original script-lettered signs. Sales rebounded, but with double-digit interest rates in the early 1980s, it took years to pay off the buyout debt, leaving little for expansion.

To grow revenues, the company relied mainly on franchising "associate" stores, opening a few new company-owned stores—all in the southeastern United States—and boosting store volume through off-premises sales. Associate stores operated under a 15-year licensing agreement that permitted them to use the Krispy Kreme system within a specific geographic territory. They paid royalties of 3 percent of on-premises sales and 1 percent of all other branded sales (to supermarkets, convenience stores, charitable organizations selling doughnuts for fund-raising projects, and other wholesale buyers); no royalties were paid on sales of unbranded or private-label doughnuts. The primary emphasis of the associate stores and many of the company stores was on wholesaling both Krispy Kreme doughnuts and private-label doughnuts to local groceries and supermarkets. Corporate revenues rose gradually to $117 million in 1989 and then flattened for the next six years.

New Leadership and a New Strategy

In the early 1990s, with interest rates falling and much of the buyout debt paid down, the company began experimenting cautiously with expanding under Scott Livengood, the company's newly appointed president and chief operating officer. Livengood, 48, joined Krispy Kreme's human relations department in 1978 three years after graduating from the University of North Carolina at Chapel Hill with a degree in industrial relations and a minor in psychology. Believing strongly in the company's product and long-term growth potential, he rose through the management ranks, becoming president and chief operating officer in 1992, a member of the board of directors in 1994, president and CEO in 1998, and president, CEO, and chairman of the board in 1999.

Shortly after becoming president in 1992, Livengood became increasingly concerned about stagnant sales and shortcomings in the company's strategy: "The model wasn't working for us. It was more about selling in wholesale channels and less about the brand." He and other Krispy Kreme executives, mindful of the thousands of "Krispy Kreme stories" told by passionate customers over the years, concluded that the emphasis on off-premises sales did not adequately capitalize on the enthusiasm and loyalty of customers for Krispy Kreme's doughnuts. A second shortcoming was that the company's exclusive focus on southeastern U.S. markets unnecessarily handcuffed efforts to leverage the company's brand equity and product quality in the rest of the U.S. doughnut market. The available data also indicated that the standard 7,000-plus-square-foot stores were uneconomic to operate in all but very high-volume locations.

By the mid-1990s, with fewer than 100 franchised and company-owned stores and corporate sales stuck in the $110–$120 million range for six years, company executives determined that it was time for a new strategy and aggressive expansion outside the Southeast. Beginning in 1996, Krispy Kreme began implementing a new strategy to reposition the company, shifting the focus from a wholesale bakery strategy to a specialty retail strategy that promoted sales at the company's own retail outlets and emphasized the "hot doughnut experience" so often stressed in customers' Krispy Kreme stories. Doughnut sizes were also increased. The second major part of the new strategy was to expand the number of stores nationally using both area franchisees and company-owned stores. In preparing to launch the strategy, the company tested several different store sizes, eventually concluding that stores in the 2,400- to 4,200-square-foot range were better suited for the company's market repositioning and expansion plans.

The franchising part of the strategy called for the company to license territories, usually defined by metropolitan statistical areas, to select franchisees with proven experience in multi-unit food operations. Franchisees were expected to be thoroughly familiar with the local area market they were to develop and also to have the capital and organizational capability to open a prescribed number of stores in their territory within a specified period. The minimum net worth requirement for franchise area developers was $750,000 per store or $5 million, whichever was greater. Area developers paid Krispy Kreme a franchise fee of $20,000 to $40,000 for each store they opened. They also were required to pay a 4.5 percent royalty fee on all sales and to contribute 1.0 percent of revenues to a company-administered advertising and public relations fund. Franchisees were expected to strictly adhere to high standards of quality and service.

By early 2000, the company had signed on 13 area developers operating 33 Krispy Kreme stores and committed to open another 130 stores in their territories within five years. In addition, the company was operating 61 stores under its own management. Sales had zoomed to $220 million, and profits were a record $6 million.

After a decision was made to take the company public in April 2000, Krispy Kreme spent much of late 1999 and early 2000 preparing for an initial public offering (IPO) of the company's stock. The old corporate structure, Krispy Kreme Doughnut Corporation, was merged into a new company, Krispy Kreme Doughnuts Inc. The new company planned to use the proceeds from its IPO to remodel or relocate older company-owned stores, to repay debt, to make joint venture investments in franchised stores, and to expand its capacity to make doughnut mix.

The IPO of 3.45 million shares was oversubscribed at $21 per share, and when the stock began trading in April under the ticker symbol KREM, the price quickly rose. Krispy Kreme was the second-best-performing stock among all IPO offerings in the United States in 2000. The company's stock began trading on the New York Stock Exchange in May 2001 under the symbol KKD.

Between early 2000 and early 2004, the company increased the number of Krispy Kreme stores from 144 to 357, boosted doughnut sales from an average of 3 million a day to an average of 7.5 million a day, and began the process of expanding internationally—opening its first factory store in Europe, located in the world-renowned department store Harrods of Knightsbridge, London (with plans for another 25 stores in Britain and Ireland by 2008), and continuing expansion in Australia, Canada, and Mexico. In fiscal 2004, Krispy Kreme captured an estimated 30.6 percent of the market for packaged doughnut sales, compared with 23.9 percent in fiscal 2003 and 6.4 percent in fiscal 2002. In December 2005, the total number of company stores domestically stood at 349.

Exhibit 1 presents a summary of Krispy Kreme's financial performance and operations for fiscal years 2000–2004.

KRISPY KREME'S BUSINESS MODEL AND STRATEGY

Krispy Kreme's business model involved generating revenues and profits from three sources:

- Sales at company-owned stores.
- Royalties from franchised stores and franchise fees from new store openings.
- Sales of doughnut mixes, customized doughnut-making equipment, and coffees to franchised stores.

Exhibit 1   **Financial Statement Data for Krispy Kreme Doughnuts, Fiscal Years 2000–2004 (dollar amounts in thousands, except per share)**

	Fiscal Years Ending				
	Jan. 30, 2000	Jan. 28, 2001	Feb. 3, 2002	Feb. 2, 2003	Feb. 1, 2004
Statement of operations data					
Total revenues	$220,243	$300,715	$394,354	$491,549	$665,592
Operating expenses	190,003	250,690	316,946	381,489	507,396
General and administrative expenses	14,856	20,061	27,562	28,897	36,912
Depreciation and amortization expenses	4,546	6,457	7,959	12,271	19,723
Arbitration award	—	—	—	9,075	(575)
Income from operations	$ 10,838	$ 23,507	$ 41,887	$ 59,817	$102,086
Interest expense, (income), net, and other adjustments	1,232	(276)	(659)	5,044	7,409
Income (loss) before income taxes	9,606	23,783	42,546	54,773	94,677
Provision for income taxes	3,650	9,058	16,168	21,295	37,590
Net income	$ 5,956	$ 14,725	$ 26,378	$ 33,478	$ 57,087
Net income per share:					
Basic	$0.16	$0.30	$0.49	$0.61	$0.96
Diluted	0.15	0.27	0.45	0.56	0.92
Shares used in calculation of net income per share (in 000s):					
Basic	37,360	49,184	53,703	55,093	59,188
Diluted	39,280	53,656	58,443	59,492	62,388
Balance sheet data					
Current assets	$ 41,038	$ 67,611	$101,769	$141,128	$138,644
Current liabilities	29,586	38,168	52,533	59,687	53,493
Working capital	11,452	29,443	49,236	81,441	85,151
Total assets	104,958	171,493	255,376	410,487	660,664
Long-term debt, including current maturities	22,902	—	4,643	60,489	137,917
Total shareholders' equity	$ 47,755	$125,679	$187,667	$273,352	$452,207
Cash flow data					
Net cash provided by operating activities	$ 8,498	$ 32,112	$ 36,210	$ 51,036	$ 95,553
Net cash used for investing activities	(11,826)	(67,288)	(52,263)	(94,574)	(186,241)
Net cash provided by (used for) financing activities	(398)	39,019	30,931	53,837	79,514
Cash and cash equivalents at end of year	3,183	7,026	21,904	32,203	21,029

Source: Company SEC filings and annual reports.

Exhibit 2 shows revenues, operating expenses, and operating income by business segment.

The company was drawn to franchising because it minimized capital requirements, provided an attractive royalty stream, and put responsibility for local store operations in the hands of successful franchisees who knew the ins and outs of operating multi-unit chains

efficiently. Krispy Kreme had little trouble attracting top-quality franchisees because of the attractive economics of its new stores (see Exhibit 3).

Krispy Kreme had developed a vertically integrated supply chain whereby it manufactured the mixes for its doughnuts at company plants in North Carolina and Illinois and also manufactured proprietary

Exhibit 2   **Krispy Kreme's Performance by Business Segment, Fiscal Years 2000–2004 (in thousands)**

	Fiscal Years Ending				
	Jan. 30, 2000	Jan. 20, 2001	Feb. 3, 2002	Feb. 2, 2003	Feb. 1, 2004
Revenues by business segment					
Company store operations	$164,230	$213,677	$266,209	$319,592	$ 441,868
Franchise operations	5,529	9,445	14,008	19,304	23,848
KK manufacturing & distribution	50,484	77,593	114,137	152,653	193,129
Total	$220,243	$300,715	$394,354	$491,549	$ 665,592*
Operating income by business segment (before depreciation and amortization)					
Company store operations	$ 18,246	$ 27,370	$ 42,932	$ 58,214	$ 83,724
Franchise operations	1,445	5,730	9,040	14,319	19,043
KK manufacturing & distribution	7,182	11,712	18,999	26,843	39,345
Total	$ 10,838	$ 23,507	$ 41,887	$ 59,817	$ 102,086*
Unallocated general and administrative expenses	$ (16,035)	$ (21,305)	$ (29,084)	$ (30,484)	$ (38,564)
Depreciation and amortization expenses					
Company store operations	$3,059	$4,838	$5,859	$ 8,854	$14,392
Franchise operations	72	72	72	108	173
KK manufacturing & distribution	236	303	507	1,723	3,006
Corporate administration	1,179	1,244	1,521	1,586	1,653
Total	$4,546	$6,457	$7,959	$12,271	$19,723*

*Totals include operations of Montana Mills, a business which was acquired in April 2003 and divested during fiscal 2005.
Source: Company SEC filings and annual reports.

doughnut-making equipment for use in both company-owned and franchised stores. The sale of mixes and equipment, referred to as "KK manufacturing & distribution" by the company, generated a substantial fraction of both revenues and earnings (Exhibit 2).

Many of the stores built prior to 1997 were designed primarily as wholesale bakeries, and their formats and site locations differed considerably from the newer stores being located in high-density areas where there were lots of people and high traffic counts. In order to improve on-premises sales at these older stores, the company was implementing a program to either remodel them or close and relocate them to sites that could better attract on-premises sales. In new markets, the company's strategy was to focus initial efforts on on-premises sales at its stores and then leverage the interest generated in Krispy Kreme products to secure supermarket and convenience store accounts and grow packaged sales.

So far, the company had spent very little on advertising to introduce its product to new markets, relying instead on local media publicity, product giveaways, and word of mouth. In almost every instance, local newspapers had run big features headlining the opening of the first Krispy Kreme stores

Exhibit 3   **Estimated Krispy Kreme Store Economics as of 2001**

Store revenues	$3,600,000
Cash flow (after operating expenses)	960,000
Cash flow margin	27%
Owner's equity investment to construct store	$1,050,000
Cash flow return on equity investment	91%

Source: As estimated by Deutsche Banc Alex. Brown.

in their area; in some cases, local radio and TV stations had sent news crews to cover the opening and conduct on-the-scene interviews. The grand opening in Austin, Texas, was covered live by five TV crews and four radio station crews (there were 50 people in line at 11:30 p.m. the night before the 5:30 a.m. store opening). At the first San Diego store opening, there were five remote TV trucks on the scene; radio reporters were out interviewing customers camped out in their pickup trucks in the parking lot; and a nationally syndicated radio show broadcast "live" at the site. It was common for customers to form lines at the door and at the drive-through window well before the initial day's 5:30 a.m. grand opening, when the HOT DOUGHNUTS NOW sign was first turned on. In a number of instances, there were traffic jams at the turn in to the store—a Buffalo, New York, traffic cop said, "I've never seen anything like this . . . and I mean it." As part of the grassroots marketing effort surrounding new-store openings, Krispy Kremes were typically given away at public events as a treat for participants—then, as one franchisee said, "the Krispy Kremes seem to work their own magic and people start to talk about them."

Krispy Kreme had originally financed its expansion strategy with the aid of long-term debt. However, the April 2000 IPO raised enough equity capital to completely pay off the long-term debt outstanding as of fiscal 2001. Since then the company had borrowed about $50 million on a long-term basis to help fund its rapid growth during 2002–2004. When the company went public, it ceased paying dividends to shareholders; currently all earnings were being retained and reinvested in growing the business.

COMPANY OPERATIONS

Products and Product Quality

Krispy Kreme produced nearly 50 varieties of doughnuts, including specialty doughnuts offered at limited times and locations. By far the biggest seller was the company's signature "hot original glazed" doughnut made from Joe LeBeau's original yeast-based recipe. Exhibit 4 shows the company's doughnut varieties as of December 2005. Exhibit 5 indicates the nutritional content for a representative selection of Krispy Kreme doughnuts.

Company research indicated that Krispy Kreme's appeal extended across all major demographic groups, including age and income. Many customers purchased doughnuts by the dozen for their office, clubs, and family. According to one enthusiastic franchisee:

> We happen to think this is a very, very unique product which has what I can only describe as a one-of-a-kind taste. They are extremely light in weight and texture. They have this incredible glaze. When you have one of the hot original doughnuts as they come off the line, there's just nothing like it.

In 2003, Krispy Kreme ranked number one in Restaurants and Institutions' Choice in Chains category, beating number-two-ranked Starbucks.

The company received several thousand e-mails and letters monthly from customers. By all accounts, most were from customers who were passionate about Krispy Kreme products, and there were always some from people pleading for stores to be opened in their area. Exhibit 6 presents sample comments

Exhibit 4   Varieties of Krispy Kreme Doughnuts, 2005

- Original Glazed
- Glazed Cinnamon
- Chocolate Iced
- Chocolate Iced with Sprinkles
- Maple Iced
- Chocolate Iced Kreme Filled
- Glazed Kreme Filled
- Traditional Cake
- Apple Fritter
- Powdered Strawberry Filled
- Key Lime Pie

- Chocolate Iced Custard Filled
- Raspberry Filled
- Lemon Filled
- Cinnamon Apple Filled
- Powdered Blueberry Filled
- Chocolate Iced Cake
- Dulce de Leche
- Sugar Coated
- New York Cheesecake

- Glazed Cruller
- Powdered Cake
- Glazed Chocolate Cake
- Chocolate Iced Cruller
- Cinnamon Bun
- Glazed Blueberry
- Glazed Sour Kream
- Caramel Kreme Crunch
- Cinnamon Twist

Source: www.krispykreme.com, December 7, 2005.

Exhibit 5   **Nutritional Content of Selected Varieties of Krispy Kreme Doughnuts, 2005**

Product	Calories	Calories from Fat	Total Fat		Saturated Fat		Carbohydrates		Sugars
			Grams	% Daily Value*	Grams	% Daily Value*	Grams	% Daily Value*	
Original Glazed	200	100	12g	18%	3g	15%	22g	7%	10g
Chocolate Iced Glazed	250	110	12	19	3	15	33	11	21
Maple Iced Glazed	240	100	12	18	3	15	32	11	20
Powdered Blueberry Filled	290	150	16	25	4	20	33	11	14
Chocolate Iced Kreme Filled	350	180	20	32	5	25	38	13	23
Glazed Kreme Filled	340	180	20	31	5	24	38	13	23
Traditional Cake	230	120	13	20	3	15	25	8	9
Glazed Cruller	240	130	14	22	3.5	17	26	9	14
Cinnamon Bun	260	140	16	24	4	20	28	9	13
Glazed Chocolate Cake	340	140	15	23	3.5	18	41	14	26

*Based on a 2,000-calorie diet.

Source: www.Krispykreme.com, December 7, 2005.

from customers and franchisees. According to Scott Livengood:

> You have to possess nothing less than a passion for your product and your business because that's where you draw your energy. We have a great product . . . We have loyal customers, and we have great brand equity. When we meet people with a Krispy Kreme story, they always do it with a smile on their faces.

Coffee   Krispy Kreme had recently launched strategic initiatives to improve the caliber and appeal of its on-premises coffee and beverage offerings, aligning them more closely with the hot doughnut experience in its stores. The first move came in early 2001 when Krispy Kreme acquired Digital Java Inc., a small Chicago-based coffee company that sourced and roasted premium quality coffees and that marketed a broad line of coffee-based and noncoffee beverages. Scott Livengood explained the reasons for the acquisition:

> We believe the Krispy Kreme brand naturally extends to a coffee and beverage offering that is more closely aligned with the hot doughnut experience in our stores. Vertical integration of our coffee business provides the capability to control the sourcing and roasting of our coffee. Increasing control of our supply chain will help ensure quality standards, recipe formulation, and roast consistency. With this capability, one of our first priorities will be the research and benchmarking necessary to develop premier blends and roasts of coffee which will help make Krispy Kreme a coffee destination for a broader audience. Beyond coffee, we intend to offer a full line of beverages including espresso-based drinks and frozen beverages. We believe we can substantially increase the proportion of our business devoted to coffee specifically and beverages generally by upgrading and broadening our beverage offering.

Since the acquisition of Digital Java, coffee sales at Krispy Kreme stores had increased nearly 40 percent due to expanded product offerings and upgraded quality. In 2003, Krispy Kreme was marketing four types of coffee: Smooth, Rich, Bold, and Robust Decaf—all using coffee beans from the top 5 percent of the world's growing regions. Beverage sales accounted for about 10 percent of store sales, with coffee accounting for about half of the beverage total and the other half divided among milk, juices, soft drinks, and bottled water. In the years ahead, Krispy Kreme hoped to increase beverage sales to about 20 percent of store sales.

Exhibit 6 **Sample Comments from Krispy Kreme Customers and Franchisees**

Customer Comments

- "I ate one and literally it brought a tear to my eye. I kid you not."
- "Oh my gosh, this is awesome. I wasn't even hungry, but now I'm going to get two dozen."
- "We got up at 3 o'clock this morning. I told them I would be late for work. I was going to the grand opening."
- "They melt in your mouth. They really do."
- "Krispy Kreme rocks."
- It's hot, good and hot. The way a doughnut should be."
- "The doughnut's magnificent. A touch of genius."
- "I love doughnuts, but these are different. It's terrible for your weight because when you eat just one, you feel like you've barely tasted it. You want more. It's like popcorn."*
- When you bite into one it's like biting into a sugary cloud. It's really fun to give one to someone who hasn't had one before. They bite into one and just exclaim."†

Franchisee Comments

- "Krispy Kreme is a 'feel good' business as much as it is a doughnut business. Customers come in for an experience which makes them feel good—they enjoy our doughnuts and they enjoy the time they spend in our stores watching the doughnuts being made."
- "We're not selling doughnuts as much as we are creating an experience. The viewing window into the production room is a theater our customers can never get enough of. It's fun to watch doughnuts being made and even more fun to eat them when they're hot off the line."
- "Southern California customers have responded enthusiastically to Krispy Kreme. Many of our fans first came to Krispy Kreme not because of a previous taste experience but rather because of the "buzz" around the brand. It was more word of mouth and publicity that brought them in to sample our doughnuts. Once they tried them, they became loyal fans who spread the word that Krispy Kreme is something special . . . We witness the excitement every day, especially when we're away from the store and wearing a hat or shirt with the Krispy Kreme logo. When people see the logo, we get the big smile and are always asked, 'When will we get one in our neighborhood?' . . . The tremendous local publicity coupled with the amazing brand awareness nationwide has helped us make the community aware of our commitment to support local charities. Our fund-raising program, along with product donations to schools, churches, and other charitable organizations have demonstrated our real desire to give back. This commitment also impacts our employees who understand firsthand the value of supporting the needy as well as the worthy causes in our neighborhoods."
- "In all my many years of owning and operating multiple food franchise businesses, we have never been able to please—until Krispy Kreme—such a wide range of customers in the community. Its like an old friend has come to town when we open our doors: we're welcomed with open arms . . . Quite frankly, in my experience, publicity for Krispy Kreme is like nothing I have ever seen. It is truly unprecedented."
- We happen to think this is a very, very unique product which has what I can only describe as a one-of-a-kind taste. They are extremely light in weight and texture. They have this incredible glaze. When you have one of the hot original doughnuts as they come off the line, there's just nothing like it.

*As quoted in "Winchell's Scrambles to Meet Krispy Kreme Challenge," *Los Angeles Times,* September 30, 1999, p. C1.
†As quoted in Greg Sukiennik, "Will Dunkin' Donuts Territory Take to Krispy Kreme?" Associated Press State & Local Wire, April 8, 2001.
Source: Krispy Kreme's 2000 and 2001 annual reports, except for the two quotes noted above.

Store Operations

Each store was designed as a "doughnut theater" where customers could watch the doughnuts being made through a 40-foot glass window (see Exhibit 7). New stores ranged in size between 2,400 and 4,200 square feet. Stores had a drive-through window and a dining area that would seat 50 or more people—a few of the newer and larger stores had special rooms for hosting Krispy Kreme parties. Store decor was a vintage 1950s look with mint green walls and smooth metal chairs; some of the newest stores had booths (see Exhibit 8). A typical store employed about 125 people, including about 65 full-time positions. Approximately half of on-premises sales occurred in the morning hours and half in the afternoon and

Exhibit 7 **Making the Doughnuts**

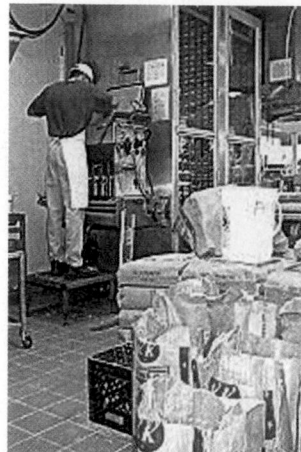

Mixing Ingredients

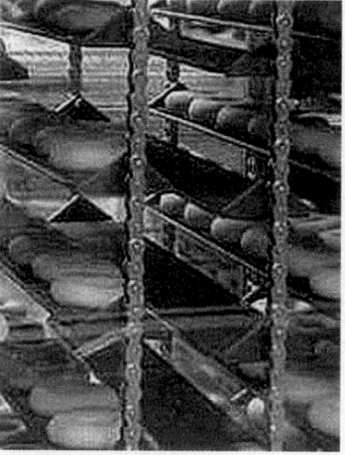

Rising

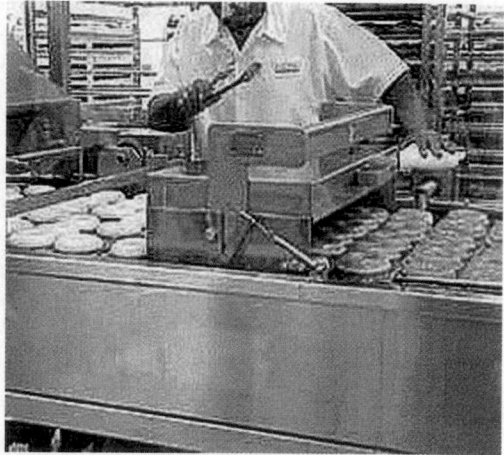

Frying and Flipping

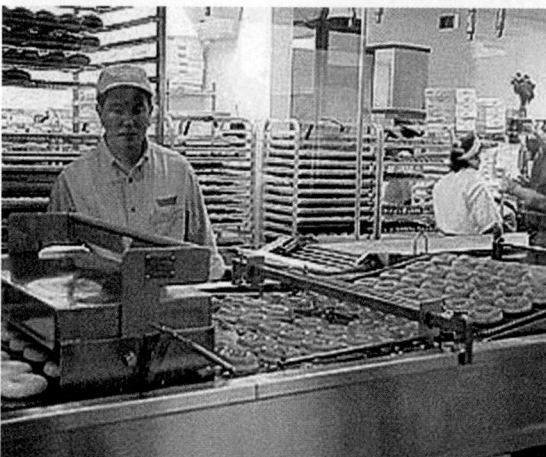

Inspection and Draining

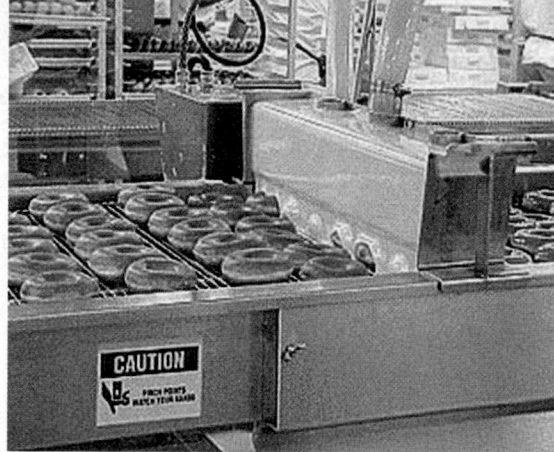

Drying and Entering Glazing

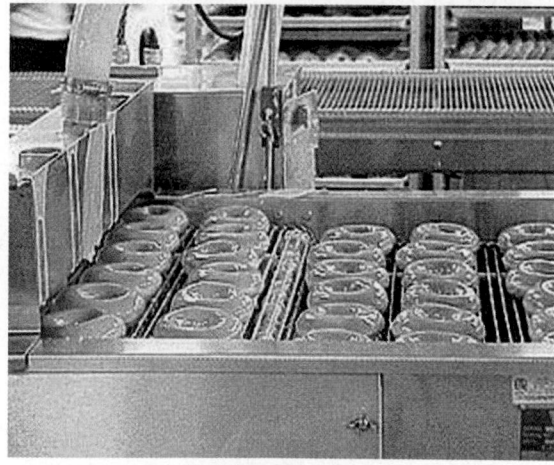

Exiting Glazing

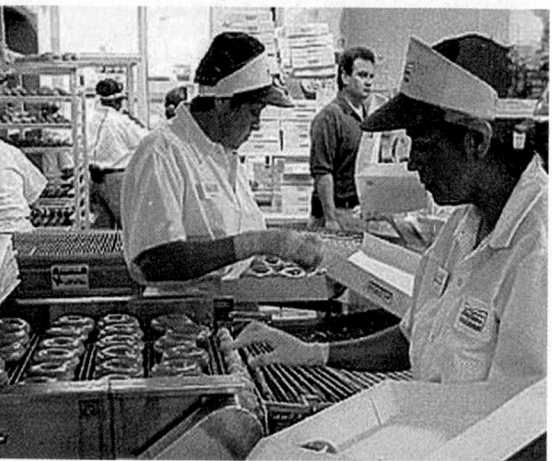

Packaging

Exhibit 8   **Representative Krispy Kreme Stores and Store Scenes**

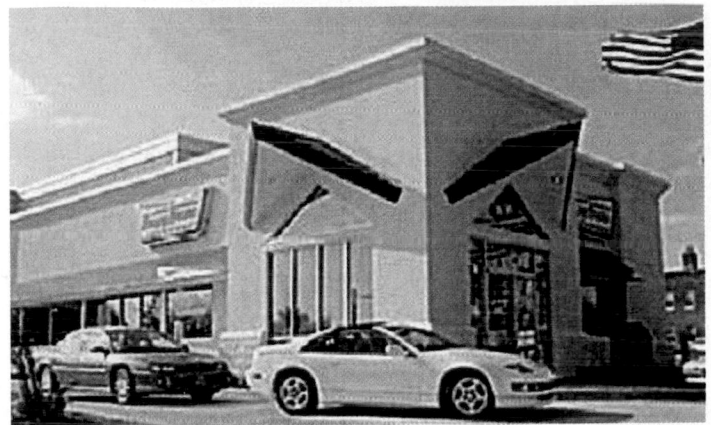
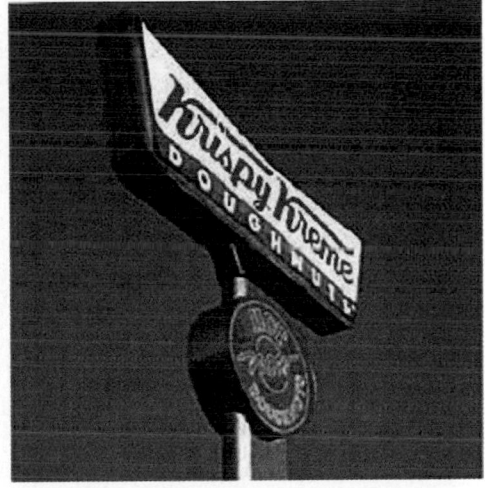
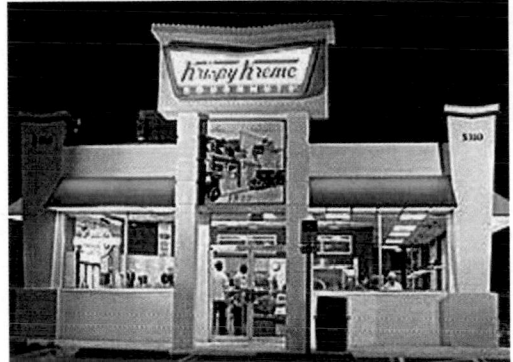
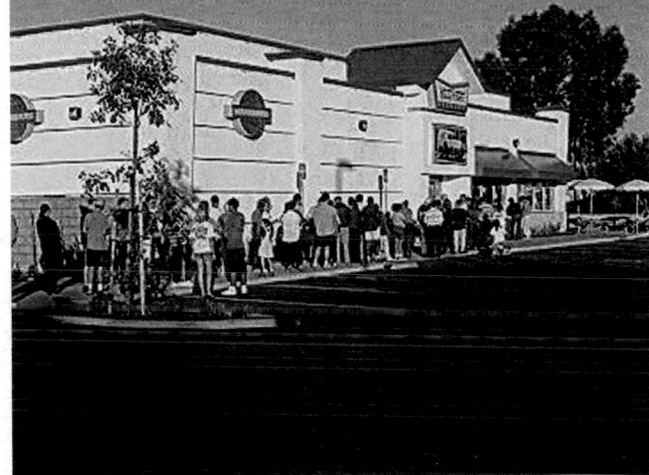
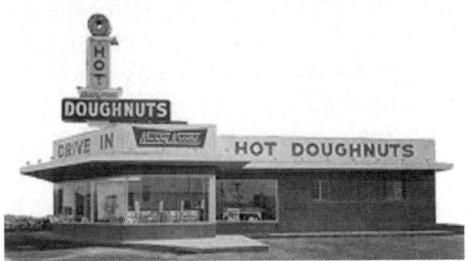
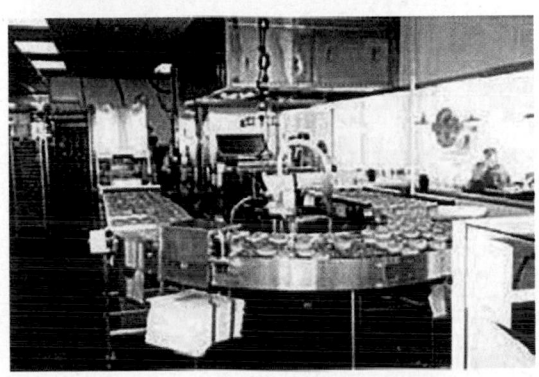
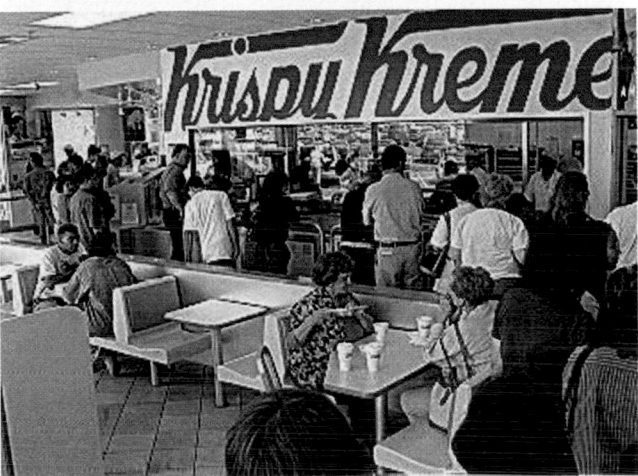

evening. Many stores were open 24 hours a day, with much of the doughnut making for off-premises sales being done between 6:00 p.m. and 6:00 a.m. Production was nearly always under way during peak in-store traffic times. In several large metropolitan areas, however, the doughnut making for off-premises sales was done in a central commissary specially equipped for large-volume production, packaging, and local-area distribution.

Each doughnut took about one hour to make. After the ingredients were mixed into dough, the dough was rolled and cut. The pieces went into a 12-foot-tall machine where each piece rotated on a wire rack for 33 minutes under high humidity and a low heat of 126 degrees to allow the dough to rise. When the rising process was complete, the doughnuts moved along a conveyor to be fried on one side, flipped, fried on the other side, and drained. Following all this came inspection. Doughnuts destined to be glazed were directed through a waterfall of warm, sugary topping; the others were directed to another part of the baking section to be filled and/or frosted. Exhibit 8 depicts the mixing, rising, frying, draining, and glazing parts of the process. Depending on store size and location, a typical day's production ranged between 4,000 and 10,000 dozen doughnuts.

Each producing store featured a prominent HOT DOUGHNUTS NOW neon sign (Exhibit 8) signaling customers that freshly made original glazed doughnuts were coming off the bakery conveyor belt and were available for immediate purchase. Generally, the signs glowed from 6:00 to 11:00 a.m. and then came on again during the late afternoon into the late-night hours.

Depending on the store location, Krispy Kreme's original glazed doughnuts sold for 60 to 75 cents each, or $4.50 to $7.50 per dozen; a mixed dozen usually sold for about 50 cents extra. Some stores charged a small premium for hot doughnuts coming right off the production line. Customers typically got a $1.00 per dozen discount on purchases of two or more dozen.

Stores generated revenues in three ways:

- On-premise sales of doughnuts.
- Sales of coffee and other beverages.
- Off-premise sales of branded and private-label doughnuts to local supermarkets, convenience stores, and fund-raising groups. Krispy Kreme stores actively promoted sales to schools, churches, and civic groups for fund-raising drives.

The company had developed a highly effective system for delivering fresh doughnuts, both packaged and unpackaged, to area supermarket chains and convenience stores. Route drivers had the capability to take customer orders and deliver products directly to retail accounts, where they were typically merchandised either from Krispy Kreme branded displays or from bakery cases (as unbranded doughnuts). The popularity of Krispy Kreme's stores had prompted many area supermarkets to begin stocking a selection of Krispy Kreme products in either branded display cases or in dozen and half-dozen packages.

The franchisee for Krispy Kreme stores in San Francisco had arranged to sell a four-pack of Krispy Kremes for $5 at San Francisco Giant baseball games at Pacific Bell Park—Krispy Kreme sold out of 2,100 packs by the third inning of the first game and, despite increasing supplies, sold out again after the fourth and sixth innings of the next two games; stadium vendors were supplied with 3,450 four-packs for the fourth game. The franchisee of the Las Vegas stores had a Web site that allowed customers to place orders online before 2:00 p.m. and have them delivered to their place of work by a courier service.

A Texas franchisee built a new 18,000-square-foot production and distribution center to supply Metroplex supermarkets, convenience stores, and other area retailers with Krispy Kreme 12-packs because newly opened Krispy Kreme stores did not have the baking capacity to keep up with both on-premises and off-premises demand; there were similar franchiser-operated wholesale baking and distribution centers in Nashville, Cincinnati, Atlanta, Chicago, and Philadelphia. Several of these centers had established delivery capability to supply Krispy Kremes to retailers in outlying areas deemed too small to justify a stand-alone Krispy Kreme store.

In 2004, about 20,000 supermarkets, convenience stores, truck stops, and other outside locations sold Krispy Kreme doughnuts. A growing number of these locations had special Krispy Kreme display cases, stocked daily with trays of different varieties for shoppers to choose from; these stand-alone cases could be placed in high-traffic locations at the end of an aisle or close to the check-out register.

The cost of opening a new store was around $2 million (including the standard package of equipment purchased from Krispy Kreme), but new store construction could range as high as $2.5 million in locations with high land and/or building costs. The initial franchise fee per unit was $40,000. Site selection was based on household density, proximity to both daytime employment and residential centers, and proximity to other retail traffic generators. A record number of new stores were opened in fiscal 2004—28 company-owned stores and 58 franchised stores (the net gain in stores was only 81 because 5 older stores were closed). Plans were in place to open 75 new stores in the upcoming fiscal 2005 year.

Weekly sales at newly opened stores could run anywhere from $100,000 to $500,000 the first couple of weeks a new store was open. Weekly sales tended to moderate to around $40,000 to $50,000 after several months of operation, but Krispy Kreme management expected new stores to have annual sales averaging more than $3 million in their first year of operation. In fiscal 2003, sales at all of the company's 276 stores (which included those open less than a year) averaged $2.82 million. In fiscal 2004, sales at all 357 stores averaged $2.76 million—slightly lower than in 2003, chiefly because of the larger number of new store openings (roughly half of the 86 new stores were open less than six months). Exhibit 9 provides data on store operations.

Krispy Kreme Manufacturing and Distribution

All the doughnut mix and equipment used in Krispy Kreme stores was manufactured and supplied by the company, partly as a means of ensuring consistent recipe quality and doughnut making throughout the chain and partly as a means of generating sales and profits from franchise operations. Revenues of the Krispy Kreme Manufacturing and Distribution (KKM&D) unit had averaged about 30 percent of total Krispy Kreme revenues for the past three years and contributed 38 to 45 percent of annual operating income (see Exhibit 2). The company's line of custom stainless-steel doughnut-making machines ranged in capacity from 230 to 600 dozen doughnuts per hour. Franchisees paid Krispy Kreme about $770,000 for the standard doughnut-making equipment package in 2003–2004 (up from about $500,000 in the late 1990s); the price increase was due partly to increased equipment capacity and partly to longer equipment durability. Increased doughnut sales at franchised stores also translated into increased revenues for KKM&D from sales of mixes, sugar, and other supplies to franchisees.

Krispy Kreme had recently opened a state-of-the-art 187,000-square-foot manufacturing and distribution facility in Effingham, Illinois, dedicated to the blending and packaging of prepared doughnut mixes and to distributing mixes, equipment, and other supplies to stores in the Midwest and the western half of North America. This facility had significantly lowered Krispy Kreme's unit costs and provided triple the production capacity of the older plant in Winston-Salem.

Exhibit 9   **Store Operations Data, Krispy Kreme Doughnuts, Fiscal Years 1998–2004**

	1998	2000	2001	2002	2003	2004
Systemwide sales	$203,439	$318,854	$448,129	$621,665	$778,573	$984,895
Number of stores at end of period:						
Company-owned	58	58	63	75	99	141
Franchised	62	86	111	143	177	216
Systemwide total	120	144	174	218	276	357
Increase in comparable store sales						
Company-owned	11.5%	12.0%	22.9%	11.7%	12.8%	13.6%
Franchised	12.7%	14.1%	17.1%	12.8%	11.8%	10.2%
Average weekly sales per store:						
Company-owned (000s)	$42	$54	$69	$72	$76	$73
Franchised (000s)	23	38	43	53	58	56

Source: Company annual reports and 10-K reports.

Training

Since mid-1999, Krispy Kreme had invested in the creation of a multimedia management and employee training curriculum. The program included classroom instruction, computer-based and video training modules, and in-store training experiences. The online part of the training program made full use of graphics, video, and animation, as well as seven different types of test questions. Every Krispy Kreme store had access to the training over the company's intranet and the Internet; employees who registered for the course could access the modules from home using their Internet connection. Learners' test results were transferred directly to a Krispy Kreme human resources database; learners were automatically redirected to lessons where their test scores indicated that they had not absorbed the material well on the first attempt. The online course was designed to achieve 90 percent mastery from 90 percent of the participants and could be updated as needed.

KKD'S BRIGHT GROWTH PROSPECTS

In 2003 and continuing into early 2004, Krispy Kreme management expressed confidence that the company was still in its infancy. The company's highest priority was on expanding into markets with over 100,000 households; management believed these markets were attractive because the dense population characteristics offered opportunities for multiple store locations, gave greater exposure to brand-building efforts, and afforded multi-unit operating economies. However, the company believed that secondary markets with fewer than 100,000 households held significant sales and profit potential—it was exploring smaller-sized store designs suitable for secondary markets. In 2002, Krispy Kreme CEO Scott Livengood stated, "We are totally committed to putting full factory stores in every town in the U.S." Krispy Kreme's management further believed the food-service and institutional channel of sales offered significant opportunity to extend the brand into colleges and universities, business and industry facilities, and sports and entertainment complexes. Management had stated that the company's strong brand name, highly differentiated product, high-volume production capability, and multichannel market penetration strategy put the company in a position to become the recognized leader in every market it entered.

Expansion into Foreign Markets

In December 2000, the company hired Donald Henshall, 38, to fill the newly created position of president of international development; Henshall was formerly managing director of new business development with the London-based Overland Group, a maker and marketer of branded footwear and apparel. Henshall's job was to refine the company's global strategy, develop the capabilities and infrastructure to support expansion outside the United States, and consider inquiries from qualified parties wanting to open Krispy Kreme stores in foreign markets. Outside of the United States, Krispy Kreme stores had opened in Canada, Australia, Mexico, the United Kingdom, and the Republic of South Korea. Krispy Kreme and its franchisees planned to open 39 new stores in Canada, 30 in Australia and New Zealand, 20 in Mexico, and 25 in Great Britain and Ireland in the coming years. So far, sales had been very promising at the foreign locations that had been opened, and franchise agreements were in the works for further global expansion.

As of May 2001, the company had stopped accepting franchise applications for U.S. locations, indicating that there were no open territories. By 2003, it had stopped accepting franchise applications in Canada, Mexico, Western Europe, and Australia, indicating that franchise contracts were already under way and that Krispy Kreme would be opening in these areas soon. According to Scott Livengood, "Krispy Kreme is a natural to become a global brand. Looking at our demographics, we appeal to a very broad customer base. We receive lots of interest on a weekly basis to expand into international locations and we are confident our brand will be received extremely well outside the U.S."

THE MONTANA MILLS ACQUISITION

Krispy Kreme's chief strategic move in 2003 was to acquire Montana Mills Bread Company, a bakery operation based in Rochester, New York, with 11 retail locations. The acquisition price was 1.2 million shares of Krispy Kreme stock (worth roughly $50 million). The Montana Mills chain of neighborhood bakeries featured fresh stone-ground flour, a highly visual presentation of the baking process in full view of the customer, and customer sampling with large slices of a variety of fresh-baked breads. In explaining why the acquisition was made, Scott Livengood said:

> This acquisition is a natural outgrowth of the development of Krispy Kreme over the past five years. As I have indicated previously, we view Krispy Kreme Doughnuts, Inc., first and foremost as a set of unique capabilities which include the abilities to explore and nurture our customers' passion for and connection to a brand, create an effective franchise network, vertically integrate to provide a complete range of products and services to a system-wide store network serving flour-based, short shelf life products, and deliver these products daily across multiple channels. Applying these core organizational competencies to the development of a second concept has the potential to create significant leverage.
>
> The opportunity to create a wholesome, fresh-baked bakery and cafe concept the 'Krispy Kreme way' is obviously unique to Krispy Kreme. I have long considered how to capitalize on this opportunity. In Montana Mills, we found the perfect foundation for this new concept—passionate bread bakers who have created a fiercely loyal customer following around a wide variety of fresh-baked goods, bread-baking theater and sampling of large slices of bread. I have personally observed this passion that each Montana Mills employee carries for their customers and their breads. This is a great platform on which to build. We will work closely with the Montana Mills team as we try to add value to an already outstanding concept.
>
> I expect we will spend in the range of two years fully developing the concept I described. As we have indicated regarding our international expansion, we will always try to prepare for any type of expansion well before we need the growth. We want the time to do it right. For this concept, I think that time is now.

In fiscal 2004, Montana Mills generated revenues of $6.7 million and had operating expenses of $8.7 million, thus resulting in an operating loss of $2.0 million.

INDUSTRY ENVIRONMENT

By some estimates, the U.S. doughnut industry was a $5 to $6 billion market in 2003–2005. Americans consumed an estimated 10 to 12 billion doughnuts annually—over three dozen per capita. In 2002, doughnut industry sales rose by about 13 percent. According to a study done by Technomic, a marketing research specialist in foods, doughnut shops were the fastest-growing dining category in the country in 2002–2003.

Prior to the excitement over Krispy Kreme's doughnuts, growth in packaged doughnut sales at supermarkets, convenience stores, and other retail outlets had been quite small. The proliferation of bakery departments in supermarkets had squeezed out many locally owned doughnut shops and, to some extent, had constrained the growth of doughnut chains. Doughnuts were a popular item in supermarket bakeries, with many customers finding it more convenient to buy them when doing their regular supermarket shopping as opposed to making a special trip to local bakeries. Doughnut aficionados, however, tended to pass up doughnuts in the grocery store, preferring the freshness, quality, and variety offered by doughnut specialty shops. Most patrons of doughnut shops frequented those in their neighborhoods or normal shopping area; it was unusual for them to make a special trip of more than a mile or two for doughnuts.

Small independent doughnut shops usually had a devoted clientele, drawn from neighborhood residents and regular commuters passing by on their way to and from work. A longtime employee at a family-owned shop in Denver said, "Our customers are very loyal to us. Probably 80 percent are regulars."[1] Owners of independent shops seemed to believe that new entry by popular chains like Krispy Kreme posed little competitive threat, arguing that the market was big enough to support both independents and franchisers, that the Krispy Kreme novelty was likely to wear off, and that unless a doughnut franchiser located a store close to their present location the impact would be minimal at worst. A store owner in Omaha said, "Our doughnut sales increased when Krispy Kreme came to town. We benefit every time they advertise because doughnuts are as popular as ever."[2]

As of early 2004, there was little indication that the low-carbohydrate weight-watching craze that had swept the United States and other countries in recent years had cut much into sales. Industry observers and company officials attributed this in part to doughnuts being an affordable indulgence, easy to eat on the run, and in part to the tendency of many people to treat themselves occasionally. Doughnuts were readily available almost anywhere.

KRISPY KREME'S CHIEF COMPETITORS

The three leading doughnut chains in North America were Krispy Kreme, Dunkin' Donuts, and Tim Hortons.

Dunkin' Donuts

Dunkin' Donuts was the largest coffee and baked-goods chain in the world, selling 4.4 million donuts and 1.8 million cups of coffee daily. The quick-service restaurant chain was owned by British-based Allied Domecq PLC, a diversified enterprise whose other businesses included the Baskin-Robbins ice cream chain, ToGo's Eateries (sandwiches), and an assortment of alcoholic beverage brands (Kahla, Beefeater's, Maker's Mark, Courvoisier, Tia Maria, and a host of wines). Allied Domecq traded on the London Stock Exchange under the symbol ALLD. In 2004, Allied Domecq's Dunkin' Donuts chain had total sales approaching $4 billion, almost 6,200 franchised outlets in 40 countries (including 4,418 in the United States), and comparable store sales growth of 4.4 percent in the United States. About 83 percent of the chain's total sales were in the United States. In New England alone, Dunkin' Donuts operated 1,200 stores, including 600 in the Greater Boston area, where the chain was founded in 1950. Starting in 2000, Dunkin' Donuts franchisees could open co-branded stores that included Baskin Robbins and ToGo. Dunkin' Donuts ranked 9th in *Entrepreneur* magazine's annual Franchise Top 500 for 2005.

The key thrust of Dunkin' Donuts' strategy was to expand into those geographic areas in the United States where it was underrepresented. In areas where there were clusters of Dunkin' Donuts outlets, most baked items were supplied from centrally located kitchens rather than being made on-site. Despite its name, Dunkin' Donuts put more emphasis on coffee and convenience than on doughnuts. According to one company executive, "People talk about our coffee first. We're food you eat on the go. We're part of your day. We're not necessarily a destination store." Roughly half of all purchases at Dunkin' Donuts included coffee without a doughnut.[3] Dunkin' Donuts menu included doughnuts (50 varieties), muffins, bagels, cinnamon buns, cookies, brownies, Munchkins doughnut holes, cream cheese sandwiches, nine flavors of fresh coffee, iced coffees, and a lemonade Coolatta.

In 2004, Coolatta was being promoted in collaboration with MTV in a campaign called "Route to Cool." Dunkin' Donuts also had a new "Express Donuts" campaign to promote the sale of boxed donuts—12-packs containing the top six flavors. This campaign was being supported by advertising based on the theme "Who brought the donuts?" In addition, the chain was emphasizing coffee sales by the pound and had recently broadened its coffee offerings to include cappuccino, latte, espresso, and iced coffees.

With regard to nutritional content, Dunkin' Donuts' 50 doughnut varieties ranged between 200 and 340 calories, between 8 and 19 grams of fat, between 1.5 and 6 grams of saturated fat, and between 9 and 31 grams of sugars; its cinnamon buns had 540 calories, 15 grams of fat, 4 grams of saturated fat, and 42 grams of sugars. Whereas Krispy Kreme's best-selling original glazed doughnuts had 200 calories, 12 grams of fat, 3 grams of saturated fat, and 10 grams of sugar, the comparable item at Dunkin' Donuts had 180 calories, 8 grams of fat, 1.5 grams of saturated fat, and 6 grams of sugar. Several Dunkin' Donuts customers in the Boston area who had recently tried Krispy Kreme doughnuts reported that Krispy Kremes had more flavor and were lighter.[4]

Dunkin' Donuts had successfully fended off competition from national bagel chains and Starbucks. When national bagel chains, promoting bagels as a healthful alternative to doughnuts, opened new stores in areas where Dunkin' Donuts had stores, the company responded by adding bagels and cream cheese sandwiches to its menu offerings. Dunkin' Donuts had countered threats from Starbucks by adding a wider variety of hot-and-cold coffee beverages—and whereas coffee drinkers had to wait for a Starbucks barista to properly craft a $3 latte, they could get coffee and a doughnut on the fly at Dunkin' Donuts for less money. Quick and consistent service was a Dunkin' Donuts forte. Management further believed that the broader awareness of coffee created by the market presence of Starbucks stores had actually helped boost coffee sales at Dunkin' Donuts. In markets such as New York City and Chicago where there were both Dunkin' Donuts and Krispy Kreme stores, sales at Dunkin' Donuts had continued to rise.

In commenting on the competitive threat from Krispy Kreme, a Dunkin' Donuts vice president said:

> We have a tremendous number of varieties, a tremendous level of convenience, tremendous coffee and other baked goods. I think the differentiation that Dunkin' enjoys is clear. We're not pretentious and don't take ourselves too seriously, but we know how important a cup of coffee and a donut or bagel in the morning is. Being able to deliver a great cup of coffee when someone is on their way to something else is a great advantage.[5]

In 2003, Couche-Tard, Canada's largest convenience store operator, bought control of the Dunkin' Donuts name in Quebec as well as the 104 Dunkin' Donuts outlets located there. Couche-Tard planned to double the number of outlets within five years to better compete with Tim Hortons and Krispy Kreme.

Tim Hortons

Tim Hortons, a subsidiary of Wendy's International, was one of North America's largest coffee and fresh-baked-goods chains, with almost 2,400 restaurants across Canada and a steadily growing base of 200 locations in key markets within the United States. In April 2004, Tim Hortons acquired 42 Bess Eaton coffee and doughnut restaurants throughout Rhode Island, Connecticut, and Massachusetts, which it planned to convert to the Tim Hortons brand and format. Tim Hortons had systemwide sales of around $3 billion in 2003, equal to annual sales of about $1.3 million per store. Same store sales were up about 4.7 percent in 2003 and, during the first nine months of 2004, were up 10.1 percent in the United States and 7.7 percent in Canada. In Canada, the Tim Hortons chain was regarded as something of an icon—it was named for a popular Canadian-born professional hockey player who played for the Toronto Maple Leafs, Pittsburgh Penguins, and Buffalo Sabers; Horton was born in 1930, started playing hockey when he was five years old, and died in an auto accident while playing for the Buffalo Sabers. A recent survey of Canadian consumers rated Tim Hortons as the best-managed brand in Canada.

The Tim Hortons division of Wendy's relied heavily on franchising— only 57 of the 2,527 Tim Hortons outlets at year-end 2003 were company owned. Franchisees paid a royalty of 3 to 6 percent of weekly sales to the parent company, depending on whether they leased the land and/or buildings from Tim Hortons and on certain other conditions; in addition, franchisees paid fees equal to 4 percent of monthly gross sales to fund advertising and promotional activities undertaken at the corporate level. Franchisees were also required to purchase such products as coffee, sugar, flour, and shortening from a Tim Hortons subsidiary; these products were distributed from five warehouses located across Canada and were delivered to the company's Canadian restaurants primarily by its fleet of trucks and trailers. In the United States, both company and franchised stores purchased ingredients from a supplier approved by the parent company.

Tim Hortons used outside contractors to construct its restaurants. The restaurants were built to company specifications as to exterior style and interior decor. The standard Hortons restaurant being built in 2003–2004 consisted of a freestanding production unit ranging from 1,150 to 3,030 square feet. Each included a bakery capable of supplying fresh baked goods throughout the day to several satellite Tim Hortons within a defined area. Tim Hortons locations ranged from full-standard stores with in-store baking facilities; to combo units with Wendy's and Tim Hortons under one roof; to carts and kiosks in shopping malls, highway outlets, universities, airports, and hospitals. Most full-standard Tim Hortons locations offered 24-hour drive-through service. Tim Hortons promoted its full-standard stores as neighborhood meeting places and was active in promoting its products for group fund-raisers and community events.

The menu at each Tim Hortons unit consisted of coffee, cappuccino, teas, hot chocolate, soft drinks, soups, sandwiches, and fresh baked goods such as doughnuts, muffins, pies, croissants, tarts, cookies, cakes, and bagels. In recent years, the chain had expanded its lunch menu to include a bigger variety of offerings. One of the chain's biggest drawing cards was its special blend of fresh-brewed coffee, which was also sold in cans for customers' use at home. About half of the purchases at Tim Hortons included coffee without a doughnut. Tim Hortons was number one in market share in Canada during breakfast, was number one in the afternoon/early-evening snack category, and had a strong number two position at lunch with a menu featuring six sandwiches.

Executives at Tim Hortons did not feel threatened by Krispy Kreme's expansion into Canada and those parts of the United States where it had stores (Michigan, New York, Ohio, Kentucky, Maine, and West Virginia). According to David House, Tim Horton's president, "We really welcome them. Anyone who draws attention to doughnuts can only help us. It is a big market and a big marketplace. I would put our doughnut up against theirs any day."[6] A Canadian retailing consultant familiar with Tim Hortons and Krispy Kreme said, "This is the Canadian elephant and the U.S. mouse. Listen, if there's anything where Canadians can kick American butt, it is in doughnuts."[7] Another Canadian retailing consultant said, "It [Krispy Kreme] is an American phenomenon. These things are sickeningly sweet."[8]

Canada was reputed to have more doughnut shops per capita than any other country in the world. Aside from Tim Hortons, other chains in Canada featuring doughnuts included Dunkin' Donuts, Robin's Donuts, Country Style, and Coffee Time. Tim Hortons management had a goal of opening 500 Tim Hortons stores in the United States over the next three years, mostly in the Northeast and Great Lakes regions, and a longer-term goal of growing to about 3,500 outlets in Canada.

Winchell's Donut House

Winchell's, founded by Verne Winchell in 1948, was owned by Shato Holdings Ltd., of Vancouver, Canada. In 2000, there were approximately 600 Winchell's units located in 10 states west of the Mississippi River, along with international franchises in Guam, Saipan, Korea, Egypt, Saudi Arabia, and New Zealand. Since then, Winchell's Doughnut House had lost steam and closed two-thirds of its locations. In 2003, there were 200 units in 12 states, plus locations in Guam, Saipan, New Zealand, and Saudi Arabia. Winchell's was the largest doughnut chain on the West Coast. To combat Krispy Kreme's entry into Southern California, where Winchell's had a brand awareness of 97 percent, Winchell's had launched a Warm 'n Fresh program for all outlets in 2000. The program entailed having display cases full of fresh glazed doughnuts that were replaced every 15 to 20 minutes between 6:00 and 9:00 a.m. daily. A flashing red light on display cases signaled that a fresh batch of glazed doughnuts was available. Winchell's was offering customers a Warm 'n Fresh doughnut between 6:00 and 11:00 a.m. daily.

As of September 2003, a "Winchell's dozen" of 14 doughnuts sold for $5.99 and a double dozen (28) sold for $9.99—a single donut sold for about 60 cents, and many stores regularly ran a special of two donuts and a cup of coffee for $1.99. Winchell's bakery offerings included 20 varieties of doughnuts and 14 flavors of muffins, as well as croissants, bagels (breakfast bagel sandwiches were available at select locations), éclairs, tarts, apple fritters, and bear claws. It served three varieties of its "Legendary" coffees—Dark Roast Supreme, Legendary Blend, and Legendary Decaf—all using only 100 percent arabica beans (considered by many to be the finest coffee beans in the world). Other beverages included regular and frozen cappuccino, soft drinks, milk, and juices.

Winchell's corporate goal for the next five years was to triple its sales. In 2003–2004 it was actively seeking franchisees in 14 western and midwestern states. Winchell's charged a franchise fee of $7,500 and required franchisee to be able to invest $75,000 of unborrowed funds; the cost of new stores depended on such factors as store size, location, style of decor, and landscaping. A 5 percent royalty and a 3 percent advertising fee were charged on net sales.

LaMar's Donuts

Headquartered in Englewood, Colorado, LaMar's was a small, privately held chain that had 32 corporate-owned and franchised doughnut shops open or under development in 10 states; 8 stores were in the Denver area. Ray LaMar opened the original LaMar's Donuts in 1960 on Linwood Avenue in Kansas City and quickly turned the shop into a local institution. On a typical day, lines started forming before 6:00 a.m., and by closing time about 11,000 donuts would be sold. Based on the doughnut shop's success and reputation, Ray and his wife, Shannon, decided in the early 1990s to franchise LaMar's. Hundreds of LaMar's devotees applied for the limited number of franchises made available in the Kansas City area; 15 were granted over a few months. But little became of the initial franchising effort, and, in 1997, Franchise Consortium International, headed by Joseph J. Field, purchased a majority interest in LaMar's Franchising, renamed the company LaMar's Donuts International, moved the company's headquarters to a Denver suburb, and began laying the groundwork for a national expansion program.

LaMar's stores were typically located along neighborhood traffic routes. Average unit sales were $500,000 in 2003, and management expected the average to increase to $750,000 in a few years.

At one point, Fields expressed an objective of having 1,200 stores in operation by 2013, but so far LaMar's expansion was far slower than had been anticipated.

LaMar's used a secret recipe to produce "artisan-quality" doughnuts that were handmade daily with all-natural ingredients and no preservatives. Day-old doughnuts were never sold at the shops but were donated at day's end to the needy. In addition to 75 varieties of doughnuts, LaMar's menu included gourmet coffee and cappuccino. LaMar's had recently partnered with Dazbog Coffee Company in Denver, Colorado, and created over a dozen customized specialty coffee blends under the LaMar's Old World Roast label. Beans were handpicked from Costa Rica and then slow-roasted in an authentic Italian brick oven. Coffee products at LaMar's shops included cappuccinos, espressos, lattes, iced coffee drinks, and chai teas.

The company used the tag line "Simply a better doughnut." Joe Fields said, "People come in and try the product and they are surprised. They are wowed, in a very different way than Krispy Kreme. They say, 'Oh my God, this is the best doughnut I've had in my life.' " The Zagat Survey, a well-known rater of premier dining spots nationwide, described LaMar's Donuts as "extraordinary; fit for kings." *Gourmet* magazine, in search of the country's favorite doughnut, conducted a nationwide poll; the winner was a LaMar's doughnut. LaMar's Donuts has been named Best in the Country by the *John Walsh Show,* a one-hour daily nationally syndicated television program. Several newspapers had named LaMar's doughnuts as tops in their market area.

UNEXPECTED DEVELOPMENTS AT KRISPY KREME IN 2004

In March 2004, KKD management announced that it expected the company to have diluted earnings per share of $1.16 to $1.18 for fiscal 2005 (up from $0.92 in fiscal 2004) and systemwide comparable store sales growth in the mid-to-high single digits. Executives estimated that systemwide sales would increase approximately 25 percent in fiscal 2005 (ending January 29, 2005) and that approximately 120 new stores would be opened systemwide, including 20 to 25 smaller doughnut-and-coffee-shop stores, during the next 12 months. But as 2004 progressed, Krispy Kreme's business prospects went from rosy to stark within a matter of months.

Developments at Krispy Kreme in May 2004

In a May 7, 2004, press release that caught investors by surprise, CEO Scott Livengood said:

> For several months, there has been increasing consumer interest in low-carbohydrate diets, which has adversely impacted several flour-based food categories, including bread, cereal and pasta. This trend had little discernable effect on our business last year. However, recent market data suggests consumer interest in reduced carbohydrate consumption has heightened significantly following the beginning of the year and has accelerated in the last two to three months. This phenomenon has affected us most heavily in our off-premises sales channels, in particular sales of packaged doughnuts to grocery store customers.

Sales at Krispy Kreme's franchised stores were approximately evenly split between on-premises and off-premises sales, while approximately 60 percent of company-owned store sales were off-premises. As a consequence of the falloff in sales at external outlets, sales at Krispy Kreme stores open at least 18 months grew by only 4 percent, well below the 9 percent realized in preceding quarter. Due to the lower than expected off-premises sales at company stores, Livengood said the company was lowering its earnings guidance for the first quarter of fiscal 2005 to about $0.23 per share, down from about $0.26 per share. The company went on to announce in the same press release that it was:

- Divesting its recently acquired Montana Mills operation. The plan was to close the majority of the Montana Mills store locations, which were underperforming, and pursue a sale of the remaining Montana Mills stores. Management indicated the Montana Mills divesture would entail write-offs of approximately $35–$40 million in the first quarter on its Montana Mills investment and would likely involve further write-offs of $2–$4 million in subsequent quarters.

- Closing six underperforming factory stores—four in older retail locations in below-average retail trade areas and two commissaries.

- Lowering its guidance for fiscal 2005 diluted earnings per share from continuing operations, excluding asset impairment and other charges described below, to between $1.04 and $1.06, approximately 10 percent lower than prior forecasts. Including the Montana Mills charges, diluted earnings per share from continuing operations were estimated to be between $0.93 and $0.95 for fiscal 2005.

In the hours following the announcement, the company's stock price was hammered in trading—dropping by about 20 percent.

On May 25, 2004, Krispy Kreme reported a $24.4 million loss for the first quarter of fiscal 2005, blaming (1) trendy low-carb diets such as Atkins and South Beach for a decline in its sales in grocery stores and (2) a $34 million write-off of its investment in Montana Mills. The stock price was down 37 percent since the May 7 lower earnings announcement and was trading at about $20.

At the company's annual stockholders' meeting on May 26, 2004, executives said the company was slowing down expansion plans and had plans to counter consumer interest in low-carbohydrate foods by adding a sugar-free doughnut to its product lineup. Management also announced that the company would soon (1) introduce a chocolate-flavored glazed doughnut, mini rings that were 40 percent smaller, and crushed-ice drinks in raspberry, latte, and double chocolate flavors and (2) begin selling bags of the company's own brand of coffee in whole-bean and ground form in grocery stores alongside Krispy Kreme doughnut displays. The company said it planned to go forward with overseas expansion. The overseas expansion was concentrated in Asia; 25 new stores were being planned for South Korea and on the horizon were stores in Japan, China, Indonesia, the Philippines, and the Persian Gulf.

Developments at Krispy Kreme in July–August 2004

In late July 2004, the company announced that the Securities and Exchange Commission was launching an inquiry into the company's accounting practices regarding certain franchise buybacks. A *Wall Street Journal* article in May had detailed questionable accounting in the $32.1 million repurchase of a struggling seven-unit franchise in Michigan that was behind on its payments for equipment, ingredients, and franchise fees, along with questionable accounting for another reacquired franchise in southern California.

In late August 2004, Krispy Kreme reported its second-quarter fiscal 2005 results:

- Systemwide sales increases of 14.8 percent as compared with the prior year's second quarter.

- An 11.5 percent increase in company revenue to $177.4 million (versus $159.2 million in the second quarter of the prior year)—company store sales increased by 18.7 percent to $123.8 million, revenues from franchise operations grew by 13.7 percent to $6.8 million, and KKM&D revenues decreased by 4.1 percent to $46.9 million (principally because of lower equipment sales to franchisees opening new stores).

- Very small comparable store sales increases—sales at company-owned stores increased by 0.6 percent and systemwide sales (at both company-owned and franchised stores) increased by only 0.1 percent.

- A decline in operating income from continuing operations for the second quarter of fiscal 2005 to $6.2 million, or $0.10 per diluted share, versus $13.4 million, or $0.22 per diluted share, in the second quarter of fiscal 2004.

- The opening of 22 new Krispy Kreme factory/retail stores in 12 new markets, and 10 doughnut-and-coffee-shop stores. Six company-owned factory/retail stores and three doughnut-and-coffee shops were closed during the quarter.

Commenting on the Krispy Kreme's second-quarter performance, Scott Livengood, said:

Although we are disappointed with the second-quarter financial results, we are optimistic about the long-term growth potential of the business. We are focusing our efforts and resources on initiatives that improve long-term business prospects. We have core strategies with supporting initiatives, a leading consumer brand and great people to address the current challenges. Krispy Kreme has proven over its 67-year history an ability to overcome challenges, and I am confident in our ability to restore our business momentum.[9]

Top management indicated that systemwide sales should grow by approximately 15 percent for fiscal 2005 and approximately 10 percent in the last two quarters of the year but declined to provide updated earnings estimates. The company said it had scaled back expansion plans and would only open approximately 75 new stores systemwide (60 factory/retail stores and 15 doughnut-and-coffee shops) during fiscal 2005.

Developments at Krispy Kreme in November–December 2004

In November 2004, Krispy Kreme reported that the company lost $3 million in the third quarter of fiscal 2005. Total revenues for the quarter, which included sales from company stores, franchise operations, and KKM&D, were up by only 1.4 percent to $170.1 million (versus $167.8 million in the third quarter of fiscal 2004). Third-quarter systemwide sales at both company-owned and franchised stores were up by 4.7 percent over the third quarter of fiscal 2004. The sales increases were well below the 10 percent gains that management had forecast in August.

During the quarter, 13 company-owned factory/retail stores and two doughnut-and-coffee shop stores were opened, and 7 company-owned factory/retail stores and two doughnut-and-coffee shop stores were closed. There were 429 Krispy Kreme stores systemwide at the end of October 2004, consisting of 393 factory/retail stores and 36 doughnut-and-coffee shops. There were plans to open approximately 10 new stores systemwide in the fourth quarter of fiscal 2005.

Exhibit 10 shows the declining performance of Krispy Kreme's stores during the first three quarters of fiscal 2005. Exhibits 11 and 12 show selected financial statistics for Krispy Kreme Doughnuts during the first nine months of fiscal 2005 compared to the first nine months of fiscal 2004.

Management declined to provide systemwide sales and earnings guidance for the fourth quarter of fiscal 2005 and withdrew its previous estimates of 10 percent systemwide sales growth made in August. Commenting on the company's performance, Scott Livengood said, "Clearly we are disappointed with our third-quarter results. We are focused on addressing the challenges facing the Company and regaining our business momentum." Early in the fourth fiscal quarter, Krispy Kreme sold its remaining Montana Mills assets for what management described as "a modest amount."

In December 2004, Krispy Kreme announced that it had identified accounting errors related to its acquisition of two franchises that could reduce net income for fiscal 2004 by 2.7 percent to 8.6 percent. It was, as yet, unclear whether it would have to restate its results for fiscal year 2004. A special committee of the company's board of directors was investigating the accounting problems. The company's outside auditor, PricewaterhouseCoopers LLP, said it refused to complete reviews of Krispy Kreme's financial performance for the first six months of 2005 until the special committee completed its probe of the bookkeeping problems. In late December 2004, Krispy Kreme's stock

Exhibit 10   Quarterly Operating Performance of Krispy Kreme Stores, Fiscal Years 2004–2005

	Fiscal Year 2004				Fiscal Year 2005		
	Q1	Q2	Q3	Q4	Q1	Q2	Q3
Average sales per week							
Company stores	$77.4	$74.4	$73.0	$69.1	$67.9	$63.1	$58.4
Area developer stores	58.0	61.2	60.3	58.7	59.2	54.3	49.9
Associate stores	52.4	48.7	45.9	42.6	46.7	43.9	41.7
Franchised store average	56.2	57.3	56.3	54.3	56.0	51.6	47.9
Systemwide average	64.1	63.7	62.7	60.1	60.7	56.3	52.2
Change in comparable store sales							
Company stores	15.4%	15.6%	13.3%	10.7%	5.2%	0.6%	−6.2%
Systemwide	11.2	11.3	9.5	9.1	4.0	0.1	−6.4
Increase in systemwide sales	24.4%	27.6%	28.6%	25.5%	24.2%	14.8%	4.7%

Source: Company press releases of quarterly earnings results.

Exhibit 11   **Financial Statement Data for Krispy Kreme Doughnuts, First Nine Months of Fiscal 2004 Versus First Nine Months of Fiscal 2005 (dollar amounts in thousands, except per share)**

	Nine Months Ending November 2, 2003	Nine Months Ending October 31, 2004
Statement of operations data		
Total revenues	$475,598	$531,941
Operating expenses	359,820	430,613
General and administrative expenses	27,362	34,928
Depreciation and amortization expenses	13,473	19,496
Arbitration award	(525)	—
Impairment charge and store closing costs	—	14,865
Income from operations	$ 75,468	$ 32,039
Interest expense, (income), net, and other expenses and adjustments	6,410	5,424
Income (loss) from continuing operations before income taxes	69,058	26,615
Provision for income taxes	27,488	11,543
Income from continuing operations	41,570	15,072
Discontinued operations	(907)	(36,741)
Net income (loss)	$ 40,663	$ (21,669)
Diluted earnings (loss) per share		
Income (loss) from continuing operations	$ 0.67	$0.24
Discontinued operations	(0.01)	(0.58)
Net income (loss) per share	0.66	(0.34)
Diluted shares outstanding (in 000s)	61,975	63,441
Balance sheet data		
Cash and cash equivalents	$ 39,287	$ 17,213
Receivables	62,454	73,416
Inventories	29,717	32,287
Payables and accrued expenses	52,101	67,820
Long-term debt and other long-term obligations, including current maturities	149,142	170,509
Total assets	629,431	675,897
Total shareholders' equity	$428,188	$437,568

Source: Company press releases, November 21, 2003, and November 22, 2004.

was trading in the $10–$13 range, well below the $40 high attained in March 2004.

KRISPY KREME IN 2005

In mid-January 2005, Krispy Kreme's board of directors took steps indicating that the company's deteriorating sales and financial problems were worse than expected. The company's board of directors forced Scott Livengood to retire. The board hired two outsiders with noted expertise in turning around troubled companies; Stephen Cooper was named CEO, and Steven Panagos was named president and chief operating officer. Both executives came to KKD from Kroll Zolfo Cooper (KZC), a company best known for presiding over the remains of Enron and rejuvenating Sunbeam and Polaroid; Cooper was chairman of KZC, and Panagos was a managing director. The two new executives were assisted by a team of professionals from KZC. Along with the management changes, Krispy Kreme also announced that average

Exhibit 12 **Krispy Kreme's Performance by Business Segment, First Nine Months of Fiscal 2004 Versus First Nine Months of Fiscal 2005 (in thousands)**

	Nine Months Ending November 2, 2003	Nine Months Ending October 31, 2004
Revenues by business segment		
Company store operations	$317,158	$369,593
Franchise operations	17,555	20,060
KK manufacturing & distribution	140,885	142,288
Total	$475,598*	$531,941
Operating income by business segment (before depreciation and amortization)		
Company store operations	$ 61,969	$ 41,797
Franchise operations	13,721	14,694
KK manufacturing & distribution	27,824	26,706
Total	$103,514*	$ 83,197
Unallocated general and administrative expenses	$ (28,571)	$ (36,293)

*Totals do not include operations of Montana Mills, a business which was acquired in April 2004 and divested during fiscal 2005; nine month revenues for Montana Mills were $4,481,000 and the operating loss at Montana Mills was $1,408,000.
Source: Company press releases, November 21, 2003, and November 22, 2004.

weekly sales per factory store were down 18 percent systemwide and down 25 percent at company stores for the eight weeks ended December 26, 2004 (compared to the corresponding weeks of 2003).

In early 2005, Krispy Kreme announced workforce reductions of about 25 percent; it was estimated that the reduced employment levels would result in annual pretax savings of about $7.4 million The company also divested its corporate airplane, realizing annual pretax savings of $3 million. In an unrelated development, employees of Krispy Kreme filed a class action lawsuit accusing Krispy Kreme of not sharing information that resulted in losses in employees' retirement accounts. The lawsuit, if won by the employees, asked that the money lost on the investments be repaid personally by four of the board members, including former CEO Scott Livengood, who allegedly withheld the needed information from the employees.

In April 2005, Krispy Kreme completed a deal that provided $225 million in new financing. The proceeds were used to repay $90 million in debt and to provide cash for operations. Management believed the move greatly strengthened the company's balance sheet and provided the cash needed to turn the company's operations around.

Also in April, Krispy Kreme asked the Securities and Exchange Commission for permission to delay submitting its 10-K report for 2005 since it was still analyzing the need to restate its financial results for fiscal years 2001, 2002, 2003, and the first nine months of 2005; the company had recently discovered further need to revise its fiscal 2004 financials by $5.2 to $6.2 million (apart from adjustments previously announced in December 2004) and determined that its financial statements for 2001 through the first nine months of fiscal 2005 should no longer be relied on. On a positive note, management said that it expected to report fiscal 2005 revenues of approximately $685 million (up about 4 percent over the $665.6 million reported in fiscal 2004). However, a big portion of the sales gains came from store sales of reacquired franchisees that were financially distressed, and management said that it expected to report a loss for the fourth quarter of fiscal 2005.

In June 2005, Krispy Kreme announced that its special committee of independent directors had concluded that six of the company's officers—including four senior vice presidents—should be discharged. The six executives were in the areas of operations, finance, business development, and manufacturing and distribution—five of the executives resigned and one retired. A new chief accounting officer, who had been a consultant with the company since December 2004 and had spent 17 years at Pricewaterhouse-Coopers, was appointed in July.

In August, Krispy Kreme and Kroll Zolfo Cooper agreed to the terms of the success fee under which KZC was providing management services. The success fee entitled KZC to purchase 1.2 million shares of Krispy Kreme's common stock at a cash exercise price of $7.75 per share. KZC monthly fees had averaged $800,000 per month since being hired in January.

The Report of the Special Committee of the Board of Directors

In August 2005, the Special Committee of Krispy Kreme's board of directors completed its studies and issued the following statement:

> The Krispy Kreme story is one of a newly-public company, experiencing rapid growth, that failed to meet its accounting and financial reporting obligations to its shareholders and the public. While some may see the accounting errors . . . as relatively small in magnitude, they were critical in a corporate culture driven by a narrowly focused goal of exceeding projected earnings by a penny each quarter.
>
> In our view, Scott A. Livengood, former Chairman of the Board and Chief Executive Officer, and John W. Tate, former Chief Operating Officer, bear primary responsibility for the failure to establish the management tone, environment and controls essential for meeting the Company's responsibilities as a public company. Krispy Kreme and its shareholders have paid dearly for those failures, as measured by the loss in market value of the Company's shares, a loss in confidence in the credibility and integrity of the Company's management and the considerable costs required to address those failures.
>
> The number, nature and timing of the accounting errors strongly suggest that they resulted from an intent to manage earnings. All those we interviewed have repeatedly and firmly denied having any intent to manage earnings or having given or received any instruction (explicit or otherwise) to do so. But we never received credible explanations for transactions that appear to have been structured or timed to allow for the improper recognition of revenue or improper reduction of expense . . .
>
> All officers or employees who we believe had any substantial involvement in or responsibility for the accounting errors have left the Company . . .
>
> Also . . . the Special Committee has concluded that it is in the best interests of the Company (i) to reject the demands by shareholders that the Company commence litigation against present and former directors and officers of the Company and the sellers of certain franchises to the Company, (ii) to seek dismissal of shareholder derivative litigation against the outside directors, the sellers of certain franchises and current and former officers other than Scott Livengood, John Tate and Randy S. Casstevens, the Company's former Chief Financial Officer, and (iii) not to seek dismissal of shareholder derivative litigation against Messrs. Livengood, Tate and Casstevens, although the Company will not assist or participate in such litigation.[10]

At the same time, top management announced that its investigation of the company's internal controls over financial reporting under Livengood, Tate, and Casstevens revealed four material weaknesses:

- The Company failed to maintain an effective control environment, including failure of former senior management to set the appropriate tone at the top of the organization and to ensure adequate controls were designed and operating effectively.

- The Company failed to maintain a sufficient complement of personnel with a level of accounting knowledge, experience and training in the application of generally accepted accounting principles [GAAP] commensurate with the Company's financial reporting requirements and the complexity of the Company's operations and transactions.

- The Company failed to maintain effective controls over the documentation and analysis of acquisitions to ensure they were accounted for in accordance with GAAP.

- The Company failed to maintain effective controls over the selection and application of accounting policies related to leases and leasehold improvements to ensure they were accounted for in accordance with GAAP.

It was as yet unclear whether the company's outside auditors, PricewaterhouseCoopers, shared any responsibility for the numerous accounting and financial reporting deficiencies discovered at Krispy Kreme during the 2001–2005 period.

Financial Statement Adjustments

In August 2005, Krispy Kreme announced that it expected to make adjustments to its prior financial statements for fiscal years 2001–2005 that would have the effect of decreasing pretax income through the third quarter of fiscal 2005 by an estimated $25.6 million. In December 2005, these adjustments were increased to an estimated $35.1 million. The latest adjustments called for decreases in pretax income of $1.6 million, $3.7 million, $4.0 million, $16.5 million, and $5.4 million for fiscal 2001, 2002, 2003, and 2004 and the first nine months of fiscal 2005, respectively, plus decreases of $3.9 million for periods prior to fiscal 2001. However, the estimates were subject to further revision and the results of the audit of the company's annual financial statements. Management said that the results of operations for both fiscal 2005 and 2006 would be adversely affected by adjustments to recognize the financial difficulties faced by certain franchisees.

In mid-December 2005, the company indicated that it would be unable to provide restated financial statements much before a recently extended deadline of April 2006.

The Latest Available Operating Results

Despite not issuing financial statements, Krispy Kreme indicated that the company lost money in the fourth quarter of fiscal 2005 and the first three quarters of fiscal 2006 (through October 31, 2005). Average weekly sales at company-owned and franchised stores, however, appeared to have stabilized at around $45,000 to $50,000 weekly (see Exhibit 13).

The company expected to report revenues of approximately $130 million for the third quarter of fiscal 2006 (which ended October 30, 2005), compared to revenues of approximately $170 million previously reported for the third quarter of fiscal 2005.

Stephen Cooper, the company's CEO, believed the company's prospects for a turnaround were good:

> While a number of challenges remain, I am pleased to report that we continue to make progress with the Company's turnaround. We have closed approximately 30 underperforming Company stores, significantly reduced overhead costs, made progress in strengthening the senior management team and are taking steps to deal with certain troubled franchisees.
>
> Our plan is simple. We are focusing on excellence in Company and franchise operations and on what makes Krispy Kreme a great brand: delivering the highest quality doughnuts and coffee and other beverages to our retail and wholesale customers. While the Company still faces serious challenges, we believe we are addressing the critical issues.[11]

Following the lead of Krispy Kreme's new management team to weed out unproductive stores, several franchisees had closed some of their worst-performing stores. And some factory stores had been converted into "satellite" stores that emphasized retail sales of doughnuts and coffee (satellite stores made few, if any, doughnuts for off-premises sales) Cooper believed that Krispy Kreme needed urban stores that were smaller on average and that focused on increasing sales of coffee and other beverages as well as doughnuts. Krispy Kreme had also restructured the

Exhibit 13   Selected Operating Results for Krispy Kreme, Fourth Quarter 2005 Through Third Quarter 2006

	Q4, FY 2005	Q1, FY 2006	Q2, FY 2006	Q3, FY 2006
Krispy Kreme's revenues	$153 million	n.a.	n.a.	$130 million
Decrease from prior year quarter	17.5%	n.a	n.a.	23.5%
Number of Krispy Kreme factory stores systemwide	400	400	400	360
Number of associate and/or satellite stores	n.a.	n.a.	50	50
Average weekly sales, systemwide	$48,000	$48,000	$46,000	$43,000
Decrease from prior year	20%	21%	18%	14%
Average weekly sales, company-owned stores	$50,000	$50,000	$49,000	$47,000
Decrease from prior year	27%	26%	20%	19%

n.a. = Not announced.

Source: Company press releases.

operations of its Canadian subsidiary, KremeKo, and was working with troubled franchisees—in some cases reacquiring their operations. In October 2005, Krispy Kreme's Philadelphia franchisee, Freedom Rings, filed for Chapter 11 bankruptcy. Krispy Kreme owned 70 percent of Freedom Rings and acquired the remaining 30 percent, prior to filing, for a nominal price; Freedom Rings owed Krispy Kreme approximately $24.1 million.[12] In November, the company announced the approval of restructuring of KremeKo. KremeKo and Krispy Kreme announced in November 2005 that KremeKo would become a wholly owned subsidiary. In December, Krispy Kreme completed the acquisition of KremeKo Inc., which had six factory stores in eastern and central Canada. KremeKo had been operating under Chapter 11 since April 2005.[13]

Going into 2006, there were 330 Krispy Kreme factory stores and 80 satellites operating systemwide in 44 U.S. states, Australia, Canada, Mexico, the Republic of South Korea, and the United Kingdom. The only new Krispy Kreme factory store in calendar year 2005 was opened in November in Missoula, Montana, by a franchisee that had 14 stores in Idaho, Nevada, Montana, and Utah.

In late 2005 Krispy Kreme named Jeff Jervik as executive vice president of operations, responsible for all company-owned operations, franchisee operations, and wholesale operations. Jervik had been national vice president of operations for Pizza Hut, with responsibility for the operations of over 1,000 Pizza Hut restaurants, having sales of approximately $800 million and over 25,000 employees. Krispy Kreme had hired an executive search firm with experience placing top executives in companies such as Starbucks, Sara Lee, Dean Foods, and Gillette, to assist in the search for a permanent chief executive officer. The company's board wanted to identify and retain a CEO as soon as possible. Krispy Kreme's stock traded in the $5–$9 range for most of 2005 and was trading around $6 in late December 2005.

Sometime in April 2006, Krispy Kreme expected to issue its first financial statements since November 2004 (at which time the financials for the third quarter of fiscal year 2005 were released).

Endnotes

[1] As quoted in "Dough-Down at the Mile High Corral," *Rocky Mountain News,* March 25, 2001, p. 1G.

[2] As quoted in "Hole-ly War: Omaha to Be Battleground for Duel of Titans," *Omaha World Herald,* September 7, 1999, p. 14.

[3] According to information in Hermione Malone, "Krispy Kreme to Offer Better Coffee as It Tackles New England," *Charlotte Observer,* March 16, 2001.

[4] "Time to Rate the Doughnuts: Krispy Kreme Readies to Roll into N.E. to Challenge Dunkin' Donuts," *Boston Globe,* February 21, 2001, p. D1.

[5] As quoted in Malone, "Krispy Kreme to Offer Better Coffee."

[6] As quoted in "Can Krispy Kreme Cut It in Canada?" *Ottawa Citizen,* December 30, 2000, p. H1.

[7] As quoted in ibid.

[8] As quoted in ibid.

[9] Company press release, August 26, 2004.

[10] Company press release, August 10, 2005.

[11] Company press releases, August 10, 2005, and December 13, 2005.

[12] Company press release, October 17, 2005.

[13] Company press release, November 14, 2005, and December 19, 2005.

Kodak at a Crossroads: The Transition from Film-Based to Digital Photography

Boris Morozov
University of Nebraska at Omaha

Rebecca J. Morris
University of Nebraska at Omaha

It's not clear with Kodak if they can successfully compete in the digital world. Are they a buggy whip manufacturer?[1]—**David Winters, chief investment officer, Franklin Mutual Advisers, Inc.**

It's a challenging strategy, there's no question about it. This is about our belief in where the company can go, and in our ability to bring growth back to the company in the next three or four years.[2]—**Daniel Carp, CEO, Eastman Kodak Company**

On September 25, 2003, Eastman Kodak Company's CEO, Daniel Carp, announced to investors that, after a three-year decline in sales, the company would stop making major investments in its consumer film business and devote its resources to becoming a "digital-oriented growth company." By the end of trading on the day of the announcement, Kodak's stock fell to an 18-year low. Institutional investors criticized Kodak's announced strategy, expressing annoyance at the company's intention to invest in ink-jet printing, a business dominated by Hewlett-Packard.[3] People at the company's meeting said that Carp did not provide enough detail on how the strategy would affect earnings before 2006.[4] Investment analyst Shannon Cross expressed the concerns of many investors, saying, "There are so many questions with regard to Kodak's future

strategy . . . The track record we've seen out of management in terms of being able to hit targets and implement a strategy has been pretty spotty."[5]

Since January 1, 2000, when Carp took over as chief executive of Kodak, the company's revenues and net income had declined, its shares had dropped by 66 percent, and Standard & Poor's (S&P) had cut Kodak's credit rating by five grades.[6] Kodak had reduced its workforce by 49 percent since 1989, cutting 7,300 employees in 2002.[7] Plans were announced to eliminate up to 6,000 jobs in 2003 to stem future losses, cutting Kodak's traditional photography divisions in Rochester, New York, to fewer workers than the firm had employed during the Great Depression.[8] Kodak's income statements for 1993 through 2003 are presented in Exhibit 1. The company's balance sheets for the 11-year period ending 2003 are presented in Exhibit 2.

Despite investing over $4 billion in digital research and related technologies since the early 1990s, Kodak was characterized as a firm struggling to find its footing in the world of digital photography. Analysts gave Kodak only two to three years to find its way or find itself fading into history. "The question is, can Kodak come up with the new products, the new insights that make sense out of digital?" asked a marketing professor from the Rochester Institute of Technology. "They have to be able to execute fast. They've got to differentiate themselves because they're going very heavily into a commodity market." [9]

Exhibit 1 **Eastman Kodak's Income Statement, 1993–2003 ($ in millions except per share data)**

	2003	2002	2001	2000	1999	1998	1997	1996	1995	1994	1993
Sales	$13,317	$12,835	$13,234	$13,994	$14,089	$13,406	$14,538	$15,968	$14,980	$13,557	$16,364
Cost of goods sold	8,130	7,391	7,749	7,105	6,731	6,372	6,986	7,423	7,046	6,442	6,952
Gross profit	5,187	5,444	5,485	6,889	7,358	7,034	7,552	8,545	7,934	7,115	9,412
SG&A expense	3,339	3,260	3,333	3,747	3,986	4,119	4,956	5,438	5,039	4,570	6,290
Operating income before depreciation	1,848	2,184	2,152	3,142	3,372	2,915	2,596	3,107	2,895	2,545	3,122
Depreciation and amortization	830	818	919	889	918	853	828	903	916	883	1,111
Operating profit	1,018	1,366	1,233	2,253	2,454	2,062	1,768	2,204	1,979	1,662	2,011
Interest expense	148	173	219	178	142	110	131	112	108	177	635
Nonoperating income (expense)	(23)	(66)	(29)	96	141	210	57	209	109	(143)	18
Special Items	(651)	(164)	(888)	(39)	(344)	(56)	(1,641)	(745)	(54)	(340)	(538)
Pretax income	196	963	97	2,132	2,109	2,106	53	1,556	1,926	1,002	856
Total income taxes	(66)	153	32	725	717	716	48	545	674	448	381
Minority interest	24	17	(11)	—	—	—	—	—	—	—	—
Income before extraordinary items	238	793	76	1,407	1,392	1,390	5	1,011	1,252	554	475
Extraordinary items	0	0	0	0	0	0	0	0	0	(266)	(2,182)
Discontinued operations	27	(23)	0	0	0	0	0	277	0	269	192
Adjusted net income	$ 265	$ 770	$ 76	$ 1,407	$ 1,392	$ 1,390	$ 5	$ 1,288	$ 1,252	$ 557	($1,515)
EPS excluding extraordinary items and discontinued operations	$0.83	$2.72	$0.26	$4.62	$4.38	$4.30	$0.01	$3.00	$3.67	$1.65	$1.44
EPS including extraordinary items and discontinued operations	0.92	2.64	0.26	4.62	4.38	4.30	0.01	3.82	3.67	1.66	(4.62)
EPS diluted; excluding extraordinary items and discontinued operations	0.83	2.72	0.26	4.59	4.33	4.24	0.01	3.00	3.58	1.63	1.44
EPS diluted; including extraordinary items and discontinued operations	0.92	2.64	0.26	4.59	4.33	4.24	0.01	3.82	3.58	1.63	(4.62)
EPS basic from operations	2.37	2.77	2.37	4.73	5.09	4.42	3.52	4.50	3.77	2.40	2.60
EPS diluted from operations	2.37	2.77	2.37	4.70	5.03	4.37	3.46	n.a.	n.a.	n.a.	n.a.
Dividends per share	$1.15	$1.80	$1.77	$1.76	$1.76	$1.76	$1.76	$1.60	$1.60	$1.60	$2.00
Common shares for basic EPS (in millions)	286.5	291.5	290.6	304.9	318.0	323.3	327.4	337.4	341.5	335.7	328.3
Common shares for diluted EPS (in millions)	286.6	291.7	291.0	306.6	321.5	327.8	331.9	n.a.	n.a.	n.a.	n.a.

Source: Eastman Kodak 2003 annual report.

Exhibit 2   Eastman Kodak's Balance Sheet, 1993–2003 ($ in millions)

	2003	2002	2001	2000	1999	1998	1997	1996	1995	1994	1993
Assets											
Cash and equivalents	$ 1,261	$ 578	$ 451	$ 251	$ 393	$ 500	$ 752	$ 1,796	$ 1,811	$ 2,068	$ 1,966
Net receivables	2,389	2,234	2,337	2,653	2,537	2,527	2,271	2,738	3,145	3,064	3,463
Inventories	1,075	1,062	1,137	1,718	1,519	1,424	1,252	1,575	1,660	1,480	1,913
Other current assets	730	660	758	869	995	1,148	1,200	856	693	1,071	679
Total current assets	5,455	4,534	4,683	5,491	5,444	5,599	5,475	6,965	7,309	7,683	8,021
Gross property and equipment	13,277	13,288	12,982	12,963	13,289	13,482	12,824	12,585	12,652	12,299	13,311
Accumulated depreciation	8,183	7,868	7,323	7,044	7,342	7,568	7,315	7,163	7,275	7,007	6,945
Net property and equipment	5,094	5,420	5,659	5,919	5,947	5,914	5,509	5,422	5,377	5,292	6,366
Investments at equity	426	382	360	0	2	3	25	31	74	@CF	@CF
Other investments	310	53	85	—	—					338	187
Intang'bles	1,678	981	948	947	982	1,232	548	581	536	616	4,312
Deferred charges	1,147	972	482	0	0	0	0	0	0	0	0
Other assets	708	1,027	1,145	1,855	1,995	1,985	1,588	1,439	1,181	1,039	1,439
Total assets	$14,818	$13,369	$13,362	$14,212	$14,370	$14,733	$13,145	$14,438	$14,477	$14,968	$20,325
Liabilities and shareholder equity											
Long-term debt due in one year	$ 457	$ 387	$ 156	$ 150	$ 2	$ 78	$ 3	$ 245	$ 0	$ 0	$ 350
Notes payab'e	489	1,055	1,378	2,056	1,161	1,440	608	296	586	371	305
Accounts payable	834	720	674	817	940	947	943	966	799	703	737
Taxes payable	654	584	544	572	612	593	567	603	567	1,701	420
Accrued expenses	1,696	1,739	1,635	1,358	1,460	1,289	1,080	1,160	731	616	609
Other current liabilities	1,177	892	967	1,262	1,594	1,831	1,976	2,147	1,960	2,344	2,489
Total current liabilities	5,307	5,377	5,354	6,215	5,769	6,178	5,177	5,417	4,643	5,735	4,910
Long-term debt	2,302	1,164	1,666	1,166	936	504	585	559	665	660	6,853
Deferred taxes	81	52	81	61	59	69	64	102	97	95	79
Minority interest	45	70	84	93	98	128	24				
Other liabilities	3,819	3,929	3,283	3,249	3,596	3,866	4,134	3,626	3,951	4,461	5,127
Total liabilities	$11,554	$10,592	$10,458	$10,784	$10,458	$10,745	$ 9,984	$ 9,704	$ 9,356	$10,951	$16,969
Common stock, at per value	$ 978	$ 978	$ 978	$ 978	$ 978	$ 978	$ 978	$ 978	$ 974	$ 966	$ 948
Additional paid in capital	842	849	849	871	889	902	914	910	803	515	213
Retained earnings	7,296	6,840	6,834	7,387	6,850	6,052	5,141	6,006	5,277	4,493	4,234
Less: treasury stock	(5,852)	(5,890)	(5,767)	(5,808)	(4,805)	(3,944)	(3,872)	(3,160)	(1,933)	(1,957)	(2,039)
Total shareholders' equity	3,264	2,777	2,894	3,428	3,912	3,988	3,161	4,734	5,121	4,017	3,356
Total liabilities and equity	$14,818	$13,369	$13,362	$14,212	$14,370	$14,733	$13,145	$14,438	$14,477	$14,968	$20,325

Source: Eastman Kodak 2003 annual report.

The switch by consumers to digital photography was coming much faster than expected, and Kodak's traditional film, papers, and photofinishing businesses were declining. By the end of 2003, analysts expected that digital cameras would begin to outsell film cameras for the first time in the United States. The digital photography industry was fast-paced and crowded, offering razor-thin profit margins. Kodak was clearly at a crossroads. Would the strategy announced on September 25, 2003, position the company for growth, or would the company continue to decline?

KODAK'S CHALLENGES IN 2003

With the slogan "You press the button, we do the rest," George Eastman put the first simple camera into the hands of consumers in 1888. In so doing, he changed an awkward and intricate process into something easy to use and accessible to nearly everyone. Since that time, the Eastman Kodak Company had led the way with an abundance of new products and processes to make photography simpler, more useful, and more enjoyable. However, in 2003, Kodak's CEO, Daniel Carp, faced challenges similar to those George Eastman faced over a century before: How to make the process of printing the picture even easier in an era of digital technologies.

The economy was in a recession in 2003, major market indexes were still at a low level, and investors were cautious. As a result of an unfavorable economic situation, shareholder wealth had been cut to a portion of what it was during the phenomenal technology-based run-up of the market in the late 1990s. The bursting of the technology bubble proved that the absence of a strong profit-generating business model could not be replaced with information technology solutions.

Kodak's moves paralleled those at many companies whose comfortable business models were threatened by rapid changes in information technology. When asked whether Kodak had moved into digital photography soon enough, Carp replied, "I saw my first digital camera inside Kodak in 1982. Today, we're arguably one of the top three providers of digital cameras in the U.S. So we did the right thing. At the same time, we shouldn't have walked away from the

historical film businesses before they turned down, because it would have destroyed value."[10]

Under slumping economic and competitive market conditions, Kodak faced tough pressure from its existing competitors as well as from new rivals in the area of digital photography. Kodak coined the term *infoimaging* to describe the use of technology to combine images and information—a development that held the potential to profoundly change how people and businesses communicated.[11] Infoimaging was a $385 billion industry composed of devices (digital cameras and personal data assistants); infrastructure (online networks and delivery systems for images); services; and media (software, film, and paper) that enabled people to access, analyze, and print images.

Although the company had invested $4 billion in digital research and related technologies and spent many years perfecting its digital cameras,[12] Kodak's status as an iconic brand was threatened by the technological shift away from its cash-cow business of traditional film and film processing. In July 2003, Kodak reported flat sales and a 60 percent drop in second-quarter profits.

When announcing the latest rounds of workforce reductions in July 2003, Carp expressed his perspective on Kodak's challenges: "I think we're at the point where we have to get on with reality. The consumer traditional business is going to begin a slow decline, though it's not going to fall off a cliff." Was Kodak closer to the edge of the cliff than Carp thought? Could Kodak survive and thrive in the digital shift? Or would Kodak fade from history like a piece of film exposed to the light?

GROWTH IN DIGITAL PHOTOGRAPHY

Three years into the 21st century, the digital camera market was expanding at a fast pace. This was a major transfer from the previous decade of consumer photography as a largely mature market. Color film photography (also known as traditional photography) was a technology rich in history and closely tied to the art world. Eastman Kodak popularized color photography after the introduction of Kodachrome slide film in 1935.[13] Color print photography using 35-millimeter film grew rapidly in 1961 after the introduction of Kodacolor II print film.[14]

Exhibit 3   **Number of Households Owning Cameras, 1996–2003 (in millions)**

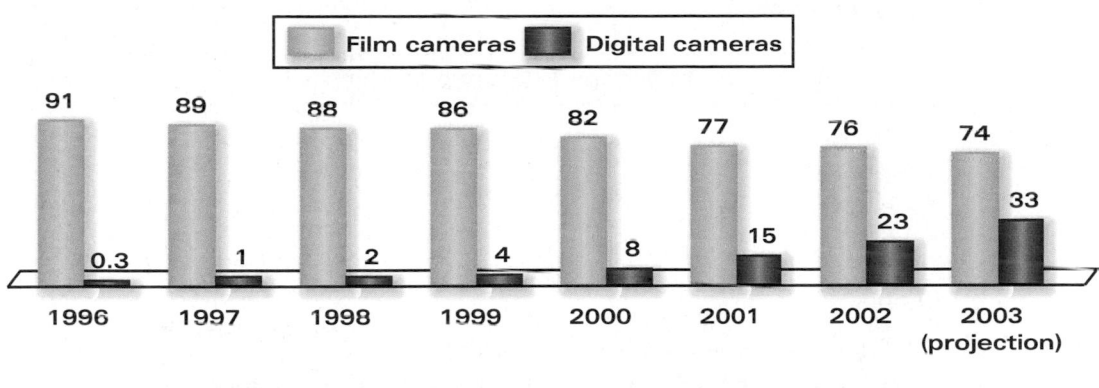

Number of U.S. households in March 2003 = 108.7 million

Source: PMA Marketing Research.

Demand for Digital Cameras

Digital photography was catching on fast in mainstream America as digital camera prices fell and image quality increased. The number of U.S. households owning a digital camera passed 1 million in 1997. By 2002, more than 23 million households owned digital cameras—this represented a 57 percent increase over 2001. Demand for digital cameras was expected to continue to increase, with more than 33 million households expected to own a digital camera in 2003. Exhibit 3 shows the growth in digital cameras and the decline in the number of households owning traditional film cameras. The 2.6 percent decline in traditional film cameras in 2002 was attributed in part to the growing demand for digital cameras and the rising popularity of one-time-use cameras. Market research projected continued further declines in traditional camera ownership.[15] Declines were also projected for sales of traditional film (down by 4 percent) and film processing (down by 3 percent) in 2003.

Although digital photography was making significant inroads with the mass market, technically sophisticated users were adopting digital technology at a higher rate. Among Internet-connected U.S. households, the estimate was that 60 percent had converted to digital cameras by the end of 2002.

Digital cameras generated a significant portion of industry revenues, accounting for $2.96 billion in revenues for 2002. This figure represented an increase of 22 percent over 2001 revenues. Revenues for traditional film, film processing, and traditional cameras had declined during this same period, as shown in Exhibit 4.

Industry experts predicted that the consumer shift to digital photography would be nearly complete by 2008, with sales of digital cameras nearly replacing sales of traditional film cameras such as 35-millimeter film cameras.[16] One-time-use cameras would continue to be popular, thus providing continued, although reduced, demand for film processing services.

What made digital cameras so attractive for consumers? Digital cameras gave users capabilities that were not possible with traditional cameras. Experts attributed the growth in digital photography to four factors—instant preview, sleek design, features, and price.[17] The technology of digital cameras allowed users to instantly view the shots they had taken and reshoot until they were satisfied with the results. The sleek design of many digital cameras made carrying one a fashion statement or a must-have item for teenagers and young professionals. Camera features also allowed digital users to capture short movies and to manipulate the images using photo-editing software that often came bundled with the camera. Price declines had made digital cameras much more affordable.

Michelle Slaughter, director of digital photography trends at InfoTrends Research Group, described digital cameras as an "essential communications device" for consumers.[18] "Consumers are becoming accustomed to the immediacy of digital photography

Exhibit 4   **Consumer Photographic Market Revenue, 2000–2002 (in billions of $)**

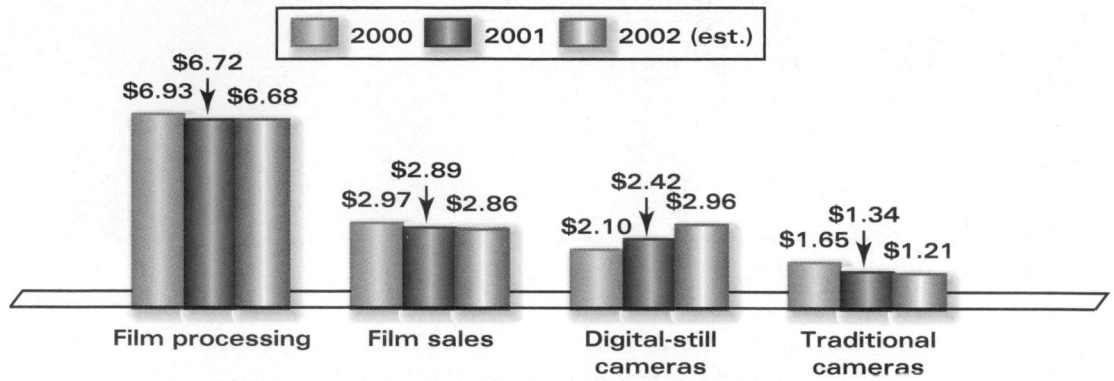

Source: PMA Marketing Research; www.pmai.org/pdf/0403_pixels_to_prints.pdf.

and are integrating digital photos into their daily communications with friends and family and for work. As a result, digital cameras have a higher intrinsic value to consumers than film cameras. This, in turn, paves the way for digital camera sales to exceed film camera sales," predicted Slaughter.

Although the price of digital cameras had declined sharply, the average price of a digital camera was still significantly more expensive than for 35-millimeter cameras. In 2002, the average price for a digital camera was $328.[19] When compared with an average price of $137 for a 35-millimeter camera, it was no surprise that more than half of digital camera buyers were in households where the annual income was $75,000 or more. Half of the digital camera buyers in 2002 were between the ages of 35 and 54. Buyers in this age group and income bracket were in the prime segment for capturing family photos and often traveled more frequently than those in other age groups and income brackets. Age and income statistics for digital camera buyers in 2002 are shown in Exhibit 5.

Although market research showed that men tended to purchase digital cameras more frequently than women (58 percent versus 42 percent), women tended to be the primary users of the equipment.[20] Women were described as the preservers of family memories and were increasingly using digital cameras to capture birthday parties, holiday celebrations, or family vacations. Women were becoming more likely to spur the decision to buy a digital camera for the household.[21] Women with children were described as the "most photo active consumers"[22]

and were expected to lead the demand for services such as digital printing.

Digital Printing Trends

Early adopters of digital photography consistently cited sending photos by e-mail as the number one reason for taking pictures with digital cameras.[23] Although mothers might e-mail friends and family the latest batch of baby photos, showing them off to a crowd gathered around a computer screen did not

Exhibit 5   **Percentage of Consumers Who Bought Digital Cameras in 2002**

By Age	
Age Group	Percent
18–24	9%
25–34	25
35–54	50
55 or older	17

By Income	
Household Income	Percent
Less than $25,000	6%
$25,000–$49,999	19
$50,000–$74,999	23
$75,000 or more	52

Source: American Demographics, July 1, 2003, p. 6.

Exhibit 6   **Destination of Digital Pictures after Capture**

| | Year | | |
Picture Destination	2000	2001	2002
Save, store, or keep	63%	68%	71%
E-mail	16	13	13
Print	12	14	20

Source: Photomarketing Association International, April 2003.

provide the same gratification and ease of use as looking at photos in an album. Consumers saw the ability to preview digital photos and to print only those they wanted as one of the strengths of the medium.

Few digital images were ever actually printed on paper. In 2000, only 12 percent of all digital images taken were printed. By 2002, this had increased to 20 percent of images taken.[24] Trends in the destination for digital images are shown in Exhibit 6.

The low ratio of printed photos to digital images was a big problem for companies wanting to profit from the printing process. According to analysts' estimations, companies such as Hewlett-Packard (HP), Lexmark, Canon, Seiko Epson, Olympus, and Eastman Kodak made almost nothing on the printers they sold. The money and profits were in the materials used to make prints. For instance, in summer 2003, HP saw profit margins of about 65 percent on ink-jet paper and ink, and roughly 30 percent margins on laser printing supplies.[25]

Consumers had a wide variety of options to choose from in obtaining prints from digital images. Digital photographers printed 2.1 billion images from digital cameras in 2003. Of these, 77 percent were printed with home printers, 6.4 percent were ordered from online photo services, 8.7 percent were made at a local retailer, and 3.6 percent were made using digital self-service kiosks. Consumers reported using "some other means" to produce 4.2 percent of all digital prints in 2003.[26]

Most consumers used their personal computers and home printers for printing their digital pictures; however, these were often perceived as lower-quality, more time-consuming, and more expensive than traditional film prints. More than half of digital camera users indicated they would print more digital images if they could make high-quality prints on their home printers.[27] Almost as many also indicated the printing

of digital images at home would need to be easier and less time-consuming. Consumers often got confused while transferring pictures from their digital cameras to their computers. "There are so many ways for people to get into trouble when they try to print photos at home," said Kristy Holch, a principal at InfoTrends Research Group.

Online photo services provided another option. Services such as Snapfish, Shutterfly, and Ofoto allowed consumers to upload their photos; preview, crop, and manipulate them; and obtain high-quality snapshots by mail. Pictures could further be shared online with friends and relatives via online albums. Custom calendars, cards, books, and mouse pads could be ordered with the customer's photos. Prints were priced significantly less than those printed at home at 19–29 cents per print versus the 62-cent cost of a print made on a Kodak Easyshare printer.[28] Disadvantages to online photo services included slow photo uploads (especially for consumers with dial-up Internet connections) and the four to six days it took to receive the prints by mail.

In September 2003, 18.4 million people visited online photography sites that could be used for sharing and printing, according to Nielsen//Net Ratings. Yahoo! Photos had 4.7 million unique visitors, followed by the Time Warner AOL unit, You've Got Pictures, with 2.7 million. Ofoto and Snapfish each had 1.67 million users, and Kodak's online site drew 1.5 million.

Local retailers such as Costco, Wal-Mart, and Walgreens provided another option for obtaining prints of digital images; however, these services failed to catch on with consumers. Many consumers did not realize that they could drop off their digital camera's memory card at the photo counter for printing. Others were reluctant to entrust the expensive memory cards to film processors. Retailers attempted to resolve these problems by adding self-service photo printing kiosks in their stores. Consumers could use the kiosks to edit photos and make their own prints from digital memory cards. Retailers launched advertising emphasizing ease of use and the immediacy of prints from the kiosks to overcome consumer's lack of awareness of this option. Expectations for growth in print volume at self-service kiosks were strong. "As digital camera users begin to use photo kiosks, print volumes on photo kiosks will increase dramatically," reported Kerry Flatley, a research analyst.[29] "Digital camera customers . . . will use photo kiosks as a high-volume source for their original photo prints," Flatley stated.

Impact on Demand for Traditional Film

The widespread adoption of digital photography had taken a toll on demand for traditional film and film processing. The volume of prints made from traditional films in 2002 declined by 700,000 over 2001 volumes. During the same time, digital prints grew by 1.3 million units. Digital images accounted for 6.1 percent of the total volume of prints made in 2002, up from only 2.4 percent in 2001.[30] Film sales were expected to decline by 4 percent in 2003, as shown in Exhibit 7.

One-time-use cameras were popular with consumers due to their convenience and low price, although the growth had slowed from 25 percent in 1999 to 8 percent in 2003. Film processing, which included both film rolls and one-time-use cameras, had declined significantly over the period from 1999 to 2003 due to the decrease in the use of traditional film among digital camera owners and the economic slowdown.

Other Digital Imaging Options

Another interesting market situation was developing—photo-capable cell phones. According to a survey done by experts in September 2003, more cell phones with integrated digital cameras than other types of digital cameras were sold in the first half of the year.[31] The research group Strategy Analytics stated that 25 million camera phones were purchased by consumers worldwide in the first half of 2003, compared with only 20 million digital still cameras.

"This is a milestone event, but it is just the first step towards the industry goal of getting a camera phone in every pocket," said Neil Mawston, senior analyst at Strategy Analytics' Global Wireless Practice. Mobile operators wanted to get customers to send picture messages regularly over their recently enhanced networks, in hopes of replicating the surprise success of text messaging. As the market for voice calls was becoming more competitive, non-voice data revenues could prove vital for operators' profitability.

However, security and privacy concerns among companies represented one potential problem for the camera phone market. Besides, Strategy Analytics said, camera phones represented no major threat to the digital still camera market because the difference in picture quality between the two technologies was too great. A Canon marketing director expressed the view of most camera manufacturers when it called even the two-megapixel camera phone just a "distraction." "It's good to have mobile phone cameras," the marketing director said, "but their functionalities are limited in terms of storage, picture quality, zooming

Exhibit 7   **Annual Change in Unit Sales of Film Rolls, One-Time-Use Cameras, and Film Processing, 1999–2003**

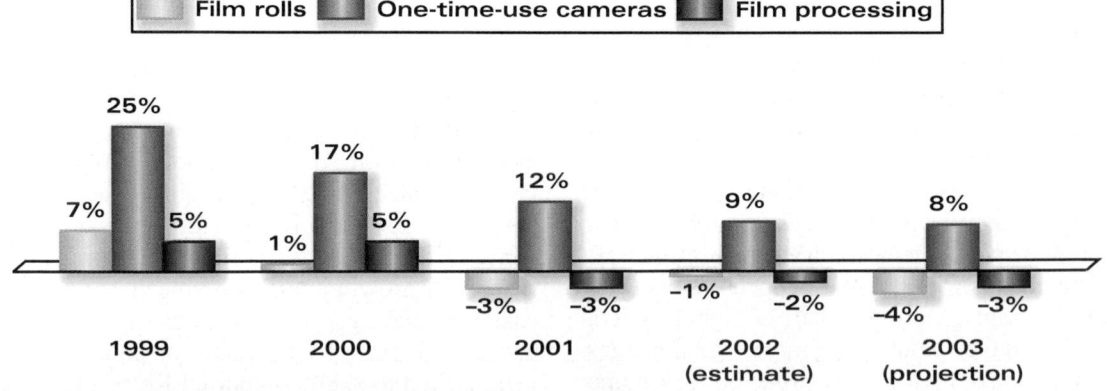

Note: Film processing includes both film rolls and one-time-use cameras.
Source: PMA Monthly Processing Surveys.

functionality, and power supply. Consumers will still go for the 'real camera' even though they have camera phones. Cameras on phones are just add-ons to give phones more functionalities."[32]

The Economist reported that camera phones might create a "nightmare scenario" for the traditional photography industry by hastening the decline of printed photos.[33] As camera phones improved, consumers might view on-screen images on phones, PCs, televisions, or even by beaming photos to a wireless-enabled picture frame. If this came to pass, "printing could become a niche, like film is expected to," said Chris Chute of the telecommunications consulting firm IDC.[34] Increased popularity of on-screen photo viewing would prove damaging for the photography industry, which depended on revenues from film processing and printing. Digital photography was threatening the first source of revenue. If camera phones caught on, cell phone operators could capture the second source, earning revenues by charging users for transmitting images.

GLOBAL TRENDS IN PHOTOGRAPHY

Income distribution among countries influenced the sales of the cameras around the world. While sales of digital cameras were booming in developed countries like the United States and Japan, consumers from emerging economies such as China bought more traditional cameras.

China was developing into a center of photography—and was doing so more rapidly than anyone would have expected only a few years ago. More than 5 million cameras were sold in China in 2002, and 400,000 of those were digital models (see Exhibit 8). This figure was set to increase, and Chinese consumers were expected to buy more than 3 million digital cameras by 2005. However, there were also other reasons why China was so important for the photographic and imaging sector, since every market segment was still growing in this country, not just the one for digital devices.

A large amount of additional sales potential remained unexploited in China. China's per capita consumption of film in 2003 was a mere 0.1 a year, compared to an average of 3.1 in Europe and 3.6 in the United States. China was still a long way from reaching market saturation even though film sales were rapidly increasing. Revenues from digital camcorders, photographic paper, data projectors, scanners, and printers were growing rapidly as well.

COMPETITIVE STANDINGS AND DIGITAL STRATEGIES

In the segment of traditional photography, Kodak's main brand competitors were Canon, Sony, and Fuji,

Exhibit 8   **Camera Sales in China, 2000–2002, with Projections for 2003–2005**

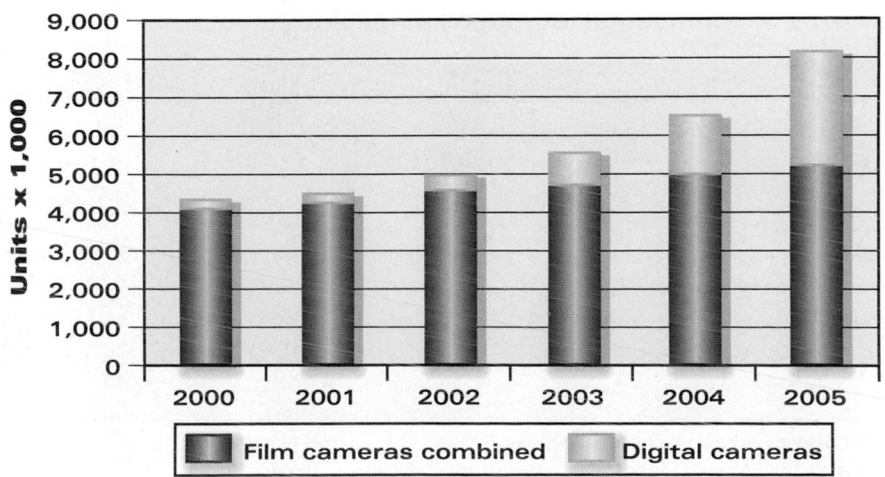

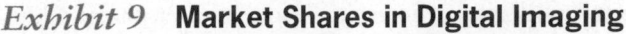

Exhibit 9 **Market Shares in Digital Imaging**

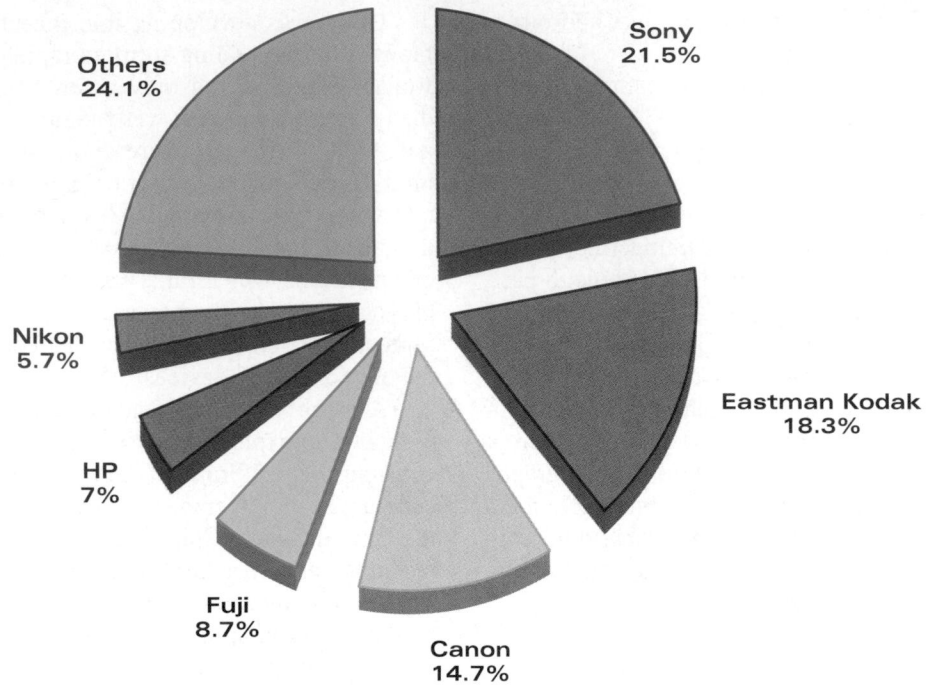

Source: "Digital Imaging's Winners and Losers," *Forbes,* August 9, 2004.

with Fuji being the biggest competitor. According to analysts' estimations, Kodak's competitors in the digital photography industry were Sony, HP, and Fuji.

Eastman Kodak captured 18.3 percent of the digital market, compared with the 15.3 percent share it had captured in the first six months of 2003. Sony led the market with a 21.5 percent share, with Canon, Fuji, HP, and Nikon following, with 14.7 percent,

8.7 percent, 7 percent, and 5.7 percent, respectively.[35] The market shares are shown in Exhibit 9.

Although Kodak was a major player in the photography market (both digital and traditional), it was far from being the biggest (see Exhibit 10). Eastman Kodak's earnings before interest, taxes, depreciation, and amortization (EBITDA) of $1.2 billion were just a fraction of its closest competitor

Exhibit 10 **Competitor Comparison for 2003**

	Kodak	Canon	Fuji	Sony
Market capitalization	$8.32 billion	$43.19 billion	$15.80 billion	$36.56 billion
Employees	70,000	98,873	72,569	161,100
Revenue growth	−3.00%	11.80%	0.4%	9.10%
Gross margin	32.17%	50.31%	41.64%	25.28%
EBITDA	$1.20 billion	$6.05 billion	$3.11 billion	$7.06 billion
Operating margins	2.79%	14.21%	6.20%	1.25%
Net income	$238 million	$2.62 billion	$532 million	$170 million
Earnings per share	$0.83	$2.948	$1.036	$0.09
Price/earnings ratio	35x	17x	30x	440x

Source: Company annual reports and Web sites.

Fuji's of $3.11 billion. Competitors Sony and Canon had EBITDA figures of $7.06 and $6.05 billion, respectively.

Sony

Sony had been on the digital wave since the mid-1990s, when it introduced its first PlayStation.[36] Nobuyuki Idei, chairman and CEO, played a key role in moving Sony into the digital network era by emphasizing the integration of audiovisual and information technology products. He was responsible for Sony's image campaign "Do you dream in Sony?" and helped coin the term "digital dream kids."[37]

Sony was a Japanese consumer electronics and multimedia giant. The firm produced music, movies, and television shows as well as the devices to bring them to the consumer. The electronics division produced video game consoles, personal digital assistants, DVD and MP3 players, digital camcorders, digital cameras, computers, and car audio products.

A team of developers gathered at a Sony laboratory in 1995 to "develop a digital still camera filled with enjoyment."[38] Sony's Cyber-Shot cameras were developed as the first "self-shooting" digital still cameras. Unburdened by a legacy in traditional film, developers relied on Sony's experience as a leading consumer technology company to develop a full line of digital cameras targeted to men and women between the ages of 25 and 55. Sony positioned its cameras at a premium or fair price based on cutting-edge technology and design. "You'll never see Sony offer a $99 camera," predicted one senior digital imaging analyst.[39] Sony's digital cameras ranged from about $180 for a point-and-shoot model to just under $1,000 for an advanced-featured Pro model.

Canon

Japan's Canon Inc. had come a long way since its days as a producer of cheap cameras. Much of Canon's success against its archrival had come on the watch of the company's president, Fujio Mitarai. A nephew of a Canon founder, Mitarai spent 23 years working in New York before returning to Japan in 1995 to head the company. Canon operated in the document reproduction markets producing copiers, fax machines, and scanners. Canon's optical segment produced diverse products such as television broadcast lenses and semiconductor manufacturing equipment. The camera division produced camcorders, binoculars, lenses, and digital cameras. Canon was relatively late to the market with its digital products, but the products it had introduced were hits.[40]

On November 21, 2001, Canon U.S.A. Inc., a subsidiary of Canon Inc., launched a marketing campaign featuring its PowerShot digital cameras and Bubble Jet printers working in concert to showcase Canon's leadership in digital photo solutions for the 2001 holiday season.[41] "The camera and printer are the stars of this 'production' number from beginning to end. Canon has a 60-year history in optics/lens technology for cameras, as well as creating its own printing technology—a combination our competitors cannot claim. By showcasing the 'digital duet' of our digital cameras and printers, we show the viewer that Canon products create picture perfect results that are unmatched by our competition," said Rick Booth, assistant director of advertising for the Canon Photographic Products Group.

Canon offered digital cameras for a wide variety of users at different price points. A simple point-and-shoot model was priced at slightly less than $200, while a professional-level digital single-lens reflex (SLR) camera sold for almost $8,000.

Fuji

Fuji, a longtime rival of Kodak, offered a complete portfolio of imaging, information, and document products, services, and e-solutions to retailers, consumers, professionals, and business customers. Fuji had been digital since 1998, when it introduced the first digital camera. "Fuji's solution was to start a suite of online options to share, order, pay for and collect digital photos," Dane Anderson of IDC, pointed out. By the summer of 2003, Fuji had developed a program for digital photography called Image Intelligence. This integrated system of digital image-processing software technologies came from the culmination of nearly 70 years of imaging expertise.

Fuji's traditional film, photo paper, developing chemicals, and nondigital printers accounted for 42 percent of the firm's 2003 sales. Experts expected the percentage of sales due to traditional photography to shrink to 31 percent by 2006.[42]

Fuji had introduced digital minilabs in the market. A minilab offered a service similar to that of traditional picture printing—consumers could print their digital photos by dropping off their digital memory cards and returning later to pick up finished prints. With more than 5,000 labs in the marketplace, Fuji had about 60 percent of the U.S. digital mini-lab market, including deals to put machines in 2,500 Wal-Mart and about 800 Walgreens outlets. Those two chains handled about 40 percent of the U.S. photo-processing market.

Hewlett-Packard (HP)

HP provided consumer and business customers with a full range of technology-based products, including personal computers, servers, storage devices, net-working equipment, and software. The company also included an information technology service organization that was among the world's largest. Known primarily by consumers for its dominance in com-puter printers, HP expanded into the digital imaging segment as a way to continue to fuel demand for HP printers and ink cartridges.

HP's breadth also provided an important advan-tage to consumers, according to HP vice president Chris Morgan. "We think consumers are going to want their products to be interoperable. Digital photography is a natural extension given our strength in computing and image processing," said Morgan. Consumers will "want to move content from camera to computer to email or DVD, from camcorder to computer to TV, or just skip the computer and go directly from device to playback system. That plays to our advantage. Not only are we the No. 1 consumer computer company in the world, we think that our understanding of big-business ecosystems will be a powerful advantage in helping us develop these solutions," he continued.[43]

Prices for HP's digital cameras ranged from about $100 to $400. As part of the firm's strategy to provide interoperable solutions that allowed consum-ers to connect various devices, HP offered several different camera and photo printer bundles and cam-era and docking station bundles.[44]

HP had a personal computer dubbed Photo Smart, which had a built-in docking slot for upload-ing photos only from HP's latest digital cameras and unified photo software that handled downloading, storing, exchanging, and printing photos.

HP was also trying to get more people to share digital pictures electronically because that got more

people making prints. HP's Instant Share software allowed consumers to preprogram e-mail addresses and photo-sharing Web sites into their cameras. After making pictures, users specified where they wanted the images sent, and the pictures were mailed the next time the camera was connected to the PC.

Nikon

Nikon was well known for its traditional photography products—35-millimeter cameras, lenses, and other consumer optical products. Nikon also produced equipment used in the manufacturing of semicon-ductors and a broad range of other optical products such as binoculars, microscopes, eyewear, and sur-veying equipment. Imaging products such as camera equipment comprised 57.6 percent of Nikon's net sales in 2003.[45]

Nikon targeted amateur photographers with its line of Coolpix cameras. These cameras ranged in price from about $140 to $850. The Coolpix line of-fered a full range of stylish and simple-to-use cam-eras designed to appeal to the first-time user and the more advanced photography hobbyist. Nikon also offered a line of digital single lens reflex (SLR) cam-eras that targeted advanced and professional pho-tographers who wanted multifeatured, easy-to-use digital cameras. Digital SLR cameras permitted the use of interchangeable lenses and were designed to provide sharper, clearer images at faster shutter speeds than other digital cameras. Nikon digital SLR cameras ranged in price from $900 (camera body only) to well over $1,200. Nikon used the trademarked phrase "Nikon . . . If the picture mat-ters, the camera matters" in the marketing of its cameras.[46]

KODAK'S PHOTOGRAPHY UNIT

Eastman Kodak was primarily engaged in develop-ing, manufacturing and marketing traditional and digital imaging products, services, and solutions for consumers, professionals, health care providers, and other commercial customers. The company oper-ated in four segments: components, health imaging (18 percent of company's total revenue), commercial imaging (11 percent of total sales), and photography (70 percent of revenue).

The photography segment included traditional and digital product offerings for consumers, professional photographers, and the entertainment industry. This segment combined traditional and digital photography and photographic services in all its forms—consumer, advanced amateur, and professional. Kodak manufactured and marketed various components of these systems, including films (consumer, professional, and motion picture); photographic papers; processing services; photofinishing equipment; photographic chemicals; and cameras (including one-time-use and digital).

Product and service offerings included kiosks and scanning systems to digitize and enhance images, digital media for storing images, and a network for transmitting images. In addition, other digitization options were available to stimulate more pictures in use, adding to the consumption of film and paper. These products served different groups of customers, including amateur photographers as well as professional, motion picture, and television customers. Technically, Eastman Kodak provided the services of picture creation to everyone who requested it, adjusting these services for specific groups of consumers.

Since Kodak's bread-and-butter unit was its photography unit, the company's stock price heavily depended on this unit's performance. The firm's stock price declined from more than $80 to $20 per share (see Exhibit 11) as revenues from traditional photography declined. In June 2003, Standard & Poor's (S&P) Rating Service placed Kodak on a CreditWatch, with negative implications, expressing concerns that economic, competitive, and leisure travel pressures would continue to impair Kodak's sales and earnings.[47] S&P analysts expressed concern that Kodak's transition to digital imaging would hurt future profitability for the firm by reducing high-margin film sales. Kodak's migration to digital technologies might also require additional restructuring as the firm adapted to evolving market conditions.

Kodak's restructuring actions prior to 2003 were primarily of a tactical nature. Three modifications between 1999 and 2003 indicated that the company's traditional film and photography businesses, while still hugely important as a source of cash, were becoming less of a central focus in a world where images were increasingly captured as bytes and bits. These modifications signaled management's attempt to keep up with the market, meaning that Eastman Kodak was losing the role of market maker.

Exhibit 11   **Eastman Kodak's Stock Price, January 1999–September 2003**

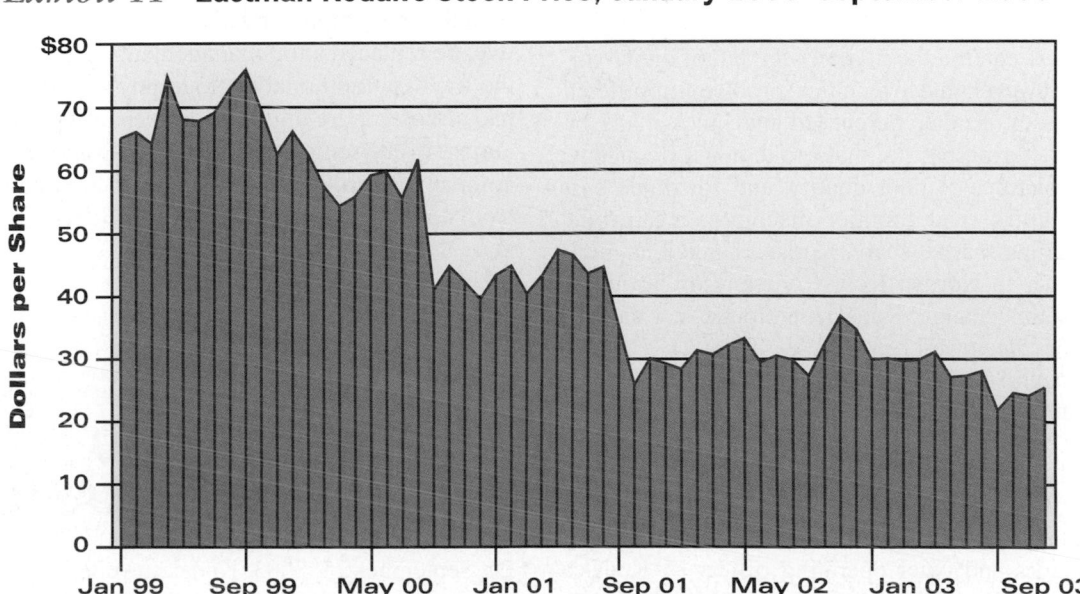

TOUGH CHOICES FOR A TRADITIONAL PHOTOGRAPHY COMPANY

Although it did not announce a change to a digital strategy until 2003, Eastman Kodak was moving toward this objective through acquisitions of smaller companies successful in the digital area. "Digital imaging is going to be like the cellular telephone business," George Fisher, Kodak's then CEO, predicted in 1997. "Highly competitive, very high growth, good profits for the leader, but not for the followers."[48]

In general, Kodak's performance in the new market conditions was varied. In some areas it was successful; in others it was not. Kodak's president and chief operating officer, Antonio Perez, had conceded that the company was behind the curve in printers, an area it regarded as key to its future digital profits. This was not for lack of effort. A joint attempt in 2000 to introduce a desktop photo inkjet printer with Lexmark flopped, partly because the product's direct-to-camera interface never caught on. Most consumers made their digital prints via PC-to-printer links. Kodak said its newly introduced system for docking a thermal printer with a PC, designed for greater ease of use, was faring much better, and would generate a respectable $100 million in sales in 2003, its first year.

Kodak entered the market segment of digital minilabs. However, due to technical problems, it suffered some losses. Kodak purchased machines made by a manufacturing partner that broke down frequently, printed pictures of poor quality, and frustrated customers. Fuji's rival Frontier machines, meanwhile, were gaining market share. Kodak changed its minilab partner to Noritsu Koki Company of Japan. As result of this change, Kodak mentioned that the machines had been well received.

Phogenix, a joint venture between HP and Kodak to develop smaller digital photo printers for retail outlets, crumbled in May 2003 because the technology had already become obsolete by the time the machines were brought to market. In a joint statement, Matthias Freund, chairman of the Phogenix board of directors and chief operating officer of Kodak's Consumer Imaging Products and Services business, and Mary Peery, member of the Phogenix board of directors and senior vice president of HP's Digital Imaging & Publishing business, said, "Both HP and Kodak believe the technology being developed by Phogenix continues to offer a viable solution for on-site digital photo processing. However, based on the anticipated return on invested capital for the parent companies, each company has separately decided to focus its own investments on other opportunities."[49]

The Phogenix labs, small enough to fit in stores typically unequipped to house typical automated film-developing machines, would have cost retailers about $40,000 but could produce only about 250 prints an hour, compared with more than 1,000 for Fuji's Noritsu minilab. Fuji's system cost $139,000 to $245,000, analysts estimated.

Kodak had had some notable digital successes. Kodak's popular EasyShare cameras were the second best-selling digital cameras in the United States in the first half of 2003, behind only those of Sony. After successfully focusing on the lower end of the camera market, Kodak was planning to begin selling more-expensive digital cameras aimed at tech-savvy shutterbugs. The company was diversifying its product line's depth and width, aiming at new segments of the market.

Finally, Kodak believed it had a strong management team. CEO Daniel Carp was considered to have good leadership skills. He was helped by other specialists, known for their extensive experience in the digital photography industry. Executive by executive, he replaced a top management cadre steeped in the ways of traditional photography with a team that had almost a pure digital pedigree. Except for Carp, almost every senior executive was from outside the company. Carp's management team was composed from new hires from Lexmark, HP, General Electric, and Olympus Optical.

SHIFT FROM TRADITIONAL PHOTOGRAPHY TO DIGITAL PHOTOGRAPHY

On September 25, 2003, Kodak unveiled its digitally oriented strategy. "We are acting with the knowledge that demand for traditional products is declining, especially in developed markets," Carp said. "Given this reality, we are moving fast—as digital markets demand—to transform our business portfolio, with an emphasis on digital commercial markets. The digital world is full of opportunity for Kodak, and we intend to lead it, as we have led innovation in the imaging industry for more than a century."[50]

Kodak was among the last photographic giants to announce its digital plans. The truly global scale of Kodak's operations represented an additional complexity for Kodak. While some parts of the world were outgrowing the shoes of traditional photography (e.g., developed countries like the United States, western European countries, and Japan), other parts of the world still exhibited growth opportunities for old film production.

Kodak recognized that, on the one hand, there were growth opportunities in areas that provided 30 percent profit margins (traditional film). These opportunities were in unstable emerging economies of countries like China, India, and the Russian Federation. On the other hand, opportunities in new digital photography looked better than those in traditional photography. The expected growth rate of the digital photography industry was about 26 percent until 2012. However, pursuing these opportunities would require substantial capital investment of up to $3 billion (according to stock analysts).

Daniel Carp's PowerPoint presentation for the September announcement showed that Kodak's new strategy would be based on three pillars—commercial imaging, health imaging, and consumer imaging.[51] Additional pillars under construction were ink-jet printers, commercial workflow management, and flat-panel displays.

The digital and film imaging strategy focused on four components:[52]

1. Manage the traditional film business for cash and manufacturing share leadership.
2. Lead in distributed output.
3. Grow the digital capture business.
4. Expand digital imaging services.

Under the first of these components, Kodak planned to reduce costs in its traditional film businesses and cut back on marketing expenditures for film (shifting instead to processing). The firm would continue to offer premium, high-margin products such as Perfect Touch processing and High Definition film in developing markets, while establishing leadership in emerging markets such as China and Russia.

Leading in distributed output referred to Kodak's plan to capture more of the demand for digital prints, whether produced in retail locations or at home. Kodak's plan called for the development of improved minilabs and kiosks that could print images faster, and for an increase of 50,000 kiosks by 2004. Kodak's home output strategy centered on the printer dock that allowed Kodak EasyShare users to transfer images directly from their cameras to a printer through a docking station. Users could then select and print images without a PC. Increasing use of Kodak's online photo service, Ofoto, was also a part of this strategy.

The digital capture business component referred to the further development of Kodak's digital cameras. Kodak intended to obtain a top-three worldwide market position for digital cameras by 2006. This goal would be reached by becoming the industry standard for ease of use and by moving to more sophisticated cameras.

Kodak planned to expand its digital imaging services by expanding the products and services offered through Ofoto to include items such as picture frames, calendars, and photo albums. Kodak also planned to develop kiosks that could print images from mobile phones. Rollout of this product had already begun in Asia and Europe and was expected to be ready for the U.S. market by the end of the fourth quarter of 2003.

On October 22, 2003, about 60 institutional shareholders met in New York City to examine other strategy alternatives, objecting to Carp's "risky" strategy of investing $3 billion into emerging digital markets.[53] Investors attending the meeting controlled about 25 percent of Kodak's stock. They felt that Kodak had been struggling with the transition to digital photography for almost 10 years and that, while it had enjoyed some success, the progress had not been enough, especially given the billions of dollars that had already been spent. Investors pushed for radical cost cuts to quickly boost earnings but had not yet come to an agreement about any long-term strategies for Kodak.

Carp argued that the cost-cutting plans touted by the investors "really aren't viable, practical options" and that Kodak had few alternatives other than slashing its dividends and pouring its resources into digital technologies.[54] Herbert A. Denton, president of Providence Capital, the host for the meeting, said, "We want them [Kodak] to let us under the tent and really show us why this strategy is best."[55] Was Carp's strategy best? Would Kodak's transition to a digital strategy be enough to help it reach its goal of becoming a $20 billion company by 2010?[56]

Endnotes

[1]C. Wolf, "Kodak Stock Plummets as Dividend Cut: Slashed by 72%," *Bloomberg News,* September 26, 2003, p. FP03.

[2]Ibid.

[3]C. H. Deutsch, "Some Positive News Aside, Kodak's Quarterly Profit Falls 63%," *New York Times,* October 23, 2003, p. C9.

[4]Wolf, "Kodak Stock Plummets."

[5]B. Dobbin, "Kodak Works Through Profit Drop," *Times Union,* October 23, 2003, p. E4.

[6]Wolf, "Kodak Stock Plummets."

[7]Ibid.

[8]Ibid.

[9]Dobbin, "Kodak Works Through Profit Drop."

[10]"What It 'Boils Down To' for Kodak," *BusinessWeek,* November 23, 2003.

[11]www.kodak.com.

[12]"Kodak Struggles to Find Its Focus," *Leader-Post,* July 28, 2003, p. B5.

[13]"Milestones—The Chronology," http://kodak.com/US/en/corp/kodakHistory/1930_1959.shtml (accessed December 6, 2004).

[14]A. Mutz, "Digital Photography Fundamentals and Trends," www.codesta.com/knowledge/technical/digital_photography/printable_version.aspx, March 26, 1993 (accessed December 6, 2004).

[15]Photo Marketing Association International, "The Path From Pixels to Print: The Challenge of Bringing Digital Imaging to the Mass Market," from www.pmai.org/pdf/0403_pixels_to_prints.pdf, April 2003 (accessed November 22, 2004).

[16]InfoTrends Research Group, "Digital Cameras Will Nearly Replace Film Cameras by 2008," press release, www.infotrends-rgi.com/home/Press/itPress/2003/6.25.03.html, June 25, 2003 (accessed November 29, 2004).

[17]I. Ismail, "Digital Photography Is Hot," *New Straits Times Press* (Malaysia), June 7, 2004, p. 9.

[18]InfoTrends Research Group, "Worldwide Consumer Digital Camera Sales to Reach Nearly 53 Million in 2004," press release, www.infotrends-rgi.com/home/press/itPress/2003/11.19.03.html, November 19, 2003 (accessed November 29, 2004).

[19]S. Yin, "Picture This," *American Demographics,* July 1, 2003, p. 6.

[20]Photo Marketing Association International, "The Path From Pixels to Print."

[21]"Digital Camera Ownership Moving Deeper into Mainstream Market, According to New InfoTrends/CAP Ventures Study," *Business Wire,* October 12, 2004.

[22]Photo Marketing Association International, "The Path From Pixels to Print."

[23]Ibid.

[24]Ibid.

[25]A. Ferrari, "The Push for More Digital Photo Prints," www.forbes.com/2003/10/30/cx_af_1030printing.html, October 30, 2003 (accessed December 6, 2004).

[26]R. A. Dalton Jr., "In a Tech World, It's a Snap," *Newsday,* September 26, 2004, p. E6.

[27]Photo Marketing Association International, "The Path From Pixels to Print."

[28]Dalton, "In a Tech World, It's a Snap."

[29]InfoTrends Research Group, "New Wave of Photo Kiosk and Digital Print Solutions Driven by Digital Photography," press release, www.infotrends-rgi.com/home/Press/itPress/2002/5.20.02.html, May 20, 2002 (accessed November 30, 2004).

[30]Photo Marketing Association International, "The Path From Pixels to Print."

[31]"Camera Phones Outselling Digital Cameras—Report," www.forbes.com/newswire/2003/09/26/rtr1092489.html, September 26, 2003 (accessed December 6, 2004).

[32]Ismail, "Digital Photography Is Hot."

[33]"Mobile Snaps," *The Economist,* July 3, 2003.

[34]Ibid.

[35]A. Ferrari, "Digital Imaging's Winners and Losers," www.forbes.com/infoimaging/2004/08/09/cx_af_0809imagingupdate_ii.html, August 9, 2004 (accessed December 3, 2004).

[36]"Sony History," www.sony.ca/sonyca/view/english/corporate/corporate_sonyhistory1.shtml (accessed December 6, 2004).

[37]"Executive Biographies," www.sony.com/SCA/bios/idei.shtml (accessed December 6, 2004).

[38]"Cybershot: The Roots," www.sony.net/Products/cybershot/the_roots_01.html (accessed December 6, 2004).

[39]B. S. Bulik, "Sony, Kodak Lead U.S. Battle for Share in Digital Cameras," *Advertising Age* 75, no. 22 (May 31, 2004).

[40]P. Klebinkov and B. Fulford, "Canon on the Loose," www.forbes.com/global/2001/0723/036_3.html, July 23, 2001 (accessed December 6, 2004).

[41]"New Canon Marketing Campaign Highlights 'Digital Duet' of Digital Cameras and Printers," *Business Wire,* November 21, 2001 (accessed via Lexis/Nexis November 30, 2004).

[42]"Fuji's Digital Picture Is Developing Fast," www.businessweek.com/print/magazine/content/04_08/b3871064.htm, February 23, 2004 (accessed November 29, 2004).

[43]"HP's Strategy: Connect 'Device Islands, '"www.businessweek.com/technology/content/dec2003/tc2003129_2679_tc137.htm, December 9, 2003 (accessed November 29, 2004).

[44]"Digital Cameras," www.shopping.hp.com (accessed November 29, 2004).

[45]"Nikon Portfolio," www.nikon.co.jp/main/eng/portfolio/index.htm (accessed November 29, 2004).

[46]Nikon Web site, www.nikonusa.com/home.php (accessed November 29, 2004).

[47]"Kodak Debt Placed on CreditWatch Negative," www.businessweek.com/print/investor/content/jun2003/pi20030619_9134_pi036.htm?chan=pi&, June 19, 2003 (accessed November 29, 2004).

[48]S. N. Chakravarty, "How an Outsider's Vision Saved Kodak," www.forbes.com/forbes/1997/0113/5901045a_3.html, January 13, 1997 (accessed December 6, 2004).

[49]"HP, Kodak to Dissolve Phogenix Venture," www.printondemand.com/MT/archives/000142.html, May 23, 2003 (accessed December 6, 2004).

[50]Kodak press release, www.kodak.com/eknec/PageQuerier.jhtml?pq-path=2709&pq-locale=en_US&gpcid=0900688a8022df48, September 25, 2003 (accessed November 29, 2004).

[51]"Kodak Strategy Review," http://media.corporate-ir.net/media_files/IROL/11/115911/Reports/Carp_Sept25.pdf, September 25, 2003 (accessed December 6, 2004).

[52]"Kodak Strategy Review: Digital and Film Imaging," http://media.corporate-ir.net/media_files/IROL/11/115911/Reports/Masson_sept25.pdf, September 25, 2003 (accessed December 6, 2004).

[53]W. Symonds, "Not Exactly a Kodak Moment," *BusinessWeek,* November 24, 2003, p. 44.

[54]Ibid.

[55]C. H. Deutsch, "Some Positive News Aside, Kodak's Quarterly Profit Falls 63%," *The New York Times,* October 23, 2003, p. C9.

[56]Kodak press release, www.kodak.com/eknec/PageQuerier.jhtml?pq-path=2709&pq-locale=en_US&gpcid=0900688a8022df48, September 25, 2003 (accessed November 29, 2004).

Adam Aircraft

Carl Hedberg
Babson College

John Hamilton
Babson College

William Bygrave
Babson College

As the sleek, six-seat Adam A500 performed a graceful arc overhead, Babson College MBA John Hamilton, vice president of marketing for Adam Aircraft Industries (AAI), had to smile. Earlier that morning, he had read an article describing the difficulties and pitfalls associated with designing, building, and certifying new aircraft. In the last 30 years, there were countless examples of start-up aircraft manufacturers that had tried and failed to deliver new products to the small and midsized aircraft markets. In fact, the only two start-up companies that had recently succeeded had been builders of very basic, single-engine aircraft.

Like most MBAs, John had been taught to analyze companies based on all the standard metrics: the management team, product viability and appeal, market demand, capitalization, and financing potential. While Adam Aircraft appeared to be a winner on all counts—including the progress it was making in the lengthy and complex certification process—the

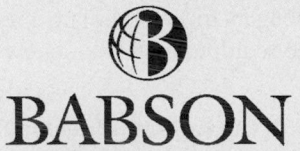

Carl Hedberg and John Hamilton prepared this case under the supervision of Professor William Bygrave, Babson College, as a basis for class discussion rather than to illustrate either effective or ineffective handling of an administrative situation. Funding provided by the F. W. Olin Graduate School and the gift of the class of 2003, and the Frederic C. Hamilton Chair for Free Enterprise.

company did not have the many millions of dollars it would need to bring its products to market and reach positive cash flow.

Talking with some of his peers in venture capital, John had come to understand that private equity investors were a fickle bunch. The vast majority preferred to invest in biotechnology, telecommunications, and other industries with historically well-defined harvest potential. Following the market correction in 2000, the flow of venture capital had significantly diminished, and investments outside of these core industries had all but ceased.

John had grown up in a family of aviators. He had been a licensed pilot for over 18 years. Since flying machines were not only his vocation but also his passion, he had to wonder whether this love was clouding his analysis. The market was clearly desperate for products like the plane performing flawlessly overhead, but did Adam Aircraft have what it took to succeed where so many had failed? Could it continue to advance toward certification and full-production capability, or would the challenges that lay ahead slow it down enough to increase its burn rate to a level that would discourage even the most ardent investor?

John did know that in less than five years company founder Rick Adam had orchestrated the fabrication of two flying prototypes—the A500 twin piston and the A700 jet—at a speed of design and production that had turned heads in all sectors of the aviation industry. Certification on both models was expected in the coming year—two years ahead of a number of well-funded competitors. With their third product—the A600 twin turboprop—nearly ready to fly, Adam Aircraft had become the one to watch in 2004.

John zipped up against the cold December wind and tracked the A500 as it snapped a sharp wing-turn on its approach to their home field at Centennial Airport in Englewood, Colorado. Another successful flight test. He smiled; definitely the one to watch . . .

THE ENTREPRENEUR

George Adam Sr. had been a career Air Force officer who had flown B-17 and B-29 bombers during World War II. His son Rick, born in 1946, grew up on Air Force bases and had always expected to follow his father into the military cockpit. When a color-vision deficiency kept him out of the Air Force Academy flight program, he joined the Army, attended West Point Academy, and then switched his commission to the Air Force.

Rick specialized in computer science, and as an Air Force captain he ran the Real Time Computer Centers at the Kennedy Space Center and at Vandenberg Air Force Base. During that time he earned his MBA at Golden Gate University, and later, as a civilian, he found his way to Wall Street. At Goldman Sachs he ran the IT department as a general partner. In 1993, Rick left Goldman to start his own business: New Era of Networks, an enterprise application integration software developer. The wildly successful company went public and grew to a market capitalization of over $1 billion. It was later acquired by the Sybase Corporation.

All the while, Rick had never lost sight of his first love, and in the early 1990s he learned to fly. Since his business required lots of travel, he was able to log over a thousand pilot-hours in just a few years by flying himself to meetings. He started in an old Skymaster, moved into a 1978 Mitsubishi MU2, and ultimately got type-rated in a 1993 Citation jet. While Rick had the opportunity and the personal wealth to progress quickly as a pilot, he recognized that the majority of owner-operators weren't as fortunate:

> As a pilot you have to go in steps; you can't get ahead of yourself. So, as you log more and more hours in the air, you can begin to fly increasingly more complex airplanes. The problem is that when you are ready to make the move from a single to a twin-engine aircraft, there are very few products to choose from. Most of the aircraft are based on old designs, which makes them tough to fly and expensive to own and operate.

One of the most popular production twin-engine planes on the market is the Beechcraft Baron—introduced in 1961! Because they quit building their more capable pressurized twins in the mid-80s, and stopped innovating at the same time, the old Baron is still their frontline light twin—and a new one costs over a million dollars. See, as the volume of orders has gone down, the prices have continued to climb (see Exhibit 1).

Rick added that the alternative to buying a new version of an old design was far worse:

> Demand for used planes is huge, because they are cheaper than new ones, and, since nothing has changed in the industry, pilots can buy something that may have been manufactured in the 70s or 80s, but it looks like a new plane. Right now the average age of a general aviation[1] aircraft is over 30 years (see Exhibit 2), and it's getting one year older every year.
>
> And frankly, these airplanes become unsafe. If you look at the accident rate in aircraft, it climbs dramatically with age. So even though there are strict regulations on maintaining these aircraft, it's hard to keep an old plane in good shape. Systems like the wiring just get to a point where they are too old to be reliable.

The more Rick thought about this aging factor, the more certain he became that the only solution would be an entirely new generation of general aviation products. It wasn't long before he had begun to evaluate the commercial viability of such a venture.

SPOTTING THE OPPORTUNITY

Almost immediately upon joining the ranks of experienced aviators, Rick began to contemplate the type of effort that would be required to deliver a new plane to the marketplace:

> Every time I went to a cocktail party or barbeque, all the pilots would go off into a corner and start talking pilot stuff. And since everybody was moaning about the lack of new products, I became convinced that there was a huge demand. So in the early 90s I started developing strategies for launching a new aircraft company.
>
> Now, I have launched a few entrepreneurial ventures, and when you think there is a big opportunity, you make sure to stop and evaluate why it hasn't been

Exhibit 1   **Annual New U.S. Manufactured General Aviation Unit Shipments/Billings, 1974–2002**

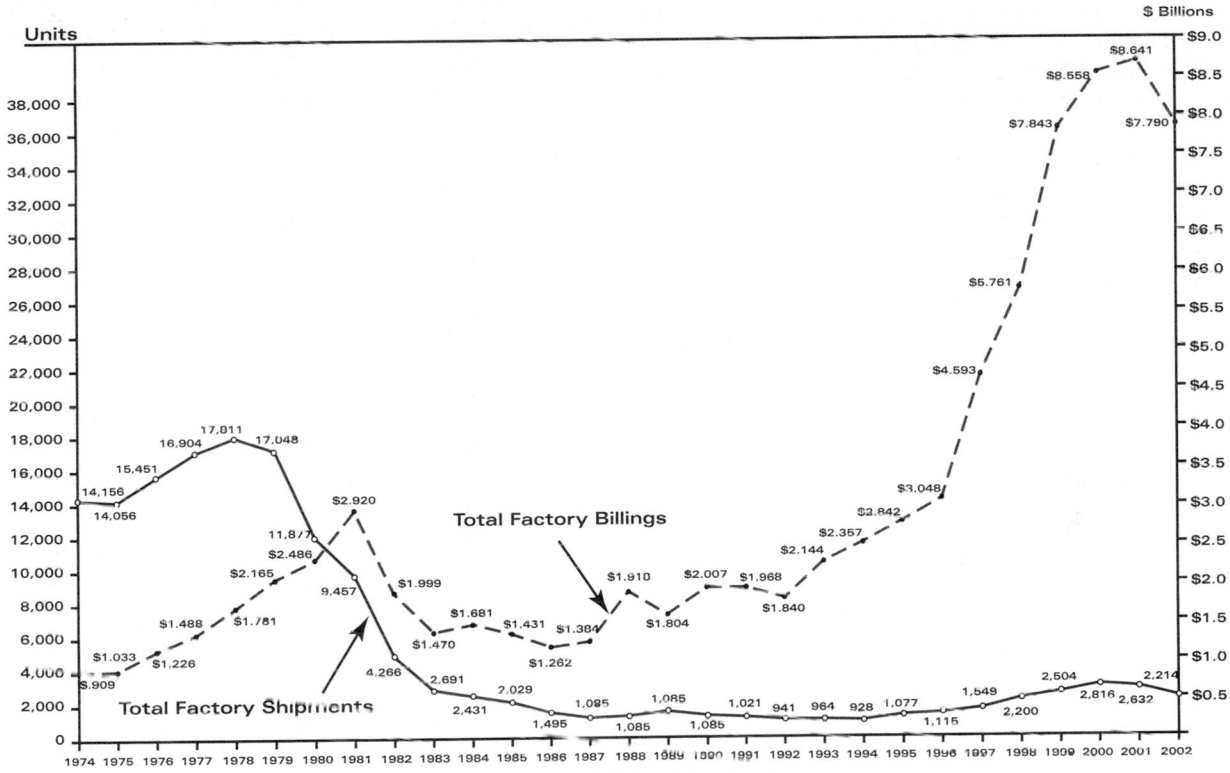

Source: General Aviation Manufacturers Association (GAMA) Statistical Databook 2002.

Exhibit 2   **Average Age of U.S. General Aviation Fleet in 2002**

Aircraft Type	Engine Type	Seats	Average Age in Years
Single-engine	Piston	1–3	36
		4	33
		5–7	28
		8+	43
	Turboprop	All	12
	Jet	All	31
Multi-engine	Piston	1–3	36
		4	33
		5–7	33
		8+	37
	Turboprop	All	26
	Jet	All	28
All aircraft			31

Source: General Aviation Manufacturers Association (GAMA) Statistical Databook 2002.

done before. Why isn't anyone pursuing this opportunity? What do I know, or what do I see that nobody else is seeing? Very often, entrepreneurial opportunities occur when a series of prior developments makes it possible to accomplish the once unachievable. You reach a point where you finally have all the ingredients to make it happen.

To illustrate, Rick referred to the electronic organizer on the table:

> There were at least a dozen attempts to bring out handheld devices ahead of the PalmPilot. The most notable was Jerry Kaplan's GO Corporation. Kaplan saw the opportunity, had the right idea, and raised $50 million in funding back in the early 90s. But since the chips weren't small enough, the displays weren't big enough, and the batteries weren't powerful enough, his product looked like a brick. He spent 50 million bucks and failed, simply because his great idea was ahead of the prevailing technology.

In a similar way, the Beechcraft Corporation was ahead of its time when, in the late 1970s, it set out to develop a new class of business aircraft. The five-and-a-half-year, $300-million development program resulted in the federally certified Starship (see Exhibit 3). The futuristic craft was the world's first pressurized, all-composite business turboprop.[2] Many in the industry had high hopes that the Starship would usher in a new age of modern propeller-driven aircraft, but that was not to be.

Developed by Scaled Composites, a cutting-edge aircraft design enterprise founded by visionary Burt Rutan,[3] the Starship project brought about the development of Federal Aviation Authority (FAA) standards for the construction of composite aircraft. Unfortunately for Beechcraft, this was a very long and difficult process resulting in an aircraft that was heavier and more expensive than predicted. As a result, the Starship's performance was only marginally better than the existing fleet—and yet its price was far higher. Despite its commercial failure, this project was the first in a series of events that would begin to spark new life into the long-ailing general aviation aircraft industry in America.

Exhibit 3   **The Beechcraft Starship**

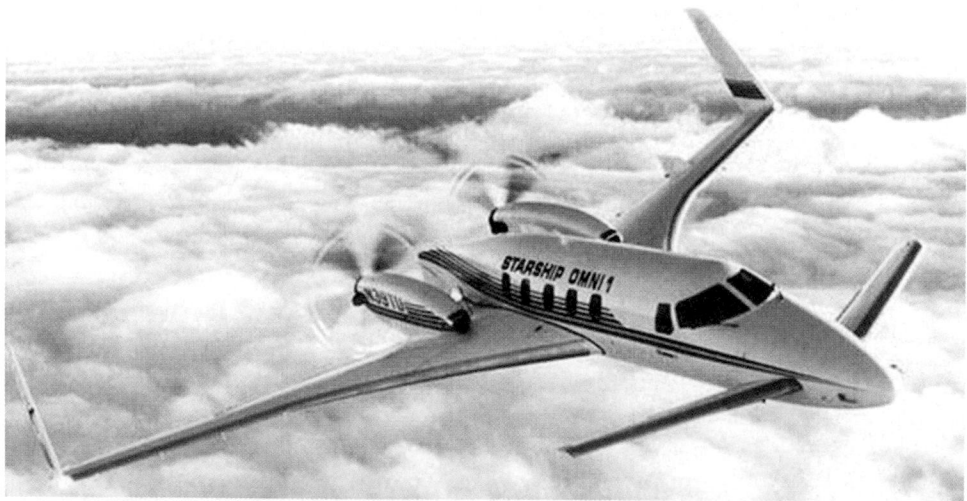

The Beechcraft Starship, a twin-turboprop pusher design, was the first all-composite pressurized airframe ever certified by the FAA. The task was larger than simply developing an all-new aircraft. Beech had to master an innovative technology, work hand-in-hand with FAA regulators, build a new manufacturing facility, and train a specialized workforce. Much of this effort was concentrated on areas the industry had not addressed before. The company built 53 Starships in all before ceasing production in the early 1990s.

A CONVERGENCE OF FACTORS

Between 1978 and 1992, the general aviation industry had suffered a 95 percent unit sales decline and the loss of over 100,000 jobs. Over that same period, general aviation (GA) manufacturers had spent as much to defend product liability suits as they had spent to develop new aircraft in the 30 years following the Second World War.

When Congress enacted the General Aviation Revitalization Act (GARA) in 1994 to protect aircraft builders from lawsuits on planes that were older than 18 years, it revitalized an industry nearly wiped out by two decades of what lawmakers were calling lawsuit abuse and trial lawyer profiteering.

The 1990s also brought about enormous advances in computing power and computer-aided design and modeling (CAD/CAM) software. Airframe geometry could now reside in the computer, with all of its internal structures defined electronically as three-dimensional models. By the end of that decade, expensive wind tunnels and physical scale models were being replaced by computational fluid dynamics software. Manufacturing and tooling capabilities had made great strides as well.

Rick said that after a couple of kit manufacturers[4] managed to achieve commercial certification for their composite designs, he figured that the time was right:

> In the early 90s, all the innovation was being done in composites and kits. Then Lancair and Cirrus announced that they were going to take what they had learned and build production airplanes. Everybody who loves flying was rooting for them, hoping they would make it, and sure enough, they both got certified.
>
> I'm watching this process and realizing that while there were quite a few single-engine, nonpressurized, fixed-gear start-ups out there, nobody had yet brought an innovative product into the middle market. It was real clear to me that pilots wanted a new twin, and once I had seen the success that the composite guys had down in single engines, I came to the conclusion it could be done in the twin-engine area.

By the latter half of the 1990s, a number of well-financed firms were competing to introduce a personal jet into this middle-market space by 2006.

Rick looked at these projects and wondered: Would it be possible to design a single airframe that could accommodate jet engines as well as twin pistons? He didn't have the answer, but he knew who would.

THE PROJECT BEGINS

Although he was still running his software venture, in 1998 Rick decided to put up a million dollars to get into the aviation business. At the same time, he brought in a talented partner: former FAA trial attorney John Knudsen, an experienced aviator with a career in the U.S. Navy as a carrier-based attack pilot. Understanding that a commercially viable new design—whether it was a jet or a twin piston—would have to blend superior performance capabilities with curb appeal, Rick said that they contacted the best in the business:

> We met with Burt Rutan and showed him some requirements, definitions, and preliminary designs for a twin piston. Since carbon fiber lends itself to much more aerodynamic shapes than you can get with aluminum construction—I told him to make it look as much like a jet as possible.
>
> As always, he had some wild stuff and he had some stuff that was more middle of the road. We narrowed four or five design concepts down to an inline, front and back engine configuration, with twin booms to get to the tail.

If this plane was going to be the step up for single-engine pilots that Rick was envisioning, they understood that ease of operation would be critical. With this in mind, they chose a centerline thrust arrangement, since, compared to twins with the power plants mounted on the wings, the push-pull design significantly reduced the difficulty of flying with one engine not functioning. Having settled on what he felt was an exciting airframe, Rick noted that they had no desire to conquer more than one frontier at a time:

> The Eclipse 500 project has raised $400 million so far in its effort to build a light business jet. They tried to develop a new airframe and a new engine at the same time. The engine didn't work, and now they are two years off schedule.
>
> I'm a raging incrementalist; the way to innovate is to take one step at a time. We chose power plants, avionics, and construction methods that had

previously been certified by the FAA for other planes; our only major innovation initially will be with the shape of the airframe. I figured that once we had that done, we could innovate on something else later on. It's just so tough to bring a certified new airplane to market; we had to be very careful to avoid adding layers of complexity—and lots of time and money.

The team at Scaled Composites began work on the conceptual designs for Adam Aircraft in May of 1999, and cut the first tool in late August.[5] When the M-309 (see Exhibit 4) lifted off on its maiden flight in March 2000, it marked the most rapid manned-aircraft development program in the company's history.

Despite the price tag, Rick understood that this "experimental" was a one-of-a-kind, hand-built model that would serve only as a research vehicle. Conventional evidence suggested that the development of

an FAA-certified version of the M-309 would take a few years, at least a couple more flying test planes, millions of engineering man-hours, and hundreds of millions of dollars. Rick was determined, however, to make sure that his aircraft company was anything but conventional.

RESEARCH AND INNOVATION

With the M-309 outfitted with an array of data collection equipment, the AAI team proceeded to log over 300 flight hours in 2000 as they scrutinized the full range of the craft's aerodynamic characteristics and performance capabilities. Rick explained that with regard to understanding the commercial viability of

Exhibit 4   **The M-309**

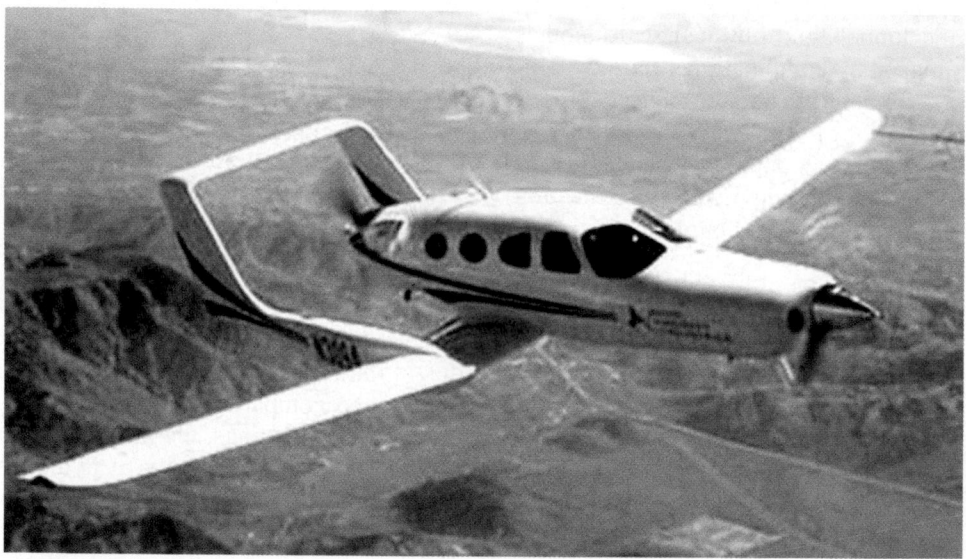

Named for Burt Rutan's 309th completed design, the Model 309 was built with the aim of delivering a very safe twin-engine aircraft that would give good performance and benign single engine handling qualities. The pressurized cabin was designed to carry a pilot and five passengers.

The central goal of this program was to develop an aerodynamically refined aircraft. However, there were several features that were more representative of a full-production airplane. For example, there were several major structural components that had been produced as single-cure parts. The outboard wings, horizontal tail, elevator, rudders, and flaperons had no secondary bonds in their primary structure. This allowed for a lighter, stronger, and safer structure due to the significant elimination of fasteners and secondary bonds.

Source: www.scaled.com.

the plane, their destinations were often just as important as their in-flight calculations:

> We collected aerodynamic data as we flew the M-309 to air shows around the country, and that gave us the opportunity to survey the market and listen to what potential customers had to say. We completely reengineered the original design. For example, we increased the size of the empennage,[6] and also moved the door for easier access to the cabin. By the fall of 2000, I had come to the conclusion that there was a significant market for this kind of aircraft.

Rick, who was self-funding most of the start-up costs, had been busy recruiting a top-tier management group. Nearly everyone on his 10-member executive staff was an accomplished pilot, and collectively they had many years of experience from all corners of the aviation industry, including Boeing, Beechcraft, Martin Marietta, Cirrus, Lancair, Scaled Composites, Eclipse, the U.S. military, and the FAA.

In December, Adam Aircraft established its home base at Centennial Field, just south of Denver. As they got down to the business of fitting the factory in advance of tooling design for the first production model, now called the Adam A500, Rick said that because of the direct relationship between time to market and project cost, they had no choice but to innovate:

> I had recently heard from an industry expert that the standard budget for a new airplane project is about $250 million. Since there has been so little success in this industry to date, it would be nearly impossible to raise that kind of money for a start-up airplane company like ours. That's a long way from $250 million, but still, we knew that the only way we could make financing achievable was by cutting development costs by at least 75 percent.

He added that to accomplish such a feat would require not only brilliant engineering but also the development of a culture unheard of in aviation manufacturing:

> Being a lifetime computer guy, speed and innovation seem very natural to me. We knew right off that time was not our friend; either we get this plane up and certified quickly, or we'd attract competitors and run out of money. One of the first things we did was to institute the kind of 24-hour scheduling that we had used to run our data centers and networks.
>
> Our people now work 12-hour, overlapping shifts; three-day weeks, with voluntary overtime on Sundays. So while our competitors are putting in five shifts in a calendar week, we are getting up to 21—in addition to high morale and very low attrition.

Over the past few decades, powerful aircraft builders like McDonnell Douglas, Lockheed, and Boeing had developed highly sophisticated modeling design tools that were powered by multimillion-dollar mainframe computers. The PC age had put those capabilities into the hands of small shops like Adam Aircraft. For an off-the-shelf cost of about $3,000 per system, the company was able to set up a 40-station CAD/CAM engineering center with all the capabilities of the big guys. Rick said that by tying this powerful design architecture into the tooling mill downstairs (see Exhibit 5), the company was able to add efficiencies by keeping the entire design process in-house:

> With aluminum technology, you design the part, and then you bid it out for tooling. You award the tooling—which typically costs over a million dollars—and

Exhibit 5   Five Axis Tooling Mill

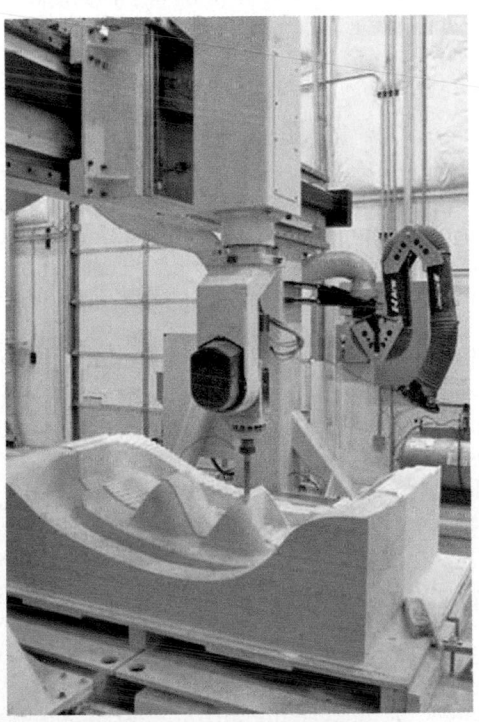

Fabricating the Air-Stair door tool out of dense foam material six to nine months later, the tool comes back. If it's wrong or you want to make a design change, you have to start all over, Because we have our own tooling mill, we can do it fast the first time, and more importantly, continue to modify the tool quickly until we get it right.

The management team understood that merely coupling rapid application development with a 24/7 working environment would not provide enough of an edge to develop the full line of airplanes they were envisioning. Rick explained that for that to happen, they would need to adopt a computer industry concept that, if successful, would change the face of general aviation manufacturing forever:

> PCs are developed around a common set of rules as to how the parts interact with each other. That way, you can change the keyboard, the disc drive, the screen, whatever you want, and it won't tear up your memory or your software; that's called modular architecture.
>
> There has been little progress in modular architecture in airplanes—until now. We are building enormous modularity into our design so we can do things like move the wing location, modify the cabin size, change the power plants; all kinds of things. What that means is that we will bring this first plane to certification status for about 50 million bucks. For another 10 million, we'll adjust the modules slightly and get a jet. For another 5 million, we'll get a turboprop.[7]

Detractors felt that this was wishful thinking, and pointed out that the modular architecture approach could potentially compromise performance. Some noted that since each power plant system would have different weight and structural characteristics, installing all three on essentially the same airframe could cause center-of-gravity problems. In addition, critics felt that using a single-wing and empennage design would mean that two of the planes, or maybe even the whole line of products, would fly at less than optimum performance.

The AAI team felt that they were on top of those challenges with innovations like their "smart tunnel," a device that enabled engineers to shift the wing location on the fuselage in order to control the range of the aircraft's center of gravity. The team felt that this technology and other specialized systems they were devising would give AAI engineers the means to modify the underlying airframe to accommodate a wide range of engine choices and configurations.

In addition, they felt that this engineering strategy would enable them to leverage their research and development spending over at least three commercially viable aircraft designs. Time would tell.

WORKING WITH THE FAA

Throughout 2001, all manner of government and industry groups had visited the plant to witness the A500 project as it came together very nearly on schedule, and on budget. Predictably, the one group that would not be offering praise or extra points for speed of design and assembly was the Federal Aviation Authority (FAA).

The task of the FAA was to see to it that the Type Certification (TC) approval process (see Exhibit 6) proceeded in a careful and thorough manner. The complex system of inspections and testing was similar to what health care companies faced with the Federal Drug Administration (FDA). Like the FDA, the FAA required exhaustive proof that products were safe before they could be marketed to consumers. In the aviation industry, that regulatory oversight translated into lots of time and money. While it was true that successful new entrants like Lancair and Cirrus had helped pave the way for subsequent efforts, Rick said that getting through the regulatory process would still be one of AAI's greatest challenges:

> Although the FAA is constantly working to improve the aircraft certification process, for good reason it is designed to be extremely arduous. Nevertheless, we do have a number of advantages over our predecessors. For example, as opposed to submitting aircraft designs on paper, we can now send designs to the FAA electronically. By doing this, we save a ton of time and, most importantly, are assured of the highest degree of accuracy in our documentation process.

By the time the A500 had been cleared for its inaugural flight in July of 2002, a second test aircraft was already under construction (see Exhibit 7), and fabrication of parts for a third had begun as well. Comprising the entire testing fleet, these three aircraft would each undergo a series of exhaustive flight and static tests—many requiring the construction of customized systems and fixtures (see Exhibit 8). If all proceeded as planned, AAI expected to achieve certification for the A500 by the first half of 2004.

THE CUSTOMERS

When AAI flew its A500 to the Experimental Aircraft Association's (EAA) AirVenture Convention in Oshkosh, Wisconsin, that summer, the company brought along a full-size mockup of the plane's cockpit and fully appointed interior. Vice President of Marketing John Hamilton noted that Oshkosh was an excellent show since it attracted buyers from all the major markets for its $895,000 twin piston:

There are two basic markets for aircraft like the A500; owner-flown, and professionally flown. The owner-flown market is just that. The owner of the aircraft is also the pilot in command. In the professionally flown market, non-owners fly the aircraft. It sounds like a silly distinction but it makes a difference in how you market the aircraft.

I would say between 70 and 80 percent of our A500 customers will be owner-operators. These folks are evaluating our aircraft from the pilot's seat. They will be very tuned in to things like the performance of the aircraft, its handling characteristics, and the

Exhibit 6   **FAA Type Certification Process**

Familiarization Meeting

Meeting to establish a partnership with the applicant. It is an opportunity to develop mutual understanding of the type certification process as it applies to the applicant's design. It's highly recommended as a beginning point in the process.

Formal Application

Applicant's formal application for a Type Certification (TC) includes a cover letter, Form 8110-2, and a three-view drawing.

Preliminary Type Certification Board

At this initial formal meeting, the project team collects data about the technical aspects of the project and the applicant's proposed certification basis and identifies other information needed to start developing the Certification Program Plan. Special-attention items are also identified at this time.

Certification Program Plan (CPP)

A key document, the Certification Plan addresses:

- The proposed FAA certification basis.
- Noise and emission requirements.
- Issue papers.
- Special conditions, exemptions, and equivalent level of safety findings.
- Means of compliance.
- Compliance checklists and schedules.
- Use of delegations/designees.

Technical Meetings

Held throughout the project, technical meetings (e.g., specialist and interim TC meetings) cover a variety of subjects. Team members may:

- Approve test plans and reports.
- Review engineering compliance findings.
- Close out issue papers.
- Review conformity inspections.
- Review minutes of board meetings.
- Revise the Certification Program Plan.
- Issue new FAA policy guidance.
- Review airworthiness limitations.
- Review instructions for continued airworthiness.

(Continued)

Exhibit 6   **Continued**

Preflight Type Certification Board

Discussions at the preflight TC board center on the applicant's flight test program, including conformity inspections and engineering compliance determinations.

Type Inspection Authorization (TIA)

Prepared on FAA Form 8110-1, the TIA authorizes conformity and airworthiness inspections and flight tests to meet certification requirements. The TIA is issued when examination of technical data required to TC is completed or has reached a point where it appears that the product will meet pertinent regulations.

Conformity Inspections and Certification Flight Tests

Conformity inspections ensure that the product conforms with the design proposed for type certification. Flight tests are conducted in accordance with the requirements of the TIA.

Aircraft Evaluation Group (AEG) Determinations

The AEG works with certification engineers and FAA flight test pilots to evaluate the operational and maintenance aspects of certified products through such activities as:

Flight Standardization Board (FSB)
- Pilot type rating.
- Pilot training checking, currency requirements.
- Operational acceptability.

Flight Operations Evaluation Board (FOEB)
- Master minimum equipment list (MMEL).

Maintenance Review Board (MRB)
- Maintenance instructions for continued airworthiness.

Final Type Certification Board

When the applicant has met all certification requirements, the ACO schedules the final formal TC board. The board wraps up any outstanding items and decides on the issuance of the TC.

Type Certificate

The certifying ACO issues the TC when the applicant completes demonstration of compliance with the certification basis. The TC data sheet is part of the TC and documents conditions and limitations to meet FAR requirements.

Postcertification Activities

This includes the Type Inspection Report (TIR)—to be completed within 90 days of issuance of the unique technical requirements and lessons learned—the Certification Summary Report (CSR), and the Postcertification Evaluation, which closes out the TC project and provides the foundation for continued FAA airworthiness monitoring activities such as service bulletins, revisions to type design, malfunction/defect reports, and Certificate Management for the remainder of the aircraft's life cycle.

electronic systems in the instrument panel. In addition, because they also manage the scheduled maintenance requirements, they will be very sensitive to serviceability.

Marketing to the professionally flown segment is a bit different since they are more focused on the needs of their client-passengers. They'll be interested in things like how comfortable the seating is, how much baggage area is available, whether the plane has a toilet or an entertainment system. They'll also want a pressurized cabin so they can fly over weather, a plane that looks and feels safe and substantial—and a plane that is appealing to the eye.

In addition, John emphasized that aviation consumers of all types demanded top service and easily maintainable aircraft:

You've got to have absolute first-rate service. Customers can't have difficulty getting parts or finding somebody to work on their airplane.

Pilots are also hesitant to adopt something that is new. We're not Cessna, we're not Beechcraft, and we're not Piper. Those guys have been around forever, and they've built a ton of airplanes.

That's why with everything we do—from delivery, to flight training, to service and parts—we

Exhibit 7   **Fuselage Construction of the A-500 SN002**

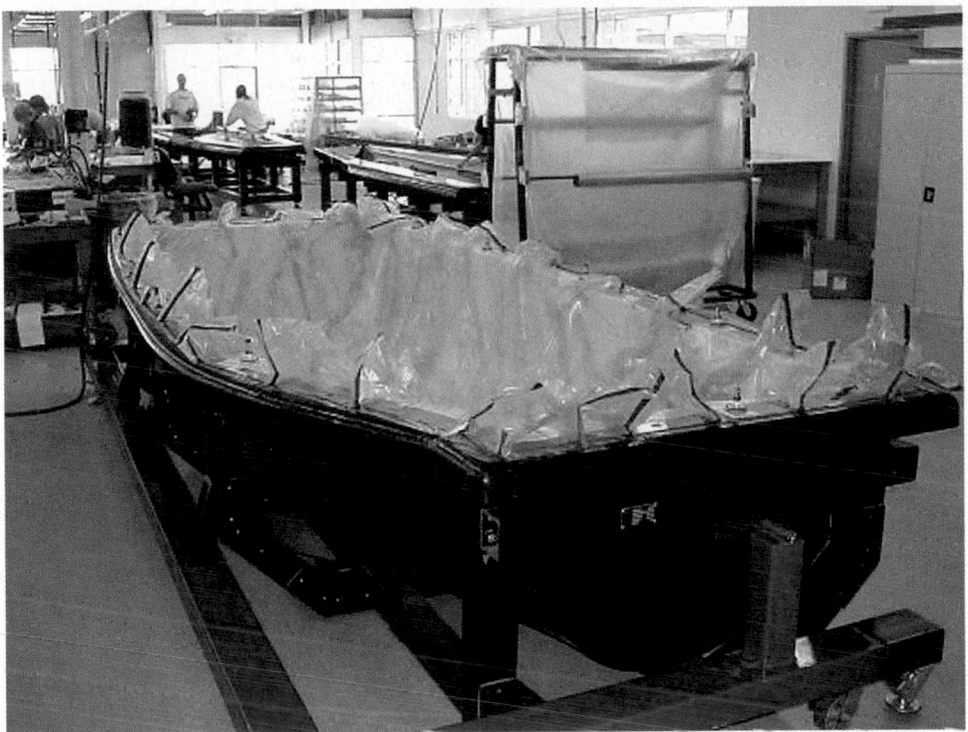

Vacuum bag on fuselage tool

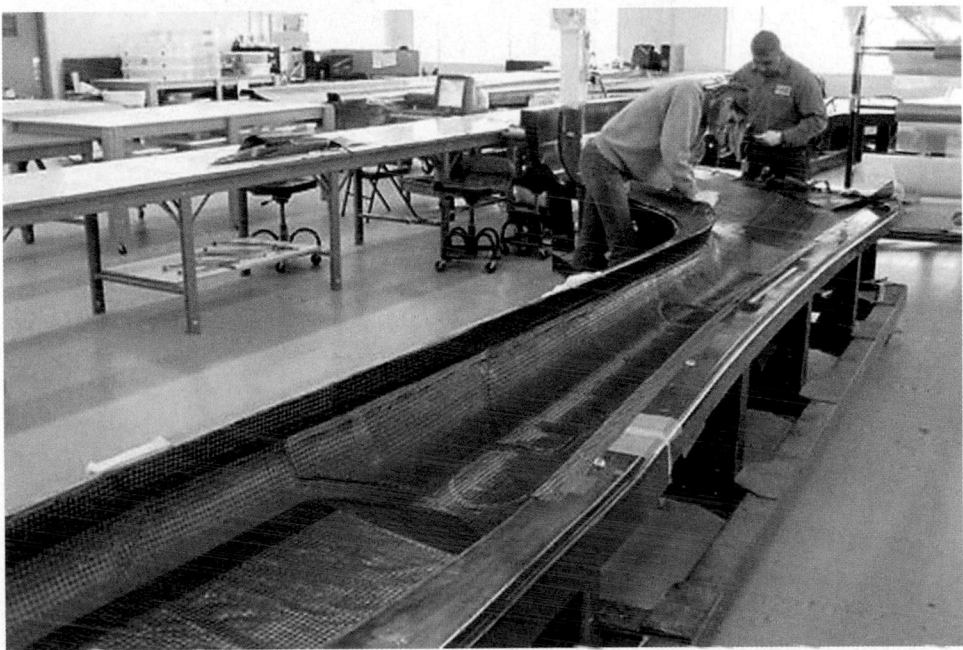

Laying up the carbon material into the tail boom tool

Exhibit 8   **Custom-Built Static Test Rig**

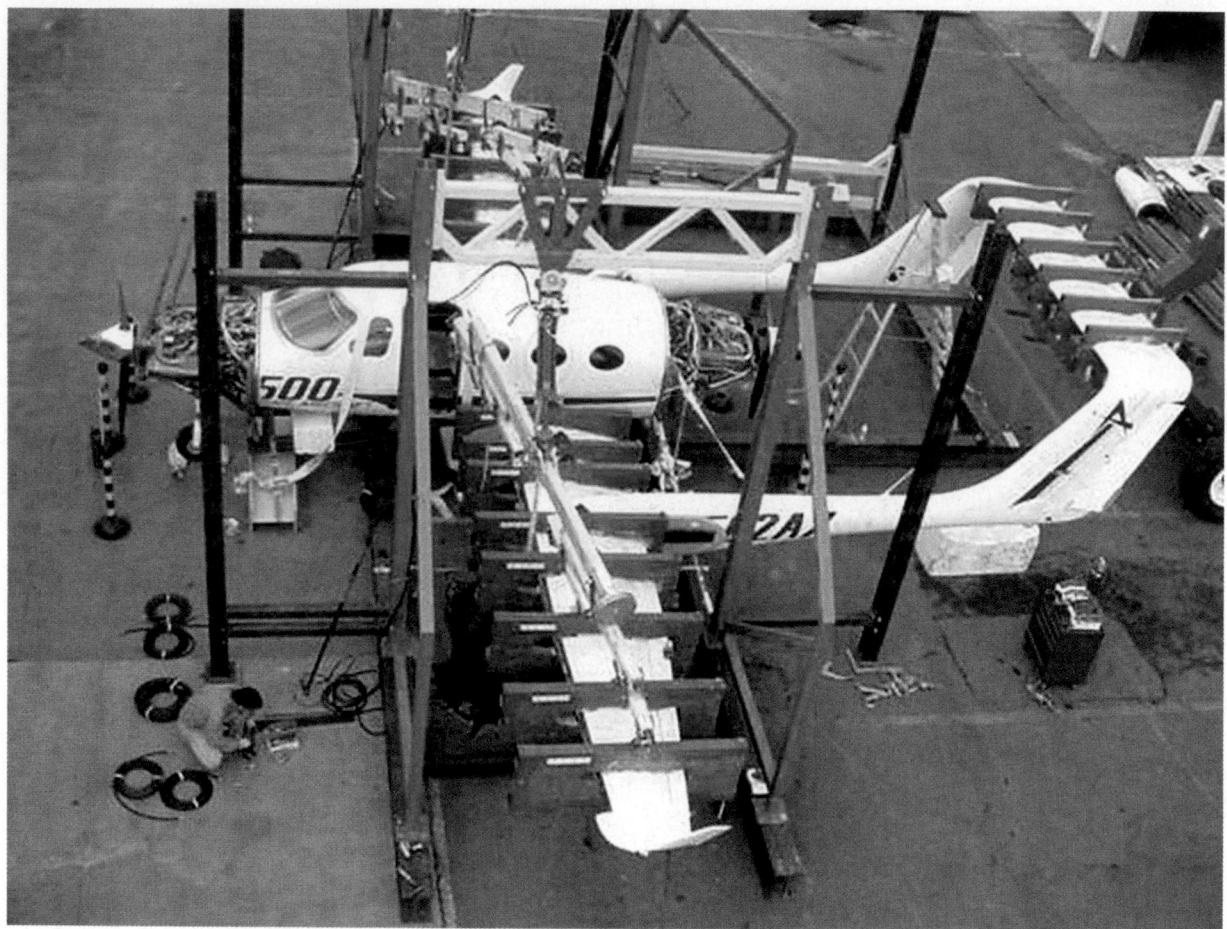

have to prove to our customers that there is a very compelling reason why they should adopt this new aircraft.

John added that the company's unique design modularity would play an important role in serviceability:

One feature of the A500 that customers will love is how easy it is to access the systems on the aircraft that need to be inspected and/or replaced. A great deal of engineering work has been performed to dramatically reduce the amount of time it takes maintenance personnel to complete the necessary service tasks. This will result in reduced downtime and lower costs of operation. Going the extra mile for owners in this area will pay substantial dividends in customer satisfaction.

EYEING THE FUTURE

In October 2002, the company announced its plan to introduce the next aircraft. The company also indicated that due to the modular systems, the A700, a six- to eight-seat stretched-fuselage twin-jet, would share 80 percent part commonality with the A500. Some critics doubted Rick's assertion that since the A700 would present only an incremental development challenge for his talented engineers, AAI would be able to build a flying model within a year.

Ten months after completing preliminary design work, the A700 jet shocked and amazed the general aviation world by making a surprise appearance at the 2003 EAA AirVenture event. Industry dignitaries such as Secretary of Transportation Norman Minetta and FAA administrator Marion Blakey welcomed the aircraft with words of support and congratulations. The aviation press was buzzing; if the company was able to hold to its schedule and achieve FAA certification for the A700 in the fourth quarter of 2004, the $1.995 million craft would be the first to market in this emerging, closely watched segment (see Exhibit 9).

John explained that this keen interest in light jets was directly related to the need for more efficient transportation solutions:

> The average mission is less than a two-hour flight, with three and a half people on board—meaning nearly every business jet in America is oversized for what it does.
>
> This emerging personal jet segment is based on the same concept that Japanese automakers used to take on Detroit 30 years ago. With gas prices going up, why not build a car which was more suitably sized to the average driver's need? Reducing the size and weight of the machine dramatically improved its operating efficiency. We're building a smaller and lighter aircraft designed for the most common trip length and passenger load to deliver optimal efficiency in the twin-jet category.

In addition to the benefits of an incremental improvement in the efficiency of twin-engine jets, personal jet aircraft were being viewed by some as the solution to the gridlock in the hub-and-spoke airline system. Rick Adam described one official's views on the subject:

> Dr. Bruce Holmes at NASA[8] has performed extensive studies of the transportation system and has concluded that the best way to increase capacity in the air is by directing more traffic to the 5,000 underutilized regional airports in this country. Regional travelers would fly point-to-point out of small airports and never enter the hub and spoke system unless they plan to fly across the country or abroad.
>
> Because this air taxi system would require a massive fleet of aircraft to achieve network coverage, the price of the aircraft and its operating cost are critical components to the success of the system. Aircraft like the A700 could get the cost per seat mile down to a level where the average business traveler could afford the service.
>
> We don't need the air taxi model to take off for the A700 to be a successful project, but it would certainly provide a fantastic upside to our company.

With two distinct models flying, Rick and his company now had a real story to tell. CFO Mike Smith observed that for outside investors and municipal development groups, one of the most attractive aspects of the AAI plan was that the economics seemed entirely within the range of possibility:

> We could break even right out of this facility [at Centennial Field] by adding roughly 100 production people to our current staff of 150. With the A500, the current overhead breaks even at somewhere between 35 and 40 planes a year, and the jet would be roughly a third of that. We have a component capacity for about 100 planes a year, and an assembly capacity for about 40 or 50. The great thing about this company is at just 50 airplanes a year, we're making money. So far we have taken deposits for over 50 twin pistons.[9] Once we are certified, we anticipate a surge in orders.

By late 2003 the planes had appeared on a host of aviation magazine covers (see Exhibit 10) and in a wide range of business publications including the *New York Times, The Wall Street Journal,* and *Forbes* magazine. Nearly all seemed to be anticipating a significant American success story.

THE CRITICAL JUNCTURE

Heading out for a meeting over in Boulder, John fired up his twin-engine Beechcraft as the A500 crossed his path on its way back to the hanger for further testing. As he taxied out in preparation for take-off, John recalled an earlier meeting with a reporter from an aviation magazine. When she had asked him whether he thought much about the possibility of failure, he prefaced his response with a story:

> You know, we were speaking with some guys in the airborne fire-fighting business. They currently use airplanes that are roughly in the A500 class to fly lead-in for fire-fighting tankers. These spotter planes fly low and left of the tankers, and tell those pilots where to make the drop.
>
> They asked if we could put a window overhead on the A500 so their lead pilots could have good visibility of the tanker high and right. They told us that none of the established competitors they had spoken with would even consider that kind of modification. Our engineers told him that it would take us about a week to figure that out.
>
> The point is, that's why I don't spend much time thinking about the business risk of this venture. Adam Aircraft has been surprising the experts and our potential customers from the very beginning; there is no reason to assume we won't continue to do so.

Exhibit 9 **Very Light Jet Segment: Competitor Profiles**

Manufacturer	Product	List Price ($000)	Seats	Cruise Speed	First Delivery	Orders to Date (11/03)	Home Base
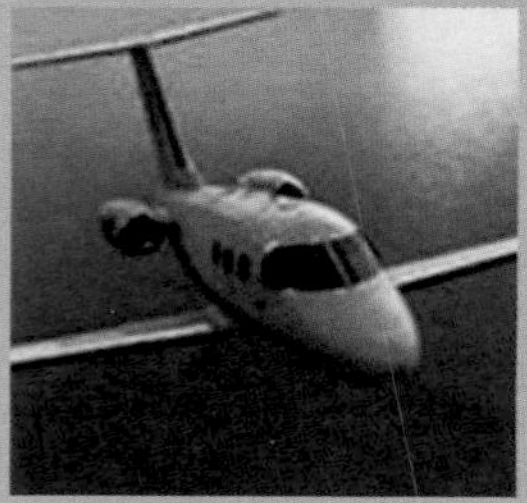 Avocet	Pro-Jet	$2,000	6–8	420	Late 2006	200	Westport, Connecticut
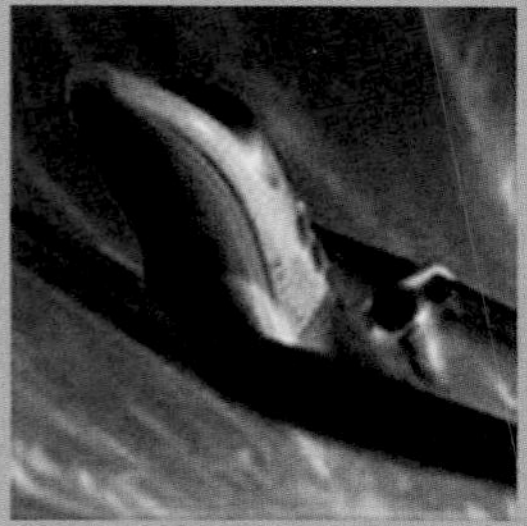 Cessna	Citation Mustang	$2,295	6	391	Late 2006	300+	Wichita, Kansas
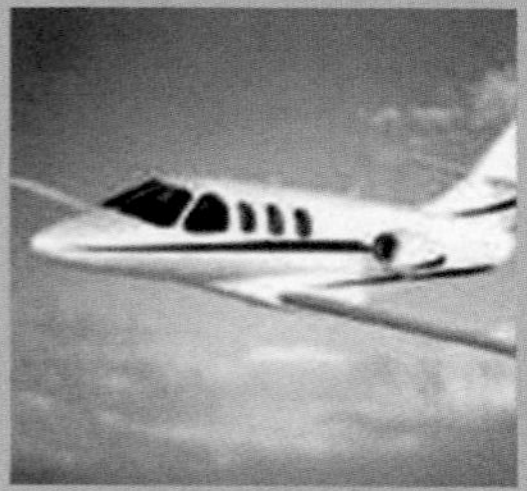 Safire	Safire Jet	$1,395	6	437	2006	300+	Miami, Florida
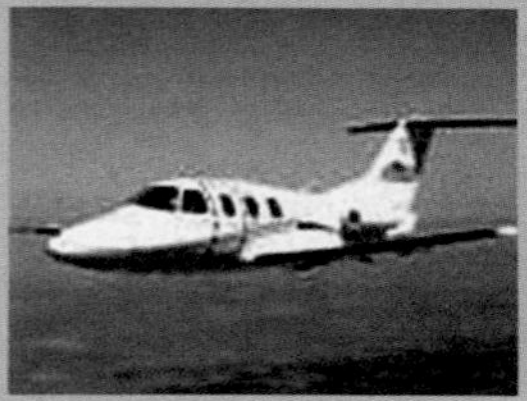 Eclipse	Eclipse 500	$ 950	3–6	432	2006	2,060	Albuquerque, New Mexico

Exhibit 10   **Magazine Cover: AAI's A700 and A500**

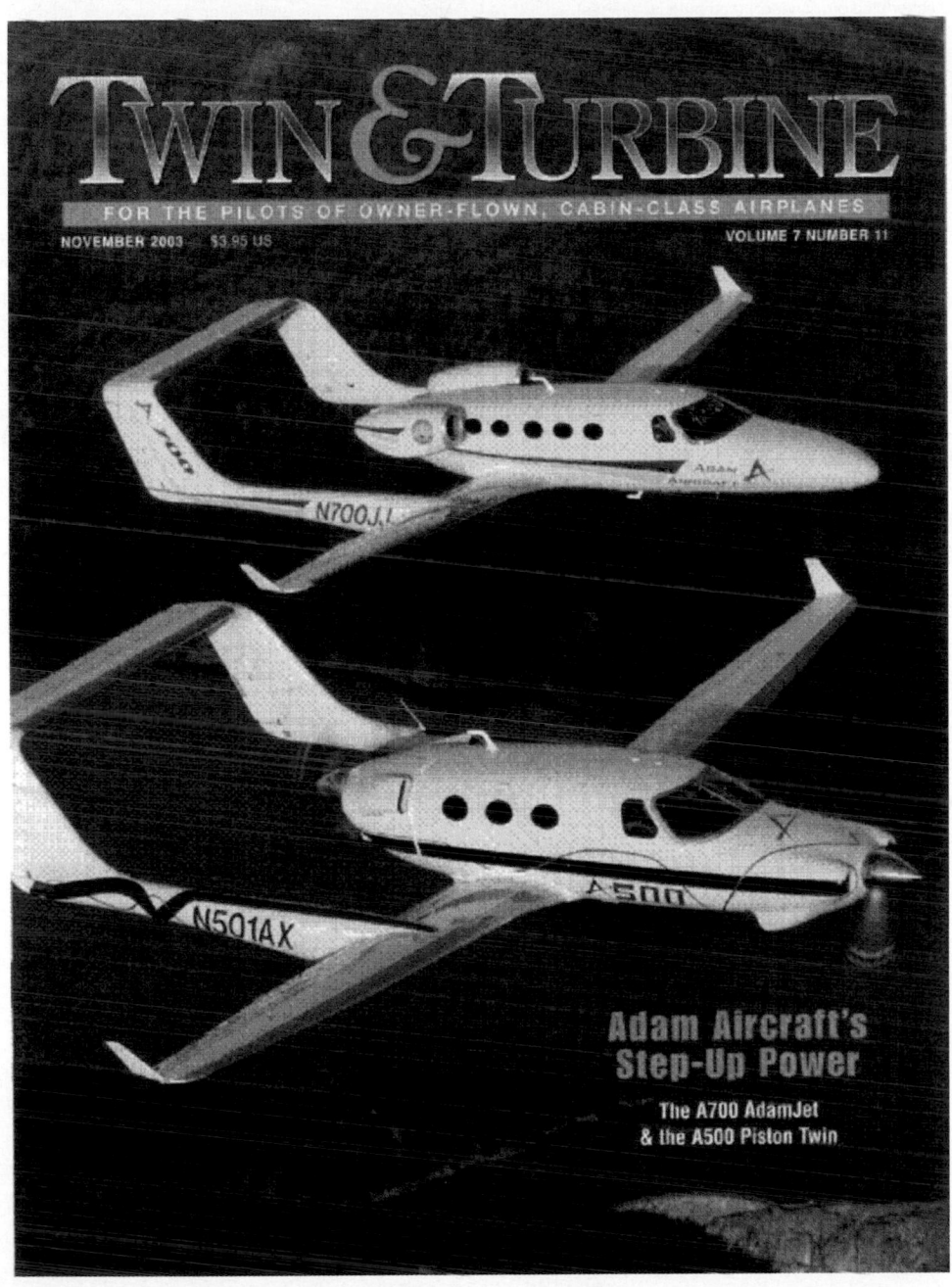

As John lifted off and banked north toward Boulder, he realized that his thrill of flying had never waned since he was a kid. Although he loved his 30-year-old Beech, he knew it wouldn't last forever—and there were a bunch of pilots just like him out there waiting for something new. He felt certain that Adam Aircraft would be the one to answer that call.

Endnotes

[1]General aviation (GA) is a term comprising all of aviation other than government and scheduled air transport (commercial airlines), and includes privately owned aircraft, charter services, business-owned aircraft, and many more types of working aircraft that are not, strictly speaking, for transportation. Although a large part of GA consists of recreational flying, an equally large part involves important commercial activities such as flight training, shipping, surveying, agricultural application, air taxi, charter passenger service, corporate flying, emergency transport, and firefighting.

[2]An easy-to-understand composite material would be an adobe brick; wet mud and straw—mixed together and dried. The result is a material stronger than either mud or straw. Composite airframes typically consisted of a carbon, graphite, or glass fiber reinforcing material, and an epoxy resin binder. Alone, these substances had very little strength, but when combined and properly cured, they became a composite structure that was very strong. Since this construction process lent itself to fluid design, composite airframes were often sleeker and more pleasing to the eye than their aluminum counterparts.

[3]As a schoolboy, Burt Rutan had designed award-winning model aircraft, and by age 16 had learned to fly. After receiving a bachelor's degree in aeronautical engineering from Cal Poly, he worked for the U.S. Air Force as a Flight Test Project Engineer at Edwards Air Force Base in California. In 1972, at age 29, he founded Rutan Aircraft Factory, which sold plans and kits for Rutan-designed aircraft. His science-fiction-like aircraft designs were considered risky by established aircraft manufacturers, who made sure that the regulators of the Federal Aviation Administration were aware of their concerns. While he successfully sold a number of different unique designs, he became frustrated by the litigious regulatory environment and substantial liability claims that had put many private aircraft manufacturers out of business. In 1982, Rutan chose to leave the homebuilt industry in favor of larger-scale designs for companies. His new firm was Scaled Composites.

[4]Kit planes were considered experimental by the Federal Aviation Administration. This designation was originally intended for aircraft designers who wanted to do research, or for amateur pilots who wanted to learn about aerodynamics as they built their own planes. Because these aircraft were barred from commercial use, the FAA felt that there was no need to impose its exhaustive and very expensive certification process on this class of aircraft.

[5]In composite engineering, a tool was the master mold that the composite material was layered into before being vacuum-compressed, and then oven-cured—a process known as thermosetting—at 240 degrees.

[6]The empennage, commonly called the tail assembly, was the rear section of the body of the airplane. Its main purpose was to provide stability to the aircraft.

[7]Turboprops were designed to carry high passenger (or cargo) loads over relatively short distances (under 300 miles or so). Short-field take-off and landing capabilities, and the ability to use kerosene instead of aviation fuel, had contributed to the popularity of turboprops, particularly in developing countries.

[8]Dr. Bruce Holmes led the Small Aircraft Transportation System Program (SATS) unit at NASA. SATS was a driving force in the incubation of innovative technologies necessary to bring affordable, on-demand flight service by small aircraft in near-all-weather conditions to small community airports.

[9]Initial deposits to secure a delivery position for an A-500 were between $50,000 (non-escrowed) and $100,000 (escrowed). An additional $50,000 progress payment would be due at aircraft type certification, with an additional $100,000 progress payment due six months prior to the scheduled delivery date of the aircraft. The balance would be due upon delivery.

KRCB Television and Radio: The Canary in the Coal Mine?

Armand Gilinsky Jr.
Sonoma State University

Teresa M. Shern
Sonoma State University

Robert H. Girling
Sonoma State University

The October 2003 board meeting had been difficult for Nancy Dobbs, president and CEO of KRCB Television and Radio in California's Sonoma County, and for her board of directors. KRCB had always run on an extremely thin financial margin, and things were not improving. The national Public Broadcasting System (PBS) funding model, based on pledge drives, appeared to be floundering at stations across the country. PBS and the Corporation for Public Broadcasting (CPB) were working against the clock to make necessary, and as yet unknown, course corrections. All PBS stations, particularly those small stations competing with larger public broadcast stations in major markets, were scrambling to find answers. The KRCB-FM pledge drive had significantly missed its goal, as had pledge drives at other National Public Radio (NPR) stations across the San Francisco Bay Area. On the television side, KRCB faced increased fixed operating costs to support its new digital transmitter. Meanwhile, noncommercial and commercial television stations alike were in danger of losing their audiences because the fundamental television broadcast model of distribution was changing. TiVo and other devices with the ability to cut out commercials and pledge drives had already come into widespread use.

This case was presented at the annual meeting of the North American Case Research Association, October 7–9, 2004, Sedona, Arizona, and also was published in the Winter 2005 issue of the *Case Research Journal.* Copyright © 2005 by the case authors. All rights reserved by the case authors and NACRA.

Walking from the portable building that housed the station to her car, Dobbs turned to her business manager, Jane Kirchman, and said:

> KRCB is my "second family," but how long can we continue to stay together? Support from the business community, especially in the form of program underwriting by local businesses, has taken a serious hit across the system in the past year. TiVo is a major threat to our fund raising model. And now we are facing competition from other Bay Area public broadcasters who really should be working together with us, instead of vying for our members and underwriting support. It's becoming increasingly likely that our station will need to undertake an expensive purchase of our leased land or move the broadcasting studios and offices within the next three to four years. We are like the canary in the coal mine. If smaller stations like ours cannot survive, then what will happen to the entire public broadcasting system?

Contributing to Dobbs's stress at the board meeting had been the irrefutable fact that the operating budget was precariously lean. The station did not have any cash reserves; it was operating hand to mouth, according to the preliminary year-end financial reports that Kirchman had prepared. Dobbs felt strongly that these budget weaknesses needed to be addressed and reconciled if the station was to survive. The precarious financial situation, in particular with respect to support for the radio station, also prompted Dobbs to reassess KRCB's current strategy. As Dobbs opened the door of her 1987 Volvo and wearily sank into the driver's seat, she wondered which challenge she needed to tackle first.

PUBLIC BROADCASTING: MARKETS AND COMPETITION

KRCB was an affiliate of PBS, which consisted of 170 noncommercial television stations in the United States, and NPR, which comprised 730 noncommercial radio stations nationwide. The station transmitted both television and FM radio programming. Its television signal was available to cable and satellite TV subscribers throughout the North Bay and the greater San Francisco Bay Area. Due to "must-carry" laws that required KRCB-TV to be carried over cable, EchoStar's Dish Network, and DIRECTV, station management believed it had an opportunity to widen both its audience and its potential membership and underwriting base. On June 1, 2003, Comcast, the local cable provider, began carrying KRCB-TV in San Francisco; as a result, KRCB did indeed witness an increase in its membership base.

The station competed directly with four educational TV broadcast stations and 15 public radio stations. Indirect competitors in the Bay Area, the nation's fifth-largest commercial media market, consisted of 15 commercial television stations and 21 commercial radio stations, according to Nielsen Media Research. KRCB-TV (cable, satellite, and broadcast Channel 22) aired a mix of local programs and those produced by other public and international television stations (see www.krcb.org/television/index.html for TV programming information). Prominent local public television competitors included KCSM-TV in San Mateo, KTEH-TV in San Jose, and KQED-TV in San Francisco (see Exhibit 1). Although each public television station felt it had a distinct programming niche, all were affiliated with PBS, airing at least the "marquee" PBS-produced programs, such as *Sesame Street* and *The NewsHour with Jim Lehrer,* as well as independently made programs. These stations competed for similar viewing audiences, and an increasing portion of their viewing audience markets overlapped.

On the radio side, KRCB-FM broadcast on 91.1 and 90.9. Its blend of locally produced and national programming reflected an eclectic format, ranging from news to classical to jazz to bluegrass to rock

music (see www.krcb.org/radio/index.htm for radio programming information). The station competed for listeners and members with KCSM-FM (91.1, primarily jazz); KQED-FM (88.5 and 88.3, exclusively news and talk); and nonprofit Pacifica Radio's Berkeley station, KPFA-FM (94.1, wide range of music and news). The latter two stations had broadcast signals strong enough to reach most of Northern California. KRCB's radio station also competed with 16 other local FM radio stations in Sonoma County, five of which were locally owned and one of which was a college station.

KRCB-FM had filed applications with the Federal Communications Commission (FCC) in 1997 and 1998 for a new broadcast license that would enable it to transmit at a higher level of power. The intent was to move broadcasts from 91.1 to 88.3 FM, the latter a "clear" frequency in Santa Rosa, the largest city in Sonoma County. Stockton Christian College won the license and then sold it in 2001 to KQED-FM, which received permission from the FCC to erect a new transmitter in Santa Rosa, thus enabling its San Francisco–based broadcasts to reach the entire North Bay.

In February 2003, KQED-FM announced that it had acquired a Sacramento public FM station, KQEI (89.3), for $3 million, boosting its coverage area to the rapidly growing counties in California's Central Valley (see Exhibit 2).[1] Subsequently, in July 2003, KQED announced a budget reduction of $4 million, layoffs of 10 percent of its staff, and a reduction of workweeks from 40 to 36 hours for its remaining 234 employees. According to a report in the *San Francisco Chronicle,* these layoffs, hour reductions, and other changes were expected to trim KQED's operating budget from $44.7 million in 2002 to $40.5 million in 2003.

KRCB-FM's radio broadcast signal did not reach beyond Sonoma and Marin counties (the latter via cable). Dobbs still hoped to boost the signal via a translator on Sonoma Mountain, the highest peak in Sonoma County. "Our application to the FCC for the translator has been pending for a number of years, but the slowness with which the FCC moves has been a big roadblock to improving our signal." Meanwhile, plans were under way to begin offering radio broadcasts to a potentially vast audience via streaming audio online in November 2003. On the air, however, the station's broadcasts often overlapped with those of San Mateo Community College's radio station, KCSM-FM. Both radio stations broadcast on 91.1 FM.

As a stopgap, KRCB-FM tried to improve its signal to reach a greater number of Sonoma County

Exhibit 1   **Profiles of Public TV and Radio Broadcasters in the San Francisco Bay Area**

	KRCB	KCSM	KTEH	KQED
Nonprofit organization	Yes	Yes	Yes	Yes
TV station	Yes	Yes	Yes	Yes
Broadcasting debut	1984	1964	n/a	1954
Areas served (counties)	• Alameda • Contra Costa • Marin • Mendocino • Napa • San Francisco • San Mateo • Solano • Sonoma	• Alameda • Contra Costa • Marin • Napa • San Francisco • San Mateo • Santa Clara • Santa Cruz • Solano • Sonoma	• San Francisco • San Jose	• North to Mendocino • South to Monterey • East to Lake Tahoe • Portions of Nevada
PBS programming	Yes	Yes	Yes	Yes
Programming focus	• Child and adult viewers • GED courses • PBS, BBC, APT programs • Local programs	• Adult viewers • College-level telecourses • PBS programs • Local programs	• Child and adult viewers • Community outreach • PBS, nationwide distributors • Local programs	• Child and adult viewers • PBS, nationwide distributors • Local programs
Number of viewers	n/a	500,000	n/a	5,000,000
Digital broadcasting?	November 2003	November 2003	November 2003	May 2000
Radio station	Yes	Yes	No	Yes
Broadcasting debut	1990	1964		1969
Areas served (counties)	• Sonoma • Marin	• San Francisco • Peninsula • South Bay Area		• North coast of CA • South to Monterey • East to the Sierra Nevada mountains
NPR programming	Yes	Yes		Yes
Programming focus	• Classical music • NPR news • Local music • Local information shows	• Jazz music • Jazz education • NPR news		• News and information • NPR, PRI, BBC
Number of listeners	n/a	200,000		745,000
Web streaming	November 2003	Yes (1999)		Yes (2000)
Operations				
Headquarters	Rohnert Park	San Mateo	San Jose	San Francisco
Web site	www.krcb.org	www.kcsm.org	www.kteh.org	www.kqed.org
Membership program	Yes	Yes	Yes	Yes
Volunteer program	Yes	Yes	Yes	Yes
For-profit ventures	No	n/a	Yes (partnership with barnesandnoble.com)	n/a

n/a = Not available or not applicable.

Sources: Information posted at www.krcb.org, www.kcsm.org, www.kteh.org, and www.kqed.org.

Exhibit 2   **Forecast Population Growth in Northern California, 2000–2040**

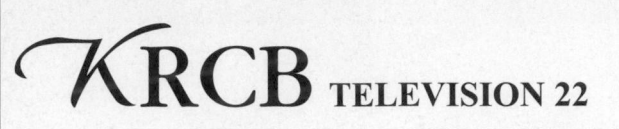

Television Coverage Map

Comcast Cable in Santa Rosa - Cable Channel 8
Sonoma, Napa, Marin, SF, Contra Costa, Solano & Almeda
Counties - Cable Channel 22
Satellite: EchoStar - 8233 & DirectTV - Channel 22

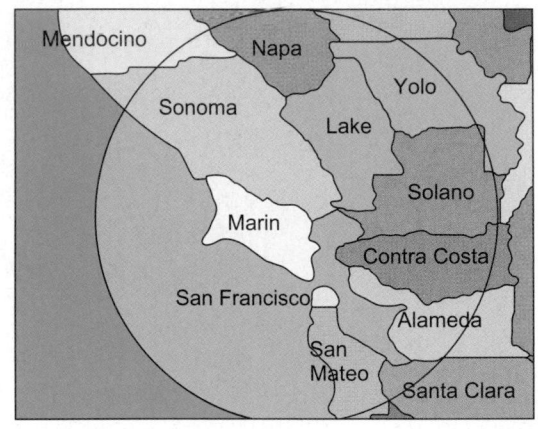

KRCB Public Television 22 and Radio 91
5850 Labath Avenue, Rohnert Park, CA 94928
707-585-8522   www.krcb.org

County	Forecast Population Change 2000–2040	County	Forecast Population Change 2000–2040
Alameda	41%	San Francisco	(−14)%
Contra Costa	36	San Joaquin	116
Lake	113	San Mateo	26
Marin	20	Santa Clara	47
Mendocino	66	Santa Cruz	91
Merced	114	Solano	75
Monterey	113	Sonoma	64
Napa	51	Stanislaus	118
Sacramento	75	Yolo	82
San Benito	122		

Source: Association of Bay Area Governments, www.abag.ca.gov/abag/overview/pub/p2000/intro.html.

listeners by installing a second signal (with its own transmitting antenna) on 90.9 FM. Even then, the radio station was only licensed to broadcast at 125 watts (effective radiated power) on either 90.9 or 91.1. At 125 watts, KRCB's signal was roughly the amount of power one might get from a common lightbulb. The station's low power had been mandated by the FCC's licensing rules and regulations, which remained in place to protect KCSM-FM's much stronger signal. Other regional, low-power noncommercial FM radio stations included KWMR, broadcasting from Point Reyes Station and Bolinas (Marin County); KMUD (broadcasting in Humboldt, Northern Mendocino, and Western Trinity counties); and KZYX (serving Mendocino County and beyond).

Emerging Technologies

In addition to rival broadcasters, print media, and other formats for news, education, arts, and culture, KRCB faced competition from the Internet and digital transmission via satellite. By July 2003, 80 percent of Americans had access to the Internet from at least one location. Edison Media Research estimated that the weekly Internet broadcast TV and radio audience had reached 30 million, or 30 percent of all Americans.[2] According to Edison Media Research, approximately 50 million Americans, or 21 percent of the adult population, watched video online or listened to audio online in 2003. Listeners tuned in most frequently to the Internet to hear radio formats such as alternative rock, urban, contemporary hit radio, and public radio (see Exhibit 3).

On the television side, the Internet video audience experienced significant gains in 2003, growing to 12 percent of the total video audience, according to the Nielsen Television Index (NTI). Movie trailers and music videos were the most-watched online video programming in 2003. In addition to Internet video, the penetration of subscriber satellite television had grown steadily from 18 percent in July 2001 to 22 percent in July 2003.[3]

Satellite radio represented a more distant threat to traditional "terrestrial" radio broadcasters.[4] The two leading satellite radio companies were XM Satellite Radio Holdings Inc. (partly owned by General Motors and Honda Motor) and Sirius Satellite Radio

Inc. Each satellite station provided about 100 channels of music and other uninterrupted, static-free programming with limited commercials. Unlike terrestrial radio, however, satellite radio services depended on a subscription model. As of June 2003, XM (70 music channels) and Sirius (61 music channels) had approximately 692,000 and 105,000 subscribers, respectively, charging monthly rates of $9.99 and $12.95. Both companies believed that building strong ties with automobile manufacturers would be critical to establishing satellite radio as a potential alternative to terrestrial broadcasting. Both GM and Honda had plans to add factory-installed XM satellite radios in select 2003–2004 models; Sirius already had deals with DaimlerChrysler, Ford, and BMW.

Government Regulation and Digital Conversion

Upon congressional passage of the Telecommunications Act of 1996, the FCC required all commercial broadcasters to convert from "legacy" analog systems to all-digital programming known as high-definition television (HDTV). Digitalization enabled the transmission of either HDTV signals or multiple program streams. With up to 10 times the resolution of standard analog television signals, digital formats generated much sharper picture quality. However, optimal HDTV picture clarity required that digitalization be used throughout the system. HDTV also required using the entire digital broadcast bandwidth as a single program stream, which precluded broadcasters from transmitting multiple digital program streams. TV stations must broadcast in digital format, programs must be transmitted digitally via cable or satellite, and reception must be digital (see Exhibit 4 for a schematic diagram).

The deadline for commercial broadcasters to convert to HDTV was May 2002, and for noncommercial broadcasters, May 2003. Since not all of the estimated 1,300 commercial TV stations could meet the original deadline set by the FCC, the build-out deadline was extended to May 1, 2003. Of the estimated 900 noncommercial stations, 215 applied for extensions to convert from analog to digital beyond the May 1, 2003, deadline; 212 extensions were granted, and KRCB-TV's was among them. A new deadline for noncommercial stations was set

Exhibit 3   **Media Usage by U.S. Internet Users, July 2000–July 2003**

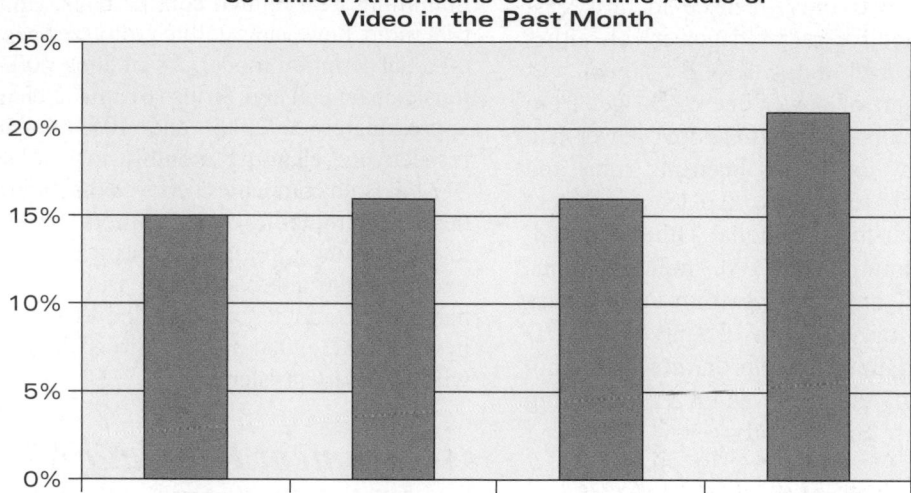

50 Million Americans Used Online Audio or Video in the Past Month

. . . and they listened to:		. . . and they listened to:	
Contemporary hit radio	26%	Other	13%
Public radio	22	Country	13
Alternative rock	20	Oldies	11
Urban	18	Big band	8
Religious	18	Jazz	7
News/talk	18	Classical	7
AOR	17	Spanish programming	6
AC	15		

Source: Internet and Multimedia II: New Media Enters the Mainstream (Arbitron/Edison Media Research).

for November 7, 2003. After that date, noncompliant stations faced fines or revocation of licenses.

Aside from picture quality, one of the most important benefits of HDTV was that it freed up parts of the broadcast spectrum and allowed its return to the government for other important uses such as public safety, police, and fire. Congress hoped to auction off the returned analog channels to help balance the federal budget, and subsequently introduced legislation to force a return of the analog spectrum to the government by December 31, 2006. However, to get the full benefits of HDTV after 2006, consumers would have to buy HDTV-ready receivers and monitors. Retail prices in 2003 for HDTV-ready receiving equipment ranged from $1,500 to $2,000. As a consequence,

penetration of this technology was projected to reach about 5 million HDTV units, or only 5 percent of all U.S. TV households in that year, according to data reported by Standard & Poor's in November 2003.

Radio was also going digital. In October 2002, the FCC endorsed a technology for radio stations to begin the conversion from analog to digital broadcasting. The commission's decision opened a transition path for public radio stations to expand and enhance their service to listeners, using digital broadcast technology to carry two or more streams of programming on the same channel, or frequency. Dobbs commented, "One of the promises of digital conversion [in radio] is that you can broadcast several streams, that is, separate channels. KCSM-FM has

Exhibit 4   **Schematic of Sample HDTV Receiving Apparatus**

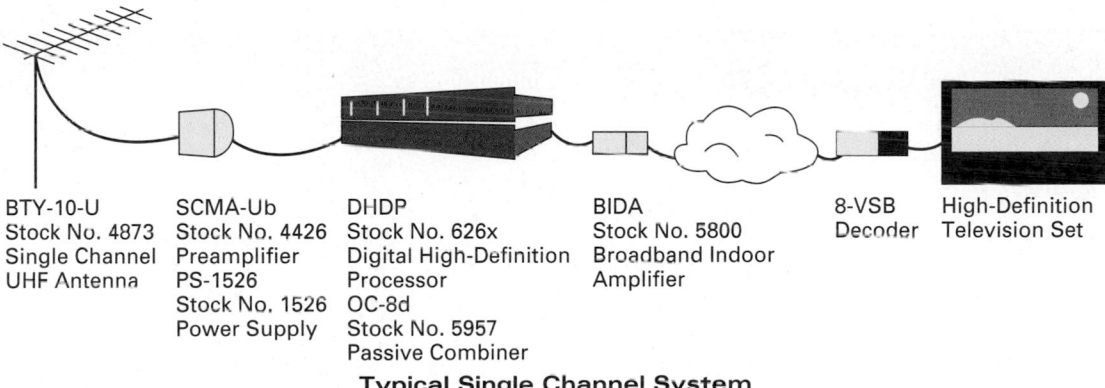

BTY-10-U	SCMA-Ub	DHDP	BIDA	8-VSB	High-Definition
Stock No. 4873	Stock No. 4426	Stock No. 626x	Stock No. 5800	Decoder	Television Set
Single Channel	Preamplifier	Digital High-Definition	Broadband Indoor		
UHF Antenna	PS-1526	Processor	Amplifier		
	Power Supply	OC-8d			
	Stock No. 1526	Stock No. 5957			
		Passive Combiner			

Typical Single Channel System

Source: www.blondertongue.com/pages/products/HDTV-processor_DHDP.php.php.

called us to ask if we want them to carry our signal on their second channel but the problem is that no one has digital radios, yet."

Kevin Klose, president and CEO of National Public Radio, estimated that the average cost of converting public radio stations to digital programming would be about $150,000. By comparison, the cost of providing the 90 public radio FM stations serving 25 top U.S. markets with another signal in the traditional but more burdensome fashion of acquiring a new channel was estimated by Klose to be between $250 and $300 million. The high cost of new station purchases enhanced the appeal of digital radio to public radio broadcasters, as that technology promised to be more affordable and cost-efficient.[5]

Viewer and Listener Demographics

Reliable and current demographic data regarding KRCB's members and audiences were not available to KRCB's management team. The station could not afford to buy ratings reports—at a cost of approximately $45,000 per year—from either of the two major media ratings services, Nielsen (a New York–based television ratings service) or Arbitron/Scarborough Research (a New York–based radio tracking and market data service). On an interim basis, KRCB hired a local survey research firm to gather data on demographics and viewing habits. The results

of this survey indicated that KRCB's audience tended to closely mirror the audiences of PBS and NPR, which reflected the social and economic makeup of the nation.

Exhibit 5 provides a breakdown of the full-day public TV audience for an average week from October to December 2002.[6] On the radio side, National Public Radio (NPR) attracted an audience that it perceived as thoughtful and discerning consumers, savvy business leaders, and influential and active community members.[7] The most recent national NPR audience profile is shown in Exhibit 6.

To reach and serve an estimated 250,000 people in the community who could not receive PBS programs from other stations, KRCB staff and volunteers worked hard to dispel the notion that the station targeted only the elite and highly educated segments of the population. KRCB sought to make culture and education more accessible to everyone in its signal range, and to broadcast local programs that met the unique needs of its North Bay community, including Spanish-language programming, quality children's programming, college courses, and adult literacy programming.[8]

KRCB'S HISTORY

Early in 1981, the North Bay counties of Sonoma, Marin, and Napa enjoyed the largest population growth spurt in their collective histories. At that time, a small group of citizens banded together to create a

Exhibit 5   **The Public Television Audience in the United States (average week, October–December 2002)**

Characteristic	Percentage of U.S. TV Households Watching Public TV	Percentage of Total TV Audience Watching Public TV
Race*		
Black	12.0%	10.7%
Spanish origin	9.1	8.5
Education*		
Less than 4 years of high school	14.9%	14.6%
4 years of high school	30.5	29.1
1–3 years of college	27.6	27.4
4+ years of college	27.0	28.9
Occupation*		
Professional/owner/manager	25.8%	25.1%
Clerical and sales	16.3	15.9
Skilled and semiskilled	26.7	23.9
Not in labor force	31.2	35.2
Household Income*		
Less than $20,000	20.0%	19.7%
$20,000–$39,999	23.9	23.3
$40,000–$59,999	18.2	18.0
$60,000+	37.9	39.0
Age—Children		
2–5	5.7%	9.0%
6–11	9.0	8.3
12–17 (teenagers)	9.1	4.7
Age—Women		
18–34	12.0%	8.3%
35–49	12.0	11.8
50–64	8.7	10.1
65+	7.1	11.3
Age—Men		
18–34	11.8%	7.4%
35–49	11.5	11.3
50–64	8.0	9.7
65+	5.1	8.2

*Head of household.
Source: Nielsen Television Index, March 2003.

Public Broadcasting station as a means to preserve, shelter, and protect their sense of community and local identity. In January 1981, the Rural California Broadcasting Corporation (KRCB) was incorporated in Rohnert Park, California, as a 501(c)(3) nonprofit organization.[9]

According to Dobbs, "The City of Rohnert Park was bemused by us. A non-profit organization didn't make sense in a city that had been developed and run primarily by leaders from the business sector." Once the land was secured, the next issue became how to get buildings on the

Exhibit 6   **National Public Radio (NPR), Nationwide Audience Profile, 2002**

	Demographics*		Lifestyles†
54%	**Men**	**76%**	**Public involvement**
	46% women		62% vote
67%	**Aged 25 to 54**		15% fund-raising
	24% aged 18 to 34	**51%**	**Theater/concert/dance**
	50% aged 35 to 54		31% attend live music performances
58%	**College degree or beyond**		65% dine out
	28% graduate school attended/degree		55% read books
73%	**Household income $50,000+**	**55%**	**Regular fitness program**
	49% HHI $75,000+		26% swim
	(mean HHI $85,675)		45% walk for exercise
64%	**Married**	**41%**	**Own financial securities**
	22% single		30% own stock/bond mutual funds
76%	**Employed**		20% own common/preferred stocks
	28% professional	**86%**	**Household owns computer**
	16% managerial		92% use online service
	35% business purchases	**74%**	**Domestic travel**
	57% view job as "career"		40% foreign travel over past 3 years

Base: Adults 18+ who listen to an NPR station.
*Reads: Over half (54%) of NPR listeners are men, etc.
†Past-year activities.
Source: MRI, Fall 2002.

property. Station funding was non-existent, and this meant that a creative solution was in order. Through legwork and strong community ties, a staff member identified a former drug rehabilitation center located just to the south in Marin County that had gone bankrupt. This company had several portable buildings and since their need for them had run out, they donated them to the station. These portables formed the core of the station's infrastructure. In 1983, the station obtained a 40-year lease from the City of Rohnert Park, with an option to purchase the land should the city eventually decide to sell.

President and CEO of the station since its founding, Dobbs had moved to Sonoma County in 1972 and worked in health care and as a legislative staffer during her previous careers. A former field representative for California legislator Barry Keane, Dobbs had left her position as house committee analyst and come to KRCB at age 35, bringing with her extensive experience in legislature, government, the media, and fund-raising. Paula Wrenn, writing in *North Bay Biz,* noted: "As the station had yet to grow grassroots or construct even a ground floor, her

[Dobbs's] skills were far more important than broadcast experience during the planning stages."[10]

Dobbs and her founding team considered the launch of the television station opportunistic. Because a frequency was immediately available for television in Sonoma County, KRCB-TV had gone on the air before the FM radio station. Dobbs recalled, "Shortly after KRCB-TV signed on the air in December 1984, we received our first donation. It was 35 cents taped on a piece of cardboard from a little boy in Glen Ellen, California. 'Finally,' he wrote, 'I can see *Sesame Street.*' We should have saved it but we needed the money."

KRCB-TV had been created to serve three specific purposes. Its primary purpose was to extend public television to 250,000 people in the region who had previously been unable to receive a signal from distant Public Broadcasting System (PBS) stations. Its secondary purpose was to extend an educational television signal to the many schools then outside the existing signal range of the other public stations. Finally, KRCB intended to provide as much local programming as possible. Volunteer producers, directors, and camera people stepped forward to run the television station and produce the local programming that would be the hallmark of the station's early years.

During the next decade, as the television station grew and achieved financial stability, the station's board of directors started to plan for a sister radio station. "It was quite remarkable that a county the size of Sonoma County did not have its own public radio station," Dobbs recalled. When a noncommercial frequency became available in 1991, the board set to work putting together a radio station to fill this void. Almost on the very day KRCB-FM signed on the air, a popular Bay Area classical station signed off the air, leaving the greater Bay Area without a source for classical music. Seizing the opportunity, the station began to offer classical music as its core program schedule, bracketed by NPR news feeds and local music and information shows. Once again, as with its television launch, volunteers helped build and staff the radio station.

KRCB-FM positioned itself as the North Bay's classical music station; Dobbs assumed that the station's listeners were expected to be similar to the NPR classical audience profile shown in Exhibit 7. Just 50 miles north of San Francisco, Sonoma County was best known for its agriculture (dairy and grapes), tourism, and technology in Telecom Valley, a spin-off of the famed Silicon Valley. Rohnert Park, where KRCB was based, was a town with a population of 42,000, in the growing and increasingly affluent Sonoma County region. Exhibit 8 shows recent population data for Sonoma County in comparison to other counties in the KRCB's viewing audience area.

Operations and Staffing

KRCB's portable buildings housing its studios and offices in Rohnert Park were old and modest, surrounded by vacant fields. Originally, the station shared a parcel of land that was also used by the minor league baseball team, the Sonoma County Crushers. The Crushers dissolved after the 2002 season, and the fate of the stadium and surrounding land was in the hands of the City of Rohnert Park. The city signed an exclusive option that would permit the development of additional big-box retailers on the site. Costco had in 2002 completed

Exhibit 7   **National Public Radio (NPR), Classical Music Audience Profile, 2002**

	Demographics*		Lifestyles†
51%	**Men**	83%	**Public involvement**
	49% women		69% vote
61%	**Aged 25 to 54**		14% fund-raising
	16% aged 18 to 34	56%	**Theater/concert/dance**
	51% aged 35 to 54		37% attend live music performances
63%	**College degree or beyond**		70% dine out
	32% graduate school attended/degree		64% read books
80%	**Household income $50,000+**	56%	**Regular fitness program**
	54% HHI $75,000+		29% swim
	(mean HHI $91,933)		49% walk for exercise
71%	**Married**	53%	**Own financial securities**
	16% single		37% own stock/bond mutual funds
74%	**Employed**		23% own common/preferred stocks
	30% professional	87%	**Household owns computer**
	17% managerial		94% use online service
	33% business purchases	81%	**Domestic travel**
	58% view job as "career"		44% foreign travel over past 3 years

Base: Adults 18+ who listen to an NPR classical station.
Reads: Over half (51%) of NPR classical music listeners are men, etc.
† Past-year activities.
Source: MRI, Fall 2002.

Exhibit 8   **Bay Area Population Estimates as of January 1, 2003**

Bay Area County	Population
Alameda (Oakland/Berkeley)	1,496,200
Contra Costa	994,900
Marin	250,400
Napa	129,800
San Francisco	791,600
San Mateo	717,000
Sonoma*	472,700

*Since 1980, Sonoma County had enjoyed an average annual increase in population of 7,923 (2.1%). From 1993 to 2002, the county witnessed a population growth of 14.7%; from 2001 to 2002, its population increased by 6,700 (1.4%). The population of Sonoma County was expected to increase to 498,600 (1.7%) in 2005, and to 541,100 (1.6%) in 2010.

In 2000, those who attended some college but did not graduate were the majority in both Sonoma County and California, at 27.9% and 24.3%, respectively.

In 2002, 40–49-year-olds accounted for 17.0% of the county's population, more than any other age group. The 40–49 age group was expected to account for 12.7% of the county's population in 2005, and 16.9% in 2010.

In 2002, Sonoma County's population by race/ethnicity could be described as largely white (80.7%) followed by Hispanic (13.3%), Asian (3.6%), African American (1.5%), and American Indian (0.92%). Hispanics were forecast to represent 28.3% of Sonoma County's population by 2005, and 41.7% by 2010.

The median household income in Sonoma County in 1999 was $53,076, compared to $47,493 in California statewide.

Source: California Department of Finance, Demographic Research Unit.

a new store opening just to the east of the stadium and the station's facilities. Due to Costco's success and in light of a budgetary crisis in 2003, the City of Rohnert Park was publicly reviewing the option to sell the land to developers known to be planning more big-box stores, which would, in turn, lead to increased retail tax revenues. Once the property was appraised, KRCB had a contractual right of first refusal to purchase the land if sufficient financing could be found.

The station's main building conveyed a sense of community, family, and pride. Paintings of Sonoma Mountain by local artist Jack Stuppin decorated the walls. The waiting area was modest, the ceilings were low, and the hallways were maze-like, lending a sense of mystery and curiosity. It was apparent that this organization was running lean financially. A station volunteer commented, "I couldn't help but notice the telephone lines hanging down from the ceiling and the old equipment people were expected to use every day to complete their work. I wonder how KRCB entices people to work there." The station's transmission facility was located in nearby Santa Rosa, on the northernmost fringe of the San Francisco Bay Area.

Station staff consisted of 20.5 full-time equivalent (FTE) employees for television and 9 FTE employees for radio. While several staff members had been with the station since its inception, Dobbs considered volunteers to be a key component of daily operations. The volunteer staff size varied between 3 and 10, depending on the activities occurring at the station at any given time. Volunteers assisted with programming, filing, writing public service announcements, and acting as program hosts ("DJs"). The station also had four to five volunteers who helped with various functions such as landscaping, facilities work, mailing, filing, fielding phone calls, and general office duties. The production department also had a group of volunteers who worked exclusively on special events such as election nights and pledge drives. These volunteers operated cameras, directed programming, and switched programming between live studio action and taped footage.

Coordinating volunteers was vital to the station's operations. Volunteers performed myriad duties at the station; they staffed its television and radio pledge drives, the annual televised auction in April, the wine auction in September, and the travel auction in November. Vanessa Bergamo, KRCB's volunteer and outreach manager explained, "Television has three auctions and four pledge drives per year. They each require phone and support teams as well as production volunteers. Last year we logged 10,000 volunteer hours, the year before 25,000, and this year we are tracking to about 12,000." For each auction, the station needed 21 phone volunteers, 15 support volunteers, and 13 production volunteers over six nights. This was a total of 294 volunteers for one auction. TV station pledge drives required eight phone volunteers, two support volunteers, and six production volunteers over four nights, for a total of 64 volunteers. In addition, two FM radio pledges per year also required volunteer support. Yet recruiting volunteers had become more difficult following the onset of the war in Iraq and the weakened U.S. economy. According to Bergamo, "People were less interested in volunteering due to the war. What I was hearing were people who wanted to 'take care of their own' in a time of uncertainty."

The station was also plagued by turnover of its paid staff. The development director had left one year earlier to pursue other interests, and that position had remained unfilled. In the interim and as part of a cost-savings initiative, Dobbs had assumed those duties on a part-time basis. In early October 2003, just as KRCB was about to enter its fall season for fund-raising, Bergamo, the volunteer coordinator, had given her two weeks' notice.

The station's organization chart, as of November 2003, is shown in Exhibit 9. Dobbs was curious to see the organization charts of other small public broadcast stations to compare staff turnover rates and also how full- and part-time employees were split between television and radio. Dobbs was also interested in other stations' staff sizes versus dollars raised, or versus numbers of members. "I think we're lean and mean because we work like crazy, but are we organized in the best possible way? I just don't know," she lamented.

Leadership and Governance

The station's mission had remained unchanged since its inception: "In order to encourage full participation in society and community, KRCB provides educational, informational, and cultural telecommunication services in partnership with our community." Three key goals associated with the mission statement focused on programming, education, and finances. The station's board of directors sought to promote community awareness of cultural richness and human diversity through the production and broadcast of local, national, and regional programs. The station hoped that its broadcast and nonbroadcast resources would serve students in various and diverse settings. The station's financial objective was to remain a stable and enduring institution by exercising sound financial management.

The station's board of directors functioned as part of the top management team. The board was responsible for setting station policy through strategic planning and tackling tough issues such as radio signal quality, differentiation among stations, and underwriting as a means to raise money (see Exhibit 10). As in most nonprofit organizations, the board was comprised of professionals who were active in the local community (see Exhibit 11). Board members were not required to have any specific qualifications. A passion for public broadcasting and the ability to

attend the board meetings were the only two requirements. Dobbs reflected, "This is a good board. We've had very few times when the situation has been difficult enough that we've actually needed to vote on something. Each member has his or her own style."

Board members served two-year terms with no limit to the number of terms that could be served. When board members joined, Dobbs spoke to them about "the need to be supportive to the station in a level that was clearly meaningful for them." Dobbs expected the board members to act as ambassadors between the station and their respective business and social networks. She appreciated introductions by the board to members of the business community and was comfortable putting herself in the position of asking for donations. Since staffing resources to properly train the board were not available, few board members were actively involved in fund-raising. Unlike many nonprofit boards, KRCB's required no fixed level of personal contribution from board members, and no individual fund-raising quotas had been set. Still, the station's board members had contributed $45,000 from their own pockets over a period of three years for the Capital Campaign, which raised money for the digital conversion.

Dobbs herself was one of only two women on the station's board of directors, which consisted solely of white, upper-income professionals. Dobbs felt that finding a board that was passionate about public broadcasting was the most important factor and that everything else would fall into place. However, when the station applied for certain types of grants, the ethnic makeup of its board was occasionally a hindrance. Dobbs had looked for people from the minority community who were passionate about public broadcasting and could join the team, but had had only limited success. At one point there had been two Hispanic board members, but they had departed by 2003.

Fund-raising

With an annual operating budget of $2.1 million for television and radio, KRCB was considered a small station in the realm of public broadcasting. Statements of activities for fiscal years ended September 30, 2000–2002, are shown in Exhibit 12. Preliminary estimates of revenue and expenses for fiscal year 2003 are shown in Exhibit 13. Approximately 30 percent of KRCB's budget came from membership dollars (about $750,000 per year), 30 percent

Exhibit 9 **KRCB's Organization Chart**

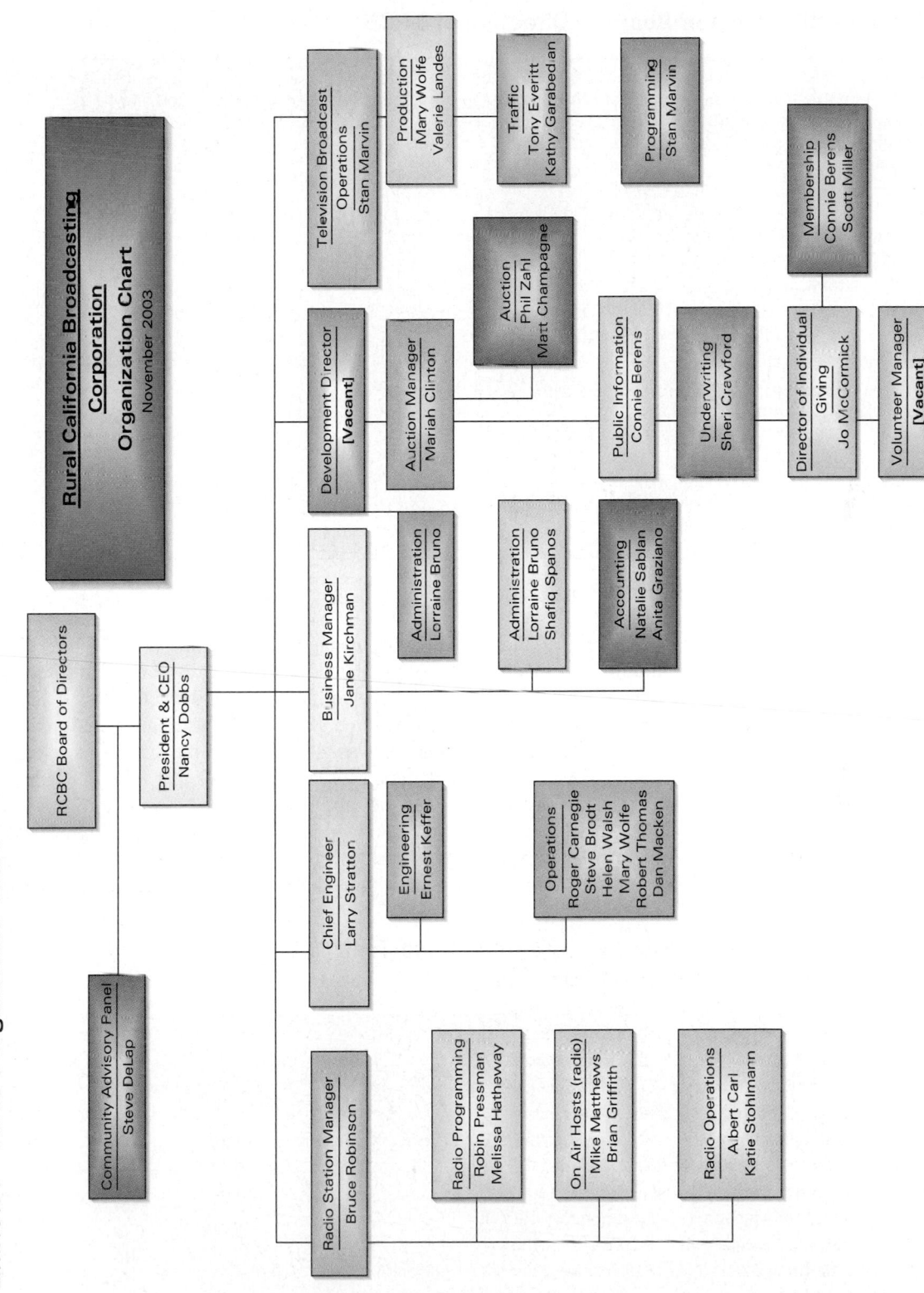

Rural California Broadcasting
Corporation
Organization Chart
November 2003

RCBC Board of Directors

President & CEO
Nancy Dobbs

Community Advisory Panel
Steve DeLap

Television Broadcast
Operations
Stan Marvin

Production
Mary Wolfe
Valerie Landes

Traffic
Tony Everitt
Kathy Garabedian

Programming
Stan Marvin

Development Director
[Vacant]

Auction Manager
Mariah Clinton

Auction
Phil Zahl
Matt Champagne

Public Information
Connie Berens

Underwriting
Sheri Crawford

Membership
Connie Berens
Scott Miller

Director of Individual
Giving
Jo McCormick

Volunteer Manager
[Vacant]

Business Manager
Jane Kirchman

Administration
Lorraine Bruno

Administration
Lorraine Bruno
Shafiq Spanos

Accounting
Natalie Sablan
Anita Graziano

Chief Engineer
Larry Stratton

Engineering
Ernest Keffer

Operations
Roger Carnegie
Steve Brodt
Helen Walsh
Mary Wolfe
Robert Thomas
Dan Macken

Radio Station Manager
Bruce Robinson

Radio Programming
Robin Pressman
Melissa Hatheway

On Air Hosts (radio)
Mike Matthews
Brian Griffith

Radio Operations
Albert Carl
Katie Stohlmann

Source: KRCB, November 2003.

C-263

Exhibit 10   **Statement of Board of Directors of KRCB**

Service on the Board of Directors of Rural California Broadcasting Corporation allows individuals to make a significant contribution to the community of Northern California through development and shaping of telecommunications resources available to and owned by the public (more commonly known as "public broadcasting"). The Board, through stations and resources of which it is the steward, is truly creating the voice and vision of our community.

While the responsibility and satisfaction are notable, Board membership carries no financial remuneration. It is important for all members to understand the particulars of those responsibilities as well as the general mutual expectations that accompany membership with RCBC. In addition to the following points, Board Members should familiarize themselves with the corporate by-laws.

- As with any non-profit Board of Directors, Members are fiscally and legally responsible and liable for the conduct of the corporation. Adequate and timely information will be provided by management as to allow the BOD to make informed decisions. The station carries Officers and Directors Liability Insurance.
- Board Members are expected to attend all Board meetings, serve on Board committees and participate annually in KRCB fundraising and other activities. Board activities normally require four to five hours per month.
- Board Members are expected to support the fundraising efforts of RCBC. Each Member will contribute what is, for them, a substantial donation annually. Each will also actively support the fundraising of the organization in whatever way is best suited to each one.
- Underlying all aspects of participation is of course a strong belief in the purpose and mission of RCBC, and the good-faith assumption that all Members of the Board are operating with the same commitment, concern and level of involvement.

Source: KRCB.

from underwriting, and 30 percent from federal and CPB grants (the State of California did not provide ongoing government funding to public television or radio stations). Revenues from the televised live auctions rounded out the last 10 percent of the budget.

Membership contributions accounted for nearly one-third of station operating revenues. These covered membership expenses such as direct mail pieces (developing, printing, and mailing), telemarketing, thank-you gifts, software, and salaries (administration,

volunteer manager, and graphic artist). The station's nonprofit status meant that all membership fees and donations qualified for tax deductions as charitable contributions. KRCB-FM estimated that its radio audience was 20 percent of the size of its television audience. Moreover, the fact that KRCB-FM's radio signal did not reach beyond Sonoma County and often overlapped with KCSM-FM's signal within the populous southern section of Sonoma County posed a huge challenge in growing the membership

Exhibit 11   **KRCB Board Members and Their Affiliations (as of October 2003)**

Steve De Lap	Santa Rosa Community Access Center, staff
Nancy Dobbs	President and CEO, KRCB
Mark Epstein	California Financial Services, owner
Paul Ginsberg	Attorney
John Kramer	Professor, Sonoma State University, station cofounder
Dan Lanahan	Attorney at law
Carol Libarle	Community volunteer
Michael Musson	Linkenheimer LLP, CPA
Howard Nurse	Engineer (retired)
Marshall Taxer	Flex Products Inc., manager of information systems
David Wolf	The Accrediting Commission for Community & Junior Colleges, retired executive director

Source: KRCB.

Exhibit 12 **KRCB Television & Radio's Statement of Activities, Fiscal Year Ending September 30, 2003, with Comparisons for Fiscal Years 2000-2002**

| | Unrestricted | | Temporarily | | | | |
	Television	Radio	Restricted	2003	2002	2001	2000
Changes in net assets:							
Support and revenue:							
Grants:							
Corporation for Public Broadcasting	$ 322,382	$ 118,013	—	$ 440,395	$ 432,356	$ 423,300	$ 351,319
Corporation, foundation, government, and other	51,820	4,430	—	56,250	544,113	364,152	23,340
Underwriting contributions	400,787	139,755	—	540,542	412,749	359,050	393,978
Membership contributions	538,968	163,902	—	702,870	653,064	677,705	618,611
Capital campaign	—	—	$ 9,722	9,722	40,521	644,592	—
Annual auction and other fundraising activities	218,642	—	—	218,642	228,916	180,231	261,252
Services and other revenues	136,664	24,865	—	161,529	151,161	147,976	156,516
Interest and dividends	6,877	16	7,677	14,570	10,401	8,880	8,967
Net unrealized and realized gains (losses) on endowment	—	—	—	—	—	(5,125)	17,052
Donated goods and services	139,437	31,739	—	171,176	103,159	138,244	169,875
Total support and revenue	1,815,577	482,720	17,399	2,315,696	2,576,440	2,939,005	2,000,910
Net assets released from restrictions	890,826	—	(890,826)	—	—	—	—
Total support, revenue, and net assets released from restrictions	$2,706,403	$ 482,720	$(873,427)	$2,315,696	$2,576,440	$2,939,005	$2,000,910
Expenses:							
Program services:							
Programming and production	$ 315,854	135,082	—	450,936	404,856	463,676	434,786
Broadcasting	404,016	136,818	—	540,834	575,566	471,819	485,508
Program information and promotion	209,921	70,637	—	280,558	168,940	120,806	140,887
Supporting services:							
Management and general	509,037	139,865	—	648,902	587,238	557,530	570,214
Fundraising	462,856	70,302	—	533,258	488,157	464,983	401,294
Total expenses	$1,901,684	$ 552,704	$ —	$2,454,388	$2,224,757	$2,078,814	$2,032,689
Increase (decrease) in net assets	804,719	(69,984)	(873,427)	(138,692)	351,683	860,191	(31,779)
Net assets, beginning of year	639,970	(446,153)	1,386,611	1,580,428	1,228,745	368,554	400,333
Net assets, end of year	$1,444,689	$ (516,137)	$ 513,184	$1,441,736	$1,580,428	$1,228,745	$ 368,554

Source: KRCB.

Exhibit 13   **KRCB TV & Radio's Preliminary Statement of Revenues and Expenses, Fiscal Year Ending September 30, 2003**

	Actual			Annual Budget	Budget Variance	Capital Campaign
	TV	Radio	Total			
Revenue						
Grants—CPB	$ 322,382	$118,013	$ 440,395	$ 413,780	$ 26,615	$116,666
Grants—Other	59,510	4,430	63,940	77,200	(13,260)	0
Underwriting—cash	116,565	67,363	183,928	313,410	(129,482)	0
Underwriting—trade	276,046	71,527	347,573	249,559	98,014	0
Open air—advertising	6,400	1,600	8,000	42,000	(34,000)	0
Membership	511,156	155,182	666,338	714,297	(47,959)	0
Major donors	27,813	8,720	36,533	40,520	(3,987)	450,117
Auction	260,603	0	260,603	301,400	(40,797)	0
Special events	0	4,618	4,618	6,500	(1,882)	0
Creative services	124,072	16,701	140,773	134,600	6,173	0
Miscellaneous	10,782	3,012	13,794	5,220	8,574	7,677
In-kind services	37,294	11,289	48,583	18,282	30,301	0
In-kind goods	5,039	14,595	19,634	700	18,934	0
Total revenue	$1,757,662	$477,050	$2,234,712	$2,317,468	$(82,756)	$574,460
Expense						
Employee expense	$ 723,667	$283,886	$1,007,553	$1,075,500	$(67,947)	$ 35,127
Advertising	176,454	59,784	236,238	192,660	43,578	0
Commissions	5,980	495	6,475	0	6,475	0
Fundraising/events	108,931	11,424	120,355	151,924	(31,569)	0
Insurance	25,122	5,743	30,865	34,416	(3,551)	0
Interest expense	46,389	5,738	52,127	43,400	8,727	0
Land lease	20,033	8,109	28,142	29,136	(994)	0
Maintenance—facility	17,997	4,493	22,490	19,992	2,498	0
Maintenance—equipment	15,503	5,335	20,838	57,108	(36,270)	0
Meetings, travel, mileage	8,969	3,299	12,268	11,250	1,018	0
Miscellaneous	5,814	2,384	8,198	2,400	5,798	0
Office supplies	10,898	2,428	13,326	11,880	1,446	0
Postage & shipping	38,548	7,179	45,727	45,821	(94)	0
Printing	39,634	4,744	44,378	41,075	3,303	0
Production	19,685	0	19,685	4,300	15,385	0
Professional services—L&A	58,636	11,034	69,670	48,399	21,271	0
Professional services—Other	80,360	12,064	92,424	73,744	18,680	0
Program acquisition	148,031	50,780	198,811	205,116	(6,305)	0
Program guide	30,550	7,638	38,188	42,000	(3,812)	0
Pub/sub/dues/fees	21,573	5,737	27,310	24,546	2,764	0
Rental equipment	1,730	319	2,049	3,776	(1,727)	0
Recording materials	7,755	1,243	8,998	27,201	(18,203)	0
Telephone	49,103	19,929	69,032	63,205	5,827	0
Utilities	49,704	6,278	55,982	44,304	11,678	0
Total expense	$1,711,066	$520,063	$2,231,129	$2,253,153	$(22,024)	$ 35,127
Excess of revenue over expense	$ 46,596	$ (43,013)	$ 3,583	$ 64,315	$(60,732)	$539,333

(Continued)

Exhibit 13 **Continued**

	Actual			Annual Budget	Budget Variance	Capital Campaign
	TV	Radio	Total			
Capital expenditures:						
Principal payments			$ 66,482	$63,587	$2,895	
Equipment acquisition			10,219	0	10,219	
Software			0	3,200	(3,200)	
Building/construction			0	0	0	
Total capital expenditures			$ 76,701	$66,787	$9,914	
Cash needed (cumulative)			$ (73,118)	$ (2,472)	$ (70,646)	
Digital capital expenses			$458,464	$ 0	$458,464	$458,464

at KRCB-FM. A related membership challenge was how to retain current members.

New members joined for two reasons: first, because they were excited about a current offer and wanted to take advantage of it while it lasted, and, second, because they were committed to being part of their community and supporting a public institution. This second group of members was much easier to retain. Jo McCormick, KRCB's director of individual giving, believed that most members felt that "civic duty [was] the right thing to do." McCormick had been pleased with the results of the summer and fall pledge drives, but was concerned about retaining these new members. Pledge drives involved special programming on radio and TV as well as teams of volunteers working the phones, in order to take information from callers who wished to join as members or renew their memberships. Local chains such as Deaf Dog Coffee and High Tech Burrito provided coupons for free mochas or burritos as incentives for members to join. Other local firms or anonymous donors provided dollar-for-dollar matches to encourage new members to join.

Annual live fund-raising auctions on KRCB-TV were scheduled three times per year. Fall auctions featured a harvest theme, showcasing locally produced wine and dining. Companies were solicited to donate goods and services for the auctions. Winter auctions featured travel packages to resorts and other destinations near and far. Spring auctions featured leisure and personal pampering products and services, such as spas, massage, and personal care products. Auctions were televised Friday through Sunday nights; as goods and services were introduced, viewers were encouraged to place bids on auction items via telephone. During the live auctions, volunteers from local businesses and other community organizations worked the phone banks, receiving bids and handing those to "runners," who would post the bids on various whiteboards visible to viewers. As the evening progressed and once individual bid boards had closed, another volunteer team called winning bidders to obtain payment information. McCormick explained further, "We're hoping our annual wine and holiday auctions will bring additional bidders from our new broadcasting area. We just don't have the PR budget to get our name out in new markets. At this time, the best we can do is trade air time to make up for the current lack of advertising dollars." Despite this, McCormick stressed that the growing donor base would be a major benefit, in particular to the station's public television audience, as it would eventually provide funds to produce local television programming.

Corporate giving or underwriting provided another third of the station's revenues. In addition to tax incentives, underwriting provided several nonmonetary benefits for its donors. First, public broadcasting members and loyal viewers and listeners who appreciated the broadcasting alternative provided by the station tended to support the businesses and organizations that supported Public Broadcasting. Second, unlike commercial stations, KRCB's non–program content constituted less than five minutes per hour, thereby retaining viewer/listener attention. Third, an organization's presence in local public broadcasting distinguished that organization as one that cared about and supported its community. Finally, for an underwriter, its continued on-air presence helped build name recognition and a positive association in the minds of existing and potential new customers, associates, and employees. The key challenge with underwriting was making organizations recognize these benefits so that they were willing to make sustained contributions.

The remaining third of revenues came from federal grants, separate for television and radio. The largest annual source of grant money was the Corporation for Public Broadcasting (CPB), created by Congress in 1967. The CPB was a private, nonprofit organization that funded over 1,000 public television and radio stations nationwide using an annual appropriation of funds from Congress, which in turn represented 12 percent of public broadcasting's revenues. The CPB provided the largest source of funds for radio programming and television programming for broadcast on NPR and PBS. CPB also led the way for public broadcasting's transition to digital service and digital programming and funded production of innovative educational programming.

According to Dobbs, "KRCB-TV would not have converted if it had not been required." KRCB's cost to get its digital TV transmitter operational was approximately $800,000. Most of this money had been raised from a Capital Campaign that had been launched in 2001, specifically to pay for the digital conversion. The remainder of funding for the project had come from grants provided by the CPB, PBS, and the State of California. In 2001, the State of California had distributed $7 million among 14 public television stations statewide to help fund the digital conversion. In return for state funds, KRCB had promised the state's Office of Emergency Services to make any unused new digital capacity available to the state in the event of emergency.

Larry Stratton, KRCB's chief engineer, said he was unsure "whether [or not] there would be a significant long-term future [for KRCB] in the digital arena." Still, Stratton had been concerned about the state of the station's aging transmission technology for some time. With the exception of an air-conditioning unit, KRCB-TV had already purchased all of the equipment required to broadcast a digital signal, but sufficient funds had not been available to upgrade the entire studio to digital all at once. As old analog equipment broke down, it was being replaced with new digital equipment. So far, the studio equipment had been installed, configured, and operational as the link to the transmitter. By mid-October 2003, the major installation of equipment at the transmitter site was expected to be complete. KRCB-TV scheduled signing on to its new digital signal for November 3, 2003.

In addition to completing the retrofits of new equipment, KRCB's technical staff had to cope with the challenge of learning how to use new technology and master the potential marketing opportunities that accompanied its use. Digital transmission technology not only could offer KRCB potential new revenue streams from licensing unused broadband capacity to other broadcasters but also could incur higher fixed operating costs and unknown variable costs associated with managing those licensed channels.

The station was also exploring the prospects of banding together with other local public broadcasters to help California with some of the projects on the statewide agenda in return for funds. One such mandate was Proposition 10, which provided funds for the education of young people about the dangers of smoking. Dobbs commented, "We're looking to partner to use our air time in a way we have never done before, realizing that we don't want to all look the same. Still, we ought to be speaking with the same voice about the value of public broadcasting in Sacramento [the state capital], San Francisco, and Los Angeles—if we want to get some of these monies."

Underwriting

An underwriter was a third party, typically a local company or foundation, that voluntarily contributed cash or trade (such as printing, mailing, or food for volunteer staff at auctions and pledge drives). Underwriting financed the production and transmission of programming. Underwriters received on-air recognition for their support. Yet tax-deductible donation patterns from underwriters with respect to nonprofit organizations were changing, and not necessarily to the station's advantage. Dobbs had read that one radio station in Los Angeles experienced a 30 percent decline in underwriting during the first nine months of 2003. She believed that the decline in revenues from underwriting was a direct result of the poor state and regional economy; as a result, local businesses did not have excess cash to spend on charitable causes. Dobbs noted that several companies who had funded KRCB-TV for nearly 20 years had decided not to renew their underwriting, instead contributing to other vital community services that had suffered from draconian State of California budget cuts.

Nationwide trends compiled by the Corporation for Public Broadcasting (CPB) showed that the public radio system's "net" revenue had declined since 1999 (see Exhibit 14). Reflecting these trends, on the radio side, KRCB-FM was operating at a loss greater than projected in the budget for 2003. The station's fund balances to fiscal year end September 30, 2003, are shown in Exhibit 15.

Exhibit 14   **Corporation for Public Broadcasting, Systemwide Financial Data, Fiscal Years 1999–2002 ($ in millions)**

	FY 1999	FY 2000	FY 2001	FY 2002
System operating revenue*†	$523	$581	$626	$654
System operating expenses*	509	567	619	655
System net revenue‡	$ 14	$ 14	$ 7	$ (1)
Number of licensees "in the red"	133			142
Number of licensees "in the black"	181			172
Average loss ($000)	$168			$257
Median loss ($000)	$ 67			$ 78
Number of licensees with losses >$1 million	4			7
Number of licensees with profits >$1 million	5			7
Four-year growth (%)				
Operating Revenue				25%
Operating Expense				29%
Programming (two-thirds of expense)				28%
Fund-raising (one-fifth of expense)				37%
Expense growth by function ($ millions)				
Programming				$ 86
Production				58
Broadcasting				21
Promotion				7
Fund-raising and underwriting				34
Management and general				20
Other				5

*Data compiled from 314 CPB radio licensees receiving annual grants of $65,000 or greater.

†Total operating revenue includes reported "in-kind" and "indirect" support.

‡Net operating revenue equals total operating revenue minus total operating expenses, but excludes capital, securities income and endowments.

Source: Corporation for Public Broadcasting, Public Radio Futures Project, www.cpb.org, July 31, 2004.

Still, noncash or trade underwriting (trading on-air acknowledgements for donated goods and services) was running well above what had been budgeted for 2003. Dobbs made a mental note that she would need to work with the KRCB underwriting staff to promote the station in such a way that when the economy turned around, they would be in front of all potential underwriters.

STRATEGIC PLANNING CHALLENGES

As KRCB-TV approached its 20th anniversary and KRCB-FM its 10th anniversary on the air, Dobbs reflected back on the events that had taken place over the years and contemplated the future of KRCB and her role in shaping and guiding that future:

> It's so easy given my upbringing to say, "Aw, shucks, I can't do that." I guess I'm not using the connections in the community as effectively as I could be. The investment the community has made in me the past 20 years needs to be utilized and built upon for expanding the station. This organization has invested in me and has a right to have a payoff, too. False modesty has not got much place here at KRCB. When all is said and done, you have to be able to live with yourself and come to terms with your own strengths and weaknesses.

As Dobbs pulled her car out of the parking lot, she pondered the challenges the station was facing. While locally KRCB had been known as "the little station that could," it was in need of a new strategy and direction.

Exhibit 15   **KRCB Television & Radio's Statements of Financial Position, Fiscal Years 2003 Versus 2002**

| | Unrestricted | | | | |
	Television	Radio	Temporarily Restricted	2003 Total	2002 Total
Assets					
Current assets:					
Cash	$ 53,214	$ —	$ —	$ 53,214	$ 86,457
Accounts receivable	9,358	—	—	9,358	16,393
Grants receivable	—	—	50,000	50,000	501,000
Contributions receivable (net of allowance for uncollectibles of $2,000)	37,159	15,818	—	52,977	55,598
Unconditional promises to give, current portion	—	—	108,100	108,100	118,849
Program license agreements	87,792	23,348	—	111,140	83,314
Prepaid expenses	162,699	23,027	—	185,726	105,184
Inventory	33,565	—	—	33,565	17,346
Total current assets	383,787	62,193	158,100	604,080	984,141
Capital campaign fund	—	—	482,277	482,277	671,450
Unconditional promises to give, net of current portion	—	—	—	—	96,312
Structures and equipment	1,151,459	100,072	—	1,251,531	733,415
Broadcast licenses	908	6,490	—	7,398	10,931
Total assets	$1,536,154	$168,755	$640,377	$2,345,286	$2,496,249
Liabilities and net assets					
Current liabilities:					
Accounts payable	$ 268,499	$ 62,754	$127,193	$ 458,446	$ 370,174
Accrued expenses	51,785	17,629	—	69,414	61,478
Deferred revenue	9,029	—	—	9,029	—
Inter-company payable	(604,509)	604,509	—	—	—
Line of credit	—	—	—	—	50,000
Current portion of long-term debt	28,062	—	—	28,062	57,603
Current portion of obligation under capital lease	1,751	—	—	1,751	9,523
Total current liabilities	(245,383)	684,892	127,193	566,702	548,778
Long-term debt, less current	336,848	—	—	336,848	365,292
Obligation under capital lease, less current	—	—	—	—	1,751
Total liabilities	91,465	684,892	127,193	903,550	915,821
Net assets	1,444,689	(516,137)	513,184	1,441,736	1,580,428
Total liabilities and net assets	$1,536,154	$168,755	$640,377	$2,345,286	$2,496,249

Back in 1997, station management and the board developed the "KRCB Television and Radio 20 Point Strategic Plan," summarized in Exhibit 16. That plan was later revised in March 1998, but had not been revisited since then. Dobbs hoped that a meeting with station staff in early 2004 to update the strategic plan, facilitated by an independent consultant, would be sufficient to satisfy the needs of KRCB and its board. The external facilitator had come highly recommended by one of the board members.

Exhibit 16 **Summary of the "KRCB-TV and KRCB-FM 16 Point Strategic Plan"**

In June 1996, the Board of Directors of KRCB began the process of strategic planning for the next three to five years. The original version of the strategic plan was published on June 7, 1997 and a revision was published on March 4, 1998.

The strategic planning committee arrived at two goals and 16 points or objectives as listed below.

Goal 1: Strengthen the quality, quantity, visibility and support of KRCB's local programs and services.

1. Establish KRCB-TV and KRCB-FM as the cultural voice and educational resource of the North Bay.
2. Establish a highly visible on-air local presence for both TV and radio which differentiates KRCB from other public television and public radio services in our area.
3. Develop KRCB-FM into a full service county-wide station.
4. Serve the programming needs/interests of diverse audiences in our coverage area.
5. Promote KRCB to build audiences, and to secure audience loyalty and support.
6. Expand KRCB's sphere of influence, community connections, and alliances, including possible collaborations.
7. Strengthen KRCB's image.
8. Develop the Board of Directors.
9. Enhance workplace professionalism.
10. Develop volunteer support.
11. Develop membership and increase fundraising capabilities to achieve financial stability.
12. Intensify ties between KRCB-TV and KRCB-FM.

Goal 2: Enhance KRCB's options in providing and responding to new technologies.

13. Prepare KRCB to change from analog to digital (DTV) transmission.
14. Position KRCB to take advantage of its technological assets by means including collaborations and partnerships.
15. Enhance technical facilities and equipment.
16. Establish profit making services.

Source: KRCB.

On the other hand, perhaps the process would be better served by developing an entirely new plan, as if the station were starting from scratch. Either way, Dobbs needed to set a strategic plan in motion in order to ensure KRCB's future as a resource to the community.

Bibliography

Arbitron.com, "Radio Today: How America Listens to Radio." Available at www.arbitron.com/home/content.stm.

Arbitron Radio Research Consortium, Inc., "Top 30 Public Radio Subscribers—Spring 2003." Available at www.RRConline.org.

California Department of Finance, Demographic Research Unit, "California City/County Estimates with Annual Percentage Change, January 1, 2002 and 2003." Available at www.dof.ca.gov/HTML/FS_DATA/profiles/pf_home.htm.

Competitor profiles, 2003, available at www.krcb.org, www.kcsm.org, www.kteh.org, www.kqed.org.

Corporation for Public Broadcasting, "Public Radio Futures Project," July 31, 2004. Available at www.cpb.org.

Digital Television FAQ, DTV Tower Siting Fact Sheet, and RF Guide. Available at www.fcc.gov/mb/policy/dtv.

Dobbs, Nancy. "KRCB: Expanding the Voice and Vision of the North Bay." KRCB handout, 2003.

———, and KRCB staff. Author interviews, August 2003–March 2004, Rohnert Park, CA.

Hand, M., and S. Harmon. "A Most Deliberate Rush for Frequencies." *Current: The Newspaper about Public TV & Radio,* July 26, 2004.

Klose, Kevin. Testimony to House Appropriations Subcommittee on Labor, Health and Human Services, Education and Related Agencies, February 25, 2004. Available at http://appropriations.house.gov/_files/KevinKloseTestimony.pdf

"KRCB Board Members and Their Affiliations." KRCB company information, 2003.

"KRCB/Channel 22 Program Schedule." Available at www.pbs.org/tvschedules/?station=KRCB.

"KRCB Mission Statement." Available at www.krcb.org/inside/mission/htm.

"KRCB Organization Chart." KRCB company information, November 2003.

"KRCB Statement of Board of Directors." KRCB company information, 2003.

"KRCB TV and FM 20 Point Strategic Plan." KRCB company information, 1998.

MRI, "NPR Audience Profile," Fall 2002.

Nielsen Television Index. "Public Television Audience in the United States," March 2003.

"Open Air." KRCB monthly program guide for members, October 2003. Available at www.krcb.org/radio/new schedule.htm.

"The Public Broadcasting Service: An Overview." Available at www.pbs.org/insidepbs/facts/faq1.html.

Rose, B., and L. Rosin. *Internet and Multimedia II: New Media Enters the Mainstream* (Arbitron Internet Broadcast Services and Edison Media Research, 2003).

Sonoma County Economic Development Board, "2003 Sonoma County Economic and Demographic Profile," available at www.sonoma-county.org/edb/Reports.htm.

Standard & Poor's. "Broadcasting and Cable Industry Survey," November 20, 2003, pp. 13–14.

"Who Owns What in the Bay Area." *San Francisco Chronicle,* June 3, 2003, p. A1.

Wrenn, P. "KRCB Turns 20!" *North Bay Biz* 28, no. 8 (July 2003), pp. 62–64.

Endnotes

[1] Opportunities to buy radio stations could be scarce and expensive. There were few or no vacant frequencies left in major radio markets. One reason was that, since the early 1990s, noncommercial religious broadcasters had outpaced public radio's growth and outbid public radio for vacant frequencies. Another reason was cost. In the top 50 markets, single commercial FM stations had sold for an average of about $22.5 million in the three years prior to 2003. In contrast, single AM stations in those same markets sold for an average of about $5.5 million. Noncommercial FM stations were selling in the range of $500,000 to $5,500,000, according to M. Hand, and S. Harmon, "A Most Deliberate Rush for Frequencies," *Current: The Newspaper about Public TV & Radio,* July 26, 2004.

[2] Edison Media Research, based in Somerville, New Jersey, conducted survey research and provided strategic information to radio stations, television stations, Internet companies, newspapers, cable networks, record labels and other media organizations. See www.edisonresearch.com/aboutus.htm.

[3] Nielsen Television Index, *Public Television Audience in the United States, 2003* (March 2003).

[4] Standard & Poor's, *Broadcasting and Cable Industry Survey,* November 20, 2003, p. 13.

[5] Testimony of Kevin Klose, president and CEO, National Public Radio, to House Appropriations Subcommittee on Labor, Health and Human Services, Education and Related Agencies, February 25, 2004, available at http://appropriations.house.gov/_files/KevinKloseTestimony.pdf.

[6] Most recent estimates from Nielsen showed that 70.9 percent of all American television-owning families watched public television in October 2002, with the average home tuning in for approximately eight hours a month. From October to December 2002, 88 million viewers in 50.6 million households watched public TV each week. This represented 47.4 percent of America's 106.7 million TV households. During the October–December 2002 period, public TV's average prime-time rating was 1.7. This rating compared with 1.4 for Lifetime, 1.3 for USA, 1.3 for Nick at Nite, 1.2 for TBS, 1.0 for Fox News, 0.8 for Discovery Channel, 0.7 for CNN, 0.7 for A&E, and 0.6 for the History Channel. Cable TV, available only to subscribers who paid about $600 per year, could be seen by only 82 percent of television owners. Public TV was freely available to 99 percent of all U.S. homes.

[7] According to Arbitron/Scarborough Research, Americans spent about 20 hours per week on average listening to their favorite radio stations in 2002. Radio listening peaked most noticeably during wake-up and commute times at 7:00 a.m. on weekdays and listening remained strong through 6:00 p.m., after which it began to taper off. On weekends, listening was at its highest between the hours of 9:00 a.m. and 3:00 p.m. In general, radio was an out-of-home medium for adults ages 18–64, while those over 65 tended to spend more time listening at home. Adults over 55 accounted for 57 percent of all commercial and noncommercial classical station listeners in the United States. By contrast, about one-third of all news/talk/information listeners nationwide were adults over 65 and over 59 percent were men. The news/talk/information format performed best in the Pacific and New England regions, where 40 percent of listeners had college degrees and 34.6 percent earned more than $75,000 per year.

[8] P. Wrenn, "KRCB Turns 20!" *North Bay Biz* 28, no. 8 (July 2003), p. 63.

[9] 501(c)(3) organizations: This section of the IRS Code exempted corporations and certain trusts from federal income tax. Organizations with 501(c)(3) status were also called *public charities.* Those who contributed money, services, or materials to a recognized 501(c)(3) organization could usually deduct the value of that contribution from their taxable income. The restrictions on deductibility of contributions were less restrictive with 501(c)(3) organizations, than they were with private foundations. The code prohibited the private inurnment from net earnings of any shareholder or private individual. The code also severely limited the activities of 501(c)(3) organizations that were directed at influencing legislation or political campaigns.

[10] Wrenn, "KRCB Turns 20!"

Western States Insurance Agency

Jeffrey Shay
University of Montana

Tony Crawford
University of Montana

Keith Jakob
University of Montana

Sally Baack
San Francisco State University

Ed Kirby, a 38-year-old professor of entrepreneurship and a management consultant, did not know what to expect as he drove into the country club in Missoula, Montana, on March 5, 2003. Larry Gianchetta, dean of the business school where Kirby worked, had asked Kirby to meet with Dennis Toussaint to discuss a potential consulting project. Toussaint was the president and chief executive officer (CEO) of Combined Benefits Management Inc. (CBMI), a wholly owned subsidiary of Blue Cross and Blue Shield of Montana (BCBS-MT) with managing responsibilities for a group of subsidiary companies that included Western States Insurance Agency (WSI). Toussaint had previously been the president and CEO of WSI.

As Kirby approached the table, Gianchetta and Toussaint rose to their feet. Gianchetta shook Kirby's hand and proceeded to make the introductions. The three ordered their lunch, discussed the approaching golf season, and became acquainted. Shortly after finishing their lunch, Gianchetta stood up and said, "Well, I'm going to leave you guys to discuss business here. I have a few appointments that I need to get back for, so I'll see you both later." After Gianchetta left the table, the conversation quickly turned to the impending consulting project. Toussaint described the parameters of the project to Kirby:

> Larry [Gianchetta] suggested that I approach you to do some consulting for us. With the rapidly changing health care environment, Blue Cross and Blue Shield

This case was presented at the Fall 2005 meeting of the North American Case Research Association, October 27–29, 2005, North Falmouth, Massachusetts. Copyright © 2005 by the case authors. All rights reserved.

is concerned about our overreliance on this segment. Therefore, we are exploring other opportunities for diversifying our risk while continuing to grow the company as a whole. Western States Insurance, the agency that I ran a few years ago before selling it to Blue, is seen by our president, Peter Babbin, as the vehicle for that growth. Peter has asked me to examine the possibility of growing Western States Insurance to the revenue level needed to raise additional capital through an initial public offering. This target revenue level not only would allow Western States to go public but also would bring in the capital necessary to continue its growth through acquisition strategy, and in turn allow Blue to underwrite its own insurance policies. That's where you come in. I'd like you to conduct an analysis of our ability to grow from our $21 million revenue level in 2002 to our target revenue level. Here are a few of the parameters for the project. First, in our recent discussions with investment bankers, we were told Western States would need annual revenues of at least $100 million in order to be considered a viable candidate for an IPO. Second, given the rapid changes in the health care industry and Peter's desire to leave the company in good shape when he retires in five years, we'd like to explore completing the IPO in five years. So . . . is this something that you'd be able to do for us? We have board meetings in June and will be discussing our options at that time.

Kirby and Toussaint continued to discuss the project's parameters, access to the appropriate managers to conduct the research, and the fee schedule for the consulting project. Kirby agreed to take on the project, and Toussaint took notes about the materials that Kirby requested to get started. The two agreed to meet again in a few weeks.

BLUE CROSS/BLUE SHIELD MONTANA

Through the subsidiaries of Blue Cross and Blue Shield of Montana (BCBS-MT), customers had the convenience of one-stop shopping for a broad range of insurance, employee benefits, and related services that complemented the company's health care benefit plans. BCBS-MT subsidiaries included Combined Benefits Management Inc. (CBMI), Western States Insurance Agency (WSI), Combined Benefits Insurance Company (CBIC), Health-e-Web, and Insurance Coordinators of Montana Inc. (ICMI). CBMI was set up as a BCBS-MT holding company for several of its Montana businesses, including all those listed above. WSI was a full-service insurance agency with offices located in 17 communities throughout Montana and Oregon (see Exhibit 1). It employed over 145 professionals and served over 60,000 customers. CBIC specialized in providing policyholder services to other insurance carriers and reinsurers. Health-e-Web was an electronic claims clearinghouse for physicians, clinics, hospitals, other health care providers, and third-party administrators. ICMI offered employee benefits including life insurance, long-term and short-term disability, and nursing home/long-term care plans.

WESTERN STATES INSURANCE AGENCY

At the end of 1995, WSI was an insurance agency with nine locations throughout the state of Montana. That would change over the next eight years, with the company acquiring eight agencies. Four of the newly acquired agencies were located in Montana (Kalispell, Stevensville, Great Falls, and Helena). The additional four agencies were located in Oregon and represented the first time that WSI had competed in another state

Exhibit 1   **Western States Insurance Agency Locations in Oregon and Montana, Spring 2003**

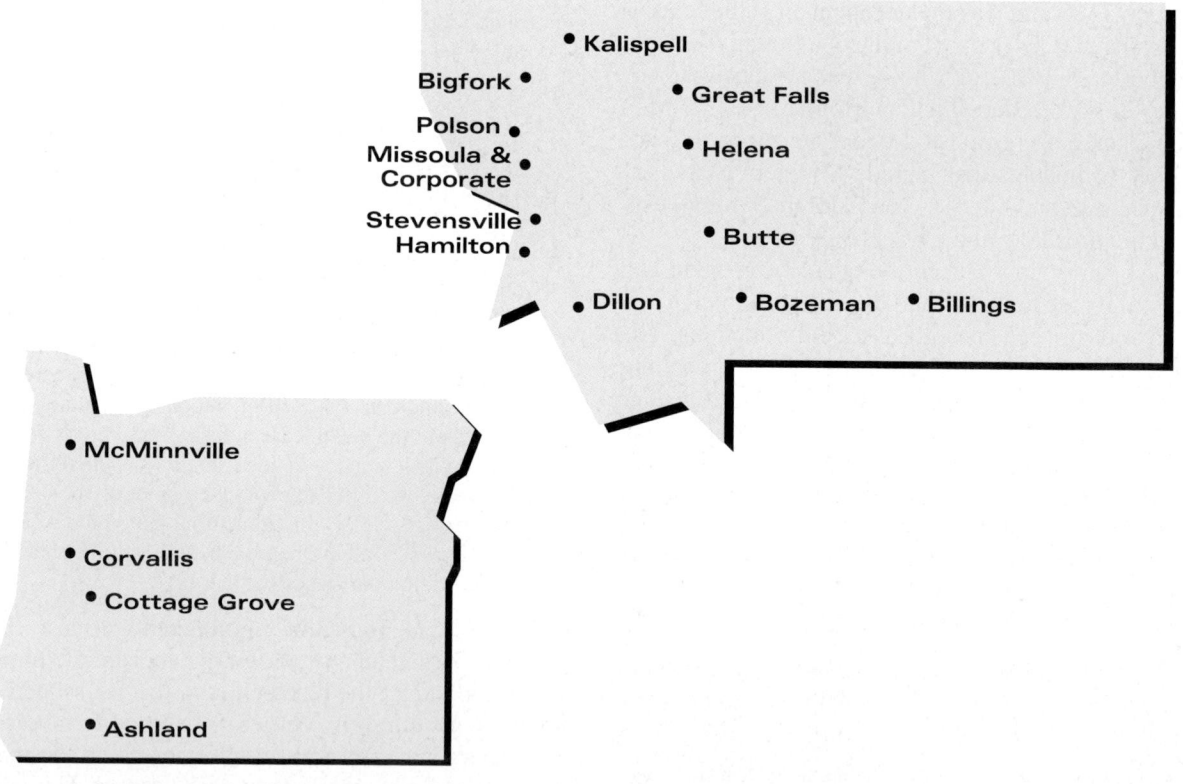

Exhibit 2   **Western States Insurance Agency's Acquisitions, 1996–2003**

Year	Number of Acquisitions	Acquisitions
1996	2	Kalispell and Helena, Montana
1997	0	
1998	1	Great Falls, Montana
1999	0	
2000	0	
2001	2	McMinnville, Oregon, and Stevensville, Montana
2002	2	Cottage Grove and Ashland, Oregon
2003*	1	Corvallis, Oregon

*WSI had already completed the Corvallis transaction, and executives felt they would close the deal on two additional acquisitions by the end of 2003.

(see Exhibit 2 for acquisitions). Though still only a regionally based agency, by 2003 the company had over 200 employees, was in the top 100 largest insurance agencies in the United States, and was the top employees benefits broker in Montana.

The company's Web site stated that WSI was "a growing and diversified insurance agency, focused on a technology enabled, fully integrated delivery of commercial & personal property/casualty insurance, group & individual life & health insurance, employee benefits and retirement planning." The regionally focused agency was capable of delivering high-quality insurance and financial products and services throughout the United States. WSI

executives emphasized the following characteristics to describe what the company was known for:

- Providing exceptional products and services.
- Offering linked solutions to protect and grow clients' assets with insurance, risk management, financial management, and employee benefits.
- Maximizing the value of the total client relationship.
- Using its status as a regional insurance agency with over $100 million in annual premium volume to form strategic alliances with insurance carriers.
- Recruiting top-caliber producers and managers.

The company Web site claimed that WSI's branches were characterized by "strong management, strong market relationships, strong local presence and community involvement, specialized areas of expertise, a history of growth, and broad financial services capabilities." WSI's management structure blended a centralized financial, administrative, and technical structure with a decentralized operating structure that was designed to allow the local branches to respond to the day-to-day needs of their clients. These centralized controls encompassed broad initiatives, such as regional sales strategy and financial reporting that were balanced by the preservation of hometown ethics and entrepreneurial drive.

Over the years, WSI had configured mix of commercial insurance, personal insurance, and financial services that was designed to fully meet its clients' needs. Exhibit 3 illustrates the mix of WSI's products and services. This range of products and services allowed WSI to offer single-source professional services for client insurance, risk management, financial management, and employee benefits programs, including property and casualty insurance; employee benefits; retirement plans; and life, health, and disability plans.

Exhibit 3   **WSI Service and Product Mix**

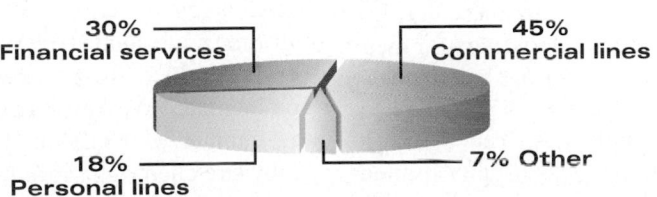

30% Financial services

45% Commercial lines

18% Personal lines

7% Other

WSI'S COMPETITIVE ENVIRONMENT

WSI executives considered the insurance agency industry to be very competitive due to the diversity of competitors and high degree of product and service differentiation. This left the end consumer with a variety of agencies and products (health, property, home, business, life, automobile, etc.) to choose from. Insurance customers also came in a wide variety. For example, large corporations that purchased health care plans for employees and had the ability to negotiate lower rates per individual than the rates available to individual customers. Individual customers had recently gained some advantages as a result of the information available on the Internet. However, customers were still left with few alternatives to the products offered by insurance agencies (e.g., depositing money into a bank account to cover unforeseeable future losses).

Although the industry had recently undergone some consolidation as a result of agencies pursuing acquisition strategies similar to WSI's, there were very few that possessed dominant positions in regional markets. This left many agencies scanning the competitive landscape to see if smaller companies were gaining market presence or if larger companies were expressing an interest in entering their market. After all, getting started required gaining the necessary professional qualifications, establishing a network with larger insurance underwriters, and making capital investments (e.g., renting office space, furnishing it, purchasing computers, and hiring a few employees).

For agencies that were unable to reach the critical mass necessary to underwrite their own insurance policies, securing a larger underwriter was an important first step to starting the agency. The amount of negotiating leverage that an individual agency possessed with these larger underwriters was highly dependent on the size of the agency. As the size of the agency increased, so did its ability to negotiate more favorable terms with underwriters. Smaller agencies often relied on several different underwriters for their policies in order to maintain competitive pricing.

Expansion beyond an agency's established market presented many challenges. The agency's name recognition, for example, was usually limited to its established markets. In addition, agencies were limited by access to underwriters that traditionally focused on specific regions. For example, an agency such as WSI had established relationships with carriers in its region, but many of these carriers did not provide their products and services in other markets. This was primarily because underwriters focused on specific products and services that they knew best. For example, underwriters focusing on the Midwest had expertise in providing insurance for homeowners who faced the threat of tornadoes while underwriters in the Southeast focused on providing homeowner coverage for hurricanes. The focus of these underwriters therefore made it difficult for agencies to penetrate markets in which their underwriters had no market presence because such expansion required establishing a new network with regional underwriters.

WSI'S GROWTH THROUGH ACQUISITIONS

Although the company had undergone rapid growth (from nearly $5 million in revenues in 1995 to just over $21 million in 2003), WSI executives felt that they had maintained the organizational culture. These executives believed they had worked hard and had a vested interest in maintaining the organizational culture they helped create. Accomplishing this while pursuing an aggressive growth through acquisition strategy was considered risky by executives, but they were proud of their success thus far. Bruce Mahelish, president of WSI, explained his philosophy on maintaining the culture as follows: "We try to recruit strong agencies to bring into the WSI family. These agencies usually have highly qualified, experienced employees . . . the type that fit well in our culture and will also help us continue with our growth plans."

WSI's acquisition team included Mahelish; the chief financial officer, Craig Stahlberg; and usually one or two additional senior-level executives. Mahelish estimated that in total approximately two full-time equivalent (FTE) executives were currently being allocated to the acquisition process, but he commented, "We know that we'll need to increase the number of FTEs in the future because we're really stretched right now. I can't imagine increasing our growth rate much more without adding qualified members to our [acquisition] team."

Prospective new branch managers came under close scrutiny by the acquisition team and vice versa. Smaller agency managers typically sought long-term security for themselves and wanted to see their agency survive and thrive beyond their own work lives. WSI offered these managers economies of scale in purchasing and back-office functions, as well as advanced technologies and automation of many labor-intensive procedures. Existing WSI branch managers, in contrast, primarily needed to be assured that the high level of service and support to which they became accustomed would not degenerate as new branches were brought into the fold.

WSI's parent company, BCBS-MT, had its own unique needs with respect to the company's growth plans. BCBS-MT needed WSI to act as the point of its comprehensive strategy. The strategic plan was based on increasing WSI's customer base to the point where BCBS-MT could launch its own underwriting and reinsurance services. BCBS-MT executives believed that this would increase the company's stability and make it better prepared to face any further changes to the industry.

BCBS-MT also had to be concerned with the motives behind the investment bankers that were interested in facilitating the initial public offering (IPO) and accompanying process. Although WSI had a history of growth and a time-proven model of acquisition-fueled growth, the investment bankers needed WSI to be a significantly larger company before entering the IPO process in order for the offering to be attractive on the financial markets. One crucial aspect that investment bankers considered highly important was that WSI needed to establish a presence beyond its current geographic scope (i.e., Montana and Oregon).

WSI'S TARGET MARKET FOR ACQUISITIONS

The market that WSI targeted for acquisitions was small insurance agencies ($500,000 to $2 million) in the northwestern United States. These agencies were small relative to those found in other regional markets and were basing their decisions of whether to be acquired on what was best for them and their company. These agency owners were usually looking for a good exit strategy for their business. "Agency owners have often spent their whole life building up their business,

and it is very difficult to let go. To them, the most important thing is knowing that they are selling the business to a company that will take care of their employees. They need to know that they are leaving the agency in good hands. Of course they are also looking for a fair price for their business because they are often looking at using the money for their own retirement."

Some agency owners were not ready to exit the business right away, so it was very important to them that WSI could offer a smooth transition and still maintain the steady flow of business. Aside from the money, agency owners were looking for extra benefits that they could not get on their own, such as high-tech information systems and economies of scale.

The insurance industry in the United States, and more specifically the Northwest, was fairly fragmented but becoming increasingly consolidated. Medium-sized companies, like WSI, that were acquiring smaller companies, were now being acquired themselves by larger companies like Brown & Brown. In turn, companies the size of Brown & Brown were being acquired by industry leaders such as Aon.

There was an increasing number of large competitors in the Northwest. For example, in 2001, Brown & Brown, based in Tampa, Florida, acquired Raleigh Schwarz & Powell of Seattle, Washington. Raleigh Schwarz & Powell had about $170 million in premiums.[1] Most of the largest competitors that were acquiring agencies in the Northwest were not based in the region.

WHAT WSI OFFERED PROSPECTIVE AGENCY OWNERS

WSI executives felt that they offered value to prospective agency owners in two principal ways. First, WSI offered back-office support activities that it performed for the agency. These support activities involved functional support in areas such as human resources and information technology that smaller agencies often did not have the resources to perform on their own. Second, WSI offered formalized activities designed to support the individual agency's primary, front-office operations such as operations, marketing, and sales.

WSI was able to perform back-office functions on behalf of its agencies because of the economies of scale inherent in an organization of its size. The human resources support helped agencies attract and retain qualified producers and helped facilitate active employee participation in the WSI benefit programs. The types of programs included a generous employee referral program, producer scholarships, various employee education programs and e-access to human resources information by employees.

In the area of technology, WSI often brought a level of automation that a smaller independent agency could not easily achieve or afford on its own. This level of automation enhanced the productivity of an agency's employees and decreased the amount of time it took for a newly acquired agency to be integrated into the WSI family. In addition to a Web-based enrollment system for L&B producers and clients and innovative online training via WebEx, WSI was developing telecommunications solutions that were on the cutting edge of the telecom world. These included building the infrastructure for a Voice over Internet Protocol (VoIP) telecom system for use by distributed customer service centers and developing an e-accounting system for future use in regionalized accounting centers.

WSI was also able to offer its agencies support in their primary activities such as operations, marketing, and sales. Some of these activities existed behind the scenes in the work that the company did to instill the WSI culture into its agencies, the management of its computer network security, and the database-mining support functions that it performed. Other activities such as the formalized sales training program (called CRISP) and the cross-selling program (called Treble-Hook) served to enhance the profitability of the agency and the firm as a whole.

One last set of support functions that WSI performed on behalf of its agencies was its management of its carrier relationships. WSI was able to ensure that an agency could offer a wider range of carriers at more favorable rates than a smaller independent agency. Similarly, a WSI agency could offer its customers a greater variety of ancillary products, which enabled the agency to differentiate itself from its smaller competitors.

Executives noted that the value of these propositions to a given agency is inversely proportionate to the size of agency being considered. Smaller agencies possessed fewer of links in the value chain that WSI offered to them. They likely had no formalized sales or human resource programs and none of the technological automation features that made a WSI agency so efficient. WSI sold prospective agencies

on the idea that they could derive competitive advantage by joining the WSI family. Mahelish noted, "The owners of these smaller agencies are typically less likely to 'shop' their agency to other potential buyers because of the time required for and costs associated with engaging in these activities." These agencies were thus easier to acquire relative to the acquisition of a larger agency that might possess the resources to shop their agency around.

Larger agencies, in contrast, already possessed many of the advantages that WSI had to offer. As such, they generally possessed the resources necessary to use information technology and human resource staff members to enhance the productivity of their employees. For these agencies, the prime motivating factor in an acquisition was cash. As such, these agencies were much more likely to "shop" their agency to several potential buyers, looking for the best overall monetary settlement. This dynamic made an acquisition of larger agencies more difficult, time-consuming, and expensive relative to the acquisition of a smaller agency. "The larger the agency," Mahelish commented, "the more difficult it is for us to get them interested in being acquired by us. The main reason is that we just don't have as much to offer them as we can offer to smaller agencies."

WSI'S COMPETITORS FOR ACQUISITIONS

WSI broke its competitors for acquisitions into two different groups: primary and secondary competitors. Primary competitors consisted of banks and other insurance agencies that competed in the western region of the United States. Banks presented serious concerns for WSI, as they were known to offer 3 to 3.5 times agency revenues for acquisitions, while WSI usually offered between 1.4 and 2 times agency revenues. According to Bruce Mahelish, "Banks have recently realized that they may be overpaying, and we expect them to lower their offering prices soon." When competing with banks for acquisitions, WSI tried to emphasize that it offered significant opportunities for improving the acquired agency, paid producers a much higher commission, and spent a great deal of time and effort courting potential acquisitions to make sure that it represented a strong fit with the organization that they were growing. Mahelish argued that "banks generally have little to offer because they do not understand the agency business. As a result, we think we are in a better position to offer the acquired agency much more than banks can."

A second source of primary competition for acquiring agencies was from other agencies that competed in the potential acquisition's market. WSI's acquisition team believed that this was due to the potential acquisition's desire to sell its business to someone it knew locally. "When we try to make acquisitions outside of our region," Mahelish commented, "we're really at a disadvantage and often end up very frustrated. We'll spend a significant amount of time courting an agency and even reach the stage where we place a deal in front of the owner. Then, the owner will often shop the offer with agencies in their market. If the local agency can come close to matching the bid that we've made, then they'll sign with the local [owner]. This is because we're seen as an unknown . . . as an outsider." As a result, members of WSI's acquisition team believed that they had to stress the technological and economies of scale advantages that WSI had to offer the potential acquisition—something that most local agencies could not offer.

Regardless of whether WSI faced competition from banks or local agencies, the company realized that this type of competition increased significantly as it went into markets outside of its current geographic area. Without brand recognition in a specific market and established trust-based relationships, many agency owners would consider WSI to be an outsider and might choose to sell to local banks or agencies.

In the search for possible acquisitions, WSI also recognized that it was increasingly facing competition from larger companies such as Aon, Marsh & McLennan, Brown & Brown, and Arthur Gallagher (competitors identified by WSI executive team). These competitors were billion-dollar companies that had a great deal of power in the insurance industry. For example, Aon and Marsh & McLennan reported $8.8 billion and $10.4 billion in sales for 2002, respectively. These companies completed acquisitions in the past that ranged from $1 million to billions of dollars. In 1997, Marsh & McLennan acquired Johnson & Higgins for $1.8 billion; and a year later became the largest insurance brokerage company when it acquired Sedgwick Group for $2.2 billion (see Exhibit 4).

Aon was an international company that made acquisitions worldwide. Competitors like Aon also had an advantage over smaller companies like WSI because they had their own in-house consulting divisions. Aon's consulting segment evaluated mergers and acquisitions for its customers.

The amount of competition WSI faced in acquiring agencies differed depending on the agency's size. If WSI wanted to acquire a $3 million (or larger) agency, it faced competition with larger, more powerful companies such Aon and Brown & Brown. In addition, the larger the agency was, the more complicated the acquisition became. Some larger prospective agencies already had many of the benefits WSI offered so they would be drawn to the extra benefits that companies like Aon possessed.

Larger prospective acquisition agencies were also more likely to hire lawyers and consultants that could impede or stop the acquisition process. Competitors such as Brown & Brown, with a large staff and acquisition team, were much better equipped to deal with these lawyers and consultants. Smaller agencies, worth $1 million or less, were not courted by the bigger competitors, especially if they were not the largest player in their market.

WSI'S ACQUISITION PROCESS

The acquisition process for WSI required a continuous effort throughout the year. More than 100 possible agencies were considered in a given year, with new agencies being added to the list as others were dropped. WSI narrowed the pool of 100 to approximately 10 agencies that seemed to have a good fit (see Exhibit 5). Of the 10, about 4 agencies prequalified and signed confidentiality agreements. Once WSI selected its first choice, it assessed the fit of the company and started preliminary discussions.

Conducting due diligence, the next step in the the process, usually took six months. It often took longer because some agencies did not share financials until later in the process. If the evaluation went well, WSI started financial negotiations with the agency. After the initial deal was made, it went to the WSI and CBIC boards for approval. This process could take three to four months, depending on whether the deal needed to be renegotiated. After an announcement was made, the companies closed the deal and moved on to the orientation and integration processes. The entire process to this point took approximately two years.

The orientation/integration process took anywhere from two to eight years, depending on the agency involved. After the deal was closed, operational integration began with an immediate office visitation, welcoming employees to the fold. Automation

Exhibit 4   **WSI's Secondary Competitors for Acquisitions**

Aon	Marsh & McLennan	Brown & Brown Inc.	Arthur Gallagher
Second largest insurance brokerage company in the industry	Largest insurance brokerage company in the industry		
Business Segments • Commercial brokerage • Consulting service • Consumer insurance • Underwriting	**Business Segments** • Reinsurance (Guy Carpenter) • Insurance • Program/management services (Seabury & Smith) • Insurance industry investment and advisory services (Seabury & Smith) • Human resources and management consulting (Mercer Consulting)	**Business Segments** • Insurance agency • Brokerage firm	**Business Segments** • Insurance brokerage and risk management
2002 sales: $8,822 million	2002 sales: $10,440 million	2002 sales: $455.7 million	2002 sales: $1,052 million
2002 net income: $466 million	2002 net income: $1,365 million	2002 net income: $83.1 million	2002 net income: $1,052 million
2002 employees: 55,000	2002 employees: 59,500	2002 employees: 3,384	2002 employees: 7,100
Acquisitions • Acquires companies worldwide • Consults for other companies doing acquisitions	**Acquisitions** • In 1997 acquired Johnson & Higgins for $1.8 billion in cash and stocks • In 1998 acquired UK broker Sedwick Group for $2.2 billion	**Acquisition** • The purchase of Schwarz & Powell, a company with a premium volume of $170 million	

was usually the step that took the longest because of producer/employee resistance to the new learning curve. One of the final steps was the orientation of branch managers. These training sessions spanned from 6 to 12 months. Finally, trainers were sent to the new branch to teach employees proper work flows and establish a sales culture and focus that was in line with WSI's sales.

PARAMETERS FOR WSI'S STRATEGIC ALTERNATIVES

Between March and April, Ed Kirby gathered a vast amount of data regarding the parameters for the alternatives WSI was exploring. Most of the parameters were consistent with Kirby's experience and research, but others required much more thought. The first parameter was in regard to the revenue benchmark that WSI needed to reach before going public through the initial public offering (IPO) process. In Kirby's initial meeting with Dennis Toussaint, the revenue benchmark for WSI was set at $100 million. However, a second benchmark of $50 million for WSI plus the acquisition of a similar-sized agency that could reach $50 million was added to Kirby's project a few weeks later, after senior executives discussed alternative methods to reach the $100 million target. WSI executives had already developed a plan to reach $50 million in revenue by penetrating a number of new markets.

Exhibit 5   **WSI's Acquisition Process**

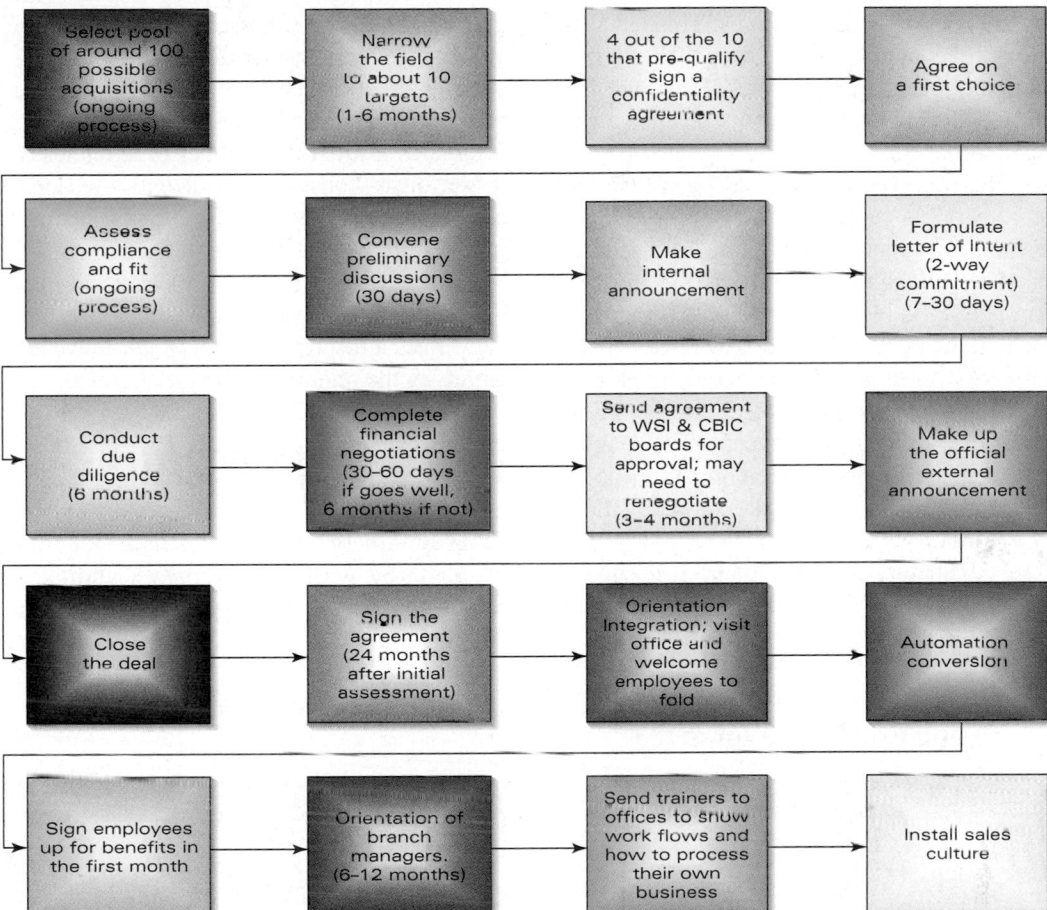

In mid-April, a third revenue target was added. The latest revenue target was reached after Terry Cosgrove, Sherry Cladouhos, Wayne Knutson, Dennis Toussaint, and Peter Babin (all senior executives with BCBS-MT)visited with investment bankers in New York City. In their discussions the investment bankers suggested that the benchmark be raised to $250 million. As a result, Kirby now had three alternatives to consider in his study:

1. Expand WSI to $50 million in revenues while simultaneously acquiring a similar-sized agency and expanding it to $50 million.
2. Expand WSI to $100 million in revenues.
3. Expand WSI to $250 million in revenues.

The second parameter that required more thought was that BCBS-MT indicated that it wanted WSI to complete the IPO in five years. That meant that the IPO would have to be completed by 2007. WSI had completed 11 acquisitions in the past eight years and would have to increase the number of acquisitions per year considerably if the company was to reach the target revenue level by 2007. Kirby was told to use $1 million as the average for each acquired agency in his forecasting to determine the number of acquisitions per year to reach the target. Based on the time frame and the average sales of acquired firms, Kirby wondered whether it was reasonable for the company to complete the number of acquisitions needed.

Kirby's initial research concluded that the time frame that the company had to reach the target revenue level needed to be considered. The IPO process takes a minimum of six months, and can take up to two years or more. Therefore, the time horizon for reaching the revenue target was actually between

3 and 4.5 years. Since it was already nearing the midyear mark of 2003, Kirby needed to take an additional six months off the time frame. This left WSI with 2.5 to 4 years as the window in which the firm had to reach the revenue target. Thus, Kirby felt that WSI would need to be at or above its revenue target by the end of 2005.

During the time frame specified, WSI also had to realize constraints regarding the time it takes to complete each individual acquisition. As discussed earlier, it takes WSI approximately two years from the time an agency is identified as a potential match to the time that the acquisition actually closes. Thus, in order for WSI to complete the acquisitions necessary for 2004, it would have needed to begin the acquisition process in 2002 for those specific agencies. Kirby wondered whether the company was far enough along in the process to make the acquisitions necessary in 2004.

A third parameter that had not been discussed by the executives at BCBS-MT or WSI concerned the population of agencies that were attractive acquisition targets. In order to increase the chance that integration of acquired agencies was successful, WSI needed to consider the product mix, market position, market size and potential, and possible cultural match of its pool of acquisition targets. These characteristics limited the number of agencies that could be seriously considered. Currently WSI develops a pool of approximately 100 potential acquisition targets and narrows it down to a field of four for closer evaluation. From the group of four, one is selected. Kirby felt that WSI needed to recognize the fact that there were a discrete number of attractive acquisition targets in the region in which it operated.

WSI'S FINANCIALS

Craig Stahlberg, WSI's chief financial officer, provided Kirby with the company's audited financial statements from 1998 to 2002 (Exhibits 6 and 7).

Exhibit 6   **WSI's Historical Consolidated Income Statements, 1998–2002 and Pro Forma for 2003**

	1998	1999	2000	2001	2002	2003 (est.)
Number of agencies	13	13	13	15	17	20
Net revenues	$ 9,509,906	$11,347,194	$12,369,457	$16,491,614	$21,279,562	$26,103,744
Total compensation	6,127,002	6,959,641	7,827,001	10,185,876	12,975,053	16,281,794
Selling & administrative expenses	443,060	477,298	461,534	539,551	804,340	940,834
Total operating expenses	1,546,879	1,656,656	1,771,101	2,055,184	2,525,016	3,583,618
EBITDA	$ 1,392,965	$ 2,253,599	$ 2,309,821	$ 3,711,002	$ 4,975,153	$ 5,297,498
Depreciation and amortization	629,544	633,000	644,123	649,852	653,165	717,876
EBIT (operating profits)	$ 763,421	$ 1,620,599	$ 1,665,698	$ 3,061,150	$ 4,321,988	$ 4,579,622
Other expenses	1,634,951	1,986,126	1,113,997	1,326,703	1,763,023	1,897,925
EBT	$ (871,530)	$ (365,527)	$ 551,700	$ 1,734,447	$ 3,212,130	$ 3,399,573
Income tax expense	283,962	213,000	(387,000)	(755,106)	(1,279,531)	(1,353,886)
Net profit	$ (587,568)	$ (152,527)	$ 164,700	$ 979,341	$ 1,932,599	$ 2,045,686

*As of March 2003 WSI had acquired one new agency (Corvallis, Oregon) but predicted that it would complete two additional acquisitions by year-end. The 2003 figures represent management's projections and reflect the completion of three acquisitions in the year.

Exhibit 7   **WSI's Historical Consolidated Balance Sheets 1998–2002 and Pro Forma for 2003**

Assets	1998	1999	2000	2001	2002	2003 (est.)
Current assets						
Cash and cash equivalents	$ 658,748	$ 416,507	$ 405,884	$ 956,081	$ 2,692,121	$ 6,144,638
Accounts receivable	2,242,934	2,382,911	2,535,739	3,298,323	3,773,361	5,054,617
Other current assets	235,867	226,944	247,389	329,832	390,947	408,003
Total current assets	$3,137,549	$ 3,026,362	$ 3,189,012	$ 4,584,236	$ 6,856,429	$11,607,258
Property plant and equipment, net	2,182,383	2,496,383	2,721,281	3,628,155	4,834,458	5,813,209
Other assets	4,190,425	4,879,293	5,318,867	7,091,394	9,281,567	10,926,783
Total assets	$9,510,357	$10,402,038	$11,229,159	$15,303,785	$20,972,454	$28,347,250
Liabilities and stockholders' equity						
Current liabilities						
Accounts payable	$1,886,383	$2,609,855	$2,844,975	$3,628,155	$ 4,963,052	$ 6,053,563
Current maturities long-term debt	712,647	737,568	804,015	659,665	933,562	967,270
Operating line of credit	150,000	—	—	—	—	—
Deferred compensation	189,902	113,472	123,695	82,458	34,545	26,045
Taxes payable	272,749	567,360	680,320	907,039	1,291,083	1,542,029
Total current liabilities	$3,211,681	$4,028,254	$4,453,005	$5,277,316	$ 7,222,242	$ 8,587,907
Long-term debt	2,994,680	2,450,000	2,253,720	2,628,516	2,974,360	3,752,902
Other	1,386,891	1,531,871	1,608,029	2,061,452	2,570,470	3,906,919
Total liabilities	$7,593,252	$8,010,125	$8,314,754	$9,967,284	$12,767,072	$16,247,728
Stockholders' equity						
Common stock	566,269	566,269	566,269	566,269	566,269	566,269
Additional paid-in capital	3,344,183	3,971,518	4,329,310	5,772,065	7,169,183	8,339,183
Treasury stock	(1,431,105)	(1,431,105)	(1,431,105)	(1,431,105)	(1,431,105)	(1,431,105)
Retained earnings	(562,242)	(714,769)	(550,068)	429,273	2,361,872	4,407,558
Accumulated other comprehensive income (loss)	—	—	—	—	(460,837)	217,617
Total shareholders' equity	$1,917,105	$ 2,391,913	$ 2,914,406	$ 5,336,501	$ 8,205,382	$ 12,099,522
Total liabilities and equity	$9,510,357	$10,402,038	$11,229,159	$15,303,785	$20,972,454	$ 28,347,250

Over the four-year period WSI acquired four additional agencies and revenues grew from $9.5 million in 1995 to more than $21 million in 2002. The company's profits had also grown from a net loss of $587,568 in 1998 to profits of more than $1.9 million in 2002. Stahlberg also provided Kirby with pro forma statements for 2003 reflecting management's estimates for the remainder of the year. The projections for 2003 included the acquisition of three additional agencies, one of which was completed and two of which were in process. The pro forma statements estimated revenues of more than $27 million and profits of more than $2 million in 2003. Stahlberg estimated that *organic* growth for existing agencies ranged between 7 and 10 percent. Additional growth during the period from 1998 to 2002 was attributed to its recent acquisitions, increasing the number of locations from 13 to 17, and sales, including organic growth, from $9.5 million to $21 million.

Kirby collected some current performance ratios for WSI's primary competitors and the industry as a whole (see Exhibit 8). He planned to evaluate WSI's performance relative to the performance of its peers, especially those it was competing against in the acquisition market.

As he prepared to perform his analysis, Kirby remembered that Toussaint had indicated that Kirby's financial analysis should assume that the average revenue for acquired agencies would be $1 million and that WSI would pay 1.4 times revenue for each acquisition. Thirty-three percent of the price would be paid in cash, with the remaining 67 percent coming from a seven-year loan with a 7 percent interest rate. WSI provided Kirby with forecasted revenues for existing locations that included organic growth (see Exhibit 9) and suggested that organic growth for new acquisitions would be 15 percent for the first year after acquisition, 10 percent for the second and third years, and 8 percent for the fourth year and beyond. WSI expected to complete one more acquisition in the remainder of 2003, and all other components of the income statement were expected to remain constant as a percentage of revenues. WSI executives believed that they could generate $10 million in cash internally, and BCBS-MT had already committed a minimum of $5 million to foster acquisitions during the next five years.

Exhibit 8   Western States Insurance Peer Performance Ratios, 2002

	Marsh & McLennan	Aon	Brown & Brown	Arthur Gallagher	Peer Average	Industry Average
Profit margin	−0.97%	5.79%	19.82%	5.10%	7.44%	4.27%
Asset turnover	0.72	0.36	0.58	0.47	0.52	0.48
Return on assets (ROA)	−0.70%	2.11%	11.58%	2.42%	3.85%	2.05%
Equity multiplier	3.64	5.64	1.95	4.43	3.92	2.92
Return on equity (ROE)	−2.55%	11.91%	22.59%	10.73%	10.67%	5.99%
Dividend payout ratio	0.00%	32.99%	15.28%	124.10%	43.09%	27.36%
Internal growth rate	−0.70%	1.43%	10.88%	−0.58%	2.24%	1.51%
Sustainable growth rate	−2.49%	8.67%	23.67%	−2.52%	6.46%	4.55%
P/E ratio (TTM)	NM	14.16	23.71	34.73	24.20	20.60
Price to sales (TTM)	1.26	0.82	4.7	1.72	2.41	1.56
Price to book (MRQ)	3.01	1.62	4.82	3.71	3.38	2.85

KIRBY PREPARES THE REPORT

By the middle of May 2003, Kirby had gone through the volumes of information provided by WSI and BCBS-MT and additional information gathered from a variety of resources. Now Kirby had to organize the information into a cohesive report that analyzed the three strategic alternatives presented to him. He realized that he faced a challenging situation. On the one hand, his report might show that the company was poised for reaching the revenue targets; on the other hand, his report might have to tell the executives something they didn't want to hear.

Exhibit 9 **WSI Forecasted Revenues by Existing Agency Location**

	2003	2004	2005	2006	2007
Kalispell	$ 2,721,600	$ 2,939,328	$ 3,174,474	$ 3,428,432	$ 3,702,707
Helena	3,043,691	3,287,186	3,550,161	3,834,174	4,140,908
Great Falls	1,764,000	1,905,120	2,057,530	2,222,132	2,399,903
McMinnville	1,254,400	1,354,752	1,463,132	1,580,183	1,706,597
Stevensville	892,600	981,860	1,060,409	1,145,242	1,236,861
Cottage Grove	931,000	1,024,100	1,126,510	1,216,631	1,313,961
Ashland	579,000	636,900	700,590	756,637	817,168
Corvallis	1,488,218	1,711,451	1,882,596	2,070,855	2,236,524
Hamilton	703,000	759,240	819,979	885,578	956,424
Polson	747,600	807,408	872,001	941,761	1,017,102
Bozeman	1,451,000	1,567,080	1,692,446	1,827,842	1,974,069
Big Fork	962,190	1,039,165	1,122,298	1,212,082	1,309,049
Butte	502,445	542,641	586,052	632,936	683,571
Billings	2,801,000	3,025,080	3,267,086	3,528,453	3,810,730
Missoula	3,789,000	4,092,120	4,419,490	4,773,049	5,154,893
Dillon	453,500	489,780	528,962	571,279	616,982
Corporate	2,019,500	2,181,060	2,355,545	2,543,988	2,747,507
Total from existing locations	$26,103,744	$28,344,271	$30,679,261	$33,171,254	$35,824,954

Endnotes

[1] http://seattle.bizjournals.com/seattle/stories/2001/07/02/daily8.html.

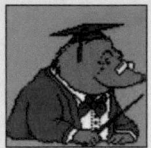

eBay: Facing the Challenge of Global Growth

Louis Marino
The University of Alabama

Patrick Kreiser
Ohio University

At the beginning of 2006, the eBay name was synonymous with the online auction industry. The company had been the dominant player in the online auction industry since its inception in 1995. On September 20, 2000, eBay surprised the financial community and announced ambitious growth objectives including yearly revenue of $3 billion by year-end 2005. Given that the company's annual sales at the time were only $400 million, the $3 billion goal would require annualized growth of 50 percent from the end of 2000 to 2005, an objective that some analysts criticized as being too aggressive. However, the company was able to meet those ambitious goals—a year early! The company's 2004 revenues were over $3.2 billion, and its expected revenues for 2005 were well over $4 billion. By most any account, eBay's record of financial and competitive success had been rather impressive (see Exhibit 1).

Building on the vision of its founder, Pierre Omidyar (pronounced oh-*mid*-ee-ar), eBay was initially conceived as a marketplace that would facilitate a person-to-person trading community based on a democratized, efficient market in which everyone could have equal access through the same medium, the Internet. Leveraging a unique business model and the growing popularity of the Internet, eBay has dominated the market since its beginning, growing to include over 168 million registered users heading into 2006. This diverse base of registered users ranged from high school and college students looking to make a few extra dollars, to Fortune 500 companies such as IBM selling excess inventory, to large

government agencies like the U.S. Postal Service selling undeliverable parcels. This differed greatly from the individuals and small companies from the United States that comprised eBay's original user base.

However, eBay's continued growth was unable to completely mask several emerging threats the company needed to address. In recognition of these challenges, Standard & Poor's had classified eBay as a "hold" stock throughout all of 2005, citing potential domestic market saturation and concern over the pace and size of the company's recent acquisitions. Why was a company that had been so financially successful, and that had been number one in terms of market share in its industry for the past decade, drawing the concern of investors? Two main issues were primarily responsible: (1) increased competition and market saturation facing eBay's domestic business, and (2) concerns over eBay's ability to compete successfully over the long term in global markets. The company readily acknowledged that it saw both of these issues as significant threats. In regard to domestic competition, eBay noted the relative lack of entry barriers into the industry and expected "competition to intensify in the future."[1] The company also acknowledged its potential difficulties in competing globally, citing its lack of experience in adapting its service to local customs, the large amount of resources required to compete globally, and the existence of established competitors in many foreign markets.[2] The company claimed that "even if we are successful, we expect the costs of operating new sites to exceed our net revenues for at least 12 months in most countries."[3] In fact, eBay had to discontinue its operations in the Japanese market in

Exhibit 1   **Selected Indicators of eBay's Growth, 1996–2005 (in millions)**

	1996	1997	1998	1999	2000	2001	2002	2003	2004	2005
Number of registered users	.041	.341	2.2	10.0	22.0	42.4	61.7	94.9	135.5	168.1
Active users	NA	NA	NA	NA	NA	18.0	27.7	41.2	56.1	68.0
Gross merchandise sales	$7	$95	$745	$2,800	$5,400	$9,300	$14,900	$24,000	$34,200	$43,067*
Number of auctions listed	0.29	4.4	33.7	129	264	423	638	971	1,412.6	1,774*

*The gross merchandise sales and number of auctions listed for 2005 are projections based on eBay estimates and on third-quarter actual results.

2002 due to rising costs and a lack of profits. Yet if the company was going to continue to experience the same levels of financial success it had enjoyed during its first 10 years of operation, it needed to develop strategies that would allow it to negate both of these potential threats.

THE GROWTH OF E-COMMERCE AND ONLINE AUCTIONS

The concepts underlying the Internet were first conceived in the 1960s, but it wasn't until the 1990s that the Internet garnered widespread use and became a part of everyday life. International Data Corporation (IDC) estimated that in 2004 there were approximately 700 million Internet users worldwide in over 150 countries, and it estimated that number would grow to 1.1 billion users worldwide by 2007, with a compound annual growth rate of 12 percent. While the top 15 countries accounted for more than 70 percent of the computers in use, slightly less than one-fourth of these Internet users (160 million) resided in the United States, whose share as a percentage of total Internet users worldwide was falling. In the United States, 87 percent of households were expected to have Internet access in 2009, and the number of households with a broadband connection was expected to be 60 percent at that time. However, the highest areas of Internet usage growth were expected to be in developing countries, where Internet penetration was currently low, such as Asia, Latin America, and Eastern Europe due to increasing access through new technologies such as Web-enabled cell phones.

IDC predicted that the worldwide market for business-to-consumer Internet spending would increase from $216.2 billion in 2003 to $759.4 billion in 2007. Forrester Research forecasted a similar increase in the online auction market, from $13 billion in revenues in 2002 to $54 billion in revenues in 2007. North America accounted for approximately 50 percent of total e-commerce sales in 2004, with the Asia-Pacific region accounting for approximately 25 percent, Western Europe accounting for approximately 20 percent, and Latin America accounting for over 10 percent of total sales. Within the business-to-consumer segment, where eBay primarily operated, U.S. e-commerce accounted for over 65 percent of all Internet transactions in 1999 but accounted for less than 40 percent in 2003 and potentially less in the future, due to rapid expansion in other parts of the world. Asia was expected to grow especially rapidly with the 2001 decision to include China in the World Trade Organization. According to IDC in 2005, the Asia-Pacific region (excluding Japan) was expected to experience a strong annual growth rate of 25 percent for Internet devices, 19 percent for online users, and 46 percent for Internet buyers. European markets were also expected to experience rapid growth in 2006 and beyond. In 2002, Germany, the United Kingdom, France, and Italy accounted for 70 percent of the e-commerce revenues in Western Europe, but this share was expected to decline as business-to-business e-commerce in Europe was expected to triple from 2003 to 2006.

KEY SUCCESS FACTORS IN ONLINE RETAILING

While it was relatively easy to create a Web site that functioned like a retail store, the more significant challenge was for an online retailer to generate traffic to the site in the form of both new and returning customers. To reach new customers, some online retailers partnered with shopping search engines (such as Google, MySimon, or StreetPrices) that allowed customers to compare prices for a given product from many retailers. Other tactics employed to build traffic included direct e-mail, online advertising at portals and content-related sites, and some traditional advertising such as print and television advertising. Once customers found their way to a site, most online retailers endeavored to provide extensive product information, include pictures of the merchandise, make the site easily navigable, and have enough new things happening at the site to keep them coming back. (A site's ability to generate repeat visitors was known as "stickiness.") Retailers also had to overcome new users' nervousness about using the Internet itself to shop for items they generally bought in stores. Web sites had to appease concerns about sending credit card numbers over the Internet and the possible sale of personal information to marketing firms. Online retailing had severe limitations in the case of those goods and services people wanted to see in person to verify their quality. From the retailer's perspective, there was the issue of collecting payment from buyers who wanted to use checks or money orders instead of credit cards.

ONLINE AUCTIONS

The first known auctions were held in Babylon around 500 BC. In AD 193, the entire Roman Empire was put up for auction after the emperor Pertinax was executed. Didius Julianus bid 6,250 drachmas per royal guard and was immediately named emperor of Rome. However, Julianus was executed only two months later, suggesting that he may have been the first-ever victim of the winner's curse (bidding more than the good would cost in a nonauction setting).

Auctions have endured throughout history for several reasons. First, they give sellers a convenient way to find a buyer for something they would like to dispose of. Second, auctions are an excellent way for people to collect difficult-to-find items, such as Beanie Babies or historical memorabilia that have a high value to them personally. Finally, auctions are one of the "purest" markets that exist for goods, in that they bring buyers and sellers into contact to arrive at a mutually agreeable price. As technological advances led to the advent and widespread adoption of the Internet, this ancient form of trade found a new medium.

Online auctions worked in essentially the same way as traditional auctions, the difference being that the auction process occurred over the Internet rather than at a specific geographic location with buyers and sellers physically present. There were three basic categories of online auctions:

1. Business-to-business auctions, typically involving equipment and surplus merchandise.
2. Business-to-consumer auctions, in which businesses sold goods and services to consumers via the Internet. Many such auctions involved companies interested in selling used or discontinued goods, or liquidating unwanted inventory.
3. Person-to-person auctions, which gave interested sellers and buyers the opportunity to engage in competitive bidding.

Online auction operators could generate revenue in four principal ways:

1. Charging sellers for listing their good or service.
2. Charging a commission on all sales.
3. Selling advertising on their Web sites.
4. Selling their own new or used merchandise via the online auction format.

More recently, however, online auction sites had also added a new revenue-generation option:

5. Selling their own goods or allowing other sellers to offer their goods in a fixed-price format.

Most sites charged sellers either a fee or a commission and sold advertising to companies interested in promoting their goods or services to users of the auction site.

Online Auction Users

Participants in online auctions could be grouped into six categories: (1) bargain hunters, (2) hobbyists and collectors, (3) professional buyers, (4) casual sellers, (5) hobbyist and collector sellers and (6) corporate and power sellers.

Bargain Hunters Bargain hunters viewed on-line auctions primarily as a form of entertainment; their objective usually was to find a great deal. Bargain hunters were thought to make up only 8 percent of active online users but 52 percent of eBay visitors. To attract repeat visits from bargain hunters, industry observers said, sites must appeal to them on both rational and emotional levels, satisfying their need for competitive pricing, the excitement of the search, and the desire for community.

Hobbyists and Collectors Hobbyists and collectors used auctions to search for specific goods that had a high value to them personally. They were very concerned with both price and quality. Collectors prized eBay for its wide variety of product offerings.

Professional Buyers As the legitimacy of on-line auctions grew, a new type of buyer began to emerge: the professional buyer. Professional buyers covered a broad range of purchasers ranging from purchasing managers acquiring office supplies to antique and gun dealers purchasing inventory. Like bargain hunters, professional buyers were looking for a way to help contain costs; and, like hobbyists and collectors, some professional buyers were seeking unique items to supplement their inventory. The primary difference between professional buyers and other types, however, was their affiliation with commercial enterprises. With the growth of online auction sites dedicated to business-to-business auctions, professional buyers were becoming an increasingly important element of the online auction landscape.

Casual Sellers Casual sellers included individuals who used eBay as a substitute for a classified ad listing or a garage sale to dispose of items they no longer wanted. While many casual sellers listed only a few items, some used eBay to raise money for a specific project or other undertaking.

Hobbyist and Collector Sellers Sellers who were hobbyists or collectors typically dealt in a limited category of goods and looked to eBay as a way to sell selected items in their collections to others who might want them. Items ranged from classic television collectibles, to hand-sewn dolls, to coins and stamps. The hobbyists and collectors used a range of traditional and online outlets to reach their target markets. A number of the sellers used auctions to supplement their retail operations, while others sold exclusively through online auctions and in fixed-price formats such as Half.com.

Power and Corporate Sellers Power sellers were typically small to medium-sized businesses that favored eBay as a primary distribution channel and often sold tens of thousands of dollars' worth of goods every month on the site. One estimate suggested that while these power sellers accounted for only 4 percent of eBay's population, they were responsible for 80 percent of eBay's total business.[4] Individuals who were power sellers could often make a full-time job of the endeavor.

As with the evolution of buyers, commercial enterprises were becoming an increasingly important part of the online auction industry. These commercial enterprises generally achieved power-seller status relatively rapidly. On eBay, for example, some of the new power sellers were familiar names such as IBM, Compaq, and the U.S. Postal Service (which sells undeliverable items on eBay under the user name usps-mrc).

PIERRE OMIDYAR AND THE FOUNDING OF eBAY

Pierre Omidyar was born in Paris, France, to parents who had left Iran decades earlier. The family emigrated to the United States when Pierre's father began a residency at Johns Hopkins University Medical Center. Pierre attended Tufts University, where he met his future wife, Pamela Wesley, who came to Tufts from Hawaii to get a degree in biology. Upon graduating in 1988, the couple moved to California, where Pierre, who had earned a bachelor's degree in computer science, joined Claris, an Apple Computer subsidiary in Silicon Valley, and wrote a widely used graphics application, MacDraw. In 1991, Omidyar left Claris and cofounded Ink Development (later renamed eShop), which became a pioneer in online shopping and was eventually sold to Microsoft in 1996. In 1994,

Omidyar joined General Magic as a developer services engineer and remained there until mid-1996, when he left to pursue full-time development of eBay.

Internet folklore has it that eBay was founded solely to allow Pamela to trade Pez dispensers with other collectors. While Pamela was certainly a driving force in launching the initial Web site, Pierre had long been interested in how one could establish a marketplace to bring together a fragmented market. Pierre saw eBay as a way to create a person-to-person trading community based on a democratized, efficient market where everyone could have equal access through the same medium, the Internet. Pierre set out to develop his marketplace and to meet both his and Pamela's goals. In 1995 he launched the first online auction under the name of Auctionwatch at the domain name of www.eBay.com. The name eBay stood for "electronic Bay area," coined because Pierre's initial concept was to attract neighbors and other interested San Francisco Bay area residents to the site to buy and sell items of mutual interest. The first auctions charged no fees to either buyers or sellers and contained mostly computer equipment (and no Pez dispensers). Pierre's fledgling venture generated $1,000 in revenue the first month and an additional $2,000 the second. Traffic grew rapidly, however, as word about the site spread in the Bay area, and a community of collectors emerged, using the site to trade and chat—there were even some marriages that resulted from exchanges in eBay chat rooms.[5]

By February 1996, the traffic at Pierre Omidyar's site had grown so much that his Internet service provider informed him that he would have to upgrade his service. When Omidyar compensated for this by charging a listing fee for the auction, and saw no decrease in the number of items listed, he knew he was on to something. Although he was still working out of his home, Omidyar began looking for a partner and in May asked his friend Jeffrey Skoll to join him in the venture. While Skoll had never cared much about money, his Stanford MBA degree provided the firm with the business background that Omidyar lacked. With Omidyar as the visionary and Skoll as the strategist, the company embarked on a mission to "help people trade practically anything on earth."

Their concept for eBay was to "create a place where people could do business just like in the old days—when everyone got to know each other personally, and we all felt we were dealing on a one-to-one basis with individuals we could trust."

In eBay's early days, Omidyar and Skoll ran the operation alone, using a single computer to serve all of the pages. Omidyar served as CEO, chief financial officer, and president, while Skoll functioned as co-president and director. It was not long until Omidyar and Skoll grew the company to a size that forced them to move out of the Omidyars' living room, due to the objections of Pamela, and into Skoll's living room. Shortly thereafter, the operations moved into the facilities of a Silicon Valley business incubator for a time until the company settled in its current facilities in San Jose, California. Exhibits 2 and 3 present eBay's recent financial statements.

eBAY'S TRANSITION TO PROFESSIONAL MANAGEMENT

From the beginning, Pierre Omidyar intended to hire a professional manager to serve as the president of eBay: "[I would] let him or her run the company so . . . [I could] go play."[6] In 1997, both Omidyar and Skoll agreed that it was time to locate an experienced professional to function as CEO and president. In late 1997, eBay's headhunters came up with a candidate for the job: Margaret Whitman, then general manager for Hasbro Inc.'s preschool division. Whitman had received her bachelor of arts degree in economics from Princeton and her master of business administration from the Harvard Business School; her first job was in brand management at Procter & Gamble. Her experience also included serving as the president and CEO of FTD, the president of Stride Rite Corporation's Stride Rite Division, and as the senior vice president of marketing for the Walt Disney Company's consumer products division.

When first approached by eBay, Whitman was not especially interested in joining a company that had fewer than 40 employees and less than $6 million in revenues the previous year. It was only after repeated pleas that Whitman agreed to meet with Omidyar in Silicon Valley. After a second meeting, Whitman realized the company's enormous growth potential and agreed to give eBay a try. According to Omidyar, Meg Whitman's experience in global marketing with Hasbro's Teletubbies, Playskool, and Mr. Potato Head brands made her "the ideal choice to build upon eBay's leadership position in the

Exhibit 2   **eBay's Income Statements, 2000–2005 (in thousands of $, except per share figures)**

	2000	2001	2002	2003	2004	First Nine Months of 2005
Net revenues	$431,424	$748,821	$1,214,100	$2,165,096	$3,271,309	$3,223,542
Cost of net revenues	95,453	134,816	213,876	416,058	614,415	578,584
Gross profit	$335,971	$614,005	$1,000,224	$1,749,038	$2,656,894	$2,644,958
Operating expenses:						
Sales and marketing	166,767	253,474	349,650	567,565	857,874	852,239
Product development	55,863	75,288	104,636	159,315	240,647	224,309
General and administrative	73,027	105,784	171,785	304,703	415,725	410,016
Patent litigation expense				29,965		
Payroll taxes on stock options	2,337	2,442	4,015	9,590	17,479	9,582
Amortization of acquired intangibles	1,443	36,591	15,941	50,659	65,927	77,516
Merger-related costs	1,550	0	0	0	0	0
Total operating expenses	$300,977	$473,579	$ 646,027	$1,119,797	$1,597,652	$1,573,662
Income (loss) from operations	$ 34,994	$140,426	$ 354,197	$ 629,241	$1,059,242	$1,071,296
Interest and other income (expense), net	46,337	41,613	49,209	37,803	77,867	85,585
Interest expense	−3,374	−2,851	−1,492	−4,314	−8,879	−2,556
Impairment of certain equity Investments	0	−16,245	−3,781	−1,230	0	0
Income before income taxes and minority interest	$ 77,957	$162,943	$ 398,133	$ 661,500	$1,128,230	$1,154,325
Provision for income taxes	−32,725	−80,009	−145,946	−206,738	−343,885	−351,455
Minority interests in consolidated companies	3,062	7,514	−2,296	−7,578	−6,122	−48
Net income	$ 48,294	$ 90,448	$ 249,891	$ 447,184	$ 778,223	$ 802,822
Net income per share:						
Basic	$0.19	$0.34	$0.43	$0.69	$0.59	$0.59
Diluted	0.17	0.32	0.43	0.67	0.57	0.58
Weighted average shares:						
Basic	251,776	268,971	574,992	638,288	1,319,458	1,350,836
Diluted	280,346	280,595	585,640	656,657	1,367,720	1,383,024

Source: Company financial documents.

one-to-one online trading market without sacrificing the quality and personal touch our users have grown to expect."[7] In addition to convincing Whitman to head eBay's operations, Omidyar had been instrumental in helping bring in other talented senior executives and in assembling a capable board of directors. Notable members of eBay's board of directors included Scott Cook, the founder of Intuit, a highly successful financial software company, and

Fred D. Anderson, executive vice president and chief financial officer of Apple.

HOW AN eBAY AUCTION WORKED

eBay endeavored to make it very simple to buy and sell goods. In order to sell or bid on goods, users first

Exhibit 3   **eBay's Consolidated Balance Sheets, 2000–2005 (in thousands of $)**

	Period Ending					
	12/31/00	12/31/01	12/31/02	12/31/03	12/31/04	9/30/05
Assets						
Current assets:						
Cash and cash equivalents	$ 201,873	$ 523,969	$1,109,313	$1,381,513	$1,330,045	$2,180,598
Short-term investments	354,166	199,450	89,690	340,576	682,004	888,783
Accounts receivable, net	67,163	101,703	131,453	225,871	240,856	274,238
Funds receivable	—	—	41,014	79,893	123,424	210,593
Other current assets	52,262	58,683	96,988	118,029	534,820	436,781
Total current assets	$ 675,464	$ 883,805	$1,468,458	$2,145,882	$2,911,149	$3,990,993
Long-term investments		286,998	470,227	934,171	1,266,289	827,191
Restricted cash and investments		129,614	134,644	127,432	1,418	—
Property and equipment, net	125,161	142,349	218,028	601,785	709,773	762,413
Goodwill		187,829	1,456,024	1,719,311	2,709,794	3,529,895
Investments	—	—	—	—	—	—
Deferred tax assets	—	21,540	84,218	—	—	—
Intangible and other assets, net	23,299	26,394	292,845	291553	392,628	515,551
Total assets	$1,182,403	$1,678,529	$4,040,226	$5,820,134	$7,991,051	$9,626,043
Liabilities and Stockholders' equity						
Current liabilities:						
Accounts payable	$ 31,725	$ 33,235	$ 47,424	$ 64,633	$ 37,958	$ 42,726
Funds payable and amounts due to customers	—	—	50,396	106,568	331,805	517,309
Accrued expenses and other current liabilities	60,882	94,593	199,323	356,491	421,969	523,584
Deferred revenue and customer advances	12,656	15,583	18,846	28,874	50,439	44,222
Debt and leases, current portion	15,272	16,111	2,970	2,840	124,272	—
Income taxes payable	11,092	20,617	67,265	87,870	118,427	138,951
Deferred tax liabilities, current	—	—	—	—	—	—
Other current liabilities	5,815	—	—	—	—	—
Total current liabilities	$ 137,442	$ 180,139	$ 386,224	$ 647,276	$1,084,870	$1,266,792
Debt and leases, long-term portion	11,404	12,008	13,798	124,476	75	—
Deferred tax liabilities, long-term	—	3,629	27,625	79,238	135,971	298,197
Other liabilities	6,549	15,864	22,874	33,494	37,698	33,690
Minority interests	—	37,751	33,232	39,408	4,096	—
Total liabilities	$ 168,643	$ 249,391	$ 483,753	$ 923,892	$1,262,710	$1,598,679
Series B redeemable convertible preferred stock and Series B warrants	—	—	—	—	—	—
	1,013,760	1,429,138	3,556,473	4,896,242	6,728,341	8,027,364
Total stockholders' equity	$1,182,403	$1,678,529	$4,124,444	$5,820,134	$7,991,051	$9,626,043

Source: Company financial documents.

had to register at the site. Once they registered, users selected both a user name and a password. Unregistered users were able to browse the Web site but were not permitted to bid on any goods or list any items for auction.

On the Web site, search engines helped customers determine what goods were currently available. When registered users found an item they desired, they could choose to enter a single bid or to use automatic bidding (called proxy bidding). In automatic bidding, the customer entered an initial bid sufficient to make him or her the high bidder; the bid would be automatically increased as others bid for the same object until the auction ended and either the bidder won or another bidder surpassed the original customer's maximum specified bid. Regardless of which bidding method they chose, users could check bids at any time and either bid again, if they had been outbid, or increase their maximum amount in the automatic bid. Users could choose to receive e-mail notification if they were outbid.

Once the auction had ended, the buyer and seller were both notified of the winning bid and were given each other's e-mail address. The parties to the auction would then privately arrange for payment and delivery of the good.

Fees and Procedures for Sellers

Buyers on eBay were not charged a fee for bidding on items on the site, but sellers were charged an insertion fee and a "final value" fee; they could also elect to pay additional fees to promote their listing. Listing, or insertion, fees ranged from 30 cents for auctions with opening bids, minimum values, or reserve prices of between $0.01 and $0.99, to $4.80 for auctions with opening bids, minimum values, or reserve prices of $500 and up. Final value fees ranged from 1.25 to 5 percent of the final sale price and were computed according to a graduated fee schedule in which the percentage fell as the final sales price rose. As an example, in a basic auction with no promotion, if the item had brought an opening bid of $200 and eventually sold for $1,500, the total fee paid by the seller would be $35.48—the $3.60 insertion fee plus $31.88. The $31.88 was based on a fee structure of 5 percent of the first $25 (or $1.25), 2.5 percent of the additional amount between $25.01 and $1,000 (or

$24.38), and 1.25 percent of the additional amount between $1,000.01 and $1,500 (or $6.25). Auction fees varied for special categories of goods such as passenger vehicles in eBay Motors, which were charged a $40 transaction fee when the first successful bid was placed, and residential, commercial, and other real estate, which carried a $100 insertion fee.

Sellers could also customize items by adding photographs and featuring their item in eBay's Gallery section. Sellers could indicate a photograph in the item's description if the seller posted the photograph on a Web site and provided eBay with the appropriate Web address. Items could be showcased in the Gallery section with a catalog of pictures rather than text. A seller who used a photograph in his or her listing could have this photograph included in the Gallery section for 25 cents or featured there for $19.95. A Gallery option was available in all categories of eBay, but fees varied among categories and according to the prominence of the Gallery. For example, a simple Gallery listing cost 25 cents, whereas a featured Gallery listing, which included a periodic listing in the featured section above the general Gallery, cost $19.95. In the eBay Motors Gallery, options could cost as much as $99.95.

To make doing business on eBay more attractive to potential sellers, eBay introduced several features. To ensure receiving a minimum price for an auction, the seller could either specify an opening bid or set a reserve price on the auction. If the bidding did not top the reserve price, the seller was under no obligation to sell the item to the highest bidder and could relist the item at no extra cost. For items with a reserve price between $0.01 and $49.99, the fee was $1.00; for prices between $50.00 and $199.99, the fee was $2.00; and for prices over $200, the fee was 1 percent of the reserve price. If the seller wished, he or she could also set a "buy-it-now" price that allowed bidders to pay a set amount for a listed item. The fee for this service was $1.00. If the buy-it-now price was met, the auction would end immediately.

As of June 11, 2001, new sellers at eBay were required to provide both a credit card number and bank account information. While eBay admits that these requirements are extreme, it argues that they help protect everyone in the community against fraudulent sellers and ensure that sellers are of legal age and are serious about listing an item on eBay.

How Transactions Were Completed

Under the terms of eBay's user agreement, if a seller received one or more bids above the stated minimum, or reserve, price, the seller was obligated to complete the transaction, although eBay had no enforcement power beyond suspending a noncompliant buyer or seller from using eBay's service. In the event the buyer and seller were unable to complete the transaction, the seller notified eBay, which then credited the seller the amount of the final value fee.

When an auction ended, the eBay system validated that the bid fell within the acceptable price range. If the sale was successful, eBay automatically notified the buyer and seller via e-mail; the buyer and seller could then work out the transaction details independent of eBay, or they could use eBay's checkout service and eBay's payment service to complete the transaction. In its original business model, eBay did not take possession of either the item being sold or the buyer's payment at any point in the process. In an effort to increase revenues, eBay expanded its offerings to facilitate buyers paying for auctions by first offering services that accepted credit card payments and electronic funds transfers on behalf of the seller and then, in 2003, purchasing PayPal, the leading third-party online payment facilitator. To make selling easier, eBay also had alliances with two leading shippers, the U.S. Postal Service (USPS) and UPS. Both of these shippers had centers on eBay that would allow sellers to calculate postage and to print postage-paid labels. However, the buyer and seller still had to independently arrange shipping terms, with buyers typically paying for shipping. Items were sent directly from the seller to the buyer unless an independent escrow service was arranged to help ensure security.

To encourage sellers to use eBay's ancillary services, the company offered an automated checkout service to help expedite communication, payment, and delivery between buyers and sellers.

FOSTERING COMMUNITY AFFINITY

From its founding, eBay considered developing a loyal, vivacious trading community to be a cornerstone of its business model. This community was nurtured through open and honest communication and was built on five basic values that eBay expected its members to honor:

> We believe people are basically good.
>
> We believe everyone has something to contribute.
>
> We believe that an honest, open environment can bring out the best in people.
>
> We recognize and respect everyone as a unique individual.
>
> We encourage you to treat others the way that you want to be treated.[8]

The company recognized that these values could not be imposed by fiat. According to Omidyar, "As much as we at eBay talk about the values and encourage people to live by those values, that's not going to work unless people actually adopt those values. The values are communicated not because somebody reads the Web site and says, 'Hey, this is how we want to treat each other, so I'll just start treating people that way.' The values are communicated because that's how they're treated when they first arrive. Each member is passing those values on to the next member. It's little things, like you receive a note that says, 'Thanks for your business.' "[9] Consistent with eBay's desire to stay in touch with its customers and be responsive to their needs, the company flies in 10 new sellers every few months to hold group meetings known as Voice of the Customer; 75–80 percent of new features are originally suggested by community members.

An example of eBay values in action took place when eBay introduced a feature that referred losing bidders to similar auctions from other eBay sellers, eliciting a strong outcry from the community. Sellers demanded to know why eBay was stealing their sales, and one longtime seller even went so far as to auction a rare eBay jacket so that he could use the auction as a forum to complain about "eBay's new policy of screwing the folks who built them."[10] This caught the attention of Omidyar and Whitman, who met with the seller in his home for 45 minutes. After the meeting, eBay changed its policy.

Recognizing that many new users may not get the most out of their eBay experience, and hoping to introduce new entrepreneurs to the community, the company created eBay University in August 2000. The university travels across the country and holds two-day seminars in various cities. These seminars attract between 400 and 500 people who each pay $25 for the experience. Courses range from freshmen-level classes that offer an introduction to buying and selling to graduate classes that teach the intricacies of bulk listing and competitive tactics. The eBay University has been so successful that the company has partnered with Evoke Communications to offer an online version of the classes. While community members gain knowledge from these classes, so does eBay. The company keeps careful track of questions and concerns and uses them to uncover areas that need improvement.

A second important initiative to make the eBay community more inclusive was aimed at the fastest-growing segment of the U.S. population, adults ages 50 and over. In an effort to bridge the digital divide for seniors, eBay launched its Digital Opportunity Program for Seniors and set a goal of training and bringing online 1 million seniors by 2005. Specific elements of this plan included partnering with SeniorNet, the leading nonprofit computer technology trainer of seniors, and donating $1 million to this organization for training and establishing 10 new training facilities by 2005, developing a volunteer program for training seniors, and creating a specific area on eBay for senior citizens (www.ebay. com/seniors).

To foster a sense of community among eBay users, the company employed tools and tactics designed to promote both business and personal interactions between consumers, to foster trust between bidders and sellers, and to instill a sense of security among traders. Interactions between community members were facilitated through the creation of chat rooms based on personal interests. These chat rooms allowed individuals to learn about their chosen collectibles and to exchange information about items they collected.

To manage the flow of information in the chat rooms, eBay employees went to trade shows and conventions to seek out individuals who had knowledge about and a passion for either a specific collectible or a category of goods. These enthusiasts would act as community leaders or ambassadors; they were never referred to as employees but were compensated $1,000 a month to host online discussions with experts.

Feedback Forum

Although personal communication between members fostered a sense of community, as eBay's community grew from "the size of a small village to a large city" additional measures were necessary to ensure a continued sense of trust and honesty among users.[11] One of eBay's earliest trust-building efforts

was the 1996 creation of the Feedback Forum, which encouraged individuals to record comments about their trading partners. At the completion of each auction, both the buyer and seller were allowed to leave positive, negative, or neutral comments about each other. Individuals could dispute feedback left about them by annotating any comments in question.

As users assigned values of +1 for a positive comment, 0 for a neutral comment, and −1 for a negative comment, each trader earned a ranking that was attached to his or her user name. A trader who had developed a positive reputation over time had a color-coded star symbol displayed next to his or her user name to indicate the amount of positive feedback. The highest ranking a trader could receive was "over 100,000," indicated by a red shooting star. Well-respected, high-volume traders could have rankings well into the thousands.

Traders who received a sufficiently negative net feedback rating (typically a −4) had their registrations suspended and were thus unable to bid on or list items for sale. Users could review a person's feedback profile before deciding to bid on an item listed by that person or before choosing payment and delivery methods. A sample user profile is shown in Exhibit 4.

The terms of eBay's user agreement prohibited actions that would undermine the integrity of the Feedback Forum, such as leaving positive feedback about oneself through other accounts or leaving multiple negative comments about someone else through other accounts. The Feedback Forum system had several automated features designed to detect and prevent some forms of abuse. For example, feedback posted from the same account, positive or negative, could not affect a user's net feedback rating by more than one point, no matter how many comments an individual made. Furthermore, a user could only make comments about his or her trading partners in completed transactions. Prior to 2004, a feedback comment could not be altered once it was made. However, as of February 9, 2004, the system was changed in response to suggestions by community members for all users to be able to mutually withdraw feedback. Withdrawn feedback would no longer impact a user's feedback rating.

The company believed its Feedback Forum was extremely useful in overcoming users' initial hesitancy about trading over the Internet, since it reduced the uncertainty of dealing with an unknown trading partner. However, there was growing concern among sellers and bidders that feedback could be positively

Exhibit 4   **A Sample Feedback Forum Profile**

Member Profile: nuggett12 (109 ☆)

| Feedback Score: | 109 |
| Positive Feedback: | 100% |

Members who left a positive:	109
Members who left a negative:	0
All positive feedback received:	118

Learn about what these numbers mean.

Recent Ratings:		Past Month	Past 6 Months	Past 12 Months
⊕	positive	4	18	34
⊙	neutral	0	0	0
⊖	negative	0	0	0

Bid Retractions (Past 6 months): 0

Member since: May-17-99
Location: United States

- ID History
- Items for Sale
- Add to Favorite Sellers
- View my Reviews & Guides

[Contact Member]

| **Feedback Received** | **From Buyers** | **From Sellers** | **Left for Others** |

118 feedback received by nuggett12 (0 ratings mutually withdrawn)   Page 1 of 5

Comment	From	Date / Time	Item #
⊕ BUY IT NOW-PAID IT NOW-w/PAY-PAL WAY TO GO !!!!!! Thank You Much !	Seller krystalriver (2930 ★)	Dec-07-05 12:19	6233794219
⊕ Verrrrrrrrrrrrrry quick payment. A credit to ebay. AAAAAAAAAAAA+++++++++++++++	Seller thegoodpackage (3859 ★)	Dec-07-05 04:23	6586487441
⊕ Great ebayer! Lightning quick shipping and kept his word about everthing!	Buyer ngun0003 (34 ☆)	Nov-27-05 07:12	8236266960
⊕ Prompt payment, ****** WWW.STORES.EBAY.COM/COMPUTERMEMORYSTORE *******	Seller mwdusa (13146 ☆)	Nov-26-05 15:13	6823044281
⊕ GoGamers.Com - A+++ Great eBayer. Transaction was a breeze!	Seller gogamerscom (57249 ☆)	Oct-28-05 08:00	8228611496
⊕ A pleasure dealing with. Smooth transaction.	Seller bkhtrains (532 ★)	Aug-03-05 05:23	5790615702
⊕ Perfectly Smooth transaction. A Credit to eBay ! A++++	Seller nup (1500 ★)	Aug-03-05 04:29	6788040863
⊕ Customers like you are *priceless* Excellent eBay member! A+ Thanks	Seller dans_cellular_accessories (55137 ☆) no longer a registered user	Aug-03-05 00:21	5789528933
⊕ Successful completion. Great customer. Thank you from THE SHARPER IMAGE!	Seller the_sharper_image (138164 ★)	Jul-25-05 05:33	5791564203
⊕ Good buyer, prompt payment, valued customer, highly recommended.	Seller vcom (9318 ☆)	Jul-21-05 16:17	5789130422
⊕ FAST PAYMENT! GREAT BIDDER. THANKS!!! AAAAA +++++++	Seller allbest4u (17890 ☆)	Jul-16-05 14:53	5788315854
⊕ Great buyer, awesome ebayer, and thank you from ECBURBANK	Seller ecburbank (14787 ☆)	Jul-16-05 14:52	5788869114
⊕ Great buyer, awesome ebayer, and thank you from ECBURBANK	Seller ecburbank (14787 ☆)	Jul-16-05 14:52	5777441953
⊕ Great buyer, awesome ebayer, and thank you from ECBURBANK	Seller ecburbank (14787 ☆)	Jul-16-05 14:52	5777441968
⊕ excellent customer, fast payment, A++	Seller ericapaul (14274 ☆)	Jul-05-05 22:42	8201576635
⊕ Great communication. A pleasure to do business with.	Seller p_accessory (187 ★) no longer a registered user	Jul-01-05 19:21	5785729365
⊕ great seller--excellent communication--very helpful. would recommend! A+A+A+A+A+	Buyer faye608 (20 ☆)	Jun-23-05 18:59	3981329520
⊕ GREAT BUYER AND VERY QUICK PAYMENT ! A REAL PLEASURE !	Seller bug_n_y2k (private)	Jun-23-05 18:50	8197028457
⊕ Top Notch Buyer - It doesn't get any better than this!!	Seller swdiscounters (12886 ☆)	Jun-17-05 19:10	8195154724
⊕ THANKS FOR YOUR ORDER	Seller jagktbs (397 ★)	Jun-17-05 14:59	243802489476
⊕ Nice ebayer. Easy smooth transaction. Thanks!	Seller 1blue1browncody (131 ☆)	Jun-07-05 12:49	4385815724
⊕ Great communication. A pleasure to do business with.	Seller amazon-books (15683 ☆)	May-22-05 06:53	4544184186
⊕ Fast shipping, great comunication...	Buyer ctrfreak (35 ☆)	May-16-05 08:18	5770942373
⊕ Excellent Buyer! A Pleasure To Do Business With. A++++	Seller businessbagsonline (1671 ★)	May-09-05 11:19	8184800507
⊕ Great Ebay buyer!! A++++++++++++++	Seller cleanpureice (827 ★)	May-08-05 19:44	4373083958

Source: www.ebay.com, December 19, 2005.

skewed, as many eBayers were afraid to leave negative feedback for fear of unfounded retribution that could damage their carefully built reputations. This concern was heightened by the fact that buyers and sellers could agree to mutually withdraw negative feedback and thus expunge evidence of a failed transaction as if it never occurred.

Unfortunately, eBay's Feedback Forum was not always sufficient to ensure honesty and integrity among traders. The company estimated that far less than 1 percent of the millions of auctions completed on the site involved some sort of fraud or illegal activity, but some users, like Clay Monroe, disagreed. Monroe, a Seattle-area trader of computer equipment, estimated that "ninety percent of the time everybody is on the up and up . . . [but] . . . ten percent of the time you get some jerk who wants to cheat you." Fraudulent or illegal acts perpetrated by sellers included misrepresentation of goods; trading in counterfeit goods or pirated goods that infringed on others' intellectual property rights; failure to deliver goods paid for by buyers; and shill bidding, whereby sellers would use a false bidder to artificially drive up the price of a good. Buyers could manipulate bids by placing an unrealistically high bid on a good to discourage other bidders and then withdraw their bid at the last moment to allow an ally to win the auction at a bargain price. Buyers could also fail to deliver payment on a completed auction.

SafeHarbor

Recognizing that fraudulent activities represented a significant danger to eBay's future, management took the Feedback Forum a step further in 1998 by launching the SafeHarbor program to provide guidelines for trade, provide information to help resolve user disputes, and respond to reports of misuse of the eBay service. The SafeHarbor initiative was expanded in 1999 to provide additional safeguards and to actively work with law enforcement agencies and members of the trading community to make eBay more secure. New elements of SafeHarbor included:

- Free insurance, with a $25 deductible for transactions under $200 and further protection for buyers and sellers who used PayPal.
- Cooperation with local, national, and international law enforcement agencies to identify and prosecute fraudulent buyers and sellers.
- Enhancements to the Feedback Forum such as listing whether the user was a buyer or a seller in a transaction.

- A partnership with SquareTrade, an online dispute resolution service.
- A partnership with Escrow.com to promote the use of escrow services on purchases over $500.
- A new class of verified eBay users with an accompanying icon.
- Easy access to escrow services.
- Tougher policies relating to nonpaying bidders and shill bidders.
- Clarification of which items were not permissible to list for sale (such as items associated with Nazi Germany or organizations such as the Ku Klux Klan that glorify hate, racial, intolerance, or racial violence).
- A strengthened antipiracy and anti-infringement program known as the Verified Rights Owner (VeRO) program, and the introduction of dispute resolution services.

The use of verified buyer and seller accounts was viewed as especially significant because it allowed eBay to ensure that suspended users did not open new eBay accounts under different names. User information was verified through Atlanta-based Equifax Inc. To further ensure that suspended users didn't register new accounts with different identities, eBay partnered with Infoglide to use a similarity search technology to examine new registrant information.

To implement these new initiatives, eBay increased the number of positions in its SafeHarbor department from 24 to 182, including full-time employees and independent contractors. It also organized the department around the functions of investigations, community watch, and fraud prevention. The investigations group was responsible for examining reported trading violations and possible misuses of eBay. The fraud prevention group mediated customer disputes over such things as the quality of the goods sold. If a written complaint of fraud was filed against a user, eBay generally suspended the alleged offender's account, pending an investigation. Despite all of these initiatives, innovative thieves were developing new ways to cheat honest bidders and sellers as quickly as eBay could identify and ban them from the system, and many eBayers still viewed this as one of the most significant threats to the eBay community.

The community watch group worked with over 100 industry-leading companies, ranging from software publishers to toy manufacturers to apparel makers, to protect intellectual property rights. To ensure that illegal items were not being sold and sale items listed did not violate intellectual property rights, this SafeHarbor group automated daily keyword searches on auction content. Offending auctions were closed and the seller was notified of the violation. Repeated violations resulted in suspension of the seller's account.

As eBay expanded its categories to include Great Collections and the new automobile categories, safeguards were introduced to meet the unique needs of these areas. In the eBay Great Collections category, the company partnered with Collector's Universe to offer authentication and grading services for specific products such as trading cards, coins, and autographs. In the automobile area, one of eBay's fastest-growing segments, eBay partnered with Saturn to provide users with access to a nationwide automobile brand and offered a free limited one-month or 1,000-mile warranty, free purchase insurance up to $20,000 with a $500 deductible, and a special escrow service (Secure Pay) designed for the needs of automotive buyers and sellers.

eBAY'S STRATEGY TO SUSTAIN ITS MARKET DOMINANCE

Meg Whitman assumed the helm of eBay in February 1998 and began acting as the public face of the company. In an effort to stay in touch with her customers, Whitman hosted an auction on eBay herself. She found the experience so enlightening that she then required all of eBay's managers to sell on eBay. Pierre Omidyar stepped back to become chairman of eBay's board of directors and focused his time and energy on overseeing eBay's strategic direction and growth, business model and site development, and community advocacy. Jeff Skoll, who became the vice president of strategic planning and analysis, concentrated on competitive analysis, new business planning and incubation, the development of the organization's overall strategic direction, and supervision of customer support operations.

The Move to Go Public

On September 24, 1998, eBay's initial public offering (IPO) began at a price of $18 per share. The IPO closed the day up 160 percent at $47, generated $66 million in new capital for the company, and was recognized by several investing publications. The success of the offering led eBay to issue a follow-up offering in April 1999 that raised an additional $600 million. As a qualification to the IPOs, eBay's board of directors retained the right to issue as many as 5 million additional shares of preferred stock with no further input from the current shareholders in case of a hostile takeover attempt.

eBay's Business Model

According to eBay's Meg Whitman, the company could best be described as a dynamic, self-regulating economy. Its business model was based on creating and maintaining a person-to-person trading community in which buyers and sellers could readily and conveniently exchange information and goods. The company's role was to function as a value-added facilitator of online buyer–seller transactions by providing a supportive infrastructure that enabled buyers and sellers to come together in an efficient and effective manner. Success depended not only on the quality of eBay's infrastructure but also on the quality and quantity of buyers and sellers attracted to the site; in management's view, this entailed maintaining a compelling trading environment, a number of trust and safety programs, a cost-effective and convenient trading experience, and strong community affinity. By developing the eBay brand name and increasing the customer base, eBay endeavored to attract a sufficient number of high-quality buyers and sellers necessary to meet the organization's goals. The online auction format meant that eBay carried zero inventory and could operate a marketplace without the need for a traditional sales force.

The eBay business model was built around three profit centers: the domestic business (auction operations within the United States), international business (auction operations outside of the United States) and payments (e.g., PayPal). For the first nine months of 2005, the company's U.S. operations accounted for 40.7 percent of revenue growth, the international share was 37.0 percent, and the remaining 22.3 percent was from payments (see Exhibit 5).

Specific elements of eBay's business model that the company particularly recognized as key to the company's success included:[12]

1. The fact that eBay was the world's largest online trading forum, with a critical mass of buyers, sellers, and items listed for sale.

Exhibit 5   **Sources of eBay's Revenue Growth, 2001–2005**

	2001	2002	2003	2004	2005 (3 quarters)
U.S. auctions	62.8%	48.0%	49.1%	42.8%	40.7%
International auctions	32.6	36.9	30.7	35.9	37.0
Payment fees (Pay Pal)	4.7	15.1	20.2	21.3	22.3

2. The compelling and entertaining trading environment, which had strong values, established rules, and procedures that facilitated communication and trade between buyers and sellers.
3. Established trust and safety programs such as SafeHarbor.
4. Cost-effective convenient trading.
5. Strong community affinity.
6. An intuitive user experience that was easy to use, arranged by topics, and fully automated.

In implementing its business model, eBay employed three main competitive tactics. First, it sought to build strategic partnerships in all stages of its value chain, creating an impressive portfolio of over 250 strategic alliances with companies such as America Online (AOL), Yahoo, IBM, Compaq, and Walt Disney. Second, it actively sought customer feedback and made improvements on the basis of this information. Third, it actively monitored the environment, both externally and internally, for developing opportunities. Two ways eBay executives keep in touch with internal trends were by hosting online town hall meetings and by visiting cities with large local markets. The feedback gained from these meetings and visits was used to adopt and adjust practices to keep customers satisfied.

eBay's Strategy

eBay's strategy to sustain growth rested on three key elements:[13]

1. *Categories:* Broaden the existing trading platform within existing product categories, across new product categories, and through geographic expansion, both local and international.
2. *Formats:* Continue to introduce additional pricing formats such as fixed-price sales, Dutch auctions (which allow a seller to sell multiple identical items to the highest bidders), eBay stores, and classified listings. Also, expand value-added

services in order to offer end-to-end personal trading service by offering a variety of pretrade and posttrade services to enhance the user experience and make trading easier.
3. *Geographies:* Continue to develop U.S. and international markets that employ the Internet to create an efficient trading platform in local, national, and international markets that can be transformed into a seamless, truly global trading platform.

Categories

Efforts intended to broaden the eBay trading platform concentrated on growing the content within current categories, broadening the range of products offered according to user preferences, and developing regionally targeted offerings. Growth in existing product categories was facilitated by deepening the content within the categories through the use of content-specific chat rooms and bulletin boards as well as targeted advertising at trade shows and in industry-specific publications.

To broaden the range of products offered, eBay developed new product categories, introduced specialty sites, and developed eBay stores. Over 2,000 new categories were added between 1998 and 2000; by 2005, eBay offered over 50,000 categories of items (greatly expanded from the original 10 categories in 1995). Projected over all of 2005, 12 of these categories had gross merchandise sales of over $1 billion, including eBay Motors ($14.3 billion), Clothing and Accessories ($3.3 billion), Consumer Electronics ($3.2 billion), Computers ($2.9 billion), Home and Garden ($2.5 billion), Books/Movies/Music ($2.4 billion), Sports ($2.1 billion), Collectibles ($2.0 billion), Toys ($1.6 billion), Jewelry and Watches ($1.5 billion), Business and Industrial ($1.5 billion), and Cameras and Photo ($1.3 billion). As of June 2005, over 55 million items were available on eBay worldwide and approximately 5 million items were being added per day.[14]

Significant new product categories and specialty sites developed since eBay's early days included:

- The eBay Motors category, which was developed when eBay noticed that an increasing number of automobile transactions were taking place on its site. In 2002, eBay Motors sold more than $3 billion worth of vehicles and parts and was currently the largest online marketplace for buying and selling autos, with over $14 billion in sales expected in 2005. According to Whitman, "One month, we saw the miscellaneous category had a very rapid growth rate, and someone said we have to find out what's going on. It was the buying and selling of used cars. So we said, maybe what we should do is give these guys a separate category and see what happens. It worked so well that we created eBay Motors."[15] In partnership with AutoTrader.com, this category was later expanded to a specialty site.

- The LiveAuctions specialty site, which allows live bidding via the Internet for auctions occurring in brick-and-mortar auction houses around the world. Through an alliance with Icollector.com, eBay users had access to more than 300 auction houses worldwide. Auction houses that participated in this agreement were well rewarded as more than 20 percent of their sales went to online bidders. One auction broadcast on the LiveAuctions site was held in February 2001 and featured items from a rare Marilyn Monroe collection, including a handwritten note from Monroe that listed her reasons for divorcing her first husband.

- The eBay Business marketplace, launched in 2002, which allowed business-related items to be sold in one location. Items such as office technology, wholesale lots, and marketplace services were offered at this destination. By the end of 2002, over 500,000 items were listed in eBay Business per week and more than $1 billion in annualized gross merchandise sales occurred across these categories. The Business and Industrial category of eBay's Web site was expected to generate $1.5 billion in revenues in 2005.

- The eBay Real Estate category was launched to foster eBay's emerging real estate marketplace. The offerings within this category were significantly enhanced by eBay's August 2001 acquisition of Homesdirect, which specialized in the sale of foreclosed properties owned by government agencies such as Housing and Urban Development and the Department of Veterans Affairs (formerly known as the Veterans Administration). The company estimated that a parcel of land was sold through the Real Estate category every 45 minutes. In February 2005, eBay also completed the acquisition of Rent.com, a leading online listing service in the apartment and rental housing industry.

Other notable moves to broaden the platform included:

- Launching the Application Program Interface (API) and Developers Program, which allowed other companies to use eBay's commerce engine and technology to build new sites.

- Launching, as of 1999, over 60 regional sites to give a more local flavor to eBay's offerings. These regional sites focused on the 50 largest metropolitan areas in the United States. Regional auction sites were intended to encourage the sale of items that were prohibitively expensive to ship, items that tended to have only a local appeal, and items that people preferred to view before purchasing. To supplement the regional sites, in mid-2001 eBay began offering eBay sellers the option of having their items listed in a special eBay seller's area in the classified sections of local newspapers. Sellers could highlight specific items, their eBay store, or their user ID in these classifieds.

- Reaching an agreement with Accenture, in May 2002, to develop a service intended to allow large sellers to more efficiently sell their products. These sellers were able to use a wide range of tools, such as high-volume listing capabilities, expanded customer service and support, and payment and fulfillment processes.

Formats

eBay also concentrated on expanding the number of formats in which its auctions were available. The company claimed that "in addition to our more established eBay Marketplace formats, we are continually looking for ways to better enable members of our community to interact and transact with one another online."[16] The company continued to develop additional pricing formats such as fixed-price sales, Dutch auctions, eBay stores, and classified listings. While eBay was primarily known for its traditional auction format, the company generated 29 percent of its gross merchandise volume through fixed-price auctions during the second quarter of 2005.[17]

Initiatives to create and develop new auction formats included:

- The establishment of a fixed-price format through the acquisition of Half.com that allowed eBay to compete more directly with competitors such as Amazon.com. Half.com was a fixed-price, person-to-person format that enabled buyers and sellers to trade books, CDs, movies and video games at prices starting at generally half of the retail price. Like eBay, Half.com offered a feedback system that helped buyers and sellers to build a solid reputation. eBay intended to eventually fully integrate both Half.com's listings and the feedback system into eBay's current site.

- The June 2001 eBay introduction of eBay stores to complement new offerings, to make it easier for sellers to build loyalty and for buyers to locate goods from specific sellers, and to prevent sellers from driving bidders to the seller's own Web site. In an eBay store, the entirety of a seller's auctions would be listed in one convenient location. These stores could also offer a fixed-price option from a seller and the integration of a seller's Half.com listings with his or her auction listings. While numerous sellers of all sizes moved to take advantage of eBay stores, the concept was especially appealing to the larger retailers such as IBM, Hard Rock Café, Sears, and Handspring, which were moving to take advantage of eBay's reach and distribution power. As of June 2005, the company had approximately 299,000 stores worldwide, with approximately 173,000 of these stores in the United States and the other 126,000 stores hosted on international sites.

- The August 2004 acquisition of a minority share in Craigslist, a company that offered online classifieds and forums. Of particular concern to eBay was penetrating international markets with classified listings. In February 2005, eBay launched online classifieds Web sites in select international markets. The international Web site was launched under the brand name Kijiji, which means "village" in Swahili. As of March 2005, Kijiji was available in over 50 cities in Canada, China, France, Germany, Italy, and Japan. Alex Kazim, eBay's senior vice president of new ventures, claimed that "Kijiji builds local communities online, giving neighbors a way to come together around local needs and interests. We're excited about making Kajiji the online neighborhood meeting place for local residents in cities across the world."[18]

- In August 2005, eBay completed the acquisition of shopping.com. Shopping.com, which had over 50 million unique visitors per month in the United States, the United Kingdom, and France, was the world's third-largest Internet shopping destination. eBay saw this as an opportunity to acquire a leading company in online comparison shopping and consumer reviews.[19]

Since its earliest days, eBay had realized that in order to be successful, its service had to be both easy to use and convenient to access. In September 2005, the company introduced member-generated product reviews and buying guides, in order to facilitate the dissemination of buying information to users. The company also sought to add services to fill these needs by offering a variety of pretrade and posttrade services to enhance the user experience and provide an end-to-end trading experience.

Early efforts in this direction included alliances with:

- Leading shipping services (USPS and UPS).
- Two companies that helped guarantee that buyers would get what they paid for (Tradesafe and I-Escrow).
- The world's largest franchiser of retail business, communications, and postal service centers (Mailboxes, Etc.).
- The leader in multicarrier Web-based shipping services for e-commerce (iShip.com).

To facilitate person-to-person credit card payments, eBay acquired PayPal, a company that specialized in transferring money from one cardholder to another, in October 2002. Using the newly acquired capabilities of PayPal, eBay was able to offer sellers the option of accepting credit card payments from other eBay users. As of the second quarter 2005, PayPal had over 78 million user accounts in 56 countries.

eBay's objective was to make credit card payment a "seamless and integrated part of the trading experience."[20] The total value of transactions on PayPal was $18.9 million in 2004. During the second quarter of 2005, over 35 percent of PayPal's revenues were from international business.

Developing International Markets

As competition increased in the online auction industry, eBay began to seek growth opportunities in international markets in an effort to create a global trading community. As of June 2005, eBay had a presence in 33 countries including Australia, Austria, Belgium, Canada, China (through an investment in the Chinese company Eachnet), France, Germany, Hong Kong, India, Ireland, Italy, Malaysia, the Netherlands, New Zealand, the Philippines, Singapore, South Korea, Spain, Sweden, Switzerland, Taiwan, Great Britain, and Latin America (through an investment in MercadoLibre.com). Through the first three quarters of 2005, 37 percent of eBay's revenues came from its international sources and over half of eBay's registered users were from countries outside the United States (82 million out of 157 million total registered users). Growth opportunities were especially appealing in Asia (due to rapid increases in Internet access) and Europe. In entering international markets, eBay considered three options: building a new user community from the ground up, acquiring a local organization, or forming a partnership with a strong local company. In realizing its goals of international growth, eBay employed all three strategies.

In late 1998, eBay's initial efforts at international expansion into Canada and the United Kingdom relied on building new user communities. The first step in establishing these communities was to create customized home pages for users in those countries. These home pages were designed to provide content and categories locally customized to the needs of users in specific countries, while providing them with access to a global trading community. Local customization in the United Kingdom was facilitated through the use of local management, grassroots and online marketing, and participation in local events.[21] In February 1999, eBay partnered with PBL Online, a leading Internet company in Australia, to offer a customized Australian and New Zealand eBay home page. When the site went live in October 1999,

transactions were denominated in Australian dollars, and, while buyers could bid on auctions anywhere in the world, they could also search for items located exclusively in Australia. Further, local chat boards were designed to facilitate interaction between Australian users, and country-specific categories, such as Australian coins and stamps as well as cricket and rugby memorabilia, were offered.

To further expand its global reach, eBay acquired Germany's largest online person-to-person trading site, Alando.de AG, in June 1999. Management handled the transition of service in a manner calculated to be smooth and painless for Alando.de's users. While users would have to comply with eBay rules and regulations, the only significant change for Alando.de's 50,000 registered users was that they would have to go to a new Web address to transact their business.

To establish an Asian presence, in February 2000 eBay formed a joint venture with NEC to launch eBay Japan. According to the new CEO of eBay Japan, Merle Okawara, an internationally renowned executive, NEC was pleased to help eBay in leveraging the tried-and-trusted eBay business model to provide Japanese consumers with access to a global community of active online buyers and sellers. In customizing the site to the needs of Japanese users, eBay wrote the content exclusively in Japanese and allowed users to bid in yen. The site had over 800 categories ranging from internationally popular categories (such as computers, electronics, and Asian antiques) to categories with a local flavor (such as Hello Kitty, Pokémon, and pottery). The eBay Japan site also debuted a new merchant-to-person concept known as Supershops, which allowed consumers to bid on items listed by companies. However, eBay discontinued its operations in the Japanese market in 2002 due to rising costs.

In 2001, eBay expanded into South Korea through an acquisition of a majority ownership position in the country's largest online trading service Internet Auction Company Ltd., and into Belgium, Brazil, Italy, France, the Netherlands, Portugal, Spain, and Sweden through the acquisition of Europe's largest online trading platform, iBazar. Further expansion in 2001 included the development of a local site in Singapore, and an equity-based alliance with the leading online auction site for the Spanish- and Portuguese-speaking communities in Latin America, MercadoLibre.com. By the end of 2004, eBay was using MercadoLibre.com to reach nine markets: Argentina, Brazil, Chile, Colombia, Ecuador, Mexico, Peru, Uruguay, and Venezuela.

Due to increasing saturation in their domestic market during 2004 and 2005, eBay implemented aggressive international expansion plans in an effort to increase the company's global presence. Among the strategic moves that the company implemented during this time were:

- The acquisition in September 2005 of Skype Technologies, a global Internet communications company. At the time of the acquisition, Skype had 54 million members in over 225 countries. eBay believed that this move would allow it to develop an enhanced global marketplace and payments platform.[22]

- The 2004 launch of a European Business Center in Dublin, Ireland, to serve as PayPal's European headquarters. This was PayPal's first facility outside the United States and hosted its European customer service and fraud prevention operations. This facility was expected to have over 400 employees by the end of 2005.

- The November 2004 launch of eBay Philippines. IDC expected business-to-consumer e-commerce in the Philippines to increase from $828 million in 2004 to $2.9 billion in 2007.[23]

- The December 2004 launch of eBay Malaysia. IDC reported that business-to-consumer e-commerce in Malaysia would increase from $1.1 billion to $3.0 billion between 2005 and 2008.[24]

- The launch of eBay Poland in April 2005. IDC predicted that business-to-consumer e-commerce would grow by over 400 percent in Poland between 2005 and 2008.[25]

- The August 2004 acquisition of Baazee.com, the largest online marketplace in India with over 1 million confirmed registered users. At that time, there were 17 million Internet users in India, and that number was expected to increase to more than 30 million by 2006.[26]

- The September 2004 acquisition of Internet Auction Company, an online trading company based in Korea.

- The November 2004 acquisition of Marktplaats.nl, the leading classifieds site in the Netherlands.

- The acquisitions in May 2005 of Gumtree.com and LoQUo.com. These two companies had classified sites in international cities. Gumtree.com offered multiple sites in countries including the United Kingdom, Australia, New Zealand, and South Africa. LoQUo.com offered a classifieds site to the Spanish market.

- The acquisition in June 2005 of Opusforum, a leading German classifieds site. Opusforum had over 1 million visitors in May 2005 and advertised jobs, housing, and services to the German market. This followed the April 2004 acquisition of Mobile.de, the leading classifieds Web site for vehicles in Germany.

HOW eBAY'S AUCTION SITE COMPARED WITH THAT OF RIVALS

Auction sites varied in a number of respects: their inventory, the bidding process, extra services and fees, technical support, functionality, and sense of community. Since its inception, eBay had gone to great lengths to make its Web site intuitive, easy to use by both buyers and sellers, and reliable. Efforts to ensure ease of use ranged from narrowly defining categories (to allow users to quickly locate desired products) to introducing services designed to personalize a user's eBay experience. Two specific services developed by eBay and launched in 1998 to increase personalization were My eBay and About Me. My eBay gave users centralized access to confidential, current information regarding their trading activities. From his or her My eBay page, a user could view information pertaining to his or her current account balances with eBay; feedback rating; the status of any auctions in which he or she was participating, as either a buyer or a seller; and auctions in favorite categories. In October, eBay introduced the About Me service, which allowed users to create customized home pages that could be viewed by all other eBay members and could include elements from the My eBay page such as user ratings or items the user had listed for auction, as well as personal information and pictures. This service not only increased customer ease of use but also contributed to the sense of community among the traders; one seller stated that the About Me service "made it easier and more rewarding for me to do business with others."[27] New features and services added in 2000 included new listing functions that could make an auction standout including Highlight and Feature Plus as well as the ability for sellers to cross-list their products in two categories, a tool to set prequalification guidelines for bidders, a new imaging and photo hosting service that made it easier for sellers to include pictures of their goods, and the introduction of the Buy It Now tool.

Throughout its history, eBay had struggled to balance its explosive growth with its technological infrastructure. To counter several significant service outages the company had faced in its early days, eBay hired Maynard Webb, a premier software engineer and troubleshooter who was working at Gateway Computer. Webb took swift action, forming alliances with key vendors such as Sun, IBM, and Microsoft, and outsourcing its technology and Web site operations to Exodus Communications and Abovenet. These outsourcing agreements were intended to allow Exodus and Abovenet to "manage network capacity and provide a more robust backbone" while eBay focused on its core business.[28] While eBay still experienced minor outages when it changed or expanded services (for example, a system crash coincided with the introduction of the original 22 regional Web sites), system downtime decreased. However, the stability of the system under eBay's explosive growth and continuous introduction of new features was a continuing management concern, especially as competitors continued to strengthen their competencies.

eBay's Main Competitors

The ability to attract buyers, the volume of transactions and selection of goods, customer service, and brand recognition were among the competitive factors eBay considered most important in the online auction industry. In October 2005, eBay introduced the "It" broadcasting campaign, in an effort to draw attention to the expansive amount of product variety offered by the company. The campaign used the slogan "Whatever It is that you are looking for, you can find It on eBay." In addition to factors such as variety and brand image, eBay was also attempting to compete along several other dimensions: sense of community, system reliability, reliability of delivery and payment, Web site convenience and accessibility, low levels of service fees, and efficient information exchange.[29]

Early in eBay's history, the company's main rivals could be considered classified advertisements in newspapers, garage sales, flea markets, collectibles shows, and other venues such as local auction houses and liquidators. As eBay's product mix and selling techniques evolved, the company's range of competitors did as well. The broadening of eBay's product mix beyond collectibles to include practical household items, office equipment, toys, and so on brought the company into more direct competition with brick-and-mortar retailers, import/export companies, and catalog and mail order companies. Further, with the acquisition of Half.com, the introduction of eBay stores, and the growing percentage of fixed-price and Buy It Now sales as a percentage of eBay's revenue, eBay considered itself to be competing in a broad sense with a number of other online retailers, such as Wal-Mart, Kmart, Target, Sears, JCPenney, and Office Depot. In competing with these larger sellers, eBay began to adopt some of their tools, such as the use of gift certificates. The company also felt that it was competing with a number of specialty retailers, such as Christie's (antiques), KB Toys (toys), Blockbuster (movies), Dell (computers), Foot Locker (sporting goods), Ticketmaster (tickets), and Home Depot (tools).[30] Exhibit 6 displays eBay's customer service rankings as compared to a variety of rivals.

Management saw traditional competitors as inefficient because their fragmented local and regional nature made it expensive and time-consuming for buyers and sellers to meet, exchange information, and complete transactions. Moreover, they suffered from three other deficiencies: (1) They tended to offer limited variety and breadth of selection as compared to the millions of items available on eBay, (2) they often had high transactions costs, and (3) they were information-inefficient in the sense that buyers and sellers lacked a reliable and convenient means of setting prices for sales or purchases. Management saw eBay's online auction format as competitively superior to these rivals because (1) it facilitated buyers and sellers meeting, exchanging information, and conducting transactions; (2) it allowed buyers and sellers to bypass traditional intermediaries and trade directly, thus lowering costs; (3) it provided global reach to greater selection and a broader base of participants; (4) it permitted trading at all hours and provided continuously updated information; and (5) it fostered a sense of community among individuals with mutual interests.

Exhibit 6   **Customer Service Rankings for Selected Companies, 2000–2004 (scores out of 100)**

Company/Sector	2000	2001	2002	2003	2004
Online Auctions					
Online auctions overall	72	74	77	78	77
eBay	80	82	82	84	80
uBid	67	69	70	73	73
Priceline.com	66	69	71	71	73
All others	73	75	78	79	76
Internet Retail					
Internet retail overall	75.2	74.3	77.6	80.8	78.6
Barnesandnoble.com	77	82	87	86	87
Amazon.com	84	84	88	88	84
Buy.com	78	78	80	80	80
1-800-Flowers.com	69	76	78	76	79
General Retail					
General retail overall	78	77	83	84	80
Target	73	77	78	77	75
Wal-Mart	73	75	74	75	73
Sears	73	76	75	73	74
Kmart	67	74	70	70	67

Source: American Customer Satisfaction Index, www.theacsi.org.

The most significant competitors to eBay's auction business included Amazon Auctions, Yahoo Auctions, uBid, and Overstock.com. Two of the smaller competitors in the online auction industry included Bidville (an auction site with no listing fees and no final value fees) and ePier (over 60,000 members as of 2004). Both of these had closely copied eBay's look and feel and touted themselves as "alternatives to eBay."

Amazon.com Auctions

Amazon.com's business strategy was to be "Earth's most customer-centric company, where customers can find and discover anything they may want to buy online, and [we] endeavor to offer customers the lowest possible prices."[31] With its customer base of 35 million users in over 220 countries and a well-known brand name, Amazon.com was considered the closest overall competitive threat to eBay, especially as eBay expanded its business model beyond is traditional auction services. Created in July 1995 as an online bookseller, Amazon had rapidly transitioned into a full-line, one-stop-shopping retailer with a product offering that included books, music, toys, electronics, tools and hardware, lawn and patio products, video games, software, and a mall of boutiques (called zShops). Amazon.com was the Internet's number one music, video, and book retailer. One of the distinctive features customers appreciated about Amazon.com was the extensive reviews available for each item. These product reviews were written both by professionals and by regular users who had purchased a specific product. The company's 2004 net income was over $440 million, which was an increase of over 600 percent from 2002 (see Exhibit 7). One significant weakness analysts noted in Amazon's financials was that the company's free shipping policies, put in place to draw more customers, had a significant negative impact on net income.

By 2003 Amazon's management felt that it was in a position that would allow it to balance demands of both cost control and growth in executing a strategy intended to enhance Amazon's position as leader in retail e-commerce. As an indication of the company's success in executing its strategy, its customer base rose from 14 million to 20 million during 2000 and to 35 million by 2004. The company invested

Exhibit 7 **Operating Income (Loss) for Amazon.com, 1996–2004**

Year	Income or (Loss) from Operations (in millions)
1996	$(6.2)
1997	(31.0)
1998	(124.5)
1999	(720.0)
2000	(863.9)
2001	(412.3)
2002	64.1
2003	270.5
2004	440.4

more than $300 million in infrastructure in 1999 and opened two international sites, Amazon.co.uk (the United Kingdom) and Amazon.de (Germany), and later added Amazon.ca (Canada), Amazon.co.jp (Japan), and Amazon.fr (France). These sites, along with Amazon.com, were among the most popular online retail domains in Europe. By 2004 international sales had grown to over $2 billion from just $168 million in 1999 and accounted for 38 percent of all Internet sales.

Some analysts felt that, in expanding its position both internationally and abroad, Amazon had conceded the top spot in online auctions to eBay and was looking for other avenues to expand its business. Amazon was continually looking for innovative ways to expand its product offering and often used strategic alliances to support these initiatives. For example, the company had agreements with Borders Books to allow customers to pick up Amazon.com book orders in-store, as well as e-commerce partnerships with Ashford.com, Drugstore.com, CarsDirect.com, and Sotheby's (a leading auction house for art, antiques, and collectibles), and opened a co-branded toy and video game store online with Toysrus.com. During 2003, the company announced an agreement with the band Pearl Jam to sell the group's music directly to fans through Amazon's Advantage program. By 2003, Amazon.com had over 550,000 active third-party sellers on its site and 350 branded sellers, most of them selling through shops rather than auctions. These third-party sellers accounted for over 22 percent of U.S. sales. To further expand its reach, in September 2003 Amazon established an independent

unit called A9 that was charged with creating the best shopping search tool for Amazon's use and for use by other companies and third-party Web sites. To compete with eBay's fixed-price formats, Amazon began including links on product pages that allowed customers to view identical new and used items from third-party sellers.

Yahoo Auctions

Yahoo.com, the first online navigational guide to the Web, launched Yahoo Auctions in 1998. Yahoo.com offered services to nearly 200 million users every month in North America, Europe, Asia, and Latin America. The Web site was available in 24 countries and 12 languages. Yahoo had entered into numerous alliances and marketing agreements to generate additional traffic at its site and was investing in new technology to improve the performance and attractiveness of its site. Its auction services were provided to users free of charge in the early days, and the number of auctions listed on Yahoo increased from 670,000 to 1.3 million during the second half of 1999. However, when Yahoo decided to start charging users a listing fee in January 2001, listings fell from over 2 million to about 200,000.[32] In recognition of the fall in listings due to the listing fee instituted in January, Yahoo! Auctions announced a revamped performance-based pricing model for its U.S. auctions in November, 2001. In this system, which was relatively similar to eBay's, listing fees were reduced and sellers were charged according to the value of an item sold. In response to this change, the number of listings rose to more than 500,000 by December 7, 2001. In an effort to gain even greater market share in the online auction industry, Yahoo Auctions stopped charging fees for any of its auction services on June 6, 2005. Yahoo Auctions also offered many extra services to its users. For example, the Premium Sellers Program was designed to reward the sellers that were consistently at the top of their category. These Premium Sellers were allowed enhanced promotions, premium placement, and direct access to customer support.

While Yahoo had significant reach throughout the world, including over 25 local auction sites internationally, Yahoo Auctions had, by 2004, reduced its international operations from 16 countries to 7 (Brazil, Canada, Hong Kong, Japan, Mexico, Singapore, and Taiwan). In 2002 alone, Yahoo conceded its auction sites in France, Germany, Italy, Spain, the United Kingdom, and Ireland and promoted eBay's sites in each of those countries via banner ads and text links. In 2003, Yahoo sold its Australian site as well. In 2004, however, Yahoo began offering auctions in China through a joint venture with the dominant Chinese Web portal Sina, indicating that it had not completely abandoned the international auction market. Further reinforcing its commitment to online retail, in July 2003 Yahoo acquired Overture, which was the leading provider of commercial search as of the end of the first quarter of 2003 with more than 88,000 advertisers globally as well as an extensive affiliate distribution network. Many of the sellers who advertised on Overture also advertised on eBay, and some analysts estimated that the amount of sales by merchants through the combination of Yahoo's and Overture's offerings would total between one-half to two-thirds of that available on eBay. In August 2005, Yahoo further strengthened its position in China by paying $1 billion in cash for a 40 percent stake in Alibaba.com, an e-commerce company that was one of the largest Internet companies in China, and turned its Chinese operations over to Alibaba.com. Alibaba's Chinese online auction company, TaoBao (which means "searching for treasure"), claimed to be the largest in the country, with 41 percent of the market.[33] The deal was brokered by Softbank, a Japanese broadband Internet provider that aggressively invested in new technologies and successfully paired with Yahoo in 2002 to drive eBay out of Japan. Yahoo believed that this partnership clearly showed Yahoo's long-term commitment to the region, and that the agreement represented the "best approach for Yahoo! to win in this region."[34]

uBid.com

The auction site uBid was founded in April 1997 and offered an initial public offering on the Nasdaq in December 1998. According to its mission statement, uBid was to "be the most recognized and trusted business-to-consumer marketplace, consistently delivering exceptional value and service to its customers and supplier partners."[35] As of 2005, uBid believed that its core values of integrity, agility, execution, caring, and innovation would allow the company to deliver competitive success in the online auction industry and to build valuable relationships with its customers, employees, and suppliers.[36] As

such, uBid considered itself to be in direct competition with eBay, although the company had difficulty denting the portion of eBay's business that was derived from large corporations and smaller companies wanting to sell their products through an auction format. As a company, uBid had experienced increased revenues almost every year since its inception; however, it had never captured the share of the auction market that its founders hoped was possible, although it at one time had a 14.7 percent share of revenues in the online auction market. The company was sold to CGMI Networks in mid-2000, and then it was sold again to Petters Group Worldwide in 2003. With each sale, the number of workers employed by uBid fell and the product mix was changed in an attempt to find a niche market that would insulate the company from the competitive power of eBay.

The business model uBid chose centered on offering brand-name (often refurbished and close-out) merchandise at a deep discount in a relatively broad range of categories from over 1,000 leading manufacturers such as Sony, Hewlett-Packard, IBM, Compaq, AMD, and Minolta. Categories included Computer and Office, Consumer Electronics, Music Movies & Games, Jewelry & Gifts, Travel & Events, Home & Garden, Sports, Toys & Hobbies, Apparel, Collectibles, and Everything Else. The merchandise was offered in both an online auction format in which prices started at $1.00 and through uBid's fixed-price superstore. The merchandise was sourced from corporate partners and from uBid's own operations, which included a 400,000-square-foot warehouse and refurbishment center, and its current parent company Petters Group Worldwide, and from small and medium-sized companies that were members of uBid's Certified Merchant Program. Although uBid had offered consumer-to-consumer auctions at one time, the company had discontinued this option as of 2002 due to the costs associated with policing fraud and concerns over product quality.

Overstock.com

Overstock.com was another online auction company that was beginning to compete more directly with eBay. Founded in 1999, the company was emerging as a growing competitive threat in the online auction industry. Overstock.com specialized in selling excess inventory via the Internet. However, it also enacted an auction feature on its Web site. Sellers listed the opening bid price, the duration of the auction, and the Make It Mine price (which was optional). As evidence of its growing importance in the industry, Overstock's revenues had increased from $1.8 million in 1999 to over $540 million in 2004. The company also claimed to have over 650,000 products listed on its Web sites as of June 2005.

eBAY'S NEW CHALLENGES

Throughout its history, eBay faced each new challenge with an eye on its founding values and an ear for community members. Omidyar stated,

> What we do have to be cautious of, as we grow, is that our core is the personal trade, because the values are communicated person-to-person. It can be easy for a big company to start to believe that it's responsible for its success. Our success is really based on our members' success. They're the ones who have created this, and they're the ones who will create it in the future. If we lose sight of that, then we're in big trouble.[37]

The company applied this perspective in response to significant customer concerns regarding the growing presence of corporate sellers on eBay.

Omidyar and Whitman recognized the importance of eBay's culture and were aware of the potential impact rapid growth and the evolution of the product line could have on this valued asset. When asked about the importance of the culture, Omidyar said, "If we lose that, we've pretty much lost everything."[38] Whitman agreed with Omidyar about the importance of eBay's culture, but she did not see the influx of larger retailers and liquidators as a significant problem. Even as these sellers grew to account for 5 percent of eBay's total business in 2004 (from 1 percent in 2001), these large sellers received no favorable treatment. Whitman stated, "There are no special deals. I am passionate about creating this level playing field."[39] While this view was applauded by the smaller sellers, some larger sellers viewed these policies as overly restrictive and were searching for additional sales outlets.

Heading into 2006, eBay faced two fundamental challenges:

1. How could eBay continue to maintain strong international growth, which was necessary given the maturing of its domestic market?

2. As eBay's business model evolved to include more fixed-price sales in an effort to combat the saturation of its domestic market, could the company transfer its competitive advantage in the online auction industry into the more general area of online retail?

Continued International Growth

While eBay had been able to secure a significant market share in many of the countries in which it was operating, the company was still well aware of its failed venture into the Japanese market. The company had decided to pull out of Japan in 2002 as a result of stiff competition from Yahoo and eBay's unwillingness to cede decision-making authority to local Japanese managers. The Japanese experience was especially salient as it appeared that the primary battleground in the online auction industry for the foreseeable future would be another Asian market— China—and that its main competition would be the Yahoo-backed competitor TaoBao. As early as 2000, eBay had begun to cautiously build its presence in the Chinese online auction industry. However, there were a number of significant challenges in penetrating the Chinese market, including the fact that many Chinese consumers were suspicious of online transactions, many of these consumers did not have credit cards, and the Chinese transportation system was not sufficient to guarantee timely delivery of items won in online auctions.[40] In 2002, eBay bought a 33 percent stake in Eachnet, a Chinese online auction company patterned after eBay, and then purchased the remaining 67 percent of the company in 2003. By the end of 2005, eBay was still losing money in its Chinese operations despite having 13.2 million registered Chinese users.

The company's position in China was especially troubling, given Amazon.com's recent announcement that it had made the Chinese market a top priority and the new partnership between Yahoo and Alibaba. Alibaba's online auction subsidiary (Tao Bao) was overseen by Alibaba's CEO, Jack Ma, who had a reputation as a scrappy competitor. Since its founding in 2003, TaoBao had been an aggressive challenger to eBay's Eachnet. In an attempt to build a large user base, TaoBao did not charge any fees for its services and did not plan to do so until 2006 at the earliest. Additionally, the company claimed to have tailored its offerings particularly well to the Chinese market by offering services such as instant messaging between users and having online forum managers take the names of heroes from Chinese literature. In order to complete the business model, the company established AliPay, an online payment service, in 2003. In an effort to attract customers, it had shunned TV advertising such as that used by eBay in China and instead relied on word of mouth, which many analysts believed was the key to Chinese marketing, and it had also directly targeted eBay's users through a variety of unconventional means.[41] In one guerrilla marketing campaign, a contingent from TaoBao disrupted an eBay user seminar by hanging a TaoBao sign in the conference room, having the waitstaff hand out TaoBao flyers to seminar attendees, and then offering to reimburse the attendees for their registration fees and inviting them to dinner.[42]

By the end of 2005, TaoBao had established itself as a legitimate contender for the Chinese online auction industry and had developed strong customer loyalty among its user base. In fact, TaoBao claimed to be the largest Chinese online auction company, with 7.2 million registered users and $200 million in sales during the second quarter of 2005, as compared to eBay's 13.2 million registered users and $100 million in sales in China. However, the Chinese online auction industry was still in its early stages, with less than 8 percent of China's population of 1.3 billion people using the Internet. As such, experts believed there was still significant room for growth in the Chinese market. While Whitman and eBay had learned a lesson from eBay's failure in the Japanese market and had given more authority to local Chinese managers, Ma felt that TaoBao would prevail due to his personal knowledge of the Chinese market and that the company would be profitable 18 months after it started charging fees.[43] Not willing to surrender in the Chinese market as it had in Japan, eBay had consistently reaffirmed its commitment to the market and had even used phone calls and special promotions to pursue individual power sellers who had moved to TaoBao.

Evolution of the Business Model

By virtually any measure, eBay's growth had been outstanding. However, this impressive track record, coupled with the progress the company had made in reaching its stated goals, had created high expectations among investors. These lofty expectations began to cause some concern among analysts as eBay's domestic core market of online auction sales began to show some warning signals. In many categories, as the number of sellers grew supply was beginning to outstrip demand. Almost half of eBay's registered users were from the United States and represented almost one-third of all U.S. Internet users. With the U.S. online auction market maturing and eBay's dominant market share, analysts were concerned with how much more penetration eBay could achieve.

In response to these concerns, eBay cited new trends indicating that even in the United States the company was reaching new customers and had room to grow. One of the trends eBay saw as particularly promising was the increasing use of eBay's more than 50,000 registered Trading Assistants and the emergence of drop-off eBay consignment services. Trading Assistants were experienced eBay sellers who, for a fee, would help users sell their items on eBay. Extending this service, drop-off consignment services begin to spring up as early as 2000. These consignment services, such as AuctionDrop, QuickDrop, and Picture-It-Sold, would take physical possession of a customer's items, typically those with an eBay value of over $50, and sell them on eBay for a fee equal to between 30 and 40 percent of the item's final sale price. The company was encouraged by these activities, which allowed it reach sellers who would not normally use the Internet.

There was little concern that anyone would seriously threaten eBay in its core auction business in the near future. However, the increasing use of tools such as gift certificates, the growing importance of fixed-price sales, the purchase of Half.com, and the growing popularity of Buy It Now put eBay into more direct competition with retailers such as Amazon.com, with e-commerce solutions, and with the likes of Microsoft. When asked about how the evolution of its business model influenced eBay's sphere of competition, Whitman said,

> If we were a retailer, we'd be the 27th-largest in the world. So our sellers are competing [with retailers] for consumer dollars. If you're thinking about buying a set of golf clubs or a tennis racket or a jacket or a pair of skis, you decide whether you're going to do that at eBay, at Wal-Mart, a sporting-goods store, or Macy's. I would define our competition more broadly than ever before.[44]

The threat of these competitors increased as fixed-price sales comprised an ever-increasing percentage of eBay's total sales and growth. In mid-2005, fixed-price trading accounted for 29 percent of eBay's gross merchandise sales (the dollar value of merchandise sold) and was expected to experience continued growth throughout the foreseeable future.

THE FUTURE

Ten years since its inception, eBay had continued to enjoy heightened levels of financial success and was the dominant player in the online auction industry. However, there were several emerging issues that clouded the company's future, and this was reflected in the volatility of its stock price (see Exhibit 8). The recent downgrades of eBay's stock seemed to indicate that Wall Street analysts were not as optimistic about eBay's ability to sustain its phenomenal growth rate and to extend its dominance to the global online auction industry. The company's executives needed to address several questions: Should additional expansion in the international markets be the highest priority? If so, in what countries should expansion efforts be focused? Alternatively, should eBay strive to broaden its offerings to include more categories, more specialty sites, and more sellers? And how much emphasis should be put on fixed-price options? If management opted to continue expanding eBay's fixed-price offerings and put the company into greater head-to-head competition with established online retailers, what competitive advantage could it hope to achieve? Would it be able to compete successfully against new, more diverse competitors such as paid search engines?

Exhibit 8   **eBay's Stock Price Performance, December 2004–December 2005**

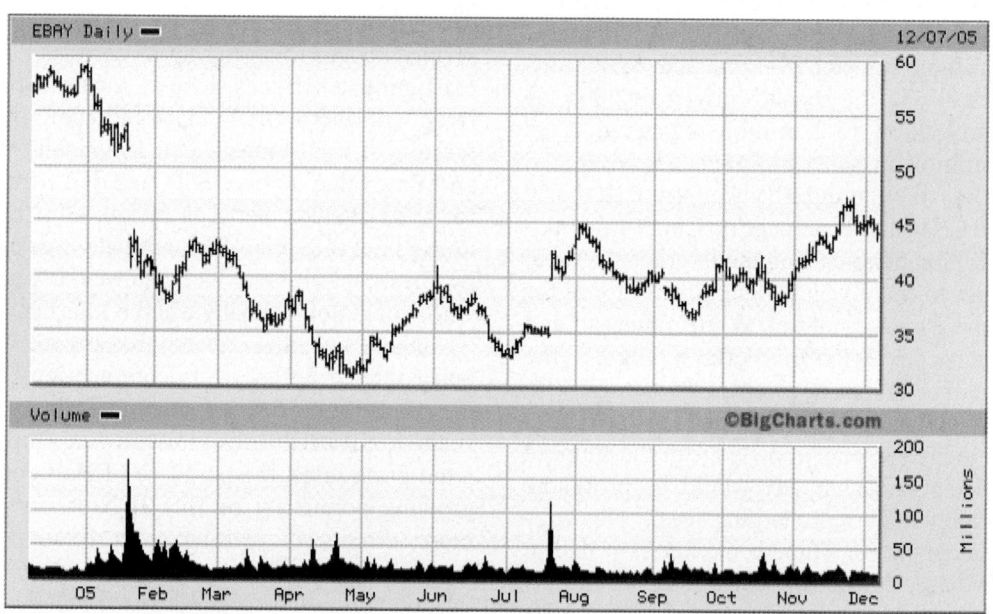

Note: A stock split occurred on February 17, 2005.
Source: www.bigcharts.com, December 8, 2005.

Endnotes

[1] 2004 eBay annual report.

[2] Ibid.

[3] Ibid.

[4] Claire Tristram, " 'Amazing'Amazon," www.contextmag.com, November 1999.

[5] Quentin Hardy, "The Radical Philanthropist," *Forbes,* May 1, 2000, p. 118.

[6] "Billionaires of the Web," *Business 2.0,* June 1999.

[7] eBay press release, May 7, 1998.

[8] http://pages.ebay.com/help/community/values.html, December 18, 2005.

[9] "Q&A with eBay's Meg Whitman," *BusinessWeek E. Biz,* December 3, 2001.

[10] Ibid.

[11] Claire Tristram, "'Amazoning' Amazon," www.contextmag.com, November 1999.

[12] 2000 eBay annual report.

[13] 2004 eBay annual report.

[14] Company press release, September 12, 2005.

[15] "Q&A with eBay's Meg Whitman."

[16] 2004 eBay annual report.

[17] Company press release, September 12, 2005.

[18] Company press release, March 8, 2005.

[19] Company press release, August 30, 2005.

[20] Company press release, May 18, 1999.

[21] 1999 eBay annual report.

[22] Company press release, September 12, 2005.

[23] Company press release, November 16, 2004.

[24] Company press release, December 1, 2004.

[26] Company press release, April 22, 2005.

[26] Company press release, June 22, 2004.

[27] Ann Pearson, in an eBay press release dated October 15, 1998.

[28] eBay press release, October 8, 1999.

[29] 2004 eBay annual report.

[30] eBay 10Q Annual Report, November 14, 2001.

[31] 2004 Amazon annual report.

[32] Troy Wolverton, "eBay Seeks to Sail into New Territory," CNET News.com, July 19, 2001.

[33] "Hot Bidding: In a Challenging China Market, eBay Confronts a Big New Rival; Yahoo Backs a Local Firm; An Online-Auction Duel Stirs Memories of Japan; Mr. Ma's Plans for Alibaba," *The Wall Street Journal,* August 12, 2005, p. A1.

[34] Yahoo company press release, August 10, 2005.

[35] www.ubid.com/about/companyinfo.asp, December 18, 2005.

[36] Ibid.

[37] "Q&A with eBay's Pierre Omidyar," *BusinessWeek E. Biz,* December 3, 2001.

[38] "The People's Company," *BusinessWeek E. Biz,* December 3, 2001.

[39] "Queen of the Online Flea Market," Economist.com, December 30, 2003.

[40] "Can Eachnet Become an eBay in China's Image?" *BusinessWeek Online,* March 27, 2000.

[41] "Hot Bidding."

[42] Ibid.

[43] Ibid.

[44] "Meg Whitman on eBay's Self-Regulation," *BusinessWeek Online,* August 18, 2003.

Google Inc. in 2006: Can the Strategy Support the Lofty Stock Price?

John E. Gamble
University of South Alabama

In 2005, Internet searches were the second most common online activity after e-mail. Advertisers spent an estimated $12 billion on paid search Internet ads in 2005—375 percent more than spending for such ads in 2004. Advertisers believed that search-based ads were particularly effective because they were highly targeted to what Internet users were immediately searching for. In 2005, Google was the leading search engine on the Web and the leading provider of search-based ads because of Internet users' faith in the search engine. The company did not collect information on search users, placed ads discreetly on its page listing search results, and did not intersperse paid search results with nonpaid search results. Perhaps Google's most important feature was its capability to retrieve highly relevant results to search queries that was made possible by its innovative PageRank technology.

When an Internet user entered a search query at Google.com, from a Google toolbar or deskbar, or from a Web site that licensed Google's search appliance, the search engine performed a computation of an equation involving 500 million variables and 2 billion terms to generate a list of best-matching search results. The results were generated in a fraction of a second and pulled from billions of Web sites that were constantly downloaded onto Google's farm of an estimated 250,000 PCs. The reason many Internet users found Google's search results more relevant than results generated by competing search engines was based on this equation, which assessed

how well the search terms matched and, most important, how many other Web sites pointed to a site. Google cofounder Larry Page suggested that Google's technology, which counted the number of "votes" for various Web sites that might match search requests, was superior to other search technologies, saying, "You're asking the whole Web who's the greatest site to ask about this subject."[1]

Internet users' preference for Google's search results allowed the company to establish hundreds of thousands of accounts with advertisers, which had produced 2004 revenues of nearly $3.2 billion and profits of more than $399 million. The company executed a successful initial public offering (IPO) in August 2004 that brought in an investment of $1.7 billion and made a subsequent offering of shares in September 2005 that added nearly $4.3 billion to its coffers. The company's cash and cash equivalents stood at $5.5 billion at the end of its third quarter of fiscal 2005. At year-end 2005, Google seemed poised to repeat its stellar 217 percent growth rate in revenues and 377 percent growth rate in net income between 2003 and 2004, since its revenues and net income for the first nine months of the fiscal year stood at $4.2 billion and $1.1 million, respectively. Google's highly scalable business model delivered profits for the first nine months of 2005 of more than $500,000 per employee.

Google's stock price had risen from its $85 IPO price in August 2004 to over $443 at year-end 2005. In late December 2005, the shares traded at a price/earnings multiple of 95—pushing its market capitalization over $131 billion. In comparison, the market capitalization for General Motors was $12 billion, the market value of Chevron's shares was $129 billion, and Intel's market cap was $159 billion. Some analysts still saw Google as a "strong buy" since as much as 30 percent of consumers' exposure to media was through the Internet and, as of 2005, only a small fraction of the $300–$400 billion spent on advertising in the United States was allocated to Internet ads.

Others considered Google's stock to be highly overvalued—pointing to a business model that relied almost exclusively on revenue from search-based ads. Over time, such ads might prove to be less effective than other forms of advertising or might reach more Internet users if provided by a rival search engine. Clearly, Web portals such as Yahoo and MSN were working furiously to improve search functionality to lure Google's loyal users to their sites. Yahoo had developed its own search capabilities in 2003 and severed its three-year agreement with Google to provide search results and ads for its own Web portal in July 2004. Microsoft had spent more than $150 million and taken 18 months to build a search engine in an effort to match Google feature for feature. MSN Search was launched in the winter of 2005 and provided direct links to MSN Encarta and other sites for searches written in plain language. In addition, MSN search users could search image files, music files, news stories, e-mails, and files residing on their PCs; they could also narrow search results locally and pull up satellite-based street maps for almost any part of the world.

Perhaps the biggest threat Microsoft posed to Google's dominance in search was its ability to embed MSN Search into Outlook, Internet Explorer, and Office applications. In fact, Microsoft had a long track record of exploiting Windows integration to upset incumbents as the market leader. During the late 1980s and early 1990s, Excel surpassed Lotus 1-2-3 as the market leader in spreadsheets within four years of its launch. Lotus held a 70 percent market share prior to Excel's development. Similarly, Word beat out WordPerfect as the dominant word processing program, and Netscape proved to be no match for Microsoft in the war for market share in the browser category.

Also of concern to some analysts was the mysterious nature of Google's cash reserves. International expansion and the development of new features such as Voice over Internet Protocol (VoIP) telephone service were obvious strategic initiatives Google should pursue, but the company had made no comments regarding the specific use of its $5.5 billion cash balance. The company also held $2.1 billion in marketable securities at the end of its third quarter of 2005. Google's management itself seemed uncertain what might drive future growth. The company's two founders, Sergey Brin and Larry Page, wrote in the company's IPO prospectus, "We would fund products that have a 10% chance of earning a billion dollars over the long term. Don't be surprised if we place smaller bets in areas that seem very speculative or even strange." The company's cash reserves had spawned hordes of Mountain View, California, entrepreneurs with the end goal of being acquired by Google. However, as of late 2005, Google had been a tough sell for those making pitches, having completed only five modestly sized acquisitions. The company's expanded advertising partnership with America Online (AOL) announced in December 2005 that involved Google acquiring a 5 percent stake in AOL for $1 billion was by far its most ambitious financial investment.

COMPANY HISTORY

The development of Google's search technology began in January 1996 when Stanford University computer science graduate students Larry Page and Sergey Brin collaborated to develop a new search engine they named BackRub. The name BackRub was chosen because of the engine's ability to rate Web sites for relevancy by examining the number of back links pointing to them. The approach for assessing the relevancy of Web sites to a particular search query used by other Web sites at the time was based on examining and counting metatags and keywords included on various Web sites. By 1997, the search accuracy of BackRub had allowed it to gain a loyal following among Silicon Valley Internet users. Yahoo cofounder David Filo was among the converted, and in 1998 he convinced Sergey Brin and Larry Page to leave Stanford to focus on making their search technology the backbone of a new Internet company.

BackRub would be renamed Google, which was a play on the word *googol*—a mathematical term for a number represented by the numeral 1 followed by 100 zeros. Brin and Page's adoption of the new name reflected their mission to organize a seemingly infinite amount of information on the Internet. In August 1998, a Stanford professor arranged for Brin and Page to meet at his home with a potential angel investor to demonstrate the Google search engine. The investor, who had been a founder of Sun Microsystems, was immediately impressed with Google's search capabilities but was too pressed for time to hear much of the informal presentation. The investor stopped the two during the presentation and suggested, "Instead of us discussing all the details, why don't I just write you a check?"[2] The two partners held the investor's $100,000 check made payable to Google Inc. for two weeks while they scrambled to set up a corporation named Google Inc. and open a corporate bank account. The two officers of the freshly incorporated company went on to raise a total of $1 million in venture capital from family, friends, and other angel investors by the end of September 1998.

Even with a cash reserve of $1 million, the two partners ran Google on a shoestring budget, with its main servers built by Brin and Page from discounted computer components and its four employees operating out of a garage owned by a friend of the founders. By year-end 1998 Google's beta version was handling 10,000 search queries per day and *PC Magazine* had named the company to its list of "Top 100 Web Sites and Search Engines for 1998."

The new company recorded successes at a lightning-fast pace, with the search kernel answering more than 500,000 queries per day and Red Hat agreeing to become the company's first search customer in early 1999. Google attracted an additional $25 million in funding from two leading Silicon Valley venture capital firms by midyear 1999 to support further growth and enhancements to Google's search technology. Google began to add employees, bringing the total number up to 39 by the end of 1999, and to add key customers for its search functionality—including AOL and Virgilio, the leading online portal in Italy—which helped push search requests to more than 3 million per day.

In 2000, Google Inc. grew to 60 employees, introduced wireless search technology, provided search services for new Web portal customers in the United States, Europe, and Asia, launched search capabilities in 10 non-English languages, expanded its index of ranked Web sites to 1.3 billion, was called the "Best Bet Search Engine" by *PC World,* and was named by *Yahoo Internet Life* magazine as the "Best Search Engine on the Internet." Yahoo also signed an agreement to make Google its default search

provider, which helped make Google the largest search engine on the Web, with more than 100 million daily searches. During 2000, the company also introduced the Google Toolbar browser plug-in, which allowed computer users to search the Internet without first visiting a Google-affiliated Web portal or Google's homepage. Among its most important innovations in 2000 was the development of keyword-targeted advertising, which provided the company with an additional revenue source beyond fees for licensing its search appliance to other Web sites.

In 2001, Google signed agreements with such wireless providers as Sprint PCS, Cingular, and AT&T that gave mobile phone users access to Google's index of Web pages. Also that year, the company acquired Deja.com, which provided Google with the Internet's largest archive of searchable messages posted on Usenet discussion boards. In other developments, Google expanded its search capabilities to 28 languages—allowing it to establish licensing agreements with 130 Web portals and destination sites in Latin American, Asian, Middle Eastern, and European countries; introduced new capabilities that enabled Google users to search an index of 250 million images, review and search daily news, search more than 1,100 mail order catalogs, and search for any published phone number in the United States; and expanded its search-based advertising program to include small businesses and individuals with a self-service advertising system that gave small advertisers the capability to set up ads online and pay Google by credit card on a per click basis. The expansion of advertising-based revenue allowed Google to increase annual revenues from $220,000 in 1999 to more than $86 million in 2001 and end the year with a profit of nearly $7 million.

Google's rapid growth in services and revenues made it obvious to Sergey Brin and Larry Page that the company needed executive-level management with experience in managing a large, rapidly growing company. In March 2001, the two asked Novell CEO and chairman Eric Schmidt to chair Google's board of directors. Four months later, Google's founders and board asked Schmidt to become CEO of the company, which moved Page to president of products and Brin to president of technology. Schmidt was brought in to introduce formal processes, procedures, and financial systems to the almost anarchic business environment that resulted from the company's unorthodox corporate culture. Employees at the company's Googleplex headquarters in Mountain View, California, were encouraged to work on pet projects that might be unrelated to work assignments, bring dogs to work, and engage in twice-a-week hockey games where checking higher-ups was fair game. Also, prior to Schmidt's arrival, important strategy and operating issues were settled by upper-level management during weekly two-hour meetings that rarely had an agenda and wandered from topic to topic. Google's board wanted Schmidt to bring a sufficient level of structure to the company to prepare it for an IPO, but avoid a cumbersome bureaucracy that would limit Google's ability to sustain its technological advantage. Schmidt commented just prior to Google's registration for a public offering that his instruction from the board was "Don't screw this up now, Eric. This is a really, really good starting point . . . So it doesn't require some gross change."[3]

In a March 2004 interview with *The Wall Street Journal,* Eric Schmidt stated, "You do not want to take big-company structures and apply them to small companies. You want to evolve small-company structures on a need-appropriate basis."[4] Even though Schmidt was made Google's CEO, both Page and Brin were deeply involved in strategy making, forming what was described by the three as a "triumvirate."[5] When asked about the roles of the two founders in decision making, Schmidt, who many business journalists suggested should have been given the title of chief operating officer instead of CEO, commented, "Whenever we have something important, two people have to agree . . . Now, often the two are the founders. When it's managerial things, things Larry and Sergey aren't as focused on, we try to get two of the vice presidents to agree."[6] Under Eric Schmidt's leadership as CEO, Google continued to add new features such as Google Compute, parcel tracking, flight information, vehicle identification number searches, Google News, Froogle, Google Deskbar, Local Search, and Gmail. A complete list of Google services and tools at year-end 2005 is presented in Exhibit 1. Exhibit 2 provides an overview of free software downloads from Google at year-end 2005.

THE INITIAL PUBLIC OFFERING

Two and a half years after Eric Schmidt arrived at Google to institute formal policies, procedures, and controls to ensure that Google did not collapse under the pressures of its accelerated growth rate, the company filed its Form S-1 Registration Statement for an initial public offering (IPO) of common stock. Google's April 29, 2004, IPO registration became the most-talked-about planned offering involving an Internet company since the dot-com bust of 2000. The registration announced Google's intention to raise as much as $3.6 billion from the issue of 25.7 million shares through an unusual Dutch auction.

One of the 10 key beliefs that comprised Google's philosophy (presented in Exhibit 3) was "You can make money without doing evil."[7] The choice of a Dutch auction stemmed from this belief since Dutch auctions allowed potential investors, regardless of size, to place bids for shares. Small investors were typically locked out of participating in IPOs since brokers handling such trades favored institutional investors or individual investors with large portfolio balances or frequent trades. After a period when investors could bid for Google shares over the Internet, the Dutch auction set the clearing price for Google shares at the lowest bid that allowed all shares to be sold. On the day the IPO was finalized, any potential investor bidding the clearing price or higher was granted shares at the clearing price. A Dutch auction would also be favorable to Google since it involved considerably lower investment banking and underwriting fees and little or no commissions for brokers.

Google's financial advisers initially believed the company's shares would fetch between $108 and $135 per share, but the clearing price was ultimately set at $85 after it became apparent that the Dutch auction process would not generate sufficient demand for the company's shares. The poor demand was caused by a number of factors, which included institutional investors' uneasiness with placing a bid absent satisfactory pricing guidance; individual investors' unfamiliarity with the auction process; and even though 28 brokerage firms were involved in the underwriting syndicate, brokers' unwillingness to help clients purchase shares when few or no commissions were involved.

Regardless of the shortcomings of the Dutch auction process, Google's initial offering was the 25th-largest U.S. IPO of all time. Google's shares appreciated by 18 percent during first day trading, making both Brin and Page about $600 million richer by the end of the day and each worth approximately $3.8 billion. Also, an estimated 900 to 1,000 Google employees were worth at least $1 million, with 600 to 700 holding at least $2 million in Google stock. On average, each of Google's 2,292 staff members held approximately $1.7 million in company stock, excluding the holdings of the top five executives.

Exhibit 1   **List of Google Services and Tools at Year-End 2005**

 Alerts
Receive news and search results via email

 Answers
Ask a question, set a price, get an answer

 Blog Search
Find blogs on your favorite topics

 Book Search
Search the full text of books

 Catalogs
Search and browse mail-order catalogs

 Directory
Browse the web by topic

 Froogle
Shop smarter with Google

 Groups
Create mailing lists and discussion groups

 Images
Search for images on the web

 Labs
Try out new Google products

 Blogger
Express yourself online

 Code
Download APIs and open source code

 Desktop
Info when you want it, right on your desktop

 Earth
Explore the world from your PC

 Gmail
A Google approach to email

 Local
Find local businesses and services

 Maps
View maps and get directions

 Mobile
Use Google on your mobile phone

 News
Search thousands of news stories

 Scholar
Search scholarly papers

 SMS
Use text messaging for quick info

 Special Searches
Search within specific topics

 University Search
Search a specific school's website

 Web Search
Search over billions of web pages

 Web Search Features
Do more with search

 Local for mobile
View maps and get directions on your phone

 Picasa
Find, edit and share your photos

 Talk
IM and call your friends through your computer

 Toolbar
Add a search box to your browser

 Translate
View web pages in other languages

Source: Google.com.

Exhibit 2   **Free Software Downloads from Google at Year-End 2005**

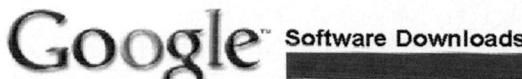 **Software Downloads**

Upgrade your computer with free Google downloads
Google can improve more than just your search experience. The free software on this page makes it easier to get the most out of your computer. Currently available for Windows® computers only (Gmail Notifier also available for Mac OS X).

Google Talk
- Make free calls and send IMs through your computer
- Talk anytime, anywhere and for as long as you want
- More info...

By downloading and installing, you agree to the Terms of Service and Privacy Policy.

[Down nload Now]

Google Toolbar
- Add a search box to your browser
- Block annoying pop-ups
- Automatically fill in online forms
- *For Internet Explorer 5.5+ (Firefox version also available)*
- More info...

[Down nload Now]

Google Desktop 2
- Find all your email, files, photos, web history, and more
- Get all your personalized info in one place with Sidebar
- More info...

By downloading and installing, you agree to the Terms & Conditions and Privacy Policy.

[Down nload Now]

Picasa Photo Organizer
- Find photos on your computer
- Edit photos and remove red-eye
- Create and share albums
- Print your photos at home
- More info...

Google Earth (BETA)
- Fly over a 3D model of the globe
- Search for hotels, dining, and more
- Get directions and fly the route
- Tilt, rotate for 3D terrain and buildings
- More info...

Gmail Notifier (BETA)
- Get alerts of new messages
- Preview email in the alerts window
- Works with any Gmail account
Get a free account (US only)
- Now available for Mac OS X
- More info...

 Blogger for Word   Post from Microsoft Word 2000+ to your blog   More info...

Source: Google.com.

Stanford University realized a $179.5 million windfall from its stock holdings granted for its early investment in Brin and Page's search engine. Some of Google's early contractors and consultants also profited handsomely from forgoing fees in return for stock options in the company. One such contractor was Abbe Patterson, who took options for 4,000 shares rather than a $5,000 fee for preparing a PowerPoint presentation and speaking notes for one of Brin and Page's first presentations to venture capitalists. After two splits and four days of trading, her 16,000 shares were worth $1.7 million.[8]

The company executed a second public offering of 14,159,265 shares of common stock in September 2005. The number of shares issued represented the first eight digits to the right of the decimal point for the value pi (π). The issue added more than $4 billion to Google's liquid assets and, as with the proceeds from the company's IPO, its management offered no specific use for the cash infusion. In its filing with the U.S. Securities and Exchange Commission, the company's management triumvirate stated that the proceeds would be for "general corporate purposes, including working capital and capital expenditures,

Exhibit 3   **The Google Philosophy: "Ten things Google has found to be true"**

1. Focus on the user and all else will follow.

From its inception, Google has focused on providing the best user experience possible. While many companies claim to put their customers first, few are able to resist the temptation to make small sacrifices to increase shareholder value. Google has steadfastly refused to make any change that does not offer a benefit to the users who come to the site:

- The interface is clear and simple.
- Pages load instantly.
- Placement in search results is never sold to anyone.
- Advertising on the site must offer relevant content and not be a distraction.

By always placing the interests of the user first, Google has built the most loyal audience on the web. And that growth has come not through TV ad campaigns, but through word of mouth from one satisfied user to another.

2. It's best to do one thing really, really well.

Google does search. With one of the world's largest research groups focused exclusively on solving search problems, we know what we do well, and how we could do it better. Through continued iteration on difficult problems, we've been able to solve complex issues and provide continuous improvements to a service already considered the best on the web at making finding information a fast and seamless experience for millions of users. Our dedication to improving search has also allowed us to apply what we've learned to new products, including Gmail, Google Desktop, and Google Maps.

3. Fast is better than slow.

Google believes in instant gratification. You want answers and you want them right now. Who are we to argue? Google may be the only company in the world whose stated goal is to have users leave its website as quickly as possible. By fanatically obsessing on shaving every excess bit and byte from our pages and increasing the efficiency of our serving environment, Google has broken its own speed records time and again.

4. Democracy on the web works.

Google works because it relies on the millions of individuals posting websites to determine which other sites offer content of value. Instead of relying on a group of editors or solely on the frequency with which certain terms appear, Google ranks every web page using a breakthrough technique called PageRank™. PageRank evaluates all of the sites linking to a web page and assigns them a value, based in part on the sites linking to them. By analyzing the full structure of the web, Google is able to determine which sites have been "voted" the best sources of information by those most interested in the information they offer.

5. You don't need to be at your desk to need an answer.

The world is increasingly mobile and unwilling to be constrained to a fixed location. Whether it's through their PDAs, their wireless phones or even their automobiles, people want information to come to them.

6. You can make money without doing evil.

Google is a business. The revenue the company generates is derived from offering its search technology to companies and from the sale of advertising displayed on Google and on other sites across the web. However, you may have never seen an ad on Google. That's because Google does not allow ads to be displayed on our results pages unless they're relevant to the results page on which they're shown. So, only certain searches produce sponsored links above or to the right of the results. Google firmly believes that ads can provide useful information if, and only if, they are relevant to what you wish to find. Advertising on Google is always clearly identified as a "Sponsored Link." It is a core value for Google that there be no compromising of the integrity of our results. We never manipulate rankings to put our partners higher in our search results. No one can buy better PageRank. Our users trust Google's objectivity and no short-term gain could ever justify breaching that trust.

7. There's always more information out there.

Once Google had indexed more of the HTML pages on the Internet than any other search service, our engineers turned their attention to information that was not as readily accessible. Sometimes it was just a matter of integrating new databases, such as adding a phone number and address lookup and a business directory. Other efforts required a bit more creativity, like adding the ability to search billions of images and a way to view pages that were originally created as PDF files. The popularity of PDF results led us to expand the list of file types searched to include documents produced in a dozen formats such as Microsoft Word, Excel and PowerPoint. For wireless users, Google developed a unique way to translate HTML formatted files into a format that could be read by mobile devices. The list is not likely to end there as Google's researchers continue looking into ways to bring all the world's information to users seeking answers.

(Continued)

Exhibit 3 **Continued**

---

8. The need for information crosses all borders.

Though Google is headquartered in California, our mission is to facilitate access to information for the entire world, so we have offices around the globe. To that end we maintain dozens of Internet domains and serve more than half of our results to users living outside the United States. Google search results can be restricted to pages written in more than 35 languages according to a user's preference. We also offer a translation feature to make content available to users regardless of their native tongue and for those who prefer not to search in English, Google's interface can be customized into more than 100 languages.

9. You can be serious without a suit.

Google's founders have often stated that the company is not serious about anything but search. They built a company around the idea that work should be challenging and the challenge should be fun. To that end, Google's culture is unlike any in corporate America, and it's not because of the ubiquitous lava lamps and large rubber balls, or the fact that the company's chef used to cook for the Grateful Dead. In the same way Google puts users first when it comes to our online service, Google Inc. puts employees first when it comes to daily life in our Googleplex headquarters. There is an emphasis on team achievements and pride in individual accomplishments that contribute to the company's overall success. Ideas are traded, tested and put into practice with an alacrity that can be dizzying. Meetings that would take hours elsewhere are frequently little more than a conversation in line for lunch and few walls separate those who write the code from those who write the checks. This highly communicative environment fosters a productivity and camaraderie fueled by the realization that millions of people rely on Google results. Give the proper tools to a group of people who like to make a difference, and they will.

10. Great just isn't good enough.

Always deliver more than expected. Google does not accept being the best as an endpoint, but a starting point. Through innovation and iteration, Google takes something that works well and improves upon it in unexpected ways. Google's point of distinction however, is anticipating needs not yet articulated by our global audience, then meeting them with products and services that set new standards. This constant dissatisfaction with the way things are is ultimately the driving force behind the world's best search engine.

Source: Google.com.

---

and possible acquisitions of complementary businesses, technologies or other assets." The team added that the company had "no current agreements or commitments with respect to any material acquisitions."[9] Exhibit 4 tracks the performance of Google's common shares between August 19, 2004, and December 16, 2005.

GOOGLE'S BUSINESS MODEL

Google's business model generated revenue from only two sources: (1) the licensing fees it charged to supply search capabilities to corporations, other Internet sites, and wireless telephone companies, and (2) the advertising fees it charged for providing highly targeted text-only sponsor links adjacent to its search results. Page and Brin insisted that the company would only sell discreet text ads placed near search results and never mix paid keyword-based ads with legitimate search results even though the practice was standard among search engine companies. Also, Google would not place banner ads on its Web site, nor would it sell pop-up ads.

Google's founders also had no interest in the search engine evolving into a Web portal such as Yahoo, MSN, or AOL.com.

Google Search Appliance

Google's search technology could be integrated into a third party's Web site or intranet if search functionality was important to the customer. The Google search appliance could be installed in one day and could search both public Web pages and local intranets to return relevant results for search users. The search appliance was available in four models tailored to the size of the organization and its search requirements. The Google Mini allowed small businesses to search up to 100,000 documents stored on local PCs and servers. The Google Mini hardware and software package could be licensed online for $2,995. The model GB-1001 was designed for departments or midsized companies and could be licensed at prices beginning at $30,000. The GB-5005 was developed for companies needing searches for companywide intranets or customer-facing Web sites, with pricing beginning at $230,000. The GB-8008 was best suited for global business units and could be implemented at licensing fees beginning at $600,000.

Exhibit 4 **Performance of Google Inc.'s Stock Price, August 19, 2004, to December 19, 2005**

(a) Trend in Google Inc.'s Common Stock Price

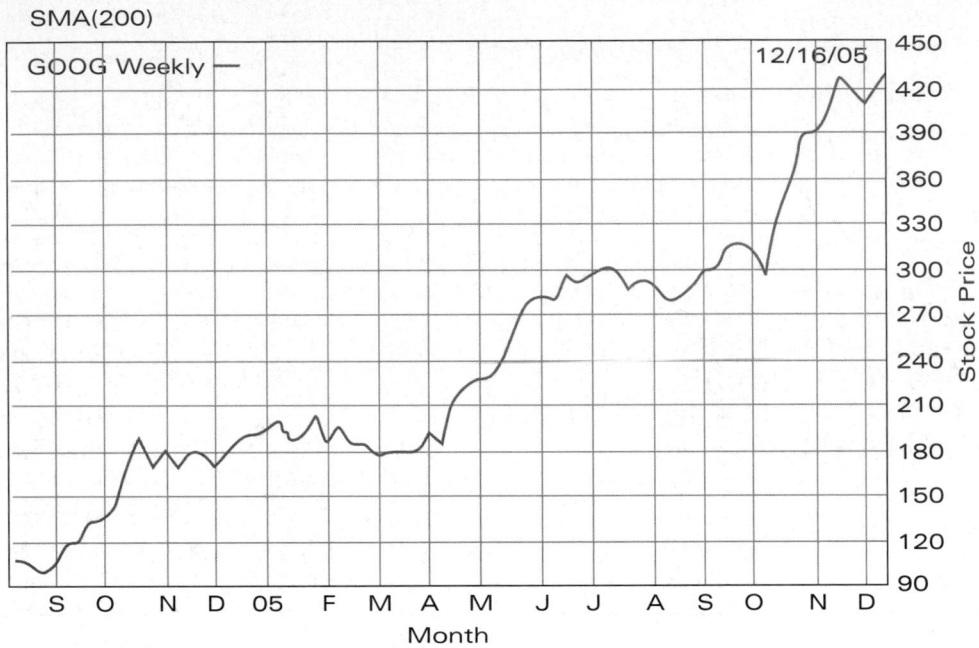

(b) Performance of Google Inc.'s Stock Price versus the S&P 500 Index

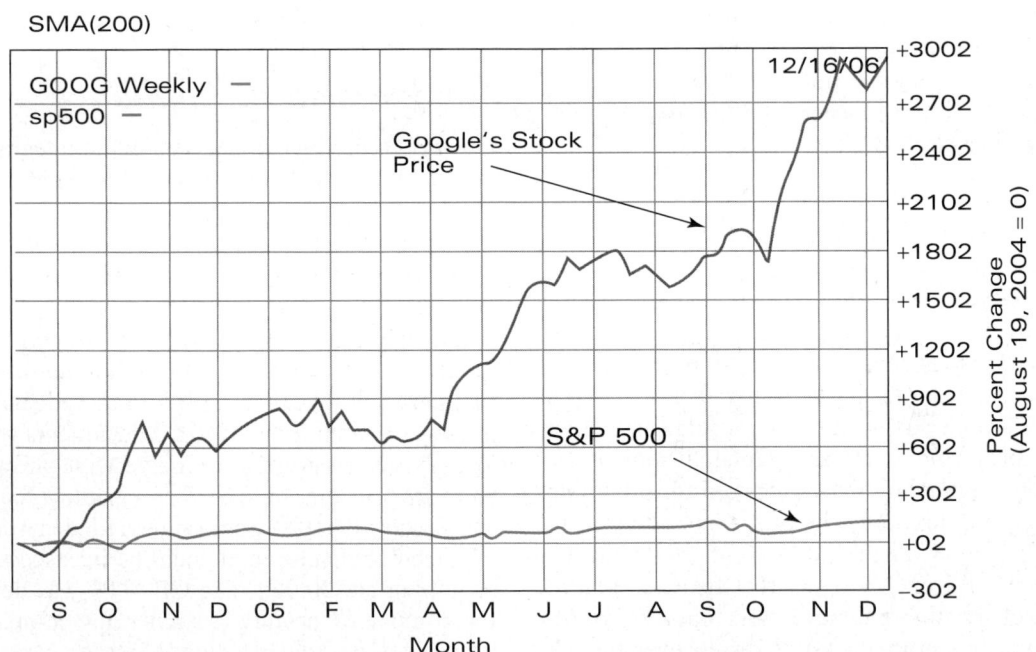

AdWords

Google AdWords allowed advertisers to, either independently through Google's automated tools or with the assistance of Google's marketing teams, create text-based ads that would appear alongside Google search results. AdWords users could evaluate the effectiveness of their advertising expenditures with Google through the use of performance reports that tracked the effectiveness of each ad. Google also offered a keyword targeting program that suggested synonyms for keywords entered by advertisers, a traffic estimator that helped potential advertiser anticipate cost-per-click (CPC) charges, and multiple payment options that included charges to credit cards, debit cards, and monthly invoicing. Google accepted payment for ads in 48 currencies.

Larger advertisers were offered additional services to help run large, dynamic advertising campaigns. Such assistance included the availability of specialists with expertise in various industries to offer suggestions for targeting potential customers, offer suggestions in identifying relevant keywords, and help develop ads that would increase click-through rates and purchase rates. Google also offered its large advertising customers bulk posting services that helped launch and manage campaigns including ads using hundreds or thousands of keywords.

Even though all advertisers were allowed to bid on keywords to achieve a more prominent placement, ads that were infrequently selected by Internet users moved to a less visible placement—regardless of the amount of the advertiser's bid for a keyword. Ads that were frequently clicked on by Internet users moved up the list, ensuring that the most relevant ads always had a good placement on Google's site.

Google also allowed users to pay a CPC rate lower than their bid price if their bid was considerably more than the next highest bid. For example, an advertiser who bid $0.75 per click for a particular keyword would only be charged $0.51 per click if the next highest bid was only $0.50. The AdWords discounter ensured that advertisers paid only 1 cent more than the next highest bid, regardless of the actual amount of their bid.

AdSense

Google's AdSense program allowed Web publishers to share in the advertising revenues generated by Google's CPC text ads. The AdSense program served content-relevant Google text ads to pages of Google Network Web sites. For example, an Internet user reading an article about the shortage of Splenda, an artificial sweetener popularized by the Atkins diet, at Foxnews.com would see two Google text ads from mail order sellers of Splenda embedded in the article. Google Network members did not pay a fee to participate in the program and received the majority of advertising dollars generated from the ads. Owners of dormant domain names could also participate in the AdSense program. During the first nine months of fiscal 2005, 79 percent of advertising revenue generated from such ads was paid to Google Network Web publishers.

The breakdown of Google's revenues by source is presented in the table below:

	Nine Months Ending September 30, 2005	2004	2003	2002	2001
Advertising revenues:					
Google Web sites	$2,278,848	$1,589,032	$772,192	$306,977	$66,932
Google Network Web sites	1,889,369	1,554,256	144,411	12,278	—
Total advertising revenues	4,168,217	3,143,288	916,603	319,255	66,932
Licensing and other revenues	51,251	45,935	45,271	28,593	19,494
Net revenues	$4,419,468	$3,189,223	$961,874	$347,848	$86,426

Source: Google Inc., Form S-1, filed April 29, 2004; 2004 Form 10-K; Form 10-Q, November 10, 2005.

GOOGLE'S COMPETITIVE POSITION AND STRATEGY GOING INTO 2006

Google's ability to sustain its competitive advantage among Internet search companies was a function of its ability to maintain strong relationships with Internet users, advertisers, and Web sites. In 2005, Internet users searching for information went to Google more often than to any other site with search capabilities. The breakdown of U.S. Internet searches among Web sites offering search capabilities in April 2005 is shown in the following table:

Search Company	% of Searches
Google	47%
Yahoo	21
MSN	14
AOL	—
Others	18
Total	100%

Source: Nielsen/NetRatings as reported by *Fortune Online,* April 18, 2005.

There was nothing that would prevent Internet users from abandoning Google to use a better search technology. Google's status in 2005 as the search engine of choice for most Internet users allowed its AdWords program to attract advertisers and its AdSense program attract Network members that would display Google ads. The development of a better search engine by a rival could lead to rapid erosion of advertising revenues for Google. Google management believed its primary competitors were Yahoo and Microsoft.

Google's Internet Rivals

Yahoo   Yahoo, founded in 1994, was the leading Internet destination worldwide in 2005, with 123 million unique visitors each month. Almost any information available on the Internet could be accessed through Yahoo's Web portal. Visitors could anonymously access content categorized by Yahoo or set up an account with Yahoo to maintain a personal calendar and e-mail account, check the latest news, check local weather, obtain maps, check TV listings, track a stock portfolio, maintain a golf handicap, keep an online photo album, or search personal ads or job listings. Yahoo's 2005 agreements with popular authors to write financial columns for its Web site was the company's first move into original content. Prior to the agreement, all Yahoo content was provided by public domain Internet sources. Also in 2005, the company also had launched a plan with the Open Content Alliance to scan out-of-copyright books that would be available on Yahoo.

Yahoo hosted Web sites for small businesses and Internet retailers and had established an alliance with SBC Communications to offer dial-up and broadband access to Internet users. SBC and Yahoo were developing a wireless telephone service that would allow users to access all Yahoo content from their wireless telephones. The company's broad range of services made it a key rival to just about any company with an Internet presence. Internet service providers, business-to-consumer e-commerce sites, business-to-business e-commerce companies, content providers, Web portals, and those who provided paid search advertising were all directly affected by the competitive moves of Yahoo.

Yahoo was among Google's earliest customers for its search appliance, but it initiated moves to distance itself from Google when it acquired Inktomi for $235 million in December 2002 and Overture Services for $1.6 billion in July 2003. Both Inktomi and Overture were developers of search technologies that would allow Yahoo to internally control its search capabilities. Yahoo began to replace Google with its own search capabilities in February 2004, and the two partners officially became rivals in July 2004 when they formally ended their relationship. After its acquisition of Overture, Yahoo filed a lawsuit against Google claiming the rival had infringed on certain Overture patents. The two parties settled the patent infringement case in August 2004, with Google acquiring the disputed technology rights in return for 2.7 million shares of Google stock.

Yahoo recorded revenues and earnings of $3.6 billion and $839.6 million, respectively, during 2004. The company's revenues and net earnings for the first nine months of 2005 were $3.8 billion and $1.2 billion, respectively. The revenue growth represented a 150 percent increase over the same period in 2004, while Yahoo's net income grew by 260 percent between the two nine-month periods.

MSN Search   After 18 months in development, Microsoft launched a preview version of its search engine in November 2004. Microsoft had spent more than $150 million developing Microsoft's MSN Search (www.search.msn.com) to enter the market for search-based advertising. MSN Search was closely modeled after Google with the appearance of its home page similar to the uncluttered, clean look of Google. Also, Microsoft's search engine returned results and text-only ads in 11 languages that looked like those offered by Google. MSN Search could perform some tasks Google was unable to carry out, such as answering plain-language questions like "When did Virginia become a state?," linking to Microsoft's online Encarta encyclopedia to answer questions, and linking to MSN Music for those wishing to purchase MP3s of specific songs. MSN Search matched Google features such as local searching, had a calculator built into its search box, and performed measurement conversions.

Microsoft's quest to overcome Google was led by its chairman and chief software architect, Bill Gates. Gates's concern over Google became heightened in 2003 when, while perusing Google's Web site, he noticed that many of the Google job postings on its site were nearly identical to Microsoft job specifications. Recognizing that the position announcements had more to do with operating-system design than search, Gates e-mailed key Microsoft executives, warning, "We have to watch these guys. It looks like they are building something to compete with us."[10] Gates later commented that Google was "more like us than anyone else we have ever competed with," and by mid-2005 Microsoft had lost more than 100 employees to Google, including the chief architect of Windows.[11]

Gates believed that Google's long-term strategy involved the development of software applications comparable to Word, Excel, PowerPoint, and other Microsoft products that could be accessed free of charge by Internet users. Under Gates's envisioned scenario, Google would record revenue from ads placed on the screens of Google application users. Microsoft's strategy to compete with Google was keyed to making MSN Search more effective than Google and integrating MSN Search into all Microsoft applications. In December 2005, the company matched Google's satellite-based mapping capabilities and began an alliance with MCI to add Voice over Internet Protocol (VoIP) capabilities to MSN Search. The VoIP service would allow MSN Search users to make local and long-distance telephone calls using a PC for as little as two cents per minute. Microsoft's ability to integrate search functionality into Outlook, Internet Explorer, and other Microsoft applications posed the greatest competitive hazard to Google. Gates believed that Microsoft could move computer users away from "Googling" topics to having search results "naturally available, based on the task they want to do."[12]

AOL   AOL, owned by Time Warner Inc., generated 2004 revenues of $8.8 billion from its Internet service provider (ISP), business, advertising sales, and sales of services to its ISP customers. More than 20 million households in the United States and 6 million European households subscribed to AOL, Netscape, or CompuServe in 2005 to gain dial-up access to the Internet. AOL also offered a service for broadband users with third-party broadband access. The company also owned destination sites such as Moviefone.com, ICQ.com, Mapquest.com, AOL Instant Messenger, and Love.com, which together attracted over 110 million unique visitors each month. In addition, AOL's sites were among the Internet's "stickiest" sites, with users averaging five hours per month on them. Yahoo users averaged just over four hours per month on the Yahoo site, while MSN users averaged slightly more than three hours per month on Microsoft's portal. AOL's exposure to vast numbers of Internet users allowed it to market banner ads and other forms of advertising to large companies that might also advertise on Time Warner cable channels or magazines. AOL accounted for 21 percent of Time Warner's 2004 revenues of $42 billion. The operating profit contributed by the AOL business unit in 2004 was $934 million. AOL's agreement with Google for search services on AOL's vast network of Web destinations generated more than $300 million in revenues during 2004.

Google's Strategy to Sustain Growth

Google's Cash Reserves   With Google's influx of cash generated from the proceeds of its 2004 IPO and successive 2005 offering, Internet companies beyond its key search rivals became concerned with the company's growth. It was believed that Google's Froogle feature would decrease traffic to Internet retailers like Amazon.com and eBay since users could perform price comparisons from Google. Amazon.com replaced Google with a search engine called A9 for searches on its site just prior to Google's IPO. Exhibit 5 presents a financial summary for Google that includes income statements and selected balance sheet and cash

Exhibit 5 **Financial Summary for Google, Inc., 2001 through First Nine Months of 2005 (in thousands, except per share amounts)**

	First Nine Months of 2005	Fiscal Year-End			
		2004	2003	2002	2001
Income statement data:					
Revenues	$4,219,468	$3,189,223	$1,465,934	$439,508	$86,426
Costs and expenses:					
Cost of revenues	1,796,128	1,457,653	625,854	131,510	14,228
Research and development	326,906	225,632	91,228	31,748	16,500
Sales and marketing	284,972	246,300	120,328	43,849	20,076
General and administrative	221,268	139,700	56,699	24,300	12,275
Stock-based compensation*	142,555	278,746	229,361	21,635	12,383
Nonrecurring portion of settlement of disputes with Yahoo	—	201,000	—	—	—
Total costs and expenses	2,771,829	2,549,031	1,123,470	253,042	75,462
Income (loss) from operations	1,447,639	640,192	342,464	186,466	10,964
Interest income (expense) and other, net	54,205	10,042	4,190	−1,551	−896
Income (loss) before income taxes	1,501,844	650,234	346,654	184,915	10,068
Provision for income taxes	408,655	251,115	241,006	85,259	3,083
Net income (loss)	$1,093,189	$ 399,119	$ 105,648	$ 99,656	$ 6,985
Net income (loss) per share:					
Basic	$4.04	$2.07	$0.77	$0.86	$0.07
Diluted	$3.80	$1.46	$0.41	$0.45	$0.04
Number of shares used in per share calculations:					
Basic	270,665	193,176	137,697	115,242	94,523
Diluted	287,841	272,781	256,638	220,633	186,776

(*Continued*)

Cash flow and balance sheet data:

Net cash provided by operating activities	$1,800,988	$ 977,044	$ 395,445	N/A
Net proceeds from public offerings	4,287,621	1,161,466	—	—
Cash and cash equivalents	5,518,569	426,995	148,995	N/A
Marketable securities	2,111,578	1,705,424	185,723	N/A
Total current assets	8,382,685	2,693,465	560,234	N/A
Total assets	$9,451,001	$3,313,351	$ 871,458	N/A
Total current liabilities	559,848	340,368	235,452	N/A
Total stockholders' equity	8,793,068	2,929,056	588,770	N/A
Total liabilities and stockholders' equity	$9,451,001	$3,313,351	$ 871,458	N/A

*Stock-based compensation, consisting of amortization of deferred stock-based compensation and the fair value of options issued to non-employees for services rendered, is allocated as follows:

Cost of revenues	$ 3,925	$ 11,314	$ 8,557	$ 876
Research and development	82,733	169,532	138,377	4,440
Sales and marketing	20,549	49,449	44,607	1,667
General and administrative	35,348	48,451	37,820	5,400
	$142,555	$278,746	$229,361	$12,383

Source: Google Inc. From S-1 filed April 29, 2004; Google Financial Release, October 21, 2004; Google Inc. 2004 10-k; Google Inc. 10-Q, November 10, 2005.

flow items for 2001 through the first nine months of fiscal 2005.

Continuing International Expansion   By 2005, Google's 112 international domains allowed 380 million unique users worldwide search billions of Web pages each month. More than 50 percent of Google searches originated outside the United States. However, at the end of Google's third quarter of 2005, only 39 percent of Google's advertising revenues originated from accounts located outside the United States. Google management opened an operation center in Brazil and Mexico in late 2005 to improve sales and services to Latin American advertisers. The company also hired one of Microsoft's most valuable employees in China in late 2005 to aid the company in its expansion efforts in China. Google had been slow to enter the world's second largest market of Internet users because the founders believed China's restrictions on speech and information conflicted with key principals of its corporate philosophy. A 2005 event seemed to confirm the founders' worst fears when the Chinese government forced Yahoo to turn over e-mail records of a journalist suspected of writing unflattering remarks about the government. The e-mail records from the journalist's Yahoo account were used to convict him and sentence him to 10 years in prison. Yahoo began conducting business in China in 1999.

Google had offered Chinese-language search results since 2000, but its site was blocked from Chinese Internet users in 2002. Google's site was reinstated in China after two weeks, but users could no longer access sites listed among Google search results that the Chinese government had found politically sensitive. In June 2004, Google became more involved in the Chinese market when it acquired a 2.6 percent stake in Baidu—the number one search engine in China. Google believed it was essential to develop a local presence in China if it were to aggressively pursue search-based advertising customers in that market since the Chinese language was so complex (for example, there were 38 different ways to say the pronoun "I" in Chinese) and since only 50 percent of Chinese Internet users who were familiar with Google could spell "Google."[13] In late 2005, Google was moving forward with its strategy in China by recruiting employees for an office located in China, developing a separate brand name for the Chinese market, and launching a Chinese ".cn" site. Adding a .cn suffix would establish Google as a Chinese site and make it subject to censorship by Chinese authorities. Google intended to give Chinese search users the "greatest amount of information possible."[14]

Google Feature Additions   Among Google's most controversial new features was its Book Search addition. The plan to digitally scan millions of books from the libraries of Harvard, Stanford, the University of Michigan, and the University of Oxford as well as from the collections of the New York Public Library brought copyright infringement lawsuits soon after the company announced the new feature. A suit filed by McGraw-Hill, Pearson, Viacom, Simon & Schuster, and John Wiley & Sons, along with a suit filed by a group of 8,000 authors, attempted to require Google to obtain permission to scan books before instructing libraries to do so. Even though the suits were still pending, Google scaled back its initiative to include only public domain works—such as classic novels, government documents, and historical books—when the feature went live in November 2005.

Google Earth allowed Internet users to view satellite images of any location in the world and create maps using satellite images. The feature could give users close-up aerial views of the Eiffel Tower, the Taj Mahal, the Grand Canyon, or their own residence. The images were not real-time images but rather were taken by commercial satellites within the past few years. However, many governments were concerned with the availability of such information to anyone with access to Google. India's secretary of science and technology stated that the feature "could severely compromise a country's security," while a Russian security agency analyst suggested, "Terrorists don't need to reconnoiter their target. Now an American company is working for them."[15] However, image resolution varied greatly across locations and the dated nature of the images made them less useful for reconnaissance. A private security analyst in the United States discounted the strategic importance of the images with the comment, "You can get imagery to determine whether there is a military base or airfield, but if you want to count aircraft, or determine there are troops there at a particular time, it is very difficult to do. It's not video."[16]

Google Talk was a new Google feature that caused great concern among those in the telecom and cable industries. Google Talk provided instant messaging services to Google users, along with free local and long-distance telephone service in some areas. For example, users might run a Google search for the phone number of a merchant locally or in another state. If a telephone icon was displayed by the merchant's phone number, the Google user could click on the icon to make a toll-free call to the merchant. Users were asked to enter their phone number once they clicked on the icon so that their phone could be called as soon as the merchant's number was dialed. Neither party incurred any phone charges using Google's VoIP technology. Google also made Google Wi-Fi service available to the entire city of San Francisco in September 2005. Google Wi-Fi not only allowed users to make free VoIP local or long-distance telephone calls but also allowed Wi-Fi-enabled users to do so without an ISP or broadband provider. Both telephone companies and cable companies alike were worried that Google Wi-Fi could dramatically affect their revenue streams. Google management said that it did not have intentions to make the service available outside San Francisco, but many analysts believed that Google would roll out the program to all major U.S. cities that could be serviced with wireless networks. Commenting on emerging technologies such as VoIP, News Corporation's Rubert Murdoch stated in September 2005,

"I believe that free voice is going to be ubiquitous not in 10 years [but] within two or three years."[17]

Google's Investment in AOL   Google's largest investment since its IPO was its proposed strategic alliance with AOL that would give Google a 5 percent stake in AOL in return for a $1 billion cash payment. The terms of the partnership would allow AOL not only to host Google ads and share in advertising revenues but also to sell search-based ads directly to advertisers and share in revenues generated from those ads when they appeared on Google Network partner Web sites. In addition, the agreement called for Google to promote content featured on AOL in its search results. The move was in large part defensive since Microsoft was very close to signing an agreement with AOL that would make MSN Search its search provider. Microsoft sought the alliance to expand the availability of MSN Search beyond MSN.com, which had approximately 100 million unique users each month. Microsoft believed it would be much easier to sell text-based advertising if its search results were available to AOL's 100 million monthly unique visitors as well as those visiting MSN.com each month.

Endnotes

[1]As quoted in "High-Tech Search Engine Google Won't Talk about Business Plan," *The Wall Street Journal Online,* June 14, 1999.
[2]As quoted in Google's Corporate Information, www.google.com/corporate/history.html.
[3]As quoted in "The Grownup at Google," *The Wall Street Journal Online,* March 29, 2004, p. B1.
[4]Ibid.
[5]Google Inc. Form S-1, ii.
[6]Ibid.
[7]As listed under "Our Philosophy," Google Corporate Information, www.google.com/corporate/tenthings.html.
[8]As reported in "For Some Who Passed on Google Long Ago, Wistful Thinking," *The Wall Street Journal Online,* August 23, 2004.

[9]As quoted in "Slice of Pi: New Google Mystery Centers on $4 Billion Share Sale," *The Wall Street Journal Online,* August 19, 2005.
[10]As quoted in "Gates vs. Google," *Fortune,* April 18, 2005.
[11]Ibid.
[12]Ibid.
[13]As reported in "As Google Pushes into China, It Faces Clashes with Censors," *The Wall Street Journal Online,* December 16, 2005, p. 1.
[14]Ibid.
[15]As quoted in "Governments Tremble at Google's Bird's-Eye View," *New York Times,* December 20, 2005.
[16]Ibid.
[17]As quoted in "Google's Wireless Plan Underscores Threat to Telecom," *The Wall Street Journal Online*, October 3, 2005, p. 1.

Copperfield's Books Inc.

Armand Gilinsky
Sonoma State University

Tom Scott
Sonoma State University

When I started in this business, it was the heyday of independent booksellers. The national corporations had not yet discovered the mass market. We could make some serious mistakes and still make money. We were a very loose company, certainly founded on business principles, but it was more like a community than a corporation. We had a lot of fun doing our jobs then. We didn't get as stressed out. —**Tom Montan, CEO of Copperfield's Books**

In late October 2004, Tom Montan, CEO of Copperfield's Books, stood in the middle of a vacant 9,700-square-foot space in Napa, California's Bel Aire Plaza shopping center. Copperfield's employed 120 people and operated six stores in Sonoma and Napa counties, located about 50 miles north of San Francisco. (See Exhibit 1 for a map of Copperfield's retail store locations.) Montan's dilemma was how to achieve his primary goals: to grow Copperfield's revenues from approximately $8 million in 2003 to $15 million by 2007, and to improve the chain's profitability. He considered the possibility of opening two or more new stores in local markets that lacked national chain penetration. While imagining how a new Bel Aire Plaza store would look full of holiday book shoppers, Montan agonized over the quarter-million-dollar annual cost of leasing the new space, located about two miles from the existing downtown Napa Copperfield's bookstore. Just then, his cell phone rang. It was Joel Jaman from Keegan & Coppin, a leading local commercial realtor.

"Tom, it's true! Borders Books is going into that new shopping center just off Highway 101. It's only a mile away from your Petaluma store," Jaman said.

"Thanks for the heads-up, Joel," Montan replied. At the moment, I'm in Napa looking at the Bel Aire Plaza site you suggested. I'll get back to you with a definite 'yes' or 'no' on this new store location by the end of next week. I'd better call Matt Brown, our Petaluma store manager, right away and give him the news about Borders."

Montan then called Brown to bring him up to date. "Matt, what are we going to do about Borders?"

"Maybe we should just work with the stores we already have, Tom," Brown said crisply. "If we could reduce our administrative overhead further, we could be much more cost-competitive with Borders."

Montan reminisced with Brown about a location they had once considered in Novato, about 10 miles south of the Petaluma store but in neighboring Marin County. A Novato outlet would have provided Copperfield's with its first entry into the affluent Marin County market. "The rent [there] was so high, Matt, but the demographics were spot-on and there was no other bookstore within 10 miles." Then he told Brown, "Maybe we'd be better off betting the farm on a 25,000-square-foot superstore format, and go after the chains where they live. After all, Matt, if we prove this Napa market with a nearly 10,000-square-foot store, what's to stop Barnes & Noble or Borders from swooping in and trying to steal what we've built? We could lose everything!"

The idea of competing head-to-head with the superstores spurred Montan's thinking about Copperfield's competitive advantage in used and rare books. "The chains can't compete with us in that market," he told Brown. "Perhaps we should work harder on a used and antiquarian megastore concept. If we did it right, we could draw bibliophiles from 50 miles in all directions. We could use it as a *monster* Internet fulfillment center for used and rare books as well. Isn't

Exhibit 1 Copperfields' Books Inc.—Store Locations as of October 2004

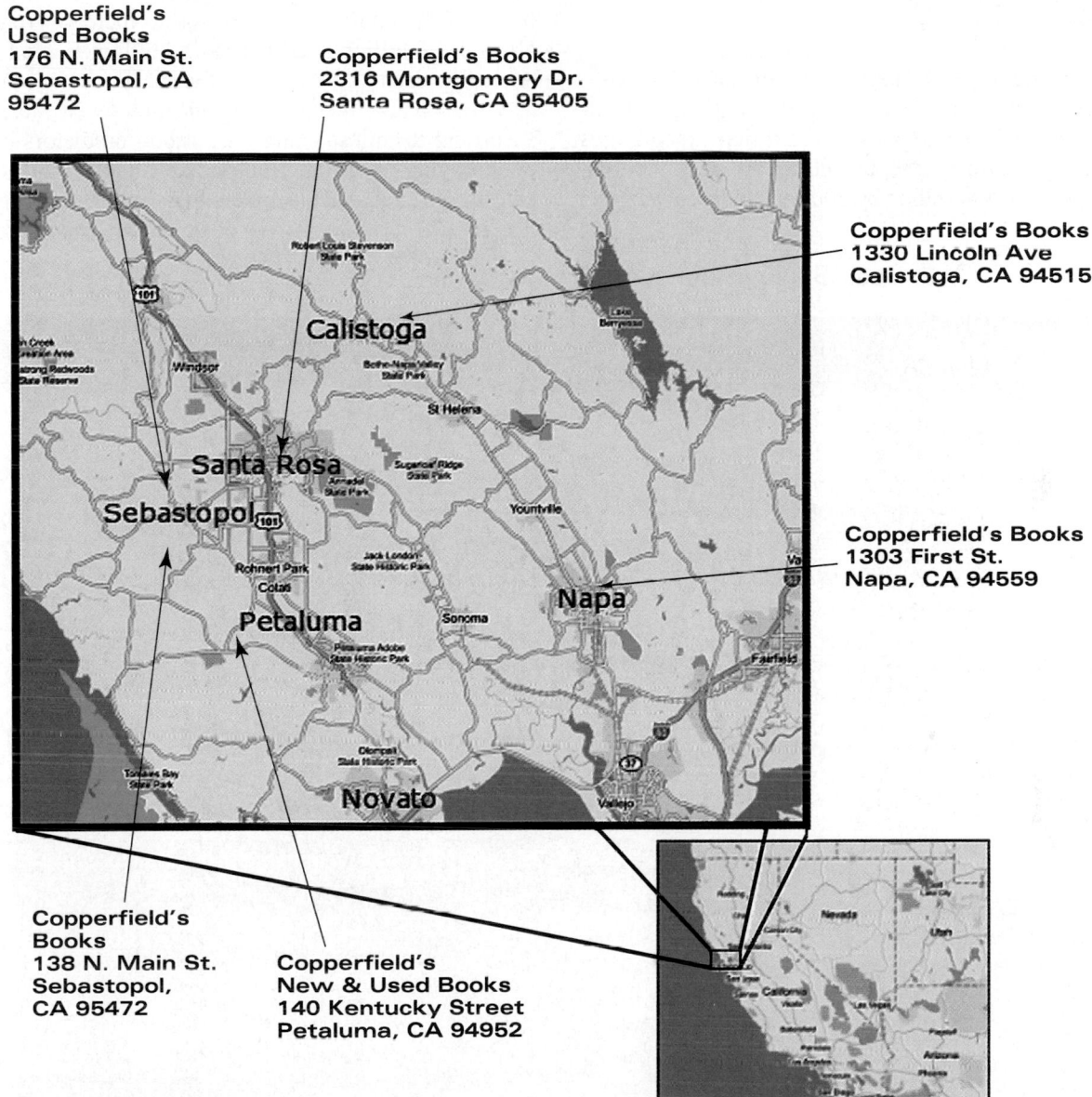

Copperfield's
Used Books
176 N. Main St.
Sebastopol, CA
95472

Copperfield's Books
2316 Montgomery Dr.
Santa Rosa, CA 95405

Copperfield's Books
1330 Lincoln Ave
Calistoga, CA 94515

Copperfield's Books
1303 First St.
Napa, CA 94559

Copperfield's
Books
138 N. Main St.
Sebastopol,
CA 95472

Copperfield's
New & Used Books
140 Kentucky Street
Petaluma, CA 94952

Source: Map adapted by case writers from www.abag.ca.gov/abag/overview/datacenter/maps/region2.gif.

the Internet, after all, where the action is in bookselling these days? See you at the store managers' team meeting tomorrow morning."

Turning off his cell phone, Montan walked around the vacant building, internally debating whether an independent bookstore chain like Copperfield's even *had* a future in a market that was now dominated by national chain superstores and Internet retailers. In his

two years as CEO, Montan had downsized Copperfield's warehouse operations and made some progress in reducing the company's administrative overhead. Still, the addition of two high-performing stores like the Montgomery Village store, he felt, could provide the scale necessary to be competitive with the national chains, or the answer might be found in a new, as yet undetermined format.

THE U.S. BOOKSELLING INDUSTRY

According to *Book Industry Trends 2004,* U.S. consumer expenditures on books exceeded $37.9 billion in 2003.[1] Analysts forecasted that expenditures would increase by 2.9 percent in 2004 to $39 billion and grow to $44 billion by 2008. In addition, analysts predicted that consumer expenditures on general trade books, commonly considered the bread-and-butter of the retail bookstores, would increase from about $11.8 billion in 2003 to $12.2 billion in 2004.[2] Annually, each U.S. household spent an average of $185 on books.[3] Income and education levels were, according to industry analysts, strong predictors of book-buying behavior. Booksellers relied on affluent, highly educated customers.[4] (Exhibit 2 presents

Exhibit 2   **U.S. Book-Buying Habits and Trends**

Compound Annual Growth Rates, 1992–2002			
Years	1992–2002	1992–1996	1997–2002
Unit growth	2.4%	3.6%	1.3%
Dollar growth	4.0	6.6	1.3
Population growth	1.1	0.9	1.2

Household Book Buying Trends, 1998–2002					
	1998	1999	2000	2001	2002
Total U.S. households (millions)	102.5	103.9	104.7	111.3	111.3
Buying households (millions)	59.7	59.5	57.4	58.6	58.2
% of total U.S. households	59.3%	58.7%	56.0%	56.1%	55.1%
Units/buying household	17.4	18.0	18.8	18.7	19.3
Dollars/buying household	$168	$174	$182	$180	$185

Book Buyer Purchasing Trends by Channel, 1992, 1995, and 1999–2002 (% units sold, by retail format)						
	1992	1995	1999	2000	2001	2002
Independent/small chain bookstores	24.9%	19.5%	15.1%	14.8%	14.8%	15.5%
Large chain superstores	5.0	9.5	12.4	14.7	14.2	13.9
Large chain other	19.1	16.0	12.2	9.0	9.2	8.6
Book clubs	16.8	18.1	17.7	18.6	19.9	19.2
Internet	—	—	5.5	7.1	7.5	8.1
Warehouse clubs	4.7	6.1	6.5	6.6	6.6	6.8
Mass merchandisers	4.4	5.6	6.2	5.9	5.6	5.8
Mail order catalogs	3.9	4.9	4.4	3.4	3.1	2.5
Variety stores	2.7	1.9	3.0	3.2	2.6	2.3
Food/drugstores	5.2	4.6	3.5	3.1	3.3	3.1
Used bookstores	4.9	4.0	3.0	2.9	3.3	4.8
Other	8.4	9.8	10.5	10.7	9.9	9.4
Total	100.0%	100.0%	100.0%	100.0%	100.0%	100.0%

(Continued)

Exhibit 2   **Continued**

Household Book-Buying Habits by Household Income, 2002			
	Units Sold (%)	Buying HH (%)	$ Purchases per Buying HH
Less than $30,000	25.7%	32.5%	$160
$30,000 to $49,999	21.9	24.8	159
$50,000 to $74,999	19.3	18.7	154
Over $75,000	33.1	24.0	230
Total	100.0%	100.0%	$185

Household Book-Buying Habits by Level of Educational Attainment, 2002			
	Units Sold (%)	Buying HH (%)	$ Purchases per Buying HH
Less than high school	6.9%	9.9%	$149
High school grad/some college	54.7	61.9	164
College grad	21.4	17.7	209
Post college	16.9	10.6	256
Total	100.0%	100.0%	$185

Note: Numbers in percentages may not add up to 100% due to rounding. The base for all of the data is general trade print books, which excludes children's books and audio and digital purchases.

Sources: IPSOS-Insight, *BookTrends, 2002* (most recent year available), www.ipsosinsight.com/knowledgeconter/syndicatedreports/bookstoadult.aspx, and the *Statistical Abstract of the United States,* www.census.gov/statab/www.

demographic and channel share data regarding U.S. customers' book-buying habits.) Meanwhile, adult readership in the United States had been on the decline for over 20 years (see Exhibit 3). Some book lovers expressed concerns regarding the power held by mass-market chains to act as "content gatekeepers" for book buyers. In 2003, the mass-market portion of the retail supply chain "often accounted for more than 40 percent of a best selling book."[5] Book publishers began issuing books with content targeted

Exhibit 3   **Trends in Domestic Literary Reading**

	1982	1992	2002
% of U.S. adult population reading literature	56.9	54.0	46.7
Number of literary readers (in millions)	96	100	96

Source: National Endowment for the Arts, *Reading at Risk: A Survey of Literary Reading in America, 2004.*

to sell in these stores. Book publishers also often self-censored books and started Christian imprints and other lines that would appeal to the religious, small-town, family values of the patrons of those stores.[6]

Nationwide, there were 10,900 bookstores in 2002; however, the industry was consolidating, as the number of retail establishments decreased by 11.9 percent between 1997 and 2002.[7] Consolidation was more acute among independent booksellers. Between 1993 and 2004, the number of independent retailers belonging to the American Booksellers Association (ABA), a trade group representing independent bookstores, decreased from 4,700 to 1,885.[8] These trends were, in part, attributed to the proliferation of national chain superstores, which offered vastly broader selections than did independent booksellers or mall chain outlets. Independent booksellers and mall chain stores had dominated the bookselling industry between 1970 and 1990, whereas superstores began to dominate in the 1990s.

Superstores ranged from 20,000 to 25,000 square feet of retail space and offered as many as 200,000 titles. Larger stores generated stronger foot traffic, which typically translated into higher sales, because 50 percent of adult trade book purchases were impulse purchases.[9] Superstore formats varied by operator but typically offered value pricing as well as a large assortment of music, magazines, newspapers, cards, and stationery in addition to books. Superstores provided inviting and comfortable environments designed to encourage browsing, and many included cafés. The trend toward superstores appeared to be driving industry growth: Barnes & Noble had opened 31 superstores in 2003, increasing its total to 647, and Borders had opened 41 new superstores in the same year, increasing its total to 445.[10] Favorable local government regulations promoted the expansion of retail tax bases by encouraging big-box development alongside freeways at the outskirts of major towns. Barnes & Noble reported that each new store opening, on average, cost about $1.9 million; this figure included $900,000 for fixtures and leasehold improvements, $700,000 for inventory, and $300,000 in pre-opening expenses.[11]

Supply Chain

Retail booksellers purchased books directly from publishing houses, which owned the distribution rights to a current, or front list, of titles. Demand for front-list titles offered by different houses was determined by consumer demand and merchandising placement at the retail level. While federal law precluded exclusive supply agreements in the publishing industry, publishing houses offered volume discounts that favored larger chains. Publishers shipped books in minimum quantities, enabling major chains to negotiate large discounts based on volume and merchandising commitments. As supplies of new titles on bestseller lists could be in short supply, publishing houses tended to supply their highest-volume retail customers first. Smaller independent retail booksellers like Copperfield's acquired merchandise from wholesale distributors that charged premium prices for acting as the intermediary but sold in smaller quantities than publishing houses. Wholesaler distributors, in turn, had developed proprietary technology interfaces that could reduce their throughput costs for smaller transaction volumes but could, in time, become a barrier to independent booksellers that wished to purchase from other wholesalers.

"Either you have to be very 'niche' or you need a physical presence that says you're significant," said Michael Powell, owner of Powell's Books in Portland, Oregon, which operated a 70,000-square-foot downtown store as well as three smaller stores that specialized in technical books, travel books, and gardening books.[12] Exhibit 4 presents comparative financial and operating data for Amazon, Barnes & Noble, and Borders Books covering the years 2001–2003.

Changing Dynamics

Accompanying the rise of national chain superstores, the emergence of Internet-based retailers like Amazon.com and the growth of book sales at mass-market retailers like Wal-Mart and Costco had dramatically changed the dynamics of the bookselling industry. Between 1992 and 2000, the independent and small chain bookstores' share of the domestic book market decreased from 24.9 to 14.8 percent.[13] During that same period, mass-market retailers' shares increased from 9.1 to 12.6 percent, and Internet retailers captured 8.1 percent of the market. However, large chain bookstores' market share decreased slightly from 24.1 to 22.5 percent between 1992 and 2000. Industry observers attributed this decline to the fact that the market-share increases produced by chains' superstores had been offset by losses at their legacy, mall-based outlets. For example, since 1989, Barnes & Noble had closed 772 of its B. Dalton subsidiary locations in shopping malls.[14] Moreover, erosion of independent booksellers' market share began to plateau after 2000. By 2003, independent and small chain sellers claimed 16 percent of the domestic market.[15]

The Book Industry Study Group reported that overall consumer spending for general trade books, which was $11.3 billion in 2002, declined by 2.7 percent to $11 billion in 2003, despite the fact that Americans purchased an approximately equivalent number of books (1.18 billion) during the same period. Between April and December 2003, consumers purchased 5 percent more books than in the same period in 2002.[16]

Emerging retail channels increased the depth of selection available to consumers: For example, Barnes & Noble's largest superstore carried 200,000 titles and Amazon.com carried an inventory of over 2 million titles, whereas Copperfield's largest store offered 72,000 titles.[17] Industry analysts credited an increased availability of obscure titles as a major driver of demand: by 2003, Amazon's sold 59 percent of all books from *outside* its list of 130,000 top titles.[18]

Used Books

In addition to discounting on new hardcover books, the growing popularity of used books contributed to the decline in dollar expenditures per book. Typically, used books were purchased through four main channels: used bookstores, independent bookstores, online retailers, and others (libraries, churches, garage sales, thrift shops, etc.). Price was a key motivator for used-book purchases. A 2003 survey of the used-book market stated that, of the purchase motivators across the four main channels, price prompted at least one out of every five used-book purchases by consumers; however, cover art, reviews, and readers' endorsements also prompted used-book buying. The survey also noted that the Internet was rapidly becoming a convenient resource for collectors of antiquarian (rare and first edition) books, which tended to fetch higher resale prices in comparison to other used books and even to some new titles.[19] Exhibit 5 presents profiles of selected Internet and storefront used booksellers. Exhibit 6 highlights recent trends in the used book segment of the bookselling industry, excerpted from a PowerPoint presentation prepared by two analysts for the Book Industry Study Group.

Digital Books

The emergence of digital content books (e-books) at the beginning of the new millennium posed a more distant threat to retail booksellers. Consumers could now download e-books directly to their computers or to a portable e-book device. Digital content downloading had already significantly changed the business model for the retail music industry, costing music retailers $700 million in sales in 2002.[20] By 2004, the bookselling industry still lacked a commercially viable platform, similar to Apple's iPod in the music industry, which could make using e-books user-friendly, for example, replicating the ease of page turning. Digital-content literature thus remained relatively user-unfriendly, lacking the tactile pleasures that many readers associated with book enjoyment. Susan Kevorkian, of IDC, an independent research firm, reported that "e-book devices remain[ed]

expensive and e-book titles [had] yet to provide readers with a broad selection of current reading material."[21] Analysts estimated the industry would sell 1.7 million e-book devices worldwide in 2004.[22]

Another potential threat posed by digital content to booksellers was emerging at Web sites like Gutenberg.org, which offered free electronic book downloads of public-domain literature. Gutenberg offered 13,000 e-books consisting primarily of books originally published prior to 1923 and including classics. In 2004, Google announced that it had begun working with university libraries to digitize books in their collections and make them accessible via Google Print.[23]

Key Industry Metrics

Profit margins in the bookselling industry reached historical lows in 2003, as large chains achieved net before-tax profit margins of approximately 5 percent.[24] Profitability among independent booksellers varied widely. A 2003 survey of 179 American Booksellers Association members revealed net before-tax profit margins ranging from 5.3 percent to −11.1 percent, with an average of 0.2 percent.[25] Exhibit 7 shows U.S. independent booksellers' average 2003 operating expenses grouped by store size in total dollar sales. Exhibit 8 shows U.S. independent booksellers' average 2003 operating expenses grouped by store size in sales per square foot.

The bookselling business was highly seasonal. With the possible exception of summer releases of blockbuster titles such as J. K. Rowling's HarryPotter series, the majority of book sales generally took place in the fourth quarter, due to the confluence of fall releases of major new titles and the holiday buying season. Borders Group Inc. reported that it realized 35.5 percent of its sales for 2003 in the fourth quarter.[26] By comparison, approximately 50 percent of Copperfield's 2003 annual sales occurred during the fourth quarter of that year. Also, sales of books were historically dependent on discretionary consumer spending, which was often affected by fluctuations in the business cycle. An equally important dynamic underlying book-buyer behavior was the hit-driven nature of the industry's merchandising strategy. Bookstore revenue and financial performance could fluctuate dramatically, depending on the number of blockbuster titles available for sale during a given time.

Exhibit 4 **Comparative Financial and Operating Highlights for Amazon.com, Barnes & Noble, and Borders Books, 2001–2003**

	Amazon.com			Barnes & Noble			Borders Books		
	12/31/03	12/31/02	12/31/01	1/31/04	2/1/03	2/2/02	1/25/04	1/26/03	1/27/02
Income statements ($ millions)									
Net sales	$ 5,263.7	$ 3,932.9	$3,122.4	$5,951.0	$ 5,269.3	$4,870.4	$3,731.0	$3,513.0	$3,387.9
Cost of sales*	4,006.5	2,940.3	2,323.9	4,323.8	3,855.8	3,560.0	2,682.6	2,439.2	2,439.2
Gross profit	1,257.2	992.6	798.6	1,627.2	1,413.5	1,310.4	1,048.4	1,073.8	948.7
Operating expenses									
Marketing and fulfillment	599.8	517.9	512.5						
Selling, general, and administrative	88.3	79.0	89.9	1,124.6	965.1	904.3	820.0	745.2	744.8
Depreciation and amortization	2.8	5.5	181.0	163.6	148.7	147.8	11.5	14.9	25.4
Other	295.7	326.1	427.4	8.8	35.6	12.5	11.3	119.8	21.5
Total Operating Expenses	986.6	928.5	1,210.8	1,297.0	1,149.4	1,064.6	842.8	879.9	791.7
Operating profit (loss)	270.6	64.1	(412.3)	330.3	264.1	245.8	205.6	193.9	157.0
Interest expense	130.0	142.9	139.2	20.1	21.5	36.3	8.7	12.6	14.4
Other non-operating expenses (income)	104.9	67.0	(25.1)	14.3	43.3	100.1	0.0	0.0	0.0
Income (loss) before tax	35.7	(145.8)	(526.4)	295.8	199.3	109.3	196.9	181.3	142.6
Taxes	—	—	—	(120.6)	(80.2)	(45.4)	(74.8)	(69.6)	(55.2)
Net income (loss)	35.7	(145.8)	(526.4)	175.3	119.1	64.0	122.1	111.7	87.4
Net income (loss), as reported†	$ 35.3	($149.1)	($567.3)	$ 151.9	$ 99.9	$ 64.0	$ 120.0	$ 111.7	$ 87.4
Total number of employees, year-end	7,800	7,500	7,800	43,000	50,000	45,000	32,300	32,700	32,000
Selected balance sheet data ($ millions)									
Current assets									
Cash and marketable securities	$ 1,394.8	$ 1,301.0	$ 996.6	$ 487.2	$ 267.6	$ 108.2	$ 378.8	$ 269.1	$ 190.2
Accounts receivable—trade	132.1			60.5	66.9	98.6	98.3	88.9	73.1
Accounts receivable—other				74.5	55.2				
Inventories	293.9	202.4	202.4	1,526.2	1,395.9	1,285.0	1,235.6	1,183.3	1,178.8
Other				119.6	101.2	99.2			
Total current assets	1,820.8	1,503.4	1,199.0	2,193.5	1,886.9	1,591.0	1,712.7	1,541.3	1,442.1
Fixed assets, net of depreciation	224.3	239.4	271.8	686.6	622.3	595.8	577.7	553.8	529.4
Other assets	116.9	247.7	166.8	627.2	486.3	436.5	175.8	173.1	207.8
Total assets	$ 2,162.0	$ 1,990.4	$1,637.5	$3,507.3	$2,995.4	$2,623.2	$2,466.2	$2,268.2	$2,179.3

(Continued)

Current liabilities	$1,106.7	$1,087.6	$1,164.1	$1,140.2	$1,231.4	$1,441.8	$921.4	$1,066.0	$1,252.7
Long-term debt		50.0	57.2	449.0	300.0	300.0	2,156.1	2,277.3	1,945.4
Deferred taxes and other	122.7	100.0	90.2	145.9	235.2	278.5			
Total liabilities	1,229.4	1,237.6	1,311.5	1,735.1	1,766.7	2,020.3	3,077.5	3,343.3	3,198.1
Minority Interest			1.7		201.0	227.3			
Shareholders' equity									
Common stock & paid-in capital	692.2	661.2	669.8	596.4	636.1	716.2	1,420.6	1,656.9	1,938.3
Retained earnings (accum. deficit)	257.7	369.4	483.2	291.7	391.7	543.5	(2,860.6)	(3,009.7)	(2,974.4)
Total shareholders' equity (deficit)	949.9	1,030.6	1,153.0	888.1	1,027.8	1,259.7	(1,440.0)	(1,352.8)	(1,036.1)
Total liabilities and shareholders' equity	$2,179.3	$2,268.2	$2,466.2	$2,623.2	$2,995.4	$3,507.3	$1,637.5	$1,990.4	$2,162.0
Selected financial ratios									
Profitability									
Gross profit margin	28.0%	30.6%	28.1%	26.9%	26.8%	27.3%	25.6%	25.2%	23.9%
Operating profit margin	4.6	5.5	5.5	5.0	5.0	5.6	−13.2	1.6	5.1
Net profit margin	2.6	3.2	3.2	1.3	1.9	2.6	−18.2	−3.8	0.7
Operating profit as % of total assets (ROA)	7.2	8.5	8.3	9.4	8.8	9.4	−25.2	3.2	12.5
Net income as a % of year-ending shareholders' equity (ROE)	9.2%	10.8%	10.4%	7.2%	9.7%	12.1%	nmf	nmf	nmf
Sales per employee	$72,083	$71,583	$76,025	$70,585	$72,680	$87,515	n/a	$344,994	$455,732
Activity									
Total asset turnover (sales/total assets)	1.6	1.5	1.5	1.9	1.8	1.7	1.9	2.0	2.4
Inventory turnover (cost of goods sold/inventory)	2.1	2.1	2.2	2.8	2.8	2.8	11.5	14.5	13.6
Fixed asset turnover (net sales/fixed assets)	6.4	6.3	6.5	8.2	8.5	8.7	11.5	16.4	23.5
A/R collection period, days	7.9	9.2	9.6	7.4	4.6	3.7	nmf	nmf	9.2
Leverage									
Total liabilities as a % of total assets	56.4%	54.6%	53.2%	66.1%	59.0%	57.6%	187.9%	168.0%	147.9%
Total liabilities as a % of shareholders' equity	129.4%	120.1%	113.7%	195.4%	171.9%	160.4%	nmf	nmf	nmf
Long-term debt as a % of shareholders' equity	12.9%	14.6%	12.8%	67.0%	52.1%	45.9%	nmf	nmf	nmf
Times interest earned ratio	10.9	15.4	23.6	6.8	12.3	16.4	(3.0)	nmf	2.1
Liquidity									
Net working capital ($ millions)	$335.4	$453.7	$548.6	$450.8	$655.4	$751.6	$277.6	$437.4	$568.1
Current ratio	1.3	1.4	1.5	1.4	1.5	1.5	1.3	1.4	1.5
Quick ratio	0.2	0.3	0.4	0.3	0.4	0.5	1.1	1.2	1.2

*Includes occupancy costs for Barnes & Noble and Borders.

†Includes adjustments for changes in accounting principles (Amazon, Borders) and minority interests (Barnes & Noble).

nmf = Not meaningful figure; n/a = Not available or not applicable.

Sources: Calculated by case writers from data provided by Mergent On-Line, company annual reports, and SEC filings; all ratios calculated based on year-end figures except where noted.

Exhibit 5 **Profiles of Selected Internet and Used Booksellers**

Company Name	Web Site	Year Founded	HQ	Ownership	Latest Sales ($ millions)	Latest Net Inc. ($ millions)	Number of Employees	Key Characteristics
Advanced Book Exchange	www.abebooks. com	1995	Victoria, BC (Canada)	Private	WND	WND	WND	>70 million new, used, rare, and out-of-print titles listed at over 13,000 independent booksellers; 5 global Web sites. Acquired BookFinder.com (Berkeley, CA) in 11/05. Partners include Alibris, Amazon. com, Barnes & Noble.com, Biblio. com, Buy.com, ILAB (International League of Antiquarian Booksellers), Overstock.com, and Powell's Books.
Alibris*	www.alibris.com	1998	Emeryville, CA	Private	$45.5	($4.8)	49	Offers >50 million used, new, & out-of-print titles from >10,000 sellers. Backed by venture capital firms. Recently postponed initial public offering.
Bookcrossing	www. bookcrossing.com	2001	Sandpoint, ID	Private	WND	WND	WND	Free paperback book swapping service. "Read, register on the Web, and release into the wild" business model. 2.6 million books "released" to 12/05.
Books-A-Million†	www.bamm.com	1917	Birmingham, AL	Public (Nasdaq: BAMM)	$475.2	$10.2	4,900	#3 U.S. book chain with 170 Books-A-Million and Books & Co. stores in 18 southeastern states. Runs 35 smaller Bookland & Books-A-Million stores. Web site inaugurated in 1998. Owns Joe Muggs' Newsstands & American Wholesales Books.

(Continued)

Company	Website	Year	Location	Ownership				Notes
Half Price Books	www.halfpricebooks.com	1972	Dallas, TX	Private	WND	WND	WND	85 Stores in 13 states, primarily in Texas. About 30% of merchandise is new.
Paperbackswap.com	www.paperbackswap.com	2004	Clermont, FL	Private	WND	WND	WND	One-for-one used book exchange. Fee free. 6,000–10,000 books per day.
Powells Books	www.powells.com	1971	Portland, OR	Private	WND	WND	WND	Web site started 1994 now accounts for >40% of total sales. Offers more than 1.5 million books. Supplies used books to Amazon.com.
Tattered Cover Book Store	www.tatteredccver.com	1974	Denver, CO	Private	WND	WND	WND	Stocks over 500,000 titles at 3 locations Runs Fourth Story restaurant at Cherry Creek location.

WND = Would not disclose.

* 2003 fiscal year data from *Hoovers Company Reports*; 1-year sales growth was 43.4% and employee growth was 8.9%.

† 2004 fiscal year data from *Hoovers Company Reports*; 1-year sales growth was 3.3%; net income growth was 41.7%; employee growth was 2.1%.

Sources: Hoover's Company Reports; company Web sites (accessed 12/20/05), and N. Lewin, "The Book Trade," Public Radio International's *Marketplace*, December 19, 2005, http://marketplace.publicradio.org/shows/2005/12/19/pm.html.

Exhibit 6   **The U.S. Used-Book Market in 2004**

- $2.2 billion in used-book sales; 11.1% growth over 2003
  —$1.6 billion in education and $600 million in other genres
- 111.2 million used-book units
  —38.6 million units in education and 72.6 million units in other genres
- Online used-book sales = $609 million; 33.3% growth over 2003
  —Bookstores (point-of-sale) = $1.57 billion; 4.6% growth over 2003
  —Other locations = $46 million and 19 million units; 1% growth over 2003
- Bookstores
  —Independents (used, new), national, college, religious, other
  —11,036 establishments per Census Bureau
  —22,321 per *Information Today* (7,131 are various retail stores)
  —Industry consensus of around 15,000 to 17,000 total bookstores
  —We estimate around 11,600 sell used books
- Online
  —*Retailers:* Barnes & Noble, Books-A-Million, Powells—emphasize new & used; tied into online specialists and marketplaces
  —*Marketplaces:* Abebooks, Alibris, Amazon, Biblio, eBay—portal for the industry inventory, transaction systems for e-commerce
  —*Online specialists* (1,000+): Individuals working out of home and selling through marketplaces, ex-used-book dealers, part-time businesses ($10K, <10,000 books/year)
  —Rapid growth in segment (30% + year over year)
  —Transforming the adult trade and professional used-book segments
  —Expanding into textbooks
  —Achieving significantly higher prices and margins than other channels
- College bookstores
  —4,650 stores serving 4,168 institutions in the United States, 200 in Canada
  —2,500 university-owned, 2,150 managed or privately owned
  —$10.9 billion revenue (North America)
  —$5.0 billion new textbooks, $220 million course packs, $440 million trade books
  —$1.75 billion used books
  —Sales via Web around $275 million
  —Facing increased competition from third parties
- Other locations: book fairs, Friends of the Library, Goodwill and thrift stores, yard sales

Source: J. Abraham and J. Hayes, "Used Book Market Analysis: Initial Preview," *Book Industry Study Group,* 2005, www.bisg.org.

Trade Area Characteristics

Copperfield's operated four store locations in Sonoma County, California, and two in neighboring Napa County. Sonoma and Napa counties were world-renowned wine-producing regions and boasted personal income levels and property values that exceeded state and national averages. According to the 2000 census, the median family household income in these counties was $61,812, about 14 percent higher than California at large.[27] (Exhibit 9 provides 2003 demographic information.) Higher *per capita* income levels were a result of a diverse local economy, itself driven by the growing wine, tourism, telecommunications, and medical equipment industries. The local economy weakened in the early 2000s due to post-9/11 fears, declining wine prices, and a major downturn for high-technology companies.

Despite the economic uncertainty, the retail segment of the local economy continued to expand

Exhibit 7   **Average Operating Expenses for U.S. Independent Booksellers by Store Size (in Sales), 2003**

| | Store Sales Volume[1] | | | | | | |
	<$250K	$250K–$500K	$500K–$1 MM	$1 MM–$2.5 MM	$2.5 MM–$5 MM	>$5 MM	Averages[2]
Sales per square feet	$122.00	$209.00	$337.00	$370.00	$456.00	$436.00	$321.67
Gross profit margin	39.5%	21.7%	39.2%	39.7%	41.6%	37.7%	39.9%
Payroll expense as a % of sales	20.9%	41.5%	20.8%	21.6%	23.4%	20.4%	21.5%
Occupancy expense as a % of sales	12.0%	10.0%	7.2%	7.0%	7.4%	8.0%	8.6%
Advertising as a % of sales	4.1%	1.9%	1.8%	1.5%	1.3%	1.0%	1.9%
Other expenses as a % of sales	12.8%	11.8%	10.0%	7.5%	9.2%	6.5%	9.6%
Net income as a % of sales	−10.3%	−2.9%	0.4%	2.1%	0.2%	1.7%	−1.5%

[1]N = 197 respondents, or 11% of ABA member booksellers.
[2]Unweighted means.
Source: Adapted and compiled by case writers from American Booksellers Association, *ABACUS Survey, 2003,* available from http://news.bookweb.org/news/2858.html.

between 2000 and 2004.[28] This expansion resulted in a shortage of supply of retail space in local trade area. In June 2004, the supply of available retail space in Sonoma County was less than 5 percent.[29] As a result of the shortage of supply and high area income levels, trade area commercial rents were among the highest in the state. In late 2004, commercial rents for Sonoma County averaged between $2.00 and $3.50 per square foot (on a monthly basis) depending on a number of variables, including location, tenant mix, and footprint of the leased premise. See Exhibit 10 for more detail and selected comparisons to market data for neighboring Marin and Napa Counties.

In addition to six Copperfield's stores, Sonoma and Napa Counties were home to over 30 independent

Exhibit 8   **Comparative Expenses for U.S. Independent Booksellers Based on Sales per sq. ft., 2003**

| | Store Sales per Square Foot | | | | |
	≤$100	$100–$200	$200–$300	$300–$400	>$400
Sales	100.0%	100.0%	100.0%	100.0%	100.0%
Gross profit margin	46.7	39.4	39.8	38.8	39.2
Salaries, wages, and benefits	24.4	20.6	21.2	21.4	21.4
Occupancy costs (including utilities and maintenance)	14.8	9.3	7.2	6.1	6.8
Advertising	3.2	2.1	2.0	1.6	1.1
Depreciation	0.6	1.4	0.8	0.4	0.8
Other expenses	53.5	36.2	30.8	27.2	27.8
Net income before tax	−10.4%	−2.6%	0.6%	2.4%	2.4%

Note: Numbers may not add to 100% due to rounding.
Source: American Booksellers Association, *ABACUS Survey, 2003,* available from http://news.bookweb.org/news/2858.html.

Exhibit 9   **Copperfield's Books Inc., Population Demographics Analysis, 2003**

	5-Mile Trade Area*				State of California[†]	United States[‡]
	Napa	**Santa Rosa**	**Petaluma**	**Sebastopol**		
Household income						
Less than $15,000	8.46%	6.60%	8.50%	14.20%	14.29%	8.87%
$15,000–$24,999	8.79	8.00	7.40	12.40	11.77	10.82
$25,000–$34,999	11.11	9.30	8.30	10.90	10.25	11.20
$35,000–49,999	15.57	17.40	13.70	15.40	14.14	15.21
$50,000–74,999	19.44	22.80	22.70	25.40	17.42	20.59
$75,000–$99,999	13.82	16.00	16.10	9.00	11.83	10.21
Over $100,000	22.81	19.90	23.30	12.70	20.31	23.11
Estimated mean household income	$77,169	$74,640	$73,615	$54,608	$66,915	n/a
Estimated median household income	$57,791	$56,945	$61,679	$46,436	$49,320	$53,991
Educational attainment for population 25 and older						
Less than high school grad	20.72%	8.30%	14.10%	11.60%	18.73%	16.38%
High school grad (income equivalent)	20.69	18.50	19.30	16.50	21.29	29.80
Some college, no degree	25.56	26.80	27.30	28.70	27.68	20.29
Associate degree	8.66	11.10	9.20	7.70	n/a	6.99
Bachelor's degree	15.47	23.30	20.80	22.80	21.21	16.89
Graduate degree	8.90	12.00	9.30	12.70	10.47	9.65
High school grad or higher	79.28%	91.70%	85.90%	88.40%	81.27%	83.62%
Bachelor's degree or higher	24.37%	35.30%	30.10%	35.50%	31.68%	26.54%
Hispanic or Latino						
Not Hispanic or Latino	70.54%	91.20%	85.40%	90.70%	67.60%	87.45%
Hispanic or Latino	29.46	8.80	14.60	9.30	32.40	12.55

n/a = Not available.

*Napa and Sonoma data for a 5-mile radius Copperfield's store locations, obtained from www.clusterbigip1.claritas.com/claritas/Default.jsp?ti=3&ci=1&pn=freeinfo (accessed October 20, 2004).

[†]Demographic data for State of California obtained from State of California, Department of Finance Demographic Research Unit, *California Population Survey Basic Report,* March 2004 Data, Tables 14 and 15, www.dof.ca.gov/HTML/DEMOGRAP/DRU_datafiles/DRU_DataFiles.asp (accessed December 27, 2005).

[‡]Demographic data for United States obtained from U.S. Census Bureau, *Statistical Abstract of the United States, 2006 edition,* Tables 37 and 45, www.census.gov/prod/www/statistical-abstract.html (accessed December 27, 2005).

bookstores and two chain superstores. Copperfield's stores were the largest independent bookstores in its trade area; its Montgomery Village and Petaluma stores each comprised more than twice the square footage as the next largest independent local competitor, thus Montan perceived chain superstores as his primary direct competitors. Exhibit 11 lists rival retail book-sellers in Napa and Sonoma.

COPPERFIELD'S HISTORY

In 1981, Barney Browne and Paul Jaffe founded Copperfield's Books in Sebastopol, California. Their first store was located in a century-old brick storefront on Sebastopol's Main Street. The store's business grew steadily by focusing on customers' needs and community service. In 1985, Copperfield's

Exhibit 10   **Late 2004 Market Data for San Francisco North Bay Area Commercial Retailers: Inventories, Vacancy Rates, and Rents**

County/Submarket	Inventory (sq. ft.)	Available Space (sq. ft.)	Vacancy Rate	Rent Range ($/sq. ft.)
Sonoma County*				
Petaluma	1,644,432	22,773	1.4%	$1.65–2.50
Rohnert Park	1,946,365	29,131	1.5	1.25–2.25
Santa Rosa	5,665,973	101,664	1.8	1.70–3.30
Windsor	632,000	13,720	2.2	1.85–2.95
Total	9,888,770	167,288	1.7	1.25–3.30
Marin County*				
Southern/Central Marin	1,832,986	52,867	2.9	1.85–4.00
San Rafael	1,517,961	25,627	1.9	1.75–3.25
Novato	1,218,459	64,390	5.3	1.45–2.25
Total	4,569,406	142,884	3.1	1.45–4.00
Napa County†				
Napa	8,800,000	290,000	3.3	1.25–2.25
Total	8,800,000	290,000	3.3	1.25–2.25

*Orion Commercial Real Estate Services, www.orionre.com.

†Napa Valley Economic Development Corporation, www.nvedc.org/nvedc/default.asp?idPage = 1031.

opened a second store in Santa Rosa, and in a 50 percent partnership with Paul's brother, Dan Jaffe, a third store in Petaluma. The Santa Rosa store was located in Montgomery Village, an older but prestigious regional shopping center. The Petaluma store was located in the heart of downtown Petaluma, in a century-old brick storefront, linking it aesthetically to the Sebastopol store. The first three stores thrived during the mid-1980s, benefiting from strong population growth in Sonoma County, the affluent educated demographics surrounding their locations, and a general lack of direct competition in the trade area.

By the mid-1990s, Copperfield's decided to establish a more traditional corporate hierarchy. Dan Jaffe became the director of operations, Paul the chief executive officer, and the two brothers embarked on a bold growth plan. They moved two stores into bigger spaces: Montgomery Village and Petaluma. Dozens of volunteers did most of the work of moving the stores. A year later, Copperfield's purchased the assets of Books Inc., a regional chain that had recently filed for bankruptcy protection, and took over its lease in the Coddingtown Center, a regional shopping mall in Santa Rosa. Copperfield's transferred inventory and personnel

from Rohnert Park to the new location and opened a second used and rare bookstore in Sebastopol, down the street from its original location. See Exhibit 12 for a list of Copperfield's store openings and closings.

In 2004, Copperfield's closed its downtown Santa Rosa location, finally succumbing to the competitive forces set in play a decade earlier when Barnes & Noble had first come to town and set up shop across the street. "We had grown out of that business model in that location," Montan told the *Santa Rosa Press Democrat.*[30] The Santa Rosa downtown store property was sold to an investment group in spring 2004 for about $826,000 after taxes, a substantial profit. Copperfield's board distributed the after-tax proceeds from the sale to shareholders, foregoing the opportunity to reinvest the proceeds in the chain. In an attempt to capture emerging Internet channel as well as the recent growth in demand for used books, Copperfield's transferred its Santa Rosa store's inventory to an unused portion of the Petaluma store's basement, which formed the foundation for a nascent Internet fulfillment center. Consolidated 1998–2003 financial statements for Copperfield's are shown in Exhibits 13 and 14. Exhibits 15 and 16

Exhibit 11   **Competing Retail Booksellers in Sonoma and Napa Counties**

Company	Location	Estimated Size	Type
Barnes & Noble	Santa Rosa	Estimated sales $2.5 mm–$ 5.0 mm	New
Bookends Napa	Napa	Estimated sales $500K–$1 mm	New
Bookends Sonoma	Sonoma	Estimated sales $500K–$1 mm	New
Book Market Inc.	Santa Rosa	Estimated sales $250K–$500K	New
Book Outlet Store	Napa	Estimated sales $250K–$500K	New
Book Warehouse	Petaluma	Estimated sales $250K–$500K	New
Borders	Santa Rosa	Estimated sales >$5 mm	New
Calistoga Books	Calistoga	Estimated sales $250K–$500K	New
Campus Textbooks	Santa Rosa	Estimated sales $250K–$500K	College
Cover to Cover	Cloverdale	Estimated sales $250K–$500K	New
Full Circle Books	Cotati	Estimated sales <$250K	Used
Gramma Queenies	Penngrove	Estimated sales <$250K	Used
Knight's Books	Santa Rosa	Estimated sales <$250K	Used
Lakeside Village Bookstore	Santa Rosa	Estimated sales <$250K	Used
Liberia Christiana	Rohnert Park	Estimated sales $250K–$500K	Religious
Liberia Christiana	Santa Rosa	Estimated sales $250K–$500K	Religious
Many Rivers Books and Tea	Sebastopol	Estimated sales $250K–$500K	New
Napa Booktree	Napa	Estimated sales $250K–$500K	New
North Light Books	Cotati	Estimated sales <$250K	New/College
Occidental Books	Occidental	Estimated sales <$250K	Used
Pages Books	Windsor	Estimated sales $250K–$500K	New
Paperbacks Unlimited	Santa Rosa	Estimated sales <$250K	Used
Parsons Books	Napa	Estimated sales <$250K	Used
Petaluma Paperbacks	Petaluma	Estimated sales <$250K	Used
Readers Books	Sonoma	Estimated sales $500K–$1 mm	New
River Reader	Guerneville	Estimated sales $250K–$500K	New
Sonoma State Bookstore	Rohnert Park	Estimated sales $500K–$1 mm	College
Stepping Stones	Occidental	Estimated sales <$250K	New
Treehorn Books	Santa Rosa	Estimated sales $250K–$500K	Used
Twice Told Books	Guerneville	Estimated sales <$250K	Used
Vicarious Experience	Cotati	Estimated sales <$250K	Used
Waldenbooks	Santa Rosa	Estimated sales $250K–$500K	New
Waldenbooks	Napa	Estimated sales $250K–$500K	New
Western Christian Bookstore	Cotati	Estimated sales <$250K	Religious

Source: Copperfield's Books Inc. and casewriters' estimates.

Exhibit 12   **Copperfield's Books: Store Openings and Closings, 1981–2004**

New Book Stores	County	Type of Location	Date Opened	Date Closed
138 N. Main Street, Sebastopol	Sonoma	Downtown	1981	
140 Kentucky Avenue, Petaluma*	Sonoma	Downtown	1985	
Montgomery Village, 2316 Montgomery Drive, Santa Rosa	Sonoma	Upscale mall	1985	
1303 First Street, Napa	Napa	Downtown	1996	
540 Raley's Town Center, Rohnert Park	Sonoma	Shopping center	1996	2001
Coddingtown Center, 2402 Magowan Drive, Santa Rosa	Sonoma	Mall	1996	2001
650 Fourth Street, Santa Rosa	Sonoma	Downtown	1996	2001
1330 Lincoln Ave., Calistoga	Napa	Downtown	2001	
Used and Rare Book Stores				
140 Kentucky Avenue, Petaluma†	Sonoma	Downtown	1995	
176 N. Main Street, Sebastopol	Sonoma	Downtown	1996	

*Petaluma store was moved in 1995 to a new, larger location on the same street.

†Used bookstore located in basement of Petaluma store.

Source: Copperfield's Books Inc.

present comparative store revenue and expense data by location for 2003 and 2002, respectively.

Marketing

Copperfield's had earned a reputation for being Sonoma County's hometown bookseller. Active in the local community, Copperfield's was instrumental in promoting local authors, hosting cultural events, and providing a venue for writers across the country to meet Northern California literati. Special events were the cornerstone of Copperfield's marketing efforts, and these were advertised in the local press, including the daily *Press Democrat* newspaper and weekly free *Bohemian* magazine. Fall 2004 literary readings and book-signing events featured Leonard Nimoy, Newt Gingrich, George Carlin, Mo Willems (Emmy Award–winning writer for *Sesame Street*), former U.S. secretary of labor Robert Reich, and Pulitzer Prize–winning poet Gary Snyder. In addition, the chain's online newsletter promoted upcoming book signings with local authors including historian Simone Wilson and photographer Richard Blair. Copperfield's also published *The Dickens,* a free journal dedicated to literature of quality: poems, stories, and creative nonfiction that gave voice to the talents of writers from Northern California.

Newly released, or front-list, book titles were sold at list prices, though individual store managers had some discretion to match the 10–20 percent discounts off cover prices offered by the larger chains. Store layouts contained a simple, casual, down-to-earth quality that differentiated them from other chain booksellers. Shelving units were made of simple unfinished fir boards. Seating was limited or nonexistent in most stores. Store signage consisted primarily of poster-board placards with hand-drawn calligraphic lettering that described major sections of the store. Lighting in the stores was simple, primarily derived from ambient ceiling sources. Music in the stores consisted of new age, classical, and jazz selections. Front-list titles and sideline merchandise targeted upscale, liberal-minded customers.

Operations

Each Copperfield's store manager controlled the merchandising, staffing, and back-list (older new-book titles) inventory for his or her store. Store layouts and product offerings varied significantly throughout the chain; the Petaluma and Sebastopol new-book stores contained special children's sections, replete with colorful fixtures and huge butterflies, while other stores did not. Some managers placed magazines in the front, while others placed them in the rear of the store. Consequently, each store had its own flavor, but common fixtures, signage, and front-list selections gave the chain continuity and branding among store locations. Front-list inventories were controlled centrally, but Montan delegated the

Exhibit 13 **Copperfield's Books Inc. Comparative Statements of Income and Expenses, 1998–2003**

	Fiscal Year Ended December 31					
	2003	2002	2001	2000	1999	1998
Revenue*	$ 8,124,422	$ 5,865,625	$ 6,002,434	$ 6,632,445	$ 6,495,758	$ 6,499,505
Cost of goods sold	4,643,866	3,489,448	3,531,834	3,972,392	3,958,974	3,918,764
Gross profit	$ 3,480,556	$ 2,376,177	$ 2,470,600	$ 2,660,053	$ 2,536,784	$ 2,580,741
Operating Expenses						
Salaries and wages	$ 1,651,299	$ 1,203,163	$ 1,252,290	$ 1,353,143	$ 1,298,109	$ 1,267,844
Benefits	248,448	171,357	183,328	192,096	182,389	176,750
Occupancy	542,519	382,073	331,438	382,571	378,692	337,008
Advertising	88,953	67,069	51,621	71,659	(5,336)	54,333
Utilities	177,812	139,789	125,277	160,237	139,981	154,562
Depreciation and amortization	123,797	115,142	123,763	112,807	111,649	86,411
Repairs and maintenance	72,389	62,070	52,361	72,498	62,956	48,723
Other costs	448,540	253,660	259,631	276,173	237,837	239,361
Total expenses	$ 3,353,757	$ 2,394,323	$ 2,379,709	$ 2,621,184	$ 2,406,277	$ 2,364,992
Income from operations	126,799	(18,146)	90,891	38,869	130,507	215,749
Income from Petaluma	(77,670)	72,630	128,957	77,796	85,936	73,704
Other income†	915,876	41,345	(180,287)	64,526	(71,164)	(51,813)
Income before taxes	$ 965,005	$ 23,199	$ (89,396)	$ 103,395	$ 59,343	$ 163,936
Provision for income taxes	14,500	1,700	2,318	4,829	4,829	3,236
Net income	$ 950,505	$ 21,499	$ (91,714)	$ 98,566	$ 54,514	$ 160,700

*In 2003, Copperfield's changed the way it accounted for its 50% interest in the Petaluma store due to the death of one of the founders, Dan Jaffe. Prior to 2003, revenues excluded sales from Petaluma, and the firm's share of the Petaluma store's net income was shown as other income to reflect the fact that Jaffe had held 50% interest in that store location. In 2003, revenue from the Petaluma store was included as company revenue, and Jaffee's heirs' shares of earnings from the Petaluma store were charged against revenues. Revenues from the Petaluma store were $2,296,561 in 2003.

†2003 income reflects a one-time $826,414 gain net of income taxes on disposal of the downtown Santa Rosa store, which was closed in June 2004. Proceeds from the sale were distributed to Copperfield's shareholders.

Source: Copperfield's Books Inc.

Exhibit 14 **Copperfield's Books Inc., Comparative Balance Sheets, 1998–2003**

			Fiscal Year Ended December 31			
	2003	**2002**	**2001**	**2000**	**1999**	**1998**
Assets						
Current assets						
Cash	$ 38,720	$ 296,582	$ 53,776	$ 147,539	$ 204,998	$ 220,509
Accounts receivable	66,204	79,133	78,695	99,806	88,211	71,158
Accounts receivable—related party	6,988	264,750	234,566	60,956	41,442	156,047
Inventory	2,030,342	1,305,012	1,525,310	1,695,389	1,643,615	1,509,409
Note receivable	6,000	6,000	7,653	8,330	15,921	16,179
Other current assets	—	6,612	5,584	25,517	30,688	25,915
Total current assets	2,148,254	1,958,089	1,905,584	2,037,537	2,024,875	1,999,217
Property and equipment	654,503	1,371,765	1,461,084	1,470,262	1,428,181	1,372,840
Other assets	35,996	23,192	27,130	28,645	36,788	41,998
Investment in Petaluma store	—	113,903	147,816	181,098	153,756	106,734
Total assets	$ 2,838,753	$ 3,471,949	$ 3,541,614	$ 3,717,542	$ 3,648,600	$ 3,520,789
Liabilities and equity						
Current liabilities						
Accounts payable	$ 976,527	$ 1,043,131	$ 1,107,049	$ 1,257,228	$ 1,181,073	$ 1,077,431
Current maturities of long-term debt	162,142	105,029	106,186	114,595	178,054	196,631
Total current liabilities	1,138,669	1,148,160	1,213,235	1,371,823	1,359,127	1,274,062
Long-term debt*	180,077	901,212	978,338	961,907	999,494	992,409
Other commitments	4,800	5,700	7,400	4,100	8,791	15,130
Stockholders' equity						
Capital stock	204,002	204,002	204,002	204,002	204,002	204,002
Retained earnings	1,157,988	1,212,875	1,138,639	1,175,710	1,077,186	1,035,136
Related party interest in affiliate†	153,217	—	—	—	—	—
Total stockholders' equity	1,515,207	1,416,877	1,342,641	1,379,712	1,281,188	1,239,188
Total liabilities and equity	$ 2,838,753	$ 3,471,949	$ 3,541,614	$ 3,717,542	$ 3,648,600	$ 3,520,789

*Decrease in Long-Term Debt from 2002 to 2003 reflects debt retirement from the sale of the Santa Rosa store, net of taxes, for $826,414.

†Jeffe family's 50% ownership stake in Petaluma store.

Source: Copperfield's Books Inc.

Exhibit 15 **Copperfield's Books Inc., Comparative Store Data, 2003**

				Fiscal Year Ended December 31			
	Petaluma New & Used *	Santa Rosa Montgomery Village	Downtown Santa Rosa	Napa	Calistoga	Sebastopol	Sebastopol Used & Rare
Revenue	$ 2,296,561	$ 2,762,670	$ 514,271	$ 418,548	$ 646,056	$ 1,265,567	$ 199,470
Cost of goods sold	1,268,712	1,679,629	255,021	240,364	371,599	744,831	67,512
Gross margin	1,027,849	1,083,040	259,250	178,183	270,417	520,736	131,958
Salaries and wages	458,040	252,953	126,119	87,608	93,031	149,727	73,291
Benefits	37,049	27,799	12,837	1,439	6,664	9,938	4,819
Occupancy	115,005	181,699	39,080	34,019	60,000	66,321	14,526
Advertising	17,430	37,273	6,506	3,317	4,434	19,152	758
Utilities	32,425	67,280	23,122	10,495	14,107	9,945	5,230
Depreciation and amortization	21,035	20,503	15,058	4,923	29,065	10,091	2,702
Repairs and maintenance	17,151	10,175	6,121	4,669	6,796	11,049	2,300
Other costs	131,825	107,420	36,900	28,288	38,431	51,378	19,277
Total expenses	829,960	705,101	265,743	174,757	252,528	327,600	122,901
Income from operations	197,889	377,939	(6,493)	3,426	17,888	193,136	9,057
Other income	19,069	126	305	—	54	—	1,930
Other expense	61,618	150	8,446	—	3,258	—	300
Overhead allocation	—	276,020	38,326	39,033	64,129	124,789	9,325
Income before taxes	$155,340	$101,894	$ (52,961)	$ (35,606)	$ (49,445)	$ 68,347	$ 1,361
Employees	19	21	N/A	8	12	15	8
% of sales nonbooks	3.7%	8.4%	N/A	1.2%	10.3%	5.5%	N/A
Total selling square feet	6,900	9,750	N/A	3,400	5,000	3,850	2,800
Leasehold cost per square foot	$1.19	$1.55	N/A	$0.83	$1.00	$1.44	$0.43

N/A = Not available.

* Petaluma store 50% owned by Copperfield's Books Inc. and by heirs of Dan Jaffee. Petaluma statements include both new and used operations. Petaluma statements also reflect administration overhead allocation of $10,245 in 2003.

Source: Copperfield's Books Inc.

Exhibit 16 **Copperfield's Books Inc., Comparative Store Data, 2002**

	Petaluma (Both New & Used)	Santa Rosa Montgomery Village	Downtown Santa Rosa	Napa	Calistoga	Sebastopol	Sebastopol Used & Rare
				Fiscal Year Ended December 31			
Revenue	$ 2,190,608	$ 2,677,781	$ 631,382	$ 403,880	$ 581,382	$ 1,271,123	$ 224,659
Cost of goods sold	1,277,229	1,675,832	319,195	227,524	334,940	801,045	82,970
Gross margin	913,379	1,001,950	312,187	176,355	246,442	470,078	141,689
Salaries and wages	453,572	303,091	143,794	85,463	80,538	170,508	66,950
Benefits	72,160	45,851	24,684	10,437	12,303	23,489	10,680
Occupancy	95,919	174,080	12,298	32,871	60,000	62,906	21,343
Advertising	21,503	31,367	8,180	3,008	5,232	18,440	673
Utilities	28,158	17,755	23,097	10,600	11,355	10,837	5,230
Depreciation and amortization	14,649	18,039	30,084	5,169	26,125	11,367	4,926
Repairs and maintenance	14,584	9,030	7,954	5,858	4,173	12,757	2,732
Other costs	73,015	60,812	21,603	13,464	22,284	34,239	7,045
Total expenses	773,560	660,024	271,693	166,868	222,011	344,542	119,578
Income from operations	139,819	341,925	40,494	9,487	24,432	125,536	22,111
Other income	20,758	223	260	176	30	1,027	21,876
Other expense	42,855	808	33,627	—	5,179	—	21,080
Overhead allocation	—	269,246	50,820	37,824	59,651	127,148	10,329
Income before taxes	$ 117,722	$ 72,094	$ (43,693)	$ (28,162)	$ (40,369)	$ (585)	$ 12,578

Note: Petaluma store 50% owned by Copperfield's Books, Inc. and by heirs of Dan Jaffee. Petaluma statements include both new and used operations. Petaluma statements also reflect administration overhead allocation of $35,969 in 2002.

Source: Copperfield's Books Inc.

placement and arrangement of front-list titles to the respective store managers. "We are working to get a handle on how product should be merchandised in our stores," stated Montan. "I have been studying the use of 'plan-o-grams' in other industries and trying to develop metrics for how to position our inventory to produce optimal sales."

Montan attributed decentralized control to helping attract and retain good employees. "We do have much more loyal employees than the chains do because we give more autonomy and creativity to our staff," Montan opined. "This creates an undefined yet very noticeable level of ownership toward the individual's store, and this attitude gets filtered down." Most of Copperfield's employees had been with the company since the 1980s, and their longevity was considered by Montan to be a key component in connecting Copperfield's to customers.

In conjunction with decentralized operations at the store level, the company invested heavily in front-office infrastructure. The corporate office provided general administrative support for the stores, which included centralized purchasing, accounting, marketing, information technology management, and special event coordination. Many of the firm's administrative employees were long tenured and had developed personal relationships with the company's founders. In 2003, approximately 22 percent of Copperfield's payroll was attributable to the corporate office, and overall corporate administration expenses cost approximately 7 percent of net sales. Corporate book buyers' salaries alone amounted to approximately 2 percent of new book sales. Exhibit 17 shows Copperfield's administrative cost structure.

Information Technology

In part, the need for front-office personnel had arisen from inefficiencies related to the company's antiquated information system based on MS-DOS, an operating system that had been in use since the

Exhibit 17   Copperfield's Books Inc., Comparative Statements of Administrative Expenses, 2001–2003

	2003		2002		2001	
Salaries and wages—executive/ general administration	$ 93,668	16.7%	$ 104,835	17.7%	$ 134,739	22.6%
Salaries and wages—accounting	72,574	12.9	65,445	11.1	70,631	11.8
Salaries and wages—advertising/ promotion	40,370	7.2	45,762	7.7	49,804	8.4
Salaries and wages—information technology	13,085	2.3	—	0.0	—	0.0
Salaries and wages—purchasing	104,917	18.7	103,465	17.5	100,623	16.9
Salaries and wages—warehouse	52,040	9.3	65,203	11.0	56,435	9.5
Salaries and wages—maintenance/ special events	2,109	0.4	6,768	1.1	9,943	1.7
Benefits	42,656	7.6	43,756	7.4	47,193	7.9
Occupancy	31,868	5.7	30,874	5.2	27,192	4.6
Utilities	16,611	3.0	18,596	3.1	18,460	3.1
Depreciation and amortization	13,623	2.4	19,020	3.2	17,684	3.0
Repairs and maintenance	10,881	1.9	28,441	4.8	7,333	1.2
Travel and business entertainment	16,722	3.0	16,634	2.8	11,008	1.8
Professional services	29,788	5.3	28,441	4.8	17,333	2.9
Other costs	20,956	3.7	13,747	2.3	28,026	4.7
Total administrative expenses	$ 561,868	100.0%	$ 590,987	100.0%	$ 596,404	100.0%

Note: Percentages may not add up to 100% due to rounding.
Source: Copperfield's Books Inc.

mid-1980s. The system issued purchase orders, created receiving documents, and maintained a perpetual inventory for the stores. It also suggested which books should be returned to the publisher or wholesaler and generated figures necessary to calculate "open-to-buy" budgets. However, the system's drawbacks were significant, according to Montan. Other chains had developed software that allowed for more connectivity with wholesalers. Different levels in the supply chain could share information to reduce costs. For example, the chains were able to receive shipments by box (instead of by individual book title, as was Copperfield's practice). Box book orders allowed other chains added efficiencies when fulfilling orders as well as receiving them. Montan believed that wholesalers would soon require this technology, or would charge a premium to ship merchandise on a per book basis, as currently required by existing software.

"There's just no new software available for us independent bookstores," Montan commented. "Because of the [consolidating] trends in the business, no one is writing software for independent bookstores." Montan related that a leading wholesaler, Ingram, was developing a proprietary software package that a bookseller could use to manage product purchased through its supply channel, but this product would not likely be comprehensive enough to meet all of Copperfield's needs for tracking inventory. Sales of new books accounted for 60 percent of chainwide revenues in 2003.

Copperfield's buyers procured new book inventory from a variety of sources. A large percentage of the backlist titles came from Ingram, which required smaller minimum purchases and shorter lead times. Copperfield's staff placed customers' special orders through Ingram. Corporate buyers also ordered directly from publishers like Random House, Penguin, and Houghton-Mifflin. Gross margins on books bought directly from publishers ranged from 41 to 43 percent, while margins on books from wholesalers averaged between 37 and 39 percent.

Copperfield's had explored outsourcing its buying functions to Ingram, which, in turn, could fill the role of a wholesaler/jobber for Copperfield's stores. Ingram purchased books from all major publishing houses and provided services to many independent booksellers that were not large enough to deal directly with publishers. Ingram offered to write all of Copperfield's orders and manage all returns, in exchange for an exclusive contract for all of the company's purchases. Montan and his team decided to turn down Ingram's offer, due to the risks of being associated with a one-source jobber, not to mention what might happen if Ingram itself should fail. Some team members were concerned that an exclusive contract would shift the retailer/supplier power balance to Copperfield's detriment. Others were worried about protecting the jobs of Copperfield's book buyers.

Copperfield's also purchased remainder books directly from publishers. Remainder books were overstocked older titles of new books that publishers sold to bookstores for "pennies on the dollar," according to Montan. The larger gross margins helped offset additional handling costs associated with remainder books. Montan said, "We have had to be careful. Remainder books have been addictive [to us] because of their higher margins and [to customers] because of their low prices."

As early as 2000, Montan had begun to worry about the decline of the downtown business districts where five of Copperfield's stores were located. The primary reason for Montan's concern arose from the flight from downtown areas of dynamic businesses that had previously helped to create a critical mass for attracting customers. This flight was a response to the development of malls in Copperfield's communities that offered free parking, security, and attractive store layouts. Montan believed that high parking fees, the rise in vacant storefronts, and a lack of after-dark foot traffic had restricted the downtown stores' performance. Meanwhile, retail development accelerated along major arterial highways, in all cases far removed from the downtown business districts. These developments were buoyed by declining state government budget allocations to local communities as well as regulations rewarding municipalities that fostered big-box retail development as a means of generating local tax revenue.

Leadership Style

Montan started working for Copperfield's in 1986, after earning a bachelor's degree in sociology. His first job was as a bookseller in the firm's Petaluma store, advancing to director of marketing in 1988. Copperfield's promoted him to be director of operations in 2002, shortly after the unexpected death of

Dan Jaffe, the preceding director of operations. He ascended to the position of CEO when founder and preceding CEO, Paul Jaffe, decided to step down from day-to-day operations.

Copperfield's mission statement emphasized customer service, respect for employees' contributions, community, independence, and free expression (see Exhibit 18). Montan stated:

> We were founded on ideals of being independent and creating a forum for ideas to be exchanged, but this path becomes more and more restricted as time goes on. So, we try to bend and adapt. The core values of the company are changing, too. I am continually frustrated with many within our industry who are very high on ideals but lack business models to support these ideals.

Montan believed that Copperfield's would have to upgrade its technology and improve organizational efficiencies. "Our goal is to make the bookstore experience increasingly exciting and locally focused with a supercharged back end that makes it easier for our stores to connect to their unique communities," he said. He created a slogan encompassing these beliefs: "Creating community, connecting with you."

Copperfield's board of directors gave Montan broad discretionary powers. His first order of business was to develop a vision for the company's growth and to make that vision a reality. During his first two years, he decentralized many of the buying functions, downsized the firm's warehouse operation, and cut staff. He standardized many human resource functions such as job descriptions and staff training programs, and implemented time and attendance controls. Montan also increased corporate communication through regular meetings with store management and weekly memos to all store employees.

Montan's management style inspired loyalty among his staff. "He really stepped up, and made it happen," exclaimed Aaron Smith, manager of the Montgomery Village store. "I had reservations when he was promoted, but now we all have a high level of trust in his intentions as well as his vision for the company. He impressed all of us in the way he dealt with the warehouse issue."

'[Standardizing human resource procedures] was something that had needed to happen for a long time," recalled Noreen Roberts, Copperfield's human resource manager. "He saw the opportunity and took it. I think he earned a lot of respect for that."

Governance and Corporate Structure

Copperfield's Inc. was organized as a subchapter S corporation at its inception with two founding stockholders: Barney Brown and Paul Jaffe. As the company grew, the board issued additional shares and sold them to members of the founders' families. As of October 2004, Copperfield's Inc. remained closely held by the Brown and Jaffe families, with the Brown family controlling a majority interest. The board of directors consisted of three members of the Brown family, one member of the Jaffe family, and one nonequity holding adviser.

Exhibit 18   **Copperfield's Books Inc. Mission Statement**

Our Intention
To create an extraordinary bookstore that is the pride of our community and staff.

Our Commitment
Service: *We strive to provide great customer service and recognize that it is only in our ability to uniquely serve our customers that we will succeed as a business.*

Responsibility: *We are committed to providing a forum for readers and writers that encourages the free expression of ideas. We are committed to remaining an independently owned and operated bookstore. We take personal responsibility for respecting one another and valuing the contributions we all make. We are committed to running a profitable business.*

Environment: *To carry a selection of books and gifts that nurtures the spirit and feeds the mind. To be a fun place to work.*

Source: Copperfield's Books Inc.

Internet

Capitalizing on the opportunities promised by the Internet posed a great challenge. Depth of selection, customized recommendations fueled by algorithms tracking previous purchasing behavior, discount pricing, and other value-added services provided by online retailers were all difficult—if not impossible—to duplicate in a storefront retail environment. While the setup costs for developing a presence on the Web were minimal and hundreds of people were selling used and rare books over the Internet, some via Web sites such as eBay, Bookfinder.com, the used-books division of Amazon.com, or Half.com, to name just a few sites, incumbent Internet booksellers erected barriers to fledgling online rivals through intensive capital investment and technical expertise. According to Montan:

> The independent book industry as a whole missed the Internet market per se [for new books]. Amazon just came and chose books as its ideal marketplace for Internet retailing. They were quite wise to do so; books are easily definable, you can have a lot of customer interactivity in terms of ratings and reviews, and it's a one-size-fits-all product that's not perishable. There are a lot of things going for books that makes a lot of sense to sell online.

As a way of providing value-added services for its existing customer base, Copperfield's used a Web site template developed by the American Booksellers Association (ABA). Through the site, customers could order books 24 hours a day. In addition, Copperfield's offered the value-added service of allowing in-store returns for online purchases, a service also offered by other retail stores that had Internet operations. Staff at the Montgomery Village store transmitted orders to a third-party wholesaler who fulfilled the orders, shipping directly to customers. Access to the ABA template cost $250 annually. Copperfield's earned a 5 percent finder's fee on sales through the site. "It's sort of a minimal cost, minimal work solution, that is certainly not the best," said Montan. In the 12 months ending in June 2004, Copperfield's posted revenues of $4,655 via this distribution channel.

Opportunities for selling used books online nevertheless appeared to be promising. Montan's belief that the Internet would be important to Copperfield's future competitiveness in the used-book market spurred his decision in 2004 to move staff and inventory of the abandoned downtown Santa Rosa location to the Petaluma store. Montan hoped to complete the first phase of operations in the new location by the end of 2004. He estimated that Copperfield's would receive one dollar in revenue per month for each title listed online. He hoped to list 10,000 titles by the end of 2004, estimating that should it achieve approximately $120,000 per year in Internet book sales, Copperfield's could then cover the online operation's overhead, realize a small profit, and begin to develop metrics for operating an online fulfillment operation. "We're learning how to do this business, but we are a long way from breakeven," Montan noted.

One problem with the fulfillment center was that there was no coordination between the other business units within the firm. Both of Copperfield's used bookstores sold online independently of the fulfillment center. There was no plan to integrate online sales of new books. Moreover, books inventoried in the fulfillment center were not available for sale in the stores. There were no mechanisms to coordinate the inventories between the used bookstores and the fulfillment center. It was possible that a customer looking for a particular book at one of the stores could be turned away, despite the fact that the book was inventoried in the fulfillment center. Conversely, shoppers looking for a particular book online did not have access to the inventories in the stores. Montan's long-range vision for the fulfillment center included "creating a 'mega-warehouse' used bookstore that could act as a warehouse for Internet sales, while developing large enough girth to attract customers from around the San Francisco Bay Area."

Used and Rare Books

Copperfield's primarily targeted the upper strata of the used-book market, that is, books valued at $20 or higher. Montan reflected:

> Used-book customers represent a different breed from new book people. They don't care about best sellers. They want what they want. They want the best copy. They are bibliophiles to the nth degree. They curmudgeonly want to get into the stacks so they can climb up the ladder and find that rare dusty "whatever" on the back shelf.

Copperfield's inventory of used and rare books was considered to be the largest in Sonoma County. The collection included a large percentage of antiquarian books and first editions, which were merchandised conspicuously throughout the stores to provide a sense of weight and refinement.

Copperfield's acquired its used books primarily from existing customers, junk dealers, and book scouts, but occasionally buyers went beyond these supply channels. In 2003, for example, the firm purchased an entire library in the Midwest. Determining the value of used books required specialized knowledge and experience. Art Kusnetz, manager of Copperfield's Petaluma Used and Rare Bookstore, had over 20 years' experience as a book scout and working with antiquarian book dealers. The need for expert employees was a significant barrier to expansion, as qualified, expert book buyers were scarce. Because kcy personnel were vital to success in the used-book business, Montan had considered equity sharing with managers of Copperfield's two used bookstores. Montan felt that owning a stake in the operation might increase their drive to grow the used-book business while protecting Copperfield's from the cost of replacing employees with rare skill sets.

THE NAPA OPPORTUNITY

After 10 years of disappointing operations in Copperfield's Napa store, Montan had begun looking for another way to access what he believed was an underserved market for books in Napa. "The fact that we secured what we felt was a sweetheart lease, [at] 80 cents per square foot, afforded us the ability to be patient," he said. "I think we had a distant hope that this area would explode, and we would be left holding the bag o' gold. But the trend currently is that this downtown space is flatter than flat." Early in 2004, Montan decided to give up on the Napa store and scheduled it for closure when the lease expired at the end of the year.

"We need to develop a store that will create a compelling gravity to attract customers," Montan said. He hoped to replicate his previous experience in Montgomery Village, consistently the most profitable store in the chain, which unlike its downtown locations, did not suffer from the lack of adequate parking, the impact of loitering transients that deterred customers from browsing, or a lack of evening foot traffic. Montan believed that new stores in regional lifestyle shopping centers with ample free parking could generate sales between $2.5 and $3 million annually, assuming that chain superstores refrained from entering into the same trade area.

Montan had located a space in a regional lifestyle center located at the intersection of two major arterial highways in Napa. The center had attracted other strong tenants like Trader Joe's, Cost Plus, and Orchard Hardware, retailers that could complement Copperfield's and help attract impulse purchasers and book browsers. To assess the market opportunity for a new Napa location, Montan pored over the demographic information for the Napa trade area, which, compared to Copperfield's current locations, had significantly larger Hispanic/Latino populations. His analysis suggested that the trade area was underserved, with over half of the area's potential book sales revenue "leaking" out of the trade area (see Exhibit 19). Yet his analysis also suggested that the surrounding area's demand could, at best, marginally support the additional retail space, because the levels of educational attainment in the Napa trade area appeared to be significantly lower than in the areas surrounding Copperfield's more successful stores (see Exhibit 20).

Copperfield's planned to recycle fixtures salvaged from the recent closure of the downtown Santa Rosa store along with those that would be transferred from the existing Napa store. By reusing fixtures, Montan felt that he could dramatically decrease the cost of opening a new store, which would still include $150,000 in tenant improvements (including $60,000 provided by the landlord), $450,000 in inventory ($150,000 of which would be transferred from the existing Napa location), and $30,000 in pre-opening expenses. An estimated total capital investment of nearly $500,000 would represent a level far exceeding any new store development Copperfield's had undertaken. The company would finance the project through bank loans collateralized by a company-owned building in Sebastopol.

The Future

When asked about the realism of his goal to grow Copperfield's Books from $8 million to $15 million in four years, Montan replied, "The biggest issue facing our company is growing to a size where we can develop a level of efficiency. We will need to develop this level of scale quickly to cover prospective increases in [administration] costs."

Exhibit 19   **Copperfield's Books Inc., Potential New Sales Analysis for Proposed Napa Store**

(1) Total trade area households*		31,885
(2) Annual average household spending at bookstores†		$162
(3) Total annual trade area potential [= (1) × (2)]		$5,165,370
(4) Existing supply‡		
Readers' Books	$600,000	
Copperfield's	420,000	
Napa Booktree	250,000	
Bookends Bookstore	550,000	
Waldenbooks	372,000	
Book Outlet Store	372,000	
(5) Total existing annual trade area sales		$2,564,000
(6) Current annual trade area "leakage" (potential sales) [= (3) − (5)]		$2,601,370
(7) Expressed as percentage of total annual trade area potential [= (6)/(3)]		50.36%

*Claritas, a marketing information resources company www.clusterbigip1.claritas.com/claritas/Default.jsp?ti=3&ci=1&pn=freeinfo (accessed October 2004).

†Represents average spending for *all* households on books, excluding children's, audio, and digital books. Household bookstore expenditures provided by *Press Democrat* and U.S. Census data from *Statistical Abstract of the United States, 2006.*

‡Supply data provided by Copperfield's; Waldenbooks and Book Outlet volumes reflect industry average per square foot; Copperfield's volume based on estimate using 2003 sales data.

Exhibit 20   **Copperfield's Books Inc., Demographic Analysis for Proposed Napa Store**

(1) Total trade area households*		31,885
(2) Annual average household spending at bookstores†		$102
(3) Total annual trade area potential [= (1) × (2)]		$5,165,370
(4) Average annual independent bookstore sales/sq. ft.‡		$248
(5) Supportable trade area bookstore space, sq. ft. [= (3)/(4)]		20,828
(6) Existing supply, sq. ft.§		
Readers' Books	3,000	
Copperfield's	3,400	
Napa Booktree	1,500	
Bookends Bookstore	4,000	
Waldenbooks	1,500	
Book Outlet Store	1,500	
(7) Total existing trade area supply, sq. ft.		14,900
(8) Additional supply trade area will support, sq. ft. [= (5) − (6)]		5,928
(9) Proposed Copperfield's store in Bel Aire Plaza, sq. ft.	9,700	
Existing Copperfield's store in downtown Napa, sq. ft.	(3,400)	
Net expansion, sq. ft.		6,300
(10) Trade area deficit after expansion, sq. ft. [= (8) − (9)]		(372)

*Claritas, a marketing information resources company, www.clusterbigip1.claritas.com/claritas/Default.jsp?ti=3&ci=1&pn=freeinfo (accessed October 2004).

†Represents average spending for *all* households on books, excluding children's, audio, and digital books. Household bookstore expenditures provided by *Press Democrat* and U.S. Census data from *Statistical Abstract of the United States, 2006.*

‡American Booksellers Association, *ABACUS Survey,* 2003.

§Supply data provided by Copperfield's; Waldenbooks and Book Outlet square footage estimated by using industry average per square foot.

The offer on the retail space in Napa expired in a week. Montan decided to take a few days with his management team and review several alternative strategies he had considered. These alternatives included opening as many as two 10,000-square-foot stores in North Bay markets, such as the proposed Napa location and perhaps also Novato (in neighboring Marin County to the south) within the next four years. Other options included increasing Copperfield's focus on the growing used- and rare-books segments, or accelerating its investment in Internet sales to complement its retail stores' sales.

Bibliography

Abraham, J., and J. Hayes. (2005). "Used Book Market Analysis: Initial Preview," Book Industry Study Group, www.bisg.org, preliminary report released September 2005.

Amazon.com, 2003 annual report.

American Booksellers Association. *ABACUS Survey 2003.*

Anderson, C. (2004, October). "The Long Tail." *Wired.*

Anonymous. (2003, September 10). "Adult Book Purchases Up Two Percent in 2002." *Bookselling This Week,* http://news.bookweb.org/news/1782.html.

Anonymous. (2004, May 6). "BookTrends Study Shows Independents Buck Trend and Gain Market Share." *Bookselling This Week,* http://news.bookweb.org/news/2514.html.

Anonymous. (2004, May 19). "BISG's Trends Predicts $44 Billion Book Market in 2008." *Bookselling This Week,* http://news.bookweb.org/news/2548.html.

Anonymous. (2004, August 24). "Independent Sellers Gain with Size, Service." *The Wall Street Journal (Eastern Edition),* Section A1.

Barnes & Noble. 2003 annual report.

Bernoff, J., C. Charron, A. Lonian, C. Stohm, and G. Fleming. (2004). "From Discs to Downloads." Forrester Research, www.forrester.com/ER/Research/Report/Summary/0,1338,16076,00.html.

Borders Group Inc., 10-K report filed with the Securities and Exchange Commission, FYE January 25, 2004.

Claritas, a Market Research Company. www.claritas.com/claritas/Default.jsp?ti = 3&ci = 1&pn = freeinfo (accessed October 20, 2004).

Howell, K. (2004, September 20). "Tattered Cover Expands to the Burbs," *Publishers Weekly.*

IPSOS-Insight. "BookTrends." www.ipsos-insight.com (accessed October 19, 2004).

Kirch, C. (2004, July 26) ."Creating an Experience." *Publisher's Weekly.*

Lewin, N. (2005, December 19). "The Book Trade," Public Radio International's *Marketplace,* http://marketplace.publicradio.org/shows/2005/12/19/pm.html.

Mariano, G. (2001, May 2). "E-book Devices Yet to Hit Bestseller's List." *CNET,* http://news.com.com/2100-1023-256938.html.

National Endowment for the Arts. (2004, June). "Reading at Risk: A Survey of Literary Reading in America." *National Endowment for the Arts,* www.arts.gov.

Patterson, W. (2004, June 6). "Retail Grows, with Vacancies under 5%," *Santa Rosa Press Democrat,* Outlook Section.

Patterson, W. (2004, June 24). "Copperfield's Moves On." *Santa Rosa Press Democrat,* p. E1.

Price, G. (2004). "Google Partners with Oxford, Harvard & Others to Digitize Libraries." *SearchEngineWatch,* http://searchenginewatch.com/searchday/article.php/3447411.

Rappaport, B. (2003, Fall). "The Used Book Marketplace: Fact or Fiction?" *Publishing Research Quarterly,* pp. 3–12.

Small Business Administration. www.onlinewbc.gov/docs/finance/fs_ratio1.html.

Trachtenberg J. (2004, August 24). "Plot Twist: To Compete with Book Chains, Some Think Big; Independent Sellers Gain with Size, Service." *The Wall Street Journal (Eastern Edition),* p. A1.

U.S. Census Bureau. (2000). *Income Distribution in 1999 of Households and Families: 2000,* QT-P32, http://factfinder.census.gov/servlet/QTTable?_bm= y&-geo_id=D&-qr_name=DEC_2000_SFAIAN_ QTP32&-ds_name=D&-_lang=en.

U.S. Department of Commerce. (2004). "Sector 44: Retail Trade: Industry Series: Comparative Statistics for the United States (1997 NAICA Basics): 2002 and 1997." *2002 U.S. Economic Census* (Release Date: July 29, 2004), www.census.gov/econ/census02/guide/INDRPT44.HTM.

Endnotes

[1]Anonymous. (2004, May 19). "BISG's Trends Predicts $44 Billion Book Market in 2008." *Bookselling This Week,* http://news.bookweb.org/news/2548.html.

[2]Ibid.

[3]IPSOS. (2003). "Book Industry Struggles with Slow Growth." www.ipsos-ideas.com/article.cfm?id=2148

[4]According to one industry observer, "The trade book industry is faced with the need to develop a strategic marketing plan that will excite customers and bring them back into the stores. Programs designed to attract the affluent, educated customer without alienating the remaining customer base are key." Rappaport, B. (2003, Fall) "The Used Book Marketplace: Fact or Fiction?" *Publishing Research Quarterly,* p. 5.

[5]Anonymous. (2003, June 22). "Wal-Mart and Other Discounters: Cultural Oligopsony?" *Oligopoly Watch,* www.oligopolywatch.com/2003/06/22.html.

[6]Ibid.

[7]"Sector 44: Retail Trade: Industry Series: Book Stores," *2002 U.S. Economic Census* (release date: July 29, 2004), www.census.gov/ccon/concuc02/guide/INDRPT44.HTM.

[8]Trachtenberg J. (2004, August 24). "Plot Twist: To Compete with Book Chains, Some Think Big; Independent Sellers Gain with Size, Service." *The Wall Street Journal (Eastern Edition),* p. A1.

[9]Anonymous. (2003, September 10). "Adult Book Purchases Up Two Percent in 2002." *Bookselling This Week,* http://news.bookweb.org/news/1782.html.

[10]Borders Group Inc., form 10-K for the fiscal year ended January 25, 2004, p. 9.

[11]Milevoj, A., Manager of Investor Relations, Barnes & Noble, e-mail message to authors, October 18, 2004.

[12]Trachtenberg, J. op. cit.

[13]Anonymous. (2004, May 6). "BookTrends Study Shows Independents Buck Trend and Gain Market Share." *Bookselling This Week,* http://news.bookweb.org/news/2514.html.

[14]Barnes & Noble, 2003 annual report, p. 10.

[15]Anonymous. (2004, May 6), op. cit.

[16]Ibid.

[17]Anderson, C. (2004, October). "The Long Tail." *Wired,* pp. 171–77.

[18]Ibid.

[19]Rappaport, B. (2003). op. cit., pp. 9–10.

[20]Bernoff, J. et. al. (2004). "From Discs to Downloads." Forrester Research, www.forrester.com/ER/Research/Report/Summary/0,1338,16076,00.html.

[21] Mariano, G. (2004). "E-book Devices Yet to Hit Bestseller's List," *CNET,* http://news.com.com/2100-1023-256938.html.

[22]Ibid.

[23]Price, G. (2004). "Google Partners with Oxford, Harvard & Others to Digitize libraries." SearchEngineWatch.com, http://searchenginewatch.com/searchday/article.php/3447411.

[24]Borders Group Inc., form 10-K for the fiscal year ended January 25, 2004, p. 17; Barnes & Noble, 2003 annual report, p. 13.

[25]American Booksellers Association, *ABACUS Survey 2004.*

[26]Borders Group Inc., form 10-K for the fiscal year ended January 25, 2004, p. 9.

[27]U.S. Census Bureau. (2000). *QT-P32. Income distribution in 1999 of households and families: 2000,* http://factfinder.census.gov/servlet/QTTable?_bm=y&-geo_id=D&-qr_name=DEC_2000_SFA-IAN_QTP32&-ds_name=D&-_lang=en.

[28]Patterson, W. (2004, June 6). "Retail Grows, with Vacancies Under 5%." *Santa Rosa Press Democrat,* Outlook Section.

[29]Ibid.

[30]Patterson, W. (2004, June 24). "Copperfield's Moves On." *Santa Rosa Press Democrat,* p. E1.

Harley-Davidson in 2004

John E. Gamble
University of South Alabama

Roger Schäfer
University of South Alabama

Harley-Davidson's management had much to be proud of as the company wrapped up its Open Road Tour centennial celebration, which began in July 2002 in Atlanta, Georgia, and ended on the 2003 Memorial Day Weekend in Harley's hometown of Milwaukee, Wisconsin. The 14-month Open Road Tour was a tremendous success, drawing large crowds of Harley owners in each of its five stops in North America and additional stops in Australia, Japan, Spain, and Germany. Each stop along the tour included exhibits of historic motorcycles, performances by dozens of bands as diverse as Lynyrd Skynyrd, Earl Scruggs, and Nickelback, and brought hundreds of thousands of Harley enthusiasts together to celebrate the company's products. The Ride Home finale brought 700,000 biker-guests from four points in the United States to Milwaukee for a four-day party that included concerts, factory tours, and a parade of 10,000 motorcycles through downtown Milwaukee. The company also used the Open Road Tour as a platform for its support of the Muscular Dystrophy Association (MDA), raising $7 million for the MDA during the 14-month tour. Photos from the Open Road Tour and Harley's new V-Rod model are presented in Exhibit 1.

Harley-Davidson's centennial year was also a year to remember for the company's being named to *Fortune*'s annual list "The 100 Best Companies to Work For" and judged third in automotive quality behind Rolls-Royce and Mercedes-Benz by Harris Interactive, a worldwide market research and consulting firm best known for the Harris Poll. Consumer loyalty to Harley-Davidson motorcycles was unmatched by almost any other company. As

a Canadian Harley dealer explained, "You know you've got strong brand loyalty when your customers tattoo your logo on their arm."[1] The company's revenues had grown at a compound annual rate of 16.6 percent since 1994 to reach $4.6 billion in 2003—marking its 18th consecutive year of record revenues and earnings. In 2003, the company sold more than 290,000 motorcycles, giving it a commanding share of the market for motorcycles in the 651+ cubic centimeters (cc) category in the United States and the leading share of the market in the Asia/Pacific region. The consistent growth had allowed Harley-Davidson's share price to appreciate by more than 15,000 percent since the company's initial public offering in 1986. In January 2004, the company's CEO, Jeffrey Bleustein, commented on the centennial year and the company's prospects for growth as it entered its second century:

> We had a phenomenal year full of memorable once-in-a-lifetime experiences surrounding our 100th Anniversary. As we begin our 101st year, we expect to grow the business further with our proven ability to deliver a continuous stream of exciting new motorcycles, related products, and services. We have set a new goal for the company to be able to satisfy a yearly demand of 400,000 Harley-Davidson motorcycles in 2007. By offering innovative products and services, and by driving productivity gains in all facets of our business, we are confident that we can deliver an earnings growth rate in the mid-teens for the foreseeable future.[2]

However, not everyone was as bullish on Harley-Davidson's future, with analysts pointing out that the company's plans for growth were too dependent on aging baby boomers. The company had achieved its record growth during the 1990s and

Exhibit 1   **Photos from Harley-Davidson's Open Road Tour and Its VRSC V-Rod**

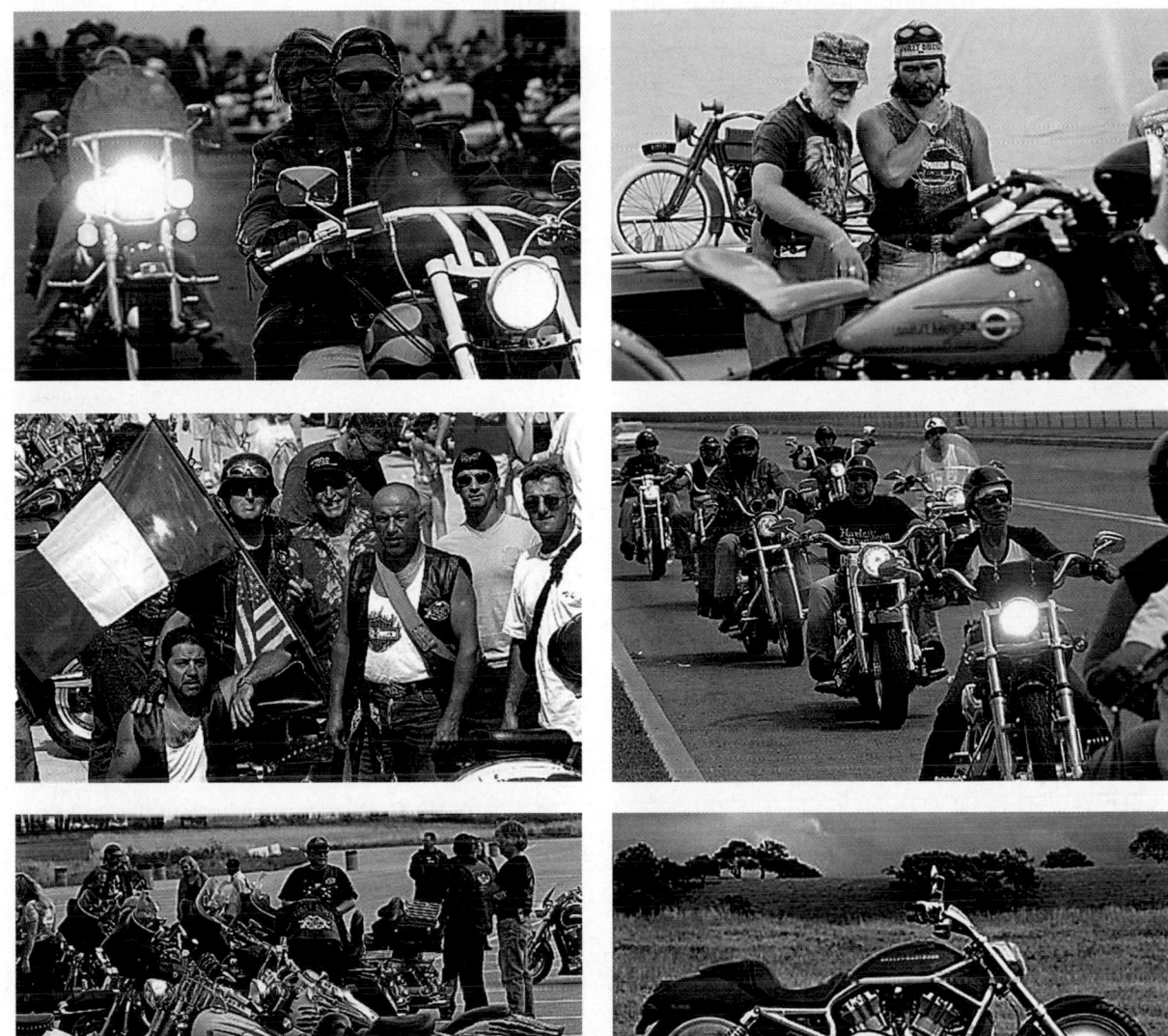

Source: Harley-Davidson Web site.

early 2000s primarily through the appeal its image held for baby boomers in the United States. Some observers wondered how much longer boomers would choose to spend recreational time touring the country by motorcycle and attending motorcycle rallies. The company had yet to develop a motorcycle that appealed in large numbers to motorcycle riders in their 20s or cyclists in Europe, both of whom preferred performance-oriented bikes over cruisers or touring motorcycles. Another concern of analysts watching the company was Harley Davidson's short-term oversupply of certain models

Exhibit 2   **Summary of Harley-Davidson's Financial Performance, 1994–2003 (in thousands, except per share amounts)**

	2003	2002	2001
Income statement data			
Net sales	$4,624,274	$4,090,970	$3,406,786
Cost of goods sold	2,958,708	2,673,129	2,253,815
Gross profit	1,665,566	1,417,841	1,152,971
Operating income from financial services	167,873	104,227	61,273
Selling, administrative and engineering	(684,175)	(639,366)	(551,743)
Income from operations	1,149,264	882,702	662,501
Gain on sale of credit card business	—	—	—
Interest income, net	23,088	16,541	17,478
Other income (expense), net	(6,317)	(13,416)	(6,524)
Income from continuing operations before provision for income taxes and accounting changes	1,166,035	885,827	673,445
Provision for income taxes	405,107	305,610	235,709
Income from continuing operations before accounting changes	760,928	580,217	437,746
Income (loss) from discontinued operations, net of tax	—	—	—
Income before accounting changes	760,928	580,217	437,746
Cumulative effect of accounting changes, net of tax	—	—	—
Net income (loss)	$ 760,928	$ 580,217	$ 437,746
Weighted average common shares:			
Basic	302,271	302,297	302,506
Diluted	304,470	305,158	306,248
Earnings per common share from continuing operations:			
Basic	$ 2.52	$ 1.92	$ 1.45
Diluted	2.50	1.90	1.43
Dividends paid	0.195	0.135	0.115
Balance sheet data			
Working capital	$1,773,354	$1,076,534	$ 949,154
Current finance receivables, net	1,001,990	855,771	656,421
Long-term finance receivables, net	735,859	589,809	379,335
Total assets	4,923,088	3,861,217	3,118,495
Short-term finance debt	324,305	382,579	217,051
Long-term finance debt	670,000	380,000	380,000
Total debt	$ 994,305	$ 762,579	$ 597,051
Shareholders' equity	$2,957,692	$2,232,915	$1,756,283

Source: Harley-Davidson Inc. 2003, 2002, and 1998 10-K reports.

brought about by the 14-month production run for its 100th anniversary models. The effect of the extended production period shortened the waiting list for most models from over a year to a few months and left some models on showroom floors for immediate purchase. The combined effects of a market focus on a narrow demographic group, the difficulty experienced in gaining market share in Europe, and short-term forecasting problems led to a sell-off of Harley-Davidson shares going into 2004. Exhibit 2 presents a summary of Harley-Davidson's financial and operating performance for 1994–2003. Its market performance for 1994 through January 2004 is presented in Exhibit 3.

2000	1999	1998	1997	1996	1995	1994
$2,943,346	$2,482,738	$2,087,670	$1,762,569	$1,531,227	$1,350,466	$1,158,887
1,979,572	1,666,863	1,414,034	1,176,352	1,041,133	939,067	800,548
963,774	815,875	673,636	586,217	490,094	411,399	358,339
37,178	27,685	20,211	12,355	7,801	3,620	
(485,980)	(427,701)	(360,231)	(328,569)	(269,449)	(234,223)	(204,777)
514,972	415,859	333,616	270,003	228,446	180,796	153,562
18,915	—	—	—	—	—	—
17,583	8,014	3,828	7,871	3,309	96	1,682
(2,914)	(3,080)	(1,215)	(1,572)	(4,133)	(4,903)	1,196
548,556	420,793	336,229	276,302	227,622	175,989	156,440
200,843	153,592	122,729	102,232	84,213	64,939	60,219
347,713	267,201	213,500	174,070	143,409	111,050	96,221
—	—	—	—	22,619	1,430	8,051
347,713	267,201	213,500	174,070	166,028	112,480	104,272
—	—	—	—	—	—	—
$ 347,713	$ 267,201	$ 213,500	$ 174,070	$ 166,028	$ 112,480	$ 104,272
302,691	304,748	304,454	151,650	150,683	149,972	150,440
307,470	309,714	309,406	153,948	152,925	151,900	153,365
$ 1.15	$ 0.88	$ 0.70	$ 1.15	$ 0.95	$ 0.74	$ 0.64
1.13	0.86	0.69	1.13	0.94	0.73	0.63
0.098	0.088	0.078	0.135	0.110	0.090	0.070
$ 799,521	$ 430,840	$ 376,448	$ 342,333	$ 362,031	$288,783	$189,358
530,859	440,951	360,341	293,329	183,808	169,615	—
234,091	354,888	319,427	249,346	154,264	43,829	—
2,436,404	2,112,077	1,920,209	1,598,901	1,299,985	980,670	676,663
89,509	181,163	146,742	90,638	8,065	—	—
355,000	280,000	280,000	280,000	250,000	164,330	—
$ 444,509	$ 461,163	$ 426,742	$ 391,572	$ 285,767	$185,228	$ 10,452
$1,405,655	$1,161,080	$1,029,911	$ 826,668	$ 662,720	$494,569	$433,232

COMPANY HISTORY

Harley-Davidson's history began in Milwaukee, Wisconsin, in 1903 when 20-year-old Arthur Davidson convinced his father to build a small shed in their backyard where Arthur and 21-year-old William Harley could try their hand at building a motorcycle. Various types of motorized bicycles had been built since 1885, but the 1901 development of a motorcycle with an integrated engine by a French company inspired Davidson and Harley to develop their own motorcycle. The two next-door neighbors built a two-horsepower engine that they fit onto a

Exhibit 3 **Yearly Performance of Harley-Davidson Inc.'s Stock Price, 1994 to January 2004**

(a) Trend in Harley-Davidson Inc.'s Common Stock Price

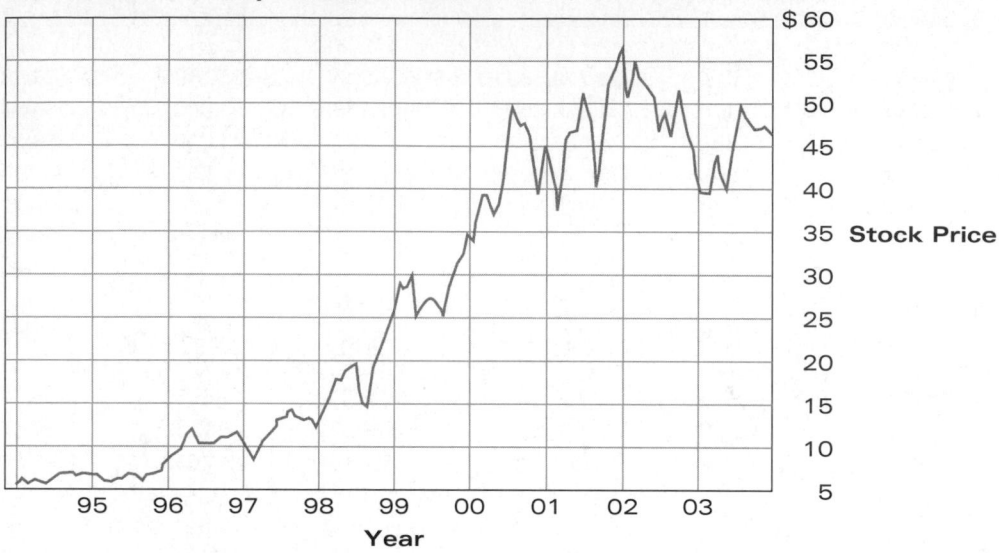

(b) Performance of Harley-Davidson Inc.'s Stock Price versus the S&P 500 Index

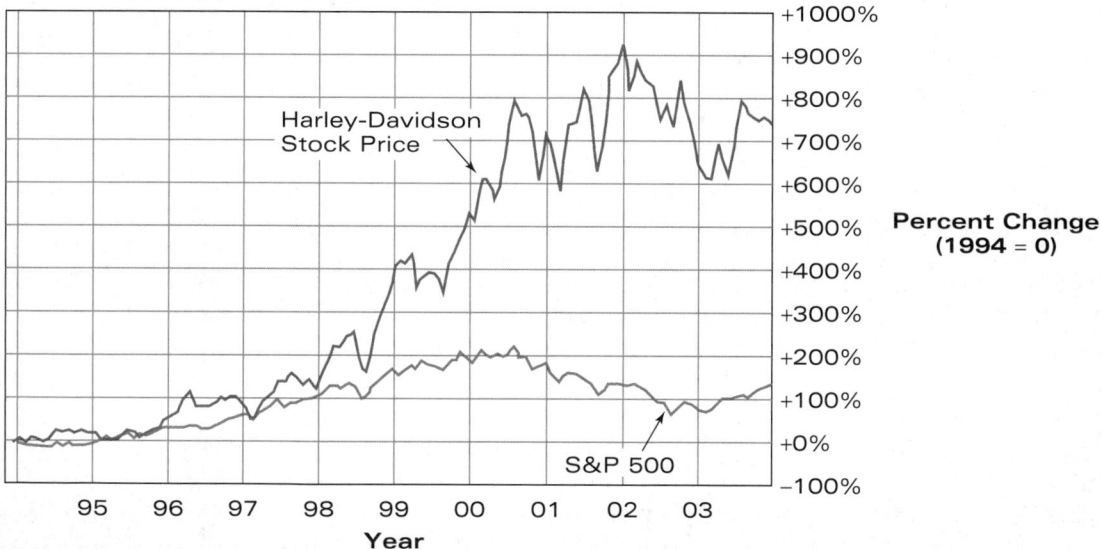

modified bicycle frame. At first the motorcycle could not pull itself and a rider up a steep hill, but after some additional tinkering, the first Harley-Davidson motorcycle could run as fast as 25 miles per hour. Milwaukee residents were amazed as Harley and Davidson rode the motorcycle down local streets, and by the end of the year the partners were able to produce and sell three of their motorcycles. Walter Davidson joined his brother and William Harley during the year to help assemble and race the company's motorcycles. In 1905, a Harley-Davidson motorcycle won a 15-mile race in Chicago with a time of 19:02, and by 1907 the company had developed quite a reputation in motorcycle racing with numerous wins in Milwaukee-area races. In 1907, another Davidson brother, William, joined the company and the company began adding dealers. Harley-Davidson's dealers helped the company sell 150 motorcycles in 1907.

In 1909, Harley-Davidson developed a more powerful seven-horsepower motorcycle engine to keep its edge in racing, an innovation that turned out to define the look of the company's motorcycles for the next century. Twin cylinders joined at a 45-degree angle became a trademark Harley-Davidson engine design characteristic and created a distinctive "potato-potato-potato" sound. Harley designed his V-twin engine with two pistons connected to a single crankpin, whereas later designs used crankpins for each piston. The single-crankpin design had been called an inferior design because it caused the pistons to come into firing positions at uneven intervals, which produced an uneven cadence in sound and excessive vibrations. Nevertheless, the vibrations and distinctive rumble of a Harley engine were accepted by the market in the early 1900s and continued to appeal to motorcyclists in the early 2000s.

The stronger engine allowed the company to produce 17,000 motorcycles for the U.S. military during World War I and become the largest motorcycle producer in the world in 1920, with 2,000 dealers in 67 countries. A number of features that make up Harley-Davidson's image originated during the 1920s, including the teardrop gas tank, the "Hog" nickname, and the "Flathead" engine design. Harley-Davidson was one of two U.S. motorcycle companies to survive the Great Depression—the other being Indian—by relying on exports and sales to police departments and the U.S. military. The 1930s saw Harley-Davidson win more races and develop additional elements of its differentiated image, including the art deco eagle design painted on its gas tanks, three-tone paint, and the "Knucklehead" engine rocker boxes. Harley-Davidson's 1936 EL model, or "Knucklehead," became its first highly styled motorcycle and formed the foundation of style elements that remained present in the highly demanded 2004 Softail Fat Boy. The company suspended production of civilian motorcycles in 1941 to produce almost 90,000 motorcycles for the U.S. military during World War II.

The recreational motorcycle market grew dramatically after World War II, as ex-GIs purchased motorcycles and led enthusiasm for riding. Harley-Davidson introduced new models for enthusiasts, including the Hydra-Glide in 1949, the K-model in 1952, the Sportster in 1957, and the Duo-Glide in 1958. The combination of racing success (Harley-Davidson riders won 18 of 24 races and set six new racing records in 1950 alone) and innovative new Harley-Davidson models led to rival company Indian's demise in 1953. Harley-Davidson would remain the sole U.S. manufacturer of motorcycles until 1998, when the Indian brand was revived.

Harley-Davidson continued to win races throughout the 1960s, but its reputation began to erode soon after its acquisition by American Machine and Foundry Company (AMF) in 1969. Harley-Davidson under AMF was known for its leaking engines, unreliable performance, and poor customer service. At one point during AMF's ownership of the company, more than one-half of its bikes had to be repaired before leaving the factory. The company attempted to offset its declining sales of road bikes with the introduction of dirt bikes and snowmobiles in the early 1970s, but by the late 1970s AMF lost faith in the acquisition and slated it for divestiture. When no buyers for the company emerged, 13 executives engineered a leveraged buyout of Harley-Davidson in 1981. Harley-Davidson struggled under the heavy debt load and came within four hours of bankruptcy in 1985, before then-CEO Richard Teerlink was able to convince new creditors to step in and restructure Harley with less costly financing terms. Teerlink also launched a restructuring program that updated manufacturing methods, improved quality, and expanded the model line.

U.S. tariffs imposed on 651+cc Japanese motorcycles also aided Harley-Davidson in gaining financial strength and competitiveness in the heavyweight segment of the U.S. motorcycle industry. Harley-Davidson completed an initial public offering in 1985 and petitioned the International Trade Commission to terminate tariffs on Japanese heavyweight motorcycles in 1987 when its market share in the U.S. heavyweight category had improved to 25 percent from 16 percent in 1985. In 1998, the company purchased Wisconsin-based Buell Motorcycle, a performance brand using Harley-Davidson engines that began as a venture between Erik Buell and Harley-Davidson in 1992. Harley-Davidson opened its 358,000-square-foot Kansas City, Missouri, plant in 1998 to produce Sportster, Dyna Glide, and V-Rod models and built an assembly plant in Brazil in 1999 to aid in its Latin American expansion. The new capacity allowed Harley-Davidson to set production records each year during the early 2000s to reach 290,000 units by year-end 2003.

OVERVIEW OF THE MOTORCYCLE INDUSTRY

Demand for motorcycles in developed countries such as the United States, Germany, France, Spain, and Great Britain, grew dramatically at the end of World War II as veterans who enjoyed riding motorcycles during the war purchased their own bikes upon return to civilian life. Groups of enthusiasts began to form motorcycle clubs that allowed them to socialize and participate in rallies and races. Two of the earliest motorcycle rallies in the United States were the Daytona Bike Week and the Sturgis Rally. The first Daytona 200, which occurs during Bike Week, was run in 1937 on a 3.2-mile beach and road course. The first Sturgis, South Dakota, race took place in 1938 when nine participants raced a half-mile track and performed such stunts as jumping ramps and crashing through plywood walls. These and other such events grew dramatically in popularity beginning in the 1970s, with both Daytona Bike Week and the Sturgis Rally each drawing over 200,000 bikers in 2003. The Sturgis Rally was said to be among the most raucous motorcycle rallies in the United States, with plenty of public drunkenness and lewd behavior accompanying the seven days of races. Such behavior was common enough that the Rally Web site (www.sturgis.com) provided the fines and bonds associated with such offenses as indecent exposure, disorderly conduct, open container in public, and possession of controlled substances.

The rowdy and rebellious image of bikers is traced to some of the motorcycle clubs that began after World War II. The outlaw image of cyclists first developed in 1947 when *Life* magazine photographers captured images of an impromptu rally at Hollister, California, by a motorcycle group calling themselves the Boozefighters. The group became quite rowdy during their motorcycling exhibition, but *Life* reporters embellished the story significantly, claiming the Boozefighters descended on the town and proceeded to terrorize its residents by drag-racing down the main street, tossing beer bottles, and riding motorcycles through the front doors of the town's saloon. The imagery of the drunken Fourth of July attack on the town became etched deeper into the minds of the world when the story became the subject of *The Wild One,* a 1954 movie starring Marlon Brando. When asked by a local resident what

he was rebelling against, Brando's character, Johnny, replied, "Whaddya got?"[3] The general public came to dislike bikers because of incidents like the one in Hollister and because of the Hollywood treatment of the event, but the Hells Angels made many people fearful of bikers and put motorcycle gangs under the close scrutiny of law enforcement at local, state, and federal levels.

The Hells Angels were established in 1948 in Fontana, California, by a group of young cyclists who had read of the Hollister rampage and wished to start their own outlaw biker group. The Hells Angels, who took their name and symbols from various World War II flying units, became notorious during the 1960s when they became linked to drug trafficking and other organized crime activities. Sonny Barger, a founder of the Oakland, California, chapter in the late 1950s, became the United States' most infamous biker after organizing a disastrous security effort for the 1969 Rolling Stones concert in Altamont at which one concertgoer was stabbed and killed by Hells Angels members. Barger, who had been convicted of attempted murder, possession of narcotics with intent to sell, and assault with a deadly weapon, commented in an interview with the British Broadcasting Corporation (BBC) that he pressed a pistol into Keith Richards' ribs and ordered him to continue to play after the Rolling Stones' guitarist threatened to end the show because of Hells Angels' rough tactics with fans.[4]

The Hells Angels and rival motorcycle clubs like the Pagans, the Banditos, and the Outlaws, rode only Harleys, which hurt Harley-Davidson's image with the public in the 1960s. Honda successfully exploited Harley's outlaw image with the slogan "You meet the nicest people on a Honda" to become the largest seller of motorcycles in the United States during the late 1960s and early 1970s.[5] The image of the Hells Angels had spilled over to the entire industry and contributed to declines in motorcycle demand in the United States and Europe during the 1960s before a new Hollywood film resurrected interest in motorcycles. *Easy Rider* (1969) portrayed bikers as less villainous rebels and appealed greatly to young people in the United States and Europe. The movie eventually gained cult status and helped charge a demand for motorcycles that began in the 1970s and continued through 2003. The red-white-and-blue 1951 Harley "Captain America" chopper ridden by Peter Fonda's Wyatt character helped

Harley-Davidson break the outlaw image and come to represent less malevolent rebellion.

Industry Conditions in 2003

In 2003, more than 950,000 motorcycles were sold in the United States and 28 million motorcycles were in operation worldwide. The industry was expected to grow by approximately 5 percent annually through 2007 with light motorcycles, Mopeds, and scooters accounting for most of the expected growth. A general increase in incomes in such emerging markets as China, India, and Southeast Asia was the primary force expected to drive industry growth. Demand growth for the heavyweight motorcycle category had outpaced smaller motorcycles in the United States during the 1990s and into 2003, but analysts projected that demand for larger motorcycles would decline as the population aged and became less able to travel on two-wheelers. In 2002, demand for heavyweight motorcycles in the United States grew by 17 percent compared to an industrywide growth rate of 10 percent.

The industry was segmented into various groups on the basis of engine size and vehicle style. Mopeds, scooters, and some small motorcycles were equipped with engines having displacements of 50 cubic centimeters (cc) or less. These motorbikes were best suited for urban areas where streets were narrow and parking was limited or for developing countries where personal incomes were limited and consumers could make only small investments in transportation. Motorcycles used for basic transportation or for motocross events were typically equipped with engines ranging from 125cc to 650cc. Larger street bikes required more power and usually had engines over 650cc. Large motorcycles with engine displacements greater than 651cc accounted for the largest portion of demand in North America and Europe as riders increasingly chose motorcycles with more horsepower and better performance. Exhibit 4 presents registrations of 651+cc motorcycles in the United States, Europe, and Asia-Pacific for 1998–2003. Even though Europe had fewer registrations of 651+cc motorcycles than the United States, it was the world's largest market for motorcycles, with 1.1 million registrations of 125+cc motorcycles in 2002. Registrations of motorcycles with engine displacements greater than 125cc in the largest European markets are presented in Exhibit 5.

Segmentation within the 651+cc Category

Motorcycles in the 651+cc segment were referred to as heavyweights and were grouped into four categories. Standard heavyweight motorcycles were designed for low-cost transportation and lacked many of the features and accessories of more expensive classes of heavyweights. Performance bikes had streamlined styling, low-profile fairings, and seat and handlebar configurations that required the rider to lean forward; they were characterized by responsive handling, rapid acceleration, and high top-end speeds. Custom motorcycles ranged from motorcycles with a custom paint scheme to highly personalized bikes painted with murals or other designs, chromed frames and other components, and accessories not found on stock motorcycles. The chopper, among the more unusual custom styles, was limited only by designers' imaginations but typically had extended forks, high handlebars, a narrow front tire, and a rigid "hardtail" frame design that lacked rear shocks and was stretched longer than normal motorcycles. Another notable feature of custom choppers was that they were almost always built from stock Harley-Davidson motorcycles, sometimes retaining only the engine.

Custom bikes were the largest segment of the U.S. heavyweight market for motorcycles and had become a curiosity for noncyclists. The Discovery Channel regularly aired two programs dedicated to the topic of choppers and other custom vehicles. The names of two custom motorcycle shops, West Coast Choppers (WCC) and Orange County Choppers, frequently made the Internet search engine Lycos's list of 50 most-searched terms. Jesse James, a descendent of the famous American Old West outlaw and owner of West Coast Choppers, also made Lycos's list of most-searched terms. WCC charged between $60,000 and $150,000 for its custom motorcycles, which were usually sold to celebrities such as movie stars, professional athletes, and rock musicians.

Touring bikes were set apart from other categories by creature comforts and accessories that included large fairings, storage compartments, CD players, cruise control, and other features typically found on cars rather than on motorcycles. Touring bikes were popular in the United States since many baby boomers wished to enjoy biking, but with some

Exhibit 4   **Market Shares of the Leading Producers of Motorcycles by Geographic Region for the Heavyweight Segment, 1998–2003 (engine displacement of 651+cc)**

	2003	2002	2001	2000	1999	1998
New U.S. registrations (thousands of units)						
Total market new registrations	461.2	442.3	394.3	340	275.6	227.1
Harley-Davidson new registrations	228.4	209.3	177.4	155.1	134.5	109.1
Buell new registrations	3.5	2.9	2.6	4.2	3.9	3.2
Total company new registrations	231.9	212.2	180.0	159.3	138.4	112.3
Percentage market share						
Harley-Davidson motorcycles	49.5%	47.5%	45.0%	45.6%	48.8%	48.1%
Buell motorcycles	0.8	0.7	0.7	1.2	1.4	1.4
Total Harley-Davidson	50.3%	48.2%	45.7%	46.8%	50.2%	49.5%
Honda	18.4%	19.8%	20.5%	18.5%	16.4%	20.3%
Suzuki	9.8	9.6	10.8	9.3	9.4	10.0
Kawasaki	6.7	6.9	8.0	9.0	10.3	10.1
Yamaha	8.5	8.9	7.9	8.4	7.0	4.2
Other	6.3	6.6	7.1	8.0	6.7	5.9
Total	100.0%	100.0%	100.0%	100.0%	100.0%	100.0%
New European registrations (thousands of units)						
Total market new registrations	323.1	303.5	292.1	293.4	306.7	270.2
Total Harley-Davidson new registrations	26.3	20.1	19.6	19.9	17.8	15.7
Percentage market share						
Total Harley-Davidson	8.1%	6.6%	6.7%	6.8%	5.8%	5.8%
Honda	16.7	21.0	17.4	21.8	22.2	24.1
Yamaha	16.0	17.7	16.4	17.3	18.0	16.3
BMW	15.3	15.1	15.1	13.0	13.0	13.4
Suzuki	15.5	14.8	16.5	14.3	15.4	17.2
Other	28.4	24.8	27.9	26.8	25.6	23.2
Total	100.0%	100.0%	100.0%	100.0%	100.0%	100.0%
New Asia-Pacific registrations (thousands of units)						
Total market new registrations	58.9	63.9	62.1	62.7	63.1	69.2
Total Harley-Davidson new registrations	15.2	13.0	12.7	12.2	11.6	10.3
Percentage market share						
Total Harley-Davidson	25.8%	21.3%	20.4%	19.5%	18.5%	14.8%
Honda	17.8	19.1	17.3	20.4	22.4	28.0
Kawasaki	13.8	15.8	15.6	18.9	19.0	22.1
Yamaha	11.4	13.6	15.8	17.0	19.0	16.0
Suzuki	10.7	10.1	12.8	10.4	9.3	7.9
Other	20.5	20.1	18.1	13.8	11.8	11.2
Total	100.0%	100.0%	100.0%	100.0%	100.0%	100.0%

Source: Harley-Davidson Inc. 10-K reports and annual reports.

Exhibit 5   **Registrations of New Motorcycles in Major European Markets, 1998–2003 (engine displacement of 125+cc)**

Country	1998	1999	2000	2001	2002	2003
Germany	175,937	187,192	170,636	158,270	145,369	138,712
Italy	79,400	103,800	122,085	126,400	129,261	130,224
France	88,500	109,105	103,900	106,802	113,852	N/A
Great Britain	84,500	98,186	93,634	91,543	93,557	N/A
Spain	35,600	39,200	38,052	31,829	35,252	N/A

N/A – Not available.

Sources: Association des Constructeurs Europeens de Motocycles, Brussels; Industrieverband Motorrad Deutschland e.V.

comfort. Comfortable saddles, upright riding positions, and other features found on touring bikes were especially welcomed by those who took cross-country or other long-distance journeys on their motorcycles. Custom and touring motorcycles were less popular outside of the United States since cyclists in other countries were more likely to travel only short distances and did not necessarily identify with the individualist or outlaw image associated with heavyweights in the United States. The largest segment of the heavyweight motorcycle category outside the United States was the performance bike category since most riders in other countries preferred sleek styling and were more interested in speed and handling rather than in comfort and tradition. In addition, motorcyclists in Europe and Asia tended to choose performance bikes over motorcycles in the custom and touring categories because of the high relative prices of such motorcycles. Exhibit 6 presents a regional comparison of motorcycle registrations by heavyweight category for 1998 through 2002.

Competition in the Global Motorcycle Industry

Rivalry in the motorcycle industry centered on performance, styling, breadth of product line, image and reputation, quality of after-the-sale service, and price. Most motorcycle manufacturers had good reputations for performance and styling with the greatest variance between brands occurring in pricing, variety of models, and quality of dealer service. Most cyclists preferred not to purchase specific brands, even if they were attracted to specific models, if the company's dealers did not have trained mechanics or had a reputation for shoddy workmanship or poor parts availability. There was also a great degree of price variability in the industry with comparable models of Japanese motorcycles typically carrying retail prices far below that of U.S.- or European-made motorcycles.

Exhibits 7 and 8 illustrate the difficulty U.S. and European manufacturers had experienced in attracting price-sensitive buyers in Europe. The Japanese producers were able to offer high-performance motorcycles at prices below those of Harley-Davidson, Ducati, Triumph, or Moto Guzzi. BMW had achieved considerable success in Europe, especially in Germany, because of exceptional performance and reputation, a strong dealer network, and regional loyalty to the brand.

Motorcycle manufacturers, like automobile manufacturers, maintained relationships with suppliers to produce or assemble components such as upholstery, tires, engine parts, brake parts, wiring harnesses, shocks, and rims. Almost without exception, the manufacturer designed and manufactured its engines and frames. Design and assembly of motorcycles took place in the manufacturers' home country, and completed motorcycles were exported to country markets where dealer networks had been established.

Consumers typically evaluated brands by talking to other cyclists, reading product reviews, perusing company Web sites, noting ads in print and other media, and noting a manufacturer's performance in competitive events. Typically, consumers had some

Exhibit 6   **Regional Comparison of the 651+cc Motorcycle Market by Segment,* 1998–2002 (percent of units registered)**

	1998	1999	2000	2001	2002
United States					
Custom	58.4%	57.7%	56.6%	58.9%	60.3%
Touring	20.4	21.7	21.1	20.3	20.2
Performance	19.4	18.9	20.4	19.1	17.3
Standard	1.8	1.8	2.0	1.7	2.2
	100.0%	100.0%	100.0%	100.0%	100.0%
Europe					
Custom	22.8%	20.2%	17.6%	17.8%	13.8%
Touring	5.3	5.5	5.2	5.2	4.8
Performance	59.8	58	61.7	59.8	61.2
Standard	12.1	16.3	15.5	17.2	20.2
	100.0%	100.0%	100.0%	100.0%	100.0%
Asia-Pacific					
Custom	18.3%	28.6%	26.7%	23.9%	n/a
Touring	3.9	4.7	3.7	7.2	n/a
Performance	76.1	64.5	66.2	65.5	n/a
Standard	1.7	2.2	3.5	3.4	n/a
	100.0%	100.0%	100.0%	100.0%	n/a

*Category definitions:

Custom: Characterized by "American styling." Often personalized by accessorizing.

Touring: Designed primarily for long trips, with an emphasis on comfort, cargo capacity, and reliability. Often have features such as two-way radios (for communication with passenger), stereo, and cruise control.

Performance: Characterized by quick acceleration, top speed, and handling. Commonly referred to as "sport bikes."

Standard: A basic, no-frills motorcycle with an emphasis on low price.

Source: Harley-Davidson Inc. 2003 and 2002 10-K reports.

ability to negotiate prices with dealers, but most preferred to buy from dealers with good service departments, large parts inventories, and attractive financing programs. Similarly, strong motorcycle dealers preferred to represent manufacturers with good reputations and strong consumer demand, responsive customer service and parts delivery, formal training programs for service technicians, and financing divisions that offered competitive rates and programs.

Consumers purchased motorcycles for various reasons. Some individuals, especially in developing countries, were looking for low-cost transportation. Lightweight motorcycles, mopeds, and scooters were priced inexpensively compared to cars and used far

less gasoline. However, motorcycles provided no protection from the elements and were used only for fair-weather transportation by most riders who also owned a car. In the United States and Europe, most consumers who purchased a motorcycle also owned a car and preferred to travel by motorcycle on weekends or other times they were not working. Some in Europe did choose to commute to and from work on motorcycles when weather permitted because of limited parking available in large European cities and the high cost of fuel. Many motorcycle owners, particularly so in the United States, looked at riding as a form of recreation and had given up other sports or hobbies to spend time touring on motorcycles. Many middle-aged bikers in the United States had

Exhibit 7   **Market Shares of the Leading Sellers of Motorcycles in Germany, 2001–2003 (engine displacement of 125+cc)**

Brand	2001 Market Share	2002 Market Share	2003 Market Share
BMW	16.0%	18.1%	19.5%
Suzuki	21.7	20.3	19.2
Yamaha	16.3	16.0	15.9
Honda	16.8	17.3	15.5
Kawasaki	11.1	10.7	10.6
KTM	3.1	3.8	4.4
Harley-Davidson	3.6	3.7	4.2
Ducati	2.8	2.8	2.9
Triumph	2.5	1.8	2.0
Aprilia	1.7	1.5	1.4
Moto Guzzi	0.6	0.7	0.9
Buell	0.4	0.3	0.6
MV/Cagiva	1.2	0.8	0.6
MZ	0.5	0.4	0.3
Sachs	0.3	0.2	0.2
Other	1.4	1.6	1.9
Total	100.0%	100.0%	100.0%

Sources: Kraftfahrtbundesamt; Industrieverband Motorrad Deutschland e.V.

Exhibit 8   **Best-Selling Motorcycle Models in Germany, November 2003**

Rank	Brand	Model	Manufacturers' Recommended Price ($ US)	Year-to-Date 2003 Registrations	Heavyweight Classification
1	BMW	R 1150 GS	$14,500	6,242	Enduro/Touring
2	Suzuki	GSF 1200 (KL)	7,399	4,023	Performance
3	BMW	F 650 GS	8,190	3,524	Enduro/Touring
4	Suzuki	SV 650	6,299	3,444	Standard
5	Yamaha	FZS 600	6,499	3,294	Standard
6	Suzuki	GSF 600	6,299	3,182	Standard
7	Suzuki	GSX-R 1000	10,599	2,836	Performance
8	Kawasaki	Z1000	8,499	2,825	Performance
9	BMW	R 1150 RT	16,290	2,607	Touring
10	BMW	R 1150 R	9,990	2,539	Performance

Sources: Kraftfahrtbundesamt; Industrieverband Motorrad Deutschland e.V.

purchased motorcycles after giving up sports and activities requiring more athleticism or endurance.

REGULATION AND LEGAL CHALLENGES

The motorcycle industry was subject to laws and regulations in all countries where motorcycles were operated. The European Parliament and the European Council included motorcycles in their agreement to reduce exhaust gas values during their March 2002 meeting. The agreement required producers of motorcycles and scooters to reduce pollutants by 60 percent for all new cycles produced after April 2003. A further 60 percent reduction would be required for motorcycles produced after January 2006. Demand for motorcycles in Europe was impacted to a great degree by the implementation of the euro in 2002; prices of motorcycles increased substantially in some countries when the currency exchange took effect. For instance, because Germany's currency was much stronger than that of many other European Union countries, prices of most products and services increased in Germany after the change to the euro since the euro attempted to equalize the differences between currencies. The difficulty in obtaining a driver's license for motorcycles in some European countries also affected demand for motorcycles. German laws required separate automobile and motorcycle licenses for riders of motorcycles larger than 125cc, and France required those applying for motorcycle licenses to have first held an automobile license for two years. Austria's licensing laws were the most restrictive, requiring applicants to first hold an automobile license for five years and to complete six training sessions prior to obtaining a motorcycle license. Motorcycles that produced excessive noise were also under attack in most European countries.

In the United States, motorcycle producers were subject to certification by the Environmental Protection Agency (EPA) for compliance with emission and noise standards, as well as agencies in some states imposing more stringent noise and emission standards. The California Air Resources Board (CARB) had outlined new tailpipe emission standards that would go into effect in 2004 and 2008. The EPA developed new emission standards that would go into effect in 2006 and 2010 to match national standards with those in California. Motorcycle producers in the United States were also required to meet the product safety standards imposed by the National Highway Traffic Safety Administration (NHTSA).

Also in the United States, many motorcyclists found that their health insurance providers excluded coverage for any injuries sustained while on a motorcycle. The American Motorcyclists Association (AMA) had successfully petitioned the U.S. Senate to pass a bill in October 2003 that would prohibit insurance companies from denying coverage to someone hurt while riding a motorcycle, a snowmobile, or an all-terrain vehicle. Insurance companies had based their policies on NHTSA statistics that found motorcycling to be much more dangerous than traveling by car. While traffic fatalities per 100 million vehicle miles traveled hit a historic low in 2002, motorcycle fatalities had increased for a fifth consecutive year, to reach 3,244 deaths. There were 42,815 traffic fatalities in 2002 involving occupants of automobiles. Fatalities involving motorcyclists ages 50 and older increased by 26 percent during 2002—a higher rate of increase than any other age demographic. State legislatures in some states where helmets were optional had attempted to force motorcyclists who chose not to wear helmets to become mandatory organ donors. However, the AMA and its membership had successfully stopped all such attempts to pass mandatory organ donor laws.

HARLEY-DAVIDSON'S STRATEGY FOR COMPETING IN THE MOTORCYCLE INDUSTRY

Harley-Davidson was reincorporated in 1981 after it was purchased from AMF by 13 of its managers through a leveraged buyout (LBO). The management team's main focus at the time was to preserve jobs, but its members soon realized the company would need to be rebuilt from the ground up to survive. The company's market share in the United States had fallen to 3 percent, primarily because its products were unreliable and had poorer performance relative to less-expensive Japanese motorcycles. In addition, its network of dealers ran greasy, run-down shops that many people didn't feel comfortable visiting. Upon assessing the company's situation, the management team concluded that a strong allegiance to the Harley brand by many bikers was the company's only resource strength. However, when managers began to meet with customers, they found that long-time Harley riders felt cheated by the company and were angry about the lack of attention to product quality and customer service under AMF ownership. Some of the most loyal Harley riders refused to call models produced in the 1970s Harleys, preferring to label them as AMFs. After the LBO, Harley management tried to win over previous customers by attending any function at which motorcyclists congregated. The company's director of communications at the time commented in a 2003 interview with a trade publication, "At first we found that our customers didn't like us, and they didn't trust us."[6] However, the distrust subsided when Harley owners saw their suggestions being implemented by the company.

Harley-Davidson's turnaround strategy including improving product quality by adopting Japanese management practices, abandoning a reliance on advertising in favor of promotions at motorcycle rallies, and improving its dealer network to broaden its appeal to new customers. After hearing complaints about dealers from Harley riders at rallies and other bike events, Harley-Davidson conducted a pilot program with two dealers in Milwaukee that called for the dealers to build clean, attractive stores to showcase the company's improved motorcycles and display apparel and other merchandise that cyclists might wish to purchase. The two dealerships recaptured their investments within 18 months, while other dealers struggled. The pilot program led to new or remodeled dealerships across the Harley-Davidson network and helped the company enter into a new product category. Harley showrooms offered a large assortment of clothing items and accessories—for example, leather jackets, T-shirts, helmets, and boots—in addition to new motorcycles. In 2003 Harley-Davidson introduced 1,200 new clothing items and licensed its name to more than 100 manufacturers making everything from Harley-Davidson Edition Ford F-150 pickups to Harley Barbie dolls. Apparel and accessories were so important

to the company and its dealers that in 2003 every dealer had a fitting room.

Cultivating Loyalty Through HOG Membership

After Harley-Davidson's product quality issues had been resolved, the company focused on cultivating the mystique of Harley ownership. The company formed Harley Owners Groups (HOGs) in 1983 to provide Harley owners with local chapters through which they could socialize and ride with other owners. Harley-Davidson established HOGs in cities where dealers were located, but did not interfere with HOG operations or try to use the organization in a self-serving way. The company's primary interest in setting up the chapters was to give motorcycle buyers a sense of community. Management understood that once new owners came to feel they belonged to the Harley community, they would bring new buyers to the company without any encouragement from Harley-Davidson.

The company provided each new Harley buyer with a free membership to a HOG where they could not only meet other area bikers but also learn the ins and outs of the biker world. HOGs also organized rides, raised money for charities, and participated in nationwide HOG events. Owners were required to renew their free memberships each year to ensure that only active participants would be on chapter roles. The HOG organization started with 33,000 members in 1983 and had grown to 793,000 members in 1,200 chapters in 2003. The company sponsored about 100 HOG rallies in 2003, with thousands of additional events organized by local chapters.

Harley's Image and Appeal with Baby Boomers

Even though Harley sold many motorcycles to construction workers, mechanics, and other blue-collar workers, Harley riders included a great many accountants, lawyers, bankers, and corporate executives. In 2003, Harley-Davidson's typical customer was a 46-year-old male earning $78,000 per year. The company had successfully added upscale consumers to its list of customers without alienating traditional bikers. Some of the more traditional bikers did complain about the new breed of "bean counter Harley owners," sometimes calling them "rubbers"—rich urban bikers. Such concern had been calmed to some degree by William G. Davidson's continuing involvement with the company. "Willie G." was the grandson of the company's cofounder and, as chief designer, had designed every motorcycle for the company since the 1960s. Willie G. was an "old-school" biker himself and rationalized the company's alliance with upscale baby boomers with comments such as "There's a lot of beaners, but they're out on the motorcycles, which is a beautiful thing."[7]

Part of the appeal of HOG membership was that new motorcyclists could experience freedom of the open road, much like a Hells Angel might, if only during occasional weekends when the weather was nice. Some middle-aged professionals purchased Harleys because riding was an opportunity to recreate and relax without being reminded of their daily responsibilities. Belonging to a HOG or other riding group was different from joining a country club or other club dominated by upper-income families; as the CEO of a Fortune 500 company explained, "Nobody cares what anybody else does. We share a common bond of freedom on a bike." This same Harley owner claimed that after a few hours of riding, he forgets he's a CEO.[8] Another affluent Harley owner suggested that Harley owners from all walks of life shared the brotherhood of the open road: "It doesn't matter if you make $10,000 a year or $300,000."[9] Others suggested that Harley ownership gave you an identity and provided you with a close group of friends in an increasingly anonymous culture.

However, other Harley owners were lured by the appeal of Harley-Davidson's outlaw image. The editor of *AARP Magazine* believed that baby boomers purchased Harleys because of a desire to feel "forever young."[10] The *AARP Magazine* editor said that riding a Harley helped take boomers back to a time when they had less responsibility. "You saw 'Easy Rider.' As a kid, you had a bit of a wild period in the '70s and you associate the motorcycle with that. But you got married. You had kids and a career. Now you can afford this. It's a safe way to live out a midlife crisis. It's a lot safer than running off with a stewardess."[11] In fact, many of Harley-Davidson's competitors have claimed that Harley sells lifestyles, not motorcycles. Harley-Davidson CEO Jeffrey Bleustein commented on the appeal of the company's motorcycles by stating, "Harley-Davidson stands for freedom, adventure, individual expression and being a little on the edge, a little bit naughty. People are drawn to the brand for those reasons."[12]

The desire to pose as a Hells Angel, Peter Fonda's Wyatt character, or Brando's Johnny helped Harley-Davidson sell more than 290,000 motorcycles and over $200 million in general merchandise in 2003. Many of Harley-Davidson's 1,400 dealers dedicated as much as 75 percent of their floor space to apparel and accessories, with most suggesting that between 25 and 40 percent of their annual earnings came from the sale of leather jackets, chaps, boots, caps, helmets, and other accessories. One dealer offered her opinion of what drove merchandise sales by commenting, "Today's consumer tends to be a little more affluent, and they want the total look."[13] The dealer also said that approximately 5 percent of the dealership's apparel sales were to non–bike owners who wanted the biker image. Even though some high-income baby boomers wanted to be mistaken from a distance for Hells Angels' "1 percenters"—the most rebellious 1 percent of the population—for most it was all show. When looking out at the thousands of leather-clad bikers attending Harley-Davidson's 2003 Memorial Day centennial celebration in Milwaukee, a Harley owner said, "The truth is, this is mostly professional people . . . People want to create an image. Everybody has an alter side, an alter ego. And this is a chance to have that."[14]

Another Harley owner who had ridden his Heritage Softail from his home in Sioux Falls, South Dakota, to attend the centennial event commented on his expectations for revelry during the four-day celebration by pointing out, "Bikers like to party pretty big. It's still a long way to go before you forget the image of the Hells Angels."[15] However, weekend bikers were quite different from the image they emulated. The Hells Angels continued to be linked to organized crime into 2003, with nine Hells Angels members being convicted in September 2003 of drug trafficking and murdering at least 160 people, most of whom were from rival gangs.[16] Similarly, Hells Angels organizations in Europe had been linked to drug trafficking and dozens of murders.[17] Fifty-seven Angels in the United States were arrested in December 2003 for crimes such as theft of motorcycles, narcotics trafficking, and firearms and explosives trafficking following a two-year investigation of the motorcycle club by the Bureau of Alcohol, Tobacco, Firearms and Explosives.[18]

Harley-Davidson balanced its need to promote freedom and rebellion against its need to distance the company from criminal behavior. Its Web site pointed out that "the vast majority of riders throughout the history of Harley-Davidson were law-abiding citizens," and the company archivist proposed, "Even those who felt a certain alienation from society were not lawless anarchists, but people who saw the motorcycle as a way to express both their freedom and their identity."[19] When looking at the rows of Harleys glistening in the sun in front of his Southern California roadside café, the longtime proprietor of one of the biggest biker shrines in the United States commented, "There used to be some mean bastards on those bikes. I guess the world has changed."[20] A Harley-Davidson dealer commented that dealers considered hardcore bikers "1 percenters" because they made up less than 1 percent of a dealer's annual sales. The dealer found that very affluent buyers made up about 10 percent of sales, with the remainder of customers making between $40,000 and $100,000 per year.[21]

Harley-Davidson's Product Line

Unlike Honda and Yamaha, Harley-Davidson did not produce scooters and mopeds, nor did it manufacture motorcycles with engine displacements less than 651cc. In addition, Harley Davidson did not produce dirt bikes or performance bikes like those offered by Kawasaki and Suzuki. Of the world's major motorcycle producers, BMW produced bikes that most closely resembled Harley-Davidson's traditional line, although BMW also offered a large number of performance bikes. In 2004, Harley-Davidson's touring and custom motorcycles were grouped into five families: Sportster, Dyna Glide, Softail, Touring, and the VRSC V-Rod. The Sportster, Dyna Glide, and VRSC models were manufactured in the company's Kansas City, Missouri, plant, while Softail and Touring models were manufactured in York, Pennsylvania. Harley-Davidson considered the Sportster, Dyna Glide, and VRSC models custom bikes, while Softails and Touring models fell into the Touring industry classification. Sportsters and Dyna Glides each came in four model variations, while Softails came in six variations and Touring bikes came in seven basic configurations. The VRSC V-Rod came in two basic styles. Harley-Davidson produced three models of its Buell performance bikes in its East Troy, Wisconsin, plant. In 2004, Harley Sportsters carried retail prices ranging from $6,495 to $8,675; Dyna Glide models sold at price points between $11,995 and $16,580; VRSC V-Rods sold between $16,895 and $17,995; Softails were offered between $13,675 and $17,580; and the Road King and Electra Glide touring models sold at prices between $16,995 and $20,405. Consumers could also order custom Harleys through the company's Custom Vehicle Operations (CVO) unit, started in 1999. Customization and accessories on CVO models could add as much as $10,000 to the retail price of Harley-Davidson motorcycles. Images of Harley-Davidson's five product families and CVO models can be viewed at www.harley-davidson.com.

Honda, Kawasaki, Suzuki, and Yamaha had all introduced touring models that were very close replicas of Harley Sportsters, Dyna Glides, Road Kings, and Electra Glides. The Japanese producers had even copied Harley's signature V-twin engine and had tuned their dual-crankpin designs in an attempt to copy the distinctive sound of a Harley-Davidson engine. However, even with prices up to 50 percent less on comparable models, none of the Japanese producers had been able to capture substantial market share from Harley-Davidson in the United States or in their home markets. (Refer back to Exhibit 4 for a breakdown of market shares in the heavyweight segment in the U.S., European, and Asia-Pacific regions.) Indian Motorcycle Corporation had experienced similar difficulties gaining adequate market share in the U.S. heavyweight segment and ceased its operations for a second time in September 2003.

Harley-Davidson's difficulties in luring buyers in the performance segment of the industry were similar to challenges that Japanese motorcycle producers had encountered in their attempts to gain market share in the custom and touring categories of the U.S. heavyweight motorcycle segment. Harley-Davidson had co-developed and later purchased Buell to have a product that might appeal to motorcyclists in the United States who were in their 20s and did not identify with the *Easy Rider* or Hells Angels images or who did not find Harley-Davidson's traditional styling appealing. Harley management also believed that Buell's performance street-racer-style bikes could help it gain market share in Europe, where performance bikes were highly popular. The Buell brand competed exclusively in the performance category against models offered by Honda, Yamaha, Kawasaki, Suzuki, and lesser-known European brands such as Moto Guzzi, Ducati, and Triumph. Buell prices began at $4,595 for its Blast model to better compete with Japanese motorcycles on price as well as on performance and styling. Buell's Lighting and Firebolt models were larger, faster motorcycles and retailed for between $9,000 and $11,000. The VSRC V-Rod, with its liquid-cooled, Porsche-designed engine, was also designed to appeal to buyers in the performance segment of the industry, both in the United States and Europe.

As of 2004, Harley-Davidson had not gained a significant share of the performance motorcycle segment in the United States or Europe. Some industry analysts criticized Harley-Davidson's dealers for the lackluster sales of V-Rod and Buell models since most dealers did little to develop employees' sales techniques. Demand for Harleys had exceeded supply since the early 1990s, and most dealers' sales activities were limited to taking orders and maintaining a waiting list. In addition, most Harley-Davidson dealers had been able to charge $2,000 to $4,000 over the suggested retail price for new Harley-Davidson motorcycles, although most dealers had begun to sell Harleys at sticker price in 2003. Harley-Davidson's revenues by product group are shown below:

Harley-Davidson Revenues by Product Group (in millions)

	2003	2002	2001
Harley-Davidson motorcycles	$3,621.5	$3,161.0	$2,671.3
Buell motorcycles	76.1	66.9	61.7
Total motorcycles	$3,697.6	$3,227.9	$2,733.0
Motorcycle Parts and Accessories	712.8	629.2	509.6
General Merchandise	211.4	231.5	163.9
Other	2.5	2.4	0.3
Net revenue	$4,624.3	$4,091.0	$3,406.8

Source: Harley-Davidson Inc. 2002 and 2003 annual reports.

The number of Harley-Davidson and Buell motorcycles shipped annually between 1998 and 2003 is presented in Exhibit 9.

Distribution and Sales in North America, Europe, and Asia-Pacific

Harley-Davidson's dealers were responsible for operating showrooms where motorcycles could be examined and test-ridden, stocking parts and accessories that existing owners might need, operating service departments, and selling biking merchandise such as apparel, boots, helmets, and various Harley-Davidson-branded gift items. Some Harley owners felt such strong connections to the brand that they either gave or asked for Harley gifts for birthdays, weddings, and anniversaries. Some Harley owners had even been married at Harley-Davidson dealerships or at HOG rallies. Harley-Davidson dealers were also responsible for distributing newsletters and promoting rallies for local HOG chapters. The 10,000-member Buell Riders Adventure Group (BRAG) was also supported by Harley-Davidson dealers.

Harley mechanics and other dealership personnel were trained at the Harley-Davidson University (HDU) in Milwaukee, where they took courses in such subjects as retail management, inventory control, merchandising, customer service, diagnostics, maintenance, and engine service techniques. More than 17,000 dealership employees took courses at the company's university in 2002. Harley-Davidson also provided in-dealership courses through its Web-based distance learning program. In 2002, HDU held 665 instructor-led classes, 115 online classes, and had participation in their courses by 96 percent of the company's dealers.

The company also held demo rides in various locations throughout the United States, and many Harley dealers offered daily rentals designed to help novices decide whether they really wanted a motorcycle. Some dealers also rented motorcycles for longer periods to individuals who wished to take long-distance trips. Harley-Davidson motorcycles could

Exhibit 9   **Annual Shipments of Harley-Davidson and Buell Motorcycles, 1998–2003**

	2003	2002	2001	2000	1999	1998
Harley-Davidson						
Sportster	57,165	51,171	50,814	46,213	41,870	33,892
Custom*	151,405	141,769	118,303	100,875	87,806	77,434
Touring	82,577	70,713	65,344	57,504	47,511	39,492
	291,147	263,653	234,461	204,592	177,187	150,818
Domestic	237,656	212,833	186,915	158,817	135,614	110,902
International	53,491	50,820	47,546	45,775	41,573	39,916
	291,147	263,653	234,461	204,592	177,187	150,818
Buell						
Buell (exc. Blast)	8,784	6,887	6,436	5,043	7,767	6,334
Buell Blast	1,190	4,056	3,489	5,416	—	—
	9,974	10,943	9,925	10,189	7,767	6,334

*Custom includes Softail, Dyna Glide, and VRSC.

Source: Harley-Davidson Inc. 2002 and 2003 annual reports.

also be rented from third parties like EagleRider—the world's largest renter of Harleys, with 29 locations in the United States and Europe. Harley-Davidson's Riders Edge motorcycle training courses were also offered by quite a few dealers in North America, Europe, and Asia-Pacific. The company had found that inexperienced riders and women were much more likely to purchase motorcycles after taking a training course. Harley-Davidson management believed the 25-hour Riders Edge program had contributed to the company's increased sales to women, which had increased from 2 percent of total sales prior to the adoption of the program to 9 percent in 2003.

In 2003, Harley-Davidson motorcycles were sold by 644 independently owned and operated dealerships across the United States. Buell motorcycles were also sold by 436 of these dealers. There were no Buell-only dealerships, and 81 percent of Harley dealers in the United States sold Harley-Davidson motorcycles exclusively. The company also sold apparel and merchandise in about 50 nontraditional retail locations such as malls, airports, and tourist locations. The company's apparel was also available seasonally in about 20 temporary locations in the United States where there was significant tourist traffic. The company also had three nontraditional merchandise outlets in Canada, where it had 76 independent dealers and one Buell

dealership. Thirty-two of its Canadian Harley dealers also sold Buell motorcycles.

Harley-Davidson had 161 independent dealers in Japan, 50 dealers and three distributors in the Australia/New Zealand market and seven other dealers scattered in smaller East and Southeast Asian markets. Only 73 of Harley Davidson's Asia-Pacific also sold Buell motorcycles. The company also had two dealers that sold Buell but not Harley-Davidson motorcycles. Harley-Davidson motorcycles were sold in 17 Latin American countries by 32 dealerships. The company did not have a dealer for its Buell motorcycles in Latin America, but had 13 retail stores carrying only apparel and merchandise in the region.

The company's European distribution division based in the United Kingdom served 32 countries in Europe, the Middle East, and Africa. The European region had 436 independent dealers, with 313 choosing to also carry Buell motorcycles. Buell motorcycles were also sold in Europe by 10 dealers that were not Harley dealers. Harley-Davidson also had 26 nontraditional merchandise retail locations in Europe.

Exhibit 10 presents the company's revenues by geographic region, along with the division of assets in the United States and abroad and a breakdown of financial services revenues by region. The company's financial services unit provided retail financing

Exhibit 10   **Harley-Davidson's Net Revenues and Long-Lived Assets
by Business Group and Geographic Region, 2000–2003**

	2003	2002	2001	2000
Motorcycles net revenue				
United States	$3,807,707	$3,416,432	$2,809,763	$2,357,972
Europe	419,052	337,463	301,729	285,372
Japan	173,547	143,298	141,181	148,684
Canada	134,319	121,257	96,928	93,352
Other foreign countries	89,649	72,520	57,185	57,966
	$4,624,274	$4,090,970	$3,406,786	$2,943,346
Financial services income				
United States	$ 260,551	$ 199,380	$ 172,593	$ 132,684
Europe	8,834	4,524	1,214	655
Canada	10,074	7,596	7,738	6,796
	$ 279,459	$ 211,500	$ 181,545	$ 140,135
Long-lived assets				
United States	$1,400,772	$1,151,702	$1,021,946	$ 856,746
Other foreign countries	41,804	36,138	33,234	27,844
	$1,442,576	$1,187,840	$1,055,180	$ 884,590

Source: Harley-Davidson Inc. 2002 and 2003 10-K reports.

to consumers and wholesale financial services to dealers, including inventory floor plans, real estate loans, computer loans, and showroom remodeling loans.

CHALLENGES CONFRONTING HARLEY-DAVIDSON AS IT ENTERED ITS SECOND CENTURY

As Harley-Davidson entered its second century in 2004, the company not only celebrated a successful centennial celebration that brought more than 700,000 of Harley's most loyal customers to Milwaukee but also a successful year with record shipments, revenues, and earnings. New capacity had allowed the company's shipments to increase to more than 290,000 units, which drove annual revenues to $4.6 billion and net earnings to nearly $761 million. The company's planned 350,000-square-foot expansion of its York, Pennsylvania, plant would allow the

company to increase production to 400,000 units by 2007. However, there was some concern that the company might not need the additional capacity.

Some market analysts had begun to believe Harley-Davidson's stock was approaching its apex because of the aging of its primary baby boomer customer group. Between 1993 and 2003, the average age of the company's customers had increased from 38 to 46. The average age of purchasers of other brands of motorcycles in 2003 was 38. Some analysts suspected, that within the next 5 to 10 years, fewer baby boomers would be interested in riding motorcycles and Harley's sales might begin to decline. Generation X buyers were not a large enough group to keep Harley's sales at the 2003 level, which would cause the company to rely on Generation Y (or echo boomer) consumers. However, most Generation Y motorcyclists had little interest in the company's motorcycles and did not identify with the *Easy Rider* or outlaw biker images that were said to appeal to baby boomers. The company's V-Rod motorcycle had won numerous awards for its styling and performance, but its $17,000-plus price tag kept most 20-year-olds away from Harley showrooms. Similarly, Buell motorcycles were critically acclaimed in terms of performance and styling but had been unable to draw performance-minded consumers in the United States or Europe away from Japanese street-racing-style bikes to any significant degree.

Europe was the largest market for motorcycles overall, and the second largest market for heavyweight motorcycles, but Harley-Davidson had struggled in building share in the region. In some ways the company's 6+ percent market share in Europe was impressive since only 4.8 percent of motorcycles purchased in 2002 were touring cycles and custom cycles accounted for only 13.8 percent of motorcycles sold in Europe during 2002. The V-Rod's greatest success was in Europe, but neither the V-Rod nor any other HD model had become one of the top-10 best-selling models in any major European market.

There was also some concern that Harley-Davidson's 14-month production run had caused an unfavorable short-term production problem since the company's waiting list, which required a two-year wait in the late 1990s, had fallen to about 90 days beginning in mid-2003. The overavailability of 2003 models had caused Harley-Davidson's management to adopt a 0 percent down payment financing program that began at midyear 2003 and would run through February 2004. When asked about the program during a television interview, Harley-Davidson CEO Jeffery Bleustein justified it by noting, "It's not zero percent financing, as many people understood it to be, its zero dollars down, and normal financing. The idea there was to get the attention of some of the people who aren't riding Harleys and are used to a world of other motorcycles where there's always a financing program of some sort going on. We just wanted to get their attention."[22] By year-end 2003, dealer inventories had declined to about 2,000 units and many dealers again began charging premiums over list price, but not the $2,000–$4,000 premiums charged in prior years.

Endnotes

[1]As quoted in "Analyst Says Harley's Success Had Been to Drive into Buyers' Hearts," *Canadian Press Newswire,* July 14, 2003.

[2]As quoted In January 21, 2004, press release.

[3]As quoted in "Wings of Desire," *The Independent,* August 27, 2003.

[4]As quoted in "Born to Raise Hell," *BBC News Online,* August 14, 2000.

[5]"Wheel Life Experiences," *Whole Pop Magazine Online.*

[6]As quoted in "Will Your Customers Tattoo Your Logo?" *Trailer/Body Builders,* March 1, 2003, p. 5.

[7]As quoted in "Will Harley-Davidson Hit the Wall?" *Fortune,* July 22, 2002.

[8]As quoted in "Even Corporate CEOs Buy Into the Harley-Davidson Mystique, *Milwaukee Journal-Sentinel,* August 24, 2003.

[9]As quoted in "Harley-Davidson Goes Highbrow at Annual Columbia, S.C., H.O.G. Rally," *The State,* September 26, 2003.

[10]As quoted in "Even Corporate CEOs."

[11]Ibid.

[12]As quoted in "Milwaukee-Based Harley-Davidson Rides into Future with Baby Boomers Aboard," *The News-Sentinel,* August 5, 2003.

[13]As quoted in "Harley-Davidson Fans Sport Motorcycle Style," *Detroit Free Press,* August 28, 2003.

[14]As quoted in "Bikers Go Mainstream 100 Years On," *Global News Wire,* September 11, 2003.

[15]Ibid.

[16]"Nine Montreal Hells Angels Sentenced to 10 to 15 Years in Prison," *CNEWS,* September 23, 2003.

[17]"Hells Angels: Easy Riders or Criminal Gang?," *BBC News,* January 2, 2004.

[18]"Feds Raid Hells Angels' Clubhouses," *CBSNews.com,* December 4, 2003.

[19]As quoted in "Wings of Desire," *Global News Wire,* August 27, 2003.

[20]Ibid.

[21]Interview with Mobile, Alabama, Harley-Davidson dealership personnel.

[22]As quoted in a CNNfn interview conducted on *The Money Gang,* June 11, 2003.

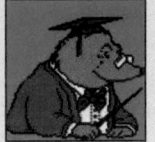

adidas: Will Restructuring Its Business Lineup Allow It to Catch Nike?

John E. Gamble
University of South Alabama

Adidas's 1998 acquisition of diversified sporting goods producer Salomon was expected to allow the athletic footwear company to vault over Nike to become the leader of the global sporting goods industry. Salomon had several businesses that adidas's management viewed as attractive—its Salomon ski division was the leading producer of ski equipment; TaylorMade Golf was the second-largest seller of golf equipment; and Mavic was the leading producer of high-performance bicycle wheels and rims. Other Salomon businesses included Bonfire snowboard apparel and Cliché skateboard equipment. Adidas had been the best-selling brand of sporting goods throughout the 1960s and 1970s, but Nike had overtaken adidas as leader of the athletic footwear industry in the late 1980s and had grown to three times the size of adidas by 1997.

Almost as soon as the deal was consummated, it looked doubtful that the €1.5 billion acquisition of Salomon would boost the corporation's performance. Chief concerns with the acquisition were the declining attractiveness of the winter sports industry and integration problems between the adidas footwear and apparel business and Salomon's business units. Not until 2003, five years after the acquisition, had adidas's earnings per share returned to the level that shareholders enjoyed in 1997. In addition, the company's stock price failed to return to its 1998 trading range until 2004. The Salomon winter sports business had contributed very little operating profit to the company's overall financial performance since its acquisition and the TaylorMade-adidas Golf

division had struggled at various times to deliver good earnings. However, TaylorMade seemed to have turned the corner in 2005, with sales and operating earnings improving by 12 percent and 185 percent, respectively, during the first six months of 2005. Salomon's operating loss of €54 million during the first six months of 2005 was 7 percent greater than its €50 million loss during the same period in 2004.

The company announced near the end of its second quarter 2005 that it would divest its winter sports brands and Mavic bicycle components business before the end of the year. In May 2005, Amer Sports Corporation, the maker of Atomic skis and Wilson sporting goods, agreed to acquire the winter sports and bicycle wheel businesses for €485 million. Adidas's October 2005 announcement that it would acquire Reebok International Ltd. for €3.1 billion ($3.8 billion) was the final component of a restructuring initiative that would focus the company's business lineup primarily on athletic footwear and apparel and golf equipment by 2006. Reebok also designed, marketed, and sold Rockport footwear, Ralph Lauren footwear, Greg Norman apparel, and CCM, Koho, and Jofa hockey equipment. In 2004, Rockport and Reebok's hockey brands contributed $377.6 million and $146.0 million, respectively, to the company's total sales of $3.8 billion. Reebok did not disclose the sales contributions of its Ralph Lauren or Greg Norman product lines. The acquisition would increase adidas's annual revenues to nearly €9 billion ($11 billion) and give the company a much stronger presence in North America, which accounted for 50 percent of the global

Exhibit 1   **Net Sales by Product Type and Geographic Region for Reebok International, 2002–2004**

	2004	2003	2002
Reebok International's net sales by product type			
Footwear	$2,430,311	$2,226,712	$2,060,725
Apparel	1,354,973	1,258,604	1,067,147
	$3,785,284	$3,485,316	$3,127,872
Reebok International's net sales by geographic region			
United States	$2,069,055	$2,021,396	$1,807,657
United Kingdom	474,704	444,693	416,775
Europe	810,418	692,400	607,381
Other countries	431,107	326,827	296,059
	$3,785,284	$3,485,316	$3,127,872

Source: Reebok International Ltd. 2004 10-K report.

sporting goods market. In addition, the new mix of businesses would draw adidas closer to overtaking Nike, which had 2004 revenues of $13.7 billion. Reebok's sales by product line and geographic region for 2002 through 2004 are presented in Exhibit 1.

COMPANY HISTORY

In 1920, a 20-year-old German baker-by-trade named Adolph Dassler began making simple canvas shoes in the rear of his family's small bakery in the North Bavarian town of Herzogenaurach. Dassler, a sports enthusiast, had little interest in working as a baker and wanted to make shoes for athletes competing in soccer, tennis, and track-and-field events. Adolph (nicknamed Adi) Dassler thought that proper footwear might improve an athlete's performance and began to study ways to improve athletic shoe design to give athletes wearing his shoes an edge in competitive events.

In 1924, Adi Dassler's brother, Rudolph, joined him in shoemaking to establish Gebrüder Dassler Schuhfabrik (Dassler Brothers Shoe Factory)—a new company specializing in innovative sports shoes. The two brothers realized that athletes should have shoes designed specifically for their respective sport and developed a variety of styles. In 1925, the Dasslers made their first major innovation in athletic shoe design when they integrated studs and spikes into the soles of track-and-field shoes. The Dassler brothers also developed other key innovations in footwear such as the arch support. Many of the standard features of today's athletic footwear were developed by Dassler brothers, with Adi Dassler alone accumulating 700 patents and property rights worldwide by the time of his death in 1978.

The Dasslers were also innovators in the field of marketing—giving away their shoes to German athletes competing in the 1928 Olympic Games in Amsterdam. By the 1936 Olympic Games in Berlin, most athletes would compete only in Gebrüder Dassler shoes, including Jesse Owens, who won four gold medals in the Berlin games. By 1937, Dassler was making 30 different styles of shoes for athletes in 11 sports. All of the company's styles were distinguished from other brands by two stripes applied to each side of the shoe.

The Dasslers' sports shoe production ceased during World War II when Gebrüder Dassler Schuhfabrik was directed to produce boots for the armed forces of Nazi Germany. Adi Dassler was allowed to remain in Herzogenaurach to run the factory, but Rudolph (or Rudi) Dassler was drafted into the army and spent a year in an Allied prisoner-of-war camp after being captured. Upon the conclusion of the war, Rudi Dassler was released by the Allies and returned to Herzogenaurach to rejoin his family. The Dasslers returned to production of athletic shoes in 1947, but the company was dissolved in 1948 after the two brothers entered into a bitter feud. Rudi Dassler moved to the other side of the small village to establish his own shoe company, Puma Schuhfabrik Rudolph Dassler. With the departure of Rudi Dassler, Adi renamed the company adidas—a combination of the first three letters of his nickname and the first three letters of his last name. Adi Dassler also applied an additional stripe to the sides of adidas shoes and registered the three-stripe trademark in 1949.

The nature of the disagreement between the Dassler brothers was not known for certain, but the two never spoke again after their split and the feud became the foundation of both organizations' cultures while the two brothers were alive. The two rival companies were highly competitive, and both discouraged employees from fraternizing with cross-town rivals. An adidas spokesperson described the seriousness of the feud by stating, "Puma employees wouldn't be caught dead with adidas employees," and continuing, "It wouldn't be allowed that an adidas employee would fall in love with a Puma employee."[1]

Adi Dassler kept up his string of innovations with molded rubber cleats in 1949 and track shoes with screw-in spikes in 1952. He expanded the concept to soccer shoes in 1954 with screw-in studs, an innovation that has been partially credited for Germany's World Cup Championship that year. By 1960, adidas was the clear favorite among athletic footwear brands, with 75 percent of all track-and-field athletes competing in the Olympic Games in Rome wearing adidas shoes. The company began producing soccer balls in 1963 and athletic apparel in 1967. The company's dominance in the athletic footwear industry continued through the early 1970s with 1,164 of the 1,490 athletes competing in the 1972 Olympic Games in Munich wearing adidas shoes. In addition, as jogging became popular in the United States during in the early 1970s, adidas was the leading brand of consumer jogging shoe in the United States. Also, T-shirts and other apparel bearing adidas's three-lobed trefoil logo were popular wardrobe items for U.S. teenagers during the 1970s.

At the time of Adi Dassler's death in 1978, adidas remained the worldwide leader in athletic footwear, but the company was rapidly losing market share in the United States to industry newcomer Nike. The first Nike shoes appeared in the 1972 U.S. Olympic Trials in Eugene, Oregon, and had become the best-selling training shoe in the United States by 1974. Both Adi Dassler and his son, Horst, who took over as adidas's chief manager after Adi Dassler's death, severely underestimated the threat of Nike. With adidas perhaps more concerned with cross-town adversary Puma, Nike pulled ahead of its European rivals in the U.S. athletic footwear market by launching new styles in a variety of colors and by signing recognizable sports figures to endorsement contracts. Even though Nike was becoming the market leader in U.S. athletic footwear market, adidas was able to retain its number one ranking among competitive athletes, with 259 gold medal winners in the 1984 Olympic Summer Games in Los Angeles wearing adidas products. Only 65 Olympic athletes wore Nike shoes during the 1984 Summer Games, but the company signed up-and-coming NBA star Michael Jordan to a $2.5 million endorsement contract after adidas passed on the opportunity earlier in the year. At the time of Horst Dassler's unexpected death in 1987, Nike was the undisputed leader in the U.S. athletic footwear market, with more than $1 billion in annual sales.

Adidas's performance spiraled downward after the death of Horst Dassler, with no clear direction from the top and quality and innovation rapidly deteriorating. By 1990, adidas had fallen to a number eight ranking in the U.S. athletic footwear market and held only a 2 percent share of the market. A number of management and ownership changes occurred between Horst Dassler's death in 1987 and 1993, when a controlling interest in the company was acquired by a group of investors led by French advertising executive Robert Louis-Dreyfus. Louis-Dreyfus launched a dramatic turnaround of the company—cutting costs, improving styling, launching new models such as the Predator soccer shoe, and creating new promotional events like the adidas Predator Cup tournament for young soccer players in Germany. The turnaround was also aided by a trend among teenagers that repopularized 1970s styles and teens' preference for niche brands that weren't likely to be purchased by adults. At year-end 1994, adidas had increased its annual sales in the United States by 75 percent from the prior year and improved its market share enough to become the third largest seller of athletic footwear in the United States, trailing only Nike and Reebok.

The company's turnaround continued in 1995 with it going public and recording annual sales of nearly €1.8 billion. In 1996, adidas outfitted more than 6,000 athletes in the Olympic Games held in

Atlanta and supplied the Official Match Ball for the European Soccer Championship. Louis-Dreyfus's turnaround also included a push in 1997 to sign athletes such as Kobe Bryant, Anna Kournikova, and David Beckham to offset the appeal of Nike's Michael Jordan with athletic footwear and apparel consumers in the United States. The company's mid-1990s image revival was also aided when celebrities such as Madonna and Elle MacPherson appeared in magazines or on television wearing adidas shoes without any prompting from the company.

Even though the company's turnaround had produced outstanding results, with sales and earnings growing at annual rates of 38.3 percent and 37.5 percent, respectively, between 1995 and 1997, the company was a distant number three in the worldwide athletic footwear and apparel industry. Nike's 1997 revenues of $9.2 billion were nearly three times greater than those of adidas, and Nike continued to grow at a fast pace as it expanded into more international markets. In addition, Nike had begun to diversify outside of athletic footwear and apparel with the 1988 acquisition of Cole-Haan and the 1995 acquisition of Bauer hockey equipment. In 1997, it was rumored that Nike was eyeing French ski maker Skis Rossignol SA. (Nike did not acquire Rossignol, but it did acquire Converse basketball shoes and Hurley skateboard equipment in 2003 and Starter athletic apparel in 2004.) In late 1997, Louis-Dreyfus and the family owners of Salomon SA, a French sports equipment manufacturer, agreed to a €1.5 billion buyout that would diversify adidas beyond footwear and apparel and into ski equipment, golf clubs, bicycle components, and winter sports apparel. The acquisition would also give adidas a stronger sales platform in North America and Asia—two markets where adidas was still struggling.

THE SALOMON SA ACQUISITION

Adidas's €1.5 billion acquisition of Salomon allowed it to surpass Reebok to become the world's second-largest sporting goods company, with projected 1998 sales of nearly €5.1 billion. Nike remained the leader of the $90 billion global sporting goods industry, but the acquisition added the number one winter sports equipment producer, the second-largest golf equipment company, and the leading producer of performance bicycle wheels and rims to adidas's lineup of businesses. The acquisition was a move toward achieving CEO Robert Louis-Dreyfus's vision of building "the best portfolio of sports brands in the world."[2]

The price of adidas's shares fell upon the announcement of the acquisition over concerns about the price adidas agreed to pay for Salomon and how the company might finance the acquisition. There was also some concern among investors that adidas did not have expertise in manufacturing sports equipment since its apparel and footwear were produced by contract manufacturers. A Merrill Lynch analyst suggested that the Salomon acquisition might prove troublesome for adidas since other athletic shoe companies had "dabbled in the hard goods segment, but they have been unsuccessful to date in making inroads."[3]

Louis-Dreyfus used 100 percent debt financing to create adidas-Salomon but was not concerned with the merged company's ability to service the debt since adidas's annual free cash flow in 1997 was projected to be more than €200 million. Adidas's 1997 results (prior to the integration of Salomon) reached record levels, with the company's annual revenues increasing 42 percent from the prior year as a result of footwear sales growing by 32 percent and apparel sales increasing by 55 percent. Gains were recorded for all geographic regions, with North American sales increasing by 66 percent during 1997, sales in Europe increasing by 31 percent, and Asia-Pacific revenues growing by 38 percent between 1996 and 1997.

Louis-Dreyfus expected the new business units to boost adidas's pretax profits by 20–25 percent in 1998 and by an additional 20 percent in 1999. He believed 2000 would be the first year shareholders would see the full potential of the acquisition. However, Louis-Dreyfus's projections never materialized, with adidas taking control of Salomon just as the winter sports equipment and golf equipment industries were becoming less attractive. The poor performance of Salomon and TaylorMade in 1998 led to a net loss of $164 million for adidas-Salomon during the first nine months of its fiscal year. To make matters worse, the integration of Mavic, Salomon, Bonfire, Cliché, and TaylorMade were not going as smoothly as Louis-Dreyfus and adidas's shareholders had expected.

Adidas's core footwear and apparel business performed commendably during 1998 to contribute to a net profit of €205 million for the fiscal year. In early 1999, adidas-Salomon's management announced that synergies from the merger would amount to less than one-half of what was initially projected. By the summer of 1999, adidas-Salomon's share price had declined by more than a third from its early 1998 high, and most large investors believed that adidas had bitten off more than it could chew with the acquisition.[4] Robert Louis-Dreyfus announced in early 2000 that he would step down from adidas-Salomon and rejoin his family's business France in early 2001. Herbert Hainer, the company's head of marketing in Europe and Asia, was tapped as his replacement to run the diversified sporting goods company.

Under Hainer's leadership, the company cut costs, introduced new apparel and footwear products, increased the company's advertising, signed additional athletes to endorsement contracts, and supplied apparel, equipment, and footwear to more than 3,000 athletes competing in 26 sports during the 2000 Olympic Games in Sydney. Also, the company expanded into company-owned retail stores in 2001 with its first adidas Originals store opening in Berlin in September, followed by stores in Tokyo, Amsterdam, and Paris by year-end. In December 2001, Hainer added to the company's lineup of sports businesses with the acquisition of Arc'Teryx, the producer of technical winter sports apparel. Adidas-Salomon recorded sales of €6.1 billion in 2001 and ended the year as the top performer in the DAX 30. The performance of adidas-Salomon's common shares is presented in Exhibit 2.

ADIDAS-SALOMON'S CORPORATE STRATEGY IN EARLY 2005

In early 2005, adidas-Salomon's businesses were organized under three units based around the company's core brands—adidas, Salomon, and TaylorMade-adidas Golf. Innovation and excellence in strategy execution were common themes in all of adidas-Salomon's three business segments. The company expected its product design teams to develop at least one major product innovation per year in each product category. In 2004, TaylorMade Golf introduced its r7 Quad driver, which was a first-of-its-kind product that incorporated four movable weights. The movable weights allowed golfers to make adjustments to the club that could produce six different ball flight trajectories. TaylorMade extended the movable weight concept to irons and hybrid clubs in 2005. The adidas Sport Performance group introduced its Roteiro soccer ball, which was the industry's first thermal-bonded soccer ball. Also, the adidas Sport Performance group and the Salomon group collaborated to develop footwear featuring a Ground Control System that adjusted for uneven ground. Adidas T-MAC HUG laceless shoes and the adidas 1 were shoe innovations developed in 2004 and 2005. The $250-per-pair adidas 1 was the first running shoe with an embedded microprocessor. The microprocessor evaluated the runner's weight, the terrain, and speed to vary the compression in the heel of the shoe with the use of mechanical shock-absorbing components.

Adidas-Salomon also relied heavily on ongoing brand-building activities to further differentiate adidas, TaylorMade, and Salomon from competing brands of sporting goods. Partnerships with major sporting events around the world and with notable athletes competing in winter sports, track and field, soccer, basketball, tennis, and golf were critical to creating a distinctive image with consumers. The company also attempted to provide its retailers with superior customer service, including on-time deliveries, since the retailer was a crucial element of the sporting goods industry value chain. Efficient supply chain management and manufacturing efficiencies were also vital to the success of the company since poor product quality might discourage repeat sales to consumers. Even though the majority of adidas-Salomon products were produced by contract manufacturers, the company employed more than 100 quality control officers to monitor supplier standards.

Adidas-Salomon management expected visible improvements in operating margins each year and anticipated that the company would achieve an overall 10 percent operating profit margin in 2006. Increased profitability in Europe, strong top-line and bottom-line growth in Asia, and steady growth in North America were expected to deliver sought-after gains in operating profit margins. The company's chief managers believed that operational efficiency coupled with product innovation would allow it to

Exhibit 2   Performance of adidas-Salomon's Stock Price, 1999–2005

(a) Trend in adidas-Salomon's Common Stock Price

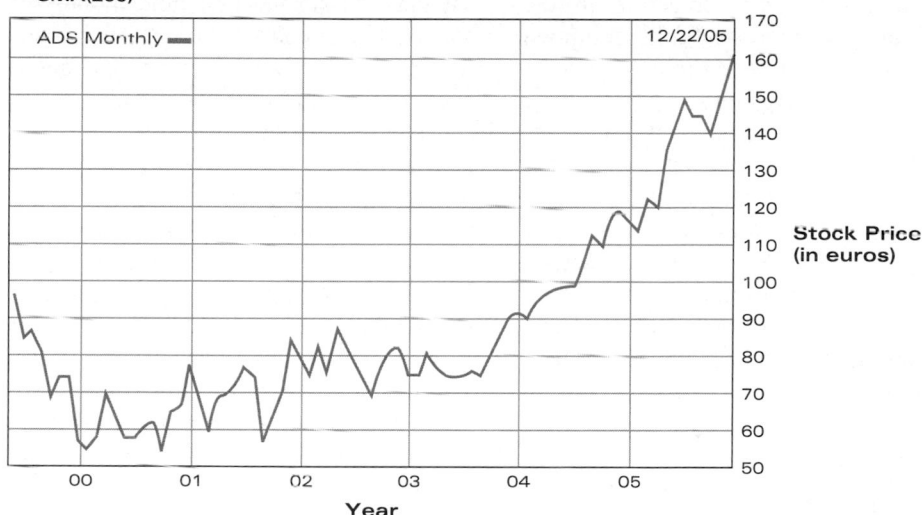

(b) Performance of adidas-Salomon's Stock Price versus the DAX 30 Index

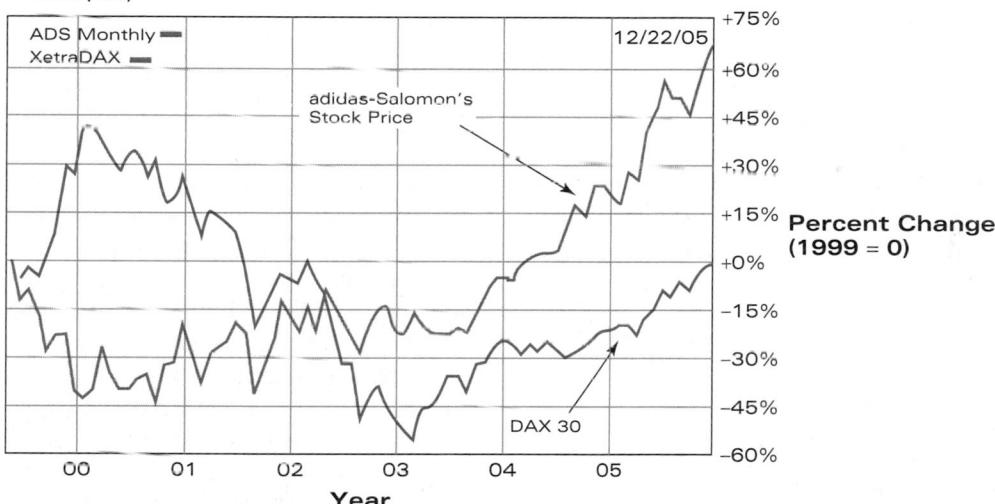

attain number one or number two positions in each sporting goods segment in which it competed.

Adidas Footwear and Apparel

Adidas footwear and apparel was organized under three categories based on the clothing needs of the consumer. The adidas Sport Performance group developed sports shoes and attire suitable for use by athletes in running, football and soccer, basketball, tennis, and general training. Adidas held number one or number two positions globally in these athletic

categories and maintained its advantage primarily through innovations like its ClimaCool 360-degree footwear ventilation system, its a³ energy management system, and endorsements by individual athletes or league sponsorships. Tim Duncan, Kevin Garnett, and Tracy McGrady were among the latest NBA athletes to endorse adidas footwear and apparel. In soccer, players such as David Beckham and Zinedine Zidane, and even entire clubs, endorsed adidas soccer shoes and clothing. Adidas was the official sponsor for the German national women's team and the UEFA European soccer league teams in Munich,

Amsterdam, Milan, and Madrid. Also, the adidas Roteiro was the Official Match Ball for all UEFA games. Adidas was also the official supplier to 18 National Olympic Committees competing in the 2004 Olympic Games in Athens and fully equipped athletes from 45 nations competing in 26 of the 28 disciplines included in the Olympics.

The company's Sport Heritage group was established in 2000 and designed new styles of shoes and apparel that were similar to the performance-oriented styles of the 1970s. Although athletes in the early 2000s would not compete in products based on 1970s technology, many teenagers and urban trend-followers liked the look of adidas's older products. Adidas limited distribution of its Sport Heritage products to avoid dilution of the brand.

As with Sport Heritage products, few purchasers of adidas Sport Style products were likely to wear such products while engaged in athletic endeavors. The Y-3 collection of sportswear, which was designed by Yohji Yamamoto, was based on athletic styles but would be only marginally suitable for sports. Most of the Y-3 line was best suited for consumers looking for trendy and comfortable casual wear with a mild sports influence. The line was launched in 2003, and adidas-Salomon management believed the division could eventually account for €100 million in sales. The company also believed that its Stella McCartney performance apparel line, David Beckham Sport Style line, and Mohammad Ali and Missy Elliott Heritage lines would prove successful.

North America   The North American market for sporting goods showed virtually no growth between 2000 and 2004 and was characterized by fierce competition among manufacturers and deep promotional discounting by retailers. All of adidas's brand-building efforts and product innovations were directed toward building on its number four ranking in North America, which was the company's weakest region in the $33 billion global athletic footwear market. In 2004, adidas held an 8.9 percent market share—behind Nike, with 36 percent market share; Reebok, with a 12.2 percent market share; and New Balance, with an approximate 11 percent market share.

In late 2004, adidas held a 55 percent market share in soccer shoes in the United States compared to Nike's 33 percent market share. However, in the overall U.S. cleated shoe segment, Nike led adidas by a 48 to 23 percent margin. Adidas was not a contender in the $3 billion basketball category, where Nike held a 70 percent market share. Adidas, Nike, and New Balance were all tied, with about 20 percent market share each in the tennis category. Nike, asics, New Balance, and Reebok all recorded gains in the running category during the first nine months of 2004, but analysts suggested that adidas missed out on growth in the category because its new technologies had not been a hit with consumers. Sales of casual sports shoes similar to those included in the adidas Heritage and adidas Sport Style lines were up 30 percent during the first nine months of 2004, but adidas did not make the list of top four brands in the category. The category was expected to grow by 40 percent in 2005 to displace running as the second-largest category of athletic shoes in the United States.

To achieve its revenue growth objectives of 10 percent annually in 2005 and 2006, adidas developed new styles and models offered in all three adidas segments, placed a strong emphasis on basketball, established marketing partnerships with college sports teams, major league soccer, and major league baseball teams, and improved retailer relations. Also, adidas expanded distribution to additional sporting goods stores, mall-based stores, department stores, urban distribution locations, and company-owned stores. Adidas also hoped to encourage retailers to create shop-within-a-shop merchandising sections and provide permanent wall space for adidas shoes. In 2004, Foot Locker agreed to give adidas's Kevin Garnett shoes permanent wall space in its best locations and feature the sub-brand in its television and print ads. Adidas also planned to expand distribution into additional urban retail stores that might not be a part of a large chain but were close to urban consumers. Adidas estimated the U.S. urban retail market for athletic footwear and apparel to be over $6 billion. Adidas also opened company-owned retail stores in Las Vegas, New York, Chicago, and San Francisco in 2005. Store openings in Portland, Boston, Washington, Philadelphia, Los Angeles, and Atlanta were planned for 2006.

Europe   Growth plans in Europe were focused on building on adidas's number one ranking in the region through its sponsorship of youth and professional soccer and continued support for running. The European athletic footwear and apparel market was growing at a modest rate, but retailers in Europe had relied even more on promotional pricing than retailers in North America. Prices for children's apparel had declined by 10 percent during 2004, and prices of adult apparel had decreased by 8.5 percent between 2003 and 2004. Adidas believed that its emphasis on product innovation and its strong brand loyalty would help protect the company from margin erosion due to price competition. Adidas also planned to increase its number of retailers in Europe by 25 percent between 2004 and 2006, with most new locations coming in emerging country markets. Adidas also intended to open additional company-owned stores in Europe during 2005 and 2006.

Asia   In 1999, adidas held a 6 percent market share in Japan, but its market share had grown to 18 percent in 2004 and its management expected a 20–24 percent market share in Japan by 2006. Adidas's increase in market share had come mainly at the expense of local brands such as asics and Mizuno. In 2004, Japan accounted for 50 percent of athletic apparel sales in Asia, but adidas and other consumer goods companies were directing considerable efforts to building brand awareness in China and other emerging Asian markets. The region's growth in gross domestic product was projected to be the highest in the world between 2005 and 2010, with much of the growth resulting from domestic-driven demand rather than exports. The size of the middle class in the region was also expected to grow dramatically in the region by 2010, with China's middle class growing from 60 million in 2002 to 160 million by 2010. Adidas's management estimated that every 1 percent increase in consumption by China's population translated into a $70 billion increase in sales of consumer goods. Adidas expected the 2008 Olympic Games in Beijing to generate interest in athletic footwear and apparel in China.

The company was rapidly adding retail stores to ensure that its products were available for purchase by China's growing consumer base. The company was adding more than 40 stores per month in urban locations in China since 55 percent of the country's population was expected to migrate from the countryside to cities by 2012. In 2004, adidas had more than 150 retail locations in only 1 province of China but expected to have more than 150 retail locations in 10 provinces by the 2008 Olympics. In 2004, adidas's revenues of more than €100 million made it the number two brand of athletic footwear and apparel in China. Nike was the leading seller of athletic goods in China. Adidas's management expected the company to double its sales in China by 2008.

Salomon

Like athletic footwear and apparel, the winter sports industry was mature, with the market declining by 3.1 percent during the 2003–2004 ski season. The 2003–2004 decline followed a 3.6 percent decline during the 2002–2003 season and a 1.8 percent decline in the 2001–2002 season. Some categories within the winter sports industry were declining at a more rapid pace, with the snowboard industry falling from €428.9 million in 2000–2001 to €344.5 million in 2003–2004. Nordic (cross-country) skiing was the only bright spot in the industry, with a 3.1 percent growth rate during the 2003–2004 ski season. The total value of worldwide winter sports equipment market in 2004 was €1.5 billion.

Revenue increases for most winter sporting goods producers had come from adding summer outdoor-inspired apparel and footwear to their product lines. Salomon was the number one producer of winter sports equipment, with a number one position in alpine (downhill) ski boots and high-end skis, a number two position in alpine skis overall and snowboard boots, and a number three position in snowboards. The company held an 80 percent market share in nordic (cross-country) ski systems. The Salomon business group also included Mavic, which was the number one brand of performance bicycle wheels and rims. The performance bicycle category was also mature, but growing a modest rate because of the popularity of road racing in the United States and Europe. Other businesses in the portfolio included Bonfire, a producer of snowboard apparel; Arc'Teryx, which produced technical winter sports apparel; and Cliché, a maker of skateboard equipment and apparel.

The businesses included in the Salomon division utilized competitive approaches similar to those of adidas-branded products. The division was committed to innovation in products in its snow, outdoor, and asphalt categories and attempted to benefit from synergies with the core adidas business when feasible. An example of such cross-division strategic fit was Salomon and adidas's collaboration on the development of the Ground Control System running shoe. Shoes using the design were marketed under both the adidas and Salomon brand names and were sold in different retail channels. The division also exploited adidas's apparel design expertise in its development of winter sports, cycling, and skateboard apparel. The collaboration between adidas and Salomon brands in apparel design had contributed to a 400 percent increase in soft goods sales for the division since 1995.

In 2004, sales for the Salomon group were nearly evenly split between winter sports hard goods and other products. The Salomon group was undertaking efforts to increase soft goods sales to 50 percent of the group's sales by expanding apparel lines, developing dedicated soft goods sales forces for each brand, and developing advertising targeting women since studies had shown that a large percentage of winter sports apparel purchases were made by women.

Improvement in operating margins was also a strategic priority at Salomon since top-line growth was limited. Since 2001, the division had shifted hardware production from France to Eastern Europe and Asia, developed a new production process in skis that lowered materials costs, reduced production time, and lowered labor costs per unit. In addition, Salomon had reduced total employment between 2002 and 2004 through early retirements and an increased number of temporary employees.

Even with Salomon management's efforts to improve operating margins for the division, there were some characteristics of the winter sports industry that precluded options that might be pursued in other industries. When asked by an investment banker why Salomon didn't shift all production to Asia, the head of Salomon, Christian Finell, responded, "The reason for this is that the main part of our business in winter sports is done in Europe. We believe it makes much more sense to have our production close to our customers. Also most of the relevant raw materials are found in Europe and not in Asia. And lead times are relatively long in this business. So by adding both the lead time and additional transportation costs it doesn't make sense to shift the production to Asia."[5]

TaylorMade-adidas Golf

TaylorMade Golf was the second largest producer of golf equipment in the $5.5 billion industry. The golf equipment industry had experience little growth since 1999 when golf's chief governing body in the United States began to ban golf clubs that it deemed performed too well. Golf equipment sales had grown dramatically during the mid- to late-1990s as golf equipment manufacturers like Callaway Golf Company, Titleist, Ping, and TaylorMade Golf introduced better-performing clubs that were more forgiving of recreational golfers' poor swing characteristics. Professional golfers using the technologically advanced equipment saw improvements in their games as well—particularly in driving distance. The United States Golf Association (USGA) began to believe that these new high-tech clubs provided a springlike effect and developed a coefficient of restitution (COR) limitation that would prevent any such effect

for golf equipment sold in the United States. Golf equipment manufacturers scoffed at the idea that clubs could produce a timed springlike or trampoline effect that could help propel the ball forward but were nevertheless obliged to discontinue research and development projects that would produce clubs exceeding a COR of 0.83.

By 2000, most golf club manufacturers had reached the 0.83 COR limitation and were compelled to find new approaches to innovation. In 2004, there was little differentiation among golf clubs until TaylorMade developed its r7 Quad driver. The driver was unique in that it allowed golfers to reposition movable weights screwed into the clubhead. The golfer could move the weights to provide a higher or lower launch angle and cause the flight path to pull to the left or fade to the right. The new innovation created 8 percent growth in driver sales for the year and made TaylorMade the number one producer of drivers and metalwoods. Prior to TaylorMade's introduction of the r7 Quad driver, Callaway Golf had held the number one position in the industry since 1991. The r7 lost its number one ranking in 2005 to Ping's G5 driver.

In 2005, the golf equipment industry had seemingly reached maturity as a sport, with the number of new participants each year barely exceeding the number who were giving up the sport. Asia's 2–3 percent annual growth in the number of new golfers made it the only geographic region to experience growth between 1999 and 2003. Poor economic conditions in the United States during 2000 caused many frequent golfers to scale back their participation levels that year, but the number of core golfers had rebounded in 2001 through 2004. However, the overall number of rounds played by golfers had declined until 2004, when the number of rounds played increased by nearly 7 percent. Exhibit 3 provides the retail value, number of units sold, and average selling price for various golf equipment categories for 1997 through 2004.

TaylorMade-adidas Golf management expected to increase sales primarily through market share gains since they had concluded that it would be unwise to count on growth of the game. TaylorMade believed it could increase market share through endorsement contracts with touring professionals on the Professional Golf Association (PGA) Tour and other professional tours and through new product innovations like the movable weight system used in its r7 driver. TaylorMade management also wished to

Exhibit 3 **Retail Value, Units Sold, and Average Selling Price of Golf Equipment in the United States, 1997–2004**

	Year	Retail Value	Units Sold	Average Selling Price
Metalwoods	1997	$676.8 million	2.93 million	$231.00
	1998	601.1	2.81	214.00
	1999	583.8	2.91	201.00
	2000	599.1	2.94	204.00
	2001	626.6	2.99	210.00
	2002	608.7	3.09	197.00
	2003	660.4	3.28	201.00
	2004	654.1	3.56	184.00
Irons	1997	$533.4 million	7.12 million	$ 74.90*
	1998	485.4	6.87	70.71
	1999	447.9	6.97	64.28
	2000	475.3	7.14	66.57
	2001	459.3	7.17	64.06
	2002	456.4	7.42	61.50
	2003	461.4	7.66	60.23
	2004	482.6	8.06	59.88
Golf balls	1997	$458.7 million	19.97 million	$ 22.97†
	1998	487.4	20.06	24.30
	1999	518.1	20.46	25.32
	2000	530.8	20.80	25.52
	2001	555.6	21.32	26.06
	2002	529.9	20.81	25.46
	2003	496.4	19.85	25.01
	2004	506.3	19.98	25.34
Footwear (pairs)	1997	$214.3 million	2.48 million	$ 86.49
	1998	204.3	2.43	84.13
	1999	206.9	2.47	83.77
	2000	220.8	2.52	87.68
	2001	217.8	2.57	84.62
	2002	211.7	2.68	78.95
	2003	217.1	2.82	76.97
	2004	234.4	3.00	78.22

*Per club.
†Per dozen.
Source: Golf Datatech.

achieve revenue growth by increasing sales in Asia. The company had successfully increased its sales in Asia from 13 percent of sales in 1999 to 31 percent of sales in 2004, and the United States accounted for only 52 percent of sales in 2004 versus 69 percent of sales in 1999. TaylorMade CEO Mark King designated Asia as a high-priority market: "Asia is very, very profitable as a region. The main reason is because the selling prices in Asia for golf equipment are higher than in any other place in the world. So the margins there are very, very strong. Profitability in North America is also very strong. The only area that we are struggling in right now a little bit is in Europe."[6] In addition, USGA rules did not apply to play in Asia and most golf club manufacturers produced models with high COR ratings for sale in Asia.

Even though TaylorMade had achieved the number one ranking in metalwoods during 2004, its market share in irons was about one-half that of industry leader, Callaway Golf Company, and its market share in putters was negligible. The division's sales of Maxfli golf balls, which was acquired by adidas-Salomon in 2002, had yet to earn profits and accounted for less than 5 percent of industry sales in 2005. Segment leader Titleist had held a 70 percent or greater market share in golf balls for decades. TaylorMade-adidas Golf's share of the metalwoods, irons, and golf footwear for January 2002–July 2004 is presented in Exhibit 4.

Like Salomon, TaylorMade-adidas Golf division attempted to benefit from adidas's core competencies in footwear and apparel design. The company offered a full line of golf apparel and footwear that was sold

in golf shops in North America, Europe, and Asia. The division expected double-digit annual growth rates in apparel and footwear revenues. Exhibit 5 presents key financial data for each of adidas-Salomon's operating divisions between 1998 and 2004. The company's financial information by geographic region for 1998–2004 is presented in Exhibit 6. Income statements for and balance sheets for 2003–2004 are provided in Exhibits 7 and 8, respectively.

ADIDAS'S DIVESTITURE OF SALOMON BUSINESS UNITS AND ITS PLANNED ACQUISITION OF REEBOK

With the Amer's acquisition of Salomon's business units completed in October 2005, adidas was able to report that its revenues and earnings for the first nine months of 2005 were quite improved when compared

Exhibit 4   **Market Shares of Leading Sellers of Golf Equipment for Metalwoods, Irons, and Footwear, January 2002–July 2004**

Metalwoods

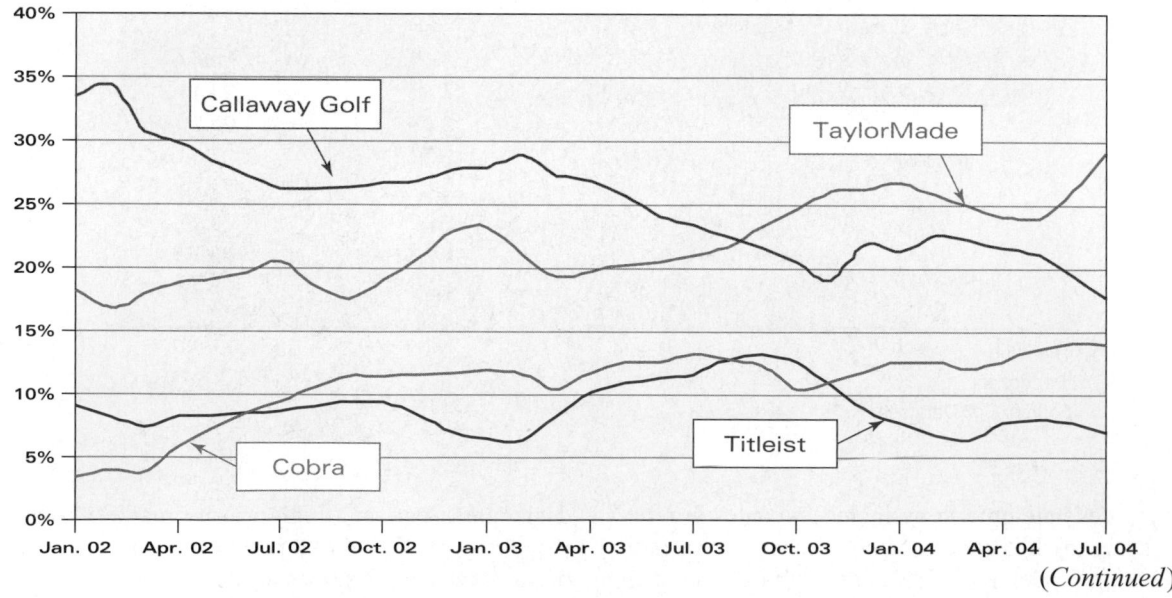

(*Continued*)

Exhibit 4   **Continued**

Irons

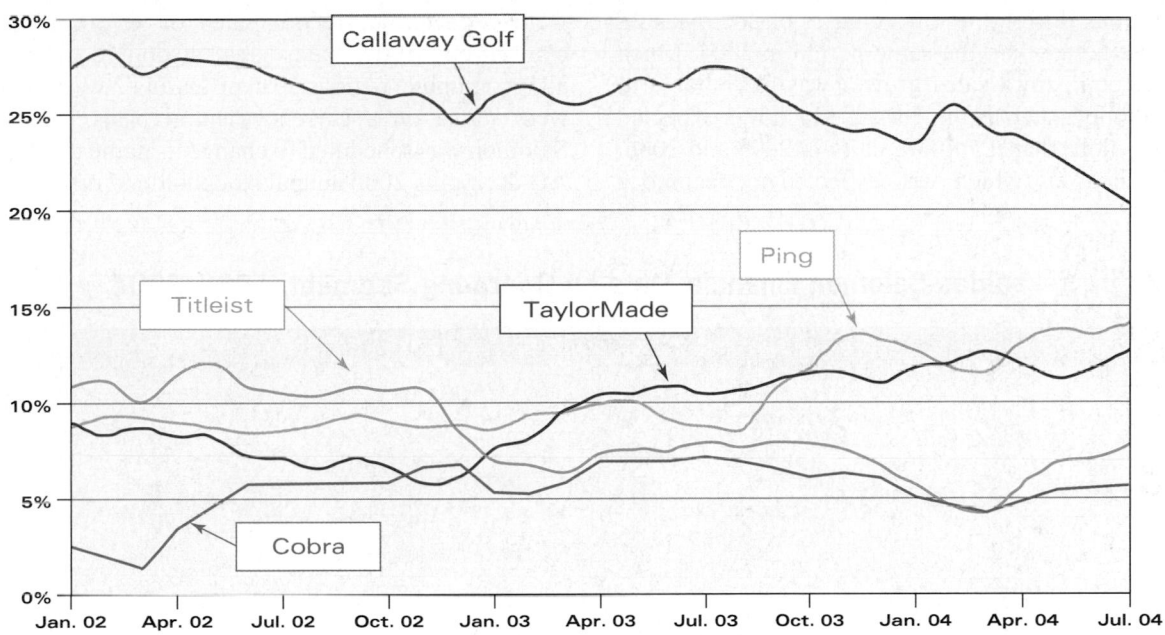

Footwear

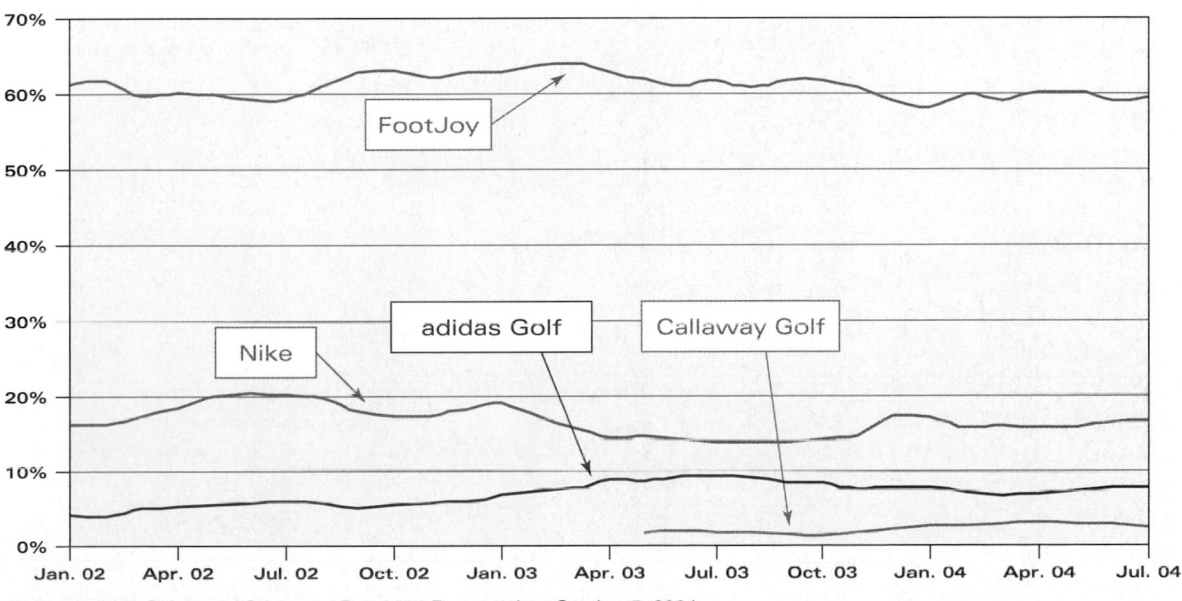

Source: adidas-Salomon AG Investor Day 2004 Presentation, October 5, 2004.

to the first nine months of 2004. The company's revenues had increased by 10 percent on a currency-neutral basis, its operating profits had increased by 12 percent, and its net income from continuing operations during the third quarter of 2005 was 28 percent better than the same period in 2004. Much of the company's sales growth was attributable to new models such as the T-Mac, which was expected to sell more than 1 million pairs in 2005 and 2006, and adidas 1, which was expected to become a

€20 million product line addition by 2006. Also, adidas's Sport Heritage line was expected to account for €1 billion in sales during 2005 and the company's 680 company-owned retail stores were expected to record sales of €750 million by year-end 2005. Sales grew at double digits in all geographic regions except Europe, were sales were stable on a currency-neutral basis. Adidas-Salomon was scheduled to change its name to adidas AG during its 2006 annual stockholders' meeting.

Exhibit 5   **adidas-Salomon Financial Data by Operating Segment, 1998–2004**

	2004	2003	2002	2001	2000	1999	1998
Adidas							
Net sales	€5,174	€4,950	€5,105	€4,825	€4,672	€4,427	€4,316
Gross profit	2,284	2,008	2,004	1,845	1,907	1,827	1,818
Operating profit	523	365	343	352	391	431	412
Operating assets	1,393	2,172	2,294	1,954	2,286	1,987	1,730
Capital expenditures	85	63	84	113	93	105	102
Amortization and depreciation, excluding goodwill amortization	56	63	57	52	45	48	38
Salomon							
Net sales	€653	€658	€684	€714	€703	€587	€487
Gross profit	259	264	279	313	296	233	188
Operating profit	9	35	39	63	61	32	6
Operating assets	505	521	581	679	566	533	598
Capital expenditures	19	18	18	38	24	17	20
Amortization and depreciation, excluding goodwill amortization	7	7	7	7	7	5	7
TaylorMade-adidas Golf							
Net sales	€633	€637	€707	€545	€441	€327	€263
Gross profit	298	290	345	281	221	160	118
Operating profit	60	67	74	63	44	30	20
Operating assets	335	391	433	316	219	156	99
Capital expenditures	9	12	49	16	12	10	16
Amortization and depreciation, excluding goodwill amortization	11	9	7	6	4	4	2
Headquarters/consolidation							
Net sales	€ 18	€ 22	€ 27	€ 28	€ 19	€ 10	—
Gross profit	218	252	191	162	104	—	—
Operating profit	(12)	23	21	(3)	(59)	(14)	(22)
Operating assets	1,648	1,104	953	1,234	947	903	782
Capital expenditures	27	29	22	20	16	—	—
Amortization and depreciation, excluding goodwill amortization	28	17	26	25	23	6	6

Source: adidas-Salomon annual reports.

Exhibit 6   **adidas-Salomon Financial Data by Geographic Region, 1998–2004**

	2004	2003	2002	2001	2000	1999	1998
Europe							
Net sales	€3,470	€3,365	€3,200	€3,066	€2,860	€2,723	€2,774
Gross profit	1,573	1,383	1,268	1,153	1,171	1,133	1,127
Operating profit	644	534	471	444	454	382	357
Operating assets	1,461	1,428	1,396	1,419	1,107	1,167	1,114
Capital expenditures	46	44	56	74	55	40	35
Amortization and depreciation, excluding goodwill amortization	30	30	27	24	22	20	19
North America							
Net sales	€1,486	€1,562	€1,960	€1,818	€1,907	€1,826	€1,784
Gross profit	534	552	742	697	729	731	713
Operating profit	79	92	162	161	177	234	276
Operating assets	768	778	969	945	862	848	666
Capital expenditures	27	22	82	68	54	26	29
Amortization and depreciation, excluding goodwill amortization	21	21	20	17	16	12	11
Asia							
Net sales	€1,251	€1,116	€1,166	€1,010	€875	€663	€383
Gross profit	615	525	562	481	416	301	156
Operating profit	244	191	189	170	129	96	26
Operating assets	480	447	505	743	455	390	201
Capital expenditures	23	12	16	15	17	18	9
Amortization and depreciation, excluding goodwill amortization	16	14	15	12	10	5	3
Latin America							
Net sales	€224	€179	€163	€178	€171	€126	€112
Gross profit	87	70	65	73	72	50	43
Operating profit	38	25	24	16	23	15	11
Operating assets	56	93	79	98	109	75	66
Capital expenditures	1	1	1	2	3	3	2
Amortization and depreciation, excluding goodwill amortization	1	1	1	2	2	1	1
Headquarters/ consolidation							
Net sales	€ 47	€ 45	€ 34	€ 40	€ 23	€ 34	€ 12
Gross profit	248	284	182	197	140	—	—
Operating profit	(426)	(352)	(369)	(316)	(346)	(239)	(254)
Operating assets	1,601	1,442	1,312	978	1,485	1,108	1,162
Capital expenditures	43	43	15	28	16	45	63
Amortization and depreciation, excluding goodwill amortization	34	30	34	35	29	25	19

Source: adidas-Salomon annual reports.

Exhibit 7   **adidas-Salomon Income Statements, 2003–2004 (in thousands except per share data)**

	2004	2003
Net sales	€6,478,072	€6,266,800
Cost of sales	3,419,864	3,453,132
Gross profit	3,058,208	2,813,668
Selling, general and administrative expenses	2,376,266	2,228,135
Depreciation and amortization (excluding goodwill)	101,764	95,519
Operating profit	580,178	490,014
Goodwill amortization	46,352	44,809
Royalty and commission income	43,166	42,153
Financial expenses, net	56,832	49,170
Income before taxes	520,160	438,188
Income taxes	196,691	166,712
Net income before minority interests	323,469	271,476
Minority interests	(9,221)	(11,391)
Net income	€ 314,248	€ 260,085
Basic earnings per share (in euros)	€6.88	€5.72
Diluted earnings per share (in euros)	€6.54	€5.72
Dividends per share (in euros)	€1.30	€1.00
Number of shares outstanding (Basic)	46,649,560	45,452,361
Number of shares outstanding (Diluted)	49,669,346	45,469,366

Source: 2004 adidas-Salomon annual report.

The Reebok acquisition, which was announced in August 2005 and was expected to be finalized sometime during the first half of 2006, would give the company pro forma aggregate 2004 revenues of €8.9 billion ($11.1 billion) and allow it to more than double its sales in North America to €3.1 billion ($3.9 billion). In addition, adidas expected to capture annual cost-sharing benefits of approximately €125 million ($150 million) within three years of the closing date. The company placed 4,531,250 shares with institutional investors in November 2005 to raise approximately €648 million to contribute to the financing of the Reebok acquisition.

Perhaps the greatest opportunity presented by the planned Reebok acquisition was the company's ability to position adidas as a technologically superior shoe designed for serious athletes, while Reebok could be positioned as leisure shoe that would sell at middle price points. In addition, the company could maintain its strategy of signing respected athletes to adidas endorsement contracts, while gaining endorsements from more edgy Reebok celebrities such as Allen Iverson, Jay-Z,

and Fifty Cent. In addition, Reebok would retain its founder and CEO Paul Fireman to lead Reebok after the acquisition.

Even though the restructured lineup of businesses offered adidas an improved chance of catching Nike in its race to be the world's largest sporting goods company, some observers were not convinced the move would prove to be any more successful than the company's 1998 acquisition of Salomon. The president of a sports marketing firm and former New Balance executive said he doubted that adidas's "German mentality of control, engineering, and production" would prove to be compatible with Reebok's "U.S. marketing-driven culture" and added, "In reality, I don't think [the merged company] is going to dent the market, because Nike is already too far ahead."[7] New Balance's CEO, Jim Davis, concurred with his former colleague's assessment by commenting, "You can try to take on Nike, but . . . Nike is Nike and will continue to be Nike.[8] A Goldman Sachs analyst added, "We fail to see how this combo will erode Nike's franchise as the global brand leader."[9]

Exhibit 8 **adidas-Salomon Balance Sheets, 2003–2004 (in thousands)**

	December 31	
Assets	**2004**	**2003**
Cash and cash equivalents	€ 195,997	€ 189,503
Short-term financial assets	258,950	89,411
Accounts receivable	1,046,322	1,075,092
Inventories	1,155,374	1,163,518
Other current assets	378,303	259,427
Total current assets	€3,034,946	€2,776,951
Property, plant and equipment, net	367,928	344,554
Goodwill, net	572,426	591,045
Other intangible assets, net	96,312	103,797
Long-term financial assets	93,134	88,408
Deferred tax assets	160,135	178,484
Other noncurrent assets	102,599	104,569
Total noncurrent assets	€1,392,534	€1,410,857
Total assets	€4,427,480	€4,187,808
Liabilities, minority interests and shareholders' equity		
Short-term borrowings	€ 185,837	€ —
Accounts payable	591,689	592,273
Income taxes	167,334	157,764
Accrued liabilities and provisions	558,121	454,573
Other current liabilities	184,332	139,095
Total current liabilities	€1,687,313	€1,343,705
Long-term borrowings	862,845	1,225,385
Pensions and similar obligations	111,321	105,264
Deferred tax liabilities	77,951	65,807
Other noncurrent liabilities	30,784	35,278
Total noncurrent liabilities	€1,082,865	€1,431,734
Minority interests	28,850	56,579
Shareholders' equity	€1,628,452	€1,355,790
Total liabilities, minority interests and shareholders' equity	€4,427,480	€4,187,808

Source: 2004 adidas-Salomon annual report.

Endnotes

[1] As quoted in "The Brothers Dassler Fight On," *Deutsche Welle,* dw-world.de.

[2] As quoted in "Adidas Foots $1.5B to Buy Sporting Firm," *USA Today,* September 17, 1997.

[3] As quoted in "Sporting Goods Consolidation Off to the Races," *Mergers & Acquisitions Report,* November 10, 1997.

[4] As quoted in "Sports Goods/Shareholders Criticize Salomon Takeover," *Handelsblatt,* May 21, 1999.

[5] Ibid.

[6] Ibid.

[7] As quoted in "Reebok and adidas: A Good Fit," *BusinessWeek Online,* August 4, 2005.

[8] Ibid.

[9] Ibid.

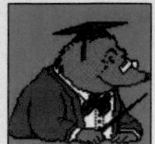

Procter & Gamble's Acquisition of Gillette

John E. Gamble
University of South Alabama

Between 2001 and 2005, Procter & Gamble's revenues increased by more than 40 percent to reach $56.7 billion; its profits more than doubled to approach $7.3 billion; and its number of billion-dollar brands such as Crest, Bounty, Charmin, Tide, Ivory, and Folgers increased from 10 to 16. The company's outstanding financial performance during the four-year period generated adequate free cash flows to fund dividend payments of $11 billion and allowed its market capitalization to increase by more than 100 percent. The company also utilized free cash flows to build its lineup of marquee brands through the acquisitions of Clairol in 2001 and Wella hair care products in 2003.

At the close of its fiscal year ending September 30, 2005, Procter & Gamble executed its largest acquisition ever with the $57 billion takeover of the Gillette Company. The acquisition delivered five additional billion-dollar brands to Procter & Gamble's business mix and made it the global leader in the market for razors and blades. In addition, Gillette's Duracell business unit was the world's number-one seller of alkaline batteries to consumers, its Oral B business was the worldwide leader in manual and electric toothbrushes, and the Braun unit produced and marketed the best-selling brand of foil electric shavers for men and the number-one hair epilator for women. The Gillette Company's sales of Gillette, Foamy, Satin Care, Right Guard, Soft & Dri, and Dry Idea also made it a leading producer of personal care products.

The $57 billion acquisition price represented a 20 percent premium over Gillette's market

capitalization one week prior to the January 28, 2005, merger announcement and would allow Gillette shareholders to exchange each Gillette share held for 0.975 shares of Procter & Gamble (P&G) stock. P&G planned to buy back $18 billion to $22 billion of its outstanding common shares within 12 to 18 months of the completion of the October 1, 2005, merger. The share buyback plan would have the effect of financing the acquisition with 60 percent equity and 40 percent debt.

P&G management expected a 1 + 1 = 3 effect from the merger since the acquisition of Gillette would give P&G a stronger business lineup and brand portfolio and provide significant cost-sharing opportunities between the two companies' businesses. Procter & Gamble's ability to introduce Gillette brands to new country markets served by its distribution system caused management to increase its near-term annual sales growth objective from 4–6 percent to 5–7 percent. In addition, P&G management had identified approximately $1 billion in annual cost savings resulting from value chain synergies between P&G businesses and Gillette business units. The company planned an immediate workforce reduction of 6,000 employees who would no longer be needed because of duplication of responsibilities and activities.

By all appearances, the Gillette acquisition seemed to offer P&G attractive new consumer products segments and ample strategic-fit opportunities that would benefit the overall performance of both business groups, but P&G shareholders had reason to question whether the company's bid for Gillette was too rich. According to an analysis by Goldman Sachs and UBS, the 20 percent purchase-price premium P&G offered to Gillette shareholders was within the range offered in other recent consumer goods mergers, but the acquisition price seemed high when comparing the merger price sales and earnings before interest and taxes (EBIT) multiples to those of other recent mergers. The $57 billion price offered for Gillette was 5.5 times greater than Gillette's most recent sales and 18.8 times greater than its most recent EBIT. The sales multiple for other acquisitions examined by Goldman Sachs/UBS ranged from 1.1 to 4.1. EBIT multiples for previous consumer goods acquisitions included in the investment firms' analysis ranged from 8.4 to 17.6. Projections that the addition of Gillette's business units to P&G's lineup would dilute P&G's EPS for up to three years was also worrisome to investors who believed the 0.975 exchange ratio was overly generous. However, as Procter & Gamble closed its first quarter as a merged company on December 31, 2005, the company was performing at the high end of analysts' expectations. In addition, the merged company's ample free cash flows had allowed it to acquire four leading detergent brands sold in Southeast Asia from Colgate-Palmolive. The new brands would dramatically improve P&G's market share in its weakest region in Asia.

COMPANY HISTORIES AND OVERVIEW OF THE MERGER

Procter & Gamble

The Procter & Gamble Company (P&G) was begun when immigrants William Procter and James Gamble settled in Cincinnati, Ohio, in 1837 and soon thereafter married sisters. At the urging of their father-in-law, the two men, one a candle maker and other a soap maker, created a partnership to manufacture and market their products in the Cincinnati area. The company's sales reached $1 million in 1859, but the company had yet to produce and market a national brand until 1879, when James Norris Gamble, son of the founder and a trained chemist, developed Ivory soap. Ivory quickly transformed Procter & Gamble into a national consumer products company with 30 brands and production facilities across the United States and Canada by 1890. The company added a food products division in 1911 when it introduced

Crisco and began a chemicals division to formalize research procedures and develop new products in 1917. P&G entered the hair care business in 1934 when it developed the first detergent-based shampoo. The company introduced popular-selling brands like Tide, Crest, Pampers, and Downy throughout the 1940s, 1950s, and 1960s.

The company expanded its presence in the cosmetics, fragrances, and toiletries industry in the 1980s with the acquisitions of Richardson-Vicks and Noxell. Richardson-Vicks was the producer of Oil of Olay and Pantene products, and Noxell manufactured and marketed Cover Girl, Noxema, and Clarion products. The company acquired Old Spice in 1990, Max Factor in 1991, Giorgio Beverly Hills in 1994, and Tambrands in 1997. Acquisitions during the 2000s included Clairol in 2001 and Wella shampoos and hair care products in 2003. In 2005, the company sold more than 300 brands in 160 countries. The company's business lineup included 16 billion-dollar brands, and P&G was the global market share leader in 7 of the 12 product categories in which it competed. Its closest rival was the market share leader in only two global markets.

P&G's businesses were organized into three product-based segments: Household Care; Health, Baby, and Family Care; and Beauty Care. The company's Household Care segment included fabric care, home care, snacks, coffee, and commercial services businesses. The Health, Baby, and Family Care division businesses included oral care, personal health care, pharmaceuticals, and pet health and nutrition. Beauty Care businesses manufactured and marketed retail and professional hair care products, feminine care products, cosmetics, fine fragrances, and personal cleansing products. The company's best-known brands in each of its business units are presented in Exhibit 1.

The Gillette Company

The history of shaving dates back to at least 3000 BC, when the first copper-bladed razors were fashioned. Razors through the 1800s were knifelike in their appearance and were prone to leaving gashes or nicks in the skin. The razor of the 21st century can be traced to the efforts of King C. Gillette and William Nickerson, who collaborated to invent the first razor with a safe, inexpensive, disposable blade. The invention

Exhibit 1   **P&G's Best-Known Brands Prior to Gillette Acquisition**

Household Care		
Brand Name	**Product Categories**	**Markets**
Ariel	Laundry detergent	Latin America, Europe, Middle East, Africa
Bounce	Dryer sheets	North America, Latin America, Asia
Dawn	Dishwashing liquid	North America, Latin America
Downy	Fabric softener	North America, Latin America, Europe, Middle East, Africa
Folgers	Whole bean, ground, and instant coffees	North America, Latin America
Gain	Laundry detergent	North America
Millstone	100% premium arabica bean coffees with over 65 varieties	North America
Mr. Clean	Multipurpose cleaner	North America, Asia
Pringles	Snack foods	North America, Latin America, Europe, Middle East, Africa, Asia
Swiffer	Sweeper system	North America, Latin America, Europe, Middle East, Africa
Tide	Laundry detergent	North America, Latin America, Europe, Middle East, Africa, Asia

Beauty Care		
Brand Name	**Product Categories**	**Markets**
Always	Sanitary pads	North America, Latin America, Europe, Middle East, Africa
Aussie	Shampoo and styling products	North America, Europe, Middle East, Africa
CoverGirl	Full line of beauty products for face, lips, eyes, and nails	North America, Latin America, Europe, Middle East, Africa, Asia
Giorgio	Fragrances	North America, Latin America, Europe, Middle East, Africa, Asia
Head & Shoulders	Shampoo	North America, Latin America, Europe, Middle East, Africa, Asia
Herbal Essences	Line of shampoos, conditioners, styling aids, and body washes	North America, Europe, Middle East, Africa, Latin America, Asia
Hugo Boss	Fragrances	North America, Latin America, Europe, Middle East, Africa, Asia
Infusium	Line of therapeutic, premium hair care products	North America, Latin America
Ivory	Line of detergent, dishwashing liquid, and body soap	North America, Latin America, Europe, Middle East, Africa, Asia
Max Factor	Full line of beauty products for face, lips, eyes, and nails	North America, Latin America, Europe, Middle East, Africa, Asia
Miss Clairol	Permanent hair color	North America, Europe, Middle East, Africa, Latin America, Asia
Nice 'n Easy	Permanent hair color	North America, Europe, Middle East, Africa, Latin America, Asia
Noxzema	Line of skin care products	North America, Latin America, Europe, Middle East, Africa
Olay	Line of skin care and cleansing products	North America, Latin America, Europe, Middle East, Africa, Asia

(Continued)

Exhibit 1   **Continued**

Beauty Care		
Brand Name	**Product Categories**	**Markets**
Old Spice	Line of shaving and fragrance products for men	North America, Latin America, Europe, Middle East, Africa, Asia
Pantene	Shampoos, conditioners, hairsprays, and styling aids	North America, Latin America, Europe, Middle East, Africa, Asia
Pert Plus	2-in-1 shampoo/conditioner, individual shampoos and conditioners	North America, Latin America, Europe, Middle East, Africa, Asia
Scope	Mouthwash	North America, Latin America
Secret	Antiperspirant	North America, Latin America, Europe, Middle East, Africa
Tampax	Tampons	North America, Latin America, Europe, Middle East, Africa, Asia
Vidal Sassoon	Hair washes, therapies, stylers, and specialty products	North America, Latin America, Europe, Middle East, Africa, Asia

Family Care		
Brand Name	**Product Categories**	**Markets**
Bounty	Paper towels	North America, Latin America
Charmin	Bathroom tissue	North America, Latin America, Europe, Middle East, Africa
Iams	Complete line of premium dog and cat foods	North America, Europe, Middle East, Africa, Latin America
Puffs	Facial tissues	North America, Latin America
PUR	Water filtration systems, including pitchers and faucet mounts	North America

Baby Care		
Brand Name	**Product Categories**	**Markets**
Luvs	Disposable diapers and wipes	North America, Latin America
Pampers	Disposable diapers, wet wipes, and bibs	North America, Latin America, Europe, Middle East, Africa, Asia

Health Care		
Brand Name	**Product Categories**	**Markets**
Crest	Toothpastes and toothbrushes	North America, Latin America, Europe, Middle East, Africa, Asia
NyQuil	Nighttime relief for temporary relief of cold/flu symptoms	North America, Latin America, Europe, Middle East, Africa
Pepto-Bismol	Antacidum that relieves most common stomach discomforts	North America, Latin America
Prilosec OTC	Over-the-counter medication used to treat frequent heartburn	North America
Vicks	Line of temporary cold symptom relief products and throat drops	North America, Latin America, Europe, Middle East, Africa, Asia

Source: www.pg.com.

led to the founding of the Gillette Company in 1901, which sold its first razors in 1903. The double-edged safety razor proved so popular with men that Gillette began to expand abroad in 1905, with the company opening a European headquarters in London. On the company's 25th anniversary in 1926, King C. Gillette heralded the success of the company's safety razor by stating, "There is no other article for individual use so universally known or widely distributed. In my travels, I have found it in the most northern town in Norway and in the heart of the Sahara Desert."[1]

In 2005, Gillette had expanded into five business segments: Blades and Razors, Duracell, Oral Care, Braun, and Personal Care. The company has maintained manufacturing operations in 14 countries and sold its products in over 200 countries. Five of Gillette's brands each accounted for more than $1 billion in annual sales. In addition to its blades and razors business unit holding the number-one position worldwide, Duracel was the global leader in alkaline battery sales to consumers, Oral B was the worldwide leader in manual and electric toothbrushes, and Braun was the best-selling brand of foil electric shavers for men and the number-one hair epilator for women. The company's Personal Care segment sold shaving creams, skin care products, and antiperspirants under the Gillette, Foamy, Satin Care, Right Guard, Soft & Dri, and Dry Idea brand names.

Rationale for Merger

Both P&G and Gillette management agreed that a merger between the two companies would offer four key benefits: (1) The companies had complementary strengths in product innovation and selling activities, (2) the merger would result in a stronger lineup of brands, (3) a merged company would generate additional opportunities for scale economies, and (4) a stronger lineup of brands would enhance relationships and bargaining power with retail buyers. Immediately upon consummation of the merger, management was to take Gillette products into developing markets such as China that were served by P&G, but not by Gillette. In addition, company managers planned to share R&D costs between P&G and Gillette products and to reduce more than $1 billion in non-value-adding costs in both business groups through synergies in purchasing and asset utilization. The companies' managers also agreed that both companies had similar cultures, visions, and values, which should facilitate their integration.

The acquisition would also better balance P&G's sales between Beauty Care, Health Care, Baby Care, Family Care, and Household Care, with approximately 50 percent of the combined company's revenues originating from the sales of Beauty and Health and 50 percent coming from the sales of Baby, Family, and Household. Also, the acquisition would give P&G 10 billion-dollar brands in Beauty and Health and 12 billion-dollar brands in Baby, Family, and Household. The merged company's nearly $2 billion R&D budget would be more than most of P&G's direct rivals combined, which should allow it to turn some if its 13 $500 million brands into billion-dollar brands. The combination of merger benefits led P&G management to increase its annual sales growth objectives through 2010 from 4–6 percent to 5–7 percent.

COMPETITIVE POSITION AND PERFORMANCE OF P&G AND GILLETTE BUSINESS UNITS

Procter & Gamble

In 2005, P&G's five business units held an average global market share of 30 percent and held 50–60 percent market shares in the Western Europe Baby Care and Feminine Care markets and the North American Fabric Care market. The company's management believed that P&G had a $15 billion opportunity for organic growth in its existing lineup of brands through continued international expansion. In 2005, emerging markets accounted for only 23 percent of P&G's sales, but accounted for 86 percent of the world's population. The combined GDPs of emerging markets represented 25 percent of the global GDP, but were expected to grow to 30 percent of global GDP by 2009.

P&G Beauty Care sales grew by 14 percent based on volume and 12 percent based on revenues in fiscal 2005, with its net earnings increasing by 22 percent for the year. The Beauty Care division held five billion-dollar brands. Pantene was the world's leading hair care brand in 2005, with sales of more than $2 billion and a 10 percent global share of the market. Head & Shoulders was the world's second best-selling brand of shampoo, with just under

10 percent of the market in 2005. P&G's fragrance lines had also experienced notable growth with the sales of Hugo Boss and Lacoste, each growing by more than 1,000 percent since 2001. Overall, the division's net sales had increased from $12.2 billion in fiscal 2003 to $19.5 billion in fiscal 2005, while net earnings for the division grew from $1.9 billion to $2.9 billion during the three-year period.

Net sales grew by 11 percent and net earning grew by 28 percent in fiscal 2005 for P&G's Family Care and Baby Care divisions. The Baby Care division held a 37 percent global market share in the category with products such as its Pampers line of disposable diapers and baby wipes. Billion-dollar brands in the Family Care division included Crest, Bounty, Charmin, and Iams. Health Care sales grew by 11 percent as well during fiscal 2005, but net income for the business segment increased by only 8 percent during the year. The company's best-known pharmaceutical products were Actonel and Prilosec OTC. Prilosec OTC held 35 percent of the U.S. heartburn treatment market, while Actonel had achieved a 33 percent global market share in the osteoporosis prevention market. The combined sales of all Baby, Family, and Health products increased from $15.7 billion in 2003 to $19.7 billion in 2005. Net income attributable to the divisions increased from $1.6 billion in fiscal 2003 to $2.3 billion in fiscal 2005.

The company's Household Care division recorded sales and earnings of $18.4 and $2.5 billion in fiscal 2005, respectively. The division's sales had grown from $15.2 billion in 2003, while net earnings contribution had increased from $2.3 billion. The company's top 10 household care products in 2005 were Folgers, Tide, Ariel, Downy, Pringles, and Dawn—all bringing in sales of more than $1 billion each. Gain, Ace, Mr. Clean, and Swiffer were other best-selling P&G household products brands.

Approximately 52 percent of P&G's fiscal 2005 sales were from outside North America, with 24 percent originating in Western Europe, 5 percent coming from Northeast Asia, and 23 percent originating from developing geographies. The company's gross margins had improved from 49.0 percent in 2003 to 51.0 percent in 2005. Free cash flow and free cash flow productivity (the ratio of free cash flow to net income) had declined slightly between 2004 and 2005. Exhibit 2 presents a financial summary for Procter & Gamble.

The Gillette Company

The strong competitive position of Gillette's business units in their respective consumer segments was among the most enticing attributes of the company as an acquisition target for P&G. Gillette held the number-one position in each of its primary product categories in 2005, including a 70 percent market share in the global razor and razor blade market, a 40 percent global market share in alkaline

Exhibit 2   **Financial Summary for Procter & Gamble, Fiscal 2000–Fiscal 2005 (in millions, except per share amounts)**

	Year Ended June 30					
	2005	2004	2003	2002	2001	2000
Net sales	$56,741	$51,407	$43,377	$40,238	$39,244	$39,951
Operating income	10,927	9,827	7,853	6,678	4,736	5,954
Net earnings	7,257	6,481	5,186	4,352	2,922	3,542
Diluted net earnings per common share	$ 2.66	$ 2.32	$ 1.85	$ 1.54	$ 1.03	$ 1.23
Dividends per common share	1.03	0.93	0.82	0.76	0.70	0.64
Total assets	61,527	57,048	43,706	40,776	34,387	34,366
Long-term debt	12,887	12,554	11,475	11,201	9,792	9,012
Free cash flow*	6,541	7,338	7,218	6,063	3,318	1,657
Free cash flow productivity†	90.1%	113.2%	139.2%	139.3%	113.6%	46.8%

*Free cash flow represents operating cash flow less capital spending.

†Free cash flow productivity is the ratio of free cash flow to net earnings.

Source: Procter & Gamble 2002 and 2005 10-Ks and 2005 S-4.

batteries, a 36 percent market share of the world-wide market for manual and electric toothbrushes. Net sales for the entire company grew by 13 percent to $10.5 billion in 2004, while gross profit increased by 16 percent and net income grew by 22 percent in 2004. In 2004, 37.8 percent of Gillette's sales were in North America, 33.8 percent came from European markets, 11.2 percent originated in Africa and the Middle East, 9.6 percent came from Asia, and 7.4 percent were in Latin America.

The Gillette Company's management believed that its growth and margin opportunities were better than those available to other consumer staple producers because of consumers' preference for branded products. The overall private-label market share for consumer staple items in the United States was 15 percent, according to a 2003 ACNielsen survey. Some categories experienced even greater pricing pressure from private-label brands, with store brands capturing 18 percent of U.S. food and beverage sales in 2003. Sales of private-label razor blades represented only 5.3 percent of the market in 2003, private-label toothbrushes held only a 6.5 percent market share, and private-label alkaline batteries had captured only 12.7 percent of the U.S. market in 2003. P&G was similarly protected from private-label brands in many categories, with private-label antiperspirants accounting for just 0.4 percent of U.S. sales of such products in 2003.

Gillette had also been successful in urging consumers to trade up to higher-price-point personal care items. For example, the company sold low-cost Gillette double-edged blades for safety razors, entry-level shaving systems like the Gillette Sensor 3, and premium shaving systems such as the battery-powered M Power Mach 3. Consumers in developed markets such as the United States were increasingly trading up to higher-priced and higher-margin personal care products. In 2004, 56 percent of the U.S. blade market was held by brands charging more than $1.50 per blade, 37 percent of the market sold at price points between $0.45 and $1.50, and only 7 percent of the market was held by brands selling at less than $0.45 per blade. Gillette saw great opportunity for higher-end shaving systems in emerging markets since such shavers held only 8 percent of sales in regions such as Asia, Latin America, and Africa–Middle East. The company saw similar opportunities in the markets for power toothbrushes, alkaline batteries, and electric shavers. The transition

to higher-priced personal care products was already evident in growing economies such as Russia, where the sales of blades priced over $1.50 grew by 33 percent in 2004 to account for 41 percent of all blade sales. The sales of the lowest-priced blades declined by 19 percent in Russia during 2004.

Buyers of premium personal care products also tended to be highly loyal, with only 23 percent of Mach3 users indicating in a 2003 NCS-USA survey that they would try another brand if Mach3 shavers were out of stock during their trip to the supermarket. Seventy-two percent of men using less expensive disposable shavers indicated that they would purchase whatever brand was available. Women surveyed in the NCS-USA survey were equally loyal to Gillette shavers, with only 22 percent of Venus users suggesting they would purchase a different brand if no Venus blades were in stock.

The company had recorded its second consecutive year of record results in 2004, with its turnaround that began in 2000 fully completed. The company's net sales had grown at a 9 percent compounded annual growth rate between 2001 and 2004, while earnings per share had grown at a 19 percent compounded annual growth rate during the four-year period. The company's gross margins had also improved by 350 basis points between 2001 and 2004, and free cash flow had improved dramatically after the turnaround began in 2000. The company's total free cash flow between 1997 and 2000 was only $1.9 billion, while free cash flow generated between 2001 and 2004 exceeded $7 billion. Exhibit 3 presents a financial summary for the Gillette Company.

P&G'S SHARE PRICE OFFER

Most analysts understood the attractiveness of a Gillette acquisition for P&G. The two companies both enjoyed strong market positions and competed in relatively attractive consumer goods segments. Also, both companies had achieved outstanding recent financial performance—including the generation of free cash flows that would support further growth. In addition, the two companies management teams believed that P&G and Gillette had similar organizational cultures, which should prove to aid in the integration of the two companies and help P&G

Exhibit 3   **Financial Summary for the Gillette Company, 2000–2004 (in millions, except per share amounts)**

	2004	2003	2002	2001	2000
Net sales	$10,477	$ 9,252	$8,453	$8,084	$8,310
Operating income	2,465	2,003	1,809	1,498	1,512
Net earnings	1,691	1,385	1,216	910	392
Diluted net earnings per common share	1.68	1.35	1.15	0.86	0.37
Dividends per common share	0.65	0.65	0.65	0.65	0.65
Total assets	10,731	10,041	9,883	9,961	10,246
Long-term debt	2,142	2,453	2,457	1,654	1,650
Free cash flow*	1,630	2,232	1,672	1,468	811
Free cash flow productivity†	96.4%	161.2%	137.5%	161.3%	206.9%

*Free cash flow represents operating cash flow less capital spending.
†Free cash flow productivity is the ratio of free cash flow to net earnings.
Source: Gillette 2001 and 2004 10-Ks.

deliver its expected $1 billion–plus cost savings from cross-business strategic fits. There was also reason to believe that the combined company's key product categories would grow at high enough rates to support future increases in shareholder value. Gillette's calculation of compounded annual growth rates for consumer goods categories between 2000 and 2004 is presented in Exhibit 4. Exhibit 5 provides perpetuity growth rates for selected consumer product categories as prepared by Merrill Lynch for P&G shareholders evaluating the merger.

Merrill Lynch analysts expected the integration of the two companies and the elimination of duplicate value chain activities to take as long as three years, which might have a dilution effect on P&G's earnings per share (EPS). Specifically, Merrill Lynch's analysis indicated P&G's EPS might be higher between 2006 and 2008 if it were to continue to operate without the inclusion of Gillette's products. Merrill Lynch also suggested P&G's EPS might show positive effects from the merger if integration went quicker than expected and cost savings from synergies between

Exhibit 4   **Gillette's Compounded Annual Growth Rates for Consumer Products Categories, 2000–2004**

Consumer Product Category	Growth Rate for Global Market (CAGR for 2000–2004)
Blades and razors	8.2%
Oral care—toothbrushes	7.3
Skin care	6.8
Chocolate confectionery	6.5
Pet food/pet cares	6.5
Baked goods	4.9
Hair care	4.4
Alkaline batteries	3.7
Oral care—toothpaste	3.5
Laundry detergent	3.4
Carbonated soft drinks	3.4

Source: Gillette presentation to the CAGNY Conference, February 24, 2005.

Exhibit 5   **Gillette's Perpetuity Growth Rates for Selected Consumer Product Categories**

Consumer Product Category	Perpetuity Growth Rate Range
Blades and razors	2.8%–3.8%
Personal care	1.5%–2.5%
Duracell	(0.1%)–0.9%
Oral care	2.4%–3.4%
Braun	0.5%–1.5%

Source: P&G 2005 S-4.

brands were captured in fewer than three years. The projected impact of the Gillette acquisition on P&G's financial performance as calculated by Merrill Lynch is shown in Exhibit 6.

The $57 billion price P&G's board of directors agreed to pay for Gillette would give Gillette shareholders a 20.1 percent premium over Gillette's trading price one week prior to the January 28, 2005, merger announcement. P&G believed that the 20.1 percent share price premium would provide Gillette's board of directors with an adequate incentive to approve the merger and prevent outsiders from interfering with the outright purchase of the company. The $57 billion deal also represented a 5.5 multiple of Gillette's 2004 net sales and an 18.8 multiple of the company's 2004 earnings before interest, taxes, depreciation, and amortization (EBITDA). A comparison of purchase-price multiples and stock-price premiums for selected consumer goods acquisitions as prepared for Gillette shareholders by Goldman Sachs and UBS is presented in Exhibit 7. While the 20.1 percent per share purchase-price premium is within the range for other acquisitions examined by

Exhibit 6   **Projected Range of Impact on P&G Performance by Gillette Acquisition**

	Fiscal Year Ending June 30		
	2006E	2007E	2008E
Earnings per share	$(0.25)–$(0.30)	$(0.10)–$0.05	$(0.05)–$0.15
Earnings per share excluding one-time charges	$(0.21)–$(0.26)	$(0.09)–$0.06	$(0.05)–$0.15
Earnings per share excluding one-time charges and new amortization	$(0.16)–$(0.21)	$(0.03)–$0.12	$ 0.00–$0.20

Source: P&G 2005 S-4.

Exhibit 7   **Gillette's Purchase-Price Multiples and Stock-Price Premiums for Selected Consumer Goods Acquisitions**

	Purchase-Price Multiples for Selected Consumer Goods Acquisitions		Per Share Purchase-Price Premium based on Stock Price
	Sales	EBITDA	One Week Prior to Announcement
Median	2.2x	13.0x	19.30%
Mean	2.2x	13.2x	29.10%
Range	1.1x–4.1x	8.4x–17.6x	5.3%–92.6%
Gillette at $54.05	5.5x	18.8x	20.1%*

*Relative to closing price on Wednesday, January 19, 2005.
Source: P&G 2005 S-4.

Exhibit 8   **Transaction Value and Per Share Purchase-Price Premiums Paid in Selected Consumer Goods Acquisitions, 1994–2004**

Announcement Date	Acquirer	Target	Transaction Value (in billions)	Premium to Share Price One Week Prior to Announcement
6/2000	Phillip Morris	Nabisco	$19.2	103.2%
8/1994	Johnson & Johnson	Neutrogena	1.0	76.3
11/2004	Constellation Brands	Robert Mondavi	1.4	52.3
3/2003	Procter & Gamble	Wella	7.0	47.3
10/2003	Tchibo	Beiersdorf	13.0	45.7
6/2000	Unilever	Bestfoods	23.7	39.9
12/2000	PepsiCo	Quaker Oats	15.1	24.0
				Average 55.5%

Source: P&G 2005 S-4.

UBS and Goldman Sachs, the purchase-price multiple exceeds that of prior acquisitions.

Merrill Lynch's analysis of the per share purchase-price premiums paid to acquire selected consumer goods between 1994 and 2004 left room for debate as to whether P&G's 20.1 percent offer was fair to Gillette shareholders. Merrill Lynch's purchase-price evaluation based on Gillette's January 26, 2005, closing price indicates the price might be considered low, although calculations based on Gillette's 52-week low and three-year average stock price was near the average paid in other acquisitions (see Exhibits 8 and 9).

Exhibit 9   **Multiples and Premium for P&G's Share Price Offer for Gillette as Calculated by Merrill Lynch**

	Gillette at Offer Price
2004 sales	5.5x
2004 EBITDA	18.8
Premium to:	
1 day (based on Gillette closing price of ($45.00 on 1/26/05)	20.1%
52-week high	18.7%
52-week low	45.9
3-year average	52.4

Source: P&G 2005 S-4.

Since P&G's shares traded for a higher price at the time of the merger than Gillette shares, Gillette shareholders received a fraction of a P&G share in exchange for their Gillette holdings. The relationship between P&G's prevailing stock price and Gillette's price resulted in an exchange ratio of 0.975. For example, a Gillette stockholder owning 1,000 Gillette shares would receive 975 P&G shares upon the completion of the merger. Fractional shares were not awarded, so a Gillette shareholder owning 100 shares would receive only 97 P&G shares.

Merrill Lynch also calculated a range of appropriate exchange ratios based on Gillette's expected contribution to the combined company's net income and the amount of levered free cash flow provided by Gillette brands (see Exhibit 10). Levered free cash flow represents free cash flow less additional debt service taken on as a result of the acquisition of Gillette. Based on the analysts' estimates of net income contributed by Gillette brands, P&G would be required to capture at least two-thirds of the expected synergies between the company's brands to approach the 0.975 exchange ratio offered to Gillette shareholders. Using the estimates based on levered free cash flow, the 0.975 exchange ratio could be justified if at least some expected synergies were achieved.

Exhibit 11 shows the financial projections used in Merrill Lynch's exchange ratio calculations to estimate the importance of Gillette's brands to the combined company's performance through 2008.

Exhibit 10   **Merrill Lynch's Estimation of Appropriate Exchange Ratios**

	Assuming No Expected Synergies Are Achieved	
	Low Estimate	High Estimate
Exchange ratio based on net income contribution for Gillette brands	0.654	0.684
Exchange ratio based on levered free cash flow provided by Gillette brands	0.848	0.875

	Assuming 50% of Expected Synergies Are Achieved	
	Low Estimate	High Estimate
Exchange ratio based on net income contribution for Gillette brands	0.876	0.886
Exchange ratio based on levered free cash flow provided by Gillette brands	1.108	1.152

	Assuming 2/3 of Expected Synergies Are Achieved	
	Low Estimate	High Estimate
Exchange ratio based on net income contribution for Gillette brands	0.941	0.963
Exchange ratio based on levered free cash flow provided by Gillette brands	1.190	1.252

Source: P&G 2005 S-4.

Exhibit 11   **Financial Projections**

	Procter & Gamble's Contribution to Combined Company	Gillette's Contribution to Combined Company
Sales		
CY* 2004E	83.6%	16.4%
CY 2005E	83.8	16.2
EBITDA		
CY 2004E	80.0	20.0
CY 2005E	79.1	20.9
EBIT		
CY 2004E	80.9	19.1
CY 2005E	79.7	20.3
Net Income		
CY 2004E	80.3	19.7
CY 2005E	78.9	21.1
CY 2006E	78.4	21.6
CY 2007	78.3	21.7
CY 2008	78.3	21.7

*Contributions based on calendar year (CY), since P&G's fiscal year ends June 30 and Gillette's fiscal year ends December 31.
Source: P&G 2005 S-4.

P&G'S EARLY POSTMERGER PERFORMANCE

As the 2005 calendar year ended and P&G closed out its first quarter as a merged company, its managers were pleased that the company's performance seemed to be exceeding analysts' predictions. The company anticipated that its audited reports would show sales growth for the quarter ending December 31, 2005, to come in at 25–26 percent. Prior to the consummation of the merger, the company's managers and financial advisers had projected sales growth for the quarter to be in the 23–26 percent range. The company's managers attributed the increase in revenues to 6–7 percent organic sales growth in its Household Care and Beauty Care business units. Much of that increase was attributable to the performance of Gillette's blades and razors, Duracell, and Braun brands, which had grown by an estimated 17 percent during the quarter. Prior to the merger, Gillette's brands had been expected to grow at a low-single-digit rate.

Procter & Gamble managers also expected that final tabulations for the quarter would report a quarterly EPS of $0.68–$0.69, which was at the very top end of the $0.66–$0.69 projected for the quarter. The achievement of best-case quarterly EPS estimate led P&G managers to predict EPS dilution for the 2006 fiscal year to be no more than $0.20 to $0.26 per share. In assessing the impact of the merger on P&G performance for 2006, Merrill Lynch analysts had expected EPS dilution to fall between $0.25 and $0.30 per share.

P&G announced on January 4, 2006, that it would acquire the Fab, Trojan, Dynamo, and Paic laundry detergent brands marketed in Hong Kong, Singapore, Thailand, and Malaysia from Colgate-Palmolive. The new brands would boost P&G's market share in the category from 2.1 percent to 12.9 percent in Singapore, from 0.3 percent to 7.9 percent in Thailand, from 0.3 percent to 12.5 percent in Malaysia, and from 1.2 percent to 12.5 percent in Hong Kong. The company's market performance relative to the S&P 500 from January 1996 to December 2005 is presented in Exhibit 12. The exhibit also provides a comparison of P&G's stock performance relative to the S&P 500 for the January–December 2005 period.

Exhibit 12 Performance of Procter & Gamble's Stock Price, January 1996–December 2005

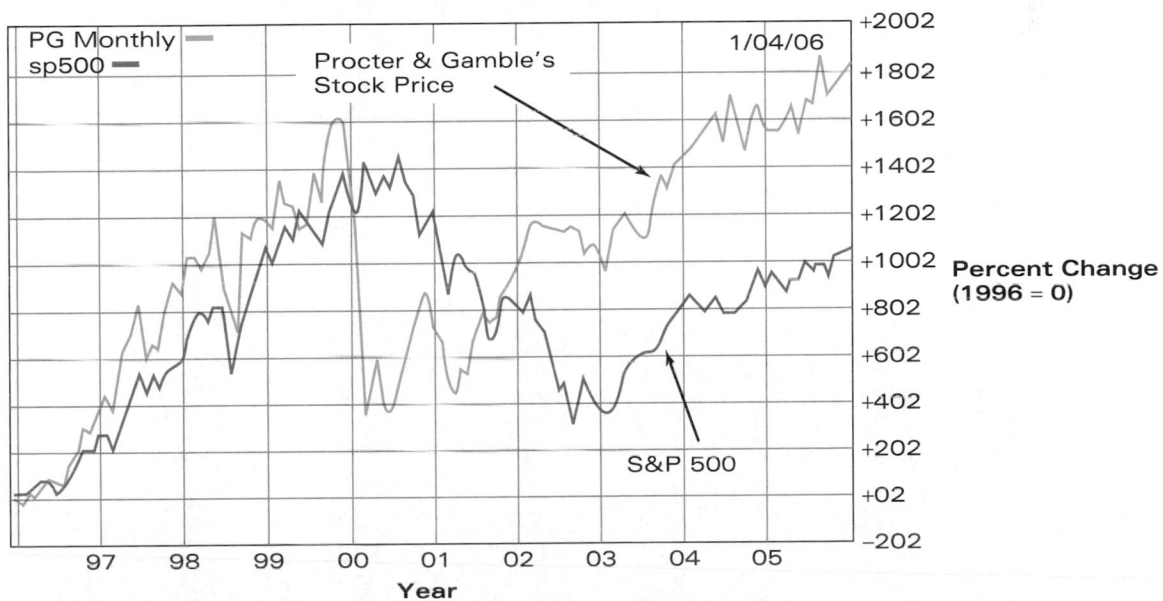

(a) Performance of Procter & Gamble's Stock Price versus the S&P 500.

(Continued)

Exhibit 12   **Continued**

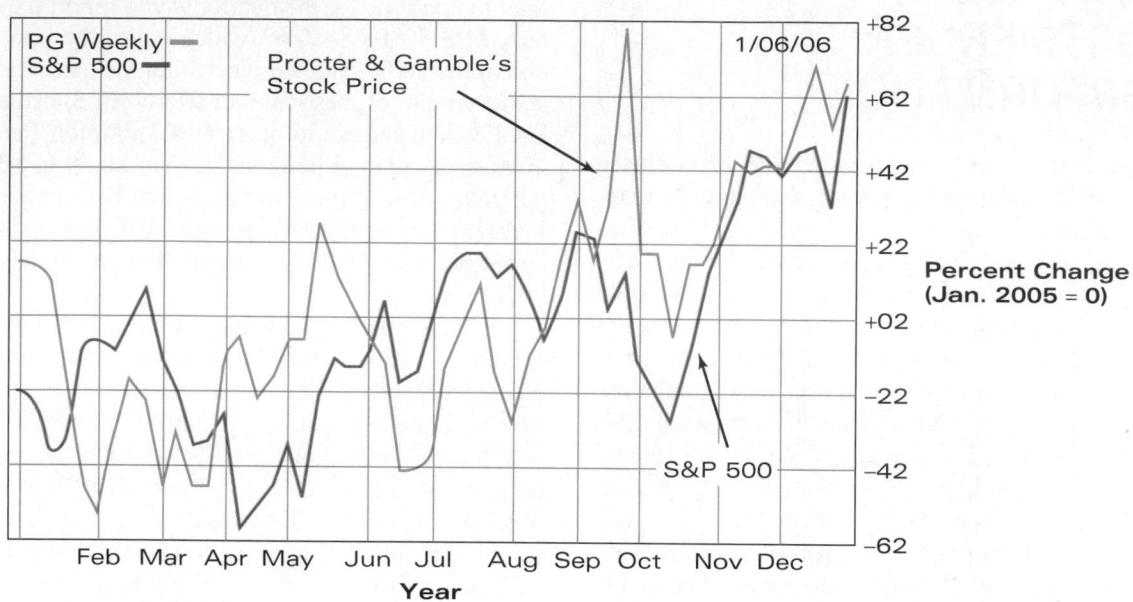

(b) Performance of Procter & Gamble's Stock Price versus the S&P 500 between January 2005 and December 2005.

Endnotes

[1]As quoted in "Gillette at a Glance," http://www.gillette.com/company/
gilletteataglance.asp

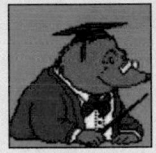

Robin Hood

Joseph Lampel
New York University

It was in the spring of the second year of his insurrection against the High Sheriff of Nottingham that Robin Hood took a walk in Sherwood Forest. As he walked he pondered the progress of the campaign, the disposition of his forces, the Sheriff's recent moves, and the options that confronted him.

The revolt against the Sheriff had begun as a personal crusade. It erupted out of Robin's conflict with the Sheriff and his administration. However, alone Robin Hood could do little. He therefore sought allies, men with grievances and a deep sense of justice. Later he welcomed all who came, asking few questions and demanding only a willingness to serve. Strength, he believed, lay in numbers.

He spent the first year forging the group into a disciplined band, united in enmity against the Sheriff and willing to live outside the law. The band's organization was simple. Robin ruled supreme, making all important decisions. He delegated specific tasks to his lieutenants. Will Scarlett was in charge of intelligence and scouting. His main job was to shadow the Sheriff and his men, always alert to their next move. He also collected information on the travel plans of rich merchants and tax collectors. Little John kept discipline among the men and saw to it that their archery was at the high peak that their profession demanded. Scarlock took care of the finances, converting loot to cash, paying shares of the take, and finding suitable hiding places for the surplus. Finally, Much the Miller's son had the difficult task of provisioning the ever-increasing band of Merrymen.

The increasing size of the band was a source of satisfaction for Robin, but also a source of concern. The fame of his Merrymen was spreading, and new recruits were pouring in from every corner of England. As the band grew larger, their small bivouac became a major encampment. Between raids the men milled about, talking and playing games. Vigilance was in decline, and discipline was becoming harder to enforce. "Why," Robin reflected, "I don't know half the men I run into these days."

The growing band was also beginning to exceed the food capacity of the forest. Game was becoming scarce, and supplies had to be obtained from outlying villages. The cost of buying food was beginning to drain the band's financial reserves at the very moment when revenues were in decline. Travelers, especially those with the most to lose, were now giving the forest a wide berth. This was costly and inconvenient to them, but it was preferable to having all their goods confiscated.

Robin believed that the time had come for the Merrymen to change their policy of outright confiscation of goods to one of a fixed transit tax. His lieutenants strongly resisted this idea. They were proud of the Merrymen's famous motto: "Rob the rich and give to the poor." "The farmers and the townspeople," they argued, "are our most important allies. How can we tax them, and still hope for their help in our fight against the Sheriff?"

Robin wondered how long the Merrymen could keep to the ways and methods of their early days. The Sheriff was growing stronger and becoming better organized. He now had the money and the men and was beginning to harass the band, probing for its weaknesses. The tide of events was beginning to turn against the Merrymen. Robin felt that the campaign must be decisively concluded before the Sheriff had a chance to deliver a mortal blow. "But how," he wondered, "could this be done?"

Robin had often entertained the possibility of killing the Sheriff, but the chances for this seemed increasingly remote. Besides, killing the Sheriff might satisfy his personal thirst for revenge, but it would not improve the situation. Robin had hoped that the perpetual state of unrest, and the Sheriff's failure to collect taxes, would lead to his removal from office. Instead, the Sheriff used his political connections to obtain reinforcement. He had powerful friends at court and was well regarded by the regent, Prince John.

Prince John was vicious and volatile. He was consumed by his unpopularity among the people, who wanted the imprisoned King Richard back. He also lived in constant fear of the barons, who had first given him the regency but were now beginning to dispute his claim to the throne. Several of these barons had set out to collect the ransom that would release King Richard the Lionheart from his jail in Austria. Robin was invited to join the conspiracy in return for future amnesty. It was a dangerous proposition. Provincial banditry was one thing, court intrigue another. Prince John had spies everywhere, and he was known for his vindictiveness. If the conspirators' plan failed, the pursuit would be relentless, and retributions swift.

The sound of the supper horn startled Robin from his thoughts. There was the smell of roasting venison in the air. Nothing was resolved or settled. Robin headed for camp promising himself that he would give these problems his utmost attention after tomorrow's raid.

Dilemma at Devil's Den

Allen Cohen
Babson College

Kim Johnson
Babson College

My name is Susan, and I'm a business student at Mt. Eagle College. Let me tell you about one of my worst experiences. I had a part-time job in the campus snack bar, The Devil's Den. At the time, I was 21 years old and a junior with a concentration in finance. I originally started working at the Den in order to earn some extra spending money. I had been working there for one semester and became upset with some of the happenings. The Den was managed by contract with an external company, College Food Services (CFS). What bothered me was that many employees were allowing their friends to take free food, and the employees themselves were also taking food in large quantities when leaving their shifts. The policy was that employees could eat whatever they liked free of charge while they were working, but it had become common for employees to leave with food and not to be charged for their snacks while off duty as well.

I felt these problems were occurring for several reasons. For example, employee wages were low, there was easy access to the unlocked storage room door, and inventory was poorly controlled. Also, there was weak supervision by the student managers and no written rules or strict guidelines. It seemed that most of the employees were enjoying freebies, and it had been going on for so long that it was taken for granted. The problem got so far out of hand that customers who had seen others do it felt free to do it whether they knew the workers or not.

The employees who witnessed this never challenged anyone because, in my opinion, they did not care and they feared the loss of friendship or being frowned upon by others. Apparently, speaking up was more costly to the employees than the loss of money to CFS for the unpaid food items. It seemed obvious to me that the employees felt too secure in their jobs and did not feel that their jobs were in jeopardy.

The employees involved were those who worked the night shifts and on the weekends. They were students at the college and were under the supervision of another student, who held the position of manager. There were approximately 30 student employees and 6 student managers on the staff. During the day there were no student managers; instead, a full-time manager was employed by CFS to supervise the Den. The employees and student managers were mostly freshmen and sophomores, probably because of the low wages, inconvenient hours (late weeknights and weekends), and the duties of the job itself. Employees were hard to come by; the high rate of employee turnover indicated that the job qualifications and the selection process were minimal.

The student managers were previous employees chosen by other student managers and the full-time CFS day manager on the basis of their ability to work and on their length of employment. They received no further formal training or written rules beyond what they had already learned by working there. The student managers were briefed on how to close the snack bar at night but still did not get the job done properly. They received authority and responsibility over events occurring during their shifts as manager, although they were never actually taught how and when to enforce it! Their increase in pay was small, from a starting pay of just over minimum wage to an additional 15 percent for student managers. Regular employees received an additional nickel for each semester of employment.

Although I only worked seven hours per week, I was in the Den often as a customer and saw the problem frequently. I felt the problem was on a large enough scale that action should have been taken, not only to correct any financial loss that the Den might have experienced but also to help give the student employees a true sense of their responsibilities, the limits of their freedom, respect for rules, and pride in their jobs. The issues at hand bothered my conscience, although I was not directly involved. I felt that the employees and customers were taking advantage of the situation whereby they could "steal" food almost whenever they wanted. I believed that I had been brought up correctly and knew right from wrong, and I felt that the happenings in the Den were wrong. It wasn't fair that CFS paid for others' greediness or urges to show what they could get away with in front of their friends.

I was also bothered by the lack of responsibility of the managers to get the employees to do their work. I had seen the morning employees work very hard trying to do their jobs, in addition to the jobs the closing shift should have done. I assumed the night managers did not care or think about who worked the next day. It bothered me to think that the morning employees were suffering because of careless employees and student managers from the night before.

I had never heard of CFS mentioning any problems or taking any corrective action; therefore, I wasn't sure whether they knew what was going on, or if they were ignoring it. I was speaking to a close friend, Mack, a student manager at the Den, and I mentioned the fact that the frequently unlocked door to the storage room was an easy exit through which I had seen different quantities of unpaid goods taken out. I told him about some specific instances and said that I believed that it happened rather frequently. Nothing was ever said to other employees about this, and the only corrective action was that the door was locked more often, yet the key to the lock was still available upon request to all employees during their shifts.

Another lack of strong corrective action I remembered was when an employee was caught pocketing cash from the register. The student was neither suspended nor threatened with losing his job (nor was the event even mentioned). Instead, he was just told to stay away from the register. I felt that this weak punishment happened not because he was a good worker but because he worked so many hours and it would be difficult to find someone who would work all those hours and remain working for more than a few months. Although a customer reported the incident, I still felt that management should have taken more corrective action.

The attitudes of the student managers seemed to vary. I had noticed that one in particular, Bill, always got the job done. He made a list of each small duty that needed to be done, such as restocking, and he made sure the jobs were divided among the employees and finished before his shift was over. Bill also stared down employees who allowed thefts by their friends or who took freebies themselves; yet I had never heard of an employee being challenged verbally, nor had anyone ever been fired for these actions. My friend Mack was concerned about theft, or so I assumed, because he had taken some action about locking the doors, but he didn't really get after employees to work if they were slacking off.

I didn't think the rest of the student managers were good motivators. I noticed that they did little work themselves and did not show much control over the employees. The student managers allowed their friends to take food for free, thereby setting bad examples for the other workers, and allowed the employees to take what they wanted even when they were not working. I thought their attitudes were shared by most of the other employees: not caring about their jobs or working hard, as long as they got paid and their jobs were not threatened.

I had let the "thefts" continue without mention because I felt that no one else really cared and may even have frowned upon me for trying to take action. Management thus far had not reported significant losses to the employees so as to encourage them to watch for theft and prevent it. Management did not threaten employees with job loss, nor did they provide employees with supervision. I felt it was not my place to report the theft to management, because I was just an employee and I would be overstepping the student managers. Also, I was unsure whether management would do anything about it anyway—maybe they did not care. I felt that talking to the student managers or other employees would be useless, because they were either abusing the rules themselves or were clearly aware of what was going on and just ignored it. I felt that others may have frowned upon me and made it uncomfortable for me to continue working there. This would be very difficult for me, because I wanted to become a student manager the next semester and did not want to create any waves that might have prevented me from doing so. I recognized the student manager position as a chance to gain some managerial and leadership skills, while at the same time adding a great plus to my resume when I graduated. Besides, as a student manager, I would be in a better position to do something about all the problems at the Den that bothered me so much.

What could I do in the meantime to clear my conscience of the freebies, favors to friends, and employee snacks? What could I do without ruining my chances of becoming a student manager myself someday? I hated just keeping quiet, but I didn't want to make a fool of myself. I was really stuck.

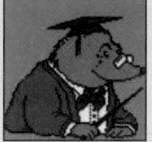

Wal-Mart Stores Inc.: Combating Critics and Sustaining Growth

Arthur A. Thompson
The University of Alabama

Throughout 2005, Wal-Mart executives were engaged in a charm offensive to combat growing outcries from the company's critics. Numerous journalists, union leaders, community activists, and so-called cultural progressives were uniting in a campaign to bash Wal-Mart on a variety of fronts and turn public opinion against the company and its seemingly virtuous business model of relentlessly wringing cost efficiencies out of its supply chain and providing customers with everyday low prices. At the center of the crusade to cast Wal-Mart in a bad light were Wal-Mart Watch and Wake Up Wal-Mart.[1] Wal-Mart Watch was founded by Andrew Stern, president of the Service Employees International Union. Wake Up Wal-Mart was a project of the United Food and Commercial Workers International Union (UFCW). Wal-Mart Watch had an e-mail utility that visitors could use to direct the recipient to anti–Wal-Mart "facts"; the e-mail had the tag line, "I thought you might enjoy this story from Wal-Mart Watch, a group who is starting to expose Wal-Mart for their bad labor standards, political corruptness and overall bad citizenship. It's getting a lot of attention in the press. Take a look."[2]

The biggest complaint of critics was that Wal-Mart's zealous pursuit of low costs had resulted in substandard wages and insufficient medical benefits for Wal-Mart's 1.3 million U.S. employees. Others opposed Wal-Mart on the grounds that it sourced too much of its merchandise from Chinese suppliers (about $18 billion), thus costing jobs for American workers and hastening the decline of the U.S. manu-

facturing sector. Some said the "Beast of Bentonville" was too big and too powerful.

Community activists in California, New York, Vermont, Massachusetts, and several other areas were vigorously opposing the company's attempts to open big-box stores in their locales, claiming that they were unsightly and detracted from the small-merchant atmosphere they wanted to preserve. Wal-Mart's low prices tended to attract customers away from apparel shops, general stores, pharmacies, sporting goods stores, shoe stores, hardware stores, supermarkets, and convenience stores operated by local merchants. It was common for a number of local businesses that carried merchandise similar to Wal-Mart's lines to fail within a year or two of Wal-Mart's arrival—this phenomenon, known as the "Wal-Mart effect," was so potent that it had spawned sometimes fierce local resistance to the entry of a new Wal-Mart among both local merchants and area residents wanting to preserve the economic vitality of their downtown areas.

Union leaders at the UFCW, which represented workers at many supermarket chains, were adamant in their opposition to the opening of Wal-Mart Supercenters that had a full-sized supermarket in addition to the usual merchandise selection. The UFCW and its Wake Up Wal-Mart organization were exerting all the pressure they could to force Wal-Mart to raise its wages and benefits for associates to levels that would be comparable to union wages and benefits at unionized supermarket chains. A UFCW spokesperson said:

> Their productivity is becoming a model for taking advantage of workers, and our society is doomed

if we think the answer is to lower our standards to Wal-Mart's level. What we need to do is to raise Wal-Mart to the standard we have set using the supermarket industry as an example so that Wal-Mart does not destroy our society community by community.[3]

Wal-Mart's labor costs were said to be 20 percent less than those at unionized supermarkets.[4] In Dallas, 20 supermarkets had closed once Wal-Mart had saturated the area with its Supercenters. According to one source, for every Wal-Mart Supercenter opened in the next five years, two other supermarkets would be forced to close.[5] A trade publication had estimated that Wal-Mart's plans to open more than 1,000 Supercenters in the United States in the 2004–2008 period would boost Wal-Mart's grocery and related revenues from $82 billion to $162 billion, thus increasing its market share in groceries from 19 percent to 35 percent and its share of pharmacy and drugstore-related sales from 15 percent to 25 percent.[6]

Wal-Mart's public image had also taken a hit in late 2003 when federal agents had arrested nearly 250 illegal immigrants after cleaning shifts at 61 Wal-Mart stores in 21 states. Agents had searched a manager's office at Wal-Mart's Bentonville headquarters and taken 18 boxes of documents relating to cleaning contractors dating back to March 2000.[7] Federal officials reportedly had wiretaps showing that Wal-Mart officials knew its janitorial contractors were using illegal cleaning crews. Wal-Mart, however, was indignant about the charges, saying that Wal-Mart had cooperated with federal authorities in the investigations for almost three years, helped agents tape conversations between some of its store managers and employees of the cleaning contractors suspected of using illegal immigrants, and revised its cleaning contracts in 2002 to include language that janitorial contractors comply with all federal, state, and local employment laws (because of the information developed in 2001), and begun bringing all janitorial work in-house because outsourcing was more expensive— at the time of the arrests, fewer than 700 Wal-Mart stores used outside cleaning contractors, down from almost half in 2000. In March 2005, Wal-Mart settled the charges with the Justice Department.

Wal-Mart had been criticized for refusing to stock CDs or DVDs with parental warning stickers (mostly profanity-laced hip-hop music) and for either pulling certain racy magazines (*Maxim, Stuff,* and *FHM*) from its shelves or obscuring their covers. Critics contended that Wal-Mart made no effort to survey shoppers about how they felt about such products but rather that it responded in ad hoc fashion to complaints lodged by a relative handful of customers and by conservative outside groups.[8] Wal-Mart had also been the only one of the top 10 drugstore chains to refuse to stock Preven, a morning-after contraceptive introduced in 1999, because company executives did not want its pharmacists have to grapple with the moral dilemma of abortion.

Moreover, Wal-Mart's high profile had made it a lightning rod for lawsuits. It was confronting roughly 6,000 lawsuits on a variety of issues, including one that it discriminated against female employees and another that claimed Wal-Mart forced employees to work beyond their shifts.

Initially, H. Lee Scott, Wal-Mart's CEO, and other top Wal-Mart executives had shrugged off the criticism and concentrated their full attention on running the business and expanding the company's operations into more countries and more communities. But in 2004–2005, Scott started to see that all the Wal-Mart bashing was taking a toll on the company's sales growth and throwing up roadblocks to its expansion plans. He decided that Wal-Mart ought to reach out to its critics, see if their concerns had merit, and explore whether Wal-Mart ought to alter some of its practices. But, while it made good business sense for Wal-Mart to be responsive to societal expectations, he knew that the company could not simply abandon doing things that were the keys to its success.[9]

COMPANY BACKGROUND

Wal-Mart's journey from humble beginnings in the 1960s as a folksy discount retailer in the boondocks of Arkansas to a global retailing juggernaut in 2006 was unprecedented among the companies of the world:

	1962	1970	1980	1990	2000	2005
Sales	$1.4 million	$31 million	$1.2 billion	$26 billion	$191 billion	$285 billion
Profits	$112,000	$1.2 million	$41 million	$1 billion	$6.3 billion	$10.3 billion
Stores	9	32	276	1,528	4,188	5,289

Wal-Mart grew its sales by $29 billion in 2004 and by $30 billion in 2005; sales were expected to reach $315 billion in fiscal 2006. It was the largest retailer in Canada and Mexico, as well as in the United States and the world as a whole. According to a 2003 report by the prominent Boston Consulting Group, "The world has never known a company with such ambition, capability, and momentum."

Just as unprecedented was Wal-Mart's impact on general merchandise retailing and the attraction its stores had to shoppers in locations where it had stores. In 2005, about 140 million people in 16 countries shopped Wal-Mart's 5,300 stores every week. More than half of American shoppers visited a Wal-Mart at least once a month, and one-third went once a week—in 2002 an estimated 82 percent of American households made at least one purchase at Wal-Mart.[10] Since the early 1990s, the company had gone from dabbling in supermarket sales to number one in grocery retailing worldwide. In the United States, Wal-Mart was the biggest employer in 21 states. The company employed about 1.7 million people worldwide and was expanding its workforce by about 120,000 new jobs annually.[11]

Wal-Mart's performance and prominence in the retailing industry had resulted in numerous awards. It had been named "Retailer of the Century" by *Discount Store News,* made the *Fortune* magazine lists of "Most Admired Companies in America" (it was ranked first in 2003 and 2004 and fourth in 2005) and "100 Best Companies to Work for in America," and been included on *Financial Times*' "Most Respected in the World" list. In 2005, Wal-Mart was ranked second on *Fortune*'s list of the "Global Most Admired Companies." In 2002, 2003, 2004, and 2005, Wal-Mart was number one on the Fortune 500 list of the largest companies in America and also on the Fortune Global 500 list. Wal-Mart received the 2002 Ron Brown Award, the highest presidential award recognizing outstanding achievement in employee relations and community initiatives. In 2003, American Veterans Awards gave Wal-Mart its Corporate Patriotism Award. Wal-Mart was the largest corporate contributor to charitable causes in the United States, with 2005 contributions of over $200 million.

Exhibit 1 provides a summary of Wal-Mart's financial and operating performance for the 1993–2005 fiscal years. Wal-Mart's success had made the Walton family (Sam Walton's heirs and living relatives) exceptionally wealthy—in 2005, five

Walton family members controlled about 1.73 billion shares of Wal-Mart stock worth about $87 billion. Increases in the value of Wal-Mart's stock over the years had made hundreds of Wal-Mart employees, retirees, and shareholders millionaires or multimillionaires. Since 1970, when Wal-Mart shares were first issued to the public, the company's stock had split 11 times. A 100-share investment in Wal-Mart stock in 1970 at the initial offer price of $16.50 equated to 204,800 shares worth $10.2 million as of December 2005.

Sam Walton, Founder of Wal-Mart

Sam Walton graduated from the University of Missouri in 1940 with a degree in economics and took a job as a management trainee at J. C. Penney Company. His career with Penney's ended with a call to military duty in World War II. When the war was over, Walton decided to purchase a franchise and open a Ben Franklin retail variety store in Newport, Arkansas, rather than return to Penney's. When the lease on the Newport building was lost five years later, Walton decided to relocate his business to Bentonville, Arkansas, where he bought a building and opened Walton's 5 & 10 as a Ben Franklin–affiliated store. By 1960, Walton was the largest Ben Franklin franchisee, with nine stores. But Walton was becoming concerned about the long-term competitive threat to variety stores posed by the emerging popularity of giant supermarkets and discounters. An avid pilot, he took off in his plane on a cross-country tour studying the changes in stores and retailing trends, then put together a plan for a discount store of his own because he believed deeply in the retailing concept of offering significant price discounts to expand sales volumes and increase overall profits. Walton went to Chicago to try to interest Ben Franklin executives in expanding into discount retailing; when they turned him down, he decided to go forward on his own.

The first Wal-Mart Discount City opened July 2, 1962, in Rogers, Arkansas. The store was successful, and Walton quickly began to look for opportunities to open stores in other small towns and to attract talented people with retailing experience to help him grow the business. Although he started out as a seat-of-the-pants merchant, he had great instincts, was quick to learn from other retailers' successes and failures, and was adept at garnering ideas for

Exhibit 1   **Financial and Operating Summary, Wal-Mart Stores, Fiscal Years 1993–2005 (dollar amounts in billions, except earnings per share data)**

	Fiscal Year Ending January 31					
	2005	2004	2003	2002	2000	1993
Financial and operating data						
Net sales	$285.2	$256.3	$229.6	$204.0	$156.2	$55.5
Net sales increase	11.3%	11.6%	12.6%	12.8%	19.7%	26.0%
Domestic comparable store sales increase*	3%	4%	5%	6%	8%	11%
Cost of sales	219.8	198.7	178.3	159.1	121.8	44.2
Operating, selling, general and administrative expenses	51.1	44.9	40.0	35.1	26.0	8.3
Interest costs, net	1.0	0.8	0.9	1.2	0.8	0.3
Net income	$ 10.3	$ 8.9	$ 8.0	$ 6.4	$ 5.3	$ 2.0
Earnings per share of common stock (diluted)	$2.41	$2.07	$1.79	$1.47	$1.19	$0.44
Balance sheet data						
Current assets	$ 38.5	$ 34.2	$ 29.5	$ 26.6	$ 23.5	$10.2
Net property, plant, equipment, and capital leases	68.6	55.2	51.4	45.2	35.5	9.8
Total assets	120.2	104.9	92.9	81.5	69.0	20.6
Current liabilities	42.9	37.4	32.2	26.7	25.5	6.8
Long-term debt	20.1	17.5	16.6	15.7	13.7	3.1
Long-term obligations under capital leases	3.6	3.0	3.0	3.0	3.0	1.8
Shareholders' equity	49.4	43.6	39.5	35.2	25.9	8.6
Financial ratios						
Current ratio	0.9	0.9	0.9	1.0	0.9	1.5
Return on assets	9.3%	8.6%	9.2%	8.4%	9.8%	11.1%
Return on shareholders' equity	22.1%	20.6%	20.9%	19.4%	22.9%	25.3%
Other year-end data						
Number of domestic Wal-Mart discount stores	1,353	1,478	1,568	1,647	1,801	1,848
Number of domestic Wal-Mart Supercenters	1,713	1,471	1,258	1,066	721	34
Number of domestic Sam's Clubs	551	538	525	500	463	256
Number of domestic Neighborhood Markets	85	64	49	31	7	—
Number of international stores	1,587	1,355	1,272	1,154	991	10

*Based on sales at stores open a full-year that have not been expanded or relocated in the past 12 months.
Source: Wal-Mart annual reports for 2003 and 2005.

improvements from employees and promptly trying them out. Sam Walton incorporated his business as Wal-Mart Stores in 1969, with headquarters in obscure Bentonville, Arkansas—in 2005, the Wal-Mart-related traffic into and out of Bentonville was sufficient to support daily nonstop flights from New York City and Chicago. When the company went public in 1970, it had 38 stores and sales of $44.2 million. In 1979, with 276 stores, 21,000 employees, and operations in 11 states, Wal-Mart became the first company to reach $1 billion in sales in such a short period of time.

As the company grew, Sam Walton proved an effective and visionary leader. His folksy demeanor and his talent for motivating people, combined with a hands-on management style and an obvious talent for discount retailing, produced a culture and a set of values and beliefs that kept Wal-Mart on a path of continuous innovation and rapid expansion. Moreover, Wal-Mart's success and Walton's personable style of leadership generated numerous stories in the media that cast the company and its founder in a positive light. As Wal-Mart emerged as the premier discount retailer in the United States in the 1980s, an uncommonly large cross-section of the American public came to know who Sam Walton was and to associate his name with Wal-Mart. Regarded by many as "the entrepreneur of the century" and "a genuine American folk hero," he enjoyed a reputation of being concerned for employees, community-spirited, and a devoted family man who epitomized the American dream and demonstrated the virtues of hard work. People inside and outside the company held him in high esteem.

Just before Sam Walton's death in 1992, his vision was for Wal-Mart to become a $125 billion company by 2000. But his handpicked successor, David D. Glass, beat that target by almost two years. Under Glass's leadership (1988–2000), Wal-Mart's sales grew at an average annual compound rate of 19 percent, pushing revenues up from $20.6 billion to $156 billion. When David Glass retired in January 2000, Lee Scott was chosen as Wal-Mart's third president and CEO. In the five years that Lee Scott had been CEO, Wal-Mart's sales had grown over $145 billion, almost matching the company's growth in its first 30 years. Even though there were Wal-Mart stores in all 50 states and 15 foreign countries in 2005, Scott and other senior executives believed there were sufficient domestic and foreign growth opportunities to permit the company to grow at double-digit rates for the foreseeable future and propel Wal-Mart's revenues past $500 billion by 2010. Wal-Mart had only a 3 percent share of global retail sales in the merchandise lines it stocked.

WAL-MART'S STRATEGY

The hallmarks of Wal-Mart's strategy were multiple store formats, low everyday prices, wide selection, a big percentage of name-brand merchandise, a customer-friendly store environment, low operating costs, innovative merchandising, a strong emphasis on customer satisfaction, disciplined expansion into new geographic markets, and the use of acquisitions to enter foreign country markets. On the outside of every Wal-Mart store in big letters was the message "We Sell for Less." The company's advertising tag line reinforced the low-price theme: "Always low prices. Always." Major merchandise lines included housewares, consumer electronics, sporting goods, lawn and garden items, health and beauty aids, apparel, home fashions, paint, bed and bath goods, hardware, jewelry, automotive repair and maintenance, toys and games, and groceries.

Multiple Store Formats

In 2005, Wal-Mart was seeking to meet U.S. customers' needs with four different retail concepts: Wal-Mart discount stores, Supercenters, Neighborhood Markets, and Sam's Clubs:

- *Discount stores*—These stores ranged from 40,000 to 125,000 square feet, employed an average of 150 people, and offered as many as 80,000 different items, including family apparel, automotive products, health and beauty aids, home furnishings, electronics, hardware, toys, sporting goods, lawn and garden items, pet supplies, jewelry, housewares, prescription drugs, and packaged grocery items. Discount stores had sales in the $30 to $50 million range, depending on store size and location.

- *Supercenters*—Supercenters, which Wal-Mart started opening in 1988 to meet a demand for one-stop family shopping, joined the concept of a general merchandise discount store with that of a full-line supermarket. They ranged from 109,000 to 220,000 square feet, employed between 200 and 550 associates, had about 36 general merchandise departments, and offered up to 150,000 different items, at least 30,000 of which were grocery products. In addition to the value-priced merchandise offered at discount stores and a large supermarket section with more than 30,000 items, Supercenters contained such specialty shops as vision centers, tire and lube expresses, fast-food restaurants, portrait studios, one-hour photo centers, hair salons, banking, and employment agencies. Typical Supercenters had annual sales in the $80–$100 million range.

- *Sam's Clubs*—A store format that Wal-Mart launched in 1983, Sam's was a cash-and-carry, members-only warehouse that carried about 4,000 frequently used, mostly brand-name items in bulk quantities along with some big-ticket merchandise. The product lineup included fresh, frozen, and canned food products, candy and snack items, office supplies, janitorial and household cleaning supplies and paper products, a selection of apparel, CDs and DVDs, and an assortment of big-ticket items (TVs, tires, large and small appliances, watches, jewelry, computers, camcorders, and other electronic equipment). Stores were approximately 110,000 to 130,000 square feet in size, with most goods displayed in the original cartons stacked in wooden racks or on wooden pallets. Many items stocked were sold in bulk quantity (five-gallon containers, bundles of a dozen or more, economy-size boxes). Prices tended to be 10–15 percent below the prices of the company's discount stores and Supercenters since merchandising costs and store operation costs were lower. Sam's was intended to serve small businesses, churches and religious organizations, beauty salons and barber shops, motels, restaurants, offices, local schools, families, and individuals looking for great prices on large-volume quantities or big-ticket items. Annual member fees were $30 for businesses and $35 for individuals—there were 46 million members in 2003. Sam's stores employed about 125 people and had annual sales averaging $67 million. A number of Sam's stores were located adjacent to a Supercenter or discount store.

- *Neighborhood Markets* Neighborhood Markets, launched in 1998, were designed to appeal to customers who just needed groceries, pharmaceuticals, or general merchandise. They were always located in markets with Wal-Mart Supercenters so as to be readily accessible to Wal-Mart's food distribution network. Neighborhood Markets ranged from 42,000 to 55,000 square feet, employed 80–100 people, and featured fresh produce, deli foods, fresh meat and dairy items, health and beauty aids, one-hour photo and traditional photo developing services, drive-through pharmacies, stationery and paper goods, pet supplies, and household supplies—about 28,000 items in total.

During 2005 and 2006, Wal-Mart expected to open about 70 new discount stores, 525 new Supercenters,

45 new Neighborhood Markets, and 75 new Sam's Clubs in the United States. Approximately 300 of the planned new U.S. Supercenters were expansions or relocations of existing discount stores, and approximately 35 of the Sam's Clubs were relocations or expansions. Internationally, Wal-Mart planned to open 390 units in the 15 countries where it already had stores; of these, 50 were expected to be relocations or expansions. In February 2005, it had 660 million square feet of selling space in its almost 5,300 retail stores across the world; it expected to add 55 million square feet of retail space in 2005 and another 60 million square feet in 2006. Wal-Mart was expanding most aggressively in Mexico, Brazil, and China. Since 2003, Wal-Mart had opened 18 new stores in China, a country where French retailer Carrefour (the world's second-largest retailer behind Wal-Mart) and Germany's Metro AG had stores.

Exhibit 2 shows the number of Wal-Mart stores in each state and country as of January 2005. There were still many locations in the United States that were underserved by Wal-Mart stores. Inner-city sections of New York City had no Wal-Mart stores of any kind because ample space with plenty of parking was unavailable at a reasonable price. Wal-Mart's first Supercenter in all of California opened in March 2004, and the whole state only had three Supercenters in early 2005. There were no Supercenters in New Jersey, Rhode Island, Vermont, and Hawaii, and only 2 in Massachusetts and 2 in Connecticut (versus 219 in Texas, 116 in Florida, 88 in Georgia, 75 in Tennessee, 71 in Alabama, and 70 in Missouri). Lee Scott believed that opportunities existed to have at least 5,500 Supercenters in the United States alone. Wal-Mart's various domestic and international stores were served by about 120 regional general merchandise and food distribution centers.

Wal-Mart's Geographic Expansion Strategy

One of the most distinctive features of Wal-Mart's domestic strategy in its early years was the manner in which it expanded into new geographic areas. Whereas many chain retailers achieved regional and national coverage quickly by entering the largest metropolitan centers before trying to penetrate less-populated markets, Wal-Mart always expanded into adjoining geographic areas, saturating each area with

Exhibit 2 **Wal-Mart's Store Count, January 2005**

State	Discount Stores	Supercenters	Sam's Clubs	Neighborhood Markets
Alabama	18	71	11	2
Alaska	7	0	3	0
Arizona	18	33	11	5
Arkansas	26	54	5	6
California	149	3	33	0
Colorado	15	40	15	0
Connecticut	28	4	3	0
Delaware	3	4	1	0
Florida	53	116	38	6
Georgia	23	88	21	0
Hawaii	7	0	2	0
Idaho	3	14	1	0
Illinois	78	45	28	0
Indiana	31	56	15	4
Iowa	20	33	7	0
Kansas	19	34	6	3
Kentucky	26	52	5	2
Louisiana	26	56	12	1
Maine	11	11	3	0
Maryland	33	6	13	0
Massachusetts	42	2	3	0
Michigan	41	30	24	0
Minnesota	33	16	13	0
Mississippi	14	51	6	1
Missouri	46	70	14	0
Montana	4	7	1	0
Nebraska	8	16	3	0
Nevada	9	12	5	4
New Hampshire	19	7	4	0
New Jersey	38	0	9	0
New Mexico	3	24	5	0
New York	53	27	18	0
North Carolina	41	65	19	0
North Dakota	8	0	2	0
Ohio	69	45	27	0
Oklahoma	33	49	8	14
Oregon	20	7	0	0
Pennsylvania	49	60	21	0
Rhode Island	7	1	1	0
South Carolina	16	45	9	0
South Dakota	5	5	2	0
Tennessee	21	75	15	4
Texas	80	219	69	28
Utah	4	24	7	5
Vermont	4	0	0	0

(Continued)

Exhibit 2   **Continued**

State	Discount Stores	Supercenters	Sam's Clubs	Neighborhood Markets
Virginia	22	56	13	0
Washington	24	13	3	0
West Virginia	6	23	4	0
Wisconsin	38	37	11	0
Wyoming	2	7	2	0
U.S. totals	1,353	1,713	551	85
International/Worldwide				
Argentina	0	11	0	0
Brazil	118*	17	12	2*
Canada	256	0	6	0
China	0	38	3	2
Germany	0	91	0	0
South Korea	0	16	0	0
Mexico	529†	89	61	0
Puerto Rico	9	4	9	32**
United Kingdom	263†	19	0	0
International totals:	942	285	91	37
Grand totals:	2,510	1,998	642	121

*Brazil includes 2 Todo Dias, 118 Bompreco.
†Mexico includes 162 Bodegas, 50 Suburbias, 48 Superamas, 269 Vips.
**Puerto Rico includes 32 Amigos.
‡United Kingdom includes 256 ASDA stores, 6 George stores, and 1 ASDA Living store.
Source: 2005 annual report.

stores before moving into new territory. New stores were usually clustered within 200 miles of an existing distribution center so that daily deliveries could be made cost-effectively; new distribution centers were added as needed to support store expansion into additional areas. In the United States, the really unique feature of Wal-Mart's geographic strategy had involved opening stores in small towns surrounding a targeted metropolitan area before moving into the metropolitan area itself—an approach Sam Walton had termed *backward expansion.* Wal-Mart management believed that any town with a shopping-area population of 15,000 or more was big enough to support a Wal-Mart discount store and that towns of 25,000 could support a Supercenter. Once stores were opened in towns around the most populous city, Wal-Mart would locate one or more stores in the metropolitan area and begin major market advertising. By clustering new stores in a relatively small geographic area, the company could share advertising expenses for breaking into a new market across all the area stores, a tactic Wal-Mart used to keep its advertising costs under 1 percent of sales (compared to 2 or 3 percent for other discount chains).

In recent years, Wal-Mart had been driving hard to expand its geographic base of stores outside the United States largely through acquisition and partly through new store construction. Wal-Mart's entry into Canada, Mexico, Brazil, Japan, Puerto Rico, China, Germany, South Korea, and Great Britain had all been accomplished by acquiring existing general merchandise or supermarket chains. In December 2005, Wal-Mart expanded its store base in Brazil by purchasing Portuguese retailer Sonae's 140-store Brazilian operations for $757 million; the acquisition boosted Wal-Mart's store portfolio in Brazil to 295 stores in 17 of Brazil's 26 states with sales totaling about $5 billion. In Mexico, Wal-Mart had sales of $12.5 billion in fiscal 2005 and had recently expanded its operations to a total of 756 stores with 112,000 employees. In late 2005, Wal-Mart had 47 stores and 27,000 employees in 20 China cities;

some of these stores had the highest traffic counts of any stores in the world. Wal-Mart China was ranked 8th among China's Top 50 Most Admired Companies by *Fortune China* in July 2004.

Wal-Mart also owned a 42 percent interest in Seiyu Ltd., Japan's fifth-largest supermarket chain, with 405 locations, and a 33⅓ percent interest in Central American Retail Holding Company (CARHCO), with 363 stores in Costa Rica, El Salvador, Guatemala, Honduras, and Nicaragua. Wal-Mart's entry into Japan via minority ownership of Seiyu had stirred a retailing revolution among Japanese retailers to improve their merchandising, cut their costs, lower their prices, and streamline their supply chains. Prior to buying the stake in Seiyu in 2002 (with an option to increase its ownership to 67 percent by 2007), Wal-Mart had studied the Japanese market for four years. Wal-Mart had a team of 15 people in Japan working with Seiyu to transition its operation to a low-cost, low-price retail structure. In late 2005, with Seiyu struggling to reduce its costs, Wal-Mart assumed control of Seiyu and stepped up efforts to bring down costs and integrate Seiyu into Wal-Mart's global procurement system and global data network.

Sales at Wal-Mart's international stores averaged over $35 million per store in fiscal 2005; the company's international division had fiscal 2005 sales of $56.3 billion (up 18.3 percent over fiscal 2004) and operating profits of $3.0 billion (up almost 26 percent). International sales accounted for nearly 20 percent of total sales in fiscal 2005, and the percentage was expected to rise in the coming years. Wal-Mart had more than 400,000 employees in its international operations.

Wal-Mart's international strategy was to "remain local" in terms of the goods it merchandised, its use of local suppliers where feasible, and in some of the ways it operated. Management strove to adapt the company's standard operating practices to be responsive to local communities and cultures, the needs and merchandise preferences of local customers, and local suppliers. Most store managers and senior managers in its foreign operations were natives of the countries where Wal-Mart operated; many had begun their careers as hourly employees. Wal-Mart did, however, have a program in which stores in different areas exchanged best practices.

Everyday Low Prices

While Wal-Mart had not invented the concept of everyday low pricing strategy, it had done a better job than any other discount retailer in executing the concept. Consumers widely saw the company as having the lowest everyday prices among general merchandise retailers. Studies showed that prices of its grocery items were 5 to 48 percent below such leading supermarket chain competitors as Kroger (which used the City Market brand in the states west of the Mississippi), Safeway, and Albertson's, after making allowances for specials and loyalty cards.[12] On average, Wal-Mart offered many identical food items at prices averaging 15 to 25 percent lower than traditional supermarkets. In-store services were also bargain-priced—customers could wire money for a flat $12.95 (versus a fee of $50 to wire $1,000 at Western Union) and could purchase money orders for 46 cents (versus the 90 cents charged by the U.S. Postal Service). Wal-Mart touted its low prices on its storefronts ("We Sell for Less"), in advertising, on signs inside its stores, and on the logos of its shopping bags.

Some economists believed that Wal-Mart's everyday low prices had reduced inflationary pressures economywide, allowing all U.S. consumers to benefit from the "Wal-Mart effect." Warren Buffet said, "You add it all up and they have contributed to the financial well-being of the American public more than any other institution I can think of."[13] A 2005 study showed that the competitive effect of Wal-Mart's low prices saved each American household an average of $2,329 in 2004.[14] The presence of Wal-Mart stores in a new geographic area created a direct price effect by offering a lower-price option to consumers and an indirect price effect stemming from lower prices on the part of nearby retailers to better compete with Wal-Mart.

Merchandising Innovations

Wal-Mart was unusually active in testing and experimenting with new merchandising techniques. From the beginning, Sam Walton had been quick to imitate good ideas and merchandising practices employed by other retailers. According to the founder of Kmart, Sam Walton "not only copied our concepts; he strengthened them. Sam just took the ball and ran with it."[15] Wal-Mart prided itself on its "low threshold for change," and much of management's time was spent talking to vendors, employees, and customers to get ideas for how Wal-Mart could improve. Suggestions were actively solicited from employees. Most any reasonable idea was tried; if it worked well in stores where it was first tested, then it was quickly implemented in other stores. Experiments in store layout, merchandise displays, store color schemes, merchandise selection (whether to add more upscale lines or shift to a different mix of items), and sales promotion techniques were always under way. Wal-Mart was regarded as an industry leader in testing, adapting, and applying a wide range of cutting-edge merchandising approaches. In 2005 Wal-Mart began upgrading the caliber of the merchandise it stocked in certain departments so as to be more competitive with Target, its major rival in discount retailing.

Advertising

Wal-Mart relied less on advertising than most other discount chains. The company distributed only one or two circulars per month and ran occasional TV ads, relying primarily on word of mouth to communicate its marketing message. Wal-Mart's advertising expenditures ran about 0.3 percent of sales revenues, versus 1.5 percent for Kmart and 2.3 percent for Target. Wal-Mart's spending for radio and TV advertising was said to be so low that it didn't register on national ratings scales. Most Wal-Mart broadcast ads appeared on local TV and local cable channels. Wal-Mart did no advertising for its Sam's Club stores. The company often allowed charities to use its parking lots for their fund-raising activities.

WAL-MART'S COMPETITORS

Discount retailing was an intensely competitive business. Competition among discount retailers centered around pricing, store location, variations in store format and merchandise mix, store size, shopping atmosphere, and image with shoppers. Wal-Mart's primary competitors were Kmart and Target. Like Wal-Mart, Kmart and Target had general merchandise stores and superstores (Super Target and Super Kmart) that also had a full-line supermarket on one side of the store. Wal-Mart also competed against category retailers like Best Buy and Circuit City in electronics; Toy "R" Us in toys; Goody's in apparel; Bed, Bath, and Beyond in household goods; and Kroger, Albertson's, and Safeway in groceries.

Wal-Mart's rapid climb to become the largest supermarket retailer via its Supercenters had triggered heated price competition in the aisles of most supermarkets. Wal-Mart's three major rivals—Kroger, Albertson's and Safeway—along with a host of smaller regional supermarket chains were scrambling to cut costs, narrow the price gap with Wal-Mart, and otherwise differentiate themselves so as to retain their customer base and grow revenues. Continuing increases in the number of Wal-Mart Supercenters meant that the majority of rival supermarkets would be within 10 miles of a Supercenter by 2010. Wal-Mart had recently concluded that it took fewer area residents to support a Supercenter than it had thought; management believed that Supercenters in urban areas could be as little as four miles apart and still attract sufficient store traffic.

The two largest competitors in the warehouse club segment were Costco and Sam's Clubs; BJ's Wholesale Club, a smaller East Coast chain, was the only other major U.S. player in this segment.[16] In 2005 Costco had sales of $51.9 billion at 464 stores versus $37.1 billion at 551 stores for Sam's. The average Costco store generated annual revenues of $112 million, over 65 percent more than the $67 million average at Sam's. Costco catered to affluent households with upscale tastes and located its stores in mostly urban areas. Costco's 45.3 million members averaged 11.4 store visits annually and spent an average of $94 per visit, which compared favorably with averages of 8.5 visits and expenditures of $78 at Sam's. Costco was the United States' biggest retailer of fine wines ($600 million annually) and roasted chickens (55,000 rotisserie chickens a day). While its product line included food and household items, sporting goods, vitamins, and various other merchandise, its major attraction was big-ticket luxury items (diamonds and plasma TVs) and the latest gadgets at bargain prices (Costco capped its markups at 14 percent). Costco had beaten Sam's in being the first to sell fresh meat and produce (1986 versus 1989), to introduce private-label items (1995 versus 1998), and to sell gasoline

(1995 versus 1997). Costco offered its workers good wages and fringe benefits (full-time hourly workers made about $40,000 after four years).

Internationally, Wal-Mart's biggest competitor was Carrefour, a France-based retailer with nearly 12,000 stores of varying formats and sizes across much of Europe and in such emerging markets as Argentina, Brazil, China, South Korea, and Taiwan. Both Wal-Mart and Carrefour were expanding aggressively in Brazil and China, going head-to-head in an increasing number of locations. In 2005, Carrefour had 1,330 stores in Asia and Latin America with sales approximating €12 million; there were 69 Carrefour hypermarkets in China. Overall, Carrefour had sales close to €95 billion in 2005.

WAL-MART'S APPROACHES TO STRATEGY EXECUTION

To profitably execute its everyday-low-price strategy, Wal-Mart put heavy emphasis on getting the lowest possible prices from its suppliers, forging close working relationships with key suppliers in order to capture win–win cost savings throughout its supply chain, keeping its internal operations lean and efficient, paying attention to even the tiniest details in store layouts and merchandising, making efficient use of state-of-the art technology, and nurturing a culture that thrived on customer service, hard work, constant improvement, and low prices.

Relationships with Suppliers

Wal-Mart was far and away the biggest customer of virtually all of its suppliers. Wal-Mart's scale of operation (see Exhibit 3) allowed it to bargain hard with suppliers and get their bottom prices. During part of 2005, Wal-Mart's requirements for PCs for the holiday sales season was so big that Hewlett-Packard devoted 3 of its 10 PC plants operated by contract manufacturers to turning out products solely for Wal-Mart. Wal-Mart looked for suppliers that were dominant in their category (thus providing strong brand-name recognition), could grow with the company, had full product lines (so that Wal-Mart buyers could both cherry-pick and get some sort of limited exclusivity on the products it chose to carry), had the long-term commitment to R&D to bring new and better products to retail shelves, and had

Exhibit 3   **The Scale of Wal-Mart's Purchases from Selected Suppliers and Its Market Shares in Selected Product Categories**

Supplier	Percent of Total Sales to Wal-Mart	Product Category	Wal-Mart's U.S. Market Share*
Tandy Brands Accessories	39%	Dog food	36%
Dial	28	Disposable diapers	32
Del Monte Foods	24	Photographic film	30
Clorox	23	Shampoo	30
Revlon	20–23	Paper towels	30
RJR Tobacco	20	Toothpaste	26
Procter & Gamble	17	Pain remedies	21
		CDs, DVDs, and videos	15–20
		Single-copy sales of magazines	15
Although sales percentages were not available, Wal-Mart was also the biggest customer of Disney, Campbell Soup, Kraft, and Gillette		Although market shares were not available, Wal-Mart was also the biggest seller of toys, guns, diamonds, detergent, video games, socks, and bedding.	

*Based on sales through food, drug, and mass merchandisers.

Sources: Jerry Useem, "One Nation Under Wal-Mart," *Fortune,* March 3, 2003, p. 66, and Anthony Bianco and Wendy Zellner, "Is Wal-Mart Too Powerful?" *BusinessWeek,* October 6, 2003, p. 102.

the ability to become more efficient in producing and delivering what they supplied. But it also dealt with thousands of small suppliers (mom-and-pop operations, small farmers, and minority businesses) that could furnish particular items for stores in a certain geographical area. Many Wal-Mart stores had a "Store of the Community" section that showcased local products from local producers; in addition, Wal-Mart had set up an export office in the United States to help small and medium-sized businesses export their American-made products (especially to Wal-Mart stores in foreign countries).

Wal-Mart buyers literally shopped the world for merchandise suitable for the company's stores—they purchased goods from 61,000 U.S. suppliers and 7,000 foreign suppliers in 2005; the purchases from U.S. suppliers totaled $150 billion. Procurement personnel spent a lot of time meeting with vendors and understanding their cost structure. By making the negotiation process transparent, Wal-Mart buyers soon learned whether a vendor was doing all it could to cut down its costs and quote Wal-Mart an attractively low price. Wal-Mart's purchasing agents were dedicated to getting the lowest prices they could, and they did not accept invitations to be wined or dined by suppliers. The marketing vice president of a major vendor told *Fortune* magazine:

> They are very, very focused people, and they use their buying power more forcefully than anybody else in America. All the normal mating rituals are verboten. Their highest priority is making sure everybody at all times in all cases knows who's in charge, and it's Wal-Mart. They talk softly, but they have piranha hearts, and if you aren't totally prepared when you go in there, you'll have your ass handed to you.[17]

All vendors were expected to offer their best price without exception; one consultant that helped manufacturers sell to retailers observed, "No one would dare come in with a half-ass price."[18]

Even though Wal-Mart was tough in negotiating for absolute rock-bottom prices, the price quotes it got were still typically high enough to allow suppliers to earn a profit. Being a Wal-Mart supplier generally meant having a stable, dependable sales base that allowed the supplier to operate production facilities in a cost effective manner. Moreover, once it decided to source from a vendor, then Wal-Mart worked closely with the vendor to find *mutually beneficial* ways to squeeze costs out of the supply chain. Every aspect of a supplier's operation got scrutinized—how products got developed, what they were made of, how costs might be reduced, what data Wal-Mart could supply that would be useful, how sharing of data online could prove beneficial, and so on. Nearly always, as they went through the process with Wal-Mart personnel, suppliers saw ways to prune costs or otherwise streamline operations in ways that enhanced their profit margins. In 1989 Wal-Mart became the first major retailer to embark on a program urging vendors to develop products and packaging that would not harm the environment. In addition, Wal-Mart expected its vendors to contribute ideas about how to make its stores more fun insofar as their products were concerned. Those suppliers that were selected as "category managers" for such product groupings as lingerie or pet food or school supplies were expected to educate Wal-Mart on everything that was happening in their respective product category.

Some 200 vendors had established offices in Bentonville to work closely with Wal-Mart on a continuing basis—most were in an area referred to locally as "Vendorville." Vendors were encouraged to voice any problems in their relationship with Wal-Mart and to become involved in Wal-Mart's future plans. Top-priority projects ranged from using more recyclable packaging to working with Wal-Mart on merchandise displays and product mix to tweaking the just-in-time ordering and delivery system to instituting automatic reordering arrangements to coming up with new products with high customer appeal. Most recently, one of Wal-Mart's priorities was working with vendors to figure out how to localize the items carried in particular stores and thereby accommodate varying tastes and preferences of shoppers in different areas where Wal-Mart had stores. Most vendor personnel based in Bentonville spent considerable time focusing on which items in their product line were best for Wal-Mart, where they ought to be placed in the stores, how they could be better displayed, what new products ought to be introduced, and which ones ought to be rotated out.

A 2005 survey conducted by Cannondale Associates found that manufacturers believed Wal-Mart was the overall best retailer with which to do business—the seventh straight year in which Wal-Mart was ranked number one.[19] Target was ranked second and Costco was ranked sixth. The criteria for the ranking included such factors as clearest company strategy, store branding, best buying teams, most innovative consumer marketing/merchandising, best supply chain management practices, overall business fundamentals, and best practice management of individual product categories. One retailing consultant said, "I think most [suppliers] would say Wal-Mart is their most profitable account."[20] While this might seem surprising because of Wal-Mart's enormous bargaining clout, the potentially greater profitability of selling to Wal-Mart stemmed from the practices of most other retailers to demand that suppliers pay sometimes steep slotting fees to win shelf space and their frequent insistence on supplier payment of such extras as in-store displays, damage allowances, handling charges, penalties for late deliveries, rebates of one kind or another, allowances for advertising, and special allowances on slow-moving merchandise that had to be cleared out with deep price discounts. Further, most major retailers expected to be courted with Super Bowl tickets, trips to the Masters golf tournament, fancy dinners at conventions and trade shows, or other perks in return for their business. All of these extras represented costs that suppliers had to build into their prices. At Wal-Mart everything was boiled down to one price number, and no funny-money extras ever entered into the deal.[21]

Most suppliers viewed Wal-Mart's single bottom-line price and its expectation of close coordination as a win–win proposition, not only because of the benefits of cutting out all the funny-money costs and solidifying their relationship with a major customer but also because what they learned from the collaborative efforts and data sharing often had considerable benefit in the rest of their operations. Many suppliers, including Procter & Gamble, liked Wal-Mart's supply chain business model so well that they had pushed their other customers to adopt similar practices.[22]

Wal-Mart's Standards for Suppliers In 1992 Wal-Mart began establishing standards for its suppliers, with particular emphasis on suppliers located in foreign countries that had a history of problematic wages and working conditions. Management believed that the manner in which suppliers conducted their business regarding long work hours, the use of child labor, discrimination based on race or religion or other factors, workplace safety, and lack of compliance with local laws and regulations could be attributed to Wal-Mart and affect its reputation with customers and shareholders. To mitigate the potential for

Wal-Mart to be adversely affected by the manner in which its suppliers conducted their business, Wal-Mart had established a set of supplier standards and formed an internal group to see that suppliers were conforming to the ethical standards and business practices stated in its published standards. The company's supplier standards had been through a number of changes as the concerns of Wal-Mart management evolved over time. In February 2003, Wal-Mart took direct control of foreign factory audits; factory certification teams based in offices in Bentonville, China, Singapore, India, United Arab Emirates, and Honduras were staffed with more than 200 Wal-Mart employees dedicated to monitoring foreign factory compliance with the company's supplier standards. All suppliers were asked to sign a document certifying their compliance with the standards and were required to post a version of the supplier standards in both English and the local language in each production facility servicing Wal-Mart. In 2004, Wal-Mart conducted 12,500 audits at 7,600 plants of suppliers; in 2005, about 20 percent of the audits conducted were to be unannounced.

Distribution Center Operations

Throughout the 1980s and 1990s, Wal-Mart had pursued a host of efficiency-increasing actions at its distribution centers. The company had been a global leader in automating its distribution centers and expediting the transfer of incoming shipments from manufacturers to its fleet of delivery trucks that made daily deliveries to surrounding stores. Prior to automation, bulk cases received from manufacturers had to be opened by distribution center employees and perhaps stored in bins, then picked and repacked in quantities needed for specific stores, and loaded onto trucks for delivery to Wal-Mart stores—a manual process that was error-prone and sometimes slow. Using state-of-the-art technology, Wal-Mart had automated many of the labor-intensive tasks, gradually creating an ever-more-sophisticated and cost-efficient system of conveyors, bar-coding machines, handheld computers, and other devices with the capability to quickly sort incoming shipments from manufacturers into smaller, store-specific quantities and route them to waiting trucks to be sent to stores to replenish sold merchandise. Often, incoming goods from manufacturers being unloaded at one section of the warehouse were immediately sorted into store-specific amounts and conveyed directly onto waiting Wal-Mart trucks headed for those particular stores—a large portion of the incoming inventory was in a Wal-Mart distribution center an average of only 12 hours. Distribution center employees had access to real-time information regarding the inventory levels of all items in the center and used the different bar codes for pallets, bins, shelves, and items to pick up for store orders. Handheld computers also enabled the packaging department to get accurate information about which items to pack for which store and what loading dock to have packages conveyed.

Wal-Mart's trendsetting use of cutting-edge retailing technologies and its best-practices leadership in supply chain activities had given it operating advantages and raised the bar not only for its competitors but for most other retailers as well. Distribution centers processed over 5 billion cases through the network to Wal-Mart's stores and Sam's Clubs.

Truck Fleet Operations

Wal-Mart used a fleet of more than 3,500 company-owned trucks and a force of more than 7,800 drivers to transport goods from its 120 distribution centers to its 5,300 stores. Wal-Mart hired only experienced drivers who had driven more than 300,000 accident-free miles with no major traffic violations. Distribution centers had facilities where drivers could shower, sleep, eat, or do personal business while waiting for their truck to be loaded. A truck dispatch coordinator scheduled the dispatch of all trucks based on the available time of drivers and estimated driving time between the distribution center and the designated store. Drivers were expected to pull their truck up to the store dock at the scheduled time (usually late afternoon or early evening) even if they arrived early; trucks were unloaded by store personnel during nighttime hours, with a two-hour gap between each new truck delivery (if more than one was scheduled for the same night.

In instances where it was economical, Wal-Mart trucks were dispatched directly to a manufacturer's facilities, picked up goods for one or more stores and delivered them directly, bypassing the distribution center entirely. Manufacturers that supplied certain high-volume items or even a number of different

items sometimes delivered their products in truckload lots directly to some or many of Wal-Mart's stores.

Store Construction and Maintenance

Wal-Mart management worked at getting more mileage out of its capital expenditures for new stores, store renovations, and store fixtures. Ideas and suggestions were solicited from vendors regarding store layout, the design of fixtures, and space needed for effective displays. Wal-Mart's store designs had open-air offices for management personnel that could be furnished economically and featured a maximum of display space that could be rearranged and refurbished easily. Wal-Mart claimed that the design and aisle width at its new Supercenters would accommodate 100 million shoppers per week. Because Wal-Mart insisted on a high degree of uniformity in the new stores it built, the architectural firm Wal-Mart employed was able to use computer modeling techniques to turn out complete specifications for 12 or more new stores a week. Moreover, the stores were designed to permit quick, inexpensive construction as well as to allow for low-cost maintenance and renovation. All stores were renovated and redecorated at least once every seven years. If a given store location was rendered obsolete by the construction of new roads and highways and the opening of new shopping locations, then the old store was abandoned in favor of a new store at a more desirable site. In 2003–2005, stores were being expanded or relocated at the rate of 100–200 annually.

In keeping with the low-cost theme for facilities, Wal-Mart's distribution centers and corporate offices were also built economically and furnished simply. The offices of top executives were modest and unpretentious. The lighting, heating, and air-conditioning controls at all Wal-Mart stores were connected via computer to Bentonville headquarters, allowing cost-saving energy management practices to be implemented centrally and freeing store managers from the time and worry of trying to hold down utility costs. Wal-Mart mass-produced a lot of its displays in-house, not only saving money but also cutting the time to roll out a new display concept to as little as 30 days. It also had a group that disposed of used fixtures and equipment that could not be used at other store via auctions at the store sites where the surplus existed—a calendar of upcoming auctions was posted on the company's Web site.

Wal-Mart's Use of Cutting-Edge Technology

Wal-Mart's approach to technology was to be on the offense—probing, testing, and then deploying the newest equipment, retailing techniques, computer software programs, and related technological advances to increase productivity and drive costs down. Wal-Mart was typically a first-mover among retailers in upgrading and improving its capabilities as new technology was introduced. The company's technological goal was to provide employees with the tools to do their jobs more efficiently and to make better decisions.

Wal-Mart began using computers to maintain inventory control on an item basis in distribution centers and in its stores in 1974. In 1981, Wal-Mart began testing point-of-sale scanners and then committed to systemwide use of scanning bar codes in 1983—a move that resulted in 25–30 percent faster check-out of customers. In 1984, Wal-Mart developed a computer-assisted merchandising system that allowed the product mix in each store to be tailored to its own market circumstances and sales patterns. Between 1985 and 1987, Wal-Mart installed the nation's largest private satellite communication network; this network allowed two-way voice and data transmission between headquarters, the distribution centers, and the stores and one-way video transmission from Bentonville's corporate offices to distribution centers and to the stores; the system was less expensive than the previously used telephone network. The video system was used regularly by company officials to speak directly to all employees at once.

In 1989, Wal-Mart established a direct satellite link with about 1,700 vendors supplying close to 80 percent of the goods sold by Wal-Mart; this link allowed the use of electronic purchase orders and instant data exchanges. Wal-Mart had also used the satellite system's capabilities to develop a credit card authorization procedure that took five seconds, on average, to authorize a purchase, speeding up credit check-out by 25 percent compared to the prior manual system. In the early 1990s, through pioneering collaboration with Procter & Gamble, it instituted an automated reordering system that notified suppliers as their items moved though store check-out lanes; this allowed suppliers to track sales and inventories of their products (so they could plan production and schedule shipments accordingly).

By 2003 the company had developed and deployed sophisticated information technology systems and online capability that not only gave it real-time access to detailed figures on most any aspect of its operations but also made it a leader in cost-effective supply chain management. It could track the movement of goods through its entire value chain—from the sale of items at the cash register backward to stock on store shelves, in-store backup inventory, distribution center inventory, and shipments en route. Moreover, Wal-Mart had collaborated with its suppliers to develop data-sharing capabilities aimed at streamlining the supply of its stores, avoiding both stock-outs and excess inventories, identifying slow-selling items that might warrant replacement, and spotting ways to squeeze costs out of the supply chain. The company's Retail Link system allowed 30,000 suppliers to track their wares through Wal-Mart's value chain, get hourly sales figures for each item, and monitor gross margins on each of their products (Wal-Mart's actual selling price less what it paid the supplier).

In mid-2003 in another of its trendsetting moves, Wal-Mart informed its suppliers that they had to convert to electronic product code (EPC) technology based on radio frequency identification (RFID) systems. The EPC technology involved embedding every single item that rolled off a manufacturing line with an electronic tag containing a unique number. When brought into range, EPC tags could be read by RFID scanners, thus allowing the company to locate and track items throughout the supply chain in real time. With EPC and RFID capability, every single DVD or can of soup or screwdriver in Wal-Mart's supply chain network or on its store shelves could be traced back to when it was made, where and when it arrived in a case or pallet of goods, and where and when it was sold or turned up missing. Further, EPC tags linked to an online database provided a secure way of sharing product-specific information with supply chain partners. Wal-Mart management believed that EPC technology, in conjunction with the expanding production of RFID-capable printers/encoders, had the potential to revolutionize the supply chain by providing more accurate information about product movement, stock rotation, and inventory levels; it was also seen as a significant tool for preventing theft and dealing with product recalls. An IBM study indicated that EPC tagging would reduce stock-outs by 33 percent, while an Accenture study showed that EPC/RFID technology could boost worker productivity by 5 percent and shrink working capital and fixed capital requirements by 5 to 30 percent. In 2005, EPC/RFID technology implementation was under way for Wal-Mart's top 200 suppliers, with around 20,000 suppliers to be involved in some way by the end of 2006.

In 2005, Wal-Mart's data center was tracking over 680 million stock-keeping units (SKUs) weekly. The company had over 75,000 associates in logistics and in its information systems division. The attention Wal-Mart management placed on using cutting-edge technology and the astuteness with which it deployed this technology along its value chain to enhance store operations and continuously drive down costs had, over the years, resulted in Wal-Mart's being widely regarded as having the most cost-effective, data-rich information technology (IT) systems of any major retailer in the world. It spent less than 1 percent of revenues on IT, far less than other retailers, and had stronger capabilities. According to Linda Dillman, Wal-Mart's chief information officer, "The strength of this division is, we are doers and do things faster than lightning. We can implement things faster than anyone could with a third party. We run the entire world out of facilities in this area [Bentonville] at a cost that no one can touch. We'd be nuts to outsource."[23] Wal-Mart rarely used commercial software, preferring to develop its own IT systems. So powerful had Wal-Mart's influence been on retail supply chain efficiency that its competitors (and many other retailers as well) had found it essential to follow Wal-Mart's lead and pursue "Wal-Martification" of their retail supply chains.[24]

Wal-Mart's Approach to Customer Service

Wal-Mart tried to put some organization muscle behind its pledge of "Satisfaction Guaranteed" and do things that would make customers' shopping experience at Wal-Mart pleasant. Store managers challenged store associates to practice what Sam Walton called "aggressive hospitality." A "greeter" was stationed at store entrances to welcome customers with a smile, thank them for shopping at Wal-Mart, assist them in getting a shopping cart, and answer questions about where items were located. Clerks and check-out workers were trained to be courteous and helpful and to exhibit a "friendly, folksy attitude." All store associates were called upon to display the "10-foot attitude" and commit to a pledge of friendliness: "I solemnly promise and declare that every customer that comes within ten feet of me, I will smile, look them in the eye, and greet them." Wal-Mart's management stressed five themes in training and supervising store personnel:

1. Think like a customer.
2. Sell what customers want to buy.
3. Provide a genuine value to the customer.
4. Make sure the customer has a good time.
5. Exceed the customer's expectations.

In all stores, efforts were made to present merchandise in easy-to-shop shelving and displays. Floors in the apparel section were carpeted to make the department feel homier and to make shopping seem easier on customers' feet. Store layouts were constantly scrutinized to improve shopping convenience and make it easier for customers to find items. Store employees wore blue vests with the tag line "How May I Help You?" on the back to make it easier for customers to pick them out from a distance. Fluorescent lighting was recessed into the ceiling to create a softer impression than exposed fluorescent lighting strips. Yet nothing about the decor conflicted with Wal-Mart's low-price image; retailing consultants considered Wal-Mart as being very adept at sending out an effective mix of vibes and signals concerning customer service, low prices, quality merchandise, and friendly shopping environment. Wal-Mart's management believed that the attention paid to all the details of making the stores more user-friendly and inviting caused shoppers to view Wal-Mart in a more positive light.

The Culture at Wal-Mart in 2005

Wal-Mart's culture in 2005 continued to be deeply rooted in Sam Walton's business philosophy and leadership style. Mr. Sam, as he was fondly called and remembered, not only was Wal-Mart's founder and patriarch but had also been its spiritual leader—and still was in many respects. Four key core values and business principles underpinned Sam Walton's approach to managing:[25]

- Treat employees as partners, sharing both the good and bad about the company so they will strive to excel and participate in the rewards. (Wal-Mart fostered the concept of partnership by referring to all employees as "associates," a term Sam Walton had insisted on from the company's beginnings because it denoted a partnerlike relationship.)

- Build for the future, rather than just immediate gains, by continuing to study the changing concepts that are a mark of the retailing industry and be ready to test and experiment with new ideas.

- Recognize that the road to success includes failing, which is part of the learning process rather than a personal or corporate defect or failing. Always challenge the obvious.

- Involve associates at all levels in the total decision-making process.

He practiced these principles diligently in his own actions and insisted that other Wal-Mart managers do the same. Until his health failed badly in 1991, he spent several days a week visiting the stores, gauging the moods of shoppers, listening to employees discuss what was on their minds, learning what was or was not selling, gathering ideas about how things could be done better, complimenting workers on their efforts, and challenging them to come up with good ideas.

The values, beliefs, and practices that Sam Walton instilled in Wal-Mart's culture and that still carried over in 2005 were reflected in statements made in his autobiography:

> Everytime Wal-Mart spends one dollar foolishly, it comes right out of our customer's pockets. Everytime we save a dollar, that puts us one more step ahead of the competition—which is where we always plan to be.

> One person seeking glory doesn't accomplish much; at Wal-Mart, everything we've done has been the result of people pulling together to meet one common goal.

> I have always been driven to buck the system, to innovate, to take things beyond where they've been.

> We paid absolutely no attention whatsoever to the way things were supposed to be done, you know, the way the rules of retail said it had to be done.

> I'm more of a manager by walking and flying around, and in the process I stick my fingers into everything I can to see how it's coming along . . . My appreciation for numbers has kept me close to our operational

statements, and to all the other information we have pouring in from so many different places.

> The more you share profit with your associates—whether it's in salaries or incentives or bonuses or stock discounts—the more profit will accrue to your company. Why? Because the way management treats the associates is exactly how the associates will then treat the customers. And if the associates treat the customers well, the customers will return again and again.

> There's no better way to keep someone doing things the right way than by letting him or her know how much you appreciate their performance.

> The bigger we get as a company, the more important it becomes for us to shift responsibility and authority toward the front lines, toward that department manager who's stocking the shelves and talking to the customer.

> We give our department heads the opportunity to become real merchants at a very early stage of the game . . . we make our department heads the managers of their own businesses . . . We share everything with them: the costs of their goods, the freight costs, the profit margins. We let them see how their store ranks with every other store in the company on a constant, running basis, and we give them incentives to want to win.

> We're always looking for new ways to encourage our associates out in the stores to push their ideas up through the system . . . Great ideas come from everywhere if you just listen and look for them. You never know who's going to have a great idea.

> A lot of bureaucracy is really the product of some empire builder's ego . . . We don't need any of that at Wal-Mart. If you're not serving the customers, or supporting the folks who do, we don't need you.

> You can't just keep doing what works one time, because everything around you is always changing. To succeed, you have to stay out in front of that change.[26]

Walton's success flowed from his cheerleading management style, his ability to instill the principles and management philosophies he preached into Wal-Mart's culture, the close watch he kept on costs, his relentless insistence on continuous improvement, and his habit of staying in close touch with both consumer and associates. It was common practice for Walton to lead cheers at annual shareholder meetings, store visits, managers' meetings, and company events. His favorite was the Wal-Mart cheer:

Give me a W!
Give me an A!
Give me an L!
Give me a squiggly! (Here, everybody sort of does the twist.)
Give me an M!
Give me an A!
Give me an R!
Give me a T!
What's that spell?
Wal-Mart!
Whose Wal-Mart is it?
My Wal-Mart!
Who's number one?
The Customer! Always!

In 2005, the Wal-Mart cheer was still a core part of the Wal-Mart culture and was used throughout the company at meetings of store employees, managers, and corporate gatherings in Bentonville to create a "whistle while you work" atmosphere, loosen everyone up, inject fun and enthusiasm, and get sessions started on a stimulating note. While the cheer seemed corny to outsiders, once they saw the cheer in action at Wal-Mart, they came to realize its cultural power and significance. And much of Sam Walton's cultural legacy remained intact in 2005, most especially among the company's top decision makers and longtime managers. As a *Fortune* writer put it:

> Spend enough time inside the company—where nothing backs up a point better than a quotation from Walton scripture—and it's easy to get the impression that the founder is orchestrating his creation from the beyond.[27]

The Three Basic Beliefs Underlying the Wal-Mart Culture in 2005   Wal-Mart's top management stressed three basic beliefs that Sam Walton had preached since 1962:[28]

1. *Every individual deserves to be treated with respect and dignity.* Management consistently drummed the theme that dedicated, hardworking, ordinary people who teamed together and who treated each other with respect and dignity could accomplish extraordinary things. Throughout company literature, comments could be found referring to Wal-Mart's "concern for the individual." Such expressions as "Our people make the difference," "We care about people," and "People helping People" were used repeatedly by Wal-Mart executives and store managers to create and nurture a family-oriented atmosphere among store associates.

2. *Service to customers is the top priority.* Management stressed that the company was nothing without its customers. To satisfy customers and keeping them coming back again and again, management emphasized that customers had to trust in Wal-Mart's pricing philosophy and to always be able to find the lowest prices with the best possible service. One of the standard Wal-Mart mantras preached to all associates was that the customer was number one and that the customer was boss. Associates in stores were urged to observe the rule regarding the "10-foot attitude."

3. *We must strive for excellence.* The concept of striving for excellence stemmed from Sam Walton's conviction that prices were seldom as low as they needed to be and that product quality was seldom as high as customers deserved. The thesis at Wal-Mart was that new ideas and ambitious goals made the company reach further and try harder—the process of finding new and innovative ways to push boundaries and constantly improve made the company better at what it did and contributed to higher levels of customer satisfaction. Wal-Mart managers at all levels spent much time and effort motivating associates to offer ideas for improvement, and to function as partners. It was iterated over and over that every cost counted and that every worker had a responsibility to be involved.

These three beliefs were supplemented by several supporting cultural themes and practices:

- *Go all out to exceed customers' expectations, and make sure that customers have a good time shopping at Wal-Mart.* Every associate repeatedly heard, "The customer is boss and the future depends on you."

- *Practice Sam Walton's 10 rules for building a business.* Management had distilled much of Sam Walton's business philosophy into 10 rules (see Exhibit 4); these were reiterated to associates and used at meetings to guide decision making and the crafting and executing of Wal-Mart's strategy.

- *Observe the Sundown Rule.* Answer requests by sundown on the day they are received. Management believed this working principle had to be taken seriously in a busy world where people's job performance depended on cooperation from others.

Wal-Mart's culture had unusually deep roots at the headquarters complex in Bentonville. The numerous journalists and business executives who had been to Bentonville and spent much time at Wal-Mart's corporate offices uniformly reported being impressed with the breadth, depth, and pervasive power of the company's culture. Jack Welch, former CEO of General Electric and a potent culture builder in his own right, noted that "the place vibrated" with cultural energy. There was little evidence that the culture in Bentonville was any weaker in 2005 than it had been 15 years earlier when Sam Walton personally led the culture-building, culture-nurturing effort. An atmosphere of frugality continued to prevail—Wal-Mart associates, including executives, flew coach, shared hotel rooms, and emptied their own trash. The philosophy was, "If we can go without something to save money, we do. It's the cornerstone of our culture to pass on our savings. Every penny we save is a penny in our customers' pockets."[29]

But Wal-Mart executives nonetheless were currently facing a formidable challenge in sustaining the culture in the distribution centers and especially in the stores. Annual turnover rates at Wal-Mart stores ran about 40 percent in 2002–2005 and had run as high as 70 percent in 1999 when the economy was booming and the labor market was tight. Such high rates of turnover among the company's 1.6 million worldwide workforce, coupled with the fact that Wal-Mart was adding about 120,000 additional associates annually to staff its new stores and distribution centers, made keeping the culture intact outside Bentonville a Herculean task. No other company in all of business history had been confronted with cultural indoctrination of so many new employees in so many locations in such a relatively short time.

Soliciting Ideas from Associates

Associates at all levels were expected to be an integral part of the process of making the company better. Wal-Mart store managers usually spent a portion of each day walking around the store checking on how well things were going in each department, listening to associates' comments, soliciting suggestions and discussing how improvements could be made, and praising associates who were doing a good job. Store managers frequently asked associates what needed to be done better in their department and what could be changed to improve store operations. Associates who believed a certain policy or procedure detracted from operations were encouraged to challenge and change it. Task forces to evaluate ideas and plan out future actions to implement them were common, and it was not unusual for the person who developed the idea to be appointed the leader of the group.

Listening to employees was a very important part of each manager's job. All of Wal-Mart's top executives relied on management by walking around; they visited stores, distribution centers, and support facilities regularly, staying on top of what was happening and listening to what employees had to say about how things were going. Senior managers at Wal-Mart's Bentonville headquarters believed that visiting stores and listening to associates was time well spent because a number of the company's best ideas had come from Wal-Mart associates—Wal-Mart's use of people greeters at store entrances was one of those ideas.

Compensation and Benefits

In 2005, Wal-Mart's average hourly wage for regular full-time associates in the United States was $9.68 an hour (the federal minimum wage was $5.15, and the average hourly wage of retail workers was $12.28—Costco, one of Wal-Mart's rivals paid its hourly workers an average of $16.00 per hour).[30] The average was higher in certain urban areas, for example, Chicago ($10.69), Atlanta ($10.80), and Los Angeles ($9.99).[31] Store clerks generally earned the lowest wage; workers who unloaded trucks and stocked store shelves could earn anywhere from $25,000 to $50,000. New hourly associates in the United States were paid anywhere from $1 to $6 above the minimum wage, depending on the type of job, and could expect to receive a raise within the first year at one or both of the semiannual job evaluations. Typically, at least one raise was guaranteed in the first year if Wal-Mart planned to keep the individual on the staff. The other raise depended on how well the associate worked and improved during the year. At the store level, only the store manager was salaried; all other associates, including the department managers, were considered hourly employees. Store managers generally had six-figure incomes.

Exhibit 4   **Sam Walton's Rules for Building a Business**

Rule 1: Commit to your business. Believe in it more than anybody else. I think I overcame every single one of my personal shortcomings by the sheer passion I brought to my work. I don't know if you're born with this kind of passion, or if you can learn it. But I do know you need it. If you love your work, you'll be out there every day trying to do it the best you possibly can, and pretty soon everybody around will catch the passion from you—like a fever.

Rule 2: Share your profits with all your Associates, and treat them as partners. In turn, they will treat you as a partner, and together you will all perform beyond your wildest expectations. Remain a corporation and retain control if you like, but behave as a servant leader in a partnership. Encourage your Associates to hold a stake in the company. Offer discounted stock, and grant them stock for their retirement. It's the single best thing we ever did.

Rule 3: Motivate your partners. Money and ownership alone aren't enough. Constantly, day-by-day, think of new and more interesting ways to motivate and challenge your partners. Set high goals, encourage competition, and then keep score. Make bets with outrageous payoffs. If things get stale, cross-pollinate; have managers switch jobs with one another to stay challenged. Keep everybody guessing as to what your next trick is going to be. Don't become too predictable.

Rule 4: Communicate everything you possibly can to your partners. The more they know, the more they'll understand. The more they understand, the more they'll care. Once they care, there's no stopping them. If you don't trust your Associates to know what's going on, they'll know you don't really consider them partners. Information is power, and the gain you get from empowering your Associates more than offsets the risk of informing your competitors.

Rule 5: Appreciate everything your Associates do for the business. A paycheck and a stock option will buy one kind of loyalty. But all of us like to be told how much somebody appreciates what we do for them. We like to hear it often, and especially when we have done something we're really proud of. Nothing else can quite substitute for a few well-chosen, well-timed, sincere words of praise. They're absolutely free—and worth a fortune.

Rule 6: Celebrate your successes. Find some humor in your failures. Don't take yourself so seriously. Loosen up, and everybody around you will loosen up. Have fun. Show enthusiasm—always. When all else fails, put on a costume and sing a silly song. Then make everybody else sing with you. Don't do a hula on Wall Street. It's been done. Think up your own stunt. All of this is more important, and more fun, than you think, and it really fools the competition. "Why should we take those cornballs at Wal-Mart seriously?"

Rule 7: Listen to everyone in your company. And figure out ways to get them talking. The folks on the front lines—the ones who actually talk to the customer—are the only ones who really know what's going on out there. You'd better find out what they know. This really is what total quality is all about. To push responsibility down in your organization, and to force good ideas to bubble up within it, you must listen to what your Associates are trying to tell you.

Rule 8: Exceed your customers' expectations. If you do, they'll come back over and over. Give them what they want—and a little more. Let them know you appreciate them. Make good on all your mistakes, and don't make excuses—apologize. Stand behind everything you do. The two most important words I ever wrote were on that first Wal-Mart sign, "Satisfaction Guaranteed." They're still up there, and they have made all the difference.

Rule 9: Control your expenses better than your competition. This is where you can always find the competitive advantage. For 25 years running—long before Wal-Mart was known as the nation's largest retailer—we ranked No. 1 in our industry for the lowest ratio of expenses to sales. You can make a lot of different mistakes and still recover if you run an efficient operation. Or you can be brilliant and still go out of business if you're too inefficient.

Rule 10: Swim upstream. Go the other way. Ignore the conventional wisdom. If everybody else is doing it one way, there's a good chance you can find your niche by going in exactly the opposite direction. But be prepared for a lot of folks to wave you down and tell you you're headed the wrong way. I guess in all my years, what I heard more often than anything was: a town of less than 50,000 population cannot support a discount store for very long.

Source: www.walmartstores.com (accessed December 19, 2005).

In fiscal 2005, nearly 11,000 hourly associates in the United States were promoted to management positions; 76 percent of those in management positions in Wal-Mart's stores had been promoted from hourly jobs. The company's U.S. workforce included 220,000 seniors 55 and older, 775,000 women, 139,000 Hispanics, and 208,000 African Americans.

A majority of Wal-Mart's hourly store associates in the United States worked full-time—at most U.S. retailers, the percentage of full-time employees ranged between 20 and 40 percent. Part-time jobs at Wal-Mart were most common among sales clerks and check-out personnel in the stores where customer traffic varied appreciably during days of the week and months of the year. New full-time and part-time associates became eligible for health care benefits after a six-month wait and a one-year exclusion for preexisting conditions.

As of 2005, about 620,000 of Wal-Mart's 1.3 million associates in the United States (48 percent) had signed up for health insurance coverage in a Wal-Mart-sponsored plan (compared with an average of 72 percent for the whole retailing industry). Many Wal-Mart associates did not sign up for health coverage because another household member already had family coverage at his or her place of employment. Worker premiums for coverage were as little as $11 per month for individuals and 30 cents per day for children (no matter how many children an associate had). There were several plans that workers could choose from; usually, the lower the premium, the higher the annual deductible. The health benefit package covered 100 percent of most major medical expenses above $1,750 in employee out-of-pocket expenses and entailed no lifetime cap on medical cost coverage (a feature offered by fewer than 50 percent of employers).[32] The company's health benefits also included dental coverage, short- and long-term disability, an illness protection plan, and business travel accident insurance. But to help control its health costs for associates, Wal-Mart's health care plan did not pay for flu shots, eye exams, child vaccinations, chiropractic services, and certain other treatments allowed in the plans of many companies; further, Wal-Mart did not pay any health care costs for retirees. Due to Wal-Mart management's recent efforts to control costs for health benefits, the company's health care costs compared very favorably with those of other organizations:[33]

	Average Cost per Eligible Employee	
	2001	2002
U.S. employees of a cross-section of large, medium, and small companies	$4,924	$5,646
Employees of wholesale/retail stores	4,300	4,834
Wal-Mart employees (estimated)	3,000	3,500

However, critics assailed Wal-Mart's health care offering on grounds that the coverage was skimpier than that of many employers and that far too few Wal-Mart employees were eligible for coverage. According to 2005 data, 5 percent of Wal-Mart associates were on Medicaid, compared to an average for national employers of 4 percent, and 27 percent of associates' children were on such programs, compared to a national average of 22 percent. In total, 46 percent of associates' children were either on Medicaid or were uninsured.[34] Wal-Mart recognized that its critics had made valid points regarding the shortcomings of the company's health care offering. Starting in January 2006, Wal-Mart began providing health insurance to more than 1 million of its 1.7 million associates and offering up to 18 different plans.

Wal-Mart's package of fringe benefits for full-time employees (and some part-time employees) also included:

- Vacation and personal time.
- Holiday pay.
- Jury duty pay.
- Medical and bereavement leave.
- Military leave.
- Maternity/paternity leave.
- Confidential counseling services for associates and their families.
- Child care discounts for associates with children (through four national providers).
- GED reimbursement/scholarships for associates and their spouses.
- Discounts on selected merchandise (Sam's Club associates received a Sam's membership card at no cost).

In fiscal 2005, Wal-Mart spent $4.2 billion on benefits for its associates (equal to 1.9 percent of revenues), up from $2.8 billion in 2002 (1.5 percent of revenues). The company's benefit expenses were growing by 15 percent annually due to a combination of factors: growing workforce size, increased age and average tenure of associates, and rising cost trends for benefits, particularly health care. Top management and the board of directors were actively looking at strategies to contain the rising costs of the company's fringe benefit package, while at the same time preserving employee satisfaction with the benefit package and avoiding outcries from critics—in late 2005, a Wal-Mart executive provided the board of directors with a 12-page memo outlining "limited-risk" and "bold step" options for revising the company's benefits strategy.[35] Recent surveys of associates indicated overall satisfaction with the current benefit package (although this varied by benefit and associate demographics), but there was opposition to higher deductibles. Interestingly, the least healthy, least productive employees tended to be the most satisfied with their benefits and expressed interest in longer careers with Wal-Mart.

The Profit Sharing Plan   Wal-Mart maintained a profit-sharing plan for full and part-time associates; individuals were eligible after one year and 1,000 hours of service. Annual contributions to the plan were tied to the company's profitability and were made at the sole discretion of management and the board of directors. Employees could contribute up to 15 percent of their earnings to their 401(k) accounts. Wal-Mart's contribution to each associate's profit-sharing account became vested at the rate of 20 percent per year beginning the third year of participation in the plan. After the associate had been employed for seven continuous years, the company's contribution became fully vested; however, if the associate left the company prior to that time, the unvested portions were redistributed to all remaining employees. The plan was funded entirely by Wal-Mart, and most of the profit-sharing contributions were invested in Wal-Mart's common stock. In recent years, the company's contribution to profit sharing and the 401(k) plan had averaged 4 percent of an associate's eligible pay and amounted to $756 million in fiscal 2005 and $662 million in fiscal 2004; more than $4 billion had been contributed to associates' profit-sharing and 401(k) accounts since 1972. Associates could begin withdrawals from their account upon retirement or disability, with the balance paid to family members upon death.

Stock Purchase and Stock Option Plans   A stock purchase plan was adopted in 1972 to allow eligible employees a means of purchasing shares of common stock through regular payroll deduction or annual lump-sum contribution. Prior to 1990, the yearly maximum under this program was $1,500 per eligible employee; starting in 1990, the maximum was increased to $1,800 annually. The company contributed an amount equal to 15 percent of each participating associate's contribution. Longtime employees who had started participating in the early years of the program had accumulated stock worth over $100,000. About one-fourth of Wal-Mart's employees participated in the stock purchase plan in 1993, but this percentage had since declined, as many new employees opted not to participate.

In addition to regular stock purchases, certain employees qualified to participate in stock option plans; options expired 10 years from the date of the grant and could be exercised in nine annual installments. In 2005 over 80 million shares, with an estimated value of $3.8 billion, were reserved for issuance under the stock option plan.

Training

Top management was committed to providing all associates state-of-the-art training resources and development time to help achieve career objectives. The company had a number of training tools in place, including classroom courses, computer-based learning, distance learning, corporate intranet sites, mentor programs, satellite broadcasts, and skills assessments. In November 1985 the Walton Institute of Retailing was opened in affiliation with the University of Arkansas. Within a year of its inception, all Wal-Mart managers from the stores, the distribution facilities, and the general office were expected to take part in special programs at the Walton Institute to strengthen and develop the company's managerial capabilities.

Management Training   Wal-Mart store managers were hired in one of three ways. Hourly associates could move up through the ranks from sales to department manager to manager of the check lanes into store management training—more than 65 percent of Wal-Mart's managers had started out as hourly associates. Second, people with outstanding merchandising skills at other retail companies were recruited to join the ranks of Wal-Mart managers. And third, Wal-Mart recruited college graduates to enter the company's training program. Store management trainees went through an intensive on-the-job training program of almost 20 weeks and were then given responsibility for an area of the store. Trainees who progressed satisfactorily and showed leadership and job knowledge were promoted to an assistant manager, which included further training in various aspects of retailing and store operations. Given Wal-Mart's continued store growth, above-average trainees could progress to store manager within five years. Through bonuses for sales increases above projected amounts and company stock options, the highest-performing store managers earned well into six figures annually.

Associate Training   Wal-Mart did not provide a specialized training course for its hourly associates. Upon being hired, an associate was immediately placed in a position for on-the-job-training. From time to time, training films were shown in associates' meetings. Store managers and department managers were expected to train and supervise the associates under them in whatever ways were needed. As one associate put it, "Mostly you learn by doing. They tell you a lot; but you learn your job every day."

Special programs had been put in place to ensure that the company had an adequate talent pool of women and minorities who were well prepared for management positions. If company officers did not meet their individual diversity goals, their bonuses were cut 15 percent.

Meetings and Rapid Response

The company used meetings both as a communication device and as a culture-building exercise. In Bentonville, there were Friday merchandising meetings and Saturday morning meetings at 7:30 a.m. to review the week. The weekly merchandising meeting included buyers and merchandising staff headquartered in Bentonville and various regional managers who directed store operations. David Glass, Wal-Mart's former CEO explained the purpose of the Friday merchandise meeetings:

> In retailing, there has always been a traditional, head-to-head confrontation between operations and merchandising. You know, the operations guys say, "Why in the world would anybody buy this? It's a dog, and we'll never sell it." Then the merchandising folks say, "There's nothing wrong with that item. If you guys were smart enough to display it well and promote it properly, it would blow out the doors." So we sit all these folks down together every Friday at the same table and just have at it.
>
> We get into some of the doggonedest, knock-down drag-outs you have ever seen. But we have a rule. We never leave an item hanging. We will make a decision in that meeting even if it's wrong, and sometimes it

is. But when the people come out of that room, you would be hard-pressed to tell which ones oppose it and which ones are for it. And once we've made that decision on Friday, we expect it to be acted on in all the stores on Saturday. What we guard against around here is people saying, "Let's think about it." We make a decision. Then we act on it.[36]

At the Saturday-morning meetings—a Wal-Mart tradition since 1961—top officers and other key personnel gathered to exchange ideas on how well things were going and talk about any problems relating to the week's sales, store performance, special promotion items, store construction, distribution centers, transportation, supply chain activities, and so on. Management described the nature and purpose of the Saturday meetings as follows:

> Created with a sense of the unpredictable and intended to entertain as well as inform, the Saturday morning meeting lets everyone know what the rest of the company is up to.
>
> The agenda constantly changes, so each meeting has an element of spontaneity. Sometimes we'll bring associates from the field in to Bentonville to praise them in front of the whole meeting. Other mornings, an associate may get a standing ovation as he receives a 20-year service award.
>
> On any given Saturday, we may invite special guests to promote product launches or just to share insights. We've had CEOs of other Fortune 500 companies, musicians, actors, journalists, authors, athletes, politicians, and children's characters . . . That kind of unpredictability keeps things interesting.
>
> But beyond focusing on giving good news, entertaining special guests, and having a good time, we use that valuable time to critique our business. We review what we could do better and encourage suggestions about correcting those weaknesses. If the solution is obvious, we can order changes right then and carry them out over the weekend, while almost everyone else in retail business is off.
>
> The meeting is where we discuss and debate management philosophy and strategy. It's the focal point of our communication efforts, where we share ideas. We look at what our competition is doing well and look for ways to improve upon their successes in our own business. Often, it's the place where we decide to try things that seem unattainable, and instead of shooting those ideas down, we try to figure out how to make them work.
>
> The Saturday morning meeting remains the pulse of our culture.

As with the Friday merchandise meetings, decisions were made about what actions needed to be taken.

The store meetings and the Friday/Saturday meetings in Bentonville, along with the in-the-field visits by Wal-Mart management, created a strong bias for action. A *Fortune* reporter observed, "Managers suck in information from Monday to Thursday, exchange ideas on Friday and Saturday, and implement decisions in the stores on Monday."[31]

WAL-MART'S FUTURE

Sam Walton had engineered the development and rapid ascendancy of Wal-Mart to the forefront of the retailing industry—the discount stores and Sam's Clubs were strategic moves that he directed. His handpicked successor, David Glass, had directed the hugely successful move into Supercenters and grocery retailing, as well as presiding over the company's growth into the world's largest retailing enterprise; the Neighborhood Market store format also came into being during Glass's tenure as CEO. Lee Scott, Wal-Mart's third CEO, had the challenge of sustaining the company's growth, globalizing Wal-Mart's operations, continuing the long-term process of saturating the U.S. market with Supercenters, overseeing Wal-Mart's ever-larger business operations, and most recently, figuring out how to counteract the anti-Wal-Mart campaign being orchestrated by the company's critics and adversaries. Some of the issues that had come to his desk were embarrassing:

- In December 2005, Wal-Mart became the subject of a criminal investigation in Los Angeles over how it handled merchandise classified as hazardous waste. Wal-Mart apparently transported the materials from stores in California to a return center in Las Vegas before dumping them at a disposal site. But federal prosecutors said that process violated the U.S. Resource Conservation and Recovery Act. Instead of going to the return center in Vegas, the materials should have gone straight to the disposal site.

- Wal-Mart was ordered to compensate a number of former employees in Canada after it was ruled that the retail giant closed a store as a reprisal against unionization attempts. In Colorado, the United Food and Commercial Workers Union had accused Wal-Mart of harassing workers to keep them from joining its local in Denver and elsewhere; the number of such complaints had grown in recent years. A Wal-Mart board member, a high-level executive, and two Wal-Mart associates were dismissed following an internal investigation of improper expense account charges, improper payment of third-party invoices, and improper use of gift cards (some of which, according to critics, entailed efforts to finance anti-union activities and defeat unionization efforts at various Wal-Mart stores).

- An internal memo to Wal-Mart's board of directors, leaked to Wal-Mart Watch and the *New York Times,* proposed ways to control Wal-Mart's health care costs, including changing the benefits package in ways that would attract a healthier workforce and dissuade unhealthy people from coming to work at Wal-Mart. The memo stated that Wal-Mart associates spent an average of 8 percent of their incomes on heath care (premiums plus deductibles plus out-of-pocket expenses), an amount about twice the national average; the 8 percent number rose to as high as 13 percent on some of the plans that the company offered to employees. In 2004, 38 percent of Wal-Mart associates spent more than 16 percent of their Wal-Mart income on health care costs. Furthermore, the memo stated that Wal-Mart associates on the Family Plan for heath care sometimes had to spend 74 to 150 percent of annual income on health care costs before insurance took over the remaining costs of a serious health problem. All this was said to be a prime reason for Wal-Mart's expansion of health insurance coverage to more of its workforce as of January 2006.

- Wal-Mart had to temporarily stop selling guns at its 118 stores across California following what California's attorney general said were hundreds of violations of state laws. Investigations by California authorities revealed that six Wal-Mart stores had released guns before the required 10-day waiting period, failed to verify the identity of buyers properly, sold illegally to felons, and allowed other violations. Wal-Mart cooperated with governmental officials and agreed to immediately suspend firearm sales until correction action could be taken and store associates properly trained on state firearms laws.

- In New York state, Wal-Mart had run afoul of New York's 1988 toy weapons law. The toy guns Wal-Mart sold had an orange cap at the end of the barrel but otherwise looked real, thus violating New York laws banning toy guns with realistic colors such as black or aluminum and not complying with New York's requirement that toy guns have unremovable orange stripes along the barrel. Investigators from the state attorney general's office shopped 10 Wal-Marts in New York state from Buffalo to Long Island and purchased toy guns that violated the law at each of them. Wal-Mart had sold more than 42,000 toy guns in the state.

- In December 2005, federal agents executed search warrants on trailers belonging to five subcontracting companies working at the construction site of a new Wal-Mart distribution center in Pennsylvania. The warrants sought evidence of possible money laundering and using illegal immigrants to work on the project; 125 illegal aliens from Costa Rica, El Salvador, Guatemala, Honduras, and Mexico were detained shortly after they arrived to work at the construction site and placed into deportation proceedings.

- The discrimination lawsuit filed in 2003 by six female employees claimed that the company discriminated against women in pay, promotions, training, and job assignments—plaintiffs' attorneys asked for class action status for the lawsuit on behalf of all past and present female workers at Wal-Mart's U.S. stores. According to data from various sources, while two-thirds of Wal-Mart's hourly employees were women, less than 15 percent held store manager positions. There were also indications of pay gaps of 5–6 percent between male and female employees doing similar jobs and with similar experience levels; the pay gap allegedly widened higher up the management ladder. Male management trainees allegedly made an average of $23,175 a year, compared with $22,371 for women trainees.

- A 98-minute documentary entitled *Wal-Mart: The High Cost of Low Price* premiered in November 2005 and bashed the company for destroying once-thriving downtowns, running local merchants out of business, paying meager wages, selling goods produced in sweatshops in third world countries, and assorted other corporate sins. It showed testimony from ex-employees describing seedy practices and clips of individuals, families, and communities that had struggled to fight the company on various issues. Canadian unions had urged their 340,000 members to take time to see the documentary and, where possible, to arrange screenings at local meetings and other union events. Anti-Wal-Mart journalists had praised the documentary. The *San Francisco Bay Guardian* said the movie "will make you fear and loathe [Wal-Mart] even more. The unscrupulous megaretailer is exposed from every angle: its devastating effect on small businesses and communities; its inadequate health care plans; its rabid antiunion stance; the racism and sexism sprinkled throughout its ranks; its blatant disregard for environmental issues; its practice of importing nearly all of its goods (churned from company sweatshops in countries like China, Bangladesh, and Honduras); and—perhaps most offensively— its faux-homespun television advertisements, which cast a golden glow on a corporation that clearly cares not for human beings, but for cold, hard cash."[38]

But Wal-Mart was beginning to fight back. It had hired a public relations firm that had put a staff of seven professionals in Bentonville to assist Wal-Mart's own PR staff to get the company's story out and respond within hours to any new blast of criticism.[39] Since mid-2004, Lee Scott had done nine interviews on TV, met with the editorial boards of *The Wall Street Journal* and the *Washington Post,* been interviewed by numerous newspaper journalists, and spoken to business and community leaders in Chicago, Los Angeles, Istanbul, and Paris. The company was striving to build relationships with congressional delegations, governors, mayors, community leaders, and activists in key locations. It had run ads in more than 100 newspapers. And it created a Web site (walmartfacts.com) to help set the record straight about what Wal-Mart did and did not do.

Wal-Mart had received favorable publicity in the media following hurricane Katrina, when its response with food, supplies, and cash assistance was faster than the U.S. government's effort; Wal-Mart had also donated $15 million to the Katrina relief effort. And there was growing interest on the part of academic researchers over whether Wal-Mart had a positive or negative effect on the economy. A New York University economist reported that a Wal-Mart store opening in Glendale, Arizona, received 8,000 applications for 525 jobs. A University of Missouri economist in an article published in the prestigious

Review of Economics and Statistics found that the entry of a Wal-Mart store increased a county's retail employment by 100 jobs in the first year and over time led to the elimination of 50 jobs at less-efficient retailers. Studies also showed that new businesses quickly sprang up near Wal-Mart stores; both new and existing stores along the routes leading to a Wal-Mart tended to flourish because of the heavy traffic flow to and from the company's stores.

But heading into 2006, stories in the media continued to be critical of Wal-Mart's operating practices and of the company in general. It was unclear whether the company's charm offensive was having the desired impact on public opinion and whether Wal-Mart's growth and profitability would be adversely affected by its critics and adversaries.

Endnotes

[1]Kevin Haslett, "Unions Wage Vicious, Misguided War on Wal-Mart," December 19, 2005, posted at www.bloomberg.com (accessed December 20, 2005).

[2] www.walmartwatch.com (accessed December 20, 2005).

[3]As quoted in Lorrie Grant, "Retail Giant Wal-Mart Faces Challenges on Many Fronts," *USA Today,* November 11, 2003, p. B2.

[4]Anthony Bianco and Wendy Zellner, "Is Wal-Mart Too Powerful?" *BusinessWeek,* October 6, 2003, p. 103.

[5]Ibid.

[6]Ibid., p. 108.

[7]Ann Zimmerman, "After Huge Raid on Illegals, Wal-Mart Fires Back at U.S.," *The Wall Street Journal,* December 19, 2003, pp. A1, A10.

[8]Bianco and Zellner, "Is Wal-Mart Too Powerful?" pp. 104, 106.

[9]As quoted in "Can Wal-Mart Fit into a White Hat?" *BusinessWeek,* October 3, 2005, p. 94.

[10]Anthony Bianco and Wendy Zellner, "Is Wal-Mart Too Powerful?" *BusinessWeek,* October 6, 2003, p. 102.

[11]Jerry Useem, "One Nation Under Wal-Mart," *Fortune,* March 3, 2003, p. 66.

[12]The most recent study was done by Jerry Hausman (Ph.D. from MIT) and Ephraim Leibtag (from U.S. Department of Agriculture) in a paper entitled "Consumer Benefits from Increased Competition in Shopping Outlets: Measuring the Effect of Wal-Mart." The paper was presented at the Economic Impact Research Conference: An In-Depth Look at Wal-Mart and Society, held in Washington, D.C., on November 4, 2005.

[13]As quoted in Jerry Useem, "One Nation Under Wal-Mart," *Fortune,* March 3, 2003, p. 68.

[14]Global Insight, *The Economic Impact of Wal-Mart,* November 2005.

[15]As quoted in Bill Saporito, "What Sam Walton Taught America," *Fortune,* May 4, 1992, p. 105.

[16]The information in this paragraph is drawn from John Helyar, "The Only Company Wal-Mart Fears," *Fortune,* November 24, 2003, pp. 158–66.

[17]As quoted in *Fortune,* January 30, 1989, p.53.

[18]As quoted in Useem, "One Nation Under Wal-Mart;" p. 68.

[19]Cannondale Associates, 2005 PoweRanking Results, November 2, 2005; press release at www.cannondaleassoc.com (accessed December 15, 2005).

[20]As quoted in Useem, "One Nation Under Wal-Mart," p. 74.

[21]Ibid.

[22]Ibid.

[23]As quoted in "Wal-Mart's Way," *Information Week,* September 27, 2004,

[24]Paul Lightfoot, "Wal-Martification," *Operations and Fulfillment,* June 1, 2003, posted at www.opsandfulfillment.com.

[25]Sam Walton with John Huey, *Sam Walton: Made in America* (New York: Doubleday, 1992), p. 12.

[26]Ibid., pp. 10, 12, 47, 63, 115, 128, 135, 140, 213, 226–29, 233, 246, 249–54, and 256.

[27]Useem, "One Nation Under Wal-Mart," p. 72.

[28]Information posted at www.walmartstores.com (accessed December 19, 2005).

[29]Quote taken from the section on Wal-Mart Culture, posted at www.walmartstores.com (accessed December 19, 2005).

[30]Data for Wal-Mart are from company sources; the wage data for retail workers and Costco workers were cited in a May 3, 2005, article appearing in the *New York Times* that was quoted in part at www.walmartwatch.com (accessed December 20, 2005).

[31]Information posted at www.walmartstores.com (accessed December 10, 2005).

[32]Bernard Wysocki and Ann Zimmerman, "Wal-Mart Cost-Cutting Finds Big Target in Health Benefits," *The Wall Street Journal,* September 30, 2003, pp. A1, A16.

[33]Ibid.

[34]Based on an internal memo by Susan Chambers to Wal-Mart's board of directors that was leaked to Wal-Mart Watch and posted at www.walmartwatch.com (accessed December 20, 2005).

[35]The contents of the memo were obtained by Wal-Mart Watch and posted at www.walmartwatch.com (accessed December 2005).

[36]Walton with Huey, *Sam Walton,* pp. 225–26.

[37]Saporito, "What Sam Walton Taught America," p. 105.

[38]*San Francisco Bay Guardian,* November 23–29, 2005, posted at www.sfbg.com (accessed December 20, 2005).

[39]Robert Berner, "Can Wal-Mart Fit into a White Hat?" *BusinessWeek,* October 3, 2005, p. 94.

Outback Steakhouse

Sarah June Gauntlett
The University of Alabama

In the wake of changing executive leadership and rising energy and commodity costs, Outback Steakhouse Inc. was struggling to retain and increase market share in the casual-dining segment of the restaurant industry. Additionally, the 2005 hurricane season was devastating—15 percent of Outback restaurants were located in the areas hit by the hurricanes. From its inception, Outback had experienced tremendous growth, adding 30–65 new locations a year domestically and internationally, but the company had experienced soft revenue growth in 2004 as same-store sales did not increase. In response, Outback reinvented its menu by focusing on core specialties and introducing smaller portions for health-conscious consumers. Despite numerous obstacles and challenges, the company remained focused on its "Recipe for Success," which included preparing each meal from scratch and treating people as individuals. Outback's goal was to succeed one restaurant, one person at a time.

To help drive company growth, management had diversified into eight different restaurant formats and menus that spanned both casual and upscale dining:

- *Outback Steakhouse*—From the signature "Bloomin' Onion" to the full-flavored steaks, chops, ribs, chicken, and seafood, Outback Steakhouse offered quality food in a casual, Australian-themed atmosphere. Outback's service was defined by a promise of "No Rules. Just Right."

- *Carrabba's*—Carrabba's Italian Grill featured warm Italian hospitality; authentic aromas from a lively exhibition kitchen; and flavorful, hearty, handmade dishes prepared from original Carrabba family recipes.

- *Lee Roy Selmon's*—Lee Roy Selmon's was a family sports restaurant featuring heartwarming hospitality and generous portions of soul-satisfying comfort food. It was a favorite place to eat, drink, relax, and be with friends and family.

- *Cheeseburger in Paradise*—At Cheeseburger in Paradise, Jimmy Buffet's famous song came to life with the signature cheeseburger in a Key West–style setting. Great food, cool cocktails, and live music every night of the week combined for the ultimate experience in an escape to paradise.

- *Bonefish Grill*—Bonefish Grill specialized in market-fresh fish from all over the world, prepared over a wood-burning grill to ensure a tasty, even flavor. A tantalizing array of sauces and original toppings was offered to enhance the flavor of the fish, each in a fun and different way.

- *Fleming's Prime Steakhouse and Wine Bar*—Fleming's offered the best in steakhouse dining in a stylish, contemporary setting. Featuring the finest prime steaks, chops, fresh grilled fish, seafood and chicken, the menu was complemented by a unique and notable wine list featuring 100 fine wines by the glass.

- *Roy's*—Founded by James Beard Award winner Chef Roy Yamaguchi, Roy's exciting and innovative Hawaiian fusion cuisine incorporated the freshest local ingredients, European sauces, and bold Asian spices, with a focus on fresh seafood.

- *Paul Lee's Chinese Kitchen*—Friends and family delighted in traditional favorites and new specialties at Paul Lee's Chinese Kitchen, where only the freshest meats, fish, and vegetables are prepared in Chinese woks. For those too busy to dine in a warm, relaxed setting, there was a second kitchen dedicated solely to take-out.

AUSSIE BEGINNING

One evening in late 1987, Chris Sullivan, Bob Basham, and Tim Gannon gathered at a jazz club in Tampa, Florida, to brainstorm the name of their new restaurant venture. Their objective was to create a dining "experience" offering high-quality food and service, generous portions at moderate prices, and a casual atmosphere entrenched with an Australian theme. After the young men had downed several brews, the name Outback emerged as a suggestion and was unanimously agreed on. Shortly thereafter, Trudy Cooper joined the team and plans were made to open the very first Outback Steakhouse on Henderson Boulevard in Tampa, Florida. Tim Gannon, known as the "Food Guy," brought in world-renowned chef Warren Larue to design and create the menu for the new restaurant venture. Larue created bold, distinctive spices and a unique flavor for each dish. Originally, the Outback business plan consisted of four restaurants, one for each respective founder. The cofounders' intent was to have fun, earn a nice income, and enjoy a Florida lifestyle. The first restaurant, which opened in 1988, met with tremendous success. Word spread quickly among consumers and industry peers regarding the quality of food, with its bold flavors, and the "no rules" service style. The number of Outback Steakhouses grew rapidly: One restaurant soon became 4, then 10, then 20, and so on (see Exhibits 1 and 2).

Exhibit 2   **International Locations of Outback Restaurants, 2004**

Australia	Japan
Bahamas	Korea
Brazil	Malaysia
Canada	Mexico
China	Philippines
Costa Rica	Puerto Rico
Dominican Republic	Singapore
Guam	Thailand
Hong Kong	United Kingdom
Indonesia	Venezuela

Source: Outback Steakhouse Inc. 2004 annual report.

The Outback Steakhouse concept was clearly well accepted by customers, Outbackers (i.e., employees), and industry peers. Company-owned restaurants consisted of restaurants owned by partnerships (with the company as the general partner) and joint ventures (with the company as one of the two members). The company's ownership interests in partnerships and joint ventures generally ranged from 50 to 90 percent. Unique to the restaurant industry, Outback provided the opportunity for true ownership and self-responsibility, cutting the managing partner a 10 percent share of ownership in his or her restaurant. Company-owned restaurants also included restaurants owned by Roy's consolidated venture, in which the company had less than a majority ownership. The rationale for consolidating this venture was that Outback Steakhouse Inc. controlled the executive committee

Exhibit 1   **Outback Steakhouse Inc. Locations, 2004**

Outback Steakhouse Inc. and Affiliates	Outback Steakhouse (Domestic)	Outback Steakhouse (International)	Carrabba's Italian Grill	Bonefish Grill	Fleming's	Roy's	Other	Total
Company-owned	652	69	168	59	31	18	14	1,011
Development joint venture	1	12	—	—	—	—	—	13
Franchise	103	44	—	4	—	—	—	151
Total	756	125	168	63	31	18	14	1,175

Source: Outback Steakhouse Inc. 2004 annual report.

and had control through representation on the committee by related parties, enabling the company to direct management and daily operations. The company was responsible for 50 percent of the costs of new restaurants operated under this consolidated venture, and the joint venture partner was responsible for the other 50 percent. Restaurants with no direct investment from the company operated under franchise agreements with the company, receiving a specified percentage of net income. The results of company-owned restaurants were included in the consolidated statements of income, and the results of development-joint-venture restaurants were accounted for under the equity method of accounting.

FINANCIAL POSITION

Outback management periodically brainstormed options for funding capital to grow. On June 18, 1991, Outback Steakhouse Inc. held an initial public offering (IPO) for its common stock, selling 1.57 million shares at a price of $15 per share; the stock began trading on the Nasdaq. Between December 1991 and March 1999, Outback's stock split four times; in April 2000, the company moved trading from the Nasdaq to the New York Stock Exchange (NYSE). Chris Sullivan, Outback's chief executive officer, felt the move would benefit the shareholders by providing greater visibility and a broader investor base. The NYSE presented lower price volatility and smaller order execution costs that benefited investors. On October 23, 2002, the company declared its first quarterly dividend of $0.12 per share of common stock.

Beginning in December 2004, Outback started revising its accounting lease practices to include option renewals reasonably assumed to be exercised resulting in the restatement of the financial statements for the years ended December 31, 2004, 2003, and 2002. The restatement reflected estimated reductions of net income of approximately $3,346,000, $2,951,000, and $2,855,000 for the years ended December 31, 2004, 2003, and 2002, respectively. These restatement adjustments were noncash and had no impact on revenues or net operating cash flow. The company also changed its accounting method for partnership programs to the "stock compensation" model from the "minority interest" model that was previously used. As a result, partnership cash flow distributions to general managers and area operating partners were treated as compensation expense instead of minority interest profit. Moreover, company purchases of partnership interests from area operating partners were treated as compensation expense instead of being recorded as an intangible asset. On July 26, 2000, the company initiated a program to repurchase up to 4 million shares of the company's stock with the timing, price, quantity, and manner of the purchases to be made at management's discretion dependent on market conditions. On July 23, 2003, the company initiated a second program to repurchase 2.5 million additional shares on a regular basis to offset shares issued due to the exercise of stock options. The company funded these repurchase programs with available cash and bank credit facilities. As of year-end 2004, 11,819,000 shares of common stock had been repurchased for approximately $400,259,000. Exhibits 3–5 show the company's restated financial statements for 2002–2004. Exhibit 6 gives details about restaurant operations during the same period.

NEW EXECUTIVE SUITE

On March 8, 2005, Outback announced that long-time chairman and CEO Chris Sullivan was stepping down immediately, turning over the reins to Bill Allen. Concurrently, the company announced that Paul Avery, who had been president, was transitioning into a co-chair role. Allen had previously headed up Outback's West Coast Concepts division. Becoming co-chair was a huge step up, as the West Coast Concepts division had fewer than 100 restaurants under its domain, whereas Outback Steakhouse Inc. had over 1,000 company-owned restaurants. Chris Sullivan and Bob Basham remained as co-chairs of the board to ensure an effective transition to new leadership. As with any company that experienced executive management transitions, Outback Steakhouse faced some level of execution risk from its changes. Even skilled executives and high-achieving companies stumbled a bit during a management transition. Although all signs indicated that Allen was a talented and motivated executive, even exceptional managers encountered a learning curve when taking on greatly expanded responsibilities.

Six weeks after Sullivan resigned, Bob Merritt, chief financial officer, announced his retirement. Merritt had been with the company since 1990 and justified his retirement decision on frustration with

Exhibit 3   **Statement of Operations, Outback Steakhouse Inc. and Affiliates, 2002–2004 (in thousands)**

	2004	2003	2002
Revenues			
Restaurant sales	$3,183,297	$2,647,991	$2,276,599
Other revenue	18,453	17,786	17,915
Total revenue	$3,201,750	$2,665,777	$2,294,514
Cost of revenue	1,193,262	983,362	856,951
Gross profit	$2,008,488	$1,682,415	$1,437,563
Operating expenses			
Selling, general, and administrative	1,562,467	1,273,478	1,078,107
Depreciation and amortization	104,310	84,876	73,294
Other	89,680	65,143	58,819
Total operating expenses	$1,756,457	$1,423,497	$1,210,220
Operating income	252,031	258,918	227,343
Total other income/expenses	(4,384)	(1,431)	(2,110)
Elimination of minority partners' interest	9,415	2,532	(1,580)
Income before tax	$ 238,232	$ 254,955	$ 226,813
Provision for income tax	82,175	87,700	78,838
Cumulative effect of a change in accounting principle	—	—	(740)
Net income	$ 156,057	$ 167,255	$ 147,235

Source: Outback Steakhouse Inc. 2004 annual report.

overzealous regulators, accounting rules bordering on "lunacy," and "growing public perception that all businesspeople were dishonest." Merritt complained about the legal and regulatory burdens associated with the Sarbanes-Oxley Act of 2002. He said that those burdens left executives with little time for strategic planning or profit building and that he spent most of his time trying to comply with arcane rules and avoid making mistakes. What sent him over the edge were the accounting rules concerning the payment of rent and improvements to leased property. Although lease-accounting rules had changed little since 1976, public accountants made cautious after Sarbanes-Oxley began to question the way in which restaurants reported leases. Outback's accountants advised the company to restate prior earnings based on changing interpretations of existing lease-accounting rules. Merritt vowed to never work for a publicly traded company again but admitted he was willing to serve on public company boards if invited. Merritt was later invited to be an independent director on the board of directors for Cosi Inc., an operator and franchisor of bakery-café stores. In October 2005, Outback named Dirk Montgomery

as Merritt's successor. Montgomery had over 15 years' experience in the food and retail industry; he had previously served as retail senior financial officer for ConAgra Foods and chief financial officer of Express.

RESTAURANT PORTFOLIO

To capitalize on the growing popularity of casual dining, Outback decided in 1993 to begin expanding its restaurant portfolio, mainly through joint-venture partnerships. The company engaged in the ownership, development, and operation of casual-dining restaurants (primarily in the United States) that served lunch and dinner, featuring menus consisting of steaks, prime rib, pork chops, ribs, chicken, seafood, and pasta. The company's provision of capital and real estate expertise, procurement services, and unit-level engineering, as well as legal and financial support, allowed partners and management of each concept to focus on the basics of their business. Outback prided itself on having the most stable young brands, with the most growth

Exhibit 4 **Balance Sheet, Outback Steakhouse and Affiliates, 2003–2004 (in thousands)**

	2004	2003
Assets		
Current assets		
Cash and cash equivalents	$ 87,977	$ 102,892
Short-term investments	1,425	20,824
Inventories	63,448	59,608
Deferred income tax asset	12,969	11,757
Other current assets	53,068	37,529
Total current assets	$ 218,887	$ 232,610
Property, plant, and equipment, net	1,235,151	1,049,546
Investments in and advances to unconsolidated affiliates, net	16,254	31,209
Intangible assets	21,683	—
Goodwill	107,719	86,745
Other assets	78,098	74,008
Notes receivable collateral for franchisee guarantee	30,239	—
Total assets	$1,708,031	$1,474,118
Liabilities and stockholders' equity		
Current liabilities		
Accounts payable	$ 74,162	$ 58,533
Accrued expenses	97,124	80,248
Current portion of long-term debt	54,626	48,901
Unearned revenue	100,895	82,670
Other current liabilities	40,383	44,177
Total current liabilities	$ 367,190	$ 314,529
Deferred rent	44,075	37,454
Partner deposit and accrued buyout liability	63,102	42,628
Long-term debt	59,900	9,550
Other long-term liabilities	36,457	6,607
Total liabilities	$ 570,724	$ 410,768
Commitments and contingencies		
Interest of minority partners in consolidated partnerships	$ 48,905	$ 58,126
Stockholders' equity		
Common stock	788	788
Treasury stock	(206,824)	(161,808)
Additional paid-in capital	271,109	254,852
Retained earnings	1,025,447	913,470
Accumulated other comprehensive loss	(2,118)	(2,078)
Total stockholders' equity	$1,088,402	$1,005,224
Total liabilities and stockholders' equity	$1,708,031	$1,474,118

Source: Outback Steakhouse Inc. 2004 annual report.

potential, among the major multichain operators within the casual-dining segment. As of March 31, 2005, the company operated 888 Outback Steakhouses, 176 Carrabba's Italian Grills, 72 Bonefish Grills, 32 Fleming's Prime Steakhouse and Wine Bars, 19 Roy's, 2 Lee Roy Selmon's, 3 Paul Lee's Chinese Kitchens, and 14 Cheeseburger in Paradise restaurants in 50 states and 21 countries. In

Exhibit 5   **Statement of Cash Flows, Outback Steakhouse
and Affiliates, 2002–2004 (in thousands)**

	2004	2003	2002
Cash flow from operating activities			
Net cash provided by operating activities	$ 322,265	$ 269,082	$ 294,000
Cash flow from investment activities			
Net cash used for investing activities	(290,860)	(230,061)	(168,066)
Cash flow from financing activities			
Net cash used in financing activities	(46,320)	(123,707)	(54,284)
Net change in cash and equivalents	(14,915)	(84,686)	71,650
Cash at beginning of period	102,892	187,578	115,928
Cash at end of period	$ 87,977	$ 102,892	$ 187,578

Source: Outback Steakhouse, Inc. 2004 Annual Report

August 2005, the company was approved by the U.S. Bankruptcy Court for the District of Delaware as the successful bidder for the rights to 76 properties of Chi-Chi's and its affiliates. Outback's objective for acquiring these rights was to have access to restaurant sites for conversion to one of its own concepts. The company's overall strategy focused on offering consumers an array of dining alternatives suited for differing needs or occasions.

Carrabba's Italian Grill

In April 1993, Outback purchased a 50 percent interest in the cash flows of two Carrabba's Italian Grill restaurants located in Houston, Texas, and entered into a 50–50 joint venture with the founders to develop more Carrabba's restaurants. Outback acquired sole ownership of this venture in early 1995. Johnny Carrabba and Damian Mandola, Carrabba's cofounders, both possessed immense passion for Carrabba's and kept their Italian roots and traditions at the forefront of the business. Carrabba's grasped diners' attention immediately with eye-catching rooftopgardens and a warm ambiance that featured handmade Italian dishes prepared in an exhibition-style kitchen. In addition to traditional Italian entrées, the menu featured fresh fish, seafood, wood-fired pizza, meats smothered in special seasonings, and an extensive wine list featuring wide selections of midrange to high-end wines. Each Carrabba's location offered a chef's daily special menu, in part to allow managing partners to accommodate local tastes and preferences.

In 2004, there was encouraging progress in the redesign of Carrabba's restaurants. The new stores were smaller and less expensive to operate. Average store sales volumes for the smaller units kept pace with the larger units, gaining the company's confidence that unit-level returns on invested capital justified widespread national expansion. In acknowledgment of emerging lifestyles, Carrabba's implemented a carside carry-out service and planned to continue enhancing this service. Advertising had also made a positive impact on revenues. Television commercials captured Johnny Carrabba and Damian Mandola's generous Italian spirit and passion for fresh, quality ingredients. Carrabba and Mandola snagged a spot on the PBS cooking show *Cucina Amore,* which aired in more than half of all TV markets. Carrabba's had a total of 168 restaurants domestically in 2004 and planned to open an additional 25 stores in 2005.

Bonefish Grill

To fill the niche between formal, upscale seafood restaurants and family-style seafood eateries, Outback formed a joint venture with Bonefish Grill. Bonefish was positioned as a casual-dining concept featuring fresh, high-quality seafood served in an upbeat environment with distinctive artwork inspired by Florida's natural coastal setting. The casual-dining seafood segment was ripe for a concept to go national. The menu featured a "cosmic" collection of finfish cooked over an oak-burning grill and hand-cut beef, pasta, and chicken dishes garnished with special sauces. Menu selections featured quality ingredients, including hearts of palm, pine nuts, artichokes, goat cheese, and sun-dried tomatoes. Bonefish showed its commitment to serving fresh food by receiving,

Exhibit 6 **Restaurant Operations, 2002–2004**

	2004	2003	2002
Average unit volumes for restaurants opened for one year or more (in thousands):			
Outback Steakhouse	$ 3,465	$ 3,375	$ 3,311
Carrabba's Italian Grill	3,108	3,103	3,050
Fleming's Prime Steakhouse and Wine Bar	4,783	3,893	4,197
Roy's	3,496	3,157	3,364
Bonefish Grill	3,220	3,124	N/A
Average unit volumes for restaurants opened for less than one year (in thousands):			
Outback Steakhouse	$ 3,179	$ 3,212	$ 3,058
Carrabba's Italian Grill	2,939	2,964	2,901
Fleming's Prime Steakhouse and Wine Bar	3,492	3,995	3,209
Roy's	3,414	3,195	2,764
Bonefish Grill	2,965	3,022	3,069
Operating weeks:*			
Outback Steakhouse	33,304	31,058	28,897
Carrabba's Italian Grill	8,228	5,327	4,221
Fleming's Prime Steakhouse and Wine Bar	1,302	1,010	711
Roy's	941	826	640
Bonefish Grill	2,234	1,070	309
Year-to-year percentage change:			
Menu price increases:†			
Outback Steakhouse	2.4%	0.8%	1.6%
Carrabba's Italian Grill	1.5	0.9	1.0
Bonefish Grill	3.0	0.3	N/A
Same-store sales (stores open 18 months or more):			
Outback Steakhouse	2.7	1.9	−0.1
Carrabba's Italian Grill	3.3	1.8	1.7
Fleming's Prime Steakhouse and Wine Bar	17.1	12.7	10.2
Roy's	11.5	10.0	11.0
Bonefish Grill	7.5	2.0	N/A

*Represents the combined number of weeks that all units in each restaurant chain were in operation and open for business; existing units were typically open all 52 weeks, but newly-opened units were open only a portion of the 52 weeks.

†Reflected nominal amounts of menu price changes, prior to any change in product mix because of price increases, and may not reflect amounts effectively paid by the customer. Menu price increases were not provided for Fleming's and Roy's as a significant portion of their sales come from specials, which fluctuate daily.

Source: Outback Steakhouse Inc. 2004 annual report.

inspecting, and hand-cutting its fish daily and preparing its dishes with modern culinary techniques. It cultivated relationships with suppliers to distribute seafood daily to the restaurant. Bonefish had 63 locations by the end of 2004 and planned to develop 35 to 40 more locations in 2005. It possessed great growth potential, evidenced by the success and acceptance of the original restaurants and new locations.

The Upscale-Dining Segment: Fleming's Prime Steakhouse and Roy's

In 1998, Outback identified upscale casual dining as a new target segment. This segment was attractive because of its revenue potential. Outback decided to break into this new segment through forming joint ventures with two proven winners: Fleming's Prime Steakhouse and Wine Bar and Roy's. Paul Fleming and Bill Allen, founders of Fleming's, had a long and successful track record in the restaurant industry, especially with restaurant chains such as P. F. Chang's China Bistro. Fleming's was embedded as a high-end prime steakhouse whose contemporary style featured light woods, high ceilings, and 100 quality wines by the glass.

The vast selection of high-end wines and the shape of its crystal glasses differentiated Fleming's from competitors. Fleming's offered an exceptional wine list featuring boutique vintages from California, Oregon, and Washington, augmented by selections from France, Italy, Australia, and South Africa. Fleming's served only the finest in USDA prime beef. USDA prime beef came from corn-fed cattle (to keep the meat tender, these cattle were given no grazing privileges). To achieve distinctive taste, Fleming's aged its steaks up to four weeks for flavor and texture, then hand-cut and broiled them at 1,600 degrees to seal in the juices. Fleming's menu featured flavorful dishes ranging from fresh seafood such as ahi tuna, swordfish, and lobster tails to chicken, pork, and lamb specialties in addition to its superior prime beef. *Nation's Restaurant News* gave Fleming's its "Hot New Concept" award in May 2000. Fleming's was the strongest earnings performer in Outback's restaurant portfolio, achieving a 10.7 percent growth of average sales volume in 2004. The company exercised its option in September 2004 to purchase an additional 39 percent interest in Fleming's from the concept's founders. As of March 31, 2005, Fleming's had 32 locations in areas such as Las Vegas, Newport Beach, Houston, El Segundo, Birmingham, and North Scottsdale, and was expected to open 9 more new locations later in the year.

In 1999, Outback established a joint venture with Roy Yamaguchi to develop and operate Roy's restaurants worldwide. Chef Roy Yamaguchi had won many prestigious awards, including the James Beard Award and admittance to the Fine Dining Hall of Fame, and Roy's had garnered acclaim as the "crown jewel of East-West eateries." Yamaguchi acted as a tireless ambassador for his cuisine and inspired and motivated chef partners while investing time visiting each restaurant location. Roy's Hawaiian fusion cuisine fit nicely in the high-end seafood segment, where attention was focused heavily on the food: textures, colors, and bold flavors appealing to all the senses. Roy's dishes were complemented well by exclusive wines blended solely for Roy's by some of the finest winemakers in the world. The menu incorporated a variety of fish and seafood, beef, short ribs, pork, lamb, and chicken with blends of flavorful sauces and Asian spices. Roy's created an upscale casual-dining experience featuring spacious dining rooms, an expansive lounge area, and an exhibition-style kitchen finished in stainless steel and appointed with copper accents. Guests of Roy's were often well-traveled individuals seeking an upscale yet casual ambiance, and they wanted the convenience of reservations. Roy's experienced a sales momentum push beginning in 2003 and lasting through 2004. Average store sales volumes grew by 10.3 percent in 2004, making Roy's a sturdy revenue contributor in Outback's portfolio.

PRINCIPLES AND BELIEFS

While Outback was growing rapidly, the founders felt that the company's fun and caring culture was eroding as more managers and hourly Outbackers came in from other restaurants. A positive aspect of the influx was that the newcomers brought with them their previous experience, but they also brought ingrained habits. In 1990, the founders knew that they needed to take action quickly to uphold Outback's unique culture and business style. Thus, the four spent nine months in 1990 contemplating and verbalizing the values, beliefs, goals, keys to success, guiding principles, and direction of the company. They hoped to recapture the original flare of Outback's culture. During this process, they started over from the beginning to figure out what had been lost.

When the "visioneering" process was complete in 1999, the leadership team produced a document called the Principles and Beliefs (P&Bs). This five-and-a-half-page document quickly became Outback's operating manifesto and gained momentum over the years. The P&Bs outlined the founders' prescribed "recipe for success"; it defined Outback to its stakeholders and explained how the company's identity was to be created. Stakeholders included Outbackers, customers, purveyors, neighbors, and partners. The P&Bs incorporated Outback's core principles, commitments to Outbackers (see Exhibit 7) and other

Exhibit 7   **Outback Steakhouse Commitment to Outbackers**

We keep our nine commitments to Outbackers, guided by our five principles.
Our purpose is to prepare Outbackers to exercise good judgment and live our *Principles and Beliefs.*
There are no probationary Outbackers.
Because of our *Serious Food, Concentrated Service,* and *No Rules,*
Outbackers approach our Customers with confidence and a sense of ownership while demonstrating our principles of Hospitality and Quality. They are proud to be Outbackers. Outback's environment requires people to be tough on results, but kind with people.
It is an environment where managers are focused on serving Customers and supporting their Outbackers.
Outbackers know they are valued and that situations special to them will be handled with respect and concern.
How we take care of Outbackers is embodied in the details of our nine commitments to them.
Clear Direction, Preparation, Involvement, Affecting One's Own Destiny, A Fair Hearing, Sharing in the Success, Making a Commitment, Having a Good Time, and *Compassion.*

stakeholders, and connections to exemplify that living the P&Bs was a source of happiness, remarkable success, and personal commitment to Outback. The leadership team recognized early that Outbackers were the faces, hearts, and hands of the company. The company considered its employees—approximately 80,000 Outbackers were employed by the company in 2004—to be its most valuable resource. They were the ones customers saw when visiting the restaurant, and the ones who established a connection with the customer. The first sentence of the P&Bs read, "We believe that if we take care of Our People, then the institution of Outback will take care of itself." Management believed that, if the P&Bs were followed, Outback would be in position to achieve the five following goals:

- *For Outbackers, A great place to work, have fun, and make money;*
- *For Customers, Favorite place to eat, drink, relax, and be with friends;*
- *For Purveyors, A great customer and source of comfort and pride;*
- *For Neighbors, A valued corporate citizen and neighbor; and*
- *For Partners, A superior financial and emotional investment opportunity.*

DAILY OPERATIONS AT OUTBACK

A typical day at an Outback Steakhouse began around nine in the morning with the arrival of the prep crew.

All signature ingredients, sauces, and soups were prepared from scratch daily. Food was delivered daily to the store and immediately placed in the preparation process. Management negotiated directly with food suppliers to ensure uniform quality and adequate supplies. The crew promptly began making salad dressings. Each dressing marinated for an extended time to ensure that the proper flavor was achieved, and croutons took three hours to season and toast. Outback used quality blends of freshly grated cheeses from Wisconsin, imported Parmesan cheese, and imported Swiss Gruyere. Outback prepared "Aussie chips," its version of French fries, in-house to guarantee quality by extensively rinsing the potatoes to remove excess starches and sugars. Desserts, including brownies and chocolate and caramel sauces—were prepared daily as well.

Outback used only top-grade USDA center-cut Choice steaks from Nebraska or Colorado and seasoned them with Outback seasoning, which consisted of a blend of various spices and 19 different peppers. To maintain quality, Outback required its beef suppliers to provide written documentation confirming that the cattle used for Outback steaks were raised and fed in compliance with U.S. government regulations designed to prevent bovine spongiform encephalopathy (mad cow disease). Additionally, the company prohibited suppliers from using mammal protein by-products in cattle feed. All chicken, beef, and fish were fresh, never frozen. About one hour before opening time, a line check took place, which consisted of tasting all the sauces, dressings, and soups to ensure quality for the customers. A heavy emphasis was placed on food quality, and extra cost was always absorbed to provide "serious food" to customers.

OUTBACK'S STRATEGY

In 2005, Outback was a well-established brand name among consumers worldwide. With 881 locations, customers knew they could dine in any Outback restaurant and receive a top-quality meal for a reasonable price. While continually growing, Outback reached consumers in new markets through creative television and radio advertising and sports affiliations. When Outback entered a new market, customers lined up to taste the beloved Bloomin' Onion. Although beef and steak items comprised a large portion of the menu, Outback restaurants also offered a variety of chicken, rib, seafood, and pasta dishes. The company's philosophy of "No Rules, Just Right" allowed customers to personalize their dining experience by choosing how menu selections were prepared. Outback chose to differentiate itself by offering generous portions of high-quality food and superior service in a casual Australian outback atmosphere.

Marketing and Advertising

In 2005, Outback's innovative, edgy advertisements drew the criticism that the company was trying too hard to be funny. The particular commercial that received the most criticism showed a man on one knee holding his beloved's hand, about to propose, when a boomerang thwacked him on the head. Instead of asking the woman to marry him, the man asked her to take him to Outback. When the boomerang returned and conked the woman on the head, she agreed. Widespread consumer disapproval caused Outback to stop using its "humor message" in core Outback brand marketing. The new advertising strategy, expected to launch around the beginning of 2006, would focus more on food and taste.

Outback engaged in a variety of promotional activities, such as contributing goods, time, and money to charitable, civic, and cultural programs. The Outback brand was attached to events ranging from NCAA college football, to Donald Trump's television show *Apprentice,* to NASCAR. Starting in 1994, the Outback Bowl attracted a national ESPN audience for the New Year's Day college football bowl game. The Outback Bowl was the sixth-highest-paying bowl game, with a matchup between the Big Ten and the Southeastern Conference. Outback's relationship with NASCAR consisted of an alliance with driver Dale Jarret and in-store driver appearances.

Broadcaster John Madden, who had an ongoing partnership with the company, traveled to his Monday-night football games in the Outback Steakhouse Madden Cruiser, providing exposure and promotional opportunities for the company. Also, the *Bloomin' Onion I,* the Outback blimp, traveled across the country providing coverage for ABC sports events, including Professional Golfers' Association tournaments, the Little League World Series, and National College Athletic Association football. The blimp aided in further enhancing awareness of Outback nationwide.

Focus on Customer and Customer Satisfaction

Outback went all out to guarantee that customers had a positive, fun dining experience. As customers walked up to the restaurant, they were greeted with a smiling face and a door that opened especially for them. Those who incurred a wait found many activities to engage in—magazines, children's toys, and free samples of Bloomin' Onion helped them pass the time. To help reduce wait times, Outback implemented call-ahead seating. This initiative increased the number of customer visits by regulating table turnover.

To address emerging consumer preferences and lifestyles, Outback began offering curbside takeaway. Following this implementation, food-to-go sales represented a larger proportion of the company's total sales compared to prior years—nearly one out of three consumers used curbside take-away. Upon calling the neighborhood Outback, the customer was greeted by a warm, friendly voice and asked to place an order. The take-away server made sure to document the color and type of car the customer would be driving. As soon as the customer arrived and parked in a specially designated spot, the server brought the food directly to the car. This process provided Outback customers with a hassle-free way to obtain a quick, high-quality dinner.

Outback was convinced that its "Commitments to Customers" were the key to having a competitive advantage (see Exhibit 8). Outbackers worked hard to personalize each customer's experience, treating all customers as individuals and responding to their unique needs. Outbackers interacted with patrons in a friendly, energized, and extroverted manner and always gave an enthusiastic yes to special requests. For example, it was routine for Outback to make an

Exhibit 8   **Outback Steakhouse Commitment to Customers**

We take care of our Customers.
We totally indulge you with *Serious Food, Concentrated Service,* and *No Rules* in an environment that is welcoming, friendly, warm, energetic, and fun.
During a wait, drinks are offered and food is shared.
The menu is broad, the portions are generous, and the drinks poured full.
Our serious food means freshness, flavors, attractive food, just-right temperatures.
It is food prepared from scratch, using the finest ingredients, and to exacting standards.
We are thick-cut steaks, fresh-cut fries, homemade croutons and salad dressings, fresh-baked brownies and meticulously prepared chocolate sauce.
We have an intense desire to please you.
You dictate the pace of service, from a quick meal to a relaxing evening with friends.
We respect your privacy and tailor our service to your wants and needs.
We delight customers one at a time ensuring everything is as you want it.
We invite you to enjoy anything you want prepared any way you like it.
We will please you, provide perfection your way, and enthusiastically say yes to your requests.
We provide a hassle-free, personalized, and totally enjoyable experience.
We do whatever it takes to deliver great food, drink, and services, are not distracted by the latest fads in the industry, and have the courage to put quality ahead of cost.

extraordinary effort to address special needs of customers who might not have otherwise been comfortable dining in public, kept special dietary items on hand for regular customers, pureed food for patrons who could not chew, sent an Outbacker to the nearest McDonald's in order to buy a Happy Meal for a customer's child, and sat customers ahead of the wait when it was obvious that waiting would have been a physical hardship. Overall, the philosophy was to treat people "Just Right."

Other Strategic Elements

- *Dinner-only hours at most locations.* Outback pioneered the strategy of having the vast majority of its restaurants open for dinner only during much of the week. In turn, this enhanced Outbackers' lifestyles by allowing them time to pursue personal interests in addition to work. Outback had the lowest labor turnover rate in the industry, which lessened its need to spend money on training replacement employees.

- *Limited seating.* The typical Outback restaurant was approximately 6,200 square feet with a seating capacity of around 220. The 220-person seating arrangement was chosen because it was considered the optimum seating capacity to guarantee a quality steak. Chris Sullivan and Bob Basham argued that an optimal facility was

more efficient and effective than a gigantic one and decided to build more Outbacks in new locations to keep up with demand.

- *Good pay for Outbackers.* Outbackers saw substantial monetary compensation as well as intangible rewards. One of the company's precepts was "Sharing in the Success of Outback." This was achieved through celebrations, recognizing individual Outbackers for their performance, and other bonus incentive programs. Overall, Outbackers earned a lot of money; a server typically left a shift with around $125 after working a three-table station.

- *Quality steaks and ingredients.* Outback's fine cuts of steak and bold, flavorful seasonings made customers crave and love their steaks. Emphasizing freshness and quality, Outback used specific methods for aging, cutting, seasoning, and searing its steaks. Outback knew that if it served a first-rate steak prepared with good seasoning, customers would be willing to wait two hours to get a seat.

- *Strong signature menu items.* The Bloomin' Onion was the menu item customers requested most often upon sitting down at a table. Many craved the zesty and bold seasonings. Approximately 35 percent of all customers ordered a Bloomin' Onion when dining in the restaurant. As for the drink menu, the Wallaby Darned proved to be a strong signature item unmatched by competitors. The bartenders mixed the drink daily from DeKuyper Peachtree schnapps, champagne, Smirnoff vodka, and secret mixers.

- *Fun and relaxed atmosphere.* Outback's lighting and ceiling reflected the unusual colors found at Ayers Rock, a formation that was a popular Australian tourist attraction. At sunset, the rock turned a burnt orange and the sky turned a deep purple. Outback replicated this scenery by painting the ceiling purple and the walls burnt orange and using pink lighting. Various Australian artifacts, such as boomerangs, surfboards, maps, and hats were hung on the walls. The floors and tables were made of a deep-colored wood with a glossy finish. Outback employed formula facilities so that a customer could walk into any Outback Steakhouse and feel at home. Customers came to recognize the green roof with red lettering as a place to dine casually and unwind.

- *Managing partner ownership.* To attract great, qualified, and motivated people—and to promote ownership and responsibility—Outback required each managing partner to purchase a 10 percent equity stake in his or her restaurant for $25,000. This interest gave the partner the right to receive a percentage of his or her restaurant's annual cash flows for the duration of the agreement. Additionally, managing partners signed a five-year employment agreement, which contributed to a stable environment and a low turnover of both managers and hourly Outbackers. During the employment term, managing partners were prohibited from selling or transferring the ownership interest; upon termination of employment, the partner was required to sell the ownership interest back to the company.

- *Large portions at reasonable prices.* Outback provided great value to its customers by serving generous portions of high-quality food at reasonable prices. The average ticket price for an adult at dinnertime was between $19 and $21. Outback customers never left the restaurant hungry.

OUTBACK'S CULTURE

Many companies' policy statements claimed that the customer came first. Outback, in contrast, realized that its employees were the company's most valuable asset and resource, so it fostered a culture that developed, recognized, and rewarded people. The founders discovered that the company had to show that it was as serious about taking care of Outbackers as it was about taking care of customers. In addition, the company recognized that Outbackers could not be asked to take care of customers if they were not being cared for themselves. The company's goal was to make work an enjoyable experience; the hope was that each Outbacker would look forward to coming in each day. Outback promised all Outbackers clear direction, extensive training, a fair hearing when a complaint arose, and a fun workplace environment (see again Exhibit 7).

A prominent feature of Outback's culture was caring. Outbackers showed compassion for one another and were always willing to help another in need. One story exemplified the nature of Outbackers: A dishwasher had his bicycle stolen during a shift. While thousands of bikes are stolen each year, this was the dishwasher's only means of transportation. Before the shift ended, the Outbackers at this particular location collected enough money among themselves to replace the bicycle. An Outbacker was sent to a nearby store to purchase a new bicycle and had it ready, including ribbons, by the end of the shift. Outback had a culture of respect and camaraderie that bred enthusiasm for helping others.

Recruitment, Screening, Promotion, and Hiring

Outback did not maintain internal or external recruiters and never created a human resource department but still boasted the lowest management and hourly turnover rate in the industry. Outback always accepted applications for employment because it believed another dedicated, fun-loving Outbacker would make a positive addition. It strove to hire people from different backgrounds to create synergy that came from great diversity. After completing an application, an individual was required to take a personality test to determine whether he or she would fit with Outback's culture and an analytical math test designed to measure quick thinking. An external third party scored the tests to prevent bias. Once hired, every new Outbacker was immediately welcomed as an integral member of the team; there were no probationary Outbackers.

Instead of requiring experience, Outback hired friendly people and provided training for work-related skills. Outback sought to hire people with enthusiasm, a positive outlook, and a winning attitude because it believed it was easier to add competence to friendliness than the reverse. The company defined a "Quality Hire" as an individual who performed the job, fit in with Outback's culture, and planned to stick around. It sought ambitious individuals who had a surplus of energy that drove them to achieve their goals and who understood that going the extra mile was the norm rather than exception.

Each Outbacker affected his or her own destiny through work ethic and commitment to the company's Principles and Beliefs. Outback initiated programs such as "Five for Our Future," in which management at all levels identified five or more Outbackers of underrepresented groups (i.e., minorities and women) with strong leadership potential and developed mentoring programs designed to help them earn more responsibility in the workplace. Outback sourced all managers internally from hourly Outbackers. These Outbackers knew what it took to be successful the Outback way. The internal promotion policy helped keep the fun-loving, generous culture alive on the management level.

Training

Outback believed that training was an essential component of providing opportunities for individuals and that exceptional training translated routine challenges in the restaurant into solutions because Outbackers felt empowered to perform their jobs. Every Outbacker underwent an intensive on-the-job training program in addition to classroom instruction. Each one-week training period on-the-job supervision by an experienced Outbacker. Classroom training programs were designed to teach Outbackers how to live the P&Bs and exercise good judgment. "Serious Food" seminars were conducted every month in each store to emphasize the importance of food quality to all Outbackers. The managing partner, front-of-house manager, and kitchen manager conducted mini-classes with groups of Outbackers to discuss how to achieve Outback's commitment to quality food. These mini-classes included kitchen tours, education regarding cuts of beef, tasting sessions, and discussions of the Outback way for food preparation. Quarterly, each restaurant held a "Concentrated Service" meeting to revisit the purpose and implementation of the P&Bs.

For managers, the Better Yourself Through Education (BYTE) program was established to enhance the skills of the management team. BYTE was a self-directed, 12-week, distance-learning program consisting of 16 classes focusing on business needs. The classes encompassed business skills, communication skills, human resources, and self-management skills. The classes were in workbook format and took roughly 10 to 32 hours to complete. In BYTE, each managing partner served as a "Working Mentor" for their managers taking the classes. The partner assisted the manager when he or she came across difficult material or sought advice on how to handle various situations. Outback's goal for the BYTE program was to prepare its managers by providing them with the resources they needed to achieve the next level of excellence.

The Outbacker Trust

Established in 1999, the Outbacker Trust was funded primarily through Outbackers. The purpose of the program was to financially support Outbackers experiencing significant hardships in life. Money was raised through voluntary contributions from Outbackers; a donor of $20 or more received a collector's pin designed for that particular year. Contributions were not solicited from suppliers, customers, or friends. Requests for disbursements from the Outbacker Trust funneled through the area joint-venture partner and were then presented to a trust committee in Tampa, Florida. The Outbacker Trust covered such cases as funeral and burial costs of loved ones; loss of housing and possessions by fire, flood, and other causes; costs of surgery; income loss during life-threatening operations; and other life-altering challenges. Outback's philosophy for this program was as follows:

> We all travel different journeys in life, all of which are filled with different hurdles along the way. It is comforting to know that even when we are faced with the most difficult times, we are surrounded by, at the very least, our incredible family of Outbackers.

The STARS Program

Outback instituted a bonus program called Sharing the Actions, Responsibilities and Success (STARS) to encourage Outbackers to live the P&Bs. The STARS program shared 25 percent of the restaurant's increase in quarterly profitability as compared to the same quarter of the prior year. Sales had to experience an increase, and cash flow had to be up a minimum of $4,000 for the quarter. Hourly Outbackers who worked a minimum average of 10 hours per week per quarter qualified for one share of the STARS bonus, and hourly Outbackers who worked a minimum average of 25 hours per week per quarter qualified for two shares. Outbackers had to be employed the entire quarter to qualify. A share of the bonus was calculated by taking the total bonus and dividing it by the total number of shares of all qualifying Outbackers. Overall, STARS encouraged Outbackers, with a sense of ownership, to support the team in building sales and profits in their respective restaurants while putting extra money in their pockets.

Community Involvement

Outback's culture strongly emphasized community involvement. Each year, Outback organized and contributed to more than 10,000 community events across the United States. The company strove to create a source of strength in times of crisis and could always be counted on to enhance the quality of life in the neighborhoods where its restaurants operated. This was achieved through continually identifying and acting on opportunities to give back to the community and to make it a better place to live, have fun, and conduct business. Outback took pride in supporting many meaningful organizations ranging from civic and charitable groups, to youth sports, to community restoration efforts, to parent teacher organizations.

Mission Outback was a program implemented to support the U.S. military and coalition troops while at war in Iraq. For the brave men and women overseas, an Outback meal was a taste of home and a reminder of how much they were appreciated. Outback sent 15 Outbackers in June 2002 to Kandahar, Afghanistan, to feed over 6,000 members of the military. An additional 15 were sent in January 2003 to Kandahar and Bagram to provide food for more than 13,000 troops, and an additional 21 Outbackers were sent in January 2004 to Al Asad, Baqubah, and Mosul (see Exhibit 9). Nearly 41,000 men and women of the military were served a dinner of Bloomin' Onions, Victoria's Filets, Rockhampton Rib-eyes, Grilled Shrimp on the Barbie, Aussie Chips, Jacket Potatoes, Mixed Veggies, and Cheesecake Olivia. The troops were overwhelmingly pleased and excited to see Outback Steakhouse in the middle of the desert. Outback received numerous letters and e-mails regarding Mission Outback. A retired veteran wrote,

Exhibit 9   **Mission Outback**

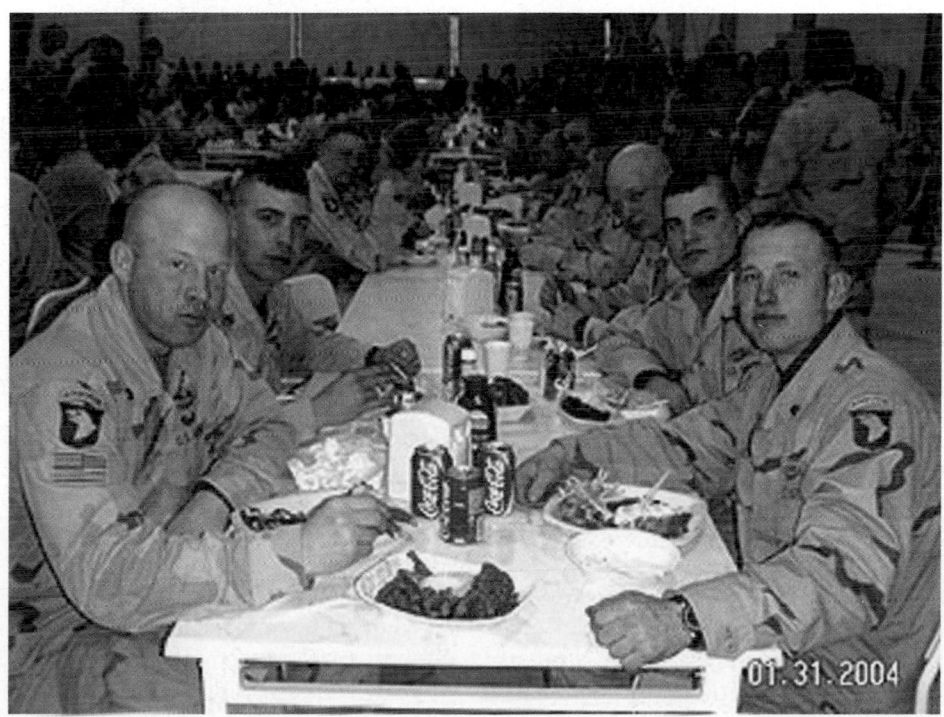

"The effort and sacrifice you and your supporters have made for our troops gladdened the hearts of numerous old vets who remember what it is like to be away from home for an extended tour and missing familiar foods." Mission Outback was a successful effort showing Outbackers' gratitude and appreciation for the men and women who risked their lives to protect freedom.

A nationwide coalition of restaurants, including Outback, designated October 5, 2005, as Dine Out for America Day. This industrywide fund-raising event raised money to aid the victims of Hurricanes Katrina and Rita. The initiative involved a record-setting 17,115 restaurants, which committed resources by designating up to 100 percent of daily sales for that day. The proceeds directly benefited the American Red Cross Disaster Relief Fund specifically earmarked for hurricane relief efforts. All Outback Steakhouse Inc. concepts contributed 100 percent of their sales on this day. Restaurants Unlimited generated the idea and was a leading force behind Dine Out for America Day in hopes the restaurant industry could cooperatively make a significant contribution to the hurricane survivors.

COMPETITORS

Lone Star Steakhouse & Saloon

Lone Star Steakhouse & Saloon positioned itself as a "destination restaurant" in the midpriced, full-service, casual-dining segment with a menu similar to that of Outback Steakhouse, but also lunchtime hours. Lone Star restaurants had a Texas-style ambiance with Texas artifacts and upbeat country-and-western music. Each restaurant was approximately 5,500 square feet with a seating capacity of 220 people featuring planked wooden floors, dim lighting, and flags and other Texas memorabilia to enhance the casual atmosphere. Moreover, Lone Star limited its menu to focus on high-quality USDA Choice-graded steaks, which were hand-cut daily, to create a competitive advantage. Generous "Texas-sized" portions were served for an average ticket price per customer of $12 for lunch and $18.50 for dinner in 2004.

Lone Star began operations in October 1989 in Winston-Salem, North Carolina. In March 1992, it became a public company traded on the Nasdaq. Through seasoned public offerings, the company satisfied all debt obligations through equity financing. In 2005, Lone Star had a total of 251 locations in the United States. In 2003, Lone Star divested its Australian operations to concentrate on domestic operations. Furthermore, the company suspended development of new stores in 2003 and 2004 to reduce the demand for additional managers, to focus on improving operations and guest relations in current stores, and to improve the quality of management. The company had plans to develop new stores in 2005. In January 2004, the company made a significant acquisition of the Texas Land & Cattle restaurants. The acquisition gave the company a stronger presence in Texas, where it also operated three Sullivan's and two Del Frisco's Double Eagle Steak Houses. Lone Star was met with intense competition from a variety of competitors, including locally owned, regional, and national restaurants. The company recognized that its ability to compete would depend on attraction and retention of loyal clientele, strong employees, experienced management, a continued offering of high-quality food, competitive prices, and an attractive dining atmosphere.

Texas Roadhouse

Founded in 1993, Texas Roadhouse was an up-and-coming competitor whose commitment to its customers was "Legendary Food, Legendary Service." Texas Roadhouse was a full-service, casual-dining restaurant chain offering an assortment of specially seasoned and aged steaks hand-cut daily on the premises and cooked to order over gas-fired grills. Guests were also offered a selection of rib, fish, chicken, and vegetable plates, and a variety of hamburgers, salads, and sandwiches, showcasing great menu diversity from hearty meals to leaner selections. Most entrées were accompanied by two made-from-scratch side items. The average dinner entrée prices ranged from $7.99 to $18.99.

Texas Roadhouse's operating strategy was designed to position each restaurant as the local hometown destination for a broad segment of customers seeking high-quality, affordable meals and friendly, attentive service. The key components to its operating strategy included high-quality, freshly prepared food; a focus on dinner only; moderate menu prices; performance-based management compensation; and a comfortable ambiance. The company successfully grew from 67 restaurants in 1999 to 193 by the end of 2004, representing a 23.6 percent compounded

Exhibit 10   **Lone Star's Statement of Income and Operating Ratios ($ thousands)**

	2004	2003	2002
Total revenue	$669,527	$591,617	$593,617
Cost of revenue	579,293	509,946	491,963
Gross profit	$ 90,234	$ 81,671	$101,654
Selling, general, and administrative expenses	45,269	43,346	45,085
Operating income	44,965	38,109	56,569
Net income from continuing operations	31,282	26,902	39,840
Net income	$ 31,213	$ 18,245	$ 38,667
Ratios			
Return on equity	7.73%	4.40%	8.75%
Return on assets	6.25	3.73	7.61
Gross profit margin	13.48	13.80	17.12
Net profit margin	4.66	3.08	6.51
Working capital	39,332	68,369	41,000
Current ratio	1.53	2.16	0.96
Debt to equity ratio	0	0	0

Source: Lone Star Steakhouse & Saloon 2004 annual report.

annual growth rate. The plan was to open 26 new restaurants in 2005. The focus remained primarily on midsize markets, where population size, income levels, and nearby shopping had proved to be fertile ground for expanding growth.

By any measure, 2004 was an exciting year for Texas Roadhouse due to achievement of significant milestones and goals. The company's initial public offering (IPO) in October 2004 was considered another way to prove itself to new partners who entrusted it with financial support. By the end of the closing bell on the day of Texas Roadhouse's IPO, the stock price had increased by 28 percent. As a result of the IPO, the company's balance sheet was stronger and more flexible. As for financial performance, total revenue increased by 27 percent in 2004 over the prior year, while comparable sales increased by 7.6 percent.

Exhibit 11   **Texas Roadhouse Financial Data ($ thousands)**

	2004	2003	% Change
Revenue:			
Restaurant sales	$354,190	$279,519	27%
Franchise royalties and fees	8,821	6,934	27
Total revenue	$363,011	$286,453	27
Income from operations	38,682	34,258	13
Total assets	276,663	148,193	87
Long-term debt including current portion	13,285	64,313	−79
Total stockholders' equity	$173,211	$ 37,902	357
Company restaurants			
Number open at end of period	107	87	23
Average unit volumes	$ 3,679	$ 3,401	8
Comparable restaurant sales growth	7.6%	3.4%	N/A

Source: Texas Roadhouse 2004 annual report.

INDUSTRY ENVIRONMENT

Revenue for the U.S. restaurant industry was $1 trillion in 2004 and was expected to reach $1.2 trillion in 2005. This included revenues from related industries such as agriculture, transportation, wholesale trade, and food manufacturing. Food-and-drink revenues were projected to be $476 billion, with operations in 900,000 locations. This industry was complex and fragmented, with different types of establishments ranging from full-service restaurants to snack bars. On a typical day in 2005, the restaurant industry posted average sales of nearly $1.3 billion. Sales were forecasted to advance 4.9 percent in 2005 and to equal 4 percent of the U.S. gross domestic product. The major growth drivers for the industry included unit expansion, same-store sales, and efforts to increase margins.

Excluding the government, the restaurant industry, a labor-intensive environment, was the nation's largest employer, with an estimated 12.2 million employees. The industry provided work for more than 9 percent of the workforce in the United States. More than 4 out of 10 adults worked in the restaurant industry at some point in their lives, and 27 percent of adults got their first job experience in a restaurant. A typical employee in food service in 2005 was a single female under 30 years of age working an average of 25 hours a week and living in a household with two or more wage earners. Restaurant industry employment was expected to reach 13.3 million by 2012. The number of food-service managers was projected to increase by 11 percent from 2005 to 2015. The industry employed more minority managers than any other; more than two-thirds of supervisors were women, 16 percent were African Americans, and 13 percent were Hispanic.

In 2002, the typical American household spent an average of $2,276 (or $910 per person) on food away from home, according to the National Restaurant Association's *Restaurant Spending* report. Every dollar spent by consumers in restaurants generated an additional $1.98 spent in other industries allied with the restaurant industry. In 2004, the U.S. Department of Agriculture estimated the average annual per capita consumption of beef was 66.3 pounds, up 2.1 pounds from 2003. More than 50 percent of all consumers visited a restaurant on their birthday, therefore making it the most popular occasion to dine out, followed by Mother's Day and Valentine's Day. Researchers had determined that more customers dined out during the month of August than any other month, while Saturday was the most popular day to dine out. Demographic characteristics dictating restaurant spending included household income, head of household's age, and household composition. Restaurant patronage was strongly correlated with increases in household income. Consumers were driven to frequent restaurants for entertainment, convenience, socialization, and nutrition. The largest spenders in the industry had a household income of over $70,000, with the household head between the ages of 45 and 54 and children older than 18.

Issues and Conditions

Characterized by tight margins and a high failure rate, the restaurant industry witnessed incredibly intense competition. The measures on which restaurants competed included price, location, and food quality, and there was a large number of well-established competitors. The industry was highly fragmented and subject to risks from food cost and wage inflation, lifestyle trends, seasonality, and shifts in investor sentiment. These external forces—including the price and availability of commodities and consumer preferences—dictated how each restaurant conducted operations. Furthermore, the fast pace of society required companies to develop efficient take-out services to accommodate working families. With fitness and health issues on the forefront of consumers' minds, restaurants had to develop new menu additions to retain health-conscious customers. In 2004, nearly two out of three restaurants added low-carbohydrate menu items as a result of the low-carb diet trend. In the steakhouse restaurant industry, emerging concerns over the ever-present rising costs of meat and decrease in U.S. cattle supply was drastically decreasing profit margins. Since the mid-1970s, the U.S. cattle headcount had declined from 130 million to 95 million, representing a 28 percent decrease despite the rising average annual per capita consumption of beef. Macroeconomic challenges became an evolving problem for the industry as gas and energy prices were rapidly increasing, with no indication of slowing down; in response, consumers frequented restaurants less often. Annually, many companies entered the industry, creating an atmosphere in which each restaurant competed on the basis of food and service quality, ambiance, location, and price–value relationship.

With demand for the best beef up and supply down, some restaurants began cutting corners. As the steakhouse industry rapidly expanded at a time of record shortages of top-quality beef, many steakhouses changed the way they did business. Some used lower-quality meats; others raised prices, shrunk steaks, and designed menus steering diners to higher-margin cuts. Finding top-quality meat became a tough challenge due to the rapid growth of the steakhouse industry beyond its traditional base of business meals and corporate accounts. The industry began trying to attract a new clientele—women—by rolling out fruity cocktails and adding more fish to the menu. In 2004, sales were up 10.7 percent from the previous year. The menus in many steakhouses were misleading to consumers. They declared at the top of the menu that their meat was either "USDA prime" or "dry-aged" or both, even if those terms did not apply to all steaks on the list. This meant that steakhouses were charging prime meat prices while quietly serving lesser grades.

In 2005, amid the worst hurricane season to date in the United States, Hurricanes Katrina and Rita devastated the restaurant industry along the Gulf Coast. Although this region was braced for the storms, these hurricanes delivered a massive punch, closing some restaurants permanently. Hurricane Katrina resulted in the temporary closure of 26 and indefinite closure of 2 Outback Steakhouse locations in Florida, Alabama, Louisiana, and Mississippi. The company reported hurricane-related losses of approximately $2.2 million in revenues. Outback also incurred costs for financial and housing assistance to Outbackers displaced by the catastrophe. The 2004 hurricane season resulted in the permanent closure of Outback's operations in the Cayman Islands. Hurricane Katrina forced Ruth's Chris Steakhouse to relocate its headquarters to Orlando from its home in Metairie, Louisiana, near the historical heart of the wind-and-flood-ravaged New Orleans. The decision was a tough one but was necessary, company executives said, amid the uncertainty that surrounded the entire Gulf Coast area.

The restaurant industry was subject to various federal, state, and local laws. Each restaurant was subject to licensing and regulation by a number of government authorities such as the alcoholic beverage control and health and safety agencies. If a restaurant wanted to sell alcoholic beverages, it was required to apply to a state authority for a license or permit to sell alcoholic beverages on the premises and to open for extended hours. In addition, control regulations were in place for daily operations including minimum age of patrons and employees, hours of operations, advertising, wholesale purchasing, and inventory control. To protect patrons, "dram-shop" statutes were in place to provide a person injured by an intoxicated person to recover damages from the established that wrongfully served alcoholic beverages to the intoxicated person.

Despite operating in a challenging cost environment (the commodities market was the worst in history, particularly the prices of beef and dairy products), Outback was able to maintain its market share. Furthermore, higher gasoline prices, labor costs, and interest rates dampened industry sales and raised the operating costs of food supplies, which were often passed on to Outback. In addition, changing lifestyles and health concerns dictated change. Outback had to adapt to changing market conditions to sustain the growth experienced throughout the years by continuing to indulge customers with top-quality ingredients that were perfectly prepared; having well-trained Outbackers to provide customers with "Concentrated Service" and "No Rules" in a welcoming, friendly, warm, energetic, and fun environment; keeping the physical plant updated; and living the Principles and Beliefs every day to remain focused on the company's commitments to its stakeholders.

Moses at the Red Sea

Mark Meckler
University of Portland

Howard Feldman
University of Portland

Michele Snead
University of Portland

Moses sat on a rock that overlooked the shores of the Red Sea. The three-day journey by pack mule, east from his home in the Nile River valley, had brought him a full week of solitary contemplation on this windswept coast. He was considering his options, knowing he must make some decisions and act on them soon.

The situation had become untenable. It had been over a year since he assumed leadership of the Israelites. The initial nine miracles he performed had long since lost their luster—after all, the Israelites were all still slaves, still living in abject poverty. Their masters, as a result of the "plagues" strategy, had become angry and brutal. Since the first of the plagues occurred, the beatings by the guards had been applied more harshly and more randomly. Moses believed that if he unleashed his 10th and final plague, the Egyptian pharaoh would finally let his people go. But how could he kill the firstborn of anyone, let alone the firstborn of the whole kingdom? And what would his people do when they arrived here at the shores of the Red Sea?

The whole tribe seemed to be bickering. The expectations of imminent freedom since the arrival of Moses over a year ago had everyone impatient, wondering what was taking so long. The heads of some of the more powerful families, who had been so supportive just a year ago, were now talking about the lack of results they had experienced, about how they were worse off than ever before, and about the possible need for a change in leadership.

Aaron[1] had come to Moses some days earlier with news that after four years of work, enough boats had been built to carry about half of his people across the sea. "Half ?" Moses questioned aloud to the sea. "How can I live with myself if I only lead half of us to freedom?" It would take another three years to build enough boats to save everyone. Cash flow was too low to purchase boats from the Africans to the south. Perhaps the women could secretly work in the papyrus scroll works after their Egyptian masters had left for the night. Papyrus scrolls, a product invented by the Egyptians, were highly prized outside of the empire and could easily be sold on the black market. Such a tactic would allow the Israelites to leave in perhaps a year and a half. However, the men couldn't do it; they were exhausted from their daily working in the mud pits and from the other hard duties forced on them by their Egyptian masters. The women might be able to do it, but the great majority had never worked anywhere but in the home or in the fields, and the conservative elders would fight this idea adamantly. Furthermore, if anyone was caught, there was no doubt the punishment would be severe.

Joshua's idea of a "ferry barge" that could carry 10 times the number of people that even the largest boat could carry was another option, but many criticized it as outlandish. Joshua had proposed to sail across the Red Sea with 15,000 paces of woven oiled rope that he would anchor at both this side and the other side so that barges could be pulled across. It was physically possible—Joshua had demonstrated

This case was presented at the fall 2005 meeting of the North American Case Research Association, October 27–29, 2005, North Falmouth, Massachusetts. All rights are reserved to the authors and NACRA. Copyright © 2005 by Mark Meckler and Howard Feldman.

the technology by pulling a boat across the Nile and back again—so perhaps men on these huge barges could pull themselves hand over hand across the Red Sea. Joshua had calculated that if they dedicated all of their extra resources to manufacturing rope, they could leave on barges within six months. However, should the rope break or a storm hit, the barges would be incapable of navigating themselves safely. They would have to leave before the beginning of the rainy season.

During secret meetings with a captain of a Hittite trade mission to the pharaoh, Moses had been offered passage for his people in exchange for helping the Hittites annex the promised land of Canaan into the Hittite empire. The Hittites had been harsh lords in the past, taxing their subjects to near poverty, but at least they promised that none of the tribes of Israel would be slaves. However, the Hittite captain made no such promises of freedom to their long-lost siblings, the Hebrews, who had remained behind in Canaan hundreds of years ago. Moses dreamed of returning and joining together with his Hebrew brethren to form one empire. He hoped for the Hebrews' welcome and help, not their enmity. Moses was also very reluctant to turn over their birthright, their promised land of Canaan waiting for them by the sea, to Hittite governance in exchange for their freedom.

Then Moses once again pondered the waking dream he had had in which the Almighty, Great Creator of All, ensured the Israelites safe passage through the Red Sea to the far shores *if they could come up with no better solution of their own*. Moses also knew from his dream that if they used this miracle to obtain freedom, it would come at a guaranteed cost of wandering the desert for 40 years before finding their way home, a home that Moses would never live long enough to see.

The food supply was even more miserable than usual; and with more and more mouths to feed, it would be only a matter of time before people began to starve. The growing chaos made Moses feel nervous and uncomfortable. "Can I do this?" he asked aloud in desperation to the sky, his feelings of inadequacy surfacing again. He knew that he needed a way to get everyone to pull together, to cooperate. We have indeed grown into a great nation, thought Moses, but how do I manage to bring my people to freedom?

Appendix: The Exodus Story from the Old Testament

The Wheel of Time turns, and Ages come and pass, leaving memories that become legend. Legend fades to myth. —Robert Jordan, *The Eye of the World*

The story of the Exodus takes place about 1445 BC. Originally, the Israelites had prospered in Egypt. Joseph, of the coat of many colors, had even become the prime minister of the country. Those days, however, were long forgotten. Over many generations, the Israelites had become slaves to the pharaohs of Egypt. The current pharaoh feared the strength of their numbers (estimated at 2 million). Moses was the firstborn of an Israelite slave family, who saved his life from a "slaying of the firstborn" edict by the pharaoh when they put him in a basket and floated him in the Nile River. Moses, found as an infant by a royal family member, was raised in the pharaoh's court. He later fell out of favor with the pharaoh, exiled from Egypt, and ended up living as a shepherd in the desert.

As he was tending his flocks in the desert, Moses saw a burning bush that was not consumed by the flames. He went to the bush, and God spoke to him from it: "Come now therefore, and I will send thee unto Pharaoh, that thou mayest bring forth my people the children of Israel out of Egypt" (Exodus 3:10). God instructed Moses on what to do when he arrived in Egypt, and Moses agreed to speak to the pharaoh and demand that he release the Israelites.

Moses was initially reluctant to take on this task. He was not a good speaker and feared that he would not be able to present God's case to the pharaoh. God told Moses' brother Aaron to meet Moses in the desert and travel into Egypt with him. God sent Aaron with Moses to act as Moses' voice: "And Aaron spake all the words which the LORD had spoken unto Moses, and did the signs in the sight of the people" (Exodus 4:30).

In Egypt, Moses, through Aaron, told the pharaoh to free the Israelites by command of the Lord. The pharaoh refused, saying he didn't know the Lord that Moses spoke of, and told the taskmasters to increase the labor burden on the Israelites. The Israelites blamed Moses and Aaron for their worsened conditions. Moses despaired and complained to God. God answered Moses and the Israelites: "Wherefore say unto the children of Israel, I am the LORD, and I will bring you out from under the burdens of the Egyptians, and I will rid you out of their bondage, and I will redeem you with a stretched out arm, and with great judgments" (Exodus 6:6).

Moses went before the pharaoh again and demanded the release of his people. The pharaoh laughed, and God, through Moses, turned all of the waters to blood. Another demand was made, another refusal, and another disaster followed. Plagues of frogs, gnats and flies, disease that killed their livestock, disease that caused the Egyptians boils, hailstones, locusts, and days of pitch darkness befell Egypt. The pharaoh promised to let the Israelites go if only Moses would bring an end to the plagues, but he didn't make good on the promise when the plagues were stopped.

Again, Moses and Aaron begged the pharaoh to capitulate and free the Israelites. Again he refused. Then the Lord told Moses that the next plague would take the firstborn of every Egyptian and the firstborn of all the Egyptians' animals. So that the Israelites would avoid the same fate, God instructed them through Moses to each sacrifice a lamb, prepare a special meal, and mark their doorposts with the blood of the lamb. Seeing the blood on the door, the angel of death would pass over their houses.

When the angel of death killed all the firstborn of Egypt, the pharaoh and the Egyptians begged the Israelites to leave. The Egyptians gave them all of their remaining wealth to speed them on their way. Moses led them into the wilderness and God showed them the way to go: "And the LORD went before them by day in a pillar of a cloud, to lead them the way; and by night in a pillar of fire, to give them light; to go by day and night" (Exodus 13:21).

By the time the Israelites reached the Red Sea, the pharaoh had changed his mind about setting them free. He sent his armies after them and trapped them against the sea. The Israelites railed against Moses, thinking their death was certain. Despite all the disasters the Lord had brought against Egypt on the behalf of His people, they still doubted His ability and willingness to save them. Yet God was faithful to the Israelites: "And Moses stretched out his hand over the sea; and the LORD caused the sea to go back by a strong east wind all that night, and made the sea dry land, and the waters were divided." And the children of Israel went into the midst of the sea upon the dry ground: and the waters were a wall unto them on their right hand, and on their left." (Exodus 14:21-22) The Israelites passed safely through the Red Sea with the Egyptians on their trail. When all the Israelites passed through, the walls of water collapsed in and the Egyptians were drowned. God's people were free from Egypt. Ultimately, it took the Israelites 40 years of wandering until they found their way back to their historical home, and were reunited with the Hebrews living in the promised land of Canaan.

THE HITTITES

The Hittites ruled a great empire that stretched from Mesopotamia to Syria and Palestine. Their empire was at its greatest from 1600 to 1200 BC, and even after the Assyrians gained control of Mesopotamia after 1300 BC, the Hittite cities and territories thrived independently until 717 BC, when the territories were finally conquered by other peoples.

The Hebrew scriptures have little to say about the Hittites, and the Egyptians regarded them as barbarians. In fact, from 1300 to 1200 BC, the Hittites waged a war against Egypt that drained both empires tragically. The Hittites were perhaps one of the most significant peoples in Mesopotamian history. Because their empire was so large and because their primary activity was commerce—trading with all the civilizations and peoples of the Mediterranean—the Hittites were the people primarily responsible for transmitting Mesopotamian thought, law, political structure, economic structure, and ideas around the Mediterranean, from Egypt to Greece.

PAPYRUS

The writing surface papyrus, named after the plant from which it is made, was manufactured as early as the first Egyptian dynasty, circa 3100 BC. The emergence of writing and the concomitant use of papyrus appear to have been a necessary outcome of the imperial bureaucracy. Papyrus was invariably used by the Egyptians until the AD 800–1000, that is, for 4,000 years. The papyrus product was made by tearing off the "skin" of the papyrus reed. The strips thus formed were first beaten and dried in the sun and then were laid lengthwise and crosswise to attain strength, perhaps with the aid of some glue (made of plants). Finally, the papyrus was stretched and smoothed to be fit for use.

ROPE

There is evidence of rope being made as far back as 17,000 BC. These early ropes were twisted by hand or braided. The earliest indication of any type of mechanical advantage in making rope comes from early Egyptian evidence relating to the craft. The Egyptians tied rope-making material to a piece of finished rope that was weighted and tied to a stick; the material was then spun around the stick. The spinning imparted a twist to the strand. Three twisted strands would then be twisted together in the opposite direction. Finished rope was oiled for use in water.

Endnotes

[1] Aaron helped his brother Moses speak to the Israelites and the Pharaoh. Moses had a lifelong speech impediment. As a child, Moses had been put to a test by the court magicians. Two braziers—one full of gold and the other hot coals—were put before him to see which he would take. If Moses took the gold, he would have to be killed. An angel guided his hand to the coals, and he put one in his mouth, saving his life but ruining his ability to speak clearly.

Implementing Strategic Change: Monica Ashley's Experience

Allen R. Cohen
Babson College

David L. Bradford
Stanford University

Monica Ashley was stunned. Just as she was successfully completing a complex two-year project that could be a major contributor to the future growth of Health Equipment and Laboratories Inc. (HEAL-INC), her boss, Dan Stella, removed her as program manager.

Although Dan, vice president for design and manufacture of one of the top lines of HEAL-INC machines, asked her to stay on in his division, Monica felt that personal defeat had been snatched from the jaws of victory. The glory from her massive effort to enable HEAL-INC to adapt its hospital-oriented, technically driven products and strategies to much wider usage would go elsewhere. It wasn't that she was hung up on glory, but it didn't seem fair to be pulled out of this incredible accomplishment just as it was finally about to overcome the ferocious opposition that had made it even more difficult than it naturally was. And she feared—correctly as it turned out—that over a year would be lost in replacing her and getting a replacement up to speed.

HEAL-INC was a rapidly growing company making a wide range of advanced diagnostic and treatment equipment. Utilizing many complex technologies, from lasers to powerful magnets to semiconductors and signal processors, the company had thrived on the enormous latitude given its very bright employees to take initiatives and pursue opportunities.

Since its inception, HEAL-INC had found great success by creating equipment that appealed to the same kinds of technically sophisticated hospital researchers and technicians it employed. Early on, top management decided that creating an atmosphere of maximum freedom would be worth the waste and duplicated effort, since it would tap the creativity and energy of smart employees. The strategy had worked, and HEAL-INC's meteoric growth had been a source of pride to management and employees—and sometimes a source of puzzlement to those who had been taught to revere order and efficiency above all else. (See Exhibit 1 for a partial organization chart.)

MORE TECH, MORE TOUCH: NEW USERS AND THEIR NEEDS

In recent years, however, the market had begun to shift, along with the technology in the industry. The equipment was increasingly going to be used in doctors' offices, small clinics, and storefront test labs, rather than exclusively in teaching hospitals. New users of the equipment were less technical and more patient-oriented than the hospital staffers who had been the company's original customers.

Furthermore, in order to make the equipment easier for less sophisticated personnel to use, the technology had grown more complicated; thus, far

Exhibit 1   **Partial Organization Chart**

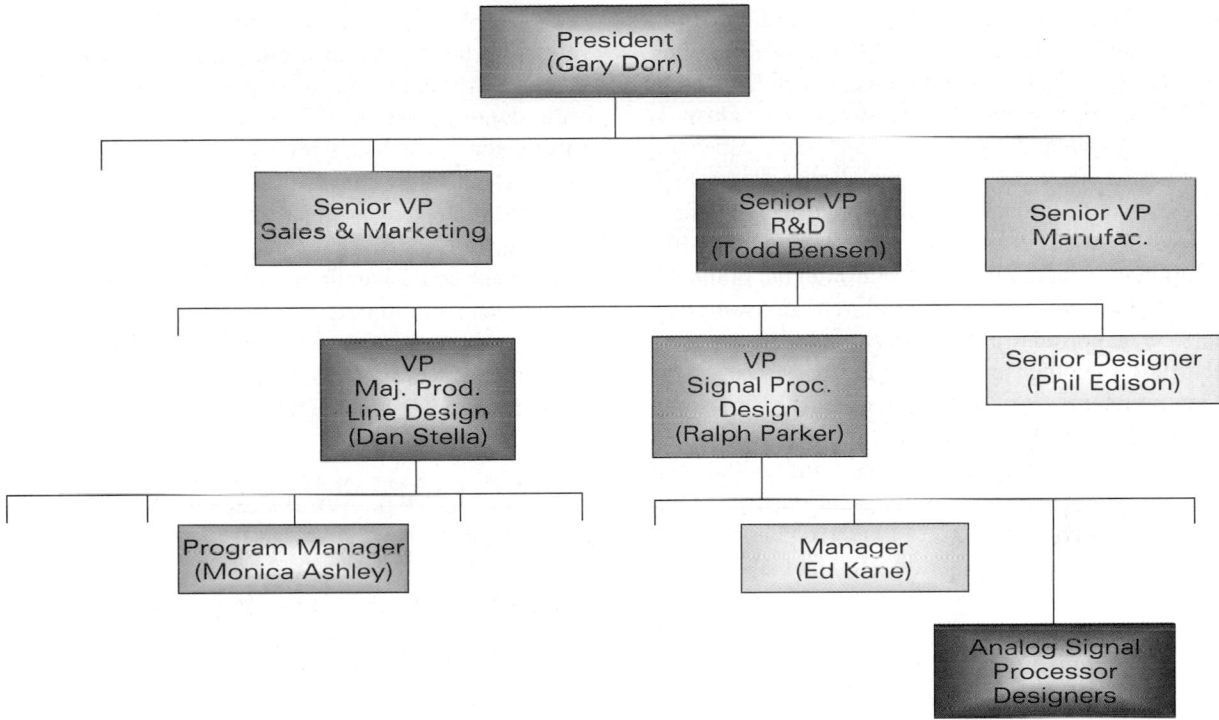

greater coordination and teamwork in design and manufacture became necessary. Many different, but interrelated, components had to be designed by teams of contributors, rather than be developed for special purposes by solo "geniuses." There were pressures for some key components to shift from analog to digital electronics. And purchasers were becoming more selective, so their interests had to be taken into account at an earlier stage of product design. Finally, it was increasingly difficult for any one company, no matter how big, to custom design all the components of the equipment. The industry leaders were beginning to form strategic alliances and purchase components from outside sources.

All of this caused considerable tension at HEAL-INC and entrepreneurial companies like it. The original ways of doing things had brought huge success, and the company was young enough so that many of those who had grown with it were still entrenched. They had a big stake in their hard-won lessons about growth, decentralization, encouragement of initiative, technical orientation, and the virtues of inventing everything within the company. The voices

of those arguing the urgent strategic need for greater ease of operation, more coordination of previously autonomous units, and purchasing components and subsystems elsewhere were not readily heard.

THE PRESIDENT OF HEAL-INC RECRUITS MONICA FOR PROJECT HIPPOCRATES

Monica had been squarely in the middle of just such issues. She had taken on Project Hippocrates reluctantly, because, even though she was ready for a line job after many successful years in important staff positions, she knew there would be major opposition. Over her years at HEAL-INC, she had developed a special relationship with Gary Dorr, the president and founder, which began at a meeting early in her career when she caught his attention by challenging his conclusions. He liked her spirit and the hard work that had enabled her to back up her views with data when he asked why she disagreed. After that, Dorr had periodic long talks with Monica and once told her that he thought of her as his HEAL-INC daughter. So, before taking the assignment as program manager of Project Hippocrates, Monica went to see Dorr.

She explained to him her concerns, especially in relation to a key manager, Ralph Parker, the vice president in charge of designing the key signal processor used in several lines of HEAL-INC equipment. Monica had heard through the grapevine that Parker, who was in a different division from hers, was politically aggressive and had not been helpful on another project that her boss, Dan Stella, had pioneered. A different approach to signal processing—from analog to digital—would likely be needed for Project Hippocrates; and, as the main designer of HEAL-INC's original analog signal processors, Parker could be a major roadblock.

So many people in her division had talked about Parker's legendary resistance to new approaches and to customer input that Monica took their views as fact and didn't bother to talk with Parker directly. She just decided that she wouldn't be another in the long line of people she knew complaining about their inability to move him; she would set out to demonstrate overwhelmingly the correctness of the need for a new signal processor design. Dorr told Monica that he knew about the problem with Parker, and that he was working on it. He told her not to take Parker on directly, but to accept the program manager role, since she would "be protected." Before Monica could reply with her continuing concerns, Dorr ended the meeting by saying, "Monica, congratulations to the new program manager."

A WHIRLWIND OF ACTIVITIES

Monica plunged in, tackling the project with the same focused intensity that she brought to everything she did. She first interviewed the new kinds of purchasers to understand their very different needs; created a task force; recruited members from other parts of HEAL-INC; introduced to HEAL-INC for the first time to the Taguchi method, a highly disciplined product design process she had learned in Japan; and initiated a series of studies on just what would be

needed to alter HEAL-INC's equipment to make it more viable for new applications. All of this activity made people uncomfortable, because the structured Taguchi process was far more rigorous than anyone was used to; and it led to something that had never been done before at HEAL-INC: a total system outline for the product revisions, including all the elements and how they would have to fit together. She created a cross-department signal-processor study group to investigate whether the existing component could handle the redesigned equipment. As Monica had intuited, the study group determined that no in-house analog product could do the job and recommended the purchase from an outside vendor of the necessary digital signal processor.

JUST ONE MORE STUDY: DIFFICULTIES WITH OUTSIDE PURCHASE OF SIGNAL PROCESSORS

This recommendation set off many months of problems. The decision was made, restudied, made again, restudied, and remade four times. Twice Monica gave presentations before the senior management staff, with competing presentations given by the signal-processor design group under Parker. Parker was nasty to her and made numerous accusations, including one that the technical people she had used in her study group were not competent (even though some had come from lower levels of Parker's organization and two had been loaned by Phil Edison, the most respected technical person in the company). Parker had publicly declared that any kind of signal processor would be purchased outside only "over my dead body." And even after the senior management staff gave the go-ahead, Parker accused Monica of proceeding without permission. So still another independent task force was created to evaluate the decision; once again, the outcome was in Monica's favor.

At the first senior management staff meeting, Gary Dorr surprised Monica by being more critical and less friendly than Monica had ever experienced. He had often complained in the past about the need at HEAL-INC to define measures that would spell out the performance of an entire diagnostic and treatment system, not just its components. Worried about the common HEAL-INC problem of components being optimized but the complete system ending up suboptimized (the whole being less than the sum of its parts), Monica had developed detailed, integrated plans, but Dorr seemed annoyed rather than pleased. At the meeting, he criticized Monica for the comprehensive approach.

Monica was confused, then flabbergasted at Dorr's continued critical tone. At first she couldn't say anything, she was so taken aback. Then as the meeting went on, she realized that Dan Stella, her boss, wasn't speaking up and defending the massive amount of work she had done to ensure that components would not be suboptimized at the expense of the total equipment systems. Assuming that her past relationship with Dorr legitimized disagreement with him, she defended the decisions. She knew that customers used different criteria for measuring overall equipment performance than the designers of each component, and she wanted that recognized.

Parker had attended the meetings of the Project Hippocrates group, during which he challenged Monica constantly and, in her view, tried to provoke her. Because Dan Stella had advised Monica to keep cool, she avoided taking Parker's bait. Then, during one meeting at which Monica asked Parker a question, he accused her of being angry. She coolly replied, "It seems to me that you're the one who is angry." Parker exploded. Monica just let him yell, and then proceeded with the meeting.

After the meeting, all who attended, including Dan, congratulated Monica for "humiliating Parker," which had not been her intent at all. She was just trying to head off a fight, as she had been advised. But the battle lines hardened further. From then on, Parker assigned one of his managers, Ed Kane, to attend Project Hippocrates task force meetings on his behalf.

At one of the subsequent meetings, Kane heatedly accused Monica of not listening and of excluding signal processor people. She was embarrassed by the attack and unhappy about being falsely accused; but, as was her custom, she handled the unjust attacks by providing more accurate information. Thinking, "If he knows the truth, he'll cool off," she told Kane the history of how the original cross-functional design team, including people from his own organization, had agreed unanimously on the need for a switch to digital signal processing, and the requisite acquisition of an outside product.

There was so much conflict at that meeting that, as it broke up, Monica's boss, Dan Stella, called a spontaneous meeting of his own managers in a nearby conference room. Because Kane was standing outside the room and he was available to attend, Stella invited him "to c'mon in and help us plan."

Once inside, an obviously outraged Kane shouted, "Who the hell do you think you are, going to an outside vendor!" and called Stella a "traitor and a renegade." Stella retorted that if anyone was a traitor it was Kane, because the signal processor department of which Kane was a member had said to go ahead, and now he was trying to subvert their decision. In Monica's eyes, the confrontation was particularly brutal ("like dinosaurs slugging it out"), especially since she knew that Stella did not particularly like conflict.

Soon after, friends of Monica began to tell her that Kane was spreading nasty personal rumors about her, including innuendoes that she was having an affair with Stella. Stunned and hurt, she decided there was nothing she could do about it. Her friends would know how absurd the rumors were, and she believed that telling others she was innocent would only help dignify the rumors. She persevered in the project.

A month later, Parker once again challenged the outside purchase decision. Monica was called to an extended senior management staff meeting where she was given one day to make a presentation of the complete program; Parker was given the next day for his rebuttal.

TWISTING IN THE WIND: ABANDONED BY THE PRESIDENT

Monica was shocked by what happened at the meeting. She had barely started her presentation when Gary Dorr began to attack her. He said that no one person was going to be in control, that Monica in particular was trying to overcontrol things—"like an Imperial Chinese Emperor" was how he phrased it—and that central control was totally inappropriate for the company. Seeing Parker smirking in the background and feeling extraordinarily jittery after the attack by the president, Monica mustered her courage and told Dorr that she was only giving the complete system overview he had asked for. Every time she tried to give a detailed calculation, Dorr broke in again with criticism. Monica and her group were devastated; they were certain that Dorr had been totally prejudiced by Parker.

When Parker made his presentation the following day, Dorr was very receptive to him. In Monica's eyes, however, Parker had no solid data, and his presentation was devoid of content and filled with glib assertions and pronouncements. The main theme of his argument was "Haven't we always met hospital needs? Just look at our original analog signal processor: it's the best in the business, and it can be adapted to any need our customers have."

As she sat there in disbelief, Monica recalled a comment Dorr had once made to her privately. He had told her that there was no way the company could do without Parker because of his signal processor contributions. After Parker finished, the people in his group were slapping each other on the back; and Kane walked over to sneer, "Ha, ha, you lose!" at Monica. She was upset that Parker and his supporters had done so much behind-closed-doors political maneuvering and it absolutely infuriated her that "politics could beat out substance" in the company. Only Dorr's earlier warning about not confronting Parker kept her from retaliating.

Sticking the knife in was not enough for Parker. He had to twist it. At the end of the meeting, Parker again brought up Monica's negotiation for the digital processor with an outside company. Dorr exploded, and yelled at Monica, "How dare you negotiate on behalf of the company? You are a renegade and an empire-builder!"

Although by this point Monica was down for the count, she defended what had happened, explaining that she acted upon a decision that had been cleared by many groups. But then, when Dorr turned to Edison, the most respected technical expert, and asked him if it had gone through the review committee he headed, Edison claimed he did not remember. Monica was amazed and shocked, since the technical guru had always been friendly to her, and he certainly was present when his review committee had made the decision.

Dorr then said that he was going to go around the room and take a vote on going outside. He said that he personally would vote if there were a tie. As fate would have it, there was a tie. Dorr turned to Monica and asked her how she would interpret the tie.

Monica had been sitting near Dorr at the meeting. After his attack, he acted conciliatory, and they even exchanged whispered comments several times, so Monica was feeling a bit restored in relationship with him. Although she was scared of how it would be taken, she summoned up a sense of humor that she was rarely able to use when tense and deadpanned, "I would say that there was an overwhelming sentiment for going ahead with the outside negotiations." Dorr laughed and agreed. Monica was enormously relieved.

At the next senior management staff meeting, Dorr wanted one more vote on the issue of negotiating with an outside vendor. When the results were in, only one person had voted against the outside purchase: Parker. One of the executive vice presidents then turned to Parker and said, "You will have to speak now or forever hold your peace." Parker finally retorted that the move was against his better judgment and that, when it proved to be a giant mistake, it would be on the heads of Monica and her boss, Dan Stella.

HEAT IN THE KITCHEN: PUT OUT THE FIRE

Monica felt herself constantly being drawn into conflict even though she had wanted to accomplish the whole project by building consensus. In part, she had been driven by her assumptions about her relationship with Dorr. She had assumed that he still wanted her to stand up for what she believed in.

Upset, she went to talk to him about what had happened at various meetings. He told her that she was no longer behaving appropriately; because she was acting like a "hot competitor" when she came to the senior management staff, she was disturbing the company's once-peaceful and productive environment.

In her defense, she tried to explain that it was not she who was causing the problems but Kane and Parker. She reminded Dorr that he himself had said Parker was a problem, but Dorr replied, "That is none of your business." She knew that Dorr admired her for having the drive to complete her advanced studies and other complex company assignments, and that he counted on her as somebody who could carry things through, but she had overestimated the amount of support she would get from him in Project Hippocrates.

Throughout Monica's career at HEAL-INC, Dan Stella had phoned her on Sunday evenings to review the previous week and discuss what was coming up. As the infighting increased at the senior staff meetings, Stella told Monica in one of these Sunday-night phone conversations that she was going too fast and causing conflict. When things got very hot, he called her into his office and tried to slow her down. She said, "Don't these people understand we have all this work to do?"

Stella replied, "Don't you understand you have to build all these relationships and deal with the politics at the top?"

Nevertheless, caught up in the need to master enormous numbers of interrelated issues, Monica pressed on. She had set a date for bringing Project Hippocrates to market, and she was determined to meet it. She knew the external competition was getting increasingly tougher, and that it would be a severe strategic blow to HEAL-INC if the company missed the deadline.

Over the ensuing several months, a new team, which included many signal processor people, was formed to begin the technology transfer process and overcome all not-invented-here feelings in preparation for a contract with an outside vendor. Parker's people chose not to help specify the features of the digital signal processor. Technical experts from Stella's organization did the work, along with some people from sales and marketing. Exhaustive effort went into design and product specification documents to pave the way for a smoother-than-usual product introduction. During this period, there were vague promises from Parker's organization about modifying the existing analog signal processor to meet the new demands, but nothing tangible happened.

ONE MORE TIME: HARD DECISIONS ABOUT THE SIGNAL PROCESSOR

While plans to educate the sales force went forward, Parker stirred up a great deal of tension around the decision to purchase signal processors. He used every meeting he attended to say negative things about Project Hippocrates. Several important customers even told Monica that Parker and his people had visited them to say that their analog signal processor was being enhanced to adapt to new uses, and that the digital processor that HEAL-INC was thinking of purchasing outside was "a pile of crap."

This immobilized Monica at first, because she couldn't understand how top management could allow this malicious behavior to go on. She got Stella to talk to Dorr about it, but she saw nothing happen to stop it. Eventually, it just spurred her into redoubling efforts and pushing her project group to work harder. "I'd have gone crazy if I had paid attention to all that nasty political stuff, so I just poured more energy into the project," she reported later.

As a result of Parker's continued complaining, Dorr formed another committee chaired by a new engineering manager, who, because he had recently been hired away from a competitor, was assumed to be unbiased. Unbeknownst to Monica, the new manager began a series of secret meetings involving most of the same people who had been part of Monica's original task force to work on what the criteria should be for making the decision.

Within the next month, the company signed a contract with an outside vendor. Shortly thereafter, Monica learned of the secret study committee and found out it was still evaluating outside purchase. She warned that the company now had a legal obligation and could be sued if it did not go ahead with the new contract.

In spite of her troubles, Monica was proud of the negotiation and the amount of continuing vendor support that she had managed to get the vendor to include in the contract. In fact, her negotiation eventually became a model for the company to purchase components from outside.

Three months after the contract was signed, the "secret" committee announced that it was ready to hear a debate on the merits of the outside digital signal processor versus the existing HEAL-INC analog product. Kane and Monica made presentations.

Another three months went by before the committee announced its decision, which was to go ahead with the outside purchase. Meanwhile, people working on the project were completely confused;

they didn't know which side to support. Monica told them to forget politics because there was work to do, but she had to keep encouraging people to get them to do what was needed.

SUDDEN DEATH: MONICA LOSES HER POSITION

Two days before a major national meeting, which Monica had organized for HEAL-INC people from around the country to finalize the support strategy for implementing Project Hippocrates, she was called to a meeting with Dan Stella and a new personnel manager. There she was told that she would no longer be managing the program.

Crushed, Monica asked why. Stella told her that the secret committee had recommended that a more technical person replace her, but that he had removed her because he thought she might have a nervous breakdown as a result of all the intensity of her involvement. He believed that she had failed to read the signals he had sent her to slow down, build relationships more, hold back her angry opinions in meetings, and, in general, learn to act "more like a top executive." To him that meant fighting battles off-line rather than in public, and learning to sit quietly through public attacks, even when they were wrong. He told her that as long as she did not understand all of that, there was no place for her in Project Hippocrates. He told her, however, he wanted to keep her on and he gave her some time to think about what her new job might be. For almost a year after that, Monica worked on minor projects as part of Stella's group.

Subsequent events made Monica feel simultaneously vindicated and regretful. Following another eight months of study, the new program manager concluded that Monica's plans were correct; he proceeded with Project Hippocrates using the innovative strategy Monica had developed for HEAL-INC. Kane was removed from Parker's staff and was having trouble getting anyone in the company to take him on in a new position. The scope of Parker's job was eventually reduced considerably, and he lost control of the most important part of the signal processor design area. And, after a year in limbo, Monica

began to acquire significant assignments again. Yet the way in which the project had lived but the leader of it had been killed off—or at least buried alive for a year—left wounds that still ached; and Monica was determined to learn from her experiences.

MONICA REFLECTS ON HER EXPERIENCES

In retrospect, and with a year to contemplate what had happened, Monica analyzed her own problems as follows:

I was very data-oriented in my approach to the project, which carried the day; but I didn't develop the interpersonal contacts to solidify my influence. Not being from the signal processor department, I was out of the design mainstream, yet there were many complex issues to deal with. I still haven't figured out why they allowed a female—especially one without an engineering background—to manage the project and whether they were setting me up for a big fall.

I know I could have had Parker's support if I hadn't challenged the sacred cow of their analog signal processor product, but I didn't see how to avoid that once we determined that the technology was too limited. When I invited the signal processor people in early in the process, they were surprised because, in their own organization, they couldn't get heard if they were not part of the original analog cult. Most of them had been trying to get the company to consider a move to digital technology for some time, but they were shot down from within their own organization.

I had heard that Parker was an authoritarian who could not be influenced and that no one dared challenge him, and I guess I was scared. There was so much work to be done and so much market opportunity that I focused on achieving the goals without trying to directly influence Parker. He had a much higher power position in the organization and was a formidable player, so I was afraid to challenge him.

I wanted Parker's people to recognize on their own that Project Hippocrates needed new signal processing capacity, but I see now that I should have dealt with Parker directly if I wanted to be treated as a senior executive.

Furthermore, I have to build my confidence; I still feel like a little kid from the sticks, despite all my success. Others see me as overconfident and aggressive, but I probably act that way to overcome my own fears of somehow being "found out." My peers tell me that they are afraid of me and don't argue with me because they know I would bowl them over with my arguments or my intensity. They see me as angry; but I feel that I am just intense. It surprises me when they act laid-back even when they have intense feelings about something; when I feel intensely, I show it.

I now see that the content of what I was doing—the plans, strategies, decisions—was the least important part. The most important is mobilizing support and resources. If the content is wrong, you can always change it; but if there is no support, you don't have a foundation. I was trying to work without a foundation under me.

Ironically, I'm getting *more* done now without having to push so hard. In the past, I thought I had to speak up and give lots of facts to prove I was credible and confident, but I no longer think that way. I don't want to be so personally exposed and vulnerable that I overreact to attacks or assume I'm being attacked when I'm not. When Dan pushed me to do some relationship building, I made excuses for why I couldn't take the time to do it. I see now that was wrong.

I did ask Phil Edison for his help on technical issues; and as evidence of his support and confidence, he gave me two key people early on. It is easier for me to ask for help when I feel that the person is supportive. Because Edison is calm and laid back, I was too. I felt I had to stay low-key or I would lose him. I didn't see how that same approach might have worked with others. Even when Edison and I disagreed, I would try to be calm and talk slowly, which is very hard for me. I would try not to fight too hard; instead I would go away and come back to him when I had the data.

Edison likes being "stroked," which was easy to do because his early support made me feel very positive toward him. It wasn't artificial at all. The two people he gave me were reputed to be very tough and ready to eat alive anyone who made a technical mistake. When they joined me, I went to them and told them I was not a technical expert and would need their help. They were great after that.

Even when Edison challenged my ideas, I would never feel personally attacked. I would just want to figure out what the right answer was. When Kane attacked me, however, he would intimidate me both verbally and physically. He would even stand much too close, and when I tried to back off, he would follow me around, trying to dominate, to win, both organizationally and technically. As an engineer, Kane had no sense of how to work through a problem taking many views and business needs into account. With him it was all or nothing; if I didn't accept his position immediately, he would fight until I did. There was no sense of compromise or mutual learning. I got the impression that he would accept nothing short of complete acquiescence on my part, which I couldn't do, because the data I had simply didn't support his position. I also felt that I had to protect those people who had come to me from his organization. They appreciated my protecting them, of course; but he didn't.

He spent lots of time building interpersonal bridges. For example, he worked hard to influence Todd Benson, my division's senior vice president, who was a longtime supporter of mine. Although I knew what Kane was doing, I didn't bother to go talk to Todd. I figured that we had data on our side, so why spend time with somebody I already knew. And he had plenty else on his plate.

In the long run, Kane's position and strategy didn't help him any more than mine helped me. He lost his job, too. We were opposite sides of the coin—he had relationships and I had data, but we both lost. Both data and relationships, together, were necessary for success.

I never lobbied anyone, even when I knew the person that Kane had gone to. For example, an outside member of our board of directors went out of his way to congratulate me every time I made any kind of presentation on Project Hippocrates. Although, in retrospect, it is clear that he could have been a strong ally, I never followed up with him.

I had nothing to offer Kane to get him to back off, except to voluntarily disappear into the woodwork. Although people had told me he was a bad apple and I should leave him alone, Dan Stella had said that I shouldn't get down to Kane's level of behavior, so I didn't know how exactly to respond when he attacked me in meetings.

I suppose that I could have gone to Kane directly after his first nasty attack and warned him that if he didn't cut it out I would expose his behavior publicly. Then, when he acted up in a meeting, I could have said something like, "You're doing it again, Kane; you're being personal about the issues instead of using data. That's just what you do when you spread rumors about me instead of dealing with the issues. Let's deal with the issues here." If I had said it calmly, I probably wouldn't have been seen as descending to his level, and that might have stopped him.

I wish I could learn to use humor instead of just being a fighter. But if someone like Kane says (and he did), "You'll do this over my dead body," should

I say, "Lie down"? I suppose if I had said something like, "Anybody here know where I can find a gun to give Mr. Kane?" I might have broken the tension. When I am not feeling uptight and tense, I can inject humor. I see now that it works very well on senior executives here, but I haven't been able to joke when I am tense.

I could have stayed quiet when Dorr attacked me; maybe it was immature to take him on in front of witnesses. I could have done it later in private; but I don't like seeing my people attacked, and I think it is my role to publicly defend them.

I've seen Dorr get furious with his people, and they just seem to take it. I thought I could get away with challenging him not only because of the old relationship but also because he expected that of me.

Maybe when he attacked me, I could have replied quietly, "That's not how I see it," or, "We have to talk; I have a different view of the facts." That might have been a more mature way to do it.

I forget to take the long-term view because I feel I have to win every battle. I need to learn to roll with the punches. I haven't been savvy about when to speak and when to be quiet. It looks as if laying low is more effective.

I guess it never occurred to me that putting a senior executive in a bad light in front of others is not such a great idea. Dorr might have liked me for challenging him when I was junior, but I guess what I didn't realize was that, as you get nearer the top, you have to play by different rules.

Dan Stella didn't support me as much as I wanted him to. He claimed that he did, but I didn't see it. And sometimes he thinks he is helpful when he is not. For example, after I complained that my ideas weren't being listened to at his management committee meetings, he would make a special point of acknowledging my contribution after I said something. But, since he didn't do that for others, it was seen as an unfair advantage. So he thought he was helping when he wasn't. Similarly, he thought that removing me from Project Hippocrates was the best thing "for my health." I needed his support, not his protection. I'm not a delicate flower. He could have handled the whole conversation much better.

At the senior management staff meeting at which Dorr attacked me, Dan said nothing. He believes in working the tough issues in private. I know now that he was trying to work behind the scenes to back Parker and Kane off, but I would have appreciated something more visible. I got the program through for him and then got shit for it. He avoids conflict until there is a major explosion.

I believe Dan changed as he got to the vice-president level. He used to welcome and solicit direct feedback, but now he doesn't. He tells us, "Be senior managers; that is, be quiet and circumspect and don't engage in direct confrontation." In the old days, there was healthy disagreement, but now it is hard to get people stirred at his meetings.

I find Dan and I can no longer have the kind of conversations we used to have when he was more congenial and collegial. Now I have to agree wholeheartedly or disagree very gently and tentatively. When I perceived that Dan was threatened by my conversations with Dorr, I learned not to tell anybody about them. But now that Dan has his own conversations with the president, I don't think he is threatened by my closeness to Dorr.

I guess I must have given Dan fits because, in his eyes, I became unpredictable and seemingly uncontrollable, and therefore potentially embarrassing. I guess that doesn't help him look good when he wants to win the respect of the senior managers. I don't want to embarrass him; I want to learn how to function in a better way.

Dan has been pushing me to work more with other members of his management committee and not rely on him as my sole contact. I have been doing that, and I find that I now do feel more effective and comfortable with them.

One of HEAL-INC's senior executives kept telling me in regards to Project Hippocrates that I didn't have to own it all. He said that the more you give away, the more will be given to you; and I'm starting to understand that. Dan tells me the same thing. Before, I was volunteering for everything. Had I volunteered for less, I would have had time for more activities, including more relationship building.

It's a curse to see the big picture and have a strict, self-imposed deadline, because you know how much has to be done. Dan and Dorr would tell me that they knew I was right but they couldn't handle everything I was throwing at them in the moment. When they didn't know the overall strategic plan, how could they worry about one subsidiary issue that I was pushing at them? I made people feel overwhelmed early on, which wasn't useful, nor intended. I felt my team was being clever and comprehensive to think of all the angles; but Dan and Dorr—most of the senior staff, in fact—just felt that I was throwing too much at them. I needed to show them an overview rather than a step-by-step plan laid out in the minutest detail.

I guess what I really need to do is persuade myself that I am bright enough so that I can focus on what is important to others rather than on proving that I am really smart. I don't know what has to happen for me to finally accept that I am. Because I was taught to be self-critical and humble, it's been difficult for me to accept this positive view of myself, although deep down I know it's true.

STELLA LOOKS BACK

Dan Stella had his own views of what had happened, and the lessons for Monica:

Monica took Kane's attacks on her too personally. She should have stepped back and let him hang himself. Furthermore, when he was out doing countermarketing to the ideas of Project Hippocrates, Monica should have been selling the project; but she didn't. We're still repairing the damage.

I agree that there was no way to deal with Parker. He does not and will not understand the needs of customers other than hospital technicians. Because he had position power, the only battle strategy to use with him was to go underground. All you can do is neutralize him, using other people. You need to practice "octopus management": Get others to see that there's a problem, and get them to raise the issue with top management. If it comes from many sides, it can be effective eventually. But you have to be cautious how you word your concerns. The trick is to get marketing to do a full-court press, since they won't be able to sell machines that are not suited to other kinds of customers.

If Monica had been patient, others would have blocked Parker, but I couldn't back her off. She set a launch date and wouldn't budge. I kept trying to slow her down, but she wasn't having that. I was angry with Parker and Kane too, but I didn't want to add to Monica's boiling. Remember the old saying: In war, if there is no chance that you will lose your life waiting, patience wins.

I gave Monica a card that says "Listen; Remove the Urgency; Trust," but it didn't get through to her at the time. That's the hardest thing for a data-driven person to do! I know, because that's the way I am too; neither of us suffers fools gladly. We just want to pile more data on.

She became a bulldozer, which got her in trouble with Dorr. He wasn't comfortable with a woman being so aggressive and tenacious, refusing to grovel. Although I think he learned from that experience, he was not happy at the time. That hurt me a lot. I've had a 10-year relationship as Monica's boss and sponsor, and I wanted to help, but I couldn't. She's rarely wrong about data, so it was extremely frustrating. I keep telling her, "Give it away; it'll come back with interest."

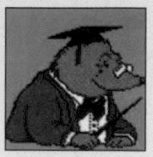

Starbucks' Global Quest in 2006: Is the Best Yet to Come?

Amit J. Shah
Frostburg State University

Arthur A. Thompson
The University of Alabama

Thomas F. Hawk
Frostburg State University

In early 2006, Howard Schultz, Starbucks' founder, chairman of the board, and global strategist, could look with satisfaction on the company's phenomenal growth and market success. Since 1987, Starbucks had transformed itself from a modest nine-store operation in the Pacific Northwest into a powerhouse multinational enterprise with 10,241 store locations, including some 2,900 stores in 30 foreign countries (see Exhibit 1). During Starbucks' early years when coffee was a 50-cent morning habit at local diners and fast-food establishments, skeptics had ridiculed the notion of $3 coffee as a yuppie fad. But the popularity of Starbucks' Italian-style coffees, espresso beverages, teas, pastries, and confections had made Starbucks one of the great retailing stories of recent history and the world's biggest specialty coffee chain. In 2003, Starbucks made the Fortune 500, prompting Schultz to remark, "It would be arrogant to sit here and say that 10 years ago we thought we would be on the Fortune 500. But we dreamed from day one and we dreamed big."[1]

Having positioned Starbucks as the dominant retailer, roaster, and brand of specialty coffees and coffee drinks in North America and spawned the creation of the specialty coffee industry, management's long-term objective was now to establish Starbucks as the most recognized and respected brand in the world. New stores were being opened at the rate of roughly 32 per week in 2005, and management

expected to have 15,000 Starbucks stores open worldwide going into 2006. Believing that the scope of Starbucks' long-term opportunity had been underestimated, Schultz had recently increased the targeted number of stores from 25,000 to 30,000 worldwide by 2013, at least half of which were to be outside the United States.[2] He noted that Starbucks had only an overall 7 percent share of the coffee-drinking market in the United States and perhaps a 1 percent share internationally. According to Schultz, "That still leaves lots of room for growth. Internationally, we are still in our infancy."[3] Although coffee consumption worldwide was stagnant, coffee was still the second-most-consumed beverage in the world, trailing only water.[4]

Starbucks reported revenues in fiscal 2005 of $6.4 billion, up 205 percent from $2.1 billion in fiscal 2000; after-tax profits in 2005 were $494.5 million, an increase of 423 percent from the company's fiscal 2000 net earnings of $94.6 million.

COMPANY BACKGROUND

Starbucks got its start in 1971 when three academics, English teacher Jerry Baldwin, history teacher Zev Siegel, and writer Gordon Bowker—all coffee aficionados—opened Starbucks Coffee, Tea, and Spice in touristy Pikes Place Market in Seattle. The three partners shared a love for fine coffees and exotic teas and believed they could build a clientele in Seattle that would appreciate the best coffees and

Exhibit 1   **Number of Starbucks Store Locations Worldwide, 1987–2005**

Fiscal Year	Number of Store Locations at End of Fiscal Year	Fiscal Year	Number of Store Locations at End of Fiscal Year
1987	17	1997	1,412
1988	33	1998	1,886
1989	55	1999	2,135
1990	84	2000	3,501
1991	116	2001	4,709
1992	165	2002	5,886
1993	272	2003	7,225
1994	425	2004	8,569
1995	676	2005	10,241
1996	1,015		

Licensed Locations of Starbucks Stores, 2005

Asia-Pacific		Europe–Middle East–Africa		Americas	
Japan	572	Spain	39	United States	2,435
China	185	Saudi Arabia	38	Canada	118
Taiwan	153	Greece	38	Mexico	60
South Korea	133	United Arab Emirates	37	Hawaii	51
Philippines	83	Kuwait	32	Puerto Rico	11
Malaysia	62	Turkey	24	Peru	6
New Zealand	41	Switzerland	21	The Bahamas	2
Indonesia	32	France	16		2,683
	1,261	Lebanon	10		
		Austria	9		
		Qatar	8		
		Bahrain	8		
		Cyprus	7		
		Oman	4		
		Jordan	4		
		United Kingdom	2		
			297		

Source: 2005 10-K report.

teas, much like what had already emerged in the San Francisco Bay area. They each invested $1,350 and borrowed another $5,000 from a bank to open the Pikes Place store. The inspiration and mentor for the Starbucks venture in Seattle was a Dutch immigrant named Alfred Peet, who had opened Peet's Coffee and Tea, in Berkeley, California, in 1966. Peet's store specialized in importing fine coffees and teas and dark-roasting its own beans the European way to bring out the full flavors. Customers were encouraged to learn how to grind the beans and make their own freshly brewed coffee at home. Baldwin, Siegel, and Bowker were well acquainted with Peet's expertise, having visited his store on numerous occasions and listened to him expound on quality coffees and the importance of proper bean-roasting techniques.

The Pikes Place store featured modest, hand-built, classic nautical fixtures. One wall was devoted to whole-bean coffees, while another had shelves of coffee products. The store did not offer fresh-brewed coffee by the cup, but tasting samples were sometimes available. Initially, Siegel was the only paid employee. He wore a grocer's apron, scooped out beans for customers, extolled the virtues of fine, dark-roasted coffees, and functioned as the partnership's retail expert. The other two partners kept their day jobs but came by at lunch or after work to help out. During the start-up period, Baldwin kept the books and developed a growing knowledge of coffee; Bowker served as the "magic, mystery, and romance man."[5] The store was an immediate success, with sales exceeding expectations, partly because of interest stirred by a favorable article in the *Seattle Times*. For most of the first year, Starbucks ordered its coffee-bean supplies from Peet's, but then the partners purchased a used roaster from Holland, set up roasting operations in a nearby ramshackle building, and developed their own blends and flavors.

By the early 1980s, the company had four Starbucks stores in the Seattle area and had been profitable every year since opening its doors. But then Zev Siegel experienced burnout and left the company to pursue other interests. Jerry Baldwin took over day-to-day management of the company and functioned as chief executive officer; Gordon Bowker remained involved as an owner but devoted most of his time to his advertising and design firm, a weekly newspaper he had founded, and a microbrewery that he was launching known as the Redhook Ale Brewery.

Howard Schultz Enters the Picture

In 1981, Howard Schultz, vice president and general manager of U.S. operations for a Swedish maker of stylish kitchen equipment and coffeemakers, decided to pay Starbucks a visit—he was curious about why Starbucks was selling so many of his company's products. The morning after his arrival in Seattle, he was escorted to the Pikes Place store by Linda Grossman, the retail merchandising manager for Starbucks. A solo violinist was playing Mozart at the door (his violin case open for donations). Schultz was immediately taken by the powerful and pleasing aroma of the coffees, the wall displaying coffee beans, and the rows of coffeemakers on the shelves. As he talked with the clerk behind the counter, the clerk scooped out some Sumatran coffee beans, ground them, put the grounds in a cone filter, poured hot water over the cone, and shortly handed Schultz a porcelain mug filled with freshly brewed coffee. After only taking three sips of the brew, Schultz was hooked. He began asking the clerk and Grossman questions about the company, about coffees from different parts of the world, and about the different ways of roasting coffee.

A bit later, he was introduced to Jerry Baldwin and Gordon Bowker, whose offices overlooked the com-pany's coffee-roasting operation. Schultz was struck by their knowledge about coffee, their commitment to providing customers with quality coffees, and their passion for educating customers about the merits of dark-roasted coffees. Baldwin told Schultz, "We don't manage the business to maximize anything other than the quality of the coffee."[6] The company purchased only the finest arabica coffees and put them through a meticulous dark-roasting process to bring out their full flavors. Baldwin explained that the cheap robusta coffees used in supermarket blends burned when subjected to dark roasting. He also noted that the makers of supermarket blends preferred lighter roasts, which allowed higher yields (the longer a coffee was roasted, the more weight it lost).

Schultz was also struck by the business philosophy of the two partners. It was clear that Starbucks stood not just for good coffee but also for the dark-roasted flavor profiles that the founders were passionate about. Top-quality, fresh-roasted, whole-bean coffee was the company's differentiating feature and a bedrock value. It was also clear to Schultz that Starbucks was strongly committed to educating its customers to appreciate the qualities of fine coffees. The company depended mainly on word of mouth to get more people into its stores, then built customer loyalty cup by cup as buyers gained a sense of discovery and excitement about the taste of fine coffee.

On his trip back to New York the next day, Howard Schultz could not stop thinking about Starbucks and what it would be like to be a part of the Starbucks enterprise. Schultz recalled, "There was something magic about it, a passion and authenticity I had never experienced in business."[7] The appeal of living in the Seattle area was another strong plus. By the time he landed at Kennedy Airport, he knew in his heart he wanted to go to work for Starbucks. At the first opportunity, Schultz asked Baldwin whether there was any way he could fit into Starbucks. While Schultz and Baldwin had established an easy, comfortable personal rapport, it still took a year, numerous meetings at which Schultz presented his ideas, and a lot of convincing to get Baldwin, Bowker, and their silent partner from San Francisco to agree to hire him. Schultz pursued a job at Starbucks far more vigorously than Starbucks pursued hiring Schultz. There was some nervousness about bringing in an outsider, especially a high-powered New Yorker who had not grown up with the values of the company. Nonetheless, Schultz continued to press his ideas about the tremendous potential of expanding the Starbucks enterprise outside Seattle and exposing people all over America to Starbucks coffee. He argued that there had to be more than just the few thousand coffee lovers in Seattle who would enjoy the company's products.

At a meeting with the three owners in San Francisco in the spring of 1982, Schultz once again presented his ideas and vision for opening Starbucks stores across the United States and Canada. He thought the meeting went well and flew back to New York, believing a job offer was in the bag. However, the next day Jerry Baldwin called Schultz and indicated that the owners had decided against hiring him because geographic expansion was too risky and they did not share Schultz's vision for Starbucks. Schultz was despondent, seeing his dreams of being a part of Starbucks' future go up in smoke. Still, he believed so deeply in Starbucks' potential that he decided to make a last-ditch appeal; he called Baldwin back the next day and made an impassioned, reasoned case for why the decision was a mistake. Baldwin agreed to reconsider. The next morning Baldwin called Schultz and told him the job of heading marketing and overseeing the retail stores was his. In September 1982, Howard Schultz took over his new responsibilities at Starbucks.

Starbucks and Howard Schultz: The 1982–1985 Period

In his first few months at Starbucks, Howard Schultz spent most of his waking hours in the four Seattle stores—working behind the counters, tasting different kinds of coffee, talking with customers, getting to know store personnel, and learning the retail aspects of the coffee business. By December, Jerry Baldwin concluded that Schultz was ready for the final part of his training, that of actually roasting the coffee. Schultz spent a week getting an education about the colors of different coffee beans, listening for the telltale second pop of the beans during the roasting process, learning to taste the subtle differences among Baldwin and Bowker's various roasts, and familiarizing himself with the roasting techniques for different beans.

Schultz made a point of acclimating himself to the informal dress code at Starbucks, gaining credibility and building trust with colleagues, and making the transition from the high-energy, coat-and-tie style of New York to the more casual, low-key ambience of the Pacific Northwest (see Exhibit 2 for a rundown on Howard Schultz's background). Schultz made real headway in gaining the acceptance and respect of company personnel while working at the Pikes Place store one day during the busy Christmas season that first year. The store was packed and Schultz was behind the counter ringing up sales of coffee when someone shouted that a shopper had just headed out the door with some stuff—two expensive coffeemakers it turned out, one in each hand. Without thinking, Schultz leaped over the counter and chased the thief up the cobblestone street outside the store, yelling, "Drop that stuff! Drop it!" The thief was startled enough to drop both pieces and run away. Howard picked up the merchandise and returned to the store, holding the coffeemakers up like trophies. Everyone applauded. When Schultz returned to his office later that afternoon, his staff had strung up a banner that read: "Make my day."[8]

Schultz was overflowing with ideas for the company. Early on, he noticed that first-time customers sometimes felt uneasy in the stores because of their lack of knowledge about fine coffees and because store employees sometimes came across as a little arrogant or superior to coffee novices. Schultz worked with store employees on customer-friendly sales skills and developed brochures that made it easy for customers to learn about fine coffees. However, Schultz's biggest inspiration and vision for Starbucks' future came during the spring of 1983 when the company sent him to Milan, Italy, to attend an international housewares show. While walking from his hotel to the convention center, he spotted an espresso bar and went inside to look around. The cashier beside the door nodded and smiled. The

Exhibit 2 **Biographical Sketch of Howard Schultz**

- His parents both came from working-class families residing in Brooklyn, New York, for two generations. Neither completed high school.
- He grew up in a government-subsidized housing project in Brooklyn, was the oldest of three children, played sports with the neighborhood kids and developed a passion for baseball, and became a die-hard Yankees fan.
- His father was a blue-collar factory worker and taxicab driver who held many low-wage, no-benefits jobs; his mother remained home to take care of the children during their preschool years, then worked as an office receptionist. The family was hard pressed to make ends meet.
- He had a number of jobs as a teenager—paper route, counter job at luncheonette, an after-school job in the garment district in Manhattan, a summer job steaming yarn at a knit factory. He always gave part of his earnings to his mother to help with family expenses.
- He saw success in sports as his way to escape life in the projects; he played quarterback on the high school football team.
- He was offered a scholarship to play football at Northern Michigan University (the only offer he got) and he took it. When his parents drove him to the campus to begin the fall term, it was his first trip outside New York. It turned out that he didn't have enough talent to play football, but he got loans and worked at several jobs to keep himself in school. He majored in communications, took a few business courses on the side, and graduated in 1975 with a B average—the first person in his family to graduate from college.
- He went to work for a ski lodge in Michigan after graduation, then left to go back to New York, landing a sales job at Xerox Corporation. He left Xerox to work for Swedish coffee-equipment maker Hammarplast, U.S.A., becoming vice president and general manager in charge of U.S. operations and managing 20 independent sales representatives.
- He married Sheri Kersch in July 1982 and later became the father of two children.
- His father contracted lung cancer in 1982 at age 60 and died in 1988, leaving his mother with no pension, no life insurance, and no savings.
- He became a principal owner of Seattle SuperSonics NBA team in 2001 and also a principal owner of Seattle Storm of WNBA.
- He owned about 32 million shares of Starbucks worth about $950 million in December 2005.

Source: Howard Schultz and Dori Jones Yang, *Pour Your Heart Into It* (New York: Hyperion, 1997).

barista behind the counter greeted Howard cheerfully and moved gracefully to pull a shot of espresso for one customer and handcraft a foamy cappuccino for another, all the while conversing merrily with those standing at the counter. Schultz thought the barista's performance was "great theater." Just down the way on a side street, he entered in an even more crowded espresso bar where the barista, whom he surmised to be the owner, was greeting customers by name; people were laughing and talking in an atmosphere that plainly was comfortable and familiar. In the next few blocks, he saw two more espresso bars. That afternoon, when the trade show concluded for the day, Schultz walked the streets of Milan to explore more espresso bars. Some were stylish and upscale; others attracted a blue-collar clientele. Most had few chairs, and it was common for Italian opera to be playing in the background. What struck Schultz was how popular and vibrant the Italian coffee bars were.

Energy levels were typically high, and they seemed to function as an integral community gathering place. Each one had its own unique character, but they all had a barista who performed with flair and maintained a camaraderie with the customers.

Schultz remained in Milan for a week, exploring coffee bars and learning as much as he could about the Italian passion for coffee drinks. Schultz was particularly struck by the fact that there were 1,500 coffee bars in Milan, a city about the size of Philadelphia, and a total of 200,000 in all of Italy. In one bar, he heard a customer order a caffe latte and decided to try one himself—the barista made a shot of espresso, steamed a frothy pitcher of milk, poured the two together in a cup, and put a dollop of foam on the top. Schultz liked it immediately, concluding that lattes should be a feature item on any coffee bar menu even though none of the coffee experts he had talked to had ever mentioned them.

Schultz's 1983 trip to Milan produced a revelation: The Starbucks stores in Seattle completely missed the point. There was much more to the coffee business than just selling beans and getting people to appreciate grinding their own beans and brewing fine coffee in their homes. What Starbucks needed to do was serve fresh-brewed coffee, espressos, and cappuccinos in its stores (in addition to beans and coffee equipment) and try to create an American version of the Italian coffee bar culture. Going to Starbucks should be an experience, a special treat, a place to meet friends and visit. Re-creating the authentic Italian coffee bar culture in the United States could be Starbucks' differentiating factor.

Schultz Becomes Frustrated

On Howard Schultz's return from Italy, he shared his revelation and ideas for modifying the format of Starbucks' stores with Jerry Baldwin and Gordon Bowker. But instead of winning their approval for trying out some of his ideas, Schultz encountered strong resistance. They argued that Starbucks was a retailer, not a restaurant or coffee bar. They feared that serving drinks would put them in the beverage business and diminish the integrity of Starbucks' mission as a purveyor of fine coffees. They pointed out that Starbucks had been profitable every year and there was no reason to rock the boat in a small, private company like Starbucks. But a more pressing reason not to pursue Schultz's coffee bar concept emerged shortly—Baldwin and Bowker were excited by an opportunity to purchase Peet's Coffee and Tea. The acquisition was finalized in early 1984, and to fund it Starbucks had to take on considerable debt, leaving little in the way of financial flexibility to support Schultz's ideas for entering the beverage part of the coffee business or expanding the number of Starbucks stores. For most of 1984, Starbucks managers were dividing their time between operations in Seattle and the Peet's enterprise in San Francisco. Schultz found himself in San Francisco every other week supervising the marketing and operations of the five Peet stores. Starbucks employees began to feel neglected and, in one quarter, did not receive their usual bonus due to tight financial conditions. Employee discontent escalated to the point where a union election was called. The union won by three votes. Baldwin was shocked at the results, concluding that employees no longer trusted him. In the months that followed, he began to spend more of his energy on Peet's operation in San Francisco.

It took Howard Schultz nearly a year to convince Jerry Baldwin to let him test an espresso bar. Baldwin relented when Starbucks opened its sixth store in April 1984. It was the first store designed to sell beverages, and it was the first store located in downtown Seattle. Schultz asked for a 1,500-square-foot space to set up a full-scale Italian-style espresso bar, but Jerry agreed to allocating only 300 square feet in a corner of the new store. As a deliberate experiment to see what would happen, the store opened with no fanfare. By closing time on the first day, some 400 customers had been served, well above the 250-customer average of Starbucks' best-performing stores. Within two months the store was serving 800 customers per day. The two baristas could not keep up with orders during the early-morning hours, resulting in lines outside the door onto the sidewalk. Most of the business was at the espresso counter, while sales at the regular retail counter were only adequate.

Schultz was elated at the test results, expecting that Jerry's doubts about entering the beverage side of the business would be dispelled and that he would gain approval to pursue the opportunity to take Starbucks to a new level. Every day he went into Baldwin's office to show him the sales figures and customer counts at the new downtown store. But Baldwin was not comfortable with the success of the new store, believing that it felt wrong and that espresso drinks were a distraction from the core business of marketing fine arabica coffees at retail. Baldwin rebelled at the thought that people would see Starbucks as a place to get a quick cup of coffee to go. He adamantly told Schultz, "We're coffee roasters. I don't want to be in the restaurant business . . . Besides, we're too deeply in debt to consider pursuing this idea."[9] While he didn't deny that the experiment was succeeding, he didn't want to go forward with introducing beverages in other Starbucks stores. Schultz's efforts to persuade Baldwin to change his mind continued to meet strong resistance, although to avoid a total impasse Baldwin finally did agree to let Schultz put espresso machines in the back of possibly one or two other Starbucks stores.

Over the next several months, Schultz made up his mind to leave Starbucks and start his own company. His plan was to open espresso bars in high-traffic downtown locations, serve espresso drinks and coffee by the cup, and try to emulate the friendly, energetic atmosphere he had encountered in Italian espresso bars. Baldwin and Bowker, knowing how frustrated Schultz had become, supported his efforts to go out on his own and agreed to let him stay in his current job and office until definitive plans were in place. Schultz left Starbucks in late 1985.

Schultz's Il Giornale Venture

With the aid of a lawyer friend who helped companies raise venture capital and go public, Howard Schultz began seeking out investors for the kind of company he had in mind. Ironically, Jerry Baldwin committed to investing $150,000 of Starbucks' money in Schultz's coffee bar enterprise, thus becoming Schultz's first investor. Baldwin accepted Schultz's invitation to be a director of the new company, and Gordon Bowker agreed to be a part-time consultant for six months. Bowker, pumped up about the new venture, urged Schultz to take pains to make sure that everything about the new stores—the name, the presentation, the care taken in preparing the coffee—be calculated to elevate customer expectations and lead them to expect something better than competitors offered. Bowker proposed that the new company be named Il Giornale Coffee Company (pronounced *il jor NAHL ee*), a suggestion that Schultz accepted. In December 1985, Bowker and Schultz made a trip to Italy, where they visited some 500 espresso bars in Milan and Verona, observing local habits, taking notes about decor and menus, snapping photographs, and videotaping baristas in action.

About $400,000 in seed capital was raised by the end of January 1986, enough to rent an office, hire a couple of key employees, develop a store design, and open the first store. But it took until the end of 1986 to raise the remaining $1.25 million needed to launch at least eight espresso bars and prove that Schultz's strategy and business model were viable. Schultz made presentations to 242 potential investors, 217 of whom said no. Many who heard Schultz's hour-long presentation saw coffee as a commodity business and thought that Schultz's espresso bar concept lacked any basis for sustainable competitive advantage (no patent on dark roast, no advantage in purchasing coffee beans, no ways to bar the entry of imitative competitors). Some noted that coffee couldn't be turned into a growth business—consumption of coffee had been declining since the mid-1960s. Others were skeptical that people would pay $1.50 or more for a cup of coffee, and the company's unpronounceable name turned some off. Being rejected by so many of the potential investors he approached was disheartening (some who listened to Schultz's presentation didn't even bother to call him back; others refused to take his calls). Nonetheless, Schultz maintained an upbeat attitude and displayed passion and enthusiasm in making his pitch. He ended up raising $1.65 million from about 30 investors; most of the money came from nine people, five of whom became directors.

The first Il Giornale store opened in April 1986. It had 700 square feet and was located near the entrance of Seattle's tallest building. The decor was Italian, and there were Italian words on the menu. Italian opera music played in the background. The baristas wore white shirts and bow ties. All service was stand-up—there were no chairs. National and international papers were hung on rods on the wall. By closing time on the first day, 300 customers had been served—mostly in the morning hours. But while the core idea worked well, it soon became apparent that several aspects of the format were not appropriate for Seattle. Some customers objected to the incessant opera music, others wanted a place to sit down, and many did not understand the Italian words on the menu. These "mistakes" were quickly fixed, but an effort was made not to compromise the style and elegance of the store. Within six months, the store was serving more than 1,000 customers a day. Regular customers had learned how to pronounce the company's name. Because most customers were in a hurry, it became apparent that speedy service was essential.

Six months after opening the first store, Schultz opened a second store in another downtown building. A third store was opened in Vancouver, British Columbia, in April 1987. Vancouver was chosen to test the transferability of the company's business concept outside Seattle. Schultz's goal was to open 50 stores in five years, and he needed to dispel his investors' doubts about geographic expansion early on to achieve his growth objective. By mid-1987, sales at the three stores were running at a rate equal to $1.5 million annually.

Il Giornale Acquires Starbucks

In March 1987 Jerry Baldwin and Gordon Bowker decided to sell the whole Starbucks operation in Seattle—the stores, the roasting plant, and the Starbucks name. Bowker wanted to cash out his coffee business investment to concentrate on his other enterprises; Baldwin, who was tired of commuting between Seattle and San Francisco and wrestling with the troubles created by the two parts of the company, elected to concentrate on the Peet's operation. As he recalls, "My wife and I had a 30-second conversation and decided to keep Peet's. It was the original and it was better."[10]

Schultz knew immediately that he had to buy Starbucks; his board of directors agreed. Schultz and his newly hired finance and accounting manager drew up a set of financial projections for the combined operations and a financing package that included a stock offering to Il Giornale's original investors and a line of credit with local banks. While a rival plan to acquire Starbucks was put together by another Il Giornale investor, Schultz's proposal prevailed—and within weeks Schultz had raised the $3.8 million needed to buy Starbucks. The acquisition was completed in August 1987. The new name of the combined companies was Starbucks Corporation. Howard Schultz, at the age of 34, became Starbucks' president and CEO.

STARBUCKS AS A PRIVATE COMPANY: 1987–1992

The following Monday morning, Howard Schultz returned to the Starbucks offices at the roasting plant, greeted all the familiar faces, and accepted their congratulations. Then he called the staff together for a meeting on the roasting plant floor:

> All my life I have wanted to be part of a company and a group of people who share a common vision . . . I'm here today because I love this company. I love what it represents . . . I know you're concerned . . . I promise you I will not let you down. I promise you I will not leave anyone behind . . . In five years, I want you to look back at this day and say "I was there when it started. I helped build this company into something great."[11]

Schultz told the group that his vision was for Starbucks to become a national company with values and guiding principles that employees could be proud of. He indicated that he wanted to include people in the decision-making process and that he would be open and honest with them.

Schultz believed that building a company that valued and respected its people, inspired them, and shared the fruits of success with those who contributed to the company's long-term value was essential, not just an intriguing option. His aspiration was for Starbucks to become the world's most respected brand name in coffee and for the company to be admired for its corporate responsibility. In the next few days and weeks, Schultz came to see that the unity and morale at Starbucks had deteriorated badly in the 20 months he had been at Il Giornale. Some employees were cynical and felt unappreciated. There was a feeling that prior management had abandoned them and a wariness about what the new regime would bring. Schultz decided to make building a new relationship of mutual respect between employees and management a priority.

The new Starbucks had a total of nine stores. The business plan Schultz had presented investors called for the new company to open 125 stores in the next five years—15 the first year, 20 the second, 25 the third, 30 the fourth, and 35 the fifth. Revenues were projected to reach $60 million in 1992. But the company lacked experienced management. Schultz had never led a growth effort of such magnitude and was just learning what the job of CEO was all about, having been the president of a small company for barely two years. Dave Olsen, a Seattle coffee bar owner Schultz had recruited to direct store operations at Il Giornale, was still learning the ropes in managing a multistore operation. Ron Lawrence, the company's controller, had worked as a controller for several organizations. Other Starbucks employees had only the experience of managing or being a part of a six-store organization. When Starbucks' key roaster and coffee buyer resigned, Schultz put Dave Olsen in charge of buying and roasting coffee. Lawrence Maltz, who had 20 years' experience in business and eight years' experience as president of a profitable public beverage company, was hired as executive vice president and charged with heading operations, finance, and human resources.

In the next several months, a number of changes were instituted. To symbolize the merging of the two companies and the two cultures, a new logo was created that melded the designs of the Starbucks logo and the Il Giornale logo. The Starbucks stores were equipped with espresso machines and remodeled to look more Italian than Old World nautical. Il Giornale green replaced the traditional Starbucks brown. The result was a new type of store—a cross between a retail coffee-bean store and an espresso bar/café that has now become Starbucks' signature.

By December 1987, the mood of the employees at Starbucks had turned upbeat. They were buying into the changes that Schultz was making and began to trust management. New stores were on the verge of opening in Vancouver and Chicago. One Starbucks store employee, Daryl Moore, who had started working at Starbucks in 1981 and who had voted against unionization in 1985, began to question the need for a union with his fellow employees. Over the next few weeks, Moore began a move to decertify the union. He carried a decertification letter around to Starbucks' stores securing the signatures of employees who no longer wished to be represented by the union. He got a majority of store employees to sign the letter and presented it to the National Labor Relations Board, which then decertified the union representing store employees. Later, in 1992, the union representing Starbucks' roasting plant and warehouse employees was also decertified.

Market Expansion Outside the Pacific Northwest

Starbucks' entry into Chicago proved far more troublesome than management anticipated. The first Chicago store opened in October 1987 and three more stores were opened over the next six months. Customer counts at the stores were substantially below expectations. Chicagoans did not take to dark-roasted coffee as fast as Schultz had anticipated. The first downtown store opened onto the street rather than into the lobby of the building where it was located; in the winter months, customers were hesitant to go out in the wind and cold to acquire a cup of coffee. It was more expensive to supply fresh coffee to the Chicago stores out of the Seattle warehouse (the company solved the problem of freshness and quality assurance by putting freshly roasted beans in special FlavorLock bags that used vacuum packaging techniques with a one-way valve to allow carbon dioxide to escape without allowing air and moisture in). Rents were higher in Chicago than in Seattle,

and so were wage rates. The result was a squeeze on store profit margins. Gradually, customer counts improved, but Starbucks lost money on its Chicago stores until, in 1990, prices were raised to reflect higher rents and labor costs, more experienced store managers were hired, and a critical mass of customers caught on to the taste of Starbucks products.

Portland, Oregon, was the next market Starbucks entered, and Portland coffee drinkers took to its products quickly. By 1991, the Chicago stores had become profitable and the company was ready for its next big market entry. Management decided on California because of its host of neighborhood centers and the receptiveness of Californians to high-quality, innovative food. Los Angeles was chosen as the first California market to enter. L.A. was selected principally because of its status as a trendsetter and its cultural ties to the rest of the country. L.A. consumers embraced Starbucks quickly, and the *Los Angeles Times* named Starbucks as the best coffee in America even before the first area store opened. The entry into San Francisco proved more troublesome because San Francisco had an ordinance against converting stores to restaurant-related uses in certain prime urban neighborhoods; Starbucks could sell beverages and pastries to customers at stand-up counters but could not offer seating in stores that had formerly been used for general retailing. However, the city council was soon convinced by café owners and real estate brokers to change the code. Still, Starbucks faced strong competition from Peet's and local espresso bars in the San Francisco market.

Starbucks' store expansion targets proved easier to meet than Schultz had originally anticipated, and he upped the numbers to keep challenging the organization. Starbucks opened 15 new stores in fiscal 1988, 20 in 1989, 30 in 1990, 32 in 1991, and 53 in 1992—producing a total of 161 stores, significantly above the 1987 objective of 125 stores.

From the outset, the strategy was to open only company-owned stores; franchising was avoided so as to keep the company in full control of the quality of its products and the character and location of its stores. But company ownership of all stores required Starbucks to raise new venture capital to cover the cost of new store expansion. In 1988, the company raised $3.9 million; in 1990, venture capitalists provided an additional $13.5 million; and in 1991, another round of venture capital financing generated $15 million. Starbucks was able to raise the needed funds despite posting losses of $330,000 in 1987,

$764,000 in 1988, and $1.2 million in 1989. While the losses were troubling to Starbucks' board of directors and investors, Schultz's business plan had forecast losses during the early years of expansion. At a particularly tense board meeting where directors sharply questioned Schultz about the lack of profitability, Schultz said:

> Look, we're going to keep losing money until we can do three things. We have to attract a management team well beyond our expansion needs. We have to build a world-class roasting facility. And we need a computer information system sophisticated enough to keep track of sales in hundreds and hundreds of stores.[12]

Schultz argued for patience as the company invested in the infrastructure to support continued growth well into the 1990s. He contended that hiring experienced executives ahead of the growth curve, building facilities far beyond current needs, and installing support systems laid a strong foundation for rapid, profitable growth on down the road. His arguments carried the day with the board and with investors, especially since revenues were growing by approximately 80 percent annually and customer traffic at the stores was meeting or exceeding expectations.

Starbucks became profitable in 1990; profits had increased every year since 1990 except for fiscal year 2000 (because of $58.8 million in investment write-offs in four dot-com enterprises). Exhibit 3 provides a financial and operating summary for 2000–2005. Exhibit 4 shows the performance of the company's stock price. The stock had split 2-for-1 five times. In September 2005, Starbucks' board of directors approved the repurchase of up to 5 million shares of common stock; a total of 35.7 million shares had been repurchased since the company went public.

HOWARD SCHULTZ'S STRATEGY TO MAKE STARBUCKS A GREAT PLACE TO WORK

Howard Schultz deeply believed that Starbucks' success was heavily dependent on customers having a very positive experience in its stores. This meant having store employees who were knowledgeable about the company's products, who paid attention to detail in preparing the company's espresso drinks, who eagerly communicated the company's passion for coffee, and who possessed the skills and personality to deliver consistent, pleasing customer service. Many of the baristas were in their 20s and worked part-time, going to college on the side or pursuing other career activities. The challenge to Starbucks, in Schultz's view, was how to attract, motivate, and reward store employees in a manner that would make Starbucks a company that people would want to work for and that would generate enthusiastic commitment and higher levels of customer service. Moreover, Schultz wanted to send all Starbucks employees a message that would cement the trust that had been building between management and the company's workforce.

One of the requests that employees had made to the prior owners of Starbucks was to extend health care benefits to part-time workers. Their request had been turned down, but Schultz believed that expanding health care coverage to include part-timers was the right thing to do. His father had recently passed away with cancer and he knew from his own experience of having grown up in a family that struggled to make ends meet how difficult it was to cope with rising medical costs. In 1988, Schultz went to the board of directors with his plan to expand the company's health care coverage to include part-timers who worked at least 20 hours per week. He saw the proposal not as a generous gesture but as a core strategy to win employee loyalty and commitment to the company's mission. Board members resisted because the company was unprofitable and the added costs of the extended coverage would only worsen the company's bottom line. But Schultz argued passionately that it was the right thing to do and wouldn't be as expensive as it seemed. He observed that if the new benefit reduced turnover, which he believed was likely, then it would reduce the costs of hiring and training—which equaled about $3,000 per new hire; he further pointed out that it cost $1,500 a year to provide an employee with full benefits. Part-timers, he argued, were vital to Starbucks, constituting two-thirds of the company's workforce. Many were baristas who knew the favorite drinks of regular customers; if the barista left, that connection with the customer was broken. Moreover, many part-time employees were called upon to open the stores early, sometimes at 5:30 or 6:00 a.m.; others had to work until closing, usually 9:00 p.m. or later. Providing these employees with health care benefits, he argued, would signal that the company honored their value and contribution.

The board approved Schultz's plan, and part-timers working 20 or more hours were offered the same health coverage as full-time employees starting in late 1988. Starbucks paid 75 percent of an employee's health care premium; the employee paid 25 percent. Over the years, Starbucks extended its health coverage to include preventive care, crisis counseling, dental care, eye care, mental health, and chemical dependency. Coverage was also offered for unmarried partners in a committed relationship. Since most Starbucks' employees were young and comparatively healthy, the company had been able to provide broader coverage while keeping monthly payments relatively low. The value of Starbucks' health care program struck home when one of the company's store managers and a former barista walked into Schultz's office and told him he had AIDS:

> I had known he was gay but had no idea he was sick. His disease had entered a new phase, he explained, and he wouldn't be able to work any longer. We sat

Exhibit 3 **Financial and Operating Summary for Starbucks Corporation, Fiscal Years 2000–2005 (dollars in 000s)**

	Fiscal Years Ending[1]					
	October 2, 2005	October 3, 2004	September 30, 2003	September 29, 2002	September 30, 2001	October 1, 2000
Results of operations data						
Net revenues:						
Retail	$5,391,927	$4,457,378	$3,449,624	$2,792,904	$2,229,594	$1,823,607
Specialty	977,373	836,869	625,898	496,004	419,386	354,007
Total net revenues	$6,369,300	$5,294,247	$4,075,522	$3,288,908	$2,648,980	$2,177,614
Cost of sales and related company costs	2,605,212	2,191,440	1,681,434	1,350,011	1,112,785	961,885
Store operating expenses	2,165,911	1,790,168	1,379,574	1,109,782	867,957	704,898
Other operating expenses	197,024	171,648	141,346	106,084	72,406	78,445
Depreciation and amortization expenses	340,169	289,182	244,671	205,557	163,501	130,232
General and administrative expenses	357,114	304,293	244,550	234,581	179,852	110,202
Income from equity ventures	76,745	59,071	36,903	33,445	27,740	20,300
Operating income	$ 780,615	$ 606,587	$ 420,850	$ 316,338	$ 280,219	$ 212,252
Internet-related investment losses[2]					2,940	58,792
Gain on sale of investment[3]				13,361		
Net earnings	$ 494,467	$ 388,973	$ 265,355	$ 210,463	$ 178,794	$ 94,564
Net earnings per common share—diluted[4]	$0.61	$0.49	$0.34	$0.54	$0.46	$0.24
Cash dividends per share	0	0	0	0	0	0
Balance sheet data						
Current assets	$1,209,334	$1,350,895	$ 924,029	$ 772,643	$ 593,925	$ 459,819
Current liabilities	1,226,996	746,259	608,703	462,595	445,264	313,251
Working capital[5]	(17,662)	604,636	335,767	328,777	165,045	146,568
Total assets	3,514,065	3,386,541	2,776,112	2,249,435	1,807,574	1,491,546
Long-term debt (including current portion)	3,618	4,353	5,076	5,786	6,483	7,168
Shareholders' equity	$2,090,634	$2,470,211	$2,068,689	$1,712,456	$1,366,355	$1,148,399

(Continued)

Exhibit 3   **Continued**

	Fiscal Years Ending[1]					
	October 2, 2005	October 3, 2004	September 30, 2003	September 29, 2002	September 30, 2001	October 1, 2000
Store operations data						
Percentage change in comparable store sales[6]						
United States	9%	11%	9%	7%	5%	9%
International	6	6	7	1	3	12
Consolidated	8	10	8	6	5	9
Systemwide stores opened during the year[7,8]						
United States						
Company-operated stores	574	514	506	503	498	388
Licensed stores	596	417	315	264	268	342
International						
Company-operated stores	161	141	124	117	151	96
Licensed stores	341	272	256	293	291	177
Total	1,672	1,344	1,201	1,177	1,208	1,003
Systemwide stores open at year-end[8]						
United States[9]						
Company-operated stores	4,867	293	3,779	3,209	2,706	2,208
Licensed stores	2,435	1,839	1,422	1,033	769	501
International						
Company-operated stores	1,133	972	801	707	590	411
Licensed stores	1,806	1,465	1,193	937	644	381
Total	10,241	8,569	7,225	5,886	4,709	3,501

[1]The company's fiscal year ends on the Sunday closest to September 30. All fiscal years presented include 52 weeks, except fiscal 2004, which includes 53 weeks.

[2]In fiscal 2000, the company wrote off most of its investment in four ill-fated dot-com businesses. In fiscal 2001, the company wrote off an additional $2.9 million in Internet-related investments.

[3]On October 10, 2001, the company sold 30,000 of its shares of Starbucks Coffee Japan Ltd. at approximately $495 per share, net of related costs, which resulted in a gain of $13.4 million.

[4]Earnings per share data for fiscal years presented above have been restated to reflect the 2-for-1 stock splits in fiscal 2006 and 2001.

[5]Working capital deficit as of October 2, 2005, was primarily due to lower investments from the sale of securities to fund common stock repurchases and increased current liabilities from short-term borrowings under the revolving credit facility.

[6]Includes only Starbucks company-operated retail stores open 13 months or longer. Comparable store sales percentage for fiscal 2004 excludes the extra sales week.

[7]Store openings are reported net of closures.

[8]International store information has been adjusted for the fiscal 2005 acquisitions of licensed operations in Germany, southern China, and Chile by reclassifying historical information from licensed store to company-operated stores.

[9]United States stores open at fiscal 2003 year end included 43 SBC and 21 Torrefazione Italia Company–operated stores and 74 SBC franchised stores.

Source: 10-K reports for 2005, 2004, 2003, 2002, and 2000. Notes reflect 2005 10-K report.

together and cried, for I could not find meaningful words to console him. I couldn't compose myself. I hugged him.

At that point, Starbucks had no provision for employees with AIDS. We had a policy decision.

Because of Jim, we decided to offer health-care coverage to all employees who have terminal illnesses, paying medical costs in full from the time they are not able to work until they are covered by government programs, usually twenty-nine months.

Exhibit 4   **The Performance of Starbucks' Stock, 1992–2005**

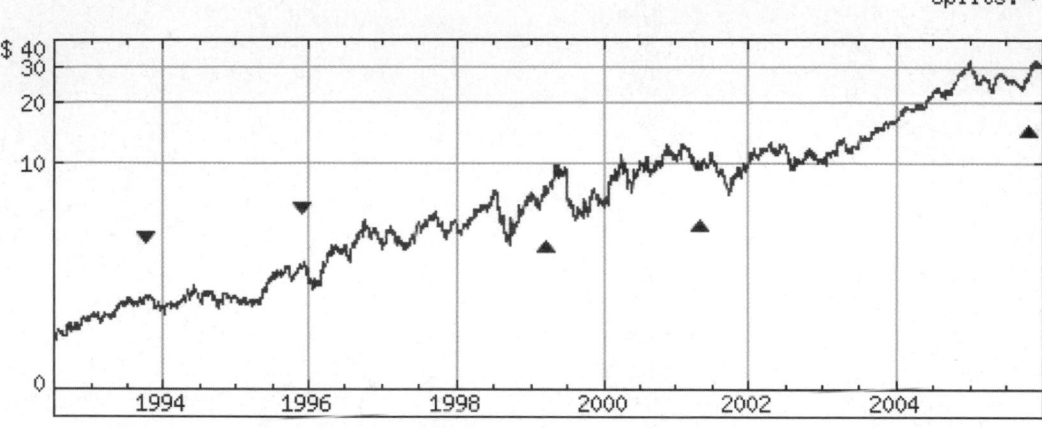

Source: http://finance.yahoo.com (accessed December 28, 2005).

After his visit to me, I spoke with Jim often and visited him at the hospice. Within a year he was gone. I received a letter from his family afterward, telling me how much they appreciated our benefit plan.[13]

In 1994 Howard Schultz was invited to the White House. He met one-on-one with President Bill Clinton to brief him on the Starbucks' health care program.

The Creation of an Employee Stock Option Plan

By 1991 the company's profitability had improved to the point where Schultz could pursue a stock option plan for all employees, a program he believed would have a positive, long-term effect on the success of Starbucks.[14] Schultz wanted to turn all Starbucks employees into partners, give them a chance to share in the success of the company, and make clear the connection between their contributions and the company's market value. Even though Starbucks was still a private company, the plan that emerged called for granting stock options to all full-time and part-time employees in proportion to their base pay. The plan, dubbed Bean Stock, was presented to the board in May 1991. Though board members were concerned that increasing the number of shares might unduly dilute the value of the shares of investors who had put up hard cash, the plan received unanimous approval. The first grant was made in October 1991, just after the end of the company's fiscal year in September; each partner was granted stock options worth 12 percent of base pay. Each October since then, Starbucks has granted employees options equal to 14 percent of base pay, awarded at the stock price at the start of the fiscal year (October 1). When the Bean Stock program was presented to employees, Starbucks dropped the term *employee* and began referring to all of its people as *partners* because everyone, including part-timers working at least 20 hours per week, was eligible for stock options after six months. At the end of fiscal year 2004, Starbucks' employee stock option plan included 38.4 million shares in outstanding options; new options for about 9 million shares were being granted annually.[15]

Starbucks Stock Purchase Plan for Employees

In 1995, Starbucks implemented an employee stock purchase plan. Eligible employees could contribute up to 10 percent of their base earnings to quarterly purchases of the company's common stock at 85 percent of the going stock price. As of fiscal 2005, about 14.8 million shares had been issued since inception of the plan, and new shares were being purchased at a rate close to 1 million shares annually by some 18,800 active employee participants (out of almost 55,100 employees who were eligible to participate).[16] During fiscal 2004, the U.K. Share Incentive Plan, a new employee stock purchase plan was introduced, discontinuing the original plan established in 2002. As of fiscal 2005, 10,732 shares had been issued.[17]

The Workplace Environment

Starbucks' management believed the company's pay scales (around $9–$12 per hour) and fringe benefit package allowed it to attract motivated people with above-average skills and good work habits. Store employees were paid several dollars above the hourly minimum wage. Whereas most national retailers and fast-food chains had turnover rates for store employees ranging from 150 to 400 percent a year, the turnover rates for Starbucks baristas ran about 65 percent. Starbucks' turnover for store managers was about 25 percent, compared to about 50 percent for other chain retailers. Starbucks executives believed that efforts to make the company an attractive, caring place to work were responsible for its relatively low turnover rates. One Starbucks store manager commented, "Morale is very high in my store among the staff. I've worked for a lot of companies, but I've never seen this level of respect. It's a company that's very true to its workers, and it shows. Our customers always comment that we're happy and having fun. In fact, a lot of people ask if they can work here."[18]

Starbucks' management used annual "Partner View" surveys to solicit feedback from the company's workforce of over 115,000 people worldwide, learn their concerns, and measure job satisfaction. In the latest sample survey of 1,400 employees, 79 percent rated Starbucks' workplace environment favorably relative to other companies they were familiar with, 72 percent reported being satisfied with their present job, 16 percent were neutral, and 12 percent were dissatisfied. But the 2002 survey revealed that many employees viewed the benefits package as only "average," prompting the company to increase its match of 401(k) contributions for those who had been with the company more than three years and to have these contributions vest immediately.

Exhibit 5 contains a summary of Starbucks' fringe benefit program. Starbucks was named by *Fortune* magazine as one of the "100 Best Companies to Work For" in 1998, 1999, 2000, 2002, 2003, 2004, and 2005. In 2005, Starbucks was ranked 11th, up from 34th in 2004. In October 2005, Starbucks had approximately 115,000 employees worldwide, of which 97,500 were in the United States. It had 91,200 employees in its U.S. company-owned stores. Employees at 10 stores in Canada were represented by a union.

Starbucks' Corporate Values and Business Principles

During the early building years, Howard Schultz and other Starbucks' senior executives worked to instill some key values and guiding principles into

---

Exhibit 5   **Elements of Starbucks' Fringe Benefit Program**

• Medical insurance	• Sick time
• Dental and vision care	• Paid vacations (first-year workers got one vacation week and two personal days)
• Mental health and chemical dependency coverage	• 401(k) retirement savings plan—the company matched from 25% to 150%, based on length of service, of each employee's contributions up to the first 4% of compensation.
• Short- and long-term disability	• Stock purchase plan—eligible employees could buy shares at a discounted price through regular payroll deductions
• Life insurance	• Free pound of coffee each week
• Benefits extended to committed domestic partners of Starbucks employees	• 30% product discounts
• Stock option plan (Bean Stock)	• Tuition reimbursement program

Source: Compiled by the case researchers from company documents and other sources.

the Starbucks culture. The cornerstone value in the effort "to build a company with soul" was that the company would never stop pursuing the perfect cup of coffee—it would continue buying the best beans and roasting them to perfection. Schultz remained steadfastly opposed to franchising; he wanted the company to be able to control the quality of its products and build a culture common to all stores. He was adamant about not selling artificially flavored coffee beans: "We will not pollute our high-quality beans with chemicals." If a customer wanted hazelnut-flavored coffee, Starbucks would add hazelnut syrup to the drink, rather than adding hazelnut flavoring to the beans during roasting. Running flavored beans through the grinders would result in chemical residues being left behind to alter the flavor of beans ground afterward; plus, the chemical smell given off by artificially flavored beans was absorbed by other beans in the store. Furthermore, Schultz didn't want the company to pursue supermarket sales because it would mean pouring Starbucks' beans into clear plastic bins where they could get stale, thus compro-mising the company's legacy of fresh, dark-roasted, full-flavored coffee.

Starbucks' management was also emphatic about the importance of employees paying attention to what pleased customers. Employees were trained to go out of their way—even to take heroic measures if necessary—to make sure customers were fully satisfied. The theme was "Just say yes" to customer requests. Further, employees were encouraged to speak their minds without fear of retribution from upper management—senior executives wanted employees to be straight with them, verbalizing what Starbucks was doing right, what it was doing wrong, and what changes were needed. Management wanted employees to be involved in and contribute to the process of making Starbucks a better company.

A values-and-principles crisis arose at Starbucks in 1989 when customers started requesting nonfat (skim) milk in making cappuccinos and lattes. Howard Schultz, who read all customer comments cards, and Dave Olsen, head of coffee quality, conducted taste tests of lattes and cappuccinos made with nonfat milk and concluded they were not as good as those made with whole milk. Howard Behar, recently hired as head of retail store operations, indicated that management's opinions didn't matter; what mattered was giving customers what they wanted.

Schultz said, "We will never offer nonfat milk. It's not who we are." Behar, however, stuck to his guns, maintaining that use of nonfat milk should at least be tested—otherwise, it appeared as if all the statements management had made about the importance of really and truly pleasing customers were a sham. A fierce internal debate ensued. One dogmatic defender of the quality and taste of Starbucks' coffee products buttonholed Behar outside his office and told him that using nonfat milk amounted to "bastardizing" the company's products. Numerous store managers maintained that offering two kinds of milk was operationally impractical. Schultz found himself in a quandary, torn between the company's commitment to quality and its goal of pleasing customers. Then, one day after visiting one of the stores in a residential neighborhood and watching a customer leave to go to a competitor's store because Starbucks did not make lattes with nonfat milk, Schultz authorized Behar to begin testing.[19] Within six months, all 30 stores were offering drinks made with nonfat milk. Currently, about half the lattes and cappuccinos Starbucks sells are made with nonfat milk.

Schultz's approach to offering employees good compensation and a comprehensive benefits package was driven by his belief that sharing the company's success with the people who made it happen helped everyone think and act like an owner, build positive long-term relationships with customers, and do things efficiently. He had vivid recollection of his father's employment experience—bouncing from one low-paying job to another, working for employers who offered few or no benefits and who conducted their business with no respect for the contributions of the workforce—and he had no intention of Starbucks being that type of company. He vowed that he would never let Starbucks employees suffer a similar fate, saying:

> My father worked hard all his life and he had little to show for it. He was a beaten man. This is not the American dream. The worker on our plant floor is contributing great value to the company; if he or she has low self-worth, that will have an effect on the company.[20]

The company's employee benefits program was predicated on the belief that better benefits attract good people and keep them longer. Schultz's rationale, based on his father's experience of going from one low-wage, no-benefits job to another, was that if you treat your employees well, they in turn will treat customers well.

STARBUCKS' MISSION STATEMENT

In early 1990, the senior executive team at Starbucks went to an off-site retreat to debate the company's values and beliefs and draft a mission statement. Schultz wanted the mission statement to convey a strong sense of organizational purpose and to articulate the company's fundamental beliefs and guiding principles. The draft was submitted to all employees for review and several changes were made based on employee comments. The resulting mission statement, which remained unchanged in 2005, is shown in Exhibit 6.

Following adoption of the mission statement, Starbucks' management implemented a "Mission Review" to solicit and gather employee opinions as to whether the company was living up to its stated mission. Employees were urged to report their concerns to the company's Mission Review team if they thought particular management decisions were not supportive of the company's mission statement. Comment cards were given to each newly hired employee and were kept available in common areas with other employee forms. Employees had the option of signing the comment cards or not. Hundreds of cards were submitted to the Mission Review team each year. The company promised that a relevant manager would respond to all signed cards within two weeks. Howard Schultz reviewed all the comments, signed and unsigned.

STARBUCKS' STORE EXPANSION STRATEGY

In 1992 and 1993 Starbucks developed a three-year geographic expansion strategy that targeted areas that not only had favorable demographic profiles but also could be serviced and supported by the company's operations infrastructure. For each targeted region, Starbucks selected a large city to serve as a hub; teams of professionals were located in hub cities to support the goal of opening 20 or more stores in the hub in the first two years. Once stores blanketed the hub, then additional stores were opened in smaller, surrounding spoke areas in the region. To oversee the expansion process, Starbucks created zone vice presidents to direct the development of each region and to implant the Starbucks culture in the newly opened stores. All of the new zone vice presidents Starbucks recruited came with extensive operating and marketing experience in chain store retailing.

Starbucks' strategy in major metropolitan cities was to blanket the area with stores, even if some stores cannibalized another store's business.[21] While a new store might draw 30 percent of the business of an existing store two or so blocks away, management believed its "Starbucks everywhere" approach cut down on delivery and management costs, shortened customer lines at individual stores, and increased foot traffic for all the stores in an area.

In 2002, new stores generated an average of $1.2 million in first-year revenues, compared to $700,000 in 1995 and only $427,000 in 1990. The steady increases in new-store revenues were due partly to growing popularity of premium coffee drinks and

Exhibit 6 **Starbucks' Mission Statement**

Establish Starbucks as the premier purveyor of the finest coffee in the world while maintaining our uncompromising principles while we grow.

The following six guiding principles will help us measure the appropriateness of our decisions:

- Provide a great work environment and treat each other with respect and dignity.
- Embrace diversity as an essential component in the way we do business.
- Apply the highest standards of excellence to the purchasing, roasting, and fresh delivery of our coffee.
- Develop enthusiastically satisfied customers all of the time.
- Contribute positively to our communities and our environment.
- Recognize that profitability is essential to our future success.

partly to Starbucks' growing reputation. In more and more instances, Starbucks' reputation reached new markets even before stores opened. Moreover, existing stores continued to post sales gains in the range of 2–10 percent annually. In 2005, Starbucks posted same-store sales increases averaging 8 percent (refer back to Exhibit 3), the 14th consecutive year the company had achieved sales growth of 5 percent or greater at existing stores. Starbucks' revenues had climbed an average of 20 percent annually since 1992.

One of Starbucks' core competencies was identifying good retailing sites for its new stores. The company was regarded as having the best real estate team in the coffee bar industry and a sophisticated system for identifying not only the most attractive individual city blocks but also the exact store location that was best; it also worked hard at building good relationships with local real estate representatives in areas where it was opening multiple store locations. The company's site location track record was so good that, as of 1997, it had closed only 2 of the 1,500 sites it had opened; its track record in finding successful store locations was still intact as of 2005 (although specific figures were not available).

International Expansion

In markets outside the continental United States (including Hawaii), Starbucks had a two-pronged store expansion plan: Either open company-owned and company-operated stores, or else license a reputable and capable local company with retailing know-how in the target host country to develop and operate new Starbucks stores. In most countries, Starbucks used a local partner/licensee to help it recruit talented individuals, set up supplier relationships, locate suitable store sites, and cater to local market conditions. Starbucks looked for partners/licensees that had strong retail/restaurant experience, had values and a corporate culture compatible with Starbucks', were committed to good customer service, possessed talented management and strong financial resources, and had demonstrated brand-building skills.

Starbucks had created a new subsidiary, Starbucks Coffee International, to orchestrate overseas expansion and begin to build the Starbucks brand name globally via licensees. (Refer back to Exhibit 1 for the number of licensed international stores in each country.) Starbucks' management expected to have a total of 10,000 stores in 60 countries by the end of 2005. As of August 2005, Starbucks was located in 34 countries, with 1,049 company-operated stores and 1,734 licensed locations outside the United States. The company's first store in France opened in early 2004 in Paris. China was expected to be Starbucks' biggest market outside the United States in the years to come. Thus far, Starbucks' products were proving to be a much bigger hit with consumers in Asia than in Europe. In 2003, the Starbucks Coffee International division was only marginally profitable, with pretax earnings of only $3.8 million on sales of $603 million. However, the profitability picture improved in 2004, with pretax profits rising to $51.7 million on sales of $803 million. And it did even better in fiscal 2005, with pretax earnings of $86.4 million on sales of $1.03 billion.

So far, Starbucks had avoided franchising, preferring licensing because it permitted tighter controls over the operations of licensees. Often, Starbucks opened foreign stores as a minority partner with local companies. In 2005, Starbucks assumed 100 percent equity ownership of previously licensed operations in Germany and Chile (where it had been a 20 percent equity partner), and it boosted its ownership of stores in southern China from 20 percent to 51 percent.

In May 2005, Starbucks announced the first step into expanding its consumer products channel in the South Pacific region by launching the sales of its Frappuccino line in Japan and Taiwan. The combined ready-to-drink markets in these countries represented more than $10 billion in annual sales.[22] Marketing of Frappuccino products also began in South Korea through agreements with leading local distributors; the ready-to-drink coffee segment in South Korea represented $320 million in annual consumer sales.[23]

Employee Training and Recognition

To accommodate its strategy of rapid store expansion, Starbucks put in systems to recruit, hire, and train baristas and store managers. Starbucks' vice president for human resources used some simple guidelines in screening candidates for new positions, "We want passionate people who love coffee . . . We're looking for a diverse workforce, which reflects our community. We want people who enjoy what they're doing and for whom work is an extension of themselves."[24]

Every partner/barista hired for a retail job in a Starbucks store received at least 24 hours training in his or her first two to four weeks. The topics included classes on coffee history, drink preparation, coffee knowledge (four hours), customer service (four hours), and retail skills, plus a four-hour workshop titled "Brewing the Perfect Cup." Baristas spent considerable time learning about beverage preparation—grinding beans, steaming milk, learning to pull perfect (18- to 23-second) shots of espresso, memorizing the recipes of all the different drinks, practicing making the different drinks, and learning how to customize drinks to customer specifications. There were sessions on operating the cash register, cleaning the milk wand on the espresso machine, explaining the Italian drink names to unknowing customers, selling home espresso machines, making eye contact with customers, and taking personal responsibility for the cleanliness of the store. Everyone was drilled in the Star Skills, three guidelines for on-the-job interpersonal relations: (1) maintain and enhance self-esteem, (2) listen and acknowledge, and (3) ask for help. And there were rules to be memorized: Milk must be steamed to at least 150 degrees Fahrenheit but never more than 170 degrees; every espresso shot not pulled within 23 seconds must be tossed; never let coffee sit in the pot more than 20 minutes; always compensate dissatisfied customers with a Starbuck coupon that entitles them to a free drink.

In response to feedback through 2003 Partner View Survey, Starbucks expanded its training and career development offerings by adding the following:[25]

Coffee Masters Program: A set of courses in which partners deepen their coffee knowledge and expertise. More than 7,000 partners have taken advantage of this training either partially or fully.

Servant Leadership Workshop: A workshop that emphasizes trust, collaboration, people development, and ethics. Approximately 6,200 partners attended this workshop.

Career Power and Career Power for Coaches Workshop: A workshop designed to provide partners and their managers with an opportunity to reflect on their personal values,

career dreams, and development through coaching and feedback. More than 200 partners in Seattle attended the workshop.

Management trainees attended classes for 8 to 12 weeks. Their training covered not only the coffee knowledge and information imparted to baristas but also the details of store operations, practices and procedures as set forth in the company's operating manual, information systems, and the basics of managing people. Starbucks' trainers were all store managers and district managers with on-site experience. Among their major objectives were to ingrain the company's values, principles, and culture and to pass on their knowledge about coffee and their passion about Starbucks.

When Starbucks opened stores in a new market, it launched a major recruiting effort. Eight to 10 weeks before opening a store, the company placed ads to hire baristas and begin their training. It sent a Star team of experienced managers and baristas from existing stores to the area to lead the store-opening effort and to conduct one-on-one training following the company's formal classes and basic orientation sessions at the Starbucks Coffee School in San Francisco.

To recognize the partner contributions, Starbucks had created 19 different awards programs ranging from frequent awards to high-level cash awards. Some of the high-level awards included Manager of the Quarter for store manager leadership, Green Apron Awards for outstanding customer service, and Green Bean Awards for exceptional support for company's environmental mission.

Real Estate, Store Design, Store Planning, and Construction

Starting in 1991, Starbucks created its own in-house team of architects and designers to ensure that each store would convey the right image and character. Stores had to be custom-designed because the company didn't buy real estate and build its own free-standing structures like McDonald's or Wal-Mart; rather, each space was leased in an existing structure, making each store differ in size and shape. Most stores ranged in size from 1,000 to 1,500 square feet and were located in office buildings, downtown and suburban retail centers, airport terminals, university campus areas, and busy neighborhood shopping areas convenient for pedestrian foot traffic and/or drivers. Only a select few were in suburban malls.

Over the years, Starbucks had experimented with a broad range of store formats. Special seating areas were added to help make Starbucks a desirable gathering place where customers could meet and chat or simply enjoy a peaceful interlude in their day. Flagship stores in high-traffic, high-visibility locations had fireplaces, leather chairs, newspapers, couches, and lots of ambience. The company also experimented with drive-through windows in locations where speed and convenience were important to customers and with kiosks in supermarkets, building lobbies, and other public places.

A "stores of the future" project team was formed in 1995 to raise Starbucks' store design to a still higher level and come up with the next generation of Starbucks stores. The vision of what a Starbucks store should be like included such concepts as an authentic coffee experience that conveyed the artistry of espresso making, a place to think and imagine, a spot where people could gather and talk over a great cup of coffee, a comforting refuge that provided a sense of community, a third place for people to congregate beyond work or the home, a place that welcomes people and rewards them for coming, and a layout that could accommodate both fast service and quiet moments. The team researched the art and literature of coffee throughout the ages, studied coffee-growing and coffeemaking techniques, and looked at how Starbucks' stores had already evolved in terms of design, logos, colors, and mood. The team came up with four store designs—one for each of the four stages of coffeemaking: growing, roasting, brewing, and aroma—each with its own color combinations, lighting scheme, and component materials. Within each of the four basic store templates, Starbucks could vary the materials and details to adapt to different store sizes and settings (downtown buildings, college campuses, neighborhood shopping areas). In late 1996, Starbucks began opening new stores based on one of four formats and color schemes. But as the number of stores increased rapidly in 2000–2003, greater store diversity and layout quickly became necessary. Exhibit 7 shows the diverse nature of Starbucks stores.

To better control average store opening costs, the company centralized buying, developed standard contracts and fixed fees for certain items, and consolidated work under those contractors who displayed good cost control practices. The retail operations group outlined exactly the minimum amount of equipment each core store needed so that standard items could be ordered in volume from vendors at 20 to 30 percent discounts, then delivered just-in-time to the store site either from company warehouses or the vendor. Modular designs for display cases were developed. And the whole store layout was developed on a computer, with software that allowed the costs to be estimated as the design evolved. All this cut store opening costs significantly and reduced store development time from 24 to 18 weeks.

In August 2002, Starbucks teamed up with T-Mobile USA, the largest U.S. carrier-owned Wi-Fi service, to experiment with providing Internet access capability and enhanced digital entertainment to patrons at over 1,200 Starbucks locations. The objective was to heighten the "third-place" Starbucks experience, entice customers into perhaps buying a second latte or espresso while they caught up on e-mail, listened to digital music, put the finishing touches on a presentation, or accessed their corporate intranet. Since the August 2002 introduction of Wi-Fi at Starbucks, wireless Internet service had been added at over 1,700 more stores. Internal research showed that the average connection lasted approximately 45 minutes and that more than 90 percent of accesses were during the off-peak store hours.

During the early start-up years, Starbucks avoided debt and financed new stores entirely with equity capital. But as the company's profitability improved and its balance sheet strengthened, Schultz's opposition to debt as a legitimate financing vehicle softened. In 1996 the company completed its second debt offering, netting $161 million from the sale of convertible debentures for use in its capital construction program. This debt was successfully converted into common stock in 1997. Over the next eight years, strong internal cash flows allowed Starbucks to finance virtually all of its store expansion with internal funds; in 2005, the company had less than $3 million in long-term debt on its balance sheet despite having $1.8 billion in net investment in facilities and equipment, but it did have long-term liabilities of $193.6 million associated with lease obligations at its stores.

Store Ambience

Starbucks management viewed each store as a billboard for the company and as a contributor to

Case 29   Starbucks' Global Quest in 2006: Is the Best Yet to Come?

C-487

Exhibit 7   **Scenes from Starbucks Stores**

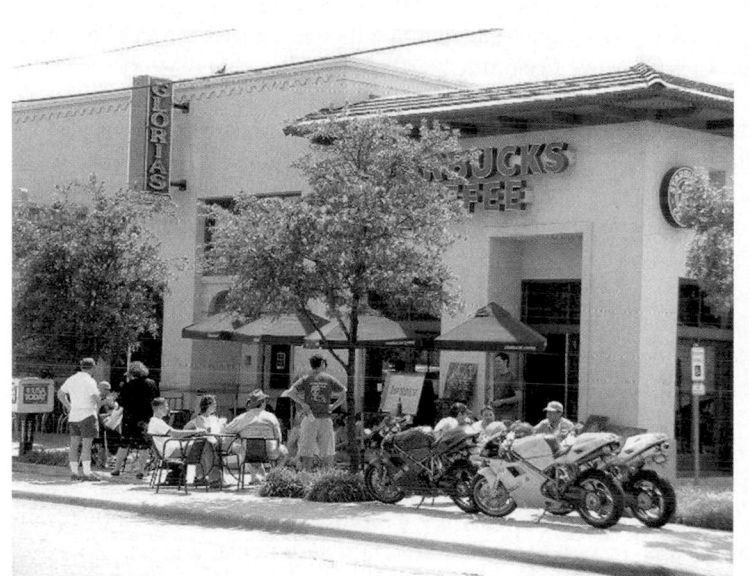
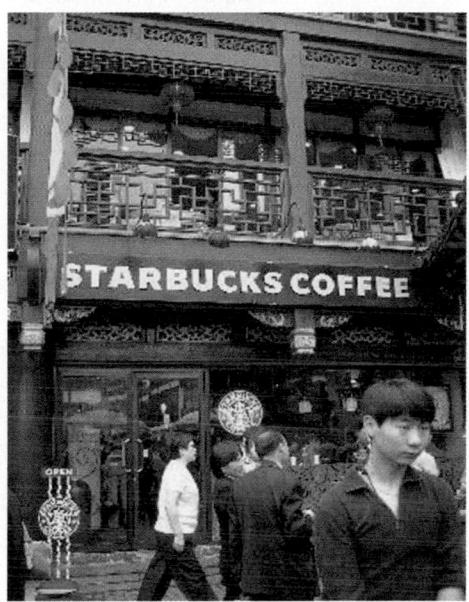
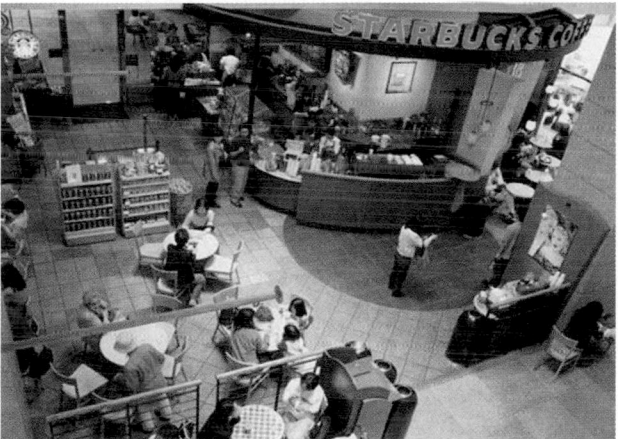
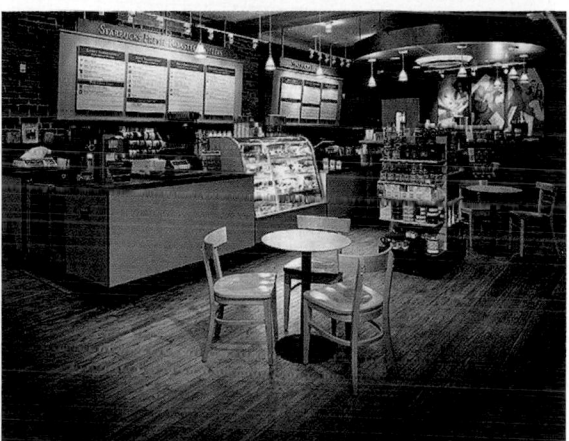
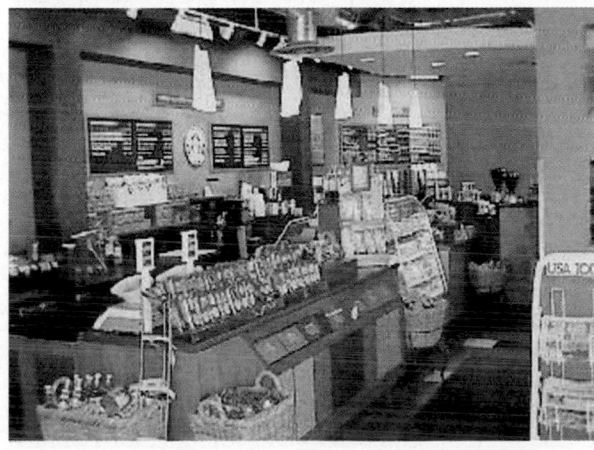
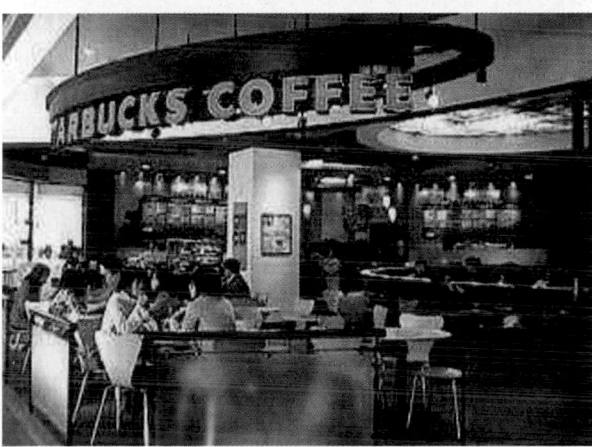

building the company's brand and image. Each detail was scrutinized to enhance the mood and ambience of the store, to make sure everything signaled "best-of-class" and reflected the personality of the community and the neighborhood. The thesis was "Everything matters." The company went to great lengths to make sure the store fixtures, the merchandise displays, the colors, the artwork, the banners, the music, and the aromas all blended to create a consistent, inviting, stimulating environment that evoked the romance of coffee, that signaled the company's passion for coffee, and that rewarded customers with ceremony, stories, and surprise. Starbucks was recognized for its sensitivity to neighborhood conservation with the Scenic America's award for excellent design and "sensitive reuse of spaces within cities."

To try to keep the coffee aromas in the stores pure, Starbucks banned smoking and asked employees to refrain from wearing perfumes or colognes. Prepared foods were kept covered so that customers would smell coffee only. Colorful banners and posters in tune with seasons and holidays kept the look of Starbucks stores fresh. Company designers came up with artwork for commuter mugs and T-shirts in different cities that were in keeping with each city's personality (peach-shaped coffee mugs for Atlanta, pictures of Paul Revere for Boston and the Statue of Liberty for New York). To make sure that Starbucks' stores measured up to standards, the company used "mystery shoppers" who posed as customers and rated each location on a number of criteria.

THE PRODUCT LINE AT STARBUCKS

Starbucks stores offered a choice of regular or decaffeinated coffee beverages, a special "coffee of the day," and an assortment of made-to-order Italian-style hot and cold espresso drinks. In addition, customers could choose from a wide selection of fresh-roasted whole-bean coffees (which could be ground or not on the premises for take-home in distinctive packages), fresh pastries, juices, hot and iced teas, coffeemaking equipment, coffee mugs and other accessories, and music CDs. From time to time, stores ran special promotions touting the company's special Christmas Blend coffee, shade-grown coffee from Mexico, organically grown coffees, and various

rare and exotic coffees from across the world. In 2003, Starbucks began offering customers a choice of using its exclusive Silk soymilk specifically designed to accentuate its handcrafted beverages using espresso roast coffee and Tazo chai teas; the organic, kosher soymilk appealed to some customers as a substitute for milk or skim milk in various coffee and tea beverages.

The company's retail sales mix in 2005 was 77 percent beverages, 15 percent food items, 4 percent whole-bean coffees, and 4 percent coffeemaking equipment and accessories.[26] The product mix in each store varied, depending on the size and location of each outlet. Larger stores carried a greater variety of whole coffee beans, gourmet food items, teas, coffee mugs, coffee grinders, coffeemaking equipment, filters, storage containers, and other accessories. Smaller stores and kiosks typically sold a full line of coffee beverages, a limited selection of whole-bean coffees, and a few hardware items.

The idea for selling music CDs (which, in some cases, were special compilations that had been put together for Starbucks to use as store background music) originated with a Starbucks store manager who had worked in the music industry and selected the new "tape of the month" Starbucks played as background in its stores. He had gotten compliments from customers wanting to buy the music they heard and suggested to senior executives that there was a market for the company's music tapes. Research through two years of comment cards turned up hundreds asking Starbucks to sell the music it played in its stores. The Starbucks CDs proved a significant seller and addition to the product line; some of the CDs were specifically collections designed to tie in with new blends of coffee that company was promoting. Starbucks had also co-produced a Ray Charles CD, *Genius Loves Company,* which became a multiplatinum album with significant sales from Starbucks stores.

In 2000, Starbucks acquired Hear Music, a San Francisco–based company, to give it added capability in enhancing its music CD offerings. In 2004, Starbucks introduced Hear Music media bars, a service that offered custom CD burning at select Starbucks stores, and it opened several Starbucks Hear Music Coffeehouses—a first-of-its-kind coffee and music establishment where customers could enjoy a freshly brewed cup of coffee while downloading music from the company's 200,000-plus song library and, if they wished, have the downloaded songs burned onto a CD for purchase.

In 2005, in an average week, an estimated 30 million-plus customers patronized Starbucks, up from about 5 million in 1998. U.S. stores did about half of their business by 11:00 a.m. Loyal customers patronized a Starbucks store 15 to 20 times a month, spending perhaps $50–$75 monthly. Some customers were Starbucks fanatics, coming in daily. Baristas became familiar with regular customers, learning their names and their favorite drinks. Christine Nagy, a field director for Oracle Corporation in Palo Alto, California, told a *Wall Street Journal* reporter, "For me, it's a daily necessity or I start getting withdrawals."[27] Her standard order was a custom drink: a decaf grande nonfat no-whip no-foam extra-cocoa mocha; when the barista saw her come through the door, she told the reporter, "They just say 'We need a Christine here.' " Since the inception of Starbucks Cards in 2001, 52 million Starbucks customers had purchased the reloadable cards that allowed them to pay for their purchases with a quick swipe at the cash register and also to earn and redeem rewards. The use of Starbucks Cards was a growing means of payment in Starbucks stores. In fiscal 2004, the company reached approximately $1 billion in total life-to-date activations and reloads on Starbucks cards. Due to its success in the United States the Starbucks Card was being launched internationally, with the initial rollouts starting in Japan and Greece.

In the fall of 2003, Starbucks, in partnership with Bank One, introduced the Duetto Visa card, which added Visa card functionality to the reloadable Starbucks Cards. By charging purchases to the Visa account of their Duetto card anywhere Visa credit cards were accepted, cardholders earned 1 percent back in Duetto Dollars, automatically loaded on their Starbucks card account after each billing cycle. Duetto Dollars could be used to purchase beverages, food, and store merchandise at any Starbucks location. The Duetto card was an example of the ongoing effort by Starbucks' management to introduce new products and experiences for customers that belonged exclusively to Starbucks; senior executives drummed the importance of always being open to reinventing the Starbucks experience.

So far, Starbucks had spent very little money on advertising, preferring instead to build the brand cup-by-cup with customers via word of mouth and the appeal of its storefronts. The company spent a total of $87.7 million on advertising in fiscal 2005, up from $49.6 million in fiscal 2003.

Joint Ventures and Acquisitions

In 1994, after months of meetings and experimentation, PepsiCo and Starbucks entered into a joint venture to create new coffee-related products for mass distribution through Pepsi channels, including cold coffee drinks in a bottle or can. Howard Schultz saw this as a major paradigm shift with the potential to cause Starbucks' business to evolve in heretofore unimaginable directions; he thought it was time to look for ways to move Starbucks out into more mainstream markets. Cold coffee products had historically met with poor market reception, except in Japan, where there was an $8 billion market for ready-to-drink coffee-based beverages. Nonetheless, Schultz was hoping the partners would hit upon a new product to exploit a good-tasting coffee extract that had been developed by Starbucks' recently appointed director of research and development. The joint venture's first new product, Mazagran, a lightly flavored carbonated coffee drink, was a failure; a market test in southern California showed that some people liked it and some hated it. While people were willing to try it the first time, partly because the Starbucks name was on the label, repeat sales proved disappointing. Despite the clash of cultures and the different motivations of PepsiCo and Starbucks, the partnership held together because of the good working relationship that evolved between Howard Schultz and Pepsi's senior executives. Then Schultz, at a meeting to discuss the future of Mazagran, suggested, "Why not develop a bottled version of Frappuccino?"[28] Starbucks had come up with Frappuccino in the summer of 1995, and the cold coffee drink had proved to be a big hot-weather seller; Pepsi executives were enthusiastic. After months of experimentation, the joint venture product research team came up with a shelf-stable version of Frappuccino that tasted quite good. It was tested in West Coast supermarkets in the summer of 1996; sales ran 10 times projections, with 70 percent being repeat business. Sales of Frappuccino reached $125 million in 1997 and achieved national supermarket penetration of 80 percent. Starbucks' management believed that the market for Frappuccino would ultimately exceed $1 billion.

In October 1995 Starbucks partnered with Dreyer's Grand Ice Cream to supply coffee extract for a new line of coffee ice cream made and distributed by Dreyer's under the Starbucks brand. The new line, featuring such flavors as Dark Roast Expresso Swirl, JavaChip, Vanilla MochaChip, Biscotti Bliss, and Caffe Almond Fudge, hit supermarket shelves in April 1996, and by July 1996 Starbucks' coffee-flavored ice cream was the top-selling superpremium brand in the coffee segment. In 1997, two new low-fat flavors were added to complement the original six flavors, along with two flavors of ice cream bars; all were well received in the marketplace.

The partnerships with Pepsi and Dreyer's produced about $20 million in revenues for Starbucks in fiscal 2005 (equal to about 2 percent of total specialty sales).

In 2004, Starbucks teamed with Jim Beam Brands to invent a Starbucks Coffee Liqueur that would be sold in bars, liquor stores, and restaurants; projections were for systemwide gross sales of over $8 million annually. Launched in February 2005, Starbucks Coffee Liqueur was the top-selling new spirit product through August 2005, according to Nielsen. In October 2005, again collaborating with Jim Beam Brands, Starbucks introduced Starbucks Cream Liqueur, a blend of cream, spirits, and a hint of Starbucks coffee. With 22 million cordial consumers in the U.S. market, the cream liqueur category was nearly three times the size of coffee liqueur category. Both Starbucks Coffee Liqueur and Starbucks Cream Liqueur were packaged in a 750-milliliter bottle priced at $22.99.

In April 2005, Starbucks purchased Ethos Water for $8 million in cash. The acquisition was made to expand the line of beverages in Starbucks' stores in the United States.

Licensed Stores and Specialty Sales

Starbucks had a licensing agreement with Kraft Foods to market and distribute Starbucks whole-bean and ground coffees in grocery and mass-merchandise channels across the United States. Kraft managed all distribution, marketing, advertising, and promotions and paid a royalty to Starbucks based on a percentage of net sales. The coffee that Starbucks sold in supermarkets featured distinctive, elegant packaging, prominent positions in grocery aisles, and the same premium quality as that it sold in its stores. Product freshness was guaranteed by Starbucks' FlavorLock packaging, and the price per pound paralleled the prices in Starbucks' retail stores. Flavor selections in supermarkets were more limited than those at Starbucks stores. Going into 2006, Starbucks coffees were available in some 31,300 grocery and warehouse clubs (such as Sam's and Costco) with 30,000 in the United States and 1,300 in the international markets. Revenues from this category comprised 24 percent of specialty revenues in fiscal 2005.

Starbucks executives recognized that supermarket distribution entailed several risks, especially in exposing Starbucks to first-time customers. Starbucks had built its reputation around the unique retail experience in its stores where all beverages were properly prepared—it had no control over how customers would perceive Starbucks when they encountered it in grocery aisles. A second risk concerned coffee preparation at home. Rigorous quality control and skilled baristas ensured that store-purchased beverages would measure up, but consumers using poor equipment or inappropriate brewing methods could easily conclude that Starbucks packaged coffees did not live up to their reputation.

Starbucks had also entered into a limited number of licensing agreements for store locations in areas where it did not have ability to locate its own outlets. The company had an agreement with Marriott Host International that allowed Host to operate Starbucks retail stores in airport locations, and it had an agreement with Aramark Food and Services to put Starbucks stores on university campuses and other locations operated by Aramark. Starbucks received a license fee and a royalty on sales at these locations and supplied the coffee for resale in the licensed locations. All licensed stores had to follow Starbucks' detailed operating procedures, and all managers and employees who worked in these stores received the same training given to Starbucks managers and store employees. As of 2005, there were 2,435 licensed or franchised stores in the United States and 1,806 licensed stores in other countries. Licensing revenues increased from $241 million in fiscal 2001 to $673 million in fiscal 2005; domestic stores accounted for $515 million of the revenues from licensing in 2005.

Starbucks had a specialty sales group that provided its coffee products to restaurants, airlines, hotels, universities, hospitals, business offices, country clubs, and select retailers. One of the early users of Starbucks coffee was Horizon Airlines, a regional carrier based in Seattle. In 1995, Starbucks entered into negotiations with United Airlines to serve Starbucks coffee on all United flights. There was much internal debate at Starbucks about whether such a move made sense for Starbucks and the possible damage to the integrity of the Starbucks brand if the quality of the coffee served did not measure up (since there was different coffeemaking equipment on different planes). It took seven months of negotiations for Starbucks and United to arrive at a mutually agreeable way to handle quality control on United's various types of planes.

In recent years, the specialty sales group had won the coffee accounts at Hyatt, Hilton, Sheraton, Radisson, and Westin hotels, resulting in packets of Starbucks coffee being in each room with coffee-making equipment. Starbucks had entered into an agreement with Wells Fargo to provide coffee service at some of the bank's locations in California. A 1997 agreement with U.S. Office Products gave Starbucks an entrée to provide its coffee to workers in 1.5 million business offices. In addition, Starbucks supplied an exclusive coffee blend to Nordstrom's for sale only in Nordstrom stores, operated coffee bars in Barnes & Noble bookstores, and, most recently, had begun coffee bar operations in Chapters bookstores (Chapters was a Toronto book retailer that had sites throughout Canada) and Borders bookstores that had cafés. Starbucks also had an alliance with SYSCO Corporation to service the majority of its food-service and restaurant accounts. In fiscal 2005, Starbucks was supplying its coffees to 15,500 food-service accounts worldwide, producing fiscal 2005 revenues of $304 million, up from $179 million in 2001.

Other Starbucks initiatives included a 24-hour Starbucks Hear Music digital music channel available to all XM satellite radio subscribers and the availability of wireless broadband Internet service in company-owned stores in the United States and Canada. Collectively, these other initiatives accounted for 3 percent of specialty revenue in fiscal 2005.

Starbucks experimented with a mail order catalog and with online sales at its Web site, but it discontinued those operations in 2003 when sales fell off (chiefly because of the growing availability of Starbucks coffees in supermarkets and the company's expanding number of store locations).

STARBUCKS COFFEE PURCHASING STRATEGY

Starbucks personnel traveled regularly to coffee-producing countries— Colombia, Sumatra, Yemen, Antigua, Indonesia, Guatemala, New Guinea, Costa Rica, Sulawesi, Papua, Kenya, Ethiopia, Java, and Mexico—building relationships with growers and exporters, checking on agricultural conditions and crop yields, and searching out varieties and sources that would meet Starbucks' exacting standards of quality and flavor. The coffee-purchasing group, working with personnel in roasting operations, tested new varieties and blends of beans from different sources.

Coffee was grown in 70 tropical countries and was the second-most-traded commodity in the world after petroleum. The global value of the 2000–2001 coffee bean crop was about $5.6 billion. By World Bank estimates, some 25 million small farmers made their living growing coffee. Commodity-grade coffee, which consisted of robusta and commercial quality arabica beans, was traded in a highly competitive market as an undifferentiated product. Coffee prices were subject to considerable volatility due to weather, economic and political conditions in the growing countries, new agreements establishing export quotas, and periodic efforts to bolster prices by restricting coffee supplies. Starbucks used fixed-price purchase commitments to limit its exposure to fluctuating coffee prices in upcoming periods and, on occasion, purchased coffee futures contracts to provide price protection. In years past, there had been times when unexpected jumps in coffee prices had put a squeeze on Starbucks' margins, forcing an increase in the prices of the beverages and beans sold at retail.

Starbucks sourced approximately 50 percent of its beans from Latin America, 35 percent from the Pacific Rim, and 15 percent from East Africa. Sourcing from multiple geographic areas not only allowed Starbucks to offer a greater range of coffee varieties to customers but also spread the company's risks regarding weather, price volatility, and changing economic and political conditions in coffee-growing countries.

During 2002, a global oversupply of more than 2 billion pounds drove the prices of commodity coffees to historic lows of $0.40–$0.50 per pound. The specialty coffee market, which represented about 10 percent of worldwide production, consisted primarily of high-quality arabica beans. Prices for specialty coffees were determined by the quality and flavor of the beans and were almost always higher than prevailing prices for commodity-grade coffee beans. Starbucks purchased only high-quality arabica coffee beans, paying an average of $1.20 per pound in 2004. Its purchases represented about 1 percent of the world's coffee bean crop. The company's green coffee costs reached a historic low in 2002 and had gradually increased since then. Given the price volatility risk, the company entered into fixed-price purchase commitments in order to secure an adequate supply of quality green coffee. As of October 2005, the company had over $375 million in fixed-price purchase commitments, which along with existing inventory was expected to provide an adequate supply of green coffee through fiscal 2006.[29]

Believing that the continued growth and success of its business depended on gaining access to adequate supplies of high-quality coffees year-in and year-out, Starbucks had been a leader in promoting environmental and social stewardship in coffee-origin countries. Starbucks' coffee sourcing strategy was to contribute to the sustainability of coffee growers and help conserve the environment. In sourcing green coffee beans, Starbucks was increasingly dealing directly with farmers and cooperatives, and its policy was to pay prices high enough to ensure that small coffee growers, most of whom lived on the edge of poverty, were able to cover their production costs and provide for their families. About 40 percent of Starbucks purchases were made under three-to five-year contracts, which management believed enabled the company to purchase its future coffee bean requirements at predictable prices over multiple crop years. Coffee purchases negotiated through long-term contracts increased from 3 percent in 2001 to 36 percent in 2002. Farmers who met important quality, environmental, social, and economic criteria, which Starbucks had developed with the support of Conservation International's Center for Environmental Leadership in Business, were rewarded with financial incentives and preferred supplier status. In fiscal 2004, the company opened its Farmer Support Center in Costa Rica to support existing and potential Starbucks coffee suppliers and their communities.

Starbucks had $375 million in fixed-price purchase commitments in October 2005 but was not planning to increase this commitment in the near future due to a significant jump in the prices of green coffee beans (in some cases the going prices for green beans were above the fixed purchase prices). The high commodity prices for coffee beans made farmers less willing to enter into fixed-price arrangements.

Fair Trade Certified Coffee

A growing number of small coffee growers were members of democratically run cooperatives that were registered with the Fair Trade Labeling Organizations International; these growers could sell their beans directly to importers, roasters, and retailers at favorable guaranteed "Fair Trade" prices. The idea behind guaranteed prices for Fair Trade coffees was to boost earnings for small coffee growers enough to allow them to afford basic health care, education, and home improvements. Starbucks marketed Fair Trade Certified coffee at most of its retail stores and through other locations that sold Starbucks coffees. In October 2005, Starbucks introduced Café Estima Blend Fair Trade Certified Coffee as the coffee of the week to support Fair Trade Month 2005. Starbucks expected to purchase 10 million pounds of Fair Trade Certified coffee in 2005, and it planned to purchase 12 million pounds in 2006.

Environmental Best Practices

Since 1998, Starbucks had partnered with Conservation International to promote coffee cultivation methods that protected biodiversity and maintained a healthy environment. A growing percentage of the coffees that Starbucks purchased were grown "organically" without the use of pesticides, herbicides, or chemical fertilizers; organic cultivation methods resulted in clean groundwater and helped protect against degrading of local ecosystems, many of which were fragile or in areas where biodiversity was under severe threat. Another environmental conservation practice involved growing organic coffee under a natural canopy of shade trees interspersed with fruit trees and other crops; this not only allowed farmers to get higher crop yields from small acreages but also helped protect against soil erosion on mountainsides.

COFFEE ROASTING OPERATIONS

Starbucks considered the roasting of its coffee beans to be something of an art form, entailing trial-and-error testing of different combinations of time and temperature to get the most out of each type of bean and blend. Recipes were put together by the coffee department, once all the components had been tested. Computerized roasters guaranteed consistency. Each batch was roasted in a powerful gas oven for 12 to 15 minutes. Highly trained and experienced roasting personnel monitored the process, using both smell and hearing, to help check when the beans were perfectly done—coffee beans make a popping sound when ready. Starbucks' standards were so exacting that roasters tested the color of the beans in a blood-cell analyzer and discarded the entire batch if the reading wasn't on target. After roasting and cooling, the coffee was immediately vacuum-sealed in bags with one-way valves that let out gases naturally produced by fresh-roasted beans without letting oxygen in—one-way valve technology extended the shelf life of packaged Starbucks coffee to 26 weeks. As a matter of policy, however, Starbucks removed coffees on its shelves after three months, and, in the case of coffee used to prepare beverages in stores, the shelf life was limited to seven days after the bag was opened.

At the end of fiscal 2005, Starbucks had roasting plants in Kent, Washington; York, Pennsylvania; Minden, Nevada; and the Netherlands. In addition to roasting capability, the Kent, York, Minden, and Netherlands plants also had additional space for warehousing and shipping coffees. The roasting plants and distribution facilities in Kent supplied stores west of the Mississippi and in the Asia-Pacific region. The newly constructed Minden plant and distribution center was used to supply stores in the Mountain West and Midwest. The roasting and distribution facility in York, which could be expanded to 1 million square feet, supplied stores mainly east of the Mississippi. The 94,000-square-foot facility in the Netherlands supplied stores in Europe and the Middle East.

STARBUCKS' CORPORATE SOCIAL RESPONSIBILITY STRATEGY

Howard Schultz's effort to "build a company with soul" included broad-based initiatives to contribute positively to the communities in which Starbucks had stores and to the environment. The guiding theme of Starbucks' social responsibility strategy was "Giving back to our communities is the way we do business." The Starbucks Foundation was set up in 1997 to orchestrate the company's philanthropic activities. Since 1991 Starbucks had been a major contributor to CARE, a worldwide relief and development organization that sponsored health, education, and humanitarian aid programs in almost all of the third world countries where Starbucks purchased its coffee supplies. Stores featured CARE in promotions and had organized concerts to benefit CARE. A second major philanthropic effort involved providing financial support to community literacy organizations. In 1995 Starbucks began a program to improve the conditions of workers in coffee-growing countries, establishing a code of conduct for its growers and providing financial assistance for agricultural improvement projects. In 1997, Starbucks formed an alliance with Appropriate Technology International to help poor, small-scale coffee growers in Guatemala increase their income by improving the quality of their crops and their market access; the company's first-year grant of $75,000 went to fund a new processing facility and set up a loan program for a producer cooperative.

Starbucks had an Environmental Committee that looked for ways to reduce, reuse, and recycle waste, as well as contribute to local community environmental efforts. There was also a Green Store Task Force that looked at how Starbucks stores could conserve on water and energy usage and generate less solid waste. Customers who brought their own mugs to stores were given a 10-cent discount of beverage purchases (in 2002, customers used commuter mugs in making purchases about 12.7 million times). Coffee grounds, which were a big portion of the waste stream in stores, were packaged and given to customers, parks, schools and plant nurseries as a soil amendment. Company personnel purchased paper products with high levels of recycled content and unbleached fiber to help Starbucks minimize its environmental footprint. Stores participated in Earth Day activities each year with in-store promotions and volunteer efforts to educate employees and customers about the impacts their actions had on the environment. Suppliers were encouraged to provide the most energy-efficient products within their category and eliminate excessive packaging; Starbucks had recently instituted a Code of Conduct for suppliers of noncoffee products that addressed standards for social responsibility, including labor and human rights. No genetically modified ingredients were used in any food or beverage products that Starbucks served, with the exception of milk. (U.S. labeling requirements do not require milk producers to disclose the use of hormones aimed at increasing the milk production of dairy herds.)

Starbucks stores participated regularly in local charitable projects of one kind or another, donating drinks, books, and proceeds from store-opening benefits. Employees were encouraged to recommend and apply for grants from the Starbucks Foundation to benefit local community literacy organizations.

Exhibit 8   Starbucks' Environmental Mission Statement

Starbucks is committed to a role of environmental leadership in all facets of our business.

We fulfill this mission by a commitment to:

- Understanding of environmental issues and sharing information with our partners.
- Developing innovative and flexible solutions to bring about change.
- Striving to buy, sell, and use environmentally friendly products.
- Recognizing that fiscal responsibility is essential to our environmental future.
- Instilling environmental responsibility as a corporate value.
- Measuring and monitoring our progress for each project.

On the Fourth of July weekend in 1997, three Starbucks employees were murdered in the company's store in the Georgetown area of Washington, D.C.; Starbucks offered a $100,000 reward for information leading to the arrest of the murderer(s). The company announced it would reopen the store in early 1998 and donate all future net proceeds of the store to a Starbucks Memorial Fund that would make annual grants to local groups working to reduce violence and aid the victims of violent crimes. In 2005, Starbucks made a $5 million, five-year commitment to long-term relief and recovery efforts for victims of Hurricane Katrina and committed $5 million to support educational programs in China.

Starbucks felt so deeply about its responsibilities that it even developed an environmental mission statement to expand on its corporate mission statement (see Exhibit 8). In 2002, Starbucks also began issuing an annual Corporate Social Responsibility Report (the reports for recent years can be viewed in the Investors section at www.starbucks.com). Going into 2004, Starbucks had received 20 awards from a diverse group of organizations for its philanthropic, community service, and environmental activities.

THE SPECIALTY COFFEE INDUSTRY

While the market for traditional commercial grade coffees had stagnated since the 1970s, the specialty

coffee segment had expanded, as interested, educated, upscale consumers became increasingly inclined to upgrade to premium coffees with more robust flavors. Whereas retail sales of specialty coffees amounted to only $45 million in 1969, by 1994 retail sales of specialty coffees had increased to $2 billion, much of which stemmed from sales in coffee bars or the shops of coffee bean retailers (like Peet's). The increase was attributed to wider consumer awareness of and appreciation for fine coffee, the emergence of coffee bars featuring a blossoming number of premium coffee beverages, and the adoption of a healthier lifestyle that prompted some consumers to replace alcohol with coffee. Coffee's image changed from one of just a breakfast or after-dinner beverage to a drink that could be enjoyed at any time in the company of others. Many coffee drinkers took to the idea of coffee bars where they could enjoy a high-caliber coffee beverage and sit back and relax with friends or business associates.

Some industry experts expected the gourmet coffee market in the United States would be saturated by 2005. But the international market was much more wide open as of early 2004. The United States, Germany, and Japan were the three biggest coffee-consuming countries.

COMPETITORS

Starbucks' primary competitors were restaurants, specialty coffee shops, doughnut shops, supermarkets, convenience stores, and others that sold hot coffee and specialty coffee drinks. In 2003, there were an estimated 14,000 specialty coffee outlets in the United States, with some observers predicting there would as many as 18,000 locations selling specialty coffee drinks by 2015.

Starbucks' success was prompting a number of ambitious rivals to scale up their expansion plans. Still, no other specialty coffee rival had as many as 400 stores, but there were at least 20 small local and regional chains that aspired to compete against Starbucks in their local market arenas, most notably Caribou Coffee (337 stores in 14 states and the District of Columbia), Tully's Coffee (98 stores in 4 states), Gloria Jean's (280 mall locations in 35 states and several foreign countries), New World Coffee (30 locations), Brew HaHa (13 locations in Delaware and Pennsylvania), Bad Ass Coffee (about 60 locations in 18 states, Japan, and South Korea),

Second Cup Coffee (the largest chain based in Canada), and Qwiky's (India). Caribou Coffee went public in late 2005, with a stock offering that raised about $68 million. McDonald's had begun opening McCafés. While it had been anticipated in the late 1990s that local and regional chains would merge in efforts to get bigger and better position themselves as an alternative to Starbucks, such consolidation had not occurred as of 2003. But numerous retail entrepreneurs had picked up on the growing popularity of specialty coffees and opened coffee bars in high-pedestrian-traffic locations to serve espresso, cappuccino, latte, and other coffee drinks. Growing numbers of restaurants were upgrading the quality of the coffee they served.

Starbucks also faced competition from nation wide coffee manufacturers—such as Kraft General Foods (the parent of Maxwell House), Procter & Gamble (the marketer of Folger's and Millstone brands), and Nestlé—that distributed their coffees through supermarkets. Both General Foods and Procter & Gamble had introduced premium blends of their Maxwell House and Folgers coffees on supermarket shelves, pricing them several dollars below Starbucks' offerings. But Starbucks' most important competitors in supermarkets were the increasing numbers of rival brands of specialty coffees—Green Mountain, Allegro, Peaberry, Brothers, and dozens of other brands. Because many consumers were accustomed to purchasing their coffee supplies at supermarkets, it was easy for them to choose whatever specialty coffee brand or brands were featured in their local supermarkets over Starbucks.

FUTURE CHALLENGES

In fiscal 2006, Starbucks planned to open 1,800 new stores globally. Top management believed that it could grow revenues by about 20 percent annually and net earnings by 20–25 percent annually for the next three to five years. Howard Schultz and CEO Jim Donald viewed China as a huge market opportunity, along with Brazil, India, and Russia. Howard Schultz believed that, to sustain its growth and make Starbucks one of the world's preeminent global brands, the company had to challenge the status quo, be innovative, take risks, and adapt its vision of who it was, what it did, and where it was headed. If the challenge was met successfully, in all likelihood the company's best years lay on the strategic road ahead.

Endnotes

[1] As quoted in Cora Daniels, "Mr. Coffee," *Fortune,* April 14, 2003, p. 139.
[2] 2004 annual report, letter to shareholders.
[3] 2002 annual report, letter to shareholders.
[4] Ibid.
[5] Howard Schultz and Dori Jones Yang, *Pour Your Heart Into It* (New York: Hyperion, 1997), p. 33.
[6] Ibid., p. 34.
[7] Ibid., p. 36.
[8] As told in ibid., p. 48.
[9] Ibid., pp. 61–62.
[10] As quoted in Jennifer Reese, "Starbucks: Inside the Coffee Cult," *Fortune,* December 9, 1996, p. 193.
[11] Schultz and Yang, *Pour Your Heart Into It,* pp. 101–2.
[12] Ibid., p. 142.
[13] Ibid., p. 129.
[14] As related in ibid., pp. 131–36.
[15] 2004 annual report, p. 36.
[16] Ibid.
[17] 2005 Starbucks 10-K report, p. 67.
[18] Ben van Houten, "Employee Perks: Starbucks Coffee's Employee Benefit Plan," *Restaurant Business,* May 15, 1997, p. 85.
[19] As related in Schultz and Yang, *Pour Your Heart Into It,* p. 168.
[20] As quoted in Ingrid Abramovitch, "Miracles of Marketing," *Success* 40, no. 3, p. 26.
[21] Daniels, "Mr. Coffee," p. 140.
[22] Company press release, May 31, 2005, and October 25, 2005
[23] Company press release, October 25, 2005.
[24] Kate Rounds, "Starbucks Coffee," *Incentive* 167, no. 7, p. 22.
[25] CSR annual report, Starbucks, fiscal 2004.
[26] Fiscal 2005 annual report, p. 14.
[27] David Bank, "Starbucks Faces Growing Competition: Its Own Stores," *The Wall Street Journal,* January 21, 1997, p. B1.
[28] As related in Schultz and Yang, *Pour Your Heart Into It,* p. 224.
[29] Starbucks 2005 form 10-K report, p. 6.

Leadership at TDC sunrise: "Always a Smile" or "Communication Is Life"?

Preston Bottger
International Institute for Management Development

George Rädler
International Institute for Management Development

Early 2001: Although the Danish telecom company TDC increased its net income by 142% [y-on-y], the share price dropped by 17% following the announcement of the annual results. One reason for this is the concern about the newly acquired Swiss operation [sunrise]—*Neue Zürcher Zeitung (NZZ)*, **Swiss newspaper, February 23, 2001**

Early 2004: For the first time ever, sunrise [TDC's Swiss operation] recorded a net income in 2003. The numbers (. . .) show that sunrise has reached normal operating temperatures—*Neue Zürcher Zeitung (NZZ)*, **Swiss newspaper, March 2, 2004**

Leadership is about breaking rules—**Georg Baselitz, Artist**

Leadership is not about getting things done, but about getting the *right* things done!

December 2000: sunrise—initially a telecom operator for fixed line and Internet services—had just merged with an operator with a mobile/wireless license. The new company kept the sunrise name, but the ownership changed. TDC, the former Danish telephone monopoly who already held a minority share in the old sunrise, increased its stake from 19.5 percent to 78.5 percent of the new company.

In this merger, the typical harmonious "get to know each other phase" was very short. The desig-nated CEO decided to leave less than one month after the merger. On December 15, TDC sent Kim Frimer, 41, to take over as CEO and president of sunrise. His job was "to fix" what was the biggest ever foreign takeover by a Danish company. Challenges came from many sides. While the whole telecom industry was suffering from massive overspending, sunrise in particular was also facing operational difficulties: The mobile division was losing 9% of its customers per month; operations had to be merged and a new company culture had to be established. The local press forecast an annual loss of up to 27 percent of sales for the year 2001.

So, how was sunrise able to reach very respectable profit levels by 2003—a year earlier than initially expected?

THE TELECOM INDUSTRY: FROM BOOM TO BUST

Since its invention in 1876, the telephone has seen many innovations on a sequential basis, some of which have been technical revolutions. Direct dialing (without an operator), touchtone instead of pulse, digital instead of analogue, caller ID, etc., have become integral parts of our daily life.

This was a high fixed-cost industry and asset utilization was key. Telecom companies were mostly operating as state monopolies and could easily cross-subsidize unprofitable operations with profits from other divisions, such as long-distance calls. However, starting in the early 1990s, several large shifts suddenly impacted the global telecom industry at once: (1) ownership changes due to privatization, (2) massive price drops due to deregulation, and (3) major changes in consumer behavior due to the arrival of mobile telephones.

The stock market hype catapulted the share prices of many newly listed, former state monopolies sky-high. For example, during their peak in 2000 France Telecom and Deutsche Telekom's shares reached €156 and €84, respectively, before beginning their decline into single digit figures.

The Swiss Market

Switzerland had always been a highly attractive market for telephone companies. High GDP levels, a considerable base of multinational companies and organizations, as well as a good private market accounted for telecom expenditure reaching 3.3 percent of GDP in 2000—the highest in Europe (refer to Exhibit 1 for key data on the Swiss telecommunications market).

In January 1998 Switzerland became the last telecommunication market in Europe to open its voice market to private enterprises (the data sector in Switzerland had been deregulated since 1992; the Internet market since 1995). State-run Swisscom, the incumbent player, traded its status of a government-owned monopoly for that of a corporation. However, the government still owned/controlled 66 percent of Swisscom.

KIM FRIMER: EARLY DAYS

While studying economies with a focus on marketing and HR in Denmark, Kim Frimer set up and operated a trucking company which grew to 20 trucks before he sold it at the end of his studies. He recalled: "In my early days, I learned a lot about accounting, processes, how to earn money and above all, I learned to be disciplined."

After graduation, Frimer joined one of the regional telephone companies that later became part of TDC. Frimer: "I joined for practical reasons. The job was close to home." His job was to develop market strategies which "was easy, as it was still a monopoly." He became increasingly bored and decided to quit. However, the company wanted to keep him and offered him a job marketing new technologies. He rose through the ranks and became CEO of data networking. The division grew rapidly from 200 people in 1992 to 1,400 in 1995.

In 1997 he moved to Switzerland for the first time, where he oversaw the launch of sunrise as chief commercial officer. In this function, he had to lobby against heavy opposition from "all sides" for the sunrise name. Initially, it was seen as a good name for a travel agency, but for a telephone company? In the end, Frimer got his "sunrise" and

Exhibit 1   Overview—The Swiss Market for Telecommunications (1998–2003)

	1998	1999	2000	2001	2002	2003
Population (millions)	7.2	7.2	7.2	7.2	7.2	7.2
Telecommunications revenue ($ billion)	7.7	8.7	8.2	8.7	9.6	9.6
Main lines in service (thousands)	4,273.6	4,153.1	4,108.2	4,101.1	4,093.6	4,081.4
Main lines (% change y-o-y)	−8.8	−2.8	−1.1	−0.2	−0.2	−0.3
Main line penetration (%)	59.6	57.9	57.3	57.2	57.1	57
Mobile subscribers (thousands)	1,698.6	3,057.5	4,638.5	5,275.8	5,747	6,436.6
Mobile subscribers (% change y-o-y)	62.6	80	51.7	13.7	8.9	12
Mobile penetration (%)	23.7	42.6	64.7	73.6	80.2	89.9
Estimated Internet users (thousands)	939	1,473	2,096	2,224	2,556	2,878
Internet users (% change y-o-y)	71.4	56.9	42.3	6.1	14.9	14.9
Internet penetration (%)	13.1	20.5	29.2	31	35.7	40.2

Source: World Markets Research Center. "Country Report Switzerland (Telecoms)," May 21, 2004.

the company put great emphasis on being ready for the first day of liberalization—January 1, 1998—to challenge the incumbent. Competitor diAx later said, "sunrise favored speed over quality," but the marketing campaign on New Year's Day worked well. A company source explained:

> December 31, 1997, PM: With the countdown to liberalization only few hours away, Swisscom [state-owned telephone monopoly in Switzerland] decided to flaunt its market dominance in a way that no one could misunderstand. The people of Zurich were invited to a huge party at a central spot in downtown Zurich, where there were to be outstanding fireworks, music and drinks. The rockets were to have been set off on the dot of half past midnight, and literally all of Zurich was watching. Suddenly, however, something completely unexpected happened. The crowds spotted someone scaling the façade of Zurich's main church. And then a huge screen was unfurled and the band hired by Swisscom fell silent, as the power was needed for the "sunrise" laser show instead. The message [on the screen] was clear: "Today is the beginning of the end of telecommunism."[1]

Frimer later remembered:

> In order to use sunrise, people had to sign up by either sending or faxing us their application. Our campaign "end telecommunism" [on December 31] got us a lot of attention in the media. I had to send out my employees to buy fax machines. It seemed like wherever we hooked up the fax machines, they were spitting out applications. The success of the launch was huge. Within just three days, we exceeded the target we had set for the whole year.

The other newcomer, diAx, however, was not ready for service by early 1998 as it "was committed to the provision of top quality services, even at the cost of losing a certain amount of market share." Once it was operational—about five months after sunrise—it found that it was not attracting as many customers as initially planned.

Originally, sunrise only offered long-distance calls (on the fixed line), at around 25 percent less than the incumbent. In 1999, it started offering local calls and Internet service. Initially Frimer ran the marketing department before taking over as interim CEO for 10 months. After spending exactly two years in Switzerland, he left sunrise in April 1999 to run a telecom company owned by TDC in Germany. However, by the end of the following year, he was back in Switzerland.

FRIMER RETURNS TO ZURICH

When Frimer arrived at sunrise's headquarters in Zurich on December 15, 2000, it was his second time at sunrise but this time as president and CEO. However, the company was barely recognizable from the one he had left only two years earlier.

First Assessment

There was a considerable migration from wireline/fixed line calls to mobiles during that period. Mobile telephony was *the* major growth and profit driver[2] in this industry but sunrise had failed to secure an operating license for mobile telephony from the government. This was pretty much a death sentence since mobile communication was expected to dominate the future. However, sunrise merged with diAx, which had successfully secured a mobile license in addition to its fixed line business.

Frimer's employer, the former Danish incumbent TDC, decided to acquire the shares or parts thereof of the former partners and thereby raised its stake in the merged company from 19.5 percent to 78.5 percent, making it the biggest Danish foreign takeover ever. The plan was to float sunrise or parts thereof on the stock market within the next few years. At HQ in Denmark the thinking was that "a Swiss company should have a Swiss CEO." However, sunrise's Swiss CEO, who was also supposed to run the merged company, decided to step down a month after the merger was announced, and hence Frimer was sent back to Switzerland.

diAx's aim was "to make some money" from the deregulation. It was a consortium headed by the six biggest Swiss utilities, two insurance companies (Swiss Re and Winterthur) and SBC, from the United States as technical partner. However, diAx was facing serious problems:

- Mobile phone operations and fixed line services were operating as standalone businesses, resulting in very different marketing and advertising strategies, etc.
- After a difficult start in the fixed line business, the launch of mobile services needed to be a success. Within four months of mobile operations, the company already had 100,000 customers. This

was much faster than in neighboring countries, but was not without a price: it turned out that the handsets were heavily subsidized by diAx with contract lengths of only six months versus. the industry norm of either 12 or 24 months. Losses occurred with every mobile phone sold.

- While the company received positive press coverage for creating many jobs (900 in 1999), some of the initial marketing tools failed miserably. For example, a free concert tour around Switzerland was intended to create awareness and goodwill among the public. However, the band selection mostly covered the taste of punks,

while the Swiss public in general disapproved of the noise levels.

When diAx initially started its mobile operations, it only covered half of the country. By late 2000, 90 percent of the country was covered. The overall mobile market in Switzerland grew by 51.7 percent in 2000 (down from 80 percent in 1999). Orange, the other entrant into mobiles, added 473,000 new users in 2000, while diAx added less than 190,000 new mobile users over the same period (refer to Exhibit 2 for the sales data for mobile phones). Customer acquisition was deteriorating in the last quarter of 2000: diAx recorded net losses of around 30,000

Exhibit 2   Swiss Market for Mobile Telephony, 1997–2003

General Data on the Swiss Mobile Market

	1997	1998	1999	2000	2001	2002	2003
Coverage (as a % of the population)	14.7%	23.8%	42.7%	64.4%	72.7%	78.4%	84.4%
Number of customers (millions)	1.044	1.698	3.058	4.639	5.276	5.736	6.177
Growth rate	57.5%	62.6%	80.1%	51.7%	13.7%	8.7%	7.7%
Postpaid customers as a % of total	80	65.3	65.5	63.2	59.2	59.6	58.0
Prepaid customers as a % of total	20	34.7	34.5	36.8	40.8	40.1	42.0

Competition in the Swiss Mobile Market

	1997	1998	1999	2000	2001	2002	2003
Number of subscribers (thousands)	1,044	1,698	3,058	4,639	5,276	5,736	6,177
Swisscom	1,044	1,672	2,282	3,168	3,373	3,605	3,792
sunrise		26	463	653	944	1,134	1,260
Orange			313	786	925	963	1,085
Others				32	33	34	40
Subscriber growth (%)	57.5%	62.6%	80.1%	51.7%	13.7%	8.7%	7.7%
Swisscom	57.5	60.2	36.5	38.8	6.5	6.9	5.2
sunrise				41.0	44.7	20.0	11.1
Orange					17.7	4.1	12.7
Others					3.1	3.0	17.6
Market shares (%)							
Swisscom	100.0%	98.5%	74.6%	68.3%	63.9%	62.8%	61.4%
sunrise		1.5	15.1	14.1	17.9	19.8	20.4
Orange			10.2	16.9	17.5	16.8	17.6
Others				0.7	0.6	0.6	0.8

Source: Swiss Federal Office of Communications (Ofcom), "Sammlung aus diversen Quellen," May 2004: 11 & 12.

users in Q4, 2000 (equivalent to a monthly churn of 9 percent), while Orange added 60,000 users in the same quarter.

Incumbent Swisscom had a real first-mover advantage in mobile phones with about 1.6 million customers before competitors began to enter in 1998. Many of these were the very best customers (high usage, price insensitive business people). Before Frimer returned to Switzerland, the mobile market became a lot tougher. Swisscom sold a 25 percent stake of its mobile division to Vodafone and subsequently had access to Vodafone's technology as well as its 295 million customers.

Can Former Competitors Work Together?

In the past both sunrise and diAx were competitors in the fixed line business. Suddenly, former enemies had to work together. Frimer remembered the beginning:

> The following Monday, I was on the plane to Zurich to head right into a management meeting. What I saw was huge frustration and two companies desperately looking to move forward. I told the people in the room that I did not care where they came from, as long as they did a good job.

The diAx brand was well known since the company had spent much more on building the brand. Unfortunately, the brand perception was not always positive due to the weak network coverage.

Frimer was surprised by the general feeling among employees that the "whole thing was seen as a license to print money." Frimer and his team were not only facing an industry problem after the tech bubble, but also management problems. There was a lot of duplication between both companies, price plans had to be adjusted, managers had to be selected. And time was running out—newspapers reported

that sunrise was expected to record losses equivalent to around 27 percent of sales.

In the process of raising its stake to 78.5 percent, TDC paid SFr 3.53 billion[3] in cash and promissory notes, and fully consolidated sunrise's and diAx' debt of SFr 1.2 billion. In the new set-up, diAx holding, a holding company for Swiss Reinsurance, Winterthur Insurance and the six utilities, reduced its holdings to 16.7 percent, and UBS (Union Bank of Switzerland) reduced its stake to 2.6 percent while the Swiss Federal Railways kept 2.2 percent of the new company respectively (refer to Exhibit 3 for the initial set-up of both consortia).[4]

Some insiders have described sunrise in 2000 as being a "paralyzed company." Based on the scale of the issues, Frimer brought with him 25 colleagues from Denmark. Within TDC, there was a strong feeling that Frimer's skills combined with those of a strong CFO would be the right solution for sunrise. Klaus Pedersen, TDC's vice president, Group Accounting & Tax was a natural choice for this position. This was the first time he would be working with Frimer.

HISTORY OF TDC (FORMERLY TELE DANMARK)

TDC A/S (TDC) was the former state monopoly for telephones in Denmark. It resulted from a merger in 1990 between four regional Danish telephone companies and the international operations. TDC was formed with the clear aim to strengthen the telecommunications industry. The merger of the various companies was seen as a response to a recommendation from the European Union (EU). In a 1989 report the regulators saw no reason for the telecommunications market to be protected by

Exhibit 3   **Original Ownership Structure in 1998**

Sunrise	Ownership	diAx	Ownership
Swiss Federal Railways	11.8%	SBC	40%
UBS Bank	9.8	diAx Holding (Swiss Reinsurance,	60
TDC	44.0	Winterthur Insurance, utilities)	
British Telecom	34.4		

state monopolies. The EU suggested that telecom companies should become part of the private competition.

The integration of the various networks and the IT platforms took several years. But the efforts paid off in 1994. TDC had its initial public offering (IPO) on the stock market and thereby government ownership went down to 51 percent. It was also one of the European pioneers to list on the New York Stock Exchange. Some saw this as a first indicator of internationalization.

Growing by Leaving Denmark

The IPO started a rapid internationalization process drive with regard to international activities and ownership. TDC began to invest in consortia outside Denmark —initially with small investments in the Ukraine and Poland. The Danish market was fully deregulated and as early as 1993, two mobile operators were chasing customers in a country with 5.4 million inhabitants. Denmark was widely considered as one of the most deregulated markets in

Exhibit 4   **Overview of TDC's International Operations**

Country	Company	Businesses	TDC's Ownership Stake in 2003 (year-end)	TDC's Ownership Stake Initially and Year of Entry
Austria	Connect Austria-One	Mobile	15%	15.00% 1997
Belgium	Belgacom	Full service telecom provider	15.9	16.50% 1996
Czech Republic	Ceske Radiokommunikace	Fixed telephony & Internet	0	20.79% 1997
	Contactel	Fixed telephony & Internet	100	16.67% 1999
Finland	TDC Hakemistot	Directories	100	100.00% 2002
Germany	Talkline	Mobile	100	100.00% 1997
Hungary	HTCC	Fixed telephony & Internet	31.9	19.00% 1997
Norway	TDC Norway	Fixed telephony & Internet	100	51.00% 1999
Lithuania	Bite	Mobile	100	17.00% 1995
Poland	Polkomtel	Mobile	19.6	19.25% 1995
	TDC Internet Polska	Internet	0	51.00% 2001
Sweden	TDC Internordia AB	Fixed telephony & Internet	100	50.00% 1995
Switzerland	TDC Switzerland	Full service telecom provider	100	44.00%* 1997
Ukraine	UMC	Mobile	0	16.33% 1993

*The acquisition in 1997 relates to sunrise Communications AG. In January 2001 this company was merged with diAx to form a new company named TDC Switzerland.

Source: TDC.

Exhibit 5   **TDC's Net Revenues and Earnings Before Interest, Taxes, Depreciation and Amortization (EBITDA)**

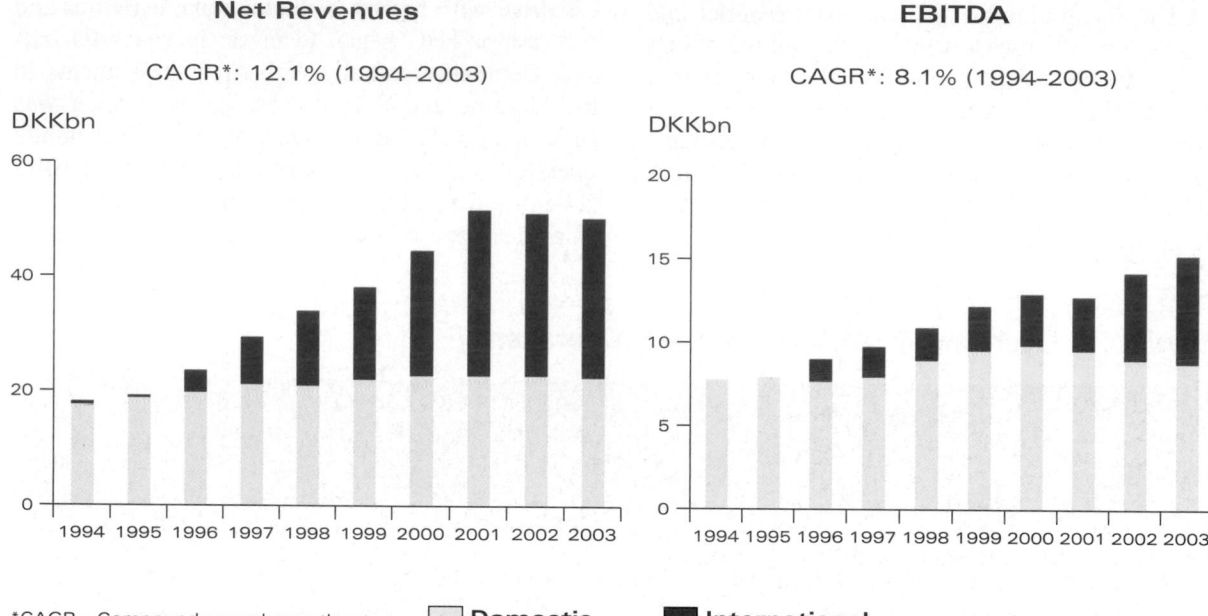

*CAGR = Compound annual growth rate   ☐ **Domestic**   ■ **International***

Source: TDC.

Europe with very low price levels. Over the years, TDC made more investments in Europe (refer to Exhibit 4 for an overview of international operations). But by 1998, the strategy changed. Torben V. Holm, TDC's senior VP corporate business development, clarified:

> Until 1998, the strategy was to go abroad, plant flags and get some experience. This was followed by swapping assets. After 1998, the question was how to get control. [We] realized that with consortia it was impossible to realize synergies between the companies due to the limited sharing potential.

In fact, between 1998 and 2003 TDC kept investments in a total of 13 companies, but direct control

increased from 1 to 8. By 1999, international sales accounted for 40% of total (up from 2% in 1995) and two years later they surpassed domestic sales for the first time (refer to Exhibit 5 for net revenues from internationalization).

While TDC's sales grew rapidly in the ten years up to 2003 (refer to Exhibit 6), its ownership also became more international. In 1997 34 percent of the Danish government's 51 percent stake in TDC was sold to Ameritech of the United States, and the remaining 17 percent was bought back in a share buy-back program. Ameritech, which later raised its stake in TDC to 42 percent, was later sold to SBC, a company that held a share in diAx.[5]

Exhibit 6   **10-Year Performance of TDC ($ in millions)**

	1993	1994	1995	1996	1997	1998	1999	2000	2001	2002	2003
Sales	$2,693	$3,256	$3,400	$4,407	$4,474	$5,336	$5,173	$5,556	$6,457	$7,546	$8,770
Sales growth		20.9%	4.4%	29.6%	1.5%	19.3%	(3.1%)	7.4%	16.2%	16.9%	16.2%
Net income	$230	$423	$630	$523	$226	$630	$476	$1,133	$(88)	$641	$305
Employees	N/A	16,678	16,476	16,763	17,268	16,410	17,464	18,363	19,130	22,263	22,429

Note: Exchange rates fluctuated over the same period.

Source: Hoover's Profile.

In a move to improve TDC's competitive position and focus more clearly on high potential growth areas, TDC restructured its operations in 2000. Three core divisions emerged (refer to Exhibit 7 for further details on the organization). Within the group, TDC Switzerland was the largest foreign operation, accounting for around 19 percent of TDC's revenues. Part of the reorganization was the introduction of the "TDC" name to replace the Tele Danmark brand.

Managing at TDC

TDC's CEO, Henning Dyremose, a former Danish finance minister, joined the company in 1998. He remembered the early days:

> Our international expansion put us in the position of being a portfolio manager. Management was not ready for this [new environment] of competition and privatization.

As a result of this, TDC developed its vision model (refer to Exhibit 8 for the vision model). But with it, Dyremose believed in rotating his top managers. He explained:

> Over the years, only three out of the 100 top managers maintained the same position—including the legal counsel and CFO. I select people based on their intellectual capacity, honesty, capability to create results, loyalty and operational skills.

Dyremose continued:

> With this [selection] criteria, I'm out for trouble. This system attracts very skilled, but at the same time also

somewhat difficult managers. In the case of Frimer, he is someone who delivers on time, is always well-prepared, sharp and precise, and employees are proud to work for him. He motivates them to go the extra mile.

TDC had a very small executive committee (three members) plus a senior management team which consisted of the six CEOs from the largest subsidiaries. They met monthly to exchange knowledge and business ideas.

The financial reporting system was clear. Karsten Hetland, executive vice president HR, clarified, "We lead by targets—both financial and operational. If we put more structure on there, this would not work." Managers in the various companies realized the importance of the financial controls and there was strong emphasis to adhere to these processes. Dyremose and his CFO, Hans Munk Nielsen, held monthly review updates with the CEOs and CFOs of the various subsidiaries. Nielsen, the CFO, explained his role:

> My role is to make sure that the figures are correct and evaluate forward-looking statements. In the case of sunrise, the critics said that TDC overpaid, the company was performing poorly and telecom was not necessarily a portable business. They were questioning TDC's business model. But time has shown that the sunrise business case was correct.

With rapid internationalization, leadership became a top priority. As part of the new vision, TDC reorganized its HR functions by combining various functions (compensation, performance, leadership development, succession management) into one

Exhibit 7   **TDC's Structure, 2003 sales in millions of $**

Division	Services Offered	Sales (% of total)	Customers (millions)	Employees
TDC Solutions	Full range of communications services for customers in Denmark and neighboring Nordic countries	$3,245 (37%)	4.4	11,675
TDC Mobile International	All mobile operations including the domestic operation	2,719 (31%)	6.1 (pro rata)	
TDC Switzerland	Fixed line, mobile, Internet services in Switzerland	1,666 (19%)	2.6	2,380
TDC Cable TV	TV network and broadband Internet access	263 (3%)	0.9	733
TDC Directories		248 (3%)		1,091
Other	TDC Service (billing and internal IT services)	629 (7%)		2,093
Total		$8,770(100%)		22,429

Source: TDC.

Exhibit 8   **TDC Vision Model and TDC Values**

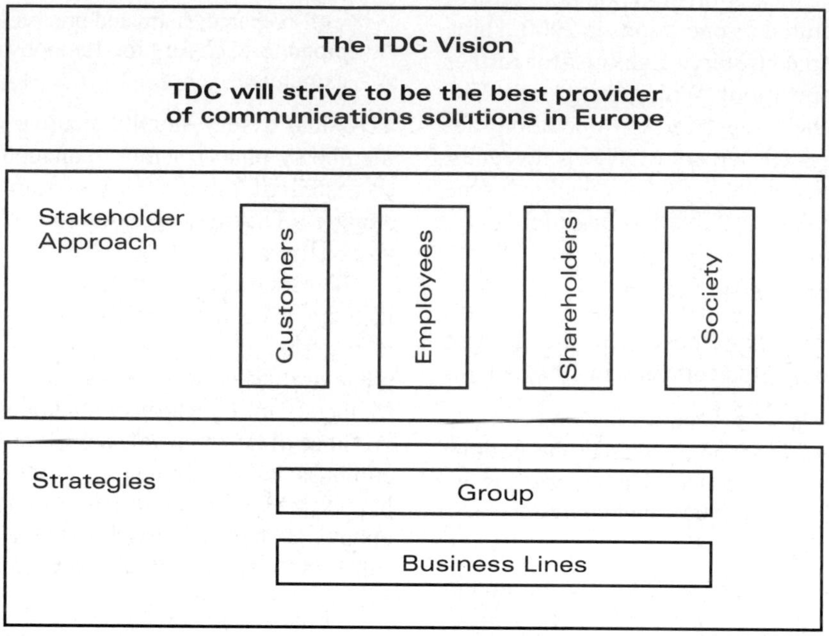

The TDC Vision

**TDC will strive to be the best provider
of communications solutions in Europe**

Stakeholder
Approach

Customers | Employees | Shareholders | Society

Strategies

Group

Business Lines

The TDC Values

We center our actions around the **customers**
We **demand the most of ourselves**
We are **trustworthy** in every context
We value **teamwork**
We **respect** the individual

We center our actions around the customers:

▸ We strive to understand our customers' requirements—and to meet these in the best possible way
▸ We encourage initiative and entrepreneurship
▸ We treat every customer as if they are our only customer

We demand the utmost of ourselves:

▸ We focus on execution and act with a sense of urgency
▸ We respect decisions taken
▸ We treat everyone like we wish to be treated
▸ We eliminate activities that are not creating value
▸ We live the values

We are trustworthy in every context:

▸ We are reliable
▸ We are good citizens

We value teamwork:

▸ We create good teams through cooperation
▸ We share knowledge across teams
▸ We secure orderly and fair decision making processes

We respect the individual:

▸ We evaluate on the basis of results
▸ We are fair to each other
▸ We seek a balance between work and private life
▸ We respect diversities and provide all with equal opportunity

Source: TDC.

department. In total, the department catered to the needs of over 100 expats.

The impact of the vision on daily jobs was measured by the climate survey. This survey consisted of 52 parameters, which measured how the focus areas of the vision model and the values were incorporated in the daily life of employees. Hetland explained, "This serves as a discussion and action tool and is the key tool for changing the company culture."

BACK TO SWITZERLAND—EARLY 2004: "SUNRISE REACHED OPERATING TEMPERATURE"[6]

Deregulation in Switzerland saw prices tumbling beyond expectations. According to Bakom, the local authorities, prices for domestic long-distance calls on fixed lines dropped by up to 83 percent between 1998 and 2003 while international calls dropped by up to 77 percent over the same period.[7] The price decreases for mobile phones were less drastic, on average between 5 percent and 19 percent over the same period. Overall, the price index for telephony fell from a base of 100 in 1998 to 68.8 in 2003.

Complete Recovery Shows in the Results

While the company increased its revenues by 9.8 percent to SFr 1.937 billion in 2003, it increased its EBITDA[8] by 79.9 percent to SFr 451 million and net income reached SFr 171 million. Interestingly, sunrise was able to return to profitability one year earlier than expected (refer to Exhibits 9 and 10 for full financial details). Sunrise's profitability was impressive on different accounts. Net income came in at 8.8 percent of sales, even beating Swisscom (7.88 percent), France Telecom (6.94 percent), and Deutsche Telekom (2.33 percent).

More important, Swisscom's growth, still around 27 percent in 2000, almost came to a halt between 2001 and 2003 (refer to Exhibit 11 for further details). Orange, after a strong launch, had lost its 2nd

Exhibit 9   **Financial Overview of Sunrise, 2001–2003**

	2001	Change (in %)	2002	Change (in %)	2003	Change (in %)
Net sales (SFr million)	1,652		1,764	6.8%	1,937	9.8%
Mobile Communication	818		904	10.4	1,042	15.3
Fixed Line Communication	718		744	3.6	765	2.9
Internet & ADSL	117		117	0.5	130	11.4
Cost of Sales (SFr million)	(1,675)		(1,534)	(8.4)	(1,486)	(1.8)
Transmission Cost and Raw Materials (includes subsidized mobile phones)	(807)		(741)	(8.2)	(789)	6.5
Other External Expenses	(626)		(542)	(13.4)	(449)	(17.1)
Salaries, wages and pension payments	(242)		(251)	3.7	(248)	(1.2)
EBITDA	(23)		251	na	451	79.9
Net Income (SFr million)	na*		(93)		171	
Customer structure						
Mobile Communications	944,000	62%	1,100,000	20	1,260,000	11.1
Fixed Line Communications	786,000	15	852,000	8.4	824,000	(3.3)
Internet & ADSL	499,000	25	518,000	3.8	526,000	1.5
Employees	2,465		2,200	(12)	2,500	12

*Note: *Neue Zürcher Zeitung* (NZZ) estimated losses of SFr 400–450 million for 2001. See NZZ, "sunrise mit Verlust," June 7, 2002.
Source: sunrise, IMD Research.

Exhibit 10   **TDC Switzerland's Financial Performance (EBITDA)**

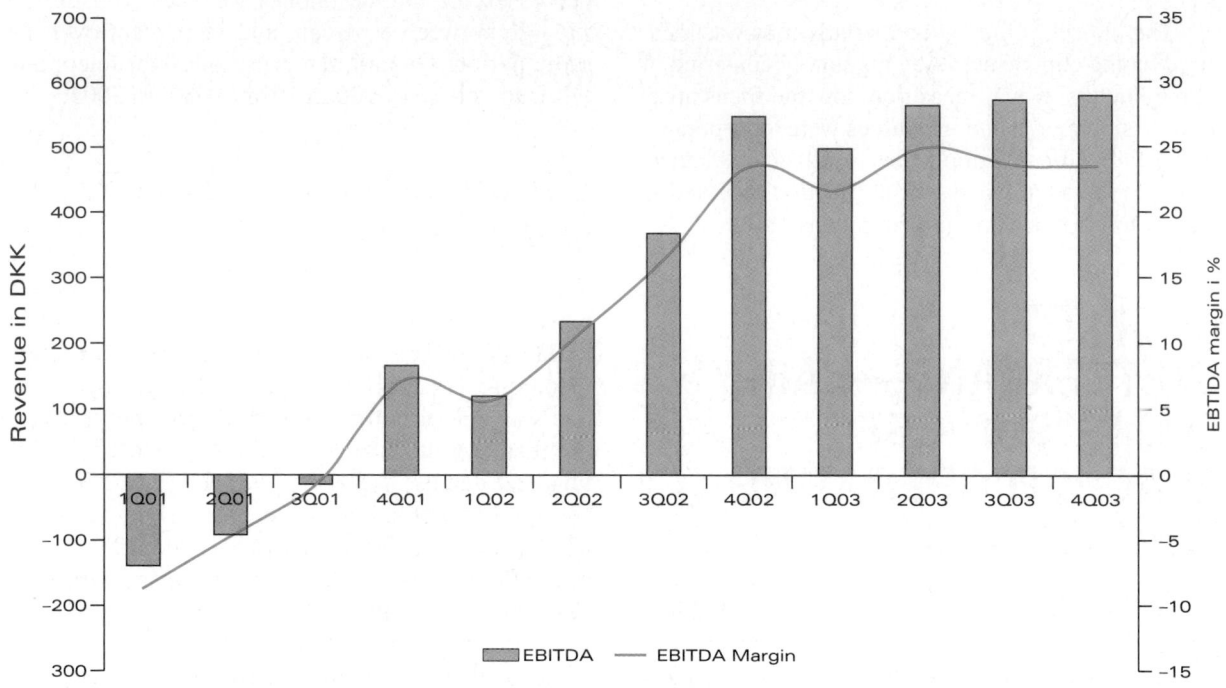

Source: TDC.

place position for mobile phones to sunrise, after Frimer and his team decided to drop the diAx brand altogether.

What did sunrise do to have such a successful turnaround?

STARTING THE TURNAROUND AT SUNRISE

Given the situation at sunrise when Frimer arrived in December 2000, he decided to call a management board[9] meeting without delay. For the board members, it sounded like a peculiar setup: The meeting was to be held in a chalet in the Swiss mountains over the weekend, and when they requested an agenda they were simply told "there is no agenda." At first they were reluctant since "there could not be a board meeting without an agenda." However, the meeting took place and Frimer began by raising two issues he wanted to discuss over the weekend: "Firstly, how to increase revenue and secondly how to reduce cost?" After the two days in the mountains, the management

board had a clear understanding of the turnaround strategy. Moreover, it set the basis for creating a "we" feeling among the top team.

The management team soon discovered that the merged company was "definitely not a license to print money" and personnel costs had to be cut. One round of layoffs was necessary and 240 employees (10 percent of the workforce) were asked to leave. However, the top management team made it clear that this was the last round of layoffs and that things would subsequently pick up.

From the beginning, Frimer and his team were worried that the wrong people were leaving. The newspapers reported an employee fluctuation rate of 32 percent.[10] Fast decisions had to be made. Frimer explained:

> I have seen it in the past, I don't care how we are organized, just get things done. I find people and then I design a structure around them. After one week, the management team was in place. This was an emergency and we did not have time to look for six months for an outsider to fill a position. We could take care of the wrong selections later on. When hiring people I look for commercial sense, people skills and operational focus. I have seen a lot of intelligent people with no people skills. It does not work.

Exhibit 11   **Competitive Data (General Data & Swiss Market)**

General Data (2003)				
	France Telecom	**Deutsche Telekom**	**Swisscom**	**sunrise**
Revenue	€46.1 billion	€55.8 billion	SFr 14.6 billion	SFr 1.937 billion
Net income	€ 3.2 billion	€ 1.3 billion	SFr 1.15 billion	SFr 0.171 billion
Net income as a % of revenue	6.94%	2.33%	7.88%	8.83%

Note: see also Appendix I.
Source: Annual reports, investor presentations.

Swiss Market: Revenues of Swisscom (SFr million)					
	1999	**2000**	**2001**	**2002**	**2003**
Net revenue	11,052	14,060	14,174	14,526	14,581
EBITDA	4,192	4,034	4,409	4,413	4,641
Net income	2,391	3,156	4,964	824	1,569
Number of mobile customers (in millions)	2.282	3.168	3.373	3.605	3.792

Note: 2001 net income includes a gain of SFr 3.8 billion from selling 25% of Swisscom's mobile division to Vodafone.

Swiss Market: Revenues of Orange (SFr million)					
	1999	**2000**	**2001**	**2002**	**2003**
Net revenue			886	1,018	1,169 (14.8%)
EBITDA		(523.7)	10.5	81	296
Number of mobile customers	313,000	786,000	925,000	962,733	1,085,000 (+12.7%)

Source: Press clippings.

In order to deal with the uncertainty among employees, HR decisions were communicated on a daily basis to all personnel via e-mail at 17:00. Communication between management and employees continued during the turnaround, and employees were closely involved both in the turnaround and the return to profitability. Early on, there was a decision that there "would be no consultants." The employees alone would be accountable for their actions. The new organizational structure was developed within just two weeks—in fact, fast decision making became a symbol of the turnaround—and it catered to the needs of Frimer's team (refer to Exhibit 12 for sunrise's structure). Legally the merger was completed on January 23, two months after the announcement.

There were some new faces on the board (refer to Exhibit 13 for the background of board members). Frimer was known for his open-door policy. He explained, "I hate [office] politics and I want to keep political infighting to a minimum by keeping discussions on a level of what helps customers." This customer orientation made the board members realize the shortcomings of their existing structure. The product groups had to join forces to serve business customers, since they often required several services at once. As a result, a key account management system was set up for business customers. These key accounters would handle all contact with sunrise. In addition, a business marketing board was set up to coordinate the various functions and this was later followed by a customer marketing board, too.

The targets for each division were ambitious. With the arrival of the Danish delegation at sunrise, it soon became clear that targets had to be met, "apologies were not accepted anymore." Board members also felt this desire to succeed. Klaus Pedersen, CFO, explained

Exhibit 12   **Organizational Chart—TDC Switzerland, May 2004**

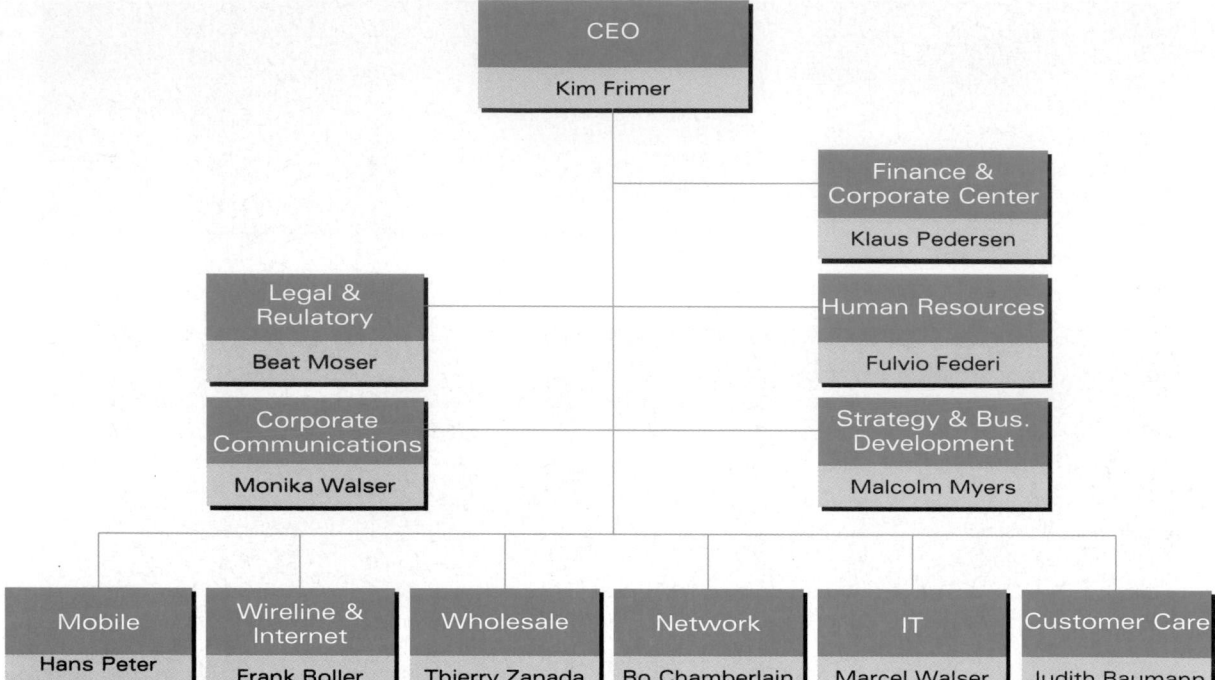

Source: Company information.

Mergers are difficult, but you can get people excited. The management board was extremely motivated, as everyone really felt part of sunrise. Failure was not an option for us.

sunrise: The Most Human Telecom Provider?

In line with "picking the low hanging fruit first," the management streamlined operations with the elimination of double functions, sunrise merged back-office functions including networks, call centers, IT, billing operations, corporate functions (HR, legal, strategy, communications), reduced office locations and fewer externals/contractors. This led to considerable cost savings, e.g., IT functions were reduced by SFr 12.5 million. Marketing budgets were cut by 25 percent. Expensive sponsoring engagements, such as the Swiss National Exhibition (Expo 2002), were stopped. Following the board meeting in the chalet, long lists were made up showing where costs could be cut. Growing the revenue was possible, too, since there was little overlap in the customer base. Only 15 percent of diAx's customers were also customers of sunrise and hence the potential was considerable.

Within two months, the management had decided on the new strategy. Sunrise was going to be the "most human telecom provider," easy, friendly, smart solutions for reasonable prices. This was quite different from the competition, which normally differentiated themselves based on hard facts such as network power and tradition (refer to Exhibit 14 for the product positioning). Some of the first advertising campaigns read: "we are here to stay," "you can hear the smile," "easy & understandable," "quality and reliability," "value for money." Although there were several entrants in the Swiss market for telecommunications, sunrise was the only alternative operator in Switzerland to offer mobile, fixed and Internet services.

The new positioning translated into the three pillars of strategy: excellent marketing and sales, cost consciousness, and customer loyalty (refer to Exhibit 15 for the strategy overview). The merged company was to fade out the diAx brand name.

Making Sure Employees Understand the Strategy

Sunrise's management put great effort into ensuring that employees understood the strategy: "We strive

Exhibit 13   **Background of Board Members**

Name	Age	Position	In This Position Since	Previous Professional Experience
Judith Baumann	39	Customer Care	2000	• Vice Director in the IT Customer Support/Private Banking division of UBS bank
Hans Peter Baumgartner	45	Mobile	2004	• Various management positions at Sony (1989–2004)
Frank Boller	46	Wireline & Internet	2003	• CEO of diAx
Bo Chamberlain	39	Network	2001	• Managing Director Technology and Network Operations at Talkline GmbH, Hamburg • Various positions within TDC incl. Manager at Switching Technology; Project Leader Central and Eastern Europe
Fulvio Federi	55	Human Resources	2004	• Various management positions in customer services/sales, HR Development
Klaus Pedersen	36	Finance	2000	• Vice President Group Accounting & Tax, TDC
Beat Moser	34	Legal & Regulatory	2000	• Attorney-at-law
Malcolm Myers	38	Strategy & Business Development	1999	• Product Manager at sunrise (1997–1999) • Senior Associate at Booz Allen & Hamilton • Marketing Manager Belgacom Mobile
Marcel Walser	44	IT	2000	• CIO Novartis Nutrition • Various senior IT positions at UBS bank
Monika Walser	38	Corporate Communications	2000	• Head of Marketing Communications at Computer 2000, a computer distributor (1998–2000) • Managing Director of a company producing traditional clothing for children (1994–1998)
Thierry Zanada	38	Wholesale	2000	• Manager at Interconnect

Source. Company information.

to be Switzerland's No. 1 or No. 2 communications provider for residential, business and wholesale customers in the product areas we are in." In practical terms, this was much easier. For mobile phones, the slogan was:

> We will beat Orange [main competitor] in mobiles.

By June 2001, the product offerings and price plans were harmonized, sunrise's new slogan was launched the same day—"Communication is life." In some cases, the slogan was used with the addition "sunrise: always a smile."

In order for the employees to get a better understanding of the strategy, Frimer and his team also set up special events. During 2001, the goal was to get a better utilization of its mobile network (after all, it was a high fixed-cost business). Frimer explained that this could be achieved with better marketing, but to some extent marketing is just "hot air." So, since the achievement of any strategic goal was generally

Exhibit 14 **Product Positioning**

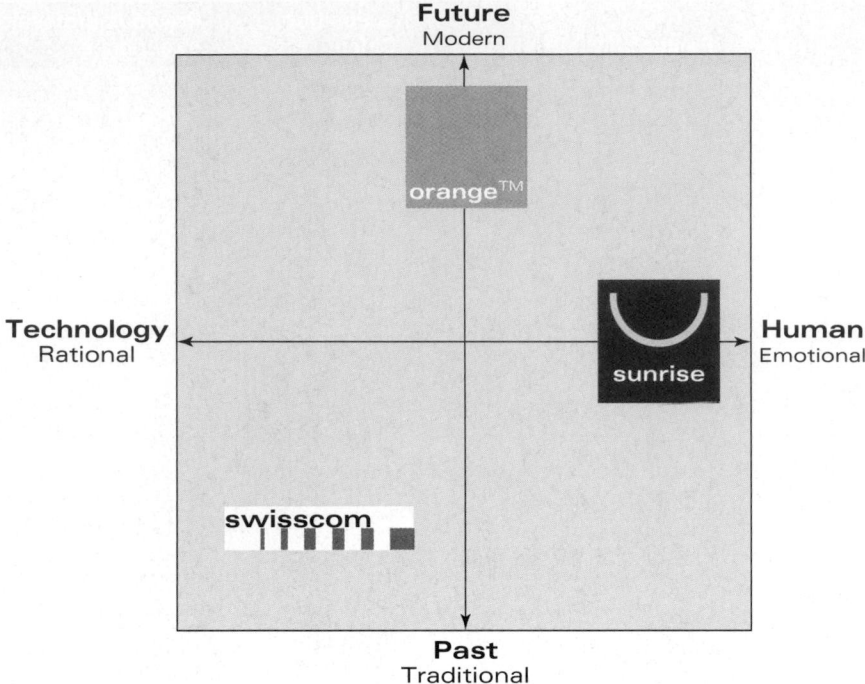

Exhibit 15 **Strategy Overview**

Excellent marketing & sales

- focus on being the most innovative in the market
- make sunrise the most appealing choice for each of our target customer segments

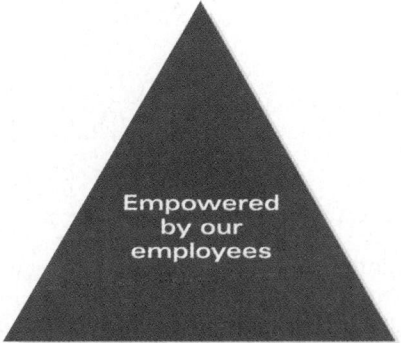

Cost consciousness

- take out cost by being smarter and more creative about how we do our work
- think "must have" rather than "nice to have" when spending the company's money

Customer loyalty

- put ourselves in our customers' shoes
- make sunrise number 1 in satisfaction

Source: Company information.

Exhibit 16 **sunrise's Year 2001 in Review (number of customers)**

	Q1 2001	Q2 2001	Q3 2001	Q4 2001
Postpaid mobile (in 000s)	376	391	407	421
Prepaid mobile (in 000s)	292	354	426	523
Fixed line (in 000s)	714	740	751	786
Internet (in 000s)	445	447	471	499

Source: sunrise Presentation to Investors, 2003, p. 10.

celebrated in style, they decided to install a hot-air balloon in the staircase of sunrise's HQ. Depending on the level of new acquisitions for mobile phone customers per week, they would lower or raise the balloon (refer to Exhibit 8 for the actual developments). sunrise was able to stop the high churn for mobiles, extend the contract length to a minimum of 12 months and grow by 62 percent in a market that was only growing at 14 percent (the slowest since 1993). Thanks to a boom in mobile phones, sunrise was adding customers fast. It was especially successful in pushing "prepaid" customers, i.e., mobile phones without a contract. These phones relied on "prepaid" cards, which were available in many different stores, and were particularly popular among teenagers. (refer to Exhibit 16).

By the end of 2001, sunrise had beaten Orange in numbers of subscribers—a cause for great celebration at the sunrise HQ! This was a celebration people would not forget in a long time and at a cost in excess of SFr 1 million for one day. But top management thought that this money was well invested. They gave short presentations on sunrise's strategy, the plan forward and organized games for employees to interact with each other.

Products, Products, Products

Over the years, sunrise remained innovative by adding new products or changing the rules of the game. For mobile phones, sunrise decided to sell packages of minutes (e.g., 75 minutes per month) at a fixed price, rather than mobile phone minutes. Other popular innovations included myzone, which was a mobile phone that would link to the local network at home. This implied that people could use their mobile phone (and pay local charges) while calling from their home zone. In 2002 sunrise was also the first in Switzerland to launch a multimedia service for mobile phones. This enabled customers to send pictures via their mobile phones.

For fixed-line customers, sunrise offered 60 minutes free of charge, but customers then had to sign up for 12 months. Also, sunrise was the first company to offer a flat rate for domestic telephone calls. This service was expected to start in mid-2004.

Streamlining Operations

Over the years, there was tremendous pressure to reduce cost. As sunrise was a smaller operator in comparison to some of the large players such as France Telecom (the owner of Orange), it could not reap similar economies of scale. Instead, it decided to start a new international alliance with smaller operators from Spain, Austria, Hungary, Norway and Italy. The goal was to reduce sourcing prices, with a combined purchasing volume of close to 40 million units.

While sunrise was reducing costs on the one hand, at the same time it was opening its own stores across Switzerland. The so-called sunrise centers were dedicated exclusively to selling sunrise products— a total of 20 shops were opened in 2003 with another 18 scheduled for 2004.

MANAGING INSIDE SUNRISE

Sunrise kept its promise of no further lay-offs. Since employees were actively engaged in the 2001 restructuring processes, they started to identify closely with sunrise. A member of the call center for business customers explained:

> Our internal processes and systems are designed to have maximum efficiency. For example, all customer contacts, such as e-mails, calls, voice messages and even letters are all available electronically, that makes it possible to deliver good value to customers.

As employees had a lot of contact with end customers, they needed not only technical skills, but also social competencies. For this, sunrise offered a considerable number of courses, including IT, sales, product infos, personality development, leadership and social competence, and project management. Overall, the company offered over 200 courses in 2002.

In fact, employees were even encouraged to air their opinions and regularly received an online employee survey aimed at measuring feelings among employees. Frimer explained:

> The frustration was huge initially, but now it has improved a lot. I use this survey widely and when it is very negative, you normally have a management problem.

"Communication Is Life" for Employees: Keeping in Touch with the Top

Sunrise's 2,500 employees had access to various methods of communication with top management. The most frequent, the "CEO News" e-mail, was sent out every four to five weeks. It was written by Frimer himself and outlined recent developments and major achievements by employees.

Employees were also able to have personal encounters with Frimer. Every six weeks his team organized a "power breakfast." Anyone could apply to attend these breakfast meetings which all followed the same format. The invited employees represented a wide pool of experiences and were first asked to introduce themselves before Frimer asked his question, "If you were CEO of sunrise for a week—what would you do?" This served as a platform for making improvements and it was not uncommon for employees to receive a personal letter from Frimer after highlighting important issues.

Since the number of places for the power breakfasts was limited, the top management team would actually visit the various locations, too. All the employees were invited to the "EMT [executive management team] on tour" event, which took place twice a year at each location. Normally, anywhere between 20 and 300 employees at each location attended the EMT on tour. There, the CEO would explain sunrise's overall strategy before two other board members clarified recent developments in their field. The board members accompanying Frimer rotated so that employees could get to know different board members. These meetings were set up in such a way that employees had enough time to ask questions. One board member commented: "A lot of good ideas come from down in the organization."

MANAGEMENT AT THE TOP: "I TRY TO DELEGATE"

Frimer was clear that "if you delegate, you have to make sure you control." Although sunrise transformed itself from a start-up to a "real" company, the delegation was key. In his approach, Frimer gave a lot of autonomy and trust, but he made it clear that his employees understood the rules: not to betray him. A member of the sunrise management board explained:

> This approach gives employees a real job: you feel you have a real job, your experience/knowledge is welcomed and you are a valued team member. This approach could only work with a level of discipline. There were very clear guidelines of what was needed/expected from the managers for "getting things done."

For board members, setting goals was a real dialogue, not a command. But once they committed, it was their job to achieve the goals! And goals become very visible. Frimer explained his style:

> There are so many systems, structures, PowerPoint presentations, and people forget what the value drivers are. My approach is to ask questions and then we will develop the conclusions together, rather than me saying you should do this . . . But sometimes you still have to say, this is not good enough.

Employees around Frimer said that they could feel the trust he placed in them. Another board member remarked: "As long as you deliver, you will not hear from him. If you are not delivering, you are told by him. If you are not delivering, it is not that much fun."

DECISION MAKING AND INFO GATHERING ON THE MANAGEMENT BOARD

Weekly Management Board Meeting on Monday   This was the major decision-making body within sunrise. Initially, the board members managing product lines also had their own commercial meeting, but this was soon stopped since there was too much overlap between the two. The meetings on Monday were seen as "holy" and board members were expected to be present. If they were unable to attend, there was a clear understanding that they had to respect the decisions taken by their colleagues.

1-on-1   These bi-weekly meetings were forums for exchange between Frimer and individual members of the board. There was no pre-arranged agenda except that the meeting would last for up to one hour. Board members would decide the issues to be discussed. Typical issues included brainstorming, operational issues or "things you do not need to discuss in a big group," e.g., at the Monday board meetings. One board member commented: "I have to tell him what I need, how it is running and where I expect help from him." If neither the board member nor the CEO had anything to discuss, then the meeting could be canceled.

Information Gathering in the Company

Business Unit Strategy Review Meetings ("Drill Down Meetings")   This was the informal meeting between Frimer and key managers (not only board members) of the various divisions. Although informal, the impact should not be underestimated as it was here that strategy discussions took place. Depending on the size of the division, these meetings would take place between once—for small units—and up to three times per year for large units. The meetings would start at 12 o'clock and be open ended. In the course of the afternoon, the responsible board members and their top managers would explain "what they were doing, what challenges and issues they were facing."

Project Board   When the new management team arrived in Switzerland they soon discovered that there was a lot of cash outflow leading to real "cash burn." Equipment was being purchased without any prior internal discussion. Now, every purchase valued at more than SFr 400,000 had to be discussed at this forum. Employees had to present their planned purchases together with a net present value (NPV) analysis. Although this board initially met with a lot of resistance, it soon became a forum for "selling ideas." The project board was jointly headed by the CEO and the following board members:

- Strategy & business development: Malcolm Myers
- Information technology (IT): Marcel Walser
- CFO: Klaus Pedersen
- COO Mobile: Geert Rieder (later replaced by Hans Peter Baumgartner)
- COO Wireline and Internet: Martin Staub (later replaced by Frank Boller)
- COO Wholesale: Thierry Zanada

Relations between CEO and Top Management

The IT system was quite detailed including a lot of data regarding performance measurement. Senior managers could have access to the performance data of sunrise from their PC at all times. This transparency also helped to highlight performance issues. In serious cases of non-performance, Frimer would, as a last resort, send in a task force. Once a problem was identified, board members were expected to fix it. If this did not happen, they would receive a warning. If the problem was not solved within the next three to four months, then Frimer would send in a task force. This team would then directly report to the CEO until the problem was fixed.

FRIMER'S DELEGATION: COMBINING THE OPPOSITES

Sunrise employees remembered well one of the first meetings with Frimer when he described the merger process. He explained that there were only two ways of pulling off a Band-Aid—slowly or fast. Frimer was very clear: "In any case it hurts, so let's pull it off fast."

For employees it soon became clear what it meant working for sunrise. Frimer's first bill to his private home read: "Frau Kim Frimer" [Mrs. Kim Frimer]. It was soon understood that there should be "no mistakes when dealing with customers." However, in other parts of the business, the management team was not averse to risk. If employees could provide the board with some hard data proving the potential of their initiatives (e.g., product launches), such as market research or surveys, then the board was willing to take the risk.

People within sunrise were constantly being challenged to take the customers' point of view, however, they were also strongly reminded of the profitability expectations from "up north"—a widely used term for referring to TDC's HQ. The reference to "up north" was a good indication that the EBITDA or net present values were too low.

Overall, employees enjoyed the trust and freedom they received from the board of management. A staff member working closely with Frimer explained his approach:

> You agree with him on what has to be done and then he leaves you all the freedom in the world. How you get it done is your responsibility.

However, a board member added:

> No one should misunderstand this freedom. Frimer did not like it if you did not think things through.

Sunrise was proud of its flexible and tolerant work environment. At the same time, it was clear to the managers that they "had to deliver" on whatever they agreed upon. While Frimer was perceived as a fun guy, everyone around him "definitely knew who the boss was." Going to his office with bad results was no fun.

While managers at various levels enjoyed the freedom, the possible threat of task forces put pressure on them to perform. After it became clear in various drill down meetings that there were operational problems in one division, this particular board member was asked to resign. In general, members of the management board were concerned not only about being overworked, but also about the general pressure to perform. Frimer commented: "Keep the pressure up and never be satisfied with the current situation!"

Also, Frimer was not afraid of taking positions. As internal communication became difficult in some instances when employees would communicate in German, although not all 56 Danes were able to read German, it was time for a message from the CEO: Starting immediately, the new official language was English, and only English.

Within sunrise, the structure remained mostly unchanged with only a few adjustments including the consumer and business marketing boards. The internal meeting structure did not change over time. However, a board member explained: "Frimer likes to disturb the balance."

While Frimer agreed with the statement about disturbing the balance, he also wondered how to maintain the balance. He was generally against organizational changes, which he believed should only be carried out if they were definitely adding value. Referring to the band aid example, it was clear that in the 2001 crisis situation, the band aid had to be removed quickly. Would Frimer take the same approach in 2003?

While sunrise reported a successful year for 2003, the pressure was going to continue. Dyremose explained:

> In Europe, our operations continue to thrive and contribute increasingly to our positive financial performance. TDC Switzerland has achieved a solid position as the second-largest telecom provider in the Swiss market. Its continued progress is illustrated by an increasing EBITDA margin and a positive net income development. We are very pleased to have been able to exploit the good growth opportunities outside Denmark.

But for Frimer, the question was how to maintain momentum. He believed in improving daily and for employees, this meant constantly moving forward.

Appendix: The Telecom Industry

HISTORIC OVERVIEW

In 1876 Graham Bell, a Scotsman in Boston, Massachusetts, succeeded in making the first "telephone" operational and started the Bell Telephone Company the following year. Bell's invention allowed sounds to be transmitted electrically via the telephone. "Tele"—the Greek word for afar—and "phone"—meaning voice or sound—soon started to replace the Morse code. For the first time, it was possible to send multiple messages over the same wireline, thereby reducing cost per call. By 1915, American telephone companies offered transcontinental service and by 1927, it was possible to make intercontinental calls to London.

Over the years, various innovations around the telephone became part of everybody's life. Direct dialing (without a switchboard operator) was followed by Touchtone in the 1960s. The 1980s saw the arrival of caller ID, the move from analogue to digital and the arrival of fiber optics. Demand from private households and corporations continued to increase, with corporations investing heavily in data networks linking various locations around the world. However, two massive shifts in the telephone industry changed the fundamentals of the industry starting in the early to mid-1990s:

1. *Privatization and deregulation*: Governments around the globe sold off their telephone companies. At the same time, they deregulated markets thereby prompting many companies and entrepreneurs to enter this "gold rush." Massive price reductions followed, especially on international calls, which often subsidized local calls. Within only a few years, the former state monopolies had to adapt to customer-driven markets.

2. *Arrival of mobile telephony*: Starting in the early 1990s, it was the arrival of mobile phone technology that truly revolutionized the industry. Annual sales of mobile handsets had reached 100 million units by 1997, before quadrupling to 400 million units in the following three years. Operators were required to invest heavily in infrastructure for mobile communications, but the price levels remained relatively high.

These shifts had far-reaching consequences: For decades this industry was seen as a commodity, utility type business with stable earnings and revenues. However, suddenly it was seen as a growth industry. Mobile telephony gave the industry a high-tech image, mobile penetration was skyrocketing and during the late 1990s, the growth phantasm of mobile operators could only be topped by Internet companies. This actual growth was for real—household expenditures on telecom have grown by more than 50 percent and revenues doubled.

However, this required massive investments in new infrastructure for mobile phones and other applications. A massive overestimation of the future demand led to overspending in capital-intensive infrastructure.

THE BUSINESS MODEL

Customers were mostly segmented across three groups: consumer, business accounts and multinational/global accounts. While consumer segments tended to be price sensitive, the corporate accounts were more interested in quality of the network, reliability, competence, innovation, partnership, one-stop-shopping and trustworthiness.

In terms of product offering, it remained difficult for telephone operators to differentiate the product offering due to "commoditization." The migration from fixed lines to mobile telephony was for real in developed countries, with revenues dropping due to the migration and decreasing price levels. Given these pressures, operators invested heavily in branding (e.g, Vodafone or T-Mobile), finer segmentation and scale.

EUROPEAN TELECOMS: FROM BOOM TO BUST

For many companies, the M& A boom was seen as a way to "create scale" and deregulation greatly facilitated such moves. In addition, European telecom companies were caught paying fictitious sums for acquiring future operating licenses for mobiles frequencies (UMTS) in 2000. They were estimated to have paid €109 billion for the next generation of mobile phone licenses.[11] Deutsche Telekom, invested €8.2 billion for acquiring such a UMTS license in its German home market—the equivalent of almost seven annual net incomes. In many cases, telecom operators overstretched their balance sheets and stock prices collapsed accordingly. Between March 2000 and September 2002, the share prices of former monopolies such as France Telecom, Deutsche Telekom and British Telecom collapsed from €156 to €6, from €84 to €8.7 and from €13.7 to €2.6, respectively. Given these adverse conditions, the strategies for telephone operators post-2001 were clear—tighten belts by reducing debt and cost, clean balance sheets (including writing off bad investments) and removing management of non-performing units and becoming more customer-oriented. Many companies maintained heavy debt levels even in 2003 (refer to Exhibit 17 for a financial overview of European telecom operators).

After the bubble in the telecom industry, many industry executives identified mobile telephony, broadband Internet connections (ADSL) and business customers as growth markets. But the profitability dynamics in the various segments was very different:

- For mobile phones it was critical to keep a good balance of network coverage and utilization without spending too much on customer acquisition. In the European market, customers were used to receiving highly subsidized mobile phones in return for 12-month contracts. In some European markets, the subsidies would reach €250 per mobile phone.

- The profitability of high-speed Internet connections was based on the transfer pricing for the so-called "last mile." The term referred to the actual access to customers, which was in many countries still controlled by the incumbent.

Exhibit 17   **Key Financial Indicators for Former State Monopolies**

Company	Country	2003 Revenue (€ billion)	2003 Total Liabilities (€ billion)	Market Capitalization in Mid-2004 (€ billion)	Free Float (percentage of shares listed on the market)
Belgacom	Belgium	€ 5.377	€ 2.368	€ 8.6	€ 42.3%
BT Group	UK	27.696	35.112	24.0	100.0
Deutsche Telekom	Germany	55.838	82.268	59.5	57.2
France Telecom	France	46.121	73.914	50.2	45.5
KPN	Netherlands	11.870	14.917	14.7	80.7
Portugal Telecom	Portugal	5.217	8.564	11.0	90.3
TDC	Denmark	6.750	8.122	5.2	83.4
Telecom Italia	Italy	30.850	59.649	36.9	83.0
Telefonica	Spain	25.704	31.576	58.7	89.8

Note: BT publishes its numbers for year end March 31.
Source: Rossana Bird and Mike Jeremy, "TDC—To Be or Not to Be," ING Financial Markets Report, June 17, 2004: 6; Thomson Analytics.

- Business customers represented large markets, but "lack of reputation/credibility/experience of newcomers" was often the main reason for keeping the business with the incumbents.

- An executive summed up the key success factors in the industry: "What do customers want, how easily can they be contacted and what are they willing to pay for?"

Endnotes

[1]"Thinking at the Speed of Light," sunrise Publication 2003: 37.

[2]In telecommunications the earnings before interest, taxes, depreciation and amortization (EBITDA) is one of the key financial drivers. Mobile telephony generally records the highest EBITDA contributions. In 2002 Swisscom reported EBITDA margins of 48.1 percent for mobile and 29.9 percent for fixed line [*Neue Zürcher Zeitung* (NZZ), November 21, 2003].

[3]Exchange rate: SFr 1 = US$0.83 on November 2, 2004.

[4]In 2003 TDC eventually took over the minority shareowners of sunrise.

[5]TDC bought back the SBC shares in 2004, thereby gaining full control.

[6]*Neue ZürcherZeitung (NZZ)*, March 2, 2004.

[7]Price declines were not a concern as long as usage was increasing faster.

[8]EBITDA = earings before interest, taxes, depreciation and amortization (see also Footnote 2).

[9]Companies in Switzerland operated on a two-tier board system: the management board took care of the operational issues; the supervisory board supervised the management board. In this case, we focus on the management board.

[10]*Neue Zürcher Zeitung (NZZ)*, December 16, 2000.

[11]See "Beyond the Bubble," supplement to *The Economist*, October 11, 2003: 109.

Merck and the Recall of Vioxx

Arthur A. Thompson
The University of Alabama

On September 30, 2004, officials at Merck & Company Inc., the sixth-largest pharmaceutical firm in the United States and a respected blue-chip company, announced that Merck was withdrawing its pain reliever Vioxx from the market because a new study indicated that the drug doubled the risks of heart attacks and strokes in patients taking it longer than 18 months. Merck's stock immediately plunged 27 percent and continued to fall further in upcoming weeks, in response to the $2.5 billion annual revenue loss from Merck's second best-selling drug and a rapidly mounting potential for costly lawsuits. An estimated 20 million Americans and another 60 million people in 80 foreign countries had taken Vioxx, primarily for relief of arthritis and acute pain, since it had been introduced in May 1999. Merck estimated that 105 million U.S. prescriptions were written for Vioxx from May 1999 through August 2004. An estimated 2 million people in the United States were taking Vioxx at the time of the recall.

As early as 2000, there had been warning signs of problems with Vioxx. Prior to the recall, roughly 30 lawsuits alleging that Vioxx was unsafe and had caused patients to suffer heart attacks and strokes, some resulting in death, had been filed in state and federal courts. In the weeks following the recall, the number of lawsuits multiplied quickly, reaching close to 700 by some counts. Some of these were class-action suits filed by high-profile trial lawyers on behalf of all potential claimants. Wall Street analysts estimated that Merck's legal costs associated with the Vioxx claims could range as high as $18 billion over the next decade.

As of 2004, the largest drug-product liability case on record involved Wyeth's recall of weight-loss remedies Redux and Pondimin in 1997, which contained a compound known as fen-phen and were estimated to cause heart-valve damage in as many as 30 percent of the people who took the pills. Some 6 million Americans had taken Redux or Pondimin; Wyeth's payouts to date had exceeded $13 billion of the $16.6 billion in reserves that the company had set aside to cover settlement costs.

Five weeks after the Vioxx recall, Standard & Poor's (S&P), which had placed a triple-A rating on Merck's debt since 1975, announced that it had put Merck's ratings on its watch list. Merck was one of only seven companies outside the financial services industry that had a triple-A S&P debt rating. The week following S&P's credit watch announcement, Moody's Investors Service lowered the rating of Merck's long-term debt two notches, to Aa2 from Aaa (its highest rating), and said it was keeping Merck's rating under review for a possible further downgrade. Moody's cited the loss in revenues and Merck's Vioxx litigation exposure as reasons for the downgrade. The Moody's downgrade and the threat of an S&P downgrade had little immediate impact on Merck—the company had $7 billion in cash and short-term investments and $10 billion in current assets to apply against its current liabilities of $2.2 billion and long-term debt of only $4.4 billion at the time of the recall, putting it in a position of strong liquidity. Nonetheless, the actions of the two credit rating agencies signaled concerns about the extent to which legal settlements would sap the company's financial resources down the road.

Moreover, the company's reputation as the gold standard of the pharmaceutical industry and one of the bluest of the blue-chip companies took a huge hit as the circumstances surrounding the recall came to light over the next several months. Internal e-mails, training aids sent to Merck salespeople, and pressures that Merck put on outside medical experts suggested that Merck personnel knew of or at least suspected Vioxx's dangers well before the recall. A front-page *Wall Street Journal* story on November 1, 2004, was headlined "E-Mails Suggest Merck Knew Vioxx's Dangers at Early Stage."

MERCK'S SITUATION IN 2004

In 2004, Merck & Company Inc., was a global research-driven company with annual sales of $22.5 billion; profits of $6.8 billion; 59,000 employees; 12 major drug research centers in the United States, Canada, Europe, and Japan; 32 manufacturing facilities; and a broad range of human and animal health care products marketed in 150 countries. Exhibit 1 shows the company's mission and core values.

MERCK'S STRATEGY

For the past 10 years or so, Merck's strategy had been to concentrate its considerable scientific and research expertise on developing blockbuster new drugs. The research-grounded strategy had three core elements:

- Develop a core competence in drug research by supporting the efforts of the best and brightest scientists and medical researchers Merck could assemble.

- Do very thorough clinical studies of promising drugs discovered in Merck's research labs to determine their effectiveness on patients and to explore the nature and extent of side effects.

- Seek to gain speedy regulatory approval of newly discovered medicines by using the results of the previously done research and clinical studies

Exhibit 1   **Merck's Mission and Core Values, 2004**

Our Mission

The mission of **Merck** is to provide society with superior products and services by developing innovations and solutions that improve the quality of life and satisfy customer needs, and to provide employees with meaningful work and advancement opportunities, and investors with a superior rate of return.

Our Values

1. **Our business is preserving and improving human life.** All of our actions must be measured by our success in achieving this goal. We value, above all, our ability to serve everyone who can benefit from the appropriate use of our products and services, thereby providing lasting consumer satisfaction.

2. **We are committed to the highest standards of ethics and integrity.** We are responsible to our customers, to Merck employees and their families, to the environments we inhabit, and to the societies we serve worldwide. In discharging our responsibilities, we do not take professional or ethical shortcuts. Our interactions with all segments of society must reflect the high standards we profess.

3. **We are dedicated to the highest level of scientific excellence and commit our <u>research</u> to improving human and animal health and the quality of life.** We strive to identify the most critical needs of consumers and customers, and we devote our resources to meeting those needs.

4. **We expect profits, but only from work that satisfies customer needs and benefits humanity.** Our ability to meet our responsibilities depends on maintaining a financial position that invites investment in leading-edge research and that makes possible effective delivery of research results.

5. **We recognize that the ability to excel—to most competitively meet society's and customers' needs—depends on the integrity, knowledge, imagination, skill, diversity and teamwork of our employees, and we value these qualities most highly.** To this end, we strive to create an environment of mutual respect, encouragement and teamwork—an environment that rewards commitment and performance and is responsive to the needs of our employees and their families.

Source: www.merck.com (accessed November 29, 2004).

to thoroughly document the benefits and safety of the drugs submitted for approval. Rapid approval to market new drugs could produce a significant competitive edge by not only allowing Merck to get its drug discoveries into the marketplace ahead of rivals but also giving it more time to sell the drug before patent expirations.

Merck's resource strengths in executing this strategy over the years had been a major factor in the company's success and in developing and fortifying what had come to be a storied reputation for first-rate scientific research and for having the best research personnel and research capabilities in the business. During the past two decades, Merck personnel had published more scientific papers than personnel at any other drug company, and Merck had patented more compounds than any of its competitors.[1] And the company's track record in getting new drugs approved expeditiously was excellent in comparison to other pharmaceutical manufacturers.

The central figure in executing Merck's research-based drug discovery strategy was Edward M. Scolnick, a graduate of Harvard Medical School who had published roughly 200 scientific papers and risen through the ranks at Merck to become its chief of research. Scolnick was reputed to have a superior intellect, and his persistent drive for research excellence permeated Merck's research activities. According to a former Merck cancer researcher, "You never went before him unprepared. He would begin probing very directly and very quickly. He would often identify some controlled experiment

that should have been done and wasn't."[2] For at least a decade before he retired in 2003, Scolnick was considered the de facto number two person at Merck (after CEO Raymond V. Gilmartin).[3] Scolnick was appointed to Merck's board of directors in 1997; he was the only inside executive on Merck's board besides the CEO. Merck's newest research lab, dedicated in October 2004—a multimillion-dollar building in Boston not far from Harvard Medical School—was named for Scolnick.

Under Scolnick's drug research leadership, Merck had racked up dazzling successes. Zocor, a cholesterol-reducing drug introduced in the early 1990s, soon became the market-leading prescription for lowering cholesterol and Merck's best-selling drug. Zocor had annual sales in 2003 of $5 billion. During the 1995–2001 period, Merck won approval from the U.S. Federal Drug Administration (FDA) for 15 new drugs, many of which became big market successes—Singulair (asthma), Fosamax (osteoporosis), Cozarr and Hyzarr (hypertension), Procepia (baldness), Vioxx (arthritis and pain relief), and Crixivan (HIV). These successful new drug introductions helped drive Merck's stock price to an all-time high of $95 per share in the fall of 2000. A breakdown of Merck's drug sales by category is shown in Exhibit 2.

But just as important to Merck's strategic success as a research-based drug-discovery organization was Scolnick's oversight of the process of gaining regulatory approval to introduce new drugs and the resulting competitive edge that accrued to Merck.

Exhibit 2   Merck's Sales by Drug Category, 2001–2003 (in millions)

Drug Category	2003	2002	2001
Atherosclerosis	$ 5,077.9	$ 5,552.1	$ 5,433.3
Hypertension/heart failure	3,421.6	3,477.8	3,584.3
Anti-inflammatory/analgesics (includes Vioxx)	2,677.3	2,587.2	2,391.1
Osteoporosis	2,676.6	2,243.1	1,629.7
Respiratory	2,009.4	1,489.8	1,260.3
Vaccines/biologicals	1,056.1	1,028.3	1,022.5
Antibacterial/antifungal	1,028.5	821.0	750.4
Ophthalmologicals	675.1	621.5	644.5
Urology	605.5	547.3	545.4
Human immunodeficiency virus (HIV)	290.6	294.3	380.8
Other	2,967.3	2,783.4	3,556.7
Total	$22,485.9	$21,445.8	$21,199.0

Source: Merck, 2003 10-K report.

The research-and-approval process for new drugs was known for being risky and tedious, both because of the need to conduct lengthy and convincing studies of drug effectiveness and safety (a high proportion of chemical compounds under investigation never survived this step) and because regulatory approval was rife with bureaucracy and sometimes contentious review procedures that could take several years. Scolnick's approach to dealing with the regulatory approval process was for Merck to submit fastidious supporting documentation for the new drugs it asked the FDA to approve, an approach that had worked well for Merck.

During the 1995–2001 period, Merck's vaunted scientific reputation, high-caliber clinical studies, and solid supporting documentation allowed the company to gain approval for all 13 new drugs it submitted to the FDA, with an average review time of 11 months. Vioxx won approval following a six-month review.[4] At Pfizer, the world's largest pharmaceutical firm in 2004, the new drug submissions during the same period had an average review time of two years. Analysts at Merrill Lynch estimated that Merck's drug research documentation capabilities and short approval times allowed the company to achieve extra sales of $3.3 billion during 1995–2001.[5]

MERCK'S RECORD OF CORPORATE SOCIAL RESPONSIBILITY AND GOOD CITIZENSHIP

Merck was strongly committed to being a solid corporate citizen and conducting its business in an ethical manner. This commitment had long been guided by the vision of the company's modern-day founder, George W. Merck, who said in 1950:

> We try never to forget that medicine is for the people. It is not for the profits. The profits follow, and if we have remembered that, they have never failed to appear.
>
> We cannot step aside and say that we have achieved our goal by inventing a new drug or a new way by which to treat presently incurable diseases, a new way to help those who suffer from malnutrition, or the creation of ideal balanced diets on a worldwide scale. We cannot rest till the way has been found, with our help, to bring our finest achievement to everyone.[6]

The two chief components of Merck's social responsibility strategy were charitable contributions and its actions to further the cause of public health by making its drugs more widely available. In 2003, Merck's philanthropic contributions totaled $843 million, consisting of cash contributions ($54 million), its patient assistance program ($393 million), and product donations ($396 million). Exhibit 3 shows Merck's recent record of charitable contributions.

Merck's efforts to live up to its commitment to make its drugs available to everyone are demonstrated in the following four examples of actions that the company had recently taken:[7]

1. Merck announced in February 2004 that the company would provide its medicines free for low-income Medicare beneficiaries who exhaust their $600 transitional assistance allowance in Medicare-endorsed drug discount cards. This action was consistent with Merck's long-standing Patient Assistance Program, which provided free medicine to patients who lacked drug coverage and could not afford Merck's drugs.

2. Since 1987, Merck had donated more than 300 million doses of its Mectizan drug to treat people in developing and third world countries who were suffering from onchocerciasis, a ravaging disease more commonly known as river blindness. Mectizan was a highly effective medicine that not only controlled and prevented river blindness but also helped limit the agonizing and disfiguring skin infections caused by the disease. The Mectizan Donation Program, a public/private partnership regarded as one of the world's most successful global health care collaborations, and funded in part by Merck, had long worked to improve the lives and prevent blindness for millions of people in Africa, Latin America, and Yemen. In 2004, doses of Mectizan reached more than 40 million people in 34 countries.

3. In poor African countries that had been hard hit by the AIDS epidemic, Merck had arranged to provide two of its HIV-fighting drugs, Stocrin and Crixivan, at prices at which it made no profit. Merck had also granted a royalty-free license to a South African pharmaceutical company to manufacture and sell a generic version of its HIV/AIDS drug Efavirenz.

4. In 2003, Merck launched the Merck Vaccine Network–Africa, an initiative designed to

Exhibit 3   **Merck's Corporate Philanthropy Contributions, 1998–2003**

Total Merck Contributions/Donations

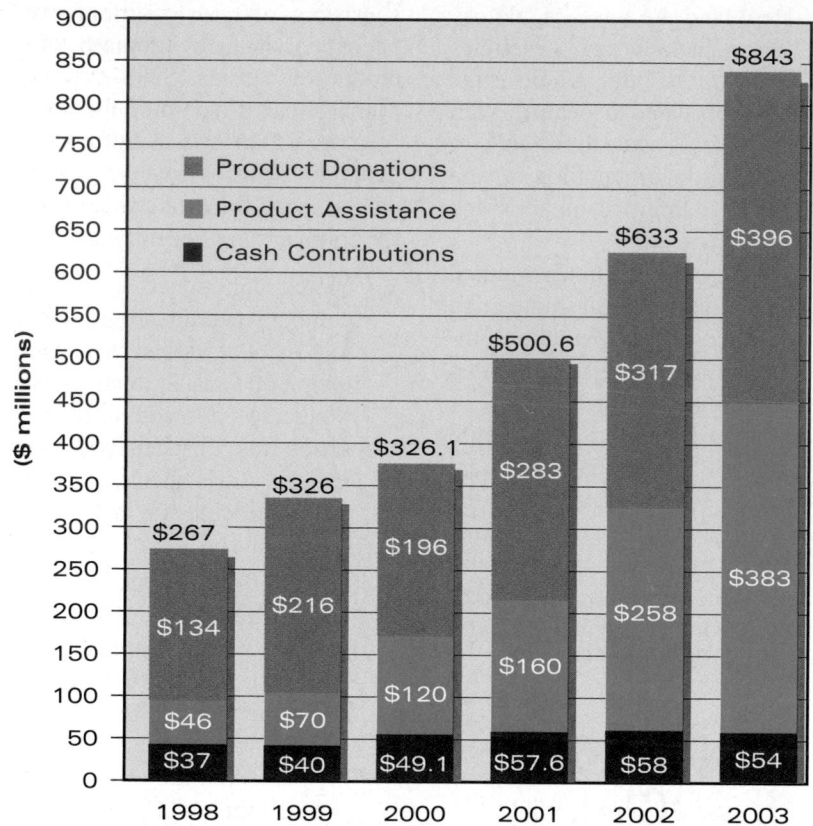

Legend:
- Product Donations
- Product Assistance
- Cash Contributions

Year	Cash Contributions	Product Assistance	Product Donations	Total
1998	$37	$46	$134	$267
1999	$40	$70	$216	$326
2000	$49.1	$120	$196	$326.1
2001	$57.6	$160	$283	$500.6
2002	$58	$258	$317	$633
2003	$54	$383	$396	$843

(*$ millions*)

*Total Merck cash contributions are the sum of contributions from The Merck Company Foundation, Merck & Co., Inc., and Merck Genome Research Institute.

Source: www.merck.com, accessed November 30, 2004.

contribute to improving the immunization infrastructure in Africa. Merck's initiative involved funding the establishment of a network of vaccination training centers at academic institutions in Kenya and Mali to provide a sustainable source of skilled health care workers in those countries and across the region. Africa had the highest per capita incidence of vaccine-preventable diseases in the world, with only half of all children in sub-Saharan Africa getting basic life-saving vaccinations during their first year of life.

In 1999 Merck developed a lengthy code of conduct entitled "Our Values and Standards: The Basis of Our Success" and distributed it to Merck employees. The company's Web site postings, in elaborating on the company's core values (see Exhibit 1) and the conduct expected of Merck employees, said:

- Every Merck employee is responsible for adhering to business practices that are in accordance with the letter and spirit of the applicable laws and with ethical principles that reflect the highest standards of corporate and individual behavior.

- Improper behavior cannot be rationalized as being in the company's interest. No act of impropriety advances the interest of the Company.

In May 2004, *Business Ethics* magazine named Merck one of its "100 Best Corporate Citizens" for the fifth consecutive year. Merck, ranked 48, was the only pharmaceutical company to gain a spot on the list in each of the five years that *Business Ethics* had published it and was also one of only two pharmaceutical companies to make the list.

MERCK'S TROUBLES IN 2004 PRIOR TO THE VIOXX RECALL

Since 2001, Merck had been struggling to maintain its earlier momentum of growing sales via a stream of new product introductions. None of its recently introduced drugs had generated annual sales of $1 billion or more. During the 1999–2001 period, Merck had lost its patent protection on five of its best-selling drugs—Vasotec (hypertension), Pepcid (ulcers), Mevacor (cholesterol), Prilosec (ulcers), and Prinivil (hypertension). The company's market-leading treatment for high cholesterol, Zocor, which generated annual sales revenues of about $5 billion, was coming off patent in 2006 and, like most other drugs without patent protection, was expected to experience sharp sales erosion when lower-priced generic imitations came onto the market. In 2003, Merck had to cancel work on four major new drugs, which were in big, costly Phase III trials. All four were thought to have real promise and had been touted by management as having major revenue potential. One of the four drugs, for depression, failed a pivotal clinical trial, and a second, for diabetes, was found in animal studies to pose a risk of cancer.

As a consequence, Merck's sales had flattened (Exhibit 2) and its net profits had eroded from the all-time peak of $7.3 billion and earnings per share (EPS) of $3.14 in 2001 to $6.8 billion and an EPS of $3.03 in 2003. Investors were fully aware of Merck's struggling condition—the company's stock price, after having risen 475 percent from 1994 to its all-time high of $95 per share in the fall of 2000, had trended downward and was trading at around $45 per share in the weeks prior to the Vioxx recall. Shareholders were restless, having suffered a loss in market capitalization of over $130 billion during the past four years. While Merck still had a number of new products in the pipeline that it expected to be able to release in upcoming years—treatments for diabetes, shingles, and assorted viruses—most analysts did not believe

the new drugs had the sales potential to overcome the anticipated falloff of Zocor's sales in 2006–2007.

However, Merck was not alone in its struggle to discover and introduce new blockbuster drugs; virtually the whole pharmaceutical industry worldwide was finding the discovery of new drugs with big sales potential tough sledding. New drugs in the pipeline at a number of major pharmaceutical companies were disturbingly low from the standpoint of boosting future revenue growth and profitability—a condition that had already prompted several large mergers and acquisitions (to try to gain better scale economies in research), as well as strategy changes. New strategy elements already in place at Merck involved cost reduction, partnering with small innovative companies on new drug discovery, and licensing promising compounds.

EVENTS AT MERCK LEADING UP TO THE INTRODUCTION OF VIOXX

Vioxx was the last of Merck's multibillion-dollar drugs under Scolnick's leadership. Discovered in laboratory experiments by Merck researchers in 1994, the drug was one of a new class of painkillers, called Cox-2 inhibitors, that reduced pain and inflammation without such side effects as ulcers and gastrointestinal bleeding. Some people had experienced such side effects while taking daily doses of aspirin, ibuprofen (the painkiller in Advil and Motrin), and naproxen (the painkiller in Aleve) for chronic pain relief. Pain relievers containing aspirin, ibuprofen, and naproxen were designated nonsteroidal anti-inflammatory drugs (NSAIDs). By some estimates, intestinal bleeding associated with long-term use of NSAIDs was responsible for the deaths of 10,000 Americans annually.

Internal e-mails at Merck indicated that the company was well aware that Vioxx had limited market potential unless it could gain acceptance in the mass market for painkillers and be preferred to cheap over-the-counter NSAIDs. A November 1996 memo by a Merck official indicated that company personnel were wrestling with this marketing dilemma.[8] There was discussion of conducting a trial to demonstrate that Vioxx was gentler on the stomach than over-the-counter painkillers. To show the difference, takers of

Vioxx could not take any aspirin, which some arthritis patients took because of its blood-thinning and cardio-protective benefits. But the necessity of excluding aspirin raised concerns at Merck. The author of the memo noted that "there is a substantial chance that significantly higher rates" of cardiovascular problems would occur in the group taking only Vioxx. A February 1997 e-mail by another Merck official said that unless patients in the Vioxx group also took aspirin "you will get more thrombotic events and kill the drug."[9] In response, a Merck vice president for clinical research indicated the company was in a "no-win situation" because giving study subjects both Vioxx and aspirin could result in gastrointestinal problems and not giving them aspirin raised "the possibility of increased CV [cardiovascular] events."[10]

It is not clear what came out of the discussion Merck officials had about the study in 1996–1997.[11] But in early 1999, around the time that Merck won FDA approval to market Vioxx, Merck began an 8,000-person clinical trial that compared people taking a high dose of Vioxx against those taking naproxen. The patients taking Vioxx were not allowed to take aspirin.

In 1998 medical researchers at the University of Pennsylvania reported findings that Cox-2 inhibitors *might* interfere with enzymes thought to play key roles in warding off cardiovascular disease; the findings were communicated to the companies developing Cox-2 inhibitors and were also published.[12] In Merck's first round of clinical trials, patients taking Vioxx had about the same rate of heart attacks and strokes as did patients who took NSAIDs or a sugar placebo. An unpublished 1998 Merck clinical trial called "Study 090," which involved 978 patients, showed that serious cardiovascular events, including heart attack and stroke, occurred about six times more often in patients taking Vioxx than in patients taking another arthritis drug or a placebo.[13] Merck said that study was too small and the results were not statistically significant enough to allow the company to draw any conclusions.

Merck's application to the FDA for Vioxx approval in November 1998 included data on approximately 5,400 osteoarthritis patients who participated in eight studies. In these studies, there were similar rates of thrombotic cardiovascular adverse events with Vioxx, placebos, and three NSAIDs (ibuprofen, diclofenac, and nabumetone). After a six-month review, Vioxx gained FDA approval on May 21, 1999, despite apparent reservations on the part of some reviewers about its possible blood vessel effects.

But the studies of Vioxx reportedly did not establish that it was a more effective painkiller than NSAIDs. The real selling proposition for Vioxx—and the main basis for its approval by the FDA—was simply a lower incidence of stomach bleeding and gastrointestinal problems, as compared to conventional pain relievers like aspirin, Tylenol, Aleve, Advil, and other over-the-counter remedies (which cost about five cents a pill versus several dollars a pill for Vioxx).[14] Thus, the chief basis for Vioxx's approval by the FDA rested mainly on its relevance for the estimated 15 percent of arthritis sufferers who could not take over-the-counter pain relievers on a sustained basis because of the resulting gastrointestinal side effects.[15]

MERCK'S DIRECT-TO-CONSUMER MARKETING CAMPAIGN FOR VIOXX

When Vioxx won FDA approval in 1999, Merck's marketing strategy included sales pitches to doctors about the drug's benefits (along with the usual free samples they could try out on patients) and an aggressive direct-to-consumer advertising campaign. The cover of Merck's 1999 annual report headlined that Vioxx was the company's "biggest, fastest, and best launch ever." In the five or so years that arthritis pain reliever Vioxx was on the market, Merck spent roughly $100 million annually for television, newspaper, and magazine ads touting Vioxx's benefits and appealing to pain suffers to ask their doctor about Vioxx.[16] Sales of Vioxx climbed steadily from 1999 to 2004, and the drug became a $2.5 billion annual revenue source for Merck. It was the second best-selling Cox-2 inhibitor when it was pulled from the market, trailing only Celebrex, which had $3 billion in annual sales. Pfizer had become the marketer of Celebrex when it acquired rival drugmaker Pharmacia in 2003.

Vioxx was one among many blockbuster drugs that had benefited from direct-to-consumer advertising opportunities that opened up in 1997 when, during the Clinton administration, the FDA loosened regulations on how pharmaceutical companies could advertise to a general audience. Since then, drugs that were originally meant to treat specific medical problems had become used in far broader populations—partly because doctors had been willing to prescribe them when requested by patients (who presumably were intrigued by the newly allowed ads for prescription drugs) and partly because the costs of such prescriptions were paid for by patients' health insurance programs. A study by Bruce Stuart at the University of Maryland showed that the biggest determinant of whether a patient took a prescription Cox-2 inhibitor or a far cheaper over-the-counter pain reliever like Aleve, Motrin, or Advil was whether the patient had health insurance that would cover much of the prescription costs.[17]

WARNING SIGNS OF TROUBLE PRIOR TO THE RECALL

In March 2000, Merck found surprising results from an 8,000-person clinical trial it had initiated in early 1999 to see if Vioxx posed fewer gastrointestinal risks than NSAIDs. The trial showed that arthritis patients taking Vioxx had more than two times as many serious cardiovascular events as those on naproxen, an NSAID sold under the Aleve brand, among other brand names (see Exhibit 4). A total of 45 serious cardiovascular thrombotic events oc-curred among the 4,047 patients taking Vioxx, whereas only 19 had occurred among the 4,029 patients taking naproxen. According to Merck, the higher number was largely due to a difference in the incidence of *nonfatal* heart attacks: 18 for Vioxx and 4 for naproxen. The number of *fatal* cardiovascular thrombotic events was similar in patients treated with Vioxx ($n = 7$) compared to naproxen ($n = 6$). Deeper analysis, however, showed that the heart-attack rate in the Vioxx group appeared to be four times as high as the naproxen group. Something akin to these results had been seemingly anticipated in the 1996–1997 memos and e-mails.

In a March 9, 2000, e-mail with the subject line "Vigor"—the name Merck gave to the Vioxx–naproxen clinical trial—Merck's chief of research, Ed Scolnick, wrote that the results showed that the cardiovascular events "are clearly there. It is a shame but it is a low incidence and it is mechanism based as we worried it was." He compared Vioxx to other drugs with known side effects, writing, "There is always a hazard."[18] Scolnick went on to say that he wanted other data available before the Vioxx–naproxen results were made public, so that it would be "clear to the world" that hazard was a characteristic of all Cox-2 inhibitors, not just Vioxx.[19]

Medical experts outside Merck who were familiar with the Vioxx–naproxen study hypothesized that the results raised valid concerns that Vioxx could indeed be causing cardiac problems. Merck took the position that the differential risks could be attributable to the added side benefits of taking naproxen rather than to problems with Vioxx. Merck personnel reportedly believed that known properties of naproxen were responsible for the differential. Nonetheless, Merck immediately put out a press release describing the Vioxx–naproxen results and informed the FDA.

But, for unknown reasons, it was not until February 8, 2001, that the FDA Arthritis Advisory Committee met to discuss concerns about the potential cardiovascular risks associated with Vioxx. On May 22, 2001, a little over three months after the FDA advisory committee meeting, Merck issued a press release entitled "Merck Reconfirms Favorable Cardiovascular Safety of Vioxx"; this effort to address doubts about Vioxx was complemented by numerous papers in peer-reviewed medical literature by Merck employees and their consultants.[20] The company sponsored continuing medical "education" symposiums at national meetings in an effort to temper concerns about the adverse cardiovascular effects of Vioxx.[21] The essence of Merck's message was that Vioxx had no cardiovascular toxicity but, rather,

Exhibit 4 **Summary-Results of Vioxx–Naproxen Study in 2000**

	People Taking Vioxx	People Taking Naproxen
Total number of people in clinical trial	4,047	4,029
Number of adverse cardiovascular events	101	46
Number of digestive system adverse events	48	97

Source: FDA's analysis of the clinical trial results, as reported in Anna Wilde Mathews and Barbara Martinez, "E-Mails Suggest Merck Knew Vioxx's Dangers at Early Stage," *The Wall Street Journal,* November 1, 2004, p. A10.

naproxen was cardio-protective. (The FDA, however, has said there is no conclusive evidence that naproxen protects the heart.)[22] In response to Merck's pro-Vioxx campaign, the FDA sent an eight-page warning letter to the company in September 2001 saying that sales representatives "have engaged in false or misleading promotional activities," and that the company's promotional campaign "minimizes the potentially serious cardiovascular findings" about Vioxx and "discounts the fact [that] patients on Vioxx were observed to have a four to five-fold increase" in heart attacks, compared with patients on naproxen.[23]

But it was not until two years later, in April 2002, that the FDA instructed Merck to include certain precautions about cardiovascular risks in its package insert. At about the same time, the FDA also decided to go a step further and do its own follow-up study of Vioxx safety, opting to sponsor a study of the medical records of 1.4 million patients insured by Kaiser Permanente, the nation's largest nonprofit health maintenance organization (HMO), serving 8.2 million members in nine states and the District of Columbia.

In November 2000, the results of the Vioxx–naproxen study were published in the *New England Journal of Medicine;* the article was co-authored by Merck employees and by academics who had received consulting contracts or research grants from Merck. But the Vioxx–naproxen trial also spurred Merck to do further clinical studies on the possible links between Vioxx and heart trouble. Shortly after learning of the Vioxx–Naproxen cardiovascular differential, Merck embarked on a long-term study called APPROVe to see whether Vioxx would lead to a reduction of colon polyps (which if shown to be the case would give doctors another reason to prescribe Vioxx). APPROVe, which involved 2,600 patients, was a true controlled trial that compared Vioxx with a placebo instead of another drug, thereby providing a more definitive test of whether Vioxx increased blood vessel risk.

MERCK'S "DODGE BALL VIOXX" TRAINING DOCUMENT

To help its sales personnel deal with questions doctors were asking about Vioxx's safety, Merck developed a sales aid entitled "Dodge Ball Vioxx." The 16-page document, addressed to "all field personnel" was intended as an "obstacle handling guide"; each of the first 12 pages listed one "obstacle" or concern that doctors might have about Vioxx, such as "I am concerned about the cardiovascular effects of Vioxx" and "The competition has been in my office telling me the incidence of heart attacks is greater with Vioxx than Celebrex."[24] Suggested responses for each obstacle were provided. The final four pages each contained a single word in capital letters: DODGE.[25] A former Merck sales representative told *60 Minutes* that when a doctor expressed concerns about the cardiovascular effects of Vioxx, "We were supposed to tell the physician that Vioxx did not cause cardiovascular events, that instead, in the studies, naproxen has aspirin-like characteristics which made naproxen a heart-protecting type of drug where Vioxx did not have that heart-protecting side."[26]

MERCK'S OFFENSIVE TO COMBAT THE CONCERNS OF ACADEMIC RESEARCHERS ABOUT VIOXX'S SAFETY

In 2000–2001, Merck took actions to combat the concerns of several academic researchers who were openly questioning the safety of Vioxx. A Stanford University professor who regularly gave prescription drug–related lectures sponsored by Merck and other drug companies pressed Merck for additional data about Vioxx.[27] When Merck failed to provide it, the professor added a slide to his lectures showing a man (representing the missing data) hiding under a blanket. Merck then canceled its sponsorship of several lectures by the professor, and a Merck official called Stanford Medical School, complaining that the professor's presentations were "irresponsibly anti-Merck and specifically anti-Vioxx." The Merck official suggested that if the lectures continued, the professor would "flame out" and there would be consequences for Stanford (presumably in the form of fewer Merck-sponsored research grants).

A professor at the University of Minnesota who had given Merck-sponsored lectures also got a call from Merck complaining about what was being said about Vioxx, as did a rheumatologist at Beth Israel Deaconess Medical Center in Boston who had worked on research with rival Celebrex but who had also worked with Merck on occasion. In the summer of 2002, a professor at the Catalan Institute of Pharmacology in Barcelona, Spain, edited a publication that repeated criticisms of Merck's handling of Vioxx that had been published in *The Lancet*, a respected British medical journal.[28] Merck approached the professor on three occasions to print a Merck-authored rebuttal. When the professor refused, Merck sued the professor and the Catalan Institute under a Spanish law that allowed plaintiffs to demand a public correction of inaccurate published information. In January 2004, the judge ruled in favor of the defendants and ordered Merck to pay the court costs. In March 2004, the professor was asked to give a featured presentation to a conference of 1,000 Spanish family physicians—a conference that Merck had helped sponsor for eight straight years. When Merck learned of the invitation, it called the conference organizer and indicated that it "preferred" that the professor not be on the program. When the organizer refused to delete the professor's presentation, Merck withdrew its $140,000 funding for the conference.[29]

OTHER EXTERNAL WARNING SIGNS OF TROUBLE WITH VIOXX

While Merck's multiyear APPROVe study was under way, several developments outside Merck further signaled there might be cardiovascular problems with Vioxx:

- An article by three medical researchers, published in the *Journal of the American Medical Association* on August 22, 2001, reviewed four studies with a total of about 18,000 patients and concluded that "the available data raise a cautionary flag about the risk of cardiovascular events with Cox-2 inhibitors."[30] One of the researchers communicated the results of the study to Merck's CEO, Ray Gilmartin, offering to visit Merck and present their findings. Neither Gilmartin nor anyone else at Merck responded to the researcher's phone calls. Merck reportedly asked the *New England Journal of Medicine* to run a Merck-authored rebuttal, but the journal editors refused.[31]

- *The Wall Street Journal* ran a front-page story on the heart risks of Vioxx and other Cox-2 inhibitor drugs on August 22, 2001, citing the concerns of several medical researchers and the Vioxx–naproxen results.

- The National Trial Lawyers Guild formed a "Cox-2 litigation group" in early 2002 and at their national convention in 2003 devoted a session to Vioxx.

- Before the Vioxx recall, more than 400 lawsuits had been filed on behalf of Vioxx patients.[32]

- A Merck-sponsored analysis, conducted by researchers at Harvard and Merck, found that Vioxx was "associated with an elevated relative risk" of heart attacks compared to the use of Pfizer's painkiller Celebrex or no similar painkiller. When Merck asked the researchers to tone down the conclusion about the no-painkiller group and the Harvard researcher refused, Merck removed the name of the Merck researcher prior to the article's publication in *Circulation* in May 2004.[33]

- A book published in the summer of 2004 by John Abramson, a family doctor and clinical instructor at Harvard Medical School, concluded that even people who did not have a history of heart problems doubled their risk of developing a cardiovascular problem by taking Vioxx instead of naproxen.[34]

All of these developments served to switch the debate on Vioxx from whether it lacked some of the cardiac-related benefits of NSAIDs to whether it was inherently risky from a cardiac-stroke perspective.

Meanwhile, in the summer of 2004, the earlier study of the medical records of 1.4 million people insured by Kaiser Permanente was producing important findings. The study, financed by the FDA and conducted by David J. Graham, associate director for science and medicine in the FDA's Office of Drug Safety, compared the outcomes of 40,405 patients who took Celebrex and 26,748 patients who took Vioxx. The results, which were reported at a conference in France on August 25, 2004, showed two significant facts:

- Patients taking the typical starting dose of Vioxx had a 50 percent greater chance of heart attacks and sudden cardiac death than patients taking Celebrex.

- Patients taking the highest recommended daily dosage of Vioxx had nearly 2.7 times the risk of heart attack and sudden cardiac death as patients taking Celebrex.

Merck issued a press release saying it strongly disagreed with the FDA study's conclusions.[35]

THE RECALL DECISION

On Thursday afternoon, September 23, 2004, almost four and a half years after the APPROVe study began, Peter Kim, who had taken over as Merck's chief of research when Scolnick retired, met with Ray Gilmartin to inform him that the results of the APPROVe study were showing that patients on Vioxx longer than 18 months had begun experiencing heart attacks and strokes at about double the rate of the control group taking placebos. Results for the first 18 months of the study did not show an increased risk of cardiovascular problems with Vioxx; these results were similar to those of two prior placebo-controlled studies described in the current U.S. labeling for Vioxx. The decision to recall Vioxx came seven days later. Exhibit 5 presents a time line of Vioxx-related actions and events at Merck up to the recall.

THE FALLOUT FOLLOWING MERCK'S VOLUNTARY WITHDRAWAL OF VIOXX

A torrent of criticism was directed at Merck in the days and weeks following the withdrawal of Vioxx from the market. Some outsiders objected strongly to the company's hyped-up marketing tactics. With Merck's share price dropping from about $45 to the $27–$29 range, equal to a $42 billion loss in market capitalization, shareholders expressed concerns about management's handling of Vioxx, arguing that a better option to the recall was to (1) immediately inform doctors writing Vioxx prescriptions for patients of the above-average risks of heart attacks and strokes, and (2) seek FDA approval to amend the warning label on Vioxx to state that patients with heart-attack and stroke risk should not take Vioxx

for longer than 18 months. Indeed, the majority of the outside clinicians Merck consulted between September 23 and September 30, 2004, advised Merck to go to the FDA and other regulatory authorities and have the prescribing information for Vioxx updated with the new findings of increased cardiovascular risk, especially since millions of people were benefiting from use of Vioxx.

Medical experts opined that Merck should have done more studies when doubts about Vioxx first surfaced. William Castelli, former director of the Framingham Heart Study, which investigated cardiac risk factors, told *Fortune* that since Cox-2 inhibitors reduce inflammation (one of the risk factors for cardiac disease), a red flag should have immediately gone up when some studies suggested that Vioxx raised the risk of heart attacks instead of reducing them.[36]

Eric J. Topol, chairman of cardiology at the Cleveland Clinic and a vocal Merck critic, said in a commentary concerning Merck's withdrawal of Vioxx that was published in the October 21, 2004, issue of the *New England Journal of Medicine*, "Had the company not valued sales over safety, a suitable trial could have been initiated rapidly at a fraction of the cost of Merck's direct-to-consumer advertising campaign." Topol believed that the early estimates of 28,000 heart attacks that might be attributable to Vioxx were low and estimated that the number of people injured by Vioxx could be as high as 160,000 (a number Merck believed was far too high). But it was pretty clear that every person who took Vioxx during 1999–2004 and subsequently had a heart attack or stroke was a potential litigant.

A month after the Vioxx recall, on November 2, 2004, the FDA announced that David J. Graham's study of the Kaiser Permanente data indicated that Vioxx may have contributed to an additional 27,785 heart attacks, strokes, or deaths that might have been avoided if patients had taken Celebrex instead. Three days later, in a study published online by *The Lancet*, Swiss researchers at the University of Berne publicly reported their conclusions that Vioxx should have been "withdrawn several years earlier."[37] Their study, funded by the Swiss National Science Foundation, analyzed 18 randomized controlled Vioxx trials and 11 related observational studies; much of the information for the study was based on prior data and study results obtained primarily from the FDA. Merck posted a strongly worded rebuttal of the *Lancet* article on its Web site, citing a variety of problems with the analysis done by the Swiss researchers.

Exhibit 5   Timeline of Information about Vioxx, as Compiled by Merck

1998	April: Results of FitzGerald study first presented. Among the results of the study were indications that Cox-2 inhibitors may increase the risk of cardiovascular events.
	April: Trial of Vioxx versus placebo in the prevention of Alzheimer's in patients with mild cognitive impairment (MCI) begins.
1999	January: Vioxx–naproxen trial initiated; patients taking aspirin for cardiac protection were excluded from the study.
	February: First trial of Vioxx versus placebo for the treatment of Alzheimer's disease begins.
	April: Public meeting of FDA Arthritis Advisory Committee on Vioxx's approval.
	May: Vioxx approved by the FDA.
	October: Terms of APPROVe trial finalized, with enrollment of 2,600 patients, ages 40–96, beginning in February 2000. Purpose was to determine ability of Vioxx to reduce colon polyps over a period of three years, with cardiovascular events to be closely monitored. Patients were allowed to take aspirin.
2000	March: Preliminary results from Vioxx–naproxen study become available to Merck. News release on preliminary results of Vioxx–naproxen results issued by Merck; preliminary Vioxx–naproxen results submitted to the FDA. Two ongoing Alzheimer's studies—one for prevention and one for treatment—show no difference in cardiovascular event rates between Vioxx and placebo.
	April: Second trial of Vioxx versus placebo for the treatment of Alzheimer's begins.
	May: Article discussing preliminary Vioxx–naproxen data submitted to the *New England Journal of Medicine* for review and publication. Vioxx–naproxen preliminary results presented at Digestive Disease Week.
	June: Final Vioxx–naproxen study data submitted to FDA in a supplemental new drug application, which included a draft prescribing new disclosure information regarding uses and possible side effects.
	November: Vioxx–naproxen findings published in the *New England Journal of Medicine.* First Vioxx versus placebo trial in the treatment of Alzheimer's disease ends; second interim analysis of safety data from Alzheimer's prevention and treatment trials shows no difference in cardiovascular event rates between Vioxx and placebo.
2001	February: Public meeting of FDA Arthritis Advisory Committee on Vioxx–naproxen results.
	May: Second trial of Vioxx versus placebo for treatment of Alzheimer's disease stopped.
	September: Merck and Oxford University sign letter of intent to conduct a randomized, double-blind, placebo-controlled, international, multicenter study of Vioxx in 7,000 colorectal cancer patients following potentially curative therapy (designated as the VICTOR trial). The primary hypothesis to be tested in the study was that Vioxx administered for two years would result in greater overall survival compared with placebo. Cardiovascular events were to be monitored.
	October: Pooled analysis of cardiovascular data from Phase II/III studies published in *Circulation,* the journal of the American Heart Association. Analysis demonstrated that Vioxx was not associated with excess cardiovascular thrombotic events compared with either placebo or non-naproxen NSAIDs.
	November: APPROVe enrollment completed.
2002	April: U.S. prescribing information for Vioxx updated as a consequence of the Vioxx–naproxen study information and data from two placebo-controlled studies. First patient is enrolled in VICTOR trial.
	June: Pooled analysis of placebo-controlled studies in patients with Alzheimer's and MCI presented to European League Against Rheumatism. The incidence of serious cardiovascular adverse events in this population was similar for both Vioxx and placebo.
2003	March: Design of a study to test ability of Vioxx to reduce incidence of prostate cancer in 15,000 patients (named Vioxx in Prostate Cancer, or ViP, trial) finalized; adverse cardiovascular events were to be monitored.
	April: Trial of Vioxx versus placebo in MCI ends.
	June: ViP trial enrollment begins. Updated pooled analysis of Alzheimer's treatment and MCI data presented to European League Against Rheumatism. The cardiovascular event rate in patients taking 25-milligram doses of Vioxx continued to be similar to the rate in patients taking a placebo; mean duration of treatment was 1.2 years in Vioxx group and 1.3 years in placebo group.
	October: Updated pooled analysis published in the *American Heart Journal* demonstrated that Vioxx was not associated with excess cardiovascular thrombotic events compared with either placebo or non-naproxen NSAIDs.
2004	September: APPROVe External Data Safety Monitoring Board notifies Merck of its recommendation to end APPROVe trial due to high Vioxx incidence of cardiovascular problems. APPROVe, ViP, and VICTOR trials also terminated early. Merck voluntarily withdraws Vioxx from the market.

Source: Information posted at www.merck.com (accessed December 4, 2004).

REACTION AND RESPONSE IN REGULATORY CIRCLES

European prescription drug regulators launched investigations of other Cox-2 inhibitor drugs, such as Pfizer's Celebrex and Bextra. On November 30, 2004, Swiss pharmaceutical manufacturer Novartis announced that it was temporarily withdrawing its application for European Union approval of its new Cox-2 painkiller Prexige in order to gather more detailed data—Prexige had already been approved in Britain and 20 other countries. Novartis was also working with the FDA on what documentation was needed to win approval to market Prexige in the United States. It was unclear to what extent Merck's next big drug, Arcoxia, would be delayed at the FDA following the FDA's request for further safety and benefit data in October 2004.

Members of Congress, as well as prominent doctors, had recently called for an investigation of the FDA, its drug approval procedures, and whether the relationship between the pharmaceutical firms and FDA officials was too cozy to produce independent oversight and adequately protect the public interest. In a congressional hearing on November 18, 2004, the FDA's David J. Graham testified that the agency downplayed mounting negative data on Vioxx and that it "seriously undervalues, disregards and disrespects drug safety" in general. Graham listed five other potentially dangerous medications currently on the market—Accutane, Bextra, Crestor, Meridia, and Serevent. Exhibit 6 lists drugs that *Forbes* magazine identified as targets for litigation. In early 2005, concerns about the safety of Celebrex began to multiply.

In response to its critics, the FDA announced that it was moving to modify its system for evaluating the safety of drugs, particularly those already on the market and those applications where there was disagreement among FDA scientists reviewing new drug applications. Under the proposed new system, when FDA reviewers failed to reach consensus, an ad hoc panel would be convened, with the panel

Exhibit 6   **Other Drugs That Could Be the Target of Litigation**

Drug	Manufacturer	Global Sales	Possible Problems
Zyprexa	Eli Lilly	$4.3 billion	A group convened by the American Diabetes Association says that this drug, used to treat schizophrenia, raises diabetes risk relative to other drugs—75 lawsuits have been filed.
Paxil	GlaxoSmithKline	$3.1 billion	This antidepressant (and others) may be linked to suicidal thoughts in children.
Neurontin	Pfizer	$2.7 billion	In May 2004, a Pfizer subsidiary paid $430 million to promote this epilepsy drug for unapproved uses; a class-action lawsuit has been filed.
Prempro	Wyeth	$1.3 billion	Almost 2,000 lawsuits involving 3,136 women who took estrogen replacement drugs Premarin or Prempro have been filed following medical trials showing that both drugs raise the risk of heart attack and that Prempro raises the risk of breast cancer. Wyeth says the increased risk of breast cancer was disclosed.
Bextra	Pfizer	$990 million	Bextra, like Vioxx, was a Cox-2 inhibitor and was being scrutinized by trial lawyers because of two studies showing it raised risks in heart surgery patients. However, Bextra was not an approved drug for heart surgery patients.
Accutane	Roche	$410 million	This acne drug has been linked to causing birth defects and has alleged links to suicide. Roche says birth defect links were prominently disclosed.
Crestor	AstraZeneca	$130 million	Public Citizen, an advocacy group, is claiming possible liver and muscle side effects; one lawsuit is pending in Mississippi.

Source: "Merck's Mess," *Forbes*, November 1, 2004, p. 51.

consisting of scientists who were not involved in the original decision-making process, including some from outside the agency. The panel would have 30 days to make a recommendation to the director of FDA's Center for Drug Evaluation & Research. However, Senate Finance Committee chair Charles E. Grassley (R-Iowa) and other knowledgeable FDA observers believed that more far-reaching changes were needed to prevent another Vioxx debacle. At the close of the November 18 hearing, Grassley said he would be pushing for an autonomous board at the FDA to track the safety of drugs after they go on the market. The board would have the power to make label changes and to withdraw drugs from the market. Advocates of an independent board argued that it was unreasonable to expect that the same agency responsible for approval of drug licensing and labeling also be committed to the task of actively seeking evidence that might indicate its decisions to approve the drug or its warning label were wrong.[38]

Since adoption of the 1992 Prescription Drug User Fee Act, the FDA had received approximately $825 million in "user fees" from drug and biologic manufacturers from fiscal years 1993 through 2001 to augment its budget and help pay for the costs of streamlining its new drug-review-and-approval process.[39] During that time, median approval times for standard, or nonpriority, drugs decreased from 27 months in 1993 to 14 months in 2001. However, drug recalls following approval increased from 1.56 percent during 1993–1996 to 5.35 percent during 1997–2001. In addition, an investigation of 18 FDA expert advisory panels revealed that more than half of the members of these panels had direct financial interests in the drug or topic they were evaluating and for which they were making recommendations.[40]

THE SPECTER OF LITIGATION AND MERCK'S EXPOSURE

As of December 2004, trial lawyers in the United States and elsewhere were still taking calls from potential clients daily in regard to Vioxx. Several prominent law firms with expertise in product liability were in the process of (1) soliciting and interviewing potential clients who believed they

had been harmed by taking Vioxx, (2) preparing and/or filing lawsuits of one kind or another, and (3) identifying and working with medical experts who might be called to testify about Vioxx's causal connections to clients' health problems. While every person who took Vioxx and subsequently suffered a heart attack or stroke could be a potential litigant, the science seemed to indicate that the cardiovascular risks of Vioxx began after 18 months of usage (which could significantly limit the number of legitimate plaintiffs and Merck's litigation exposure). Moreover, a successful plaintiff would have to prove that it was Vioxx and not any of a myriad of other reasons— smoking, poor eating habits, excess weight, lack of exercise—that *caused* the health problem.

On the other hand, lawyers for the plaintiffs believed they could introduce documents and testimony showing that Merck swept adverse evidence about Vioxx's safety under the rug. In litigation in New Jersey and Alabama, where over 150 Vioxx cases were pending, plaintiffs' lawyers had successfully gotten discovery rights from the courts and obtained some 3 million Merck documents and e-mails relating to Vioxx.[41] In the New Jersey cases, plaintiffs' lawyers were also expected to claim that Merck's direct-to-consumer advertising campaign had induced patients to ask their doctors for Vioxx— in New Jersey (and other jurisdictions), a drugmaker that employed direct-to-consumer marketing lost the protection of a legal rule that says it need only provide safety warnings sufficient to alert doctors (not patients) to a drug's risks.

Some of the plaintiffs' lawyers were seeking to have their pending cases consolidated and transferred to jurisdictions where jury awards for damages were quite generous. Merck was trying to get many of the federal cases transferred to courts in Maryland, where it believed the judicial climate was more favorable to its position.[42]

MERCK'S POSITION ON ITS DECISION TO WITHDRAW VIOXX FROM THE MARKET

When Merck pulled Vioxx from the market on September 30, 2004, CEO Raymond Gilmartin said that the new study findings prompting Merck's decision were "unexpected" and that Merck's voluntary withdrawal was "really putting patient safety first"—needy patients could readily switch to other Cox-2 inhibitors such as Celebrex or NSAIDs.

Merck's position right up until it withdrew Vioxx was that the evidence about Vioxx's cardiovascular effects was inconclusive. For example, in the first round of clinical trials, patients who took Vioxx had about the same rate of heart attacks and strokes as patients who took NSAIDs or a sugar-pill placebo.[43] Merck said that it had conducted a number of studies before and after FDA approval that did not show the heart risk seen in the Vioxx–naproxen study.[44]

And management believed it had done the right things, pointing out that:[45]

- It had extensively studied Vioxx before seeking regulatory approval to market it.

- After it saw the results of the Vioxx–naproxen trial, it immediately put out a press release.

- It added warning language to its Vioxx label and prescription usage information.

- When questions arose, it took additional steps, including conducting further studies to gain more clinical information. For example, it voluntarily and ethically initiated the APPROVe study, which ultimately identified the increased cardiovascular risks of long-term use of Vioxx.

- When information from the additional clinical trials became available, Merck had put patient safety first and promptly recalled Vioxx rather than amend the prescription warnings.

According to Merck general counsel Kenneth Frazier:

We communicated appropriately about the product, we monitored it appropriately, we studied it appropriately, and in the end we took the actions that benefited patients.[46]

Endnotes

[1] John Simons and David Stipp, "Will Merck Survive Vioxx?" *Fortune,* November 1, 2004, p. 96.

[2] Ibid.

[3] Ibid., p. 94.

[4] Ibid., p. 96.

[5] As cited in ibid., pp. 96–97.

[6] Quotes posted at www.merck.com (accessed November 30, 2004).

[7] These examples are based on information in company press releases posted at www.merck.com (accessed November 30, 2004).

[8] Anna Wilde Mathews and Barbara Martinez, "E-Mails Suggest Merck Knew Vioxx's Dangers at Early Stage," *The Wall Street Journal,* November 1, 2004, p. A10.

[9] Ibid.

[10] Ibid.

[11] Ibid.

[12] Simons and Stipp, "Will Merck Survive Vioxx?" p. 102.

[13] "Prescription for Trouble," a *60 Minutes* documentary posted at www.cbsnews.com, November 14, 2004 (accessed December 4, 2004).

[14] Holman W. Jenkins Jr., "Was Withdrawing Vioxx the Right Thing to Do?" *Wall Street Journal,* November 10, 2004, p. A17.

[15] Ibid.

[16] Amy Isao, "Drug Ads—Without Harmful Side Effects," *Business Week Online,* posted November 8, 2004.

[17] Jenkins, "Was Withdrawing Vioxx the Right Thing to Do?" p. A17.

[18] Mathews and Martinez, "E-Mails Suggest Merck Knew," p. A10.

[19] Ibid.

[20] Eric J. Topol, "Failing the Public Health—Rofecoxib, Merck, and the FDA," *New England Journal of Medicine* 351, no. 17 (October 21, 2004), p. 1707.

[21] Ibid.

[22] "Prescription for Trouble."

[23] Ibid.

[24] Mathews and Martinez, "E-Mails Suggest Merck Knew," p. A10, and "Prescription for Trouble."

[25] Mathews and Martinez, "E-Mails Suggest Merck Knew," p. A10.

[26] "Prescription for Trouble."

[27] Mathews and Martinez, "E-Mails Suggest Merck Knew," p. A10.

[28] Ibid.

[29] Ibid., p. A11.

[30] Debabrata Mukherjee, Steven E. Nissen, and Eric J. Topol, "Risk of Cardiovascular Events Associated with Selected Cox-2 Inhibitors," *Journal of the American Medical Association* 286, no. 8 (August 22, 2001), pp. 954–59.

[31] Mathews and Martinez, "E-Mails Suggest Merck Knew," p. A10.

[32] According to LexisNexis "Mealey Reports," and cited in "Merck's Mess," *Forbes,* November 1, 2004, p. 51.

[33] Mathews and Martinez, "E-Mails Suggest Merck Knew," p. A11.

[34] John Abramson, *Overdosed America: The Broken Promise of American Medicine* (New York: HarperCollins, 2004); and Mathews and Martinez, "E-Mails Suggest Merck Knew," p. A10.

[35] Mathews and Martinez, "E-Mails Suggest Merck Knew," p. A11.

[36] Simons and Stipp, "Will Merck Survive Vioxx?" p. 104.

[37] Peter Jüni, Linda Nartey, Stephan Reichenbach, Rebekka Sterchi, Paul A Dieppe, and Matthias Egger, "Risk of Cardiovascular Events and Rofecoxib: Cumulative Meta-Analysis," *The Lancet* 364, no. 9450 (November 5, 2004), pp. 2021ff.

[38] Phil B. Fontanarosa, Drummond Rennie, and Catherine D. DeAngelis, "Postmarketing Surveillance—Lack of Vigilance, Lack of Trust," *Journal of the American Medical Association* 292, no. 21 (December 1, 2004), p. 2649.

[39] Ibid., p. 2647.

[40] Ibid., p. 2647.

[41] Roger Perloff, "How Bad Will the Lawsuits Get?" *Fortune,* November 1, 2004, p. 97.

[42] Barbara Martinez, "Preparing for Vioxx Suits, Both Sides Seek Friendly Venues," *The Wall Street Journal,* November 17, 2004, p. B1.

[43] Simon and Stipp, "Will Merck Survive Vioxx?" p. 102.

[44] "Prescription for Trouble."

[45] "An Open Letter from Merck," appearing in many newspapers, November 12, 2004.

[46] As quoted in Perloff, "How Bad Will the Lawsuits Get?" p. 96.

Kimpton Hotels: Balancing Strategy and Environmental Sustainability

Murray Silverman
San Francisco State University

Tom Thomas
San Francisco State University

Michael Pace faced a dilemma. He was Kimpton Hotels' West Coast director of operations and environmental programs, general manager of its Villa Florence Hotel in San Francisco, and the main catalyst for implementing its EarthCare program nationally. He was determined to help the boutique hotel chain walk the talk regarding its commitment to environmental responsibility, but he also had agreed not to introduce any new products or processes that would be more expensive than those they replaced. Now that the first phase of the program had been implemented nationwide, he and the company's team of "eco-champions" were facing some difficult challenges with the rollout of the second, more ambitious phase.

For example, the team had to decide whether to recommend the purchase of linens (towels, sheets, pillowcases, etc.) made of organic cotton, which vendors insisted would cost at least 50 percent more than standard linens. It would cost an average of $100,000 to $150,000 to switch out all the linens in each hotel. If Kimpton couldn't negotiate the price down, was there some way it could introduce organic cotton in a limited but meaningful way? All linens are commingled in the laundry, so they can't be introduced one floor at a time. Maybe the company could start with pillowcases—though the sheets wouldn't be organic, guests would be resting their heads on organic cotton. Would it even be worth spending so much on linens? From a public relations perspective,

would it make that much of a difference? Should the company wait and see, phase organic cotton in over time, or drop the idea altogether? Similar issues would arise when the company had to decide whether to recommend environmentally friendly carpeting or furniture.

And then there was recycling. The program had been field-tested at Kimpton hotels in San Francisco, a singular city in one of the most environmentally progressive states in the United States. Now the eco-champions team had to figure out how to make it work in cities like Chicago, which didn't even have a municipal recycling program in place. In Denver, recycling actually cost more than waste disposal to a landfill, due to the low cost of land in eastern Colorado. Pace knew that the environmental initiatives most likely to succeed would be those that could be seamlessly implemented by the general managers and employees of the 39 unique Kimpton hotels around the country. The last thing he wanted to do was to make their jobs more difficult by imposing cookie-cutter standards.

Kimpton had recently embarked on a national campaign to build brand awareness by associating its name with each unique property. Pace knew that the success of Kimpton's strategy would rest heavily on its ability to maintain the care, integrity, and uniqueness that customers had come to associate with its chain of boutique hotels. Other hotel companies had begun investing heavily in the niche that Kimpton had pioneered. To differentiate itself, the company had to continue to find innovative ways to offer services that addressed the needs and values of its customers, and EarthCare was a crucial part of its plans. But could Pace find a way to make it happen within Kimpton's budget, and without adversely affecting the customer experience? Would Kimpton be able to keep the promises made by its new corporate brand?

THE U.S. HOTEL INDUSTRY

By the summer of 2005, the absence of any major terror attacks since September 11, 2001, had encouraged Americans to begin traveling again. Buoyed by a rebound in business travel and continued growth in leisure related spending, the lodging industry had shown steady growth since mid-2003. In 2004, the industry posted impressive gains in room occupancy levels, revenue per available room (REVPAR), and average room rates (see Exhibit 1). In the previous year, demand had been dampened by the outbreak of the war with Iraq and the soft U.S. economy. Industry pretax profit increased in 2004 to $14.5 billion over $12.8 billion in 2003 but was still far below the recent peak of $22.5 billion in 2000.

The U.S. hotel industry was comprised of 55,000 properties and 4.5 million rooms. Its $112 billion in revenues in 2004 included room sales (75 percent), food and beverage sales (18 percent), and miscellaneous such as phone charges and movie rentals (7 percent). Revenues in 2003 were $105 billion. There were many large hotel chains (see Exhibit 2); however, no single lodging company accounted for more than 15 percent of all U.S. hotel rooms. Hotels were segmented into luxury (Four Seasons, Fairmont, Carlton); upscale (Embassy, Sheraton, Radisson, Courtyard); midmarket (Holiday Inn, Ramada, Comfort Inn); and economy (Motel 6, Days Inn, Red Roof). Within the upscale segment there were two strategic niches: (1) boutique hotels in urban areas, which differentiated themselves through unique decor, amenities and service, and (2) bed and breakfasts (B&Bs), which were typically small, independent properties featuring unique settings and decor.

Kimpton Hotels had built a portfolio of unique properties in the upscale segment of the industry and had been credited with inventing the boutique hotel segment in 1981.[1] By 1999, boutique hotels accounted for about 15 percent of San Francisco's estimated 31,000 rooms, according to PKF Consulting. Boutique hotels constituted about 1 percent of the industry nationwide, and the segment was growing. The Starwood Hotel chain entered the segment with its W hotels, and Continental Hotels PLC entered with Hotel Indigo. In San Francisco, Kimpton was the recognized market leader, with 67 percent of the city's boutique hotels. Joie de Vivre Hotels had 20 percent of the local market, and Personality Hotels on Union Square had 12 percent. With 2004 sales of $400 million, up from $350 million in 2003, Kimpton planned to add at least three to five properties per year in major markets such as New York, Boston, Washington, D.C., and Miami.

Approximately 55 percent of hotel customers were individuals attending a business meeting, conference, or group meeting. Foreign travelers contributed significantly to room demand, especially in major cities. Competition for these customers was based on many factors, including price, location, brand loyalty, customer service, and value-added services. It appeared that the industry's earnings recovery had been limited by consumer price shopping on the Internet and by cost pressures driven by rising health care costs, energy costs, and property taxes. Companies were intensifying efforts to win customer loyalty. Efforts included establishing reward

Exhibit 1   **Hotel and Lodging Industry Trends**

	2000	2001	2002	2003	2004
Average room rates	$85.43	$85.35	$83.48	$83.41	$86.70
Occupancy rate	65.3%	61.9%	60.9%	60.8%	63.1%
Average revenue per available room per night*	$55.78	$52.83	$50.84	$50.71	$54.70
Estimated pretax income, industrywide (in billions)	$ 22.5	$ 16.2	$ 14.2	$ 12.8	$ 14.5

*Equal to the average room rate multiplied by the occupancy rate.
Source: Smith Travel Research.

Exhibit 2   **Large Hotel Companies (based on number of affiliated rooms worldwide)**

Company	Major Chains	Number of Properties	Number of Rooms
Cendant Corporation	Days Inn, Ramada (U.S.), Super 8, Howard Johnson, Travel Lodge	6,399	518,435
InterContinental Hotels Group	Holiday Inn, Inter-Continental	3,500	538,000
Marriott International	Marriott, Marriott Courtyard, Residence Inn, Fairfield Inn, Renaissance, Ramada (outside U.S.)	2,753	496,920
Arcor SA	Motel 6, Mercure, Ibis, Novotel, Red Roof Inns, Hotel Sofitel, Formule 1	3,950	455,000
Choice Hotels International	Comfort Inn, Quality Inn, Econo Lodge	4,678	375,859
Hilton Hotels	Hilton (U.S.), Hampton Inns, Doubletree, Embassy Suites, Homewood Suites	2,157	345,141
Best Western International	Best Western	4,105	312,329
Starwood Hotels & Resorts	Sheraton, Westin	736	227,815
Carlson Hospitality Group	Radisson, Country Inns & Suites by Carlson, Regent International Hotels	885	147,000
Hyatt Corporation	Hyatt Regency	121	59,000
Total		29,494	3,498,423

Source: Standard & Poors Industry Surveys, Lodging & Gaming (New York: McGraw-Hill, December 2004).

programs for frequent visitors and targeting a hotel's best customers for direct marketing programs.

The longer-term outlook for the industry seemed positive. U.S. demographic trends were highly favorable. Baby boomers, then in their peak earning years, would be seeking elaborate or expensive vacations. In addition, more and more Americans would be retiring and traveling in their leisure time.

THE GREENING OF THE U.S. HOTEL INDUSTRY

The U.S. hotel industry—with its 4.5 million rooms and its common areas, lobbies, convention rooms, restaurants, laundry facilities, and back offices—had a significant environmental impact. According to the American Hotel and Lodging Association, the average hotel toilet was flushed seven times per day per guest, an average shower was 7.5 minutes long, and 40 percent of bathroom lights were left on as nightlights. A typical hotel used 218 gallons of water per day per occupied room. Energy use was pervasive, including lighting in guest rooms and common areas, heating and air-conditioning, and washing and drying towels and linens. The hotel industry spent $3.7 billion per year on electricity.[2]

Guestrooms generated surprisingly large amounts of waste, ranging from 0.5 pound to 28 pounds per day, and averaging 2 pounds per day per guest. In California, 2 percent of all food waste came from the hotel and lodging industry. A short list of other environmental impacts of the hotel industry included the following:

- Non refillable amenity bottles (shampoos, etc.) generated large amounts of plastic waste.
- Products used to clean bathrooms and furniture contained synthetic additives.

- Paints contained high levels of volatile organic compounds.

- Back-office and front-desk activities generated large amounts of wastepaper.

- Furniture, office equipment, and kitchen and laundry appliances were usually not selected for their environmental advantages.

Opportunities for reducing a hotel's environmental footprint were plentiful, and many could yield bottom-line savings. Reduced laundering of linens, at customer discretion, had already been adopted enthusiastically across the spectrum of budget to luxury hotels, to the point that 38 percent of hotels had linen reuse programs. Low-flow showerheads could deliver the same quality shower experience using half the water of a conventional showerhead. Faucet aerators also could cut the water requirements by 50 percent. A 13-watt compact fluorescent bulb gave the same light as a 60-watt incandescent, lasted about 10 times longer, and used about 70 percent less energy. Waste costs also could be significantly reduced. For many hotels, 50–80 percent of their solid waste stream was compostable, and a significant part of the remaining waste was recyclables such as paper, aluminum, and glass.

Fairmont Hotels & Resorts, a Canadian-based hotel chain, had generated considerable savings since implementing its environmental programs in the early 1990s. While concern for the environment drove Fairmont's program, many of its initiatives resulted in bottom-line benefits. Examples of the types of environmental initiatives and their associated savings at the Fairmont Hotels & Resorts are listed in Exhibit 3. Fairmont Hotels also pursued initiatives and made investments that did not produce readily apparent bottom-line benefits. For example, one of its hotels purchased 20 percent of their energy as renewable energy (solar, wind, and hydro) even though the cost was higher. The company supported the expense of a corporate office of environmental affairs and a manager of environmental affairs. It also financially supported efforts related to habitat restoration and preservation of endangered species.[3]

In addition to bottom-line savings, environmental programs held the potential to generate new business. Governmental bodies, nongovernmental organizations, corporations, and convention/meeting planners were showing increased interest in selecting hotels using environmental criteria. California had recently launched its Green Lodging Program (GLP). State employees were encouraged to select from the GLP's list of certified hotels. The state's $70 million annual travel budget was an incentive for hotels to be certified by the program. The criteria for certification included recycling, composting, energy- and water-efficient fixtures and lighting, and nontoxic or less toxic alternatives for cleaning supplies. State governments in Pennsylvania, Florida, Vermont, and Virginia also had developed green lodging programs.

Exhibit 3 **A Sampling of Fairmont Hotels & Resorts' Environmental Cost-Saving Initiatives**

- The Fairmont Royal York Hotel in Toronto recycled over 212,000 pounds of cardboard and paper annually, saving 2,025 trees and $79,000 in landfill fees.

- Prior to establishing a recycling program for kitchen grease, the Fairmont Winnepeg spent over $1 million to have its sewer system cleared of kitchen grease buildup. Kitchen grease was now picked up and recycled free of charge.

- The breakfast buffet at Fairmont Tremblant eliminated individual servings of jams in 22-milliliter glass jars. Instead, the kitchen prepared seven varieties of homemade jams and served them in large attractive jars with serving spoons. With over 49,500 breakfasts served annually, the restaurant saved over $19,000 per year.

- The Fairmont Royal York had over 34,000 light fixtures. The hotel switched 1,920 bulbs in the guest bathrooms and 5,500 bulbs in the guestrooms from incandescent to compact fluorescent bulbs, saving $57,135 annually. In public areas and staircases, over 773 bulbs had been switched, generating additional savings of $23,095 per year.

- The staff at the Fairmont Hotel Vancouver separated organic waste (from room service, meetings, and conference meals) from its regular waste stream. The organic waste was picked up from the hotel (free of charge) and used to make a rich organic fertilizer. This produced a 50 percent reduction in landfill wastes and an annual savings of $11,000.

Source: Fairmont Hotels & Resorts, *The Green Partnership Guide*, 2nd ed., 2001.

CERES, a well-respected environmental nonprofit organization, had developed the Green Hotel Initiative, designed to increase and demonstrate demand for environmentally responsible hotel services. Some major corporations endorsed the initiative, including Ford Motor Company, General Motors, Nike, American Airlines, and Coca-Cola. The Coalition for Environmentally Responsible Conventions (CERC) and the Green Meetings Industry Council were encouraging meeting planners to "green" their events by, among other things, choosing environmentally friendly hotels for lodging and meeting sites. This trend toward booking lodging and meeting sites based on green criteria was in its very early stages. Industry insiders believed that environmentally driven demand was extremely limited at this point, and the ultimate impact of this movement was uncertain.

Environmental progress in the U.S. hotel industry had been limited. With a few exceptions, most hotels were doing little beyond pursuing the low-hanging fruit, in the form of easy-to-implement cost-saving initiatives. Those hotels had been reducing their environmental footprint as a welcome consequence of their cost-cutting efforts, but they were not necessarily committed to a comprehensive environmental program. During a 1998 effort by Cornell University's School of Hotel Administration to identify hotels employing environmental best practices, researchers were "surprised by the dearth of nominations." The four U.S. hotels selected as champions—Colony Hotel, Hotel Bel Air, Hyatt Regency Chicago, and Hyatt Regency Scottsdale— were primarily focused on cost savings in energy and waste streams.[4] In contrast to those in the United States, hotels in Canada and Europe seemed to be embracing the hotel greening process, as exemplified by the Fairmont Hotel & Resorts' effort to institutionalize innovative approaches to reducing its environmental footprint throughout its operations.

KIMPTON'S BUSINESS PHILOSOPHY AND STRATEGY

Kimpton Hotels was founded in 1981 by Bill Kimpton, who once said, "No matter how much money people have to spend on big, fancy hotels, they're still intimidated and unsettled when they arrive. So the psychology of how you build hotels and restaurants is very important. You put a fireplace in the lobby and create a warm, friendly restaurant, and the guest will feel at home." By 2005, Kimpton had grown to include 39 hotels throughout North America and Canada, each one designed to create a unique and exceptional guest experience (see Exhibit 4). Every hotel lobby had a cozy fireplace and plush sitting area, where complimentary coffee was served every morning, and wine every evening. Guest rooms were stylishly decorated and comfortably furnished, offering amenities such as specialty suites that included Tall Rooms and Yoga Rooms. Every room offered high-speed wireless Internet access and desks with ample lighting. Rather than rewarding customer loyalty with a point program, Kimpton offered customization and personalization. "We record the preferences of our loyal guests," said Mike Depatie, Kimpton's CEO of real estate, "Someone may want a jogging magazine and a Diet Coke when they arrive. We can get that done."

Business travel (group and individual) accounted for approximately 65 percent of Kimpton's revenues, and leisure travel (tour group and individual) the other 35 percent. The selection of hotels for business meetings and conferences was through meeting and conference organizers. Around 35 percent of all rooms were booked through the company's call center, 25 percent through travel agents, and 25 percent through the company's Web site; the remainder of customers "came in off the street." The Internet portion of Kimpton's business continued to grow, but the company didn't cater to buyers looking for the steal of the century. Rather, Kimpton was increasingly being discovered by the 25 percent of the customer pool that market researchers called "unchained seekers," many of whom used the Internet to search for unique accommodations that matched their particular needs or values.

Steve Pinetti, senior vice president for sales and marketing, noted, "If I were to drive a customer to the airport after their stay and ask them what their experience was like, the right answer would be, 'It felt great.' They don't have to know why, it could be the bed, the room, the wine, or the friendly employees. The next time they want to book a room, though, they'll come to us." Kimpton's REVPAR tended to meet or exceed norms within its upscale segment, due primarily to its relatively high occupancy rates. Occupancy rates rose to 68 percent in the fourth quarter of 2004, up from 63 percent during the same

Exhibit 4   **List of Kimpton Hotels**

	Style/Theme	Rooms	Year
Aspen, Colorado			
• Sky Hotel	Play & Action	90	2001
Boston, Massachusetts			
• Onyx Hotel	Emerging Art	112	2004
Cambridge, Massachusetts			
• Hotel Marlowe	Discovery	236	2003
Chicago, Illinois			
• Hotel Allegro Chicago	Be a Star	483	1998
• Hotel Monaco Chicago	Indulge Your Senses via Body, Mind & Soul	192	1998
• Burnham Hotel	Architecture	122	1999
Cupertino, California			
• Cypress Hotel	Good Life: Body, Mind & Soul	224	2002
Denver, Colorado			
• Hotel Monaco Denver	Adventure	189	1998
Miami			
• Mayfair Hotel & Spa	Tranquility and Sensuality	179	2005
New Orleans, Louisiana			
• Hotel Monaco New Orleans	Indulge Your Senses via Exotic Pleasures	250	2001
New York, New York			
• 70 Park Avenue Hotel	Private Residence	205	2004
Portland, Oregon			
• Hotel Vintage Plaza	Italian Romance	107	1992
• Fifth Avenue Suites Hotel	Patron of the Arts	221	1996
Salt Lake City			
• Hotel Monaco Salt Lake City	Indulge Your Senses via Guilty Pleasures	225	1999
San Diego, California			
• Solamar	Art Lies Within	235	2005
San Francisco, California			
• Villa Florence Hotel	Celebration of Italy	183	1986
• Monticello Inn	Literary	91	1987
• Prescott Hotel	Private Residence	164	1989
• Tuscan Inn	Family	221	1990
• Harbor Court Hotel	Energy & Well-being	131	1991
• Hotel Triton	Art, Music and Eco	140	1991
• Sir Francis Drake Hotel	Classic San Francisco	417	1994
• Hotel Monaco San Francisco	Sophisticated World Travel	201	1995
• Serrano Hotel	Fun & Games	236	1999
• Palomar Hotel	Art in Motion	198	1999
• Argonaut Hotel	Adventure	252	2003

(Continued)

Exhibit 4   **Continued**

	Style/Theme	Rooms	Year
Seattle, Washington			
• Alexis Hotel	Art of Living	109	1992
• Hotel Vintage Park	Washington Wine	126	1992
• Hotel Monaco Seattle	Animals	189	1997
Tacoma, Washington			
• Sheraton Tacoma Hotel	Business, conference center	319	1984
Vancouver, British Columbia			
• Pacific Palisades	Fun, Fresh and in the Now	233	2000
Washington, D.C.			
• Hotel Rouge	Playful Interactions	137	2001
• Topaz Hotel	Wellness	99	2001
• Hotel Monaco DC	Indulge Your Senses	184	2002
• Hotel Madera	Home Away From Home	86	2002
• Hotel Helix	Your 15 Minutes	178	2002
• Hotel George	George Washington w/contemporary flair	139	2003
Whistler, British Columbia			
• Summit Lodge	Romance, premier ski resort	81	2000

quarter in 2003. REVPAR during the same period rose from $87 to $102.[5]

Historically, Kimpton prospered by purchasing and renovating buildings at a discount in strategic nationwide locations that were appropriate for its niche segment. The hotel industry in general had been slow to enter the boutique niche, and Kimpton enjoyed a substantial edge in experience in developing value-added services for guests. "All hotels are starting to look alike and act alike, and we are the counterpoint, the contrarians," said Tom LaTour, Kimpton president and CEO. "We don't look like the brands, we don't act like the brands, and as the baby boomers move through the age wave, they will seek differentiated, experience-oriented products."

Kimpton's top executives took pride in their ability to recognize and develop both undervalued properties and undervalued people. Kimpton's hotel general managers were often refugees from large branded companies who did not thrive under hierarchical, standardized corporate structures. At Kimpton, they were afforded a great deal of autonomy, subject only to the constraints of customer service standards and capital and operating budgets.

This sense of autonomy and personal responsibility was conveyed down through the ranks to all 5,000 Kimpton employees. Kimpton's flexible corporate structure avoided hierarchy, preferring a circular structure where executives and employees were in constant communication.[6] Steve Pinetti liked to tell the story of a new parking attendant who had to figure out how to deal with a guest who felt that he had not been adequately informed of extra charges for parking his car at the hotel. The attendant decided on the spot to reduce the charges and asked the front desk to make the necessary adjustments. He had heard his general manager tell employees that they should feel empowered to take responsibility for making guests happy, but he fully expected to be grilled by his general manager, at the very least, about his actions. A sense of dread took hold as he was called to the front of the room at a staff meeting the very next day, but it dissipated quickly when his general manager handed him a special award for his initiative.

ESTABLISHING THE KIMPTON BRAND

While Kimpton was known for designing hotels that reflected the energy and personality of its distinct locations, by 2004 the company's top executives realized that uniting its hotel portfolio under a single recognizable brand could add considerable value. Cross-selling of hotel rooms in different cities, for instance, would be easier for salespeople handling corporate accounts if the properties all shared the Kimpton name. So the company launched what it called the Lifestyle Hotel Collection, with the theme "Every Hotel Tells a Story." One aspect of the branding effort was to add the Kimpton name to each property, as in Hotel Monoco San Francisco, a Kimpton Hotel. According to CEO LaTour, "We think of our hotels as a family, all having their own first names and sharing the last name Kimpton. We are ready to tell the world the Kimpton story."[7]

The distinctive value proposition associated with the Kimpton brand guaranteed the customer a unique and satisfying experience along five different dimensions, what the company referred to as Care, Comfort, Style, Flavor, and Fun:

- *Care*—Just as Kimpton treated its guests with a strong dose of friendly personal attention and tender loving care, its culture also emphasized concern and responsibility for the communities in which it did business, and the people it employed. Each hotel's general manager and staff expressed this sense of care by engaging in their own forms of community outreach, employee diversity, and environmental quality initiatives.

- *Comfort*—Kimpton focused intently on making its guests feel comfortable, their plush rooms and intimate public spaces providing a home away from home. It kept overhead costs in check by limiting the range of services it provided, forgoing the gyms, spas, swimming pools, and other space-hungry amenities that larger chains regularly offered.

- *Style*—No two Kimpton hotels were alike. Each attempted to draw on the distinctive character of the city and neighborhood in which it was located. Interiors tended to be upscale and stylish rather than opulent or ornate.

- *Flavor*—The restaurants located in each hotel were designed to stand on their own, catering to local clientele rather than rely on hotel guests for the bulk of their business.

- *Fun*—Employees were encouraged to bring their personalities to work, and to make sure that guests enjoyed their stay. According to Mike Depatie, "We don't try to make people Kimpton people. We want them to express the best of what they are."

An important part of Kimpton's story was its long-standing commitment to social responsibility. Staff at each hotel had always been encouraged to engage with local community nonprofits that benefited the arts, education, the underprivileged, and other charitable causes. Kimpton maintained these local programs even in periods of falling occupancy rates and industry downturns. These local efforts evolved into the companywide Kimpton Cares program in 2004, as part of the company's corporate branding effort, expanding its social and environmental commitments to the national and global arenas. At the national level, Kimpton supported the National AIDS Fund's Red Ribbon Campaign and a program called Dress for Success (which assisted economically disadvantaged women struggling to enter the workforce) by allotting a share of a guest's room fee to the charity. At the global level, Kimpton embarked in a partnership with Trust for Public Land (TPL), a nonprofit dedicated to the preservation of land for public use. In July 2005, Kimpton committed to raising $15,000 from its total room revenues to introduce the TPL's Parks for People program, and created eco-related fund-raising events in each of its cities to further support the campaign. Kimpton's EarthCare program was designed to be instituted through a comprehensive environmental program rolled out to all of Kimpton's hotels. "As business leaders, we believe we have a responsibility to positively impact the communities we live in, to be conscious about our environment and to make a difference where we can," said Niki Leondakis, Kimpton's chief operating officer.

Kimpton's top executives considered the Kimpton Cares program, and its EarthCare component, essential parts of the company's branding effort. Steve Pinetti noted, "What drove it was our belief that our brand needs to stand for something. What do we want to stand for in the community? We want to draw a line in the sand. We also want our impact to be felt as far and wide as it can. Hopefully, through our good deeds, we'll be able to influence other companies."

The early evidence suggested that the branding effort also had financial payoffs. Kimpton was receiving significant public relations coverage of its EarthCare program in local newspapers and travel publications. According to Pinetti, "The number of people who visit our Kimpton Web site has tripled in the year since we began the branding effort. Membership in the company's 'InTouch' guest loyalty program, which markets to previous guests via e-mail, rose from 86,000 in the 1st quarter of 2004 to 112,000 in the 4th quarter."[8] Consumer surveys showed big gains in awareness that each hotel is part of a bigger organization, with properties in other cities." As for the firm's Kimpton Cares program and its new EarthCare initiative, anecdotal evidence pointed to top-line benefits. "We've booked almost half a million dollars in meetings from a couple of corporations in Chicago because of our ecological reputation," said Pinetti. "Their reps basically told us, 'Your values align with our values, and we want to spend money on hotels that think the way we do.' " Kimpton believed that companies that identified with being socially responsible would look for partners like Kimpton that shared those values, and that certifications like the California Green Lodging program would attract both individuals and corporate clientele.

However, Pinetti noted, "The cost-effectiveness wasn't clear when we started. I thought we might get some business out of this, but that's not why we did it. We think it's the right thing to do, and it generates a lot of enthusiasm among our employees." Kimpton's real estate CEO, Mike Depatie, believed that incorporating care for communities and the environment into the company's brand had been a boon to hiring: "We attract and keep employees because they feel that from a values standpoint, we have a corporate culture and value system that's consistent with theirs. They feel passionate about working here." While the hotel industry was plagued with high turnover, Kimpton's turnover rates were lower than the national averages.

THE HOTEL TRITON

Kimpton's environmental consciousness reached back to 1985, when the company introduced the Galleria Park Hotel in San Francisco as an urban retreat with an open-space "park" within the hotel. In 1995, Kimpton's commitment picked up steam as it converted an entire floor of the 140-room Triton Hotel in San Francisco into an "eco-floor." With assistance from Green Suites International, a supplier of environmental solutions for the lodging industry, the Triton introduced the following initiatives in the 24 rooms on its eco-floor:

- Energy-efficient lighting solutions, including compact fluorescent bulbs and sensor nightlights (cutting energy costs by 75 percent).
- Bathroom amenity dispensers using biodegradable hypoallergenic soaps, lotions, and shampoos.
- Programmable digital thermostats to control guestroom energy consumption.
- Low-flow/high-pressure showerheads and sink aerators, and toilets that reduced water use.
- A linen and towel reuse program.
- Nontoxic, nonallergenic, all-natural cleaning products.
- Facial and bathroom tissues made from 100 percent recycled materials with at least 30 percent postconsumer wastepaper.
- Recycling receptacles.
- Bedding and bath towels made from organically grown cotton. (On average, 1.5 pounds of agricultural chemicals were used to produce the conventionally grown cotton in a single set of queen-size sheets.)
- Water filters to improve water quality and air filters to improve air quality.
- Low-volatile-organic-compound (VOC) paints used to paint walls and ceilings.

For Michael Pace, the sustainability lightbulb came on when he was general manager of the Monticello Hotel, prior to taking over as general manager of the Triton. At first, his interest was piqued by recycling efforts at the Monticello. But one day, he said, "I had a personal epiphany, where I realized how lucky I am. I'm living the American Dream, and I pass by a dozen homeless people on my way to work every day. I just realized that I wanted to do more than focus on myself and my job. The more I got involved, the more I saw the positive impact these efforts could have."

When Pace became general manager of the Triton in 2003, he felt that the eco-floor concept should be expanded throughout the Triton hotel's rooms and common areas. He immediately began to institute most of the eco-floor initiatives in the hotel's other guestrooms. He worked closely with the hotel staff to sort the hotel's entire waste stream and was able to reduce waste-hauling expenses from $2,200 to $600 per month.

As a result of Pace's conservation efforts, in 1994, the Triton was recognized as one of four properties in Northern California to qualify at the

Leadership Level for the State's new Green Lodging program. More important, the Triton was ready to serve as the template for the EarthCare program and the rest of Kimpton's hotels.

PLANNING THE EARTHCARE PROGRAM ROLLOUT CAMPAIGN

Pinetti and Pace realized that they were too busy to handle all the planning and operational details of the national rollout, so they turned to Jeff Slye, of Business Evolution Consulting, for help. Slye was a process management consultant who wanted to help small and medium-sized business owners figure out how to "ecofy" their companies. He knew that entrepreneurs were typically far too busy to do much about the resources they didn't like to overuse, and the waste they didn't like to generate. He had heard that Kimpton was trying to figure out how to make its operations greener and integrate this effort into its branding. When they first met in October 2004, Pinetti and Pace handed Slye a 10-page document detailing their objectives and a plan for rolling out the initiative in phases. Kimpton's program was to have the following eco-mission statement:

> Lead the hospitality industry in supporting a sustainable world by continuing to deliver a premium guest experience through non-intrusive, high quality, eco-friendly products and services.
>
> Our mission is built upon a companywide commitment towards water conservation; reduction of energy usage; elimination of harmful toxins and pollutants; recycling of all reusable waste; building and furnishing hotels with sustainable materials; and purchasing goods and services that directly support these principles.

Slye worked with Pinetti and Pace to fill various gaps in their plan and develop an "ecostandards program," a concise report outlining a strategy for greening the products and operational processes that Kimpton used to deliver a superior experience to its guests. In December 2004, Pinetti asked Slye to present the report to Kimpton's chief operating officer, Niki Leondakis. Leondakis greeted the proposal enthusiastically, but noted that it needed an additional component: a strategy for communicating the program both internally (to management

and staff) and externally (to guests, investors, and the press). As important as these external audiences were, Slye knew that the internal communications strategy would be particularly crucial, given the autonomy afforded each Kimpton hotel, each with its own set of local initiatives. Getting everyone on board would require a strategy that respected that aspect of Kimpton's culture. Slye kept that in mind as he worked with Pace to draft a communications strategy.

They decided to create an ad hoc "eco-champions" network throughout the company. The national "lead" (Pace) and "co-lead" (Pinetti) would head up the communications effort and would be accountable for its success. Each of five geographic regions (Pacific Northwest; San Francisco Bay Area; Central United States; Washington, D.C.; and Northeast/Southeast), covering six or seven hotel properties, would also have a lead and co-lead who would help communicate the program to employees, and be the local point-person in the chain of command. One of their key roles would be to solicit employee suggestions regarding ways to make products and processes greener.

In addition, a team of national eco-product specialists (EPSs) would be key components of the network. These specialists would be responsible for soliciting staff input and identifying and evaluating greener products as potential substitutes for existing ones. Products would be tested for effectiveness and evaluated on the basis of their environmental benefits, effect on guest perceptions, potential marketing value, and cost. Pinetti and Pace determined that specialists would be needed initially for six product categories: beverages, cleaning agents, office supplies, engineering, information technology, and room supplies.

Pinetti and Pace knew that the various regional leads and national product specialists would have to be selected carefully. The program's success would depend largely on the enthusiasm and capability that team members would bring to the task. They faced a dilemma: Ask for volunteers, or handpick preferred candidates? They decided to identify likely candidates and invite them to participate, an approach made possible by Kimpton's tractable size and intimate culture. As they anticipated, everyone they approached responded enthusiastically and volunteered on the spot.

Meanwhile, Pace and Pinetti asked all general managers to report on their existing environmental initiatives, to get baseline feedback on what individual hotels were doing already. They turned the results into a matrix they could use to identify gaps and monitor progress for each hotel.

They also sent out to all Kimpton directors of operations (regional managers) a briefing that laid out the communications strategy, including the mission statement, a description of the new eco-champions network, an overview of the phased roll-out of products and processes (see Exhibit 5), and a "talking points" document that explained to employees the benefits of the new program (see Exhibit 6).

NATIONAL ROLLOUT OF THE EARTHCARE PROGRAM

By February 2005, Kimpton's new network of eco-champions was in place, and everyone had agreed on the two basic ground rules for the transition: New

initiatives couldn't cost more than what was already budgeted for operations and capital improvements, and they couldn't adversely affect customer perceptions or satisfaction. The ground rules also mandated that any new product or service could not cost more than the product or service it replaced. All leads, co-leads, and product specialists began meeting via conference call every Friday morning to discuss the greening initiative and share accounts of employee suggestions, progress achieved, and barriers encountered. One revelation that emerged early in the process was that, due to the uniqueness of each hotel and autonomous nature of the organization, all plans and proposals would have to be presented in a clear, concise package in order to ensure effective implementation.

To help communicate the program's goals and achievements, and help motivate employees seeking recognition, the team began to post regular updates and success stories in Kimpton's internal weekly newsletter, *The Word*, which was distributed throughout the organization and read by all general

Exhibit 5   **Rollout of Kimpton's EarthCare Program**

Phase I:

Phase I initiatives are designed to make hotel staff comfortable with the concept of greener management by introducing non-disruptive and cost-reducing operational practices.

- Recycling program ("Back of house")—Bottles, cans, paper, cardboard.
- Cleaning chemicals—Tub & tile cleaners, glass cleaners, deoderizers, and disinfectants all have to be switched to non-toxic, natural products.
- Promotional materials printed on recycled paper, using soy-based inks.
- Complimentary coffee served in lobbies every morning must be organically grown.
- Towel/linen reuse—Sheets and towels are replaced only at guest's request.

Phase II:

Hotels that successfully complete their implementation of Phase I initiatives will then move to Phase II, which focuses on investments in water and energy conservation, organically-grown cottons, and extending Phase I initiatives.

- Water conservation—Install 2.0 GPM sink aerators, 2.5 GPM showerheads, and phase in 1.6 GPF toilets.
- Energy conservation—Install motion sensors in rooms, fluorescent bulbs in corridors and back-of-house.
- Use recycled content paper for copying and notepads back-of-house, toilet paper and tissues in-room.
- Serve organic coffee in rooms and meeting rooms, organic tea in lobby.
- Switch to organic linens and towels, if feasible.

Phase III:

The most fundamental changes are anticipated when hotels are renovated and new hotels are acquired and converted. In addition to implementing Phases I and II, this will require extensive investment in building materials, labor, and appliances. The good news is that rooms can be designed, rather than retrofitted, to be more energy efficient, and green building materials can be ordered in larger quantities, thus lowering costs.

- Install only Energy Star rated appliances, computers, and electronic.
- Use only low-VOC paints.
- Install energy efficient lighting, heating, and air conditioning.

Exhibit 6   **Internal Talking Points Document**

Quick Facts on the Difference You Will Make . . .

Printing on 35% post consumer recycled paper: Kimpton will save:

- 24,000 pounds (12 tons) of wood
- 3,720 pounds (1.75 tons) of solid waste
- 7,260 pounds (3.6 tons) of CO_2 emissions
- 58,230,000 BTUs of total energy
  (Assumes 30 hotels participate using 1 case/5,000 sheets per month)

Using Green/Eco friendly cleaning products: Kimpton will:

- Improve worker productivity by between 0.5 percent and 5 percent by reducing cleaning supply toxins (U.S. institutions spend more than $75 million a year on medical expenses and lost time wages due to chemical-related injuries).
- Reduce environmental pollution as traditional cleaning products are responsible for approximately 8% of total non-vehicular emissions of volatile organic compounds (VOCs).

Recycling waste: Recycling 50% of hotel waste Kimpton properties will:

- Save over $250,000 per year in waste disposal costs.
- Reduce unnecessary landfill waste by over 100,000 gallons per year.
  (Assumes 30 hotels participate)

Recycling glass: Recycling 100 glass bottles/month, Kimpton will:

- Save the equivalent of powering one hundred 100-watt light bulbs for 1,440 hours (60 days).

Recycling aluminum: Recycling 20 Aluminum cans/day, Kimpton will:

- Save the equivalent of nearly 1,500 gallons of gas—enough to run a car for nearly three years.

managers. They also ran an EarthCare contest to further galvanize interest, which generated over 70 entries for categories such as "Best Eco-Practice Suggestion," "Most EarthCare Best Practices Adopted," and "Best Art and Humor Depicting EarthCare."

Potential benefits of the program became clear when the team of eco-product specialists began researching the availability of nontoxic cleaning agents. Common cleaning products such as furniture polish, carpet cleaner, spot remover, air fresheners, disinfectants and bleach can contain hazardous compounds such as toluene, naphthalene, trichloroethylene, benzene and nitrobenzene, phenol, chlorine, and xylene. These and other hazardous ingredients found in many cleaning products are associated with human health concerns including cancer, reproductive disorders, respiratory ailments, and eye or skin irritation. An EPA-funded study by the Western Regional Pollution Prevention Network found that 41 percent of all standard cleaning products they tested were potentially hazardous to the health of individuals using them. Cleaning chemicals could also include ozone-depleting substances and toxic materials that can accumulate in the environment and harm plant and animal life. The health

and environmental consequences for Kimpton were substantial, as one of its suppliers (Sierra Environmental) estimated that every housekeeping worker handled 60 pounds of cleaning agents per year. With an average of 15 room cleaners, times 39 hotels, it added up.

The eco-specialists learned that one of Kimpton's incumbent vendors did have a Green Seal–certified nontoxic line, but the products were selling at a 10–15 percent premium over standard products. They discovered that virtually every product they were interested in was more expensive than those currently used. At the extreme, eco-friendly paper products were priced 50 percent above standard products.

The eco-specialists knew that this would not satisfy the imperative that the greening initiative should not increase operating costs. Determined, they just kept going back to the vendors and asking them to keep working on it until they could supply a greener product of the same quality at the same, or lower, price. Eventually, existing or new vendors were able to meet these criteria, and now the typical hotel used eco-friendly products such as organic coffee and tea, air fresheners, and cleaning agents at no extra cost, and saved thousands of dollars a month by recycling waste materials that were previously shipped to landfills.

By 2005, the Internet had become a popular supply channel, with BuyEfficent.com emerging as the major online catalog from which hotels purchased their products. Assisting the eco-product specialists, consultant Jeff Slye discovered that it could be a nightmare getting the Web site to add new eco-vendors; more than once he had to personally obtain and supply vendor and product codes in order to purchase greener products through the site. While efforts such as these were time-consuming, part of the long-term payoff for the company and its eco-champions was knowing that they'd made it easier for the entire industry to follow in their footsteps.

The team of eco-champions also quickly learned that the national roll-out effort would have its share of potential operational risks and challenges which would need to be addressed. Among them:

- *Resistance by general managers to centralized imperatives*—Kimpton's culture of uniqueness and autonomy might be threatened by a green management program mandated by corporate headquarters. General managers might chafe at what they saw as corporate intrusion on their autonomy. They might see it as just the first step in a trend that would ultimately lead to centralization of the firm as a result of its rebranding effort. Local vendors and distributors might not offer green products. Search and acquisition costs might increase if general managers had to work with a broader range of vendors.

- *Resistance by hotel staff to new products and procedures*—Kimpton's relatively low turnover meant that some employees had been working there for many years, and had become accustomed to familiar ways of doing things. (Informal queries by management, for example, revealed that many cleaning staff equated strong chemical odors with cleanliness.) Also, many of the service staff did not speak English fluently and potentially had difficulty understanding and accepting management's rationales for switching to new procedures or greener cleaning products.

- *Few tangible benefits, a slow payback period, or a low rate of return*—Unless informed, guests would not be aware that their rooms had been painted with low-VOC paints. Likewise, organic cottons were not likely to feel or look

superior to traditional materials. The gains in operating costs achieved by installing longer-life and more energy-efficient fluorescent lighting could take years to pay off, while higher acquisition costs could inflate short-term expenses. The same logic applied to water conservation investments. Would general managers be around to enjoy the benefits? Would corporate executives and investors be patient? What if consumer tastes or Kimpton's branding strategies changed before investments had paid off?

- *Investments that exceeded existing budgets or failed to meet the cost parity criterion*—Linens and towels made from organic cotton could cost at least 50 percent more than conventional products, and the initial cost of converting an average Kimpton hotel to organic cotton linens would run between $100,000 and $150,000. Other environmentally friendly products, such as environmentally friendly carpeting and draperies and sustainable flooring, would also have a price premium. Would additional budget be provided? Would savings in other areas be allowed to pay for it?

- *Marketing challenges*—How should the Earth-Care program be promoted, given customer concerns regarding the impact of some environmental initiatives on the quality of their guest experience? Guests might be concerned, for example, about whether low-flow showerheads or fluorescent lighting would meet their expectations. Environmental awareness and concern varied considerably by geographic region, from very high on the West Coast and in the Northeast, to considerably lower in the South and Midwest. Would this affect customer perceptions and demand? Would the program affect the quality rating of Kimpton's hotels? According to the American Automobile Association's Diamond Rating Guidelines, some water-saving showerheads and energy-saving lightbulbs could lower a hotel's diamond rating.[9] Eventually, information about the EarthCare program was to be disseminated through Kimpton's Web site, guest directory, and sales brochures that would go to travel agents, corporate travel planners, and meeting planners. Should the program be marketed more aggressively?

- *Regional differences in recycling infrastructure and regulatory environment*—California had a mandated recycling program requiring

70 percent recycling of solid waste by 2007, so San Francisco's disposal service provided free recycling containers. Other localities might not be so generous.

Even in the face of these challenges, Kimpton executives believed that the EarthCare program was the smart, as well as the right, thing to do. According to Tom LaTour, chairman and CEO:

> It's good business. It's not just because we're altruistic, it's good for business. Otherwise the investors would say, what are you guys doing? A lot of people think it's going to cost more. It's actually advantageous to be eco-friendly than not.

Niki Leondakis, chief operating officer, saw the program's impact on marketing and employee retention:

> Many people say we're heading toward a tipping point: If you're not environmentally conscious, your company will be blackballed from people's choices. Also, employees today want to come to work every day not just for the paycheck but to feel good about

what they're doing. . . . It's very important to them to be aligned with the values of the people they work for, so from the employee retention standpoint, this helps us retain and attract them so we can select from the best and the brightest.[10]

Investors appeared to be happy with Kimpton's efforts to manage their properties in a more sustainable manner, as the firm announced a new round of financing in June 2005. Private investors poured $157 million into the company for a new wave of expansion and renovation. Yale University put up most of the funds, making an investment valued at close to 1 percent of its $12.7 billion endowment.

By July 2005, Phase I of the EarthCare initiative had been successfully implemented at all Kimpton hotels. The percentage of waste materials recycled at its hotels in San Francisco had gone from 10–20 percent to over 50 percent (by volume) since the program's inception. Chemical cleaning agents were no longer used in any of Kimpton's hotel rooms. Every hotel served organic coffee in its lobby and printed promotional materials on recycled paper with soy-based ink. The challenges of Phase II lay ahead.

Endnotes

[1]Gene Sloan, "Let the Pillowfights Begin," *USA Today,* August 27, 2004.

[2]California Green Lodging Program, www. Ciwmb.ca.gov/epp.

[3]Fairmont Hotels & Resorts, *The Green Partnership Guide,* 2nd ed., 2001.

[4]Cathy A. Enz, and Judy A. Siguaw, "Best Hotel Environmental Practices," *Cornell Hotel and Restaurant Administartion Quarterly,* October 1999.

[5]Robyn Parets, National Real Estate Investor, www.nreionline.com, March 2005.

[6]Liz French, Americanexecutive.com, December 2004.

[7]"Boutique Meets Lifestyle as Kimpton Hotels Let the Secret Out with Launch of National Brand Campaign," Kimpton Hotels press release.

[8]Ryan Tate, "Kimpton Hotels Remakes Its Beds," *San Francisco Business Times,* January 28, 2005.

[9]*AAA Lodging Requirements & Diamond Rating Guidelines* (Heathrow, FL: AAA Publishing, June 2001).

[10]Carlo Wolff, "Environmental Evangelism: Kimpton Walks the Eco-Walk," *Lodging Hospitality,* March 1, 2005.

Monsanto and the Genetic Engineering of Agricultural Seeds

Lisa Johnson
The University of Puget Sound

"This field's planted in mustard. That field's planted in oats," Percy Schmeiser explained on the windy summer 2005 day. "We can't plant canola anymore, on account of the volunteer plants. Our entire fields are contaminated with Monsanto's patent, so we just don't grow that anymore." As Schmeiser gazed over his fields in central Saskatchewan, he continued, "I remember in 1947 when a chemical representative came out here and met with my father. I was right there in that meeting. He told us if we would use his chemical herbicide, why, we'd never have to worry about weeds again. Those were in the days when chemical farming was just unheard of, and we all farmed using the traditional knowledge that had been accumulated over the years. No one needed chemicals. Today, our fields are so saturated with chemicals that a field requires a fair bit of preparatory work before it is even suitable for planting from year to year."

Schmiser continued: "With the introduction of genetically modified crops, Monsanto tells the young farmers when to spray, what to spray, what to plant, when to plant. The younger generation doesn't know anything of the farming methods of their fathers. There's a young farmer in this community who follows Monsanto's instructions and I said to him, 'Your father was one of the best farmers that this province had ever seen. Why don't you just follow

what you learned from him?' He doesn't know how to answer that. I asked him, 'Does Monsanto also tell you when it's going to rain?' He didn't like that comment too much." Percy chuckled.[1]

While Percy Schmeiser checked on his fields, Monsanto Company's legal department was wrestling with another suspected case of patent infringement. The company, which was a leading producer of genetically engineered agricultural products with 2005 revenues of approximately $6.3 billion, was highly committed to protecting its patents. The company's managers believed that farmers who had paid a technology fee for the use of patented products expected Monsanto to prevent other farmers from growing crops from Monsanto seeds without paying a fee. Even though there were cases of farmers deliberately acquiring and growing patented genetically modified organisms (GMOs) without paying a technology fee, there were unintentional natural causes of farmers improperly possessing patented Monsanto plants. Studies had shown that seeds from some types of patented plants could drift as far as 13 miles in heavy winds. In addition, some legal scholars had suggested that the existence of stray seeds constituted trespass or negligence on the part of the patent holder.

The decision to sue farmers was not taken lightly. "It is . . . [an] uncomfortable [position] for us," said Scott Baucum, Monsanto's chief intellectual property protector. "They are our customers, and they are important to us."[2] With 70 percent of all processed food in the United States being grown from genetically engineered plants and the percentage increasing each year, it seemed that Baucum and other chief managers at Monsanto would be forced to either pursue patent infringement cases on an increasingly regular basis or develop less aggressive patent protection measures.

PLANT HUSBANDRY: A BRIEF PRIMER

Civilizations historically relied on open-germination seeds to propagate the food supply in subsequent horticultural generations. Seeds could be saved from year to year, and since open-pollination plants had large gene pools, they were known for their stability and disease resistance. Hybridization, developed in the late 19th century, improved the reliability of food production by making plants stronger and more resistant and provided ownership interests in portions of the food supply. Genetically modified (GM) agricultural products were a relatively new technology, appearing in North American markets in the 1990s. GM agricultural technology provided resistance to herbicides, increased yield, and improved appearance of food. Developers of GM agricultural products were granted patents that provided a legal monopoly of the patented product and created incentives for further advancements in agricultural research and development. However, despite technological advances in agricultural production, one child died every five seconds from hunger and related causes.[3]

GENETICALLY MODIFIED ORGANISMS AND THE GLOBAL FOOD SUPPLY

In 2005, 85 percent of all soybeans in the United States were genetically engineered and subject to patent ownership.[4] Seventy percent of all processed food consumed by Americans and virtually all domestic animal feed in the United States came from genetically modified products.[5] At least 25 percent of all corn and 60 percent of all soybeans harvested in the United States, and more than 100 million acres of farmland worldwide were planted in genetically modified crops.[6] At least 200 million acres of biotech crops were planted in 2004, and the percentage of farmland in bioengineered crops had increased sharply every year.[7]

Much of the world's population relied on local farmers to save seeds from year to year. Annually, more than 1.4 billion people were fed from the food resulting from seed-saving farmers. Opponents of GM agricultural products feared that patent ownership may have threatened the rights of farmers worldwide to save seed. Many seed-saving farmers could not afford the technology fee or defend against lawsuits brought by patent-owning corporations.

Many countries that had resisted genetically modified crops had been pressured by the United States, and in some cases bribed by GM plant patent owners, to rethink their positions. Lifting the European Union (EU) ban on genetically modified plants had become a matter of U.S. national strategic priority, and, through pressure exerted by the United States, the EU reluctantly lifted the ban in 2004.[8] After the repeal of its ban on GMOs, the EU also unenthusiastically demanded that Austria, Luxembourg, France, Germany, and Greece all lift national bans.[9] The European commissioners felt they had "no alternative" but to "fulfill their legal obligations" and force through the decision to lift the ban, despite widespread opposition among its members' populations.[10] India, reluctantly, and Brazil had allowed this technology into their countries as well.[11] In 2005, Monsanto was fined $1.5 million by the U.S. Securities and Exchange Commission for bribing an Indonesian environmental official to permit genetically modified crops in Indonesia.[12]

MONSANTO AND ROUND-UP READY PATENTS

Monsanto was a global supplier of agricultural products whose revenues of $6.3 billion in 2005 were generated by two primary business units. Its Seeds and Genomics business unit developed, produced, and marketed DEKALB, Asgrow, Bollgard, and Roundup Ready brands of genetically engineered

Exhibit 1   **Financial Summary for Monsanto Company, Fiscal 2000–Fiscal 2005 (dollar amounts in millions, except per share and pro forma share amounts)**

	12 Months Ended Aug. 31,			Eight Months Ended Aug. 31,*		Year Ended Dec. 31,		
	2005	**2004**	**2003**	**2003**	**2002**	**2002**	**2001**	**2000**
Operating results								
Net sales	$ 6,294	$ 5,423	$ 4,924	$ 3,378	$ 3,129	$ 4,674	$ 5,450	$ 5,457
Income from operations	742	603	676	483	151	344	672	567
Income from continuing operations	157	266	98	—	48	146	318	196
Income (loss) on discontinued operations	98	1	(18)	(11)	(11)	(17)	(23)	(21)
Cumulative effect of a change in accounting principle	—	—	(12)	(12)	(1,822)	(1,822)	—	(26)
Net income (loss)	255	267	68	(23)	(1,785)	(1,693)	295	149
Basic earnings (loss) per share and per pro forma share								
Income from continuing operations	$ 0.59	$ 1.01	$ 0.37	$ —	$ 0.18	$ 0.56	$ 1.23	$ 0.76
Income (loss) on discontinued operations	0.37	—	(0.06)	(0.04)	(0.04)	(0.07)	(0.09)	(0.08)
Cumulative effect of accounting change	—	—	(0.05)	(0.05)	(7.00)	(6.99)	—	(0.10)
Net income (loss)	0.96	1.01	0.26	(0.09)	(6.86)	(6.50)	1.14	0.58
Diluted earnings (loss) per share and per pro forma share								
Income from continuing operations	$ 0.58	$ 0.99	$ 0.37	$ —	$ 0.18	$ 0.56	$ 1.21	$ 0.76
Income (loss) on discontinued operations	0.36	—	(0.06)	(0.04)	(0.04)	(0.07)	(0.09)	(0.08)
Cumulative effect of accounting change	—	—	(0.05)	(0.05)	(6.92)	(6.94)	—	(0.10)
Net income (loss)	0.94	0.99	0.26	(0.09)	(6.78)	(6.45)	1.12	0.58
Financial position at end of period								
Total assets	$10,579	$ 9,164	$ 9,536	$ 9,536	$ 9,175	$ 8,949	$11,454	$11,731
Working capital	2,485	3,037	2,920	2,920	2,804	2,537	2,373	2,213
Current ratio	2.15:1	2.60:1	2.45:1	2.45:1	2.62:1	2.36:1	1.99:1	1.80:1
Long-term debt	1,458	1,075	1,258	1,258	1,148	851	893	962
Debt-to-capital	24%	22%	23%	23%	27%	19%	19%	19%
Other data (applicable for periods subsequent to IPO)								
Dividends per share	$0.68	$0.68	$0.49	$0.25	$0.24	$0.48	$0.48	$0.09

(Continued)

Exhibit 1 **Continued**

	12 Months Ended Aug. 31,			Eight Months Ended Aug. 31,*		Year Ended Dec. 31,		
	2005	2004	2003	2003	2002	2002	2001	2000
Stock price per share:								
High	$69.23	$38.50	$26.35	$26.35	$33.29	$33.290	$38.800	$27.380
Low	34.15	23.08	13.55	13.55	13.01	13.010	26.875	19.750
End of period	63.84	36.60	25.71	25.71	18.37	19.130	33.800	27.060
Basic shares outstanding	266.8	264.4	261.6	261.7	260.3	260.7	258.1	258.0
Diluted shares outstanding	272.7	269.2	261.8	262.1	263.2	262.6	263.6	258.5

*Monsanto Company changed its fiscal year end from December 31 to August 31, effective August 31, 2003. Year-to-year comparisons between 2002 and 2003 should be done using the eight month ending data for those two years.

Source: Monsanto Company 2005 10-K report.

seeds. Monsanto's Agricultural Productivity business segment created and sold herbicides such as Roundup and genetically engineered products that, for instance, increased milk production in dairy cows. Exhibit 1 presents a summary of Monsanto's financial performance between 2000 and 2005. Exhibits 2 and 3 show the revenue and gross profit contributions of each business unit and key product categories.

Monsanto sold GM canola seeds in Canada and GM soybean seeds in the United States. Its patents in Canada covered genetically modified cells and genes contained in canola plants, and U.S. patents protected all GM soybeans produced from biolistics, which is a technique for inserting GM genes into cells. The Canadian canola patents specifically covered "the gene and the process for its insertion . . . and the cell

Exhibit 2 **Sales and Gross Profit Contributions for Monsanto's Seeds and Genomics Business Segment, Fiscal 2001–Fiscal 2005 (in millions)**

	12 Months Ended Aug. 31,			Eight Months Ended Aug. 31,		Year Ended Dec. 31,	
	2005	2004	2003	2003	2002	2002	2001
Net sales							
Corn seed and traits	$1,494	$1,145	$ 959	$ 592	$ 366	$ 734	$ 688
Soybean seed and traits	889	699	591	270	251	572	670
Vegetable and fruit seed	226	—	—	—	—	—	—
All other crops seeds and traits	643	476	371	322	247	295	375
Total net sales	$3,252	$2,320	$1,921	$1,184	$ 864	$1,601	$ 1,733
Gross profit							
Corn seed and traits	$ 825	$ 638	$ 505	$ 282	$ 117	$341	$ 298
Soybean seed and traits	613	429	334	127	103	310	384
Vegetable and fruit seed	113	—	—	—	—	—	—
All other crops seeds and traits	431	302	234	213	156	176	174
Total gross profit	$1,982	$1,369	$1,073	$ 622	$ 376	$ 827	$ 856
EBIT	$ 374	$ 196	$ 182	$ 17	$(2,254)	$(2,088)	$ (241)

Source: Monsanto Company 2005 10-K report.

Exhibit 3   **Sales and Gross Profit Contributions for Monsanto's Agricultural Productivity Business Segment, Fiscal 2001–Fiscal 2005 (in millions)**

	12 Months Ended August 31			Ended August 31		Year Ended December 31	
	2005	**2004**	**2003**	**2003**	**2002**	**2002**	**2001**
Net sales							
Roundup and other glyphosate-based herbicides	$2,049	$2,005	$1,844	$1,349	$1,393	$1,888	$ 2,488
All other agricultural productivity products	993	1,098	1,159	845	872	1,185	1,229
Total net sales	$3,042	$3,103	$3,003	$2,194	$2,265	$3,073	$ 3,717
Gross profit							
Roundup and other glyphosate-based herbicides	$ 637	$ 703	$ 695	$ 533	$ 661	$ 823	$ 1,234
All other agricultural productivity products	385	455	505	397	389	496	500
Total gross profit	$1,022	$1,158	$1,200	$ 930	$1,050	$1,319	$ 1,734
EBIT	$ (27)	$ 249	$ (24)	$ (33)	$ 353	$ 362	$ 760

Source: Monsanto Company 2005 10-K report.

derived from that process," which were glyphosate-resistant.[13] In Canada, Monsanto did not claim protection for the entire GM plant, but only for those genes and cells.[14] In the United States, Monsanto's patent covered the entire plant.

Roundup, an herbicide manufactured by Monsanto, contained glyphosate. Many generic herbicides also contained glyphosate. Unless they were genetically modified to be glyphosate-resistant, plants died when they were sprayed with Roundup. Monsanto Roundup Ready GM plants had increased resistance to glyphosate. Indeed, this was a stated object of the patented invention.[15] Genetically modified plants could not be distinguished from other plants on sight, but plants that did not die after being sprayed with Roundup were presumed to contain the patented GM cells or genes.[16] Monsanto marketed GM canola plants as Roundup Ready Canola and GM soybean plants as Roundup Ready Soybeans. Those names aptly implied that canola and soybean plants that emerged from seeds containing the patented gene or cell would survive a Roundup spraying, and that plants that did not contain the Roundup Ready patented gene or cell would die. Roundup Ready Canola and Roundup Ready Soybean plants were open-pollination plants. Their seeds could be saved from year to year and their progeny would display the same characteristics of the parent plants. In addition,

genetically modified plants such as Roundup Ready Canola or Roundup Ready Soybean plants could cross-pollinate with non-GM plants and the progeny would be genetically modified.

Farmers who wished to plant Roundup Ready Canola were required to sign a limited-use license agreement with Monsanto. This agreement allowed a one-time planting, prohibited seed saving, and allowed Monsanto to inspect farmers' fields to take samples for three years after the expiration of the agreement.[17] Similarly, Monsanto's Technology Use Guide expressly allowed Monsanto and its agents to enter on farmers' lands to take samples to verify compliance with the licensing agreement.[18] Monsanto contended that its licensing agreements protected its patents and ensured a return on its $400 million annual research expense.[19]

MONSANTO'S APPROACH TO PATENT PROTECTION

In 2005, Monsanto dominated large portions of the agricultural seed market with genetically modified seeds that gave rise to plants that were more resistant to disease and herbicides and provided higher yields than naturally occurring plants. The company had pressed its ownership claims successfully through the courts against both Canadian and U.S. farmers who had been found in possession of the GM agricultural products without a license. Courts in both countries had concluded that patented plants, and plants containing a patented gene or cell, were owned by the patent holder regardless of how those plants happened to arrive on private land, and regardless of whether the owner of that land consented or even had knowledge of their presence.

Given those court decisions, it appeared that intellectual property rights had trumped common law rights over agricultural products. Common law property rights supported the customary and age-old practice of seed saving for food security. Yet patent holders had effectively usurped this right with the introduction of patented plants, genes, and cells that contaminated the lands of farmers who did not wish for that technology to be present on those lands. Courts had upheld patent holders' claims against unsuspecting farmers for patent infringement, at great financial and emotional costs to the farmers. The courts had been reluctant to address those controversies through the lens of common law property rights or tort analysis, and favored as a threshold inquiry the intellectual property analysis. In other words, if there was a patent owner, then that was the end of the analysis, and the patent owner's legal monopoly over that product was protected.

Patent owners, like Monsanto, solicited information from members of farming communities about suspected patent infringement. In exchange for promotional items or free agricultural products, farmers who suspected that other farmers in their area were using agricultural products containing the patent were encouraged to call a hotline and report their suspicions.[20] This report would launch an inquiry by investigators hired by the patent owner—frequently retired police officers or retired Royal Canadian Mounted Police in Canada. Those investigations would include visiting the suspect farmers' homes, taking plants out of the farmers' fields—with or without permission of the farmer—and sending settlement letters to the farmer. Settlement terms demanded a payment for damages, frequently ranging from $25,000 to $50,000. These figures far exceeded the resources of most farmers, who often owed mortgages and other secured debts on their farm equipment.

Monsanto's patent protection policy had serious effects on farming communities. Built on generations of trust and long histories of family relationships, farming communities were suddenly divided by suspicion and fear. Sometimes farmers would report other farmers out of spite from some long-standing dispute unrelated to genetically modified crops, not out of factual evidence.

Farmers also were aware of the great financial and personal consequences suffered by the few farmers who had chosen to fight the legal charges leveled against them by Monsanto. Reports of serious health effects—such as stress-induced heart attacks and injuries resulting from lack of sleep—were not uncommon. Many defendant farmers who had equity in their property eventually mortgaged their homes, lands, and equipment simply to fight the lawsuit. The farmers' fears of losing their homes, health, and lands encouraged farmers accused of patent infringement to settle rather than to argue against Monsanto's contention.

PERCY SCHMEISER'S LEGAL TROUBLES WITH MONSANTO

Monsanto tested the validity of its Roundup Ready Canola patent under Canadian law in 1998 with a case against Percy Schmeiser. Schmeiser had farmed his land in Saskatchewan, Canada, for more than 50 years and was known as a seed saver and seed developer in his community.[21] He also used open-pollination seed on his land.[22, 23] Mr. Schmeiser primarily grew canola commercially, but he also kept some acreage in peas and wheat.[24] He farmed conventionally, not organically.[25] Schmeiser not only farmed but also had served as a member of the Canadian Parliament, as the mayor of his community, and on several federal and provincial agricultural committees.[26]

In 1996, five other farmers in Schmeiser's area planted Roundup Ready Canola.[27] Schmeiser did not plant Roundup Ready Canola but instead planted his own seed saved from prior harvests in his fields, which had been his practice for many decades. His own seed had been developed over his many years of farming, and was unique, hardy, and disease-resistant.[28] Schmeiser was proud of the superior performance of the seed he had developed.[29]

In the spring of 1997, he planted seeds saved from his 1996 harvest. As was customary, he sprayed approximately three acres in ditches and around power poles with Roundup and was puzzled by the number of "volunteer" plants, or plants that did not die. The power company paid Schmeiser approximately $120 to perform that service each year. He estimated that 60 percent of the canola plants were unaffected by the Roundup spraying.[30] Schmeiser did not spray to isolate any GM plants, but instead sprayed because it is a common practice among Saskatchewan canola farmers to chemically burn off, or "chem fallow," the field before spring planting or between growing seasons.[31]

In 1997, Monsanto agents heard a rumor that Schmeiser might have grown Roundup Ready Canola without a license.[32] An investigator hired by Monsanto took samples from the public road allowance bordering Schmeiser's land after that area had been sprayed with Roundup, and confirmed that those plants were Roundup Ready.[33] Monsanto put Schmeiser on notice of its belief that he had grown Roundup Ready Canola without a license. Schmeiser denied the allegation, stating that he had never purchased[34] and never intended to grow Roundup Ready Canola.

In 1998, Schmeiser planted his acreage with those seeds saved from his 1997 harvest.[35] He did not spray his crop with Roundup. Monsanto again took samples from the public road allowance bordering Schmeiser's land, and because Roundup Ready Canola was found, Monsanto filed a complaint against Schmeiser alleging patent infringement.[36] The lawsuit against Schmeiser eventually depleted all of his retirement funds of $200,000.[37] Exhibit 4 describes the lawsuit, including the Federal Court of Appeals and the Supreme Court of Canada's reasoning and the holding.

MONSANTO'S LEGAL PURSUIT OF PATENT INFRINGEMENT

After the Schmeiser case, many American farmers who saved genetically modified seeds settled with or had judgments entered in favor of Monsanto. According to the Center for Food Safety's *Monsanto v. U.S. Farmer Report of 2005,*[38] several cases have resulted in judgments and settlements against farmers totaling in the millions of dollars. For example, a judgment in excess of $3 million was entered against Richard Anderson, a Texas farmer. A judgment against Ray Dawson, a Missouri farmer, was entered for more than $2.5 million. Not only was a judgment of more than $2 million entered against Kem Ralph, a Tennessee farmer, but Ralph was also sentenced to eight months in prison after he was caught lying about a hidden truckload of cottonseed. This was the first criminal prosecution associated with Monsanto's "seed wars." Interestingly, in *Monsanto Co. v. Mc-Farling,*[39] the liquidated damages clause requiring farmers to pay 120 times the technology fee was held to be unenforceable under Missouri law because it was a penalty rather than damages.[40] That farmer would likely end up paying Monsanto about $10,000 instead of $780,000 after the lower court computed the actual damages the farmer caused Monsanto.[41]

By 2005, Monsanto had filed multiple lawsuits in half of the U.S. states involving 147 farmers and 39 small farm businesses.[42] It maintained an annual budget of $10 million and 75 full-time employees "devoted solely to investigating and prosecuting farmers."[43] The company had won more than $15 million in judgments against farmers in the United States, ranging from $5,000 to more than $3 million and annually investigated about 500 tips that farmers were illegally using its seed.[44, 45] Exhibits 5 and 6 provide an overview of U.S. and Canadian Patent Law regarding genetically modified organisms.

THE NATURAL SPREAD OF GENETICALLY ENGINEERED PLANTS

In 2005, the Montana legislature considered the Farmer Limited Liability for Genetically Engineered Wheat Act, which ultimately failed. This bill would have shielded Montana wheat farmers from lawsuits and would have prevented patent holding companies from suing farmers for patent infringement if genetically engineered wheat drifted across property lines

Exhibit 4   **Background on the *Monsanto v. Schmeiser* Case**

Monsanto filed a complaint against Percy Schmeiser alleging patent infringement.[a] The trial court rejected Schmeiser's argument that the Roundup Ready Canola was the result of a natural occurrence, such as wind, because of the concentration of the Roundup Ready Canola discovered. It also noted that Schmeiser should have known that it was Roundup Ready Canola when he discovered that some plants on his land were Roundup tolerant.[b] The court also rejected Schmeiser's argument that the patent was invalid because the subject of its protection—i.e., entire plants—was not patentable. The trial court ruled in favor of Monsanto by concluding that the patent was valid, and that Schmeiser committed patent infringement because he knew, or should have known, that he saved and planted seed containing the patented genes and cells of Roundup Ready Canola.

After the Federal Court of Appeal upheld the trial court's ruling, Schmeiser appealed.[c] The Supreme Court of Canada held that the patent was valid, and that Schmeiser committed patent infringement when he saved and planted the seed, then harvested and sold the plants that contained the patented cells and genes.[d]

The Supreme Court found that it was irrelevant whether Schmeiser intended to infringe on the patent or whether Schmeiser knew about the patented product on his land, because "it is a settled issue in Canadian patent law that intention is irrelevant to infringement,"[e] though the presumption of use is rebuttable.[f] The court acknowledged that the plants containing the patented product could have been the result of pollen that blew onto Schmeiser's land but found that the manner in which the Roundup Ready Canola product got onto Mr. Schmeiser's land was irrelevant. The Court specifically declined to address the "innocent discovery by farmers of "blow-by" patented plants on their land or in their cultivated fields . . . [or] . . . the scope of the . . . patent or the wisdom and social utility of the genetic modification of genes and cells."[g]

Since Canada's Patent Act confers on the patent owner "the exclusive right, privilege and liberty of making, constructing and using the invention and selling it to others to be used,"[h] the only relevant inquiry was whether Schmeiser "used" the genetically modified plants and seeds and whether Schmeiser's acts interfered with the exclusive rights granted by the patent.[i] The Supreme Court found that Mr. Schmeiser "used" the patent and interfered with the exclusive rights granted by the patent to Monsanto, and affirmed the lower courts' rulings. The court held that "by cultivating a plant containing the patented gene and composed of the patented cells without license, [Schmeiser] deprived the respondents of the full enjoyment of the monopoly" created by the patent.[j] However, the damages awarded to Monsanto by the lower court were reversed, because Schmeiser did not earn profit from the use of the patented product, since he did not use Roundup herbicide on those plants.

According to the Court, despite the fact that Monsanto's patent only protects the genetically modified cell or gene, infringement does not require use of the cell or gene in isolation.[k] Indeed, if a plant containing a genetically modified cell or gene propagates, grows and is used by a nonlicensee farmer—even though the presence of the plant is unknown to the farmer—the farmer has committed patent infringement. Also, even though the object of the patent is to provide glyphosate-resistance, lack of use of Roundup herbicide is irrelevant. In other words, patent infringement can exist whether or not the unauthorized "user" of the patent utilizes the patent for its purpose.

When addressing whether a volunteer plant could appropriately fall under the patent's protection even though the Canadian patent was not intended to protect whole plants, the Court noted that "infringement is possible . . . [when] the patented invention is [only] part of . . . a broader unpatented structure or process." The Court was persuaded by the firm principle that "the main purpose of patent protection is to prevent others from depriving the inventor, even in part and even indirectly, of the monopoly that the law intends to be theirs: only the inventor is entitled, by virtue of the patent and as a matter of law, to the full enjoyment of the monopoly conferred."[l]

[a]*Monsanto Canada, Inc. v. Schmeiser* [2001] FTC 256.

[b]Ibid.

[c]*Schmeiser v. Monsanto Canada* [2004] SCC 34.

[d]Ibid.

[e]Ibid., The court also cites *Stead v. Anderson* (1847), 4 C.B. 806, 136 Eng. Rep. 724 (C.P.), at p. 736. The issue is "what the defendant does, not . . . what he intends," at para. 49.

[f]Ibid. at para. 56.

[g]Ibid. at para. 2.

[h]Ibid. at para. 25.

[i]Ibid.

[j]Ibid.

[k]Ibid.

[l]Ibid. at para. 43.

Exhibit 5   **Overview of Canadian Patent Law**

Canada stands virtually alone among developed countries in its nonrecognition of the patentability of higher life forms. However, Canada is well within its international rights to exclude the patentability of higher life forms. The World Trade Organization's Agreement on Trade-Related Aspects of Intellectual Property (TRIPs) allows the exclusion of animals and plants from patentability.[a] Not only does Canada exercise this right of exclusion, but this right is also typically embraced by developing nations, while other countries, notably the United States, may wish to limit or eliminate the exclusion.[b]

Despite the fact that Canada does not allow higher life forms to be patented, the Schmeiser decision, by a 5–4 majority, suggests that patent holders of components of higher life forms have found a way around this barrier. This decision does an apparent end run around the prohibition against patenting higher life forms by finding patent infringement in cases where a nonlicensee possesses a whole that contains a patented part. This effectively provides monopolistic protection of the whole to patent holders of the part, even though such patents are not permitted under law. The Schmeiser dissent astutely noted that "allowing gene and cell claims to extend patent protection to plants renders this provision of TRIPs meaningless. To find that possession of plants, as the embodiment of a gene or cell claim, constitutes a "use" of that claim would have the same effect as patenting the plants."[c] Aside from the Schmeiser decision, commentators have noted that the Canadian practice of issuing patents to protect the cells of plants, instead of the entire plant, has the same effect as patenting the entire plant.[d]

[a]World Trade Organization, Agreement on Trade-Related Aspects of Intellectual Property, Art. 27.3 (b).

[b]"Patenting of Higher Life Forms and Related Issues: Report to the Government of Canada Biotechnology Ministerial Coordinating Committee" June 2002, available at http://cbac-cccb.ca/epic/internet/incbac-cccb.nsf/en/ah00213e.html (accessed April 15, 2005).

[c]*Schmeiser v. Monsanto Canada* [2004] SCC 34, at para 167.

[d]Lenni Carreiro, "The Supreme Court of Canada Finds Higher Life Forms Not Patentable Subject Matter," March 19, 2003, available at www.dww.com/articles/higher_life_forms.htm (accessed April 15, 2005).

and was found on the land of farmers who did not intentionally grow it.

The *New York Times* reported that a study by the Environmental Protection Agency (EPA) found that genetically engineered creeping bentgrass could spread for miles, could pollinate test plants of the same species as far away as measured (which was 13 miles downwind), and could pollinate natural wild grass of a different species nine miles away. Previous studies indicated it could only pollinate between different varieties no more than one mile away. The Bureau of Land Management and the Forest Service opposed this product because it "ha[d] the potential to adversely impact all 175 national forests and grasslands." The Department of Agriculture had decided to complete an environmental impact statement to determine whether or not to allow the plant to be commercialized.[46] However, advocates of genetically modified agricultural plants argue that soybeans and canola do not contain the same risk, because the creeping bentgrass of the study had extraordinarily light pollen.

A large-scale study conducted in Great Britain concerning its largest crop, winter rape, indicated

that wildlife suffered as a result of GM crops. The herbicide sprayed on the crops that killed the weeds resulted in one-third fewer seeds for birds and wildlife to eat than the seeds available after a conventional crop. Even when the herbicide was not sprayed again, there were still 25 percent fewer seeds for wildlife.[47]

TERMINATOR SEED TECHNOLOGY AND PATENT PROTECTION

Sterile seed technology or "terminator seed"— self-destructs after one generation. That invention effectively would prohibit farmers from saving their seed from year to year, because the seed of the harvest would not be fertile, and it would protect the patent owners from patent infringement by protecting its patented invention and limiting the use of its invention to licensees only.

The danger of terminator seeds lay in the fact that genetically modified organisms had not been contained to only licensee farmers' lands. The GMO

Exhibit 6   **Overview of U.S. Patent Law**

The United States allows patents on higher life forms, including both plants and animals.[a] For example, a patent was granted by the U.S. Patent and Trademark Office (PTO) for the OncoMouse,[b] a genetically modified cancer-prone mouse, as early as 1988. Indeed, patents have been granted over many higher life forms.[c]

Those decisions were not made in a legal void. Since the 1980 Supreme Court decision in *Diamond v. Chakrabarty,*[d] inroads have been laid to allow the patentability of higher life forms in the United States. In that case, the subject matter was a bacteria engineered to break down crude oil components. Patent protection was allowed, after the PTO initially denied the patent because U.S. patent protection, at that time, did not extend to living things. The Patent Appeals Court reversed, and proclaimed that "the fact that microorganisms are alive is a distinction without legal significance for patent law." The Supreme Court affirmed, stating that "a live, human-made microorganism is patentable subject matter . . . [The inventor's] discovery is not nature's handiwork, but his own . . . [and] anything under the sun that is made by man" is patentable.[e]

After *Chakrabarty,* seeds were subsequently deemed patentable subject matter.[f] In 1987, the PTO announced that "non-naturally occurring, non-human, multi-cellular living organisms, including animals" were patentable subject matter.[g]

In 2001, the Supreme Court held in *J.E.M. Ag Supply v. Pioneer Hi-Bred International* that farmers could not save seed that is the subject matter of a general utility patent, including genetically modified seed. That decision effectively invalidated the protections afforded under the Plant Variety Protection Act of 1970, which allowed farmers to save the seed from sexually reproducible plants without violating the rights held by the developers of new plant varieties.[h]

U.S. courts have consistently upheld patent infringement claims against farmers who have saved GM seeds intentionally, or who unknowingly possessed GM plants on their land. However, interesting dicta in the concurring opinion in *Smithkline Beecham Corp. v. Apotex,*[i] indicates perhaps a willingness by some members of the judiciary to rethink the legal implications of wholesale patent protection for products resulting from the escape of genetically modified organisms. "[T]he implication—that the patent owner would be entitled to collect royalties from every farmer whose cornfields contained even a few patented . . . stalks . . . cannot possibly be correct."[j]

[a]"Patenting Higher Life Forms Report."

[b]Granted in 1988 to Harvard geneticist Philip Leder and Timothy Steward of the University of California, San Francisco.

[c]See e.g., *Ex Parte Allen* 2 U.S.P.Q.2d (BNA) 1425 (Bd. Pat. App. & Int. 1987), *aff'd,* 846 F.2d 77 (Fed. Cir. 1988) (oysters)

[d]*Diamond v. Chakrabarty,* 447 US 303 (1980).

[e]Ibid.

[f]*Ex parte Hibberd,* 227 U.S.P.Q. (BNA) 443 (Bd. App. & Int., 1985).

[g]L. J. Deftos, "Patenting Life: Mighty OncoMouse Squeaks About the Ethics of Biopatents," *Endocrine News* 29, no. 1 (February 2004), available at www.endo-society.org/news/endocrine_news/2004/EthicsCorner-Feb2004.cfm (accessed April 15, 2005).

[h]*J.E.M. Ag Supply v. Pioneer Hi-Bred Int'l,* 534 U.S. 124 (2001).

[i]*Smithkline Beecham Corp. v. Apotex,* 365 F.3d 1306 (Fed. Cir. 2004).

[j]Ibid.

technology had contaminated neighboring farms, and destroyed those farms' own lines of open-pollination seed with the GM gene or cell. Terminator seed technology could threaten nonlicensee seed-saving farmers' future crops by effectively sterilizing the seeds of harvests from which seeds would normally be saved.

The world had not yet embraced terminator technology, despite lobbying by large agricultural companies and trade associations. Some countries had also pressed forward with their support. For example, Canada favored terminator seed technology, but at the March 2005 United Nations Conference in Bangkok, the technology was narrowly shelved for more research.[48]

LEGAL AND ETHICAL DEFENSES TO CHARGES OF PATENT INFRINGEMENT BY FARMERS

Intellectual property rights have seemingly trumped common law property rights in the area of GM plants. The intellectual property threshold question of patent infringement had effectively foreclosed analyses under common-law property rights and tort claims. However, nonlicensee or seed-saving farmers facing patent infringement litigation could consider counterclaims and legal defenses under common law theories. For a farmer to be successful in a tort claim, he or she must show some type of physical harm. Genetic contamination of nonlicensee farmers' land could constitute trespass or negligence among other claims.

The Stray Bull Theory

Landowners had the right to claim ownership over what is found on their land. This was an ancient tradition firmly rooted and recognized at common law. What was attached to one's land could not belong to another. Historically, for example, crops, which were part of the land, could not be "lost" or "wrongfully withheld" from another because they were attached to the land. Consequently, an action to recover those goods would not stand.[49]

Commentators had argued that straying genetic material from genetically modified plants and their progeny was analogous to the progeny of a straying bull. Under settled common law, when a straying male animal wandered in another's land to breed other female animals on that land, the owner of the female owned the progeny.[50] This theory for recovery was advanced on the premises that the law of straying animals promoted neighborliness, and was stable, predictable, and grounded in common sense.[51]

Federal Court of Appeal judge W. Andrew McKay, who presided over *Monsanto v. Schmeiser,* disagreed with the stray bull analogy because "Monsanto does have ownership in its patented gene and cell and . . . has the exclusive use of its invention," apparently distinguishing the non-ownership of the product of a straying bull's libido by the bull's owner.[52] The Supreme Court of Canada simply rejected the stray bull argument without discussion, stating tersely that the issue "is not [one of] property rights, but patent protection. Ownership is no defense to a breach of the patent act."[53]

Trespass

Genetically modified agricultural product contamination was a physical entry upon land, resulting in the use or interference with the owner's exclusive possession of the land, because patent owners were entitled to the profits derived from nonlicensee use of the patent, and when genetically modified agricultural product contamination occurred on nonlicensee land, it interfered with the owner's exclusive possession. Similarly, when a licensee terminated his agreement with the patent owner, but the patented product remained on the land, trespass had occurred because the patented product had remained after the agreed upon period had ended. In either case, the intent element could be met in the genetically modified agricultural product context if the patent owner knew that genetic contamination was likely to occur because the technology was uncontainable.

Some states had enacted statutes to protect farmers from patent owners accessing land to take samples without the farmer's knowledge and consent, which would provide additional statutory protection in the event that agents of patent owners entered land without permission.[54]

Negligence

Since genetically modified organism containment was impossible, patent owners could foresee the possibility that nonlicensee land would be contaminated with the patented product. Therefore, patent owners had a duty to protect against risk. Since nonlicensee farmers' crops were being contaminated with the patented product, this duty had been breached. The causal connection was clear, and the resulting injury could be measured in lost opportunity costs due to interference with exclusive use of land, damage or destruction of personal property, and other related injuries.

Percy Schmeiser's wife, Louise, filed a small claims complaint of negligence against Monsanto seeking $140 in damages for the cost of removing Roundup Ready Canola plants from her organic garden and a grove of trees on her property. Since the Supreme Court of Canada ruled that Monsanto owns plants that contain the patented cell and gene, and that any plant that survives Roundup spraying is a Monsanto-owned plant, then Monsanto must remove the plant. As of late 2005, Monsanto had failed to do so and the small claims court decision was still pending.[55]

Endnotes

[1]Interview with Percy Schmeiser, in Bruno, Saskatchewan, Canada, June 4, 2005.

[2]Roger Snyder, "Seed Police Sue Farmers for High Tech Piracy," January 18, 2005, available at http://printsho.station193.com/php/wordpress/archives/2005/01/18/seed-police-sue-farmers-for-high-tech-piracy (accessed September 13, 2005).

[3]Information from the U.N. World Food Programme, available at www.wfp.org (accessed June 1, 2005).

[4]Paul Elias and Anne Fitzgerald, "Monsanto Sues Farmer Customers Over Piracy Issues," Des Moines Register, January 30, 2005, available at www.mindfully.org/GE/2005/Monsanto-Sues-Farmers30jan05.htm.

[5]William Engdahl, "Seeds of Destruction: The Geopolitics of GM Food," Current Concerns, March 6, 2005, www.currentconcerns.ch/archive/2004/05/20040505.php.

[6]Martin Lee, "Food Fight—International Protests Mount Against Genetically Engineered Crops," San Francisco Bay Guardian, June 25, 2001, available at www.sfbg.com/reality/28.html.

[7]Elias and Fitzgerald, "Monsanto Sues Farmer."

[8]"European Union Lifts GM Food Ban," BBC News World Edition, May 19, 2004, available at http://news.bbc.co.uk/2/hi/europe/3727827.stm (accessed April 15, 2005).

[9]Paul Brown and David Gow, "Damning Verdict on GM Crop," The Guardian, March 22, 2005.

[10]Ibid.

[11]"Monsanto Chalks Up Crop of Global Biotech Victories," Associated Press, March 19, 2005, available at www.mindfully.org/GE/2005/Monsanto-Biotech-Victories19mar05.htm (accessed March 22, 2005).

[12]William Baue, "Monsanto $1.5 Million Fines for Genetic Engineering Bribe Illustrates Risks of GE Strategy," Social Funds.com, January 19, 2005, available at www.mindfully.org/GE/2005/Monsanto-$1_5M-Fines19jan2005.htm (accessed March 22, 2005).

[13]Schmeiser v. Monsanto Canada [2004] SCC 34, at para. 60.

[14]Ibid., at para. 17.

[15]Ibid., at para. 18.

[16]Ibid.

[17]2005 Monsanto Technology/Stewardship Agreement (limited-use license).

[18]Monsanto 2005 Technology Use Guide.

[19]Elias and Fitzgerald, "Monsanto Sues Farmer."

[20]Monsanto 2005 Technology Use Guide.

[21]Percy Schmeiser, address at the University of Texas at Austin, October 10, 2001, transcribed by Paul Goettlich, "Heartbreak in the Heartland: The True Cost of Genetically Engineered Crops," available at www.mindfully.org/GE/GE4/Heartbreak-In-The-Heartland21jul02.htm (accessed March 22, 2005).

[22]Ibid.

[23]Schmeiser v. Monsanto Canada [2004] SCC 34, at para 60.

[24]Schmeiser, address.

[25]Schmeiser v. Monsanto Canada [2004] SCC 34, at para. 60.

[26]Schmeiser, address.

[27]Schmeiser v. Monsanto Canada [2004] SCC 34, at para. 60.

[28]Brief for defendants at paras. 5, 9, Schmeiser v. Monsanto Canada, Inc. [2002] FCA 209. (Fed Court of Appeal, Court File No. T-L593-98).

[29]Ibid. at para. 10.

[30]Ibid. at para. 26.

[31]Ibid. at para. 12.

[32]Ibid. at para. 38, citing deposition of Mr. Mitchell, Monsanto's lead investigator in the Schmeiser case.

[33]Ibid at paras. 60–66.

[34]Schmeiser v. Monsanto Canada [2004] SCC 34, at para. 6.

[35]Schmeiser v. Monsanto Canada [2004] SCC 34, at para. 63.

[36]Monsanto Canada, Inc. v. Schmeiser [2001] FTC 256.

[37]Schmeiser, address.

[38]The Center for Food Safety, "Monsanto vs. U.S. Farmer," 2005.

[39]Monsanto Co. V. McFarling, 363 F.4d 1336, 1344 (Fed. Cir. 2004), petition for cert. filed, No. 04-31 (U.S. July 6, 2004).

[40]Ibid.

[41]David R. Moeller and Michael Sligh, "Farmers' Guide to GMOs," 2004, citing Robert Schubert, "Mississippi Farmer Gets Big Break from Appeals Court in Monsanto Biotech Seed Case," CropChoice, April 27, 2004, available at www.cropchoice.com/leadstry.asp?recid+2540.

[42]Center for Food Safety Report, "Monsanto vs. U.S. Farmer," p. 6.

[43]Ibid.

[44]Ibid., cited in A. V. Krebs, "Monsanto Charged with Using U.S. Patent Laws to Control Staple Crop Seeds," Agribusiness Examiner, January 19, 2005, available at www.mindfully.org/GE/2005/Monsanto-Patent-Control19jan05.htm.

[45]Jane Roberts, "Farmers Take on Monsanto over Seed Fines," Knight Rider/Tribune Business News, September 26, 2004, available at www.cropchoice.com/leadstry5eaa.html?recid+2777 (accessed April 15, 2005).

[46]Andrew Pollack, "Genes from Engineered Grass Spread for Miles, Study Finds," New York Times, September 21, 2004.

[47]Brown and Gow, "Damning Verdict."

[48]Stephen Leahy, "Ban Endures on Terminator Seeds," February 11, 2005, available at www.mindfully.org/GE/2005/Canada-Terminator-Seeds11feb05.htm.

[49]W. Page Keeton, Prosser and Keeton on Torts 91, 5th ed. (West Publishing, 1984).

[50]Drew L. Kershen, "Of Straying Crops and Patent Rights," Washburn Law Journal 42 (2004), citing E. G. Ark Valley Land & Cattle Co. 130 US at 62.

[51]Ibid.

[52]Cited in Ibid.

[53]Schmeiser v. Monsanto Canada [2004] SCC 34, at para. 96.

[54]See e.g., S.D. Codified Laws section 38-1-45., N.D. Cent. Code section 4-24-13 (H.B. 1442), available at www.state.nd.us/lr/cencode/t04c24.pdf

[55]"Monsanto Facing Another Schmeiser Suit," Canadian Broadcasting Corporation, October 19, 2004.

ENDNOTES

Chapter 1

[1]Costas Markides, "What Is Strategy and How Do You Know If You Have One?" *Business Strategy Review* 15, no. 2 (Summer 2004), pp. 5–6.

[2]For a discussion of the different ways in which companies can position themselves in the marketplace, see Michael E. Porter, "What Is Strategy?" *Harvard Business Review* 74, no. 6 (November–December 1996), pp. 65–67.

[3]For an excellent treatment of the strategic challenges posed by high-velocity changes, see Shona L. Brown and Kathleen M. Eisenhardt, *Competing on the Edge: Strategy as Structured Chaos* (Boston: Harvard Business School Press, 1998), Chapter 1.

[4]See Henry Mintzberg and Joseph Lampel, "Reflecting on the Strategy Process, *Sloan Management Review* 40, no. 3 (Spring 1999), pp. 21–30; Henry Mintzberg and J. A. Waters, "Of Strategies, Deliberate and Emergent," *Strategic Management Journal* 6 (1985), pp. 257–72; Costas Markides, "Strategy as Balance: From 'Either-Or' to 'And,'" *Business Strategy Review* 12, no. 3 (September 2001), pp. 1–10; Henry Mintzberg, Bruce Ahlstrand, and Joseph Lampel, *Strategy Safari: A Guided Tour through the Wilds of Strategic Management* (New York: Free Press, 1998), 7; and C. K. Prahalad and Gary Hamel, "The Core Competence of the Corporation," *Harvard Business Review* 70, no. 3 (May–June 1990), pp. 79–93.

[5]Joseph L. Badaracco, "The Discipline of Building Character," *Harvard Business Review* 76, no. 2 (March–April 1998), pp. 115–24.

[6]Joan Magretta, "Why Business Models Matter," *Harvard Business Review* 80, no. 5 (May 2002), p. 87.

Chapter 2

[1]For a more in-depth discussion of the challenges of developing a well-conceived vision, as well as some good examples, see Hugh Davidson, *The Committed Enterprise: How to Make Vision and Values Work* (Oxford: Butterworth Heinemann, 2002), Chapter 2; W. Chan Kim and Renée Mauborgne, "Charting Your Company's Future," *Harvard Business Review* 80, no. 6 (June 2002), pp. 77–83; James C. Collins and Jerry I. Porras, "Building Your Company's Vision," *Harvard Business Review* 74, no. 5 (September–October 1996), pp. 65–77; James C. Collins and Jerry I. Porras, *Built to Last: Successful Habits of Visionary Companies* (New York: HarperCollins, 1994), Chapter 11; and Michel Robert, *Strategy Pure and Simple II*

(New York: McGraw-Hill, 1998), Chapters 2, 3, and 6.

[2]Davidson, *Committed Enterprise,* pp. 20, 54.

[3]Ibid., pp. 36, 54.

[4]Jeffrey K. Liker, *The Toyota Way* (New York: McGraw-Hill, 2004), and Steve Hamm, "Taking a Page from Toyota's Playbook," *BusinessWeek,* August 22/29, 2005, p. 72.

[5]As quoted in Charles H. House and Raymond L. Price, "The Return Map: Tracking Product Teams," *Harvard Business Review* 60, no. 1 (January–February 1991), p. 93.

[6]Robert S. Kaplan and David P. Norton, *The Strategy-Focused Organization* (Boston: Harvard Business School Press, 2001), p. 3.

[7]Ibid., p. 7. Also, see Kevin B. Hendricks, Larry Menor, and Christine Wiedman, "The Balanced Scorecard: To Adopt or Not to Adopt," *Ivey Business Journal* 69, no. 2 (November–December 2004), pp. 1–7; and Sandy Richardson, "The Key Elements of Balanced Scorecard Success," *Ivey Business Journal* 69, no. 2 (November–December 2004), pp. 7–9.

[8]Information posted on the Web site of the Balanced Scorecard Institute, www.balancedscorecard.org (accessed August 22, 2005).

[9]Darrell Rigby, "Management Tools Survey 2003: Usage Up as Companies Strive to Make Headway in Tough Times," *Strategy & Leadership* 31, no. 5 (May 2003), p. 6.

[10]Information posted on the Web site of Balanced Scorecard Collaborative, www.bscol.com (accessed August 22, 2005). This Web site was created by the co-creators of the balanced scorecard concept, Professors Robert S. Kaplan and David P. Norton, Harvard Business School.

[11]The concept of strategic intent is described in more detail in Gary Hamel and C. K. Prahalad, "Strategic Intent," *Harvard Business Review* 89, no. 3 (May–June 1989), pp. 63–76; this section draws on their pioneering discussion. See also Michael A. Hitt, Beverly B. Tyler, Camilla Hardee, and Daewoo Park, "Understanding Strategic Intent in the Global Marketplace," *Academy of Management Executive* 9, no. 2 (May 1995), pp. 12–19.

[12]For a fuller discussion of strategy as an entrepreneurial process, see Henry Mintzberg, Bruce Ahlstrand, and Joseph Lampel, *Strategy Safari: A Guided Tour through the Wilds of Strategic Management,* (New York: Free Press, 1998), Chapter 5. Also see Bruce Barringer and Allen C. Bluedorn, "The Relationship Between Corporate Entrepreneurship and Strategic Management," *Strategic Management*

Journal 20 (1999), pp. 421–444, and Jeffrey G. Covin and Morgan P. Miles, "Corporate Entrepreneurship and the Pursuit of Competitive Advantage," *Entrepreneurship: Theory and Practice* 23, no. 3 (Spring 1999), pp. 47–63.

[13]The strategy-making, strategy-implementing roles of middle managers are thoroughly discussed and documented in Steven W. Floyd and Bill Wooldridge, *The Strategic Middle Manager* (San Francisco: Jossey-Bass Publishers, 1996), Chapters 2 and 3.

[14]"Strategic Planning," *Business Week,* August 26, 1996, pp. 51–52.

[15]For an excellent discussion of why a strategic plan needs to be more than a list of bullet points and should in fact tell an engaging, insightful, stage-setting story that lays out the industry and competitive situation as well as the vision, objectives, and strategy, see Gordon Shaw, Robert Brown, and Philip Bromiley, "Strategic Stories: How 3M Is Rewriting Business Planning," *Harvard Business Review* 76, no. 3 (May–June 1998), pp. 41–50.

[16]For a discussion of what it takes for the corporate governance system to function properly, see David A. Nadler, "Building Better Boards," *Harvard Business Review* 82, no. 5 (May 2004), pp. 102–5; Cynthia A. Montgomery and Rhonda Kaufman, "The Board's Missing Link," *Harvard Business Review* 81, no. 3 (March 2003), pp. 86–93; and John Carver, "What Continues to Be Wrong with Corporate Governance and How to Fix It," *Ivey Business Journal* 68, no. 1 (September–October 2003), pp. 1–5. See also Gordon Donaldson, "A New Tool for Boards: The Strategic Audit," *Harvard Business Review* 73, no. 4 (July–August 1995), pp. 99–107.

Chapter 3

[1]There are a large number of studies of the size of the cost reductions associated with experience; the median cost reduction associated with a doubling of cumulative production volume is approximately 15 percent, but there is a wide variation from industry to industry. For a good discussion of the economies of experience and learning, see Pankaj Ghemawat, "Building Strategy on the Experience Curve," *Harvard Business Review* 64, no. 2 (March–April 1985), pp. 143–49.

[2]The five-forces model of competition is the creation of Professor Michael Porter of the Harvard Business School. For his original presentation of the model, see Michael E. Porter, "How Competitive Forces Shape Strategy," *Harvard Business Review* 57, no. 2

(March–April 1979), pp. 137–45. A more thorough discussion can be found in Michael E. Porter, *Competitive Strategy: Techniques for Analyzing Industries and Competitors* (New York: Free Press, 1980), Chapter 1.

[3]Many of these indicators of whether rivalry produces intense competitive pressures are based on Porter, *Competitive Strategy,* pp. 17–21.

[4]The role of entry barriers in shaping the strength of competition in a particular market has long been a standard topic in the literature of microeconomics. For a discussion of how entry barriers affect competitive pressures associated with potential entry, see J. S. Bain, *Barriers to New Competition* (Cambridge: Harvard University Press, 1956); F. M. Scherer, *Industrial Market Structure and Economic Performance* (Chicago: Rand McNally, 1971), pp. 216–20, 226–33; and Porter, *Competitive Strategy,* pp. 7–17.

[5]Porter, "How Competitive Forces Shape Strategy," p. 140, and Porter, *Competitive Strategy,* pp. 14–15.

[6]For a good discussion of this point, see George S. Yip, "Gateways to Entry," *Harvard Business Review* 60, no. 5 (September–October 1982), pp. 85–93.

[7]Porter, "How Competitive Forces Shape Strategy," p. 142, and Porter, *Competitive Strategy,* pp. 23–24.

[8]Porter, *Competitive Strategy*, p. 10.

[9]Ibid., pp. 27–28.

[10]Ibid., pp. 24–27.

[11]For a more extended discussion of the problems with the life-cycle hypothesis, see ibid., pp. 157–62.

[12]Ibid. p. 162.

[13]Most of the candidate driving forces described here are based on the discussion in ibid., pp. 164–83.

[14]Ibid., Chapter 7.

[15]Ibid., pp. 129–30.

[16]For an excellent discussion of how to identify the factors that define strategic groups, see Mary Ellen Gordon and George R. Milne, "Selecting the Dimensions That Define Strategic Groups: A Novel Market-Driven Approach," *Journal of Managerial Issues* 11, no. 2 (Summer 1999), pp. 213–33.

[17]Porter, *Competitive Strategy,* pp. 152–54.

[18]Strategic groups act as good reference points for predicting the evolution of an industry's competitive structure. See Avi Fiegenbaum and Howard Thomas, "Strategic Groups as Reference Groups: Theory, Modeling and Empirical Examination of Industry and Competitive Strategy," *Strategic Management Journal* 16 (1995), pp. 461–76. For a study of how strategic group analysis helps identify the variables that lead to sustainable competitive advantage, see S. Ade Olusoga, Michael P. Mokwa, and Charles H. Noble,

"Strategic Groups, Mobility Barriers, and Competitive Advantage," *Journal of Business Research* 33 (1995), pp. 153–64.

[19]Porter, *Competitive Strategy,* pp. 130, 132–38, and 154–55.

[20]For a discussion of legal and ethical ways of gathering competitive intelligence on rival companies, see Larry Kahaner, *Competitive Intelligence* (New York: Simon & Schuster, 1996).

[21]Ibid., pp. 84–85.

[22]Some experts dispute the strategy-making value of key success factors. Professor Pankaj Ghemawat has claimed that the "whole idea of identifying a success factor and then chasing it seems to have something in common with the ill-considered medieval hunt for the *philosopher's stone,* a substance which would transmute everything it touched into gold." Pankaj Ghemawat, *Commitment: The Dynamic of Strategy* (New York: Free Press, 1991), p. 11.

Chapter 4

[1]Many business organizations are coming to view cutting-edge knowledge and intellectual resources of company personnel as a valuable competitive asset and have concluded that explicitly managing these assets is an essential part of their strategy. See Michael H. Zack, "Developing a Knowledge Strategy," *California Management Review* 41, no. 3 (Spring 1999), pp. 125–45, and Shaker A. Zahra, Anders P. Nielsen, and William C. Bogner, "Corporate Entrepreneurship, Knowledge, and Competence Development," *Entrepreneurship Theory and Practice,* Spring 1999, pp. 169–89.

[2]In the past decade, there's been considerable research into the role a company's resources and competitive capabilities play in crafting strategy and in determining company profitability. The findings and conclusions have coalesced into what is called the resource-based view of the firm. Among the most insightful articles are Birger Wernerfelt, "A Resource-Based View of the Firm," *Strategic Management Journal,* September–October 1984, pp. 171–80; Jay Barney, "Firm Resources and Sustained Competitive Advantage," *Journal of Management* 17, no. 1 (1991), pp. 99–120; Margaret A. Peteraf, "The Cornerstones of Competitive Advantage: A Resource-Based View," *Strategic Management Journal,* March 1993, pp. 179–91; Birger Wernerfelt, "The Resource-Based View of the Firm: Ten Years After," *Strategic Management Journal* 16 (1995), pp. 171–74; Jay Barney, "Looking Inside for Competitive Advantage," *Academy of Management Executive* 9, no. 4 (November 1995), pp. 49–61; Christopher A. Bartlett and Sumantra Ghoshal, "Building Competitive Advantage through People,"

MIT Sloan Management Review 43, no 2, (Winter 2002), pp. 34–41; and Danny Miller, Russell Eisenstat, and Nathaniel Foote, "Strategy from the Inside Out: Building Capability-Creating Organizations," *California Management Review* 44, no. 3 (Spring 2002), pp. 37–54.

[3]George Stalk Jr. and Rob Lachenauer, "Hard Ball: Five Killer Strategies for Trouncing the Competition," *Harvard Business Review* 82, no. 4 (April 2004), p. 65.

[4]For a more extensive discussion of how to identify and evaluate the competitive power of a company's capabilities, see David W. Birchall and George Tovstiga, "The Strategic Potential of a Firm's Knowledge Portfolio," *Journal of General Management* 25, no. 1 (Autumn 1999), pp. 1–16, and Nick Bontis, Nicola C. Dragonetti, Kristine Jacobsen, and Goran Roos, "The Knowledge Toolbox: A Review of the Tools Available to Measure and Manage Intangible Resources," *European Management Journal* 17, no. 4 (August 1999), pp. 391–401. Also see David Teece, "Capturing Value from Knowledge Assets: The New Economy, Markets for Know-How, and Intangible Assets," *California Management Review* 40, no. 3 (Spring 1998), pp. 55–79.

[5]See Barney, "Firm Resources," pp. 105–9, and David J. Collis and Cynthia A. Montgomery, "Competing on Resources: Strategy in the 1990s," *Harvard Business Review* 73, no. 4 (July–August 1995), pp. 120–23.

[6]Donald Sull, "Strategy as Active Waiting," *Harvard Business Review* 83, no. 9 (September 2005), p. 121–122.

[7]Ibid., p. 122.

[8]Ibid., pp. 124–26.

[9]See Jack W. Duncan, Peter Ginter, and Linda E. Swayne, "Competitive Advantage and Internal Organizational Assessment," *Academy of Management Executive* 12, no. 3 (August 1998), pp. 6–16.

[10]The value chain concept was developed and articulated by Professor Michael Porter at the Harvard Business School and is described at greater length in Michael E. Porter, *Competitive Advantage* (New York: Free Press, 1985), Chapters 2 and 3.

[11]Ibid., p. 36.

[12]Ibid., p. 34.

[13]The strategic importance of effective supply chain management is discussed in Hau L. Lee, "The Triple-A Supply Chain," *Harvard Business Review* 82, no. 10 (October 2004), pp. 102–112.

[14]M. Hegert and D. Morris, "Accounting Data for Value Chain Analysis," *Strategic Management Journal* 10 (1989), p. 180; Robin Cooper and Robert S. Kaplan, "Measure Costs Right: Make the Right Decisions," *Harvard Business Review* 66, no. 5 (September–October, 1988), pp. 96–103; and John K. Shank and Vijay

Govindarajan, *Strategic Cost Management* (New York: Free Press, 1993), especially Chapters 2–6, 10.

[15] For more on how and why the clustering of suppliers and other support organizations matter to a company's costs and competitiveness, see Michael E. Porter, "Clusters and the New Economics of Competition," *Harvard Business Review* 76, no. 6 (November–December 1998), pp. 77–90.

[16] For discussions of the accounting challenges in calculating the costs of value chain activities, see Shank and Govindarajan, *Strategic Cost Management,* especially Chapters 2–6, 10, and 11; Cooper and Kaplan, "Measure Costs Right"; and Joseph A. Ness and Thomas G. Cucuzza, "Tapping the Full Potential of ABC," *Harvard Business Review* 73, no. 4 (July–August 1995), pp. 130–38.

[17] For more details, see Gregory H. Watson, *Strategic Benchmarking: How to Rate Your Company's Performance Against the World's Best* (New York: John Wiley, 1993); Robert C. Camp, *Benchmarking: The Search for Industry Best Practices That Lead to Superior Performance* (Milwaukee: ASQC Quality Press, 1989); Christopher E. Bogan and Michael J. English, *Benchmarking for Best Practices: Winning through Innovative Adaptation* (New York: McGraw-Hill, 1994); and Dawn Iacobucci and Christie Nordhielm, "Creative Benchmarking," *Harvard Business Review* 78 no. 6 (November–December 2000), pp. 24–25.

[18] Jeremy Main, "How to Steal the Best Ideas Around," *Fortune,* October 19, 1992, pp. 102–3.

[19] Shank and Govindarajan, *Strategic Cost Management,* p. 50.

[20] Some of these options are discussed in more detail in Porter, *Competitive Advantage,* Chapter 3.

[21] An example of how Whirlpool Corporation transformed its supply chain from a competitive liability to a competitive asset is discussed in Reuben E. Stone, "Leading a Supply Chain Turnaround," *Harvard Business Review* 82, no. 10 (October 2004), pp. 114–21.

[22] James Brian Quinn, *Intelligent Enterprise* (New York: Free Press, 1993), p. 54.

[23] Ibid., p. 34.

Chapter 5

[1] This classification scheme is an adaptation of a narrower three-strategy classification presented in Michael E. Porter, *Competitive Strategy: Techniques for Analyzing Industries and Competitors* (New York: Free Press, 1980), Chapter 2, especially pp. 35–40 and 44–46. For a discussion of the different ways in which companies can position themselves
in the marketplace, see Michael E. Porter, "What Is Strategy?" *Harvard Business Review* 74, no. 6 (November–December 1996), pp. 65–67.

[2] Porter, *Competitive Advantage*, p. 97.

[3] Iowa Beef Packers' value chain revamping was first reported in ibid., p. 109. Since then the company has successfully extended its efforts to reconfigure the meat industry value chain, including an entry into the pork segment. IBP was acquired in 2001 by Tyson Foods after a heated bidding war with Smithfield Foods drove Tyson's acquisition price up to $14 billion. Tyson is now applying many of the same value chain revamping principles in chicken, beef, and pork.

[4] Ibid., pp. 135–38.

[5] For a more detailed discussion, see George Stalk, Philip Evans, and Lawrence E. Schulman, "Competing on Capabilities: The New Rules of Corporate Strategy," *Harvard Business Review* 70, no. 2 (March–April 1992), pp. 57–69.

[6] The relevance of perceived value and signaling is discussed in more detail in Porter, *Competitive Advantage,* pp. 138–42.

[7] Ibid., pp. 160–62.

[8] Gary Hamel, "Strategy as Revolution," *Harvard Business Review* 74, no. 4 (July–August 1996), p. 72.

Chapter 6

[1] Yves L. Doz and Gary Hamel, *Alliance Advantage: The Art of Creating Value through Partnering* (Boston: Harvard Business School Press, 1998), pp. xiii, xiv.

[2] Jason Wakeam, "The Five Factors of a Strategic Alliance," *Ivey Business Journal* 68, no. 3 (May–June 2003), pp. 1–4.

[3] Jeffrey H. Dyer, Prashant Kale, and Harbir Singh, "When to Ally and When to Acquire," *Harvard Business Review* 82, no. 7/8 (July–August 2004), p. 109.

[4] Salvatore Parise and Lisa Sasson, "Leveraging Knowledge Management across Strategic Alliances," *Ivey Business Journal* 66, no. 4 (March–April 2002), p. 42.

[5] David Ernst and James Bamford, "Your Alliances Are Too Stable," *Harvard Business Review* 83, no. 6 (June 2005), p. 133.

[6] An excellent discussion of the portfolio approach to managing multiple alliances and how to restructure a faltering alliance is presented in ibid., pp. 133–41.

[7] Michael E. Porter, *The Competitive Advantage of Nations* (New York: Free Press, 1990), p. 66. For a discussion of how to realize the advantages of strategic partnerships, see Nancy J. Kaplan and Jonathan Hurd, "Realizing the Promise of Partnerships," *Journal of Business Strategy* 23, no. 3 (May–June 2002), pp. 38–42; Parise and Sasson,
"Leveraging Knowledge Management," pp. 41–47; and Ernst and Bamford, "Your Alliances Are Too Stable," pp. 133–41.

[8] A. Inkpen, "Learning, Knowledge Acquisition, and Strategic Alliances," *European Management Journal* 16, no. 2 (April 1998), pp. 223–29.

[9] For a discussion of how to raise the chances that a strategic alliance will produce strategically important outcomes, see M. Koza and A. Lewin, "Managing Partnerships and Strategic Alliances: Raising the Odds of Success," *European Management Journal* 18, no. 2 (April 2000), pp. 146–51.

[10] Doz and Hamel, *Alliance Advantage,* Chapters 4–8; Patricia Anslinger and Justin Jenk, "Creating Successful Alliances," *Journal of Business Strategy* 25, no. 2 (2004), pp. 18–23; Rosabeth Moss Kanter, "Collaborative Advantage: The Art of the Alliance," *Harvard Business Review* 72, no. 4 (July–August 1994), pp. 96–108; Joel Bleeke and David Ernst, "The Way to Win in Cross-Border Alliances," *Harvard Business Review* 69, no. 6 (November–December 1991), pp. 127–35 and Gary Hamel, Yves L. Doz, and C. K. Prahalad, "Collaborate with Your Competitors—and Win," *Harvard Business Review* 67, no. 1 (January–February 1989), pp. 133–39.

[11] This same 50 percent success rate for alliances was also cited in Ernst and Bamford, "Your Alliances Are Too Stable," p. 133; both co-authors of this *HBR* article were McKinsey personnel.

[12] Doz and Hamel, *Alliance Advantage,* pp. 16–18.

[13] Dyer, Kale, and Singh, "When to Ally and When to Acquire," p. 109.

[14] For an excellent discussion of the pros and cons of alliances versus acquisitions, see ibid., pp. 109–15.

[15] For an excellent review of the strategic objectives of various types of mergers and acquisitions and the managerial challenges that different kinds of mergers and acquisitions present, see Joseph L. Bower, "Not All M&As Are Alike—and That Matters," *Harvard Business Review* 79, no. 3 (March 2001), pp. 93–101.

[16] For a more expansive discussion, see Dyer, Kale, and Singh, "When to Ally and When to Acquire," pp. 109–10.

[17] See Kathryn R. Harrigan, "Matching Vertical Integration Strategies to Competitive Conditions," *Strategic Management Journal* 7, no. 6 (November–December 1986), pp. 535–56; for a more extensive discussion of the advantages and disadvantages of vertical integration, see John Stuckey and David White, "When and When Not to Vertically Integrate," *Sloan Management Review* (Spring 1993), pp. 71–83.

[18] The resilience of vertical integration strategies despite the disadvantages is discussed in

Thomas Osegowitsch and Anoop Madhok, "Vertical Integration Is Dead or Is It?" *Business Horizons* 46, no. 2 (March–April 2003), pp. 25–35.

[19]This point is explored in greater detail in James Brian Quinn, "Strategic Outsourcing: Leveraging Knowledge Capabilities," *Sloan Management Review* 40, no. 4 (Summer 1999), pp. 9–21.

[20]Dean Foust, "Big Brown's New Bag," *BusinessWeek,* July 19, 2004, pp. 54–55.

[21]"The Internet Age," *BusinessWeek,* October 4, 1999, p. 104.

[22]For a good discussion of the problems that can arise from outsourcing, see Jérôme Barthélemy, "The Seven Deadly Sins of Outsourcing," *Academy of Management Executive* 17, no. 2 (May 2003), pp. 87–100.

[23]For an excellent discussion of aggressive offensive strategies, see George Stalk Jr. and Rob Lachenauer, "Hardball: Five Killer Strategies for Trouncing the Competition," *Harvard Business Review* 82, no. 4 (April 2004), pp. 62–71. A discussion of offensive strategies particularly suitable for industry leaders is presented in Richard D'Aveni, "The Empire Strikes Back: Counterrevolutionary Strategies for Industry Leaders," *Harvard Business Review* 80, no. 11 (November 2002), pp. 66–74.

[24]George Stalk, "Playing Hardball: Why Strategy Still Matters," *Ivey Business Journal* 69, no. 2 (November–December 2004), pp. 1–2.

[25]Ian C. MacMillan, "How Long Can You Sustain a Competitive Advantage?" in *The Strategic Planning Management Reader,* ed. Liam Fahey (Englewood Cliffs, NJ: Prentice Hall, 1989), pp. 23–24.

[26]Ian C. MacMillan, Alexander B. van Putten, and Rita Gunther McGrath, "Global Gamesmanship," *Harvard Business Review* 81, no. 5 (May 2003), pp. 66–67; also, see Askay R. Rao, Mark E. Bergen, and Scott Davis, "How to Fight a Price War," *Harvard Business Review* 78, no. 2 (March–April, 2000), pp. 107–16.

[27]Stalk and Lachenauer, "Hardball," p. 64?

[28]Stalk, "Playing Hardball," p. 4.

[29]Stalk and Lachenauer, "Hardball," p. 67.

[30]For an interesting study of how small firms can successfully employ guerrilla-style tactics, see Ming-Jer Chen and Donald C. Hambrick, "Speed, Stealth, and Selective Attack: How Small Firms Differ from Large Firms in Competitive Behavior," *Academy of Management Journal* 38, no. 2 (April 1995), pp. 453–82. Other discussions of guerrilla offensives can be found in Ian MacMillan, "How Business Strategists Can Use Guerrilla Warfare Tactics," *Journal of Business Strategy* 1, no. 2 (Fall 1980), pp. 63–65; William E. Rothschild, "Surprise

and the Competitive Advantage," *Journal of Business Strategy* 4, no. 3 (Winter 1984), pp. 10–18; Kathryn R. Harrigan, *Strategic Flexibility* (Lexington, MA: Lexington Books, 1985), pp. 30–45; and Liam Fahey, "Guerrilla Strategy: The Hit-and-Run Attack," in *The Strategic Management Planning Reader,* ed. Liam Fahey (Englewood Cliffs, NJ: Prentice Hall, 1989), pp. 194–97.

[31]The use of preemptive strike offensives is treated comprehensively in Ian MacMillan, "Preemptive Strategies," *Journal of Business Strategy* 14, no. 2 (Fall 1983), pp. 16–26.

[32]W. Chan Kim and Renée Mauborgne, "Blue Ocean Strategy," *Harvard Business Review* 82, no. 10 (October 2004), pp. 76–84.

[33]Philip Kotler, *Marketing Management,* 5th Edition (Englewood Cliffs, N.J.: Prentice Hall, 1984), p. 400.

[34]Michael E. Porter, *Competitive Advantage* (New York: Free Press, 1985), p. 518.

[35]For an excellent discussion of how to wage offensives against strong rivals, see David B. Yoffie and Mary Kwak, "Mastering Balance: How to Meet and Beat a Stronger Opponent," *California Management Review* 44, no. 2 (Winter 2002), pp. 8–24.

[36]Stalk, "Playing Hardball," pp. 1–2.

[37]Porter, *Competitive Advantage,* pp. 489–94.

[38]Ibid., pp. 495–97. The list here is selective; Porter offers a greater number of options.

[39]For a more extensive discussion of how the Internet impacts strategy, see Michael E. Porter, "Strategy and the Internet," *Harvard Business Review* 79, no. 3 (March 2001), pp. 63–78.

[40]Porter, *Competitive Advantage,* pp. 232–33.

[41]For research evidence on the effects of pioneering versus following, see Jeffrey G. Covin, Dennis P. Slevin, and Michael B. Heeley, "Pioneers and Followers: Competitive Tactics, Environment, and Growth," *Journal of Business Venturing* 15, no. 2 (March 1999), pp. 175–210 and Christopher A. Bartlett and Sumantra Ghoshal, "Going Global: Lessons from Late-Movers," *Harvard Business Review* 78, no. 2 (March–April 2000), pp. 132–45.

[42]For a more extensive discussion of this point, see Fernando Suarez and Gianvito Lanzolla, "The Half-Truth of First-Mover Advantage," *Harvard Business Review* 83, no. 4 (April 2005), pp. 121–27.

[43]Gary Hamel, "Smart Mover, Dumb Mover," *Fortune,* September 3, 2001, p. 195.

[44]Ibid., p. 192.

[45]Costas Markides and Paul A. Geroski, "Racing to be 2nd: Conquering the Industries of the Future," *Business Strategy Review* 15, no. 4 (Winter 2004), pp. 25–31.

Chapter 7

[1]For an insightful discussion of how much significance these kinds of demographic and market differences have, see C. K. Prahalad and Kenneth Lieberthal, "The End of Corporate Imperialism," *Harvard Business Review* 76, no. 4 (July–August 1998), pp. 68–79.

[2]Joseph Caron, "The Business of Doing Business with China: An Ambassador Reflects," *Ivey Business Journal* 69, no. 5 (May–June 2005), p. 2.

[3]Extrapolated from 2002 statistics reported by the U.S. Department of Labor.

[4]Michael E. Porter, *The Competitive Advantage of Nations* (New York: Free Press, 1990), pp. 53–54.

[5]Ibid., p. 61.

[6]For more details on the merits of and opportunities for cross-border transfer of successful strategy experiments, see C. A. Bartlett and S. Ghoshal, *Managing Across Borders: The Transnational Solution,* 2nd ed. (Boston: Harvard Business School Press, 1998), pp. 79–80 and Chapter 9.

[7]H. Kurt Christensen, "Corporate Strategy: Managing a Set of Businesses," in *The Portable MBA in Strategy,* ed. Liam Fahey and Robert M. Randall (New York: Wiley, 2001), p. 42.

[8]Porter, *Competitive Advantage,* pp. 53–55.

[9]Ibid., pp. 55–58.

[10]C. K. Prahalad and Yves L. Doz, *The Multinational Mission* (New York: Free Press, 1987), p. 60.

[11]Porter, *Competitive Advantage,* p. 57.

[12]Ibid., pp. 58–60.

[13]Several other types of strategic offensives that companies have occasionally employed in select foreign market situations are discussed in Ian C. MacMillan, Alexander B. van Putten, and Rita Gunther McGrath, "Global Gamesmanship," *Harvard Business Review* 81, no. 5 (May 2003), pp. 63–68.

[14]Canadian International Trade Tribunal, findings issued June 16, 2005 and posted at www.citttcce.gc.ca (accessed September 28, 2005).

[15]George Stalk, "Playing Hardball: Why Strategy Still Matters," *Ivey Business Journal* 69, no. 2 (November–December 2004), pp. 1–2.

[16]For two especially insightful studies of company experiences with cross-border alliances, see Joel Bleeke and David Ernst, "The Way to Win in Cross-Border Alliances," *Harvard Business Review* 69, no. 6 (November–December 1991), pp. 127–35, and Gary Hamel, Yves L. Doz, and C. K. Prahalad, "Collaborate with Your Competitors—and Win," *Harvard Business Review* 67, no. 1 (January–February 1989), pp. 133–39.

17See Yves L. Doz and Gary Hamel, *Alliance Advantage* (Boston, MA: Harvard Business School Press, 1998), especially Chapters 2–4; Bleeke and Ernst, "The Way to Win," pp. 127–33; Hamel, Doz, and Prahalad, "Collaborate with Your Competitors," pp. 134–35; and Porter, *Competitive Advantage,* p. 66.

18Christensen, "Corporate Strategy," p. 43.

19For an excellent presentation on the pros and cons of alliances versus acquisitions, see Jeffrey H. Dyer, Prashant Kale, and Harbir Singh, "When to Ally and When to Acquire," *Harvard Business Review* 82, no. 7/8 (July–August 2004), pp. 109–15.

20For additional discussion of company experiences with alliances and partnerships, see Doz and Hamel, *Alliance Advantage,* Chapters 2–7, and Rosabeth Moss Kanter, "Collaborative Advantage: The Art of the Alliance," *Harvard Business Review* 72, no. 4 (July–August 1994), pp. 96–108.

21Details are reported in Shawn Tully, "The Alliance from Hell," *Fortune,* June 24, 1996, pp. 64–72.

22Jeremy Main, "Making Global Alliances Work," *Fortune,* December 19, 1990, p. 125.

23Prahalad and Lieberthal, "The End of Corporate Imperialism," p. 77.

24Ibid.

25This point is discussed at greater length in Prahalad and Lieberthal, "The End of Corporate Imperialism," pp. 68–79; also see David J. Arnold and John A. Quelch, "New Strategies in Emerging Markets," *Sloan Management Review* 40, no. 1 (Fall 1998), pp. 7–20. For a more extensive discussion of strategy in emerging markets, see C. K. Prahalad, *The Fortune at the Bottom of the Pyramid: Eradicating Poverty through Profits* (Upper Saddle River, NJ: Wharton, 2005), especially Chapters 1–3.

26Brenda Cherry, "What China Eats (and Drinks and . . .)," *Fortune,* October 4, 2004, pp. 152–53.

27Prahalad and Lieberthal, "The End of Corporate Imperialism," pp. 72–73.

28Tarun Khanna, Krishna G. Palepu, and Jayant Sinha, "Strategies That Fit Emerging Markets," *Harvard Business Review* 83 no. 6 (June 2005), p. 63.

29Prahalad and Lieberthal, "The End of Corporate Imperialism," p. 72.

30Khanna, Palepu, and Sinha, "Strategies That Fit Emerging Markets," pp. 73–74.

31Ibid., p. 74.

32Ibid., p. 76.

33Niroj Dawar and Tony Frost, "Competing with Giants: Survival Strategies for Local Companies in Emerging Markets," *Harvard Business Review* 77, no. 1

(January–February 1999), p. 122; see also Guitz Ger, "Localizing in the Global Village: Local Firms Competing in Global Markets," *California Management Review* 41, no. 4 (Summer 1999), pp. 64–84.

34Dawar and Frost, "Competing with Giants," p. 124.

35Ibid., p. 125.

36Steve Hamm, "Tech's Future," *BusinessWeek,* September 27, 2004, p. 88.

37Dawar and Frost, "Competing with Giants," p. 126.

30Hamm, "Tech's Future," p. 89.

Chapter 8

1Michael E. Porter, *Competitive Strategy: Techniques for Analyzing Industries and Competitors* (New York: Free Press, 1980), pp. 216–23.

2Phillip Kotler, *Marketing Management,* 5th ed. (Englewood Cliffs, NJ: Prentice Hall, 1984), p. 366, and Porter, *Competitive Strategy,* Chapter 10.

3Several of these were pinpointed and discussed in Charles W. Hofer and Dan Schendel, *Strategy Formulation: Analytical Concepts* (St. Paul, MN: West, 1978), pp. 164–65.

4Ibid., pp. 164–65.

5Porter, *Competitive Strategy,* pp. 238–40.

6The following discussion draws on ibid., pp. 241–46.

7Kathryn R. Harrigan and Michael E. Porter, "End-Game Strategies for Declining Industries," *Harvard Business Review* 61, no. 4 (July–August 1983), pp. 112–13.

8R. G. Hamermesh and S. B. Silk, "How to Compete in Stagnant Industries," *Harvard Business Review* 57, no. 5 (September–October 1979), p. 161, and Kathryn R. Harrigan, *Strategies for Declining Businesses* (Lexington, MA: Heath, 1980).

9Hamermesh and Silk, "How to Compete," p. 162; Harrigan and Porter, "End-Game Strategies," p. 118.

10Hamermesh and Silk, "How to Compete," p. 165.

11Harrigan and Porter, "End Game Strategies," pp. 111–21; Harrigan, *Strategies for Declining Businesses;* and Phillip Kotler, "Harvesting Strategies for Weak Products," *Business Horizons* 21, no. 5 (August 1978), pp. 17–18.

12The strategic issues companies must address in fast-changing market environments are thoroughly explored in Gary Hamel and Liisa Välikangas, "The Quest for Resilience," *Harvard Business Review* 81, no. 9 (September 2003), pp. 52–63; Shona L. Brown and Kathleen M. Eisenhardt, *Competing on the Edge: Strategy as*

Structured Chaos (Boston: Harvard Business School Press, 1998); and Richard A. D'Aveni, *Hyper-Competition: Managing the Dynamics of Strategic Maneuvering* (New York: Free Press, 1994). See also Richard A. D'Aveni, "Coping with Hypercompetition: Utilizing the New 7S's Framework," *Academy of Management Executive* 9, no. 3 (August 1995), pp. 45–56, and Bala Chakravarthy, "A New Strategy Framework for Coping with Turbulence," *Sloan Management Review* (Winter 1997), pp. 69–82.

13Brown and Eisenhardt, *Competing on the Edge,* pp. 4–5.

14Ibid., p. 4.

15For deeper insight into building competitive advantage through R&D and technological innovation, see Shaker A. Zahra, Sarah Nash, and Deborah J. Bickford, "Transforming Technological Pioneering into Competitive Advantage," *Academy of Management Executive* 9, no. 1 (February 1995), pp. 32–41.

16Brown and Eisenhardt, *Competing on the Edge,* pp. 14–15. See also Kathleen M. Eisenhardt and Shona L. Brown, "Time Pacing: Competing in Markets That Won't Stand Still," *Harvard Business Review* 76, no. 2 (March–April 1998), pp. 59–69.

17The circumstances of competing in a fragmented industry are discussed at length in Porter, *Competitive Strategy,* Chapter 9; this section draws on Porter's treatment.

18What follows is based on the discussion in Eric D. Beinhocker, "Robust Adaptive Strategies," *Sloan Management Review* 40, no. 3 (Spring 1999), p. 101.

19Gary Hamel, "Bringing Silicon Valley Inside," *Harvard Business Review* 77, no. 5 (September–October 1999), p. 73.

20Beinhocker, "Robust Adaptive Strategies," p. 101.

21Kotler, *Marketing Management,* Chapter 23; Michael E. Porter, *Competitive Advantage* (New York: Free Press, 1985), Chapter 14; and Ian C. MacMillan, "Seizing Competitive Initiative," *Journal of Business Strategy* 2, no. 4 (Spring 1982), pp. 43–57. For a perspective on what industry leaders can do when confronted with revolutionary market changes, see Richard D'Aveni, "The Empire Strikes Back: Counterrevolutionary Strategies for Industry Leaders," *Harvard Business Review* 80, no. 11 (November 2002), pp. 66–74.

22The value of being a frequent first-mover and leading change is documented in Walter J. Ferrier, Ken G. Smith, and Curtis M. Grimm, "The Role of Competitive Action in Market Share Erosion and Industry Dethronement: A Study of Industry Leaders and Challengers," *Academy of Management Journal* 42, no. 4 (August 1999), pp. 372–88.

23George Stalk Jr. and Rob Lachenauer, "Five Killer Strategies for Trouncing the Competition," *Harvard Business Review* 82, no. 4 (April 2004), pp. 64–65.

24Ibid., pp. 67–68.

25For more details, see R. G. Hamermesh, M. J. Anderson, and J. E. Harris, "Strategies for Low Market Share Businesses," *Harvard Business Review* 56, no. 3 (May–June 1978), pp. 95–96.

26Porter, *Competitive Advantage*, p. 514.

27Some of these options are drawn from Kotler, *Marketing Management,* pp. 397–412; Hamermesh, Anderson, and Harris, "Strategies for Low Market Share Businesses," pp. 97–102; and Porter, *Competitive Advantage,* Chapter 15.

28William K. Hall, "Survival Strategies in a Hostile Environment," *Harvard Business Review* 58, no. 5 (September–October 1980), pp. 75–85. See also Frederick M. Zimmerman, *The Turnaround Experience: Real-World Lessons in Revitalizing Corporations* (New York: McGraw-Hill, 1991), and Gary J. Castrogiovanni, B. R. Baliga, and Roland E. Kidwell, "Curing Sick Businesses: Changing CEOs in Turnaround Efforts," *Academy of Management Executive* 6, no. 3 (August 1992), pp. 26–41.

29A study performed by Crest Advisors, a boutique investment firm and reported in Leigh Gallagher, "Avoiding the Pitfalls of Orphan Stocks," www.forbes.com, April 24, 2003.

30Phillip Kotler, "Harvesting Strategies for Weak Products," *Business Horizons* 21, no. 5 (August 1978), pp. 17–18.

Chapter 9

1For a further discussion of when diversification makes good strategic sense, see Constantinos C. Markides, "To Diversify or Not to Diversify," *Harvard Business Review* 75, no. 6 (November–December 1997), pp. 93–99.

2Michael E. Porter, "From Competitive Advantage to Corporate Strategy," *Harvard Business Review* 45, no. 3 (May–June 1987), pp. 46–49.

3Michael E. Porter, *Competitive Strategy: Techniques for Analyzing Industries and Competitors* (New York: Free Press, 1980), pp. 354–55.

4Ibid., pp. 344–45.

5Yves L. Doz and Gary Hamel, *Alliance Advantage: The Art of Creating Value through Partnering* (Boston: Harvard Business School Press, 1998), Chapters 1 and 2.

6Michael E. Porter, *Competitive Advantage* (New York: Free Press, 1985), pp. 318–19 and pp. 337–53, and Porter, "From Competitive Advantage," pp. 53–57. For an empirical study confirming that strategic fits are capable of enhancing performance (provided the resulting resource strengths are competitively valuable and difficult to duplicate by rivals), see Constantinos C. Markides and Peter J. Williamson, "Corporate Diversification and Organization Structure: A Resource-Based View," *Academy of Management Journal* 39, no. 2 (April 1996), pp. 340–67.

7For a discussion of the strategic significance of cross-business coordination of value chain activities and insight into how the process works, see Jeanne M. Liedtka, "Collaboration across Lines of Business for Competitive Advantage," *Academy of Management Executive* 10, no. 2 (May 1996), pp. 20–34.

8"Beyond Knowledge Management: How Companies Mobilize Experience," *Financial Times,* February 8, 1999, p. 5.

9For a discussion of what is involved in actually capturing strategic fit benefits, see Kathleen M. Eisenhardt and D. Charles Galunic, "Coevolving: At Last, a Way to Make Synergies Work," *Harvard Business Review* 78, no. 1 (January–February 2000), pp. 91–101. Adeptness at capturing cross-business strategic fits positively impacts performance; see Constantinos C. Markides and Peter J. Williamson, "Related Diversification, Core Competences and Corporate Performance," *Strategic Management Journal* 15 (Summer 1994), pp. 149–65.

10Peter Drucker, *Management: Tasks, Responsibilities, Practices* (New York: Harper & Row, 1974), pp. 692–93.

11While arguments that unrelated diversification are a superior way to diversify financial risk have logical appeal, there is research showing that related diversification is less risky from a financial perspective than is unrelated diversification; see Michael Lubatkin and Sayan Chatterjee, "Extending Modern Portfolio Theory into the Domain of Corporate Diversification: Does It Apply?" *Academy of Management Journal* 37, no. 1 (February 1994), pp. 109–36.

12For a review of the experiences of companies that have pursued unrelated diversification successfully, see Patricia L. Anslinger and Thomas E. Copeland, "Growth through Acquisitions: A Fresh Look," *Harvard Business Review* 74, no. 1 (January–February 1996), pp. 126–35.

13Of course, management may be willing to assume the risk that trouble will not strike before it has had time to learn the business well enough to bail it out of almost any difficulty. But there is research that shows this is very risky from a financial perspective; see, for example, Lubatkin and Chatterjee, "Extending Modern Portfolio Theory," pp. 132–33.

14For research evidence of the failure of broad diversification and trend of companies to focus their diversification efforts more narrowly, see Lawrence G. Franko, "The Death of Diversification? The Focusing of the World's Industrial Firms, 1980–2000," *Business Horizons* 47, no. 4 (July–August 2004), pp. 41–50.

15For an excellent discussion of what to look for in assessing these fits, see Andrew Campbell, Michael Gould, and Marcus Alexander, "Corporate Strategy: The Quest for Parenting Advantage," *Harvard Business Review* 73, no. 2 (March–April 1995), pp. 120–32.

16Ibid., p. 128.

17Ibid., p. 123.

18A good discussion of the importance of having adequate resources, and also the importance of upgrading corporate resources and capabilities, can be found in David J. Collis and Cynthia A. Montgomery, "Competing on Resources: Strategy in the 90s," *Harvard Business Review* 73, no. 4 (July–August 1995), pp. 118–28.

19Ibid., pp. 121–22.

20Drucker, *Management,* p. 709.

21See, for example, Constantinos C. Markides, "Diversification, Restructuring, and Economic Performance," *Strategic Management Journal* 16 (February 1995), pp. 101–18.

22For a discussion of why divestiture needs to be a standard part of any company's diversification strategy, see Lee Dranikoff, Tim Koller, and Antoon Schneider, "Divestiture: Strategy's Missing Link," *Harvard Business Review* 80, no. 5 (May 2002), pp. 74–83.

23Drucker, *Management,* p. 94.

24See David J. Collis and Cynthia A. Montgomery, "Creating Corporate Advantage," *Harvard Business Review* 76, no. 3 (May–June 1998), pp. 72–80.

25Drucker, *Management,* p. 719.

26Evidence that restructuring strategies tend to result in higher levels of performance is contained in Markides, "Diversification, Restructuring," pp. 101–18.

27Company press release, October 6, 2005.

28Dranikoff, Koller, and Schneider, "Divestiture," p. 76.

29C. K. Prahalad and Yves L. Doz, *The Multinational Mission* (New York: Free Press, 1987), p. 2.

30Ibid., p. 15.

31Ibid., pp. 62–63.

32For a fascinating discussion of the chess match in strategy that can unfold when two DMNC's go head-to-head in a global marketplace, see Ian C. MacMillan, Alexander B. van Putten, and Rita Gunther McGrath, "Global Gamesmanship," *Harvard Business Review* 81, no. 5 (May 2003), pp. 62–71.

Chapter 10

[1]James E. Post, Anne T. Lawrence, and James Weber, *Business and Society: Corporate Strategy, Public Policy, Ethics,* 10th ed. (Burr Ridge, IL: McGraw-Hill/Irwin, 2002), p. 103.

[2]For research on what are the universal moral values (six are identified—trustworthiness, respect, responsibility, fairness, caring, and citizenship), see Mark S. Schwartz, "Universal Moral Values for Corporate Codes of Ethics," *Journal of Business Ethics* 59, no. 1 (June 2005), pp. 27–44.

[3]See, for instance, Mark S. Schwartz, "A Code of Ethics for Corporate Codes of Ethics," *Journal of Business Ethics* 41, nos. 1–2 (November–December 2002), pp. 27–43.

[4]For more discussion of this point, see ibid., pp. 29–30.

[5]T. L. Beauchamp and N. E. Bowie, *Ethical Theory and Business* (Upper Saddle River, NJ: Prentice Hall, 2001), p. 8.

[6]Based on information in U.S. Department of Labor, "The Department of Labor's 2002 Findings on the Worst Forms of Child Labor," www.dol.gov/ILAB/media/reports, 2003.

[7]ILO-IPEC (SIMPOC), *Every Child Counts: New Global Estimates on Child Labour,* www.ilo.org/public/english/standards/ipec/simpoc/others/globalest.pdf, April 2002. The estimate of the number of working children is based on the definition of the "economically active population," which restricts the labor force activity of children to "paid" or "unpaid" employment, military personnel, and the unemployed. The definition does not include children in informal work settings, non-economic activities, "hidden" forms of work, or work that is defined by ILO Convention 182 as the worst forms of child labor.

[8]W. M. Greenfield, "In the Name of Corporate Social Responsibility," *Business Horizons* 47, no. 1 (January–February 2004), p. 22.

[9]For a study of why such factors as low per capita income, lower disparities in income distribution, and various cultural factors are often associated with a higher incidence of bribery, see Rajib Sanyal, "Determinants of Bribery in International Business: The Cultural and Economic Factors," *Journal of Business Ethics* 59, no.1 (June 2005), pp. 139–45.

[10]For a study of bribe-paying frequency by country, see Transparency International, *2003 Global Corruption Report,* p. 267; this report can be accessed at www.globalcorruptionreport.org.

[11]Roger Chen and Chia-Pei Chen, "Chinese Professional Managers and the Issue of Ethical Behavior," *Ivey Business Journal* 69, no, 5 (May/June 2005), p.1.

[12]Thomas Donaldson and Thomas W. Dunfee, "When Ethics Travel: The Promise and Peril of Global Business Ethics," *California Management Review* 41, no. 4 (Summer 1999), p. 53.

[13]John Reed and Erik Portanger, "Bribery, Corruption Are Rampant in Eastern Europe, Survey Finds," *Wall Street Journal,* November 9, 1999, p. A21.

[14]See Transparency International, *Global Corruption Report* for 2003, 2004, and 2005; these reports can be accessed at www.globalcorruptionreport.org.

[15]For a study of "facilitating" payments to obtain a favor (such as expediting an administrative process, obtaining a permit or license, or avoiding an abuse of authority), which are sometimes condoned as unavoidable or are excused on grounds of low wages and lack of professionalism among public officials, see Antonio Argandoña, "Corruption and Companies: The Use of Facilitating Payments," *Journal of Business Ethics* 60, no. 3 (September 2005), pp. 251–64.

[16]Donaldson and Dunfee, "When Ethics Travel," p. 59.

[17]Thomas Donaldson and Thomas W. Dunfee, *Ties That Bind: A Social Contracts Approach to Business Ethics* (Boston: Harvard Business School Press, 1999), pp. 35, 83.

[18]Based on a report in M. J. Satchell, "Deadly Trade in Toxics," *U.S. News and World Report,* March 7, 1994 p. 64, cited in Donaldson and Dunfee, "When Ethics Travel," p. 46.

[19]Chen and Chen, "Chinese Professional Managers," p. 1.

[20]Two of the definitive treatments of integrated social contracts theory as applied to ethics are Thomas Donaldson and Thomas W. Dunfee, "Towards a Unified Conception of Business Ethics: Integrative Social Contracts Theory," *Academy of Management Review* 19, no. 2 (April 1994), pp. 252–84, and Donaldson and Dunfee, *Ties That Bind,* especially Chapters 3, 4, and 6. See also Andrew Spicer, Thomas W. Dunfee, and Wendy J. Bailey, "Does National Context Matter in Ethical Decision Making? An Empirical Test of Integrative Social Contracts Theory," *Academy of Management Journal* 47, no. 4 (August 2004), p. 610.

[21]P. M. Nichols, "Outlawing Transnational Bribery through the World Trade Organization," *Law and Policy in International Business* 28, no. 2 (1997), pp. 321–22.

[22]Donaldson and Dunfee, "When Ethics Travel," pp. 55–56.

[23]Archie B. Carroll, "Models of Management Morality for the New Millennium," *Business Ethics Quarterly* 11, no. 2 (April 2001), pp. 367–69.

[24]Ibid., pp. 369–70.

[25]John R. Wilke and Don Clark, "Samsung to Pay Fine for Price-Fixing," *The Wall Street Journal,* October 14, 2005, p. A3.

[26]For survey data on what managers say about why they sometimes behave unethically, see John F. Veiga, Timothy D. Golden, and Kathleen Dechant, "Why Managers Bend Company Rules," *Academy of Management Executive* 18, no. 2 (May 2004), pp. 84–89.

[27]For more details see Ronald R. Sims and Johannes Brinkmann, "Enron Ethics (Or: Culture Matters More Than Codes)," *Journal of Business Ethics* 45, no. 3 (July 2003), pp. 244–46.

[28]As reported in Gardiner Harris, "At Bristol-Myers, Ex-Executives Tell of Numbers Games," *The Wall Street Journal,* December 12, 2002, pp. A1, A13.

[29]Ibid., p. A13.

[30]Veiga, Golden, and Dechant, "Why Managers Bend the Rules," p. 36.

[31]The following account is based largely on the discussion and analysis in Sims and Brinkmann, "Enron Ethics," pp. 245–52. Perhaps the definitive book-length account of the corrupt Enron culture is Kurt Eichenwald, *Conspiracy of Fools: A True Story* (New York: Broadway Books, 2005).

[32]Chip Cummins and Almar Latour, "How Shell's Move to Revamp Culture Ended in Scandal," *The Wall Street Journal,* November 2, 2004, p. A14.

[33]Gedeon J. Rossouw and Leon J. van Vuuren, "Modes of Managing Morality: A Descriptive Model of Strategies for Managing Ethics," *Journal of Business Ethics,* 46, no. 4 (September 2003), pp. 389–400.

[34]Empirical evidence that an ethical culture approach produces better results than the compliance approach is presented in Terry Thomas, John R. Schermerhorn, and John W. Dienhart, "Strategic Leadership of Ethical Behavior," *Academy of Management Executive* 18, no. 2 (May 2004), p. 64.

[35]Anna Wilde Mathews and Barbara Martinez, "E-Mails Suggest Merck Knew Vioxx's Dangers at Early Stage," *The Wall Street Journal,* November 1, 2004, pp. A1 and A10.

[36]Archie B. Carroll, "The Four Faces of Corporate Citizenship," *Business and Society Review* 100/101 (September 1998), p. 6.

[37]Business Roundtable, "Statement on Corporate Responsibility," New York, October 1981, p. 9.

[38]Sarah Roberts, Justin Keeble, and David Brown, "The Business Case for Corporate Citizenship," a study for the World Economic Forum, www.weforum.org/corporatecitizenship, October 14, 2003, p. 3.

[39]N. Craig Smith, "Corporate Responsibility: Whether and How," *California Management Review* 45, no. 4 (Summer 2003), p. 63.

[40]Jeffrey Hollender, "What Matters Most: Corporate Values and Social Responsibility," *California Management Review* 46, no. 4 (Summer 2004), p. 112. For a study of the

corporate social responsibility reports of leading European companies, see Simon Knox, Stan Maklan, and Paul French, "Corporate Social Responsibility: Exploring Stakeholder Relationships and Program Reporting across Leading FTSE Companies," *Journal of Business Ethics* 61, no. 1 (September 2005), pp. 7–28.

[41] World Business Council for Sustainable Development, "Corporate Social Responsibility: Making Good Business Sense," www.wbscd.ch, January 2000 (accessed October 10, 2003), p. 7. For a discussion of how companies are connecting social initiatives to their core values, see David Hess, Nikolai Rogovsky, and Thomas W. Dunfee, "The Next Wave of Corporate Community Involvement: Corporate Social Initiatives," *California Management Review* 44, no. 2 (Winter 2002), pp. 110–25, and Susan Ariel Aaronson, "Corporate Responsibility in the Global Village: The British Role Model and the American Laggard," *Business and Society Review,* 108, no. 3 (September 2003), p. 323.

[42] www.chick-fil-a.com (accessed November 4, 2005).

[43] Smith, "Corporate Responsibility," p. 63. See also World Economic Forum, "Findings of a Survey on Global Corporate Leadership," www.weforum.org/corporatecitizenship, (accessed October 11, 2003).

[44] Roberts, Keeble, and Brown, "The Business Case," p. 6.

[45] Ibid., p. 3.

[46] Wallace N. Davidson, Abuzar El-Jelly, and Dan L. Worrell, "Influencing Managers to Change Unpopular Corporate Behavior through Boycotts and Divestitures: A Stock Market Test," *Business and Society,* 34, no. 2 (1995), pp. 171–196.

[47] Tom McCawley, "Racing to Improve Its Reputation: Nike Has Fought to Shed Its Image as an Exploiter of Third-World Labor, Yet It Is Still a Target of Activists," *Financial Times,* December 2000, p. 14, and Smith, "Corporate Social Responsibility," p. 61.

[48] Based on data in Amy Aronson, "Corporate Diversity, Integration, and Market Penetration," *BusinessWeek,* October 20, 2003, pp. 138 ff.

[49] Smith, "Corporate Social Responsibility," p. 62.

[50] See Social Investment Forum, *2001 Report on Socially Responsible Investing Trends in the United States* (Washington, DC: Social Investment Forum, 2001).

[51] Smith, "Corporate Social Responsibility," p. 63.

[52] See James C. Collins and Jerry I. Porras, *Built to Last: Successful Habits of Visionary Companies,* 3rd ed. (London: HarperBusiness, 2002); Roberts, Keeble, and Brown, "The Business Case," p. 4; and Smith, "Corporate Social Responsibility," p. 63.

[53] Roberts, Keeble, and Brown, "The Business Case," p. 4.

[54] Smith, "Corporate Social Responsibility," p. 65; Lee E. Preston and Douglas P. O'Bannon, "The Corporate Social-Financial Performance Relationship," *Business and Society* 36, no. 4 (December 1997), pp. 419–29; Ronald M. Roman, Sefa Hayibor, and Bradley R. Agle, "The Relationship between Social and Financial Performance: Repainting a Portrait," *Business and Society* 38, no. 1 (March 1999), pp. 109–25; and Joshua D. Margolis and James P. Walsh, *People and Profits* (Mahwah, NJ: Lawrence Erlbaum, 2001).

[55] Smith, "Corporate Social Responsibility," p. 71.

[56] Business Roundtable, "Statement on Corporate Governance," Washington, DC, September 1997, p. 3.

[57] Henry Mintzberg, Robert Simons, and Kunal Basu, "Beyond Selfishness," *MIT Sloan Management Review* 44, no. 1 (Fall 2002), p. 69.

[58] For a good discussion of the debate between maximizing shareholder value and balancing stakeholder interests, see H. Jeff Smith, "The Shareholders versus Stakeholders Debate," MIT *Sloan Management Review* 44, no. 4 (Summer 2003), pp. 85–91.

[59] Smith, "Corporate Social Responsibility," p. 70.

[60] Based on information in Edna Gundersen, "Rights Issue Rocks the Music World," *USA Today,* September 16, 2002, pp. D1, D2.

[61] This information is based on Charles Gasparino, "Salomon Probe Includes Senior Executives," *The Wall Street Journal,* September 3, 2002, p. C1; Randall Smith and Susan Pulliam, "How a Star Banker Pressed for IPOs," *The Wall Street Journal,* September 4, 2002, pp. C1, C14; Randall Smith and Susan Pulliam, "How a Technology-Banking Star Doled Out Shares of Hot IPOs," *The Wall Street Journal,* September 23; 2002, pp. A1, A10; and Randall Smith, "Goldman Sachs Faces Scrutiny for IPO-Allocation Practices," *The Wall Street Journal,* October 3, 2002, pp. A1, A6.

Chapter 11

[1] As quoted in Steven W. Floyd and Bill Wooldridge, "Managing Strategic Consensus: The Foundation of Effective Implementation," *Academy of Management Executive* 6, no. 4 (November 1992), p. 27.

[2] Jack Welch with Suzy Welch, *Winning* (New York: HarperBusiness, 2005), p. 135.

[3] For an excellent and very pragmatic discussion of this point, see Larry Bossidy and Ram Charan, *Execution: The Discipline of Getting Things Done* (New York: Crown Business, 2002), Chapter 1.

[4] For an insightful discussion of how important staffing an organization with the right people is, see Christopher A. Bartlett and Sumantra Ghoshal, "Building Competitive Advantage through People," *MIT Sloan Management Review* 43, no. 2 (Winter 2002), pp. 34–41.

[5] The importance of assembling an executive team with exceptional ability to see what needs to be done and an instinctive talent for figuring out how to get it done is discussed in Justin Menkes, "Hiring for Smarts," *Harvard Business Review* 83, no. 11 (November 2005), pp. 100–9 and Justin Menkes, *Executive Intelligence* (New York: HarperCollins, 2005), especially Chapters 1–4.

[6] Welch with Welch, *Winning,* p. 139.

[7] See Bossidy and Charan, *Execution: The Discipline of Getting Things Done,* Chapter 1.

[8] Menkes, *Executive Intelligence,* pp. 68, 76.

[9] Bossidy and Charan, *Execution;* Chapter 5.

[10] Welch with Welch, *Winning,* pp. 141–42.

[11] Menkes, *Executive Intelligence,* pp. 65–71.

[12] Jim Collins, *Good to Great* (New York: HarperBusiness, 2001), p. 44.

[13] John Byrne, "The Search for the Young and Gifted," *BusinessWeek,* October 4, 1999, p. 108.

[14] James Brian Quinn, *Intelligent Enterprise* (New York: Free Press, 1992), pp. 52–53, 55, 73–74, 76. Also see Christine Soo, Timothy Devinney, David Midgley, and Anne Deering, "Knowledge Management: Philosophy, Processes, and Pitfalls," *California Management Review* 44, no. 4 (Summer 2002), pp. 129–51, and Julian Birkinshaw, "Why Is Knowledge Management So Difficult?" *Business Strategy Review* 12, no. 1 (March 2001), pp. 11–18.

[15] Robert H. Hayes, Gary P. Pisano, and David M. Upton, *Strategic Operations: Competing through Capabilities* (New York: Free Press, 1996), pp. 503–7. Also see Jonas Ridderstråle, "Cashing in on Corporate Competencies," *Business Strategy Review* 14, no. 1 (Spring 2003), pp. 27–38, and Danny Miller, Russell Eisenstat, and Nathaniel Foote, "Strategy from the Inside Out: Building Capability-Creating Organizations," *California Management Review* 44, no. 3 (Spring 2002), pp. 37–55.

[16] Quinn, *Intelligent Enterprise,* p. 43.

[17] Quinn, *Intelligent Enterprise,* pp. 33, 89; James Brian Quinn and Frederick G. Hilmer, "Strategic Outsourcing," *Sloan Management Review* 35, no. 4 (Summer 1994), pp. 43–55; Jussi Heikkilä and Carlos Cordon, "Outsourcing: A Core or Non-Core Strategic Management Decision," *Strategic Change* 11, no. 3 (June–July 2002), pp. 183–93; and James Brian Quinn, "Strategic Outsourcing: Leveraging Knowledge Capabilities," *Sloan Management Review* 40, no. 4 (Summer 1999), pp. 9–22. A strong case for outsourcing is presented in

C. K. Prahalad, "The Art of Outsourcing," *The Wall Street Journal,* June 8, 2005, p. A13. For a discussion of why outsourcing initiatives fall short of expectations, see Jérôme Barthélemy, "The Seven Deadly Sins of Outsourcing," *Academy of Management Executive* 17, no. 2 (May 2003), pp. 87–98.

[18] Quinn, "Strategic Outsourcing," p. 17.

[19] For a more extensive discussion of the reasons for building cooperative, collaborative alliances and partnerships with other companies, see James F. Moore, *The Death of Competition* (New York: HarperBusiness, 1996), especially Chapter 3; Quinn and Hilmer, "Strategic Outsourcing"; and Quinn, "Strategic Outsourcing."

[20] Quinn, *Intelligent Enterprise,* pp. 39–40; also see Barthélemy, "The Seven Deadly Sins."

[21] The importance of matching organization design and structure to the particular needs of strategy was first brought to the forefront in a landmark study of 70 large corporations conducted by Professor Alfred Chandler of Harvard University. Chandler's research revealed that changes in an organization's strategy bring about new administrative problems that, in turn, require a new or refashioned structure for the new strategy to be successfully implemented. He found that structure tends to follow the growth strategy of the firm—but often not until inefficiency and internal operating problems provoke a structural adjustment. The experiences of these firms followed a consistent sequential pattern: new strategy creation, emergence of new administrative problems, a decline in profitability and performance, a shift to a more appropriate organizational structure, and then recovery to more profitable levels and improved strategy execution. See Alfred Chandler, *Strategy and Structure* (Cambridge, MA: MIT Press, 1962).

[22] The importance of empowering workers in executing strategy and the value of creating a great working environment are discussed in Stanley E. Fawcett, Gary K. Rhoads, and Phillip Burnah, "People as the Bridge to Competitiveness: Benchmarking the 'ABCs' of an Empowered Workforce," *Benchmarking: An International Journal* 11, no. 4 (2004), pp. 346–60.

[23] Iain Somerville and John Edward Mroz, "New Competencies for a New World," in *The Organization of the Future,* ed. Frances Hesselbein, Marshall Goldsmith, and Richard Beckard (San Francisco: Jossey-Bass, 1997), p. 70.

[24] Exercising adequate control over empowered employees is a serious issue. For example, a prominent Wall Street securities firm lost $350 million when a trader allegedly booked fictitious profits; Sears took a $60 million write-off after admitting that employees in its automobile service departments recommended unnecessary repairs to customers. Several makers of memory chips paid fines of over $500 million when over a dozen of their employees conspired to fix prices and operate a global cartel—some of the guilty employees were sentenced to jail. For a discussion of the problems and possible solutions, see Robert Simons, "Control in an Age of Empowerment," *Harvard Business Review* 73 (March–April 1995), pp. 80–88.

[25] For a discussion of the importance of cross-business coordination, see Jeanne M. Liedtka, "Collaboration across Lines of Business for Competitive Advantage," *Academy of Management Executive* 10, no. 2 (May 1996), pp. 20–34.

[26] Michael Hammer and James Champy, *Reengineering the Corporation* (New York: HarperBusiness, 1993), pp. 26–27.

[27] Ibid. Although functional organization incorporates Adam Smith's division-of-labor principle (every person/department involved has specific responsibility for performing a clearly defined task) and allows for tight management control (everyone in the process is accountable to a functional department head for efficiency and adherence to procedures), *no one oversees the whole process and its result.*

[28] Rosabeth Moss Kanter, "Collaborative Advantage: The Art of the Alliance," *Harvard Business Review* 72, no. 4 (July–August 1994), pp. 105–6.

[29] For an excellent review of ways to effectively manage the relationship between alliance partners, see Kanter, "Collaborative Advantage," pp. 96–108.

Chapter 12

[1] For a discussion of the value of benchmarking in implementing strategy, see Christopher E. Bogan and Michael J. English, *Benchmarking for Best Practices: Winning Through Innovative Adaptation* (New York: McGraw-Hill, 1994), Chapters 2 and 6; Mustafa Ungan, "Factors Affecting the Adoption of Manufacturing Best Practices," *Benchmarking: An International Journal* 11, no. 5 (2004), pp. 504–20; and Paul Hyland and Ron Beckett, "Learning to Compete: The Value of Internal Benchmarking," *Benchmarking: An International Journal* 9, no. 3 (2002), pp. 293–304; and Yoshinobu Ohinata, "Benchmarking: The Japanese Experience," *Long-Range Planning* 27, no. 4 (August 1994), pp. 48–53.

[2] Michael Hammer and James Champy, *Reengineering the Corporation* (New York: HarperBusiness, 1993), pp. 26–27.

[3] Gene Hall, Jim Rosenthal, and Judy Wade, "How to Make Reengineering Really Work," *Harvard Business Review* 71, no. 6 (November–December 1993), pp. 119–131.

[4] For more information on business process reengineering and how well it has worked in various companies, see James Brian Quinn, *Intelligent Enterprise* (New York: Free Press, 1992), p. 162; Ann Majchrzak and Qianwei Wang, "Breaking the Functional Mind-Set in Process Organizations," *Harvard Business Review* 74, no. 5 (September–October 1996), pp. 93–99; Stephen L. Walston, Lawton R. Burns, and John R. Kimberly, "Does Reengineering Really Work? An Examination of the Context and Outcomes of Hospital Reengineering Initiatives," *Health Services Research* 34, no. 6 (February 2000), pp. 1363–88; and Allessio Ascari, Melinda Rock, and Soumitra Dutta, "Reengineering and Organizational Change: Lessons from a Comparative Analysis of Company Experiences," *European Management Journal* 13, no. 1 (March 1995), pp. 1–13. For a review of why some company personnel embrace process reengineering and some don't, see Ronald J. Burke, "Process Reengineering: Who Embraces It and Why?" *TQM Magazine* 16, no. 2 (2004), pp. 114–19.

[5] For some of the seminal discussions of what TQM is and how it works written by ardent enthusiasts of the technique, see M. Walton, *The Deming Management Method* (New York: Pedigree, 1986); J. Juran, *Juran on Quality by Design* (New York: Free Press, 1992); Philip Crosby, *Quality Is Free: The Act of Making Quality Certain* (New York: McGraw Hill, 1979); and S. George, *The Baldrige Quality System* (New York: Wiley, 1992). For a critique of TQM, see Mark J. Zbaracki, "The Rhetoric and Reality of Total Quality Management," *Administrative Science Quarterly* 43, no. 3 (September 1998), pp. 602–36.

[6] For a discussion of the shift in work environment and culture that TQM entails, see Robert T. Amsden, Thomas W. Ferratt, and Davida M. Amsden, "TQM: Core Paradigm Changes," *Business Horizons* 39, no. 6 (November–December 1996), pp. 6–14.

[7] For easy-to-understand overviews of Six Sigma, see Peter S. Pande and Larry Holpp, *What Is Six Sigma?* (New York: McGraw-Hill, 2002); Jiju Antony, "Some Pros and Cons of Six Sigma: An Academic Perspective," *TQM Magazine* 16, no. 4 (2004), pp. 303–6; Peter S. Pande, Robert P. Neuman, and Roland R. Cavanagh, *The Six Sigma Way: How GE, Motorola and Other Top Companies Are Honing Their Performance* (New York: McGraw-Hill, 2000); and Joseph Gordon and M. Joseph Gordon Jr., *Six Sigma Quality for Business and Manufacture* (New York: Elsevier, 2002). For how Six Sigma can be used in smaller companies, see Godecke Wessel and Peter Burcher, "Six Sigma for Small and Medium-sized Enterprises," *TQM Magazine* 16, no. 4 (2004), pp. 264–72.

[8] Based on information posted at www.isixsigma.com, November 4, 2002.

9Kennedy Smith, "Six Sigma for the Service Sector," *Quality Digest Magazine,* May 2003, posted at www.qualitydigest.com (accessed September 28, 2003).

10Del Jones, "Taking the Six Sigma Approach," *USA Today,* October 31, 2002, p. 5B.

11Pande, Neuman, and Cavanagh, *The Six Sigma Way,* pp. 5–6.

12Smith, "Six Sigma for the Service Sector."

13Jones, "Taking the Six Sigma Approach," p. 5B.

14Terry Nels Lee, Stanley E. Fawcett, and Jason Briscoe, "Benchmarking the Challenge to Quality Program Implementation," *Benchmarking: An International Journal* 9, no. 4 (2002), pp. 374–87.

15For a recent study documenting the imperatives of establishing a supportive culture, see Milan Ambroz, "Total Quality System as a Product of the Empowered Corporate Culture," *TQM Magazine,* 16, no. 2 (2004), pp. 93–104. Research confirming the factors that are important in making TQM programs successful in both Europe and the United States is presented in Nick A. Dayton, "The Demise of Total Quality Management," *TQM Magazine,* 15, no. 6 (2003), pp. 391–96.

16Judy D. Olian and Sara L. Rynes, "Making Total Quality Work: Aligning Organizational Processes, Performance Measures, and Stakeholders," *Human Resource Management* 30, no. 3 (Fall 1991), pp. 310–11, and Paul S. Goodman and Eric D. Darr, "Exchanging Best Practices Information through Computer-Aided Systems," *Academy of Management Executive* 10, no. 2 (May 1996), p. 7.

17Thomas C. Powell, "Total Quality Management as Competitive Advantage," *Strategic Management Journal* 16 (1995), pp. 15–37. See also Richard M. Hodgetts, "Quality Lessons from America's Baldrige Winners," *Business Horizons* 37, no. 4 (July–August 1994), pp. 74–79; and Richard Reed, David J. Lemak, and Joseph C. Montgomery, "Beyond Process: TQM Content and Firm Performance," *Academy of Management Review* 21, no. 1 (January 1996), pp. 173–202.

18Based on information at www.utc.com and www.otiselevator.com (accessed November 14, 2005).

19Fred Vogelstein, "Winning the Amazon Way," *Fortune,* May 26, 2003, pp. 70, 74.

20*BusinessWeek,* November 21, 2005, pp. 87–88.

21Such systems speed organizational learning by providing fast, efficient communication, creating an organizational memory for collecting and retaining best practice information, and permitting people all across the organization to exchange information and updated solutions. See Goodman and Darr, "Exchanging Best Practices Information," pp. 7–17.

22*BusinessWeek,* November 21, 2005, pp. 85–90.

23Vogelstein, "Winning the Amazon Way," p. 64.

24For a discussion of the need for putting appropriate boundaries on the actions of empowered employees and possible control and monitoring systems that can be used, see Robert Simons, "Control in an Age of Empowerment," *Harvard Business Review* 73 (March–April 1995), pp. 80–88.

25Ibid. Also see David C. Band and Gerald Scanlan, "Strategic Control through Core Competencies," *Long Range Planning* 28, no. 2 (April 1995), pp. 102–14.

26The importance of motivating and empowering workers so as to create a working environment that is highly conducive to good strategy execution is discussed in Stanley E. Fawcett, Gary K. Rhoads, and Phillip Burnah, "People as the Bridge to Competitiveness: Benchmarking the 'ABCs' of an Empowered Workforce," *Benchmarking: An International Journal* 11, no. 4 (2004), pp. 346–60.

27Jeffrey Pfeffer and John F. Veiga, "Putting People First for Organizational Success," *Academy of Management Executive* 13, no. 2 (May 1999), pp. 37–45; Linda K. Stroh and Paula M. Caligiuri, "Increasing Global Competitiveness through Effective People Management," *Journal of World Business* 33, no. 1 (Spring 1998), pp. 1–16; and articles in *Fortune* on the 100 best companies to work for (various issues).

28As quoted in John P. Kotter and James L. Heskett, *Corporate Culture and Performance* (New York: Free Press, 1992), p. 91.

29For a provocative discussion of why incentives and rewards are actually counterproductive, see Alfie Kohn, "Why Incentive Plans Cannot Work," *Harvard Business Review* 71, no. 6 (September–October 1993), pp. 54–63.

30See Steven Kerr, "On the Folly of Rewarding A While Hoping for B," *Academy of Management Executive* 9, no. 1 (February 1995), pp. 7–14; Steven Kerr, "Risky Business: The New Pay Game," *Fortune,* July 22, 1996, pp. 93–96; and Doran Twer, "Linking Pay to Business Objectives," *Journal of Business Strategy* 15, no. 4 (July–August 1994), pp. 15–18.

31Kerr, "Risky Business," p. 96.

Chapter 13

1Joanne Reid and Victoria Hubbell, "Creating a Performance Culture," *Ivey Business Journal* 69, no.4 (March–April 2005), p. 1.

2John P. Kotter and James L. Heskett, *Corporate Culture and Performance* (New York: Free Press, 1992), p. 7. See also Robert Goffee and Gareth Jones, *The Character of a Corporation* (New York: HarperCollins, 1998).

3Kotter and Heskett, *Corporate Culture and Performance,* pp. 7–8.

4Ibid., p. 5.

5John Alexander and Meena S. Wilson, "Leading across Cultures: Five Vital Capabilities," in *The Organization of the Future,* ed. Frances Hesselbein, Marshall Goldsmith, and Richard Beckard (San Francisco: Jossey-Bass, 1997), pp. 291–92.

6Terrence E. Deal and Allen A. Kennedy, *Corporate Cultures* (Reading, MA: Addison-Wesley, 1982), p. 22. See also Terrence E. Deal and Allen A. Kennedy, *The New Corporate Cultures: Revitalizing the Workplace after Downsizing, Mergers, and Reengineering* (Cambridge, MA: Perseus, 1999).

7Vijay Sathe, *Culture and Related Corporate Realities* (Homewood, IL: Richard D. Irwin, 1985).

8Kotter and Heskett, *Corporate Culture and Performance,* Chapter 6.

9See Kurt Eichenwald, *Conspiracy of Fools: A True Story* (New York: Broadways, 2005).

10Reid and Hubbell, "Creating a Performance Culture," pp. 2, 5.

11This section draws heavily on the discussion of Kotter and Heskett, *Corporate Culture and Performance,* Chapter 4.

12There's no inherent reason why new strategic initiatives should conflict with core values and business principles. While conflict is always possible, most strategy makers lean toward choosing strategic initiatives that are compatible with the company's character and culture and that don't go against ingrained values and beliefs. After all, the company's culture is usually something that strategy makers have had a hand in building and perpetuating, so they are not often anxious to undermine core values and business principles without serious soul searching and compelling business reasons.

13Kotter and Heskett, *Corporate Culture and Performance,* p. 52.

14Ibid., p. 5.

15Avan R. Jassawalla and Hemant C. Sashittal, "Cultures That Support Product-Innovation Processes," *Academy of Management Executive* 16, no. 3 (August 2002), pp. 42–54.

16Kotter and Heskett, *Corporate Culture and Performance,* pp. 15–16. Also see Jennifer A. Chatham and Sandra E. Cha, "Leading by Leveraging Culture," *California Management Review* 45, no. 4 (Summer 2003), pp. 20–34.

17Judy D. Olian and Sara L. Rynes, "Making Total Quality Work: Aligning Organizational Processes, Performance Measures, and Stakeholders," *Human Resource Management* 30, no. 3 (Fall 1991), p. 324.

[18]Information posted at www.dardenrestaurants. com (accessed November 25, 2005); for more specifics, see Robert C. Ford, "Darden Restaurants' CEO Joe Lee on the Importance of Core Values: Integrity and Fairness," *Academy of Management Executive* 16, no. 1 (February 2002), pp. 31–36.

[19]For several perspectives on the role and importance of core values and ethical behavior, see Joseph L. Badaracco, *Defining Moments: When Managers Must Choose between Right and Wrong* (Boston: Harvard Business School Press, 1997); Joe Badaracco and Allen P. Webb, "Business Ethics: A View from the Trenches," *California Management Review* 37, no. 2 (Winter 1995), pp. 8–28; Patrick E. Murphy, "Corporate Ethics Statements: Current Status and Future Prospects," *Journal of Business Ethics* 14 (1995), pp. 727–40; and Lynn Sharp Paine, "Managing for Organizational Integrity," *Harvard Business Review* 72, no. 2 (March–April 1994), pp. 106–17.

[20]For a study of the status of formal codes of ethics in large corporations, see Emily F. Carasco and Jang B. Singh, "The Content and Focus of the Codes of Ethics of the World's Largest Transnational Corporations," *Business and Society Review* 108, no. 1 (January 2003), pp. 71–94, and Murphy, "Corporate Ethics Statements." For a discussion of the strategic benefits of formal statements of corporate values, see John Humble, David Jackson, and Alan Thomson, "The Strategic Power of Corporate Values," *Long Range Planning* 27, no. 6 (December 1994), pp. 28–42. An excellent discussion of whether one should assume that company codes of ethics are always ethical is presented in Mark S. Schwartz, "A Code of Ethics for Corporate Codes of Ethics," *Journal of Business Ethics* 41, nos. 1–2 (November– December 2002), pp. 27–43.

[21]See Schwartz, "A Code of Ethics," p. 27.

[22]Ford, "Darden Restaurants' CEO Joe Lee."

[23]For excellent discussions of the problems and pitfalls in leading the transition to a new strategy and to fundamentally new ways of doing business, see Larry Bossidy and Ram Charan, *Confronting Reality: Doing What Matters to Get Things Right* (New York: Crown Business, 2004); Larry Bossidy and Ram Charan, *Execution: The Discipline of Getting Things Done* (New York: Crown Business, 2002), especially Chapters 3 and 5; John P. Kotter, "Leading Change: Why Transformation Efforts Fail," *Harvard Business Review* 73, no. 2 (March–April 1995), pp. 59–67; Thomas M. Hout and John C. Carter, "Getting It Done. New Roles for Senior Executives," *Harvard Business Review* 73, no. 6 (November–December 1995), pp. 133–45; and Sumantra Ghoshal and Christopher A. Bartlett, "Changing the Role of Top Management: Beyond Structure to Processes," *Harvard Business Review* 73, no. 1 (January–February 1995), pp. 86–96.

[24]For a pragmatic, cut-to-the-chase treatment of why some leaders succeed and others fail in executing strategy, especially in a period of rapid market change or organizational crisis, see Bossidy and Charan, *Confronting Reality.*

[25]Fred Vogelstein, "Winning the Amazon Way," *Fortune,* May 26, 2003, p. 64.

[26]For a more in-depth discussion of the leader's role in creating a results-oriented culture that nurtures success, see Benjamin Schneider, Sarah K. Gunnarson, and Kathryn Niles-Jolly, "Creating the Climate and Culture of Success," *Organizational Dynamics,* Summer 1994, pp. 17–29.

[27]Jeffrey Pfeffer, "Producing Sustainable Competitive Advantage through the Effective Management of People," *Academy of Management Executive* 9, no.1 (February 1995), pp. 55–69.

[28]For some cautions in implementing ethics compliance, see Robert J. Rafalko, "A

Caution about Trends in Ethics Compliance Programs," *Business and Society Review* 108, no. 1 (January 2003), pp. 115–26. A good discussion of the failures of ethics compliance programs can be found in Megan Barry, "Why Ethics and Compliance Programs Can Fail," *Journal of Business Strategy* 26, no. 6 (November–December 2002), pp. 37–40.

[29]For documentation of cross-country differences in what is considered ethical, see Robert D. Hirsch, Branko Bucar, and Sevgi Oztark, "A Cross-Cultural Comparison of Business Ethics: Cases of Russia, Slovenia, Turkey, and United States," *Cross Cultural Management* 10, no. 1 (2003), pp. 3–28, and P. Maria Joseph Christie, Ik-Whan G. Kwan, Philipp A. Stoeberl, and Raymond Baumhart, "A Cross-Cultural Comparison of Ethical Attitudes of Business Managers: India, Korea, and the United States," *Journal of Business Ethics* 46, no. 3 (September 2003), pp. 263–87.

[30]James Brian Quinn, *Strategies for Change: Logical Incrementalism* (Homewood, IL: Richard D. Irwin, 1980), pp. 20–22.

[31]Ibid., p. 146.

[32]For a good discussion of the challenges, see Daniel Goleman, "What Makes a Leader," *Harvard Business Review* 76, no. 6 (November–December 1998), pp. 92–102; Ronald A. Heifetz and Donald L. Laurie, "The Work of Leadership," *Harvard Business Review* 75, no. 1 (January–February 1997), pp. 124–34; and Charles M. Farkas and Suzy Wetlaufer, "The Ways Chief Executive Officers Lead," *Harvard Business Review* 74, no. 3 (May–June 1996), pp. 110–22. See also Michael E. Porter, Jay W. Lorsch, and Nitin Nohria, "Seven Surprises for New CEOs," *Harvard Business Review* 82, no. 10 (October 2004), pp. 62–72.

PHOTO CREDITS

P1.1   Chapter 1   ©Cary Henrie/CORBIS
P2.1   Chapter 2   ©Rob Colvin/CORBIS
P3.1   Chapter 3   ©John S. Dykes/CORBIS
P4.1   Chapter 4   ©Leon Zernitsky/CORBIS
P5.1   Chapter 5   DigitalVision/Getty Images/MGH-DIL
P6.1   Chapter 6   ©Eric Westbrook/CORBIS
P7.1   Chapter 7   DigitalVision/Getty Images/MGII-DIL
P8.1   Chapter 8   DigitalVision/Getty Images/MGH-DIL
P9.1   Chapter 9   ©Rob Colvin/CORBIS
P10.1   Chapter 10   DigitalVision/Getty Images/MGH-DIL
P11.1   Chapter 11   ©Rob Colvin/CORBIS
P12.1   Chapter 12   ©Rob Day/CORBIS
P13.1   Chapter 13   ©Paul Anderson/CORBIS

ORGANIZATION

A. J. Gallaher & Company, 329
A. T. Kearney, 117
A&E network, 314
A&W restaurants, 247
AARP Magazine, C-370
ABC network, 148, 314, C-124, C-140
ABC Outdoor, 170
Abercrombie & Fitch, 193
Abovenet, C-304
Accenture, 117, 167, 219, C-300
Accuvue, 277
ACE Ltd., 329
Acer Computers, 244, C-90, C-100
Ackerley Group, 170
Acqua della Madonna bottled water, C-24
Acushnet Company, C-83, C-85
Adam Aircraft Industries, C-235 to C-250
Adams Golf, C-69, C-79
Adams Media Research, C-153, C-154
Adelphia Communications, 11, 327, 328,
    424, 449
adidas, 33, C-376 to C-391
adidas Golf, C-85
adidas-Salomon, C-69, C-81
Advanced Book Exchange, C-336
Advanced International Multitech
    Company, C-73
Advanced Micro Devices, 56 57, 178,
    253–254, C-307
Aerospatiale, 219, 375
AES, 420
Agilent Technologies, 303
Ahold USA, C-5
AIG, 329, 449
Airborne Express, 401, C-98
Airbus Industrie, 219, C-48, C-53, C-62
AirTran Airways, C-54, C-55, C-58, C-65
AirTran Holdings, C-65
Alando.de AG, C-302
Alaska Airways, C-54, C-55, C-56, C-58, C-65
Alberto-Culver, 416, 417, 432, 433
Albertson's, 103, C-4, C-5, C-35, C-36, C-38,
    C-42, C-46, C-418, C-419
Alcan Aluminum, 240, 397
Alcatel, 219
Aldila, C-73
Alibaba.com, C-307, C-308
Alibris, C-336
AliPay, C-309
Allied Domecq PLC, C-208
Allied Signal, 397
Alpha Beta stores, C-42
Altria Group, 298, 305, 333
Amazon Auctions, C-305 to C-306
Amazon.com, 6, 103, 110, 185, 186, 188, 193,
    248, 366, 367, 401–402, 403, 407, 426,

440, C-102, C-153, C-301, C-308, C-323,
    C-332, C-333 to C-334, C-351
AMC, 180
Amerada Hess, C-103
American Airlines, 166, C-51, C-54, C-55,
    C-56, C-58, C-65, C-66, C-537
American Association of Retired People, 47
American Automobile Association, C-545
American Booksellers Association, C-331,
    C-335, C-351
American Brands, C-85
American Eagle, C-54, C-55
American Express, 176
American Hotel & Lodging Association, C-535
American Machine and Foundry Company,
    C-361
American Motorcyclists Association, C-368
American Productivity and Quality Center,
    117, 118, 395
American Red Cross, C-61
American Standard, 281
American Tobacco, 256
America Online, 169, 171, 188, C-149, C-299,
    C-313, C-314, C-319, C-323, C-327
America West, C-54, C-55, C-57, C-58,
    C-63, C-65
AmeriHost, 305
Ameritech, C-502
Amersham, 307
Amer Sports Corporation, C-376
AMF, C-368 to C-369
AM-FM Inc., 170
Amgen, 407
AmSouth, 104
Anaheim Angels, 314
Andy's Produce, C-38
Anheuser-Busch Companies, 71, 251
Animal Planet, 152
AOL-Time Warner, 171
Aon Corporation, 329, C-279, C-284
Applebee's, C-190
Apple Computer, 59, 103, 112, 128, 256, 259,
    326, C-90, C-116, C-118, C-119, C-120,
    C-121, C-122, C-124, C-126, C-127,
    C-130 to C-147, C-161, C-289
Apple iPod, C-91, C-108, C-118, C-119,
    C-123, C-127, C-140 to C-141
Apple Market, C-46
Appropriate Technology International, C-493
Aprilia, C-367
Aramark Food and Services, C-490
Arbitron/Scarborough Research, C-257
Archos, C-119, C-120, C-121, C-124 to C-125
ArcorSA, C-535
Arc'Teryx, C-383
Arsenal Digital Solutions, 219

Arthur Andersen, 29, 339
Arthur Gallagher, C-279, C-280, C-284
Artisan, C-160
Asahi Glass, 240
Ashford.com, C-306
AstraZeneca, C-530
ATA Airlines, C-54, C-55, C-65
AT&T, 64, 269, 297, C-314
AT&T Broadband, 5
AT&T Canada, 32
Atlantic Express, C-66
Atlantic Southeast, C-54, C-55
Au Bon Pain, C-190
Audi, 103, 152, 165
Audible, C-123
AudioFeast, C-123
AutoTrader.com, C-300
Avid Technology, 152
Avis, 305
Avis Europe, C-162, C-163
Avocet, C-248
Avon Products, 13, 36, 85, 128–131, 147, 196

B. Dalton Bookstores, C-332
Baazee.com, C-303
Baccarat, 256
Bad Ass Coffee, C-494
Bahama Breeze, 277, 434
Baja Fresh, C-190 to C-191
Bajaj Auto, 225
Bally shoes, 256
Bally Total Fitness, C-55
Banana Republic, 83
Bandag, 152
Band-Aids, 277
B&Q (UK), 344
Bank of America, 104, 168–169, 170
Bank of Scotland Corporate Banking, C-165
Bank One, 409, C-489
Barnes & Noble, 64, C-332, C-333 to
    C-334, C-491
Baskin-Robbins, C-208
BB&T Insurance Services, 104, 329
BEA, 166, 219
Beaird-Poulan, 143, 275
Beatrice Foods, C-195
Bed, Bath, and Beyond, C-419
Beechcraft Corporation, C-236, C-238,
    C-241, C-244, C-247
Belgacom, C-516
Bell companies, 190, 331
Bell Labs, 304
Bell's Market, C-28, C-43, C-46
Bellsouth, 64
Ben & Jerry's Homemade, 93, 101, 155, 240,
    301, 348, C-22

Note: Page numbers in *italics* indicate material in illustrations; page numbers followed by t indicate material in tables; page numbers followed by n indicate notes; page numbers preceded by C- indicate material in Cases.

Benchmark Exchange, 117, 395
BenchNet, 117, 395
Ben Franklin stores, C-412
Ben Hogan Golf, C-79, C-80
Berkshire Hathaway, 315
Berol, 314
Berry's, C-38
Bertelsmann, 354
Bess Eaton, C-209
Best Buy, 70, 171, C-92, C-114,
    C-153, C-419
Bestfoods, 302
Best Practices LLC, 117, 395
Best Western International, C-535
Bic, 143
Bidville, C-305
Big John's, C-38
Biotherm, 277
Birkenstock, 176
BitTorrent, 138
BJ's Wholesale Club, C-419
Black & Decker, 143, 251, 275
Blockbuster Entertainment, 24, 112, 185,
    C-148, C-151, C-153, C-154 to
    C-158, C-304
Blowout Entertainment, C-159
Blue Cross & Blue Shield of Montana,
    C-273, C-274, C-277, C-281, C-282,
    C-284 to C-285
Blue Diamond, 256
Blue Ice, 314
BMW Group, 6, 25, 32, 103, 145, 152, 159,
    165, 171, 196, 219, 232, 397, C-119,
    C-255, C-364, C-365, C-367, C-371
Body Shop, 348
Boeing Company, 219, 375, C-49, C-53,
    C-241
Bombardier, 275
Bonefish Grill, C-436, C-437, C-440, C-441
    to C-442
Bonehead's Seafood, C-191
Bonfire, C-376, C-379, C-383
Bookcrossing, C-336
Book Industry Study Group, C-332, C-335
Books-A-Million, C-336
Borders Group Inc., 303, C-306, C-332,
    C-333 to C-334, C-335
Boston Consulting Group, C-412
BP Amoco, 202
Braun, 301, C-392
Bravo, 307
Bread & Circus, C-9
Bread of Life, C-9
Brew HaHa, C-494
Bridgestone, 112–113
Bridgestone/Firestone, 70
Briggs & Stratton, 143
Bristol-Myers Squibb, 327, 331
British Aerospace, 219
British Airways, C-66
British Broadcasting Corporation, C-362
British Petroleum, 403
British Telecom, 269, 344, C-500, C-516

Broadcom, 376
Brown & Brown, C-277, C-279, C-280, C-284
Bruno's, C-5
Brute, 314
BT Group, C-516
BTR, 297
Budget Rent-a-Car, 305
Buell Motorcycles, C-361, C-364, C-365,
    C-371 to C-372, C-373
Buffalo Sabres, 328, C-209
Buick, 206
Business Evolution Council, C-542
Business Roundtable, 342, 350
Buy.com, 185, 187

CableLabs, 190
Cadillac, 103, 152
Café Express, C-189
California Green Lodging program, C-541
California Pizza Kitchen, 303
Callaway Golf Company, 251, C-69, C-72,
    C-73, C-74, C-75, C-76 to C-81, C-82,
    C-83, C-84, C-85, C-86, C-87, C-384,
    C-386, C-387
Calphalon, 314
Campbell's Soup, 145, 251, 302, C-5
Cannondale Associates, 152, 256, C-421
Canon Inc., 33, 153, 273, C-225, C-226,
    C-227, C-229
Canon U.S.A. Inc., C-229
Capers Community Markets, C-22
CARE, C-493
Carefree, 277
Caribou Coffee, C-494, C-495
Carl's Jr., C-43
Carlson Hospitality Group, C-535
Carlton Hotels, C-534
Carrabba's Italian Grill, C-436, C-437,
    C-440, C-441
Carrefour, 122, 213, 251, C-420
Carrier heating, 281
Carroll Farms, C-175
CarsDirect.com, C-306
Cartier, 147
Casio, C-139
Castrol, 202, 206
Catalan Institute of Pharmacology, C-527
Caterpillar Inc., 23, 47, 145, 199, 228, 397
CBS network, 148
CCM, C-376
Cdigix, 128
CDW Computer Centers, 441
Cendant Corporation, 305–306, C-535
Central American Retail Holding
    Company, C-418
Century 21, 305
CERES, C-537
Cessna, C-244, C-248
CGA Inc., 152
CGMI Networks, C-307
Chanel, 6, 83, 84, 153
Charles Schwab, 26, 145, 187
Charmin, 275

Chase Manhattan Bank, C-50
Cheap Tickets, 305
Cheeseburger in Paradise, C-436
Chemical Bank, 32
Chevron, 238, 375, C-313
Chicago Cutlery, 256
Chicago Express, C-65
Chi-Chi's, C-441
Chick-Fil-A, 346, C-184
Chili's Grill, C-190
Chinese Academy of Sciences, C-113
Chipotle Mexican Grill, C-189
Choice Hotels International, C-535
Christie's, C-304
Chrysler Corporation, 168, 171
Chubb fire detection, 281
Ciba Specialty Chemicals, 368
CIGNA, 32
Cingular Wireless, C-139, C-314
Circuit City, 64, 184, C-114, C-153, C-419
Cirque du Soleil, 180
Cirrus, C-239, C-241, C-242
Cisco Systems, 169, 177, 196, 219, 226, 302,
    366, 367, 376, 426, C-91, C-104
Citibank, 104
Citicorp, 327
Citigroup, 301, 354, 356
Claris, C-289
Classic Sports Network, 314
Clear Channel Communications, 170
Clear Channel Worldwide, 170
Cleveland Golf, C-77
Cliché, C-376, C-379, C-383
CNBC, 7, 307
CNN, 147
Coalition for Environmentally Responsible
    Conventions, C-537
Cobra Golf, C-77, C-79, C-80, C-83 to C-86,
    C-85, C-386, C-387
Coca-Cola Company, 25, 58, 103, 145, 169,
    209, 221, 222, 238, 298, 303, 344, 350,
    C-5, C-537
Coffee Time, C-210
Coldwell Banker, 305
Cole-Haan, C-379
Colony Hotel, C-537
Comair, C-54, C-55
Combined Benefits Insurance Company,
    C-274
Combined Benefits Management Inc.,
    C-273, C-274
Comcast, 4–5, 17, 252, C-154
Comcast Digital Voice, 5
Comfort Inn, C-534, C-535
Community Coffee, 151–152
Community Pride Food Stores, 346
Compaq Computer, 171, 225, 244, C-89,
    C-90, C-96, C-98, C-104, C-109 to
    C-110, C-133, C-289, C-299, C-307
Compass, 104
CompUSA, C-92, C-114
CompuServe, C-323
ComPysch, C-65

ConAgra Foods, C-439
Conde Nast Traveler, C-48
Conrad Hotels, 156
Conservation International's Center for
    Environmental Leadership in
    Business, C-492
Continental Airlines, 166, 403, 410–411, C-51,
    C-54, C-55, C-56, C-58, C-65, C-66
Continental Hotels PLC, C-534
Continental tires, 70
Contract Poultry Growers Association, C-174
Cookware Europe, 314
Coors, 71
Copperfield's Books Inc., C-328 to C-355
Corel, 171
Corner Bakery, C-185, C-187
Corporation for Public Broadcasting,
    C-251, C-268
Cosi Inc., C-187, C-439
Costco, 13, C-5, C-30, C-35, C-36, C-38,
    C-39, C-46, C-114, C-225, C-261, C-332,
    C-419, C-420, C-421, C-428
Cost Plus, C-352
Cotati Farmer's Market, C-28
Couche-Tard, C-209
Country Inns & Suites by Carlson, C-535
Country Style, C-210
Courtyard by Marriott, 156, C-534
Covent Garden Soup, 240
Craftsman, 63
Craigslist, C-301
Cray Computer, 370
Creative Labs, C-139 to C-140,
    C-141 to C-143
Creative Technology, C-119, C-120, C-121,
    C-124, C-125, C-127
Credit Suisse First Boston, 330, 354, 356–357
Crest toothbrush, 240
Cuddledown, 256
CVS Pharmacies, 246

Daimler-Benz, 168, 171
Daimler-Benz Aerospace, 219
DaimlerChrysler, 32, 71, 165–166, 168, 206,
    219, 232, 373, C-255
D&M Holdings Inc., C-118, C-145
Dannon Yogurt, C-5
Darden Restaurants, 277, 434–435
Darrell Survey, C-72
Dasani, 169
Dassler Brothers Shoe Factory, C-377
Days Inn, 247, 305, C-534, C-535
Dazbog Coffee Company, C-211
DBC Communications, C-502
Deaf Dog Coffee, C-267
Dean Foods, C-5, C-218
Deja.com, C-314
Del Frisco Double Eagle Steak Houses, C-450
Delhaize, C-5
Dell Direct Store kiosks, C-100
Dell Inc., 13, 68, 71–72, 119, 121, 142, 164,
    177, 179, 196, 206, 207, 219, 222, 225,
    226, 244, 275, 326, 367, 368, 373, 375,

426, 449, C-89 to C-115, C-119, C-120,
    C-121 to C-122, C-125 to C-126, C-127
    to C-128, C-137, C-143, C-304
Deloitte & Touche, 211, C-60
Delta Air Lines, 166, 401, C-53, C-54, C-55,
    C-56, C-58, C-63, C-65
Delta Song, C-58
Deutsche Telekom, C-505, C-516
Development Dimensions International,
    C-61
DHL Air Group, C-66
Diamond Multimedia, C-116
DiaSorin, 281
diAx, C-498, C-499, C-500, C-502, C-508
Digital Equipment Corporation, C-109
Digital Java Inc., C-200
Digital Networks North America, C-118
Dillard's, 83
DirecTV, 5, 252, C-155, C-252
Discount Store News, C-412
Discovery Channel, C-363
Dish Network, C-252
Disney Channel, 314, C-140
Disney Cruise Line, 314
Disney Radio, 314
Doc Green's Gourmet Salads, C-191
Dollar General, 256
Domino's Pizza, 110, 152, 246, C-43
Doubletree Hotels, 156, C-535
Dow Jones & Company, 315, 373
Dreyer's Grand Ice Cream, C-489 to
    C-490
Dr Pepper, 145, 256
Drugstore.com, C-306
Dry Idea, 301
Ducati, C-365, C-367, C-371
Duke Children's Hospital, 32
Dunkin' Donuts, 66, C-190, C-208 to
    C-209, C-210
DuPont Corporation, 28, 32, 397
Duracell, 275, 301, C-392

E. & J. Gallo Winery, 374
Eastman Kodak, 28, 103, 375, 376, 423,
    C-219 to C-234
easyCar.com, C-162 to C-170
easyCinema, C-170
easyGroup, C-162, C-165, C-167, C-170
easyJet, 103, C-162
eBay, 7, 23, 36, 155, 180, 185, 188, 357,
    402, 426, C-77, C-102, C-286 to
    C-311, C-351
eBay Japan, C-302
eBay Philippines, C-303
Eberhard Faber, 314
EBSCO, 387
EchoStar, 5, C-252
Eckhoff Accountancy Corporation, C-42
Eclat Consulting, C-63
Eclipse, C-241, C-248
Econo Lodge, 247, C-535
Edison Media Research, C-255
eDonkey, 128

Edward Jones, 441
Edwin Watts stores, C-73
Eiger Labs, C-116, C-140
Electronic Arts, 209, 252
Electronic Data Systems, 37, 366,
    C-94
Eli Lilly, C-530
Eller Media Company, 170
E-Loan, 186
eMachines Inc., C-113 to C-114, C-138
Embassy Suite Hotels, 156, C-534, C-535
Embraer, C-53, C-66
EMC, 440, C-91
Emerson Electric, 275, 397
EMI/Virgin, 354
E! network, 314
Enron Corporation, 11, 29, 327, 328, 330,
    332–333, 339, 354, 424
Enterprise Command Centers, C-101
Enterprise Rent-a-Car, 152
ePier, C-305
Epson, 13, 153
Equifax Inc., C-297
ERA, 305
Ernst & Young, 211, 346, 355
E*Service, 401
ESPN, 252, 314, C-140
ESPN: The Magazine, 252
ESPN Motion, 252
ESPN360, 252
Ethos Water, C-490
eToys, 188
Europcar, C-163
European Business Center, C-303
Evoke Communications, C-295
Exertris Interactive Bikes, 248, 265
Exodus Communications, C-304
Expedia, 166
Experimental Aircraft Association, C-243
Express Jet, C-54, C-55
ExxonMobil, 32, 202, 375

Fairfield Inn, 156
Fairmont Hotels and Resorts, C-534, C-536
Fair Trade Labeling Organization
    International, C-492
Fanta, 169
Fast Company magazine, C-151
Federal Express, 7, 139, 145, 149, 181, 373,
    401, 418
Fendi, 83, 84
Ferrara's New York cheesecake, C-24
FGI Research, C-151
Fiesta, C-38
Financial Times, C-412
FiOS Internet Service, C-160
First Automotive Works, 219
Fleet Boston Financial, 169
Fleming's Prime Steakhouse and Wine Bar,
    C-436, C-437, C-440, C-442 to C-443
Flextronics, 376
Flyi Incorporated, C-65
Foamy, 301

Folgers Coffee, 275, C-495
Food 4 Thought, C-9
Food Lion, C-5
FoodMaxx, C-38, C-39, C-46
Foot Joy, C-85, C-387
Foot Locker, C-304, C-382
Ford Motor Company, 20, 24, 33, 71, 145, 171, 219, 221, 232, 265, 357, 373, 375, C-165, C-255, C-537
ForeSee Results, C-151
Formule 1 Hotels, C-535
Forrester Research, C-108, C-287
Fortune Brands, C-77, C-85, C-86
Four Seasons Hotels, 7, 256, C-534
Fox Broadcasting, 252
Fox Network, 148, 307
Fox News, 147, 169
Fox Sports, 169
Fox Studios, 169
France Telecom, C-505, C-516
Freedom Rings, C-218
Fresh & Wild, C-9
FreshDirect, C-35
Fresh Fare, C-4
Fresh Fields Markets, C-9
Fresh Market, C-22, C-23 to C-24
Frito-Lay, 303, 418
Frontier Airlines, C-58, C-65
Fuji, C-227 to C-228, C-229 to C-230, C-232
Fujikura, C-73, C-74
Fujitsu, C-99
Fujitsu-Siemens, C-90, C-109
Fuji-Xerox, 116–117
Future Shop, C-114
FX, 169

Galleria Park Hotel, C-541
Game Crazy stores, C-158, C-159
Gamestation, C-155
G&G supermarkets, C-38, C-46
Gap, Inc., 83
Gardenia, 314
Garner, 277
Gartner Research, C-107, C-116 to C-117, C-139
Gateway Computer, 244, C-89, C-90, C-98, C-109, C-113 to C-114, C-138, C-304
Gatorade, 169
Gebrüder Dassler Schuhfabrik, C-377
Genentech, 164
General Electric, 36, 143, 263, 275, 281, 296, 307, 314, 366, 395, 397, 406, 416, 420, 440, 442, C-86, C-99, C-232, C-428
General Electric Capital Mortgage, 397
General Electric Healthcare, 307
General Electric Medical Systems, 307
General Magis, C-290
General Mills, 302, 346, C-5
General Motors, 33, 165–166, 193, 206, 207, 219, 226, 232, 237, 256, 265, 371, 373, 423, C-255, C-313, C-537
General Nutrition, C-26

Geneva Motor Show, C-165
Genji Express, C-14
Genworth Financial, 307
Gerber, 251
Giant Foods, C-5
Gillette Company, 13, 275, 301, C-218, C-392 to C-404
Giorgio Armani, 277
Giorgio Beverly Hills, C-393
GlaxoSmithKline, 120, 344, C-530
Gloria Jean's, C-494
GO Corporation, 238
Godiva Chocolates, 153
Gol Airlines, 140
Goldman Sachs, 330, 354, 356, 357, C-236, C-392 to C-393, C-400
Golfcraft Inc., C-83
Golfsmith.com, C-73
Goodyear, 70, 112–113, 147, 193
Goody hair accessories, 314
Goody's, C-419
Google Inc., 24, 152, 155, 192, 238, 366, 367, 407, 413, 416, 417, 426, 449, C-102, C-161, C-288, C-312 to C-327, C-335
Google Scholar, 387, 413
Graco strollers, 314
Graffaloy, C-73, C-74
Granite Construction, 392, 441
Graphic Design, C-73 to C-74
Greater Boston Food Bank, C-48
GreenCine, C-148, C-153, C-160 to C-161
Greenmarket farmers' market, C-12
Green Meeting Industry Council, C-537
Green Mountain Coffee Roasters, 345, C-5
Greenpeace, 26
Greg Norman apparel, C-376
Grokster, 128
Groupe Danone, C-5
Gucci, 83, 84, 147, 153
Gumtree.com, C-303

H. J. Heinz Company, 23, 28, 33, 47, 71, C-5
Häagen-Dazs, 6, 93, 153, 240
Hain Celestial Group, 256, C-5
Half.com, C-301, C-309, C-351
Half Price Books, C-337
Hamilton Sunstrand, 281
Hammarplast U.S.A., C-472
Hampton Inns, 66, 156, C-535
H&H bagels, C-24
Handspring, C-301
Handy Dan Home Improvement, 179
Hannaford Bros. stores, C-5
Hanson PLC, 307
Hard Rock Café, C-301
Harley-Davidson Inc., 6, C-356 to C-375
Harley-Davidson University, C-372
Harley Owners Group, C-369
Harris Corporation, 390
Harris Interactive, C-356
Harrison Drape, 314
Harris Teeter, C-4
Harrods, C-196

Harry's Farmers Market, C-7, C-9, C-11
Hasbro Inc., C-290
Hawaiian Airlines, C-54, C-55, C-65
Hawaiian Holdings, C-65
Head & Shoulders, 275
Health-e-Web, C-274
HealthSouth, 11, 327, 424, 449
Health Valley, 256
Helena Rubenstein, 277
Hellman's, 302
Hells Angels, C-362, C-370
Henry's Marketplace, C-22
Herman Miller Company, 448
Hero Group, 225, 228
Hertz, C-163, C-168
Hewlett-Packard, 13, 29, 142, 153, 164, 166, 171, 177, 179, 219, 225, 226, 251, 303, 326, 393, C-50, C-89, C-90, C-91, C-100, C-102, C-104, C-105, C-109, C-109 to C-111, C-112, C-119, C-124, C-130, C-137 to C-138, C-219, C-225, C-228, C-230, C-232, C-307, C-420
Hi-C, 169
Hickory Stick USA, C-77
High Tech Burrito, C-267
Hillenbrand, 179
Hilton Garden Inns, 156
Hilton Hotels Corporation, 23, 156, 202, 204, C-491, C-535
History Channel, 152
Hitachi, 73, C-99, C-117, C-122
Holiday Autos, C-163
Holiday Inn, C-534, C-535
Hollinger International, 424
Hollywood Entertainment, C-158, C-159
Hollywood Video stores, C-158
Home Depot, 13, 28, 70, 104, 138, 145, 179, 180, 193, 223, 344, 387, C-304
Homewood Suites, 156, C-535
Honda lawn mowers, 213
Honda motorcycles, C-364, C-367, C-371
Honda Motors, 63, 71, 145, 219, 232, 273, 310, 370, 371, C-255, C-362
Horizon Airlines, C-490
Hotel Bel Air, C-537
Hotel.com, 186
Hotel Indigo, C-534
Hotel Sofitel, C-535
Hotmail, 189
Houghton-Mifflin, C-349
Howard Johnson, 305, C-535
Huawei, 226
Hummer, 256
Hyatt Corporation, C-491, C-535
Hyatt Regency Chicago, C-537
Hyatt Regency Scottsdale, C-537
Hynix Semiconductor, 326

iBazar, C-302
Ibis Hotels, C-535
IBM, 7, 73, 164, 176, 177, 219, 225, 226, 402, 423, C-89, C-90, C-91, C-96, C-99, C-100, C-102, C-103, C-109, C-131,

C-133, C-286, C-289, C-299, C-301, C-304, C-307, C-425
IBM Global Services, C-111
IBM/Lenovo, C-111 to C-113
ICQ.com, C-323
I-Escrow, C-301
Il Giornale Coffee Company, C-474 to C-475, C-476
IMC Global, 240
Independence Air, C-54, C-55
Indian Motorcycle Corporation, C-371
Infineon Technologies, 326
InfoTrac, 387
InfoTrends Research Group, C-223, C-225
Ingram, C-349
Inktomi, C-322
Insurance Coordinators of Montana Inc., C-274
Intel Corporation, 26, 27, 57, 66, 164, 169, 178, 198, 249, 253–254, 366, 368, 426, C-131
InterContinental Hotels Group, C-535
International Data Corporation, C-107 to C-108, C-287
International House of Pancakes, C-190
Internet Auction Company Ltd., C-302, C-303
Internet Security Systems, 219
Intuit, C-291
Iowa Beef Packers, 140–142
iRiver Inc., C-119, C-120, C-122, C-128, C-139, C-143 to C-144
iShip.com, C-301
Ivory soap, 275

J. D. Power & Associates, 152
J. M. Smucker, 37
J. W. Marriott Hotels, 156
Jack in the Box Inc., C-189, C-190
Jaguar, 171
Jani-King International, 204
JCPenney Company, 71, C-304, C-412
Jeep Grand Cherokee, 206
JetBlue Airways, 103, C-48 to C-67
Jif, 275
Jiffy Lube International, 7
Jim Beam Brands, C-490
JM Family Enterprises, 407
Jofa, C-376
John Deere, 63
John Reuter Jr. Inc., C-83
Johnson & Higgins, C-279
Johnson & Johnson, 6, 145, 166, 277, 302, 303, 343, 344, 448
John Wiley & Sons, C-326
Joie de Vivre Hotels, C-534
Jollibee Foods, 225
JPMorgan Chase, 104, 409
J-Rag Inc., C-183
Juvenile Diabetes Research Foundation, C-24

Kagan Research, C-154
Kaiser Permanente, 402, C-57, C-526, C-528

Karastan, 145
Karsten Manufacturing, C-86 to C-87
Kash 'n Karry, C-5
Kawasaki, C-364, C-367, C-371
Kazaa, 128
KB Toys, C-304
Keegan & Copin, C-328
Kellogg, 222, C-5
Kentucky Fried Chicken, 204, 247, 303, C-43
Kerastase Paris, 277
Keybank, 104
Kiehl's, 277
Kimberly Clark, 315
Kimpton Hotels, C-533 to C-546
Kinko's, 441
Kirsch, 314
KLM Royal Dutch Airlines, 218
Kmart, 6, 83, 84, 171, 275, 303, C-304, C-418, C-419
Knights Inn, 305
Knorr's, 302
Kohl's, 83
Koho, C-376
Komatsu, 199
KPMG, 211, 355, 424
KPN, C-516
Kraft General Foods, 169, 256, 298, 302, 305, C-5, C-495
KRCB Television and Radio, C-251 to C-272
KremeKo Inc., C-218
Krispy Kreme Doughnuts, 172, C-190, C-193 to C-218
Kroger, 66, 70, 103, 141, C-4, C-5, C-28, C-35, C-36, C-38, C-43, C-418, C-419
Kroll Zolfo Cooper, C-214, C-216
KTM, C-367

L. L. Bean, 6, 71, 147, 256
LaMar's Donuts, C-210 to C-211
Lancair, C-239, C-241, C-242
Lancaster Colony, 281
Lancôme, 277
Lands' End, 256
La Roche-Posay, 277
La-Z-Boy, C-48
Lee Roy Selmon's, C-436
Lenovo Group Ltd., 226, C-89, C-90, C-99, C-100, C-111 to C-113
Lenscrafters, 441
Le Roy Selmon's, C-440
Levi Strauss & Company, 17, 25, 251
Levolor, 314
Lexmark, 13, 138, 153, C-105, C-225, C-232
Lexus, 103, 151, 152, 171
Lifetime network, 314
Lincoln automobile, 84, 103, 152
Lincoln Electric, 143, 407
Linux, 238
Liquid Paper, 314
Listerine, 145
Lite House, C-5
Little League World Series, C-445
Little Tikes toys, 314

LiveTV LLC, C-52, C-62
Loblaw, C-5
Lockheed, C-241
Lola's, C-46
Lone Star Steakhouse & Saloon, C-450
Long John Silver's, 247
Long's Drugs, C-43
LoQUo.com, C-303
L'Oréal, 277
Lowe's, 104
Lucent Technologies, 303, 304, 321
Lucent Worldwide Services, 304
Lucky's supermarkets, C-41
Lycos, C-363

MacWorld Boston, C-132
Macy's Department Stores, 71, 83, C-309
Magnavox, 212
Mailboxes, Etc., C-301
Mama Fu's Asian House, C-191
Mapquest, C-323
Marks & Spencer, 298
Marktplaats, C-303
Marriott Hotels, 156, 202
Marriott International, 441, C-535
Marriott Residence Inns, 156
Marsh & McLennan Companies Inc., 327, 329, 339, 354, 424, C-279, C-280, C-284
Martin Marietta, C-241
Maruti-Suzuki, 221
Mary Kay Cosmetics, 85, 147, 193, 256, 432, 442
Match.com, 152
Matrix, 277
Matsushita, C-99
Mavic, C-379
Max Factor, C-393
Maxwell House, 152, C-495
Maybelline, 277
Mayo Clinic, 26
Maytag, 164
Mazola, 302
MBNA, 169–170
McAfee, 7
McCafés, C-495
McDonald's Corporation, 12, 25, 33, 66, 104, 204, 213, 222, 223, 225, 251, 343, 375, 392, 441, 442, C-5 to C-6, C-49, C-189, C-190, C-446, C-485, C-495
McDonnell Douglas, C-241
McGraw-Hill Companies, C-326
MCI Communications, 64, 330, 331, C-323
McKinsey & Company, 167, 250, 308, 366, 367, 406
McKinsey Quarterly, C-185
McWane, 424
Mectizan Donation Program, C-521
Medaire Inc., C-60
Media Play, 171
MercadoLibre.com, C-302 to C-303
Mercedes-Benz, 6, 84, 103, 145, 152, 171, 206, C-165, C-356
Mercer Consulting, 329

Merchant of Vino, C-9

Merck & Company Inc., 166, 339, 405,
    C-518 to C-532

Merck Vaccine Network—Africa,
    C-521 to C-522

Mercure Hotels, C-535

Merrill Lynch, 354, 375, C-379, C-399,
    C-400, C-401, C-402, C-521

Metro-Goldwyn-Mayer Studios, 5,
    C-160

Michelin, 70, 112–113, 145

Micro Center, C-114

Micron Technology, 326

Microsoft Corporation, 13, 14, 17, 24, 33, 58,
    63, 66, 128, 147, 164, 166, 188, 219, 225,
    238, 251, 253, 309, 343, 366, 367, 371,
    390, 418, C-113, C-121, C-122, C-132,
    C-135, C-138, C-139, C-142, C-147,
    C-148, C-289, C-304, C-309, C-313,
    C-322 to C-323

Microsoft Office, 145, 171

Microsoft Windows, 145

Microsoft Word, 171

Microsoft Xbox, 178

Midwest Airlines, C-58

Mighty Ducks, 314

Miller Brewing, 298

Millstone Coffee, C-495

Minolta, C-307

Minute Maid, 169

Miramax, C-160

Mitsubishi, 164, C-236

Mobile.de, C-303

Mobile ESPN, 252

Moe's Southwestern Grill, C-191

Molsberry, C-38

Monistat, 277

Monsanto, C-547 to C-558

Montana Mills Bread Company, C-206 to
    C-207, C-211, C-213, C-215

Montecito Markets, C-42

Monticello Hotel, C-541

Moody's Investor Services, 259, C-518

More Group, 170

Morris Air, C-49, C-50, C-51

Motel 6, 154, C-534, C-535

Motion Picture Association of America,
    C-160

Moto Guzzi, C-365, C-367, C-371

Motorola, Inc., 32, 145, 164, 225, 397, C-119
    to C-120, C-131, C-139

Moviefone.com, C-323

Movie Gallery Inc., C-153, C-154,
    C-158 to C-159

MovieLink, C-148, C-154, C-160

Moyer Packing Company, C-171

Mr. Coffee, 275

Mrs. Gooch's, C-9

MSN, C-313, C-319

MSNBC, 307

MSN Search, C-322 to C-323, C-327

Murphy-Brown LLC, C-171

Murphy Family Farms, C-177 to C-178

Muscular Dystrophy Association, C-356

Musicland, 112, 171

Musicmatch, 128

MV/Caviga, C-365

Myopia Hunt Club, C-86

MySimon, C-288

MZ, C-365

Nabisco Foods, 305, C-40

Napster, 128

NASCAR, 209

Nasdaq, C-6

National AIDS Fund's Red Ribbon Campaign,
    C-540

National Airlines, C-52

National Association for the Specialty Food
    Trade, C-37

National Basketball Association, 209, C-161

National Cash Register Systems, C-111

National College Athletic Association, C-445

National Football League, 209

National Golf Foundation, C-75, C-76

National Olympic Committees, C-382

National Public Radio, C-251, C-252, C-257,
    C-259, C-260, C-268

National Restaurant Association, C-452

National Semiconductor, C-132

National Trial Lawyers Guild, C-527

National Tyre Services, 297

NationsBank, 169

Natural Abilities Inc., C-9

Nature's Heartland, C-9

NBC network, 148, 307, C-140

NBC Universal, 281

NBGI Private Equity, C-165

NCR, C-111

NEC, C-99, C-100

Neiman Marcus, 83, 84

Nestlé, 169, 196, 256, 302, 309, C-495

Netflix, C-148 to C-161

Netscape Communications, C-323

Neutrogena, 277

Nevada Bob's, C-73

New Balance, C-382, C-390

Newell Rubbermaid, 314

New Era of Networks, C-236

News Corporation, 169, 252, 315, C-327

New World Coffee, C-494

NeXT Software Inc., C-132

Nielsen Media Research, C-252

Nielsen/Net Ratings, C-225

Nielsen Television Index, C-255

Nike, Inc., 25, 33, 184, 213, 348, 351, 366,
    376, C-376, C-378, C-379, C-382, C-387,
    C-390, C-537

Nike Golf, C-72, C-77, C-79, C-85, C-87 to
    C-88

Nikki, 202

Nikon, C-228, C-230

Nintendo, 25, 63, 309, 311, C-147

Nissan Motors, 33, 110, 145, 219

Nokia, 25, 145, 164, 196, 225, 397, 426

Nordstrom, 83, 393, 407, 416, 418, C-62, C-491

Noritsu Koki Company, C-232

North Carolina National Bank, 169

Northwest Airlines, 166, 218, 401, C-50,
    C-54, C-55, C-57, C-58, C-63, C-65

Northwest Water (UK), 395–396

Nova Scotia Power, 32

Novell, 171, C-314

Novotel, C-535

Noxell, C-393

NPD Foodworld, C-186

NPD Group, C-126, C-186

NRT, 305

NTT Communications, 219, 269

Nucor Corporation, 77, 121, 135, 136, 240,
    409, 410–411, 431

Oakley sunglasses, C-118

Oasis Day Spa, C-58

Occidental Petroleum, 416

Odwalla, 169

Office Depot, 77, 185, 186, C-114, C-153,
    C-304

Office Max, 77, 185, 186, 303

Oldsmobile, 237

Old Spice, C-393

Olive Garden, 277, 434

Oliver's Markets, C-28 to C-47

Olympus, C-225

Olympus Optical, C-232

Omega-3, 256

On Cue, 171

Opusforum, C-303

Oracle Corporation, 166, 219, C-150, C-489

Oral-B toothbrush, 275, 301

Orange, C-499, C-505

Orange County Choppers, C-363

Orbitz, 166, 305

Orchard Hardware, C-352

Organic Trade Association, C-4

Orsini cheese, C-24

Orvis, 256

Otis Elevator, 281, 401

OtisLine, 401

Outbacker Trust, C-448

Outback Steakhouse, C-436 to C-453

Overland Group, C-206

Overstock.com, 185, C-305, C-307 to C-308

Overture Services, C-307, C-322

Owens Corning, 397

P. F. Chang's China Bistro, C-443

Packerland Holdings, C-171

Palm Inc., 305, C-91

PalmPilot, 305

Panasonic, 259

Panera Bread, 187, C-185, C-187, C-190

Papa John's International, 246

Paperbackswap.com, C-337

Paper Mate, 314

Paramount Pictures, C-160

Parker Pens, 314

Parmalat, 327, 424

Patagonia, 256

Paul Lee's Chinese Kitchen, C-436 to C-437
Pavillions supermarkets, C-47n
Paxton Communications, 170
PayPal, C-294, C-298, C-301, C-302, C-303
PBL Online, C-302
PC Magazine, C-107, C-141, C-314
PCs Limited, C-91
PC World, C-107, C-314
Peapod, 188, C-23, C-35
Pearson, C-326
Peets Coffee and Tea, C-469, C-473
Pemex, 327
Penguin, C-349
Pennzoil, 202
Penske truck leasing, 281
Pep Boys, 30
Pepcid AC, 166, 277
PepsiCo, 58, 103, 145, 169, 221, 277, 298,
     303, 350, 366, C-131, C-489 to C-490
PerkinElmer, 307
Personality Hotels, C-534
Petaluma, C-38
Petters Group Worldwide, C-307
Pfizer, Inc., 344, 405, C-521, C-527, C-530
PGA Merchandise Show, C-87
Philadelphia 76ers, 252
Philip Morris USA, 298, 305, 333, 334
Philips Electronics, 207, 212, C-122
Phogenix, C-232
Pigeon Cove Seafood, C-11, C-18, C-19
Pineapple Express, C-49
Ping Golf, C-72, C-73, C-77, C-80, C-81,
     C-84, C-86 to C-87, C-384, C-387
Pinnacle Golf, C-85
Piper aircraft, C-244
Piper Jaffray & Company, C-135
Pirelli tires, 70
Pittman Financial Partners, C-182
Pittsburgh Penguins, C-209
Pixar Studios, 167
Pizza Hut, 66, 204, 246, 247, 303, C-218
PJ's Coffee, C-191
PKF Consulting, C-534
Planet Smoothie, C-191
PNC, 104
Polaroid Corporation, 376
Polo Ralph Lauren, 83, 93
Porsche, 152, 165
Portugal Telecom, C-516
PotashCorp, 240
Powell Books, C-332, C-337
Powerade, 169
PowerPoint, 8
Pratt & Whitney, 281
Predator soccer shoes, C-378
Prestage Farms, Inc., C-174
Price Club, C-92
Price/Costco, C-92
Priceline.com, 185, 188
PricewaterhouseCoopers, 211, 355, C-213,
     C-215, C-216
Primaris Airlines, C-66
Procter & Gamble, 25, 71, 110, 141, 169, 240,

     251, 275, 301, 302, 366, 368, C-290,
     C-392 to C-404, C-422, C-424, C-495
Professional Golfers' Association, C-69,
     C-384, C-445
Progressive Insurance, 154, 155
Providian Financial Corporation, 330
Prudential Securities, 330, 354
Public Broadcasting System, C-251,
     C-252, C-259
Publix Super Markets, 441, C-4, C-5
Puma Schuhfabrik Rudolph Dassler,
     C-378
Pure Software, C-149
Putnam Investments, 329

Qdoba Mexican Grill, C-190
Quaker Oats, 169, 277
Quaker State, 202
Qualcomm, 448
Qualilty Inn, C-535
Quality Assurance International, C-3
Qualserve Benchmarking Clearinghouse,
     117, 118
Qwest Communications, 64, 331, 424
Qwicky's, C-495

R. J. Reynolds Tobacco, 305, 333
Radio Shack, C-43
Radisson Hotels, C-491, C-534, C-535
Raleigh Schwarz & Powell, C-277
Raley's, C-38, C-46
Ralph Lauren, 145, 147, 277, C-376
Ralph's Fresh Fare, C-4
Ralph's Supermarkets, C-28, C-38,
     C-43, C-46
Ramada Inn, 305, C-534, C-535
Random House, C-349
Rational Software, C-149
Raving Brands, C-191
RCA, C-120, C-144 to C-145
RealNetworks, 253, C-118
Recording Artists' Coalition, 354
Recording Industry Association of America,
     128, C-116
Red Hat Linux, 13, 14, 17, 23, 58, C-314
Redhook Ale Brewery, C-470
Redken, 277
Red Lobster, 277, 434
Red Roof Inns, C-534, C-535
Reebok International, C-377, C-378, C-382,
     C-386, C-390
Refco, 424
Regency, C-116
Regent International Hotels, C-535
ReignCom Ltd., C-122, C-144
Remote Solutions, C-116
Renaissance Hotels, C-535
Renault, 219, C-165
Renault-Nissan, 219
Revlon, C-80
Rhapsody, C-123
Richardson-Vicks, C-393
Right Guard, 301

Ringling Brothers and Barnum and Bailey, 180
Rio Inc., C-118, C-120, C-124, C-126, C-127,
     C-128, C-144, C-145
Rite Aid, 246, 327, 424
Ritz Carlton Hotels, 7, C-62
Robin's Donuts, C-210
Roche, C-530
Rockport, C-376
Rockwell Automation, 164
Rodale Institute, C-4
Rolex, 6, 84, 145, 147
Rolls-Royce, 147, 153, C-356
Ronald McDonald House program, 343–344
Roto-Rooter, 204
Roughneck storage, 314
Royal Ahold, 70, 297
Royal & Ancient Golf Club of Saint Andrews,
     C-68, C-74
Royal Dutch/Shell, 249, 327, 333, 345,
     348, 424
Roy's restaurants, C-436, C-440, C-442 to
     C-443
Rural California Broadcasting Corporation,
     C-258
Ruth's Chris Steakhouse, C-453
Ryanair, 103, 140, 179

Saab, 237
Saatchi & Saatchi, 32
Sachs, C-365
SaeHan information systems, C-116
Safety Components International, 240
Safeway, 66, 70, 103, 141, C-4, C-5, C-35,
     C-36, C-38, C-39, C-40, C-46, C-47n,
     C-418, C-419
Safire, C-248
Saint Louis Bread Company, C-190
Saks Fifth Avenue, 83, 84
Sally Beauty Company, 416
Salomon SA, C-81, C-376, C-379, C-383 to
     C-384, C-390
Salomon Smith Barney, 301, 330, 357
Sam Goody, 171
Sam's American Choice, 71
Sam's Clubs, C-5, C-30, C-92, C-414 to
     C-415, C-419, C-423, C-430
Samsung Electronics, 145, 164, 225, 259, 309,
     326, C-117, C-122
Samuel Adams, 256
SanDisk, C-119, C-120, C-123, C-127, C-128,
     C-139 to C-140, C-145 to C-146
Sanford highlighters, 314
SAP, 166, 219
Sara Lee, C-218
SAS, 219
Saturn Motors, 193
Save-a-Lot, C-4, C-5, C-22, C-25 to C-26
SBC Communications, 190, C-322
Scaled Composites, 238, C-240, C-241
Schiller Del Grande Restaurant Group, C-189
Sci-Fi Channel, 307
Seagate Technology, 33
Sears, 32, 64, 83, 171, 423, C-301

Sears/Kmart, 84
Seasons restaurants, 434
Seattle Storm, C-472
Seattle Supersonics, C-472
Second Cup Coffee, C-495
Sedgwick Group, C-279
Sega, 309, 311
Seiko Epson, C-225
Seiyu Ltd., C-418
Select Fish, C-11, C-18
SeniorNet, C-295
Service Employees International
    Union, C-410
7-Eleven Stores, 204, C-23
SFX Entertainment, 170
SGI, 177
Shane's Rib Shack, C-191
Shareasa, 128
Sharp, 259, C-99, C-139
Sharpie markers, 314
Shato Holdings, C-210
Shell Oil, 25, 202, 424
Sheraton Hotels, 202, C-491, C-534, C-535
Sherwin-Williams, 171
Shopping.com, C-301
Shu Uemura, 277
Siebel, 166
Siemens, 32, 309
SigmaTel Inc., C-145
Sikorsky Helicopters, 281
Silicon Graphics, 177
Simon & Schuster, C-326
Sirius Satellite Radio, 84, C-255
Six Sigma Academy, 396
Sixt, C-163
Skippy peanut butter, 302
Skis Rossignol SA, C-379
Skymaster, C-236
Skype Technologies, C-303
Skywest, C-54, C-55
SlimFast, 301
Smithfield Foods, C-171 to C-181
Smokey Bones Barbecue & Grill, 434
Snapple, 63
Snicker's, 275
Soft & Dry, 301
Softbank, C-307
Soft Sheen/Carson, 277
Soft Warehouse Superstores, C-92
Solectron, 376
Sony Corporation, 5, 63, 110, 128, 142, 164,
    184, 196, 206, 251, 259, 265, 273,
    308–309, 310, 311, 354, 355, C-98,
    C-99, C-109, C-116, C-119, C-120,
    C-123, C-126, C-128 to C-129, C-144,
    C-146, C-147, C-227 to C-228, C-229,
    C-307
Sony Pictures Entertainment, C-160
Sony PlayStation, 178, 273, 309, 310
Sotheby's International, 305, C-306
Soundbuzz, C-122
Southland Corporation, C-23
Southwest Airlines, 6, 103, 117, 121, 138,

140, 142, 179, 366, 367, 401, 419, C-50,
    C-51, C-53, C-54, C-55, C-57, C-58,
    C-59, C-63, C-65
Sports Authority, 303
Sports Illustrated, 252
Sprint PCS, C-314
Stagnito's New Products Magazine, C-184
Stain Shield, 314
Standard & Poor's, 259, C-6, C-63, C-219,
    C-231, C-286, C-518
Staples, 70, 77, 185, 186, C-92, C-153
Starbucks Coffee International, C-484
Starbucks Corporation, 7, 33, 36, 102, 110,
    145, 152, 177, 235–236, 251, 345, 347,
    380, 441, C-5, C-190, C-199, C-208,
    C-468 to C-495
Starbucks Foundation, 345, C-493
Starbucks Hear Music Coffeehouses,
    C-488, C-491
STAR satellite TV, 223
Starwood Hotels and Resorts, C-534, C-535
Starz Entertainment Group, C-154
State Street, 104
Stayfree, 277
Stonyfield Farm, 346, 348
Stop & Shop, C-23
Strategic Planning Institute's Council on
    Benchmarking, 117
Strategy Analytics Global Wireless
    Practice, C-226
StreetPrices, C-288
Stride Rite Corporation, 143, C-290
Subaru, 84
Subway, 104, C-189, C-190
Sullivan's restaurants, C-450
Summers Group, 297
Sunbeam, 275
Suncoast, 171
Sundaram Fasteners, 226
Sunflower Markets, C-22, C-25
Sun Harvest, C-22
Sun Microsystems, 219, C-102, C-304,
    C-314
Super 8 motels, 247, C-535
Super Kmart, C-419
Super Target, C-419
Supervalu, C-4, C-5, C-22, C-25 to C-26
Sure & Natural, 277
Suzuki, 223, C-364, C-367, C-371
Swish, 314
Swisscom, C-500, C-505
Swiss Federal Railways, C-500
Swiss National Exhibition, C-508
Swiss Reinsurance, C-500
Sybase Corporation, C-236
Sylvan Learning Centers, 66
Synovus, 407
SYSCO Corporation, C-491

T. J. Maxx, 83
Taco Bell, 104, 204, 247, 303, 375
Taiwan Semiconductor, 376
TakeAlongs, 314

Tambrands, C-393
Tandem Computer, C-109
TaoBao, C-307, C-308, C-309
Target Stores, 6, 13, 83, 84, 275, 303, 402,
    C-304, C-419, C-421
Tattered Cover Book Store, C-337
TaylorMade-adidas Golf, C-81 to C-83, C-384
    to C-386
TaylorMade Golf, C-69, C-72, C-77, C-79,
    C-80, C-84, C-85, C-86, C-376, C-379,
    C-380
TDC Sunrise, C-496 to C-514, C-516
Telecom Italia, C-516
Tele Danmark, C-500
Telefonica, C-516
Televisa, 225
Tennessee Valley Authority, 32
Texas Instruments, 376, C-122
Texas Land & Cattle restaurants, C-450
Texas Roadhouse, C-450 to C-451
TGW.com, C-73
Thomson Worldwide, C-144
3Com, 305
3M Corporation, 33, 101, 145, 245, 442
    Dental Products Division, 23
Ticketmaster, C-304
Tiffany, 147, 256
Time Warner AOL, C-225
Time Warner Inc., 169, 170, 171, 297, 307,
    354, C-323
Timex, 84
Tim Hortons, C-209 to C-210
Titleist, C-72, C-77, C-79, C-80, C-81, C-83
    to C-86, C-384, C-386, C-387
TiVo, C-251
T-Mobile USA, C-486
ToGo's Eateries, C-208
Tommy Hilfiger USA, 424
Toon Disney, 314
Top-Flite Golf, C-79, C-80
Toro, 63
Toronto Maple Leafs, C-209
Toshiba, 36, 142, C-99, C-100, C-109,
    C-117, C-139
Towers Perrin, 117
Toyota Motor Corporation, 7, 28, 33, 102,
    122, 145, 151, 152, 164, 177, 179, 196,
    206, 219, 265, 368, 371, 372, 373, 407,
    C-165
Toyota Production System, 372
Toys "R" Us, 346, 402, C-419
Toysrus.com, C-306
Trader Joe's, 24, 153–154, C-22, C-24 to C-
    25, C-28, C-35, C-38, C-40, C-46, C-352
Tradesafe, C-301
Trane furnaces, 281
Transparency International, 320, 325
Travelers Group, 301
Travel Lodge, C-535
Travelocity, 166
Travelodge, 305
Tree of Life, 256, C-22
Trio cable channel, 307

Triton Hotel, C-541
Triumph, C-365, C-367, C-371
Trust for Public Land, C-540
Tully's Coffee, C-494
Tupperware, 442
Twentieth Century Fox, 169, C-160
Tyco International, 11, 263, 302–303, 327, 330, 424
Tylenol, 277
Tyson Foods, 140, C-5

UAL Corporation, C-63
uBid.com, C-305, C-307
UBS (Union Bank of Switzerland), C-30, C-392, C-400, C-500
Ukrop's Super Markets, 407
Unilever, 101, 169, 222, 256, 301, 302, C-22
United Airlines, 166, C-54, C-55, C-57, C-58, C-63, C-65, C-66, C-490
United Food and Commercial Workers International Union, C-410, C-433
United Natural Foods, C-18
United Parcel Service, 32, 149, 176, 401, C-98, C-301
United States Golf Association, C-68 to C-69, C-74, C-79, C-86, C-384
United States Postal Service, 78, 401, C-286, C-289, C-294, C-301
United Technologies, 281
Universal Outdoor, 170
Universal Studios, 307, 354, C-160
UPS Store, 204
US Airways, C-54, C-55, C-57, C-58, C-62, C-63
USA Network, 307
USA Today, 193, C-107
UST, C-73, C-74

Vauxhall Corsa, C-165
Verio, 219
Verizon Communications, 190, 352, 375, 445
Verizon Online, C-160
VHQ Entertainment, C-159

Viacom, 307, C-155, C-326
Viacom/CBS, 170
Vichy Laboratories, 277
Video Update, C-159
Virgilio, C-314
Virgin, C-118
Virgin America, C-66
Vist, 225
Vitamin World, C-26
Vivendi Universal Entertainment, 307
Vodafone, C-500
Volkswagen, 145, 165, 219, 373, 397, C-49
Volkswagen-Porsche, 232
Vons supermarkets, C-47n

W. L. Gore & Associates, 37, 153, 407, 441
W. Newell & Company, C-26
Wachovia, 104, 169
Walgreens, 185, 246, C-225
Wall Street Journal, C-107
Wal-Mart Discount City, C-412
Wal-Mart Neighborhood Markets, C-414, C-415
Wal-Mart Stores Inc., 6, 12–13, 66, 70, 71, 83, 84, 103, 121, 138, 140, 141, 143, 177, 184, 196, 211–212, 251, 275, 303, 333, 397, 415–416, 431, 440, 441, C-4, C-30, C-35, C-36, C-37, C-38, C-47n, C-92, C-118, C-151, C-153, C-225, C-304, C-309, C-332, C-410 to C-435, C-485
Wal-Mart Supercenters, C-5, C-410, C-411, C-414, C-415, C-417, C-419
Wal-Mart Watch, C-410, C-433
Walt Disney Company, 7, 164, 167, 170, 232, 307, 314, 368, 441, C-124, C-290, C-299
Walt Disney Pictures, C-160, C-161
Walton Institute of Retailing, C-431
Warner Brothers Studios, C-160
Waterman pens, 314
Weather Channel, 7, 180
Webvan, 188, C-35
Wells Fargo, 23, 32, 104, 168, 329, C-491

Wendy's International, 32, 104, C-189, C-190, C-209
West Coast Choppers, C-363
Western Digital, 33
Western States Insurance Agency, C-273 to C-285
Western Union, C-418
Westin Hotels, C-491, C-535
WestJet, C-50
Weston Presidio, C-50
Whirlpool, 143, 207, 211, 213, 397, 398
White Rain, 301
Whole Foods Market, 7, 103, 345, 348, 405, C-2 to C-27, C-29, C-36, C-38, C-46
Wild Oats Markets, C-22 to C-23, C-25, C-26
Winchell's Donut House, C-210
Windows Media Player, 253
Winterthur Insurance, C-500
WordPerfect, 171
WorldCom, 11, 29, 330, 331, 354, 356, 424
Wyeth, C-518, C-530
Wyndam motels, 305

Xerox Corporation, 33, 116–117, 188, 397, C-92, C-472
    Palo Alto Research Center, C-130
Xilinx, 407
XM digital radio, C-48
XM Satellite Radio Holdings Inc., 84, C-255

Yahoo!, 29, 30, 164, 185, 187, 188, 265, 357, 367, C-102, C-299, C-313, C-319, C-322
Yahoo Auctions, C-305, C-306 to C-307, C-308
Yahoo Internet Life, C-314
Yahoo! Photos, C-225
Yamaha, C-364, C-367
You've Got Pictures, C-225
Yum! Brands, 204

Zagat Survey, C-211
Zoës Kitchen, C-182 to C-192

NAME INDEX

Aaron, C-454, C-457n
Aaronson, Susan Ariel, EN-8
Abraham, J., C-338, C-354
Abramovitch, Ingrid, C-495n
Abramson, John, C-532n
Abruzzo, Roxanne "Rocky," C-39, C-41
Adam, George, Sr., C-236
Adam, Rick, C-235 to C-242, C-246, C-247
Adams, Gary, C-81
Agle, Bradley R., EN-8
Ahlstrand, Bruce, EN-1
Alexander, John, EN-10
Alexander, K. L., C-67n
Alexander, Marcus, 266, EN-6
Aleyne, Adrian, 115
Ali, Mohammed, C-382
Allen, Bill, C-438, C-443
Alonso-Zaldivar, R., C-66n
Ambroz, Milan, EN-10
Amelio, Gil, C-132
Amsden, Davida M., EN-9
Amsden, Robert T., EN-9
Anderson, C., C-354, C-355n
Anderson, Dane, C-229
Anderson, Fred D., C-132, C-291
Anderson, M. J., EN-6
Anderson, Richard, C-553
Anslinger, Patricia L., EN-3, EN-6
Antonico, John, C-157, C-158
Antony, Jiju, EN-9
Arensman, Russ, C-129n
Argandoña, Antonio, EN-7
Armstrong, D., C-67n
Arnold, David J., EN-5
Aronson, Amy, EN-8
Ascari, Allessio, EN-9

Baack, Sally, C-273
Babbin, Peter, C-273, C-281
Badaracco, Joseph L., EN-1, EN-11
Bailey, Wendy J., EN-7
Bain, J. S., EN-2
Baker, C., C-67n
Baker, William, C-80
Baldwin, Jerry, C-468 to C-470, C-471,
     C-473, C-474, C-475
Baliga, B. R., EN-6
Bamford, James, EN-3
Band, David C., EN-10
Bane, Dan, C-24
Bank, David, C-495n
Barger, David, C-51, C-62
Barger, Mike, C-62
Barger, Sonny, C-362
Barney, Jay, EN-2
Barrett, Amy, 302
Barringer, Bruce, EN-1
Barry, Megan, EN-11
Barthélemy, Jérome, EN-4, EN-9

Bartlett, Christopher A., EN-2, EN-4, EN-8,
     EN-11
Baselitz, Georg, C-496
Basham, Bob, C-437, C-438, C-446
Basu, Kunal, 316, EN-8
Baucom, Scott, C-547 to C-548
Baue, William, C-558n
Baumann, Judith, C-509
Baumgartner, Hans Peter, C-509, C-513
Baumhart, Raymond, EN-11
Beauchamp, T. L., EN-7
Beckard, Richard, EN-9, EN-10
Beckett, Ron, EN-9
Beckham, David, C-379, C-381, C-382
Behar, Howard, C-482
Beinhocker, Eric D., 250, EN-5
Bell, Alexander Graham, C-515
Bellman, Eric, 221
Bentley, S., C-170n
Berens, Connie, C-263
Bergamo, Vanessa, C-261
Bergen, Mark E., EN-4
Berner, Robert, C-435n
Bernick, Carol Lavin, 433
Bernoff, J., C-354, C-355n
Berry, Ray, C-23 to C-24
Bezos, Jeff, 403, 440
Bhide, Amar, 160, 414
Bianco, Anthony, C-420, C-435n
Bickford, Deborah J., EN-5
Birchall, David W., EN-2
Bird, Rosanna, C-516
Birinyi, Laszlo, 48
Birkenshaw, Julian, EN-8
Blair, Richard, C-343
Blakey, Marion, C-247
Blank, Arthur, 179
Bleeke, Joel, EN-3, EN-4, EN-5
Bleustein, Jeffrey, C-356, C-370, C-375
Bluedorn, Allen C., EN-1
Bogan, Christopher E., EN-3, EN-9
Bogner, William C., EN-2
Boller, Frank, C-509, C-513
Bommer, Fred, C-83
Bontis, Nick, EN-2
Booth, Rick, C-229
Bossidy, Lawrence, 358, 388, EN-8, EN-11
Bottger, Preston, C-496
Bower, Joseph L., EN-3
Bowie, N. E., EN-7
Bowker, Gordon, C-468 to C-470, C-471,
     C-473, C-474, C-475
Bradford, David L., C-458
Brandenburger, Adam M., 160
Brando, Marlon, C-362, C-370
Branson, Richard, C-66
Brin, Sergey, 417
Brinkman, Johannes, EN-7
Brinston, Woody, C-178

Briscoe, Jason, EN-10
Brodt, Steve, C-263
Bromiley, Philip, EN-1
Brown, Barney, C-350
Brown, David, EN-7, EN-8
Brown, E., C-67n
Brown, Matt, C-328
Brown, Michael E., 316
Brown, Paul, C-558n
Brown, Robert, EN-1
Brown, Shona L., 243, EN-1, EN-5
Browne, Barney, C-340
Bruno, Anthony, C-129n
Bruno, Lorraine, C-263
Bryant, Kobe, C-379
Bucar, Branko, EN-11
Buell, Erik, C-361
Buettner, Shane C., C-161n
Buffet, Warren, C-418
Buffett, Jimmy, C-436
Bulik, B. S., C-234n
Burcher, Peter, EN-9
Burd, Steve, C-47n
Burke, Ronald J., EN-9
Burleson, Kasey, C-187
Burnah, Phillip, EN-9, EN-10
Burns, Lawton R., EN-9
Burrows, Peter, C-115n, C-129n
Burt, T., C-170n
Bygrave, William, C-235
Byrne, John A., 366, EN-8
Byrnes, Nanette, 334

Caliguiri, Paula M., EN-10
Callaway, Eli, C-70, C-75, C-77 to C-78
Cameron, Scotty, C-85
Camo, Robert C., EN-3
Campailla, F., C-67n
Campbell, Andrew, 266, EN-6
Carasco, Emily F., EN-11
Carey, S., C-67n
Carl, Albert, C-263
Carlin, George, C-343
Carnegie, Roger, C-263
Caron, Joseph, EN-4
Carp, Daniel, C-219, C-222, C-232,
     C-233, C-234
Carrabba, Johnny, C-441
Carreiro, Lenni, C-555
Carroll, Archie B., EN-7
Carter, John C., EN-11
Carver, John, EN-1
Casper, Billy, C-88
Cassimus, John, C-182 to C-184, C-192
Cassimus, Marcus, C-182
Cassimus, Zoë, C-182
Casstevens, Randy S., C-218
Castelli, William, C-528
Castrogiovanni, Gary J., EN-6

Note: Page numbers in *italics* indicate material in illustrations; page numbers followed by t indicate material in tables; page numbers followed by n indicate notes; page numbers preceded by C- indicate cases; page numbers preceded by EN- indicate endnotes.

Cavanagh, Roland R., EN-9, EN-10
Cha, Sandra E., EN-10
Chakravarthy, Bala, EN-5
Chakravarty, S. N., C-234n
Chamberlain, Bo, C-509
Chambers, Susan, C-435n
Champagne, Matt, C-263
Champy, James, EN-9
Chandler, Alfred, EN-9
Chao, Julie, C-115n
Charan, Ram, 358, EN-8, EN-11
Charles, Ray, C-488
Charron, C., C-354
Chatham, Jennifer A., EN-10
Chatterjee, Sayan, EN-6
Chen, Chia-Pei, EN-7
Chen, Ming-Jer, EN-4
Chen, Roger, EN-7
Cherry, Brenda, EN-5
Chisholm, Shirley, 316
Chowdhury, Neel, C-115n
Christensen, H. Kurt, EN-4, EN-5
Christie, P. Maria Joseph, EN-11
Chue, Chris, C-227
Cladouhos, Sherry, C-281
Clark, Don, EN-7
Clinton, Bill, C-50, C-480
Clinton, Mariah, C-263
Cohen, Allen, C-407, C-458
Cohen, Ben, 155
Collins, James C., 358, 392, EN-1,
    EN-8
Collins, John, 230
Collis, David A., EN-2, EN-6
Cook, Scott, C-291
Cook, Timothy D., C-133
Cooper, Peter, EN-3
Cooper, Robin, EN-2
Cooper, Stephen, C-214, C-217
Cooper, Trudy, C-437
Copeland, Thomas E., EN-6
Cordon, Carlos, EN-8
Cosgrove, Terry, C-281
Covin, Jeffrey G., EN-1, EN-4
Crawford, Sheri, C-263
Crawford, Tony, C-273
Crockett, Roger O., C-129n
Crosby, Philip, EN-9
Cross, Shannon, C-219
Cucuzza, Thomas G., EN-3
Cummins, Chip, EN-7
Currie, Neil, C-47
Curtis-McIntyre, Amy, C-60
Cusamano, Michael A., 230

Dahm, Lori, C-184
Dalton, R. A., Jr., C-234n
Daly, John, C-74, C-86
Daniel, C., C-67n
Darr, Eric D., EN-10
Dassler, Adolph, C-377 to C-378
Dassler, Horst, C-378

Dassler, Rudolph, C-377 to C-378
D'Aveni, Richard A., C-47, EN-4, EN-5
Davidson, Arthur, C-359 to C-361
Davidson, Hugh, 22, EN-1
Davidson, Wallace N., EN-8
Davidson, William G., C-359 to C-360,
    C-370
Davis, Jim, C-390
Davis, Scott, EN-4
Dawar, Niraj, 194, 224, EN-5
Dawson, Ray, C-553
Dayton, Nick A., EN-10
Deal, Terrence E., EN-10
Dechant, Kathleen, EN-7
Deering, Anne, EN-8
Deftos, L. J., C-558
Delaney, Kevin J., C-161n
DeLap, Steven, C-164, C-263
Dell, Michael, C-89, C-91, C-92 to C-95,
    C-97, C-98, C-102, C-103, C-104, C-105
    to C-106, C-107, C-114 to C-115
De Lollis, B., C-67n
Denton, Herbert A., C-234
Depatie, Mike, C-537, C-540, C-541
Deutsch, C. H., C-234n
Devinney, Timothy, EN-8
Dickinson, C. J., C-67n
Didius Julianus, C-288
Dienhart, John W., 339, EN-7
Dieppe, Paul A., C-532n
Dillman, Linda, C-425
DiMarco, Chris, C-88
Dixie Chicks, 355
Dobbin, B., C-234n
Dobbs, Nancy, C-251, C-252, C-256, C-258,
    C-259, C-260, C-261, C-262, C-263,
    C-264, C-268, C-269, C-270, C-271
Donald, Jim, C-495
Donaldson, Gordon, EN-1
Donaldson, Thomas, EN-7
Donnelly, S. B., C-66n, C-67n
Doz, Yves L., 219, EN-3, EN-4, EN-5, EN-6
Dragonetti, Nicola C., EN-2
Dranikoff, Lee, EN-6
Drapeau, Ron, C-76, C-78, C-79 to C-80
Drucker, Peter F., EN-6
Duncan, Jack W., EN-2
Duncan, Tim, C-381
Dunfee, Thomas W., EN-7, EN-8
Dutta, Soumitra, EN-9
Dwyer, R., C-67n
Dye, Pete, C-86
Dyer, Jeffrey H., EN-3, EN-5
Dyremose, Henning, C-503, C-513

Eastman, George, C-222
Ebbers, Bernard, 356
Edmondson-Jones, Gareth, C-58
Egger, Mathias, C-532n
Eichenwald, Kurt, EN-7, EN-10
Eisenhardt, Kathleen M., 243, EN-1,
    EN-5, EN-6

Eisenstat, Russell, EN-2, EN-8
El-Jelly, Abuzar, EN-8
Elias, Paul, C-558n
Emerson, Ralph Waldo, 16
Engdahl, William, C-558n
English, Michael J., EN-3, EN-9
Enz, Cathy A., C-546n
Epstein, Mark, C-164
Ernst, David, EN-3, EN-4, EN-5
Evans, Philip, EN-3
Everitt, Tony, C-263

Fahey, Liam, EN-4
Farkas, Charles M., EN-11
Fastow, Andrew, 328
Fauber, Bernard, 160
Fawcett, Stanley E., EN-9, EN-10
Federi, Fulvio, C-509
Feldman, Howard, C-454
Feldman, J. M., C-67n
Fellows, George, C-80
Felsted, A., C-170n
Ferrari, A., C-234n
Ferratt, Thomas W., EN-9
Fiegenbaum, Avi, EN-2
Field, Joseph J., C-210 to C-211
Fifty Cent, C-390
Finell, Christian, C-384
Finn, B., C-67n
Fiorina, Carly, C-110, C-111
Fireman, Paul, C-390
Fisher, George, C-232
Fitzgerald, Anne, C-558n
Fitzmaurice, Andrew, C-168
Flatley, Kerry, C-225 to C-226
Fleming, G., C-354
Fleming, Paul, C-443
Flint, P., C-67n
Floyd, Steven W., EN-1, EN-8
Fonda, Peter, C-362, C-370
Fontanarosa, Phil B., C-532n
Foote, Nathaniel, EN-2, EN-8
Ford, Henry, 20
Ford, Robert C., EN-11
Foust, Dean, EN-4
Francese, Peter, C-47
Francis, Theo, 329
Franko, Lawrence G., EN-6
Frazier, Kenneth, C-532
French, Liz, C-546n
French, Paul, EN-8
Freund, Matthias, C-232
Friedman, Milton, 316
Frimer, Kim, C-496, C-497 to C-499, C-500,
    C-506 to C-507, C-509, C-512, C-513,
    C-514
Frost, Tony, 194, 224, EN-5
Fulford, B., C-234n

Gallagher, Leigh, EN-6
Galunic, D. Charles, EN-6
Gamble, James, C-393

Gamble, James Norris, C-393
Gamble, John E., C-48, C-68, C-89, C-312,
    C-356, C-376, C-392
Gannon, Tim, C-437
Garabedian, Kathy, C-263
Garnett, Kevin, C-381
Gasparino, Charles, EN-8
Gates, Bill, C-131
Gauntlett, Sarah June, C-436
George, S., EN-9
Ger, Guitz, EN-5
Geroski, Paul A., EN-4
Ghemawat, Pankaj, EN-1, EN-2
Ghoshal, Sumantra, EN-2, EN-4,
    EN-8, EN-11
Gianchetta, Larry, C-273
Gilinsky, Armand, Jr., C-28, C-251, C-328
Gillette, King C., C-393 to C-396
Gilliland, Mike, C-22, C-25, C-26
Gilmartin, Raymond V., C-520, C-527,
    C-528, C-531
Gingrich, Newt, C-343
Ginovsky, J., C-67n
Ginsberg, Paul, C-164
Ginter, Peter, EN-2
Girling, Robert H., C-251
Glass, David D., C-414, C-432, C-433
Goffee, Robert, EN-10
Golden, Thomas D., EN-7
Goldsmith, Marshall, EN-9, EN-10
Goleman, Daniel, EN-11
Goll, David, C-47
Gomez, Alain, 194
Goodman, Paul S., EN-10
Goold, Michael, 266, EN-6
Gordon, Joseph, EN-9
Gordon, M. Joseph, Jr., EN-9
Gordon, Mary Ellen, EN-2
Govindarajan, Vijay, EN-2 to EN-3
Gow, David, C-558n
Graham, David J., C-527, C-528, C-530
Graham, Jefferson, 407
Grant, Peter, 190, C-161n
Grassley, Charles E., C-531
Graziano, Anita, C-263
Greenberg, Jeffrey, 329
Greenfield, Jerry, 155
Greenfield, W. M., EN-7
Griffith, Brian, C-263
Grimm, Curtis M., EN-5
Grove, Andrew S., 26, 27, 194
Grubman, Jack, 356
Guiliani, Rudolph, C-51
Gundersen, Edna, EN-8
Gunnarson, Sarah K., EN-11
Gunter, Marc, 5
Gupta, Anil K., 48

Hachman, Mark, C-129n
Haglock, Travis, C-27n
Hainer, Herbert, C-380
Haji-Ioannou, Stelios, C-162, C-165, C-168,
    C-169, C-170n

Hall, Gene, EN-9
Hall, William K., EN-6
Hambrick, Donald C., EN-4
Hamel, Gary, 132, 219, 230, EN-1, EN-3,
    EN-4, EN-5, EN-6
Hamermesh, R. G., EN-5, EN-6
Hamilton, John, C-235, C-236, C-243, C-244
    to C-247, C-249
Hamm, Steve, EN-1, EN-5
Hammer, Michael, 388, EN-9
Hand, M., C-271, C-272
Hansell, Paul, C-129n
Hardee, Camilla, EN-1
Harding, Mike, C-195
Hardy, Quentin, C-311n
Harley, William, C-359 to C-360
Harmon, S., C-271, C-272
Harrigan, Kathryn R., EN-3, EN-4, EN-5
Harris, Gardiner, EN-7
Harris, J. E., EN-6
Harris, R., C-66n
Haslett, Kevin, C-435n
Hastings, Reed, C-148, C-149, C-161
Hathaway, Melissa, C-263
Hattaway, John, C-130
Hauser, Robert, C-190
Hausman, Jerry, C-435n
Hawk, Thomas F., C-468
Hayes, J., C-338, C-354
Hayes, Robert H., 94, EN-8
Hayibor, Sefa, EN-8
Hedberg, Carl, C-235
Heeley, Michael B., EN-4
Hegert, M., EN-2
Heifetz, Ronald A., EN-11
Heikkilä, Jussi, EN-8
Heller, Walter, C-47
Helmstetter, Richard C., C-74 to C-75, C-78
Helyar, John, C-435n
Hendricks, Kevin B., EN-1
Henshall, Donald, C-206
Herzberg, Frederick, 388
Heskett, James L., EN-10
Hess, David, EN-8
Hesselbein, Frances, EN-9, EN-10
Hetland, Karsten, C-503, C-505
Hill, Ronald Paul, 343
Hilmer, Frederick G., EN-8, EN-9
Hirsch, Robert D., EN-11
Hitt, Michael A., EN-1
Hodgetts, Richard M., EN-10
Hodgson, N., C-170n
Hofer, Charles W., EN-5
Holch, Kristy, C-225
Holder, Larry, C-174
Hollender, Jeffrey, EN-7
Holm, Torben V., C-502
Holmes, Bruce, C-247, C-250n
Holpp, Larry, EN-9
Hookham, M., C-170n
Horton, Tim, 209
Hosmer, LaRue T., C-171
House, Charles H., EN-1

Hout, Thomas M., EN-11
Howe, Peter J., C-147n
Howell, K., C-354
Hubbell, Victoria, EN-10
Huey, John, C-435n
Humble, John, EN-11
Hurd, Jonathan, EN-3
Hurd, Mark, C-111
Hyde, J., C-170n
Hyland, Paul, EN-9

Iacobucci, Dawn, EN-3
Iansiti, Marco, 141
Idei, Nobuyuki, C-229
Immelt, Jeffrey R., 36, 307, 316, 414
Inkpen, A., EN-3
Inouye, Wayne, C-113
Ismail, I., C-234n
Iverson, Allen, C-390

Jackson, Katy Beth, C-116, C-130
Jacobsen, Kristine, EN-2
Jaffe, Dan, C-341, C-344, C-346,
    C-347, C-350
Jaffe, Paul, C-340, C-350
Jakob, Keith, C-272
Jaman, Joel, C-328
James, Jesse, C-363
James II of Scotland, C-68
James III of Scotland, C-68
James IV of Scotland, C-68
James VI of Scotland/I of England, C-68
James VII of Scotland, C-68
Jarret, C-445
Jassawalla, Avan R., EN-10
Jay-Z, C-390
Jenk, Justin, EN-3
Jenkins, Holman W., Jr., C-532n
Jeremy, Mike, C-516
Jervik, Jeff, C-218
Jobs, Steven, C-130, C-131, C-132,
    C-133, C-140
Johnson, Kim, C-407
Johnson, Lisa, C-547
Johnson, William R., 47
Jones, Del, EN-10
Jones, Gareth, EN-10
Jones, Kathryn, C-115n
Jordan, Michael, C-378, C-379
Joshua, C-454 to C-455
Judge, P., C-67n
Jung, Andrea, 36
Jüni, Peter, C-532n
Juran, Joseph, EN-9

Kageyama, Yuri, 259
Kahaner, Larry, EN-2
Kahn, Gabriel, 221
Kale, Prashant, EN-3, EN-5
Kami, Michael, 2
Kane, Louis, C-190
Kanter, Rosabeth Moss, EN-3, EN-5, EN-9
Kaplan, Jerry, C-238

Kaplan, Nancy J., EN-3
Kaplan, Robert S., EN-1, EN-2, EN-3
Kaufman, Rhonda, EN-1
Keane, Barry, C-259
Keeble, Justin, EN-7, EN-8
Keeton, W. Page, C-558n
Keller, Ernest, C-263
Kelly, Thomas, C-51
Kennedy, Allen A., EN-10
Kennedy, R., C-67n
Kerr, Steven, 411, EN-10
Kersh, Sheri, C-472
Kevorkian, Susan, C-335
Khanna, Tarun, EN-5
Kidwell, Roland E., EN-6
Kim, Peter, C-528
Kim, W. Chan, 94, EN-1, EN-4
Kim, Young Se, C-126
Kimberly, John R., EN-9
Kimpton, Bill, C-537
King, Mark, C-385
Kipling, Rudyard, 316
Kirby, Ed, C-273, C-280 to C-285
Kirch, C., C-354
Kirchman, Jane, C-251, C-263
Klebinkov, P., C-234n
Klose, Kevin, C-257, C-271
Knight, Phil, 348
Knox, Simon, EN-8
Knudsen, John, C-239
Knutson, Wayne, C-281
Kohn, Alfie, EN-10
Koller, Tim, EN-6
Kotler, Philip, EN-4, EN-5, EN-6
Kotter, John P., 22, EN-10, EN-11
Kournikova, Anna, C-379
Kovacevich, Richard M., 358
Koza, M., EN-3
Kramer, John, C-164
Krebs, A. V., C-558n
Kreiser, Patrick, C-286
Kress, Donald, 94
Kusneta, Art, C-352
Kwak, Mary, EN-4
Kwan, Ik-Whan G., EN-11

Lachenauer, Rob, 132, EN-2, EN-4, EN-6
LaMar, Ray, C-210
LaMar, Shannon, C-210
Lampel, Joseph, C-405, EN-1
Lanahan, Dan, C-164
Landes, Valerie, C-263
Langley, Monica, 329
Lanzolla, Gianvito, EN-4
Larue, Warren, C-437
Lasher, William, C-47
Lashinsky, Adam, C-115n
Latour, Almar, EN-7
LaTour, Tom, C-539, C-546
Laurie, Donald L., EN-11
Lawrence, Anne T., EN-7
Lawrence, John J., C-162

Lawrence, Ron, C-475
Leahy, Stephen, C-558n
LeBeau, Joe, C-194
LeDuff, Charlie, C-181n
Lee, Elizabeth, C-27n
Lee, Hau L., EN-2
Lee, Louise, C-115n
Lee, Martin, C-558n
Lee, Terry Nels, EN-10
Leibowitz, Mitchell, 30
Leibtag, Ephraim, C-435n
Lemak, David J., EN-10
Leonard, Wayne, 414
Leondakis, Niki, C-540, C-542, C-546
Leuchter, Miriam, 366
Levering, Robert, 392
Levien, Roy, 141
Levinsohn, Peter, C-160
Levy, Steven, C-129n
Lewandowski, Joe, C-27n
Lewin, A., EN-3
Lewin, N., C-337, C-354
Libarle, Carol, C-164
Lieberthal, Kenneth, EN-4, EN-5
Liedtka, Jeanne M., EN-6, EN-9
Lightfoot, Paul, C-435n
Liker, Jeffrey K., EN-1
Lincoln, Abraham, 18
Livengood, Scott, C-193, C-195, C-200, C-206, C-207, C-211 to C-216
Lloyd, M. E., C-27n
Lombardi, Vince, 358
Lonian, A., C-354
Lorek, Laura, 186
Lorsch, Jay W., EN-11
Lott, S., C-67n
Louis-Dreyfus, Robert, C-378 to C-379, C-380
Lowry, Tom, 252
Lubatkin, Michael, EN-6
Luter, Joseph W., III, C-172, C-173, C-174
Lynyrd Skynyrd, C-356

Ma, Jack, C-308, C-309
Maass, Ruch, C-28 to C-29
Maass, Steve Oliver, C-28 to C-29, C-38, C-40, C-42, C-43
Machrone, Bill, C-147n
Macintosh, J., C-170n
Macken, Dan, C-263
Mackey, John, C-2, C-6 to C-7, C-11 to C-12, C-16, C-19, C-27n
MacMillan, Ian C., EN-4, EN-5, EN-6
MacPherson, Elle, C-379
Madden, John, C-445
Maddox, Braxton, C-148, C-182
Madhok, Anoop, EN-4
Madonna, C-379
Magglos, Jim, C-190
Magglos, Linda, C-190
Magretta, Joan, C-115n, EN-1
Mahelish, Bruce, C-276, C-278, C-279
Maich, Steve, C-129n

Main, Jeremy, EN-3, EN-5
Majchrzak, Ann, EN-9
Maklan, Stan, EN-8
Maldutis, Julius, C-66
Malone, Hermione, C-218n
Maltz, Lawrence, C-475
Malugen, Joe, C-159
Mandola, Damian, C-441
Mann, P., C-66n
Marcus, Bernie, 179
Margolis, Joshua D., EN-8
Mariano, G., C-354, C-355n
Marino, Louis D., C-116, C-130, C-286, C-311
Markides, Costas C., 2, 94, 230, 358, EN-1, EN-4, EN-6
Markkula, Mike, C-130, C-131
Marr, Melissa, C-161n
Martinez, Barbara, C-525, EN-7
Marvin, Stan, C-263
Mathews, Anna Wilde, C-525, C-532n, EN-7
Matthews, Mike, C-263
Mauborgne, Renée, EN-1, EN-4
Mawston, Neil, C-226
Maynard, M., C-67n
Mays, Lowry, 170
McAleer, Joseph, C-195
McBride, Sarah, C-161n
McCartney, Scott, C-58
McCawley, Tom, EN-8
McCline, Richard L., C-28
McCombs, Joe, 170
McCormick, Jo, C-263, C-267
McDonald, D., C-67n
McDonald, Ian, 329
McGrady, Tracy, C-381
McGrath, Rita Gunther, 132, 155, EN-4, EN-6
McKay, W. Andrew, C-557
McMillan, Ian C., 132, 155
McTaggart, Jenny, C-47
Meckler, Mark, C-454
Mehta, Stephanie N., 5
Menkes, Justin, EN-8
Menor, Larry, EN-1
Merritt, Bob, C-438 to C-439
Meuse, Eric, C-41, C-42
Meyerson, Morton, C-94
Michaels, D., C-67n
Mickelson, Phil, C-72, C-80
Midgley, David, EN-8
Miles, Morgan P., EN-1
Miller, Anthony, C-190
Miller, Danny, EN-2, EN-8
Miller, Scott, C-263
Milne, A. A., 358
Milne, George R., EN-2
Minietta, Norman, C-246
Mintzberg, Henry, 316, EN-1, EN-8
Mitarai, Fujio, C-229
Moeller, David R., C-558n
Mohammed, 321
Mokwa, Michael P., EN-2

Monroe, Clay, C-297
Montan, Tom, C-328, C-329, C-341,
    C-343 to C-348, C-349, C-350, C-351,
    C-352, C-354
Montgomery, Cynthia A., EN-1, EN-2, EN-6
Montgomery, Dirk, C-439
Montgomery, Joseph C., EN-10
Moore, Daryl, C-476
Moore, Gordon, 27
Moore, James F., EN-9
Moore, John, C-28
Morgan, Chris, C-230
Morozov, Boris, C-219
Morris, D., EN-2
Morris, Mark, C-66
Morris, Rebecca J., C-219
Moser, Beat, C-509
Moses, C-454 to C-457
Moskowitz, Milton, 392
Mossberg, Walter S., C-147n
Mouawad, J., C-67n
Mowat, Jennifer, C-168
Mroz, John Edward, EN-9
Much, Marilyn, C-27n
Mukherjee, Debabrata, C-532n
Murdoch, Rupert, 252
Murphy, Patrick E., EN-11
Murphy, Wendell H., C-177, C-178
Musson, Michael, C-164
Mutz, A., C-234n
Myers, Malcolm, C-509, C-513

Nadler, David A., EN-1
Nagy, Christine, C-489
Nalebuff, Barry J., 160
Nartey, Linda, C-532n
Nartinez, Barbara, C-532n
Nash, Sarah, EN-5
Naumes, Margaret J., C-47
Neeleman, David, C-48 to C-52, C-59 to
    C-60, C-62, C-63, C-66n, C-67n
Neman, Robert P., EN-10
Ness, Joseph A., EN-3
Neuman, Robert P., EN-9
Newman, R., C-66n
Nichols, P. M., EN-7
Nickelback, C-356
Nickerson, William, C-393
Nielsen, Anders P., EN-2
Nielsen, Hans Munk, C-503
Niles-Jolly, Kathryn, EN-11
Nimoy, Leonard, C-343
Nissen, Steven E., C-532n
Noble, Charles H., EN-2
Noddle, Jeff, C-26
Nohria, Nitin, EN-11
Nordheim, Christie, EN-3
Norton, David P., EN-1
Nurse, Howard, C-164

O'Bannon, Douglas P., EN-8
Odak, Perry, C-22, C-23
Ohinata, Yoshinobu, EN-9

Ohmae, Kenichi, 48
Ohno, Taiichi, 372
Okawara, Merle, C-302
Olian, Judy D., EN-10
Olsen, Dave, C-475, C-482
Olusaga, S. Ade, EN-2
Omidyar, Pierre, C-286, C-289 to C-290,
    C-291, C-294, C-298, C-308
Oppenheimer, Peter, C-133
Osegowitsch, Thomas, EN-4
Oster, Christopher, 329
Oster, Sharon, 2
Overby, S., C-66n, C-67n
Owen, John, C-51
Oztark, Sevgi, EN-11

Pace, Michael, C-533, C-541, C-542
Page, Larry, 417
Paine, Lynn Sharp, EN-11
Palenchar, Joseph, C-129n
Palepu, Krishna G., EN-5
Palmer, Arnold, C-75
Panagos, Steven, C-214
Pande, Peter S., EN-9, EN-10
Par, Terence P., 116
Parets, Robyn, C-546n
Parise, Salvatore, EN-3
Park, Daewoo, EN-1
Parker, Doug, C-63
Parrish, Harrison, C-159
Patterson, George, C-68
Patterson, W., C-354, C-355n
Pearl Jam, C-306
Pedersen, Klaus, C-500, C-507,
    C-509, C-513
Peery, Mary, C-232
Peet, Alfred, C-469
Perez, Antonio, C-232
Perloff, Roger, C-532n
Pertinax, C-288
Peteraf, Margaret A., EN-2
Peters, J. W., C-67n
Pfeffer, Jeffrey, EN-10, EN-11
Pinetti, Steve, C-537, C-540 to C-541, C-542
Pisano, Gary P., 94, EN-8
Pollack, Andrew, C-558n
Porras, Jerry I., EN-1, EN-8
Portanger, Erik, EN-7
Porter, Michael E., 55, 111, 114, 132, 134,
    C-47, EN-1, EN-2, EN-3, EN-4, EN-5,
    EN-6, EN-11
Post, James E., EN-7
Powell, Michael, C-332
Powell, Thomas C., EN-10
Prahalad, C. K., 132, EN-1, EN-3, EN-4,
    EN-6, EN-9
Prasso, S., C-66n
Pressman, Robin, C-263
Preston, Lee E., EN-8
Price, G., C-354, C-355n
Price, Raymond L., EN-1
Procter, William, C-398
Pulliam, Susan, EN-8

Quelch, John A., EN-5
Quinn, James Brian, EN-3, EN-4, EN-8,
    EN-9, EN-11

Rädler, George, C-496
Rafalko, Robert J., EN-11
Ralph, Kem, C-553
Ramstad, Evan, C-129n
Randall, Robert M., EN-4
Rao, Askay R., EN-4
Rappaport, B., C-354, C-355n
Raskin, Jeff, C-130, C-131
Reed, D., C-67n
Reed, John, EN-7
Reed, Richard, EN-10
Reese, Jennifer, C-495n
Reich, Robert, C-343
Reichenbach, Stephan, C-532n
Reid, Joanne, EN-10
Rhoades, Ann, C-51, C-60, C-61
Rhoads, Gary K., EN-9, EN-10
Richards, Keith, C-362
Richardson, Sandy, EN-1
Ridderstråle, Jonas, EN-8
Rieder, Geert, C-513
Rigby, Darrell, EN-1
Rives, Karen Schill, C-27n
Robert, Michel, 22, 160, EN-1
Roberts, Jane, C-558n
Roberts, Noreen, C-350
Roberts, Sarah, EN-7, EN-8
Robinson, Bruce, C-263
Rock, Melinda, EN-9
Rogovsky, Nikolai, EN-8
Rojas, Peter, C-147n
Rolling Stones, C-362
Rollins, Kevin, C-95, C-102, C-104,
    C-105, C-115n
Roman, Ronald M., EN-8
Roos, Goran, EN-2
Rose, B., C-272
Rosenthal, Jim, EN-9
Rosin, L., C-272
Ross, Joel, 2
Rothmuller, Ken, C-130
Rothschild, William E., EN-4
Rounds, Kate, C-495n
Roussouw, Gedeon J., 335, EN-7
Rovenpor, Janet, C-48
Rowling, J. K., C-335
Rudolph, Vernon, C-194 to C-195
Rutan, Burt, C-238, C-239, C-240,
    C-250n
Rynes, Sara L., EN-10

Sablan, Natalie, C-263
Salter, C., C-66n, C-67n
Sanger, E., C-67n
Santero, Renay, C-39, C-41, C-42
Sanyal, Rajib, EN-7
Saporito, Bill, C-435n
Sapsford, Jathon, 219
Sashittal, Hemant C., EN-10

Sasson, Lisa, EN-3
Satchell, M. J., EN-7
Sathe, Vijay, EN-10
Sauer, Patrick J., C-161n
Scanlan, Gerald, EN-10
Schäfer, Roger, C-356
Schendel, Dan, EN-5
Scherer, F. M., EN-2
Schermerhorn, John R., 339, EN-7
Schmal, Michele, C-186
Schmeiser, Louise, C-557
Schmeiser, Percy, C-547, C-552 to
    C-557, C-558n
Schneider, Antoon, EN-6
Schneider, Benjamin, EN-11
Schulman, Lawrence E., EN-3
Schultz, Howard, 36, C-470 to C-483, C-486,
    C-489, C-493, C-495
Schumer, Charles, C-51
Schwartz, Mark S., EN-7, EN-11
Scolnick, Edward M., C-520, C-525,
    C-528
Scott, H. Lee, C-411, C-414, C-433, C-434
Scott, Michael, C-130, C-131
Scott, Tom, C-28, C-39, C-40, C-41, C-42,
    C-43, C-328
Scruggs, Earl, C-356
Sculley, John, C-131
Selby, Richard W., 230
Shah, Amit J., C-193, C-468
Shaich, Ron, C-190
Shank, John K., EN-2, EN-3
Shaw, Gordon, EN-1
Shaw, Hollie, C-27n
Shay, Jeffrey, C-273
Shern, Teresa M., C-251
Sherwood, B., C-170n
Shirouzu, Norihiko, 219
Siegel, David, C-63
Siegel, Zev, C-468 to C-470
Siguaw, Judy A., C-546n
Silk, S. B., EN-5
Silverman, Murray, C-533
Simons, John, C-532n
Simons, Robert, 316, EN-8, EN-9, EN-10
Simpkins, E., C-170n
Sims, Ronald R., EN-7
Singh, Harbir, EN-3, EN-5
Singh, Jang B., EN-11
Sinha, Jayant, EN-5
Skoll, Jeffrey, C-290, C-298
Slaughter, Michelle, C-223
Slevin, Dennis P., EN-4
Sligh, Michael, C-558n
Sloan, Gene, C-546n
Slye, Jeff, C-545
Smith, Aaron, C-350
Smith, Adam, EN-9
Smith, H. Jeff, EN-8
Smith, Iain, 343
Smith, Kennedy G., EN-5, EN-10
Smith, Mike, C-247
Smith, N. Craig, EN-7, EN-8

Smith, Randall, EN-8
Smith, Steve, C-129n, C-147n
Smothers, R., C-67n
Snead, Michele, C-454
Snyder, Gary, C-343
Snyder, Roger, C-558n
Solheim, Karsten, C-86 to C-87
Solis, Luis, C-162
Sommerville, Iain, EN-9
Soo, Christine, EN-8
Soros, George, C-50
Spanos, Shafiq, C-263
Spindler, Michael, C-131 to C-132
Spurlock, David, C-66
Stabile, Vincent, C-61, C-62
Stahlberg, Craig, C-276, C-282
Stalk, George, Jr., 132, EN-2, EN-3,
    EN-4, EN-6
Stanton, J., C-170n
Staub, Martin, C-513
Stephens, Debra, 343
Stephens, Greg, C-174, C-175
Sterchi, Rebekka, C-532n
Stipp, David, C-532n
Stith, Pat, C-181n
Stoeberl, Phillip A., EN-11
Stohlman, Katie, C-263
Stohm, C., C-354
Stone, Reuben E., EN-3
Stratton, Larry, C-263, C-268
Strickland, A. J., III, C-148, C-436
Stringer, Howard, 259, C-123
Stroh, Linda K., EN-10
Stuart, Bruce, C-525
Stuckey, John, EN-3
Stuppin, Jack, C-261
Suarez, Fernando, EN-4
Sudhaman, Arun, C-129n
Sukiennik, Greg, C-201
Sull, Donald, EN-2
Sullivan, Chris, C-437, C-438, C-446
Sun Zi, 414
Swayne, Linda E., EN-2
Symonds, W., C-234n

Tahmincioglu, E., C-67n
Tarnowski, Joseph, C-47
Tate, John W., C-218
Tate, Ryan, C-546n
Taxer, Marshall, C-164
Taylor, A., C-67n
Teece, David, EN-2
Teerlink, Richard, C-361
Teets, John W., 18
Terry, Robert J., 266
Thomas, Howard, EN-2
Thomas, Robert, C-263
Thomas, Terry, 339, EN-7
Thomas, Tom, C-533
Thompson, Arthur A., C-2, C-89, C-148,
    C-193, C-410, C-468, C-518
Thomson, Alan, EN-11
Tichy, Noel, 414
Topol, Eric J., C-532n

Torvalds, Linus, 14
Toussaint, Dennis, C-273, C-281, C-284
Tovstiga, George, EN-2
Trachtenberg, J., C-354, C-355n
Traywick, Jennifer, C-182
Treviño, Linda K., 316
Tristram, Claire, C-311n
Trump, Donald, C-445
Tucci, Joe, 440
Tully, Shawn, EN-5
Turock, Art, C-47
Tuxhorn, Laurie, C-39, C-40
Twer, Doran, EN-10
Tyler, Beverly B., EN-1

Uihlein, Wally, C-86
Ungan, Mustafa, EN-9
Upton, David M., 94, EN-8
Useem, Jerry, C-420, C-435n

Välikangas, Lissa, 230, EN-5
Van Houten, Ben, C-495n
Van Putten, Alexander B., 155, EN-4,
    EN-6
Van Vuuren, Leon J., 335, EN-7
Veiga, John R., EN-7, EN-10
Very, Philippe, 266
Vickers, Marcia, 329
Vilaga, Jennifer, C-129n
Vogelstein, Fred, 407, EN-10, EN-11

Wade, Judy, EN-9
Wademan, D., C-67n
Waitt, Ted, C-113
Waleam, Jason, EN-3
Walker, Daryl, C-178
Walker, Lee, C-92 to C-94
Walker, M., C-67n
Walser, Marcel, C-509, C-513
Walser, Monika, C-509
Walsh, Helen, C-263
Walsh, James P., EN-8
Walston, Stephen L., EN-9
Walton family, C-412
Walton, M., EN-9
Walton, Sam, 440, C-412 to C-414, C-417,
    C-418, C-425 to C-429, C-428, C-435n
Wambold, Richard, 266
Wang, Qianwei, EN-9
Warrick, Joby, C-181n
Waters, J. A., EN-1
Watson, Gregory H., EN-3
Webb, Allen P., EN-11
Webb, Maynard, C-304
Weber, James, EN-7
Welch, Jack, 2, 266, 307, 316, 366, 388, 440,
    C-428, EN-8
Welch, Suzy, EN-8
Wells, John R., C-27n
Wells, M., C-67n
Wendlandt, A., C-170n
Wernerfelt, Birger, EN-2
Wesley, Pamela, C-289 to C-290

Wessel, Godecke, EN-9
Wetlaufer, Suzy, EN-11
Whelan, D., C-67n
White, Dan, C-186, C-187
White, David, EN-3
Whitman, Margaret, 36, C-290 to C-291,
    C-298, C-300, C-308, C-309
Wie, Michelle, C-88
Wilke, John R., EN-7
Willems, Mo, C-343
William IV of England, C-68
Williams, A., C-67n
Williamson, Peter J., 94, EN-6
Wilson, John J., C-27n
Wilson, Meena S., EN-10
Wilson, Simone, C-343
Winchell, Verne, C-210

Wingfield, Nick, C-161n
Winters, David, C-219
Wolf, C., C-234n
Wolf, David, C-164
Wolfe, Mary, C-263
Wolff, Carlo, C-546n
Wolverton, Troy, C-311n
Wong, E., C-67n
Woodberry, W., C-67n
Woods, Tiger, 368–369, C-72, C-74,
    C-87, C-88
Woodyard, C., C-66n
Woolridge, Bill, EN-1, EN-8
Worrell, Dan L., EN-8
Wozniak, Steven, C-130
Wrenn, Paula, C-259, C-272
Wysocki, Bernard, C-435n

Yamaguchi, Roy, C-436, C-443
Yang, Dori Jones, C-472, C-495n
Yin, S., C-234n
Yip, George S., EN-2
Yoffie, David B., EN-4
Young, Phil, C-83
Young, Shawn, 190, 304

Zack, Michael H., EN-2
Zahl, Phil, C-263
Zahra, Shaker A., EN-2, EN-5
Zanada, Thierry, C-509, C-513
Zbaracki, Mark J., EN-9
Zellner, Wendy, C-66n, C-420, C-435n
Zidane, Zinedine, C-381
Zimmerman, Ann, C-435n
Zimmerman, Frederick M., EN-6

SUBJECT INDEX

AARP Magazine, C-370
Ability, developing, 369, 385
Accounting; *see also* Sarbanes-Oxley Act
  activity-based vs. traditional, 116t
    Big Four firms, 211
    financial statement adjustments,
      C-216 to C-217
    internal controls failure, C-216
Accounting scandals, 327–332, 424
Achievement, 100, 408–410, 441
Acid-test ratio, 98t
Acquisitions; *see* Mergers and acquisitions
Action agenda; *see also* Strategic actions
  for changing problem cultures, 428–432
  for embedding values and ethics, 436
  for implementing strategy, 42–43
  for strategy execution, 361, 362–363
Action plan, 3–4
Activist groups, 347–348, C-410 to C-411
Activity-based accounting, 112, 114–115
  compared to traditional accounting, 116t
Activity ratios, 99t
Actual value, 147
Adaptive corporate cultures, 425–426
Added-value tests for diversification, 270
Administrative expenses, 136
Administrative support activities
  outsourcing, 374, 375
  strategic fit in, 276
  in value chain, 111
Advertising
  celebrity endorsements, C-72, C-87 to C-88
  costs for low-cost providers, 137–138
  in kiosks, C-100
  by Krispy Kreme, C-198 to C-199
  low-cost leadership and, C-419
  by Outback Steakhouse, C-445
  PC industry, C-107
Advertising manager, 40
African Americans
  buying power, 348
  golf players, C-76
Agents of change, 394
Aggressive moves, 262
Aggressive pricing strategy, C-162
Aggressive promotional strategies, C-23
Aircraft industry, C-235 to C-250
Airline industry, C-48 to C-67
Alliances; *see* Strategic alliances
American Demographics, C-30
American Veterans Awards, C-412
Amoral managers, 324, 334–336, 338,
  352–353
Anti-Bribery Convention, 320
Anticorruption legislation, 338
Antitrust action, 252, 253
Asian Americans
  buying power, 348
  golf players, C-76

Assets
  competitive, 98–100, 290
  selling off, 257
Attractiveness strength matrix, 292–294, 293t
Audit committee, 45
Authoritarian structure, 379, 383–384
Authority
  delegating, 378–381, C-512
  placing limits on, 380–381
Automobile insurance business, 155
Average collection period, 99t
Awards and celebrations
  Best of CES Award, C-142
  Corporate Patriotism Award, C-412
  as incentive, 407
  Master Entrepreneur of the Year,
    C-173 to C-174
  national awards, 392, 433
  for operational excellence, 442
  in results-oriented climate, 442
  role in corporate culture, 432, 433
  Ron Brown Award, C-412

Backward expansion, C-417
Backward integration, 68, 71, 171, 172–173
Balanced scorecard approach
  example, 33
  financial/strategic objectives, 31
  long- and near-term objectives, 32
  performance measures, 31–32
  strategic intent, 32–34
  team effort, 34
  top-down objective setting, 34–35
  users of, 32
Bargaining leverage, 290
Bargaining power
  of buyers, 69–72
  company vs. suppliers, 138
  to lower prices, 143
  from outsourcing, 175
  of suppliers, 66–68
Barriers to entry
  capital requirements, 62
  cost/resource disadvantages, 61
  customer loyalty, 62
  distribution channel challenges, 62
  diversification and, 270
  economies of scale, 60–61
  in emerging industries, 232–233
  high vs. low, 63
  incumbent obstacles, 62–63
  regulatory policies, 62
  rising or falling, 63–64
  strong brand preferences, 62
  supply-side fragmentation and, 246
  trade restrictions, 62
Benchmarking, 116–118
  competitive strengths, 122
  consulting organizations, 117

Benchmarking—*Cont.*
  for continuous improvement, 393,
    394–395, 400
  corporate culture and, 423
  cost disadvantages and, 117–120
  ethics and, 118
  for operational excellence, 442
  on workforce diversity, 347
Best-cost provider strategies, 157t
  compared to low-cost providers, 150
  competitive advantage, 150–151
  contrasted with other strategies, 156–158
  example, 152
  key points, 159
  optimum conditions for, 150–151
  risks of, 151
  target market for, 151
Best of CES Award, C-142
Best practices, 43, 238
  and benchmarking, 116
  continuous improvement programs for
    benefits of initiatives, 399–401
    business process reengineering, 395–396
    identifying best practices, 393–395
    Six Sigma quality control, 396–399
    total quality management, 396, 399
  corporate culture and, 423
  cultural climate for, 438
  definition, 393–394
  environmental, C-492, C-542 to C-546
Better-off test, 270
Big Four accounting firms, 211
Blue ocean strategy, 180–181, 192
Board of directors
  and chief executive officers, 44–45
  decision making and information
    gathering, C-513
  independence of, 45–46
  negligence by, 45
  public radio, C-264
  report on operations, C-216
  role in crafting strategy, 44–46, 47
  shareholder revolt, C-157
Book Industry Trends, C-330
Booksellers, C-328 to C-355
Bottom-up objective-setting, 34–35
Boundaryless company, 366
Brand awareness, C-533 to C-534
Brand loyalty, 59, 233, C-356
  cultivating, C-369
Brand name, exploiting, 273
Brand portfolio, Procter & Gamble, C-394
  to C-395
Brand preferences, 62
Brand reputation (image)
  competitive asset, 290
  hotel industry, C-539 to C-541
Brands, private label, C-40
Brand switching, 58–59

Note: Page numbers in *italics* indicate material in illustrations; page numbers followed by t indicate material in tables; page numbers followed by n indicate notes; page numbers preceded by C- indicate material in Cases.

Brazil, 199–200
Bribery
  ethical relativism and, 319–320
  in global business, 325–327
  Global Corruption Report, 326t, 327t
Brick-and-click strategies, 184–185, 186
Brick-and-mortar operations, 75, 185
Broadband service, 190
Broadcasting industry, C-251 to C-272
Broad differentiation strategies; *see*
  Differentiation strategies
Broadly diversified companies, 284
Budget
  reallocation, 390
  strategy-driven, 389
Budget-conscious buyers, 151
Build-to-order manufacturing, C-95 to C-97,
  C-109, C-114
Build-to-stock value chain model, C-109
Bureaucracies, 374, 375
  change-resistant, 423
Bureau of Land Management, C-555
Business base
  expanding, 300–303
  narrowing, 303–306
Business Builder Awards, 433
Business case
  for ethical strategy, 338–341
  for social responsibility, 347–349,
    353–354
Business environment
  competent analysis of, 92–93
  competitive forces, 51, 52, 54–74, *55,* 91
    profitability and, 72–74
    rivalry among sellers, 55–60, *57*
    seller–buyer relationships, 69–71
    substitute products, 64–65, *65*
    supplier–seller relationships, 66–69
    threat of new entrants, 60–64, *61*
  competitive intelligence, 85, 92
    monitoring rivals, 85–86
    predicting rivals' moves, 86–87
  diagnosis for strategy making, 49
  dominant economic features, 52–54, 53t,
    90–91
  driving forces, 52, 91
    assessing impact of, 80–81
    concept, 74
    identifying, 74–79
    link with strategy, 81
    most common forces, 80t
  factors influencing, 49–50
  fast-changing, 426
  in foreign markets, 198–199
  industry outlook, 52, 89–90, 92
  key success factors, 52, 87–89, 88t, 92
  macroenvironment, 49–51, *51*
  market position, 52, 81–84, 91–92
    evaluating strategic group maps, 83–84
    rivalry effect, 56
    strategic group mapping, 81–83, *83*
  strategically relevant components, 49–51
  strategy corrections, 43–44
  thinking strategically about, *50,* 51–52

Business ethics, 316–342, 352–353; *see also*
  Ethical *entries;* Social responsibility
  in benchmarking, 118
  business case for, 338–341
  codes of ethics, 434t, 435
    on bribes/kickbacks, 320
    genuineness of, 341–342
    worldwide enforcement, 323
  company approaches, 333–338, 335t
    compliance approach, 336–337
    damage control approach, 336
    ethical culture approach, 337
    reasons for changing, 338
    unconcerned/nonissue approach, 334–336
  company strategies, 327–338
  compliance and enforcement, 443–444
  core values and, 27–29
  corporate culture and, 434–437
  definition, 317
  drivers of unethical strategies
    company culture, 332–333
    earnings targets, 330–332
    pursuit of personal gain, 328–330
  leadership in, 443–444
  management morality
    amoral managers, 324–325
    immoral managers, 324
    moral managers, 323
  managerial immorality in global
    markets, 325–327
  moral case for, 338
  recent scandals, 327–332
  schools of thought
    ethical relativism, 319–322
    ethical universalism, 318
    integrative social contracts theory,
      322–323
  strategy and, 10–12
  strategy/core values and, 341–342
  test of, 340
  universal vs. local norms, 321–322
Business Ethics, C-19, C-522 to C-523
Business model, 12–13
  car rental business, C-162
  at eBay, C-298 to C-299, C-309 to C-310
  for emerging markets, 225–226
  example, 14
  at Google Inc., C-319 to C-321
  Krispy Kreme, C-196 to C-199
  PC industry, C-95 to C-107, C-113 to C-114
  Smithfield Foods, C-173 to C-174
  telecommunications industry, C-515 to
    C-516
Business principles, 416
Business process reengineering,
  395–396, 442
Business purpose, 24
Business risk
  first movers, 191
  industry attractiveness and, 287
  of multiple strategy horizons, 250–251
  in outsourcing, 177
  reduced by outsourcing, 176
  reduction in, 79

Business risk—*Cont.*
  unrelated diversification, 280
  from vertical integration, 173–174
Business Roundtable, 342, 350
Business strategy, 38, *39,* 267; *see also*
  Strategy *entries*
  at eBay, C-299 to C-302
  golf equipment industry, C-77 to C-88
  hotel industry, C-537 to C-539
  impact on rivals, C-108 to C-109
  and organization structure, 377–378
  rules for running a business, C-429
  single-business enterprise, 40, 95–97, *96*
  strategy cohesion, 41
  in strategy-making hierarchy, 37–40, *39*
Business-to-business relationships, 71–72
Business units
  competitive strength
    calculating scores, 289–291, 291t
    interpreting scores, 291–292
    nine-cell matrix, 292–294, 293t
  cross-business strategic fits, 381
  cross-unit coordination, 381–383
  degree of authority in, 378–381
  Eastman Kodak, C-230 to C-231
  performance targets, 408
  ranking performance prospects,
    298–299, 299t
  strategy execution and, 377–378
BuyEfficient.com, C-545
Buyer bargaining power, 69–72, *72,* 143
Buyer demand, 76
  fall-off in, 58
  increase in, 57–58
  seasonal or cyclical, 287
  slow-down, 236
Buyer demographics, 76
Buyer diversity, 151
Buyer needs and requirements
  differentiation strategies and, 148
  product use, 143
Buyer perceptions, 147, 148
Buyer preferences; *see also* Customers
  competitive advantage and, 6
  dealing with cross-country
    variations, *205*
  diversity of, 148
  as driving force, 78–79
  in foreign markets, 197–198
  in fragmented industries, 246
  outsourcing and, 176
  supply-side fragmentation and, 246
Buyer-related activities, dispersed, 210–211
Buyers; *see also* Customers
  best-cost provider strategy and, 151
  budget-conscious, 151
  competitive pressure on sellers, 69–72, *72*
  number of, 53t
  price-sensitive, 135
  seller–buyer partnerships, 71–72
  social responsibility and, 347–348
  switching brands, 58–59
  value-conscious, 151
  view of product attributes, 149

Buyer segments, 153, 156
Buyers' market, 70
Buying power, 348

Cable television industry, 5
California Air Resources Board,
    C-368
Canada, patent law, C-555
Capability-related KSFs, 88t
Capacity-matching problems, 174
Capacity utilization, 137
Capital formation, C-476 to C-477
Capital-intensive business, 137
Capital investment
    fortify-and-defend strategy,
        252–253
    priorities, 268
    unrelated diversification, 279–280
Capital requirements
    barrier to entry, 62
    for export strategy, 203
    technological requirements and, 77
Carbon-copy strategies, 4
Car rental business, C-162 to C-170
Cash cows, 294–296
Cash flow
    differences in, 294–296
    generating, 260
Cash hogs, 294–296
Cell manufacturing techniques,
    C-96
Centralized decision making,
    378–379, 378t
Champions, 441
Change; see also Resistance to change
    adapting to, 261
    in adaptive cultures, 425–426
    anticipating, 242
    driving forces, 74–81
    in high-velocity markets, 241–245
    in industry environment, 9
    leading, 242
    reacting to, 242
Change-resistant cultures, 422
Channel conflict, avoiding, 183–184
Channel stuffing, 331
Charitable contributions, 343–344, 351
Chief executive officer, 36
    and board of directors, 44–45
    compensation of, 352
    ethical leadership, 443
    leading culture change, 429, 430
    role in crafting strategy, 35–36
    social responsibility initiatives, 445
    and top management, C-513
Chief financial officer, 45
Child labor, 319
China
    counterfeit products from, C-77
    Dell Inc. in, C-99
    as emerging market, 221
    Google Inc. in, C-326
    partnership agreements, 165
Circulation, C-527

Codes of ethical conduct
    bribes/kickbacks and, 320
    corporate culture and, 434t, 435
    culture-building role, 435–436
    genuineness, 341–342
    Smithfield Foods, C-181
    worldwide enforcement, 323
Coffee bar industry, C-468 to C-495
Collaboration in crafting strategy, 37
Collaborative partnerships, 68–69, 161, 191
    advantages, 164–166
    capturing benefits of, 166–167
    dangers of relying on, 167–168
    definition, 163
    examples, 164
    factors in making, 163
    in foreign markets, 217–220
    MP3 player industry, C-410
    PC industry, C-97 to C-98
    picking a good partner, 166
    with suppliers, 383
    with suppliers/buyers, 290
    unstable, 167
    in video rental business, C-148
Combination strategies
    in diversification, 284–285
    turnaround strategies, 259
Command-and-control paradigm, 379,
    383–384
Commitment
    to customers, C-446
    to low costs and quality, C-53 to C-58
    in strategic alliances, 166
Commodity products, 143
Communicating strategic vision
    motivational value, 25
    payoffs, 26
    resistance to change and, 25
    in slogans, 25–26
    strategic inflection points, 26, 27
    by top-level executives, 41
Community activists, C-410
Community citizenship, C-18 to C-19
Community involvement, 343, C-9,
    C-449 to C-450
Companies, 14
    business model, 12–13
    changes in environment, 26, 27
    coping with rapid change, 242
    evaluating business prospects, 3
    evolution of strategy, 8–9
    indicators of strategy, 7–8
    managing ethical conduct, 335t
        compliance approach, 335t, 336–337
        damage control approach, 336
        ethical culture approach, 335t, 337
        reasons for changing approaches, 338
        unconcerned/nonissue approach,
            333–338, 335t
    menu of strategy options, *162*
    strategic intent, 32–34
    strategy choices, 4
    strategy effectiveness, 95–97, *96*
    strategy-focused, 15

Companies—*Cont.*
    strategy-making hierarchy, 37–40
    winning strategies for, 13
Company culture; *see* Corporate culture
Company opportunity, 106
Company reputation (image)
    appeal of, C-369 to C-371
    low-cost leadership and, C-411
    rehabilitating, 339–340
    social responsibility and, 347–348
Company subcultures, 419–420
Company values, 27–29
Company Web sites; *see* Web site strategies
    bookselling, C-351
    brick-and-click strategies, 184–185, 186
    Dell Inc., C-101 to C-102
    of manufacturers, 75
    minor distribution channel, 184
    online enterprises, 184–187
    outsourcing design of, 375
    for price comparisons, 70–71
    product information only, 183–184
Company-wide objectives, 34
Compensation
    airline industry, C-62 to C-63
    culture change and, 431
    designing systems of, 410–411, 412
    of executives, 44–45, 352
    in food retailing, C-41 to C-42
    401(k) plans, C-17
    fringe benefits, 405, C-431, C-481
    low-cost leadership strategies,
        C-428 to C-431
    nonmonetary rewards, 404–405
    organic food retailing, C-17 to C-18
    profit sharing plan, C-431
    stock option plan, C-17, C-431, C-480
    stock purchase plan, C-17, C-431,
        C-480 to C-481
    team-based system, 136
    for top executives, 409
Compensation committee, 45
Competencies, 165; *see also* Core
        competencies; Distinctive competence
    compared to core competence, 102
    cross-border transfer, 211–212
    definition, 100–101
    differentiation strategies and, 147
    SWOT analysis, 100–102
Competition; *see also* Five-forces model of
        competition
    booksellers, C-342
    building a picture of, 54
    coffee house business, C-494 to C-495
    contending on global level, 226
    in digital photography industry,
        C-227 to C-230
    in DVD rental business, C-148 to C-159
    for eBay, C-304 to C-308
    fast-casual dining, C-188 to C-191
    food industry, C-46
    from foreign markets, 196
    in fragmented industries, 246–247
    globalization and, 75

Competition—*Cont.*
  global vs. international, 196
  golf equipment industry, C-68 to C-88
  key success factors, 87–89, 88t, 92
  for Krispy Kreme, C-208 to C-211
  leapfrogging, 178
  for low-cost leadership, C-419 to C-420
  in maturing industries, 236
  motorcycle industry, C-365 to C-368
  MP3 player industry, C-119 to C-129,
      C-141 to C-147
  multicountry vs. global, 201–202
  organic foods industry, C-20 to C-26
  for Outback Steakhouse, C-450 to C-451
  in PC industry, C-109 to C-114, C-137
      to C-138
  price cuts and, 59
  from product innovation, 76
  profit sanctuaries and, 213–215
  in public broadcasting, C-252 to C-257
  quantitative strength ratings, 122
  from substitute products, 64–65, 65
  threat of new entrants, 60–64, 61t
  weakened rivalry, 58
Competitive advantage
  best-cost provider strategy, 150–151
  from blue ocean strategy, 180–181
  building core competencies, 386
  from core competencies, 373
  in cross-business opportunities, 268
  of cross-business strategic fits, 294, 295t
  differentiation-based, 172–173
  in differentiation strategies, 144
  focused differentiation strategy, 153–154
  focused low-cost strategy, 153
  in foreign markets, 227
      cross-border coordination, 212–213
      cross-border transfers, 211–212
      locational advantages, 198–199, 209–211
  key success factors, 89
  of multinational corporations, 308–311
  from offensive strategies, 177–182
  online enterprises, 185
  outsourcing and, 176
  in related diversification, 276–277
      economies of scope, 277
      shareholder value, 277
  strategy and, 6–7, 13
  sustainable, 6, 13
  unrelated diversification, 284
  from value chain analysis, 120–122, 121
Competitive assets, 100–102, 104, 290
Competitive attack
  choosing basis for, 181–182
  choosing rivals for, 181
Competitive capabilities, 363, 385, 386
  access from merger or acquisition, 169
  from backward integration, 172–173
  building
      competitive advantage, 372, 373
      cross-functional work groups, 369
      customer needs, 370
      emergence of, 369–370

Competitive capabilities—*Cont.*
  building—*Cont.*
      employee training, 371–373
      role of leadership, 442–443
      three-stage development, 368–371
  of business units, 290
  costly to emulate, 373
  cross-border transfer, 211–212
  from cross-unit collaboration, 381–382
  differentiation strategies and, 147
  examples, 368
  from forward integration, 173
  golf equipment industry, C-72
  identifying, 105t
  of mature industries, 238
  mergers and acquisitions for, 370–371
  outsourcing, 370
  resource fit and, 297
  strengthening, 108
  SWOT analysis, 97–104
  traits, 369–370
  updating and remodeling, 371
Competitive conditions, 370
Competitive deficiencies, identifying, 104, 105t
Competitive edge, 56, 373
Competitive environment, 51–52
  insurance business, C-276
Competitive forces; *see* Five-forces model of
      competition
Competitive intelligence
  on foreign markets, 165
  monitoring rivals, 85–86
  predicting moves of rivals, 86–87
Competitive liabilities, 104
  reducing, 108
Competitive position, 95–96, 201, 244, 261
  Gillette Company, C-397 to C-398
  Google Inc., C-322 to C-327
  Procter & Gamble, C-396 to C-397
  strengthened by diversification, 268
Competitive power of resource strengths,
      102–104
Competitive pressures, 55, 84
  buyer bargaining power, 69–72
  in five-forces model, 54
  jockeying among rival sellers, 55–60
  new entrant threat, 60–64
  profitability and, 72–74
  from substitute products, 64–65
  supplier bargaining power, 66–69
Competitive rivalry; *see also* Five-forces
      model of competition
  among competing sellers, 55–60, 55t, 63t
  among industry leaders, 251–254
  cross-group rivalry, 84
  cutthroat or brutal, 60
  in declining industries, 239–241
  in emerging markets, 231–234
  factors influencing, 56–60
  in fragmented industries, 245–249
  golf equipment industry, C-72 to C-74
  in high-velocity markets, 241–245
  in macro environment, 53t

Competitive rivalry—*Cont.*
  in maturing industries, 236–239
  moderate, 60
  MP3 player industry, C-119 to C-129
  in rapid-growth businesses, 249–251
  in rapidly growing markets, 234–235
  runner-up firms and, 254–257
  scope of, 53t
  threat of new entrants, 60–64, 61t
  weak, 60
  weak/crisis-ridden businesses, 257–261
  weakened, 58
  weapons in, 56, 57t
Competitive rivals
  commodity products, 143
  competitive advantage and, 6–7, 370
  cross-border rivals, 60
  defensive strategies against, 182
  few differentiators among, 148
  global vs. multicountry competition,
      201–202
  golf equipment industry, C-77 to C-88
  for Google Inc., C-322 to 323
  identifying strategies of, 85–86
  in low-cost leadership, C-419 to C-420
  maneuvering by, 369–370
  market position of, 81–82, 91–92
  MP3 player industry, C-141 to C-147
  number of, 53t
  offensive strategies against, 177–182
  online auction business, C-303 to C-308
  organic foods industry, C-20 to C-26
  PC industry, C-89, C-90, C-108 to C-109,
      C-109 to C-114
  predicting next moves of, 86–87
  price competition, 143
  resource strengths of, 103
  resource strengths/weaknesses, 85–86
  strategy choices, 4
  strengths or weaknesses versus, 122–125
  underestimating, 262
  value chain differences, 112–113
Competitive scope, 95–96
Competitive strategies, 132–159, 134, 157t
  best-cost provider strategies, 150–151
  contrasting features, 156–158
  definition and purpose, 133
  differentiation strategies, 144–150
  for emerging industries, 233–234
  five distinct approaches, 134–135
  focused (market niche) strategies, 151–156
  in foreign markets, 204–209, 208
  functional-area strategy for, 187
  key points, 158–159
  low-cost provider strategies, 135–144
  multibrand strategies, 156
  stuck-in-the-middle strategies versus, 158
Competitive strength, 262
  relative market share, 289–290
Competitive strength assessment, 122–125,
      123t, 127
  of business units
      measures, 289–292

Competitive strength assessment—*Cont.*
 of business units—*Cont.*
  nine-cell matrix for, 292–294, 293t
 interpreting, 124–125
 unweighted rating system, 122–124, 123t
 weighted rating system, 123t, 124
Competitive superiority, 101–102, 103
Competitive weakness, 262
 attacking, 179
Competitive weapons, 56, 57t
Competitors
 for acquisitions, C-278 to C-279, C-280
 cooperation among, C-500
 costs of, 290
 identifying strategy of, 85–86
 increase in diversity of, 59–60
 increase in number of, 56–57
Complementary strategic options, *162*
Compliance
 approach, 335t, 336–337
 with ethical standards, 443–444
 notices of violations, C-179 to C-181
Compromise strategies, 262
Conservative strategies, 4
Consolidated financial statements, 129–131
Consumer electronics market, C-138 to C-147
Consumerism, C-433
Consumer Protection Distance Selling
  Regulations (UK), C-169
Consumer tastes, 202
Content follower strategy, 256–257
Continuous improvement programs
 benchmarking for, 393, 394–395
 benefits of, 399–401
 business process reengineering, 395–396
 comparison of, 399
 for operational excellence, 442
 Six Sigma quality control, 366, 396–399
 total quality management, 396, 399
Contract farming, C-174 to C-175
Control
 in decentralized structure, 380–381
 over empowered employees, 403–404
 flawed, C-216
 information systems for, 402–403
 Six Sigma program, 395, 396–399, 412
 total quality management, 396
Convenience stores, C-29
Core competencies, 363, 385, 386
 attacking, 217
 building
  competitive advantage, 372, 373
  employee training, 371–373
  role of leadership, 442–443
  three-stage development, 368–371
 compared to competencies, 102
 as competitive advantage, 120–121
 costly to emulate, 373
 from cross-unit collaboration, 381–382
 definition, 101
 examples, 368
 foreign markets and, 196
 to identify retail sites, C-484

Core competencies—*Cont.*
 mergers and acquisitions for, 370–371
 outsourcing and, 370, 374–375
 traits, 369–370
 updating and remodeling, 371
Core values
 versus actual practice, 29
 business principles and, C-481 to C-483
 case study, C-2 to C-27, C-6 to C-7, C-8
   to C-9
  community citizenship, C-18 to C-19
  company background, C-6
  compensation/incentives, C-17 to C-18
  competitors, C-20 to C-26
  facilities, C-7 to C-11
  financial performance, C-19 to C-20
  growth strategy, C-7
  marketing and customer service,
    C-14 to C-16
  merchandising, C-12 to C-14
  organic foods industry, C-2 to C-4
  product line, C-11 to C-12
  purchasing and distribution, C-18
  quality standards, C-13
  retailing organic foods, C-4 to C-6
  slogan, C-6 to C-7
  store operations, C-16 to C-17
  values statement, C-8 to C-9
 in company subcultures, 419–420
 in corporate culture, 416, 447–448
 grounding culture in
  benefits, 436–437, 437t
  codes of ethics, 434t
  cultural norms, 436
  culture-building role of values, 435–436
 JetBlue Airways, C-60 to C-61
 linked to strategy, 341–342
 linking vision with, 27–29, 30
 Merck & Company, C-519
 strategy–culture fit and, 427
 in strong-culture companies, 420–421
 telecommunications industry, C-504
 in weak-culture companies, 421–422
Corporate culture, 416–438, 447–448
 adaptive, 425–426
 as ally or obstacle, 426–428
 change approaches, 428–432, 429t
  making case for change, 429–430
  substantive actions, 430–431
  symbolic actions, 431–432
  time factor, 432
 definition, 415
 ethical, 337
 ethical failures and, 332–333
 evolution of, 419
 examples, 417, 433
 grounded in core values/ethics, 434–437
  benefits of cultural norms, 426–427, 437t
  culture-building role, 435–436
  transforming values and ethics, 436
 high-performance, 424–425
 identifying key features, 416–420
 JetBlue Airways, C-59 to C-61

Corporate culture—*Cont.*
 multinational strategy–culture fit, 437–438
 Oliver's Markets, C-40 to C-41
 Outback Steakhouse, C-447 to C-450
 perpetuating, 418–419
 psyche of, 415–416
 results-oriented, 438
 role of stories, 418
 at Starbucks, C-481 to C-483
 strategy execution and, 43
  perils of strategy–culture conflict, 428
  promoting better execution, 426–428
 strong vs. weak
  strong-culture company, 420–421
  weak-culture company, 421–422
 subcultures, 419
 unhealthy
  change-resistant culture, 422–423
  insular/inwardly focused, 423–424
  politicized culture, 422
  unethical/greed-driven culture, 424
 values-based, 438
 at Wal-Mart, C-425 to C-428
Corporate downsizing, 168, 384
Corporate governance, 44–46, 47, C-216
 booksellers, C-350
 public broadcasting, C-262
Corporate intrapreneurship, 37
Corporate Patriotism Award, C-412
Corporate restructuring; *see* Restructuring
Corporate social responsibility; *see* Social
  responsibility
Corporate strategy, 38, *39*, 267
 single-business enterprise, 40
 strategy cohesion, 41
Corrective adjustments, 19, 43–44, 47
 leadership in making, 445–446
 process, 446
Corruption Perception Index, 325t
Cost advantages, 61
 of direct selling, 139
 economies of scope, 278
 focused low-cost strategy, 153
 in foreign markets, 198
 in low-cost provider strategies
  cost-efficient value chain, 137–139
  example, 140–142
  revamping value chain, 139–140
 of online technology, 139–140
 of outsourcing, 138
 pitfalls, 144
 of price cutting, 178, 262
 steel industry, 136
 of vertical integration, 138
Cost-based competitive advantage, 6
Cost changes, 78
Cost cutting
 in declining industries, 240
 fixation on, 144
 by low-cost providers, 137–138
 in rapidly growing markets, 235
 revenue-increasing turnaround strategy, 248
 by runner-up companies, 255

Cost disadvantages
    from forward channel allies, 119–120
    internal, 119
    remedying, 117–120
    supplier-related, 119
Cost efficiency
    build-to-order manufacturing, C-95 to C-97
    from mergers, 168
    in value chain analysis, 121–122
Cost-efficient management of value chain
        activities, 137–139
Cost estimates, 115
Cost-of-entry test, 270
Costs
    competitive, 109–122, 127
    versus competitor costs, 290
    of ethical failure, 338–340, 339t
    expense categories, 114–115
    locational advantages, 211
    in online auctions, C-293 to C-294
    trimming, 238
Cost-saving efficiencies, 67
Counterfeit products, C-76 to C-77
Coverage ratio, 99t
Crafting strategy; see Strategy crafting;
        Strategy making
Credit rating, 297
Crisis-ridden businesses; see Weak
        businesses
Cross-border alliances, 217–220
Cross-border coordination, 212–213
Cross-border cultural change, 437–438
Cross-border markets, transfer of expertise
        to, 225
Cross-border rivals, 60
Cross-border transfer, 211–212
Cross-business collaboration, 273, 310
Cross-business economies of scope, 308–309
Cross-business strategic fit, 274–278, 294,
        295t, 381
    example, 302
Cross-business subsidization, 311
Cross-business value chain relationships, 268
Cross-country collaboration, 310
Cross-country differences
    competing in foreign markets, 197–201
        customization vs. standardization,
                197–198
        host government policies, 200–201
        locational advantages, 198–199
        market growth rates, 197
        multicountry vs. global strategy,
                204–209, 205, 208
        product design, 197
        risk of exchange rate changes, 199–200
    in cross-border alliances, 218–220
Cross-country subsidization, 311
Cross-functional work groups, 369, 395
Cross-group competitive rivalry, 84
Cross-industry strategic fits, 287
Cross-market subsidization, 214–215,
        227–228
Cross-subsidization tactics, 311–312

Cultural differences, 197
    in cross-border alliances, 218–220
    sensitivity to, 166
Cultural fit, 304–305
Cultural imperatives, 433
Cultural norms, 421, 430
    grounded in core values, 436–437
    strictly enforced, 436
Culture and lifestyle
    compensation and, 410
    cross-cultural variability, 320–321
    in global community, 325–327
    incentive pay, 411–412
    multinational operations and, 419–420
Culture-changing actions, 428–432, 429t, 447
    example, 433
    leadership factor, 429, 430
    making case for, 429–430
    substantive actions, 430–431
    symbolic actions, 431–432
    time factor, 432
Cultures
    ethical relativism in, 319–322
    moral agreement across, 318
Culture training, 438
Current ratio, 98t
Customer-based sales focus, C-99
Customer commitments, C-13
Customer forums, C-102 to C-103
Customer loyalty, 62
Customer needs, changes in, 370
Customers; see also Buyers
    aircraft industry, C-243 to C-246
    bargaining leverage with, 290
    book-buying habits, C-330 to C-331
    cultural differences, 197
    feedback from, 382
    in foreign markets, 196
    increasing sales to, 238
    Internet use, 75
    lifestyle changes, C-117 to C-118
    for low-cost leadership, C-412
    for online auctions, C-289
    for organic foods, C-6
    pressuring, 253
    shopping patterns, C-35
    value chain, 113
Customer satisfaction, C-8, C-445 to C-446
    airline industry, C-55 to C-58
    DVD rental business, C-151
    examples, C-201
    MP3 players, C-120, C-142
    short-pay policy, 392
Customer service activities
    in best-cost provider strategy, 150
    in differentiation strategies, 146, 148
    in distinctive-image strategy, 256
    in food retailing, C-40
    in low-cost leadership, C-425
    in maturing industries, 238
    organic foods retailing, C-8
    organic foods sales, C-14 to C-16
    PC industry, C-101 to C-103

Customer service activities—Cont.
    personalized, 253
    Six Sigma analysis, 399
Customer type specialization, 247–248
Cycle time, 375
Cyclical factors, 287

Damage control approach, 335t, 336
Data sharing, 138
Days of inventory ratio, 99t
Debt overload, 257
Debt-to-assets ratio, 98t
Debt-to-equity ratio, 99t
Decentralized corporate structure,
        C-16 to C-17
Decentralized decision making, 379–380
Decentralized organization
    capturing strategic fits, 381
    decision-making authority, 379–380
    maintaining control in, 380–381
    trends to, 383–384
Decision making
    by board of directors, C-513
    centralized vs. decentralized, 378–381
    speeding up, 375
    in strategic alliances, 166
Declining industries
    decline in demand and, 239
    end-game strategies
        fast exit, 241
        slow exit, 241
    strategy alternatives, 240–241
    strategy choices, 239–240
Defensive strategies, 125, 192
    blocking challengers, 182
    for emerging markets
        contending on global level, 226
        home-field advantages, 224–225
        new business models, 225–226
        transfer of expertise, 225
    signaling retaliation, 182–183
Demand
    decline in, 239
    seasonal or cyclical, 287
Demand conditions, 53t
Demographics
    of buyers, 76
    differences, 197
    radio-television audiences, C-257
Department of Agriculture, C-4
    Food and Safety Inspection Service, C-2
    National Organic Program, C-3, C-4
Department of Defense, C-60
Departments, 377
Deregulation, 79
Differentiation-based competitive advantage,
        172–173
Differentiation strategies, 6, 144–150, 157t, 262
    buyer preferences and, 78–79
    contrasted with other strategies, 156–158
    in declining industries, 240
    definition, 134
    easy-to-copy features and, 145

Differentiation strategies—*Cont.*
  focused, 153–156
  in golf equipment industry, C-73
  key points, 158
  mistakes in, 149–150
  optimum conditions for, 148
  perceived value, 147
  pitfalls, 148–150
  in rapidly growing markets, 235
  reward systems, 408
  routes to competitive advantage, 146–147
  by runner-up companies, 255
  signaling value, 147
  successful, 144–145
  types of themes, 145
  value chain activities, 145–146
Digital conversion requirement,
    C-255 to C-257
Digital photography industry, C-219 to C-234
Digital subscriber line, 190
Direct sales strategy, C-91 to C-92, C-95 to
    C-97, C-99 to C-100, C-114
Direct selling, 139
Direct-to-consumer marketing,
    C-524 to C-525
Discount Store News, C-412
Discount supermarkets, C-30
Distinctive competence, 101–102, 104,
    120–121, 147, 369, 370, 374–375, 385
Distinctive image, 262
Distinctive-image strategy, 256
Distribution activities
  collaborative partnerships, 383
  in differentiation strategies, 146
  DVD rental business, C-150 to C-151
  expansion into, C-205
  gold equipment, C-73 to C-74
  low-cost leadership, C-422 to C-423
  motorcycle industry, C-372 to C-374
  organic foods industry, C-18
  strategic fit in, 275
  truck fleet operations, C-423
  in value chain, *111*
Distribution channels
  as barrier to entry, 62
  Internet use
    brick-and-click strategies, 184–185, 186
    minor distribution channel, 184
    online enterprises, 185–187
    product information only, 183–184
  low-cost, 139
  in rapidly growing markets, 235
Distribution-related KSFs, 88t
Diverse strategy portfolio, 249–251
Diversification, 266–315; *see also* Related
    diversification; Unrelated diversification
  added-value tests
    better-off test, 270
    cost-of-entry test, 270
    industry attractiveness test, 270
  building shareholder value, 269–270
  candidates for, 268
  combination strategies, 284–285

Diversification—*Cont.*
  key points, 312–313
  post-diversification strategies
    broadening business base, 300–303, 301t
    divestiture strategies, 303–306
    multinational diversification, 308–312
    restructuring, 306–308
  related vs. unrelated, 272
  in restaurant business, C-436 to C-437
  strategic alternatives, *273*
  strategic analysis, 285–300, 312–313
    business-unit competitive strengths,
        289–294
    cross-business strategic fits, 294
    industry attractiveness, 286–289
    new strategic moves, 299–300
    performance prospects, 298–299
    resource allocation priorities,
        298–299, 299t
    resource fit, 294–298
  strategies for, 270–272
    acquisition, 271
    internal start-up, 271
    joint ventures, 271–272
  strategy-making facets, 267–268
  when to diversify, 269
Diversified companies
  building blocks of, 377–378
  cross-business strategic fits, 381
  decentralized decision making, 379
  identifying strategy of, *285*
  strategy-making authority, 267–268
  strategy options, 301t
    broader business base, 300–303
    divestiture, 303–306
    multinational diversification, 308–312
    restructuring, 306–308
Diversified multinational corporations,
    308–312
Divestiture
  adidas-Reebok, C-386 to C-390
  aimed at retrenching, 303–306
  candidates for, 303, 306–307
  of cash hogs, 296
  cultural fit and, 304–305
  of marginal businesses, 299
  in MP3 player industry, C-145
  PC industry, C-112 to C-113
  by selling off, C-211
  selling or spinning off, 305–306
Dividend payout ratio, 99t
Dividend yield on common stock, 99t
Divisional units, 377
DMADV Six Sigma process, 396
DMAIC Six Sigma process, 396–399
  components, 397
  example, 398
  for performance variations, 399
"Do-good" executives, 349–351
Domestic companies
  basic offensive strategies, 177–181
  basis of competitive attack, 181–182
  choosing rivals to attack, 181

Domestic companies—*Cont.*
  cross-market subsidization, 214–217
  defensive strategies, 182–183
  profit sanctuary potential, *214,* 215
  strategies for emerging markets, 224–226
    contending on global level, 226
    home-field advantages, 224–225
    new business markets, 225–226
    transferring expertise, 225
Domestic-only companies, *214*
Dominant-business enterprises, 284
Dominant technology, 233
Dot-com enterprises, 185–187
Doughnut industry, C-207
Dow Jones Global Index, 348
Downsizing, 168, 384
Driving forces
  assessing impact of, 80–81
  concept, 74
  identifying, 74–80
  most common, 80t
  for outsourcing, 175
  strategic group mapping, 84
  strategy and impact of, 81
  technological innovation, 275
Dumping strategies, 216
DVD rental business, C-148 to C-159

Earnings management, 331
Earnings per share, 98t
Earnings targets, 330–332
EarthCare program, C-540 to C-546
Easy Rider, C-362, C-371, C-374
Easy-to-copy features, 145
E-commerce, 183–187, 192, 383, C-105,
    C-106; *see also* Internet *entries;*
    Web site strategies
  case study, C-286 to C-311
    business model, C-298 to C-299
    business operation, C-292 to C-294
    business purpose, C-286
    community affinity, C-294 to C-298
    company background, C-289 to C-290
    completing transactions, C-294
    developing international markets, C-302
        to C-303
    evaluation of business model, C-309 to
        C-310
    feedback forum, C-295 to C-297
    fees and procedures, C-294
    formats, C-300 to C-302
    going public, C-298
    growth of online auctions, C-287 to
        C-288
    international growth, C-308 to C-309
    maintaining market dominance, C-298
        to C-303
    nature of online auctions, C-288 to C-289
    new challenges, C-308 to C-310
    online auction success factors, C-288
    professional management, C-290 to
        C-291
    range of categories, C-299 to C-300

E-commerce—*Cont.*
  case study—*Cont.*
    recent challenges, C-286 to C- 287
    rivals and competitors, C-303 to C-308
    safe harbor, C-297 to C-298
    stock performance, C-310
    strategy elements, C-299
  growth of, C-287 to C-288
  retailing, C-351
Economic value added, C-18
Economies of scale, 53t
  as barrier to entry, 60–61
  compared to economies of scope, 277
  locational advantages, 210
  of low-cost providers, 137
  in multinational diversification, 308
  from outsourcing, 176
  product standardization and, 198
  supply-side fragmentation and, 246
Economies of scope
  in multinational diversification, 308–309
  in related diversification, 277
Edge, 366
Efficiency changes, 78
Electronic product code technology,
    C-424 to C-425
Electronic scorecards, 403
E-mail, 75
Emerging industries, 79
  strategic hurdles, 234
  strategies for competing in, 231–234
  strategy options, 233–234
  unique characteristics, 232–233
Emerging markets, 220–226, 228
  local company strategies
    contending on global level, 226
    home-field advantages, 224–225
    new business models, 225–226
    transferring expertise, 225
  market growth rates, 197
  opportunities in, 220–221
  strategy options for, 222–223, *224*
  tailoring products for, 221–222
Emerging threats; *see* Threats
Employees; *see also* Workforce
  access to management, C-512
  child labor issue, 319
  in coffee bar business, C-477 to C-480
  with company values, C-61
  constructive pressure on, 441–442
  degree of authority, 378–381
  discrimination lawsuit, C-434
  in high-performance cultures, 424–425
  of high-tech companies, 367
  as intellectual capital, 367–368
  interaction with managers, 416
  job satisfaction survey, C-17
  linked to performance, 408–411
  performance tracking, 402–403
  promotion policy, C-447 to C-448
  recruitment and retention, 347, 365–368,
      C-447 to C-448
  recruitment and selection, C-61 to C-62

Employees—*Cont.*
  rewards and incentives
    balancing rewards and punishments,
      406–408
    motivational practices, 404–406, 407
  screening, 418–419, C-447 to C-448
  sharing information with, 405–406
  in slaughterhouses, C-175
  social responsibility and, 347
  soliciting ideas from, C-428
  strategy execution by, 359–360
  in strong-culture companies, 420–421
  understanding strategy, C-508 to C-511
  in weak-culture companies, 421–422
  work environment, 344, 346
  workforce diversity, 344–345
Employee stock option plan, C-480
Employee suggestions, 405
Employee training, 392, 441
  airlines industry, C-62
  costs of, 347
  culture training, 438
  in ethics and values, 444
  expansion into, C-206
  inadequate, C-407 to C-409
  leadership development, 364–365, 366
  in low-cost leadership, C-425, C-431 to C-432
  Outback Steakhouse, C-478
  at Starbucks, C-484 to C-485
  for strategy execution, 367–368, 371–373
Empowered employees, 372, C-8
  agents of change, 394
  in decentralized decision making,
      379–380
  exercising control over, 403–404
  Outback Steakhouse, C-478
  policies and procedures and, 393
  for quality improvement, 400
  work teams, 379–380
End-game strategy, 241, 257
Energy, 366
Energy conservation, C-66
Enforcement of ethical standards, 443–444
Enterprise resource planning, 138
Entrepreneurship, 35
  at Adam Aircraft, C-236 to C-238, C-239
      to C-240
  in airline industry, C-49 to C-50
  PC industry, C-91 to C-95
Entry barriers; *see* Barriers to entry
Entry of major firms, 77
Entry of new competitors, 312
  means of entry, 267, 270–272
  shareholder value tests, 270
  unrelated diversification, 280
Environmental best practices, C-492
Environmental issues
  case study, C-533 to C-546
    brand awareness, C-533 to C-534
    brand establishment, C-539 to C-541
    business strategy, C-537 to C-539
    cost-saving initiatives, C-536
    EarthCare program, C-542 to C-546

Environmental issues—*Cont.*
  case study—*Cont.*
    greening of hotel industry, C-535 to C-537
    recycling, C-533
    Triton Hotel concept, C-541 to C-542
  industry attractiveness and, 287
  organic foods, C-2 to C-3
  social responsibility and, 344, 346, 348,
      445, C-493 to C-494
  vertical integration as, C-171 to C-181
Environmental management systems, C-179
Environmental mission statement, C-494
Environmental policy statement, C-180
Environmental protection, 344
Environmental Protection Agency,
    C-368, C-555
Ethical culture approach, 335t, 337
Ethical failures, 11–12
  accounting scandals, 424
  business costs, 338–340, 339t
  and core values, 29
  counterfeit products, C-76 to C-77
  drivers of unethical strategies
    company culture, 332–333
    earnings targets, 330–332
    pursuit of personal gain, 328–330
    responses to, 333–336
  in ethical relativism
    bribes and kickbacks, 319–320
    child labor, 319
    multiple ethical standards, 320–321
    rudderless ethics, 321–322
  Global Corruption Report, 325–327
  managerial immorality in global business,
      325–327
  recent scandals, 327–332
  reporting infractions, 444
Ethical norms, 321–322
Ethical relativism, 352
  breakdown of, 321–322
  bribery and kickbacks, 319–320
  child labor issue, 319
  definition, 319
  multiple ethical standards, 320–321
Ethical standards, 416
  core values and, 341–342
  multiple sets of, 320–321
  origin of, 319–323
  rudderless, 321–322
  schools of thought, 352
Ethical strategy
  business case for, 338–340
  moral case for, 338
Ethical universalism, 318, 352
Ethics; *see* Business ethics
European car rental industry, C-163 to C-164
European Council, C-368
European Parliament, C-368
European Union, C-548
Everyday low prices, C-418
Excess capacity, 58
Exchange rate fluctuations, 199–200
Execution, 366

Executive compensation, 409
   linked to social responsibility, 352
   top-level executives, 409
Exercise equipment industry, 248
Exit of major firms, 77
Exit strategies, MP3 player industry,
   C-118 to C-119
Exodus story, C-455 to C-457
Expansion strategies
   airline industry, C-52 to C-53
   coffee bar industry, C-476 to C-477
   food industry, C-43 to C-47
   insurance business, C-276
   by Krispy Kreme, C-194, C-196, C-206
   by low-cost leadership, C-415 to C-418
   opposition to, C-172 to C-178
   PC industry, C-99 to C-100, C-103 to C-105
   restaurant industry, C-183 to C-184
   at Starbucks, C-483 to C-488
Expense categories, 114–115
Experience curve effects; see Learning
   curve effects
Expertise, 7, 99–100, 101
   in diversification, 310
   transfer of, 225
   transfers in diversification, 272
Export strategies, 203
External environment; see Macroenvironment

Facilities
   appealing, 406
   car rental business, C-165 to C-166
   coffee bar business, C-485 to C-488
   construction and maintenance,
      C-423 to C-424
   doughnut retailing, C-201 to C-205
   foreign markets
      concentrated, 209–210
      dispersed, 210–211
   formula facilities, 247
   in low-cost leadership, C-414 to C-415,
      C-416 to C-417
   organic food retailers, C-7 to C-11, C-12
      to C-14
   PC manufacturing, C-95 to C-97
   relocating, 140
   topping-out problem, 236
Fast-casual dining restaurants, C-182
   to C-192
Fast-exit strategy, 241, 257
Federal Aviation Administration, C-242,
   C-243 to C-244
Federal Communications Commission, 170,
   C-138, C-252, C-255
Financial accounting practices, 45
Financial incentives, 404–405
Financial objectives
   achieving, 35
   kinds of, 31
   success indicators, 96–97
Financial performance, 31–32
   adidas-Solomon, C-388 to C-391
   Amazon.com, C-306

Financial performance—Cont.
   Apple Computer, C-119, C-132, C-134,
      C-135
   Blockbuster, C-156, C-157
   Callaway Golf, C-82, C-83
   Copperfield's Books, C-344 to C-348
   decline in, C-211 to C-215
   Dell Inc., C-92, C-93, C-105,
      C-107, C-137
   Eastman Kodak, C-220 to C-221
   easyCar, C-162
   at eBay, C-291 to C-292
   Gillette Company, C-399
   Google Inc., C-324 to C-325
   Harley-Davidson, C-358 to C-359, C-372
   Hewlett-Packard, C-112
   JetBlue Airways, C-33, C-64
   KRCB ratio/television, C-265 to
      C-267, C-270
   Krispy Kreme, C-197 to C-198
   mass market booksellers, C-333 to C-334
   Monsanto Company, C-549 to C-551
   Netflix, C-151 to C-153
   Outback Steakhouse, C-438, C-440
   Procter & Gamble, C-397
   Smithfield Foods, C-171
   Starbucks, C-478 to C-479
   TDC, C-502
   Wal-Mart, C-412 to C-413
   Western States Insurance, C-282 to C-283
   Whole Foods Market, C-20 to C-21
Financial ratios, 98t–99t
Financial reporting practices, 45
Financial resources
   allocation options, 299t
   cash hogs vs. cash cows, 294–296
   credit rating, 297
   of public broadcasting, C-262 to C-269
   resource fit and, 294–296
   star businesses, 296
   unrelated diversification and, 280
Financial statement adjustments, C-216 to
   C-217
Financial Times, C-412
First-follower advantage, 188
First-mover advantage, 188–191
   decisions about, 189–191
   example of, 190
   versus late-mover advantage, 189
   for runner-up companies, 255
   sustaining the advantage, 188
   timing of, 188
Five forces model of competition, 54–74,
   55t, 91
   buyer bargaining power, 69–72
   competitive pressures in, 54
   jockeying among rival sellers, 55–60
   picturing competition, 54
   profitability and, 72–74
   sellers of substitute products, 64–65
   supplier bargaining power, 66–69
   threat of new entrants, 60–64
Focus, 244

Focused (market niche) strategies, 6–7,
   151–156
   contrasted with other strategies, 151–152,
      156–158
   in declining industries, 240
   definition, 135
   differentiation strategy, 153–154, 157t
   example, 155
   hotel industry, C-533 to C-546
   key points, 159
   low-cost strategy, 153, 157t
   risks, 156
Food and Drug Administration, C-242, C-520,
   C-524, C-526, C-528, C-530 to C-531
   Arthritis Advisory Committee, C-525
Food retailing, C-30 to C-37
Forbes, C-530
Foreign Corrupt Practices Act, 320
Foreign markets
   cross-country differences, 197–201
      buyer preferences, 197–198
      in cross-border alliances, 218–220
      gaining competitive advantage, 198–199
      global vs. multicountry strategies,
         204–209, 205, 208
      host government policies, 200
      market differences, 198
      risks of exchange rate changes, 199–200
   cross-market subsidization, 214–215,
      227–228
   emerging market strategies, 220–226
      defending against global giants, 224,
         224–226
      example of, 221
      local company strategies, 224, 224–226
      strategy options, 222–223
      tailoring products for, 221–222
   entry into, 79
   expansion into
      by eBay, C-302 to C-303
      by Google Inc., C-326
      Harley-Davidson, C-372 to C-374
      by Krispy Kreme, C-206
      low-cost leadership, C-417 to C-418
      by mature industries, 238
      reasons for, 196
      by strategic alliances, 165
   international vs. global competition, 196
   key points, 226–228
   multicountry vs. global competition,
      200–201
   offensive strategies, 215–217
   PC industry expansion, C-99 to C-100
   profit sanctuaries, 213–214, 227
   purchasing power variations, 197,
      221–222
   quest for competitive advantage, 209–213
      cross-border coordination, 212–213
      cross-border transfers, 211–212
      locational advantages, 209–211
   strategic alliances, 217–220
      examples, 219
      motivations for, 217–218

Foreign markets—*Cont.*
strategic alliances—*Cont.*
questionable need for, 220
risks of, 218–220
strategic issues, 195, 226
strategy options, 202–209, *205*
examples, 209
export strategies, 203
franchising strategies, 204
licensing strategies, 203–204
localized vs. global, 204–209, *208*
Forest Service, C-555
Formula facilities, 247
Fortify-and-defend strategy, 252–253, 257
Fortune, 392, C-16, C-358, C-412, C-421, C-528
Fortune China, C-418
Forward channel allies
cost disadvantages from, 119–120
value chains of, 113
Forward integration, 171, 173
401(k) plans, C-17
Fragmented industries
competitive conditions, 246–247
examples, 245
illustration of, 248
strategy options, 247–249
supply-side fragmentation, 245–246
Franchising
by Krispy Kreme, C-196, C-198
restaurant business, C-191
strategies, 204
Frills-free products, 140
Fringe benefits, 405, C-430 to C-431, C-481
Full-capacity operation, 137
Full integration, 171–172
Functional-area strategies, 38–40, *39, 162,* 192
choosing, 187–188
strategy cohesion, 41
Functional organization structure, 377
weaknesses, 382
Funding, 389

Gain-sharing program, C-17
General administration, *111*
General Aviation Revitalization Act, C-239
Generally accepted accounting principles, 45, C-216
General managers, C-42 to C-43
Generic competitive options, *162*
Genetically modified organisms, C-547 to C-558
Geographic coverage
Dell Inc., C-94
in fragmented industries, 248–249
low-cost leadership, C-416 to C-418
from mergers and acquisitions, 168–169
in rapidly growing markets, 235
supply-side fragmentation and, 246
Geographic expansion, by low-cost leadership, C-415 to C-418
Geographic organizational units, 377

Global companies, *214*
strategy–culture fit, 437–438
subcultures in, 419–420
Global competition, 227; *see also* International competition
case study
company background, C-468 to C-471
competitive environment, C-494 to C-495
employee training/recognition, C-484 to C-485
environmental best practices, C-492
facilities, C-485 to C-488
growth strategy, C-495
international expansion, C-484
joint ventures/acquisitions, C-489 to C-490
licensed stores, C-490 to C-491
mission statement, C-483
operations, C-492 to C-493
product line, C-488 to C-489
purchasing strategy, C-491 to C-492
social responsibility, C-493 to C-494
specialty sales, C-490 to C-491
store ambience, C-486 to C-488
store expansion strategy, C-483 to C-488
work environment, C-477 to C-483
worldwide store locations, C-469
versus international competition, 196
versus multicountry competition, 201–202
Global Corruption Report, 320, 325–327, 325t–326t
Global food supply, C-548
Globalization
case study, C-286 to C-311
as driving force, 75
of photography, C-227
strategic alliances and, 163
strategy options from, 225–226
technology transfer and, 78
Global market leadership
illustration of, 170
strategic alliances for, 163, 165
Global markets, 201
ethical relativism and, 321–322
management immorality in, 325–327
Global strategy, 204–209
low-cost leadership and, C-418
Golf equipment industry, C-68 to C-88
Government policies, 200–201
Government regulation
as barrier to entry, 62
of broadcasting, C-255 to C-257
as driving force, 79
against dumping, 216
Foreign Corrupt Practices Act, 320
foreign markets and, 200–201
industry attractiveness and, 287
of motorcycles, C-368
Organic Food Production Act, C-3
Sarbanes-Oxley Act, 338, 341
Greed-driven cultures, 424
Green Lodging Program, C-536
Gross profit margin, 98t

Growth
by acquisition, 255
slowing rate of, 236–237
Growth development leaders, 433
Growth rate potential, 286
Growth strategies
adidas, C-382 to C-383
airline industry, C-52 to C-53
car rental business, C-163 to C-164
coffee house business, C-495
DVD rental business, C-151
earnings targets, 330–332
food management, C-180
in food retailing, C-43 to C-47
by Krispy Kreme, C-194, C-206
by merger, C-276 to C-277
organic foods retailing, C-7
for rapid company growth, 249–251
restaurant business, C-191 to C-192
Guerrilla offensive, 179

Harvesting strategies, 260–261
High-definition television (HDTV), 5, C-255 to C-257
High-end differentiators, 151
High-performance cultures, 424–425
High-tech companies, 367
High-velocity change, 9
High-velocity markets, 241–245
coping with rapid change, 242
strategy options, 242–245, *243*
Hispanics
buying power, 348
golf players, C-76
Hit-and-run warfare, 179
Home-field advantages, 224–225
Host government policies, 200–201
Hotel industry, C-533 to C-546
Human assets, 100
Human resource management, *111*
airline industry, C-61 to C-63
at Oliver's Markets, C-41 to C-42
Human rights activists, 348
Hurricane Katrina, C-434, C-450, C-453
Hurricane Rita, C-450

Illegal immigrants, C-411
Immoral managers, 324, 334–336, 352
Inc. magazine, C-22, C-161
Incentive programs, 404–411; *see also* Rewards and incentives
Independent supermarkets, C-29
Industries; *see also* Declining industries; Emerging industries; Fragmented industries; Maturing industries
competitive attractiveness, 73
convergence of, 169
diversification strategy-making, 267–268
emerging, 79
global competition, 201–202
key success factors, 87–89, 88t, 92
learning/experience curve effects, 54
multicountry competition, 201

Industries—*Cont.*
in rapidly growing markets, 234–235
strategic alliances, 164
strategic groups, 82
topping-out problem, 236
types of market space, 180
value chain system, 113–*114*
Industry attractiveness
competitive conditions, 73
conditions for, 89–90, 92
in diversification
calculating scores, 277t, 286–288
difficulties in scoring, 288–289
interpreting scores, 288
measures of, 286–287
nine-cell matrix for, 292–294, 293t
performance prospects and, 298
Industry attractiveness test
attractiveness-strength matrix, 292–294, 293t
for diversification, 270
Industry conditions, 53t
booksellers, C-335 to C-342
buyer bargaining power, 69–72
competitive forces, 54–74
dominant economic features, 52–54
driving forces, 74–81
European car rentals, C-163 to C-164
golf equipment industry, C-69 to C-77
information technology industry,
C-107 to C-108
market position of rivals, 81–84, 91–92
monitoring rivals, 85–87
motorcycle industry, C-363
outlook, 89–90, 92
PC industry, C-133 to C-137
rivalry indicators, 56
supplier bargaining power, 66–68
supply-side fragmentation, 245–246
threat of new entrants, 60–64, 61t
union vs. nonunion, 66–67
Industry demand, 260
Industry environment; *see also* Business
environment
case study, C-48 to C-87
base of operations, C-51 to C-52
company background, C-48 to C-50
compensation, C-62 to C-63
corporate culture, C-59 to C-61
entrepreneurial spirit, C-49 to C-50
financial performance, C-63
human resource management,
C-61 to C-63
industry position, C-62 to C-66
innovative technology, C-58 to C-59
low costs/quality service, C-53 to C-58
management team, C-51
rapid expansion, C-52 to C-53
strategic vision, C-50
training, C-62
changing circumstances, 9
doughnut industry, C-207
for focused (market niche) strategies,
154–155

Industry environment—*Cont.*
relative attractiveness, 89–90, 92
restaurant business, C-452 to C-453
strategic thinking about, 51–52
strategy options in, 263
Industry growth
digital photography, C-222 to C-227
rate of, 53t, 75–76
Industry leaders
examples, 251
illustration of, 252
insular corporate culture, 423–424
strategies for, 251–254
supermarket chains, C-4 to C-5
Industry life cycle, 74
Industry newcomers, 143–144
Industry opportunity, 106
Industry position, 263
Industry profitability, 287
Industry uncertainty, 287
reduction in, 79
Infoimaging, C-222
Information
for benchmarking, 117
for board of directors, C-513
for leadership, 439–440
rapid dissemination of, 383
shared with employees, 405–406
statistical, 403
Information systems
areas covered by, 402
for control over empowered employees,
403–404
installing, 401–404
performance tracking, 402–403
real-time, 403
Information technology, C-348 to C-349
in low-cost leadership, C-424 to C-425
market conditions, C-107 to C-108
Initial public offering, C-196, C-298, C-315
to C-319
Innovation in merchandising, C-418 to C-419
Inputs, 67
lower specifications, 138–139
substitutes, 138
Inside the USGA, C-86
Insular/inwardly-focused cultures, 423–424
Insurance business, C-273 to C-285
Intangible assets, 100
Integrative social contracts theory, 322–323, 352
Intellectual capital, 100, 101, 367, 370
Internal cash flow, 99t
Internal controls, C-216
Internal cost disadvantage, 119
Internal cross-unit coordination, 381–383
Internal start-up, 271
Internal weaknesses, 104
International competition, 196; *see also*
Global competition; Multinational
corporations/enterprises
global vs. multicountry, 201–202
in maturing industries, 236
International expansion, 238, C-484

International Labor Organization, 319
Internet
conducting business via, 382
as driving force, 74–75, 91
media usage, C-256
for price comparisons, 70–71
Web site strategies, 192
brick-and-click strategies, 184–185, 186
minor distribution channel, 184
online enterprises, 185–187
product information only, 183–184
Internet-based phone networks, 76–77
Internet retailing, C-351
Internet sales, C-102
Internet technology applications, 235
broadband service, 5, 190
direct selling, 139
e-commerce, 383
leadership in, C-105, C-106
radio formats, C-255
search engines, C-312 to C-327
supply chain management, 139–140
Voice over Internet Protocol, 5, 74–75,
76–77, 231–233, 327, C-323
Intrapreneurship, 37
Inventory control
just-in-time systems, C-98 to C-99
in low-cost leadership, C-424 to C-425
Inventory turnover, 99t
Invest-and-expand strategy, 296
Investment priorities, 268

Japan, Dell Inc. in, C-99
Jet fuel prices, C-63 to C-66
Job applicant screening, 418–419
Job satisfaction survey, C-17
Joint marketing agreements, 165
Joint ventures
case study, C-489 to C-490
for diversification, 271–272
in foreign markets, 217–220
Journal of the American Medical Association,
C-527
Just-in-time systems, 140, C-96, C-98 to C-99

Kaizen, 396
Key financial indicators, C-516
Key success factors, 87–89
common types, 88t
competitive strength assessment,
122–124, 123t
identifying, 89
online retailing, C 288
resource fit and, 297
Kickbacks, 319–320, 326
Kiosks, C-100
Knowledge diffusion, 78
KSFs; *see* Key success factors

Labor costs, C-35 to C-37, C-59, C-411
in foreign markets, 198
national differences, 75
union vs. nonunion, 66–67

Labor-saving operating methods, 138
Lagging indicators, 31–32
Lancet, The, C-527, C-528
Late-mover advantages, 189
Lawsuits
  car rental business, C-168 to C-169
  employee discrimination, C-434
  low-cost leadership, C-411, C-433 to C-434
  patent infringement, C-553 to C-557
  potential drug targets, C-530
  product liability, C-518, C-525 to C-532
  product quality, C-141
Leadership; *see also* Global market
    leadership; Industry leaders; Market
    leaders
  airline industry, C-48 to C-51, C-59 to C-61
  by board of directors, 44–46
  bookselling, C-349 to C-350
  case study, C-405 to C-406
  changes in, C-438 to C-439
  in changing corporate culture, 429, 430
  in e-commerce, C-105, C-106
  by example, 431–432, 443
  failures, C-407 to C-409
  in global competition, C-470 to C-475
  golf equipment industry, C-77 to C-88
  growth development leaders, 441–442
  by local managers, 438
  new strategy and, C-195 to C-196
  office conflict and, C-458 to C-467
  PC industry, C-92 to C-95
  public broadcasting, C-262
  in strategy execution, 359–360, 448
    characteristics, 439
    constructive pressure, 441–442
    development of competencies, 442–443
    ethics, 443–444
    focus on excellence, 441–442
    information sources for, 439–440
    internal leadership, 43
    making corrective adjustments, 445–446
    managing by walking around, 440
    social responsibility, 445
    tests of leadership, 446–447
  in telecom industry, C-496 to C-514
Leadership development programs, 366
Leading indicators, 31–32
Leapfrogging competitors, 178
Learning curve effects, 53t, 54
  in emerging industries, 233
  locational advantages, 210
  of low-cost providers, 137
  in multinational diversification, 308
  product standardization and, 198
Leveraged buyout, C-368 to C-369
Leverage ratios, 98t–99t
Licensed stores, C-490 to C-491
Licensing strategies, 203–204
Life magazine, C-362
Lifestyle changes, 79–80, C-117 to
  C-118, C-187
Lifestyle differences, 197
Liquidation of weak business, 261

Liquidity ratios, 98t
Local circumstances
  accommodating, 222–223
  unacceptable, 223
Local content rules, 200
Local firms, 181
Localized multicountry strategies, 204–209
Locational advantages
  booksellers, C-329
  car rental business, C-165 to C-166
  in foreign markets, 198–199, 209–211
  organic food retailers, C-7 to C-11
  restaurant business, C-192, C-437
"Long-jump" strategic initiatives, 249, *250*
Long-term debt-to-equity ratio, 99t
Long-term objectives, 32
Low-cost leadership, 6
  airline industry, C-53 to C-58
  car rental business, C-167 to C-168
  case study, C-410 to C-435
    advertising, C-419
    awards for, C-412
    backward expansion, C-417
    company background, C-411 to C-414
    compensation and benefits,
      C-428 to C-431
    competitors, C-419 to C-420
    corporate culture, C-425 to C-428
    customer service, C-425
    cutting-edge technology, C-424 to C-425
    distribution activities, C-422 to C-423
    employee input, C-428
    employee training, C-431 to C-432
    everyday low prices, C-418
    favorable publicity, C-434 to C-435
    financial performance, C-413
    geographic expansion strategy,
      C-415 to C-418
    legal challenges, C-433 to C-434
    meetings and rapid response, C-432 to
      C-433
    merchandising innovations, C-418 to
      C-419
    multiple store formats, C-414 to C-415
    organized opposition to, C-410 to C-411
    response to Hurricane Katrina, C-434
    rules for building a business, C-429
    store construction/maintenance, C-423
      to C-424
    store count, C-416 to C-417
    strategy approaches, C-420 to C-433
    strategy execution, C-414 to C-419
    supplier relationships, C-420 to C-422
    truck fleet operations, C-423
  in declining industries, 240
  in foreign markets, 210
  industry leadership and, 251
  keys to achieving, 142–143
  PC industry, C-92, C-109
Low-cost provider strategies, 6, 135–144, 157t
  achieving cost advantages with, 135–142
    cost efficient management of value chain,
      137–139

Low-cost provider strategies—*Cont.*
  achieving cost advantages with—*Cont.*
    examples, 140–142
    illustration of, 136
    revamping value chain, 139–140
  airline industry, C-53 to C-58, C-66
  company options, 135
  compared to best-cost providers, 150
  compared to focused low-cost strategy, 153
  contrasted with other strategies, 156–158
  definition, 134
  focused (market niche), 153, 154–156
  in foreign markets, 210
  in fragmented industries, 247
  key points, 158
  keys to success, 142–143
  optimum conditions for, 143–144
  pitfalls, 144
  reward systems, 408

Macroenvironment, 49–51, *51*
  competitive environment, 51–52
  competitive forces, 54–74
  industry attractiveness, 89–90
  industry changes, 75–81
  industry environment, 51–52
  industry's economic features, 52–54
  ket success factors, 87–89
  key points, 90–93
  market position of rivals, 81–84
  relevant components, 49–*51*
  strategic moves by rivals, 85–87
Malcolm Baldrige National Quality Award, 392
Management
  action plan, 3–4
  employee access to, C-512
  of ethical conduct, 333–338
  in food retailing, C-42 to C-43
  in low-cost leadership, C-425 to C-426
  online auction business, C-290 to C-291
  in unrelated diversification, 283–284
  values, principles, and standards, 416
Management morality, 323–325
  amoral managers, 324
  immorality in global business, 325–327
  immoral managers, 324
  moral managers, 323
Management team
  airline industry, C-51
  at General Electric, 366
  at Lenovo, C-113
  staffing, 364–365, 366
  for strategy execution, 360
Management training, C-431 to C-432
  at Starbucks, C-485
Managerial requirements, 283–284
Managerial skills, 359–360, 361
Managers
  business strategy role, 38
  crafting and executing strategy, 15–16
  ethics and, 10–12
  four Es of, 366
  functional-area strategies, 38–40

Managers—*Cont.*
  grading of, 366
  interaction with employees, 416
  internal transfer, 366
  local, 438
  proactive vs. reactive, 9–10
  role in crafting strategy, 35–37
  strategic fit, 276
  strategic issues and problems, 125–126
  strategy execution tasks, 359–360, 361
  unified strategic moves, 40–41
  winning strategies, 13
Managing by walking around, 440
Manufacturers
  backward integration, 71
  buyer bargaining power and, 70–71
  export strategies, 203
  franchising strategies, 204
  licensing strategies, 203–204
  online buying groups, 71
  power over retailers, 66
  revamping value chain, 139–142
  strategic alliances by, 165–166
  supplier bargaining power, 67–68
  value chain cost efficiency, 137–139
  Web sites, 75
Manufacturing activities
  build-to-order production, C-95 to C-97,
    C-109, C-114
  business process reengineering,
    395–396, 412
  cell manufacturing, C-96
  concentrated, 209–210
  cross-border coordination, 212–213
  cycle time, 375
  in differentiation strategies, 146
  dispersed, 210–211
  exchange rate fluctuations and, 199–200
  expansion into, C-205
  in foreign markets, 198–199
  globalization and, 75
  gold equipment industry, C-73
  innovation in, 76–77
  self-manufacturing, 68
  Six Sigma quality control, 396–399, 412
  strategic fit in, 275
  total quality management, 396, 399, 412
  vertical integration drawbacks, 173–174
Manufacturing costs, 198, 209–210
Manufacturing executive system software, 138
Manufacturing-related KSFs, 88t
Market(s); *see also* Foreign markets
  as competitive battlefield, 55–56
  high-velocity, 241–245
  in public broadcasting, C-252 to C-257
  rapidly growing, 234–235
  slow- vs. fast-growing, 57–58
Market advantage, 100
Market base, 196
Market capitalization, C-312 to C-313
Market conditions
  adapting to changes in, 261
  dealing with cross-country variations, *205*

Market conditions—*Cont.*
  DVD rental business, C-153 to C-154
  in foreign markets, 197–201
  future, 106
  information technology industry,
    C-107 to C-108
  with slowing growth, 236–237
  volatility, 106
Market demand, 239
Market dominance, sustaining, C-298 to
  C-303, C-323 to C-327
Market growth, 197, 234
Marketing activities
  by booksellers, C-343
  in differentiation strategies, 146
  direct-to-consumer, C-524 to C-525
  innovation in, 77
  at Oliver's Markets, C-39 to C-40
  online enterprises, 187
  organic foods sales, C-14 to C-16
  by Outback Steakhouse, C-445
  PC industry, C-99 to C-100
  strategic fit in, 276
  in value chain, *111*
Marketing-related KSFs, 88t
Marketing strategy, 38
Marketing survey, C-184
Market leaders, 169–170, 254, 295–296
  in MP3 player industry, C-119
  vulnerable, 181
Market niche, for emerging markets, 225–226
Market niche strategies; *see* Focused (market
  niche) strategies
Market opportunities
  identifying, 104–106, 105t
  priority, 109
Market-penetration curve, 189
Market position
  in business environment, 81–84
  cash cows and, 295–296
  key success factors, 89, 92
  nine-cell matrix, 293t
  from offensive strategies, 177–182
  from product innovation, 76
  rivalry and, 58
  strategic group mapping, 81–84, *83,* 91–92
  strengthening, 301–302
Market reconnaissance, 106
Market segments
  blue ocean strategy, 180
  motorcycle industry, C-363 to C-365
  offensive strategies for, 179
Market share
  antitrust policy and, 252, 253
  Dell Inc., C-106
  in digital imaging, C-228
  exchange rates and, 199
  in fortify-and-defend strategy, 252–253
  gold equipment industry, C-84 to C-85
  from guerrilla offensive, 179
  head-to-head competition for, 236
  motorcycle industry, C-364
  PC industry, C-89, C-90, C-110, C-137

Market share—*Cont.*
  from potent brand name, 273
  from product innovation, 178
  in rapidly growing markets, 234–235
  relative, 289–290
  small, 254
  strategies to build, 254–255
Market shocks, 107
Market size, 53t, 286
Market space, types of, 180
Market territory, uncontested, 179
Maturing industries
  definition, 236
  from slow growth, 236–237
  strategic pitfalls, 238–239
  strategies for, 237–238
Measurement; *see* Performance measures
Measurement of objectives, 29–30
Media companies, 170
"Medium-jump" strategic initiatives, 249, *250*
Merchandising
  innovation in, C-418 to C-419
  meetings, C-432 to C-433
  organic foods sales, C-12 to C-14
Mergers and acquisitions, 161, 168–171, 191
  access to competitive capabilities, 169
  access to new technologies, 169
  adidas-Reebok, C-390
  adidas-Salomon, C-379 to C-380
  bargain-prices, 238
  case study, C-393 to C-404
    business units performance,
      C-396 to C-398
    company histories, C-393 to C-396
    company performance, C-392 to C-393
    early postmerger performance,
      C-403 to C-404
    product lines, C- 394 to C-395
    share price offer, C-398 to C-402
  company subcultures and, 419–420
  competitors for, C-278 to C-279, C-280
  cost-efficient, 168
  definition, 168
  for diversification, 271
  by eBay, C-303
  examples, 169–171, C-9
  to expand geographic coverage, 168–169
  failures, 171
  fast-exit strategy and, 241
  in financial industry, 301
  to get core competencies, 370–371
  insurance business, C-276 to C-277
  to invent new industry, 169
  by Krispy Kreme, C-206 to C-207
  leveraged buyout, C-368 to C-369
  for market leadership, 60
  in maturing industries, 237
  new product categories from, 169
  number of, 168
  PC industry, C-110 to C-111,
    C-113 to C-114
  PG/Gillette, C-392 to C-404
  process, C-279 to C-280

Mergers and acquisitions—*Cont.*
  by runner-up companies, 255
  Smithfield Foods, C-171
  in target industry, 302–303
  work environment after, C-513 to C-514
Minimum wage, C-428
Mission statement, 23–25
  coffee bar business, C-483
  Copperfield Books, C-350
  environmental, C-494
  JetBlue Airways, C-50
  Merck & Company, C-519
  Oliver's Markets, C-40 to C-41
  organic foods industry, C-2, C-3
  Trader Joe's, C-24 to C-25
  Western States Insurance, C-275
Mobile phone industry, C-496 to C-517
Monetary rewards, 404–405
Monsanto Co. v. McFarley, C-553
Monsanto v. Schmeiser, C-554, C-557
*Monsanto v. U.S. Farmer Report of
  2005,* C-553
Moral case
  for ethical strategy, 338
  for social responsibility, 346–347, 353
Moral managers, 323, 336–337, 352
Moral scrutiny, 10–12
Moral standards, 318
Motivation; *see also* Rewards and incentives
  for strategic alliances, 217–218
  in strategic vision, 25
  in strategy execution, 43
Motorcycle industry, C-362 to C-368
Mover-and-shaker offensives, 255
MP3 player industry, C-116 to C-129,
  C-138 to C-147
Multibrand strategies, 156
Multicountry companies, *214*
Multicountry competition, 201–202, 227
Multicountry strategies, 204–209, *205, 208*
Multicultural companies, 419–420
Multinational competition, 195
Multinational corporations/enterprises
  changing local markets, 223
  company subcultures and, 419–420
  ethical relations in, 321–323
  lack of need for alliances, 220
  performance-based incentives in, 411–412
  post-diversification strategies
    appeal of, 308–309
    combined effects of, 311–312
    global scope of, 308–309
    strategy–culture fit, 437–438
Multinational diversification strategies
  appeal of, 308–311
  characteristics, 308
  combined effect of, 311–312
Multiple strategy horizons, 250–251
Muscle-flexing strategy, 253–254
Mutual funds, 350

Narrowly diversified companies, 284
National Highway Traffic Safety
  Administration, C-368

National Organic Program, C-3, C-4
Natural foods industry, C-2 to C-27
Near-term objectives, 32
Negligence, C-557
Net competitive advantage, 122
Net competitive disadvantage, 124
Net profit margin, 98t
Net return on sales, 98t
New England Journal of Medicine, C-526,
  C-527, C-528
New entrants, threat of, 60–61, 61t
New product categories, 169
New product introduction, 382
New products, C-103 to C-105
New York Times, C-175, C-433, C-555
Next-generation products, 56, 375
Next-generation technology, 178
No-layoff policy, 392, C-511 to C-512
Nonissue approach, 334–336, 335t
Nonmonetary rewards, 405, 411, 412
Nonunion workforce, 66–67, 136, C-42, C-59
North Carolina Department of Environment
  and Natural Resources, C-179 to C-180

Objectives, 19, 29–35
  examples, 33
  financial, 31
  quantifiable, 29
  short- vs. long-term, 32
  strategic, 31
  and strategic plan, 41–42
Objective setting, 46
  balanced scorecard approach
    company-wide objectives, 34
    examples, 33
    financial vs. strategic objectives, 31
    performance measures, 31–32
    short-term vs. long-term objectives, 32
    strategic intent, 32–34
    top down vs. bottom-up, 34–35
  nature of objectives, 20–30
  restaurant business, C-444
  for sales, 34–35
  in strategy making, 29–35
  stretch objectives, 30–31
Occupational Safety and Health
  Administration, 24
Offensive strategies, 4, 125, 177–182, 192
  basis for attack, 181–182
  behaviors and principles, 177–178
  blue ocean strategy, 180–181
  to build market share, 254–255
  choosing targets, 181
  against competitive strengths, 178
  cross-market subsidization, 214–215
  for foreign markets, 215–217
  mover-and-shaker offensives, 255
  pharmaceutical industry, C-526 to C-527
  stay-on-the-offense strategy, 251–252
  time needed for, 178
  types of, 178–180
Office of Fair Trading (UK), C-168 to C-169
Office supply industry, 186
Oil price increases, C-63 to C-66

Olympic Games, C-377
Online buying groups, 71
Online enterprises, 185–187, C-286 to C-311
Online marketing, 77
Online technology, 139–140
On-site customer service, C-102
Operating costs, C-56 to C-57
Operating efficiencies
  eliminating unnecessary work, 140
  labor-saving methods, 138
  outsourcing, 138
  software for, 138
  vertical integration, 138
Operating excellence, 441–442
Operating performance, C-63, C-64
Operating profit margin, 98t
Operating strategies, *39,* 40
  by booksellers, C-343 to C-348
  doughnut retailing, C-199 to C-206
  strategy cohesion, 41
Operating systems
  installing, 401–404
  restaurant business, C-444
  streamlining, 375
Operations activities, in value chain, *111*
Opportunities, 106
  cross-business, 268
  emerging, 286
Order-filling, 186–187, 382
Organic Food Production Act, C-3
Organic foods industry, C-2 to C-27
Organizational assets, 100
Organizational bridge-building, 383
Organizational building blocks, 377
Organizational design tools, 384
Organizational flexibility, 176
Organizational learning
  airline industry, C-62
  competitive advantage and, 120
  internal universities, 371–373
Organization building
  collaboration with suppliers, 383
  competitive capabilities, 363, 368–373
  core competencies, 363, 368–373
  current trends, 383–384
  internal cross-unit coordination, 381–383
  staffing, 363, 364–368
  for strategy execution, 363–364
  structure and work effort, 373–381, 383
Organization for Economic Cooperation and
  Development, Anti-Bribery
  Convention, 320
Organization structure, 385, C-350
  centralized vs. decentralized, 378–379,
    378t
  current trends in, 383–384
  to fit strategy, 363
  flattening, 375
  modified to fit strategy, 377–378
  strategy-critical activities, 376–378
  strategy execution and, 373–383
    collaboration and alliances, 383
    cross-unit coordination, 381–383
    delegating authority, 378–381

Organization structure—*Cont.*
  strategy execution and—*Cont.*
    strategy-critical activities, 376–378
    value chain activities, 373–376
  streamlining, 384
  supply chain management in, 383
  in telecommunications industry, C-503
Outsourcing, 192
  advantages, 175–177
  of core competencies, 370
  cost advantages, 138
  definition, 175
  drivers of, 175
  in high-velocity markets, 244
  order fulfillment, 186
  protests against, 348
  risks of, 177
  supply chain management and, 175
  of value chain activities
    benefits, 374–375
    dangers of excess in, 376
    versus internal performance, 373–376
    partnering, 375
Overdifferentiation, 149

Partial integration, 171–172
Partial ownership, 305
Partnerships, 375
Patent infringement litigation, C-553 to C-557
Patent law, Canada, C-555
Patent protection, C-551 to C-552
Patents, C-103
Payoffs of vision statement, 26
Peer pressure
  in corporate culture, 416
  for ethical standards, 337
People management policies, 406, 416
Perceived value, 147
Performance
  consistent, 369
  DVD rental business, C-151 to C-153
  near- or long-term, 32
  outclassing rivals, 374–375
  post-merger, C-403 to C-404
Performance evaluation, 19, 43–44, 47
Performance indicators
  lagging vs. leading, 31–32
  strategy and, 13
  tracking, 403
Performance measures, 29–30
  financial ratios, 98t–99t
  stock prices, 348–349
  strategic vs. financial, 31–32
  SWOT analysis, 97–109
Performance outcomes, linked to rewards,
    407–410
  compensation system design, 410–411
  example of, 409
  importance of results, 408–410
  in multinational enterprises, 411
Performance prospects, 298–299, 299t, 313
Performance targets, 29–30
  airline industry, C-59 to C-61
  companywide, 35

Performance targets—*Cont.*
  in continuous improvement programs,
    400–401
  heavy pressure to meet, 330–332
  linked to compensation, 408–410
  resource fit and, 296
  shortfalls, 96–97
  social responsibility and, 345
  strategic moves to achieve, 299–300
  in strategic plan, 42
Performance tracking, 402–403
Perks, 405
Personal computer industry, 164, C-89 to
    C-115, C-130 to C-147
Personal digital assistants, C-138 to C-139
Personal gain, 328–330
Pharmaceutical industry, C-518 to C-523
Philanthropy, 343–344, 351, C-522
Photography trends, C-227
Physical assets, 100
Pirated music and movies, C-160
Plant manager, 40
Policies and procedures for strategy execution,
    390–393, *391*, 412
  consistency, 391
  example, 392
  top-down guidance, 391
  work climate, 391–393
Politicized corporate cultures, 422
Portfolio restructuring
  case study, C-36 to C-391
    acquisition, C-379 to C-380
    company background, C-377 to C-379
    corporate strategy, C-380 to C-386
    divestiture, C-386 to C-390
    financial performance, C-385, C-388 to
      C-391
  restaurant business, C-439 to C-443
  by unrelated diversification, 280
Preemptive strike, 179–180
Prescription Drug Use Fee Act, C-531
Pressure groups, 347–348
Price competition, 56
  airline industry, C-52
  car rental business, C-167 to C-168
  commodity products, 143
  in emerging markets, 222
  in food retailing, C-39 to C-40
  golf equipment industry, C-69
  by industry newcomers, 143–144
  low-cost leadership, C-418
  in mature market, 238
  organic food sales, C-12
  substitute products, 64–65
  union critics, C-410
Price-cost comparisons, 109–122, 127
  activity-based costing, 114–116
  assessing cost competitiveness, 114–116
  benchmarking value chain costs,
    116–117, 118
  components of cost structure, 110–112
  industry value chain, 113–114
  need for, 109–110
  remedying cost disadvantages, 117–120

Price-cost comparisons—*Cont.*
  translating performance into competitive
    advantage, 120–122, *121*
  value chain concept, 110–112, *111*
  value chain variations, 112–113
Price cutting
  aggressive, 144
  by competitors, 59
  cost advantages and, 262
  by dumping, 216
  by industry newcomers, 143–144
  in low-cost provider strategies, 135
  offensive strategy, 178
Price/earnings ratio, 99t
Price-fixing, 326
Price premium, 149
Primary value chain activities, *111*, 111–112
Private-label brands, 71, 153, C-40
Proactive (intended) strategy, 9–10
Process departments, 377, 382
Product(s)
  broad or narrow offering, 186
  competitor imitation of, 148–149
  counterfeit, C-76 to C-77
  customization versus standardization,
    197–198
  diversity of, C-511
  doughnut retailing, C-199 to C-200
  easy-to-copy features, 145
  frills-free, 140
  in low-cost leadership, C-414 to C-415
  next-generation, 178
  noneconomic features, 147
  overdifferentiated, 149
  pruning, 237
  standardized vs. differentiated, 78–79
  substitutes, 64–65
  supply-side fragmentation and, 245
  tailored for emerging markets, 221–222
  tie-in, 244
  unbranded, C-106 to C-107
  user applications
    in emerging industries, 232–233
    in maturing industries, 236
    in rapidly growing markets, 235
    in runner-up firms, 256
  user requirements, 143
Product attributes, 146, 149, 232
  matching or beating, 290
Product boycotts, 347–348
Product customization
  gold equipment, C-73 to C-74
  motorcycles, C-363
  PC industry, C-96 to C-97
Product design, 197–198
Product development strategy, 38
Product differentiation, 53t, 59, 143, C-73;
  see also Differentiation strategies
  weak vs. strong, 149–150
Product information, 183–184
Product innovation, 53t, C-103 to C-105
  aircraft industry, C-240 to C-242
  in declining industries, 240
  as driving force, 76

Product innovation—*Cont.*
  in maturing industries, 236
  new product categories, 169
  as offensive strategy, 178
  in rapidly growing markets, 235
Production procedures; *see* Manufacturing
    activities
Product line
  Apple Computer, C-135 to C-136
  Dell Inc., C-91
  expansion of, 235, C-103 to C-105
  at Harley-Davidson, C-371 to C-372
  limited, 140
  natural/organic food stores, C-26
  organic food retailers, C-11 to C-12
  at Starbucks, C-488 to C-489
Product modifications, 382
Product performance, 146
Product positioning, C-510
Product quality; *see also* Quality control
  customer commitment and, C-13
  doughnut retailing, C-199 to C-200
  improving, 382
  natural and organic foods, C-2 to C-4
Product recall, C-525 to C-532
Product research and development, *111*
Product standardization, 59
  buyer preferences and, 78–79
  versus customization, 197–198
Product type specialization, 247
Profit, 25
  in core values, C-9
  in cost-of-entry test, 270
  overall prospects, 90
Profitability
  backward integration and, 172–173
  business model and, 12–13
  of business units, 290
  competitive advantage and, 7
  erosion in differentiation strategy, 149
  in five-forces model, 72–74
  identifying threats to, 106–107
  industry attractiveness and, 287
  in maturing industries, 237
  related diversification and, 278
  in unrelated diversification, 282
Profitability ratios, 98t
Profit sanctuaries, 213–215, *214,* 227, 311
Profit sharing plan, C-431
Promotional activities
  car rental business, C-168
  in food retailing, C-40
Promotion from within, 405
Promotion policy, C-448 to C-449
Proprietary technology, 232
Public broadcasting, C-252 to C-257
Punishment, rewards and, 406–408
Purchasing, C-18, C-491 to C-492
Purchasing power variations, 197,
    221–222

Quality, commitment to, C-53 to C-58
Quality control
  PC industry, C-97

Quality control—*Cont.*
  Six Sigma quality control, 396–399, 412
  total quality management, 396, 399, 412
Quality of life, 344
Quantifiable objectives, 29–30
Quick ratio, 98t
Quick-response capability, 244

Radio frequency identification systems,
    C-424 to C-425
Raleigh News & Observer, C-174 to C-178
Rapid company growth
  danger of multiple strategies, 250–251
  strategic initiatives, 249–250
  sustaining, 249–251
Rapidly growing markets, 234–235
Reactive (adaptive) strategy, 9–10
  in high-velocity markets, 242
Real-time information systems, 403
Recruitment and selection
  airline industry, C-61 to C-62
  capable employees, 365–367
  ethical values in, 436
  Outback Steakhouse, C-447 to C-448
  role in corporate culture, 416
  staffing procedures, 363–365
Recycling, C-533
Regional firms, 181
Related diversification, 312
  case for, 272–278
  competitive advantage and, 277–278
    cautions on, 278
    economies of scope, 278
    profitability, 278
    shareholder value, 278
  cross-business strategic fits
    in administrative support, 276
    in distribution, 275
    examples, 277
    in manufacturing, 275
    R&D and technology, 274–275
    in sales and marketing, 276
    in supply chain activities, 275
  strategic appeal, 274
  strategic fit
    characteristics, 272–274, *274*
    competitive advantage, 277–278
    economies of scope, 277–278
    identifying, 274–277
    profitability, 278
    shareholder value, 278
  strategy options, *273*
  versus unrelated diversification, 272
  with unrelated diversification, 284–285
Relationship managers, 383
Relative market share, 289–290
Religions, 323
Research and development, *111*
  aircraft industry, C-240 to C-242
  costs of, 137–138
  customer-driven, C-103
  in differentiation strategies, 145–146
  in high-velocity markets, 243–244
  strategic fit in, 274–275

Research and development departments, 381
Resistance to change, C-545
  communicating strategic vision and, 26
  in corporate culture, 422–424
Resource advantages, 61
Resource allocation, 42, 298–299, 299t
Resource Conservation and Recovery
    Act, C-433
Resource fit
  caution on resource transfer, 298
  competitive capabilities, 297
  credit rating, 297
  definition, 294
  financial resources, 294–296
  managerial resources, 297–298
  performance targets, 296
Resource requirements, 287
Resources for strategy execution, 389–390;
    see also Financial resources
Resource strengths, 313
  combinations of, 104
  competencies, 100–102
  competitive power of, 102–104
  of competitive rivals, 85–86
  cornerstone of strategy, 109
  cross-border transfer, 211–212
  forms of, 97–100
  in high-velocity markets, 244
  identifying, 105t
  locational advantages, 210
  resource fit and, 297
  specialist strategy, 256
  strategy based on, 7
  SWOT analysis, 97–104
Resource weaknesses
  of competitive rivals, 85–86
  identifying, 104, 105t
Restaurant industry, C-436 to C-453
  fast-casual dining, C-182 to C-192
  ten fastest growing chains, C-190
  in United States, C-184 to C-188
Restructuring, reasons for, 306–308
Results-oriented corporate culture, 438
Results-oriented work climate, 441–442
Retail channels, 62
Retailers; *see also* Sales
  booksellers, C-328 to C-355
  food retailing, C-30 to C-37
  golf equipment, C-70 to C-71,
      C-73 to C-74
  low-cost leadership, C-412
  natural and organic foods, C-4 to C-6
  online, C-288
  online buying groups, 71
  online vs. brick-and-mortar, 184–185
  organic foods industry, C-16 to C-17
  private-label brands, 71
Retaliation, 182–183
Retrenchment, 258, 303–306
Return on sales, 98t
Return on stockholders' equity, 98t
Return on total assets, 98t
Revenue-increasing turnaround strategy, 248
Review of Economics and Statistics, C-435

Rewards and incentives, 404–411, 412
  balancing rewards and punishments,
    406–408
  economic value added, C-18
  examples, 407
  linked to performance
    design of compensation system,
      410–411
    importance of results, 408–410
    in multinational enterprises, 411
  low-cost leadership, C-428 to C-431
  as management tool, 408
  for operational excellence, 442
  organic food retailing, C-17 to C-18
  at Outback Steakhouse, C-448 to C-449
  at Starbucks, C-485
  in strategy execution, 43
  strategy-facilitating motivational practices,
    404–406, 407
Risk-averse companies, 4
Rivalry; see Competitive rivalry
Rivals; see Competitive rivals
Ron Brown Award, C-412
Runner-up firms, 181, 254–257
  market share strategies, 254–255
  obstacles for, 254
  strategic approaches, 255–257
    content follower strategy, 256–257
    distinctive-image strategy, 256
    growth by acquisition, 255
    specialist strategy, 256
    superior product strategy, 256
    vacant-niche strategy, 256

Safety concerns, 79–80
Salary cap, C-17 to C-18
Sales; see also Retailers
  brick-and-click strategies, 184–185, 186
  in differentiation strategies, 146
  direct sales, 139
  e-stores, 184
  low-cost leadership and, C-412, C-418
  in mature market, 238
  online enterprises, 185–187
  PC industry, C-91 to C-92, C-95 to C-97,
    C-99 to C-100, C-107 to C-108, C-114
  pharmaceutical industry, C-520
  setting objectives, 34–35
  stagnating, 76
  strategic fit in, 276
Sales and marketing activities, 111
Sales volume, 137–138
San Francisco Bay Guardian, C-434
Sarbanes-Oxley Act, 338, 341
Satellite radio, C-255
Screening applicants, 418–419
Search engines, C-312 to C-327
Seasonal factors, 287
Secondary value chain activities,
  110–112, 111
Securities and Exchange Commission, 330,
  341, 424, C-215, C-548
Selfish interests, 328–330
Self-manufacturing, 68

Seller–buyer relationships
  collaboration, 383
  competitive pressures from, 68–72
Sellers' market, 70
Selling businesses, 305–306
Selling costs, low-cost providers, 137–138
Sell-out-quickly strategy, 241
Service activities, 111
Shareholder interests, 44–45
Shareholders, 350
Shareholder value
  in core values, C-9
  diversification and, 272
    related diversification, 278
    tests for, 269–270
    unrelated diversification, 282–283
  DVD rental business, C-157 to C-158
  social responsibility and, 348–349, 351
"Short-jump" strategic initiatives, 249, 250
Short-pay policy, 392
Short-term objectives, 32
Signaling value, 147
Single-business enterprise, 40
  business strategy-making, 267
  strategic action plan, 263–264
  strategy effectiveness, 95–97, 96
Six Sigma quality control, 366, 395,
  396–399, 412
  capturing benefits of, 399–301
  DMADV process, 396
  DMAIC process, 396–399
  for operational excellence, 442
Skills, 99–100, 101, 165, 174, 369–370
Skills-related KSFs, 88t
Slogans, 25–26
Slow-exit strategy, 241, 257
Small firms, 181
Smart Money, C-76
Social activism, C-18 to C-19
Social causes, 351
Social conscience
  components, 342–345, 343t
  demonstrating, 345–346
Social contract, 322–323, 352
Social factors, 287
Social forces, 79–80
Social responsibility, 342–354
  actions and behaviors for, 353
  business case for
    buyer patronage, 347–348
    internal benefits, 347
    shareholder value, 348–349
  charitable contributions, 343–344, 351
  in corporate culture, C-493 to C-494
  crafting strategy for, 345–346
  "do-good" executives and, 349–351
  environmental protection, 344
  evading social harms and, 349
  extent of, 351
  leading initiatives in, 445
  linked to executive compensation, 352
  meaning of, 342–345
  moral case for, 346, 353–354
  origin of concept, 342

Social responsibility—Cont.
  pharmaceutical industry, C-521 to C-523
  shareholder value and, 342, 351
  social causes, 351
  social conscience and, 342–345
  at Whole Foods Market, C-18 to C-19
  work environment, 344
  workforce diversity, 344–345
Social responsibility strategy, 345–346
Software companies, 14
Specialists, 175–176
Specialist strategy, 256
Specialization strategy
  customer type, 247–248
  in high-velocity markets, 244
  product type, 247
Specialty coffee industry, C-494
Specialty stores, C-490 to C-491
Spinning off businesses, 305–306
Sporting goods industry, C-376 to C-391
SS United States, 321
Staffing, 42, 385
  capable employees, 365–368
  management team, 360, 364–365, 366
  procedures, 363–365
  public broadcasting, C-260 to C-262
Stagnant industries, 239–241
Stakeholder interests, 44–45, 346–347,
  417–418, 425–426, 434
  social responsibility and, 350
Stakeholders, C-443 to C-444
Standardized components, C-103
Standardized products; see Product
  standardization
Star businesses, 296
Start-up companies
  emerging industries, 231–234
  internal start-up, 271
Statement on Corporate Responsibility, 342
Statistical information, 403
Stay-on-the-offense strategy, 251–252
Stock-keeping units, C-425
Stock option plan, C-17, C-431, C-480
Stock prices, 348–349
Stock purchase plan, C-17, C-431,
  C-480 to C-481
Stock trading, 350
Store buyers, C-421
Store sizes and locations, C-7 to C-11
Stories, in corporate culture, 418
Strategic action plan format, 263–264
Strategic actions, 161; see also Competitive
  strategies
  backward expansion, C-417
  at Blockbuster, C-155
  decisions about, 161
  defensive strategies
    blocking avenues, 182
    signaling retaliation, 182–183
  for emerging industries, 233–234
  ethical standards and, 341–342
  ethics of, 10–12
  first-mover advantages, 188–191
  functional-area strategies, 161, 187–188

Strategic actions—*Cont.*
  golf equipment industry, C-77 to C-88
  to improve performance, 299–300
  key points, 191–192
  late-mover advantages, 189
  for maturing industries, 237–238
  mergers and acquisitions, 161, 168–171
  offensive strategies, 161, 177–182
    basis for competitive attack, 181–182
    blue ocean strategy, 180–181
    choosing rivals to attack, 181
    principles and behaviors, 177–178
    types of, 178–180
  outsourcing strategies
    advantages, 175–177
    definition, 175
    risks, 177
  predicting, 86–87
  questions for, 263
  for rapid-growth companies, 249–251
  for runner-up firms, 254–257
  strategic alliances, 161, 163–168
    advantages, 164–166
    capturing benefits of, 166–167
    dangers of relying on, 167–168
    definition, 163
    factors in making, 163
    unstable, 167
  Sunflower Markets, C-25
  from SWOT analysis, 108–109
  vertical integration
    advantages, 172–173
    backward, 172–173
    definition, 171
    disadvantages, 173–174
    forward, 173
    partial vs. full, 171–172
    pros and cons, 175
  Web site strategies
    brick-and-click strategies, 184–185, 186
    e-stores, 184
    online enterprises, 185–187
    product information only, 183–184
Strategic alliances, 100, 191
  advantages, 164–166
  capturing benefits of, 166–167
  dangers of relying on, 167–168
  definition, 163
  for diversification, 271–272
  in emerging industries, 233
  examples, 164
  factors in making, 163
  in foreign markets, 227
    examples, 219
    motivation for, 217–218
    questionable need for, 220
    risks of, 218–220
  for global market leadership, 165
  by Google Inc., C-327
  in high-velocity markets, 244
  for industry position, 165–166
  in MP3 player industry, C-122
  organizational bridge-building, 383
  picking a good partner, 166

Strategic alliances—*Cont.*
  Starbucks Corporation, C-498 to C-490
  with suppliers, C-97 to C-98
  with suppliers/buyers, 290
  unstable, 167
Strategic analysis of diversification, 285–300,
    312–313
  business-unit competitive strength
    calculating scores, 289–291
    interpreting scores, 291–292
    nine-cell matrix, 292–294, 293t
  cross-business strategic fit, 294, 295t
  industry attractiveness
    calculating scores, 288–296
    difficulties of calculating scores, 288–289
    interpreting scores, 288
  new strategic moves, 299–300
  performance prospects, 298–299
  resource fit
    cautions, 298
    competitive capabilities, 297
    credit rating, 297
    financial resources, 294–296, 299t
    managerial resources, 297–298
    performance targets, 296
Strategic balance sheet, 104
Strategic coordination, 310
Strategic fit, 313
  of business units, 290
  competitive advantage and, 294, 295t
  cross-business, 381
  cross-industry, 287
  in decentralized organization, 381
  example, 302
  in related diversification
    administrative support, 276
    characteristics of, 272–274, *273, 274*
    competitive advantage and, 277–278
    in distribution, 275
    examples, 277
    in manufacturing, 275
    in research and development, 274–275
    in sales and marketing, 276
    in supply chain activities, 275
    in technology, 274–275
Strategic group, 82
Strategic group mapping, 81–84, *83,* 91–92
  construction of map, 82–83
  learning from, 83–84
Strategic inflection points, 26, 27, 189
Strategic initiatives, portfolio of, 249–250
Strategic intent, 32–34
Strategic issues
  about foreign markets, 195, 226
  for online enterprises, 185–187
Strategic issues "worry list," 125–126, 127
Strategic mistakes, 238–239
  case study, C-407 to C-409
  by Krispy Kreme, C-195 to C-196
  pharmaceutical industry, C-52
Strategic objectives
  achieving, 35
  kinds of, 31
  success indicators, 96–97

Strategic partnerships, 68–69
Strategic performance, 31–32, 95–97, *96*
Strategic plan, 47
  action agenda for, 42–43
  development of, 41–42
  for public broadcasting, C-269 to C-271
Strategic vision, 19, 46
  characteristics, 21–23
  common shortcomings, 22
  communicating, 25–27
  definition, 20
  developing, 20–39
  distinctive and specific, 20–21
  example of, C-155
  examples, 23
  external/internal considerations, 21
  at Google Inc., C-318 to C-319
  as incentive, 405
  linked with company values, 27–29, 30
  in low-cost leadership, C-414
  as managerial tool, 21
  versus mission statements, 23–25
  Outback Steakhouse, C-443 to C-444
  resistance to change and, 25
  and strategic plan, 41–42
  telecommunications industry, C-504
Strategy, 2–17; *see also* Business strategy;
    Competitive strategies
  business model and, 12–13, 14
  competitive advantage and, 6–7
  of competitive rivals, 85–86
  crafting and executing, 15–16
  criteria for judging, 13
  customer-based, C-99
  definition, 3–4
  drivers of unethical behaviors, 330–333
  effectiveness, 95–97, *96*
  ethics and, 10–12
  evolution, 8–9
  example of, 5
  identifying, 7–8
  key components, 95–97, *96*
  key points, 16–17
  Krispy Kreme, C-196 to C-199
  linked to ethics and core values, 340–341
  matched to competitive conditions, 73–74
  of multinational diversification, 311–312
  offensive vs. conservative, 4
  proactive vs. reactive, 9–10
  resource strengths and, 109
  restaurant business, C-445 to C-446
  results of changes in, 390
  rules for running a business, C-429
  for social responsibility, 345–346
  steps in crafting, 35
  and strategic plan, 41–42
  success factors, 4, 7
  to sustain market dominance,
      C-298 to C-303
  tailored to circumstances
    commandments for success, 261–262
    emerging industries, 231–234
    fragmented industries, 245–249
    high-velocity markets, 241–245

Strategy—*Cont.*
  tailored to circumstances—*Cont.*
    industry leaders, 251–254
    key points, 262–264
    maturing industries, 236–239
    rapid-growth companies, 249–251
    rapidly growing markets, 234–235
    runner-up firms, 254–257
    stagnant/declining industries, 239–241
    weak/crisis-ridden businesses, 257–261
  temporary and fluid, 9
  for unrelated diversification, 280
  winning strategy, 13, 17
Strategy cohesion, 41
Strategy crafting; *see also* Strategy making
  delegating authority, 37
  importance of, 15–16
  participants, 35–37
  phases, 19–20
  process, 35–42
  strategic plan, 41–42
  strategy-making hierarchy, 37–40
  uniting strategy-making effort, 40–41
Strategy-critical activities, 376–378, 385
  cross-unit collaboration, 382
  dangers of outsourcing, 376
  examples, 376–377
  functional departments, 377
  geographic units, 377
  internal performance, 374–376
  organizational building blocks, 377
Strategy–culture clash, 421
Strategy–culture fit, 421, 426–428, 447
  core values and, 427
  for multinational enterprises, 437–438
Strategy execution, 20, 358–387, 388–412;
    see also Corporate culture
  adidas-Salomon, C-380 to C-386
  airline industry, C-49 to C-52
  benchmarking for, 394–395
  car rental business, C-166 to C-167
  in coffee bar business, C-477 to C-483
  continuous improvement programs
    benefits of initiatives, 399–401
    business process reengineering, 395–396
    identifying best practices, 393–395
    Six Sigma quality control, 396–399
    total quality management, 396
  Copperfield Books, C-346 to C-349,
    C-351 to C-352
  core competencies and
    competitive advantage, 372, 373
    employee training, 371–373
    three-stage development, 368–371
  corporate governance and, 44–46
  corrective adjustments, 43–44, 47
  DVD rental business, C-150 to C-153
  framework for, 361
  at Harley-Davidson, C-368 to C-374
  hog processing industry, C-174 to C-178
  hotel industry, C-539 to C-541
  impact on rivals, C-108 to C-109
  implementation phase, 42–43
  importance of, 15–16

Strategy execution—*Cont.*
  information and operating systems,
    401–404
  key points, 46–47
  leadership in, 439–447
    constructive pressure, 441–442
    developing competencies, 442–443
    ethics, 443–444
    focus on excellence, 441–442
    information sources for, 439–440
    making corrective adjustments, 445–446
    social responsibility, 445
  long-term, 261
  low-cost leadership, C-420 to C-433
  management skills for, 359–360
  management team for, 360
  managerial components, 262–263, 362
  marshaling resources for, 389–390
  in MP3 player industry, C-119 to C-129,
    C-141 to C-147
  with new leadership, C-195 to C-196
  online auctions, C-294 to C-298
  organization building for, 363–364
  organizing work effort, 373–383, 374t
    collaboration and alliances, 383
    cross-unit collaboration, 382
    delegating authority, 378–381
    internal cross-unit coordination, 381–383
    strategy-critical activities, 376–378
    value chain activities, 373–376
  PC industry, C-95 to C-107, C-131 to C-133
  performance evaluation, 43–44, 47
  pharmaceutical industry, C-519 to C-521
  phases, 19–20
  policies and procedures, 390–393
  principal aspects, 42–43
  rewards and incentives for, 404–411
  staffing for
    employee recruitment and retention,
      365–368
    management team, 364–365, 366
  video-on-demand, C-159 to C-161
  video rentals, C-155 to C-158
  in weak-culture companies, 422
Strategy-facilitating motivational practices,
  404–406
Strategy-focused enterprise, 15
Strategy horizons for rapid growth
  kinds of, 249, 250
  risks of, 250–251
Strategy implementation
  case study, C-458 to C-467
  challenge of, 360
  as companywide crusade, 361
  first steps, 361
  low-cost leadership, 6
Strategy makers, 35
Strategy making, 20
  airline industry, C-50 to C-53
  car rental business, C-164 to C-165
  corporate governance and, 44–46
  crafting strategy, 35–42
  developing strategic vision, 20–29
  for diversified companies, 267–268

Strategy making—*Cont.*
  driving forces and, 81
  ethical, 338–340
  in foreign marketing, 208
    think-global, act-global, 206–207
    think-global, act-local, 207–209
    think-local, act-local, 204–206
  implementation phase, 42–43
  key points, 46–47
  key success factors, 89, 92
  at Netflix, C-149 to C-150
  organic foods market, C-7 to C-17
  PC industry, C-113 to C-114
  phases, 19–20
  role of intrapreneurship, 37
  setting objectives, 29–35
  supermarket chains, C-39 to C-40
  uniting, 40–41
Strategy-making hierarchy, 37–40, 39
  business strategy, 38, 39
  corporate strategy, 38, 39
  functional-area strategies, 38–40, 39
  operating strategies, 39, 40
Strategy management process
  and corporate governance, 44–46
  corrective adjustments, 43–44
  crafting strategy, 35–42
  implementation phase, 42–43
  key points, 46–47
  performance evaluation, 43–44
  setting objectives, 29–35
  strategic vision, 20–29
  strategy-making hierarchy, 37–40
Strategy options
  airline fuel prices and, C-66
  case study, C-405 to C-406, C-454 to C-455
  company menu of, 162
  for competitors, 4
  complementary, 162
  Copperfield Books, C-352 to C-354
  for declining industries, 240–241
  for diversification, 270–272
    acquisition, 271
    internal start-up, 271
    joint venture, 271–282
  of diversified companies, 301t
    broader business base, 300–303
    divestiture, 303–306
    multinational diversification, 308–312
    restructuring, 306–308
  Eastman Kodak, C-232 to C-234
  for emerging industries, 233–234
  emerging markets
    avoiding some markets, 223
    changing local markets, 223
    local circumstances, 222–223
    price competition, 222
  in foreign markets, 227
    dealing with cross-country variations, 205
    exporting, 203
    franchising, 204
    generic strategies, 202–203
    licensing, 203–204
    localized or global, 204–209

Strategy options—*Cont.*
  for fragmented industries, 247–249
  generic, *162*
  from globalization pressures, 225–226
  in high-velocity markets, 242–245, *243*
  to improve corporate performance,
      299–300
  pitfalls to avoid, 263
  for resource allocation, 299t
  Western States Insurance, C-280 to C-282
Strategy revision, 258
Stray bull theory, C-557
Stretch objectives, 30–31, 406, 442
Strong-culture companies, 420–421
Struggling enterprises, 181
Stuck-in-the-middle strategy, 158, 239
Subcultures, 419–420
Substantive culture-changing actions,
    430–431
Substitute inputs, 138
Substitute products, 64–65
Sudden-death threat, 107
Supercenters, C-29
Superior product strategy, 256
Supermarket chains, C-4 to C-5
Supermarket terminology, C-29
Supplier bargaining power, 66–69, *69*
Supplier-related cost disadvantage, 119
Suppliers, 67–68
  bargaining leverage with, 290
  category managers, C-421
  collaboration with, 383, C-97 to C-98
  company bargaining power and, 138
  to golf equipment industry, C-73
  organic foods industry, C-18
  outsourcing and, 175
  relocating facilities, 140
  standards for, C-422
  strategic partnerships with, 68–69, 244
Supplier–seller relationships
  creating competitive pressures
      examples, 66–67
      seller–supplier partnerships, 68–69
      supplier bargaining power, 66–68
  low-cost leadership, C-420 to C-422
Supply chain activities
  in differentiation strategies, 145
  strategic fit in, 275
Supply chain management, *111*
  booksellers, C-332, C-348 to C-349
  cross-unit collaboration, 382
  example, C-198 to C-199
  improving efficiency, 138
  with Internet, 139–140
  in low-cost leadership, C-424 to C-425
  in organization structure, 383
  outsourcing and, 175
  remedying cost disadvantages, 119
  vertical integration and, 173–174
Supply conditions, 53t
Supply-side fragmentation, 245–246
Support activities
  strategic fit in, *274*
  in value chain, 110, *111*

Sustainable competitive advantage
  outsourcing and, 176
  significance of, 261–262
  strategy for, 6–7, 13
Switching costs
  alternative suppliers, 67
  barrier to entry, 62
  buyer bargaining power and, 70
  low, 143
  product differentiation and, 59
  rivalry and, 58–59
  substitute product and, 64–65, *65*
SWOT analysis, 97–109, 126–127
  competitive deficiencies, 104, 105t
  on competitive strengths, 122
  drawing conclusions from, 107–109, *108*
  identifying market opportunities, 104–106,
      105t
  identifying threats to profitability, 106–107
  implications for strategic action, 108–109
  key financial ratios, 98t–99t
  questions for, 107–108
  resource strengths and capabilities, 97–104
      competencies and capabilities, 100–102
      power of resource strengths, 102–104
      resource weaknesses, 104, 105t
Symbolic culture-changing actions, 431–432
Systems development, *111*

Target market
  for acquisition, C-277
  best-cost provider strategy, 150–151
  competitive strategies for, 134–135
  DVD rental business, C-151
  focused low-cost strategy, 153
Tariffs, 62
Tax burdens, 200
Team-based incentive compensation system, 136
Team effort, 34, 36, 360, C-16 to C-17
Technical know-how, 78
Technical support activities, C-101 to C-103
Technological innovation
  airline industry, C-58 to C-59
  at Apple Computer, C-130 to C-133
  case study, C-219 to C-234
      business shift, C-232 to C-234
      challenges, C-222
      company problems, C-219 to C-222
      competitors, C-227 to C-230
      global trends, C-337
      growth of digital photography,
          C-222 to C-227
      photography unit, C-230 to C-231
      stock price decline, C-231
      strategy options, C-232
  differentiation strategies and, 148
  driver of diversification, 275
  as driving force, 76–77
  genetically modified foods, C-547 to C-558
  golf equipment industry, C-72, C-74 to
      C-75, C-77 to C-88
  at Google Inc., C-326, C-327
  in high-velocity markets, 243–244
  improved by outsourcing, 176

Technological innovation—*Cont.*
  limitations on, C-74 to C-75
  in low-cost leadership, C-424 to C-425
  motorcycle industry, C-361
  in MP3 player industry, C-117, C-124 to
      C-129, C-142 to C-147
  at Netflix, C-150
  pace of, 53t
  in public broadcasting, C-255
  reason for strategic alliances, 164–165
  restructuring and, 306
  by runner-up companies, 255
Technology
  access from merger or acquisition, 169
  in diversification, 272
  dominant, 233
  franchising strategies, 204
  licensing strategies, 203–204
  in low-cost leadership, C-424 to C-425
  next-generation, 178
  proprietary, 232
  standardized, C-103
  strategic fit in, 274–275
  in value chain, *111*
Technology branching, 246
Technology-related KSFs, 88t
Technology sharing, 167
Technology transfer, 78
Telecommunications Act of 1996, C-255
Telecommunications industry
  boom and bust, C-496 to C-497, C-516 to
      C-517
  history of, C-515
  Swiss market, C-497
Ten commandments for strategy, 261–262
Terrorist attack of 2001, 107, C-50, C-60
Think-global, act-global strategy making,
    206–207
Think-global, act-local strategy making,
    207–209
Think-local, act-local strategy making,
    204–206
Threats, external
  emerging threats, 286
  identifying, 106–107
  new entrants, 60–64, 61t
Tie-in products, 244
Times interest earned, 99t
Timing of strategic actions, 102
  first movers, 188, 189
  offensive strategies, 178
Top-down guidance, 391
Top-down objective setting, 34–35
Top-level executives
  action agenda, 362–363
  and company values, 29
  compensation, 409
  corporate strategy role, 38
  crafting diversification strategy, 267–268
  decentralized decision making, 380
  directing strategy execution, 359–360,
      384–385
  ethical leadership, 443
  leading culture change, 429, 430

Top-level executives—*Cont.*
  managing ethical conduct, 333–338
  role in crafting strategy, 35–36
  setting objectives, 34–35
  social responsibility and, 349–351
  social responsibility initiatives, 445
  strategic vision, 20
  strategy cohesion, 41
  strategy–culture fit and, 427–428
  weak, 364–365
Topping-out problem, 236
Total quality management, 399, 442
  capturing benefits of, 399–401
  characteristics, 395, 396
Trade restrictions, 62
Traditional accounting, 114, 116t
Traditional functional departments, 377
Traditions, company, 417
Trespass, C-557
Truck fleet operations, C-423
Turnaround strategies, 59
  adidas, C-378 to C-379
  Gateway Computer, C-113 to C-114
  at Harley-Davidson, C-369
  Krispy Kreme, C-214 to C-218
  results from, C-505 to C-511
  in unrelated diversification, 282
  for weak businesses, 257–258

Unbranded products, C-106 to C-107
Uncertainty, 79
Unconcerned approach, 334–336, 335t
Underage labor, 319
Underpricing competitors, 135
Unethical behavior; *see* Ethical failures
Unethical/greed-driven cultures, 424
Unhealthy corporate cultures, 422–424
Unionism, C-410 to C-411
Unions, 66–67, C-59
Unit costs, 290
Unrelated diversification, 279–284, 312
  basic premise, 279
  criteria for, 279–280
  drawbacks
    demands on management, 283–284
    limited competitive advantage, 284
  examples, 281
  mergers and acquisitions, 280
  merits of
    general merits, 280–282
    shareholder value, 282–283
  portfolio building, 280
  versus related diversification, 272
  with related diversification, 284–285
  strategy options, *273*
Unweighted rating system, 122–124, 123t
Up-and-out policy, 406

Vacant-niche strategy, 256
Value
  in best-cost provider strategy, 150
  buyer perceptions, 148
  created for buyers, 110
  perceived vs. actual, 147

Value—*Cont.*
  signaling, 147
Value-added services, C-101
Value chain
  concept, 110–112, *111*
  cross-business relationships, 268
  for entire industry, 113–*114*
  PC vendors, C-97
  reinventing, 237
  supply-side fragmentation and, 246
  system for entire industry, 171–175
  variations in, 112–113
  in vertical integration, 377
Value chain activities, 385
  benchmarking costs, 116–117
  competitive advantage, 120–122, *121*
  cost disadvantages and, 117–120
  cost efficiency in performing, 121–122
  dangers of excessive outsourcing, 376
  in differentiation strategies, 145–146
  expense categories, 114–115
  in-house, 175
  internal vs. outsourced, 373–376
  linked, 113 *114*
  in low-cost provider strategies
    cost-management of, 137–139
    examples of revamped activities, 140–142
    revamping, 139–140
  in organizing work effort, 373–376
  primary, 110–112, *111*, 114
  reengineering, 396
  related diversification, 273
  secondary, 110–112, *111*
  strategic fit and, 273, *274*, 274–278
  support activities, 110, *111*
  unrelated diversification, 279
Value-conscious buyers, 151
Values; *see* Core values
Vertical integration, 53t, 161, 171–175, 191–192
  advantages, 172–173
  backward, 171, 172–173
  cost advantages, 138
  disadvantages, 173–174
  divisional units, 377
  as environmental issue, C-171 to C-181
  forward, 171, 173
  full vs. partial, 171–172
  pros and cons, 175
Videoconferencing, 75
Video-on-demand, 5, C-159 to C-161
Vioxx recall, C-518 to C-532
Vision statements, 21, C-2; *see also* Mission statement; Strategic vision
  common shortcomings, 22
Voice over Internet Protocol, 5, 74–75, 76–77, 231–233, 235, 327, C-323

Wall Street Journal, 319–320, C-161, C-434, C-527
Wal-Mart: The High Cost of Low Prices, C-434
Washington Post, C-434
Weak businesses
  harvesting strategies, 260–261

Weak businesses—*Cont.*
  liquidation of, 261
  strategies for, 257–261
  turnaround strategies, 258–259
    boosting revenues, 258
    chances of success, 259
    combination efforts, 259
    cutting costs, 258
    example, 259
    selling off assets, 258
    strategy revision, 258
Weak-culture companies, 421–422
Weak executives, 364–365
Web site strategies
  avoiding channel conflict, 183–184
  brick-and-click strategies, 184–185, 186
  minor distribution channel, 184
  online enterprises, 185–187
  product information only, 183 184
Weighted competitive strength scores, 291t
Weighted industry attractiveness scores, 288t, 289
Weighted rating system, 123t, 124
Wholesale channels, 62
Wholesale clubs, C-29
Wild One, C-362
Winning strategy, 13, 17
Wireless Fidelity networking, C-108
Women, buying power, 348
Work climate/environment
  corporate culture and, 416
  high-energy, 346
  as incentive, 405
  after merger, C-513 to C-514
  monitoring, 351
  organic food retailing, C-16 to C-17
  politicized, 424
  quality of life and, 344
  results-oriented, 441–442
  at Starbucks, C-481
  for strategy execution, 391–393
  Toyota Production System, 372
Work effort, 363, 385
  organizing, 373–383, 374t, 386
    collaboration and alliances, 383
    delegating authority, 378–381
    internal cross-unit coordination, 381–383
    strategy-critical activities, 376–378
    value chain activities, 373–376
  reengineering, 395
Workforce; *see also* Employees; Labor *entries*
  child labor issue, 319
  no-layoff policy, 392, C-511 to C-512
  nonunion, 66–67, 136
  people-first strategy, 346
Workforce diversity, 344–345, 347
Workforce retention, 347
Working capital, 98t
Workout process, 366
Work teams
  empowerment, 379–380
  management team, 360, 364–365, 366
World Trade Organization, 200, 216
Worry list, 126, 127